Zaoutis & Chiang's Comprehensive Pediatric Hospital Medicine

Zaoutis & Chiang's Comprehensive Pediatric Hospital Medicine

Third Edition

Editors

Vincent W. Chiang, MD
Chief Medical Officer
Boston Children's Hospital
Associate Professor of Pediatrics and Emergency Medicine
Harvard Medical School
Boston, Massachusetts

Samir S. Shah, MD, MSCE, MHM
Vice Chair, Clinical Affairs and Education
Departmental Endowed Chair
Attending Physician in Hospital Medicine & Infectious Diseases
Cincinnati Children's Hospital Medical Center
Professor, Department of Pediatrics
University of Cincinnati College of Medicine
Cincinnati, Ohio

Associate Editors

Amanda S. Growdon, MD
Clinical Chief, Hospital Medicine
Assistant Professor, Harvard Medical School
Boston, Massachusetts

Sanjay Mahant, MD, FRCPC, MSc
Staff Paediatrician, Division of Paediatric Medicine
Professor
Department of Paediatrics
University of Toronto
Hospital for Sick Children
Toronto, Ontario, Canada

Erin Shaughnessy, MD, MSHCM
Division Director and Beth Gordy Dubina Endowed Chair,
Pediatric Hospital Medicine
Executive Vice Chair and Professor of Pediatrics
University of Alabama at Birmingham
Birmingham, Alabama

Joanna Thomson, MD, MPH
Associate Professor, Department of Pediatrics
University of Cincinnati College of Medicine
Attending Physician
Division of Hospital Medicine
Cincinnati Children's Hospital Medical Center
Cincinnati, Ohio

Mc Graw Hill

Zaoutis & Chiang's Comprehensive Pediatric Hospital Medicine, Third Edition

1 2 3 4 5 6 7 8 9 DSS 30 29 28 27 26 25

ISBN 978-1-264-84932-1
MHID 1-264-84932-X

This book was set in Minion Pro by KnowledgeWorks Global Ltd.
The editors were Timothy Y. Hiscock and Kim J. Davis.
The production supervisor was Richard Ruzycka.
Project management was provided by Radhika Jolly of KnowledgeWorks Global Ltd.
The cover designer was W2 Design.

This book is printed on acid-free paper.

Library of Congress Cataloging-in-Publication Data

Names: Chiang, Vincent W., editor. | Shah, Samir S., editor.
Title: Zaoutis & Chiang's comprehensive pediatric hospital medicine / editors, Vincent W. Chiang, Samir S. Shah ; associate editors, Amanda S. Growdon, Sanjay Mahant, Erin Shaughnessy, Joanna Thomson.
Other titles: Comprehensive pediatric hospital medicine | Zaoutis and Chiang's comprehensive pediatric hospital medicine
Description: Third edition. | New York : McGraw Hill, [2025] | Preceded by Comprehensive pediatric hospital medicine / editors, Lisa B. Zaoutis, Vincent W. Chiang ; associate editors, Samir S. Shah, Brian Alverson, Sanjay Mahant. Second edition. [2018]. | Includes bibliographical references and index. | Summary: "This textbook serves as a resource, providing the fundamental knowledge and skills required to care for the hospitalized child"—Provided by publisher.
Identifiers: LCCN 2023057576 (print) | LCCN 2023057577 (ebook) | ISBN 9781264849321 (hardcover ; alk. paper) | ISBN 9781264849741 (ebook)
Subjects: MESH: Pediatrics—methods | Hospital Medicine—methods | Child, Hospitalized
Classification: LCC RJ45 (print) | LCC RJ45 (ebook) | NLM WS 100 | DDC 618.92—dc23/eng/20240401
LC record available at https://lccn.loc.gov/2023057576
LC ebook record available at https://lccn.loc.gov/2023057577

For my dear friends and colleagues with whom I have had the privilege to work... especially the lunch crew and Alcove 2.

For Molly, Grace and Aidan...who put up with me and of whom I could not be more proud.

And especially for Susanne...the best partner a person could have.

–Vinny

To my children—Siddharth, Avani, and Ace—who constantly remind me the importance of bravery, curiosity, and kindness.

To my friends and colleagues at Cincinnati Children's, for helping make the world a better place for children.

To our patients for teaching us and to their families for trusting us.

–Samir

Contents

Section Editors

Jessica L. Bettenhausen, MD [Part I]
Professor of Pediatrics
University of Missouri Kansas City School of Medicine
Associate Chair, Department of Pediatrics
Children's Mercy Kansas City
Kansas City, Missouri

Lauren G. Solan, MD, MEd [Part I]
Associate Professor of Pediatrics
University of Rochester Golisano Children's Hospital
Rochester, New York

Derek J. Williams, MD, MPH [Part I]
Professor of Pediatrics
William R. Long Director of Child Health Research
Department of Pediatrics
Monroe Carell, Jr. Children's Hospital at Vanderbilt, University Medical Center
Vanderbilt University School of Medicine
Nashville, Tennessee

Kris P. Rehm, MD, MMHC [Part II]
Professor of Pediatrics
Vanderbilt University School of Medicine
Monroe Carell Jr Children's Hospital at Vanderbilt
Nashville, Tennessee

Erinn O. Schmit, MD, MEd [Part II]
Associate Professor of Pediatrics
University of Alabama at Birmingham Heersink School of Medicine
Children's of Alabama
Birmingham, Alabama

Jennifer Smith, BMBS, MSc, FRCPC [Section A]
Pediatrician
Department of Pediatrics
The Hospital for Sick Children
Toronto, Ontario, Canada

Michael J. Tchou, MD, MSc [Section B]
Associate Professor of Pediatrics
University of Colorado School of Medicine
Children's Hospital Colorado
Aurora, Colorado

Waheeda Samady, MD, MSCI [Section C]
Associate Professor of Pediatrics
Hospital-Based Medicine
Northwestern University Feinberg School of Medicine
Chicago, Illinois

Vineeta Mittal, MD [Section D]
Professor of Pediatrics
University of Texas Southwestern Medical Center
Children's Medical Center
Dallas, Texas

Christine L. Schuler, MD, MPH [Section E]
Associate Professor of Pediatrics
University of Cincinnati College of Medicine
Division of Hospital Medicine
Cincinnati Children's Hospital Medical Center
Cincinnati, Ohio

Stephanie Berger, MD [Section F]
Professor of Pediatrics, Division of Pediatric Hospital Medicine
Director of Pediatric Clerkship
University of Alabama Heersink School of Medicine
Birmingham, Alabama

Michelle M. Kelly, MD, PhD [Section G]
Professor
Department of Pediatrics
University of Wisconsin School of Medicine and Public Health
Madison, Wisconsin

Rebecca D. Ganetzky, MD [Section H]
Assistant Professor of Pediatrics
Children's Hospital of Philadelphia
Philadelphia, Pennsylvania

Michelle W. Parker, MD [Section I]
Division of Hospital Medicine
Cincinnati Children's Hospital Medical Center
University of Cincinnati College of Medicine
Cincinnati, Ohio

Nichole Samuy, MD, MSHI [Section I]
Associate Professor of Pediatrics
University of Alabama at Birmingham Heersink School of Medicine
Children's of Alabama
Birmingham, Alabama

Marie E. Wang, MD, MPH [Section J]
Clinical Professor of Pediatrics
Division of Pediatric Hospital Medicine
Stanford University School of Medicine
Lucile Packard Children's Hospital Stanford
Palo Alto, California

Charu Gupta, MD, MBBS, MPH [Section K]
Children's National Medical Center
Washington, DC

Lisa E. Herrmann, MD, MEd [Section L]
Associate Professor of Pediatrics
University of Cincinnati College of Medicine
Cincinnati Children's Hospital
Cincinnati, Ohio

Neera Goyal, MD, MSc [Section M]
Associate Professor of Pediatrics
Nemours Children's Health and Sydney Kimmel College of Medicine at Thomas Jefferson University
Philadelphia, Pennsylvania

Susan Wu, MD [Section N]
Associate Professor of Clinical Pediatrics
Children's Hospital Los Angeles
University of Southern California Keck School of Medicine
Los Angeles, California

Stephanie K. Doupnik, MD, MSHP [Section O]
Director, Division of Pediatric Hospital Medicine
William R. Long Director in Health Policy
Assistant Professor of Pediatrics
Vanderbilt University Medical Center
Nashville, Tennessee

Susan Chu Walley, MD, MHCM, NCNTT, FAAP [Section P]
Professor of Pediatrics
George Washington University School of Medicine
Children's National Hospital
Washington, DC

Melissa M. Hazen, MD [Section Q]
Assistant Professor of Pediatrics
Harvard Medical School
Program in Rheumatology
Department of General Pediatrics
Boston Children's Hospital and Harvard Medical School
Boston, Massachusetts

Katie Meier, MD [Section R]
Assistant Professor of Pediatrics
University of Cincinnati College of Medicine
Division of Hospital Medicine
Cincinnati Children's Hospital Medical Center
Cincinnati, Ohio

Yemisi Jones, MD, MEd [Section S]
Associate Professor of Pediatrics
University of Cincinnati College of Medicine
Cincinnati Children's Hospital Medical Center
Cincinnati, Ohio

Catherine Diskin, MB, BCh, MRCPI, MSc [Section T]
Assistant Professor and Staff Paediatrician
Division of Paediatric Medicine (Complex Care)
University of Toronto
Hospital for Sick Children
Toronto, Ontario, Canada

Eyal Cohen, MD [Section T]
Professor of Paediatrics and Health Policy, Management and Evaluation
University of Toronto
Hospital for Sick Chilldren
Toronto, Ontario, Canada

Alexander W. Hirsch, MD [Part IV]
Instructor of Pediatrics
Harvard Medical School
Division of Emergency Medicine, Boston Children's Hospital
Boston, Massachusetts

Contributors

Mayssa Abuali, MD [24]
Attending Physician
Einstein Medical Center Philadelphia
Associate Professor of Pediatrics
Thomas Jefferson University
Philadelphia, Pennsylvania

Ellen Overson, MD [75]
Division of Hospital Medicine
Internal Medicine/Pediatrics
University of Minnesota Medical School
Minneapolis, Minnesota

Aisha Ahmed, MD [47]
Assistant Professor of Pediatrics
Northwestern University Feinberg School of Medicine
Attending Physician
Division of Allergy/Immunology
Ann & Robert H. Lurie Children's Hospital
Chicago, Illinois

Bridget C. Allard, DO [147]
Attending Physician, Children's National Hospital
Division of Hospital Medicine
Assistant Professor of Pediatrics,The George Washington University School of Medicine and Health Sciences
Washington, DC

Ann Allen, MD [168]
Department of Pediatrics
University of Wisconsin School of Medicine and Public Health
Madison, Wisconsin

Francisco Alvarez, MD [61]
Clinical Professor of Pediatrics
Division of Pediatric Hospital Medicine
Stanford School of Medicine
Associate Chief, Regional Pediatric Hospital Medicine Programs
Pediatric Hospitalist
Lucile Packard Children's Hospital
Stanford, California

Bakri J. Alzarka, MD, MS [110]
Department of Pediatrics
Division of Nephrology and Hypertension
University of Maryland School of Medicine
Baltimore, Maryland

Rasheda Z. Amin, MBBS, MSHS [117]
Pediatric Nephrologist
Inova Children's Specialists
Fairfax, Virginia
Inova L. J. Murphy Children's Hospital
Falls Church, Virginia
Assistant Professor
George Washington School of Medicine
Washington, DC

James W. Antoon, MD, PhD, MPH [46]
Division of Hospital Medicine
Monroe Carell Jr. Children's Hospital at Vanderbilt
Department of Pediatrics
Vanderbilt University Medical Center
Nashville, Tennessee

Stephanie Bousquet Arar, MD [51]
University of Texas Southwestern
Dallas, Texas

Yousef Arar, MD, MPH [51, 52]
University of Texas Southwestern
Dallas, Texas

Paul L. Aronson, MD, MHS [91]
Associate Professor of Pediatrics and Emergency Medicine
Deputy Director, Pediatric Residency Program
Yale School of Medicine
New Haven, Connecticut

Erin Avondet, MD [180]
Assistant Professor of Pediatrics
University of Utah School of Medicine
Primary Children's Hospital
Salt Lake City, Utah

Jill Azok, MD [86]
Assistant Dean for Student Affairs
Assistant Professor of Pediatrics
Case Western Reserve University School of Medicine
Cleveland, Ohio

Elaine B. Barfield, MD [76]
Clinical Associate Professor of Pediatrics
Department of Pediatrics
Weill Cornell Medicine
New York, New York

Lindsay S. Baron, MD [185]
Chief of Radiology
Tufts Medicine—Lowell General Hospital
Lowell, Massachusetts

Ebony Beaudoin, MD [127]
Associate Professor of Pediatrics
University of Texas—Health Science Center at Houston
Houston, Texas

Andrew F. Beck, MD, MPH [6]
Professor of Pediatrics
Cincinnati Children's Hospital Medical Center
University of Cincinnati College of Medicine
Cincinnati, Ohio

Carolyn E. Beck, MD, MSc [93]
Division of Paediatric Medicine
Department of Paediatrics
The Hospital for Sick Children
University of Toronto
Toronto, Ontario, Canada

Deanna Bell, MD [9]
Associate Professor of Clinical Pediatrics
Division of Pediatric Hospital Medicine
Vanderbilt University School of Medicine
Monroe Carell Jr. Children's Hospital at Vanderbilt
Nashville, Tennessee

Christina Bemrich-Stolz, MD [87]
Assistant Professor
Division of Hematology-Oncology
Department of Pediatrics
University of Alabama School of Medicine
Birmingham, Alabama

Kathleen J. Berg, MD [2]
Children's Mercy Kansas City
Associate Professor, Department of Pediatircs
University of Missouri-Kansas City School of Medicine
Kansas City, Missouri

Stephanie Berger, MD [69]
Associate Professor of Pediatrics
University of Alabama at Birmingham Heersink School of Medicine
Children's of Alabama
Birmingham, Alabama

Ajay Bhasin, MD [48]
Assistant Professor of Internal Medicine and Pediatrics
Northwestern University Feinberg School of Medicine
Ann & Robert H. Lurie Children's Hospital
Northwestern Memorial Hospital
Chicago, Illinois

Zia Bismilla, MD, MEd, FRCPC [187]
Division of Paediatric Medicine
Department of Paediatrics
Universitiy of Toronto
Hospital for Sick Children
Toronto, Ontario, Canada

Ari Bitnun, MD, MSc, FRCPC, FIDSA [104]
Professor of Pediatrics
Division of Infectious Diseases, Hospital for Sick Children (SickKids)
Department of Pediatrics
University of Toronto
Toronto, Ontario, Canada

Amanda Bogart, MD [43]
Assistant Professor of Pediatrics, Adolescent Medicine
University of Colorado School of Medicine
Aurora, Colorado

Benjamin S. Bolser, MD [65]
Staff Physician
Division of Hospital Medicine
Cincinnati Children's Hospital and Medical Center
Cincinnati, Ohio

Marie-Hélène Bourassa, MD [141]
Montreal Children's Hospital
McGill University
Montreal, Quebec, Canada

Adam E. Bracken, MD [40]
Assistant Professor, Departments of Medicine and Pediatrics
University of Rochester
Rochester, New York

Patrick W. Brady, MD, MSc [4]
Professor and Director, Division of hospital Medicine
James M. Anderson Center for Health System Excellence
Cincinnati Children's Hospital Medical Center
Department of Pediatrics
University of Cincinnati College of Medicine
Cincinnati, Ohio

Tonia Branche, MD, MPH [195]
Division of Neonatology
Ann & Robert H. Lurie Children's Hospital
Department of Pediatrics
Northwestern University Feinberg School of Medicine
Chicago, Illinois

Kathleen G. Brimsek, MD [156]
University of Colorado
Children's Hospital Colorado
Aurora, Colorado

Rebeccah L. Brown, MD [155]
Division of Pediatric General and Thoracic Surgery
Cincinnati Children's Hospital Medical Center
Department of Surgery
University of Cincinnati College of Medicine
Cincinnati, Ohio

Natasha Brownrigg, BScN, MN, NP-Pediatrics [165]
The Hospital for Sick Children
Faculty of Nursing
University of Toronto
Toronto, Ontario, Canada

Celina Brunson, MD [109]
Pediatric Nephrology
Children's National Hospital
Washington, DC

Michael Bryant, MD [14]
Division Head, Hospital Medicine
Vice Chair for Pediatric Diversity, Equity, and Inclusion
Clinical Professor
Keck School of Medicine
University of Southern California
Los Angeles, California

April Buchanan, MD [25]
Professor of Pediatrics
Pediatric Hospitalist
Associate Dean for Medical Education
University of South Carolina School of Medicine Greenville/ Prisma Health
Greenville, South Carolina

Alina G. Burek, MD [190]
Children's Wisconsin
Department of Pediatrics
Medical College of Wisconsin
Milwaukee, Wisconsin

Alicia Caldwell, MD [88]
Division of Hospital Medicine
Cincinnati Children's Hospital Medical Center
Department of Pediatrics
University of Cincinnati College of Medicine
Cincinnati, Ohio

Tara N. Calhoun, MD, MS [174]
Assistant Professor of Pediatrics
University of Cincinnati College of Medicine
Division of Hospital Medicine
Cincinnati Children's Hospital Medical Center
Cincinnati, Ohio

Rebecca Cantu, MD, MPH [69]
Associate Professor of Pediatrics, Division of Pediatric Hospital Medicine
Section Chief, Pediatric Hospital Medicine
Program Director, PHM Fellowship
University of Arkansas for Medical Sciences College of Medicine
Little Rock, Arkansas

Robert Casey, MD [16]
Medical Director, Pediatric Hospital Medicine
Clerkship Director, Pediatrics
Associate Residency Program Director
Joe DiMaggio Children's Hospital
Florida Atlantic University Schmidt College of Medicine
Hollywood, Florida

Angela Castellanos, MD [33]
Pediatric Hospital Medicine Fellow
Boston Children's Hospital
Clinical Fellow in Pediatrics
Harvard Medical School
Boston, Massachusetts

Cynthia E. Castiglioni, MD, MS [45]
Ann & Robert H. Lurie Children's Hospital of Chicago
Northwestern University Feinberg School of Medicine
Chicago, Illinois

Mary Wu Chang, MD [60]
Associate Professor of Dermatology and Pediatrics
University of Connecticut School of Medicine
Farmington, Connecticut

Pearl W. Chang, MD [130]
Assistant Professor of Pediatrics
University of Washington & Seattle Children's Hospital
Seattle, Washington

Rabia A. Cheema, MD [156]
University of California, Los Angeles
Mattel Children's Hospital
Los Angeles, California

Laura P. Chen, MD [73]
Division of Hospital Medicine
Department of Pediatrics
University of Wisconsin School of Medicine and Public Health
Madison, Wisconsin

Jackie K. Chiang, MD, MA, FRCPC [182]
Pediatric Pulmonologist
Hospital for Sick Children
University of Toronto
Toronto, Ontario, Canda

Romy Cho, MD, FRCPC, DRCPSC (Child Maltreatment Paediatrics) [35]
Assistant Professor, Faculty of Medicine
University of Toronto
Division of Paediatric Medicine
The Hospital for Sick Children
Toronto, Ontario, Canada

Eric Choy, MD, MPH [85]
Assistant Professor, Department of Pediatrics
Section of Pediatric Hospital Medicine
Baylor College of Medicine
Houston, Texas

Erica Chung, MD [26]
Department of Pediatrics
Hasbro Children's Hospital
The Warren Alpert Medical School of Brown University
Providence, Rhode Island

Alexandra M. Clark, MD [146]
Loma Linda University Children's Hospital
Division Chief of General Pediatrics, Medicine-Pediatrics, and Pediatric Hospital Medicine
Assistant Professor of Pediatrics
Loma Linda, California

Jamie L. Clute, MD, FHM, FAAP [20]
Pediatric Hospitalist
Senior Lecturer, University of Queensland, School of Medicine-Ochsner Health
Faculty, Ochsner Pediatric Residency Program
Ochsner Children's Hospital
Jefferson, Louisiana

Megan E. Coe, MD, FAAP [64]
Section of Hospital Pediatrics
Nationwide Children's Hospital
Assistant Professor of Pediatrics
The Ohio State University College of Medicine
Columbus, Ohio

Craig J. Conard, MD [34]
Tulane School of Medicine
Pediatric Hospital Medicine
Assistant Professor of Pediatrics
New Orleans, Louisiana

Evelyn Constantin, MD, CM, MSc(Epi), FRCPC [141]
McGill University
Montreal, Quebec, Canada

Michael Contarino, MD [84]
Associate Professor of Medicine and Pediatrics
University of North Carolina School of Medicine
Chapel Hill, North Carolina

Anthony Cooley, MD [151]
Associate Professor Emeritus of Pediatrics
Emory University School of Medicine
Atlanta, Georgia
Newborn and Pediatric Hospitalist
Mission Children's Hospital
Asheville, North Carolina

Emma Cory, MD, FRCPC, DRCPSC (Child Maltreatment Pediatrics) [39]
Assistant Professor
University of Toronto
Co-Director, Suspected Child Abuse and Neglect (SCAN) Program
Hospital for Sick Children
Toronto, Ontario, Canada

Melissa Cossey, MD [121]
Associate Chief Medical Officer
Dell Children's Medical Center
Associate Professor of Pediatrics
Dell Medical School, University of Texas at Austin
Austin, Texas

Diana L. Culbertson, PA-C, MMSc, MS [77]
Division of Pediatric Emergency Medicine
University of Washington
Seattle Children's Hospital
Seattle, Washington

John D'Orazio, MD, PhD [86]
Professor of Pediatrics
Chief, Division of Pediatric Hematology/Oncology
University of Kentucky College of Medicine
Lexington, Kentucky

Evan Dalton, MD, MSHP [138]
Assistant Professor of Pediatrics
Section of Pediatric Hospital Medicine
Texas Children's Hospital
Department of Pediatrics
Baylor College of Medicine
Houston, Texas

Ria Dancel, MD, SFHM, FACP, FAAP [186]
Professor of Medicine and Pediatrics
Division of Hospital Medicine
Departments of Internal Medicine and Pediatrics
University of North Carolina at Chapel Hill
Chapel Hill, North Carolina

Yasmeen N. Daud, MD [184]
Associate Professor of Pediatrics
Department of Pediatrics
Division of Pediatric Hospital Medicine
Washington University School of Medicine
St. Louis, Missouri

Stephanie R. Davis-Rodriguez, MD, MS [110]
Department of Pediatrics
Division of Hospital Medicine
Cincinnati Children's Hospital Medical Center
University of Cincinnati School of Medicine
Cincinnati, Ohio

Michael T. Del Vecchio, MD [179]
Professor, Clinical Pediatrics
Division Director, Temple Pediatric Hospitalist Division
Department of Pediatrics
Lewis Katz School of Medicine at Temple University
Philadelphia, Pennsylvania

Sarah F. Denniston, MD [160]
Assistant Professor of Pediatrics
Department of Pediatrics, Division of Pediatric Hospital Medicine
Tufts University School of Medicine
Attending Physician, Tufts Children's Hospital
Associate Designated Institutional Official, Tufts Medical Center
Pediatric Hospital Medicine Fellowship Director, Tufts Children's Hospital
Boston, Massachusetts

Arti D. Desai, MD, MSPH [11]
Associate Professor of Pediatrics
University of Washington School of Medicine
Seattle Children's Hospital
Seattle, Washington

Jennifer E. deSante-Bertkau, MD, MBE [12]
Assistant Professor
Division of Hospital Medicine
Cincinnati Children's Hospital Medical Center
Assistant Professor
Department of Pediatrics
University of Cincinnati College of Medicine
Cincinnati, Ohio

Joseph DiCara, MD, MPH [189]
Associate Professor
Northwestern Feinberg School of Medicine
Ann & Robert H. Lurie Children's Hospital
Chicago, Illinois

Emilee Dobish, MD, MS [57]
Associate Professor
University of Tennessee Health Science Center
Le Bonheur Children's Hospital
Memphis, Tennessee

Julia R. Donner, MD [26]
Department of Pediatrics
Hasbro Children's Hospital
The Warren Alpert Medical School of Brown University
Providence, Rhode Island

Joana Dos Santos, MD, MHSc, FRCPC [165]
Medical Urologist
Division of Urology
The Hospital For Sick Children
Assistant Professor of Paediatrics
University of Toronto
Toronto, Ontario, Canada

Christine N. Duncan, MD [134]
Associate Professor of Pediatrics
Harvard Medical School
Boston Chidlren's Hospital
Dana Farber Cancer Institute
Boston, Massachusetts

Martin Duncan, MD [18]
Clinical Assistant Professor of Pediatrics
Division of Hospital-Based Medicine
Ann & Robert H. Lurie Children's Hospital of Chicago
Department of Pediatrics
Northwestern University Feinberg School of Medicine
Chicago, Illinois

Katherine Dyer, DO, FAAP [55]
Assistant Clinical Professor, Child Health
University of Arizona College of Medicine—Phoenix
Phoenix Children's Hospital Medicine
Phoenix, Arizona

Jodi Ehrmann, MD [93]
Division of Hospital Medicine
Department of Pediatrics
Mott Children's Hospital
University of Michigan
Ann Arbor, Michigan

Scott A. Elisofon, MD [75]
Division of Gastroenterology, Hepatology and Nutrition
Center for Childhood Liver Disease
Boston Children's Hospital
Harvard Medical School
Boston, Massachusetts

Marina M. Eskandar, MD [118]
Assistant Professor
Division of Child Neurology
Children's National Hospital
Washington, DC

Kelly N. Evans, MD [166]
University of Washington School of Medicine
Associate Professor, Department of Pediatrics
Division of Craniofacial Medicine
Seattle Children's Craniofacial Center
Seattle, Washington

Uchenna C. Ewulonu, MD [42]
Pediatric Hospitalist
Ann & Robert H. Lurie Children's Hospital of Chicago
Assistant Professor
Northwestern Feinberg School of Medicine
Chicago, Illinois

Melissa Clemente Fabrega, MD, FAAP [50]
Nicklaus Children's Hospital
Miami, Florida

Richard A. Falcone, MD, MPH, MMM [157]
Professor of Clinical-Affiliate
Division of Pediatric and Thoracic Surgery
Cincinnati Children's Hospital Medical Center
Department of Surgery
University of Cincinnati College of Medicine
Cincinnati, Ohio

Yaron Finkelstein, MD, FACMT [169]
Divisions of Emergency Medicine and Clinical Pharmacology and Toxicology
Department of Pediatrics
Hospital for Sick Children
Departments of Pediatrics and Pharmacology and Toxicology
University of Toronto
Toronto, Ontario, Canada

Erin Finn, MD, FAAP [186]
Assistant Professor of Medicine and Pediatrics
Division of Hospital Medicine
Departments of Internal Medicine and Pediatrics
University of North Carolina at Chapel Hill
Chapel Hill, North Carolina

Todd A. Florin, MD, MSCE [97]
Division of Emergency Medicine
Ann & Robert H. Lurie Children's Hospital of Chicago
Department of Pediatrics
Northwestern University Feinberg School of Medicine
Chicago, Illinois

Eleanor Floyd, MD [44]
Instructor of Medicine and Pediatrics
Division of General Internal Medicine
Department of Medicine
University of Colorado School of Medicine
Aurora, Colorado

Dana M. Foradori, MD, MEd [119]
Department of Pediatric Hospital Medicine
Cleveland Clinic Children's
Cleveland, Ohio

Catherine S. Forster, MD, MSc [100]
Department of Pediatrics
University of Pittsburgh School of Medicine
Pittsburgh, Pennsylvania

Kristine Fortin, MD, MPH [36]
Associate Professor of Pediatrics
Perelman School of Medicine at the University of Pennsylvania
Children's Hospital of Philadelphia
Philadelphia, Pennsylvania

Cristin Q. Fritz, MD, MPH [6]
Vanderbilt University School of Medicine
Vanderbilt University Medical Center
Nashville, Tennessee

Jennifer Fuchs, MD [68]
Pediatric Hospitalist
UNC Children's Hospital
Pediatric Hospital Medicine Fellowship Director
Assistant Professor of Pediatrics
University of North Carolina Chapel Hill School of Medicine
Chapel Hill, North Carolina

Megan M. Gaffey, MD [159]
Clinical Assistant Professor
Department of Otolaryngology-Head and Neck Surgery
New York University Grossman School of Medicine
Hassenfeld Children's Hospital at NYU Langone
New York, New York

Sandra L. Gage, MD, PhD, FAAP, SFHM [145]
Pediatric Hospitalist
Director of Professional Development
Phoenix Children's Hospital
Associate Professor of Pediatrics
University of Arizona College of Medicine-Phoenix
Phoenix, Arizona

Beth D. Gamulka, MDCM, FRCPC [107]
Staff Physician, Division of Paediatric Medicine
The Hospital for Sick Children
Assistant Professor, Department of Paediatrics
Temerty Faculty of Medicine
University of Toronto
Toronto, Ontario, Canada

Rebecca D. Ganetzky, MD [82]
Assistant Professor of Pediatrics
Children's Hospital of Philadelphia
Philadelphia, Pennsylvania

Hannah M. Gardner, MD, MSHQS [70]
Assistant Professor of Pediatrics
Department of Pediatrics, Section of Hospital Medicine
University of Colorado School of Medicine
Children's Hospital of Colorado
Aurora, Colorado

Jeffrey S. Gerber, MD, PhD [90]
Professor of Pediatrics and Epidemiology
University of Pennsylvania School of Medicine
Division of Infectious Diseases, Children's Hospital of Philadelphia
Philadelphia, Pennsylvania

Timothy Gibson, MD [194]
Clinical Associate Professor of Pediatrics
UMass Chan Medical School
Worcester, Massachusetts

Peter J. Gill, MD, DPhil [95]
The Hospital for Sick Children
Department of Pediatrics, University of Toronto
Child Health Evaluative Sciences, SickKids Research Institute
Institute of Health Policy, Management and Evaluation
The University of Toronto
Toronto, Ontario, Canada

Courtney A. Gilliam, MD [175]
Assistant Professor of Pediatrics
Division of Hospital Medicine
Cincinnati Children's Hospital Medical Center
Cincinnati, Ohio

Mirna Giordano, MD [28, 160]
Associate Professor of Pediatrics
Department of Pediatrics
Division of Pediatric Critical Care & Hospital Medicine
Columbia University Vagelos College of Physicians and Surgeons
Attending Physician
New York-Presbyterian Morgan Stanley Children's Hospital
New York, New York

Laurie Glader, MD [181]
Professor of Pediatrics
The Ohio State University College of Medicine
Division of Complex Care
Nationwide Children's Hospital
Columbus, Ohio

Elliott S. Gordon, MD, MSc [76]
Division of Pediatric Gastroenterology, Hepatology, and Nutrition
New York-Presbyterian/Weill Cornell Medicine
New York, New York

Craig H. Gosdin, MD, MSHA [13]
Associate Professor of Pediatrics
University of Cincinnati College of Medicine
Division of Hospital Medicine
Cincinnati Children's Hospital Medical Center
Cincinnati, Ohio

Neera Goyal, MD, MSc [124]
Associate Professor of Pediatrics
Nemours Children's Health and Sydney Kimmel College of Medicine at Thomas Jefferson University
Philadelphia, Pennsylvania

Cori Grant, MD [158]
Instructor, Division of Pediatric Hospital Medicine
Washington University in St. Louis School of Medicine
St. Louis, Missouri

Elena C. Griego, MD [177]
Department of Pediatrics
Division of Hospital Medicine
University of Washington School of Medicine
Seattle, Washington

Karisa Grizzle, MD [31]
Assistant Professor of Clinical Pediatrics
Monroe Carell Jr. Children's Hospital at Vanderbilt
Nashville, Tennessee

Jacqueline Guay, MD [195]
Division of Hospital-Based Medicine
Ann & Robert H. Lurie Children's Hospital
Department of Pediatrics
Northwestern University Feinberg School of Medicine
Chicago, Illinois

Thomas Guggina, MD [194]
Assistant Professor of Pediatrics
UMass Chan Medical School
Worcester, Massachusetts

Kanika Gupta, MD [49]
Nemours Children's Hospital, Delaware
Wilmington, Delaware
Clinical Assistant Professor of Pediatrics
Sidney Kimmel Medical College
Thomas Jefferson University
Philadelphia, Pennsylvania

Nirupama Gupta, MD [114]
BlueJay Pediatrics
Leesburg, Virginia

Herodes Guzman, MD, MPH [82]
Clinical Genetics, Medical Biochemical Genetics & Endocrinology Fellow
Children's Hospital of Philadelphia
Philadelphia, Pennsylvania

Hilary Haimes, MD [58]
Department of Dermatology
Boston Children's Hospital
Harvard Medical School
Boston, Massachusetts

David E. Hall, MD [181]
Adjunct Professor of Pediatrics
Medical University of South Carolina
Professor of Clinical Pediatrics (Retired)
Founder, Program for Children with Medically Complex Needs
Vanderbilt University School of Medicine
Monroe Carell Jr. Children's Hospital at Vanderbilt
Nashville, Tennessee

Jennifer S. Hall, MD, FAAP [145]
Pediatric Hospitalist
Phoenix Children's Hospital
Clinical Assistant Professor
University of Arizona, College of Medicine-Phoenix
Clinical Assistance Professor
Creighton University School of Medicine
Phoenix, Arizona

Laurie Seidel Halmo, MD, FAAP [167]
Assistant Professor of Pediatrics and Medical Toxicologist
Section of Hospital Medicine, Department of Pediatrics
University of Colorado School of Medicine
Aurora, Colorado

HyoJeong Han, MD [89]
Assistant Professor of Pediatrics
Division of Hematology/Oncology
Texas Children's Hospital
Baylor College of Medicine
Houston, Texas

Beth Harper, MD [188]
Boston Children's Hospital
Harvard Medical School
Boston, Massachusetts

Andrew Haynes, MD [102]
University of Colorado School of Medicine
Department of Pediatrics
Section of Pediatric Infectious Diseases
Aurora, Colorado

Melissa M. Hazen, MD [152, 153]
Assistant Professor of Pediatrics
Harvard Medical School
Program in Rheumatology
Department of General Pediatrics
Boston Children's Hospital
Harvard Medical School
Boston, Massachusetts

Kayla Heller, MD, MHPE [56]
Assistant Professor of Pediatric Hospital Medicine
Children's Mercy Hospital
Kansas City, Missouri

Jennifer Henningfeld, MD [144]
Associate Professor of Pediatrics
Division of Pulmonary Medicine
Medical College of Wisconsin
Children's Wisconsin
Milwaukee, Wisconsin

Daniel Herchline, MD, MSEd [178]
Cincinnati Children's Hospital Medical Center
Cincinnati, Ohio

Alison C. Herndon, MD, MSPH [135]
Assistant Professor of Clinical Pediatrics
Section Head, Division of Hospital Medicine
Assistant Director, Pediatric Residency Program
Medical Director, Pediatric Medicine & Acute Care
Department of Pediatrics
Vanderbilt Univ School of Medicine
Monroe Carell Jr Children's Hospital at Vanderbilt
Nashville, Tennessee

Adriana Herrera, MD, MPH [173]
Assistant Professor of Pediatrics
Division of Pediatric Hospital Medicine
University of North Carolina School of Medicine
Chapel Hill, North Carolina

Kathryn C. Hines, MD [87]
Assistant Professor
Division of Pediatric Hospital Medicine
Department of Pediatrics
University of Tennessee College of Medicine Chattanooga
Chattanooga, Tennessee

Kim Hoang, MD [79]
Division of Hospital Medicine
Department of Pediatrics
Stanford University School of Medicine
Palo Alto, California

Jennifer A. Hoefert, MD [70]
Assistant Professor of Pediatrics
Division of General Academic Pediatrics, Section of Hospital Medicine
Saint Louis University School of Medicine
SSM Health Academic Medical Group
Cardinal Glennon Children's Hospital
St. Louis, Missouri

Erik R. Hoefgen, MD [63]
Assistant Professor of Pediatrics
Washington University in St. Louis
St. Louis, Missouri

Meghan E. Hofto, MD, MPH [98]
Associate Professor of Pediatrics
Department of Pediatrics, Division of Hospital Medicine
University of Alabama at Birmingham
Children's of Alabama
Birmingham, Alabama

Merranda D. Holmes, MD [140]
Assistant Professor of Clinical Internal Medicine and Pediatrics
Division of Hospital Medicine
Vanderbilt Monroe Carell Children's Hospital
Vanderbilt University Medical Center
Nashville, Tennessee

Mark D. Hormann, MD [125]
Professor of Pediatrics and Assistant Dean for Clinical Education
Office of Educational Programs
UTHealth McGovern Medical School
Attending Physician
Children's Memorial Hermann Hospital
Houston, Texas

Christine Hrach, MD, SFHM, FAAP [16]
Associate Professor of Pediatrics
Division of Hospitalist Medicine
Co-Interim Pediatric Residency Program Director
Washington University School of Medicine
St. Louis Children's Hospital
St. Louis, Missouri

Jonathan D. Hron, MD [21]
Assistant Professor
Harvard Medical School
Pediatric Hospitalist
Boston Children's Hospital
Boston, Massachusetts

Gary Hsich, MD [119]
Cleveland Clinic Foundation
Center for Pediatric Neuroscience
Cleveland, Ohio

Brittany M. Hunter, MD [42]
Pediatric Hospital-Based Medicine Fellow
Ann & Robert H. Lurie Children's Hospital
Chicago, Illinois

Samar A. Hussein, MD, FAAP [111, 112]
Pediatrics-Hospital Medicine
HSC Pediatric Center
Washington, DC

Dena Ibrahim, MD [23]
Assistant Professor of Clinical Pediatrics
Department of Pediatrics
Vanderbilt University School of Medicine
Monroe Carell Jr Children's Hospital at Vanderbilt
Nashville, Tennessee

Lana Ismail, MD [116]
Children's National Hospital
Washington, DC

Kristyn Jeffries, MD, MPH [176]
Arkansas Children's Hospital
Hospital Medicine, Department of Pediatrics
University of Arkansas for Medical Sciences
University of Arkansas for Medical Sciences
Little Rock, Arkansas

Karen E. Jerardi, MD, MEd [95]
Professor and Director, Hospital Medicine
Cincinnati Children's Hospital Medical Center
University of Cincinnati School of Medicine
Cincinnati, Ohio

David P. Johnson, MD [3]
Associate Professor
Division of Hospital Medicine, Department of Pediatrics
Vanderbilt University School of Medicine
Director of Quality
Department of Pediatrics
Medical Director of Inpatient Quality and Patient Safety
Monroe Carell Jr. Children's Hospital at Vanderbilt
Vanderbilt University Medical Center
Nashville, Tennessee

Kelsey Johnson, MD [133]
Division of Hospital Medicine
Children's Hospital Los Angeles
Los Angeles, California

Leah Jones, MD [56]
Assistant Professor of Pediatric Hospital Medicine
Children's Mercy Hospital
Kansas City, Missouri

Neha Shirish Joshi, MD, MS [128]
Clinical Scholar, Pediatrics
Stanford University School of Medicine
Stanford, California

Valerie Jurgens, MD [143]
Hospital Medicine Division
Children's National Hospital
The George Washington University School of Medicine and Health Sciences
Washington, DC

Benjamin Kalm, MD, FAAP [180]
Assistant Professor of Pediatrics
University of Utah School of Medicine
Salt Lake City, Utah

Tammy I. Kang, MD, MSCE, FAAHPM [183]
Professor of Pediatrics
Division Chief, Palliative Care
Baylor College of Medicine
Houston, Texas

Malika Kapadia, MD [134]
Dana Farber Cancer Institute
Boston, Massachusetts

Rachna Kapoor, MD, MS [162]
Academic General Pediatrics
Nemours Children's Hospital of Delaware
Wilmington, Delaware

Parisa Kaviany, MD [147]
Assistant Professor of Pediatrics
Children's National Hospital | Pulmonary & Sleep Medicine
George Washington University School of Medicine & Health Sciences
Washington, DC

Allysa L. Kehring, MD [23]
Pediatric Medicine Specialist
Phoenix, Arizona

Louisa Keith, MD [121]
Assistant Professor
Department of Neurology
Courtesy Assistant Professor
Department of Pediatrics
Dell Medical School, University of Texas at Austin
Austin, Texas

Chén Kenyon, MD, MSHP [142]
Attending Physician
General Pediatrics and Complex Care
Children's Hospital of Philadelphia
Associate Professor of Pediatrics
Perelman School of Medicine
University of Pennsylvania
Philadelphia, Pennsylvania

Alisa Khan, MD, MPH [5]
Pediatric Hospital Medicine
Boston Children's Hospital
Harvard Medical School
Boston, Massachusetts

Amina Khan, MD, MPH [114]
Children's National Hospital
Washington, DC

Heidi A. Kim, MD [53]
Division of Cardiology, Department of Pediatrics
University of Texas Southwestern Medical Center and Children's Health
Dallas, Texas

Juliann Lipps Kim, MD, FAAP [32]
Department Chair, Pediatric Hospitalists
Palo Alto Medical Foundation
Adjunct Clinical Associate Professor of Pediatrics
Stanford University
Palo Alto, California

Susan Kim, MD, MMSc [150]
Professor of Pediatrics
Benioff Children's Hospital, University of California
San Francisco, California

Erin King, MD [28]
Adjunct Associate Professor of Pediatrics
Director of Graduate Medical Education
Children's Minnesota
Associate Program Director
University of Minnesota Pediatric Residency Program
Minneapolis, Minnesota

Sarah Kitts, MD [62]
University of Cincinnati Dermatology
University of Cincinnati Department of Dermatology
Cincinnati, Ohio

Heather Kreth, PsyD [140]
Clinical Director of Inpatient Behavioral Health
Associate Professor of Clinical Pediatrics
Divisions of Hospital Medicine and Psychology
Vanderbilt Monroe Carell Children's Hospital
Vanderbilt University Medical Center
Nashville, Tennessee

Matthew P. Kronman, MD, MSCE [101]
Section of Infectious Diseases
Department of Pediatrics
University of Washington
Seattle Children's Hospital
Seattle, Washington

Kiran Kulkarni, MD, MS [48]
Assistant Professor of Pediatrics
Ann & Robert H. Lurie Children's Hospital
Northwestern University Feinberg School of Medicine
Chicago, Illinois

Anika Kumar, MD [24]
Staff Physician
Cleveland Clinic Children's
Assistant Professor of Pediatrics
Cleveland Clinic Lerner College of Medicine of Case Western Reserve University
Cleveland, Ohio

Amethyst C. Kurbegov, MD, MPH [71]
Division of Gastroenterology, Hepatology, and Nutrition
Department of Pediatrics, Vanderbilt University Medical Center
Monroe Carell Jr. Children's Hospital at Vanderbilt
Nashville, Tennessee

Jared Kusma, MD [78]
Pediatric Hospital Medicine Fellow
Phoenix Children's Hospital
Phoenix, Arizona

William Kwan, MD, FAAP [186]
Assistant Professor of Medicine and Pediatrics
Division of Hospital Medicine
Departments of Internal Medicine and Pediatrics
University of North Carolina at Chapel Hill
Chapel Hill, North Carolina

Joseph Lazar, MD [198]
Boston Children's Hospital
Boston, Massachusetts

Diana S. Lee, MD [148]
Mount Sinai Kravis Children's Hospital
New York, New York

Jennifer Lee, MD [136]
Columbia University Irving Medical Center
New York, New York

Ashley N. Lepse, MD [120]
Child Neurology
University of Missouri-Kansas City School of Medicine
University of Kansas School of Medicine
Children's Mercy Kansas City
Kansas City, Missouri

Emilee Colella Lewis, MD [68]
Assistant Professor of Pediatrics
University of North Carolina Chapel Hill School of Medicine
Pediatric Hospitalist
UNC Children's Hospital
Chapel Hill, North Carolina

JoAnna K. Leyenaar, MD, PhD, MPH [136]
Associate Professor of Pediatrics
The Dartmouth Institute for Health Policy & Clinical Practice
Geisel School of Medicine, Dartmouth Health
Lebanon, New Hampshire

Danni Liang, MD [92]
Pediatric Hospital Medicine Fellow
Stanford University School of Medicine
Palo Alto, California

Marilyn G. Liang, MD [58]
Department of Dermatology
Boston Children's Hospital
Harvard Medical School
Boston, Massachusetts

Nancy Liao, MD [54]
Assistant Professor of Pediatrics
The Ohio State University
Interim Associate Chief
Section of Hospital Pediatrics
Nationwide Children's Hospital
Program Director
Pediatric Hospital Medicine Fellowship
Columbus, Ohio

Carrie Lind, MD [14]
Associate Professor
Monroe Carell Junior Children's Hospital at Vanderbilt
Associate Director of Utilization Management
Pediatric Chair
Monroe Carell Junior Children's Hospital at Williamson Medical Center
Nashville, Tennessee

Matthew T. Lister, MD [30]
Department of Surgery
Division of Otolaryngology
University of Wisconsin School of Medicine and Public Health
Madison, Wisconsin

Huay-Ying Lo, MD [89]
Associate Professor of Pediatrics
Division of Pediatric Hospital Medicine
Texas Children's Hospital
Baylor College of Medicine
The Woodlands, Texas

Mindy S. Lo, MD, PhD [154]
Division of Immunology
Boston Children's Hospital
Assistant Professor
Harvard Medical School
Boston, Massachusetts

Michael Lopez, MD, FAAP [50]
Nicklaus Children's Hospital
Miami, Florida

Jeffrey P. Louie, MD [175]
Associate Professor of Pediatrics
Division of Emergency Medicine
University of Minnesota Masonic Children's Hospital
Minneapolis, Minnesota

Nicholas A. Lunig, MD [197]
Medical Director, Hospitalist Physician Team
Children's Hospital of Philadelphia
Philadelphia, Pennsylvania

Joseph D. Lynch, MD, FAAP, CHSE [170]
Assistant Professor of Pediatric Hospital Medicine
West Virginia University School of Medicine
Morgantown, West Virginia

W. G. Stuart Mackenzie, MD [162]
Orthopedics, Nemours Children's Hospital of Delaware
Wilmington, Delaware

Katherine MacKrell, MD [103]
Division of Pediatric Hospital Medicine
Children's Hospital & Medical Center
Department of Pediatrics
University of Nebraska Medical Center
Omaha, Nebraska

Paul E. Manicone, MD [118]
Division of Pediatric Hospital Medicine
Children's National Hospital
Washington, DC

W. Aaron Manning, MD [44]
Assistant Professor of Medicine and Pediatrics
Division of Hospital Medicine
Department of Medicine
Section of Pediatric Hospital Medicine
Department of Pediatrics
University of Colorado School of Medicine
Aurora, Colorado

Kalyani Marathe, MD, MPH [62]
Cincinnati Children's Dermatology
Associate Professor of Dermatology and Pediatrics
University of Cincinnati
Division of Dermatology
Cincinnati Children's Hospital
Cincinnati, Ohio

Arwen Marker, PhD [9]
Pediatric Psychology Fellow
Primary Children's Hospital
Salt Lake City, Utah

Jessica L. Markham, MD, MSc [1, 96]
Department of Pediatrics
Children's Mercy Kansas City
University of Missouri-Kansas City School of Medicine
Kansas City, Missouri
University of Kansas School of Medicine
Kansas City, Kansas

Julia A. Marlow, MD, MS [97]
Division of Pediatric Hospital Medicine
University of California, Davis School of Medicine
Sacramento, California

Abbey Masonbrink, MD, MPH [41]
Associate Professor of Pediatrics
Children's Mercy Hospital
University of Missouri School of Medicine
Kansas City, Missouri

Roshni Mathew, MD [106]
Department of Pediatrics, Division of Infectious Diseases
Center for Academic Medicine
Stanford University School of Medicine
Stanford, California

Brian May, MD, Med [69]
Assistant Professor of Pediatrics
Division of Pediatric Hospital Medicine
Assistant Professor of Internal Medicine
Division of Hospital Medicine
Assistant Director
Combined Internal Medicine and Pediatrics Residency Program
University of Alabama Heersink School of Medicine
Birmingham, Alabama

Jennifer McAllister, MD, IBCLC [131]
Associate Professor of Pediatrics
Department of Pediatrics
University of Cincinnati College of Medicine
Perinatal Institute
Cincinnati Children's Hospital Medical Center
Medical Director, NOWS Follow-Up Clinic
Cincinnati Children's Hospital Medical Center
Medical Director, Newborn Nursery
University of Cincinnati Medical Center
Cincinnati, Ohio

Sarah C. McBride, MD [33]
Director, Pediatric Hospital Medicine Fellowship Program
Boston Children's Hospital
Assistant Professor of Pediatrics
Harvard Medical School
Boston, Massachusetts

Russell McCulloh, MD [103]
Division of Pediatric Hospital Medicine
Children's Hospital & Medical Center
Department of Pediatrics
University of Nebraska Medical Center
Omaha, Nebraska

Vanessa McFadden, MD, PhD [171]
Department of Pediatrics
Pediatric Hospital Medicine
Medical College of Wisconsin
Milwaukee, Wisconsin

Jennifer L. McLaren, MD [136]
Dartmouth Health
Dartmouth Hitchcock Medical Center
Department of Psychiatry
Lebanon, New Hampshire

Heather S. McLean, MD [3]
Professor of Pediatrics
Division of Hospital Medicine
Department of Pediatrics
Duke University School of Medicine
Vice Chair for Quality
Interim Chief, Division of Emergency Medicine
Department of Pediatrics
Durham, North Carolina

Kaitlyn McQuistion, MD [115]
Children's National Hospital
Washington, DC

Katie Meier, MD [165]
Associate Professor of Pediatrics
University of Cincinnati College of Medicine
Division of Hospital Medicine
Cincinnati Children's Hospital Medical Center
Cincinnati, Ohio

Amanda Messer, MD [29, 66]
Assistant Professor of Pediatrics
Louisiana State University Health Sciences Center
New Orleans, Louisiana

Elizabeth Messer, MD [158]
Assistant Professor
Division of Pediatric Hospital Medicine
Washington University in St. Louis
School of Medicine
St. Louis, Missouri

Talene A. Metjian, PharmD [90]
Antimicrobial Stewardship Program, Manager
Children's Hospital of Philadelphia
Philadelphia, Pennsylvania

Amy E. Miller, MD [63]
Pediatric Hospital Medicine Fellow
Washington University in St. Louis
St. Louis, Missouri

Adolfo Molina, MD, MSHQS [84]
Associate Professor of Pediatrics
University of Alabama at Birmingham
Birmingham, Alabama

Nawal Momani, MD [46]
Division of Hospital-Based Medicine
Ann & Robert H. Lurie Children's Hospital of Chicago
Department of Pediatrics
Northwestern University Feinberg School of Medicine
Chicago, Illinois

Kimberly K. Monroe, MD, MS [137, 196]
Clinical Associate Professor
C. S. Mott Children's Hospital
University of Michigan
Ann Arbor, Michigan

Stephanie Moss, MD [88]
Department of Hospital Medicine
Cleveland Clinic Community Care
Department of Pediatric Hospital Medicine
Pediatrics Institute
Cleveland, Ohio

Mark Murphy, DO [105]
Assistant Professor
Department of Pediatrics
University of Cincinnati College of Medicine
Division of Pediatric Infectious Diseases
Cincinnati Children's Hospital Medical Center
Cincinnati, Ohio

Melinda S. Murphy, MD, FAAP [163]
Associate Professor of Pediatrics
University of South Florida Morsani College of Medicine
Tampa, Florida

Liza Murray, MD [37]
University of Arkansas for Medical Sciences
Arkansas Children's Hospital
Little Rock, Arkansas

Rene P. Myers, MD [166]
Associate Professor
Department of Surgery, Neurosurgery, and Otolaryngology
University of Alabama at Birmingham Heersink School of Medicine
Birmingham, Alabama

Aleisha Nabower, MD, MHPTT [99]
Children's Hospital and Medical Center
University of Nebraska Medical Center
Omaha, Nebraska

Nassr Nama, MD, MSc, FAAP [19]
Assistant Professor
Hospital Medicine, Department of Pediatrics
Seattle Children's Hospital, University of Washington
Seattle, Washington

Lauren B. Nassetta, MD [94]
Professor of Pediatrics
Department of Pediatrics
Division of Hospital Medicine
University of Alabama at Birmingham
Children's of Alabama
Birmingham, Alabama

Dena Nazer, MD [39]
Associate Professor of Pediatrics
Wayne State University
Medical Director
Kids TALK Children's Advocacy Center
Detroit, Michigan

Anika Nelson, MD [71]
Division of Hospital Medicine
Department of Pediatrics
Medical College of Wisconsin
Children's Hospital of Wisconsin
Milwaukee, Wisconsin

Thomas B. Newman, MD, MPH [130]
Professor Emeritus of Epidemiology & Biostatistics and Pediatrics
University of California, San Francisco
San Francisco, California

Roger K. Nicome, MD [138]
Associate Professor of Pediatrics
Baylor College of Medicine
Texas Children's Hospital
Division of Pediatric Hospital Medicine
Houston, Texas

Alison E. Niebanck, MD [161]
Associate Professor of Pediatrics
Mercer University School of Medicine—Savannah
Memorial Health University Medical Center
Dwaine and Cynthia Willett Children's Hospital of Savannah
Savannah, Georgia

Kathleen Nolan, MD, FRCP(C), DRCPSC (Child Maltreatment) [36]
Assistant Professor of Pediatrics at McMaster University
McMaster Children's Hospital
Hamilton, Ontario, Canada

Chloë E. Nunneley, MD [152]
University of Texas Southwestern Medical Center
Children's Medical Center
Dallas, Texas

Sean O'Brien, MD [72]
Division of Hospital Medicine
Department of Pediatrics
University of Minnesota Masonic Children's Hospital
University of Minnesota Medical School
Minneapolis, Minnesota

Daniel M. O'Connell, MD [73]
Division of Gastroenterology, Hepatology and Nutrition
Department of Pediatrics
University of Wisconsin School of Medicine and Public Health
Madison, Wisconsin

Katherine O'Connor, MD [8]
Pediatric Hospitalist
Children's Hospital at Montefiore
Bronx, New York

Kimberly O'Hara, MD [102]
Department of Pediatrics
Section of Pediatric Hospital Medicine
University of Colorado School of Medicine
Aurora, Colorado

Laura O'Neill, MD, MS, MEd [81, 108]
Assistant Professor of Pediatrics
Children's National Hospital
George Washington University School of Medicine and Health Sciences
Washington, DC

Andrew P. J. Olson, MD [7]
Attending Physician
Department of Pediatrics
Department of Medicine
University of Minnesota Medical Center
Associate Professor of Medicine & Pediatrics
University of Minnesota Medical School
University of Minnesota
Minneapolis, Minnesota

Tracy Omoegbele, MD [29]
Fellow, Pediatric Hospital Medicine
Louisiana State University Health Sciences Center
New Orleans, Louisiana

Mary M. Orr, MD, MPH [30]
Associate Professor of Pediatrics
University of Alabama at Birmingham Heersink School of Medicine
Department of Pediatrics, Division of Hospital Medicine
Children's of Alabama
Birmingham, Alabama

Rachel R. Osborn, MD [91]
Assistant Professor of Pediatrics
Director, Pediatric Residency Program
Yale School of Medicine
New Haven, Connecticut

Snezana Nena Osorio, MD, MS [11]
Department of Pediatrics
Weill Cornell Medicine
New York, New York

Yuliya Oumarbaeva-Malone, MD [116]
Children's National Hospital
Washington, DC

Margot A. Paisley, MD [47]
Attending Physician
Division of Hospital Based Medicine
Ann & Robert H. Lurie Children's Hospital of Chicago
Assistant Professor of Pediatrics
Northwestern University Feinberg School of Medicine
Chicago, Illinois

Brandon Palmer, MD [101]
Section of Hospital Medicine
Department of Pediatrics
Medical College of Wisconsin
Children's Wisconsin
Milwaukee, Wisconsin

Shannon B. Palombo, MD [34]
Louisiana State University New Orleans School of Medicine
Pediatric Hospitalist Medicine
Assistant Professor of Pediatrics
New Orleans, Louisiana

Michelle W. Parker, MD [72]
Division of Hospital Medicine
Cincinnati Children's Hospital Medical Center
University of Cincinnati College of Medicine
Cincinnati, Ohio

Chase Parsons, DO, MBI [17]
Pediatric Hospitalist
Interim Chief Medical Information Officer
Boston Children's Hospital
Instructor of Pediatrics
Harvard Medical School
Boston, Massachusetts

Robert F. Pass, MD [94]
Professor Emeritus
Department of Pediatrics
Division of Hospital Medicine
University of Alabama at Birmingham and Children's of Alabama
Birmingham, Alabama

Anuj Patel, MD [22]
Assistant Professor
Vanderbilt Children's Hospital
Nashville, Tennessee

Reina Patel, DO, FAAP [55]
Associate Clinical Professor, Child Health
University of Arizona College of Medicine—Phoenix
Phoenix Children's Hospital Medicine
Phoenix, Arizona

Kamakshya P. Patra, MD, MMM [20]
Associate Professor, Dept. of Pediatrics
WVU School of Medicine
Pediatric Hospitalist
WVU Medicine Children's Hospital
Morgantown, West Virginia

Grant Paulsen, MD [105]
Assistant Professor
Department of Pediatrics
University of Cincinnati College of Medicine
Division of Pediatric Infectious Diseases
Cincinnati Children's Hospital Medical Center
Cincinnati, Ohio

Anuradha Pavuluri, MD [67]
Pediatric Hospitalist
Assistant Professor of Pediatrics
Director of the Pediatric Accelerated Track
Atrium Health Navicent
Beverly Knight Olson Children's Hospital
Mercer University School of Medicine
Macon, Georgia

Karine Pepin, MD [37]
University of Montreal
Centre Hospitalier Universitaire (CHU) Sainte-Justine
Montreal, Quebec, Canada

Rachel J. Peterson, MD [44]
Assistant Professor of Clinical Medicine & Clinical Pediatrics
Departments of Medicine & Pediatrics
Indiana University School of Medicine
Medical Director & Associate Division Chief of Pediatric Hospital Medicine
Riley Hospital for Children at Indiana University Health
Indianapolis, Indiana

Elizabeth W. Pingree, MD [109]
Department of Medicine
Boston Children's Hospital and Department of Pediatrics
Harvard Medical School
Boston, Massachusetts

Laura Piper, MD [172]
Hospitalist, Assistant Professor of Pediatrics
University of Cincinnati
Cincinnati Children's Hospital Medical Center
Cincinnati, Ohio

Carlos Plancarte, MD, MSc [8]
Pediatric Hospitalist
Monroe Carell Jr. Children's Hospital at Vanderbilt
Nashville, Tennessee

Jacqueline Ponczek, MD, MS [18]
Clinical Instructor of Pediatrics
Division of Hospital-Based Medicine
Ann & Robert H. Lurie Children's Hospital of Chicago
Department of Pediatrics
Northwestern University Feinberg School of Medicine
Chicago, Illinois

Jillian Popel, MD, FRCPC [38]
Division of Pediatric Hospital Medicine
The Stollery Children's Hospital
Department of Pediatrics
University of Alberta
Edmonton, Alberta, Canada

Sampath Prahalad, MD, MSc [151]
Marcus Professor and Chief, Division of Pediatric Rheumatology
Children's Healthcare of Atlanta
Professor of Pediatrics and Human Genetics
Emory University School of Medicine
Atlanta, Georgia

Jessica R. C. Priestley, MD, PhD [83]
Biochemical Genetics
Corewell Health
Grand Rapids, Michigan

Amy Prudhomme, DO [29, 66]
Associate Professor of Pediatrics
Louisiana State University Health Sciences Center
New Orleans, Louisiana

Henry T. Puls, MD [12]
Associate Professor of Pediatrics
Children's Mercy Kansas City
University of Missouri-Kansas City School of Medicine
Kansas City, Missouri

Katherine Pumphrey, MD, MHA, MSHP [142]
Department of Pediatrics, Boston Children's Hospital
Harvard Medical School
Boston, Massachusetts

Maria Quidgley-Martin, MD [191]
Pediatric Emergency Fellow
Children's Hospital of Philadelphia
Philadelphia, Pennsylvania

Bianca N. Quiñones-Pérez, MD [74]
Division of Hospital Medicine
Boston Children's Hospital
Harvard Medical School
Boston, Massachusetts

Katherine Rakoczy, MD [27]
Assistant Professor
Department of Pediatrics
Section of Pediatric Hospital Medicine
New York University Grossman School of Medicine
New York, New York

Suchitra Rao, MBBS, MSCS [10]
Associate Professor of Pediatrics – Hospital Medicine and Infectious Diseases
University of Colorado School of Medicine
Aurora, Colorado

David I. Rappaport, MD [49, 162]
Nemours Children's Hospital
Delaware, Wilmington, Delaware
Professor of Pediatrics
Sidney Kimmel Medical College
Thomas Jefferson University
Philadelphia, Pennsylvania

Leah Rappaport, MD [137]
Clinical Instructor
Boston Children's Hospital
Boston, Massachusetts

Irit R. Rasooly, MD, MSCE [7]
Attending Physician
Department of Pediatrics
Department of Biomedical & Health Informatics
Children's Hospital of Philadelphia
Assistant Professor
Perelman School of Medicine
University of Pennsylvania
Philadelphia, Pennsylvania

Daniel A. Rauch, MD, FAAP [15]
Professor of Pediatrics
Tufts University School of Medicine
Boston, Massachusetts

Robin Ray, MD [161]
Vitreoretinal Service
Georgia Eye Institute of the Southeast
Savannah, Georgia

Lisa M. Remer, MD [65]
Assistant Professor of Pediatrics
Division of Pediatric Hospital Medicine
University of Cincinnati School of Medicine
Cincinnati Children's Hospital and Medical Center
Cincinnati, Ohio

Kyung E. Rhee, MD, MSc, MA [40]
Professor, Department of Pediatrics
University of California, San Diego
San Diego, California

Katherine M. Richardson, MD [96]
Department of Pediatrics
Division of Pediatric Infectious Diseases
Prisma Health
University of South Carolina School of Medicine
Shriners Hospital for Children
Greenville, South Carolina

Lisa M. Rickey, MD [153]
Fellow, Pediatric Hospital Medicine
Department of Pediatrics
Boston Children's Hospital
Harvard Medical School
Boston, Massachusetts

Raymond Rios-Nieves, MD, FAAP [163]
Assistant Professor of Pediatrics
University of South Florida Morsani College of Medicine
Tampa, Florida

Hayley Ron, MD [80]
Attending Physician and Assistant Professor
Hackensack University Medical Center
Rutgers, The State University of New Jersey
Hackensack, New Jersey

Rebecca E. Rosenberg, MD, MPH, FAAP [159]
Associate Professor of Pediatrics
New York University Grossman School of Medicine
Hassenfeld Children's Hospital at NYU Langone
New York, New York

Amy Rule, MD, MPH [123]
Assistant Professor
Department of Pediatrics
Divisions of Neonatology and Hospital Medicine
Emory University School of Medicine
Children's Healthcare of Atlanta
Atlanta, Georgia

Margaret Rush, MD [115]
Children's National Hospital
Washington, DC

Anne Daley Ryan, MD [192]
Instructor of Pediatrics (Hospital-Based Medicine)
Northwestern University Feinberg School of Medicine
Ann & Robert H. Lurie Children's Hospital of Chicago
Chicago, Illinois

Joshua K. Schaffzin, MD, PhD [10]
Associate Professor of Pediatrics
University of Ottawa Faculty of Medicine
Staff Physician
Pediatric Infectious Diseases
Children's Hospital of Eastern Ontario
Ottawa, Ontario, Canada

Sarah Schmidt, MD [80]
Metabolic Disease Program and Division of Human Genetics, Children's Hospital of Philadelphia
Philadelphia, Pennsylvania

Hayden T. Schwenk, MD, MPH [106]
Department of Pediatrics
Division of Infectious Diseases
Center for Academic Medicine
Stanford University School of Medicine
Stanford, California

Kristin Shadman, MD [168]
Department of Pediatrics
University of Wisconsin School of Medicine and Public Health
Madison, Wisconsin

Neha H. Shah, MD, MPH [143]
Hospital Medicine Division
Children's National Hospital
The George Washington University School of Medicine and Health Sciences
Washington, DC

Nader Shaikh, MD, MPH [100]
Department of Pediatrics
University of Pittsburgh School of Medicine
Pittsburgh, Pennsylvania

Akshay Sharma, MBBS [86]
Assistant Member
Bone Marrow Transplantation and Cellular Therapy
St. Jude Children's Research Hospital
Memphis, Tennessee

Eleanor A. Sharp, MD, MS [177]
Department of Pediatrics
Division of Pediatric Hospital Medicine
University of Pittsburgh School of Medicine
UPMC Children's Hospital of Pittsburgh
Pittsburgh, Pennsylvania

Marni Shear, DO [132]
Harbor UCLA Medical Center
David Geffen School of Medicine at UCLA
Torrance, California

Yi Shi, MD, PharmD [108]
Assistant Professor of Pediatric Nephrology
New York-Presbyterian Morgan Stanley Children's Hospital
Columbia University Vagelos College of Physicians and Surgeons
New York, New York

Blair Simon, MD [192]
Neonatology Fellow
Ann & Robert H. Lurie Children's Hospital of Chicago
Chicago, Illinois

Blair E. Simpson, MD [155]
Division of Hospital Medicine
Cincinnati Children's Hospital Medical Center
Department of Pediatrics
University of Cincinnati College of Medicine
Cincinnati, Ohio

Gwenn Skar, MD [99]
Children's Hospital and Medical Center
University of Nebraska Medical Center
Omaha, Nebraska

Grace Slater, MD [183]
Assistant Professor of Pediatrics
Anesthesiology and Pain Management
UT Southwestern, Children's Health
Dallas, Texas

Alla Lescure Smith, MD [193]
Assistant Professor of Pediatrics
Harvard Medical School
Boston Children's Hospital, Division of Medical Critical Care
Boston, Massachusetts

Karen L. Smith, MD, MEd [81]
Professor of Pediatrics
Children's National Hospital
George Washington University School of Medicine and Health Sciences
Washington, DC

Cassi Smola, MD [27, 166]
Associate Professor of Pediatrics
Department of Pediatrics
Division of Pediatric Hospital Medicine
University of Alabama at Birmingham Heersink School of Medicine
Birmingham, Alabama

Kathleen D. Snow, MD [21]
Clinical Fellow
Pediatric Hospital Medicine
Boston Children's Hospital
Boston, Massachusetts

Joy L. Solano, MD, MHPE [5, 120]
Pediatric Hospital Medicine
University of Missouri-Kansas City School of Medicine
University of Kansas School of Medicine
Children's Mercy Kansas City
Kansas City, Missouri

Courtney Solomon, MD [52]
University of Texas Southwestern
Dallas, Texas

Tina Sosa, MD, MSc [4]
Division of Pediatric Hospital Medicine
Golisano Children's Hospital
UR Medicine Quality Institute
University of Rochester Medical Center
Department of Pediatrics
University of Rochester School of Medicine and Dentistry
Rochester, New York

Katherine S. Spencer, PsyD, HSP [135]
Assistant Professor of Clinical Pediatrics
Divisions of Pediatric Hospital Medicine and Pediatric Psychology
Department of Pediatrics
Monroe Carell Jr Children's Hospital at Vanderbilt
Nashville, Tennessee

Stephanie S. Squires, MD [79]
Division of Hospital Medicine
Department of Pediatrics
Stanford University School of Medicine
Palo Alto, California

Nivedita Srinivas, MD [92]
Clinical Associate Professor
Stanford University School of Medicine
Palo Alto, California

Mythili Srinivasan, MD, PhD [184]
Professor of Pediatrics
Department of Pediatrics
Division of Pediatric Hospital Medicine
Washington University School of Medicine
St. Louis, Missouri

Nicole E. St Clair, MD [30]
Professor of Pediatrics
Department of Pediatrics
Division of Pediatric Hospital Medicine
University of Wisconsin School of Medicine and Public Health
Madison, Wisconsin

Deborah R. Stein, MD [113]
Division of Nephrology
Boston Children's Hospital
Harvard Medical School
Boston, Massachusetts

John R. Stephens, MD [1]
Departments of Internal Medicine and Pediatrics
University of North Carolina School of Medicine
Chapel Hill, North Carolina

Rebecca Steuart, MD, MS [144]
Assistant Professor of Pediatrics
Medical College of Wisconsin
Physician, Complex Care Program
Children's Wisconsin
Milwaukee, Wisconsin

Patricia A. Stoeck, MD [139]
Instructor in Pediatrics
Department of Pediatrics
Harvard Medical School
Division of General Pediatrics
Boston Children's Hospital
Boston, Massachusetts

Brooke Surran, MD [122]
Northern Light Eastern Maine Medical Center
Bangor, Maine

Arsala Syed, DO, MS, MA [179]
PGY3 Pediatric Resident
St. Christopher's Hospital for Children
Philadelphia, Pennsylvania

David C. Synhorst, MD, MPA [59]
Division of Hospital Medicine
Helen DeVos Children's Hospital
Michigan State College of Medicine
Grand Rapids, Michigan

Ellen Szydlowski, MD [191]
Associate Professor of Clinical Pediatrics
Perelman School of Medicine at the University of Pennsylvania
Director of Procedural Education
Division of Emergency Medicine
Children's Hospital of Philadelphia
Philadelphia, Pennsylvania

Khoon-Yen Tay, MD [176]
Division of Emergency Medicine
Children's Hospital of Philadelphia
Department of Pediatrics
University of Pennsylvania Perelman School of Medicine
Philadelphia, Pennsylvania

W. Michelle Terry, MD [13]
Department of Pediatrics
University of Washington
Seattle, Washington

Joel Tieder, MD, MPH, FAAP [19]
Seattle Children's Hospital
University of Washington
Seattle, Washington

Lauren L. Titus, MD [171]
Department of Pediatrics
Pediatric Hospital Medicine
Medical College of Wisconsin
Milwaukee, Wisconsin

Gunjan Tiyyagura, MD, MHS [35]
Associate Professor of Pediatrics and Emergency Medicine
Yale University School of Medicine
New Haven, Connecticut

Indi Trehan, MD, MPH, DTM&H [77]
Departments of Pediatrics
Divisions of Emergency Medicine and Infectious Diseases
Global Health, and Epidemiology
University of Washington
Seattle Children's Hospital
Seattle, Washington

Janice Tsai, MD [146]
Loma Linda University Children's Hospital
Program Director of Categorical Pediatric Residency
Assistant Professor of Pediatrics, Pediatric Hospitalist
Loma Linda, California

Venée N. Tubman, MD, MMSc [85]
Assistant Professor, Department of Pediatrics
Section of Pediatric Hematology/Oncology
Baylor College of Medicine
Houston, Texas

Amy Turner, MD [74]
Division of Gastroenterology
Boston Children's Hospital
Harvard Medical School
Boston, Massachusetts

Amanda Ullman, RN, PhD [190]
Centre for Children's Health Research
Children's Health Queensland Hospital and Health Service
South Brisbane, Queensland, Australia
School of Nursing, Midwifery and Social Work
The University of Queensland
Brisbane, Queensland, Australia

Ndidi I. Unaka, MD, MEd [6]
Professor of Pediatrics
Chief Health Equity Officer, Lucille Packard Children's Hospital
Stanford University School of Medicine
Cincinnati, Ohio

Hayato Unno, MD [124]
Clinical Instructor of Pediatrics
Nemours Children's Health
Sydney Kimmel College of Medicine at Thomas Jefferson University
Philadelphia, Pennsylvania

Anna Valentine, MD [43]
Instructor, Pediatric Endocrinology
University of Colorado School of Medicine
Colorado Springs, Colorado

Kristi H. Vito, MD [45]
Ann & Robert H. Lurie Children's Hospital of Chicago
Northwestern Feinberg University School of Medicine
Chicago, Illinois

Lauren A. Wagner, DO [67]
Pediatric Hospitalist
Assistant Professor of Pediatrics
Associate Program Director of Pediatric Residency
Atrium Health Navicent
Beverly Knight Olson Children's Hospital
Mercer University School of Medicine
Macon, Georgia

Gita Wahi, MD, PhD [2]
McMaster Children's Hospital
Associate Professor
Department of Pediatrics
McMaster University
Hamilton, Ontario, Canada

Jillian Wall, MD, MPH [78]
Division of Hospital Medicine
Phoenix Children's Hospital
Phoenix, Arizona

Terry Wall, MD, MPH [129]
Professor of Pediatrics
Division of Academic General Pediatrics
University of Alabama at Birmingham
Birmingham, Alabama

G. Joy Walton, MD [181]
Associate Program Director of Internal Medicine Residency
OhioHealth Doctors Hospital in (Previously) Complex Healthcare Physician
with Nationwide Children's Hospital
Columbus, Ohio

Dane C. Warner, MD, MPH [157]
Instructor
Division of Hospital Medicine
Cincinnati Children's Hospital Medical Center
Department of Pediatrics
University of Cincinnati College of Medicine
Cincinnati, Ohio

Mollie Wasserman, MD [149]
Instructor of Pediatrics
Harvard Medical School
Boston Children's Hospital
Boston, Massachusetts

Kirstin Weerdenburg, MD, FRCPC [169]
Department of Emergency Medicine and Pediatrics
IWK Health
Department of Emergency Medicine and Pediatrics
Dalhousie University
Halifax, Nova Scotia, Canada

Michael Weinstein, MD [182]
Associate Professor of Paediatrics
University of Toronto
Division of Paediatric Medicine
Hospital for Sick Children
Toronto, Ontario, Canada

Gillian Weston, MD [60]
Assistant Professor of Dermatology and Dermatopathology
University of Connecticut School of Medicine
Farmington, Connecticut

Kathryn Westphal, MD [54]
Pediatric Hospital Medicine Fellow
Nationwide Children's Hospital
Columbus, Ohio

Maria C. Widmann, MD, FAAP [64]
Medical Director for Hospital Pediatrics
Big Lots Behavioral Health Pavilion
Section of Hospital Pediatrics
Nationwide Children's Hospital
Assistant Professor of Pediatrics
The Ohio State University College of Medicine
Columbus, Ohio

Allison E. Williams, MD [164]
UPMC Children's Hospital of Pittsburgh
University of Pittsburgh
Pittsburgh, Pennsylvania

Kelly E. Wood, MD [126]
Clinical Professor of Pediatrics
University of Iowa Stead Family Children's Hospital
Stead Family Department of Pediatrics
Iowa City, Iowa

Charles R. Wulff, MD [139]
Instructor in Psychiatry
Department of Psychiatry
Boston Children's Hospital
Harvard Medical School
Boston, Massachusetts

Jeremy Yardley, MD, FAAP [122]
Brown University
Hasbro Children's Hospital
Barrington, Rhode Island

Frances Yeung, MD, FRCPC, DRCPSC [38]
Division of Pediatric Medicine
The Hospital for Sick Children
Department of Pediatrics
University of Toronto
Toronto, Ontario, Canada

Rae S. M. Yeung, MD, PhD, FRCPC [107]
Hak-Ming and Deborah Chiu Chair in Paediatric Translational Research
Professor of Paediatrics
Immunology and Institute of Medical Science
The Hospital for Sick Children
University of Toronto
Toronto, Ontario, Canada

Andrew G. Yu, MD [53]
Division of Hospital Medicine
Department of Pediatrics
University of Texas Southwestern Medical Center and Children's Health
Dallas, Texas

Eric Zwemer, MD [173]
Associate Professor of Pediatrics
Division of Pediatric Hospital Medicine
University of North Carolina School of Medicine
Chapel Hill, North Carolina

Foreword

The first edition of *Comprehensive Pediatric Hospital Medicine* was published in 2007, and it helped to define the field of during its childhood. Pediatric hospital medicine (PHM) has continued to develop and mature and now stands as a board-certifiable subspeciality within the American Board of Pediatrics. The field continues to evolve to face challenges that could not even be imagined more than a decade and a half ago. The COVID pandemic that rocked our planet is now devolving into a strangely familiar hazard of modern life despite its ongoing impact on mortality and morbidity. COVID's waves of infections continue to cause casualties to populations, healthcare systems, education systems, and economies, while also creating new and deeper schisms in societies and politics. There is a growing awareness and attention to the disparities in healthcare which have been revealed in glaring clarity.

Struggles with mental health are increasing in the patients we care for and in their families. Hospitalists remain well poised to recognize, bring attention to, and help address these very real mental health challenges. Pediatric patients with mental health needs are hospitalized in a range of healthcare settings and hospitalists are stepping up to support these patients, whether it is the primary reason for admission or when they are important co-morbidities. Skill building and creative collaboration with mental health professionals are crucial next steps to provide this essential care that our patients deserve.

Burnout among physicians, other healthcare workers, and among medical trainees continues to rise. The resultant increase in attrition in our workforce, especially among our most experienced coworkers, further increases the stress on the system and staff, and could affect the quality of patient care. As hospitalists strive to meet the evolving demands of our patients, we must also focus on creating a sustainable professional model for ourselves. Our field is past the point of proving its value, and now can and should take responsibility for establishing work standards and support systems to promote career satisfaction, longevity, and well-being. Attending to these concerns is critical to recruit and retain an engaged PHM workforce. In this way we can remain vital, dynamic, and inspired to meet the ever-changing needs of the children and families entrusted to us.

Pediatric hospital medicine has grown into a well-established and well-respected field, with firm footing in a dynamic healthcare environment. This textbook continues to serve as a resource, providing the fundamental knowledge and skills required to care for the hospitalized child. It also has a role in supporting hospitalists to drive positive change and become leaders in healthcare systems. From this vantage, we can continue to shape the healthcare systems for the benefit of healthcare providers and healthcare recipients more broadly.

Lisa B. Zaoutis, MD

Preface

Twenty years ago to the day (-ish), a group of us had just finished dinner and decided to take an evening stroll to check out the Alamo. We had all come to San Antonio for a meeting sponsored by the (then) Ambulatory Pediatric Association for the first group of practitioners who were calling themselves pediatric hospitalists. This gathering of about 130 physicians was the genesis of what we now affectionately know as the annual PHM Conference. While we were all still experiencing the high from that first day of meetings (as well as the churros for dessert), none of us had any idea what the next 20 years would bring.

But bring it did. That meeting turned out to be the springboard for what would become the fastest growing subspecialty in the history of pediatrics. The first board exam was offered in 2019. And now, after only two exam cycles, over 2,500 certifications have been awarded, which makes Pediatric hospital medicine the fifth largest pediatric subspecialty. It's not just the growth in the number of practitioners that has been notable. The heights of the achievements of the individual members has been impressive as well. Pediatric hospitalists are now Division Chiefs and Department Chairs, Deans and Directors, and virtually almost every role within the alphabet soup of the C-suite. Simply stated, it has been astounding.

We are so excited to bring you all the third edition of *Comprehensive Pediatric Hospital Medicine*. When you get to number three, there is this sense that you might actually have a good thing going and will stick around for a while. To get to this point in the journey, the list of people to acknowledge gets pretty long.

Being hospitalized is a time of great vulnerability. We are most thankful for the privilege of being able to care for all of our patients and families along the way. Hospital medicine is most definitely a team sport. We appreciate all of you as our peers and colleagues who understand the joys and lows of practicing pediatric hospital medicine. We are grateful for all of the other providers (consultants, nurses, pharmacists, therapists, etc.) with whom we partner in our care journey. And for many of us, we are fortunate enough to work with trainees (fellows, residents, and students) represent the future of our field.

More specifically to this edition though, we want to thank the folks at McGraw Hill, especially Tim Hiscock, who have been great partners and so supportive of this effort. But most importantly, we want to recognize our four associate editors: Amanda, Erin, Joanna and Sanjay—it truly has been a pleasure and a privilege. We could not have asked for a more dedicated, capable, and understanding group. Thank you for putting up with us!

Vincent W. Chiang, MD

Samir S. Shah, MD, MSCE

PART I

Inpatient Pediatric Medicine

Part Editors

Lauren G. Solan, MD, MEd, Derek J. Williams, MD, MPH, and Jessica L. Bettenhausen, MD

CHAPTER 1 Variation in Healthcare

Jessica L. Markham, MD, MSc and John R. Stephens, MD

INTRODUCTION

Variation in the structures, processes, and organization of healthcare services occurs commonly in the United States. Understanding variation is essential to improving the safety, efficiency, effectiveness, and equity of healthcare delivery. Contributions from hospitalists and others in the fields of health services research and quality improvement remain instrumental in advancing our understanding of the drivers of variation and their impacts on the cost, quality, and outcomes of care delivered to hospitalized children.

HISTORICAL PERSPECTIVES ON VARIATION

The first population-based study of variation in pediatric healthcare was published by British researcher J. Allison Glover in the *Proceedings of the Royal Society of Medicine* in 1938. In this seminal work, Glover observed that early in the 20th century, rates of tonsillectomies among school children in England and Wales rose dramatically. By 1931, tonsillectomies made up three-quarters of all procedures performed on children in the United Kingdom. Glover observed the proportion of children undergoing tonsillectomy varied by as much as tenfold across boroughs, even among neighboring boroughs and areas with similar populations. However, neither socioeconomic status nor any other population characteristics explained why a child living in one borough had a higher probability of getting their tonsils removed than a similar child in a different borough. Glover concluded that the variation "defie[d] explanation."

In the 1960s, John Wennberg coined the term "unwarranted variation" to describe variation in healthcare service utilization that cannot be explained by patient illness, patient preference, or evidence, suggesting differences in health system performance. Taking advantage of newly implemented health data systems, Wennberg and his colleagues at Dartmouth and Johns Hopkins analyzed healthcare utilization patterns among neighboring hospital service areas throughout New England. In what would become a highly influential series of publications, the Dartmouth group reported wide geographic variation in hospital admissions, diagnostic testing, and surgical procedures—including high variability in rates of tonsillectomies. These findings persisted after adjustments for disease prevalence, patient demographics, socioeconomic factors, and medical practice differences. From these groundbreaking studies, Wennberg and colleagues founded the Dartmouth Atlas Project (http://www.dartmouthatlas.org), a publicly available resource providing comprehensive information about how healthcare resources (and healthcare quality) vary across the United States. Publications arising from the Dartmouth Atlas have played a significant role in efforts to standardize delivery and improve overall healthcare value. Perhaps the most significant Dartmouth Atlas finding, reported by Yasaitis et al, is that greater healthcare spending does not always correlate with higher quality of care and, in some cases, may be associated with suboptimal care (*Health Affairs Project Hope*, 2009).

VARIATION STUDIES IN PEDIATRICS

The Dartmouth Atlas shaped our understanding of pediatric healthcare variation. The initial analyses using the Dartmouth Atlas were largely limited to investigations of adult populations using Medicare data though subsequently this work was leveraged to investigate geographic variation in pediatric healthcare. For example, using data from commercial insurers and Medicaid, *The Dartmouth Atlas of Children's Health Care in Northern New England* reported rates of inpatient and outpatient healthcare utilization across regions and hospitals. Among other findings, the authors observed that emergency room visits varied threefold across the region and were inversely correlated with rates of office visits.

In parallel with the growth of the Dartmouth Atlas, pioneers in pediatric hospital medicine utilized health data systems in Boston (MA), Rochester (NY), and other US cities to uncover wide variation in the management of inpatient conditions such as asthma, gastroenteritis, and lower respiratory tract infections. For example, Perrin et al studied variation in hospitalization rates for common conditions across three urban areas and found two to three times higher relative risks of hospitalization for head injury and asthma in Boston (MA) and New Haven (CT) compared with Rochester (NY). More recently, publicly available (e.g., Agency for Healthcare Research and Quality [AHRQ] Healthcare Cost and Utilization Project [HCUP] databases, including the Kids' Inpatient Database [KID]) and proprietary administrative databases (e.g., Pediatric Health Information Systems [PHIS] Database), have provided researchers with the opportunity to examine variation within large, sometimes nationally representative, pediatric patient samples. As an example, Pati et al used the KID database to study variation in length of stay based on insurance status among children hospitalized with pneumonia and found significantly longer stays for those with public insurance versus private or no insurance (*Journal of Hospital Medicine*, 2012).

CONCEPTUAL FRAMEWORK FOR VARIATION

The challenge of studying practice variation lies in defining what constitutes "unwarranted" differences in care. Variation in practice can occur for many legitimate reasons, leading some to argue that variation is only unwarranted if it deviates from evidence-based standards or has a significantly negative impact on health outcomes. By these definitions, much of the observed variation in healthcare could be considered "unexplained" as opposed to unwarranted. This is especially the case for care provided to children, as there are few conditions with indisputable standards of care. On the other hand, if clinical outcomes are demonstrated to be similar for varied practices, the practices that use more resources likely involve overuse or waste and are thus unwarranted. Regardless of whether it is considered unwarranted or unexplained, a general framework for understanding variation and generating hypotheses about its sources and significance involves grouping care into three major categories: (1) supply-sensitive, (2) preference-sensitive, and (3) effective (**Table 1-1**).

Supply-sensitive care refers to healthcare services that are utilized at higher rates in areas where there is greater resource availability, contributing to higher per capita healthcare expenditures. Unfortunately, this high utilization is rarely associated with better outcomes or patient satisfaction, and often represents waste of healthcare dollars and lost opportunity costs. In Wennberg's early studies, this was demonstrated by observations that patients living in areas with greater bed capacity were

TABLE 1-1 Framework for Understanding Healthcare Variation

Category of Variation	Definition	Example
Supply-sensitive	Variation based on relative availability of specific types of care.	Variation rate of hospitalization based on proximity to hospital. Wennberg et al, *New England Journal of Medicine*, 1989
Preference-sensitive	Variation based on having two or more options for care without specific evidence demonstrating superiority of one option.	Choice of initial surgical versus initial medical treatment for conditions possibly amenable to either, such as retropharyngeal abscess. Lipsett et al, *Hospital Pediatrics*, 2021
Effective	Variation based on variable application of best available evidence for a particular condition.	High rates of and variation in use of electrolyte testing for children with gastroenteritis despite several guideline statements that it is unnecessary. Nabower et al, *Hospital Pediatrics*, 2020

more likely to be hospitalized, patients living in areas with more surgeons were more likely to have a surgical procedure, and patients living in areas with more radiology services were more likely to have imaging studies performed. The primary driver of this type of variation is felt to be the subtle influence of service availability on clinician decision-making in cases where the tradeoffs are not as well defined and choices to admit or test are at the discretion of the physician.

Preference-sensitive care entails the management of conditions for which there are several justifiable options for diagnosis and treatment. In some cases, there may be no evidence to support any single option. In others, evidence does exist, but each option may involve important tradeoffs that need to be considered on a patient-by-patient basis. One similarity between supply-sensitive and preference-sensitive care is the hypothesis that variation in physician practice styles, as opposed to differences in patient preferences, is the major driver of variation in care. While patient preferences will produce some degree of variation in care, management decisions such as whether to perform surgical procedures are unlikely to be driven by patient preference alone. As an example, Lipsett et al found that surgical versus medical treatment for children with deep neck infections varies widely by specific children's hospital, suggesting significant influence by providers in decision-making (*Hospital Pediatrics*, 2021). The unbalanced influence of the physician on clinical decision-making has also been demonstrated for elective pediatric procedures. In a 2012 study by Fox et al (*Academic Pediatrics*), the decision to proceed with a fundoplication in children with severe reflux was rarely based on definitive testing, and most physicians perceived that family decisions to proceed with surgery were more strongly influenced by subspecialist preference than by counseling from their primary provider. Since there is little evidence to guide the treatment of severe reflux, these decisions were likely guided by anecdotal experiences and the physicians' own interpretation of existing literature rather than informed family preferences.

Effective care involves the management of conditions for which there is strong scientific evidence to support best practices. Inpatient conditions including asthma, bronchiolitis, urinary tract infection, fever in young infants, and community-acquired pneumonia have evidence-based guidelines to support clinical decision-making. Most providers can agree that adherence to these guidelines is of great clinical importance and value to their patients, yet a high proportion of children receive non-guideline concordant care. Though a variety of factors can contribute to these deviations, many are too large to be attributed to patient differences alone. For example, despite several guidelines recommending against routine electrolyte testing for pediatric gastroenteritis, Nabower et al found that 85% of children hospitalized at children's hospitals had that testing performed (*Hospital Pediatrics*, 2020). As a second example, Stephens et al reported that over half of children hospitalized for skin and soft tissue infections had blood cultures drawn, despite guidelines stating they are generally unnecessary (*Hospital Pediatrics*, 2020).

STRATEGIES FOR ADDRESSING EACH CATEGORY OF VARIATION

Supply-sensitive care. Fee-for-service payment systems traditionally used in US healthcare may contribute to unchecked overuse of supply-sensitive care. Accordingly, proposed strategies for reducing variation and lowering costs involve alternative payment models, including population-based (e.g., accountable care organizations [ACOs]) and episode-based payment models (e.g., bundled payments for specific conditions). In the ACO model, healthcare organizations contract to provide comprehensive care to a population of patients for a fixed per-member price, and payments for each hospitalization are shared across all members of the hospital system's medical staff, including inpatient and outpatient providers responsible for the care of the child. ACOs are paid on a capitated basis and/or for achieving certain quality/cost targets, and thus are incentivized to manage the quality and utilization of care more responsibly. In their early stages of development, some ACOs appear to be successful at reducing cost while improving quality, as shown in 2017 work by Perrin et al (*Pediatrics*), but more needs to be learned about which organizational factors most contribute to a successful ACO model. In episode-based models, single bundled payments are made to cover all costs for a specific healthcare episode, such as a surgery or hospitalization. Episode-based models have been most extensively studied in the surgical care of adult patients and show some promise for containing costs while maintaining quality for certain procedures (e.g., total joint replacement surgery) as demonstrated in a systematic review by Agrawal et al (*Health Affairs Project Hope*, 2020).

Preference-sensitive care. A general approach to reducing the influence of the "individual" provider/institution within preference-sensitive care variation is to establish and disseminate evidence-based best practices and the use of provider feedback (e.g., audit and feedback). Where guidelines are lacking, prioritizing the development of best practices for the most prevalent and costly inpatient conditions, such as those reported by Gill et al (JAMA Network Open, 2021), may aid in developing best practices to further address preference-sensitive care. Another strategy is to define when variable approaches result in similar clinical outcomes, which would then support that the less expensive or invasive option should be preferred. As an example, in the aforementioned study by Lipsett et al on variation in management of deep neck infections, children initially managed medically versus surgically had no differences in readmissions but had lower costs and shorter length of stay, suggesting that medical management should be pursued.

Effective care. The first hurdle in reducing variation in effective care is overcoming the gap between scientific discovery and clinical practice, which according to some estimates, can take decades to effectively implement. For conditions with high variation in effective care such as febrile urinary tract infections and community acquired pneumonia, clinical practice guidelines (CPGs) have been an important tool for educating providers on evidence-based practice. Specifically, use of CPGs has resulted in improvements in adherence to care, reduced lengths of stay, and lower resource utilization. Even with CPGs, though, variation in adherence to effective care persists indicating that these interventions alone are not always enough to change physician behavior.

Additional tools have been developed to support implementation of CPGs and reduce variation in effective care in clinical settings. The most widely studied CPG support tools are protocols and clinical pathways. Unlike CPGs, which typically only *describe* best practice and reference-supporting evidence, protocols and pathways are designed to enhance evidence-based care delivery and coordination of care and may be integrated as active decision support tools in electronic medical records. Protocols are most appropriate for systematically guiding individual providers through treatment decisions by outlining the specific evidence-based criteria under which a clinician would or would not choose a course of treatment (e.g., phototherapy vs. exchange transfusion for neonates with hyperbilirubinemia). Alternatively, clinical pathways promote coordination of care within interdisciplinary care teams, by describing specific steps in care by individual care team members. A strength of pathways is that they often contain a built-in component for measuring defined outcomes (cost, treatment success, adherence) and providing feedback to clinicians.

The literature contains numerous examples of both successful and unsuccessful applications of CPGs, protocols, and pathways for reducing variation in effective care, and it is likely that there is no one-size-fits-all strategy. As one example, Desai et al reported increased timely administration of corticosteroids and reductions in CXR utilization, emergency department length of stay, and antibiotic prescriptions after implementing pediatric asthma pathways (*Pediatric Quality and Safety*, 2020). Implementation science itself is a burgeoning field of study, seeking to optimize methods for implementing (or de-implementing) clinical pathways. Multiple frameworks have been developed to assist clinicians in pathway implementation such as the Consolidated Framework for Implementation Research (CFIR, https://cfirguide.org). One important example of de-implementation is the work by Bonafide et al (*Pilot and Feasibility Studies*, 2019) focused on eliminating overuse of pulse oximetry monitoring within bronchiolitis.

On a national policy level, hospitals are being encouraged to learn from variation in effective care by forming partnerships with neighboring health centers. Using what is called a *positive deviance* approach, the CMS-sponsored Hospital Engagement Networks (HENs) have committed to exploring factors that facilitate high-quality care. By sharing information on care processes, quality improvement tools, and implementation strategies, HENs work to collectively identify and implement standardized practices that consistently produce better outcomes. A pediatric example of a HEN is Solutions for Patient Safety (https://www.solutionsforpatientsafety.org). To date, HEN collaborations have minimized variation in care across networks and led to dramatic reductions in adverse events (http://www.jcrinc.com/CMS-Hospital-Engagement-Network).

VARIATION AND COMPARATIVE EFFECTIVENESS RESEARCH

Even in the case of effective care, it may be difficult to determine what degree of variation is truly unwarranted, emphasizing the need to continuously monitor both processes and outcomes of care to understand what does and does not work. In this way, existing variation creates new opportunities for comparative effectiveness research (CER). With resources and tools such as nationally representative administrative datasets, clinical registries, and evolving statistical methods, CER can address clinical questions that previously would have been too costly and infeasible to study.

As CER in pediatric hospital medicine has grown, efforts have been made to define research priorities. Due to growing funding constraints and other challenges inherent to pediatric research (e.g., small sample sizes, relatively rare outcomes), the research community has a responsibility to focus CER efforts on conditions for which the opportunity to impact patient outcomes and/or resource utilization is greatest. Strategies for determining high priority conditions requires knowledge of current disease prevalence, burden of illness, cost, gaps in evidence, feasibility of study, and importance of outcomes to patients. As previously described, Gill et al ranked the priority of inpatient conditions using the PHIS database and a standardized costing method to identify the 50 most costly and prevalent pediatric inpatient conditions. Not surprisingly, conditions such as asthma and dehydration were found to be among the highest priority conditions. Also identified were conditions for which variation and the potential for clinical impact may have been underappreciated, such as scoliosis surgery, and acute appendicitis.

The development of achievable benchmarks of care (ABCs) is another method for defining CER priorities and also a method for identifying goals for implementation/de-implementation. ABCs utilize a data-driven approach to define performance goals/targets using the top performers among at least 10% of the studied population. Notably, ABCs may change over time as evidence evolves. As an example, Ralston et al developed updated ABCs for care of children with bronchiolitis, reflecting reductions in non-evidence-based care interventions following publication of national bronchiolitis guidelines (*Pediatrics*, 2021).

National strategies including Choosing Wisely (https://www.choosingwisely.org) have been initiated to address the dissemination and implementation of evidence-based practices and CER. The Choosing Wisely campaign identifies common areas of unnecessary medical use by specialty. Priorities are based on recommendations from experts in the field and guided by available evidence. Notably, the Choosing Wisely recommendations have been combined with ABC metrics for some conditions as demonstrated in the work by Reyes et al (Hospital Pediatrics, 2017) to allow healthcare entities to further refine targets for improvement.

CONTRIBUTIONS FROM HOSPITAL MEDICINE

Given their understanding of complex hospital systems, pediatric hospitalists are well suited to study variation, identify best practices, and to design system-level interventions to improve healthcare quality and safety. Groups such as the Pediatric Research in Inpatient Settings (PRIS) Network and the AAP's Value in Inpatient Pediatrics (VIP) Network have made significant progress in these domains. As the field advances, pediatric hospitalists involved in research and operational efforts to reduce and study variation have several important challenges to address.

First, providers and hospital leaders need to advocate for payment reforms that incentivize high-value care and reduce unwarranted variation in supply-sensitive care. Second, given diminishing availability of support from federal funders, hospitalists need to prioritize the subjects of their research efforts, focusing on conditions for which innovations in care will have a large impact on value and outcomes. Third, networks of researchers and providers need to continue to develop reliable and transparent data sources with which to longitudinally monitor processes and outcomes across health systems. Such data will promote a collective sense of accountability as well as encourage collaborative efforts to disseminate guidelines and reduce variation in effective care. Fourth, the scope of comparative effectiveness research needs to be broadened to account for the diversity and complexity of healthcare systems and gain a deeper understanding of the unique organizational barriers and facilitators to implementing effective and more patient-centered care. Finally, CER conducted by hospitalists needs to be methodologically rigorous, utilizing advanced methods for risk adjustment and subpopulation analyses of observational data and publishing rigorous systematic reviews and meta-analyses on existing data from the literature.

SUMMARY

It is well known that healthcare services, resource utilization, quality, and outcomes vary tremendously across the United States. In some cases, this variation may be the result of appropriate decision-making and consideration of differing patient preferences, but much of this variation is likely unwarranted and not based on patient preferences or evidence-based practice. The consequences of unwarranted variation are profound and include uncontrolled healthcare spending and large disparities in quality of care. Payment system reform, better tools for shared decision-making, public reporting of outcomes, and implementation of CPGs, protocols, and pathways are needed to reduce variation, control cost, and optimize quality. Investigating variation provides opportunities to learn how we can improve care delivery and offers many opportunities for comparative effectiveness research. Understanding the driving factors and consequences of variation—warranted and unwarranted—will be essential to improving value and reducing disparities in the care of hospitalized children in the US healthcare system.

SUGGESTED READINGS

Fisher ES, Welch HG. Avoiding the unintended consequences of growth in medical care: how might more be worse? *JAMA*. 1999; 281(5):446-453.

Gill PJ, Anwar MR, Thavam T, et al. Identifying conditions with high prevalence, cost, and variation in cost in US children's hospitals. *JAMA Netw Open*. 2021;4(7):e2117816.

Goodman DC, Morden NE, Ralston SL, Chang C. The Dartmouth Atlas of Children's Health Care in Northern New England. http://www.dartmouthatlas.org/downloads/atlases/NNE_Pediatric_Atlas_121113.pdf.

Moen A, Goodman DC. Unwarranted geographic variation in paediatric health care in the United States and Norway. *Acta Paediatr*. 2022;111(4):733-740.

Pasquali SK, Thibault D, Hall M, et al. Evolving cost-quality relationship in pediatric heart surgery. *Ann Thorac Surg*. 2022;113(3):866-873.

Perrin JM, Homer CJ, Berwick DM, et al. Variations in rates of hospitalization of children in three urban communities. *N Engl J Med*. 1989; 320(18):1183-1187.

Reyes M, Paulus E, Hronek C, et al. Choosing wisely campaign: report card and achievable benchmarks of care for children's hospitals. *Hosp Pediatr*. 2017;7(11):633-641.

Wennberg JE. Time to tackle unwarranted variations in practice. *BMJ*. 2011;342:d1513.

Yasaitis L, Fisher ES, Skinner JS, Chandra A. Hospital quality and intensity of spending: is there an association? *Health Aff Proj Hope*. 2009;28(4):w566-572.

CHAPTER 2

Evidence-Based Practice

Gita Wahi, MD, PhD and Kathleen Berg, MD

INTRODUCTION

Ideal clinical care integrates a healthcare professional's clinical experience, individual patient preferences and values, and current best evidence. How this evidence is applied to individual patients and integrated into clinical care systems is the art of evidence-based practice (EBP). In 2003, a consensus statement conceived by the delegates of the second international conference of Evidence-Based Health Care Teachers and Developers in Sicily, Italy, stated that EBP "requires that decisions about health care are based on the best available, current, valid, and relevant evidence. These decisions should be made by those receiving care, informed by the tacit and explicit knowledge of those providing care, within the context of available resources" (*BMC Med Educ*, 2005). This chapter provides practical guidance on efficiently and effectively formulating questions, appraising literature, and applying evidence.

FORMULATING THE QUESTION

Asking clinical questions is fundamental to EBP. A well-formulated and specific question allows for an efficient, manageable literature search that yields valuable resources for analysis. Before asking a specific foreground question, it may be necessary to gather background information, such as in a review article. A solid comprehension of the disease process in question serves as the basis for a successful examination of the evidence.

The "PICO" mnemonic, developed in 1995, facilitates identifying evidence to address a focused clinical question. There are four parts: patient Population, Intervention or exposure being considered, Comparison intervention or exposure, and the measurable Outcome of interest. While there are variations on the mnemonic with the addition of Time when outcomes are measured relative to intervention or exposure and Study design (i.e., PICOT or PICOTS), the basic purpose of the tool remains to craft a focused question for the clinical problem at hand. For example, while caring for a 10-month-old admitted with pyelonephritis, decisions on empiric treatment while awaiting urine culture and susceptibilities may prompt you to ask the following question:

1. Patient population (includes patient problem)—*In otherwise healthy children 2 months to 2 years of age with pyelonephritis*
2. Intervention (treatment or diagnostic test) or exposure—*does empiric use of first-generation cephalosporins (e.g., cefazolin)*
3. Comparison or control intervention—*compared with third-generation cephalosporins (e.g., ceftriaxone)*
4. Measurable outcome—*affect length of stay or readmissions?*

POPULATION

Clearly defining the patient population is important. For example, exclusion of neonates may be appropriate if the question involves diagnoses associated with fever for which neonates would be managed differently. Qualifiers such as "previously healthy" or "with complex medical conditions" may be important to the search strategy. When evidence on the pediatric population is not available, the scope may be expanded, when appropriate, to include adults; in such cases, the results should be carefully considered before potentially extrapolating to the care of children.

INTERVENTION

While the intervention is often a therapy, it can also be a diagnostic test, a medical device, or a patient, provider, program, or health system characteristic. For example, the presence or absence of leukocyte esterase on urinalysis could be compared using urine culture as the gold standard for diagnosing urinary tract infection. Alternatively, the intervention may be an exposure as in the following: In patients 2 months to 2 years of age with pyelonephritis, is the presence of urinary tract dilation class 1 to 2 compared with no dilation associated with risk of recurrent urinary tract infection? It is also important to consider that the intervention may be to intervene less, provide supportive care, or simply observe; for example, in patients without complex medical conditions diagnosed with cystitis, is a 5-day course of antibiotics compared to >5-day course associated with risk of treatment failure? This type of question is essential when considering de-implementation strategies in the context of high-value care.

COMPARISON

The comparison is often the standard of care or most common practice or the absence of an intervention or exposure. It serves as a benchmark to the alternative intervention being considered. For prognostic questions, the comparison may be a different patient population.

OUTCOME

The measurable outcome reflects the current clinical concerns, values, and preferences of both the clinician and patient. Common outcomes in hospital medicine include treatment success, care escalation, length of stay, adverse events, and cost or other resource utilization. These outcomes are of interest to hospitals, clinicians, patients, and families. Some important outcomes are more patient-specific, such as number of venipuncture events, frequency of sleep interruptions, or quality of communication with the medical team. The outcome may also be the reliability or validity if the intervention is a diagnostic test.

The PICO framework may not be appropriate for all types of clinical questions. It is most applicable to "which" questions, comparing one intervention to another. While still possible, it can be more challenging to fit prognostic questions into its framework. It is of little utility for "how" or "why" questions. True to EBP principles, other strategies have been evaluated in comparison to PICO and pursuit of the optimal framework is ongoing.

SEARCHING THE LITERATURE

PRIMARY SOURCES

After formulating a question and reviewing background material, searching primary literature sources, including journal articles and conference proceedings, is typically required. Databases for medical literature include MEDLINE, a National Library of Medicine bibliographic database derived from more than 5200 journals, including over 29 million citations in 40 different languages. With frequent and regular addition of new citations and sources, this database continues to steadily grow. There are multiple ways to access MEDLINE including but not limited to PubMed and Ovid.

Before beginning a search, it is helpful to understand how articles are indexed in MEDLINE. One method of limiting the number of articles you wade through is by attaching suffixes to the keyword. These suffixes allow you to search one journal, search by author, look for words in a title or abstract, or restrict the search by year of publication. Some useful suffixes are listed in **Table 2-1**.

TABLE 2-1 Suffixes for Medline Searches

.ab	Word in Abstract
.au	Author
.jn	Journal
.ti	Word in title
.tw	Word in title or abstract
.yr	Year of publication

TABLE 2-2 Subheadings for Medline Searches

/ae	Adverse effects
/co	Complications
/di	Diagnosis
/dt	Drug therapy
/ep	Epidemiology
/hi	History
/th	Therapy

MEDLINE is also indexed using Medical Subject Headings (MeSH) terms. The keyword will be mapped automatically to one or more subject headings. For example, if searching for the term *bronchiolitis*, it will automatically be mapped to the MeSH terms: bronchiolitis, bronchiolitis obliterans, and bronchiolitis viral. If you are only interested in viral bronchiolitis, including *viral bronchiolitis* will limit your search to more relevant articles. Finally, using subheadings may further narrow search results. Some helpful subheadings are listed in **Table 2-2**. A librarian with knowledge in medical literature searches would be an expert resource in this area for more extensive searches.

SECONDARY SOURCES

Once articles have been identified through Medline, the quality of the studies and validity of the conclusions must be considered. One approach is to use secondary sources, such as databases with summaries of literature that have been reviewed. Examples of such databases include: American College of Physicians (ACP) Journal Club; Database of Abstracts of Reviews of Effects (DARE); Cochrane Central Register of Controlled Trials (CCTR); and Cochrane Database of Systematic Reviews (CDSR). If you find articles on the topic of interest in one of these four databases, the quality of the article or articles will be assessed for you. Each of the four databases is described in **Table 2-3**.

OTHER WEB SOURCES

Other resources on the web include The National Guideline Clearinghouse (www.guidelines.gov). This is a database of evidence-based clinical practice guidelines (CPG) and related documents originally developed by the Agency for Healthcare Research and Quality (AHRQ). UpToDate (www.uptodate.com), an easily accessible electronic textbook that is frequently revised is another popular web resource. Google Scholar (scholar.google.com) may allow for broad retrieval of information, though often requires additional scrutiny to ascertain the quality of search results.

ASSESSING THE EVIDENCE

The above databases and web sites will help to find relevant articles, but it is also important to have a basic understanding of levels of evidence and the components of various study designs when considering an article investigating a prognostic factor, a treatment, or a diagnostic test **(Figure 2-1)**.

TABLE 2-3 Databases for Secondary Sources

American College of Physicians (ACP) Journal Club	A database of commentary on clinically relevant, methodologically sound articles
Database of Abstracts of Reviews of Effects (DARE)	A database of critical assessments of systematic reviews covering diagnosis, prevention, rehabilitation, screening, and treatment
Cochrane Central Register of Controlled Trials (CCTR)	A database of definitive controlled trials in the literature
Cochrane Database of Systematic Reviews (CDSR)	A database of updated systematic reviews about therapy, intervention, or prevention

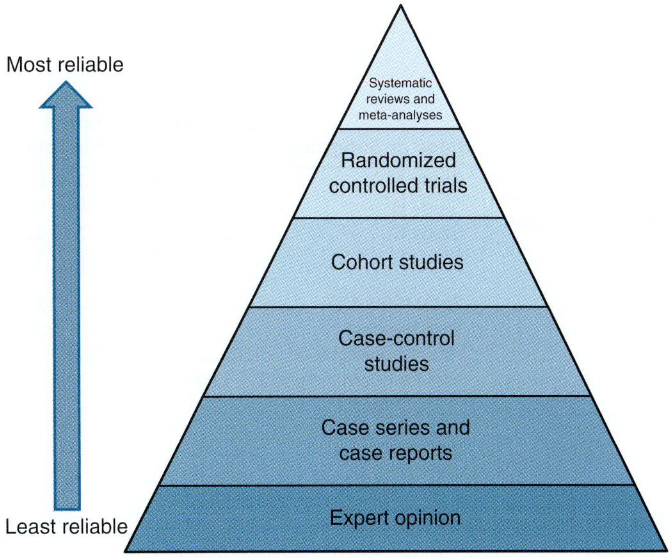

FIGURE 2-1. Hierarchy of the quality of evidence. (Reproduced with permission from Sherer JT, Aparasu RR, Bentley JP, eds. Principles of Evidence-Based Medicine: *Principles of Research Design and Drug Literature Evaluation*, 2nd ed. New York, NY: McGraw-Hill; 2020.)

META-ANALYSES AND SYSTEMATIC REVIEWS

Meta-analyses and systematic reviews sit first and second, respectively, atop the evidence hierarchy (see Figure 2-1). Both use explicit methodology to search, appraise, and synthesize other literature. Each begins with the identification of a specific research question with formulation of inclusion and exclusion criteria, followed by a search for and selection of appropriate studies. The quality of each individual study is assessed, then either data are extracted, combined, and reanalyzed in the case of a meta-analysis or results are described in the case of a systematic review.

Meta-analyses synthesize results of multiple studies to yield a quantitative summary, often presented as summary odds ratios, relative risks, or number needed to treat. It is particularly useful to be familiar with the forest plots commonly used to display such results. **Figure 2-2** details the components of a typical forest plot. The diamond near the x-axis represents the combined effect of study results, with statistical significance if the diamond does not cross the vertical "line of null effect." The I^2 statistic is a measure of heterogeneity (i.e., inconsistency) between studies, preferably <50%.

The quality of a meta-analysis or systematic review depends, in part, on transparent and complete description of the methodology. PRISMA (Preferred Reporting Items for Systematic Reviews and Meta-Analyses) is a widely used guideline to facilitate and standardize reporting. This tool, updated in 2020, includes a 27-step checklist including assessments of risk of bias, heterogeneity of included studies, and certainty of the evidence. Meta-analyses often include Summary of Findings tables for each intervention comparison and most commonly follow the GRADE (Grading of Recommendations Assessment, Development, and Evaluation) approach. This includes not only the estimate of effect, but also appraisal of risk of bias, inconsistency, indirectness, and imprecision. Together these inform the certainty, or quality, of the evidence (high, moderate, low, or very low).

RANDOMIZED CONTROLLED TRIALS

Randomized controlled trials (RCTs) sit high on the evidence hierarchy just after systematic reviews and meta-analyses (see Figure 2-1). In clinical settings, RCTs answer questions of efficacy, effectiveness, and/or safety of a treatment on the outcome of a patient's condition. A RCT allocates participants randomly to intervention or control groups. The participants are followed prospectively for a set period with measurement of the outcome of the trial. The simplest RCT design is a parallel

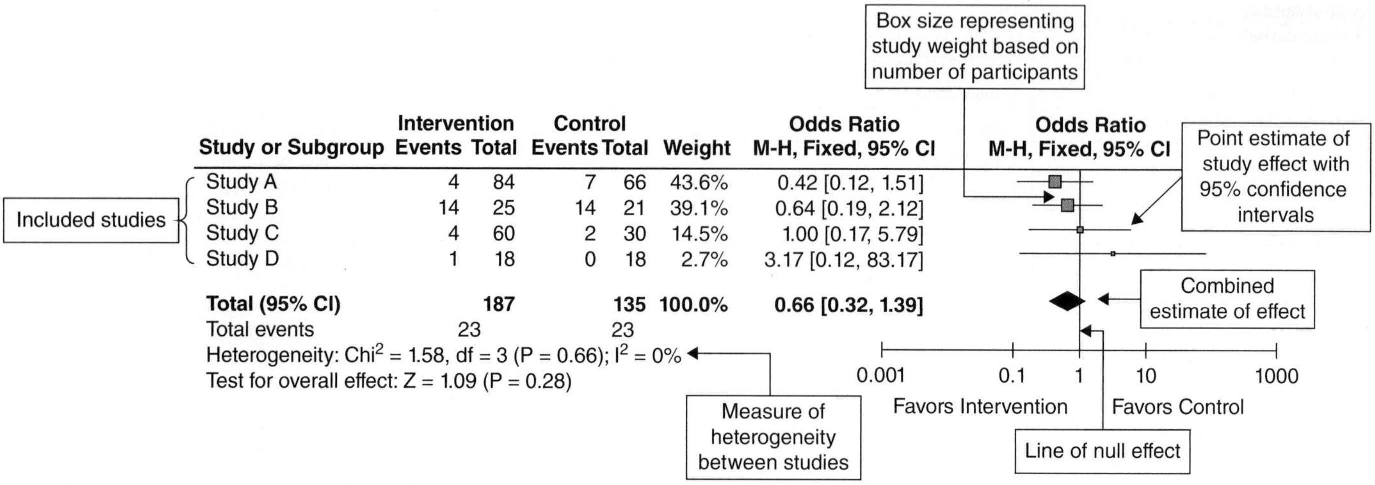

FIGURE 2-2. Anatomy of a forest plot.

group design where individual participants are randomized to the intervention or control. Other RCT designs include factorial designs, where varying levels of intervention or multiple interventions are evaluated, and cross-over designs where participants alternate between intervention and control groups. In RCTs randomization reduces bias by controlling for measured and unmeasured confounders. Another way to reduce bias is blinding. Blinding occurs when the participants, researchers, and or outcome adjudicators are not aware, or "blinded," to the group allocation of the participant. Further, while traditional RCTs are often highly selective and seek to answer efficacy of interventions under a set of ideal, tightly controlled conditions, pragmatic RCTs focus on evaluating the efficacy of interventions in real-world settings.

RCTs are reported using standard guidelines from the CONsolidated Standards of Reporting Trials 2010 guideline (CONSORT). The CONSORT guideline standardizes RCT reporting and promotes transparency, including reporting of the design, analysis, and interpretation. The CONSORT guidelines cover a variety of RCT designs, such as cluster RCTs and pilot RCTs as well as many others.

OBSERVATIONAL STUDIES

Observational study designs sit lower on the evidence hierarchy and include cohort studies and case control studies (see Figure 2-1). Similar to RCTs, observational studies are held to a reporting standard. Most often observational studies will be reported with the Strengthening the Reporting of Observational Studies in Epidemiology (STROBE) Statement.

Cohort studies are longitudinal studies, where participants are selected based on their exposure, and then followed over time to observe if they develop the outcome of interest. Cohort studies can be designed prospectively as well as retrospectively and are helpful in studying rare exposures. Challenges with cohort studies which place them lower on the evidence hierarchy are selection bias and confounding.

Case control studies help determine if an exposure is associated with an outcome. In case control studies a group of study participants are identified based on whether or not they have the outcome of interest, often designated as cases and controls. The study team then looks retrospectively at each group to determine the main exposures, comparing the frequency of the exposure in the case group to the control group. Case control studies are particularly helpful in studying rare diseases or outcomes but are more subject to bias compared to cohort studies.

Other observational study designs include cross-sectional studies which give a prevalence of a condition in a population at a particular time or the association between an exposure and an outcome. However, since measured a one point in time, the sequence events cannot be assumed. Case reports or case series provide description of a single case or a series of cases and provide descriptive information.

APPLICABILITY

How valid information is integrated into the care of individual patients is the art of EBP. For example, a RCT may determine that for patients with mild to moderate asthma exacerbation, dexamethasone is as effective as a 5-day course of prednisone without increasing the need for return medical visits. You determine the study is valid, but question if whether it applies to your individual patient. Does the population in the trial sufficiently match the age, medical complexity, and severity of illness of your patient? Are there other factors such as health literacy or access to medical care to consider? Does the favored intervention align with your patient's and their family's preferences and values? The Evidence to Decision framework is a tool within the GRADE methodology that prompts assessment of additional variables before applying study results. It includes consideration of risks and benefits, value, resource utilization, cost effectiveness, equity, acceptability, and feasibility. This framework is often used by expert panels developing clinical practice guidelines but can also be valuable to teams of clinicians reviewing best practices in their care settings.

While the practice of EBP is essential to the care of individual patients, evidence should also be applied within systems of care. This is where EBP and quality improvement intersect. Early in the quality improvement framework, EBP should inform aims and intervention methods. With this foundation, improvement methodology can serve to implement best practices solidly grounded in evidence.

TEACHING EVIDENCE-BASED PRACTICE

In addition to incorporating EBP methodology into clinical practice, pediatric hospitalists may also be expected to teach it to medical students, residents, fellows, and colleagues. The use of EBP is an essential skill for trainees, included as an Accreditation Council for Graduate Medical Education (ACGME) competency for both General Pediatrics and Pediatric Hospital Medicine. A variety of curricula have improved trainee competency in EBP methodology and increased citing of evidence on rounds. Educational strategies often include longitudinal didactics and activities to provide foundational knowledge followed by advancement to application, then integration. However, it is also helpful to model, for learners, your evidence-based approach to care during bedside teaching. It is important for learners to see that even the most experienced clinicians rely on the evidence-gathering process to make informed patient care decisions. In addition to knowledge-based learning, skill-based learning with transparent discussions about your clinical questions, resources and search strategies is key to your learners' long-term success. Many of the clinical pearls trainees learn will change throughout their careers. With the fundamental tools to appraise and apply new literature, they can continue to practice high value, evidence-based care as recommendations continually evolve.

SUGGESTED READINGS

Accreditation Council for Graduate Medical Education. Pediatrics. Program Requirements. Published July 1, 2022. Program Requirements and FAQs and Applications (acgme.org). Available at: https://www.acgme.org/specialties/pediatrics/program-requirements-and-faqs-and-applications/. Accessed September 23, 2022.

Alonso-Coello P, Oxman AD, Moberg J, et al. GRADE Evidence to Decision (EtD) frameworks: a systematic and transparent approach to making well informed healthcare choices. 2: Clinical practice guidelines. *BMJ*. 2016;353:i2089.

Chitkara MB, Boykan R, Messina CR. A longitudinal practical evidence-based medicine curriculum for pediatric residents. *Acad Pediatr*. 2016;16(3):305-307.

Dasgupta MN, Kirkey DC, Weatherly JA, Kuo KW, Rassbach CE. Using self-determination theory to drive an evidence-based medicine curriculum for pediatric residents: a mixed methods study. *Acad Pediatr*. 2022;22(3):486-494.

Dawes M, Summerskill W, Glasziou P, et al. Sicily statement on evidence-based practice. *BMC Med Educ*. 2005;5(1):1.

Guyatt G. *Users' Guides to the Medical Literature: A Manual for Evidence-Based Clinical Practice*. 3rd ed. New York: McGraw Hill; 2015.

Kuzma N, Kersten HB, Thompson ED. Evidence-based medicine in the clinical learning environment of pediatric hospital medicine. *Pediatr Clin North Am*. 2019;66(4):713-724.

Li SA, Alexander PE, Reljic T, et al. Evidence to decision framework provides a structured "roadmap" for making GRADE guidelines recommendations. *J Clin Epidemiol*. 2018;104:103-112.

Moyer V, Elliott E, Davis R, et al., eds. *Evidence Based Pediatrics and Child Health*. London: BMJ Books; 2000.

Page MJ, Moher D, Bossuyt PM, et al. PRISMA 2020 explanation and elaboration: updated guidance and exemplars for reporting systematic reviews. *BMJ*. 2021;372:n160.

Richardson WS, Wilson MC, Nishikawa J, Hayward RS. The well-built clinical question: a key to evidence-based decisions. *ACP J Club*. 1995;123(3):A12-A13.

Schulz KF, Altman DG, Moher D; CONSORT Group. CONSORT 2010 statement: updated guidelines for reporting parallel group randomised trials. *BMJ*. 2010;340:c332.

Schünemann HJ, Higgins JPT, Vist GE, et al. Chapter 14: Completing 'Summary of findings' tables and grading the certainty of the evidence. In: Higgins JPT, Thomas J, Chandler J, et al. (eds). *Cochrane Handbook for Systematic Reviews of Interventions* version 6.3 (updated February 2022). Cochrane, 2022. Available at: www.training.cochrane.org/handbook.

Straus SE, Glasziou P, Richardson WS, Hayes RB. *Evidence-Based Medicine: How to Practice and Teach EBM*. 5th ed. Elsevier; 2018.

von Elm E, Altman DG, Egger M, et al. The Strengthening the Reporting of Observational Studies in Epidemiology (STROBE) statement: guidelines for reporting observational studies [published correction appears in Ann Intern Med. 2008;148(2):168]. *Ann Intern Med*. 2007;147(8):573-577.

CHAPTER 3

Quality Improvement

David P. Johnson, MD and Heather S. McLean, MD

INTRODUCTION

Members of the Pediatric Hospital Medicine (PHM) community influence patient care from the bedside to the boardroom. In recent years, the growth in quality improvement (QI) knowledge and skills in the PHM community combined with these positions of influence have provided an environment ripe to improve patient care. QI involves systematic, rigorous, data-driven activities that seek to bring about rapid improvements in healthcare delivery and outcomes. Like the field of PHM, the introduction of QI into healthcare is a relatively recent phenomenon. Many of the QI methods that we utilize now were developed in industry and have been adapted to healthcare in recent decades. Walter Shewhart developed Statistical Process Control Charts in the 1920s as a means to provide a statistically rigorous method to define and represent a system. W. Edwards Deming utilized this new data representation tool as one of the cornerstones to his improvement theory which eventually became known as his Theory of Profound Knowledge and reshaped the Japanese auto industry.

The desire to create immediate change in our systems stems from ever-rising healthcare costs and known quality gaps. In the early 2000s, The National Academy of Medicine (formerly the Institute of Medicine) provided a jolt to healthcare workers everywhere with the release of *To Err is Human* and *Crossing the Quality Chasm* which together represented a sobering assessment of healthcare quality in the United States. More recently, recognized gaps in the quality of care led to the creation of the Choosing Wisely® campaign by the American Board of Internal Medicine which has spread to many other specialties. To date, two PHM-specific lists have been created by leaders in the field. Each list includes five recommendations encouraging more targeted use of resources such as radiography in bronchiolitis and asthma, and phototherapy in neonatal jaundice. Socioeconomic factors and structural racism also contribute to poor outcomes. Such factors are associated with disparities in infant mortality and outcomes in many conditions including children with Type 1 diabetes mellitus and children requiring access to mental healthcare.

Pediatric hospitalists are well positioned to influence improvement within our healthcare system. While most QI work goes unpublished, the medical literature has representative examples in which pediatric hospitalists led or participated in teams focused on improving care delivery. Patient safety can be improved by reducing emergency transfers, improving hand hygiene, and reducing physical restraint use in children experiencing mental health crises. Clinical practice guidelines for common conditions such as asthma can improve outcomes and reduce hospital resource use. Targeted approaches can reduce unnecessary laboratory tests. Hospitalists also work on projects to improve patient experience such as reducing the time patients are fasting before sedation or reducing sleep interruptions in the hospital.

To address issues of quality, value, and health equity, rigorous quality improvement methods must be used. This chapter will share proven frameworks and methods. We introduce the Model for Improvement and Lean Six Sigma, along with other helpful tools to drive improvement. To highlight the importance of analyzing data over time, we also discuss run and control charts which are paramount to understanding the impact of improvement work on a system.

THE MODEL FOR IMPROVEMENT

The Model for Improvement has proven useful in many environments, including healthcare. This model is simple in its concept, comprised of three questions followed by the well-known (but often misunderstood) Plan-Do-Study-Act (PDSA) cycle (**Figure 3-1**). Answering the three questions ("What are we trying to accomplish?", "How will we know that a change is an improvement?," and "What changes can we make that will result in an

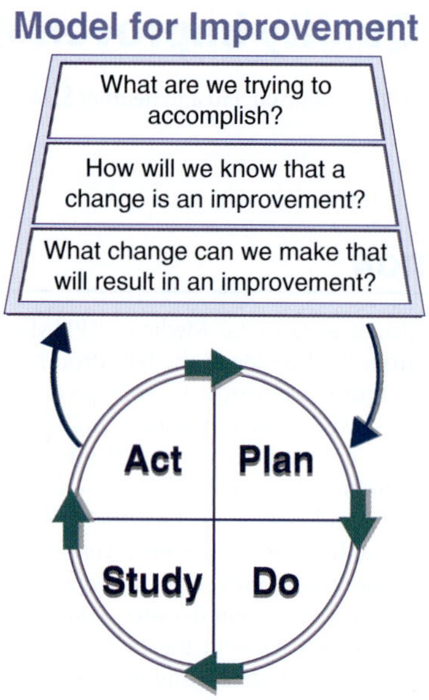

FIGURE 3-1. The Model for Improvement, developed by the Associates in Process Improvement. (Reproduced with permission from Lloyd Provost, Associates in Process Improvement. Available at: http://www.apiweb.org. Accessed June 21, 2022.)

improvement?") provides teams with the ability to reflect and begin building knowledge about their systems through specific, targeted tests of change via PDSA cycles. The Model for Improvement's simplicity, effectiveness, and diverse potential applications has led to its adoption by leading professional organizations such as the Institute for Healthcare Improvement.

QUESTION 1: WHAT ARE WE TRYING TO ACCOMPLISH?

We have likely all been part of teams which set out to tackle a problem that is discussed in very abstract terms—like improving the "patient experience." In many of these scenarios, team members might feel they know what needs to be done, but if we were to ask each person to define what exactly the team is setting out to do, there would likely be many different answers. Addressing the first question of the Model for Improvement to specify what the team is trying to accomplish helps create a shared mental model among team members and can accelerate change. This is often done using a concise SMART (Specific, Measurable, Achievable, Relevant, Timely) aim and may be supplemented by a team charter for formal projects. Creating an aim can be more difficult than one might expect, but the time spent clearly framing the goal often saves time and frustration during the project.

QUESTION 2: HOW WILL WE KNOW THAT A CHANGE IS AN IMPROVEMENT?

Identifying improvement in our QI work is important to both teams and patients. For smaller tests of change, qualitative data from front-line team members or families may tell us if we are on the right track toward our improvement goal. However, almost all improvement projects will have at least one objective data measure (often defined in the "Measurable" aspect of the SMART aim) and many projects will have a portfolio of measures, including the primary outcome measure and related process and balancing measure(s). Since, by definition, change happens over time, teams should have methods in place to extract the data frequently and plot the measures over time. This allows the team to understand how specific interventions are affecting the process and bolsters the degree of belief that objective improvements are a result of their work.

QUESTION 3: WHAT CHANGES CAN WE MAKE THAT WILL RESULT IN AN IMPROVEMENT?

Team members may feel like they know what needs to happen for improvement to occur, but healthcare systems are complex and seemingly obvious interventions often do not affect change the way teams would expect. If teams take the time to answer the first two questions using the Model for Improvement, they will find themselves in a vastly different mindset and are poised to identify small tests of change that will guide their subsequent improvement work. Because the Model for Improvement encourages iterative small-scale testing, teams need not have total consensus on what exactly to test. These potential changes are simply hypotheses upon which teams will build knowledge through this disciplined approach.

PLAN-DO-STUDY-ACT CYCLES

Once teams have answered all three questions within the Model for Improvement, they are ready to begin testing these changes through PDSA cycles. This well-known QI acronym for healthcare teams is often misunderstood and misused. Frequently, teams will use the terms PDSA cycles and interventions interchangeably. Even published QI manuscripts often use the term PDSA cycle when the methods were simply studying the effect of one or more interventions. In reality, PDSA cycle testing utilizes the scientific method to test the team's hypotheses. Teams must **Plan** their initial test of change which includes who is going to perform the test, where it is going to happen, and what data will be collected. It is often helpful to also have team members **P**redict what may happen, especially if opinions vary on what the outcome may be. The team will then **Do** the test and document how it went. Together, the team can then **Study** the results. How did it go? Were the results expected? What did the team learn? With this newfound knowledge about the system, the team now has information to **A**ct and can decide to adapt, adopt, or abandon the change altogether. These PDSA cycles inform the answers to the first three questions of the Model for Improvement and build on each other in size and scope until the team has a high degree of belief that the changes are resulting in the desired improvement. Thereafter, the change can be implemented and made part of the desired everyday workflow. This process is vastly different from simply performing an intervention such as an education campaign or a change to the electronic health record without the disciplined, rapid, iterative learning to understand whether and how the outcome is impacted.

LEAN AND SIX SIGMA

In healthcare, it is commonplace to see a blend of methods used in quality improvement which can differ depending on the preference of the organization. The various improvement methods are similar because they are rooted in the scientific method and can be thought of as a set of tools or concepts that can be applied to a particular problem. Lean and Six Sigma began as two separate methodologies that have merged into one way of thinking in its application to healthcare. Originally, Lean focused on the reduction of waste in the process steps of a production schema, while Six Sigma was invented by Motorola as a statistical method for describing how many defects per million were produced. (Six Sigma takes its name from the sixth standard deviation on a normalized curve and corresponds to a defect ratio of 1 in 1,000,000 opportunities.) Lean is used to make a process more efficient, while Six Sigma designs a process with fewer defects.

Improved efficiency and fewer defects are both laudable goals in delivering care in a hospital setting, and thus Lean Six Sigma has been combined into one overarching strategy in many healthcare organizations. In general, the Lean part of a project focuses on what is known as a "value stream map," which organizes all parts of the process into "value added" and "non-value added" steps. Steps that do not add value are considered waste, and attempts are made to eliminate or minimize those steps using a standard group of solutions that are often effective in process redesign. The Six Sigma part of a project focuses on the rate of defects in the product. The Six Sigma method can be used within the Define, Measure, Analyze, Improve and Control (DMAIC) or Model for Improvement frameworks that are used to organize the work. An in-depth explanation of Six Sigma and high-reliability concepts is beyond the scope of this chapter but understanding of how Lean and Six Sigma complement each other and how they can be used within one of these frameworks is valuable to those pursuing quality improvement. For example, improving processes such as hospital throughput or medication handling in a pharmacy might lend themselves well to a Lean Six Sigma approach as both are working to reduce waste and focusing on high-reliability systems.

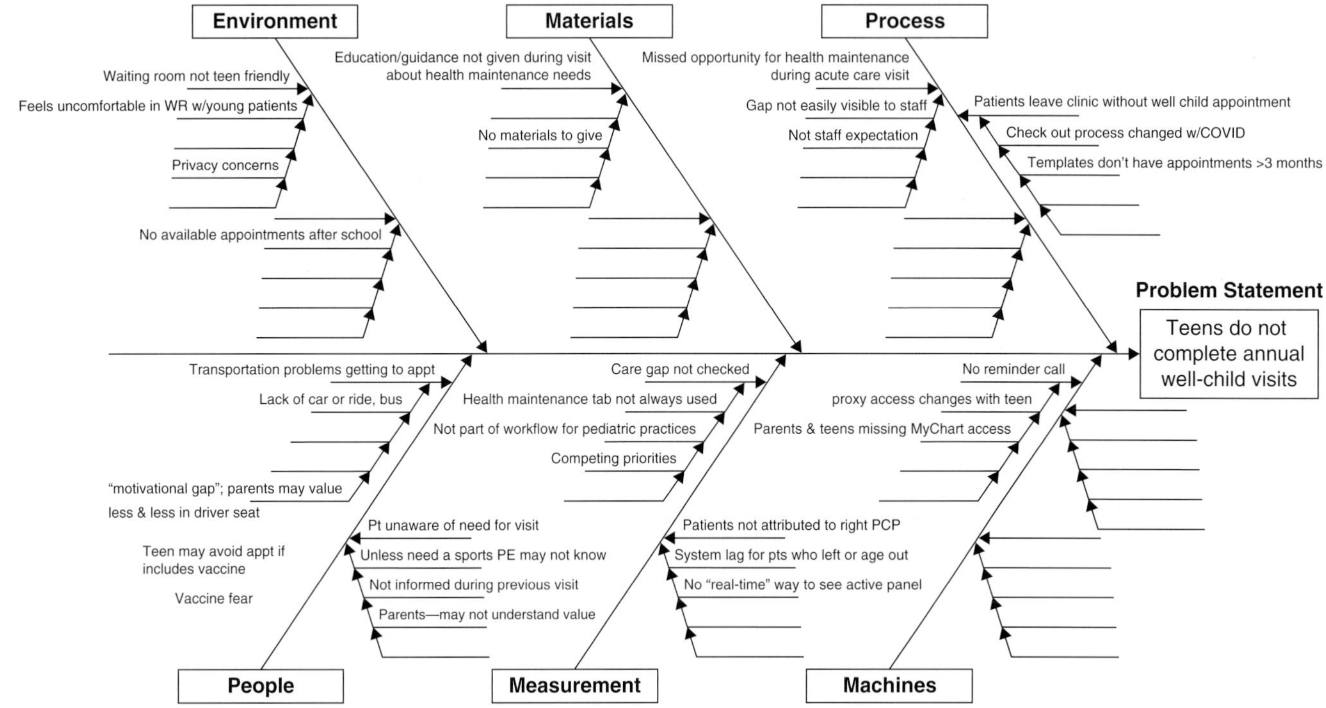

FIGURE 3-2. Fishbone diagram from a project team learning why teens do not complete annual adolescent well visits.

QUALITY IMPROVEMENT TOOLS (FISHBONE, PROCESS MAP, PARETO, KEY DRIVER DIAGRAM)

Quality improvement tools used in projects can be grouped into six categories: viewing systems and processes, gathering information, organizing information, understanding variation, understanding relationships, and managing projects. Examples of commonly used tools that help teams understand the system or process, get to the root of the problem, and organize the theory for improvement will be described in this section.

The key to success in improvement work is to spend ample time understanding the system and problem at hand before making changes. A common error is to propose solutions based on assumptions before understanding the process and problem in depth. Strategic use of QI methods and tools is critical to avoid this pitfall. For example, a fishbone cause-and-effect diagram is used to collect and organize knowledge based on the "5 Whys" from a diverse group of stakeholders to systematically understand a problem. **Figure 3-2** displays a Fishbone diagram from a project that used this problem-solving tool to learn why adolescents were not coming in for routine care visits. The "head" of the fish is the problem statement and the "bones" represent the components of the system. The details are completed by asking a series of "Why does that happen?" until the root of the problem is identified.

A process map provides a visual depiction of the process using direct observations with or without measured time intervals to identify waste in the system (**Figure 3-3**). A Pareto chart or diagram prioritizes problems for the team to work on using a vertical bar graph in which values or categories are plotted in decreasing order of relative frequency from left to right. By applying the Pareto principle, teams can identify the "vital few" effects to focus their efforts. The example Pareto chart in **Figure 3-4** was used to help a team prioritize which hospital-acquired conditions (HAC) had the most frequent harm events so resources could be allocated to those conditions to have the largest impact.

Finally, organizing the project into a key driver diagram is critical for the team to visualize the theory for improvement with the aims, drivers, and proposed interventions summarized in a single figure. Each of the diagram's sections should logically connect from change concepts to drivers in the system to the goal or aims of the project as shown in **Figure 3-5**.

MEASUREMENT IN QUALITY IMPROVEMENT – RUN & STATISTICAL PROCESS CONTROL CHARTS

Regardless of the framework a team chooses to drive their improvement work, measuring data over time is vital to understand the impact of changes on complex systems. Run charts and statistical process control (SPC) charts are both graphical displays of data over time that can help teams answer this question. Both plot time along the *x*-axis and the chosen measure along the *y*-axis. Because teams should be looking for frequent feedback as to the impact of their changes, plotting data in short time intervals such as days or weeks is often most useful.

Run charts use the median as a measure of central tendency and use specific rules to identify a "signal of change," such as six consecutive data points above or below the median. SPC charts are based on the work of statistician Walter Shewhart and are often referred to as Shewhart

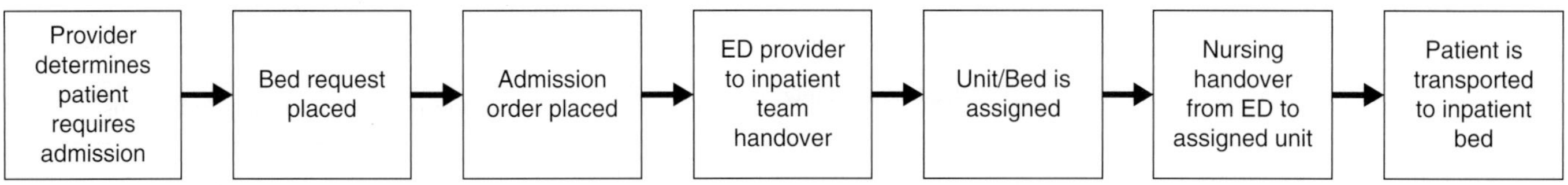

FIGURE 3-3. High-level process map that may be used when trying to improve ED (Emergency Department) throughput by looking at the time from the decision to admit to patient transport. Teams can begin with similarly high-level process maps and then get as granular as needed as they learn about their systems and plan interventions by breaking down each step into even smaller parts.

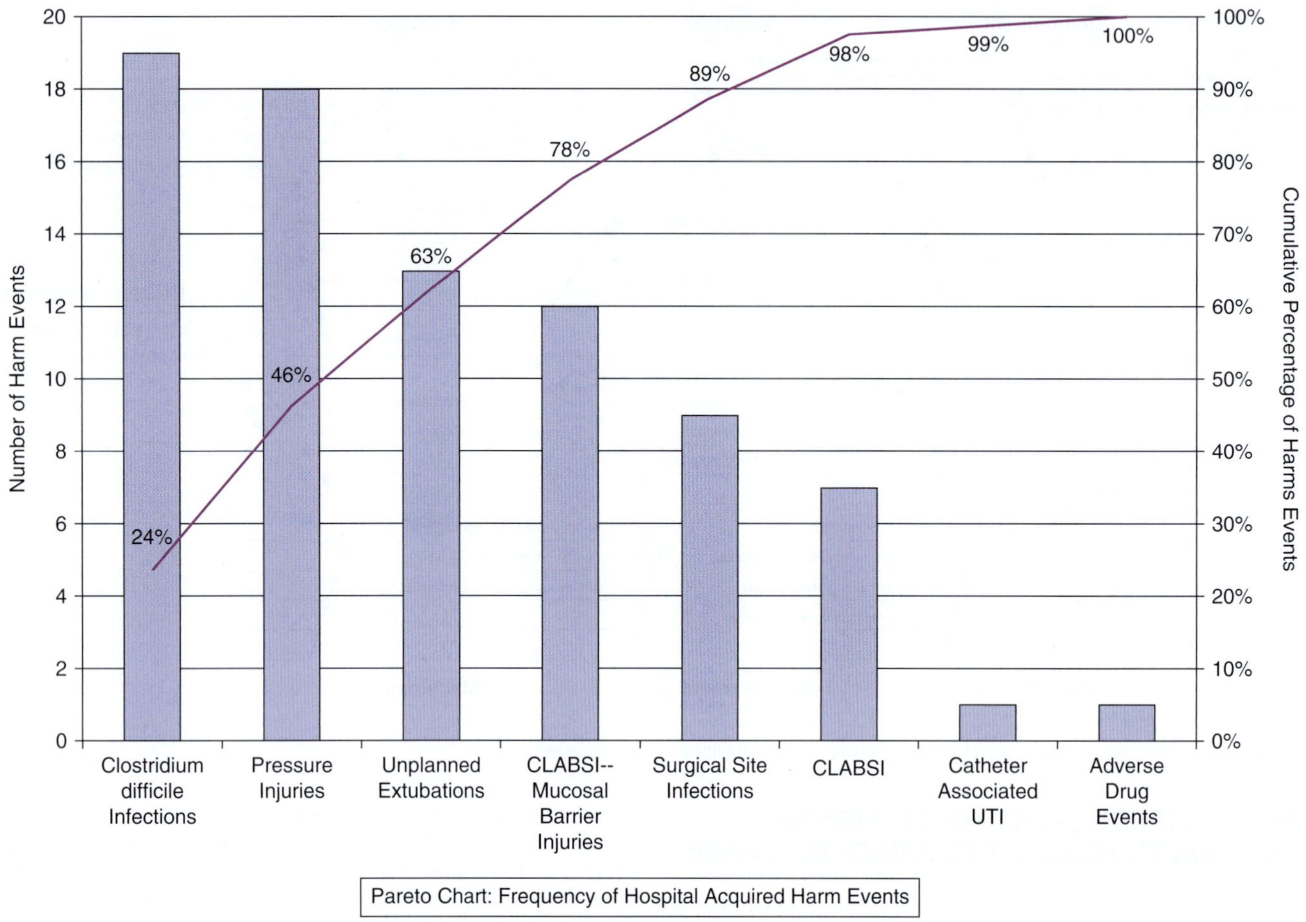

FIGURE 3-4. Example of a Pareto chart used to prioritize the frequency of Hospital-Acquired Harm Events by the condition category.

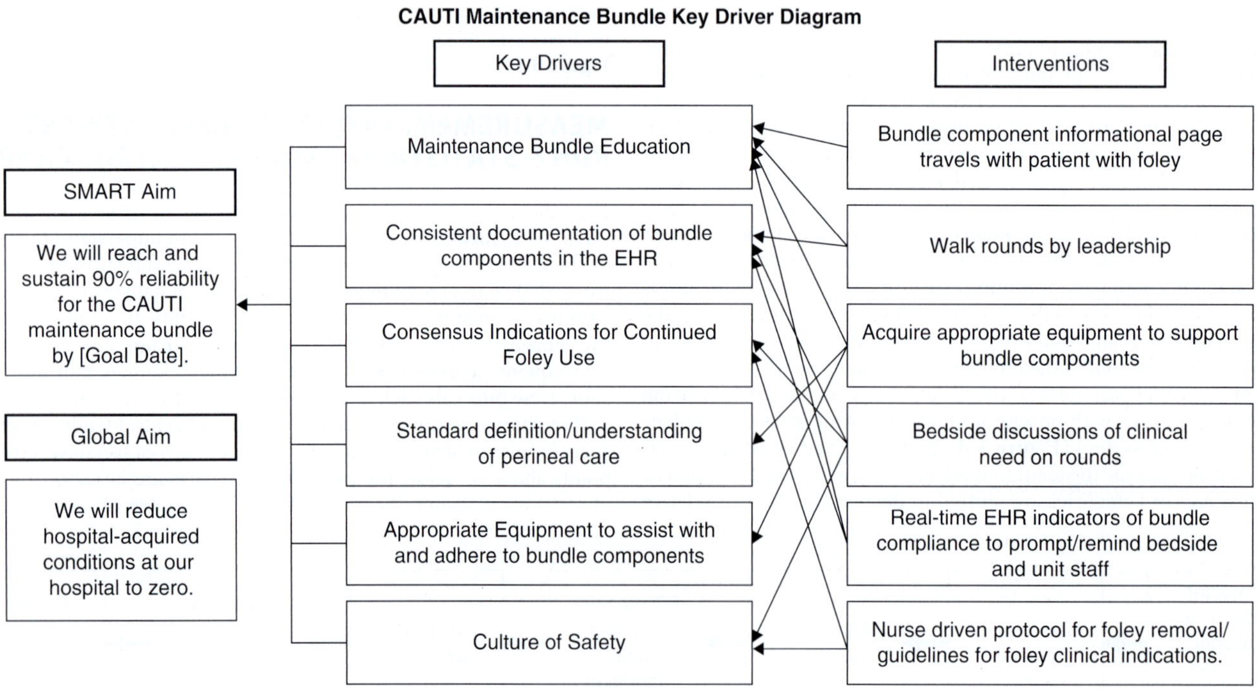

FIGURE 3-5. Example key driver diagram that a hospital might use to reduce Catheter Associated Urinary Tract Infections (CAUTI). The SMART AIM should directly address the first question in the Model for Improvement. Key drivers are hypotheses or theories that should help drive toward the aim and can also serve as process measures. Interventions are the specific activities the team undertakes to affect change in the system that will directly affect the key drivers, and ultimately the aim.

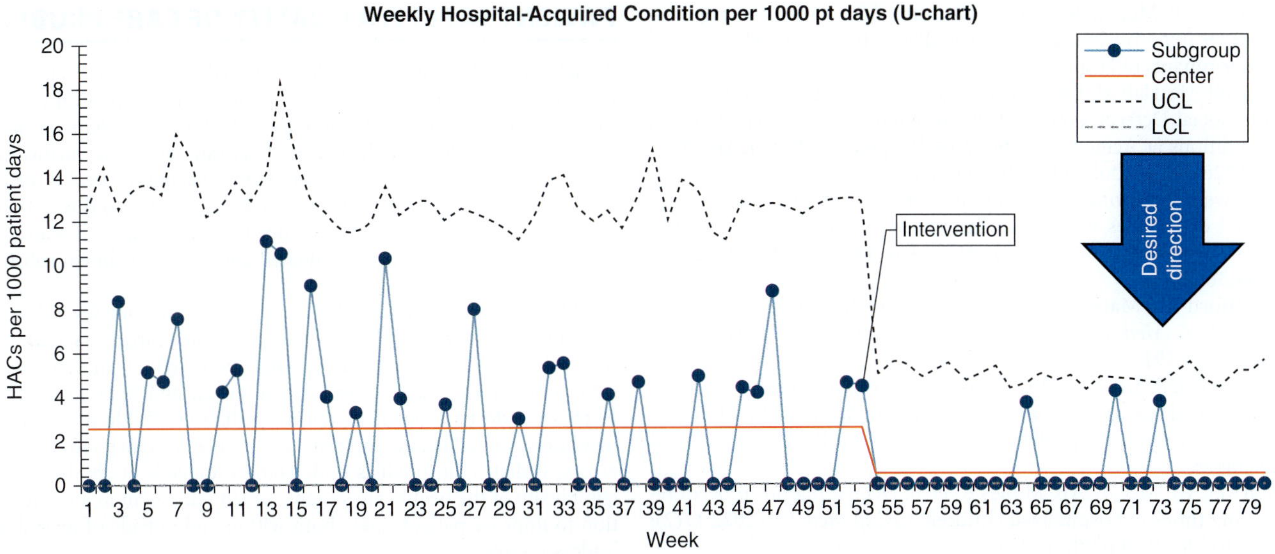

FIGURE 3-6. Statistical Process Control Chart indicating a successful reduction in the weekly rate of a hypothetical hospital-acquired condition. Following the intervention, special cause variation represented by 8 consecutive points below the mean line were observed allowing a shift in the mean line to a new lower rate. (Chart generated using QI Charts, Process Improvement Products; Austin, TX)

control charts. These charts include visual representations of statistical calculations for a measure of central tendency, usually the mean, along with upper and lower control limits. These visual displays provide more robust information for teams and the ability to identify common and special cause variation, whereas run charts only identify a signal of change. Common cause variation is variation that teams should expect in their data due to the inherent nature of the system being measured while special cause variation represents fluctuations in data that occur due to factors that are not routinely part of the system. Proper use of these charts can provide teams useful, real-time information into whether their changes are making the intended difference and prevent teams from wasting resources and energy by reacting to variations that simply reflect common cause. **Figure 3-6** represents a hypothetical example of a SPC chart illustrating a successful project to reduce the weekly rate of a hospital-acquired condition following a specific intervention.

CONCLUSION

Pediatric hospitalists work in environments that are rich in opportunities for improvement work that will benefit our patients. While teams may be able to improve some systems and processes through increased vigilance and education campaigns, much of the important, patient-centered outcomes that we strive for require the use of rigorous QI methods. We have introduced frameworks and concepts in this chapter that can lead teams to improved success when the concepts are understood deeply and utilized effectively. These skills will likely require some formal training or mentorship in addition to exploring some of the suggested readings at the end of this chapter followed by continued practice by participating in multiple QI endeavors. To this end, many institutions have developed internal QI training programs to formally train a critical mass of people to accelerate improvement work. Rigorous utilization of these frameworks and data analysis helps our patients through faster improvements and, when we share through publication, what we learn at our own institution or multi-site QI projects can spread to others to impact children on a much larger scale.

SUGGESTED READINGS

1. Arthur J, ed. *Lean Six Sigma for Hospitals: Improving Patient Safety, Patient Flow and the Bottom Line.* 2 ed. McGraw Hill; 2018.
2. Baily MA, Bottrell M, Lynn J, et al. The ethics of using QI methods to improve health care quality and safety. *Hastings Cent Rep.* Jul-Aug 2006;36(4):S1-40. doi:10.1353/hcr.2006.0054
3. Center for Medicare & Medicaid Services. National Health Expenditures 2020 Highlights. Accessed June 13, 2022. https://www.cms.gov/files/document/highlights.pdf
4. Chassin MR. Is health care ready for Six Sigma quality? *Milbank Q.* 1998;76(4):565-91, 510. doi:10.1111/1468-0009.00106
5. de Koning H, Verver JP, van den Heuvel J, et al. Lean six sigma in healthcare. *J Healthc Qual.* Mar-Apr 2006;28(2):4-11. doi:10.1111/j.1945-1474.2006.tb00596.x
6. Deming WE. *The new economics: for industry, government, education.* 2nd ed. MIT Press; 2000:xvi, 247 p.
7. George ML. *The lean Six Sigma pocket toolbook: a quick reference guide to nearly 100 tools for improving process quality, speed, and complexity.* McGraw-Hill; 2005:vi, 282 p.
8. Kohn LT, Corrigan J, Donaldson MS. *To err is human: building a safer health system.* National Academy Press; 2000:xxi, 287 p.
9. Langley GJ, Moen RD, Nolan KM, et al. *The improvement guide: a practical approach to enhancing organizational performance.* 2nd ed. Jossey-Bass; 2009:xxi, 490 p.
10. Institute of Medicine (U.S.). Committee on Quality of Health Care in America. *Crossing the quality chasm: a new health system for the 21st century.* National Academy Press; 2001:xx, 337 p.
11. Ogrinc GS, Joint Commission Resources Inc., Institute for Healthcare Improvement. *Fundamentals of health care improvement: a guide to improving your patient's care.* 2nd ed. Joint Commission; Institute for Healthcare Improvement; 2012:xvii, 190 p.
12. Quinonez RA, Garber MD, Schroeder AR, et al. Choosing wisely in pediatric hospital medicine: five opportunities for improved healthcare value. *J Hosp Med.* Sep 2013;8(9):479-485. doi:10.1002/jhm.2064
13. Shewhart WA. Economic quality control of manufactured product. *Bell Syst Tech J.* Apr 1930;9(2):364-389. doi:DOI 10.1002/j.1538-7305.1930.tb00373.x
14. Taylor MJ, McNicholas C, Nicolay C, et al. Systematic review of the application of the plan-do-study-act method to improve quality in healthcare. *BMJ Qual Saf.* Apr 2014;23(4):290-298. doi:10.1136/bmjqs-2013-001862
15. Tchou MJ, Schondelmeyer AC, Alvarez F, et al. Choosing Wisely in Pediatric Hospital Medicine: 5 New Recommendations to Improve Value. *Hosp Pediatr.* Nov 2021;11(11):1179-1190. doi:10.1542/hpeds.2021-006037
16. Perla RJ, Provost LP, Parry GJ. Seven propositions of the science of improvement: exploring foundations. *Qual Manag Health Care.* Jul-Sep 2013;22(3):170-86. doi:10.1097/QMH.0b013e31829a6a15 https://accessmedicine.mhmedical.com/content.aspx?bookid=2309&sectionid=180042695

17. Provost LP, Murray SK. *The health care data guide: learning from data for improvement.* 1st ed. Jossey-Bass; 2011:xxviii, 445 p. Social Determinants of Health
18. Carroll AR, Hall M, Brown CM, et al. Association of Race/Ethnicity and Social Determinants with Rehospitalization for Mental Health Conditions at Acute Care Children's Hospitals. *J Pediatr.* Jan 2022; 240:228-234 e1. doi:10.1016/j.jpeds.2021.08.078
19. Maxwell AR, Jones NY, Taylor S, et al. Socioeconomic and racial disparities in diabetic ketoacidosis admissions in youth with Type 1 diabetes. *J Hosp Med.* Aug 18 2021; doi:10.12788/jhm.3664
20. Pettiford B. Maternal and infant mortality in North Carolina. *N C Med J.* May-Jun 2021;82(3):191-194. doi:10.18043/ncm.82.3.191
21. Williams DR, Lawrence JA, Davis BA. Racism and health: evidence and needed research. *Annu Rev Public Health.* Apr 1 2019;40: 105-125. doi:10.1146/annurev-publhealth-040218-043750 Published PHM QI examples
22. Carroll AR, McCoy AB, Modes K, et al. Decreasing pre-procedural fasting times in hospitalized children. *J Hosp Med.* Feb 2022;17(2): 96-103. doi:10.1002/jhm.12782
23. Dalton EM, Herndon AC, Cundiff A, et al. Decreasing the use of restraints on children admitted for behavioral health conditions. *Pediatrics.* Jul 2021;148(1). doi:10.1542/peds.2020-003939
24. McLean HS, Carriker C, Bordley WC. Good to Great: Quality-improvement initiative increases and sustains pediatric health care worker hand hygiene compliance. *Hosp Pediatr.* Apr 2017;7(4):189-196. doi:10.1542/hpeds.2016-0110
25. Johnson DP, Arnold DH, Gay JC, et al. Implementation and improvement of pediatric asthma guideline improves hospital-based care. *Pediatrics.* Feb 2018;141(2). doi:10.1542/peds.2017-1630
26. Johnson DP, Lind C, Parker SE, et al. Toward high-value care: a quality improvement initiative to reduce unnecessary repeat complete blood counts and basic metabolic panels on a pediatric hospitalist service. *Hosp Pediatr.* Jan 2016;6(1):1-8. doi:10.1542/hpeds.2015-0099
27. Lin HM, Macias C, McGee C, et al. "Help Me Sleep": a quality initiative to reduce overnight vital signs. *Hosp Pediatr.* Feb 1 2022;12(2):142-147. doi:10.1542/hpeds.2021-006250
28. Sosa T, Sitterding M, Dewan M, et al. Optimizing situation awareness to reduce emergency transfers in hospitalized children. *Pediatrics.* Oct 2021;148(4). doi:10.1542/peds.2020-034603
29. Tchou MJ, Tang Girdwood S, Wormser B, et al. Reducing electrolyte testing in hospitalized children by using quality improvement methods. *Pediatrics.* May 2018;141(5). doi:10.1542/peds.2017-3187

CHAPTER 4

Patient Safety

Tina Sosa, MD, MSc and Patrick W. Brady, MD, MSc

INTRODUCTION

Hospitalists play a critical role in hospital operations, including quality and safety. Hospital-based safety initiatives encompass many broad areas of focus, including quality improvement, quality assurance, and regulatory efforts. Improvement science describes a framework of learning from both adverse events and safety successes to drive improved outcomes and decreased harm for both patients and employees. This chapter provides an overview of key safety concepts with a focus on the inpatient system of care.

PATIENT SAFETY: A QUALITY OF CARE PROBLEM

As defined by the National Academy of Medicine (NAM), patient safety is "freedom from accidental injury" acquired from medical care leading to harm or death. The landmark report *To err is human: building a safer health system,* published in 2000, estimated that medical error contributed up to 98,000 deaths annually—placing medical error as the sixth leading cause of death. While the study that led to this estimate of deaths due to medical error has not been repeated, rates of medical error and patient harm have been evaluated and have not shown substantial improvement.

Children are more susceptible to error and harm for several reasons, including developmental level, reliance on adult caregivers, and unique medical conditions. It is estimated that about 70,000 children hospitalized annually experienced an adverse event, and approximately 60% of these could be prevented. Within pediatrics, children with chronic conditions or medical complexity experience a higher rate of medical errors. Pediatric hospitalists understand the needs of children and the complexity of the healthcare system, which puts them in a unique position to improve patient safety both within and outside of formal safety leadership roles.

Reason's Swiss cheese model of error is helpful in understanding how risks persist even in the face of systems established to prevent harm (**Figure 4-1**). When an error occurs, there are multiple protective barriers in place within the system to block the error from reaching the patient and causing harm. For example, if a physician writes an erroneous order, a nurse, the computer physician order entry system, pharmacist, or parent of a patient may interrupt it before it reaches the patient. None of these barriers are flawless, and sometimes an error reaches the patient and causes harm. Incident reporting and safety learning systems should not only focus on errors that reach the patient but also learn from "near miss error events" that are caught and do not cause harm, but often reveal system vulnerabilities.

MEDICAL ERROR

ORIGINS AND EPIDEMIOLOGY

Understanding the etiologies and magnitude of adverse events is one of the first steps in developing improvements. Excluding birth-related events, children most frequently experience adverse events related to medications and diagnostic errors (including delayed or wrong diagnosis or management), with surgical adverse events occurring at a significant but far lower rate. Medication errors emerged as a specific focus for improvement efforts following the NAM report; however, this work has largely focused on the adult population. Research conducted

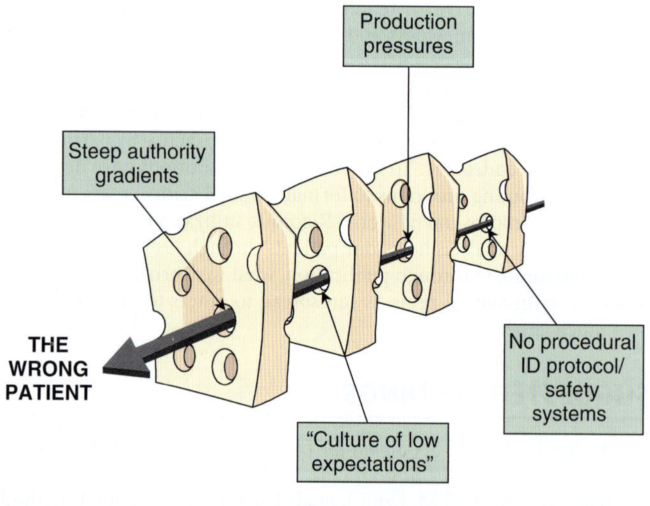

FIGURE 4-1. James Reason's Swiss cheese model of organizational accidents. (Adapted from Reason JT. *Human Error*. New York, NY: Cambridge University Press; 1990.)

on medication errors in children is limited primarily to the domain of prescribing errors, including admission medication reconciliation, rather than the dispensing, administering, and documenting of medication administration. In addition to medication errors, diagnostic errors are common, with over half of pediatricians endorsing at least one per month. Fortunately, far fewer incidents of diagnostic error lead to harm. Recent studies on diagnostic error and diagnostic uncertainty have proposed both cognition-based and system-based improvement interventions, including diagnostic checklists, closed-loop diagnostic feedback, diagnostic teams, and informatics-based decision support systems.

While medication errors and diagnostic errors are common causes of harm in pediatric patients, other hospital-acquired conditions also contribute to the overall scope of harm. Central-line associated blood stream infection, catheter-associated urinary tract infection, surgical site infection, and ventilator-associated pneumonia are examples of hospital-acquired infections which lead to increased morbidity and mortality. Falls, pressure ulcers, and venous thromboembolism acquired in the hospital are some other hospital-acquired conditions contributing to patient harm.

IDENTIFYING HARM EVENTS

Systems to detect harm in individual hospitals are critical to improving patient safety. Current trends have encouraged the use of event reporting systems by providing timely feedback to those who submit reports and utilizing reports to develop systematic solutions to promote a safer patient care environment. However, voluntary reporting of incidents underestimates the actual number of medical errors, including both near misses and harm events. Regardless, hospitalists should continue to emphasize the need to report errors. To further quantify harm, some hospitals have used retrospective review with the Institute for Healthcare Improvement's (IHI's) Global Trigger Tool or a pediatric version of this trigger tool. Trained reviewers such as nurses, pharmacists, and physicians review charts to identify signs or "triggers" which prompt further review of the patient's medical record to identify whether harm occurred. Further review of findings from trigger tools can help guide hospital efforts to reduce harm.

DISCLOSURE AND DEBRIEFING

Disclosure refers to communication directed from healthcare personnel to the affected patient and family about an adverse event. Disclosure and open communication with patients and their families may provide benefit to the patient and to the healthcare provider through the promotion of trust, reduction in guilt, improved event follow-up, and the advancement of a positive safety culture. Patients and families often desire full disclosure and may be less likely to pursue litigation against the healthcare system if timely and complete disclosure occurs.

In addition to adverse event disclosure, event debriefs are critically important for two primary reasons: (i) to facilitate a systems-based approach to identifying medical errors, their contributing factors, and possible solutions and (ii) to provide emotional support for the involved individuals in order to promote resiliency, recovery, and well-being. Morbidity and mortality conferences at a division, department, and/or institutional level provide a structured forum for error and risk analysis. Small-scale clinical event debriefings are also used to achieve similar goals, with an emphasis on participant engagement, generation of an improvement plan for system leaders, and psychological safety. Psychological safety is defined as the ability to raise concerns and ask questions without the fear of negative consequences for self-image, status, or career.

RAPID RESPONSE SYSTEMS

Clinical deterioration is a critical aspect of patient safety for hospitalists and has been a key focus of research and improvement initiatives over the past two decades. The deterioration of hospitalized patients is rarely sudden or unpredictable, and leveraging preceding factors including vital sign abnormalities and family or clinician concern is critical to preventing morbidity and mortality. Rapid response systems are designed to predict, detect, and respond to deterioration as early as possible, and deploy teams with critical care expertise to aid in management or escalate care to the critical care setting. All United States children's hospitals have a rapid response system, although they vary in operational logistics including activation protocol and staffing structure. Importantly, rapid response systems are associated with a significant reduction in codes outside of the intensive care unit and mortality. Given that codes outside of the intensive care unit are increasingly rare, validated proximal metrics to cardiopulmonary arrest were developed to evaluate the success of rapid response systems in identifying and mitigating clinical deterioration and adverse patient outcomes. Critical deterioration events and emergency transfers are two validated metrics associated with adverse outcomes (e.g., increased length of stay and mortality) which have been reduced through situation awareness and rapid response system optimization (**Figure 4-2**).

EMPLOYEE SAFETY

Occupational safety is an increasingly prominent focus of hospital-based medicine. Employee injury rates in healthcare are significant, and efforts to reduce preventable staff harm have increased in magnitude over the past several years. Historically, the focus of occupational safety efforts included injuries such as needlesticks, blood-borne pathogen exposures, slips, trips, and falls, and overexertion injuries. Violence and patient interaction injuries, including from children with neuropsychiatric disease or developmental disabilities, are a growing source of harm to both ambulatory and hospital-based staff. Improvement efforts are currently focused on the comprehensive incorporation of employee safety event reporting and wellness into safety culture, as well as the development of systematic processes for de-escalation of violent and aggressive behavior in the inpatient setting.

CRITICAL COMPONENTS OF PATIENT SAFETY INITIATIVES

SYSTEMATIC APPROACH TO HARM REDUCTION

Reducing harm and improving patient safety for pediatric patients is imperative for many reasons. Some hospitals have conducted wide-scale cultural and system initiatives using quality improvement methodology to decrease serious harm events in children, and significant reductions in serious safety event rates have been demonstrated. In 2019, the American Academy of Pediatrics released a policy statement about patient safety and decreasing harm due to medical care. The committee recommended several key strategies. One necessary, but not sufficient, step is to increase patient safety knowledge among pediatricians. Patient safety-focused sessions at conferences and learning collaboratives at the local, regional, and national levels (e.g., the >145 children's hospital Solutions for Patient Safety Network) are ways to accomplish this. Through these sessions and initiatives, hospitalists can learn from one another and commit to sharing this knowledge with their practice group and institutions in which they care for patients. Another key strategy is to promote patient safety by focusing on the unique safety risks which exist for pediatric patients; importantly, this is an area of expertise for pediatric hospitalists. Development of pediatric-specific error reporting systems, enhancing family-centered care, adhering to evidence-based pediatric practices, targeting medication safety, and implementing pediatric-specific electronic health record improvements are all important examples of critical improvement initiatives in which hospitalists can and should be engaged.

An additional recommendation is the use of standardized protocols of care, or "bundles," to decrease harm. The IHI describes bundle theory as a set of evidence-based interventions applied to a certain population of patients that when used together will result in better outcomes than if the interventions were applied separately. Initiatives focused on the implementation of bundles often employ high reliability organization (HRO) principles. HROs are organizations such as aviation or the nuclear power industry which operate under high-risk conditions daily but achieve exemplary safety records. Weick and Sutcliffe described five characteristics that HROs share: sensitivity to operations, preoccupation

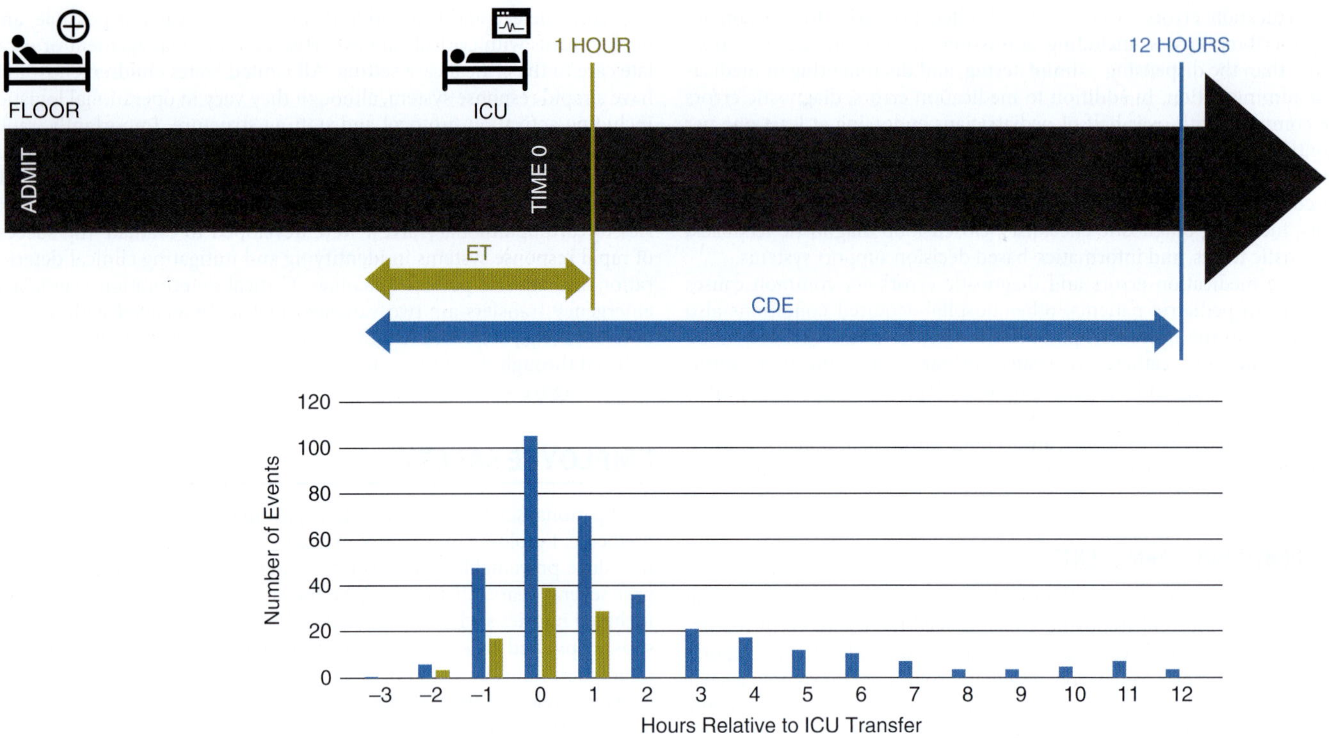

FIGURE 4-2. Two validated measures of unrecognized clinical deterioration in children. ET = Emergency Transfer, defined as a patient undergoing intubation, receiving vasopressors, or receiving three or more fluid boluses within one hour of transfer to the intensive care unit (ICU). CDE = Critical Deterioration Event, defined as a patient receiving non-invasive positive pressure ventilation, intubation, or vasopressor initiation within twelve hours of ICU transfer. (Reproduced with permission from Sosa T, et al. Comparing two proximal measures of unrecognized clinical deterioration in children. *J Hosp Med.* 2020;15(11):673-676.)

with failure, deference to expertise, resilience, and reluctance to simplify (**Table 4-1**). These organizations rely on all members of the organization to have a focus on safety by constantly looking for risk points and ways to mitigate risk. There are several examples of hospital-based initiatives which successfully utilized bundle theory and HRO principles to reduce harm, including projects to reduce the rates of hospital-acquired conditions such as central-line associated bloodstream infections and ventilator-associated pneumonia. Another groundbreaking example involved implementation of the I-PASS mnemonic—illness severity, patient summary, action list, situation awareness and contingency planning, and synthesis by receiver—which led to significant improvements in resident-to-resident shift handoff in teaching hospitals. Implementation of this process was associated with a 23% reduction in medical errors and a 30% reduction in preventable adverse events in a multicenter study. While just a few examples of systematic, hospital-based improvement initiatives and care bundles are provided here, hospitalists can play a critical role in leading and participating in all inpatient-focused improvement teams.

TABLE 4-1 Five Characteristics of High Reliability Organizations

Preoccupation with Failure	Encourage the reporting of small errors and create a plan to address errors
Reluctance to Simplify Interpretations	Encourage diversity in experience, perspective, and opinion
Commitment to Resilience	Errors do not disable
Deference to Expertise	Decision-making is deferred to workers with the most knowledge and expertise, not the highest rank
Sensitivity to Operations	Find loopholes in the system's defenses, embed safeguards on the front lines, and maintain situation awareness

Source: Weick KE, Sutcliff KM. *Managing the Unexpected: Resilient Performance in an Age of Uncertainty.* 2nd ed. San Francisco, CA: Jossey-Bass; 2007.

EQUITY

While the importance of focusing on equity to provide the highest quality healthcare has been acknowledged for decades, there is an urgent need for quality improvement and safety efforts to critically examine existing disparities based on social determinants of health and intentionally focus on designing interventions to eliminate these disparities. Over twenty years ago, the NAM Committee on Quality of Health Care in America identified equity as one of the six target aims for improvement. The inadequate progress made in this area was highlighted nearly two decades later by Derek Feely, former president of the IHI, in an article entitled *There Can Be No Quality Without Equity*. The persistent, pervasive, and unacceptable impact of inequities due to structural racism, implicit bias, resource allocation, insurance status, preferred language, and other social determinants is widespread, affecting all healthcare settings across pediatric and adult populations. Worse outcomes are reported for Black and Latino populations and patients from lower income households in the rate of misdiagnosis, surgical approach, post-operative complications and mortality, and perforation rate for appendicitis. Furthermore, there is evidence of an increased odds of death for Black children as compared to white children in the setting of severe sepsis. Another recent multicenter study described higher rates of adverse events for hospitalized Latino children as compared with non-Latino white children, as well as higher rates of preventable events for children who are publicly insured. One retrospective study reported a twofold increased risk of serious medical events for Spanish-speaking pediatric patients as compared to patients who do not require an interpreter. With increasing awareness of these differences in safety and quality of care, leaders in hospital-based pediatrics are calling for research and improvement initiatives to both further understand and target potential etiologies.

PATIENT AND FAMILY ENGAGEMENT

Patients and caregivers represent an often underutilized but critical resource for knowledge and expertise on how to provide safe care to hospitalized children. An increasing body of research describes the importance of, and strategies to facilitate, the partnership between clinicians, patients, and caregivers to improve the safety and quality of care, both at the bedside and as part of hospital-based improvement teams. This point deserves particular emphasis for the growing population of children with medical complexity in pediatric hospital medicine, for whom caregivers are invaluable in providing insight on deviations from baseline in their children. One important example of patient and family involvement in an inpatient safety initiative is the incorporation of patients and families as activators of the rapid response system, to directly and independently activate critical care outreach teams with concerns about the patient's clinical status. As described by the Institute for Patient- and Family-Centered Care's Framework for Family Involvement in Quality Improvement, patient safety initiatives should involve patients and families in a systematic and escalating manner ranging from engaging in evaluative activities as respondents to serving as fully integrated co-leaders of improvement initiatives.

SUGGESTED READINGS

Ahuja N, Zhao W, Xiang H. Medical errors in US pediatric inpatients with chronic conditions. *Pediatrics*. 2012;130(4):e786-93.

Bonafide CP, et al. Impact of rapid response system implementation on critical deterioration events in children. *JAMA Pediatr*. 2014; 168(1):25-33.

Burrus S, et al. Factors related to serious safety events in a children's hospital patient safety collaborative. *Pediatrics*. 2021;148(3).

Committee on Medical Liability and Risk Management, Council on Quality Improvement and Patient Safety, et al. Disclosure of adverse events in pediatrics. *Pediatrics*. 2016;138(6):e20163215.

Crisis Prevention Institute. Cited 2022 August. Available from: https://www.crisisprevention.com/.

Feely D. There can be no quality without equity. *Australian Health Review*. 2020;5(4):503.

Galligan MM, et al. Implementation of a multidisciplinary debriefing process for pediatric ward deterioration events. *Hosp Pediatr*. 2021;11(5):454-461.

Ingram ME, et al. Systematic review of disparities in care and outcomes in pediatric appendectomy. *J Surg Res*. 2020;249:42-49.

Institute of Medicine, Committee on Quality of Health Care in America. *Crossing the Quality Chasm: A New Health System for the 21st Century*. Washington, DC: National Academy Press; 2001.

Khan A, et al. Engaging families as true partners during hospitalization. *J Hosp Med*. 2018;13(5):358-360.

Kirkendall ES, et al. Measuring adverse events and levels of harm in pediatric inpatients with the Global Trigger Tool. *Pediatrics*. 2012;130(5):e1206-14.

KohnLT, Corrigan JM, Donaldson MS, eds. *To Err Is Human: Building a Safer Health System*. National Academy Press; 2000.

Lockwood JM, et al. Characteristics of pediatric rapid response systems: results from a survey of PRIS Hospitals. *Hosp Pediatr*. 2021;11(2): 144-152.

Marshall TL, et al. Diagnostic error in pediatrics: a narrative review. *Pediatrics*. 2022;149(Suppl 3).

Miller MR, et al. Medication errors in paediatric care: a systematic review of epidemiology and an evaluation of evidence supporting reduction strategy recommendations. *Qual Saf Health Care*. 2007;16(2): 116-26.

Mitchell HK, et al. Hospital outcomes for children with severe sepsis in the USA by race or ethnicity and insurance status: a population-based, retrospective cohort study. *Lancet Child Adolesc Health*. 2021;5(2):103-112.

Mueller BU, et al. Principles of pediatric patient safety: reducing harm due to medical care. *Pediatrics*. 2019;143(2).

Nafiu OO, et al. Race, postoperative complications, and death in apparently healthy children. *Pediatrics*. 2020;146(2).

Peterson TH, Teman SF, Connors RH. A safety culture transformation: its effects at a children's hospital. *J Patient Saf*. 2012;8(3):125-30.

Ramazani S, et al. The value of family advisors as coleaders in pediatric quality improvement efforts: a qualitative theme analysis. *J Patient Exp*. 2020;7(6):1708-1714.

Resar R, Griffin FA, Haraden C, Nolan TW. Using care bundles to improve health care quality. IHI Innovation Series White Paper. Cambridge, MA: Institute for Healthcare Improvement; 2012.

Sharek PJ, et al. Effect of a rapid response team on hospital-wide mortality and code rates outside the ICU in a Children's Hospital. *JAMA*. 2007;298(19):2267-2274.

Sosa T, et al. Comparing two proximal measures of unrecognized clinical deterioration in children. *J Hosp Med*. 2020;15(11):673-676.

Sosa T, et al. Optimizing situation awareness to reduce emergency transfers in hospitalized children. *Pediatrics*. 2021;148(4).

Starmer AJ, et al. Changes in medical errors after implementation of a handoff program. *N Engl J Med*. 2014;371(19):1803-1812.

Stockwell DC, et al. Racial, ethnic, and socioeconomic disparities in patient safety events for hospitalized children. *Hosp Pediatr*. 2019;9(1):1-5.

Weick KE, Sutcliff KM. *Managing the Unexpected: Resilient Performance in an Age of Uncertainty*. 2nd ed. San Francisco, CA: Jossey-Bass; 2023.

Woods D, et al. Adverse events and preventable adverse events in children. *Pediatrics*. 2005;115(1):155-160.

CHAPTER 5 Patient- and Family-Centered Care

Joy L. Solano, MD, MHPE and Alisa Khan, MD, MPH

INTRODUCTION

"Nothing about me without me" conveys a powerful message of patients' active involvement in healthcare decisions. The approach to the hospitalized child and family has changed dramatically over the last two decades. Physicians are rarely the sole decision-makers, and patients and families expect to be actively involved in medical decision-making. This expectation is strongly supported by leaders in healthcare and government.

Patient- and family-centered care (PFCC) is fundamental to pediatric hospital medicine and has been long endorsed by several organizations, including the American Academy of Pediatrics (AAP) and the National Academy of Medicine. PFCC involves collaboration among multiple key partners including patients, families, physicians, nurses, and other healthcare professionals in order to plan, deliver, and evaluate pediatric healthcare. The Picker Institute, a foundation dedicated to establishing partnerships between patients and healthcare systems, identified the following eight dimensions of "person-centered care" (originally termed as "patient-centered care"), which are easily applied to PFCC: (i) Faster access to reliable healthcare advice; (ii) Effective treatment by trusted professionals; (iii) Continuity of care and smooth transitions; (iv) Involvement and support for family and caregivers; (v) Clear information, communication, and support for self-care; (vi) Involvement in decisions and respect for preferences; (vii) Emotional support, empathy, and respect; and (viii) Attention to physical and environment needs.

The core principles of PFCC described in the AAP Policy Statement on Patient- and Family-Centered Care and the Pediatrician's Role align with these eight dimensions and include honoring diverse patient and family experiences; tailoring services to the needs of each individual patient and family; sharing complete, honest and unbiased information; collaborating with patients and families in all aspects of healthcare; and empowering patients and their families to participate in making decisions about their healthcare. In the inpatient setting, pediatric hospitalists promote PFCC by conducting rounds at the bedside and engaging patients and their families in shared decision-making, modeling and teaching PFCC principles to trainees, and involving patients and families in the design and implementation of research, quality improvement initiatives, advocacy projects and healthcare system improvements.

FACILITATING PATIENT- AND FAMILY-CENTERED CARE

CO-PRODUCTION

The partnership between healthcare professionals and healthcare recipients is embodied in the concept of co-production. Co-production of healthcare services requires civil discourse with open and respectful communication between patients/families and healthcare professionals, leading to effective co-planning and co-execution of services to achieve high-value healthcare and promote good healthcare for all. This process invites patients/families and healthcare professionals to develop a deeper understanding of each other's expertise and values and create a high level of mutual trust. This facilitates the development of shared goals, responsibility, and accountability to ensure high-quality healthcare services.

Co-production is broken into four tenets: (i) co-commissioning, (ii) co-design, (iii) co-delivery, and (iv) co-assessment. Co-commissioning addresses policy planning and prioritizing agendas. In the pediatric hospital medicine setting, this approach can be applied to deciding which quality improvement projects to prioritize, for instance. Patient-centered outcomes research is another prime example and emphasizes including patients and families in setting research agendas. Co-design refers to planning healthcare services that encompass all clinical care. This includes shared decision-making where patients/families and clinicians partner in making healthcare decisions by reviewing the best evidence together and taking joint ownership of decisions made. In the pediatric hospital medicine setting, this can also include shared decision-making on rounds and partnering with patients/families in executing research and quality improvement projects together. Co-delivery involves co-managing and co-performing services (e.g., appointments, procedures). Medical education is another example of a service that can be co-delivered with patients/families. For instance, patients/families can be included in trainee education and curriculum development (e.g., including family advisors in resident training about family-centered rounds). Co-assessment refers to monitoring and evaluation of all aspects of healthcare services, including research, quality improvement, process improvement, patient care, hospital operations, and safety. Involving patients and families in the evaluation of these areas ensures the patient/family experience is considered when monitoring for problems that need to be addressed or assessing the quality of current services.

HEALTH LITERACY

A key aspect of PFCC is communicating with patients and their families in a manner they can understand. Personal health literacy refers to an individual's ability to gather, understand, and use resources to make appropriate health-related decisions for themselves or those they care for. Organizational health literacy refers to how well organizations equitably enable people to do this. Employing principles of health literacy, such as the use of universal health literacy precautions (practicing clear communication for all patients/families with the assumption that everyone benefits from clear communication), is essential to the humanistic success of PFCC. Clinicians are strongly encouraged to assume that health literacy is a "state," not a "trait," and can vary with time, place, and context (e.g., sleep deprivation or stress). Therefore, hospitalists must recognize that all patients/families may have difficulty finding, understanding, and using health-related information and services; this may result in difficulty partnering with clinicians in healthcare decision-making in the inpatient setting. By using health literacy best practices, hospitalists can ensure all patients and families have the opportunity to understand, navigate, and meaningfully partner in their own healthcare. Tips to promote understanding by all patients/families are found in **Table 5-1**. Of note, these principles are applicable to family-centered rounds and other communication interactions between hospitalized pediatric patients and families and their clinicians, including at the time of admission, transfer, and discharge.

DIVERSITY, EQUITY, & INCLUSION (DEI)

PFCC demands a healthcare system that provides diverse, equitable, and inclusive care to patients and their families. Implicit bias impairs professionals' ability to provide such care. Implicit bias has been defined by the National Institutes of Health as "a form of bias that occurs automatically and unintentionally, that nevertheless affects judgements, decisions, and behaviors." Poor self-awareness of such bias inhibits healthcare's ability to provide equitable healthcare to all persons, no matter of one's insurance status, gender or gender identity, race, ethnicity, primary language, sexual orientation, socioeconomic status, religion, or ability. Hospitalists must be aware of ways in which they may perpetuate implicit and explicit bias (e.g., addressing comments to a patient's White mother instead of their Black father on rounds) and ways in which they can serve as upstanders (e.g., intervening if a patient or other staff member perpetuates a microaggression against a trainee). Intentional hospital-based interventions must be undertaken to integrate DEI efforts in the inpatient setting with advance the PFCC agenda. PFCC cannot exist in hospital medicine without a culture that embraces DEI.

Hospitalists are also uniquely poised to address the needs of patients and families who use languages other than English for care. They can ensure that "communication shortcuts" are not taken (e.g., using rudimentary high-school Spanish language skills to "get by" or asking teenage patients to interpret for family members). Instead, hospitalists can ensure that certified interpretation is used with every communication encounter, including admission, rounds, ad hoc afternoon updates, and discharge communications. They can also ensure they build trust and rapport with patients and families who speak languages other than English. Building trust has been shown to increase psychological safety and willingness to speak up and partner in care. Hospitalists should also ensure discharge materials are translated into the family's language of choice, which may involve advanced planning early in the admission and working with their hospital to expand availability of translation services. These actions will help ensure that patients who use languages other than English are able to meaningfully experience PFCC.

TABLE 5-1 Tips to Promote Understanding by All Patients and Families

1. **Use plain language**
   a. Avoid medical jargon. Use simple, non-technical "living room language" in all communication with patients/families.
2. **Chunk information**
   a. Limit information to 3-5 key points.
3. **Be specific and concrete**
   a. Avoid language that is too general.
4. **Demonstrate**
   a. Draw pictures to give visual representation of information provided. Show how something is done (e.g., how to use an inhaler with spacer).
5. **Repeat and summarize frequently**
   a. Consider doing this after delivering 3-5 key points.
6. **Use teach-back**
   a. Test your communication skills by asking the family to repeat back what you have discussed using their own words to make sure you have done a good job explaining things.

Source: Adapted from the AHRQ Health Literacy Universal Precautions Toolkit.

HOSPITAL CARE

ORIENTATION TO THE HOSPITAL

Hospitalization can be an incredibly stressful event for both children and their families. They may experience feelings ranging from fear of the unknown to complete loss of control. These feelings complicate the clinical situation and detract from a healing environment. Physicians and other healthcare professionals should address these stresses directly and provide an environment designed to preserve patient and family control. Sample scripting can be helpful (e.g., "we know it can be stressful to be in the hospital," "you're an expert on your child and we invite you to speak up to share your questions, concerns, and thoughts so together we can take the best care possible of your child."). When admitting children to the hospital, processes must be in place to orient patients and families to the flow of the wards. Hospitals often provide typical orientation such as visiting hours and restrictions, cafeteria access, availability of interpreter services, patient relations, and parking. Information should also be provided about daily routines, including nursing shift change, timing and process of rounds, presence and role of learners in providing care, ways to report safety concerns, and access to special services such as child life, social work, and pastoral care. In addition, patients and families should be oriented to limitations of hospital care processes in order to better manage patient/family expectations (e.g., medication timing may vary by around 30 minutes each day, shared rooms, expectations around response time to call bells). The amount of information given may be overwhelming, so multiple methods of communication, including printed materials or pre-recorded videos available in multiple languages, may be helpful in educating patients and families.

ORIENTATION TO THE PATIENT AND FAMILY ROLE

Hospitalists must encourage patients and families to take an active role in the hospitalization. Hospitalists can affirm that patients and families are experts in care and proactively solicit their input. This requires an established patient- and family-centered culture within the hospital and extends beyond active participation on rounds. However, because rounds are a primary venue for daily medical decision-making, families should be encouraged to be present to provide their input and participate in decision-making for their child. Some families are unable to be present due to work obligations, inability to find childcare, transportation, or other barriers. Measures should be taken to include families who cannot be physically present at the bedside in discussions via phone or video conferencing to ensure medical decision-making remains shared, recognizing that the ability to be present at the bedside during hospitalization may not be feasible for all families. Additionally, it should not be assumed that all families will participate without prompting. Instead, patients and families should be intentionally invited. An introduction to rounds should be provided upon admission and communication preferences (for on and outside of rounds) elicited. Families have endorsed that participating on rounds gives them more confidence in the healthcare team, reduces anxiety, and improves the care their children receive.

PATIENT- AND FAMILY-CENTERED ROUNDS

Pediatric hospitalists are strongly encouraged to conduct rounds at the bedside to facilitate transparent communication and shared decision-making with patients and their families. Patient- and family-centered rounds (PFCRs) have traditionally been defined as rounds which take place in patients' rooms at their bedsides and involve active participation from the patient and family in decision-making. However, family-centered rounds do not always occur "at the bedside." Eliciting patient and family communication preferences for rounds is important and conducting rounds in any location with a family member actively involved still meets family-centered criteria (e.g., outside the room with the family member if the family member expresses this preference given patient anxiety, via phone/video conferencing if families are unable to be at the bedside). PFCRs ideally involve the multi-disciplinary care team in medical decision-making, communication, teaching, discharge planning, and coordination of care. At a minimum, the physician care team (e.g., attending, residents, and medical students), the bedside nurse, and the patient/family should be actively involved. This shift in medical culture from physician-centered care to patient-centered care has taken decades to occur but remains at the heart of pediatric hospital medicine.

Decision-making should be transparent to all involved. The family is often the best source of information about a child but can be frequently overlooked. Actively considering the family's values, background, and preferences, as well as family members' unique knowledge of the patient can assist in decision-making. All diagnostic and treatment decisions should be made with the full participation of the family unless families have stated otherwise. Healthcare team members must be willing to work constructively with families even when their decisions do not align with the advice of the medical team.

Communication that recognizes the patient's family as the driving force is central to their empowerment. A simple gesture, such as asking patients or families about their preferences regarding rounds, allows the family to regain a sense of control and involvement. Honest and open communication between medical professionals and families is vital to the success of the hospitalization. Total transparency in all aspects of hospitalization is necessary to maintain optimal lines of communication.

Best practices for PFCRs include patients/families speaking first, setting goals, healthcare providers speaking in a language understood by families (through use of plain language instead of medical jargon and with support of an interpreter when the family speaks a language other than English), conducting shared decision-making, asking open-ended questions, and assessing patient/family understanding. The Patient and Family Centered I-PASS framework for PFCRs embraces these practices. This intervention was co-produced with parents, nurses, and physicians in an effort to improve family-centeredness of and communication effectiveness during rounds. A structured communication framework was developed that emphasized patient/family engagement (patients/families were asked to share first on rounds), nurse engagement (nurses were encouraged to speak early on rounds), health literacy (plain language was strongly encouraged), bidirectional communication (teach-back was used to assess patient/family understanding). This communication occurred around the organizing framework of I-PASS (Illness severity, Patient summary, Action items, Situation awareness, and Synthesis by Receiver) (**Table 5-2**). Implementation of this intervention at seven pediatric hospitals across the United States and Canada was associated with a 38% decrease in harmful medical errors and improvements in aspects of family experience.

In addition to communication and patient care, PFCRs also present a venue for medical education and assessment. Trainees appreciate bedside teaching of physical exam skills and value attending physician role modeling. Role modeling can help trainees learn about core aspects of communication, compassion, accountability, and respect toward diverse patient populations. Observing trainees interact with each other, nursing staff, and with patients/families during rounds also allows for direct observation and real-time feedback. Trainees report that having a visual impression of a patient or a disease condition and seeing how different physicians interact and respond to family questions is a valuable learning experience. Learner autonomy has sometimes been reported by trainees to be at odds with PFCRs. However, creating a psychologically safe learning environment that encourages both trainees and patients/families to speak up and share their thoughts freely can help promote effective and educational rounds. PFCRs should allow for a simultaneous integration of patient care with medical education. While the PFCR model is often applied to teaching teams, it should apply to all patient care teams, including those without trainees.

Conducting PFCRs can be challenging in certain situations and may require modifications. Hospitals with double rooms, patients on isolation precautions, patients with non-accidental injuries, psychiatric illnesses, or sensitive diagnoses requiring confidentiality (e.g., sexually transmitted diseases) pose unique challenges. PFCRs can still be performed in these instances, but may require adjustments (e.g., huddling beforehand about how to discuss sensitive topics).

CHILD LIFE SERVICES

Partnering with child life can be a way to promote PFCC in the pediatric hospital medicine setting. The overall objectives of child life services are to recognize and address developmental issues related to healthcare experiences and respond to fears and concerns of hospitalized children and their families. Child life professionals meet these objectives through a variety of activities, including creating opportunities for play and enhanced self-esteem, providing inpatient schoolwork, assessing coping responses, minimizing stress, preparing children and families for healthcare experiences, facilitating family celebrations, and communicating these goals to the healthcare team. These activities can be crucial for the hospitalized child.

The way a child plays often communicates his or her interpretation of medical care or illness in a manner that may be inaccessible to other healthcare professionals. Child life may correct misunderstandings that

TABLE 5-2 Example PFCR Presentation in Patient- and Family-Centered I-PASS Format

Element	Definition	Example Presentation
Illness Severity	Whether patient is better, worse, or same	1. "How is Maria today compared to yesterday? Better, worse or the same?" (to family) 2. "What questions or worries do you have that you want to make sure we talk about today on rounds?"........."Great question; I'll make sure to talk about it" (to family) 3. "What concerns or issues are there from nursing?" (to nurse)
Patient Summary	Summary of overnight events, assessment, plan (Can be in "SOAP" format); directed at family and rest of team	• [Subjective] "Last night, Maria had a fever to 101 degrees, lower than the last 2 days so that's good. We sent another blood culture to be sure there's no infection in her blood. She was drinking better so we stopped her fluids through the IV." • [Objective] "As far as numbers, her vital signs were normal other than a high heart rate to 120 when she had the fever, which can happen with fever. She drank 720 ml (or 24 ounces) yesterday and was peeing very well (2 ml/kg/hr) which is great news! As far as her exam, heart, lungs, belly, and skin all looked good. I wasn't concerned about dehydration because her lips were moist, and she made tears when she cried. For labs, her blood culture did not grow any bacteria yet, which is good." • [Assessment] "In summary, Maria is 2 years old, came in with 3 days of fever, and was found to have a urinary tract infection or UTI. She is doing better overall, which we can tell because she is eating and drinking better, and her fevers are coming down. She needs to stay in the hospital till her fevers are better and we know exactly what bacteria is causing her infection." • [Plan] "Our plan for today is: 1) We'll keep checking her urine (pee) cultures to figure out exactly what bacteria is causing her urine infection. 2) Until then, we will continue her on the antibiotic called ceftriaxone and keep watching her fevers and how much she is eating and drinking."
Action Items	To dos for day (checkboxes)	• "So big to dos for today are to keep checking her blood and urine cultures. We may change her antibiotics once her urine test comes back." (to family and team)
Situation Awareness	Things to look out for/things that may change	• "As far as things to look out for, if she does not drink enough (18 ounces today), we may need to give her some fluids through her IV. Please watch her drinking closely and let us know how she is doing." (to family and nursing)
Synthesis by Receiver	Teach-back/readback of key point(s)	• "I know we went over a lot today. Just so I know I'm doing a good job explaining things, can you tell me what you'll be looking out for with Maria today?" (to family)

Source: Reproduced with permission from the Patient and Family-Centered I-PASS Study Group.

arise during play or relay critical developmental concerns to the family and other professionals on the child's healthcare team. In addition, play is a method of coping in the unfamiliar environment of the hospital. Therapeutic play can include dramatic play, artistic activity, pet therapy, sensory play (e.g., making dough), games, and attending special events such as musical performances. Medical play provides children with an open-ended opportunity to act, draw, or otherwise use creative media to explore medical equipment, situation, or themes. These activities familiarize children with their surroundings and help them better understand their own medical experiences.

Child life specialists also provide educational resources and environments for family members to help them cope with a child's illness. In-hospital libraries for families, educational video broadcasting in-hospital, and setting aside specific time for siblings in child life rooms can help alleviate a family's anxiety during a child's illness or hospitalization. Each child life specialist is a member of the comprehensive medical team caring for the patient and can serve as a valuable liaison between the family and child and healthcare professionals and can thereby help promote PFCC.

QUALITY AND OUTCOMES

Hospitals strive to improve quality of care and patient outcomes. Family/patient experience correlates directly with physician and nursing communication. Involving patients and families in every aspect of hospitalization and having clear and open communication can help improve patient outcomes. Maintaining transparency in care and using lay language to improve family understanding of medical conditions may further help communication and family satisfaction. In addition, patients and families can be partners in improving and measuring quality and outcomes, in accordance with principles of co-production.

DISCHARGE PLANNING AND TRANSITION TO THE MEDICAL HOME

An orderly transition from the inpatient to the outpatient setting can ensure continuity of clinical care. Discharge planning and goals should be established as soon as possible after admission. These goals should be reviewed and updated at least daily and explicitly discussed on rounds with patients/families and nurses. The more specific the discharge goals, the more helpful they are to patients/families and other team members. Once established, discharge goals facilitate ongoing care and discharge planning. Understanding discharge criteria and the role of care coordination is a valuable learning experience for trainees. Well-designed care systems are needed to facilitate discharges. Use of care coordinators or discharge planners may assist the primary medical team in accessing necessary outpatient services and proactively dealing with insurance-related and care coordination issues (e.g., arranging home intravenous infusions or supplies for nasogastric tube feeds). Communication with primary care providers (PCPs) is also necessary before discharge and sets the stage for safe handoff of care and closes the communication loop. Gaining the support and cooperation of PCPs facilitates effective transition. Important items to discuss include discharge diagnosis, results of diagnostic testing, outstanding tests that need follow-up, discharge medications, follow-up appointments, family concerns, and things to look out for. This communication should supplement and not replace a written discharge summary and should optimally occur before the patient's discharge from the hospital. Finally, hospitalization summaries, follow-up instructions, and anticipatory guidance should be provided to families both verbally and in writing using plain language (e.g., saying to watch for "trouble breathing" rather than "respiratory distress"). Readability assessments of written material can be performed in common word processing programs to ensure they are at the recommended 5th grade reading level. Translation of written information should also be performed for patients/families who speak a language other than English, which may take advance planning. For further detail on discharge planning and transitions, see Chapter 11.

CONCLUSION

A PFCC approach to the hospitalized child honors dimensions of care that patients and families value. These dimensions of care include honoring patient's and families' preferences, showing respect, using effective communication techniques (including health literacy best practices), developing shared goals, acknowledging biases, and being transparent about care processes and outcomes. PFCC includes evidence-based clinical care and addresses issues of timeliness, access, efficiency, safety, and equity. Care that is systems-based and accounts for these aims will produce more satisfactory clinical outcomes. Pre-hospital preparation, orientation to hospital and the unit (and its limitations), and robust child life services can further enhance family comfort and the experience of hospitalization. Conducting daily PFCRs to involve families in decision-making, improving communication, educating trainees, and facilitating discharge timeliness are crucial. Attention must be paid to discharge planning and the transition from inpatient to ambulatory settings. Good communication among healthcare providers and with patients and families supports a safe transition and handoff of care. Co-production by involving *all* patients and their families—particularly those with language or other barriers—at all levels of healthcare services can improve the quality, safety, experience, and equity of pediatric hospital care in a manner that is patient- and family-centered.

SUGGESTED READINGS

Ahmed A, Chu D, Wang S. Current caregiver perspectives and effects of demographics on family-centered rounds. *Clinical Pediatrics*. 2018;57(6):694-699.

AHRQ health literacy universal precautions took kit. Agency for Healthcare Research and Quality. https://www.ahrq.gov/health-literacy/improve/precautions/index.html. Content last reviewed September 2020. Accessed July 14, 2022.

Baker A. Crossing the quality chasm: a new health system for the 21st century. British Medical Journal Publishing Group; 2001.

Batalden M, Batalden P, Margolis P, et al. Coproduction of healthcare service. *BMJ Quality & Safety*. 2016;25(7):509-517.

Committee on Hospital Care and Institute for Patient-and Family-Centered Care. Patient-and family-centered care and the pediatrician's role. *Pediatrics*. 2012;129(2):394-404.

Everhart JL, Haskell H, Khan A. Patient-and family-centered care: leveraging best practices to improve the care of hospitalized children. *Pediatric Clinics*. 2019;66(4):775-789.

Fernandes AK, Wilson S, Nalin AP, et al. Pediatric family-centered rounds and humanism: a systematic review and qualitative meta-analysis. *Hospital Pediatrics*. 2021;11(6):636-649.

Glick AF, Goonan M, Kim C, Sandmeyer D, Londoño K, Gold-von Simson G. Factors associated with parental participation in family-centered rounds. *Hospital Pediatrics*. 2021;11(1):61-70.

Health Literacy in healthy people 2030. U.S. Department of Health and Human Services. https://health.gov/healthypeople/priority-areas/health-literacy-healthy-people-2030. Accessed July 14, 2022.

Implicit bias. U.S. Department of Health & Human Services: National Institutes of Health. https://diversity.nih.gov/sociocultural-factors/implicit-bias#:~:text=Implicit%20bias%20is%20a%20form,retaining%20a%20diverse%20scientific%20workforce. Page last updated June 3, 2022. Accessed July 14, 2022.

Khan A, Spector ND, Baird JD, et al. Patient safety after implementation of a coproduced family centered communication programme: multicenter before and after intervention study. *BMJ*. 2018;363.

Morrison AK, Glick A, Yin HS. Health literacy: implications for child health. *Pediatr Rev*. 2019;40(6):263-277.

Rea KE, Rao P, Hill E, Saylor KM, Cousino MK. Families' experiences with pediatric family-centered rounds: a systematic review. *Pediatrics*. 2018;141(3).

The Picker Principles of Person Centred Care. Picker Institute. https://picker.org/who-we-are/the-picker-principles-of-person-centred-care. Published 2022. Accessed July 8, 2022.

Vara T, Anderson M, Baird JD, Calaman,S. O'Toole JK. We Are All Learning, Together: An imperative for patient-and family-centered rounds from the patient and family perspective. *Hospital Pediatrics*. 2021;11(7):e117-e119.

CHAPTER 6

Health Equity and the Social Determinants of Health

Cristin Q. Fritz, MD, MPH, Andrew F. Beck, MD, MPH, and Ndidi I. Unaka, MD, MEd

INTRODUCTION

Optimal health of all individuals, households, communities, and populations is the ideal state; and yet its achievement remains elusive often on account of social determinants of health. In this chapter, we highlight key terms of central relevance to the pursuit of optimal health and health equity across care settings, review mechanisms by which the social determinants influence health outcomes, and identify action steps for pediatric hospitalists to optimize the health and well-being of their patients and, by extension, their households and communities.

TERMINOLOGY

Healthy People 2030 defines social determinants of health as "the conditions in the environments where people are born, live, learn, work, play, worship, and age that affect a wide range of health, functioning, and quality-of-life outcomes and risk" (**Table 6-1**). These conditions, which include economic stability, education access and quality, neighborhood and built environment, social and community context, and healthcare access and quality, can enhance or inhibit health and well-being in profound ways. For example, variation exists across communities regarding access to reliable and efficient public transportation, grocery stores, and affordable housing. This variation, in turn, affects individual- and household-level social risk factors, needs, and assets that influence outcomes across care settings, including for those admitted to pediatric hospital medicine services.

Social factors influencing health and structural processes inform the distribution of resources of pertinence to health; the social determinants of health can be thought of as byproducts of a range of structural factors which promulgate health inequities. Structural determinants of health are the "causes of the causes" or the context (shaped by social norms and policies) and mechanisms that configure social hierarchy and gradients (e.g., inequitable power, classism, racism, sexism, exclusion). These structural factors reinforce the wide chasms between the experiences of individuals, households, communities, and populations of varying social identities and resources, chasms shaped by the reality that some have seemingly endless opportunities and others seemingly insurmountable burdens.

An understanding of racism as a structural determinant of health is foundational to our pursuit of health equity. Race is a social construct—it has no biological basis but has significant political and social implications. Racism is a system fortified by the social construct of race. Racism in all its forms (intrapersonal, interpersonal, institutional, and structural) insidiously works to structure advantage and disadvantage based on the interpretation of physical characteristics (i.e., skin color) and flawed assumptions regarding inherent attributes of racialized individuals and populations. For example, structural racism is at the root of residential segregation. Discriminatory practices such as redlining, rooted in policy decisions in the 1930s that led to the systematic denial of services to residents of certain areas based on their race or ethnicity, have resulted in chronic disinvestment in marginalized communities which, in turn, contributes to a current lack of access to vital resources. Indeed, evidence suggests a clear relationship between systemic practices such as denying mortgages or other financial investments to individuals in historically redlined neighborhoods and both subsequent residential segregation and downstream health effects (e.g., diminished life expectancy). Additionally, social and structural determinants of health, and related social risk factors and needs (e.g., food insecurity, housing instability), are connected to adverse childhood experiences (ACEs) and the subsequent

TABLE 6-1 Glossary of Key Terms

Term	Definition
Social risks or risk factors	"Specific, individual adverse social conditions associated with poor health."[a] Examples include food insecurity, housing instability. **Screening tools identify social risks.**
Social needs	"Social risk factors that individuals identify and prioritize."[a]
Social determinants of health	"The conditions in the environments where people are born, live, learn, work, play, worship, and age that affect a wide range of health, functioning, and quality-of-life outcomes and risk."[b]
Structural determinants of health	"Societal norms, macroeconomic, social and health policies; and the structural mechanisms that shape social hierarchy and gradients (e.g., power, racism, sexism, classism, exclusion) and in turn the distribution, quality, and chronicity of social determinants of health and social needs."[a]
Adverse Childhood Experiences	Potentially traumatic events that children experience that can impact health and well-being. ACEs include aspects of a child or adolescent's environment that threaten their sense of safety and stability. Examples include physical or emotional abuse, neglect, intimate partner violence, having an incarcerated parent, and parental substance abuse
Population Health	"The health outcomes of a group of individuals, including the distribution of such outcomes within the group."[c]
Social Construct	A concept created or invented by individuals of a society, culture, or institution that exists solely based on a society's acceptance of it. Social constructs depend on historical, political, and economic conditions which means they can evolve and change. Race is a social construct and has no biological basis.
Racism	"An umbrella concept that encompasses specific mechanisms that operate at the intrapersonal, interpersonal, institutional, and systemic levels of a socioecological framework."[d] The four levels of racism: • Intrapersonal (internalized): acceptance of negative messages about one's self worth and abilities (e.g., self-devaluation, stereotype threat) • Interpersonal (personally mediated): prejudice, implicit/explicit bias which are differential assumptions about the abilities, motives, and intentions of others often rooted in stereotypes • Institutional racism: differential access to goods, services, and opportunities based on race that exists in specific institutional or organizational policies and practices • Systemic (or structural racism): "ways in which societies foster racial discrimination, via mutually reinforcing inequitable systems (e.g., in housing, education, employment, earnings, benefits, credit, media, healthcare, criminal justice, etc.) that in turn reinforce discriminatory beliefs, values, and distribution of resources, reflected in history, culture, and interconnected institutions"
Inequality	State or instances in which individuals and communities have access to different resources and opportunities regardless of their unique needs or assets.
Inequity	A disparity or difference that is unfair, unjust, and avoidable. Health inequities are "systematic differences in the opportunities groups have to achieve optimal health, leading to unfair and avoidable differences in health outcomes."[d]
Equality	State or instances in which individuals or communities are given the same resources and opportunities regardless of their unique needs or assets.
Equity	Based on the principle of distributive justice; the allocation of resources, benefits, and burdens across society that is informed by the social conditions of individuals and communities. Health equity is the absence of socially unjust, unfair, and avoidable health disparities.

[a] Health Begins. Upstream communication toolkit. HealthBegins-Upstream-Communications-Toolkit-Feb-2022.pdf (netdna-ssl.com). Published 2019.

[b] Office of Disease Prevention and Health Promotion, Office of the Assistant Secretary for Health, Office of the Secretary, U.S. Department of Health and Human Services. Social Determinants of Health. Healthy People 2030 Website. https://health.gov/healthypeople/priority-areas/social-determinants-health. Published 2022.

[c] Kindig D, Stoddart G. What is population health? *Am J Public Health.* 2003;93(3):380-383.

[d] Baciu A, Negussie Y, Geller A, et al. *Communities in Action: Pathways to Health Equity.* Washington (DC); 2017.

[e] Bailey ZD, Krieger N, Agenor M, et al. Structural racism and health inequities in the USA: evidence and interventions. *Lancet.* 2017;389(10077):1453-1463.

toxic stress and trauma that ensues. ACEs such as physical, emotional, and sexual abuse, incarceration, and substance abuse are common and have far reaching implications on health opportunities throughout the life course and across generations.

The social and structural determinants of health also influence the distribution of health outcomes across populations. A state of health equity can only be achieved when everyone has a fair and just opportunity to be as healthy as possible. Achieving equity requires meeting the specific needs of individuals and communities through the just distribution of resources and burdens. Unlike equality, which focuses on sameness, equity and justice center on the unique context, assets, and needs of specific individuals, households, communities, and/or populations. Equity in health cannot be achieved by solely focusing on the healthcare sector. Rather, a concerted, coordinated effort across sectors should address upstream factors, such as economic stability, stable housing within healthy and safe neighborhoods, and access to quality education, that influence overall health and well-being. Likewise, the pursuit of equity cannot occur within one phase of care within single healthcare organizations. That is, the pursuit of equity is not solely the responsibility of primary care providers. Instead, pediatricians, including pediatric hospitalists, must seize upon available opportunities to address social needs through awareness, adjustment, assistance, alignment, and advocacy to achieve our collective goal of excellent and equitable health outcomes for all individuals, households, communities, and populations.

MECHANISMS BY WHICH SOCIAL DETERMINANTS INFLUENCE HEALTH EQUITY & OUTCOMES FOR THE HOSPITALIZED CHILD

The socioecological model illustrates potential mechanisms through which social and structural determinants influence patient and population outcomes. This model frames factors at the individual, household, and community levels that influence outcomes for populations, including those pertinent to pediatric hospital medicine (Bronfenbrenner, 1979).

Using this model, example pathways through which social and structural determinants may act are illustrated in **Table 6-2**. Different individuals, households, communities, and populations have very different lived experiences. These "upstream" differences can promote (or prevent) illnesses that might result in hospitalization. Consider what may precede a hospitalization in the case of a child with asthma, a common chronic disease that causes significant morbidity and frequently results in the hospitalization of children. Economic instability linked to a range of competing priorities (e.g., food insecurity, challenging work schedules, inconsistent childcare) can lead to suboptimal adherence to preventive routines and care visits. This child may also live in a home with poor-quality indoor air or in a community near a busy thoroughfare spewing pollutants. The map in **Figure 6-1** illustrates this concept: a community

TABLE 6-2 Example Mechanisms by Which the Social Determinants of Health* Influence Likelihood of Hospitalization, Severity of Hospitalization, and Transition Back to Home

	Individual	Household	Community
Economic Stability	• Limited access to healthy foods prompting poorer baseline health	• Parent(s) do not make enough money to make ends meet making health-promoting purchases difficult	• Gentrification that displaces certain populations into communities with less opportunity for upward mobility
Education Access and Quality	• Negative educational environment can have negative effect on mental health (and adherence to preventive regimen)	• Limited health literacy and numeracy affect ability to adhere to treatment guidance	• Certain communities are characterized by lower performing schools, with fewer health-promoting supports (e.g., nurses, social workers)
Healthcare Access and Quality	• Difficulty accessing routine primary care prompting shift of care to the acute setting	• Parent(s) work odd hours, multiple jobs making it hard to bring child to preventive visit	• Differential access to primary and subspecialty care based solely on health insurance carrier
Neighborhood and Built Environment	• Adverse in-home exposures exacerbating respiratory health	• Rights affronted by unresponsive, predatory landlord leading to unstable housing, threat of eviction	• Community located by busy roadway with poorer outdoor air quality
Social and Community Context	• Heightened exposure to stress impairing immune response	• Limited support networks for household in times of need (e.g., a child's hospitalization)	• Policies that propagate racist structures and systems; widen inequities

*Social determinants of health domains as defined by Healthy People 2030.

with substantial variability in measures like poverty, a household within that community with unhealthy living conditions, a child within that household who ends up hospitalized. The reality is that such a petri dish of economic, educational, healthcare, environmental, and social factors can make hospitalizations more likely for some than others. These factors can also prolong hospitalizations and influence the transition from hospital to home and the transition from illness back to health.

Multiple studies have assessed the prevalence and impact of these determinants (**Table 6-3**). Quantitative studies have highlighted the predominance of social needs on inpatient settings—hospitalized families frequently experience financial stress and/or caregiver mental health concerns. Family substance abuse, legal circumstances, economic strain, and foster care involvement have each been shown to be independently associated with longer lengths of stay. Such factors also influence the experience of care during hospitalization. For example, barriers to care (e.g., distrust in healthcare system or team, lack of perceived partnership with team, insufficient confidence in skills needed to care for child) have been associated with longer length of stay and increased 30-day rehospitalizations. Barriers more commonly occur among those families of greater social disadvantage, including those with public insurance, those identifying as a minoritized race/ethnicity, and those who speak a language other than English.

Further, qualitative studies have highlighted the "fog" families find themselves in during the shock of an inpatient stay. This "fog" can be particularly severe for those struggling with more than just an acute physical or mental illness. Although all families "took a hit" from the stress of a hospitalization, those from more impoverished communities were more likely to describe logistical challenges, limited support networks impacting their transition from hospital to home, and less buffer with which they could withstand that hit. That is, different populations experience pediatric hospitalizations, inpatient hospital care, and transitions back to home in different ways. In many cases, these differences are driven by the contextual factors that influence a child's likelihood of exacerbating a chronic condition, being afflicted by an acute condition, and returning to their baseline state of health.

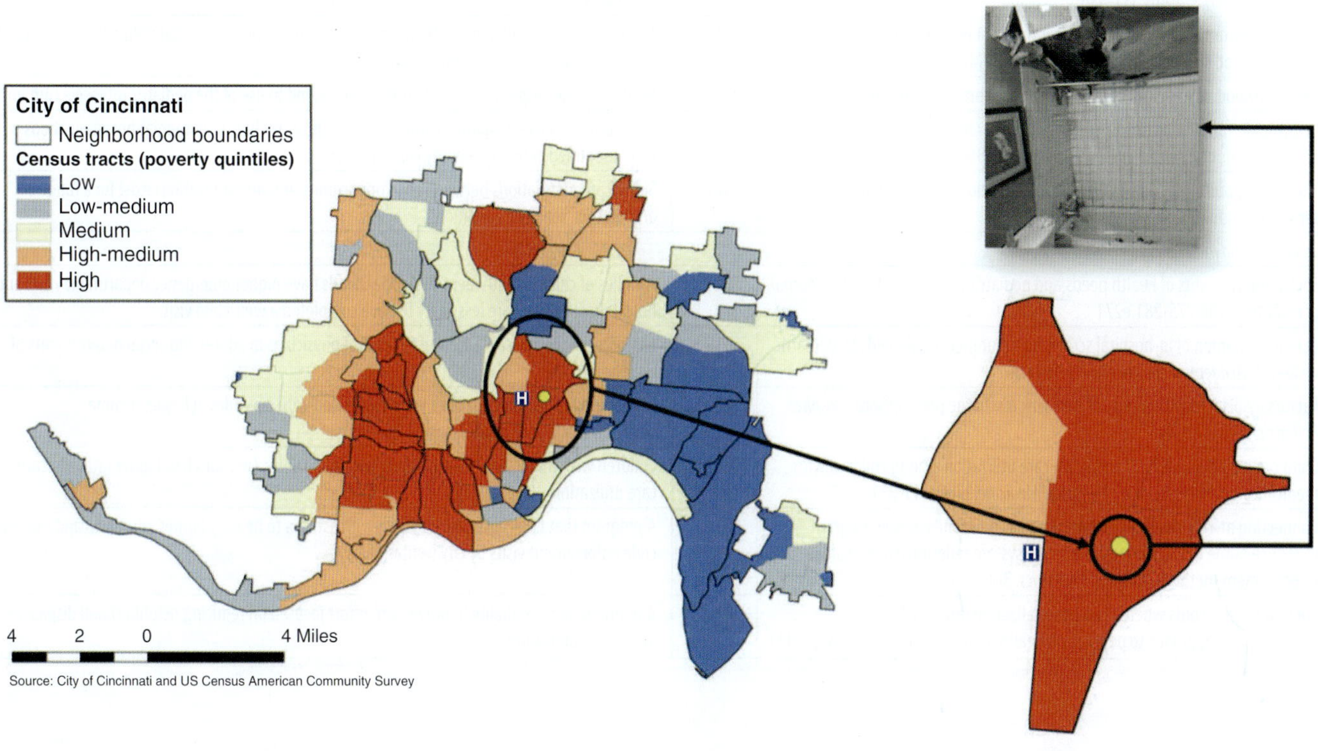

FIGURE 6-1. Illustrative map of the intersection between social and structural determinants of health and the lived reality within neighborhoods. The primary map is of the City of Cincinnati. The dark black boundaries represent city neighborhoods, colored according to underlying rates of poverty. One high-poverty neighborhood is called out. Imagine a child living within that neighborhood, with accordant risks and assets felt within that community. Now imagine that child hospitalized to an inpatient service.

TABLE 6-3 Published Work Addressing Healthy Equity and Social Determinants of Health Among Hospitalized Children

Manuscript and Reference	Year	Summary of Study
Mechanisms by Which Social Determinants Influence Health Equity & Outcomes for the Hospitalized Child		
Identification of caregiver-reported social risk factors in hospitalized children. *Hospital Pediatrics*. 10(1):20-28	2020	Social risk screening is feasible in the inpatient setting and positive screens are common.
Associations between social factor documentation and hospital length of stay and readmission among children. *Hospital Pediatrics*.10(1):12-19	2020	Social International Classification of Diseases (ICD) codes are not frequently used in the inpatient setting but are associated with prolonged hospitalizations and readmissions.
Identifying modifiable health care barriers to improve health equity for hospitalized children. *Hospital Pediatrics*. 10(1):1-11	2020	Nine out of 10 barriers to care associated with at least 1 worse hospital outcome. System barriers, skill barriers, cultural distance, and marginalization were significantly associated with cumulative social disadvantage.
Socioeconomic status influences the toll paediatric hospitalisations take on families: a qualitative study. *BMJ Quality and Safety*. 26(4):304-311	2017	Families of lower socioeconomic status (SES) experience stress and challenges (e.g. financial strain) related to their child's hospitalization that are distinct from families of higher SES
Differential Exposures Widening Equity Gaps in Experienced Morbidity		
Explaining racial disparities in child asthma readmission using a causal inference approach. *JAMA Pediatrics*.170(7):695-703	2016	The majority of racial disparity in asthma-related readmissions is "explained" by social, economic, and environmental factors.
Medical home quality and readmission risk for children hospitalized with asthma exacerbations. *Pediatrics*.131(1):64-70	2013	Poor access to a medical home was associated with increased readmission in hospitalized children with asthma
Inequalities in neighborhood child asthma admission rates and underlying community characteristics in one US county. *The Journal of Pediatrics*.163(2):574-580	2013	Substantial neighborhood-to-neighborhood disparities exist in asthma admission rates.
The child opportunity index and disparities in pediatric asthma hospitalizations across one Ohio Metropolitan Area, 2011-2013. *The Journal of Pediatrics*. 190:200-206 e201	2017	Lower opportunity measured at the neighborhood level is associated with increased asthma hospitalizations.
Areas with high rates of police-reported violent crime have higher rates of childhood asthma morbidity. *The Journal of Pediatrics*.173:175-182 e171	2016	Associations exist between exposure to violent crime and asthma hospitalizations.
Housing code violation density associated with emergency department and hospital use by children with asthma. *Health Affairs*. 33(11):1993-2002	2014	Associations exist between housing code violations measured by local municipalities and asthma emergency department visits and hospitalizations.
Financial and social hardships in families of children with medical complexity. *The Journal of Pediatrics*. 172:187-193 e181	2016	Financial and social hardship is common among families with children with medical complexity.
Socioeconomic and racial disparities in diabetic ketoacidosis admissions in youth with type 1 diabetes. *Journal of Hospital Medicine*. doi:10.12788/jhm.3664	2021	Significant links exist between area-level measures of socioeconomic status and suboptimal outcomes for youth with type 1 diabetes mellitus.
Challenges following hospital discharge for children with medical complexity. *Hospital Pediatrics*. 10(6):531-536	2020	Discharge challenges (e.g. follow up appointments, medications) were commonly reported by caregivers of children with medical complexity.
Pervasive income-based disparities in inpatient bed-day rates across conditions and subspecialties. *Health Affairs*. 37(4):551-559	2018	There is substantial variability, by socioeconomic measures, in hospital utilization across nearly every condition cared for in the hospital.
Neighborhood poverty and pediatric intensive care use. *Pediatrics*.144(6)	2019	Socioeconomic disparities in acute utilization extend to use of the pediatric intensive care unit.
Geographic variation in hospitalization for lower respiratory tract infections across one county. *JAMA Pediatrics*.169(9):846-854	2015	"Hot spots" of lower respiratory tract infection (bronchiolitis, pneumonia) hospitalizations were identified in higher poverty communities.
The child opportunity index 2.0 and hospitalizations for ambulatory care sensitive conditions. *Pediatrics*. 148(2)	2021	Significant associations between child opportunity and hospitalizations exist for a range of ambulatory-sensitive conditions.
Screening and Intervening		
Social determinants of health needs and pediatric health care use. *The Journal of Pediatrics*. 238:275-281.e271	2021	Families of children with identified social needs have higher emergency department visits and hospitalizations and are less likely to have completed a well-child visit.
Caregiver opinion of in-hospital screening for unmet social needs by pediatric residents. *Academic Pediatrics*.16(2):161-167	2016	Caregivers have a positive view of the role of physicians in addressing social determinants of health.
Factors associated with pickup of pediatric discharge prescriptions. *Hospital Pediatrics*. 9(6):440-446	2019	Higher medication pick-up rates were associated with zip codes in higher income neighborhoods and privately insured patients.
Child opportunity index 2.0 and acute care utilization among children with medical complexity. *Journal of Hospital Medicine*.17(4):243-251	2022	Children with medical complexity from low opportunity ZIP codes had higher rates of acute care utilization
Connecting at-risk inpatient asthmatics to a community-based program to reduce home environmental risks: care system redesign using quality improvement methods. *Hospital Pediatrics*. 3(4):326-334	2013	A program that links hospitalized youth with asthma to healthy homes education and housing code enforcement visits by city sanitarians.
Cooling the hot spots where child hospitalization rates are high: a neighborhood approach to population health. *Health Affairs*. 38(9):1433-1441	2019	A multidisciplinary quality improvement effort focused on reducing neighborhood disparities in hospital utilization.

DIFFERENTIAL EXPOSURES WIDENING EQUITY GAPS IN EXPERIENCED MORBIDITY

The term *population health* is defined as "the health outcomes of a group of individuals, including the distribution of such outcomes within the group." The distribution of hospital medicine outcomes for youth are influenced by the context in which a child is born, lives, learns, works, plays, worships, and ages.

CHRONIC CONDITIONS

Asthma is one of the most common chronic conditions of childhood, resulting in thousands of pediatric hospitalizations every year. Hospitalization and rehospitalization rates are significantly greater among youth who identify as a minoritized race compared with their majority peers. Asthma-related morbidity is exacerbated by socioeconomic hardship, limited functional access to preventive care, and adverse environmental exposures in one's home (e.g., cockroaches, mold) and in one's community (e.g., traffic-related pollutants). These social determinants of health influence the degree to which children with asthma require hospitalization. Links between patient-level asthma hospitalization risk and the social determinants also extend to populations. Communities with higher hospitalization rates are significantly more likely to be characterized by more poverty, housing code violations, and crime, and by less educational and socioeconomic opportunity, pharmacy access, and availability of reliable transportation.

This pattern extends to other chronic conditions. Youth with type 1 diabetes who live in higher poverty neighborhoods are significantly more likely to be admitted for diabetic ketoacidosis than their peers who reside in more affluent neighborhoods. Similar patterns occur for those with public compared with private insurance. Additionally, nearly all families of children with medical complexity experience at least one financial or social need, or hardship. These hardships, and the context from which children with medical complexity are hospitalized and to which they are discharged, influence their health and well-being. As a result, care models that are truly multi-disciplinary, inclusive of those capable of identifying and addressing health-related social risks and needs, have shown promise on the inpatient side. This is true for teams focused on supporting children with medical complexity and likely extends to general hospital medicine teams as well.

ALL-CAUSE INPATIENT BED-DAYS, AMBULATORY CARE SENSITIVE CONDITIONS, AND ACUTE ILLNESSES

Health inequities experienced by hospitalized individuals extend from chronic to acute conditions. There exists a graded relationship between all-cause inpatient bed-days and area-level poverty. Bed-day rates—the number of days children from a given community spent hospitalized divided by a population denominator—increase as community poverty rates increase. Moreover, graded relationships are present for nearly every diagnosis cared for in the hospital, including acute conditions (e.g., lower respiratory tract infections) and ambulatory care sensitive conditions (e.g., cellulitis, gastroenteritis and dehydration, seizure, and urinary tract infection). Similar graded relationships are present for days that youth spend in intensive care. These health inequities, influenced by the social and structural determinants of health, do not need to be a foregone conclusion. There is a role for pediatricians in general, and multidisciplinary, integrated pediatric hospital medicine teams more specifically, in the pursuit of equitable outcomes.

SCREENING AND INTERVENING

The American Academy of Pediatrics (AAP) recommends screening for social risks during patient encounters to identify social needs and link families to supportive services as early as possible. Connection to resources from healthcare settings can decrease a family's number of social risks, increase community resource enrollment, and improve caregiver-reported child health. Inpatient screening for social risks and needs serves an important role. Hospitalized children have higher rates of social risks than the general population. Additionally, new social needs may develop during hospitalization due to the financial and emotional stress associated with hospitalization. Finally, hospitalizations provide a unique opportunity to identify risks and address needs among a population who may not receive coordinated care in an outpatient medical home and more often rely on acute care for medical issues. Fortunately, families are receptive to social risk screening in the inpatient setting (**Table 6-4**).

The National Academy of Sciences, Engineering, and Medicine (NASEM) released a landmark Consensus Study Report that provides a framework for healthcare systems to utilize as they seek to integrate social and medical care. The foundation of social care integration is *Awareness*, a hospital's ability to identify the social needs of its patient

TABLE 6-4 Pediatric-Focused Screening Tools

Tool Name	Number of Social Needs Questions	Domains Included	Literacy Level	Languages Available	Reference
FAMNEEDS	22	Childcare Access, Education, Employment, Food Insecurity, Health Insurance, Health Literacy, Housing Insecurity, Legal, Mental Health, Public Benefits, Social Support, Substance Use, Transportation, Utilities	Not Reported	English; Spanish; Haitian Creole; Urdu; Punjabi; Hindi; Arabic	Uwemedimo OT, May H. Disparities in utilization of social determinants of health referrals among children in immigrant families. *Front Pediatr.* 2018;6:207.
iScreen	23	Child Care Access, Education, Financial Strain, Food Insecurity, Health Care Access, Health Insurance, Housing safety, Housing Stability, Immigration, Legal Needs, Mental Health, Neighborhood safety, Public Benefits, School Safety, Transportation,	7th grade	English, Spanish	Gottlieb L, Hessler D, Long D, et al. A randomized trial on screening for social determinants of health: the iScreen study. *Pediatrics.* 2014;134(6):e1611-1618.
iHelp	14	Education, Financial Strain, Food Insecurity, Health Care Access, Housing Insecurity, Housing Quality, Immigration status, Intimate Partner Violence, Power of Attorney	7th grade	English	Colvin JD, Bettenhausen JL, Anderson-Carpenter KD, et al. Multiple behavior change intervention to improve detection of unmet social needs and resulting resource referrals. *Academic Pediatrics.* 2016;16(2):168-174
SEEK	9	Food Insecurity, Intimate Partner Violence, Mental Health, Social Support, Stress, Substance Use	4th-5th grade	Spanish, Chinese, Swedish, Vietnamese	Dubowitz H, Feigelman S, Lane W, et al. Pediatric primary care to help prevent child maltreatment: the Safe Environment for Every Kid (SEEK) Model. *Pediatrics.* 2009;123(3):858-864.
We Care	6 or 15	Childcare Access, Education, Employment, Food Insecurity, Housing Insecurity, Mental Health, Substance Use, Utilities	9th grade	English, Spanish	Garg A, Toy S, Tripodis Y, et al. Addressing social determinants of health at well child care visits: a cluster RCT. *Pediatrics.* 2015;135(2):e296-304.

population. Interventions may focus on the individual patient through *Adjustment* (a change in clinical practice to accommodate existing barriers) or *Assistance* (connecting individuals or households to resources directly through referral). Hospitals may also work for change at the community level through *Alignment* (engaging with stakeholders to enhance social care outside the hospital walls) and *Advocacy* (promoting policy changes that will improve health and address social needs for communities and populations). The remainder of this section will explore how hospitalists and hospitals can apply the concepts of Awareness, Adjustment, Assistance, Alignment, and Advocacy to develop an approach to augmenting positive and mitigating negative social determinants that influence health outcomes.

AWARENESS

Universally recommended screening tools (**Table 6-4**) or uniform approaches to screening within the hospital do not currently exist. However, hospitals, and hospitalists, can incorporate universal best practices into their inpatient screening programs. First, families are more likely to disclose needs when given a tablet or paper-based screening forms as they avoid discussion of sensitive information aloud. Additionally, care teams are more likely to fit completion of electronic health record (EHR)-based, automated screening templates into their busy clinical workflow. Specific screening approaches and implementation plans can be tailored to fit the needs of patients and populations, existing EHR tools, clinical infrastructure, and resource networks, aided by the NASEM framework and report.

ADJUSTMENT

Families of lower socioeconomic status, and those with more social needs, frequently express increased difficulty navigating the transition from hospital to home. Thus, adapting care around the time of discharge to better support families is important. For instance, families with lower income have decreased rates of medication pick up from off-site pharmacies. In response, hospitals may consider programs developed to deliver discharge medications to the bedside to combat transportation difficulties. Interventions to provide additional support and care coordination at the time of discharge for children with medical complexity residing in high poverty, low opportunity communities may also be relevant given the higher rate of hospital admission within this population.

ASSISTANCE

Interventions to directly connect patients and their families to resources may be implemented at various time points during hospitalization, starting at the time of admission. For instance, identification of food insecurity, or hunger, early on may be addressed through guest trays, meal vouchers, or gift cards that help families obtain food during hospitalization. During the hospital stay, inpatient teams may focus interventions on connecting families to resources at the time of discharge though referrals to community organizations. A "warm" hand-off (i.e., direct referral communication between a hospital provider and community organization) for families with food insecurity with community organizations that can provide emergency food resources and assist with enrollment in federal nutrition programs may be a prudent course of action. Co-location of resources, such as an on-site food pantry or pharmacy is another model within hospitals. Inpatient teams can continue to support families after discharge by addressing social and structural factors that contribute to hospital utilization for a subset of patients, including environmental risk factors. For example, connections to community-based programs capable of providing healthy homes education and action may be appropriate for those hospitalized with respiratory diagnoses.

ALIGNMENT

Hospitals can use data from inpatient social risk screening to guide non-healthcare-based interventions such as partnerships between the hospital and surrounding community organizations focused on improving the health of the hospital's population. Community partners can include faith-based organizations, community development organizations, nonprofits, public health departments, and local school districts. Geospatial mapping of social risk factors and health outcomes can be used to direct interventions to communities with high rates of poverty and morbidity in order to improve outcomes and narrow equity gaps. Multidisciplinary teams that share data, coordinate on the pursuit of shared outcomes, and address needs across the medical-social continuum can lead to better outcomes and narrowed gaps for shared populations.

ADVOCACY

Pediatric hospitalists must address the structures and systems that influence child health and well-being. Evidence increasingly suggests a link between civic engagement and health outcomes across the life course, including for the hospitalized child. As such, there are things that clinician-citizens can do inside and outside of the healthcare setting. Clinicians should make sure that they are registered to vote and ready to cast their ballot on each and every election day. Clinicians should encourage their eligible patients and household members to exercise their own right to vote. Voter registration is an evidence-based action that has a role in the hospital as well as the community. Pediatric hospital medicine providers should maintain an awareness of policies relevant to the profession and to the patients they treat. Pediatric hospitalists can seize opportunities to highlight evidence in policy debates, engage with civic leaders (local, state, and federal) on topics of central importance, and write and speak in support of policies that could meaningfully improve child health outcomes. For some, running for office may prove an attractive option for enacting lasting change.

CONCLUSION

The social and structural determinants of health are relevant to the care of the hospitalized child. They influence health outcomes for individuals, households, communities, and populations. As such, there is a role for clinicians as they seek to understand and address such factors before, during, and after a hospitalization as they join in the movement toward optimal and equitable health outcomes.

SUGGESTED READINGS

AAP Council on Community Pediatrics. Poverty and child health in the United States. *Pediatrics*. 2016;137(4).

Baciu A, Negussie Y, Geller A, Weinstein JN, eds. *Communities in Action: Pathways to Health Equity*. Washington (DC); 2017.

Bailey ZD, Krieger N, Agenor M, et al. Structural racism and health inequities in the USA: evidence and interventions. *Lancet*. 2017; 389(10077):1453-1463.

Beck AF, Cohen AJ, Colvin JD, et al. Perspectives from the Society for Pediatric Research: interventions targeting social needs in pediatric clinical care. *Pediatr Res*. 2018;84(1):10-21.

Braveman P, Arkin E, Orleans T, et al. What is Heatlh Equity? Robert Wood Johnson Foundation. https://www.rwjf.org/en/library/research/2017/05/what-is-health-equity-.html Published 2017.

Bronfenbrenner U. *The Ecology of Human Development: Experiments by Nature and Design*. Cambridge, MA: Harvard University Press; 1979.

Felitti VJ, Anda RF, Nordenberg D, et al. Relationship of childhood abuse and household dysfunction to many of the leading causes of death in adults. The Adverse Childhood Experiences (ACE) Study. *Am J Prev Med*. 1998;14(4):245-258.

Gottlieb LM, Hessler D, Long D, et al. Effects of social needs screening and in-person service navigation on child health: a randomized clinical trial. *JAMA pediatrics*. 2016;170(11):e162521.

Health Begins. Upstream communication toolkit. HealthBegins-Upstream-Communications-Toolkit-Feb-2022.pdf (netdna-ssl.com). Published 2019.

Huang SJ, Sehgal NJ. Association of historic redlining and present-day health in Baltimore. *PLoS One*. 2022;17(1):e0261028.

Kindig D, Stoddart G. What is population health? *Am J Public Health*. 2003;93(3):380-383.

McKinlay JB. A Case For Refocusing Upstream: The Political Economy of Illness. IAPHS Occasional Classics Web site. https://iaphs.org/wp-content/uploads/2019/11/IAPHS-McKinlay-Article.pdf. Published 2019.

National Academies of Sciences Engineering and Medicine. *Integrating social care into the delivery of health care: Moving upstream to improve the nation's health.* Washington, DC: The National Academies Press; 2019.

Office of Disease Prevention and Health Promotion, Office of the Assistant Secretary for Health, Office of the Secretary, U.S. Department of Health and Human Services. Social Determinants of Health. Healthy People 2030 Website. https://health.gov/healthypeople/priority-areas/social-determinants-health. Published 2022.

Taylor LA, Tan AX, Coyle CE, et al. Leveraging the social determinants of health: what works? *PLoS One.* 2016;11(8):e0160217.

Wall M, Hayes R, Moore D, et al. Evaluation of community level interventions to address social and structural determinants of health: a cluster randomised controlled trial. *BMC Public Health.* 2009;9:207.

CHAPTER 7

Diagnostic Uncertainty

Irit R. Rasooly, MD, MSCE and Andrew P. J. Olson, MD

UNCERTAINTY, AN INHERENT ELEMENT OF THE DIAGNOSTIC PROCESS

Uncertainty is inherent in medical diagnosis, prognosis, and treatment. Diagnostic uncertainty has been conceptualized by Bhise et al as the *subjective (and often appropriate) perception of an inability to provide an accurate explanation of the patient's health problem.* Uncertainty is contextual and takes many forms.

There is potential for uncertainty at every phase of the diagnostic process, with different manifestations and consequences for patients, their families, and clinicians (**Figure 7-1**). Hospitalized patients and their families may experience uncertainty about the diagnostic process itself (about if, when, why, how, and by whom diagnoses are formed), about when to request care/evaluation, about what constitutes abnormal symptoms, about what historical information is relevant, about the significance of laboratory or imaging findings, about when to seek additional opinions, about how to navigate differing clinical opinions, and about the finality, accuracy, meaning, and implication of diagnoses. For hospital medicine clinicians, uncertainty may result from unsettled science (and the resulting imperative of maintaining clinical equipoise), from an incomplete knowledge base, or about the accuracy and patient-specific context of information (e.g., Is the caregiver or patient report reflective of the actual condition? How much do these symptoms deviate from the patient baseline?). Moreover, there is a difficulty to quantify degree of uncertainty deriving from inherent human variability and from the unpredictable, complex clinical care environment. Clinicians may be uncertain about whether sufficient information has been gathered, about when subspecialty consult is beneficial, about test characteristics including accuracy and precision, about significance and relevance of test findings, about when diagnoses can be safely excluded and when it might be appropriate to consider rare or unusual conditions, and about how to communicate and document the degree of uncertainty that exists.

Individual patients, families, and clinicians can have different reactions to and tolerance of uncertainty, ranging from curiosity and wonder to stress about "not knowing." Moreover, responses to uncertainty vary depending on context. Variation in how people experience and make sense of uncertainty can have marked influence on clinical interactions. Responses to uncertainty are modifiable contributors to the quality of care. Recognition of uncertainty, communication about diagnostic reasoning and uncertainty within the care team, framing the degree and nature of uncertainty to patients/caregivers, and taking appropriate steps to resolve uncertainty are hallmarks of safe, high-quality hospital care.

FORMS OF UNCERTAINTY

Uncertainty is an aspect of daily life. In medicine, resolving uncertainty is a defining responsibility and navigating uncertainty contributes to the *art* of medicine.

Recent efforts in medicine have sought to categorize and define diagnostic uncertainty in order to understand its impact on clinical care. Three such classification schemes are addressed here. One approach classifies uncertainty as either *informational or intrinsic/existential. Informational uncertainty* is the result of knowledge deficits; such deficits can result from lack of information about the patient, gaps in medical knowledge or inability to apply such knowledge to a clinical scenario, or an absence of scientific data about a particular topic. *Intrinsic or existential uncertainty* stems from the limited human ability to make decisions in a complex, variable system where multiple factors contribute to patient outcomes. A second approach classifies uncertainty as either *epistemic or aleatoric. Epistemic uncertainty* relates to inadequate data and/or knowledge in a given situation (e.g., "are these symptoms signs of infection?"), while *aleatoric uncertainty* relates to uncertainty which arises from inherent variability in complex systems (e.g., "why did this happen to me now?" "what else might happen?"). A third approach of uncertainty relates to diagnosis and the diagnostic process: we sometimes use an *etiologic/specific diagnosis* (e.g., pneumonia due to *Streptococcus pneumoniae*), while in other similar situations we may be working with a *descriptive or syndromic diagnosis* (e.g., respiratory distress or respiratory failure). This distinction is helpful in differentiating between what is known and what is important to know; one may be uncertain about *what* caused a neonate to become febrile, while being very certain that the patient with fever in the neonatal period requires admission for evaluation and monitoring. In fact, the goal of many pediatric hospitalizations is not to determine a specific etiologic diagnosis, but rather to reduce the risk associated with uncertainty by evaluating for potentially serious and/or progressive conditions. Said differently, "what it isn't" is sometimes more important that "what it is."

These classification schemes help define the goals in a given situation of uncertainty (within and across teams) as well as what actions should be taken in the face of uncertainty. Effective and adaptive reactions to the different types of uncertainty in each of these frameworks varies. For example, more data and knowledge can help reduce epistemic uncertainty, while aleatoric uncertainty is unlikely to be completely resolved with more information. When trying to resolve aleatoric or existential uncertainty, adding data may waste time, waste resources, and lead to frustration; instead, adding empathy may be more effective in helping patients, their families, and the healthcare team navigate uncertainty. Further, these frameworks are helpful when describing the nature of uncertainty to patients and families (e.g., "we are admitting you to determine what caused you to have a seizure" [*etiologic* framework] vs. "we are admitting you because your seizures aren't under control and are really impacting your life" [*descriptive* framework]).

NEGATIVE REACTIONS TO UNCERTAINTY

Diagnostic uncertainty is often a source of discomfort and vulnerability for a care team as well as patients and their families. The culture of medicine can suppress diagnostic uncertainty in conscious and unconscious ways; in a 2016 *New England Journal of Medicine* editorial Simpkin and Schwartzstein argue that the emphasis on standardized protocols and checklists contribute to a culture that obscures and ignores uncertainty. At a more individual level, overconfidence (which may be subconscious) can lead individual clinicians to not recognize or acknowledge the presence of uncertainty, fail to access knowledge/information resources, or make cognitive errors (such as premature closure and anchoring). Trainees in particular report higher anxiety due to uncertainty, more concern about bad outcomes when faced with uncertainty, greater reluctance to disclose uncertainty to patients/families, and burnout symptoms associated with navigating uncertainty. Encouraging trainees to acknowledge and accept uncertainty is an

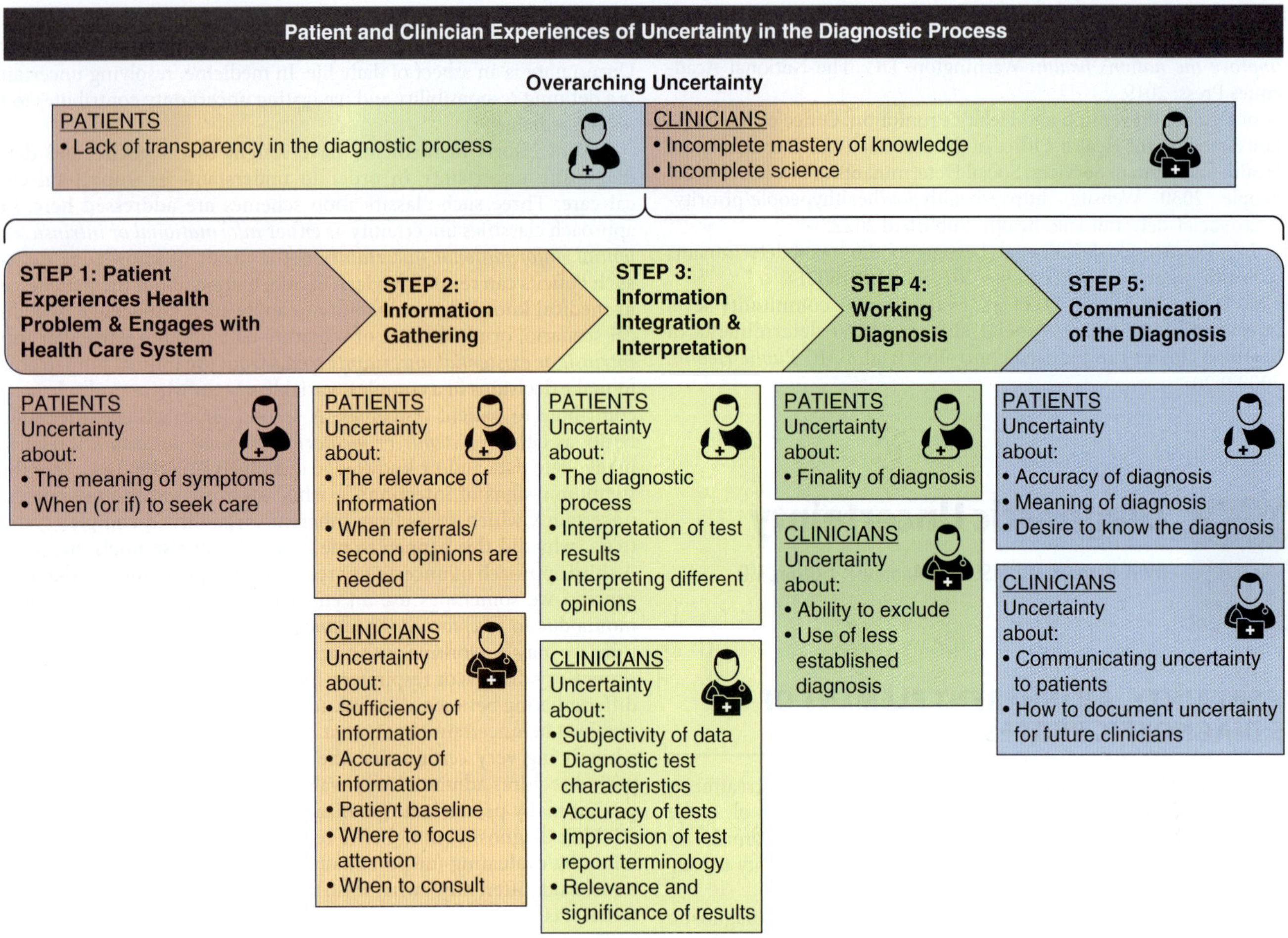

FIGURE 7-1. Patient and clinician experiences of uncertainty in the diagnostic process. (Reproduced with permission from Meyer AND, Giardina TD, Khawaja L, Singh H. Patient and clinician experiences of uncertainty in the diagnostic process: Current understanding and future directions. *Patient Educ Couns*. 2021;104(11):2606-2615.)

important aspect of medical education with important implications for patients, learners, and teams.

When uncertainty is obscured, buried, or ignored, clinicians and clinical teams are vulnerable to cognitive bias; for example, the team may anchor on provisional working diagnosis or give undue weight to hidden assumptions and biases, creating potential for diagnostic error. In 2022, the Joint Commission recognized diagnostic overshadowing, the harm that comes from cognitive bias, as an important threat to diagnostic safety and contributor to health disparities.

RECOGNITION OF UNCERTAINTY

Many strategies allow individual clinicians and clinical teams to recognize diagnostic uncertainty, prompt reflection, and expose and potentially counteract the negative effects of cognitive bias. Examples of these strategies include the "diagnostic pause," "diagnostic timeout," or "deliberate reflection" which serve to force transition from automatic to analytic thinking through structured questions (**Table 7-1**). Deliberate reflection, for instance, builds upon decades of cognitive psychology and guides individuals through consideration of potential diagnoses and how a given case's features do or do not align with each diagnosis. Several studies and narrative reports have explored application of standardized questions, huddles, and protocols to promote recognition of uncertainty and improve diagnostic reasoning in pediatric hospital medicine. Organizations like the Children's Hospital Association have published "timeout templates" to be used in clinical practice to support deliberate reflection. The effectiveness and sustainably of these tools and interventions is not yet clear.

COMMUNICATION OF DIAGNOSTIC REASONING AND UNCERTAINTY AMONG CARE TEAM MEMBERS

The diagnostic process is iterative and complex, involving information gathering (from multiple sources), information integration/interpretation, and formulation of provisional diagnoses to be reevaluated in light of response to time and treatment (Figure 7-1). In the hospital

TABLE 7-1 Questions to Prompt Reflection on Diagnosis

1. What *else* could this be?
2. What information *doesn't fit*?
3. Is it possible that *more than one* thing is going on?
4. Is this a case where I need to *slow down* my thinking?
5. If I changed *one piece of information* (e.g., if the patient developed a fever; if the patient was 8 years old instead of 8 months old) would that change my thinking?
6. How many diagnoses did I *consider* on my differential?
7. When was the last time I got a *second opinion* from a colleague or thought out loud to my team?
8. How am I going to relate the story *without bias*?
9. When was the last time I spoke with my pathology or radiology consultants instead of just reading the report?
10. Does the patient know when/how to *follow up* if things change or symptoms do not resolve?

environment, where teams are dynamic, large, and interprofessional, shared communication of uncertainty allows the team to recognize clinical status changes, identify opportunities to refine diagnoses, or reconsider diagnoses altogether. A fulsome shared mental model that is co-constructed by all members of the team (including patients and families) and includes an understanding of the existing and emerging uncertainty in a case is fundamental for enabling high-quality decision-making.

More broadly, communication of both a diagnostic label and diagnostic reasoning (explicit identification of both the findings that support the diagnosis and the information that does not fit or is not yet known) helps teams work together to iteratively refine the diagnosis. Handovers, consults, progress notes, and rounds are all opportunities for refinement, correction, and clarification to reduce/resolve uncertainty. Transitions of care are often discussed in terms of the safety vulnerabilities they present, but they also provide an opportunity to review and reconsider diagnoses. Even simply asking *What aspects of this diagnosis are uncertain?* can prompt important reconsideration and bring uncertainty to light for members of the team. Such reconsideration provides an important safeguard against cognitive bias in cases where decompensation and/or new signs or symptoms arise after a handover; absent explicit identification of uncertainty, subsequent providers may not reconsider diagnoses even when presented with new clinical information. For example, worsening respiratory failure in a patient admitted on a pneumonia pathway might prompt broadening of anti-microbial coverage. Yet if there is some uncertainty about the etiology of the patient's respiratory failure, further imaging or other testing for conditions like heart failure might be warranted. Communication of diagnostic uncertainty as part of a handover opens the door for diagnostic reconsideration by subsequent members of the care team.

In a training environment, where calibration of clinical reasoning contributes to development of clinical competence, structured feedback on clinical reasoning may promote identification of cognitive biases and communication about uncertainty.

FRAMING THE DEGREE AND NATURE OF UNCERTAINTY TO PATIENTS

For pediatric patients and their caregivers, hospitalization is often stressful and disorienting and uncertainty associated with medical diagnosis can be an added challenge. Identifying, framing, characterizing, and resolving (or not) uncertainty are fundamental aspects of hospital care. Effective communication about uncertainty empowers patients and caregivers to participate in the diagnostic process by recognizing clinical changes, providing relevant history, monitoring response to therapy, and ensuring a longitudinal perspective on disease course. While expressions of clinician uncertainty are associated with greater patient satisfaction, clinicians are inconsistent in their discussions about uncertainty, often omitting discussions of uncertainty entirely.

Patients and caregivers are heterogeneous. Responses and reactions to uncertainty are dynamic and vary across patients/caregivers and across time within a hospitalization or illness. For instance, parents of a medically complex and frequently hospitalized patient who presents with fever in the presence of a central venous catheter have different experiences, knowledge, and expectations of a conversation about uncertainty than the parents of a neonate who presents with fever. Responses to uncertainty may be informed by prior experiences with healthcare. Minoritized families, patients vulnerable to health disparities, and those who have experienced diagnostic error may be skeptical of certainty as a sign of medical hubris or, conversely, interpret uncertainty negatively as a sign of ignorance. Conversations may be interpreted through culturally bound conceptions of the clinician/patient relationship and are informed by prior experiences with healthcare. Moreover, the acuity and context of diagnosis may frame what patients and caregivers need and want to know. For example, the response to uncertainty for a patient with ear pain and fever in the clinic is likely to be different than for a patient admitted to the hospital for evaluation of chronic fever, weight loss, and lymphadenopathy. Risk and risk tolerance are key determinants in the experience and understanding of uncertainty. As risk changes throughout a hospital stay, conversations about diagnostic uncertainty are iterative and must occur throughout a hospitalization. Transparency, humility, and respect for patient experience and autonomy are important characteristics of effective conversations about uncertainty. Further, it is important to share when uncertainty is not likely to be resolved during a hospitalization so that shared expectations are set, and the importance of follow-up is emphasized.

RESOLVING UNCERTAINTY—OR NOT

Contextual factors that define and influence uncertainty include the people involved in a given situation (including both members of the professional healthcare team and patients/caregivers), the clinical environment (and associated resources and constraints), and the risk (or perception of risk) associated with the patient's situation. While framing and describing uncertainty is essential, it is also important to identify when reducing uncertainty may not improve care. For example, in a child admitted to the hospital with bronchiolitis, the addition of a positive polymerase chain reaction test for Respiratory Syncytial Virus *does* reduce uncertainty about etiology, but *does not* change management in typical risk, previously healthy patients. Further, time is often the most important diagnostic test and management tool in hospital medicine; and after immediately actionable diagnoses have been eliminated, it is often appropriate to "watch and wait." In such situations, empathy in the face of unresolved—or even unresolvable—uncertainty is important for building trust between clinicians and patients, ensuring appropriate follow-up, and setting proper expectations.

APPROPRIATE MANAGEMENT OF UNCERTAINTY PROVIDES HIGH VALUE CARE

Appropriate management and communication of diagnostic uncertainty delivers "high value care," which has been conceptualized by National Academies of Medicine as "the best care for the patient, with the optimal result for the circumstances, delivered at the right price."

Inappropriate management of uncertainty can take multiple forms including both acceptance of cognitive biases (e.g., confirmation bias, anchoring) that result in dismissal of or failure to recognize uncertainty. For example, if uncertainty is dismissed in the evaluation of an infant presenting with a BRUE (brief, resolved, unexplained event), clinicians may jump to explaining to families the symptoms with gastro-esophageal reflux, trialing medications, or ordering specialist speech language pathology consults and miss critical data collection that points to alternative etiologies. Over-testing not only imposes financial and logistic burdens on the patient and healthcare system, but also adds to the cognitive burden associated with diagnosis by introducing additional, extraneous, and potentially distracting information into an already overloaded information system. For instance, consider how much more complicated it is to discern which lab values point to an actionable diagnosis when sifting through results of a dozen "routine daily labs," as compared to a scenario in which you have explicitly ordered a particular test or study to better understand a specific condition. Moreover, clinicians run the risk of being falsely reassured by "normal," but irrelevant or inappropriate, tests. Diagnosis is, to some degree, an exercise in signal detection amid the "noisiness" of our information systems and the addition of extraneous tests ("noise") can further obfuscate diagnosis.

FUTURE DIRECTIONS

As diagnostic performance gains acceptance as a domain of hospital safety and quality, attention to diagnostic uncertainty (and its communication and resolution) has increased. Key research and quality improvement priorities include: (i) Developing tools to proactively identify uncertainty through automated means in hospitalized patients to prompt further investigations and intervention; (ii) Identifying how individual and collective perceptions of, and reactions to, uncertainty impact diagnosis and disparities in care; and (iii) Establishing, implementing, and teaching empathetic, effective communication of uncertainty among a care team (including patients and families). Effective engagement of patients and families, as collaborators in diagnosis and members of effective diagnostic teams, is essential to moving this work forward. Uncertainty is a defining nature of medicine and life, and further understanding it will make a substantial difference in the lives of clinicians and patients.

SUGGESTED READINGS

Balogh E, Miller BT, Ball J, Institute of Medicine (U.S.), eds. *Improving Diagnosis in Health Care*. The National Academies Press; 2015.

Berner ES, Graber ML. Overconfidence as a cause of diagnostic error in medicine. *Am J Med*. 2008;121(5 Suppl):S2-23.

Bhise V, Rajan SS, Sittig DF, Morgan RO, Chaudhary P, Singh H. Defining and measuring diagnostic uncertainty in medicine: a systematic review. *J Gen Intern Med*. 2018;33(1):103-115.

Child Health Patient Safety Organization. Team diagnostic timeout template. Accessed September 29, 2022. https://media.childrenshospitals.org/images/pso/Diagnostic_Timeout_Template_Poster.pdf.

Committee on the Learning Health Care System in America, Institute of Medicine. Smith M, Saunders R, Stuckhardt L, McGinnis JM, eds. *Best Care at Lower Cost: The Path to Continuously Learning Health Care in America*. National Academies Press (US); 2013. http://www.ncbi.nlm.nih.gov/books/NBK207225/. Accessed September 29, 2022.

Croskerry P. The importance of cognitive errors in diagnosis and strategies to minimize them. *Academic Medicine*. 2003;78(8).

Dahm MR, Cattanach W, Williams M, Basseal JM, Gleason K, Crock C. Communication of diagnostic uncertainty in primary care and its impact on patient experience: an integrative systematic review. *J Gen Intern Med*. 2023;38(3):738-754.

Gordon GH, Joos SK, Byrne J. Physician expressions of uncertainty during patient encounters. *Patient Educ Couns*. 2000;40(1):59-65.

Graber ML. Educational strategies to reduce diagnostic error: can you teach this stuff? *Adv Health Sci Educ*. 2009;14(S1):63-69.

Graber ML, Kissam S, Payne VL, et al. Cognitive interventions to reduce diagnostic error: a narrative review. *BMJ Qual Saf*. 2012;21(7):535-557.

Iezzoni LI. Dangers of diagnostic overshadowing. *N Engl J Med*. 2019; 380(22):2092-2093.

Ipsaro AJ, Patel SJ, Warner DC, et al. Declaring uncertainty: using quality improvement methods to change the conversation of diagnosis. *Hosp Pediatr*. 2021;11(4):334-341.

Johnson MW, Gheihman G, Thomas H, Schiff G, Olson APJ, Begin AS. The impact of clinical uncertainty in the graduate medical education (GME) learning environment: a mixed-methods study. *Med Teach*. 2022;44(10):1100-1108.

The Joint Commission. Diagnostic overshadowing among groups experiencing health disparities. *Sentinel Event Alert*. June 22, 2022:1-7.

Kasick RT, Melvin JE, Perera ST, et al. A diagnostic time-out to improve differential diagnosis in pediatric abdominal pain. *Diagnosis (Berl)*. 2021;8(2):209-217.

Lane KP, Chia C, Lessing JN, et al. Improving resident feedback on diagnostic reasoning after handovers: the LOOP project. *J Hosp Med*. 2019;14(10):622-625.

Lian OS, Nettleton S, Wifstad Å, Dowrick C. Negotiating uncertainty in clinical encounters: a narrative exploration of naturally occurring primary care consultations. *Soc Sci Med*. 2021;291:114467.

Mamede S, Schmidt HG. Deliberate reflection and clinical reasoning: founding ideas and empirical findings. *Med Educ*. 2023;57(1):76-85.

Mamede S, Schmidt HG. The structure of reflective practice in medicine. *Med Educ*. 2004;38(12):1302-1308.

Marsicek SM, Odom B, Woodard A, Hopkins A. Time for a time-out: the value of a diagnostic time-out in prolonged fever and lymphadenopathy. *Hospital Pediatr*. 2019;9(2):139-141.

Meyer AND, Giardina TD, Khawaja L, Singh H. Patient and clinician experiences of uncertainty in the diagnostic process: current understanding and future directions. *Patient Educ Couns*. 2021; 104(11):2606-2615.

Olson ME, Borman-Shoap E, Mathias K, Barnes TL, Olson APJ. Case-based simulation empowering pediatric residents to communicate about diagnostic uncertainty. *Diagnosis (Berl)*. 2018;5(4):243-248.

Perry MF, Melvin JE, Kasick RT, et al. The diagnostic error index: a quality improvement initiative to identify and measure diagnostic errors. *J Pediatr*. 2021;232:257-263.

Simpkin AL, Schwartzstein RM. Tolerating uncertainty—the next medical revolution? *N Engl J Med*. 2016;375(18):1713-1715.

Trowbridge RL. Twelve tips for teaching avoidance of diagnostic errors. *Medical Teach*. 2008;30(5):496-500.

Wray CM, Loo LK. The diagnosis, prognosis, and treatment of medical uncertainty. *J Grad Med Educ*. 2015;7(4):523-527.

Yale S, Cohen S, Bordini BJ. Diagnostic time-outs to improve diagnosis. *Crit Care Clin*. 2022;38(2):185-194.

CHAPTER 8 Medical Consultation and Co-Management

Carlos Plancarte, MD, MSc and Katherine O'Connor, MD

INTRODUCTION

Consultation and co-management roles are continuously evolving for the pediatric hospitalist. Historically, hospitalists provided direct care for inpatients, seeking consultation from specialty colleagues as needed. However, hospitalists have increasingly been called upon to provide medical consultation or to co-manage patients with another subspecialty provider or service. Pediatric hospitalists provide a pediatrician's view of global issues such as child development, pain management, and home healthcare to patients admitted for surgical procedures or diagnoses managed primarily by pediatric specialists, as well as to aid in the diagnosis and management of children with medical complexity. The hospitalist can offer "anticipatory guidance" that includes counseling for acute illness course and complications, addressing relevant aspects of preventive care, and planning and executing post-acute care. Children with chronic complex conditions account for a growing proportion of pediatric admissions and stand to benefit most from well-developed co-management or consultative care models. For hospitalists to provide optimal service to patients and providers in these consultant and co-management roles, definitions, expectations, and goals should be clear. This chapter reviews consultation and co-management in the current literature, defines goals of each, explores existing models, and examines future directions.

The co-management model of care, which is distinct from consultation, has grown substantially. *Consultation* is defined as a deliberation between providers on a case or its treatment to address a problem that has emerged. This care model applies when the hospitalist as consultant provides a primary subspecialty service with diagnostic or treatment recommendations. *Co-management*, on the other hand, refers to a more comprehensive approach between providers to deliver care to patients through synergistic means. Co-management requests are often initiated at the onset of a care episode; co-managers are typically involved at time of hospital admission and provide direct medical care as well as offer specific advice. In some cases, a pediatric hospitalist may be consulted for a specific question but asked to interact daily in a broader capacity including longitudinal care and/or coordination of patient care needs; the latter scenario is a request for co-management.

Both care models (i.e., consultation and co-management) are prevalent in pediatric hospital medicine (PHM). The 2021 PHM National Workforce Survey found that pediatric hospitalists were frequently consulted in the Emergency Department (ED) with about half of community PHM programs and about one-fifth of university PHM programs providing ED consultation. There was also a high reported prevalence of co-management with nearly a third of university PHM programs and nearly half of community PHM programs offering surgical co-management.

EVOLUTION OF HOSPITALISTS AS CONSULTANTS AND CO-MANAGERS

EVOLUTION OF CONSULTATION MODELS

The literature regarding the use of pediatric hospitalists as consultants remains limited. While this gap in the literature provides many opportunities for future research, it also limits the ability to assess the impact of consultant hospitalists on patient care. Frequently, adult studies are used to extrapolate potential impact in pediatrics. Adult hospitalist literature has focused on the impact of curbside (i.e., being asked for advice, often verbally, without request to see the patient) or electronic (i.e., documenting recommendations within the health record without seeing the patient) consultation with little data on the more traditional consultative model. Notably, the literature on both curbside and electronic consults are mixed and while there are described benefits, caution must be taken with this type of interaction given that recommendations are being provided without seeing the patient; thus, any guidance may be based on incomplete information or knowledge of the patient and their conditions. This limitation may result in fragmented communication, sharing of partial information, and the potential to complicate or confuse patient care recommendations.

EVOLUTION OF CO-MANAGEMENT MODELS

Though still limited in number outside of the surgical co-management realm, studies of co-management models address hospitalist and non-hospitalist provider experiences, opportunities and barriers, and impact on patient care outcomes. Results from studies of co-management models have shown mixed effects on cost-effectiveness, and patient/provider satisfaction, while generally showing positive outcomes in terms of patient safety and hospitalization outcomes. Studies assessing surgeon's opinions and satisfaction with pediatric co-management models have varied. One recent national survey of pediatric general and orthopedic surgeons demonstrated that while most perceived a positive impact on coordination of care and co-morbidity management, few perceived any positive impact on length of stay or pain management. Some adult studies have shown no difference in patient satisfaction, but improved provider perceptions of quality of care and length of stay. Perhaps the strongest evidence to support the pediatric co-management model lies in the results of hospitalist-driven quality improvement initiatives and the beneficial impact of these initiatives on patient outcomes. For example, such initiatives have demonstrated decreased length of supplemental oxygen use after orthopedic surgery in children with complex chronic conditions, improved venous thromboembolism risk screening and prophylaxis implementation, and standardized processes of care to facilitate earlier post-operative discharges. Future research should focus on the impact of the co-management model on cost-effectiveness and provider/patient satisfaction while also continuing to describe patient outcomes.

RECOMMENDED PRACTICES FOR THE PEDIATRIC HOSPITALIST AS CONSULTANT

By definition, a pediatric hospitalist acting as consultant focuses on a specific question involving a given patient. Most consultations involve a single interaction. The goal should be to provide either diagnostic and therapeutic treatment options or a single comprehensive pediatric screening examination. Basic tenets of effective consultation include determining the question, establishing the urgency, gathering data, generating succinct and specific recommendations that include solutions to anticipated problems, tactful communication, personal verbal or direct contact, and daily follow-up until the issue is no longer active or can be managed by the primary service. To bill for consultation services, documentation must include three elements: a request for the hospitalist to consult, a reason by the service asking for the consult, and a report by the hospitalist. Discussion of evaluation and management options with the requesting provider as well as communication with the patient/family after that discussion are essential. Pediatric hospitalist consultation commonly addresses one or more of the following questions:

1. Is this child stable for the planned procedure or intervention? This is answered by performing a global screening assessment and plan.
2. Is the current evaluation and treatment appropriate? This requires a review of the plan of care.
3. What is the cause of and treatment for a specific problem? This requires a problem-focused assessment and plan.

Each of these situations requires a thorough history and physical exam, but with a different emphasis. Even for the problem-focused question, however, the pediatric hospitalist should include relevant issues that are at the heart of general pediatrics and may not be thoroughly considered by requesting services, such as nutrition, pain management, opportunities for catching up on healthcare maintenance concerns, psychosocial factors, and developmental needs.

Certain trends for pediatric hospitalist consultation have emerged. In particular, surgeons and specialists with limited pediatric expertise may benefit from consistent, planned pediatric inpatient consultation for their patients. Consultation may also be requested on a case-by-case basis (e.g., previously healthy patient develops hypoxia post-operatively), or there may be an agreement that all patients in a particular group or setting will have a single initial consultation (e.g., all patients less than 16 years of age on the physical rehabilitation and medicine unit receive consultation by a pediatric hospitalist upon admission). Institutional guidelines and expectations can also guide the pediatric hospitalist's level of involvement in acute care settings; each hospital system must determine the best approach for their patients, community, and facility.

As with many subspecialties, hospital medicine providers may be asked diagnostic and treatment plan questions about patients not under their care. This educational and often uncompensated "curbside" consultation is generally discouraged because research in the adult literature found that curbside consultation can result in inaccurate information with frequent changes to the plan of care. However, while acknowledging the risk and taking caution with this model, it is worth highlighting that remote consultation, usually done by phone, can be an effective way to support colleagues and enable safe management of pediatric patients in their home community. In this remote consultative role, clinical issues can vary from discussion of need for admission to highly complex emergency transport requirements. Pediatric hospitalists involved in coordinating and directing care teams for community wide emergency transport offer a unique and critical form of remote consultation. As the practice of telemedicine continues to grow, many of these remote consultations may become more formal and include virtual examination of patients.

Regardless of the model used, guidelines should be developed for the hospitalist's role as a consultant to optimize patient care, remove redundancies, and ensure clear and comprehensive communication. When establishing guidelines, key issues to consider include defining roles and establishing communication expectations.

RECOMMENDED PRACTICES FOR THE PEDIATRIC HOSPITALIST AS CO-MANAGER

Co-management can be defined as a situation in which two or more providers are involved in the ongoing care of a patient. Coordination of care is considered by many to be a significant strength of the pediatric hospitalist. In addition to addressing specific acute and/or chronic pediatric conditions or problems, the hospitalist may coordinate care by improving discharge planning, enhancing communication with the primary care provider, and ensuring family-centered care. The goals of any co-management relationship should include providing a comprehensive evaluation of all the patient's needs, increasing team communication and patient engagement, decreasing errors and delays in decision-making, and ensuring accountability to the patient. The models for co-management may have similarities to those described for hospitalist consultation and should be developed to fit individual community and hospital needs.

As with consultation, guidelines must be established if co-management is to succeed. It is important to define which provider is the "captain of the ship." Defining lines of authority is crucial, and these should be established upon assuming care. Other expectations must also be addressed, including who will write orders (or specific types of orders) for the patient and who will communicate with the primary care provider, the family, the patient, other consultants, nursing staff, and (in teaching institutions) the residents involved in the patients care. A collaborative approach is also required when involved providers have differing clinical management recommendations (including decisions to involve other consultants), or when there are conflicts with the family's wishes.

Many models can be successful if expectations are clear, however a lack of co-management agreements can lead to confusion in roles, dissatisfaction, and burnout. Additionally, hospitalists should beware of creep of scope of practice as hospitalists take over more aspects of patient care. Guidelines for communication and responsibilities can help prevent hospitalists from taking on responsibilities that are not aligned with training and expertise. If a patient with a past medical history of cerebral palsy and a ventriculoperitoneal shunt presents with fever and renal failure, the hospitalist might serve as the primary attending provider, with the patient's neurosurgeon co-managing. The decision to consult nephrology or infectious diseases is the hospitalist's decision as the primary attending. If a patient with diabetes is admitted with fever and joint swelling, the patient's endocrinologist may serve as primary attending managing the diabetes while the hospitalist co-manages all other aspects of diagnostic and therapeutic evaluation, including the decision to consult orthopedics, if needed.

The Society for Hospital Medicine white paper provides guidance for successful co-management and suggested metrics for measuring the success of a co-management program. Metrics focus on: quality (e.g., medication reconciliation accuracy, readmissions, hospital-acquired infection [HAI] reduction, order set compliance, timing to surgical intervention), engagement (e.g., provider satisfaction, ancillary services satisfaction, recruitment and retention [for both specialists and hospitalists] and patient satisfaction), and finances to track for the purpose of program sustainability in a time of value-based care and limited resources (e.g., clinical documentation accuracy, length of stay, and resource utilization).

OTHER CONSIDERATIONS

While the current state of data on consultation and co-management leaves room for more study, there is also a gap in provider training and education about consultation and co-management. Although advanced communication skills and leading a healthcare team are part of the PHM core competencies, specific expectations for and/or training on how to function as a consultant and co-manager are poorly described. Implementing a formal curriculum on consultation and co-management with specific competencies may be a valuable consideration.

Billing issues may also arise when the hospitalist serves as a consultant or co-manager. Knowledge of initial consultation and follow-up codes will prevent billing confusion and delays. Only one provider per medical group can be the attending of record, requiring that other providers bill as "consultants" (regardless of whether they are serving as consultants or co-managers of care, according to the definitions provided earlier). Any co-management billing in which the hospitalist is not the primary attending of record is done as follow-up visits without initial consult visit codes, admission, or discharge codes. These issues have important implications for the financial stability of PHM programs; it is important to discuss financial aspects with relevant department or hospital leadership to ensure the success of hospitalist consultant and co-management models.

Pediatric hospitalists may benefit from leadership skills to resolve differences of opinion regarding clinical care and/or effectively collaborate with other specialties, which may be particularly relevant in the arena of co-management. These skills may also be used at an organizational level to institute consultation and co-management policies and related changes, improve patient safety, streamline processes, advocate for new technology and services, and control costs.

FUTURE DIRECTIONS

The pediatric hospitalist's role as consultant and as partner in co-management is growing rapidly and is needed to ensure seamless care. Whether providing a consultative or co-management hospitalist model, goals should focus on the triple aim: improving population health, improving the patient experience of care (including quality and satisfaction), and reducing per capita costs of healthcare. The Accountable Care Organization model for healthcare challenges providers to bring coordinated care to the patient in a cost-conscious manner. Hospitalists should be accountable to these aims and challenges by consulting and co-managing with an acute and chronic view.

More studies are needed to demonstrate the variety and sources of consultations and co-management in the pediatric population, as well as effects on cost-effectiveness, provider/patient/staff perceptions, and patient outcomes. Methods should include surveys of those involved as well as studies of length of stay, cost, and clinical outcome data by disease type and acuity level. Multicenter data collection will be necessary to validate results in varied hospital settings. The impact on the hospitalist intensity of service, autonomy, feeling of being valued and respected, schedules, and burnout should also be studied. Training for current and future hospitalists should include lessons learned from these studies and from mature systems outside the United States. Current pediatric hospitalist task forces, with the leadership of the Joint Council of Pediatric Hospital Medicine and supporting groups—the Academic Pediatric Association, American Academy of Pediatrics and the Society of Hospital Medicine, Pediatric Research in Inpatient Settings (PRIS) Research Network, and the Value in Inpatient Pediatrics (VIP) Quality Improvement—are well positioned to study and refine expectations for the hospitalist as consultant and co-manager in the ever-evolving healthcare system.

SUGGESTED READINGS

Bal BS, Teo W, Brenner LH. Medicolegal sidebar: getting sued by someone else's patient-when does a curbside consultation carry medicolegal jeopardy? *Clin Orthop Relat Res.* 2019;477(10):2204-2206.

Brower LH, Kremer N, Meier K, et al. Quality initiative to introduce pediatric venous thromboembolism risk assessment for orthopedic and surgery patients. *Hospital Pediatrics.* 2017;7(10):595-601.

Burden M, Sarcone E, Keniston A, et al. Prospective comparison of curbside versus formal consultations. *J Hosp Med.* 2013;8(1):31-35.

Ettinger NA, Hill VL, Russ CM, et al. Guidance for structuring a pediatric intermediate care unit. *Pediatrics.* 2022;149(5).

Fromme HB, Ruch-Ross HS, Marks M, Barone L, Shaughnessy E. The 2021 Pediatric Hospital Medicine Workforce: Results of a National Survey of Program Leaders. *Hospital Pediatrics.* 2022;12(5):456-463.

Gill PJ, Anwar MR, Thavam T, et al. Identifying conditions with high prevalence, cost, and variation in cost in US Children's Hospitals. *JAMA Network Open.* 2021;4(7):e2117816-e2117816.

Hardik Vora BA, Stephen Behnke, Chris Cockerham, O'Neil Pyke, Roy Sittig. The Evolution of Co-management. Society Of Hospital Medicine. https://www.hospitalmedicine.org/globalassets/practice-management/practice-management-pdf/pm-19-0004-co-management-white-paper_minor-update-m.pdf. Published 2017. Accessed August 28, 2022.

Hsu BS, Hill V, Frankel LR, et al. Executive summary: criteria for critical care of infants and children: PICU Admission, Discharge, and Triage Practice Statement and Levels of Care Guidance. *Pediatrics.* 2019;144(4).

Levine DM, Chalasani R, Linder JA, Landon BE. Association of the patient protection and affordable care act with ambulatory quality, patient experience, utilization, and cost, 2014-2016. *JAMA Netw Open.* 2022;5(6):e2218167.

Lopez MA, Campbell J. Developing a communication curriculum for primary and consulting services. *Med Educ Online.* 2020;25(1):1794341.

Luu BC, Davis MJ, Raj S, Abu-Ghname A, Buchanan EP. Cost-effectiveness of surgical comanagement: A systematic review. *Surgeon.* 2021;19(2):119-127

Matsuo T, Hayashi K, Uehara Y, Mori N. Essential consultants' skills and attitudes (Willing CONSULT): a cross-sectional survey. *BMC Med Educ.* 2021;21(1):366.

Najaf N, Harrison JD, Duong J, Greenberg A, Cheng HQ. It all just clicks: development of an inpatient E-Consult program. *J Hosp Med.* 2017;12(5):332-334.

Nandiwada DR, Kohli A, McNamara M, et al. High-value consults: a curriculum to promote point-of-care, evidence-based recommendations. *J Grad Med Educ.* 2017;9(5):640-644.

Obucina M, Harris N, Fitzgerald JA, et al. The application of triple aim framework in the context of primary healthcare: a systematic literature review. *Health Policy.* 2018;122(8):900-907.

Pavitt S, McHugh A, Chi K, et al. Improving inpatient consult communication through a standardized tool. *Pediatrics.* 2021;147(5).

Pordes E, Gordon J, Sanders LM, Cohen E. Models of care delivery for children with medical complexity. *Pediatrics.* 2018;141(Suppl 3): S212-S223

Rauch DA, CARE COH, MEDICINE SOH, et al. Physician's role in coordinating care of hospitalized children. *Pediatrics.* 2018;142(2).

Roche SD, Johansson AC, Giannakoulis J, et al. Patient and clinician perceptions of factors relevant to ideal specialty consultations. *JAMA Netw Open.* 2022;5(4):e228867.

Rohatgi N, Weng Y, Ahuja N. Surgical comanagement by hospitalists: continued improvement over 5 years. *J Hosp Med.* 2020;15(4):232-235.

Rosenberg RE, Abzug JM, Rappaport DI, et al. Collaborations with pediatric hospitalists: national surveys of pediatric surgeons and orthopedic surgeons. *J Hosp Med.* 2018;13(8):566-569.

Shaughnessy EE, Meier KA, Kelleher K. The Value of the Pediatric Hospitalist in Surgical Co-Management. *Curr Treat Options Pediatr.* 2018;4(2):247-254.

Stucky ER, Maniscalco J, Ottolini MC, et al. The pediatric hospital medicine core competencies supplement: a framework for curriculum development by the society of hospital medicine with acknowledgement to pediatric hospitalists from the american academy of pediatrics and the academic pediatric association. *J Hosp Med.* 2010;5 Suppl 2:i-xv, 1-114.

Vimalananda VG, Orlander JD, Afable MK, et al. Electronic consultations (E-consults) and their outcomes: a systematic review. *J Am Med Inform Assoc.* 2019;27(3):471-479.

Yang CJ, Bottalico D, Philips K, et al. Improving the pediatric floor discharge process following tonsillectomy. *Laryngoscope.* 2022;132(1):225-233.

CHAPTER 9 Child Development: Implications for Inpatient Medicine

Deanna Bell, MD and Arwen Marker, PhD

UNDERSTANDING CHILD DEVELOPMENT

Child development is the process of cognitive, emotional, language, motor, and social changes that occur from the perinatal period to young adulthood. Development usually occurs as a progressive and predictable sequence of milestones, within ranges of individual variation. Environmental, genetic, biological, social, and demographic factors participate in a complex interplay affecting trajectory of development. Knowledge of child development aids the pediatric hospitalist in explaining diagnosis and care to patients and families, aids parents in helping their children adapt to hospitalization, and promotes health and well-being for young patients. Furthermore, a child's participation in cares is dependent on physical ability, as well as attitudes, beliefs, and understanding of their illness that are impacted by developmental status.

Risks for developmental delay are compounded in children with chronic illness and medical complexity, who are more likely to present for care in the hospital medicine setting. This increased risk is multifactorial. Children with chronic illness are at increased risk of developmental vulnerability in all developmental domains, regardless of number or type of illnesses. Vulnerability stems not only from physiological impact of illness but from limitation of age-appropriate environmental interaction and socialization imposed by disability and hospitalization. Furthermore, children and youth with special healthcare needs (CYSHCN) are very likely to suffer from adverse social determinants. Specifically, CYSHCN are much more likely than their peers to live in poverty, suffer from malnutrition, endure all forms of abuse, and develop difficulties in attachment.

Impacts extend beyond the patient to the patient's support system as well. Families of CYSHCN report difficulty maintaining long-term employment due absences associated with medical care, and many report they are unable to work due to inability to secure medically appropriate childcare. This not only compounds poverty but leads to difficulty with access as well. Families of CYSHCN are more likely to report unmet medical needs and inadequate or discontinuous insurance coverage, with less continuous coverage reported in families financially ineligible for Medicaid. In addition, families of children with medical complexity are more likely to endorse poor mental health and unmet vital resource needs. Finally, families of CYSHCN are more likely than peers to miss developmental screening opportunities, underscoring the need for screening at every care opportunity.

IMPORTANCE OF SCREENING

Clinician knowledge of typical developmental trajectory and developmental screening tools enables early detection of variations in development. Knowledge of developmental status of the child and of relative strengths and weaknesses of the family unit can guide clinicians' communication, education, and support for self-management, making compliance more likely and lessening medical trauma. Furthermore, developmental delay or plateau is often the first sign of either underlying medical pathology or toxic stress in the child's environment.

Toxic stress refers to strong, frequent, or prolonged activation of the body's stress response system, occurring in the absence of appropriate socioemotional nurturing. Prolonged activation of the body's stress response system alters the chemical milieu of the brain, impacting genetic expression at the cellular level and changing anatomy of the prefrontal cortex. Such changes alter neurochemical processing leading to detrimental developmental changes in cognition, executive function, resiliency, and social-emotional skills in childhood and are associated with poorer health outcomes in childhood and adulthood.

A variety of adverse childhood experiences and social determinants have been linked with toxic stress response. Toxic stresses such as poverty, parental stress, substance use, and maltreatment particularly predispose children to adverse impacts on development. Children who suffer most developmental impact are those enduring toxic stimulus over time, with a dose-dependent effect that carries forward to adult behavior and health. These effects have been shown to be partially or fully reversible when toxic stimuli are identified and reversed. While evidence-based standards for toxic stress and developmental screening have been published, over one-third of children and adolescents are delinquent in Early Periodic Screening, Diagnosis, and Treatment services in a given year. The acute care setting presents unique opportunities for delineation of developmental problems and risk factors when they may be more apparent. It is now suggested practice for subspecialty pediatricians and those in acute care settings to play a larger role in screening for developmental delay and developmental risk factors.

Many advances have been made with the design of new screening tools for age-appropriate developmental milestones and risk factors. It is important clinicians utilize these tools, as subjective assessment in isolation has been shown to miss many patients with delays. Many clinicians report feeling overwhelmed by new screening recommendations, and feel it is difficult to use these tools regularly. However, comprehensive screening for all children with all tools is not necessary. Clinicians should familiarize themselves with a range of screening tools and apply these in a targeted fashion. Quality improvement science reveals better screening success when screens are implemented with the help of clinical decision support, when processes are embedded in the practice flow, and shared by all members of the clinical team. The American Academy of Pediatrics has developed helpful toolkits on use of screening tools for various indications. Most of these are categorized by developmental age or indication, are available in the open domain, and can be replicated for non-commercial use with attribution. **Table 9-1** includes a list of screening tools freely accessible with attribution that are likely helpful to the pediatric hospitalist.

TABLE 9-1 Behavioral Health and Developmental Screening Tools

Tool	Functions	Age
Early childhood and developmental screening		
Early Childhood Screening and Assessment (ECSA) [1]	emotional, behavioral, maternal distress	18-60 months
Survey of Well-being of Young Children (SWYC) [2,3,4]	development, temperament, emotional, behavioral, autism, environmental and family stress	2-65 months
Brief Early Childhood Screening Assessment[5]	emotional and social assessment	1.5-6 years
Modified Checklist for Autism in Toddlers (Revised with Follow-up) (MCHAT-R)[6]	autism screening	16-30 months
Preschool Feelings Checklist[7]	depression in young children	36-66 months
Broadband behavioral health screening		
HEADSSS,[8] HEEADS4[9]	home environment, education and employment, eating, peer-related activities, drugs, sexuality, suicide/depression, and safety from injury and violence, media use	Adolescents
SSHADESS [10]	strengths, school, home, activities, drubs, emotions/eating, sexuality, safety	Adolescents
Pediatric Symptom Checklist -35 (PSC-35)[11,12]	attention, externalizing symptoms, internalizing symptoms	4-16 years
Pediatric Symptoms Checklist-17 (PSC-17)[13]	attention, externalizing symptoms, internalizing symptoms	4-16 years
Strengths and Difficulties Questionnaires (SDQ)[14]	positive and negative psychosocial attributes, function in home, educational and play domains	3-17 years
NIH Toolbox[15]	individual measures of cognitive, sensory, motor, and emotional function	3-85 years
PROMIS Measures[16]	individual measures of global, mental, physical, and social health	5-17 years
Social determinants and toxic stress		
IHELP[17]	Income, Housing, Education, Literacy, Legal status, and Personal safety	parents, caregivers
WE CARE[18]	parental educational attainment, employment, childcare, risk of homelessness, food security, and household heat and electricity	parents, caregivers of children 2 months -10 years
Pediatric Aces and Related Life -Events Screener (PEARLS)[19]	adverse childhood experiences	0-19 years
Health Leads[20]	food, housing, utility, financial, transportation stability; exposure to violence; sociodemographic	all ages
Hunger Vital Sign[21]	food insecurity and related social determinants	Birth-3 years
Abuse Assessment Screen (AAS)[22]	domestic violence	adolescent girls and women
Parents and caregivers		
Parental Stress Scale (PSS)[23]	parent/caregiver stress	caregivers of all ages
Multidimensional Scale of Perceived Support (MSPSS) Parents Stress Inventory[24]	parent/caregiver social support	adults
Edinburgh Postnatal Depression Scale (EPDS)[25]	parent/caregiver depression	perinatal
Substance use		
Screening to Brief Intervention (S2BI) and CRAFFT [26,27]	substance use	adolescents
Brief Screener for Adolescent Tobacco, Alcohol, and other Drugs (BSTAD)[28]	alcohol, marijuana, tobacco use	12-17 years
National Institute on Alcohol Abuse and Alcoholism Youth Alcohol Screening[29]	individual and peer alcohol use	adolescents
Alcohol Use Disorders Identification Test (AUDIT)[30]	risky alcohol use	10-21 years
Mental health		
Pediatric Health Questionairre-9 (PHQ-9)[31]	depression	11-17 years
Center for Epidemiological Studies Depression Scale for Children (CES-DC)[32]	depression	6-17 years
Short Mood and Feelings Questionnaire (SMFQ)[33]	depression	8-16 years
Generalized Anxiety Disorder Assessment (GAD-7)[34]	generalized anxiety	13 years-adult
Screen for Child Anxiety Related Disorders (SCARED)[35]	anxiety	8-18 years
Brief Impairment Scale (BIS), multidimensional[36]	function in interpersonal relations, self-care, and school/work domains	4-17 years
AAP Brief Mental Health Update[37]	selected open-ended questions for a variety of mental health symptoms	birth-21 years
Pediatric Medical Traumatic Stress, A Comprehensive Toolkit for Medical Providers[38,39]	pediatric medical traumatic stress screening tools and treatment resources	various
Ask Suicide-Screening Questions (ASQ)[40]	suicide risks in youth with psychiatric concerns	10-24 years
Suicide Assessment Five Step Evaluation (SAFE-T)[41]	suicide risk and protective factors, risk level, intervention needs	children and adolescents
SCOFF[42,43]	disordered eating	11 years-adult
Eating Disorder Examination Questionnaire (EDE-Q)[44]	disordered eating	14 years-adult

(Continued)

TABLE 9-1 Behavioral Health and Developmental Screening Tools (*Continued*)

[1]Gleason MM, Zeanah CH, Dickstein S. Recognizing young children in need of mental health assessment: development and preliminary validity of the early childhood screening assessment. *Infant Mental Health J.* 2010;31(3):335-357.

[2]Sheldrick RC, Perrin EC. Evidence-based milestones for surveillance of cognitive, language, and motor development. *Acad Pediatr.* 2013;13(6):577-586.

[3]Sheldrick RC, Henson BS, Neger EN, Merchant S, Murphy JM, Perrin EC. The baby pediatric symptom checklist: development and initial validation of a new social/emotional screening instrument for very young children. *Acad Pediatr.* 2013;13(1):72-80.

[4]Sheldrick RC, Henson BS, Merchant S, Neger EN, Murphy JM, Perrin EC. The preschool pediatric symptom checklist (PPSC): development and initial validation of a new social/emotional screening instrument. *Acad Pediatr.* 2012;12(5):456-467.

[5]Fallucco EM, Wysocki T, James L, Kozikowski C, Williams A, Gleason MM. The brief early childhood screening assessment. *J Dev Behav Pediatr.* 2017;38(2):89-98.

[6]Robins DL, Casagrande K, Barton M, Chen CMA, Dumont-Mathieu T, Fein D. Validation of the modified checklist for autism in toddlers, revised with follow-up (M-CHAT-R/F). *Pediatrics.* 2013;133(1):37-45.

[7]Luby JL, Heffelfinger A, Koenig-McNaught AL, Brown K, Spitznagel E. The preschool feelings checklist: a brief and sensitive screening measure for depression in young children. *J Am Acad Child Adolesc Psychiatry.* 2004;43(6):708-717.

[8]Doukrou M, Segal TY. Fifteen-minute consultation: Communicating with young people—how to use HEEADSSS, a psychosocial interview for adolescents. *Arch Dis Child Educ Pract Ed.* 2017;103(1):15-19.

[9]Clark DL, Raphael JL, McGuire AL. HEADS4: social media screening in adolescent primary care. *Pediatrics.* 2018;141(6):e20173655.

[10]Ginsburg KR. Ch. 32: The SSHADESS screening: A strength-based psychosocial assessment. In Ginsberg KR, Ramirez McClain, Brett Z, American Academy of Pediatrics, eds. *Reaching Teens: Strength-Based, Trauma-Sensitive, Resilience-Building Communication Strategies Rooted in Positive Youth Development.* 2nd ed. American Academy of Pediatrics; 2020.

[11]Jellinek MS, Murphy JM, Little M, Pagano ME, Comer DM, Kelleher KJ. Use of the pediatric symptom checklist to screen for psychosocial problems in pediatric primary care. *Arch Pediatr Adolesc Med.* 1999;153(3).

[12]Hacker KA, Myagmarjav E, Harris V, Suglia SF, Weidner D, Link D. Mental health screening in pediatric practice: factors related to positive screens and the contribution of parental/personal concern. *Pediatrics.* 2006;118(5):1896-1906.

[13]Gardner W, Lucas A, Kolko DJ, Campo JV. Comparison of the PSC-17 and Alternative Mental Health Screens in an At-Risk Primary Care Sample. *J Am Acad Child Adolesc Psychiatry.* 2007;46(5):611-618.

[14]Goodman R, Ford T, Simmons H, Gatward R, Meltzer H. Using the Strengths and Difficulties Questionnaire (SDQ) to screen for child psychiatric disorders in a community sample. *Br J Psychiatry.* 2000;177(06):534-539.

[15]Gershon RC. NIH Toolbox. www.healthmeasures.net. Published 2017. Accessed August 31, 2022. https://www.healthmeasures.net/explore-measurement-systems/nih-toolbox.

[16]Hanmer J, Jensen RE, Rothrock N. A reporting checklist for Health Measures' patient-reported outcomes: ASCQ-Me, Neuro-QoL, NIH Toolbox, and PROMIS. *J Patient Rep Outcomes.* 2020;4(1).

[17]KenyonC, Sandel M, Silverstein M, Shakir A, Zuckerman B. Revisiting the social history for child health. *Pediatrics.* 2007;120(3):e734-e738.

[18]Garg A, Toy S, Tripodis Y, Silverstein M, Freeman E. Addressing social determinants of health at well child care visits: a cluster RCT. *Pediatrics.* 2015;135(2): e296-e304.

[19]Koita K, Long D, Hessler D, et al. Development and implementation of a pediatric adverse childhood experiences (ACEs) and other determinants of health questionnaire in the pediatric medical home: a pilot study. *PLoS One.* 2018;13(12):e0208088.

[20]The Health Leads Screening Toolkit. Health Leads. Published 2022. https://healthleadsusa.org/resources/the-health-leads-screening-toolkit. Accessed July 30, 2022.

[21]Gundersen C, Engelhard EE, Crumbaugh AS, Seligman HK. Brief assessment of food insecurity accurately identifies high-risk US adults. *Public Health Nutr.* 2017;20(8):1367-1371.

[22]Reichenheim ME. Comparison between the abuse assessment screen and the revised conflict tactics scales for measuring physical violence during pregnancy. *J Epidemiol Community Health.* 2004;58(6):523-527.

[23]Berry JO, Jones WH. The parental stress scale: initial psychometric evidence. *J Social Pers Relat.* 1995;12(3):463-472.

[24]Canty-Mitchell J, Zimet GD. Psychometric Properties of the Multidimensional Scale of Perceived Social Support in Urban Adolescents. *Am J Community Psychol.* 2000;28(3):391-400.

[25]Gibson J, McKenzie-McHarg K, Shakespeare J, Price J, Gray R. A systematic review of studies validating the Edinburgh Postnatal Depression Scale in antepartum and postpartum women. *Acta Psychiatr Scand.* 2009;119(5):350-364.

[26]Kelly SM, Gryczynski J, Mitchell SG, Kirk A, O'Grady KE, Schwartz RP. Validity of brief screening instrument for adolescent tobacco, alcohol, and drug use. *Pediatrics.* 2014;133(5):819-826.

[27]Knight JR, Sherritt L, Shrier LA, Harris SK, Chang G. Validity of the CRAFFT substance abuse screening test among adolescent clinic patients. *Arch Pediatr Adolesc Med.* 2002;156(6):607.

[28]Chung T, Smith GT, Donovan JE, et al. Drinking frequency as a brief screen for adolescent alcohol problems. *Pediatrics.* 2012;129(2):205-212.

[29]*Alcohol Screening and Brief Intervention for Youth a Practitioner's Guide 1 in 3 Children Starts Drinking by the End of 8th Grade.* National Institutes of Health, National Institute on Alcohol Abuse and Alcoholism. https://pubs.niaaa.nih.gov/publications/Practitioner/YouthGuide/YouthGuide.pdf.

[30]Johnson JA, Lee A, Vinson D, Seale JP. Use of AUDIT-based measures to identify unhealthy alcohol use and alcohol dependence in primary care: a validation study. *Alcohol Clin Exp Res.* 2012;37(Suppl. 1):E253-E259.

[31]Richardson LP, McCauley E, Grossman DC, et al. Evaluation of the patient health questionnaire-9 item for detecting major depression among adolescents. *Pediatrics.* 2010;126(6):1117-1123.

[32]Garrison CZ, Addy CL, Jackson KL, McKeown RE, Waller JL. The CES-D as a screen for depression and other psychiatric disorders in adolescents. *J Am Acad Child Adolesc Psychiatry.* 1991;30(4):636-641.

[33]Rhew IC, Simpson K, Tracy M, et al. Criterion validity of the Short Mood and Feelings Questionnaire and one- and two-item depression screens in young adolescents. *Child Adolesc Psychiatry Ment Health.* 2010;4(1).

[34]Spitzer RL, Kroenke K, Williams JBW, Löwe B. A brief measure for assessing generalized anxiety disorder. *Arch Intern Med.* 2006;166(10):1092.

[35]Birmaher B, Brent DA, Chiappetta L, Bridge J, Monga S, Baugher M. Psychometric Properties of the Screen for Child Anxiety Related Emotional Disorders (SCARED): A Replication Study. *J Am Acad Child Adolesc Psychiatry.* 1999;38(10):1230-1236.

[36]Bird HR, Canino GJ, Davies M, et al. The Brief Impairment Scale (BIS): a multidimensional scale of functional impairment for children and adolescents. *J Am Acad Child Adolesc Psychiatry.* 2005;44(7):699-707.

[37]Foy JM. Enhancing pediatric mental health care: algorithms for primary care. *Pediatrics.* 2010;125(Supplement 3):S109-S125.

[38]Dyregrov A, Yule W. Screening measures—the development of the UNICEF screening battery. Paper presented at the Fourth European Conference on Traumatic Stress. Paris, May 7–11. In: *Fourth European Conference on Traumatic Stress;* 1995.

[39]*Pediatric Medical Traumatic Stress a Comprehensive Guide.* National Institutes of Health, National Institute on Alcohol Use and Alcoholism; 2019. Accessed July 28, 2022. https://www.nctsn.org/sites/default/files/resources//pediatric_toolkit_for_health_care_providers.pdf

[40]Ballard ED, Cwik M, Van Eck K, et al. Identification of at-risk youth by suicide screening in a pediatric emergency department. *Prev Sci.* 2016;18(2):174-182.

[41]Jacobs D, US Department of Health and Human Resources. Suicide Assessment, Five-Step Evaluation and Triage (SAFE-T). 2009.

[42]Morgan JF, Reid F, Lacey JH. The SCOFF questionnaire: assessment of a new screening tool for eating disorders. *BMJ.* 1999;319(7223):1467-1468.

[43]Perry L, Morgan J, Reid F, et al. Screening for symptoms of eating disorders: reliability of the SCOFF screening tool with written compared to oral delivery. *Int J Eat Disord.* 2002;32(4):466-472.

[44]Serier KN, Smith JE, Yeater EA. Confirmatory factor analysis and measurement invariance of the Eating Disorder Examination Questionnaire (EDE-Q) in a non-clinical sample of non-Hispanic White and Hispanic women. *Eat Behav.* 2018;31:53-59.

PEDIATRIC MEDICAL TRAUMA

Of particular concern to the pediatric hospitalist is toxic stress leading to medical trauma. Pediatric medical traumatic stress (PMTS) refers to a set of psychological and physiological responses of children and their families to pain, injury, serious illness, medical procedures, and invasive or frightening treatment experiences. Approximately 30% of children and families experience PMTS over the course of treatment, and approximately 3% to 10% go on to develop post-traumatic stress disorder (PTSD). Risk factors for PMTS include prior PMTS, negative affectivity, preexisting psychosocial dysfunction, parent and child perception of threat to life, pain, degree of injury, and frequency of invasive medical procedures. PMTS is associated with poorer psychosocial outcomes, treatment adherence, and health in both short and long term.

Regular screening for risk factors and signs of PMTS is currently recommended in all stages of illness recovery, starting with the acute phase of illness. Preventative measures are based on providing trauma informed care, age-appropriate procedural preparation, and pain management. Caregiver involvement and trauma-informed cognitive behavioral therapy have shown the most promising findings in reducing risk for PMTS. Brief, self-guided, online interventions have shown promise in preventing or ameliorating trauma associated with medical care. Pediatric hospitalists can play a critical role in reducing the developmental impact of PMTS and should familiarize themselves with screening tools and treatment resources, referring parents and children at high risk for PMTS early in disease. Safe, stable, and nurturing environments, caregiver engagement and response to child, structured environments for education and play, and trauma-focused cognitive behavioral therapy are examples of interventions which decrease the impact of toxic stress. Pediatric clinicians should maintain a working knowledge of community, education, and mental health resources so that prompt referrals can be placed when positive screening results are obtained.

DEVELOPMENTAL IMPLICATIONS FOR THE HOSPITALIZED CHILD

PARENTS AND CAREGIVERS

Medical diagnoses and hospitalizations in childhood can negatively impact quality of life, mental and physical health for parents and caregivers. Specifically, parents of youth with acute or chronic illness endorse higher levels of anxiety, depression, distress, sleep disruption, and post-traumatic stress symptoms than parents of healthy youth. Parents in the perinatal period are at particular risk for anxiety and depression with increased rates of depression among caregivers with newborns who are premature, low birth weight, or require neonatal intensive care. Factors which negatively impact parent responsiveness leave children at increased risk for developing social, emotional, and behavioral concerns. Screening for perinatal depression, parenting stress, and acute stress symptoms allows providers to refer families to receive early intervention, reducing long-term adverse effects on both parents/caregivers and young children. Referral to cognitive behavioral therapy or interpersonal therapy, antidepressant medications, and physical activity interventions demonstrate benefits for reducing perinatal parental depression. Additionally, education on acute stress symptoms and referral to trauma-focused cognitive behavioral therapy interventions have demonstrated effectiveness for treating post-traumatic stress symptoms for parents.

INFANTS

Within the first months of life, infants start to recognize familiar caregivers, and caregivers can learn to differentiate infant needs based on their behavior. Consistent parent responsiveness helps the infant to feel safe, secure, and trusting, all important components of secure attachment formation. Infants are at risk for negative developmental and psychological impacts, as well as future risk of maltreatment, when separated from their primary caregivers during hospitalization. Premature and low birth weight infants are particularly at risk, due to the need for technological interventions that limit typical contact with parents/caregivers. Although infants cannot describe their symptoms, parents/caregivers can learn to recognize infant pain, distress, and delirium by noticing changes in crying, irritability/fussiness, sleep disruption, vigorous movements/agitation, physical symptoms (e.g., diarrhea), and vitals (e.g., tachycardia).

Parent/caregiver inclusion in care is necessary to develop appropriate parent responsivity to infant cues and foster infant development in the hospital setting. When families are fully integrated into care teams, it reduces parental stress, increases parent recognition of infant stress responses, improves infant weight gain, and reduces length of hospital stay. Specific interventions include frequent opportunities for parents to provide skin-to-skin contact, comfort and feed their baby, and receive direct instruction recognizing and responding to infant distress. Access to neonatal providers, developmental specialists, lactation consultants, social work, and psychology can help parents establish routines around feeding, sleep, play, and treatment regimens. Finally, peer mentoring support can provide families with non-judgmental acceptance and validation of their experiences, and help families develop advocacy skills to communicate their infant's needs to the medical team.

UNDERSTANDING ILLNESS AND HOSPITALIZATION

Child understanding of their illness and hospitalization is largely impacted by developmental status. Toddlers and preschoolers display magical thinking styles, tend to confuse cause and effect, and have a poor perception of time, which can result in inaccuracies and inconsistencies regarding their understanding of illness. Children often develop their own causal explanations for illness and their role in it (e.g., "I was bad, so I got sick. If I am good, I will get better."). Children as young as 5 to 8 years become aware of body sensations that help them communicate symptoms and understand care needs. At this age, children can follow simple directions, understand rules, and start to learn more complex coping skills. However, there is a great deal of variability in both knowledge and application of logic in school-aged children, and they have their own priorities in health, which are not always recognized by clinicians and parents. At middle school age, children typically have an accurate understanding of illness causality and reversibility and grasp the relationships between symptoms and body systems.

For young children, medical information should be simple, concise, and use age-appropriate language, as increased details and complexity interfere with comprehension. It is important for clinicians to explain to their preschool-aged patients that body state, germs, or accidents may be the cause of their current illness, rather than more proximal causes (e.g., the doctor or being in the hospital). Medical providers should consider rounding outside patient rooms when discussing more detailed medical information and aid parents and caregivers in developing appropriate language to relay information to their young child. As children progress through middle childhood and into adolescence, they should be increasingly included in conversations about their illness and treatment planning. Parents and caregivers who foster communication directly between their child and the medical team are more likely to have children with more independence and initiative in their care. However, providers should be mindful that communication styles should still be tailored to the individual child, with some children and adolescents appreciating detailed information and advance warning of medical cares, whereas for others detailed information may disproportionately increase anticipatory anxiety.

BEHAVIORAL ISSUES

As children get older and start to increase their independence, this can result in frustration for both families and medical teams. Young children may start to resist or refuse medical interventions that are painful or aversive, such as procedures, pokes, and swallowing medications. Young children also develop age-appropriate separation anxiety and stranger fears. As children progress through middle childhood, greater self-regulation of emotions and use of problem-solving strategies increases engagement in medical cares. However, avoidance of unpleasant side effects, oppositional behaviors, and busy family schedules continue to be barriers to medical care across age groups.

To mitigate fears, the presence of familiar caregivers at the hospital should be encouraged, and parents should be allowed to accompany children to procedures when possible. When caregivers have to be away from the hospital, providing clear explanation of where caregivers are going, when they will return, and encouraging use of transitional objects can ease separation fears. Providers can take advantage of young children's natural curiosity and desire for independence by offering forced choices (e.g., "Do you want to take your medicine with applesauce or pudding?"), including them in care (e.g., holding equipment, pushing buttons, picking a finger), and offering immediate praise and tangible rewards to increase compliance. Distraction is often the best pain coping tool for very young children. Older children can learn various strategies, including problem-solving, social support, secondary control (e.g., cognitive reappraisal, acceptance, distraction), and passive/avoidant coping. While passive and avoidant strategies are often viewed as less beneficial for coping with medical illness than active coping. However, Tailoring coping strategies to the patient's level of perceived control may be appropriate. For example, passive coping strategies may be preferred for patients who have limited control over their illness and symptoms. Access to child life specialists and developmentally appropriate medical play can improve child understanding of and coping with procedures across age groups. Parents and caregivers can also promote security for their child by modeling calm and avoiding excessive reassurance.

IMPACT ON FUNCTIONING AND HEALTHY LIFESTYLES

For children with developmental delays, hospitalization can overshadow developmental screening and cause potential issues to be missed. Functioning in typical areas of child development can also be delayed or regress during hospitalization, including sleeping, feeding, dressing, and toileting. Learning early self-feeding skills may be disrupted for children with medical complexity early in life, with resulting oral-motor and behavioral feeding problems negatively impacting nutrition and growth. In fact, most children with developmental delays and medical complexity experience feeding difficulties. Almost all hospitalized children demonstrate some level of sleep disruption, including changes to typical day-night schedule, frequent nighttime awakenings, and reduced sleep quality. Sleep disruptions may be due to environmental (e.g., noise, light) or medical/individual factors (e.g., pain, medical cares, anxiety). Patients receiving certain medications (e.g., benzodiazepines, narcotics) or intensive care (e.g., mechanical ventilation, sedation), as well as oncology patients and premature infants, are particularly at risk for sleep disruption and delirium. The majority of adolescents already obtain less than the recommended amount of sleep at baseline, and thus are at increased risk for disordered sleep during hospitalization. Finally, recent findings have highlighted the negative effects of media exposure that is pervasive in hospitalized youth. With excess screen time, young children are at increased risk for behavioral problems and developmental delays, and adolescents report increased psychosomatic symptoms, decreased physical activity, and declines in mental well-being. Hospitalized youth may also demonstrate difficulty meeting general guidelines for exercise, diet, and weight, given time burdens and activity restrictions related to their treatment regimens.

Children with feeding difficulties may benefit from access to feeding therapy and dietary interventions to reduce reliance on enteral feeding, develop safe chewing and swallowing techniques, and increase food volume/variety to meet nutritional goals. Frequent screening for sleep disruption, confusion, and disorientation can identify patients at risk. Medications, sleep hygiene interventions, and environmental precautions (e.g., minimizing noise, cycled lighting, clustered cares) can all improve sleep. Providers should be aware of the detrimental impact of excessive media exposure and guide appropriate screen time limits for hospitalized patients. Hospital visits may also provide opportunities for education, brief intervention, and support to help pediatric patients engage in broader healthy lifestyle behaviors. Physical activity interventions specifically hold promise for broad positive effects in those with chronic illness.

Finally, screening for neurodevelopmental disorders, including autism, attention deficit hyperactivity disorder, intellectual and learning problems, should be a priority during hospitalization to best understand supports the child may need during and after hospitalization. While hospitalized, setting clear expectations and implementing differential attention techniques (e.g., ignoring complaints/refusal, praising eating behavior, earning rewards) can help children re-engage in age-appropriate behaviors. For older children, behavioral incentives and token economy systems may be helpful to motivate participation in a variety of daily tasks. For children with severe functional deficits, referral to more intensive behavioral therapy or Applied Behavior Analysis (ABA) therapy may be indicated.

ACADEMICS AND SOCIALIZATION

Youth with chronic health conditions demonstrate lower school performance and higher school drop-out rates than their healthy peers. Frequent hospital visits, prolonged hospital stays, complex treatment regimens, and cognitive impacts of treatment can significantly disrupt school routines. Youth with certain medical conditions (e.g., cancer, diabetes, epilepsy) and co-occurring depression are most at risk for school absenteeism and subsequent academic underachievement. Hospitalization and treatment can also limit time available for typical social interactions and undermine social development. Visible symptoms or treatment, "feeling different," bullying, stigmatization, and peer rejection due to medical illness can be sources of social-emotional distress. Unfortunately, pediatric chronic illness disruptions to socialization and academics have long-term impacts on educational and employment attainment into adulthood. Hospital school liaisons can improve family understanding of their child's needs and advocacy for appropriate school supports to improve educational outcomes. Depending on the severity of medical care, access to schoolteacher supports in the hospital, online, or home-based schooling options may be useful. Combined support from parents/caregivers and peers can improve outcomes for hospitalized youth.

RISKY BEHAVIORS AND MENTAL HEALTH

Adolescence is commonly associated with increased desire for autonomy, reliance on peer influences, and risk-taking behavior. Experimentation with substances, sexual activity, violence, and incomplete development of higher executive functions contribute to unintentional injuries and homicide being leading causes of mortality and morbidity for this age group. In addition, the United Nations International Children's Emergency Fund (UNICEF) estimates, in *The State of the World's Children 2021,* that one in seven adolescents, or 166 million adolescents globally, meet criteria for a mental health disorder. Rates of mental health disorders, such as depression, anxiety, and disordered eating, increase throughout adolescence, with suicide being the second leading cause of death for 10 to 24-year-olds. Substance use in adolescents is often comorbid with other psychiatric concerns; current screening for substance in hospital settings is likely insufficient. Fortunately, validated screening tools exist to assess for the risky behaviors, substance use, and mental health concerns that are particularly apparent during adolescence (see Table 9-1). Early identification of safety concerns can help refer adolescent patients to appropriate levels of mental healthcare.

ADHERENCE

For youth with chronic illness, adolescence is a time of documented declines in adherence to medical treatment. Cognitive development changes rapidly throughout adolescence from more concrete thinking styles focused on immediate consequences in early adolescence, to increased self-awareness and acknowledgement of long-term consequences of behavior in late adolescence and early adulthood. Declines in adherence during adolescence have been linked to increased desire for autonomy, transition of responsibility for care from parents to teens, and parent-child communication style. Beliefs about treatment play a unique role in non-adherence on both ends of the spectrum, from a perceived lack of consequences due to non-adherence in patients with minimal symptoms to avoidance of time-consuming treatments for patients with a bleak view of their disease prognosis. An approach that balances adolescents expressed needs with parent and provider involvement, with focus on shared responsibility for medical cares, is likely to improve adolescent motivation and adherence. For those struggling with adherence, behavioral interventions (e.g., problem-solving, parent training) and multi-component interventions (e.g., social support, skills training, education) result in the best outcomes.

TRANSITION

Preparation for transition to adult care is an important consideration for adolescents with chronic illness. Important aspects of transition to adult care include patient-focused, strengths-based approaches that stress the importance of early preparation, effective communication, and shared accountability and decision-making. There is a significant literature on medical communication in this transitional period. Respectful communication includes using the patient's correct name and pronouns, age-appropriate opportunities for private discussion of sensitive topics, and non-judgmental regard for patients. Providers should focus on open-ended questions and transparency about confidentiality with this age group to promote honest disclosure and open discourse. Joint recommendations from the American Academy of Pediatrics, the American Academy of Family Physicians, and the American College of Physicians for successful transition from pediatric to adult care include assessing readiness for transition, creating a transition plan that adequately prepares youth for adult approaches to care, monitoring progress, and obtaining feedback to confirm the patient has seen their new adult provider.

CONCLUSION

A developmental approach to patients is essential to the well-being and appropriate diagnosis of the hospitalized child. Developmental screening guides the clinician in communication and treatment planning with the patient and family and helps identify modifiable threats to typical development in the child's environment. Hospitalists play a crucial role in identifying toxic stress and referring families to appropriate interventions to minimize adverse childhood experiences that impact both child and adult health outcomes. Furthermore, a developmentally informed approach assists the clinician in reducing PMTS and reducing medical trauma for the child and family.

SUGGESTED READINGS

Anderson E, Durstine JL. Physical activity, exercise, and chronic diseases: A brief review. *Sports Med Health Sci.* 2019;1(1):3-10.

Berger J, Zaidi M, Halferty I, Kudchadkar SR. Sleep in the hospitalized child: a contemporary review. *Chest.* 2021;160(3):1064-74.

Boyce WT, Levitt P, Martinez FD, McEwen BS, Shonkoff JP. Genes, environments, and time: the biology of adversity and resilience. *Pediatrics.* 2021;147(2).

Chua WD, Pipan M, Rosen AR. Neurologic and developmental considerations in children with medical complexity. *Curr Probl Pediatr Adolesc Health Care.* 2021;51(9):101073.

Committee on Hospital Care, Institute for Patient- and Family-Centered Care. Patient-and family-centered care and the pediatrician's role. *Pediatrics.* 2012;129(2):394-404.

Compas BE, Jaser SS, Dunn MJ, Rodriguez EM. Coping with chronic illness in childhood and adolescence. *Annu Rev Clin Psychol.* 2012; 8:455.

Craig J, Glick C, Phillips R, Hall S, Smith J, Browne J. Recommendations for involving the family in developmental care of the NICU baby. *J Perinatol.* 2015;35(1):S5-S8.

Crump C, Rivera D, London R, Landau M, Erlendson B, Rodriguez E. Chronic health conditions and school performance among children and youth. *Ann Epidemiol.* 2013;23(4):179-84.

Dean AJ, Walters J, Hall A. A systematic review of interventions to enhance medication adherence in children and adolescents with chronic illness. *Arch Dis Child.* 2010;95(9):717-23.

De Young AC, Paterson RS, Brown EA, et al. Topical review: Medical trauma during early childhood. *J Pediatr Psychol.* 2021;46(7):739-46.

Dosman C, Andrews D. Anticipatory guidance for cognitive and social-emotional development: Birth to five years. *Paediatr Child Health.* 2012;17(2):75-80.

Ewulonu UC. Utility of a psychosocial assessment during an acute care hospitalization. *Curr Probl Pediatr Adolesc Health Care.* 2021;51(5): 100998.

Earls MF, Foy JM, Green CM. *Addressing Mental Health Concerns in Pediatrics: A Practical Resource Toolkit for Clinicians.* American Academy of Pediatrics; 2021.

Finkelstein-Fox L, Park CL. Control-coping goodness-of-fit and chronic illness: a systematic review of the literature. *Health Psychol Rev.* 2019;13(2):137-62.

Forkey H, Szilagyi M, Kelly ET, et al. Trauma-informed care. *Pediatrics.* 2021;148(2).

Foy JM, Green CM, Earls MF, et al. Mental health competencies for pediatric practice. *Pediatrics.* 2019;144(5).

Garner A, Yogman M, Committee on Psychosocial Aspects of Child and Family Health. Preventing childhood toxic stress: partnering with families and communities to promote relational health. *Pediatrics.* 2021;148(2).

Heron M. National vital statistics reports. *Natl Vital Stat Rep.* 2021;70(3).

Kahana S, Drotar D, Frazier T. Meta-analysis of psychological interventions to promote adherence to treatment in pediatric chronic health conditions. *J Pediatr Psychol.* 2008;33(6):590-611.

Keeley B. *The State of the World's Children 2021: On My Mind–Promoting, Protecting and Caring for Children's Mental Health*: ERIC; 2021.

Khan A, Lee E-Y, Rosenbaum S, Khan SR, Tremblay MS. Dose-dependent and joint associations between screen time, physical activity, and mental wellbeing in adolescents: an international observational study. *Lancet Child Adolesc Health.* 2021;5(10):729-38.

Lerch MF, Thrane SE. Adolescents with chronic illness and the transition to self-management: A systematic review. *J Adolesc.* 2019;72:152-61.

Lipkin PH, Macias MM, Norwood KW, et al. Promoting optimal development: identifying infants and young children with developmental disorders through developmental surveillance and screening. *Pediatrics.* 2020;145(1).

Pardhan S, Parkin J, Trott M, Driscoll R. Risks of digital screen time and recommendations for mitigating adverse outcomes in children and adolescents. *J Sch Health.* 2022.

Phalen JA. Managing feeding problems and feeding disorders. *Pediatr Rev.* 2013;34(12):549-57.

Shaw RJ. Treatment adherence in adolescents: Development and psychopathology. *Clin Child Psychol Psychiatry.* 2001;6(1):137-50.

Shonkoff JP, Garner AS, Child CoPAo, et al. The lifelong effects of early childhood adversity and toxic stress. *Pediatrics.* 2012;129(1):e232-e46.

Smith JR, Hazen EP, Kaminski TA, Wilens TE. Literature review: Substance use screening and co-morbidity in medically hospitalized youth. *Gen Hosp Psychiatry.* 2020;67:115-26.

Weitzman C, Wegner L, Developmental So, et al. Promoting optimal development: Screening for behavioral and emotional problems. *Pediatrics.* 2015;135(2):384-95.

White PH, Cooley WC, Boudreau ADA, et al. Supporting the health care transition from adolescence to adulthood in the medical home. *Pediatrics.* 2018;142(5).

CHAPTER 10 Infection Control for Pediatric Hospitalists

Joshua K. Schaffzin, MD, PhD and Suchitra Rao, MBBS, MSCS

The goals of the disciplines of hospital medicine (HM) and infection prevention and control (IP&C) have considerable overlap. Hospitalists play a vital role in IP&C activities such as preventing healthcare-associated infections, supporting antimicrobial and diagnostic stewardship, and advocating for high value and safe care for patients and families. In this chapter, we will summarize what IP&C encompasses, review IP&C principles, and outline how hospitalists impact IP&C efforts.

INFECTION PREVENTION & CONTROL IN HOSPITAL SETTINGS

The goal of an IP&C program is to prevent transmission of any infectious agent within the healthcare facility in which it operates, encompassing patients, families, employees, and visitors. The Centers for Medicare and Medicaid Services require that a hospital have an Infection Control Plan that details how standards are met and an Infection Control Officer (typically a Director of Infection Prevention and Control or a Hospital Epidemiologist) to oversee plan execution through IP&C staff, known as Infection Preventionists. Infection preventionists employ several methods to prevent transmission, including surveillance, outbreak investigation, education and policy creation, risk assessment and supporting institutional functions and efforts around vaccination, public reporting, and biocontainment (**Figure 10-1**).

The conduct of these activities varies between institutions, and programs can report through hospital operations, academic divisions (typically Infectious Diseases), patient services, safety, or a combination of these.

SURVEILLANCE

IP&C conducts disease surveillance to monitor community and healthcare-associated infection trends. IP&C is often responsible for an institution's public reporting (see later), and following community trends of respiratory diseases (e.g., RSV, influenza, pertussis), vaccine-preventable diseases (e.g., measles, mumps), and other pathogens informs testing and management approaches throughout a medical center and its community. Additionally, IP&C monitors for healthcare-associated infections (HAI) to identify outbreaks (e.g., cases of norovirus on an inpatient unit), unplanned exposures (e.g., legionellosis), and track device-related HAIs (e.g., catheter-associated urinary tract infection) using the Centers for Disease Control and Prevention's (CDC) National Healthcare Safety Network (NHSN) defined processes.

Disease surveillance typically begins with review of positive microbiological testing (e.g., cultures and molecular diagnostics), followed by chart review and/or direct interview when indicated.

IP&C also conducts surveillance of adherence to institutional processes such as hand hygiene or transmission-based precautions (also known as isolation precautions), cleaning and disinfection of equipment, and regular evaluation of infection control processes in sensitive areas (e.g., sterile processing division, clean pharmacy rooms). This most often also involves direct observation and engagement of stakeholders. Recently, a greater emphasis has been placed on risks that derive from the constructed environment, including air, water, fomites, and areas where construction or renovation are occurring. Infection preventionists often participate in surveillance related to these risks, including reviewing airflow measurements and testing to mitigate airborne pathogen spread; reviewing waterborne pathogen surveillance such as regular *Legionella* testing; evaluating environmental services activities; and rounding to evaluate proper containment of construction projects.

EDUCATION & POLICIES

Infection preventionists utilize education and policies to provide a framework for expectations and guidance for prevention. Education occurs directly through group presentations or while rounding and indirectly through signage and messaging. Policies include CMS conditions of participation adherence and institutional standards by which processes are evaluated. Examples include routine cleaning and disinfection of equipment, hand hygiene, transmission-based precautions, employee illness and exposure, and outbreak investigation and control.

RISK ASSESSMENT

Given the wide range and depth of IP&C coverage, programs often employ formal risk assessments to prioritize activities that maximize benefits and match available resources. For example, in a hospital that experienced a *Legionella* outbreak, priority may be given to development and enforcement of a water safety program. A hospital that changed laundry providers may choose to allocate time and effort to assure the new provider adheres to the required standards. During the COVID-19 pandemic, IP&C resources were utilized to lead and/or support numerous different efforts such as contact tracing, PPE requirements and utilization, vaccine requirements, patient isolation, visitation policy, exposure risk stratification, practice around services like child life and school, hospital policy for screening and testing, and internal and external messaging. Risk assessments can be performed for any type of hospital-based activity and are often categorized by service or location such as dialysis, home care, and ambulatory services. Risk assessments may be conducted annually with a high-level overview, or with more granularity and frequency for specific projects or events. For example, when renovation is undertaken in patient care areas, an Infection Control Risk Assessment that outlines how they will contain and prevent pathogen exposure during the project is often required.

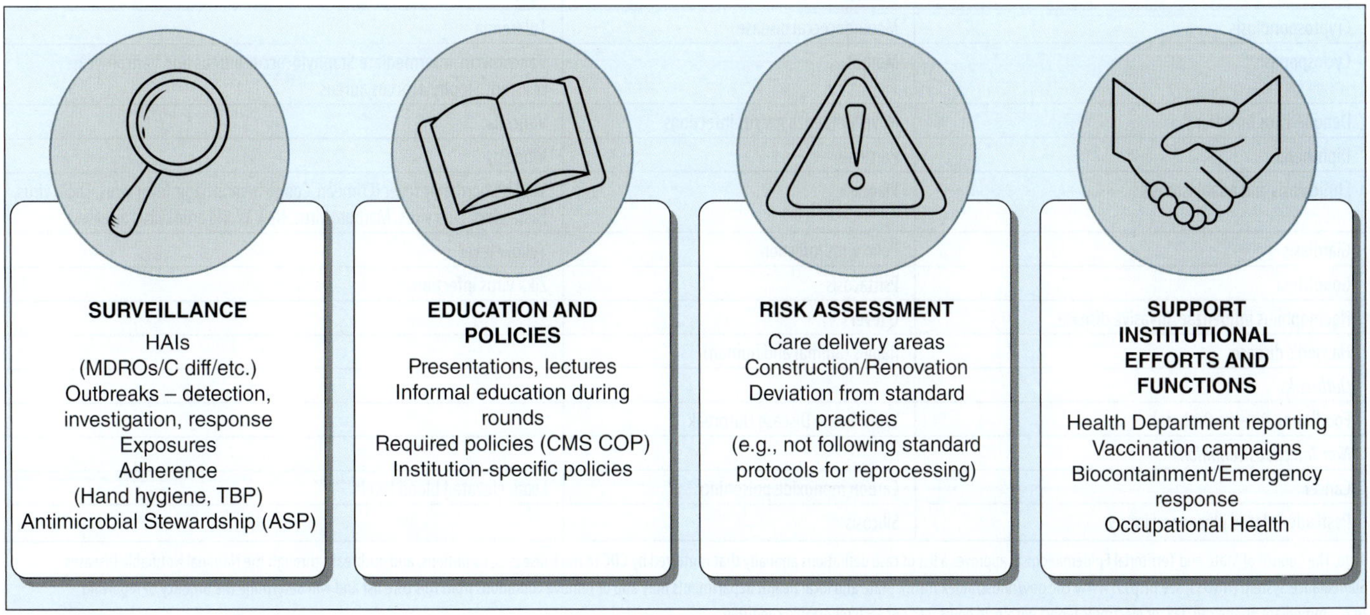

FIGURE 10-1. Role of infection preventionists.

ALIGNMENT WITH INSTITUTIONAL FUNCTIONS & EFFORTS

Clinicians should notify their local or state health department of any reportable condition (the full list of reportable conditions and their timeline for reporting differs by state and locality, see **Table 10-1**). Rather than expecting clinicians to report individual cases, IP&C often takes responsibility for all reporting at a given institution. IP&C is positioned well for reporting since they are connected to public health agencies directly through various collaborations, and they have centralized data sources that facilitate efficient and timely reporting. IP&C teams often collaborate closely with Occupational Health, and in some facilities, the medical director of IP&C will also serve as the medical director of Occupational Health. This ensures consistency in policies and recommendations for staff and patients alike. For example, infection preventionists often support institutional efforts to vaccinate employees, patients, and families for the prevention of seasonal influenza and other infectious diseases. Infection preventionists are often trained in emergency management and response and participate in efforts that involve communicable conditions like Ebola viral disease or COVID-19. Because of their broad reach and partnerships with many team members in an institution, IP&C will often be the first group to be notified of any exposure or safety risk, ultimately handing off the next steps in risk assessment to other staff members for continued management. For example, IP&C can bridge between clinical and facilities teams to help address a water intrusion and remediation.

INFECTION PREVENTION & CONTROL PRINCIPLES

Despite the active role hospitalists play in IP&C, there is no national requirement for IP&C education or training in medical school, residency, or fellowship (except for Infectious Diseases fellows who are required to rotate through IP&C). General overviews are often covered during an orientation, but the likelihood of retention of IP&C principles from one-time educational sessions is low. Nonetheless, it is important for hospitalists to understand IP&C principles including modes of disease transmission and interventions to disrupt transmission, in order to optimize the safety for patients, staff, and families.

CHAIN OF TRANSMISSION

While not comprehensive or free of exception, the general process of an infectious agent entering an environmental reservoir (another person,

TABLE 10-1 Nationally Notifiable Disease List (2022)

Infectious Conditions		
Anthrax	Hantavirus infection	Rubella
Arboviral diseases (California serogroup virus, Chikungunya virus, Eastern equine encephalitis virus, Powassan virus, St Louis encephalitis virus, and West Nile virus diseases)	Hemolytic uremic syndrome, post-diarrheal	Salmonellosis
Babesiosis	Hepatitis A	*Salmonella* Paratyphi or *Salmonella* Typhi infection
Botulism	Hepatitis B	Severe acute respiratory syndrome-associated coronavirus disease
Brucellosis	Hepatitis C	Shiga toxin-producing *Escherichia coli*
Campylobacteriosis	HIV infection	Shigellosis
Candida auris	Influenza-associated pediatric mortality	Smallpox
Carbapenemase Producing Carbapenem-Resistant Enterobacteriaceae (CP-CRE)	Invasive pneumococcal disease	Spotted fever rickettsiosis
Chancroid	Legionellosis	Streptococcal toxic shock syndrome
Chlamydia trachomatis infection	Leptospirosis	Syphilis
Cholera	Listeriosis	Tetanus
Coccidioidomycosis	Lyme disease	Toxic shock syndrome (other than streptococcal)
Congenital syphilis	Malaria	Trichinellosis
Coronavirus Disease 2019 (COVID-19)	Measles	Tuberculosis
Cryptosporidiosis	Meningococcal disease	Tularemia
Cyclosporiasis	Mumps	Vancomycin-intermediate Staphylococcus aureus and Vancomycin-resistant Staphylococcus aureus
Dengue virus infections	Novel influenza A virus infections	Varicella
Diphtheria	Pertussis	Vibriosis
Ehrlichiosis and anaplasmosis	Plague	Viral hemorrhagic fever (Crimean-Congo hemorrhagic fever virus, Ebola virus, Lassa virus, Lujo virus, Marburg virus, New World arenavirus diseases)
Giardiasis	Polio virus infection	Yellow fever
Gonorrhea	Psittacosis	Zika virus infection
Haemophilus influenzae, invasive disease	Q fever	
Hansen's disease	Rabies (animal and human)	
Outbreaks		
Foodborne Disease Outbreak	Waterborne Disease Outbreak	
Non-Infectious Conditions		
Cancer	Carbon monoxide poisoning	Lead, elevated blood levels
Pesticide-related Illness and Injury	Silicosis	

Note: The Council of State and Territorial Epidemiologists approves a list of case definitions annually that is utilized by CDC to track diseases, conditions, and outbreaks through the National Notifiable Diseases Surveillance System (NNDSS, see https://www.cdc.gov/nndss/index.html). State and local health departments may add or remove conditions from this core list and will determine the urgency of reporting (e.g., immediate phone call, fax, or electronic report within 24 hours, etc.) of each reportable condition.

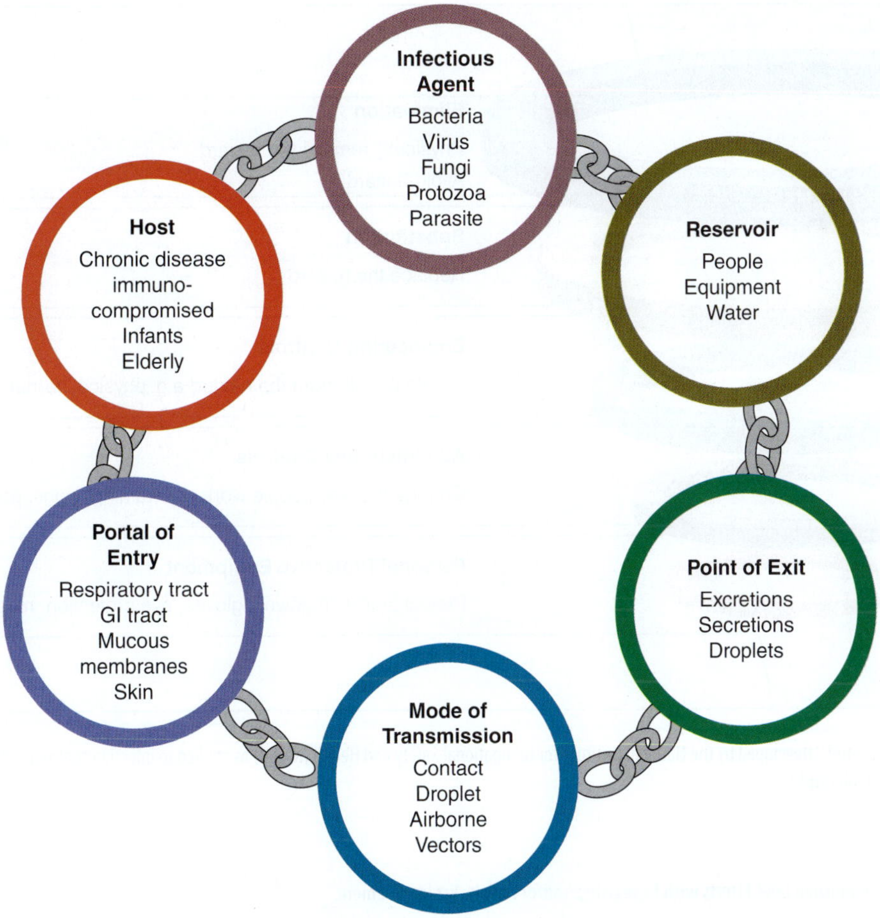

FIGURE 10-2. Chain of infection transmission. (Adapted from Centers for Disease Control and Prevention. Principles of Epidemiology, 3rd ed. Atlanta: U.S. Department of Health and Human Services; 2011.)

an animal, air, water, surfaces, etc.), and finding its way to a host who becomes infected and restarts the cycle, is how IP&C conceptualizes nosocomial transmission and identifies risks in need of mitigation. Put simply, IP&C's goal is to break the chain between these three groups to prevent transmission (**Figure 10-2**).

While any infectious agent could be transmitted, viral or bacterial agents are most common and often targeted by hospital-based IP&C activities. Further, while an agent may demonstrate a predominant mode of transmission, no agent is thought to be transmitted exclusively by a single mode. Respiratory syncytial virus, for example, can be transmitted through infectious respiratory droplets and by contact with contaminated surfaces, so it requires both Droplet and Contact precautions. Finally, even though certain hosts may be more susceptible to an infection when exposed (e.g., a patient with prolonged neutropenia who develops aspergillosis), any host can be susceptible to most pathogens. This principle is important to remember when considering exposure of otherwise healthy healthcare providers to patients with communicable diseases.

HIERARCHY OF EXPOSURE CONTROLS

Hazards exist in every workplace; two Federal agencies, the Occupational Safety and Health Administration (OSHA) and the National Institute for Occupational Safety and Health (NIOSH), are responsible for creating standards and guidance to protect against these risks. Some of these are clear safety enhancements and welcomed by all (e.g., fire escapes, eyewash stations), while some are less apparent (e.g., prohibition of drinks in clinical areas). NIOSH has published a list of measures that can be taken to prevent exposure to hazards that they have prioritized into a hierarchy (**Figure 10-3**).

The broadest interventions (Elimination and Substitution) are the most effective and reliable, but also require the greatest amount of system-level change. Facilities will often utilize these high-level measures when designing new spaces, which may incur significant costs, while individual stakeholders may engage in personal measures which are less costly but require ongoing education. Tuberculosis (TB) is often used as a case study for the NIOSH hierarchy, because the mandated Respiratory Protection Plan is designed to prevent TB introduction and transmission. For TB, as with many infectious agents, Elimination and Substitution are not currently possible. Plans therefore rely on Engineering Controls (airborne isolation rooms), Administrative Controls (signage requiring N95 Airborne precautions), and Personal Protective Equipment (N95-level respiratory protection when providing care). It is important to recognize that both PPE and education are low-reliability interventions, requiring greater effort to make each effective (e.g., through repeated training and auditing with feedback).

HOW HOSPITALISTS CAN MINIMIZE HEALTHCARE-ASSOCIATED INFECTION TRANSMISSION RISK

Hospitalists can affect IP&C efforts meaningfully both at system and individual levels while engaged in their daily clinical practice. Reports of the impact of hospitalists in IP&C domains are abundant in the published literature. Some examples are summarized in **Table 10-2**.

Specific areas in which hospitalists can have an impact are listed in **Table 10-3**. As advocates for safe optimal care, hospitalists can ensure interventions are used only when indicated, such as antibiotics, catheters, and transmission-based precautions. As system thinkers and leaders, hospitalists are in a position to ensure IP&C is aligned with institutional safety and educational efforts, and that higher reliability interventions can be considered and/or implemented during design processes.

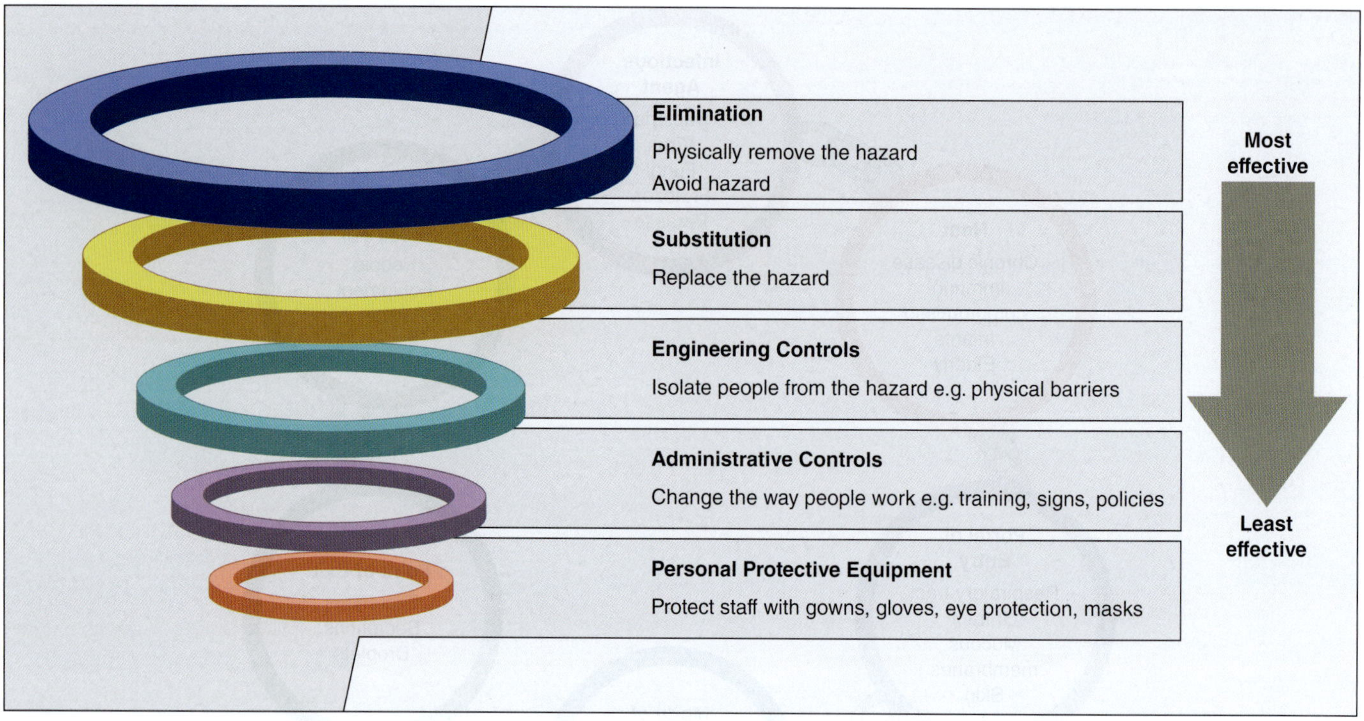

FIGURE 10-3. Hierarchy of controls. Developed by the National Institute for Occupational Safety and Health (NIOSH) as applied to infection control practices. (Adapted from https://www.cdc.gov/niosh/topics/hierarchy/default.html.)

TABLE 10-2 Examples of Published IP&C Efforts with Leadership and/or Hospitalist Involvement

Manuscript and Reference	Year	Summary of study
HAI prevention		
A Program to Prevent Catheter-Associated Urinary Tract Infection in Acute Care N Engl J Med 374(22):2111-9	2016	Led a national prevention program (Comprehensive Unit-based Safety Program or CUSP) that successfully reduced urinary catheter use in non-ICUs (incidence rate ratio 0.68, 95% confidence interval [CI] 0.56-0.82) and catheter-associated infection in both ICUs (incidence rate ratio 0.86, 95% CI 0.76-0.96) and non-ICUs (incidence rate ratio 0.93, 95% CI 0.90-0.96)
"Lose the Tube": A Choosing Wisely initiative to reduce catheter-associated urinary tract infections in hospitalist-led inpatient units Am J Infect Control 45(3):333-5	2017	Hospitalist-led effort using an EMR identification tool, daily interdisciplinary query, and education to reduce urinary catheter days (mean 3.3-2.9 per person), catheter-related infections (2.85-0.32 per 1000 catheter days), and cost (estimated $32,245).
Engaging Frontline Staff in Central Line-Associated Bloodstream Infection Prevention Practice in the Wake of Superstorm Sandy Jt Comm J Qual Patient Saf 41(10):462-8	2015	Utilized hospital shutdown 'downtime' to improve CLABSI prevention efforts yielding improved bundle reliability and decreased CLABSI rates (2.7-0.5 per 1000 catheter days).
Risk factors for first cerebrospinal fluid shunt infection: findings from a multi-center prospective cohort study J Pediatr 164(6):1462-8.e2.	2014	Epidemiologic analysis of ventricular shunt infections to guide prevention efforts that found infection risk was most significantly associated with previous shunt revision (1 revision vs none, hazards ratio 3.9, 95% CI, 2.2, 6.5; ≥2 revisions, hazards ratio 13.0, 95% CI, 6.5, 24.9).
Standardizing preoperative preparation to reduce surgical site infections among pediatric neurosurgical patients J Neurosurg Pediatr 19:399–406	2017	Standard pre-operative protocol implementation for elective neurosurgical procedure that reduced surgical site infection rates (risk ratio 0.21, 95% CI 0.08-0.56).
Assessment of Federal Value-Based Incentive Programs and In-Hospital Clostridioides difficile Infection Rates JAMA Network Open 4(10):e2132114	2021	Evaluation of the effect of CMS value-based incentive program (designed to promote prevention) for healthcare facility-onset Clostidioides difficile infection (HO-CDI) that found rates decreased following program implementation (adjusted quarterly incidence rate ratio 0.96, 95% CI 0.95-0.97).
Transmission-based precautions (Isolation)		
Do physicians examine patients in contact isolation less frequently? A brief report Am J Infect Control 31(6):354-6	2003	Direct observation of morning rounds noting which patients were in transmission-based precautions and which were examined by senior residents and attending physicians that found attending physicians were half as likely to examine patients in contact precautions vs those who were not (relative risk 0.49, 95% CI 0.30-0.79).
Care of Children Isolated for Infection Control: A Prospective Observational Cohort Study Pediatrics 122(2):e411-5	2008	No difference in quantity (direct observation of time spent in room and number of organ systems examined) or quality (parental completion of the Pediatric Family Satisfaction Questionnaire) of care provided to patients in isolation precautions on an inpatient pediatric ward.

(Continued)

TABLE 10-2 Examples of Published IP&C Efforts with Leadership and/or Hospitalist Involvement (*Continued*)

Manuscript and Reference	Year	Summary of study
Antimicrobial Stewardship		
Accelerating Initiation of Adequate Antimicrobial Therapy Using Real-Time Decision Support and Microarray Testing Pediatr Qual Saf 4(4):e191	2019	Utilized automated notification of culture results to guide use of proper antimicrobial therapy, reducing time of improper coverage by 87% (38-4.7 hours).
Automated identification of antibiotic overdoses and adverse drug events via analysis of prescribing alerts and medication administration records J Am Med Inform Assoc 24(2):295-302	2017	Evaluated user response to automatic medication dosing alerts and found <1% resulted in true overdose administrations. Revising thresholds to match accurate dosing decreased alert frequency and improved alert salience.
Decreasing Duration of Antibiotic Prescribing for Uncomplicated Skin and Soft Tissue Infections Pediatrics 137(2):e20151223	2016	Quality improvement initiative to increase the proportion of discharges with short course prescription for uncomplicated SSTIs (23% to 74% over 23 months), found no significant change in readmissions or treatment failures.
Hand Hygiene		
Utilizing improvement science methods to improve physician compliance with proper hand hygiene Pediatrics 129(4):e1042-50	2012	Quality improvement initiative to increase physician hand hygiene adherence that utilized learners to observe and conduct immediate mitigation of failures and improved adherence from 68% to >95% within 6 months.
Good to Great: Quality-Improvement Initiative Increases and Sustains Pediatric Health Care Worker Hand Hygiene Compliance Hosp Pediatr 7(4):189-196	2017	Hospital Medicine-led QI effort using high-reliability human-factor interventions increased adherence to ≥95% within 9 months and sustained for over 2 years.
Advocacy		
Vaccine Administration in Children's Hospitals Pediatrics 149(2):e2021053925	2022	Administrative database (Pediatric Health Information Systems) analysis that found ≥1 vaccine administration in 12.9% of all admissions (range 1% to 45% among 49 children's hospitals), but only 1.9% were not the hepatitis B birth dose or influenza.
Be inFLUential: Evaluation of a multifaceted intervention to increase influenza vaccination rates among pediatric inpatients Vaccine. 2020;38(6):1370-1377	2020	Multifaceted intervention to promote influenza vaccine for inpatients yielded increased likelihood of proper admission screening (odds ratio 1.23, 95% CI 1.11-1.35), vaccine order (odds ratio 2.27, 95% CI 2.01-2.56), and evidence of influenza vaccination at discharge (odds ratio 1.39 95% CI 1.27-1.53).

TABLE 10-3 Steps Hospitalists Can Take to Minimize Infections in the Hospital Setting

Principle	Examples
Education	Education to learners and other staff on IP&C best practices, modeling hand hygiene, appropriate isolation procedures, and PPE
Collaboration with IP&C	Notification to IP&C teams of suspected outbreaks Research and quality improvement work involving IP&C efforts
Leadership and Teamwork	Serving on committees, developing policies to prevent infection transmission Incorporating IP&C into process and structural design efforts
Vigilance and patient advocacy	Antimicrobial stewardship Vaccine advocacy Minimizing HAI through judicious use and prompt removal of indwelling catheters, lines Rounding checklists
Personal and patient-focused practices	Correct donning and doffing of PPE Adhering to PPE and other IP&C policies Staying home when sick Reporting absence due to illness Sharps safety Aseptic technique for procedures

In academic settings, hospitalists can have a direct impact on best practices and educating learners on the rationale behind IP&C practices, including hand hygiene and transmission-based precautions, HAI prevention, and antimicrobial stewardship. They can also serve as role models on proper practices for patients, families, and clinical teams.

SUGGESTED READINGS

Association of Professionals in Infection Control and Epidemiology (APIC). Education for the Prevention of Infection (EPI®) Education Series (excellent and thorough overview designed for IPs, cost associated). Available at https://apic.org/education-and-events/epi-education-series/.

Guidelines for Environmental Infection Control in Health-Care Facilities. Available at https://www.osha.gov/sites/default/files/CDC's_Guidelines_for_Environmental_Infection_Control.pdf.

Hierarchy of Controls. The National Institute for Occupational Safety and Health. Available at https://www.cdc.gov/niosh/topics/hierarchy/default.html.

Improving Patient and Worker Safety. Available at https://www.jointcommission.org/-/media/tjc/documents/resources/patient-safety-topics/patient-safety/tjc-improvingpatientandworkersafety-monograph.pdf.

Infection Control. Centers for Disease Control and Prevention. Available at https://www.cdc.gov/infectioncontrol/index.html

SHEA—Guidelines and Expert Guidance Documents. Available at https://shea-online.org/guidance/.

SHEA—Prevention CHKC (practical training module, cost associated). Available at https://learningce.shea-online.org/content/prevention-chkc.

Society for Healthcare Epidemiology of America (SHEA). Primer on Healthcare Epidemiology, Infection Control & Antimicrobial Stewardship (educational series on principles and practices, cost associated). Available at https://learningce.shea-online.org/content/primer-healthcare-epidemiology-infection-control-antimicrobial-stewardship-1.

WHO Hand Hygiene Guidelines (2009). Available at https://www.who.int/publications/i/item/WHO-IER-PSP-2009.07.

CHAPTER 11

Transitions, Communication, Transport and Discharge Planning

Snezana Nena Osorio, MD MS and Arti D. Desai, MD, MSPH

INTRODUCTION

Care transitions for hospitalized children are a vulnerable time for patients and families. These transitions include home-to-hospital, interfacility transfers and transports, transitions between different hospital units (e.g., emergency department [ED] to intensive care unit [ICU] to general medical ward), and the transition from hospital-to-home or to a sub-acute care facility. As the care of the child shifts between different provider teams, clear communication, and information exchange are critical components for seamless transitions. However, miscommunication and gaps in care are prevalent during these care transitions resulting in a high incidence of adverse events. For example, a study by Heath et al. demonstrated that one in five pediatric patients experience a post-discharge issue requiring intervention. Thus, supporting patients and families through each of these care transitions is a key issue for hospitalists. This chapter summarizes an important body of work on transitions of care, communication, transport, and discharge planning; notable studies are summarized in **Table 11-1**.

COMMUNICATION DURING TRANSITIONS

As care of the child shifts between provider teams, care transitions can result in the loss of essential information. For example, a summary of the literature conducted by the Society of Hospital Medicine and the Society of General Internal Medicine found that discharge summaries were only available at 12% to 34% of first post-discharge visits; further, many discharge summaries lacked elements important to continue patient care. Communication gaps can result in a variety of negative outcomes—some relatively benign, but others potentially life-threatening. With excellent communication between providers, this loss of information can be minimized across all care transitions.

Several efforts are underway to improve communication during care transitions. Perhaps the most well-known of these is the IIPE-PRIS Accelerating Safe Sign-outs (I-PASS) program. Across nine pediatric residency training programs, I-PASS implementation reduced medical errors by 23% and preventable adverse events by 30%. Innovative modes of communication are also being developed to promote efficiency and information exchange beyond traditional modes of telephone conversations or fax. These include the utilization of secure electronic mail, secure messaging systems within and outside the electronic health record (EHR), and telemedicine for children with medical or social complexity (see Table 11-1). Pediatric hospitalists are leading research to understand the most effective modes of communication for promoting seamless transitions, patient safety, and enhancing family experiences with care (see Table 11-1). Furthermore, in the past 5 years, there has been a growth of new measures to assess the quality of communication during care transitions in pediatrics, which can be utilized to rigorously assess ongoing quality improvement (QI) work (see Table 11-1).

HOME-TO-HOSPITAL TRANSITIONS

While much work to improve care transitions for hospitalized patients focuses on the discharge process and hospital-to-home transitions, how to provide high-quality care as patients are transitioning *into the hospital* in the setting of an acute illness is also important. Few studies have examined communication between primary care providers (PCPs) and ED providers; though Beamon et al. found that communication was absent between these two teams for most patients presenting to a pediatric ED. There is a growing body of research to understand effective practices for home-to-hospital transitions including the value of direct admissions in facilitating more seamless transitions. Given 25% of unscheduled pediatric hospital admissions occur via direct admission, the American Academy of Pediatrics released a policy statement in 2023 highlighting recommendations to optimize the quality and safety of this hospital admission approach. Additionally, shared care plans for children with medical complexity (CMC) may help ensure that ED providers have critical information about the patient's unique management needs at the point-of-care to reduce adverse events and enhance patient experiences for this heterogeneous population.

The transition from home-to-hospital often involves care transitions between community EDs and tertiary care centers. Although there are some insights into potential standardized processes around the flow, communication, and information exchange during these transitions (see Table 11-1), QI efforts to ensure the safe transport of critically ill children remain a large responsibility of many pediatric hospital medicine programs. This field has rapidly progressed over the past two decades with advances in mobile ICU care and growth of pediatric specialized transport teams as these transitions continue to expand.

TRANSITIONS WITHIN THE HOSPITAL

Care transitions within the hospital are commonplace as pediatric patients move between different units of a hospital system, such as the ED, ICU, and general medical floor. Like the literature on home-to-hospital transitions, there is a paucity of evidence supporting best practices for ED to ICU or general medical floor transitions. However, many of the same principles are also critical during these transitions including effective communication, matching of clinical workflows, understanding differing clinical cultures, and alignment of expectations. Transitioning care from the ICU to the general medicine team also requires standardizing protocols to optimize timing of patient transfers, enhancing partnerships between patients and families during the transfer process, and identifying patient populations at higher risk of clinical deterioration or those requiring additional psychosocial support. Innovative strategies to improve ICU-to-floor transitions continue to evolve and promising interventions warrant further research, such as the inclusion of an ICU liaison nurse described by Herbst et al. which was associated with reductions in discharge delays.

As alluded to previously, the most extensive body of work to improve care transitions within the hospital relates to the I-PASS program. This comprehensive program trains clinicians to exchange and synthesize relevant patient information to develop a shared mental model for each patient. The I-PASS Handoff Bundle leverages a standardized mnemonic tool including the following elements: Illness severity, Patient summary, Action list, Situation awareness and contingency plans, and Synthesis by receiver. There is also a growing body of work exploring the role of patients and families in facilitating more seamless transitions between provider teams within the hospital, as well as ensuring these interventions result in equitable improvements across patients and families with different racial and ethnic identities or preferred languages for care.

HOSPITAL-TO-HOME TRANSITIONS

Pediatric care transitions from hospital to home are complex events involving multiple microsystems. The multifaceted nature of these processes calls for a novel approach to address quality risks that have been associated with failed transitions.

EXPLORATION OF CHALLENGES AND IMPROVEMENT NEEDS FOR HOSPITAL-TO-HOME TRANSITIONS

Qualitative studies of caregivers of children with either an acute medical condition and/or CMC elucidated families' preferences, priorities, and goals for achieving seamless transitions from hospital to home (see Table 11-1). Understanding how caregivers process information about their child's diagnosis, treatment and recovery is critical to their ability to assume care at home and "feel ready" for discharge. Across all studies,

TABLE 11-1 Relevant Publications Regarding Pediatric Transitions of Care, Communication, Transport, and Discharge Planning

Publication (Title and Source)	Author (Year)	Key Findings
Examining the Quality of Inter-Facility Transfers and Transport		
Which patients and where: a qualitative study of patient transfers from community hospitals. *Med Care*	Bosk et al. (2011)	The transfer process is burdensome for community hospital staff, varies by condition, and is often not focused on optimizing patient outcomes.
Profiling interfacility transfers for hospitalized pediatric patients. *Hospital Pediatrics*	Rosenthal et al. (2016)	• 9.4% of non-neonatal, non-pregnancy hospitalizations were admitted by transfer from another hospital. • Illness severity, principal diagnosis, insurance status, and race were associated with a higher odd of admission by transfer.
Improving emergency care for children with medical complexity: parent and physicians' perspectives. *Academic Pediatrics*	Pulcini et al. (2021)	• Parents of CMC identified challenges in ED care to involved extended treatment time, communication gaps, inefficient data exchange, and emotionally and logistically burdensome. • Providers also identified challenges related to time, data accessibility/availability, and communication.
Explorations of Challenges and Improvement Needs for Hospital-to-Home Transitions		
Pediatric discharge content: a multisite assessment of physician preferences and experiences. *Hospital Pediatrics*	Coughlin et al. (2014)	Surveys of inpatient and outpatient providers helped to identify seven essential elements of discharge communication: • admission/discharge dates • discharge diagnosis • description of a brief hospital stay • medications • follow-up appointments • immunization received during hospitalization • pending labs
The Family Perspective on Hospital to Home Transitions: A Qualitative Study *Pediatrics*	Solan et al. (2015)	Four main concepts identified: • "In a fog" (barriers to processing and acting on information) • "What I wish I had" (desired information and suggestions for improvement) • "Am I ready to go home" (discharge readiness) • "I am home, now what" (confidence and post discharge care)
Pediatric primary care providers' perspectives regarding hospital discharge communication: a mixed methods analysis. *Academic Pediatrics*	Leyenaar et al. (2015)	Five themes identified capturing: • problematic aspects of communication (written vs. oral communication and lack of having a standardized communication content, if using phone call, it was unclear who will call, when to call, etc.) • push/pull (conflicting expectations about a counterpart's role and responsibilities) • perception of providers roles • post discharge care • proposed solutions (use of standardized verbal and written communication templates, Resident training, timing of verbal communication, and tapping into technology e.g., smart phones, videoconferencing)
Caregiver perceptions of hospital to home transitions according to medical complexity: a qualitative study. *Academic Pediatrics*	Desai et al. (2016)	Development of a multidimensional theoretical framework representing caregivers needs and preferences for hospital to home transitions consisting of: • "self-efficacy" for home care management • comprehensive knowledge of the care plan, and • Adequate support and resources Discharge needs varied across medical complexity
How avoidable are hospitalizations for children with medical complexity? Understanding patient perspectives. *Academic Pediatrics*	Nelson et al. (2016)	Admission may not be avoidable. Parent's decision to seek urgent or emergent care, influenced by: • susceptibility and severity of illness • health system factors (access to care) • family capacity and resources (how and when to seek help /connect with parents facing similar issues
Families' priorities regarding hospital-to-home transitions for children with medical complexity. *Pediatrics*	Leyenaar et al. (2017)	Seven domains identified: • family engagement and normalization and routine (2 overarching domains) • hospital domains (3 domains): respect for families' discharge readiness, care coordination, efficient and timely discharge processes • home domains (2 domains): self-efficacy to support recovery, development, and pain control
Socioeconomic status influences the toll paediatric hospitalizations take on families. *BMJ Qual and Saf*	Beck et al. (2017)	Identified 3 themes related to socioeconomic status, which potentially modify the hospital to home transition experience: • logistical (disruption in home life, ability to adhere to discharge instructions) • emotional (overwhelming, exhausting experience) • financial (transportation and meal costs, missed work)

(Continued)

TABLE 11-1 Relevant Publications Regarding Pediatric Transitions of Care, Communication, Transport, and Discharge Planning (*Continued*)

Publication (Title and Source)	Author (Year)	Key Findings
Improvement Efforts to Enhance the Quality of Hospital-to-Home Transitions		
Hospitalists collaborate to improve timeliness of discharge communication. *Hospital Pediatrics*	Shen et al. (2013)	Multicenter QI grass roots collaborative • Main outcome documentation of hospitalist to PCP communication within 2 calendars days of discharge (through either e-mail, fax, or telephone call) • An improvement in the outcome from 75-85% was noted during the study period; For the 7 hospitals that were able to collect >16 weeks of data before July 2010, the mean rate of communication was >90%. • Improved perceptions of quality improvement knowledge among participants were noted as well
A quality improvement collaborative to improve the discharge process for hospitalized children. *Pediatrics*	Wu et al. (2016)	Intervention: Change Package (addressing discharge planning, quality of discharge instructions and providing post discharge support by phone) • Reduced number of discharge-related care failures on follow-up phone calls • Improved readiness for discharge • No change in readmission rates
Project IMPACT pilot report: feasibility of implementing a hospital-to-home transition bundle. *Pediatrics*	Mallory et al. (2017)	Intervention: 4-element discharge bundle Transition Checklist Teach-back Handoff to PCPs Follow-up phone call Improved caregivers teach-back of key home management skills on follow-up phone call No change in readmission rate
Post-discharge nurse home visits and reuse: the hospital to home outcomes (H2O) trial. *Pediatrics*	Auger et al. (2017)	Intervention: Children randomly assigned to receive a single nurse home visit or no visit • Parents in the intervention group recalled more red flags at 14 days, while post discharge coping scores and number of days until returning to a normal routine were similar • No difference in 30-day unplanned, urgent health care reuse (readmission, ER, or urgent care visit)-per protocol analysis • Increased reuse for patients who receive a single nurse home visit- in the intention to treat analysis
Factorial analysis quantifies the effects of pediatric discharge bundle on hospital readmission. *Pediatrics*	Osorio et al. (2021)	• Effect of bundle elements varied across medical complexity groups • The single most effective element in reducing readmissions was the checklist for children with no or a single chronic condition and teach-back for children with medical complexity • Combination of teach-back plus a checklist had the greatest effect on reducing readmissions.
Innovations in Care Transitions		
Hospital to home: a quality improvement initiative to implement high-fidelity simulation training for caregivers of children requiring long-term mechanical ventilation. *J Pediatr Nurs*	Thrasher et al. (2018)	Intervention: A multi-model discharge preparedness curriculum • Instructional videos, printed handouts, cardiopulmonary resuscitation training • Two mandatory high-fidelity simulation scenarios depicting tracheostomy and ventilatory emergencies • High-fidelity training was the most useful, while post-simulation debriefing was the most helpful element of this training program • Trend in reducing 7-day readmissions was noted
Implementation of a multidisciplinary discharge videoconference for children with medical complexity: a pilot study. *Pilot Feasibility Study*	Ravid NL et al. (2020)	Intervention: a multidisciplinary discharge videoconference for CMC (the patient, caregiver, hospitalist, care coordinator PCP, and possibly public nurse) • Low adoption of intervention • Potential benefits identified by family and providers included shared understanding of patients' care plan, transparency, humanization of the care handoff, and increased PCP comfort with care of CMC Barriers: technological (quality of Internet access in PCP offices), financial and time constraints (logistics of scheduling time for an important, but non-billable activity)
User-centered design of a longitudinal care plan for children with medical complexity. *J Am Med Inform Assoc*	Desai et al. (2020)	Designs sessions with caregivers of CMC and 5 groups of healthcare providers, identified 6 design preferences for longitudinal care plans for CMC: • a familiar yet customizable layout • a problem-based organization schema • linked content between sections • a table layout for most sections • a balance between unstructured and structured data fields • use of family-centered terminology

(*Continued*)

TABLE 11-1 Relevant Publications Regarding Pediatric Transitions of Care, Communication, Transport, and Discharge Planning (*Continued*)

Publication (Title and Source)	Author (Year)	Key Findings
Simulation-based discharge education program for caregivers of children with tracheostomies. *Hospital Pediatrics*	Yuen et al. (2021)	Intervention: Simulation discharge program • Single session of simulation-based education (SBE) to teach basic skills related to routine and emergency tracheostomy care • Peer-to-peer support by family advisors (volunteers who themselves have a technology-supported child and who are trained by social workers and child life specialist on how to provide support) during and for 6 months after the SBE session • Improved both, self-reported comfort and confidence and performance of tracheostomy skills.
Feasibility of post-hospitalization telemedicine video visits for children with medical complexity. *J Pediatr Health Care*	Ming et al. (2022)	Non-randomized pilot study assigned CMC to weekly telemedicine video visits for 4 weeks post hospitalization • Feasible (half of all video visits successfully connected in 1 min), majority of patients completed at least one video visit (82%) • Parents rated acceptability, usability, and experience of video visits highly. • Parental self-reports of self-efficacy and self-management, as well as healthcare utilization were similar in both video visit and control groups
Quality Measures to Assess Care Transition Quality		
Quality measures to assess care transitions for hospitalized children. *Pediatrics*	Leyenaar et al. (2016)	Development and field testing of 3 new pediatric medical records based quality measures at children's and community hospitals: • Family discharge instruction content • Timeliness of discharge communication between inpatient and outpatient providers • ICU-to-floor transition note quality Feasible to implement, but scores varied significantly across sites
Utilizing family-centered process and outcome measures to assess hospital-to-home transition quality *Academic Pediatrics*	Desai et al. (2018)	Summary of strengths and limitations of several family-centered process and outcome experience measures to assess hospital-to-home transition quality

family engagement, self-efficacy, and care coordination emerged as important factors for achieving seamless transitions. Several distinct needs and preferences have been identified for children with CMC, including having comprehensive discharge education, access to medical staff familiar with the patient's condition, hands-on approach to learning how to care for a device of a child who is technology-supported, and peer support. Furthermore, patients from marginalized communities have unique transition challenges in terms of their ability to access follow-up care and whether they have financial support, such as food security and adequate transportation, to optimize their child's recovery.

Several studies have also elicited medical providers' views on hospital-to-home transitions (see Table 11-1). This work describes numerous problems with hospital to PCP communication at the time of hospital discharge, including perceived devaluation of the PCP and uncertainty about post-discharge responsibilities. Although, the content and format of discharge communication with PCPs have been previously identified, medical providers have expressed a need for a structured discharge template to present this information clearly and consistently via the electronic medical record when available. This approach may improve the timeliness and receipt of discharge documents by PCPs. Furthermore, direct personal communication between hospitalists and PCPs by telephone, secure/encrypted email, or videoconferences has been identified as a potential solution to improve communication and increase access to hospital staff and information (see Table 11-1).

Altogether, this exploratory body of research is highly informative to design and test QI transition interventions.

IMPROVEMENT EFFORTS TO ENHANCE THE QUALITY OF HOSPITAL-TO-HOME TRANSITIONS

QI efforts initially focused on improving communication between inpatient and outpatient providers (see Table 11-1). However, mounting evidence in the adult and pediatric literature revealed that hospital-to-home transitions require complex interventions such as discharge bundles to impact change (see Table 11-1). These bundles consist of a combination of previously described factors known to influence transitions including communication between inpatient and outpatient providers, care coordination, and family engagement. For example, communication of changes in medical management during hospitalization, follow-up plans, and outstanding labs with outpatient providers is important. To facilitate care coordination tasks, some QI initiatives introduced checklists (see Table 11-1). Likewise, to engage families in the transition process required that interventions had a mechanism to address health literacy barriers and to ensure the use of the family's preferred language during hospitalization and at hospital discharge. QI and other research efforts demonstrate that pediatric discharge bundles are effective in improving patient-centered outcomes such as caregivers' readiness for discharge and the ability to teach-back key home management skills (see Table 11-1). However, the effect on healthcare reutilization as an outcome metric has been equivocal. Most studies reported no effects on readmission rates (see Table 11-1). In one randomized controlled trial, children randomly assigned to receive a single nurse home visit after discharge had higher odds of 30-day healthcare reutilization compared with those receiving standard care (see Table 11-1).

A recent study by the Improving Pediatric Patient-Centered Care Transitions (IMPACT) team, in which a retrospective factorial analysis was used to assess the individual and combined discharge bundle elements (checklist, teach-back, handoff to PCPs and follow-up phone call) on 30-day all-cause readmission rates further supported that discharge needs may vary based on medical complexity. For example, utilization of a checklist was the single most effective bundle element in reducing readmission rates for children with no chronic conditions or children with a single chronic condition, whereas a combination of checklist and teach-back was most effective for CMC including those who are technology-supported. The value of completing a coordination task by medical providers may only be realized when caregiver education is adequately ensured (e.g., using a checklist to document that feeding tube supplies have been delivered to home while providing education to caregivers on how to use feeding tube at home using teach-back). Taken together, research using either single or combined interventions as pediatric discharge bundles seem to indicate that "advanced/tailored" pediatric discharge bundles may be needed for CMC.

INNOVATION IN CARE TRANSITIONS

Interventions such as the use of telehealth and simulation-based education have emerged as transition interventions that may further assist caregivers' self-efficacy, access to care, and care coordination (see Table 11-1). During the Covid-19 pandemic, broad health system support and payer financing led to a massive scale-up in telehealth video visits. The content of these video visits can be developed using previously described preferences of families of CMC during hospital to home including review of medications, home equipment, and direct assessment of the patient home environment (see Table 11-1). Similarly, video teleconferencing prior to hospital discharge that includes caregivers, inpatient providers, PCP, and care coordinators can be used to address previously identified communication gaps occurring at and after hospital discharge. However, the use of telehealth may be limited based on patient access to adequate technology, internet connections, and digital literacy. Therefore, efforts to reduce the "digital divide" are integral to further reducing health disparities.

Lastly, drawing on the use of simulation in medical education and the desire from caregivers for hands-on training, simulation-based education (SBE) can be used to enhance existing patient education. For example, for caregivers of children with tracheostomies, this education can be tailored to address either basic skills in tracheostomy care or device-related emergencies (see Table 11-1). To further assist caregivers of CMC, SBE can be enhanced by partnering with a network of parents facing similar challenges (see Table 11-1). These complex interventions need to be tested on a larger scale using clinical trials or multicenter QI research collaboratives to demonstrate their efficacy in improving outcomes for CMC.

PROCESS AND OUTCOME MEASURES

A variety of transition process and outcome measures including prescription fills, medication-related adverse events, readiness for discharge, caregiver knowledge and/or experience, responsiveness to outstanding labs, implementation of a home health plan, receipt of information by PCP, patient mortality, health-related quality of life, and healthcare reutilization (i.e., returns to ED and planned/unplanned readmissions) have been used to measure the quality of transitions from hospital to home. While reducing hospital reutilization is a worthy effort that can only be adequately investigated via multi-center QI research collaboratives, measuring patient and caregivers' ability to manage diseases (e.g., self-efficacy, activation), medication adherence/safety, and caregiver's transition experiences may be more suitable outcomes to assess our efforts at creating seamless transitions (see Table 11-1).

CONCLUSIONS

Care transitions will continue to remain a top priority for pediatric hospitalists and a critical area for practitioners and investigators in the pediatric hospital medicine community to engage in rigorous QI and research to advance the implementation of evidence-based practices. Patients and families must remain at the center of these efforts to ensure improvements are targeted to meet their needs, enhance their experiences, and most importantly, promote patient safety across the care continuum.

SUGGESTED READINGS

Auger K. Simon T, Cooperberg D, et al. Summary of STARNet: Seamless Transitions and (RE) admissions Network. *Pediatrics*. 2015;135-164.

Beamon BD, Cortright LM, Pawlowski CB, et al. Communication between primary care pediatricians and the pediatric emergency department. *Pediatr Emerg Care*. 2021;37(2):92-95.

Coghlin DT, Leyenaar JK, Shen M, et al. Pediatric discharge content: a multisite assessment of physician preferences and experiences. *Hosp Pediatr*. 2014;4(1):9-15.

Hamline MY, Rosenthal JL. Interfacility transfers: a process ridden with improvement opportunities. *Hosp Pediatr*. 2020;10(2):195-197.

Heath J, Dancel R, Stephens JR. Postdischarge phone calls after pediatric hospitalization: an observational study. *Hosp Pediatr*. 2015;5(5): 241-248.

Herbst LA, Desai S, Benscoter D, et al. Going back to the ward-transitioning care back to the ward team. *Transl Pediatr*. 2018;7(4):314-325.

Kornburger, C, Gibon C, Sadowski S, at al. Using "Teach-Back" to promote a safe transition from hospital to home: an evidence based approach to improving the discharge process. *J Pediatr Nurs*. 2013; 28:282–291.

Leyenaar JK, Hill V, Lam V, et al; Committee on Hospital Care. Direct admission to hospital for children in the United States. *Pediatrics*. 2023;151(3):e2022060973.

Leyenaar JK, Shevenell M, Rizzo PA, et al. Multi-stakeholder informed guidelines for direct admission of children to hospital. *J Pediatr*. 2018;198:273-278.

Leyenaar JK, Bergert L, Mallory LA, et al. Pediatric primary care providers' perspectives regarding hospital discharge communication: a mixed methods analysis. *Acad Pediatr*. 2015;15(1):61-68.

Ong MS, Coiera E. A systematic review of failures in handoff communication during intrahospital transfers. *Jt Comm J Qual Patient Saf*. 2011;37(6):274-284.

Onofri A, Pavone M, De Santis S, et al. Telemedicine in children with medical complexity on home ventilation during the COVID-19 pandemic. *Pediatr Pulmonol*. 2021;56(6):1395-1400.

Schillinger D Piette J, Grumbach K, et al. Closing the loop: physician communication with diabetic patients who have low health literacy. *Arch Intern Med*. 2003;163: 83-90.

Snow V, Beck D, Budnitz T, Miller DC, et al. Transitions of care consensus policy statement American College of Physicians-Society of General Internal Medicine-Society of Hospital Medicine-American Geriatrics Society-American College of Emergency Physicians-Society of Academic Emergency Medicine. *J Gen Intern Med*. 2009; 24(8):971-976.

Starmer AJ, Spector ND, Srivastava R, et al.; I-PASS Study Group. Changes in medical errors after implementation of a handoff program. *N Engl J Med*. 2014;371(19):1803-1812.

Starmer AJ, Spector ND, Srivastava R, et al.; I-PASS Study Group. I-pass, a mnemonic to standardize verbal handoffs. *Pediatrics*. 2012;129(2):201-204.

Stroud MH, Trautman MS, Meyer K. Pediatric and neonatal interfacility transport: results from a National Consensus Conference. *Pediatrics*. 2013;132(2):359-366.

CHAPTER 12 Ethical Issues in Pediatric Hospital Practice

Henry T. Puls, MD and Jennifer E. deSante-Bertkau, MD, MBE

INTRODUCTION

The ethical dimensions of health and medicine pervade all aspects of clinical care. Pediatric hospitalists frequently encounter situations in which ethical considerations are vital, ranging from the routine task of obtaining parental permission for medical care to dilemmas regarding refusal of necessary care or requests for futile care. Competence in handling ethically problematic situations can be enhanced by expanding knowledge of ethical frameworks, learning how to approach ethical dilemmas common to the pediatric inpatient setting, and knowing which resources are available to help resolve ethical problems.

ETHICAL FRAMEWORKS

There are multiple different approaches to analyzing ethical conflicts and dilemmas. For some ethical dilemmas, application of more than one framework may be helpful. The four principles and casuistry are two of the more commonly used ethical frameworks; the best interest standard (BIS), satisficing parentalism, and the zone of parental discretion are three theories specific to parental medical decision-making.

FOUR BIOETHICAL PRINCIPLES

Beauchamp and Childress's frequently cited core principles of bioethics (beneficence, non-maleficence, autonomy, and justice) offer a framework for how to approach an ethical dilemma. These principles speak across different demographics, professions, and backgrounds because they are valued by many different moral traditions. *Beneficence* seeks to maximize the benefits caused by our actions, whereas *nonmaleficence* seeks to minimize the harm that our actions cause. *Autonomy* seeks to enable an individual's values to guide his or her medical care; respecting a patient's autonomy is a central way we respect their dignity. Given that most pediatric medical decisions are made by surrogate decision-makers, the application of autonomy is more complicated in pediatric medical ethics and will be discussed later. Considerations of *justice* involve how the care of one person fits into the larger system of the care of all persons. Understanding how these four core principles may conflict with one another in specific situations can help elucidate why different individuals may view ethical dilemmas in different ways and may serve as a starting point for discussion and resolution of conflict.

CASUISTRY

The casuist approach to bioethics is based on the belief that ethical guidance can be found by comparing a specific situation to a classic or ideal case. This approach evolved out of Aristotle's call for practical wisdom, which states that the ethical option depends on the specifics of the situation. Using a casuist approach, similar cases should have similar resolutions and different cases are treated differently. For example, if a family is requesting access to a costly treatment for their child, it is important to compare this case to prior cases where the treatment was approved or not. Examination of cases with different resolutions can identify key differences and clarify important ethical distinctions. A casuist approach allows for a degree of consistency in how ethical conflicts and dilemmas are handled. Unfortunately, a casuist approach requires that similar cases already exist for comparison. So while this framework can be beneficial in clinical practice, it has limitations when encountering unique situations.

BEST INTEREST STANDARD

Since most pediatric patients lack the capacity to be autonomous decision-makers, parents are frequently surrogate decision-makers providing permission for medical interventions. The considerations of beneficence and nonmaleficence carry more importance when surrogates are making medical decisions. The BIS states that the surrogate decision-maker should choose the treatment option that maximizes benefits and minimizes harms to the patient. The BIS demands a narrow focus; it does not allow the surrogate to consider how this decision affects other people, only the harms and benefits to the patient. The BIS has been criticized for lacking pragmatism by imposing unrealistic demands on parents, not respecting the family, and being too narrow in scope. However, the BIS grants the surrogate the capacity to evaluate the risks and benefits and gives the surrogate wide discretion in how to weigh them against each other.

SATISFICING PARENTALISM

Where the BIS demands that parents pursue what is "best" for a child irrespective of other interests, satisficing parentalism demands that parents only do what is "good enough" or satisfactory. While "good enough" may fall short of what many strive for, satisficing parentalism serves as a complementary framework for addressing some criticisms of the BIS. Disagreements often persist when reasonable minds disagree on what is "best" and which of the patient's interests should be prioritized. By not demanding the ideal, satisficing parentalism allows for a broader consideration of contextual factors, such as family values, societal resources and inequities, and cultural differences.

TABLE 12-1 Harm Principle Conditions for Justified State Interference with Parental Decision-Making

1. By refusing to consent are the parents placing their child at significant risk of serious harm?
2. Is the harm imminent, requiring immediate action to prevent it?
3. Is the intervention that has been refused necessary to prevent the serious harm?
4. Is the intervention that has been refused of proven efficacy, and therefore, likely to prevent the harm?
5. Does the intervention that has been refused by the parents not also place the child at significant risk of serious harm, and do its projected benefits outweigh its projected burdens significantly more favorably than the option chosen by the parents?
6. Would any other option prevent serious harm to the child in a way that is less intrusive to parental autonomy and more acceptable to the parents?
7. Can the state intervention be generalized to all other similar situations?
8. Would most parents agree that the state intervention was reasonable?

Source: Reproduced with permission from Diekema D. Parental refusals of medical treatment: The harm principle as a threshold for state intervention. *Theoretical Medicine and Bioethics*. 2004:25(4);252.

ZONE OF PARENTAL DISCRETION AND HARM PRINCIPLE

Parental authority is not absolute. How then do we determine the zone of parental discretion (i.e., the range of decisions parents may make for their children, even if they are perceived to be sub-optimal). The Harm Principle can help objectively delineate an extreme margin of parental discretion. Conceived by Diekema, the Harm Principle is an ethical framework for determining when state interference in parental decision-making is justified, specifically when parents refuse to consent for medical care (i.e., medical neglect) (**Table 12-1**). Generally, the Harm Principle calls for a significant and imminent risk of harm to the child without the recommended intervention, that the recommended intervention is able to prevent the imminent harm, that there are no other options less intrusive to parental authority, and that state intervention would be generalizable and perceived by most parents as reasonable. The Harm Principle echoes portions of the federal definition for child abuse and neglect, "an act or failure to act which presents an imminent risk of serious harm", (Diekema, 2004) which is not surprising given the narrow intent of the Harm Principle. Concepts derived from both the Harm Principle and the zone of parental discretion can be useful for determining when to supersede parental authority in a broader range of situations involving either refusals or demands for care (**Table 12-2**).

TABLE 12-2 Considerations for Determining the Permissibility of Parental Decision-Making and Actions

1. Does the parental decision or action (or inaction) place their child at significant risk of serious and imminent harm?
2. Would the recommended medical intervention decrease the risk of harm with reasonable side effects?
3. How certain are the outcomes both with and without the parental decision or action?
4. What are the practical harms associated with overriding parental authority and would they exceed the harms to the child if the parental decision were supported?
5. Does the parental decision realistically function to attain their goals of care?
6. Would superseding parental authority be defensible in all other similar situations?
7. What are the capacity, competence, and degree of emerging autonomy of the child and what is their opinion?
8. Are there acceptable, if less ideal, alternatives that have not been explored?

COMMON PEDIATRIC INPATIENT SITUATIONS

Although empiric estimates are lacking, our experience suggests that hospital-based pediatricians will encounter most or all the following situations.

DETERMINING DECISION-MAKING CAPACITY

When can an adolescent consent to medical care? The laws that govern this issue vary by state, so it is prudent to check with your hospital legal counsel. In general, persons are judged to be legally competent to consent to care when they are 18 years old or when they have been emancipated from parental authority by circumstances such as being married, being pregnant or having borne a child, or living on their own. In addition, adolescents seeking care for certain conditions (e.g., reproduction, emergencies, sexually transmitted diseases, or drug and alcohol abuse) may also be legally able to consent to treatment without parental permission.

Occasionally, pediatric hospitalists may care for patients 18 years or older who have questionable decision-making capacity (e.g., due to intellectual disability) or patients less than 18 years old who display characteristics that indicate they may have capacity. Hospitalists may be expected to assess their capacity for medical decision-making. Relevant criteria to be considered when determining decision-making capacity include (i) understanding of the indications, risks, benefits, and alternatives of the treatment; (ii) appreciation for how the treatment decision will affect their specific situation; (iii) evaluation of the treatment options; and (iv) the ability to communicate a choice consistently enough for it to be enacted. Decision-making capacity is a clinical assessment; competency is a legal determination. If a patient does not have decision-making capacity, the action required varies by institution and state; some states and hospitals have procedures to identify a surrogate, while others require a legally appointed guardian. In addition to assessing decision-making capacity, it is important to know whether the patient has been declared legally incompetent and, if so, who has been specified as the surrogate decision-maker through either guardianship or durable power of attorney.

OBTAINING PERMISSION, ASSENT, OR CONSENT

According to American Academy of Pediatrics (AAP) Policy, there are three important processes by which parents or patients agree that the patient will receive certain medications, tests, or procedures. *Informed permission* is used when a pediatric patient lacks the necessary decision-making capacity and legal empowerment to make an autonomous decision, requiring the parent or designated surrogate to do so. *Assent* is sought when a child or adolescent has some ability to participate in medical decision-making but is not yet legally empowered to consent. *Informed consent* is used when an adolescent or young adult has legal authority to make decisions regarding his or her healthcare. Many states have "mature minor" statutes, which allow a judge to rule that a minor may make a legally binding decision regarding their own medical care.

The processes of obtaining informed permission and informed consent include four key components as described by Faden: (i) appropriate disclosure of information, (ii) adequate personal understanding of the information, (iii) emotional capacity to decide, and (iv) voluntariness or freedom from coercion. The process of seeking assent translates these elements into a developmental framework applicable to pediatric patients.

Adolescents should participate in their medical decision-making to the extent that they are able and interested in doing so. Compared to adults, adolescents have a limited capacity to evaluate risk, a lack of experience to inform their decisions, and a decreased ability to make voluntary decisions outside of external influence. However, involving adolescents in their medical decisions recognizes their developing autonomy, generates buy-in with their plan of care, and reduces potential psychological distress about a lack of control over their body. It is important to consider the urgency, risks, and benefits of the proposed treatment; in general, adolescents cannot dissent to life-sustaining treatment.

Necessary medical care should not be withheld because of a lack of consent if the care is likely to prevent serious harm. No evaluation of a life-threatening or emergent condition should be delayed because of a perceived problem with consent. Additionally, a parent's act of leaving his or her child with another custodian or the state may represent implied consent when the parent is not immediately available for verbal consent and nonelective medical care is needed. These situations are limited to scenarios where "the child is suffering from an emergent condition that places his or her life or health in danger." (Committee on Pediatric Emergency Medicine and Committee on Bioethics, 2011)

DISCLOSURE AND CONFIDENTIALITY

Hospitalists may encounter parents who do not want their children to be informed of a serious diagnosis or complex treatment plan. While parents may be trying to protect their children from psychological and emotional suffering by limiting disclosure of medical information, clinicians are required to be truthful in all patient discussions. There are benefits to the children of being informed about their diagnoses. For instance, children who are informed of their diagnoses and treatment plans often cope better compared to children who do not know their diagnoses. In addition, disclosure to the child may increase their adherence to the treatment plan. It is also important to consider the improbability of limiting discussions of medical information, and the associated risk of accidental disclosure, within large healthcare systems. Finally, if a child learns about medical information that has been kept from them, this can cause long-term damage to the child's trust in the healthcare system.

Hospitalists frequently wish to protect confidentiality when discussing health concerns with adolescent patients but need to understand that there are ethical and legal exceptions to patient-doctor confidentiality, including cases of abuse and the risk of harm to self or others. In addition, while pediatric hospitalists should do their best to protect a patient's confidentiality, it may be practically difficult to guarantee confidentiality in age of electronic records, insurance billing, and integrated healthcare systems.

FUTILITY AND POTENTIALLY INAPPROPRIATE TREATMENTS

Parents sometimes want an increased level of technologic support for their child beyond what healthcare providers believe to be medically appropriate or in the child's best interests. This may be stated as wanting to "do everything." Futility is often invoked as an argument against these escalations in care. However, many ethicists and medical societies discourage invoking futility arguments when determining ethical obligations or making clinical decisions. This is due to the lack of consensus definition for futility, the degrees of prognostic uncertainty, the fact that decisions are often value-based, and the clinicians' propensity for bias and underestimation of quality of life among children with medical complexity. Instead, the Society for Critical Care Medicine recommends that interventions should be withheld when they are potentially inappropriate, or "when there is no reasonable expectation that the patient will improve sufficiently to survive outside the acute care setting, or when there is no reasonable expectation that the patient's neurologic function will improve sufficiently to allow the patient to perceive the benefits of the treatment."[16] Consensus concerning the appropriateness of a medical intervention should be sought amongst the healthcare team—inclusive of multiple specialties and non-physician members of the team—based upon medical standards of care and legal precedent specific to the scenario. If the healthcare team cannot reach consensus on the appropriateness of an intervention, then that decision likely falls under the zone of parental discretion. If the healthcare team reaches consensus that a requested intervention is inappropriate, efforts should be focused on improving communication with the family, delineating goals of care, and exploring the family's values as poor communication often fuels such disputes. Failure to reach consensus at any stage of these processes may be a good indication for requesting an ethics consult.

PARENTAL REFUSAL OF CARE

In contrast to futile treatment disputes, parents sometimes refuse care that the healthcare team perceives to be necessary, perhaps instead seeking complementary and alternative therapies. In general, parental authority should be respected, so long as parents are working toward their child's interests and parental decisions do not pose a significant and imminent risk to the child. It is the policy of the AAP that all children deserve effective medical treatment that is likely to prevent substantial harm, suffering, or death. It is under this framework that the AAP supports tolerance of complementary and alternative medicine (except when the therapies both lack efficacy and are believed to be unsafe) but does not support the withholding of lifesaving blood products.

FORGOING LIFE-SUSTAINING TREATMENT

There is strong consensus within the medical ethics community that foregoing life-sustaining treatment is an ethically permissible act when the treatment no longer increases the likelihood of accomplishing the patient's therapeutic goals. There is no salient ethical difference between withholding (i.e., never starting) and withdrawing (i.e., stopping) treatment. Rather these decisions exist on a timeline during which parents can provide and retract consent for care.

Although widely held as ethically permissible and not dissimilar to the forgoing of other life-sustaining treatments, some healthcare professionals may feel less comfortable with forgoing medically provided nutrition and hydration, particularly for children who cannot consent for themselves. The AAP argues that intravenous infusions and tube feedings are no different from other forms of therapy that competent patients or their authorized surrogates have the right to refuse if the expected burden of the intervention to the patient exceeds the potential benefit. Healthcare providers should feel empowered to conscientiously object to providing care that they find conflicts with their own moral integrity, so long as they meet their professional duties by being transparent, they provide all relevant and legal treatment options as part of the informed-consent process, and their abstaining does not increase the probability of mortality or serious morbidity.

SOCIAL JUSTICE AND INDIVIDUAL DECISION-MAKING

Social justice, including the unequal distribution of social determinants of health and access to resources that positively impact health, is a critically important issue in pediatric hospital practice. At times, ethical decision-making for individual children exposes and perpetuates these inequalities. For instance, it is common, but not universal, practice to require two caregivers at home for children with a tracheostomy and if not available, seek alternative care through foster care or a long-term care facility. While requiring two caregivers is, in theory, clinically reasonable and prioritizes that individual child's safety, such a requirement may disproportionately impact populations with less social capital and connectivity, including single-parent households. While hospitalists should be mindful of these types of situations, advocate for social change at the institutional and societal level and feel empowered to be creative in conceiving unique safe discharge plans for individual families, it is advisable to keep the individual patient's needs central during the decision-making process for each patient.

KEY RESOURCES

When confronting ethically problematic situations, most pediatric physicians can draw on valuable resources within their hospitals.

KEY PEOPLE

To improve communication, build shared understanding, clarify goals, generate novel solutions, or mediate disputes, physicians may turn to professional interpreters, social workers, nurses, pastoral care staff, palliative care team members, legal counsel, mediators, or other physicians with particular skills in these areas.

INSTITUTIONAL ETHICS COMMITTEES

Institutional ethics committees develop or review hospital policies, perform clinical ethics consultations, and educate healthcare professionals and patients. Seven principles guide the process of ethics consultation (**Table 12-3**).

TABLE 12-3 Principles of Ethics Consultations

1. Any patient, parent or guardian, or family member can initiate an ethics consultation.
2. The patient and parent or guardian can refuse to participate in an ethics consultation.
3. The refusal of a patient or parent or guardian to permit an ethics consultation does not hinder the ability of an ethics committee to provide consultation services to physicians, nurses, and other concerned staff.
4. Any physician, nurse, or other healthcare provider involved in the care of the patient can request an ethics consultation without fear of reprisal.
5. The process of ethics consultation is open to all persons involved in the patient's care but is conducted in a manner that respects patient and family confidentiality.
6. Anonymous requests for ethics consultation are not accepted in the absence of an identified person who is willing to speak to the issue being raised.
7. The primary care pediatrician is invited to participate in the consultation to support existing physician–family relationships.

LEGALITY AND HOSPITAL POLICY

An ethical assessment can be rendered independent of legal considerations, but clinical practice must operate within the confines of the law. Pediatrics hospitalists should be familiar with their local and state laws on important topics, such as age of consent, reproductive health, and definitions and reporting requirements for child abuse and neglect. Hospital policy may also provide specific instructions regarding the issue at hand. For instance, hospitals typically provide guidance about when the general consent for care granted by a parent at the time of admission is inadequate and specific parental permission to perform certain diagnostic or therapeutic procedures must be obtained and documented. Such rules and policies can often be found in the medical staff bylaws or in national guidelines published by the AAP, American Medical Association, or other organizations.

SUGGESTED READINGS

American Academy of Pediatrics, Committee on Bioethics. Informed consent in decision-making in pediatric practice. *Pediatrics.* 2016; 138(2).

American Academy of Pediatrics, Committee on Bioethics. Informed consent, parental permission, and assent in pediatric practice. *Pediatrics.* 1995;95:314-317. [This policy was reaffirmed in *Pediatrics* 2012; 130(2):e467-8.]

American Academy of Pediatrics, Committee on Bioethics. Institutional ethics committees. *Pediatrics.* 2001;107:205-209. [A revision of this policy was published in Pediatrics 2019;143(5):e20190659].

American Academy of Pediatrics, Committee on Bioethics. Religious objections to medical care. *Pediatrics.* 1997;99:279-281.

Appelbaum PS. Assessment of patients' competence to consent to treatment. *N England J Med.* 2007;357:1834-1840.

Beauchamp TL, Childress JF. *Principles of Biomedical Ethics.* 6th ed. Oxford: Oxford University Press; 2009.

Bioethics Case Based Teaching Guides for Resident Training. https://www.aap.org/en/learning/bioethics-case-based-teaching-guides-for-resident-training/. Published August 24, 2021. Accessed July 28, 2022.

Blustein J. Doing the best for one's Child: satisficing versus optimizing parentalism. *Theor Med Bioeth.* 2012;33(3):199-205.

Committee on Pediatric Emergency Medicine and Committee on Bioethics. Consent for emergency medical services for children and adolescents. *Pediatrics.* 2011;128(2):427-433.

Diekema D. Parental refusals of medical treatment: the harm principle as threshold for state intervention. *Theor Med Bioeth.* 2004;25(4):243-264.

Diekema DS, Botkin JR, American Academy of Pediatrics Committee on Bioethics. Clinical report—forgoing medically provided nutrition and hydration in children. *Pediatrics.* 2009;124(2):813-822.

Diekema DS, Mercurio MR, Adam MB. *Clinical Ethics in Pediatrics: A Case-Based Textbook.* Cambridge: Cambridge University Press; 2011.

Fins JJ, Solomon MZ. Communication in intensive care settings: the challenge of futility disputes. *Crit Care Med.* 2001;29(2 Suppl):N10-N15.

Gillam L. The zone of parental discretion: an ethical tool for dealing with disagreement between parents and doctors about medical treatment for a child. *Clinical Ethics*. 2015;11(1):1-8.

Kemper KJ, Vohra S, Walls R. The use of complementary and alternative medicine in pediatrics. *Pediatrics*. 2008;122(6):1374-1386.

Kon AA, Shepard EK, Sederstrom NO, et al. Defining futile and potentially inappropriate interventions. *Crit Care Med*. 2016;44(9):1769-1774.

Lantos JD, Singer PA, Walker RM, et al. The illusion of futility in clinical practice. *Am J Med*. 1989;87(1):81-84.

Lo B. *Resolving Ethical Dilemmas: A Guide for Clinicians*. Philadelphia: Wolters Kluwer/Lippincott Williams & Wilkins; 2009.

Salter EK. Deciding for a child: a comprehensive analysis of the best interest standard. *Theor Med Bioeth*. 2012;33(3):179-198.

Weise KL, Okun AL, Carter BS, Christian CW, committee on Bioethics, Section on Hospice and Palliative Medicine, Committee on Child Abuse and Neglect. Guidance on forgoing life-sustaining medical treatment. *Pediatrics* September 2017;140(3):e20171905.

Weise KL, Okun AL, Carter BS, et al. Guidance on forgoing life-sustaining medical treatment. *Pediatrics*. 2017;140(3).

CHAPTER 13 Medicolegal Issues in Pediatric Hospital Medicine

Craig H. Gosdin, MD, MSHA and W. Michelle Terry, MD

INTRODUCTION

Pediatric hospital medicine providers participate in complex medical care and make critical decisions for hospitalized pediatric patients. Over the last two decades, hospitalists have become integral to hospital quality and efficiency outcomes and are clinical leaders within the hospitals and health systems. Specifically, hospitalists participate in the planning and implementation of modern medical practices along with discerning the investigation of past medical errors; educating trainees of multiple specialties; and promoting patient safety via continuous quality improvement efforts.

There has not been much data published regarding claims against board-certified pediatric hospitalists. In general, patients are less likely to sue pediatricians versus other specialists, however they have the highest average indemnity payment of all specialties. Among all pediatricians, hospital-based pediatric specialists are more likely to be sued than non-hospital-based specialists, or general pediatricians. Hospitalists may reduce malpractice claims by improving the delivery of efficient, evidence-based, high-value care that results in patient and family satisfaction.

Physicians may face legal action when pediatric patients in their care have bad medical outcomes, especially when a physician deviates from published guidelines or published clinical policies. When a lawsuit is instituted, the plaintiff must show that the physician had a duty to the patient, breached that duty, and did not meet the standard of care, which refers to the degree of care a prudent and reasonable person would exercise under the circumstances. The plaintiff must then show that this breach caused damage or injury to the patient. Certain hospital processes and situations pose a particular risk for allegations of negligence among hospitalists, including topics involving communication, informed consent, refusal of care, medical record documentation, use of consultant opinions, treatment of incidental findings, patient confidentiality, and coordination of care for a safe discharge from the hospital. The legal obligations surrounding each of these situations are described in this chapter.

COMMUNICATION AND DEVELOPING A THERAPUETIC ALLIANCE

Effective communication between a pediatric hospitalist, patient, and the parent or guardian is an essential component of patient and family satisfaction. Patients and their family must perceive a caring attitude, openness, professional integrity, and a commitment to standards of excellence in patient care. In contrast, poor communication can lead to frustration, omission, or distortion of essential information, and may result in patient harm. A direct relationship between effective communication skills and fewer malpractice allegations has been described in prior review of claims. For instance, families that sue physicians after infants suffered permanent injury or death are often dissatisfied with physician-patient communication with expressed concerns that physicians would not listen, would not talk openly, attempted to mislead them, or did not warn them about the possibility of long-term neurodevelopmental problems.

In addition, physicians must develop and maintain a therapeutic alliance with patients and families. Patients and families are not always aware of the physician's credentials and experience, however they are keenly aware of time spent with them and the physician's demeanor in conversation. Families remember how the doctor looked, acted, spoke, and listened; whether the doctor was neatly dressed; and whether the doctor was pleasant or disinterested, serious or cavalier, respectful or condescending, and polite or discourteous. Nonverbal communication such as good eye contact and relaxed body language are also important. Pediatric hospitalists have multiple opportunities to interact and optimize the relationship their relationship with families during an admission. Establishing good rapport with the patient's family can sometimes be difficult, yet it is nonetheless essential to providing optimal care for the patient. Families who have been economically marginalized by society and/or do not speak English as their preferred language may need more time to develop a therapeutic alliance, based on historical experiences.

Pediatric hospital medicine providers must also establish rapport with the patient. It is best to avoid casual teasing or joking, in conversation; One should also refrain from talking about the patient without attempting to include the patient who is able participate in the conversation. Sensitivity to patient modesty and dignity must always be maintained with the assurance of adequate personal privacy, and well-maintained and equipped hospital rooms with appropriate supplies for examination and treatment. In addition, and sheets should be available to the patient. Age-appropriate communication is also important, coupled with the knowledge that young children usually understand far more than may be spoken. Pediatric hospitalists with effective communication skills are flexible, open, and affirming, and pause for questions and freely offer statements of clarification.

Patient- and family-centered care, including rounding with families and patients, enhances communication and may reduce medical errors. An American Academy of Pediatrics (AAP) policy statement recommends that providers conduct rounds either within or just outside of the patient rooms with parents or guardians present. During patient and family-centered rounds, the inpatient team introduces themselves to the patient and family and includes their role on the healthcare team (Chapter 5).

In addition to the patient and family, communication needs to include everyone on the medical staff involved in the patient's care, including medical and surgical residents and fellows, nursing, allied professional staff, and consulting physician specialists. The members of the medical team have important roles in the care of hospitalized patients and respectful communication is essential, particularly when discussing a variation in the plan of care. Effective communication between the primary care physician and the hospitalist is also crucial. Retrospective studies of medical negligence cases often reveal a breakdown in the patient-physician relationship. Perceived communication problems included the perception that physicians were not listening to the patients' and parents' concerns, did not talk openly, did not speak of complications, or failed to mention long-term sequelae to the disease. Optimally, communication between medical staff and primary care physicians should include information about necessary procedures, suspected diagnoses, and the child's overall progress, because if allegations of negligence are made, sometimes discovery reveals that the medical teams had differing opinions, or advocated for different treatment plans, and subsequently did not reach agreement on the patient's medical plan amongst themselves. In cases when multiple medical specialists are involved, scheduling "provider only" in person conferences to discuss patient treatment options and resolve differences in care preferences may facilitate consensus in medical management. In addition, specialty teams should plan to round together in the presence of the family to show alignment of medical planning and reinforce shared communication. On hospital services where many medical staff members are involved in the care of extended stay patients; a continuity provider may be identified to monitor care progression and serve as a resource for the family. Additionally, it is important to provide updates to the patient's primary care provider and encourage the PCP to ask questions directly to the inpatient medical team; this communication is ideally done by either telephone or secure videoconferencing. The primary care medical team may help to provide important contextual history. If the family and medical teams cannot reach agreement on the plan of care using standard medical practices, an ethics consult may be helpful to identify, analyze, and help resolve the challenges presented.

Conflicts may arise when patients and families disagree with the medical treatment plan. For instance, a family may insist on tests, medications, or procedures that fall outside of evidence-based practice. In this circumstance, hospitalists must thoughtfully explain why such tests, medications, or procedures are not necessary to make a diagnosis and/or explain the risks and consequences of obtaining unnecessary laboratory and radiologic studies. Family conferences with the medical teams involved in the care, with support from a nurse case manager, social worker, or cultural navigator are preferred in these circumstances. Patient satisfaction with care is not necessarily tied to the treatment received but rather to the patient's perception of the amount of time the physicians spent explaining the illness, and the family's understanding of the diagnosis and treatment plan.

In some cases, communication with a parent may become particularly difficult. For example, a parent may predictably become angry and/or uncooperative when child welfare services begin an investigation because of specific medical findings. In all states, medical providers are considered "mandatory reporters" of suspected child abuse and neglect and are legally compelled to notify authorities of the suspicion of abuse or neglect found in children. In this situation, medical staff may acknowledge the stress that the family may feel, however state that their professional responsibility is to the child. Pediatric hospital medicine providers must also be aware that beginning in 2016, with rulemaking completed in 2022, the 21st Century Cures Act requires healthcare organizations give patients unrestricted access to their electronic medical records. Brief, pertinent notes that use accurate descriptions of the patient's medical condition and plan of care with neutral language may help to mitigate possible chart note misinterpretation. If a note must be amended or changed, please make note of the reason the note signed note is being altered. Electronic medical records keep track of all input to the patient's record and the metadata is often useful in litigation because it usually includes information when a document was created, edited and/or accessed, the documents' author(s), and all previous versions of the document, may be reviewed during legal proceedings.

An undesired outcome—even if inevitable—coupled with the parents' feeling that the physician was rushed or was not interested in the child may provoke an allegation of negligence. Thus, when meeting with families, it is advisable for the providers to introduce themselves by name and role, make sure the hospital badge is visible, hold the conversation in a private and quiet setting, and spend time asking open-ended questions. This expression of courtesy gives the parents the message that, at least for the next few minutes, they have your undivided attention, no matter how many other children are in the hospital. The perception of the time spent with the patient is doubled when a physician sits down in the presence of the patient. Finally, if a medical error is made, it is important to disclose what happened to the patient's parents/guardians as soon as it is feasible to do so while following published hospital policies and procedures. It is also important to explain to the parents/guardians about your plans to include hospital-level experts in patient safety to investigate the situation and improve processes.

Pediatric hospital medicine providers may endorse the utilization of all available resources to navigate difficult and important discussions with patients and families. Most hospitals employ patient advocates and social workers who can help clinicians effectively communicate with families, especially if the patient's parents/guardians have demonstrated frustration or significant stressors. Primary care physicians may also provide invaluable help in communicating with families in situations. In addition, consultation with the medical ethics service can help in defining common goals between the patient, family, and medical team, and lead to better communication in high acuity and high complexity cases.

INFORMED DECISION-MAKING AND INFORMED CONSENT

Prior to performing a procedure or treatment, it is necessary for patients and their families to know the diagnosis, the nature and purpose of the proposed treatment or procedure, the risks, consequences and side effects of the proposed procedure, reasonably available alternatives and their risks, and the anticipated prognosis without treatment. The medical provider obtaining informed consent must be from the medical or surgical service performing the procedure, and the parent or guardian authorizing the procedure must be given time to ask questions. If the patient, parent, or guardian's preferred language is not English, the medical provider must obtain informed consent via a certified language interpreter in the patient's preferred language to ensure that the patient, parent, or guardian understands the information presented. Federal and state regulations require healthcare organizations to provide trained interpreters for patients with limited English proficiency (LEP), a patient's family member is not an acceptable substitute for a certified language interpreter because of risk of conflict of interest, because a close family member may not translate all of the discussion accurately, and/or may omit medical information. A healthcare system must have a policy for medical interpretation and provide a combination of in person, video, and audio interpretation options that are available 24 hours per day on demand to communicate with patients and families.

Parents should have the opportunity to ask questions about the proposed treatment or procedure. **Table 13-1** summarizes procedures for assisting parents with informed decision-making. Parents have the right to be informed about their child's medical care and to give consent for treatment. Although adults may refuse treatment—even life-sustaining treatment—for themselves, it is not always the same for their children. For instance, if parents are determined to be neglectful or abusive, the courts can relieve them of medical decision-making and, if necessary, custody.

The following scenarios are common to hospitalists:

- In a true emergency, such as unconscious, severely injured, or toxic-appearing patients, informed consent prior to a procedure or treatment is not necessary. In this scenario, treating without consent is appropriate, rather than failing to provide reasonable treatment without informed consent.
- In a non-life saving scenario, informed consent for blood products should include a person legally designated to provide informed consent. In addition to complications from blood transfusions, some families have a religious objection to the use of blood products, which left unconsidered may be viewed as negligence in a non-life-threatening situation.
- In many states, adolescents may make decisions regarding mental healthcare, substance abuse treatment, and reproductive healthcare without a parent or guardian's knowledge or informed consent. In other states just the opposite is true, and parents must be informed if minor children seek certain healthcare services. It is essential that physicians are familiar with state laws to protect patient confidentiality to abide by legal statutes.

TABLE 13-1 Responsibilities for Informed Decision-Making (Informed Consent)

Assess the patient's or guardian's decision-making capacity
Provide the patient and guardian with appropriate information
Diagnosis
Nature of procedure or intervention
Purpose of procedure or treatment
Risks and benefits of procedure or treatment
Alternative treatments and associated risks and benefits
Prognosis with and without treatment
Assess the patient's or guardian's comprehension of the discussion
Ensure that the decision is made freely, not coerced
After the discussion, obtain signed consent

- Among patients undergoing an evaluation for sepsis, parents may have misperceptions about the lumbar puncture procedure employed when a diagnosis of meningitis is suspected, hospitalists should carefully explain the techniques involved in obtaining cerebral spinal fluid (CSF) and inform parents/guardians of the imprecision of the alternative treatment plan. If there is no signed informed consent document, and subsequently the CSF sample is not obtained, broad-spectrum antibiotic treatments should be initiated.

Consent forms are widely used at most hospitals and should be written at an appropriate comprehension level for most patients or parents. Although parents usually sign a general consent form at the time of presentation to the hospital that allows for a standard medical evaluation and treatment of the child, this document does not include informed consent for all treatments and medical and/or surgical procedures. It is possible that a patient or parent may claim that the risks and benefits of treatments and procedures were not adequately explained days or weeks into a hospitalization, and lack of recall may be worse under emotional stress. A signed consent form provides some legal protection, but clear documentation in the medical record, noting what was explained to the parent/guardian, is also essential.

Not all decisions by a parent or guardian are completely free of outside influences. Most parents need and want the physician's opinion to help them decide what is best for their child. Physicians have an ethical obligation to include patients in the discussion of proposed treatments or procedures, and obtain assent to care, if possible.

REFUSAL OF CARE

Despite all efforts, some patients, parents, or guardians refuse treatment or leave the hospital against medical advice (AMA). Emancipated minors have the right to refuse treatment for themselves or their child. Some may wish to leave the hospital because they are frustrated about a long wait for medical treatment, fear a prolonged or expensive hospitalization, or anticipate unnecessary and painful procedures for themselves or their child. Other patients, parents, or guardians are afraid to learn of a serious diagnosis, have competing responsibilities outside the hospital, or maybe less trusting of a hospitalist physician with whom they do not have a previous medical connection. However, an AMA discharge may result in persistent or worsening symptoms from an undertreated medical problem. Further, the hospital and physicians may be subjected to a lawsuit if the patient suffers serious morbidity or dies, even if the patient, parent, or guardian signed out AMA.

Hospitalists should attempt to keep the patient from leaving the hospital prematurely by inquiring and documenting the reasons the patient, parent, or guardian wish to leave the hospital. It is important for the hospitalist to remain courteous, concerned, and flexible with the treatment plan, in addition to maintaining excellent communication skills (e.g., allowing the parent/guardian to express concerns without interruption). Challenging parents/guardians to leave the inpatient setting AMA, or a threat to call hospital security officers is not an acceptable course of action. The duties of a hospital security officer are to protect staff, patients, and visitors while ensuring that the hospital property is secure. It is not the job of the hospital security officer to enforce a proposed medical treatment plan for a patient.

If a parent or guardian wishes to leave the hospital despite all efforts to reach an agreement, a statement releasing the doctor and the hospital from all liability should be signed by the parents/guardian prior to their departure. Although such signed documents may have limited legal usefulness because parents can later claim that they did not fully understand the risks involved in leaving AMA. However, a signed statement witnessed by one or two staff members may transfer some responsibility to the parent or guardian in the event of an adverse medical outcome. If the patient or parent/guardian decides to leave the hospital AMA, staff should make reassurances that they can always return to the hospital for reevaluation if they change their minds or if the patient's condition worsens.

Hospitalists and medical staff must document in the patient's medical record the medical care provided for the patient and the discussion of AMA discharge in detail. For instance, good documentation would include physical exam findings, the impression of what tests or treatment are needed, the parents' stated reason to leave AMA, a detailed explanation of the risks of refusing treatment, alternative care options, and the guidance to return to the hospital with worsening symptoms. These steps and documentation reflect a sincere interest in the patient. The AMA designation is used in part to provide documentation if a patient becomes sicker and needs readmission or seeks care at another health facility.

In some situations, the patient cannot be permitted to leave the hospital under any circumstances. If the parent or guardian is disoriented or intoxicated and cannot understand the consequences of refusing care, the patient should not leave the hospital until they can make informed decisions. In cases of a true emergency or if sustained treatment for a life-threatening condition is needed, hospitalists are obligated to provide prompt medical intervention even if the parent or guardian objects to the medical care or the person providing care. Similarly, if child abuse is suspected and the perpetrator is unknown, the patient should not be released from the hospital without the assistance of child social services to determine a safe discharge plan. In caring for a seriously ill child where deterioration is imminent, and the child may suffer severe morbidity or death without medical intervention a social services worker may be helpful in discerning the course of action. It is possible that engagement with hospital counsel, administrators, local law enforcement, and a judge via an emergency call to seek a verbal temporary medical hold (depending on the relevant state statutes) may be necessary. All conversations should be documented within the patient's medical record, including the specific actions authorized. Note that the procedure to obtain court permission to treat a child may vary in different locales; hospitalists should utilize the hospital's legal counsel when indicated to determine specific rules, regulations, and laws that apply to a particular situation.

MEDICAL RECORD DOCMENTATION

Clear, concise, and precise medical record documentation is important. Many years may pass before a physician is advised of malpractice litigation, due to the extended statute of limitation for children (i.e., typically three years past age 18 years). The patient's chart is always the first document reviewed by parents, attorneys, and their consulting physicians. A record that demonstrates thorough examination and testing may avoid a lawsuit at the outset. Likewise, a record that does not demonstrate conclusively whether an important test or portion of the examination was negative or positive may lead counsel to assume that it was not done. Many settlements have been offered even when good medical care was rendered but not substantiated in the medical records.

Common issues that arise during medico-legal review of Hospitalist malpractice cases include:

- Failure to include a differential diagnosis, including the clinical reasoning why certain diagnoses are less likely at the time of admission
- Failure to document clinical thought process, particularly in complex cases
- Failure to document requests for consultation and discussions with consultants
- Lacking the medical necessity for lab and radiology orders
- Failure to document procedures
- Allergies, particularly to medicines

The medical record will become public record if a lawsuit is filed. Therefore, only comments that one would be comfortable to read in front of a jury should be documented in the medical record. In situations where Electronic medical records (EMR) is not available, illegible records can compromise the quality of care and make the hospitalist appear unprofessional.

EMR are widely used in hospitals across the United States and may decrease malpractice claim payments because, if properly organized, EMRs are more complete than written records. However, errors may occur when physicians are not mindful while the temptation to copy and paste patient histories instead of taking new histories risks missing current information and perpetuates previous errors. EMRs may also affect the progression of malpractice litigation by increasing the availability of documentation with which to both defend or prove a malpractice claim.

If a physician needs to make a correction to the medical record, do so in a timely way. For hand-written notes, an amendment would be accomplished by drawing a single line through the error, with a hospitalist initial and date of correction. Within the EMR, hospitalists may be able to revise the record, or add an addendum. EMR record all electronic transactions. This metadata provides a permanent electronic footprint that tracks physician activity. Metadata validates that the electronic medical record was modified when the treatment was administered, bolstering the defendant's ability to rely on the electronic medical record when defending against a malpractice allegation. Alternatively, if the record was revised at a time incongruous to the treatment, metadata can raise a suspicion of falsification of the medical record, even in the absence of actual wrongdoing.

While discoverable in civil trials under federal law, metadata discoverability varies under state law which administers most malpractice litigation. Medical staff should never attempt to make changes to or alter in any way the medical record after the case is involved in litigation. It is likely that any change made to the record will be discovered and will be viewed as deliberate and dishonest. Especially for EMR, it is easy to determine when a late entry into the chart was made. In general, it is easier to defend missing facts or a poor record than an altered one. Credibility is a key factor in any litigation, and an altered record impugns physician's credibility. When there is a need to expand upon clinical information after an untoward event occurs, it is better to do so in a confidential communication to the physician's attorney rather than adding to the chart.

Besides resulting in the loss of a lawsuit, tampering with the record may have other consequences, including the award of "punitive damages," to cite the physician for attempting to mislead the court, or in certain states it may be considered a criminal offense. Further, malpractice policies may deny coverage if it is determined that medical records were altered to change the narrative.

State laws vary on the length of time a medical record must be retained. Guidelines state that medical records should be kept for at least ten years from the date of a patient's last visit, prescription refill, telephone contact, test or other patient contact; 21 years from the date of a minor patient's birth; six years from the date of a patient's death; or indefinitely, if the practitioner has reason to believe the patient is incompetent; there are any problems with a patient's care, or the patient may be involved in litigation. Again, in the case of an EMR, a patient's medical chart may be archived and kept indefinitely.

CONSULTANTS

No physician in the hospital works in isolation. There is often a need to consult with the primary care physician, critical care specialists, surgeons, and other physicians while caring for ill children. The hospitalist should call for consultation when the care required is beyond their scope of expertise or when another opinion will be helpful. Hospitalists should contact the consultant about the clinical concern or question, discuss the expected time and modality for the consultation (e.g., if the consultation is needed urgently or in person), and document this communication in the patient chart. Failure to consult appropriately and in a timely manner can result in an allegation of negligence should there be a poor outcome. Further, if the family insists on consultation or a second opinion (e.g., a plastic surgeon to suture a facial laceration), it is wise to comply if the request is reasonable. Last, radiology consultation ensures optimal reading of a film. If the hospitalist misreads a child's radiograph if a radiologist was available, there may be liability. The hospitalist is not held to the same standard as a radiologist, but rather whatever expertise the jury believes the hospitalist should possess.

In most instances the hospitalist will have time to compose to interview the patient and family and complete the medical database prior to consulting a specialist. However, in a true emergency, such as a surgical abdomen or an airway emergency, the hospitalist should consult specialist promptly. If the consultant does not arrive in a timely manner, consider transferring the child to another institution. If appropriate consultation is not available or available consultants do not have the expertise regarding the patient's specific diagnosis, arrange safe transport of the child to another facility after discussion with the parents.

Effective communication with the consultant is essential. Share appropriate information with the consultant and make certain that the specialist understands the questions and the reasons for consultation. The consultant should discuss their findings with the hospitalist, and the two should decide who will discuss the next steps in the treatment plan. Consultants should write complete notes and list apparent reasons for their recommendations. For radiology consultations, it is important to have a system in place so that reports of reread radiographs reach the hospitalist, especially any opinion that differs from that of the hospitalist. It should be clear to all parties who will be placing new orders so that there is no confusion or omission of desired treatment. With most consultations, the hospitalist remains responsible for the patient. If care is to be formally transferred to a consultant who evaluates a patient, document the time of transfer.

Telephone consultations without direct examination by the consultant—so called curbside consultations—may result in incomplete information and incorrect advice and pose a risk for both the consultant and hospitalist. In general, the hospitalist should not allow the specialist to deem that a formal consultation is unnecessary if the hospitalist thinks that a formal consultation is appropriate for the patient's condition.

Understandably, disagreements about patient management between a hospitalist and a consultant will occasionally arise. The hospitalist is not legally bound to accept the advice of a consultant although both physicians may be held responsible for a patient's poor outcome. An automatic acceptance of the consultant's advice without discernment may cause liability for the hospitalist and the consultant if the patient has an untoward outcome. However, it is not advisable to reject the advice of a specialist without careful consideration of the consequences. If there is a poor outcome, the consultant's views as a specialist will be given great weight in court. If there are questions about care, discuss the case personally with the consultant. Document reasons why consultant's recommendations are not followed. Do not discuss disputes about care in front of the patient or family; instead, try to resolve these disagreements amicably, away from the patient. If medical staff members cannot reach a resolution, it may be appropriate to tell the family in a nonjudgmental way about the difference in opinion. If the family accepts the opinion of the consultant rather than the hospitalist, note this in the record, and transfer care to the consultant if possible. Consult hospital conflict resolution policies, if available, and encourage cordial dialogue.

TREATMENT OF INCIDENTAL FINDINGS

If a child is admitted to the hospital to manage a specific condition and during treatment another medical problem is identified. Whether the hospitalist is responsible for the workup of incidental, non-emergent findings (e.g., hypertension, scoliosis) is unclear. However, treatment depends on whether the finding falls within the hospitalist's scope of practice. The hospitalist should clarify and document who will manage the new diagnosis and whether it needs management in an inpatient or ambulatory setting. The hospitalist is responsible for informing the patient, parent, or guardian of the new diagnosis, the need for follow-up, to facilitate the appropriate referral for care, and to document this conversation.

CONFIDENTIALITY

Confidentiality, a core duty of medical practice, requires healthcare providers to keep a patient's personal health information private unless the patient provides consent to release the information. Patients have filed many lawsuits because of breaches of confidential information. Adolescent patients are particularly sensitive about confidentiality. Older adolescents might avoid seeking necessary care to prevent their parents/guardians from finding confidential medical information.

The health insurance portability and accountability act (HIPAA) is a federal law to ensure that patient medical data remains private and secure. There are two main sections of the law, the privacy rule which addresses the use and disclosure of individuals' health information, and the security rule which sets national standards for protecting the confidentiality, integrity, and availability of electronically protected health information (PHI). These identifiers include demographic and other information relating to the past, present, or future physical or mental health or condition of an individual, or the provision to or payment of healthcare from an individual. HIPAA broadly defines PHI as any health information transmitted or maintained in electronic media. PHI includes both the transmission on electronic media and any oral communications of individually identifiable health information that constitutes PHI. For example, if a hospitalist speaks in a public place within the hospital that can be a HIPAA violation if any PHI is mentioned. Most medical records in healthcare institutions and clinics meet the definition of PHI, and care must be taken so that computer screens are locked, privacy screens are used on monitors, passwords are not shared, and printed information from the medical record is not left visible on hospital desks, counters, or other public spaces. Likewise, the communication of PHI outside of the institution is a potential violation of HIPAA. Hospitalists must take care to search only the medical records of patients in their care and not search medical records of former patients and their personal family members. In addition, e-mail has become important in the practice of medicine. However, e-mail can result in a breach of privacy if the message is inadvertently sent to the wrong person or left unattended on a computer screen, where it can be viewed by another party. E-mail is discoverable in legal proceedings. Likewise, texting a patient's name or any other personally identifiable health information (PHI) is a HIPAA violation. If communication of PHI outside of the EMR is required the use of a HIPAA compliant secure text app is preferable, where the communication is sent via encrypted and password-protected messaging channels. Under no circumstances is it ever acceptable to discuss patients via social media, communicate PHI via social media, or reply directly to various public physician rating services with a personal narrative contradicting or supporting the published statements by patients. If a violation of HIPAA is discovered via a complaint or via a routine audit, the penalties are severe. A person who knowingly obtains or discloses individually identifiable health information in violation of the HIPAA Privacy Rule may face a criminal penalty of up to $50,000 and up to 1-year in prison.

EMR can improve quality of care by compiling and centralizing all pertinent information related to the pediatric patient. The EMR system must protect the privacy of patients' health information by restricting access according to local and federal laws and policies. Electronic health record systems should also protect adolescent privacy and ideally prevent inadvertent disclosure through billing activities, although since in most instances the parents/guardians are the fiscally responsible party, there may be instances where parents/guardians infer the adolescent's patient's treatment administered via a review of the medical bill. The electronic medical record may be programmed to selectively omit or conceal sensitive information and may use sets of personal collective codes designed to alert providers or teams of providers to confidential information within a patient's record. Hospitals may designate a confidential note type, or ability to designate notes as not visible, to allow segmented access to health information within the EMR and develop a practice workflow for all staff to maintain and protect privileged information for minor adolescent patients. Specifically, mental health records are usually kept separately from the patient's medical records. Hospitalists may meet with the health informatics team and legal counsel to decide how to share entrusted information responsibly, and to understand the hospital's or health system's plan for adolescent confidentiality and its compliance with state and federal laws.

DISCHARGE FROM THE HOSPITAL

Hospital Medicine providers should review the child's problems and treatment, give directions for ongoing therapy, give a diagnosis with written discharge instructions, and review these carefully with the patient, parent, or guardian at the time of discharge. Nonspecific instructions to "give fluids" or "return as needed" and medical abbreviations do not promote understanding. Instead, it is important to give clear instructions about medications dosing and timing and how to taper medication doses, if necessary, contact information for the inpatient team, primary care physician, and specialists, and include anticipatory guidance with a few examples of worrisome signs that would warrant timely re-evaluation by the primary care physician or an immediate return to the emergency department.

Prior work describes that many patients and families do not understand their care or the discharge instructions. Using the "teach back" technique, the parents/guardians retell the discharge instructions to the physician to indicate where the physician may provide more detail so that parents/guardians fully understand the discharge plan of care. Language services (i.e., interpretation, translation) are always required for parents/guardians who do not speak or read English as their preferred language. Hospitalists should seek questions from the parents/guardians and investigate potential social challenges such as inability to obtain medications, need for transportation home, inability to be seen by the primary care physician, or other factors that may interfere with the care of the child. Finally, hospitalists must provide specific information about new diagnoses or medications that may lead to serious events or side effects after discharge. For example, concerning a new diagnosis of seizures, the hospitalist should advise the parent or guardian to only allow swimming with direct supervision. There are many cautions that are specific to diagnoses that optimally are reviewed with patients' parents/guardians prior to discharge from the hospital. Computer-generated discharge instructions are advantageous because they are thorough, legible, readable, and designed to be understood with plain language. Many electronically generated handouts can be personalized and edited and include the instructions in several languages, with larger print, and illustrations. Return visits can be avoided with careful discharge instructions and care coordination. In all cases, the patient and/or parents/guardians should acknowledge that they have received and understand the discharge instructions, and a copy of the documentation should be kept in the medical record. In addition to ensuring a proper transition from hospital to home, good discharge instructions may prevent litigation, or may mitigate negotiations and damages in the event of a lawsuit.

FOLLOW-UP CARE

The American Academy of Pediatrics (AAP) has published guidelines for the role of each physician involved in the care of a hospitalized child. The AAP states that, if not directly involved in the hospital care, the primary care physician should be notified about the patient's hospitalization and clinical course at the time of discharge. For a successful transition from the hospital to primary care, communication between pediatric hospitalists and primary care physicians must be consistent, timely, and informative, usually accomplished via the discharge summary. The primary care physician has an obligation to assume care after receiving discharge communication and to ensure follow-up in their clinic and with necessary specialists after discharge. If a patient, parent, or guardian calls the inpatient team about a change in condition, the pediatric hospitalist must share this additional information with the primary care physician. Pediatric hospitalists must also ensure that primary care physicians know of pending laboratory studies or test results expected to be received after discharge. Many hospitals assist patients and parents in making appointments with primary care providers prior to the actual hospital discharge, so there is not a lapse in care.

MALPRACTICE AND THE STATE MEDICAL BOARD

On occasion, a patient, parent, or guardian may file a complaint with the state's medical board. Each state evaluates and manages complaints differently. If a hospitalist receives notice that a complaint has been filed, it is important for the hospitalist to notify the hospital legal counsel. If the complaint is validated, and there is a corresponding claim of negligence, an expert may be hired by the state medical board to evaluate the complaint. After testimony from the physician and evaluating any supporting evidence, the state medical board may take any of several actions specific to the individual state's medical practice act which may include: an informal disposition, a reprimand, a monetary fine, a formal order detailing "finding of facts," specific educational or training requirements to fulfill, and in cases of imminent danger to the public, there may be an immediate suspension of the physician's state medical license. In many cases, the medical board closes the investigation "without findings." All malpractice payment awards, and findings of negligence and/or serious criminal acts must be reported to the National Practitioner Data Bank within the United States Department of Health and Human Services, by healthcare organizations and state and federal agencies.

CONCLUSION

Pediatric hospital medicine providers face many medicolegal obligations in providing care for children. The risk of complaints and allegations of negligence may be mitigated when hospitalist understanding communication practices, informed consent, refusal of care policies, medical record documentation, use of consultant opinions, treatment of incidental findings, patient confidentiality, and coordination of care to ensure recuperation of the patient and safe discharge from the hospital.

SUGGESTED READINGS

Adamson TE, Schann JM, Guillan DS, et al. Physician communication skills and malpractice claims: A complex relationship. *West J Med.* 1989;150:356-360.

American Academy of Pediatrics, Committee on Adolescence and Council on Clinical and Information Technology. Standards for health information technology to ensure adolescent privacy. *Pediatrics.* 2012; 130:987-990.

American Academy of Pediatrics, Committee on Hospital Care. Family-centered care and the pediatrician's role. *Pediatrics.* 2003;112(3): 691-696.

American Academy of Pediatrics, Committee on Hospital Care. Physician's Role in Coordinating Care of Hospitalized Patients. https://publications.aap.org/pediatrics/article/142/2/e20181503/37540/.

Carlson J, Goldstein R, Hoover K, et al. The 21st Century Cures Act & Adolescent Confidentiality. https://adolescenthealth.org/advocacy/advocacy-activities/the-21st-century-cures-act-adolescent-confidentiality/.

Diekema DS. Parental refusals of medical treatment: the harm principle as a threshold for state intervention. *Theor Med Bioth.* 2004;25: 243-264.

Federation of State Medical Boards, Elements of Modern Medical Board. https://www.fsmb.org/siteassets/advocacy/policies/elements-modern-medical-board.pdf.

Flores G. Language barriers and hospitalized children: are we overlooking the most important risk factor for adverse events? *JAMA Pediatr.* 2020;174(12):e203238.

Landrigan CP, Conway PH, Edwards S, Srivastava R. Pediatric hospitalists: a systematic review of the literature. *Pediatrics.* 2006;117(5): 1736-1744.

Lye P, American Academy of Pediatrics Committee on Hospital Care and Section on Hospital Medicine. Clinical report—physicians' roles in coordinating care of hospitalized children. *Pediatrics.* 2010; 126:829-832.

Mangalmurti SS, Murtagh L, Mello MM. Medical malpractice liability in the age of electronic health records. *N Engl J Med.* 2010; 363:2060-2067.

McAbee GN, Brown JL. Legal issues related to e-mail, web sites and telemedicine. In: Donn SM, McAbee GN eds. *Medicolegal Issues in Pediatrics.* 7th ed. Elk Grove Village, IL: American Academy of Pediatrics; 2012:83-94.

Miller AR, Tucker CE. Electronic Discovery and Electronic Medical Records: Does the Threat of Litigation Affect Firm Decisions to Adopt Technology? Washington, DC: Federal Trade Commission; 2009.

Mussman GM, Conway PH. Pediatric hospitalist systems versus traditional models of care: effect on quality and cost outcomes. *J Hosp Med.* 2012;7(4):350-357.

Paterick ZR, Patel NJ, Ngo E, et al. Medical liability in the electronic medical records era. *Proc (Bayl Univ Med Cent).* 2018 Sep 11; 31(4):558-561.

Percelay CM, Strong GB, American Academy of Pediatrics Section on Hospital Medicine. Guiding principles for pediatric hospitalist programs. *Pediatrics.* 2005;115:1101-1102.

Rauch DA, Committee on Hospital Care; Section on Hospital Medicine; Jewell JA, et al. Physician's role in coordinating care of hospitalized children. *Pediatrics.* 2018;142(2):e20181503.

Simon TD, Mahant S, Cohen E. Pediatric hospital medicine and children with medical complexity: past, present, and future. *Curr Probl Pediatr Adolesc Health Care.* 2012;42(5):113-119.

Trends in Pediatric Malpractice Claims 1987–2015: Results From the Periodic Survey of Fellows | Pediatrics | American Academy of Pediatrics (aap.org).

CHAPTER 14 Pediatric Hospital Medicine Systems of Care

Michael Bryant, MD and Carrie Lind, MD

HISTORY OF PEDIATRIC HOSPITAL MEDICINE

Adaptability is a core attribute for the successful pediatric hospitalist. Perhaps it is because pediatric hospital medicine (PHM) is a relatively young subspecialty and accepting and leading change seems to be woven into the pediatric hospitalist's DNA.

PHM initially evolved to address the patient care needs of the hospitalized child. The PHM model of care diverged from the traditional model where pediatricians rounded on the ward and in the nursery at the beginning and end of the day, while spending the bulk of their time in the office setting. Since the mid-1990s, care of the hospitalized child has become increasingly complex, both in terms of the nature of the underlying disease process and the number of co-morbid medical conditions of the patient. The increased acuity and complexity of inpatient pediatrics, coupled with external pressures focusing on patient safety and hospital utilization, made the traditional model untenable for most primary care pediatricians.

In 1996, Dr. Robert Wachter defined a hospitalist as a physician dedicated to the delivery of comprehensive medical care to hospitalized patients, while engaging in clinical care, teaching, research, or leadership. This definition extends to pediatric hospitalists, but in addition to providing expert care for infants and children, the pediatric hospitalist must also be proficient in providing family-centered patient care.

As of 2017, an estimated 4000 pediatric hospitalists practice in the United States and approximately 900 hospitals in the United States have pediatric hospitalists. While most children's hospitals rely on pediatric hospitalists to provide general inpatient pediatric care, more than half of the PHM workforce can be found in community hospitals.

PROFESSIONAL ORGANIZATIONS

As PHM has grown and evolved, so have the organizations that support it. The Academic Pediatric Association (APA), the American Academy of Pediatrics (AAP), and the Society of Hospital Medicine (SHM) are all strongly invested in PHM and serve as co-sponsors of the annual PHM conference, the largest national PHM gathering.

The APA's mission is to improve the health and well-being of all children and adolescents by promoting research, advancing a scholarly approach to education, developing innovations in healthcare delivery, advocating for an equitable child health agenda, and fostering leadership and career development of child health professionals. Pediatric hospitalists are considered a core constituency of the APA and serve in various roles, such as editors of the APA journal *Academic Pediatrics*. The APA is also a co-sponsor for the Advancing Pediatric Educator Excellence (APEX) Teaching Program.

The mission of the AAP is to attain optimal physical, mental, and social health and well-being for all infants, children, adolescents, and young adults. Over the last 10 years the Section on Hospital Medicine (SOHM) has been the fastest growing section of the AAP now boasting almost 2800 members. The SOHM sponsored the development of the first journal dedicated to PHM, *Hospital Pediatrics*. SOHM also sponsors the national PHM Fellows Conference, co-sponsors the national PHM conference, and co-sponsors the Advancing Pediatric Educator Excellence (APEX) Teaching Program with the APA. The AAP's commitment to advocacy, both nationally and globally, is evident in its child health efforts including healthcare access and coverage, gun violence prevention, vaccine safety and efficacy, and maternal child health.

The mission of the SHM is to promote the highest quality of care for all hospitalized patients and excellence in the practice of hospital medicine through education, advocacy, and research. Of the estimated 44,000 hospitalists in the United States, approximately 16,000 are SHM members. Of note, SHM advocates for healthcare reform nationally, including Medicare and Medicaid reform. SHM sponsors an annual meeting that includes a pediatric track and publishes the *Journal of Hospital Medicine*. The number and influence of pediatric hospitalists within SHM is growing; in fact, the organization just elected its first pediatric hospitalist as president, and a pediatric hospitalist became editor-in-chief of the *Journal of Hospital Medicine* in 2019.

Several additional organizations have moved the field of PHM forward. These include the Pediatric Research in Inpatient Settings (PRIS) network, which works to improve the health of and delivery to hospitalized children and their families through large, multi-institutional studies in areas of inpatient pediatric care. The Value in Inpatient Pediatrics (VIP) network is a grass-roots organization founded in 2008 by a group of pediatric hospitalists committed to improving the value of care for hospitalized children in the United States and Canada, both inside the walls of free-standing children's hospitals and for the 70% of hospitalized children that are cared for in non-children's hospitals. The Consortium of PHM is an organization that seeks to provide a unified home for PHM and its key stakeholders, and includes representatives from APA, AAP, and SHM.

DEVELOPMENTS SINCE LAST EDITION

In 2016, the American Board of Medical Specialties approved the petition for PHM to become the newest pediatric subspecialty, taking PHM on a divergent path from the Focused Practice in Hospital Medicine designation established for adult hospitalists. The American Board of Pediatrics (ABP) allowed experts already practicing in the discipline to access the board examination for a limited period without completing a formal fellowship program. However, in 2025, pediatric hospitalists will need to complete an accredited fellowship of 2 years or more to become board-eligible in PHM. The number of PHM fellowship programs continues to grow; for the 2023 appointment year, there were 67 PHM fellowship programs in the National Resident Matching Program, with 104 certified positions and 120 applicants.

Since the publication of the last edition, the COVID-19 pandemic has necessitated rapid changes in healthcare delivery across the United States in all fields, including the care of hospitalized children. While there was initially a major decline in the volume of hospitalized children resulting in the closure of numerous pediatric inpatient units, there has since been a robust increase in pediatric volumes nationwide with a change in the expected seasonal variation in volumes due to respiratory syncytial virus (RSV) and influenza. While most cases of COVID-19 in children are mild or asymptomatic, a small number of patients may develop severe disease. COVID-19 has brought new childhood disease processes to manage in the inpatient setting such as respiratory failure/distress associated with acute COVID-19, multisystem inflammatory syndrome in children (MIS-C), and COVID-associated neurologic complications (Chapters 106 and 107). Additionally, the pandemic has had a substantial adverse impact on healthcare worker mental health, staffing, and burnout.

PRACTICE SETTINGS

There are two major locations where pediatric hospitalists practice—the university/academic center and the community setting. Formerly, academic children's hospitals have been labeled "teaching hospitals," though community hospitals often serve as teaching hospitals for medical students, residents, fellows, and nursing students.

UNIVERSITY/ACADEMIC CENTER-BASED SETTING

The models of care in university/academic centers vary considerably among pediatric hospitalists. A key philosophical and financial consideration is whether to have 24/7 in-house coverage or not. 24/7 in-house coverage, while desirable, is costly. Historically, pediatric residents have been the lynchpin of 24/7 coverage with supervising attendings providing on-site supervision during the day and remote coverage after hours. Pediatric hospitalists have increasingly assumed the role of supervisor in this model.

In the settings where residents are not available to provide bridging care overnight, "attending-only services" have emerged. These services vary from 24/7 in-house pediatric hospitalist presence, amenable to shifts (day, swing, overnight shifts), to daytime coverage/nighttime call. In university/academic centers, the medical complexity of patients may require an in-house presence of an attending pediatric hospitalist. For the medically complex child, pediatric hospitalists often navigate multiple medical issues and orchestrate the input of multiple subspecialists. Pediatric hospitalists can also serve as partners to other subspecialists in the care of hospitalized children (Chapter 8). Finally, there are pediatric subspecialty-specific inpatient practitioners. While the term hospitalist has been used for these providers (e.g., NICU hospitalist, Hematology/Oncology hospitalist), the ABP explicitly requires that eligibility for PHM board certification necessitates exposure to a variety of hospitalized pediatric patients in various practice settings including the nursery and medical/surgical units.

In addition to the various models of care, the role of trainees and non-physician providers must be considered as an important part of the delivery of healthcare to the hospitalized child. These include medical students, residents, and fellows as well as advanced practice providers (APPs). In university/academic centers, the traditional family-centered rounding model usually includes physician trainees with a hierarchy that extends from medical student to resident to fellow, and finally, attending. With the Accreditation Council for Graduate Medicine Education (ACGME) overseeing PHM fellowship programs, fellows must be supervised by an attending pediatric hospitalist and cannot bill independently. Additionally, the role of APPs continues to evolve, and their scope of practice often varies by state and institution.

Pediatric hospitalist compensation models in university/academic settings also vary. Pay for performance (PFP) using relative value units (RVUs) has been used to assess productivity and as a compensation benchmark but the shift work of a pediatric hospitalist often creates significant disparities in the ability of providers to generate revenue. As an example, nocturnists generate significantly less revenue than their daytime counterparts. In recognition of this, many pediatric hospitalists receive a base salary with an additional "bonus structure" that is often predicated on overall division performance instead of individual metrics. This bonus structure recognizes that pediatric hospitalists do not "control" who is admitted. Finally, there are payment paradigms where "total cash compensation" is divided into a "fixed" and "variable" portion. The fixed component is a guarantee, and the variable component is based upon achievement of individualized and/or group metrics.

As PHM has evolved as a subspecialty, pediatric hospitalists have embraced the desire to not only excel in clinical care but also establish comprehensive programs that include research, education, leadership development, quality improvement, high-value care, advocacy, and mentorship. University/academic PHM divisions are seeking to nest these initiatives in their practice environments as necessary companions to the clinical care provided, though these initiatives require time, money, and mentorship.

COMMUNITY-BASED SETTING

Community-based pediatric hospitals and inpatient units offer local pediatric care close to patients' homes. Staffing community hospitals can be a challenge as patients require 24/7 coverage, often without resident support, but with smaller volumes and less revenue. Several models exist to staff community pediatric hospitals including 24/7 in-house coverage and daytime coverage with remote night call. Community hospitals often utilize the pediatric hospitalist to also help cover the newborn nursery or the emergency department (as either a fast-track emergency physician for pediatric patients or as a consultant for the adult emergency physician).

Community pediatric units often admit patients with short, anticipated hospital stays and lower illness acuity, including patients with common conditions such as asthma, hyperbilirubinemia, bronchiolitis, failure to thrive, and dehydration. To admit higher acuity patients to the community pediatric unit, community hospitals can utilize telemedicine or e-consulting services from nearby university/academic hospitals. Adult subspecialty surgical and medical services can often care for some pediatric patients in a community hospital, including those patients meeting specific weight or age criteria. These adult subspecialists may prefer to admit to the pediatric hospitalist or have the pediatric hospitalist consult or co-manage for pediatric-specific management of antibiotics, intravenous fluids, and pain control. Caring for children with medical complexity and other patients who may need subspecialty consultation often requires an infrastructure that community pediatric hospitals may not have or deem necessary to support (e.g., pediatric radiology, child life services, speech, and nutrition services).

Physician compensation can also be challenging in the community setting. RVU-based bonus structure is especially challenging for community pediatric hospitalists who do not benefit from high-volume and/or high-acuity bonus incentives. Nevertheless, community hospitals have developed creative opportunities to improve revenue for the community pediatric hospitalist, including staffing services such as infusion centers, sedation, discharge follow-up clinics, and pediatric and neonatal critical care unit coverage.

In many states, community pediatric units have survived by partnering with university/academic centers. These larger institutions often find it favorable to direct the general pediatric care to community hospitals which can provide care at lower cost and free up beds for patients requiring subspecialty expertise and consultation. Many partnership models exist including ownership of a community pediatric hospital by the children's hospital or serving as a satellite. Lease arrangements and creative partnerships also exist where the community hospital pays for services provided by the physicians and staff from a university/academic pediatric center.

In the community setting, achieving value and quality metrics and pursuing high-value care is especially essential. The community pediatric hospitalist often serves as one of the few pediatric experts in the hospital and can be well-positioned for roles in hospital administrative committees. In an adult-focused medical center, the pediatric hospitalist's role within the dynamics of the medical staff is especially important to forward pediatric-specific goals and objectives.

CHALLENGES FACED IN BOTH SETTINGS

As the models of care continue to evolve in PHM, challenges abound. While PHM is the fastest growing subspecialty field in pediatrics, there are not enough fellowship training spots to fill the growing need of pediatric hospitalists in the various practice settings. Board eligibility for those on the practice pathway will sunset in 2025, and PHM faces the prospect of a tiered system bifurcating into those who are board eligible and those who are not. Pediatric hospitalists will need to decide if board certification is required to provide inpatient pediatric care; a decision that may be influenced by insurers in the market. Mentorship also continues to be a challenge for existing and aspiring leaders. Thankfully, leadership programs have been developed by the APA, AAP, and SHM to provide support in this area.

Nationally, community children's hospitals have closed due to a lack of profitability. These closures are likely explained in part by a decrease in pediatric inpatient volume due to improving pediatric health. However, centralization of pediatric care in large referral centers and replacement of pediatric beds in community hospitals with more profitable adult units have also contributed to the closure of community pediatric units and hospitals. The reimbursement for care of children is substantially less than that for adults, exacerbating the mismatch between revenue generated and the amount available for services rendered to support compensation. Revenue challenges persist as reimbursement for the care of children and especially those with medical complexity lag woefully behind that of adults, and yet the acuity of pediatric inpatient care continues to rise. Additionally, consolidation continues to occur in the market and as community hospitals close their pediatric programs, more patients will present to university/academic institutions which have continued to expand their capacity.

Finally, physician burnout has increasingly threatened those in the field and may dissuade those who are interested in pursuing a career in PHM. Studies have sought to define the clinical load and hours of a sustainable professional profile, but there is considerable debate about what is truly "sustainable." Seeking to integrate clinical care with other roles including research, education, and quality improvement provides further challenges to the pediatric hospitalist. It is entirely reasonable to expect that the field of PHM will continue to grow, but these challenges will need to be addressed to ensure longevity.

OPPORTUNITIES IN EACH SETTING

The community setting offers the compelling advantage of keeping children near the neighborhoods in which they live. For trainees at all levels, the community environment offers a unique clinical experience that differs from that of a larger pediatric facility and can be a tremendous adjunct to their training. University/academic centers offer a centralized hub of care for patients whose care cannot be accommodated in smaller/more remote settings, allowing access to subspecialists across a broad spectrum of care. Community-academic partnerships can result in mutually beneficial scenarios fostering a more effective healthcare model for patients and healthcare organizations. Finally, opportunities in research, education, quality improvement, advocacy, mentorship, and leadership abound for pediatric hospitalists.

SUGGESTED READINGS

Forman K, Tran-viet K-N, McKnight H, Lakshminrusimha S, Hamline M. UC Davis Health, CA, Sacramento Meeting: Hospital Medicine 2020, Virtual Competition. https://shmabstracts.org/abstract/benefits-of-a-community-hospital-academic-university-pediatric-partnership/.

Ottolini M, Wohlberg R, Lewis K, Greenberg L. Using observed structured teaching exercises (OSTE) to enhance hospitalist teaching during family centered rounds. *J Hosp Med.* 2011;6(7):423-427.

Seelbach EB, Ottolini MC. Primary care physicians and hospitalists: two branches of the same tree. *Pediatr Ann.* 2010;39(2):84-88.

Simon TD, Berry J, Feudtner C, et al. Children with complex chronic conditions in inpatient hospital settings in the United States. *Pediatrics.* 2010;126(4):647-655.

Wachter RM, Goldman L. The emerging role of "hospitalists" in the American health care system. *N Engl J Med.* 1996;335:514-517.

PART II

Common Presenting Signs and Symptoms

Part Editors
Kris P. Rehm, MD, MMHC and Erinn O. Schmit, MD, MEd

CHAPTER 15

Abdominal Mass

Daniel A. Rauch, MD, FAAP, SFHM

BACKGROUND

Although evaluation of an abdominal mass can occur in an outpatient setting, pediatric hospitalists are often asked to expedite the initial assessment and coordinate the appropriate consultations. The diagnostic possibilities vary considerably, based on the patient's age and associated symptoms. The most urgent considerations are acute surgical conditions and neoplasms. A careful history and physical examination should guide a directed laboratory and imaging evaluation, leading to the diagnosis.

PATHOPHYSIOLOGY

There are many structures within the abdomen from which masses can arise (**Table 15-1**). Abdominal masses can represent abnormal tissue mass of a solid organ such as the liver, spleen, or kidney or abnormal filling of a viscous organ such as the bowel or bladder. The most common source of an abdominal mass besides constipation is kidney pathology.

HISTORY

Abdominal masses present in two distinct ways: painless or with abdominal symptoms. A painless mass is the classic sign of abdominal malignancy, particularly Wilms tumor and neuroblastoma. However, painless masses may also be completely benign, such as a fecal mass in a constipated child, a horseshoe kidney, or a wandering spleen. Painless masses are usually identified incidentally, often by parents when bathing the child, and sometimes on routine physical examinations. Systemic symptoms such as weight loss, pallor, bruising, or bleeding are suggestive of a malignant process. Diarrhea can be a sign of a vasoactive secreting tumor, while hematuria strongly suggests renal involvement. Masses may cause or be the result of gastrointestinal (GI) obstruction and can present with vomiting, abdominal pain, and constipation. Masses that are renal in origin can present with symptoms of urinary dysfunction and hematuria. Painful masses require evaluation for diagnoses requiring urgent intervention, such as ischemia secondary to processes like ovarian torsion or intussusception or the need for decompression of the bowel or bladder. Duration of the symptoms is an important consideration. Slowly growing masses are typical of some malignancies, while rapidly enlarging masses are more typical of others. Chronic abdominal pain and abnormal bowel habits may point to constipation. Periodic pain may point to a recurrent process, either acutely, as in intussusception, or chronically, such as a volvulus.

Age is an important factor to consider. Neonates can present with congenital anomalies such as cystic kidneys. Neuroblastomas and storage diseases typically present in children younger than 2 years old. Wilms tumors and other malignancies are more common in older children. Certain syndromes, such as Beckwith-Weidemann, confer increased risk of Wilms tumors.

PHYSICAL EXAMINATION

A thorough physical examination will help determine the source of the mass. Tenderness will confirm the report of pain, and rebound tenderness indicates a more severe and acute process that has evolved into peritonitis. Localization of the mass aids the differential diagnosis.

The abdomen is classically divided in four quadrants. The right upper quadrant contains the liver, gallbladder, and bowel. The liver is often palpated under the costal margin, and up to 2 to 3 cm below in infants. The liver may be displaced inferiorly with hyperaeration of the chest cavity. When the liver edge extends to the left of the midline, it is likely enlarged. Extreme hepatomegaly that extends to the right lower quadrant can be missed because the liver edge is not palpable anywhere in the right upper quadrant. The left upper quadrant contains the spleen, pancreas, stomach, and bowel. Because the spleen is a mobile structure, palpation of a mildly enlarged spleen tip may move it beyond tactile sensation. Both the right lower quadrant and the left lower quadrant contain bowel and the female reproductive organs. In young infants the bladder may be

TABLE 15-1 Possible Diagnoses of Abdominal Masses

Region	Organ or Site	Diagnosis
Epigastrium	Stomach	Distended stomach from pyloric stenosis, duplication
	Pancreas	Pseudocyst
Flank	Kidney	Hydronephrosis, Wilms tumor, dysplastic kidney, ureteral duplication
	Adrenal	Neuroblastoma, ganglioneuroblastoma, ganglioneuroma
	Retroperitoneum	Neuroblastoma, ganglioneuroblastoma, ganglioneuroma, teratoma
Lower abdomen	Ovary	Dermoid, teratoma, ovarian tumor, torsion of ovary
	Kidney	Pelvic kidney
	Urachus	Urachal cyst
	Omentum, mesentery	Omental, mesenteric, peritoneal cysts
Pelvic	Bladder, prostate	Obstructed bladder, rhabdomyosarcoma
	Uterus, vagina	Hydrometrocolpos, hydrocolpos, rhabdomyosarcoma
Right upper quadrant	Biliary tract	Cholecystitis, choledochal cyst
	Liver	Hepatomegaly from congestion, hepatitis, or tumor; mesenchymal hamartoma; hemangioendothelioma; hepatoblastoma; hepatocellular carcinoma; hepatic abscess; hydatid cyst
	Intestine	Intussusception, duplication
Left upper quadrant	Spleen	Splenomegaly from congestion, infectious mononucleosis, leukemic infiltration, or lymphoma; splenic abscess; cyst
Right lower quadrant	Appendix ileum	Appendiceal abscess
		Meconium ileus, inflammatory mass (complication of Crohn disease), intestinal duplication
	Lymphatics	Lymphoma, lymphangioma
Left lower quadrant	Colon Lymphatics	Fecal impaction
		Lymphoma, lymphangioma

Source: From Zitelli B, Davis H. *Atlas of Pediatric Physical Diagnosis*. 4th ed. Philadelphia: Elsevier; 2002.

palpable in the suprapubic area, but this structure becomes intrapelvic in later infancy. Retroperitoneal structures, such as the aorta and kidneys, are not typically palpable. Normal structures may be felt in patients who are very thin and have relaxed abdominal musculature, especially the aorta, which can be appreciated as a pulsatile midline structure, and the tip of the spleen in the left upper quadrant.

The female reproductive tract resides in the pelvis but can expand into the lower abdomen under certain circumstances. Ovarian cysts or, much less commonly, neoplasms, can become large enough to be palpable by direct abdominal examination. An engorged uterus may be palpable in the suprapubic area with congenital vaginal atresia, and is seen with hydrometrocolpos. A gravid uterus extends beyond the pelvic brim at approximately 12 weeks' gestation. Ectopic pregnancy within a fallopian tube is usually symptomatic before being palpable but should always be considered in patients with abdominal pain and a positive pregnancy test. An intravaginal-abdominal bimanual examination can facilitate palpation of the female reproductive organs.

The bladder, which is a pelvic structure after infancy, can expand into the lower abdomen when enlarged. This may occur with urinary retention.

Retroperitoneal structures such as the kidneys, adrenals, pancreas, and midline paravertebral nodes and vessels may be palpable through the abdomen when there is significant tissue bulk, as can be seen with neoplasms such as Wilms tumor, neuroblastoma, and lymphoma. Cystic kidney disease may present as an abdominal mass. Neonates may have a palpable right kidney, which may be completely normal.

Mobile masses more commonly originate from the GI tract, while fixed masses are from the liver or retroperitoneal structures. Compressible masses may be cystic. Examination of other organ systems can also provide clues as to the origin of an abdominal mass. The classic extra-abdominal finding of neuroblastoma is "raccoon eyes," and proptosis can also be observed. Aniridia is associated with Wilms tumors, as is hemihypertrophy.

DIFFERENTIAL DIAGNOSIS

Focal areas of distention can present as a mass, such as in duplication, intussusception, volvulus, and constipation. Intestinal duplications are rare and may present with obstruction or bloody diarrhea in addition to a palpable mass. Intussusception uncommonly presents with the classic triad of colicky abdominal pain, vomiting, and currant jelly stool. More typical is some combination of vomiting, lethargy, and abdominal pain, with a right upper quadrant sausage-shaped mass and an empty right lower quadrant (Dance sign) in an infant or toddler. Volvulus presents with bilious vomiting and pain associated with an acute obstruction. Constipation is the most common cause of a palpable abdominal mass in any of the quadrants; it is usually tubular, mobile, and nontender.

Hepatomegaly is a nonspecific finding that may represent primary liver pathology or myriad secondary processes. Enlargement may be due to an increase in the size or number of cells or structures in the liver, including the hepatocytes (e.g., glycogen storage diseases), biliary tree (cholelithiasis), and vascular spaces (e.g., congestive heart failure), or to an infiltrative process (e.g., neuroblastoma). A list of possible infectious causes is provided in **Table 15-2**. Other causes to consider are listed in **Table 15-3**.

The spleen can enlarge in response to a wide range of insults. Many of the infectious, metabolic, neoplastic, and inflammatory disorders that can cause hepatomegaly can also cause splenomegaly, either in isolation or in combination. Hemolytic disorders can cause chronic splenomegaly or, as in the case of acute splenic sequestration of sickle cell disease, sudden splenic enlargement with profound anemia. Serum sickness and subacute bacterial endocarditis can cause splenomegaly, with deposition of immune complexes in the spleen. Chronic granulomatous disease can cause intrasplenic granuloma formation.

Suprapubic masses can represent the bladder or the uterus. Enlarged bladders are typically painful and associated with urinary symptoms. Pregnancy should be considered in any pubertal girl.

The abdominal wall is a rare source of abdominal masses, taking the form of incarcerated hernias or sarcomas.

TABLE 15-2 Infectious Causes of Hepatomegaly
Bacteremia
Infectious hepatitis
Mononucleosis
Syphilis
Leptospirosis
Histoplasmosis
Brucellosis
Toxoplasmosis
Tuberculosis
Ascariasis
Amebiasis
Pyogenic abscess
Visceral larva migrans
Q fever
Gonococcal or chlamydial perihepatitis
AIDS
Neonatal enteroviral infection
Gianottic-Crosti syndrome
Cat-scratch disease (granuloma)

Source: Reproduced with permission from Green M, ed. The abdomen. In *Pediatric Diagnosis: Interpretation of Symptoms and Signs in Children and Adolescents*. 6th ed. Philadelphia: Saunders; 1998.

DIAGNOSTIC EVALUATION

Blood work should be directed toward the likely diagnosis. Initial tests can include a CBC looking for signs of cell line deficits, liver function tests, inflammatory markers, and oncology markers for neuroblastoma. Hematuria can be found with Wilms tumors, and urine pregnancy tests should be done in pubertal girls.

Imaging studies can help localize the mass, determine the origin, or identify the cause. Plain abdominal radiographs can identify some abnormalities (e.g., solid tumors with calcifications) but are more useful as part of an obstruction series. The additional views demonstrate the effect of gravity on the intra-abdominal structures and fluids, revealing patterns of bowel obstruction, abscess, or free air.

Ultrasonography is a readily available, nonionizing imaging modality that usually does not require the patient to be sedated. It provides information regarding the consistency of the mass (e.g., solid vs. cystic), can readily identify an abscess, and can often identify the organ of origin. Cystic masses are usually from the GI or genitourinary tract and are less likely to be malignant than solid masses.

Computed tomography and magnetic resonance imaging provide a more complete assessment and greater structural detail. Factors such as need for sedation, radiation exposure, availability, and likely yield are important considerations. In addition, when the diagnosis is likely to

TABLE 15-3 Noninfectious Causes of Hepatomegaly
Anemia (sickle cell disease)
Passive vascular congestion (congestive heart failure)
Metabolic disorders (mucopolysaccharidosis)
Cholestatic disorders (biliary atresia)
Neoplastic disease (Hodgkin disease)
Cysts (congenital hepatic cyst)
Fatty infiltration (idiopathic steatohepatitis)
Trauma (subcapsular hematoma)
Autoimmune (systemic lupus erythematosus)
Hemosiderosis
Poisoning (hypervitaminosis A)

be a malignancy and additional body areas will need to be imaged for staging purposes, studies should be coordinated to the extent possible. Further discussion of imaging is provided in Chapter 185.

MANAGEMENT

Treatment is entirely dependent on the ultimate cause of the abdominal mass and often involves coordination of care with nephrology, gastroenterology, infectious diseases, oncology, or genetics as appropriate.

SPECIAL CONSIDERATIONS

Any evaluation that includes possible malignancy or other potentially fatal entities such as the storage diseases requires extreme sensitivity toward the patient and family. Families need to be engaged in the need for a prompt workup which necessitated the hospitalization, and they should be kept abreast of the results of each study in a timely manner. Additionally, the caregivers will direct how much information can be revealed to the child. A multidisciplinary approach including social work and child life can help families cope with the process and break any potential bad news to the child and other family members.

The evaluation may require special testing that is not available at all hospitals, so prompt transfer to a tertiary care facility may be required to expedite certain tests.

KEY POINTS

- The diagnostic possibilities for abdominal masses vary considerably, based on the patient's age and associated symptoms.
- While the evaluation can often take place in an outpatient setting, pediatric hospitalists are often involved in the initial evaluation.
- Ultimate diagnosis may depend on testing that is not available at all centers, so appropriate referral may be required.

SUGGESTED READINGS

Kim HHR, Hull NC, Lee EY, Phillips GS. Pediatric abdominal masses: imaging guidelines and recommendations. *Radiol Clin North Am.* 2022;60(1):113-129.

Nicholas M. Potisek, James W. Antoon. Abdominal masses. *Pediatr Rev.* 2017;38(2):101-103.

Uzunova L, Bailie H, Murray MJ. Fifteen-minute consultation: a general paediatrician's guide to oncological abdominal masses. *Arch Dis Child Educ Pract Ed.* 2019;104(3):129-134.

Zitelli B, Davis H. *Atlas of Pediatric Physical Diagnosis.* 8th ed. Philadelphia, PA: Elsevier; 2032.

CHAPTER 16 Abdominal Pain

Christine Hrach, MD, SFHM, FAAP and Robert Casey, MD

BACKGROUND

Abdominal pain is one of the most common complaints encountered by pediatric hospitalists. Despite this, the evaluation is often exceedingly difficult, and in many cases no definitive diagnosis is made during a hospitalization. The most urgent matter for the hospitalist is to rule out a life-threatening surgical emergency. If an acute abdomen is suspected, prompt surgical consultation is imperative.

PATHOPHYSIOLOGY

Abdominal pain can be caused by inflammation of the abdominal organs themselves (or their visceral peritoneum) or by inflammation of the parietal peritoneum lying in proximity to the underlying inflammation. Irritation of the abdominal wall musculature can also lead to pain, and various extra-abdominal processes can cause abdominal pain (e.g., diabetic ketoacidosis or lower lobe pneumonia). Pain due to a process in the small intestine is usually felt in the midline around the umbilicus initially; as the inflammation progresses, the parietal peritoneum in the area of inflammation becomes involved, allowing better localization of pain. The classic example is appendicitis, with a dull periumbilical ache early in the course followed by a progressive shift of pain to the right lower quadrant as the inflammation evolves. Certain elements of the history and physical examination findings may help identify the cause of abdominal pain (**Table 16-1**).

PATIENT HISTORY

In addition to a full history, the timing, location, and progression of the pain should be elicited, as well as its quality and severity; those details may provide helpful diagnostic hints. For example: in appendicitis, the pain begins in the umbilical area and progresses to right lower quadrant. Gastric ulcer disease typically presents with burning or boring pain while the pain associated with peritonitis is sharp and stabbing. Pain that comes in waves or is colicky in nature is common in diseases that involve blockage of peristalsis of a hollow viscous, such as the small bowel, biliary

TABLE 16-1 Using History and Physical Examination Findings to Diagnose Abdominal Pain

Findings	Possible Diagnosis
History of present illness	
Sudden onset	Ovarian or testicular torsion, intussusception, volvulus, trauma
Bilious emesis	Bowel obstruction
Bloody stools	IBD (older patients), intussusception (younger patients), infectious colitis
Recent weight loss	IBD, malignancy
Travel	Infectious colitis, parasitic infection
Fevers	Infectious colitis, IBD
Rash	IgA vasculitis, IBD (erythema nodosum)
Menstrual history	Dysmenorrhea, pregnancy, mittelschmerz
Past medical history	
Pharyngitis	Mesenteric adenitis, EBV-associated splenic distention
Gastroenteritis	Intussusception, postinfectious gastroparesis
Abdominal surgery	Obstruction from adhesions
Family history	
IBD	IBD
Migraines	Abdominal migraines
Social history	
Pets, especially reptiles	Infectious colitis
Sexual history	Pelvic inflammatory disease, pregnancy, ectopic pregnancy
Physical examination	
Clubbing or pallor	IBD
Perianal skin tags	Crohn disease
Jaundice	Biliary disease
Bluish color of flank or umbilicus	Pancreatic disease, trauma
Hemorrhoids, caput medusae	Chronic liver disease

EBV, Epstein-Barr virus; IBD, inflammatory bowel disease.

tree, or ureter. Aggravating or alleviating factors of pain should be elicited as well. For example, eating a meal might cause some pain to worsen, such as in biliary disease or pancreatitis, but other pain to be relieved, such as peptic ulcer disease. If they are experiencing bilious vomiting, the patient has a surgical emergency until proven otherwise, as this sign is suggestive of a bowel obstruction distal to the sphincter of Oddi. In younger children, classically 18 to 36 months, who have abdominal pain and bilious vomiting without other symptoms, intussusception should be strongly suspected. The pain of intussusception can be intermittent and is occasionally associated with mental status changes or lethargy. Any toxic-appearing child at any age with bilious vomiting should be evaluated for malrotation with midgut volvulus.

In a verbal child, questions about urinary complaints should be included, such as dysuria, frequency, or foul-smelling urine. These symptoms may suggest a urinary tract infection, nephrolithiasis, or the nephritis of IgA vasculopathy.

A patient's stooling pattern should also be ascertained. Stools that are hard or extremely large suggest constipation. Diarrhea can be consistent with common causes, such as gastroenteritis, or more serious causes, such as inflammatory bowel disease. In patients with an upper gastrointestinal (GI) bleed, stools often appear very dark and melanotic.

It is also important to ask about systemic symptoms. Fever can be associated with many inflammatory, infectious, or malignant causes of abdominal pain. Typical red flag symptoms of weight loss, fatigue, and night sweats are associated with prolonged systemic disease, such as Crohn disease or malignant processes. Additionally, inflammatory bowel disease (IBD) can present with extra-intestinal symptoms, such as rash, arthralgias, or eye problems.

It is important to take a full family history, as many heritable disorders, such as IBD, are genetic. Also, ask about medication use. Nonsteroidal anti-inflammatory drugs can cause ulcer disease and recent antibiotic use predisposes a patient to *Clostridium difficile* infection. Social history is also crucial to the hospitalized child with abdominal pain. Sexual history needs to be asked as recent sexual activity can lead to sexually transmitted infection or pelvic inflammatory disease. Additionally, social stressors can lead to psychosomatic complaints.

PHYSICAL EXAMINATION

The physical examination starts with an evaluation of the vital signs. True abdominal catastrophes with associated abdominal pain (volvulus, perforated duodenal ulcer, splenic rupture following Epstein-Barr virus [EBV] infection, severe trauma) can quickly progress to frank shock, with accompanying changes in hemodynamics and vital signs. Fever is often found with inflammatory and infectious processes. The degree of fever is not necessarily directly related to the severity of the eventual diagnosis.

The importance of the patient's general examination on presentation cannot be overstated. A toxic child needs emergent evaluation and intervention after ensuring that circulation, airway, and breathing are maintained. A patient with normal vital signs who smiles and jokes while complaining of 10 out of 10 abdominal pain likely does not warrant admission. Examination of the acute abdomen was addressed earlier, with an emphasis on recognizing the signs of peritonitis. After inspection of the abdomen (for distension, discoloration, visible masses, etc.) bowel sounds should be assessed, because deep palpation can alter their character.

Percussion of the abdomen is invaluable. A distended or tympanitic abdomen would potentially be suggestive of increased intraluminal air proximal to an obstruction. Organomegaly or abdominal mass is associated with a fixed area of dullness. Fluid waves or shifting dullness is present in patients with ascites.

Palpation is also important in evaluating for masses and organomegaly and for eliciting pain, and should be performed after auscultation and percussion. One should always begin palpating as far away from the reported location of the patient's pain as possible. Having the child flex the hips and bend the knees is helpful to relax the abdominal musculature. Distraction of the patient during the abdominal exam, especially for younger patients, is important. The practitioner's eyes should be fixed on the patient's face, looking for even subtle signs of tenderness. The obturator sign and the psoas sign are suggestive of inflammation in or near those muscles, often secondary to organic abdominal pathology. The Rovsing sign is present when palpation in the left lower quadrant produces pain in the right lower quadrant, suggesting appendicitis. Rebound is thought to be sensitive for peritonitis, although many examiners feel that this is an unnecessarily painful maneuver that often adds little to the final evaluation. In patients where there is concern for somatization or nonorganic pain, distracting the patient by asking questions or having them talk while palpating the abdomen can be a useful technique.

All children should have a full examination in addition to the abdominal examination, with an emphasis on findings that could be causing or contributing to the abdominal pain. Controversy exists over which children need rectal examinations, which females need pelvic examinations, and which males need testicular exams. In selected cases, these examinations can be immensely informative, and the need for them is dictated by the history.

DIFFERENTIAL DIAGNOSIS

The differential diagnosis of abdominal pain is extensive (**Table 16-2**). In addition to the typical history and physical examination, epidemiologic factors are extremely helpful in narrowing the differential diagnosis, including age, sex, season, and geographic location. As stated above, a patient with peritonitis requires timely surgical evaluation. On history, these patients may report that the bumps in the road on the trip to the emergency department caused pain. These patients prefer to lie motionless and do not want their abdomen palpated. The examiner can check for signs of peritonitis immediately by "inadvertently" bumping the bed; a wince of pain from the patient is a sign that any movement at all is irritating to the inflamed parietal peritoneum. Bowel sounds may be hypoactive or absent at this late stage, reflecting an ileus. The abdomen may be rigid, and the patient may have voluntary or involuntary guarding, a mechanism to prevent painful manipulation of the underlying enflamed peritoneum. Patients with peritonitis are likely to have rebound tenderness, when the pain that is felt when the examiner releases the abdomen is greater than that caused by the palpation itself. Patients of any age who fit this classic description of an acute abdomen are highly likely to require surgical intervention.

Unfortunately for physicians, most cases of abdominal pain are not this clear cut. For each disease process in the differential diagnosis, there is a wide range of severity. For example, a patient with severe constipation may be in extremis, whereas a patient with early appendicitis may have so little pain (or such a high tolerance for pain) that he or she is sent home without having had further workup. A full history and physical examination are paramount to determine the cause of the pain. It must be kept in mind that common benign diagnoses (e.g. viral gastroenteritis and constipation) occur commonly, but depending on the presentation are often diagnoses of exclusion. It is the examiner's job to triage these patients appropriately while recognizing the red flags that point to less common entities or those that need more urgent evaluation or intervention.

DIAGNOSTIC EVALUATION

As stated earlier, a patient with an obvious surgical abdomen often needs no further evaluation before surgical exploration is undertaken. For other patients, the question is whether and when to perform radiologic studies and/or laboratory tests.

RADIOLOGY

The simplest and most widely available initial study is a supine plain radiograph of the abdomen (also known as a kidney, ureter, and bladder [KUB] study). Most findings are nonspecific and merely confirm the findings elicited by physical examination. Exceptions include a renal or ureteral calculus, the finding of a fecalith in the right lower quadrant, or a large amount of stool suggesting constipation. A fecalith is a

TABLE 16-2 Differential Diagnosis of Abdominal Pain

Gastrointestinal	Surgical
Viral gastroenteritis	Appendicitis
Bacterial infectious colitis	Intussusception
Parasitic infection	Malrotation with midgut volvulus
Constipation	Incarcerated inguinal hernia
Colic	Trauma with associated hematoma
Functional abdominal pain	Postsurgical obstruction
Abdominal migraine	Psoas (or other) abscess
Acute cholecystitis, cholelithiasis	Toxicologic
Ulcer disease (gastric, peptic)	Heavy metal poisoning
Pancreatitis	Food (toxin-mediated) poisoning
Hepatitis	Infectious
Inflammatory bowel disease	Tuberculosis
Gastroesophageal reflux	Zoster
Esophagitis	Mesenteric adenitis
Gastroparesis, ileus	Mononucleosis
Lactose intolerance	Sepsis
Toxic megacolon	Pulmonary
Meckel diverticulum	Lower lobe pneumonia
Hirschsprung disease	Meconium ileus equivalent
Urologic	Endocrinologic
Urinary tract infection	Diabetic ketoacidosis
Urolithiasis	Hematologic
Testicular torsion	Vaso-occlusive crisis
Gynecologic	Porphyria
Ovarian torsion, cyst	Oncologic
Pregnancy, ectopic pregnancy	Tumor (e.g. Wilms)
Pelvic inflammatory disease	Renal
Dysmenorrhea	Nephrosis
Endometriosis	Spontaneous bacterial peritonitis
Hematocolpos	Hemolytic uremic syndrome
Ovarian neoplasm	Cardiovascular
Rheumatologic	Abdominal aortic aneurysm
IgA vasculitis	Psychiatric
Familial Mediterranean fever	Somatic symptoms and related disorders

small, radiodense mass of hardened stool that obstructs the lumen of the appendix, preventing the outflow of intestinal bacteria and predisposing the patient to appendicitis. Distended loops of bowel are a common and nonspecific finding. The addition of a second abdominal view in the upright or left lateral decubitus allows for effect of gravity on air and fluid to be examined. Air–fluid levels may be visible within bowel secondary to ileus or obstruction. Free air may be visible on the upright film, but these patients often have peritoneal signs on examination. Patients subsequently diagnosed with intussusception often have a paucity of air in the ascending colon, as this is the most common site for an intussusception to occur.

The radiologic evaluation of patients with suspected appendicitis has changed over the years. Ultrasonography is a preferred initial modality, owing to the lack of radiation and its specificity for appendicitis. An added advantage of ultrasonography is the ability to assess blood flow in real time, which is particularly helpful in female patients with right lower quadrant pain, for whom ovarian torsion is in the differential diagnosis. Ultrasound can also be used in the evaluation of suspected intussusception to identify a target sign (the intussusceptum within the lumen of the intussuscipiens). Air-contrast enema has the advantage of being able to both diagnose and treat intussusception, but because there is a small risk of perforation, this procedure should be performed only in centers staffed by surgeons competent in the care of small children.

Computed tomography, especially when done with contrast, has high specificity for appendicitis, and is often undertaken if an initial ultrasound is equivocal. The radiologist can see signs of inflammation in the right lower quadrant, including free fluid and stranding in the pericecal fat. With effective contrast, an appendix that does not fill is presumed to be obstructed, confirming the diagnosis of appendicitis.

Other imaging studies that may be encountered in the evaluation of abdominal pain include upper GI series (effective for the evaluation of malrotation with intermittent volvulus and for IBD) and, rarely, nuclear medicine studies for GI bleeding with associated abdominal pain. Magnetic resonance enterography is a modality that is effective at finding and monitoring the small bowel inflammation in patients with IBD.

LABORATORY STUDIES

As with radiologic studies, the history and physical examination guide the practitioner regarding laboratory studies. The result of all laboratory testing needs to be taken in context and cannot supersede physical findings or discount the importance of serial physical examinations.

In patients with abdominal pain, a complete blood count (CBC) with differential is helpful in the evaluation for inflammation, infection, or anemia. In general, an elevated high white blood cell (WBC) count with a neutrophilic predominance is more suspicious for an acute infectious or inflammatory cause of the patient's pain. However, a normal WBC count does not rule out infection, and an elevated WBC count does not confirm it. Anemia, if observed, can be very helpful in pointing the practitioner toward a chronic disease such as IBD or a disease associated with bleeding. A low mean corpuscular volume (MCV) with a high RDW suggests iron deficiency. Sudden acute blood loss may present with evidence of hemodynamic compromise before there is a fall in the hemoglobin level on an initial CBC.

A basic chemistry panel with serum electrolytes, glucose, creatinine, and BUN can help evaluate hydration status, acid-base balance, and electrolyte derangements, especially if vomiting, diarrhea, or inadequate oral intake is part of the clinical picture. These studies are typically less helpful in identifying the etiology of abdominal pain but are often needed for appropriate management.

Evaluation of serum hepatic enzymes and bilirubin levels, often referred to as liver function tests, are useful for patients with right upper quadrant pain or tenderness, or with jaundice. These tests usually include alanine aminotransferase (ALT), aspartate aminotransferase (AST), alkaline phosphatase, γ-glutamyl transferase (GGT), and levels of both the conjugated and unconjugated fractions of serum bilirubin (see Chapter 71 for further discussion of these tests). Concern for mononucleosis should prompt testing for EBV with EBV serology. Elevations of pancreatic enzymes, including amylase and lipase, are concerning for pancreatitis, and these studies would be warranted in patients with epigastric pain or tenderness or prominent vomiting (see Chapter 78).

Markers of inflammation, including erythrocyte sedimentation rate (ESR) and C-reactive protein (CRP) are usually elevated with chronic diseases like IBD, but are nonspecific and therefore can be elevated in many infectious, inflammatory, or malignant conditions. Newer serologic tests for IBD may be helpful in patients with a suggestive clinical picture, such as fecal calprotectin but definitive diagnosis still requires endoscopy with confirmatory tissue biopsy (see Chapter 76).

Urinalysis can provide information regarding hydration status (specific gravity) as well as indications of genitourinary involvement (e.g. red blood cells secondary to ureteral calculus or IgA vaculopathy) or infection (e.g. nitrates and white blood cells secondary to pyelonephritis). Patients with appendicitis may have sterile pyuria if the inflamed appendix settles on the wall of the bladder. All stools for any child with abdominal pain should be tested for blood, and if there is concern for infectious gastroenteritis or colitis. Appropriate samples may be sent to evaluate for the bacteria, toxins, parasites, or viruses of concern.

MANAGEMENT

The treatment of abdominal pain depends on the results of the initial workup or diagnosis. Patients thought to have surgical pathology are given nothing by mouth and often need resuscitation with intravenous fluids before definitive surgical intervention. Particular attention should be paid to pain control. Surgery is undertaken when the patient is stable for anesthesia, or occasionally before this point if the patient is toxic and deteriorating. If bowel perforation is suspected, the patient is started on broad-spectrum antibiotics to cover enteric pathogens, including anaerobes. Patients who are admitted without a definitive diagnosis require close monitoring, and serial abdominal exams. Recent literature suggests that serial examinations by pediatric surgeons are as effective as radiologic evaluation in patients with suspected early appendicitis. Diligent monitoring of fluid intake and output, along with vital signs, can provide an early clue that a disease is progressing. If there are stigmata of systemic GI disease, consultation with a pediatric gastroenterologist is appropriate. A child with viral gastroenteritis needs fluid resuscitation and time to improve oral intake.

As stated earlier, many patients who present with abdominal pain never receive a definitive diagnosis. In these instances, the goal of the hospitalization is to evaluate for potential life threatening or emergent conditions. When a symptomatic patient has been fully evaluated and organic disease has been ruled out, the goal of treatment is to control the patient's symptoms and reassure the patient and family prior to discharge. A child must be able to tolerate enough by mouth to stay hydrated and prevent weight loss. A school-age child must be able to attend school on most days. Most importantly, a patient with pain and a negative workup needs close follow-up, sometimes with a specialist, but always with the primary care physician. Literature increasingly suggests that patients with depression or anxiety may present with abdominal pain. In this case, a psychiatrist and/or psychologist may need to be involved, both for the evaluation of pain and for the teaching of coping strategies.

For patients discharged to home without a definitive diagnosis, it should be stressed to parents that the workup is ongoing and will continue in the outpatient setting.

SUGGESTED READINGS

Baker RD. Acute Abdominal Pain. *Pediatr Rev.* 2018;39:130-139.

Smith J, Fox S. Pediatric abdominal pain an emergency medicine perspective. *Emerg Med Clin N Am* 2016;34:341-361.

CHAPTER 17 Acidosis

Chase Parsons, DO, MBI

BACKGROUND

Acidosis is a common finding in many childhood disease states, ranging from self-resolving diarrheal illnesses to progressively degenerative mitochondrial disorders to severe sepsis and septic shock. Given the broad range of underlying illnesses and their distinct clinical consequences, identifying the specific etiology of acidosis can be crucial to a child's hospital care. In circumstances where there is relative diagnostic certainty, appropriate identification and characterization of acidosis can contribute important clinical evidence for or against a prevailing diagnostic theory or management strategy. For patients whose illnesses have not been fully characterized, a rational approach to the interpretation of acidosis can help direct more specific diagnostic testing and further clinical evaluation.

In this chapter, we discuss the pathophysiology, differential diagnoses, and evaluation strategies for acidosis, focusing primarily on metabolic acidosis. We include a section on respiratory acidosis in Special Considerations.

PATHOPHYSIOLOGY

Acidosis is a metabolic state characterized by a relative excess of hydrogen ions (H^+). This relative excess can result from a number of processes: (i) an increase in H^+ generation, (ii) a decrease in H^+ elimination via the kidneys, (iii) a decrease in basic buffer molecules, or (iv) a combination of the three. These processes reflect imbalances in the various counterregulatory systems involved with acid-base homeostasis.

A growing child generates a net of 1 to 3 mEq/kg/day of acid through normal metabolic processes. To maintain the optimal conditions for enzymatic activity (a pH between 7.35 and 7.45), the body must efficiently eliminate this and any additional acid load. Three primary mechanisms are responsible for maintaining this balance: the blood buffer system, respiratory ventilation, and renal excretion. Immediately upon exposure to excess acid, circulating buffers, including bicarbonate (HCO_3^-), bind excess H^+, diminishing its concentration in the extracellular space. The excess H^+ that binds to bicarbonate forms the "volatile" carbonic acid, which can then dissociate into carbon dioxide (CO_2) and water. Assuming sufficient H^+ excess and effective pulmonary ventilation, excess CO_2 is then removed from circulation through pulmonary capillaries and alveoli. In response to persistently low pH, peripheral chemoreceptors and central respiratory centers increase minute ventilation to augment this process. Lastly, proximal tubules in the kidney respond to excess H^+ by increasing bicarbonate reabsorption and ammonia synthesis, the latter of which assists with renal hydrogen ion elimination in the form of ammonium ions (NH_4^+).

Acidemia, defined as an arterial pH of less than 7.35, occurs when the body's numerous compensatory mechanisms to address an acid load are overwhelmed or compromised. The compensatory mechanisms can be overwhelmed in the setting of excess "non-volatile" acid production, as occurs acutely in lactic acidosis, diabetic ketoacidosis (DKA), or more indolently in the organic acidopathies. The body's buffer system can be compromised when there is a reduction in circulating bicarbonate from gastrointestinal losses (e.g., prolonged diarrheal illness) or renal losses as in proximal renal tubular acidosis. Compromised ventilation diminishes the body's ability to readily eliminate volatile acid in the form of CO_2, leading to retained H^+. Defects in the kidney's ability to appropriately acidify urine, as occurs with distal renal tubular acidosis (RTA), comprises the last set of conditions that lead to imbalances of this intricate homeostatic system.

DEFINITIONS

Acidosis: A state of relative excess of hydrogen ions.

Acidemia: Arterial pH less than 7.35.

Metabolic Acidosis: An acute or chronic state resulting from excess non-volatile H^+ production, decreased H^+ elimination via the kidneys, or diminished buffering capacity.

Respiratory Acidosis: An acute or chronic state of excess H^+ resulting from inadequate removal of volatile acid in the form of CO_2 via the lungs.

PATIENT HISTORY

Generally, the symptoms of acidosis are non-specific and therefore history should be targeted toward identifying the source of the acidosis. Common features of acute metabolic acidosis are tachypnea and hyperpnea (deep breathing). Other symptoms may include vomiting, fatigue, lethargy, seizures, and alterations in mental status. Children with diarrheal illness may have acidosis but this is not a symptom of the acidosis, rather the precipitant. Similarly, children with respiratory acidosis may present with decreased respiratory rate or respiratory failure, also conditions which led to the acidosis. History of ingestion is particularly important, as is history of medical conditions that may predispose the patient to acidosis. Among others, these include diabetes mellitus, prior diagnosis of metabolic disorder, seizure disorder on a ketogenic diet or anti-epileptic medication (AED), and systemic lupus erythematosus (which can be associated with a distal RTA). Several medications are associated with iatrogenic acidosis, specifically acetazolamide and other medications that can inhibit carbonic anhydrase (i.e., some AEDs) and amphotericin B or amiloride, that may mimic RTAs.

PHYSICAL EXAMINATION

Physical examination findings for children with acidosis are similarly nonspecific. Signs of hypovolemia (tachycardia, hypotension, delayed capillary refill, etc.) are often present in children with a diarrheal cause of excess bicarbonate loss or in those with lactic acidosis or DKA. Tachypnea and hyperpnea are common findings in acute metabolic acidosis in children due to respiratory compensation. Children presenting with DKA may present with fruity-smelling breath from increased acetone ventilation, and while signs of volume depletion are common in these patients, they may be less than expected given that intravascular volume may be maintained secondary to increased intravascular osmolality from hyperglycemia. Patients with severe acidosis may present with alterations in level of consciousness or obtundation.

DIFFERENTIAL DIAGNOSIS

The differential diagnosis for acidosis is broad. As with other clinical scenarios, a basic understanding of epidemiology helps to generate an ordered differential diagnosis by assessing the prior probability of a particular cause with respect to the individual characteristics, symptoms, and signs of the child before you. Etiologies such as diarrheal illness and lactic acidosis are most probable from the general population perspective. However, certain groups require special consideration, including toddlers, where ingestions are particularly common, and newborns, where undiagnosed inherited disorders of metabolism are more prevalent. While Bayesian logic helps to order the possible diagnostic options, several well-established and relatively formulaic strategies can assist in the characterization of a child's acidosis and are valuable in guiding further evaluation. One such strategy is detailed in **Figure 17-1**.

The initial step in categorization is to determine whether acidemia (pH <7.35) is present. In the non-emergent, non-intensive care setting, serum bicarbonate concentration is often used as a proxy for acidemia. While low bicarbonate concentration is reflective of acidosis, this is not equivalent to acidemia, which is important when considering whether there is appropriate compensation or a mixed disorder. An important rule of thumb is that the body's normal compensatory mechanisms will never overcome the primary process.

The second consideration is the primary source of the acidosis, which can usually be determined by assessing HCO_3^- and pCO_2. HCO_3^- of <22 mEq/L in the setting of acidemia indicates a metabolic acidosis, whereas a pCO_2 of >45 mm Hg on an appropriately collected and processed arterial blood gas indicates a respiratory acidosis.

Upon identification of a metabolic acidosis, the third consideration is to determine whether there is an anion gap. Based on the concept of electrochemical neutrality, total serum cation concentration must equal total serum anion concentration, so in normal metabolic states a fixed number should be derived when subtracting the sum of commonly measured serum cations from the sum of commonly measured anions. The most frequently used equation for anion gap is:

$$\text{anion gap} = [Na^+] - ([Cl^-]+[HCO_3^-]) = 12 \pm 2 \text{ mEq/L}$$

While there is never a "real" anion gap, a calculated gap of >14 mEq/L provides the clinician with evidence of both the presence and quantity of unmeasured anions, although gaps of up to 16 mEq/L may be normal in newborns. These unmeasured anions are generated through the buffering action of HCO_3^- in the presence of excess acid, as depicted in the following equilibrium:

$$H^+anion^- + NaHCO_3 \Leftrightarrow H_2O + CO_2 + Na^+anion^-$$

In this equilibrium, H^+anion^- represents the excess acid, such as keto-acids, lactic acid, and organic acids. Through this reaction, HCO_3^- is metabolized, and the anion salt of the excess acid remains and serves to maintain serum electrochemical neutrality. When HCO_3^- is metabolized at a greater rate than the acid salt is eliminated and new HCO_3^- generated, an unmeasured anion is detected when calculating the anion gap. Etiologies of anion gap and non–anion gap acidosis are presented in **Table 17-1**, and the diagnostic evaluation of these categories is discussed in the next section. Of note, the calculated anion gap may be inappropriately low in the presence of unmeasured cations, as with lithium toxicity and hypermagnesemia, or in the setting of hypoalbuminemia, which is a potent contributor to the normal anion gap. In the setting of low albumin, an adjusted AG can be calculated using the following formula:

$$\text{adjusted anion gap (mEq/L)} = \text{calculated AG (mEq/L)} + 2.5 \times [\text{normal albumin (g/dL)} - \text{measured albumin (g/dL)}]$$

A non–anion gap acidosis indicates either the loss of HCO_3^- through the kidney or gastrointestinal tract, with the subsequent retention of Cl^-, or the addition of an acid, with the subsequent consumption of HCO_3^- and a rapid renal excretion of the accompanying anion and replacement with Cl^-. In both cases, HCO_3^- is effectively replaced by Cl^-, which maintains a normal anion gap. Because of this tendency for Cl^- to replace HCO_3^-, non–anion gap acidosis is also known as hyperchloremic metabolic acidosis.

After determining whether there is an anion gap, the next consideration is whether the respiratory system is appropriately compensating for the acidosis. Winter's formula is a traditional approach to assessing respiratory compensation in acute metabolic acidosis.

$$([HCO_3^-] \times 1.5) + 8 \pm 2 = pCO_2$$

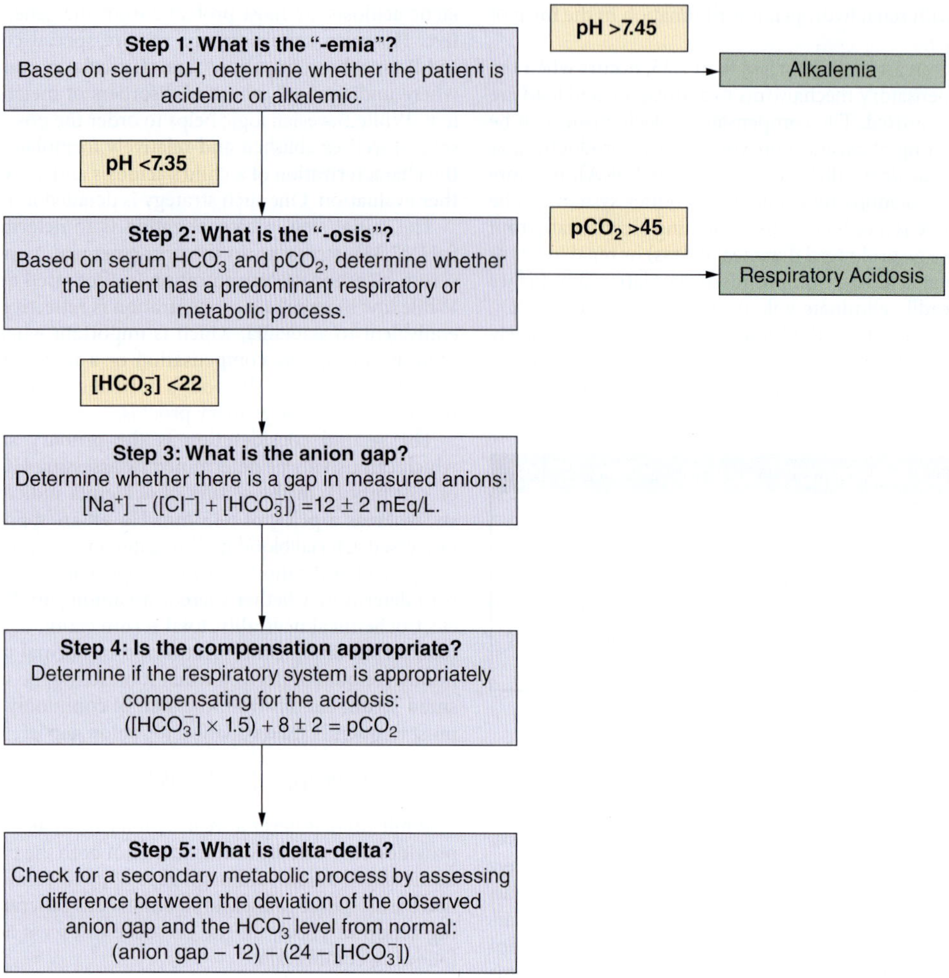

FIGURE 17-1. Step-wise approach to evaluation of metabolic acidosis.

Using this approach, if the pCO_2 does not have the above relationship with $[HCO_3^-]$, either the respiratory compensation is not appropriate for an acute acidosis or there is a secondary process. Additional general guidelines exist to help to assess appropriate respiratory compensation for both acute and chronic metabolic acidosis (**Figure 17-2**).

Last, assess for a second metabolic process in patients with an elevated anion gap by calculating the delta-delta.

$$\text{delta-delta} = (\text{anion gap} - 12) - (24 - [HCO_3^-])$$

This formula represents the difference between the observed anion gap and a normal anion gap and the observed decrease in bicarbonate buffer. The underlying principle of this formula is that the addition of an acid to the serum should result in an equimolar change in the bicarbonate and the unmeasured anion. Given this, in a pure metabolic acidosis one would expect this value to be zero. A value > 6 suggests the presence of a mixed disorder, such as the concomitant respiratory alkalosis in salicylate toxicity. Exceptions to this rule include lactic acidosis, where the increase in the anion gap can be as much as 1.6 to 1.8 times the decrease in serum bicarbonate, and diabetic ketoacidosis, where it is often less than 1:1, as ketoacids are lost in the urine.

DIAGNOSTIC EVALUATION

The most important initial labs in the evaluation of metabolic acidosis are a basic metabolic panel and an arterial, venous, or capillary blood gas. While the latter three are highly correlated on all parameters except pO_2, an appropriately collected and processed sample is critical in properly evaluating the nature of the acidosis. Using a systematic approach to interpretation of these tests, like the method described above, a clinician can determine whether further diagnostic evaluation is necessary, and if so, engage in a rational and targeted approach. Depending upon the acuity of the child's illness and the suspected causes, an evaluation may be relatively extensive and consultation with appropriate subspecialists may be warranted.

EVALUATION OF ANION GAP ACIDOSIS

As described above, an anion gap of >14 usually suggests the presence of unmeasured anions and may warrant further investigation. An anion gap of 20 or greater is more than 4 standard deviations above the mean and in this scenario, a metabolic acidosis is likely to be present, regardless of whether the pH or serum HCO_3^- are within the normal range. In those with an anion gap greater than 20, a specific cause for the metabolic acidosis will likely be discerned from the usual screening tests (**Table 17-2**).

Depending on clinical suspicion as to the cause of the acidosis, specific studies should be considered. A complete blood count may be abnormal in the setting of lactic acidosis from distributive shock secondary to infection or systemic illness. Elevated liver enzymes and abnormal function test results might indicate hepatic failure/dysfunction. In an infant or toddler with a history of poor growth or delayed development, recurrent vomiting or lethargy, or acidosis or hypoglycemia with illness, a metabolic disorder should be considered, and appropriate screening studies should be performed in consultation with a metabolism specialist (**Table 17-3**). An electrocardiogram should be performed if there is evidence of severe acidosis or other electrolyte abnormalities such as hyperkalemia. Serum or urine toxicology screening can be obtained if there is concern for ingestion or if interpretation of the initial labs reveals a second metabolic process.

TABLE 17-1 Etiologies of Anion Gap and Non–Anion Gap Metabolic Acidosis

- **Anion Gap Acidosis**
  - Ketoacidosis
    - Diabetic ketoacidosis
    - Alcoholic ketoacidosis
    - Starvation
  - Lactic acidosis
    - Tissue hypoxia
      - Shock
      - Dehydration
      - Hypoxia
      - Carbon monoxide poisoning
  - Increased production or decreased clearance of lactate
    - Leukemia, lymphoma, large tumors
    - Liver or renal failure
  - Renal failure (especially if GFR <15 mL/min/1.73 m^2; uremia and lactic acidosis)
  - Toxins or drugs
    - High osmolal gap
      - Ethylene glycol
      - Ethanol
      - Methanol
    - Normal osmolal gap
      - Salicylate
      - Ibuprofen
      - Toluene inhalation
      - Isoniazid
      - Iron
      - Metformin
  - Inborn errors of metabolism
- **Non–Anion Gap Acidosis**
  - Gastrointestinal loss of HCO_3^-
    - Diarrhea
    - Enteric fistulas (e.g., pancreatic) or enterostomies
    - Ureterosigmoidostomy (Cl^-/HCO_3^- exchanger)
      - Drugs (e.g., calcium chloride, cholestyramine, magnesium sulfate)
  - Renal acidosis
    - Loss of HCO_3^-
      - Proximal RTA (type 2)
      - Drugs (e.g., acetazolamide)
    - Failure to excrete H^+
      - Distal RTA (type I)
      - Drugs (e.g., potassium-sparing diuretics, amphotericin B)
    - Decreased ammoniagenesis
      - Generalized distal nephron dysfunction (type 4 RTA)
      - Early and moderate renal insufficiency (GFR 20–50 mL/min/1.73 m^2)
  - Acid load
    - Hyperalimentation
  - Dilutional
    - Rapid saline administration

GFR, glomerular filtration rate; RTA, renal tubular acidosis.

In the setting of an elevated anion gap and concern for ingestion, calculating the serum osmolal gap can be useful. Serum osmolality is calculated according to the following equation:

$$\text{osmolality}_{calc}\ (\text{mOsm/kg}) = 2 \times Na^+\ (\text{mEq/L}) + \text{blood urea nitrogen (mg/dL)}/2.8 + \text{glucose (mg/dL)}/18$$

The osmolal gap (the difference between measured osmolality and calculated osmolality) is normally 10 to 15 mOsm/kg. If the measured osmolality exceeds the calculated osmolality by more than 15 to 20 mOsm/kg, this indicates an accumulation of osmolytes other than the sodium salts, urea, and glucose, as seen with ingestion of ethylene glycol or methanol.

Metabolic Acidosis

Winter's formula: $([HCO_3^-] \times 1.5) + 8 \pm 2 = pCO_2$

Rule of thumb: Last 2 digits of pCO_2 should equal last 2 digits of pH

Respiratory Acidosis

For every 10 mm Hg increase in pCO_2, expect:

Acute: 1 mEq/L increase in $[HCO_3^-]$ and .08 decrease in pH

Chronic: 3.5 mEq/L increase in $[HCO_3^-]$

FIGURE 17-2. Appropriate compensation for metabolic and respiratory acidosis.

EVALUATION OF NON–ANION GAP ACIDOSIS

The urine anion gap (UAG) can be useful in differentiating between two common causes of non–anion gap acidosis: gastrointestinal losses and renal tubular acidosis (RTA). The UAG is calculated by obtaining spot measurements of urinary Na^+, potassium (K^+), and Cl^- (all units mEq/L):

$$UAG = (Na^+ + K^+)_{urine} - (Cl^-)_{urine}$$

The UAG is an indirect measure of urinary ammonium (NH_4^+), the precursor of which (ammonia = NH_3) is generated in the proximal tubules in the setting of acidosis. NH_4^+ is assumed to be present if the sum of the major urinary cations ($Na^+ + K^+$) is less than the major anion (Cl^-); because electrochemical neutrality must exist in the urine, some cation must be balancing the apparent surplus in measured Cl^-. In a metabolic acidosis from chronic diarrhea, the functioning kidneys increase proximal tubule NH_3 synthesis, thus providing more urinary buffer. In RTA, the urinary NH_4^+ is low because of the kidney's intrinsic inability to compensate for acid loads. A negative UAG usually suggests an extrarenal cause of non–anion gap acidosis (but can be negative with a proximal RTA), whereas a positive UAG suggests a renal cause (specifically distal RTA) of non–anion gap acidosis. The UAG should be interpreted with caution in the setting of hypovolemia, as adequate distal delivery of Na^+ is necessary for appropriate distal acidification, and when urinary pH >6.5, as HCO_3^- is likely present in the urine.

With specific regard to RTA, the acidosis in a distal RTA is usually more profound than with proximal RTA. A urine pH >5.5 in the setting

TABLE 17-2 Initial Laboratory Evaluation for Metabolic Acidosis

- Standard
  - Arterial blood gas
  - Electrolytes (Na^+, K^+, Cl^-, HCO_3^-)
  - Blood urea nitrogen, creatinine
  - Glucose
  - Urine pH
  - Consider urine electrolytes
- Based on clinical suspicion
  - Serum toxicology screen or measurement of specific drug if suspected
  - Complete blood count
  - Bacterial cultures
  - Hepatic enzymes and albumin determinations
  - Prothrombin time
  - Screening tests for suspected metabolic disorder (see Table 18-3)
  - Electrocardiogram

TABLE 17-3 Laboratory Studies for Suspected Inborn Error of Metabolism

Blood
Complete blood count with differential
Blood gas
Serum electrolytes
Glucose
Ammonia, lactate, and pyruvate
Amino acid quantification
Acylcarnitine profile
Free and total carnitine
Urine
Urinalysis, including ketones
Organic acids
Acylglycines

of acidosis may indicate impaired acidification of the urine, pointing toward a distal RTA. The urine pH in proximal RTA is variable, depending on the threshold of bicarbonate reabsorption. In general, children with proximal RTA can appropriately acidify the urine to <5.3 in the setting of acidosis, but the pH can be >5.3 if above the child's bicarbonate resorptive threshold. If proximal RTA is suspected based on above evaluation, other features of proximal tubular dysfunction (Fanconi syndrome) may be present, such as glucosuria, hypokalemia, hypophosphatemia, and generalized aminoaciduria.

MANAGEMENT

Management of metabolic acidosis is directed to treatment of the underlying cause. In general, treating the causes of anion gap acidosis can regenerate bicarbonate within hours; however, non–anion gap acidosis can take days to resolve and may require exogenous bicarbonate therapy. Insulin, hydration, and electrolyte repletion will correct the acidosis in diabetic ketoacidosis. Lactic acidosis will resolve with increasing tissue oxygenation using crystalloid, blood products, inotropic agents, and oxygen. Renal failure may require dialysis. Ethylene glycol and methanol ingestion can be treated with fomepizole, ethanol, and hemodialysis. Management of salicylate ingestion may include repeated doses of activated charcoal, alkalization of urine to optimize excretion, correction of metabolic derangements such as hypoglycemia and hypokalemia, and hemodialysis for severe ingestion. For acidosis secondary to metabolic disorders, the basic principle is to reverse counter-regulation and tissue catabolism with appropriate energy substrate (see Chapter 83). Diarrhea can be managed with fluid and electrolyte repletion. Bicarbonate supplementation and management of calcium and potassium homeostasis are effective in managing RTA, regardless of type.

The use of sodium bicarbonate in the treatment of severe metabolic acidosis is controversial. Once considered a mainstay of acute therapy for severe acute metabolic acidosis, studies have failed to demonstrate benefit of sodium bicarbonate in a number of scenarios, including severe diabetic ketoacidosis, neonatal resuscitation, and preterm metabolic acidosis. This has led some to question whether it has any role in acute metabolic acidosis therapy, especially given the list of potential side effects. Most notably, in the setting of suboptimal ventilation, bicarbonate infusion can lead to increase intracellular pCO_2, as HCO_3^- undergoes rapid conversion to carbonic acid and dissociation to H_2O and CO_2, which will diffuse into the tissue without adequate elimination via ventilation.

Despite accumulating evidence for lack of clear benefit, sodium bicarbonate is frequently used in the setting of severe acidosis (pH <7.0), where there are theoretical benefits to myocardial contractility, pulmonary vascular resistance, and arteriolar dilation and treatment options are limited. Clinicians may have a lower threshold (pH <7.2) to administer sodium bicarbonate for patients with compromised renal acid excretion, such as those with acute kidney injury or chronic kidney disease.

SPECIAL CONSIDERATIONS

RESPIRATORY ACIDOSIS

Respiratory acidosis is an abnormal clinical process that causes the arterial pCO_2 to increase to greater than 45 mm Hg. Increased CO_2 concentration in the serum may be secondary to increased CO_2 production or decreased ventilation. For example, administration of bicarbonate (which the body converts to CO_2) without adequate ventilation can result in respiratory acidosis. Decreased ventilation can result from depressed central respiratory drive, abnormalities in the chest wall or respiratory muscles, or alveolar hypoventilation. **Table 17-4** describes clinical scenarios in which respiratory acidosis may occur. When it does occur, cellular buffering begins within minutes. Renal compensation is optimized in 3 to 5 days.

The history and physical examination should focus on assessing the severity of respiratory symptoms, detecting consequences of acidemia, and identifying the underlying cause. The clinician should elicit any history of trauma, ingestion, or preceding illness, as well as any pertinent past medical history (e.g., severity of asthma exacerbations). The patient's general appearance, mental status, respiratory effort and drive, and cardiovascular examination are particularly relevant.

The arterial blood gas should be measured. As depicted in Figure 17-1, a decreased pH and high pCO_2 indicate respiratory acidosis. Expected metabolic compensation for respiratory acidosis can be calculated using the following rule: for every 10 mm Hg increase in pCO_2, serum HCO_3^- is expected to increase by 1 mEq/L acutely and 3.5 mEq/L chronically (Figure 17-2). Compensation for chronic respiratory acidosis rarely exceeds HCO_3^- of 38 mEq/L. If the pH or HCO_3^- is different from what was expected, a mixed acid-base disorder should be suspected.

The arterial blood gas results should be interpreted in their clinical context. For example, a normal pCO_2 in a patient with increased work

TABLE 17-4 Clinical Scenarios Causing Respiratory Acidosis

Acute central nervous system depression
Drug overdose
Benzodiazepines
Narcotics
Barbiturates
Head trauma
Cerebrovascular accident
Central nervous system infection
Acute neuromuscular disease
Guillain-Barré syndrome
Spinal cord injury
Myasthenia gravis
Toxin mediated (e.g. botulism, tetanus)
Acute pleural or chest wall disease
Pneumothorax
Hemothorax
Flail chest
Weakness secondary to electrolyte disturbances (hypophosphatemia, hypomagnesemia, hypokalemia)
Acute airway disease
Status asthmaticus
Upper airway obstruction
Acute parenchymal and vascular disease
Cardiogenic pulmonary edema
Acute lung injury
Multilobar pneumonia
Massive pulmonary embolism
Severe pneumonitis

Source: Data from Palmer BF, Clegg DJ. Respiratory Acidosis and Respiratory Alkalosis: Core Curriculum 2023 [published online ahead of print, 2023 Jun 20]. *Am J Kidney Dis.* 2023;S0272-6386(23)00610-8.

of breathing and tachypnea may indicate relative hypoventilation and respiratory fatigue. If available, an end-tidal CO_2 monitor can be helpful in following pCO_2 and detecting significant changes. In addition to arterial blood gas, the clinician should consider a chest radiograph, toxicology screen, electrolytes, lumbar puncture, and head computed tomography, based on clinical suspicion.

Acute respiratory acidosis can be a medical emergency that may require emergent airway intubation and mechanical ventilation. Otherwise, the underlying disease should be treated, and supportive care should be provided as necessary. Oxygen should be administered if the patient is hypoxemic. If the patient is unable to ventilate or oxygenate adequately, or if respiratory acidosis is severe, mechanical ventilation with continuous positive airway pressure, bilevel positive airway pressure, or intubation may be indicated. It is important not to correct acidosis too quickly if prolonged hypercapnia is suspected. Rapid correction can cause cerebrospinal fluid alkalization, which can result in seizures. Medications that suppress respiratory drive, such as narcotics, should be avoided until adequate assistance with ventilation is achieved. Electrolytes, particularly phosphate, magnesium, and potassium, should be maintained within normal ranges to optimize respiratory muscle function. Bicarbonate is not typically used to treat respiratory acidosis because it generates more CO_2.

INBORN ERRORS OF METABOLISM

Inborn errors of metabolism typically present from the neonatal period to early childhood, but they can present later, even in adolescence. Because the clinical presentation is varied and non-specific, metabolic disorders are often mistaken for another illness, such as sepsis. Signs and symptoms suggesting a metabolic disorder are listed in **Table 17-5**.

A child with a metabolic disorder may come to medical attention in several ways. State-mandated newborn screening often detects certain metabolic disorders before newborns are symptomatic. However, each state tests for a limited number of metabolic disorders, and false-negative results may occur if the test is done too early (i.e., within 24 hours of life) or before the newborn is feeding well. A child may also present to the primary pediatrician with a history of suggestive signs and symptoms, and the pediatrician might pursue a laboratory workup. Finally, a child might present to urgent care or the emergency department with an intercurrent illness, and laboratory abnormalities such as hypoglycemia, acidosis, hyperammonemia, or liver dysfunction might be discovered, suggesting a metabolic disorder.

When a metabolic disorder is suspected, the clinician should obtain the laboratory studies listed in Table 17-3. The likelihood of these studies detecting an inborn error of metabolism is higher if samples are taken at the time of illness and before treatment is delivered. In the setting of metabolic acidosis, hypoketotic hypoglycemia is highly suggestive of a fatty acid oxidation disorder. Hyperammonemia can occur with fatty acid oxidation disorders or with organic acidemias. When lactate levels are elevated, the clinician can calculate the lactate-to-pyruvate ratio (**Figure 17-3**). Other than severe acidosis, the initial laboratory results for organic acidemias are variable. Therefore, diagnosis is based on the characteristic pattern of urine organic acids and urine acylglycines.

Because clinical manifestations occur secondary to toxic metabolites formed during tissue catabolism, the general principle of therapy in cases of a suspected metabolic disorder is to reverse counter-regulation and tissue catabolism and to promote an anabolic state. This is accomplished by meeting the body's metabolic needs with energy substrates that can be used by the patient. For example, in cases of suspected organic acidemia or a fatty acid oxidation disorder, this can be achieved by correcting existing hypoglycemia with a bolus of 0.25 to 0.5 g/kg dextrose and then providing basal glucose needs at 10 mg/kg per minute. Practically, this can be accomplished with a 10% dextrose solution at a rate of 1.5 times maintenance, or its enteral equivalent. Other methods of lowering counter-regulatory hormones include ensuring an adequate circulating volume, controlling vomiting, recognizing and treating any infection or precipitating event, aggressively treating fever, and minimizing pain, stress, and agitation.

TABLE 17-5 Signs and Symptoms of a Metabolic Disorder

Severe presentation of simple illness
Lethargy with illness or fasting
Irritability
Poor feeding
Recurrent vomiting
Failure to thrive
Seizure disorder
Loss of developmental milestones or developmental delay
Hypotonia
Apnea or tachypnea
Hepatosplenomegaly

KEY POINTS

- Acidosis is commonly encountered in the setting of systemic illness and can be easily characterized using a systematic approach to basic laboratory evaluation.
- A basic understanding of acid-base homeostasis and the principle of electrochemical neutrality reveal important clinical distinctions and diagnostic branch points.
- Appropriate interpretation of basic labs by will help facilitate a rational diagnostic evaluation or obviate the need for additional testing and consultation.
- Treatment of metabolic acidosis should be directed to the treatment of the underlying cause.

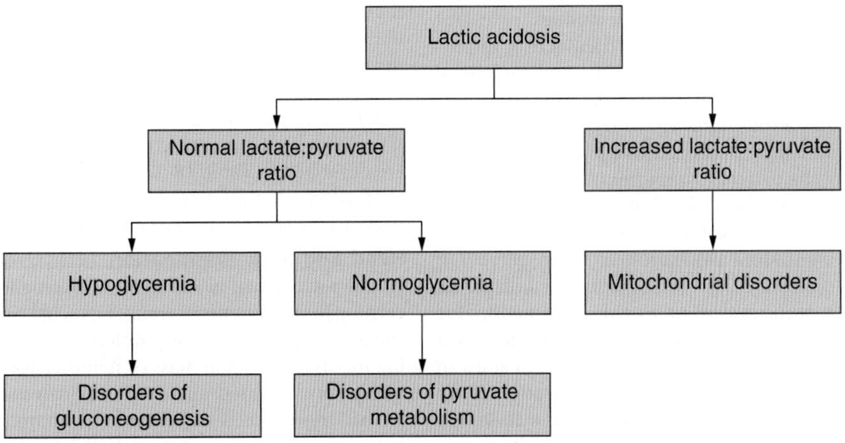

FIGURE 17-3. Further metabolic evaluation for lactic acidosis.

SUGGESTED READINGS

Aschner JL, Poland RL. Sodium bicarbonate: basically useless therapy. *Pediatrics*. 2008;122(4):831-835.

Beveridge CJ, Wilkinson AR. Sodium bicarbonate infusion during resuscitation of infants at birth. *Cochrane Database Syst Rev*. 2006;2006(1):CD004864.

Danhauser K, Smeitink JA, Freisinger P, et al. Treatment options for lactic acidosis and metabolic crisis in children with mitochondrial disease. *J Inherit Metab Dis*. 2015;38(3):467-475.

Haber RJ. A practical approach to acid-base disorders. *West J Med*. 1991;155(2):146.

Koves IH, Neutze J, Donath S, et al. The accuracy of clinical assessment of dehydration during diabetic ketoacidosis in childhood. *Diabetes Care*. 2004;27(10):2485-2487.

Kraut JA, Madias NE. Metabolic acidosis: pathophysiology, diagnosis and management. *Nat Rev Nephrol*. 2010;6(5):274-285.

Lawn CJ, Weir FJ, McGuire W. Base administration or fluid bolus for preventing morbidity and mortality in preterm infants with metabolic acidosis. *Cochrane Database Syst Rev*. 2005;2005(2):CD003215.

Loh TP, Metz MP. Trends and physiology of common serum biochemistries in children aged 0-18 years. *Pathology*. 2015;47(5):452-461.

Lopez-Garcia SC, Emma F, Walsh SB, et al. Treatment and long-term outcome in primary distal renal tubular acidosis. *Nephrol Dial Transplant*. 2019;34(6):981-991.

Lorenz JM, Kleinman LI, Markarian K, Oliver M, Fernandez J. Serum anion gap in the differential diagnosis of metabolic acidosis in critically ill newborns. *J Pediatr*. 1999;135(6):751-755.

Viallon A, Zeni F, Lafond P, et al. Does bicarbonate therapy improve the management of severe diabetic ketoacidosis? *Crit Care Med*. 1999;27(12):2690-2693.

Yıldızdaş D, Yapıcıoğlu H, Yılmaz HL, Sertdemir Y. Correlation of simultaneously obtained capillary, venous, and arterial blood gases of patients in a paediatric intensive care unit. *Arch Dis Child*. 2004;89(2):176-180.

CHAPTER 18 Altered Mental Status

Jacqueline Ponczek, MD, MS and Martin Duncan, MD

BACKGROUND

Altered mental status (AMS) is a broadly applied term used to describe any change in a patient's baseline behavior, cognitive abilities, or awareness of and interaction with the environment. In particular, it is important to understand the patient's baseline mental status and individual development. The presentation of AMS in a pediatric patient encompasses a wide variety of manifestations, ranging from confusion to lethargy, stupor, obtundation, and coma. Approach to the child with AMS requires careful assessment of the patient's symptoms and physical exam as well as eliciting a detailed medical and developmental history along with prodromal symptoms, potential exposures (environmental and pharmacologic), and preceding trauma. Evaluation and management of children with AMS is often complicated by a broad differential diagnosis and potentially limited ability of the patient to provide information due to their impaired mental status or developmental age. Clinicians must often rely on parents or caregivers to elicit contextual details to assist in the assessment. Initial management should focus on stabilization of the circulation, airway, and breathing, followed by completing a thorough interview and physical examination, and determining further diagnostic evaluations.

PATIENT HISTORY

In the acute setting, providers should take a focused history prioritizing initial interventions to reduce morbidity and mortality. When appropriate, providers should elicit a detailed history if possible from the patient, parent, guardian, or caregiver. The history should focus on the following elements:

1. Baseline behavior, developmental age, and neurologic state: This is particularly important given the functional variations among different pediatric age groups, and those observed among children with developmental and intellectual disabilities.
2. Onset/Timing: Obtain information on the acuity, timing, and course of the symptoms. The impairments may be described as acute, intermittent, fluctuating, persistent, recurrent, or progressive.
3. Associated symptoms: Providers should perform a full review of systems. Providers should pay special attention to any concurrent, preceding, or prodromal symptoms including fever, headache, nausea, vomiting, seizure, or changes in bowel or bladder habits.
4. Trauma: Inquire about trauma or other observed injuries such as bruising, especially if no clear mechanism of injury exists or if the suggested mechanism is inconsistent with the clinical presentation.
5. Past medical history: Obtain immunization status in addition to existing medical and psychiatric conditions (acute or chronic), surgeries, or other recent procedures.
6. Medications: Obtain a detailed delineation of any prescription or over-the-counter medication (OTC) changes, including new medications, recent dose adjustments, or discontinuation of medications. Also collect a list of medications belonging to other household members to which the patient may have access including both prescription and OTCs or supplements.
7. Social history: Obtain a history of access to or risk for recreational drug or alcohol use by both the patient and family members or household contacts. Assess stressors in the home or at school. In the adolescent population, complete a HEADSS assessment (Home, Education, Activities, Drugs, Sex, Suicide) if patient's mental status allows.
8. Travel history/exposures: Obtain an account of recent domestic and international travel. Assess outdoor activities and potential exposures to disease vectors such as tick or mosquito bites. Obtain a history of environmental exposure, such as access to household cleaning items, chemicals, or risks for lead exposure. Assess for any other close contacts with similar symptoms.
9. Family history: Obtain a family history with special focus on autoimmune disease, migraines, coagulopathies, stroke, seizure disorders, and psychiatric illness.

PHYSICAL EXAM

Following initial stabilization, the patient's clinical features including their vital signs and physical exam can frequently offer clues to help narrow the differential diagnosis and direct the diagnostic workup to uncover underlying etiologies.

Taking a systematic approach allows simultaneously for a rapid assessment for initial stabilization and an organized approach to the differential diagnosis. Common etiologies for specific vital sign abnormalities are described in **Table 18-1**.

In addition, a physical examination focusing on the head, neck, and nervous systems can be particularly helpful during the initial assessment.

Head and neck examination Ecchymoses suggest possible trauma, whether accidental or inflicted. A bulging fontanelle in an infant is concerning for meningitis or trauma. Nuchal rigidity in an older child would suggest meningitis. An asymmetric pupillary examination is concerning for an intracranial mass or hemorrhage, while symmetric mydriasis, miosis, or decreased pupillary responsiveness would be consistent with a toxic ingestion. If papilledema is appreciated, the evaluation should focus on causes of increased ICP including meningitis, CNS masses, or intracranial hemorrhage. If signs of orbital cellulitis or sinusitis are

TABLE 18-1 Clinical Features

Temperature	Hyperthermia	Infection Autoimmune process Drug overdose/Adverse reaction • Anticholinergics • Sympathomimetics • Neuroleptic malignant syndrome • Serotonin syndrome
	Hypothermia	Toxic ingestion exposure (e.g., alcohol) Hypothyroidism Hypoglycemia Infection Exposure (prolonged cold environment)
Heart Rate	Bradycardia	Toxic ingestion exposure: • Beta-blockers • Calcium channel blockers • Carbamates Hypothyroidism Hypoglycemia Increased intracranial pressure
	Tachycardia	Infections Hyperthyroidism Ingestion (e.g., sympathomimetics, anticholinergics)
Respiratory Rate	Tachypnea	Infection Toxic ingestion • Salicylates • Ethylene glycol Carbon monoxide poisoning Methemoglobinemia
	Bradypnea or Hypopnea	Toxic ingestions (e.g., opioids) Increased intracranial pressure • CNS masses • Infections • Hemorrhage
Blood Pressure	Hypertension	Hypertensive encephalopathy Intracranial hemorrhage Posterior reversible encephalopathy (PRES) Toxic ingestion (e.g., sympathomimetics)
	Hypotension	Infections Toxic ingestions (e.g., opioids or benzodiazepines) Shock

present, the differential should include cavernous venous thrombosis or an epidural abscess.

Neurological examination The neurological examination should first focus on a patient's level of consciousness as compared to a developmentally appropriate level of awareness and alertness. For children with developmental or intellectual disabilities, caregiver input is critical to ascertain differences from baseline. The most commonly used terms to describe impaired levels of consciousness are described in **Table 18-2**. The Glasgow Coma Scale, including a modified version for the pediatric population, is frequently used to provide an objective measure of the level of impairment both on initial evaluation and during subsequent examinations (**Table 18-3**).

Most of the diagnoses on the differential for AMS can occur with any of the levels of impairment described in **Table 18-2**, depending on the severity or duration of symptoms. However, more significant impairment (e.g., stupor and coma) should result in a more expeditious and broader initial differential diagnosis and subsequent diagnostic evaluation.

TABLE 18-2 Definitions of Altered Levels of Consciousness

Confusion	A state of disorientation: patient often has difficulty following commands, patient may be agitated or drowsy
Lethargy	A state of mildly depressed consciousness: patient fully awakens with mild external stimuli, can remain alert for brief periods of time before falling back asleep
Obtundation	A state of moderately reduced consciousness with slow response to moderate external stimuli: patient remains drowsy without ever becoming fully alert, patient will fall back asleep if not repeatedly stimulated
Stupor	A state of significantly reduced consciousness: patient requires significant vigorous stimuli to respond, responds by grimacing or withdrawing from stimuli without becoming fully awake, returns immediately to sleep
Coma	A state of unarousable unresponsiveness: patient has no response to vigorous external stimuli

Patients who present without changes in consciousness or only mild impairments can be assessed more fully for changes in behavior and cognitive abilities. Agitation may be a sign of a drug or toxic ingestion, withdrawal, psychosis, or hyperthyroidism. Cognitive dysfunctions—including disorientation or difficulties with speech or memory—may also be due to a toxic exposure, infection, CNS mass, traumatic brain injury, or intracranial hemorrhage.

Additional examination findings, such as hyperreflexia or asymmetric reflexes, as well as hemiplegias suggest a CNS infection, intracranial mass, or stroke. Psychomotor slowing or rigidity would suggest neuroleptic malignant syndrome (NMS) or a primary psychiatric illness.

DIFFERENTIAL DIAGNOSIS AND DIAGNOSTIC EVALUATION

AMS is used to describe a patient's symptoms rather than a definable disease and can be the presenting symptom in a multitude of disease processes that range from benign to life-threatening. It is important to analyze the history and constellation of symptoms to determine diagnosis. Most etiologies fall within a number of broad categories as outlined in **Table 18-4**. The most commonly obtained diagnostic studies, including laboratory evaluations and imaging studies are also outlined in **Table 18-4**. Creating a framework based on age and broad categories of disease may be a useful initial approach. For example, primary

TABLE 18-3 Glasgow Coma Scale (including Pediatric Modifications)

Activity	Modified for Pediatrics		Score
Eye opening	Spontaneous	Spontaneous	4
	Response to verbal stimuli	Response to verbal stimuli	3
	Response to painful stimuli	Response to painful stimuli	2
	No response	No response	1
Verbal response	Cooing, babbling	Oriented, appropriate response	5
	Irritable, crying	Confused	4
	Cries with painful stimuli	Inappropriate words	3
	Moans with painful stimuli	Incomprehensible or non-specific words	2
	No response	No response	1
Motor response	Spontaneous and purposeful movements	Obeys commands	6
	Withdraws to touch	Localizes pain	5
	Withdraws to painful stimuli	Withdraws to painful stimuli	4
	Decorticate posturing in response to painful stimuli	Decorticate posturing in response to painful stimuli	3
	Decerebrate posturing in response to pain		2
	No response	No response	1

TABLE 18-4 Common Etiologies of Altered Mental Status and Initial Diagnostic Approach

Category	Diagnoses	Common Diagnostic Studies
Infections	**Meningitis and Infectious Encephalitis** *Bacterial* *Viral* *Fungal*	**CBC with Differential** **Blood culture** **Inflammatory Markers** *(ESR, CRP, Procalcitonin)* **CSF Analysis** *(Cell count, gram stain, culture, viral testing)*
	Sepsis *Bacterial* *Viral* *Fungal*	**CBC with Differential** **Blood culture** **Inflammatory Markers** *(ESR, CRP, Procalcitonin)* **Urinalysis** **Urine culture**
	Other CNS Infection and Postinfectious Entities *(e.g., CNS abscess, MIS-C, ADEM)*	**Neuroimaging** *(CT/MRI)*
Neurology	**Seizure** **Paroxysmal Non-epileptiform Disorders** **Migraine**	**Neuroimaging** *(CT/MRI)* **EEG**
Structural	**Vascular Abnormality** **Stroke Syndromes** *(Ischemic Stroke--AIS, CSVT vs. hemorrhagic stroke)* **Space-occupying Lesion** *(e.g., tumor)* **Device Malfunction**	**Neuroimaging** *(CT/MRI with dedicated vascular imaging)* **Xray Shunt Series (if shunt present)**
Trauma	**Traumatic Brain Injury** **Concussion** **Intracranial Hemorrhage/Hematoma**	**Neuroimaging** *(CT/MRI)*
Metabolism/Endocrine	**Thyroid dysfunction**	**Thyroid function tests** *(TSH, FT4, T3)*
	Hypoglycemia/Hyperglycemia	**Point-of-care glucometer (immediate evaluation)** **BMP/CMP** **Urinalysis** **Serum ketones or beta-hydroxybutyrate**
	Electrolyte Disturbances *(Hypernatremia, hyponatremia, hypophosphatemia, hypercalcemia)*	**BMP/CMP** *with serum magnesium, ionized calcium, and phosphorus* **Urinalysis**
	Metabolic Disturbances *(Hyperammonemia, uremia, metabolic acidosis, metabolic alkalosis, hypercapnia)* **Hepatic Dysfunction** **Renal Dysfunction**	**Blood Gas and pH Analysis (arterial preferred)** **BMP/CMP** **LFTs/HFP** **Urinalysis** **Serum Ammonia** **Serum Lactate** **Serum and Urine Amino Acids** **Serum and Urine Organic Acids** **Serum Free Fatty Acids** **Serum Acylcarnitine Profile**
Autoimmune	**Autoimmune Encephalitis** **Lupus Cerebritis** **Multiple Sclerosis**	**Neuroimaging** *(CT/MRI)* **EEG** **Specific Autoantibodies**
Cardiovascular	**Syncope** *(i.e., arrythmia, hypotension, structural or functional heart disease, vasovagal episode)* **Hypertensive Encephalopathy**	**EKG** **Echocardiogram** **Blood Pressure Monitoring** **BMP/CMP** *with serum magnesium, ionized calcium, and phosphorus*
Toxins, Drugs, and Environmental Exposures	**Medication Overdose** **Medication Underdose** **Polypharmacy and Medication Interaction** **Medication/Drug Withdrawal** **Medication Adverse Effect** **Recreational Drugs/Alcohol Intoxication** **Environmental Toxins**	**Serum Toxicology Screen** **Urine Toxicology Screen** **Medication Drug Levels** **EKG**

(Continued)

TABLE 18-4 Common Etiologies of Altered Mental Status and Initial Diagnostic Approach (*Continued*)

Category	Diagnoses	Common Diagnostic Studies
Psychiatry	Delirium Primary Psychiatric Illness Secondary Psychiatric Illness	Neuroimaging *(CT/MRI)* Serum Toxicology Screen Urine Toxicology Screen Medication Drug Levels CSF analysis *(Cell count, gram stain, culture, viral testing, autoimmune studies)* EEG
Other	Intussusception	Abdominal Ultrasound
	PRES *(Hypertensive encephalopathy, immunosuppressive medications, renal disease)*	Neuroimaging *(CT/MRI)* Blood pressure monitoring
	Hemolytic uremic syndrome	CBC, LDH, BMP/CMP

ADEM, Acute Disseminated Encephalomyelitis; AIS, Arterial Ischemic Stroke; BMP, basic metabolic panel; CBC, complete blood count; CMP, comprehensive metabolic panel; CNS, central nervous system; CRP, C-reactive protein; CSF, cerebrospinal fluid; CSVT, Cerebral Sinovenous Thrombosis; CT, computed tomography; EEG, electroencephalogram; EKG, electrocardiogram; ESR, erythrocyte sedimentation rate; FT4, free thyroxine; HFP, hepatic function panel; LDH, lactate dehydrogenase; LFTs, liver function tests; MIS-C, Multisystem inflammatory syndrome in children; MRI, magnetic resonance imaging; T3, triiodothyronine; TSH, thyroid stimulating hormone.

neurologic, infectious, or toxin-mediated etiologies have a higher likelihood in the pediatric population when compared to adults. In the adolescent population, ingestion or toxicology may be of particularly high yield.

There is no standard approach to evaluation of AMS in children and it may vary based on initial presentation, degree of impairment, and by provider. Subspeciality consultation should be sought out as needed.

Patients who present with a more significant degree of mental status impairment (obtundation, stupor, or coma), persistently AMS, or in those cases in which the underlying etiology is not immediately identified will often undergo more extensive and emergent evaluation to rule out etiologies requiring immediate intervention. Frequently, the time-sensitive nature of the management decisions do not allow for a thorough history to be obtained. These patients should be evaluated for acute processes like CNS masses, hemorrhage, stroke, trauma, electrolyte derangements (particularly hypoglycemia), toxic ingestions, CNS infections, and shock. There should be a low threshold for obtaining emergent neuroimaging in those with persistently AMS. In the emergency setting, neuroimaging may be accomplished with head computed tomography (CT) or if available, rapid magnetic resonance imaging (MRI) of the brain may be an acceptable alternative in nontraumatic scenarios. Additional studies obtained in the acute period may also include electrocardiogram (ECG), laboratory evaluation including an extended chemistry panel (electrolytes, BUN, creatinine, calcium, magnesium, and phosphorus), point-of-care tests like glucose and blood gas, complete blood count (CBC) and urinalysis, blood and urine cultures, and blood and urine toxicology screens. Lumbar puncture with cerebrospinal fluid (CSF) analysis should only be obtained once neuroimaging has been performed in cases of suspected increased intracranial pressure such as in those patient that present with coma, papilledema, focal neurologic deficits, history of hydrocephalus, CSF shunt, recent CNS trauma or neurosurgery, or history of intracranial pathology.

Additional detail regarding common etiologies and suggested diagnostic workup are listed below.

Infections For patients presenting with signs of meningitis (acute onset of lethargy, confusion, fever, headaches, nuchal rigidity, seizures), the diagnostic workup should include CSF analysis (cell count, protein, glucose, gram stain, and culture), as well as a CBC with differential. Bacterial, viral, and rickettsial causes of meningitis should be considered. In areas where tick-borne illnesses such as Lyme and Rocky Mountain Spotted Fever are endemic, specific studies should be obtained. *Enterovirus* testing should be obtained during the summer and fall seasons. Herpes simplex virus (HSV) testing should also be considered in infants.

CSF analysis including viral studies should also be obtained for patients in whom encephalitis is suspected (initially fluctuating levels of consciousness that become persistently depressed with seizures, fevers, headaches, or a focal neurological examination). Head CT or brain MRI can also be helpful in establishing a diagnosis. Additional testing for suspected infectious causes, including Epstein-Barr virus, HSV, influenza, and mycoplasma may be helpful. In endemic regions, testing for the arboviruses should also be considered.

Special consideration should be given to patients who are immunocompromised (may benefit from CSF evaluation for fungal infections), undervaccinated patients, and travelers returning from areas with specific endemic viruses, parasites, and fungi.

Neurology Seizures are a common cause of AMS. Patients may present actively seizing (convulsive or non-convulsive) or present in a postictal state. Some etiologies of seizure include: febrile seizure (simple and complex), primary seizure disorder, CNS mass, infection, traumatic brain injury, stroke, ingestion, electrolyte derangement, or hypoglycemia. Lab evaluation may include electrolytes, glucose, and CSF analysis with infectious studies. Neuroimaging is also frequently helpful, especially when trauma, ischemic stroke, intracranial hemorrhage, or infections are suspected. EEG may be helpful if non-convulsive status epilepticus the presence of a primary seizure disorder is suspected, or if the diagnosis of a seizure is unclear. For children presenting with a simple febrile seizure and a non-focal examination, no further evaluation is generally necessary. In patients with known seizure disorders on anticonvulsant therapy, anti-epileptic drug levels should be obtained.

Structural Strokes are relatively rare in the pediatric population, but should be considered in patients presenting with AMS who are noted to have hemiparesis, headaches, ataxia, or changes in speech. Ischemic strokes in children are divided into arterial ischemic stroke or cerebral sinovenous thrombosis. Neuroimaging should be obtained emergently whenever a stroke is suspected. This includes MRI or CT with dedicated vascular imaging. Stroke should especially be considered in patients with risk factors, such as sickle cell disease, congenital heart disease, prothrombotic disorders, vasculopathy, history of prior strokes, or significant head and neck infections. Migraine may mimic ischemic stroke.

Increased ICP (regardless of etiology) can result in AMS. A high index of suspicion in the medical history and physical exam is critical to obtaining emergent neuroimaging and preventing severe morbidity and mortality. Increased ICP is frequently accompanied by a history of headaches and/or vomiting. The suspicion of a space-occupying lesion such as a tumor, arteriovenous malformation, or aneurysm should be evaluated with neuroimaging. Device failure or malfunction should always be considered in children with CNS shunts. This should be evaluated with neuroimaging and/or dedicated X-rays.

Trauma Traumatic brain injuries ranging from concussions to intracranial hemorrhages generally present with a history of trauma preceding the alteration in mental status. Patients presenting with prolonged loss of consciousness, persistent or worsening alterations in their levels of consciousness, a focal neurological examination, or a seizure should be evaluated with neuroimaging.

Children who present with any level of decreased consciousness, especially with unexplained, vague, or implausible history of trauma, bruising, scalp swelling, or bulging fontanelle, should obtain neuroimaging, as non-accidental trauma should be suspected.

Metabolism/Endocrine Hypoglycemia is a common etiology for AMS, especially in infants and younger children with a history of prolonged fasting (often due to gastroenteritis). Patients with a history of inborn errors of metabolism are also prone to hypoglycemia. Toxic ingestions (e.g., ethanol and beta-blockers) can also present with hypoglycemia. Point-of-care glucometer testing or serum glucose testing should be obtained.

Electrolyte derangements can also cause AMS and should be considered in patients with significant dehydration or renal dysfunction. An extended electrolyte panel and renal function testing should be obtained to assist in the diagnosis.

Thyroid function tests should also be obtained, although some etiologies including Hashimoto encephalitis can present with normal thyroid function. Antithyroid antibodies (microsomal and thyroglobulin) need to be sent to establish the diagnosis.

Autoimmune Autoimmune encephalitis should be suspected in a patient who presents with acute-onset neuropsychiatric symptoms including anxiety, unusual behaviors, paranoia, and delusions that devolve to decreased levels of consciousness and seizures. Some patients may also present with autonomic instability. Specific serum or CSF autoantibodies (e.g., N-methyl-D-aspartate or NMDA) should be sent for evaluation. An EEG and brain MRI are also often helpful in establishing the diagnosis.

Toxicology/Environmental Exposures Toxic ingestions (intentional or unintentional) frequently present with AMS, especially in toddlers and adolescents. Toxicology screens may be useful in assessing for the most common drugs of abuse or over-the-counter medications, but many pharmacologic agents may be missed. Extended screens or directed testing for certain medications (e.g., anti-epileptic drugs) may also be beneficial. If there is high suspicion of an illicit drug ingestion, naloxone may be administered before results of the toxicology screens are available.

Psychiatry Primary psychiatric illness is a frequent presentation to the emergency room and etiology of AMS.

Patients presenting with new and acute neuropsychiatric symptoms may require evaluation for medical etiologies of secondary psychosis. Some organic disease processes may include hyper- and hypothyroidism, autoimmune encephalitis, metabolic disorders (e.g., Wilson disease), illicit drug use, CNS masses, or seizures (e.g., temporal lobe seizures). High-quality evidence links drugs of abuse with psychosis onset and so urine or blood toxicology screens should be obtained.

Other Additional etiologies that may present with AMS as part of their constellation of symptoms should be evaluated individually as supported by the clinical history and diagnostic evaluation. For example, intussusception should be suspected in children with AMS and episodic abdominal pain, vomiting, and bloody stools and should be further evaluated with an abdominal ultrasound. Posterior reversible encephalopathy syndrome (PRES) can have various etiologies and is best evaluated with neuroimaging and frequent blood pressure monitoring.

MANAGEMENT

The management of AMS is generally determined by the most likely or identified underlying etiology and may include administration of antiepileptics, antimicrobials, antidotes, or correction of electrolyte imbalances. All patients with AMS require serial neurologic examinations to monitor for progression of symptoms. Patients with severe neurologic impairment may require additional support for vital functions including intubation for airway protection, hemodynamic support, and/or parenteral fluids.

KEY POINTS

- The chief complaint of AMS requires a careful history and physical examination to narrow an otherwise broad differential.
- In cases of significant impairment and medical instability, rapid evaluation and management is paramount to minimizing morbidity and mortality.
- When time permits, a thorough history and physical examination frequently provides the clues to generate a tailored assessment to guide practical and efficient diagnostic evaluation.

SUGGESTED READINGS

Avner JR. Altered states of consciousness. *Pediatr Rev.* 2006;27(9):331-338.

Boyer EW, Shannon M. The serotonin syndrome. *N Engl J Med.* 2005;352(11):1112-1120.

Button K, Capraro A, Monuteaux M, Mannix R. Etiologies and yield of diagnostic testing in children presenting to the emergency department with altered mental status. *J Pediatr.* 2018;200:218-224.e2.

Bykowski J, Kruk P, Gold JJ, Glaser CA, Sheriff H, Crawford JR. Acute pediatric encephalitis neuroimaging: single-institution series as part of the California Encephalitis Project. *Pediatr Neurol.* 2015;52(6):606-614.

Clinical policy for the initial approach to patients presenting with altered mental status. *Ann Emerg Med.* 1999;33(2):251-281.

Clinical policy for the initial approach to patients presenting with acute toxic ingestion or dermal or inhalation exposure. *Ann Emerg Med.* 1999;33(6):735-761.

Del Brutto OH, Rajshekhar V, White AC, et al. Proposed diagnostic criteria for neurocysticercosis. *Neurology.* 2001;57(2):177-183.

Dlamini N, Billinghurst L, Kirkham FJ. Cerebral venous sinus (sinovenous) thrombosis in children. *Neurosurg Clin N Am.* 2010;21(3):511-527.

Ferriero DM, Fullerton HJ, Bernard TJ, et al. Management of stroke in neonates and children: a scientific statement from the American Heart Association/American Stroke Association. *Stroke.* 2019;50(3):e51-e96.

Florance NR, Davis RL, Lam C, et al. Anti-N-methyl-D-aspartate receptor (NMDAR) encephalitis in children and adolescents. *Ann Neurol.* 2009;66(1):11-18.

Fortu JMT, Kim IK, Cooper A, Condra C, Lorenz DJ, Pierce MC. Psychiatric patients in the pediatric emergency department undergoing routine urine toxicology screens for medical clearance: results and use. *Pediatr Emerg Care.* 2009;25(6):387-392.

Glaser CA, Honarmand S, Anderson LJ, et al. Beyond viruses: clinical profiles and etiologies associated with encephalitis. *Clin Infect Dis.* 2006;43(12):1565-1577.

Hartman AL, Lunney KM, Serena JE. Pediatric stroke: do clinical factors predict delays in presentation? *J Pediatr.* 2009;154(5):727-732.

Jackson BF, Porcher FK, Zapton DT, Losek JD. Cerebral sinovenous thrombosis in children: diagnosis and treatment. *Pediatr Emerg Care.* 2011;27(9):874-880; quiz 881-883.

Kanich W, Brady WJ, Huff JS, et al. Altered mental status: evaluation and etiology in the ED. *Am J Emerg Med.* 2002;20(7):613-617.

Kimia A, Ben-Joseph EP, Rudloe T, et al. Yield of lumbar puncture among children who present with their first complex febrile seizure. *Pediatrics.* 2010;126(1):62-69.

Kimia AA, Ben-Joseph E, Prabhu S, et al. Yield of emergent neuroimaging among children presenting with a first complex febrile seizure. *Pediatr Emerg Care.* 2012;28(4):316-321.

Kleizen KJ, Hunck A, Wijnen MH, Draaisma JMT. Neurological symptoms in children with intussusception. *Acta Paediatr.* 2009;98(11):1822-1824.

Koita J, Riggio S, Jagoda A. The mental status examination in emergency practice. *Emerg Med Clin North Am.* 2010;28(3):439-451.

Leypoldt F, Armangue T, Dalmau J. Autoimmune encephalopathies. *Ann N Y Acad Sci.* 2015;1338(1):94-114.

MacNeill EC, Vashist S. Approach to syncope and altered mental status. *Pediatr Clin North Am*. 2013;60(5):1083-1106.

Merritt J, Tanguturi Y, Fuchs C, Cundiff AW. Medical Etiologies of Secondary Psychosis in Children and Adolescents. *Child Adolesc Psychiatr Clin N Am*. 2020;29(1):29-42.

Mick N, Brown DFM, Nadel ES. Pediatric altered mental status. *J Emerg Med*. 2003;25(2):193-196.

Moraitis E, Ganesan V. Childhood infections and trauma as risk factors for stroke. *Curr Cardiol Rep*. 2014;16(9):527.

Nigrovic LE, Malley R, Kuppermann N. Cerebrospinal fluid pleocytosis in children in the era of bacterial conjugate vaccines: distinguishing the child with bacterial and aseptic meningitis. *Pediatr Emerg Care*. 2009;25(2):112-117; quiz 118-120.

Nigrovic LE. Aseptic meningitis. *Handb Clin Neurol*. 2013;112:1153-1156.

Ramgopal S, Karim SA, Subramanian S, Furtado AD, Marin JR. Rapid brain MRI protocols reduce head computerized tomography use in the pediatric emergency department. *BMC Pediatr*. 2020;20(1):14.

Seydel KB, Kampondeni SD, Valim C, et al. Brain swelling and death in children with cerebral malaria. *N Engl J Med*. 2015;372(12):1126-1137.

Skikic M, Arriola JA. First episode psychosis medical workup: evidence-informed recommendations and introduction to a clinically guided approach. *Child Adolesc Psychiatr Clin N Am*. 2020;29(1):15-28.

Stoodley N. Neuroimaging in non-accidental head injury: if, when, why and how. *Clin Radiol*. 2005;60(1):22-30.

Sulkowski JA, Judy KD. Acute mental status changes. *AACN Clin Issues*. 1997;8(3):319-334; quiz 502-504.

Tatman A, Warren A, Williams A, Powell JE, Whitehouse W. Development of a modified paediatric coma scale in intensive care clinical practice. *Arch Dis Child*. 1997;77(6):519-521.

Teasdale G, Jennett B. Assessment of coma and impaired consciousness. *Lancet*. 1974;304(7872):81-84.

Venkatesan A, Tunkel AR, Bloch KC, et al. Case definitions, diagnostic algorithms, and priorities in encephalitis: consensus statement of the international encephalitis consortium. *Clin Infect Dis*. 2013;57(8):1114-1128.

Yu HJ, Lee J, Seo DW, Lee M. Clinical manifestations and treatment response of steroid in pediatric Hashimoto encephalopathy. *J Child Neurol*. 2014;29(7):938-942.

CHAPTER 19 Brief Resolved Explained and Unexplained Events

Nassr Nama, MD, MSc, FAAP and Joel Tieder, MD, MPH, FAAP

BACKGROUND

Infants commonly experience brief self-resolving events associated with a change in color, breathing pattern, tone, or level of consciousness. These events can appear frightening to caregivers, leading them to seek emergency care. Most of these events are related to developmental immaturity. Infrequently, however, they represent an index presentation of a more serious illness.

Increased awareness of Sudden Infant Death Syndrome (SIDS) in the 1970s led some to question whether these brief events were a precursor to SIDS. However, research has shown that these events are distinct, with no increase in mortality among babies experiencing these events compared to the general population. With improved understanding and research, the terminology of these events has evolved. Historically, these were labeled as *near-miss SIDS*, *aborted crib deaths*, or *apparent life-threatening events (ALTEs)*. The American Academy of Pediatrics (AAP) introduced the more specific term *Brief Resolved Unexplained Events* (BRUE—pronounced *brew*) in 2016, supported by mounting evidence of benign outcomes among most patients (**Table 19-1, Figure 19-1**). The clinical practice guideline focused on the specific population of well-appearing infants presenting with brief

TABLE 19-1 Definition of Brief Resolved Unexplained/Explained Events (BRUE/BREE)

Duration: Brief	<1 min; typically 20–30 s
Resolved	At the time of medical evaluation: • Patient returned to baseline • Normal vital signs • Normal appearance
Characteristics	One of the following four:
• *Color change:*	• Central cyanosis (face, gums, trunk) or central pallor. • Not including acrocyanosis, perioral cyanosis or rubor.
• *Abnormal breathing pattern:*	• Absent, decreased, or irregular breathing. • May include central or obstructive apnea. • Not including periodic breathing of the newborn or breath-holding spells.
• *Marked change in tone:*	• Hypertonia or hypotonia • Not associated with crying, choking, feeding, or breath-holding spells. • Not associated with tonic-clonic seizure, eye deviation, or infantile spasms.
• *Altered responsiveness:*	• Loss of consciousness, mental status change, lethargy, somnolence, or postictal phase.
Explanation	*BRUE*: Diagnosis of exclusion. No explanation identified. *BREE*: Symptom of an underlying disorder. Explanation identified on history, physical examination, or diagnostic testing.

Source: Adapted from Tieder JS, Bonkowsky JL, Etzel RA, et al. Brief resolved unexplained events (formerly apparent life-threatening events) and evaluation of lower-risk infants. *Pediatrics*. 2016;137(5):e20160590.

and resolved events without a clear explanation following a detailed history and physical examination. In patients whose history and physical examination reveal an explanation, these events are labeled as Brief Resolved Explained Events (BREE—pronounced *brie*). BRUE is considered a diagnosis of exclusion, while a BREE is a presenting symptom of another diagnosis.

Less than 5% of patients with events unexplained after thorough history and exam in the ED will have a serious underlying diagnosis that benefits from prompt medical evaluation and treatment.

The pediatric hospitalist may be asked to clarify the features of the presentation, discuss the risks and benefits of admission and further investigations with the caregivers, and provide an understanding of risk and reassurance as indicated.

PATHOPHYSIOLOGY

Brief periods of apnea are common and often normal in infants. Concerning apneic events are associated with physiologic compromise, as indicated by changes in oxygenation, color, muscle tone, or bradycardia. Apneic events may be obstructive, central, or mixed (see Chapter 141).

Color changes result from decreased oxygenation or differential blood flow to a portion of the body. Transient pallor may result from vasoconstriction, whereas plethora may result from hyperemia and localized vasodilation (often venous). Both tend to be mediated by autonomic activity. Cyanosis results from hemoglobin desaturation and is most reliably identified centrally by blue or purple discoloration of the lips or tongue. Acrocyanosis and circumoral cyanosis are often seen in healthy infants and are not necessarily signs of a central cyanotic state or abnormal gas exchange. As such, these do not meet the BRUE diagnostic criteria. Acrocyanosis in newborns is common and may be due to vasomotor instability or vasoconstriction due to heat-retention efforts. Circumoral cyanosis often presents as a circular blue or purple discoloration in the perioral area, not involving the lips or tongue. It is likely related to this region's congestion of the superficial venous plexus and is more easily recognized with crying, breath holding, or other Valsalva-type efforts.

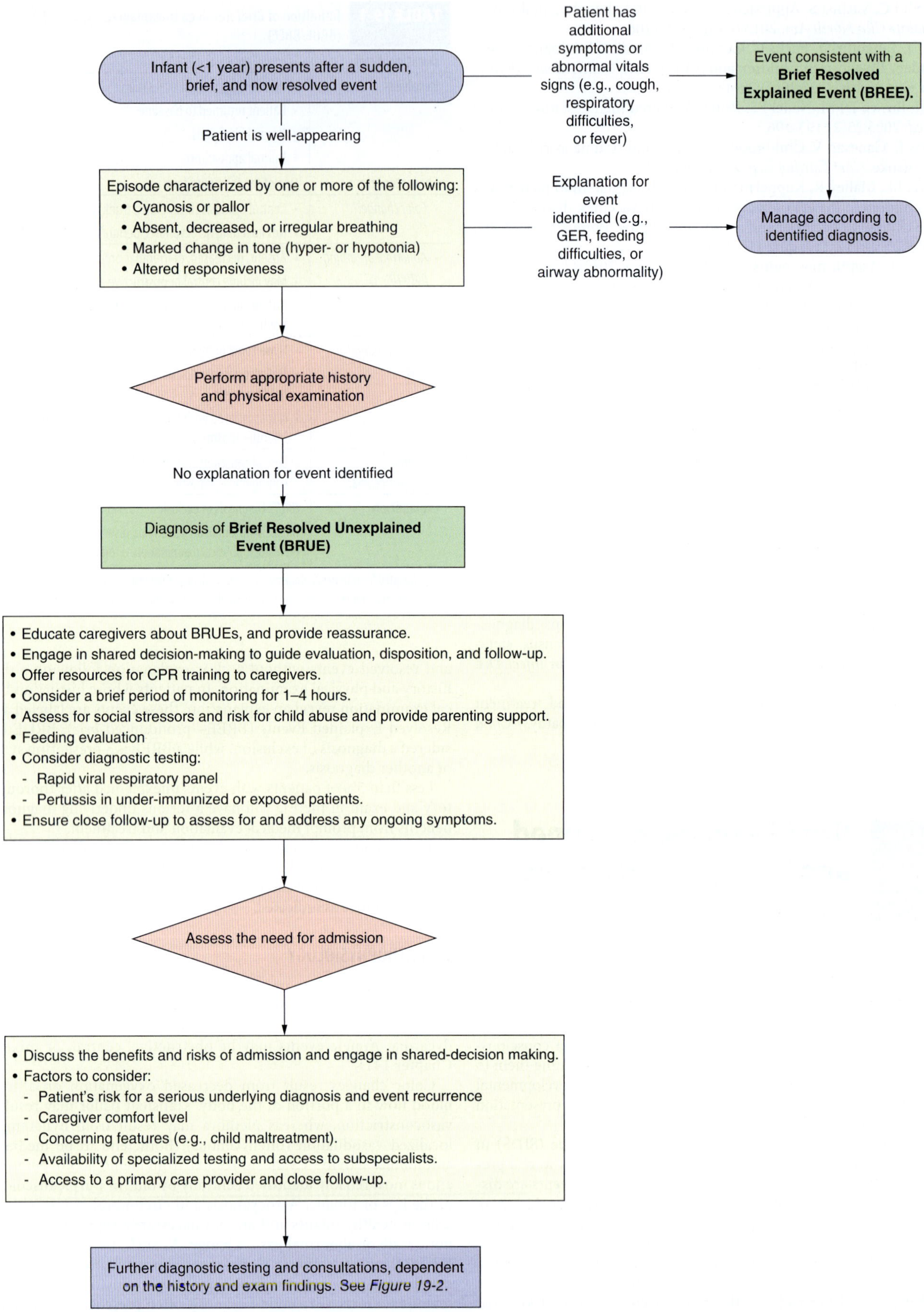

FIGURE 19-1. Diagnosis and management of infants presenting with brief resolved events and differentiating between BRUE and BREE. BREE: Brief resolved explained event; BRUE: Brief resolved unexplained event; GER: Gastroesophageal reflux; HCP: Healthcare provider; PCP: Primary care provider. (Adapted from Tieder JS, Bonkowsky JL, Etzel RA, et al. Brief resolved unexplained events (formerly apparent life-threatening events) and evaluation of lower-risk infants. *Pediatrics*. 2016;137(5):e20160590.)

Due to neurological immaturity, transient changes in tone can be normal in infants and can appear as rapid jerking movements or myoclonus. This is also seen in infantile reflexes (e.g., Startle or Moro). More concerning are tone changes that are sustained, rhythmic, unprovoked, and not suppressible, which may suggest seizures or infantile spasms (see Chapters 118 and 120).

It is challenging to document changes in the level of consciousness in infants. However, abrupt changes in the level of awareness that may be associated with apnea or cyanosis can be concerning. This may also be seen after a breath-holding episode; however, that does not meet the diagnostic criteria for a BRUE.

PATIENT HISTORY

Brief resolved events (BRUE and BREE) present commonly in the early months of life, with a reported median of 1.5 months and more than 75% of events occurring in patients under 4 months. Most presenting infants are healthy (70%), term (74%-81%) with no risk factors on family (90%) or social history (97%). Approximately a third of patients had a similar event prior to their presentation.

The most common presentation is an abnormal respiratory pattern (53%-69%), followed by color change (32%-50%), tone abnormalities (7%-45%), and altered responsiveness (9%-36%). Most events are under 1 minute, with 29% of these brief events reported by the caregiver as lasting for a minute or longer. Event clusters are noted in 30% of patients. Rarely caregivers report performing cardiopulmonary resuscitation that is later deemed appropriate by medical providers (2%).

A detailed history is the most essential element in the diagnostic evaluation of BRUE. Obtaining the history can help understand the event's nature, confirm the diagnosis of a BRUE/BREE, and identify potential causes. Hospitalists should obtain a firsthand account of the event description from caregivers and inquire about the presence of any preceding symptoms and the infant's state following the event (**Table 19-2**). Clarifying a temporal relationship to feeding or crying is essential. Additionally, hospitalists should assess whether there are any concerning features on past medical history, family history, or social history (**Table 19-3**).

TABLE 19-2 Description of the BRUE/BREE Event

Before the event
• Timing: Related to feed/emesis/spit-up, sleep, crying
• Position: Supine/prone, flat/upright, crib/floor/car seat
• Objects nearby that infant might choke on, toys, pillows, blankets
The BRUE/BREE description
• Witness
• Breathing: absent/shallow/gasping, regular/irregular, work of breathing
• Color: baseline/changed, pale/red/blue/purple, face/perioral/lips/tongue/arms/legs/trunk
• Alertness: Conscious, responsive, sleepy, interested in surroundings
• Tone: Rigid, limp/floppy
• Movement: Active/moving, quiet/flaccid, repetitive movement, focal/generalized, suppressible
• Abnormal eye movement, deviation, blank stare
• Choking/gagging, crying/irritable, distressed/alarmed
After the event
• Duration until baseline. Gradual vs. immediate return.
• Interventions to stop the event: picking up, drink/food, tapping back, mouth-to-mouth, chest compressions (pulse presence, trained provider, duration)
• Calling 911 and assessment by first responders
• Following event: baseline, quiet, fussy/crying, tired/sleepy

Source: Adapted from Tieder JS, Bonkowsky JL, Etzel RA, et al. Brief resolved unexplained events (formerly apparent life-threatening events) and evaluation of lower-risk infants. *Pediatrics.* 2016;137(5):e20160590.

TABLE 19-3 Key Elements on History for Patients Presenting with a Brief Resolved Event

Review of systems
• Prior BRUE/BREE or other concerning events
• Preceding illness or sick contacts: Details on symptoms, severity, duration, fever, oral intake, respiratory symptoms.
• Feeding: Chocking or coughing with feeds, reflux (symptoms and treatment), gagging.
• Respiratory symptoms: Noisy breathing, snoring, apneic events, or abnormal respiratory pattern.
Past medical history
• Perinatal history and complications: Prematurity, risk factors for infections, exposures, and newborn metabolic screen.
• Prior hospitalizations, surgeries.
• Medications, allergies, and immunization status (pertussis in particular).
• Abnormalities in growth (failure to thrive) or developmental delays.
Family history
• Sudden or unexpected death, SIDS
• BRUE in siblings
• Cardiac arrhythmias: Long QT syndrome
• Neurologic disorders: Infantile spasms or seizure disorder
• Genetic or metabolic conditions, developmental delays, consanguinity
Social history
• Housing, caregivers, and family structure
• Exposure to smoking, marijuana, or illicit drugs
• Caregivers' coping or other stressors
• Previous involvement of child protective services
• History of trauma or unexplained bruising

SIDS: Sudden Infant Death Syndrome.

Source: Adapted from Tieder JS, Bonkowsky JL, Etzel RA, et al. Brief resolved unexplained events (formerly apparent life-threatening events) and evaluation of lower-risk infants. *Pediatrics.* 2016;137(5):e20160590.

PHYSICAL EXAM

A thorough physical exam can also help identify a cause and differentiate a BRUE from a BREE. To diagnose a BRUE, the infant should appear well with normal vitals (Figure 19-1). Particular attention should be given to growth parameters and assessment for signs of upper airway problems, neurological problems, and child abuse (**Figure 19-2**).

DIFFERENTIAL DIAGNOSIS

Half of the patients presenting with a brief and resolved event will have a diagnosis identified before hospital discharge. History and physical examination have the highest yield in determining a diagnosis. Once a diagnosis is confirmed, the event is more appropriately labeled as a BREE.

Tables 19-4 and **19-5** provide a list of serious (4.6%) and less-serious diagnoses (43.1%) identified in a large BRUE cohort.

MANAGEMENT

RISK EVALUATION

The risks following a BRUE presentation are:

- Event recurrence in hospital estimated at 14%.
- Serious underlying illness that would benefit from prompt medical intervention in 4.6%.
- No increased risk of death when compared to healthy infants during the first year of life.

	History	Physical Examination	Diagnoses	Investigations/ Consultations
Child Maltreatment	• Inconsistent history of the event or incompatible with developmental age • Delay in seeking medical attention • Recurrent events or clusters • Prior CPS involvement • Significant family stressors • Domestic violence, substance abuse, history of mental illness	• Unexplained bruising • Torn frenulum or oral bleeding/trauma • Scleral or subconjunctival hemorrhage • Trauma on GU examination • Large head circumference • Anormal neurological exam	• Non-accidental head trauma • Smothering or suffocation • Poisoning or accidental ingestion • Factitious syndrome by proxy	• Consultation with child protection expert • Skeletal survey, head imaging, and retinal examination • Toxicology screen
Neurological	• Recurrent, paroxysmal or stereotypical events • Abnormal eye movements • Loss of consciousness or lethargy • Developmental delays/regressions • FHx: Infantile spasms, seizures, genetic or metabolic disorders, developmental delays	• Abnormal tone, reflexes, or neurological exam • Neurocutaneous findings • Dysmorphic features • Papilledema • Micro- or macrocephaly	• Seizure • Infantile spasms • CNS malformation	• EEG and neurology consultation • Consider head imaging
Airway & Respiratory	• Multiple or recurrent events • Respiratory pattern abnormalities (e.g., apnea or periodic breathing) • Work of breathing • Noisy breathing or snoring • Concern for foreign body	• Dysmorphic features • Micrognathia • Poor tone • Tachypnea or periodic breathing • Stridor, or abnormal breath sounds	**Airway abnormalities** • Choanal atresia • Laryngomalacia • Foreign body	• Otolaryngology consultation
Airway & Respiratory	• Multiple or recurrent events • Respiratory pattern abnormalities (e.g., apnea or periodic breathing) • Persistent work of breathing • Noisy breathing • Aspiration event	• Tachypnea or periodic breathing • Stridor, or abnormal breath sounds • Focality on respiratory exam	**Respiratory diseases** • Central apnea (secondary to infection, CNS, CCHS, prematurity, or trauma) • Obstructive apnea (secondary to airway abnormality or poor tone) • Mixed apnea • Foreign body • Respiratory tract infection • Breath-holding spells • Periodic breathing	• Otolaryngology and pulmonology consultation • Comprehensive polysomnography (if concerns regarding apnea) • Consider head imaging (if central apnea) • Consider CXR (if bacterial pneumonia)
Gastro-Intestinal	• Event was around feeding time • Coughing or choking with feeding • Chronic, severe, or recurrent feeding problems • Regurgitation or vomiting, irritability, feeding resistance, poor weight gain, and back arching	• Presence of milk or formula in the mouth • Vomiting or spitting up • Choking or gagging noises • Poor growth • Desaturations with feeds	• GER, GERD • Laryngospasm • Overfeeding	• Swallowing and feeding evaluation • Consider gastroenterology consultation
			• Oropharyngeal dysphagia	• Swallowing and feeding evaluation • Consider VFSS
Gastro-Intestinal	• Bloody or bilious emesis • Bloody stools or melena • Poor oral intake or urine output • Lethargy	• Pallor or lethargy • Distended abdomen, absence of bowel sounds • Signs of bowel obstruction • Abdominal mass	**GI obstruction or anomaly:** • Intussusception • Malrotation • Pyloric stenosis • Foreign Body	• Abdominal imaging (x-ray, ultrasound, UGI) • Consider surgical consultation
Metabolic	• Recurrent events or associated with stress/fasting • Severe initial event • Failure to thrive or feeding difficulties • Abnormalities on newborn screening • Developmental delay • Severe/frequent illnesses • FHx: SIDS, metabolic/genetic condition, consanguinity	• Tachycardia or tachypnea • Jittery • Abnormal level of consciousness • Dysmorphic features • Microcephaly or poor growth • Hepatosplenomegaly	• Hypoglycemia • Electrolyte abnormalities (e.g., hypocalcemia) • IEM	• Blood glucose, sodium, potassium, chloride, urea, creatinine, calcium, venous blood gas, ammonia, lactic acid • Biochemical genetics consult
Infectious	• Additional episodes of gagging, gasping, color change with respiratory pause • Fever, respiratory or URTI symptoms. • Poor oral intake or urine output. • Foul-smelling urine. • Lethargy • Prematurity, maternal GBS, PROM, maternal chorioamnionitis • Sick contacts • Under-immunized population • Previous bacterial infection	• Fever, tachycardia or tachypnea • Periods of apnea • Coryza • Irritability, lethargy or ill appearance • Poor perfusion	• Viral URTI/LRTI (e.g., RSV) • Pertussis • Bacterial pneumonia • Bacteremia, meningitis, UTI	• Viral respiratory panel and pertussis • Urinalysis and urine culture • Consider blood culture • Consider the need for lumbar puncture.
Cardiac	• Failure to thrive, diaphoresis with feeds • Recurrent cyanotic episodes • FHx: Arrhythmia (LQTS, WPW), sudden or unexpected death, SIDS, syncope	• Abnormal heart rate or rhythm • Murmur or weak pulses • Low oxygen saturation • Poor growth	• Arrhythmia: LQTS, WPW • Cardiomyopathy • Congenital heart disease	• ECG and cardiology consult • Consider an echocardiogram
Anemia	• Prematurity • No iron supplementation, when indicated • History of hemolytic disease or blood loss • Delay in introduction of iron rich solids	• Pallor • Tachycardia or murmur • Recurrent desaturations	• Anemia of prematurity • Iron deficiency anemia	• Obtain a CBC and Ferritin.

FIGURE 19-2. Signs and symptoms suggestive of common etiologies identified after a BRUE/BREE, and relevant diagnostic tests and consultations. CBC: Complete blood count; CCHS: Congenital central hypoventilation syndrome; CNS: Central nervous system; CPS: Child protection services; CXR: Chest X-ray; ECG: Electrocardiogram; EEG: Electroencephalogram; FHx: Family history; GBS: Group B streptococcus; GER/GERD: Gastroesophageal reflux (disease); GI: Gastro-intestinal; GU: Genitourinary; IEM: Inborn errors of metabolism; LQTS: Long QT syndrome; PROM: Prolonged rupture of membranes; RSV: Respiratory syncytial virus; SGA/LGA: Small/large for gestational age; SIDS: Sudden infant death syndrome; UGI: Upper gastrointestinal series; URTI/LRTI: Upper/lower respiratory tract infection; UTI: Urinary tract infection; VFSS: Videofluoroscopic swallowing study; WPW: Wolff-Parkinson-White.

TABLE 19-4 Frequency of Serious Underlying Diagnoses (*N* = 150) Identified Among a Cohort of 3283 Patients Presenting with a Brief Resolved Event (BRUE/BREE)

Serious Underlying Diagnosis	4.6% of BRUE patients
Neurological disorders	**32.7%**
Seizure and epilepsy	26.7%
Infantile spasms	2.7%
Brain malformation	1.3%
Subarachnoid hemorrhage (Non-traumatic)	0.7%
Hydrocephalus	0.7%
Developmental delay	0.7%
Infectious diseases	**17.3%**
UTI, bacteremia, or bacterial meningitis	6.7%
Bronchiolitis [moderate/severe, requiring oxygen, ventilation]	5.3%
Pertussis	4.0%
Bacterial pneumonia	1.3%
Gastrointestinal disorders	**15.3%**
Oropharyngeal dysphagia [severe]	6.0%
GER or GERD [leading to FTT]	5.3%
Intussusception	2.0%
Malrotation	0.7%
Pyloric stenosis	0.7%
Foreign Body in Esophagus	0.7%
Respiratory disorders	**10.7%**
Apnea of prematurity [requiring caffeine]	3.3%
Central apnea	3.3%
Obstructive sleep apnea	1.3%
Mixed apnea	1.3%
Near suffocation	0.7%
Cystic Fibrosis	0.7%
Airway abnormality [requiring surgical intervention]	**12.7%**
Laryngomalacia	8.7%
Choanal atresia	1.3%
Subglottic stenosis	0.7%
Mixed airway abnormality	0.7%
Choanal stenosis	0.7%
Laryngeal cleft	0.7%
Child maltreatment	**6.7%**
Cardiac disorders	**2.7%**
Supraventricular tachycardia (SVT)	1.3%
Wolff-Parkinson-White (WPW)	0.7%
Congenital heart disease (Pulmonary regurgitation)	0.7%
Other	**4.0%**
Hypoglycemia	1.3%
Hypocalcemia	0.7%
Hyponatremia and hyperkalemia	0.7%
Accidental ingestion	0.7%
Death (no identified cause)	0.7%

Note: Three patients had 2 diagnoses identified.

FTT: Failure to thrive; GER/GERD: Gastroesophageal reflux (disease); UTI: Urinary tract infection.

Source: Adapted from Nama N, Hall M, Neuman M, et al. Risk prediction after a brief resolved unexplained event. *Hosp Pediatrics*. 2022;12(9):772-785.

TABLE 19-5 Frequency of Less Serious Underlying Diagnoses (*N* = 878) Identified Among a Cohort of 2036 Patients Presenting with a Brief Resolved Event (BRUE/BREE)

Less Serious Diagnosis	43.1% of BRUE patients
Gastrointestinal disorders	**66.9%**
Gastroesophageal reflux and overfeeding	42.8%
Choke, gag, laryngospasm	18.9%
Oropharyngeal dysphagia	4.7%
Acute gastroenteritis	0.3%
Constipation	0.1%
Respiratory disorders	**27.2%**
Viral lower respiratory tract infections	10.1%
Breath holding spell	9.6%
Periodic breathing of the newborn	5.0%
Airway abnormality	2.2%
Apnea of prematurity	0.3%
Neurological disorders	**1.8%**
Seizure (not treated with anti-epileptic)	1.7%
Brain abnormality	0.1%
Other	**4.1%**
Acrocyanosis	1.7%
Normal infant movement	1.7%
Purple crying and colic	0.7%

Source: Adapted from Tieder JS, Sullivan E, Stephans A, et al. Risk factors and outcomes after a brief resolved unexplained event: a multicenter study. *Pediatrics*. 2021;148(1):e2020036095.

Two diagnostic challenges face the hospitalist when assessing an infant with an unexplained resolved event. First, the hospitalist needs to identify infants at a higher-risk for rare serious diagnoses. Second, the differential for serious diagnoses is heterogenous, making it challenging to decide which further investigations or consultations to pursue.

Based on ALTE literature, the AAP provided the first risk stratification for BRUE patients (**Table 19-6**). Studies published since have shown that only a minority of patients meet the lower risk criteria (10%-15%). Combined with the low prevalence of a serious underlying diagnosis, this stratification showed poor discrimination, with a positive predictive value of 5% (i.e., 5% of patients labeled as higher-risk will have a serious underlying diagnosis).

Recent studies have developed more accurate prediction models and risk stratification tools. Different risk factors were identified for a serious underlying diagnosis and event recurrence (**Table 19-7**). A risk calculator based on these models is available on MDCalc (https://www.mdcalc.com/calc/10400/brief-resolved-unexplained-events-2.0-brue-2.0-criteria-infants). These calculators can be used as part of the shared decision-making model. Clinicians can show families a visual representation of their child's risk to guide the discussion on the benefits and harms of admission and further investigations.

CAREGIVER EDUCATION, REASSURANCE, AND SHARED-DECISION MAKING

Following the diagnosis of a BRUE (see Figure 19-1), it is crucial to educate caregivers on this diagnosis. This can help decrease caregiver

TABLE 19-6 Higher-Risk Criteria as Per the AAP Clinical Practice Guideline

• Age ≤ 60 days
• Prematurity: Born < 32 weeks, or 32-38 weeks and corrected < 45 weeks
• Event ≥ 1 minute
• Multiple events or event clusters
• CPR by a trained medical provider
• Concerning features on history or physical examination

CPR: Cardiopulmonary resuscitation.

TABLE 19-7 Risk Factors for Serious Underlying Diagnosis and Event Recurrence Based on Clinical Prediction Rules Developed from 3283 BRUE Infants in the United States

Serious underlying diagnosis
History of similar event
Abnormal medical history (e.g., prior hospitalization, infection, etc.)
Age (risk correlates with an increase in age in days)
Event recurrence
Prematurity: Born < 32 weeks, or 32-38 weeks and corrected < 45 weeks
History of similar event, multiple events, or event clusters
Color change (cyanosis, pallor)
Absence of an abnormal respiratory pattern [1]
Absence of tone change [1]

[1]Risk of event recurrence decreases in infants presenting with an abnormal respiratory pattern or tone change.

Source: Adapted from Nama N, Hall M, Neuman M, et al. Risk prediction after a brief resolved unexplained event. *Hosp Pediatrics*. 2022;12(9):772-785.

TABLE 19-8 Potential Benefits and Risks Associated with Hospital Admission

Benefits of Hospital Admission	Risks of Hospital Admission
• Observation for recurrent events	• Alarm anxiety and detection of non-clinically significant events
• Serial assessments of breathing, sleep, and feeding.	• Nosocomial infections
• Expedite diagnostic tests and consultations when indicated	• False positive testing
• Provide reassurance that events are self-resolving.	• Iatrogenic complications
• Reassurance by monitoring and negative testing	• Financial cost to the family, in addition to the loss of income
	• Increase caregiver concerns regarding the well-being of their healthy child (vulnerable child syndrome)

anxiety and may reduce unnecessary return visits. The following handout provided by the AAP and based on the clinical practice guideline recommendations may be helpful [https://doi.org/10.1542/ppe_document103] (available in English and Spanish).

While validating the caregiver's worries regarding the presenting event, it is essential to provide reassurance that the witnessed event does not increase their child's risk for SIDS. Hospitalists should then engage in shared decision-making with the family to guide evaluation, disposition, and follow-up. This collaborative approach empowers families to make decisions congruent with their values and risk tolerance and improves families' and clinicians' satisfaction.

INITIAL MANAGEMENT

A period of observation with cardiorespiratory monitoring is reasonable to watch for recurrent events. This can also help provide reassurance if the observed events are self-resolving without any concerning features. The optimal time for monitoring is not clearly defined, but a brief period of 1 to 4 hours may be reasonable. The benefits of monitoring should be balanced with the harms of prolonged hospitalization, detection of non-clinically significant events (false positives), and alarm fatigue.

Caregivers should also be offered resources for Cardiopulmonary resuscitation (CPR) training in the community. This can empower caregivers if the event recurs.

Witnessing a BRUE may cause stress and anxiety in caregivers and a feeling that their child is vulnerable to disease. Hospitalists have the opportunity to provide support and screen for mental health conditions to target this support better. This can be done by a social worker or a trained healthcare worker. Additionally, a small percentage of patients presenting with BRUE are later diagnosed with child maltreatment, despite the absence of signs of trauma on initial assessment. As such, hospitalists must keep a high index of suspicion for child maltreatment, specifically when red flags are present (e.g., a changing story or events incompatible with the child's developmental stage).

Disorders related to swallowing and feeding are among the most frequent serious and less-serious diagnoses identified in infants evaluated after a BRUE. Therefore, patients, especially those with a history of feeding difficulties, would benefit from a feeding evaluation by a trained provider, such as an occupational therapist or a speech and language pathologist.

ADMISSION

Not all infants presenting with a BRUE (well-appearing by definition) require hospital admission, although approximately three-quarters are currently, with a decrease in admission rates since the AAP guidelines. Admission is indicated if there are significant social concerns or features worrisome for child maltreatment. Otherwise, the decision on hospital admission should be shared between the clinician and the family. Important factors to consider in this discussion:

- Patient's risk for a serious underlying diagnosis and event recurrence
- Caregiver comfort level
- Presence of concerning elements on history or physical examination
- Availability of specialized testing and access to subspecialists in hospital and as an outpatient
- Access to a primary care provider and close follow-up.

To guide this discussion, the clinician should discuss the benefits and harms of hospital admission (**Table 19-8**).

DIAGNOSTIC EVALUATION

Given the vast heterogeneity of causes of BRUE, the yield of any diagnostic test is low. Additionally, the result obtained may be nonspecific or spurious. Therefore, in patients with no symptoms or exam findings that can direct the evaluation, the provider must balance the invasiveness and cost of the test with the potential harm that could occur from missing or delaying a diagnosis. Specific red flags on history and physical examination for common diagnoses are listed in Figure 19-2.

Neurological disorders The BRUE presentation might be related to an epilepsy disorder or infantile spasms. Patients presenting with paroxysmal or stereotyped events, developmental delays or regression, concerning family history, or abnormal neurological exam would benefit from neurologic consultation and a detailed neurological examination. Patients may require an electroencephalogram (EEG) depending on the level of concern. Timing of the EEG, as inpatient or ambulatory, depends on the available resources and the index of suspicion for an underlying seizure disorder. Structural brain anomalies are rare among identified diagnoses, and the yield of head imaging is generally low. Specific patients that may benefit from imaging are those with concerns for child maltreatment or significant neurological abnormalities.

Cardiac disorders Arrhythmias or congenital heart disease are uncommon causes of BRUE (<0.1%). Recent evidence supports the low yield of the electrocardiogram (ECG), which can be limited to those with concerning features (e.g., positive family history). Similarly, the yield of an echocardiogram is low and should be limited to patients with abnormalities on history or physical examination (e.g., recurrent cyanotic episodes or growth faltering).

Gastrointestinal (GI) disorders GI disorders are commonly identified and are usually mild and self-limited. Well and thriving infants presenting with gastroesophageal reflux (GER) or associated laryngospasms can be assessed clinically, without further testing, and should not be prescribed acid suppression therapy. Patients with troublesome or persistent symptoms would be diagnosed with gastroesophageal reflux disease

(GERD). These patients may initially benefit from some non-pharmacological intervention, such as thickened feeds or slow-paced nipples, as well as a gastroenterology consultation.

Oropharyngeal dysphagia has also been commonly identified among BRUE patients. Patients would present with a history of feeding difficulties associated with choking or coughing. A bedside feeding evaluation remains the first step in the assessment. Patients with a highly suggestive history may benefit from a videofluoroscopic swallowing study (VFSS), as this can identify silent aspiration among some patients with a normal feeding evaluation. Research studies have suggested a high positive rate among BRUE patients undergoing VFSS. However, a significant proportion of these patients only show laryngeal penetration with unclear clinical significance. Additionally, it is currently unknown whether the rate of silent aspiration is increased in comparison to healthy infants (see Chapter 79).

Less commonly, the event might be caused by a serious surgical GI anomaly such as pyloric stenosis, malrotation, or intussusception. Patients with these disorders are unlikely to have a single brief resolved event and appear well at the time of assessment. Further imaging and surgical consultation are indicated when the patient's clinical presentation suggests one of these disorders (see Chapter 155).

Respiratory conditions Apnea of prematurity is a common etiology among patients with a serious underlying illness causing BRUE (see Chapter 141). Meanwhile, breath-holding spells and periodic breathing are frequently noted among the non-serious diagnoses. Airway anomalies can also lead to obstructive apnea. If history or physical exams suggest an airway abnormality, an Otolaryngology evaluation is recommended to determine the benefits of laryngoscopy.

Apneic events can also be the presenting sign of a viral illness such as RSV (respiratory syncytial virus), more commonly in those younger than two months or born prematurely. Most patients will have mild symptoms, however, obtaining a viral diagnosis may provide an opportunity for anticipatory guidance and reassure caregivers that an etiology is identified. Of note, PCR testing for some viruses might remain positive long after the acute illness has resolved, and a positive test does not imply that this has caused the BRUE presentation.

Similarly, patients with pertussis might have a BRUE-like presentation with gasping, gagging, and color change episodes, followed by apnea. Fever, cough, and other respiratory symptoms might be delayed. Testing may be warranted in underimmunized communities, visitors of endemic regions, and during outbreaks.

Chest x-rays and blood gas are of limited yield and should be reserved for patients with ongoing respiratory concerns. A brief period of monitoring (1-4 hours) on continuous oximetry is usually sufficient to detect clinically significant desaturations. However, prolonged monitoring (24 hours) may be considered in patients with recurrent events or concerning history. Polysomnography may be indicated in patients with risk factors for central apnea (prematurity, neurological abnormalities) or obstructive apnea (poor tone, abnormal airway).

Infectious diseases Rarely an invasive bacterial infection (bacteremia or meningitis) has been documented among patients presenting with a BRUE. Infants with such conditions are unlikely to have a fully resolved event and appear well. As such, in the absence of ongoing symptoms or risk factors, the yield of white blood cell count, inflammatory markers, blood culture, and lumbar puncture are low. More often, these can be falsely elevated or show contaminants, leading to prolonged empiric antibiotic coverage, lengthy admissions, and increased parental anxiety until an invasive infection is ruled out. Similarly, evidence supporting the routine use of urinalysis is lacking.

Inborn errors of metabolism (IEM) Studies on BRUE patients have shown the prevalence of metabolic conditions to be much lower than previously estimated based on the ALTE population. As such, diagnostic evaluation for IEM is of limited value. The hospitalist should confirm that a newborn screen was normal. Testing can include glucose, extended electrolytes, lactic acid, and ammonia (see Figure 19-2). (See Chapters 81 and 82.)

Anemia Anemia is an uncommon condition to be identified as a cause of BRUE. A routine hemoglobin check is not recommended and should be reserved for those with risk factors (see Figure 19-2).

SPECIAL CONSIDERATIONS

HOSPITAL DISCHARGE AND OUTPATIENT FOLLOW-UP

Studies have shown that families have mixed feelings regarding the diagnosis of BRUE. They feel reassured by the unlikelihood of a serious diagnosis; however, they remain uncomfortable with the uncertainty of the "Unexplained" diagnosis. A close follow-up with a primary care provider is crucial to support the family and reassure them that their child will continue to be assessed in the community following hospital discharge.

Beyond reassurance, appropriate follow-up is critical for several reasons. First, there is a considerable risk of event recurrence following discharge. Second, this event may represent a symptom of an underlying disorder (more commonly a less-serious one), which still requires assessment and potential therapy. Third, almost half of serious diagnoses are identified in the outpatient setting rather than the index hospitalization. Finally, investigations and consultations may be deemed safe to be arranged as an outpatient.

Families should also receive clear instructions on when to return to care if their child displays further symptoms of a serious underlying disorder.

Home cardiorespiratory monitoring is not recommended following a BRUE, as these devices have not been shown to alter clinical outcomes or prevent SIDS. Additionally, they may cause alarm anxiety and exacerbate a "vulnerable child syndrome."

KEY POINTS

- Brief self-resolving events are common in healthy infants and are not associated with increased mortality. Almost half of these events will remain unexplained and fit the diagnostic criteria for BRUE. The other half will have an etiology identified and can be labeled as a BREE.
- Identified etiologies are commonly benign and self-limited, with only 5% of patients having a serious diagnosis.
- A detailed history and physical examination are the most essential elements in the diagnostic evaluation of BRUE. Hospitalists must keep a high index of suspicion for red flags for child maltreatment.
- Infants presenting with a BRUE may benefit from a brief monitoring period, CPR training for caregivers, and a social worker and a feeding specialist assessment.
- Hospitalists should then engage in shared decision-making with the family to guide evaluation, hospital admission, and follow-up.
- Given the vast heterogeneity of serious causes of BRUE, the yield of any diagnostic test is low. No test is recommended for all patients presenting with a BRUE.
- A close follow-up with a primary care provider is crucial to support the family and reassure them that their child will continue to be assessed in the community following hospital discharge.

SUGGESTED READINGS

Ari A, Atias Y, Amir J. Long-term follow-up of infants after a brief resolved unexplained event-related hospitalization. *Pediatr Emerg Care.* 2019;35(11):765-768. doi:10.1097/pec.0000000000001816

Bochner R, Tieder JS, Sullivan E, et al. Explanatory diagnoses following hospitalization for a brief resolved unexplained event. *Pediatrics.* Published online 2021:e2021052673. doi:10.1542/peds.2021-052673

Brand DA, Fazzari MJ. Risk of death in infants who have experienced a brief resolved unexplained event: a meta-analysis. *J Pediatrics.* 2018;197:63-67. doi:10.1016/j.jpeds.2017.12.02810.

Brand DA, Mock A, Cohn E, Krilov LR. Implementing the 2016 American Academy of Pediatrics Guideline on brief resolved unexplained events: the parent's perspective. *Pediatr Emerg Care.* 2018;Publish Ahead of Print(5):1. doi:10.1097/pec.0000000000001659

Chaiyachati BH, Wood JN. Brief resolved unexplained events vs. child maltreatment: a review of clinical overlap and evaluation. *Pediatr Radiol.* 2021;51(6):866-871. doi:10.1007/s00247-020-04793-z

Duncan DR, Amirault J, Mitchell PD, Larson K, Rosen RL. Oropharyngeal dysphagia is strongly correlated with apparent life-threatening events. *J Pediatr Gastr Nutr*. 2017;65(2):168-172. doi:10.1097/mpg.0000000000001439

Duncan DR, Growdon AS, Liu E, et al. The impact of the American Academy of Pediatrics Brief Resolved Unexplained Event Guidelines on gastrointestinal testing and prescribing practices. *J Pediatrics*. 2019;211:112-119.e4. doi:10.1016/j.jpeds.2019.04.007

Haddad R, Parker S, Farooqi A, DeLaroche AM. Diagnostic evaluation low yield for patients with a lower-risk brief resolved unexplained event. *Global Pediatric Heal*. 2021;8:2333794X2096758. doi:10.1177/2333794x20967586

Khan A, Wallace SS, Sampayo EM, Falco C. Caregivers' perceptions and hospital experience after a brief resolved unexplained event: a qualitative study. *Hosp Pediatrics*. 2019;9(7):508-515. doi:10.1542/hpeds.2018-0220

Merritt JL, Quinonez RA, Bonkowsky JL, et al. A framework for evaluation of the higher-risk infant after a brief resolved unexplained event. *Pediatrics*. 2019;144(2):e20184101. doi:10.1542/peds.2018-4101

Nama N, Hall M, Neuman M, et al. Risk prediction after a brief resolved unexplained event. *Hosp Pediatrics*. 2022;12(9):772-785. doi:10.1542/hpeds.2022-006637

Ramgopal S, Noorbakhsh KA, Callaway CW, Wilson PM, Pitetti RD. Changes in the management of children with brief resolved unexplained events (BRUEs). *Pediatrics*. 2019;144(4):e20190375. doi:10.1542/peds.2019-0375

Schmitz K. Vulnerable child syndrome. *Pediatr Rev*. 2019;40(6):313-315. doi:10.1542/pir.2017-0243

Sethi A, Baxi K, Cheng D, Laffey S, Hartman N, Heller K. Impact of guidelines regarding brief resolved unexplained events on care of patients in a pediatric emergency department. *Pediatr Emerg Care*. Published online 2020. doi:10.1097/pec.0000000000002081

Tieder JS, Bonkowsky JL, Etzel RA, et al. Brief resolved unexplained events (formerly apparent life-threatening events) and evaluation of lower-risk infants. *Pediatrics*. 2016;137(5):e20160590. doi:10.1542/peds.2016-0590

Tieder JS, Sullivan E, Stephans A, et al. Risk factors and outcomes after a brief resolved unexplained event: a multicenter study. *Pediatrics*. 2021;148(1):e2020036095. doi:10.1542/peds.2020-036095

CHAPTER 20

Chest Pain

Kamakshya P. Patra, MD, MMM and Jamie L. Clute, MD

BACKGROUND

Chest pain is a common symptom in pediatrics, and often causes significant anxiety and concern for patients and families. Although cardiac etiologies are often the principal concern for families, pediatric chest pain is rarely caused by cardiac disease (0%-5%). More common causes involve the pulmonary, gastrointestinal, or musculoskeletal systems. Hospitalists caring for patients with chest pain must be able to utilize a thorough history and physical to determine benign from organic disease among the long list of differential diagnoses (**Table 20-1**).

PATIENT HISTORY

Table 20-2 outlines some of the common findings and their associated diagnoses in pediatric chest pain. It is often difficult for younger children to accurately articulate the location, severity, or quality of chest pain. For example, younger children may complain of chest pain when they are experiencing palpitations. It is important to consider pathology of the gastrointestinal organs due to the proximity of the epigastric area to the sternum. Modifying factors such as relationship to exercise, positional change, effect with inspiration, and relationship to eating or swallowing can be helpful in discerning which organ system may be involved.

Associated symptoms are particularly helpful in identifying the cause of pediatric chest pain. Fever is often associated with conditions such as lower respiratory tract infections, pericarditis, or myocarditis. Dyspnea in pediatrics is most commonly associated with disorders that involve the airway, the lung parenchyma, or the pulmonary vasculature. However, cardiac conditions such as myocarditis, dilated cardiomyopathy, and cardiac tamponade can raise the left atrial pressure, resulting in pulmonary edema and dyspnea.

Patients with acute chest pain should be evaluated for current and past medical conditions that may predispose them to important underlying pathology. Asthma exacerbation can result in chest pain from bronchospasm, pneumothorax, or pneumomediastinum. Any patient with a previous history of a cardiomyopathy or congenital heart disease should be closely evaluated for cardiac disease and should be examined by or discussed with a pediatric cardiologist. Patients with a previous history of Kawasaki disease, multisystem inflammatory syndrome in children (MIS-C), or vasculitis may have had coronary artery aneurysms that would increase their risk of myocardial ischemia. Inflammatory conditions such as systemic lupus erythematosus, inflammatory bowel disease, or other rheumatologic conditions increase the possibility of pericarditis, pleuritis, or a venous thromboembolism (VTE). Patients with central venous catheters are at particular risk for VTE, as are those with significant trauma or prolonged immobilization. Patients with a malignancy who have been exposed to chemotherapeutic agents such as anthracyclines should be evaluated for a cardiomyopathy or a pericardial effusion. Patients with sickle cell disease who develop chest pain require urgent evaluation and treatment for possible acute chest syndrome. Substance abuse, toxic exposures, and use of certain medications can trigger pathology that causes chest pain. Cocaine can induce coronary or systemic vasoconstriction that leads to myocardial ischemia or systemic hypertension. Use of methamphetamines, other stimulant medications, and synthetic cathinones like bath salts increase risk of arrhythmia. Caustic ingestions or foreign body aspiration can lead to esophageal injury or upper airway obstruction.

Family historical data regarding cardiomyopathies, sudden unexplained death, Marfan syndrome, and hypercoaguable conditions should be obtained.

PHYSICAL EXAMINATION

Ascertainment of vital signs and general appearance will help determine the required pace of an evaluation. Patients in severe distress may need treatment or stabilization concurrent with ongoing evaluation. Tachycardia will be present with many of the conditions discussed in the differential diagnosis. Tachypnea can be present with a variety of pulmonary and cardiac conditions that result in airway obstruction, lung parenchyma, or pulmonary vascular diseases. Palpation of the chest wall for costochondral tenderness can be performed while evaluating for a hyperdynamic precordium or a right ventricular heave. A complete respiratory evaluation including ausculatation and an assessment of work of breathing should be done to evaluate for lung parenchymal or pleural disease. The cardiovascular examination should include auscultation for pathologic murmurs (e.g., aortic stenosis), friction rubs, or gallops. Pulses, blood pressure, perfusion, and peripheral skin temperature should be evaluated to determine if there is any compromise in cardiac output. Hepatomegaly may be reflective of an elevated central venous pressure, while presence of abdominal tenderness raises suspicion for cholecystitis, pancreatitis, or gastritis.

DIFFERENTIAL DIAGNOSES

CARDIAC CONDITIONS

Myocardial Ischemia Based on the concern for cardiac ischemia in adults, chest pain creates significant anxiety in practitioners as well as patients. Ischemia as a result of inadequate myocardial perfusion is rare in children, however, certain congenital or acquired conditions increase this risk. Patients with a history of Kawasaki disease and resultant

TABLE 20-1 Causes of Chest Pain

Cardiovascular	**Mediastinal**
Myocardial ischemia, injury, infarction spectrum	Mediastinal air leak
Coronary anomalies	Barotrauma due to mechanical ventilation
Acute coronary syndromes	Pneumopericardium or pneumomediastinum
Kawasaki disease	Masses and malignancies
MISC	Thymoma
Vasculitides	Lymphoma
Stimulant use	Teratoma
Myocardial contusion	Mediastinitis
Aortic dissection (Marfan syndrome)	Infectious or noninfectious
Hypertensive emergency	Ruptured esophagus
Illicit substances, including cocaine and stimulants	**Gastrointestinal**
Acute or chronic kidney disease	Trauma to organs in the upper abdomen
Cardiomyopathies—hypertrophic cardiomyopathy	Esophageal causes
Congestive heart failure	Foreign body
Arrhythmias	Rupture
Valvular heart disease	Spasm
Myocarditis	Motility disorders, including achalasia
Pericarditis	Esophagitis—infectious or noninfectious
Endocarditis	Esophageal procedures
Pancarditis	Gastroesophageal reflux disease
Acute rheumatic fever	Biliary disease, including cholelithiasis and cholecystitis
Pericardial effusion	Pancreatitis
Cardiac tamponade	Hepatitis
Cardiac masses and tumors	Subdiagphragmatic processes—inflammation, infection, mass
Complications of central venous catheters, including thromboses	Referred pain from abdominal processes—splenomegaly, malignancy, mass
Substance use—cocaine, inhalants, stimulants, bath salts, marijuana	**Musculoskeletal**
Smoking, Vaping	Costochondritis and chest wall pain
Pulmonary	Tietz syndrome
Diseases of the airways	Blunt injury and trauma
Asthma	Child abuse
Bronchospasm	Fractures to bones of the chest, including ribs
Foreign body	Pectus deformities
Diseases of the parenchyma	Scoliosis
Pneumonia—nosocomial or community acquired	Myofascial pain syndromes, including fibromyalgia
Pulmonary infarction	Precordial catch syndrome
Bronchogenic cyst	Floating and slipping rib syndromes
Cystic adenomatoid malformation	Disorders of bone mineralization, including rickets
Acute chest syndrome of sickle cell crisis	Pain in and around the breasts
Diseases of the pleura	**Neuropathic and Psychiatric**
Pneumothorax	Acute anxiety and panic disorders
Hemothorax	Mood disorders, including depression and anxiety
Pleural effusion	Varicella-zoster (pain may precede vesicular eruption)
Empyema	Postherpetic neuralgia
Pleuritis of autoimmune diseases (e.g. systemic lupus erythematosus)	Chronic pain syndromes
Diseases of the vasculature	Somatization
Pulmonary embolism, air embolism	Functional esophageal disorders
Pulmonary hypertension	

coronary artery aneurysms are at higher risk for major cardiac events. Patients with anomalous origins of the coronary arteries most often present in infancy with symptoms of heart failure or shock, but those with good collateral blood flow may present later with exertional syncope or chest pain. It is important to note that patients with anomalous coronary artery origins may have a normal physical examination and electrocardiogram (ECG). Aortic stenosis and hypertrophic obstructive cardiomyopathy can result in impaired coronary blood flow when there is severe left ventricular outflow tract obstruction.

Pericarditis Pericarditis is one of the more common causes of acute cardiac chest pain in pediatrics and can result from a variety of etiologies. Idiopathic pericarditis represents the majority of cases and is thought to be a post-infectious or post-viral inflammatory condition involving the pericardium. The accompanying chest pain is often pleuritic, sharp, and worsens in the supine position. It is often accompanied by fever due to the systemic inflammation. On physical examination, patients may have tachycardia, an uncomfortable appearance, or a pericardial friction rub. Having the patient lean forward may help to elicit the friction

TABLE 20-2 Clues to the Cause of Chest Pain

Timing
Sudden onset—air embolism, pulmonary embolism, myocardial ischemia or infarction, arrhythmias, air leak during mechanical ventilation, spontaneous pneumothorax
Gradual onset—community-acquired or nosocomial pneumonia and complications such as pleural effusion and empyema
Hospital Setting
Pain on initial presentation
Toxicologic causes, including inhalants and stimulant use
Pain during the course of hospitalization
Postoperative complications
Infection at incisions
Bleeding
Barotrauma
Pneumonia
DVT-PE complex in native vessels or arising from central catheters
Myocardial ischemia
Characterization of Pain
Severe—myocardial ischemia or infarction; classically, associated symptoms include nausea, vomiting, radiation of pain to neck, jaw, and arms
Crushing—myocardial ischemia or tamponade
Sharp—pleuritic, pericardial, musculoskeletal, and gastrointestinal causes; arrhythmias
Pleuritic—pericardial or pleural disease
Associated Symptoms and Signs
Abdominal pain—lower lobe pneumonia, pancreatitis, biliary and liver disease
Bruising—nonaccidental trauma of child abuse
Central venous catheters—arrhythmias, pneumothorax, DVT-PE complex
Clubbing—chronic lung disease, such as cystic fibrosis or bronchiectasis
Cough—pneumonia, asthma, pulmonary edema, pleural effusions
Crepitus—subcutaneous air due to air leak secondary to barotrauma
Cyanosis—congenital heart disease, pneumonia, heart failure
Dyspnea—asthma, pulmonary edema, multiple cardiopulmonary causes
Extremity edema—DVT progressing to PE
Gallop—heart failure
Odynophagia—para- or retropharyngeal abscess
Pericardial rub—pericardial effusion, pneumopericardium
Pleural rub—pleural effusion due to inflammation or infection
Stridor—foreign body, occluding infectious process in the airway (e.g., epiglottitis, bacterial tracheitis, croup)
Tall and hypermobile (often with pectus excavatum)—Marfan syndrome
Wheezing—asthma, multiple cardiopulmonary causes

DVT, deep venous thrombosis; PE, pulmonary embolus.

rub. The ECG classically shows diffuse ST-segment elevations and PR-segment depressions. An echocardiogram can be performed to evaluate for the presence and size of pericardial effusion, but cardiac tamponade is a clinical diagnosis and should be evaluated for by measuring pulsus paradoxus. The mainstay of therapy for pericarditis is nonsteroidal anti-inflammatory medications, and some practitioners utilize colchicine as an adjunct. Pericardiocentesis is typically performed only in patients with signs of cardiac tamponade.

Myocarditis Myocarditis is a rare pediatric condition that may initially cause symptoms similar to more common illnesses such as a viral lower respiratory tract infection. This disease can affect children of all ages and results from an infectious or immunologic injury to the myocardium. The spectrum of disease ranges from chest pain and mild ECG changes to cardiogenic shock and death. Older patients who complain of fever and chest pain should have an ECG performed to look for signs of myocardial injury, including T-wave inversions, ST-segment changes, or conduction abnormalities. Troponins have high specificity (84%) and low sensitivity (34%) for detecting myocarditis, but have not been shown to predict outcomes (see Chapter 53).

Pulmonary Vascular Disease Pulmonary embolism (PE) is a rare, but likely underrecognized occurrence in children. The hospitalized pediatric patient may have many of the risk factors that predispose to VTE, including the presence of a central venous catheter, prolonged immobility, post-surgical or traumatic injury, or malignancy. Providers should consider VTE in the differential diagnosis for patients with these risk factors and acute chest pain, tachycardia, hypoxemia, or extremity pain and swelling. A spiral chest computed tomography scan is the diagnostic test of choice for PE.

Pulmonary hypertension (PAH) can be idiopathic, but can also be found in patients with other medical conditions including various lung diseases, obstructive sleep apnea, chronic VTE disease, and certain forms of congenital heart disease. Patients with PAH often have a loud S2 on examination and may have an S3 gallop or right ventricular heave if the right ventricle is dilated or dysfunctional.

Arrhythmias It is not unusual for younger children experiencing irregular heartbeats or arrhythmias to complain of chest or even abdominal pain. When older children or adolescents are having an arrhythmia and complaining of chest pain, this suggests that their cardiac output is compromised. The most common arrhythmia in children is supraventricular tachycardia (SVT). Compared to the general pediatric population, patients with a history of congenital heart disease and a history of cardiac surgery are at increased risk of having an arrhythmia. Common forms of SVT include atrioventricular reentrant tachycardia (AVRT), atrioventricular nodal reentrant tachycardia (AVNRT), and atrial flutter. Ventricular tachycardia is rare in pediatrics, but must be identified and treated quickly. Prompt recognition is essential and tools such as an ECG or a cardiac monitor can help make a diagnosis quickly and accurately. A hospitalist must be able to discern a narrow complex from a wide complex tachycardia and begin to support the circulation, airway, and breathing while either treating the rhythm disturbance or seeking expert consultation.

Cardiomyopathy The two most common forms of cardiomyopathy in pediatrics are dilated (DCM) and hypertrophic (HCM). Chest pain is rarely the primary complaint that brings patients to medical attention, who more often present with respiratory symptoms, exercise intolerance, a new murmur, or a family history of cardiomyopathy. Myocarditis and DCM can present similarly and echocardiography is necessary to confirm these diagnoses (see Chapter 55).

PULMONARY CONDITIONS

Respiratory disorders are fairly common causes of acute chest pain in pediatrics. The most frequent conditions include asthma, pneumonia, and respiratory tract infections. Asthmatics may develop chest pain from frequent coughing as this can cause muscular strain and soreness. Bronchoconstriction can also create a feeling of chest tightness which is often described as pain or discomfort. Signs of obstructive disease on examination include wheeze or a prolonged expiratory phase, and chest radiography may demonstrate hyperexpanded lung fields. The presence of stridor would suggest an upper airway obstruction from a foreign body or an infectious process including croup, bacterial tracheitis, or epiglottitis. Vaping and smoking in children can be associated with chest pain. Pneumonia is common in pediatrics and often presents with fever in addition to tachypnea. It can be complicated by pleuritis or a parapneumonic effusion (empyema), which can cause significant chest pain and discomfort. Pneumothorax should be considered in the patient with acute chest pain and respiratory distress. Patients suffering from coughing paroxysms who have the tall and lean body type that puts them at risk for spontaneous pneumothoraces may also be at risk for the development of pneumomediastinum.

MUSCULOSKELETAL CONDITIONS

Children and adolescents with chest pain must be asked about chest wall trauma, as rib fractures or muscle contusions may be the etiology of their pain. A history of weightlifting or other isometric chest exercises may suggest muscle strains and injuries to the chest wall. The incidence of chest pain caused by conditions of the musculoskeletal system has been reported to be as high as 31%. Costochondritis is common and is often described as a unilateral sharp pain that typically lasts for minutes. This is an inflammatory condition that should have reproducible pain on palpation of the chest and will often respond to nonsteroidal anti-inflammatory therapy. Tietz syndrome is a benign self-limited cause of chest pain characterized by inflammatory swelling and tenderness of second and third costal cartilages. Precordial catch syndrome is a similar sharp, stabbing chest pain that is very well localized with a fingertip. The pain is usually of quite short duration, self resolving, and does not require any medical therapy. The etiology of this disorder is unknown, but some believe it is related to poor posture. Slipping rib syndrome has also been reported as a cause of chest pain in children. In this condition, the floating ribs are attached to the sternum by hypermobile fibrous connections that allow slipping of the cartilage and impingement on the intercostal nerves.

GASTROINTESTINAL CONDITIONS

Discomfort in the epigastric area can be construed as chest pain, and intra-abdominal diseases can sometimes manifest referred pain to the shoulders due to phrenic innervation. A complete abdominal examination is necessary to evaluate for some of these common conditions. Gastroesophageal reflux disease and esophagitis are the most common causes of gastrointestinal-induced chest pain and may be described as burning in character. Hepatic or biliary conditions can result in right-sided chest and shoulder pain from hepatic capsular distention or diaphragmatic irritation. Pancreatitis and cholecystitis are less common than in the adult population, but do occur and can be evaluated with laboratory tests. Esophageal spasm and other motility disorders have also been reported as causes of pediatric chest pain, but often require invasive manometry studies to make this diagnosis. Chest pain can be frequently seen following esophageal procedures.

NEUROLOGIC AND PSYCHIATRIC CONDITIONS

The presence of underlying depression has been reported in adolescents and young adults with chronic pain syndromes, and is a significant risk factor for affecting daily functioning. Rarely, children or adolescents present with burning pain preceding the eruption of vesicles in a dermatomal distribution that allows for a clinical diagnosis of varicella-zoster. Radicular pain can result from spinal cord compression or the presence of an epidural abscess or other mass. Functional esophageal disorders can present with chest pain and globus.

MISCELLANEOUS

Patients with sickle cell disease who present with chest pain need to be simultaneously evaluated and treated for presumed acute chest syndrome (see Chapter 85). Aortic dissection is often described as a severe tearing type of chest pain, but is exceedingly rare in pediatrics. It should be considered in the differential in patients who suffered a high-velocity traumatic injury or in those patients with Marfan, Ehlers-Danlos, Loeys-Dietz, or Turner syndromes presenting with acute chest pain.

DIAGNOSTIC EVALUATION

ELECTROCARDIOGRAM

High-risk patients complaining of acute chest pain should undergo a 12-lead ECG, and inpatients with a new complaint of chest pain should also be placed on a monitor to help detect arrhythmia. Rate and rhythm are particularly important when entertaining the possibility of a rhythm disturbance. ST-segment and T-wave abnormalities may be present in conditions such as pericarditis (diffuse ST-segment elevations), myocarditis (heart block, tachycardia, ST-T wave flattening, or inversions), hypertrophic cardiomyopathy (left ventricular hypertrophy, T-wave inversions), or pulmonary embolic disease (RV strain, S1Q3T3). The accuracy of reading ECGs is variable among hospitalists and proficiency in ECG interpretation is warranted.

CHEST RADIOGRAPHY

Patients with fever, cough, dyspnea, tachypnea, respiratory distress, or abnormal lung sounds in addition to their complaint of chest pain should have a chest x-ray performed. A chest x-ray may allow for identification of a pneumonia, pneumothorax, pleural effusion, pulmonary vascular congestion, and cardiomegaly. Point of care ultrasound can be a helpful bedside tool for evaluation of chest pain in children to rule out certain pathologies.

LABORATORY TESTING

Rarely is lab testing helpful in the diagnosis of chest pain. An increased white blood cell count may be suggestive of an intercurrent infectious condition such as pneumonia. Evaluating for a troponin leak is not routinely indicated in pediatrics. Troponins have been shown to be sensitive for myocarditis and are helpful when evaluating for myocardial ischemia in adults, but are rarely elevated in pediatric patients with chest pain when they are afebrile and/or had a normal ECG. D-Dimer is used in the adult population to help rule out pulmonary embolism in low-probability patients. Its use is not recommended in the evaluation of adult inpatients suspected of having a PE. Also, the ability of this test to help risk stratify in pediatric patients is unknown and if routinely obtained, may result in excessive use of computed tomography scans.

MANAGEMENT

Children with the acute onset of chest pain are more likely to have an underlying disease process and may need to have treatment delivered quickly. A thorough and complete history and physical will often determine the cause or identify the patients that require further diagnostics or immediate treatments. Some evidence-based guidelines and algorithms, based on history and physical exam, have been utilized to target management and referral, and implementing a tiered approach may substantially reduce charges. Please refer to the specific chapters regarding the treatment options for the working diagnosis. For patients who do not have any abnormalities on their physical examination or concerning aspects of their history, it is unlikely that they have serious underlying pathology. It becomes very important to be able to reassure patients and families, since chest pain often results in self-restriction from athletics and other activities. Education and reassurance are two critical components in the successful treatment of pediatric chest pain.

KEY POINTS

- Acute chest pain can be an anxiety-provoking symptom for both families and physicians.
- Differential diagnosis is broad and includes cardiac and non-cardiac etiologies, benign and potentially serious conditions.
- Chest pain is usually benign in children. Most common cause of chest pain in children imusculoskeletal.
- A careful history and physical examination is crucial to guiding further diagnostic evaluation.

SUGGESTED READINGS

Abman SH, Ivy DD. Recent progress in understanding pediatric pulmonary hypertension. *Curr Opin Pediatr.* 2011;23(3):298-304.

Agnelli G, Becattini C. Acute pulmonary embolism. *N Eng J Med.* 2010;363:266-274.

Anderson BR, Vetter VL. Arrhythmogenic causes of chest pain in children. *Pediatr Clin N Am*. 2010;57:1305-1329.

Basso C, Maron BJ, Corrado D, et al. Clinical profile of congenital coronary artery anomalies with origin from the wrong sinus leading to sudden death in young competitive athletes. *J Am Coll Cardiol*. 2000;34:1493-1501.

Berezin S, Medow MS, Glassman MS, et al. Chest pain of gastrointestinal origin. *Arch Dis Child*. 1988;63:1457.

Brown RT. Costochondritis in adolescents. *J Adolesc Health Care*. 1981; 1:198.

Centers for Disease Control and Prevention (CDC). Emergency department visits after use of a drug sold as "bath salts"—Michigan, November 13, 2010-March 31, 2011. *MMWR Morb Mortal Wkly Rep*. 2011;60(19):624-627.

Friedman KG, Alexander ME. Chest pain and syncope in children: a practical approach to the diagnosis of cardiac disease. *J Pediatr*. 2013;163(3):896-901.e1-3.

Glassman MS, Medow MS, Berezin S, et al. Spectrum of esophageal disorders in children with chest pain. *Dig Dis Sci*. 1992;37(5): 663-666.

Harahsheh AS, O'Byrne ML, Pastor B, Graham DA, Fulton DR. Pediatric chest pain-low-probability referral: a multi-institutional analysis from Standardized Clinical Assessment and Management Plans (SCAMPs®), the Pediatric Health Information Systems Database, and the National Ambulatory Medical Care Survey. *Clin Pediatr (Phila)*. 2017;56(13):1201-1208.

Kane DA, Fulton DR, Saleeb S, et al. Needles in hay: chest pain as the presenting symptom in children with serious underlying cardiac pathology. *Congenit Heart Dis*. 2010;5:366-373.

Kudo Y, Yamasaki F, Doi Y, et al. Clinical correlates of PR-segment depression in asymptomatic patients with pericardial effusion. *J Am Coll Cardiol*. 2002;39(12):2000-2004.

Lauer B, Niederau C, Kuhl U, et al. Cardiac troponin T in patients with clinically suspected myocarditis. *J Am Coll Cardiol*. 1997;30: 1354-1359.

Liesemer K, Casper RC, Korgenski K, et al. Use and misuse of serum troponin assays in pediatric practice. *Am J Cardiol*. 2012;110: 284-289.

Lipshultz SE, Sleeper LA, Towbin JA, et al. The incidence of pediatric cardiomyopathy in two regions of the United States. *N Engl J Med*. 2003;348:1647-1655.

Mahle WT, Campbell RM, Favaloro-Sabatier J. Myocardial infarction in adolescents. *J Pediatr*. 2007;151(2):150-154.

Meeus M, Nijs J, Van Mol E, et al. Role of psychological aspects in both chronic pain and in daily functioning in chronic fatigue syndrome: a prospective longitudinal study. *Clin Rheumatol*. 2012;31(6): 921-929.

Mooney DP, Shorter NA. Slipping rib syndrome in childhood. *J Pediatr Surg*. 1997;32:1081-1082.

Pantell RH, Goodman BW Jr. Adolescent chest pain: a prospective study. *Pediatrics*. 1983;71:881.

Parasuraman S, Goldhaber SZ. Venous thromboembolism in children. *Circulation*. 2006;113:e12-e16.

Rowe BH, Dulberg CS, Peterson RG, et al. Characteristics of children presenting with chest pain to a pediatric emergency department. *CMAJ*. 1990;143:388-394.

Selbst SM, Ruddy RM, Clark BJ, et al. Pediatric chest pain: a prospective study. *Pediatrics*. 1988;82:319-323.

Selbst SM. Approach to the child with chest pain. *Pediatr Clin N Am*. 2010;57:1221-1234.

Son MF, Sundel RP. Musculoskeletal causes of pediatric chest pain. *Pediatr Clin N Am*. 2010;57:1385-1395.

Soongswang J, Durongpisitkul K, Nana A, et al. Cardiac troponin T: a marker in the diagnosis of acute myocarditis in children. *Pediatr Cardiol*. 2005;26:45-49.

Verghese GR, Friedman KG, Rathod RH, et al. Resource utilization reduction for evaluation of chest pain in pediatrics using a novel Standardized Clinical Assessment and Management Plan (SCAMP). *J Am Heart Assoc*. 2012;1(2):jah3-e000349.

CHAPTER 21

Cyanosis and Hypoxemia

Jonathan D. Hron, MD and Kathleen D. Snow, MD

BACKGROUND

Hypoxia and hypoxemia are common reasons for hospital admission, usually in the context of a primary respiratory illness. An understanding of the evaluation, diagnosis, and monitoring of patients with hypoxemia can improve patient care and resource utilization.

DEFINITIONS

Hypoxia: A relative or absolute deficiency of oxygen.

Hypoxemia: A relative or absolute deficiency of oxygen in the blood.

Cyanosis: Bluish discoloration of the skin or mucus membranes due to reduced fraction of oxygenated hemoglobin.

Respiratory failure: Inability to properly oxygenate and/or ventilate, resulting in hypoxemia and/or hypercapnia (CO_2 retention).

PATHOPHYSIOLOGY

The fundamental role of the cardiovascular, pulmonary, and hematology systems is to deliver oxygen (O_2) to tissues to enable oxidative phosphorylation and to remove carbon dioxide (CO_2), the gaseous waste product of aerobic metabolism. O_2 always moves down its partial pressure gradient from dry atmospheric air (partial pressure of O_2 [PO_2] 160 mmHg at sea level) to the mitochondria in tissues (PO_2 3-20 mmHg).

First, oxygen is inspired and diffuses across the alveolar-capillary membrane into the blood. The alveolar-arterial gradient (A-a gradient) represents the difference between the partial pressure of oxygen in the alveoli (PAO_2) and the partial pressure of oxygen in the artery (PaO_2). PaO_2 can be easily obtained by a blood gas test. PA_{O2} can be estimated using the alveolar gas equation: $PA_{O2} = (P_{ATM} - PH_2O)\ FIO_2 - (Pa_{CO2}/RQ)$ where P_{ATM} is the barometric pressures (primarily a function of altitude), PH_2O is the water vapor pressure (usually 47 mmHg), FIO_2 is the fraction of inspired O_2, Pa_{CO2} is the partial pressure of CO_2 and RQ is the respiratory quotient (~0.8). Diseases altering diffusion, lung ventilation, pulmonary perfusion, ventilation-perfusion (V/Q) matching, and fixed shunt fraction can impact PaO_2.

Next, the oxygen is transported from the lungs into the circulatory system. Once O_2 crosses the alveolar-pulmonary capillary membranes, a minimal amount is dissolved in plasma (0.003 mL per dL of blood for each mmHg of PaO_2). The majority is transported bound to hemoglobin reversibly as oxyhemoglobin. When 100% of the O_2 binding sites are occupied, hemoglobin carries 1.34 mL (at standard temperature and pressure [STP]) of O_2 per gram. The arterial oxygen content (CaO_2) can be expressed as $CaO_2 = (1.34 \times \text{hemoglobin} \times SaO_2) + (0.003 \times PaO_2)$. The rate of oxygen delivery to tissues is a product of cardiac output (a function of stroke volume and heart rate) and the arterial content of oxygen (CaO_2).

The O_2 binding relationship with hemoglobin tetramers is complex, generating an S-shaped curve of O_2 percent saturation of hemoglobin binding sites when viewed graphically (**Figure 21-1**). This hemoglobin saturation-desaturation relationship facilitates increased O_2 uptake at alveolar-pulmonary capillary membranes where the PAO_2 is high (~100 mmHg) and the release of O_2 in tissues, where PO_2 is low (3-20 mmHg). Several substances and conditions can "shift" the oxyhemoglobin saturation curve rightward, toward decreased pulmonary O_2 uptake and improved tissue release, or leftward, leading to improved pulmonary O_2 uptake and inhibited tissue release (see legend, Figure 21-1).

Understanding these processes of oxygenation and oxygen delivery aids in understanding clinical physiologic responses to hypoxia (hyperventilation/tachypnea, increased cardiac output/tachycardia, polycythemia, V/Q matching, etc.) and pathophysiologic disequilibrium (V/Q mismatch,

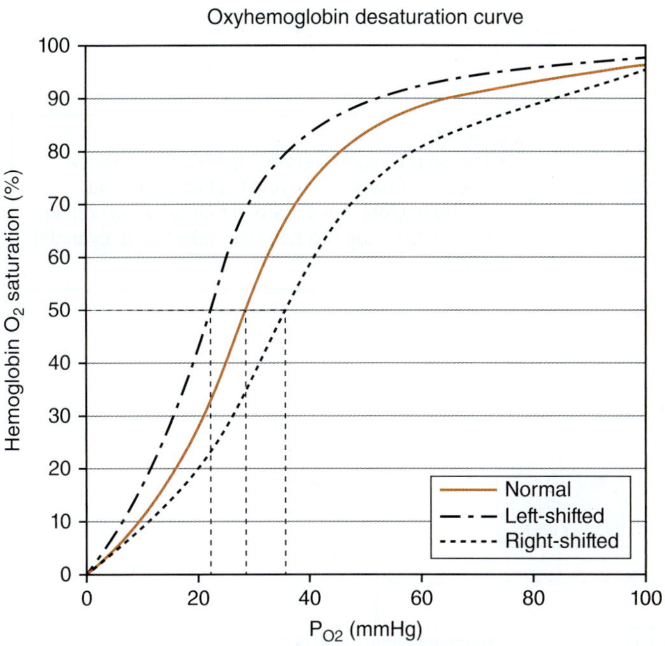

FIGURE 21-1. Oxyhemoglobin saturation-desaturation curve. The normal curve for adult hemoglobin is depicted, as are examples of left-shifted (poor tissue O_2 unloading) and right-shifted (improved tissue O_2 unloading) curves. The curve is shifted to the left by alkalemia, carboxyhemoglobinemia, hypocarbia, hypothermia, methemoglobinemia, high fetal hemoglobin content, and low 2,3-diphosphoglycerate (2,3-DPG). The curve is shifted to the right by acidemia, hypercarbia, hyperthermia, sulfhemoglobinemia, and high levels of 2,3-DPG, an end product of red cell metabolism. Note the Po_2 at which 50% of the O_2 is unloaded for each curve.

increased shunt fraction, shock, hyperventilation, respiratory failure, etc.). The most common clinical manifestations of disease resulting in a risk for tissue hypoxia result in blood hypoxemia as well, although important exceptions exist.

DEFINITIONS

Categories of Hypoxia:

1. Hypoxemic hypoxia: low blood O_2 levels from pulmonary or environmental causes (e.g., pneumonia with V/Q mismatch, high altitude, interstitial lung disease, shunting from congenital heart disease).
2. Anemic hypoxia: decreased blood O_2-carrying capacity (e.g., anemia, carbon monoxide poisoning, methemoglobinemia).
3. Stagnant hypoxia (hypoperfusion): decreased tissue O_2 delivery (e.g., shock, arterial occlusive disease).
4. Histotoxic hypoxia: reduction in ATP production by mitochondria (e.g., cyanide poisoning).

PATIENT HISTORY

A careful and complete history and physical examination are essential in the evaluation of hypoxemia and cyanosis. Review of the history with regard to underlying lung disease, cardiovascular disease, medication use, prior thoracic surgery, chest wall deformity or restriction (e.g., scoliosis), allergy, prior or current O_2 baseline use, and prior need for artificial ventilatory support are essential. If cyanosis is present, the history should focus on a detailed description of the areas of the body involved, timing, and severity, and associated symptoms. Changes in cyanosis with crying, choking, vomiting, or postural changes may help identify the underlying cause.

PHYSICAL EXAMINATION

The physical examination should start with a critical evaluation of the patient's vital signs based on norms for age. Tachypnea and tachycardia are common compensatory measures for hypoxemia and should raise concern for respiratory failure.

Pulse oximetry, often considered the "fifth vital sign," is a quick and convenient tool to measure peripheral oxygen saturation (SpO_2). Pulse oximetry utilizes the principles of spectrophotometry to determine the proportion of oxygenated and deoxygenated hemoglobin in the blood. Several factors can affect the validity and accuracy of pulse oximetry, and studies have highlighted racial bias in pulse oximetry measurement. Despite its limitations, pulse oximetry clearly exceeds the ability to detect hypoxemia by clinical examination as evidence of cyanosis does not develop until deoxyhemoglobin reaches 5g/dL or an arterial oxygen saturation around 67%. Physicians should be thoughtful about their use of pulse oximetery as the presence or absence of hypoxemia impacts healthcare resource use.

A careful and complete physical exam should be performed to help localize the etiology of hypoxemia **(Table 21-1)**. A thorough pulmonary exam should look for signs of respiratory distress (e.g., grunting, nasal flaring, retractions) and abnormal breath sounds (e.g., rales, wheezes, rhonchi). The cardiovascular examination should evaluate for abnormal heart sounds or signs of hypoperfusion. A neurologic evaluation is important to consider respiratory drive, strength of the muscles of respiration, and level of consciousness (as the brain is the most sensitive tissue to hypoxia).

Cyanosis is generally classified as either central or peripheral. Central cyanosis is associated with arterial desaturation and involves the skin, mucous membranes, lips, tongue, and nail beds. Peripheral cyanosis occurs when there is increased oxygen uptake in peripheral tissues; it is not associated with arterial desaturation. Peripheral cyanosis often involves only the extremities. Differential cyanosis, in which the upper extremities are pink and the lower extremities are cyanotic, is associated with conditions such as coarctation of the aorta and interrupted aortic arch when there is a right-to-left shunt through a patent ductus arteriosus. In newborns, acrocyanosis, or blueness of exposed extremities, is common and is typically insignificant. Similarly, isolated circumoral cyanosis due to prominent venous plexuses in the skin is insignificant, as long as cardiac output is normal.

DIFFERENTIAL DIAGNOSIS

The differential diagnosis of hypoxemia is broad and can be divided into categories based on the underlying pathophysiology:

1. Decreased inspired oxygen content (FIO_2)—e.g., smoke inhalation, high altitude
2. Decreased respiratory rate or apnea—e.g., toxin ingestion, traumatic brain injury
3. Increased right-to-left shunt—e.g., congenital heart disease, pulmonary arteriovenous malformation
4. Increased ventilation-perfusion mismatch—e.g., small airways disease, atelectasis
5. Diffusion abnormality—e.g., restrictive lung disease
6. Decreased affinity of hemoglobin for oxygen—e.g., methemoglobinemia

DIAGNOSTIC EVALUATION

Figure 21-2 provides an algorithm for the evaluation of a patient with evidence of hypoxia. The first steps in the evaluation should include pulse oximetry to determine if the patient is hypoxemic. Next, one should obtain a blood gas sample to assess acid-base status and ventilation. Arterial blood gases (ABG) if properly obtained and handled, can also yield information about oxygenation. Depending on IV access and available resources, a venous blood gas (VBG) or capillary blood gas

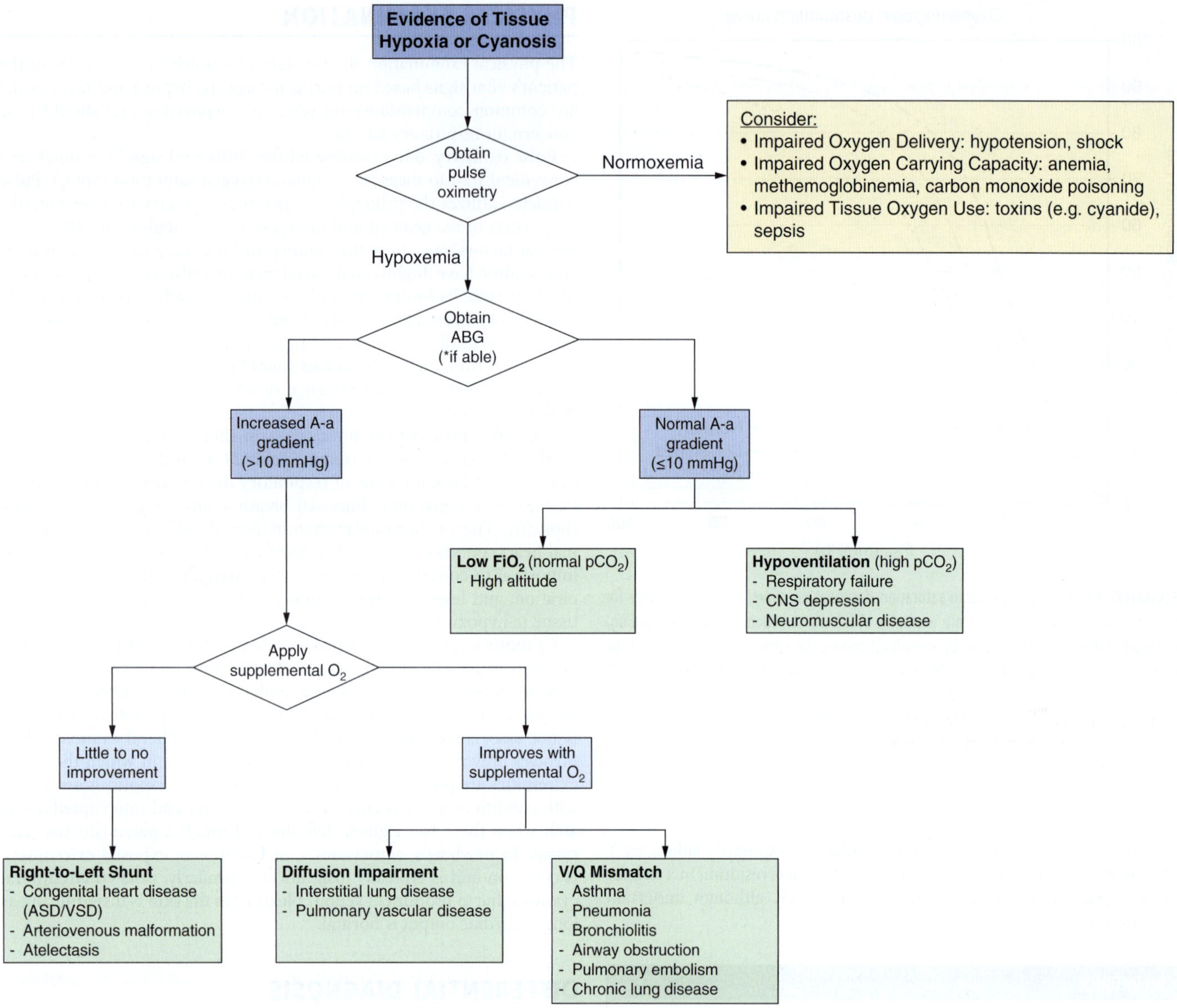

FIGURE 21-2. Diagnostic algorithm for the patient with hypoxia or cyanosis. With evidence of tissue hypoxia, pulse oximetry will help distinguish between hypoxemic hypoxia and other less common causes of hypoxia. A properly obtained arterial blood gas (ABG) can provide information about oxygenation (PaO_2), ventilation ($PaCO_2$), hemoglobin level, and acid-base status of the patient. Calculation of the Alveolar-arterial (A-a) gradient and application of supplementation oxygen can help narrow the broad differential diagnosis for hypoxemia.

(CBG) may be more feasible to obtain and contain reliable estimates of pH and $PaCO_2$. When combined with an accurate FiO_2, an A-a gradient can be calculated. Hypoxia in the setting of a normal A-a gradient suggests hypoventilation or decreased FiO_2 as the cause, whereas an elevated A-a gradient points to right-to-left shunting, ventilation-perfusion mismatch, or diffusion abnormality. One may also consider a hyperoxygenation test, which is a repeat arterial PO_2 determination after the patient has been inhaling 100% oxygen via mask or plastic hood for 20 minutes. If there is significant improvement of the arterial PO_2 or if it rises to greater than 150 mmHg with 100% oxygen, cardiac causes are unlikely. If there is little or no improvement, cyanotic congenital heart disease is suggested.

Additional workup should be guided by the history and physical examination findings. Chest radiographs are helpful in evaluating heart size, pulmonary blood flow, and pulmonary parenchymal disease. Electrocardiography and echocardiography should be performed if a cardiac cause is suggested. Other laboratory studies to consider are a complete blood count, glucose level, electrolytes, surrogate markers of hypoperfusion such as lactate, and evidence of end-organ dysfunction such as kidney (blood urea nitrogen and creatinine) and liver function tests.

MANAGEMENT

INITIAL STABILIZATION

As always, circulation, airway, and breathing should be addressed immediately. Supplemental oxygen should be administered. Assisted ventilation or intubation may be necessary if there is cardiorespiratory or neurologic compromise. Intravenous access, continuous pulse oximetry, and continuous cardiac monitoring are indicated. If possible, a blood gas should be obtained; however, treatment should not be delayed to obtain these studies. Once the patient is stabilized, a more complete history and physical examination are indicated to guide further evaluation and treatment.

OXYGEN ADMINISTRATION

Supplemental oxygen is an important intervention for many causes of hypoxemia and can be delivered in a variety of fashions (**Table 21-2**). The impact on FiO_2 of a particular O_2 delivery technique can vary based on a patient's size, respiratory rate, and tidal volume per breath. Nasal cannula provides the lowest levels of oxygen supplementation, with flow rates in children typically <5 L/min. The amount of FiO_2 delivered via

TABLE 21-1 Physical Examination

Vital signs, including temperature and blood pressures in the right arm and right leg
Right lower extremity systolic blood pressure 10 mmHg lower than that in right upper extremity suggests coarctation of the aorta or interrupted aortic arch
General
Dysmorphic features may indicate syndrome with other congenital anomalies
Poor growth indicates chronic underlying pathology
Cyanotic changes with crying or feeding
Skin
Degree and location of cyanosis; evaluate nail beds; jaundice may indicate underlying liver disease
Head, eyes, ears, nose, and throat
Foreign body or anatomic anomaly causing upper airway obstruction
Plethoric sclera with CHD
Cyanosis of oral mucosa, tongue, and lips with central cyanosis
Neck
Meningismus suggests meningitis
Mass causing possible obstruction
Respiratory
Rales, wheezing, grunting, or flaring suggests pulmonary pathology
Unequal air entry (e.g., pneumothorax or foreign body aspiration)
Stridor with upper airway obstruction or laryngeal irritation due to severe gastroesophageal reflux
Significant retractions and labored breathing indicate pulmonary pathology
Shallow, irregular respirations or apnea may indicate CNS depression
Tachypnea is common with CHD
Breathing is often minimally affected with CHD unless congestive heart failure, acidosis, or pulmonary edema is present
Cardiovascular
Hyperactive precordium with CHD
Arrhythmia may cause congestive heart failure with pulmonary edema and cyanosis
Murmur is suggestive of CHD, although the absence of murmur does not rule it out (e.g., transposition of the great arteries may have no murmur or only a soft murmur)
Single, loud S_2 may indicate CHD
Gallop
Unequal peripheral pulses or pulse lag suggests coarctation of the aorta or interrupted aortic arch
Poor peripheral perfusion may indicate sepsis, shock, or low cardiac output
Gastrointestinal
Hepatosplenomegaly or ascites may indicate congestive heart failure or underlying hepatic disease
Extremities and musculoskeletal
Clubbing signifies long-standing hypoxemia and cyanosis
Peripheral edema may indicate heart failure
Scoliosis is seen with chronic cyanosis and CHD, notably tetralogy of Fallot
Restrictive chest deformities
Neurologic
Abnormal head circumference may indicate hypoxic injury or other CNS pathology
Weakness may suggest neuromuscular disease
Hypotonia and lethargy may indicate CNS depression
Inconsolability may indicate meningitis
Unusual movements or seizures

CHD, congenital heart disease; CNS, central nervous system.

nasal cannula can be estimated using the equation FIO_2 = 21% + (Nasal cannula flow L/min × 3). A simple face mask delivers oxygen at flow rates from 5 to 10 L/min, yielding FIO_2 values between 30% and 65%. Partial re-breather masks and nonrebreather masks utilize an attached reservoir bag to increase FIO_2 delivery.

Depending on your clinical setting and facility capacity, other oxygen delivery devices with positive pressure support may be available. High flow nasal cannula provides humidified air at high flow rates (up to 60 L/min) with adjustable amounts of FIO_2. In small children especially, these high flow rates may provide significant positive pressure to aid in ventilation. Noninvasive positive pressure respiratory support (CPAP and BiPAP) allows for oxygen delivery in combination with positive airway pressure to overcome alveolar collapse and increase functional residual capacity. Ultimately, if the response to O_2 is inadequate despite escalating O_2 delivery, intubation should be considered.

FURTHER TREATMENT

Ongoing treatment is guided by the underlying cause. In neonates with suspected cyanotic congenital heart disease, pulmonary blood flow is often dependent on shunting through a patent ductus arteriosus. In these patients, an intravenous infusion of prostaglandin E_1 should be started, typically at a dose of 0.05 to 0.1 μg/kg per minute, to keep the ductus open while the evaluation progresses. If airway obstruction is suspected, laryngoscopy or bronchoscopy may be indicated. Other pulmonary therapies are directed at the underlying cause (e.g., bronchodilators for asthma). If there is evidence of pneumonia or sepsis, appropriate intravenous antibiotic therapy should be initiated. Shock should be treated with fluid resuscitation and blood pressure support as needed. Electrolyte abnormalities, hypoglycemia, and acidosis should be corrected. Warming or bundling may be effective in peripheral cyanosis secondary to cold exposure.

SPECIAL CONSIDERATIONS

BRIEF RESOLVED UNEXPLAINED EVENT

A brief resolved unexplained event (BRUE), formerly known as apparent life-threatening event (ALTE), is defined by the American Academy of Pediatrics as a brief, sudden, and resolving episode in an infant <1 year old with observed cyanosis, irregular or absent breathing, changes in tone, or altered level of responsiveness. The term is intended to be used for asymptomatic infants who present with an event without a clear etiology after a detailed history and physical exam are obtained. Evidence-based guidelines exist to help the provider differentiate between low- and high-risk infants and determine need for further diagnostic workup (see Chapter 19).

CYANOTIC SPELLS

Cyanotic spells are associated most frequently with tetralogy of Fallot and occur due to a sudden increase in right ventricular outflow tract obstruction and resultant increase in right to left shunt. These "tet spells" in infants are characterized by uncontrolled crying with rapid, deep breathing, worsening cyanosis and disappearance of the heart murmur. Toddlers with tetralogy of Fallot may squat to increase systemic vascular resistance and decrease, or temporarily reverse, the shunt thereby increasing pulmonary blood flow. This can be achieved by the healthcare provider as well, by placing the child in a knee-to-chest position. Untreated, these episodes can lead to limpness, convulsions, or death. Treatment is emergent and initially includes calming, oxygen administration, and morphine for sedative effect (see Chapter 51).

METHEMOGLOBINEMIA

Methemoglobin is hemoglobin with the iron in the ferric state (Fe^{3+}) as opposed to normal hemoglobin where iron is in the ferrous state (Fe^{2+}). In the ferric state, methemoglobin is unable to bind O_2 and shifts the oxyhemoglobin dissociation curve to the left for the remaining hemoglobin molecules in the tetramer (see Figure 21-1). Only about 1.5 g/dL methemoglobin in the circulation results in clinical cyanosis. A small amount of methemoglobin (1%) is normal, and there are cellular mechanisms to reduce iron back to the ferrous state, although these can be

TABLE 21-2 Oxygen Delivery Systems

O_2 Delivery Device	Flow Rate (L/min)	Theoretical F_{IO_2} Delivered (%)	Advantages	Disadvantages
Nasal cannula	<1-5	22-40	Ease of use, comfortable, inexpensive, able to eat without removal	Higher flow rates dry out mucous membranes; cannula easily dislodged
High Flow Nasal cannula	4-60	Adjustable, up to 100%	Capable of providing positive airway pressure and humidification, washout of CO_2 in dead space	Cost, may cause discomfort due to high flow rates
Simple mask	5-10	30-65	Can deliver higher flow rates than nasal prongs	Must remove to eat and drink and for airway care; insufficient flow rates may cause CO_2 retention
Partial rebreather†	6-15	60-95	Higher F_{IO_2} with lower flow rates	Same as above; risk of atelectasis and O_2 toxicity with prolonged use
Nonrebreather†	6-15	Approaches 100	Same as above	Same as above
Venturi mask†	4-10	Fixed F_{IO_2} set by mask design and flow rate	More predictable F_{IO_2} delivered	Same as above; also, high-flow systems are noisy; if backpressure develops on the jet, less room air enters, and F_{IO_2} can elevate unpredictably
Reservoir nebulizer†	Up to 80	Approaches 100	Can deliver humidification, and positive pressure	As for masks above; noisy; risk of O_2 toxicity and barotrauma
Oxygen Hood/head box	>10	Approaches 100	High F_{IO_2} possible	Insufficient flow can lead to CO_2 retention; O_2 gradients develop within the box; patient must be removed for care and feeding; significant temperature effect possible
Oxygen Tent	>10	About 50	Can provide humidification	Same as above; also, combustion hazard; claustrophobia

†Mask with reservoir bags attached. A nonrebreather mask-bag set up with sufficient flow to prevent complete collapse of the bag and a tight mask seal will deliver 100% F_{IO_2}.

CO_2, carbon dioxide; F_{IO_2}, fraction of inspired oxygen; O_2, oxygen.

genetically absent (e.g., cytochrome b_5 reductase deficiency). Exogenous agents such as nitrites, phenacetin, sulfonamides, lidocaine (including topical absorption), and aniline dyes are known to cause methemoglobinemia. Pulse oximetry is not adequate to recognize methemoglobinemia; a blood gas sample (arterial, capillary, or venous) with co-oximetry will confirm the diagnosis. In most cases, discontinuation of the offending agent is adequate treatment. Intravenous methylene blue at a typical dose of 1 to 2 mg/kg promptly removes methemoglobin and resolves cyanosis. In severe cases of methemoglobinemia, transfusion and hyperbaric O_2 have been used.

PULMONARY EMBOLISM

Although rare in children, rates of venous thromboembolism (VTE) are increasing, perhaps secondary to more frequent use of indwelling lines and catheters in hospitalized pediatric patients. In this population, it remains important to consider thrombus or infectious emboli for patients who become acutely hypoxemic, particularly in the absence of other signs of respiratory distress. Other risk factors for pulmonary embolism include recent surgery, immobility, use of estrogen-containing contraceptives and malignancy.

KEY POINTS

- Hypoxemia is a low arterial O_2 level and is one of four major categories of hypoxia.
- History, physical examination, and blood gas studies can add significantly to the understanding of a clinical presentation of hypoxemia.
- Clinically, pulmonary infection, chronic lung disease, or both are the most common causes of hypoxemia, with V/Q mismatch the most common pathophysiology.
- V/Q mismatch responds to O_2 administration, which is the mainstay of treatment.
- Pulse oximetry can detect and monitor hypoxemia in most situations, and is adequate for titrating O_2 therapy but has limitations that must be understood by the pediatric hospitalist.

SUGGESTED READINGS

Bonafide CP, Xiao R, Brady PW, et al. Prevalence of continuous pulse oximetry monitoring in hospitalized children with bronchiolitis not requiring supplemental oxygen. *JAMA*. 2020;323(15):1467-1477.

Carpenter SL, Richardson T, Hall M. Increasing rate of pulmonary embolism diagnosed in hospitalized children in the United States from 2001 to 2014. *Blood Advances*. 2018;2(12):1403-1408.

Hall JE, Hall ME. Principles of Gas Exchange; Diffusion of Oxygen and Carbon Dioxide Through the Respiratory Membrane. In: *Guyton and Hall Textbook of Medical Physiology*. 14th ed. Philadelphia, PA. Elsevier; 2021: 40; 511-520.

Lee JH, Rehder KJ, Williford L, et al. Use of high flow nasal cannula in critically ill infants, children, and adults: a critical review of the literature. *Intensive Care Med*. 2013;39(2):247-257.

Park MK, Salamat M. Pathophysiology of cyanotic congenital heart defects. In: *Pediatric Cardiology for Practitioners*. 7th ed. St Louis, MO: Mosby-Year Book; 2020;11: 107-118.

Rengasamy S, Nassef B, Bilotta F, et al. Administration of supplemental oxygen. *N Engl J Med*. 2021;385(3):e9. doi:10.1056/NEJMvcm2035240

Ross PA, Newth CJL, Khemani RG. Accuracy of pulse oximetry in children. *Pediatrics*. 2014;133(1):22-29.

Sarnaik AP, Clark JA, Heidemann SM. Respiratory Distress and Failure. In: Kleigman RM, St Gemell JW, eds. *Nelson Textbook of Pediatrics*. 21st ed. Philadelphia, PA: Elsevier; 2020:583-601.

Sjoding MW, Dickson RP, Iwashyna TJ, et al. Racial Bias in Pulse Oximetry Measurement. *N Engl J Med*. 2020;383(25):2477-2478.

Snider HL. Cyanosis. In: Walker HK, Hall WD, Hurst JW, eds. *Clinical Methods: The History, Physical, and Laboratory Examinations*. Boston, MA: Butterworth; 1990.

Tieder JS, Bonkowsky JL, Etzel RA, et al. Brief resolved unexplained events (formerly apparent life-threatening events) and evaluation of lower-risk infants. *Pediatrics*. 2016;137(5):e20160590.

Vesoulis Z, Tims A, Lodhi H, et al. Racial discrepancy in pulse oximeter accuracy in preterm infants. *J Perinatol*. 2022;42(1):79-85.

Vo P, Kharasch VS. Respiratory failure. *Pediatr Rev*. 2014;35(11):476-486.

CHAPTER 22

Diarrhea

Anuj Patel, MD

INTRODUCTION

Worldwide, diarrhea remains one of the leading causes of morbidity and mortality among the pediatric population, especially in children under 5 years of age. Over the past decade, rates of diarrhea-associated mortality have fallen, but it remains a top five cause of mortality in this age range, alongside prematurity, birth trauma/complications, pneumonia, and congenital anomalies. Access to clean water, sanitation initiatives, and the increased adoption of the rotavirus vaccine have significantly reduced morbidity and mortality, yet despite the progress, it is estimated that there are greater than 1.5 million deaths annually worldwide, and approximately a third of those cases (~ 500,000) are in children under the age of five.

BACKGROUND

Diarrhea is the condition of passing loose or liquid stools, usually three or more per day (or more frequently than is normal for an individual). The condition requires both an increase in frequency and liquidity of stools. Normal daily stool volumes vary by age and size of the child. Neonates and infants have a normal daily stool weight of 5 g/kg/day. For preschool-age children, average stool weights range from 50 to 75 g/day. Older children and adults have stool weights up to 250 g/day. Diarrhea typically results in stool volumes >10 g/kg/day in children younger than 3 years and >200 g/day in children older than 3 years. Diarrheal episodes are typically classified into acute and chronic, based on duration. Acute diarrhea is defined as an episode of diarrhea that is acute in onset and lasts less than 14 days. Chronic diarrhea is defined as an episode that lasts equal to or longer than 14 days. This distinction has implications for etiology, management, and prognosis.

In the United States, Pediatric diarrhea accounts for approximately 1.7 million outpatient visits. While many of these illnesses resolve with anti-emetics and oral rehydration therapy, approximately 70,000 children are hospitalized annually, with fewer than 300 deaths. The median cost of an acute gastroenteritis hospitalization is estimated at $3210, with a total yearly healthcare cost of $225 million dollars.

PATHOPHYSIOLOGY

In the normally functioning gastrointestinal tract, nutrients are absorbed via active, carrier-mediated transport across the intact mucosal lining. Electrolytes such as sodium, potassium, chloride, and bicarbonate are transported via both active and passive mechanisms, with sodium transport creating the most significant gradient. This sodium gradient is responsible for promoting the passive transport of water across the mucosal lining. Under normal circumstances, there is a balance between the absorptive and secretory functions, which are the opposing unidirectional electrolyte fluxes. This results in a net water absorption, with 90% of the absorption occurring in the small intestine.

Altered pathophysiologic mechanisms resulting in diarrhea can be divided into four categories: osmotic, secretory, inflammatory, and motility disorders. Osmotic diarrhea occurs when excessive amounts of solutes are retained in the lumen of the intestine, resulting in decreased water absorption. Osmotic diarrhea will typically cease with fasting or withholding of the poorly absorbed solute. Secretory diarrhea occurs when secretion of water into the lumen of the intestine exceeds absorption. In most cases, the diarrhea is not affected by alterations in enteral intake. Inflammation can cause diarrhea when there is mucosal damage resulting in decreased water absorption and increased fluid secretion. Inflammatory diarrhea may be associated with mucus, blood, and protein losses in the stool. This type of diarrhea is most commonly associated with inflammatory bowel disease and toxin-producing bacterial gastroenteritis. Lastly, motility disorders cause either increased or decreased transit time in the intestine, leading to altered water absorption. An increase in gut motility leads to decreased transit times and thus diarrhea.

PATIENT HISTORY

The frequency, duration, volume, associated symptoms, and character of the diarrhea (including odor, color, and presence of mucus or blood) should be determined during history-taking. Relation to vomiting can help differentiate infectious from other causes. It is important to understand the patient's normal bowel habits to determine the degree of change from baseline. A careful diet history may help identify inciting factors contributing to osmotic diarrhea, as well as identify foods associated with food- or water-borne pathogens (*Salmonella*, *Shigella*, *Campylobacter*, *Escherichia coli*, *Giardia*). Daycare attendance, sick contacts, recent medication changes, exposures to pets/farm animals, and recent travel history should all be explored. Viral causes, such as Rotavirus, enteric Adenovirus, and Norovirus, are the most common cause of infectious diarrhea and commonly spread in communal settings like daycares. One should inquire about exposure to animal vectors such as reptiles, which can be associated with *Salmonella*, as well as travel to areas with common endemic parasitic or bacterial infections. A history of recent antibiotic use should be obtained. Antibiotic-associated diarrhea typically resolves with cessation of medication, but *Clostridium difficile* can be associated with persistent diarrhea or blood in stool following recent antibiotic use.

It is also important to elicit any accompanying systemic symptoms. Fever is often associated with viral and bacterial infections. Rash or wheezing may accompany allergy-mediated diarrhea. Seizure activity associated with diarrhea in an otherwise healthy child can be seen with *Shigella* infection.

Post-infectious carbohydrate intolerance, a form of acquired lactose intolerance, can result in osmotic diarrhea in an otherwise well patient with recent acute gastroenteritis. Both nonspecific diarrhea of childhood and post-infectious carbohydrate intolerance may be related to ingestion of excessive amounts of sugary fluids (juice, soda). Constipation with encopresis should also be considered in children with chronic diarrhea, which represents leakage of watery stool around a blockage in a dilated colon.

Growth history and nutritional status should be obtained, especially when considering the cause of chronic diarrhea. One of the most common causes of chronic diarrhea in toddler-age children is a disorder of small intestinal motility called *nonspecific diarrhea of childhood* ("toddler's diarrhea"). Plotting a careful growth curve can assist in making a diagnosis in children with chronic diarrhea. Patients with cystic fibrosis, abetalipoproteinemia, or other metabolic conditions often have poor growth beginning soon after birth. Newborn state screens should be obtained and reviewed in all newborns with poor weight gain. In contrast, children with celiac disease typically exhibit poor growth after 4 to 6 months of age, coincident with the introduction of gluten-containing solids to the diet.

PHYSICAL EXAMINATION

The physical examination should first focus on the patient's hemodynamic stability and hydration status to determine whether immediate fluid resuscitation is needed. Comparison of premorbid weight to the weight at presentation is the most reliable method of determining the degree of dehydration, but this is not always feasible. Mild dehydration occurs when the patient is 3% to 5% dehydrated. Clinical signs are usually evident at ~3%. Moderate dehydration results from 6% to 9% body weight lost. Severe dehydration occurs when the patient is greater than or equal to 10% dehydrated and can be fatal. Fluid status should also be assessed by examination of mental status, mucous membranes, anterior fontanelle, tear production, skin turgor, capillary refill, and urine output. Because chronic diarrhea may represent underlying systemic illness as well as lead to the loss of calories, protein, and other minerals and vitamins (including zinc and vitamin B_2), the physical examination should also look for evidence of these deficiencies (**Table 22-1**).

TABLE 22-1 Selected Physical Findings Consistent With Evidence of Malnutrition or Systemic Illness

Area of Examination	Finding	Nutritional Deficiency/ Systemic Illness
General	Underweight	↓ Calories
	Edematous	↓ Protein
Hair	Easily pluckable, sparse	↓ Protein, zinc
Skin	Generalized dermatitis	↓ Zinc
	Erythema nodosum	Inflammatory bowel disease
Subcutaneous tissue	Decreased	↓ Calories
Muscles	Decreased mass	↓ Calories, protein
Mouth/tongue	Glossitis, angular stomatitis	↓ Vitamin B_2
	Oral ulcers	Inflammatory bowel disease
Extremities	Digital clubbing	Cystic fibrosis
Anus/rectum	Rectal prolapse	Cystic fibrosis
	Perianal tags, fissures, fistulas	Inflammatory bowel disease

DIFFERENTIAL DIAGNOSIS

The list of possible causes of diarrhea is extensive (**Table 22-2**). Distinguishing acute diarrhea from chronic diarrhea can be helpful in creating a differential. Most commonly, the cause of acute diarrhea is infectious. Viral infections (rotavirus, enteric adenovirus, caliciviruses, astrovirus) account for most cases of acute diarrhea. Other infectious causes include bacterial pathogens (*E. coli*, *Salmonella*, *Shigella*, *Campylobacter*) and parasites (*Giardia*, *Entamoeba*, *Cryptosporidium*).

Chronic diarrhea involves a broad list of possible causes. When evaluating chronic diarrhea, the age of the patient is helpful in narrowing the differential. In children under 1 year of age, intractable diarrhea of infancy is a common diagnosis comprised of a heterogenous group of illnesses. This entity is associated with diffuse mucosal injury resulting in persistent diarrhea, malabsorption, possible hematochezia, and malnutrition beginning before the age of 6 months. Chronic diarrhea is most commonly related to either cow milk allergy, soy protein intolerance, or prolonged post-infectious mucosal injury. Between the ages of 1 and 5 years, post-infectious enteritis, giardiasis, and celiac disease are more common diagnoses. In children older than 5 years, inflammatory bowel disease, constipation with encopresis, and acquired lactose intolerance are more likely. It is also important to remember that chronic diarrhea may be a presenting symptom of an immune deficiency, including HIV.

DIAGNOSTIC EVALUATION

In most cases of viral gastroenteritis, laboratory evaluation is not necessary. The laboratory evaluation for patients presenting with diarrhea is individualized, with attention paid to the acute versus chronic nature of the diarrhea. For some patients, the search for a specific cause should be explored, including hospitalized patients with nosocomial exposure, immunocompromised patients, young infants, and in those presenting with high fever, toxic appearance, grossly bloody stools, and with recent antibiotic use.

TABLE 22-2 Causes of Diarrhea

Infectious	Inflammatory bowel disease
Viruses	Monosaccharide deficiencies
Rotavirus	Disaccharide deficiencies
Caliciviruses (Norovirus & Sapovirus)	Post-infectious enteropathy
Enteric adenovirus	Motility disorders
Astrovirus	Irritable bowel syndrome
Bacteria	Late-stage intussusception
Salmonella	Allergic or intolerance
Shigella	Eosinophilic enteropathy
Campylobacter jejuni	Cow milk or soy protein intolerance
Escherichia coli	Systemic
Staphylococcus aureus	Hemolytic uremic syndrome
Clostridium difficile	Hyperthyroidism
Aeromonas hydrophila	α_1-Antitrypsin deficiency
Plesiomonas shigelloides	Immune deficiency
Vibrio cholera	Intestinal lymphangiectasia
Vibrio parahaemolyticus	Acrodermatitis enteropathica
Yersinia enterocolitica	Pancreatic insufficiency
Parasites	Hormone-secreting tumors
Giardia lamblia	Adrenal insufficiency
Entamoeba histolytica	α-lipoproteinemia
Cryptosporidium	Carcinoid tumor
Congenital	Abetalipoproteinemia
Congenital microvillus atrophy	Protein calorie malnutrition
Autoimmune enteropathy	Miscellaneous
Hirschsprung disease	Toddler's diarrhea
Congenital chloride-losing diarrhea	Constipation with encopresis
Intractable diarrhea of infancy	Poisoning (organophosphate or mushrooms)
Short-bowel syndrome	Iatrogenic
Malabsorptive	Antibiotic associated
Celiac disease	Laxative induced
Cystic fibrosis	Neonatal abstinence syndrome

When a diagnosis is necessary, stool should be sent for any or all of the following: occult blood, presence of fecal leukocytes, fecal fat, bacterial culture, ova and parasites, rotavirus antigen testing, *C. difficile* toxin, and *Giardia* antigen assay. If there is concern for a particular bacterial pathogen, this should be communicated to the laboratory so that the specimen can be plated on the appropriate media. If carbohydrate malabsorption is suspected, acidic stool pH (<5.5) and detection of reducing substances may be helpful in making a diagnosis. Stool calprotectin or lactoferrin are useful screening tools to identify children likely to need endoscopy for possible inflammatory bowel disease. Depending on the severity of the illness, serum laboratory studies may be necessary. In patients with severe dehydration, evaluation of electrolytes and renal function may be warranted. The hemoglobin can identify the presence of anemia associated with acute or chronic hematochezia. If an underlying immunodeficiency is suspected, complete blood count with differential may be helpful. Measurement of erythrocyte sedimentation rate, C-reactive protein, and procalcitonin are nonspecific but may be elevated in an infectious or inflammatory process. Total protein, albumin, and prealbumin levels may reflect the extent or chronicity of malnutrition if present. Vitamin and mineral deficiencies can be identified with further laboratory investigation, if indicated. If celiac disease is suspected in patients presenting with chronic diarrhea, tests for antigliadin, antiendomysial, and tissue transglutaminase antibodies should be performed. A sweat chloride test should be obtained when cystic fibrosis is a concern.

In recent years, the popularity and availability of multiplex-PCR-based stool panels has increased. These tests are accurate, faster than conventional cultures, and have reduced the need for additional intervention (imaging, antibiotic prescriptions, and endoscopy). To avoid excessive healthcare cost, they should be ordered for patients with bloody diarrhea, immunocompromised populations, chronic or severe illnesses, or those younger than 3 months old with fever and diarrhea. History, exam, and clinical judgment should guide the use of such testing. Cultures remain the gold standard and should be obtained concurrently if the history remains consistent with an illness not tested on the panel, a need to test for antibiotic sensitives arises, or if PCR testing is not available.

Imaging studies are rarely helpful or indicated in the evaluation of patients with acute diarrhea. Plain films of the abdomen will typically reveal a nonspecific bowel gas pattern, with or without air-fluid levels. Constipation or encopresis should be evident from stool load on a plain film but is also frequently apparent by history and physical examination. Radiographs, computed tomography, or endoscopy may be warranted to evaluate other diagnostic considerations, especially if the symptoms are severe or prolonged.

MANAGEMENT

Management of diarrheal illness depends on identification of the underlying cause and institution of appropriate therapy. Because most cases of acute diarrhea are caused by viral infections and are self-limited, the role of the physician is to rule out other causes that may be more serious or require more specific treatment. Pediatric patients with diarrhea are most commonly hospitalized because of dehydration and the need for intravenous fluid. Most cases of mild or moderate dehydration due to diarrhea can be managed with oral rehydration therapy. Once a patient is able, oral intake should be initiated as soon as possible, with advancement to solid intake as tolerated. For patients who are unable to tolerate adequate enteral hydration, have underlying illnesses that complicate management, or need rapid fluid resuscitation for severe dehydration, intravenous boluses of an isotonic solution should be administered and repeated until the patient's intravascular volume has been restored. Replacement of any remaining fluid deficits, continued fluid maintenance requirements, and ongoing fluid losses should be handled with infusions of appropriate intravenous solutions (see Chapter 116).

There is no medical reason to delay solid food intake secondary to persistent diarrhea. Although intestinal absorption of nutrients may be somewhat compromised in the presence of diarrhea, 80% of dietary carbohydrates and 50% of dietary proteins continue to be absorbed. Some studies suggest that early initiation of dietary nutrients may help decrease output or promote the resolution of diarrhea. Avoidance of cow milk protein is not typically warranted with acute diarrheal illnesses, because clinically significant acquired lactase deficiency is uncommon in this setting. In severe cases of malnutrition, nasogastric or nasojejunal feeds or even parenteral nutrition may need to be considered, especially in those with an associated underlying systemic illness.

Pharmacologic treatment is rarely needed for acute diarrhea, although appropriate antibiotic therapy should certainly be given for specific infectious causes (see Chapter 99). Antidiarrheal agents should be avoided in young children. Although adsorbents (including activated magnesium aluminum silicate and bulk-forming fibers) act to absorb fluid within the intestine, they do not decrease overall fluid losses or the risk of dehydration. Antimotility agents should never be used in the presence of bloody diarrhea or when an infectious cause is suspected; they may prolong the carrier state. Probiotic agents continue to gain increased popularity in the management of diarrhea. *Lactobacillus GG* and *Saccharomyces boulardii* function to alter the intestinal flora, resulting in a modest decrease in stool output. Specifically, *Lactobacillus GG* has been associated with decreased severity of rotavirus infection. A 2019 Cochrane review revealed modest benefit in probiotic usage with antibiotic associated diarrhea. Yet, the specifics of probiotic administration (duration, dosage, timing) remain unclear and will require further research for widespread recommendation. Zinc replacement therapy, on the other hand, has been recommended by the WHO since 2004 in the reduction of acute diarrhea. Recent data has shown noninferiority of 5 or 10 mg daily for 10 to14 days as compared to the original WHO study of 20 mg daily. Lastly, antiemetic therapy may be helpful for patients with associated vomiting.

SPECIAL CONSIDERATIONS

While most cases of diarrhea self-resolve with supportive management, severe and serious complications must be considered. In particular, hemolytic uremic syndrome, toxic megacolon, reactive arthritis, Guillen-Barre, or sepsis are possibilities that must be kept in mind after a positive associated bacterial causative agent is identified.

KEY POINTS

- Most pediatric patients with diarrhea have acute viral illness and do not need further workup beyond the history and physical examination.
- The search for a specific cause should be explored in hospitalized patients with nosocomial exposure, immunocompromised patients, and young infants, and in those presenting with high fever, toxic appearance, grossly bloody stools, or with recent antibiotic use.
- Pediatric patients with diarrhea are most commonly hospitalized because of dehydration and the need for intravenous fluid.

SUGGESTED READINGS

Akhondi H, Simonsen KA. Bacterial Diarrhea. [Updated 2022 May 6]. In: StatPearls [Internet]. Treasure Island (FL): StatPearls Publishing; 2022 Jan-. Available from: https://www.ncbi.nlm.nih.gov/books/NBK551643/?report=classic.

Axelrad JE, Freedberg DE, Whittier S, Greendyke W, Lebwohl B, Green DA. Impact of gastrointestinal panel implementation on health care utilization and outcomes. *J Clin Microbiol.* 2019;57(3).

CaJacob NJ, Cohen MB. Update on diarrhea. *Pediatr Rev.* 2016;37(8): 313–322.

Child Health and Development. (2004, December 8). *Clinical management of acute diarrhoea: WHO/Unicef joint statement.* World Health Organization. Retrieved July 31, 2022, from https://www.who.int/publications/i/item/WHO_FCH_CAH_04.7.

Child mortality (under 5 years). (2022, January 28). World Health Organization. https://www.who.int/news-room/fact-sheets/detail/levels-and-trends-in-child-under-5-mortality-in-2020/

Dadonaite B. (2019, August 26). *More than half a million children die from diarrhea each year. How do we prevent this?* Our World in Data. Retrieved July 31, 2022, from https://ourworldindata.org/childhood-diarrheal-diseases.

Dhingra U, Kisenge R, Sudfeld CR, et al. (2020). Lower-dose zinc for childhood diarrhea—a randomized, multicenter trial. *N Engl J Med.* 2020;383(13):1231-1241.

Duggan C, Nurko S. "Feeding the gut": the scientific basis for continued enteral nutrition during acute diarrhea. *J Pediatr.* 1997;131:801-808.

Guandalini S, Dhawan A. *Textbook of Pediatric Gastroenterology, Hepatology and Nutrition: A Comprehensive Guide to Practice.* 2nd ed. Springer; 2021.

Guo Q, Goldenberg JZ, Humphrey C, El Dib R, Johnston BC. Probiotics for the prevention of pediatric antibiotic-associated diarrhea. *Cochrane Database Syst Rev.* 2019;4(4):CD004827.

King CK, Glass R, Bresee JS, Duggan C, Centers for Disease Control and Prevention. Managing acute gastroenteritis among children: oral rehydration, maintenance, and nutritional therapy. *MMWR Recomm Rep.* 2003;52(RR-16): 1-16.

Leshem E, Tate JE, Steiner CA, Curns AT, Lopman BA, Parashar UD. National Estimates of Reductions in Acute Gastroenteritis–Related Hospitalizations and Associated Costs in US Children After Implementation of Rotavirus Vaccines. *J Pediatric Infect Dis Soc.* 2017; 7(3):257-260.

Nagler J, Hsu DC. Diarrhea. In: Chamberlain J, Shook JE, Pereira F, eds. *Fleisher & Ludwig's Textbook of Pediatric Emergency Medicine.* 8th ed. LWW; 2020:152-158.

Sethi G, Sankaranarayanan S, Sukhija M. Low lactose in the nutritional management of diarrhea: case reports from India. *Clin Epidemiol Glob Health.* 2018;6(4):160-162.

CHAPTER 23

Growth Faltering

Dena Ibrahim, MD and Allysa L. Kehring, MD

BACKGROUND

Growth faltering is among the most common diagnostic and therapeutic challenges facing pediatric hospitalists. Growth faltering is not a diagnosis, but rather a description of undernutrition and deficient growth over time. The previously used term Failure to Thrive (FTT) has fallen out of favor secondary to its vagueness, as well as the implied presumption that a caregiver has failed or that a child is not thriving globally. Many have suggested that FTT be replaced by a term such as "growth deficiency," "undernutrition," or "growth faltering."

There is no uniformly accepted definition for growth faltering and therefore prevalence can only be estimated. In high-risk populations (low-birth weight infants, children living in poverty, and children with special healthcare needs), estimates run as high as 5% to 10%. Growth faltering can occur at any age. Young children and those with special healthcare needs are particularly vulnerable due to their complete dependence on caregivers for nutrition. Over 95% of patients with growth faltering are under the age of 2, with approximately 80% of these cases involving infants less than 6 months of age.

While this condition is primarily managed in the outpatient setting, more severely affected patients or those whose safety is in question may require hospitalization. The interaction of psychosocial, behavioral, and physiologic factors can be tremendously complex, thus it is critical for pediatric hospitalists to have a clear approach to this diagnostic challenge.

PATHOPHYSIOLOGY

The etiology of growth faltering is most frequently multifactorial. Psychosocial and behavioral factors play a predominant role in the majority of cases, but pathologic medical reasons for poor growth must also be considered. Historically, etiologies of growth faltering were dichotomized into organic versus inorganic subcategories. This is an outdated framework due to its disregard for the dynamic interplay between multiple etiologies that often occur simultaneously.

It is useful to recognize that inadequate growth can be caused by any combination of three factors: (i) abnormally low caloric intake, (ii) inadequate digestion and/or absorption of ingested calories, and (iii) abnormally high metabolic demands or impaired utilization of calories.

In the early stages, undernutrition may have little obvious consequence to the child. However, longstanding cases may lead to short stature, reduced muscle mass, impaired brain growth, and behavioral or developmental abnormalities. Refractory cases can progress to severe weight deficiency (marasmus) and protein deficiency (kwashiorkor); marasmus and kwashiorkor are seen rarely in the United States secondary to a generally steady food supply.

DEFINITIONS

There is no consensus definition for growth faltering.

In practice, this is a child with inadequate growth over time relative to standardized growth charts after considering genetic background.

Growth faltering is commonly defined as:

- patient weight below the 5th percentile
- a decline in growth rate that results in the crossing of two major percentile lines for weight
- weight-for-height or height-for-age below the 10th percentile

These rigid criteria greatly oversimplify the complex task of identifying children in whom growth is truly a problem.

For example, as many as 25% of normal infants will cross major percentile lines during their first 2 years of life, then maintain growth consistently along their new curve. In the absence of other signs of illness, these children should not be categorized as having growth faltering.

Similarly, there are healthy children who track consistently along a specific growth curve at or below the 5th percentile, usually due to genetic factors such as diminutive parental height. By definition such children represent 5% of the normal population and should not be labelled as growth restricted.

PATIENT HISTORY

Few conditions better illustrate the value of a careful history than growth faltering (**Table 23-1**). Because so many cases are attributable to behavioral and psychosocial factors, the first step in evaluating the condition is to obtain a detailed feeding history.

Important diet history details include:

- Frequency—grazing vs. dedicated feed/meal times
- Content—typical day's meals, formula mixing recipe, excessive juice/milk intake, following a special diet (e.g., vegan)
- Route—oral vs. tube fed
- Feeding environment—supervision, distractions, feeding position, bottle propping
- Feeding behaviors—distractibility, food refusal, early satiety, vomiting/spit-up

For breastfed infants, it is important to assess the frequency and duration of feedings and whether the baby is latching well, audibly swallowing, and showing signs of satiety. After completion of a feeding, a mother should typically note that her breasts feel softer and less full. The frequency and volume of urine and stool output also lend insight to the quantity of intake.

For tube fed children, it is important to assess if they are fed via gravity from a feed bag, via syringe pushed directly into the tube, or via a pump. If pump fed then further questions detailing the pump rate, duration, and amount of formula left in the bag after a feed can help in identifying potential equipment errors.

Familial growth patterns should be assessed. In addition, a detailed social history is critical. Key areas to explore include major stressors in the home, financial difficulties including food insecurity, depression,

TABLE 23-1 Focused History

Focused History
Dietary History
• Details of everything the child eats
• For formula-fed infants, assess if formula is prepared properly
• For breastfed infants, assess duration and frequency of feedings and for signs of adequate milk transfer (e.g., softer breasts post-feed)
• Quantify caloric intake (preferably from a diet log)
• History of excessive juice, soft drinks, or cow's milk
• Vegetarian or other dietary preference
Feeding History
• When, where, and with whom the child eats
• For infants, feeding/breastfeeding position
• Does the patient make eye contact while feeding (especially infants)
• Distractions during feeding (TV, toys, siblings, etc.)
• Duration of each feeding
• Does the patient seem hungry at feeding time
• Does the infant or child resist eating
Family History
• History of delayed growth in either parent or in siblings
• Obtain height and weight of both parents
• Family history of major systemic disease (CF, IBD, rheumatic disease, etc.)
Social History
• How does the patient interact with the family
• Parental description of patient's temperament
• Financial stressors including food insecurity
• Identify all caregivers, especially those who feed the patient
• Parental history of depression or other mental illness
• Indicators of substance abuse in the family
• Indicators of domestic violence
• History of Child Protective Services involvement with the family
History suggestive of underlying medical disease
• Difficulty initiating suck
• Sputtering or choking during feeding
• Spitting up, vomiting, or signs of pain after feeding
• Early satiety (patient starts feeding eagerly but stops prematurely)
• Abnormal stools (watery, bloody, mucusy, foul-smelling)
• Indicators of neurodevelopmental delay
• History of birth trauma, asphyxia, or postnatal head injury
• For infants, sweating or shortness of breath when feeding
• Chronic shortness of breath, labored breathing, stridor, or snoring
• Chronic/recurrent fevers
• HIV risk factors

substance abuse, domestic violence, and any history of prior Child Protective Service reports. The remainder of the history is directed toward eliciting symptoms suggestive of underlying pathologic disease including a complete review of systems.

PHYSICAL EXAMINATION

A directed physical examination (**Table 23-2**) should begin with an accurately obtained weight, length, and head circumference. For children from 0 to 2 years old, these measurements should be plotted on the 2006 WHO Child Growth Standards charts which were developed using longitudinal data from breastfed children in several developed countries. For children over 2 years old, the data can be plotted on the 2002 CDC growth charts. Several syndrome-specific growth charts are available on which to plot anthropometric measurements for children with known inherited disorders (e.g., trisomy 21).

TABLE 23-2 Directed Physical Examination

Directed Physical Examination
Vital Signs
• Bradycardia, hypothermia (concerning for critical malnutrition)
General
• Plot height, weight, head circumference, and BMI on appropriate growth charts
• Calculate mid-parental height*
• Inspect for lack of subcutaneous fat, temporal or thenar wasting
• Poor hygiene, dental caries, other possible signs of neglect
• Dysmorphic features suggestive of genetic syndrome
HEENT
• Markedly enlarged tonsils
• Stridor
• Craniofacial anomalies (include digital examination for occult cleft palate)
• Chronic TM changes or posterior dental caries which might suggest gastroesophageal reflux
Chest
• Increased work of breathing
• Chest wall deformities
Cardiovascular
• Signs of increased cardiac work (tachycardia, hyperdynamic precordium)
• Pathologic murmur
Abdomen
• Hepatomegaly or jaundice
Extremities
• Clubbing
Skin
• Pallor
• Cyanosis
Neurologic
• Abnormal tone or reflexes
• Developmental delay
• Abnormal affect or social interactions

*Mid-parental height calculation: boys: (maternal height + paternal height + 13 cm)/2; girls: (maternal height + paternal height - 13 cm)/2.

Longitudinal comparison of the growth measurements may provide insight into the chronicity or etiology of the process. Initially, undernutrition causes an isolated slowing of weight gain. With more longstanding nutritional deficiency, height velocity also slows while head growth is typically spared until the problem has become severe and longstanding. Isolated microcephaly in the setting of poor weight gain may also indicate an underlying endocrinopathy, metabolic or neurological disorder.

The physical examination should be targeted to identify any craniofacial anomalies or features suggestive of a chromosomal abnormality, signs of chronic cardiac or pulmonary disease, hepatic enlargement, or neurodevelopmental abnormalities. Close attention should also be paid to any potential signs of abuse or neglect (bruising, oral injury, injury inappropriate for child's developmental abilities, etc.). Particular note should be made of the quantity of subcutaneous fat, and the temporal and thenar areas should be inspected for wasting.

DIFFERENTIAL DIAGNOSIS

Many processes can contribute to growth faltering. The underlying causes are summarized in **Table 23-3**.

Inadequate caloric intake is commonly caused by one or more psychosocial or behavioral factors that inhibit appropriate feeding. Through this process the infant or child may lose or fail to develop appropriate hunger-satiety cues and inadequate intake may become entrenched in the child's behavior. In the tube fed population, inadequate calories may stem from formula measurement errors and mechanical pump malfunctions.

TABLE 23-3 Major Etiologies of Growth Faltering
Inadequate Intake
• Disturbance of parent-child relationship
• Neglect
• Food aversion, behavioral problem
• Incorrectly mixed formula
• Insufficient breast milk intake
• Improper food choices, inadequate food
• Oromotor dyscoordination
• Gastroesophageal reflux
• Pyloric stenosis
• Delayed gastric emptying
• Cleft palate
Malabsorption
• Cow's milk allergy
• Cystic fibrosis
• Celiac disease
• Villous atrophy
• Hepatobiliary disease
• Acrodermatitis enteropathica
Increased Metabolic Demands
• Congestive heart failure
• Chronic hypoxemia
• Bronchopulmonary dysplasia
• Cystic fibrosis
• Restrictive lung disease
• Upper airway obstruction
• Chronic anemia
• Chronic infection (HIV, TB, others)
• Renal tubular acidosis
• Chronic renal failure
• Chronic inflammatory disease (IBD, others)
• Malignancy
• Thyroid disease
• Spasticity
Defective Utilization of Calories
• Inborn error of metabolism
• Chromosomal anomaly
• Diabetes mellitus

Anatomic abnormalities can interfere with feeding. Cleft palate or other undetected oropharyngeal anomalies may inhibit an infant's normal suck-swallow mechanism. Brain injury or in utero drug exposure may impair the development of an organized feeding pattern or result in slowed gastrointestinal motility. Delayed gastric emptying may cause early satiety and contribute to gastroesophageal reflux. Gastroesophageal reflux often causes pain immediately after eating and may lead to feeding aversion or habitual early cessation of feeding. Slow intestinal motility can lead to chronic constipation with resultant feeding intolerance presenting with abdominal distension and emesis.

Inadequate absorption of ingested calories may stem from inherited or acquired gastrointestinal conditions. Such conditions result in inadequate growth despite appropriate caloric intake. Malabsorption syndromes typically cause abnormal stool character, with malodorous, bulky stools (cystic fibrosis), bloody or mucus-filled stools (cow's milk protein allergy), or watery, unformed stools persisting after a bout of infectious diarrhea (villous atrophy).

Increased metabolic demands can stem from multiple conditions. Common causes of increased metabolic demand include cardiac disease (e.g. congestive heart failure), pulmonary disease resulting in chronically increased work of breathing (e.g., bronchopulmonary dysplasia), chronic hypoxemia, severe chronic anemia, chronic acidosis (e.g., Renal Tubular Acidosis [RTA]), chronic inflammation (e.g., inflammatory bowel disease), malignancy, inborn errors of metabolism causing impaired utilization of calories (e.g., mitochondrial disease), and chronic infection (e.g., HIV).

DIAGNOSTIC EVALUATION

Often, the most informative evaluation is to directly observe a feeding after confirming a detailed history. Multiple feedings should be evaluated, and the environment should be as similar to the home environment as possible. Consultation with a certified lactation specialist may be particularly helpful in the evaluation of breastfed infants, and comparison of pre- and post-breastfeeding weights can more precisely quantify breast milk intake.

With infants in particular, careful attention must be paid to the interaction between the infant and caregiver during feedings as psychosocial disruption may contribute to feeding difficulties. An infant with disorganized early feeding behavior, or one who becomes easily distracted or fussy during feeding may pose a challenge to a caregiver's ability to feed them. It is particularly notable if, under these circumstances, the parent prematurely stops feeding the baby.

As part of the evaluation, consultation with a feeding specialist should be considered whenever possible. In addition to observing the caregiver's approach to feeding, these professionals will feed the patient themselves and can often identify abnormalities in oromotor coordination or swallowing. During their evaluation sessions they can experiment with subtle variations in positioning, timing of feeds, nipple types, and feeding environment to determine if a successful feeding routine can be established.

With young children beyond infancy, the initial evaluation also involves close observation of feeding behavior. Key elements to evaluate include the child's overall temperament, the ability of the child to focus during mealtimes, issues with textures, food choices, attitudes toward eating and food, and emotional struggles with caregivers regarding food. Specific attention should be paid to consistent food refusal, as this is the hallmark of behavioral causes of growth faltering in a toddler.

Even when behavioral or psychosocial issues are identified, and feeding disturbances are clearly present, it often remains unclear if these factors represent the sole explanation for poor growth. In these circumstances, or in cases when no clear feeding disturbance can be identified, the next step should be to carefully monitor daily weights during a period when caloric intake is closely monitored. If appropriate weight gain is shown with adequate caloric intake, the focus of care can remain on feeding, and reinforcing a feeding schedule that will set parents up for success at home.

If appropriate caloric intake does not result in adequate weight gain, a more comprehensive workup should be undertaken to look for causes of either malabsorption or increased metabolic demands. It should be noted that when growth restriction affects length and head circumference along with weight, it is substantially more likely that an underlying medical condition is present. Laboratory evaluations for underlying medical conditions are best reserved for cases where feeding disturbances and psychosocial factors have been ruled out. Historical data suggest that without specific evidence for an underlying medical condition, laboratory testing is helpful in approximately only 2% of cases of growth faltering. If underlying medical disease is strongly suspected, laboratory evaluation should include Complete Blood Count, Basic Metabolic Panel, and stool samples for occult blood, pH, and reducing substances. These tests can help rule out anemia, chronic acidosis, renal disease, carbohydrate malabsorption, or cow's milk intolerance. Many practitioners will also include erythrocyte sedimentation rate, thyroid function tests, sweat chloride, and fecal fat quantitation as part of the initial laboratory evaluation.

MANAGEMENT

INITIAL STABILIZATION

Figure 23-1 outlines a general approach to diagnostic evaluation and management of children with growth faltering. The initial assessment should focus on ruling out life-threatening causes (e.g., developing heart

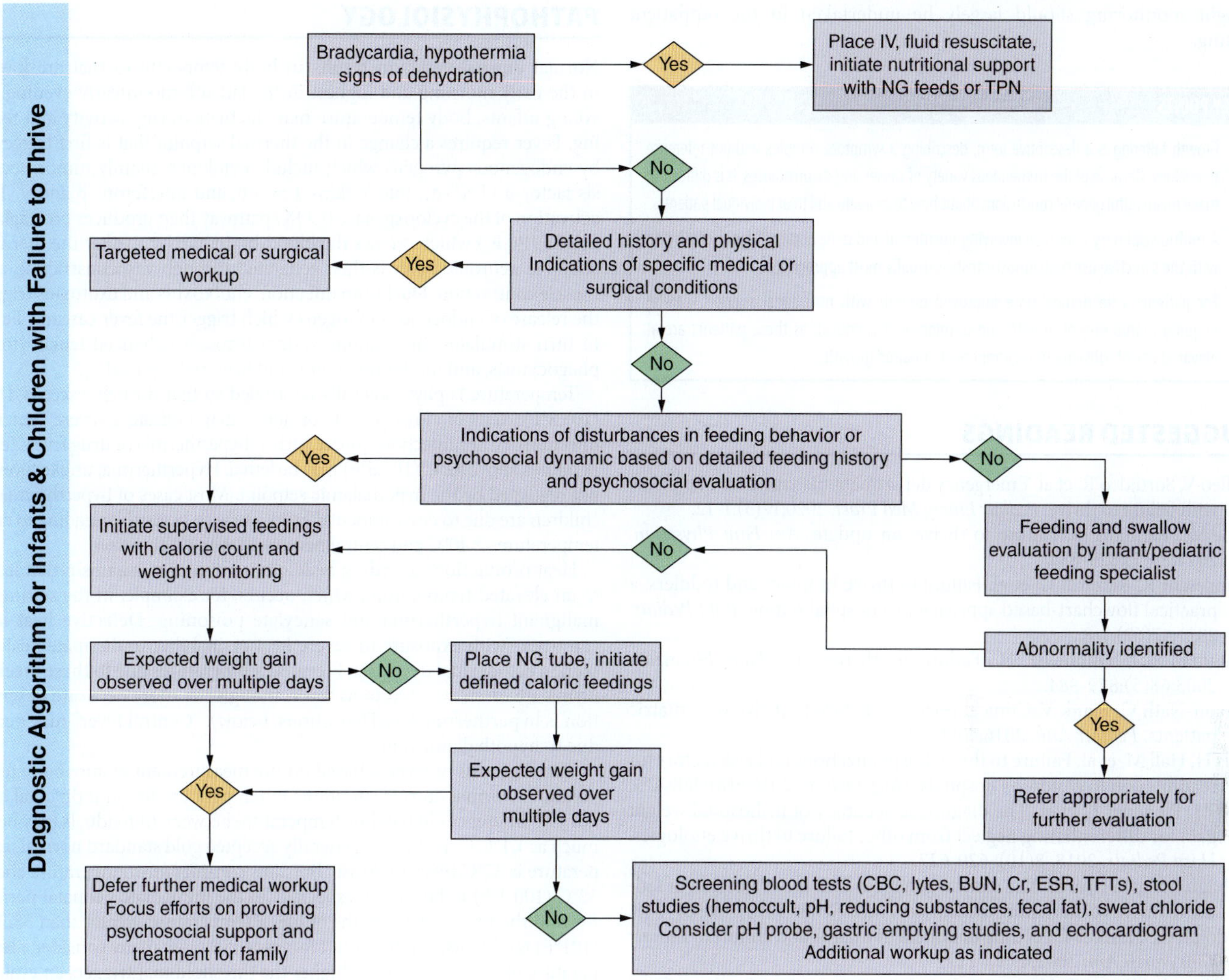

FIGURE 23-1. Algorithm outlines a general approach to diagnostic evaluation and management of children with failure to thrive.

failure in a neonate). With rare exception, the majority of patients typically present clinically stable. Concerning signs for critical malnutrition include bradycardia, hypothermia, electrolyte imbalances, hypoglycemia, and altered mental status. If any of these signs are present, the acute management should focus on stabilization. Subsequently, enteral nutrition should be reintroduced slowly to avoid the complications of refeeding syndrome.

SUBSEQUENT TREATMENT

Through detailed history and exam, potential underlying causes of poor weight gain should be identified and corrected if possible. Treatment of known chronic medical conditions should be optimized. Behavioral and psychosocial problems should be addressed, with ongoing family counseling and social work support as indicated.

Regardless of etiology, all patients with growth faltering need caloric supplementation to promote catch-up growth. Caloric requirements will vary with the age of the infant, the degree of undernutrition, and the presence or absence of underlying medical disease. Infants should be placed on a feeding schedule with defined volume goals. Many will require hypercaloric formula or fortified breastmilk (24-30 calories per ounce) to obtain catch-up growth. For toddlers and children, caloric intake may be increased through dietary counseling and use of high-calorie liquid supplements. In all cases it is advisable that dietary changes be made under the supervision of a pediatric nutritionist when accessible. In cases of malabsorption, parenteral nutrition may be indicated.

Despite dietary modifications, it is not uncommon for weight gain to fall short of expectations. Patients who have experienced chronic undernutrition often experience early satiety. In these cases, placement of a nasogastric (NG) tube for supplementation is often effective to ensure adequate intake. It is generally preferable to deliver the NG supplementation at night so as not to interfere with daytime appetite. Of note, a child with nighttime positive pressure ventilation (CPAP, BiPAP) for obstructive sleep apnea should alternatively receive post-pyloric NJ feeds to reduce the risk of aspiration.

Hospitalization may be indicated in cases of severe malnutrition, rapid weight loss, poor response to prolonged outpatient intervention trials or indicators leading to concern for the child's safety. Nearly half of children hospitalized for growth faltering have at least one complex chronic condition and those with prematurity-related conditions as well as families with low median household incomes have been found to be at risk for subsequent readmission. Admission should not be performed purely to document the ability of the child to gain weight as this has not been found to accurately differentiate neglect from other etiologies.

Growth faltering is particularly challenging to address in the typical hospital setting. Hospital rooms can be noisy and distracting, and busy hospital staff may de-prioritize infants who are not acutely ill. Weight trends are better followed over weeks than days, which makes a primarily hospital-based evaluation problematic. In order to facilitate a productive hospital stay, it is preferable for the patient to stay in a private room with the primary caregiver. Typical hospital interruptions such as monitors and nighttime vital signs should be minimized as medically able based on the child's chronic health conditions. Goals for a hospitalization should include the identification and treatment of any underlying disease, establishing a feeding regimen that will deliver adequate calories, and educating parents about appropriate feeding techniques. Long-term weight monitoring should largely be undertaken in the outpatient setting.

KEY POINTS

- Growth faltering is a descriptive term, describing a symptom complex without reference to etiology. Because of the tremendous variety of causes and circumstances, it is difficult to make meaningful general conclusions about how to evaluate and treat individual patients.
- A multidisciplinary approach involving nutritional and behavioral guidance combined with the selective use of diagnostic tests is usually most appropriate.
- For patients who demonstrate improved growth with nutritional support, careful ongoing monitoring of growth and development is critical, as these patients are at elevated risk of subsequent recurrences of impaired growth.

SUGGESTED READINGS

Calleo V, Surujdeo R, et al. Emergency department management of patients with failure to thrive. *Pediatr Emerg Med Pract*. 2020;17(3):1-12.

Cole SZ, Lanham JS. Failure to thrive: an update. *Am Fam Physician*. 2011;83(7):829-834.

Franceschi R, Rizzardi C, et al. Failure to thrive in infant and toddlers: a practical flowchart-based approach in a hospital setting. *Ital J Pediatr*. 2021;47(62):1-8.

Krugman SD, Dubowitz H. Failure to thrive. *Am Fam Physician*. 2003;68(5):879-884.

Larson-Nath C, Biank V. Clinical review of failure to thrive in pediatric patients. *Pediatr Ann*. 2016;45(2):e46-e49.

Puls H, Hall M, et al. Failure to thrive hospitalizations and risk factors for readmission to children's hospitals. *Hosp Pediatr*. 2016;6(8):468-475.

Puls H, Plencner L, et al. The diagnostic accuracy of in-hospital weight gain for differentiating neglect from other failure to thrive etiologies. *Hosp Pediatr*. 2018, 8(10): 620-627.

Robago J, Marra K, et al. The clinical geneticist and the evaluation of failure to thrive versus failure to feed. *Am J Med Genet*. 2015;169:337-348.

Rudolph CD, Link DT. Feeding disorders in infants and children. *Pediatr Clin North Am*. 2002;49:97-112.

Scholler, I, Nittur, S. Understanding failure to thrive. *Paediatr Child Health*. 2012;22(10):438-442.

Schwartz D. Failure to thrive: an old nemesis in the new millennium. *Pediatr Rev*. 2000;21:257.

Shields, B, Wacogne, I, Wright, CM. Weight faltering and failure to thrive in infancy and early childhood. *BMJ*. 2012;345:e5931.

Tang A, Adolphe S, Rogers S, Frank D. Failure to thrive or growth faltering: medical, developmental/behavioral, nutritional and social dimensions. *Pediatr Rev*. 2011;42(11):591-603.

CHAPTER 24 Fever

Mayssa Abuali, MD and Anika Kumar, MD

BACKGROUND

Fever is an increase in body temperature, outside of the normal diurnal variation that is regulated by the hypothalamus in response to endogenous pyrogens.

The epidemiology of infection as a cause of fever has significantly changed with routine vaccination against pneumococcal and Haemophilus influenzae Type b disease. Viral infections remain the most common cause of fever in children. Occult bacteremia is now rare, and gram-negative bacteria (*Escherichia coli* in particular) have emerged as the leading cause of bacterial illness (urinary tract infections [UTI]) in febrile children.

PATHOPHYSIOLOGY

Normal diurnal variation results in body temperatures that are lowest in the early morning and highest in the late afternoon/early evening. In young infants, body temperature may fluctuate during activity and feeding. Fever requires a change in the thermal setpoint that is first triggered by endogenous pyrogens which include cytokines, mainly tumor necrosis factor-α (TNF-α), interleukins 1 and 6, and interferons β and γ. The activation of the cyclooxgenase (COX) pathway then produces prostaglandin E2 (PGE_2) which crosses the blood-brain barrier to alter the thermosensitive neurons. Fever is then generated through vasoconstriction and muscle contraction. During an infection, endotoxins and exotoxins trigger the release of endogenous pyrogens which trigger the fever cascade. Fever in turn stimulates the immune system through enhanced leukocytosis, phagocytosis, and inhibition of viral and bacterial replication.

Temperature is physiologically controlled so that it rarely exceeds 41°C (105.8°F). Temperatures at 41°C or above may indicate a severe bacterial infection or a noninfectious source such as hyperthermia or drug fever. Temperatures above 42°C (107.6°F) may be lethal. Hyperthermia, unlike fever, is not regulated by the hypothalamic setpoint. Most cases of hyperthermia in children are due to environmental exposure with heatstroke leading to core temperatures ≥ 40°C and central nervous system dysfunction.

Heat production exceeding heat loss is another mechanism that leads to an elevated temperature, which occurs, for example, in the setting of malignant hyperthermia and salicylate poisoning. Defective heat loss can occur with exposure to severe heat or inability to dissipate heat, as seen in ectodermal dysplasia. Elevated temperatures due to these mechanisms are often referred to as fever, though the more accurate description is hyperthermia (see Definitions, below). "Central fever" may occur due to hypothalamic injury.

The diagnosis of fever is based on the measurement of core body temperature. Normal diurnal variations in temperature for an individual and normal differences in baseline temperature between individuals may be as much as 1.1°C (2°F), but the generally accepted gold standard normal temperature is 37°C (98.6°F). Most clinicians consider any temperature above 38°C (100.4°F) to be a fever, especially in the immediate neonatal period. Beyond the first 2 to 3 months of life, a temperature greater than 38.3°C (101°F) is often used as the cutoff for fever, although many consider a temperature of 39°C (102.2°F) or higher the threshold that triggers an evaluation for a serious bacterial illness. The most accurate method of obtaining core body temperature is by a rectal thermometer. Oral temperatures are also considered accurate, although may result in readings that are lower than rectal by about 0.5°C. Axillary temperatures are typically 0.5°C to 1°C lower than rectal temperatures and may be considered abnormal if above 37.5°C. Tympanic and infrared temperature readings taken at home are less accurate but should be considered when taking a history.

DEFINITIONS

Fever: Elevation of body temperature that occurs as part of a specific physiologic response that is mediated and controlled by the central nervous system by increasing the hypothalamic set point. Fever does not cause brain damage. It is uncommon for temperature to exceed 41°C (105.8°F) without some element of concomitant hyperthermia.

Hyperthermia: Abnormal elevation of body temperature that occurs without a change in the thermoregulatory set point in the hypothalamus. This failure of normal homeostasis results in heat production that exceeds the body's capacity for dissipation. Can be rapidly fatal; adverse physiologic effects begin to occur at temperatures >41°C (105.8°F).

PATIENT HISTORY

A detailed and targeted history provides the most important clues in determining the cause of fever, which can range from self-limited conditions to life-threatening illness. A careful history functions to narrow the differential diagnosis, thus helping the clinician avoid overtesting. Important historical clues include the duration and pattern of fever, and associated symptoms such as rash. While children with UTIs may not present with localizing exam findings, dysuria or other urinary symptoms may be

TABLE 24-1 Patterns of Fever

Fever Type	Description
Intermittent	Exaggerated circadian rhythm that includes normal temperatures on most days
Septic	Wide fluctuation in temperatures
Sustained	Persistent fever that does not fluctuate by more than 0.5°C in 24 hours
Remittent	Persistent fever that varies by more than 0.5°C in 24 hours (e.g., tuberculosis, viral fever, many bacterial infections)
Relapsing	Febrile periods separated by intervals of normal temperature (e.g., *Borrelia* infection, syphilis, histoplasmosis, Behcet disease, systemic lupus erythematosus)
Biphasic	Illness with two distinct periods of fever over ≥1 week (e.g., poliomyelitis, enteroviral infections)
Periodic	Recurring illnesses with some periodicity (e.g., cyclic neutropenia, Periodic fever aphthous stomatitis pharyngitis adenopathy [PFAPA], familial Mediterranean fever)
Double Quotidian	Fever that peaks twice in 24 hours (classically associated with inflammatory arthritis)
Tertian	Fever that occurs on the first and third days (malaria caused by *Plasmodium vivax*)
Quartan	Fever that occurs on the first and fourth days (malaria caused by *Plasmodium malariae*)

elicited. Other important questions include exact temperature reading and mode the temperature was obtained (tactile vs. thermometer), the last timing of an antipyretic dose, along with travel, animal exposure, tick or mosquito bite history, and swimming history with location (freshwater etc.). Certain historical features are unique to specific underlying infectious diseases such as anosmia and dyguesia seen with SARS-CoV-2 infection.

Viral infections typically are associated with a slow decline in fever over a week, whereas uncomplicated bacterial infections are associated with prompt resolution of fever within 24 to 48 hours of effective antibiotic administration. **Table 24-1** describes common fever patterns and the associated diseases. Since the fever pattern is so important, a home fever diary is an extremely valuable tool when evaluating a patient with prolonged fever. The past medical history of a patient with fever should include immunization status, history of immunodeficiencies, previous major illnesses, recent hospitalizations, and presence of hardware or recent dental work. Additional information that is important to elucidate are sick contacts, daycare or school attendance, medications currently used (including prescriptions, over-the-counter medications, and alternative remedies), and any family history of recurrent fever syndromes.

PHYSICAL EXAMINATION

A thorough physical examination is crucial to determining the etiology of fever. The general appearance of the patient must be assessed (i.e., does the patient appear toxic or well?) in addition to a complete examination with attention to possible signs of infection (pain, erythema, swelling, tenderness). The skin should be closely examined, as rashes with fever may be diagnostic (e.g., erythema migrans in Lyme, involvement of palms and soles with Rocky Mountain Spotted fever or Hand Foot Mouth disease). A full lymph node examination should also be performed as many infectious diseases (e.g., Ebstein Barr virus, cytomegalovirus, and Bartonella) present with characteristic lymphadenopathy, and certain rheumatic conditions (e.g., Kawasaki disease) may present with lymphadenopathy as a presenting symptom. An examination of the joints for arthritis may point to a rheumatological disorder or an infectious source (e.g., Lyme or septic arthritis). Warning signs of serious bacterial infection may include tachycardia, petechial/purpuric rash, bloody diarrhea, nuchal rigidity/meningismus, bulging fontanelle, tachypnea/respiratory distress, mucocutanenous findings, or cardiac dysfunction (e.g., Multisystem Inflammatory Syndrome in Children [MIS-C]).

A complete set of vital signs including pulse oximetry is necessary for evaluation of a febrile child. The relationship between the patient's pulse rate and fever may also aid diagnosis. It is normal for a fever to raise the heart rate by 10 beats/min for each 1°C degree rise in temperature, but relative tachycardia, in which the pulse rate is elevated out of proportion to temperature, is suggestive of a noninfectious process or an infectious toxin-mediated illness. Relative bradycardia, when the pulse rate is low despite the temperature elevation, suggests typhoid fever, brucellosis, or leptospirosis.

When a patient has a fever greater than 41°C, noninfectious conditions should be considered, including central fever resulting from central nervous system dysfunction, drug fever, cocaine or methylenedioxymethamphetamine ingestion, serotonin syndrome, malignant neuroleptic syndrome, heatstroke, and malignant hyperthermia.

DIFFERENTIAL DIAGNOSIS

The differential diagnosis of fever is broad and generally falls into one of four categories: infectious disease, rheumatic disease, malignancy, or miscellaneous (drug reaction, heat disorders, etc.). A complete history and physical provides essential information needed to narrow the differential diagnoses being considered for each patient and identify if further workup is necessary. For example, a post-operative patient may develop fever from a number of causes, most commonly including atelectasis, deep vein thrombosis, wound infection, and bacteremia. Patients who have had urinary bladder catheters in place are at increased risk for developing a UTI. Further, any procedure involving the surgical placement of a device such as a catheter, shunt, rod, or other hardware carries a risk of infection (see Chapter 103).

DIAGNOSTIC EVALUATION

The evaluation of fever is often dependent upon the specific characteristics and circumstances of the child presenting with fever. Most febrile episodes in a normal host can be diagnosed by a thorough history and physical exam requiring few, if any, laboratory, or radiographic tests. However, in children with fever and no apparent source, additional testing may be warranted on a case-by-case basis. Chapter 91 discusses fever in infants and toddlers, and Chapter 92 discusses illnesses associated with prolonged fever and fever of unknown origin. Fever in an immunocompromised host is discussed in Chapter 105. Elevations in body temperature that occur without an inflammatory trigger, as seen in heat disorders, are discussed in Chapter 174.

MANAGEMENT

Management should focus on treating the underlying cause of the fever or condition that incited the increased cytokine production. Fever due to specific underlying etiologies resolves with appropriate treatment of the disease. Examples include administration of antibiotics for bacterial infections or administration of intravenous immunoglobulin to treat Kawasaki disease.

Antipyresis for decreasing the elevated temperature is controversial among clinicians, scientists, caregivers, and patients. Many caregivers believe that fever is a disease (rather than a symptom) or that fever itself may have life-threatening effects. There is no evidence that children with fever as a result of endogenous and exogenous pyrogens are at increased risk of adverse outcomes such as brain damage. There is some evidence that the same pyrogenic cytokines responsible for fever have potentially detrimental effects, including increased oxygen consumption, carbon dioxide production, and cardiac output, all of which can worsen the condition of children in shock or with chronic diseases such as cardiac insufficiency, pulmonary insufficiency, sickle cell anemia, diabetes mellitus, or inborn errors of metabolism. The drawbacks to treating fever include the concerns that lowering a fever may impair the body's ability to fight off infection, remove important diagnostic clues regarding the pattern of fever, and interfere with the interpretation of the response to therapy for the inciting condition. The benefits of fever reduction include patient comfort, improved oral intake, decreased insensible fluid loss, and improved ability to assess the patient's demeanor. However, a fever's response to antipyretics is not diagnostic and does not provide information about its cause. Of note, there is no evidence that antipyretic therapy decreases the recurrence of febrile seizures.

International recommendations for fever management are based on the patient's level of distress or discomfort and not degree of temperature. For most healthy children with temperatures <39°C (101.2°F), therapeutic antipyresis is not required. However, as temperatures become higher, children may become more uncomfortable.

Most parents expect their children to be treated for fever. The consensus amongst international guidelines is for clinicians to counsel families to assess the child's sleep cycle, appetite, motor activity, mood, and overall appearance when deciding to treat fever. Families should also be counseled that providing symptomatic relief does not change the course of the underlying disease. It is important that the goals of treating fever are discussed with families, emphasizing the therapeutic endpoints for maximizing the child's comfort and fluid intake rather than focusing on achieving normothermia. Families should be counseled to observe for signs of serious illness and discouraged from focusing on the fever alone.

Fever is most commonly treated pharmacologically. PGE_2, which is central to the production of fever, is synthesized from arachidonic acid, mediated by the COX enzyme. There are two isoforms of the enzyme, COX-1 and COX-2. COX-1 is expressed throughout the body constitutively and is thought to be important in maintaining homeostasis. COX-2 is inducible by several pyrogenic cytokines and is thought to be the key mediator of PGE_2 during febrile and inflammatory responses.

Acetaminophen and ibuprofen are the two most commonly used antipyretic medications in pediatrics. Despite its worldwide popularity, acetaminophen's mechanism of action is not completely understood. It is a weak inhibitor of COX, but its effect may be based on tissue-specific COX inhibitors. Acetaminophen penetrates the blood-brain barrier and causes a fall in central nervous system PGE_2 production. Thus, acetaminophen has good systemic antipyretic activity with weak local anti-inflammatory effects. Nonsteroidal anti-inflammatory drugs (NSAIDs), such as ibuprofen, interfere with prostaglandin production through non-selective COX inhibition and downregulation of the expression of COX enzymes. As a result, NSAIDs have both antipyretic and anti-inflammatory effects.

Acetaminophen (10-15 mg/kg every 4-6 hours) and/or ibuprofen (10 mg/kg every 6 hours in children over 6 months of age) are the mainstays of treatment. Aspirin should not be used due to the risk of Reye syndrome. Tepid sponge baths are not recommended to reduce fever because data have shown that they are no more effective than antipyretics alone and significantly increase patient discomfort scores. Alcohol baths are also discouraged because there have been reported adverse events associated with systemic absorption of alcohol.

Some clinicians recommend using acetaminophen and ibuprofen in an alternating or combined fashion. While there are some studies that show lower temperatures, lower stress scores, and less time missed from childcare in the combination treatment groups versus single-agent treatment groups, questions remain regarding the safety of this practice due to potential dosing confusion and whether it improves the comfort of the child. Regardless of whether a single medication or alternating antipyretics are used, caregivers should be counseled on proper formulation, weight-based dosing, dosing intervals, and safe storage of these medications. Children should not receive cough and cold medications at the same time as antipyretics because there are often additional antipyretic medications in the cough and cold formulations. Families do not need to wake children for the purpose of administering antipyretic medications. It is often helpful for families, especially those with multiple caregivers, to keep a medication log to include the type of antipyretic, dose, and time given to avoid inadvertent overdosing.

KEY POINTS

- Fever is a common presenting complaint prompting medical evaluation in children.
- Fever is a sign of an underlying pathology, not a disease itself.
- History and physical examination play an important role in determining diagnostic evaluation and management options.
- The differential diagnosis of fever is broad and generally falls into one of four categories: infectious disease, rheumatic disease, malignancy, or miscellaneous.
- Antipyresis using COX inhibition is the mainstay of treatment.
- The goal of treatment is patient comfort, not normothermia.
- Fever due to specific underlying etiologies resolves with the appropriate treatment of the disease.

SUGGESTED READINGS

Barbi E, Marzuillo P, Neri E, Naviglio S, Krauss BS. Fever in children: pearls and pitfalls. *Children (Basel)*. 2017;4(9):81.

Cioffredi LA, Jhaveri R. Evaluation and management of febrile children: a review. *JAMA Pediatr*. 2016;170(8):794-800.

Doria M, Careddu D, Ceschin F, et al. Understanding discomfort in order to appropriately treat fever. *Int J Environ Res Public Health*. 2019; 16(22):4487.

Grom AA. Fever and the Inflammatory Response. In Long S, Pickering LK, Prober CG, ed. *Principles and Practice of Pediatric Infectious Diseases*. 4th ed. Churchill Livingstone; 2012:91-95.

Hashimoto R, Suto M, Tsuji M, et al. Use of antipyretics for preventing febrile seizure recurrence in children: a systematic review and meta-analysis. *Eur J Pediatr*. 2021;180(4):987-997.

Kumar V, Abbas AK, Aster JC, eds. *Inflammation and Repair. In Robbins & Cotran Pathologic Basis of Disease*. 10th ed. Elsevier Health Sciences; 2021.

Nield LS, Kamat D. Fever. In: Kliegman R, Stanton B, St Gemell J, Schor N, eds. *Nelson Textbook of Pediatrics*. 20th ed. Elsevier Health Sciences; 2016.

Section on Clinical Pharmacology and Therapeutics, Committee on Drugs, Sullivan JE, Farrar HC. Fever and antipyretic use in children. *Pediatrics*. 2011;127(3):580-587.

CHAPTER 25

Gastrointestinal Bleeding

April Buchanan, MD

BACKGROUND

Gastrointestinal (GI) bleeding produces alarm and anxiety in parents and physicians. Most causes of GI bleeding do not result in significant blood loss, and many cases of GI bleeding cease spontaneously. Larger volume bleeding can lead to hemodynamic compromise that requires aggressive resuscitation and intervention. Thus, a systematic approach to diagnosis is required.

DEFINITIONS

Hematemesis: Vomiting of either fresh or altered blood (such as coffee grounds emesis). Implies recent or continuing bleeding proximal to the ligament of Treitz.

Hematochezia: Bright red blood per rectum or maroon-colored stools. Usually originates in the colon. Upper GI hemorrhage can also present with hematochezia secondary to decreased transit time in infants or with brisk bleeding. Blood-streaked stools suggest a bleeding source in the rectum or anal canal.

Melena: Dark or black, tarry stools with a characteristic odor. Indicative of blood that has been in the GI tract for a long time, allowing the denaturation of hemoglobin by bowel flora. Melenic stools are typically from a hemorrhage originating proximal to the ileocecal valve.

Occult blood: Presence of blood in the stool that is not visible but is confirmed by chemical testing (i.e., guaiac)

PATIENT HISTORY

The history can be helpful in identifying the cause and location of bleeding in the GI tract (**Table 25-1**). Quantifying the volume and acuity of blood loss is important in understanding the risk of hemodynamic compromise. The character of the blood may indicate a more likely location of bleeding, with bright red blood usually from the colon and rectum, though brisk bleeding from an upper GI source can cause hematochezia. Fever, recent travel, or known sick contacts may implicate an infectious

TABLE 25-1 Focused History
Characteristics of Bleeding
Quantity: volume of blood (few drops vs. a cup)
Duration: intermittent bleeding, isolated episode, ongoing bleeding
Character: bright red blood, coffee grounds emesis, melena, hematochezia
Abdominal Complaints
Bowel patterns: diarrhea (infectious) or constipation (fissures), change in stool color
Abdominal pain: indicates inflammation or ischemia of bowel wall
Painless bleeding: indicates Meckel diverticulum, duplication, vascular malformation, or polyps
Abdominal distention: possible bowel obstruction
Tenesmus or urgency to defecate: consider IBD or infectious colitis
Dietary History
Cow milk or soy formula: consider allergic colitis
Breastfeeding: consider ingested maternal blood
Ingestion of products mistaken for hematemesis: artificial food coloring, gelatin, artificial fruit drinks, certain antibiotics, and cough syrups
Ingestion of products mistaken for melena: beets, iron supplements, dark chocolate, bismuth, spinach, blueberries, grapes, licorice, others
Review of Systems
General: fever, weight loss or gain, anorexia
Skin: rash, vascular malformations, edema, jaundice, lymphadenopathy, easy bruising
Extremities: arthralgia, arthritis, clubbing
Genitourinary: hematuria
Abdomen: distention, pain, bowel patterns, vomiting
Ears, nose, and throat: pharyngitis, epistaxis
Past Medical History
Previous GI bleeding
Liver disease: indicates possible variceal bleeding or coagulopathy
Previous or recent hospitalization: stress gastritis
Medications or ingestions: NSAIDs, aspirin, steroids, anticoagulants, alcohol, toxins (rat poison)
Umbilical artery catheterization: risk for portal vein thrombosis
Coagulopathy
Recent antibiotic exposure: pseudomembranous colitis
Presence of gastrostomy or nasogastric tube
Family History
IBD, peptic ulcer disease, polyposis, bleeding diatheses
Social History
Immediate contacts with similar symptoms: may indicate infectious cause
Travel, camping, or daycare: consider infectious causes

GI, gastrointestinal; IBD, inflammatory bowel disease; NSAID, nonsteroidal anti-inflammatory drug.

source, while longer-standing symptoms and associated weight loss may indicate a more serious underlying cause such as inflammatory bowel disease (IBD). A complete medication history is essential, including recent use of nonsteroidal anti-inflammatory drugs (NSAIDs) or antibiotics. Certain foods or medications can also cause a red discoloration of GI fluids and be mistaken for hematemesis or melena.

PHYSICAL EXAMINATION

The physical examination can be helpful in determining the etiology of GI bleeding (**Table 25-2**). The first priority is a quick assessment to identify patients with hemodynamic compromise or shock who need immediate resuscitation. Vital signs should be monitored closely. Patients may lose up to 15% of blood volume without evidence of hemodynamic compromise, and the blood pressure may be maintained until the patient has lost as much as 30% of the blood volume. Once the patient is determined to be stable, a comprehensive history and physical examination should be pursued.

TABLE 25-2 Directed Physical Examination Findings and Associated Diseases
Vital Signs
Fever: infectious causes or inflammatory diseases (IBD or IgA vasculitis)
Weight loss: chronic diseases (IBD, cystic fibrosis, liver disease)
Tachypnea: hemodynamic compromise or acidosis
Tachycardia: earliest sign of hemodynamic compromise
Hypotension: present with significant blood volume loss
General
Distressed or toxic-appearing patient: hemodynamic compromise from significant hemorrhage or underlying process causing systemic illness (toxic colitis, intussusception, ischemic bowel, necrotizing enterocolitis)
Well-appearing patient: less urgent causes of bleeding
Failure to thrive: malnutrition from chronic diseases (IBD, cystic fibrosis, liver disease)
Head, Eyes, Ears, Nose, and Throat
Nose: evidence of epistaxis
Eyes: scleral icterus (liver disease), iritis (IBD)
Oropharyngeal: mucosal trauma or bleeding from posterior pharynx
Cardiovascular
Evidence of hemodynamic compromise: tachycardia, gallop rhythm, delayed capillary refill, poor perfusion
Abdominal
Abdominal tenderness: nonspecific but indicates inflammation or ischemic injury of the bowel
Abdominal mass: intussusception, intestinal duplication may result in right lower quadrant masses
Evidence of portal hypertension: hepatosplenomegaly, ascites
Rectal examination: stool specimen for hemoccult testing, palpable polyp
Perineal and anal inspection: skin tags (IBD), fissures, superficial skin breakdown or inflammation (streptococcal cellulitis)
Extremities
Clubbing: chronic diseases (cystic fibrosis, IBD, liver disease)
Arthritis: IBD
Skin
Vascular malformations: syndromes with associated GI vascular malformations (e.g., Klippel-Trénaunay syndrome, Rendu-Osler-Weber syndrome)
Cutaneous or oral pigmentation: Peutz-Jeghers syndrome
Purpura or petechiae: IgA vasculitis or bleeding diathesis
Erythema nodosum: IBD

GI, gastrointestinal; IBD inflammatory bowel disease.

DIFFERENTIAL DIAGNOSIS

The differential diagnosis of GI hemorrhage can be divided into upper and lower GI bleeding. Although certain causes are more likely in certain ages, there is considerable overlap between age groups. Patients with complex medical issues have special diagnostic considerations in the evaluation of GI bleeding. The causes of upper and lower GI bleeding are summarized in **Tables 25-3** and **25-4**, respectively.

UPPER GASTROINTESTINAL BLEEDING

Some causes of upper GI bleeding are unique to neonates and young infants. Swallowed maternal blood from the birth process or from breastfeeding may cause hematemesis. To differentiate between maternal and fetal blood, an Apt test may be performed. Adult hemoglobin is reduced to a brown-yellow color, whereas fetal hemoglobin is resistant to reduction and remains pink.

Esophagitis can lead to upper GI bleeding and may manifest with symptoms of dysphagia, regurgitation, cough, arching, or growth faltering. It may be acid related, traumatic, infectious, associated with a caustic ingestion, or allergic, as in the case of eosinophilic esophagitis.

TABLE 25-3 Causes of Upper Gastrointestinal Bleeding

Neonates and Young Infants	Older Infants, Children, and Adolescents
Ingested maternal blood	Gastritis/ gastroduodenal ulceration
At delivery	Sepsis
During breastfeeding	Stress
Milk protein allergy	Medications
Trauma (nasogastric tube)	Ingestion
Gastritis	Burns
Overwhelming illness	Increased ICP±
Medications	Ischemia
Idiopathic	Acidosis
Ischemia	*Helicobacter pylori**
Acidosis	Esophagitis
Esophagitis	Reflux
Reflux	Infectious
Infectious	Ingestion
	Eosinophilic
Necrotizing enterocolitis	Esophageal foreign body
Coagulopathy	Gastroesophageal varices
Congenital malformations	Cirrhosis
Duplication cyst	Extrahepatic portal vein thrombosis†
Vascular malformation	Budd-Chiari syndrome
	Nasopharyngeal bleeding source
	Epistaxis
	Tonsils
	Tooth extraction
	Coagulopathy
	Hemobilia
	Hepatic injury
	Trauma to intestinal mucosa
	Nasogastric tube
	Gastrostomy tube
	Mallory-Weiss tear
	Prolapse gastropathy
	Vascular anomalies†
	Hemangioma
	Dieulafoy lesion
	Telangiectasia
	Other
	IgA vasculitis
	Crohn disease
	Pulmonary hemorrhage
	Congenital malformations†
	Duplication cyst

*More common in older children and adolescents.

†More common in infants and young children.

±ICP, intracranial pressure.

TABLE 25-4 Causes of Lower Gastrointestinal Bleeding

Neonates and Infants	Young Children	Older Children and Adolescents
Necrotizing enterocolitis	Anal fissure	inflammatory bowel disease
Anal fissure	Intussusception	Vasculitis
Allergic colitis	Juvenile polyps (>4 y)	IgA vasculitis
Milk protein	Vascular lesions	Juvenile or inflammatory polyps
Soy protein	Hirschsprung enterocolitis	Colonic or rectal varices
Swallowed maternal blood	Intestinal duplication	Hemorrhoids
Meckel diverticulum	Infectious enterocolitis	Anal or rectal fissure
Hirschsprung enterocolitis	Inflammatory bowel disease (>4 y)	Infectious enterocolitis
Infectious enterocolitis	Meckel's diverticulum	Colonic or rectal ulceration
Malrotation or volvulus	Perianal streptococcal cellulitis	Bleeding diathesis
Intestinal duplication	IgA Vasculitis	Eosinophilic gastroenteropathy
Bleeding diathesis	Hemolytic uremic syndrome	Rectal trauma
	Typhlitis*	Typhlitis*
	Eosinophilic gastroenteropathy	
	Bleeding diathesis	
	Colonic or rectal varices	
	Lymphoid nodular hyperplasia	
	Colonic or rectal ulceration	
	Rectal trauma	

*Immunocompromised patients.

Children with neuromuscular diseases are more prone to severe gastroesophageal reflux disease that leads to esophagitis.

Esophageal varices can cause sudden, massive hematemesis, which can lead to hemodynamic compromise. Varices are associated with portal hypertension from both intrahepatic and extrahepatic causes. Portal vein thrombosis may be associated with umbilical artery catheterization or omphalitis, but it usually occurs in young, previously healthy children, and the cause is not identified. Thrombosis of the hepatic veins (Budd-Chiari syndrome) is usually associated with hypercoagulable states. Portal hypertension is most commonly caused by cirrhosis associated with chronic biliary diseases such as biliary atresia, cystic fibrosis, sclerosing cholangitis, and parenteral nutrition-induced cholestasis. Endoscopic evaluation of patients with known cirrhosis and esophageal varices is important, because the source of bleeding is commonly from gastric and duodenal ulcerations rather than varices. Patients with liver failure may develop GI bleeding from other mechanisms, such as associated coagulopathy.

Forceful vomiting or retching may lead to a Mallory-Weiss tear or cause prolapse gastropathy, a phenomenon in which the gastric fundus is prolapsed into the esophagus, resulting in injury to the mucosa. Trauma to the esophageal or gastric mucosa may occur with nasopharyngeal suctioning or from nasogastric or gastrostomy tubes, which can lead to local irritation or laceration.

Gastritis may be induced by many commonly used medications, including NSAIDs and steroids. *Helicobacter pylori* may cause gastritis and subsequent ulceration in children. Stress gastritis can occur in any age group and may be a complication of an overwhelming or life-threatening illness. Gastric or duodenal ulceration may also accompany head trauma, increased intracranial pressure (Cushing ulcer), or significant burns (Curling ulcer).

LOWER GASTROINTESTINAL BLEEDING

Similar to upper GI bleeding, neonates and young infants have some unique causes of lower GI bleeding. In premature or young infants, necrotizing enterocolitis is a significant cause of morbidity and mortality and is an important diagnosis to exclude when evaluating hematochezia. Necrotizing enterocolitis typically presents with bloody stools, vomiting, abdominal distention, temperature instability, and discoloration or erythema of the abdominal wall. Volvulus is another diagnostic consideration when evaluating lower GI bleeding in neonates and infants. Volvulus leads to ischemic injury of the bowel and can cause active bleeding;

it is a surgical emergency. Hirschsprung colitis may also cause severe illness in young infants. A more common cause of bloody stools in well-appearing infants is allergic colitis, which is usually due to cow milk protein allergy or soy protein intolerance.

Infectious enterocolitis can lead to bloody stools in infants and children. The classic pathogens include *Salmonella, Shigella, Yersinia, Escherichia coli* (enteroinvasive or enterohemorrhagic), *Campylobacter jejuni*, and *Entamoeba histolytica*. Viral pathogens such as rotavirus, Norwalk virus, and adenovirus 40/41 can also cause bloody stools. Antibiotic therapy puts patients at risk for the development of *Clostridium difficile* colitis; this should be considered in any patient who develops bloody stools with a history of recent antibiotic exposure.

Meckel diverticulum is a remnant of the omphalomesenteric duct that can present with painless rectal bleeding. The rule of twos applies to Meckel diverticulum: it occurs in approximately 2% of the population, is located within 2 feet of the ileocecal junction, is around 2 inches long and 2 cm in diameter, has two types of ectopic mucosa (gastric and pancreatic), and has a 2:1 male-to-female ratio. In addition, Meckel's presents before 2 years of age in 50% of patients. Bleeding is caused by ulceration of the ileal mucosa adjacent to the secretion-producing ectopic tissue. Duplications of the bowel may also contain ectopic mucosa and present with bleeding from a similar mechanism, or act as lead points for intussusception and subsequent ischemic injury.

Painless, intermittent rectal bleeding may be caused by juvenile polyps, which are non-neoplastic inflammatory lesions found in the rectosigmoid region of school-age children. Bleeding diatheses are another cause of painless rectal bleeding in any age group.

IgA vasculitis (formerly referred to as Henoch-Schoenlein Purpura) is a systemic vasculitis that affects primarily small vessels of the skin, joints, kidneys, and GI tract. The GI manifestations can precede the skin manifestations or occur days after. Bloody stools can result from diffuse mucosal hemorrhage or from intussusception resulting from IgA vasculitis. Rarely, IgA vasculitis may result in massive hemorrhage.

IBD is an important diagnostic consideration in older children and adolescents with hematochezia. Ulcerative colitis is a diffuse mucosal inflammation limited to the colon. In contrast, Crohn disease may occur in any segment of the GI tract. Both may present with bloody mucopurulent diarrhea, abdominal pain, and weight loss, as well as extraintestinal manifestations.

DIAGNOSTIC EVALUATION

LABORATORY STUDIES

Laboratory studies are directed at determining both the extent of blood loss and the underlying cause. An initial complete blood count should be followed by serial hemoglobin measurements to assess ongoing bleeding. Thrombocytopenia can be associated with multiple systemic illnesses that cause GI bleeding, such as necrotizing enterocolitis, sepsis, idiopathic thrombocytopenic purpura, and hypersplenism. Eosinophilia may be present in allergic colitis or parasitic infections (**Table 25-5**).

TABLE 25-5 Labs and Imaging/Studies to Be Considered in the Diagnostic Evaluation of GI Bleeding

Labs	Imaging/Studies
Apt or Downey test	Abdominal radiograph
CBC with differential and serial testing	Abdominal ultrasound
Coagulation studies	Meckel scan
Type and Cross	CT
Chemistries, including LFTs and ESR	Barium or air-contrast enema
Blood culture	Angiography
Hemoccult or gastroccult	Esophagogastroduodenoscopy (EGD)
Stool studies	Colonoscopy
	Upper GI
	Capsule endoscopy

Clotting studies should be performed to rule out a bleeding diathesis. Blood typing and cross-matching are necessary if there is any suggestion of profuse or ongoing bleeding or hemodynamic compromise. Routine chemistries, including renal and hepatic function, should be checked. Elevated blood urea nitrogen in the setting of a normal creatinine level may indicate a large amount of intraluminal blood in the small intestine with blood resorption. Azotemia may be present with hemolytic uremic syndrome or IgA vasculitis. Elevated liver transaminases or bilirubin may indicate hepatic failure or cirrhosis, raising the suspicion for varices. In an ill-appearing neonate with bloody stools, a blood culture should be obtained. Inflammatory markers such as the erythrocyte sedimentation rate and C-reactive protein may be elevated in inflammatory diseases such as IBD or IgA vasculitis. Infectious causes may also lead to increased inflammatory markers.

Red dyes, fruit juices, tomato skins, and beets can cause the vomitus or stool to look reddish in color. In addition, grapes, spinach, blueberries, licorice, and iron can cause the stool to look dark. A stool guaiac test uses a leukodye that has an oxidative reaction in the presence of hemoglobin, producing a blue color. False positives can occur in the presence of certain ingested foods such as rare meat, turnips, radishes, tomatoes, horseradish, cantaloupe, cauliflower, broccoli, grapes, and cherries. False negatives can occur due to the consumption of vitamin C. The Hemoccult test is accurate on stool but is inactivated by acid; therefore, gastric contents should be tested with the Gastroccult test. Stool studies should include fecal leukocytes, eosinophils, bacterial culture, ova and parasites, viral studies, and screening for *C. difficile* toxin A and B when appropriate.

IMAGING

Imaging may be an important in the workup of GI hemorrhage to define the pathology or pinpoint the bleeding site. Some centers may offer interventional options as well. A barium study can detect abnormalities associated with infectious esophagitis, esophageal varices, or an esophageal foreign body. An upper GI study may demonstrate abnormalities associated with profound reflux, obstructive causes such as malrotation with midgut volvulus, or gastric or duodenal ulcers. Plain abdominal radiographs are helpful in the evaluation of GI bleeding to assess for an obstructive bowel gas pattern, intraperitoneal free air, and pneumatosis coli in necrotizing enterocolitis or typhlitis. However, computed tomography is the preferred imaging modality to confirm the diagnosis of typhlitis in immunocompromised children. A barium enema can reveal mucosal abnormalities associated with IBD and can demonstrate polyps. Extraluminal complications of Crohn disease, such as adhesions or abscess formation, are better evaluated with computed tomography or magnetic resonance imaging. An air-contrast enema can be diagnostic and therapeutic for intussusception.

Nuclear medicine imaging using a tagged red blood cell scan can be helpful in pinpointing the location of bleeding. In one method, the patient's blood is drawn, labeled with a marker, and then reinjected. The images are evaluated in 5-minute frames for up to 2 hours to localize a bleeding source. Another valuable nuclear medicine technique is the Meckel scan, which is designed to demonstrate the presence of ectopic gastric mucosa within the diverticulum. Technetium 99m pertechnetate is injected intravenously and concentrates in gastric mucosa. Serial images are then obtained in 5-minute intervals to determine the presence of ectopic mucosa within a Meckel diverticulum. Capsule endoscopy can be beneficial for obscure sources of GI bleeding in the small intestine; however, sites can be missed if there is no active bleeding and the location may be difficult to pinpoint.

In specialized centers, angiography of the celiac or superior mesenteric artery can be performed in cases of brisk bleeding that cannot be diagnosed with other approaches. Arteriography may allow for transcatheter therapy with vasopressin or embolization.

MANAGEMENT

INITIAL STABILIZATION

Patients with GI bleeding who present with evidence of hemodynamic compromise should have circulation, airway, breathing assessed

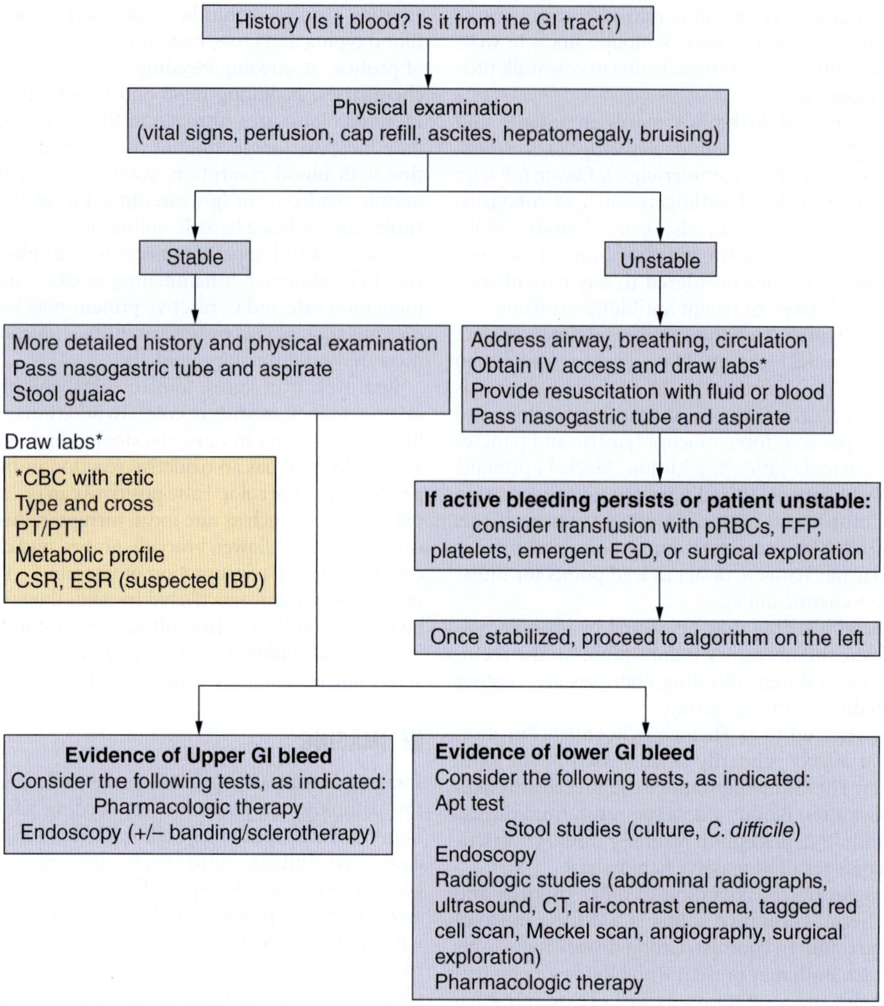

FIGURE 25-1. Diagnostic and treatment algorithm for GI bleeding.

(**Figure 25-1**). Once the airway and respiratory status are stabilized, the volume status should be addressed. Aggressive fluid resuscitation may be necessary, initially with crystalloid. Significant blood loss may require transfusion of blood products (red blood cells or fresh frozen plasma). In the case of any significant GI bleeding episode, a nasogastric tube should be placed and gastric lavage performed to assess for ongoing bleeding. Presence of blood in the nasogastric aspirate can confirm an ongoing upper GI bleed in patients with hematemesis or melena. The absence of blood in the nasogastric aspirate does not exclude upper GI bleeding from the postpyloric region in patients with hematochezia or melena with brisk bleeding. A gastroenterology consultation should be obtained for upper and/or lower endoscopy in cases of ongoing or severe bleeding or if a diagnosis cannot be established by other imaging modalities.

PHARMACOLOGIC THERAPY

Gastritis and peptic ulcer disease in children is effectively treated with H_2-antagonists and proton pump inhibitors. Early use of acid-suppressive medications in critically ill patients or those on high-dose steroids or anti-inflammatory medications may be prudent. *H. pylori* infection in children is treated similarly to that in adults, with antibiotics, acid suppression, and bismuth preparation.

C. difficile colitis requires antibiotic therapy. However, many bacterial pathogens causing bloody diarrhea do not require antibiotic treatment, and appropriate therapy should be reviewed on a case-by-case basis.

For esophageal varices, intravenous or intra-arterial continuous infusions of ocreotide or vasopressin may be administered. These therapies work by reducing splanchnic arterial blood flow, therefore reducing the amount of bleeding from the varices.

There are many pharmacologic therapies available for the management of IBD. Use of these medications should be guided by a gastroenterologist (see Chapter 76).

ENDOSCOPY

Upper GI endoscopy is the preferred procedure for the diagnosis and evaluation of acute, severe upper GI hemorrhage or persistent or recurrent upper GI bleeding. Endoscopy is sensitive and specific and may allow for immediate therapy. Endoscopic interventions are available for active bleeding ulcers and varices, and tissue specimens can be obtained by biopsy. Endoscopic sclerotherapy and elastic band therapy have been used successfully for esophageal varices in children.

Lower GI bleeding that is persistent or recurrent can also be effectively evaluated and possibly intervened upon by endoscopy. Flexible sigmoidoscopy is usually sufficient to evaluate for colitis and polyps. Colonoscopy reaching the level of the terminal ileum may be needed to evaluate more proximal lesions. Lower endoscopy is a valuable diagnostic modality to detect vascular lesions. Polyps can frequently be removed with electrocautery through an endoscope.

SURGERY

Surgical indications include bowel perforation, ischemic bowel from obstructive causes including irreducible intussusception, as well as ongoing or massive bleeding not amenable to control with endoscopy or interventional radiology. In cases of ulcerative colitis refractory to medical management, the disease can be cured with a total colectomy. Complications of Crohn disease, such as adhesions or fistula formation, may require surgical intervention. There are several surgical treatment options for portal hypertension and esophageal varices, including esophageal transection, portosystemic shunts, and transjugular intrahepatic portosystemic shunts, which are most often used in children with extrahepatic portal vein obstruction. Candidates for these procedures should be determined by consultation with a gastroenterologist and a surgeon.

SPECIAL CONSIDERATIONS

Immunocompromised patients may develop GI bleeding from some unique causes. They are at risk for esophagitis secondary to cytomegalovirus and fungi, as well as chemically induced mucositis from chemotherapeutic agents. Typhlitis is an important diagnostic consideration in immunocompromised patients with abdominal pain and lower GI bleeding. Immunocompromised patients with bloody diarrhea should be evaluated for opportunistic infections as well as cytomegalovirus colitis.

KEY POINTS

- GI bleeding can present from infancy through adolescence, and the differential diagnosis changes with age.
- The most important initial step is hemodynamic stabilization, followed by a thorough evaluation of the likely location and source of bleeding.
- Evaluation and treatment is guided by patient age, the acuity of the presentation, and presence or absence of continued bleeding.
- Treatment modalities include pharmacologic therapy, radiologic intervention, endoscopy, and surgical management.

SUGGESTED READINGS

Baker RD, Baker SD. Gastrointestinal bleeds. *Pediatr Rev.* 2021;42:546-557.

Karrer F, Narkewicz M. Esophageal varices: current management in children. *Semin Pediatr Surg.* 1999;8:193-201.

Lykavieris P, Gauthier F, Hadchouel P, et al. Risk of gastrointestinal bleeding during adolescence and early adulthood in children with portal vein obstruction. *J Pediatr.* 2000;136:805-808.

Liacouras CA, Piccoli DA, Bell LM, eds. *Pediatric Gastroenterology: The Requisites in Pediatrics.* Philadelphia, PA: Mosby; 2008:87-97.

Owensby S, Taylor K, Wilkins T. Diagnosis and management of upper gastrointestinal bleeding in children. *J Am Board Fam Med.* 2015;28 (1): 134-145.

Rodgers B. Upper gastrointestinal hemorrhage. *Pediatr Rev.* 1999;20: 171-174.

CHAPTER 26

Hypoglycemia

Julia R. Donner, MD and Erica Chung, MD

BACKGROUND

PATHOPHYSIOLOGY

Normal plasma glucose is maintained by the complex interaction of hormones that regulate the production and utilization of glucose. Glucose is produced from the breakdown of glycogen stores or from conversion of alternate substrates to glucose.

The clinical manifestations of hypoglycemia can be divided into two categories: those associated with activation of the autonomic nervous system and those associated with decreased glucose utilization by the brain. At blood glucose levels below 50 to 60 mg/dL, adrenergic symptoms including tachycardia, tremulousness, and weakness, and cholinergic symptoms including dizziness, nausea, and hunger are generally found. At blood glucose levels less than 50 mg/dL, neuroglycopenic symptoms, including lethargy, irritability, confusion, seizure, and coma can be seen. Recurrent episodes of hypoglycemia with plasma glucose less than 50 mg/dL may lead to severe neurologic outcomes including developmental delays, learning disabilities, and behavioral problems.

DEFINITION

The definition of hypoglycemia is controversial and dependent on various factors, including the age of the patient and the temporal relationship to meals. Clinical hypoglycemia has been defined as the blood glucose level at which autonomic symptoms appear. For purposes of this chapter, *hypoglycemia* is defined as blood glucose less than 50 mg/dL.

PATIENT HISTORY

The history in a hypoglycemic patient can provide important clues to the underlying cause of abnormal glucose homeostasis. First, it is critical to determine whether the hypoglycemia occurs during a fed or a fasting state. If the child develops hypoglycemia just after eating, the specific contents of the preceding meal may provide clues to the underlying problem. For example, children with galactosemia, hereditary fructose intolerance, or defects of organic acid metabolism may develop hypoglycemia shortly after consuming milk products, fructose, or protein, respectively. Inquiring about food aversions may be helpful, as many children learn to avoid foods that make them sick. Given the predictability of the processes that maintain plasma glucose based on duration of fast (**Table 26-1**), one can gain additional diagnostic clues based on the time since the previous meal. A notable increase in the typical duration of fasting occurs as infants consolidate their overnight sleep; infants may present with new-onset hypoglycemia during this transition period.

The child's past medical history should also be thoroughly explored. Birth history should be gathered, as being large for gestational age or having experienced perinatal stress suggests hyperinsulinemia. If prior episodes of hypoglycemia have occurred, it is important to determine the age of onset. Inborn errors of metabolism generally present within the first 2 years of life, whereas ketotic hypoglycemia, cortisol deficiency, and growth hormone deficiency generally present after 1 year of age. The possibility of past hypoglycemic episodes that were not diagnosed as such should also be considered; a history of unexplained seizures or recurrent respiratory infections (hyperventilation secondary to metabolic acidosis) may, in fact, represent episodes of hypoglycemia. Children who are hypoglycemic after an overnight fast may awaken irritable or lethargic or request juice upon awakening. A careful developmental history should be obtained, because recurrent or prolonged hypoglycemia may manifest as delayed acquisition of milestones.

The patient's family history may provide clues to a hereditary cause of hypoglycemia. A history of Reye syndrome, sudden infant death syndrome (or unexplained childhood death), and other family members with hypoglycemia may suggest an inborn error of metabolism.

Finally, a history of ingestions should also be considered, particularly in young children. Hypoglycemia can be secondary to the consumption of alcohol, oral hypoglycemic agents, β-adrenergic blockers, aspirin, or other substances.

TABLE 26-1 Primary Energy Source Relative to Duration of Fast

Duration of Fast (hour)	Primary Energy Source
0-2	Ingested food
2-6	Glycogen
6-12	Gluconeogenesis
12-24	Fatty acid oxidation

TABLE 26-2 Physical Findings in Disorders Associated With Hypoglycemia

Finding	Disorder
Short stature	Hypopituitarism, growth hormone deficiency, glycogen storage disorder
Tall stature	Beckwith-Wiedemann syndrome, Sotos Syndrome
Failure to thrive	Disorders of carbohydrate, organic acid, or amino acid metabolism, ACTH deficiency, primary adrenal insufficiency
Tachypnea	Inborn errors of metabolism
Midline facial defect	Hypopituitarism, growth hormone deficiency
Nystagmus	Hypopituitarism, growth hormone deficiency
Cryptorchidism, microphallus	Hypopituitarism, growth hormone deficiency
Hyperpigmentation	Adrenal insufficiency
Macrosomia, macroglossia, umbilical hernia	Beckwith-Wiedemann syndrome
Hepatomegaly	Glycogen storage disease, galactosemia, disorders of gluconeogenesis, fructose intolerance

PHYSICAL EXAMINATION

In addition to performing a thorough physical examination, clinicians should pay particular attention to specific physical findings that can provide diagnostic clues in children with hypoglycemia. **Table 26-2** highlights some of these physical findings.

DIFFERENTIAL DIAGNOSIS

Hypoglycemia can be caused by the body's inability to absorb or mobilize carbohydrates or convert alternative energy sources into glucose. Causes include accelerated glucose utilization, absent or abnormal hormone signaling, ingestions, or inadequate glucose stores. The most common cause of hypoglycemia in toddlers and young children without diabetes is idiopathic ketotic hypoglycemia. This is most often precipitated by viral illness. **Table 26-3** lists the differential diagnosis of hypoglycemia.

TABLE 26-3 Differential Diagnosis of Hypoglycemia

Disorders of carbohydrate metabolism
Glycogen storage diseases
Galactosemia
Pyruvate carboxylase deficiency
Phosphoenolpyruvate carboxykinase deficiency
Hereditary fructose intolerance
Liver failure
Disorders of amino acid metabolism
Maple syrup urine disease
Methylmalonic acidemia
Propionic acidemia
Glutaric aciduria
Tyrosinemia
Disorders of fat metabolism
Fatty acid oxidation defects
Carnitine deficiency
Hormone deficiencies
Growth hormone deficiency
Adrenocorticotropic hormone deficiency
Cortisol deficiency
Panhypopituitarism
Glucagon deficiency
Ingestions/Drugs
Ethanol
Salicylates
Quinine
Oral hypoglycemics
Exogenous insulin [diabetes, factitious hyperinsulinism]
β-Adrenergic blocking agents
Ackee fruit
Unripe lychee
Increased glucose utilization
Persistent hyperinsulinemic hypoglycemia of infancy
Beckwith-Wiedemann syndrome
Infection [Gastroenteritis, Sepsis, Malaria]
Burns
Hyperthyroidism
Malignancy
Inadequate glucose stores
Severe malnutrition
Prematurity
Miscellaneous
Idiopathic ketotic hypoglycemia
Dumping syndrome
Insulinoma
Liver failure

DIAGNOSTIC EVALUATION

Blood samples should be obtained prior to the administration of glucose if feasible and if the patient is stable. This critical sample should be sent for plasma glucose, free fatty acids, β-hydroxybutyrate, lactate, total and free carnitine, acylcarnitine, insulin, C-peptide, cortisol, and growth hormone (**Table 26-4**). Other blood tests to consider include electrolytes, liver function tests, ammonia, toxicology studies, and specific metabolic screens based on suspected diagnoses. The patient's first voided urine should also be sent for ketones and reducing substances. Other urine tests to consider include toxicology studies and organic acids.

If a critical sample was not obtained prior to administration of glucose, once the patient is medically stabilized, a controlled elective fast may be performed, and critical sample obtained when hypoglycemia is achieved. However, fatty acid oxidation disorders should be excluded first, as hypoglycemia in these disorders can provoke severe encephalopathy. Fasting should be timed such that the period of hypoglycemia is most likely to occur when symptoms can be observed (i.e., when patient is awake) and adequate staff is available for evaluation. The fast should be stopped if neurogenic symptoms appear.

In a normal host, hypoglycemia induces counterregulatory hormones to stimulate the production of alternative fuels, resulting in ketosis. When interpreting the data collected from a patient with hypoglycemia, the first step is to determine whether the patient has appropriately developed ketones. Patients who do not produce ketones in response to hypoglycemia are likely to have either hyperinsulinism (endogenous or exogenous) or a disorder of fatty acid oxidation. Appropriate ketosis, in contrast, suggests signal dysregulation or a disorder of carbohydrate or amino acid metabolism. An algorithm to guide the interpretation of laboratory data is provided in **Figure 26-1**.

When the evaluation points to a specific disease, confirmatory testing may be possible. For example, fructose tolerance tests can be performed if hereditary fructose intolerance is suspected, or DNA analysis can be done for disorders in which a gene mutation has been identified. In some patients, the cause of hypoglycemia may remain undiagnosed despite obtaining all the history, physical examination, and laboratory data noted above. In this setting, additional studies such as glucagon challenge testing or monitored fasting may prove useful. Finally, liver biopsy may be necessary to evaluate for hepatic enzyme deficiencies.

TABLE 26-4 Blood and Urine Tests Useful in the Evaluation of Hypoglycemia

Test	Test increased (↑) or decreased (↓)	Associated Diagnosis
Blood tests		
Insulin (plus C peptide)	↑	Hyperinsulinism, exogenous insulin overdose
C peptide	↑	Hyperinsulinism
	↓	Exogenous insulin overdose
Cortisol	↓	Cortisol deficiency, adrenal Insufficiency
ACTH	↑	Adrenal Insufficiency (primary)
	↓	Adrenal Insufficiency (secondary or central)
Growth hormone	↓	Growth hormone deficiency
Free fatty acids	↑	Fatty acid oxidation defect
β-hydroxybutyrate, acetoacetate	↓	Fatty acid oxidation defect
Amino acids (glycine)	↑	Organic acidemia
Lactate, pyruvate	↑	Glycogen storage disease, disorders of gluconeogenesis
Carnitine, acylcarnitine	↓	Fatty acid oxidation defect
Electrolytes (with calculated anion gap)	Electrolyte imbalances, can see elevated anion gap	Organic acidemia, maple syrup urine disease, glycogen storage disease, disorders of gluconeogenesis
Ammonia, Urea	↑	Organic acidemia, urea cycle defects
Toxicology screen (alcohol, salicylates)	↑	Ingestions
Venous blood gas	metabolic acidosis	Organic acidemia, maple syrup urine disease, glycogen storage disease, disorders of gluconeogenesis
Urine tests		
Ketones	↑	Fructose intolerance
	↓	Hyperinsulinism, fatty acid oxidation defect
Glucose, reducing substance	↑	Galactosemia, fructose intolerance
Organic acids	↑	Organic acidemia
Acylglycine	↑	Fatty acid oxidation defect

MANAGEMENT

The initial management of a hypoglycemic patient is to ensure the adequacy of the patient's circulation, airway and breathing, and to raise serum glucose levels. Treatment of symptomatic hypoglycemia should not be delayed; however, if possible, blood samples should be obtained prior to the administration of glucose. If the patient is conscious and can safely consume by mouth, then 15 grams (or 0.2 grams/kilogram for infants) of a fast-absorbing carbohydrate such as glucose tablets/gel, fruit juice, or table sugar may be administered enterally. Otherwise, an intravenous bolus of 10% dextrose at a dose of 0.2 grams/kilogram should be given. This should be followed by a 10% dextrose infusion to prevent recurrent hypoglycemia at a rate of 5 to 6 milligrams/kilogram/minute in infants or a 5% dextrose infusion at 2 to 3 milligrams/kilogram/minute in older children. The plasma glucose level should be monitored closely (initially every 15-20 minutes) and the dextrose infusion should be titrated accordingly (increasing in increments of 0.5 to 1 milligram/kilogram/minute) until the goal plasma glucose of 70 mg/dL or greater is achieved. When the goal plasma glucose level is reached, the frequency of the glucose checks can be spaced to hourly, and then

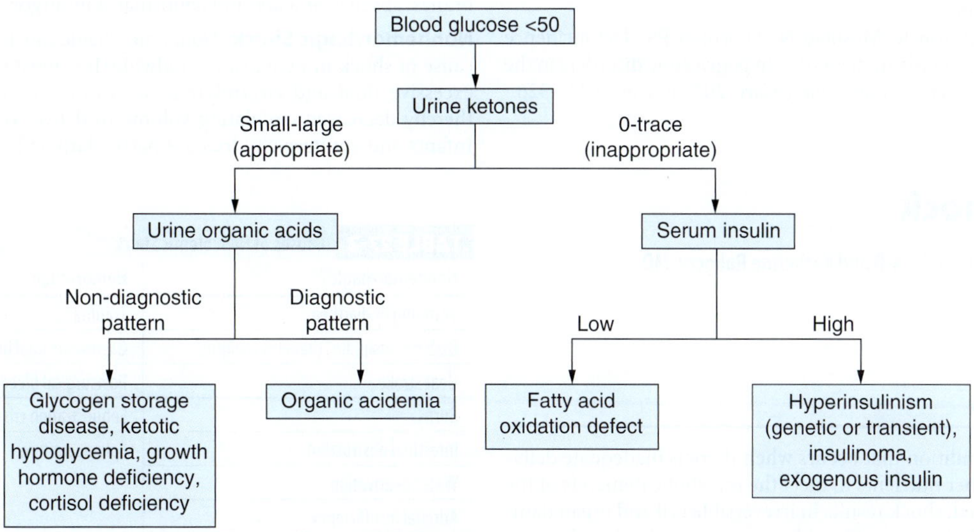

FIGURE 26-1. Algorithm for the interpretation of laboratory data in the evaluation of hypoglycemia.

to every 3 to 4 hours thereafter. If intravenous access or dextrose is not immediately available or mental state is altered, then intramuscular or subcutaneous glucagon can be administered. Glucagon can be expected to raise blood sugar within 10 to 15 minutes but is only effective in patients with insulin-mediated hypoglycemia.

Long-term treatment is driven by the final diagnosis and may include dietary therapy (i.e., avoidance of branched-chain amino acids in maple syrup urine disease), medical or surgical management of hyperinsulinism, or consumption of sustained-release forms of carbohydrates (corn starch) for patients with glycogen storage diseases.

KEY POINTS

- Normal plasma glucose is maintained by a complex interplay of hormones that regulate the production and utilization of glucose and is dependent on the ability to metabolize alternate sources of fuel in the fasting state.
- Recurrent hypoglycemia can cause devastating neurological consequences and must therefore be recognized and treated promptly.
- Treatment of symptomatic hypoglycemia should not be delayed; however, if possible, blood samples for diagnostic testing should be obtained prior to the administration of glucose.

SUGGESTED READINGS

Casertano A, Rossi A, Fecarotta S, et al. An overview of hypoglycemia in children including a comprehensive practical diagnostic flowchart for clinical use. *Front Endocrinol.* 2021;12:684011.

De Leon-Crutchlow DD, Lord K. Approach to hypoglycemia in infants and children. In: UpToDate, Wolfsdorf JI (ed). *UpToDate*, Waltham, MA. (Accessed on July 30, 2022)

Ghosh A, Banerjee I, Morris AAM. Recognition, assessment and management of hypoglycaemia in childhood. *Arch Dis Child.* 2016; 101(6):575-580.

Haymond MW, Sunehag A. Controlling the sugar bowl: regulation of glucose homeostasis in children. *Endocrinol Clin North Am.* 1999; 28:663.

Mayatepek E, Hoffmann B, Meissner T. Inborn errors of carbohydrate metabolism. *Best Pract Res Clin Gastroenterol.* 2010;24:607-618.

Straussman S, Levitsky LL. Neonatal hypoglycemia. *Curr Opin Endocrinol Diabetes Obes.* 2010;17:20-24.

Thornton PS, Stanley CA, De Leon DD, et al. Recommendations from the pediatric endocrine society for evaluation and management of persistent hypoglycemia in neonates, infants, and children. *J Pediatr* 2015;167:238.

Weinstein DA, Steuerwald U, De Souza CFM, Derks TGJ. Inborn errors of metabolism with hypoglycemia: glycogen storage diseases and inherited disorders of gluconeogenesis. *Pediatr Clin North Am.* 2018 Apr;65(2):247-265.

White K, Truong L, Aaron K, Mushtaq N, Thornton PS. The incidence and etiology of previously undiagnosed hypoglycemic disorders in the emergency department. *Pediatr Emerg Care.* 2020 Jul;36(7): 322-326.

CHAPTER 27

Shock

Cassi Smola, MD and Katherine Rakoczy, MD

BACKGROUND

Shock is a clinical condition that occurs when there is inadequate delivery of oxygen and other nutrients to meet the metabolic demands of the tissues. If left untreated, shock results in irreversible cell and organ damage and death. The clinician must be able to recognize shock early, initiate therapy rapidly, and possibly arrange safe transport of the patient to an intensive care facility. These lifesaving tasks require that the clinician have a fundamental knowledge of the causes, presentations, therapies, and complications of shock.

TABLE 27-1 Hypotension Parameters

Age	Minimum Systolic Blood Pressure (mmHg)
Term neonate (0-28 days)	60
Infant (1-12 months)	70
Child (1-10 years)	70 + (2 × age in years)
Older than 10 years	90

Physiologically, shock can be classified as *compensated*, when the patient is able to maintain a normal blood pressure for age, or *decompensated*, when deterioration has led to hypotension. In general, compensated shock progresses to decompensated shock if left untreated, which emphasizes the importance of early recognition and intervention. Children can generally maintain a normal blood pressure until advanced stages of shock; therefore, hypotension (see **Table 27-1** for age-based definitions of hypotension) in a pediatric patient is an ominous sign of impending circulatory collapse. When measuring blood pressure with a sphygmomanometer, it is important to select the smallest cuff that covers two-thirds of the upper arm or leg.

PATHOPHYSIOLOGY: CATEGORIES OF SHOCK

Shock is classified by cause: hypovolemic, distributive, cardiogenic, or obstructive. The mechanisms may differ, but inadequate tissue perfusion is the common final pathway.

HYPOVOLEMIC SHOCK

Hypovolemic shock is the most common type of shock in children; the two main types are *non-hemorrhagic* and *hemorrhagic*, and examples of each are provided in **Table 27-2**. Hypovolemic shock occurs when there is a decrease in intravascular volume secondary to fluid or blood loss. This leads to decreased venous return, and causes decreased preload and subsequently, decreased stroke volume. To maintain cardiac output, the heart rate increases in compensation, according to the formula: Cardiac output = Heart rate × Stroke volume. However, cardiac output decreases when this compensatory response is inadequate, leading to decreased delivery of oxygen and other substrates to the tissues.

In the early stage of hypovolemic shock, autoregulatory mechanisms shunt blood flow preferentially to the brain, heart, and adrenal system thus preserving blood pressure. Because flow is diverted from less critical organs, patients may present initially with cool or mottled extremities and decreased urine output. Other signs may include dry mucous membranes, absence of tears, and abnormal skin turgor.

Nonhemorrhagic Shock Nonhemorrhagic shock is the most common cause of shock in pediatrics worldwide. It is most commonly caused by excessive fluid and electrolyte losses from vomiting or diarrhea, and thereby decreased circulating volume to deliver oxygen and nutrients. Infants and younger children are particularly vulnerable to this type of

TABLE 27-2 Causes of Hypvolemic Shock

Nonhemorrhagic	Hemorrhagic
Vomiting or diarrhea	Trauma
Diabetes insipidus, diabetes mellitus	Gastrointestinal bleeding
Heat stroke	Postsurgical bleeding
Burns	Sequestration crisis
Intestinal obstruction	Splenic rupture
Water deprivation	
Adrenal insufficiency	
Hypothyroidism	

TABLE 27-3 Causes of Distributive Shock

Septic shock
Anaphylaxis
Medications
Foods
Envenomations or stings
Blood products
Latex
Neurologic
Head injury
Spinal shock
Drugs

shock because they rely on caregivers to manage their fluid intake, and because of their unique physiology including higher body water content and basal metabolic rate.

Hemorrhagic Shock Hemorrhagic shock is a decrease in blood volume and hemoglobin, and thereby a decrease in oxygen delivery to the body. It can often be due to trauma which is typically diagnosed at the initial presentation. It can also occur in post-operative patients. Victims of child abuse are at risk for delayed diagnosis of hemorrhagic shock because the initial history may be incomplete, inaccurate, or misleading, and symptoms may progress over time.

DISTRIBUTIVE SHOCK

Distributive shock is caused by a decrease in systemic vascular resistance. Abnormalities in vasomotor tone lead to peripheral pooling of blood, which results in a diminished effective preload, decreased cardiac output, and inadequate tissue perfusion. This process can occur without frank fluid loss. Causes of distributive shock are listed in **Table 27-3**.

Septic Shock Sepsis is a clinical syndrome that results from overwhelming infection creating a cascade of endogenous inflammatory mediators resulting in widespread tissue injury. Cytokines released during sepsis cause blood vessels to dilate. Toxins produced by bacteria cause damage to blood vessels, which leads intravascular fluid to leak into surrounding tissue. This results in intravascular volume depletion, decreased flow to vital organs including the heart, and ultimately metabolic derangements at the cellular level. It is important to consider septic shock early, because a seemingly stable patient with minimal findings of infection can quickly progress to sepsis. In the early (compensated) phase, often designated as "warm shock," septic shock may present with a hyperdynamic state including decreased vascular resistance, widened pulse pressure, increased cardiac output, tachycardia, tachypnea, warm extremities, and normal urine output. As it progresses to the decompensated phase, patients develop intravascular volume depletion due in part to capillary leak, cool extremities, thready pulses, central nervous system changes, respiratory distress, and decreased cardiac output, often denoted as "cold shock."

Although anyone can develop septic shock, risk factors include young age, chronic medical condition, the presence of central intravenous (IV) catheters, immunocompromised state, burns, and malnutrition. Septic shock can result from bacterial, viral, or fungal infection. It is important to note that septic shock can occur when cultures or other diagnostic tests do not yield a definitive organism. Shock can also develop from localized bacterial infections that produce toxins; this is referred to as toxic shock. This form of shock is most commonly associated with toxin-producing strains of *Group A Streptococci* and *Staphylococcus aureus*.

Anaphylactic Shock Anaphylactic shock occurs when an exogenous stimulus causes an allergic systemic immunoglobulin E–mediated response that triggers the release of histamine and other vasoactive factors from mast cells, with resulting vasodilation (see Chapter 45).

Neurogenic Shock Neurogenic shock may occur with spinal cord transection above the first thoracic level, with severe injuries to the brainstem or with isolated intracranial injuries. An injury to the cervical cord may result in unopposed parasympathetic tone and subsequent vasodilation.

TABLE 27-4 Causes of Cardiogenic Shock

Cardiomyopathies
Familial
Infectious
Infiltrative
Idiopathic
Arrhythmias
Ventricular fibrillation
Supraventricular tachycardia
Bradycardia
Complete heart block
Mechanical defects
Congenital heart disease
Coarctation of the aorta
Cardiac tumor
Ischemia or infarction
Anomalous coronary artery
Kawasaki disease

CARDIOGENIC SHOCK

Cardiogenic shock occurs when there is decreased cardiac output caused by pump failure. The main causes are listed in **Table 27-4**. Children with congenital heart disease can be at increased risk of developing cardiogenic shock depending on their structural or electrical defect. Myocarditis can also lead to cardiogenic shock. Myocarditis is inflammation of the myocardium, most commonly caused by a viral infection. Undiagnosed or untreated myocarditis can devolve to cardiogenic shock. Cardiogenic shock should be strongly considered in the following clinical scenarios: no history of fluid losses, physical examination reveals hepatomegaly or rales, chest radiograph demonstrates cardiomegaly, and when there is no clinical improvement despite oxygenation and volume expansion. Providers should have heightened suspicion for possible cardiogenic shock if a patient experiences worsening tachycardia or shortness of breath during volume resuscitation.

Management of cardiogenic shock should focus on correcting arrhythmias if present, improving preload and cardiac contractility, and reducing afterload. The stress on the heart can be minimized by decreasing metabolic demand including achieving normothermia; correction of anemia if present; and sedation, intubation, and mechanical ventilation if necessary.

Although cardiogenic shock is uncommon as the primary cause of shock in children, it may be a late manifestation of other forms of shock.

OBSTRUCTIVE SHOCK

Obstructive shock occurs when blood is prevented from circulating normally. In obstructive shock, there is a barrier to blood either being delivered to or leaving from the heart or great vessels. This causes a decrease in cardiac output, decreased peripheral circulating blood volume, and hypotension. Obstructive shock is an emergency, and requires immediate recognition and treatment. It is a rare cause of shock, accounting for about 1% to 2% of all pediatric patients with shock. Examples include pulmonary embolism, tension pneumothorax, constrictive pericarditis, and pericardial tamponade.

PATIENT HISTORY: PROGRESSION OF SHOCK

In compensated shock, pediatric patients are able to maintain cardiac output and blood pressure by increasing the heart rate and peripheral vascular resistance. With further compromise of cardiac function, the

TABLE 27-5 Organ Dysfunction in Shock

Cardiovascular
- Decreased BP <5th %
- Need for vasoactive agent to maintain normal BP
  - metabolic acidosis (bicarbonate <19)
  - lactate >4
  - urine output <0.5 mL/kg/h
  - capillary refill >5 seconds

Respiratory
- Non-invasive or invasive mechanical ventilation
- >50% FiO_2 needed for sat >92%
- CO_2 >65 mm Hg on blood gas
- PaO_2/FiO_2 <300 (without cyanotic CHD)

Neurologic
- GCS ≤11 or ≥3 decrease from baseline

Hematologic
- Platelet <80,000/mm³ or 50% decrease from highest over past 3 days (oncology patients)
- INR >2

Renal
- Creatinine >2 × upper limit of normal or 2-fold increase in baseline

Hepatic
- bilirubin ≥4 mg/dL (not for newborns)
- ALT 2 × upper limit of normal

Abbreviations: ALT, Alanine Transaminiase; BP, Blood Pressure; CHD, Congenital Heart Disease; CO_2, Carbon Dioxide; FiO_2, Fraction of inspired oxygen; GCS, Glasgow Coma Scale; INR, International Normalized Ratio; PaO_2, Partial pressure of oxygen in arterial blood.

compensatory tachycardia is insufficient to maintain cardiac output. Decreased perfusion affects many systems, causing metabolic acidosis, oliguria, elevated transaminases from hepatocellular hypoperfusion, cool extremities, mottling of the skin, and ileus. Tachypnea develops to increase the elimination of carbon dioxide, which helps compensate for the metabolic acidosis.

In the late stages of shock, end-organ failure may manifest as central nervous system depression (ranging from confusion and agitation to sleepiness and ultimately coma), anuria, uremia, hyperkalemia, acute respiratory distress syndrome, and coagulopathies. Specific organ dysfunctions that are the result of shock are outlined in **Table 27-5**.

Early recognition of shock is important. Providers should elicit whether patients have an underlying factor that increases their risk for shock including but not limited to immunocompromised status, chronic diseases, or implanted hardware. Additional questions should be directed at recent exposures through travel, trauma or infectious agents; recent therapies such as medications, fluids, and procedures; and allergies to medications, foods, and environmental chemicals.

PHYSICAL EXAMINATION

The physical examination (**Table 27-6**) should focus on aspects that will help the clinician distinguish among the different causes of shock.

DIFFERENTIAL DIAGNOSIS

Shock, once recognized, should be treated immediately and attention to specific underlying causes should be pursued only after the basic resuscitation needs are met. Shock in a neonate may be the result of any of the previously mentioned causes, but the differential diagnosis of neonatal shock should also include those listed in **Table 27-7**. Likewise, the diagnosis of shock may be more challenging in chronically medically vulnerable patients as they can have abnormal vasomotor responses resulting in widely variable blood pressures and heart rates or possess implanted hardware placing them at higher risk. These patients may also be unable to mount an adequate immune response.

TABLE 27-6 Directed Physical Examination

- Vital signs
- Skin
  - Rash
  - Petechiae
  - Ecchymosis
  - Erythroderma
  - Mottling
- Head, eyes, ears, nose, and throat
  - Evidence of head trauma
  - Pupil size and reactivity
  - Conjunctival pallor
  - Central cyanosis (lips, tongue)
- Neck
  - Meningismus
  - Cervical spine tenderness
- Lungs
  - Abnormal breathing pattern (e.g., Kussmaul)
  - Retractions
  - Wheezes or rales (focal or bilateral)
  - Diminished breath sounds or dullness to percussion
- Heart
  - Hyperdynamic
  - Murmur
  - Rub
  - Gallop
- Abdomen
  - Tenderness, rebound, or guarding
  - Distention or ascites
  - Mass or organomegaly
- Extremities
  - Temperature
  - Peripheral pulses
  - Clubbing
- Neurologic
  - Mental status
  - Focal deficit

DIAGNOSTIC EVALUATION

Diagnostic tests should focus on the aforementioned organ dysfunctions and tests that may aid in identifying the inciting cause of shock (**Table 27-8**). A lactate should always be checked, though elevation often

TABLE 27-7 Special Considerations in Neonatal Shock

- Congenital adrenal hyperplasia
- Inborn errors of metabolism
- Left-sided cardiac obstructive lesions
  - Aortic stenosis
  - Hypoplastic left heart syndrome
  - Critical coarctation of the aorta
  - Interrupted aortic arch
- Blood loss at delivery
- Perinatal infection
- Abdominal catastrophe (midgut volvulus)

TABLE 27-8 Diagnostic Tests Considered for Patients in Shock

Complete blood count with differential
Serum chemistries
Electrolytes including calcium
Blood urea nitrogen
Creatinine
Glucose
Liver enzymes including bilirubin
Pancreatic enzymes
Cardiac enzymes
Lactic acid
Coagulation studies
Prothrombin time
Partial thromboplastin time
Fibrinogen
Fibrin split (degradation) products
Inflammatory Markers (CRP, ESR, and Procalcitonin)
Venous or Arterial blood gas
Type and crossmatch
Cultures
Blood
Urine
Cerebrospinal fluid
Pleural fluid
Abscess drainage
Toxicology
Urine
Serum
Urinalysis
Imaging
Chest radiograph
Abdominal radiograph or obstruction series
Electrocardiogram

occurs only late in disease course. Many pediatric patients in shock can have a normal lactate and thus the clinician should not be falsely reassured.

MANAGEMENT

A pediatric patient in shock represents a medical emergency. For this reason, identification of the precise cause of shock may be delayed while resuscitation and stabilization proceed. Attention to the CAB (circulation, airway, and breathing) remains a basic principle in the initial general assessment. In general, increasing oxygen delivery to the tissues and decreasing oxygen demand are key. General time goals and management for resuscitation are delineated in **Figure 27-1**. It is imperative that the entire care team is aware of the timing of the resuscitation interventions. Adherence to timely fluid and algorithm goals has been shown to decrease mortality as well as decrease hospital and intensive care length of stay. Using a standardized protocol is useful in ensuring all algorithm components are met. If there is suspicion of trauma, cervical spine immobilization should be maintained until the spine can be evaluated. The primary survey of a pediatric patient in shock is directed toward the rapid identification of immediately life-threatening conditions that should be addressed before a more extensive evaluation.

A stable airway should be established and maintained, and supplemental oxygen should be provided even if the saturation is normal. Hypoxemia should be corrected with oxygen supplementation to keep arterial oxygen saturation greater than 95%. Evaluating peripheral perfusion and pulses provides a rapid assessment of the circulation. Continuous cardiorespiratory monitoring and frequent blood pressure measurement are important to assess the response to intervention. The goal is to maintain reliable intravascular access through which vigorous resuscitation can proceed. If peripheral IV access is not immediately obtained, intraosseous access should be considered (see Chapter 191). Unless the patient has myocardial or known chronic renal disease, the initial therapy should be 20 mL/kg of isotonic fluid (normal saline or Lactated Ringer's) administered intravenously rapidly over the 10 to 20 minutes. This may need to be repeated one to two more times, to a total of 40 to 60 mL/kg within the first hour, with close clinical assessment of vital signs, perfusion, urine output, and mental status for improvement. In the case of hemorrhagic shock, blood products should be given as soon as possible. Until appropriate blood products are available, isotonic IV fluids are used as a temporizing measure to restore intravascular volume.

If the patient remains hypotensive and poorly perfused despite 40 to 60 mL/kg of IV fluids, termed fluid-refractory shock, inotropic support should be strongly considered while consulting with an intensivist. Depending on the type of shock different vasoactive medications may be used. For example, in septic shock epinephrine or norepinephrine can be used. Vasopressin is typically added when a patient is requiring high-dose vasoactive medications. Milrinone improves inotropy and lusitropy, therefore it can be used to augment cardiac function in cardiogenic shock. Hydrocortisone (1-2 mg/kg IV) should be considered for patients with adrenal insufficiency and those requiring daily steroids.

A chest radiograph may be helpful to assess the presence of cardiomegaly, fluid overload, pulmonary edema, pneumonia, pleural effusion, or pneumothorax.

Antipyretics should be administered to a febrile patient to decrease metabolic demand. Conversely, warming should be instituted in a hypothermic patient (see Chapter 175). Broad-spectrum antibiotics should be given intravenously or intraosseously unless it is known that infection is not the cause of the patient's condition.

In a neonate with shock in whom a duct-dependent cardiac lesion is a possible cause, prostaglandin E_1 should be considered to maintain patency of the ductus arteriosus. Preparation should be made for the possibility of intubation, because prostaglandin E_1 may cause apnea. The decision to administer prostaglandin E_1 is usually made in consultation with a neonatologist or pediatric cardiologist.

Anaphylactic shock management should include administration of intramuscular epinephrine, antihistamines such as diphenhydramine, and corticosteroids in addition to supportive measures listed earlier. Continuing monitoring is essential, as development of a biphasic reaction can occur (see Chapter 45).

SPECIAL CONSIDERATIONS: TRANSPORT OF THE PATIENT IN SHOCK

Early initiation of transport can be life- and limb-saving for patients in shock. The child may require continuous or invasive monitoring, or an advanced airway; in such cases, they will require an intensive care unit. If transfer to another institution is necessary, the clinician has the challenging task of weighing the risks and benefits of the different modes of transportation (see Chapter 11). In every case, whether the patient is transferred to another facility or from one unit to another within the same facility, it is essential that the team transporting the patient have the appropriate personnel and equipment to do so safely. Communication of the patient's condition and the interventions performed is key, and medical records, imaging studies, and laboratory results should accompany the patient whenever possible.

KEY POINTS

- Shock can be classified as hypovolemic, distributive, cardiogenic, or obstructive.
- Hypotension is often a late finding in pediatric shock.
- Early recognition of shock and rapid intervention is crucial to decreasing morbidity and mortality.

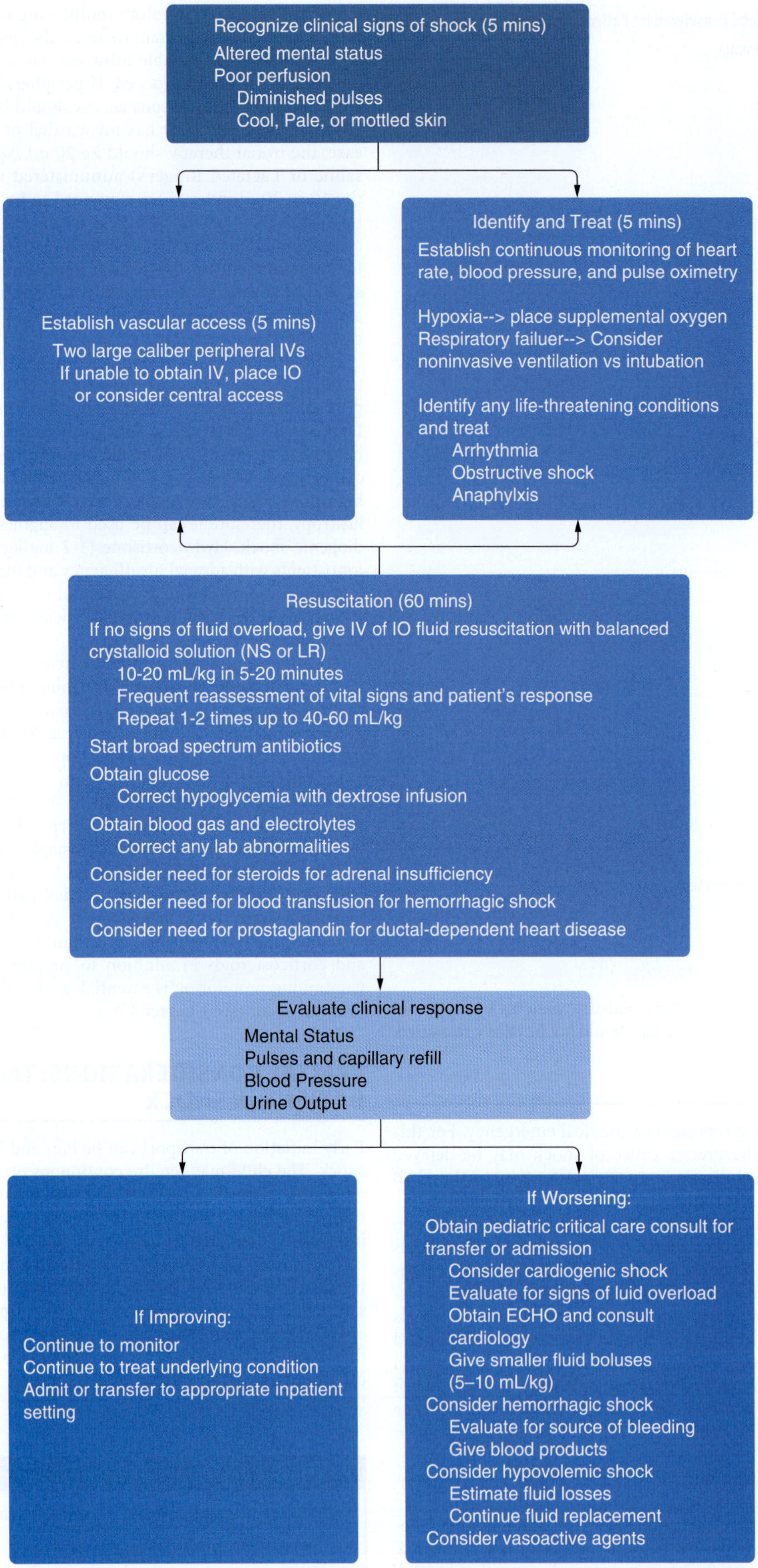

FIGURE 27-1. Initial management of pediatric shock.

SUGGESTED READINGS

Aziz K, Lee HC, Escobedo MB, et al. Part 5: Neonatal resuscitation: 2020 American Heart Association guidelines for cardiopulmonary resuscitation and emergency cardiovascular care. *Circulation.* 2020;142(16_suppl_2):S524-S550.

Brissaud O, Botte A, Cambonie G, et al. Experts' recommendations for the management of cardiogenic shock in children. *Ann Intensive Care.* 2016;6(1):14.

Davis A, Carcillo J, Aneja R, et al. American College of Critical Care Medicine Clinical Practice Parameters for hemodynamic support of pediatric and neonatal patients in septic shock. *Crit Care Med.* 2017;45(6):1061-1093.

Cruz AT, Perry AM, Williams EA, et al. Implementation of goal-directed therapy for children with suspected sepsis in the emergency department. *Pediatrics.* 2011;127:e758-766.

Fleming S, Thomson M, Stevens R, et al. Normal ranges of heart rate and respiratory rate in children from birth to 18 years of age: a systematic review of observational studies. *Lancet.* 2011;377:1011.

Larsen GY, Mecham N, Greenberg R, et al. An emergency department septic shock protocol and care guideline for children initiated at triage. *Pediatrics.* 2011;127:e1585-e1592.

Mathias B, Mira JC, Larson SD. Pediatric sepsis. *Curr Opin Pediatr.* 2016;28(3):380-387.

Mendelson J. Emergency department management of pediatric shock. *Emerg Med Clin North Am.* 2018;36(2):427-440.

Menon K, Schlapbach L, Akech S, et al. Criteria for Pediatric Sepsis—A systematic review and meta-analysis by the pediatric sepsis definition taskforce. *Crit Care Med.* 2022 Jan;50(1):21-36.

Topjian AA, Raymond TT, Atkins D, et al. Part 4: Pediatric basic and advanced life support: 2020 American Heart Association guidelines for cardiopulmonary resuscitation and emergency cardiovascular care. *Circulation.* 2020;142(16_suppl_2):S469-S523.

Weiss S, Peters M, Alhazzani W, et al. Surviving Sepsis Campaign International Guidelines for the Management of Septic Shock and Sepsis-Associated Organ Dysfunction in Children. *Pediatr Crit Care Med.* 2020;21(2):e52-e106.

CHAPTER 28 Irritability and Intractable Crying

Mirna Giordano, MD and Erin King, MD

BACKGROUND

Irritability and intractable crying may be the presenting complaint for a wide range of medical problems in infants and children, some of which are potentially serious. It has been estimated that 5% of infants presenting to the emergency department with crying have a serious underlying illness and two-thirds of these cases may be identified through careful history and physical examination. Hospital providers must be able to differentiate significant irritability and intractable crying from developmentally appropriate crying. They must be familiar with common and unusual causes of irritability/intractable crying and a stepwise approach to evaluation.

Irritability is a state of increased sensitivity to stimuli. Parents may describe children as fussy, whiny, uncomfortable, or with increased crying. Crying is the primary way that infants and young children express hunger, thirst, fear, fatigue, desire for attention, and discomfort/pain. Crying and/or expressions of pain may be similar indicators for older and developmentally delayed children. When caregivers have taken the usual measures to address needs, such as feeding, holding the child and changing the diaper, yet the child continues to cry, the child is said to be inconsolable or to have intractable crying.

The quantity as well as the quality of crying or fussy behavior should be considered. What qualifies as excessive crying varies based on the age and development of the child, as well as the clinical scenario. Typically developing infants cry most during the first 3 to 4 months of life with a peak around 6 to 8 weeks of age. During this period, serious illness may present with few or only subtle signs and symptoms, making evaluation in this age group particularly challenging. For medically complex children, those with cerebral palsy or various neuromuscular conditions, the history from the caregiver is of paramount value. A history should include whether similar behavior occurred before, and prior problems with constipation, feeding intolerance, gastroesophageal reflux (GERD), seizures etc.

Crying/pain/irritability should also be evaluated to determine whether it is appropriate for the clinical scenario, and whether the diagnosis fits the physical exam. For example, a febrile infant with a viral upper respiratory infection is likely to be irritable and may cry more than usual. However, crying with movement of the child's lower extremities should lead to suspicion of an alternative cause, such as fracture, arthritis, septic hip joint, or meningitis. Stranger anxiety—appearing around 8 to 9 months of age, peaking at 12 to 15 months, and decreasing thereafter - may manifest as inconsolable crying during examination; however, an otherwise healthy child should be comforted and calmed in the arms of a caregiver within minutes. Caregiver-directed examination may be helpful in these instances. The character of a child's cry may also be significant: louder, higher pitch, or more urgent tone or a weak, stridulous, or hoarse cry may suggest the presence of illness. For medically complex children, evaluation of tone (presence of spasticity, dystonia, seizures etc.), abdominal exam, and careful review of current medications may provide additional clues.

PATHOPHYSIOLOGY

Irritability and crying may result from pain, discomfort, fatigue, direct neurologic insult, or altered metabolic, infectious, and endocrine status. Crying in infants and young or developmentally delayed children is an involuntary action that serves physiologic and protective purposes. A newborn's first cries enable essential changes in the cardiorespiratory system during the transition to postnatal life. Crying increases to an average 3 hours daily by 6 weeks of life, decreasing thereafter. During this period of greatest crying, often referred to as the Purple period, infants cry most during the late afternoon and evening hours. Crying is also a way for infants and children to express their emotions.

DEFINITIONS

Irritability: A state of increased sensitivity to stimuli.

Intractable crying: Crying that persists despite usual efforts to comfort the child.

PATIENT HISTORY

It is important to obtain a detailed description of the irritability and crying, as delineated in **Table 28-1**. Note history of associated symptoms, including fever, malaise, feeding difficulty, respiratory symptoms, vomiting (bilious/bloody), stool pattern and composition, parents' perception of the source of pain, limping/joint discomfort, skin irritation/redness/swelling, poor weight gain, headache or perception of head pain, developmental delay or regression, and seizures or abnormal movements.

PHYSICAL EXAMINATION

When initially examining the infant/child, it is often helpful to observe respiration, movement, and behavior from across the room. This provides useful information and helps eliminate the confounding influence of stranger anxiety. With a frightened toddler or developmentally delayed

TABLE 28-1 Elements of the History Relevant to Intractable Crying/Irritability
Baseline crying/irritability behavior
Duration of presenting crying/irritability episode
Quality of crying (i.e., intensity, character, pitch)
Previous similar episodes of crying/irritability
Characteristics of crying episodes
Duration of previous crying episodes
Time of day
Circumstances or triggers
Efforts of caregivers to console child
Conditions that make crying better or worse
Associated symptoms
Exposures, including recent immunizations, immunization status, and/or travel
Caregivers' ideas regarding causes
Usual and recent feeding patterns
Usual and recent elimination patterns
Usual and recent sleep patterns
Growth pattern
Birth history, including gestational age and any history of in-utero drug exposure
Developmental history
Past medical and surgical history
Medications
Allergies

child, caregivers can assist in the physical examination by exposing areas of skin and moving the extremities to check for tenderness while the examiner stands back and observes. Use of distraction techniques can facilitate physical examination. It is essential to examine the child from head to toe and fully exposed. Growth parameters, including head circumference in infants, should be assessed.

Because of the extensive differential diagnoses, a stepwise approach is essential. The presence of fever makes an infectious, inflammatory, neurologic or endocrine process more likely. Serious bacterial infections can present without fever or with low temperature, particularly in neonates or those with significant neurological injuries, and may coexist with benign conditions such as viral upper respiratory tract infections. Most common causes of irritability and intractable crying in afebrile patients are apparent after a careful history and physical examination. A period of observation and monitoring may be helpful and could unmask new symptoms.

Bruising in non-ambulatory infants and developmentally delayed children, particularly over the trunk, ears, neck, face, or oral cavity, limb swelling, and/or other signs of unexplained injury should raise concern for non-accidental trauma (see **Figure 28-1**). Evaluation for the presence

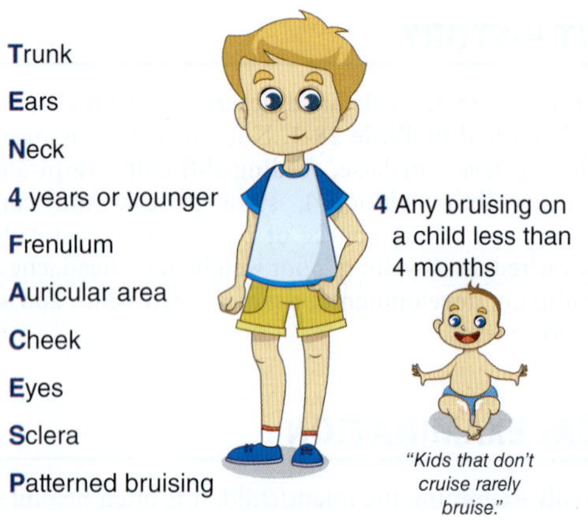

FIGURE 28-1. A mnemonic for Torso, Ears, Neck, Frenulum, Angle of the jaw, Cheeks, Eyelids, or Subconjunctivae in infants <4 months or with a pattern (TEN-4 FACES).

of ear bleeding, periorbital ecchymosis, rib bruising, crepitus, a bulging fontanelle, and retinal hemorrhages should be included.

Otitis, mastoiditis, and hair tourniquets are often found to cause pain and irritability in small children. Parents may not notice the presence of a hair tourniquet around an appendage such as a digit, penis, or clitoris, which can cause swelling and pain. The band of hair may not be visible if it is buried beneath a fold of edematous tissue. In some cases, the hair may be so tightly wound that it is difficult to release. Applying a hair removal cream to the affected area for about 5 to 10 minutes may dissolve the hair and relieve the constriction. If trying to decipher whether crying is related to otitis media, a trial of oral or topical pain relief can be attempted.

Ocular abnormalities, including corneal abrasion and acute glaucoma, are difficult to discern by history or physical examination, because tearing and conjunctival injection are difficult to appreciate in the setting of excessive crying. If suspected, consider a topical anesthetic, fluorescein stain, ultraviolet light examination of both eyes, and lid eversion to rule out corneal abrasion or foreign body in conjunction with ophthalmology consultation. If increased intraocular or intracranial pressure is a concern, ophthalmology evaluation is indicated.

The presence of tachypnea may suggest metabolic acidosis, respiratory tract infection, or cardiac dysfunction. Foreign body aspiration or other airway obstruction may produce symptoms of respiratory distress such as cyanosis, increased work of breathing, diaphoresis, drooling, stridor, stertor, wheezing, or rales.

DIFFERENTIAL DIAGNOSIS AND EVALUATION

If a child continues to cry inconsolably during a period of observation after initial examination and no reasonable cause has been identified, admission for further evaluation and monitoring should be considered as a serious occult condition may be present. It is essential for the clinician to entertain an extensive differential diagnosis, focusing first on potentially serious or life-threatening conditions (**Table 28-2**). A broad evaluation of ill-appearing infants and children at this point includes a complete blood count, inflammatory markers (C-reactive protein, procalcitonin, erythrocyte sedimentation rate [ESR]), lipase, complete metabolic panel, urinalysis, urine culture, chest radiograph/x-ray (CXR), abdominal radiograph/x-ray (AXR), stool studies/gastrointestinal polymerase chain reaction testing (GI PCR), blood culture, medication levels/toxicology analysis, and consideration of a lumbar puncture.

Evidence of recent trauma ascertained either by history or on physical examination should be investigated further. Evidence of injury in the absence of a history supporting a reasonable mechanism of injury, or different descriptions of trauma by various observers represent red flags. An assessment of the family environment and social stressors and the observation of interactions among family members are also important to identify possible non-accidental trauma, such as abusive head trauma (see Part III, Section A: Abuse and Neglect).

Symptoms of altered sensorium, such as increased somnolence, lethargy, confusion, or agitation, may suggest central nervous system infection, inflammation or injury, a metabolic disorder, drug ingestion or withdrawal, toxin exposure, or cardiopulmonary failure. It is important to inquire specifically about toxins and medications (prescription, non-prescription, traditional, and homeopathic) that the child may have ingested or have been exposed to at home/elsewhere. Loss of developmental milestones could suggest a metabolic or neurodegenerative disorder.

Constipation is a common problem that can cause irritability. Further investigation of symptoms of gastrointestinal obstruction should be done expeditiously to evaluate for ischemia. Screaming attacks are a common presenting sign of intussusception, and are particularly concerning if accompanied by vomiting and/or periods of lethargy and blood in stool. Crying associated with bilious emesis in the young infant is midgut volvulus, a surgical emergency, until proven otherwise. Additional concerns may arise with bilious vomiting in older children or those with indwelling devices (ventriculo- or spinal-peritoneal shunts). Abdominal or scrotal swelling may be a sign

TABLE 28-2 Causes of Irritability and Intractable Crying

General
- Infection/Inflammation
- Pain/Discomfort
- Dehydration/Hunger
- Anemia
- Leukemia
- Colic

Eyes, ears, nose, and throat
- Corneal abrasion
- Ocular foreign body
- Glaucoma
- Otitis media/externa, mastoiditis
- Thrush
- Herpangina
- Herpes stomatitis
- Herpes eye infections
- Teething
- Gingivitis
- Tonsillitis/pharyngitis
- Palatal burns or trauma
- Dental caries or abscess
- Nasal, oropharyngeal, or otic foreign body
- Choanal atresia

Cardiovascular
- Arrhythmia (e.g., supraventricular tachycardia)
- Myocardial ischemia or infarction
- Endocarditis/Myocarditis/Pericarditis
- Congestive heart failure or congenital heart defect
- Kawasaki disease

Respiratory
- Respiratory distress or failure
- Pneumonia
- Pneumothorax
- Upper and Lower respiratory tract infection
- Foreign body aspiration

Gastrointestinal
- Incarcerated hernia
- Cholecystitis
- Cholelithiasis
- Spontaneous perforation of bile duct
- Appendicitis
- Esophagitis/GERD
- Gastritis/Gastroenteritis
- Milk-protein allergy
- Pancreatitis
- Small or Large bowel obstruction
- Malrotation, volvulus
- Intussusception
- Henoch-Schönlein purpura
- Bowel perforation
- Constipation
- Gaseous distention, ileus
- Anal fissure
- Hemorrhoids
- Gastrostomy or gastrojejunal tube tension associated with growth/blockage

Genitourinary
- Testicular/ovarian torsion
- Epididymitis
- Urinary tract obstruction or infection
- Nephrolithiasis
- Urethritis
- Meatal ulcer
- Sexual abuse
- Incarcerated inguinal/umbilical hernia

Endocrine and metabolic
- Congenital adrenal hyperplasia
- Hyperthyroidism
- Syndrome of inappropriate antidiuretic hormone
- Diabetes insipidus
- Hypoglycemia
- Electrolyte abnormalities (sodium, calcium, potassium)
- Inborn error of metabolism
- Metabolic acidosis
- Pheochromocytoma
- Reye syndrome

Neurologic
- Central nervous system injury/Cerebral edema
- Abusive head trauma
- Increased intracranial pressure (e.g., Pseudotumor cerebri, hydrocephalus, encephalitis, hemorrhage, mass)
- Meningitis, encephalitis, brain abscess
- Pseudotumor cerebri or hydrocephalus
- Migraine
- Subdural/epidural hematoma
- VP shunt malfunction/infection

Drugs and toxins
- Neonatal abstinence or other withdrawal syndromes
- Fetal alcohol syndrome
- Poisoning (e.g., lead, mercury, iron, carbon monoxide)
- Monosodium glutamate reaction
- Drugs (e.g., antihistamines, atropines, phenothiazines, pseudoephedrine, albuterol, theophylline or other methylxanthines, metoclopramide, promethazine, barbiturates, tricyclic antidepressants, vitamin A, vitamin D, salicylates, amphetamines, cocaine, phencyclidine)
- Vaccine reaction

Skin
- Hair tourniquet
- Insect, arachnid, or arthropod bite or sting
- Burn
- HSV dermatitis, dermatitis herpetiformis (pain may precede vesicles)
- Cellulitis
- Paronychia
- Atopic dermatitis, acrodermatitis enteropathica, or other pruritic conditions
- Pressure ulcer

Orthopedic/Musculoskeletal
- Fracture
- Non-accidental trauma
- Acute arthritis (infectious, postinfectious, inflammatory)
- Dactylitis/Vaso-occlusive crisis
- Myositis
- Nursemaid's elbow or joint dislocation (i.e., hip subluxation)
- Discitis
- Osteomyelitis

of a serious acute process like obstruction, infection, testicular torsion, or epididymitis.

Medically complex children dependent on technology: baclofen pumps, vagal nerve stimulators, ventriculo-peritoneal shunts, gastrostomy tubes, gastro-jejunal tubes, various drains, and non-invasive positive pressure ventilation should be carefully examined, especially at the areas where devices attach or implant. If medications are delivered through devices, inadequate dosing or withdrawal, overdosing, malfunction, and infection should be considered by providers.

In cases of recurrent or chronic intractable crying or irritability, a broader differential may need to be considered (**Table 28-3**).

In well-appearing children, there are no standard screening laboratory tests, with the exception of urinalysis and culture in girls and uncircumcised boys younger than 2 years, and circumcised boys younger than 6 months who present with fever. Laboratory and radiographic evaluation should be guided by findings from the history and physical examination.

MANAGEMENT

A multidisciplinary, family-centered approach to care is recommended given how stressful irritability and intractable crying in infants and children can be to families. Providers should use the opportunity to educate and advise parents on the care of their child. Achieving a careful balance of not dismissing concerns as a benign condition without proper evaluation yet avoiding unnecessary testing or medical intervention can be challenging.

SPECIAL CONSIDERATIONS

One in five infants may struggle with excessive crying or regulatory problems and these infants may be at increased risk of child abuse and future behavior problems in childhood. Mothers of these infants are at increased risk of postpartum depression and early breastfeeding cessation. Consideration of a screening evaluation for postpartum depression and social determinants of health is encouraged.

TABLE 28-3 Syndromes and Conditions Associated With Chronic or Recurrent Irritability or Intractable Crying
Anomalous origin of the coronary artery
Congenital heart disease (e.g., "tet" spells of tetralogy of Fallot)
Gastroesophageal reflux, Sandifer syndrome
Colic
Milk protein intolerance
Lactose intolerance
Nutritional deficiencies (e.g., iron, zinc, vitamin C, vitamin D, hypocalcemia)
Diabetes insipidus
Sickle cell disease
Metabolic and neurodegenerative disorders (e.g., glutaric aciduria type I, acute intermittent porphyria, Pompe disease, pyridoxine deficiency, tryptophan malabsorption, hypoglycinemia, arginemia, tyrosinemia, pyruvate carboxylase deficiency, biotin deficiency, argininosuccinate lyase deficiency, Krabbe disease, lipogranulomatosis)
Genetic syndromes (e.g., Smith-Lemli-Opitz, Williams, Cornelia de Lange)
Unrecognized deafness
Epilepsy syndromes (e.g., West, Lennox-Gastaut, Benign Rolandic epilepsy, infantile spasms, non-epileptic seizures)
Status dystonicus
Movement disorders
Behavioral problems (e.g., attention-deficit hyperactivity disorder, ODD)
Parent–child interactions, problems, or stress
Mental illness (e.g., depression, anxiety, bipolar disorder)
Rheumatologic disorders (e.g., juvenile idiopathic arthritis)
Infantile cortical hyperostosis (Caffey disease)

COLIC, GASTROINTESTINAL DISTURBANCES, AND FEEDING PROBLEMS

Clinicians should be able to differentiate clinical features of infantile colic, a common cause of excessive and intractable crying in infants, from other conditions. Colic is characterized by episodes of inconsolable crying in an otherwise healthy infant and is a diagnosis of exclusion. The timing of colic parallels the normal peak of infant crying, usually beginning during the second to third week of life and resolving by 3 or 4 months of age. Colic is commonly defined by the "rule of threes": crying for more than 3 hours per day, on more than 3 days per week, in an infant 3 months or younger. The crying episodes tend to occur suddenly during the late afternoon and evening hours and are often described as more intense. The episodes may be associated with facial flushing, abdominal distention, and increased tone.

Colic likely stems from different causes in different infants. Proposed causes include immaturity of the nervous system, impaired intestinal absorption or motility, sensitivity to milk protein, or a reflection of temperament or parent-child interactions. Parental education, reassurance, and support are important aspects of management. Increased efforts to intentionally soothe the infant and limit air swallowing, improve burping, and minimize environmental stimulation may be helpful. Parents may use medications such as simethicone, but use is not supported in trials. In breastfed infants under 3 months of age, probiotic supplementation with *L. reuteri* may reduce crying episodes.

Excessive crying beyond 3 months of age might raise suspicion for a gastrointestinal disorder. While crying in infants is frequently attributed to GERD by both parents and clinicians, objective evidence that GERD underlies symptoms or that acid-suppressive medications are beneficial in this group are lacking. Some children may have increased spit-up, vomiting, and crying surrounding feeding time.

Food allergies, primarily cow milk protein allergy in infants, may present in both formula-fed and breastfed infants with irritability, eczema, bloody stools, and less commonly, vomiting, diarrhea, feeding difficulties, or poor growth. Protocols for allergen-elimination diets in breastfeeding mothers have been published, and some evidence suggests that use of hypoallergenic formula may reduce crying in formula-fed infants.

Congenital lactase deficiency is extremely rare, although secondary lactose intolerance may result from damage to intestinal villa, such as from gastroenteritis. Use of lactose-free formula in non-breastfed infants may have a role in managing symptoms. Functional lactose overload in breastfed infants may produce excessive crying accompanied by poor satiety and frothy or explosive stools as a result of low milk fat content and rapid gastrointestinal transit, such as in instances of oversupply. Lactation consultation may be helpful in such instances.

NEW IRRITABILITY OR EXCESSIVE CRYING IN A HOSPITALIZED PATIENT

Although the approach to irritability or inconsolability that develops in a hospitalized patient is similar, additional causes must be considered. Dietary, environmental, and sleep-wake schedule changes should be reviewed. For example, restricting oral intake before or after procedures could result in crying due to hunger. Patients with prolonged exposure during examination and monitoring may become cold, or infants under warmers may become overheated. Intravenous catheter sites should be inspected for any evidence of thrombophlebitis, and the locations of other catheters, tubes, and probes should be examined for skin irritation, skin breakdown, excessive traction, discharge, and infection. Adverse effects and interactions of medications should also be considered as possible contributors. Appropriate prevention and treatment of procedural pain must also be considered, including use of breastfeeding/breast milk, sucrose, and non-nutritive sucking in infants or other analgesics in older children.

NEW IRRITABILITY OR EXCESSIVE CRYING IN A TECHNOLOGY-DEPENDENT CHILD WITH MEDICAL COMPLEXITY

History, examination, and evaluation of the child with medical complexity who presents with apparent new pain or crying should be performed in concert with the child's caregiver. It is known that pain behaviors occur much more frequently in this population compared with typically developing children. Validated tools exist to assist in evaluation of pain (i.e., r-FLACC or INRS) and overall evaluation of the child (i.e., GRASP). Consideration of factors such as dysautonomia, spasticity, neuropathic pain, seizures, dystonia, and side effects of prior treatments, medications, and indwelling devices should be made (see Table 28-3). Once a possible source has been identified, both pharmacologic and non-pharmacologic strategies should be employed. For this population, consideration of palliative care consultation may also be helpful.

KEY POINTS

- Crying that is concerning to parents in infancy and childhood is a frequent reason for seeking care.
- A careful history and physical examination should identify most of the serious underlying causes of irritability and crying.
- Diagnostic examination should be directed based on results of the history and physical exam.

SUGGESTED READINGS

Academy of Breastfeeding Medicine. ABM clinical protocol # 24: allergic proctocolitis in the exclusively breastfed infant. *Breastfeed Med.* 2011;6(6):435-440.

Barr R. (2022, June 20) *What Is the Period of Purple Crying?* The Period of Purple Crying. http://www.purplecrying.info/

Crellin DJ, Harrison D, Santamaria N, Babl FE. Systematic review of the Face, Legs, Activity, Cry and Consolability scale for assessing pain in infants and children: is it reliable, valid, and feasible for use? *Pain.* 2015;156(11):2132-2151.

Dickstein DP, Barthelemy CM, Jenkins GA, et al. This is your brain on irritability: a clinician's guide to understanding how we know what we know now, and what we need to know in the future, about irritability in children and adolescents. *Child Adolesc Psychiatr Clin N Am.* 2021;30(3):649-666. doi:10.1016/j.chc.2021.04.013

Douglas PS, Hiscock H. The unsettled baby: crying out for an integrated, multidisciplinary primary care approach. *MJA.* 2010;193(9):533-536.

Feldman KW, Tayama TM, Strickler LE, et al. A prospective study of the causes of bruises in premobile infants. *Pediatr Emerg Care.* 2020;36(2):e43-e49.

Freedman SB, Al-Harthy N, Thull-Freedman J. The crying infant: diagnostic testing and frequency of serious underlying disease. *Pediatrics.* 2009;123:841.

Hemmi MH, Wolke D, Schneider S. Associations between problems with crying, sleeping and/or feeding in infancy and long-term behavioral outcomes in childhood: a meta-analysis. *Arch Dis Child.* 2011:96(7):622-629.

Hauer J, Houtrow AJ, AAP Section on Hospice and Palliative Medicine, Council on Children with Disabilities. Pain assessment and treatment in children with significant impairment of the central nervous system. *Pediatrics.* 2017;139(6):e20171002.

Howard CR, Lanphear N, Lanphear BP, et al. Parental responses to infant crying and colic: the effect on breastfeeding duration. *Breastfeed Med.* 2006;1:146-155.

Johnson JD, Cocker K, Chang E. Infantile colic: recognition and treatment. *Am Fam Physician.* 2015, Oct;92(7):577-582.

Korja R, Nolvi S, Grant KA, McMahon C. The relations between maternal prenatal anxiety or stress and child's early negative reactivity or self-regulation: a systematic review. *Child Psychiatry Hum Dev.* 2017;48(6):851-869. doi:10.1007/s10578-017-0709-0

Leventhal JM, Edwards GA, Barr RG. Abusive Head Trauma and Infant Crying—A Flawed Analysis. *JAMA Pediatr.* 2021;175(11):1181. doi:10.1001/jamapediatrics.2021.2505

Reijneveld SA. Can der Wal MF, Brugman E, et al. Infant crying and abuse? *Lancet.* 2004;364(9442):1340-1342.

Roberts D, Ostapchuk M, O'Brian James. Infantile colic. *Am Fam Physician.* 2004; 70(4):735-740.

Shah PS, Herbozo C, Aliwalas LL, et al. Breastfeeding or breast milk for procedural pain in neonates (Review). *Cochrane Database Syst Rev.* 2012;12:1-24.

Sung V, D'Amico F, Cabana MD, et al. *Lactobacillus reuteri* to treat infant colic: a meta-analysis. *Pediatrics.* 2018;141(1):e20171811. doi:10.1542/peds.2017-1811

The Royal Children's Hospital Melbourne. (2022). *Unsettled or Crying Babies.* (endorsed by the Paediatric Improvement Collaborative) https://www.rch.org.au/clinicalguide/guideline_index/Crying_Baby_Infant_Distress/

Vik T, Grote V, Escribano J, et al. Infantile colic, prolonged crying, and maternal postnatal depression. *Acta Paediat.* 2009;98:1344-1348. doi:10.1016/j.chc.2021.04.013r.

Zeevenhooven J, Browne PD, L'Hoir MP, et al. Infant colic: mechanism and management. *Nat Rev Gastroenterol Hepatol.* 2018 Aug;15(8):479-496.

CHAPTER 29

Limp

Tracy Omoegbele, MD, Amanda Messer, MD, and Amy Prudhomme, MD

BACKGROUND

"Limp" is a common complaint in pediatric clinics, urgent care centers, and emergency rooms. The differential diagnosis for a limping child is broad and includes a wide spectrum of potential diseases, from benign and self-resolving to emergent and limb-threatening. A diagnosis can often be narrowed down with a thorough history and physical evaluation. Knowledge of possible limp etiologies can prevent further complications. This chapter reviews the approach to a child with limp and topics relevant to the pediatric hospitalist.

PATHOPHYSIOLOGY

The American Academy of Pediatrics defines "limp" as "a deviation from the normal pattern of gait." Understanding normal walking patterns by age can aid in assessing a child who limps. Most toddlers appear to have a wide-based gait with a degree of bowing. By 7 years of age, children usually achieve adult gait and posture.

Limp can be further described by gait pathology, which can help provide clues about the diagnosis.

HISTORY

A detailed history helps identify the likely cause of limp and provides key information to guide diagnostic testing.

Some conditions are much more likely in certain age groups (**Table 29-1**), such as transient synovitis in a toddler or slipped capital femoral epiphysis (SCFE) in an older child or adolescent. The acuity vs. chronicity of symptoms also helps narrow the differential. Limps that are acute in nature are typically due to infection or trauma, whereas chronic limps are usually secondary to a neurological disorder or developmental pathology. Associated symptoms are helpful in narrowing down a differential diagnosis. For example, the presence or absence of fever could point toward an infectious and/or inflammatory cause such as

TABLE 29-1 Age-Specific Diagnosis in Patients Presenting with a Limp

Toddler (<3 years)	Child (3-10 years)	Adolescent (>10 years)
Developmental Dysplasia of the hip	Legg-Calve-Perthes disease	Slipped capital femoral epiphysis
Congenital limb deficiencies	Stress fractures	Legg-Calve-Perthes disease
Neuromuscular abnormalities	Tumors	Juvenile idiopathic arthritis
Painful gait	Osteochondrosis	Overuse syndromes
Toddler fracture	Kohler disease	Osteochondrosis
Septic arthritis	Osteochondritis dissecans	Tumors
Reactive arthritis	Osgood-Schlatter disease	Osteochondritis dissecans
Transient synovitis	Transient synovitis	Stress fractures
Osteomyelitis	Osteomyelitis	Osteomyelitis
Foreign object in knee or foot	Leg-length discrepancy	Discoid meniscus
		Tarsal coalition

osteomyelitis or septic arthritis. The character of pain is often difficult to assess, especially in children younger than 5 years of age; however, certain features of pain may help distinguish the diagnosis.

The history should also include questions about recent trauma, recent illnesses, and a thorough review of systems.

PHYSICAL EXAM

A full examination in a hospital gown is indicated to ensure no outward signs of trauma or injury are missed. Examination should include inspection and palpation for erythema, warmth, edema, asymmetry, and perfusion; active and passive range of motion while sitting and/or supine; and gait evaluation. Examination of the unaffected extremity should take place prior to examining the affected side, which may help facilitate cooperation. A thorough neurological exam may also be indicated based on history and exam.

DIFFERENTIAL DIAGNOSIS

The differential diagnoses for a child presenting with a limp is broad and includes traumatic injuries, infections, neoplasms, inflammatory conditions, and developmental causes (**Table 29-2**). Traumatic injuries, infections, and neoplasms may lead to serious complications if diagnosis and treatment are delayed. Prompt evaluation and diagnosis are important to determine if a serious condition is present.

DIAGNOSTIC EVALUATION

TRAUMA

Traumatic injuries may be explained by history alone. However, occult trauma is possible and should be considered in patients with limp or lower extremity pain without explanation. In patients with signs of traumatic injury that are unexplained or with inconsistent history, non-accidental trauma (NAT) should be considered. If NAT is suspected, a complete NAT workup should be done, which should include a skeletal survey, lab evaluation, and may include a computed tomography (CT) scan of the head if there are concerns for head trauma.

A toddler fracture occurs after minor twisting injury or fall, resulting in a spiral or oblique tibial shaft fracture. Some cases are missed given the normal exam outside of the limping and initial negative radiographs on presentation. The radiograph of the affected extremity is positive after 10 days to 2 weeks, once the healing process begins. Casting of the extremity for 4 weeks provides comfort and prevents worsening of the injury.

Puncture wounds and retained foreign bodies can also cause limp in a child. Some children may not report their foot being punctured, resulting in a retained foreign body. Although some caregivers report removal of the foreign body, fragments of the foreign body may be retained. Radiographs or ultrasonography are helpful for localizing foreign bodies for removal. If a foreign body is present on imaging or the child is unresponsive to antibiotics and local wound care, surgical exploration is indicated. Puncture wounds through sneakers raise concerns for *Pseudomonas* infections and children with such history should be re-evaluated within 48 hours after initiation with antibiotics.

INFECTION

Infections of the bones and joints can be caused by direct inoculation, hematogenous spread, or contiguous spread. Septic arthritis is inflammation of a joint due to an infection, peak age seen in those younger than 3 years old. Septic arthritis most commonly affects the knee, followed by the hip and ankle. The underlying infection is often bacterial, most commonly *Staphylococcus aureus*. *Kingella kingae* should be considered in children less than 3 years old. *Streptococcus pyogenes* and *Strepococcus pneumoniae* are also common. Less common pathogens include *Neisseria meningitidis* and *Neisseria gonorrhea* in sexually active adolescents, and *Salmonella*, which can be associated with an underlying diagnosis such as sickle cell disease. *Pseudomonas* should be considered if there is a puncture wound. Polymicrobial infections are seen in cases of intravenous (IV) drug use. Arthritis due to Lyme disease occurs secondary to tickborne infection with the spirochete *Borrelia burgdorferi* causing inflammation of one or more joints. Most often the knee is affected, but other joints can also be involved. Though uncommon, Lyme arthritis may present as monoarticular hip pain and can be difficult to distinguish from transient synovitis and septic arthritis.

Patients with septic arthritis typically present with acute pain and fever with refusal to move the joint or bear weight. A child with septic arthritis will likely have an erythematous, edematous joint, which is tender to palpation; however, when the hip is the affected joint, swelling and erythema may not be present. Children with septic arthritis may be toxic-appearing and notably in pain.

While exams are often helpful in distinguishing between septic arthritis and other diseases, such as transient synovitis, the Kocher criteria can also help determine the probability of septic arthritis when the hip is involved **(Table 29-3).** In septic arthritis, up to 40% of cases will have concurrent bacteremia. If septic arthritis is suspected, joint aspiration is indicated for diagnostic evaluation and decompression of the joint. Joint fluid studies include cell count and culture. Greater than 50,000 WBC/uL, more than 75% neutrophils, and/or positive gram stain are

TABLE 29-2 An Overview of Conditions That Cause Limping in a Child

Trauma	Infection	Inflammatory	Development	Neoplasm
• Fracture • Sprain • Contusion *Consider non-accidental trauma	• Septic arthritis • Osteomyelitis • Cellulitis • Lyme arthritis • Discitis • Pyomyositis • Reactive arthritis	• Rheumatologic conditions, including: lupus, arthritis, myositis • Enthesitis • Henoch-Schönlein purpura • Chronic Recurrent Multifocal Osteomyelitis	• Orthopedic ◦ Legg Calve Perthes disease ◦ Slipped capital femoral epiphysis (SCFE) ◦ Tarsal coalition ◦ Osteochondritis dissecans • Neuromuscular process ◦ Cerebral palsy ◦ Metabolic muscle disease	• Leukemia • Lymphoma • Benign bone or soft tissue • Malignant bone or soft tissue

TABLE 29-3 Kocher Criteria for Septic Arthritis

Kocher Criteria for Septic Arthritis of the Hip	
Criteria	**Probability for Septic Arthritis**
Non weight bearing	1. criterion – 3%
Temp > 38.5°C / 101.3°F	2. criteria – 40%
ESR > 40 mm/hr	3. criteria – 95%
WBC > 12,000 cells/mm^3	4. criteria – 99.6%

supportive of septic arthritis. Synovial fluid culture is positive in 50% to 60% of cases.

In septic arthritis, plain films may show soft tissue swelling or widened joint space. Ultrasound, technetium bone scan, or magnetic resonance imaging (MRI) may be considered for further evaluation in uncertain cases, but should not delay care in an ill-appearing patient.

Treatment for septic arthritis should begin with empiric antibiotic coverage for *S. aureus,* with consideration of methicillin-resistant *S. aureus* coverage based on local trends. Additional antibiotic treatment should be considered based on the patient's age and history, including consideration of *K. kingae, N. gonorrhea,* or *Salmonella*. Length of antibiotic treatment may vary, though is typically at least 2 to 4 weeks.

Osteomyelitis is an inflammatory disease of the bone which can occur alone or in combination with septic arthritis. The introduction of pathogens occurs similarly, and most commonly through hematogenous spread. 70% to 90% of cases are due to *S. aureus*. Consider *Streptococcus agalactiae* and gram-negative organisms in infants less than 2 months old. *K. kingae* should be considered in younger children, as well as *S. pyogenes* and *S. pneumoniae.* Less common pathogens include: *Bartonella henslae, Mycobactereium tuberculosis, Histoplasma,* and *Cryptococcus.* While *Haeomophilus influenzae type b* was previously a common cause of septic arthritis and osteomyelitis, it is now rare due to the introduction of the Hib vaccine.

For children in whom acute hematogenous osteomyelitis is a concern, a blood culture and a C-reactive protein (CRP) should be obtained. The Infectious Diseases Society of America (IDSA) does not recommend using serum procalcitonin for monitoring of acute hematogenous osteomyelitis. MRI with contrast is the diagnostic modality of choice for osteomyelitis and deep soft-tissue infections.

Treatment of osteomyelitis includes empiric antibiotics and surgical drainage and/or debridement if indicated. Surgical debridement is recommended for patients with evidence of sepsis, rapid progression, or in whom a fluid collection larger than 2 cm is present. In an ill-appearing or worsening patient, empiric antibiotics should not be delayed while awaiting surgical specimens. Initiation of antibiotics in osteomyelitis does not interfere with pathogen identification in the bone, when the specimen is collected within 24 to 48 hours. As with septic arthritis, empiric antibiotic coverage should include coverage of *S. aureus*, including methicillin-resistant strains based on local trends. Consider coverage for other bacteria based on age and history, such as *K. kingae or Salmonella spp.*

Transition to oral therapy is recommended for patients who demonstrate clinical improvement and down-trending CRP with intravenous (IV) therapy and are able to tolerate an oral regimen. For a patient clinically improving on IV therapy but oral therapy is not an option, outpatient parenteral antibiotic therapy may be pursued in order to avoid prolonged hospitalization. However, consideration of risk/benefit stratification related to long-term IV lines, such as a peripherally inserted central catheter (PICC) should be discussed. Long-term subspecialty follow-up is recommended for monitoring during and after treatment.

Discitis is an infection of the intervertebral space resulting in inflammation of the intervertebral discs, ultimately causing pain for the patient. This condition is relatively uncommon and difficult to treat due to the limited blood supply to these areas. Common pathogens identified in discitis are similar to those seen in septic arthritis. Discitis usually occurs in children younger than 5 years. Clinical findings on presentation include back pain, limp, and refusal to bear weight and bend forward, and tenderness over the involved spine. Abdominal pain and vomiting may be the only complaints at presentation. Erythrocyte sedimentation rate (ESR) is elevated in more than 90% of patients. MRI is the best modality of choice for diagnosis. Blood cultures are usually sterile and aspiration of the disc space for cultures is usually not warranted. Empiric antibiotic therapy should be started and directed against pathogens described earlier, as well as initiation of analgesics for pain control.

INFLAMMATION

Transient synovitis may present similarly to septic arthritis with a limp or refusal to bear weight, but generally patients are non-toxic appearing and there is often a history of recent viral illness such as upper respiratory symptoms, vomiting, or diarrhea.

Transient synovitis is self-limited, painful inflammation of the synovial joint lining, typically following a viral infection. It is most commonly seen in ages 3 to 10 years, though it can occur in younger or older patients. Patients usually present with monoarticular, unilateral joint involvement; some cases involve bilateral joints. Ultrasound is helpful in detecting effusion. Joint aspiration for hip pain may be considered if needed to delineate from other diagnoses in a patient with fever, elevated ESR, or severe pain. Treatment includes supportive care with non-steroidal anti-inflammatory drugs (NSAIDs) for pain control. If the diagnosis is not certain, these patients may be admitted for observation and serial exams. Patients usually demonstrate improvement in 24 to 48 hours and symptoms resolve within 7 to 10 days. Recurrence can occur in up to 20% of patients.

Benign acute childhood myositis, sometimes informally called viral myositis, is also mild, self-limited, and follows a viral illness. Patients are often school-age and median timing of onset is 3 days after resolution of the viral illness. Symptoms usually involve an acute refusal to walk and bilateral lower extremity pain. Most commonly, the lower legs are involved, though rarely other areas can be affected. Development of myoglobinuria or renal failure is very rare in these patients; laboratory evaluation (creatine phosphokinase level, urine myoglobin, renal function studies) can be obtained in severe cases to rule out rhabdomyolysis and renal injury/failure. Benign acute childhood myositis usually self-resolves within days. Management involves supportive care with rest and pain control.

Rheumatologic conditions such as Immunoglobulin A vasculitis (Henoch-Schonlein Purpura), dermatomyositis, juvenile idiopathic arthritis (JIA), and systemic lupus erythematosus should be considered in certain cases. Prolonged or recurrent symptoms may indicate an underlying rheumatologic condition. The pathophysiology and presentation of some of these conditions is discussed in Section Q: Rheumatology.

Osgood-Schlatter disease is an overuse injury usually seen in children 9 to 14 years old characterized by apophysitis of the tibial tubercle through traction. History usually involves a child participating in running or jumping sports and over time develop a limp with pain that worsens with activity. Exam findings include tenderness and swelling of the tibial tubercle that sometimes appear as a lump on exam. ROM of the hip and knee are usually normal, and radiographs are generally not indicated. Rest, ice to the affected area, and NSAIDs are first line for management. Orthopedist evaluation and physical therapy may be helpful if symptoms do not improve with symptomatic treatment.

Sever disease, also known as calcaneal apophysitis, typically affects children between 7 and 9 years of age that wear flat shoes or those active in sports that cause repetitive stress to the heel. This condition usually occurs during growth spurts. Patients usually complain of heel pain and on exam, heel tenderness with swelling, limping, and limited or painful ankle dorsiflexion. Treatment involves stretching of the Achilles tendon, rest or limiting exercising activity, NSAIDs, and a change in footwear with heel inserts.

DEVELOPMENTAL

The most common hip pathologies that cause limp in a developing child are developmental dysplasia of the hip (DDH), Legg-Calvé-Perthes Disease (LCPD), and slipped capital femoral epiphyses (SCFE). DDH is an abnormality of the hip that involves dysplasia of the acetabulum preventing the femoral head from fitting into the acetabulum. Individuals at high risk for DDH include females, firstborn children, breech presentation at birth, and those with a family history of DDH. Most cases present with an abnormal gait or painless limp when missed before walking age.

Physical examination usually displays uneven skin folds on the thigh, limping, discrepant leg length, and if both hips are affected, a waddling gait. Ultrasound of the hips and pelvis is preferred for confirming diagnosis when the patient is less than 3 months old given lack of bone ossification. When the patient is older than 3 months, radiographs are best for confirming diagnosis. Affected children should be referred to an orthopedist for further evaluation and management.

LCPD is an idiopathic avascular necrosis of the femoral head. It generally occurs in children 4 to 8 years old, with a higher incidence in males. Risk factors include a family history of LCPD, low birth weight, and abnormal birth presentation. Onset is insidious and patients usually present with intermittent hip, knee, groin, or thigh pain, and a painless limp. Physical exam findings are notable for loss of internal rotation and abduction, a limp, and, if diagnosis is delayed, limb length discrepancy. Radiograph of the hips and pelvis is the preferred method for diagnosis. Referral to an orthopedist with NSAIDs, limited activities, and physical therapy is the treatment of choice for LCPD.

SCFE is characterized by slippage of the proximal femoral epiphyses from the metaphysis of the femur. This condition is most common in adolescents, with a predominance in males that are obese and undergoing a period of growth spurt. Pain usually occurs in the hip, but there are some cases with groin, thigh, and knee pain. Patients usually present on exam with a Trendelenburg limp with external rotation of the affected hip. Some cases present with refusal to bear weight. Anterior Posterior (AP) and frog-leg lateral radiographs of both hips are diagnostic. Consider screening for endocrine and metabolic conditions if obesity is present. Orthopedic surgical consultation and management is indicated.

ONCOLOGIC

It is important to note that some cancers may present initially with bone or joint pain, or a child with a limp. In a 2016 systematic review and meta-analysis, limb pain was a presenting symptom in 43% of cases of leukemia, highlighting the need for a thorough history and physical in patients with unexplained limb pain or limp.

Bone tumors are also a consideration in a patient with pain and/or swelling of a bone or joint. Associated symptoms include systemic symptoms such as fever or weight loss, pain at nighttime, or persistence of symptoms for several weeks. The most common bone cancers in children are osteosarcoma and Ewing sarcoma. Rhabdomyosarcomas can also present with lower extremity pain, depending on the site of origin.

Osteochondroma is a benign tumor that forms over the distal femur and proximal tibia. Occurrence is usually seen in children ages 3 to 5 years who present with pain with activity and a mass near the joints. Children may also present with limp if the mass is large and near a muscle group. Radiographs usually confirm the diagnosis, but biopsy is indicated for a definitive diagnosis.

Osteoid Osteoma is also a benign tumor that causes limping and pain in a child. The lesion is a small nidus surrounded by reactive bone. Dull, aching pain worse with activity and at night are the common complaints. Osteoid Osteoma is distinguished from other tumors because of its response to anti-inflammatory medications. CT scan is the imaging modality of choice for diagnosis. Evaluation by an orthopedist is recommended for treatment and management.

Pediatric hospitalists will encounter patients admitted for limp or refusal to walk. The differential diagnosis for pediatric limp is broad and includes a wide array of diseases. A thorough history and physical exam can help narrow down potential diagnoses and guide diagnostic evaluation, if indicated.

KEY POINTS

- Musculoskeletal complaints are common in children. Many can be managed in an outpatient setting, though some will require hospitalization for evaluation and treatment.
- The differential for limp is broad. History and physical exam is especially important for narrowing the differential. Any concern for infection should be promptly evaluated.
- Subspecialty consultation may be indicated for patients with suspected serious infections, trauma, compartment syndrome, or malignancy.

SUGGESTED READINGS

Akin E, Schiffern A. Evaluating a Child Who Has a Limp. *A Pediatric Perspective*, 2013. Available from: https://www.gillettechildrens.org/assets/uploads/for-medical-professionals/A_Pediatric_Perspective_2013_Limping_Child.pdf.

Arndt CA, Rose PS, Folpe AL, Laack NN. Common musculoskeletal tumors of childhood and adolescence. Mayo Clin Proc. 2012;87(5):475-487.

Bradley JS, Woods CR. Clinical Practice Guideline by the Pediatric Infectious Diseases Society and the Infectious Diseases Society of America: 2021 Guideline on Diagnosis and Management of Acute Hematogenous Osteomyelitis in Pediatrics. *IDSA*, 5 Aug. 2021. Available from: https://www.idsociety.org/practice-guideline/bone-and-joint-infections—osteomyelitis/.

Brisca G, Mariani M, Pirlo D, et al. Management and outcome of benign acute childhood myositis in pediatric emergency department. *Ital J Pediatr*. 2021;47:57.

Castellazzi L, Mantero M, Esposito S. Update on the management of pediatric acute osteomyelitis and septic arthritis. *Int J Mol Sci*. 2016;17(6):855.

Clarke RT, Van den Bruel A, Bankhead C, Mitchell CD, Phillips B, Thompson MJ. Clinical presentation of childhood leukaemia: a systematic review and meta-analysis. *Arch Dis Child*. 2016;101(10):894-901.

Cook PC. Transient synovitis, septic hip, and Legg-Calvé-Perthes disease: an approach to the correct diagnosis. *Pediatr Clin North Am*. 2014;61(6):1109-1118.

Glotzbecker MP, Kocher MS, Sundel RP, Shore BJ, Spencer SA, Kasser JR. Primary Lyme arthritis of the pediatric hip. *J Pediatr Orthop*. 2011;31(7):787-790.

Herman MJ, Martinek M. The limping child. *Pediatr Rev*. 2015;36(5): 184-95; quiz 196-7. Available from: https://publications.aap.org/pediatricsinreview/article/36/5/184/34877/The-Limping-Child.

Kocher MS, Mandiga R, Murphy JM, et al. A clinical practice guideline for treatment of septic arthritis in children: efficacy in improving process of care and effect on outcome of septic arthritis of the hip. *J Bone Joint Surg Am*. 2003;85(6):994-9.

Magee H, Goldman RD. Viral myositis in children. *Can Fam Physician*. 2017;63(5):365-368.

Muscara JD, Blazar E. Diskitis. [Updated 2022 May 13]. In: StatPearls [Internet]. Treasure Island (FL): StatPearls Publishing; 2022 Jan-. Available from: https://www.ncbi.nlm.nih.gov/books/NBK541047/.

Whitelaw CC, Varacallo M. Transient Synovitis - Statpearls - NCBI Bookshelf. *Transient Synovitis*, 2022, https://www.ncbi.nlm.nih.gov/books/NBK459181/.

CHAPTER 30

Neck Pain and Swelling

Mary M. Orr, MD, MPH, Matthew T. Lister, MD, and Nicole E. St Clair, MD

BACKGROUND

Neck pain can be present with or without swelling. Although neck pain is a common presenting symptom, it is rarely a discharge diagnosis. The presence, absence, and location of swelling are greatly useful in determining the etiology of pain. This chapter emphasizes the most common nontraumatic diagnoses associated with neck pain and swelling that result in hospital admissions for children.

DEFINITIONS

A variety of terms deserve attention in the description and management of neck pain symptoms:

Neck stiffness: an abnormal preferred position of the neck or a normal position with restricted range of motion.

Meningismus: neck stiffness related to meningeal irritation or inflammation.

Torticollis: neck stiffness associated with the child holding his or her head to the side with the chin rotated in the opposite direction due to sternocleidomastoid muscle spasm (Latin for "twisted neck").

Trismus: limited opening of the jaw due to involuntary muscle spasm and pain.

Lymphadenopathy: enlargement of solitary lymph nodes or chains of nodes by any cause with or without a milder degree of associated pain

Lymphadenitis: an acute, painful infection of individual lymph nodes, typically by bacterial or atypical infectious agents.

Various neck spaces or potential spaces deserve description (**Figure 30-1**), as involvement of a particular space narrows the differential, determines the presentation, and may dictate treatment of the disorder.

Sublingual space: (supramylohyoid space, a subdivision of the submandibular space) space beneath the tongue, medial to the body of the mandible and superior to the myelohyoid muscle.

Peritonsillar space: a potential space between the capsule of the palatine tonsil and the superior constrictor muscle of the pharynx.

Danger space: a potential space that is bound superiorly by the skull base, anteriorly by the alar fascia, and posteriorly by the prevertebral fascia, extending down to the diaphragm.

Retropharyngeal space: anterior to the danger space and posterior to the visceral space containing the esophagus and trachea. It potentially communicates laterally with the parapharyngeal and danger spaces.

Parapharyngeal space: (also pharyngomaxillary space or lateral pharyngeal space) best described as an inverted pyramid with the base at the skull base and the apex at the greater cornu of the hyoid bone, lateral to the superior pharyngeal constrictors, medial to the parotid gland, mandible, and lateral pterygoid muscles, anterior to the prevertebral fascia, and posterior to the pterygomandibular raphe.

Masticator space: surrounds the muscles of mastication including the pterygoids, temporalis, and masseter muscles, lying anterior to the parotid, anterior and lateral to the parapharyngeal space, and both medial and lateral to the mandibular ramus. It is bound superficially by the superficial layer of the deep cervical fascia.

General definitions applicable to a description of infections anywhere in the body:

Cellulitis: a superficial infection involving skin or other surface layers without discernible fluid collection, usually with signs of pain/itching, induration, erythema, and warmth.

Phlegmon: a soft tissue infection with signs including pain, induration, and functional impairment. Imaging findings may include edema of surrounding tissues, blurring of fascial planes, and possible necrosis of tissues, but no clearly defined capsule, fluid pocket, or enhancing rim on contrast imaging. It may or may not be possible to obtain fluid from a phlegmon using needle or open techniques.

Abscess: a walled-off collection of necrotic tissue and purulence which typically exhibits an enhancing rim and hypodense fluid center on CT imaging. It is difficult to distinguish abscess from phlegmon without contrast-enhanced imaging.

PATHOPHYSIOLOGY

Neck pain and swelling can have many causes including infectious, vascular, inflammatory, neoplastic, iatrogenic, congenital, autoimmune, traumatic, neurologic, traumatic, and idiopathic etiologies. Because of the complex anatomy and diverse structures in the neck, various pathologies may present with similar symptoms. Therefore, accurate diagnosis relies heavily on examination and imaging findings.

EVALUATION

PATIENT HISTORY

A detailed history can be invaluable in determining the likely causes of neck pain and/or localized neck swelling in a pediatric patient (**Table 30-1**). A recent and past history including preceding illness, injury, procedures (including dental work), and exposures along with the location and evolution of the pain and/or swelling can help paint a general picture. Painless enlargement of isolated or clustered lymph nodes in the neck is often associated with neoplasia or congenital processes such as branchial cleft or thyroglossal duct cysts. Significant functional impairment or pain with activities, including difficulty with breathing, chewing, swallowing, speaking, or hearing may point to a specific location of swelling, inflammation, or neurologic involvement. The presence of fever, headache, mental status change, gait disturbance, vomiting, and bowel or bladder dysfunction may indicate more serious systemic or neurologic involvement. Systemic findings such as weight loss, fatigue, or night sweats may suggest chronic infectious, inflammatory, or neoplastic etiologies. Family history can be helpful in some cases of rheumatologic or vascular disease. A thorough past medical and surgical history including medication use, genetic syndromes, bleeding disorders, dysmorphologies, and immunodeficiency may point to known association with or predisposition to presenting pathology.

PHYSICAL EXAMINATION

On inspection, it is important to note the general appearance of the patient, including his or her position of comfort. Signs of respiratory distress or upper airway swelling could include difficulty managing saliva and other secretions, stridor or stertor, posturing such as tripod posture with trunk leaning forward and neck extended, retractions, and paradoxical movement of the abdomen.

Asymmetry in the neck, face, or any paired structures should be noted and investigated. Eye examination should include taking note of pupils, conjunctivae, extraocular movements, and gross visual acuity when possible. Oral examination includes assessment of jaw opening, mucous membranes, teeth and gums, the floor of the mouth for induration and edema, tongue position and mobility, tonsils, posterior oropharynx, uvula, and palate. External ear (including position with notation of auricular proptosis or mastoid erythema, fluctuance, or tenderness), ear canal, and middle ear assessment should be completed. Superficial inspection of the nasal tissues may be performed with an otoscope. Neck examination should assess for visible erythema or asymmetric swelling, torticollis, head tilt, stiffness, meningeal irritation, palpable masses, lymphadenopathy, crepitus, fluctuance, tenderness, bruits, and skin lesions or rash. Note should be taken of whether any swelling is unilateral or bilateral, and whether it involves a single lymph node, a nodal chain, or multiple chains. The extent of local erythema, induration, or fluctuance along with possible tracks or defined margins should be delineated and marked at presentation for follow-up. Any sites that drain to the involved nodes should be examined for signs of infection. A general examination for other regional swelling or hepatosplenomegaly should be performed along with cardiac and pulmonary assessment for murmurs, wheezing, and abnormal breath sounds. Finally, a complete neurologic examination is important to confirm or rule out mental status changes, nerve palsy, generalized weakness or spasticity, sensory deficit, and gait abnormality.

DIFFERENTIAL DIAGNOSIS AND TREATMENT

When neck pain or swelling is a presenting symptom, there is a broad differential that includes infectious, vascular, inflammatory, idiopathic, neoplastic, iatrogenic, congenital, autoimmune, and traumatic etiologies (**Table 30-2**). The history and physical findings applied to a broad differential should guide diagnostic studies, requests for consultation, and treatment. Given the significant variation in possible diagnostic approaches and treatments based on presenting signs and symptoms, the following sections will describe potential etiologies for nontraumatic neck pain and swelling, each paired with disease-specific diagnostic and therapeutic recommendations.

INFECTIOUS CAUSES

Cervical Lymphadenitis and Lymphadenopathy Although often used interchangeably with lymphadenopathy, the term "lymphadenitis"

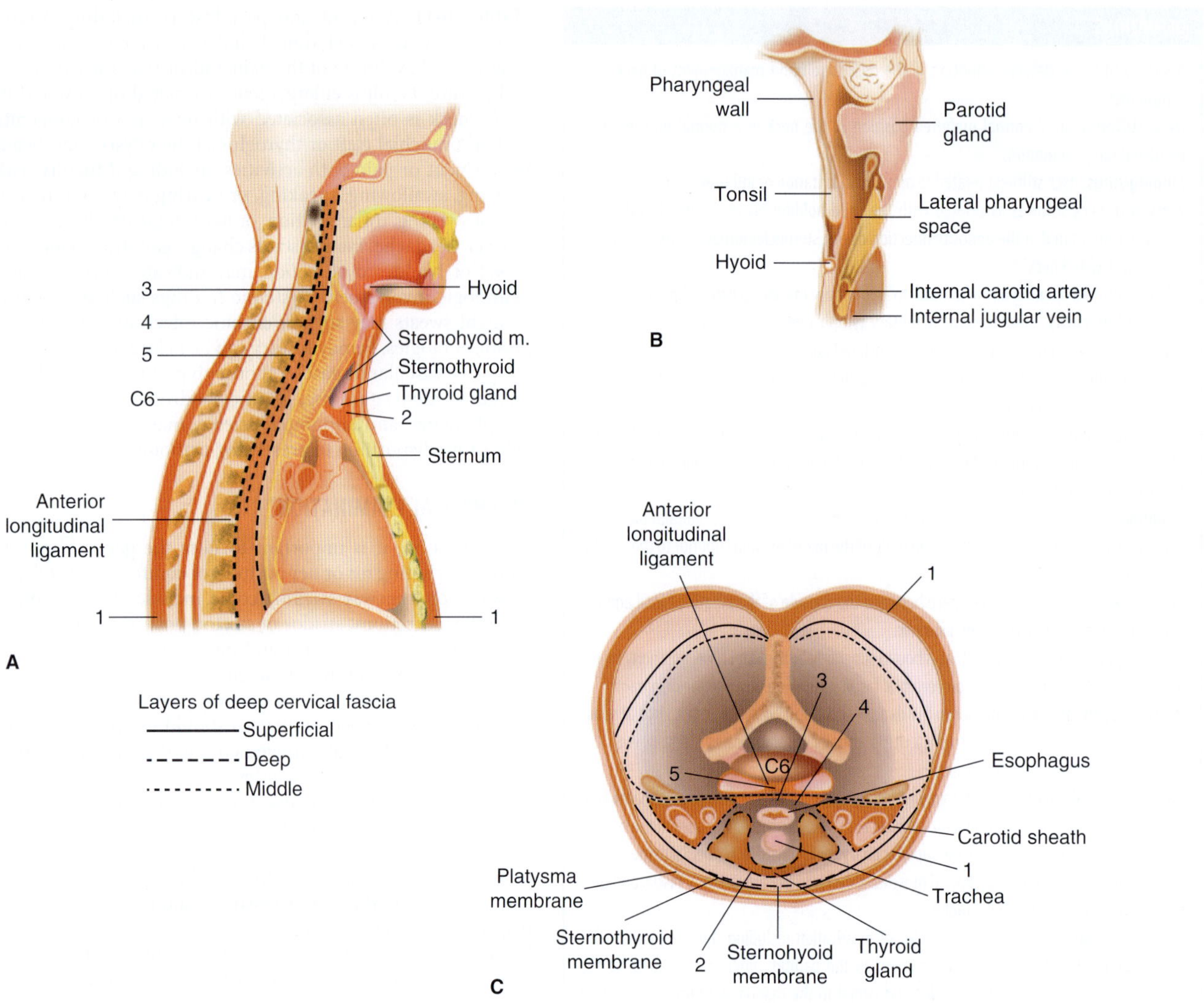

FIGURE 30-1. Lateral pharyngeal, retropharyngeal, and prevertebral spaces and their relationship with each other. (A) Midsagittal section of the head and neck. (B) Coronal section in the suprahyoid region of the neck. (C) Cross-section of the neck at the level of the thyroid isthmus. 1, superficial space; 2, pretracheal space; 3, retropharyngeal space; 4, danger space; 5, prevertebral space. (Reproduced with permission from Chow AW. Infections of the oral cavity, neck and head. In: Mandell GL, Bennett JE, Dolin R. *Principles and Practice of Infectious Diseases.* 7th ed. Churchill Livingstone Philapelphia, PA: Elsevier; 2010.)

should more properly be reserved for localized overwhelming infection of a lymph node or small group of nodes with a variety of bacterial and atypical pathogens rather than milder, more generalized inflammatory enlargement (reactive lymphadenopathy) in the course of a normal immune response to various pathogens including viruses. Although the cells in lymph nodes typically proliferate in the setting of infection, lymphadenitis results from a focal lymph node infection proceeding to tissue destruction or abscess involving the node, nearby soft tissue inflammation, and often cellulitis of the overlying skin. Because lymphatic drainage is regional, the involved node(s) may reflect a distal primary infection or a systemic illness affecting multiple lymph nodes. The differential diagnosis for involved lesions includes bacterial, mycobacterial, fungal, and viral processes, as well as noninfectious causes (**Table 30-3**). Acute, unilateral lymphadenitis is usually bacterial, while bilateral "reactive" lymphadenopathy is more often viral. The organisms most commonly responsible for lymphadenitis are the gram-positive *Staphylococcus aureus* (including methicillin-resistant strains) and group A β-hemolytic *Streptococcus* species. Other *Staphylococcus* and *Streptococcus* species (particularly group B streptococci in neonates) are implicated less frequently, but should be considered in the differential diagnosis of lymphadenitis resulting from breaks in the skin secondary to lacerations, insect bites, or dermatitis. A dental source can result in infections from gram-negative organisms such as *Bacteroides* and *Prevotella* or anaerobic bacteria such as *Actinomyces*.

Mycobacteria can also cause lymphadenitis, particularly in the cervical lymph node chains, and tends to be a more subacute or chronic presentation. *Mycobacterium tuberculosis* can cause focal lymphadenitis or generalized lymphadenopathy, but atypical mycobacteria are usually the culprit organisms in focal soft tissue infections. The most common mycobacteria species implicated in lymphadenitis is *Mycobacterium avium* complex (MAC). MAC infections typically affect preschool-aged children, most often involve the submandibular nodes, and the overlying skin can be violaceous.

Close attention should be paid to possible cutaneous sources of drainage to a regional lymph node. Lymphadenitis can result from progression of local inoculation and trauma, such as with gram-negative *Bartonella henselae*, resulting in cat-scratch disease; gram-negative *Pasteurella multocida* after a cat or dog bite; or local fungal infection such as tinea capitis. With a worrisome clinical presentation in the setting of possible arthropod or zoonotic exposure to rare organisms, the differential diagnosis should be widened to include tularemia, anthrax, and bubonic plague (*Yersinia pestis*). Although these diseases are uncommon in developed countries, timely recognition and aggressive antibiotic treatment are necessary.

TABLE 30-1 History Components

Area of Pain or Swelling
Location, prior swellings in that location
Chronology, progression, local symptoms
Recent injuries, infections, or breaks in skin distal to involved site
Review of Systems
Fever course, if present
Malaise
Bruising or bleeding
Weight loss
Exposures
Geography—residence and travel
Sick contacts
Family members or caretakers with chronic cough
Contact with prison or homeless populations
Insect bites
Exposure to pets, farm animals, or wild animals, or to their meat or carcasses
Past Medical History
Recent infections, including upper respiratory infections
History of prior infections
Past dental or surgical procedures
Major illnesses, dysmorphologies, diagnosed syndromes

TABLE 30-2 Differential Diagnosis of Neck Pain and Swelling in Children

Diagnostic Category	Diagnosis
Infectious	Cervical lymphadenitis
	Cervical lymphadenopathy
	Peritonsillar abscess
	Retropharyngeal abscess
	Parapharyngeal abscess
	Jugular septic thrombophlebitis (Lemierre syndrome)
	Dental abscess
	Submandibular space infection (Ludwig angina)
	Sialadenitis
	Meningitis
	Cervical osteomyelitis
	Suppurative thyroiditis
	Infected branchial cleft cyst
	Infected thyroglossal duct cyst
Vascular	Vertebral artery dissection
	Stroke
Inflammatory/ Idiopathic	Atlantoaxial instability
	Cervical spine stenosis
	Acute cervical disk calcification
	Relapsing polychondritis
Neoplastic	Posterior fossa, spinal canal, and neck tumors
	Osteoid osteoma
Iatrogenic	Non-traumatic atlantoaxial rotatory subluxation
	Conditions associated with surgical positioning
Congenital/CNS	Chiari I malformation
Autoimmune	Arthritis and spondyloarthropathy
Traumatic	Vertebral fracture
	Spinal epidural hematoma
	Esophageal injury
	Laryngotracheal injury

CNS, central nervous system.

Lymphadenopathy simply refers to lymph node enlargement. It is itself a symptom and/or a physical exam finding rather than a diagnosis such as lymphadenitis. Lymphadenopathy may be painless or accompanied by mild-moderate pain or discomfort due to local tissue inflammation; however, it is usually much less painful than lymphadenitis and typically lacks overlying skin erythema, induration, and cellulitis. Lymphadenopathy may be localized when secondary to an isolated infection or in certain forms of lymphoma, especially Hodgkin's disease. Generalized and symmetric lymphadenopathy is usually reactive, indicating an immune response to a variety of viral pathogens, including Epstein-Barr virus (EBV), cytomegalovirus, varicella, toxoplasma, adenovirus, coxsackievirus, herpes simplex virus, human herpesvirus 6, and human immunodeficiency virus (HIV).

Diagnostic evaluation should be guided by history and physical exam. Acute pyogenic bacterial lymphadenitis is most often caused by *Staphylococcus* or *Streptococcus*. Laboratory testing is indicated if there is suspicion of a disease other than localized *Staphylococcus* or *Streptococcus* infection, thereby affecting treatment decisions. Bacteremia can occur in pediatric patients—particularly young infants with fever—with significant focal bacterial lymph node infections, so obtaining blood cultures may help identify a bacterial organism as well as its sensitivities. A complete blood count with leukocyte differential may be helpful to determine leukocytosis and indicate possible infectious mononucleosis or oncologic processes. Infectious mononucleosis is caused by EBV and commonly presents with atypical lymphocytosis, lymphadenopathy, and fever as well as exudative pharyngitis and hepatosplenomegaly. Initial testing for EBV may include heterophile antibody testing—most sensitive in patients older than 4 years—as well as EBV serum titers for immunoglobulins M, G, and EBNA; these tests are most sensitive after 2 to 3 weeks of illness. Cytomegalovirus infections can present similarly to EBV infections and can be tested by sending titers. HIV testing should be performed if there is history of possible HIV exposure such as unprotected sex or if there is suspicion of an underlying immune deficiency. Acute retroviral syndrome can present with lymphadenopathy and advanced disease can present with opportunistic infection. Depending on the differential diagnosis for a given patient, serology for more unusual organisms may also be indicated.

If there is a history of travel to developing countries or other possible exposure to tuberculosis (TB), a Mantoux tuberculin purified protein derivative (PPD) test should be done. A negative PPD test should not be considered definitive in the setting of high clinical suspicion for TB, because 10% of immunocompetent children with culture-documented TB may have a negative PPD; this number is higher in immunocompromised patients and in those with disseminated TB. Atypical mycobacterial disease can sometimes cause a positive PPD. An interferon-gamma release assay (IGRA) has less cross-reactivity and can be useful to distinguish non-tuberculosis from *M. tuberculosis* in children 2 years and older, though cross-reactions can occur with *M. kansasii*, *M. marinum*, and *M. szulgai*.

CT with contrast can be useful in the acute setting to identify most pathologies in the differential of neck pain and swelling. To spare radiation, ultrasonography can be used if there is a palpable, fluctuant, superficial mass. MRI with and without contrast can identify anatomy and deeper pathology but may require sedation in children.

If the infection has a loculated component or an organized abscess, drainage may be therapeutic as well as diagnostic. Fine-needle aspiration, under ultrasound guidance if necessary, is a useful method of obtaining a fluid sample for bacterial, mycobacterial, and fungal stains and cultures. It is important to note that many organisms that cause lymphadenitis, especially mycobacteria, are fastidious and may not grow in culture. Incision for drainage can lead to a chronically draining sinus

TABLE 30-3 Differential Diagnosis of Lymphadenitis

Lymphadenitis due to the Following Organisms	Other Causes of Cervical Lymphadenopathy That Can Mimic Lymphadenitis
Common skin and nasopharyngeal flora	Viral infections
Staphylococcus aureus, including MRSA	Epstein-Barr virus
Streptococcus species, particularly group A	Cytomegalovirus
Bacteria from a dental source	Varicella-zoster virus
Bacteroides, *Prevotella*, other gram-negative dental organisms	Adenovirus
Actinomyces and other anaerobes	Coxsackievirus
Mycobacteria	Herpes simplex virus
Atypical mycobacteria, particularly *Mycobacterium ovium* complex	Human herpesvirus 6 (roseola)
Mycobacterium tuberculosis	Human immunodeficiency virus
Less common organisms that can infect lymph nodes after local infection	Measles
Bartonella henselae (cat-scratch disease)	Mumps
Trichophyton or *Microsporum* species (resulting in tinea capitis)	Rheumatologic causes
Sporothrix schenckii (after gardening)	Kawasaki disease
Vibrio species and other water-based organisms	Kikuchi disease
After exposure in relevant geographic regions	System lupus erythematosus
Wuchereria bancrofti or *Brugia* species (filariasis)	Juvenile rheumatoid arthritis
Histoplasma capsulatum (histoplasmosis)	Multisystem Inflammatory Syndrome in Children (MIS-C)
Francisella tularensis (tularemia)	Periodic Fever, apthous stomatitis, pharyngitis, adenitis (PFAPA)
Bacillus anthracis (anthrax)	Immune deficiencies
Yersinia pestis (bubonic plague)	Chronic granulomatous disease
Special organisms in immunocompromised patients	Hyper-IgE syndrome
Burkholderia cepacia	Leukocyte adhesion deficiency
	Inflammatory processes
Other causes of neck swelling	Sarcoidosis
Anatomic malformations	Oncologic processes
Head and neck area	Lymphoma
Thyroglossal duct cyst (midline)	Lymphoproliferative disorders
Branchial cleft cyst (lateral)	Castleman Disease
Dermoid cyst	Langerhan's cell histiocytosis
Salivary gland processes	Metastatic lymph nodes from other primary tumors
	Primary neoplastic processes
	Soft tissue neoplasms

tract, particularly in the setting of a mycobacterial infection; in these cases, excisional biopsy is the preferred approach. If there is little concern about rare or resistant organisms and if a good response to antibiotic treatment alone is expected in a given patient, treatment is often initiated presumptively. When wound cultures cannot be obtained and concerns exist for resistant organisms, swabs from the nares, axilla, and/or rectum to detect for methicillin-resistant *S. aureus* (MRSA) colonization may be performed, though concordance of nasal carriage and infectious agent is not assured.

Treatment is tailored to the most likely organism. For suspected *Staph* or *Strep* infection, recommended antibiotics are cefazolin/cephalexin, or clindamycin if allergic, for 5 to 7 days, with duration tailored by resolution of signs or symptoms. Consider MRSA coverage based on local prevalence. *Bartonella henselae* is generally a self-limited disease, resolving spontaneously in 2 to 4 months. In most cases antibiotics are not necessary, but some recommend therapy in acutely or severely ill patients with systemic symptoms and all immunocompromised patients. Azithromycin, clarithromycin, ciprofloxacin, doxycycline, trimethoprim-sulfamethoxazole, ceftriaxone, gentamicin, and rifampin have in vitro activity against the organism. There are no controlled trials of drug treatment of non-tuberculosis mycobacteria in children. Complete surgical excision is curative and limits potential spontaneous drainage that can result in scarring. If excision is incomplete, not an option, or disease recurs, clarithromycin or azithromycin plus ethambutol and/or rifampin can be used. Resolution is slow and treatment is continued for months.

Deep Neck Space Infections Peritonsillar abscess presents in patients of all ages, more commonly in older children and adolescents. There may be an antecedent tonsillar or upper respiratory infection (URI), but symptoms typically progress rapidly once unilateral throat pain begins. Symptoms include severe unilateral tonsillar pain, otalgia, odynophagia, and sometimes fevers. Signs include trismus, drooling, tender cervical adenopathy, asymmetry of tonsils with edema and intense erythema of the soft palate, and uvular deviation. Treatment includes specialty consultation with Otolaryngology for localization and drainage of the abscess and possible tonsillectomy followed by IV or oral antibiotic therapy. Peritonsillar "cellulitis" or phlegmon may have a similar presentation, but may respond to oral antibiotics and pain medication without the need for drainage. A CT scan is not always indicated, but may be helpful in cases with atypical presentation or in younger children (**Figure 30-2**).

Retropharyngeal phlegmons and abscesses occur most commonly in preschool children. They are usually the result of a suppurative lymph node infection in the retropharyngeal space. There is often an antecedent history of URI, and occasionally with the presence of neck stiffness

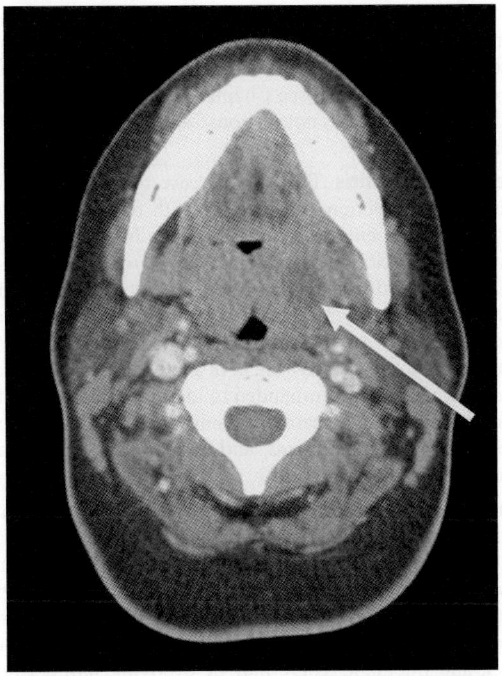

FIGURE 30-2. Computed tomography of a peritonsillar abscess. (Reproduced with permission from Children's Hospital of Wisconsin Imaging Department, David Gregg, MD.)

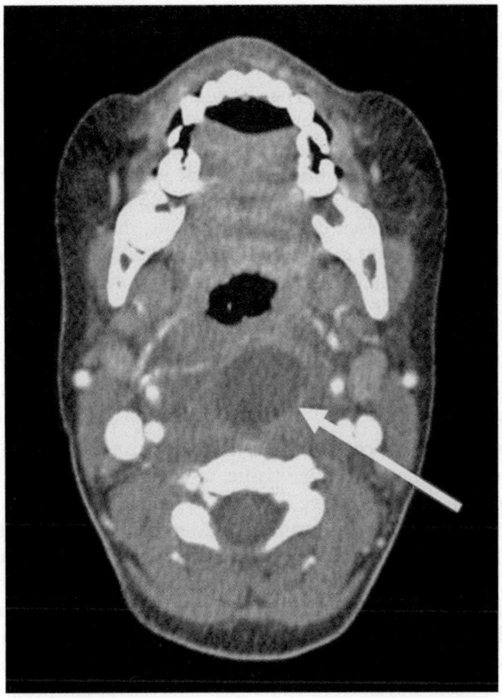

FIGURE 30-4. Computed tomography of a retropharyngeal abscess. (Reproduced with permission from Children's Hospital of Wisconsin Imaging Department, David Gregg, MD.)

and pain. Hallmarks include high fever, drooling, torticollis, dysphagia, odynophagia, edema or mass of the posterior pharyngeal wall, and airway distress. Diagnostic studies include lateral neck films, which are abnormal 90% of the time and, for more detail, CT scans (**Figures 30-3** and **30-4**). Typical pathogens include β-hemolytic streptococci, respiratory anaerobes, and *S. aureus*, though retropharyngeal swelling can also be seen with Kawasaki disease. Children with retropharyngeal infections should be hospitalized, started on empiric broad-spectrum antibiotics,

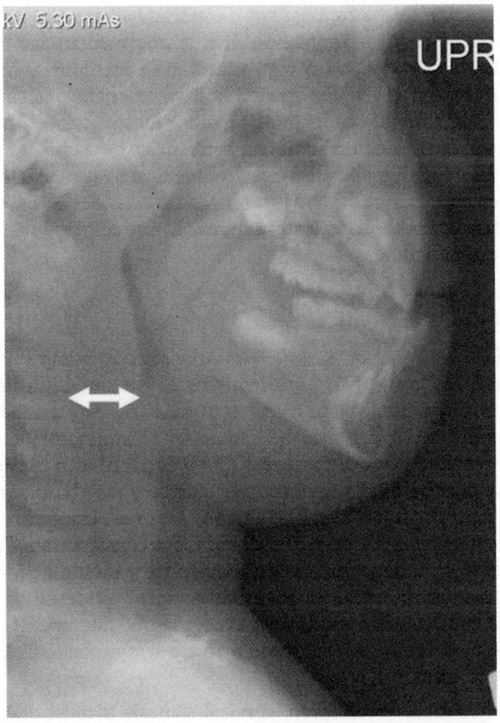

FIGURE 30-3. Enlarged retropharyngeal space secondary to soft tissue swelling anterior to the upper cervical bodies seen in a retropharyngeal abscess. (Reproduced with permission from Children's Hospital of Wisconsin Imaging Department, David Gregg, MD.)

and managed in consultation with an Otolaryngologist. Patients with airway compromise should undergo immediate airway stabilization and surgical drainage. Patients with early retropharyngeal infection without associated abscess (retropharyngeal cellulitis or phlegmon) may respond to antibiotics alone and not require surgical drainage. For stable patients with small or immature retropharyngeal abscesses, there is evidence to support initial management with antimicrobial therapy, close observation, and surgical drainage if there is not a clinical response within 24 to 48 hours. Those patients with mature retropharyngeal abscesses, particularly if >2 cm, generally require both drainage and antimicrobial therapy. The addition of corticosteroids may reduce the need for surgical drainage.

Suppurative infections can also occur in the parapharyngeal space. Patients tend to be older than those with retropharyngeal abscesses. Infections in this area often arise as a result of dental disease or procedures such as wisdom tooth extraction occurring in adolescents who have developed permanent dentition. Dysphagia and trismus are common; patients may also develop a Horner syndrome on the affected side and other unilateral cranial nerve deficits. An associated complication is septic jugular vein thrombophlebitis (Lemierre syndrome). The most useful imaging study is a CT scan with contrast to determine whether there is abscess formation. Treatment involves empirical coverage with broad-spectrum intravenous antibiotics. If there is no response to medical therapy within 24 to 72 hours, or an abscess is clearly identified, incision and drainage may be warranted.

Abscesses of the masticator space similarly occur in older children and adolescents who develop infections in their molars or have dental extractions including wisdom tooth extraction and become secondarily infected with oral pathogens. The presentation depends heavily on the location and extent of the abscess, whether it is lateral to the mandible causing primarily pain and trismus without airway effect, or medial to the mandible with pain, trismus, mass effect on the pharynx and possible airway edema. CT with contrast is the imaging study of choice and can often identify the involved source/tooth if not obvious based on dental procedure history. Broad spectrum antibiotics and intravenous steroids are an integral part of therapy at diagnosis. Consultation with Otolaryngology and Anesthesiology as well as Oral Surgery is warranted to determine the best method for abscess drainage and source control (including possible dental extraction) while minimizing risk to the airway.

Jugular Septic Thrombophlebitis (Lemierre Syndrome) Patients with Lemierre syndrome present with systemic findings concurrent with or following pharyngotonsillitis, dental infection, deep neck infection, mastoiditis, or sinusitis. The classic presentation is associated with a dental infection and foul-smelling breath. Most patients with jugular septic thrombophlebitis have unilateral neck pain below the mandibular angle along the sternocleidomastoid muscle with severe tenderness, but no discrete mass or other associated findings to account for the tenderness. Patients often present with shaking chills, spiking fevers, and possibly dyspnea. The most common organism identified is *Fusobacterium necrophorum*, although this infection is usually polymicrobial. The diagnosis is suggested if *F. necrophorum* grows from a blood culture, and it can be confirmed by contrast CT scan of the neck. Treatment is a 4- to 6-week course of broad-spectrum antibiotics to cover aerobic and anaerobic bacteria, and supportive care. Anticoagulation is recommended only if there is evidence of continued propagation of the thrombus.

Submandibular Space Infection (Ludwig Angina) Ludwig angina is a cellulitis of the connective tissue, fascia, and muscles of the submandibular space. The source is usually a dental infection. In its most severe and life-threatening form, induration of the submandibular tissues can force the tongue base to occlude the airway. It occurs most often in older children and adolescents. The clinical presentation includes a toxic-appearing patient with fever, foul breath, drooling, odynophagia; frequently the voice is affected. Physical examination characteristics include an erythematous, tender, and indurated floor of mouth, swollen and tender neck, and an elevated tongue. This is a rapidly progressive illness and represents a true airway emergency. Nearly all children require emergent intubation or tracheotomy. Treatment involves controlling the airway and administering broad-spectrum intravenous antibiotics; abscess is usually not identified, and imaging is not usually helpful in the initial assessment and management.

Dental Abscess Dental abscess is typically caused by mouth flora in the setting of dental caries. It typically presents with face or neck swelling, pain, and fever. A fluctuant area near the affected tooth or gum is sometimes palpable. The acute treatment is intravenous or oral antibiotics to cover aerobic and anaerobic organisms, followed by definitive dental treatment. For more information, see Chapter 31, Oral Lesions.

Sialadenitis Inflammation or infection of the major salivary glands may be a cause of neck pain. The most commonly affected are the parotid glands and submandibular glands. Edema, induration, tenderness, and occasionally warmth and erythema may be present and are usually unilateral. Causes of infection or inflammation include viral illnesses, ductal obstruction due to stones, dehydration leading to thickening of secretions and poor salivary flow with secondary infection, thickened secretions due to medications such as antihistamines and anticholinergics, autoimmune conditions associated with Sjogren syndrome, prior treatment with radiation or chemotherapy, and trauma to ducts. The most common pathogens are *Staphylococcus* species or other oral flora. Treatment includes aggressive oral hydration when feasible, IV hydration when necessary, IV or PO antibiotic therapy, heat over the affected gland, pressure/massage to encourage drainage of infected saliva, removal of obstructing debris or stone by an otolaryngologist if needed, and the use of sialogogues such as sour candy or lemons.

Meningitis The classic clinical presentation of meningitis is fever, meningismus, irritability, and vomiting in a toxic-appearing patient. It is usually associated with viral or bacterial infections. Diagnosis is made by evaluation of cerebral spinal fluid (CSF) from a lumbar puncture; CSF pleocytosis is present in most cases. Bacterial culture and viral studies can provide a definitive diagnosis. Appropriate treatment includes supportive care and empiric or targeted antimicrobial treatment. Please refer to Chapter 94 for further details pertaining to the evaluation and management of meningitis.

Cervical Osteomyelitis The clinical presentation of osteomyelitis of the cervical spine includes focal tenderness, limited range of motion, and fever. This infection occurs most often in children older than 8 years. The most common organism identified is *S. aureus*. Evidence of infection is supported by magnetic resonance imaging (MRI) or bone scan. Cultures of the blood or bone obtained by biopsy are useful in choosing antibiotics, but in their absence, treatment should be a prolonged course of antibiotics covering *S. aureus* and GABHS, with consideration of *Kingella kingae* for younger children (see Chapter 101). Surgical debridement is indicated if the patient does not demonstrate clinical improvement after appropriate treatment.

Suppurative Thyroiditis This rare disease typically occurs after an upper respiratory infection and presents with the acute onset of fever, chills, and a tender, enlarged thyroid gland. Infection is most often caused by *S. aureus*, *Streptococcus*, and *Enterobacter*. Diagnosis is made by ultrasound-guided needle aspiration or biopsy with culture. Thyroid function tests are rarely abnormal. Many cases may turn out to be related to a persistent thyroglossal duct, though some children have a pyriform sinus fistula. After treatment of acute infection, endoscopy, CT, or a barium swallow is recommended to identify a communication with the pyriform sinus. Initial treatment is empiric IV antibiotics to cover *S. aureus*, *Streptococcus pneumoniae*, and *Enterobacter*. Treatment can be narrowed based on culture results.

Other Infections Infections in congenital abnormalities such as a branchial cleft cyst/sinus or a thyroglossal duct cyst are not uncommon. Usually, there is a history of antecedent upper respiratory illness, followed by swelling of a midline neck cyst (in the case of a thyroglossal duct cyst) or a cyst along the sternocleidomastoid anterior border (in the case of a second branchial cleft cyst), which may then become painful, tender, and fluctuant. There may be overlying skin erythema, and drainage from a sinus tract in the case of a branchial cleft abnormality. Treatment is with needle aspiration or drainage procedures along with oral antibiotics covering *Staphylococcus* species for less severe infections. Rarely, an epidural abscess or infectious discitis in the cervical region can also present with fever and neck pain.

VASCULAR CAUSES

Spontaneous Arterial Dissection Dissection of the cervical and intracranial portions of the carotid and vertebrobasilar arteries may occur spontaneously or in association with trauma or other underlying risk factors. Classically, patients present with head and neck pain in association with ataxia, vomiting, or other focal neurologic signs. Dissection is a known cause of stroke in children. In one study of vertebral artery dissection in children, half of those who had cervical radiographs had associated cervical anomalies. They had a median age of 9 years (although it can occur at any age) with a male predominance of 6.6:1. Causes of dissection include trauma and vasculopathy; in some cases, the cause is unknown. The diagnosis is made most accurately by angiography; magnetic resonance angiography may also be useful. Limited data are available regarding the most effective medical treatment of dissection in children and young adults. Most physicians consider antiplatelet and/or anticoagulation therapy. Interventional neuroradiology may offer an approach in difficult cases.

INFLAMMATORY/IDIOPATHIC

Upper Cervical Spine Instability Atlantoaxial instability is typically caused by congenital abnormalities of the odontoid process or ligamentous hyperlaxity, and it affects as many as 15% of children with Down syndrome. It can also be caused by inflammatory conditions such as juvenile idiopathic arthritis (JIA). Patients with cervical spine instability may be totally asymptomatic or they may have severe neck pain and neurologic deficits. The diagnosis is made using plain films of the cervical spine or three-dimensional CT reconstruction. Treatment is surgical fusion; however, the decision to treat should be individualized, because many children with radiographic evidence of instability do not exhibit symptoms. Most experts agree that operative fusion should be performed only on those who are symptomatic or have neurologic symptoms.

Cervical Stenosis In children, cervical stenosis is most often associated with achondroplasia. All children with this condition have abnormal growth of the pedicles with associated spinal stenosis. One-third of patients with achondroplasia have symptomatic stenosis by age 15 years.

Patients present with pain in the lower back and legs that is exacerbated by activity. MRI is diagnostic and can identify the extent of the stenosis. The treatment is surgical decompression.

Acute Cervical Disk Calcification Disk calcification is thought to be due to a nonspecific inflammatory process. The child usually presents with fever and a painful, stiff neck. Examination reveals tenderness over the affected disk, most commonly in the cervical area. Radiographs show calcification of the intervertebral disk space 1 to 3 weeks after the onset of symptoms. Treatment is symptomatic, with a cervical collar and anti-inflammatory medication. Most cases resolve within 2 to 3 weeks.

Relapsing Polychondritis Relapsing polychondritis is a rare condition involving inflammatory changes in cartilage and other connective tissue, and can occur in both children and adults. Episodes occur with rapid onset of inflammatory symptoms and signs over cartilage in the head and neck as well as in other joints, causing pain, erythema, warmth, and tissue swelling usually involving the auricular cartilage. The inflammation may last 1 to 2 weeks and is occasionally treated with systemic steroids. Diagnosis is clinical, with laboratory testing notable only for nonspecific signs of inflammation.

AUTOIMMUNE

Lymphadenopathy Noninfectious causes of lymphadenopathy or focal neck masses include rheumatologic or immunologic disease, inflammatory syndromes, or neoplastic diseases. Kawasaki disease is a vasculitis that often presents with focal lymph node swelling and tenderness in the setting of fever—a careful history and physical examination should evaluate for other signs of Kawasaki disease that typically distinguish it from lymphadenitis. Periodic fever, aphthous stomatitis, pharyngitis, and adenopathy (PFAPA) is a syndrome that includes intermittent attacks of fever with tender cervical adenopathy. Affected children most commonly present between the ages of 2 and 5 years old and are well between episodes. A variety of immune deficiencies and inflammatory processes, such as sarcoidosis, multisystem inflammatory syndrome in children (MIS-C), Castleman disease, and Kikuchi's disease can also present with cervical lymphadenopathy.

Arthritis and Spondyloarthropathy Although uncommon, neck stiffness can be the presenting sign of diagnoses such as JIA and psoriatic arthritis. The affected joints have limited motion and are warm, tender, and swollen. The cause of most inflammatory joint diseases is unknown. With the spondyloarthropathies, involvement of the cervical spine increases with age and disease duration. The diagnosis is made by history and physical examination findings. Laboratory tests such as sedimentation rate, HLA typing, or specific antibodies may help support the diagnosis.

NEOPLASTIC

Neoplastic causes of lymph node swelling include lymphoma, lymphoproliferative disorders, and metastatic lymph nodes from regional primary tumors. The location (e.g., supraclavicular or generalized), size, quality (matted or firm), and duration (months) of swelling increase the possibility of malignancy. Focal oncologic processes such as soft tissue sarcomas may also mimic lymph node swelling.

Posterior Fossa, Spinal Canal, and Neck Tumors Tumors causing neck pain can occur in a variety of locations, and the signs and symptoms vary with location. In general, pain is a prominent symptom. Patients often have associated neurologic deficits involving the cranial nerves or motor function; sensory deficits are uncommon. Up to 25% of patients with neck or spinal tumors present with secondary scoliosis; torticollis can be seen with posterior fossa tumors. Diagnosis is usually made by CT scan or MRI. Treatment is dependent on the cause of the tumor.

Osteoid Osteoma Osteoid osteomas are benign bone tumors characterized clinically by localized pain over the affected region. They most commonly occur in the lower extremities but may occur in the spine as well, in which case a painful secondary scoliosis may be evident. The cause of these lesions is unclear. They most commonly occur in older children and adolescents, with a 2:1 male predominance. The diagnosis can be made by plain films; a bone scan or CT provides more detail if needed. Most osteoid osteomas are self-limited and gradually calcify and blend into surrounding bone. Treatment with nonsteroidal anti-inflammatory drugs is sufficient in most cases, with some requiring surgical excision of the nidus.

IATROGENIC

Nontraumatic Atlantoaxial Rotatory Subluxation (Grisel Syndrome) Grisel syndrome is rare, and presents with painful torticollis, most commonly after otolaryngologic procedures such as adenoidectomy. The cause is thought to be hyperemia of the tissues, leading to laxity of the atlantoaxial joint. The diagnosis is made by CT scan with three-dimensional reconstruction. Treatment consists of a cervical collar and anti-inflammatory medications until symptoms resolve. If reduction does not occur, cervical traction may be necessary.

Conditions Associated With Surgical Positioning In the appropriate clinical setting, disorders of the neck musculature and joints including the temporomandibular joint can present after surgery. These may be simply related to muscle strain or spasm from a period of neck rotation, flexion, or extension during a procedure or may relate to intubation or use of jaw-opening devices and retractors during surgery in the mouth or throat. Management is through the use of anti-inflammatory medications, heat, and possibly physical therapy in the case of muscle strain/spasm, with more urgent intervention if jaw dislocation is suspected.

CONGENITAL

In addition to infectious processes involving congenital cysts, some conditions may present with neck pain as a symptom of other pathology affecting the central nervous system (CNS) and spine.

Chiari I Malformation Type I Chiari malformation is defined as descent of the cerebellar tonsils more than 5 mm below the foramen magnum. The cause is unknown. Classically, it presents with occipital headache or posterior neck pain lasting seconds to minutes, which is worsened by Valsalva maneuvers. Although associated neurologic deficits are common, many patients with this malformation are asymptomatic. Up to 50% of individuals with type I Chiari malformation have an associated syrinx, or a collection of fluid caused by obstruction of CSF flow. The recognized incidence of Chiari malformation has dramatically increased with the advent of MRI scanning, the diagnostic test of choice. Treatment, if indicated, is surgical decompression.

TRAUMA

Discussion of traumatic causes of neck pain is beyond the scope of this chapter. Most significant trauma in children is managed by a trauma team. Less obvious forms of trauma, such as an unwitnessed fall from a bed or a hyperextension injury from gymnastics, are important considerations when a child presents with neck pain that does not appear to have an infectious cause. In nonverbal children, it is important to consider nonaccidental trauma as a possible issue. When neck trauma is suspected, priority should be placed on cervical spine immobilization with appropriate imaging and evaluation.

KEY POINTS

- Etiologies of neck pain in children can vary widely, but for hospitalized children the diagnoses often require prompt evaluation and management.
- For young children, neck pain can be subtle and often the only indication of pain is the presence of limited neck movement.
- Careful head, oropharyngeal, neck, and neurologic examinations are indicated, and the presence of fever should warrant exclusion of meningitis and deep neck space infections.

ACKNOWLEDGMENTS

This chapter was revised from content originally authored by Nicole Frei, MD and Amanda Growdon, MD.

SUGGESTED READINGS

Aulino, JM, Kirsch CFE, Burns J, et al. ACR Appropriateness Criteria® Neck Mass/Adenopathy. Available at https://acsearch.acr.org/docs/69504/Narrative/. American College of Radiology. Accessed August 4, 2022.

Bochner RE, Gangar M, Belamarich PF. A clinical approach to tonsillitis, tonsillar hypertrophy, and peritonsillar and retropharyngeal abscesses [published correction appears in Pediatr Rev. 2017 May;38(5):240]. *Pediatr Rev.* 2017;38(2):81-92.

Bridwell R, Gottlieb M, Koyfman A, Long B. Diagnosis and management of Ludwig's angina: an evidence-based review. *Am J Emerg Med.* 2021; 41:1-5.

Ho ML. Pediatric neck masses: imaging guidelines and recommendations. *Radiol Clin North Am.* 2022;60(1):1-14.

Committee on Infectious Diseases, American Academy of Pediatrics, Kimberlin D, Barnett E, Lynfield R, Sawyer M. Red Book: 2021-2024 Report of the Committee on Infectious Diseases. 2021.

Lipsett SC, Porter JJ, Monuteaux MC, Watters K, Hudgins JD. Variation in the management of children with deep neck infections. *Hosp Pediatr.* 2021;11(3):277-283.

Woods CR, Cash ED, Smith AM, et al. Retropharyngeal and parapharyngeal abscesses among children and adolescents in the United States: epidemiology and management trends, 2003-2012. *J Pediatric Infect Dis Soc.* 2016;5(3):259-268.

Goenka PK, Hall M, Shah SS, et al. Corticosteroids in the treatment of pediatric retropharyngeal and parapharyngeal abscesses. *Pediatrics.* 2021;148(5):e2020037010.

CHAPTER 31 Oral Lesions and Oral Health

Karisa Grizzle, MD

BACKGROUND

Pediatric dental disease is the most common chronic illness of school-aged children. It is five times more common than asthma and has lifelong health implications. Severe tooth decay can lead to bacterial infections within the tissues of the mouth, the bones surrounding the oral cavity, and the sinuses. Pediatric dental disease can lead to malnourishment and pain, and adult dental disease is associated with bacterial pneumonia, diabetes, heart disease, stroke, and poor pregnancy outcomes, including premature labor. It is important to include a close examination of the oral cavity on admission, as many children have not seen a dentist in the past and have undiagnosed pathology. Dental caries lead to more cumulative missed school hours than any other chronic disease and can lead to difficulties with eating, drinking, speaking, and attentiveness.

Children with special healthcare needs are at particularly high risk of severe tooth decay due to their underlying medical issues and barriers to accessing dental care. Dental care remains the most frequently cited unmet health need for this population of children. Pediatric hospital medicine physicians can help fill this gap by addressing oral health concerns on admission and facilitating proper dental care after discharge from the hospital.

Intraoral disease may be a primary indication for admission to the hospital (e.g., dental abscess) or may be a secondary finding on an inpatient examination (e.g., aphthous ulcers in lupus [**Table 31-1**] or delayed tooth eruption due to a genetic disorder [**Table 31-2**]). Oral lesions, commonly caused by viruses (see **Table 31-3**) or candida, may also lead to such significant difficulty with drinking and swallowing that infants and children require admission for pain control and treatment of dehydration. See Chapter 96 for a review of causes of stomatitis.

Traumatic mucosal injuries are the most common type of oral injury in infants and young children. These injuries may be caused by burns, either chemical (e.g., alkali) or thermal (e.g., hot drinks); sucking on a pacifier or finger; abrasions or lacerations resulting from sharp objects inserted into the mouth; or blunt trauma. Children presenting with mucosal trauma may also have injuries involving the teeth.

TABLE 31-1 Conditions With Oral Manifestations

Condition	Oral Signs or Symptoms
Acrodermatitis enteropathica	Angular chelitis, glossitis
Acute myelogenous leukemia	Subtypes can present with gingival hyperplasia, oral ulcers
Crohn disease	Recurrent oral abscesses, dry mouth, redness and scaling around the lips, angular chelitis
Cyclic neutropenia	Oral ulcers, early loss of primary teeth
Iron-deficiency anemia	Burning sensation of the tongue, pallor of oral mucosa, atrophy of papillae on tongue
Leukocyte adhesion deficiency disorder	Severe gingival inflammation around primary teeth, increased tooth mobility, early tooth loss
Kawasaki disease	Dry, fissured lips and "strawberry tongue"
Osler-Weber-Rendu disease	Telangiectasia of oral mucosa
Peutz-Jeghers syndrome	Melanotic spots on lips and buccal mucosa
Porphyria	Possibly reddish brown discoloration of teeth
Primary HIV infection	Oral ulcers, pharyngitis, cervical lymphadenopathy
Scarlet fever	Red "strawberry" tongue
Stevens-Johnson syndrome	Fragile mucosal bullae, shallow oral ulcers with a gray or white membrane
Systemic lupus erythematosus	Oral or nasal mucocutaneous ulcerations

HIV, human immunodeficiency virus.

PATHOPHYSIOLOGY

Dental abscesses generally result from untreated tooth decay, which leads to a deep cavity within a tooth, penetrating through the enamel and dentin into the central pulp. Abscesses can also develop after trauma causes a deep crack in a tooth. Once the pulp is exposed, bacteria can invade, causing the pulp to necrose and forming pockets of purulence at the base of the tooth (see **Figure 31-1** for tooth anatomy).

PATIENT HISTORY

Children with dental abscesses may present with excruciating pain and swelling within the mouth. Other symptoms may include fever, pain with chewing, hot or cold sensitivity, bad breath, a bitter taste in the mouth, general discomfort, or feeling unwell. The child may also have nausea, vomiting, diarrhea, chills, or sweats. If the abscess has spread, a child may present with complaints of facial swelling, trismus, symptoms

TABLE 31-2 Syndromes Associated With Delayed Tooth Eruption

Albright hereditary osteodystrophy
Apert syndrome
Cornelia de Lange syndrome
Hunter syndrome
Incontinentia pigmenti
Miller-Dieker syndrome
Osteogenesis imperfecta type I
Progeria syndrome

TABLE 31-3 Viral Stomatitis

Cause	Lesion	Site and Distribution
Primary HSV (herpes stomatitis)	Inflamed gingiva and mucosa Followed by vesicles that promptly rupture to reveal characteristic irregular, painful, superficial ulcers	Anterior: gingival, labial, lingual, and buccal mucosa; floor of mouth; extension to perioral skin and "drop" lesions Posterior: hard palate and tonsils
Recurrent HSV	Single or small clusters of vesicles	Mucocutaneous junction of lips
Varicella-zoster HHV-6	Shallow, non-painful ulcers Erythematous papules	Palate Soft palate and base of uvula
Rubeola (measles)	Mottled erythema in prodromal phase Grayish white granular lesions on pronounced erythematous mucosa (Koplik spots) on about day 10	Prodromal findings: palate Koplik spots—initially, buccal mucosa adjacent to lower molars Subsequently extends throughout oral mucosa
Enteroviruses Coxsackieviruses (including hand-foot-and-mouth disease) Echoviruses	Rapidly-ulcerating vesicles, painful	Lingual and buccal surfaces; soft palate

HHV-6, human herpesvirus 6; HSV, herpes simplex virus.

of maxillary sinusitis, or difficulty swallowing or speaking. Of note, a child with a dental abscess may also be asymptomatic, with the infection only noted on thorough examination, particularly if an abscess is draining spontaneously through a sinus tract.

Past medical history may reveal prior dental caries or trauma to the teeth. Children with a history of osteogenesis imperfecta or other conditions resulting in abnormal dentin are at higher risk of developing dental abscesses from dental caries. Spontaneous dental abscesses are also frequently noted in familial hypophosphatemia or vitamin D-resistant rickets, due to hypomineralization of the dentin and enlargement of the pulp. Children with diabetes and males are also at higher risk.

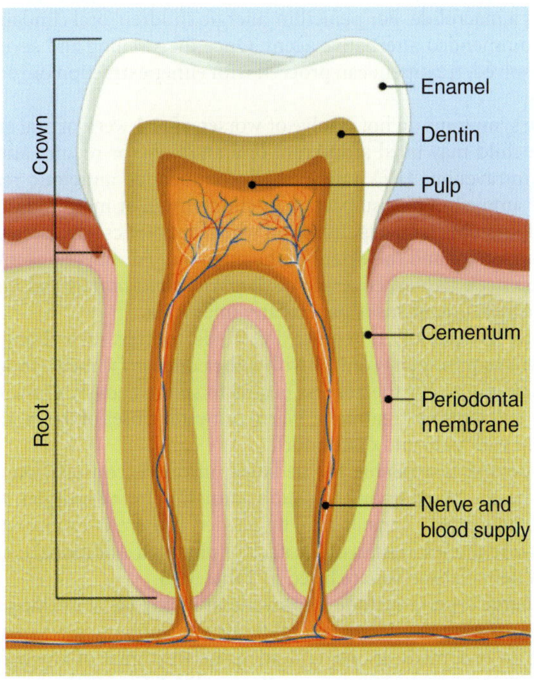

FIGURE 31-1. Tooth anatomy.

DEFINITIONS

- Enamel: Hard mineralized external layer covering the crown of the tooth (superior to the gum line)
- Cementum: Calcified substance covering the root of the tooth and assisting in tooth support in the bone, along with the periodontal membrane
- Dentin: An inner, second layer of calcified material, located deep to the enamel of the tooth (superior to the gum line) or cementum (inferior to the gum line)
- Pulp: The central inner section of the tooth, composed of connective tissue, blood vessels, and nerves
- Apical: Direction toward the root tip(s) of the tooth
- Coronal: Direction toward the crown of the tooth or something related to the crown itself
- Root canal: A canal extending from the central pulp to the root, or apex, of the tooth
- Root canal treatment: Dental procedure which removes the infected or necrosed pulp of the tooth to save the tooth from possible extraction
- Avulsion: Complete displacement of a tooth out of its socket

Soft tissue injuries within the mouth are generally quite painful and therefore noted shortly after the trauma occurs. Cuts of the lower lip or tongue are usually caused by biting down during a fall. A child who falls with an object in his mouth, such as a pencil or toothbrush, may sustain serious injuries to the posterior oral cavity or pharynx.

PHYSICAL EXAMINATION

On physical examination, the child with a dental abscess may have fever or tachycardia, and depending on the extent of illness, the child may appear sick or uncomfortable. On focused examination of the oral cavity, the gums surrounding an infected tooth are often reddened and swollen, and purulence may be expressed from the base of the tooth. Pain is often elicited on palpation of the tooth, and the tooth may feel loose. Swelling may extend along the base of several teeth. If the infection tracks into the soft tissues of the neck, it can lead to airway compromise and drooling, or a muffled voice may be noted. If the abscess has spread to involve the soft tissues of the face, the child may have notable unilateral swelling of either the jaw or the upper face, depending on whether the lower teeth or upper teeth are involved. The facial skin may be erythematous and warm, particularly when compared to the opposite side of the face. The maxillary sinus can become involved with a dental abscess of the upper teeth, and unilateral maxillary sinus tenderness may be noted on percussion. There may also be unilateral cervical lymphadenopathy, which may be the only external sign in early dental infections.

Children with thermal or chemical burns may have areas of mucosal erythema or sloughing. As healing proceeds, adherent white material may appear. The distribution may include the palate, the lips, or the peripheral areas of the tongue. These lesions may be painful, but generally heal within 2 weeks. Ulcers from sucking are usually found on the hard palate.

DIFFERENTIAL DIAGNOSIS

The differential diagnosis for dental abscesses includes inflammation or infection of the surrounding tissues (**Table 31-4**). For children with intraoral injuries, one must consider the possibility of inflicted trauma. Child abuse should be considered with any signs of facial or oral trauma, particularly with lacerations of the oral frenulae or bruising of the labial sulcus (lower border between the lip and gums) in a non-ambulatory child. The head, face, and neck are the most common sites affected by physical abuse and may be the only manifestation on physical examination. Other orofacial injuries suggestive of child abuse include swollen lips with underlying ecchymoses and dental fractures without an adequate history. Sexual abuse may present with oral findings, such as bruising of the hard and soft palates, tears of the lingual frenulum, or oral

TABLE 31-4 Differential Diagnosis for Dental Abscess
Acute inflammation of the salivary glands (e.g. parotitis, mumps)
Periorbital cellulitis
Peritonsillar abscess
Sinusitis
Burkitt's lymphoma
Unerupted tooth or impaired eruption of tooth

lesions associated with a sexually transmitted disease. Neglect may be suspected in a child with severe, untreated dental caries and oral infection, but this can be difficult to differentiate from parental unawareness of proper dental hygiene, difficulty with dental hygiene due to special healthcare needs, or difficulty with obtaining a dental care provider (e.g., lack of access or barriers to care).

DIAGNOSTIC EVALUATION

The diagnosis of a dental abscess is predominantly clinical (**Figure 31-2**). However, if there is concern for involvement of the upper airway or the spread into the lateral pharyngeal space, a CT of the neck may be helpful to determine if procedural intervention is needed. If a dentist is involved with the child's care while in the hospital, x-rays of the teeth and surrounding structures may be requested. Routine laboratory studies are not indicated. A blood culture may be considered in cases of dental abscess complicated by osteomyelitis or with signs of sepsis or endocarditis.

If the abscess is surgically drained or is spontaneously draining through a sinus tract, the material may be sent for gram stain and culture. However, with intraoral drainage, the culture can be contaminated by normal oral flora, so the utility of the results may be limited. An acute dental abscess is usually polymicrobial in origin, comprised of both facultative anaerobes (e.g., viridans group streptococci) and strict anaerobes (e.g., *Prevotella* and *Fusobacterium*) as well as possible aerobes.

For intraoral injuries, clinical examination should reveal the extent of damage, but radiographs of the teeth and surrounding bones may be indicated. Head or neck CT or CTA may be indicated to evaluate for possible retained foreign bodies or associated arterial injury. There is a small risk (studies note a 0.6% incidence) of internal carotid artery damage or thrombosis with lateral soft palate or peritonsillar injury.

In cases of suspected child abuse, radiographs may reveal multiple healed fractures of the teeth and jaw. Unexplained oral bleeding in an infant warrants investigation with a complete blood count and coagulation studies. If sexual abuse is suspected, testing for sexually transmitted infections (such as herpes, gonorrhea, or syphilis) may be indicated. (See Part III, Section A for more on child abuse injuries.)

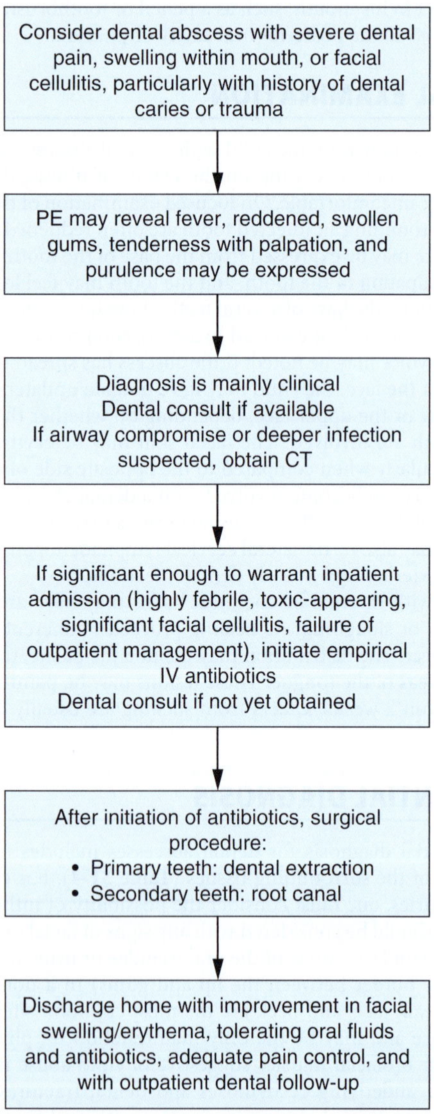

FIGURE 31-2. Suspected dental abscess: diagnostic and treatment algorithm.

MANAGEMENT

DENTAL ABSCESS

Treatment of an uncomplicated dental abscess without facial swelling, associated systemic symptoms (e.g., fever), or severe pain may be accomplished with a dental procedure alone. For an infected *primary* tooth, the treatment is extraction. For an infected *permanent* tooth, the infected pulp material is removed and root canal treatment is performed. No antibiotics are needed if the infection is limited to the tooth and its root(s).

If facial swelling or severe pain is present, oral antibiotics are given first to reduce the inflammation, followed by a dental examination in 1 week. Amoxicillin or penicillin should cover the causative organisms in most dental abscesses. However, if local epidemiologic patterns reveal a high resistance rate to amoxicillin alone, or if the child is at higher risk of resistant organisms, alternative regimens include amoxicillin with clavulanic acid, clindamycin, or a combination of metronidazole plus amoxicillin or a macrolide. For penicillin-allergic children, oral clindamycin is the recommended alternative agent. Once the swelling and severe pain have resolved, treatment can proceed with either extraction or root canal therapy.

If the symptoms do not resolve or worsen after 1 week of oral antibiotics, the child may need a different oral antibiotic or require admission for an intravenous (IV) antibiotic. Recommended antibiotic regimens include ampicillin plus sulbactam or clindamycin or metronidazole plus ampicillin/sulbactam, depending on which antibiotics have been utilized as an outpatient and the extent of the infection. For infections involving the deep neck tissues, coverage of *Staphylococcus aureus* and Group A *Streptococcus* organisms is particularly important.

Inpatients also often require IV fluids to treat dehydration, and most will require pain control with either oral or IV medications. The pain may improve if the abscess begins to spontaneously drain, but the abscess still requires treatment. Warm saltwater rinses of the mouth may also help with pain and discomfort.

If a dentist is available for pediatric inpatient consultation, he/she should be contacted upon the child's admission to the hospital. An otolaryngology (ENT) consult may be needed if there is extension of the abscess into the soft tissues of the neck or pharynx. Additional complications of dental abscesses are listed in **Table 31-5**.

Discharge criteria include improvement in any facial swelling or erythema, an ability to tolerate enteral fluids and antibiotics, adequate pain control on oral medications, and adequate treatment of any complications (e.g., deep neck infection or osteomyelitis). Close primary care and dental follow-up should be ensured prior to discharge.

TABLE 31-5 Possible Complications From Dental Abscess

Dental cyst	Septicemia
Facial cellulitis	Endocarditis
Sinusitis	Pneumonia
Osteomyelitis	Brain abscess, meningitis
Airway compromise	Cavernous sinus thrombosis
Septic thrombophlebitis (Lemierre syndrome)	Sublingual or submandibular cellulitis (Ludwig angina)

A large percentage of children lack dental insurance, and for those covered by Medicaid, it can be difficult to find a dental provider. Thus, a dentist must be identified for follow-up prior to discharging the patient home. Many children with dental abscesses suffer from generally poor oral health. Prevention is key to avoid future dental problems. (See Box, **Prevention of Dental Abscesses**.)

PREVENTION OF DENTAL ABSCESSES

- Most, if not all, dental abscesses are preventable with good dental hygiene and prompt attention to any dental trauma.
- Children should have their first visit to the dentist by age 1 and have a dental home, as well as a medical home.
- If the family's primary water source is deficient in fluoride, the child should be on daily oral fluoride supplementation.
- The risk of dental caries is increased with a diet high in sugars and with the intake of sodas and sports drinks.

ORAL TRAUMA

Treatment for children with mucosal injuries depends on the etiology but is largely supportive, and most children who seek care at the hospital are discharged from the emergency department. Bleeding from the oral mucosa often initially appears to be more significant due to mixing with saliva but should resolve within 10 minutes of direct pressure. Lacerations of the lower lip do not usually penetrate the entire lip and do not need suturing unless the outward portion is gaping or involves the vermillion border. Tongue lacerations also tend to heal on their own, provided any gaping resolves when the tongue is relaxed. Lacerations of the hard or soft palate or involving the tonsils may need surgical repair, although observation may be an option for smaller lacerations, provided no foreign body is retained.

Children with dental injuries are also typically cared for in the outpatient setting. Injuries to primary teeth involve different strategies than injuries to permanent teeth, as damaged or missing permanent teeth can have significant negative effects. A severe dental injury (e.g., an avulsed permanent tooth) requires emergent dental evaluation, whereas a loose permanent tooth or fractured permanent tooth without exposure of the pulp should be evaluated by a dentist within 24 hours. Less significant injuries, such a non-painful fracture to a primary or permanent tooth, may be followed up on a less urgent basis. If a primary tooth is slightly loose after trauma, it should be left in place, as many of these injuries will heal on their own. A soft diet is recommended for 1 to 2 weeks, and good oral hygiene is important to reduce the chance of infection. However, if the primary tooth is extremely loose, it may need to be removed to reduce the risk of aspiration of the tooth.

A primary tooth that is completely avulsed out of the socket should not be replaced, as this can damage the permanent tooth beneath the gums.

An avulsed permanent tooth is a serious dental emergency, and a dentist should be contacted immediately if the tooth is located and the child is stable. The avulsed tooth should be held by the crown, gently rinsed in saline or tap water, and then placed back into the socket and held there by the child biting down on gauze or with finger pressure. Ideally, the tooth should be replaced in the socket within 15 minutes to an hour, but the tooth may remain viable for longer if placed in a container of cold milk or tooth storage media.

Displaced permanent teeth due to luxation injuries will have the best possible outcome with urgent repositioning by a dentist within a few hours. Subluxed teeth, or loose teeth in normal position, must be followed closely and seen by a dentist as soon as possible for stabilization, ideally within 24 hours.

Permanent teeth that are fractured with exposure of the pulp should be seen by a dentist within 24 hours. Tooth fragments should be located and saved in tooth storage media or tap water. Cold milk is not necessary, as the fragments do not contain live fibroblasts, but the tooth fragments will become discolored if not kept wet. If the fracture does not involve the pulp of the tooth, the fracture is not usually painful or at high risk for infection, so dental evaluation can wait up to 7 days.

KEY POINTS

- A dental abscess can be dangerous and may cause both local and systemic complications.
- Indications for admission include dehydration, worsening facial or neck swelling, inability to handle oral secretions, concern for airway compromise, systemic involvement, or failure of outpatient therapy.
- Antibiotics should cover both anaerobes and strict aerobes. Include Group A *Strep* and *Staph aureus* coverage for neck involvement.

SPECIAL CONSIDERATIONS

During hospitalization, good oral hygiene should be taught and emphasized for all patients, with a particular focus on children with special healthcare needs. Teeth should be brushed twice daily with a small amount of water, and for children over age 2 years, a pea-sized amount of fluoridated toothpaste should be added. The teeth do not need to be rinsed after brushing, as the fluoride in the toothpaste has a beneficial topical effect. Children with tight spaces between primary teeth or with permanent teeth should also floss at least once a day.

Children who are NPO or exclusively tube-fed are at higher risk for alterations in oral pH and should receive the same oral care as other children. Bruxism in children with cerebral palsy can erode the enamel and lead to a higher chance of tooth decay. Also, children with gastroenteritis, gastroesophageal reflux disease, or bulimia need to have the stomach acids removed from their teeth to prevent decalcification. Pediatric oncology patients are at higher risk of mucositis if oral hygiene is not maintained, and saliva provides an important barrier of defense against infection. For children at risk of gum bleeding, brushing should be done gently and the use of mouthwash is encouraged.

Medications may also increase the risk of oral health problems. Some medications may decrease salivary flow, increasing the risk of dental decay (see **Table 31-6**), while others such as phenytoin may cause gingival hyperplasia, making plaque more difficult to remove. Also, many oral medications for children are given in sugar-based syrups, which lead to a higher risk of tooth decay. Children receiving these types of medications on a frequent or chronic basis may need to brush more often or use antibacterial mouthwashes.

TABLE 31-6 Medication Classes Associated With Decreased Salivary Flow

Anticholinergics	Benzodiazepines
Antidepressants	Cytotoxic drugs
Antihistamines	Diuretics
Antihypertensives	Opiates
ADHD medications	Proton pump inhibitors

ACKNOWLEDGMENT

The authors wish to acknowledge the work of Dr. Suzanne Swanson Mendez on the prior version of this chapter.

SUGGESTED READINGS

Blevins JY. Oral health care for hospitalized children. *Pediatr Nurs.* 2011; 37(5):229-235.

Bourguignon C, Cohenca N, Lauridsen E, et al. International Association of Dental Traumatology guidelines for the management of traumatic dental injuries: 1. Fractures and luxations. *Dent Traumatol.* 2020;36(4):314-330.

Brook I. Microbiology and management of endodontic infections in children. *J Clin Pediatr Dent.* 2003;28(1):13-17.

Casamassimo PS, Flaitz CM, Hammersmith K, Sangvai S, Kumar A. Recognizing the relationship between disorders in the oral cavity and systemic disease. *Pediatr Clin North Am.* 2018;65(5): 1007-1032.

Day PF, Flores MT, O'Connell AC, et al. International Association of Dental Traumatology guidelines for the management of traumatic dental injuries: 3. Injuries in the primary dentition. *Dent Traumatol.* 2020;36(4):343-359.

Fouad AF, Abbott PV, Tsilingaridis G, et al. International Association of Dental Traumatology guidelines for the management of traumatic dental injuries: 2. Avulsion of permanent teeth. *Dent Traumatol.* 2020; 36(4):331-342.

Hong CHL, Dean DR, Hull K, et al. World Workshop on Oral Medicine VII: Relative frequency of oral mucosal lesions in children, a scoping review. *Oral Dis.* 2019;25(S1):193-203.

Khan L. Dental care and trauma management in children and adolescents. *Pediatr Ann.* 2019;48(1):e3-e8.

Lebrun-Harris LA, Canto MT, Vodicka P, Mann MY, Kinsman SB. Oral health among children and youth with special health care needs. *Pediatrics.* 2021;148(2):e2020025700.

Lewis CW. Dental care and children with special health care needs: a population-based perspective. *Acad Pediatr.* 2009;9(6):420-426.

Macedo GV, Diaz PI, De O Fernandes CA, Ritter AV. Reattachment of anterior teeth fragments: a conservative approach. *J Esthet Restor Dent.* 2008;20(1):5-18; discussion 19-20.

Randall DA, Kang DR. Current management of penetrating injuries of the soft palate. *Otolaryngol Head Neck Surg.* 2006;135(3): 356-360.

Robertson D, Smith AJ. The microbiology of the acute dental abscess. *J Med Microbiol.* 2009;58(2):155-162.

Section on Oral Health. Maintaining and improving the oral health of young children. *Pediatrics.* 2014;134(6):1224-1229.

Seow WK. Review: diagnosis and management of unusual dental abscesses in children. *Aust Dent J.* 2003;48:(3):156-168.

Soose RJ, Simons JP, Mandell DL. Evaluation and management of pediatric oropharyngeal trauma. *Arch Otolaryngol Head Neck Surg.* 2006; 132(4):446-451.

US Department of Health and Human Services. Oral Health in America: A Report of the Surgeon General–Executive Summary. Rockville, MD: US Department of Health and Human Services, National Institute of Dental and Craniofacial Research, National Institutes of Health; 2000.

US Department of Health and Human Services. Oral Health in America: Advances and Challenges–Executive Summary. Rockville, MD: US Department of Health and Human Services, National Institute of Dental and Craniofacial Research, National Institutes of Health; 2020.

CHAPTER 32

Respiratory Distress

Juliann Lipps Kim, MD, FAAP

BACKGROUND

Respiratory distress is one of the most common reasons for a child to present to the emergency department or a practitioner's office. Respiratory distress can result from disorders in the respiratory system or in organ systems that control or influence respiration. Young children have an increased risk for respiratory distress because of their anatomy and physiology. Nearly 20% of all emergency department visits for children younger than 2 years are for respiratory disease. The causes of respiratory distress are vast, and practitioners caring for children should have a systematic approach to its diagnosis and management. Cardiopulmonary arrest in children is largely due to respiratory failure (in adults, cardiac causes are most common). Rapid evaluation and management of severe pediatric respiratory disease may be necessary to prevent respiratory failure.

PATHOPHYSIOLOGY

Understanding respiratory physiology can aid the practitioner in diagnosing the cause of respiratory symptoms. The main goals of respiration are oxygen uptake and elimination of carbon dioxide. Secondary goals include acid-base buffering, hormonal regulation, and host defense. To achieve the goals of respiration, three main functional components of the respiratory system are used: (1) mechanical structures (including chest wall, respiratory muscles, and pulmonary circulation), (2) membrane gas exchanger (interface between airspace and pulmonary circulation), and (3) regulatory system (network of chemical and mechanical sensors throughout the circulatory and respiratory systems). All three components are tightly integrated, and dysfunction of one can lead to respiratory distress or failure.

Respiratory function is tightly controlled by a complex network of central and peripheral chemoreceptors and mechanoreceptors responding to information from the body about the status of the respiratory system. This network modulates the neural output to the respiratory muscles, affecting the timing and force of respiratory effort. Central chemoreceptors in the ventral reticular nuclei of the medulla are sensitive to changes in pH and partial pressure of carbon dioxide (PCO_2) of cerebrospinal fluid. The intrinsic brain-stem function of the dorsal and ventral respiratory centers of the medulla controls inspiration and expiration, respectively. The apneustic center in the pons increases the depth and duration of inspiration, whereas the pneumotaxic center decreases depth and duration. The cerebellum, hypothalamus, motor cerebral cortex, and limbic system also play a role in mediating respiration. Carotid and aortic bodies are peripheral chemoreceptors sensitive to the partial pressure of oxygen (PO_2), PCO_2, and pH in arterial blood. Mechanoreceptors (stretch, juxtacapillary, and irritant reflex) distributed along the airways, lung parenchyma, and chest wall respond to lung volume, changes in pulmonary microvasculature, chest wall muscle activity, and environmental irritants.

Information from central and peripheral receptors is integrated in the brainstem, and efferent impulses are transmitted to alter respiratory function and maintain homeostasis. Even slight alterations in arterial pH, PO_2, or PCO_2 stimulate the respiratory centers to modify the respiratory pattern. Increased arterial PCO_2 and decreased arterial PO_2 lead to an increase in respiratory drive and increased neural output to respiratory muscles. The resulting increase in ventilation can be achieved by increases in tidal volume or respiratory rate, because the product of these two factors determines the minute ventilation. Respiratory insufficiency or the more severe entity, respiratory failure, occurs when regulatory systems or the effector organs (lungs, respiratory muscles) are impaired or overwhelmed. This results in diminished oxygenation (decreased arterial PO_2), retention of carbon dioxide (increased arterial PCO_2), and acidosis (decreased arterial pH).

Disruption of the mechanics of the lung or chest wall results in the majority of respiratory disease in children. Obstructive or restrictive disease leads to increased work of breathing and increased energy demands on the respiratory muscles to meet the body's needs. This increased work manifests itself clinically as respiratory distress, evidenced by increased work of breathing. When demand exceeds capability, the result is respiratory insufficiency, which can progress to respiratory failure. In respiratory muscle dysfunction, neural output is sent to the respiratory muscles, but they are unable to respond adequately to increase respiratory effort. The physical signs of respiratory failure in this setting are more subtle, and the signs of increased work of breathing may not be present. When the difficulty involves the control of breathing, there is an inadequate neural response to hypoxemia or hypercarbia. Arterial hypoxemia or hypercarbia without an increase in respiratory effort should lead one to suspect an anomaly in the neural control of breathing caused by central nervous system injury, drug-induced inhibition, or dysfunction of spinal motor neurons or nerve fibers innervating the respiratory muscles.

INITIAL ASSESSMENT

Rapid assessment and intervention for the child with respiratory distress can prevent the progression from respiratory compromise to respiratory failure. To assess the airway, determine whether it is patent, stable, and maintainable. If not, such an airway must be established (e.g., repositioning, instrumentation). Once these three criteria are met, the breathing process is evaluated by determining the respiratory rate, oxygen saturation, adequacy of breath sounds, and quality of respiratory effort (e.g., labored, use of accessory muscles). Determination of arterial blood gas levels may be needed if there is evidence of respiratory insufficiency or failure. If spontaneous ventilation is inadequate, assisted breathing with positive pressure, initially via a bag-mask device, is indicated. Assessment of the patient's circulation and mental status are other key aspects of the initial evaluation. Based on this rapid assessment, the clinician obtains information about the severity of the patient's condition and how rapidly interventions must be performed.

Providing supplemental oxygen is an important first step for a child presenting in distress, especially with hypoxemia demonstrated by oximetry. Oxygen can be delivered by multiple devices, and the choice depends on the child's clinical status and oxygen needs. Some of these devices can agitate a child further, worsening respiratory compromise and increasing the metabolic demand for oxygen. Allow the child to remain with the parent as much as possible and use the least noxious form of oxygen delivery necessary. In a small number of children, airway adjuncts such as a nasopharyngeal airway, oropharyngeal airway, or assisted ventilation are needed. An oropharyngeal airway holds the tongue forward to prevent airway obstruction, so it will not be tolerated in a conscious or semiconscious patient with an intact gag reflex, and it may induce vomiting. A nasopharyngeal airway can be used in a conscious or unconscious patient but should be avoided in those with facial trauma. Continuous positive airway pressure may assist inspiratory efforts as well as provide positive end-expiratory pressure (PEEP). PEEP provides resistance to expiration, which may help expand atelectatic portions of the lung and thereby reduce ventilation-perfusion mismatch. Bilevel positive airway pressure provides inspiratory and expiratory pressure via a firmly fitting facemask, which may be uncomfortable and not well tolerated in infants or young children (see Chapter 193).

Careful reevaluation after every intervention is critical to the care of a child with respiratory compromise. This confirms proper application of the intervention and monitors the patient's response.

PATIENT HISTORY

Therapeutic interventions in an ill child should not be delayed to perform a detailed history. A focused history includes an assessment of respiratory and systemic symptoms (**Box 32-1**). The history will guide the practitioner toward the diagnostic possibilities and appropriately focus the management. For children with complex medical history or chronic respiratory problems, ask about the child's baseline respiratory status, how this episode is different, and what interventions have been successful in the past.

Box 32-1 Components of a Focused History

- Onset, duration, chronicity, character of symptoms
- Alleviating and provoking factors
- Treatment to date
- Activity level
- Respiratory symptoms
  - Cold symptoms
  - Cough (wet, dry, time of day)
  - Trouble breathing (rapid breathing, retractions, abdominal muscle use, "seesaw" respirations, positional distress)
  - Noise with respiration (Stridor, stertor)
  - Color change (pale, cyanotic)
  - Altered pattern of breathing (periodic, shallow or deep, bradypnea, apnea)
  - Inability to clear upper respiratory tract because of weakness or poor gag
- Systemic symptoms
  - Fever
  - Poor feeding, fluid intake
  - Urine output
  - Weight loss or failure to gain weight
  - Emesis or diarrhea
- Past medical history
  - Special healthcare needs or preexisting medical conditions (complex heart disease, chronic infections, prematurity)
  - Respiratory disease (asthma, cystic fibrosis)
- Family history of atopy, cardiac or respiratory disease
- Medications (respiratory treatments, oral medications, herbal supplements)
- Allergies (medications, foods, environment)
- Immunization status
- Last oral intake (in case airway management becomes necessary)

PHYSICAL EXAMINATION

Certain features of the physical examination are particularly important in determining the severity of respiratory distress and localizing the primary cause (**Box 32-2**). Vital signs help determine cardiopulmonary status but may be influenced by various factors. Fever increases the respiratory rate by approximately three to seven breaths per minute for each degree Celsius above normal. Tachycardia commonly occurs as a response to the increased sympathetic tone in a child with respiratory distress; sympathetic tone is also increased with fever. Bradycardia is a late and ominous sign of severe hypoxia. Pulsus paradoxus (>10 mmHg decrease in blood pressure during inspiration) can occur with severe pulmonary disease. Cyanosis is not evident until more than 5 g of hemoglobin are desaturated, which correlates with an oxygen saturation of less than 70% to 75%. Central cyanosis is evidenced by blue, gray, or dark purple discoloration of mucous membranes, most reliably assessed at the lips and tongue. Perioral cyanosis is not indicative of central cyanosis and likely represents local venous congestion. It is often seen with Valsalva-like maneuvers (e.g., crying) in fair-skinned infants. Acrocyanosis is often present in healthy newborns; in older children, it may be more suggestive of cardiovascular status (e.g., peripheral vasoconstriction secondary to hypotension). Pulse oximetry is a useful, noninvasive means of assessing hypoxia, but it has some limitations. It can be unreliable with low blood pressure, movement, or arterial PO_2 less than 50 mmHg, if hemoglobin is bound to molecules other than oxygen (e.g., carbon monoxide), or if significant methemoglobinemia is present.

Restlessness or anxiety is associated with early hypoxia ("air hunger"), but the mental status can progress to somnolence and lethargy with hypercarbia and severe hypoxemia. The position of comfort can provide information about the location of dysfunction. Children with upper

Box 32-2 Directed Physical Examination

- General
  - Level of consciousness (alertness, responsiveness)
  - Preferred position of child
  - Color
  - Failure to thrive
  - Signs of prematurity or trauma
- Vital signs
- Respiratory
  - Airway
    - Nasal flaring
    - Inspiratory or expiratory noises: seal-like barking, sonorous (nasal or pharyngeal), harsh (tracheal), high pitched (intrathoracic), stertor (gurgling)
    - Symmetry of palate and tonsils
    - Prominence of posterior pharynx
    - Drooling, dysphagia
  - Inspection
    - Depth and quality of respirations
    - Retractions (subcostal, supraclavicular, intercostal)
    - Accessory muscle use
    - Symmetry of chest wall movement
    - Shape of chest (scoliosis, pectus excavatum or carinatum)
  - Auscultation
    - Air entry
    - Inspiration-to-expiration ratio
    - Rales or crackles
    - Wheezing (inspiratory or expiratory)
    - Symmetry of breath sounds
    - Presence of pleural rub
  - Cardiac
    - Murmur
    - Rhythm
    - Heart sounds
    - Thrill, rub, gallop
    - Quality of pulses
    - Capillary refill time
    - Color
  - Abdomen
    - Hepatomegaly
    - Splenomegaly
    - Mass
    - Ascites
  - Extremities
    - Clubbing
    - Deformities
  - Neurologic
    - Focal deficit
    - Cranial nerves
    - Muscle tone and strength
    - Evidence of increased intracranial pressure

airway obstruction often sit upright with the neck extended to open the airway. Infants with laryngomalacia have more pronounced stridor in the supine position compared with the prone position. Inspiratory and expiratory noises can help localize the underlying process and may suggest the cause. Stridor is a predominantly inspiratory monophasic noise indicating an extrathoracic airway obstruction. Upper airway obstruction can lead to acute deterioration and severe morbidity and mortality. Expiratory wheezing or stridor usually reflects intrathoracic obstruction; however, biphasic stridor may suggest a fixed lesion at any point along the airway. Grunting represents a child's attempt to increase the PEEP and raise the functional residual capacity by closing the glottis during expiration.

Auscultation along the entire airway, including the nose, mouth, neck, and chest, may provide localizing information. The presence of rales, wheezing, or asymmetrical breath sounds and the duration of inspiration versus expiration are particularly noteworthy. The ratio of inspiration to expiration (I/E) is normally 1:1. Extrathoracic obstruction tends to prolong the inspiratory phase (e.g., I/E ratio of 3:1), whereas lower airway obstructive pathology, such as asthma or bronchiolitis, produces a prolonged expiratory phase (e.g., I/E ratio of 1:3).

Respiratory distress may be caused by nonrespiratory pathology or may have an impact on other organ systems. Detailed cardiac, abdominal, musculoskeletal, skin, and neurologic examinations should be performed.

DIFFERENTIAL DIAGNOSIS

Respiratory difficulties may result from abnormalities within the respiratory system or from the dysfunction of organ systems influencing the respiratory system. Within the respiratory system, problems can arise from upper airway obstruction, lower airway obstruction, changes in gas diffusion from the alveolus to the capillary, abnormal pulmonary blood flow, or alterations in nerves and muscles that control breathing. Disease in other organ systems can compromise respiratory function directly or may induce compensatory respiratory mechanisms (**Tables 32-1** and **32-2**).

DIAGNOSTIC EVALUATION

Further workup may be indicated to evaluate the severity of illness or its cause and should be guided by the clinical assessment. In children with chronic disease, compare laboratory studies and radiographs to previous studies, if available.

Pulse oximetry can detect hypoxemia but does not provide direct information about the adequacy of ventilation. Exhaled carbon dioxide levels can be measured with noninvasive devices, but this determination is used most often in the setting of endotracheal intubation. Arterial blood gas analysis can assess oxygenation (arterial PO_2) and ventilation (arterial PCO_2) and detect metabolic derangements of pH, bicarbonate, and base excess. Venous and capillary blood samples can provide some information about ventilation but are less useful for assessing oxygenation. The utility of obtaining other laboratory studies depends on the clinical setting and the diagnostic considerations.

Radiographs may be an important adjunct in the evaluation of a child with respiratory disease. Chest radiographs (anteroposterior and lateral views) are performed upright and on full inspiration whenever possible. Quality images can assist in the identification of airspace disease, hyperinflation, effusion, mass, foreign body, chest wall deformity or trauma, or cardiac abnormality. If an effusion is suspected, decubitus films may be helpful to determine whether the fluid shifts with gravity ("layers out"). Inspiratory and forced expiratory or bilateral decubitus chest films are useful to evaluate for the presence of a foreign body or other localized lower airway obstruction. An obstructing lesion can cause air trapping distal to the site. On an expiratory film, the unobstructed lung tissue decreases in volume and appears denser, whereas the obstructed region is relatively hyperlucent. With decubitus films, the dependent (inferiorly positioned) lung should decrease in volume and appear denser, except for an obstructed region that remains inflated due to air trapping. When the patient's position is switched, the affected lung is superior and appears fully aerated, making the

TABLE 32-1 Differential Diagnosis of Respiratory Distress

Respiratory System	Other Organ Systems
Upper airway (nasopharynx, oropharynx, larynx, trachea, bronchi)	Central nervous system
Anatomic: craniofacial abnormalities, choanal atresia, tonsillar hypertrophy, macroglossia, midface hypoplasia, micrognathia, laryngomalacia, tracheomalacia, hemangioma, webs, cysts, laryngotracheal cleft, papilloma, subglottic stenosis, vocal cord paralysis, tracheal stenosis, fistula, bronchomalacia, bronchogenic cyst	Structural abnormality: agenesis, hydrocephalus, mass, arteriovenous malformation Infectious: meningitis, encephalitis, abscess, poliomyelitis Dysfunction or immaturity: apnea, hypoventilation, hyperventilation Inherited degenerative disease: spinal muscular atrophy
Infectious: nasal congestion, peritonsillar abscess, tonsillitis, croup, epiglottitis, retropharyngeal abscess, tracheitis, bronchitis	Intoxication or toxins: alcohol, barbiturates, benzodiazepines, opiates, tetanus Seizure
Environmental or traumatic: chemical or thermal burn, aspiration of foreign body	Trauma: hemorrhage, birth asphyxia, spinal cord injury, anoxic encephalopathy
Mass, including malignancy	Other: transverse myelitis, acute paralysis, myopathy
Inflammatory: angioneurotic edema, anaphylaxis	Peripheral nervous system
Lower airway (bronchioles, acini, interstitium)	Phrenic nerve injury
Inflammatory: asthma, allergy, angioneurotic edema, meconium aspiration, near drowning, gastroesophageal reflux, aspiration	Environmental or toxins: tick paralysis, heavy metal poisoning, organophosphates, botulism, snakebite
Infectious: bronchiolitis, pneumonia (bacterial, viral, atypical bacterial, *Chlamydia*, *Pertussis*, fungal, *Pneumocystis*), abscess, empyema	Metabolic: inborn errors of metabolism, carnitine deficiency, porphyria Inflammatory: dermatomyositis, polymyositis
Congenital malformation: congenital emphysema; cystic adenomatoid malformation; sequestration; pulmonary agenesis, aplasia, or hypoplasia; pulmonary cyst	Other: Guillain-Barré syndrome, multiple sclerosis, myasthenia gravis, muscular or myotonic dystrophy, muscle fatigue
Environmental or traumatic: thermal or chemical burn, smoke, carbon monoxide, hydrocarbon, drug-induced pulmonary fibrosis, bronchopulmonary traumatic disruption, pulmonary contusion	Cardiovascular Structural: congenital heart disease, pericardial effusion, pericardial tamponade, aortic dissection or rupture, mass, coronary artery dilation or aneurysm, pneumopericardium, great vessel anomalies
Other: bronchiectasis, interstitial lung disease, bronchopulmonary dysplasia, cystic fibrosis, pulmonary edema, hemorrhage, embolism, atelectasis, mass	Other: arrhythmia, myocarditis, myocardial ischemia or infarction, congestive heart failure
Chest wall and intrathoracic	Gastrointestinal
Pneumothorax, tension pneumothorax	Abdominal pain
Pneumomediastinum	Appendicitis
Pleural effusion	Ascites
Empyema	Mass (including hepatomegaly, splenomegaly)
Chylothorax	Necrotizing enterocolitis
Hemothorax	Obstruction
Diaphragmatic hernia	Perforation, laceration
Cyst, mass	Hematoma
Spinal deformity (kyphoscoliosis)	Contusion
Pectus excavatum or carinatum	Esophageal foreign body
Rib fracture, flail chest	Metabolic and endocrine
	Acidosis: fever, hypothermia, dehydration, sepsis, shock, inborn errors of metabolism, liver disease, renal disease, diabetic ketoacidosis, salicylates

obstructed portion difficult to appreciate. If the obstruction is longstanding, the obstructed portion may become atelectatic or fluid filled and appear as a persistent density in the various views.

Lateral and anteroposterior radiographs of the neck are useful for the evaluation of upper airway obstruction, allowing the visualization of retropharyngeal, supraglottic, and subglottic spaces. These films may be useful to diagnose retropharyngeal abscess, epiglottitis, croup, foreign body aspiration, or tracheitis. Ill children with suspected upper airway obstruction should not be sent to the radiology department unattended or should have films deferred until they are stabilized.

TABLE 32-2 Common Causes of Respiratory Distress

Neonate	Infant or Child
Transient tachypnea of the newborn	Bronchiolitis
Sepsis	Pneumonia
Respiratory distress syndrome	Asthma
Pneumonia	Croup
Nasal obstruction or airway anomalies	Foreign body aspiration
Congenital heart disease	Fever
	Sepsis
	Metabolic derangements
	Allergy

Other imaging modalities to consider are computed tomography (CT), magnetic resonance imaging (MRI), airway fluoroscopy, and barium swallow studies. CT evaluates cervical and thoracic structures in greater detail and may help identify areas of intrinsic or extrinsic compression. Mediastinal, pleural, and pulmonary parenchymal abnormalities are well identified with CT. MRI is particularly helpful to delineate hilar and vascular anatomy. Airway fluoroscopy provides dynamic pictures of the respiratory system, including the airways and diaphragm. Barium swallow studies are helpful in the evaluation of patients with recurrent pneumonia, persistent cough, stridor, or wheezing. The anatomy of the gastrointestinal tract from the mouth to the stomach is revealed, and compression along the esophagus may suggest a lesion that is compressing the airway as well. Contrast material is mixed with substances of different consistencies and textures, ranging from thin liquids to thick liquids to solids. Barium swallow studies evaluate swallowing mechanics and the presence of vascular rings, tracheoesophageal fistulas, and gastroesophageal reflux.

MANAGEMENT

Acute interventions should not be delayed in a child with respiratory distress, regardless of the underlying cause. Restoration of oxygenation and ventilation is the main priority. Airway patency should be established and maintained, followed by a rapid assessment of breathing and circulation. Oxygen delivery should be initiated using the least noxious form possible that provides an adequate fraction of inspired oxygen (FIO_2), and the child should be placed on cardiopulmonary monitors, including pulse oximetry. Airway adjuncts may be necessary to maintain patency. If these are unsuccessful, or if oxygenation and ventilation are inadequate, endotracheal intubation may be indicated. Breathing treatments (albuterol, racemic epinephrine, ipratropium bromide) may be useful in certain clinical situations, including asthma, bronchiolitis, or croup. Further therapies are determined by the underlying cause of respiratory distress.

KEY POINTS

- Do not delay the management of a compromised child to perform detailed history and physical examination.
- Clinical history and physical examination are critical to determining likely etiologies of respiratory compromise.
- Respiratory difficulties may arise from causes other than abnormalities within the respiratory system.

SUGGESTED READINGS

Gadomski AM, Permutt T, Stanton B. Correcting respiratory rate for the presence of fever. *J Clin Epidemiol.* 1994;47(9):1043.

Infosino A. Pediatric upper airway and congenital anomalies. *Anesthesiol Clin North Am.* 2003;20:4.

Messinger AI, Kupfer O, Hurst A, Parker S. Management of pediatric community-acquired bacterial pneumonia. *Pediatr Rev* September 2017;38(9):394-409.

O'Dempsey TJ, Laurence BE, McArdle TF, Todd JE, Lamont AC, Greenwood BM. The effect of temperature reduction on respiratory rate in febrile illnesses. *Arch Dis Child.* 1993;68(4):492.

Patel SJ, Teach SJ. Asthma. *Pediatr Rev* November 2019;40(11):549-567.

Perez Fontan JJ, Haddad GG. Respiratory pathophysiology. In: Behrman RE, Kliegman RM, Jenson HB, eds. *Nelson Textbook of Pediatrics.* Philadelphia: WB Saunders; 2004:1376-1379.

Ralston SL, Lieberthal AS, Meissner HC, et al. Clinical practice guideline: the diagnosis, management, and prevention of bronchiolitis. *Pediatrics.* 2014;134(5):e1474-e1502.

Ruddy RM. Evaluation of respiratory emergencies in infants and children. *Clin Pediatr Emerg Med.* 2002;3:156-162.

Ryu J, Hagood JS, Haddad GG. Diagnostic approach to respiratory disease. In: Kliegman RM, St. Geme JS, eds. *Nelson Textbook of Pediatrics.* Philadelphia: WB Saunders; 2021:2150-2161.

Sarnaik AP, Clark JA, Heidemann SM. Respiratory Distress and Failure. Kliegman RM, St. Geme JS, eds. *Nelson Textbook of Pediatrics.* Philadelphia: WB Saunders; 2021:583-601.

Stevenson MD, Gonzalez del Rey JA. Upper airway obstruction: infectious cases. *Clin Pediatr Emerg Med.* 2002;3:163-172.

Weiner DL, Deanehan JK. Respiratory distress. In: Fleisher GR, Ludwig S, eds. *Textbook of Pediatric Emergency Medicine.* 8th ed. Philadelphia, PA: Lippincott Williams & Wilkins; 2021:478-490.

CHAPTER 33

Syncope

Sarah C. McBride, MD and Angela Castellanos, MD

BACKGROUND

Syncope, often described as "fainting" or "blacking out," is defined as a transient period of unconsciousness that is brief, abrupt in onset and resolves spontaneously to a restored level of function. It is a symptom rather than a diagnosis and does not necessarily indicate disease. The causes of syncope in children are heterogeneous and are most often benign in nature. Nevertheless, syncopal events can cause distress among patients, families, school personnel, and physicians. Since it is a relatively common occurrence in childhood, hospitalists should have a practical approach to the evaluation of pediatric syncope, focusing on identification of those individuals who are at risk for serious underlying disease.

PATHOPHYSIOLOGY

Patients experience syncope when inadequate cerebral perfusion results in a transient loss of consciousness and postural tone. Presyncope describes a similar event without full loss of consciousness. Syncope most often occurs during adolescence with a peak incidence between 13 and 19 years of age. Most pediatric syncope is autonomic in origin, isolated, and benign. In fact, the risk of sudden death among pediatric patients with prior syncopal events has been found to be equivalent to the risk of sudden death in the general population.

PATIENT HISTORY

History and physical examination can provide valuable clues to the probable cause of a syncopal episode and may curtail or circumvent the need for further diagnostic evaluation. Important historical features of a patient presenting with syncope are included in **Table 33-1**. Recent circumstances and those immediately preceding the syncopal event should be thoroughly explored. Because patients are often unable to provide details of an episode, witnesses to the event are important. Past medical history, especially with regard to previous syncopal episodes, cardiac or neurologic conditions, and medications, should always be obtained. Specific inquiries about family history should include sudden death, syncope, sudden infant death syndrome, congenital heart disease, seizures, and congenital deafness (associated with a variant of long-QT syndrome). A patient's baseline level of health should also be ascertained, including any overall changes in energy level, exercise tolerance, nutritional status, or the development of new respiratory symptoms, chest pain, palpitations, or emotional stressors.

TABLE 33-1 Directed Patient History for Syncope
Environmental factors/triggers (posture, temperature, hydration status, fatigue, illness)
Frequency and duration of syncope
Level of activity just prior to syncopal episode (exertion*)
Elements of history from any witnesses (cyanosis*)
Medication history (potential for lengthening QTc or arryhthmogenic*)
Generalized symptoms of concern (fatigue, cough, weight loss, shortness of breath, chest pain*)
Personal or family history of any of the following conditions*
congenital heart disease
sudden cardiac death
Long-QT syndrome
sensorineural hearing loss
other familial heart diseases

*Increased concern for cardiac causes.

PHYSICAL EXAMINATION

Although the findings are often normal, a thorough physical examination should be performed. Mental status should be evaluated and compared to the patient's baseline level of function. Blood pressure measurements and evaluation of distal pulses in both the supine and upright positions and from both upper extremities and a lower extremity should be obtained. Cardiac examination may reveal a gallop, murmur, or click and there may be hepatomegaly or crackles on lung examination. Any of these examination findings raises the concern for cardiac disease. In addition, a complete neurologic examination is indicated. In young children and infants, a thorough skin and musculoskeletal examination should be performed to assess for signs of trauma.

DIFFERENTIAL DIAGNOSIS

A differential diagnosis of pediatric syncope is listed in **Table 33-2**. Etiologies of childhood syncope can be divided into three major categories: (1) cardiac, (2) autonomic, and (3) metabolic. Regardless of the cause, syncope is the end result of inadequate cerebral perfusion, oxygenation, or glucose delivery.

AUTONOMIC SYNCOPE

Autonomic syncope is the most common cause of syncope in pediatrics and can be further described as either reflex or dysautonomic. Of these two types, reflex syncope is more common. Although their exact mechanisms of action are not clearly understood, physical stressors such as anemia, dehydration, hunger, illness, heat, and physical exhaustion can trigger autonomic syncopal episodes. Orthostatic hypotensive syncope occurs during an excessive or prolonged decrease in blood pressure when an individual suddenly assumes an upright position or after prolonged standing. Patients with high basal vagal tone are at higher risk for autonomic syncope.

Neurocardiogenic syncope (often referred to as vasovagal or vasodepressor syncope) is the most common type of reflex syncope and can usually be diagnosed by gathering a careful and complete history, performing a thorough physical examination, and with minimal use of diagnostic testing (**Figure 33-1**). Postural changes and variation in cardiac output or blood volume are triggers for pressure sensors that send signals to the medulla by vagal C fibers. This signaling causes compensatory changes in heart rate, ventricular contractility, and blood vessel compliance by neurohormonal transmitters as a way to maintain cerebral perfusion. A common clinical presentation begins with a prodrome lasting seconds to minutes, followed by a brief period of unconsciousness, after which the patient returns to a previous level of alertness. The premonitory symptoms may include lightheadedness, dizziness, nausea, pallor, shortness of breath, diaphoresis, and visual changes. **Figure 33-2** depicts one hypothesized mechanism for neurocardiogenic syncope, called the hypotensive cardioinhibitory response.

Dysautonomic syncope is caused by dysfunction of the autonomic nervous system and can occasionally lead to syncope in children. Pediatric causes for autonomic failure include familial dysautonomia, toxin exposure, and infectious or inflammatory disease. Syncope caused by a more variable dysfunction of the autonomic nervous system than is seen with neurocardiogenic syncope, without serious underlying disease, has been termed "postural orthostatic tachycardia syndrome" (POTS). Children and adolescents with more constant symptoms and disability related to orthostatic intolerance fall into this category. Although the complete pathophysiology of POTS is not well understood, a hallmark finding is tachycardia during upright posture.

CARDIAC SYNCOPE

Syncope may occur when there is obstruction to cardiac outflow, myocardial dysfunction, or a cardiac arrhythmia. Patients who have a prior history of surgery for congenital cardiac lesions are often at increased risk for acquired and residual structural lesions, myocardial dysfunction, and arrhythmias. Therefore, a cardiologist should evaluate any patient with a prior cardiac history who presents with syncope. Cardiac syncope that is caused by an obstruction to blood flow usually occurs in association with exertion or exercise. It is often related to a fixed or dynamic obstruction to cardiac output due to a structural lesion or related to pulmonary vascular disease. Myocardial dysfunction can also result in syncope when the dysfunction is severe enough to lessen stroke volume and the cardiac output is inadequate to meet increased physical demands (e.g., exertion). Cardiac arrhythmias may also cause associated myocardial dysfunction and result in syncope.

Bradycardia and tachycardia can lead to syncope if effective stroke volume is detrimentally affected. Syncope due to isolated bradycardia in pediatrics is uncommon and is usually due to a medication effect, cardiac manifestations of severe anorexia, or central nervous system trauma. Sinus node pauses and first- and second-degree heart block do not commonly cause syncope. Tachycardia, originating from the sinus node or from an ectopic supraventricular focus, may lead to syncope and is often associated with chest pain, palpitations, lightheadedness, pallor, or nausea.

Ventricular arrhythmias with congenital causes such as Long-QT syndrome and Brugada syndrome or acquired causes such as prolonged QTc due to medication effect can occur in the absence of structural heart disease. Long-QT syndrome is characterized by a prolonged QT interval due to a genetic defect in cardiac potassium or sodium channels with a resultant delay in repolarization. Syncope among patients with Long-QT syndrome is an ominous finding and is presumed to relate to an episode of torsades de pointes that resolves spontaneously. Brugada syndrome is caused by a genetic defect in cardiac sodium channels, which can lead to polymorphic ventricular tachycardia. ST segment elevation may be seen in the anterior precordial leads by electrocardiogram (ECG) in Brugada syndrome, but these findings may also be intermittent. An increased incidence of behavioral health issues among pediatric patients has led to greater use of QTc-prolonging medications which necessitate monitoring, particularly among patients with associated risk factors.

TABLE 33-2 Differential Diagnosis of Syncope

Cardiac
Obstruction to blood flow
Hypertrophic cardiomyopathy
Valvular aortic stenosis
Primary pulmonary hypertension
Eisenmenger syndrome
Myocardial dysfunction
Dilated cardiomyopathy
Arrhythmogenic right ventricular dysplasia/cardiomyopathy (ARVD/C)
Mitral valve prolapse (with severe mitral valve regurgitation)
Neuromuscular disorders (e.g., Duchenne, Becker muscular dystrophies)
Inflammatory disease (e.g., COVID-associated Multisystem Inflammatory Syndrome in Children, Kawasaki disease, viral myocarditis)
Ischemia (e.g., anomalous coronary artery)
Arrhythmias
Long QT syndrome (congenital or acquired)
Supraventricular tachycardia
Sinus node dysfunction
Atrioventricular block
Arrhythmogenic right ventricular dysplasia
Brugada syndrome
Autonomic
Reflex (neurocardiogenic, situational)
Dysautonomic (familial dysautonomia, drugs/toxins, immune-mediated)
Metabolic
Hypoglycemia
Electrolyte imbalances
Endocrine disorders
Toxins and drugs

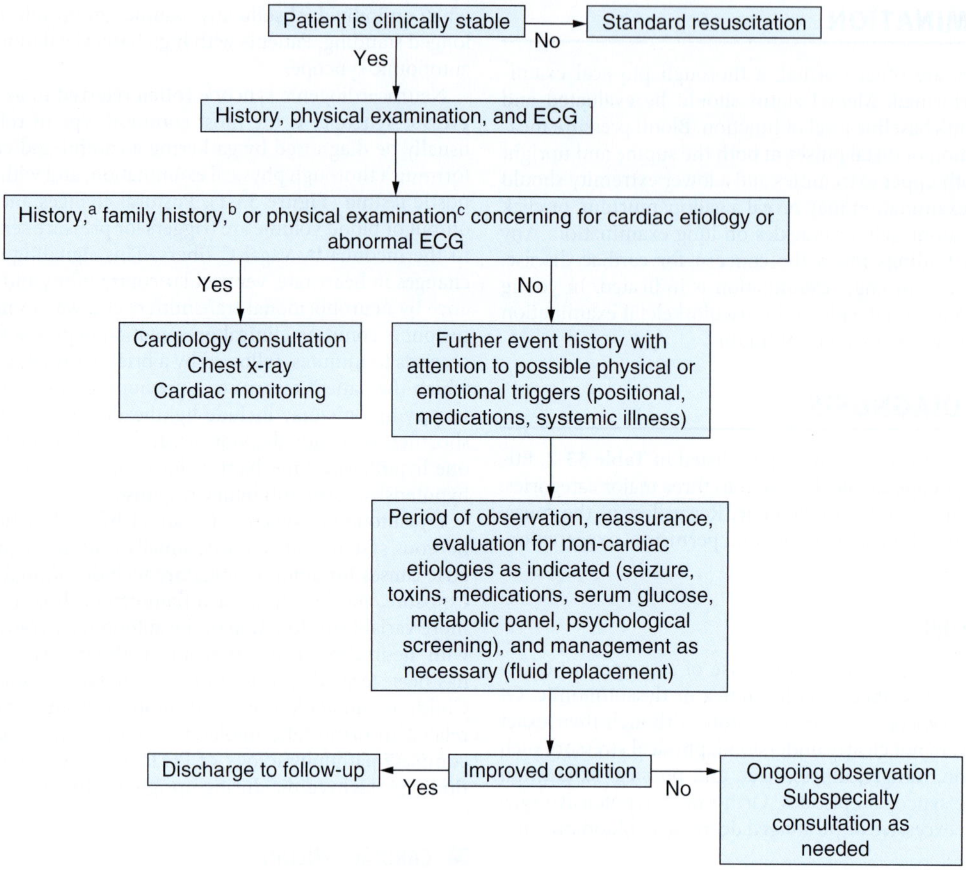

FIGURE 33-1. Neurocardiogenic syncope algorithm. [a]: exertional syncope, history of cardiac surgery, palpitations, chest pain, or shortness of breath; [b]: first-degree relative or multiple family members with sudden death before age 50 years, cardiomyopathy, pulmonary hypertension, or familial arrhythmia; [c]: pathological murmur, gallup, rub, loud or single S_2, toxic appearance, marked tachycardia, tachypnea, peripheral edema, crackles on lung examination, hepatomegaly, or irregular heart rhythm.

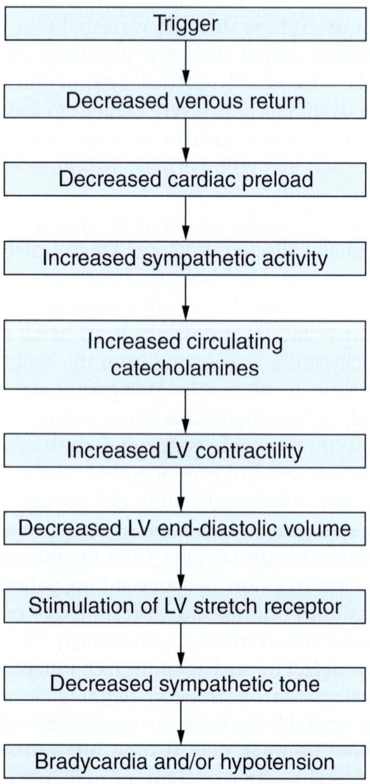

FIGURE 33-2. Autonomic syncope cascade. LV, left ventricular.

Even though mitral valve prolapse is generally asymptomatic in the pediatric population, it is worth mentioning because of its prevalence. It is now believed that when syncope occurs in patients with mitral valve prolapse, the causes are multifactorial and may involve either autonomic dysfunction or arrhythmia, depending on the nature and severity of mitral valve dysfunction.

METABOLIC SYNCOPE

Metabolic derangements associated with syncope include hypoglycemia, hypoxia, and hyperventilation. In general, these conditions produce persistent symptoms that require medical intervention and are usually unaffected by position or activity. Clinical presentation may include a depressed level or loss of consciousness and seizure activity. Diaphoresis, tremor, and altered mental status may precede an episode of hypoglycemic syncope. Hypoxia leading to syncope may initially present with agitation and progress to somnolence. Hyperventilation may lead to a loss of consciousness if cerebral vasoconstriction occurs due to resultant hypocapnia. Drugs and toxin exposure can cause syncope or altered consciousness due to metabolic derangement. Hypoxia and hypocapnia are thought to be significant factors that lead to loss of consciousness in these instances.

A number of conditions that can mimic true syncope are listed in **Table 33-3**. For example, a seizure may mimic a syncopal episode but generally lasts longer than several seconds and may include a preceding aura, abnormal movements, and a postictal period. Atypical migraines can present with syncope-like spells and may include a preceding aura or severe headache. Psychogenic episodes such as panic attacks or hyperventilation can mimic true syncope and occur most often among adolescent patients. A detailed history of the event usually supports the diagnosis and may include a preceding period of stress or hyperventilation while in the presence of others. Patients who have a full recollection of the event are less likely to have suffered a full loss of consciousness. Although

TABLE 33-3 Conditions That Mimic Syncope

Neurologic
Seizure
Migraine
Psychogenic
Panic attacks
Breath-holding
Conversion disorder
Malingering
Munchausen syndrome
Munchausen syndrome by proxy
Trauma

uncommon, malingering, Munchausen syndrome, or Munchausen syndrome by proxy may present with a history of a syncope-like episode. Features that support these diagnoses include the patient's or caregiver's strong desire for extensive or invasive evaluation or therapy.

DIAGNOSTIC EVALUATION

Diagnostic evaluation of the patient with syncope is aimed at detecting those few individuals with serious underlying cardiac or non-cardiac disease. The diagnosis of myocardial dysfunction can usually be achieved by clinical examination, ECG, and echocardiography.

An ECG should be performed as part of all initial evaluations for syncope, with special attention paid to the QT interval corrected for heart rate (QTc) and T-wave morphology for evidence of Long-QT syndrome. In addition, voltage criteria for ventricular hypertrophy suggestive of an obstructive lesion, the pre-excitation of Wolff-Parkinson-White syndrome, and ectopy and conduction disturbances should be ruled out during ECG interpretation. In a patient with a normal ECG but a history suspicious for cardiac arrhythmia, a 24-hour ambulatory Holter monitor may aid in the diagnosis if the episodes are frequent. In a patient whose episodes are isolated or less frequent, an event monitor that can be turned on to record symptomatic events may be more appropriate. In general, a more extensive cardiovascular evaluation is indicated if syncope occurs with exertion and in cases in which there is chest pain preceding the loss of consciousness, recurrent syncope, or an abnormal cardiac examination. It is important to realize that cardiac causes of syncope may be accompanied by seizures that result from global cerebral hypoperfusion. Supraventricular arrhythmias generally cause palpitations rather than syncope. However, atrioventricular nodal bypass tracts, which occur in Wolff-Parkinson-White syndrome, may cause rapid conduction of atrial flutter or fibrillation to the ventricles, resulting in syncope or sudden death.

Ventricular arrhythmias occur more frequently in postoperative patients with congenital heart disease but may also be seen in patients with structurally normal hearts. Long-QT syndrome predisposes patients to ventricular arrhythmias by its characteristic prolongation of the QTc, which places patients at risk for a polymorphic ventricular tachycardia known as torsades de pointes. If prolonged, torsades de pointes can lead to cardiac arrest or death as it degenerates into ventricular fibrillation. In some patients, an ECG demonstrating borderline QTc prolongation may be consistent with the upper range of normal but should be put into context with other features of the syncopal event and past medical history. Some ECG abnormalities may become more exaggerated with an increased heart rate as the QTc fails to shorten appropriately with the R-R interval. Brief and self-resolving periods of rhythm disturbances causing syncope may be precipitated by exercise or a startling experience. Genetic causes of Long-QT syndrome are due to either a defect in cardiac potassium or sodium channels. Acquired causes of prolonged QTc include electrolyte disturbances (e.g., hypokalemia, hypocalcemia, hypomagnesemia), increased intracranial pressure, and medications (e.g., atypical antipsychotics, tricyclic antidepressants, phenothiazines, antiarrhythmics) and should be considered based on laboratory data, neurologic examination, or by medication history.

Laboratory testing for metabolic or endocrine derangements associated with syncope can include a blood glucose level, electrolyte panel, and complete blood count when indicated by the patient's history. If a toxic ingestion is suspected, a serum and urine toxicology screen should be obtained. Anemia can predispose to syncope when it is severe or more acute in onset. Because hypoxia due to carbon monoxide poisoning can lead to syncope, co-oximetry with a carboxyhemoglobin level should be considered when indicated by circumstances. A pregnancy test is also indicated in postmenarchal adolescents with syncope.

An electroencephalogram or imaging of the central nervous system is often part of an evaluation when epilepsy or other neurologic causes for syncope are being considered.

The diagnostic accuracy of upright tilt table testing has not been validated during the general evaluation of pediatric syncope, or for guiding management or prognosis.

MANAGEMENT

Therapeutic intervention to prevent or treat recurrent syncope depends on the pathogenic cause and the frequency and severity of the episodes. Standard resuscitative interventions should be instituted for acute syncopal events. Patients who have known structural heart disease or other cardiac disease should be admitted to the hospital and evaluated by a cardiologist. The treatment of cardiogenic syncope is generally overseen by a cardiologist and is based on a careful and thorough diagnostic evaluation to determine the underlying abnormality. Suppression of symptomatic supraventricular arrhythmias is often managed with medication, but treatment varies based on the inciting or propagating feature of the disorder. Patients with Long-QT syndrome may benefit from alpha-adrenergic antagonists to prevent exercise-induced ventricular arrhythmia, but pacemakers or implanted cardiac defibrillators are necessary in some cases. Surgical intervention may be needed for structural abnormalities, and intensive care interventions are required for those with progressive or unstable conditions.

Autonomic syncope is considered a benign illness, and in most cases, prophylaxis against presyncope or "near syncope" is sufficient intervention. Educating patients and families generally results in earlier awareness of symptoms and the ability to abort episodes by assuming a recumbent posture. Additional measures for prophylaxis include the avoidance of dehydration and a salt-enriched diet. When these prevention strategies are not effective, treatment with medications such as beta-blockers, fludrocortisone, and midodrine may be trialed. No single pharmacologic agent has been shown to be consistently efficacious and often a combination of therapeutic strategies is necessary to manage symptoms effectively. Atrioventricular pacing has been used in some patients with frequent episodes of symptomatic bradycardia, but this is reserved for refractory cases when pharmacologic agents are unsuccessful.

The treatment of metabolic or other systemic causes of syncope focuses on the underlying process, both in the acute resuscitation phase and in the prevention stage. Identification of a causative entity often allows patients and families to prevent future syncopal events or to manage such events safely if and when they reoccur.

SPECIAL CONSIDERATIONS

The diagnosis of heritable conditions during an evaluation for syncope necessitates genetic counseling for family members.

When heart disease is identified as a cause for syncope, evaluation and management should address both the underlying condition and the potential for an associated life-threatening arrhythmia.

Cerebrovascular events are rare in children but should be considered in patients with underlying disease affecting the peripheral vasculature who present with syncope.

KEY POINTS

- Syncope in children is most often benign and self-limited.
- History and physical examination are the most important initial diagnostic tools in the evaluation of syncope.
- Evaluation of a patient presenting with syncope is geared toward identifying those few patients who are at high risk for serious underlying disease.

SUGGESTED READINGS

Anderson JB, Czosek RJ, Cnota J, et al. Pediatric syncope: National Hospital Ambulatory Medical Care Survey results. *J Emerg Med.* 2012; 43:575-583.

Boudoulas H, Wooley CF. The floppy mitral valve, mitral valve prolapse, and mitral valvular regurgitation. In: Allen HD, Gutgesell HP, Clark EB, Driscoll DJ, eds. *Moss and Adam's Heart Disease in Infants, Children, and Adolescents.* 6th ed. Philadelphia, PA: Lippincott Williams & Wilkins; 2001:964.

Bryarly M, Phillips L, Fu Q, Vernino S, Levine B. Postural orthostatic tachycardia syndrome: JACC focus seminar. *J Am Coll Cardiol.* 2019;73(10):1207-1228.

Driscoll DJ, Jacobsen SJ, Porter CJ, Wollan PC. Syncope in children and adolescents. *J Am Coll Cardiol.* 1997;29:1039-1045.

Jensen KG, Juul K, Fink-Jensen A, Correll C, Pagsberg AK. Corrected QT changes during antipsychotic treatment of children and adolescents: a systematic review and meta-analysis of clinical trials. *J Am Acad Child Adolesc Psychiatry.* 2015;54(1):25-36.

Paris Y, Toro-Salazar OH, Gauthier NS, et al. Regional implementation of a pediatric cardiology syncope algorithm using standardized clinical assessment and management plans (SCAMPS) methodology. *J Am Heart Assoc.* 2016;5:e002931.

Rennette Z, Metais B, Tuckfield L, DelVecchio M, Aronoff S. Pediatric syncope: a systemic review. *Pediatr Emerg Care.* 2020;36:442-445.

Schunk PC, Ruttan T. Pediatric syncope: high-risk conditions and reasonable approach. *Emerg Med Clin North Am.* 2018;36(2): 305-321.

Sheldon R, Grubb B, Olshansky B, et al. 2015 heart rhythm society expert consensus statement on the diagnosis and treatment of postural tachycardia syndrome, inappropriate sinus tachycardia and vasovagal syncope. *Heart Rhythm.* 2015;12(6):e41-63.

Shen WK, Sheldon RS, Benditt DG, et al. 2017 ACC/AHA/HRS guideline for the evaluation and management of patients with syncope: a report of the American College of Cardiology/American Heart Association Task Force on Clinical Practice Guidelines and the Heart Rhythm Society. *J Am Coll Cardiol.* 2017; *70*(5): e39-e110.

Stewart J, Boris J, Chelimsky G, et al. Pediatric disorders of orthostatic intolerance. *Pediatrics.* 2018;141(1):e20171673.

Strickberger SA, Benson DW, Biaggioni I, et al. AHA/ACCF Scientific Statement on the evaluation of syncope: from the American Heart Association Councils on Clinical Cardiology, Cardiovascular Nursing, Cardiovascular Disease in the Young, and Stroke, and the Quality of Care and Outcomes Research Interdisciplinary Working Group; and the American College of Cardiology Foundation: in collaboration with the Heart Rhythm Society: endorsed by the American Autonomic Society. *Circulation.* 2006;113:316.

CHAPTER 34

Vomiting

Craig J. Conard, MD and Shannon B. Palombo, MD

BACKGROUND

Vomiting is a common chief complaint for hospitalized pediatric patients and can be a presenting sign of illness in nearly every organ system. Evaluation based on history, examination, and ancillary testing can help identify the etiology of vomiting, contribute to appropriate interventions, and avoid or minimize related complications.

PATHOPHYSIOLOGY

Vomiting is a highly coordinated, centrally mediated reflex. It occurs when the contents of the stomach are forcefully expelled out of the mouth. Descent of the diaphragm and constriction of abdominal musculature occur simultaneously with relaxation of the gastric cardia, forcing the contents of the stomach retrograde into the esophagus.

The vomiting centers of the brain, which reside in the reticular formation of the medulla, receive sensory input from a number of sources that trigger vomiting. These include afferent signals from the gastrointestinal (GI) tract arising from the vagus nerve and other parasympathetic nerves and afferent signals from outside the GI tract originating from organs located in the thorax and abdomen. Additionally, the chemoreceptor zone in the brainstem detects chemical abnormalities in the body, such as uremia or ketoacidosis, which can stimulate vomiting. In the setting of cerebral trauma, extramedullary centers in the brain receive afferent signals from injured areas that can cause vomiting. Erratic motion can alter perception of body position and stimulate vomiting via the vestibular system. Based on the complexity of pathophysiology, vomiting therefore can be a manifestation of disease from multi-organ system inputs, necessitating a broad differential diagnosis.

PATIENT HISTORY

A thorough history should be conducted in all children presenting with vomiting. A few key questions can guide the patient's history.

- What is the age of the patient?
- What is the character of the emesis (bilious or nonbilious? bloody or non-bloody? projectile?)
- When was the onset? Duration? Associated time of day? Is it cyclical?
- Is it associated with the act of eating or triggered by specific types of food?
- Are there recent exposures to new foods, drugs, or environments? Recent travel?
- Are there associated complaints within the GI tract (weight loss, abdominal pain, change in stool)?

Finally, completing a comprehensive review of systems is a useful adjunct in identifying patterns of illness that can point toward an appropriate workup and diagnosis.

PHYSICAL EXAMINATION

The physical examination in the evaluation of the vomiting child begins with an initial assessment of the patient to gauge the acuity of illness with close attention given to the vital signs based on age-appropriate normal ranges. This includes a plotted assessment of growth as well. A head-to-toe physical evaluation can then be performed with emphasis on a focused examination of the abdomen in each quadrant, including epigastric and suprapubic areas. Exam techniques include inspection, auscultation, percussion, and palpation. Notable findings could include:

- abdominal distention
- skin changes
- abnormal bowel sounds
- tenderness, guarding, or rebound pain
- masses, organomegaly
- radiating or referred pain
- fluid shifts or ascites

Of note, bowel obstruction causes abdominal distention, high-pitched bowel sounds, a taut abdominal wall, and abdominal pain with palpation. Absence of bowel sounds suggests an ileus. Rebound pain is seen in conditions causing peritonitis.

Based on the patient's history, careful examination of associated systems is needed to correlate exam features that may narrow the differential diagnosis and direct next steps for evaluation.

Lastly, vomiting frequently causes dehydration; therefore, assessment of hydration status based on the physical exam is important to guide appropriate treatment interventions.

DIFFERENTIAL DIAGNOSIS

The differential diagnosis of vomiting can be organized in terms of gastrointestinal versus non-gastrointestinal pathologies as well as by age of the patient.

GASTROINTESTINAL CAUSES

The causes of vomiting within the GI tract are numerous and can be stratified by age and by obstructive versus non-obstructive causes.

Obstructive Vomiting in the first few days of life can signify serious pathology. Nonbilious emesis is a sign that an obstruction is proximal to the ampulla of Vater. Esophageal atresia presents with nonbilious emesis in an infant. Characteristic findings include the inability to pass a nasogastric tube into the stomach and a paucity of bowel gas on an abdominal plain film. The caveat to this radiographic finding would be if there is the presence of a tracheoesophageal fistula in addition to esophageal atresia. Duodenal atresia can present with nonbilious emesis depending on the level of atresia. It usually presents within hours of birth and rarely is associated with abdominal distension due to the proximal nature of the obstruction. A classic radiographic finding would show a "double bubble" appearance due to air within the stomach as well as in the first portion of the duodenum proximal to the atresia.

Bilious emesis is indicative of more distal obstructive GI malformations requires urgent evaluation to avoid bowel strangulation and ischemia. The differential diagnosis includes duodenal or jejunal atresias, intestinal duplication, malrotation with midgut volvulus, meconium plug or ileus, colonic atresia or stenosis, imperforate anus, microcolon, or Hirschsprung disease. More distal jejunal obstructions usually present within the first 24 hours of life and are associated with abdominal distension. Malrotation with midgut volvulus most typically presents with bilious emesis within the first week of life, though can also occur outside of the newborn period secondary to lack of mesenteric anchoring to the retroperitoneum. A meconium plug or ileus can cause bilious emesis that either resolves as the meconium passes or may require surgical intervention. This diagnosis should raise clinical suspicion for cystic fibrosis. A history of failure to pass meconium can also be seen in Hirschsprung disease. Contrasted abdominal radiographs will show marked dilation throughout the bowel proximal to the "transition zone."

Complications such as bowel strangulation and ischemia can occur outside the newborn period in the setting of malrotation due to increased risk of volvulus secondary to lack of mesenteric anchoring to the retroperitoneum.

Beyond the immediate newborn period, nonbilious emesis can be a sign of pyloric stenosis. The classic history includes that of projectile vomiting in a hungry infant who continues to desire to feed despite persistent emesis. A palpable "olive" on examination in the epigastric region due to pyloric hypertrophy is often a late finding. Lactobezoars, a conglomeration of milk and mucous, can be a rare cause of gastric outlet obstruction and nonbilious emesis in milk-fed infants.

Obstructive pathologies beyond infancy can include malrotation with midgut volvulus, intussusception, achalasia, cricopharyngeal incoordination, esophageal webs and strictures, hiatal and diaphragmatic hernias, duodenal webs, duodenal hematomas, intestinal strictures, and vascular rings and slings. Pediatric patients with midgut volvulus present with bilious emesis, abdominal distension, electrolyte abnormalities, irritability, lethargy, and even shock due to bowel ischemia and acidosis. Stridor can be present in the setting of a vascular ring, as the aberrant vessel compresses the trachea in addition to the esophagus. Superior mesenteric artery syndrome should be considered in a patient who has had rapid weight loss resulting in the loss of the fat pad that normally is situated between the superior mesenteric artery and the duodenum, causing compression of the duodenum and eventual obstruction and emesis. Intussusception should be suspected in patients presenting with paroxysms of severe abdominal pain, vomiting, and lethargy. Currant jelly stools are a late finding indicative of bowel ischemia and necrosis. A torsed Meckel diverticulum, incarcerated hernias, and adhesions in the setting of prior abdominal surgeries should be on the differential of vomiting due to obstruction. A history of abdominal trauma should raise suspicion for a duodenal hematoma, pancreatic pseudocyst, or other abdominal organ injury that could lead to an obstructive process. Ingestion of foreign bodies can obstruct the pylorus or esophagus in toddlers, including coins, batteries, or other nonfood items, as well as bezoars that build up over time due to chronic ingestion of hair, carpet, or other unusual items.

Non-obstructive Non-obstructive causes of vomiting within the GI tract in the immediate newborn and infant period include necrotizing enterocolitis, inborn errors of metabolism, milk or soy protein allergy, gastroesophageal reflux, overfeeding, and improper mixing of formula. Necrotizing enterocolitis can present with bilious or nonbilious emesis and should be suspected in a toxic-appearing infant with abdominal distension and radiographic evidence of pneumatosis intestinalis or air in the bowel wall with possible hepatic portal venous gas if perforation has occurred. Although rare, inborn errors of metabolism should be suspected in the vomiting, acidotic, and/or hypoglycemic infant.

Gastroesophageal reflux can affect children of any age. A history of emesis, back arching, crying with feeds, or symptoms that intensify with supine positioning should raise the suspicion for gastroesophageal reflux disease. Complications of gastroesophageal reflux disease include Sandifer syndrome, a condition characterized by back arching that may mimic seizure activity gastritis and gastric or duodenal ulcers.

In infancy and beyond the early childhood period, protein intolerance can be an etiology of emesis, diarrhea, bloody stools, irritability, and poor weight gain. Commonly implicated proteins include milk, soy, and egg. Allergic reactions to foods or medications can also manifest as emesis, especially if accompanied by urticaria, respiratory distress, edema, abdominal pain, or anaphylaxis. Food protein-induced enterocolitis syndrome (FPIES) is characterized by delayed development of severe vomiting and diarrhea in the hours following ingestion of a food trigger. Eosinophilic esophagitis or enteritis is often associated with food allergens and can present with emesis, abdominal pain, reflux, and food refusal. Celiac disease is caused by gluten sensitivity and leads to villous atrophy and malabsorption, the sequelae of which include vomiting, diarrhea, and poor weight gain in infants and children.

Most often seen in older children, inflammatory bowel disease can also cause emesis along with other symptoms including hematochezia, weight loss, and abdominal pain. Biliary pathologies such as cholecystitis, cholethiasis, and choledocholithiasis tend to present with nausea, vomiting, and

TABLE 34-1 Causes of Vomiting by Gastrointestinal System

Esophageal	Necrotizing enterocolitis
Stricture	Intestinal stenosis or adhesions
Web	Incarcerated hernia
Ring	Meckel's diverticulum
Atresia	**Colon**
Tracheoesophageal fistula	Hirschsprung disease
Achalasia	Meconium plug or ileus
Foreign body	Microcolon
Stomach	Imperforate anus
Pyloric stenosis	Bezoar
Web	Foreign body
Duplication	**Other**
Gastroesophageal reflux disease	Celiac disease
Gastritis	Milk/soy protein allergy
Ulcer	Lactose intolerance
Hiatal Hernia	Food allergies
Small Intestine	Eosinophilic enteritis
Duodenal atresia	Inflammatory bowel disease
Malrotation with midgut volvulus	Pancreatitis
Duplication	Annular pancreas
Intussusception	Hepatitis
Bezoar	Cholelithiasis, choledocholithiasis
Foreign body	Abdominal trauma
Pseudo-obstruction	

TABLE 34-2 Causes of Vomiting by Organ Systems (Non-Gastrointestinal)

Neurologic	**Infectious**
Intracranial mass lesion	Viral gastroenteritis
Hydrocephalus	Bacterial gastroenteritis
Intracranial bleed	Post-viral gastroparesis
Cerebral edema	Appendicitis
Pseudotumor cerebri	Cholecystitis
Migraine headache	Helicobacter pylori
Cyclic vomiting syndrome	Pneumonia
Abdominal migraine	Bronchiolitis
Seizure	Pertussis
Meningitis	Sinusitis
Kernicterus	Otitis
Vestibular system disruption	Pharyngitis
Concussion	Meningitis
Genitourinary	Encephalitis
Obstructive uropathy	Sepsis
Pyelonephritis	**Cardiac**
Renal insufficiency	Arrhythmias
Renal tubular acidosis	Heart failure
Glomerulonephritis	**Psychiatric**
Ovarian or testicular torsion	Anorexia nervosa
Pregnancy	Bulimia
Metabolic	Hyperventilation
Hypercalcemia	Anxiety
Hypokalemia	Rumination
Hyperammonemia	**Benign**
Urea cycle defects	Overfeeding
Amino acidopathies	Aerophagia
Organic acidopathies	Innocent spitting
Glycogen storage disease	Excessive handling in newborn
Fatty acid oxidation defects	**Miscellaneous**
Galactosemia	Ingestions
Lysosomal storage diseases	Drug toxicities
Peroxisomal disorders	Medications
Endocrine	Child abuse
Diabetic ketoacidosis	
Congenital adrenal hyperplasia	
Adrenal insufficiency	

right upper quadrant abdominal pain that is colicky in nature and associated with meals, and is more frequent in children with rapid red blood cell turnover, those with prolonged parenteral nutrition, or taking certain medications. Pancreatitis can occur in children secondary to viral infection, trauma, drug ingestion, structural abnormality, genetic or autoimmune predisposition, or idiopathic causes. The hallmark of pancreatitis is nausea, emesis, and severe epigastric abdominal pain. Hepatitis secondary to viruses, toxins, drugs, metabolic or autoimmune causes presents with emesis, jaundice, and right upper quadrant abdominal pain.

NON-GASTROINTESTINAL CAUSES

Neurologic Vomiting may be a presenting sign of serious neurologic sequelae. Increased intracranial pressure (ICP) can cause vomiting, headache, and vision changes. Late findings indicative of impending herniation are cranial nerve palsies and vital sign changes consistent with Cushing's triad of hypertension, bradycardia, and abnormal respirations. Increased ICP may be due to a mass lesion, hydrocephalus, vascular malformations, hematomas such as in the setting of head trauma, or idiopathic intracranial hypertension (IIH). These conditions may lead to intractable vomiting and headaches that awaken a child from sleep or worsen with Valsalva maneuvers. IIH can stimulate nausea and vomiting as well as positional headaches and visual field deficits. Vomiting can also occur in association with seizure activity, or can indicate intracranial infection such as meningitis or encephalitis when associated with fever, neck stiffness, and headache.

Nausea and vomiting are commonly associated with migraine headaches. Cyclic vomiting syndrome and abdominal migraines are thought to share similar pathophysiologic mechanisms. The former is characterized by recurrent episodes of nausea and vomiting where no alternative cause is identified. For diagnosis, the patient must have at least three episodes of rapid onset, recurrent vomiting that lasts for hours to days followed by intervals of normal health. Abdominal migraines involve episodic abdominal pain and emesis associated with nausea, anorexia, photophobia, headache, and pallor; and they usually occur in the setting of a family history of migraines. Interval periods of normal health between episodes also exist.

Disruption of the vestibular system as seen in labyrinthitis, motion sickness, benign paroxysmal positional vertigo, and even otitis media can cause vomiting.

Genitourinary Emesis is a prevalent feature in all types of genitourinary pathologies, including structural abnormalities, infections, and organ dysfunction caused by genetic or metabolic conditions. More common diagnoses include pyelonephritis, nephrolithiasis, ureteropelvic junction obstruction, acute renal failure, and testicular and ovarian torsions. Vomiting in adolescent females should prompt pregnancy testing.

Metabolic An underlying metabolic or mitochondrial process should be considered in an infant or young child with persistent emesis and electrolyte abnormalities. Hypercalcemia, hypokalemia, hypoglycemia, and hyperammonemia can all cause vomiting. Urea cycle defects, amino- and organic acidopathies, fatty acid oxidation disorders, and glycogen storage diseases are among the metabolic conditions that can present with vomiting. Mitochondrial diseases are often associated with intestinal dysmotility or pseudo-obstruction. In addition, these children often have a long history of gastroesophageal reflux, feeding intolerance, abdominal pain, constipation or diarrhea, and failure to thrive.

Endocrine Diabetic ketoacidosis can lead to intractable vomiting in the setting of ketosis. Salt-wasting congenital adrenal hyperplasia should be suspected in a vomiting female infant with signs of virilization. Male infants with this condition usually have normal genitalia, often leading to a delayed diagnosis. Adrenal insufficiency can present with emesis during an acute crisis. Hypothyroidism and associated constipation may also lead to vomiting.

Infectious Infectious etiologies of vomiting are numerous. The majority of cases are caused by acute gastroenteritis (AGE) from viral and bacterial sources. Most AGEs are self-limited and require supportive care only, although treatment should be considered for at-risk age groups and immunocompromised patients with select infections. Bacterial causes of emesis should be considered in a history consistent with certain food, animal, or environmental exposures. Examples include *Staphylococcus aureus*, *Bacillus cereus*, *Shigella*, *Salmonella*, *Escherichia coli*, *Yersinia enterocolitica*, and *Campylobacter jejuni*. Parasitic infections such as ascariasis or giardiasis can lead to vomiting, diarrhea, and obstructive pathologies. A child presenting with emesis in the setting of a preceding viral illness may have post-viral gastroparesis leading to delayed gastric emptying and emesis, which can take days to weeks to resolve.

Appendicitis should be considered in the child presenting with fever, anorexia, nausea, emesis, and periumbilical pain that migrates to the right lower quadrant. Viral or bacterial meningitis can present with vomiting in addition to headache, vision changes, and altered mentation. Sinusitis or pharyngitis can also present with emesis, as can infections such a pertussis or bronchiolitis that cause excessive coughing and post-tussive emesis. It is important not to overlook lower lobe pneumonia as an etiology of abdominal pain and emesis associated with fever, tachypnea, and cough.

Cardiac Cardiovascular etiologies of vomiting generally involve arrhythmias such as supraventricular tachycardia in the irritable infant, or heart failure in an infant with feeding intolerance and poor weight gain. Myocarditis may also present with vomiting.

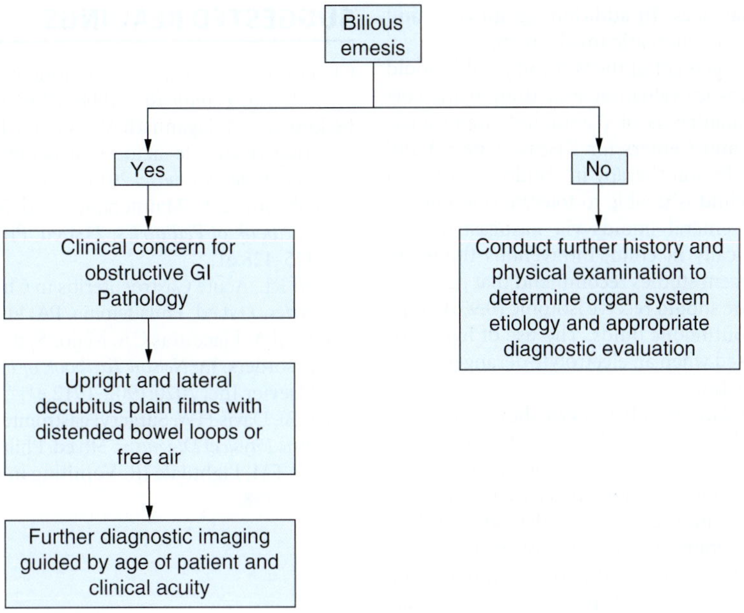

FIGURE 34-1. Approach to diagnosis of vomiting.

Psychiatric Psychiatric etiologies of emesis should be considered when the history supports a behavioral diagnosis. For example, emesis is a key feature of anorexia nervosa-purging type and bulimia nervosa. Although the pathophysiology differs from emesis, rumination syndrome or the act of regurgitating undigested food can be seen in pediatric patients with severe stress, developmental delay, and autism spectrum disorder. Anxiety and other heightened emotions can contribute to visceral hyperalgesia, nausea, and emesis, the long-term effects of which may precipitate development of functional abdominal pain syndromes.

Drug-Induced Drug-induced emesis is common and can include intentional or unintentional ingestions. Emesis is also a well-known side effect of chemotherapy agents. Similarly, post-operative nausea and vomiting can be triggered by anesthesia. Cannabis hyperemesis syndrome is caused by excessive or long-term use of marijuana.

DIAGNOSTIC EVALUATION AND MANAGEMENT

The management of vomiting is dependent on the etiology and pathophysiology of the organ system(s) involved (**Figures 34-1** and **34-2**). A thorough history and physical examination will guide a focused, diagnostic evaluation of the vomiting infant or child.

If clinical concern for obstruction exists, a nasogastric tube should be placed immediately, followed by abdominal radiographs and appropriate contrasted imaging to evaluate gastrointestinal anatomy. Furthermore, urgent surgical consultation is key to preventing continued bowel ischemia. Ultrasound is helpful if there is concern for abdominal or pelvic organ pathology. A complete blood count and inflammatory markers can be useful to determine if there is infection or inflammation. A complete metabolic profile will assess kidney and liver function

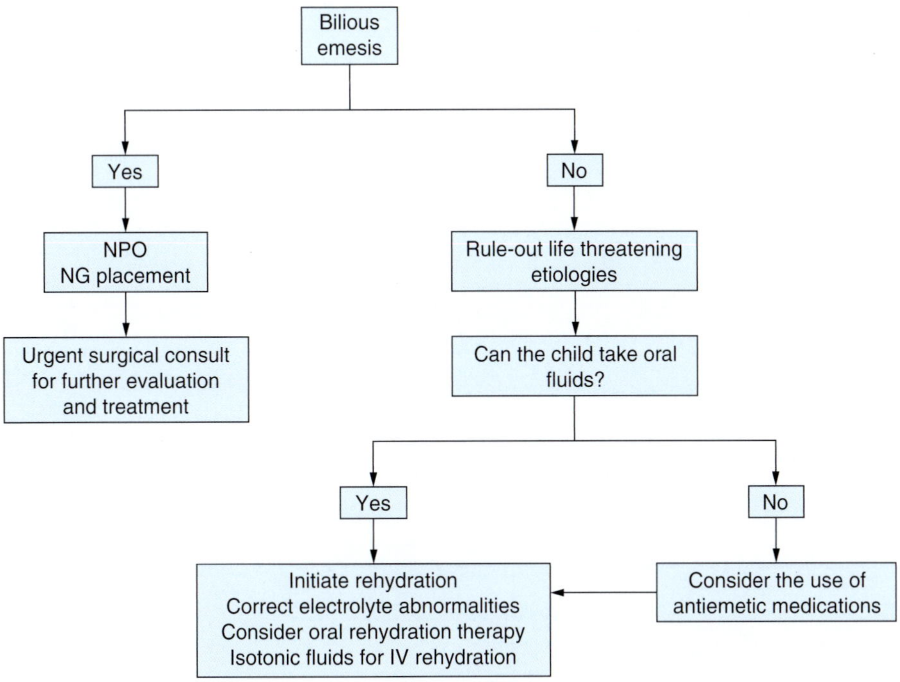

FIGURE 34-2. Approach to treatment for vomiting.

and evaluate for electrolyte imbalances. In addition, an amylase and lipase can be considered to rule out pancreatic involvement.

Stabilization and symptom management of the vomiting child should occur concomitantly with a diagnostic evaluation. Rehydration and correction of any electrolyte abnormalities is of paramount importance. The World Health Organization and Centers for Disease Control and Prevention recommend oral rehydration therapy in children with mild to moderate dehydration. If the child is unable to tolerate oral liquids, options for rehydration include enteral liquids via nasogastric tube or intravenous fluid. In the critically ill child, intravenous fluids are needed for initial stabilization. Recent studies recommend that pediatric patients greater than 1 month of age should receive isotonic (0.9%) saline for all intravenous boluses and continuous fluids. The use of hyper- or hypotonic fluids should only be used when an electrolyte derangement is present and warrants urgent correction.

Antiemetic therapies such as ondansetron have been shown to reduce vomiting, improve tolerance of oral fluids, and reduce hospital admissions and length of stay in children with gastroenteritis. Additional medication regimens, procedural interventions, and behavioral practices may be considered in the setting of refractory vomiting or specific diagnoses such as cyclic vomiting syndrome, chemotherapy, and chronic gastroparesis.

Primary care physicians should be considered partners in managing chronic, recurrent, or refractory emesis. Subspecialty referrals may include gastroenterology, surgery, endocrinology, genetics, and neurology as appropriate.

KEY POINTS

- Vomiting is a common presenting symptom in children, and can be an indicator of pathology in nearly every organ system.
- A thorough history and physical examination should be conducted in every child presenting with vomiting to narrow the differential diagnosis and guide an evaluation.
- Bilious emesis can be a sign of bowel obstruction and should prompt imaging and urgent surgical consultation.
- Management of vomiting should focus on rehydration and correction of electrolyte abnormalities.
- Antiemetic medications are useful for treatment of vomiting due to acute gastroenteritis.
- Subspecialty referral should be considered in the setting of chronic, recurrent, and refractory emesis.

SUGGESTED READINGS

Chandran L, Chitkara M. Vomiting in children: reassurance, red flag, or referral? *Pediatr Rev.* 2008; 29(6):183-192.

Fedorowicz Z, Jagannath VA, Carter B. Antiemetics for reducing vomiting related to acute gastroenteritis in children and adolescents. *Cochrane Database.* 2011;9:CD005506.

Greenbaum, LA. Maintenance and Replacement Therapy. In: *Nelson Textbook of Pediatrics.* 21st ed. Philadelphia, PA: Elsevier Inc; 2020: 425-428.e1.

Kotloff KL. Acute Gastroenteritis in Children. In: *Nelson Textbook of Pediatrics.* 21st ed. Philadelphia, PA: Elsevier Inc; 2020:2012-2033.e2.

Maqbool A, Liacouras CA. Major Symptoms and Signs of Digestive Tract Disorders. In: *Nelson Textbook of Pediatrics.* 21st ed. Philadelphia, PA: Elsevier Inc; 2020:1902-1912.e1.

Zitelli BJ, Davis HW. Surgery: gastrointestinal obstruction. In: *Atlas of Pediatric Physical Diagnosis.* 5th ed. Philadelphia, PA: Mosby; 2007: 632-641.

Shields TM, Lightdale JR. Vomiting in Children. *Pediatr Rev.* 2018;39(7): 342-358.

PART III

Systems Approach

SECTION A

Abuse and Neglect

CHAPTER 35 Cutaneous Injuries of Concern for Child Maltreatment

Romy Cho, MD, FRCPC, DRCPSC and
Gunjan Tiyyagura, MD, MHS

BACKGROUND

Pediatric providers are uniquely positioned to identify situations concerning for child maltreatment and intervene accordingly. Child maltreatment may present with a wide array of signs and symptoms which may seem medically inconsequential (e.g., frenum injury or bruising in a pre-mobile infant), but are sentinel injuries concerning for child physical abuse.

According to the US Department of Health and Human Services in 2019, 618,000 children were determined to be victims of abuse and neglect by child protective services in the United States. While a majority of children are victims of neglect, 16.5% are victims of physical abuse (child maltreatment 2019). For the purpose of this section, we will concentrate on the various aspects of child physical abuse (Chapters 35-39), as well as the legal issues which are inherent in all cases of child maltreatment (Chapter 39).

Cutaneous injuries are often the most noticeable findings suggesting that a child may have been physically abused. They should be documented and carefully considered in the context of the child's overall history and presentation. Although the presence of a cutaneous injury is not necessarily specific for child physical abuse, particular characteristics of skin findings, such as bruises, burns/thermal injuries, and bite marks, can raise concerns for an abusive etiology.

CLINICAL PRESENTATION

The clinical presentation of the child with cutaneous lesions can vary widely. Regardless of whether the child is presenting with a stated concern for a skin injury or one is detected as an incidental finding, the medical provider should be prepared to seek additional information if the child's injury is not in keeping with the history provided.

BRUISES

Bruises are a common physical finding in child physical abuse, but often missed as a sentinel injury in about one-third of serious abusive injuries. When present in the pre-mobile child who is not yet cruising, crawling, or walking (usually children <6 months of age), bruises should raise concern for possible physical abuse or an underlying medical condition. However, bruising from normal activity is frequently found in toddlers and school-aged children. Accidental bruises correlate with the child's level of independent mobility and usually occur from typical childhood injuries, such as falling forward onto the ground or falling from furniture. These bruises are usually small and typically occur over anterior surfaces or over bony prominences, such as the anterior tibia or knee, head, and forehead.

In contrast, bruises due to abuse are more commonly located on the ears, soft portions of the face, neck, trunk, and buttocks. Compared with bruises from accidental causes, these bruises are typically found on soft and cushioned parts of the body without underlying bony prominences (e.g., fleshy part of the cheek instead of the forehead). Abusive bruises are also more often extensive in terms of size and number of bruises. Clustered bruises are unusual in routine activities, and disclosures from abused children have revealed that the bruising can be the result of a defensive mechanism (e.g., when children flex their legs and wrap their arms around their bodies to protect themselves) on the upper arms or outer thighs. Patterned bruises that are the result of impact with an object with corresponding surface features and orientation are also concerning for abuse. Linear bruising is caused by contact with an object with a linear edge (e.g., rods, rulers, belts). Likewise, flexible objects (e.g., ropes, cords, chains) can leave a loop-configured bruise at the site of contact. Slap marks may appear as a negative image such that an outline of the handprint is created on the skin as a result of blood extravasating from vessels into the surrounding interstitial space. Patterned bruising is uncommon with routine childhood activities and should raise concern for inflicted injury.

Pierce et al. examined bruising characteristics that differentiated abused from non-abused children presenting to 5 children's hospital emergency departments (EDs) and 2,161 children <4 years old with bruising were identified through deliberate examination. Authors found bruising on the torso (T) which includes chest, abdomen, back, buttocks, and genitourinary area, ears (E), neck (N), bruising to frenulum (F), angle of jaw (A), soft part of the cheek (C), eyelid (E), sclera (S), patterned bruising, or any bruising in a child < 4.99 months was predictive of abuse. More than two-thirds of abuse patients in this study presented without any initial history of trauma. This clinical decision rule (called TEN-4 FACES-P) had a sensitivity of 95.6% and specificity of 87.1% for distinguishing abusive from non-abusive trauma. These test characteristics did not vary significantly by skin tone.

Finally, authors have also examined whether it was possible to determine the age of bruising in children. In a systematic review by Maguire et al, results of the included studies revealed that any color could be present in fresh, intermediate, and old bruises. These findings demonstrate that the age of a bruise cannot be accurately determined from clinical assessment or from photographs.

BURNS

A systematic review by Loos et al reported pooled data of 10 incidence studies which estimated that approximately 9.7% of burns in children were concerning for physical abuse. Clinical features can help calibrate one's level of concern for child maltreatment regarding a burn and include the child's developmental abilities, the location and extent of the burn, the presence of bilateral injuries, a delay in presentation for medical care, and whether the overall appearance of the burn is compatible with the explanation being provided by caregivers. As with bruising, burns in premobile infants are generally more concerning than burns in ambulatory children, as well as burns located on posterior surfaces or protected areas of the body, such as the buttocks or genitalia. Burns concerning for child maltreatment tend to be deeper and associated with additional injuries, such as other cutaneous injuries, bruises, and fractures.

In the pediatric population, scald burns from contact with a hot liquid are the most frequently encountered type of burn injury and may be produced by a hot liquid flowing across the skin or by immersing part of the body into a hot liquid. When a scald burn is caused by an accidental injury from a hot flowing liquid, the burn tends to be deepest at the initial site of contact where contact with the hot liquid is the longest. As the hot liquid travels down the body, heat dissipates and the liquid cools resulting in variable burn depths and a flow pattern with irregular borders. Kemp et al reported that the most common agents of scald burns were hot beverages from pull-down injury in children < 5 years old and spill injuries in children 5 to 16 years old.

In contrast, an immersion burn, more often due to abusive injury, is caused by submerging part of the body below the surface of a hot liquid and characteristically has a uniform burn depth as the burned area is exposed to the hot liquid for the same duration of time. These burns are typically circumferential and are associated with a sharp demarcation line between burned and normal skin. When the extremities are involved, the child can present with localized glove (i.e., hand/arm) or stocking (i.e., feet/leg) distribution of burned skin.

In scald burns, areas of sparing indicate that there was no contact with hot liquid and can be informative regarding a child's positioning at the time of a burn injury or contact with a surface. For example, a child sustaining an immersion burn while seated in a bathtub will have burns to the skin exposed to the hot liquid with sparing of the buttocks in contact with the bathtub surface. The presence or absence of splash marks on the skin does not typically provide additional information in the interpretation of burn injuries. The appearance of a burn can also be influenced by the temperature of the water, subsequent burn treatment measures and the presence of clothing, which may offer some protection to the skin.

Contact burns are the second most common type of paediatric burn injury presenting for medical attention. In a study by Kemp et al, contact burns most commonly affected the hands and accidental burns usually occurred in children <5 years old (71%), often as a result of touching irons, hair straighteners, or stovetops. It can be difficult to differentiate between accidental and inflicted contact burns, but as described above, any burns that present in pre-mobile infants, are located on posterior or protected areas of the body, present with bilaterality, a delay in seeking medical care or an incompatible explanation should raise concerns for child maltreatment. In addition, contact burns with a recognizable shape are caused by contact with a hot object with corresponding orientation and surface features and should raise concerns for inflicted injury.

Other types of burns less frequently encountered include flame, electrical, and chemical burns. Obtaining a detailed medical history can be helpful in discerning their etiology.

BITE MARKS

Human bite marks on the skin have typically been described as interrupted ovoid-shaped lesions with or without surrounding skin swelling or bruising. However, there are limitations to the analysis of bite marks that have made them challenging to interpret in the context of child maltreatment cases. Human skin may not be an accurate registration material for recording bite marks as there is distortion caused by postural or anatomical factors. The degree of distortion associated with the bite mark depends on whether the bite is located on skin over fatty tissue, muscle, or bone as there is variability in skin tension with these locations. This was demonstrated in a study by Pretty and Sweet involving ink-stamping and human cadaveric skin where dentition was applied to the skin using a clamp. Therefore, features that were previously felt to be forensically significant, such as the uniqueness of human dental impressions and the ability to differentiate between adult-child bite marks or human-animal bite marks, have been challenged. A child abuse pediatrician or a forensic odontologist, if available, can be consulted and may be able to provide further assistance in the examination and interpretation of concerning bite marks.

DIFFERENTIAL DIAGNOSIS

A broad differential diagnosis of medical conditions and cultural practices should be considered for all cutaneous injuries for which child maltreatment is a concern. For example, hematologic conditions, congenital conditions, infections, and oncologic processes can all mimic the appearance of abusive injuries (**Table 35-1**).

DIAGNOSTIC EVALUATION

A comprehensive medical evaluation is essential for the child presenting with a cutaneous finding concerning for abuse. An organized, systematic approach will lessen the likelihood of an inaccurate diagnosis leading to additional injury or death if an abused child is discharged to the caregiver without any interventions or inappropriate involvement of the child protective services (CPS) agency in the case of an accidental injury.

TABLE 35-1 Common Mimickers of Abusive Cutaneous Injuries

	Bruising	Burn	Patterned appearance
Accidental Events			
Car seat burns		X	X
Liquids		X	
Contact		X	X
Congenital Conditions			
Hemangiomas	X		
Dermal melanosis (Mongolian spots)	X		
Connective Tissue Disorders			
Ehlers-Danlos	X		
Striae distensae (stretch marks)	X		X
Chemical Contact			
Hair relaxers and dye		X	
Household chemicals		X	
Toxic substances		X	X
Cultural Practices			
Coining/spooning	X		X
Cupping	X	X	X
Moxibustion		X	
Complementary and alternative therapies	X	X	X
Dermatologic Conditions			
Eczema		X	
Epidermolysis bullosa		X	
Irritant diaper dermatitis		X	X
Hematologic Conditions			
Coagulation disorders	X		
Hemophilia	X		
Platelet disorders	X		
Von Willebrand disease	X		
Vitamin K deficiency	X		
Hemolytic uremic syndrome	X		
Disseminated intravascular coagulation	X		
Hypersensitivity Syndromes			
Erythema multiforme	X		
Allergic contact dermatitis	X	X	X
Panniculitis	X		
Erythema nodosum	X		
Perniosis (chilblains)	X		
Angioedema			X
Infections			
Impetigo		X	X
Ecthyma		X	X
Tinea corporis		X	X
Oncologic disorders	X		
Pigmentation Disorders			
Nevus of ota/nevus of ito	X		
Incontinentia pigmenti	X		
Urticaria pigmentosa	X		
Vasculitic Disorders			
Henoch-Schönlein purpura	X		
Hypersensitivity vasculitis	X		
Other Conditions			
Phytophotodermatitis	X		X
Ink/dye staining	X		
Maculae ceruleae	X		
Valsalva effect	X		

HISTORY

Pediatricians face many barriers in recognizing child maltreatment. First, child maltreatment disproportionately affects young, nonverbal children who are unable to provide a reliable history. Second, caregivers, who providers rely on to provide an accurate history, may be motivated in these cases to provide a false history or no history at all. Finally, provider biases may prevent providers from considering maltreatment on the differential diagnoses, even when it is the likely cause. Thus, providers should carefully document the full history as provided by the caregivers, including the mechanism of injury, onset of symptoms, and the child's developmental abilities. Providers should obtain a detailed medical history (not a forensic one) and elicit specific information describing the circumstances surrounding the event. For example, information needed for a child presenting with a bruise after an alleged fall would include location/position of child prior to the fall, height of the fall, fall surface, landing position, and surrounding objects in the vicinity of the fall. If no trauma history is provided, providers should ask how the child might have sustained the cutaneous injury and consider whether the injury is in keeping with both the mechanism provided and the child's developmental ability. A complete medical and family history should also be obtained to determine other possible medical etiologies of the cutaneous findings (see "Differential Diagnosis" section above). Shum et al describes the acronym, MORE, which may aid providers in obtaining a history in a systematic fashion. M stands for *mechanism of injury*, O is for *others present*, and reminds the provider to identify others who may be able to corroborate the history, R is for *review of development*, and E is for *examination details* and reminds the provider to perform a fully disrobed assessment to examine for other injuries.

EVALUATION

Any cutaneous injury suggestive of possible abuse should prompt further workup for a possible underlying medical condition and for occult abusive trauma, which is trauma that cannot be diagnosed by physical examination alone. Infants < 6 months of age, even in the setting of a normal neurological exam, should have screening head imaging with CT or MRI, with fast MRI protocol if available, to identify occult intracranial injury. A complete skeletal survey, which includes x-rays of the entire skeleton, should be performed in children <2 years of age to identify occult fractures. Follow-up skeletal surveys should be performed 2 weeks after the initial test for children with high-risk cutaneous injury. The utility and yield of the skeletal survey declines significantly after 24 months of age as the physical exam becomes more reliable in the diagnosis of trauma.

Cutaneous injuries concerning for child maltreatment should also trigger additional laboratory evaluation including liver transaminases (AST/ALT) and lipase. Using a threshold of 80 IU/L for either AST or ALT, Lindberg and colleagues showed that an elevated AST or ALT had a high sensitivity (77%) and specificity (82%) for predicting occult intra-abdominal injury. Therefore, abdominal imaging (i.e., abdominal CT) should be strongly considered for children presenting with liver transaminases above 80 IU/L in whom abuse is a concern.

Finally, the presence of a coagulopathy must be considered as a cause of bruising in children. Obtaining a careful family history, history of previous easy or frequent bleeding, and history of bruising or petechiae at pressure sites (e.g., from clothing lines or infant seat fasteners) will guide further evaluation. If concerns of coagulopathy persist, evaluation with laboratory studies, including a complete CBC with platelets, PT/PTT, von Willebrand factor antigen and activity, factor VIII, and Factor IX should be performed and consultation with a pediatric hematologist pursued in the setting of any abnormal results. It is important to note that not all children with cutaneous injuries need an evaluation for a bleeding diathesis, such as when an abusive event leading to bruising is independently witnessed, a child provides a direct and clear history of the event, or a bruise is present in the exact configuration of an object such as a belt or a hand.

Whenever possible, photographing cutaneous lesions is highly recommended, as most skin findings will resolve or change in appearance over time. Images should be properly labeled and a measuring device should be placed near the finding. If a ruler is not available, an object of universal size (e.g., a coin) may be used instead. Providers should be compliant with institutional policies governing the permission to obtain images as well as the process for safe storage and release of the images.

MANAGEMENT

Hospital admission may be required to facilitate medical evaluation of cutaneous injuries concerning for child maltreatment. Depending on the cutaneous injury and the extent, subspecialist involvement may be required, for example, extensive burns may require surgical intervention and management by a Plastic Surgery or Burns specialist.

Additionally, in both the United States and Canada, healthcare providers are mandated by law to report to CPS with any suspicion or reasonable cause to believe that a child is being abused or neglected. Although the local resources available to CPS may vary, in most regions CPS has the capability of conducting an investigation, which may involve visiting the home, examining the scene where the alleged incident occurred, and making outreach to other individuals known to the child (e.g., daycare providers, teachers, neighbors, family members), in an effort to obtain a more comprehensive understanding of the child's injury.

CONSULTATION

Effective case management of the child suspected to have been abused is best achieved using a multidisciplinary approach. Collaboration with relevant subspecialty services may help clarify the diagnosis, identify possible underlying medical conditions which may account for findings, and lend further understanding to the mechanism contributing to the findings. Given the challenges presented by some cutaneous lesions, it is not uncommon to obtain consultation from Dermatology, Hematology, Genetics, or Dentistry. Child protection teams, frequently composed of child abuse pediatricians, nurses, social workers, psychologists, and specialists with expertise in managing individuals involved in relationships characterized by interpersonal violence, serve as a critical asset for frontline providers to aid in case formulation, communication with CPS, and as a source of continued consultation to law enforcement, attorneys, and CPS even after the child has been discharged. Opinions provided by consultation services should be formally documented in the patient's medical record, as the views of curbside consults are not verifiable in future discussions of the case with external agencies or during legal proceedings.

KEY POINTS

- Correlate the history of presentation with the examination findings and the developmental stage of the child. Remember that "children who do not cruise rarely bruise."
- Bruising in the TEN-4 FACES P configuration, which stands for the torso (T) including chest, abdomen, back, buttocks, and genitourinary area, ears (E), neck (N), bruising to frenulum (F), angle of jaw (A), soft part of the cheek (C), eyelid (E), sclera (S), patterned bruising (P) , or any bruising in a child < 4.99 months has been found to be predictive of abuse and requires further evaluation. Likewise, cutaneous injuries characterized by a patterned configuration are atypical and should prompt further query for suspected abuse.
- When possible, photograph cutaneous findings. Follow hospital protocol regarding issues around consent, storage, and release of photographic images.
- In the evaluation of children with concerns of suspected physical abuse, a skeletal survey should be completed in children less than 2 years of age and brain imaging performed for pre-mobile children (<6 months old).
- A multidisciplinary approach enhances the management of suspected child abuse cases; therefore, actively engage your child abuse pediatrician, hospital-based child protection team, and other subspecialty services.

SUGGESTED READINGS

Anderst JD, Carpenter SL, Abshire TC, Section on HO, Committee on Child A, Neglect of the American Academy of P. Evaluation for bleeding disorders in suspected child abuse. *Pediatrics*. 2013;131(4): e1314-1322.

Children's Bureau AfCaF, US Department of Health and Human Services. Child Maltreatment. 2019.
Christian CW, Committee on Child A, Neglect AAoP. The evaluation of suspected child physical abuse. *Pediatrics*. 2015;135(5):e1337-1354.
Kemp AM, Jones S, Lawson Z, Maguire SA. Patterns of burns and scalds in children. *Arch Dis Child*. 2014;99(4):316-321.
Loos MHJ, Almekinders CAM, Heymans MW, de Vries A, Bakx R. Incidence and characteristics of non-accidental burns in children: a systematic review. *Burns*. 2020;46(6):1243-1253.
Lindberg DM, Shapiro RA, Blood EA, Steiner RD, Berger RP, Ex Si. Utility of hepatic transaminases in children with concern for abuse. *Pediatrics*. 2013;131(2):268-275.
Maguire S, Mann MK, Sibert J, Kemp A. Are there patterns of bruising in childhood which are diagnostic or suggestive of abuse? A systematic review. *Arch Dis Child*. 2005;90(2):182-186.
Maguire S, Mann MK, Sibert J, Kemp A. Can you age bruises accurately in children? A systematic review. *Arch Dis Child*. 2005;90(2):187-189.
McNamara CR, Panigrahy A, Sheetz M, Berger RP. The likelihood of an occult fracture in skeletal surveys obtained in children more than 2 years old with concerns of physical abuse. *Pediatr Emerg Care*. 2022;38(2):e488-e492.
Pierce MC, Kaczor K, Lorenz DJ, et al. Validation of a clinical decision rule to predict abuse in young children based on bruising characteristics. *JAMA Netw Open*. 2021;4(4):e215832.
Pretty IA, Sweet D. A paradigm shift in the analysis of bitemarks. *Forensic Sci Int*. 2010;201(1-3):38-44.
Sheets LK, Leach ME, Koszewski IJ, Lessmeier AM, Nugent M, Simpson P. Sentinel injuries in infants evaluated for child physical abuse. *Pediatrics*. 2013;131(4):701-707.
Shum M, Asnes A, Leventhal JM, Bechtel K, Gaither JR, Tiyyagura G. The use of experts to evaluate a child abuse guideline in community emergency departments. *Acad Pediatr*. 2021;21(3):521-528.
Ward MG, Ornstein A, Niec A, Murray CL; Canadian Paediatric Society, Child and Youth Maltreatment Section. The medical assessment of bruising in suspected child maltreatment cases: A clinical perspective. *Paediatr Child Health*. 2013 Oct;18(8):433-42. Erratum in: Paediatr Child Health. 2013;18(9):456.

CHAPTER 36

Abusive Head Trauma

Kristine Fortin, MD, MPH and
Kathleen Nolan, MD, FRCP(C), DRCPSC

BACKGROUND

The terms abusive head trauma (AHT) or traumatic head injury due to child maltreatment (THI-CM) are used to describe the spectrum of injuries to the head (skull and/or brain and/or intracranial structures) which may also be accompanied by injury to the face, scalp, eye, neck, spine, or other extracranial injuries, as a result of the external application of force from child maltreatment.

EPIDEMIOLOGY

AHT can affect children of any age but is most common in the first year of life, with a peak incidence in the first few months of life and is the leading cause of child physical abuse mortality. Narang et al reported the estimated incidence of AHT in children less than one year of age in the United States is 32 to 38 cases per 100,000 children per year while in Canada, Bennet et al reported an incidence of 14.1 per 100,000 children per year; however, these are likely underestimates due to cases going unrecognized, particularly in children with mild injuries. Jenny et al reported that AHT may be more commonly missed in children with caregivers who are married, white, and/or economically stable.

NOMENCLATURE

The nomenclature of this entity continues to evolve as scientific data advance. Previous nomenclature included battered child syndrome, whiplash shaken infant syndrome, shaken impact syndrome, shaken baby syndrome, and inflicted childhood neurotrauma. The American Academy of Pediatrics adopted the term Abusive Head Trauma in 2009, recognizing that inflicted head injury of children can involve a variety of biomechanical forces, including shaking. In 2020 the Public Health Agency of Canada in partnership with the Canadian Paediatric Society recommended "Traumatic Head Injury due to Child Maltreatment" as the preferred term in Canada for research, public health, policy, and prevention. They suggested that clinicians who suspect THI-CM document a diagnosis of Traumatic Head Injury, along with a list of key medical findings and followed by a statement of concern for THI-CM as a possible cause, with the understanding that in Canada the determination of THI-CM as a final opinion must be made based on combined information from the medical, child welfare, and/or legal sectors.

PATHOPHYSIOLOGY/MECHANISMS

Mechanisms of injury vary among children with AHT and can include inertial forces, blunt impact, or a combination of both. Impact can cause no visible injury, or can result in scalp injury, skull fractures, and/or direct injury to the intracranial structures. Subdural hemorrhages (SDH) are the most common intracranial injury in AHT and can be associated with parenchymal injury. SDH can result from acceleration/deceleration forces, direct contact, or crush injury. Direct trauma to the parenchyma from rapid acceleration/deceleration with or without impact may result in contusions, lacerations, and/or shearing injuries. Pathophysiology can also include secondary brain injury from a cascade of injury events. Brain edema may lead to midline shift and possible herniation of brain tissue. The edema may also compress smaller blood vessels which provide oxygen and nutrients to brain tissue. Children who have experienced AHT are thought to be at higher risk of hypoventilation and apnea, contributing to poor oxygenation of parenchymal tissue and worsening injury. They are also at high risk for convulsive and non-convulsive seizures, which may further exacerbate brain injury. As mechanisms of injury and patient characteristics vary, so do injuries among children with AHT. **Table 36-1** outlines injuries that may be observed.

CLINICAL PRESENTATION

There is variability in how children with abusive head trauma present to care. Factors including the nature of injuries sustained impact presenting signs and symptoms. Neurological impairment can range from mild or asymptomatic to severe, and extracranial injuries can range from absent to obvious injuries on physical exam. While some children present to care soon after injuries are sustained, others, especially those with mild or nonspecific symptoms, may not present to care while their injuries are acute or may be misdiagnosed on initial presentation. Studies by Jenny et al and Letson et al found that close to 1/3 of children ultimately diagnosed with abusive head trauma had a prior missed opportunity for diagnosis. Presentation for mild and nonspecific symptoms such as irritability or vomiting was associated with missed detection. Consideration of abusive head trauma on the differential diagnosis and careful attention to clinical findings such as head circumference growth trajectory and skin injuries could facilitate detection when children present with nonspecific symptoms.

While signs of blunt impact are not always present as outlined above, scalp swelling or palpable skull deformities may be noted in some patients. When increased intracranial pressure is present due to injuries such as space occupying intracranial hemorrhages or cerebral edema clinical signs can include bulging fontanels, splayed sutures, and increasing head circumference. Vital signs could also be altered; signs of increased intracranial pressure (ICP) can include hypertension, bradycardia, and irregular respiration. Other signs and symptoms of head injury that can be observed or reported include loss of consciousness, seizures, and apnea/hypoventilation. Some children present only with symptoms that are not specific to head trauma such as vomiting and fussiness; the broad differential diagnosis for these symptoms can make recognition challenging.

TABLE 36-1 Examples of Injuries That May Be Seen in Patients With AHT

Head
Scalp and skull
• Scalp swelling / hematoma
• Scalp laceration
• Skull fracture
• Bruising
• Traumatic alopecia
Extra-axial space
• Subdural hemorrhage
• Subpial hemorrhage
• Subarachnoid hemorrhage
• Epidural hemorrhage
Brain
• Contusions / parenchymal lacerations
• Shear injuries
• Hypoxic ischemic injury
• Edema
Eye
Outer
• Subconjunctival hemorrhage
Inner
• Retinal hemorrhages
• Retinal fold
• Retinoschisis
Spine
• Soft tissue edema
• Ligamentous injury
• Subdural / epidural hematoma
• Spinal cord injury
Skin
• Skin injuries
Skeleton
• Factures including rib and classic metaphyseal lesions
Other
• Oral injuries including frenular tears
• Intra-abdominal injuries

It is also important to discuss clinical presentation of extracranial injuries. Retinal hemorrhages are present in up to approximately 75% of children with abusive head trauma, and dilated indirect fundoscopy by an ophthalmologist is the optimal method for assessment. Eye findings that may be present on direct physical exam include subconjunctival hemorrhage and findings related to increased intracranial pressure (downward gaze, sixth nerve palsy). In a study by Adamsbaum et al, approximately one-third of patients with confessed abusive head trauma had bruising and approximately one-third had fractures. Of note, some fractures associated with abusive head trauma such as rib and classic metaphyseal fractures (planar fracture through the metaphysis) may be clinically occult. When present, skin injury and signs of fracture (limb disuse, deformity, and swelling) can alert clinicians to the differential diagnosis of trauma. However, many children with abusive head trauma present without visible injuries on external exam.

Hospitalists may also encounter children with abusive head trauma when they present for management of sequelae of their injuries.

DIFFERENTIAL DIAGNOSIS

The differential diagnosis for AHT will depend on the specific injuries present and generally includes inflicted injury, birth injury, accidental trauma, and nontraumatic medical or congenital etiologies. Careful consideration of differential diagnoses with systematic evaluation of other potential causes for the observed findings are critical component of evaluation of suspected AHT.

Clinicians must first ensure an accurate understanding of the specific intracranial findings identified in the child. Hospitalists may wish to consult with radiology colleagues to clarify radiologic findings and ophthalmology to understand retinal findings.

Depending on the age of the child and the clinical findings, the differential diagnosis could include birth injury, which can result in certain patterns of subdural and retinal hemorrhages. Studies of birth-related subdural hemorrhages in asymptomatic infants provide insights into typical characteristics and course, including resolution of most asymptomatic birth-related SDH by 4 to 6 weeks of age. Similarly, birth-related retinal hemorrhages have been studied and most resolve by 2 weeks of age. The primary differential diagnosis in suspected AHT is accidental traumatic brain injury. Short falls are a common historical explanation for injuries. Severe intracranial injuries from short falls are rare, but some fall characteristics including from significant heights or involving a higher degree of force can lead to greater injury. If a history of a fall is provided it should be carefully considered with reference to the most current peer-reviewed literature and possible collaboration with a child maltreatment specialist.

The differential diagnosis of AHT may also include inherited and acquired coagulopathies, structural causes such as arteriovenous malformations and benign enlargement of the subarachnoid space, neoplasms, infectious causes such as meningitis, and genetic/metabolic conditions like Menke's disease and Glutaric Aciduria type I. Most of these conditions have other classic associated findings and can be ruled out with further testing and subspecialist consultation as required.

In addition to the above diagnoses, hospitalists should also be aware of the emergence of scientifically unsupported theories to explain abuse, particularly in the courtroom.

Consultation with a child maltreatment specialist can be helpful to review the most current literature and understand findings expected as a result of traumatic and medical causes.

DIAGNOSTIC EVALUATION

History As with other conditions, history and physical exam are key components of the evaluation that inform the differential diagnosis. When a trauma event is reported, detailed information about context (where, when, who was present), what happened, and child and caregiver responses can be elicited. Information about the nature, onset, and progression of symptoms starting from when the child was last well can be obtained even when no trauma event is reported. Components of the past medical history include a detailed birth history, prior injuries, and known underlying medical conditions. Information about hereditary conditions that could predispose to the child's findings such as bleeding disorders can be collected on family history. Developmental history is important to assess what types of self-initiated accidents could be possible as well as to identify significant developmental delays that could be associated with underlying medical conditions such as glutaric aciduria. The review of systems could identify symptoms of associated injuries or of underlying medical conditions such as bleeding disorders. A vital component of social history for patients with abusive head trauma is the presence of other children in the same care environments who may also have been harmed. Components of social history in addition to household members and childcare arrangements include prior child protective services involvement, interpersonal violence, substance abuse, mental illness, and family stressors. While social factors may be important for identifying family needs, healthcare providers should be mindful that the presence or absence of population-based risk factors should not influence the medical opinion regarding injury plausibility and specific findings, as this can increase the risk of cognitive errors.

Physical Examination While not always present, signs of head and extracranial injuries noted in the clinical presentation section above may be detected on physical exam. The skin exam can be informed by the bruising clinical decision rule TEN-4-FACESp, as described by Pierce et al. This rule highlights bruising characteristics that signal potential abuse: building on the torso, ear, neck, frenulum, angle of the jaw, cheek (fleshy part), eyelids, subconjunctivae, bruising anywhere in a child ≤4.99 months and patterned bruising. Cursory skin exams could miss critical signs of trauma so an unclothed exam is important. The physical exam could also detect stigmata of underlying medical conditions.

Neuroimaging Workup to evaluate head injuries, extracranial injuries, and differential diagnoses can be informed by clinical evaluation and recommendations from professional associations including the American Academy of Pediatrics. Computed tomography (CT), magnetic resonance imaging (MRI), or both are recommended neuroimaging modalities. Noncontrast CT is the most sensitive modality for skull fracture detection and is also sensitive for injuries requiring intervention. MRI is the best modality for detecting and fully assessing intracranial injury but is usually not as readily accessible as CT and often requires sedation. Therefore, noncontrast CT can be used as the initial study in acutely ill children, and MRI can be used for further evaluation. There is evolving literature on spinal imaging, and current practice with respect to universal imaging of the cervical and whole spine varies across centers. Spinal injury is present in some but not all cases of abusive head trauma (Henry and Wood reported that the incidence of cervical spinal injury ranges across studies from 15% to 78%). MRI of the spine can be used to assess for spinal extra-axial hemorrhage and bony, ligamentous, and cord injuries.

Ophthalmology Evaluation Evaluation for retinal hemorrhages is done through ophthalmology consultation. Dilated indirect examination as soon as possible, medical condition permitting, is ideal as some hemorrhages could resolve quickly. It is important not only to note whether retinal hemorrhages are present but also their number, type, location, and pattern. Some ophthalmology findings such as too many to count, multi-layered retinal hemorrhages that extend to the periphery, retinoschisis and retinal folds have a high specificity for inflicted trauma while other patterns such as few intraretinal hemorrhages isolated to the posterior pole have a broader differential diagnosis.

Investigations for Extracranial Injury Recommendations for occult extracranial injury workup also include skeletal survey per American College of Radiology protocol in children <2 years and in some children aged 2 to 5 years. Follow-up skeletal survey approximately 2 weeks after initial imaging is recommended in cases of physical abuse for reasons including detection of injuries that were radiographically occult at the time of initial presentation. Liver and pancreatic enzymes (AST, ALT, amylase, lipase) have been studied as screening tests for occult abdominal trauma. Considerations for workup of siblings and other young household contacts of children injured from physical abuse include physical exam and skeletal survey for contacts aged < 2 years.

Investigations for Underlying Medical Conditions Evaluation for medical conditions that could explain findings is also a component of the workup. The American Academy of Pediatrics published a clinical report on evaluation for bleeding disorders in suspected abusive head trauma that outlines indications for and components of workup (CBC, PT, aPTT, factor VIII level, factor IX level, if neurologic compromise D-dimer and fibrinogen, hematology consultation as needed). Clinical evaluation and local practices such as content of newborn screens can inform need for additional workup for other possible underlying medical conditions including genetic/metabolic conditions.

MANAGEMENT

Management of abusive head trauma involves a multidisciplinary approach to address medical and psychosocial needs. Head injury treatment depends on factors such as injury types and clinical status including vital signs and Glasgow Coma Scale (GCS). Neurosurgery colleagues can assist in determining when surgical intervention is necessary. Medical management to prevent secondary injury can include seizure treatment and prophylaxis, maintaining electrolyte balances with attention to sodium and glucose, intubation plus mechanical ventilation and medical treatment of increased intracranial pressure as indicated. Specialists and settings that may be needed include level 1 trauma center, neurologists, neurosurgeons, and intensivists. When there is concern for abuse rising to the level of a mandated report to Child Protective Services, information to be shared with caregivers honestly and respectfully without blame includes identified injuries, medical plan for workup and management, need for mandated report, and anticipatory guidance.

Children with abusive head trauma often have ongoing medical needs. Long-term neurological outcomes among survivors can range from complete recovery to severe disability with need for tracheostomy to support respiration. An AAP clinical report on ongoing healthcare after maltreatment notes that approximately 60% to 80% of children have some neurologic impairment. Sequelae can include visual impairment, cerebral palsy, feeding difficulties with need for feeding tube and speech delays. Close developmental monitoring is indicated. It is also important to monitor endocrine status. In addition to short-term effects like syndrome of inappropriate antidiuretic hormone secretion and diabetes insipidus, children can experience ongoing pituitary hormone issues including growth hormone deficiency.

ADMISSION AND DISCHARGE CRITERIA

Children with suspected abusive head trauma need admission for workup, monitoring, treatment, and social needs assessment. Rehabilitation specialists can help determine which children would benefit from inpatient rehabilitation. In addition to medical readiness, Child Protective Services determination of a safe discharge plan is also needed prior to discharge.

CONSULTATIONS

Cases of AHT are often best managed by a multidisciplinary team. If a hospital-based child protection team with child abuse/maltreatment pediatricians is available, they can be consulted. Depending on the specific findings, subspecialty consultation with radiology, ophthalmology, neurosurgery, neurology, intensivists, trauma surgery, orthopedics, endocrinology, hematology, genetics, and/or rehabilitation specialists may be warranted. When available, social work staff can provide support to caregivers and the medical team.

All jurisdictions in the United States and Canada require physicians to report to a child protection agency when they suspect or believe that a child has been harmed or is at risk of harm due to abuse or neglect. Reporters are not expected to provide proof that abuse or neglect has occurred. Physicians should understand the legislation in their jurisdiction with respect to disclosure of personal health information to law enforcement and others. Physicians should be prepared to interface with outside agencies and provide accurate medical information and clear, objective documentation (within the bounds of what is permitted by personal health information and mandatory reporting legislation).

KEY POINTS

- The preferred terminology is Abusive Head Trauma (AHT) in United States and Traumatic Head Injury due to Child Maltreatment (THI-CM) in Canada.
- Clinical presentation varies with injury mechanisms and injury types and can range from severe neurologic impairment to asymptomatic or nonspecific symptoms such as fussiness or vomiting.
- The diagnosis may be missed, particularly when children present with milder symptoms and absent external injuries. A thorough history and physical examination is important in all patients where AHT is on the differential diagnosis.
- Differential diagnoses to carefully consider, informed by child and injury characteristics, can include birth injury, accidental injury, and nontraumatic medical causes.
- Workup of head injuries, extracranial injuries including those that are clinically occult, and underlying medical conditions can be informed by clinical evaluation and professional society recommendations.
- Hospitalists can collaborate with hospital and community-based professionals for evaluation and management; United States and Canadian physicians are mandated to report suspected abuse to child protection agencies.

SUGGESTED READINGS

Adamsbaum C, Grabar S, Mejean N, Rey-Salmon C. Abusive head trauma: judicial admissions highlight violent and repetitive shaking. *Pediatrics*. 2010;126(3):546-55.

American College of Radiology. ACR-SPR practice parameters for the performance and interpretation of skeletal surveys in children. 2021. Available at: https://www.acr.org/-/media/ACR/Files/Practice-Parameters/Skeletal-Survey.pdf.

Anderst J, Carpenter SL, Abshire TC, Killough E, AAP Section on Hematology/Oncology, American Society of Pediatric Hematology/Oncology, AAP Council on Child Abuse and Neglect. Evaluating for bleeding disorders in suspected child abuse. *Pediatrics*. 2022; 150(4):e2022059726.

Bennet S, Ward M, Moreau K, Fortin G, King J, Mackay M, Plint A. Head injury secondary to suspected child maltreatment: results of a prospective Canadian national surveillance program. *Child Abuse Negl*. 2011;35(11)930-6.

Christian CW, Levin AV, Council on Child Abuse and Neglect, Section on Ophthalmology, American Association of Certified Orthoptists, American Association for Pediatric Ophthalmology and Strabismus, American Academy of Ophthalmology. The eye examination in the evaluation of child abuse. *Pediatrics*. 2018;142(2):e20181411.

Christian CW, Committee on Child Abuse and Neglect. The evaluation of suspected child physical abuse. *Pediatrics*. 2015;135(5):e1337-54.

Choudhary AK, Servaes S, Slovis TL, Palusci VJ, Hedlund GL, Narang SK, et al. Consensus statement on abusive head trauma in infants and young children. *Pediatr Radiol*. 2018;48:1048-65.

Flaherty E, Legano L, Idzerda S, Council on Child Abuse and Neglect. Ongoing pediatric health care for the child who has been maltreated. *Pediatrics*.2019;143(4):e20190824.

Henry MK, Wood JN. Advanced cervical spine imaging in abusive head trauma: an update on recent literature and future directions. *Acad Pediatr*. 2018;18(7):733-35.

Jenny C, Hymel KP, Ritzen A, et al. Analysis of missed cases of abusive head trauma. *JAMA*. 1999;281(7):621-626.

Laskey, A. Cognitive Errors: Thinking clearly when it could be maltreatment. *Pediatric Clin N Am*. 2014;61(5):997-1005.

Letson MM, Cooper JN, Deans KJ et al. Prior opportunities to identify abuse in children with abusive head trauma. *Child Abuse Negl*. 2016; 60:36-45.

Narang SK, Fingarson A, Lukefahr J, AAP Council on Child Abuse and Neglect. Abusive head trauma in infants and children. *Pediatrics*. 2020;145(4):e20200203

Pierce MC, Kaczor K, Lorenz DJ, et al. Validation of a clinical decision rule to predict abuse in young children based on bruising characteristics. *JAMA Netw Open*. 2021;4(4):e215832.

Public Health Agency of Canada. Joint Statement on Traumatic Head Injury due to Child Maltreatment: An update to the Joint Statement on Shaken Baby Syndrome. Feb 2020.

CHAPTER 37

Skeletal Injuries Concerning for Child Maltreatment

Karine Pepin, MD and Liza Murray, MD

BACKGROUND

Skeletal injuries are frequent in childhood but also represent one of the most common presentations of physical abuse. Estimates indicate that fractures are the second most common abusive injury in toddlers after soft tissue injuries and are found in up to a third of children being investigated for inflicted trauma. Among children hospitalized with fractures in the United States, the proportion of skeletal injuries attributable to abuse averages 12% with an overall incidence of abusive fractures of 15.3 cases per 100,000 children under the age of 36 months, as demonstrated in a study by Leventhal et al. Abusive fractures are more prevalent in infants and toddlers than in older children. It is therefore crucial for the clinician to distinguish accidental from inflicted skeletal trauma in order to prevent ongoing harm and identify children requiring the intervention of child protection services.

When assessing a child with an unexplained fracture, a thorough history with a particular attention to any reported trauma event should be taken and a careful clinical examination should be conducted. The possibility of abuse should always be kept in mind. Laboratory testing and imaging can be helpful in identifying pathological fractures or patients at increased risk of fracture.

CLINICAL PRESENTATIONS

FRACTURE TYPES AND SPECIFICITIES

Any bone or type of fracture can be involved with physical abuse, although some fractures are more commonly seen in accidental trauma whereas others are more specific to abuse (**Table 37-1,** Kleinman, 1998). In every situation, clinical correlation with the reported mechanism is required.

1. High specificity fractures: classic metaphyseal lesions (CML) and rib fractures

   CML were initially described by John Caffey and were thought to be avulsion fractures of the extremity of the long bones. They have now been recognized as being a planar fracture occurring through the metaphyses and predominantly affecting the immature growing bones of infants, as described by Kleinman, et al, 1986. Classic metaphyseal lesions can be identified on simple radiographs and will typically produce a "bucket-handle" or a "corner" fracture. Healing of CMLs is variable and less predictable than other types of fractures.

   Classic metaphyseal lesions are caused by the application of tractional or shearing forces to the limb. Although CMLs have been reported with specific accidental mechanisms, there is a high association between this type of fracture and abusive traumatic events. Classic metaphyseal lesions generally cause subtle to no symptoms

TABLE 37-1 Specificity of Radiologic Findings for Abuse

High specificity*
Metaphyseal lesions
Posterior rib fractures
Scapular fractures
Spinous process fractures
Sternal fractures
Moderate specificity
Multiple fractures, especially bilateral
Fractures of different ages
Epiphyseal separations
Vertebral body fractures and subluxations
Digital fractures
Complex skull fractures
Pelvic fractures
Common but low specificity
Subperiosteal new bone formation
Clavicular fractures
Long bone shaft fractures
Linear skull fractures

*Highest specificity applies in infants.

Source: Reproduced With permission from Kleinman PK. *Diagnostic Imaging of Child Abuse*. 2nd ed. St. Louis, MO: Mosby-Year Book; 1998.

after the initial injury event and therefore might not be recognized by a non-offending caregiver.

Rib fractures can occur at different locations on the rib, either in the posterior position (next to the transverse process of the vertebra), anterior position (near the costochondral junction), or antero-laterally (on the side of the chest). Kleinman and Schlesinger reported that biomechanical and animal models studies have shown that posterior rib fractures are caused by levering of the rib with the transverse process of the adjacent vertebra when a child is held by the chest, for example. Anterior or lateral rib fractures, on their part, are caused by antero-posterior compression of the rib cage or direct impact to the chest. Posterior rib fractures are recognized as highly specific fractures for abuse (Table 37-1), but anterior and lateral rib fractures are also associated with abusive mechanisms.

Rib fractures can be difficult to diagnosis when they are acute and are sometimes identified only with the formation of a visible callus. They can also be an incidental finding on a chest radiograph obtained for another clinical indication than trauma. Radiographic dating of rib fractures is limited. Rib fractures generally cause minimal to no symptoms after the initial injury event and therefore might not be recognized by a non-offending caregiver.

2. Low specificity fractures: long bones and skull

   Long bone fractures are common accidental injuries but can also occur with abuse, requiring knowledge and understanding of forces involved in the various fracture types. Spiral fractures require a torque or twist of the bone around its longitudinal axis and this type of mechanism can be found in household falls or falls from a child's standing height. In the ambulatory child, spiral or oblique fractures of long bones such as the femur or tibia are common accidental injuries and not specifically indicative of abuse. Transverse fractures result from a combination of bending and tensile forces, with a direct or indirect application of a force to the bone. Transverse fractures can become comminuted when the bone is submitted to a higher energy mechanism. Buckle or torus fractures result from axial loading forces. These fractures unique to the growing bone are common in children, particularly after a fall on an extremity.

   Skull fractures have a low specificity for abuse as they are commonly seen after accidental trauma but can also be the result of abuse. Skull fractures can be categorized as being simple linear or complex. Simple linear skull fractures consist of a single fracture line with minimal diastasis and often affect one bone, whereas complex fractures can present as multiple fracture lines, cross a suture, or be depressed. Complex skull fractures are generally considered to be the result of higher energy mechanisms. Simple linear skull fractures are non-specific fractures and can occur after accidental trauma or a fall from a height.

   Skull fractures might not be recognized immediately after the injury event and might only come to medical attention when the swelling and size of the associated hematoma peaks, or when caregiving activities involve handling the scalp, such as hair washing.

   Despite being non-specific and frequent, careful assessment of each case is warranted. Age of the child and level of mobility seem to be the predominant factors determining the likelihood of finding supplemental injuries in these children.

DIAGNOSTIC EVALUATION

Accurate detection of pediatric fractures concerning for abuse requires evaluation with evidence-based imaging modalities and interpretation by a trained pediatric radiologist. Fractures with high specificity for abuse can be subtle and difficult to detect, particularly in the acute phase and no single imaging modality has 100% sensitivity and specificity to detect all fractures.

The x-ray skeletal survey is the primary imaging modality to detect fractures concerning for abuse and is recommended for all suspected victims of physical abuse less than 2 years old. Skeletal surveys are not universally recommended in older children but may be considered in children between the ages of 2 and 5 years for evaluation of suspected victims with extensive injury or inability to localize pain. Per the American College of Radiology, skeletal survey consists of frontal and lateral views of the skull; lateral views of the cervical spine and thoracolumosacral spine; single frontal views of the long bones, hands, feet, chest, and abdomen; and oblique views of the ribs. The skeletal survey can be limited in detection of subtle fractures in the acute phase and a follow-up skeletal survey is recommended for suspected victims of physical abuse at about 2 weeks for improved detection of fractures and clarification of equivocal findings. It is recommended that skeletal surveys be interpreted by a pediatric radiologist with consideration of a double read, or second review, to minimize false positive and negative interpretations.

Additional imaging studies to detect fractures may be considered for cases in which a skeletal survey and follow-up skeletal survey are unable to provide timely and necessary information for diagnosis and safety assessment. Bone scintigraphy may assist in the detection of fractures not confirmed by skeletal survey, particularly rib fractures, but has several limitations. Bone scintigraphy requires additional radiation exposure, is insensitive in the identification of classic metaphyseal lesions, may remain positive for up to a year, requires correlation with the skeletal survey for a fracture diagnosis and does not eliminate the need for a follow up skeletal survey. Chest CT can increase the detection of rib fractures not identified on skeletal survey but also requires additional radiation exposure. Whole-body MRI can identify some fractures without additional radiation exposure and provides additional information regarding soft tissue swelling and injury but is insensitive for the detection of all fractures and may require sedation. This study can be considered for young patients who may be undergoing head or spine MRI as an add-on test to provide timely information regarding bone lesions and soft tissue injuries in addition to the skeletal survey. Ultrasound is not a first-line study for fracture evaluation but may be beneficial in evaluating an equivocal finding of a classic metaphyseal lesion identified by skeletal survey.

Children with abusive fractures are also at risk for other types of abusive injury and additional radiologic and laboratory studies are recommended based on the patient's age, developmental level, and presentation. A comprehensive injury evaluation may include a head CT or a head and spine MRI to evaluate for head and spine injury, as well as liver enzymes and consideration of an abdominal CT to evaluate for intra-abdominal trauma. All young children with a fracture should also undergo a complete skin examination to evaluate for any suspicious bruising.

DIFFERENTIAL DIAGNOSIS

The evaluation of a fracture in a young child requires consideration of abusive, accidental and medical causes of fractures based on the patient's age, development, history, exam, and laboratory and radiographic studies. There are multiple medical conditions which are known to predispose infants and children to fracture **(Table 37-2)**. Genetic, metabolic, or other medical conditions contributing to fracture susceptibility are often associated with recognizable clinical, laboratory, or radiographic abnormalities and consultation with experts in pediatric radiology, genetics, endocrinology, and child abuse can be helpful for an accurate diagnosis particularly in cases with atypical presentations.

Initial evaluation for any fracture should include a comprehensive history and examination. A detailed explanation of the presenting injury should include any available trauma history and symptoms associated with the fracture. Medical history for infants should include birth history, including any difficulties with the delivery or complications requiring a prolonged stay in the NICU, as well as other chronic medical

TABLE 37-2 Conditions With Increased Fracture Susceptibility[a]

Rickets	Caffey Disease
Osteogenesis Imperfecta	Hypophosphatasia
Cholestatic Liver Disease	Alagille Syndrome
Job Syndrome	Osteopenia of Prematurity
Leukemia	Osteomyelitis
Bruck Syndrome	Cole-Carpenter Syndrome
Menkes disease	Copper deficiency

[a]Not a comprehensive list.

problems, medications, and supplements. Dietary history should highlight sources of dietary calcium and vitamin D. Family history should include exploration of any family members with known or suspected fracture susceptibility. A detailed examination should be performed to identify additional injuries such as bruising as well as any other physical abnormalities on exam. Abnormal exam or historical findings suggestive of an underlying genetic or metabolic condition may include abnormal facial features, blue-gray sclera, contractures, developmental delays, short stature, seizures, prolonged jaundice, or a family history of multiple fractures. Radiologic studies may demonstrate osteopenia, bowing of long bones, Wormian bones, metaphyseal cupping, or other atypical findings and laboratory evaluation may demonstrate evidence of metabolic bone disease.

Initial laboratory evaluation for fractures can include evaluation for metabolic bone disease with alkaline phosphatase, parathyroid hormone (PTH), calcium, phosphate, and 25-OH Vitamin D. In isolation, vitamin D deficiency is not known to contribute to fractures in infants and toddlers and a diagnosis of rickets requires supportive laboratory or radiologic evidence of bony involvement. If there are laboratory or radiologic abnormalities suspicious for a metabolic, genetic, or medical condition contributing to fracture susceptibility, further consultation with a geneticist, endocrinologist, or other appropriate pediatric subspecialist is recommended.

In addition to medical conditions contributing to fracture susceptibility, accidental mechanisms of injury and, in young infants, birth trauma should be considered during the evaluation of a fracture. While clavicle fractures are commonly recognized as birth-related, other types of fractures can be associated with birth including skull fractures, long bone fractures, and rarely rib fractures. A history of a difficult delivery is often associated with birth-related fractures. Careful consideration of the birth history in consultation with a pediatric radiologist to evaluate fracture healing can be useful in determining the likelihood of a fracture being related to birth. There is no singular type of fracture which is exclusively caused by abuse or accidental mechanisms and consideration of the history, age and developmental level of the child is required to determine if a fracture is suspicious for abuse. Any unexplained fracture in an infant or toddler should be considered for the possibility of abuse.

SUGGESTED READINGS

Aldana Sierra MC, Christian CW. Vitamin D, rickets and child abuse: controversies and evidence. *Pediatr Radiol.* 2021;51(6):1014-1022.

Bronicki LM, Stevenson RE, Spranger JW. Beyond osteogenesis imperfecta: causes of fractures during infancy and childhood. *Am J Med Genet C Semin Med Genet.* 2015;169(4):314-327.

Caffey J. Some traumatic lesions in growing bones other than fractures and dislocations: clinical and radiological features: The Mackenzie Davidson Memorial Lecture. *Br J Radiol.* 1957;30(353):225-238.

Flaherty EG, Perez-Rossello JM, Levine MA, et al. Evaluating children with fractures for child physical abuse. *Pediatrics.* 2014;133(2):e477-89.

Kemp AM, Dunstan F, Harrison S, et al. Patterns of skeletal fractures in child abuse: systematic review. *BMJ.* 2008;337:a1518.

Kleinman PK, Marks SC, Blackbourne B. The metaphyseal lesion in abused infants: a radiologic-histopathologic study. *AJR Am J Roentgenol.* 1986;146(5):895-905.

Kleinman PK, Schlesinger AE. Mechanical factors associated with posterior rib fractures: laboratory and case studies. *Pediatr Radiol.* 1997; 27(1):87-91.

Kleinman PK. *Diagnostic Imaging of Child Abuse.* 2nd ed. St. Louis, MO: Mosby-Year Book; 1998. Copyright © Elsevier.

Kleinman PK, Rosenberg AE, Tsai A. Skeletal trauma: general considerations. In: Kleinman PK. *Diagnostic Imaging of Child Abuse.* 3rd ed. Cambridge, UK: Cambridge University Press; 2015:23-52.

Leventhal JM, Martin KD, Asnes AG. Incidence of fractures attributable to abuse in young hospitalized children: results from analysis of a United States database. *Pediatrics.* 2008;122(3):599-604.

Marine MB, Forbes-Amrhein MM. Fractures of child abuse. *Pediatr Radiol.* 2021;51(6):1003-1013.

Paine CW, Wood JN. Skeletal surveys in young, injured children: a systematic review. *Child Abuse Negl.* 2018;76:237-249.

Pierce MC, Bertocci GE, Vogeley E, Moreland MS. Evaluating long bone fractures in children: a biomechanical approach with illustrative cases. *Child Abuse Negl.* 2004;28(5):505-24.

Wood JN, Fakeye O, Feudtner C, Mondestin V, Localio R, Rubin DM. Development of guidelines for skeletal survey in young children with fractures. *Pediatrics.* 2014;134(1):45-53.

Wootton-Gorges SL, Soares BP, Alazraki AL, et al. ACR appropriateness criteria® suspected physical abuse—child. *J Am Coll Radiol.* 2017;14(5):S338-S349.

CHAPTER 38 Medical Child Abuse: Caregiver Fabricated Illness and Other Manifestations

Jillian Popel, MD, FRCPC and
Frances Yeung, MD, FRCPC, DRCPSC

BACKGROUND

Caregiver fabricated illness (CFI) is a complex, harmful, and potentially fatal form of child maltreatment that can be difficult for the pediatrician to recognize and manage. CFI, as defined by the American Academic of Pediatrics (AAP), refers to "maltreatment that occurs when a child has received unnecessary and harmful or potentially harmful medical care because of the caregiver's fabricated claims or signs and symptoms induced by the caregiver." However, there have been and continue to be many other terms to refer to CFI, which reflects our growing understanding of this form of child maltreatment.

CFI was first described by Dr. Roy Meadows in 1977, who coined the term Munchausen Syndrome by Proxy. Since then, various other names have been used, each with its own definition and focus (**Table 38-1**). CFI is the currently recommended term by AAP 2013, whereas FII and FIIC are used in UK and Australia, respectively. This chapter will continue to use CFI given the North American context. This chapter addresses typical features that should raise concerns for CFI and outlines an approach for the general community or hospital-based pediatrician, including when to involve child maltreatment pediatricians or local child protection agencies.

TABLE 38-1 Various Terms Used to Describe Caregiver Fabricated Illness

Term	How This Term Is Used
Munchausen syndrome by proxy Factitious disorder by proxy Pediatric condition falsification **Factitious disorder imposed on another (FDIA)**	Diagnoses to be given to the caregiver. Requires verified deception by the caregiver. FDIA is the current DSM-5[a] and ICD-11[b] diagnosis and refers to the falsification of psychological or physical signs or symptoms, or induction of disease or injury in another, associated with identified deception.
Fabricated or induced illness (FII) Fabricated or induced illness in a child (FIIC) **Caregiver fabricated illness (CFI)**	Diagnoses to be given to the child. Focuses on the harm and experiences of the child. May be diagnosed by a pediatrician, as it does not require understanding of caregiver motives or verifying purposeful deception. May include cases that are motivated by caregivers' anxieties or strongly held beliefs.
Medical child abuse	Reflects the medical setting, role of the healthcare professionals and how the child is being harmed

[a]DSM-5: Diagnostic and Statistical Manual of Mental Disorders, 5th edition.

[b]ICD-11: International Classification of Diseases, 11th revision.

EPIDEMIOLOGY

The prevalence of CFI is widely accepted to be significantly underestimated due to confusion with various terminology and under-recognition and under-reporting of CFI. Jenny and Metz suggested that most primary care pediatricians report seeing at least one case of CFI in their career, but this can increase up to 20 to 30 cases per year at large academic pediatric hospitals. The age range of affected children spans infancy to adolescence, though cases cluster in early childhood and the time to detection of abuse is typically lengthy (months-years). Siblings are also at increased risk for CFI. Flaherty and Macmillan reported that mortality rates have been estimated to be 6% to 9%, with greatest risk in cases of illness induction. Morbidity includes long-term physical disabilities, psychological harm, and social and school disruption.

Importantly, it has been suggested that modern healthcare systems, increased access to medical information on the Internet, and increased online social connectivity may be contributing to rising prevalence of CFI. Current electronic medical records allow for easy "copy and pasting" of medical diagnoses and requesting extensive testing through standardized "order sets." Furthermore, without a unified healthcare record, caregivers can easily "doctor shop" between physicians and provide different accounts of medical history. Caregivers may request specific testing or suggest certain diagnoses for their child to physicians that they have read about on the Internet. Finally, it has been noted that some caregivers garner extensive social attention, sympathy, and even crowd-funded donations by reporting their child's illnesses online. This may provide motivation for some to exaggerate or escalate the severity of their child's illness.

PATHOPHYSIOLOGY

To understand CFI, one must understand the complex interactions between the caregiver, healthcare provider, and child.

CAREGIVER

The caregiver typically initiates the harm indirectly by exaggerating, falsifying or inducing symptoms and/or signs in the child, causing the medical provider to order unnecessary testing or treatments. Examples include claiming there has been an increase in seizure frequency or falsifying bloody stools by putting blood from another source into a child's diaper. This can be taken further if the caregiver has involved multiple physicians and withholds or falsifies information to each. In some cases, the induction of symptoms can directly physically harm child, for example by contaminating a central line to induce bacteremia, or suffocation to induce apnea.

The motives behind the caregiver's actions are complex and thought to involve the psychosocial gain of placing their child in the "sick role." The caregiver may then be viewed in a positive light and gain attention, sympathy, and even sponsored or crowd-funded donations. They may achieve a closer relationship with their child or may have excitement from interacting with the medical system. Tully et al suggested that the analogy of addiction may help to understand the caregiver's persistence of fabrication despite the seriousness of harm coming to the child.

HEALTHCARE PROVIDER

The healthcare provider plays the role in repeatedly seeing and examining the child, ordering medical investigations, and initiating treatments. Despite best intentions, all of this may be unnecessary and only causing harm to the child. It is essential to recognize that CFI by its nature involves the medical system. Medical interventions may be prompted by an unreliable or false history; however, decisions are made and orders placed by the physician caring for the patient.

Recognizing CFI can be challenging for pediatricians, as the core of our work relies on an implicit trust between physician and caregiver. The caregiver is relied upon to accurately report their concerns with the child. When this does not occur, the physician must overcome the cognitive bias and question whether harm is coming to the child at the instigation of the caregiver. The physician's intense commitment to providing care and investment in finding an organic cause for the patient's symptoms may present an additional barrier to early recognition of medical child abuse.

Furthermore, the diagnosis is not as simple as whether there is the presence or absence of an underlying organic disease. Many children with CFI have pre-existing medical conditions. Thus, it is always important to keep CFI on your differential diagnosis when there are unusual or medically unexplained signs and symptoms in a child. CFI should be considered while medical workup is ongoing, otherwise this may result in further delay in diagnosis. Finally, it is important to note that making the diagnosis of CFI hinges simply on whether harm has occurred to the child or is likely to occur. The motives of the perpetrator, as in other forms of child abuse, are not relevant to the diagnosis and can be a distraction from the primary goal of protecting the patient from further harm.

CHILD

Due to the instigation from the caregiver, and the role of the healthcare provider, the child may undergo harm in the following ways:

1. **Physical harm**
   - Unnecessary medical testing (blood draws, radiation from imaging, sedation for imaging)
   - Unnecessary procedures (gastrostomy-tube insertions, central line insertions, endoscopies)
   - Unnecessary medications, treatments, and their side effects
   - Illness induction (suffocation, poisoning, withholding food or medication, confining them to a wheelchair)
2. **Psychological harm**
   - Distress from repeated medical interactions and examinations
   - Anxiety or confusion about their health
   - Developing false beliefs that they are actually sick, adopting the "sick role"
   - Beginning to collude with the caregiver. This may develop into factitious disorder imposed on self
   - Developing anxiety, depression, or other mental health disorders
3. **Social and educational concerns**
   - Prolonged absences from school due to hospitalizations or being kept at home
   - Social isolation, limited peer relationships
   - Disruption of normal daily life

CLINICAL PRESENTATION

PRESENTING CONDITIONS IN THE CHILD

Due to the medical complexity and multiple specialists involved by the time CFI is recognized, CFI most often presents in the pediatric in-patient setting. Furthermore, many children with CFI have underlying medical conditions or developmental disabilities. Thus, the fabricated symptoms or signs may be new for the child or may be exaggerated prior symptoms (e.g., increasing seizure frequency). Common presentations of CFI include seizure, apnea, diarrhea, vomiting, altered level of consciousness, fever, bleeding, allergies and rash. Fabricated developmental or behavioral problems have been described as well. It must be noted that this is not an exhaustive list and CFI continues to have expansive and varied presentations.

COMMON FEATURES IN THE CAREGIVER

Recently, research has focused on commonalities in the caregiver. Jenny and Metz identified that it has been reported that in 85% to 98% of cases the caregiver is female and often the mother. The father is often absent or has limited involvement. The caregiver commonly has a background in healthcare, which may contribute in them appearing confident and competent in navigating healthcare systems. The caregiver may have their own history of child maltreatment or psychiatric conditions including anxiety, somatization, personality disorders (borderline, histrionic, sociopathic), or factitious disorder imposed on self.

Putting this together, **Table 38-2** lists features in the child and caregiver that may suggest a concern for CFI (adapted from Glaser, and Tully et al).

TABLE 38-2 Features Raising Concern for Caregiver Fabricated Illness

Child
Reported symptoms and signs not independently observed
Symptoms and signs, reported or observed, cannot be explained by a medical condition or by medical assessments
Symptoms and signs improve when the caregiver is absent
Multiple diagnoses involving different organ systems
Reported diagnosis of underlying organic disease in the absence of medical verification
Unexpected or poor response to standard treatments
Unexplained functional impairment, including feeding, use of mobility aids and social isolation
Caregiver
One caregiver is the sole source of information—not allowing child to be seen alone, talks for the child, other caregivers absent
Ongoing reporting of new symptoms that may be unusual or atypical
Insists/demands more clinically unwarranted tests, referrals, opinions, and treatments
Cannot be reassured by normal tests, resists positive change to health status, insists that something is wrong
Repeated presentations for medical care and/or repeatedly not bringing the child to medical attention or cancelling certain appointments
Doctor shopping, firing of certain doctors
Objection to communication or information sharing between healthcare professionals
Positive interactions with doctors who comply but may escalate or disengage if challenged. May become litigious
Splitting of providers: Intense involvement of or special relationship with a particular healthcare professional and frequent complaints of other healthcare professionals

Source: Adapted from Glaser D. Fabricated or induced illness: From "Munchausen by proxy" to child and family-oriented action. *Child Abuse Negl.* 2020;108:104649 and Tully J et al. Fabricated or induced illness in children: a guide for Australian health-care practitioners. *Pediatr Child Health.* 2021;57(12):1847-1852.

It must be remembered that these should not be used as diagnostic criteria, but rather red flags that should raise concern for possible CFI and require further investigation for such.

DIAGNOSTIC EVALUATION

If there are features concerning for possible CFI, one must consider additional workup and possible collaboration with local child abuse pediatrics teams and/or child protection agencies. Considering CFI on the differential diagnosis is the first key step toward diagnosis. **Figure 38-1** from Tully et al demonstrates where CFI lies on the spectrum of healthcare seeking behaviors by parents and **Table 38-3** (Tully et al) suggests differential diagnoses for CFI and methods of intervention for each.

The diagnosis of CFI is very challenging and time consuming. A literature review by Sheridan found that the average time from onset of symptoms to the diagnosis of CFI is almost 22 months. The diagnosis of CFI includes information gathering and medical record review, as well as working with local child protection agencies and child abuse pediatricians. Roesler and Jenny stated that considering the following questions can be helpful in making a diagnosis of CFI. (i) Are the history, signs, and symptoms of disease credible? (ii) Is the child receiving unnecessary and harmful or potentially harmful medical care? (iii) If so, who is instigating the evaluation and treatment?

INFORMATION GATHERING

As there are often several different healthcare providers involved in suspected CFI cases, it is important to gather information directly from all those involved in the child's care. It is often helpful to first identify all healthcare providers involved and arrange an interdisciplinary meeting to discuss the concerns around CFI. Early consultation with a local Child Abuse Pediatrician is also beneficial, for advice around the diagnosis and workup of suspected CFI cases. An inpatient admission for direct observation of the child may also be beneficial. If a child is admitted, it is important to have clear communication around the goals for the hospital admission among the care team. Medical providers should be responsible for administering all medications and feeds, or directly supervising the caregivers doing these tasks. Clear and objective documentation should be done during the hospitalization of objective signs and symptoms observed in the child, and what is reported by the caregiver. It is also important to gather information from community sources when possible, such as the child's school, including attendance, emotional and behavioral concerns, mobility, and any necessary supports or aids which the child is receiving and on what basis.

MEDICAL RECORDS REVIEW

After identifying the healthcare providers involved in a child's medical care, a thorough review of all medical records should be undertaken. The aim of reviewing the medical records is to document the signs and symptoms being reported and compared with the objective findings from clinical visits and testing that the child has received. As these cases typically involve a large volume of medical records, it is recommended to use a standardized chart review template. Key information in the

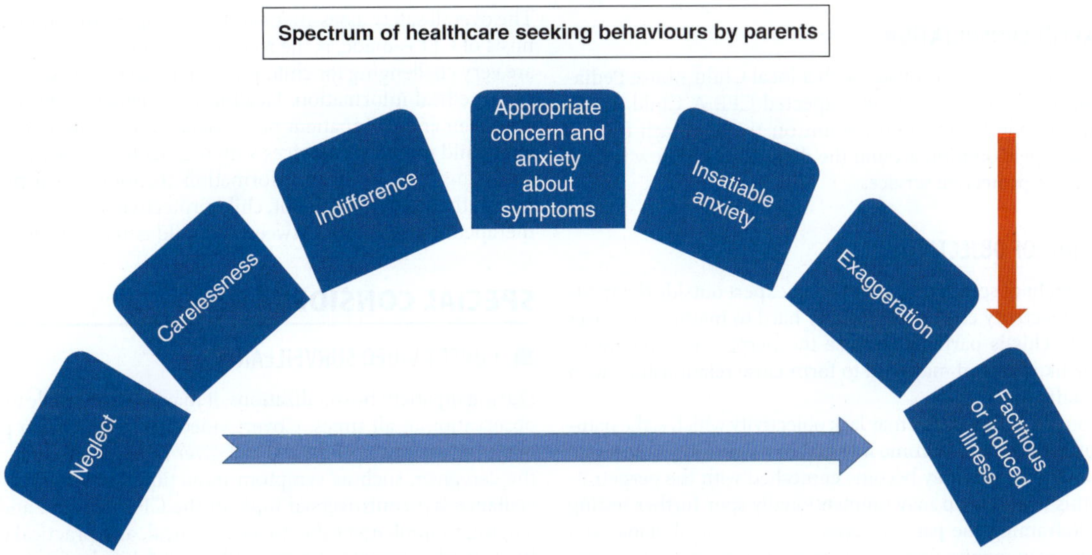

FIGURE 38-1. Spectrum of healthcare seeking behaviors by parents. (Reproduced with permission from Tully J, Hopkins O, Smith A, Williams K. Fabricated or induced illness in children: A guide for Australian health-care practitioners. *Pediatr Child Health.* 2021; 57(12): 1847-1852.)

TABLE 38-3 Differential Diagnosis of Over-Medicalization Phenomena

Carefully distinguish fabricated illness from…	Intervene by…
The over-anxious or misguided parent, genuine misunderstanding, and unintentional misattribution	*Reassuring, educating,* and *redirecting parents*—parents acknowledge and comply
The diagnostic dilemma	Identifying the *rare medical diagnosis*
The Medically Unexplained Symptoms (functional disorders, somatisation)	*Collaborative work* to achieve health, psychological intervention to manage symptoms driven by the *child's anxiety* or *mental state*—underlying factors are acknowledged by the parents
Malingering	Identifying a *defined material gain* or *positive avoidance* and acting to stop it continuing
Maternal delusional psychosis	Providing *psychiatric assessment and treatment* of carer
Over-anxious clinician or clinician unwilling to refuse parental request or unwarranted demand for tests, medication, completion of forms, and referrals to specialists	Practising *responsibly, ethically* and having the *courage* to say "no" when it is in the child's best interest

Source: Reproduced with permission from Tully J, Hopkins O, Smith A, Williams K. Fabricated or induced illness in children: A guide for Australian health-care practitioners. *Pediatr Child Health.* 2021;57(12): 1847–1852.

review would be date, location, reason for contact/visit type, provider, reported signs/symptoms per caregiver, objective observation by the medical provider, conclusion/diagnosis, and treatment/interventions. The chart review should also focus on subjective signs and symptoms reported by the caregivers, which are difficult for medical providers to objectively verify. In reviewing prescribed medications, it is important to document response to those medications, and if objective testing was done to assess medication adherence (e.g., certain antiepileptic levels). See Figure 42-2 from Jenny and Metz in the "Suggested Readings" section for an example of a template for medical chart review. A meticulous medical chart review is very time consuming in cases of suspected CFI, and it is often not feasible for the primary care physician or inpatient pediatrician to complete a comprehensive review of all records. This review may be completed with assistance by the Child Abuse Pediatrics team, and/or local child protection agencies. When involved, child protective services may also review other sources of information, such as social media sites, and fundraising activities.

SEEKING EXPERT CONSULTATION

If available, it is often helpful to consult with a local Child Abuse Pediatrician when concerns are raised about suspected CFI. A Child Abuse Pediatrician can provide helpful information on the approach to suspected CFI cases, expert opinion around the diagnosis, and how to best liaise with local child protective services.

THE CHALLENGE OF OBJECTIVITY

The additional benefit of seeking the input of an expert outside the treating team is that objectivity can be particularly hard to maintain in cases of suspected CFI. This is partially because the perpetrating parent or caregiver may be likeable and may tend to form close relationships with physicians and staff.

Another reason the treating team may lack objectivity which is the natural inclination of physicians to become invested in diagnosing an unusual or rare condition. Physicians may become enmeshed with the perpetrating parent and this relationship may unintentionally spur further testing and treatment. Reframing the patient's presentation as attributable to a non-organic cause may require providers to engage in honest self-assessment and develop a willingness to recognize and understand their role in perpetuating unnecessary and potentially harmful medical care.

REPORTING CONCERNS TO CHILD PROTECTION AGENCIES

When CFI is suspected, medical providers are mandated to report their concerns to child protective services in order to prevent ongoing harm to the child. Reporting is required when a physician or other healthcare provider has reasonable and probable grounds to believe at child has been harmed or is being harmed due to suspected CFI. A report to the local child protective services should be made when there are concerns that a child is being harmed, or potentially being harmed by unnecessary medical care. Due to the medical complexity of these cases, it is often challenging for child protective services to understand the concerns. Having objective information and input from several different members of the healthcare team can be helpful for child protective services. However, waiting for the full completion of the medical record review, an inter-disciplinary meeting, or further confirmation of the diagnosis should not delay a report to Child Protective Services. In making a report to child protective services, the healthcare provider should focus on clearly communicating the harm done to the child, including physical harm, psychological harm, and social and educational concerns. The medical team and child protective services should also be aware that the time of highest risk to the child may be at the time of reporting, due to escalation of caregiver actions to "prove" their child's diagnosis.

MANAGEMENT

Once the diagnosis of CFI is made, a coordinated interdisciplinary approach between healthcare providers and child protective services is essential in the management. It is important that all members of the healthcare team agree to stop all unnecessary medical treatment and diagnostic workup, and steps are taken to discuss the diagnosis of CFI with the family. Roesler and Jenny discuss that an "informing session" rather than a "confrontation" should be conducted between the medical team and the family. The goals of the session should be to discuss the child's medical condition and dispel any false claims of diagnoses as well as expressing concern over the caregiver's distorted perception of the child's health. It is also helpful to provide a written summary that can be placed in the child's medical record clearly outlining which medical diagnoses have been confirmed, ruled-out, and which treatments are no longer indicated. In complex cases, consideration can be made of admitting the child to hospital to work on de-medicalizing their care and removing treatments in a safely observed place.

DISCHARGE CRITERIA

The overall safety assessment and planning for the child in which a diagnosis of CFI is made, is the role of child protective services. These cases are very challenging for child protective service workers, due to the complex medical information. Healthcare providers, especially the primary physician and/or inpatient pediatrician, are essential in communicating with child protective services with regards to the harms to the child, and also translating medical information to nonmedical professionals. As part of the safety assessment, child protective services may also enforce a therapeutic separation between the child and caregiver.

SPECIAL CONSIDERATIONS

COVERT VIDEO SURVEILLANCE

During inpatient hospitalizations, it may not be feasible to have 1:1 direct observation at all times. Covert video surveillance can provide further observations of the child and caregiver interactions and actions done by the caregiver, such as symptom induction. However, covert video surveillance is a controversial topic in the CFI literature and is often challenging to implement due to legal, ethical, and practical considerations. In particular, covert video surveillance is felt to be forensic in nature and thus, having hospital staff monitor for symptom induction is often outside their role. Additionally, if the level of concern for CFI is high enough that covert video surveillance is being considered, then a report should be made to child protective services rather than watching and waiting for further harm to occur.

RECORD KEEPING

An additional important consideration in cases of medical child abuse is creating a thorough and accurate record of the patient's hospital course, including any events that raised concerns for exaggerated, falsified, or induced symptoms. Concerns for the possibility of CFI should be made explicit in the assessment even if certainty is lacking. Records should be kept with the expectation that they may be reviewed at some point in the future by subsequent medical providers, because a parent or caregiver who has already sought care from multiple providers in different jurisdictions is likely to continue this pattern. Parents who retain custody of the child will also have continued access to the medical record. Therefore, documentation should be comprehensive, yet objective and clear.

LEGAL CONSIDERATIONS

Finally, due to the complexity and high-risk nature of these cases, the treating team would be well served by notifying the hospital's risk management, general counsel, or equivalent administrative entity of their concerns for CFI in the patient's hospital course.

KEY POINTS

- The complex nature of caregiver fabricated illness often hampers diagnosis. It is necessary to maintain a high index of suspicion in order to diagnose this under-recognized but potentially serious or fatal condition.
- Cases of caregiver fabricated illness are complex and challenging. Both review of prior records and objective verification of symptoms during the hospitalization are essential. Early consultation with the hospital-based child protection team can ensure early diagnosis and proper management.
- Treatment of caregiver fabricated illness is beyond the scope of the medical team alone. A multidisciplinary approach that prioritizes close collaboration with the local Child Abuse Pediatrician and child protective services offers the best chance of successfully protecting the child.

SUGGESTED READINGS

Cardona L, Asnes A. Disclosure of caregiver-fabricated illness to a child: a team-based approach to communicating with pediatric patients. *Clin Child Psychol Psychiatry*. 2019;24(3):494-502.

Flaherty EG, Macmillan HL. Caregiver-fabricated illness in a child: a manifestation of child maltreatment. *Pediatr*. 2013;132(3):590-597.

Glaser D. Fabricated or induced illness: from "Munchausen by proxy" to child and family-oriented action. *Child Abuse Negl*. 2020;108:104649.

Jenny C, Metz B. Medical child abuse and medical neglect. *Pediatr Rev*. 2020;41(2):49-60.

Roesler TA, Jenny C. *Medical Child Abuse: Beyond Münchausen Sydrome by Proxy*. Elk Grove Village, Illinois, IL: American Academy of Pediatrics Press; 2009.

Sheridan MS. The deceit continues: an updated literature review of Munchausen syndrome by proxy. Child abuse & neglect. 2003 Apr 1; 27(4):431-451.

Tully J, Hopkins O, Smith A, Williams K. Fabricated or induced illness in children: a guide for Australian health-care practitioners. *Pediatr Child Health*. 2021;57(12):1847-1852.

CHAPTER 39 Legal Issues

Emma Cory, MD, FRCPC, DRCPSC (Child Maltreatment Pediatrics) and Dena Nazer, MD

BACKGROUND

The role of the pediatrician and hospitalist in child advocacy and protection extends well beyond the inpatient hospitalization. When a concern of child maltreatment arises, it is the physician's legal responsibility to report suspected child abuse and neglect and, on occasion, to subsequently provide ethical testimony when required. In cases of suspected abuse, a pediatric hospitalist may also share their specific expertise by participating in case reviews and as a member of a multidisciplinary team such as the child death review team.

A number of chapters in this book focus on recognition and the appropriate medical evaluation when child maltreatment is suspected. This chapter, however, focuses on the legal responsibilities of the physician including mandated reporting of child protection concerns. It provides a basic understanding of how the legal system works in order to be more comfortable and competent. This chapter also includes general recommendations for chart documentation and verbal communication in the setting of a child abuse concern, including guidelines for ethical testimony in legal proceedings.

REPORTING CHILD MALTREATMENT

In North America, each state, province or territory has established definitions to inform regional and community efforts to prevent, identify, and manage child abuse and neglect. It is important for inpatient pediatricians to be familiar with the laws and definitions of the various types of maltreatment in their local practice context. In general, across North America, there is regional legislation that requires certain professionals to report incidents of suspected child abuse and neglect to their local child protective services (CPS) agency. Common mandated reporters are physicians, nurses, teachers, psychologists, social workers, and law enforcement personnel. Despite the variability in local laws and mandated reporter specifications, physicians are considered mandated reporters in all regions. The reader is advised to access more information, resources, and tools covering topics on child welfare and child abuse and neglect from the Child Welfare Information Gateway (https://www.childwelfare.gov) and from their local child welfare resources.

Only a reasonable level of concern or suspicion of abuse is typically required to mandate a report to the local child protection services; a person does not need evidence or definitive confirmation of abuse or neglect to make a report (Case example 39.1). In general, if the report to a CPS agency has been made in good faith, the mandated reporter is generally protected from any civil or criminal liability in the case if the report is investigated and deemed erroneous or unsubstantiated. In contrast, failure of a mandated reporter to report suspected child abuse may result in a fine, malpractice suit, or criminal sanctions. More importantly, it may result in the child and caregiver remaining in a situation with risk of further maltreatment.

Case example 39.1: A 2-month-old baby boy presents with pain and swelling of his left leg. Imaging reveals a transverse femur fracture. There is no history provided to explain the fracture. Considering the baby's age and the absence of any history of trauma, the pediatrician is concerned for possible physical abuse. The pediatrician is a mandated reporter of child maltreatment and needs to report appropriately to the local CPS agency.

As an inpatient pediatrician caring for a patient with a concern for child maltreatment, it is essential to confirm that a report has been made according to the local duty to report legislation. It is also essential to become familiar with internal policies within their hospital or practice setting. While institutional policies may address the process of reporting and need to be reviewed, they do not relieve the physician from the responsibility to report. As mandated reporting requirements may vary by region, pediatric providers should become knowledgeable about the reporting requirements within their local area and consult as needed regarding specific local legislation. If another person or institution has filed a report about the same episode of abuse, no other professionals are required to duplicate that report. However, if a new indicator of potential abuse is observed, an additional report must be filed (Case example 39.2).

Case example 39.2: The 2-month-old baby with an unexplained femur fracture is transferred to another hospital. The referring physician appropriately initiated a report to the local CPS agency due to the lack of history to explain the fracture. Subsequent medical evaluation identifies multiple posterior rib fractures. The accepting physician at the second hospital is mandated to make a supplementary report regarding the rib fractures as part of their ongoing duty to report additional child protection concerns.

Unfortunately, some physicians continue to be uncertain or experience reluctance about the legal mandate to report and may fail to initiate a report when indicated. Pediatricians are accustomed to practicing in a family-centered care model. When faced with the recognition of a child abuse concern, the pediatrician may experience tension between their typical family-centered approach and the necessity to make a child-focused mandated report to child protection services. Physicians may be influenced by factors such as their pre-existing relationship with a family and their knowledge of risk or protective factors in the family unit. In addition, physicians may lack confidence in the investigative process, and may fear negative personal consequences including the loss of patients from their practice and the possibility of formal complaints.

When a report is made to CPS, it is important to provide as much information as possible regarding the child and the incident or circumstances that led to the suspicion of maltreatment. In certain circumstances, an individual may choose to make an anonymous report to CPS. However, especially in the hospital setting, it is recommended that parents or guardians be notified when a medical professional is going to make a report to preserve (to the extent possible) an open, honest relationship. The most effective means of notifying parents or guardians is to express concern that the child may have been harmed, rather than directly accuse the caregiver of maltreatment. Although the physician-parent relationship may become strained, parents generally respond better to honesty and transparency. This should facilitate a more comfortable working relationship while the child remains in the hospital and may encourage appropriate follow-up care.

RACE AND BIAS IN CHILD MALTREATMENT REPORTING AND DIAGNOSIS

Race/ethnicity and poverty have been shown to be factors for CPS reports during a child maltreatment-related hospitalization. Concern has also arisen regarding the over-representation of Black and Indigenous children in the foster care system. As described by Palusci and Botash, 2021, it is necessary to implement programs and policies that mitigate implicit bias to prevent ongoing inequities regarding which children receive child protection reports and system intervention (Case example 39.3). In addition to the medical professional offering culturally sensitive care and being respectful to ethnic diversity, one needs to be aware of specific rules, for example, the Indian Child Welfare Act (ICWA) which has particular implications in child neglect and abuse cases.

Case example 39.3: As the physician considers reporting to CPS, they may reflect on whether unconscious bias is affecting their level of concern. Developing a process to peer review cases can provide quality assurance to mitigate bias and ensure a standardized approach to cases.

MEDICAL HISTORY AND DOCUMENTATION OF CHILD ABUSE CONCERNS

It is always important for physicians to be complete, accurate, and legible when documenting events in a patient's medical records. In the setting of a child maltreatment concern, the importance of detailed documentation is magnified as there is the potential for the medical records to be submitted as evidence during a legal proceeding. Correct, thorough, decipherable medical records can help the treating physician recall their findings when preparing to testify in a legal proceeding which may occur months to years after the physician's initial involvement with the patient. The medical records when entered into evidence may assist the fact-finder (i.e., judge or jury) in their understanding of a child's injuries and may be an important factor in the legal proceeding.

Interviewing of a child by the medical care team in the context of a suspicious injury is generally discouraged as forensic interviewing follows a specific protocol and is typically the role of investigators or forensic medical team members. However, during routine history taking from an older child with injury concerns, a hospitalist pediatrician may encounter circumstances when a child makes a disclosure regarding an injury mechanism or an alleged perpetrator. All hospital staff must clearly document a child's statements describing the history of the illness or injury and the presenting symptoms, as they may be admissible in legal proceedings. When a child makes a disclosure to a medical team member, it is recommended that the provider document precisely using quotations when able. It is also recommended that the provider documents their own statements before and after the disclosure so that the context of the conversation can be understood by other relevant parties. Without careful documentation of exactly what questions were asked and exactly what the child said, the professional will likely not remember months or years later if called as a witness.

Careful documentation of physical examination findings is also required in the context of a child abuse concern. Body diagrams and accurate measurements of skin findings are recommended. Photography of skin findings may be an important adjunct to the written documentation. Hospitalist pediatricians are encouraged to know their institutional policies surrounding patient photography including consent and secure storage of sensitive photographs.

On occasion, child protection workers and law enforcement may request that a member of the healthcare team provide copies of health records or photographs to inform their investigation. Typically, it is best practice to redirect the investigators to the institutional health records department to ensure that the medical records are released in the appropriate context with the necessary documentation on file.

CHILD PROTECTIVE SERVICES

Child Protective Services (CPS) is a governmental agency responsible for investigating reports of child maltreatment, determining whether child abuse or neglect has occurred, and providing interventions to ensure a safe environment for the child. In most cases, CPS agencies assist families in finding appropriate support services to protect and improve the well-being of their children. When it is deemed necessary, these agencies also secure alternative placements of safety for children or, in rare cases, pursue the termination of parental rights. Although CPS agencies vary by location, professional standards of practice have been widely accepted and implemented.

CHILD PROTECTIVE SERVICES AND POLICE INVESTIGATION

Once a report is made, the CPS staff determines whether the report meets criteria to be accepted as an investigation or assessment and is thus "screened in." Reports that do not meet the criteria may be "screened out" with suggestions made for referral to other support services. When the CPS worker reviews the information contained within a report and makes an assessment that the referral meets threshold, then an investigation is initiated. The CPS investigation begins by gathering all the relevant information about the case. Many laws and regulations outline the investigative procedure in great detail. The CPS report is typically triaged according to urgency and the level of concern. Certain high-concern circumstances will require contact with the child and family within 24 hours and other circumstances will generate a response within 2 to 7 days. Interviews are conducted with the child, the parents, other family members, and other individuals who might have knowledge about the specific allegations or about the risk and protective factors in the family environment.

There are regional variations in whether a physician is mandated or permitted to make a referral to law enforcement. Pediatricians are encouraged to seek consultation and be aware of their local regulations related to communication with police. Typically, consent, warrant, or subpoena is required for a physician to release confidential health information about a patient. In some regions, CPS and law enforcement have joint investigation protocols that guide their investigative process.

A CPS and police investigation in the context of a concern for physical abuse may involve the examination of similar information but with a different focus. CPS is investigating with a focus on the safety of the involved child. The police investigation is focused on establishing whether a criminal act has occurred and whether it can be established that a single person had the exclusive opportunity to commit the offense. The burden of proof is higher for criminal charges to be laid. The child protection system may have to make a safety plan with consideration that a child's injuries could have been produced by multiple individuals within a family unit when a single individual of concern cannot be identified.

CHILDREN'S ADVOCACY CENTERS

Many jurisdictions have children's advocacy centers in place to assist and guide the child interview process. Children's advocacy centers provide a multidisciplinary team approach to investigations of child abuse, including forensic interviews, therapeutic interventions, victim support and advocacy, and case management. Such facilities provide a safe, child-friendly environment to conduct forensic interviews of a neutral, fact-finding nature. Often these agencies work in collaboration with law enforcement and CPS to minimize the number of times the child victim is interviewed.

DISPOSITION AFTER THE INVESTIGATION

Regulations require that the CPS agency conclude the investigative process by arriving at a disposition or a formal finding of whether child abuse or neglect has occurred within a given time frame. A number of terms, including *indicated*, *supported*, *confirmed*, or *substantiated*, may be used when CPS has determined that a child was a victim of maltreatment; words such as *unfounded* or *unsubstantiated* indicate that there was insufficient evidence to conclude that child maltreatment occurred.

A finding that abuse or neglect has been substantiated frequently requires further action by the child protection agency and the family. The child protection agency is mandated to explore options to maintain a child safely within the family home or in an appropriate kin placement rather than placing the child in foster care. Thus, the next step often involves the formulation of a safety case plan by CPS and the guardian, with the main goals of ensuring the child's safety and strengthening the family system. The case plan reflects the expectations and responsibilities of family members as well as the role and contributions of the CPS agency. The safety plan is then monitored at regular intervals to determine whether the CPS file remains open or is closed.

A minority of substantiated cases of child maltreatment result in some type of child protection court proceeding. This occurs when the child is thought to be in imminent danger of repeated maltreatment or when attempts to maintain safety within the family unit have not been successful.

Cases investigated by CPS become "closed" for a variety of reasons, ranging from the conclusion that the child is safe in so far as can be determined, to the termination of parental rights and placement of the child in a permanent alternate care environment.

EMERGENCY REMOVAL

In certain cases when the child is judged to be in imminent danger, CPS has the ability to take the child into the care of the CPS agency. The child may be placed with a protective family member in a kinship arrangement or may be placed in a foster home or group home setting. Additional protective orders may also be subsequently issued by the court against the individuals alleged to be responsible for the child's maltreatment, such as orders for those individuals to vacate the home and restrictions on the nature of the access between the child and individuals of concern.

LEGAL PROCEEDINGS AND TESTIMONY

Medical testimony may be required in a variety of legal proceedings in both civil and criminal courts, including a child protection hearing, the criminal prosecution of an alleged perpetrator of child maltreatment, and a civil action for damages from injuries. From the perspective of a pediatrician involved in court testimony, the expectations are similar across different legal proceedings. The lawyer involved in a court proceeding needs to provide the pediatrician more information regarding the specifics of the legal proceeding.

A pediatrician is notified of the requirement to participate in a legal proceeding by the receipt of a summons or subpoena. Receiving a subpoena to testify in a legal proceeding is naturally an anxiety-producing experience for a pediatrician. Physicians may receive support and advice from an experienced colleague, institutional supports, or resources available through their licensing body. A preparation session with the lawyer involved in the proceeding may also provide relevant information to assist the pediatrician in understanding the context and preparing to participate in a legal hearing (Case example 39.4).

Case example 39.4: The pediatrician receives a subpoena to testify in criminal court in the case of the 2-month-old infant with a femur fracture and multiple rib fractures. A parent has been charged related to the traumatic injuries. The pediatrician feels anxious about appearing in a legal proceeding for the first time and wonders if their medical care will be criticized. They are unsure where to seek guidance related to the subpoena.

CHILD PROTECTION COURT

In child protection proceedings the focus is on the child—whether they have been subjected to abuse or neglect, and if so, what intervention is needed not only to protect the child but also to strengthen the family unit. It is not always necessary to prove that a specific parent or guardian injured a child. In child protection legal proceedings, the standard of proof is less than that required in criminal court. Decisions may be made in a child protection proceeding based on the balance of probabilities or based on a "preponderance of the evidence that it is more likely than not that the allegations are true."

CRIMINAL COURT

In some cases, the conclusion of a law enforcement investigation may involve criminal charges laid against an individual. Criminal cases involve the prosecution of an individual to establish their guilt or innocence of particular criminal charges and to determine appropriate sentences for those found guilty. In contrast to the balance of probabilities in child protection, criminal cases require a higher degree of certainty—"beyond a reasonable doubt"—to establish guilt.

EXPERT AND NON-EXPERT TESTIMONY

A hospitalist pediatrician may be subpoenaed to appear in a court proceeding to provide either material (fact) or expert (opinion) evidence. A material or fact witness provides factual testimony based on personal knowledge and is not to express an opinion based on that knowledge. A pediatrician may be requested to provide fact-based testimony of what they did, what they saw, and what was said during the assessment of a child with abuse concerns. In contrast, an expert witness may testify about the medical and scientific concepts of the case in the form of an opinion or otherwise. For example, in the case of a child with physical injuries, an expert in child maltreatment may provide an opinion on whether the findings are the result of inflicted injury, accidental injury, or a medical condition that is mimicking injury. An expert witness can formulate a professional opinion on the matter at hand, assist the factfinder (typically a judge) in understanding the evidence, or answer a hypothetical question. Prior to the testimony, the judge hears information regarding the proposed expert's curriculum vitae and makes the decision whether a witness has sufficient knowledge, education, training, skill, and experience applicable to the case to qualify as an expert witness.

Organizations including the American Academy of Pediatrics (AAP), the Helfer Society, and the Society for Pediatric Radiology Ethics Committee drafted recommendations for ethical expert legal testimony (see Suggested Reading). The statement by the AAP applies to medical expert witness consultation or testimony in all legal venues and provides new guidance on ways to prevent irresponsible testimony in child abuse cases.

PREPARING TO TESTIFY

Testifying in a court hearing can be stressful, even for the most experienced professionals. It is crucial to be well prepared to ease anxiety, decrease the risk of surprises, and ensure that the court is provided with the most accurate information possible. When dealing with pretestimony anxiety it is also helpful to remember that the legal system is designed as an adversarial process to allow the most appropriate decision to be made by the judge or jury. Anxiety may be lessened by the understanding that the lawyers from each side are there to ask questions from differing perspectives to create the most nuanced understanding of the case. The physicians themselves are not on trial. This understanding may assist the physician to maintain a calm demeanor in the face of the expected critique of aspects of their testimony during cross-examination.

Communication in advance with the attorney is crucial. It is important for the physician to meet in advance with the attorney who subpoenaed them. This preparation meeting allows the physician to share their knowledge and involvement in the case as well as any review, any questions, or past experiences. The attorney will provide information regarding court expectations and process which may provide reassurance to a physician unfamiliar with court testimony. The attorney should provide the physician with the framework of court testimony and a list of anticipated questions.

A preparation meeting is important to clarify whether the physician is anticipated to testify as a fact or expert witness. The physician should inquire whether documents will be admitted partially or entirely into evidence and whether they will be permitted to refer to chart documentation as part of their testimony. Practical issues such as whether photographs or radiology studies will be reviewed in court are also important items for discussion. It is critical that the attorney be aware of the strength of the physician's medical opinion and understand the reasoning behind that opinion. It is equally important for the physician to be transparent about the limitations or scope of both their factual testimony and opinions. If there are controversies in the medical field related to an aspect of the case, it is important for a medical expert to provide an explanation of the controversy and how it was considered in relation to the case on trial. A preparation discussion with an attorney can also clarify whether a physician would defer to the expertise of another subspecialist involved on some aspects of the case and can clarify if other medical providers also need to be subpoenaed. In rare circumstances, the preparation meeting and a discussion of limitations of the medical opinion may lead a lawyer to elect not to proceed with the case.

TESTIFYING IN COURT

On the day of the trial, the physician should dress professionally, arrive early, and notify the attorney of their presence. A brief check-in with the lawyer allows an opportunity to clarify any new issues that may have arisen since the last contact. Of note, witnesses often are sequestered, meaning that they are allowed in the courtroom only during their own testimony.

While on the witness stand, it is imperative that the physician listen to and understand each question. If the question is not fully heard or comprehended, the physician should ask the attorney to repeat the question or rephrase it. It is appropriate to pause to carefully consider the response to the question. Questions should be answered with truthfulness, precision, and clarity. As the audience in the courtroom is nonmedical, it is often necessary to define unfamiliar terminology and explain medical concepts. It is optimal for the physician to always attempt to answer questions in language that is understandable to lay-people. When the physician is asked a question to which they do not know the answer, it is important that the physician clearly responds that they do not know. Guessing or speculating outside their knowledge or expertise can have negative effects on the physician's credibility and more importantly can lead to an incorrect legal outcome.

The initial part of expert testimony involves qualifications if the physician is expected to testify as an expert witness. The attorney begins by asking a series of questions regarding the physician's professional education and experience. In some instances, the physician's curriculum vitae will be admitted as an exhibit. The opposing counsel then has an opportunity to ask further questions if they plan to refute this qualification.

Once the physician is qualified as an expert, testimony can take one of three forms: an opinion, an answer to a hypothetical question, or a lecture that provides background information for the judge or jury. Most often the expert is asked to render an opinion based on the facts of the case. Sometimes the expert's testimony is in the form of an answer to a hypothetical question that includes significant facts relevant to the case at hand. On occasion, an expert may testify in the form of a lecture that provides the factfinder (i.e., judge or jury) with background information on technical, clinical, or scientific issues.

Whatever the form of question and answer, it is important that the answer be well thought out, accurate, and clearly articulated. The physician should explain all conclusions and analyses in terms that are understood by the factfinder and ensure that they do not exceed the bounds of their expertise or exaggerate in any manner. In formulating an opinion, an expert may rely on all relevant clinical, scientific, historical, and factual information. Experts are not permitted to express an opinion on legal issues such as the guilt or innocence of a defendant.

During cross-examination, the opposing counsel will attempt to show the factfinder that the expert's testimony is flawed in some way. This may involve trying to discredit the expert's knowledge of the relevant evidence or posing other theories to explain the child's condition. An expert who has thoroughly reviewed all medical documents and relies on up-to-date knowledge in the field should be well equipped for cross-examination. The expert should also be prepared to explain the nature of possible differential diagnoses, their manifestations, and whether they could be a plausible explanation for the findings in the patient. It is important that a physician maintain a neutral and objective approach during all aspects of court testimony including cross-examination. This may be facilitated by remembering that a medical expert has a duty to the court rather than any particular side in the matter. The physician has an obligation to explain medical concepts and the findings in a case to the judge and/or jury so that they may make an appropriate assessment. The physician should maintain neutrality and objectivity without a position of the outcome of the case on trial.

In conclusion, it is the pediatrician's ethical and legal responsibility to suspect, medically assess and report child maltreatment concerns. As physicians seek to further their clinical knowledge, they also need to further their knowledge of the laws and regulations in their state or province regarding child maltreatment. Preparation, communication, and collaboration with other disciplines are essential to ensure an objective investigation and safe outcomes for children.

KEY POINTS

- Physicians should familiarize themselves with their regional laws, hospital practice procedures, and venues for support services with regard to child maltreatment.
- If there is "reasonable cause" to suspect that a child has been maltreated, the physician must file a report with the local CPS agency.
- Ensure complete, accurate, legible documentation in medical records, especially when dealing with cases of suspected child maltreatment. Those records may be subpoenaed by a court of law.
- Physicians should be well prepared before testifying in court, whether as a factual witness or an expert witness. This includes reviewing all medical records and conferring with the attorney who subpoenaed the physician.

ACKNOWLEDGMENT

The authors wish to acknowledge the contributions of Lisa Santos Spector in writing the original version of the chapter.

SUGGESTED READINGS

Canadian Medical Protective Association. (Revised 2022) Testifying: What it involves and how to do it effectively. https://www.cmpa-acpm.ca/en/advice-publications/browse-articles/2018/testifying–what-it-involves-and-how-to-do-it-effectively.

Narang SK, Melville JD. Legal issues in child maltreatment. *Pediatr Clin North Am.*2014;61(5):1049-1058.

Narang SK, Paul SR, Committee on Medical Liability and Risk Management. Expert witness participation in civil and criminal proceedings. *Pediatrics.* 2017;139(3):e20164122.

Palusci VJ, Botash AS. Race and bias in child maltreatment diagnosis and reporting. *Pediatrics.* 2021;148(1):e2020049625.

Strouse PJ, Callahan MJ, Annam A, et al. Guidelines for expert testimony in pediatric radiology. *Pediatr Radiol.* 2021;51(7):1275-1280.

Strouse PJ, Moreno JA, Dias MS, Narang SK. Preparing for court testimony. *Pediatr Radiol.*2021;51(6):1084-1092.

SECTION B
Adolescent Medicine

CHAPTER 40 Eating Disorders

Kyung E. Rhee, MD, MSc, MA and Adam E. Bracken, MD

BACKGROUND

Eating disorders are defined by the American Psychiatric Association as a set of neurobiological/behavioral conditions characterized by severe and persistent disturbance in eating behaviors and its associated distressing thoughts and emotions. Eating disorders are common and can be associated with severe medical and psychiatric morbidity. They affect millions of Americans with a lifetime prevalence estimated at 8.4% for women and 2.2% for men. Eating disorders are increasing in incidence and prevalence among adolescents. Although most patients with eating disorders are managed in an outpatient setting, this chapter provides a practical framework for the pediatric hospitalist to stabilize and initiate management of a patient hospitalized for an eating disorder.

The five major subgroups of eating disorders described in the literature are defined in the fifth edition of the *Diagnostic and Statistical Manual of Mental Disorders* (DSM-5) as anorexia nervosa, bulimia nervosa, binge-eating disorder, avoidant/restrictive food intake disorder (ARFID), and other specified feeding or eating disorder.

The prevalence of anorexia nervosa and bulimia nervosa is estimated to be up to 4% and 3% respectively in adolescents, with a growing incidence among children <15 years old. While females account for most of the cases, these disorders also occur in males. In fact, eating disorders are increasing in prevalence in males and is reported to occur in up to 10% to 25% of identified cases. Eating disorders also occur across all races and socioeconomic strata. Although the exact etiology of these disorders is unknown, they are thought to be multifactorial in origin, with strong evidence for neurobiological predispositions and gene-environment interactions. In addition to eating disorders that meet DSM-5 criteria, disordered eating behaviors are very common in adolescents. Up to 25% of high school girls and 11% of boys report disordered eating behaviors (e.g., dieting, fasting, skipping meals, using diet pills or laxatives) that are severe enough to warrant evaluation, and 9% of high school girls and 4% of boys induce vomiting to control their weight.

CLINICAL PRESENTATION

A patient presenting with weight loss, poor growth, pubertal cessation, restrictive attitudes about weight, unexplained vomiting, or abnormal eating behaviors should prompt a consideration of the diagnosis of eating disorder. The consequences of severe weight loss or purging activity can lead to medical instability requiring hospitalization. Presenting signs and symptoms (**Table 40-1**) may include syncope, orthostatic hypotension, chest pain, hematemesis, menstrual irregularities or other symptoms of hypogonadism, and constipation. Preconceived notions about what a patient with an eating disorder "looks like" may delay diagnosis in patients with obesity or adolescent males. Younger patients (e.g., preteens) with eating disorders may present in a less typical manner; some may not lose weight but may instead fail to grow in either weight and/or height. While anorexia nervosa and bulimia nervosa are the most frequently diagnosed eating disorders, and can have the most severe medical complications, all eating disorders can cause significant medical and psychiatric morbidity. Early medical and psychological intervention is associated with improved outcomes.

ANOREXIA NERVOSA

Patients with anorexia nervosa restrictive type usually present with (i) restriction of energy intake leading to a significantly low body weight (<85% of expected weight), (ii) an intense fear of gaining weight or becoming fat even though they are underweight, and (iii) a disordered body image, or unrealistic perception of what their body should look like. They often display little concern over their weight loss and report that they "feel fine" and still need to lose more weight. The presence of amenorrhea, a prior criterion, is no longer necessary to diagnosis anorexia nervosa. Patients who meet the above criteria for anorexia nervosa but also engage in binge eating and purging-type behaviors are diagnosed as having anorexia nervosa binge-purge type. These patients are significantly underweight, but engage in behaviors that persistently sabotage weight gain, such as self-induced vomiting, excessive exercise, or use of laxatives or diuretics.

Parents and caregivers may not always recognize that their child is restricting their nutritional intake because they appear to be interested or involved in the cooking process; many patients exhibit elaborate rituals pertaining to food or an intense interest in para-eating behaviors, such as collecting recipes, preparing food for the family, or watching food-related television programs. They often display traits of perfectionism or behavioral rigidity, which can be seen in varying eating rituals (e.g., only eating one brand of yogurt because of the ingredients, not allowing certain foods to touch on the plate), or as excellence in school and overachievement in extracurricular activities, sports, or the arts. These behaviors can mask the underlying eating disorder and sometimes lull parents into thinking that their children are navigating adolescence well. However, when patients do eat, they frequently complain of early satiety, abdominal bloating, post-prandial discomfort, pain, and/or nausea. Some patients will vomit to relieve this discomfort. As patients lose more weight and become severely malnourished, they will develop other symptoms—dizziness or fainting, cold intolerance, constipation, dry or yellow skin, fatigue, weakness, or muscle cramps. Post-menarchal females with anorexia nervosa may develop secondary amenorrhea; pre-menarchal children may have delayed linear growth.

While most people equate anorexia nervosa with extreme underweight, there are some patients who engage in all of the above behaviors but are not low weight. These patients are classified as having atypical anorexia nervosa because they have lost significant weight and have disordered body image thoughts, but do not meet the criteria of being severely underweight. Instead, they are in the normal weight or overweight range. These patients typically have a history of obesity and have successfully lost weight but want to lose more and are not satisfied with their current weight status or body image. They are also consumed by food- or weight-related thoughts throughout the day and may have developed rigid eating rituals as well. Despite being in the normal weight range, they may have similar symptoms as patients with typical anorexia nervosa, including constipation, dizziness, fainting, weakness, and loss of menses.

BULIMIA NERVOSA

Bulimia nervosa classically presents as recurrent episodes of binge eating followed by unhealthy behaviors (e.g., self-induced vomiting, laxative abuse, excessive exercise) to alleviate the distress caused by the excessive consumption of food and prevent weight gain. Binge eating episodes are characterized by the consumption of an amount of food in a fixed period (usually within 2 hours) that is larger than what most people would eat and a sense of loss of control over that eating episode. In response to an episode of bingeing, the individual may display maladaptive behaviors to prevent weight gain. These behaviors take one of two forms: (i) purging: the patient engages in self-induced vomiting or the use of laxatives,

TABLE 40-1 Potential Signs and Symptoms in Patients With Eating Disorders

Related to Nutritional Restriction	Related to Purging
Cardiac	
Bradycardia	Bradycardia
Arrhythmia, Palpitations	Arrhythmia, Palpitations
Orthostasis, Dizziness	Orthostasis, Dizziness
Pitting edema of extremities (more frequent with refeeding)	Pitting Edema
Cardiac murmur (one third have mitral valve prolapse)	
Dyspnea	
Endocrine/Metabolism	
Oligomenorrhea or Amenorrhea	Oligomenorrhea
Low Libido	Low Libido
Hypothermia, Cold Intolerance	Hypothermia
Thinning scalp hair	
Ear, Nose, and Throat	
Sunken Cheeks	Dental enamel erosion
	Parotitis
	Mouth sores and Pain
	Palatal or tonsillar pillar scratches
Dermatologic/Musculoskeletal	
Sallow, yellowish skin	Dry Skin
Lanugo	Russell sign
Bone Pain	Bone Pain, Muscle Cramping
Stress Fractures	Stress Fractures
Cold Extremities, acrocyanosis	
Gastrointestinal	
Abdominal Pain, Nausea, Early Satiety, Abdominal Distention	Abdominal Pain, Heart Burn, Abdominal Distention
Constipation	Constipation
Dysphagia	Rectal Prolapse
	Diarrhea
Psychologic	
Anxiety, Apathy, Depression	Anxiety, Apathy, Depression
Flat affect	
Neurologic	
Headaches	Headaches
Seizures	Seizures
Peripheral Polyneuropathy	Paresthesia
Poor Concentration	Poor Concentration
Fatigue and Weakness	Weakness

*Callused knuckles from inducing gagging or vomiting by pushing fingers down throat.

Source: Data adapted from American Academy of Pediatrics, Committee on Adolescence. Identifying and treating eating disorders. *Pediatrics*. 2003;111:204-211.

enemas, or diuretics, or (ii) nonpurging: the patient engages in excessive exercise as compensatory methods. To be formally diagnosed with bulimia nervosa, these behaviors occur at least once per week for 3 months. An individual with bulimia is usually aware that his or her eating pattern is abnormal and may go to great lengths to conceal it.

BINGE-EATING DISORDER

Binge-eating disorder is characterized by binge-eating episodes as defined in the criterion for bulimia nervosa, but without any episodes of purging. Binge-eating disorder, while a debilitating and common disorder, rarely requires inpatient medical stabilization, so is not discussed in detail in this chapter.

AVOIDANT-RESTRICTIVE FOOD INTAKE DISORDER

A newer category in the DSM-5 is Avoidant-Restrictive Food Intake Disorder (ARFID). Patients with ARFID often have a fear of eating, but this fear does not involve a fear of weight gain or distorted body image cognitions. Individuals with ARFID eat insufficient calories due to (i) poor appetite, a lack of interest in eating or food, or feeling full quickly; (ii) selective eating behaviors secondary to sensory concerns or issues with taste or texture; and/or (iii) fear of consequences of eating such as choking, vomiting, or an allergic reaction. Most patients with ARFID are brought to medical attention because these fears have significantly impaired their ability to eat to the point where some are no longer meeting their nutritional requirements or eating anything by mouth, requiring NG tube feeds, or are losing significant weight. The diagnosis of ARFID requires that no other cause that would explain the eating pattern, either medically or culturally, could be identified.

OTHER SPECIFIED FEEDING AND EATING DISORDERS AND UNSPECIFIED FEEDING AND EATING DISORDERS

These two diagnostic categories ("other specified" and "unspecified") differentiate subgroups within what used to be characterized as "eating disorders not otherwise specified." Other specified feeding and eating disorders refers to a cluster of disturbed eating habits that also entail disordered body image and fear of gaining weight. However, they do not formally meet the criteria for one of the above-mentioned eating disorders. These disorders are usually categorized into the following groups: atypical anorexia nervosa, subthreshold bulimia nervosa and binge-eating disorder (occurring less than once a week and/or for less than three months duration), purging disorder (purging without binge eating), and night-eating syndrome (awakening from sleep to eat or eating an excessive amount after dinner which causes significant distress). Unspecified feeding and eating disorders include eating disorders considered to be clinically significant because they can cause significant distress or impact daily functioning, but again, do not meet diagnostic criteria of one of the above-mentioned eating disorders or fall into any of the other categories. A few examples of these include pica, chewing and spitting behaviors, and orthorexia (an obsession with "clean eating" and healthy lifestyle behaviors). These disorders can still cause significant medical compromise and psychiatric morbidity. Both the "other specified" and "unspecified" eating disorders require equally aggressive care, both medically and psychologically, because lack of treatment may lead to the development of an eating disorder that meets full diagnostic criteria. Early recognition of these disordered eating behaviors may prevent poor outcomes.

DIFFERENTIAL DIAGNOSIS

The initial assessment of a patient with a suspected eating disorder should be sufficiently complete to ensure that a thorough differential diagnosis has been considered, and no alternate cause of the symptom of concern (e.g., weight loss, vomiting) is present. **Table 40-2** provides a list of conditions that may present mimicking an eating disorder.

TABLE 40-2 Differential Diagnosis of Eating Disorders

Central nervous system condition: mass, inflammatory condition
Gastrointestinal disorders: inflammatory bowel disease, infection, celiac disease
Endocrine disorders: diabetes mellitus, thyroid disease, Addison disease, hypopituitarism
Psychiatric disorders: depression, obsessive-compulsive disorder, anxiety disorder, substance abuse
Chronic infections: tuberculosis, human immunodeficiency virus infection
Other: rheumatologic disorder, superior mesenteric artery syndrome, malignancy

Source: Adapted from Rosen DS. Identification and management of eating disorders in children and adolescents. *Pediatrics*. 2010;136(6):1240-1253.

DIAGNOSTIC EVALUATION

The diagnostic criteria for eating disorders are published in the DSM-5. In assessing an individual with a suspected eating disorder, the provider must first determine the patient's current weight, their previous weight gain trajectory, the history of weight loss (including peak weight and rate of loss), and how current weight compares with expected body weight.

There are several methods for determining how a patient's weight compares with expected body weight. One method is to examine pre-illness growth curves, and to restore patients to their previous growth trajectory. If patients were always underweight, or overweight, and the clinician feels they should therefore not return to their prior weight trajectory, or if growth records are unavailable, the 50th percentile body mass index (BMI) for age and gender published by the Centers for Disease Control and Prevention can be a helpful starting point. This BMI is then multiplied by the square of the current height to calculate a median body weight. However, this is a rough reference point, as body weight is very individualized and not everyone will need to achieve exactly the median BMI-for-age. In addition, if a patient has had significant linear growth stunting, it may be necessary to calculate a goal weight using the projected height that the patient should have achieved had she/he continued along a pre-eating disorder growth trajectory. Because of this, current guidelines recommend determining treatment goal weights by carefully incorporating patients' individual pre-illness growth and pubertal trajectories. In addition, goal weight criteria should only be used as guidelines when assessing severity of illness and whether or not the patient has reached a healthy weight. Several mental health and physical health criteria should be considered when trying to determine if the patient no longer has an eating disorder. These include return of menses and lack of disordered body image thoughts.

The evaluation of a patient with a suspected eating disorder includes a complete history and physical examination. Special attention should be paid to questions regarding dieting, body image, weight-control measures, and associated psychiatric conditions (**Table 40-3**). It is important to interview both the patient and their parents, as some adolescents with eating disorders can significantly under-report their symptoms. When speaking with parents, it is important to show empathy and emphasize that their child's illness did not occur because of something they did or did not do (i.e., "it's not your fault"). This approach can be very helpful for the parents as they often feel an enormous burden of guilt that their child became ill. Table 40-1 lists the potential physical findings in a patient with an eating disorder.

The diagnosis of an eating disorder is a clinical diagnosis; one cannot perform a confirmatory laboratory test. However, some laboratory and ancillary testing may be indicated in the evaluation of a patient with a suspected eating disorder (**Table 40-4**). While initial laboratory values are often in the normal range even in the presence of severe malnutrition, the purpose of such testing is to exclude other disease processes, detect complications of purging or vomiting, and monitor the effects of nutritional rehabilitation. For example, an erythrocyte sedimentation rate (ESR) or C-reactive protein (CRP) can be helpful in screening for chronic inflammatory diseases as the cause of weight loss. The ESR is characteristically low (usually <5 mm/hour) in patients with eating disorders. A higher value, even if within the normal range, should prompt a search for another diagnosis. Hyponatremia, which occurs if the patient is practicing water loading, is often accompanied by a low urine specific gravity. A patient who vomits frequently may have hypokalemia with elevated serum bicarbonate. A clue to laxative abuse may be a metabolic acidosis without an elevated anion gap. Electrocardiographic findings may include bradycardia or a prolonged QTc interval, even in the absence of abnormal serum electrolytes. Attention to the broad differential diagnosis (Table 40-2) of eating disorders and malnutrition should be considered throughout the diagnostic workup. For example, computed tomography or magnetic resonance imaging of the head to check for a brain tumor, or a gastrointestinal or endocrine workup to rule out inflammatory bowel, celiac, or thyroid disease, as well as occult diabetes, should be performed if clinical suspicion warrants.

TABLE 40-3 Screening Questions for Patients With Suspected Eating Disorders

What was the most you ever weighed and what was your age and height at the time?
What was the least you ever weighed (after reaching adolescence) and what was your age and height at the time?
What do you think you should weigh? What weight seems too high for comfort? What weight seems too low for comfort?
Which areas of your body cause you stress?
Is there anything you do to check your body regularly (such as weighing yourself, looking frequently in the mirror, or body pinching)?
What percent of the day do you spend thinking about food or your body?
Can you tell me what you ate over the last 24 hours?
Do you count carbohydrates, fats, or calories? Is there a limit for how much you allow?
Do you follow a special diet?
Do you ever feel out of control with your eating?
Do you ever feel fearful or guilty of eating? Would you describe yourself as a picky eater?
Are there foods you have cut out of your diet? If so, which foods?
Do you ever binge on food? If so, what foods do you binge on? How much do you eat? How often do you binge? What triggers you to binge?
Do you ever make yourself throw up to lose weight? If you vomit, how soon after eating?
Do you ever take diet pills, caffeine or laxatives, or diuretics with the intent of weight loss? If so, which types do you take and how much? How often do you take them?
Do you ever feel out of control with your eating?
How much do you exercise? What do you do for exercise? How long and intense is your exercise routine? Are you stressed if you miss a workout?
What is your past medical history?
Is there a family history of eating disorders, obesity, or mental illness? Does anyone in your family follow a special diet? Does anyone in your family struggle with substance abuse?
Does anyone in your family take any psychiatric medications?
For girls: When did you experience menarche? What is your menstrual history–menarche, regularity, date of last menstrual period?
Perform HEADSS Screening
Have you experienced any of the following (review of symptoms)?
Dizziness, syncope, weakness, or fatigue
Cold intolerance
Fevers
Vomiting, diarrhea, or constipation
Abdominal or epigastric pain, bloating or fullness
Hair loss, lanugo, or dry skin
Pallor, bleeding, or bruising
Chest pain or palpitations
Muscle cramps or joint pain
Menstrual irregularities
Excessive thirst and voiding

Source: Adapted from Hornberger LL, Lane MA, Hornberger LL, et al. Identification and management of eating disorders in children and adolescents. *Pediatrics*. 2021;147(1):e2020040279.

MANAGEMENT

The inpatient management of eating disorders requires a coordinated multidisciplinary team of individuals. The team ideally consists of a physician (hospitalist who is comfortable managing eating disorders and/or a sub-specialist specializing in eating disorders), a registered dietician, a psychiatrist and/or psychologist, and the family. Clearly defining the role of each team member can help optimize team functioning. Many inpatient facilities that treat patients with eating disorders use specific protocols. **Table 40-5** provides treatment guidelines for a patient with an eating disorder that warrants inpatient admission.

Inpatient treatment of patients with eating disorders often requires that the team address many different domains to ensure optimal treatment of the patient's physical and mental health needs. Initial management should ensure medical stabilization, which includes fluid management,

TABLE 40-4 Laboratory Evaluation in Patients With Eating Disorders

Complete blood cell count
Erythrocyte sedimentation rate and potentially CRP
Serum electrolytes with glucose
Blood urea nitrogen and creatinine
Serum calcium, magnesium, phosphorus concentrations
Liver function tests: transaminases, albumin, prealbumin
Urinalysis with specific gravity
Amylase and lipase
Pre-albumin
Fasting lipid panel: cholesterol, triglycerides, high density lipoprotein, and low-density lipoprotein
Celiac panel: IgA tissue transglutaminase and anti-endomysial antibodies
Thyroid function tests: TSH, free T4
Females: pregnancy testing, prolactin, luteinizing hormone, and follicle stimulating hormone, estradiol
Males: testosterone, prolactin, luteinizing hormone, and follicle stimulating hormone
Iron panel and ferritin
Other nutrition studies as needed: vitamin D, vitamin B_1, zinc, vitamin B_{12}
Other labs as indicated: PPD (purified protein derivative test for tuberculosis), HIV (human immunodeficiency virus antibody testing), morning cortisol, stool for occult blood, lactic dehydrogenase, uric acid
ECG with follow-up ECHO as needed
DXA and bone age (can be done in the outpatient setting)

electrolyte replacement, cardiac and vital sign stabilization, and nutritional supplementation (orally or via nasogastric tube feeding). The main goal for inpatient management is to stop or reverse any medical complications (discussed in more detail below) and demonstrate weight gain, often in the range of 1 to 2 kg per week (or 150-300 g per day). Current and pre-morbid growth curves should be reviewed to determine a treatment goal weight. While patients will not remain in the inpatient setting to reach this goal weight, parents should be informed that for females this weight should support restoration of normal menstrual cycles. For males, this weight should restore normal testicular function.

Historically, nutritional supplementation was started "low and slow" (e.g., 1000-1200 kcals/day). However, more recent data shows that refeeding can be initiated more aggressively at 1600 to 2000 kcals/day. With close electrolyte monitoring and replacement as needed, refeeding syndrome can be avoided and length of stay reduced. Caloric intake can be increased by 200 to 400 calories/day until steady weight gain is achieved. Ultimately, patients with anorexia nervosa may require 3000 to 4000 kcals/day to meet their metabolic needs and achieve their goal weight. A dietitian should be involved in care to help create a structured meal plan that includes adequate sources of fat, protein, and carbohydrates, as well as vitamins and minerals. If patients refuse to eat by mouth, nasogastric (NG) tube feeds can be used. While some may view the use of an NG tube as punitive, others view it as a means to reduce the physical and psychological pain of refeeding. Presenting this intervention in an empathic way to the patient and family may increase acceptability. Ideally, bolus feeds would be used to mimic normal eating patterns and gastric functioning. Total parenteral nutrition and surgical placement of gastrostomy or jejunostomy tubes should be avoided because of the increased risk of dependence on non-oral methods of eating and unnecessary medical complications (e.g., hepatic injury, line infections).

Intravenous fluids are typically not required unless the patient demonstrates considerable dehydration or cardiac/orthostatic instability. Depending on the severity of the patient's dehydration, fluid boluses may be used. However, the degree of malnutrition and protein depletion should be considered and limiting fluid bolus volume to 10 mL/kg may be necessary to decrease the risk of edema, fluid overload, and congestive heart failure. Intravenous glucose should also be used judiciously in maintenance fluids because of the risk of rapid insulin surges triggered by the influx of glucose, which can then initiate serious electrolyte shifts and worsen the risk of refeeding syndrome. While enteral feeding and rehydration is safer and always preferred, some patients may not tolerate this method and may require IV supplementation of fluids at a low rate to ensure that they do not get fluid overloaded.

Cardiac monitoring should be implemented for all patients when admitted to the hospital. Patients who are severely malnourished often display signs of bradycardia, especially at night. They may also have cardiac arrhythmias, prolonged QTc, or pericardial effusions. Severe bradycardia (<40 bpm) while sleeping may require additional nutrition or fluids overnight to maintain cardiac status. Over time, heart rates and abnormal cardiac rhythms typically improve with nutrition as cardiac muscle is rebuilt. Restoration of normal protein levels in the body will also assist with resolution of any pericardial effusions.

Gastrointestinal dysmotility or delayed gastric emptying often occurs with severe malnutrition or purging behaviors. Nutritional rehabilitation will often resolve any physical issues that may exist. However, in the short-term, pro-motility agents (e.g., metoclopramide) may be useful. Unfortunately, feelings of bloating and abdominal pain may not be relieved and may reflect the dysregulation in brain reward systems of patients with eating disorders and their increased sensitivity to normal gastrointestinal function. Constipation can be addressed using osmotic agents, stool softeners, or laxatives. Stimulant laxatives, suppositories, or enemas may be required in more severe cases but should only be used after careful consideration of the patient's history of laxative abuse.

TABLE 40-5 Suggested Guidelines for Inpatient Treatment of Eating Disorders

Nursing staff is essential. Their approach should be firm yet supportive, and there should be no bargaining with the patient.
Nutrition is restored through food trays planned by a nutritionist, and the patient is expected to finish each meal.
Calories are provided through three meals and snacks over the course of the day. In general, start at 1600-2000 calories/day and increase by 200-400 calories/day until the goal calorie level is achieved.
All meals are supervised; typically, supervision is initially provided by a staff member and then switches to a parent or adult caregiver. Family members are allowed in the room during mealtimes and normalizing mealtime interactions and conversations should be encouraged.
The medical team monitors electrolytes and fluid shifts, cardiac status, and other potential medical complications, with special attention to electrolytes including phosphorus over the first week when the risk of refeeding syndrome is highest.
The patient must rest for 1 hour after each meal; observation is maintained during this time.
The patient is allowed 30 minutes to finish each meal. If the patient is unable to do so, a nutritional supplement may be used to attain the allotted calories. If patient is unable to comply with the nutritional supplement, a nasogastric tube is inserted, the nutritional supplement is provided by that means, and the tube is removed.
The patient is weighed daily in a hospital gown, and a urine specific gravity is obtained around that time.
During the initial phase of hospitalization, the patient should be closely monitored to avoid excess exercise or purging.
A mental health professional is involved in the initial assessment to screen for comorbid psychiatric diagnoses and to provide ongoing care. Cognition is often limited in cases of severe malnutrition, and therapy may not begin until the patient's nutritional status improves.
Hospitalization should continue long enough for the patient to stop losing weight, establish a weight-gain trend, normalize vital signs and laboratory studies, and be able to eat adequately with a caregiver present.
Social workers and case managers should be available to help arrange for care outside the hospital, whether in an inpatient eating disorder facility, a partial hospitalization program, or outpatient treatment with adequate mental health, nutrition, and medical follow-up.

Source: Data from Rome ES, Ammerman S, Rosen DS, et al. Children and adolescents with eating disorders: the state of the art. *Pediatrics*. 2003;111:e98-e108.

To optimize bone health, vitamin D and calcium can be started during the refeeding process. Weight restoration and return of normal gonadal functioning is ultimately what is needed to prevent chronic bone disease. However, during the refeeding process, many often question whether sex hormone replacement or anti-resorptive agents can be used to prevent severe osteoporosis. Oral contraceptive pills or estrogen supplementation are not routinely recommended to improve bone mineral density, particularly among younger teens. While a few small trials have shown some effect, inducing cyclic vaginal bleeding may actually reinforce the patient's belief that they are not ill and that they can continue their restrictive or maladaptive eating behaviors without serious physiologic consequences. However, estrogen supplementation may be warranted in young adults with severe and enduring anorexia nervosa who have not been able to maintain proper nutritional intake; in this situation, it may be worth protecting against the chronic effects of malnutrition on bone density and suppression of the hypothalamic-pituitary-gonadal axis. Bisphosphonates are not generally recommended because of the lack of long-term studies on efficacy and safety in patients with eating disorders.

If the patient also displays suicidal ideation, aggressive behaviors, or impaired safety, inpatient psychiatric treatment may be required (concurrently or as soon as the patient is medically stable).

Even though many inpatient units are not able to provide intensive psychological therapy during hospitalization, it is important to know that the tenets of many of these therapies can begin during the acute hospitalization. Currently the most evidence-based treatment is family-based treatment, where a parent or caregiver is typically enlisted to oversee the refeeding process until the patient is able to participate in making appropriate nutrition-related decisions. By the time a patient is admitted to the hospital though, parents usually have not been able to feed their child adequately at home, and the inpatient team will need to act as overseer of nutritional rehabilitation, medical management of eating disorders, and facilitator of psychological treatment. Parents should be reminded that they are still the expert in their child's needs and knowledge of their child's preferences, and should not be blamed for the failure of refeeding in the outpatient setting. Parents can be allowed to participate in refeeding again during the inpatient stay when the patient is more medically stable. Shared decision-making with the patient around nutrition can occur when the patient transitions to the outpatient setting. Cognitive behavioral therapy and dialectical behavioral therapy show promise as well for some patients, typically older patients or patients where the family dynamic (because of abuse or divorce) does not support the use of family-based treatment.

MEDICAL COMPLICATIONS

Eating disorders can affect all organ systems, causing multiple serious complications, such as low bone density, cardiac arrhythmias, and liver damage (**Table 40-6**). Common complications for pediatrics hospitalists to be familiar with are detailed below.

CARDIAC COMPLICATIONS

Both malnutrition and the electrolyte abnormalities from food restriction and purging can lead to cardiac complications. Starvation can lead to blood pressure changes such as orthostasis, arrhythmias, decreased cardiac muscle and cardiac dysfunction, and pericardial effusions. Many of the cardiac vital sign changes occur due to increased vagal tone and decreased basal metabolic rate which result from reduced energy consumption and/or volume depletion. A prolonged QTc interval can be a harbinger of cardiac arrhythmias, and a baseline electrocardiogram should be considered in all patients admitted for malnutrition. One-third of patients with anorexia have mitral valve prolapse secondary to cardiac muscle wasting. Low amplitude forces (R and T waves in the electrocardiogram that are smaller in amplitude than expected) in the left ventricle are also more common in anorexia than the other eating disorders and is suggestive of cardiac muscle wasting secondary to malnutrition or pericardial effusion. Up to 35% of adolescents with anorexia have some degree of pericardial effusion, presumably from protein depletion, that often improves with refeeding. While patients may not complain of chest pain, muffled heart sounds should raise one's suspicion of an effusion.

TABLE 40-6 Medical Complications of Eating Disorders

Malnutrition-related effects
Amenorrhea
Arrested growth
Atrophic vaginitis
Breast atrophy
Cardiac muscle wasting
Constipation
Cortical atrophy
Decreased antidiuretic hormone secretion
Delayed puberty
Hypercholesterolemia
Hypercortisolemia
Hypophosphatemia
Hypokalemia, Hypomagnesemia, Hyponatremia, Hypoglycemia
Infertility
Osteopenia
Pancytopenia
Peripheral neuropathy
Vital sign abnormalities
Bradycardia: pulse <50 beats/min daytime or <45 beats/min overnight
Hypotension: systolic blood pressure <90 mm Hg or diastolic blood pressure <45 mm Hg
Orthostatic blood pressure
Hypothermia: temperature <36.3°C (<96.8°F)
Purging-related effects
Cardiac arrhythmias
Chronic hypovolemia
Dental enamel erosion
Electrolyte abnormalities
Esophagitis
Mallory-Weiss tears
Parotid gland swelling
Pneumothorax or pneumomediastinum
Pseudo-Bartter syndrome
Renal calculi
Russell sign (callused knuckles from using fingers to induce vomiting)
Vital sign abnormalities
Bingeing-related effects
Esophageal rupture
Gastric rupture

Source: Adapted from Rome ES, Ammerman S. Medical complications of eating disorders: an update. *J Adolesc Health*. 2003;33:418-426; and Becker AD, Grinspoon SK, Klibanksi A, Herzog DB. Eating disorders. *N Engl J Med*. 1999;340:1092-1098.

An echocardiogram may be warranted in patients with evidence of low amplitude forces, other abnormal ECG findings (e.g., inverted T waves, left ventricular hypertrophy, left axis deviation suggesting prolapsed valves, or regurgitation), and/or persistent hypotension despite adequate nutrition.

REFEEDING SYNDROME

When a malnourished patient is provided with sufficient energy intake, the body shifts from the catabolic state of starvation to an anabolic state. It is during this time that the patient is at risk for refeeding syndrome, characterized by fluid and electrolyte shifts, delirium, cardiovascular collapse, difficulty breathing, and possible death. The hallmark of refeeding syndrome is hypophosphatemia and resultant organ system failure. Prolonged starvation results in a decreased level of total body phosphorus. When calories, particularly in the form of glucose, are added to the patient's diet, there is a shift of extracellular phosphate to intracellular sites for incorporation into cell products and adenosine triphosphate (ATP). This may result in dangerously decreased extracellular phosphorus stores, which can lead to cardio-pulmonary collapse. Adolescents at greatest risk for refeeding syndrome are those that are severely malnourished (<65-70% of ideal body weight). The risk of refeeding syndrome is increased at the beginning of weight restoration, usually in the first 3 to 7 days of treatment.

Serum electrolytes, including phosphorus, potassium, and magnesium should be monitored at least daily during the first 7 to 10 days of refeeding. Twice-daily monitoring should be considered for extremely severe cases of malnutrition (patients who are <65%-70% of their ideal body weight). Oral phosphorus supplementation can be initiated during the first week of refeeding to help prevent complications or initiated when phosphorus is noted to be decreasing during laboratory monitoring. Supplementation with potassium and magnesium should also be initiated if declining. Thiamine supplementation has been found to be protective for the development of delirium in severely malnourished patients at high risk of refeeding syndrome. In such high-risk patients, some centers advocate using nasogastric feeds for the first week with a reduced carbohydrate containing formula. However, the majority of patients will do well with a balanced oral diet that is advanced daily as tolerated.

PSYCHIATRIC CONSIDERATIONS

Patients with eating disorders typically become very distressed during the refeeding process. They are often ambivalent about treatment and do not recognize the severity of their malnutrition and weight loss. This lack of awareness is part of the disorder, and these emotional responses to treatment are to be expected. At times, patients can become significantly emotionally dysregulated and may require medications or other behavioral limits to contain their agitation. Patients will often begin to negotiate with the treatment team to reduce caloric intake and the rate of weight gain, stating that they are in pain or too full. Weight gain may also trigger body image issues that add to the psychological distress of the patient, resulting in increased depression and/or anxiety. It may be tempting to "rescue" patients from their distress by reducing caloric intake and slowing down treatment; however, this typically lengthens the inpatient stay and backfires psychologically. By reducing the calorie level of the meals, patients' anxiety around eating decreases and the team will have inadvertently reinforced the eating disorder. Patients then do not learn how to manage feelings of distress and fear of weight gain. In these situations, the healthcare team should supportively manage the patient's pain and/or distress while maintaining firm expectations for continued caloric intake and weight gain. These actions help to model maintenance of firm boundaries for families and further teach adolescents to build distress tolerance and manage uncomfortable emotions and fears. Behavioral health consultation is important in treatment to help guide the adolescent through the psychological difficulties associated with refeeding and to detect and manage other mental health comorbidities.

Psychiatric medications may be warranted in the treatment of eating disorders, although there are few well-designed RCTs to help inform this practice. SSRIs may help decrease the number of binge and purge episodes in youth with bulimia nervosa. However, SSRIs do not appear to be effective in severely malnourished patients with anorexia nervosa. Atypical antipsychotics such as olanzapine and aripiprazole may have more promise, but most studies include small numbers of patients. These medications, which target dopamine D2 receptors, may be useful in decreasing fear and anxiety around eating and assisting with weight gain. Benzodiazepines may also be useful in the short-term, but the risk of misuse over time limits long-term use. Medications for the treatment of co-morbid depression, anxiety, or OCD should be considered, but may not be effective until patients gain more weight. Consultation with a psychiatrist should be made before initiating any of these therapies.

ADMISSION CRITERIA

Medical hospitalization of an adolescent with an eating disorder is occasionally necessary to stabilize vital signs or cardiac abnormalities, correct electrolyte abnormalities, rehydrate and carefully initiate refeeding, or complete a diagnostic workup. Inpatient admission may also be required if the patient continues to lose weight and fails outpatient management. The goal of admission is stabilization of the patient's acute medical, nutritional, or psychiatric needs. **Table 40-7** details indications for inpatient admission.

TABLE 40-7 Indications for Inpatient Medical Stabilization

Indications
Severe malnutrition: body weight <75% of median ideal body weight for age and sex
Significant hypovolemia or hypotension (BP < 90/45)
Orthostasis by blood pressure (decrease of > 20 mm Hg systolic or >10 mm Hg diastolic) or heart rate (change > 20-40 bpm)
Bradycardia (heart rate < 50 beats/min)
Cardiac dysfunction or arrhythmia (e.g., prolonged QTc interval)
Significant laboratory abnormalities: Hypokalemia, Hypomagnesemia, Hypophosphatemia, Hyponatremia
Blood glucose < 60 mg/dL
Hypothermia (<36°C, (<96.8°F)
Intractable multiple bingeing or purging episodes per day
Failure of outpatient management (e.g., no weight gain, continued weight loss, no reduction in bingeing or purging episodes)
Suicidal thoughts or gestures
Acute food refusal resulting in >2-3 lb. weight loss in a week
>10% weight loss in 6 months or >20% weight loss in 1 year
Acute medical complications of malnutrition (e.g., seizures, syncope, SMA syndrome, pancreatitis, hepatitis, severe anemia, hematemesis)

Source: Adapted from Campbell K, Peebles R. Eating disorders in children and adolescents: state of the art review. *Pediatrics*. 2014;134:582-592.

DISCHARGE CRITERIA

Most guidelines recommend that patients remain in the hospital until (i) their vital signs and electrolytes have fully stabilized, (ii) they are ingesting enough food by mouth without vomiting to demonstrate weight gain, and (iii) they meet a minimal weight criterion (usually at least 75% of ideal body weight) to transition to an intensive outpatient treatment program. These discharge goals are meant to maximize the chance of success after discharge in an outpatient program but may take weeks to achieve. Early recognition of an eating disorder and aggressive weight restoration has been associated with improved eating disorder cognitions (i.e., patient no longer endorses body image concerns) and favorable long-term health outcomes, even in patients who were severely malnourished and cognitively impaired on admission. When a patient with an eating disorder is discharged from an acute care hospital, it is essential to address their ongoing medical, nutritional, and mental health needs. If available, the standard of care for children and adolescents would involve initiating intensive outpatient treatment either at a residential treatment program that specializes in eating disorders, a partial hospitalization program, or an intensive outpatient program. Partial hospitalization programs include ~10 hours of psychiatric treatment and nutritional monitoring per day, 5 to 6 days per week. Intensive outpatient programs offer ~3 to 6 hours of similar multidisciplinary treatment 5 days per week. Parents should be involved in decisions regarding outpatient therapy plans and discussions should be initiated early in the inpatient stay to ensure minimal gaps in care. Unfortunately, many areas of the United States do not have programs or providers trained to deliver this type of treatment. If these options are not available, family-based treatment at home with a qualified team should be implemented. This team should include a pediatrician or other primary care physician for weekly medical monitoring (i.e., weight and vital signs), a dietitian for monthly nutritional monitoring, and a mental health team including psychology and psychiatry to provide therapy and psychiatric medications as needed. If safety concerns necessitate further inpatient psychiatric care, transfer to an inpatient psychiatric program or unit should be facilitated.

CONSULTATION

When an eating disorder is suspected, consultation with experienced mental health professionals is indicated to help guide behavioral support. Nutrition consultation is critical to inpatient refeeding and treatment. Psychiatric consultation is often useful to initiate medication management for co-occurring depression and/or anxiety. Finally, social work consultation is helpful in disposition planning. Other subspecialty consultation is indicated if other illnesses are suspected as part of the differential diagnosis or if complications of certain organ systems are severe and require additional expertise (e.g., superior mesenteric artery syndrome, significant liver enzyme elevation). While patients typically present with bradycardia or hypotension, routine cardiology consultation is not generally indicated and is only necessary if vital sign abnormalities are profound or if there are additional concerns such as arrhythmias or pericardial effusion.

KEY POINTS

- Eating disorders are common and carry the highest risk of mortality of all the psychiatric diagnoses.
- Common eating disorders are anorexia nervosa, bulimia nervosa, binge-eating disorders, avoidant-restrictive food intake disorder, and Other Specified Feeding or Eating Disorder.
- The role of the inpatient team is to stabilize the patient and establish medical, nutritional, and mental health support for continued treatment during hospitalization and in preparation for discharge.
- Although there are many complications related to eating disorders, cardiac dysfunction and refeeding syndrome are the major considerations in the acute inpatient setting.

SUGGESTED READINGS

Chamay-Weber C, Narring F, Michaud PA. Partial eating disorders among adolescents: a review. *J Adolesc Health*. 2005;37(5):417-427.

Friedli N, Stanga Z, Sobotka L, et al. Revisiting the refeeding syndrome: results of a systematic review. *Nutrition*. 2017;35:151-160.

Garber AK, Cheng J, Accurso EC, et al. Short-term outcomes of the study of refeeding to optimize inpatient gains for patients with anorexia nervosa: a multicenter randomized clinical trial. *JAMA Pediatr*. 2021;175(1):19-27.

Garber AK, et al. A systematic review of approaches to refeeding in patients with anorexia nervosa. *Int J Eat Disord*. 2016;49(3):293-310.

Golden NH, et al. Position paper of the society for adolescent health and medicine: medical management of restrictive eating disorders in adolescents and young adults. *J Adolesc Health*. 2015;56(1):121-125.

Hudson LD, Court AJ. What paediatricians should know about eating disorders in children and young people. *J Paediatr Child Health*. 2012;48(10):869-875.

Klein DA, Walsh BT. Eating disorders: clinical features and pathophysiology. *Physiol Behav*. 2004;81(2):359-374.

Le Grange D, et al. Eating disorder not otherwise specified presentation in the US population. *Int J Eat Disord*. 2012;45(5):711-718.

Madden S, Miskovic-Wheatley J, Wallis A, Kohn M, Hay P, Touyz S. Early weight gain in family-based treatment predicts greater weight gain and remission at the end of treatment and remission at 12-month follow-up in adolescent anorexia nervosa. *Int J Eat Disord*. 2015;48(7):919-922.

Marikar D, Reynolds S, Moghraby OS. Junior MARSIPAN (Management of Really Sick Patients with Anorexia Nervosa). *Arch Dis Child Educ Pract Ed*. 2016;101(3):140-143.

Peebles R, Collins Lyster-Mensh L, Kreipe RE. Eating Disorders. In: Ginsburg KR and Kinsman SB, ed. *Reaching Teens: Strength-Based Communication Strategies to Build Resilience and Support Healthy Adolescent Development*. Elks Grove Village IL: American Academy of Pediatrics; 2013.

Rome ES, et al. Children and adolescents with eating disorders: the state of the art. *Pediatrics*. 2003;111(1):e98-e108.

Rosen DS. Eating disorders in children and young adolescents: etiology, classification, clinical features, and treatment. *Adolesc Med*. 2003;14(1):49-59.

Rosen DS. Identification and management of eating disorders in children and adolescents. *Pediatrics*. 2010;126(6):1240-1253.

Weaver L, Sit L, Liebman R. Treatment of anorexia nervosa in children and adolescents. *Curr Psychiatry Rep*. 2012;14(2):96-100.

CHAPTER 41 Sexually Transmitted Infections in Adolescents and Young Adults

Abbey Masonbrink, MD, MPH

BACKGROUND

Each year, approximately 20 million new cases of sexually transmitted infections (STIs) are diagnosed. Adolescents and young adults (hereafter referred to as adolescents; 15-24-year-olds) comprise only one quarter of the sexually active population, yet account for almost half of all STI cases. The Centers for Disease Control and Prevention (CDC) surveillance data reveal that STI incidence in adolescents has increased in the past decade. Further, while STI testing in 2020 to 2021 decreased compared to prior years, recent studies show an increase in positivity of STI tests in adolescents, thus raising concerns of increasing prevalence of STIs in this population during the COVID-19 pandemic.

Several behavioral and psychosocial factors independently influence the disproportionately high rates of STIs in adolescents. Behavioral factors include early age of sexual activity debut, higher number of lifetime sexual partners, multiple concurrent partners, condomless sex, anal sex, or substance use. In addition, some sub-groups of adolescents may have increased risk for STIs including adolescents with mental health disorders, adolescents living in detention facilities, adolescents involved in commercial sexual exploitation, and adolescents who exchange sex for drugs, money, food, or housing, as well as transgender adolescents, young males who have sex with males, young females who have sex with females, and adolescents who have sex with both females and males. Disparities in STIs by sex, race, and ethnicity are also seen in the adolescent population with higher rates in women and racial and ethnic minorities. The difference across sex is likely attributable to increased screening of females, as well as to the often-asymptomatic presentation of infection in males. Disparities across race and ethnicity are not fully understood but are likely attributable to institutionalized racism, including differences in healthcare access.

The long-term sequelae and complications of STIs in adolescents include pelvic inflammatory disease, infertility, ectopic pregnancy, and chronic pelvic pain, in addition to mental health issues associated with shame, stigma, discrimination, and stress that may result from these diagnoses. Adolescents commonly encounter barriers to accessing preventive services for STIs, due to lack of health insurance, inability to pay, confidentiality concerns, and discomfort with adult-designed healthcare services. It is important that healthcare providers in all clinical settings, including the pediatric hospitalist, understand the epidemiology of STIs, common signs and symptoms, how to obtain a confidential sexual history, evidence-based guidelines for prevention, testing, and treatment including indications for hospitalization.

PATHOPHYSIOLOGY

While behavioral and psychosocial factors are contributors to the high prevalence of STIs in adolescents there is also a biologic basis for the increased burden. Differences in anatomy, immunology, and the role of co-infections all contribute to the high STI burden in this age group.

Changes in the cervical epithelium make young women increasingly susceptible to STIs. During puberty, the cervical columnar epithelium undergoes squamous metaplasia, during which a transformation zone is formed in the junction between the endocervical columnar and ectocervical squamous cells. As a result, columnar cells, which are more vulnerable to infection with bacteria such as *Chlamydia trachomatis* and *Neisseria gonorrhoeae,* are present in greater numbers on the exposed ectocervix. In addition, the area of higher cell turnover in the transformation zone is a prime host for viruses such as HPV. Comparatively, the ectocervix of the adult cervix is predominately composed of squamous cells, which are less susceptible to infection.

Having an STI also places adolescents at increased risk for subsequent and concurrent infections. Disruptions in the skin and mucous membranes as a result of STIs (e.g., genital ulcers) serve as entry points for additional pathogens. The inflammatory state of the infected cells also renders them easier targets for bacteria and viruses. For example, the presence of a concurrent STI makes an individual two to five times more likely to acquire and transmit HIV through unprotected sex. Treatment of STIs decreases the risk of HIV acquisition. The role of STIs in HIV transmission underscores the importance of early detection and treatment of STIs in adolescents (HIV is discussed in detail in Chapter 104).

CLINICAL PRESENTATION

Although most STIs in adolescents are asymptomatic, there are specific clinical syndromes worth noting. **Table 41-1** details differential diagnoses to consider in the context of specific clinical presentations or diagnoses.

LOWER GENITOURINARY TRACT INFECTION

Vaginitis Vaginitis typically presents with vaginal odor, discharge, vulvar irritation, and/or pruritis. *Trichomonas vaginalis* is the most common sexually transmitted cause of vaginitis. This protozoa classically causes a frothy yellow-green discharge, foul odor, and cervical petechiae (i.e., "strawberry cervix"). While *Neisseria gonorrhoeae* and *C. trachomatis* may cause vaginitis in prepubescent females, these organisms are more commonly associated with cervicitis in post-menarchal females.

Urethritis Pain and burning with urination, with or without urethral discharge, are the cardinal features of urethritis. As with cervicitis, *N. gonorrhoeae* and *C. trachomatis* are the primary causative organisms. Other less common causes of urethritis include *T. vaginalis,* herpes simplex virus, *Mycoplasma genitalium, Ureaplasma urealyticum,* and *Mycoplasma hominis.* Enteric organisms may also lead to urethritis via insertive anal sex.

Epididymitis Ascending infection from the urethra in males can lead to epididymitis, which typically presents as unilateral testicular pain, swelling, tenderness, and palpable swelling of the epididymis. There may be accompanying hydrocele. Symptoms of urethritis often accompany or precede epididymitis. The causative organisms of epididymitis are typically the same as urethritis.

Genital Ulceration A number of sexually transmitted pathogens can cause anogenital ulcerative lesions, with or without inguinal adenopathy. In the United States, herpes simplex virus (HSV) is the predominant pathogen. Primary HSV infection often presents with systemic symptoms including fever, myalgias, headache, and malaise. The lesions of HSV are classically painful, shallow, multiple, and associated with lymphadenopathy that may be bilateral (**Figure 41-1**). However, symptoms may be minimal or absent, especially with recurrent episodes. Primary HSV infection often presents with systemic symptoms including fever, myalgias, headache, and malaise. Recurrent episodes tend to have a milder presentation. Severe HSV outbreaks may also disseminate, leading to hepatitis, pneumonitis, or meningoencephalitis.

The chancre of primary syphilis is typically a solitary, painless, deep, and indurated ulcer (**Figure 41-2**). Other important ulcer-forming infections include chancroid (*Hemophilus ducreyi*), lymphogranuloma venereum (LGV), and granuloma inguinale *(Klebsiella granulomatis).* Chancroid may present with single or multiple papules evolving into painful genital ulcers with ipsilateral tender adenopathy. LGV is an invasive lymphatic disease caused by *C. trachomatis* serovars L1-L3. It is characterized by an initial ulcerative genital lesion with subsequent tender, unilateral, suppurative inguinal or femoral lymphadenopathy. Granuloma inguinale, a rare entity in the United States, is characterized by progressive beefy, red, painless ulcerative genital or perineal lesions without lymphadenopathy.

TABLE 41-1 Differential Diagnosis

Careful history-taking and physical examination can help distinguish STIs from other common illnesses with similar symptomatology.

Clinical Symptoms or Diagnosis	Diagnostic Considerations
Vaginitis	Consider candidiasis, bacterial vaginosis, foreign body, or irritant vaginitis from bubble baths, soaps, or detergents.
Urethritis	While it may be difficult to distinguish urethritis from urinary tract infection (UTI) on clinical presentation alone, hematuria, fever, and urgency are less common in urethritis.
Testicular Pain	It is crucial to distinguish epididymitis from testicular torsion, which is a true surgical emergency. A positive Prehn sign (relief of pain with elevation of the affected testis), normal testicular position, and present cremasteric reflex all suggest epididymitis instead of torsion. However, imaging with Doppler ultrasound to rule out torsion is always warranted when the diagnosis is uncertain, in order to preserve the testicle in cases of torsion.
Genital Ulceration	Ulcerative disease of the anogenital region and mucous membranes can also be caused by EBV, Behçet's disease, Crohn's disease, drug eruption, and varicella zoster virus.
Anorectal Disease	Anorectal pain, bleeding, discharge, or diarrhea can also be caused by inflammatory bowel disease or gastroenteritis.
Pelvic Inflammatory Disease (PID)	PID has a broad differential diagnosis including gastrointestinal (e.g., appendicitis, enteritis, cholecystitis, mesenteric lymphadenitis, inflammatory bowel disease, constipation), gynecologic (e.g., ectopic pregnancy, ruptured ovarian cyst, ovarian torsion, endometriosis), and urinary causes (e.g., pyelonephritis, UTI, urinary calculus).
Pharyngitis	Nongonococcal causes of exudative pharyngitis include group A streptococcus, adenovirus, Epstein-Barr virus, and cytomegalovirus.
Disseminated Disease	Disseminated gonococcal infections and syphilis may be confused with a host of other disorders. The differential diagnosis for disseminated gonococcal infection includes hematogenously seeded infections from other bacteria, as well as autoimmune diseases including lupus, vasculitis, and juvenile rheumatoid arthritis. Primary syphilis is a consideration in all patients with ulcerative genital lesions. The rash of secondary syphilis may resemble pityriasis rosea, drug eruptions, viral exanthems (e.g., hand-foot-and-mouth disease secondary to coxsackievirus), and many other papulosquamous cutaneous disorders. Condyloma latum may be confused with condyloma acuminatum, and the mucous patches of syphilis may resemble thrush. Tertiary syphilis is a consideration in a wide range of cardiovascular, cerebrovascular, encephalopathic, and progressive spinal cord processes.

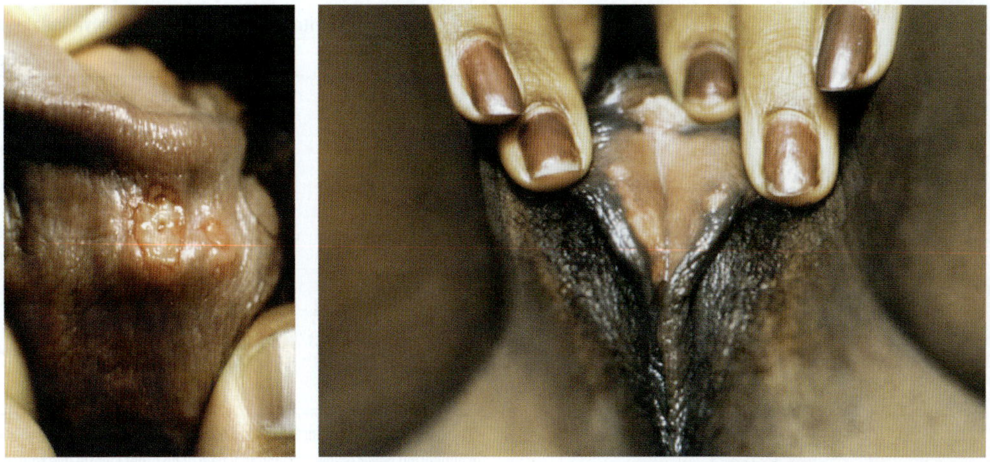

A B

FIGURE 41-1. Genital HSV. (Used with permission from CDC/ Susan Lindsley, Centers for Disease Control and Prevention.)

Genital Warts Anogenital warts (i.e., condylomata acuminata) are skin-colored flat, papillary, or pedunculated lesions with a cauliflower- or frond-like appearance (**Figure 41-3**). They can appear throughout the anogenital region. Condyloma acuminata are caused by the *Human papilloma* virus (HPV), with 90% caused by the non-oncogenic types 6 or 11. While these lesions are typically asymptomatic, they may cause itching, burning, or bleed easily when irritated.

Condyloma latum are a highly infectious, characteristic lesion of secondary syphilis. These gray-white, coalescent plaques of wart-like lesions are typically painless and occur in intertriginous areas **(Figure 41-4).**

ANORECTAL INFECTION

Patients who engage in receptive anal intercourse may present with anorectal infection.

Proctitis Proctitis is inflammation limited to the rectum. Manifestations include anorectal pain, bleeding, and/or discharge, with accompanying tenesmus. It is commonly caused by *N. gonorrhoeae*, *C. trachomatis*, *Treponema pallidum*, and HSV.

Proctocolitis Proctocolitis is inflammation of the colonic mucosa, extending to 12 cm above the anus; proctocolitis has the additional symptoms of diarrhea and bloating. In addition to the organisms that cause proctitis, *Campylobacter* species, *Shigella* species, and *Entamoeba histolytica* may cause proctocolitis. LGV can be a cause of hemorrhagic proctocolitis and may lead to anal fistulas and stricture mimicking inflammatory bowel disease.

Enteritis Enteritis manifests as abdominal cramping and diarrhea without evidence of proctitis or proctocolitis. It is often caused by *Giardia lamblia* in patients who engage in oral-anal sexual practices.

UPPER GENITOURINARY TRACT INFECTION

Cervicitis Cervicitis is characterized by purulent or mucopurulent cervical exudates and cervical friability which may manifest as vaginal bleeding, particularly postcoitally and pelvic discomfort. The most common causes of cervicitis in adolescent females are *N. gonorrhoeae* and *C. trachomatis*.

Pelvic Inflammatory Disease Pelvic inflammatory disease (PID), infection of the upper genital tract in females, is an important cause of

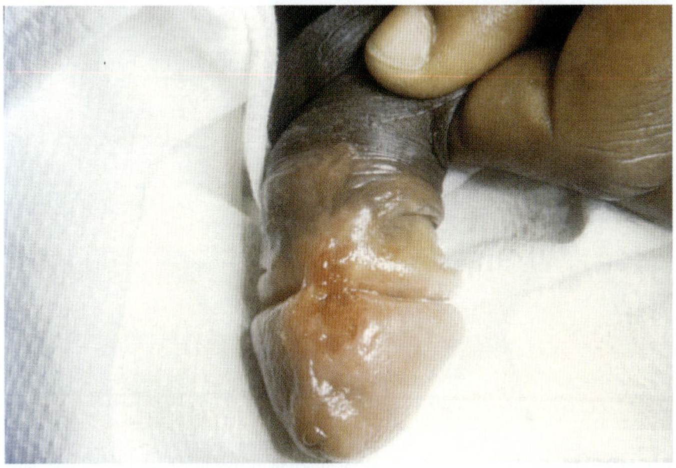

FIGURE 41-2. Chancre of primary syphilis. (Used with permission from Centers for Disease Control and Prevention.)

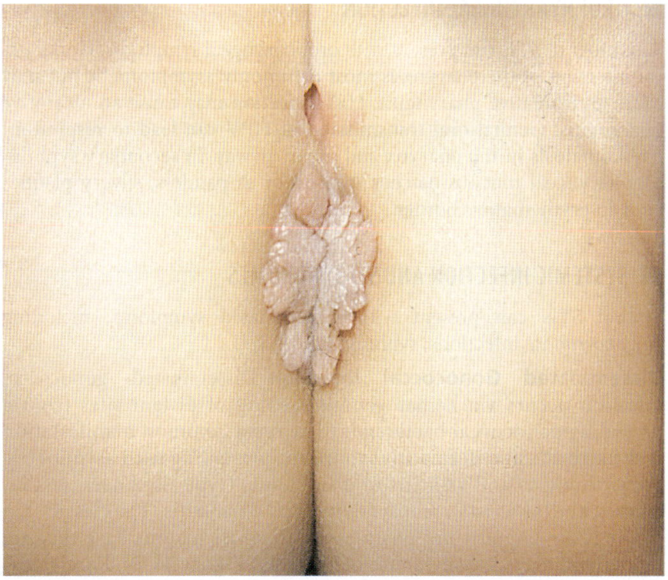

FIGURE 41-3. Condylomata acuminata. (Reproduced with permission from Prose NS, Kristal L. *Weinberg's Color Atlas of Pediatric Dermatology*. 5th ed. New York, NY: McGraw Hill; 2017, Figure 5-28.)

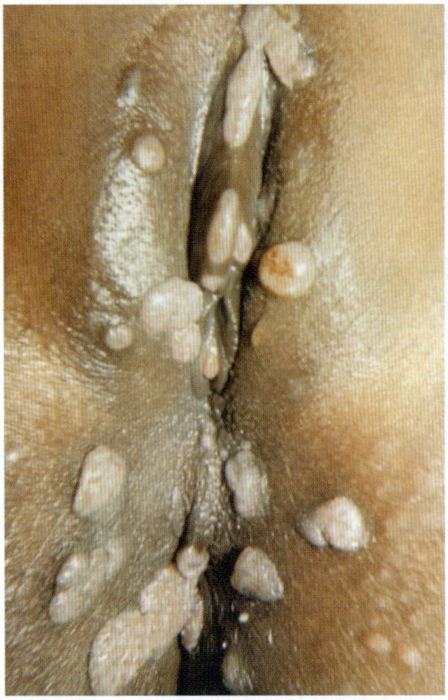

FIGURE 41-4. Conyloma lata. (Used with permission from CDC/ Joyce Ayers, Centers for Disease Control and Prevention.)

TABLE 41-2 Criteria for the Diagnosis of Pelvic Inflammatory Disease (PID)

Minimal Criteria*	Additional Criteria⁺	Definitive Criteria
Lower abdominal tenderness *and* No other identifiable source *and* ≥1 of the following: • Uterine tenderness • Adnexal tenderness • Cervical motion tenderness	Those listed under "Minimal" **plus** ≥1 of the following: • Fever (>38.3°C) • Presence of abundant WBCs on vaginal fluid microscopy • Abnormal vaginal or cervical discharge • Elevated ESR or CRP • Laboratory evidence of *Chlamydia trachomatis* or *Neisseria gonorrhoeae* cervicitis	Histopathologic evidence of endometritis on endometrial biopsy Transvaginal ultrasound or MRI that demonstrates thickened, fluid-filled fallopian tubes or tubo-ovarian abscess Laparoscopic abnormalities consistent with PID

*Presumptive treatment for PID should be initiated for sexually active young women if they are experiencing pelvic or lower abdominal pain, if no other identifiable source other than PID can be identified, or if one or more of the following three minimum clinical criteria are present on pelvic examination.

⁺One or more the additional criteria can be used to enhance the specificity of the minimum clinical criteria and support a PID diagnosis.

CRP, C-reactive protein; ESR, erythrocyte sedimentation rate.

Source: Adapted from Workowski KA, Bolan GA. Sexually Transmitted Infections Treatment Guidelines, 2021. Center for Disease Control and Prevention. *MMWR Recomm Rep.* 2021;70(No.4): 94-98.

pelvic pain in sexually active females. PID may include any combination of endometritis, salpingitis, tubo-ovarian abscess, peritonitis, or perihepatitis (Fitz-Hugh-Curtis syndrome). While most often caused by untreated ascending *C. trachomatis* and *N. gonorrhoeae* infections, in two-thirds of cases no pathogen is isolated from the lower genital tract. Other known pathogens include endogenous vaginal flora (*Gardnerella vaginalis, Haemophilus influenzae,* group B *streptococci*), *Mycoplasma hominis, M. genitalium,* and *U. urealyticum*. PID is a challenging clinical diagnosis because of the wide range of symptoms, which may be absent, vague, or nonspecific. The diagnostic criteria for PID are provided in **Table 41-2**.

OROPHYARYNGEAL INFECTION

A number of STIs can present with oropharyngeal symptoms. Gonococcal infection of the pharynx is most commonly asymptomatic but may cause an exudative pharyngitis. HSV infection may cause an ulcerative pharyngitis. Genital-oral transmission of HPV can lead to respiratory papillomatosis in the pharynx and upper airway. In secondary syphilis, oropharyngeal mucous patches may occur as painless, silvery plaques with an erythematous border.

SYSTEMIC INFECTION AND STI SYNDROMES

Several STIs can present with disseminated symptoms, including *N. gonorrhoeae* infections, syphilis, and HSV.

Disseminated Gonococcal Infection Disseminated gonococcal infection occurs via hematogenous seeding of distant sites from a preceding gonococcal bacteremia. The most common manifestation is the arthritis and dermatitis syndrome, presenting with asymmetric polyarthralgias and arthritis of distal joints (typically knees, ankles, elbows, and/or wrists), tenosynovitis, and dermatitis. The classic skin findings are papules and pustules on an erythematous base that are tender and may show evidence of necrosis (**Figure 41-5**). Rarely, disseminated gonococcal infection may cause endocarditis, meningitis, and hepatitis.

Syphilis Caused by the spirochete *T. pallidum*, syphilis can present in any of the three symptomatic phases of illness (primary, secondary, and tertiary) or may be detected during the asymptomatic latent phase. During the latent phase, patients are noninfectious except for transplacental transmission from mother to fetus. Neurosyphilis, characterized by cranial neuropathy, meningitis, stroke, altered mental status, auditory or ophthalmic abnormalities, and loss of vibratory sense, can occur at any of the stages of disease. The clinical findings in the different stages of syphilis are provided in **Table 41-3**.

Reiter Syndrome Reiter syndrome (arthritis, urethritis, and bilateral conjunctivitis) is a reactive inflammatory condition that may follow *C. trachomatis* infection.

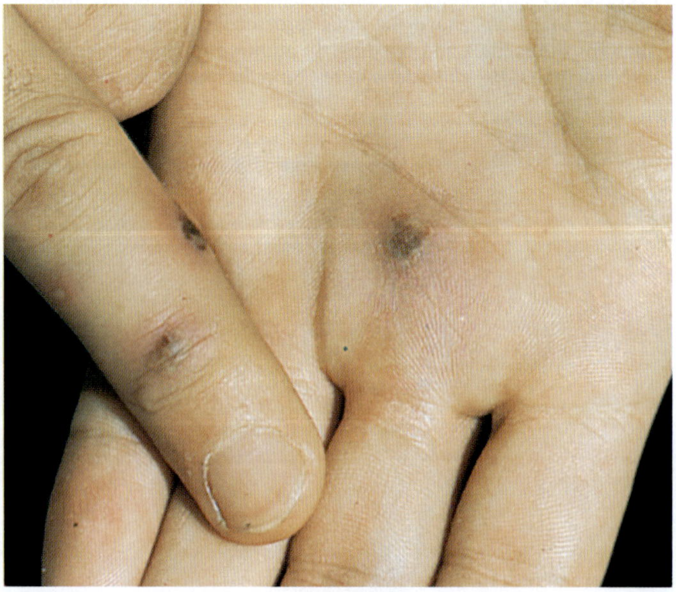

FIGURE 41-5. Disseminated gonococcal infection. (Reproduced, with permission, from Goldsmith LA, Katz SI, Gilchrest BA, Paller AS, Leffell DJ, Wolff K, eds. *Fitzpatrick's Dermatology in General Medicine*. 8th ed. New York, NY: McGraw-Hill Education; 2012, Figure 205-5.)

TABLE 41-3 Symptoms of Syphilis by Stage of Infection

	Primary	Secondary	Tertiary	Latent	Neurosyphilis
Time course	Incubation period: 1-4 wk Lesion resolves in 3-6 wk	Begins after 6-12 wk Resolution in 1-3 mo	Cardiac occurs 10-40 y after infection Destructive gummas form after 1-10 y	Early latent: acquired within the past year Late latent: acquired >1 y ago	Can occur at any stage of syphilis
Symptoms	Painless ulcer or chancre at inoculation site	Rash: salmon-pink macules progress to copper-colored papules; evolves centrifugally, involves palms and soles Adenopathy: generalized, painless Mucosa: grayish patches Condyloma latum: broad, flat macules, especially on vulva, scrotum, anus, axilla Constitutional: fever, malaise Other: patchy alopecia, arthritis, osteitis, gastritis, hepatitis, splenomegaly, nephrotic syndrome myalgias, sore throat	Cardiac: aneurysm of ascending aorta ± aortic insufficiency Gummas (granulomas) may involve skin, respiratory tract, gastrointestinal tract, bones, tabes dorsalis, general paresis	Asymptomatic infection with positive serology	Meningeal: cranial neuropathies, sensorineural deafness Meningovascular: endarteritis, stroke Tabes dorsalis: demyelination of posterior columns, Charcot joint, incontinence, ataxia General paresis Asymptomatic CSF abnormalities Uveitis, iritis, conjunctivitis, posterior interstitial keratitis, optic neuropathy, retinal vasculitis

Source: Adapted from Workowski KA, Bolan GA. Sexually Transmitted Infections Treatment Guidelines, 2021. Center for Disease Control and Prevention. *MMWR Recomm Rep.* 2021;70(No.4):39-41.

DIAGNOSTIC EVALUATION

Evaluation and diagnosis of STIs include comprehensive history taking, physical examination, and laboratory testing as appropriate.

SEXUAL HEALTH DISCUSSION

When addressing sexual health issues, providers must create a safe space and set the stage for confidentiality. Adolescents should spend at least part of the history talking privately with providers. Providers should explain what confidentiality means, detailing its protections and limitations, including mandatory reporting of physical and sexual abuse and imminent risk of harm to self or others. Adolescents should know that they may be encouraged to talk to their parents, but that they have a right to access testing and treatment for STIs and HIV confidentially in all healthcare settings within the context of legal, ethical, and professional guidelines. **Table 41-4** includes a list of questions to ask when taking a developmentally appropriate, comprehensive sexual health history.

The majority of STIs are diagnosed and treated in the outpatient setting, but hospitalists caring for adolescents need to be competent in evaluating and treating STIs. This includes considering these diagnoses as part of a differential for serious medical or surgical problems requiring hospital admission, addressing symptoms that may arise, and ensuring that teens receive evidence-based care for STIs knowing that many adolescents do not receive routine primary care.

LABORATORY TESTING

Table 41-5 provides guidance on appropriate laboratory testing for various STIs. All post-menarchal females presenting with lower abdominal or pelvic pain or other symptoms concerning for STI should also have an HCG performed to rule out pregnancy.

Vaginitis/Cervicitis When vaginal discharge is present, appropriate physical exam includes inspection of external genitalia for any lesions or mucosal changes. A sample of the discharge may be obtained for microscopy and other testing by patient- or provider-collected blind vaginal swab. A speculum examination may also be helpful to determine other causes of vaginitis or cervicitis, but usually is not necessary. Laboratory testing and/or microscopy should be performed for common causes including *C. trachomatis*, *N. gonorrhoeae*, *T. vaginalis*, yeast, and bacterial vaginosis. Testing includes either patient- or provider-collected (i.e., vaginal or cervical) swabs or first void urine for *C. trachomatis* and *N. gonorrhoeae* nucleic acid amplification test (NAAT) testing. Testing for *T. vaginalis* includes provider-collected vaginal specimen for microscopy or NAAT testing or patient- or provider-collected vaginal swab for NAAT testing. Culture can be used to test urogenital, as well as extragenital, sites although this has lower sensitivity.

Dysuria/Urethritis In female patients, urinalysis and culture should be sent to evaluate for urinary tract infection. However, dysuria is often a symptom of an STI and therefore testing for *C. trachomatis* and *N. gonorrhoeae* should also be sent. Male patients with dysuria and/or urethral discharge should be evaluated for an STI. Patients should be tested

TABLE 41-4 Sexual Health History Discussion

Consider asking about home, education, and activities as domains of adolescent social history first to develop rapport.

Don't start with Are you sexually active?

- It's important for you know that doctors and nurses have a responsibility to help young people stay healthy, which means avoiding unwanted pregnancy and STIs.
- All young people develop sexual feelings and have to make decisions about sexual behaviors as they grow up. Have you ever had a crush or a romantic relationship with a boy or girl? Are you romantically or sexually attracted to men (boys), women (girls), or both?
- Are you dating someone? Tell me about who you are dating, and what your relationship is like.
- Have you ever had any physical contact, like kissing or touching in private areas, with a boy or a girl? If touching, above or below the waist? Clothes on or off? Has any of this ever happened, even against your will?
- Have any of your friends started to have sex? What do you think about that? Can you explain how you will make decisions about when to have sex?
- Do you or have you ever had vaginal sex (meaning penis in vagina sex)? Oral sex (meaning mouth on penis or vagina sex)? Anal sex (meaning penis in rectum/anus sex)?
- How would you describe your sexual orientation? Many young people aren't sure or prefer not to use a label and that's OK, too. For example, do you consider yourself gay, lesbian, bisexual, or heterosexual (straight)? Do you have sex with men (boys), women (girls), or both?
- If you have questions about sex, what adult in your life can you talk to?
- How do you protect yourself against sexually transmitted diseases and pregnancy?
- When you use condoms for anal or vaginal sex, how many times out of ten do you use them?
- Do you have sex with anyone other than your boyfriend or girlfriend? In those situations, how often are you using condoms?
- Has anyone ever pressured you or forced you into doing something sexually that you didn't want to do?
- Have you ever needed to trade sex for money, drugs, or a place to stay?
- Are you having any pain or burning with urination or vaginal or penile discharge? Any bumps, sores, or rashes in your genital area?
- Have you ever been tested or diagnosed with a sexually transmitted infection? Have any of your partners ever been diagnosed with a sexually transmitted infection?
- Are you interested in testing for sexually transmitted infections? I recommend getting tested to all my teen patients who are might be concerned about having an infection.

TABLE 41-5 Sexually Transmitted Infection Diagnostic and Screening Tests

STI	Specimen Source	Test	M	F
Neisseria gonorrhoeae	Urine*	NAAT	✓	✓
	Cervix/vagina	NAAT	–	✓
	Meatus/urethra	NATT	✓	–
	Throat	NAAT	✓	✓
	Anus	NAAT	✓	✓
Chlamydia trachomatis	Urine*	NAAT	✓	✓
	Cervix/vagina	NAAT	–	✓
	Meatus/urethra	NAAT	✓	–
	Throat	NAAT	✓	✓
	Anus	NAAT	✓	✓
Bacterial vaginosis	Vaginal (collected by patient or provider)	Microscopy/wet mount, *or* Affirm nucleic acid probe test	–	✓
Trichomonas vaginalis	Vaginal (collected by patient or provider)	Microscopy/wet mount, *or* OSOM rapid test, *or* Affirm nucleic acid probe test	–	✓
HIV	Blood	HIV antibody, antigen/antibody combo, rapid test *or*	✓	✓
	Oral Fluid	Rapid test only	✓	✓
Syphilis	Blood	RPR with reflex treponemal test *or* EIA with reflex titer	✓	✓
Hepatitis A	Blood	Serology	✓	✓
Hepatitis B	Blood	Serology	✓	✓
Hepatitis C	Blood	Serology	✓	✓
HSV	Blood	Type specific glycoprotein G (gG)–based assay	✓	✓
	Lesion	PCR assay		

*Should be first void (no void during previous hour), No genital cleaning

EIA enzyme immunoassay; HIV, human immunodeficiency virus; HSV herpes simplex virus; NAAT, nucleic acid amplification test; PCR polymerase chain reaction; RPR rapid plasma regain.

using NAAT of first void urine sample or patient collected meatal swab or provider collected urethral swab and treated presumptively for *C. trachomatis* and *N. gonorrhoeae.*

Pharyngitis An oropharyngeal swab can be obtained and sent for *C. trachomatis* and *N. gonorrhoeae* testing if your laboratory has established appropriate performance specifications.

Ulcerative Lesions Direct sampling of lesions and testing for syphilis, HSV, chancroid, and LGV should be considered.

Anorectal Disease In patients with anorectal pain, bleeding, or discharge, inspection of the anal area for tags, fissures, and hemorrhoids is warranted and rectal examination for abnormalities and fecal occult blood testing may be indicated. Patient- or provider-collected rectal swabs for *C. trachomatis* and *N. gonorrhoeae* testing should be sent. LGV, syphilis, and general stool culture testing should also be considered.

Abdominal/Pelvic Pain in the Adolescent Female Bimanual examination should be performed to establish minimum criteria for PID treatment (Table 41-1). Urine, vaginal, or cervical specimens should be sent for *C. trachomatis* and *N. Gonorrhoeae* testing. When vaginal discharge is also present, patient- or provider-collected vaginal swabs with or without speculum examination may be considered to evaluate for other causes of vaginitis.

MANAGEMENT

Following thorough evaluation including history, physical examination, and diagnostic testing, treatment of STIs among adolescents should be prompt and err on the side of treatment. The consequences of untreated STIs can be serious, including infertility, chronic pain, and increased susceptibility to and likelihood of onward transmission of other STIs. **Table 41-6** details the most recent Centers for Disease Control STI treatment guidelines.

ADMISSION CRITERIA

Most patients with STIs do not require hospitalization; however, those with a toxic appearance and those unlikely to comply with therapy should be admitted. If urgent or emergent surgical intervention is a consideration (e.g., acute abdomen, testicular or ovarian torsion), evaluation, observation, and treatment should be performed as an inpatient.

The criteria for hospitalization for PID include lack of clinical response to oral antimicrobial therapy, inability to follow or tolerate an oral outpatient regimen, severe illness (including nausea, vomiting, or high fever), presence of tubo-ovarian abscess, and inability to exclude a surgical emergency such as appendicitis. Hospitalization is also warranted if the diagnosis is uncertain and other significant pathology has not yet been excluded.

Patients with disseminated gonococcal infection warrant admission for intravenous therapy until clinical improvement is demonstrated. Disseminated HSV infections such as pneumonitis, hepatitis, or complications of the central nervous system also require inpatient admission and intravenous therapy. Hospitalization for pain control may be necessary in cases of severe localized anogenital HSV, especially if there is concern for urinary retention.

DISCHARGE CRITERIA

Patients may be discharged when they are able to tolerate and adhere to an oral treatment regimen, are clinically improved, and able to manage their pain on oral medications.

TABLE 41-6 STI Treatment for Adolescents and Adults

DISEASE	RECOMMENDED REGIMENS	DOSE/ROUTE*	ALTERNATIVE REGIMENS* To be used if medical contraindication to recommend regimen
CHLAMYDIA TRACHOMATIS			
Uncomplicated genital/ rectal/pharyngeal infections	• Doxycycline **OR** • Azithromycin	100 mg po bid × 7 d 1 g po × 1	Levofloxacin[2] 500 mg po q day × 7 d
Pregnant women	• Azithromycin **OR** • Amoxicillin	1 g po × 1 500 mg po tid × 7 d	
NEISSERIA GONORRHOEAE: Ceftriaxone is the preferred treatment for adults and adolescents with uncomplicated *Neisseria gonorrhoeae*. Dual therapy with ceftriaxone 500 mg IM × 1 (increased from 250 mg) Plus azithromycin 1 g po × 1 or doxycycline 100 mg po bid × 7 d is recommended for all patients with *Neisseria gonorrhoeae* if *Chlamydia trachomatis* has not been ruled out.			
Uncomplicated Genital/ Rectal Infections	**Dual therapy with** • Ceftriaxone **PLUS** • Doxycycline (if *Chlamydia trachomatis* has not been excluded)	500 mg IM × 1 (< 150 kg); 1000 mg IM × 1 (> 150 kg) 100 mg PO BID × 7 d	**Dual therapy with** • If Ceftriaxone is not available: gentamicin 240 mg IM × 1 or Cefixime 800 mg po × 1 **plus** Azithromycin 2 g po × 1 • If Cephalosporin allergy: Gemifloxacin 320 mg po × 1 **PLUS** Azithromycin 2 g po **OR** Gentamicin 240 mg IM × 1 **PLUS** Azithromycin 2 g po × 1
Pharyngeal infections	**Dual therapy with** • Ceftriaxone **PLUS** Azithromycin **OR** • Doxycycline	500 mg IM × 1 (< 150 kg); 1000 mg IM × 1 (> 150 kg) 1 g po × 1 100 mg po bid × 7 d	• Azithromycin 2 g po × 1
Disseminated gonococcal disease	**Ceftriaxone** **PLUS** Doxycycline (if *Chlamydia trachomatis* has not been excluded)	1 g IM or IV* q 24hrs 100 mg PO BID × 7 d	Cefotaxime 1 g IV* q 8h Or Ceftizoxime1g IV* q 8h If *Chlamydia trachomatis* has not been excluded, providers should treat for chlamydia with doxycycline 100mg po BID × 7 d
Pregnant women	**Dual therapy with** • Ceftriaxone **PLUS** Azithromycin (if *Chlamydia trachomatis* has not been excluded)	500 mg IM × 1 (< 150 kg); 1000 mg IM × 1 (> 150 kg) 1g po × 1	
PELVIC INFLAMMATORY DISEASE	**Parenteral** Ceftriaxone or Cefotetan **or** Cefoxitin **PLUS** Doxycycline AND Metronidazole **OR** • Clindamycin **AND** Gentamicin **IM/Oral** • **Either** Ceftriaxone or Cefoxitin **PLUS** Probenecid **PLUS** Doxycycline **PLUS** Metronidazole	 1 g IV* q24h 2 g IV* q12h 2 g IV* q6h 100 mg po or IV* q 12 h 500 mg po or IV* q 12h 900 mg IV* q 8 h 2 mg/kg IV* or IM followed by 1.5 mg/kg IV* or IM q8h 500 mg IM × 1 2 g IM × 1 1 g po × 1 100 mg po bid × 14 d 500 mg po bid × 14 d	**Parenteral** • Ampicillin/Sulbactam 3 g IV* q6h **plus** Doxycycline 100 mg po or IV* q12h

(*Continued*)

TABLE 41-6 STI Treatment for Adolescents and Adults (*Continued*)

DISEASE	RECOMMENDED REGIMENS	DOSE/ROUTE*	ALTERNATIVE REGIMENS* To be used if medical contraindication to recommend regimen
CERVICITIS	Doxycycline **OR** Azithromycin	100 mg po bid × 7 d 500 mg po bid × 7 d	
NONGONOCOCCAL URETHRITIS	Doxycycline **OR** Azithromycin	100 mg po bid × 7 d 1 g po × 1	• Azithromycin 500 mg po × 1, then 250 mg qday × 4 days
EPIDIDYMITIS	Likely due to *Neisseria gonorrhoeae* or *Chlamydia trachomatis* • Ceftriaxone **plus** Doxycycline	500 mg IM × 1 100 mg po bid × 10 d	
	Likely due to enteric organisms • Levofloxacin	500 mg po qday × 10 d	
	For acute epididymitis most likely caused by sexually transmitted *Chlamydia trachomatis*, *Neisseria gonorrhoeae* or enteric organisms (men who practice insertive anal sex) • Ceftriaxone **plus** • levofloxacin	500 mg IM × 1 500 mg po qday × 10 d	
CHANCROID	• Azithromycin **OR** • Ceftriaxone **OR** • Ciprofloxacin **OR** • Erythromycin base	1 g po × 1 250 mg IM × 1 500 mg po bid × 3 d 500 mg po tid × 7 d	
LYMPHOGRANULOMA VENEREUM	• Doxycycline	100 mg po bid × 21 d	• Erythromycin base 500 mg po qid × 21 d **OR** • Azithromycin 1 g po qweek × 3 weeks
TRICHOMONAS VAGINALIS			
Non-pregnant women	• Metronidazole	500 mg po bid × 7 d	• Tinidazole 2 g po × 1
Pregnant women	• Metronidazole	500 mg po bid × 7 d	
Men	• Metronidazole	2 g po	• Tinidazole 2 g po × 1
BACTERIAL VAGINOSIS			
Adults/adolescents	• Metronidazole **OR** • Metronidazole gel **OR** • Clindamycin cream	500 mg po bid × 7 d 0.75%, one full applicator (5 g) intravaginally qday × 5 d 2%, one full applicator (5 g) intravaginally qhs × 7 d	• Tinidazole 2 g po qday × 2 d **OR** • Tinidazole 1 g po qday × 5 d **OR** • Clindamycin 300 mg po bid × 7 d **OR** • Clindamycin ovules 100 mg intravaginally qhs × 3 d • Secnidazole 2 gm po × 1
Pregnant women	• Metronidazole **or** • Metronidazole **or** • Clindamycin	500 mg po bid × 7 d 250 mg po tid × 7 d 300 mg po bid × 7 d	
ANOGENITAL WARTS			
External genital/perianal warts (Human papillomavirus)	**Patient-Applied** • Imiquimod 3.75% or 5% cream **OR** • Podofilox 0.5% solution or gel **OR** • Sinecatechins 15% ointment **Provider-Administered** • Cryotherapy **OR** • Trichloroacetic acid (TCA) 80%-90% **OR** • Bichloroacetic acid (BCA) 80%-90% **OR** • Surgical removal	Topically qhs 3 × 1 wk up to 16 wk Topically bid × 3 d followed by 4 d no tx for up to 4 cycles Topically tid, for up to 16 wk Apply once q 1-2 wk Apply once q 1-2 wk Apply once q 1-2 wk	**Alternative Regimen** • Podophyllin resin 10%-25% in compound tincture of benzoin may be considered for provider-administered treatment if strict adherence to the recommendations for application **OR** • Intralesional interferon **OR** • Laser surgery **OR** • Photodynamic therapy **OR** • Topical cidofovir

(*Continued*)

TABLE 41-6 STI Treatment for Adolescents and Adults (*Continued*)

DISEASE	RECOMMENDED REGIMENS	DOSE/ROUTE*	ALTERNATIVE REGIMENS* To be used if medical contraindication to recommend regimen
Mucosal genital warts	• Cryotherapy **OR** • TCA or BCA 80%-90% **OR** • Surgical removal	Vaginal, urethral meatus, and anal	
ANOGENITAL HERPES			
First clinical episode of anogenital herpes	• Acyclovir **OR** • Famciclovir **OR** • Valacyclovir	400 mg po tid × 7-10 d 250 mg po tid × 7-10 d 1 g po bid × 7-10 d	
Established infection			
Suppressive therapy	• Acyclovir **OR** • Famciclovir **OR** • Valacyclovir **OR** • Valacyclovir	400 mg po bid 250 mg po bid 500 mg po qday 1 g po qday	
Episodic therapy for recurrent episodes	• Acyclovir **OR** • Acyclovir **OR** • Famciclovir **OR** • Famciclovir **OR** Famciclovir • Valacyclovir **OR** • Valacyclovir	800 mg po bid × 5 d 800 mg po tid × 2 d 1000 mg po bid × 1 d 500 mg once, then 250 mg bid × 2 d 125 mg bid × 5 d 500 mg po bid × 3 d 1 g po qday × 5 d	
HIV Co-Infected			
Suppressive therapy	• Acyclovir **OR** • Famciclovir or **OR** • Valacyclovir	400-800 mg po bid or tid 500 mg po bid 500 mg po bid	
Episodic therapy for recurrent episodes	• Acyclovir **OR** • Famciclovir **OR** • Valacyclovir	400 mg po tid × 5-10 d 500 mg po bid × 5-10 d 1 g po bid × 5-10 d	
TREPONEMA PALLIDUM			
Primary, secondary, and early latent	• Benzathine penicillin G	2.4 million units IM × 1	• Doxycycline 100 mg po bid × 14 d or • Tetracycline 500 mg po qid × 14 d or • Ceftriaxone 1 g IM or IV* qday × 10 d
Late latent and latent of unknown duration	• Benzathine penicillin G	7.2 million units, administered as 3 doses of 2.4 million units IM each, at 1-week intervals	• Doxycycline 100 mg po bid × 28 d or • Tetracycline 500 mg po qid × 28 d
Neurosyphilis	• Aqueous crystalline penicillin G	18-24 million units daily, administered as 3-4 million units IV* q 4 h × 10-14 d	• Procaine penicillin G, 2.4 million units IM qday × 10-14 d **plus** Probenecid 500 mg po qid × 10-14 d
Pregnant Women			
Primary, secondary, and early latent	• Benzathine penicillin G	2.4 million unit IM	• None
Late latent and latent of unknown duration	• Benzathine penicillin G	7.2 million units, administered as 3 doses of 2.4 million units IM each, at 1-week intervals	• None
Neurosyphilis	• Aqueous crystalline penicillin G	18-24 million units daily, administered as 3-4 million units IV* q 4 h × 10-14 d	• Procaine penicillin G 2.4 million units IM qday × 10-14 d **PLUS** Probenecid 500 mg po qid × 10-14 d

*For IV treatment regimens, length of IV therapy is determined by clinical improvement. Consider changing to oral agent guided by antimicrobial susceptibility testing 24–48 hours after substantial clinical improvement and consider discussion with Infectious Disease specialist.

The complete list of recommended regimens and further treatment details can be found in Sexually Transmitted Infections Treatment Guidelines, 2021. https://www.cdc.gov/std/treatment-guidelines/default.htm.

CONSULTATION

In cases where the differential diagnosis includes an acute abdomen of unknown etiology, consultation with surgery is essential. Concerns about ectopic pregnancy or possible ovarian torsion require emergent gynecological or surgical consultation. Similarly, urology or surgery should be consulted emergently in cases of suspected testicular torsion. In cases of PID with tubo-ovarian abscess, gynecology or surgery should be consulted for assistance with management. Consultation with an HIV specialist is recommended in cases of acute HIV infection, or when a patient known to have HIV is diagnosed with another STI.

SPECIAL CONSIDERATIONS

HIV INFECTION

HIV infection is further detailed in Chapter 104. Pediatric hospitalists should consider screening adolescents for HIV and employ appropriate testing when acute HIV infection is suspected. The presentation of acute HIV infection often includes a host of nonspecific symptoms including fevers, sore throat, rash, abdominal pain, and diarrhea; it may be confused with other viral illnesses such as influenza or infectious mononucleosis. If acute HIV is suspected, NAAT testing should be sent because the patient may not have yet developed antibodies to the virus and most routine screening tests will remain negative. Additionally, for any adolescent diagnosed with one STI, HIV and syphilis testing should be recommended. For adolescents who are HIV-negative but considered high risk for subsequent HIV infection, referral for pre-exposure prophylaxis (PrEP) may be considered (Tables 104-5, 104-6, and 104-7).

SEXUAL ASSAULT

In cases of sexual assault, baseline and follow-up testing for HIV, *C. trachomatis*, *N. gonorrhoeae*, *T. vaginalis*, syphilis, and hepatitis B should be performed. As follow-up may be poor after the initial evaluation, presumptive treatment for *C. trachomatis*, *N. gonorrhoeae*, and *T. vaginalis* for women and *C. trachomatis* and *N. gonorrhoeae* for men is recommended. In addition, non-occupational HIV post-exposure prophylaxis (nPEP) may be warranted if the patient is presenting within 72 hours of the assault (Tables 104-5, 104-6, and 104-7). Consultation with an HIV or infectious disease specialist is recommended prior to prescribing an nPEP regimen. Additionally, postexposure hepatitis B vaccination (without HBIG) is recommended if the hepatitis status of the assailant is unknown and the survivor has not been previously vaccinated. HPV vaccination for female and male survivors of sexual assault aged 9 and older who have not been vaccinated or are incompletely vaccinated for HPV is recommended.

CONFIDENTIALITY AND REPORTING

While it is preferable to include parents in the care of an adolescent, adolescents have the right to confidential healthcare related to diagnosis and treatment of STIs within legal, ethical, and professional guidelines, with particular exceptions (e.g., STI prevention, HIV testing, treatment, and prophylaxis; https://www.cdc.gov/hiv/policies/law/states/minors.html). As there is variation in state laws, providers must be aware of the specific laws for the state in which they practice. In addition, many common STI diagnoses require filing a report with the state or local health department. Adolescent medicine providers or social workers can be an excellent resource for providers unfamiliar with state legal requirements for confidentiality and reporting.

PARTNER TREATMENT

When an adolescent is diagnosed with and treated for an STI, providers need to ensure that the patient's sexual partners are treated appropriately. Several strategies exist to promote partner treatment and prevent re-infection. Patients should be instructed to refer their most recent partner and all partners within the last 60 days for evaluation, testing, and treatment. If patients feel uncomfortable contacting partners directly, healthcare providers, or health departments can contact partners anonymously. Another alternative strategy which has been shown to improve partner treatment rates and reduce rates of re-infection is Expedited Partner Therapy (EPT). EPT is the treatment of the sexual partner(s) of a patient with an STI by giving medications or prescriptions to the patient to deliver directly to the partner or providing a prescription directly to the partner without physical examination. EPT can only be used for STIs that can be treated orally. EPT is legal in the majority of states; https://www.cdc.gov/std/ept includes detail by state.

RISK OF UNINTENDED PREGNANCY

When any female is diagnosed with an STI or has a history of an STI, it is important to address her risk for unintended pregnancy. Contraception and pregnancy prevention should be discussed and offered. If a young woman has had unprotected sex, had contraceptive failure, or been a victim of sexual assault within the past 120 hours, emergency contraception (e.g., levonorgestrol, ulipristal) should be offered immediately.

PREVENTION

Primary prevention of STIs includes encouraging adolescents to delay sexual intercourse until they are older, and vaccination during early adolescence to prevent HPV infection. For adolescents who engage in sexual intercourse, prevention strategies include encouragement of consistent condom use and minimizing the number of sexual partners. Routine screening of all sexually active adolescents for *C. trachomatis, N. gonorrhoeae, HIV, and T. pallidum* (depending on geographic prevalence) is one key part of a national STI control strategy in the United States.

When an adolescent is diagnosed with an STI or discloses a sexual risk behavior during hospitalization, STI prevention should be discussed and appropriate follow-up recommended. The American Academy of Pediatricians recommends that developmentally appropriate sexual education be incorporated into routine clinical practice. For prevention messages to be effective, they must be tailored to and relevant to the adolescent considering their personal risk and using personalized goal-setting strategies. Adolescents engaging in certain sexual behaviors may have a history of sexual abuse or significant mental health problems; identifying and addressing these issues can be an important component of a comprehensive risk-reduction management strategy. In addition to risk reduction, pediatricians should discuss with adolescents how they can have healthy and safe relationships. Ultimately, as pediatricians working with adolescents and their families, we have a tremendous opportunity to help adolescents grow up to be sexually healthy adults.

KEY POINTS

- Treat suspected sexually transmitted infections (STIs) empirically to reduce the risk of long-term sequelae.
- Consider STI in the differential diagnosis of adolescents presenting with acute abdominal or genitourinary symptoms.
- Hospitalization is warranted in cases of uncertain diagnosis, systemic or disseminated illness, inability to tolerate oral medications, or concerns about compliance with outpatient treatment.
- All adolescents diagnosed with an STI should be offered testing for other STIs (e.g., *Chlamydia trachomatis, Neisseria gonorrhoeae, Trichomonas vaginalis*, syphilis, HIV).

SUGGESTED READINGS

Ackers ML, Greenberg AE, Lin CY, et al. High and persistent HIV seroincidence in men who have sex with men across 47 U.S. Cities. *PLoS One*. 2012;7:E34972.

Centers for Disease Control and Prevention. Sexually Transmitted Disease Surveillance 2019. Atlanta: U.S. Department of Health and Human Services; 2021.

Committee on Adolescent Health Care. Committee Opinion No 699: Adolescent Pregnancy, Contraception, and Sexual Activity. *Obstet Gynecol.* 2017;129(5):e142-e149.

Committee on Adolescence, Braverman PK, Adelman WP, et al. Contraception for adolescents. *Pediatrics.* 2014;134(4):e1244-e1256.

Forhan SE, Gottlieb SL. Prevalence of sexually transmitted infections among female adolescents aged 14 to 19 in the United States. *Pediatrics.* 2019;124(6):10.

Hwang LY, et al. Factors that influence the rate of epithelial maturation in the cervix in healthy young women. *J Adolesc Health.* 2009;44(2):103-110.

Kester LM, BG, Blythe MJ. Sexually Transmitted Infection Syndromes. In: Long SS, ed. *Principles and Practics of Pediatric Infectious Diseases.* Elsevier; 2012.

Kreisel KM, Spicknall IH, Gargano JW, et al. Sexually transmitted infections among US women and men: prevalence and incidence estimates, 2018. *Sex Transm Dis.* 2021;48(4):208-214.

Shafii T, Levine D. Office-Based Screening for Sexually Transmitted Infections in Adolescents. *Pediatrics.* 2020;145(Supplement_2):S219-S224.

Sieving RE, McRee AL, Mehus C, et al. Sexual and Reproductive Health Discussions During Preventive Visits. *Pediatrics.* 2021;148(2): e2020049411.

Society for Adolescent Health and Medicine. Sexual and reproductive health care: a position paper of the society for adolescent health and medicine. *J Adolesc Health.* 2014;54(4):491-496.

Upadhya KK, Committee on Adolescence, Breuner CC, et al. Emergency contraception. *Pediatrics.* 2019;144(6):e20193149.

Weinstock HS, Kreisel KM, Spicknall IH, Chesson HW, Miller WC. STI prevalence, incidence, and costs in the united states: new estimates, new approach. *Sex Transm Dis.* 2021;48(4):207-207.

Workowski KA. Skin and Mucous Membrane Infections and Inguinal Lymphadenopathy. In: Long, SS, ed. *Principles and Practice of Pediatric Infectious Diseases.* Elsevier; 2012.

Workowski KA, Bachmann LH, Chan PA, et al. Sexually transmitted infections treatment guidelines, 2021. *MMWR Recomm Rep.* 2021; 70(4):1-187.

CHAPTER 42 Abnormal Uterine Bleeding

Brittany M. Hunter, MD and Uchenna C. Ewulonu, MD

BACKGROUND

Abnormal uterine bleeding, the most common gynecologic complaint of hospitalized adolescents, serves as an overarching term for any bleeding from the uterine corpus that is abnormal in volume, duration, regularity, and/or frequency in the absence of pregnancy. Heavy menstrual bleeding, the most common symptom of abnormal uterine bleeding amongst adolescents, affects over one-third of adolescents and can result in severe anemia. Abnormal uterine bleeding includes menstrual cycles that (i) occur more frequently than every 21 days or less frequently than every 45 days, (ii) occur more than 90 days apart, (iii) last for more than 7 days, and/or (iv) result in excessive blood loss that interferes with quality of life. Chronic abnormal uterine bleeding refers to abnormal bleeding that is present for the majority of the preceding 6 months. Acute abnormal uterine bleeding refers to a single episode of heavy bleeding with sufficient quantity to warrant immediate intervention, which can occur with or without chronic abnormal uterine bleeding. Abnormal uterine bleeding may indicate a serious underlying condition and therefore requires medical evaluation.

PATHOPHYSIOLOGY

It is important to understand normal menstruation in adolescence to appropriately evaluate for abnormal uterine bleeding (**Table 42-1**).

TABLE 42-1 Patterns of Menstruation in Adolescents

	Normal Pattern	Abnormal Pattern
Frequency (cycle interval[a])	21-45 days	Amenorrhea: > 90 days Infrequent: > 45 days Frequent: < 21 days
Duration (days of flow)	≤ 7 days	Prolonged: > 7 days
Regularity (cycle variation[b])	≤ 9 days	Irregular: > 9 days
Volume (heaviness of flow)	Menstrual product use: 3-6 pads or tampons per day Patient experience: Patient considers normal	Heavy: > 6 pads or tampons per day; changing soaked product every 1-2 hours; patient considers flow heavy Light: patient considers flow light

[a]Cycle length is the number of days from the first day of bleeding of one menstrual cycle to the first day of bleeding of the next menstrual cycle.

[b]Cycle variation is the difference between the shortest and longest cycle interval.

Source: Adapted from Committee Opinion No. 557: Management of Acute Abnormal Uterine Bleeding in Nonpregnant Reproductive-Aged Women. *Obstet Gynecol*. 2013;121(4):891-896 and Haamid F, Sass AE, Dietrich JE. Heavy Menstrual Bleeding in Adolescents. *J Pediatr Adolesc Gynecol*. 2017;30(3):335-340.

Menarche, the first occurrence of menstruation, begins at puberty, ranging from 10 to 16 years of age, with a median age of ~12.5 years. Menstrual cycles often vary within the first 1 to 2 years after menarche given irregularities in ovulation due to an immature hypothalamic-pituitary-ovarian axis (HPO axis). The interval between each menstrual cycle during this time ranges from 21 to 45 days. Menstrual flow typically lasts for 7 days or less and requires 3 to 6 pads or tampons per day.

The HPO axis regulates the menstrual cycle based on a complex process involving negative and positive feedback. Hormones produced through the hypothalamic-pituitary unit, gonadotropin hormone-releasing hormone (GnRH), follicle stimulating hormone (FSH), and luteinizing hormone (LH) exist in dynamic equilibrium with the hormones of the ovaries, estrogen, and progesterone. GnRH is secreted in a pulsatile fashion from the hypothalamus once puberty starts and is transported to the anterior pituitary to signal the secretion of FSH and LH. FSH and LH subsequently regulate the levels of estrogen and progesterone produced by the ovarian follicles (**Figure 42-1**).

During the first phase of the menstrual cycle, the preovulatory follicular (or proliferative) phase, estradiol (the primary form of estrogen during reproductive years) drives rapid growth of the endometrium. Variability in length of the menstrual cycle occurs due to variations in this phase of the menstrual cycle. Thereafter, progesterone drives glandular differentiation of the endometrial lining during the postovulatory luteal (or secretory) phase. If pregnancy does not occur during this time, progesterone levels fall and the endometrium becomes ischemic, resulting in shedding of the endometrial lining and menstrual bleeding. The amount of menstrual blood produced directly correlates with the thickness of the endometrium, the coagulation cascade functioning to control blood loss, and the re-exposure to estrogen at the start of a new menstrual cycle. Any disruption or abnormality in this process can result in abnormal bleeding patterns.

CLINICAL PRESENTATION

Abnormal uterine bleeding in adolescents typically presents with "skipped periods" or "too much bleeding." Abnormalities in menstrual bleeding can present as abnormalities in frequency (amenorrhea, frequent or infrequent menstrual bleeding), duration (prolonged menstrual bleeding), regularity (irregular menstrual bleeding), or volume (heavy menstrual bleeding) (Table 42-1). Heavy menstrual bleeding is defined as bleeding requiring frequent pad or tampon changes, soaking more than one product every 1 to 2 hours, or excessive bleeding interfering with the patient's physical, emotional, social, and material quality of life. Though prior definitions included quantification of blood volume loss or hemoglobin quantification, the definition of heavy menstrual bleeding now focuses on the patient's lived experience.

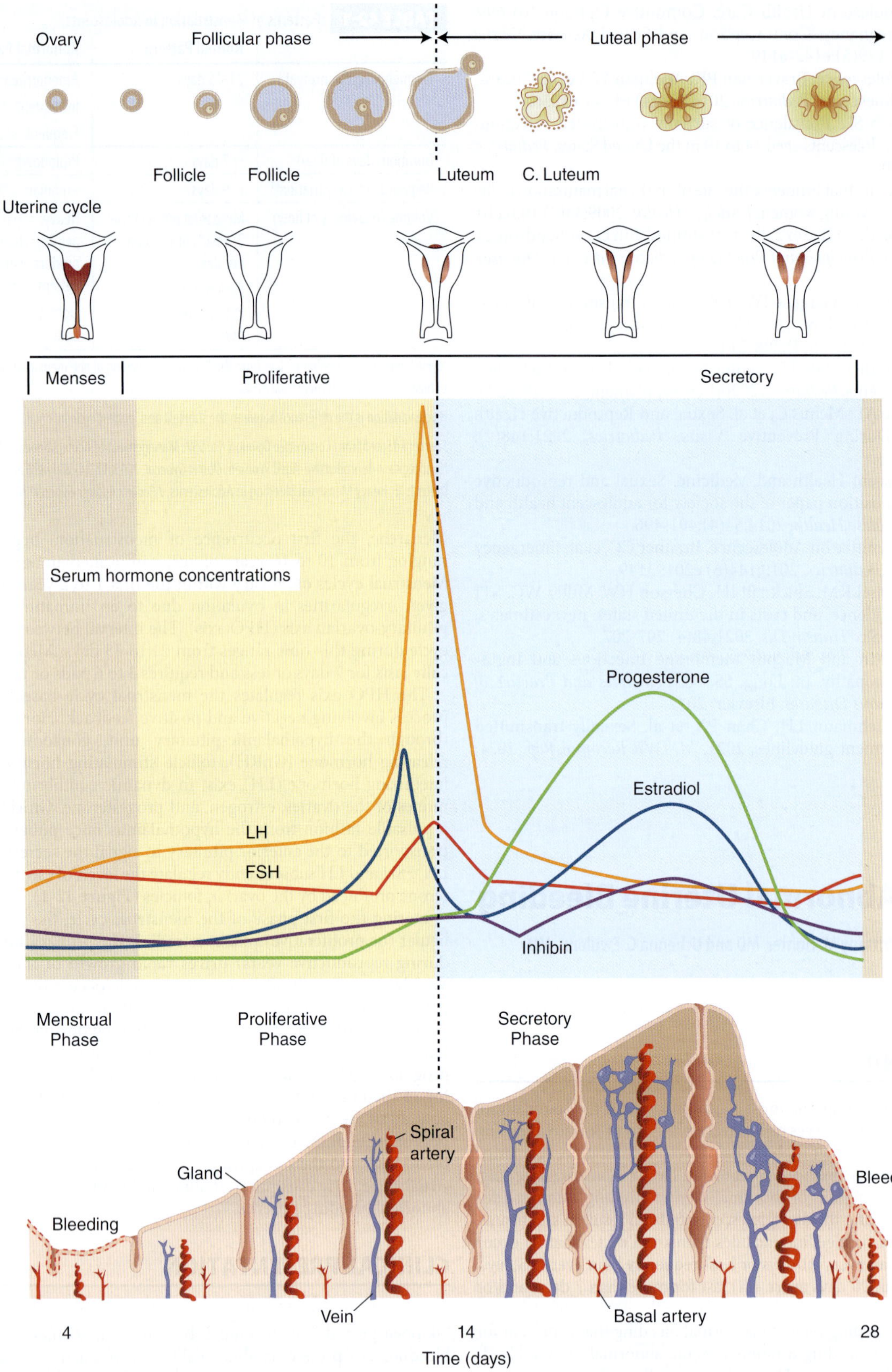

FIGURE 42-1. Normal menstrual cycle: ovarian, uterine, hormonal, and endometrial changes. (Reproduced with permission From Janson LW, Tischler ME. *The Big Picture: Medical Biochemistry.* New York, NY: McGraw Hill; 2018; Reproduced with permission from Kibble JD, Halsey CR. *The Big Picture: Medical Physiology.* New York, NY: McGraw Hill; 2009.)

Abnormal uterine bleeding can also present as intermenstrual bleeding, bleeding between cyclically regular onset of menses, and unscheduled bleeding (bleeding between menses while on hormonal therapy). Though terms such as menorrhagia, metrorrhagia, and oligomenorrhea have been traditionally used to describe abnormal uterine bleeding, the International Federation of Gynecology and Obstetrics (FIGO) recommends using the more clearly defined, standardized terminologies above.

Patients presenting with abnormal uterine bleeding can have variable associated clinical symptoms based on the severity, frequency, and chronicity of blood loss. Adolescents with acute or chronic abnormal uterine bleeding with heavy menstrual bleeding may present with anemia, fatigue, and even hemodynamic instability, though others may have normal hemoglobin levels and lack clinical symptoms. Heavy menstrual bleeding may cause psychological distress and impact quality of life which may manifest as missed school days, physical activity limitations, and need for prolonged rest. Patients may additionally have symptoms related to the underlying cause of abnormal uterine bleeding discussed later.

DIFFERENTIAL DIAGNOSIS

The differential diagnosis for abnormal uterine bleeding is extensive. The PALM-COEIN classification system, developed by FIGO and supported by the American College of Obstetrics and Gynecology (ACOG), provides standardized terminology and a framework for the various etiologies of abnormal uterine bleeding (**Table 42-2**). This classification system separates abnormal uterine bleeding into two main categories: abnormal uterine bleeding related to structural causes (PALM: Polyp, Adenomyosis, Leiomyoma, Malignancy, and hyperplasia) and abnormal uterine bleeding related to non-structural causes (COEIN: Coagulopathy, Ovulatory dysfunction, Endometrial, Iatrogenic, Not yet classified).

NON-STRUCTURAL ETIOLOGIES

Ovulatory Dysfunction Of non-structural etiologies, disorders of ovulation, specifically anovulatory uterine bleeding, are the most common cause of abnormal uterine bleeding. In the first few years following menarche, the immaturity of the HPO axis results in anovulatory cycles and unpredictable bleeding. As the complex feedback relationship between estrogen and the anterior pituitary is the last to mature during development, ovulation may not occur. Lack of ovulation subsequently limits progesterone secretion and causes an unopposed estrogenic proliferation of the endometrium leading to an unstable endometrial lining, which ultimately results in abnormal uterine bleeding.

Anovulatory cycles are common in the first two years after menarche, with most adolescents developing normal and predictable cycles within 3 years of their first menstrual cycle. Although anovulatory cycles can be physiologic in adolescents, irregular bleeding may be a symptom of disorders affecting ovulation such as endocrinopathies (e.g., polycystic ovary syndrome [PCOS], thyroid disorders, congenital adrenal hyperplasia, hyperprolactinemia, diabetes mellitus) or chronic illness (e.g., renal disease, systemic lupus erythematosus [SLE], liver disease). Anovulatory uterine bleeding should therefore be considered a diagnosis of exclusion.

Adolescents may have longer cycle intervals compared to adults; however, it is uncommon for adolescents to remain amenorrheic for more than 3 months without the use of hormonal contraception. Therefore, adolescents with more than 3 months between periods should be evaluated for amenorrhea. Pregnancy is the most common cause of amenorrhea in adolescents. Other causes of amenorrhea to consider include functional hypothalamic amenorrhea, primary ovarian insufficiency, and chromosomal abnormalities (i.e., Kallman syndrome and Turner syndrome).

Coagulopathies Bleeding disorders are the second most common etiology of abnormal uterine bleeding among adolescents. Up to 30% of adolescents presenting with heavy menstrual bleeding will have an underlying inherited bleeding disorder; thus, it is important to include bleeding disorders in the differential diagnosis of all adolescents presenting with heavy menstrual bleeding. Von Willebrand disease (VWD) is the most common of the inherited bleeding disorders. Other bleeding disorders to consider include inherited clotting factor deficiencies (e.g., hemophilia), thrombocytopenia, and other platelet disorders (e.g., idiopathic thrombocytopenic purpura, Chapter 88).

TABLE 42-2 Differential Diagnosis of Abnormal Uterine Bleeding in an Adolescent Using the FIGO Classification of Uterine Bleeding in Nongravid Women

PALM (Structural Causes)
Polyp
Adenomyosis
Leiomyoma (fibroid)
Malignancy and hyperplasia
COEIN (Nonstructural Causes)
Coagulopathy
Coagulation defect (e.g., von Willebrand disease, liver disease)
Thrombocytopenia (e.g., immune thrombocytopenic purpura, leukemia)
Platelet function disorder (e.g., Glanzmann disease)
Ovarian dysfunction
Anovulatory cycles due to immature hypothalamic-pituitary-ovarian axis
Anovulatory cycles due to endocrinopathy
Polycystic ovary syndrome
Hypothyroidism
Hyperthyroidism
Hyperprolactinemia
Adrenal disorders
Anovulatory cycles secondary to systemic disease
Chronic renal failure
Systemic lupus erythematosus
Endometrial causes
Endometritis (e.g., pelvic inflammatory disease)
Iatrogenic
Hormonal contraception
Medications
Anticoagulants
Antiplatelets
Antidepressants (e.g., SSRIs, TCAs)
Antipsychotics (e.g., risperidone)
Anticonvulsants (e.g., valproate)
Not classified

Note: Extrauterine causes of bleeding should be considered as well when approaching abnormal uterine bleeding including pregnancy, sexually transmitted infections, vaginal lacerations, vaginal foreign body, vascular malformation, ruptures ovarian cyst, Mullerian anomalies.

Source: Adapted from Committee Opinion No. 557: Management of acute abnormal uterine bleeding in nonpregnant reproductive-aged women. *Obstet Gynecol.* 2013;121(4):891-896.

Endometrial Causes Endometrial causes of abnormal uterine bleeding in adolescents are uncommon, accounting for fewer than 10% of abnormal uterine bleeding cases. When present, bleeding due to uterine pathology is usually due to endometritis secondary to pelvic inflammatory disease (PID) caused by *Neisseria gonorrhoeae* or *Chlamydia trachomatis*. Patients commonly present with pain (80% of patients) in addition to abnormal bleeding (35% of patients). As the risk of PID is 10 times higher in adolescents than adults, PID should always be considered in an adolescent with abnormal uterine bleeding. Other endometrial causes, including endometrial cancer, are exceedingly rare in adolescents.

Iatrogenic Causes Hormonal contraception use is the most common iatrogenic cause of abnormal uterine bleeding in adolescents. Amenorrhea, unscheduled bleeding, and heavy menstrual bleeding are common side effects of hormonal contraception. Abnormal uterine bleeding is most common in the first few months of use and then typically improves depending on the form of contraception. Though both combined hormonal contraceptives (CHCs) and progestin-only contraception are associated with abnormal uterine bleeding, irregular bleeding is seen more commonly with progestin-only methods.

Other medications associated with abnormal uterine bleeding include anticoagulants, antipsychotics, selective serotonin reuptake inhibitors (SSRIs), tricyclic antidepressants (TCAs), and anticonvulsants.

STRUCTURAL ETIOLOGIES

In adolescents, structural causes of abnormal uterine bleeding are rare, accounting for ~1% of abnormal uterine bleeding. Structural causes include uterine polyps, adenomyosis, leiomyomas (uterine fibroids), congenital anomalies, vascular malformations, or malignancy.

EXTRAUTERINE ETIOLOGIES

A complaint of abnormal vaginal bleeding is not always indicative of uterine bleeding. It may instead indicate bleeding in the lower genital tract (cervix, vagina, vulva) or upper genital tract (uterine corpus, fallopian tubes, ovaries). Non-uterine sources of bleeding to consider include pregnancy, sexually transmitted infections (STIs), vaginal lacerations, vaginal foreign body, vascular malformation, ruptured ovarian cyst, and Mullerian anomalies. Regardless of reported sexual history, adolescents presenting with abnormal bleeding should be evaluated for pregnancy, STIs, sexual trauma, and vaginal foreign bodies.

DIAGNOSTIC EVALUATION

Initial evaluation of a patient presenting with abnormal uterine bleeding should differentiate acute from chronic abnormal uterine bleeding. Acute abnormal uterine bleeding may require immediate intervention and patient stabilization prior to further diagnostic evaluation. Signs of hypovolemia or hemodynamic instability (tachycardia, hypotension, orthostasis) should be appropriately addressed before further evaluation.

Though anovulatory uterine bleeding due to an immature HPO axis accounts for 90% of abnormal uterine bleeding in non-pregnant adolescents, it remains a diagnosis of exclusion and other causes of abnormal uterine bleeding should be considered and excluded. All adolescents presenting with abnormal uterine bleeding should undergo a thorough history and physical with further studies obtained if indicated.

HISTORY

A thorough history with a focus on menstruation, other sources of bleeding, and family history can narrow the differential diagnosis of abnormal uterine bleeding and guide further workup (**Table 42-3**).

Menstrual history should include age at menarche, menstrual regularity, duration in days, number and size of tampons/pads per day, impact of bleeding on quality of life, and last menstrual period (LMP). Patterns of bleeding can be helpful in indicating underlying etiology. Irregular bleeding with 2 or 3 months without bleeding followed by phases of spotting, heavy bleeding, or sudden and substantial hemorrhage is consistent with anovulatory uterine bleeding. Other conditions associated with irregular bleeding include PCOS, hypothyroidism, hyperprolactinemia, and hypothalamic dysfunction due to exercise, stress, or weight. Heavy menstrual bleeding is associated with various bleeding disorders and less commonly thyroid disorders, systemic illnesses, and medication use (e.g., anticoagulants). Common causes of intermenstrual or unscheduled bleeding include use of hormonal contraception, sexually transmitted infections, trauma, or foreign body. Patients who report soaking through menstrual products every 1 to 2 hours are at risk for significant blood loss and may require more urgent evaluation. The passage of clots has been associated with underlying bleeding disorders and should be assessed on history. The presence or absence of dysmenorrhea should also be evaluated as dysmenorrhea may be an indicator of ovulatory cycles.

Screening questions for underlying disorders of hemostasis should be incorporated. Risk factors for an underlying bleeding disorder include heavy menstrual bleeding since menarche; history of postpartum hemorrhage, surgery-related bleeding, or bleeding associated with dental work; frequent bruising, epistaxis, gum bleeding; or a family history of bleeding symptoms. Family history of bleeding disorders, autoimmune disorders, and menstrual history should be obtained from first-degree relatives.

TABLE 42-3 Focused History for Evaluation of Abnormal Uterine Bleeding

Menstrual History	Age at menarche
	Duration of bleeding in days
	Regularity, bleeding frequency (cycle interval, bleeding between cycles)
	Flow volume (number and size of tampons/pads per day, how frequently soaking through products)
	Associated dysmenorrhea
	Presence of clots
	First day of last menstrual period (LMP)
	Impact on quality of life
	Symptoms of anemia (headache, palpitations, shortness of breath, dizziness, fatigue)
Medical History	Pregnancy history
	Autoimmune disorder
	Liver disease
	Renal disease
	Bleeding disorder
	Prior GU procedures
Bleeding History	Heavy menstrual bleeding since menarche
	Epistaxis
	Mucosal bleeding
	Easy bruising
	Prolonged bleeding after surgery or dental procedures
Family History	Bleeding disorders
	Autoimmune disorders
	Endocrine disorders
	Menstrual history of first-degree relatives
Social History	Sexual history
	Recent stressors
	Changes in eating patterns
	Athletic or exercise activities
Medications	Current and prior contraception use
	Anticoagulants
	Antidepressants
	Antipsychotics
	Anticonvulsants
	Herbal supplements (e.g., ginseng)
Symptoms indicating systemic etiology	Hyperandrogenism (obesity, acne, hirsutism)
	Thyroid dysfunction (weight changes, heat/cold intolerance, fatigue)
	Hyperprolactinemia (galactorrhea, vision changes, headaches)
	Hypothalamic dysfunction (weight changes, exercise patterns)
	GU Infection (fever, vaginal discharge)
Other History	Precipitating trauma
	Foreign body

In addition to the above, a full medical history, current medications (including hormonal contraception), sexual history, and review of systems should be performed. Review of systems should include recent stressors, weight changes, changes in eating, athletic activities, syncope, visual changes, headaches, gastrointestinal symptoms, hair loss, acne, hirsutism, and temperature dysregulation.

PHYSICAL EXAM

The physical examination should start with an assessment of the patient's vital signs. Tachycardia, hypotension, and orthostasis should be addressed immediately as they may indicate significant blood loss or malnutrition. Presence of a fever may indicate infection such as PID. Abnormal trends in weight or BMI, obesity, or underweight status may indicate functional hypothalamic amenorrhea or underlying endocrinopathy. Skin should be inspected for pallor (anemia), bruises, and petechiae (bleeding disorder), as well as acne, hirsutism, and acanthosis nigricans (endocrinopathy). Breast examination should be completed to evaluate sexual maturity rating and the presence of galactorrhea (hyperprolactinemia). Thyroid should be evaluated for diffuse enlargement (Hashimoto's thyroiditis, Grave's disease), consistency (firm-Hashimoto's thyroiditis, soft-Grave's disease), and tenderness (thyroiditis).

All adolescents with abnormal bleeding should have an external genital exam completed to evaluate for extrauterine bleeding (e.g., perineal trauma). Pelvic exams may be distressing for adolescents, and non-sexually active adolescents may have difficulty tolerating a full pelvic exam. Furthermore, structural lesions in adolescents are rare. Therefore, in cases of non-severe bleeding, pelvic exam may be postponed until after a trial of medical therapy is attempted. As an alternative, pelvic ultrasonography can be used to evaluate for structural lesions. When warranted, a one finger digital exam and speculum exam with an appropriate size speculum should be performed. Pelvic examination under anesthesia may need to be considered if the pelvic examination is inadequate or a diagnosis cannot be established despite imaging.

LABORATORY EVALUATION

Initial evaluation includes a pregnancy test (regardless of sexual history), hemoglobin concentration (anemia), platelet count (thrombocytopenia), and screening for sexually transmitted infections (STIs). As reported amounts of bleeding are often not a reliable predictor of blood loss, hemoglobin concentration can be used to categorize presentation severity. However, it is important to note hemoglobin levels can initially be normal in acute hemorrhage due to a concomitant loss of both red cells and plasma. Screening for iron deficiency, including ferritin (low), total iron binding capacity (high), transferrin (high), and serum iron (low), should also be considered as anemia and microcytosis develop later in the setting of iron deficiency.

In patients who are sexually active or who have symptoms consistent with a STI regardless of reported sexual history, nucleic acid amplification testing (NAAT) for *N. gonorrhea*, *C. trachomatis*, and *Trichomonas* should be performed. Vaginal or endocervical samples are preferred as first-catch urine samples are less sensitive and may miss up to 10% of infections.

For patients with a suspected underlying bleeding disorder, prothrombin time, activated partial thromboplastin time, and fibrinogen should be obtained. Adolescents presenting with acute abnormal uterine bleeding who report heavy bleeding since menarche should additionally undergo testing for von Willebrand disease including von Willebrand factor antigen, ristocetin cofactor assay, and factor VIII. Consultation with hematology is recommended to guide further evaluation.

For patients with signs or symptoms of thyroid disease, TSH should be measured and, if abnormal, free T4 obtained. For patients with signs of excess androgen production (hirsutism, acne, clitoromegaly) suggestive of PCOS or other causes of hyperandrogenism, androgen testing including total and free testosterone, dehydroepiandrosterone sulfate (DHEAS), and androstenedione (A4) should be obtained. For patients presenting with amenorrhea, headaches, or nipple discharge (i.e., galactorrhea), prolactin measurement should be obtained to evaluate for hyperprolactinemia.

MANAGEMENT

The management of abnormal uterine bleeding is based on the patient's clinical stability, acuity of symptoms, suspected underlying etiology, underlying medical conditions, and impact on quality of life. Once an underlying etiology has been identified, management should be tailored toward the specific underlying disease process. Management considerations by severity of abnormal uterine bleeding presentation can be found in **Table 42-4**.

In patients presenting with acute abnormal uterine bleeding, the main objectives in management are to control the current episode of heavy bleeding (acute therapy) and reduce menstrual blood loss in subsequent cycles (maintenance therapy). Hormonal therapy is the preferred treatment in the acute management period with dosing regimens guided by the degree of anemia, severity of bleeding, and hemodynamic stability. Once stabilized from an acute heavy menstrual bleeding event, a patient should be transitioned to maintenance therapy.

For patients presenting with chronic abnormal uterine bleeding, the primary objective is to reduce further blood loss and optimize quality of life. For patients presenting with anemia and/or iron deficiency, medical management with hormonal therapy and/or antifibrinolytics is recommended. In adolescents without anemia or iron deficiency, observation and reassurance are sufficient, though medical therapy should be discussed and offered if management is desired to optimize quality of life.

HORMONAL THERAPY

For both acute and chronic abnormal uterine bleeding, hormonal therapy with progestin alone, or in combination with estradiol, is considered first-line medical therapy. Progestins form the foundation of hormonal treatment by stabilizing the endometrial lining while estrogen provides hemostasis by inducing endometrial vascular vasospasm, increasing clotting factors, and stimulating endometrial proliferation which heals sites of endometrial bleeding. Multiple hormonal regimens have been shown to be effective with no clear consensus on the optimal approach. Hormonal regimens with both estrogen and progestin consists of combined hormonal contraceptives (CHCs), which includes combined oral contraceptives (COCs), combined vaginal rings, and combined hormonal patches. Progestin-only regimens include progestin-only pills, depot medroxyprogesterone acetate injections, etonogestrel implants, and levonorgestrel IUDs. The regimen should be individualized based on severity of presentation, acuity of bleeding, presence or absence of anemia, and potential contraindications to estrogen therapy. Example treatment regimens based on presentation severity can be found in Table 42-4. All patients should be evaluated for potential contraindications to certain hormone therapy regimens prior to initiation. For patients with contraindications to specific regimens, such as migraine with aura, SLE, high risk of recurrent deep venous thrombosis, or certain anticonvulsant use, hormone therapy should be tailored accordingly. A comprehensive list of contraindications can be found online at the CDC's U.S. Medical Eligibility Criteria for Contraceptive Use, 2016.

Abnormal Uterine Bleeding Without Acute Bleeding (Hgb 8-12) In patients with anemia that is not severe (Hgb 8-12 g/dL) and without acute bleeding, treatment with progestins alone or in combination with estradiol are recommended. Progestin-only treatments can be given cyclically to those who desire menstrual cycles or continuously for menstrual suppression. Commonly used progestin-only regimens include norethindrone, oral micronized progesterone, and medroxyprogesterone. Irregular spotting is common at initiation. For patients without contraindications to estrogen, progestins can be combined with estrogen, in the form of CHCs to allow for regular and predictable cycles and provide contraception. COCs with a minimum of 30 mcg ethinyl estradiol (to prevent breakthrough bleeding) are typically used if combination therapy is preferred.

Abnormal Uterine Bleeding With Acute Bleeding (Hgb < 12) For patients presenting with acute bleeding resulting in anemia (Hgb < 12), initial treatment should focus on the cessation of bleeding. Both high-dose progestin and high-dose estradiol therapy, in combination or alone, are quite effective with 90% of adolescents responding to treatment. Treatment options include IV conjugated equine estrogen, COCs, and oral progestins. While COCs and oral progestins typically stop bleeding within 3 days, IV conjugated equine estrogen stops bleeding within 8 hours in most patients. If using IV estrogen, it is important to initiate combined hormonal contraceptives as soon as possible to provide the progestin needed to stabilize the endometrium and prevent withdrawal bleeding upon IV estrogen discontinuation. Patients receiving high-dose estradiol may require anti-emetics for nausea and vomiting. Once current bleeding has stopped, medication should be tapered to lower dose,

TABLE 42-4 Management of Abnormal Uterine Bleeding (AUB)[a]

Management of Abnormal Uterine Bleeding (AUB)[a]
Mild (Hgb >12)
Reassurance
Menstrual calendar
Can consider treatment if patient/family desires
Consider iron supplementation
Observation with regular follow-up
Moderate without Acute Bleeding (Hgb 8-12)
Hormonal therapy with estrogen-progestin regimen or progestin-only regimen[b]
Estrogen-progestin regimen:
COC containing 30-35 µg ethinyl estradiol, one pill daily including placebo pills
Progestin-only regimens:
Medroxyprogesterone 10 mg × first 10 days of each calendar month
Norethindrone acetate 5 mg × first 5-10 days of each calendar month
Alternative non-hormonal therapy (for patients who decline hormonal treatment or hormonal therapy contraindicated):
Tranexamic acid 1,300 mg TID daily for 5 days of menses
Once symptoms controlled, other maintenance therapies can be considered including combined hormonal patches, combined hormonal rings, depot medroxyprogesterone acetate injections, etonogestrel implant, and levonorgestrel intrauterine device
Iron supplementation
Moderate with Acute Bleeding (Hgb 8-12)
High-dose hormonal therapy with estrogen-progestin regimen or progestin-only regimen until bleeding stops followed by taper[b]
Estrogen-progestin regimen:
Initial: COC containing 30-35 µg ethinyl estradiol, 1 pill every 6-8 hours until bleeding stops followed by,
Taper: 1 pill QID × 4 days, then 1 pill TID × 3 days, then 1 pill BID × 2 days, then 1 pill daily
Progestin-only regimen:
Initial: Medroxyprogesterone 10 mg (or norethindrone acetate 10 mg) every 6 hours until bleeding stops followed by,
Taper: 10 mg QID × 4 days, then 10 mg TID × 3 days, then 10 mg BID × 2 days, then 10 mg daily
Following taper, continue maintenance therapy (see regimen options for moderate AUB without acute bleeding above)
Antiemetics with high-dose estrogen
Iron supplementation
Severe with Acute Bleeding (Hgb <8)
Hospitalization required
High-dose hormonal therapy until bleeding stops followed by taper[b]
Estrogen-progestin regimen:
Initial: COC containing 35-50 µg ethinyl estradiol, 1 pill every 4-6 hours until bleeding stops followed by,
Taper: 1 pill QID × 4 days, then 1 pill TID × 3 days, then 1 pill BID × 2 days, then 1 pill daily
Progestin-only regimen:
Initial: Medroxyprogesterone 10 mg (or norethindrone acetate 10 mg) every 4-6 hours until bleeding stops followed by,
Taper: 10 mg QID × 4 days, then 10 mg TID × 3 days, then 10 mg BID × 2 days, then 10 mg daily
For patients unable to tolerate PO:
IV conjugated estrogen 25 mg every 4-6 hours until bleeding stops for up to 24 hours
As soon as able add oral progestin or transition to combined oral contraceptive regimen
If bleeding not improved within 24 hours, consider addition of hemostatic agent:
Tranexamic acid 10 mg/kg IV every 6-8 hours
Aminocaproic acid 100-200 mg/kg (max 30 g/day) IV or oral every 4-6 hours
Following taper, continue maintenance therapy (see regimen options for moderate abnormal uterine bleeding without acute bleeding above).
Skip placebo pills for one to three cycles if necessary for recovery of hemoglobin level
Antiemetics with high-dose estrogen
Iron supplementation

COC, combined oral contraceptive

[a]Significant variability exists in treatment regimens for abnormal uterine bleeding without clear consensus on an optimal regimen. The included regimens are to serve as an example. Individual patient characteristics and institutional practices should be considered when deciding treatment regimen.

[b]Hormonal therapy contraindications should be reviewed prior to initiating treatment, see the CDC U.S. Medical Eligibility Criteria for Contraceptive Use, 2016 (US MEC): https://www.cdc.gov/reproductivehealth/contraception/mmwr/mec/summary.html.

maintenance, hormone therapy. All patients presenting with acute bleeding should receive iron supplementation.

Maintenance Hormonal Therapy After the acute episode of bleeding is controlled and the initial course of hormonal therapy is completed, patients should be transitioned to a maintenance regimen. Hormonal therapy options include CHCs and progestin-only therapies. For patients who remain anemic at time of transition, menstrual suppression with continuous progestin regimens or non-placebo COC regimens can be considered. COCs can be discontinued after 6 months if anemia has resolved and if desired by the patient. For patients who desire contraception, intermittent progestin regimens should not be used. Though continuous progestin regimens can be used for contraception, they are not preferred given the need for extreme consistency in administration time which may be difficult for patient adherence.

NON-HORMONAL THERAPIES

Antifibrinolytics, such as tranexamic acid and aminocaproic acid, work by preventing fibrin degradation and have been shown to decrease bleeding alone and in conjunction with hormonal therapies. Tranexamic acid, the most commonly used antifibrinolytic, can be taken during menses for patients with chronic abnormal uterine bleeding and also be considered as adjunctive therapy in patients with severe acute abnormal uterine bleeding who do not respond to hormonal therapy within 24 to 48 hours. Increased risk of thromboembolism with the use of tranexamic acid has been reported but has been shown to be rare in short-term use and comparable to the risk attached to use of COCPs.

Nonsteroidal anti-inflammatory drugs (NSAIDs), including ibuprofen and naproxen, have been shown to reduce blood loss when compared with placebo and also treat dysmenorrhea, but are overall less effective than hormonal therapy or antifibrinolytics in treating heavy menstrual bleeding.

ADMISSION AND DISCHARGE CRITERIA

ADMISSION CRITERIA

Abnormal uterine bleeding is commonly managed safely in the outpatient setting. Indications for hospitalization include:

- Hemodynamic instability
- Severe anemia (Hgb < 8 g/dl)
- Heavy bleeding with Hgb < 10 g/dL
- Inability to tolerate oral medications
- Inadequate follow-up

DISCHARGE CRITERIA

- Hemodynamically stable, with control of excessive bleeding
- Ability to tolerate oral hormone therapy
- Reliable outpatient follow-up

CONSULTATION

Consultation with an adolescent medicine specialist is appropriate for any concerns regarding a patient with abnormal uterine bleeding. Adolescent medicine specialists are trained in and can help guide evaluation and management of abnormal uterine bleeding, using a teen-sensitive approach. This can be particularly helpful in managing abnormal uterine bleeding in patients with medical comorbidities where estrogen is contraindicated, or when patients do not respond to initial therapy.

Consultation with a hematologist is warranted in all patients with a known bleeding disorder as management may differ and include treatments such as DDAVP, antifibrinolytics, or factor replacements. In patients in which there is a strong suspicion for underlying bleeding disorder or abnormal initial screening for bleeding disorders, consultation with a hematologist is recommended to guide further evaluation and interpret results.

Gynecology consultation is indicated for patients who are hemodynamically unstable, who do not respond to medical management, or who have an underlying structural etiology. Though exceedingly rare in adolescents, surgical intervention such as dilation and curettage, or other procedures, such as hysteroscopy with polypectomy or myomectomy or uterine balloon tamponade, may be needed to control bleeding.

SPECIAL CONSIDERATIONS

POST DISCHARGE

Establishment of appropriate outpatient follow-up is essential prior to hospital discharge. Patients should be monitored closely for response to treatment, resolution of anemia, recurrence of bleeding, and medication side effects. In the immediate post-hospitalization period, patients are at risk for bleeding recurrence as hormonal therapies are tapered and may require adjustments. Long-term follow-up is required to ensure establishment of normal menstrual cycles and to re-evaluate need for continued therapy. Patients should follow-up with a provider comfortable with the management of abnormal uterine bleeding and titrating therapies including primary care clinician, adolescent medicine specialist, or adolescent gynecologist.

PREVENTION

Pediatricians should provide patients and their families with anticipatory guidance about normal pubertal development and discuss normal menstruation. Following menarche, clinicians should include a menstrual evaluation at each visit. This allows clinicians to detect abnormal menstrual pattens and identify potential underlying health concerns. Through routine evaluation of the menstrual cycle, clinicians can assist in early detection and treatment of abnormal uterine bleeding can prevent sequalae such as iron-deficiency anemia and reduced quality of life.

KEY POINTS

- Anovulatory cycles from HPO axis immaturity is the most common cause of abnormal uterine bleeding in adolescents within 3 years of menarche and most commonly presents with heavy menstrual bleeding.
- Anovulatory cycles from HPO axis immaturity remain a diagnosis of exclusion in the workup of abnormal uterine bleeding.
- It is important to perform a comprehensive history and physical examination to evaluate for any underlying medical etiologies.
- A pregnancy test is mandatory in the evaluation of any adolescent presenting with abnormal uterine bleeding.
- The primary objectives of treatment for acute and chronic abnormal uterine bleeding are to control current bleeding, minimize future blood loss, and improve quality of life.
- Treatment for abnormal uterine bleeding is determined by the underlying pathology, acuity of bleeding, and degree of anemia.
- Hormonal therapy with progestin alone, or in combination with estradiol, is the most effective treatment for abnormal uterine bleeding. The CDC's U.S. Medical Eligibility Criteria for Contraceptive Use, 2016 (US MEC) should be referenced to determine contraindications to hormonal treatment.
- Antiemetics are important with high-dose estrogen therapy.

SUGGESTED READINGS

Alaqzam TS, Stanley AC, Simpson PM, Flood VH, Menon S. Treatment modalities in adolescents who present with heavy menstrual bleeding. *J Pediatr Adolesc Gynecol.* 2018;31(5):451-458.

Benjamins LJ. Practice guideline: evaluation and management of abnormal vaginal bleeding in adolescents. *J Pediatr Health Care.* 2009; 23(3): 189-193.

Borzutzky C, Jaffray J. Diagnosis and management of heavy menstrual bleeding and bleeding disorders in adolescents. *JAMA Pediatr.* 2020; 174(2):186.

Committee Opinion No. 557: Management of acute abnormal uterine bleeding in nonpregnant reproductive-aged women. *Obstet Gynecol.* 2013;121(4):891-896.

Committee Opinion No. 651: Menstruation in girls and adolescents using the menstrual cycle as a vital sign. *Obstet Gynecol.* 2015;126(6): e143-e146.

Fraser I, Critchley H, Broder M, Munro M. The FIGO recommendations on terminologies and definitions for normal and abnormal uterine bleeding. *Semin Reprod Med.* 2011;29(05):383-390.

Haamid F, Sass AE, Dietrich JE. Heavy menstrual bleeding in adolescents. *J Pediatr Adolesc Gynecol.* 2017;30(3):335-340.

Hernandez A, Dietrich JE. Abnormal uterine bleeding in the adolescent. *Obstet Gynecol.* 2020;135(3):615-621.

Kabra R, Fisher M. Abnormal uterine bleeding in adolescents. *Curr Probl Pediatr Adolesc Health Care.* 2022;52(5):101185.

Munro MG, Critchley HOD, Broder MS, Fraser IS, for the FIGO Working Group on Menstrual Disorders. FIGO classification system (PALM-COEIN) for causes of abnormal uterine bleeding in nongravid women of reproductive age. *Int J Gynecol Obstet.* 2011;113(1):3-13.

Munro MG, Critchley HOD, Fraser IS, the FIGO Menstrual Disorders Committee. The two FIGO systems for normal and abnormal uterine bleeding symptoms and classification of causes of abnormal uterine bleeding in the reproductive years: 2018 revisions. *Int J Gynecol Obstet.* 2018;143(3):393-408.

Practice Bulletin No. 128: Diagnosis of abnormal uterine bleeding in reproductive-aged women. *Obstet Gynecol.* 2012;120(1):197-206.

CHAPTER 43 Care of Gender Diverse Youth

Amanda Bogart, MD and Anna Valentine, MD

BACKGROUND

Gender diverse youth are children and adolescents whose gender identity does not align with their sex assigned at birth. An individual's sex assigned at birth is typically male or female, based largely on the appearance of the external genitalia, sometimes in conjunction with available testing such as sex chromosomes identified on noninvasive prenatal testing by cell-free fetal DNA. Gender identity is defined as a person's innate sense of self, which may be congruent with their sex assigned at birth (cisgender), or incongruent with or opposite of their sex assigned at birth (transgender). Many consider gender identity to exist on a spectrum, which may range from male/masculine to female/feminine, though there are gender identities that exist apart from this spectrum, such as agender (without a gender), two-spirit, or genderqueer. A nonbinary identity is often described as being between male and female or having components of both male and female gender identities. The term "transgender" may be used as an umbrella term to describe a person who does not identify as cisgender, though not all gender diverse people personally identify as transgender. Many other descriptive terms continue to emerge and evolve over time as individuals gain the tools and language to better express their identities, which is why a "+" symbol was added to the acronym LGBTQ (lesbian, gay, bisexual, transgender, queer). LGBTQ+ is considered a more inclusive acronym, which reflects the expanding diversity of identities within the community.

A recent national survey reported 1.8% of American high school students identify as transgender, with an additional 1.6% responding that they were not sure if they identify as transgender. As the number of gender diverse youth accessing gender-affirming care increases, it is critical that pediatric hospitalists have familiarity with gender diversity, and awareness of gender-affirming treatments and their effects.

COMORBIDITIES

Some, but not all, gender diverse youth have gender dysphoria, which is the psychological distress that stems from having a gender identity that differs from one's sex assigned at birth, as defined by the Diagnostic and Statistical Manual of Mental Disorders (DSM), 5th edition. Gender diverse youth are three to four times more likely to experience clinically significant symptoms of depression when compared with same aged peers. In a 2022 survey of LGBTQ+ youth in the United States, more than half of transgender and nonbinary youth reported seriously contemplating suicide over the preceding 12 months. The estimated rates of prior suicide attempt among transgender youth are between 35% and 40%. Notably, in studies comparing gender diverse youth with and without social support, those who reported having family or trusted adults who affirmed their identity showed significant reductions in risk of depression, suicidal thinking, and suicide attempt. The Trevor Project's 2021 National Survey on LGBTQ Youth Mental Health also found marked reductions in history of suicide attempt within the last year for youth who were able to legally change their name and gender marker on government documents.

A 2017 national report surveying high school students in 10 states and nine large urban school districts found that transgender youth were significantly more likely to experience violence victimization compared to their cisgender peers. Specifically, these youth were more likely to report harassment at school, intimate partner violence, and sexual violence. Violence victimization is a known risk factor for substance abuse, and the same study identified that use of tobacco and other substances were also increased in the gender diverse population compared to cisgender peers.

Body image dissatisfaction and disordered eating (Chapter 40) have also been noted at high rates among gender diverse youth. Similar to substance use disorders, disordered eating patterns have been associated with prior history of violence victimization. Some gender diverse youth have admitted to intentional behaviors to change their weight to address gender dysphoria (i.e., gaining weight to hide perceived feminine curves, or aggressively losing weight to reduce appearance of breasts, or to slim what they perceive as a masculine, muscular body shape.)

Additionally, there is a higher odds of autism spectrum disorder among gender diverse youth compared with cisgender peers. Awareness of these potential co-morbidities and co-occurring diagnoses may enhance the individualization of each child's care during hospitalization.

HEALTH DISPARITIES

Gender diverse youth face a number of health disparities when compared with the general pediatric and adolescent population. These youth frequently experience discrimination in their schools, places of work, and often in medical offices. As a result, many gender diverse youth face barriers to age-appropriate preventive healthcare, such as screening for sexually transmitted infections, contraceptive counseling, and prompt medical evaluation for acute health concerns. Even a routine well visit may cause apprehension and distress for families, who may fear their child's reaction to unaffirming language, staff misgendering the patient (i.e., using names and pronouns that do not align with the child's identity), or staff disparaging parents who support their child due to lack of education on, or experience with the LGBTQ+ population. In a 2021 systematic review of experiences accessing medical care by gender diverse youth from 17 countries, major themes identified included barriers to care, stigma, and invalidation by healthcare providers, and internalized fear of being mistreated while accessing medical care. Protective factors included healthcare providers who were well-educated about gender identity and gender-affirming care, with whom youth felt they could partner to improve their health outcomes.

CLINICAL MANAGEMENT

PRONOUNS AND INTRODUCTIONS

Pronouns are words that are substituted for an individual's name that allow others to reference them in the third person. Examples include she/her, he/him, they/them, ze/zir, ze/hir, and elle (Spanish). This list is not exhaustive, and like all terminology, continues to evolve over time. Some gender diverse youth may use combinations of pronouns, such as he/they, or do not use any specific pronouns, and instead prefer to be referenced by their affirmed name. The phrase "preferred pronouns" is outdated and should be avoided, as it suggests that a person's gender identity is merely a preference and not intrinsic to that individual's sense of self. A more inclusive and supportive alternative might be to simply ask, *What pronouns do you use?*

Using the correct name and pronouns can contribute to a sense of safety during a time of distress. Gender diverse youth who feel safe and supported in their identify demonstrate improved health outcomes, including lower rates of mental health symptoms when compared to unsupported peers. Providers and hospital teams can create an inclusive environment for all patients and their families by introducing themselves by name and pronouns in addition to stating their role on the team. While a patient's legal name and sex may be included on their medical chart and identification band, care teams should avoid the presumption that a patient's legal name or sex align with their gender identity, or the way they wish to be addressed by their team.

For example, upon entering the patient's room, the resident physician might say, *Hi, I'm Dr. Smith, my pronouns are she/her/hers, and I am the senior resident physician on your team. What name and pronouns are you most comfortable with me using to address each of you during this admission?* This open introduction establishes that learning a person's name and pronouns is not an experience unique to patients who might appear to be gender diverse, and informs the patient and accompanying support people that the team is interested in making every person feel safe and seen during the admission. In scenarios where a patient is in the process of exploring their gender identity, this introduction also provides an opportunity for a patient to choose to disclose or not disclose the pronouns they may use in private spaces. For children and adolescents who are exploring their gender identity but have not shared with their parents, this creates space for a patient to later inform members of the care team if they have a name or pronouns they want to be used when their guardians are out of the room.

SENSITIVITY WITH PHYSICAL EXAMINATIONS

As described earlier in this chapter, gender diverse youth are at increased risk for violence victimization, and many experience dysphoria related to particular body parts, including the chest area or genitalia. As with all pediatric physical examinations of sensitive areas, it is important to ensure patient autonomy and respect for their rights to accept or decline examinations. In order to partner with the patient to meet their healthcare needs, it is useful to explain why a physical examination of sensitive anatomy may be necessary (e.g., screening for cancer, evaluating for cause of pain). Language is important in creating safe spaces for patients, and if a particular area of anatomy will require continued evaluation or assessment, care team members can ask patients if there are medical anatomy terms that they would prefer not to be used, allowing the patient to provide an alternative, equally specific term during the examination. For patients assigned female at birth who identify as gender diverse, and may have dysphoria related to their body, there are some common alternatives to medical anatomical terms that can be helpful. These include chest tissue instead of breasts, and bleeding episode instead of periods or menstruation. Some pediatric patients and their families may already use medical terms comfortably; for those patients it might be appropriate to continue to use medical terminology such as penis, testicles, uterus, or vagina.

GENDER-AFFIRMING INTERVENTIONS

When caring for gender diverse youth in the inpatient setting, it is important to be aware of any medical, surgical, and other supportive interventions the patient receives as part of their ongoing care. Understanding these interventions contributes to a supportive treatment environment, and patient-centered care. Gender diverse youth may receive a wide range of interventions as part of their care including mental health services, nonmedical interventions, medications, and in rare cases, surgeries. Importantly, while some youth will pursue gender-affirming hormone therapy and/or surgery, many do not pursue any medical interventions for a wide variety of reasons. Thus, providers must not make assumptions about any previous or future medical or surgical care that gender diverse youth have had, or desire, based on their gender identity.

Many gender diverse youth access mental health services to explore their gender identity, address co-morbid conditions such as anxiety or depression, and/or to assess readiness for gender-affirming hormone therapy. The World Professional Association for Transgender Health (WPATH) has published guidelines for mental health professionals working with gender diverse youth, as well as criteria for proceeding with both reversible and irreversible medical interventions. The following sections briefly highlight potential interventions that hospitalized patients may have accessed or intend to access as part of their ongoing care.

Nonmedical Gender-Affirming Interventions Whether or not gender diverse youth pursue any medical interventions, they may utilize other supports to affirm their gender identity (**Table 43-1**). A social transition consists of changing one's name and pronouns to align with their gender identity and may also involve changing one's outward appearance such as in hair, clothing, and makeup to align their gender expression with their gender identity.

Chest dysphoria, or the distress caused by the presence of breast tissue in a person who does not identify as female, can lead to social isolation, inconsistent bathing practices to avoid seeing their body, and weight gain due to discomfort exercising in public. While chest dysphoria can be irreversibly treated with gender-affirming chest surgery, reversible treatment options for patients who are either not of age to receive the surgery, or not planning to pursue surgery, can

TABLE 43-1 Nonmedical Interventions for GDY

Non-medical Intervention	Description	Considerations
Social transition	Changing to gender identity-aligned name and pronouns in social settings (school, home, work, peer groups)	Parents, family, and peers may struggle with changes to the youth's name and pronouns In many but not all states, the school can update the child's name without a legal name change A social transition may or may not include changes in gender expression (hair style, clothing, activities, friendship groups) that align with the patient's identity. Gender expression is not the same as gender identity
Chest binding or taping	Garment or accessory that compresses breast tissue to flatten the appearance of the chest Recommended use < 8 hours per day; should not be worn in sleep or during exercise (unless using a larger size)	Should be sized appropriately to patient's chest per manufacturer guidelines Possible risks: truncal acne, itching/skin irritation, shortness of breath, musculoskeletal pain, or difficulty breathing Rib fractures are rare with appropriate use
Voice therapy	Working with a trained speech therapist to safely modulate vocal pitch	Several informal, at-home voice therapy resources exist. Professional support may reduce risk of vocal cord injury
Packing	Use of a prosthetic phallus under clothing to simulate a genital bulge	
Genital tucking	Positioning the penis behind the legs, moving the testicles upward into the inguinal canal or abdomen to reduce appearance of a bulge	Prolonged tucking or tucking tightly may increase risk of orchitis, cystitis, hernia, or testicular torsion. Case reports of lower sperm count due to elevated body temperature have been published.

include the use of a chest binder or tape. Chest binders are tight garments worn under clothing that flatten the appearance of breast tissue. Binders come in sizes based on measurements and should be appropriately fitted to a patient before use. Most patients with asthma or other chronic respiratory conditions can safely wear a binder, but should not use them during acute illnesses (e.g., asthma exacerbation, pneumonia). When safely used, binders may allow hospitalized patients to feel more affirmed during their course of treatment. Trans tape, similar to kinesiology tape, has been used by some transmasculine and nonbinary youth to similarly reduce the appearance of the chest area. If the binder or tape is too tight, or the chest is restricted beyond 8 hours per day, complications may include shortness of breath, or in rare cases, rib fracture.

Voice dysphoria is a common experience for many gender diverse youth, but may be particularly distressing for transfeminine or nonbinary patients who have experienced some or all of a masculinizing puberty. Beyond the personal distress, female presenting youth who have experienced the permanent deepening of their voice due to pubertal testosterone exposure may face discrimination or risk unintentional disclosure of their gender history. Feminizing hormone therapy does not raise a person's vocal pitch, leaving many medically transitioned patients with a voice that does not align with their gender identity. Voice therapy, which involves vocal exercises with the support of a speech therapist, has been shown to reduce voice dysphoria and reduce the risk of vocal strain or vocal cord disorders as a result of overuse.

For transmasculine youth who experience dysphoria related to the lack of male genitalia, the use of a prosthetic phallus, or genital packing, can alleviate distress by creating a bulge similar to a penis under their clothing. Devices that allow patients without a penis to urinate while standing can also help alleviate social dysphoria and contribute to safety in public, especially for youth accessing public, male-gendered bathrooms. While stalls do exist in most bathrooms, sitting down or facing forward may result in an unintentional disclosure, which has been cited as the impetus for violence and harassment of transmasculine and nonbinary youth in public.

Youth assigned male at birth who do not identify as male, may experience genital or "bottom" dysphoria, which (similarly to chest dysphoria) can impact personal hygiene, limit the clothing they can comfortably wear or their desire to socialize, and exacerbate depressive symptoms. Gender-affirming genital surgery can irreversibly address genital dysphoria for adults but may not be accessible to many patients due to lack of competent providers, the patient's age, financial barriers to the surgery, or support for recovery following the surgery. Some patients may engage in genital tucking, which is the process of reducing the appearance of the bulge from penis and testicles by pushing the penis behind the legs, and the testicles upward into the inguinal canal or abdomen. If tucked too tightly or for prolonged periods of time, tucking may increase the risk of cystitis, orchitis, or hernia. Prompt medical evaluation is recommended for patients who tuck their genitals and present with scrotal or penile pain.

Fully Reversible Medical Interventions Fully reversible medical interventions include medications used for puberty suppression, menstrual suppression, and anti-androgen therapy (**Table 43-2**). The goal of pubertal suppression is to pause and delay masculinizing or feminizing changes to a person's body to prevent the distress associated with those changes. For patients assigned female at birth, starting puberty blockers may delay or prevent the development of noticeable breast tissue and feminine body fat redistribution, as well menarche. For patients assigned male at birth, puberty blockers can delay or prevent the permanent deepening of a young person's voice, development of an Adam's apple, and the growth of coarse facial and body hair. Gonadotropin-releasing hormone agonists (GnRHas) have been used since the 1980s for treatment of central precocious puberty, and work by quieting the hypothalamic-pituitary-gonadal (HPG) axis through suppression of luteinizing hormone (LH) secretion. Similar to their use in central precocious puberty, withdrawal of the medication through discontinuation of injections or removal of the implant allows the HPG axis to reactivate and return to typical functioning with stimulation of the gonads to secrete estrogen (ovaries) or testosterone (testes). Experiencing periods can be stressful for all youth assigned female at birth but is particularly distressing for those who do not identify as female. The goal of menstrual suppression is to eliminate or significantly reduce the bleeding and cramping from menstrual cycles in patients who have already experienced menarche and are not candidates for puberty blockers. Anti-androgen medications work by blocking testosterone action at the androgen receptor, resulting in slowed facial and body hair growth in patients who were not able to access puberty suppression before these changes occurred.

TABLE 43-2 Reversible Medical Interventions for Gender Diverse Youth

Intervention	Medication	Potential Side Effects (Reversible)
Puberty suppression	GnRHa Injection (leuprolide acetate) Implant (histrelin acetate) Progesterone	Mood changes, weight gain, delayed growth spurt, decreased relative bone mineral density
Menstrual suppression	Progestin-only contraceptives Oral (norethindrone acetate) Injection (medroxyprogesterone) Implanted device (etonogestrel, levonorgestrel) Combined estrogen-progestin contraceptives Oral (multiple formulations) Patch (multiple formulations)	Mood changes, weight changes more likely with medroxyprogesterone injections. Progestin-only pills have short half-life, and late or missed doses may result in irregular spotting or bleeding.
Anti-androgen therapy	Spironolactone Finasteride, dutasteride Cyproterone acetate	Hyperkalemia, orthostatic intolerance, decreased erections, decreased sperm count, gynecomastia

Partially Reversible Interventions Partially reversible interventions include masculinizing and feminizing hormone therapy with testosterone and estradiol, respectively. Testosterone therapy can be delivered via injection or transdermal application. Estradiol is given exclusively as 17-beta estradiol when administered orally, sublingually, or transdermally, and in various formulations when administered by injection. Ethinyl estradiol is no longer recommended for use in gender-affirming hormone therapy given its association with increased risk of venous thromboembolism (VTE). Routes and frequencies of administration are noted below in **Table 43-3**. Masculinizing and feminizing effects are noted in **Tables 43-3** and **43-5**, respectively.

Irreversible Interventions Irreversible interventions include surgical procedures such as chest masculinizing surgery (mastectomy), genital feminizing (vaginoplasty) and masculinizing (phalloplasty) surgeries, facial feminizing surgery, and chondrolaryngoplasty (tracheal shave). Genital surgery is generally not available to minors but may be pursued once individuals reach the age of majority and meet the standards of care. At the time of this chapter's writing, gender-affirming chest surgeries for minors remain controversial, and access to surgery for older adolescents is limited depending on geographic access, insurance coverage, and parental support.

One common gender-affirming surgery for older adolescents assigned female at birth is chest masculinizing surgery, colloquially referred to as "top surgery." The WPATH Standards of Care do not require any length of time on gender-affirming hormone therapy prior to chest surgery, as

TABLE 43-3 Administration of Masculinizing and Feminizing Hormone Therapy

Medication	Route of Administration	Frequency of Administration
Testosterone	Injection, subcutaneous	Every 7 days
	Injection, intramuscular	Every 7-14 days
	Transdermal (gel, patch)	Daily
Estradiol	Transdermal (patch)	Change 1-2 times weekly
	Oral	Daily
	Sublingual	Daily
	Injection, intramuscular	Every 7-14 days

TABLE 43-4 Expected Effects of Masculinizing Hormone Therapy

Effect	Onset
Acne, oily skin	1-6 months
Fat redistribution	1-6 months
Clitoral enlargement*	1-6 months
Vaginal atrophy	1-6 months
Cessation of menses	1-6 months
Increased muscle mass with exercise	6-12 months
Facial/body hair growth	6-12 months
Deepening voice*	6-12 months
Androgenic hair loss	6-12 months

*Irreversible.

Source: Adapted from WPATH Standards of Care.

not all patients with chest dysphoria intend to pursue masculinizing hormone therapy as part of their medical care. While there are several technical approaches, the goal outcome of the surgery is both reduction and recontouring of the breast tissue, resulting in a masculine chest contour and appearance. Hematoma, seroma, and infection are the most common complications of the procedure. Breast cancer risk is not eliminated by the procedure due to residual breast tissue; patients who have undergone chest masculinizing surgery will still need cancer surveillance as they age but will not be able to undergo mammography due to lack of sufficient tissue.

Gender-affirming hysterectomy may be pursued by young adults assigned female at birth, to address uncontrolled vaginal bleeding that is refractory to other treatments, or dysphoria related to the presence of a uterus. Due to the importance of sex steroids in the prevention of bone disease, oophorectomy is recommended only for patients who intend to remain on lifelong testosterone, or who may be comfortable taking estrogen replacement therapy in the future. For those intending to use testosterone lifelong, bilateral salpingoophorectomy often accompanies hysterectomy, and can eliminate the risk of ovarian cancer.

Gender-affirming genital surgeries for patients assigned male at birth are generally performed in adulthood. These may include orchiectomy and vaginoplasty. Vaginoplasty requires ongoing supportive treatment for dilation and maintenance of the new vaginal canal.

CONTINUING CARE DURING HOSPITAL ADMISSION

Many electronic health records already allow for identification of patients by their affirmed (in addition to legal) names to ensure that patients feel respected by their care team. In addition, regardless of the reason for hospitalization, patients should not be denied access to their gender-affirming treatments unless contraindicated for medical reasons, as withholding these therapies could have detrimental effects on the youth's mental and physical health. If the primary team is considering withholding any gender-affirming hormone therapy during admission, consultation with child's outpatient prescribing team is recommended.

TABLE 43-5 Expected Effects of Feminizing Hormone Therapy

Effect	Onset
Decreased spontaneous erections	1-3 months
Decreased libido	1-3 months
Breast growth	3-6 months
Skin softening, decreased oiliness	3-6 months
Fat redistribution	3-6 months
Decreased muscle mass	3-6 months
Decreased testicular volume	3-6 months
Decreased facial/body hair	6-12 months
Erectile dysfunction	Variable
Scalp hair growth	Variable
Decreased sperm production	Unknown
Voice change	Does not occur

Source: Adapted from WPATH Standards of Care.

Efforts should be made to continue hormone therapy and menstrual suppression during the admission, to avoid the risk of waning hormone levels and exacerbating dysphoria during hospitalization. In cases where medication access may be a limiting factor, such as for GnRHa therapy, consideration should be given to using home medications or specialty pharmacy ordering to avoid the risk of irreversible breakthrough puberty. Short-term exceptions may be reasonable for patients hospitalized due to a complication of their treatment (i.e., VTE in a patient on estradiol for gender-affirming care). It is important to consider that unlike cisgender women on hormonal contraception, transgender women and nonbinary patients assigned male at birth may not have safe alternatives to estrogen medications to manage their dysphoria, and may still opt to continue estrogen despite significant medical complications.

Acute care for the transgender patient should be sensitively executed. A detailed history should be taken for all complaints using affirming language. Care should be taken to avoid assumptions about a patient's psychosocial experiences. An age-appropriate adolescent sexual history should include whether and how a patient engages in sex with others (oral, anal, vaginal/penile), and providers should avoid presuming a sexual partner's anatomy based on the patient's reported sexual orientation.

For example, JR is a 16-year-old transgender male who has been on testosterone for 2 years, presenting to the hospital with lower abdominal pain for 1 week. He reports having sex with only his girlfriend of 2 years. Without additional questioning, the provider may assume that JR is not at risk for pregnancy or vaginal infections. In fact, JR's girlfriend is also transgender, and still has a penis and testicles. JR is still at risk for pregnancy, cervicitis, and pelvic inflammatory disease. Patients who have a uterus and ovaries presenting with abdominal pain should be evaluated for pregnancy, STI, ovarian cysts and torsion, in addition to the gender-neutral differential diagnoses such as appendicitis, colitis, or bowel obstruction.

Youth assigned male at birth who identify as feminine or nonbinary, presenting with complaints of abdominal or pelvic pain should similarly have a thorough social history taken, and be evaluated for testicular torsion, epididymitis, orchitis, and cystitis. A history of tucking would be important to elicit if there are abdominal or genitourinary complaints.

Considerations for Continuing Estradiol During Hospitalization

Gender diverse youth on feminizing hormone therapy are prescribed 17-beta estradiol, which is more physiologic and has lower VTE and cardiovascular risk than ethinyl estradiol. While the risk of VTE is lower, attention must be paid to each individual's risk of clotting during admission. Admitted patients who are not ambulating may require consideration of VTE prophylaxis, such as sequential compression devices, physical therapy involvement, and sometimes anti-coagulation medication, depending on the unique patient scenario. Recent studies looking at perioperative risk associated with estradiol use have been inconclusive, and at this time routine discontinuation of estradiol preoperatively and during hospitalization is not recommended. If there is question regarding continued estradiol administration during hospitalization, the hospitalist team should consult the patient's outpatient specialist.

Considerations for Continuing Testosterone During Hospitalization

Testosterone increases hemoglobin/hematocrit (H/H), leading to higher reference values in males than females. Complete blood counts are often ordered during hospital admission and may reveal elevated H/H above reference values for the patient's female sex assigned at birth. Higher risk of VTE exists when hematocrit > 50%, and if this value persists outside of the setting of dehydration, the patient's outpatient prescribing team should be consulted to discuss the need for dose adjustment.

SPECIAL CONSIDERATIONS

CREATING AN INCLUSIVE HOSPITAL CULTURE

Along with individual healthcare providers and team members, hospital systems should work to create and foster an inclusive environment where gender diverse youth feel safe and validated. At the institutional level, welcoming signage to show support and inclusion of the LGBTQ+ community, along with gender neutral or all-gender bathrooms, can help offer a sense of belonging. Other specific measures can include electronic health records that prominently display the patient's affirmed name at the top of each chart, and patient wristbands that include the affirmed name and exclude sex markers. When communicating in public spaces with the patient or family, or needing to confirm the patient's name and date of birth, consider using the affirmed name or last name. Because gender disclosure can be important for medical risk and evaluation, providing a private space for safe disclosure is paramount. When surveyed, gender diverse individuals responded that they value healthcare environments where the providers and clinical team all use inclusive language, treat identity disclosure (such as pronouns) as routine, and show experience and knowledge about gender diverse people and their healthcare needs. Institutions should require training for all employees that includes the care of gender diverse youth, as education of learners, healthcare personnel, and hospital staff can foster an overall hospital culture that promotes a welcoming atmosphere. Overall, these measures not only promote a culture of inclusion, but also decrease the risk of depression and suicidality.

KEY POINTS

- Approach all youth and caregivers with open-ended questions and introductions to promote safety during hospital care.
- Consider how medical and nonmedical interventions may impact differential diagnoses and medical workup in hospital care of gender diverse youth.
- When safe and possible, continue all gender-affirming care during hospitalization.

SUGGESTED READINGS

Chong LSH, Kerklaan J, Clarke S, et al. Experiences and perspectives of transgender youths in accessing health care: a systematic review. *JAMA Pediatr.* 2021;175(11):1159-1173.

Coleman E, Radix AE, Bouman WP, et al. Standards of care for the health of transgender and gender diverse people, Version 8. *Int J Transgend Health.* 2022 S;23(Suppl 1):S1-S259.

Hembree WC, Cohen-Kettenis PT, Gooren L. Endocrine treatment of gender-dysphoric/gender-incongruent persons: an endocrine society clinical practice guideline. *J Clin Endocrinol Metab.* 2017;102(11):3869-3903.

Johns MM, Lowry R, Andrzejewski J, et al. Transgender identity and experiences of violence victimization, substance use, suicide risk, and sexual risk behaviors among high school students—19 states and large urban school districts, 2017. *MMWR Morb Mortal Wkly Rep.* 2019; 68(3):67-71.

Rafferty J, Committee on Psychosocial Aspects of Child and Family Health, Committee on Adolescence, Section on Lesbian, Gay, Bisexual, and Transgender Health and Wellness, et al. Ensuring comprehensive care and support for transgender and gender-diverse children and adolescents. *Pediatrics.* 2018;142(4):e20182162.

Wiepjes CM, Nota NM, de Blok CJM, et al. The Amsterdam cohort of gender dysphoria study (1972-2015): trends in prevalence, treatment, and regrets. *J Sex Med.* 2018;15(4):582-590.

CHAPTER 44 Care of Young Adults

W. Aaron Manning, MD, Eleanor Floyd, MD, and Rachel J. Peterson, MD

BACKGROUND

Medical advancements for treating pediatric illness have progressed significantly over the past several decades. As a result, patients with complex medical conditions of childhood are living longer and developing more typical "adult" conditions as well. These patients are often followed by pediatric subspecialists well into their third decade of life or longer and are thus frequently admitted to pediatric institutions. Accordingly, the number of transitional age (18-21 years) and older (>22 years) patients admitted to children's hospitals has increased. A recent study of 30 tertiary care children's hospitals in the United States showed that 4.4% of patients discharged from 2004 to 2019 were age 18 or older, and that the number of these adult discharges is increasing yearly. Pediatric hospitalists, therefore, need to know how to provide high-quality care for young adults and should be familiar with medical conditions commonly encountered in hospitalized adults.

ADULT MEDICAL CONDITIONS

CHEST PAIN

The differential diagnosis for chest pain in the adult patient is broad and is often grouped into common and "can't miss" diagnoses, where missing a diagnosis can lead to a high risk of morbidity or mortality. Common etiologies include many diagnoses already familiar to most pediatricians, including musculoskeletal chest pain, gastroesophageal reflux disease, anxiety, pericarditis, and pneumonia. Conversely, many of the "can't miss" diagnoses, including acute coronary syndromes (ACS), pulmonary embolism (PE), arrythmia, spontaneous pneumothorax, and aortic dissection, range from uncommon to extremely rare in the pediatric population.

Acute Coronary Syndrome (ACS) When evaluating an adult patient with chest pain, first determine whether the chest pain is typical for ACS. Typical chest pain is substernal, brought on by exertion, and resolves with rest or nitroglycerin. Any patient with typical chest pain warrants prompt evaluation for ACS. Other historical features that make ACS more likely are radiation of the pain to the left arm, right arm, or the jaw (with the radiation to the right arm having the highest likelihood ratio for ACS at 4.7), and association with nausea, vomiting, or diaphoresis. Exam findings that increase the likelihood of ACS include hypotension, a third heart sound, and pulmonary crackles. Conversely, certain characteristics make ACS less likely, including pleuritic or "sharp" pain, pain reproduced by movement or palpation, discomfort that can be localized with one finger, and pain that is short in duration (**Table 44-1**).

TABLE 44-1 Diagnosis of ACS

Signs, Symptoms, and Exam Findings

ACS MORE Likely	ACS LESS Likely
Substernal chest pain	Pleuritic or sharp chest pain
Chest pain brought on by exertion	Chest pain reproduced by movement or palpation
Chest pain resolves with rest or nitroglycerine	Chest pain can be localized with one finger
Chest pain radiates to the left arm, right arm, or jaw	Chest pain is short in duration (seconds to a few minutes)
Chest pain associated with nausea, vomiting, or diaphoresis	
Hypotension present	
Pulmonary crackles present	
Third heart sound present	

Importantly, women, older adults, and patients with diabetes may have atypical presentations.

Hospitalists should have a very low threshold to obtain an electrocardiogram (ECG) and high-sensitivity troponin in an adult patient who develops acute chest pain not easily explained by an alternate etiology. Troponin levels may not become elevated until a few hours after symptom onset. If the initial troponin is negative and a high suspicion for ACS remains, then the troponin should be repeated 2 to 3 hours after symptom onset. Similarly, an initial ECG obtained shortly after symptom onset may be nondiagnostic and should be repeated every 15 minutes if clinical suspicion remains high. Treatment of ACS varies significantly depending on the specific coronary syndrome present and should be guided by a cardiologist. Thus, early involvement of cardiology when ACS is suspected (high clinical suspicion based on presentation, elevated troponin, >1 mm ST-segment elevation in two anatomically contiguous leads, new left bundle branch block, or ST-segment depression on ECG) is critical to help guide workup and management. A normal troponin and/or ECG should not delay cardiology consultation when clinical suspicion for ACS is high, as again these tests may be normal when obtained shortly after symptom onset.

If the suspicion for ACS is high, a dose of aspirin 325 mg should be administered orally or rectally while awaiting cardiology input if there is no absolute contraindication to this medication such as a life-threatening bleed. Patients should also be given supplemental oxygen to keep oxygen saturation greater than 90%. For chest discomfort, sublingual nitroglycerin 0.4 mg may be given every 5 minutes for up to three doses if the patient is not taking a phosphodiesterase inhibitor (e.g., sildenafil used for erectile dysfunction) and there is no evidence of hemodynamic compromise which may suggest a right ventricular infarction. Intravenous morphine 2 to 4 mg may be given for chest pain refractory to nitrates. Depending on the coronary syndrome present, patients may be treated with reperfusion therapy (percutaneous coronary intervention or fibrinolytics) or no reperfusion therapy. In both scenarios, patients are generally also treated with antiplatelet (ticagrelor, prasugrel, or clopidogrel in addition to aspirin) and anticoagulant (unfractionated heparin, enoxaparin, fondaparinux, or bivalirudin) therapy. The dosing and timing of these agents should be guided by a cardiologist.

Pulmonary Embolism Acute pulmonary embolism (PE) should also be considered in an adult patient with unexplained chest pain. Patients with acute PE typically complain of pleuritic chest pain and dyspnea on exertion. Common exam findings include tachypnea, tachycardia, and calf swelling or tenderness. Hypotension and jugular venous distention may be seen with high- or intermediate-risk PEs which cause right ventricular dysfunction.

When evaluating a patient for PE, a risk-stratification tool such as the Wells' Criteria for PE or Revised Geneva Score should be used to identify patients with a low, intermediate, or high probability of PE. For patients who are stratified as low probability, the Pulmonary Embolism Rule-Out Criteria (PERC) score should then be applied and can safely rule out PE without need for additional testing if all PERC criteria are fulfilled (**Table 44-2**).

If all PERC criteria are not fulfilled, additional testing should be pursued. In this situation most guidelines recommend obtaining a D-dimer, which is a very sensitive (but not specific) test for thromboembolism that identifies a fibrin degradation product produced during clot breakdown. A D-dimer should also be obtained in all patients with an intermediate probability of PE. In patients with a high probability of PE and patients with a low or intermediate probability who also have an elevated D-dimer, CT angiography (or a ventilation/perfusion scan if the patient has a contraindication to IV contrast) should be performed.

Once identified, PEs should be classified as high-risk (also called massive), intermediate-risk (also called sub-massive), or low-risk. PEs are classified as high-risk if associated with hemodynamic instability, generally defined as a systolic blood pressure <90 mmHg or a drop in systolic blood pressure of ≥40 mmHg from baseline. PEs are classified as intermediate-risk if there is evidence of right-ventricular strain on laboratory testing (elevated high-sensitivity troponin or B-Type Natriuretic Peptide) or echocardiography, but no hemodynamic instability. Low-risk PEs are not associated with hemodynamic instability or right-ventricular strain. Therapeutic anticoagulation is generally indicated once a PE is identified, although emerging data suggests some low-risk patients with isolated subsegmental PEs (small peripheral emboli occurring in the more distal subsegmental pulmonary arteries) may not need anticoagulation. Conversely, patients with high- or intermediate-risk PEs may warrant thrombolytic therapy. Hematology and/or pulmonology consultation is recommended to assist in the management of these patients.

SUBSTANCE USE DISORDERS

Substance use disorders (SUD) are frequently encountered in the hospitalized adult population. Management varies greatly based on the specific substance a patient is using, and so it is important to specify the known substance(s) that the patient uses to better identify potential toxicity and withdrawal symptoms. Alcohol use disorder and opioid use disorder are two of the most commonly encountered SUDs in hospitalized adult patients and should not be missed due to their significant withdrawal symptoms and associated morbidity and mortality.

Alcohol Use Disorder and Alcohol Withdrawal Alcohol use disorder (AUD) is prevalent among youth and young adults. According to the National Survey on Drug Use and Health, 1.7% of youth aged 12 to 17 and 10.1% of those aged 18 to 25 (the highest of any age group) met criteria for AUD. Some percentage of these patients will be at risk of alcohol withdrawal while hospitalized; the AUDIT-PC is a validated predictor of alcohol withdrawal in hospitalized patients.

Alcohol withdrawal symptoms typically develop between 6 and 24 hours after the last ingestion, and life-threatening withdrawal syndromes can occur after 6 to 96 hours. Initial withdrawal signs and symptoms include anxiety, agitation, hallucinations or illusions, diaphoresis, tremulousness, nausea/vomiting, tachycardia, and hypertension. If untreated, symptoms may progress to include seizures and delirium tremens, potentially resulting in death. The mainstay of alcohol withdrawal treatment is benzodiazepines, which both treat symptoms of withdrawal and prevent progression to more severe withdrawal. Some patients may require high doses of these medications, necessitating intensive care unit admission. Symptom-triggered rather than fixed-dosing of benzodiazepines improves patient outcomes. Several validated scoring systems for severity of alcohol withdrawal have been published and should be used to guide symptom-triggered treatment (**Table 44-3**). These scoring systems can be protocolized and administered by bedside nursing staff in patients at risk of alcohol withdrawal.

All patients with AUD should be treated with thiamine 100 mg (oral or IV) daily to prevent Wernicke encephalopathy and Korsakoff syndrome. If signs of Wernicke encephalopathy develop (encephalopathy, oculomotor dysfunction, and gait ataxia comprise the classic triad of symptoms), the dose should be increased to 500 mg IV three times daily for 2 days followed by 250 mg IV daily for five additional days. Additionally, all patients with AUD should be offered mediation-assisted treatment to help them achieve abstinence. Options include naltrexone 50 to 100 mg daily (preferred option but contraindicated if liver enzymes are ≥ 3 times upper limit of normal), acamprosate 666 mg three times daily, topiramate 25 mg once daily, or disulfiram 250 to 500 mg daily. Patients should also be offered any locally available resources to encourage alcohol cessation, such as outpatient or inpatient substance use treatment programs.

Opioid Use Disorder (OUD) and Opioid Withdrawal Opioid use is less common than alcohol use, but the 18 to 25 age group remains the most affected; 4.1% of this age group reported misuse of opioids in the 2020 National Survey on Drug Use and Health. Symptoms suggestive of opioid withdrawal include diaphoresis, mydriasis, rhinorrhea, yawning, piloerection, anxiety, irritability, muscle and joint aches, and gastrointestinal upset. Withdrawal symptoms may develop as soon as 6 to 12 hours after last heroin or short-acting opioid use, while patients misusing opioids with a longer half-life (such as methadone) may develop symptoms after a longer timeframe. The Clinical Opiate Withdrawal Scale (COWS) is a tool which can be used to track severity of withdrawal symptoms and to determine when treatment should be initiated (**Table 44-4**).

Although opioid withdrawal is not life-threatening, it should be identified and managed appropriately as it can cause patients significant distress during a hospitalization and can contribute to a patient's decision

TABLE 44-2 Pulmonary Embolism Risk-Stratification Scores

Scoring Tool	*Wells' Criteria for PE*	*Revised Geneva Score*	*PERC Score*
Utility	Provides an estimated pre-test probability for PE	Provides an estimated pre-test probability for PE	If low initial pre-test probability (using Wells' or Revised Geneva Scores), PERC Score can rule out PE without need for additional testing
Interpretation and Management	If 0-1 points, patient has low probability of PE. PERC Score should be used to determine need for further testing. If 2-6 points, patient has intermediate probability of PE. A D-dimer should be obtained, and CT angiography or ventilation/perfusion (V/Q) scan performed if D-dimer is elevated. If >6 points, patient has high probability of PE. CT angiography or V/Q scan should be performed.	If 0-3 points, patient has low probability of PE. PERC Score should be used to determine need for further testing. If 4-10 points, patient has intermediate probability of PE. A D-dimer should be obtained, and CT angiography or V/Q scan performed if D-dimer is elevated. If >10 points, patient has high probability of PE. CT angiography or V/Q scan should be performed.	If all of the below criteria are fulfilled, no additional testing for PE is indicated. If one or more criteria are fulfilled, a D-dimer should be obtained, and CT angiography or V/Q scan performed if D-dimer is elevated.
Score Components	Clinical signs and symptoms of DVT = 3 points	Age > 65 = 1 point	Age < 50 years
	Alternative diagnoses are less likely than PE = 3 points	Previously diagnosed thromboembolism = 3 points	Initial heart rate < 100 beats/min
	Heart rate >100 = 1.5 points	Surgery or lower limb fracture in past month = 2 points	Initial oxygen saturation >94% on room air
	Immobilization for at least 3 days OR surgery in previous 4 weeks = 1.5 points	Active malignant condition = 2 points	No unilateral leg swelling
	Previously diagnosed thromboembolism = 1.5 points	Unilateral lower limb pain = 3 points	No hemoptysis
	Hemoptysis = 1 point	Hemoptysis = 2 points	No surgery or trauma within 4 weeks
		Heart rate 75-94 (= 3 points) or greater than 94 (= 5 points)	No history of venous thromboembolism
		Pain on lower limb palpation and unilateral edema = 4 points	No estrogen use

to leave the hospital before medically ready. Additionally, offering treatment to patients with OUD is increasingly imperative given the rapidly rising number of overdose deaths nationally. If an outpatient clinic that can provide medication-assisted treatment is available on discharge, providers should consider initiating buprenorphine or methadone during the hospitalization. Typical starting doses are 2 to 4 mg for buprenorphine and 20 to 30 mg for methadone, with doses uptitrated as needed to control symptoms. Importantly, buprenorphine should not be started until the patient is in mild to moderate withdrawal, as it can precipitate withdrawal if started prior to onset of withdrawal symptoms. Additional medications should be considered to help treat acute symptoms of opioid withdrawal in the inpatient setting, including clonidine (α2-adrenergic agonist which can reduce opioid withdrawal symptoms), loperamide (to treat diarrhea), NSAIDS and acetaminophen (to treat muscle and joint aches), hydroxyzine (to treat anxiety), and ondansetron (to treat nausea). Finally, on discharge all patients with OUD should be prescribed naloxone to reverse opioid-related overdose. Patients should also be offered any locally available resources to encourage ongoing opioid abstinence, such as outpatient or inpatient substance use treatment programs.

HYPERTENSION

Hypertension in adult patients is most commonly defined as a blood pressure of 130/80 mmHg or greater on two or more occasions. While less frequently seen in the pediatric population, hypertension is very common in the hospitalized adult population. Importantly, elevated blood pressure measurements in the inpatient setting are often not indicative of true chronic hypertension. Multiple factors, including pain, anxiety, agitation, hypervolemia, and medications such as corticosteroids, can contribute to transiently elevated blood pressure. Thus, patients with elevated blood pressure readings should first be assessed for the presence of these potential factors, which should then be mitigated when possible. Even when blood pressure measurements remain elevated in the absence of, or despite appropriate mitigation of, contributing factors, acute treatment of hypertension in the inpatient setting is often not indicated. Multiple studies have shown that rapid lowering of blood pressure with antihypertensive therapy confers excess risk for cerebral ischemia, myocardial ischemia, and acute kidney injury. Additionally, studies have shown that risks associated with aggressive treatment of inpatient hypertension generally outweigh any benefits derived from this treatment. Thus, treatment of inpatient hypertension should be approached cautiously.

When treatment is desired, for example in a patient with suspected chronic hypertension presenting with blood pressure readings consistently elevated above 160/90 mmHg, there are multiple antihypertensive options available to the clinician. Typically, clinicians should start with a low dose of a medication from one of the following classes: angiotensin-converting enzyme (ACE) inhibitors such as lisinopril, angiotensin receptor blockers (ARBs) such as losartan, calcium channel blockers (CCBs) such as amlodipine, or thiazide diuretics such as hydrochlorothiazide. These medications can be gradually uptitrated over several days to target a goal blood pressure of < 140/90 mmHg. Again, care should be taken to avoid decreasing blood pressure too quickly. ACE inhibitors, ARBs, and thiazide diuretics should generally be avoided in the setting of acute kidney injury, with CCBs (or sometimes beta blockers such as labetalol) preferred in this setting. Patients who are already maintained on an antihypertensive in the outpatient setting should generally be continued on these therapies while hospitalized. Notable exceptions to this are patients presenting with sepsis, hypovolemia, or hypotension (in which case all antihypertensives should be held), and patients presenting with acute kidney injury (in which case ACE inhibitors, ARBs, and thiazide diuretics should be held until the acute kidney injury resolves).

While rare, young adult patients may occasionally present with hypertensive emergency, defined as end-organ damage due to hypertension. The blood pressure is almost always severely elevated (>180/120 mmHg) in these situations. These patients should generally be managed in an intensive care unit setting as they require close monitoring with frequent antihypertensive titration. The general goal in these patients is to reduce the blood pressure by 10% to 20% in the first hour and by an additional 5% to 15% over the next 23 hours. Most guidelines suggest using parenteral short-acting antihypertensives, such as nitroprusside, nicardipine, and esmolol.

A final important consideration for the pediatric hospitalist is the evaluation of the young adult suspected to have a new diagnosis of chronic hypertension. As is true for pediatric patients, adults under 30 years of

TABLE 44-3 Scoring Systems Used for Alcohol Withdrawal

Scoring Tool	Minnesota Detoxification Scale (MINDS)		Clinical Institute Withdrawal Assessment Alcohol Scale Revised (CIWA-AR)	
Interpretation and Management	Protocols vary by institution—please defer to your specific institution's protocol if one is available. If no protocol exists, consider: Score < 5: Treatment generally not indicated. Consider repeating score in 1 hour. Score 5-14: Consider giving diazepam 10 mg or lorazepam 2 mg PO or IV. Consider repeating score in 30 minutes. Score 15-19: Consider giving diazepam 15 mg or lorazepam 4 mg IV. Consider repeating score in 30 minutes. Score ≥ 20: Consider giving diazepam 20 mg or lorazepam 8 mg IV. Consider repeating score in 15-30 minutes. Patients requiring frequent/high benzodiazepine dosing may require transfer to an intensive care unit. Consider using lorazepam if patient is pregnant, has liver failure, or is over age 70.		Protocols vary by institution—please defer to your specific institution's protocol if one is available. If no protocol exists, consider: Score 0-8: Treatment generally not indicated. Consider repeating score in 1 hour. Score 8-10: Consider giving diazepam 10 mg or lorazepam 2 mg PO or IV. Consider repeating score in 30 minutes. Score 11-20: Consider giving diazepam 15 mg or lorazepam 4 mg IV. Consider repeating score in 30 minutes. Score ≥ 21: Consider giving diazepam 20 mg or lorazepam 8 mg IV. Consider repeating score in 15-30 minutes. Patients requiring frequent/high benzodiazepine dosing may require transfer to an intensive care unit. Consider using lorazepam if patient is pregnant, has liver failure, or is over age 70.	
Score Components	Pulse <90 = 0 points 90-110 = 1 point >110 = 2 points	Diastolic blood pressure <90 = 0 points 90-110 = 1 point >110 = 2 points	Nausea/Vomiting None = 0 points Mild nausea/no vomiting = 1 point Intermittent nausea with dry heaves = 4 points Constant nausea, frequent vomiting = 7 points	Tremor No tremor = 0 Not visible, but can be felt fingertip to fingertip = 1 point Moderate, with arms extended = 4 points Severe, even with arms not extended = 7 points
	Tremor Absent = 0 points Visible = 2 points Moderate = 4 points Severe = 6 points	Sweat Absent = 0 points Barely, moist palms = 2 points Beads visible = 4 points Drenching = 6 points	Paroxysmal sweats No sweat visible = 0 points Barely, moist palms = 1 point Beads visible = 4 points Drenching = 7 points	Anxiety None = 0 points Mild = 1 point Moderate = 4 points Severe = 7 points
	Hallucinations Absent = 0 points Mild = 1 point Moderate, intermittent = 2 points Severe, continuous = 3 points	Agitation Normal activity = 0 points Somewhat > normal = 3 points Moderately fidgety, restless = 6 points Pacing, thrashing = 9 points	Agitation Normal activity = 0 points Somewhat > normal = 1 point Moderately fidgety, restless = 4 points Pacing, thrashing = 7 points	Tactile disturbances None = 0 points Mild itching, burning, or numbness = 2 points Moderate itching, burning, or numbness = 3 points Severe hallucinations = 5 points Continuous hallucinations = 7 points
	Orientation Oriented ×3 = 0 points Oriented ×2 = 2 points Oriented ×1 = 4 points Total disorientation = 6 points Intubated = 0 points	Delusions Absent = 0 points Present = 6 points	Auditory disturbances None = 0 points Mild ability to frighten = 2 points Moderate ability to frighten = 3 points Moderately severe hallucinations = 4 points Severe hallucinations = 5 points Continuous hallucinations = 7 points	Visual disturbances None = 0 points Mild sensitivity = 2 points Moderate sensitivity = 3 points Moderately severe hallucinations = 4 points Severe hallucinations = 5 points Continuous hallucinations = 7 points
	Seizures Absent = 0 points Present = 6 points		Headache None = 0 points Mild = 2 points Moderate = 3 points Severe =5 points Extremely severe = 7 points	Orientation Oriented = 0 points Uncertain about date = 1 point Disoriented for date by ≤ 2 days = 2 points Disoriented for date by > 2 days = 3 points Disoriented to place or person = 4 points

age who are found to have chronic hypertension should be evaluated for secondary hypertension, defined as hypertension due to an identifiable underlying cause. Etiologies include renovascular disease, primary kidney disease, coarctation of the aorta, Cushing's syndrome, obstructive sleep apnea, pheochromocytoma, and primary aldosteronism. Evaluation should be guided by patient presentation but will generally include four-extremity blood pressure measurement, serum electrolyte and creatinine testing, urinalysis, renal imaging with ultrasound, and an echocardiogram. Providers should have a low threshold to consult nephrology or cardiology to guide additional workup and management.

DIABETES MELLITUS TYPE 2

As the incidence of type 2 diabetes in the young adult population increases, pediatric providers who care for young adult patients need to become familiar with the inpatient management of this condition. Unlike

TABLE 44-4 Clinical Opiate Withdrawal Scale (COWS)

Scoring Tool	COWS	
Interpretation and Management	Score <5: No active withdrawal. Score 5-12: Mild withdrawal Score 13-24: Moderate withdrawal Score 25-36: Moderately severe withdrawal Score >36: Severe withdrawal Consider initiating treatment with buprenorphine 2-4 mg once patient is in mild to moderate withdrawal (COWS score > 8-10). If methadone is preferred, it may be initiated at a dose of 20-30 mg once the patient reports any withdrawal symptoms. Buprenorphine should generally be increased by 2-4 mg every 2 hours until COWS score is ≤5, for a total dose of 12-16 mg on day 1. The dose can be further increased over the next few days as needed to achieve a typical daily dose of 16-24 mg per day. Methadone should be increased by 5-10 mg every 2-3 hours to a maximum daily dose of 40 mg on day 1. The dose can be further increased over the next few days as needed to minimize withdrawal symptoms. In addition to the above, consider initiating clonidine, loperamide, NSAIDS, acetaminophen, hydroxyzine, and ondansetron as needed to manage symptoms of withdrawal.	
Score Components	Resting Pulse Rate ≤ 80 = 0 points 81-100 = 1 point 101-120 = 2 points >120 = 4 points	Sweating None = 0 points Subjective chills or flushing = 1 point Flushed or observable moistness on face = 2 points Beads of sweat = 3 points Sweat streaming off face = 4 points
	Restlessness Able to sit still = 0 points Reports difficulty sitting still, but able to do so = 1 point Frequent shifting of extraneous movements of legs/arms = 3 points Unable to sit still for more than a few seconds 5 points	Pupil Size Pinpoint or normal size for room light = 0 points Pupils possibly larger than normal for room light = 1 point Pupils moderately dilated = 2 points Pupils so dilated that only the rim of the iris is visible = 5 points
	Bone or Joint Aches None = 0 points Mild diffuse discomfort = 1 point Severe diffuse aching of joints/muscles = 2 points Rubbing joints/muscles and unable to sit still due to discomfort = 4 points	Runny Nose or Tearing None = 0 points Nasal stuffiness or unusually moist eyes = 1 point Nose running or tearing = 2 points Nose constantly running or tears streaming down cheeks = 4 points
	GI Upset (over last 30 minutes) No GI symptoms = 0 points Stomach cramps = 1 point Nausea or loose stool = 2 points Vomiting or diarrhea = 3 points Multiple episodes of vomiting or diarrhea = 5 points	Tremor of Outstretched Hands No tremor = 0 points Tremor can be felt, but not observed = 1 point Slight tremor observable = 2 points Gross tremor or muscle twitching = 4 points
	Yawning No yawning = 0 points Yawning once or twice during assessment = 1 point Yawning 3 or more times during assessment = 2 points Yawning several times/minute = 4 points	Anxiety or Irritability None = 0 points Patient reports increasing irritability or anxiousness = 1 point Patient obviously irritable/anxious = 2 points Patient so irritable/anxious that assessment is difficult = 4 points
	Gooseflesh Skin Skin is smooth = 0 points Piloerection of skin can be felt or hairs standing up on arms = 3 points Prominent piloerection = 5 points	

patients with type 1 diabetes, patients with type 2 diabetes are often on noninsulin therapies including metformin, sulfonylureas, thiazolidinediones, glucagon-like peptide-1 receptor antagonists (GLP-1Ras), dipeptidyl peptidase 4 inhibitors (DPP4is), and sodium-glucose cotransporter-2 inhibitors (SGLT2is). Non-insulin medications cannot be titrated as rapidly as insulin, and thus may place patients at an increased risk for hypoglycemia in the setting of acute illness and interruption of nutrition. Additionally, acute illness may increase the risk of adverse effects associated with some of these medications, such as lactic acidosis and acute kidney injury. Thus, in accordance with a recently published Endocrine Society Clinical Practice Guideline, in most situations these medications should be held when patients are hospitalized, using insulin for glycemic control instead. In some cases, it may be reasonable to continue DPP4is and GLP-1Ras as these medications have been studied more extensively in the inpatient population and have a favorable side effect profile. Continuing SGLT-2is in patients who are admitted with decompensated heart failure (rare in the young adult population) may be considered, as there is data to suggest that these medications improve diuresis. It is reasonable to resume outpatient noninsulin therapies once patients are approaching discharge.

In hospitalized patients with type 2 diabetes who develop persistent hyperglycemia ≥180 mg/dL, insulin therapy should be initiated to

TABLE 44-5 ATS/IDSA Criteria for Severe CAP

Patients who meet 1 major criterion OR 3 minor criteria meet the definition for severe CAP

Major Criteria	Minor Criteria
Septic Shock with need for vasopressors Respiratory failure requiring mechanical ventilation	Respiratory rate ≥ 30 breaths/minute PaO_2 / FiO_2 ratio ≤ 250 Multilobar infiltrates Confusion/disorientation Blood urea nitrogen level ≥ 20 mg/dL White blood cell count <4000 cells/μL (due to infection alone) Hypothermia Hypotension requiring aggressive fluid resuscitation

target a glucose range of 100 to 180 mg/dL. Some experts recommend targeting a more conservative range of 140 to 180 mg/dL to avoid hypoglycemia. For patients who are not on insulin in the outpatient setting, correctional (also referred to as bolus or sliding scale) insulin using a short-acting insulin such as lispro can be used alone. In patients who continue to have hyperglycemia ≥180 mg/dL, adding scheduled (basal) insulin with a long-acting insulin is recommended. Patients who are already on insulin as an outpatient should generally have their home regimen continued, though dose adjustments may be required in setting of acute illness.

COMMUNITY ACQUIRED PNEUMONIA

Community acquired pneumonia (CAP) is another condition in which management differs in the adult population. For adult patients admitted with a diagnosis of CAP, the 2019 CAP Guideline developed by the American Thoracic Society and Infectious Diseases Society of America can be utilized. This guideline sorts patients into severe and non-severe categories based on the presence of a group of major and minor criteria (**Table 44-5**). The guideline also recommends evaluating risk factors for methicillin-resistant *Staphylococcus aureus* (MRSA) or *Pseudomonas aeruginosa*. Testing and treatment recommendations are then based on the patient's severity category and the presence of MRSA and/or *Pseudomonas* risk factors. Blood cultures, sputum cultures, and *Legionella* and pneumococcal urinary antigen testing are generally recommended only for patients with severe disease. Blood and sputum cultures should also be obtained in patients being empirically treated for MRSA or *Pseudomonas*. For patients at low risk for MRSA and *Pseudomonas* infections, the recommended inpatient regimen is a β-lactam (ampicillin + sulbactam 1.5-3 g every 6 hours, cefotaxime 1-2 g every 8 hours, ceftriaxone 1-2 g daily, or ceftaroline 1-2 g every 12 hours) in combination with a macrolide (typically azithromycin 500 mg daily), or monotherapy with a respiratory fluoroquinolone (levofloxacin 750 mg daily or moxifloxacin 400 mg daily). For all patients with prior MRSA or *Pseudomonas* respiratory infections, or for patients with severe CAP with locally validated risk factors for MRSA or *Pseudomonas*, the guideline suggests empirically initiating therapy for MRSA and/or *Pseudomonas*. Antibiotic therapy should be narrowed if testing for MRSA and/or *Pseudomonas* (nasal MRSA PCR, sputum cultures) is negative. For adult patients admitted with suspicion for aspiration pneumonia, anaerobic coverage is typically not indicated unless the patient has an abscess or empyema. A typical treatment course is 5 days of antibiotic therapy, provided the patient shows evidence of clinical improvement.

VENOUS THROMBOEMBOLISM (VTE)/DEEP VENOUS THROMBOSIS (DVT) PROPHYLAXIS

When admitting young adults, venous thromboembolism (VTE) prophylaxis should always be considered. Use a risk assessment tool such as the Padua prediction score or the IMPROVE risk score to determine if the patient is at high risk or low risk for VTE (**Table 44-6**). High-risk patients generally require VTE prophylaxis. For patients without a contraindication such as active bleeding, chemical VTE prophylaxis

TABLE 44-6 Venous Thromboembolism Risk Assessment Tools

Assessment Tool	*Padua Prediction Score*	*IMPROVE Risk Score*
Interpretation and Management	If 0-3 points, VTE risk is low. VTE prophylaxis generally not indicated. If ≥ 4 points, VTE risk is high. VTE prophylaxis is generally indicated.	If 0-1 points, VTE risk is low. VTE prophylaxis is generally not indicated. If ≥ 2 points, VTE risk is moderate to high. VTE prophylaxis is generally indicated.
Score Components	Active cancer = 3 points Previously diagnosed VTE = 3 points Reduced mobility = 3 points Known thrombophilic condition = 3 points Trauma or surgery within past month = 2 points Age ≥ 70 = 1 point Heart or respiratory failure = 1 point Acute myocardial infarction or ischemic stroke = 1 point Acute infection or rheumatologic disorder = 1 point BMI ≥ 30 = 1 point Ongoing hormonal treatment = 1 point	Previously diagnosed VTE = 3 points Known thrombophilic condition = 2 points Current lower-limb paralysis = 2 points Active cancer = 2 points Immobilization ≥ 7 days = 1 point Intensive Care Unit stay required during hospitalization = 1 point Age > 60 = 1 point

should generally be used. Commonly used regimens include subcutaneous enoxaparin 40 mg daily, subcutaneous unfractionated heparin (UFH) 5000 units two or three times daily, fondaparinux 2.5 mg daily, or a prophylactic dose of a direct-acting oral anticoagulant (DOAC) such as rivaroxaban 10 mg daily or apixaban 2.5 mg twice daily. A recent meta-analysis compared these options and concluded that enoxaparin and fondaparinux both significantly reduced the risk of VTE while conferring a lower risk of bleeding than UFH and DOACs. For high-risk patients with a contraindication to chemical VTE prophylaxis, mechanical prophylaxis with sequential compression devices should generally be used. For patients who score as low risk for VTE, no VTE prophylaxis is generally indicated.

SPECIAL CONSIDERATIONS

MEDICOLEGAL & ETHICAL ISSUES

Bodily Autonomy, Assent, and Consent Autonomy, the right of competent adults to make informed decisions about their own medical care, is considered a primary principle in an individual's health. While children may not have medical decision-making capacity for themselves, they can participate in conversations around their own medical care and should be taught from a young age that their voice is important. As patients age into adulthood, it is important to understand the shift that occurs around their bodily autonomy, from both a developmental and medicolegal perspective. For some of these patients and families, such as those with congenital conditions impacting them since childhood, the pivot toward the patient being the primary decision-maker requires resetting of expectations.

Privacy The privacy rights and ability to consent of an adolescent patient (<18 years old) varies widely by state; at age 18, patients with medical decision-making capacity have the right to privacy and access to their own medical records. All institutions should have a policy or guideline for who is permitted to access an adult patients' medical records. The care team should clarify which individuals an adult patient wishes to have involved in their care, documenting this clearly, and ensuring that the patient's wishes are followed.

TABLE 44-7 Types of Decision-Making Supports

Types of Decision-Making Support	Description
Guardian/conservator	Court-appointed proxy decision-maker Removes patient's authority to make decisions (can be limited)
Statutory supported decision-making	Legal framework for patients who need support but retain legal authority to make decisions
Medical durable power of attorney	Appointed by patient Limitations can be in place
Advance directives	Written documentation of a patient's wishes
Legal surrogate	Statutory hierarchy of decision-maker Defined by states

Decision-Making Capacity, Assessment, and Supports Capacity is defined as the ability to process information about an illness and proposed interventions to make a choice that aligns with one's own values and preferences. Some adult patients, because of a wide variety of stable or temporary conditions (e.g., intellectual disability, intoxication, critical illness) may not have capacity to make their own medical decisions. Formal evaluation of decision-making capacity can be performed by the treating physician, and at many institutions, consultation with psychiatry is available if the treating physician is not comfortable performing this assessment. In general, to have decision-making capacity a patient must be able to communicate a choice, demonstrate understanding of the information relevant to that choice, appreciate the potential consequences of the decision, and reason logically about the decision.

For patients who do not have capacity, there are a variety of frameworks for support (**Table 44-7**). These exist on a spectrum from most to least restrictive and should be used as appropriate to the patient's situation. Which of these options are available varies widely by state; providers should be familiar with the statutes in their own area.

Reporting Abuse or Neglect Physicians are mandatory reporters to state agencies if they identify a vulnerable patient who they are concerned is being abused or neglected. Vulnerable adults are defined as those individuals age 18 or older who have an inability to care for themselves functionally, mentally, or physically. In the majority of states, physicians are also mandatory reporters to Adult Protective Service (APS) agencies for these vulnerable adults. APSs are locally/regionally governed but are all guided by the National Adult Protective Services Association (NAPSA).

In situations where the adult is not considered "vulnerable" and has the capacity to make their own medical decisions, physicians can recommend a patient report abuse (such as in the case of domestic violence), but they cannot do so without the consent of that patient.

TRANSITIONS OF CARE

While it is widely recognized that transition processes should be guided by the patient's primary care physician and their primary specialists, there is still a role for hospitalists around the inpatient management of transition. This might start with the identification that a patient is nearing the age/time of transition and working with the involved specialty teams to coordinate a smooth transition process.

Guidelines outlining the ideal transition from pediatric to adult healthcare systems have been created by agencies geared toward improving this process. Six core elements of transition include: (i) Transition and Care Policy/Guide, (ii) Tracking and Monitoring, (iii) Transition Readiness, (iv) Transition Planning, (v) Transition of Care, and (vi) Transfer Completion.

Physicians should be aware of the guidelines/policies around transition that exist at their institution. This should include knowing whether there are age limits for patients that can be safely cared for at their hospital. Additionally, awareness around outpatient transition policies for various specialties can help determine when patients may need to transition care into adult medicine practices so that a patient's transition is not spread between both pediatric and adult institutions for a prolonged time. Similarly, tracking adult-aged patients in a pediatric institution can help physician teams understand the patients that are being admitted. As patients get closer to the age at which transition is expected, the inpatient team can start to discuss with the patient and family their readiness for transition into adult healthcare settings. For more complex patients, this might include assisting in creating a portable medical summary focused on the inpatient care of that individual patient. Utilizing a multidisciplinary team, a physician can address goals and develop a care plan with the family, as well as identify the time that transition might occur. Pediatric inpatient providers can also work to help the patient and their family identify and communicate to inpatient adult teams that might be best equipped to care for the patient with their medical issues. Outpatient clinics focused on this transition can also be hugely helpful partners in facilitating transition into adult care.

DISCHARGE PLANNING

Discharge planning for adults has key differences when compared with discharge planning for children. Considering the supports that a patient might have to recover from hospitalization can play an important role in determining whether a patient is safe to discharge to home. Whereas guardians are presumed to be the responsible person when children are sick, adults may have limited support networks providing challenges in safe discharge home.

When patients are typically discharged needing rehabilitation services from a children's hospital, there are two options that are commonly available: discharge home under the care of guardians with intensive outpatient therapies, or admission to an inpatient acute rehabilitation unit. Adult-aged patients have two additional options: admission to a skilled nursing facility (SNF) for a lower level of subacute rehabilitation or admission to a more intensive acute care unit known as a long-term acute care (LTAC) facility.

Case management teams caring for adults should also be familiar with supporting those adults through knowledge of Family Medical Leave Act (FMLA) forms, vocational support/rehabilitation options, and disability forms.

LEVERAGING ADULT MEDICINE RESOURCES

When caring for the young adult population, pediatric hospitalists should be aware of ancillary resources at their disposal to help care for this patient population. At the local level there may be colleagues who routinely care for this patient population, like combined internal medicine/pediatrics or family-medicine-trained physicians who are available to informally consult as needed. Some institutions may use adult-trained providers to staff a formal adult consult service or a young adult team to help care for this patient population. If these resources do not exist, pediatric hospitalists should consider reaching out to their adult-trained peers at neighboring institutions. These colleagues may be particularly helpful when subspecialty consultation is warranted, as they can provide invaluable time-sensitive treatment advice for a variety of life- or limb-threatening conditions seen more commonly in adult patients. They may also aid with decision-making regarding if and when the patient should be transferred to an adult institution.

Many pediatric hospitals regularly provide care for patients over the age of 18. These institutions should consider quality improvement initiatives to improve the care of this patient population. For example, clinical pathways are becoming more widely implemented to improve patient care in the inpatient setting. Pathways for common adult conditions can be adapted from neighboring adult institutions to improve the quality of care provided to adult patients at pediatric centers. The Electronic Health Record (EHR) can also be utilized to improve young adult care through evidence-based recommendations for adults. For example, an EHR "best practice advisory" can prompt providers to consider VTE prophylaxis for this patient population, promoting evidence-based use of prophylactic anticoagulation for high-risk adult patients as discussed earlier.

KEY POINTS

- The number of adult patients receiving care at pediatric hospitals is increasing, and so pediatric hospitalists should be familiar with common as well as potentially life-threatening medical conditions which may present in adult-aged patients.
- Scoring and evaluation tools are widely available to assist in the early diagnosis and treatment of adult-related conditions.
- Special consideration around the medicolegal care, social supports, and discharge planning of adults should be taken by medical teams.

SUGGESTED READINGS

American Academy of Pediatrics, American Academy of Family Physicians, and American College of Physicians-American Society of Internal Medicine. A consensus statement on health care transitions for young adults with special health care needs. *Pediatrics*. 2002;110(Supplement 3):1304-1306.

Allen AQ, Hall M, Goodman DM, et al. The increasing proportion of adult discharges at children's hospitals, 2004-2019. *J Hosp Med*. 2022;17(12):990-993.

Calcaterra SL, Martin M, Bottner R, et al. Management of opioid use disorder and associated conditions among hospitalized adults: a Consensus Statement from the Society of Hospital Medicine. *J Hosp Med*. 2022;17(9):744-756.

Coller RJ, Ahrens S, Ehlenbach ML, et al. Transitioning from General Pediatric to Adult-Oriented Inpatient Care: National Survey of US Children's Hospitals. *J Hosp Med*. 2018;13(1):13-20.

Eck RJ, Elling T, Sutton AJ, et al. Anticoagulants for thrombosis prophylaxis in acutely ill patients admitted to hospital: systematic review and network meta-analysis. *BMJ*. 2022;378:e070022.

Goodman DM, Hall M, Levin A, et al. Adults with chronic health conditions originating in childhood: inpatient experience in children's hospitals. *Pediatrics*. 2011;128(1):5-13.

Hollander JE, et al. State-of-the-art evaluation of emergency department patients presenting with potential acute coronary syndromes. *Circulation*. 2016;134(7):547.

Holleck JL, Merchant N, Gunderson CG. Symptom-triggered therapy for alcohol withdrawal syndrome: a systematic review and meta-analysis of randomized controlled trials. *J Gen Intern Med*. 2019;34(6):1018-1024.

Korytkowski MT, Muniyappa R, Antinori-Lent K, et al. Management of hyperglycemia in hospitalized adult patients in non-critical care settings: an Endocrine Society clinical practice guideline. *J Clin Endocrinol Metab*. 2022 Jul 14;107(8):2101-2128.

Manning WA, Bakel LA. Adaptation of adult pathways to improve the care of adult patients at pediatric hospitals. *Hosp Pediatr*. 2021;11(8): e164-e166.

Metlay JP, Waterer GW, Long AC, et al. Diagnosis and treatment of adults with community-acquired pneumonia. An official clinical practice guideline of the American Thoracic Society and Infectious Diseases Society of America. *Am J Respir Crit Care Med*. 2019;200(7): e45-e67.

O'Gara PT, et al. 2013 ACCF/AHA guideline for the management of ST-elevation myocardial infarction: a report of the American College of Cardiology Foundation/American Heart Association Task Force on practice guidelines. *Circulation*. 2013;127:e362.

Rastogi R, Sheehan MM, Hu B, et al. Treatment and outcomes of inpatient hypertension among adults with noncardiac admissions. *JAMA Intern Med*. 2021;181(3):345-352.

Stevens SM, Woller SC, Kreuziger LB, et al. Antithrombotic Therapy for VTE Disease: Second Update of the CHEST Guideline and Expert Panel Report. *Chest*. 2021;160(6):e545–e608. Erratum in: Chest. 2022;162(1):269.

Wesson DR, Ling W. The Clinical Opiate Withdrawal Scale (COWS). *J Psychoactive Drugs*. 2003;35(2):253-259.

Whelton PK, Carey RM, Aronow WS, et al. 2017 ACC/AHA/AAPA/ABC/ACPM/AGS/APhA/ASH/ASPC/NMA/PCNA Guideline for the prevention, detection, evaluation, and management of high blood pressure in adults. *J Am Coll Cardiol*. 2018;71(19):e127-e248.

SECTION C
Allergy and Immunology

CHAPTER 45 Anaphylaxis

Cynthia E. Castiglioni, MD, MS and Kristi H. Vito, MD

BACKGROUND

Anaphylaxis is an acute, potentially fatal, systemic allergic response that causes a sudden release of mast cell and basophil mediators, resulting in abnormalities in two or more organ systems. Providers must recognize the signs and symptoms of anaphylaxis and treat quickly to minimize the risk of biphasic reactions and, more importantly, to prevent morbidity and mortality.

PATHOPHYSIOLOGY

IgE-mediated anaphylaxis occurs after allergen-specific IgE antibodies bind to high-affinity mast cell and basophil receptors, causing mast cell and basophil degranulation. Non-IgE-mediated anaphylaxis can occur through several pathways: the direct release of mast cell and basophil mediators independent of receptor binding; activation of the Mas-related G protein-coupled receptor X2 (mrgprx2) on mast cells; an IgG-dependent pathway where IgG alone, or in complexes, activates the mast cell; or complement activation with release of C3a, C5a, and C5b-9 which trigger mast cells and basophils.

Common symptoms of both IgE- and Non-IgE-mediated anaphylaxis include urticaria, flushing, pruritis, throat tightness, shortness of breath, nausea, vomiting, diarrhea, and cardiovascular collapse. Typical IgE-mediated triggers include foods, insect stings, latex, and antibiotics, while non-IgE-mediated triggers include opiates, neuromuscular-blocking agents, chimeric IgG monoclonal antibodies, blood transfusions, and contrast dyes.

EPIDEMIOLOGY

The prevalence of anaphylaxis due to all causes in the general pediatric population ranges from 0.05% to 1.8%. Food-induced anaphylaxis is the most common cause of anaphylaxis in emergency rooms in the United States, with a reported incidence of 1.35 to 2.71 per million person-years. Peanuts, tree nuts, and cow's milk are the most common food allergies in children. Drug reactions are the second leading trigger for anaphylaxis, with antibiotics and non-steroidal anti-inflammatory drugs being the most common offenders. Other triggers in the inpatient setting include blood products, contrast materials, latex, and muscle relaxants. Hymenoptera stings (i.e., bees, hornets, wasps) are the most common insect-induced cause of anaphylaxis. Exercise can also induce anaphylaxis independently or in association with certain recently consumed foods. In up to 10% of pediatric cases, the cause of anaphylaxis is undetermined.

Death is rare, with prior studies showing case fatality rates ranging between 0.6% and 2%. Patients with atopy are at increased risk for anaphylaxis. Genotypic gender also appears to influence anaphylaxis risk, although the exact pathophysiology is unknown. The incidence of anaphylaxis is higher in boys until the age of 10 years. Starting at age 10 years, the incidence of anaphylaxis trends higher in girls.

CLINICAL PRESENTATION AND DIAGNOSIS

Clinical criteria for diagnosis of anaphylaxis are detailed in **Table 45-1**. Most anaphylactic reactions occur within 1 hour of exposure. More rapid symptom-onset generally correlates with higher reaction severity.

TABLE 45-1 Clinical Criteria for Diagnosing Anaphylaxis

Anaphylaxis is highly likely when any one of the following three criteria are fulfilled:

1. Acute onset of an illness (minutes to several hours) with involvement of the skin, mucosal tissue, or both *and at least one of the following:*
   a. Respiratory compromise
   b. Reduced BP or associated symptoms of end-organ dysfunction
2. Two or more of the following that occur rapidly after exposure to a likely allergen for that patient (minutes to several hours)
   a. Involvement of the skin-mucosal tissue
   b. Respiratory compromise
   c. Reduced BP or associated symptoms
   d. Persistent GI symptoms
3. Reduced BP after exposure to known allergen for that patient (>30% decrease in systolic BP)

Source: Reproduced with permission from Sampson HA, et al. *J Allergy Clin Immunol*. Elsevier. 2006; 117(2): 391–397.[9]

The most severe reactions generally have the most rapid symptom onset. Intravenous exposures generally cause more immediate and severe reactions, while oral exposure often results in more gastrointestinal symptoms and delayed presentation. Fatalities tend to occur within 30 minutes of allergen exposure due to cardiovascular collapse and/or respiratory failure. Cardiovascular collapse can occur in anaphylaxis without cutaneous or respiratory symptoms.

A biphasic reaction, which is defined as the recurrence of prior reaction or onset of new symptoms after the original presentation without further allergen exposure, can occur within 1 to 72 hours of initial anaphylaxis reaction with median times ranging from 4 to 22 hours. Delayed epinephrine administration greater than 1 hour from symptom onset and anaphylaxis requiring more than one dose of epinephrine has been shown to correlate with biphasic reactions.

The utility of tryptase levels obtained within 2 to 3 hours of reaction onset and again at least 24 hours after symptom resolution to confirm diagnosis remains unclear. The World Allergy Organization and several European medical societies recommend obtaining tryptase levels in adults and some children to assist in confirmation of anaphylaxis at follow-up. For patients with an elevated serum tryptase level at presentation, the positive predictive value for anaphylaxis is high (93%); however, a low value does not correlate to absence of anaphylaxis, with many patients with food allergies having low tryptase at time of presentation to medical care (NPV = 17%). Higher tryptase levels are associated with more severe anaphylaxis reactions and with certain food triggers, like milk protein. Hymenoptera venom anaphylaxis is more consistently associated with an elevated tryptase. The differential diagnosis for patients with elevated tryptase levels includes mast cell disorders and hereditary alpha tryptasemia. More research is needed to identify a more reliable biomarker for anaphylaxis.

DIFFERENTIAL DIAGNOSIS

Other conditions may resemble anaphylaxis or have systemic symptoms that are similar in presentation to an allergic reaction. The differential diagnosis for anaphylaxis includes autonomic dysregulation, shock syndromes, endocrine disorders, drug reactions, toxic processes, hematologic processes, immunologic disorders, infections, and psychosomatic disorders. **Table 45-2** outlines the differential for anaphylaxis.

TABLE 45-2 Differential Diagnosis for Anaphylaxis

Neurologic/autonomic dysregulation	**Immune disorders**
Vasovagal reaction	Bradykinin-mediated angioedema
Postural orthostatic tachycardia syndrome	**Psychosomatic**
Cerebral vascular event	Panic attack
Seizure	Fictitious
Drug reactions	Vocal cord dysfunction
Vancomycin	**Shock syndromes**
Niacin	Cardiogenic
General anesthetics	Hypovolemic
Endocrine disorders	Septic
Carcinoid	**Toxic ingestion**
Pheochromocytoma	Scombroidosis
Vasoactive intestinal peptide-secreting tumors	Monosodium glutamate (MSG)
Thyroid medullary carcinoma	Sulfites
Hypoglycemia	
Hematologic processes	
Systemic mastocytosis	
Urticaria pigmentosa	

Source: Modified from LoVerde D, Iweal O, Eginli A, Krishnaswamy G. Anaphylaxis. *Chest*. 2018;153(2): 536-537.

MANAGEMENT

The main and most important treatment for anaphylaxis is epinephrine, which should be given as soon as possible by IM injection to the anterior lateral thigh to maximize peak plasma concentration. Subcutaneous delivery or delivery to the deltoid muscle is no longer recommended due to slower absorption. Epinephrine is dosed 0.01 mg/kg of 1:1000 solution with a maximum dose of 0.5 mg; this may be repeated every 5 minutes until symptoms improve. Delayed administration of epinephrine has been documented in multiple anaphylactic fatalities, thus early identification of anaphylaxis and prompt administration of epinephrine remains paramount in management.

Assessment and management of the airway, breathing, and circulation are also critical, along with removing the inciting allergen(s), such as IV antibiotics, contrast dye, or latex in the inpatient setting. Some also advocate for elevating the lower extremities and placing patients supine to avoid severe complications of sudden onset hypotension and shock.

AIRWAY AND BREATHING

The effects of anaphylaxis on airway and breathing range from mild bronchospasm to more severe and life-threatening laryngeal edema and respiratory failure. Bronchodilators may help treat bronchoconstriction and nebulized racemic epinephrine may help treat upper airway obstruction, but these therapies should not be used as a substitute for repeated doses of intramuscular epinephrine in the setting of refractory symptoms. In the most severe cases, airway management can be complicated by significant laryngeal edema, and cricothyrotomy may be needed if laryngeal edema compromises the airway by preventing successful intubation.

CIRCULATION

The increased vascular permeability in anaphylaxis can cause up to 50% of intravascular volume to rapidly diffuse into the extravascular space, resulting in rapid and profound hypotension and shock. This requires aggressive management with epinephrine and intravenous fluid boluses.

For patients who already have IV access, are severely hypotensive, and are not responding to the IM doses of 1:1000 epinephrine and IV fluids, consider IV or IO epinephrine at the standard cardiac arrest dose of 0.01 mg/kg of the 1:10,000 solution. An infusion of epinephrine at 0.1 μg/kg/min can be initiated and titrated up to 1 μg/kg/min if needed in protracted anaphylaxis. Of note, patients on beta-blocking agents may have persistent hypotension during anaphylaxis despite treatment with epinephrine due to the alpha-adrenergic effects of epinephrine. Glucagon should be given to reverse the beta-blockade (0.5 mg IV/IM × 1 for patients under 20 kg and 1 mg IV/IM × 1 for patients weighing 20 kg or more). After an initial bolus of glucagon is administered, a continuous infusion of glucagon may be needed to maintain the blood pressure. Glucagon often causes vomiting, thus assuring airway protection when administering this medication is paramount.

Additional treatments for primary anaphylaxis include H1 and H2 antihistamines and oral steroids. However, these therapies have not been shown to offer clear significant benefit in preventing biphasic reactions and if given prior to epinephrine, may delay administration of this most important first-line therapy. Antihistamines may be useful in the treatment of associated symptoms of anaphylaxis, including pruritis and urticaria.

ADMISSION CRITERIA

Indications to admit a patient with anaphylaxis include hypotension, specifically a wide pulse pressure at presentation, airway obstruction, prolonged bronchospasm, and the administration of multiple doses of epinephrine. More caution is advised in patients with a co-morbid diagnosis of reactive airway disease or asthma due to greater risk of mortality.

DISCHARGE CRITERIA

There is insufficient evidence to define an optimal duration of observation following onset of anaphylaxis. Patients are eligible for discharge once symptoms have fully resolved. For patients with perceived higher risk for a biphasic reaction (severe anaphylaxis and/or >1 dose of epinephrine) or increased risk of anaphylaxis mortality due to lack of access to epinephrine and/or emergency services, an extended observation of 6 to 8 hours to monitor for biphasic anaphylaxis is reasonable.

Intramuscular injection with epinephrine is the mainstay treatment for primary or biphasic anaphylaxis reactions. After an anaphylactic episode, every patient should be prescribed an epinephrine autoinjector (EpiPen, Auvi-Q, or Adrenaclick). Prior to discharge, the patient and their caregiver should receive education on anaphylaxis and the risk of occurrence, trigger avoidance, and the use and storage of the epinephrine autoinjector. Studies have shown that only 20% to 26% of children receive epinephrine prior to receiving emergency medicine services and only 30% of individuals with food allergies and their caregivers can demonstrate appropriate use of an epinephrine autoinjector.

Based on the findings of a recent systematic review, it is no longer recommended to prescribe H1 or H2 antihistamines or glucocorticoids at time of discharge as a way to prevent biphasic reactions. The analysis demonstrates no clear benefit of treating with H1 or H2 antihistamines or glucocorticoids in preventing biphasic reactions, with the Number Needed to Treat (NNT) for H1 antihistamines and glucocorticoids being 72 and 161, respectively. In addition, there is initial evidence that glucocorticoids may actually increase the risk of biphasic reaction occurrence in children. Further research on the confounding effect of reaction severity on this finding is needed.

If a biphasic reaction were to occur and symptoms return, families should be instructed to administer epinephrine IM as first-line therapy. Families may be counseled to use antihistamines for treatment of urticaria and pruritis as needed, but only after administration of epinephrine.

An Anaphylaxis Action Plan should be provided to the family, with copies provided for additional households and school, if applicable. This emergency plan should include information on allergic triggers, presence or absence of asthma or previous anaphylaxis, and individualized medication dosing and indications for use. Use of a medical ID bracelet for patients with severe allergies is encouraged.

CONSULTATION

Patients with new-onset anaphylaxis should be referred to an allergist/immunologist for confirmation of the anaphylaxis trigger. In addition to reviewing the history, they may perform skin prick tests, serum specific IgE blood tests, or perform an oral food challenge based on the suspected allergen. Allergists/immunologists can also provide ongoing education around allergen avoidance, renew epinephrine autoinjector prescriptions, and discuss the use of desensitization protocols if clinically indicated.

PREVENTION

Avoidance of the allergen is the only true prevention for anaphylaxis. Premedication with antihistamines and glucocorticoids prior to giving specific agents in chemotherapy protocols associated with anaphylaxis or infusion-related reaction and prior to aeroallergen rush immunotherapy (RIT) is still recommended. However, neither medication is recommended to prevent anaphylaxis prior to the administration of low- or iso-osmolar, non-ionic radiocontrast media in patients with previous hypersensitivity reactions.

KEY POINTS

- Anaphylaxis is an acute and potentially fatal systemic response that requires early recognition and prompt treatment to minimize morbidity and mortality.
- Anaphylaxis can be either IgE-mediated or non-IgE-mediated. Presenting symptoms involve the cutaneous, respiratory, and/or gastrointestinal systems and can lead to cardiovascular collapse.
- Early administration of intramuscular epinephrine is essential for treatment of anaphylaxis. Surveillance and management of airway, breathing, and circulation is also necessary.
- Prior to discharge, every patient presenting with anaphylaxis should be prescribed an epinephrine autoinjector and parent education should be completed. Continuation of antihistamine and glucocorticoid therapy are no longer recommended for prevention of biphasic reactions.
- Avoidance of the inciting allergen is key to prevention of future anaphylactic episodes.

SUGGESTED READINGS

Cardona V, Ansotegui IJ, Ebisawa M, et al. World allergy organization anaphylaxis guidance 2020. *World Allergy Organ J.* 2020;13(10): 100472.

Cianferoni A. Non-IgE-mediated anaphylaxis. *J Allergy Clin Immunol.* 2021;147(4):1123-1131.

Feldweg AM. Exercise-induced anaphylaxis. *Immunol Allergy Clin North Am.* 2015;35(2):261-275.

Ko BS, Kim WY, Ryoo SM, et al. Biphasic reactions in patients with anaphylaxis treated with corticosteroids. *Ann Allergy Asthma Immunol.* 2015;115(4):312-316.

Lieberman P. Anaphylactic reactions during surgical and medical procedures. *J Allergy Clin Immunol.* 2002;110:564-569.

LoVerde D, Iweala OI, Eginli A, Krishnaswamy G. Anaphylaxis. *Chest.* 2018;153(2):528-543.

Miles LM, Ratnarajah K, Gabrielli S, et al. Community use of epinephrine for the treatment of anaphylaxis: a review and meta-analysis. *J Allergy Clin Immunol Pract.* 2021;9(6):2321-2333.

Motosue MS, Li JT, Campbell RL. Anaphylaxis: epidemiology and differential diagnosis. *Immunol Allergy Clin North Am.* 2022;42(1):13-25.

Muraro A, Worm M, Alviani C, et al. EEACI guidelines: anaphylaxis (2021 update). *Allergy.* 2022;77:357-377.

Pourmand A, Robinson C, Syed W, Mazer-Amirshahi M. Biphasic anaphylaxis: a review of the literature and implications for emergency management. *Am J Emerg Med.* 2018;36(8):1480-1485.

Sampson HA. Anaphylaxis and emergency treatment. *Pediatrics.* 2003; 111(3):1601-1608.

Shaker MS, Wallace DV, Golden DBK, et al. Anaphylaxis-a 2020 practice parameter update, systematic review, and Grading of Recommendations, Assessment, Development and Evaluation (GRADE) analysis. *J Allergy Clin Immunol.* 2020;145(4):1082-1123.

Sicherer SH. Use assessment of self-administered epinephrine among food-allergic children and pediatricians. *Pediatrics.* 2000;105: 359-362.

Simons FER. Pharmacologic treatment of anaphylaxis: can the evidence base be strengthened? *Curr Opin Allergy Clin Immunol.* 2010;10(4): 384-393.

Tanno LK, Demoly P. Anaphylaxis in children. *Pediatr Allergy Immunol.* 2020;31 Suppl 26:8-10.

Turner PJ, Campbell DE, Motosue MS, Campbell RL. Global trends in anaphylaxis epidemiology and clinical implications. *J Allergy Clin Immunol Pract.* 2020;8(4):1169-1176.

Wang J, Sicherer SH; SECTION ON ALLERGY AND IMMUNOLOGY. Guidance on Completing a Written Allergy and Anaphylaxis Emergency Plan. *Pediatrics.* 2017;139(3):e20164005.

Wang Y, Allen KJ, Suaini NHA. The global incidence and prevalence of anaphylaxis in children in the general population: a systematic review. *Allergy.* 2019;74(6):1063-1080.

Webb LM, Lieberman P. Anaphylaxis: a review of 601 cases. *Ann Allergy Asthma Immunol.* 2006;97(1):39-43.

CHAPTER 46 Drug Allergy

James W. Antoon, MD, PhD, MPH and Nawal Momani, MD

BACKGROUND

Adverse drug reactions are broadly defined by the World Health Organization as "any noxious, unintended, and undesired effect of a drug that occurs at doses used for prevention, diagnosis, or treatment." These reactions can be classified into types A and B.

Type A reactions, which account for most adverse drug reactions, are predictable, dose dependent, and related to the pharmacologic mechanism of the drug. Examples include respiratory depression with the administration of increasing amounts of opiates or cushingoid features with chronic systemic steroid use. Type B reactions are unpredictable, dose independent, and not related to the drug's pharmacologic actions. Both allergic (i.e., immune-mediated) and non-allergic (i.e., non-immune mediated) hypersensitivity reactions are included in this type.

Allergic reactions require prior sensitization and typically show signs consistent with an underlying allergic mechanism, such as angioedema, rash, wheezing, lightheadedness, and anxiety. They resolve after the implicated drug is discontinued, though the timeline to resolution may vary. Briefly, nonimmune hypersensitivity reactions, also termed pseudoallergic reactions, are clinically similar to allergic reactions but cannot be proved to be immunologic owing to a lack of detectable drug-specific antibodies or drug-specific T lymphocytes. Many causes for these reactions have been proposed and they are dependent on the implicated drug. For example, the reaction caused by radiocontrast material is believed to be primarily from nonspecific histamine release and complement activation, although immunoglobulin E (IgE)-mediated reactions may also occur. In contrast, the angioedema seen as a reaction to angiotensin-converting enzyme inhibitors is thought to be from the accumulation of bradykinin. The primary focus of the remainder of this chapter is on immune-mediated type B reactions.

PATHOPHYSIOLOGY

Immune-mediated reactions can be organized according to the Gell and Coombs classification. Drug reactions often involve a combination of mechanisms and classifying them into one of these four categories may not always be possible.

TYPE I REACTIONS

Type I reactions have a rapid onset and develop when a drug or drug metabolite interacts with preformed **specific IgE** antibodies bound to mast cells and basophils. This results in cross-linking of IgE Fc-epsilon-RI receptors on mast cells and basophils, leading to cellular degranulation and the release of histamine and leukotrienes. These released chemicals propagate urticaria, bronchospasm, vasodilation, and other manifestations of anaphylaxis. Antibiotics, particularly beta-lactams, are commonly implicated in Type 1 reactions. Uniphasic reactions are most common and account for over 85% of cases. Biphasic reactions, wherein symptoms resolve and then return after an asymptomatic period an hour or greater without further exposure to the offending drug, can occur up to 48 hours after initial reaction.

TYPE II REACTIONS

Type II reactions usually occur 5 to 8 days after drug exposure and involve binding of immunoglobulin G (**IgG**) or immunoglobulin M (**IgM**) **antibodies** to recognized cell membrane-bound drug antigens typically found on circulating blood cells. The cells become coated with antibody and are then injured via the complement system. The resulting sequela includes granulocytopenia, hemolytic anemia, and thrombocytopenia. Common offending agents include antibiotics, anticonvulsants, sulfonamides, and heparin.

TYPE III REACTIONS

Type III reactions also have a delayed onset of action occurring one or more weeks after exposure. They are due to soluble **antigen-antibody complexes** deposited in various tissues including in the walls of blood vessels, joints, and renal glomeruli, which then activate the complement cascade. Clinical manifestations include serum sickness, vasculitis, or arthus reaction. Anti-toxins (rabies, botulism, venom), immune modulating agents (such as biologics), and vaccinations are the agents most often reported in serum sickness. Arthus reactions are rare, localized hypersensitivity reactions; toxin-antitoxin (e.g. Diphtheria antitoxin), Hepatitis B vaccine, and Diptheria Tetanus and Pertuss (DTaP) vaccination have been implicated in most case reports. Other drugs implicated in Type III reactions include hydralazine, procainamide, and minocycline, which can manifest as drug-induced vasculitis or lupus.

TYPE IV REACTIONS

Type IV reactions involve **antigen-specific T-lymphocyte-mediated reactions**, such as those seen in allergic contact dermatitis, drug fever, drug rash with eosinophilia and systemic symptoms (DRESS), and Stevens-Johnson syndrome/Toxic Epidermal Necrolysis (SJS/TEN). Type IV reactions are delayed in onset, ranging from 48 hours to several weeks following drug exposure, depending on the robustness of drug-induced T-cell activation. HLA associations between specific drug and specific reactions, including DRESS and SJS/TEN, are well characterized. Certain drug-specific Type IV reactions are dose dependent, as seen with allopurinol and lamotrigine.

EPIDEMIOLOGY

It is estimated that adverse drug reactions (ADRs) affect 1.5% of pediatric outpatients and 9.5% of hospitalized children. Drug hypersensitivity reactions account for about 15% of all ADRs. The true incidence of pediatric drug allergy and drug-induced anaphylaxis is unknown, with many children being labeled as having a drug allergy without proper evaluation. Risk factors for drug hypersensitivity reactions include female gender, previous drug allergy, recurrent drug exposure, concurrent illness, and genetic factors.

SPECIFIC IMMUNE REACTIONS AND SPECIFIC DRUG CATEGORIES

ANAPHYLAXIS

Antibiotics are frequent causes of drug-induced anaphylaxis. Penicillin allergy labels are common and occur in up to 10% of children, with most labels reporting symptoms of anaphylaxis such as rash, swelling, and vomiting. However, the vast majority of these documented allergies are inaccurate; nearly 95% of children with a penicillin allergy label can safely receive penicillins. If a child has a true penicillin allergy, cross-reactivity among cephalosporins, though rare, may occur due to beta-lactam ring structure or side-R1 side-chain similarities. The most common reaction symptom with penicillin is a morbilliform rash, however these alone are not considered life threatening; caution is advised if the rash bears any similarity to urticaria and occurs within hours of the first dose of medication. Validated screenings for anaphylaxis in children are available and allow for accurate penicillin allergy risk stratification. These screenings use information on symptom reaction (typically stratified into high- and low-risk symptoms) and timing (for certain low-risk reactions: less or greater than 4-6 hours or unknown timing after first dose of the medication) based on parental report and can stratify a child as either high or low risk for a true anaphylactic reaction. Those screened as low risk may skip skin testing and undergo a direct amoxicillin oral challenge. Those who screen as high risk should receive an alternative antibiotic or undergo skin testing. Similar risk stratification for cephalosporin allergy has been developed.

In some cases, desensitization of a penicillin antibiotic may be necessary in the treatment of serious or drug-resistant infections. Desensitization is typically performed in consultation with an immunology specialist, often occurs in the intensive care unit setting, and consists of administering progressively larger doses of the medication to which the patient is allergic until the full therapeutic dose is reached. Once a patient is desensitized, consistent dosing intervals must be maintained to

TABLE 46-1 Drug Allergy Classification

Type	Mechanism	Example	Timing	Clinical Features	Most Commonly Implicated Drugs
I	IgE, mast, and/or basophil-mediated immediate reaction	Anaphylaxis	Immediate (30-60 min), less commonly 6-48 h	Pruritis, urticaria, angioedema, bronchospasm	Beta-lactams, sulfonamides, macrolides, fluroquinolones
II	Antibody-mediated cell damage	Drug-induced hemolytic anemia, thrombocytopenia, and neutropenia	Delayed (> 5 h)	Anemia, neutropenia, agranulocytosis, thrombocytopenia	Sulfonamides, rifampin, bet lactams, vancomycin
III	IgG-Drug immune complex deposition with activation of complement system	Serum Sickness, Arthus reaction	Delayed (>3 h)	Rash, arthralgia, arthritis	Beta lactams, sulfonamides, tetracyclines
IV	T-cell-mediated reaction	DRESS, SJS/TEN, AGEP, Drug Fever, morbilliform eruptions	Delayed (>24 h), up to several weeks after exposure initiation	*DRESS*: Fever, edema, lymphadenopathy, pruritic exanthem or urticarial papular, erythroderma, non-erosive mucositis, often >50% of body surface area	*DRESS*: carbamazepine, phenytoin, lamotrigine, allopurinol, sulfonamide antibiotics, allopurinol, vancomycin, minocycline
				SJS/TEN: Fever, malaise, painful macular erythema, blisters, +Nikoslky sign, erosive mucositis	*SJS/TEN:* allopurinol, anticonvulsants, sulfonamide antibiotics, NSAIDs, beta lactams

prevent re-sensitization. Once the medication is discontinued, the desensitized state will eventually be lost, and if the patient needs to receive this medication in the future, repeat desensitization will be necessary. Desensitization has no benefit and is strictly contraindicated when the mechanism is non-IgE mediated, such as in serum sickness reactions, anticonvulsant hypersensitivity syndrome, or desquamating reactions such as Stevens-Johnson syndrome or toxic epidermal necrolysis.

The mainstay of treatment for Type I reactions is epinephrine and diphenhydramine along with symptomatic care as needed with antihistamines, bronchodilators, and steroids. See Chapter 45 for greater detail about anaphylaxis.

SERUM SICKNESS AND SERUM SICKNESS LIKE REACTIONS

Serum sickness typically occurs within 1 to 2 weeks of drug exposure, sooner in patients with previous reactions. Anti-venom, vaccinations, and biologic drugs are often implicated. Classic symptoms include fever, joint involvement, lymphadenopathy, and rash. The rash may be maculopapular, purpuric, or urticarial in nature. Both arthritis and arthralgias may occur and the hands, feet, knees, ankles, and shoulders are most affected. Laboratory studies demonstrate an elevated CRP/ESR, low C3, low C4, low albumin, and proteinuria or hematuria on urinalysis. Serum sickness is a self-limited disease with resolution of symptoms typically occurring within 2 weeks of discontinuing the offending drug. Symptoms may be more prolonged in severe cases. Once the offending agent is removed, treatment is directed at symptomatic control. Nonsteroidal anti-inflammatory drugs (NSAIDs) and antihistamines are useful in mild/moderate disease. Glucocorticoids may be beneficial in more severe cases.

Serum sickness-like reactions present with similar, often milder symptoms: rash and arthralgias with or without fever. Symptoms typically appear within 7 to 10 days of exposure. It is more often seen in children than adults. Antibiotics, particularly β-lactams, are the most common triggers, with cefaclor reported to have the highest risk. The exact pathophysiology is unknown; however, it is not associated with antigen antibody complex deposition as seen in classic serum sickness and thus complement levels are usually normal. Diagnosis is largely based on history and physical exam findings as laboratory values tend to be non-specific. Aside from discontinuing the offending agent, no treatment guidelines have been established but use of NSAIDs, antihistamines, glucocorticoids, and IVIG has been reported.

ERYTHEMA MULTIFORME

Erythema multiforme is thought to be lymphocyte mediated. Up to 50% of cases are attributed to medications (the rest are thought to be due to viral infections), starting 1 to 2 weeks after drug exposure. Commonly associated medications include sulfonamides, penicillins, NSAIDs, and barbiturates. Erythema multiforme is characterized by a targetoid rash that starts distally and progresses proximally. The rash may be pruritic or elicit a burning sensation, is typically symmetrical in distribution and starts on the acral extremities and spreads centripetally. Lesions appear for up to 5 days and resolve within 3 weeks of onset. Mucosal involvement, including oral, ocular, or genital mucosa, occurs in up to 70% of cases. Prodromal symptoms of fever, fatigue, and myalgia are more common in severe cases than in milder presentations. The mainstay of treatment is removal of the offending medications and symptomatic care. Evidence for efficacy of symptom-specific treatment is low. Severe pruritis or skin discomfort may be treated with typical corticosteroids. Oral involvement may be treated with topical steroids and oral solutions containing lidocaine, diphenhydramine, and antiacids. In cases of severe oral involvement, some centers elect to treat with systemic glucocorticoid therapy. See Chapter 62 for further detail on Erythema Multiforme.

STEVENS-JOHNSON SYNDROME AND TOXIC EPIDERMAL NECROLYSIS

Stevens-Johnson Syndrome (SJS) and toxic epidermal necrolysis (TEN) are uncommon but life-threatening severe cutaneous adverse drug reactions. SJS and TEN are believed to be varying severities of the same disease process, with SJS indicating 10% body surface area (BSA) involvement, SJS/TEN overlap syndrome 10% to 30% BSA, and TEN more than 30% BSA. The overall incidence of SJS, SJS/TEN overlap, and TEN are 5.3, 0.8, and 0.4 per million children, respectively, in the United States and is higher in the hospitalized population. Risk factors for SJS/TEN include drug-specific HLA alleles, HIV, concomitant diuretic use, higher doses of medications, pre-existing renal impairment (allopurinol specific), malignancy, and systemic lupus erythematosus. Additionally, there are age-based differences in the incidence of SJS/TEN, with risk generally increasing with increasing age. The most common causative agents in children are antiepileptic drugs and sulfonamides. Though frequently prescribed medications such as aminopenicillins, cephalosporins, NSAIDs, and acetaminophen have been implicated as well. SJS/TEN generally presents with prodromal symptoms of fever, cough, and rhinorrhea followed by acute onset of blistering skin erosion with mucous membrane involvement. Any organ system can be involved including the pulmonary, ophthalmic, and genitourinary systems. There is a latency period of 1 to 4 weeks following drug exposure, with drug-specific differences in timing onset. The diagnosis of SJS/TEN is made clinically, though skin biopsy may aid in the diagnosis if uncertain. Several assessment tools are available to aid in determining the offending drug, such as the ALDEN, Naranjo, and Liverpool tools. However, none of these tools are validated in the pediatric population and there is wide inter-rater reliability in use of all three. The approach to diagnosis and treatment of SJS/TEN is typically multidisciplinary with dermatology, infectious disease, ophthalmology, burn or surgical teams, and other medical disciplines involved in the care of the patient. The mainstay of therapy for SJS/TEN is removal of the causative agent and supportive care, which typically occurs in the intensive care unit or burn care center. While there is wide variability in pharmacologic treatment, including intravenous immunoglobulin, systemic steroids, TNF inhibitors, and cyclosporin, none of these have been shown to significantly alter the disease course in children. Outcomes in children are generally better than adults, with in-hospital mortality rates of 0.13% for SJS and 3.2% for TEN. The highest mortality is found in younger children. Outcomes in those with underlying chronic conditions are uniformly worse than those without chronic conditions. Evidence of long-term complications remains sparse, but includes ophthalmologic, urinary, and respiratory morbidities. Recurrence is uncommon. For additional information on Stevens-Johnson syndrome, refer to Chapter 63.

DRUG REACTION WITH EOSINOPHILIA AND SYSTEMIC SYMPTOMS (DRESS) SYNDROME

Drug reaction with Eosinophilia and Systemic Symptoms (DRESS) syndrome, formerly known as anticonvulsant hypersensitivity syndrome, was first reported with aromatic anticonvulsants such as phenytoin, phenobarbital, and carbamazepine. It has now been associated with numerous medications including vancomycin, dapsone, sulfonamides, nevirapine, allopurinol, and minocycline. Similar to SJS/TEN, certain medications are believed to have a dose-dependent relationship with the development of DRESS. Known risk factors for DRESS include concomitant renal failure and advanced age. Symptoms of DRESS typically occur 2 to 8 weeks following drug exposure and consistent of a prodromal phase of fever, malaise, and lymphadenopathy followed by a rash that can progress to exfoliative dermatitis. Eosinophilia occurs in up to 90% of cases and there may be various organ involvement, including liver, kidney, cardiac, pulmonary, and CNS involvement. Symptoms can last several weeks with the majority of cases resolving within 8 weeks following cessation of the offending medication. Treatment of mild cases consists of supportive care with limited evidence for systemic steroids. Severe cases may be treated with systemic steroids and include second-line agents such as cyclosporin, IVIG, or biologic inhibitors. For additional information on DRESS, see Chapter 61.

VANCOMYCIN FLUSHING REACTION

Vancomycin flushing reaction is the term used to describe the generalized flushing often seen with intravenous vancomycin administration, formerly referred to as "red man syndrome." It is the most common immediate reaction reported in both adults and children, accounting for up to 16% of all hypersensitivity reactions reported. It is non-IgE mediated and a result of histamine release from mast cells and basophils.

Symptoms include flushing, pruritis, and a rash to the face, neck, and upper torso. It can be elicited in a majority of patients if the medication is given too quickly. Diagnostic tests for distinguishing vancomycin flushing reaction from anaphylaxis are lacking, although serum tryptase has been proposed which is typically normal during in a flushing reaction but elevated in anaphylaxis. Pretreatment with antihistamines and reducing the infusion rate may help avoid this reaction.

ANAPHYLACTOID REACTIONS

Anaphylactoid reactions mimic IgE-mediated reactions clinically, but prior sensitization and specific antibodies cannot be demonstrated. These reactions have been observed with the use of radiocontrast media and are for the most part dose, concentration, and rate dependent. Anaphylactoid reactions are also well recognized in the use of IV *N*-acetylcysteine (NAC) for treatment of acetaminophen overdose. Symptoms are generally reported as mild and usually develop within the first 20 minutes of exposure. Mild reactions are treated supportively. Diphenhydramine, albuterol, and epinephrine are used in moderate-to-severe reactions. Antihistamines and slower infusion rates have been used in management of NAC anaphylactoid reactions.

DIAGNOSTIC EVALUATION

The first step to identifying the offending medication in a patient presenting with a probable drug hypersensitivity reaction is a thorough history, including all medication exposures with dates of administration, dose changes, and discontinuation. Concurrent medication administration is important as it may alter the clinical presentation of drug allergy. Please see preceding sections (and reaction specific chapters) for specifics regarding diagnostic evaluations.

MANAGEMENT

Once a drug reaction has been characterized and the medication responsible has been revealed, the offending agent should be avoided. Please see preceding sections for reaction-specific management, admission, and discharge criteria (Chapters 45, 61, 62, and 63). Allergy referral should be made in many circumstances especially in cases of severe hypersensitivity reactions (e.g., DRESS, SJS, TEN, anaphylaxis).

KEY POINTS

- Allergic drug reactions can generally be classified into four categories, with Types I and IV being more common in clinical practice.
- Timing and clinical signs and symptoms may be helpful in distinguishing one reaction from another, although there can be overlap.
- Management includes identifying and discontinuing the offending agent and supportive care.
- Evidence for steroid and immunosuppression therapy in the treatment of drug allergies remains limited.

SUGGESTED READINGS

Alvarez-Arango S, Yerneni S, Tang O, et al. Vancomycin hypersensitivity reactions documented in electronic health records. *J Allergy Clin Immunol Pract.* 2021;9(2):906-912.

Antoon JW, Goldman JL, Lee B, Schwartz A. Incidence, outcomes, and resource use in children with Stevens-Johnson syndrome and toxic epidermal necrolysis. *Pediatr Dermatol.* 2018;35(2):182-187.

Antoon JW, Goldman JL, Lee BR. Severe cutaneous adverse reactions: comparing outcomes in children with and without complex chronic conditions. *J Allergy Clin Immunol Pract.* 2020;8(2):790-792 e793.

Antoon JW, Goldman JL, Shah SS, Lee B. A retrospective cohort study of the management and outcomes of children hospitalized with Stevens-Johnson syndrome or toxic epidermal necrolysis. *J Allergy Clin Immunol Pract.* 2019;7(1):244-250 e241.

Antoon JW, Grijalva CG, Grisso AG, et al. Feasibility of a centralized, pharmacy-led penicillin allergy delabeling program. *Hosp Pediatr.* 2022;12(7):e230-e237.

Antoon JW, Grijalva CG, Carroll AR, et al. Parental perceptions of penicillin allergy risk stratification and delabeling. *Hosp Pediatr.* 2023; 13(4):300-308.

Brown T, Gonzalez J, Monteleone C. Angiotensin-converting enzyme inhibitor-induced angioedema: a review of the literature. *J Clin Hypertens (Greenwich).* 2017;19(12):1377-1382.

Del Pozzo-Magana BR, Abuzgaia A, Murray B, Rieder MJ, Lazo-Langner A. Paediatric serum sickness-like reaction: a 10-year retrospective cohort study. *Paediatr Child Health.* 2021;26(7):428-435.

Delli Colli L, Gabrielli S, Abrams EM, et al. Differentiating between beta-lactam-induced serum sickness-like reactions and viral exanthem in children using a graded oral challenge. *J Allergy Clin Immunol Pract.* 2021;9(2):916-921.

Dillman JR, Trout AT, Davenport MS. Allergic-like contrast media reaction management in children. *Pediatr Radiol.* 2018;48(12):1688-1694.

Dispenza MC. Classification of hypersensitivity reactions. *Allergy Asthma Proc.* 2019;40(6):470-473.

Dykewicz MS, Lam JK. Drug hypersensitivity reactions. *Med Clin North Am.* 2020;104(1):109-128.

Fok JS, Smith WB. Hypersensitivity reactions to gadolinium-based contrast agents. *Curr Opin Allergy Clin Immunol.* 2017;17(4):241-246.

Goldman JL, Chung WH, Lee BR, et al. Adverse drug reaction causality assessment tools for drug-induced Stevens-Johnson syndrome and toxic epidermal necrolysis: room for improvement. *Eur J Clin Pharmacol.* 2019;75(8):1135-1141.

Gruchalla RS. 10. Drug allergy. *J Allergy Clin Immunol.* 2003;111(2 Suppl): S548-559.

Hsu DY, Brieva J, Silverberg NB, Paller AS, Silverberg JI. Pediatric Stevens-Johnson syndrome and toxic epidermal necrolysis in the United States. *J Am Acad Dermatol.* 2017;76(5):811-817 e814.

Kaur S, Sarkar R, Thami GP, Kanwar AJ. Anticonvulsant hypersensitivity syndrome. *Pediatr Dermatol.* 2002;19(2):142-145.

Koo G, Yu R, Phillips EJ, Stone CA, Jr. Retrospective stratification of cephalosporin allergy label risk using validated penicillin allergy frameworks. *J Allergy Clin Immunol Pract.* 2022.

Levi N, Bastuji-Garin S, Mockenhaupt M, et al. Medications as risk factors of Stevens-Johnson syndrome and toxic epidermal necrolysis in children: a pooled analysis. *Pediatrics.* 2009;123(2):e297-304.

McKenna JK, Leiferman KM. Dermatologic drug reactions. *Immunol Allergy Clin North Am.* 2004;24(3):399-423, vi.

McNulty R, Lim JME, Chandru P, Gunja N. Fewer adverse effects with a modified two-bag acetylcysteine protocol in paracetamol overdose. *Clin Toxicol (Phila).* 2018;56(7):618-621.

Norton AE, Konvinse K, Phillips EJ, Broyles AD. Antibiotic allergy in pediatrics. *Pediatrics.* 2018;141(5).

Peter JG, Lehloenya R, Dlamini S, et al. Severe delayed cutaneous and systemic reactions to drugs: a global perspective on the science and art of current practice. *J Allergy Clin Immunol Pract.* 2017;5(3): 547-563.

Rixe N, Tavarez MM. Serum sickness. In: *StatPearls.* Treasure Island (FL) 2022.

Rukasin CRF, Norton AE, Broyles AD. Pediatric drug hypersensitivity. *Curr Allergy Asthma Rep.* 2019;19(2):11.

Sheridan RL, Schulz JT, Ryan CM, et al. Long-term consequences of toxic epidermal necrolysis in children. *Pediatrics.* 2002;109(1):74-78.

Vyles D, Adams J, Chiu A, Simpson P, Nimmer M, Brousseau DC. Allergy testing in children with low-risk penicillin allergy symptoms. *Pediatrics.* 2017;140(2).

Vyles D, Antoon JW, Norton A, et al. Children with reported penicillin allergy: public health impact and safety of delabeling. *Ann Allergy Asthma Immunol.* 2020;124(6):558-565.

Yarema M, Chopra P, Sivilotti MLA, et al. Anaphylactoid reactions to intravenous N-acetylcysteine during treatment for acetaminophen poisoning. *J Med Toxicol.* 2018;14(2):120-127.

Zhu LJ, Liu AY, Wong PH, Arroyo AC. Road less traveled: drug hypersensitivity to fluoroquinolones, vancomycin, tetracyclines, and macrolides. *Clin Rev Allergy Immunol.* 2022;62(3):505-518.

CHAPTER 47

Primary Immunodeficiency Diseases

Aisha Ahmed, MD and Margot A. Paisley, MD

BACKGROUND

Primary immunodeficiency (PI) disorders affect approximately 1 in 2000 children in the United States but the age at presentation and clinical picture can vary widely. As such, the greatest challenge for the pediatric hospitalist is in making an expeditious diagnosis of PI. The most common types of PI are disorders of humoral immunity (defects in antibody production or B-cell differentiation), followed by T-cell and combined B- and T-cell defects, and finally phagocytic and complement disorders. Initial evaluation often occurs during a hospitalization for prolonged, severe, or recurrent infections. Occasionally, illnesses due to rare or unusual pathogens raise suspicion for an underlying immunodeficiency. Thus, increased awareness of the key features of PIs not only assists in management of these children when admitted, but also helps the pediatric hospitalist identify children at risk for PI. In most cases, these children benefit when the hospitalist can promptly initiate appropriate laboratory studies and obtain consultation from a pediatric immunologist.

CLINICAL PRESENTATION

HISTORY

Timely identification of children with a PI is paramount to reduce the risk of irreversible sequelae of invasive infections such as bronchiectasis, encephalitis, or kidney failure. Establishing a set of clear warning signs that indicate a PI has been challenging because of the subjective nature of what constitutes a "severe" infection or exactly what patterns constitute "recurrent" infections. A well-publicized list of ten "warning signs" of primary immunodeficiency has been promoted for years to raise awareness among both medical professionals and the lay public; the presence of *two or more* of these features should raise suspicion for PI: family history of PI, need for IV antibiotics for definitive treatment of infection, persistent fungal infections of the skin including oral thrush, infant growth failure, abscesses of the skin or organs which are recurrent, greater than or equal to two pneumonias in a year, 2 months on antibiotics (with little effect), two deep-seated infections (i.e. sepsis), two severe sinus infections in a year, and greater than or equal to four ear infections in a year. However, these warning signs largely emphasize infections as a core feature of PI and fail to identify many subjects with PI, as features of defective self-tolerance, including autoimmune and allergic diseases, and malignancies are not included. Nevertheless, the need for intravenous antibiotics, failure to thrive, or a relevant family history are the strongest predictors of PI. It is also important to note that there can be significant variability in genotype/phenotype correlation in patients with primary immunodeficiency. Even kindreds who share the same genetic mutation can have varying severity of clinical presentation.

PHYSICAL EXAMINATION

The physical examination of patients with PI should focus on sites where infections and autoimmunity can occur. General appearance is important to note, especially with regard to muscle wasting or failure to thrive. Since many syndromes can present with associated immunodeficiency, physical features of the major chromosomal syndromes, including DiGeorge syndrome and Down syndrome, should be noted. Attention to scarring of the tympanic membranes can be important for identifying a history of chronic otitis and for potentially understanding hearing loss in these patients. Patients with cellular immunodeficiency or humoral immunodeficiency such as hypogammaglobulinemia or agammaglobulinemia can have small and underdeveloped tonsils. Oculocutaneous albinism accompanies PI diseases where transport of pigments is defective (e.g., Chediak-Higashi syndrome). Pallor of the conjunctiva can indicate anemia which can be seen in patients with primary immunodeficiency and be due to varying etiology such as immune-mediated or splenic sequestration. Conical teeth are seen in NEMO syndrome. Thrush is commonly seen in T-cell deficiencies and in patients with chronic mucocutaneous candidiasis. Periodontitis is seen in patients with neutrophil deficiencies. Telangiectasias of the bulbar conjunctiva and cheeks are common in ataxia-telangiectasia after age 3, along with ataxia. Erythroderma and severe eczema are common in Omenn syndrome, IPEX, and severe combined immunodeficiency (SCID) with maternal engraftment accompanied by graft-versus-host-like disease. Severe eczema with skin infections and cutaneous abscesses are also seen in hyper-IgE syndromes. Examination of peripheral lymph nodes is important for lymphoproliferative diseases associated with PIs and for T-cell deficiencies. Hepatosplenomegaly is seen in Common variable immunodeficiency (CVID), Wiskott-Aldrich syndrome, and in disorders of lymphoproliferation (e.g., ALPS, Chediak-Higashi, BENTA). Examination of the nails is important to identify fungal diseases. Warts are commonly seen in GATA2 deficiency, DOCK8, Netherton syndrome, WHIM syndrome, and epidermodysplasia verruciformis disorders. Chronic skin infections by viruses such as molluscum contagiosum can indicate a T-cell defect such as DOCK8 deficiency (**Table 47-1**).

DIAGNOSTIC EVALUATION

NEWBORN SCREENING

A recent success in the early detection of patients with severe PI was the development of a qPCR-based assay that quantifies TRECs (T cell receptor excision circles) which are excised DNA fragments produced during T-cell receptor rearrangement. TRECs are used as a marker of successful TCR recombination and thymic output. A newly established screening program using this assay now evaluates almost all newborns in the United States and can identify newborns with T-cell lymphopenia such as SCID, ataxia-telangiectasia, partial DiGeorge syndrome, CHARGE anomalies, chromosomal breakage syndromes, secondary loss of lymphocytes, or idiopathic T-cell lymphopenia. Patients flagged by this assay may possess biologically relevant defects of immunological pathways and can be identified long before they have any typical warning signs or classical "immunological phenotypes," such as opportunistic infections. While diagnostic and treatment algorithms for these patients are not well-defined, the general pediatrician should be prepared to receive notifications for these diagnoses in otherwise well infants and refer them for full immune evaluation as early as possible.

LABORATORY EVALUATION

Apart from newborn screening, laboratory studies are the mainstay of diagnosis for PIs. These tests are heavily skewed toward evaluating circulating hematopoietic cells, which has the unintentional consequence of biasing the clinician away from thinking about innate immune pathways that are tissue resident, such as the innate defenses of the skin, GI tract, and mucosa.

Table 47-2 outlines a tier-wise approach that many immunologists will take to evaluate patients with suspected PI. Occurring in select cases at present, and likely even more so in the future, genetic testing may move up to the initial steps of evaluation.

Disorders where numerical deficiencies are the main feature (e.g., X-linked agammaglobulinemia or SCID) are diagnosed initially by flow cytometric measurement of the cells. Many labs will perform flow cytometric enumeration of the various lymphocyte subsets, where proportions and absolute counts of T-cells (CD4+ and CD8+), B-cells, and NK cells are provided. In a few cases, absolute T cell or B cell counts are not sufficient and flow cytometry for more specific cell types is required. For example, in evaluating infants for SCID, it may be very helpful to know the number of naïve T-cells, which often express the long isoform of CD45 (called CD45RA), as opposed to the total number of T-cells, which might include maternally engrafted T-cells. In diagnosing patients with CVID, the number of switched memory B-cells (that express the memory marker CD27 but lack the naïve B-cell receptor isotypes of IgM and IgD) correlates with risks of autoimmunity and splenomegaly. Aside

TABLE 47-1 Common Physical Examination Findings in Primary Immunodeficiency Disorders

System	Finding	Main Associated Immunodeficiency Disorder
GENERAL	Signs of poor growth, wasting	Multiple
FACE	Syndromic facial features	DiGeorge, Trisomy 21
EYES	1. Conjunctival pallor 2. Light colored irises 3. Telangiectasias of bulbar conjunctiva	1. Anemia in autoimmune cytopenias 2. Oculocutaneous albinism/Chediak-Higashi syndrome 3. Ataxia-telangiectasia
HAIR	1. Silver tuft of hair 2. Bamboo hair	1. Chediak-Higashi 2. Cartilage hair hypoplasia
EARS	Scarring of tympanic membranes due to chronic otitis media	Multiple
OROPHARYNX	1. Small/underdeveloped tonsils 2. Conical teeth 3. Thrush 4. Periodontitis	1. Hypogammaglobulinemia, agammaglobulinemia 2. NEMO deficiency 3. T-cell deficiency, chronic mucocutaneous candidiasis 4. Neutrophil deficiencies
GASTROINTESTINAL	Hepatosplenomegaly	CVID, Wiskott-Aldrich syndrome, disorders of lymphoproliferation
DERMATOLOGIC	1. Severe atopic dermatitis, erythroderma 2. Severe atopic dermatitis, skin abscesses 3. Warts 4. Molluscum 5. Fungal diseases of the nail 6. Albinism 7. Vitiligo, pyoderma, alopecia, petechiae 8. Telangiectasias of cheeks	1. Omenn syndrome, IPEX, SCID 2. Hyper-IgE deficiency, DOCK 8 deficiency 3. GATA2 & DOCK8 deficiencies, Netherton & WHIM syndromes, epidermodysplasia verruciformis 1&2 4. T-cell defects 5. Multiple 6. Oculocutaneous albinism/Chediak-Higashi 7. CVID 8. Ataxia-telangiectasia
LYMPHATIC	Peripheral lymph node enlargement	Lymphoproliferative diseases, T-cell deficiencies
NEUROLOGIC	Ataxia	Ataxia-telangiectasia

from lymphocytes, enumeration and phenotyping of myeloid cells may be important for identifying eosinophilia (e.g., as seen in Omenn syndrome) or neutrophilia (e.g., as seen in CD18 deficiency). When considering lymphocyte and other leukocyte counts, it is critically important for the pediatric hospitalist to remember that there are significant differences in the normal values that are dependent on age. It is also worth considering that other factors, including time of day, relationship to meals, and recent stressors can dramatically change the counts of leukocytes in the blood.

Laboratory studies are also often required to assess the functions of the cellular immune system. Activation of T-cells can be functionally assessed at multiple levels, from signals proximal to the triggering of the T-cell receptor, such as calcium flux, to downstream effects, such as proliferation and cytokine production. Defects in signaling of the cytokine receptors on lymphocytes can be assessed by measuring phosphorylation of key signaling molecules, such as STAT3 phosphorylation upon triggering of the IL-6 of IL-21 receptors. The oxidative burst of neutrophils is partially to completely inoperative in the chronic granulomatous diseases and can be assessed using flow cytometry to ascertain an oxidation-dependent fluorescent shift of the dyes dihydrorhodamine-1,2,3 (DHR) or 2′, 7′-dichlorofluorescein diacetate (DCF). B-cell function can be assessed functionally by immunizing the subject and assessing antibody responses. For T-dependent neoantigens, this kind of test would reveal the capability of naïve B-cells to trigger, receive T-cell help, undergo isotype switching, and produce antibodies. For recall antigens, this test would assess the capacity of memory B-cells to produce protective levels of antibodies. The complement pathways can be assessed by the CH50 and AH50 tests, which test the capacity of complement to lyse red blood cells or by quantifying individual complement levels.

TABLE 47-2 Tier-Wise Approach to Immunologic Testing

1. General: CBC with differential, Immunoglobulins, Lymphocyte subset, Complement levels
2. Vaccine response evaluation: T-dependent vs. T-independent responses (S. pneumo, Tetanus, Hib), Lymphocyte proliferation assays
3. Directed testing: CD40L, BTK protein expression, Neutrophil Oxidative Index (NOI), STAT phosphorylation assays etc.
4. Genetic testing: Gene panel, Whole exome, Whole genome

Of note, many immunologists favor moving toward early genetic testing rather than performing extensive laboratory evaluations. In many cases, genetic testing is a quicker and less expensive diagnostic tool that can provide clinicians with a timely diagnosis which can then direct therapy.

OVERVIEW OF SELECTED PI

SEVERE COMBINED IMMUNE DEFICIENCY

SCID refers to a collection of disorders where generation of functional T-cells is absent, due to defects in the cytokine receptors or associated signaling pathways, V(D)J recombination machinery, calcium signaling pathways, or in the T-cell receptor complex itself. Mutations in at least 20 genes have been implicated.

Many types of SCID also feature deficiency of B-cells and NK cells. Most infants with SCID will show pan-hypogammaglobulinemia as maternal antibodies wane (around 3-6 months of age). In rarer circumstances, some children with SCID-associated gene mutations develop into Omenn syndrome phenotype, with eosinophilia, erythroderma, and expansion of highly activated, oligoclonal, autoreactive T-cells.

Children with SCID present with failure to thrive in the first few months of life with recurrent, severe, or opportunistic infections such as *Pneumocystis* pneumonia. Treatment focuses on stabilization, replacement of immunoglobulins, nutritional support, and HSCT (hematopoietic stem-cell transplantation). A few SCID types have been successfully managed by autologous gene correction ("gene therapy") performed in a research setting.

Of note, the term combined immune deficiency refers to disorders where T-cells are present but in lower numbers and/or diminished function. These disorders may also affect B-cell numbers and function, either because of the effect of the mutation itself or because of poor T-cell help needed for isotype switching and germinal center activity. These disorders include SCID, Wiskott-Aldrich syndrome, Hyper IgM syndrome, DOCK8 deficiency, and many others.

COMMON VARIABLE IMMUNODEFICIENCY (CVID)

CVID is one of the most common PIs. This group is extremely heterogeneous; unifying features are low immunoglobulin levels (low IgG with low IgM or IgA), low vaccine-specific antibody levels against vaccine antigens, and history of recurrent infections (mainly upper and lower respiratory bacterial infections). Most of these patients require either prophylactic antibiotic treatment or replacement of immunoglobulins by intravenous or subcutaneous routes to decrease the frequency and severity of infections. With time, autoimmune complications may develop. Occasionally autoimmune cytopenias may precede the classic infectious CVID phenotype. It appears from a few published cases that HSCT is curative for CVID with severe autoimmunity, but the long-term outcomes for these patients remains unclear. Additionally, patients may develop granulomas in the lungs, skin, or other organs and require biological anti-inflammatory therapies to control progression of granulomatous disease. Solid organ transplantation has been utilized in cases where the granulomatous disease results in organ failure.

A growing fraction of patients previously categorized as CVID are now being identified as having diverse monogenic defects. Thus, in young children the diagnosis of CVID should be accompanied by a vigilant search for specific genetic defects, which can be important for predicting prognosis or directing therapy. As an example, recently cases of CVID were identified with chromosome telomere dysfunction (dyskeratosis congenita or telomere syndrome), which can increase risks of bone marrow failure, liver disease, and autoimmunity. With the increased availability of whole-exome sequencing, the spectrum of genetic causes of CVID will undoubtedly increase and may allow clinicians to plan specific treatments.

TRANSIENT HYPOGAMMAGLOBULINEMIA OF INFANCY

Unlike CVID, patients with transient hypogammaglobulinemia have low immunoglobulin G levels in the first years of life that improves without intervention between 2 and 6 years. These patients may need prophylactic antibiotics for a short period of time, or rarely, immunoglobulin replacement. Patients with transient hypogammaglobulinemia associated with low IgA or mildly elevated antinuclear antibodies may be more likely to develop food allergies and autoimmunity later in life.

AGAMMAGLOBULINEMIA

Although not very common, patients may have complete absence of immunoglobulins as a result of defects in early B-cell development. Depending on the specific defect, the inheritance can be X-linked or autosomal recessive. These patients are prone to enteroviral and bacterial respiratory infections early in life, and immunoglobulin replacement therapy is essential as supportive therapy. The laboratory evaluation is notable for absence (or near absence) of B-cells and of all immunoglobulin isotypes. These patients typically present early in childhood, often as early as 6 months when maternally transferred IgG has waned. Occasionally, if the mutation does not fully ablate signaling of the B-cell receptor, a few B-cells may be found in the peripheral blood. Agammaglobulinemic patients often develop autoimmunity secondary to dysregulation of this small subset of B-cells. Definitive treatment with HSCT or gene therapy has been reported.

CHRONIC GRANULOMATOUS DISEASE

Mutations in five genes that comprise the NADPH oxidase complex are known to give rise to a functional defect of neutrophils to generate a sufficient burst of reactive oxygen species to kill phagocytosed bacteria, a set of disorders called chronic granulomatous disease (CGD). The majority of cases are seen in boys due to mutations of the *Cybb* gene. Invasive infections such as pneumonias, abscesses, and lymphadenitis with organisms, including *Staphylococcus aureus*, *Burkholderia cepacia*, *Aspergillus* species, and *Serratia marcescens*, should raise the suspicion of chronic granulomatous disease or other neutrophil defects. In addition, very early onset (before age 6) or treatment refractory inflammatory bowel disease has been described in CGD patients. Diagnosis is made first by the DHR test (also known as neutrophil oxidative burst test), which screens for the production of H_2O_2 by neutrophils using flow cytometric evaluation of fluorescent shift of dihydrorhodamine (DHR) upon stimulation by PMA. Because production of H_2O_2 requires both the NADPH oxidase enzymes as well as myeloperoxidase (MPO), it should be noted that MPO deficiency leads to false identification of a defective oxidative burst. All patients with CGD should receive prophylaxis with an antibiotic (trimethoprim/sulfamethoxazole is recommended) and antifungal (itraconazazole is recommended) to protect from the common pathogens. Aggressive treatment of infections is required, and prolonged treatment may be required. Many pediatric immunologists in the United States also recommend prophylaxis with interferon gamma. Hematopoietic stem cell transplantation is curative.

INNATE IMMUNE DEFECTS

The term innate immunity refers to the first-line, nonspecific arm of the immune system designed to quickly recognize and respond to invading pathogens. There are several components of innate immunity, including pattern recognition receptors and physical barriers.

Patients with mutations in the NF-Kappa B regulator NEMO have features of ectodermal dysplasia including a failure to sweat and conical teeth and carry an increased susceptibility to viral and bacterial infections because of defective Toll-like receptor signaling and defective cytotoxic function of NK cells. They generally have variable antibody responses and poor antibody class switching. Notably, many of these children have infections early in infancy despite maternal antibodies, highlighting the failure of innate cells to be activated by opsonized bacteria. HSCT has been successful in restoring immune function in these patients.

Patients with mutations in the cytokine signaling axis that includes IL-12, interferon-gamma, and STAT1 have characteristic susceptibility to mycobacterial infections (including generally nonvirulent strains such as from the Bacille Calmette-Guerin vaccine), chronic mucocutaneous *Candida* infections, and salmonellosis. Gain-of-function mutations in STAT1 have, in addition, been associated with autoimmunity. Patients with hyper-IgE syndrome (HIES, Job syndrome), due to deficiency of STAT3, show characteristic physical features (wide nose, facial asymmetry, delayed shedding of primary teeth) and recurrent staphylococcal infections of the soft tissue. Because of the critical role of STAT3 in development of Th17 cells, the absence of these cells is a useful diagnostic marker. These patients have a significant increase in susceptibility to pneumonias with formation of pneumatoceles, and recurrent episodes of varicella zoster infection and Epstein-Barr infection.

Deficiencies of virtually every circulating complement component have been described. Patients with defects early in the complement cascade (e.g., C2 and C4) show an increased predisposition to bacterial infections and autoimmunity, including systemic lupus erythematosus and rheumatoid arthritis. In addition, these subjects and those with defects in later parts of the cascade show a characteristic susceptibility to *Neisseria* infection.

HALLMARK SIGNS IN PATIENTS WITH PI

In order to identify PI patients as early as possible and mitigate or avoid permanent sequelae, clinicians should maintain increased vigilance for hallmark signs of PI based on a detailed clinical history (failure to thrive, need for IV antibiotics and positive family history of PI being the strongest predictors). In addition, evidence of increased susceptibility to infections, autoimmunity, evidence of immune dysregulation, or cancer are other hallmark findings. We cover each of the areas next.

SUSCEPTIBILITY TO INFECTION

Pediatric hospitalists should be aware that increased susceptibility to infections is the main hallmark of PIs. Infections can be severe, persistent, invasive, and/or recurrent. Opportunistic organisms are not uncommon in situations where cellular immunity or innate defenses are compromised. Infections may not be apparent in the first few months of life due to transient passive immunity conferred from transplacental transfer of IgG from the mother, mostly during the third trimester.

Depending on the specific immunodeficiency, infants will be susceptible to particular pathogens. Infants with defects of T-cell immunity such as SCID may present with severe diarrheal illnesses due to vaccine-strain rotavirus. In addition, defects in innate or T-cell immunity can also result in local or disseminated infection from the *Mycobacterium Bovis* Bacille Calmette-Guerin vaccine strain ("BCGosis") in countries outside the United States where this vaccine is employed. Severe encephalitis in infancy due to HSV-1 may be indicative of defects of the innate TLR3 pathway. Severe candidal infections have been described in infants with defects of tolerance due to impaired selection of T-cells in the thymus. Along with unusual infections, infants with PI can have more severe courses of disease with common childhood viral infections such as RSV or EBV, often times requiring prolonged hospitalization. It may also take longer than 3 weeks for patients to clear their infection and return to baseline health.

Outside of infancy, older children and young adults may present with bacterial, viral, and fungal infections. Any serious, invasive infection in a child should at least trigger consideration of an immune defect, especially if it involves an opportunistic pathogen such as CMV, Toxoplasmosis, or Cryptoccocus. If infections are disseminated (bacteremia) or occur in uncommon locations (ex. Staphylococcus liver abscess or Neisseria meningitis), then an immunologic evaluation may be warranted.

SUSCEPTIBLITY TO AUTOIMMUNITY

Autoimmunity is increasingly noted either as a presenting sign of PI (especially in pediatrics) or as a complication of PI. It poses a great challenge to specialists, as autoimmunity in PI often is refractory to initial therapy. Further, autoimmune manifestations can broaden with time, and flares may be triggered by infections.

Curiously, the generation of autoreactive cells is a natural phenomenon throughout childhood but mechanisms of central and peripheral tolerance attenuate these cells at specific checkpoints of T- and B-cell development. In PI, the immune defect may impair these checkpoints and allow for the accumulation of autoreactive cells, priming the patient for development of clinical autoimmune disease.

In PI, autoimmune cytopenias (e.g., immune thrombocytopenia, autoimmune hemolytic anemia, and autoimmune neutropenia) are the most common autoimmune disorders. Any patient with autoimmune cytopenia who has a prolonged and complicated course or insufficient response to conventional therapy should be considered for evaluation of PI. Of note, at least 65% of cases of pediatric Evan's syndrome (development of autoimmune hemolytic anemia and immune thrombocytopenic purpura, and more rarely neutropenia) may be due to a monogenic cause; identification of the underlying genetic mutations may help guide toward targeted therapy. Autoimmune cytopenias often reflect B-cell dysregulation and therefore can be present in a wide variety of PIs where B- and T-cell tolerance is impaired such as in common variable immunodeficiency (CVID), autoimmune polyendocrinopathy candidiasis ectodermal dystrophy (APECED), immunodysregulation polyendocrinopathy enteropathy X-linked (IPEX) syndrome, or autoimmune lymphoproliferative syndrome (ALPS) with defects in apoptosis and therefore increased survival of autoreactive T-cells.

The most common PI is CVID, which is characterized by insufficient production of immunoglobulins leading to poor specific responses to vaccinations and (typically) recurrent sinopulmonary infections. Autoimmune cytopenias can be present in 10% to 30% of CVID cases; CVID patients often initially present with an autoimmune cytopenia and later develop infectious complications. Furthermore, other autoimmune complications such as vitiligo have recently been associated with CVID.

Endocrine autoimmune manifestations can occur among patients with APECED and IPEX, where infections are coupled with early onset adrenal or parathyroid disease or type 1 diabetes. APECED patients may present solely with candidiasis early in life, while autoimmune manifestations of the endocrine system may appear in later decades. On the other hand, for IPEX patients, around 75% have type 1 diabetes and 60% have autoimmune skin disease (i.e., eczematous dermatitis) as early as infancy.

Hypomorphic genetic defects in the RAG1 or RAG2 (recombinase-activating gene) genes are also associated with an autoimmune presentation, along with a recently described phenotype of combined immunodeficiency (CID). Patients in this group have fewer infections than might be expected with this genetic defect, but late-onset autoimmune disease often occurs that may include destructive granulomatous vasculitis, myasthenia gravis, Guillen-Barre syndrome, and vitiligo. Ultimately, some of these patients require HSCT for resistant cases.

Patients with DiGeorge syndrome (22q11.2 deletion syndrome which presents with hypocalcemia, immunodeficiency, cleft palate, heart defects, and other complications) will also present with autoimmune complications, including arthritis (2% in children) and autoimmune cytopenias (4%). The autoimmune phenotype of Wiskott-Aldrich syndrome patients (who commonly present with eczema, immunodeficiency and recurrent infections) is quite variable (40%-72% prevalence) and has been shown in experimental models to be due to defective tolerance of both T-cells and B-cells. Autoimmune manifestations include hemolytic anemia (~30%), arthritis, vasculitis, and inflammatory bowel disease. When associated with autoimmune manifestations, patients with Wiskott-Aldrich syndrome have poorer long-term outcomes and therefore qualify for early consideration of hematopoietic stem cell transplantation.

Currently, one of the great challenges in the treatment of autoimmune disorders is the occurrence of granulomatous conditions. These lesions are most commonly seen in the lung but may occur in any mucosal surfaces including the GI tract, skin, or brain). These lesions can occur in a variety of PIs. In the lung, function can be severely impaired, and if associated with vasculitis may result in destruction of the surrounding tissues. Treatment with anti-inflammatory and immunosuppressive medications has shown success in reducing the impact of granulomatous conditions, including the use of rituximab and azathioprine.

In addition, autoimmune enteropathies can pose additional challenges to specialists and can contribute to low immunoglobulin (mainly IgG) levels and even loss of lymphocytes. In genetically susceptible individuals, triggers of enteropathy may include infections or dietary gluten or dairy. Severe diarrhea from noninfectious enteropathy can start early in life in patients with SCID or IPEX; both immunodeficiencies are considered emergencies.

SUSCEPTIBLITY TO CANCER

In a recent meta-analysis, the prevalence of malignancy in CVID patients was found to be 8.6%, with a prevalence of lymphoma of 4.1%. The increased susceptibility to malignancy has been noted in several other primary immunodeficiencies. It is thought that chronic infection (due to inability to fully clear pathogens), along with chronic inflammation, immune dysregulation due to specific mutations as well as defective cancer surveillance by immune cells may all contribute to this increased risk.

Chronic infection from *Helicobacter pylori*, and the resulting inflammation, may underlie increased risk of developing stomach cancers. Screening for *H. pylori* is recommended for CVID patients, even if asymptomatic, though there is no consensus regarding type or frequency of screening. The most cost-effective approach is screening for the *H. pylori* antigen in the stool.

B-cell lymphomas have been described in patients with varying primary immunodeficiencies, mostly associated with Epstein-Barr virus (EBV), with most cases presenting in the 4th to 7th decades of life, more commonly in women. One risk factor identified in large cohorts is high polyclonal IgM levels. Diagnostic evaluation of persistent lymphadenopathy in CVID patients where there is a suspicion of lymphoma may require a multidisciplinary approach including Immunology, hematology/oncology, and rheumatology.

There is a significant increase in cancers among primary immune deficiencies where the underlying defect entails impaired repair of DNA damage, for example, ataxia-telangiectasia (A-T), Nijmegen breakage syndrome, Lynch syndrome (also known as hereditary nonpolyposis colorectal cancer), and MRE11 mutation (ataxia-telangiectasia-like disorder). Approximately 10% of A-T patients develop lymphoid malignancies, most commonly T-cell-derived non-Hodgkin lymphomas and leukemias. The severity of the neurological phenotype of A-T does not appear to correlate with the risk of developing lymphoid cancers. A-T patients also bear an increased risk of developing carcinomas of the stomach, breast, and parotid glands. Management of cancers in these patients is especially complex because of the systemic toxicities of radiation and chemotherapy and their poor ability to repair DNA damage.

Patients with DC-monocyte-B-NK deficiency disease, an autosomal dominant deficiency of the transcription factor *Gata2,* have an increased susceptibility to myelodysplastic syndrome and acute myeloid leukemias. This deficiency should be suspected in patients with monocytopenia along with other myeloid abnormalities, such as chronic neutropenia or refractory cytopenias. Immune deficiencies (such as complete NK cell deficiency and combined immune deficiency) where chronic inflammation can result from defective clearance of chronic viral infections (including Ebstein Barr virus) or inappropriate downregulation of immune responses, can be associated with the development of tumors. A few patients with ALPS have developed diverse lymphomas, with an average age of diagnosis around 28 years. Though at least six genes have been identified as leading to the ALPS (autoimmune lymphoproliferative syndrome) phenotype, it is not yet known if all genotypes lead to an increased risk of cancers. Patients with familial inheritance of genes that increase risk of hemophagocytic lymphohistiocytosis (HLH) are also suspected to have an increased risk of lymphomas.

SUSCEPTIBLITY TO IMMUNE DYSREGULATION

Although inflammatory conditions are often without a clear genetic defect and are primarily managed by rheumatologists, it is not uncommon to see PI cases presenting in increased states of inflammation (elevated inflammatory markers, immunoglobulin G and A levels). An elevated IgG level does not exclude an underlying antibody deficiency and evaluating the quality of antibodies by measures such as vaccine-specific titers should be strongly considered. Specifically, patients with gain-of-function mutations in STAT1 and STAT3 have significant autoinflammation including fevers, vasculitis, enteropathy, and mucocutaneous inflammation. They also have an increased susceptibility to infection. Patients with ALPS classically present with generalized lymphadenopathy, hepatosplenomegaly, increased levels of immunoglobulins, and B-cells with autoimmune manifestations that commonly include hemolytic anemia, glomerulonephritis, and idiopathic thrombocytopenic purpura. In auto-inflammatory syndromes, the presence of generalized serositis might mislead the clinician to suspect infectious arthritis. This is often accompanied by a myriad of symptoms, including elevation of acute-phase reagents, intermittent dermatitis, deafness, joint deformity, and multifocal osteomyelitis.

Hemophagocytic lymphohistiocytosis (HLH) is a rare but potentially fatal disease in which cytokine dysfunction, uncontrolled accumulation of activated T-cells and histiocytes, and the inability to terminate the immune response leads to clinical manifestations of extreme inflammation and end-organ damage. Familial forms of HLH may present late in childhood or even in adulthood. Recurrent fevers without source, with hepatomegaly and laboratory evidence of severe inflammation (highly increased ferritin levels and inflammatory markers) are warning signs of HLH.

Two recently discovered immunodeficiencies that highlight the overlap between immunodeficiency and immune dysregulation are PLCG2-associated antibody deficiency and immune dysregulation (PLAID) and B-cell expansion with NF-KB and T-cell anergy (BENTA). PLCG2 patients have a distinct history of hives that appear after sweat evaporation occurs on the skin. The constellation of symptoms includes cold urticaria and variable manifestations including atopy, granulomatous rash, autoimmune thyroiditis, presence of antinuclear antibodies, sinopulmonary infections, and common variable immunodeficiency. Along the same lines, mutations in *PLCG2* were also reported in a new inflammatory disease characterized by recurrent blistering skin lesions, bronchiolitis, arthralgias, ocular inflammation, enterocolitis, absence of autoantibodies, and mild susceptibility to infections. Additionally six patients have been diagnosed with BENTA and found to have mutations of CARD11 (also called CARMA1) which result in gain-of-function signaling of the NF-KB pathway with evidence of systemic inflammation, congenital hepatosplenomegaly, lymphadenopathy, and B-cell lymphocytosis. They also show poor T-cell proliferative responses and as a consequence, chronic EBV and other herpes viral infections.

SUSCEPTIBLITY TO ATOPIC DISEASE

Immune dysregulation in PI may also manifest with a wide array of food or environmental allergies. Severe atopic dermatitis is the hallmark of Wiskott-Aldrich syndrome and hyper-IgE syndrome with either STAT3 or DOCK8 mutations. Wiskott-Aldrich syndrome and DOCK 8 deficiency patients often have numerous food allergies with a history of anaphylaxis that may continue to adulthood. Patients with less ablative mutations associated with SCID generate T- and B-cells in low numbers but with autoreactive properties. The expansion of autoreactive T-cells on the periphery can result in hyperinflammation and severe dermatitis resembling eczema, termed Omenn syndrome. Gain-of-function mutations in STAT5b have been reported to cause eosinophilia, urticaria, and atopic dermatitis.

KEY POINTS

- The occurrence of recurrent, severe, invasive, or opportunistic infections or severe autoimmune diseases (including autoimmune cytopenias) in any child should prompt a thoughtful history, physical examination, and laboratory studies to evaluate for primary immunodeficiency.
- Need for intravenous antibiotics, failure to thrive, or a relevant family history are the strongest predictors of PI.
- Consultation with a pediatric immunologist and other pediatric subspecialists are often necessary for diagnosis and treatment of these children.

SUGGESTED READING

Bjelac JA, Yonkof JR, Fernandez J. Differing performance of the warning signs for immunodeficiency in the diagnosis of pediatric versus adult patients in a two-center tertiary referral population. *J Clin Immunol.* 2019;39:90-98.

Boyle JM, Buckley RH. Population prevalence of diagnosed primary immunodeficiency diseases in the United States. *J Clin Immunol.* 2007; 27: 497-502.

Chase NM, Verbsky JW, Hintermeyer MK, et al. Use of combination chemotherapy for treatment of granulomatous and lymphocytic interstitial lung disease (GLILD) in patients with common variable immunodeficiency (CVID). *J Clin Immunol.* 2013;33:30-39.

Dhabhar FS, Miller AH, Stein M, et al. Diurnal and acute stress-induced changes in distribution of peripheral blood leukocyte subpopulations. *Brain Behav Immun.* 1994;8:66-79.

Hadjadj J, Aladjidi N, Fernandes H, et al. Pediatric Evans syndrome is associated with a high frequency of potentially damaging variants in immune genes. *Blood.* 2019;134:9-21.

Kiaee F, Azizi G, Rafiemanesh H, et al. Malignancy in common variable immunodeficiency: a systematic review and meta-analysis. *Expert Rev Clin Immunol.* 2019;15(10):1105-13.

Krainer J, Siebenhandl S, Weinhäusel A. Systemic autoinflammatory diseases. *J Autoimmun.* 2020;109.

Ma CA, Xi L, Cauff B, et al. Somatic STAT5b gain-of-function mutations in early onset nonclonal eosinophilia, urticaria, dermatitis, and diarrhea. *Blood.* 2017;129:650-653.

MacGinnitie A, Aloi F, Mishra S. Clinical characteristics of pediatric patients evaluated for primary immunodeficiency. *Pediatr Allergy Immunol.* 2011; 22:671-675.

O'Sullivan MD, Cant AJ. The 10 warning signs: a time for a change? *Curr Opin Allergy Clin Immunol.* 2012;12:588-594.
Reda SM, El-Ghoneimy DH, Afifi HM. Clinical predictors of primary immunodeficiency diseases in children. *Allergy Asthma Immunol Res.* 2013;5:88-95.
Wen L, Atkinson JP, Giclas PC. Clinical and laboratory evaluation of complement deficiency. *J Allergy Clin Immunol.* 2004;113:585-593.
Zhou Q, Lee, G-S, Brady J, et al. A hypermorphic missense mutation in PLCG2, encoding phosolipase Cy2, causes a dominantly inherited autoinflammatory disease with immunodeficiency. *Am J Hum Gen.* 2012;91:713-720.

CHAPTER 48

Intravenous Immune Globulin (IVIg)

Kiran A. Kulkarni, MD, MS and Ajay Bhasin, MD

BACKGROUND

Intravenous immunoglobulin (IVIg) is a polyclonal mixture of immunoglobulin G (IgG) antibodies that can be administered intravenously. IVIg is used primarily as replacement therapy in a variety of disorders marked by IgG deficiency. Additionally, IVIg has anti-inflammatory and immune-modulatory functions and plays a role in the treatment of various autoimmune disorders.

Each IVIg dose is manufactured from pooled human plasma obtained from thousands of donors who are screened for infection with human immunodeficiency virus (HIV) 1 and 2, hepatitis B and C, prion disease, and syphilis. Besides donor screening, most IVIg preparations undergo multiple purification steps that further reduce the potential risk of viral contamination. All IVIg preparations have trace amounts of IgA antibodies. As with all blood products, there is theoretical but extremely low risk of transmission of viral or other pathogens.

MECHANISM OF ACTION

The mechanisms of action of IVIg are multiple, complex, and yet have not been completely elucidated. The prophylactic effects of IVIg against infection occur because IVIg provides high titer antibodies against common pathogens. Prophylaxis against infection can usually be achieved with "replacement" doses of approximately 0.4 g/kg.

The anti-inflammatory activity of IVIg is less well understood. Multiple theories have been proposed including Fc glycosylation increasing expression of inhibitory Fc receptors on antigen presenting cells reducing auto-antibody production, direct binding and sequestration of abnormal host antibodies, or potentially complement mediated antibody removal, but the true mechanism remains unknown. IVIg is typically dosed at 1 to 2 g/kg when used to control inflammation.

APPROVED USES AND DOSING

The US Food and Drug Administration (FDA) has approved seven applications of IVIg or subcutaneous immunoglobulin (SCIG): primary immunodeficiency, acute immune thrombocytopenic purpura, secondary immunodeficiency due to leukemia, prevention of infection and graft-versus-host disease in bone marrow or stem cell transplant recipients (HSCT), prevention of infection in pediatric HIV disease, chronic inflammatory demyelinating polyneuropathy, and prevention of coronary sequelae of Kawasaki disease. Though not FDA approved, IVIg use is considered standard of care in Multisystem Inflammatory Syndrome in Children (MIS-C) secondary to severe acute respiratory syndrome coronavirus 2 (SARS-CoV-2) as well. Dosing recommendations for these approved indications are provided in **Table 48-1**. There are also many other off-label uses, some of which are discussed later in this chapter.

TABLE 48-1 Approved Indications for Intravenous Immunoglobulin Therapy

FDA Indication	Suggested Dose and Regimen
Primary immunodeficiency	400-500 mg/kg every 3-4 wk
Immune thrombocytopenic purpura	0.8-1 g/kg × 1 dose (low dose) *or* 1 g/kg/day × 2 days *or* 400 mg/kg/day × 5 days
Chronic lymphocytic leukemia	400 mg/kg every 3-4 wk
Stem cell transplantation	500 mg/kg/wk prn (IgG <500)
HIV infection	400 mg/kg every 4 wk
Kawasaki disease	2 g/kg × 1-2 doses
Chronic inflammatory demyelinating polyneuropathy	2 g/kg loading dose, followed by 1 g/kg every 3 wk

FDA, Food and Drug Administration; HIV, human immunodeficiency virus; IgG, Immunoglobulin G.

PRIMARY IMMUNODEFICIENCY

Antibody replacement for primary immunodeficiency is indicated for patients with hypogammaglobulinemia and increased susceptibility to infection. Disorders in this category include severe combined immunodeficiency, agammaglobulinemia, common variable immunodeficiency, and specific antibody deficiency in addition to other disorders that may drive a lower total serum IgG.

Past studies established the benefit of keeping IgG levels above 500 mg/dL to decrease the risk of bacterial and *Pneumocystis* pneumonia. The exact target IgG level should be determined in discussion with immunologists considering the child's specific immunodeficiency and clinical condition, but dosing should start at the FDA recommended dose of 100 mg/kg/week and titrate further to achieve maximum benefit with minimal drug.

IMMUNE THROMBOCYTOPENIA

Although immune thrombocytopenic purpura (ITP) typically does not require treatment, platelet count in patients with ITP will immediately increase post IVIg infusion. Therefore, IVIg may be considered in situations where patients are at higher risk for bleeding (surgical procedures), overt bleeding, or a platelet count less than 30,000/mm^3. Though corticosteroids are often first-line therapy, IVIg may also be used as first line therapy, with steroid failure, or adjunctively with steroids. In situations with life-threatening bleeding, IVIg is administered along with corticosteroid therapy. IVIg tends to raise counts rapidly, but the effect may be temporary.

IMMUNODEFICIENCY WITH LEUKEMIA

A secondary immunodeficiency can occur with B-cell chronic lymphocytic leukemia. In such patients with hypogammaglobulinemia and a history of infections, IVIg therapy is indicated. Randomized trials have demonstrated a beneficial decrease in infections at recommended doses.

STEM CELL TRANSPLANTATION

IVIg historically was given to prevent infection, decrease rates of CMV reactivation, and decrease risk of acute graft-vs-host disease during HSCT (see Chapter 134). However, evidence has been mixed on reduction of post-transplant infectious events, and no trial has demonstrated significant mortality benefit. Further, its use has become controversial with the advent of better CMV-directed therapies (e.g., ganciclovir, valganciclovir, foscarnet, cidofovir, maribavir) and post-transplant management. The effect of IVIg seems to be greatest in patients with post-transplant hypogammaglobulinemia, but no trial has compared subsets of HSCT recipients (HLA-identical vs non-identical, high vs low IgG or formulation or administration route). Use of IVIg should be at the discretion of the treating hematologist for select indications.

KAWASAKI DISEASE

Kawasaki disease is a pediatric vasculitis of unclear cause, but recent evidence suggests a viral trigger. Though infrequent, aneurysmal damage to coronary (or other) may occur as a result of the vasculitis. Numerous studies have demonstrated that an immunosuppressive dose of IVIg in the first 7 to 10 days of the disease lowers risk of coronary artery aneurysms. While historically a second dose of IVIg was considered if fever persists >36 hours after the first dose, recent data suggests that infliximab may be superior to a second dose of IVIg for refractory disease. For more information, see Chapter 148.

MULTISYSTEM INFLAMMATORY SYNDROME IN CHILDREN (MIS-C) ASSOCIATED WITH SEVERE ACUTE RESPIRATORY SYNDROME CORONAVIRUS 2 (SARS-COV-2)

The hallmarks of MIS-C mirror those of Kawasaki disease though MIS-C affected patients have generally been older (see Chapters 106 and 107). IVIg in conjunction with methylprednisolone results in improvement in fever, reduced left ventricular dysfunction, reduced PICU stay, and reduced length of stay. Currently, no trials exist comparing efficacy of therapy; however, given the similarity to Kawasaki disease and potential aversion of poor outcomes, use of IVIg in MIS-C is recommended at a dose of 2 g/kg. For patients with refractory disease, additional biologic therapy (e.g., infliximab or anakinra) may be considered if IVIg and methylprednisolone (1-2 mg/kg IV q12 hours; can increase to 10-30 mg/kg/day [max 1000mg/day] for 1-3 days) do not abate the disease course with all up-to-date information listed on the CDC and NIH websites.

HUMAN IMMUNODEFICIENCY VIRUS INFECTION

Pediatric HIV infection (Chapter 104) is marked by frequent viral and bacterial infections. In the early 1990s, the role of IVIg in reducing rates of secondary infection was studied in large crossover, placebo-controlled, randomized, double-blind trials. These trials demonstrated benefits to children, particularly those with CD4 counts greater than 200 cells/μL. Moreover, the CD4 counts of patients receiving IVIg decreased at a slower pace than those receiving placebo.

CHRONIC INFLAMMATORY DEMYELINATING POLYNEUROPATHY

Chronic inflammatory demyelinating polyneuropathy, a rare, acquired peripheral sensory and/or motor polyneuropathy closely related to Guillain-Barré syndrome, may be treated with IVIg. IVIg (in combination with other approved therapies (plasma exchange and corticosteroids) improves disability at 1 month relative to placebo through reducing symptoms (weakness, sensory loss, imbalance, and pain) and improving functional status. Additionally, long-term treatment (every 3-4 weeks) resulted in a prolonged time to relapse.

OFF LABEL USES

IVIg may be used to treat many diseases off label. Some diseases, like Guillain-Barré syndrome and MIS-C, with similar pathophysiologic origin to those with FDA-approved treatment indications, like CIDP and Kawasaki disease, respectively, are treatable by IVIg. The role of IVIg in other disorders is controversial and is often not supported by convincing clinical evidence, especially in pediatrics.

NEUROLOGIC DISORDERS

Guillain-Barré syndrome is a polyradiculoneuritis with a presumed immune-mediated cause. It may follow viral respiratory infections and can lead to respiratory failure in children. In adults, numerous trials of IVIg have demonstrated a benefit similar to plasma exchange in hastening the recovery of walking. Consequently, use of IVIg has been incorporated into the latest American Academy of Neurology practice parameters for Guillain-Barré syndrome. Several small trials in children have also demonstrated benefits similar to plasma exchange. Dosing of 2 g/kg divided over 2 days or 5 days appears to be equally effective.

IVIg may be beneficial in other neurologic disorders like myasthenia gravis, Lambert-Eaton myasthenic syndrome, and multiple sclerosis. In children, refractory seizures as part of Lennox-Gastaut and Rasmussen syndromes have been treated successfully with several different dosing regimens of IVIg, although recommendation for general use is limited by the size and quality of the studies, and none have been repeated since the early 1990s. Notably, large-scale studies of adults with refractory seizures have failed to consistently show benefit.

IMMUNE-MEDIATED BLOOD DYSCRASIAS

IVIg has been used to treat multiple immune-mediated blood dyscrasias. Isoimmune and alloimmune hemolytic disease of the newborn increase the risk of hyperbilirubinemia and kernicterus. Severe cases may require exchange transfusion. For isoimmune hemolytic disease of the newborn, the American Academy of Pediatrics (AAP) recommends administration of IVIg if the total serum bilirubin rises despite phototherapy or is within 2 mg/dL of the exchange transfusion level. IVIg has shown no benefit for alloimmune hemolytic disease to date, though higher quality studies are needed.

IVIg may also be used to treat autoimmune hemolytic anemia (AIHA). Additionally, it is considered first-line treatment in children with Evan's syndrome (AIHA, ITP, and/or autoimmune neutropenia) when ITP or AIHA are present. It can additionally be used prophylactically in children with Evan's syndrome to maintain IgG levels.

Moreover, IVIg has been reported as a potential therapy for children with autoimmune neutropenia.

INFECTION PREVENTION AND TREATMENT

In premature infants, there is limited evidence regarding the efficacy of IVIg in prevention of nosocomial infections. Large center trials have evaluated use of IVIg in sepsis and septic shock for preterm and/or low birth weight infants and failed to show efficacy. Additionally, despite the hypothetical benefit of endotoxin-blocking antibodies in septic shock, a placebo-controlled multicenter trial including over 3000 infants did not demonstrate any difference in death, major disability at age 2 or subsequent sepsis. Therefore, current evidence does not support the routine use of IVIg in neonatal sepsis. No high-quality data exists examining the use of IVIg in sepsis for older pediatric patients; however, given the lack of benefit in adult patients and the known lack of efficacy in neonates, it can be postulated that IVIg administration will not improve outcomes. As such, routine IVIg use cannot be recommended for use in pediatric patients with sepsis.

IVIg may be used to treat certain infections. In conjunction with antivirals, it may be used to treat RSV in stem cell transplant patients, though results of its efficacy are mixed. Historically, orally administered IVIg has been used to treat gastrointestinal infections, such as rotavirus, with a single dose of orally administered IVIg at 0.3 g/kg. A placebo-controlled trial demonstrated that this dose shortened duration of diarrhea, viral shedding, and length of hospitalization for children with acute rotaviral gastroenteritis. It may be considered in the case of recalcitrant or worsening rotaviral diarrhea despite maximum supportive care.

SOLID ORGAN TRANSPLANT

IVIg is widely used in solid-organ transplant patients to both prevent and treat acute humoral rejection. Multiple case series and case reports demonstrate benefit in pediatric and adult patients for many different types of solid organ transplant. Some evidence from smaller randomized trials has demonstrated benefit; however, this has largely been limited to adults receiving renal transplants.

OTHER AUTOIMMUNE DISORDERS

Finally, IVIg may play a role in the treatment of autoimmune disorders such as autoimmune blistering skin diseases (e.g., pemphigoid diseases and epidermolysis bullosa acquisita), juvenile dermatomyositis, and catastrophic antiphospholipid antibody syndrome. Though there may not be controlled, prospective trials in children, available evidence suggests efficacy and a role for IVIg in treating these disorders in children.

ADVERSE REACTIONS

Because infectious risk is lower than other blood products, protocols for obtaining formal informed consent vary by institution. Nevertheless, patients should be counseled on theoretical infectious risks and common adverse reactions. Adverse reactions to IVIg are common: approximately 2.5% of patients experience some type of reaction.

The most common reactions include headache, fever, myalgia, chills, transient urticaria, and flushing during the infusion; these are likely related to IgG aggregates and complement activation. These effects can be diminished by reducing the rate of infusion, premedicating with diphenhydramine and acetaminophen/non-steroidal anti-inflammatories, decreasing the concentration of the IVIg solution, or changing to a different IVIg product. Hypotension can occur and should be treated with immediate cessation of the infusion, intramuscular epinephrine, and volume expansion. Anaphylaxis is extremely rare. Some case series describe anaphylaxis in patients receiving IVIg who are IgA or IgA subclass deficient. In these situations, an IVIg preparation with a low IgA content should be used if IVIg therapy is still necessary.

Renal failure following IVIg is unusual in children but can sometimes be seen in adults. To avoid this complication, patients should be well hydrated. If concern arises for potential medication-induced toxicity or in patients in whom there is elevated risk of medication-induced toxicity, sucrose-free formulations are available.

Headaches following IVIg administration can be common. Headaches typically present 6 to 12 hours after infusion and can last up to 72 hours. Some patients may develop aseptic meningitis, which classically appears within 48 hours of therapy. Few patients may develop posterior reversible encephalopathy syndrome. Typically, only supportive care is needed, and the symptoms typically resolve after 2 to 3 days. Proper hydration, antihistamines, and analgesics can help prevent and treat headaches and aseptic meningitis. Many institutions employ pre-medication protocols to help avert these side effects. Occasionally, corticosteroids may be required to treat symptoms associated with IVIg infusion.

Many less-common reactions have been described. Patients may develop asymptomatic liver enzyme (aspartate aminotransferase and alanine aminotransferase) elevations. Screening for hepatitis infection is recommended in these cases, and it may be necessary to switch products for future administration. Because IVIg contains anti-ABO blood group antibodies, transient Coombs-positive hemolytic anemia can be seen. Transient neutropenia following IVIg has been described in case reports. Serious but rare complications include thromboses, transfusion-associated acute lung injury, and arrhythmia.

SPECIAL CONSIDERATIONS

IV FORMULATIONS

Many IVIg formulations are available, and although they are labeled for specific uses by the FDA, products are often used interchangeably. This is particularly true given periodic shortages of certain IVIg products. Product choice may also be influenced by the content of other additives or contaminants. For example, products with low IgA content may be preferred in patients with undetectable IgA levels, or use of sucrose-free products may be preferred in patients with renal disease.

TROUGH LEVELS AND LABORATORY ASSESSMENT

Trough levels in primary immune deficiency should be monitored every 6 months for patients on regular therapy, or more often during periods of rapid growth. Trough levels can suggest inadequate dosing but should not be used to withhold doses if the trough level is above goal (i.e., doses should continue at the scheduled 3-4-week intervals). Doses can be adjusted for both trough levels and frequency of infections. Some patients may require higher trough levels to remain infection free, and dosing decisions should not be based on trough IgG level alone. Other routine laboratory monitoring is not required, but kidney and liver function tests and CBC may be considered for those receiving scheduled therapy.

VACCINE RESPONSE

Recent receipt of IVIg or other immunoglobulin may diminish responses to live vaccines. After a patient has received IVIg, one should avoid giving the measles-mumps-rubella vaccine (or its components) or the varicella live-virus vaccine for 8 to 11 months. There are generally no restrictions to the administration of non–live-virus vaccines following IVIg, and in fact, many practitioners routinely administer inactivated influenza vaccine to patients receiving IVIg. Vaccination information is freely available on the CDC website.

SUBCUTANEOUS IVIg

Increasingly common is the use of subcutaneous IVIg (SCIG). SCIG is equally effective in providing treatment for many of the mentioned conditions. As opposed to IVIg which attains a much higher Ig "spike" concentration owing to the dosing mechanism and frequency, the subcutaneous variant does not, leading to fewer side effects at the expense of more frequent dosing. Mild local reactions are common. Another advantage, especially in the pediatric population, is that intravenous access is not required. Because of the lower incidence of systemic side effects and the ease of administration, subcutaneous immunoglobulin has become the dominant route of immunoglobulin replacement for children with immunodeficiency.

KEY POINTS

- IVIg is a medication consisting of polyclonal IgG antibodies purified from human blood donors. The risk of infection is extremely low, but transfusion reactions are common.
- IVIg plays a major role in providing passive humoral immunity in primary immunodeficiencies, leukemia, HIV infection, and sometimes hematopoietic stem cell transplantation.
- In high doses, it can be immunosuppressive and has become a standard therapy for immune modulation in numerous pediatric diseases, both on and off label.
- IVIg is associated with some side effects which may be mitigated with pre-medication, hydration, and close observation.

SUGGESTED READINGS

Acero-Garcés DO, García-Perdomo HA. First line treatments for newly diagnosed primary immune thrombocytopenia in children: a systematic review and network meta-analysis. *Curr Pediatr Rev.* 2020;16(1):61-70.

Ahmed AR, Dahl MV. Consensus statement on the use of intravenous immunoglobulin therapy in the treatment of autoimmune mucocutaneous blistering diseases. *Arch Dermatol.* 2003;139(8):1051-1059.

Bonagura VR, Cunningham-Rundles S, Edwards BL, Ilowite NT, Wedgwood JF, Valacer DJ. Common variable hypogammaglobulinemia, recurrent Pneumocystis carinii pneumonia on intravenous gammaglobulin therapy, and natural killer deficiency. *Clin Immunol Immunopathol.* 1989;51(2):216-231.

Brocklehurst P, Farrell B, King A, et al. Treatment of neonatal sepsis with intravenous immune globulin. *N Engl J Med.* 2011;365(13):1201-1211.

Burns JC, Roberts SC, Tremoulet AH, et al. Infliximab versus second intravenous immunoglobulin for treatment of resistant Kawasaki disease in the USA (KIDCARE): a randomised, multicentre comparative effectiveness trial. *Lancet Child Adolesc Health.* 2021;5(12):852-861.

Cervera R, Rodríguez-Pintó I, Legault K, Erkan D. 16th International Congress on Antiphospholipid Antibodies Task Force Report on

Catastrophic Antiphospholipid Syndrome. *Lupus.* 2020;29(12): 1594-1600.

Chaigne B, Mouthon L. Mechanisms of action of intravenous immunoglobulin. *Transfus Apher Sci.* 2017;56(1):45-49.

Eftimov F, Winer JB, Vermeulen M, de Haan R, van Schaik IN. Intravenous immunoglobulin for chronic inflammatory demyelinating polyradiculoneuropathy. *Cochrane Database Syst Rev.* 2013;(12): CD001797.

Garcia-Lloret M, McGhee S, Chatila TA. Immunoglobulin replacement therapy in children. *Immunol Allergy Clin North Am.* 2008;28(4): 833-849, ix.

Guarino A, Canani RB, Russo S, et al. Oral immunoglobulins for treatment of acute rotaviral gastroenteritis. *Pediatrics.* 1994;93(1):12–16.

Guo Y, Tian X, Wang X, Xiao Z. Adverse effects of immunoglobulin therapy. *Front Immunol.* 2018;9:1299.

Hallek M, Cheson BD, Catovsky D, et al. iwCLL guidelines for diagnosis, indications for treatment, response assessment, and supportive management of CLL. *Blood.* 2018; 131 (25): 2745-2760.

Hughes RA, Swan AV, van Doorn PA. Intravenous immunoglobulin for Guillain-Barre syndrome. *Cochrane Database Syst Rev.* 2012;7: CD002063.

Jaime-Pérez JC, Aguilar-Calderón PE, Salazar-Cavazos L, Gómez-Almaguer D. Evans syndrome: clinical perspectives, biological insights and treatment modalities. *J Blood Med.* 2018 Oct 10;9:171-184.

Jharna N. Shah, Roy F. Chemaly; Management of RSV infections in adult recipients of hematopoietic stem cell transplantation. *Blood.* 2011; 117 (10): 2755-2763.

Jordan SC, Toyoda M, Kahwaji J, Vo AA. Clinical aspects of intravenous immunoglobulin use in solid organ transplant recipients. *Am J Transplant.* 2011;11(2):196-202.

Keogh M, Sedehizadeh S, Maddison P. Treatment for Lambert-Eaton myasthenic syndrome. *Cochrane Database Syst Rev.* 2011;2011(2): CD003279.

Lam CG, Manlhiot C, Pullenayegum EM, et al. Efficacy of intravenous Ig therapy in juvenile dermatomyositis. *Ann Rheum Dis.* 2011;70: 2089-2094.

Liew WKM, Powell CA, Sloan SR, et al. Comparison of plasmapheresis and intravenous immunoglobulin as maintenance therapies for juvenile myasthenia gravis. *JAMA Neurol.* 2014;71(5):575-580.

Martinez C, Wallenhorst C, van Nunen S. Intravenous immunoglobulin and the current risk of moderate and severe anaphylactic events, a cohort study. *Clin Exp Immunol.* 2021;206(3):384-394.

Mofenson LM, Moye J Jr, Korelitz J, Bethel J, Hirschhorn R, Nugent R. Crossover of placebo patients to intravenous immunoglobulin confirms efficacy for prophylaxis of bacterial infections and reduction of hospitalizations in human immunodeficiency virus-infected children. The National Institute of Child Health and Human Development Intravenous Immunoglobulin Clinical Trial Study Group. *Pediatr Infect Dis J.* 1994;13(6):477-484.

Narula S, Hopkins SE, Banwell B. Treatment of pediatric multiple sclerosis. *Curr Treat Options Neurol.* 2015;17(3):336.

Neunert C, Terrell DR, Arnold DM, et al. American Society of Hematology 2019 guidelines for immune thrombocytopenia. *Blood Adv.* 2019;3(23):3829-3866. Erratum in: *Blood Adv.* 2020;4(2):252.

Newburger JW, Takahashi M, Gerber MA, et al. Diagnosis, treatment, and long-term management of Kawasaki disease: a statement for health professionals from the Committee on Rheumatic Fever, Endocarditis and Kawasaki Disease, Council on Cardiovascular Disease in the Young, American Heart Association. *Circulation.* 2004; 110(17):2747-2771.

Ohlsson A, Lacy JB. Intravenous immunoglobulin for preventing infection in preterm and/or low birth weight infants. *Cochrane Database Syst Rev.* 2013;2:CD000361.

Ohmoto A, Fuji S, Shultes KC, et al . Controversies about immunoglobulin replacement therapy in HSCT recipients with hypogammaglobulinemia. *Bone Marrow Transplant.* 2022;57: 874-880.

Orange JS, Hossny EM, Weiler CR, et al. Use of intravenous immunoglobulin in human disease: a review of evidence by members of the Primary Immunodeficiency Committee of the American Academy of Allergy, Asthma and Immunology. *J Allergy Clin Immunol.* 2006; 117(4 Suppl):S525-S553.

Ouldali N, Toubiana J, Antona D, et al. Association of Intravenous Immunoglobulins Plus Methylprednisolone vs Immunoglobulins Alone With Course of Fever in Multisystem Inflammatory Syndrome in Children. *JAMA.*2021;325(9):855-864.

Visentin A, Mauro FR, Rosati S, et al. Protective Role Immunoglobulin Replacement Therapy in Chronic Lymphocytic Leukemia: FOCUS on Subcutaneous Immunoglobulin Formulations. *Blood.* 2018; 132 (Supplement 1): 4954.

Wilma Barcellini, Bruno Fattizzo; How I treat warm autoimmune hemolytic anemia. *Blood.* 2021; 137 (10): 1283-1294.

Zwiers C, Scheffer-Rath ME, Lopriore E, de Haas M, Liley HG. Immunoglobulin for alloimmune hemolytic disease in neonates. *Cochrane Database Syst Rev.* 2018;3(3):CD003313.

SECTION D
Cardiology

CHAPTER 49 The Cardiac Examination

Kanika Gupta, MD and David I. Rappaport, MD

INTRODUCTION

A detailed history and comprehensive physical examination provide invaluable information about a patient's clinical status. A thorough cardiac examination can help detect many conditions, both primary cardiac conditions and non-cardiac conditions that involve the cardiovascular system. Clinicians must consider the cardiac examination in an appropriate clinical context—for example, a murmur in an otherwise thriving child likely requires a different approach than a murmur in a child with systemic symptoms. Extracardiac physical examination findings may suggest a systemic disease that involves the heart. This chapter details the components of a thorough pediatric cardiac examination and discusses common extracardiac manifestations associated with select syndromes.

VITAL SIGNS

Vital signs are important. The assessment of vital signs in a hospitalized patient who is febrile or agitated may require monitoring over time for a more accurate assessment. Special considerations may be required for neurodivergent patients, postoperative patients, or patients with conditions such as osteogenesis imperfecta. Techniques for improving the accuracy of vital signs include establishing rapport with patients, utilizing distraction techniques, or obtaining vital signs while children are sleeping. If possible, it is always helpful to establish a patient's baseline vital signs to help with interpretation and trends.

HEART RATE

Average heart rate values vary with the patient's age. For premature infants, ranges of 120 to 170 beats per minute (bpm) are typical; for infants 0 to 6 months, 100 to 160 bpm can be appropriate, while preschool-aged children are often 80 to 120 bpm, and ages 6 and above typically range from 60 to 100 bpm.

Tachycardia is common in hospitalized patients and can be associated with many conditions including fever, sepsis, anemia, pain, hyperthyroidism, dehydration, pulmonary disease, anxiety, and agitation. Persistent tachycardia without other explanation can suggest myocarditis or myocardial dysfunction. It can also be seen in cardiac tamponade as a part of Beck's Triad: tachycardia, elevated jugular venous pressures, and hypotension. Tachycardia > 220 bpm suggests a tachyarrhythmia, most commonly supraventricular tachycardia.

Bradycardia is commonly noted in athletes and in hospitalized patients with eating disorders, hypothyroidism, heart block, or increased intracranial pressure. Patients with relatively severe hypoxia may also demonstrate bradycardia.

TEMPERATURE

A normal average temperature is 36.5°C to 37.5°C. A fever is typically defined as a temperature greater than 38°C. In patients with either hyperthermia or hypothermia, heart rate can be affected. For every one degree Celsius in temperature elevation, the heart rate typically increases by 10 bpm and the respiratory rate by 2 to 4 breaths/minute.

RESPIRATORY RATE

Normal respiratory rate ranges vary by age. Typically, infants breathe 30 to 60 breaths/minute, toddlers breathe 20 to 30 breaths/minute, and an adolescent range is typically 12 to 18 breaths/minute.

Tachypnea often occurs in patients with respiratory disease, sepsis, or acid-base disturbances but also occurs in patients with cardiac dysfunction, including large left-to-right shunts or left-sided obstructive lesions. Clinicians should be especially suspicious of a cardiac etiology for tachypnea if a patient has isolated tachypnea with clear breath sounds. Orthopnea refers to shortness of breath while supine and can indicate elevated pulmonary venous pressure from left-sided obstructive lesions, mitral regurgitation, or cardiomyopathy.

BLOOD PRESSURE

An appropriate cuff size must be used for accurate blood pressure measurement. The width of the bladder of the blood pressure cuff should be 40% of the upper arm circumference, and the length of the bladder of the cuff should encircle at least 80% of the upper arm circumference. If measurements are taken in the leg, corresponding cuff sizes relate to the calf or thigh. Falsely elevated blood pressure may occur if the cuff is too small or the patient is agitated or anxious. If hypertension is detected, repeat the measurement at the end of the examination when the patient may be more relaxed. Abnormal automated or oscillometric blood pressure readings should be confirmed with an auscultatory (manual) blood pressure reading.

For assessment of patients with suspected coarctation of the aorta, measurements are necessary in the upper and lower extremities, ideally four-extremity blood pressures. In patients without coarctation of the aorta, the systolic pressure in the lower extremity is usually 5 to 10 mmHg greater than that in the upper extremity because of a standing wave effect. Systolic pressure in the arm >10 mmHg than that in the leg suggests coarctation.

Hypertension should be diagnosed if a child or adolescent has auscultatory-confirmed BP readings ≥95th percentile at three different visits. Hypertensive urgency is elevated blood pressure without end-organ damage. Patients with acute hypertension often demonstrate symptoms such as headache, nausea, or blurry vision. Hypertensive emergency is elevated blood pressure with concomitant end-organ dysfunction such as renal failure, altered mental status, seizures, intracranial ischemia, or hemorrhage.

Hypotension is defined as BP readings ≤5th percentile. Pediatric Advanced Life Support (PALS) algorithms define neonatal hypotension as systolic BP <60 mmHg, infants aged 1 to 12 months as systolic BP <70 mmHg, and for children aged >1 year to 10 years as systolic BP $<70 + (2 \times \text{age in years})$.

Pulse pressure is the difference between systolic pressure and diastolic pressure. A widened pulse pressure (>40 mmHg) can be seen in patients with a patent ductus arteriosus, truncus arteriosus, or as an early sign of shock. A narrow pulse pressure (<25 mmHg) is seen in patients with tension pneumothorax, congenital heart disease with myocardial failure, cardiac tamponade, tachycardia, or severe hemodynamic instability.

Pulsus paradoxus is characterized by a reduction in systemic blood pressure >10 mmHg during exhalation. Pulsus paradoxus is associated with severe respiratory distress, pericarditis, or can be a feature of cardiac tamponade.

PHYSICAL EXAMINATION

GENERAL APPEARANCE

A patient's general appearance can give insight into overall wellness, interaction, activity, acuity of illness, nutritional status, and position preferences.

ILLNESS SEVERITY

An essential part of a child's evaluation is identifying whether a child is well-appearing or in distress. Identify an infant or child's level of alertness and interaction. Evaluate how interactive a child is (playing and looking around, or lethargic, laying quietly with limited movement). Evaluate for a weak cry or signs of respiratory distress such as labored breathing or tachypnea. Evaluate for any diaphoresis or edema.

COLOR

Note if the patient has evidence of cyanosis, pallor, or jaundice. Cyanosis is an important visual sign caused by cardiac, pulmonary, hematologic, or central nervous system disorders. Arterial saturation levels are usually <85% before cyanosis is detectable on physical examination. Findings can be subtle but examine areas with good vascular supply and relatively thinner skin such as lips, mucous membranes, nailbeds, hands, and feet. In patients with darker skin pigmentation, cyanosis can be more easily visualized in mucous membranes such as lips, gums, buccal mucosae, and conjunctivae. Due to the characteristics of fetal hemoglobin, which produces higher oxygen saturations for a given oxygen tension, cyanosis can be subtle in neonates. Acrocyanosis can be a normal finding in newborns. Jaundice may signify hemolysis or hepatic involvement in a variety of disease processes including right heart failure. Pallor can be subjective, so it is always important to ask parents or caregivers. Locations for evaluation for pallor include palpebral conjunctivae, oral mucosae, nail beds, or palms. Pallor can be seen in severe anemia or vasoconstriction.

GROWTH

Nutritional status can be estimated upon immediate visualization. Evaluate for signs of malnourishment such as muscle wasting and subcutaneous fat loss may be reflected by a cachectic appearance with temporal wasting, prominent ribs, or a scaphoid abdomen. Infants with congenital heart disease and large left-to-right shunts often present with failure to thrive. Correlate visual inspection with growth charts to ensure that patients are growing appropriately. In infants with congenital heart disease, weight is usually affected before height and head circumference.

CARDIAC-FOCUSED EXAMINATION

While the information in this chapter is presented in a head-to-toe order for ease of reference, note that the order can and should be changed to accommodate the child being examined.

Fontanelle A neonate's anterior fontanelle can be auscultated, and a bruit may be heard. A vein of Galen malformation, a congenital aneurysm that shunts blood from the cerebral arteries into internal cerebral veins, can result in cardiomegaly and cardiac failure.

Eyes Conjunctival pallor suggests anemia. Xanthelasma suggests hyperlipidemia. Roth spots, hemorrhagic retinal lesions with a central white spot, are associated with infective endocarditis. Colobomas may suggest CHARGE syndrome.

Mouth When evaluating mucous membranes and the oropharynx, note that poor dentition is a risk factor for infectious endocarditis. A cleft palate may be associated with other embryonic midline defects. Mucous membrane changes of the lips, tongue, and/or pharynx may suggest Kawasaki disease. Tetralogy of Fallot is associated with a "geographic," wrinkled tongue. For patients with recent pharyngitis, consider acute rheumatic fever.

Neck The jugular veins drain deoxygenated blood from the brain, face, and neck to the heart via the superior vena cava. Jugular venous distension (JVD) is difficult to assess in infants and young children. To evaluate for JVD, place the child recumbent at a 45-degree angle and have them turn the neck to the left. Identify the internal jugular vein by its double waveform pulsation and locate the top of the pulsation. Then measure the distance to the sternal notch. Generally, a measurement of >4 cm indicates elevated central venous pressures in the superior vena cava such as in right-sided heart failure, pulmonary hypertension, tricuspid regurgitation, or constrictive pericarditis.

Chest Wall Inspection Pectus excavatum, commonly referred to as "funnel chest" as the sternum develops inward, accounts for 90% of all chest wall deformities, and can compress the heart and lung. It is associated with Marfan syndrome and mitral valve prolapse. Pectus carinatum, where the anterior chest wall protrudes outward ("pigeon chest"), can be associated with Marfan syndrome, Ehlers-Danlos Syndrome, and scoliosis. Always evaluate the thorax for any surgical scars. A median sternotomy is most common for cardiac surgery, though minimally invasive cardiac surgery is becoming increasingly common.

Chest Wall Palpation Palpation of the chest may provide important clinical information. To locate a patient's point of maximum impulse (PMI), begin by evaluating chest wall pulsations. The normal point of maximum impulse (PMI) is located along the mid-clavicular line in the fifth intercostal space. In children younger than 3 years of age, the PMI may be in the fourth intercostal space and gradually migrates into the fifth intercostal space as the child ages. Since the PMI correlates to left ventricular systolic contraction, there should be a single impulse per cardiac cycle, and the size of the area of impulse should be a maximum of 2 to 3 cm. A visible, hyperdynamic PMI is associated with left ventricular volume overload conditions, including left-to-right shunts, aortic regurgitation, and mitral regurgitation or hypermetabolic states such as anemia, hyperthyroidism, and high-cardiac output. A palpable double impulse corresponds to left ventricular filling during diastole and is typically pathologic. If the PMI is displaced and a visible parasternal impulse is visualized, consider right-sided ventricular dilation or conditions with severe pulmonary regurgitation such as Tetralogy of Fallot or Ebstein's anomaly with severe tricuspid regurgitation. Thrills are palpable vibrations that signify turbulent blood flow. A thrill along the left lower sternal border can be palpated in some patients with a VSD. Similarly, thrills in the upper left sternal border often correspond to pulmonic stenosis. Upper right sternal border thrills are associated with aortic stenosis. Thrills overlying the carotid arteries can be seen in patients with carotid bruit, coarctation of the aorta, or aortic stenosis.

Respiratory Exam Auscultation of the lung fields should occur anteriorly and posteriorly. Evaluate work of breathing including tachypnea and dyspnea, which typically worsens with feeding. Tachypnea can be an early sign of left-sided heart failure.

Abdomen Evaluate the liver via palpation and percussion. Hepatomegaly is defined as a liver edge > 3.5 cm below the costal margin in newborns and >2 cm in older children. Average spleen size is age dependent. The spleen length (cm) can roughly be estimated by adding 6 cm to 1/3 cm per year of age. A palpable spleen tip >2 cm below the left costal margin is generally considered enlarged. Splenomegaly can be seen in heart failure. It is estimated that 5% of the cardiac output volume passes the spleen each minute.

Extremities Evaluate for clubbing, a sign of chronic arterial desaturations, by looking for the loss of the normal angle or diamond-shaped window between the nail and nailbed. Clubbing usually starts in the thumbs. Edema is caused by reduced oncotic pressure, increased capillary permeability, or increased blood volume related to cardiac output. It can be localized or generalized in distribution. To evaluate for pitting or non-pitting edema, push firmly into a lower extremity and determine the depth and time required for the skin to rebound to its original appearance. Edema is graded on a scale of 0 to 4 as per **Table 49-1**.

An assessment of perfusion requires evaluation of mentation, urine output, pulses, and capillary refill. Evaluate central pulses, including radial, femoral, and brachial. Pulses should be palpated simultaneously in the upper and lower extremities to assess for delays, such as radio-radial delay seen in patients with subclavian artery stenosis, Takayasu

TABLE 49-1 Grading of Peripheral Edema

Grade of Edema	Pitting Depth	Rebounding Time
0	None	N/A
1	2 mm	Immediate
2	4 mm	15 seconds
3	6 mm	30 seconds
4	Severe	>30 seconds

TABLE 49-2	The Examination of a Newborn Requires Special Considerations Due to Elevated Pulmonary Vascular Resistance in the Neonate
Normal Neonatal Findings	**Abnormal Neonatal Findings**
Acrocyanosis	Central cyanosis
Easily palpable pulses that may appear bounding, due to lack of subcutaneous fat	Decreased or weak pulses
Innocent Flow Murmur, such as PDA or Pulmonary Flow Murmur	
Single S2 (normal in first few days of life)	
PACs within the first week of life	
PMI at lower left sternal border	
	Hepatomegaly for age
	Abnormal CCHD screen

arteritis, or in aortic coarctation proximal to the left subclavian artery. A delay between radial and femoral pulses suggests aortic coarctation proximal to the left subclavian artery. Pulsus alternans is characterized by alternating variability of pulse strength and is associated with left ventricular dysfunction. Pulsus bisferiens, a double pulse noted during systole, is seen in patients with hypertrophic cardiomyopathy and aortic disease such as rheumatic heart disease, Marfan syndrome, and bicuspid aortic valve. A faster pulse with inspiration is consistent with sinus arrhythmia, a normal phenomenon.

Skin Ensure that the patient is in a well-lit room, in a gown, when possible, for optimum evaluation of skin and extremities. Identify any skin findings that could indicate an underlying cardiovascular issue. Xanthomata, yellow skin lesions in any distribution, are associated with familial hypercholesterolemia, a risk factor for developing cardiac disease. Examination of hands and fingernails is particularly important. There are several cutaneous manifestations associated with infective endocarditis (see Chapter 52). Splinter hemorrhages, longitudinal thin red-brown lines that correspond to nail bed capillaries, can be found in various conditions and trauma, but suggest bacterial endocarditis, especially if seen in multiple nails. Similarly, Janeway lesions, painless erythematous and usually flat lesions on the palms and soles, caused by septic emboli, are more specific for infective endocarditis. Osler's nodes are painful, raised, and usually located on distal fingers and toes. Sweating, especially in neonates, may suggest congestive heart failure due to excess sympathetic activity as a compensatory mechanism for decreased cardiac output.

Musculoskeletal Patients with acute rheumatic fever typically have a migratory arthritis.

The newborn exam requires special considerations due to different baseline physiology (**Table 49-2**). **Table 49-3** lists clinical exam findings that may prompt cardiac consultation.

TABLE 49-3	Physical Examination or Historical Findings Prompting Consideration of Cardiology Consultation/Referral
Physical Examination Findings	
Grade III or higher murmur	
Diastolic murmur	
Murmur with increased intensity upon standing	
Click	
Extra sounds such as S3 or S4	
Cyanosis	
Discrepancy in blood pressures > 10 mmHg across extremities	
Historical Findings	
Symptomatic neonates with unexplained poor weight gain, cyanosis with feeds	
Symptomatic bradycardia or tachycardia	
New diagnosis or suspected syndrome with cardiac involvement	
Suspected Kawasaki disease	
Unexplained hypoxia or suspected shunting	
Suspected infective endocarditis	
Suspected rheumatic fever	

AUSCULTATION AND HEART SOUNDS/MURMURS

THE CARDIAC CYCLE

The cardiac cycle can be divided into two phases: diastole and systole.

Systole The cardiac cycle starts with the firing of the SA node, stimulating the atria to depolarize and contract, resulting in an increase in atrial pressure. Blood flows into the ventricles through the atrioventricular (AV) valves (tricuspid and mitral valves). As atrial contraction completes, atrial pressure falls, and the AV valves close, producing the first heart sound, S1, and indicating the beginning of systole. S1 is best heard at the left lower sternal border. During systole, the semilunar valves (pulmonary and aortic valves) remain closed briefly as ventricular depolarization and contraction occur. This is called isovolumetric contraction, where all valves are closed, and no blood is ejected. Ventricular pressures then increase to >80 mmHg to overcome aortic pressures, and the semilunar valves open, rapidly ejecting blood from the ventricles. During ventricular relaxation, ventricular pressures drop, and the semilunar valves close, creating the second heart sound, S2, signifying the end of systole.

Diastole The aortic valve closes before the pulmonary valve, creating a normal splitting of S2. Inhalation can also widen the S2 splitting. Diastole now starts, and the ventricles relax. The atria fill with blood, and atrial pressures increase. Once the atrial pressure rises above ventricular pressures, the AV valves open and blood flows from the atria to the ventricles. A third heart sound, S3, is heard with rapid ventricular filling. While S3 can be normal in older children and athletic patients, a high index of suspicion for pathology must be maintained. Finally, a fourth heart sound, S4, at the end of diastole is rare, always pathologic, and signifies blood filling in a ventricle with poor compliance.

EVALUATION OF MURMURS AND EXTRA HEART SOUNDS

Position Positional changes can help differentiate benign from pathological murmurs. Generally, benign or innocent murmurs are produced

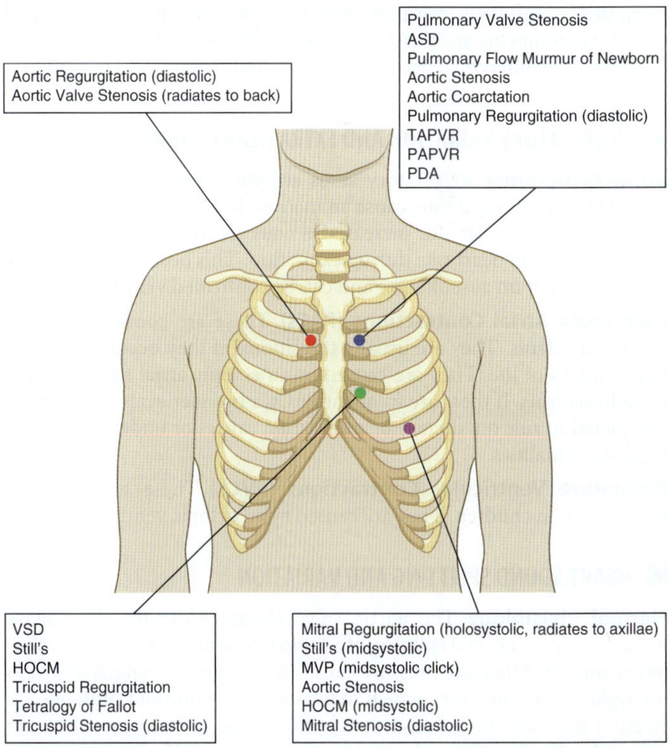

FIGURE 49-1. Location of cardiac auscultation and corresponding murmurs. Red = aortic region; right 2nd ICS (intercostal space), Blue = pulmonic region; L 2nd ICS; Green = tricuspid region left 4th ICS parasternal); Purple = mitral region, left 5th ICS mid-clavicular line. *Abbreviations*: ASD, atrial septal defect; TAPVR, total anomalous pulmonary venous return; PAPVR, partial anomalous pulmonary venous return; PDA, patent ductus arteriosus; VSD, ventricular septal defect; HOCM, hypertrophic obstructive cardiomyopathy; MVP, mitral valve prolapse.

by normal blood flow. Since positional changes affect flow, innocent murmurs typically change with positional variations. Pathologic murmurs typically do not change in intensity with Valsalva maneuvers (reduces venous blood flow to the heart) or positional changes. The one exception to note is the murmur associated with Hypertrophic Obstructive Cardiomyopathy (HOCM), detailed later.

Timing Murmurs can occur in systole, diastole, or can be continuous throughout the cardiac cycle.

Systolic Murmurs can be broken down into early, mid, or late phase; and classified as ejection or regurgitation (holosystolic) murmurs. Ejection murmurs are caused by blood traveling through a narrow vessel or an irregular valve. Several conditions including stenotic semilunar valves, stenotic intracardiac lesions (such as double-chamber right ventricle), stenotic intravascular lesions (such as supravalvular semilunar valve obstruction, coarctation, or peripheral pulmonary stenosis), regurgitant atrioventricular valves, or normal cardiac anatomy can produce ejection murmurs. Many conditions in hospitalized children, such as tachycardia and anemia, increase flow across normal semilunar valves and can create a systolic ejection murmur. Ejection murmurs often have a crescendo-decrescendo pattern, directly correlated to flow into the great vessels. Common holosystolic murmurs in children include mitral regurgitation, tricuspid regurgitation, and VSD murmurs.

Diastolic Murmurs are produced by regurgitation across semilunar valves (aortic or pulmonary) or turbulent flow across the atrioventricular (mitral or tricuspid) valves. The murmur of aortic regurgitation is higher pitched with a decrescendo pattern. Diastolic murmurs are generally considered pathologic.

Continuous Murmurs are heard throughout systole and diastole. They are produced in conditions involving connections between systemic and pulmonary circulations. These include patent ductus arteriosus, arteriovenous malformations, connections between systemic arteries and cardiac chambers such as coronary arteriovenous fistulas, and conditions associated with disturbed arterial flow in arteries (collateral circulation associated with aortic coarctation) or veins, such as a venous hum. Except for a venous hum, most continuous murmurs are pathologic. The murmur associated with a patent ductus arteriosus is classically machine-like, caused by the high-pressure differential between the aorta and pulmonary circulation.

RESPIRATORY VARIATION AND EXTRA HEART SOUNDS

Sinus Arrhythmia Respiratory sinus arrhythmia is common in children. Changes in vagal tone cause an increase in heart rate during inspiration to accommodate for increased venous return and cardiac output and a decrease in heart rate during expiration. This heart rate variability can be heard upon auscultation and can be confirmed via EKG.

Premature Atrial Contractions (PACs) These are common in neonates and infants. They are usually transitional if they occur within the first 2 weeks of life. They are caused by an ectopic atrial focus causing extra heartbeats. If there are frequent PACs, a broader evaluation can be completed to rule out dietary or medication causes or underlying structural abnormalities.

Premature Ventricular Contractions (PVCs) These are also not uncommon in children. They are caused by an ectopic ventricular focus.

HEART SOUND SPLITTING AND VARIATION

Normal Physiology The aortic valve closes before the pulmonary valve, creating a normal splitting of S2 into two sounds, A2 and P2. Inhalation (negative thoracic pressure causes an increase in venous return to the right side of the heart, which increases RV volume and prolongs RV ejection time and thus delays the closure of the pulmonary valve) can also widen the S2 splitting by an average of 0.04 to 0.05 seconds.

Split S2 Sound A widely fixed split S2 (>0.04 seconds) that does not vary with respiration or resolves with standing can be seen in conditions with an increased RV ejection time (right ventricular volume overload) or a shortened LV ejection time. These include ASD (due to increased RV volume), partial anomalous pulmonary venous return, complete RBBB (delayed complete RV ejection), mitral regurgitation, or pulmonic stenosis. A narrow split S2 can be normal but is often heard when there is delayed aortic valve closure or premature pulmonary valve closure. These include pulmonary hypertension, aortic stenosis, or a left bundle branch block (LBBB).

Isolated (Non-Split) S2 Sound This finding can occur in patients with structural heart disease when only one semilunar valve is developed, such as pulmonary atresia, truncus arteriosus, or aortic atresia.

Split S1 Sound S1 splitting can be heard in RBBB or Ebstein's anomaly. Special attention is needed to differentiate a split S1 from an extra S4 sound.

MURMUR QUALITIES

Loudness Systolic murmurs are graded from I to VI and are often louder in states of high cardiac output.

- Grade I: barely audible, softer than S1/S2 heart sounds
- Grade II: audible
- Grade III: loud, without accompanying palpable thrill
- Grade IV: murmur with palpable thrill
- Grade V: murmur can be heard with a stethoscope partially off the chest
- Grade VI: audible loud murmur without a stethoscope

Pitch When blood flows from areas of high pressure to lower pressure, it typically has high velocity, creating a higher-pitched noise that can be vibratory and musical. Murmurs originating from stenotic areas typically are harsher and lower-pitched and usually reflect pathological disease.

COMMON MURMURS IN CHILDREN

Still's Murmur Still's murmur is the most common benign murmur in children. It is characterized by a musical, soft, low-frequency, vibratory, Grade I-III systolic ejection murmur generated by normal vibrations of the left outflow tract. It is loudest while supine and decreases in intensity upon standing.

Peripheral Pulmonic Artery Stenosis (PPS) PPS is often heard in premature infants and infants younger than 6 months of age and is caused by the small size of branch pulmonary arteries. It is typically described as a Grade I-II, mid-systolic murmur, loudest at the left upper sternal border with radiation to the bilateral axillae and back.

Pulmonary Flow Murmur of Childhood This murmur is a Grade I-III mid-systolic murmur, heard best at the LUSB. It is usually heard in children older than 8 years old.

Venous Hum This is a benign, continuous murmur without radiation. It is most appreciable while upright and usually disappears while supine or with compression of the jugular vein (accomplished by turning the neck). It is described as a low-pitched, Grade I-III murmur at the right sternal border. This murmur must be distinguished from a PDA murmur.

Patent Ductus Arteriosus (PDA) This murmur is a transient, systolic murmur heard in infants on the first 1 to 2 days of life. It is caused by the closing of the ductus arteriosus and is most prominent at the LUSB and left axilla.

Ventricular Septal Defect (VSD) The murmur of a VSD is holosystolic, harsh in quality, best heard in the left lower sternal border, and obscures the closure sounds of the mitral and tricuspid valves.

Atrial Septal Defect (ASD) An ASD murmur is heard best at the location of the pulmonary region and often has a fixed S2.

Mitral Regurgitation The murmur of mitral regurgitation is a uniform, high-pitched, blowing, systolic murmur heard best at the apex with radiation to the left axilla or lower back.

Hypertrophic Cardiomyopathy (HOCM) HOCM is caused by muscular wall thickening obstructing blood from exiting the heart. When standing, venous return to the heart decreases, causing reduced left ventricular diastolic volume. As the left ventricle size decreases, the left ventricular outflow tract narrows and the outflow obstruction increases during systole, and thus the murmur increases in intensity while standing. HOCM is a leading cause of sudden death in athletes.

OTHER HEART SOUNDS

Clicks Clicks are sharp, extra heart sounds corresponding to valve pathology. Ejection clicks can be heard with bicuspid aortic valve or in aortic or pulmonary valve stenosis if the valve is mobile. A click heard shortly after S1 corresponds to pulmonic or aortic stenosis. Aortic valve stenosis can be heard best at the RUSB and can be accompanied by a palpable thrill over the carotid arteries. The click of pulmonary valve stenosis will increase in intensity with exhalation. A mid-systolic, apical, constant click is present in mitral valve prolapse. It may also accompany mitral regurgitation murmurs, typically a late-systolic murmur that intensifies when standing. An early systolic, apical, constant click is typical of a bicuspid aortic valve. An early left upper sternal border variable click occurs with pulmonary stenosis and is louder in expiration.

Rumbles If a mid-diastolic rumble is heard, consider lesions with a large left-to-right shunt, such as an ASD, VSD, or PDA that creates increased volume to the right atrium.

Pericardial Friction Rub This grating sound is created by inflamed visceral and parietal pericardial surfaces rubbing against each other. It is not typically present if there is a large pericardial effusion. The rub is accentuated in the sitting position with the patient leaning forward in inspiration, and it may occur in systole, diastole, or continuously. A pericardial rub occurs with pericarditis and in the recovery period after cardiac surgery in which the pericardial space was entered.

Muffled Heart Sounds Muffled heart sounds may be heard in patients with pericardial effusions or heart failure.

EXTRACARDIAC MANIFESTATIONS WITH GENETIC SYNDROMES

Several genetic syndromes associated with cardiac disease have extracardiac manifestations seen on physical examination.

Trisomy 21 Patients with Trisomy 21 have characteristic physical exam features such as upslanting palpebral fissures, hypotonia, single palmar creases, Brushfield spots (white spots on the iris), protruding tongue, and a flattened face. Approximately 40% to 50% of these patients have congenital heart defects, most classically endocardial cushion defects such as atrioventricular septal defects.

DiGeorge Syndrome/22q1.2 Deletion Syndrome DiGeorge syndrome is caused by a microdeletion in the long arm of chromosome 22. Typical findings in patients with DiGeorge syndrome include palatal insufficiency/cleft palate, hypocalcemia, immunodeficiency, and cardiac disease, especially interrupted aortic arch, truncus arteriosus, and Tetralogy of Fallot.

Marfan Syndrome Marfan syndrome, a connective tissue disorder, is associated with a tall, thin body habitus, high-arched palate, chest wall defects, joint laxity, and long arms, legs, and fingers (arachnodactyly). Cardiac complications associated with Marfan syndrome include mitral valve prolapse, aortic regurgitation, aortic dilation, increased risk of aortic dissection, and cardiomyopathy.

Noonan Syndrome Noonan syndrome is an autosomal dominant condition often caused by mutations in PTPN11 (protein tyrosine phosphatase) characterized by short stature, webbed neck, chest wall defects, low-set nipples, wide-spaced eyes, and low-set ears. Associated congenital heart defects include pulmonary valve stenosis, hypertrophic cardiomyopathy, and ASD.

Turner Syndrome Turner syndrome is an X chromosome deletion or partial deletion syndrome, thus affecting only females, characterized by short stature and delayed puberty. Physical exam findings in these patients include webbed neck, low hairline, and extremity swelling. Common associated cardiac conditions include bicuspid aortic valve, coarctation of the aorta, and/or aortic arch elongation.

Williams Syndrome Patients with Williams syndrome have a wide variety of physical features, most commonly including short stature, full cheeks with a wide mouth, prominent lips with a small jaw, epicanthal folds, and large ears. Cardiac disease occurs in about 75% to 80% of patients due to an elastin arteriopathy with narrowed vessels, most commonly supravalvular aortic stenosis and peripheral pulmonic stenosis.

Other Syndromes If a patient has skeletal abnormalities of the hand or carpal bones, including absent thumbs, consider Holt-Oram Syndrome, an autosomal dominant genetic condition in which 75% of patients have congenital heart malformations, including ASD and VSD. Patients with Alagille syndrome, a disorder caused by JAG1 gene mutation causing biliary dysfunction and associated with Tetralogy of Fallot, have distinctive facial features, including a prominent, broad forehead and a small, pointed chin. Newborns with evidence of CHARGE syndrome are associated with conotruncal abnormalities, including Tetralogy of Fallot, double-outlet right ventricle, and truncus arteriosus.

SUGGESTED READINGS

Etoom Y, Ratnapalan S. Evaluation of children with heart murmurs. *Clin Pediatr (Phila).* 2014;53(2):111-117.

Flynn, JT, Kaelber DC, Baker-Smith CM, et al. Clinical practice guideline for screening and management of high blood pressure in children and adolescents. *Pediatrics.* 2017;140:3: e20171904.

Gonzalez VJ, Kyle WB, Allen HD. Cardiac examination and evaluation of murmurs. *Pediatr Rev.* 2021;42(7):375-382.

Kleinman K, McDaniel L, Molloy M, eds. *The Harriet Lane Handbook.* 22nd ed. Philadelphia, PA: Elsevier; 2021.

Park MK, Salamat M. *Park's Pediatric Cardiology for Practitioners.* 7th ed. Philadelphia, PA: Elsevier; 2021.

CHAPTER 50 Electrocardiogram Interpretation

Melissa Clemente Fabrega, MD, FAAP and Michael Lopez, MD, FAAP

BACKGROUND

The electrocardiogram (ECG) is a useful, versatile, noninvasive, and inexpensive clinical test that has been used for more than a century to aid in the diagnosis of cardiac diseases including electrical disturbances, anatomical abnormalities, myocardial ischemia/infarction, electrolyte disorders and drug toxicity, among others. The ECG constitutes a time/voltage chart of the heartbeat, and it functions by way of recording cardiac electrical current through sensors placed on the surface of the body called electrodes.

It is of utmost importance that frontline medical caregivers in the hospital setting are familiar with the interpretation of this test, as they are often required to make critical decisions. Computer readings are often inaccurate, particularly in the interpretation of pediatric ECGs.

There are many subtle variations in the pediatric ECG related to age-specific changes; as the child develops from the newborn period to infancy, childhood, adolescence, and adulthood there are significant changes in the size and position of the heart relative to the body and in the cardiac physiology. For example, during intrauterine life fetal circulation relies mostly on the right side of the heart, therefore the right ventricle is thicker than the left ventricle. The changes that happen during birth and early infancy result in a shift to a left-sided predominance; such that by 6 months the left ventricle is twice the thickness of the right and by adolescence it should be at least 2.5 times the thickness of the right. As a result of these changes, the normal infant ECG changes quickly over the first few weeks of life and it is not until around the age of 3 that it begins to resemble an adult ECG pattern.

BASIC PRINCIPLES

The heart can be thought of as an electrically timed pump, where the wires that are part of the pump are the conduction system in the heart. Normally, the start of a heartbeat happens in the sinoatrial (SA)

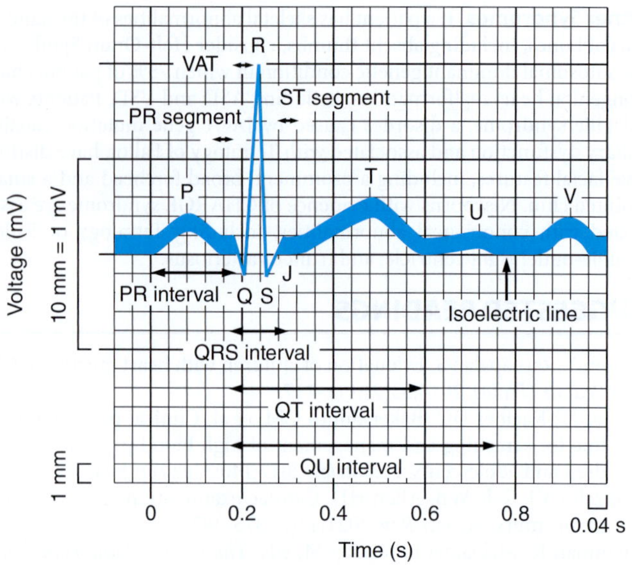

FIGURE 50-1. EKG Basics: Summary of the major components of the ECG graph: 5 waveforms: P, QRS, ST, T, and U; 4 intervals: RR, PR, QRS, and QT; and 3 segments: PR, ST, and TP. Note that the ST can be considered a waveform or a segment. (Reproduced with permission from Gomella LG, Haist SA. *Gomella and Haist's Clinician's Pocket Reference*, 12e. New York: McGraw Hill; 2023.)

node, which is located at the superior and rightward aspect of the right atrium, adjacent to the superior vena cava. From there, the signal goes through the right and left atrium to contract and pump blood through the tricuspid and mitral valves to the right and left ventricle respectively. The signal then reaches the atrioventricular (AV) junction where the atrioventricular node (AVN) is located. The AVN acts as an electrical relay connecting the atria and ventricles. The AVN inserts into the muscular portion of the interventricular septum as the Bundle of His that then divides into two main branches: the right bundle branch that stimulates the right ventricle and the left bundle branch that stimulates the left ventricle. From there the signal travels through specialized cells called the Purkinje fibers from the endocardium to the myocardium and generate ventricular contraction that will pump the blood to the pulmonary and systemic circulation through the pulmonary and aortic valve respectively.

The process by which the stimulus travels through the heart and activates it is called depolarization and the process by which the heart returns to its resting phase is called repolarization. This sequence of depolarization/repolarization traveling through the atria and ventricles generates all the electrical currents that are recorded in the ECG in the different waveforms, segments, and intervals. The depolarization process is depicted in the ECG by the P waves (atrial depolarization) and QRS waves (ventricular depolarization), and the repolarization process is depicted by the T wave and, if present, the U wave (ventricular repolarization). Atrial repolarization is masked by the larger voltage of the simultaneous ventricular depolarization (QRS). In the interpretation of ECGs, the term segment refers to parts of the ECG that start with the end of one waveform and end with the beginning of another one (example: PR and ST), and the term interval is used for parts that include at least one waveform (example: QT). See **Figure 50-1**.

TECHNICAL ASPECTS

The conventional way of depicting the electrical activity of the heart on the ECG is with the 12-lead ECG. These leads record the differences in electrical potential between the electrodes placed on the different parts of the body. By doing this, the ECG can give the clinician different views, providing a better picture of the three-dimensional electrical activity that is taking place in the heart. The conventional 12-lead ECG includes 6 limb leads: I, II, III, aVR, aVL, and aVF and 6 chest leads: V1, V2, V3, V4, V5, and V6. The correct placement of these leads is very important for an accurate interpretation of the ECG. The 6 limb leads are generated by 4 electrodes placed on each of the limbs. The arm electrodes should be placed anywhere on the arms distal to the shoulder and the leg electrodes should be placed anywhere distal to the pelvis. The 6 precordial leads are generated by 6 "unipolar" chest leads. V1 and V2 should be placed on the right and left parasternal border respectively, on the 4th intercostal space. V4, V5, and V6 should be placed in the 5th intercostal space at the left mid-clavicular line, anterior axillary line, and mid-axillary line respectively. V3 is then placed in between V2 and V4. See **Figure 50-2**.

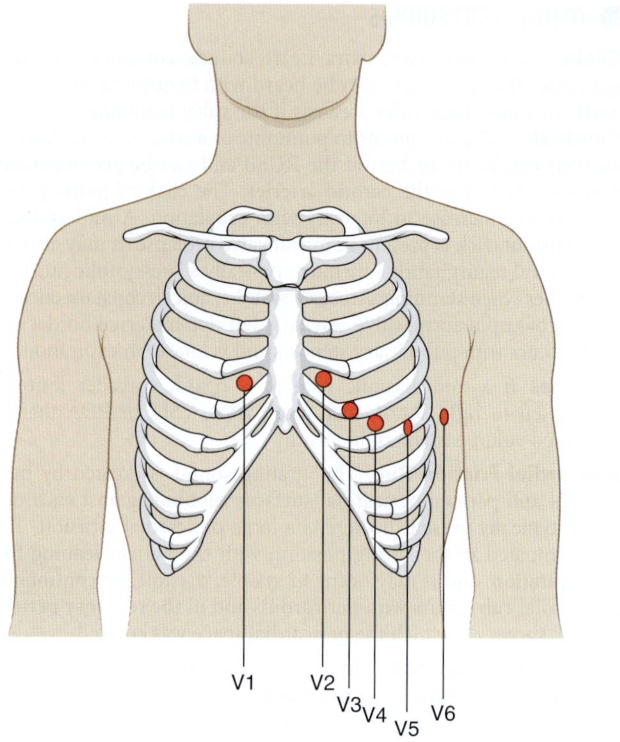

FIGURE 50-2. Correct position of electrodes: A: Position of precordial leads. (Reproduced with permission from Zimmerman FH. *ECG Core Curriculum*, New York: McGraw Hill; 2023.)

The 12 ECG leads have a specific orientation and a specific polarity. The limb leads orientation is depicted in the Einthoven's triangle and they look at the heart from a frontal plane (**Figure 50-3A**). The chest leads show the electrical current on electrodes placed along the anterior chest wall and they provide a view of the horizontal plane of the heart (**Figure 50-3B**). The polarity of the leads implies that there is a positive and a negative pole to each lead that will determine the direction of the trace in the ECG, if the electrical current is moving toward the positive pole, it will generate an upward deflection and if directed toward the negative pole it will generate a downward deflection.

The sequence of the waveforms, segments and intervals that constitute a heartbeat are recorded in a specific graph paper (see **Figure 50-4**). The standard recording rate is 25 mm/s, therefore on the horizontal axis every mm (little box) represents 0.04 second, and every 5 mm (big box) represent 0.2 second. The vertical axis indicates the voltage where 10 mm = 1mV, in a standard setting. Therefore, every waveform in the ECG can be described on the basis of its duration (horizontal axis) or voltage (vertical axis).

INTERPRETATION OF THE ECG

The best recommendation to tackle the interpretation of ECGs is the use of a systematic approach to reading ECGs that should include special attention to: rate, rhythm, axis, waveforms, segments, and intervals. In the particular case of pediatric ECGs, it should also take into account the different normal values for age (**Table 50-1**).

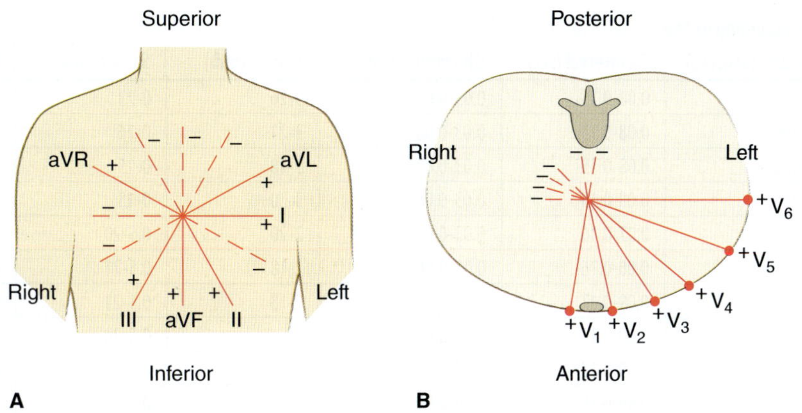

FIGURE 50-3. A. Frontal plane leads. B. Horizontal plane leads. (Reproduced with permission from Loscalzo J, Fauci A, Kasper D, Hauser S, Longo D, Jameson J. *Harrison's Principles of Internal Medicine,* 21e. New York: McGraw Hill; 2022.)

RATE

The rate refers to the number of cardiac cycles per minute. The easiest way of calculating the heart rate from an ECG is the box counting method. Using lead II, or the lead with less artifact, and counting the number of big boxes (0.2 second) in between 2 QRSs, the heart rate will be equal to 300 divided by the number of big boxes. If the heart rate is too fast the heart rate can be calculated with the little boxes (0.04 second), in this case heart rate will be equal to 1500 divided by the number of little boxes. If the heart rate is irregular, an average can be calculated by counting the number of QRSs in a time interval and then multiplying by the

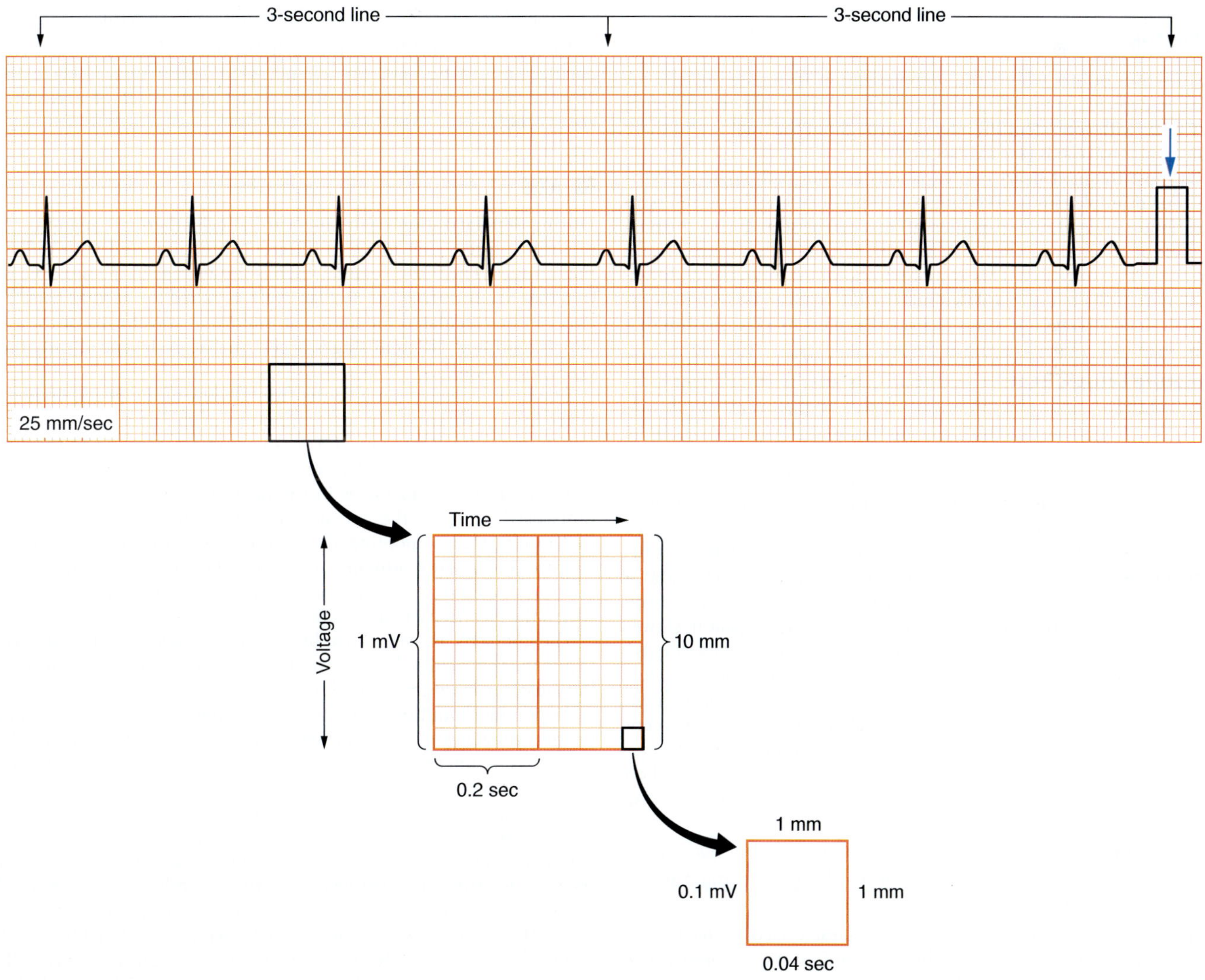

FIGURE 50-4. ECG Graph paper: Time is measured on the horizontal axis and amplitude is measured on the vertical axis. (Reproduced with permission from Zimmerman FH. *ECG Core Curriculum*, New York: McGraw Hill; 2023.)

TABLE 50-1 Normal ECG Values According to Age

Age	HR (bpm)	QRS axis (degrees)	PR interval (sec)	QRS interval (sec)	R in V1 (mm)	S in V1 (mm)	R in V6 (mm)	S in V6 (mm)
1st wk	90-160	60-180	0.08-0.15	0.03-0.08	5-26	0-23	0-12	0-10
1-3 wk	100-180	45-160	0.08-0.15	0.03-0.08	3-21	0-16	2-16	0-10
1-2 mo	120-180	30-135	0.08-0.15	0.03-0.08	3-18	0-15	5-21	0-10
3-5 mo	105-185	0-135	0.08-0.15	0.03-0.08	3-20	0-15	6-22	0-10
6-11 mo	110-170	0-135	0.07-0.16	0.03-0.08	2-20	0.5-20	6-23	0-7
1-2 yr	90-165	0-110	0.08-0.16	0.03-0.08	2-18	0.5-21	6-23	0-7
3-4 yr	70-140	0-110	0.09-0.17	0.04-0.08	1-18	0.5-21	4-24	0-5
5-7 yr	65-140	0-110	0.09-0.17	0.04-0.08	0.5-14	0.5-24	4-26	0-4
8-11 yr	60-130	−15-110	0.09-0.17	0.04-0.09	0-14	0.5-25	4-25	0-4
12-15 yr	65-130	−15-110	0.09-0.18	0.04-0.09	0-14	0.5-21	4-25	0-4
>16 yr	50-120	−15-110	0.12-0.20	0.05-0.10	0-14	0.5-23	4-21	0-4

Source: Reproduced with permission from Ra'id Abdullah, MD.

appropriate factor (example counting every 10 seconds and multiplying by 6).

Normal resting heart rates vary with age. The average heart rate peaks around 2 months of life (120-180 BPM) and then slowly declines until adolescence (50-120 bpm). When interpreting the rate on an ECG it is important to acknowledge the different normal for age.

RHYTHM

Sinus rhythm occurs when atrial depolarization is initiated by the SA node and depicted in the ECG when there is a P wave that occurs before every QRS, with consistent PR interval throughout the tracing and there is a normal P wave axis (see axis section).

The most frequent heart rate variations are not pathologic arrhythmias. For example, sinus arrythmia or respiratory arrythmia refers to the variation in heart rate (p-p interval) that can be seen during the normal cycle of respiration. The heart rate will increase with inspiration and decrease with expiration. This is more pronounced in young children. Sinus bradycardia refers to a slow sinus rhythm that can be seen in aerobically trained athletes and sinus tachycardia refers to a fast rhythm that can be seen with anxiety, crying and fever.

Premature Ectopic Beats These heartbeats arise from different locations than the SA node and can be classified as premature atrial contractions (PAC) or premature ventricular contractions [PVCs]. PACs can be identified by a p wave that occurs earlier than would be expected for a given heart rate, with a different morphology. Often, these P waves will be difficult to identify directly, but cause a disturbance in the preceding T wave. PACs are typically followed by a narrow QRS complex indistinguishable from the normal QRS. However, if the PAC is sufficiently premature there can be widening of the subsequent QRS and it can be mistaken for a PVC. PVCs are generally wide-complex as they do not originate within the normal conduction system and result in slower propagation through the myocardium. Premature ectopic beats can also be further described as frequent or infrequent. Based on these characteristics some of these will be classified as normal variants (e.g., infrequent PACs are almost always benign) or possible abnormalities (e.g., frequent PVCs can be seen in congenital heart disease or ventricular dysfunction). Patients with frequent PVCs may require further cardiac workup including echocardiogram, Holter monitoring and exercise stress testing depending on the individual case.

Tachyarrhythmias Defined as heart rates that are above the normal limit for age and can be distinguished primarily by their origin in the conduction system of the heart:

- Supraventricular tachycardia (SVT) is characterized by having an electrical circuit that includes the atria and/or the AV node. The most common forms of SVT in children are re-entry circuits that involve either an extra pathway connecting the atria and ventricle or an extra pathway within the AV node itself. These typically appear as narrow complex tachycardias with no distinguishable P wave before the QRS, and often with heart rates above 220 bpm in newborns and infants and above 180 bpm in older children.
- Other forms of SVT, such as atrial flutter and atrial fibrillation are less common in children.
- Lastly those arising below the AV node are called ventricular tachycardias and are described as wide QRS complex tachycardias.

Hospitalized children with arrhythmia, including sinus bradycardia, should be kept on telemetry to better characterize their rhythm and more easily capture onset and offset of arrhythmia recurrence.

AXIS

During depolarization of the myocardial cells there are many vectors of cardiac forces that move in different directions and with different magnitudes. The mean vector, which is the average of the multiple vectors that occur during the cardiac cycle, is called the cardiac axis. This axis can be calculated for the most important waveforms of the ECG which represent different stages of the cardiac cycle, specifically the P, QRS, and T waves.

The limb leads, which give the frontal view of the heart, divide the heart into quadrants. The determination of the axis of the different waveforms will fall into one of these quadrants depending on the direction of the waves depicted in the ECG, this represents the direction of the mean vector of forces in the heart at a given time. The quadrants used to locate the axis are derived from the hexaxial diagram that results after combining all the limb leads directions and polarity (**Figure 50-5**). This provides important information about the conduction of electricity and the sizes of the different chambers through which the electricity is conducted.

The QRS axis, is determined by a larger number of vectors that constitute the ventricular depolarization process, and it is greatly affected by the muscle mass in the ventricles.

As previously outlined, this axis will change from a right-sided axis in the neonatal period (right ventricle dominance) to a normal left-sided axis in older children and adolescents (left ventricle dominance) (**Figure 50-6**).

To estimate the QRS axis use the axes created by leads I and aVF as mentioned above to divide the plane into quadrants. Then identify in which quadrant the mean vector would be located based on whether the QRS is primarily positive or negative in both leads. For example, a negative QRS in lead I indicates the axis is on the left half of the circle, that is between +90 and +270 degrees. A positive QRS in aVF would therefore indicate that the axis would be on the lower half of the circle, that is between 0 and +180 degrees. Therefore for both to be true, the overlapping quadrant (+90 to +180 degrees) contains the cardiac axis.

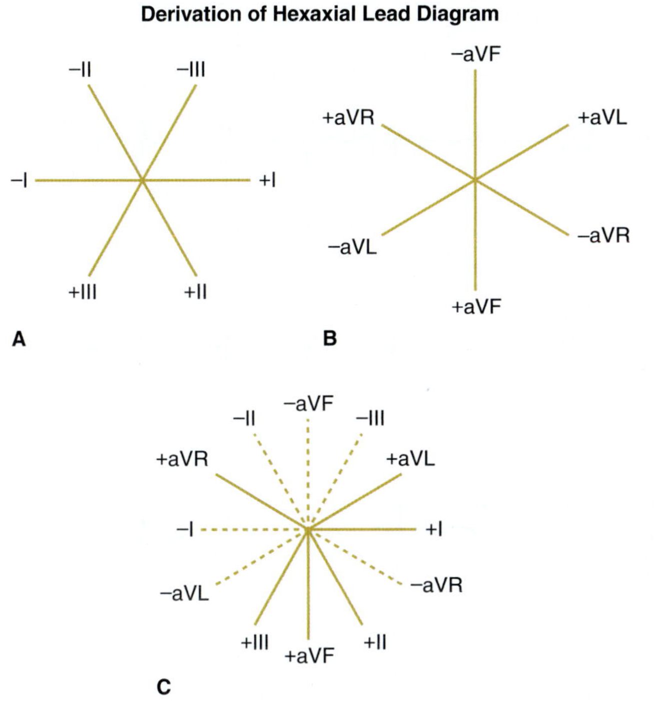

FIGURE 50-5. A. Triaxial diagram of the bipolar leads B. Triaxial diagram of the augmented limb leads C. The combination of the two triaxial diagrams constitutes the hexaxial lead diagram. (Reproduced with permission from Goldberg A, Goldberg Z, Shvilkin A. Clinical *Electrocardiograpy: A Simplified Approach*. 9th ed. Elsevier; 2018.)

In the neonate and up to 2 months of age, the rightward axis (+60° to +180°) will result in a large amplitude R wave in V1 and V2, and a small amplitude R wave in V5 and V6. As the child grows the left ventricle increases in mass and the axis moves to the left side (0° to +90°) resulting in decreasing R waves in V1 and V2 and increasing R waves in V5 and V6; similarly inverse changes will occur in the S waves in the precordial leads.

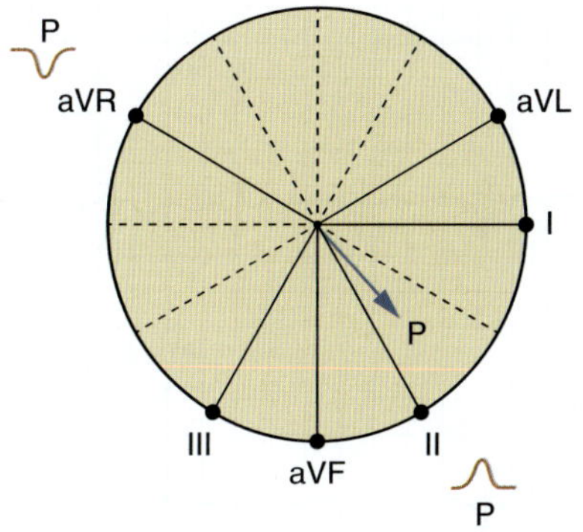

FIGURE 50-7. Normal P wave axis. (Reproduced with permission from Goldberg A, Goldberg Z, Shvilkin A. *Clinical Electrocardiograpy: A Simplified Approach*. 9th ed. Elsevier; 2018.)

A superior axis deviation (−1° to −181°) can be seen in infants with atrioventricular canal of ostium primum atrial septal defects.

P WAVE

Represents atrial depolarization and it is the first waveform depicted in the ECG. The normal P wave has an axis around +60°and should have a positive deflection in the precordial leads. The P wave axis or predominant direction of atrial depolarization should be directed downward and to the left in normal sinus rhythm, this should fall in the southeast quadrant in between 0° and 90°. It can be calculated by looking for the lead where the P wave has the biggest deflection. A normal P wave axis should always reflect a positive P wave in aVF and lead II and a negative deflection on aVR. See **Figure 50-7**.

The P wave in V1 can have an initial positive deflection which is the right atrial depolarization followed by a small negative deflection which is the left atrial depolarization that occurs later. Alterations in this pattern could represent a rhythm that is not originating in the sinus node. The normal P wave is less than 2.5 to 3 mm in amplitude and shorter than 70 ms in infants and 90 ms in children. Right atrial enlargement is seen with a P wave in lead II that is narrow and greater

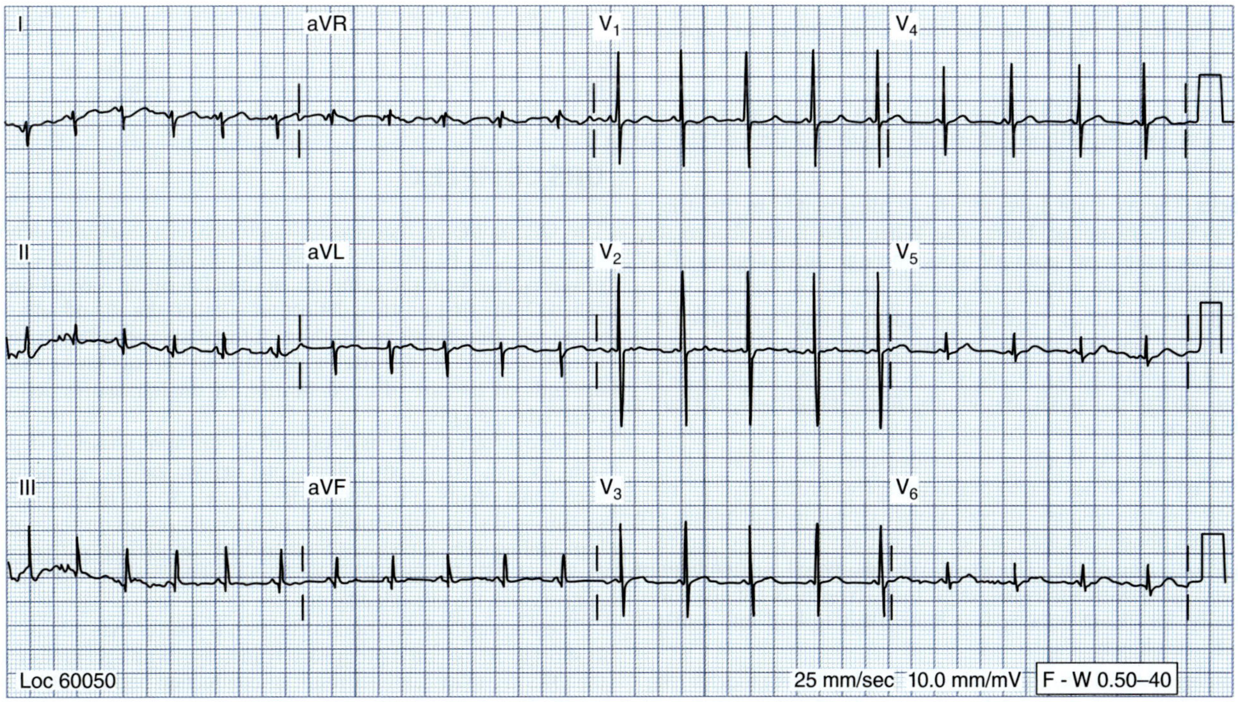

FIGURE 50-6. Right axis deviation that can de normal in the newborn. (Used with permission from Dr. Michael Saalouke.)

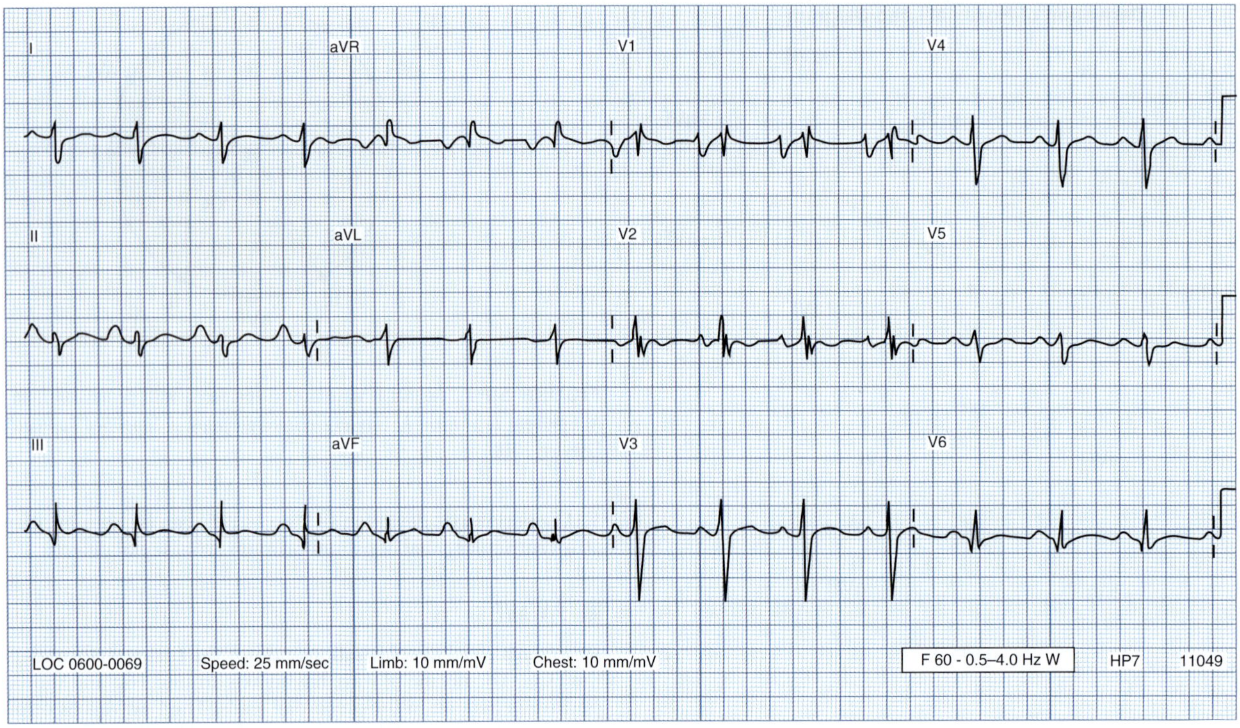

FIGURE 50-8. Left atrial enlargement. (Used with permission from Dr. Michael Saalouke.)

than 3 mm in infants up to 6 months of age and greater than 2.5 mm in older children. Left atrial enlargement will be demonstrated with a widened P wave (>120 ms) in lead II or a deep biphasic P wave on V1. See **Figure 50-8**.

PR INTERVAL

This interval is an isoelectric region that starts with the end of the P wave and ends at the beginning of the QRS complex. It is usually a reflection of the atrio-ventricular conduction. The normal PR interval varies with age, gradually increasing as the muscle mass in the heart increases. In neonates it ranges from 0.08 to 0.15 seconds and in adolescents from 0.12 to 0.20 seconds (or 80-150 ms and 120-200 ms).

Prolonged PR intervals are usually associated with atrio-ventricular (AV) conduction block, these happen as a result of a delay in the AV conduction.

AV Blocks The AV node drives the electrical current from the atria to the ventricles in the normal heart cycle. When there is any abnormality in this passage the result is an AV block; there are three degrees of AV block, all of which can happen in children:

- First-degree AV block is characterized by a fixed prologued PR interval for age. First-degree AV block can be normally present when there is high vagal tone, such as in athletes or during sleep. This is generally benign and almost never progresses to higher grade block.
- Second-degree AV block, is subdivided into two different types: Mobitz type I (Wenckebach) characterized as progressive PR prolongation until a QRS is dropped; Mobitz type II in which there are occasional nonconducted P waves without any warning or preceding prolongation of the PR interval. Whereas type I is often benign and also seen with increased vagal tone, type II is usually more clinically significant because it is more likely to lead into a third-degree heart block.
- Third-degree AV block, also known as complete heart block, is characterized by independent atrial and ventricular depolarizations with complete dissociation between the P and the QRS complexes. There are several congenital and acquired causes of third-degree blocks in children including maternal Systemic Lupus Erythematosus, muscular dystrophies, and rheumatic fever.
- In the hospital setting, children with any heart block greater than first degree would benefit from telemetry to document their ventricular rate.

Shortened PR intervals can be associated with a pre-excitation syndrome known as Wolff-Parkinson-White syndrome (WPW). This is represented by a short PR interval with a widened QRS that has a characteristic slurred upstroke that gives the appearance of a triangle with the vertical portion of the QRS. This wide upstroke is called the delta wave and is caused by early depolarization of the ventricles via a congenital bypass tract. WPW is an important clinical finding as it is associated with SVT and sudden death. See **Figure 50-9**.

QRS COMPLEX

The QRS complex represents the process of ventricular depolarization. The QRS patterns are conventionally described by the sequence of waves that form the complex: an initial negative wave, if present, is called Q; the first positive deflection is called the R; and any negative waveform after this is called the S. If there is a second positive deflection it is called R'. The use of capital letters versus lower case letters depends on the size of the deflection. A single negative deflection is referred to as a QS.

These patterns occur as a result of the different phases of depolarization: an initial interventricular septal depolarization, represented by a vector that points to the right side as the electricity moves through the septum and that will result on a positive deflection on the right-sided leads; followed by a phase of biventricular depolarization that results in a vector pointed to the left ventricle and will be represented in a positive deflection in the left-sided leads.

The normal QRS duration in children is shorter than adults, it can be as short as 30 ms and it progressively increases with age. Prolongation of the QRS complex can be a result of conduction abnormalities, such as bundle branch block.

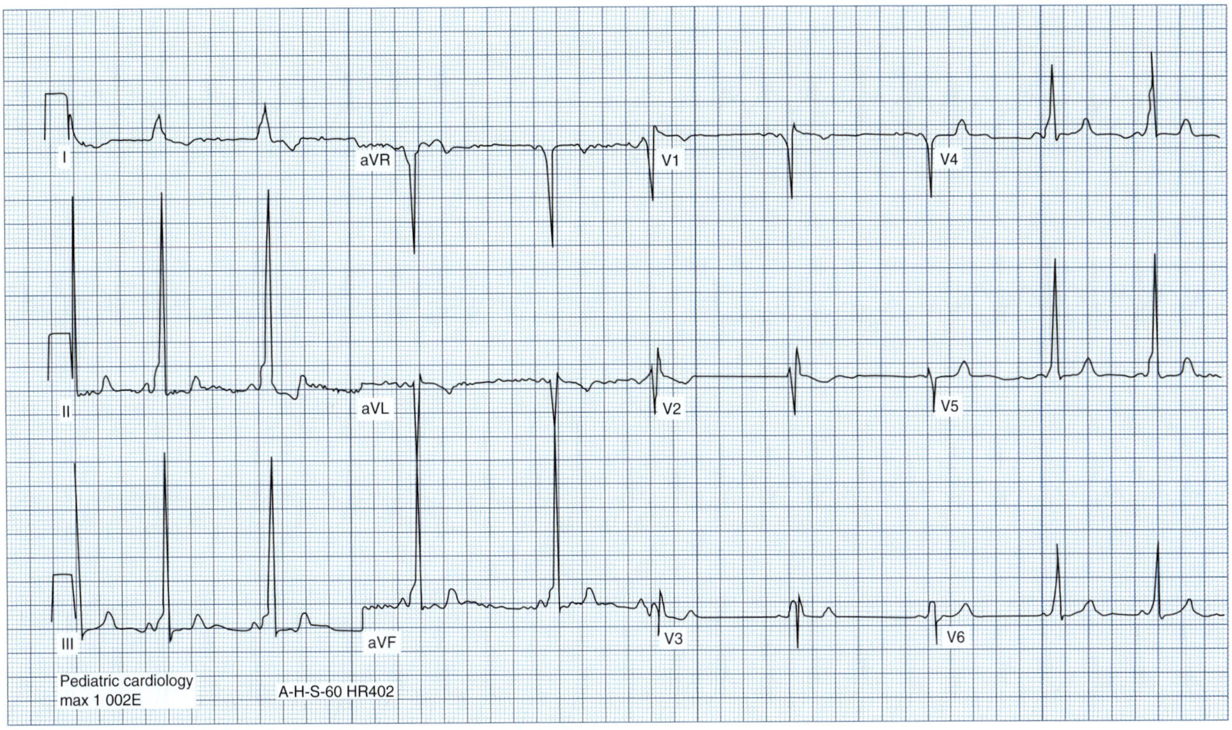

FIGURE 50-9. Delta waves in WPW. (Used with permission from Dr. Michael Saalouke.)

Bundle Branch Blocks These are specific types of intraventricular conduction disturbances and refer to abnormalities in the intraventricular propagation of the impulse generated in the AV node resulting in aberrant shapes and/or duration of the QRS complex. These may be caused by congenital structural abnormalities in the distal His-Purkinje conduction system or abnormalities in the ventricular myocardium that occur with fibrosis, calcifications, post-surgical repairs of congenital lesions, infiltrative lesions, and impaired vascular supply.

- Right Bundle Branch Block (RBBB): This is the more common of the two types of bundle branch blocks. It manifests in the ECG as a QRS duration greater than the upper limits of normal for age, or 120 ms in older children and adults as well as a characteristic QRS pattern. There is a narrow initial component followed by a slow and wider component which appears as an rS in lead I, rsR' in V1, and a rS in V6. This pattern reflects normal and rapid initial conduction via the His bundle and left bundle branches, with a slow later phase in the right ventricle due to conduction block in the RBB. A RBBB pattern can sometimes be seen in normal hearts, especially athletes, however should be investigated to confirm there is no underlying pathology (**Figure 50-10**).
- Left Bundle Branch Block (LBBB): less common in children than RBBB. It follows the same limits for duration of the QRS as the RBBB, but, as it reflects absent or slow conduction through the left bundle, it is accompanied by a broad, notched or slurred R wave in leads I, aVL, V5, and V6; absent Q waves in leads I, V5 and V6 and ST and T waves usually opposite in direction to the QRS. See **Figure 50-11**.

Ventricular Hypertrophy It can also be evaluated with the QRS complex, the muscle mass in the ventricles will determine the amplitude of the QRS complex on various leads.

Right ventricular hypertrophy is better evaluated in V1 with an R wave greater than the 98th percentile for age, an RSR' pattern, with the R' measuring more than 15 mm in infants younger than 1 year of age and more than 10 mm in children older than 1 year of age, an S wave will also be higher than the 98th percentile for age on V6, the presence of a Q wave on V1, a pure R wave in V1 after 6 months of age, or an upright T wave in V1 after 1 week of life until about 8 years of age.

On the other hand, left ventricular hypertrophy is better evaluated on V5 or V6, with an R wave that is more than the 98th percentile in V5/V6, or less than the 5th percentile in lead V1 or V2; S wave amplitude greater than the 98th percentile on V1; a Q wave that is greater than 4 mm in lead V5 or V6 and a left axis deviation.

Q WAVES

The Q wave corresponds to the first negative deflection on the QRS complex and it is a representation of the depolarization of the interventricular septum. They are usually narrow (average 0.02 second). They are usually detected in the left lateral and inferior leads.

Q waves are abnormal if they appear on the right precordial leads, usually represent right ventricular hypertrophy; if they are absent in the left precordial leads this might represent a conduction abnormality such as left bundle branch block or ventricular pre-excitation (WPW); if they are abnormally deep, they might indicate left ventricular hypertrophy and if they are abnormally deep and wide (greater than 40 ms), they can represent the presence of myocardial ischemia or infarction.

QT INTERVAL

Corresponds to the interval from the beginning of the QRS complex to the termination of the T wave and represents the whole process of ventricular depolarization and repolarization.

The QT interval varies with heart rate, shortening as the heart rate increases. Numerous formulas have been proposed to correct the QT from the rate effect. In children the most common formula used is the Bazett formula, in which the corrected QT interval (QTc) is equal to the QT measured/√ preceding RR interval, where the QT and the RR are measured in seconds. The normal QTc interval is sex dependent, with normal in males generally defined as less than or equal to 440 ms whereas in females normal is generally less than 460 ms. There is also some variability with age, as infants may have a QTc as long as 490 ms. The measurement of the QTc can vary lead to lead, and therefore should be measured in more than one lead, typically leads II and V5/V6; if the measurement will be done from one single lead, it should be from the lead that has the longest interval.

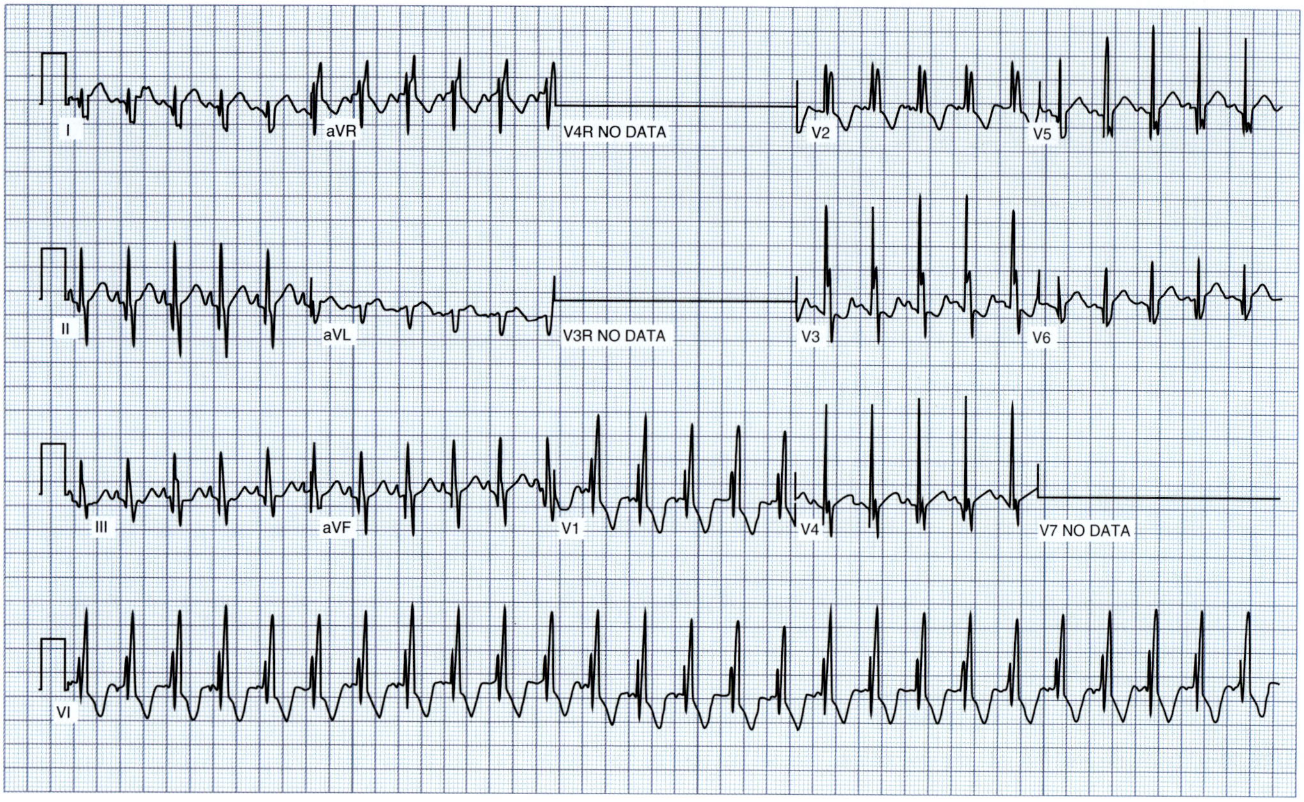

FIGURE 50-10. Right bundle branch block.

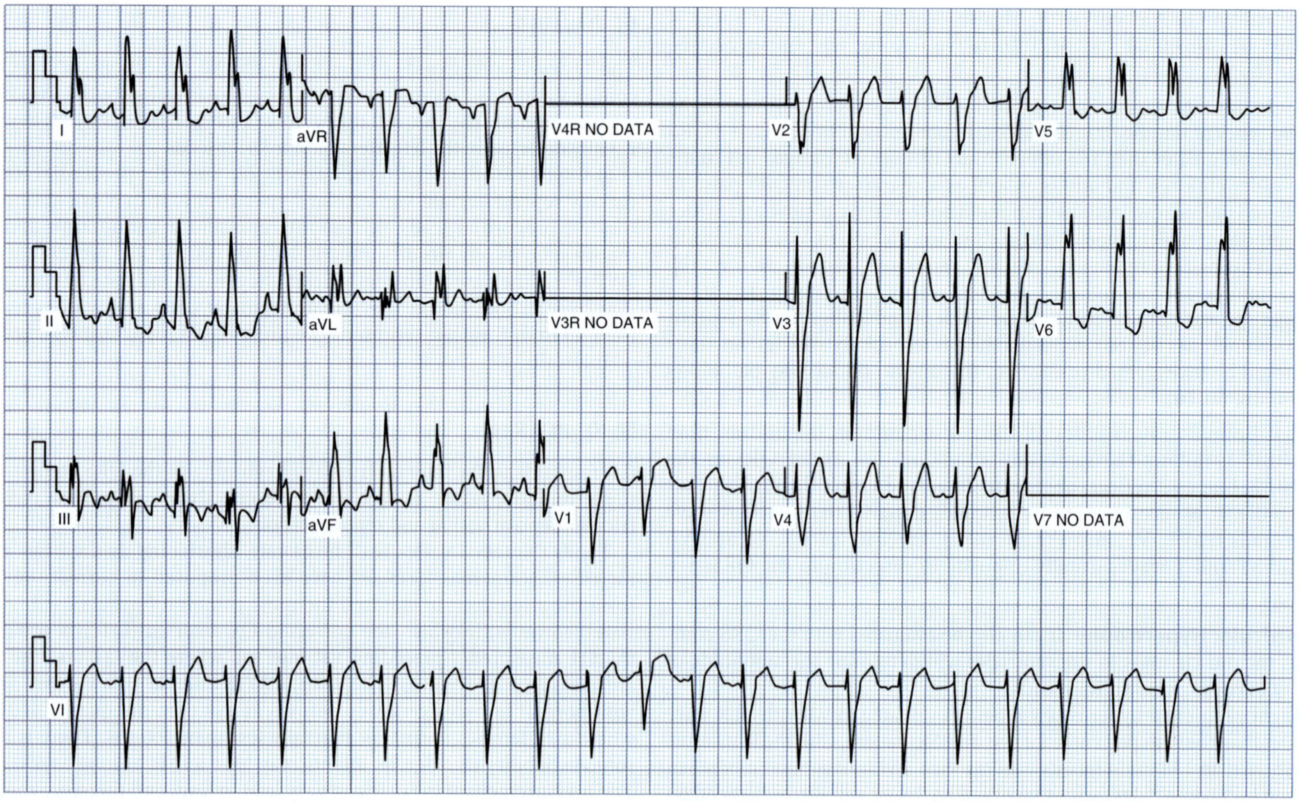

FIGURE 50-11. Left bundle branch block.

TABLE 50-2 Medications That Can Prolong QT Stratified by Risk

Medication Type	Low Risk	Moderate Risk	High Risk
Analgesics, anesthetics and sedatives	Dexmedetomidine Buprenorphine	Propofol	Methadone
Antiarrhythmic		Flecainide, pilsicainide, propafenone	Amiodarone, disopyramide, dofetilide, dronedarone, ibutilide, procainamide, quinidine, sotalol, vernakalant
Antianginal	Ranolazine		
Anticholinergic	Solifenacin		
Antimicrobials	Armenther-lumefantrine, hydroxychloroquine Itroconazole, ketoconazole (low to moderate risk) Ciprofloxacin, norfloxacin, ofloxacin (low to moderate risk) Foscarnet (low to moderate risk) Roxithromycin, telithromycin (low to moderate risk) Efavirenz, fostemsavir, lopinavir-ritonavir, rilpivirine (low to moderate risk) Metronidazole (low to moderate risk) Telavancine (low to moderate risk) Triclabendazole (low to moderate risk)	Cloroquine, halofantrine, piperaquine Fexinidazole, meglumine antimoniate, sodium stibogluconate Fluconazole, voriconazole Clofazimine Gemifloxacin, levofloxacin, moxifloxacin, sparfloxacin Azithromycin, clarithromycin, erythromycin Saquinavir Pentamidine	Delamanid, quinidine, quinine Bedaquiline

The presence of prologued QTc can predispose those patients to life-threatening arrhythmias, therefore should be routinely evaluated in all ECGs. The etiology of prolonged QTc can be congenital, for example genetic long QTc syndromes, or acquired, commonly related to electrolyte imbalances like hypocalcemia and hypokalemia, or from medication use which prolonged the QTc. See **Table 50-2**. Hospitalized patients with long QT, either congenital or acquired, should be on telemetry to monitor for arrhythmia.

ST SEGMENT

Constitutes the portion of the ECG from the end of the QRS complex to the beginning of the T wave. It represents complete depolarization of the ventricles. The beginning of the ST segment, exactly at the junction of the end of the QRS and the beginning of the ST segment is called the J point.

The normal ST segment is usually isoelectric, but it might be slightly depressed or elevated (less than 1 mm) in the limb leads and still be normal. An ST segment with a gentle upward slope (J point depression) is considered normal, as opposed to a horizontal or downward depression which is always considered pathological. Early repolarization, with notching at the J-point up-sloping elevated ST segments is normal in adolescents and young adults.

The presence of pathological ST changes is associated with pericarditis, myocarditis, or myocardial ischemia.

T WAVE

The T wave represents ventricular repolarization. At birth it is usually upright, though it can be flat or inverted in the inferior and anterior leads. After about 1 week, it should become inverted in V1 and upright in lead I and V4 to V6. The anterior T waves in V1 to V3 should remain inverted until about 8 years of age, at which time they may begin to flip upright usually starting from V3 to V1. Persistently inverted T waves in V1 to V3 is called a juvenile T wave pattern that is normal. The T wave should always be upright in V4 to V6.

Tall peaked T waves can be seen as a first ECG finding in hyperkalemia, as well as a sign of ventricular hypertrophy (**Figure 50-12**). Large, deeply inverted T waves are seen with increased intracranial pressure.

U WAVE

When present, represents the last stage of repolarization of the ventricles. It is characterized as a small, rounded deflection seen after the ending of the T wave. Normally the direction of the U wave should be the same as the direction of the preceding T wave; it is best seen in leads V1 and V2, and most often seen with slower heart rates. Prominent U waves are characteristics of hypokalemia. When the U wave is 50% of the T wave size or greater, it should be included in the QT measurement, otherwise it is ignored for purposes of QTc calculation.

ABNORMAL ECG FINDINGS

Abnormal ECG findings may help identify structural defects, conditions with abnormal function such as myocarditis, as well as electrolyte abnormalities. Each of these entities have patterns on ECG that can aid diagnosis and management. Some examples are represented in **Table 50-3**.

NORMAL VARIANTS IN PEDIATRIC ECGs

- T wave inversion: In the anterior precordial leads (V1-V3) many children over the age of 8 years old will continue to demonstrate T wave inversion as a normal variant. It is important to note, however, that

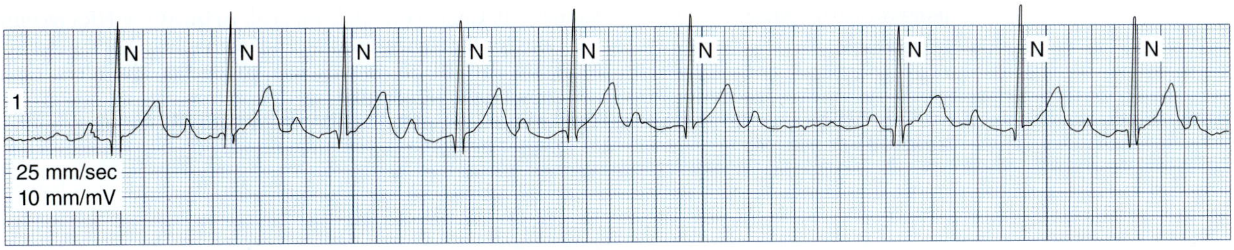

FIGURE 50-12. Tall peaked T waves in hyperkalemia. (Used with permission from Dr. Michael Saalouke.)

TABLE 50-3 Abnormal ECG Findings in Pediatric Patients

Pathology	Common ECG Findings
PDA—Patent Ductus Arteriosus	Left Ventricular Hypertrophy (older child)
ASD—Atrial Septum Defect	Right Ventricular Hypertrophy Right Atrial Enlargement Right Atrial Enlargement Right Bundle Branch Block
VSD—Ventricular Septal Defect	Right Ventricular Hypertrophy Left Ventricular Hypertrophy Left Atrial Enlargement Right Bundle Branch Block
CoA- Coarctation of the Aorta	Right Ventricular Hypertrophy (newborn) Left Ventricular Hypertrophy (older child) Right Axis Deviation (newborn)
ToF—Tetralogy of Fallot	Right Ventricular Hypertrophy Right Atrial Enlargement Right Bundle Branch Block (after repair)
TGA—Transposition of Great Arteries	Right Ventricular Enlargement Right Atrial Enlargement Left Atrial Enlargement
Tricuspid Atresia	Left Ventricle Hypertrophy Right Atrial Enlargement Left Atrial Enlargement
Pulmonary Atresia	Left Ventricular Hypertrophy
HLHS—Hypoplastic Left Heart Syndrome	Right Ventricular Hypertrophy
AS—Aortic Stenosis	Left Ventricular Hypertrophy
PS—Pulmonic Stenosis	Right Ventricular Hypertrophy Right Atrial Enlargement Right Axis Deviation
AVC—Atrioventricular canal defects	Right Ventricular Hypertrophy Left Ventricular Hypertrophy Right Atrial Enlargement Left Atrial Enlargement Left Axis Deviation Right Bundle Branch Block
HCM—Hypertrophic Cardiomyopathy	Left Ventricular Hypertrophy Left Atrial Enlargement
Myocarditis	Sinus Tachycardia Junctional Tachycardias Second or Third-degree AV Blocks T wave flattening or inversion Low QRS complex voltage
Hypercalcemia	Decreased T wave amplitude High take-off of the ST segment Abbreviation of the QT interval
Hypocalcemia	Prolongation of the QT interval
Hyperkalemia	Peaked T waves Wide QRS Decreased P wave amplitude PR prolongation ST segment elevations
Hypokalemia	Flattened T waves Increased U wave prominence

while inverted T waves in V1-V3 after the age of 8 years is a normal variant, upright T waves in V1 before the age of 8 years (and after 1 week of life) is abnormal, and indicative of RVH.

- RSR' complex: a small percentage of children can show an RSR' pattern on the right precordial leads. To be consistent with a normal variant the duration of the QRS should not be greater than 10 ms longer than the normal duration for age and the R' voltage in V1 should be less than 15 mm in infants and less than 10 mm in children older than 1 year of age.
- Elevated J point: early repolarization is commonly seen in adolescents, seen most commonly in the inferior and precordial leads. Often there is notching of the J-point.
- Presence of sinus arrythmias, with a variable P-P interval; usually related to changes in respiration.
- Short sinus pauses of <1.8 seconds.
- First Degree Atrioventricular Block/Mobitz type 1 second degree Atrioventricular Block/Junctional Rhythm; most of them associated with sleep, but can also happen in the waking state.
- Ventricular or Supraventricular Extrasystole: usually isolated and associated with periods of low heart rate, the frequency should not exceed 5% to 10% of the total QRS complexes within 24 hours (by Holter).

KEY POINTS

- The ECG is a valuable, inexpensive, readily available test that can be used in the diagnosis of multiple pathologies including cardiac structural or functional abnormalities, as well as electrolyte imbalances.
- The interpretation of pediatric ECGs requires familiarity with the normal physiological changes that happen from the newborn period through adolescence.
- There are multiple normal variants that can constitute a benign finding in the pediatric ECG.
- The recognition of certain patterns of abnormalities can aid the pediatric hospitalist in management decisions.
- The use of a systematic approach to the interpretation of ECGs is the most effective way of reading ECGs.

SUGGESTED READINGS

Benatar A. The pediatric electrocardiogram. *Ann Card Cardiovasc Dis.* 2017; 2(1).

Dickinson D. The normal ECG in childhood and adolescence. *Heart.* 2005;91:1626-1630.

Evans WN, Acherman RJ, Mayman GA, Rollins RC, Kip KT. Simplified pediatric electrocardiogram interpretation. *Clin Pediatr (Phila).* 2010; 49(4):363-372.

Goldberg A, Goldberg Z, Shvilkin A. *Clinical Electrocardiograpy: A Simplified Approach.* 9th ed. Elsevier; 2018.

O'Connor M, McDaniel N, Brady WJ. The pediatric electrocardiogram Part I: Age-related interpretation. *Am J Emerg Med.* 2008;26(4): 506-512.

Sharieff GQ, Rao SO. The pediatric ECG. *Emerg Med Clin North Am.* 2006;24(1):195-208, vii-viii.

Surawicz B, Childers R, Deal BJ, et al. AHA/ACCF/HRS recommendations for the standardization and interpretation of the electrocardiogram Part III: intraventricular conduction disorders. *Circulation.* 2009;119(10):e235-40.

Tipple M. Interpretation of electrocardiograms in infants and children. *Images Paediatr Cardiol.* 1999;1(1):3-13.

CHAPTER 51

Congenital Heart Disease

Stephanie Bousquet Arar, MD and Yousef Arar, MD, MPH

BACKGROUND

Congenital heart disease is estimated to occur in about 1% of all children. Fortunately, most of these problems are minor or self-limited and do not require intervention. About one in four children with congenital heart disease have critical congenital heart disease (CCHD) that often requires intervention. For this important group of patients with heart disease, the past 70 years have witnessed a remarkable advance in diagnostic and therapeutic techniques such that many of these children with previously lethal defects may now lead relatively normal lives. Congenital heart disease ranks among the top causes of infant death in the United States and is comparable to the death rate for sepsis and respiratory distress syndrome.

Children with congenital heart disease may be hospitalized at the time of diagnosis, after cardiac interventions (surgery or transcatheter), or for acute illness related or unrelated to their heart condition. While some congenital cardiac disease has straightforward anatomy, the hospitalist may care for children with the most complex cardiac anatomy, as these children typically spend significant time in the hospital. The pediatric hospitalist frequently plays an important role in the care of children with congenital heart disease—especially when it coexists with other disease processes.

PATHOPHYSIOLOGY

While the anatomic variation of congenital heart disease is vast, the four main elements of pathophysiology in congenital heart disease are desaturation, pulmonary overcirculation, pulmonary vascular disease, and compromised systemic perfusion. Interventions undertaken for patients with congenital heart disease are done to address or prevent one or more of these issues. These pathologies are discussed more fully in the context of the more common examples of congenital heart disease.

CLINICAL PRESENTATION

Congenital heart disease typically presents during one of three time frames: the newborn period, in early infancy, or in childhood. During the newborn period most present as CCHD. What defines these lesions as "critical" is that survival depends on patency of the ductus arteriosus or emergent surgical/catheter intervention. Typical clues to suggest CCHD in the newborn include cyanosis or signs and symptoms of decreased perfusion. Increasingly, newborns with congenital heart disease have detailed anatomic diagnoses prior to delivery due to prenatal screening by fetal echocardiography. Antenatal diagnosis allows for appropriate and anticipatory management of these infants and has led to improved outcomes for complex heart disease. Another important presentation for newborns with CCHD is the screening program endorsed by the Centers for Disease Control and now adopted by legislation in much of the United States. This simple screening uses a pulse oximeter to check saturations in the right hand and foot in newborns more than 24 hours old or immediately pre-discharge. Any reading <90%, three readings 90% to 94%, or a more than 3% difference between the hand and the foot generates the recommendation for a diagnostic echocardiogram. This test will detect most CCHD and some hypoplastic left heart syndrome and other mixing lesions. A recent meta-analysis of several published studies shows a high sensitivity of this test (76%) for CCHD and a low false positive rate (0.05%) when done >24 hours after birth. It is worthwhile to note there are many critical non-cyanotic congenital heart diseases that will not be detected by this screen, including coarctation of the aorta (CoA).

A second group of patients with congenital heart disease presents as the pulmonary vascular resistance (PVR) falls to its nadir at 8 to 12 weeks of life. This group may present with a murmur, or they could present with symptoms of congestive heart failure (tachypnea, hepatomegaly) if there is significant pulmonary overcirculation. Examples that may have this presentation include large Ventricular Septal Defects (VSD) or other significant left-to-right shunts. Late presentations associated with closure of the ductus arteriosus may also present in the weeks after birth with cyanosis, shock, or decreased femoral pulses, for example CoA.

The third common time frame for diagnosis of congenital heart disease is during childhood when a previously subtle murmur is detected. This often happens between age 2 and 5 years when the child is sufficiently cooperative with cardiac auscultation.

In addition to the more typical presentations of congenital heart disease, there are infants and children with serious cardiovascular malformations that masquerade as more common illnesses such as lung disease or laryngomalacia (**Table 51-1**).

DIFFERENTIAL DIAGNOSIS

For infants who are critically ill with low oxygen saturation and/or hypotension, the more common neonatal diagnoses are usually first to be considered. Respiratory distress syndrome, sepsis, meconium aspiration

TABLE 51-1 Examples of Congenital Heart Disease That Masquerade as Other Diseases

Masquerading Disease	Congenital Heart Disease	Hint/Clue	Definitive Diagnostic Test
Frequent lower respiratory illnesses Asthma / bronchiolitis Failure to thrive	Ventricular septal defect Patent ductus arteriosus Atrioventricular canal defect Aortopulmonary window *with* elevated pulmonary vascular resistance	Loud, single second heart sound Abnormal ECG	Echocardiogram
Croup Laryngomalacia Bronchomalacia Feeding difficulties Reflux	Vascular ring	Often right aortic arch on chest x-ray	CT scan MRI Bronchoscopy
Asthma Bronchiolitis Dilated cardiomyopathy	Anomalous left coronary artery from the pulmonary artery (ALCAPA)	Cardiomegaly on CXR Abnormal ECG (infarction pattern)	Echocardiogram (looking specifically at origin of coronary arteries)
Hypertension	Coarctation of the aorta	Decreased intensity of femoral pulses and/or radio-femoral delay	Four extremity blood pressures Echocardiogram
Severe neonatal respiratory distress	Total anomalous pulmonary venous return (with obstruction)	History not suggestive for infant at-risk for pulmonary disease	Echocardiogram (complete, but especially focusing on pulmonary veins)

TABLE 51-2 Critical Newborn Heart Disease Dependence on a Patent Ductus Arteriosus (PDA)

PDA Required to Support Pulmonary Flow	PDA Required to Support Systemic Flow	PDA Increases Mixing
Critical pulmonary stenosis	Critical aortic stenosis	d-Transposition of great arteries (d-TGA)
Pulmonary atresia/intact ventricular septum	Critical coarctation/Interrupted aortic arch	
Tricuspid atresia (normally related great arteries)	Tricuspid atresia (transposed great arteries)	
Tetralogy of Fallot (some)	Hypoplastic left heart syndrome	
Complex single ventricle with pulmonary stenosis/atresia	Complex single ventricle with systemic outflow obstruction	

syndrome, pneumonia, and others are usually first considered because their incidence is much higher. CCHD should especially be suspected when cyanosis is present without accompanying respiratory distress, or when there are signs of decreased systemic perfusion such as weak or absent femoral pulses and/or metabolic acidosis (**Table 51-2**). A high index of suspicion for cardiac pathology should be maintained for infants who appear to have severe respiratory disease and who are not improving with conventional management.

Two points are important to make at this juncture:

1. A "normal" fetal echocardiogram or ultrasound should not be reason to exclude the consideration of serious congenital heart disease. The fetal diagnosis of congenital heart disease is a very operator-dependent test and has known limitations for assessing structures such as the pulmonary veins. There are many instances of infants with "normal" in-utero testing diagnosed with congenital heart disease.
2. An echocardiogram done on a critically ill newborn is a very difficult test to perform and interpret accurately. The infant may be ventilated on an oscillator or have labile blood pressure/saturation where even brief imaging is poorly tolerated. There are numerous hemodynamic factors that make the acquisition and interpretation of images difficult. In addition, some of the most difficult diagnoses to make by echocardiogram (such as obstructed total anomalous pulmonary venous return) typically present in this scenario. While more neonatologists, radiologists, and hospitalists are acquiring advanced training in pediatric echocardiography, it is imperative that physicians caring for the critically ill infant do not overstep their degree of expertise when assessing for potential critical heart disease due to the above described factors.

DIAGNOSTIC EVALUATION FOR CONGENITAL HEART DISEASE

When critical heart disease is suspected in the neonate, diagnostic and empiric interventions should be performed simultaneously. The first step should always be obtaining a chest X-ray to evaluate for pulmonary edema, the cardiac silhouette, and evidence of various pathologies. Measurement of blood brain natriuretic peptide and troponin levels can be helpful markers whose elevation may signal cardiac pathology. For diagnosis, consultation with a pediatric cardiologist and full transthoracic echocardiogram are indicated. With such evaluation, the diagnosis of virtually all congenital heart disease in the newborn period is possible. If the index of suspicion for heart disease is lower, a chest radiograph, electrocardiogram, and hyperoxic test should be performed. The hyperoxic test is performed by placing the infant on 100% FiO_2 for 10 minutes and measuring a post-ductal arterial PO_2. A value of >150 mmHg most always excludes cyanotic congenital heart disease. An infant with a PO_2 <150 mmHg who has poor perfusion, or who remains critically ill despite usual treatment measures for other conditions should have a complete echocardiogram.

In those infants suspected of having CCHD, empiric therapy with intravenous prostaglandin E-1 (PGE) should be commenced immediately at a dose of between 0.01 μg/kg/min and 0.05 μg/kg/min. PGE will reopen a closing ductus arteriosus and restore pulmonary or systemic flow in critical heart disease, temporizing the situation and allowing time for diagnosis and planning of intervention. Side effects of prostaglandin include apnea, hypotension, tachycardia, and fever, and these resolve with discontinuation of the medication. PGE is indicated in all PDA-dependent lesions, and a positive response would be demonstrated by an increase in saturations and cardiac output.

The recognition of congenital heart disease rests on the foundation of a good clinical history and physical examination (see Chapter 49). An electrocardiogram may add supplemental information to the assessment of cardiac anatomy and is necessary for diagnosis of rhythm abnormalities. The diagnosis of congenital heart disease has been revolutionized by two-dimensional echocardiography. It provides detailed anatomic and physiologic diagnosis of congenital heart disease, is noninvasive, and is performed at the bedside. Coupled with the Doppler technique, blood velocity may also be assessed; this can be used to estimate chamber pressures, presence of heart or great vessel obstruction, and valve regurgitation. Factors that limit the usefulness of transthoracic echocardiography include obesity, obstructive lung disease, and certain chest wall deformities. Three-dimensional echocardiography is in the early stages of clinical application and may provide additional understanding of anatomy, particularly valvar morphology.

Magnetic resonance imaging (MRI) is increasingly being used for diagnostic evaluation of congenital heart disease. Advantages of cardiac MRI include excellent anatomic detail that is not limited by lung tissue (unlike echocardiography), and MRI therefore is an especially good modality for imaging the great vessels. A major disadvantage of cardiac MRI is the requirement for sedation and the relatively long post-processing and interpretation time. Functional assessment of blood flow by MRI is possible and may be more accurate than echocardiography. Implanted metal such as surgical clips or embolization coils present in many children with serious congenital heart disease can render bothersome imaging artifacts when performing cardiac/thoracic MRIs. MRI is generally contraindicated in patients with pacemakers and defibrillators. Cardiac computed tomography (CT) is being more commonly utilized due to the decreasing radiation burden and excellent spatial resolution allowing more precise anatomical diagnosis.

Cardiac catheterization with angiography was once considered the gold standard for anatomic diagnosis. However, echocardiography, CT, and MRI have now almost completely supplanted cardiac catheterization for anatomic diagnosis. Cardiac catheterization remains the gold standard for hemodynamic assessment, and increasingly it is being used as an interventional rather than diagnostic tool.

MANAGEMENT OF CONGENITAL HEART DISEASE

Definitive treatment of congenital heart disease is complex due to the wide variety of anatomy, the physiologic changes that occur over time (e.g., fall in PVR), and growth. Straightforward heart lesions are approached with surgical or transcatheter techniques that address a single problem (e.g., atrial septal defect). More complex forms of congenital heart disease are approached by cardiologists and cardiovascular surgeons by first attempting to decide if there are enough required cardiac "parts" to immediately or eventually repair the heart in such a way that it is physiologically, if not anatomically, correct. A "complete" or "two-ventricle" repair entails having separate systemic and pulmonary circuits, each with its own ventricle and atrioventricular valve able to pump deoxygenated blood to the lungs and oxygenated blood to the body. Although this type of repair is referred to as a "complete," the resulting cardiac anatomy is often very different from normal. Where possible, complete repair is generally the preferred option.

If there are insufficient "parts" to perform a complete repair (e.g., hypoplastic left heart syndrome, tricuspid atresia), then a single ventricle pathway must be pursued. The single ventricle pathway typically follows as a series of palliative surgeries that culminate with a Fontan procedure. This staged cardiac surgery ultimately results in a circulation where the venous blood return is *passively* routed to the lungs without traveling through a ventricle, and then returns to a functionally single ventricle

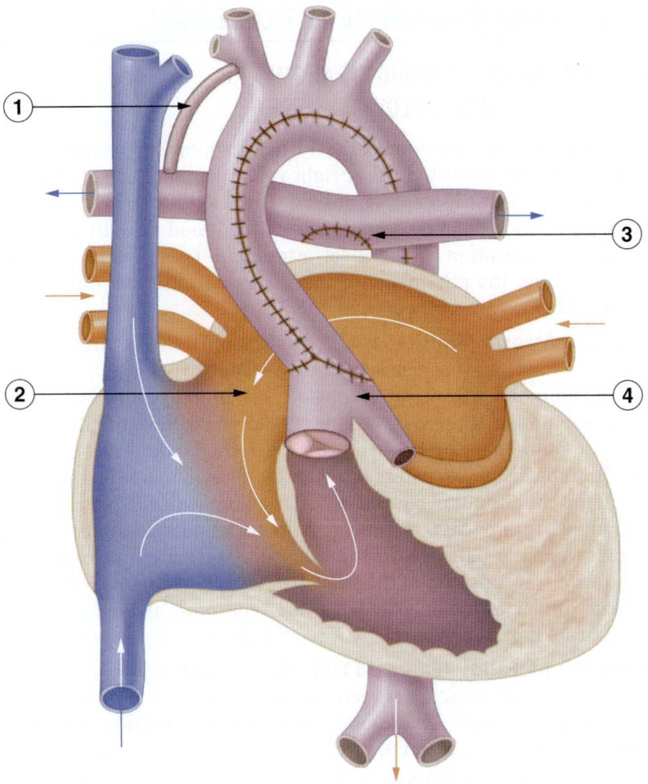

FIGURE 51-1. Stage I single ventricle pathway for hypoplastic left heart syndrome (see Figure 51-8 for unrepaired anatomy). 1. Right modified Blalock-Thomas-Taussig shunt. 2. Large (surgically created) atrial septal defect. 3. Main pulmonary artery has been detached form branch pulmonary arteries. 4. Unobstructed egress of blood from the heart to the body has been achieved by using the main pulmonary artery and native aorta with additional patch material. (Reproduced from Sinclair CM. *The Report of the Manitoba Pediatric Cardiac Surgery Inquest: An Inquiry Into Twelve Deaths at the Winnipeg Health Sciences Center in 1994.*)

that pumps to the body. For this type of repair to succeed, the patient must have a relatively competent atrioventricular valve, good systolic ventricular function, unobstructed outflow from the heart, widely patent pulmonary arteries, and low PVR. The vascular resistance of the neonatal pulmonary vascular bed is too high to accept the passive pulmonary flow of a Fontan, and so a series of operations is necessary to ultimately achieve this type of palliation.

STAGE I: SINGLE VENTRICLE PATHWAY (FIGURE 51-1)

The first stage of the single ventricle pathway provides for *adequate pulmonary blood flow* and *unobstructed systemic flow* in the newborn period. This palliation generally occurs at approximately 1 week of life.

If the original cardiac anatomy is such that there is insufficient blood flow to the pulmonary vascular bed, a shunt is placed to provide flow from the systemic circulation to the pulmonary circulation. A common surgical shunt is the modified Blalock-Thomas-Taussig (BTT) shunt, which is a synthetic tube placed from the subclavian artery to the ipsilateral pulmonary artery. Another frequently used method to provide stable pulmonary blood flow is a stent placed in the PDA. A Sano shunt is a right ventricle to pulmonary artery conduit that can also provide pulmonary blood flow. There are many types of shunts and modifications of techniques, which depend on the individual anatomy and operator preference.

The infant with an "ideal" physiology following a shunt has a systemic oxygen saturation of about 80%. Empirically this saturation has been found to be the best balance between systemic oxygen delivery and pulmonary overcirculation. Because blood circulating to the lungs is already partially saturated, shunt physiology is inefficient, and even with this "ideal" saturation of 80%, there is still about twice as much blood being circulated to the lungs as to the body.

If the original cardiac anatomy results in too much pulmonary flow such that the pulmonary pressures are high and/or the infant is in congestive heart failure, then the first stage in palliation is a pulmonary artery band (PAB). A PAB is a surgical "noose" placed around the pulmonary artery that creates an artificial stenosis and limits pulmonary flow.

Of great importance in the single ventricle pathway is the provision for an unobstructed pathway for systemic blood flow. The proximal pulmonary artery and aorta are often used together to recreate a single unobstructed outflow from the heart in this first stage (Damus-Kaye-Stansel or DKS procedure).

STAGE II: BIDIRECTIONAL GLENN (FIGURE 51-2)

At about 4 to 8 months of age, the PVR has typically decreased sufficiently to accept a portion of the venous return in a passive manner. The second step of cardiac palliation for children proceeding down the single ventricle pathway is the "bidirectional Glenn," or stage II. This involves connecting the superior vena cava directly to the pulmonary arteries and eliminating any previous shunted source of pulmonary blood flow, such as a BTT shunt, Sano, or PDA stent. The arterial saturations are usually about the same before and after the procedure (~80%); however, this type of circulation is preferable because it is more efficient. In the shunted scenario (stage I), the single ventricle pumps blood to both the body and the lungs, and the blood pumped to the lungs is already partially saturated. After the stage II repair, the heart is only pumping blood to the body, and only desaturated blood

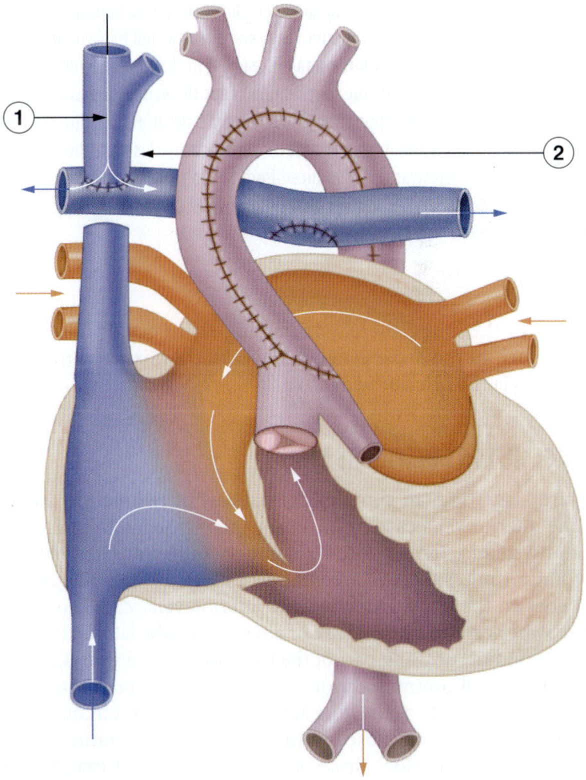

FIGURE 51-2. Stage II single ventricle pathway for hypoplastic left heart syndrome. 1, 2. The right modified Blalock-Thomas-Taussig shunt that was created at the stage 1 repair has been removed. The superior vena cava is divided and the proximal portion is attached directly to the right pulmonary artery, allowing the blood from the superior vena cava (SVC) to flow to both lungs ("bidirectional Glenn"). "Bidirectional" refers to the SVC blood flowing to both the right and left lungs. (Reproduced from Sinclair CM. *The Report of the Manitoba Pediatric Cardiac Surgery Inquest: An Inquiry Into Twelve Deaths at the Winnipeg Health Sciences Center in 1994.*)

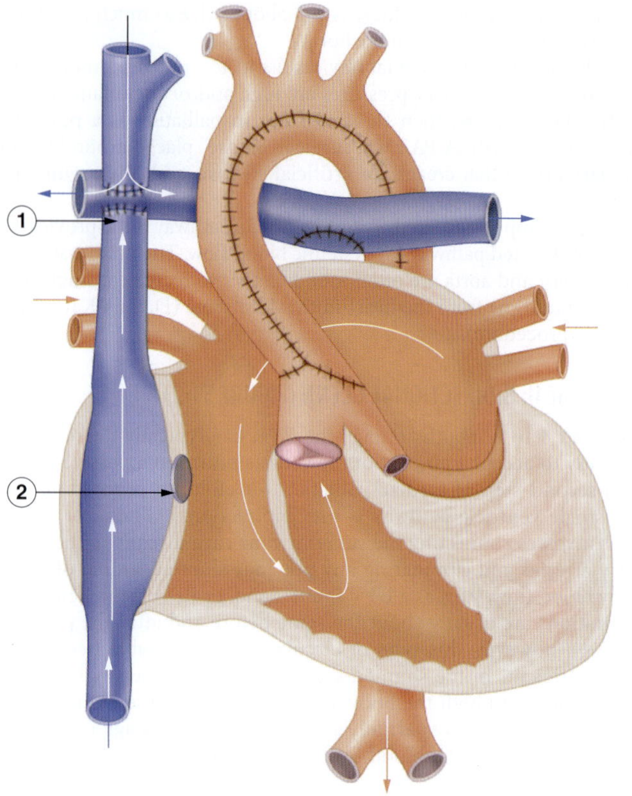

FIGURE 51-3. Stage III single ventricle pathway for hypoplastic left heart syndrome. 1. A tube has been placed within the right atrium to direct the blood from the inferior vena cava to the superior vena cava. The superior vena cava is reattached to the undersurface of the pulmonary artery. 2. Fenestration: a small hole is left in the tube to allow some of the venous blood to bypass the lungs. The fenestration keeps the venous pressure from rising too high after the Fontan operation, but results in some desaturation. The fenestration may be optional in some patients, but if desired can be easily closed in the cardiac catheterization laboratory afterward. (Reproduced from Sinclair CM. *The Report of the Manitoba Pediatric Cardiac Surgery Inquest: An Inquiry Into Twelve Deaths at the Winnipeg Health Sciences Center in 1994.*)

is flowing to the lungs, thereby increasing efficiency. It is worth noting that much of the deoxygenated blood is still mixing with systemic circulation via the inferior vena cava.

STAGE III: FONTAN (FIGURE 51-3)

The third stage (Fontan completion) consists of redirecting the blood from the inferior vena cava to the lungs, thereby separating the pulmonary and systemic circuits. After this surgery, all desaturated blood goes to the lungs (unless there is a Fontan fenestration), and all oxygenated blood goes to the body. Directing the inferior vena cava blood to the lungs may be accomplished by use of a synthetic tube lateral to the heart (external conduit) or using part of the right atrium as a wall (lateral tunnel). Often a small communication is left in the tube (fenestration) to act as a pressure "pop-off" as the lung acclimate to the new circulation. This fenestration may later be closed in the cardiac catheterization lab. After closure of the fenestration, these patients have normal oxygen saturations. Stage III is usually performed between ages 2 and 5 years, depending on center preference and technique.

Postoperative problems encountered by patients with Fontan-type repairs include early problems such as prolonged pleural effusions (serous and chylous) and late problems such as increased risk for stroke and thrombus formation in the Fontan, arrhythmia development (especially atrial flutter), and protein-losing enteropathy as well as plastic bronchitis (lymphatic insufficiency).

CRITICAL NEWBORN HEART DISEASE

PATENT DUCTUS ARTERIOSUS AUGMENTS: PULMONARY BLOOD FLOW

In this set of lesions, a portion of the normal anatomy supporting pulmonary blood flow (tricuspid valve, right ventricle, pulmonary valve, and pulmonary arteries) is small or absent. The ductus arteriosus provides pulmonary blood flow by shunting systemic blood flow to the lungs. While d-transposition of the great arteries (d-TGA) is also included in this section, the physiology of this lesion is somewhat different, as explained below.

Tricuspid Atresia (Figure 51-4) The tricuspid valve is atretic in this lesion and the right ventricle is typically severely hypoplastic.

If the pulmonary flow is inadequate, a systemic-to-pulmonary artery shunt is required. If there is too much pulmonary flow, the infant may require a pulmonary artery band to reduce the amount of pulmonary flow. In some instances, nature provides just enough pulmonary stenosis so that the child is not in congestive heart failure with adequate systemic saturations. In any case, the infant with tricuspid atresia also follows a single ventricle pathway. In some instances, tricuspid atresia is also found with transposition of the great arteries. These infants will require a repair similar to hypoplastic left heart syndrome, as the aortic valve and arch are typically hypoplastic when the great arteries are transposed.

Tetralogy of Fallot (Figure 51-5) This condition arises when the ventricular septal muscle between the aorta and the pulmonary artery is deviated anteriorly. This causes the pulmonary outflow area to be stenotic, a special type of VSD to be present under the aorta (anterior malalignment), and the aorta to then be aligned over the VSD and crest of the ventricular septum (overriding aorta). There is usually accompanying right ventricular hypertrophy, which completes the four parts of the tetralogy. While simple in its description, there is a huge variation in

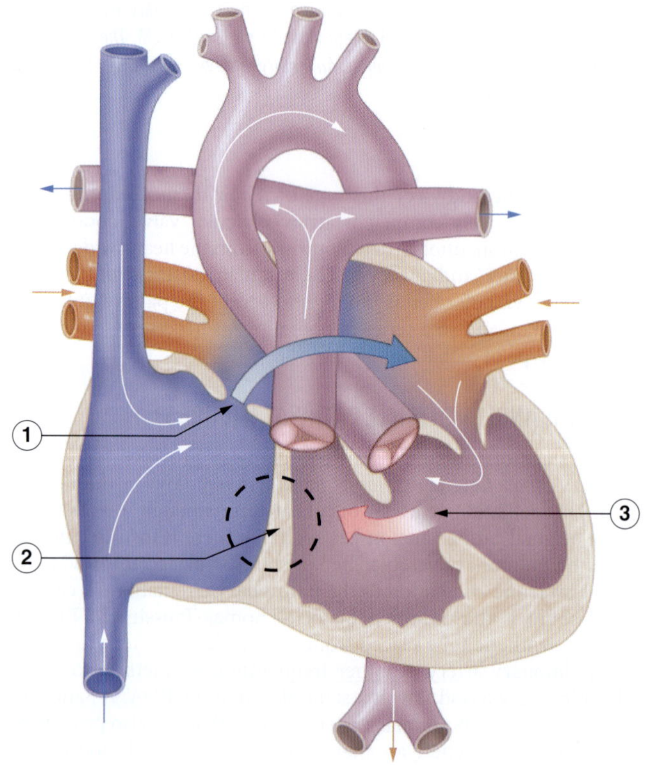

FIGURE 51-4. Tricuspid atresia (normal great arteries). 1. Patent foramen ovale with flow right to left. 2. Atretic tricuspid valve. 3. Ventricular septal defect (VSD). Size of VSD and amount of restriction is variable. (Reproduced from Sinclair CM. *The Report of the Manitoba Pediatric Cardiac Surgery Inquest: An Inquiry Into Twelve Deaths at the Winnipeg Health Sciences Center in 1994.*)

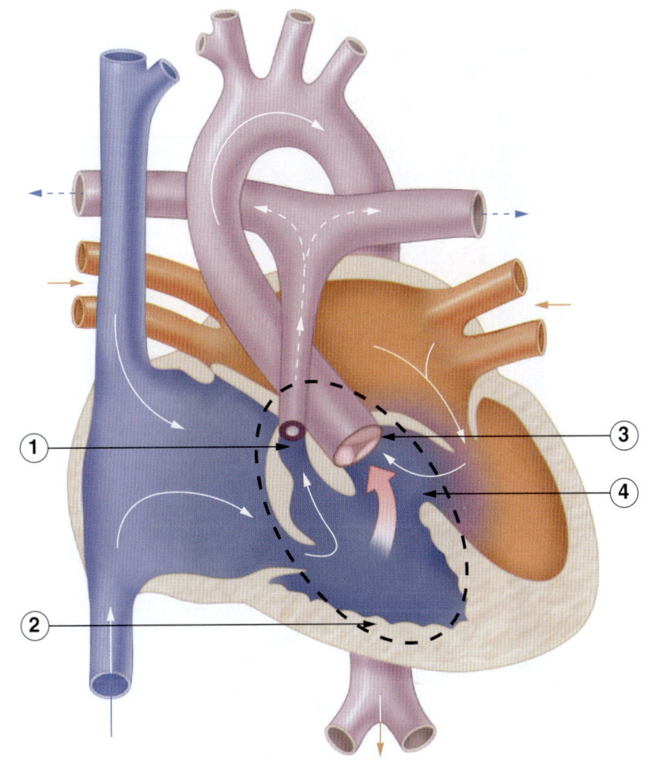

FIGURE 51-5. Tetralogy of Fallot. 1. Pulmonary valve and subvalvar stenosis. 2. Hypertrophied right ventricle. 3. Overriding aorta. 4. Ventricular septal defect. (Reproduced from Sinclair CM. *The Report of the Manitoba Pediatric Cardiac Surgery Inquest: An Inquiry Into Twelve Deaths at the Winnipeg Health Sciences Center in 1994.*)

the severity of this disease that is largely dependent upon the pulmonary artery architecture. When there are well-developed pulmonary arteries and mild or moderate pulmonary stenosis, this lesion is not critical. Systemic oxygen saturations from 80% to 95% are possible, and infants may undergo elective complete repair between 3 and 12 months of age. Surgical repair in these cases involves closing the VSD and relieving the pulmonary obstruction by patching the right ventricular outflow tract, pulmonary valve, and main pulmonary artery as needed.

More severe obstruction at the pulmonary valve and right ventricular outflow tract may lead to more profound cyanosis and ductal dependency. These infants may require a shunt to increase pulmonary flow in anticipation of a complete repair at an older age, or they may undergo complete repair as infants.

At the extreme, there may be complete atresia of the pulmonary valve, and only a thread-like main pulmonary artery. Associated with this more severe obstruction are downstream architectural abnormalities of the pulmonary arteries, with stenosis or absence of branches of the pulmonary arteries and the presence of collateral vessels from the aorta to the pulmonary arteries that may supply multiple segments of the lung. Presence of these aorto-pulmonary collateral vessels and small, stenotic pulmonary arteries makes definitive surgical repair a challenge, and is individualized for each patient's anatomy, usually requiring a series of staged operations and cardiac catheterizations for dilation of stenotic pulmonary arteries.

Important pediatric concerns of infants with tetralogy of Fallot, especially when associated with pulmonary atresia, is the association with the 22q deletion/velocardiofacial/DiGeorge syndrome complex. Infants with this heart disease should have genetic testing (fluorescence in situ hybridization (FISH)) done for the 22q deletion, and calcium levels should be monitored in the newborn period. If positive, immunologic workup and genetic and anticipatory guidance should be provided to patients and families.

Another important issue for patients with tetralogy of Fallot is the possibility of experiencing "tet-spells," which are sudden episodes of profound desaturation. The classic explanation of the pathophysiology of this condition is "spasm" of the muscle under the pulmonary valve leading to decreased pulmonary flow and increased cyanosis, though this is certainly an oversimplified mechanism. Tet-spells can be treated by increasing the systemic resistance to force more blood across the pulmonary circuit. This can be done mechanically by putting the patient in a knee-to-chest position, or pharmacologically by administering intravenous phenylephrine. Supplemental oxygen may be of some benefit (due to pulmonary vasodilation) as is the administration of subcutaneous or intravenous morphine as a sedative. Ketamine is an especially useful drug in managing tet-spells, as it provides both sedation and increased systemic vascular resistance, and it can be administered intravenously or intramuscularly. Patients who have had one or more tet-spells should be considered for surgical palliation or repair, as these spells, if prolonged, can be associated with morbidity and mortality.

d-Transposition of the Great Arteries (Figure 51-6) In d-transposition of the great arteries (d-TGA), the aorta arises from the right ventricle and the pulmonary artery arises from the left ventricle. This leads to systemic blood returning from the body, recirculating to the body, and pulmonary blood recirculating to the lungs (parallel circulations), and profound cyanosis. Survival depends on mixing of the two circulations at the atrial, ventricular, or great vessel levels. Prostaglandin E-1 temporizes this condition by increasing the amount of blood in the pulmonary system by maintaining patency of the ductus arteriosus, which encourages mixing at the atrial or ventricular level. For prostaglandin to work, there must be an atrial or ventricular septal defect. If no septal defect is present, or if mixing is inadequate as evidenced by oxygen saturation less than 80%, an atrial septal defect may need to be created, or an existing one enlarged, to stabilize the infant in anticipation of corrective surgery.

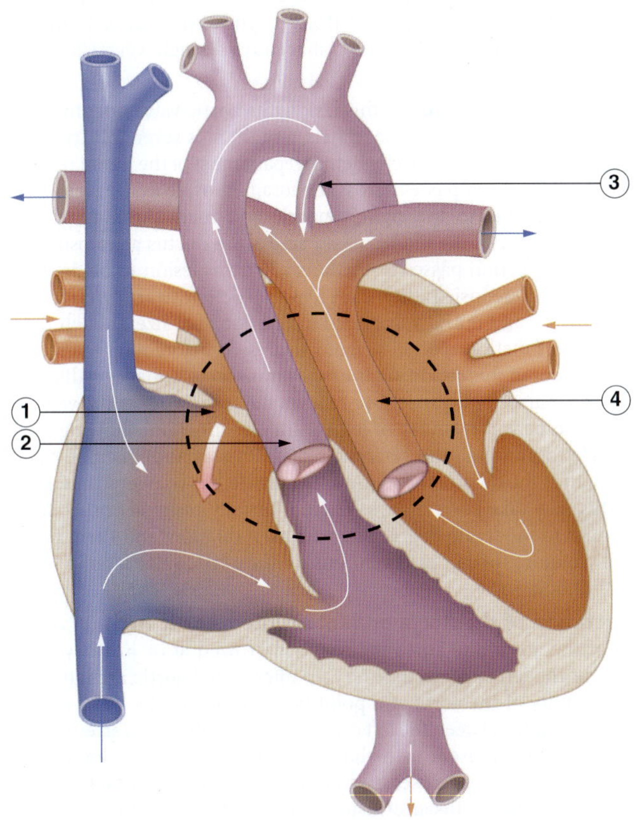

FIGURE 51-6. d-Transposition of the great arteries. 1. Patent foramen ovale with left-to-right flow. 2. Transposed great arteries. Aorta arises from right ventricle. 3. Ductus arteriosus with flow from aorta to pulmonary artery. 4. Transposed great arteries. Pulmonary artery arises from left ventricle. (Reproduced from Sinclair CM. *The Report of the Manitoba Pediatric Cardiac Surgery Inquest: An Inquiry Into Twelve Deaths at the Winnipeg Health Sciences Center in 1994.*)

This procedure (balloon atrial septostomy) is accomplished by passing a balloon catheter through the atrial septum, inflating the balloon, and pulling it back across the atrial septum to tear a hole in the atrial septum, thereby creating an atrial septal defect. This procedure can be performed at the bedside under echocardiographic guidance alone, or in the cardiac catheterization laboratory under fluoroscopic guidance.

Definitive therapy for d-TGA is surgical. Since the mid-1980s, the procedure of choice for this lesion is the "arterial switch," where the aorta and pulmonary arteries are transected above the valves and reattached to their physiologically correct ventricle. The Achilles-heel of this procedure is transfer of the coronary arteries, which must be removed separately and reattached to the aorta. The coronary artery anatomy is variable and makes preoperative definition of this anatomy important and appropriate surgical planning imperative. Associated lesions are usually corrected at the same surgery, which may include VSD and coarctation of the aorta. The prognosis for children with d-TGA is generally excellent. Postoperative problems related to coronary artery obstruction can occur, as can residual lesions related to the surgical correction.

PATENT DUCTUS ARTERIOSUS AUGMENTS: SYSTEMIC BLOOD FLOW

In this set of lesions, a portion of the normal anatomy supporting systemic blood flow (mitral valve, left ventricle, aortic valve, and aorta) is narrowed, small, or absent. The ductus arteriosus provides systemic blood flow by shunting some of the pulmonary blood through the ductus arteriosus to the aorta. Infants with these lesions often present with shock or decreased femoral pulses as the ductus arteriosus closes. Critical aortic stenosis, interrupted aortic arch, and critical coarctation of the aorta are all examples of critical left heart disease that require prostaglandin to stabilize and temporize, but can all have repairs that result in a complete repair. Hypoplastic left heart syndrome is an extreme form of left heart obstructive disease that requires a single ventricle surgical approach.

Critical Aortic Stenosis In this lesion, the aortic valve opening is narrowed by partial fusion of the leaflets, and there is severe obstruction to outflow from the left ventricle. Before repair, most of the blood returning from the left atrium passes across the foramen ovale to the right atrium and subsequently to the right ventricle and main pulmonary artery, where a portion of the blood passes across the ductus arteriosus to the body and a portion passes to the lungs. For this lesion to be defined as critical aortic stenosis rather than hypoplastic left heart syndrome, the left ventricle, and mitral valve need to be of normal size, though the left ventricular function is often severely depressed before intervention.

Treatment of this condition is usually transcatheter balloon dilation of the aortic valve. This procedure relieves the narrowing at the valve sufficiently to permit recovery of left ventricular function, allowing the left ventricle to pump all the systemic blood. Prostaglandin can be discontinued after the dilation once the left ventricle has recovered adequately, but this may take several days. There is usually residual aortic stenosis of a mild to moderate degree after neonatal dilation, and these patients usually require further interventions for the aortic valve later in infancy or childhood.

Coarctation of the Aorta and Interrupted Aortic Arch In coarctation of the aorta, the aorta is severely narrowed at or just beyond the origin of the left subclavian artery. In interrupted aortic arch, there is a discontinuity of the aorta at a point between one of the head and neck vessels (usually between the left carotid and left subclavian arteries). Both lesions typically present with shock and/or decreased femoral pulses as the ductus arteriosus closes and are temporized by prostaglandin E-1, which opens the ductus arteriosus, supplementing systemic blood flow.

The treatment of either lesion is surgical repair in the neonatal period. The surgical repair for critical coarctation usually involves removing the narrowed segment and rejoining the descending aorta to the aortic arch in an unobstructed fashion. The repair is usually done without the need for cardiopulmonary bypass. The repair of interrupted aortic arch is a much more complex arch reconstruction requiring the use of cardiopulmonary bypass. A ventricular septal defect—associated with the most common type of interrupted aortic arch—is repaired at the same surgery.

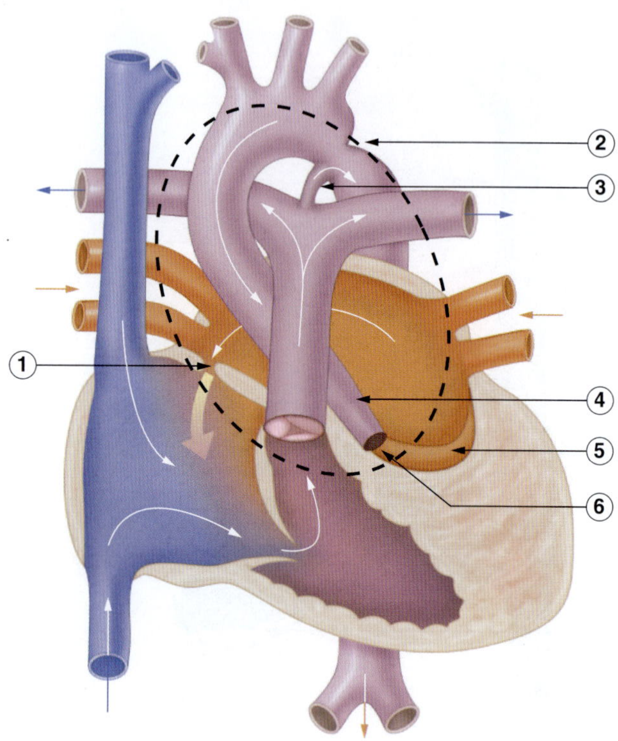

FIGURE 51-7. Hypoplastic left heart syndrome. 1. Atrial septal defect with left-to-right flow. 2. Coarctation of the aorta. 3. Patent ductus arteriosus with flow from pulmonary artery to aorta. 4. Hypoplastic ascending aorta. 5. Small mitral valve—sometimes atretic. 6. Small Aortic valve—sometimes atretic. (Reproduced from Sinclair CM. *The Report of the Manitoba Pediatric Cardiac Surgery Inquest: An Inquiry Into Twelve Deaths at the Winnipeg Health Sciences Center in 1994.*)

Interrupted aortic arch (type B) is also associated with the 22q deletion/DiGeorge complex and as with tetralogy of Fallot, these patients should have appropriate calcium monitoring, and genetic and immunologic workup.

Hypoplastic Left Heart Syndrome When the left-sided heart structures (mitral valve, left ventricle, aortic valve, and aortic arch) are too small to support the cardiac output needed for the body, the condition is referred to as hypoplastic left heart syndrome (**Figure 51-7**). The mitral or aortic valves may be so small as to be atretic. In the unrepaired state, the right ventricle pumps the combined venous return from the body and from the lungs to the pulmonary artery, where a portion of the blood passes to the lungs and a portion passes through the ductus arteriosus to supply the body. The degree of cyanosis depends on the proportion of pulmonary to systemic blood flow. As the ductus arteriosus closes, more blood is directed to the lungs and less to the body, leading to higher systemic saturations but signs and symptoms of low cardiac output and ultimately shock. Prostaglandin E-1 opens the ductus arteriosus and temporizes the situation.

Surgical repair of this condition follows the principles of the single ventricle pathway outlined in a subsequent section and involves three stages. The first stage is more involved than most other types of first-stage single ventricle palliations because the main pulmonary artery must be used along with the native (small) aorta and prosthetic patch material to refashion the aortic arch (DKS procedure). Pulmonary blood flow is provided by placing a tube graft from either a subclavian artery to pulmonary artery (modified Blalock-Thomas-Taussig or MBTTS) or from the right ventricular outflow tract to the pulmonary artery (Sano shunt).

The initial palliation strategy for hypoplastic left heart syndrome is technically difficult and even in the best centers has one of the higher mortalities for congenital heart disease surgery. As a result, the past decade has seen the development and refinement of an alternative strategy called a "hybrid stage I" (**Figure 51-8**). This technique is a hybrid surgical and transcatheter technique where a surgical noose (band) is

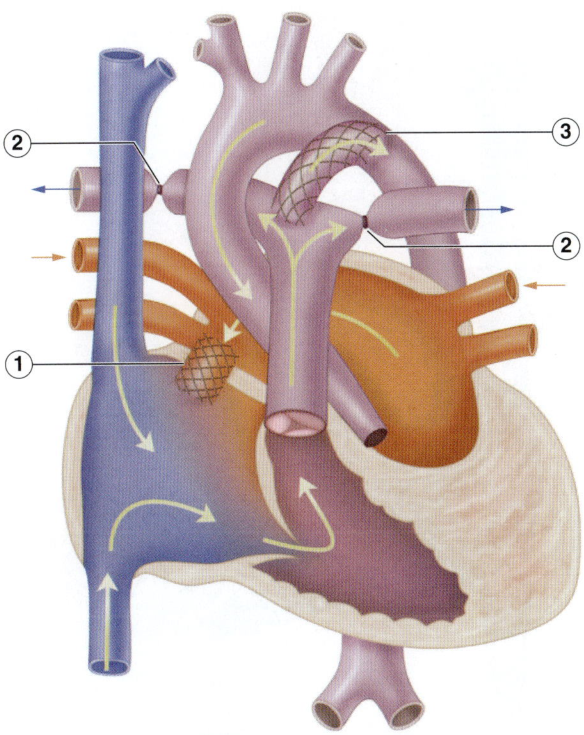

FIGURE 51-8. Hypoplastic left heart syndrome after hybrid stage I palliation. 1. Stent in atrial septum (sometimes required). 2. Pulmonary artery bands on right and left pulmonary arteries. 3. Stent across ductus arteriosus. Note that stent often covers the origin of the aortic arch. Blood traverses through the struts of the stent to reach the head and perfuse the coronary arteries. (Reproduced from Sinclair CM. *The Report of the Manitoba Pediatric Cardiac Surgery Inquest: An Inquiry Into Twelve Deaths at the Winnipeg Health Sciences Center in 1994.*)

placed on each pulmonary artery to limit pulmonary blood flow, and a stent is placed in the ductus arteriosus to maintain systemic perfusion. The atrial septum is also enlarged if needed using catheter balloon and/or stent techniques. This hybrid stage I approach results in a much more stable infant post-procedure. The infant is then adequately palliated until he/she is about 4 to 6 months of age and then undergoes a "comprehensive stage II" procedure where the ductal stent and pulmonary artery bands are removed, and then the previously described first-stage operation is performed, with the exception that a Glenn shunt (superior vena cava to pulmonary artery) is used rather than a systemic-pulmonary artery shunt. This makes for a more complex stage II procedure, but at a time when the infant is much bigger, making the procedure easier. In addition, the Glenn shunt is a more stable source of pulmonary blood flow than is a systemic-pulmonary artery shunt. The infant then continues down the single ventricle pathway to arrive at a Fontan procedure typically between 3 and 5 years of age. These two techniques in multicenter series appear to have similar outcomes, but some centers prefer one technique over the other depending on their center-specific outcomes for both approaches.

Another strategy for managing patients with hypoplastic left heart syndrome is infant heart transplantation. Despite significant advances in immunosuppressive regimens, success of the heart transplantation strategy for hypoplastic left heart syndrome has been limited by a lack of donor organs and late graft failure, which occurs over decades in virtually all transplanted hearts.

CRITICAL NEWBORN HEART DISEASE: PATENT DUCTUS ARTERIOSUS NOT REQUIRED

Total anomalous pulmonary venous return (TAPVR) with obstruction is the classic example of newborn heart disease that is not temporized by prostaglandin E-1. In this lesion, the pulmonary veins do not return to the left atrium but communicate with the systemic veins by means of a supplemental venous channel. This channel may be obstructed, leading to progressive pulmonary edema, "whiteout" on chest x-ray, and an inability to ventilate or oxygenate. This lesion is the one most often mistaken for pulmonary disease in the newborn. If a newborn has progressive pulmonary disease and is failing conventional treatment, the diagnosis of congenital heart disease—especially obstructed TAPVR—should be entertained and an echocardiogram obtained. Repair consists of reattaching the pulmonary venous chamber to the left atrium.

LESIONS PRESENTING WITH CONGESTIVE HEART FAILURE OR MURMUR IN INFANCY

As the PVR falls in the first weeks of life, lesions that permit the transmission of high flow or pressure to the lungs become manifest. These lesions include VSD, atrioventricular septal defect (AVSD), and patent ductus arteriosus (PDA).

VENTRICULAR SEPTAL DEFECT (FIGURE 51-9)

The ventricular septum is a complex anatomical structure dividing the left and right ventricles. Near the aortic valve, the septum is a thin membrane (membranous septum) whereas it is a thick muscle in other parts. A defect in the wall is called a VSD. The most common defects occur in the membranous septum, but they can occur anywhere in the wall, and may be multiple. The presentation of VSD is dependent on two factors—the size of the VSD and the PVR.

Small VSD A small muscular ventricular septal defect presents in the first days to weeks of life with a high-pitched, asymptomatic murmur. When the resistance in the pulmonary circulation falls, so too does the right ventricular pressure, creating a large pressure difference between the left and right ventricles. A small hole between the ventricles creates

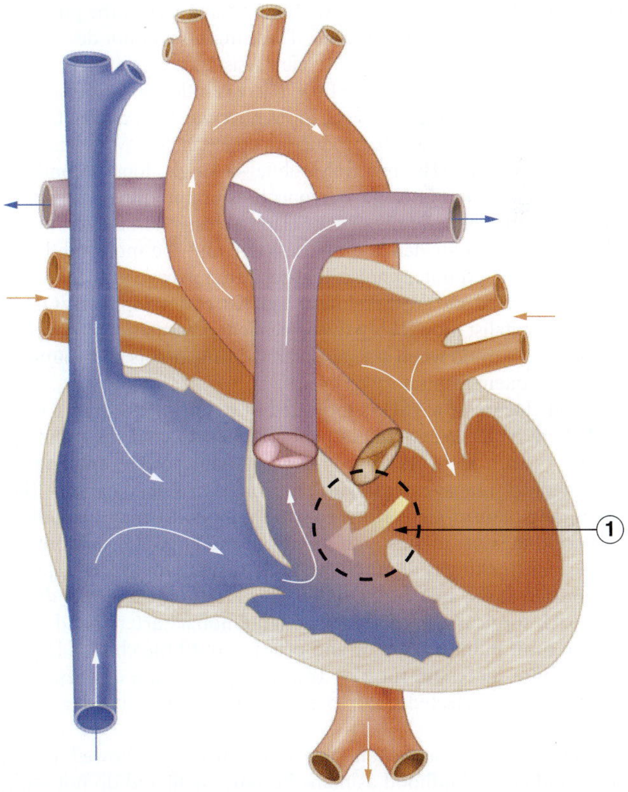

FIGURE 51-9. Ventricular septal defect. 1. Ventricular septal defect (VSD) with flow from left ventricle to right ventricle. Position of VSD in ventricular septum determines type. More common type located just underneath the aortic valve (membranous). (Reproduced from Sinclair CM. *The Report of the Manitoba Pediatric Cardiac Surgery Inquest: An Inquiry Into Twelve Deaths at the Winnipeg Health Sciences Center in 1994.*)

a turbulent left-to-right flow jet, and a loud murmur is heard. In this scenario, the total amount of blood recirculated through the lungs and back to the left ventricle is minimal.

Moderate VSD If the VSD is somewhat larger, as the pulmonary resistance falls, the VSD may still be small enough to limit the pressure transmitted to the right ventricle but large enough to admit more blood flow. In this circumstance, the amount of extra blood flow to the lungs recirculating back to the left heart may be significant, and the infant may have respiratory symptoms and perhaps some degree of congestive heart failure. A loud murmur will be present as the pressure gradient and flow are high.

Large VSD At a certain point, the VSD is so large as to be unable to limit the pressure transmitted by the left ventricle. As the pulmonary resistance falls, there is more and more blood recirculating to the lungs, but the pressure in the right ventricle and pulmonary artery remains at systemic levels (so-called unrestrictive defects). The intensity of the systolic murmur is proportional to the degree of left-to-right shunting; however, there is often (counterintuitively) only a relatively soft murmur because there is little turbulence across the large VSD. With excessive pulmonary blood flow, infants typically display failure to thrive. If left uncorrected for a prolonged period of time, these infants run the risk of developing irreversible changes to the pulmonary vasculature that progresses even after the defect is corrected. Pulmonary blood vessels when exposed to high pressure for too long develop irreversible changes called pulmonary vascular obstructive disease (PVOD), also known as Eisenmenger Complex. PVOD is averted by limiting the pressure to which the lung vasculature is exposed by either closing the VSD or applying downstream resistance to flow by placing a pulmonary artery "band." Irreversible PVOD does not usually develop until after age 1 year, although the time course after this point is remarkably variable. Patients with Down syndrome seem to be at higher risk at an earlier age and intervention is recommended before age 9 months in this subgroup.

Although most infants with large VSDs with left-to-right shunt present with congestive heart failure as the pulmonary resistance falls, there is a small group of patients with unrestrictive VSDs in whom the pulmonary resistance falls very little or not at all. These infants will not develop congestive heart failure, and if the pulmonary resistance is very high, may not have much additional pulmonary flow. There is little if any heart murmur as there is no restriction to flow at the ventricular level and not enough increase in pulmonary flow to produce an appreciable flow murmur. The only cardiac sign may be relatively subtle—a single, loud second heart sound. These children often have frequent respiratory illness, which may further limit the ability of the pediatrician to clearly auscultate the heart. With no loud murmur demanding attention, and the more subtle signs often masked by respiratory noise, these children may go undiagnosed for a prolonged period and are therefore at high risk of developing PVOD. The pediatric hospitalist should keep this infrequent presentation of congenital heart disease in mind when assessing and treating infants and young children with frequent respiratory problems.

Surgical closure of a VSD is indicated in infancy (less than 1 year of age) if there is persistent congestive heart failure, or if the pulmonary pressures remain high. As some VSDs get smaller with time and even close, medical management with anticongestive medications (lasix, digoxin, angiotensin-converting enzyme inhibitors) may be indicated for a period in some infants with moderate and large VSDs. More complex decision-making is required for VSDs that are multiple—especially those located at the apex of the heart. This location is typically difficult to approach surgically. In this instance, a pulmonary artery band may be placed to limit pulmonary flow and pressure until the child is larger to undergo more successful surgery. Transcatheter closure devices may be another option in selected children, sometimes combined with a surgical approach.

Moderate ventricular septal defects are usually followed through infancy and early childhood as many become small and do not require intervention. Closure is recommended for VSDs that remain moderate with a pulmonary to systemic flow ratio of more than about 2:1.

Transcatheter closure devices for membranous VSDs are in clinical trials. These devices need special design and delivery systems to avoid interfering with the aortic valve, which forms the superior border of the membranous septum.

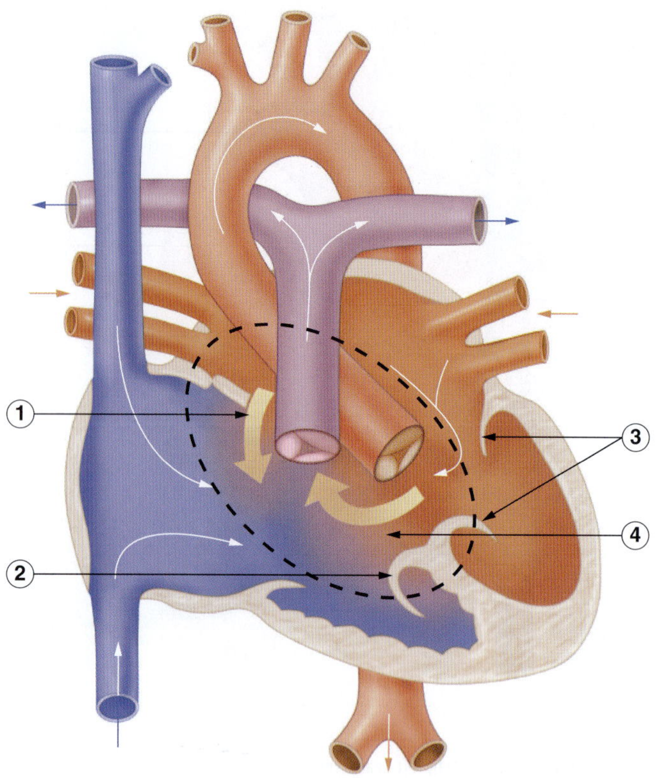

FIGURE 51-10. Atrioventricular septal defect. 1. Atrial septal defect (ostium primum type). 2. Right side of common atrioventricular valve (incompletely formed tricuspid valve). 3. Left side of common atrioventricular valve (incompletely formed mitral valve). 4. Ventricular septal defect (of "inlet" ventricular septal type). (Reproduced from Sinclair CM. *The Report of the Manitoba Pediatric Cardiac Surgery Inquest: An Inquiry Into Twelve Deaths at the Winnipeg Health Sciences Center in 1994.*)

ATRIOVENTRICULAR SEPTAL DEFECT (FIGURE 51-10)

The atrioventricular septal defect (AVSD) is a more complex form of heart disease than simply a combination of an atrial and ventricular septal defect. It involves an incomplete separation of the embryonic common atrioventricular valve into separate tricuspid and mitral components. In addition, there is both a ventricular and atrial septal defect in the portion of the septa that are immediately adjacent to the atrioventricular valve. This lesion is often associated with Trisomy 21 Presentation is similar to those patients with moderate or large ventricular septal defects. The septal defects do not close spontaneously and so all patients with AVSD will require surgical repair to partition the atrioventricular valve and close the atrial and ventricular septal defects. Partitioning the atrioventricular valve is surgically challenging so as not to produce mitral stenosis or regurgitation. Most centers perform complete repairs on these children between 3 and 6 months when the infants are somewhat larger, but soon enough to prevent the development of pulmonary vascular disease.

PATENT DUCTUS ARTERIOSUS (FIGURE 51-11)

The ductus arteriosus is the conduit for fetal blood to bypass the lungs in utero. After birth, the ductus usually closes in the first days of life. If it does not close, as PVR falls, blood shunts from the aorta into the pulmonary artery. Depending on the size of the ductus arteriosus and PVR, the ductus will shunt a variable amount of blood similar to the physiology of a ventricular septal defect, and this lesion may present with congestive heart failure if large, or a machine-like murmur if the ductus is smaller.

The treatment of a patent ductus arteriosus is surgical or transcatheter closure. Transcatheter closure is now routine in children, infants, and is now common in premature neonates. Surgical closure is indicated in those where there is other accompanying heart disease that requires surgical intervention. A small patent ductus arteriosus associated with a

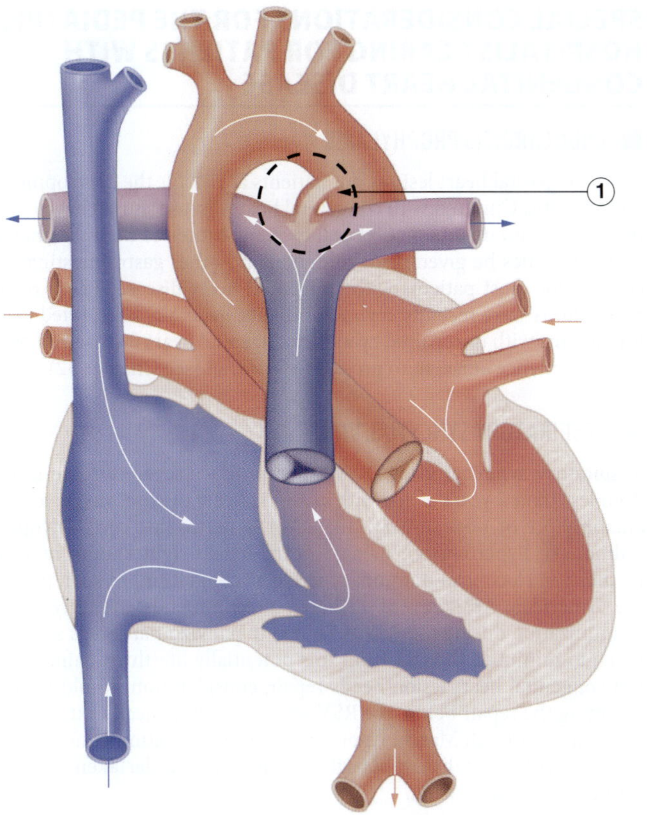

FIGURE 51-11. Patent ductus arteriosus. 1. Ductus arteriosus with flow from aorta into pulmonary artery. (Reproduced from Sinclair CM. *The Report of the Manitoba Pediatric Cardiac Surgery Inquest: An Inquiry Into Twelve Deaths at the Winnipeg Health Sciences Center in 1994.*)

murmur—even in the absence of significant shunting—is closed in the catheterization laboratory to prevent the lifelong risk of endarteritis of the ductus, which is estimated at ~0.45%/year. The general consensus is that a small ductus arteriosus found by echocardiography *without* an associated murmur should not be closed, as the risk of endarteritis does not appear to be higher than that of the general population.

COARCTATION OF THE AORTA

When severe, this lesion presents in the newborn period as a critical newborn heart lesion with shock or cyanosis. If milder, this lesion may present with a murmur, or more commonly, with the astute pediatrician noting decreased intensity of the femoral pulses. Repair of this lesion is usually done surgically. Diagnosis of coarctation later in childhood is sometimes made by the finding of upper extremity hypertension. Therapeutic options later in childhood and through adulthood include surgery or transcatheter balloon dilation with stent placement. Later diagnosis and repair of this lesion may lead to persistent hypertension even after repair.

LESIONS PRESENTING WITH A MURMUR IN CHILDHOOD

Less severe obstructions and shunts typically present with a murmur in childhood. Stenosis of the semilunar valves (aortic stenosis or pulmonary stenosis) as well as atrial septal defects may present in this time frame.

PULMONARY STENOSIS AND AORTIC STENOSIS

These lesions, when severe, present as critical heart disease in the newborn, as previously discussed. When milder, they present as a murmur. Treatment is undertaken for pulmonary stenosis when the narrowing is moderate or severe and consists of transcatheter balloon dilation of the valve. Such intervention is highly effective and typically does not need to be repeated. Treatment is undertaken for aortic stenosis when the gradient is moderate to severe. The first approach is usually balloon dilation of the valve. The success of aortic balloon dilation may be good, but relief of stenosis in many patients is often accompanied by creation of aortic regurgitation. Surgical valve repair, replacing the aortic valve with the patient's own pulmonary valve (Ross procedure), or prosthetic valve replacement are all options.

ATRIAL SEPTAL DEFECT (FIGURE 51-12)

The atrial septum divides the right and left atria. A defect in the wall is called an atrial septal defect (ASD). Blood returning to the left atrium passes from left to right across the ASD and recirculates to the lungs, placing a volume load on the right ventricle, pulmonary vascular bed, and atria. The amount of excess blood flow (or "shunt") is determined by both the size of the defect as well as the balance between the diastolic compliance of the left and right heart. In infancy, the right ventricle is relatively noncompliant, and there may be minimal flow across even a large ASD. During childhood the right ventricle becomes more compliant while the left ventricular compliance decreases, thereby increasing the amount of shunting. The consequences of an unrepaired ASD include right ventricular dysfunction and atrial arrhythmias from chronic volume load, the potentially devastating complication of pulmonary hypertension and pulmonary vascular disease—which may develop in up to 5% to 10% of these patients during adult life—and risk of paradoxical embolus.

If there is evidence of right ventricular volume overload by echocardiography, then the lesion should be closed. Usually this decision is made after age 2 years, as some ASDs will get smaller over the first years of life. If the defect is of the secundum type it may be closed in the cardiac

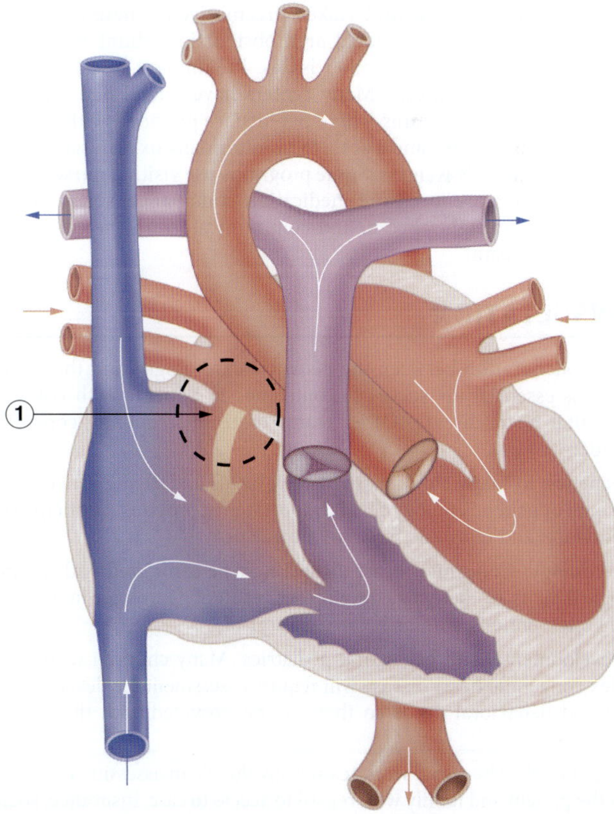

FIGURE 51-12. Atrial septal defect. 1. Atrial septal defect with flow from left atrium into right atrium. (Reproduced from Sinclair CM. *The Report of the Manitoba Pediatric Cardiac Surgery Inquest: An Inquiry Into Twelve Deaths at the Winnipeg Health Sciences Center in 1994.*)

catheterization laboratory with specially designed closure devices. If the defect is large or is located in other anatomic regions of the atrium, then surgery is required for closure.

ADMISSION AND DISCHARGE CRITERIA

Patients who present critically ill obviously require admission. Infants with congestive heart failure may require admission for initiation or optimization of medical management that may include diuretics, digoxin, and supplemental caloric addition and/or nasogastric feeding to assist with growth.

Patients with congenital heart disease may require admission for intercurrent illness such as respiratory syncytial virus and other viral or bacterial infections. Infants with congenital heart disease may have a more severe course with a higher risk of complications than other children.

Discharge of patients after congenital heart disease surgery has been evolving. There has been a greater move to "fast-track" patients with congenital heart disease after surgery with a view toward early extubation, early removal of central lines and chest tubes, and ultimately early discharge. The average length of stay in some centers for simple congenital heart disease surgery is now 1 day for atrial septal defect and 3 days for VSD repair. When properly implemented, this has been shown to not increase mortality or readmission rates. Infants and children are discharged postoperatively once all the acute surgical issues are resolved, they are able to be fed, pain is well controlled, and they are on an oral medical regimen. Early discharge, however, also mandates close early follow-up.

For infants with shunt-dependent pulmonary blood flow or those with hypoplastic left heart syndrome after conventional stage I or hybrid stage I, a significant "interstage" mortality has been recognized. Some of these children will die at home or present in extremis to the emergency department for anatomic problems that can arise insidiously. For this reason, many centers have taken the approach that a very close monitoring program will lead to decrease in interstage mortality if these children can be monitored very closely at home and appropriate intervention undertaken preemptively. These conditions include development of residual arch obstruction, shunt narrowing, atrial septal narrowing, and other issues. Preliminary research seems to support this hypothesis. Many centers have established intensive home monitoring programs where parents are provided with an oxygen saturation monitor and a scale to monitor daily oxygen saturations and at least biweekly weights. Some programs use visiting nurse checks one a week or more to ensure medication compliance, verify oxygen saturation and weight checks, and communicate with the cardiology and pediatric team.

CONSULTATION

Close collaboration between the pediatric cardiologist and the pediatrician is essential for successful outcomes in patients with complex congenital heart disease. Other teams that are frequently consulted include:

- Genetics: In many children, there may be an underlying genetic syndrome or genetic etiology that is important for prognosis, anticipatory guidance, and reproductive counseling.
- Neurology: Congenital heart disease may be associated with neurologic deficits, or these may develop as a result of neurologic injury during interventions, primarily cardiac surgical.
- Developmental and behavioral pediatrics: Many children with complex congenital heart disease will require assessment for developmental and behavioral needs so they can be provided with the needed services.
- Social work: The social work team is invaluable in assessing the needs of the patient and family with regard to access to care, insurance, social supports, ability of parents and caregivers to care for a child with additional needs, etc.

Other subspecialty consultations may be needed as indicated.

SPECIAL CONSIDERATIONS FOR THE PEDIATRIC HOSPITALIST CARING FOR PATIENTS WITH CONGENITAL HEART DISEASE

ENDOCARDITIS PROPHYLAXIS

Most congenital heart lesions put patients at risk for the development of endocarditis. Children with congenital heart disease should have regular dental care and maintain good oral hygiene. It used to be recommended that antibiotics be given prior to dental and other gastrointestinal procedures for most patients with congenital heart disease. These recommendations were recently revised and have generally been lifted except for patients with unrepaired cyanotic congenital heart disease and others with turbulence adjacent to prosthetic material (see Chapter 52).

RESPIRATORY SYNCYTIAL VIRUS

Respiratory syncytial virus (RSV) may produce severe disease in children less than 2 years of age with cyanotic heart disease, single ventricle anatomy pre or post surgery, dilated or hypertrophic cardiomyopathy, pulmonary hypertension, or significant left-to-right shunts requiring medication to control pulmonary vascular congestion. In such patients, the American Academy of Pediatrics recommends monthly passive immunization during the RSV season with palivizumab. Steps should be taken to minimize the risk from this potentially life-threatening illness. If a congenital heart lesion needs repair, consideration should be given to timing the repair before the RSV season which typically extends from November through March. Appropriate reverse isolation of hospitalized children with heart disease at high risk should be undertaken to prevent nosocomial transmission.

PACEMAKERS AND IMPLANTABLE DEFIBRILLATORS

Children with congenital heart disease may have congenital or iatrogenic surgical conduction defects that necessitate pacemaker placement. Pacemakers work by emitting an electric current that stimulates cardiac depolarization. Though pacemakers are very reliable, the interface between the pacemaker and the heart (the leads) are prone to a variety of problems. Extreme physiologic changes (e.g. acidosis) in the patient may also increase the amount of energy needed to depolarize the heart above that set by the pacemaker. In-hospital monitoring of children with pacemakers using a cardiac monitor is insufficient, as these monitors will usually detect the pacemaker impulse even when not followed by a cardiac depolarization. A physiologic monitor such as a pulse oximeter or arterial waveform should be used to confirm heat rate in paced patients. Similarly, during resuscitation, one should not mistake the pacemaker impulse as a cardiac depolarization, and physiologic parameters (e.g., palpation of a pulse) should be used to determine the cardiac rate.

Patients with pacemakers or implantable defibrillators requiring non-cardiac surgery may need the device reprogrammed prior to surgery to avoid oversensing, and electrocautery should be avoided. Patients with these devices may not undergo MRI examinations with few exceptions.

CENTRAL ACCESS AND PARADOXICAL EMBOLIZATION

Central access may be difficult in patients with congenital heart disease because of vein occlusion owing to previous long-term access lines or cardiac catheterization access. Central access in the internal jugular or subclavian veins is usually discouraged in patients who are progressing down the single ventricle pathway because of the risk of possible superior vena cava obstruction making the Fontan palliation problematic.

In children with any right-to-left shunting, bubbles or clots introduced in the venous system risk traveling to the cerebral circulation, causing strokes. Intravenous lines should be meticulously cleared of air prior to infusion to prevent this potential problem, and indwelling lines should be heparinized.

FEEDING/GROWTH ISSUES

Infants with congenital heart disease and pulmonary overcirculation have significantly increased caloric needs. Infants may require more than 160 Kcal/kg/day to grow with these increased metabolic demands. In addition, infants may be less able to tolerate normal feeding volumes due to tachypnea. Increased caloric density of feeds is usually required and tube feeding is sometimes required to assist these infants.

PREVENTION

There have been studies showing a decrease in the incidence of congenital heart defects in infants of mothers taking multivitamins with folic acid during the periconceptual period compared to a similar group of mothers who did not take supplements. A case-control study in Atlanta showed a 24% decrease in the incidence of congenital heart disease, and a study in California had similar results. These studies are not definitive, but folate appears to be a reasonable preconceptual regimen, and the additional risk-reduction of neural tube defects appears to make this recommendation compelling. Other than folate, there have been no other preventative measures identified that may decrease the risk of congenital heart disease. Fetal diagnosis may provide the option of termination for those defects with poor prognosis if the parents so choose.

KEY POINTS

- The incidence of congenital heart disease is approximately 1%, while the incidence of congenital heart disease requiring intervention is much lower. Nonetheless, congenital heart disease remains in the top 10 causes of death for children <1 year of age.
- Children with congenital heart disease may be hospitalized at the time of diagnosis if they present with critical heart disease, after cardiac interventions (surgery or transcatheter), or for acute illness related or unrelated to their heart condition.
- The four main alterations of physiology with congenital heart disease are desaturation, pulmonary overcirculation, pulmonary vascular disease, and compromised systemic perfusion.
- Newborn pre-discharge screening with right hand and foot pulse oximetry has a high sensitivity and low false positive rate for the detection of critical congenital heart disease.
- In complex congenital heart disease, the ideal goal is a repair that creates a four-chambered septated heart with the anatomic left ventricle pumping to the body. When this is not possible, the best palliation is usually a Fontan circulation, where the systemic venous return is routed passively to the lungs and the heart is used to pump the blood to the body.
- VSDs are one of the most common congenital heart lesions. Small VSDs rarely require closure. Moderate and large VSDs may become small and have three time horizons during which surgical closure is contemplated: in the first 6 months of life for failure to thrive, by 1 year of age if the VSD is not sufficiently restrictive to eliminate pressure damage to the pulmonary vascular bed, and by 3 to 5 years of age if there continues to be a large volume load on the left ventricle.
- Mortality and emergent readmission for infants with shunts and hypoplastic left heart syndrome may be reduced by adopting a discharge strategy of intensive home monitoring.

ACKNOWLEDGMENT

Barry Love contributed to this chapter in the second edition and material from that chapter has been retained here.

SUGGESTED READINGS

Donofrio MT, Moon-Grady AJ, Hornberger LK, et al. Diagnosis and treatment of fetal cardiac disease. *Circulation*. 2014;129(21):2183.

Feinstein JA, Benson DW, Dubin AM, et al. Hypoplastic left heart syndrome. *J Am Coll Cardiol*. 2012;59(1):S1-S42.

Mahle WT, Sable CA, Matherne PG, Gaynor JW, Gewitz MH. Key concepts in the evaluation of screening approaches for heart disease in children and adolescents. *Circulation*. 2012;125(22):2796.

Oster ME, Lee KA, Honein MA, Riehle-Colarusso T, Shin M, Correa A. Temporal trends in survival among infants with critical congenital heart defects. *Pediatrics*. 2013;131(5):e1502-e1508.

Thangaratinam S, Brown K, Zamora J, Khan K, Ewer AK. Pulse oximetry screening for critical congenital heart defects in asymptomatic newborn babies: a systematic review and meta-analysis. *Lancet*. 2012;379(9835):2459-2464.

CHAPTER 52

Infective Endocarditis

Courtney Solomon, MD and Yousef Arar, MD, MPH

BACKGROUND

Infective endocarditis (IE) is a rare, yet important cause of morbidity and mortality in the pediatric population. Despite major advancements in diagnostic and therapeutic modalities, the complexity in recognition and management of IE remains. Understanding risk factors, causative microorganisms, and the spectrum of clinical presentations coupled with a multidisciplinary treatment approach is key to achieving the best clinical outcome.

Historically, rheumatic heart disease was the leading predisposing condition for IE. Targeted prevention strategies for rheumatic fever led to a significant decline in rheumatic heart disease in the United States and other developed countries (although remains a prominent risk in developing countries due to poor social and environmental conditions). Along with the increasing prevalence of congenital heart disease due to increased survival rates beyond infancy, the epidemiology of risk factors has shifted over the past few decades.

The overall incidence of pediatric IE is ~ 0.43 to 0.69 cases per 100,000 children per year, compared to 15 cases per 100,000 in adults. In the pediatric population, congenital heart disease is now the leading predisposing condition for IE making up 50% to 70% of cases, 34% occurring in children with cyanotic cardiac conditions. Among those with acyanotic cardiac conditions, presence of a prosthetic valve is the highest risk for IE. In addition, children who had undergone cardiac surgery in the prior 6 months are more than five times likely to develop IE compared with those who had not undergone a cardiac surgery or intervention. See predisposing factors for infective endocarditis in children in **Table 52-1**.

There has been a growing incidence of IE in children without structural heart problems (~12%-26%), the majority of whom have underlying medical conditions. Frequent exposure to healthcare settings increases risk for IE due to likelihood of requiring invasive treatments and placement of indwelling catheters and central venous catheters

TABLE 52-1 Predisposing Factors for Infective Endocarditis in Children

	Non-Structural Heart Problems	
Structural Heart Problems	Chronic Conditions (e.g., malignancy, prematurity)	No Underlying Conditions
Cyanotic heart conditions	Indwelling catheters	*Staphylococcus aureus* bacteremia
Cardiac Surgery in prior 6 months	Central venous catheter	Older children
	Multiple invasive treatments	
Prosthetic valve		
Left-sided heart lesions		

(e.g., chemotherapy, hemodialysis, nutrition support). There has also been a rise in IE in premature neonates and children with malignancy likely for similar reasons. Congenital or acquired immunocompromised status may increase risk, although some studies demonstrated that the extent of endocardial disruption and the virulence of the causative microorganism have a greater influence on the development of IE.

Compared to children with structural heart problems, children without known structural heart problems or underlying conditions tend to be older and have poorer prognosis. Poorer outcomes may relate to *Staphylococcus aureus* being the common causative microorganism of IE in children without known structural heart problems, which tends to be more virulent compared to other microorganisms.

In the adult population, degenerative valve disease and valve replacement are the leading predisposing conditions for IE, which are uncommon in pediatrics The increasing prevalence of congenital heart disease has also led to a rise in IE in the adult population. IE in the setting of intravenous drug use is more likely to be seen in adults but should be considered in adolescents based on history and clinical presentation.

PATHOPHYSIOLOGY

Studies of animal models confirm that the development of a nidus for endocardial infection requires a locus of denuded endothelium as well as exposure to bacteria (or other microorganisms). The disrupted endothelial surface exposes collagen to the bloodstream, which leads to the deposition of fibrin and platelets and the formation of a thrombotic vegetation. Circulating microorganisms, most commonly bacteria, can become embedded in the vegetation, resulting in an endocardial infection. Additional deposits of platelets and fibrin form protective layers that shield the pathogens from host immune defenses. As the process continues, the vegetation grows, creating layers of embedded microorganisms. The organisms sequestered within the vegetation have a great potential for proliferation.

Congenital heart lesions with turbulent blood flow are most susceptible to vegetation, owing to the potential for endothelial damage on low pressure areas (e.g., atrial side of tricuspid valve and mitral valve, ventricular side of pulmonary valve and atrial valve). Adding appreciably to this risk is the presence of foreign material, which itself can offer a site prone to the development of platelet and fibrin plugs. Children with surgically placed grafts or palliative shunts (e.g., Blalock-Thomas-Taussig shunts) are thus at high risk for IE. See **Table 52-2** for common locations of vegetation formation in the heart.

In addition to host factors, a better understanding of virulent factors associated with the organisms themselves has contributed to insight into the pathogenesis of IE. Such factors include the ability to produce adhesins that facilitate binding of bacteria, to generate biofilms that cover devices such as prosthetic valves, and to stimulate platelet aggregation, which enhances the propagation of vegetations.

TABLE 52-2 Common Locations of Vegetation Formation in the Heart

Common Locations of Vegetation Formation in the Heart
Native Cardiac Valves
Prosthetic Valves
Bioprosthetic
Mechanical
Non-valvular cardiovascular structures
Unrepaired ventricular septal defect
Patent ductus arteriosus
Prosthetic materials
Patches
Shunts
Conduits
Stents
Implanted devices
Pacemaker
Leads
Ventricular assist devices

Source: Adapted from Cox DA, Tani LY. Pediatric infective endocarditis: a clinical update. *Pediatr Clin North Am*. 2020;67(5):875-888.

Gram-positive cocci remain the largest single group of organisms associated with infective endocarditis in children. Globally, *Staphylococcus aureus* predominates with viridans group streptococcus ranking second. However, with the rise in hospital-acquired IE, there has been a growing incidence of coagulase negative staphylococcus.

Less common organisms include enterococci, Gram-negative rods (the HACEK [*Haemophilus* species, *Aggregatibacter actinomycetemcomitans*, *Cardiobacterium hominis*, *Eikenella* species, and *Kingella kingae*] organisms), and fungi.

Among causes of culture-negative endocarditis, *Coxiella* and *Bartonella* species are predominant.

CLINICAL PRESENTATION

The presentation of IE may be indolent (subacute) or fulminant (acute). The clinical picture relates to the combination of systemic responses to bacteremia or fungemia, the local mechanical impact of the vegetation, and in some cases, the deleterious effects of embolic and systemic immunologic responses.

Classically, in subacute bacterial endocarditis, somatic complaints predominate. These nonspecific symptoms include low-grade fever, malaise with weakness and fatigue, anorexia (often with weight loss), intermittent diaphoresis, myalgias, and arthralgias. This group of complaints should raise the suspicion for subacute bacterial endocarditis, especially in the context of a child at risk for IE.

In addition to these general complaints, focal signs should be sought. Cardiac manifestations result from either direct valve damage or valvulitis. Thus, new murmurs may appear, such as mitral or aortic regurgitation, and symptoms of congestive heart failure may develop or worsen.

Extracardiac manifestations can also be helpful in establishing the diagnosis, although they occur less frequently in children than in adults. Skin findings such as petechiae, splinter hemorrhages in the nail beds, Janeway lesions (nontender hemorrhagic plaques on the palms and soles), and Osler nodes (tender purplish lesions on the pads of fingers and toes, thenar eminences, and lower arms) may be found on examination. Janeway lesions are thought to represent septic emboli; however, it is unclear whether Osler nodes are attributable to the same phenomenon or are due to an immune vasculitis. Roth spots are pale retinal lesions with areas of hemorrhage usually located near the optic disk. Emboli to any organs, including the heart, kidneys, lungs, brain, spleen, or liver, can cause infarction (thrombotic emboli) or abscess (septic emboli). Emboli to the central nervous system can result in stroke or mycotic aneurysm. Mycotic aneurysms develop when septic emboli cause local arterial infection and inflammation resulting in occlusion of the vessel. The damage to the muscular wall and increased pressure cause dilation of the vessel. Despite the name, these aneurysms almost always result from bacterial infection. Splenomegaly is seen in more than half of patients and can be caused by immune system activation. Both focal and diffuse glomerular nephritis have been described, with immune complex deposition noted.

Patients with rapidly progressing acute endocarditis may present in shock, with a clinical picture consistent with overwhelming sepsis. In such circumstances, the classic findings of infective endocarditis may be absent, and suspicion for this disease may be raised only by a history of cardiac lesions and persistently positive blood cultures.

IE can have varying presentations within the pediatric population. Therefore, high index of suspicion based on symptoms and risk factors will be key to diagnosis.

DIFFERENTIAL DIAGNOSIS

Alternative diagnostic considerations are extremely broad and are based on the predominant signs and symptoms. Prolonged fever should prompt evaluation for a fever of unknown origin. Neurologic features may suggest a wide range of intracranial conditions, including stroke, epilepsy, and encephalopathy. Rheumatologic and oncologic processes can mimic the nonspecific findings of fatigue, malaise, weight loss, and joint pain.

DIAGNOSTIC EVALUATION

The diagnosis of IE can be elusive and hinges on a careful assessment of risk factors in the setting of suggestive findings. In an attempt to improve the clinical diagnosis of IE, Durack and colleagues developed a scoring system. This was subsequently modified to include a greater emphasis on imaging data. These diagnostic criteria have been tested in pediatric populations and found to be useful. **Figure 52-1** outlines the definitions of and criteria for the diagnosis of infective endocarditis.

Large-volume blood cultures (ideally obtained prior to initiation of empiric antimicrobial therapy) are recommended in all children with suspected IE. This includes any child with a history of fever without an obvious explanation who has known heart disease or who has had endocarditis previously. The proper collection technique for highest yield consists of at least 3 blood cultures (1-3 mL/culture for infants, 5-7 mL/culture in older children, and 10 mL/culture for adults), from different sites, >1 hour apart. However, this may not always be feasible in clinical practice. Consider collection of anaerobic cultures to increase yield of obligate anaerobes, recognizing that obligate anaerobes are not the common causative pathogen in endocarditis.

In children who have been on antibiotics, greater numbers of cultures over an extended period may be required. It is useful to notify the laboratory that infective endocarditis is suspected so that prolonged (>2 weeks) incubation of culture specimens will be done. Gram-negative rods (the HACEK organisms), for example, are typically slowly growing organisms.

In organisms successfully cultured, testing for antibiotic susceptibility is extremely important for clinical management. Measurement of the minimum inhibitory concentration of the particular antibiotic chosen is the standard guide to therapeutic efficacy. While the minimum bactericidal concentration is not usually employed, it may be of use in particular situations, based on the advice of an infectious disease expert. Use of antibiotics may be delayed or discontinued in selected patients who are not acutely ill, in order to obtain additional blood cultures if the initial set remain negative after preliminary incubation.

Other laboratory markers of infection and inflammation can be useful, serially, as guides to therapy. Acute-phase reactants (erythrocyte sedimentation rate and C-reactive protein) are usually elevated, and hypergammaglobulinemia may be noted. Rheumatoid factor may initially be elevated and can be followed as confirmation of response to therapy. Although the presence of leukocytosis (white blood cell count >15,000) is variable, increased segmented neutrophils or other immature forms (bands) are typical. Thrombocytopenia and mild anemia can be present. Abnormal liver function tests are less common without heart failure or hepatic emboli, but abnormalities in urinary sediment are frequently present. Hematuria may represent either an embolic process or glomerular nephritis. Signs of an immune complex nephritis can include

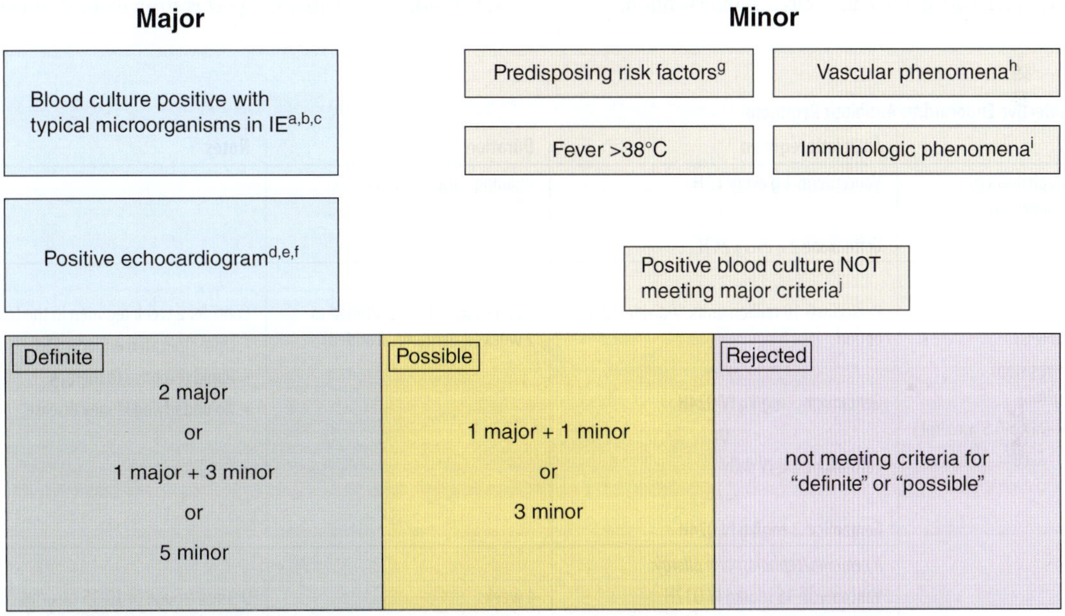

a. Two separate blood cultures: 1) viridans group streptococcus, streptococcus bovis, or HACEK; or 2) community-acquired staphylococcus aureus or enterococci (in absence of primary focus)

b. More than 2 positive cultures of blood samples drawn >12 h apart, or all of 3 or majority of >4 separate blood cultures (first and last sample drawn >1 h apart)

c. Single positive blood culture for Coxiella burnetii or phase IgG antibody titer >1:800

d. Defined as: 1) vegetation; or 2) abscess, pseudoaneurysm, or intracardiac fistula; 3) valvular perforation or aneurysm; 4) new partial dehiscence of prosthetic valve

e. Abnormal activity around the site of a prosthetic valve detected by PET/CT assuming >3 months after surgery or radiolabeled leucocyte-SPECT/CT

f. Definite paravalvular lesions by cardiac CT.

g. Predisposing heart condition or IV drug use

h. Includes major arterial emboli, septic pulmonary infarct, mycotic aneurysm, intracranial hemorrhage, Janeway lesions (including phenomena detected by imaging)

i. Includes glomerulonephritis, Osler nodes, Roth spots, and rheumatoid factor

J. Positive blood culture not meeting major criteria or serologic evidence of active infection with organism consistent with IE

FIGURE 52-1. Criteria for diagnosis of infective endocarditis. Abbreviations: CT = computed tomography; HACEK = *Haemophilus* species, *Aggregatibacter actinomycetemcomitans*, *Cardiobacterium hominis*, *Eikenella* species, and *Kingella kingae*; IE = infective endocarditis; IgG = immunoglobulin; IV = intravenous; PET = positron emission tomography; SPECT = simple-photon emission computerized tomography.

proteinuria, red cell casts, and abnormal renal function measures, including creatinine and blood urea nitrogen. Low serum complement levels support the diagnosis of glomerular nephritis, but this is not definitive.

Echocardiography with Doppler color flow mapping is the standard diagnostic modality in patients with suspected infective endocarditis. It can identify valvular vegetations as well as impaired cardiac performance, prosthetic valve dehiscence, disturbed conduit flow, and abscess. Moreover, echocardiography can define the presence of an occult structural abnormality, such as a bicuspid aortic valve, thus identifying a clinically silent risk factor. It has been well established that echocardiography can detect cardiac involvement in patients with otherwise occult infective endocarditis, and this has been confirmed in children.

For most infants and children, unlike adults, transthoracic echocardiography is usually sufficient to establish a diagnosis. In certain circumstances, however, transesophageal imaging is required, particularly in children with previous cardiothoracic surgical procedures, pulmonary problems that confound imaging windows, or substantial obesity.

A transesophageal study may be superior to a transthoracic study to detect paravalvular leakage or dehiscence, aortic root abscess development, and prosthetic valve endocarditis. Serial echocardiographic Doppler studies are also useful to gauge the response to therapy and assess for potential complications. For example, vegetation size and mobility may be an indicator of risk for embolization. Importantly, in a patient undergoing treatment for IE, the diagnosis of myocardial abscess causing a new arrhythmia or progressive aortic root enlargement could suggest the need for a shift in treatment, including surgical intervention.

In some cases, cardiac computed tomography (CT) may be used to better appreciate conduit endocarditis. If all studies are negative, then a positron emission tomography (PET) scan can be used to localize the lesion.

MANAGEMENT

There are limited studies in the pediatric population and many IE treatment strategies are inferred from adult guidelines and expert opinion. Owing to the tenacious nature of these infections, a prolonged course of parenteral antibiotics is required. Several factors contribute to the difficulty of eradicating the source of the infection. As described earlier, the microbial organisms are layered within elements of the vegetation, which sequesters them from the immune system and antibiotic exposure. Organisms with limited antibiotic susceptibilities may also require prolonged treatment for eradication. **Table 52-3** outlines antibiotic regimens for infective endocarditis in a variety of settings.

Empiric antibiotics should cover the most common pathogens of infective endocarditis, including *Staphylococcus aureus*, viridans group streptococci, and enterococci. HACEK organisms should also be considered. Typical treatment duration is at least 4 to 6 weeks based on causative pathogen, presence of prosthetic device, or associated complications. Newer studies have demonstrated potential for transition to oral antimicrobials following clinical improvement on IV therapy depending on pathogen involved and uncomplicated course. However, consultation with an Infectious Disease expert is strongly recommended.

TABLE 52-3 Infective Endocarditis Antibiotic Regimens

Microorganism	Antibiotic regimen	Duration	Notes
Empiric coverage (staphylococci, streptococci, and enterococci)	Vancomycin 1 g every 12 H + Ceftriaxone 2 g every 24 H	Pending culture results	
Viridans Streptocci • Penicillin-susceptible (MIC 0.1 mcg/mL or less) • Relative Penicillin-resistant (MIC 0.12-0.5 mcg/mL) • Penicillin resistant (MIC>0.5 mcg/mL) Or Abiotrophia species	Penicillin G 18 million units IV divided Q4H or Q6H +/– Gentamicin 3 mg/kg IV Q24H Or Ceftriaxone 2 g IV daily +/– Gentamicin 3 mg/kg IV Q24H	4 weeks (could be shortened to 2 weeks if Gentamicin added)	Consider 2 week regimen in the following: • Uncomplicated endocarditis • Rapid response to therapy • No underlying kidney disease
	If penicillin/cephalosporin allergy: Vancomycin 15 mg/kg IV Q12H	4 weeks	Desired trough of 10-15 mcg/mL
	If prosthetic valve present: Penicillin or Ceftriaxone +/– Gentamicin	6 weeks (use Gentamicin first 2 weeks if added)	
	Penicillin G 24 million U IV divided Q4H or Q6H + Gentamicin 3 mg/kg IV Q24H *Alternative (if susceptible):* Ceftriaxone	4 weeks (use Gentamicin for first 2 weeks)	
	IgE-mediated allergy to penicillin: Vancomycin 15 mg/kg IV Q12H	4 weeks	
	Prosthetic valve present: Penicillin or Ceftriaxone + Gentamicin See treatment for enterococcal endocarditis	4 weeks See treatment for enterococcal endocarditis	

(*Continued*)

TABLE 52-3 Infective Endocarditis Antibiotic Regimens (*Continued*)

Microorganism	Antibiotic regimen	Duration	Notes
Group D Streptococci (Enterococci)	Ampicillin 2 g IV every 4 H OR Penicillin G 18-30 million units IV divided Q6H + Gentamicin 1 mg/kg IV Q8H OR Ampicillin 2 g IV every 4 H + Ceftriaxone 2 g IV Q12H *Alternative if unable to tolerate or have resistance to penicillin/ampicillin:* Vancomycin + Gentamicin	4-6 weeks	Recent clinical studies demonstrated equivalent clinical outcomes for the 2 regimens. Longer duration for patients with symptoms >3 moths, relapse, or presence of prosthetic valve endocarditis.
Staphylococcus aureus • Methicillin-susceptible • Methicillin-resistant • Coagulase negative	Nafcillin (or Oxacillin) 12 g IV divided Q4H or Q6H OR Cefazolin 6 g IV divided Q8H *Prosthetic valve present:* Nafcillin or Oxacillin or Cefazolin + Rifampin + Gentamicin	6 weeks 6 weeks	If brain abscess 2/2 MSSA, Nafcillin preferred over Cefazolin. If history of immediate type hypersensitivity to B-lactams, consider a desensitization protocol. Hx of non-anaphylactoid reactions to penicillins, Cefazolin should be used.
	If unable to tolerate beta-lactam therapy: Vanc 30 mg/kg/day div Q12H or Q8H OR Daptomycin IV 8 mg/kg/day *If prosthetic valve present:* Vancomycin or Daptomycin + Rifampin + Gentamicin	6 weeks 6 weeks	Goal trough level 15-20 mcg/kg
	Prosthetic Valve present: Vancomycin 30 mg/kg/day div Q8H or Q12h + Rifampin 300 mg every 8 H + Gentamicin 3 mg/kg IV Q8H	6 weeks (Gentamicin for first 2 weeks only)	Don't use beta-lactams in CONS unless have susceptibilities (CONS frequently resistant to methicillin)
HACEK Organisms	Ceftriaxone 2 g IV Q24H (or another 3rd generation cephalosporin)	4 weeks (6 weeks if prosthetic valve present)	For penicillin allergy experience is limited, consider fluoroquinolones
Culture-negative Endocarditis	Consult with ID expert	Consult with ID expert	Consider serologic testing and coverage for Bartonella, Chlamydia, Brucella or T. whipplei species if risk factors

Source: Adapted from Boslett BA, Bystritsky R. Infective Endocarditis. In: Papadakis MA, McPhee SJ, Rabow MW, McQuaid KR. eds. *Current Medical Diagnosis & Treatment 2023*. McGraw Hill;2023. https://accessmedicine.mhmedical.com/content.aspx?bookid=3212&sectionid=269141584. Accessed August 25, 2022.

In most cases, bacteremia resolves within a few days of treatment with appropriate antibiotics. *S. aureus* may persist in the blood for longer periods—up to 5 to 10 days after therapy. It is advisable to wait until bacterial cultures are negative before placing a long-term central venous catheter.

In approximately 5% to 10% of cases, even if a vegetation is visualized on echocardiography, no specific organism grows in the laboratory from blood cultures, possibly due to previous antibiotic treatment, infection by slow-growing pathogens, or inadequate collection technique. In culture-negative endocarditis, empirical treatment is required. Consultation with an infectious disease expert can be helpful in guiding the laboratory in the search for uncommon or fastidious organisms (e.g., *Bartonella* species, *Coxiella*, *Chlamydia* species, *Brucella* species, and *Tropheryma whipplei*). Serologic testing should be performed in patients who have epidemiologic risk factors for these infections. Most commonly, therapy in children is still aimed against staphylococci or streptococci, but the HACEK organisms should also be considered.

Mortality rate in IE is estimated at 1% to 5% in the pediatric population (up to 50% in children with congenital heart disease) and 10% in adult population. Despite an ever-increasing armamentarium of powerful antibiotics for the treatment of IE, a high proportion of patients suffer some type of complication. These complications are often the result of mechanical obstruction by the vegetation or are caused by emboli, cardiac dysfunction (including arrhythmias and heart block), and congestive heart failure. Systemic infectious or immunologic issues may also be a factor resulting in complications. In addition, malnutrition has been found to be a poor prognostic factor that can lead to a greater occurrence of complications and poorer surgical outcomes. Most complications following completion of IE treatment occur within the first 12 months, with up to 30% of patients requiring surgery within the first year and a recurrence rate of ~2% to 6%.

Urgent surgical intervention in children with at least moderate congestive heart failure improves survival and quality of life. **Table 52-4** reviews the circumstances indicating an increased risk for the development of complications, and **Figure 52-2** reviews the factors related to the need for surgery. Although it is preferable to administer a prolonged course of antibiotics before proceeding with surgery, it is important not to delay surgery in the face of a changing clinical picture. It is incumbent on the hospitalist, when the leader of the management team, to consider cardiothoracic surgical consultation at an early stage and on a continuing basis when caring for children with infective endocarditis.

TABLE 52-4 Risk factors for Infective Endocarditis Complications in Children

Vegetation >1 cm
Staphylococcus aureus
Fungal Infection
No known heart disease
Left sided valvular lesions
Complex congenital heart disease
Prematurity
Persistent fever
Elevated white blood cell counts and plasma C-reactive protein

Adapted from Vicent L, Luna R, Martinez-Selles M. Pediatric infective endocarditis: a literature review. *J Clin Med*. 2022; 11(11):3217.

Anticoagulation is contraindicated in native valve endocarditis due to increased risk of intracerebral hemorrhage and remains controversial in prosthetic valve endocarditis. Discussion with a Cardiology expert is recommended for further guidance.

ADMISSION CRITERIA

- Newly diagnosed infective endocarditis.
- Newly recognized untreated intracardiac vegetation, even if asymptomatic.
- Any evidence of significant change in cardiac status or evidence of potential distant complications (e.g., embolic complication, worsening cyanosis) in a patient at risk for infective endocarditis.

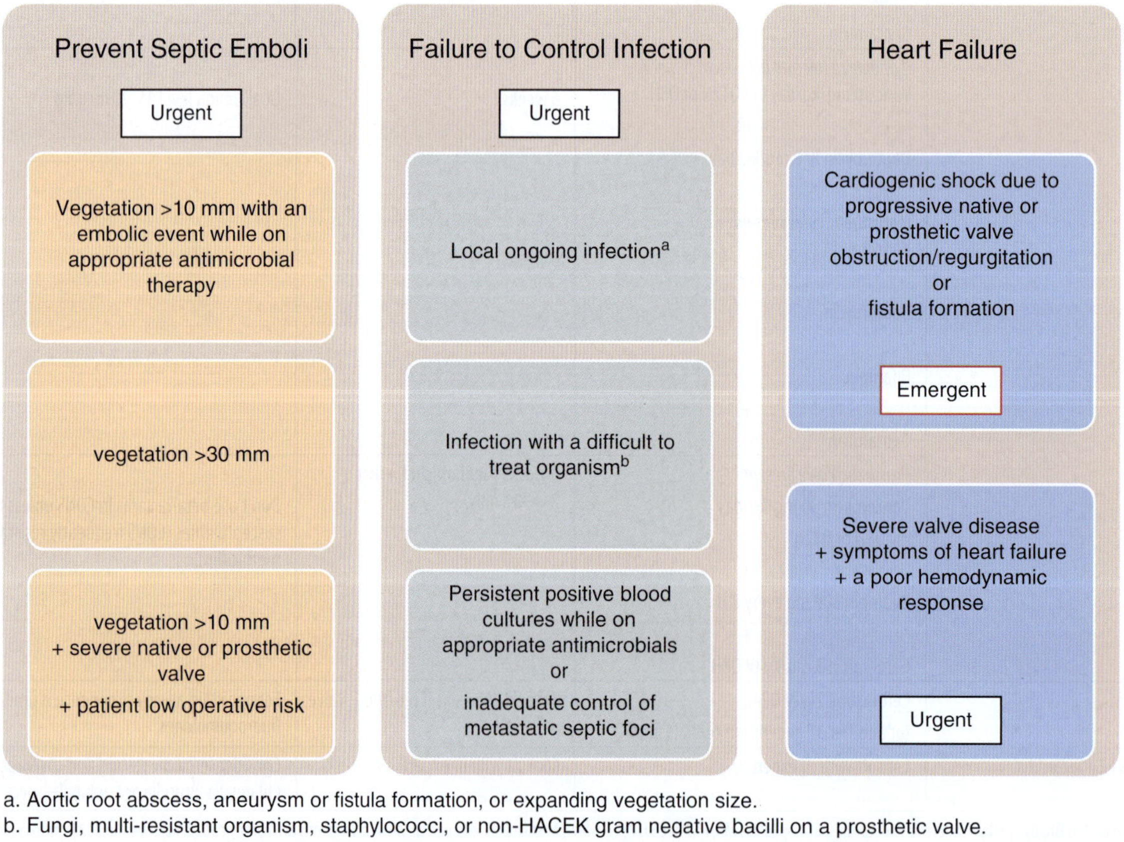

FIGURE 52-2. Indications for surgical intervention. (*Source:* Adapted from Rajani R, Klein JL. Infective endocarditis: A contemporary update. *Clin Med (Lond)*.2020;20(1): 31-35.)

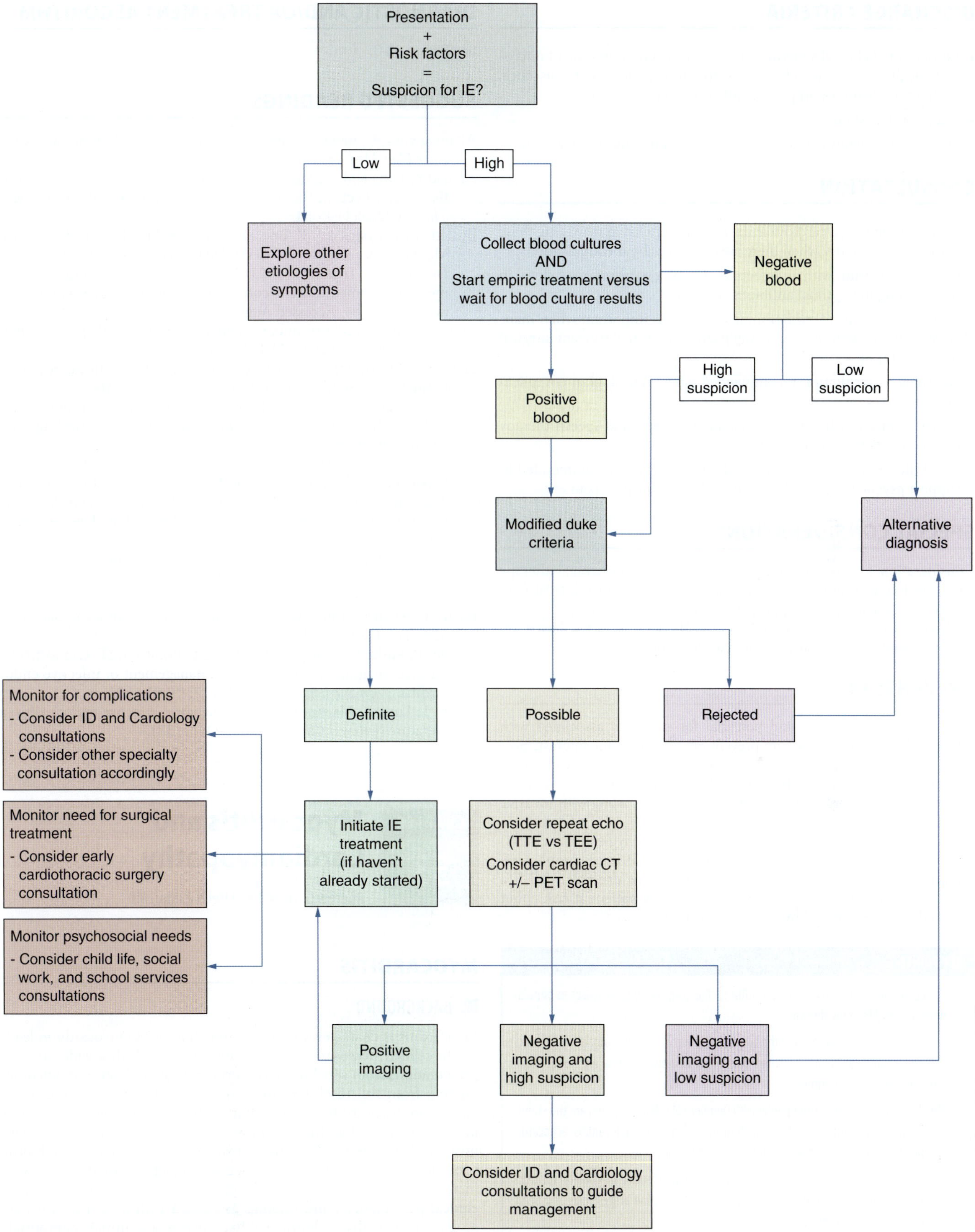

FIGURE 52-3. Multidisciplinary approach to evaluation and management of infective endocarditis. Abbreviations: CT= computerized tomography; ID = infectious disease; IF = infective endocarditis; PET= positron emission tomography; TEE = transesophageal echocardiogram; TTE = transthoracic echocardiogram.

DISCHARGE CRITERIA

- Resolution of clinical signs of active infection after initiation of microbiologically determined effective treatment (e.g., fever defervescence, bacteremia clearance, improved inflammatory markers)
- Stable cardiac status
- Decreasing vegetation size in the absence of ongoing embolization.

CONSULTATION

- Consultation with a cardiovascular expert is crucial in managing these patients, particularly when there are concerns about complications.
- Close consultation with an infectious disease expert may be helpful in determining the optimal antibiotic regimen.
- Early involvement of cardiothoracic surgery is important when managing patients who develop complications that may warrant surgical intervention.
- Neurology consultation recommended when neurological complications occur.
- Consider physical therapy, occupational therapy, and speech therapy based on deficits and deconditioning.
- Child life services, social work, and school services recommended to support psychosocial needs during prolonged hospital course.

SPECIAL CONSIDERATIONS

Consideration for outpatient completion of IV antimicrobial therapy based on initial response, confirmed ability to maintain full treatment course after discharge, and appropriate follow-up available.

Cardiac Rehabilitation (or alternative therapy services) based on deconditioning, cardiac surgery, or neurologic deficits.

PREVENTION

The important morbidity and potential for mortality associated with infective endocarditis make its prevention of significant interest. Secondary prophylaxis regimens in general have been curtailed in recent years and continue to be restrictive due to lack of clear evidence demonstrating secondary prophylaxis to be effective. Also, along with invasive dental procedures, there are other circumstances in which bacteremia occurs spontaneously (e.g. mastication, routine oral hygiene maneuvers) and for which antibiotic prophylaxis is not feasible. Primary prophylaxis (antibiotic usage at the time of cardiac surgery, for example) still is a standard of therapy. Furthermore, reminding any patient at risk about the need for excellent oral hygiene is important.

KEY POINTS

- The epidemiology of infective endocarditis is changing owing to increases in populations susceptible to the disease.
- Gram-positive bacteria represent the largest subgroup of causative organisms in infective endocarditis, although infections with gram-negative bacteria and fungi occur, especially in specific subgroups.
- Blood cultures and echocardiography with Doppler color flow mapping are the standard diagnostic modalities in patients with suspected infective endocarditis; echocardiography is also used to assess the effectiveness of therapy.
- Complications of infective endocarditis can be severe and include mechanical obstruction by vegetations or emboli, cardiac dysfunction (including arrhythmias and heart block), and systemic infection.
- High index of suspension and early treatment using a multidisciplinary approach is key to achieving beset outcomes.
- Oral health may play an important role in reducing risk of infective endocarditis, especially in high-risk groups.

DIAGNOSTIC AND/OR TREATMENT ALGORITHM

See Figure 52-3.

SUGGESTED READINGS

Akamagwuna U, Badaly D. Pediatric Cardiac Rehabilitation: a Review. *Curr Phys Med Rehabil Rep*. 2019;7(2):67-80.

Arshad V, Talha KM, Baddour LM. Epidemiology of infective endocarditis: novel aspects in the twenty-first century. *Expert Rev Cardiovasc Ther*. 2022;20(1):45-54.

Boslett BA, Bystritsky R. Infective Endocarditis. In: Papadakis MA, McPhee SJ, Rabow MW, McQuaid KR, eds. *Current Medical Diagnosis & Treatment 2023*. McGraw Hill; 2023. https://accessmedicine.mhmedical.com/content.aspx?bookid=3212&sectionid=269141584. Accessed August 25, 2022.

Cox DA, Tani LY. Pediatric infective endocarditis: a clinical update. *Pediatr Clin North Am*. 2020;67(5): 875-888.

de Loizaga SR, Beaton AZ. Rheumatic fever and rheumatic heart disease in the United States. *Pediatr Ann*. 2021;50(3):e98-e104.

Durack OT, Lukes AS, Bright DK. New criteria for diagnosis of infective endocarditis: utilization of specific echocardiographic findings. *Am J Med*. 1994;96:200-209.

Kimberlin DW, Barnett E, Lynfield R, Sawyer MH. Red Book 2021: Report of the Committee on Infectious Diseases. 32nd ed. American Academy of Pediatrics; 2021. https://search.ebscohost.com/login.aspx?direct=true&db=nlebk&AN=2939296&site=ehost-live. Accessed September 3, 2022.

Li JS, Sexton OJ, Mick N, et al. Proposed modifications to the Duke criteria for the diagnosis of infective endocarditis. *Clin Infect Dis*. 2000;30:633-638.

Rajani R, Klein JL. Infective endocarditis: a contemporary update. *Clin Med (Lond)*.2020;20(1):31-35.

Silbiger JJ, Rashed E, Chen H, Wiesenfeld E, Robinson SE, Cagliostro M. Cardiac imaging for diagnosis and management of infective endocarditis. *J Am Soc Echocardiogr*. 2022;35(9):910-924.

Vicent L, Luna R, Martinez-Selles M. Pediatric infective endocarditis: a literature review. *J Clin Med*. 2022:11(11):3217.

CHAPTER 53 Myocarditis and Cardiomyopathy

Andrew G. Yu, MD and Heidi A. Kim, MD

MYOCARDITIS

BACKGROUND

Myocarditis is characterized by inflammation of the myocardium leading to cellular necrosis and cardiac dysfunction. With a wide range of presentations from subclinical to overt cardiogenic shock and outcomes ranging from full resolution to chronic heart failure requiring transplantation, myocarditis poses a clinical challenge. Furthermore, as our understanding and definition of this disease continues to evolve, diagnosis itself presents a challenge. Histopathologic diagnosis by biopsy is becoming less common while cardiac magnetic resonance (CMR) is increasingly utilized to confirm the diagnosis. Awareness of the various clinical presentations and findings associated with myocarditis is necessary for the pediatric hospitalist to recognize and initiate appropriate management for this condition.

Pathophysiology Myocarditis is frequently caused by viral infection (enteroviruses, adenovirus, herpes viruses, and others) but may also be associated with other infectious and non-infectious etiologies (toxins, drugs, hypersensitivity reactions, autoimmune and systemic diseases). Pathogenesis is related to the host immune response. In the acute phase of viral myocarditis, infection of myocytes leads to activation of an innate immune response and release of inflammatory cytokines. Subsequently, adaptive immune system activation leads to B and T cell migration and stimulation, which contributes to ongoing inflammation and tissue injury. Autoantibodies are implicated in both infectious and autoimmune etiologies of myocarditis. Finally, in the chronic phase, some patients recover while others experience persistent inflammation, cardiac remodeling, and scar formation, which progresses to a dilated cardiomyopathy (DCM) phenotype.

CLINICAL PRESENTATION

Pediatric myocarditis has an estimated incidence of 0.8 per 100,000 children, a characteristic bimodal age distribution with peaks in infancy and late adolescence, and a male predominance. Classically, patients with myocarditis present with a poorly functioning dilated left ventricle (LV) and associated acute heart failure symptoms in the setting of a recent viral respiratory or gastrointestinal illness. An index of suspicion is required as patients may present with variable and non-specific symptoms and are frequently misdiagnosed at presentation. Signs and symptoms of heart failure in infants include fussiness, poor feeding, listlessness, diaphoresis, and respiratory distress. Other symptoms in older children may include fatigue, nausea, vomiting, abdominal pain, chest pain, lethargy, and exercise intolerance. Respiratory symptoms are frequently the predominant complaint in both infants and older children, and fever is also common. The onset of symptoms is typically days to weeks. Physical examination may reveal signs of congestive heart failure, including tachypnea with rales, tachycardia, a gallop rhythm, and hepatomegaly. For severely symptomatic patients, poor perfusion may be evident with hypotension, pallor, or an ashen appearance.

Other clinical presentations include fulminant myocarditis (sudden onset severe ventricular dysfunction with cardiogenic shock, life-threatening arrhythmias, and multi-organ failure), acute coronary syndrome mimic (acute chest pain and dyspnea with electrocardiogram changes and elevated cardiac enzymes suggestive of ischemia, typically in adolescent and young adult males), syncope, and sudden death. Chronic and recurrent forms of myocarditis have also been reported.

Early in the coronavirus disease-19 (COVID-19) pandemic, a novel form of shock with systemic inflammation, multi-organ involvement, and cardiac dysfunction in children with recent severe acute respiratory syndrome coronavirus 2 (SARS-CoV-2) infection was recognized, termed multisystem inflammatory syndrome in children (MIS-C). See Chapter 107 for more details regarding diagnosis and management of MIS-C.

SARS-CoV-2 mRNA vaccines have been associated with rare cases of myocarditis and pericarditis, predominantly in adolescent and young adult males who present with acute onset chest pain and dyspnea, abnormal electrocardiogram (ECG), and elevated troponin levels following second vaccine dose. These cases have generally been mild and self-limited, and benefit-risk analyses have determined that benefits to both individuals and populations clearly outweigh the risk of this rare complication, as COVID-19 itself is associated with myocarditis.

DIFFERENTIAL DIAGNOSIS

As children with myocarditis present with non-specific and variable signs and symptoms, myocarditis is important to keep on the differential for other common illnesses. Respiratory symptoms predominate, especially in younger children, and may initially be misdiagnosed as pneumonia, asthma, or viral illness. Abnormalities on cardiac physical examination such as hepatomegaly are not uniformly present, and appropriate consideration of chest X-ray and electrocardiogram may augment detection sensitivity.

Acute pericarditis may occur concurrently with viral myocarditis and may be caused by similar viruses. Precordial chest pain that worsens in the supine position and a friction rub are characteristic findings in pericarditis. Tamponade is uncommon in acute viral pericarditis but should be monitored for in the acute setting. Findings of cardiac tamponade may include tachypnea, respiratory distress, distant heart sounds, hypotension, elevated central venous pressure (jugular venous distension), and narrowed pulse pressure.

Table 53-1 lists many known infectious and non-infectious causes of myocarditis, which may require additional investigation in the appropriate setting based on patient characteristics, history, and physical exam. In the child presenting with acute heart failure with a dilated poorly contractile left ventricle, other causes of DCM should be rationally investigated.

DIAGNOSTIC EVALUATION

Laboratory Testing Serologic evaluation is commonly part of the initial evaluation in the child with suspected myocarditis. Elevations in white blood cell count, inflammatory markers, and aspartate aminotransferase may be observed, though are nonspecific. Troponin T and I levels may be markedly elevated in the setting of cardiac myocyte injury, though these are not specific and normal values do not exclude myocarditis. B-type natriuretic peptide is commonly elevated in the setting of heart failure, though not specific for myocarditis. Polymerase chain reaction (PCR) testing is available and sensitive for common cardiotropic viruses, though correlation between peripheral blood samples and endomyocardial biopsy in determining causative agents is not well established and complicated by high prevalence of these common viruses in the general population.

Chest X-Ray A chest x-ray is frequently performed because the child presents with some degree of respiratory distress. Radiography is often abnormal and may demonstrate cardiomegaly and increased pulmonary venous markings with or without pulmonary edema or pleural effusion.

Electrocardiogram An ECG should be obtained in all patients with suspected myocarditis, as it is frequently abnormal and may show tachycardia, low voltages, and ST-segment and T-wave abnormalities. ECG findings may mimic those of acute coronary syndrome in adolescents and young adults. A wide variety of tachyarrhythmias, bradyarrhythmias, and conduction abnormalities ranging from first-degree to complete heart block may be seen.

Echocardiogram Echocardiography is the first-line and most commonly used modality to assess LV structure and function in suspected myocarditis. Common findings include LV systolic dysfunction, dilation, changes in wall thickness, and segmental wall motion abnormalities (**Figure 53-1A, B**). A pericardial effusion or intracavitary thrombus may also be seen (**Figure 53-1C**). Ventricular dysfunction ranges from subtle to profound, which carries prognostic significance. Although a mainstay of diagnosis and monitoring, echocardiography has limitations in differentiating myocarditis from other etiologies of LV dysfunction.

Cardiac Magnetic Resonance Imaging Cardiac magnetic resonance imaging (CMR) is increasingly utilized in the diagnosis of myocarditis and can be used to distinguish acute inflammatory myocarditis from noninflammatory cardiomyopathies. In addition to being the gold standard for assessing ventricular volumes and function, CMR is particularly useful for localizing and characterizing tissue injury. In the setting of clinically suspected myocarditis, specific radiologic criteria ("Lake Louise" criteria) corresponding to myocardial edema (increased T2 intensity), hyperemia/capillary leak (early gadolinium enhancement), and myocyte injury/fibrosis (late gadolinium enhancement) may provide supportive evidence of myocarditis and may be followed over time with possible prognostic value.

Endomyocardial Biopsy Histopathologic confirmation of myocardial inflammation remains the reference standard for diagnosis of myocarditis, though recent trends include decreased use of endomyocardial biopsy (EMB) and increased use of CMR. The 1987 Dallas criteria had previously been used to establish a histologic diagnosis, but there has been increased recognition of the limitations of these criteria due to variability of interpretation and low sensitivity. Newer criteria based on immunoperoxidase staining seem to have greater sensitivity, as does testing the myocardial biopsy sample for viral genomes by PCR. Myocarditis is a patchy non-homogenous infiltrate with preferential involvement of the LV and may be missed on random sampling of the more commonly biopsied right ventricle (RV). As hemodynamic catheterization and biopsy is an invasive procedure that carries risk, endomyocardial biopsy is currently recommended on the basis of the likelihood of finding a specific treatable disorder (e.g., giant cell myocarditis).

TABLE 53-1 Causes of Myocarditis

Category	Type	Cause
Infectious		
	Viral	
		Adenoviruses
		Echoviruses
		Enteroviruses (including coxsackieviruses A and B)
		Hepatitis B and C
		Herpes viruses (including cytomegalovirus, Epstein-Barr virus, human herpes virus 6)
		Human immunodeficiency virus
		Influenza A and B
		Parvovirus B19
		Respiratory syncytial virus
		Severe acute respiratory syndrome coronavirus 2
	Bacterial	
		Brucella
		Chlamydia
		Corynebacterium diphtheria
		Legionella
		Mycobacterium tuberculosis
		Mycoplasma pneumonia
		Staphylococcus
		Streptococcus A
		Streptococcus pneumoniae
	Fungal	
		Actinomyces
		Aspergillus
		Blastomyces
		Candida
		Cryptococcus
		Histoplasma
	Rickettsial	
		Coxiella burnetii
		Rickettsia prowazekii
		Rickettsia rickettsia
	Spirochetal	
		Borrelia burgdorferi
		Leptospira
		Treponema pallidum
	Protozoal	
		Entamoeba histolytica
		Leishmania
		Toxoplasmosis gondii
		Trypanosoma cruzi
Non-Infectious		
	Autoimmune and systemic disease	
		Celiac disease
		Churg-Strauss syndrome (eosinophilic granulomatosis)
		Dermatomyositis
		Giant cell myocarditis
		Granulomatosis with polyangiitis
		Hypereosinophilic syndrome
		Inflammatory bowel disease
		Kawasaki disease
		Myasthenia gravis
		Rheumatoid arthritis
		Sarcoidosis
		Scleroderma
		Systemic lupus erythematosus
		Takayasu arteritis
		Thyrotoxicosis
	Hypersensitivity reaction	
		Benzodiazepines
		Beta-lactams
		Carbamazepine
		Clozapine
		Diuretics (loop and thiazides)
		Fluoroquinolones
		Macrolides
		Methyldopa
		Nonsteroidal anti-inflammatory drugs
		Smallpox vaccine
		Sulfonamides
		Tetanus toxoid
		Tetracyclines
		Tricyclic antidepressants
		Vancomycin
		Venom (insect, scorpion, snake, spider)
	Toxin	
		Aminophylline
		Amphetamines
		Anthracyclines
		Arsenic
		Carbon monoxide
		Chloramphenicol
		Cocaine
		Copper
		Cyclophosphamide
		Doxorubicin
		Ethanol
		Iron
		Lead
		Phenytoin
		Radiotherapy

Source: Data from Kindermann I, Barth C, Mahfoud F, et al. Update on myocarditis. *J Am Coll Cardiol*. 2012;59(9):779-792. and Law YM, Lal AK, Chen S, et al. Diagnosis and management of myocarditis in children: a scientific statement from the American Heart Association [published correction appears in Circulation. 2021;144(6):e149]. *Circulation*. 2021;144(6):e123-e135.

MANAGEMENT

Supportive care is the mainstay of management in myocarditis. Careful attention to potential complications (including development of arrhythmias or worsening cardiac function) and judicious triaging and disposition is necessary, as patients may be at risk for rapid deterioration.

Medical Management Management of heart failure due to myocarditis is similar to that caused by other etiologies. Patients with poor perfusion are often admitted to an intensive care unit and may be stabilized with inotropic medications including milrinone, while others may require mechanical circulatory support. For patients with symptoms of congestion but with adequate perfusion, diuretics and vasodilators are first-line agents used for symptomatic improvement. For stable symptomatic patients requiring chronic management, angiotensin-converting enzyme inhibitors (or angiotensin receptor blockers as an alternative), beta-blockers, and aldosterone antagonists are commonly used based on

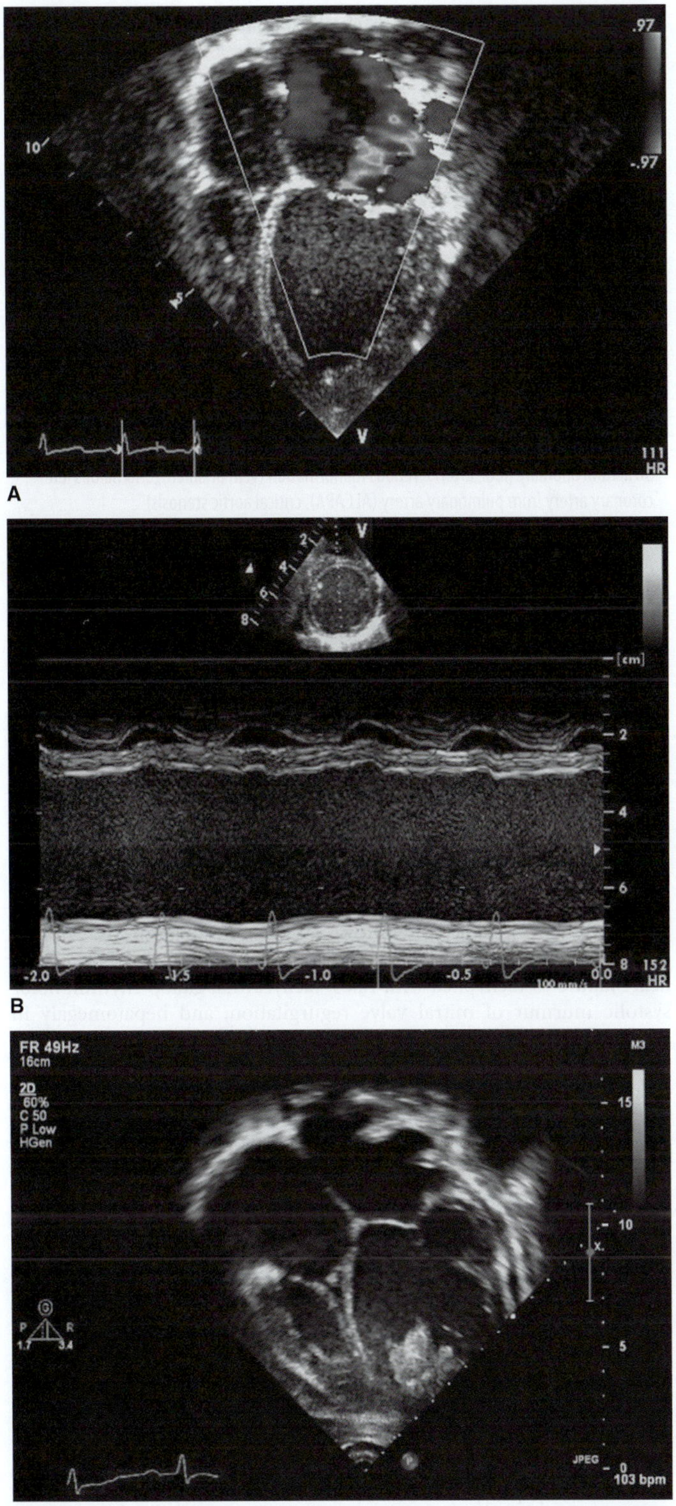

FIGURE 53-1. A. Two-dimensional echocardiogram and color Doppler of a patient with DCM, demonstrating a dilated LV cavity and mitral regurgitation. B. M-mode echocardiogram demonstrating a dilated LV cavity and poor systolic function (shortening fraction 15%, ejection fraction 28%). C. Two-dimensional echocardiogram demonstrating a large thrombus in the apex of the left ventricle.

extrapolation from adult heart failure studies that demonstrate benefits in symptoms, ventricular function, and survival, though pediatric data is more limited and has not clearly shown the same benefit.

Monitoring for and managing atrial and ventricular arrhythmias is critical in early acute myocarditis, and rhythm control may sometimes be required in the chronic phase as well. Management of arrhythmias should be done in consultation with a cardiologist and may require eventual pacemaker placement if persistent.

Nonsteroidal anti-inflammatory drugs (NSAIDs) are not recommended during acute or subacute myocarditis due to murine studies demonstrating evidence of increased inflammation and mortality. Similarly, digitalis is also not recommended due to murine models demonstrating poorer outcomes.

Mechanical Circulatory Support In patients with progressive deterioration, early consideration of mechanical circulatory support (MCS) may be lifesaving. This may be temporary, such as extracorporeal membrane oxygenation (ECMO), or more durable such as a ventricular assist device (VAD). Patients not showing improvement on mechanical support should be considered for cardiac transplantation.

Immunomodulation and Antivirals There is a paucity of data regarding immunomodulatory therapy in pediatric myocarditis, though it is commonly used at many centers. Despite numerous case reports on the treatment of myocarditis with immunosuppression, including steroids, cyclosporine, azathioprine, and OKT3, there is no longitudinal data to support this form of therapy. In a randomized adult trial using steroids with either cyclosporine or azathioprine in patients with biopsy-proven myocarditis, there was no benefit in the treated group. Based on the results of a small study, many pediatric centers routinely use intravenous gamma globulin (IVIG) (1-2 g/kg over 12-24 hours), though larger multi-site and national registry studies have failed to demonstrate improved outcomes. It is important to note that if IVIG is to be used and the child may require cardiac transplantation in the future, transplant labs should be drawn before IVIG is given.

Antiviral treatments have not been rigorously studied in myocarditis, and patients are often thought to present too late for antiviral therapy to prevent inflammatory cardiac damage. However, their use might be considered if an active infection is diagnosed, even without definitive proof of myocardial infection. Use of antiviral compounds including interferon-alpha and beta have been proposed based on adult case series. Consultation with an infectious disease expert may be helpful.

For non-infectious myocarditis, such as giant cell myocarditis, sarcoidosis, and eosinophilic myocarditis, immunosuppression is more well established and may be of benefit. Myocarditis in the setting of systemic autoimmune disease may benefit from treatment of the underlying disease. In such cases, consultation with a rheumatologist is recommended.

ADMISSION AND DISCHARGE CRITERIA

Admission A symptomatic patient with a new diagnosis of heart failure and poor LV function should be admitted to the hospital, usually to an intensive care unit, for medical therapy and observation until the course of the illness can be established, as patients can deteriorate rapidly. Monitoring of cardiovascular status, including continuous rhythm and close hemodynamic monitoring, is required at admission. Transfer to a center that can provide advanced pediatric cardiovascular care, including mechanical circulatory support and transplantation, may be necessary if such care is not available at the admitting facility. For patients with abnormal but reasonable ventricular function on oral medications who have demonstrated a stable trajectory over a period of time, observation in a non-ICU setting can be considered.

Discharge Patients who remain stable in the hospital on oral medication are ready for discharge. Newborns and infants must be able to feed and show adequate caloric intake with minimal symptoms of congestive heart failure. The older child and adolescent should be ambulatory and stable for several days on chronic medication. Patients should be arrhythmia-free or have a stable arrhythmia on or off antiarrhythmic therapy. Follow-up with a cardiologist should be ensured for both ongoing surveillance of cardiac function and possible modification or discontinuation of heart failure and/or antiarrhythmic medications pending patient course.

CONSULTATION

A pediatric cardiologist should be consulted in cases of suspected or confirmed myocarditis. Triage to an intensive care unit may be indicated at admission, particularly to a center with advanced cardiovascular support capabilities including mechanical circulatory support and transplant. Infectious disease experts may be helpful when considering antiviral or immunomodulatory treatments. A rheumatologist may provide management guidance in myocarditis in the context of systemic autoimmune disease.

SPECIAL CONSIDERATIONS

There is a risk of sudden cardiac death associated with myocarditis, especially with exercise. Families should be advised that patients should not participate in competitive sports while active inflammation is present, and a resting echocardiogram, 24-hour Holter monitor, and exercise ECG must be performed 3 to 6 months after the initial diagnosis. Ventricular function must have normalized, and clinically significant arrhythmias must be absent prior to return to training and competition.

KEY POINTS

- Myocarditis is a potentially life-threatening condition with nonspecific and variable presentations that may overlap with other common pediatric illnesses. Recognition of clinical presentations and appropriate use of diagnostic studies are necessary to make an accurate diagnosis.
- Initial management requires close attention to cardiovascular monitoring, judicious disposition, and appropriate consultation.
- Diagnostic confirmation is challenging and increasingly utilizes cardiac magnetic resonance imaging. Management is primarily supportive, though immunomodulation may be considered in certain cases.
- Clinical stability, appropriate follow-up, and activity restrictions are important discharge considerations.

DILATED CARDIOMYOPATHY

BACKGROUND

Dilated cardiomyopathy (DCM) is a myocardial disorder characterized by LV dilation and systolic dysfunction that commonly results in congestive heart failure. DCM is the most common cardiomyopathy in children with an estimated incidence of 0.57 cases per 100,000 children per year (50%-60% of all pediatric cardiomyopathy cases) and carries a high risk of morbidity and mortality.

Pathophysiology While most children have idiopathic disease, there are many heterogeneous etiologies that can lead to DCM, including myocarditis, genetic mutations, neuromuscular disease, toxin exposure, coronary artery abnormalities, tachyarrhythmias, nutritional deficiencies, and underlying syndromes. See **Table 53-2**. The "final common pathway" hypothesis posits that disruption between the cytoskeleton and sarcomere underlies the pathogenesis of the DCM phenotype.

CLINICAL PRESENTATION

The presentation of a child with dilated cardiomyopathy (DCM) depends on the acuteness of the illness. While acute viral myocarditis may present as cardiovascular collapse over a short period of time as described in the previous section, other causes of DCM may have a more progressive subacute to chronic course. A slow decrease in ventricular function over months or years may go unnoticed, whereas a rapid drop in ventricular function over several days may result in severe heart failure and cardiovascular collapse, as compensatory mechanisms have not yet taken effect. The chronic stable patient has little cardiac reserve, however, and any stressor such as an unrelated illness may result in cardiac decompensation. The history of an antecedent viral infection in the child presenting with a dilated and dysfunctional LV may therefore not necessarily indicate a diagnosis of myocarditis, as the illness may be "unmasking" a previously undiagnosed chronic compensated DCM.

TABLE 53-2 Potential Causes of Dilated Cardiomyopathy

Acquired
Infection (e.g., viral myocarditis)
Nutritional deficiency (e.g., calcium, carnitine, selenium)
Peripartum
Toxic (e.g., anthracyclines, alcohol)
Congenital
Genetic mutation
Ion channelopathy
Inborn errors of metabolism (e.g., beta-ketothiolase deficiency)
Metabolic storage disorders
Mitochondrial disease (e.g., Barth syndrome)
Muscular Dystrophy (e.g., Duchenne, Becker)
Myopathy (e.g., nemaline)
Structural anomaly (e.g., arterio-venous malformation (vein of Galen), anomalous left coronary artery from pulmonary artery (ALCAPA), critical aortic stenosis)
Mixed
Autoimmune disease (e.g., systemic lupus erythematosus)
Endocrine disorder (e.g., hypothyroidism)
Endomyocardial disease
Infiltrative disease (e.g., hemochromatosis)
Tachyarrhythmia (e.g., supraventricular tachycardia)

Source: Adapted from Jefferies JL, Towbin JA. Dilated cardiomyopathy. *Lancet*. 2010;375(9716):752-762.

The usual presentation of DCM is that of congestive heart failure and low cardiac output. Signs and symptoms of heart failure include respiratory distress, gastrointestinal symptoms (nausea, vomiting, and abdominal pain due to hepatic congestion), fatigue, and diaphoresis. Physical examination is variable and may range from normal in compensated heart failure to tachypnea with rales, tachycardia, gallop rhythm, holosystolic murmur of mitral valve regurgitation, and hepatomegaly in symptomatic heart failure. Peripheral edema is less common in infants and young children compared to adults.

In addition to recognition of heart failure, careful attention should be paid to identifying potential etiologies, including infectious (i.e., myocarditis), metabolic, acquired, or congenital causes. In infants, particular attention should be paid to investigating for underlying metabolic, mitochondrial, or other genetic syndromes. A history of developmental delay or regression, failure to thrive, seizures, metabolic decompensation with illness, or pertinent family history as well as findings of dysmorphic features, hypotonia or hypertonia, or vision or hearing loss may prompt targeted evaluation and consultation with genetic and metabolic experts. Specific nutritional deficiencies (carnitine, selenium, calcium, vitamin D) may result in cardiomyopathy that is reversible and should be investigated in the appropriate setting.

A unique pediatric population associated with cardiomyopathy is children with muscular dystrophies. Cardiac involvement is universal in Duchenne muscular dystrophy (DMD) with a median age of diagnosis of cardiomyopathy at 14 to 15 years. Patients with the milder Becker muscular dystrophy (BMD) may be more likely to develop symptoms of heart failure than patients with DMD due to preserved ambulation and associated cardiac demand. Other dystrophies with associated cardiomyopathy include myotonic muscular dystrophy, Emery-Dreifuss muscular dystrophy, and limb girdle muscular dystrophies.

DIFFERENTIAL DIAGNOSIS

Potential causes and differential diagnoses of DCM are listed in Table 53-2, grouped by acquired, congenital, and mixed etiologies. All attempts should be made to diagnose treatable causes of cardiomyopathy such as structural heart disease, underlying arrhythmias, endocrine disorders, and nutritional deficiencies. Although structural heart defects and arrhythmias are not truly diseases of the myocardium, they are listed as they may present similarly to a DCM and must be considered in the evaluation of these children.

DIAGNOSTIC EVALUATION

Table 53-3 includes an extensive list of studies that may be performed in the evaluation of a patient with newly diagnosed DCM. The extent of evaluation should be tailored to the patient based on the patient's clinical characteristics, medical history (e.g., a history of anthracycline administration), physical exam, and study results. When identifiable causes are excluded or point to a familial or inherited disorder, family screening becomes important.

Chest x-ray generally demonstrates cardiomegaly and varying degrees of pulmonary edema. ECG is usually abnormal in DCM and may demonstrate LV hypertrophy or ST-segment and T-wave changes. ECG features commonly seen in myocarditis are described in the myocarditis section. Q waves in lead I and aVL due to myocardial infarct are very suspicious of anomalous origin of the left coronary artery from the pulmonary artery (ALCAPA). Ectopic beats should raise the suspicion of poorly controlled supraventricular tachycardia or ventricular arrhythmias, although in severe cardiac dysfunction, ventricular arrhythmias may occur secondary to myocardial disease.

The echocardiogram is the modality of choice to establish the diagnosis of a dilated LV with poor systolic function (Figure 53-1A, B), while simultaneously excluding structural causes of LV dysfunction. Although ventricular dysfunction usually manifests as global hypokinesia, segmental wall motion abnormalities may be present. The evaluation should also search for the presence of a thrombus in the left atrium or ventricle (Figure 53-1C). Doppler cardiography will often demonstrate mitral as well as tricuspid insufficiency. RV size and function may be spared early on, but the RV may also dilate and demonstrate poor contractility.

CMR is increasingly utilized in the diagnosis and management of DCM and as described previously, may be useful in distinguishing myocarditis from other etiologies of DCM. Hemodynamic catheterization may be utilized to obtain baseline hemodynamics, perform an endomyocardial biopsy, or exclude structural disease not eliminated by echocardiography.

Laboratory evaluation may be useful in assessing the severity of the patient's heart failure as well as determining the underlying etiology. B-type natriuretic peptide is elevated in heart failure and may be followed over time. Evaluation for infectious myocarditis is discussed in the previous section. Specific nutritional, electrolyte, and endocrine disturbances may be assessed by serologic testing. Targeted studies (serum and urine organic acids, lactate, pyruvate, enzyme testing, etc.) may be indicated based on suspicion for metabolic or mitochondrial disorders. Genetic testing is increasingly performed for patients without a clear etiology of cardiomyopathy and represents a field of increasing priority as new genetic studies and targeted interventions with the potential to affect outcomes become available. Guidelines outlining the approach for genetic evaluation of patients and families in specific contexts have been published.

TABLE 53-3 Evaluation Considerations for Newly Diagnosed Dilated Cardiomyopathy

Imaging and Non-Invasive Testing
Chest x-ray
Electrocardiogram
Echocardiogram
Cardiac magnetic resonance imaging
Laboratory Studies
Blood
Acylcarnitine profile
Basic metabolic panel
B-type natriuretic peptide
Calcium
Carnitine
Cholesterol
Complete blood count with differential
Creatine kinase
Erythrocyte sedimentation rate
Lactic acid
Liver function tests
Magnesium
Pyruvate
Selenium
Thyroid function studies
Troponin
Plasma amino acids
Viral testing
Urine
Amino acids
Organic acids
Urinalysis
Genetic Evaluation
Genetics consultation
Metabolic / enzyme testing
Sequence-based genetic testing (e.g., cardiomyopathy, mitochondrial, muscular dystrophy panels)
Invasive Testing
Hemodynamic catheterization and angiography of structural lesions
Skeletal muscle biopsy (histology, electron microscopy, mitochondrial respiratory chain analysis)
Endomyocardial biopsy (histology, electron microscopy, viral genome PCR, mitochondrial analysis)

MANAGEMENT

Supportive care to manage symptoms of heart failure is the primary goal in both the acute and chronic setting. Medical management of heart failure is primarily symptomatic and similar to other scenarios of acute and chronic heart failure, as outlined in the myocarditis section. Management should involve consultation with a cardiologist. Mechanical circulatory support or transplantation may be required in a significant proportion of patients with a reported 5-year transplant-free survival rate of only 50% in a national registry, though prognosis differs by underlying etiology.

Disease-specific therapy is largely unavailable in both idiopathic and many known etiologies of DCM, but some important disease-specific therapies are possible (e.g., surgical repair of ALCAPA, management of underlying arrhythmia, appropriate supplementation in some inborn errors of metabolism or nutritional deficiencies), and therefore, secondary causes should always be investigated. Gene-directed therapy in Duchenne muscular dystrophy is being investigated and, if successful, may serve as a model for other genetic DCMs. Pulmonary artery banding in DCM has shown promise in small pediatric studies.

ADMISSION AND DISCHARGE CRITERIA

Patients with a new diagnosis of heart failure require admission for evaluation and stabilization. Intensive care unit admission may be required, especially in the setting of poor perfusion or a potentially unstable hemodynamic trajectory (e.g., fulminant myocarditis). Rhythm monitoring for detection of arrhythmias should be considered. Consideration of advanced pediatric cardiovascular care capabilities is warranted, including mechanical circulatory support and transplantation. For chronic stable patients with reasonable ventricular function on oral medications, observation in a non-ICU setting may be appropriate. Patients who are stable on oral medication with minimal symptoms of congestive heart failure may be discharged with appropriate follow-up with a cardiologist.

CONSULTATION

A pediatric cardiologist should be consulted in cases of suspected or confirmed DCM. Many pediatric cardiology centers now have multidisciplinary teams that specialize in the care of children with heart failure due to DCM or other etiologies and provide comprehensive and integrated care. Patients with DCM face significant morbidity and mortality, highlighting the importance of referral to and follow-up at a center with advanced cardiovascular care. Depending on the suspected etiology of DCM, specialists with expertise in genetic and metabolic disorders, neurology, infectious disease, rheumatology, or endocrinology may provide guidance on additional workup and management of the underlying cause.

SPECIAL CONSIDERATIONS

In patients with a suspected genetic or inherited DCM, the Heart Failure Society of America recommends genetic and periodic clinical screening for first-degree relatives to detect cardiac disease and decrease the risk for heart failure progression or sudden death.

Patients with Duchenne and Becker muscular dystrophies, with or without overt cardiomyopathy, can have severe complications from anesthesia, including cardiac arrest related to hyperkalemia in the setting of succinylcholine, malignant hyperthermia, and rhabdomyolysis. Caution with anesthesia is warranted.

HYPERTROPHIC CARDIOMYOPATHY

BACKGROUND

Hypertrophic cardiomyopathy (HCM) is a heterogeneous, familial disorder of cardiac muscle that affects sarcomeric proteins, resulting in myocyte and myofibrillar disorganization and fibrosis. It is the second-most common cardiomyopathy in children with an incidence of 0.47 per 100,000 children (40%-45% of pediatric cardiomyopathies). HCM has an autosomal dominant pattern of inheritance with incomplete penetrance. Mutations in genes that code for sarcomeric proteins may result in HCM; some mutations are relatively benign, whereas others are associated with early death.

Pathophysiology HCM is characterized by a thickened but non-dilated LV in the absence of other explanatory cardiac or systemic disease. Various parts of the ventricle can undergo myocytic hypertrophy, and this results in a stiff LV with impaired diastolic filling, which may lead to congestive symptoms. In addition, the cellular disarray and hypertrophy may serve as substrate for electrical instability and arrhythmias.

Patients with HCM may develop LV outflow tract obstruction when there is systolic anterior motion (SAM) of the mitral valve against the hypertrophied ventricular septum. As such, LV outflow obstruction in HCM is dynamic and worsens with conditions that increase the outflow gradient, such as low systemic vascular resistance (SVR) or hypovolemia. Interventions such as intravascular volume expansion or increasing SVR may lessen the obstruction. Coronary arteries walls may thicken, and mismatch between myocardial mass and coronary circulation can lead to episodes of ischemia and the development of scar tissue.

CLINICAL PRESENTATION

Common features of HCM include chest pain from impairment of myocardial perfusion as well as palpitations, syncope, or sudden death from arrythmias. Left-sided failure may produce dyspnea and exercise intolerance. Patients may also present with the onset of a new murmur (usually a medium-pitched systolic ejection murmur) that varies in intensity with the degree of outflow obstruction. Classically, maneuvers that decrease preload (such as Valsalva and standing) will increase the murmur, and maneuvers that increase SVR (such as handgrip) will decrease the murmur. Many asymptomatic patients are found on screening after identification of a family member with HCM.

Sudden death is often the first symptom of HCM and is thought to be due to ventricular arrhythmia. HCM is the most common cause of nontraumatic sudden death in children and adolescents, though sudden death is rare before age 10 years. In teenagers, it most commonly occurs with exercise.

DIFFERENTIAL DIAGNOSIS

Patients presenting with HCM in infancy should be evaluated for metabolic disorders and syndromes associated with or mimicking HCM, such as Noonan syndrome, Pompe disease, mitochondrial myopathies, and other metabolic storage diseases (PRKAG2, Fabry disease, LAMP2 cardiomyopathy). The treatment and prognosis for these are often different from those with sarcomeric HCM. Friedreich ataxia, an autosomal recessive neurologic condition that typically presents at puberty with discoordination, progressive ataxia, and dysarthria, may have associated LV hypertrophy that mimics HCM but does not have outflow tract obstruction, which may progress to impaired LV systolic function and dilation.

Athletic training, particularly in rowing and cycling sports, can produce physiologic and clinically benign increases in LV wall thickness and mass (so-called athlete's heart), which may pose a diagnostic dilemma in differentiation from HCM. A variety of characteristic differences in clinical, echocardiographic, and magnetic resonance findings can help distinguish these two entities.

DIAGNOSTIC EVALUATION

The 12-lead ECG is abnormal in 90% to 95% of patients with HCM, but the changes are not specific to this disorder. Common abnormalities include increased R-wave voltages in V_5 and V_6 and abnormal T waves and Q waves in the lateral precordial leads due to septal hypertrophy. Abnormal ECG findings may be present before diagnostic echocardiographic features. Echocardiography can reveal abnormal hypertrophic areas of the myocardium as well as define outflow tract obstruction and abnormalities of systolic and diastolic function. CMR has emerged as a complementary tool that provides more precise wall thickness measurements and a more complete interrogation of HCM morphology. It is important to note that up to 40% of carriers may not exhibit diagnostic criteria until later in life.

MANAGEMENT

The goals of treatment include relief of symptoms, control of complications, and prevention of sudden death. Beta-blockers reduce LV contractility and heart rate and therefore myocardial wall stress, oxygen requirements, and outflow gradients, all of which may improve symptoms of chest pain and pulmonary congestion. Verapamil, a calcium channel-blocking agent, has been demonstrated to improve exercise capacity in adults without obstruction. Relief of LV outflow obstruction is indicated in symptomatic patients with significant obstruction (gradient >50 mmHg). The most common procedure performed is surgical myotomy-myectomy, which involves resection of excess muscle from the ventricular septum, and results in symptomatic improvement and substantial reduction in the outflow gradient in a majority of patients.

Implantable defibrillators are the only treatment strategy that have been proven to alter the natural history of HCM, and with increasing experience in both children and adults, they are considered to be highly effective in preventing sudden death and decreasing the HCM mortality rate. Insertion of an implantable cardioverter defibrillator is indicated for secondary prevention after cardiac arrest. Implantation for primary prevention of sudden death is based on risk factors (**Table 53-4**).

Previous guidelines have recommended against participation in competitive sports for patients with phenotypic HCM, but more recent updates have suggested shared decision-making between providers and patients, as precisely defining the risk for cardiac death is not possible. Furthermore, multiple studies have shown a similar ventricular arrhythmia burden in those with HCM engaged in competitive sports and those who are not.

TABLE 53-4 Implantable Cardioverter-defibrillator (ICD) Placement in Hypertrophic Cardiomyopathy (HCM)

Indications for ICD for secondary prevention
Prior cardiac arrest or spontaneous sustained ventricular tachycardia
Important risk factors when evaluating ICD for primary prevention
Family history of premature HCM-related sudden death*
Extreme LV hypertrophy ≥30 mm*
Unexplained recent syncope, unlikely vasovagal by history, particularly if recurrent and exercise related*
Multiple episodes of non-sustained ventricular tachycardia (Holter)
Late gadolinium enhancement (fibrosis) on cardiac magnetic resonance comprising ≥15% of LV mass
End-stage HCM
Left ventricular apical aneurysm
Abnormal blood pressure response with exercise

*Risk factors most predictive of sudden death in children and adolescents.

Source: Adapted from Maron BJ, Desai MY, Nishimura RA, et al. Management of hypertrophic cardiomyopathy: JACC State-of-the-Art Review. *J Am Coll Cardiol*. 2022;79(4):390-414.

ADMISSION AND DISCHARGE CRITERIA

Hospitalization post-cardiac arrest is necessary to establish cardiovascular stability and for full evaluation. Most other patients can be evaluated as outpatients. Evaluation includes exam, ECG, echocardiogram, stress testing for exercise tolerance, and cardiac MRI to evaluate for scar tissue that may be a nidus for possible arrhythmia initiation. Discharge is appropriate when the patient has demonstrated clinical stability and outpatient follow-up has been established.

CONSULTATION

A pediatric cardiologist should be involved with the evaluation and management of children with suspected or confirmed HCM and should follow these patients in an outpatient setting.

SPECIAL CONSIDERATIONS

If a patient with known HCM is admitted for a non-cardiac procedure and sedation or general anesthesia is necessary, the patient should not be allowed to become intravascularly depleted, and an IV for fluids should be started early if there is a wait for the procedure. Anesthesia should be aware of the diagnosis and should use sedatives that do not decrease the SVR, as the LV outflow tract gradient will increase and cardiac output will decrease.

Family members of patients with HCM should be referred for outpatient evaluation, including genetic testing, ECG, and echocardiography to screen for undiagnosed HCM. The frequency of follow-up depends on age, with increased frequency from age 12 to 21 years due to accelerated disease progression in this age group, though ongoing surveillance into adulthood may also be prudent in some cases.

Pre-participation screening for high school and college-aged sports participants via personal and family history and physical exam is intended to detect cardiovascular abnormalities such as HCM that carry a potential risk for sudden death with intense exercise, though many cases may remain unsuspected. The routine use of ECG in pre-participation screening remains controversial and is not currently recommended.

RESTRICTIVE CARDIOMYOPATHY

BACKGROUND

Restrictive cardiomyopathy (RCM) is the least common form of cardiomyopathy, accounting for 2.5% to 5% of pediatric cardiomyopathies, and carries a significantly poorer prognosis than that of DCM or HCM.

Pathophysiology Restrictive cardiomyopathy is characterized by abnormal diastolic function due to impaired ventricular compliance and relaxation. Multiple etiologies may cause RCM including infiltrative and non-infiltrative processes, storage diseases, genetic mutations, endomyocardial diseases, myocarditis, and following cardiac transplantation, though the majority of cases are idiopathic.

CLINICAL PRESENTATION

Early on, patients with restrictive cardiomyopathy are asymptomatic. With advanced disease, dyspnea on exertion or exercise intolerance is frequently reported due to an inability to increase cardiac output during exercise. There is often a history of misdiagnoses related to pulmonary symptoms, such as recurrent lower respiratory tract infections or asthma. Weakness and shortness of breath are common, and chest pain and syncope occasionally occur. On exam, signs of right heart failure may be evident, with hepatomegaly, ascites, rales secondary to pulmonary edema, and peripheral edema. Abnormal heart sounds including a gallop rhythm and a loud P2 are commonly heard.

DIFFERENTIAL DIAGNOSIS

Causes of restrictive cardiomyopathy are summarized in **Table 53-5**. An important entity with a remarkably similar presentation is constrictive pericarditis (CP). In contrast to RCM, CP is a treatable condition that is managed with surgical removal of the pericardium. A number of laboratory, ECG, echocardiographic, MRI, and hemodynamic catheterization findings may help distinguish these two entities, though considerable overlap can occur, and occasionally endomyocardial biopsy is required.

DIAGNOSTIC EVALUATION

A 12-lead ECG is usually abnormal and shows evidence of left and right atrial enlargement, which occurs secondary to high diastolic pressures within the stiff ventricles. Arrhythmias and conduction disturbances are common. Chest x-ray reveals a normal to slightly increased heart size and signs of pulmonary venous congestion. Echocardiogram is usually diagnostic and characteristically demonstrates markedly enlarged left and right atria with normal ventricular systolic function and decreased diastolic function. In cases of infiltrative disease, ventricular walls may be thickened. Additional laboratory studies may include urine and serum protein levels, complete metabolic panel, iron studies, CBC, and BNP (which is typically elevated in restrictive cardiomyopathy but not in constrictive pericarditis). Catheterization defines the hemodynamics and can help differentiate restrictive from constrictive disease. Endomyocardial biopsy may also be useful in evaluating patients with restrictive cardiomyopathy due to amyloidosis and other specific causes (e.g., metabolic storage disease such as glycogen storage, hemochromatosis, or sarcoidosis).

MANAGEMENT

Once restrictive cardiomyopathy becomes symptomatic, it is usually progressive. Occasionally, the disease process can be slowed with treatment,

TABLE 53-5 Causes of Restrictive Cardiomyopathy

Idiopathic
Familial / Genetic
Endomyocardial fibrosis (endemic in parts of Africa, India, South and Central America, and Asia)
Löffler's disease (hypereosinophilia syndrome)
Infiltrative disorders (amyloidosis, hemochromatosis, sarcoidosis, carcinoid syndrome, systemic sclerosis)
Lysosomal disorders (Hurler, Gaucher, Fabry) and glycogen storage diseases
Iatrogenic (radiation therapy to the chest, anthracycline cardiotoxicity)
Malignant (metastatic tumors)

especially if an underlying cause can be determined and is amenable to therapy. For example, for patients with hemochromatosis, therapy aimed at iron binding may be beneficial to slow ongoing iron deposition and resultant damage to the myocardium. Symptomatic treatment generally involves the use of diuretics to treat high atrial pressures and resultant congestive symptoms. The diastolic relaxing effects of carvedilol may offer some therapeutic benefit. Vasodilators may also be used but monitoring for hypotension is vital. As the disease progresses, fibrosis of the AV valves may occur and may also involve the sinus and AV nodes, leading to arrhythmias and possibly requiring insertion of a pacemaker. Heart rate must be maintained at a rate slow enough to allow maximal ventricular filling.

The prognosis for children with RMC is poor; approximately half of children die or require transplantation within 2 to 3 years of diagnosis. With disease progression, development of pulmonary hypertension and associated morbidity and mortality is common, and cardiac transplantation is the definitive therapy.

SUGGESTED READINGS

Ghelani SJ, Spaeder MC, Pastor W, Spurney CF, Klugman D. Demographics, trends, and outcomes in pediatric acute myocarditis in the United States, 2006 to 2011. *Circ Cardiovasc Qual Outcomes*. 2012;5(5): 622-627.

Law YM, Lal AK, Chen S, et al. Diagnosis and management of myocarditis in children: a scientific statement from the American Heart Association. *Circulation*. 2021;144(6):e123-e135.

Lee TM, Hsu DT, Kantor P, et al. Pediatric cardiomyopathies. *Circ Res*. 2017;121(7):855-873.

Maron BJ, Desai MY, Nishimura RA, et al. Management of hypertrophic cardiomyopathy: JACC State-of-the-Art Review. *J Am Coll Cardiol*. 2022;79(4):390-414.

Maron BJ, Doerer JJ, Haas TS, Tierney DM, Mueller FO. Sudden deaths in young competitive athletes: analysis of 1866 deaths in the United States, 1980-2006. *Circulation*. 2009;119(8):1085-1092.

Shaddy RE, Penny DJ, Feltes TF, Cetta F, Mital S. *Moss & Adams' Heart Disease in Infants, Children, and Adolescents Including the Fetus and Young Adult*. 10th ed. Lippincott Williams & Wilkins; 2021.

Teele SA, Allan CK, Laussen PC, Newburger JW, Gauvreau K, Thiagarajan RR. Management and outcomes in pediatric patients presenting with acute fulminant myocarditis. *J Pediatr*. 2011;158(4):638-643.e1.

CHAPTER 54

Pericarditis

Kathryn Westphal, MD and Nancy Liao, MD

Abbreviations

CRP C-reactive protein
ECG electrocardiogram
ESR erythrocyte sedimentation rate
CT chest tomography
MRI magnetic resonance imaging
NSAID non-steroidal anti-inflammatory drugs
PPS post pericardiotomy syndrome
COVID-19 coronavirus disease of 2019

BACKGROUND

Pericarditis refers to inflammation of the pericardium, a fibrous sac that surrounds the heart, and is defined as acute, incessant, recurrent, or chronic. The serous pericardium consists of two main layers with the inner most layer, the visceral pericardium, adhering to the heart. The potential space between the two layers contains a small amount of serous fluid which provides lubrication during the contraction of the heart to reduce friction with surrounding structures. The pericardial sac functions as a barrier against infection from the lungs, an anchor to the mediastinum, a limit to acute myocardial distension, and a modulator of ventricular interdependence. Inflammation of the pericardium can be accompanied by an increase in the serous fluid, resulting in a pericardial effusion. If the effusion impacts cardiac filling, life-threatening cardiac tamponade may result. Furthermore, the inflammation from the pericardium may extend to the myocardium, resulting in myopericarditis. Therefore, timely identification and treatment of pericarditis may reduce complications and prevent recurrences.

EPIDEMIOLOGY

Although chest pain is a common pediatric complaint, cardiac causes are infrequent and epidemiologic data on pericarditis is limited. Several studies have reported an adolescent male predilection for pericarditis in the pediatric population. In a large retrospective cohort study, investigating emergent cardiac etiologies of chest pain in pediatric patients without a history of cardiovascular disease, pericarditis accounted for 29% (7/24) of cardiac etiologies for chest pain, but only 0.16% (7/4288) of cases of chest pain overall. In another single center study, pericarditis accounted for 42% (5/12) of cardiac causes of chest pain and 4.6% of cases of chest pain. Although pericarditis is relatively rare in pediatrics, incidence is probably underestimated due to subclinical cases (asymptomatic or mild symptoms) that go undetected.

ETIOLOGIES

Most cases of pericarditis will be considered "idiopathic" after a thorough history, physical exam, and evaluation fail to identify a specific cause. Many of these cases are attributed to an undiagnosed viral infection or an immune response to an infection. Identifiable causes of pericarditis are usually categorized as infectious or noninfectious. The most common infectious causes vary by geographic location and local epidemiology. In developed countries, infectious pericarditis is typically viral and a result of direct infection of the pericardium or a secondary immune-mediated inflammation of the pericardium. In contrast, tuberculosis pericarditis is the most common etiology in areas with endemic tuberculosis. Recent studies demonstrate changing trends in etiologies of pericarditis across all ages with post pericardiotomy syndrome (PPS) being more common than infectious pericarditis in resource-rich nations. Viral or idiopathic pericarditis remains most common etiology in recurrent pediatric pericarditis. The proposed mechanism of PPS is autoimmune inflammation of the pericardium 1 to 2 weeks after pericardial injury. PPS may be more common after atrial septal defect surgery. Other well-described etiologies in pediatric patients include autoimmune diseases, medications or post-vaccination, malignancy, and trauma. Identifiable causes of pericarditis are listed in **Table 54-1**.

CLINICAL PRESENTATION

Pericarditis can present along a wide spectrum of symptoms ranging from mild chest pain to severe cardiovascular compromise and shock, depending on the size of the effusion and the rate at which it accumulates. The most common symptom of pericarditis is chest pain, classically described as left-sided sharp pain with radiation to the neck or shoulder and worse with inspiration or supine positioning. Infants will have fussiness and poor feeding. Older children may present with fatigue or weakness, palpitations, or dizziness and syncope. Some patients with acute pericarditis will report abdominal

TABLE 54-1 Causes of Acute Pericarditis

Infectious	Medications or Post-Vaccination
Viral or post viral	COVID-19[a] and meningococcal vaccinations
Enteroviruses (Coxsachieviruses, Echovirus), Adenovirus, Parvovirus B19, Epstein-Barr, Influenza, Mumps, Varicella, Cytomegalovirus, Hepatitis B and C, Human immunodeficiency virus, Human herpesvirus 6, Severe acute respiratory syndrome coronavirus 2	Drugs causing Lupus-like syndrome
	Hydralazine, isoniazid, phenytoin
	Antineoplastic drugs
	Doxorubicin, daunorubicin, cyclophosphamide
Bacterial	Others
Staphylococcus aureus and group A *Streptococcus*	Cyclosporine, dantrolene, mesalamine, methylsergide, procainamide, rifampin
Mycobacterium tuberculosis	Metabolic
Borrelia burgdorferi	Uremia, end stage renal disease
Streptococcus pneumoniae and *Haemophilus influenzae* type B (pre-vaccination)	Hypothyroidism
Fungal	Malignancy
Protozoal	Metastatic lymphomas
Noninfectious	s/p bone marrow transplantation
Autoimmune	Trauma
Juvenile rheumatic arthritis	Blunt or penetrating trauma to the chest
Systemic lupus erythematosus	Radiation therapy
Rheumatic fever	Post-pericardiotomy syndrome
Kawasaki disease	

[a]COVID-19, coronavirus disease of 2019.

pain, either isolated or with chest pain. Cough and low-grade fever may be present in all age groups.

On physical examination, patients may be tachypneic and tachycardic. Patients with a small or moderate pericardial effusion may have a pericardial friction rub, a high-pitched sound commonly described as crinkling paper or rubbing two pieces of sandpaper together. This sound is best heard during expiration with the patient sitting and leaning forward, with the stethoscope over the third to fourth left intercostal interspace. Patients with large effusions may have distant muffled heart sounds and do not have a rub because the pericardial and epicardial surfaces do not contact each other. Patients with large effusions may show signs and symptoms of hemodynamic compromise such as pallor, prolonged capillary refill, altered mental status, and hypotension. Evidence of cardiac tamponade may include increased pulsus paradoxus, narrowed pulse pressure, jugular venous distention, and hepatomegaly.

Increased pulsus paradoxus is an early sign of cardiac tamponade. The normal changes in the blood pressure during the respiratory cycle are exaggerated in cardiac tamponade. During inspiration, there is increased filling of the right atrium and increased capacity in the pulmonary vascular bed, resulting in decreased left-sided filling and decreased cardiac output. Clinically, this produces a difference in systolic blood pressure during inspiration and expiration that is normally <10 mmHg. In patients with cardiac tamponade, this pressure difference becomes >10 mmHg. To check for pulsus paradoxus, the patient should be seated comfortably, and the blood pressure checked manually on the brachial artery. The cuff pressure should be released until the first Korotkoff sound is heard only during expiration. Once this systolic pressure is noted, the cuff pressure should be lowered until the first Korotkoff sound is heard throughout the respiratory cycle; the difference between these two systolic pressures represents the pulsus paradoxus.

DIAGNOSTIC EVALUATION

There are no guidelines that establish diagnostic criteria for acute pericarditis in pediatrics, however the European Society of Cardiology requires the presence of two out of the following four criteria in adults: chest pain, pericardial rub, changes on electrocardiogram (ECG), and new or worsening pericardial effusion. In children, diagnosis typically is made based on chest pain in conjunction with either ECG changes, physical exam findings suggestive of pericardial effusion, or imaging evidence of pericardial inflammation. Supportive findings may include elevated inflammatory markers, such as elevated erythrocyte sedimentation rate (ESR), C-reactive protein (CRP), and white blood cell count.

There are no specific biomarkers for pericarditis but elevation in troponin I or T is helpful in confirming myopericarditis. These patients may additionally have depressed ventricular function. Elevated troponins are not associated with increased complications or worse outcomes. The yield for positive troponin in patients with a normal ECG is low. Additional studies to determine etiology may include respiratory viral panels, viral titers, blood culture, thyroid screen, rheumatologic evaluation, and assessment of renal function.

ECG is abnormal in 90% to 100% of children who present to the emergency department with pericarditis. Initially there are diffuse ST changes with ST elevations in I, II, III, aVL, aVF, and V2-V6 with ST depressions in aVR and V1 (**Figure 54-1**). The PR interval may also become depressed. Several days to 2 weeks later in the disease course, the ST and PR intervals will normalize and the T waves flatten and invert. Within 4 to 6 weeks, the ECG usually normalizes but the T wave changes can become permanent. With large effusions, the ECG will have low voltages and occasionally electrical alternans due to movement of the heart within the effusion. In patients with constrictive pericarditis, there may be low voltages and nonspecific ST changes.

The chest radiograph may be normal in acute pericarditis without a significant pericardial effusion. A larger pericardial effusion is usually necessary to result in an enlarged cardiac silhouette on chest radiography (**Figure 54-2**).

Though echocardiography can be normal patients with pericarditis, it can be helpful to diagnose complications such pericardial effusions, tamponade physiology, concurrent myocarditis with cardiac dysfunction, or constrictive pericarditis. Echocardiography will show the size and distribution of pericardial effusion (**Figure 54-3**), however may not be able to visualize loculated fluid and can underestimate the size of pericardial effusions. In cardiac tamponade,

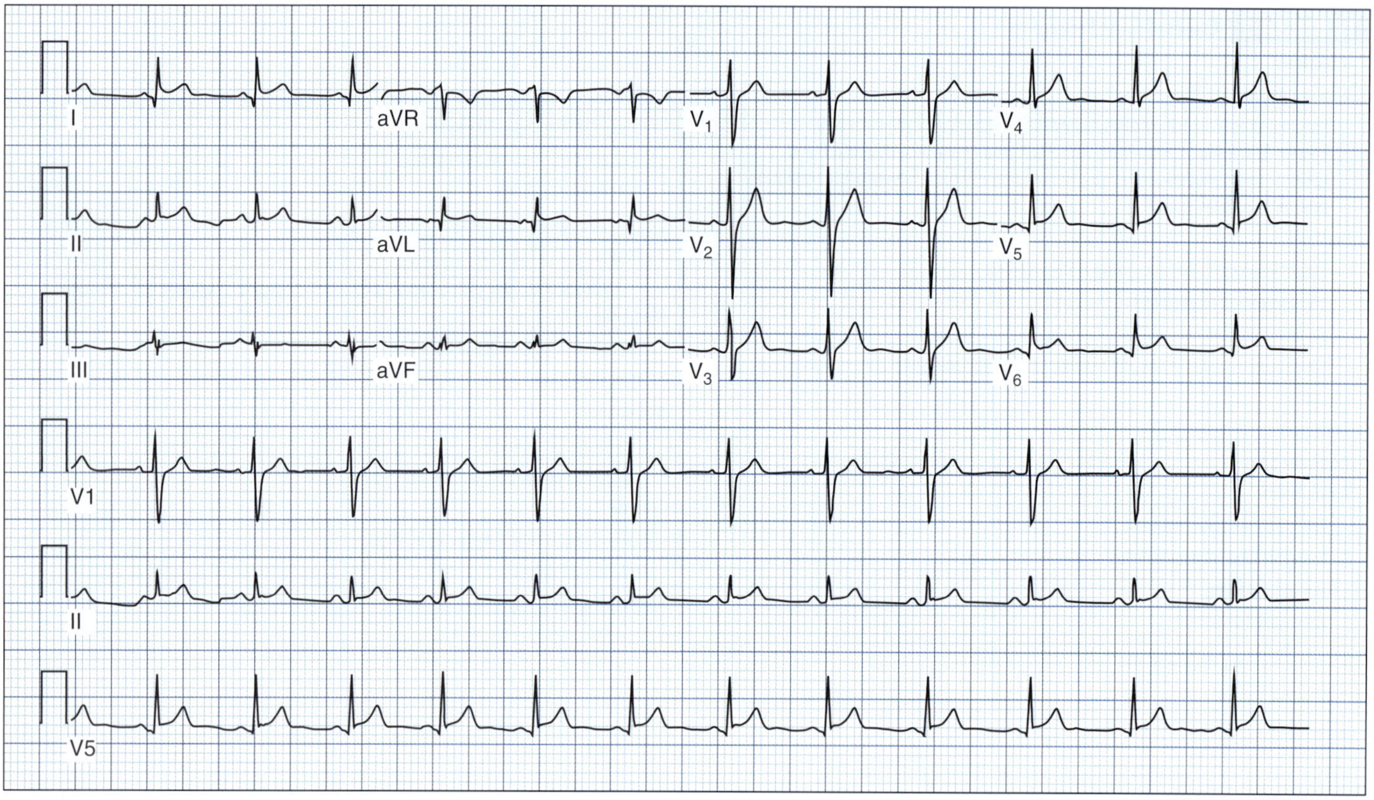

FIGURE 54-1. Electrocardiogram of a patient with acute pericarditis showing diffuse ST segment elevations in leads I, II, II and in the precordial chest leads V1-V6. There are also mild PR segment depressions seen.

there can be marked respiratory variation in peak Doppler velocity of flow across the valves, right atrial free wall collapse, or bulging of the interventricular septum toward the left ventricle. In patients with constrictive pericarditis, the echocardiogram can show pericardial thickening, and provides a method to evaluate the movement and filling of the cardiac chambers.

Chest tomography and cardiac magnetic resonance imaging (MRI) are generally not necessary in the evaluation of acute pericarditis but may be indicated with recurrent or chronic pericarditis. These tests can be helpful in the acute setting if the echocardiogram shows a loculated effusion or if pericardial thickening is suspected. Cardiac MRI can distinguish between constrictive pericarditis, restrictive cardiomyopathy, and myopericarditis.

Pericardiocentesis is generally reserved for patients with cardiac tamponade, but occasionally is performed for diagnostic purposes when purulent or malignant pericarditis is suspected or when the course of pericarditis is atypical. Tests that should be performed on the effusion include cell count with differential, protein, glucose, gram stain, acid-fast stain, triglyceride, lactate dehydrogenase, aerobic and anaerobic cultures, cultures for *Mycobacterium tuberculosis*, fungi, and viruses, and viral polymerase chain reaction.

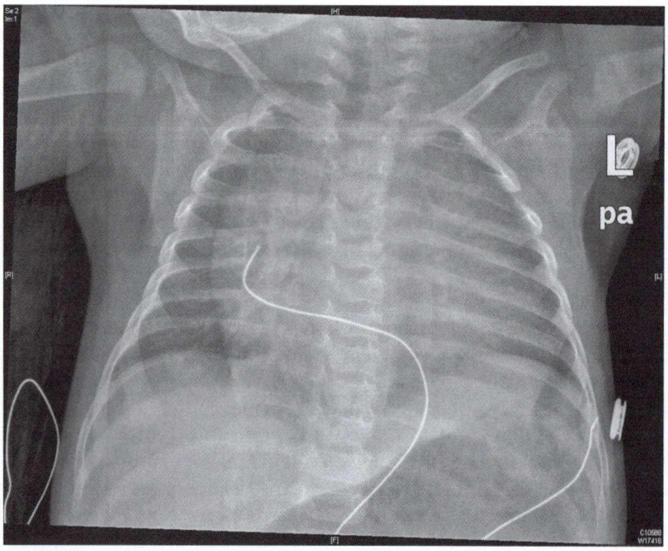

FIGURE 54-2. Chest x-ray of a patient with acute pericarditis showing an enlarged cardiac silhouette secondary to a large pericardial effusion.

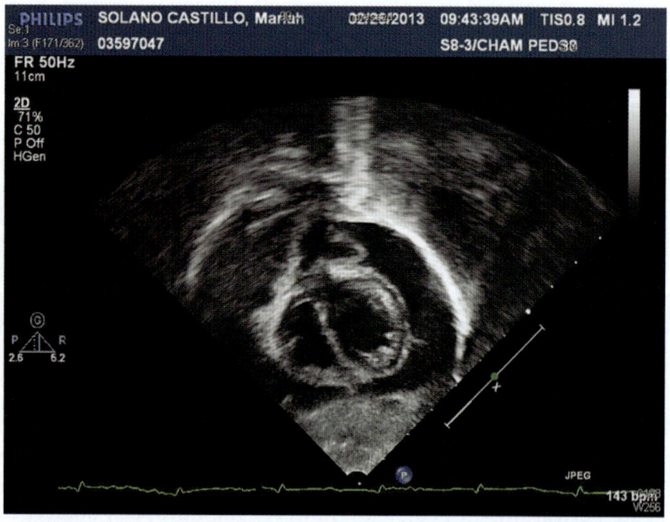

FIGURE 54-3. Echocardiogram of a patient with acute pericarditis showing a large concentric pericardial effusion.

MANAGEMENT

MEDICAL

There are no pediatric specific guidelines on the management of pericarditis and a wide practice variation exists among children's hospitals. Therefore, we recommend developing a treatment and follow-up plan in consultation with a cardiologist once pericarditis is identified. **Table 54-2** lists common medications and dosages used in treatment. Typically, patients with viral or idiopathic pericarditis respond well to oral NSAID therapy. The literature behind the use of colchicine in the pediatric population is not as robust as the adult population, however when added to the oral regimen it likely reduces the risk of a recurrent pericarditis. Corticosteroids are used less frequently in initial treatment regimens because their use has been associated with an increased risk for recurrent episodes of pericarditis.

Optimal length of treatment is not well defined, but in general the NSAID should be continued until the patient is asymptomatic and inflammatory markers have normalized, after which they are usually tapered over several weeks. Given the prolonged course, a proton pump inhibitor is useful for gastritis prophylaxis. If colchicine is used, the recommended course is 3 months. Some patients who are steroid dependent or resistant to colchicine have responded to interleukin-1β receptor antagonists. When pericarditis is secondary to another treatable cause such as an underlying autoimmune disorder (i.e., systemic lupus erythematosus) or bacterial infection (i.e., tuberculosis), treatment of the underlying disorder usually results in resolution of the pericarditis.

SURGICAL

Patients with cardiac tamponade require emergent pericardiocentesis, which can be therapeutic and diagnostic. While coordinating the procedure, consider intravenous fluid administration to support cardiac output as diastolic filling is compromised in cardiac tamponade. The complications of pericardiocentesis include cardiac perforation or injury, coronary artery laceration, cardiac arrythmias, pneumothorax or pneumopericardium, hemopericardium, aortic laceration, liver laceration, and infection. In cases of pericarditis refractory to medical management, pericardiotomy or pericardiectomy can be performed.

LIFESTYLE MODIFICATIONS

Exercise induced tachycardia and stress can exacerbate pericardial inflammation. Restricting strenuous physical activity for 1 to 3 months may minimize the risk of prolonged symptoms or recurrence.

PATIENT DISPOSITION

Patients who are clinically well with mild symptoms of pericarditis (i.e., chest pain that improves with NSAIDs, no pericardial effusion, and absence of fever) do not need to be admitted to the hospital if they have close follow-up. Patients who are clinically well but present with pericardial effusion should be admitted and started on treatment to make sure that they respond appropriately (i.e., defervesce, effusion stabilizes or improves, and chest pain resolves). Consider an intensive care unit for any patient who appears toxic or has signs of cardiac tamponade. The length of hospitalization will depend on the underlying cause of the pericarditis and response to treatment. As a general guide for discharge readiness, patients should be free from fever and chest pain, and the pericardial effusion should be resolving. Follow-up should be arranged with pediatric cardiology.

TABLE 54-2 Medications to Consider for Treatment of Acute Pericarditis in Pediatrics

Drug	Dosing
Ibuprofen	30-50 mg/kg/day divided every 8 hours; Maximum dose: 2.4 g/day
Naproxen	>2 years of age: 10 mg/kg/day divided twice daily; Maximum dose: 15 mg/kg/day
Colchicine	0.25-2 mg/day; Maximum dose of oral solution: 1.2 mg/day
Prednisone	0.25-0.5 mg/kg/day
Anakinra (interleukin-1β receptor antagonist)	1-2 mg/kg subcutaneous daily; Maximum dose: 100 mg/day

OUTCOMES

Prognosis, morbidity, and mortality depend on underlying etiology but generally are self-limited. The duration of acute pericarditis is less than 4 to 6 weeks by definition. Incessant pericarditis is present for more than 4 to 6 weeks without a period of remission. Recurrent pericarditis is defined by a symptom free interval of 4 to 6 weeks prior to new signs or symptoms of pericardial inflammation. In pediatrics, risk of recurrence has been reported up to 22% of pediatric idiopathic cases. Patients with recurrent pericarditis may have significant morbidity. Children with extra-gastroentestinal manifestations of inflammatory bowel disease and underlying rheumatologic disease such as systemic lupus erythematosus, systemic-onset juvenile idiopathic arthritis, and sarcoidosis are at higher risk for reoccurrence. Chronic pericarditis is defined by a duration of greater than 3 months.

SUGGESTED READINGS

Chiabrando JG, Bonaventura A, Vecchié A, et al. Management of acute and recurrent pericarditis: JACC State-of-the-Art Review. *J Am Coll Cardiol*. 2020;75(1):76-92.

Schwier NC, Tsui J, Perrine JA, Guidry CM, Mathew J. Current pharmacotherapy management of children and adults with pericarditis: prospectus for improved outcomes. *Pharmacotherapy*. 2021;41(12): 1041-1055.

Shakti D, Hehn R, Gauvreau K, Sundel RP, Newburger JW. Idiopathic pericarditis and pericardial effusion in children: contemporary epidemiology and management. *J Am Heart Assoc*. 2014;3(6):e001483.

Tunuguntla H, Jeewa A, Denfield SW. Acute Myocarditis and pericarditis in children. *Pediatr Rev*. 2019;40(1):14-25.

CHAPTER 55

Acute Rheumatic Fever

Katherine Dyer, DO, FAAP and Reina Patel, DO, FAAP

BACKGROUND

Acute rheumatic fever (ARF) is an inflammatory condition manifested by the nonsuppurative sequelae of a preceding group A β-hemolytic streptococcal (GAS) pharyngitis. ARF involves the heart, central nervous system, joints, and skin and is the most common cause of acquired heart disease in many regions of the world. Diagnosis of the disease relies on the identification of major and minor criteria that include clinical observations and obtaining confirmatory laboratory and imaging, an approach that has been modified since its introduction in 1944 by Jones. The greatest impact of the illness lies in its potential to cause progressive valvular heart disease, which is more likely with recurrent episodes of ARF. Secondary antibiotic prophylaxis is therefore important to minimize the likelihood of long-term sequelae including rheumatic heart disease (RHD) and reduce risk of recurrent GAS pharyngitis.

EPIDEMIOLOGY

It is well accepted that the frequency of ARF has declined in part because of the use of antibiotics to treat pharyngitis. Investigations have shown that appropriate antimicrobial therapy has led to fewer episodes of ARF in the United States and other developed countries, although the prevalence remains high in many parts of the world, especially in crowded populations in areas with lower socioeconomic resources. Endemic, high-risk areas include Asia-Pacific, Africa, and indigenous populations of Australia. Low-risk populations include Canada, Europe, and the United States. Nevertheless, sporadic outbreaks have been identified in the United States among populations at low risk. Given the frequency of ARF as well as the different clinical presentations among populations, the Jones criteria were modified in 2015 to define the two groups more precisely.

PATHOPHYSIOLOGY

Literature supports that GAS pharyngitis is rheumatogenic, and certain types of group A streptococci predispose to the development of ARF, based on the virulence of the organism. Group A streptococci with high concentrations of M-protein, a component of the cell wall, are believed to be the most virulent strains and therefore the most likely to cause ARF.

The actual pathogenetic mechanism by which GAS pharyngitis leads to ARF is still somewhat speculative. The organism adheres to the pharyngeal mucosa, with subsequent destruction of epithelial cells. The immune reaction to this interaction results in both a humoral and a cell-mediated response to streptococcal antigens of the cell membrane. These antigens mimic those of cardiac tissue, whereas M-proteins have similar antigenicity to myosin and sarcolemma, as well as cartilage and synovium. The cross-reactivity likely results in damage to these target tissues. In addition, the GAS carbohydrate components mimic antigens of cardiac valves, a possible explanation for valvular involvement in ARF. Cell-mediated involvement in the pathogenesis is supported by the presence of CD^{4+} helper cells in heart valves. It is possible that the M-protein and streptococcal pyrogenic exotoxins may act as superantigens in the immune response. A genetic basis for predisposition to development of rheumatic fever following GAS infection has been entertained for many years without definitive proof, but a 2010 report found the presence of potential rheumatic epitopes in the S2 region of human cardiac myosin.

The initial pathologic lesion in ARF is edema of the ground substance in connective tissue, with accompanying cellular infiltration of T and B lymphocytes. Degenerative deposition of eosinophils in these regions is described as fibrinoid necrosis. Although these pathologic findings are present early in the process, with the administration of anti-inflammatory therapy, they typically regress. This stage of inflammation is followed by the more chronic and pathognomonic changes known as the Aschoff body; this pathologic lesion is characterized by an area of central necrosis encircled by mononuclear and polynuclear cells.

Myocarditis is seen microscopically in ARF, with inflammatory cells noted in perivascular regions as well as near areas of Aschoff bodies. Though these changes are subclinical in many patients, other affected individuals may have pronounced heart failure in the acute phase of the disease. Pericardial inflammation is manifested as a serofibrinous reaction with pericardial fluid production. Valvular inflammation is well described, involving primarily the aortic and mitral valves. Deposition of platelet-fibrin collections is seen on the valve leaflets in the acute phase. Over many years, the leaflets may develop progressive fibrosis and contraction, as do the chordae tendineae of the mitral valve. These changes limit excursion of the valves, manifested as stenosis or a lack of coaptation of the leaflets and resultant regurgitation. The tricuspid and pulmonic valves are involved infrequently.

Joint inflammation is common in ARF, leading to the clinical manifestation of arthritis. Pathologically, a serous effusion is seen in the joint space, with inflammation of the articular surfaces; however, long-standing arthritis is not a typical sequela of the disease.

Sydenham chorea is characterized pathologically by cellular infiltration and neuronal loss of the basal ganglia, supported by findings of focal striatal enlargement by magnetic resonance imaging. Anti-basal ganglia antibodies have been demonstrated in the sera of patients with Sydenham chorea in both acute and chronic settings.

Subcutaneous nodules are composed of fibrinoid necrosis, similar to that seen in Aschoff bodies.

CLINICAL PRESENTATION

The onset of ARF occurs after a variable latent period, typically 10 to 30 days following streptococcal pharyngitis; however, many patients give no history of a preceding pharyngitis. The diagnosis is established by meeting the modified Jones criteria (**Table 55-1**). A history of appropriate therapy for streptococcal pharyngitis does not preclude the diagnosis, since ARF has occurred following GAS treatment.

Early in the disease, complaints may center on a migratory polyarthritis involving the large joints, including the knees, ankles, elbows, and wrists. Fever between 38°C and 39°C is often an accompanying sign. The cardiac examination may be notable for tachycardia at rest which is exacerbated by fever. The precordium is hyperdynamic in the face of fever-associated tachycardia, myocardial dysfunction, valvulitis with moderate mitral or aortic regurgitation, or the additive effects of mitral and aortic regurgitation producing left ventricular volume overload.

Carditis classically has been defined by auscultation of murmurs that indicate mitral and/or aortic valve regurgitation. The most common murmur is a blowing pansystolic regurgitant murmur heard best at the apex and left lower sternal border with radiation to the axilla. When the regurgitation is moderate or greater, the diastolic rumble of relative mitral stenosis (Carey Coombs murmur) is present at the apex, sometimes best heard with the patient rotated in the left lateral recumbent position using the bell of the stethoscope. High-frequency diastolic murmurs of aortic regurgitation are heard best using the diaphragm of the stethoscope with the patient seated and leaning forward, with the breath held in expiration. In patients with heart failure, an S_3 gallop is often present, heard best at the apex with the bell. A three-component

TABLE 55-1 Jones Criteria (Revised)

For patient populations with evidence of preceding Group A Streptococcal infection	
Diagnosis (initial ARF)	2 major criteria OR 1 major plus 2 minor criteria
Diagnosis (recurrent ARF)	2 major criteria OR 1 major and 2 minor OR 3 minor
Major Criteria	
Low Risk Population[a]	***Moderate and High-Risk Population***
Carditis (clinical and/or sub clinical[b])	Carditis (clinical and/or sub clinical[b])
Arthritis (polyarthritis only)	Arthritis (monoarthritis or polyarthritis; polyarthralgia[c])
Chorea	Chorea
Erythema marginatum	Erythema marginatum
Subcutaneous nodules	Subcutaneous nodules
Minor Criteria	
Low Risk Population[a]	***Moderate and High-Risk Population***
Polyarthralgia	Monoarthralgia
Fever (≥38.5°C)	Fever (≥38°C)
ESR ≥ 60 mm in first hour and/or CRP ≥3.0 mg/dL[d]	ESR ≥ 30 mm/h and/or CRP ≥3.0 mg/dL[d]
Prolonged PR interval, after accounting for age variability (unless carditis is a major criterion)	Prolonged PR interval, after accounting for age variability (unless carditis is a major criterion)

Source: Adapted from Gewitz MH, Baltimore RS, Tani LY, et al. Revision of the Jones criteria for the diagnosis of acute rheumatic fever in the era of Doppler echocardiography. A scientific statement from the American Heart Association. *Circulation.* 2015;131:1806.

ARF, acute rheumatic fever; CRP, C-reactive protein; ESR, erythrocyte sedimentation rate.

[a]Populations with ARF incidence <2 per 100,000 school-aged children (5-14 years old) or any age prevalence of rheumatic heart disease of ≤1 per 1000 population per year.

[b]Refer to Table 55-2 for echocardiographic definition.

[c]Must exclude other causes of polyarthralgia such as autoimmune, viral, or reactive arthropathies before using as a major criteria in moderate or high-risk populations. Joint manifestations can only be considered in either the major or minor categories but not both in the same patient.

[d]CRP value should be greater than upper limit of normal for laboratory. Peak ESR values should be used.

pericardial friction rub is heard in the presence of serofibrinous pericarditis, although the sound may be muted when a moderate to large effusion is present. Cardiac tamponade is extremely rare in ARF. Pulses and perfusion are well maintained, except in the unusual case of severe myocardial decompensation. Although carditis runs a spectrum of tissue involvement including pancarditis (involving the endocardium, myocardium, and pericardium), valvulitis is the most common cardiac manifestation. Subclinical valvulitis occurs when classic auscultatory findings of valvular dysfunction either are not present, or are not recognized on examination, but mitral or aortic valvulitis is noted on echocardiography/Doppler studies.

Erythema marginatum is a serpiginous, salmon-colored rash characterized by lesions with clear centers over the extremities and trunk. It is evanescent, noted more frequently during febrile episodes or after a bath or shower.

Although subcutaneous nodules were once a classic part of the description of ARF, they are now an infrequent finding, often seen in less than 5% of patients. When present, they are non-tender, knobby lesions usually palpated over the extensor surfaces of the elbows or knees, but can also occur around wrists, ankles, or spine.

Sydenham chorea is an involuntary movement disorder of the extremities and face that is exacerbated during periods of stress. Irritability and emotional lability/outbursts are common. The onset may be gradual, but the symptoms may persist for many months, making speaking or writing difficult, and thereby limiting attendance at school. The neurologic signs usually resolve over a period of months without long-term sequelae. Of note, carditis and arthritis are not typically noted in combination with chorea. In particular, when the primary manifestation of the illness is chorea, the latent period from the preceding streptococcal infection can be as long as 6 months.

DIFFERENTIAL DIAGNOSIS

The differential diagnosis of ARF is wide, given the systemic nature of its manifestations. Arthritis or polyarthralgia is present in many acute illnesses, including juvenile idiopathic (rheumatoid) arthritis, post-streptococcal arthritis, reactive arthritis, vector-borne disease such as Lyme, septic arthritis, infective endocarditis, leukemia, and sickle cell disease. Some consider post-streptococcal arthritis to be a separate entity from ARF, but others consider these two disorders to be different presentations along a common spectrum of disease. Implications for the prevention of recurrence continue to make this an important but controversial point of distinction. Additionally, in the post-SARS-CoV-2 (COVID-19) infection era, consideration should also be given to a diagnosis of acute COVID-19 or Multi-System Inflammatory Syndrome in Children (MIS-C). MIS-C has a broad clinical presentation, from mild illness to shock, includes non-specific laboratory findings supporting systemic inflammation, and may also result in carditis (although more commonly with decreased cardiac function, pericarditis or coronary involvement, rather than valvular disease) (see Chapter 107). These diagnoses can be identified by careful consideration of the constellation of history, physical exam findings, cardiac imaging, and laboratory tests, including complete blood count with smear and inflammatory markers, blood cultures, and joint aspiration where necessary.

DIAGNOSTIC EVALUATION

The diagnosis of ARF from primary streptococcal infection relies on criteria derived from the physical examination and laboratory findings. In the setting of a preceding GAS infection, patients with **2 major** manifestations or **1 major** manifestation *and* **2 minor** manifestations (Table 55-1) meet the criteria for the diagnosis of ARF. The index of suspicion for recurrent ARF should be higher in an individual with previous ARF. Diagnosis of recurrent ARF is accepted if, in the presence of a preceding streptococcal infection, **2 major**, or **1 major** *and* **2 minor** or **3 minor** manifestations are present.

Fever is present in virtually all patients with ARF and should be documented carefully during hospitalization as a marker of the inflammatory process. In addition, the erythrocyte sedimentation rate and C-reactive protein level, both nonspecific indicators of inflammation, are elevated in ARF. In a patient with chorea, however, both values might be normal, because the condition can follow the inciting event by a number of months.

TABLE 55-2 Doppler Criteria for Diagnosis of Rheumatic Valvulitis

Pathological Aortic Regurgitation (meet all 4 criteria)	Pathological Mitral Regurgitation (meet all 4 criteria)
Seen in at least 2 views	Seen in at least 2 views
Jet length ≥1 cm in at least 1 view	Jet length ≥2 cm in at least 1 view
Peak velocity >3 m/s	Peak velocity >3 m/s
Pandiastolic jet in at least 1 envelope	Pansystolic jet in at least 1 envelope

Source: Adapted from Gewitz MH, Baltimore RS, Tani LY, et al. Revision of the Jones criteria for the diagnosis of acute rheumatic fever in the era of Doppler echocardiography. A Scientific statement from the American Heart Association. *Circulation.* 2015;131:180.

In the setting of severe heart failure, the erythrocyte sedimentation rate may be within the normal range, but the C-reactive protein is usually elevated. Both values improve after the institution of anti-inflammatory therapy and are useful for following the course of the acute illness.

Laboratory tests that support the likelihood of a preceding streptococcal infection are important for establishing the diagnosis of ARF. Evidence of an antecedent GAS infection can be an elevated or rising antistreptolysin (ASO) or anti-deoxyribonuclease B (anti-DNAase B) titer, positive rapid streptococcal antigen or streptococcal throat culture. Ideally, all patients should have throat cultures to identify the presence of a GAS infection. However, because throat cultures are often negative after patients have been treated and signs of ARF may not appear until a period of time after the acute infection, streptococcal antibody tests are useful to establish a recent infection. The antistreptolysin test (ASO) identifies the presence of an antibody to streptolysin O, an extracellular product of β-hemolytic streptococci. ASO is known to rise in the first week of illness and peak 3 to 6 weeks later. There are several reference values available however ASO titers less than 250 Todd units are generally considered normal; titers of 500 Todd units or more are considered positive. Values falling between 250 and 500 units are supportive but not diagnostic of a preceding infection. Elevated titers of other serologic tests, including anti-DNAase B, anti-hyaluronidase, and anti-streptokinase suggest a preceding streptococcal infection and may be helpful when ASO titers are not definitive.

In the setting of chorea, these supportive diagnostic tests may be normal, thus, rather unhelpful, given the extended latency period between streptococcal exposure and the onset of neurologic signs.

Cardiac testing for ARF includes an electrocardiogram, which can show prolongation of the PR interval (a minor manifestation) or higher degrees of atrioventricular block, providing evidence of conduction system inflammation. Echocardiography plays a pivotal role in the assessment of a patient with presumed carditis because it can confirm the presence of mitral or aortic regurgitation by color flow Doppler interrogation of the valves, even if evidence of carditis is not picked up on clinical exam (**Table 55-2**). Use of portable echocardiography to evaluate for subclinical cases of ARF and RHD has potential benefit in endemic areas to identify patients for streptococcal prophylaxis.

RECURRENT ACUTE RHEUMATIC FEVER

The Jones criteria are intended for the first time diagnosis of ARF. The diagnosis of a recurrent bout of ARF is straightforward when the Jones criteria are met; however, the diagnosis may be elusive, given the presence of residual mitral or aortic valve disease from the first episode. In these cases, using carditis as a manifestation may not be possible in the presence of a febrile illness. In such situations, polyarthritis along with a minor criterion should be considered diagnostic, as should the presence of chorea. Given the frequency of ARF in certain populations at higher risk, additional criteria have been adopted by the Committee on Rheumatic Fever, Endocarditis, and Kawasaki Disease in an effort to capture these cases. The presence of subclinical carditis, monoarthritis, and polyarthralgia now constitute major criteria, while monoarthralgia and fever >38° are new minor categories as of 2015.

Another confounding issue is the diagnosis of poststreptococcal reactive arthritis, which tends to follow streptococcal pharyngitis by 3 to

14 days. The arthritis can be nonmigratory, unresponsive to salicylates, and persist longer than that seen with ARF. For individuals who do not explicitly meet the Jones criteria, treatment should occur if all other pertinent diagnoses have been considered and ruled out.

MANAGEMENT

All patients with the presumptive diagnosis of ARF should be hospitalized for observation and treatment until their condition stabilizes.

The therapy for ARF is predominantly supportive and preventative. The goal is to reduce inflammation, treat underlying carditis if it is hemodynamically significant, and provide secondary prophylaxis. There is not a standardized approach to managing fever, pain, and inflammation in ARF. Historically, clinicians used aspirin at a dose of 50-100 mg/kg/day divided every 6 hours as the drug of first choice. Recently, nonsteroidal anti-inflammatory (NSAID) medications have replaced aspirin as a mainstay of supportive management, usually resulting in a dramatic clinical improvement within 1 to 2 days. Naproxen, dosed at 10 to 20 mg/kg/day divided every 12 hours (max of 1000 mg per dose) for children >2 years old, is slowly becoming the preferred choice in pediatrics. These two medications have not been studied rigorously in this setting but naproxen has been found in recent pediatric studies to have less side effects including bleeding, anemia, and thrombocytopenia. Ibuprofen has also been used successfully in younger children with ARF. Regardless of NSAID choice, the anti-inflammatory medication is typically continued over several weeks and then tapered slowly. An H-2 blocker or proton pump inhibitor may be considered for children with underlying gastrointestinal concerns or those who develop gastritis while on medications for supportive management. There are limited studies available regarding the risk of intestinal side effects in otherwise healthy children on NSAID therapy, especially with short-term use. It is well established that patients who take NSAIDs frequently and/or at high doses, patients who are older than 65, have a history of stomach ulcers, take corticosteroids or blood thinners are highest risk for gastrointestinal issues.

Despite the availability of steroid therapy for the past several decades, superiority over aspirin or NSAIDs alone in reducing rheumatic heart disease has not been firmly established. An extensive meta-analysis of the treatment of rheumatic carditis failed to show a convincing superiority of steroids over NSAIDs for the reduction of rheumatic heart disease a year after the acute illness. With regard to the treatment of acute myocarditis, intravenous gamma globulin infusion has not proved to be of benefit in ARF, but a single report suggests its use may moderate the course of Sydenham chorea.

In the setting of carditis, individuals with symptoms of heart failure should be treated with diuretics under the supervision of a cardiologist, but rarely require inotropic support or afterload reduction therapy. Restraint from physical activity is mandatory; complete bed rest for several weeks-to-months was the rule for many decades. Although these restrictions are somewhat less stringent today, individuals with acute carditis should abstain from exertion and sports until the clinician is confident that the ventricular dysfunction or the degree of aortic or mitral regurgitation has stabilized, as evidenced by echocardiographic reassessments at frequent intervals. Restriction from activity is generally recommended for a time interval of 6 weeks, although natural history of disease lasts about 3 months in 90% of patients. Given the extended period needed for resolution, close communication with school teachers and childcare providers of school-aged children is necessary. If needed, home-based schooling may be considered.

In rare circumstances, acute rheumatic carditis does not respond to conventional diuretics, aggressive anti-congestive measures, anti-inflammatory therapy, or rest. Heart failure is usually the result of marked left ventricular dysfunction with accompanying mitral or aortic regurgitation. In these refractory cases, patients may benefit from care on the cardiology floor with telemetry or in the intensive care unit. Depending on the severity, cardiac surgical intervention with valvular replacement may be necessary. Continued intense medical therapy is required postoperatively until the underlying hemodynamic derangement improves.

TABLE 55-3 Discharge Criteria for Hospitalized Patients With Acute Rheumatic Fever

- Establishment or elimination of the diagnosis of ARF
- Completion of observation to confirm illness course has stabilized
- Completion of diagnostic testing to identify the severity of illness, including cardiac involvement
- Initiation of appropriate treatment for the primary GAS infection and for ARF signs and symptoms
- Institution of secondary prophylaxis regimen for prevention of subsequent GAS infection
- Education of the patient and caregivers regarding endocarditis prophylaxis
- Establishment of follow-up and communication with primary care clinician and subspecialists

Source: Reproduced with permission from Zaoutis LB, Chiang VW., eds. *Comprehensive Pediatric Hospital Medicine.*, 2nd ed. New York, NY: McGraw Hill; 2017.

ARF, acute rheumatic fever; GAS, group A streptococcal infection.

ADMISSION AND DISCHARGE CRITERIA

All patients with the presumptive diagnosis of ARF or recurrent ARF should be hospitalized. Ability to admit to a telemetry unit is preferred, in the case that carditis is identified. Discharge criteria are summarized in **Table 55-3**. Special consideration should be given to detailed communication with primary care physicians at time of discharge to ensure continuation of care, especially given the need for monthly secondary prophylaxis and potential subspecialist care coordination.

CONSULTATION

Cardiology subspecialists are routinely involved in the initial evaluation and management. They are also part of the long-term follow-up of patients after discharge. For patients presenting with chorea, Neurology subspecialists are often involved. Consider Infectious Disease and/or Rheumatology consultation in patients with recurrent acute rheumatic fever, difficult to control arthritis, or those with seemingly elusive diagnoses.

SPECIAL CONSIDERATIONS

PRIMARY PREVENTION

The prevention of ARF is based on the prompt treatment of GAS pharyngitis, the only infection known to cause ARF. Positive throat swabs for rapid antigen testing or culture for GAS in patients with pharyngitis indicate the need for antibiotic therapy. In developed countries, where the prevalence of ARF is low, a 10-day course of oral penicillin V is the routine treatment of documented GAS pharyngitis (**Table 55-4**). Many pediatric clinicians in the United States prescribe amoxicillin as an alternative. Despite reports of scattered development of resistance of GAS, penicillin is still the first-line agent for prevention of ARF. A single intramuscular injection of benzathine penicillin is recommended in areas with a high prevalence of rheumatic fever to ensure compliance. Mass prophylaxis has been implemented at military bases, successfully aborting outbreaks of ARF. Efforts to create a vaccine that targets rheumatogenic strains of group A streptococci have been underway, but there are no signs of a vaccine on the immediate horizon.

Repeat throat culture is not necessary in patients who have received adequate treatment. Despite completion of appropriate therapy, approximately 20% of patients with resolved pharyngitis may continue to test positive for group A streptococci in the throat. However, the bacteria lose

TABLE 55-4 Primary Prevention of Rheumatic Fever (Treatment of Streptococcal Tonsillopharyngitis)

Penicillins							
Antibiotic	Penicillin V (phenoxy methyl penicillin) (oral)		Amoxicillin (oral)		Benzathine penicillin G (intramuscular)		
Dosage	≤27 kg: 250 mg 2-3 times daily >27 kg, adolescents, adults: 500 mg 2-3 times daily	OR	50 mg/kg once daily (maximum dose 1 g)	OR	≤27 kg: 600,000 U >27 kg: 1,200,000 U		
Duration	10 days		10 days		Once		
Rating	IB		IB		IB		
For individuals with penicillin allergy							
Antibiotic	Narrow-spectrum cephalosporin[a] (cephalexin, cefadroxil) (oral)		Clindamycin (oral)		Azithromycin (oral)		Clarithromycin (oral)
Dosage	Variable	OR	20 mg/kg per day divided in 3 doses (maximum 1.8 g/d)	OR	12 mg/kg once daily (maximum 500 mg)	OR	15 mg/kg per day divided in 2 doses (maximum 250 mg/dose)
Duration	10 days		10 days		5 days		10 days
Rating	IB		IIaB		IIaB		IIaB

Source: Adapted from Gerber MA, Baltimore RS, Eaton CB, et al. Prevention of rheumatic fever and treatment of acute streptococcal pharyngitis: a scientific statement from the American Heart Association Rheumatic Fever, Endocarditis and Kawasaki Disease Committee of the Council on Cardiovascular Disease in the Young, the Interdisciplinary Council on Functional Genomics and Translational Biology, and the Interdisciplinary Council on Quality of Care Outcomes Research: endorsed by the American Academic of Pediatrics. *Circulation.* 2009; 119:1541.

Rating indicates classification of recommendations and level of evidence (LOE) (i.e.: IB indicates class I, LOE B).

[a]Avoid in patients with immediate (type I) hypersensitivity to penicillin.

M-proteins and virulence after treatment. In low-resource settings, once-daily treatment with amoxicillin was shown to be non-inferior to twice daily penicillin V dosing in eradicating GAS in children with pharyngitis.

SECONDARY PREVENTION

All patients with ARF should receive long-term therapy to prevent the recurrence of infection (**Table 55-5**). With regard to long-term prophylaxis, the intramuscular administration of benzathine penicillin every 3 to 4 weeks is preferred, although oral penicillin twice daily is an acceptable alternative. Keeping in mind that true penicillin allergies are rare, in this setting clindamycin is a reasonable alternative.

The risk of a first episode of ARF following untreated streptococcal pharyngitis is 1% to 3%; however, the risk of recurrent attacks of ARF with subsequent streptococcal infections increases dramatically to as high as 50%. Individuals manifesting carditis with the first attack of ARF are at significant risk for recurrent carditis during subsequent episodes, so prophylaxis is particularly critical in this group. Recommendations regarding the duration of prophylaxis have changed over the past half century. Previously, all patients were advised to take penicillin prophylaxis for life; however, if there is no carditis during the episode of rheumatic fever, current recommendations suggest discontinuing prophylaxis treatment 5 years after the last episode of ARF or after the age of 21 years, whichever is longer. If carditis is present but there is no residual heart disease, prophylaxis is recommended for 10 years since the last episode or after the age of 21 years, whichever is longer. If carditis is present and there is residual heart disease (valvular disease), prophylaxis is recommended for at least 10 years after the last episode or until age 40 years, whichever is longer; lifetime prophylaxis may be recommended if the individual is regularly exposed to populations with a high prevalence of streptococcal infections, such as teachers or daycare workers who work closely with children. In individuals with recurrence of ARF, the boundaries for prophylaxis should be extended, and the frequency of benzathine penicillin administration may need to be increased to every 3 weeks as protection wanes into the 4th week.

TABLE 55-5 Secondary Prevention of Rheumatic Fever (Prevention of Recurrent Attacks)

Antibiotic	Benzathine penicillin G (intramuscular)		Penicillin V (oral)		Sulfadiazine (oral)
Dosage	≤27 kg: 600,000 U every 4 weeks[a] >27 kg: 1,200,000 U every 4 weeks[a]	OR	250 mg twice daily	OR	≤27 kg: 0.5 g once daily >27 kg: 1.0 g once daily
Rating	IA		IB		IB
For individuals with penicillin and sulfadiazine allergy					
Antibiotic	Macrolide or azalide (oral)				
Dosage	Variable				
Rating	IC				

Source: Adapted from Gerber MA, Baltimore RS, Eaton CB, et al. Prevention of rheumatic fever and treatment of acute streptococcal pharyngitis: a Scientific statement from the American Heart Association Rheumatic Fever, Endocarditis and Kawasaki Disease Committee of the Council on Cardiovascular Disease in the Young, the Interdisciplinary Council on Functional Genomics and Translational Biology, and the Interdisciplinary Council On Quality of Care Outcomes Research: endorsed by the American Academy of Pediatrics. *Circulation.* 2009; 119:1541.

Rating indicates classification of recommendations and level of evidence (i.e.: IA indicates class I, LOE A).

[a]In high incidence populations, recommendation is to administer every 3 weeks.

TERTIARY PREVENTION

Tertiary prevention is aimed at managing individuals with decompensatory heart failure and other consequences of RHD to limit morbidity. Medical intervention includes care of heart failure, stroke, arrhythmias, and infective endocarditis. Surgical intervention includes valvular dilation, repair, or replacement; note that tissue grafts in children do often require repeat surgery within a few years. Valvular surgery also requires lifelong anticoagulation therapy with close monitoring.

PREVENTION OF ENDOCARDITIS

In patients with rheumatic heart disease, chemoprophylaxis for endocarditis for procedures such as dental work is not recommended unless the patient falls into a high-risk category by virtue of prior mechanical valve placement or a documented episode of subacute bacterial endocarditis (SBE).

KEY POINTS

- Although less common than in previous decades, ARF continues to affect children, despite the availability of therapy that could all but eliminate the presumed inciting agent, GAS.
- The diagnosis of ARF requires application of the 2015 modified Jones criteria, after which treatment of the streptococcal disease and sequelae is instituted.
- Doppler echocardiography should be performed in all suspected cases of ARF to identify the presence of subclinical valvulitis, typically mitral or aortic regurgitation.
- Long-term penicillin prophylaxis is mandatory to prevent recurrent streptococcal pharyngitis and the likelihood of episodes of recurrent ARF. Successful reduction of recurrent ARF minimizes the risk for hemodynamically significant rheumatic heart disease in the ensuing two-to-three decades.
- Anti-inflammatory therapy ameliorates the arthritis associated with ARF. Treatments vary but NSAIDs such as naproxen or ibuprofen are now more commonly used in place of aspirin due to fewer side effects. Steroids are not commonly used. The natural history of ARF symptomatology is 3 months, regardless of supportive management.
- Rest and cardiac anti-congestive medications are the mainstays of treatment for aortic or mitral carditis, which often persists for several months and should be trended by echocardiogram before return to exertional activities.
- Small outbreaks of ARF were reported in the United States in the last 2 decades of the 20th century, and the incidence remains high among children of Polynesian descent in Australia, Hawaii, and New Zealand. Cardiac screening of children with presumed ARF or RHD in endemic areas using portable echocardiographic units may better target those who would benefit from treatment to prevent recurrent episodes of ARF and is the subject of continued discussion.
- Efforts continue to create a vaccine that targets the rheumatogenic strains of group A streptococci.

SUGGESTED READINGS

Auala T, Zavale BG, Mbakwem AÇ, Mocumbi AO. Acute rheumatic fever and rheumatic heart disease: highlighting the role of Group A Streptococcus in the global burden of cardiovascular disease. *Pathogens.* 2022;11(5).

Bradley-Hewitt T, Longenecker CT, Nkomo V, et al. Trends and presentation patterns of acute rheumatic fever hospitalizations in the United States. *Cardiol Young.* 2019;29(11):1387-1390.

de Loizaga SR, Beaton AZ. Rheumatic fever and rheumatic heart disease in the United States. *Pediatr Ann.* 2021;50(3).

Gewitz MH, Baltimore RS, Tani LY, et al. Revision of the Jones criteria for the diagnosis of acute rheumatic fever in the era of Doppler echocardiography. A Scientific statement from the American Heart Association. *Circulation.* 2015;131:1806.

Gerber MA, Baltimore RS, Eaton CB, et al. Prevention of rheumatic fever and treatment of acute streptococcal pharyngitis: a scientific statement from the American Heart Association Rheumatic Fever, Endocarditis and Kawasaki Disease Committee of the Council on Cardiovascular Disease in the Young, the Interdisciplinary Council on Functional Genomics and Translational Biology, and the Interdisciplinary Council on Quality of Care Outcomes Research: endorsed by the American Academic of Pediatrics. *Circulation.* 2009; 119:1541.

Kimberlin DW, Barnett ED, Lynfield R, Sawyer MH. Group A Streptococcal Infections. In: *Red Book 2021-2024 Report of the Committee on Infectious Diseases.* 32nd ed. American Academy of Pediatrics; 2021:694-707.

Marijon E, Celermajer DS, Tafflet M, et al. Rheumatic heart disease screening by echocardiography. *Circulation.* 2009;120(8):663-668.

SECTION E
Dermatology

CHAPTER 56 Petechiae and Purpura

Leah Jones, MD and Kayla Heller, MD, MHPE

INTRODUCTION

Petechial and purpuric rashes can be a concerning presentation for parents and clinicians alike. Many underlying etiologies may contribute to petechial and purpuric rashes, and pediatric hospitalists must be able to differentiate between life-threatening etiologies, such as meningococcemia, and more benign conditions, such as viral rashes. A thorough history, physical exam, and laboratory tests are essential tools that enable hospitalists to evaluate, diagnose, and manage patients with petechiae or purpura.

Petechiae and purpura are hemorrhages seen in the skin or mucous membranes. Petechiae are nonblanching, pinpoint areas of hemorrhage that are less than 2 mm in diameter. Purpura are nonblanching hemorrhages that are greater than 2 mm in diameter that may result from extravascular, intravascular, or vascular processes. Nonpalpable purpuric lesions develop from extravascular and intravascular phenomena, whereas palpable purpura result from a vascular process. Purpura fulminans is a progressive condition in which cutaneous infarctions occur and result in extensive skin necrosis.

PATHOPHYSIOLOGY

Petechiae and purpura may develop through a variety of pathophysiologic mechanisms that interfere with the complex process of hemostasis **Table 56-1**. Thrombocytopenia, abnormal platelet function, von Willebrand factor defects, and clotting factor deficits may disrupt hemostasis and result in petechiae and purpura. Infection, inflammation, and mechanical trauma disrupt vascular integrity and contribute to the development of petechiae and purpura. For example, trauma from increased intravascular pressure may lead to endothelial injury and subsequent petechiae or purpura; coughing or vomiting are common causes of endothelial trauma. Purpura fulminans typically occurs in the setting of bacterial sepsis and disseminated intravascular coagulopathy (DIC). Intrinsically abnormal vascular components, such as collagen defects in connective tissue disorders, may predispose some patients to petechial and purpuric lesions as well.

TRAUMATIC PETECHIAE

In otherwise healthy children, petechiae occur occasionally on the face and chest after vigorous coughing or vomiting and in dependent areas after standing in place or engaging in vigorous physical activity for long periods. **Figure 56-1** illustrates postictal petechiae. In hospitalized children, traumatic petechiae may result from medical intervention, such as with vascular access, tourniquet use for blood draws, or blood pressure monitoring. These lesions are benign and are not necessarily associated with any underlying disease process.

VASCULAR PETECHIAE AND PURPURA

Vascular petechiae and purpura develop when an inflammatory process involves the vessel wall, resulting in vasculitis. Leukocytoclastic vasculitis (LCV) is mediated by immune complex formation and fibrin deposition in the vascular basement membrane zone; subsequently, there is complement activation and an influx of neutrophils. LCV and associated inflammation lead to vessel destruction and result in hemorrhagic papules and nodules referred to as palpable purpura. Lesions tend to occur in angulated and starburst patterns conforming to vessel configuration in affected areas.

TABLE 56-1 Pathophysiology of Purpura

Extravascular
Trauma
Accidental
Nonaccidental (iatrogenic, self-induced, abuse)
Defective collagen synthesis
Nutritional deficiency (vitamin C, protein, calorie)
Hereditary disorders (Ehlers-Danlos syndrome)
Intravascular
Thrombocytopenia
Autoimmune thrombocytopenic purpura
Systemic lupus erythematosus
Marrow failure (leukemia, lymphoma, aplastic anemia)
Drug induced
Infection and disseminated intravascular coagulation
Hereditary coagulation defects
Factor VIII or IX deficiency or dysfunction
Vascular
Small-vessel leukocytoclastic vasculitis
Henoch-Schönlein purpura
Drug induced
Collagen vascular disease (systemic lupus erythematosus)
Medium-sized arteritis
Polyarteritis nodosa
Lymphocytic vasculitis
Progressive pigmented purpuric dermatosis
Autoimmune (Sjögren syndrome, drug reaction)

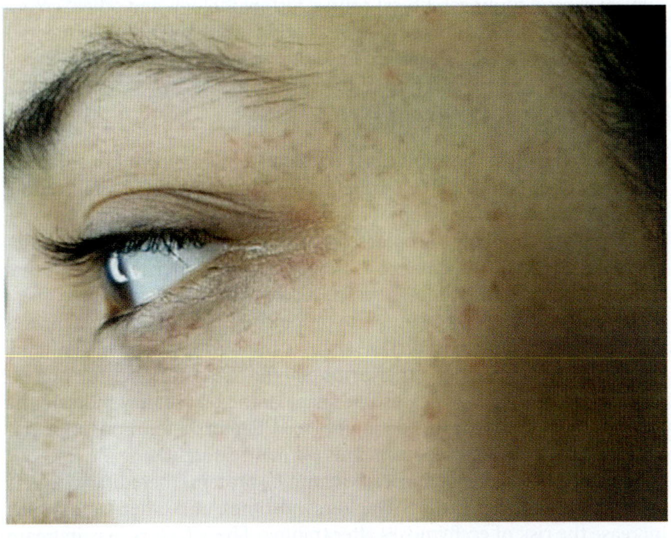

FIGURE 56-1. Postictal periorbital petechiae. (Reproduced with permission from Wali MA, MG. Postictal periorbital petechiae. *Can J Neurol Sci*. 2018;45(1):92, Figure 1.)

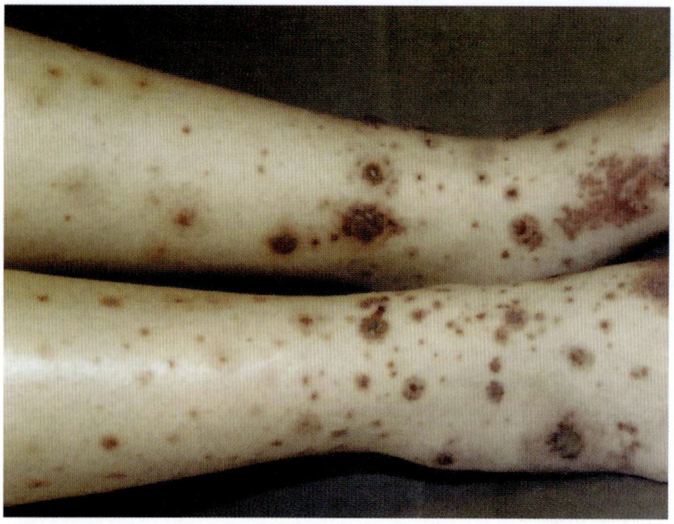

FIGURE 56-2. Henoch-Schönlein purpura.

Infectious agents, medications, autoimmune disorders, and malignancies may trigger LCV. Many drugs have been implicated as inciting factors of LCV with antibiotics, nonsteroidal anti-inflammatory drugs, anticonvulsants, and thiazide diuretics being most common. Hypersensitivity vasculitis may also be triggered by infections with hepatitis B and C and streptococcal species. Infectious agents (e.g., Rocky Mountain spotted fever, meningococcemia) may invade and damage the vascular endothelium directly and prompt leukocyte invasion. Purpura associated with infectious agents may be nonpalpable (related to DIC and sepsis), palpable (due to infectious vasculitis), or both.

Henoch-Schönlein purpura (HSP) is the most common primary systemic vasculitis process in children, and usually affects individuals between 3 and 10 years of age. In HSP, a small-vessel LCV typically results in palpable purpuric lesions less than 1 cm in diameter on the extensor surfaces of the arms and legs, buttocks, cheeks, and ears. Although early lesions may appear urticarial, confluent lesions may develop and produce areas with larger purpura, bullae, necrosis, and ulceration (**Figure 56-2**). In addition to palpable purpura, patients also often present with abdominal pain, arthralgias/arthritis, and renal involvement.

LCV in HSP involves small dermal blood vessels, usually postcapillary venules. A normal hemoglobin, platelet count, and coagulation studies may help differentiate HSP from disorders causing intravascular purpura. Further laboratory workup may include serum chemistries, stool guaiac testing, abdominal imaging, urinalysis, and kidney biopsy. Typical clinical findings, clinical course, histopathology, and other screening laboratory studies are useful in excluding lupus and other connective tissue disorders. HSP is discussed in greater detail in Chapter 149.

EXTRAVASCULAR PURPURA

Trauma is the most common cause of extravascular purpura in children. Nonblanching, nonpalpable purple patches following accidental trauma are usually located over bony prominences such as the knees, elbows, extensor surfaces of the lower legs, forehead, nose, and chin. Ecchymoses are large, confluent subcutaneous hemorrhages, greater than 1 cm, that are caused by ruptured blood vessels; ecchymoses are generally consistent with generalized bruising. The presence of purpura or ecchymoses on protected or unexposed sites, such as the buttocks, spine, genitalia, upper thighs, and upper inner arms, should raise concern for nonaccidental trauma. In some cases, the shape of the bruise may indicate the type of object used to inflict an injury (see Chapter 35 for more information on cutaneous injuries suspicious for maltreatment).

Scars, nutritional deficiencies (vitamin C, protein), hereditary defects in collagen synthesis (Ehlers-Danlos syndrome), and other factors may increase the risk of ecchymoses after trauma. These factors may increase skin fragility and decrease the tensile strength of fat and other perivascular tissues in the dermis. Children with hereditary deficiency or dysfunction of coagulation factors, most commonly factor VIII or IX, bruise easily but do not commonly develop purpura.

INTRAVASCULAR PURPURA

Intravascular purpura results from disorders that interfere with normal coagulation. In severe cases, bleeding may occur in the joints, deep soft tissues, kidneys, gastrointestinal tract, central nervous system, and other viscera. Disorders associated with intravascular purpura may result from abnormalities in platelet quantity or function, as well as from coagulation factor deficiencies. Disorders associated with intravascular purpura include autoimmune thrombocytopenic purpura, acute leukemia with thrombocytopenia, aplastic anemia, sepsis with DIC, and various coagulation factor deficiencies.

Primary immune thrombocytopenic purpura (ITP) is the most common type of intravascular purpura in previously healthy children. This condition was previously termed idiopathic thrombocytopenic purpura. Patients typically present 2 to 4 weeks after a viral illness with petechiae and purpura after minimal or no trauma (**Figure 56-3**). Occult blood may be detected in the stool or urine, but clinically significant hemorrhage is rare. Platelet counts may decrease to $<10{,}000/mm^3$ for several weeks but usually return to normal within 4 to 6 weeks. Other cell lines are unaffected, and patients appear well without fever or other systemic symptoms. Antiplatelet antibodies and thrombocytopenia may also develop in other less common disorders, including systemic lupus erythematosus, leukemia, lymphoma, and drug reactions. Other heritable coagulation defects may also be associated with nonpalpable purpura (**Figure 56-4**).

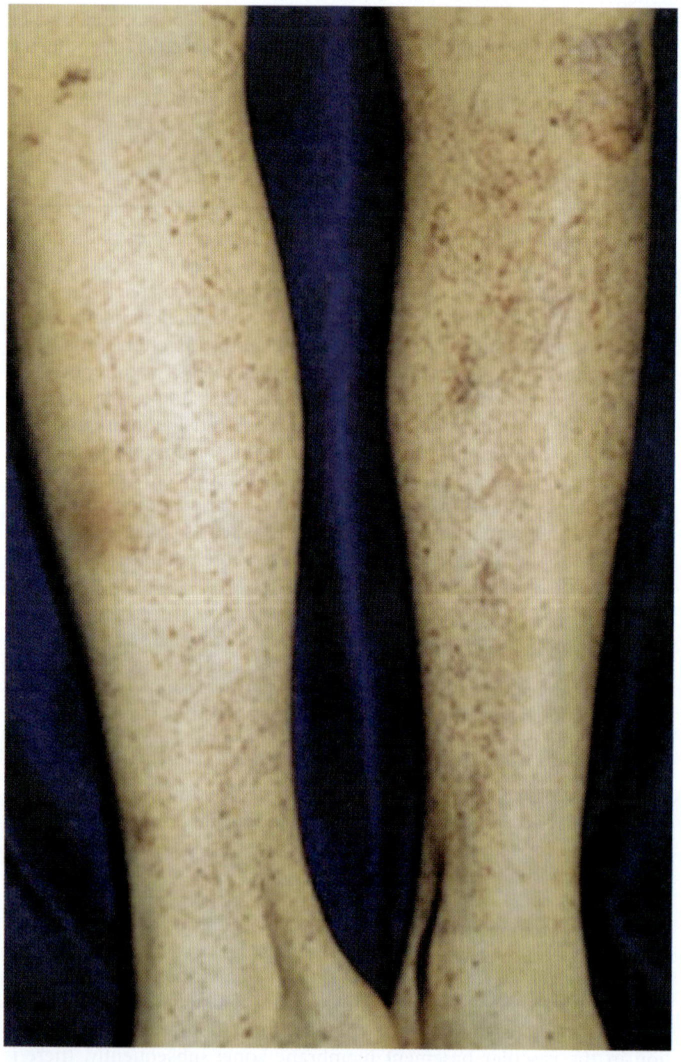

FIGURE 56-3. Immune thrombocytopenic purpura.

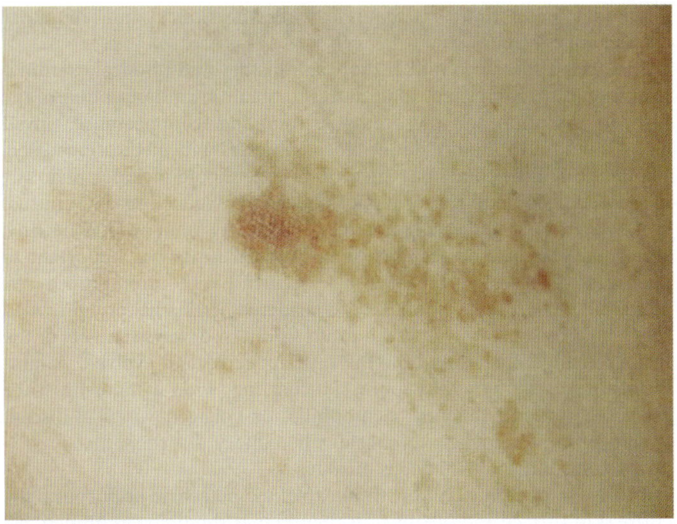

FIGURE 56-4. Pigmented purpura.

PURPURA FULMINANS

Purpura fulminans is the cutaneous manifestation of sepsis and DIC and is characterized by rapidly progressive hemorrhages that may cover large areas of skin (**Figure 56-5**). Hemorrhage into multiple organs may also occur. Purpura fulminans is associated with ischemia and large areas of necrosis can develop in patients who survive. In healthy children, meningococcal and Rocky Mountain spotted fever infections are probably the most common causes of purpura fulminans. *Streptococcus pneumoniae*, *Haemophilus influenzae*, and *Staphylococcus aureus* are common causes of sepsis in children with asplenia or splenic dysfunction. Several other bacterial, viral, and fungal organisms may lead to purpura fulminans in immunocompromised patients. Finally, DIC and purpura fulminans may be associated with acquired or inherited protein C or protein S deficiency after benign childhood infections such as varicella.

CLINICAL PRESENTATION

Key information from the history (**Table 56-2**) and physical examination (**Table 56-3**) can help determine the most likely cause of petechiae or purpura and direct further evaluation and management.

The anatomic location of skin lesions may suggest certain disease processes but often does not definitively determine diagnosis. In general, petechiae solely above the nipple line suggest a benign cause such as vomiting or coughing. These Valsalva-like maneuvers cause spikes in intravascular pressure in the venous system of the head and neck. Lesions primarily on the buttocks and lower extremities are suggestive of Henoch-Schönlein purpura. Lesions in a stocking-glove or generalized distribution are more concerning for bacterial disease, although viruses may also give rise to this pattern; for instance, a glove-and-stocking distribution may occur in the setting of parvovirus B19 infections (**Figure 56-6**).

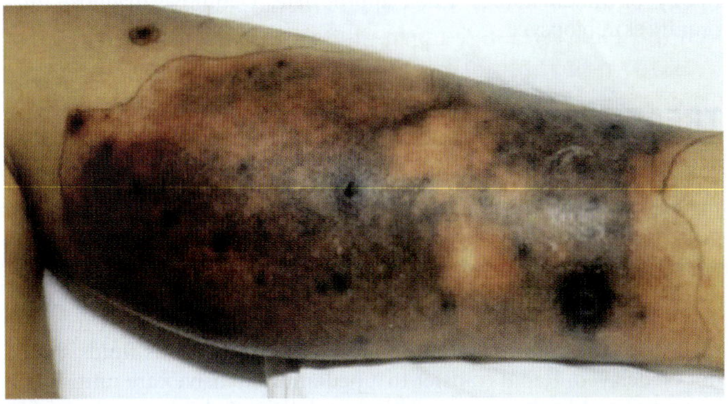

FIGURE 56-5. Purpura fulminans.

TABLE 56-2 Focused History

Characteristic	Questions
Onset and duration of lesions	Acute? Rapidly progressing? Recurrent or chronic?
Location of the lesions	Only above the nipple line? Only on the buttocks and lower extremities? In a stocking-glove distribution? Generalized? Involving the mucous membranes?
Predisposing factors	Coughing? Vomiting? Recent trauma? Recent illnesses such as an upper respiratory infection? Bloody diarrhea? Medications?
Systemic signs or symptoms	Fever? Irritability? Lethargy?
Review of systems	Headache? Stiff neck? Bleeding from other sites such as epistaxis or per rectum? Darkened urine? Joint pain or swelling? Abdominal pain? Bone pain? Myalgias?
Past medical history	Immunization status? History of prolonged bleeding?
Birth history for neonates	Was the mother ill? Did the mother have any medical conditions such as pre-eclampsia or lupus? Was the mother taking any medications?
Family history	Bleeding disorders? Siblings with conditions such as neonatal thrombocytopenia?

TABLE 56-3 Directed Physical Examination

System	Physical Examination Findings
Vital signs	Febrile? Hypotensive?
General	Well or toxic appearing? Irritable? Lethargic?
HEENT	Bulging fontanelle? Pupils equal and reactive? Photophobia? Palatal petechiae? Erythematous oropharynx? Tonsillar exudates?
Neck	Nuchal rigidity? Kernig or Brudzinski signs?
Cardiovascular	New murmur? Capillary refill and extremity perfusion?
Abdomen	Hepatomegaly or splenomegaly? Tenderness?
Musculoskeletal	Joint swelling? Joint pain on movement?
Neurologic	Mental status? Focal findings?
Skin	Location of the lesions (e.g., At the site of the blood pressure cuff? Above the nipple line only? On the buttocks and lower extremities primarily? In a stocking-glove distribution or generalized?)
	Characteristics of the lesions (e.g., Are the lesions palpable?) Quantity of lesions present?

HEENT, head, ears, eyes, nose, and throat.

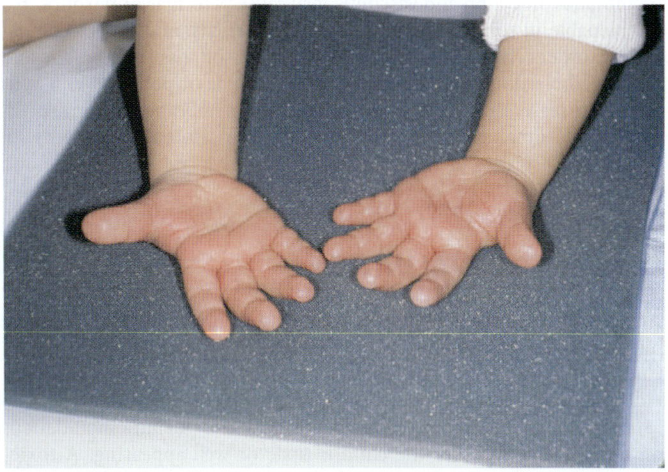

FIGURE 56-6. Papular purpura in parvovirus B19 infection. (From Shah BR, Mahajan P, Amodio J, Lucchesi M. *Atlas of Pediatric Emergency Medicine*. 3rd ed. New York, NY: McGraw Hill; 2019, Figure 3.73. Reproduced with permission from photo contributor: Binita R. Shah, MD.)

TABLE 56-4 Causes of Petechiae and Purpura

General Mechanism	Categories	Examples
Disrupted vascular integrity	Infection	Bacterial (meningococcemia, pneumococcal or *Haemophilus influenzae* sepsis, group A streptococcal infections)
		Viral (adenovirus, enteroviruses, influenza A virus, Epstein-Barr virus, parvovirus B19)
		Rickettsial (Rocky Mountain spotted fever)
	Vasculitis	Henoch-Schönlein purpura, Kawasaki disease, systemic lupus erythematosus
	Mechanical	Trauma (accidental, nonaccidental, or birth related), coughing, vomiting
	Abnormal vascular components	Collagen vascular disorders (Ehlers-Danlos syndrome), vitamin C deficiency (scurvy)
Thrombocytopenia	Decreased platelet production	Leukemia, aplastic anemia, medications (sulfonamides, carbamazepine, valproic acid), vitamin B_{12} or folate deficiency
	Increased platelet destruction	Idiopathic thrombocytopenic purpura, hemolytic uremic syndrome, thrombotic thrombocytopenic purpura
	Splenic sequestration	Hypersplenism, consumptive hemangioma (Kasabach-Merritt syndrome)
Platelet dysfunction	Hereditary	Bernard-Soulier syndrome, Glanzmann thrombasthenia, storage pool disease
	Acquired	Medications (aspirin, nonsteroidal anti-inflammatory drugs), uremia
Coagulation defects	Hereditary	Factor deficiencies, factors VIII and IX most commonly (hemophilia A and B); von Willebrand disease; fibrinogen disorders
	Acquired	Liver disease, vitamin K deficiency, medications (heparin, warfarin), disseminated intravascular coagulopathy, clotting factor inhibitors

Note: Some causes may result in petechiae or purpura by more than one mechanism.

DIFFERENTIAL DIAGNOSIS

As discussed, several different pathophysiologic mechanisms can cause petechiae or purpura, (**Table 56-4**). The clinical manifestations of petechiae or purpura vary according to the underlying defect. Thrombocytopenia and abnormal platelet function typically result in petechiae, ecchymoses, and persistent bleeding from superficial cuts and mucosal membranes. Infection and vasculitis may cause petechiae or purpura that are palpable in some cases. Clotting factor deficits, and other coagulation disorders, typically cause hemarthroses, soft tissue bleeding, and prolonged bleeding, but may also cause petechiae or purpura. Von Willebrand disease usually manifests as mucosal membrane bleeding, postsurgical bleeding, and menorrhagia, but it can also be associated with petechiae. Disorders of vascular fragility can give rise to petechiae and purpura as well.

DIAGNOSTIC EVALUATION

Any child who presents with petechia or purpura requires a complete history, review of systems, family history, and physical examination. Cutaneous finding and signs and symptoms of systemic illness may provide diagnostic clues to the underlying etiology.

The initial evaluation of a child with petechiae or purpura should focus on determining whether the child is toxic or well appearing. A toxic-appearing patient with fever, headache, hypotension, and diffuse purpura requires immediate evaluation and treatment for septicemia; DIC must be considered in this clinical scenario. Immediate cardiovascular and respiratory support, and prompt initiation of therapy (empirical antibiotics, bolus fluids) is required while the clinical and laboratory assessment continues.

In a well-appearing child, a thorough history and physical examination should be completed. In addition to obtaining a description of the rash, its evolution and the events surrounding its appearance, physicians should also inquire about recent illnesses and medications used. Exploration of the child's past medical history should include previously diagnosed coagulation disorders or collagen vascular diseases, unusual diet, weight loss, bone pain, anemia, joint laxity, poor wound healing, abnormal scarring, or easy bruising. Surgical history is important to determine if excessive bleeding has occurred with prior procedures. Nonaccidental trauma should be considered if the history provided seems inconsistent with physical exam findings, or key elements of the history change, including how the rash appeared and evolved. A family history of skin fragility, poor skin healing, wide disfiguring scars, increased bruising, anemia, hemophilia, or collagen vascular disease should prompt clinicians to consider hereditary disorders that predispose to bleeding and cutaneous purpura.

In a well-appearing child with unexplained petechiae or purpura, the entire skin surface and the mucous membranes should be examined. All findings should be carefully documented. Bruises in unusual shapes that may suggest nonaccidental trauma should prompt a thorough evaluation for other signs of occult physical trauma and child abuse; such cutaneous findings should be photographed.

Children presenting with petechiae and purpura often warrant a complete blood count (CBC), including a platelet count and white blood cell count (WBC) with differential. A peripheral blood smear, partial thromboplastin time (PTT), and prothrombin time (PT) may also be helpful.

Children who present with fever and petechiae or purpura warrant immediate attention because this can be a medical emergency. In addition to the initial screening laboratory tests mentioned above, a blood culture and cerebrospinal fluid (CSF) studies, including cell counts, glucose, protein, Gram stain, and culture, should be considered. If DIC is suspected, blood studies should be obtained to evaluate for fibrinogen and fibrin degradation products, including a D-dimer assay. If infection by group A-hemolytic streptococcus is suspected, a rapid streptococcal test and/or culture of the oropharynx is indicated. Testing for viruses, such as adenovirus and influenza, may be indicated depending on the level of clinical suspicion. Other studies such as enteroviral polymerase chain reaction assay on CSF or Rocky Mountain spotted fever antibody titers may be helpful in some settings. If a patient has multiple abnormalities on CBC, evaluation of a peripheral blood smear by a hematologist or pathologist for conditions such as leukemia is indicated.

If the child does not have a fever, does not appear acutely ill, and suspicion for an acute infection is low, the evaluation should be directed by the clinical scenario. See **Table 56-5** for suggested studies to work up various causes.

When the cause of cutaneous bleeding is not apparent, a CBC and coagulation studies can help exclude intravascular purpura. When indicated, specific quantitative and functional coagulation factor studies should be performed. Additional targeted diagnostic evaluation may be enhanced with subspecialty involvement, such as dermatology, hematology, or rheumatology when appropriate. Definitive diagnosis may require skin biopsy.

TREATMENT AND MANAGEMENT

Petechiae and purpura are typically addressed by treating the underlying cause. In most instances when hospitalists are likely to encounter petechia and purpura (e.g., associated with viral illness, coughing episodes, HSP), no specific treatment is required; supportive care may be all that is indicated. Conversely, when petechiae or purpura occur in a very ill appearing child with concerning vital signs, aggressive management with the administration of antibiotics intravenous fluids should not be delayed. Rapid transfer to a pediatric intensive care unit should be prioritized in these cases. This population of children requires frequent monitoring of vital signs, mental status, and respiratory status,

TABLE 56-5 Evaluation of Petechiae and Purpura

Condition Suspected	Recommended Studies
Acute lymphocytic leukemia	CBC with platelet count and WBC differential, peripheral blood smear, PT, and PTT
Infection	Blood culture, CSF studies, CRP; consider a rapid streptococcal antigen test or oropharyngeal culture, respiratory viral cultures, specific viral antibody titers, RMSF antibody titers
Vasculitis	ESR, CRP, ANA, anti-double-stranded DNA antibody, complement levels (C3, C4, CH50); consider other specific autoantibody titers
Mechanical	Imaging studies for trauma, including head CT scan and skeletal survey for suspected nonaccidental trauma
Abnormal vascular components	Skin biopsy for Ehlers-Danlos syndrome or other collagen vascular disorders, ascorbic acid level
Thrombocytopenia	Consider bone marrow biopsy; urinalysis, BUN, creatinine
Platelet dysfunction	Bleeding time, platelet aggregation studies, clot retraction assay, BUN, creatinine
Coagulation defect	Specific clotting factor assays, thrombin time, fibrinogen level; bleeding time, factor VIII activity, von Willebrand factor antigen level, and ristocetin cofactor activity for von Willebrand disease; liver function tests, correction of PT and PTT after administration of vitamin K, mixing studies to detect factor inhibitors

ANA, antinuclear antibody; BUN, blood urea nitrogen; CBC, complete blood count; CH50, 50% hemolyzing dose of complement; CRP, C-reactive protein; CSF, cerebrospinal fluid; CT, computed tomography; ESR, erythrocyte sedimentation rate; PT, prothrombin time; PTT, partial thromboplastin time; RMSF, Rocky Mountain spotted fever; WBC, white blood cell.

and these children are at risk of developing shock, respiratory failure, or DIC.

SPEICAL CONSIDERATIONS

NEONATAL PETECHIAE OR PURPURA

Petechiae and purpura in a neonate may be due to a number of causes in addition to those listed earlier, including birth trauma, congenitally acquired infection (i.e., toxoplasmosis, rubella, cytomegalovirus, herpes simplex virus), other infections such as syphilis or human immunodeficiency virus infection, neonatal alloimmune thrombocytopenic purpura, congenital thrombocytopenic syndromes such as thrombocytopenia-absent radius syndrome, and congenital abnormalities of platelet function. The clinical status of the neonate should direct the investigation and determine the urgency of evaluation. If the neonate is ill, sepsis and DIC must be strongly considered and proactively treated. If the neonate is well, proceeding with basic screening laboratory tests in a systematic way is appropriate. Depending on initial lab results, further investigation under the guidance of a hematologist or neonatologist may be helpful.

KEY POINTS

- Purpura can arise from intravascular, extravascular, and vascular causes. Nonpalpable lesions result from intravascular and extravascular purpura; a vascular process leads to palpable lesions.
- Treatment of petechiae and purpura is based on clinical acuity and the underlying cause. In many cases children are stable and well-appearing and require supportive care only. When sepsis is a consideration and a child is ill or toxic appearing, prompt treatment with fluids and antibiotics is necessary.
- Children who present with fever and petechiae or purpura warrant immediate attention because this can be a medical emergency.
- Trauma is the most common cause of petechiae and purpura, but nonaccidental injury should be considered when the distribution is not typical of accidental injury, or the history is not consistent with a plausible mechanism of injury.

SUGGESTED READINGS

Barut K, Sahin S, Kasapcopur O. Pediatric vasculitis. *Curr Opin Rheumatol.* 2016;28(1):29-38.

Brogan PA, Raffles A. The management of fever and petechiae: making sense of rash decisions. *Arch Dis Child.* 2000;83:506-507.

Cannon L, Wu EY. Recent advances in pediatric vasculitis. *Rheum Dis Clin North Am.* 2021;47(4):781-796.

Chalmers E, Cooper P, Forman K, et al. Purpura fulminans: recognition, diagnosis, and management. *Arch Dis Child.* 2011;96:1066-1071.

Joly BS, Coppo P, Veyradier A. Pediatric thrombotic thrombocytopenic purpura. *Eur J Haematol.* 2018;101(4):425-434.

Leung AKC, Barankin B, Leong KF. Henoch-Schönlein purpura in children: an updated review. *Curr Pediatr Rev.* 2020;16(4):265-276.

Mudd SS, Findlay JS. The cutaneous manifestations and common mimickers of physical child abuse. *J Pediatr Health Care.* 2004;18:123-129.

Nielsen HE, Anderson EA, Anderson J, et al. Diagnostic assessment of haemorrhagic rash and fever. *Arch Dis Child.* 2001;85:160-165.

Piram M, Mahr F. Epidemiology of immunoglobulin A vasculitis (Henoch-Schonlein): current state of knowledge. *Curr Opin Rheumatol.* 2013;25:171-178.

Provan D, Arnold DM, Bussel JB, et al. Updated international consensus report on the investigation and management of primary immune thrombocytopenia. *Blood Adv.* 2019;3(22):3780-3817.

Tristani-Firouzi P, Meadous KP, Vanderhooft S. Pigmented purpuric eruption of childhood. *Pediatr Dermatol.* 2001;18:299-304.

CHAPTER 57 Vesicles and Bullae

Emilee Dobish, MD, MS

BACKGROUND

The diagnosis of vesicular and bullous diseases in childhood can be a difficult task. To better understand the defining characteristics of vesiculobullous disorders, a general knowledge of skin anatomy is helpful. **Figure 57-1** illustrates normal skin histology. The numerous causes of blistering can be divided into those with neonatal versus childhood

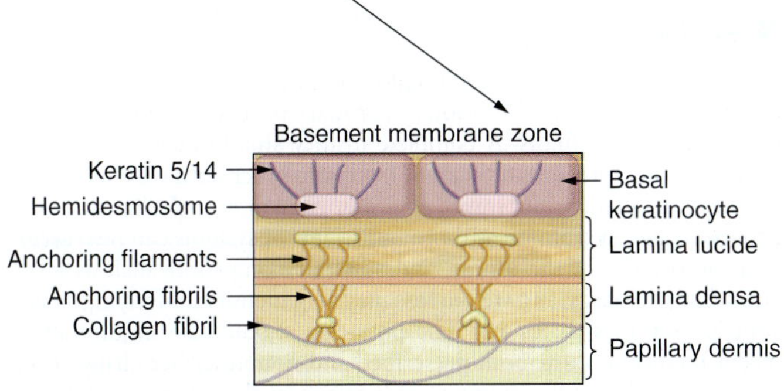

FIGURE 57-1. Normal skin histology.

TABLE 57-1 Definition of Vesiculobullous Lesions: Primary and Secondary Findings

Lesion	Definition
Primary	
Vesicle	Fluid-filled lesion <0.5 cm
Bulla	Fluid-filled lesion >0.5 cm
Pustule	Blistering lesion filled with purulent exudate
Secondary	
Erosion	Partial loss of epidermis
Ulceration	Complete loss of epidermis with extension into dermis
Excoriation	Scratched primary lesions; may be linear or crusted
Scaling	Dry, superficial accumulations of keratin
Crusting	Dried serous, hemorrhagic, or purulent exudate (i.e., scabbing)
Milia	Small 1-2-mm epidermal cysts

onsets. Additionally, secondary characteristics, such as distribution and morphology, can further limit the differential diagnosis.

It is important to have a clear understanding of the terminology used to describe vesicular or bullous lesions and their associated physical features. A *vesicle* is a fluid-filled, dome-shaped lesion of 0.5 cm or less; if such a lesion is greater than 0.5 cm, it is termed a *bulla*. The fluid inside may be clear, hemorrhagic, or serous in nature. If the material is purulent, the lesion is called a *pustule*. Secondary lesions, including crusting, excoriation, scaling, milia, and scarring, may also be noted. An *erosion* is a superficially denuded vesicle with damage confined to the epidermis. *Ulceration* is a deeper lesion, with loss of the entire depth of the epidermis. Secondary scarring does not usually result from erosion, except if secondary infection occurs. However, secondary scarring is common with ulceration given the depth of the injury (**Table 57-1**; **Figure 57-2**). Milia (small, white, superficial epidermal cysts) may result from a healing blistering process.

PATHOPHYSIOLOGY

A defining characteristic of the vesicle or bulla is whether the lesion is flaccid or tense. Nikolsky and Asboe-Hansen signs may be useful for differentiating lesions. A positive Nikolsky sign occurs when a blister is induced by rubbing normal-appearing skin with the eraser of a pencil. A positive Nikolsky sign is associated with flaccid lesions. The Asboe-Hansen sign is elicited by applying lateral pressure to the edge of a bulla away from the center. If the lesion extends, the split is higher up in the epidermis and the lesion is classified as flaccid. If the lesion does not extend, it is defined as tense. A tense bulla suggests a deeper process in which the split in the epidermis lies below the level of the lamina lucida located in the basement membrane zone. This gives the lesion enough support to hold the fluid tense under pressure. In contrast, a flaccid bulla is a more superficial process that generally occurs higher in the epidermis, where skin tension may easily disrupt the lesion's integrity (**Figure 57-3**).

CLINICAL PRESENTATION

HISTORY

Clinical presentation of vesiculobullous lesions may vary tremendously, depending on whether the lesion is a primary process or a manifestation of an underlying illness. A complete history should include the duration of disease, previous or current infection, other family or household members affected, recent travel, environmental or household exposures, and associated symptoms. A thorough review of systems can help ascertain the severity of the illness, and systemic complaints such as fever, arthralgias, lethargy, and weight loss may help identify underlying causes contributing to skin lesions. The physician should also inquire about recent medication use, both prescribed and nonprescribed drugs. Even regularly used over-the-counter medications, such as nonsteroidal anti-inflammatory drugs, can cause blistering reactions, including bullous fixed drug reactions, pseudoporphyria, or even toxic epidermal necrolysis. A detailed family history is vital to the diagnosis of many genetic vesiculobullous disorders, including various forms of epidermolysis bullosa and Hailey-Hailey disease. A positive family history of autoimmune diseases may also assist in making a diagnosis. Finally, a detailed history of the rash itself is essential. Physicians should determine the date of onset of the vesiculobullous lesions, location and spread throughout the body, and any associated factors such as pruritis. The history should reveal whether the lesions are acute, subacute, or chronic in duration. Lesions may appear simultaneously, in crops, or follow a cyclical pattern, with periods of activity followed by resolution. Special care must be taken in the evaluation of neonates, because associated symptoms are not always well defined in this age group, and occult infection can easily be missed.

PHYSICAL EXAM

Aside from identifying the nondermatologic features on physical examination, a clear description of the skin lesions is necessary, using the terms defined earlier. Delineating the nature of the lesions, the pattern of eruption, and its distribution can be invaluable in differentiating among vesiculobullous diseases. Note whether the lesions are grouped or scattered, localized to a specific area or generalized, or linear or annular in configuration; determine whether lesions follow the lines of Blaschko or occur in a dermatomal distribution. The lesions may appear to have recently erupted, resolving, or occur in a mixed pattern. A total body skin exam is often necessary, which includes the nailbeds, scalp, and mucus membranes; detailed and sequential exams over the course of days may be helpful to assess how lesions evolve. Attention to the mucosal surfaces is important because many systemic blistering disorders involve the oral, genital, or ocular mucosal surfaces.

DIFFERENTIAL DIAGNOSIS

As noted above, the age of onset of a disorder is an important clue in the diagnosis of vesiculobullous disorders. The differential diagnoses of neonatal and childhood vesiculobullous disorders are described in **Tables 57-2** and **57-3**, respectively. Lesions that appear in the neonatal period may be genetic, infectious, or even iatrogenic. For example, neonates may present with scattered or solitary bullae on the forearm, wrist, or hand secondary to vigorous sucking in utero. These sucking blisters are a diagnosis of exclusion in an otherwise well neonate and resolve in days to weeks without any intervention. Infectious causes should always be considered in a newborn with vesiculobullous findings. If the lesions are congenital, a genetic blistering disorder should be considered. Some autoimmune disorders can be transferred through the presence of maternal antibodies, up to about 6 months of age. Disorders in this category include neonatal lupus, neonatal pemphigus, and pemphigus foliaceus.

DIAGNOSTIC EVALUATION

Although in many cases the clinical picture is sufficient to determine the diagnosis, laboratory testing is indicated in certain situations. The laboratory workup of a patient with a vesiculobullous disorder should include investigations to rule out plausible causes and those that may place the patient at risk for significant morbidity or mortality. For example, vesiculobullous lesions that include mucosal surfaces should encourage the physician to consider Stevens-Johnson Syndrome, toxic epidermal necrolysis, or herpetic disorders in their differential diagnosis. Laboratory testing to consider may include a complete blood count to investigate leukocytosis or leukopenia; these findings may point to an infectious etiology. A complete metabolic panel may be warranted to assess electrolytes and hydration status in patients who are ill-appearing, have lesions involving the oral cavity preventing adequate hydration, or have extensive involvement of the skin, placing them at risk for excessive fluid losses. Physicians can consider obtaining inflammatory markers, such as C-reactive protein and erythrocyte sedimentation rate, if an inflammatory condition or autoimmune disorder is suspected. If a viral cause is suspected, a Tzanck smear, rapid fluorescent antibody stain,

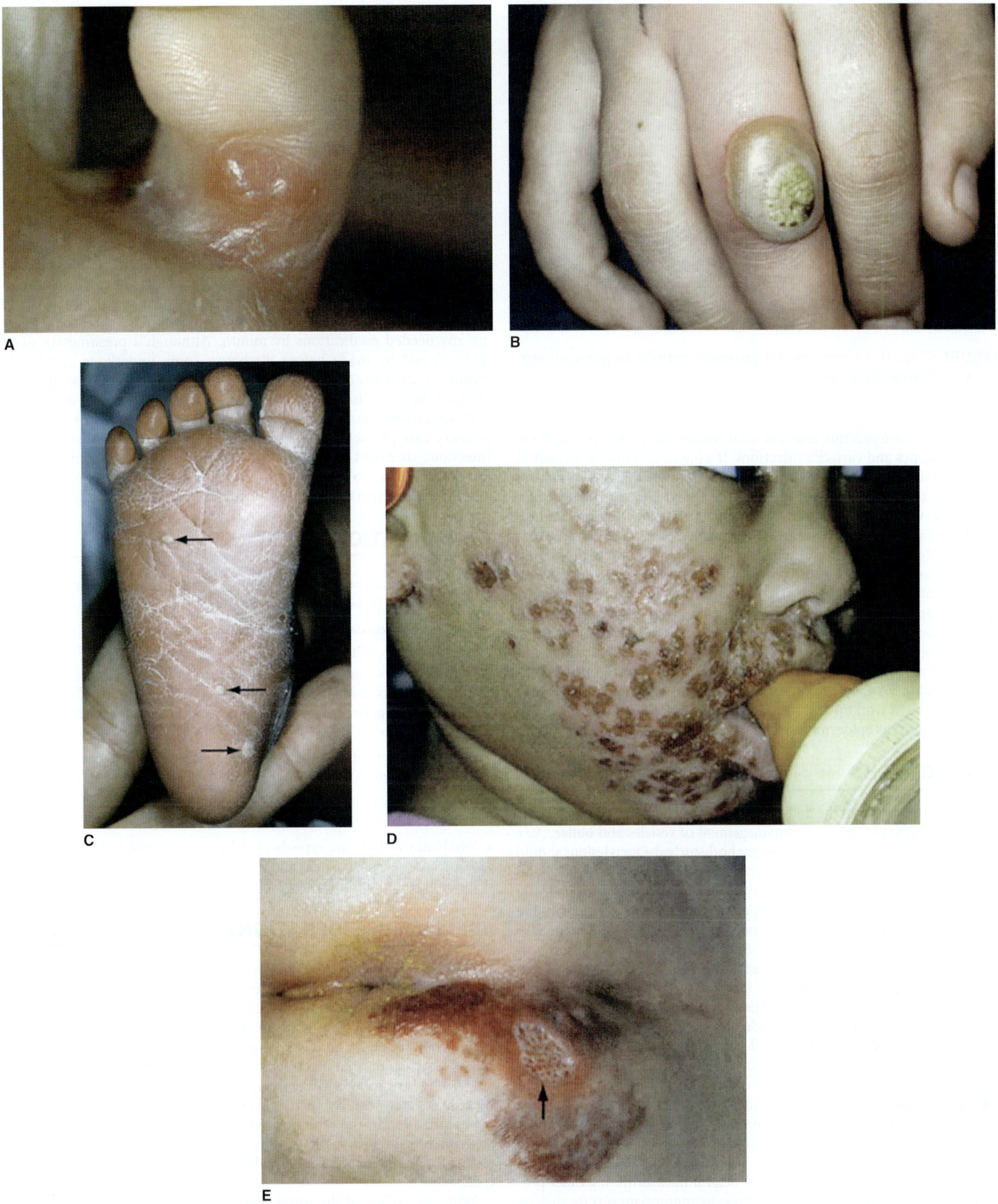

FIGURE 57-2. Clinical examples. A. Vesicle (scabies). B. Bulla (adverse reaction to topical cantharidin). C. Pustules (transient neonatal pustular melanosis). D. Erosion (eczema herpeticum). E. Ulcer (ulcerated infantile hemangioma).

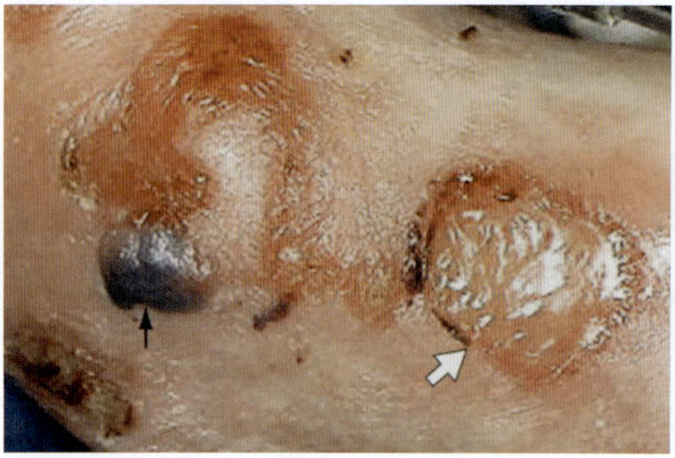

FIGURE 57-3. Flaccid (*open arrow*) and tense (*solid arrow*) bullae in a patient with recessive dystrophic epidermolysis bullosa.

polymerase chain reaction assay, or viral culture should be considered to rule out herpes and varicella infections. If a bacterial cause is suspected, a Gram stain and appropriate cultures can aid in the diagnosis of gram-positive and gram-negative bacterial infections. For suspected fungal infections, Giemsa stain or a potassium hydroxide preparation can help identify hyphal and yeast forms. Infectious diseases consultation may be warranted to help determine need for additional microbiologic testing, such as organism-specific polymerase chain reaction or organism-specific antibodies. A particularly thorough workup should be done in neonates and in immunocompromised children of all ages. Infectious diseases can present atypically in these special patients, and without timely diagnosis and treatment the outcome can be devastating. The workup of a neonate with a blistering disorder of unknown cause is outlined in **Table 57-4**. Consultation with dermatology may be warranted for assistance in workup and need for skin biopsy to confirm suspected diagnoses, such as epidermolysis bullosa.

MANAGEMENT

Aside from treatment of the underlying cause or condition, there are some general principles regarding the management of vesicles and bullae. As a rule, vesicles and small bullae should not be disturbed. Open lesions should be kept clean by gentle washing without harsh soap, coated with bland petrolatum ointment, and covered with a sterile bandage if needed. If a large bulla is intact and in an area that causes pain, or if it keeps expanding due to pressure, the fluid can be drained using a sterile large-bore needle. Alternatively, a number 11 blade can be used to make a linear incision near the base of the bulla to allow drainage of the fluid contents. The incision should be large enough to ensure that the bulla will not reform after drainage, but small enough to keep the blister roof in place; unroofed lesions are often painful. Extensively denuded lesions may be associated with increased insensible losses and could contribute to fluid and electrolyte disturbances that require intervention. Temperature control may be disrupted, especially in neonates. Pain may be significant and requires special attention. Pain control may be needed around the clock or during certain activities such as dressing changes and physical therapy. Finally, depending on the ultimate cause of the vesiculobullous lesion, infection control may be warranted including droplet, contact, and airborne precautions. Infectious diseases consultation can be helpful in determining exact precautions and any need to report the illness to appropriate entities such as local and state health departments.

ADMISSION AND DISCHARGE CRITERIA

ADMISSION

Because neonates with blistering conditions are at high risk for serious infectious or other life-threatening conditions, they require hospitalization to conduct an appropriate evaluation, initiate therapy, and manage potential complications. Infants and children with vesiculobullous eruptions warrant admission when a serious condition is suspected that requires prompt diagnosis or therapy. Such indications may include abnormal vital signs, involvement of the mucosal surfaces, extensive total body surface area involvement and alterations in mental status. Patients demonstrating rapid progression or extensive skin involvement merit hospitalization. Children unable to tolerate sufficient oral intake secondary to oral mucosal lesions or uncontrolled pain may require inpatient admission for intravenous rehydration and pain control.

DISCHARGE

Patients are eligible for discharge once vital signs are stable, medical complications associated with the lesions have been mitigated and ongoing skin care regimens have been determined, if necessary. Infants and children should be able to maintain hydration with oral intake and tolerate any needed medications by mouth. Although a presumptive diagnosis should be made before discharge, some underlying conditions require confirmation with genetic testing; results may not be available by the time patients achieve discharge criteria. All patients discharged with vesiculobullous lesions should have adequate follow-up with their primary care physician and appropriate consultants (e.g., dermatology, infectious diseases) arranged. Discharge instructions should address local wound care to promote wound healing, prevent spread to others and minimize the risk of superimposed bacterial infections.

CONSULTATION

- Dermatology as needed for assistance with diagnosis, inpatient management, and if the condition is ongoing, outpatient follow-up.
- Infectious diseases as needed for recommended testing and interpretation of results, empirical antibiotic therapy, and adjustment of therapy.
- Critical care or burn center when cardiorespiratory support is needed, the extent of bedside interventions exceeds the capacity of a noncritical care setting, or resources and expertise are unavailable at the existing institution.
- Physical or occupational therapy for maintaining or reestablishing mobility, reconditioning, or implementing medical equipment (e.g., splints).
- Plastic surgery for management of skin lesions that may require grafting or scar revision.
- Psychiatry if there are reports of changes in mental status, as associations between psychiatric and dermatologic conditions (e.g., schizophrenia and pemphigus) are well reported in the literature.

SPECIAL CONSIDERATIONS

While *Mycoplasma pneumoniae* is a well-known cause of respiratory diseases in pediatric patients, a new phenomenon of *M. pneumoniae*-induced rash and mucositis (MIRM) has been described. MIRM is a mucocutaneous eruption felt to be distinct from other mucocutaneous manifestations of *M. pneumonia* such as Stevens-Johnson syndrome (SJS), toxic epidermal necrolysis (TEN), and erythema multiforme (EM). The rash in MIRM involves painful erosions of the lips and oral mucosa covered with hemorrhagic crusting and associated conjunctival hyperemia. Rarely, the remaining skin is affected, helping to differentiate from SJS, TEN, and EM. Often, consultation with dermatology and testing for *M. pneumoniae* is helpful in making the diagnosis and guiding treatment.

With the arrival of the novel coronavirus infection and global pandemic (COVID-19), much has been learned about the dermatologic manifestations of this disease in children. In most instances, these skin changes present early in the disease course. Of the commonly reported cutaneous manifestations reported in children with COVID-19 infection, Chilblain-like lesions were the most common, followed by erythema multiforme-like and varicella-like lesions. If these lesions are noted on physical exam, COVID-19 should remain high on the differential diagnosis.

TABLE 57-2 Neonatal Vesiculobullous Disorders

Disorder	Onset and Duration	Clinical Characteristics	Diagnosis
Benign, transient erythema toxicum neonatorum	24-72 hr after birth; lasts 1 wk	Blotchy erythema with small central pustule; generalized, except palms and soles; full-term, healthy infants	Clinical, Gram stain: eosinophils
Neonatal acne	Weeks to months	Erythematous papules and pustules on face and chest; healthy neonates	Clinical, stains mostly negative, but may see yeast forms
Transient neonatal pustular melanosis	Birth; hyperpigmentation lasts months	Pustules without erythema; collarette when wiped away; heals, but hyperpigmentation lasts months; generalized, palms, and soles; healthy neonates; more common in darker pigmented skin types	Clinical, Gram stain: neutrophils
Miliaria (rubra or crystal lina)	Days to months; lasts hours to days	Small erythematous papules (rubra) to clear vesicles (crystallina) on forehead, upper chest, and back; history of fever, overheating	Clinical, all stains negative
Infantile acropustulosis	Days to months; may last 2-3 yr	Extremely pruritic vesicles and pustules occurring in crops on hands and feet	Clinical, biopsy
Eosinophilic pustular folliculitis	Birth to 1 yr; may last years	Pruritic follicular-based papules and pustules on scalp and face; very rare	Biopsy
Congenital Langerhans cell histiocytosis	Birth to days	Vesicles to crusted papules, petechiae; solitary to numerous; scalp, groin, flexures most common	Biopsy, electron microscopy
Sucking blister	Birth or later	Noninflamed blister; usually solitary; most often on hands or wrists	Clinical, all stains negative
Inflammatory mastocytosis	Birth to several months	Mastocytoma: solitary pink, tan, or brown macule to indurated plaque with overlying bullae	Clinical, all stains negative, biopsy showing mast cells
		Urticaria pigmentosa: multiple lesions as described for mastocytoma	
		Diffuse cutaneous mastocytosis: peau d'orange (indurated yellowish orange skin) with vesicles and bullae at sites of trauma	
Infectious syphilis	Birth	Vesicles and bullae, often eroded; perioralo (snuffles), hands, and feet; may be localized or generalized; associated with hepatosplenomegaly and pseudoparalysis	Serology, DFA; darkfield examination
Candidiasis, congenital	Birth to 24 hr; lasts 2 wk	Generalized erythema and pustules or vesicles	KOH: pseudohyphae
Candidiasis, neonatal	Past 1 wk of age	Erythematous macules or papules with satellite pustules; diaper area and flexures most commonly affected	Clinical, KOH: pseudohyphae
Herpes simplex	Birth to weeks	Vesicles or pustules; erosions to scarring; localized to generalized	Clinical, Tzanck (rarely done), DFA, PCR, culture, or serology
Varicella	Birth	Linear scarring, erosions; often affects extremities; fetal anomalies occur with first- or second-trimester infection	Clinical, Tzanck, DFA, PCR, culture, or serology
Scabies	Weeks	Vesicles to crusted papules, nodules with burrows; hands, feet, axilla, scalp	Clinical, Mineral oil preparation
Genetic incontinentia pigmenti	Birth	Linear and whorled vesicles along lines of Blaschko; progresses to verrucous lesions; localized to limb or generalized; may be associated with seizures, retinopathy, and eosinophilia	Biopsy, genetic testing (*NEMO* gene)
Epidermolysis bullosa	Birth to teens (for certain forms such as Weber-Cockayne)	Noninflammmatory vesicles, bullae; often eroded; milia with dystrophic forms; extremities most often affected; severity depends on type; some forms associated with pyloric atresia, GI involvement, failure to thrive	Biopsy, electron microscopy, genetic testing (keratins 5/14, plectin, laminin 5, collagen XVII, α6β4 integrin, collagen VII)
Transient bullous dermolysis of the newborn	Birth; resolves within months	Extensive blistering due to transient defect in collagen VII	Biopsy, electron microscopy
Epidermolytic hyperkeratosis (bullous congenital ichthyosiform erythroderma)	Birth	Generalized erythema and scaling with bullae and erosions; evolves to generalized ichthyosis with flexural predominance	Biopsy, genetic testing (keratins 1/10)
Ichthyosis bullosa of siemens	Birth	Milder blisters and erosions than epidermolytic hyperkeratosis; episodic superficial peeling	Clinical, biopsy; genetic testing (keratin 2e)
AEC syndrome birth (Hay-Wells)	Birth	Associated with erosive scalp dermatitis	Clinical, genetic testing (*p63* gene)
Ectodermal dysplasia; skin fragility syndrome	Birth	Generalized erythema with superimposed bullae, erosions; perioral redness and desquamation; sparse hair and dystrophic nails; abnormal sweating	Biopsy, genetic testing (plakophilin)
Congenital erosive and vesicular dermatosis	Birth; heals in weeks to months	Premature infants; diffuse vesicles, erosions, and crusting; palms, soles, face relatively spared; heals with reticulated scarring	Biopsy

(*Continued*)

TABLE 57-2 Neonatal Vesiculobullous Disorders (*Continued*)

Disorder	Onset and Duration	Clinical Characteristics	Diagnosis
Kindler syndrome	Birth to months	Acral blistering that later develops poikiloderma	Biopsy, electron microscopy
Metabolic acrodermatitis enteropathies	Birth to 6 mo	Copper-colored patches and plaques; perioral region, groin, hands, and feet; overlying vesicles and bullae	Low serum zinc level, low alkaline phosphatase
Autoimmune herpes gestationis	Birth; resolves in weeks	Very pruritic, urticarial plaques with overlying tense vesicles, bullae; results from transfer of maternal antibodies; self-limited	Biopsy, direct and indirect immunofluorescence
Neonatal pemphigus	Birth; resolves in a few weeks	Pruritic, urticarial plaques with flaccid bullae, erosions; occurs in infants of mothers with active pemphigus vulgaris or foliaceus due to transfer of maternal antibodies	Maternal history, biopsy, direct and indirect immunofluorescence

AEC, ankyloblepharon-ectodermal dysplasia-clefting; DFA, direct fluorescent antibody; GI, gastrointestinal; KOH, potassium hydroxide; NEMO, NF-kappa B essential modulator; PCR, polymerase chain reaction.

TABLE 57-3 Infantile and Childhood Vesiculobullous Disorders

Disorder	Clinical Characteristics	Diagnosis
Acquired		
Psoriasis (pustular)	Widespread erythematous, well-defined papules with overlying pustules; may be exacerbated by systemic corticosteroid use	Biopsy, Giemsa stain shows sterile neutrophils
Allergic contact dermatitis	Very pruritic; may be localized or generalized; erythematous papulovesicles to bullae; linear distribution with poison ivy	Clinical, biopsy
Dyshidrotic eczema	Erythematous papulovesicles to bullae on hands and feet; may have generalized reaction	Clinical, biopsy
Erythema multiforme	Targetoid to bullous erythematous macules or maculopapules; palms, soles, mucous membranes frequently affected; HSV most common trigger	Clinical, biopsy
Stevens-Johnson syndrome; toxic epidermal necrolysis	Generalized erythematous macules to morbilliform eruption, with frequent progression to flaccid bulla formation and widespread desquamation; mucosal involvement common; drugs, infections, vaccinations may trigger	Clinical, biopsy
Phototoxic; drug	Erythematous macules or papulovesicles with vesicle or bulla formation in photodistribution	Clinical, biopsy
Acute generalized exanthematous pustulosis	Generalized erythematous small papules or erythroderma studded with numerous small pustules; associated with sudden fever; drug, viral, mercury, immunization triggers possible	Clinical, biopsy
Burn	Well-defined to figured erythema with overlying vesicle or bulla formation; may be sign of abuse	Clinical
Friction blister	Noninflamed vesicle to bulla at site of friction	Clinical
Coma blister	Noninflamed bulla occurring in comatose patient; possible associated bruising; generally, occurs 24 hr after onset of coma	Clinical
Hydroa vacciniforme	Crusted erosions with varioliform scarring; photodistribution	Clinical
Autoimmune		
Pemphigus vulgaris	Generalized flaccid, easily eroded, crusted bullae; Nikolsky sign positive; may be drug induced	Biopsy with direct and indirect immunofluorescence
Pemphigus foliaceus	Erythematous, very superficially crusted, eroded, polycyclic plaques; most common on the head and neck	Biopsy with direct and indirect immunofluorescence
Paraneoplastic pemphigus	Generalized pemphigus lesions with severe mucosal lesions common; often refractory to treatment; may be associated with lymphoma or Castleman tumor	Biopsy with direct and indirect immunofluorescence
Epidermolysis bullosa acquista	Skin fragility to tense bulla formation; healing with scarring and milia; mucous membranes may be involved	Biopsy with immunofluorescence
Bullous pemphigoid	Urticarial plaques with overlying tense bullae; may be annular or polycyclic; facial and palmar or plantar involvement more common in children	Biopsy with direct and indirect immunofluorescence
Bullous lupus erythematosus	Generalized, pruritic, tense bullae; predominantly photodistributed; very rare in childhood	Biopsy with immunofluorescence, antinuclear antibodies
Dermatitis herpetiformis	Intensely pruritic papulovesicles to vesicles; symmetrical over extensor surfaces; often associated with gluten-sensitive enteropathy	Biopsy with immunofluorescence
Linear IgA disease (chronic bullous disease of childhood)	Abrupt onset of tense vesicles or bullae, often in string-of-pearls configuration; groin and perioral region favored; mucous membrane involvement common	Biopsy with immunofluorescence
Genetic		
Hailey-Hailey disease	Moist, erythematous, eroded plaques in flexures; may have vesicles or pustules; presents in second to fourth decades	Biopsy, family history, genetic testing (*ATP2C1* gene)
Epidermolysis bullosa	Noninflammatory bullae appearing at sites of trauma; may present from birth to teen years	Biopsy, family history, genetic testing

(*Continued*)

TABLE 57-3 Infantile and Childhood Vesiculobullous Disorders (*Continued*)

Disorder	Clinical Characteristics	Diagnosis
Pachyonychia congenita	Hypertrophic nails, hyperkeratotic palms and soles, leukokeratosis beginning in infancy to childhood; bullae may form at sites of friction usually in late childhood	Clinical, genetic testing (keratins 6/16 or 17)
Porphyrias (congenital erythropoietic porphyria, porphyria cutanea tarda, variegate porphyria)	All may have varying degrees of photosensitivity with blistering; severe types present early, porphyria cutanea tarda in childhood	Biopsy, porphyrin testing
Infectious		
Impetigo	Honey-colored, crusted, oozing vesicles with erythema; may be primary infection (common in perioral, perinasal regions) or secondary infection (atopic dermatitis, varicella); caused by *Staphylococcus*, *Streptococcus*, or both	Clinical, Gram stain, culture
Blistering distal dactylitis	Erythema with bullae on distal fingers; caused by β-hemolytic streptococci	Clinical, Gram stain, culture
Staphylococcal scalded skin syndrome	Painful erythema with localized flaccid bullae; may generalize to erythroderma; patient is ill appearing, with malaise, fever; Nikolsky sign positive; neonates most susceptible; caused by staphylococcal exfoliative toxins	Clinical, cultures from mucosal surfaces and blood
Scabies	Vesicles to crusted papules or nodules with burrows; hands, feet, axilla, scalp (in infants)	Clinical, Mineral oil preparation
Bullous arthropod reaction	Pruritic vesicles, bullae, pustules on exposed areas; causes include fleas, red ants	Clinical, biopsy
Herpes simplex	Grouped vesicles on erythematous base; erosions may heal with scarring; painful oral ulcerations in primary outbreaks; localized (perioral, genital) to generalized (eczema herpeticum)	Clinical, Tzanck,* DFA, PCR, culture, or serology
Varicella (chickenpox)	Crops of pruritic vesicles that are pustular and crusted; can heal with scarring; caused by varicella-zoster virus	Clinical, DFA, PCR, culture
Zoster	Dermatomal distribution of urticarial papules or plaques to vesicles; pain may be associated, but less than in adults	Clinical, DFA, PCR, culture
Dermatophytosis	Annular, pink, scaling pruritic plaques; often bullous on the feet or hands	Clinical, KOH
Hand-foot-and-mouth disease	Oval vesicles and bullae on hands and feet; painful erosions in mouth; most caused by coxsackievirus A16; severe blistering with A6 strain	Clinical PCR, culture

DFA, direct fluorescent antibody; HSV, herpes simplex virus; KOH, potassium hydroxide; PCR, polymerase chain reaction.

*Tzanck smear is virtually never used given widespread availability of HSV PCR tests.

At the time of this writing, an emerging number of cases of the rare zoonotic disease monkeypox are occurring. Traditionally seen in African countries, there have been increasing case reports of monkeypox viral infections in the United States. Monkeypox manifests as smallpox-like lesions with vesicular-pustular lesions predominantly on the face, but also involving the hands and soles of the feet. With the COVID-19 pandemic, recent monkeypox infections, and increasing globalization of the population, hospitalists will need to keep abreast of new and emerging infectious diseases that often initially present with a vesiculobullous rash. If patients present with a vesiculobullous rash concerning for monkeypox, consultation with infectious diseases and the local health department is prudent.

TABLE 57-4 Workup for Unidentified Vesicular or Pustular Rash in Neonates

Study	Cause
Direct preparations	
Tzanck*	Herpesviruses
Gram stain	Bacteria
Potassium hydroxide	Fungal elements
Mineral oil	Scabies
Giemsa or Wright	Inflammatory cell type
Darkfield	Syphilis
Fluorescent antibody testing	Herpes simplex virus, varicella-zoster virus, syphilis, immunobullous disorders
Histology	
Biopsy	If cause cannot otherwise be ascertained
Electron microscopy	Epidermolysis bullosa, Langerhans cell histiocytosis
Laboratory	
Complete blood count with differential	Infectious and parasitic causes, incontinentia pigmenti (eosinophils)
Zinc, alkaline phosphatase	Acrodermatitis enteropathica
Polymerase chain reaction	Herpes simplex virus, varicella-zoster virus, enterovirus
Porphyrins	Porphyria
Antinuclear antibody	Lupus erythematosus

*Virtually never used given widespread availability of HSV PCR tests.

KEY POINTS

- Vesiculobullous disorders constitute a wide variety of conditions, including some that are benign and self-limited, acute or chronic, disfiguring, debilitating, or even life-threatening.
- The clinical presentation often provides sufficient diagnostic information, but when a serious causative or underlying condition is suspected, appropriate infectious, immunologic, genetic, or autoimmune testing is indicated.
- Many vesiculobullous conditions are self-limited, but complications of the skin lesions can include scarring, deformities, recurrence, superinfection, fluid and electrolyte imbalance, and pain.
- In general, skin care involves gentle cleansing and application of bland petroleum jelly to all open areas. Any infectious causes should be treated concomitantly.
- Numerous infectious diseases and psychiatric illnesses have an association with vesiculobullous lesions, thus consultation with dermatology, infectious diseases and psychiatry may be warranted to coordinate comprehensive care for pediatric patients.

SUGGESTED READINGS

Afsar FS, Cun S, Seremt S. Neonatal sucking blister. *Dermatol Online J.* 2019;25(11).

Bunge EM, Hoet B, Chen L, et al. The changing epidemiology of human monkeypox-A potential threat? A systematic review. *PLoS Negl Trop Dis.* 2022;16(2):e0010141.

Canavan TN; Mathes EF, Fieden I, Shinkai K. *Mycoplasma pneumoniae*-induced rash and mucositis as a syndrome distinct from Stevens-Johnson syndrome and erythema multiforme: a systematic review. *J Am Acad Dermatol.* 2015;72(2):239-245.

Ferrari S, Pellegrini G, Mavilio F, De Luca M. Gene therapy approaches for epidermolysis bullosa. *Clin Dermatol.* 2005;23:430-436.

Johyr RJ, Schachner LA. Neonatal dermatologic challenges. *Pediatr Rev.* 1997; 18(3): 86-84.

Knopfel N, Noguera-Morel L, Latour I, Torrelo A. Viral exanthems in children: a great imitator. *Clin Dermatol.* 2019; 37(3): 213-226.

Kridin K, Zelber-Sagi S, Comaneshter D, Cohen AD. Association between schizophrenia and an autoimmune bullous skin disease-pemphigus: a population-based large-scale study. *Epidemiol Psychiatr Sci.* 2019;28(2):191-198.

Marathe K, Lu J, Morel KD. Bullous diseases: kids are not just little people. *Clin Dermatol.* 2015;33(6): 644-656.

Meadows KP, Egan CA, Vanderhooft S. Acute generalized exanthematous pustulosis, an uncommon condition in children: case report and review of the literature. *Pediatr Dermatol.* 2000;17:399-402.

Neto RP, Mazzo FAT, Vieira FA, et al. COVID-19 cutaneous manifestation in children and adolescents: a systematic review. *Rev Paul Pediatr.* 2022;40:e2021134.

Quddusi FI, Youssef MJ, Davis DMR. Dermatologic manifestations of systemic diseases in childhood. *Pediatr Rev.* 2021; 42(12): 655-671.

Santos RP, Silva M, Vieira AP, Brito C. Mycoplasma pneumoniae-induced rash and mucositis: a recently described entity. *BMJ Case Rep.* 2017;2017.

Sussman M, Zhai L, Morquette A, Huang S, Hsu S. Annular bullous diseases. *Clin Dermatol.* 2022;40(5):516-528.

van Doornum GJ, Guldemeester J, Osterhaus AD, Niesters HG. Diagnosing herpesvirus infections by real-time amplification and rapid culture. *J Clin Microbiol.* 2003;41:576-580.

Van Praag MCG, Van Rooij RWG, Folkers E, et al. Diagnosis and treatment of pustular disorders in the neonate. *Pediatr Dermatol.* 1997;14:131-143.

CHAPTER 58

Vascular Anomalies

Hilary Haimes, MD and Marilyn G. Liang, MD

BACKGROUND

Vascular anomalies are often benign and uncomplicated, but a minority require treatment and inpatient care. The International Society for the Study of Vascular Anomalies classifies vascular anomalies into two main categories: malformations and tumors (**Table 58-1**). The pediatric hospitalist should be able to recognize major types of vascular anomalies, have a basic understanding of the anticipated clinical course, and identify when lesions require subspecialty involvement.

VASCULAR MALFORMATIONS

INTRODUCTION AND CLINICAL FEATURES

Vascular malformations are comprised of structurally abnormal vessels with normal endothelial turnover; they are subcategorized based on their endothelial components (e.g., capillary, venous, lymphatic, and/or arteriovenous) and flow characteristics (e.g., slow-flow vs. fast-flow). These anomalies may be stable or progressive; they generally do not regress. Vascular malformations are categorized as follows: capillary, venous, lymphatic, arteriovenous, or combined.

Capillary Malformations Capillary malformations, also known as "port-wine stains," are slow-flow lesions that may be focal, regional, or diffuse. Clinically, capillary malformations are pale pink to deep red blanching patches that are present at birth and generally permanent. Over time, some lesions, particularly those on the face, may darken, thicken, and become nodular. Regional and diffuse capillary malformations may be associated with soft tissue and/or bony overgrowth or undergrowth. Capillary malformations involving the forehead may be associated with Sturge-Weber syndrome (SWS), which is characterized by seizures and/or glaucoma. Similar to other congenital midline lesions such as lipomas, tails, or dermal sinuses, capillary malformations in the midline lumbosacral region may indicate occult spinal dysraphism.

TABLE 58-1 Biological Classification of Vascular Birthmarks

Tumors	Malformations
Benign	Capillary malformation
Infantile hemangioma	Venous malformation
Congenital hemangioma	Lymphatic malformation
RICH	Arteriovenous malformation
NICH	Arteriovenous fistula
Tufted angioma	Combined malformation
Locally aggressive or borderline	Capillary-venous malformation
Kaposiform hemangioendothelioma	Capillary-lymphatic malformation
Malignant	Capillary-lymphatic-venous malformation
	Malformations associated with other anomalies
	Klippel-Trenaunay syndrome
	Parkes Weber syndrome
	Congenital Lipomatous
	Overgrowth, Vascular malformations, Epidermal nevi, and Spinal/Skeletal anomalies/Scoliosis (CLOVES)

Adapted from International Society for the Study of Vascular Anomalies classification for vascular anomalies, 2018 revision (Table 1).

Fading capillary stains/nevus simplex (also referred to as angel's kiss, stork bite, or salmon patch) are a form of capillary malformation located on the glabella, eyelids, forehead, and posterior neck. Unlike the typical vascular malformation, these lesions often fade or disappear by 1 to 2 years of life; however, some lesions, particularly those on the nape of the neck, may persist.

Venous Malformations Venous malformations are slow-flow vascular malformations comprised of irregular, dilated venous channels. Lesions are present at birth, though they may not be clinically evident. Typically, a venous malformation presents as a soft, compressible bluish papule, nodule, or mass that tends to become more prominent with age, dependency, and physical activity (**Figure 58-1**). Lesions may be confined to the skin and subcutaneous tissue or may involve deeper structures such as muscle, bone, and viscera. Diminished or stagnant blood flow within ectatic venous channels may lead to production of thrombin and conversion of fibrinogen to fibrin. This process results in chronic localized intravascular coagulation which may be associated with pain and swelling. Bleeding may occur due to consumption of clotting factors; deep vein thrombosis and pulmonary embolism may result from hematologic stasis.

Multiple cutaneous venous malformations, particularly on the palms and soles, may be associated with gastrointestinal tract venous malformations in blue rubber bleb nevus syndrome (BRBNS). Clinical manifestations may include anemia from chronic occult gastrointestinal bleeding, abdominal pain, rectal bleeding, melena, or hematemesis. Rarely, patients with BRBNS may develop intussusception and volvulus which can lead to bowel infarction.

Lymphatic Malformations Lymphatic malformations are slow-flow vascular lesions comprised of irregular, ectatic lymphatic channels. Lymphatic malformations are classified as microcystic or macrocystic based on the size of the cystic spaces present. Microcystic lesions (formerly called "lymphangioma circumscriptum") may form clear or hemorrhagic thin-walled vesicles or hyperkeratotic papules on the surface of the skin.

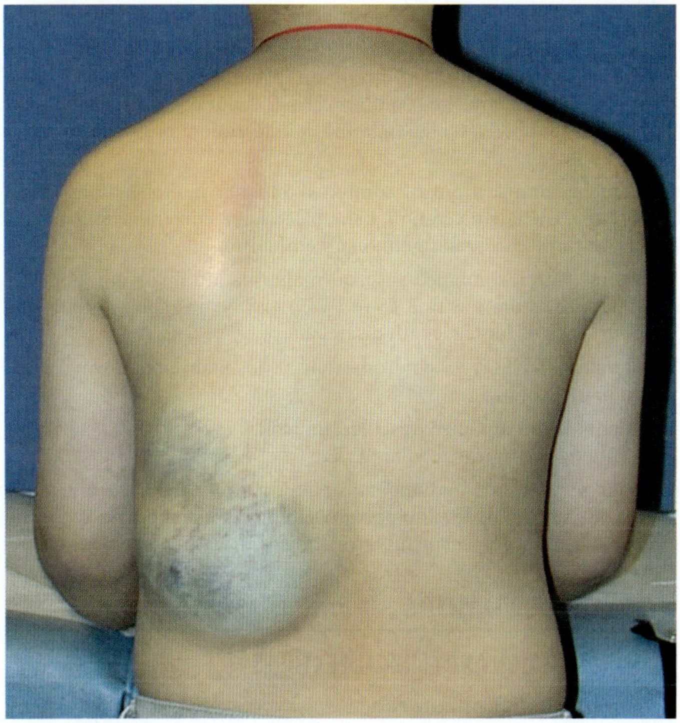

FIGURE 58-1. Venous malformation on back of a school-aged boy.

Macrocystic lymphatic malformations (formerly referred to as "cystic hygromas") are usually visible at birth, commonly occur on the neck and axilla, and are characterized by large, subcutaneous, compressible masses. Lymphatic malformations are predisposed to bacterial superinfection and may obstruct the airway. Respiratory distress may also occur due to obstruction of lymphatic channels and resultant lymphatic fluid accumulation in the lungs (chylous pleural effusions) or abdominal cavity (chylous ascites).

Arteriovenous Malformations Arteriovenous malformations (AVMs) are fast-flow lesions consisting of structurally abnormal arterial and venous vessels directly connected without an intervening capillary bed. Although present at birth, many AVMs may not be apparent until childhood. An AVM typically presents as a pink to red patch and may mimic a capillary malformation or infantile hemangioma. Lesions may have increased warmth or a palpable thrill. Over time, AVMs may expand, darken, and invade deeper structures; pregnancy, puberty, trauma, or radiologic or surgical treatment may precede such changes. Late-stage lesions may cause deep destruction with necrosis, ulceration, severe pain, and life-threatening bleeding. High output cardiac failure may occur with large lesions due to increased blood flow.

Capillary malformation-arteriovenous malformation (CM-AVM) is an autosomal dominant condition most commonly caused by mutations in *RASA1* or *EPHB4* in which patients develop multifocal capillary malformations associated with fast-flow vascular lesions. CM-AVM typically presents with multiple pink-red, small, round-to-oval macules, some of which have a pale halo. Although patients with CM-AVM generally have a benign clinical course, they do have an increased risk of developing cerebral and spinal AVMs, which may rupture and lead to hemorrhagic strokes.

Combined Malformations Combined malformations are vascular malformations that include more than one anomalous vessel type (including capillary, venous, lymphatic, and arteriovenous malformations). Examples include capillary-venous malformation, capillary-lymphatic malformation, and capillary-lymphatic-venous malformation. These are frequently associated with skeletal and soft tissue hypertrophy or hypotrophy. Combined malformations typically occur in the setting of genetic disorders delineated in the "Vascular Malformations Associated With Other Anomalies" section.

Vascular Malformations Associated With Other Anomalies Vascular malformations are often associated with other anomalies and occur in the context of genetic syndromes. PIK3CA-Related Overgrowth Spectrum (PROS) is an umbrella term for a group of genetic disorders in which patients develop overgrowth of tissue and/or vasculature resulting from a somatic mutation in the PIK3CA gene. Klippel-Trenaunay syndrome (KTS) and CLOVES (**C**ongenital **L**ipomatous **O**vergrowth, **V**ascular malformations, **E**pidermal nevi, and **S**pinal/**S**keletal anomalies/**S**coliosis) syndrome are two examples. KTS is characterized by abnormal capillary, lymphatic, and venous lesions with accompanying limb overgrowth; CLOVES syndrome consists of various cutaneous and musculoskeletal anomalies including vascular malformations such as capillary malformations, lymphatic malformations, or arteriovenous malformations.

Another genetic condition associated with vascular malformations, Parkes Weber syndrome (PWS), presents with AVMs along with overgrowth of an extremity due to mutations in the RASA1 gene (like CM-AVM). These patients are also at risk of cerebral and spinal AVMs.

DIAGNOSTIC EVALUATION

The assessment and management of vascular malformations depends on the type, location, and extent of the lesion(s). Capillary malformations are diagnosed clinically. Venous malformations, lymphatic malformations, and AVMs may be diagnosed clinically or with ultrasonography or magnetic resonance imaging (MRI).

Capillary Malformations Infants with capillary malformations involving the forehead should be considered for SWS evaluation. Capillary malformations that confer a particularly high risk for SWS include those that are hemifacial, localized to the median forehead, or extending across the bilateral forehead. Workup includes MRI with and without contrast to assess for leptomeningeal angiomatosis and an ophthalmologic examination to evaluate for choroidal vascular malformations and glaucoma.

Given the risk of occult spinal dysraphism, capillary malformations in the midline lumbosacral region may warrant further investigation with imaging studies. Paraspinal lumbosacral capillary malformations that appear in combination with a second congenital midline skin lesion present a particularly high risk for spinal anomalies. Infants less than 3 to 4 months of age should have an ultrasound to evaluate underlying structures; older infants and children may require MRI.

Patients with regional capillary malformations of the lower limb, PWS, and KTS may have overgrowth of the affected leg. Patients should be evaluated by an orthopedic surgeon for limb length discrepancy around 1 year of age and then followed over time.

Venous Malformations Given the risk of gastrointestinal venous malformations in BRBNS, patients with cutaneous venous malformations who present with signs or symptoms concerning for gastrointestinal bleeding require further workup; a complete blood count to assess for anemia and endoscopic studies may be indicated.

Lymphatic Malformations Chylous pleural effusions and chylous ascites occurring in the setting of lymphatic malformations may be more fully characterized with lymphoscintigram. If a pleurocentesis or paracentesis is performed, fluid analysis may show elevated triglycerides. An alternative approach to diagnosis is fat feeding, in which cream is administered enterally prior to obtaining a fluid sample. As triglycerides tend to accumulate in the lymphatic system, if there is a chyle leak, pleural effusions or ascites will become a characteristic milky white color.

Arteriovenous Malformations Evaluation of a potential AVM may include a Doppler exam, which may reveal a fast-flow lesion. Given that patients with CM-AVM are at risk for cerebral and spinal AVMs, further workup with an MRI/magnetic resonance angiogram (MRA) of the brain and spine may be considered.

MANAGEMENT

Capillary malformations may be treated with pulsed dye laser, which can yield partial clearance. Response varies based on location, age, and skin tone, among other factors. At least 8 to 10 treatments are required to optimize results, and touch-ups are typically required after initial treatments. Patients with SWS complicated by seizure disorder may require antiepileptic medications.

Venous malformation treatment is warranted when there is risk of disfigurement, functional impairment, pain, and swelling. Conservative management may include compression therapy to alleviate pain, reduce localized intravascular coagulation, and limit edema. Sclerotherapy and excision, alone or in combination, may be indicated for more symptomatic lesions. Low-molecular-weight heparin may improve pain resulting from localized thrombus formation. Direct oral anticoagulants may be beneficial in prophylaxis or treatment of thrombo-embolic sequelae of localized thrombus formation. Placement of an inferior vena cava filter may be warranted for patients at risk for pulmonary embolism. Finally, medical therapy with sirolimus may be beneficial in the treatment of gastrointestinal bleeding associated with BRBNS and other venous malformations.

Treatment of lymphatic malformations may be considered to preserve function, limit deformity, and minimize pain and swelling. First-line treatments for lymphatic malformations include medical therapy with sirolimus and/or sclerotherapy, depending on the size and extent of the lesions. Excision of lymphatic malformations may also be indicated in certain situations. Lastly, light-based therapies, such as pulsed dye laser (for hemorrhagic lesions) and carbon dioxide laser (a resurfacing laser), may be indicated for treatment of superficial microcystic lymphatic malformations.

Management of AVMs may be challenging. Treatment generally consists of embolization, resection, and/or medical therapy with trametinib. However, recurrence rates are high, ranging from 85% to 98%. There have also been case reports of successful treatment with trametinib, a mitogen-activated protein kinase (MEK) inhibitor. The risk of recurrence is typically lower following treatment of earlier-stage lesions.

Sirolimus targets the phosphatidylinositol 3-kinase (PI3K)/AKT signaling pathway to inhibit angiogenesis and lymphangiogenesis and has led to significant improvement in both vascular tumors and malformations. Recent evidence suggests that medical therapy with sirolimus is a safe and effective treatment for patients with a broad range of complicated vascular anomalies, including venous and lymphatic malformations as noted above.

Alpelisib, an oral medication that directly inhibits PIK3CA, was approved by the Food and Drug Administration in 2019 for the treatment patients with PIK3CA-related overgrowth syndrome (PROS), including KTS or CLOVES, with severe symptoms such as extensive vascular malformations or debilitating musculoskeletal issues due to overgrowth or scoliosis. Retrospective data indicate that alpelisib is both well-tolerated and effective in mitigating symptoms and complications related to PROS.

ADMISSION CRITERIA

Certain clinical scenarios require immediate attention and possible admission for complications of vascular malformations and/or postoperative management following necessary procedures. During admission, hospitalists may need to collaborate with vascular anomalies specialists in dermatology, hematology/oncology, orthopedics, otolaryngology, pathology, plastic surgery, radiology, and surgery.

- Patients with SWS and extensive leptomeningeal angiomatosis may require hospitalization for seizure management, and, at times, hemispherectomy. SWS patients with glaucoma and poorly controlled seizures may require admission following ophthalmologic procedures for observation of potential seizure activity.
- Patients with extensive venous malformations may have localized intravascular coagulopathy, deep venous thrombosis, and pulmonary emboli, particularly perioperatively, which may necessitate inpatient care for anticoagulation and monitoring.
- Patients with BRBNS may require inpatient stabilization or possible surgical intervention for gastrointestinal bleeding, intussusception, volvulus, or infarction.
- Patients with lymphatic malformations commonly develop bacterial superinfection and may require admission for intravenous antibiotics.
- Patients with lymphatic malformations may be hospitalized for respiratory distress in the setting of upper airway compression (usually due to infected lymphatic malformations), chylous pleural effusions, or chylous ascites. Airway compression may necessitate tracheotomy.
- Large AVMs may result in ulceration, pain, bleeding, obstruction of vital structures, and high-output cardiac failure. Admission may be required for endovascular embolization, resection, or management of heart failure.
- Potential complications of combined vascular malformations on an extremity include ulceration, pain, bleeding, recurrent cellulitis, deep venous thrombosis, and pulmonary embolism.
- Patients with a combined vascular malformation involving the lower limb (such as those with KTS or PWS) may be hospitalized following epiphysiodesis for leg length discrepancy.
- Patients with CLOVES syndrome may be hospitalized following spinal fusion for scoliosis.
- Patients with combined vascular anomalies (such as PROS) may be admitted for surgical debulking.
- Patients with venous or lymphatic malformations who have undergone sclerotherapy may develop postprocedural edema and pain requiring hospitalization (especially in the setting of airway involvement).

VASCULAR TUMORS

INTRODUCTION AND CLINICAL FEATURES

Vascular tumors arise due to endothelial hyperplasia and may be benign, borderline, locally aggressive, or sometimes malignant.

Infantile Hemangiomas Infantile hemangiomas are the most common vascular tumor of infancy, affecting 1% to 2.6% of healthy newborns. The clinical appearance of these benign tumors depends on their relative depth in the skin. Superficial lesions typically present as brightly erythematous lobulated plaques, while deep lesions are bluish to skin-colored, compressible subcutaneous nodules.

Infantile hemangiomas have a life cycle that is both predictable and unique. Infantile hemangiomas may be present at birth as a premonitory mark, such as a bruise-like lesion, erythematous patch, or area of pallor with or without telangiectasias. Infantile hemangiomas typically undergo accelerated growth in the first two months of life, followed by less rapid growth through the end of infancy, then slow involution over years.

Infantile hemangiomas in specific distributions may lead to functional sequelae or carry risk of comorbid conditions. Periorbital infantile hemangiomas (**Figure 58-2**) may cause visual obstruction or corneal deformation (astigmatism). Infantile hemangiomas involving the lower face (the preauricular region, chin, anterior neck, and lower lip) (**Figure 58-3**) are associated with subglottic infantile hemangiomas that may cause airway obstruction.

Multiple cutaneous infantile hemangiomas are associated with visceral hemangiomas, most commonly, hepatic infantile hemangiomas. Infants with five or more cutaneous infantile hemangiomas have a greater risk of accompanying hepatic hemangiomas. Patients with diffuse or multifocal intrahepatic hemangiomas may be at risk for high output cardiac failure due to arteriovenous shunting.

Patients with large infantile hemangiomas, particularly hepatic infantile hemangiomas, are at risk for hypothyroidism. Infantile hemangiomas produce type 3 iodothyronine deiodinase, which inactivates thyroxine and triiodothyronine.

Patients with regional infantile hemangiomas of the head and neck (**Figure 58-4**) are at risk for structural anomalies of cerebral vasculature, eyes, sternum, and aorta, which is denoted by the acronym PHACES (**P**osterior fossa anomalies, **H**emangioma, cervical and intracranial **A**rterial lesions, **C**ardiac abnormalities and **C**oarctation of the aorta, **E**ye abnormalities, and **S**ternal defects).

Regional infantile hemangiomas involving the lumbosacral region, perineal region, or lower extremity have been associated with urogenital anomalies, lipomas, tethered spinal cord, spinal dysraphism, bony abnormalities (such as limb length discrepancy and hip dysplasia), imperforate anus, arterial anomalies, and renal anomalies. These findings are denoted by the acronyms LUMBAR (**L**ower body hemangioma, **U**rogenital anomalies/ulceration, **M**yelopathy, **B**ony deformities, **A**norectal

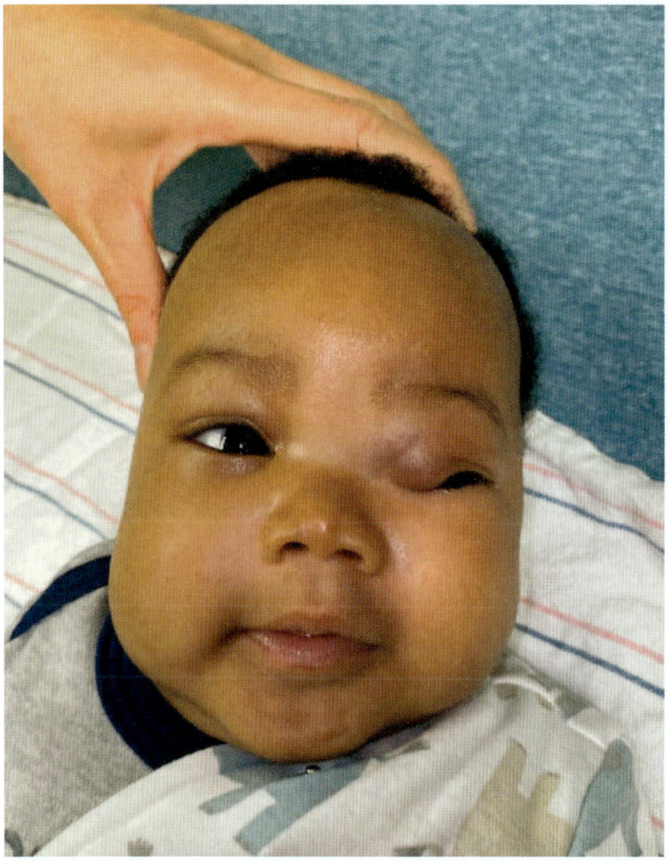

FIGURE 58-2. Infantile hemangioma of the left eyelid in an infant with astigmatism and visual obstruction.

malformations, arterial anomalies, and **R**enal anomalies), SACRAL (**S**pinal dysraphism, **A**nogenital, **C**utaneous, **R**enal and urologic anomalies, associated with an **A**ngioma of **L**umbosacral localization), and PELVIS (**P**erineal hemangioma, **E**xternal genitalia malformations, **L**ipomyelomeningocele, **V**esicorenal abnormalities, **I**mperforate anus, and **S**kin tag). Lumbar spine hemangiomas, in particular, have been associated with high risk of myelopathy. Infants with extensive lower extremity infantile hemangiomas may have underlying arterial anomalies in the affected region.

Congenital Hemangiomas Congenital hemangiomas are benign vascular tumors that, unlike infantile hemangiomas, are fully developed

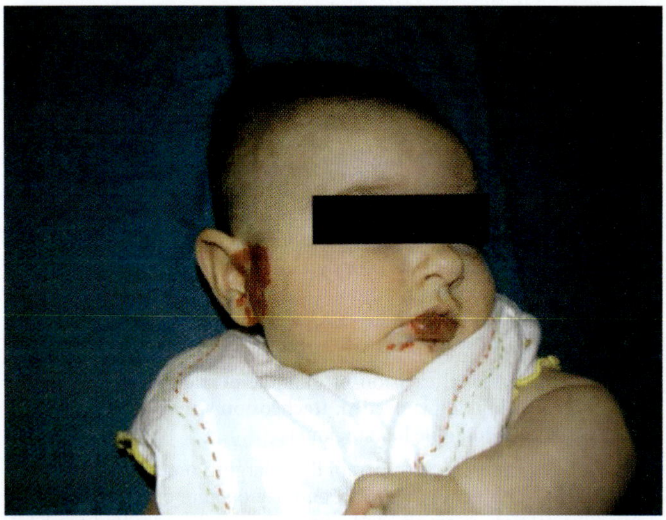

FIGURE 58-3. Lower facial infantile hemangioma in infant with subglottic hemangioma.

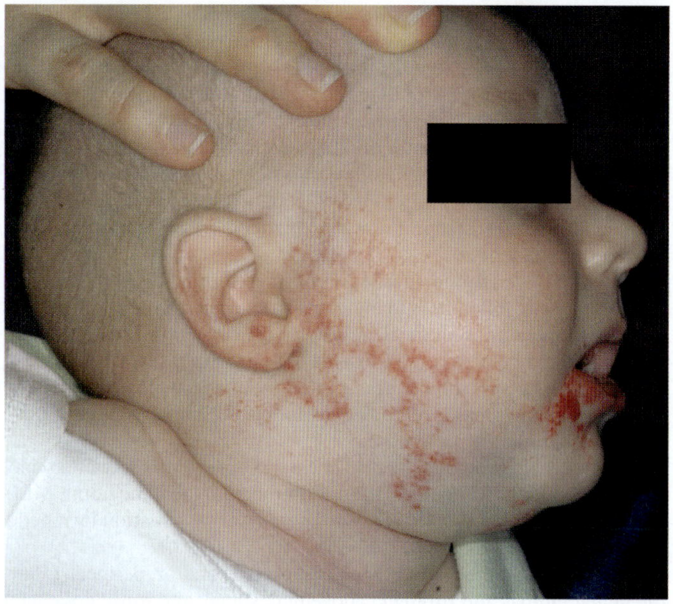

FIGURE 58-4. Regional facial infantile hemangioma in infant with PHACES association. MRI showed dysgenesis of the corpus callosum.

at birth and do not exhibit accelerated postnatal growth. Two primary variants of congenital hemangioma have been described: rapidly involuting congenital hemangiomas (RICH) and non-involuting congenital hemangiomas (NICH). RICH fully regress during infancy, while NICH tend to grow proportionately with the child and do not regress. Although variable in appearance, congenital hemangiomas are typically light blue-purple with multiple telangiectasias and sometimes surrounded by a pale halo. Hepatic RICH, which are usually discovered as palpable masses in the newborn period or incidentally on imaging, may be associated with high-output heart failure.

Tufted Angioma and Kaposiform Hemangioendothelioma Tufted angioma tend to develop in infancy or early childhood. Tufted angioma are generally ill-defined, infiltrating, firm, red to violaceous plaques. These may be associated with hyperhidrosis or hypertrichosis. Although the clinical course of tufted angioma may vary, typical progression includes slow growth over several months followed by size stabilization; spontaneous regression has occasionally been reported.

Kaposiform hemangioendothelioma (KHE) are rare infiltrative tumors that typically appear in infancy and may mimic infantile hemangiomas. Most commonly, KHE present as single, ill-defined, red to purple indurated plaques of the trunk or extremities. The clinical spectrum of KHE is broad; lesions may range from small, superficial cutaneous lesions to large, infiltrative lesions with involvement of fascia, muscle, and bone.

Tufted angioma and KHE may overlap both clinically and histologically and these tumors may exist on a continuum. Furthermore, both tufted angioma and KHE may be associated with Kasabach-Merritt phenomenon (KMP), characterized by profound thrombocytopenia and microangiopathic hemolytic anemia (resulting from intralesional trapping of platelet and clotting factors). Common presenting features of KMP include: (1) an enlarging lesion that becomes violaceous, indurated, and ecchymotic; (2) severe thrombocytopenia; (3) musculoskeletal pain or decreased function; and (4) anemia due to intravascular hemolysis.

DIAGNOSTIC EVALUATION

In most cases, vascular tumors may be diagnosed through history and physical examination. If the diagnosis is unclear, imaging studies including ultrasound and/or MRI as well as biopsy should be considered. These diagnostic studies/procedures can help distinguish between vascular tumors and mimickers, such as infantile fibrosarcoma, myofibroma, and rhabdomyosarcoma.

Periorbital infantile hemangiomas should be evaluated and monitored by a pediatric ophthalmologist to address visual obstruction or astigmatism and to prevent amblyopia. Prompt treatment is vital in this population of infants due to risk of long-term visual sequelae including ptosis, proptosis, strabismus, and permanent vision loss.

Given the risk of subglottic infantile hemangiomas in patients with lower facial infantile hemangiomas, laryngoscopy, and bronchoscopy should be pursued if stridor, barky cough, cyanosis, or hoarseness develop. Respiratory symptoms in these patients are often misdiagnosed as croup.

Abdominal ultrasound should be considered in patients with five or more cutaneous infantile hemangiomas to evaluate for hepatic involvement. If diffuse or multifocal intrahepatic hemangiomas are present, patients should be monitored for signs of high-output cardiac failure.

Thyroid function should be assessed in infants with large hepatic infantile hemangiomas given risk of hypothyroidism due to type 3 iodothyronine deiodinase production.

In patients with regional infantile hemangiomas of the face and scalp, evaluation for PHACES association should be pursued, including MRI/MRA of the brain and neck, echocardiogram, and evaluation by a pediatric ophthalmologist.

Given the association between lumbosacral and/or perineal infantile hemangiomas and urologic, anogenital, spinal, and musculoskeletal abnormalities, evaluation with imaging is indicated. Younger infants (often less than 3 months of age) may be evaluated with ultrasound of the spine. In older infants, spinal MRI should be considered, as ultrasound alone may miss spinal anomalies. All patients should have abdominal ultrasounds to evaluate for urologic abnormalities.

A lower extremity Doppler ultrasound or MRI/MRA to evaluate for arterial anomalies may be considered for infants with extensive lower extremity infantile hemangiomas.

Infants who present with a rapidly enlarging vascular lesion and signs of thrombocytopenia (e.g., bruising, petechiae, bleeding), should be evaluated for KMP. Initial laboratory workup will show severe thrombocytopenia (< 50,000/mm^3), decreased fibrinogen levels, increased fibrin split products, normal or minimally elevated prothrombin time and activated partial-thromboplastin time, and anemia. Imaging studies, such as ultrasonography, MRI, or biopsy, may be required to confirm the diagnosis.

Patients with hepatic RICH are at risk of developing high-output heart failure and should undergo cardiac workup if they develop shortness of breath, dyspnea, orthopnea, or edema.

MANAGEMENT

Infantile hemangiomas may be observed if they are small, localized, and spare vital structures. Systemic treatment is generally indicated for infantile hemangiomas associated with potential complications such as ulceration, visual impairment, airway obstruction, congestive heart failure, and disfigurement.

Propranolol is first-line therapy for infantile hemangiomas requiring systemic treatment. It is frequently initiated at a dose of 1 mg/kg/day, divided two or three times daily, with escalation to a target dose of 2 to 3 mg/kg/day, divided two or three times daily. Relative contraindications to propranolol therapy include sinus bradycardia, hypotension, heart block, and reactive airway disease. Hospitalization for initiation of propranolol has been recommended for very young infants, infants with inadequate social support, infants with comorbid cardiovascular or respiratory conditions, and those who require rapid escalation of propranolol dosing for management of high-risk hemangiomas. Reported side effects in infants taking propranolol include hypoglycemia, hypotension, wheezing, bradycardia, hyperkalemia, sleep disturbances, somnolence, cool extremities, and gastrointestinal upset. In order to avoid hypoglycemic events, propranolol should be held if a patient is ill, not feeding well, or vomiting.

Prior to 2008, when propranolol was first reported to dramatically improve infantile hemangiomas, systemic corticosteroids were considered first-line treatment for infantile hemangiomas. They are now primarily used in patients with high-risk infantile hemangiomas (e.g., vision-threatening lesions) that are rapidly growing and warrant dual therapy, or which have not responded to propranolol alone. Systemic corticosteroids may also be used when propranolol is contraindicated. Prednisolone is typically initiated at a dose of 2 mg/kg/day and is slowly tapered over months. Potential side effects include transient growth delay, gastric irritation, hyperglycemia, hypertension, Cushingoid appearance, vaccination failure, irritability, hypothalamic-pituitary-adrenal axis suppression, and increased risk of infection. Systemic corticosteroids stabilize or reduce the size of proliferating hemangiomas in approximately 85% of cases. Infantile hemangiomas that do not respond to propranolol and/or systemic corticosteroids may have a favorable clinical response to sirolimus.

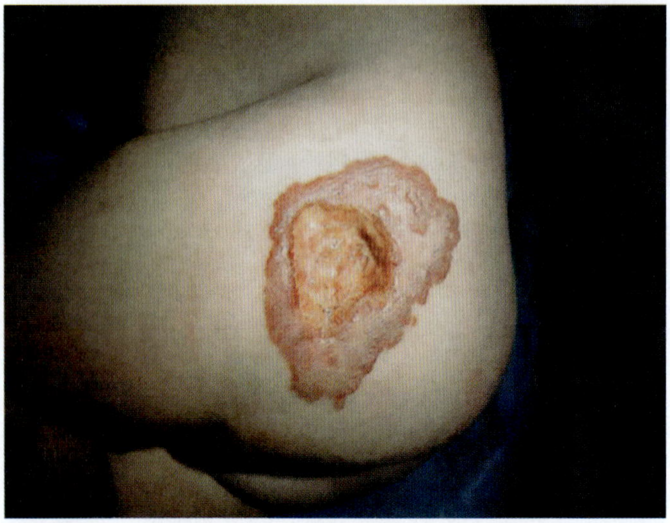

FIGURE 58-5. Ulcerated infantile hemangioma in an infant.

Large, deep, or painful ulcerations (**Figure 58-5**), particularly those that interfere with feeding, warrant referral to a specialist in vascular anomalies. Treatment options include barrier cream, topical or oral antibiotic, topical analgesic, pulsed dye laser, wound vacuum assisted closure (VAC), or systemic pharmacotherapy.

KHE and tufted angioma complicated by KMP may be associated with significant morbidity and mortality from hemorrhage, sepsis, or invasion of vital structures. Accordingly, prompt diagnosis and management are required. Treatment with sirolimus is now considered first-line therapy; systemic corticosteroids, propranolol, vincristine, cyclophosphamide, interferon alfa-2a, aspirin, ticlopidine, and radiotherapy have also been used successfully. Platelet transfusions should be avoided, except in cases of active bleeding or prior to procedures. Heparin should also be avoided.

ADMISSION CRITERIA

Occasionally, complications of vascular tumors of infancy may require immediate medical attention and admission:

- Ulcerated infantile hemangiomas may require admission for pain management, antibiotics, feeding evaluation/optimization, other pharmacologic treatment (such as propranolol or systemic corticosteroids), or excision.
- Rapidly proliferating infantile hemangiomas at risk of ulceration, functional impairment (e.g., obstruction of vision in eyelid lesions, airway obstruction in subglottic hemangiomas), or disfigurement may require admission for systemic therapy. These interventions may include rapid escalation of propranolol dosing while monitoring for hypoglycemia or, when propranolol has not yielded adequate improvement, initiation of intravenous corticosteroid.
- Patients may require hospitalization for postoperative management when total or partial excision of infantile hemangiomas is required or if urgent debulking is needed; tracheostomy may be necessary for some subglottic infantile hemangiomas.
- Patients who present with a rapidly enlarging or purpuric vascular lesion in combination with thrombocytopenia or pain/decreased range of motion of an affected extremity may be admitted for KMP management.

- Infants with large hepatic infantile hemangiomas may require admission for rapid initiation of intravenous thyroid hormone replacement therapy, management of abdominal compartment syndrome, or rarely, management of high-output cardiac failure.
- Hepatic RICH also carries the risk of high-output heart failure and admission may be required for cardiac management.

KEY POINTS

- Vascular anomalies are classified into malformations and tumors.
- Vascular malformations are composed of structurally abnormal vessels with normal endothelial turnover and can be composed of capillary, venous, lymphatic, arterial, or arteriovenous elements, alone or in combination. Vascular tumors result from endothelial hyperplasia.
- Treatment of vascular malformations is dictated by degree of functional impairment, disfigurement, pain, bleeding, or issues related to associated syndromes.
- Complications of vascular malformations warranting inpatient admission include management of seizures, coagulopathy, pain, bleeding, bacterial superinfection, chylous pleural effusions and/or ascites, airway compromise, musculoskeletal abnormalities, and rarely, high-output cardiac failure.
- Infantile hemangioma is the most common vascular tumor of infancy; it typically proliferates for the first 10 to 12 months of life, then involutes slowly over years.
- Many infantile hemangiomas may be observed or treated with topical timolol; lesions that pose risks such as ulceration, visual impairment, airway obstruction, bleeding, hypothyroidism, permanent disfigurement, and high-output cardiac failure warrant systemic treatment.
- Problematic infantile hemangiomas are typically treated with propranolol. Severe cases may require systemic corticosteroids and/or excision.
- Kasabach-Merritt phenomenon is severe thrombocytopenia secondary to platelet trapping by kaposiform hemangioendothelioma or tufted angioma and warrants urgent inpatient care. Kasabach-Merritt phenomenon does not occur with infantile hemangioma.

SUGGESTED READINGS

Adams DM, Trenor CC, Hammill AM, et al. Efficacy and safety of sirolimus in the treatment of complicated vascular anomalies. *Pediatrics.* 2016;137(2):e20153257.

Canaud G, Lopez Gutierrez J, Irvine A, et al. LBA23 - EPIK-P1: retrospective chart review study of patients (pts) with "PIK3CA"-related Overgrowth Spectrum (PROS) who have received alpelisib (ALP) as part of a compassionate use programme. 2021.

Dávila-Osorio VL, Iznardo H, Roé E, Puig L, Baselga E. Propranolol-resistant infantile hemangioma successfully treated with sirolimus. *Pediatr Dermatol.* 2020;37(4):684-686.

ISSVA classification for vascular anomalies. https://www.issva.org/classification.

Klosterman T, O TM. The management of vascular malformations of the airway: natural history, investigations, medical, surgical and radiological management. *Otolaryngol Clin North Am.* 2018;51(1):213-223.

Nicholson CL, Flanagan S, Murati M, et al. Successful management of an arteriovenous malformation with trametinib in a patient with capillary-malformation arteriovenous malformation syndrome and cardiac compromise. *Pediatr Dermatol.* 2022;39(2):316-319.

Ogu UO, Abusin G, Abu-Arja RF, Staber JM. Successful management of Blue Rubber Bleb Nevus Syndrome (BRBNS) with sirolimus. *Case Rep Pediatr.* 2018;2018:7654278.

Sabeti S, Ball KL, Bhattacharya SK, et al. Consensus statement for the management and treatment of Sturge-Weber syndrome: Neurology, neuroimaging, and ophthalmology recommendations. *Pediatr Neurol.* 2021;121:59-66.

van der Vleuten CJM, Zwerink LGJM, Klappe EM, de Jong EMGJ, Te Loo DMWM. Is there a place for prophylaxis with DOACs in Klippel-Trenaunay syndrome and other low-flow vascular malformations with intravascular coagulopathy and thromboembolic events? *Thromb Res.* 2022;213:30-33.

Zhuo KY, Russell S, Wargon O, Adams S. Localised intravascular coagulation complicating venous malformations in children: associations and therapeutic options. *J Paediatr Child Health.* 2017;53(8):737-741.

CHAPTER 59

Atopic Dermatitis

David C. Synhorst, MD, MPA

BACKGROUND

Although atopic dermatitis (AD) is often encountered and managed in the outpatient setting, hospitalists must be familiar with its presentation and management in inpatient settings. AD, or atopic eczema, is a common inflammatory skin disorder characterized by pruritus, a chronic and recurrent course, and a distinctive anatomic distribution and morphology. It is often accompanied by a personal or family history of other allergic disorders. Epidemiologic data suggest the prevalence of AD is increasing, with rates approaching 20% in the United States. Although most patients are treated in the outpatient setting, one-third to-half of the yearly expenditures for AD are directly related to the costs of hospitalization, either due to the severity of AD itself or due to secondary complications such as bacterial or viral superinfection.

PATHOPHYSIOLOGY

AD appears to be a multifactorial disease that involves dysregulation of the immune response, creating a compromised skin barrier and associated cutaneous hyperreactivity. Studies suggest that T cells, particularly those expressing markers for the Th2-response, are upregulated in acute AD. The elaboration of Th2-related cytokines, such as interleukin (IL)-4, IL-5, and IL-13, indirectly results in increased immunoglobulin E (IgE) production and eosinophilia. In the chronic phase of AD, Th1-related cytokines predominate, including IL-12 and interferon-γ. Other pathobiologic abnormalities noted in patients with AD include a genetic predisposition to atopy, disturbed essential fatty acid metabolism, increased leukocyte phosphodiesterase activity, autonomic nervous system dysregulation, pruritus, and a predisposition to infection.

Although the genetic basis of AD has yet to be elucidated, studies of twins and families clearly indicate a familial predisposition in approximately two-thirds of patients. It is unlikely that AD is the result of a single gene; rather, it appears to be the result of multiple genes interacting with environmental factors to produce the disorder. Mutations in filaggrin, kallikrein 7, and cystatin A genes may play a central role in barrier function defects.

The threefold increase in the prevalence of AD over the past three decades is likely multifactorial. However, the marked prevalence increase is likely in part explained by the hygiene hypothesis. In brief, the hygiene hypothesis suggests that improved hygiene in the modern era has decreased immune exposure to infectious agents with the unfortunate adverse effects of increased autoimmunity and dysregulation of components of the immune response.

Patients with AD are prone to colonization and infection (i.e., superinfection) by both bacterial and viral organisms, especially *Staphylococcus aureus*, herpes simplex virus (HSV), and molluscum contagiosum virus. The propensity for microbial colonization in AD patients is likely multifactorial. Impaired skin integrity creates a favorable environment for organisms to adhere to the skin while there is a concurrent decrease in antimicrobial skin properties. Naturally occurring skin peptides with antimicrobial activity, including cathelicidins and defensins, are produced less in patients with AD. These factors collectively predispose AD patients to staphylococcal superinfection, Kaposi varicelliform eruption (or, more specifically, eczema herpeticum), and extensive outbreaks with molluscum contagiosum and coxsackie viruses. Some speculate that because certain bacterial superantigens are known to bind glucocorticoid receptors, patients with significant bacterial colonization may seem steroid resistant or appear to have tachyphylaxis.

CLINICAL PRESENTATION

AD typically affects young children (under 2 years of age) and presents with markedly pruritic, erythematous papules arising from a background of dry skin, generally with notable excoriations present (**Table 59-1**). Typically, parents of the affected child will report a chronic and relapsing course with the rash noted most prominently on flexor surfaces. Nighttime itching is also commonly reported. Typically, exposed skin surfaces not covered by clothing are prone to itch, although certain rough fabrics, such as wool, may aggravate pruritus in atopic patients.

The skin in early atopic eczema may itch without obvious cutaneous findings. With continued scratching, the skin becomes erythematous, scaly, and excoriated. The term *eczema* has its origins in a Greek word meaning "boiling over," and this accurately describes the morphology of an acute lesion of atopic eczema, with exuberant oozing and crusting. Chronic excoriation may lead to thickening and altered pigmentation of the skin. Patients with significant involvement of the hands may also have nail pitting. The findings of xerosis, ichthyosis, keratosis pilaris, pityriasis alba, pruritus with sweating, perifollicular accentuation, orbital darkening, hand and foot dermatitis, conjunctivitis, white dermatographism, and nipple eczema are all associated with AD. Although these findings have low individual sensitivity and specificity for AD, the presence of multiple corroborating features may be helpful in identifying AD when the presentation is atypical.

The distribution of AD lesions evolves with age. Infants tend to show more widespread disease, with generalized involvement of the face, neck, extremities, and torso. Sparing of the nose, perinasal area, and diaper area is characteristic; this helps distinguish AD from seborrheic dermatitis and other skin disorders (**Figure 59-1**). Accentuation within the flexural creases—the wrist, antecubital, proximal posterior thigh, popliteal, and ankle areas (**Figures 59-2 and 59-3**)—may be evident in infancy but is more frequently observed in toddlers and older children. Children may also suffer from scalp pruritus, scaling, and lymphadenopathy, which may make it difficult to distinguish AD from other scalp dermatoses such as tinea capitis. Most affected adolescents and adults have limited involvement of the hands (more pronounced on dorsal aspect) or face (including eyelids).

Fortunately, 84% of affected children have mild to moderate disease and most improve with age. Those with more severe disease are less likely to have spontaneous remission. However, remission rates >90% by age 10 years for infants with AD have been reported; 10-year clearance rates appear to be closer to 50% to 70% for those who develop signs of AD later during childhood. Unfortunately, patients with AD have an increased propensity for developing other atopic diseases including asthma and allergic rhinitis. Based on clinical observations, patients sometimes progress sequentially from AD to the development of asthma and allergic rhinitis in what has been referred to as the "atopic march."

TABLE 59-1 Clinical Features of Atopic Dermatitis

Essential Features
Pruritus
Eczema (acute, subacute, chronic)—typical morphology and age-specific patterns with chronic or relapsing history
Important Features
Early age of onset
Atopy—manifested by personal or family history or immunoglobulin E reactivity
Associated Features
Atypical vascular responses—dermatographism, delayed blanch response, facial pallor
Keratosis pilaris, hyperlinear palms, ichthyosis
Ocular or periorbital changes
Other areas of change (e.g. periorbital, periauricular)
Perifollicular accentuation, lichenification, prurigo lesions

Source: Reproduced with permission From Eichenfield LF, Hanifin JM, Luger TA, et al. Consensus conference on pediatric atopic dermatitis. *J Am Acad Dermatol.* 2003; 49(6): 1088-1095.

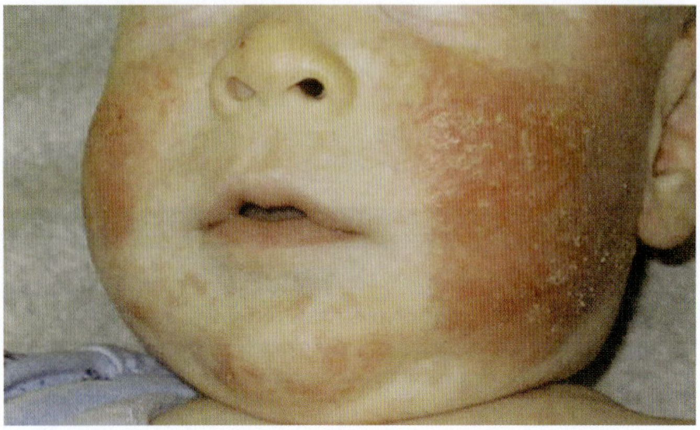

FIGURE 59-1. Atopic dermatitis of the face. Note the characteristic sparing of the perinasal areas.

SUPERINFECTION

Bacterial Superinfection Clinical signs of bacterial superinfection are likely to include worsening AD symptoms, oozing or weeping pustules, increasing erythema, warmth, pain, and failure to respond to usual AD therapies. Although patients with AD are nearly universally colonized by *S. aureus*, approximately half go on to develop frank signs and symptoms of infection at some point in their disease (**Figure 59-4**). Other skin flora such as Group A streptococcus can also cause bacterial superinfection in children with AD.

Kaposi Varicelliform Eruption Patients with AD may suffer acute superimposed eruptions of umbilicated vesicular or pustular lesions due to superinfection by HSV, coxsackievirus, vaccinia virus, and variola virus. The phenomenon has been referred to as Kaposi varicelliform eruption because of its resemblance to severe varicella infection.

When the causative agent is HSV, the condition is specifically called eczema herpeticum. As individual lesions of HSV evolve, they become hemorrhagic and then develop a more typical "punched-out" appearance (**Figure 59-5**). Often, clusters of vesicles and pustules localize to facial or flexural areas and may be superimposed on areas of existing AD. Children may be ill appearing, have fever, lymphadenopathy, and poor oral intake, especially if there is an associated gingivostomatitis.

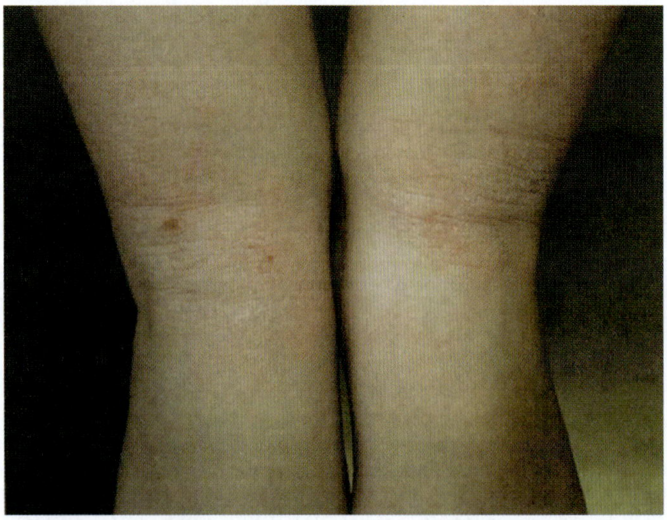

FIGURE 59-2. Atopic dermatitis involving the popliteal spaces.

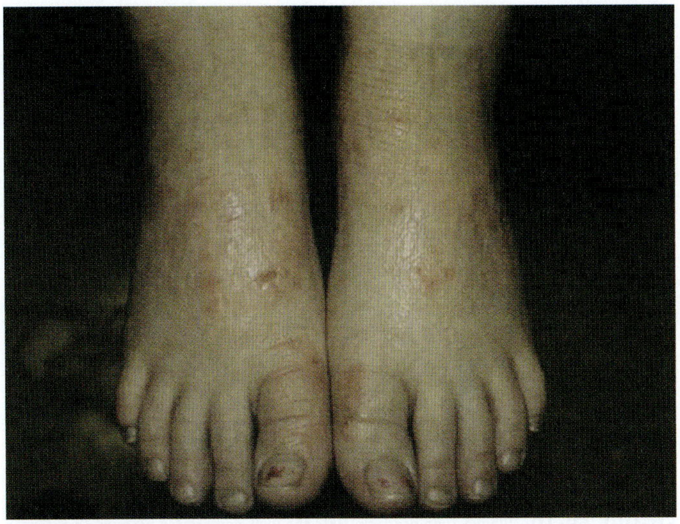

FIGURE 59-3. Atopic dermatitis involving the ankles.

Superinfection with coxsackievirus, vaccina virus, and variola virus are less common but can cause similar rashes that are painful, erythematous, and overlie areas of active AD.

DIFFERENTIAL DIAGNOSIS

A variety of conditions may have overlappying features with or complicate AD and should be considered in the differential diagnosis. Pityriasis alba is characterized by patches of indistinct hypopigmentation and scaling, often on the face or extremities. This may represent an incomplete form of AD, a feature supportive of a diagnosis of AD, or an independent phenomenon. It is often aggravated by the use of harsh soaps or cleansers.

Nummular dermatitis (nummular eczema) consists of discrete, coin-shaped areas of erythema, lichenification, and scaling (**Figure 59-6**). It may occur on extensor surfaces. This disease is often less responsive to low-potency topical agents and may require higher-potency agents. Although nummular dermatitis may represent a form of AD, some argue that it is a distinct entity.

Keratosis pilaris is identified by perifollicular keratotic papules on the face, upper arms, or legs. Although keratosis pilaris is a minor manifestation associated with AD, it is a distinct clinical disorder that is frequently mistaken for AD. The condition typically does not respond significantly to topical therapies. However, applying moisturizers, especially keratolytic moisturizers (those containing urea or lactate), can be helpful in moderating the appearance of the lesions.

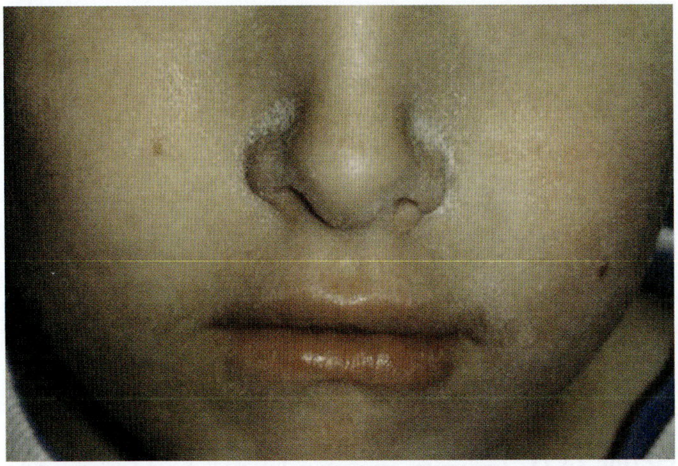

FIGURE 59-4. Atopic dermatitis associated with staphylococcal superinfection.

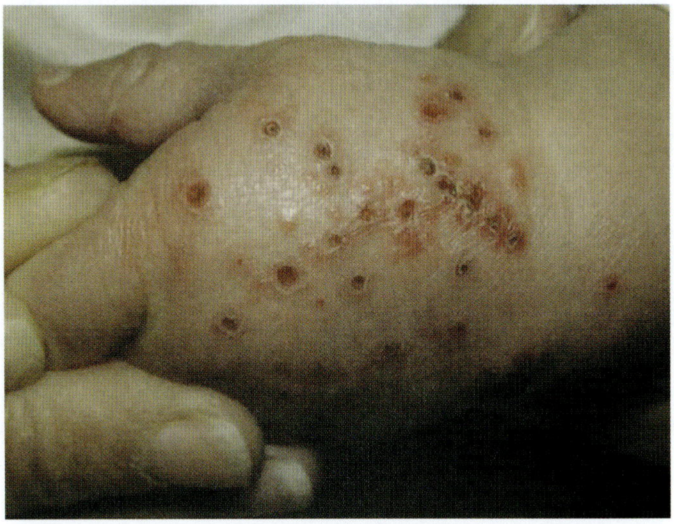

FIGURE 59-5. Note the "punched-out" erosions characteristic of eczema herpeticum.

Prurigo lesions are often lichenified or even keratotic papules and nodules, whereas lichen simplex chronicus manifests as lichenified plaques (**Figure 59-7**). Both result from chronic excoriation of an area of skin. These dermatoses may occur as a result of AD or may be initiated by some other pruritic process. They are often less responsive to low-potency topical agents and may require higher-potency agents.

Seborrheic dermatitis (seborrheic eczema) is a salmon-colored erythema and scaling of the scalp, perinasal area (**Figure 59-8**), eyebrows, ears, axillae, or diaper area; often, little pruritus occurs.

Contact dermatitis (contact eczema) consists of patterned areas of erythema, scaling, oozing, or frank vesiculation. Linear or geometric areas may be noted in response to an allergen (e.g., poison ivy, nickel, fragrances).

Scabies infestation may resemble AD due to involvement of the hands, feet, wrists, ankles, and other flexural creases. In addition, scratching may cause secondary eczematous changes. However, involvement of atypical areas such as the axillae, inguinal creases, scrotum, and inframammary areas suggests scabies (**Figure 59-9**). Also, household contacts with similar symptoms, or an initial onset outside of the typical age range, favors scabies over AD.

Although there may be some similarities between the skin lesions of AD and psoriasis, several distinguishing features may be visible on clinical examination. Psoriatic lesions typically consist of well-demarcated plaques with beefy erythema and superficial white scale (**Figure 59-10**).

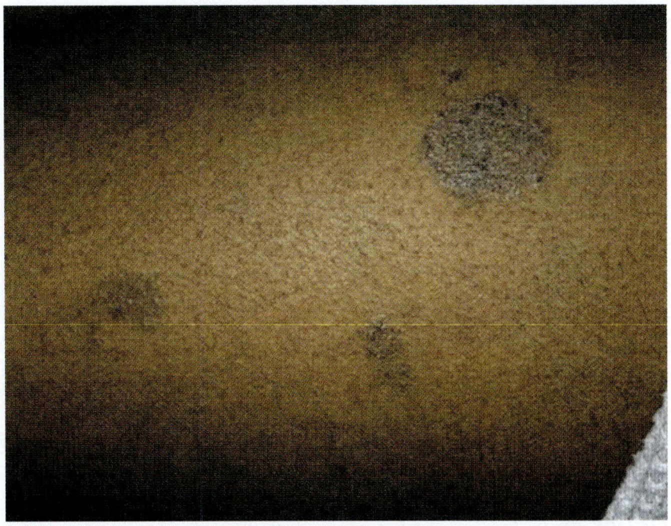

FIGURE 59-6. Coin-shaped lesions of nummular dermatitis.

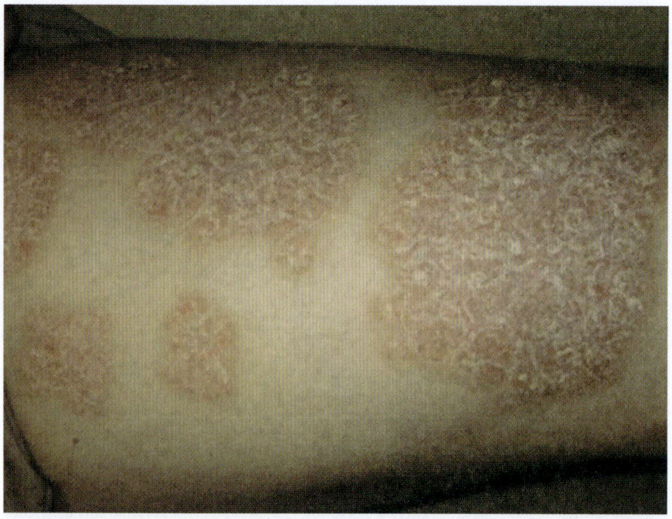

FIGURE 59-7. Areas that are chronically excoriated can evolve into lichen simplex chronicus.

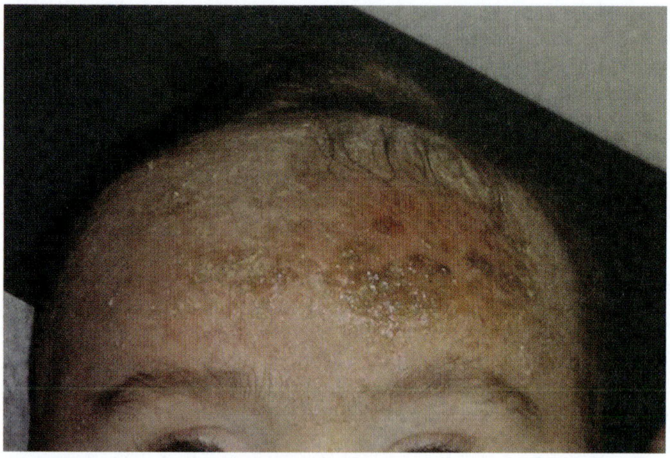

FIGURE 59-8. A patient with seborrheic dermatitis.

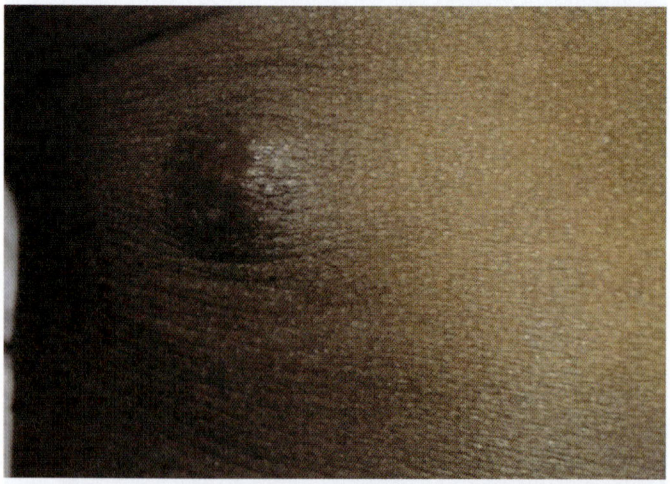

FIGURE 59-9. Scabies in an infant may manifest with vesicles and papules associated with excoriations.

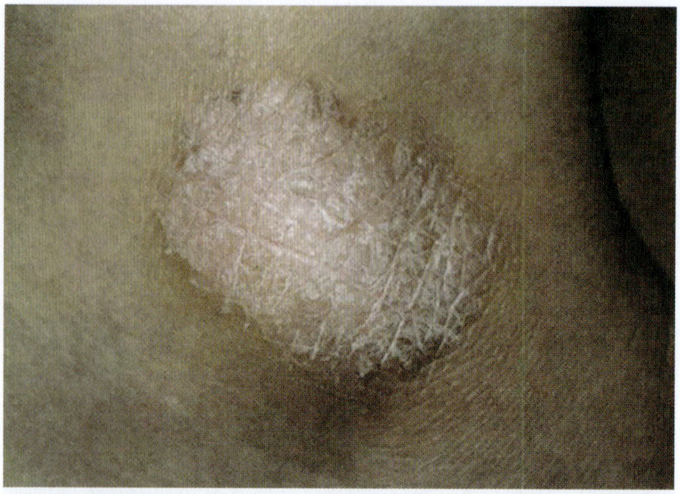

FIGURE 59-10. Plaque-type psoriasis. Note the well-demarcated plaques on extensor surfaces.

Lesions are classically located on extensor surfaces, rather than flexural creases. The scalp, palms, soles, and intertriginous (axillae, inguinal, genital, intergluteal) areas may also be involved. Nail pitting may be seen in both AD and psoriasis.

The differential diagnosis for scalp scaling includes scalp AD as well as psoriasis, seborrheic dermatitis, tinea capitis, and Langerhans cell histiocytosis.

The facial (often U-shaped area around the mouth) and acrally located dermatitis of acrodermatitis enteropathica (**Figure 59-11**) may resemble AD, though this disorder is related to zinc metabolism. However, there is typically chronic diaper-area involvement, as well as symptoms of diarrhea, hair loss, and irritability.

Wiskott-Aldrich syndrome and hyper-IgE syndrome are associated with chronic, severe AD. A number of other diseases result in an eczematous dermatitis resembling AD. These include ataxia-telangiectasia, cutaneous T-cell lymphoma, dermatophytosis, Dubowitz syndrome, gluten-sensitive enteropathy, Hartnup syndrome, histidinemia, Hurler syndrome, hypervitaminosis A, ichthyosis, kwashiorkor, Langerhans cell histiocytosis, necrolytic erythema, Netherton syndrome, phenylketonuria, selective IgA deficiency, severe combined immunodeficiency, secondary syphilis, and X-linked agammaglobulinemia.

DIAGNOSTIC EVALUATION

AD is diagnosed using characteristic clinical criteria. Although many historical factors and physical examination findings have been associated with AD, certain features are particularly helpful as they have

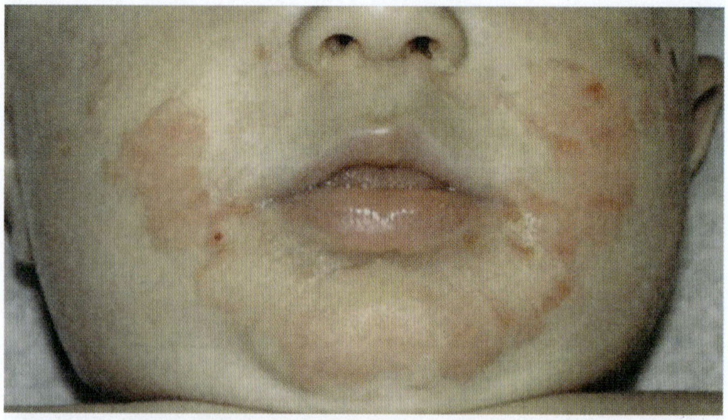

FIGURE 59-11. Acrodermatitis enteropathica. Note the U-shaped distribution of the facial dermatitis that is typical of patients with this condition.

TABLE 59-2 Criteria for the Diagnosis of Atopic Dermatitis*

Major Criteria	Minor Criteria
Typical morphology and distribution	Xerosis
Children: facial and extensor involvement	Ichthyosis, keratosis pilaris, palmar hyperlinearity
Adults: flexural lichenification or linearity	Immediate (type I) skin test reactivity
Chronic or relapsing dermatitis	Elevated serum immunoglobulin E
Personal or family history	Early age of onset
Pruritus	Tendency for skin infection (*Staphylococcus aureus*, herpes), impaired cellular immunity
	Hand or foot dermatitis
	Nipple eczema
	Conjunctivitis
	Dennie-Morgan fold
	Keratoconus
	Anterior subcapsular cataracts
	Orbital darkening
	Facial pallor, erythema
	Pityriasis alba
	Anterior neck folds
	Itch when sweating
	Intolerance to wool or lipid solvents
	Perifollicular accentuation
	Food intolerance
	Course influenced by environmental or emotional factors
	White dermatographic, delayed blanch

*Patients must have three of four major criteria and three minor criteria.

Source: Reproduced with permission from Hanifin JM, Rajka G. Diagnostic features of atopic dermatitis. *Acta Derm Venereol.* 1980; 92: 44-47.

greater sensitivity and specificity. While diagnostic criteria described for the purposes of AD research have been difficult to apply in the clinical setting, a set of practical working guidelines for the diagnosis of AD was created through a consensus conference that includes essential and supporting diagnostic criteria (**Table 59-2**). Pruritus and a chronic, relapsing skin rash with typical morphology and distribution are essential to the diagnosis of AD.

While not part of the above diagnostic criteria, most cases are also associated with an early age of onset (typically younger than 2 years) and a personal or family history of atopy (e.g., asthma, allergic rhinitis, IgE reactivity). Additional findings may help confirm the diagnosis. These guidelines emphasize that AD is principally a clinical diagnosis. Confirmatory laboratory testing or histopathologic analysis is generally not indicated or required; however, AD has been associated with some common lab findings (**Table 59-3**).

Diagnosis of superinfection is based on clinical recognition of erythema, warmth, weeping or crusting of lesions, and potentially systemic signs of illness. Because of skin colonization, routine bacterial surface swabs are generally not indicated, unless there is concern for antibiotic resistance or recurrent infection. For Kaposi varicelliform eruption, swabs of the affected area for fluorescent antibody testing (HSV), polymerase chain reaction (HSV, coxsackie, vaccinia), viral culture (HSV), or skin biopsy for histology and electron microscopy (variola) may be warranted.

TREATMENT

Most patients with AD are successfully managed in the outpatient setting. However, recalcitrant itching and scratching, associated poor sleep quality and secondary infections can be burdensome for patients and families. AD is often chronic, never "cured." Thus, the goals of AD management include: (i) optimizing skin care; (ii) reducing pruritus and cutaneous inflammation; (iii) avoiding potential aggravating factors, including environmental and food allergens; and (iv) treating secondary infection. Hospitalists should be aware that the treatments for AD are often time and labor intensive; psychosocial and socioeconomic costs of this disease are often substantial.

TABLE 59-3 Laboratory Assessment for Atopic Dermatitis

Laboratory Test*	Rationale
Complete blood count with differential; blood culture	Eosinophilia may be present; leukocytosis may be compatible with superinfection
Immunoglobulin E (IgE) levels	May be very elevated; may be associated with hyper-IgE syndrome
Serum zinc levels	Increased skin turnover may result in low serum zinc levels; patients with irritability and chronic facial and acral dermatitis may have acquired zinc deficiency, which may resemble atopic dermatitis
Skin culture	Bacterial culture may help determine the antibiotic-resistance profile of resident *Staphylococcus* species and may be useful in superinfected patients to determine optimal antibiotic therapy
Direct fluorescent antibody testing, polymerase chain reaction, or viral culture of skin lesions	May be helpful in identifying viral agents causing secondary infection or Kaposi varicelliform eruption (e.g. herpes simplex virus, coxsackievirus, vaccinia virus)
Skin biopsy	May be helpful in differentiating atopic dermatitis from other scaly skin disorders (e.g. psoriasis, ichthyosis, nutritional deficiency syndromes)
Skin testing or RAST	Food allergy may occur in up to 30% of severe cases of atopic dermatitis

*Laboratory testing not routinely required in the diagnosis or treatment of AD.

RAST, radioallergosorbent test.

ATOPIC SKIN CARE

Bathing Controversy exists regarding bathing. Some practitioners advocate for frequent, long baths to reduce exposure to environmental allergens and hydrate the skin (the "wet school"). Others argue against frequent bathing, with concern that it alters normal skin pH, reduces normal skin proteins that help maintain skin hydration, and is more laborious for families (the "dry school"). The choice of a wet versus a dry approach varies among clinicians, and patients and families may have their own preferences. A mild soap with a neutral or acidic pH, such as Dove, Oil of Olay, Cetaphil, or comparable products, is recommended for bathing.

Emollients Frequent use of emollients can improve skin barrier integrity and reduce reliance on other pharmacologic agents. Because lotions have a high alcohol content, children may complain of burning or stinging when they are applied; therefore, creams and ointments are the preferred vehicles for emollients. These include petrolatum-based moisturizers and various hydrophilic ointments such as petroleum jelly, Aquaphor, Eucerin, Absorbase, Acid Mantle cream, Cetaphil cream, Vanicream, or other comparable products. In addition, newer ceramide-containing emollients have been developed to reduce transepidermal water loss and improve barrier function.

Avoidance of Aggravating Factors Although patients may be unable to identify specific triggers for their AD flares, several environmental factors have been associated with the aggravation of AD. Wool or other abrasive fabrics, pets, dust mites, and specific foods may trigger flares in certain patients. Food allergens are associated with AD in a minority of patients (5% to 30%); though, the likelihood of a food allergy tends to increase with the severity of AD. The most common foods implicated in AD exacerbations include milk, eggs, wheat, soy, and nuts. Because it is difficult to eliminate all these foods, consultation with an allergist may be helpful when environmental or specific food allergens are suspected. In addition, contact dermatitis may coexist in patients with recalcitrant atopic dermatitis. Referral for patch testing should be considered in suspected cases.

PRURITUS AND INFLAMMATION

Children with AD often require topical anti-inflammatory agents to reduce pruritus and inflammation. When selecting topical agents, the choice of vehicle is important in terms of both efficacy and compliance. Ointments are more occlusive and tend to contain fewer ingredients and less alcohol therefore causing less stinging and burning; however, they may leave the patient feeling greasy. Creams are less occlusive, have a greater propensity to cause stinging and burning, but may be better tolerated by older children and adults. Lotions and solutions are generally less effective emollients and contain higher concentrations of alcohol, but these may be better tolerated in hair-bearing areas such as the scalp.

Topical Corticosteroids Topical corticosteroids have been used extensively for AD to reduce inflammation. Corticosteroids bind to cytoplasmic receptors, and translocate to the nucleus, where they decrease the transcription of proinflammatory cytokines. The choice of topical corticosteroid should be based on the patient's age, the anatomic site being treated, and tailored to disease severity.

Low-potency topical corticosteroids (e.g., hydrocortisone acetonide 1% or 2.5%, desonide 0.05%, alclometasone 0.05%) can be used safely on all areas of the body, including the face and intertriginous areas, for short periods of time. Medium-potency agents (e.g., fluocinolone 0.025%, hydrocortisone valerate 0.2%, triamcinolone 0.1%, fluticasone 0.05%) may be necessary for patients with more active disease. These agents should be avoided on the face and intertriginous areas and warrant closer medical supervision. High-potency corticosteroids (e.g., fluocinonide 0.05%, desoximetasone 0.25%, betamethasone dipropionate 0.05%) may be considered for short-term, supervised use for recalcitrant disease on the hands and feet. Although high-potency topical steroids are more effective than low-potency agents, their potential side effects are more notable, including cutaneous atrophy and striae, Cushing syndrome, and hypothalamic-pituitary-adrenal axis suppression.

Topical Calcineurin Inhibitors Topical calcineurin inhibitors have been approved by the Food and Drug Administration (FDA) for the treatment of AD. Tacrolimus (Protopic) 0.03% and 0.1% ointment and pimecrolimus (Elidel) 1% cream are macrolide immunosuppressive agents that reduce inflammation by decreasing the production of proinflammatory cytokines. Because these agents are nonsteroidal, they do not have the side effects of topical corticosteroids and can be used on any affected cutaneous surface, including the face, eyelids, and perineal area. In general, pimecrolimus 1% cream is indicated for the treatment of mild to moderate AD, while topical tacrolimus ointments are indicated for the treatment of moderate to severe AD. Both pimecrolimus 1% cream and tacrolimus 0.03% ointment are indicated in children 2 years and older for the treatment of acute AD flares, as well as for long-term, intermittent therapy; the more concentrated tacrolimus 0.1% ointment is approved for children 15 years and older. For both agents, application twice daily is recommended for optimal effect. Topical tacrolimus appears to have greater efficacy but may irritate the skin more than pimecrolimus.

In February 2005 the FDA issued a public health advisory regarding the use of topical calcineurin inhibitors. Specifically, the advisory cited the increased risk of lymphoma and skin cancers observed in animal studies where very high doses of the drugs were ingested. It is unclear whether clinically useful doses of topical calcineurin inhibitors pose any significant risk to humans. Population-based studies, as well as most laboratory and theoretical models, have not found an increased incidence of cancer among pediatric and adult patients using either medication. Manufacturers of both agents have established long-term patient registries to gather safety information. Both drugs continue to represent useful additions to the pharmacopeia for AD for long-term, intermittent use as a maintenance strategy in the prevention of disease flare.

Phosphodiesterase Inhibitors Crisaborole, a topical, small-molecule phosphodiesterase-4 inhibitor, reduces production of proinflammatory cytokines by increasing cyclic AMP. It also rapidly reduces pruritus in AD patients. Oral apremilast, a phosphodiesterase inhibitor currently indicated for psoriasis, may provide some benefit in AD according to case series.

Antihistamines Studies have reached conflicting conclusions regarding the efficacy of antihistamines for AD-associated pruritus. Sedating antihistamines, such as hydroxyzine, diphenhydramine, and doxepin, appear to be more effective than less sedating antihistamines. For patients complaining of nighttime itching, a sedating antihistamine at bedtime may be particularly helpful.

Systemic Corticosteroids In general, the use of systemic steroids (prednisone, prednisolone, methylprednisolone, and dexamethasone) should not be a first-line therapy for AD. If steroids are necessary for the management of other comorbid conditions such as asthma, a gradual taper over 7 to 14 days may be considered, and topical steroids should be instituted as part of the regimen to minimize the potential for AD flare with steroid withdrawal. Some clinicians have anecdotally observed that patients receiving multiple courses of systemic steroids subsequently suffer from more brittle AD; however, it is also possible that patients with more severe AD are treated with systemic steroids more often than are those with less severe disease.

Wet Wraps Wet wraps may be used to provide a semi-occlusive dressing that promotes penetration of topical steroids into the skin and supports skin hydration. This relatively easy and effective method may obviate the need for systemic corticosteroids, can be initiated during hospitalization, and continued after discharge. After the patient is bathed in lukewarm water, a low-potency topical steroid is applied to all affected areas of skin. Soft, moist, water-soaked dressing material, with excess water removed by squeezing, is applied to the skin, followed by a layer of dry dressings. This method generally works best when the dressings are left in place for many hours or worn overnight. This process can be continued for 1 to 2 weeks. At home, the child can substitute moist cotton pajamas for the water-soaked dressing.

Biologic Agents For those with more severe or refractory disease, biologic agents should be considered. The most commonly used of these is dupilumab. Dupilumab is an IL-4 antagonist and has been approved by the US Food and Drug Administration for the treatment of children 6 months and older with moderate to severe AD. Generally, this medication is administered subcutaneously with a loading dose, followed by maintenance doses every 2 weeks. Another potential biologic medication that shows promise in the treatment of AD is omalizumab, a humanized IgG antibody which binds the patient's IgE, thus reducing atopy. This medication was initially used in the treatment of severe asthma, however, given the common immune pathways between the two conditions, studies are currently underway to evaluate omalizumab's efficacy in the treatment of AD. Both medications should likely be considered in consultation with a dermatologist or allergist.

Alternative Agents Patients who suffer from severe AD may be prescribed other medications or therapeutic options. Ultraviolet (UV) light has a number of effects on the skin; in patients with AD, it reduces the presence of cutaneous inflammatory T cells. Patients on UV treatment may have tanned skin and run the risk of ultraviolet light burns, especially those receiving photosensitizing agents as part of their therapy.

Cyclosporine, a potent, broad-spectrum, systemic immunosuppressive, has been used successfully in patients with severe, recalcitrant AD. Its use is limited, however, by the potential side effects, ranging from nausea, fatigue, and hirsutism to hypertension, renal insufficiency, immune suppression, and increased risk for malignancy.

Additional studies have documented the use of the potent, broad-spectrum immunosuppressives azathioprine and mycophenolate mofetil, but they carry the side effects of immune suppression and an increased risk for malignancy. Of note, patients who are deficient in the enzyme thiopurine *S*-methyltransferase may suffer severe marrow suppression when azathioprine or its derivatives are administered.

Methotrexate, a well-known antimetabolite, anti-inflammatory agent, improves the clinical findings in some patients with severe AD. Its use is limited by potential mucositis, marrow suppression, hepatotoxicity, and, less commonly, pulmonary complications.

Allergy immunotherapy reducing sensitizations and reactions to aeroallergens is helpful in select patients. Although some patients will worsen as immunotherapy is initiated, most patients with sensitization to aeroallergens improve after treatment. As with all immunotherapy, risk of reactions including anaphylaxis should be reviewed for each patient.

SECONDARY INFECTION

Studies indicate that AD patients with secondary bacterial infection improve more rapidly when treated with antistaphylococcal antibiotics.

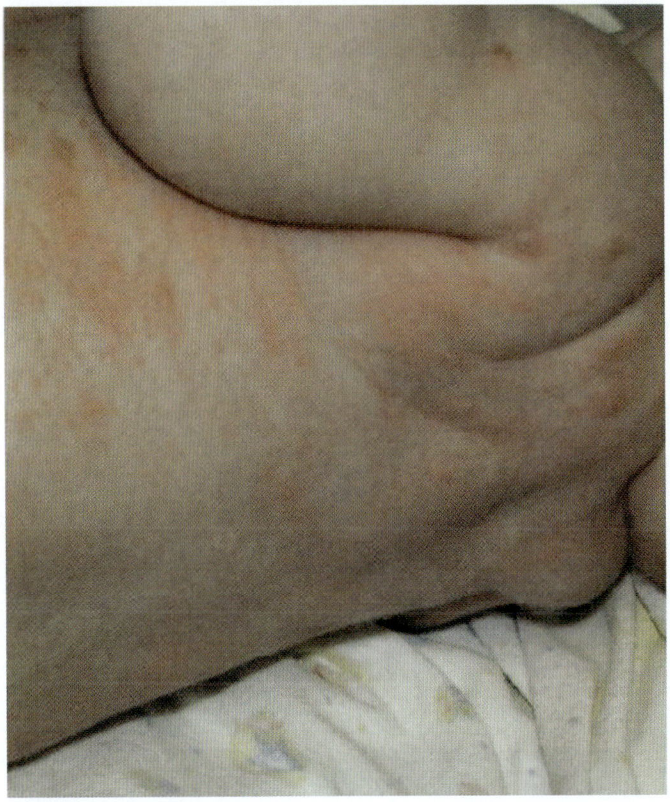

FIGURE 59-12. Atopic dermatitis complicated by methicillin-resistant staphylococcal furunculosis.

Given that only a minority of patients are infected with bacteria that are methicillin resistant, first-line therapy typically includes a penicillinase-resistant penicillin such as dicloxacillin, or a first-generation cephalosporin such as cephalexin when cellulitis or furuncles are present (**Figure 59-12**).

For more severe infections, and especially in communities where methicillin resistance is high, clindamycin, trimethoprim-sulfamethoxazole, or vancomycin should be considered. If clindamycin is used, the possibility of inducible resistance should be considered in patients who do not respond as expected to antibiotic treatment. If clindamycin resistance is suspected, a D-test can be ordered on a positive staphylococcal bacterial culture to determine whether inducible resistance is present. In instances of proven resistance, antimicrobial choice should be informed by culture results and inpatient therapy should be considered.

Patients with secondary viral infections should be treated with antivirals, such as acyclovir for eczema herpeticum, when appropriate. Ophthalmic complications of eczema herpeticum require consultation with an ophthalmologist, aggressive therapy, and probably hospitalization. Patients with severe gingivostomatitis may benefit from soothing mouth rinses commonly known as "magic mouthwash," a mixture of diphenhydramine liquid and aluminum and magnesium hydroxide (Maalox or Mylanta) or bismuth subsalicylate (Kaopectate). It is important to realize that patients with eczema herpeticum have a one in four chance of developing a reactivation of HSV on the skin within 6 months of the primary episode.

Importantly, during the acute phase of a viral or bacterial secondary infection, discontinuation of topical immunosuppressive agents such as corticosteroids or calcineurin inhibitors may be advisable. Then, as the patient improves, reintroduction of low-potency topical steroid agents, and later calcineurin inhibitors, is reasonable.

COLONIZATION

Patients who have methicillin-resistant staphylococcal carriage in reservoir areas such as the nares, fingertips, or perianal area may benefit from treatment with mupirocin applied to these reservoir areas to reduce the carrier state. The use of a diluted formulation of chlorine bleach may help reduce bacterial skin colonization. Typically, one capful per gallon of water, or approximately ¼ cup of bleach per ½ bathtub of water, is used once or twice a week for 5 minutes. It should be noted that patients may feel stinging or burning if there is fissured skin. Children should be patted dry with a white towel. Dilute bleach baths should be continued as part of maintenance routine to decrease the burden of bacterial colonization.

CONSULTATION

- Dermatology: for severe cases of atopic dermatitis unresponsive to typical outpatient therapy
- Allergy: for evaluation of food or environmental allergies
- Ophthalmology: for evaluation and management of ophthalmic complications of Kaposi varicelliform eruption
- Infectious disease: for severe complications due to secondary infections

ADMISSION CRITERIA

- Severe flare of AD unresponsive to outpatient therapy
- Secondary infection unresponsive to outpatient therapy
- Severe secondary infection—bacterial superinfection necessitating intravenous antibiotic therapy, severe Kaposi varicelliform eruption, or infection with concern for ocular involvement
- Persistent eczematous dermatitis unresponsive to outpatient therapy, necessitating further evaluation for other underlying causes and escalation of therapy

DISCHARGE CRITERIA

- Clinical improvement of AD flare
- Signs of resolving infection: for bacterial infection, resolution of fever, absence of bacteremia, and clinical improvement; for viral infection, resolution of vesicular lesions and crusting over of initial lesions
- Adequate oral intake and hydration status
- Caretakers have completed education on appropriate atopic skin care and use of pharmacologic agents such as topical corticosteroids, calcineurin inhibitors, antihistamines, emollients, and other adjuncts to therapy
- Appropriate follow-up established

KEY POINTS

- AD is an increasingly common, pruritic, inflammatory skin disorder characterized by a chronic course with intermittent, recurrent flares.
- Patients with AD may suffer from associated atopic disorders, including asthma and allergic rhinitis, and demonstrate an increased predisposition to secondary skin infection.
- Not all eczematous dermatitides are AD. Some forms of eczema may resemble AD but are associated with other systemic metabolic disorders.
- Treatment of AD should optimize the impaired skin barrier, minimize exposure to environmental allergens, reduce pruritus and inflammation, and eliminate secondary infection. A consistent care regimen is often able to control the signs and symptoms of AD.
- Biologic treatments, including dupilumab can be used to treat severe or refractory disease.
- AD patients may require hospitalization for a severe flare or superinfection by bacterial or viral pathogens.
- Empiric antibiotic therapy for bacterial superinfection should be aimed at skin flora, specifically staphylococcus aureus, with penicillinase-resistant penicillins or a first-generation cephalosporin.
- HSV superinfection requires treatment with acyclovir, pain control, and supportive care.

SUGGESTED READINGS

Cardona ID, Kempe EE, Lary C, Ginder JH, Jain N. Frequent versus infrequent bathing in pediatric atopic dermatitis: a randomized clinical trial. *J Allergy Clin Immunol Pract*. 2020;8(3):1014-1021.

Cork MJ, Danby SG, Vasilopoulos Y, et al. Epidermal barrier dysfunction in atopic dermatitis. *J Investig Dermatol*. 2009;129(8):1892-1908.

Dabade TS, Davis DMR, Wetter DA, et al. Wet dressing therapy in conjunction with topical corticosteroids is effective for rapid control of severe pediatric atopic dermatitis: experience with 218 patients over 30 years at Mayo Clinic. *J Am Acad Dermatol*. 2012;67(1):100-106.

Freitas E, Gooderham M, Torres T. New topical therapies in development for atopic dermatitis. *Drugs*. 2022;82(8):843-853.

Galli E, Neri I, Ricci G, et al. Consensus conference on clinical management of pediatric atopic dermatitis. *Ital J Pediatr*. 2016;42:26.

Langan SM, Irvine AD, Weidinger S. Atopic dermatitis. *Lancet*. 2020; 396(10247):345-360.

Matiz C, Tom WL, Eichenfield LF, Pong A, Friedlander SF. Children with atopic dermatitis appear less likely to be infected with community acquired methicillin-resistant *Staphylococcus aureus*: the San Diego experience. *Pediatr Dermatol*. 2011; 28(1):6-11.

Ong PY, Ohtake T, Brandt C, et al. Endogenous antimicrobial peptides and skin infections in atopic dermatitis. *N Engl J Med*. 2002;347(15):1151-1160.

Paller AS, Spergel JM, Mina-Osorio P, Irvine AD. The atopic march and atopic multimorbidity: Many trajectories, many pathways. *J Allergy Clin Immunol*. 2019;143(1):46-55.

Van Zuuren EJ, Fedorowicz Z, Christensen R, Lavrijsen A, Arents BW. Emollients and moisturisers for eczema. *Cochrane Database Syst Rev*. 2017;2:CD012119.

Weidinger S, Novak N. Atopic dermatitis. *Lancet (London, England)*. 2016; 387(10023):1109-1122.

Worldwide variation in prevalence of symptoms of asthma, allergic rhinoconjunctivitis, and atopic eczema: ISAAC. The International Study of Asthma and Allergies in Childhood (ISAAC) Steering Committee. *Lancet (London, England)*. 1998;351(9111):1225-1232.

CHAPTER 60 Ecthyma Gangrenosum

Gillian K. Weston, MD and Mary Wu Chang, MD

BACKGROUND

Skin lesions evolving from erythematous macules to vesicles to necrotic ulcers, in the setting of *Pseudomonas aeruginosa* septicemia, were initially described in the late 19th century. The term *ecthyma gangrenosum* was coined at that time. Although *P. aeruginosa* is the classic pathogen in ecthyma gangrenosum, other infectious organisms (**Table 60-1**) can produce clinically identical lesions. Ecthyma gangrenosum is currently considered a morphologic pattern of cutaneous necrosis secondary to blood vessel occlusion by organisms proliferating in vessel walls; this occurs due to bacteremia with *Pseudomonas* or other bacterial species or may be secondary to fungemia. Regardless of the causative organism, ecthyma gangrenosum has a predilection for immunocompromised hosts, particularly individuals with neutropenia and hematologic malignancies and may also be the initial presentation of a primary or acquired immunodeficiency. However, healthy children may also develop ecthyma gangrenosum. Ecthyma gangrenosum tends to progress rapidly and has a high mortality rate without treatment, so early recognition and prompt administration of antimicrobial therapy are essential.

TABLE 60-1 Organisms That Have Been Reported to Cause Ecthyma Gangrenosum-Like Lesions

Bacteria
Gram-negative rods
Pseudomonas aeruginosa
Pseudomonas stutzeri
Burkholderia (Pseudomonas) cepacia
Methylobacterium (Pseudomonas) mesophilica
Stenotrophomonas (Xanthomonas) maltophilia
Aeromonas hydrophila
Klebsiella pneumoniae
Serratia marcescens
Citrobacter freundii
Morganella morganii
Escherichia coli
Vibrio vulnificus
Yersinia pestis
Chromobacterium violaceum
Gram-negative cocci
Moraxella (Branhamella) catarrhalis
Moraxella nonliquefaciens
Neisseria gonorrhoeae
Gram-positive rods
Corynebacterium diphtheriae
Enterococcus Faecalis (Mariana 2019)
Gram-positive cocci
Staphylococcus aureus (including methicillin-resistant organisms)
*Streptococcus pyogenes**
Fungi
Candida spp.
C. albicans
C. tropicalis
Aspergillus spp.[†]
A. fumigatus
A. niger
Zygomycetes[†]
Mucor
Rhizopus
Absidia
Other organisms causing hyalohyphomycosis[†‡]
Fusarium solani
Pseudoallescheria boydii
Metarrhiziurn anisopliae
Organisms causing phaeohyphomycosis[†‡]
Curvularia
Exserohilum
Drechslera
Scytalidium dimidiatum
Viruses
Herpes simplex virus

*Local infection can result in ecthyma, a condition distinct from ecthyma gangrenosum (see Table 60-3).

[†]Primarily soil saprophytes found in decaying vegetation.

[‡]Representing molds with hyaline (nonpigmented) hyphae.

[§]Representing molds with dematiaceous (brown-black) hyphae.

PATHOPHYSIOLOGY

Ecthyma gangrenosum may evolve as (i) a classic bacteremic (or fungemic) form, caused by hematogenous dissemination of the organism to the skin, or (ii) a nonbacteremic form in which the skin lesions are located at a cutaneous site where inoculation occurred. Although blood cultures are initially negative in the latter scenario, secondary bacteremia and clinical decompensation may occur if treatment is delayed.

The most recognized pathogen of ecthyma gangrenosum, *P. aeruginosa*, is a gram-negative bacillus that is present in the normal intestinal flora in 10% to 15% of healthy individuals; in hospitalized populations, *P. aeruginosa* may be present in more than one-third of patients. Cancer patients are particularly prone to colonization of the oropharynx and gastrointestinal tract with *P. aeruginosa* and other potentially pathogenic microorganisms. Even in otherwise immunocompetent individuals, gastrointestinal colonization may be the source of pathogenic *P. aeruginosa*. Alternatively, preceding viral illness (respiratory syncytial virus, influenza, enteropathogenic viruses etc.) may directly impair mucosal barriers, or otherwise temporarily disrupt mucosal host defenses. Compromised barriers may permit *P. aeruginosa* and other pathogens to translocate with subsequent development of ecthyma gangrenosum.

P. aeruginosa infections manifesting as ecthyma gangrenosum in immunocompromised hosts may also originate from the skin. Although it cannot survive on intact, dry skin, *P. aeruginosa* colonizes moist, intertriginous areas, such as the groin and axillae, in approximately 2% of the population. Rarely, *P. aeruginosa* septicemia may develop in immunocompromised hosts as a result of primary cutaneous ecthyma gangrenosum.

The vascular destruction that leads to ecthyma gangrenosum lesions in septicemia due to *P. aeruginosa* is thought to be related to dissolution of the elastic lamina by pseudomonal elastase. Other bacteria (e.g., *Aeromonas maltophilia*) implicated in the development of ecthyma gangrenosum also produce elastase and various proteases. Several of the opportunistic mycoses that may also cause ecthyma gangrenosum (e.g., aspergillosis, fusariosis, zygomycosis) have a propensity to invade blood vessel walls, resulting in thrombosis and tissue necrosis.

RISK FACTORS

Conditions that have been associated with ecthyma gangrenosum in children are listed in **Table 60-2**. Approximately one-third of pediatric patients with ecthyma gangrenosum have leukemia or aplastic anemia. The occurrence of ecthyma gangrenosum usually coincides with neutropenia related to the administration of chemotherapy or myeloablative regimens for hematologic stem cell transplantation. Additional predisposing factors for the development of ecthyma gangrenosum in cancer patients, and other immunocompromised hosts, include occlusion or maceration of the skin, prior antibiotic therapy, treatment with systemic corticosteroids or other immunosuppressive medications, diabetes mellitus, and hypocomplementemia. Intravenous catheters and invasive procedures are important iatrogenic risk factors for ecthyma gangrenosum. Bacterial contamination (e.g., with *P. aeruginosa*) of moist hospital equipment and supplies, ranging from nebulizers to antiseptic solutions to bath toys, may be a source of nosocomial infections manifesting as ecthyma gangrenosum in immunocompromised patients. Finally, premature infants are also at increased risk of ecthyma gangrenosum, particularly when exposed to a high-humidity environment.

Almost half of the pediatric cases of ecthyma gangrenosum reported to date occurred in previously healthy children (**Table 60-2**). Ecthyma gangrenosum occasionally heralds the onset of leukemia in a previously healthy child. In children without a recognized predisposing condition, ecthyma gangrenosum most often presents with fever and diarrhea in the setting of acute enteritis. An especially virulent strain of *P. aeruginosa* is sometimes implicated. In addition, ecthyma gangrenosum occasionally develops in conjunction with otitis media/externa secondary to *P. aeruginosa* and/or a preceding viral respiratory tract infection. Most previously healthy patients with ecthyma gangrenosum have transient neutropenia, and approximately one-third are found to have hypogammaglobulinemia, a neutrophil disorder, or another immunodeficiency syndrome. Abnormal neutrophil function (resulting from quantitative or qualitative defects) represents the most important risk factor for both disseminated *P. aeruginosa* infection and opportunistic mycoses.

TABLE 60-2 Underlying Conditions in Pediatric Patients With Ecthyma Gangrenosum

Previously Healthy Children	Children With Known Pre-Existing Conditions
Hypogammaglobulinemia	Acute leukemia
Persistent/recurrent neutropenia or abnormal neutrophil function	Solid tumors
Transient neutropenia due to viral illness	Aplastic anemia
Recent antibiotic therapy	Severe burn/toxic epidermal necrolysis
	Prematurity
	HIV/AIDS
	Nutritional deficiency
	Recent major surgery or trauma
	Immunosuppression status post organ transplant
	Other acquired immunodeficiency
	- Hemophagocytic lymphohistiocytosis
	- Myelofibrosis
	Inherited immunodeficiency syndromes

CLINICAL PRESENTATION

Ecthyma gangrenosum typically begins as a painless, erythematous macule, often with a relatively blanched or grayish center. Over a 12- to 24-hour period, the lesion becomes indurated, and a hemorrhagic vesicle or pustule develops centrally (**Figure 60-1**). Rupture then leads to the formation of a necrotic ulcer with a gray-black eschar and a red to violaceous border. One or multiple lesions may be present, either grouped or in a scattered distribution, with sizes ranging from a few millimeters to several centimeters in diameter. Erythematous nodules may be seen adjacent to or distant from necrotic lesions.

Ecthyma gangrenosum can develop anywhere on the cutaneous surface. Ecthyma gangrenosum occasionally affects the oral, nasal, and conjunctival mucosa. Widespread ecthyma gangrenosum lesions represent "septic emboli" associated with bacteremia or fungemia. In contrast, ecthyma gangrenosum localized to moist, occluded sites (e.g., the diaper area or the skin underlying adhesive tape securing an intravenous catheter) may be due to primary inoculation of the skin. Ecthyma gangrenosum due to *P. aeruginosa* has a predilection for the groin, buttocks, and anogenital area; in children, more than 50% of all cases, and more than

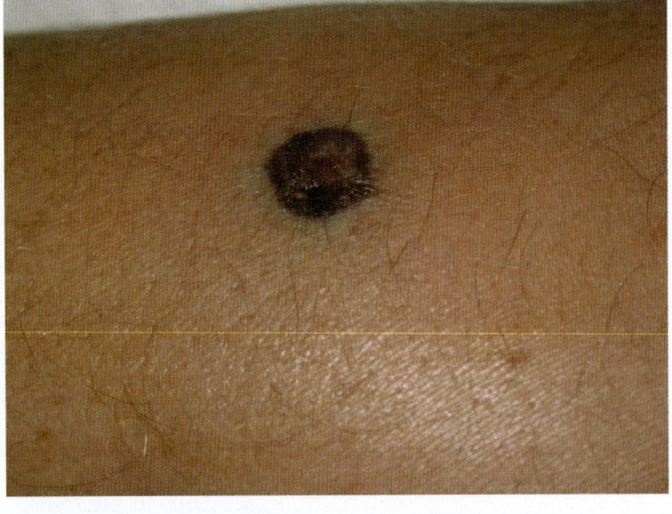

FIGURE 60-1. Hemorrhagic, necrotic papule with blanched halo in a child. (Reproduced with permission from Dr. Albert Yan.)

90% of nonbacteremic cases, involve these sites. Bacteremic patients with ecthyma gangrenosum tend to have extremity involvement, regardless of the etiologic agent.

The spectrum of cutaneous lesions that can develop in association with septicemia (due to *P. aeruginosa* as well as other bacterial and fungal organisms) also includes purpuric macules or papules (especially in thrombocytopenic patients), subcutaneous nodules, and necrotic cellulitis. Pseudomonal infections in immunocompromised hosts may have atypical presentations, such as edematous follicular papulopustules in the groin (resembling "hot tub" folliculitis) that subsequently evolve into classic ecthyma gangrenosum. Of note, the gangrenous orofacial and anogenital lesions of noma neonatorum are thought to represent a neonatal form of ecthyma gangrenosum secondary to *P. aeruginosa* infection in debilitated premature infants. Infections with some pathogens that can cause ecthyma gangrenosum-like lesions may have other characteristic manifestations in immunocompromised patients (**Table 60-3**).

In the classic bacteremic form of ecthyma gangrenosum that occurs in immunocompromised individuals, patients are critically ill and typically present with fever, hypotension, tachycardia, and altered mental status. In contrast, *P. aeruginosa* gastrointestinal infections often manifest in healthy children with fever and diarrhea alone. Pseudomonas-associated gastrointestinal infections may occur in conjunction with enteroviral gastroenteritis or ruptured appendicitis. The development of ecthyma gangrenosum in a child with a clinical presentation that

TABLE 60-3 Differential Diagnosis of Ecthyma Gangrenosum

Disorder	Distinctive Clinical Features	Distinctive Microscopic Features
Disseminated Infections Causing EG-Like Lesions in Immunocompromised Hosts		
Pseudomonas	EG favors the groin, buttocks, and anogenital area	Presence of gram-negative rods
Staphylococcus aureus	Disseminated pustular purpura	Presence of gram-positive cocci
Candida	In addition to EG, often presents with pustules (may be misdiagnosed as folliculitis) or multiple firm, pink papules with central pallor	Budding yeast and pseudohyphae in dermis*
Aspergillus	EG lesions are relatively large (>2-3 cm) and few in number; propensity for primary infections at sites of intravenous catheters	45-degree dichotomous branching of septate, medium-width, uniform hyphae in an "oriented" array in dermis
Mucor, *Rhizopus*, and *Absidia*	Cutaneous extension of an underlying fungal sinus infection can initially present as subtle, unilateral facial swelling and erythema that, without therapy, leads to extensive necrosis†; poorly controlled diabetes mellitus is a risk factor	90-degree branching of broad, nonseptate, ribbon-like hyphae in dermis
Fusarium	Widespread, painful EG lesions with high fever and severe myalgias; primary site of infection is often paronychia or insect bite	45- or 90-degree branching of septate hyphae in dermis (less uniformity and orientation than *Aspergillus*)
Herpes simplex virus	Chronic ulcers with scalloped borders in perioral, perinasal, and perianal areas (preceded by vesicles); disseminated vesicles and crusted erosions‡	Tzanck preparation reveals multinucleated giant cells (representing virally infected keratinocytes)
Other Infections§		
Ecthyma (deep form of impetigo, most often caused by *Streptococcus pyogenes*)	Round, punched-out, shallow ulcers on legs, with thick crust covering purulent base; setting of poor hygiene and minor trauma	Presence of gram-positive cocci
Necrotizing fasciitis	Rapidly spreading, dusky grayish purple erythema and tense edema, with development of bullae, malodorous watery discharge, and deep necrotic ulcers; favors extremities and perineum	Presence of gram-positive cocci or mixed flora
Bacillus cereus infection	Single necrotic bulla on extremity of neutropenic patient	Presence of gram-positive rods
Cutaneous diphtheria	Punched-out ulcer with rolled borders and grayish membrane-like eschar on acral site	Presence of gram-positive rods
Cutaneous anthrax	Painless eschar with surrounding edema and vesiculation	Presence of gram-positive rods
Atypical mycobacterial infections	Protean manifestations in immunocompromised hosts, including necrotic ulcers	Presence of acid-fast bacilli
Dimorphic fungal infections (e.g., histoplasmosis, blastomycosis, coccidioidomycosis)	Protean manifestations in immunocompromised hosts, including mucocutaneous ulcers	Characteristic yeast forms (or, in coccidioidomycosis, spherules with endospores) within neutrophilic and granulomatous infiltrates
Noninfectious Disorders		
Sweet syndrome	Painful, edematous, erythematous plaques; may be pseudovesicular or pustular; favors the face and dorsal hands; particular association with AML	Dense neutrophilic infiltrate¶
Pyoderma gangrenosum	Inflammatory pustule progressing to painful, necrotic ulcer with irregular, purple, undermined borders, and purulent base; favors the legs	Neutrophilic infiltrate in active lesions¶
Primary vasculitides	Manifestations include purpuric papules and nodules, hemorrhagic bullae, and necrotic ulcers; favors the lower legs and dependent sites	Neutrophilic infiltrate or dust and fibrin deposition within vessel walls¶
Vaso-occlusive disorders (e.g., monoclonal cryoglobulinemia)	Retiform (branching, netlike) purpura progressing to necrotic ulcers with angular shape; favor acral sites	Intravascular thrombi and erythrocyte extravasation with minimal inflammation¶
Spider bite	Single painful, edematous, inflammatory plaque progressing to necrotic ulcer	Neutrophilic infiltrate and cutaneous necrosis¶
Erythema multiforme (see Chapter 62)	Target lesions with a dusky or bullous center, pale edematous ring, and peripheral erythema; oral erosions	Vacuolar interface dermatitis with lymphocytic infiltrate¶

*Rather than in the stratum corneum, as in mucocutaneous candidiasis.

†*Aspergillus* and *Fusarium* infections may also originate from the sinuses.

‡Similar lesions may be seen in disseminated zoster.

§Additional considerations may include leprosy (Lucio phenomenon) and parasitic infections such as leishmaniasis or amebiasis.

¶Negative cultures and special stains for organisms.

AML, acute myelogenous leukemia; EG, ecthyma gangrenosum.

otherwise suggests viral gastroenteritis represents an important diagnostic clue, allowing early recognition and appropriate treatment of a potentially life-threatening bacterial infection. Last, the presence of ecthyma gangrenosum-like lesions in the context of persistent fever, prolonged neutropenia, and broad-spectrum antibiotic therapy should raise the suspicion of a fungal infection, especially in patients who are also being treated with systemic corticosteroids.

Factors associated with increased mortality in pseudomonal ecthyma gangrenosum include multiple lesions, a delay in the institution of appropriate antimicrobial therapy, and persistent neutropenia. Nonbacteremic pseudomonal ecthyma gangrenosum has a better prognosis than the bacteremic form, with mortality rates of 5% to 15% and 25% to 50%, respectively. Ecthyma gangrenosum due to opportunistic mycoses is a particularly ominous sign, with the presence of disseminated skin lesions portending mortality rates of 70% to 90%. In any situation, recovery of neutrophil-mediated immunity is imperative for survival of the patient and eventual healing of the necrotic ulcerations. Necrosis and tissue destruction in the setting of ecthyma gangrenosum may be extensive and ultimately lead to functional impairment of nearby structures (e.g., nerve palsies, impaired sucking due to oral tissue loss) long after the infection is treated.

DIFFERENTIAL DIAGNOSIS

Infectious and noninfectious entities in the differential diagnosis of ecthyma gangrenosum-like skin lesions are presented in **Table 60-3**. Although early ecthyma gangrenosum lesions can mimic insect bites, the latter differ in their prominent pruritus and inflammatory (rather than necrotic) evolution. In infants, the differential diagnosis of ecthyma gangrenosum localized to the diaper area may also include subcutaneous fat necrosis, Jacquet erosive diaper dermatitis, and an ulcerated infantile hemangioma.

DIAGNOSTIC EVALUATION

Ecthyma gangrenosum constitutes a dermatologic emergency, especially in an immunocompromised patient. In a healthy child, a high index of suspicion is required to diagnose and initiate appropriate antimicrobial therapy. When skin lesions resembling ecthyma gangrenosum are seen, particularly in immunocompromised or acutely ill patients, the evaluation (preferably before the initiation of antimicrobial therapy) should include the following:

- A deep (punch or incisional) skin biopsy specimen for culture (bacterial, mycobacterial, fungal, and viral). Obtaining a deep tissue sample for culture is particularly important in the diagnosis of invasive fungal infections, as cultures obtained by swabbing or shaving the surface of necrotic ulcerations may reveal only bacterial colonization or secondary superficial infection.
- A skin biopsy specimen for histologic examination, including special stains for bacteria (e.g., a tissue Gram stain), mycobacteria (e.g., a Fite stain), and fungi (e.g., a periodic acid–Schiff stain or Gomori methenamine silver stain).
- Examination of a Gram stain of the vesicular contents or a touch preparation from the biopsy specimen (needed to establish the presence of bacteria).
- Examination of a potassium hydroxide preparation of dermal scrapings (looking for the presence of hyphae or pseudohyphae).
- Swab of lesion drainage or ulcer base for detection of viral organisms via polymerase chain reaction (PCR) studies. Alternatively, examination of a Tzanck smear (HSV) or viral direct fluorescent antibody testing (HSV, varicella) of scrapings from the base of a vesicle or edge of an ulcer may detect viral infection when PCR is unavailable.
- Blood, urine, and (if indicated clinically) stool or cerebrospinal fluid cultures.

A complete blood count with differential, serum electrolyte panel, serum creatinine level, blood urea nitrogen level, prothrombin time, partial thromboplastin time, hepatic function panel, serum complement levels or CH50 assay, and urinalysis should also be obtained. These studies will allow the clinician to evaluate for indicators of severe infection, underlying organ dysfunction or immunocompromised state If clinically indicated, additional laboratory tests and imaging studies may be needed to rule out systemic involvement or occult underlying condition.

When ecthyma gangrenosum develops in previously healthy infants and children, the evaluation should include serum immunoglobulin levels, analysis of lymphocyte subsets, assays of neutrophil function (including a nitroblue tetrazolium reduction), and human immunodeficiency virus testing. In addition, it is important to exclude the possibility of an underlying leukemia. Because initial neutropenia may be due to toxic effects of the infecting organism, the complete blood count and differential should be followed for at least a month; this also enables the detection of cyclic neutropenia.

The typical histologic findings of ecthyma gangrenosum include cutaneous necrosis, extravasated erythrocytes, and extensive collections of organisms within the media, adventitia, and surrounding regions of dermal and subcutaneous vessels. The intima and lumina are characteristically spared, and inflammation is often minimal, especially in neutropenic patients.

MANAGEMENT

Patients with ecthyma gangrenosum require aggressive systemic antibiotic therapy. If pseudomonal ecthyma gangrenosum is suspected, administration of a combination of an antipseudomonal β-lactam antibiotic and an aminoglycoside should be initiated immediately after obtaining blood, urine, and skin samples for culture. The decision to begin treatment with a systemic antifungal or antiviral agent should be based on clinical suspicion and the findings of the aforementioned bedside evaluations. Adjustment of the antimicrobial regimen may be necessary when culture and sensitivity results are available, or sooner if the patient's clinical condition deteriorates. For neutropenic patients, administration of granulocyte colony-stimulating factor to expedite neutrophil recovery can accelerate the healing of ecthyma gangrenosum lesions. Granulocyte infusions are another therapeutic option for patients with profound, refractory neutropenia.

In most cases of ecthyma gangrenosum due to *P. aeruginosa* or other bacterial pathogens, surgical debridement is not required. However, some authors have noted that wide surgical debridement with or without the use of negative pressure wound therapy, skin grafting, or use of dermal substitutes may help to promote healing and minimize scarring, particularly in immunocompromised cancer patients. Wide surgical debridement is an important component of therapy for ecthyma gangrenosum secondary to infections with opportunistic molds, and surgical excision may be an option for localized fungal lesions. Surgical decompression has been required in rare instances of compartment syndrome due to ecthyma gangrenosum on an extremity. Nonetheless, persistent infection and extremely poor wound healing are commonly seen until neutropenia resolves.

ADMISSION AND DISCHARGE CRITERIA

Admission to the hospital is warranted in a pediatric patient with lesions suspicious for ecthyma gangrenosum and abnormal vital signs or altered mental status that may suggest severe infection or sepsis. In the absence of signs of critical illness, high risk patients including those who are immunocompromised, are neutropenic, or have widespread or atypical lesions, and those who cannot tolerate oral antibiotic formulations in the outpatient setting, may also warrant inpatient admission for prompt treatment, appropriate workup, and close monitoring. Additionally, patients with extensive or special site involvement (face, perineal/genital) who may require surgical debridement, or special wound care to prevent or reduce functional impairment, are candidates for admission.

Prior to discharge, patients with ecthyma gangrenosum should have stable vital signs, appropriate mentation, ability to maintain hydration and nutrition, improvement in existing skin lesions, and an absence of newly developing skin lesions. Patients and their caregivers should also demonstrate prior to discharge understanding that remaining antimicrobial therapy must be completed and the importance of wound care and any other treatments required at home; patients and families must be able to perform these important tasks.

CONSULTATION

Consultations by a dermatologist (to evaluate the cutaneous lesions) and an infectious disease specialist (to evaluate for systemic infection and institute appropriate antimicrobial coverage) are recommended for all patients suspected of having ecthyma gangrenosum. Depending on the clinical situation, the input of hematology-oncology or immunology teams might be helpful in the diagnosis and treatment of underlying medical conditions. The assistance of additional pediatric subspecialists may be useful for patients with multiple organ systems involved or wounds that require specialized surgical treatment.

SPECIAL CONSIDERATIONS

PREVENTION

Although pseudomonal septicemia accounted for one-quarter of life-threatening infections in cancer patients during the 1950s, it is seen less frequently today. This can be attributed to shorter durations of neutropenia (e.g., due to the use of granulocyte colony-stimulating factors) and prophylactic administration of antibiotics (e.g., fluoroquinolones). Likewise, the incidence of disseminated candidiasis has decreased significantly with the use of prophylactic fluconazole. As a result, the spectrum of pathogens that cause septicemia and ecthyma gangrenosum-like lesions in oncology patients has changed and now includes a wider variety of bacterial and fungal organisms.

Meticulous skin care, especially in the diaper area, for pediatric patients with hematologic malignancies may help prevent ecthyma gangrenosum arising from a cutaneous portal of entry. Patients should receive a thorough skin examination and treatment of preexisting dermatoses before commencing myelosuppressive regimens. During periods of profound neutropenia, exposure to potential environmental sources of *Pseudomonas* and opportunistic molds should be avoided (e.g., cut flowers in vases).

KEY POINTS

- The skin lesions of ecthyma gangrenosum evolve over 12 to 24 hours from an erythematous macule or nodule to a hemorrhagic vesicle, to a necrotic eschar.
- Ecthyma gangrenosum represents a dermatologic emergency due to its rapid progression, tissue destruction, and association with sepsis, especially in an immunocompromised host.
- Hospitalization may be required, with immediate initiation of intravenous antimicrobial therapy after cultures are obtained. Anti-pseudomonal antibiotics are necessary pending cultures; anti-fungal and antiviral agents should also be considered.
- Ecthyma gangrenosum typically occurs in immunocompromised patients due to underlying hematologic malignancy, hypogammaglobulinemia, genetic syndromes, or due to immunosuppressive agents in the setting of organ transplant.
- Otherwise healthy children with ecthyma gangrenosum should undergo workup for underlying immunodeficiency or leukemia
- Diagnosis is based on histologic examination and culture of a skin biopsy specimen, performed in conjunction with blood cultures.

SUGGESTED READINGS

Buttery JP, Alabaster SJ, Heine RG, et al. Multiresistant *Pseudomonas aeruginosa* outbreak in a pediatric oncology ward related to bath toys. *Pediatr Infect Dis J*. 1998;17:509-513.

Ceylan N, Demir N, Kocaman S, Peker E, Tuncer O. An extraordinary cause of the sucking difficulty: ecthyma Gangrenosum. *Case Rep Med*. 2016;2016:8502150.

Chuang CH, Wang YH, Chang HJ, et al. Shanghai fever: a distinct *Pseudomonas aeruginosa* enteric disease. *Gut*. 2013;63:736-743.

Cohen N, Capua T, Bilavsky E, et al. Ecthyma gangrenosum skin lesions in previously healthy children. *Acta Paediatr*. 104:e134-e138.

El Baze P, Thyss A, Vinti H, et al. A study of nineteen immunocompromised patients with extensive skin lesions caused by *Pseudomonas aeruginosa* with and without bacteremia. *Acta Derm Venereol*. 1991; 71:411-415.

Gałązka P, Kaczor P, Kałużny K, et al. Ecthyma gangrenosum as a serious complication of *Pseudomonas aeruginosa* infection in departments of paediatric oncology. *Postepy Dermatol Alergol*. 2021;38(4):537-543.

Gioacchini FM, Baccarani A, Villari D, Postacchini V, Alicandri-Ciufelli M. Ecthyma gangrenosum in a newborn causing external otitis with complete facial nerve palsy. *J Cutan Med Surg*. 2014;18(3):210-213.

Greene SL, Su WP, Muller SA. Ecthyma gangrenosum: report of clinical, histopathologic, and bacteriologic aspects of eight cases. *J Am Acad Dermatol*. 1984;11:781-787.

Hoffman MA, Finberg L. *Pseudomonas* infections in infants associated with high-humidity environments. *J Pediatr*. 1955;46:626-630.

Huang YC, Lin TY, Wang CH. Community-acquired Pseudomonas aeruginosa sepsis in previously healthy infants and children: analysis of forty-three episodes. *Pediatr Infect Dis J*. 2002;21(11): 1049-1052.

Murphy O, Marsh PJ, Gray J, et al. Ecthyma gangrenosum occurring at sites of iatrogenic trauma in pediatric oncology patients. *Med Pediatr Oncol*. 1996;27:62-63.

Reich HL, Fadeyi DW, Naik NS, et al. Nonpseudomonal ecthyma gangrenosum. *J Am Acad Dermatol*. 2004;50:S114-S117.

Vaiman M, Lazarovitch T, Heller L, et al. Ecthyma gangrenosum and ecthyma-like lesions: review article. *Eur J Clin Microbiol Infect Dis*. 2015;34(4):633-639.

CHAPTER 61

Drug-Associated Rashes

Francisco Alvarez, MD

BACKGROUND

Drug-associated rashes are very common in hospitalized patients. These rashes may be identified during the course of an admission for another indication; these rashes are often benign and do not require treatment. However, some drug-associated rashes occur as part of life-threatening condition, or in very ill children, which may warrant hospitalization for evaluation and intervention. Therefore, it is important for hospitalists to recognize the common patterns of cutaneous drug reactions, discern between benign and potentially harmful conditions, identify underlying causative agent(s), and institute appropriate therapy. Children with severe or systemic illness, or those requiring supportive care with intravenous fluids, steroids, or IVIG will likely warrant admission. Hospitalization is often not necessary for patients with common drug eruptions that are not severe and not likely to progress.

PATHOPHYSIOLOGY

Drug reactions result from both immunologic and nonimmunologic mechanisms. Nonimmunologic adverse reactions account for most drug reactions and may be related to acute overdose, cumulative toxicity, metabolic alterations, and drug-drug interactions; idiosyncratic reactions may also occur. Alternatively, many drug eruptions are mediated by immunologic mechanisms. Generally, these eruptions are hypersensitivity reactions and are classified by the Gell and Coombs classification of hypersensitivity, including types I to IV; Gell and Coombs reactions are described further in Chapter 46. Genetic polymorphisms may also play a role in the pathophysiology of drug reactions and predispose some individuals to severe adverse drug reactions.

CLINICAL PRESENTATION

Drug-related rashes may manifest in a variety of ways, ranging from maculopapular to purpuric rashes, or possibly confluent erythema; rashes may evolve or include fixed skin lesions. Skin findings may be noted in patients that are well or very ill appearing. The wide range of clinical presentations may make it difficult to accurately identify drug-related rashes since other etiologies, such as viral or tick-borne infections, may also present with skin findings. Drug-related rashes may also occur concurrently with infectious processes which may contribute to diagnostic uncertainty. Some patients may be taking multiple medications; isolating an offending agent may be more difficult in these cases. Clinical history may include use of medications that are known to cause drug dermatologic reactions such as penicillins, sulfa drugs, morphine, phenytoin, and carbamazepine.

Acuity of illness, and degree of systemic involvement, may vary considerably in children with drug-associated rashes. Hospitalists should be aware of drug-associated rashes that are typically associated with systemic findings versus those that do not generally include systemic illness; this framework may assist in narrowing the differential diagnosis and directing evaluation.

COMMON DRUG-ASSOCIATED RASHES IN SYSTEMIC ILLNESS

Drug Hypersensitivity Syndrome or Drug Rash With Eosinophilia and Systemic Symptoms (DRESS) Drug hypersensitivity syndrome, or drug rash with eosinophilia and systemic symptoms (DRESS) refers to a subset of severe drug reactions characterized by the triad of cutaneous eruption, fever, and internal organ dysfunction caused by exposure to a drug. This entity was previously known as anticonvulsant hypersensitivity syndrome but is now reported in association with several other categories of drugs. A number of medications that can cause drug hypersensitivity are commonly used in the care of hospitalized children, including anticonvulsants (phenytoin, phenobarbital, carbamazepine, and lamotrigine), sulfonamides, trimethoprim, minocycline, dapsone, azathioprine, and allopurinol.

The pathophysiology of DRESS is complex and not fully understood; underlying genetic predisposition and viral reactivation may play a role. The syndrome usually occurs from 1 to 6 weeks into therapy but may occur months after initiation. Most patients with DRESS present with fever, generalized lymphadenopathy, eosinophilia, and a rash of varying distribution and severity. DRESS should be high on the differential when a patient presents with the described multi-system involvement, whereas isolated skin involvement more commonly occurs in other drug-associated reactions. Of note, eosinophilia may not be present in all cases and therefore should not be used as a diagnostic marker when considering DRESS as a diagnosis. The rash may present as monomorphic papules favoring the trunk and proximal extremities, a morbilliform eruption, atypical targets with an acral predilection ("erythema multiforme-like"), or even as an exfoliative erythroderma with prominent desquamation (**Figure 61-1**). Mucus membrane lesions may or may not be present. Prominent facial swelling is often seen, and patients may appear quite ill.

The hallmark of DRESS is multisystem internal organ involvement; the most frequent findings include hepatitis, hematologic abnormalities, and nephritis. Pneumonitis, cardiac involvement, and hypothyroidism (sometimes delayed) may also be seen. Hematologic findings are variable in severity and frequency; the most common findings are eosinophilia and atypical lymphocytosis, although pancytopenia, agranulocytosis, thrombocytopenia, and anemia have been described. Hepatic involvement, seen in every patient in one case series, ranges from mild elevation of transaminases to frank hepatic necrosis; involvement of other systems is variable. In one DRESS case series, patients with an erythema multiforme–like rash were found to have more severe hepatic involvement. The disorder carries a 10% mortality rate, with prognosis dependent upon the extent and severity of organ involvement. Fulminant hepatic failure is the most common cause of death

Recognition of the temporal association between initiation of the drug and onset of the syndrome is key to establishing the diagnosis. If the diagnosis is in question, skin biopsy may help establish the rash as a drug reaction by revealing a dense infiltrate of eosinophils or lymphocytes in the papillary dermis. Bocquet's diagnostic criteria may be used as a diagnostic aid, requiring three features: cutaneous drug eruption, hematologic abnormalities (i.e., eosinophilia [$>1.5\times10^3/\mu L$] or atypical lymphocytes) and systemic involvement (e.g., lymphadenopathy $\geq$ 2 cm, hepatitis [liver transaminases values > twice the upper normal limit], interstitial nephritis, interstitial pneumonitis, or carditis).

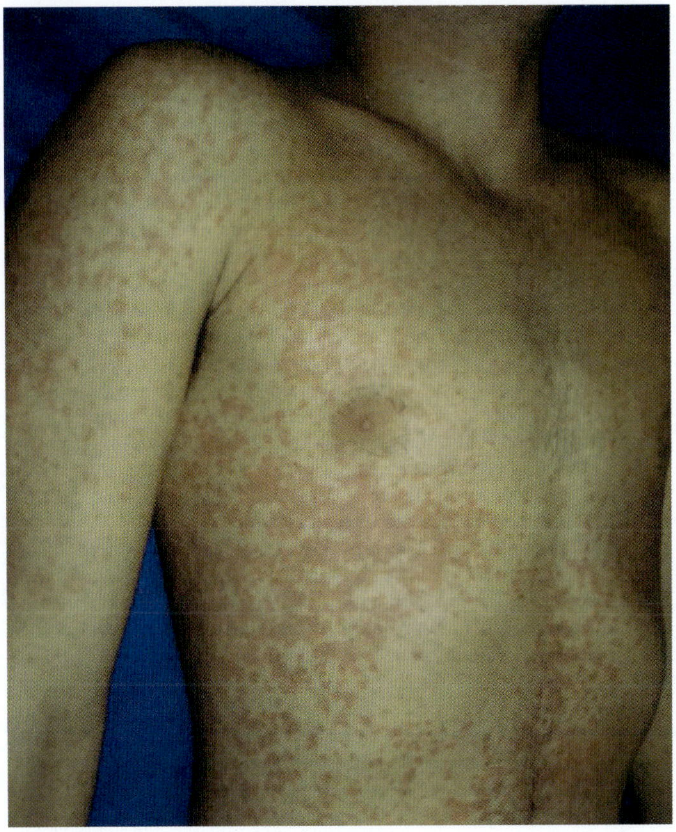

FIGURE 61-1. Morbilliform drug eruption.

Treatment begins with recognition of the diagnosis and removal of the offending agent. A delay in diagnosis may increase morbidity and mortality. The use of multiple medications may make it difficult to discern the causative agent. Consequently, the usual practice is to stop administering all possible offending drugs that are not lifesaving, especially in patients with severe reactions. Because drugs with long half-lives may be difficult to remove, dialysis may be indicated. Compromised organ function (e.g., liver or kidney dysfunction) may impact on drug clearance; monitoring of serum drug levels may be indicated when available. Cross-reactivity is common among the implicated anticonvulsants (phenobarbital, phenytoin, carbamazepine, and lamotrigine), so alternative antiepileptic therapy must be chosen carefully. Benzodiazepines, valproate, and gabapentin are among the commonly suggested alternatives, although they should be used with caution in patients with hepatic dysfunction. In certain cases, epicutaneous patch testing, performed weeks after full recovery, or lymphocyte transformation testing may be helpful in identifying the causative agent

Patients with DRESS or concern for DRESS should likely be hospitalized and closely monitored for signs of severe organ involvement, which may develop even after cessation of the offending drug. Many children become ill enough to require hospitalization, and some may require critical care. As mentioned earlier, testing should be directed toward assessing multi-organ involvement; lab studies could include, but are not necessarily limited to, complete blood count (CBC), liver function tests (LFT's), urinalysis and basic metabolic panel (BMP). Although routine monitoring of cardiac enzymes is not required, occasionally, cardiomyopathy may occur during the acute phase of the drug reaction, and clinicians should obtain a cardiology consultation in children experiencing chest pain. Intensive supportive care, including aggressive nutritional support, fluid/electrolyte replacement, and meticulous skin care, is critical. Many experts recommend that patients with DRESS and severe organ involvement are treated with systemic corticosteroids, often high dose. A number of case reports have described dramatic improvement in visceral organ dysfunction after the administration of steroids. Early administration of systemic steroids, at a minimum dose of 1 mg/kg/day of prednisone or equivalent, is recommended. Severe cases may initially be treated with pulsed methylprednisolone at 30 mg/kg intravenously for 3 days. Although systemic steroids are typically the treatment of choice for all patients presenting with DRESS, there is some evidence to support adjuvant use of intravenous immunoglobulin (IVIG); IVIG has been studied extensively in patients with toxic epidermal necrolysis. However, unlike in toxic epidermal necrolysis, IVIG should not be administered without steroids in the treatment of DRESS. Other potential treatments include cyclophosphamide, cyclosporine, interferons, mycophenolate mofetil, rituximab, *N*-acetylcysteine to aid in drug detoxification, and anti-herpesvirus medications such as valganciclovir to combat HHV-6 reactivation associated complications. In addition to systemic therapy, topical steroids may provide symptomatic relief. Additionally, plasma exchange has been used in the treatment of life-threatening cases of DRESS syndrome refractory to systemic steroids.

After the initial phase of therapy, prolonged, tapering courses of steroids over 3 to 6 months may be required, and the disease often relapses after cessation of therapy. Although steroids are the mainstay of therapy, immunosuppression may promote reactivation of viruses and can be associated with a rare, prolonged, steroid-dependent variant of DRESS. It is not uncommon for the disease to fluctuate for many months before finally resolving. Frequent monitoring of liver function tests, urinalysis, and creatinine may be necessary and may be needed on a daily or weekly basis if there are signs of multi-organ involvement progression. Children with DRESS are also susceptible to cardiomyopathy after the initial phase of disease and should be monitored for exercise intolerance or other cardiac symptoms. Additionally, as long-term thyroid complications may occur, evaluation of thyroid function tests at baseline, after 2 to 3 months, and periodically for at least 2 years is recommended.

Serum Sickness Serum sickness is an illness caused by circulating immune complexes (Type III reaction). The syndrome was initially described in the early 1900s when it was seen in association with the use of horse serum containing diphtheria antitoxin. Approximately 8 to 13 days after injection of the serum, a syndrome consisting of fever, malaise, lymphadenopathy, rash, proteinuria, and arthralgias developed. The syndrome was termed *serum sickness* and a half-century later was reported to be linked to the creation and deposition of circulating immune complexes in tissues and complement activation.

Serum sickness is now most commonly seen after the administration of animal-derived immunoglobulins such as snake antivenin. The illness usually begins 2 to 21 days after the offending medication is given. The most frequent clinical findings are fever, malaise, rash, arthralgias, gastrointestinal symptoms, and lymphadenopathy. The cutaneous findings are characterized by a fixed, polycyclic urticarial eruption, edema, and purpuric serpiginous lesions on the lateral surface of the feet and hands. Demonstration of low C3 and C4 and abnormal findings on urinalysis can be helpful in establishing the diagnosis.

Treatment is supportive because the illness is self-limited. Nonsteroidal anti-inflammatory drugs (NSAIDs) and corticosteroids may be helpful if symptoms are severe or bothersome.

Serum Sickness–Like Reactions A serum sickness–like reaction is also well described. Patients have similar symptoms (fever, rash, and arthralgias); however, immune complex deposition is not seen. Medications most commonly associated with serum sickness–like reactions include penicillins, cephalosporins (particularly cefaclor), sulfonamides, phenytoin, and salicylates. The mechanism of the syndrome is poorly understood, but it has been proposed to be due to a cytotoxic effect on cells.

The differential of a serum sickness–like reaction includes acute annular urticaria, also known as urticaria multiforme. Typical features of urticaria multiforme include annular and polycyclic urticarial lesions with or without ecchymotic skin changes (but not true targetoid lesions), pruritus, acral edema with or without face edema, absence of arthralgias and arthritis, and favorable response to antihistamines. Triggers commonly include antibiotics, immunizations, and viral illnesses.

Treatment for this is similar to other IgE-mediated reactions (Type I reaction) including discontinuation of the offending agent, oral NSAIDs, antihistamines, and addition of H_2 blockers and steroids if reaction is severe.

Drug-Induced Lupus Drug-induced lupus is a disorder characterized by a constellation of symptoms mimicking those of SLE. The most frequently implicated drugs are procainamide, hydralazine, isoniazid, lithium, phenytoin, and oral contraceptives. Clinically, patients present with fever, malaise, myalgias, polyarthritis, pleuritis, cutaneous vasculitis, or any combination of these findings. Systemic symptoms are more common than skin manifestations. Laboratory analysis will reveal antinuclear antibodies in the majority of patients, and many will also have an elevated erythrocyte sedimentation rate, hypocomplementemia, and anti-histone antibodies. Other, more specific SLE-associated antibodies, such as anti–double-stranded DNA, have been reported in tumor necrosis factor alpha inhibitor–induced lupus.

The most important initial intervention for patients with drug-induced lupus is discontinuation of the offending drug. The majority of patients will improve, albeit slowly, with this intervention alone, although occasionally persistence of symptoms necessitates therapy with immunosuppressive agents. NSAIDs can provide symptomatic relief during the resolution phase. Rheumatology consultation may be helpful in the diagnosis and management of this disorder in hospitalized patients.

LESS COMMON DRUG-ASSOCIATED RASHES IN SYSTEMIC ILLNESS

Exanthematous Drug Eruptions An exanthem is the most common type of cutaneous drug eruption. The terms *maculopapular* and *morbilliform* ("measles-like") are also often used to describe this class of drug rash. The eruption is characterized by pruritic, red- to salmon-colored macules or papules that at times coalesce into plaques (**Figure 61-2**). The lesions tend to be bilateral and symmetrical; they generally appear on the

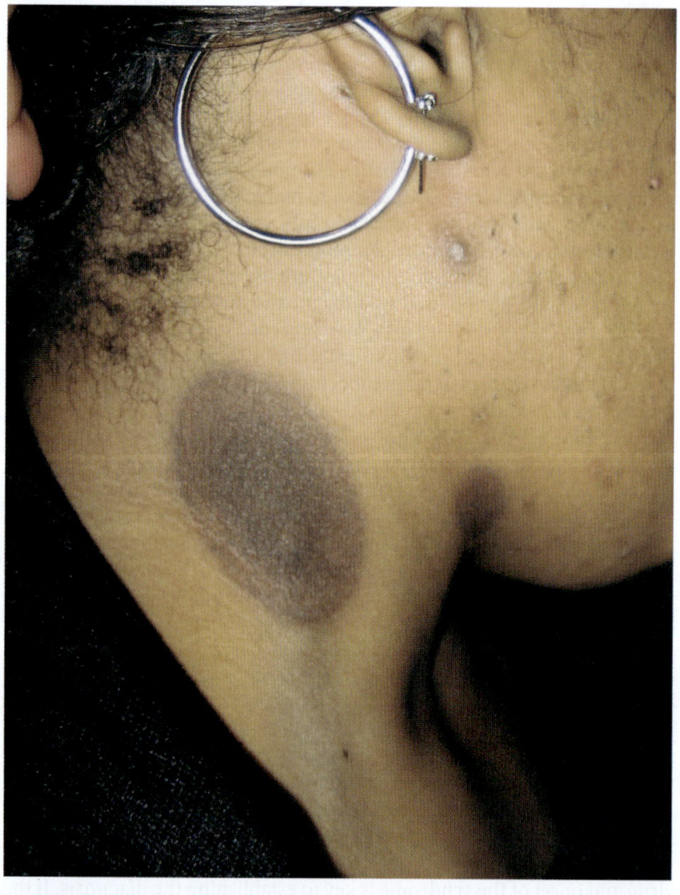

FIGURE 61-2. Fixed drug eruption with significant hyperpigmentation secondary to acetaminophen.

TABLE 61-1 Drugs Commonly Causing Exanthematous Eruptions in Children
Penicillin derivatives
Sulfonamides
Phenytoin
Carbamazepine
Barbiturates
Amphotericin B
Oral hypoglycemic agents
Thiazides
Benzodiazepines
Phenothiazines
Allopurinol
Antimalarials
Captopril
Nonsteroidal anti-inflammatory drugs
Gentamicin
Lithium

trunk initially and then spread peripherally to the extremities. They may spare the face, palms, and soles, but this is inconsistent. Many drugs may cause exanthematous eruptions (**Table 61-1**), but penicillin antibiotics are among the most frequently implicated agents. The eruption classically appears 7 to 14 days after the start of a new medication, although it may appear sooner or later. The presence of a viral infection is thought to increase the likelihood of an exanthematous drug eruption. The most well-recognized example occurs in patients with mononucleosis who experience a morbilliform eruption when exposed to aminopenicillin agents (e.g., amoxicillin).

When an exanthematous drug eruption is suspected, the differential diagnosis also includes primary viral exanthems, as well as less common etiologies, including eczematous dermatitis and graft-versus-host disease, among others. Viruses may cause rashes identical to those of drug eruptions. If histopathology is available, the presence of an eosinophilic infiltrate supports a drug etiology, but the findings are generally nonspecific. Drug hypersensitivity syndrome may also present with an exanthematous rash, although these patients typically have high fever, characteristic facial edema, eosinophilia, and other evidence of multiorgan system involvement.

The mechanism(s) underlying exanthematous drug eruptions are unclear, though a T-cell–mediated process is suspected based on the time delay between exposure and the development of symptoms. It appears, however, that such reactions may not be Gell and Coombs type IV reactions as they do not consistently occur with subsequent exposures.

Exanthematous eruptions typically last days to weeks and almost universally resolve after removal of the offending agent. Time to resolution is dependent on a variety of factors, including the half-life of the involved drug. Specific therapeutic interventions are not required, but topical corticosteroids may be useful in providing symptomatic relief and antihistamines may be helpful for relief of itching. An exanthematous reaction is not necessarily an absolute contraindication to future use of the drug, although many patients will experience recurrence of the rash with rechallenge. Therefore, in the majority of cases, the patient should be considered "allergic" to the medication. However, drug "allergies" are likely over diagnosed; oral challenge tests (OCT) following diagnosis of β lactam drug allergy from a maculopapular or delayed-onset urticarial rash are positive in less than 10% of patients. Over-diagnosis is an important issue to consider as patients labelled "allergic" may require alternative antibiotic therapy. Children with chronic conditions at increased risk for multi-drug resistant organisms may benefit from OCT to delineate true allergy to allow continued use of narrow spectrum antibiotics.

Urticarial Drug Eruptions Urticaria is among the most frequent of the drug eruptions. Urticaria may be acute or chronic. Chronic urticaria is urticaria that persists beyond 6 weeks. It may be IgE-induced (i.e., Type I reaction) and occur after antibiotic exposure, or non–IgE-induced in the case of a pseudoallergic reaction to NSAIDs or opiates. Urticarial rashes are characterized by intensely pruritic erythematous, edematous papules, and plaques (**Figure 61-3**). Lesions may occur anywhere on the body, including the palms and soles, and occasionally have a "dusky" appearance or central pallor. The rash may appear within minutes of exposure to the offending agent or several days later. Each individual hive usually persists for a period of hours, but less than 24 hours total. If lesions remain fixed for longer than 24 hours, other diagnoses should be entertained including urticarial vasculitis, erythema multiforme, or acute hemorrhagic edema of infancy. Additional diagnostic considerations include serum sickness-like reaction and acute annular urticaria. Annular urticaria, also known as urticaria multiforme, is a common variant hypersensitivity reaction in children presenting with arcuate, polycyclic annular lesions, often with acral edema. Lesions may have a dusky appearance, often causing concerns of a diagnosis of erythema multiforme, though the absence of target lesions, central blisters and necrosis will differentiate these conditions.

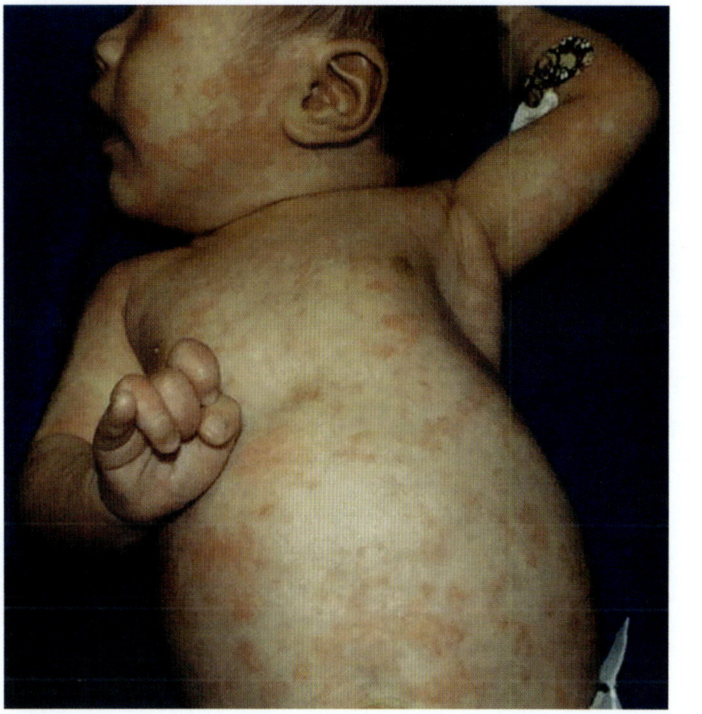

FIGURE 61-3. Diffuse urticarial drug eruption.

A number of inflammatory mediators are thought to be involved in the pathogenesis of urticaria. Histamine release from mast cells plays an important role. Additional mediators that may be involved include prostaglandins, leukotrienes, neutrophil and eosinophil chemotactic factors, platelet-activating factor, interleukin-1, and kinins. Urticarial lesions occur when these inflammatory mediators cause a local increase in the permeability of capillaries in the skin with subsequent dermal edema.

The first line of therapy is removal of the offending agent. Oral antihistamines are the recommended therapy for uncomplicated acute urticaria and are generally sufficient to control symptoms. Depending on the individual situation, both sedating and nonsedating H_1 blockers may be appropriate. There is also evidence to support adjunctive use of H_2 blockers in more severe cases or in those unresponsive to H_1 blockers. Patients with very severe acute urticaria may occasionally require systemic corticosteroids, although there is limited evidence supporting this practice and the vast majority of cases can be managed with antihistamines alone. Allergy to the medication should be documented in the medical record.

Patients with localized urticarial reactions without evidence of progression and without airway involvement often do not require admission, especially if the symptoms are stable or improving during a period of observation. The hospitalist should be aware, however, that acute urticaria may initially appear to be an isolated finding, but patients may progress and urticaria may occur in the setting of angioedema, anaphylaxis, or both. Angioedema refers to transient edema of subcutaneous or submucosal tissue. Common areas of involvement include the lips, eyelids, oropharynx, and tongue. If deeper airway structures such as the larynx become involved, stridor and airway obstruction can result. Patients may also experience nausea, emesis, and diarrhea. Anaphylaxis is defined as a hypersensitivity reaction to a substance that results in severe systemic symptoms. Anaphylaxis is a life-threatening emergency; acute management is discussed in Chapter 45.

Photosensitivity Reactions Photosensitivity reactions, including both phototoxic and photoallergic reactions, comprise up to 8% of cutaneous drug reactions. Phototoxic reactions are dose dependent and non-immunologic. Prior sensitization is not required. Commonly implicated drugs include tetracyclines (most significantly doxycycline), fluoroquinolones, retinoids, NSAIDs, griseofulvin, amiodarone, antipsychotic agents (specifically phenothiazines and thioxanthenes), and voriconazole. Clinically, this typically presents as an exaggerated sunburn in sun-exposed areas within hours to 1 day of sunlight exposure. Additionally, phototoxic reactions secondary to tetracyclines have been associated with onycholysis.

In contrast to phototoxic reactions, photoallergic reactions require sensitization and present as eczematous, pruritic eruptions, with or without papulovesicles, in sun-exposed areas 1 to 14 days after sunlight exposure. Commonly implicated medicines include thiazide diuretics (may appear lichenoid clinically), griseofulvin, sulfonamides, sulfonureas, quinidine, and pyridoxine. NSAIDs, particularly naproxen, have also been implicated in pseudoporphyria, a specific type of photosensitivity. Unlike phototoxic reactions which mainly require minimizing exposure to sunlight, photoallergic reactions require discontinuation of the offending agent in severe cases. Otherwise, treatment focuses on symptom relief, including itching and pain, as well as sun protection and sun avoidance. Anticipatory guidance on sun-related safety is particularly important for agents well-known to be associated with photosensitivity reactions.

Fixed Drug Eruption A fixed drug eruption presents as a distinct lesion or lesions after systemic drug exposure. This eruption generally appears as single or multiple sharply circumscribed, round to oval patches or plaques (**Figure 61-4**). The lesions may be red, gray, violaceous, or brown, and a central vesicle or bullae may be present. They tend to progress from erythematous to hyperpigmented. The rash may occur anywhere on the body, but the most common locations are the face, lips, hands, feet, and genitalia. The lesions are usually asymptomatic or only mildly pruritic. The eruption typically develops within 1 to 2 weeks of starting a new medication. Fixed drug eruptions are often underdiagnosed, which leads to recurrences when and if the drug is readministered. A classic characteristic of a fixed drug eruption is that when patients receive the offending medication again, the lesion(s) reappear(s) in the same anatomic location and do so rapidly, possibly within hours of exposure. The most common agents implicated in fixed drug eruptions include sulfonamides, tetracyclines, NSAIDs, laxatives containing phenolphthalein, barbiturates, and carbamazepine, although many other medications have been implicated (**Table 61-2**). Cross-reactivity may occur within a class of similar drugs. Biopsy of an early lesion of a fixed drug eruption reveals a lichenoid infiltrate, hydropic degeneration of the basal cell layer and dyskeratotic keratinocytes. A later-stage biopsy will reveal a large amount of melanin within macrophages in the upper dermis.

The differential diagnosis for a fixed drug eruption includes insect bites (when the lesion is solitary) and urticaria and erythema multiforme when multiple lesions are present. A thorough history evaluating potential exposures is key to establishing a diagnosis, though in rare cases, if the diagnosis is in question, a biopsy may be helpful. The physician may also choose to rechallenge the patient with the medication.

If a specific drug is determined to be the cause of the reaction, treatment should involve removal of the offending agent. The eruption generally resolves after discontinuation of the medication, but hyperpigmentation in the area may persist for months to years. Any future re-exposure to the offending agent leads to eruption at the same site; these types of reactions are unlikely to progress to anaphylaxis or other severe allergic reactions. The cause of the disorder is unknown. Familial cases have been described, and an association with HLA-B22 has been identified.

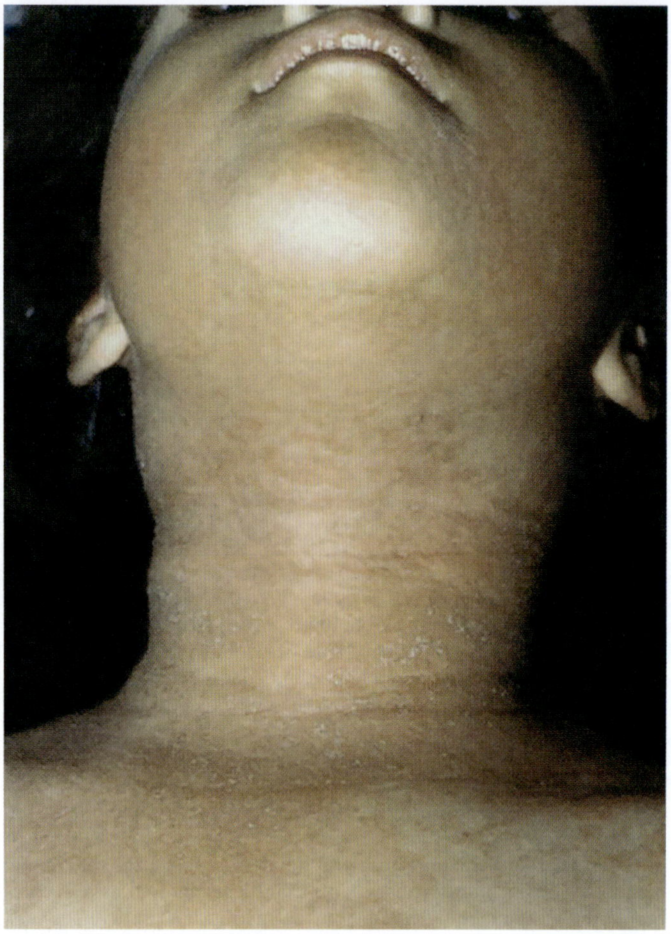

FIGURE 61-4. Exanthem and fine scaling associated with drug rash with eosinophilia and systemic symptoms (DRESS) from carbamazepine.

Acute Generalized Exanthematous Pustulosis Acute generalized exanthematous pustulosis (AGEP) is an acute drug eruption (Type IV reaction) characterized by numerous fine pustules. The pinpoint,

TABLE 61-2 Drugs Commonly Associated With Fixed Drug Eruptions in Children
Sulfonamides
Trimethoprim
Tetracyclines
Penicillin derivatives
Clindamycin
Erythromycin
Antifungal agents
Dapsone
Antimalarials
Metronidazole
Barbiturates
Opiates
Benzodiazepines Anticonvulsants
Nonsteroidal anti-inflammatory drugs (ibuprofen, paracetamol) Acetaminophen
Laxatives containing phenolphthalein
Dextromethorphan
Allopurinol
Sympathomimetics (pseudoephedrine)

nonfollicular, sterile pustules typically first appear on erythematous, slightly edematous skin on the face and in intertriginous regions before becoming more generalized. They may coalesce into sheets of subcorneal pustules which quickly peel or rupture, evolving into areas of superficial desquamation. AGEP may be due to medications, typically antibiotics, or viral infections. Mucous membranes are rarely involved. It may be associated with fever and neutrophilia. Clinically and histopathologically, AGEP can resemble pustular psoriasis; often, a family history of psoriasis is present.

Treatment includes stopping the offending agent (and including the offending agent as a listed allergy) and supportive care such as emollients and antihistamines as needed. Because there are reports of systemic steroids leading to AGEP, steroid therapy is typically limited to use of topical steroids. Typically, AGEP spontaneously resolves in a few days. However, AGEP is associated with a 5% mortality rate, most often due to secondary infection.

Drug-Induced Vasculitis Cutaneous vasculitis occurs with a number of disorders, such as Henoch-Schönlein Purpura (HSP), Kawasaki Disease, Wegener's granulomatosis, and Polyarteritis Nodosa, as well as with the systemic administration of certain drugs. It is associated with immune complex deposition in the skin, but the precise mechanism is poorly understood. Lesion morphology varies, although urticaria-like plaques and palpable purpura concentrated on the lower extremities develop in most patients (**Figure 61-5**). The plaques may blister or ulcerate. Rarely, there is progression to systemic disease involving the liver, kidney, joints, and brain. A definitive diagnosis is made by histopathologic detection of characteristic inflammation of small vessels within the dermis. A perivascular disintegrating neutrophilic infiltrate occurs with fibrin deposition and hemorrhage. Tissue eosinophilia may also be present. Immunofluorescence studies characteristically reveal deposition of immunoglobulin and complement.

The drugs most commonly implicated in cutaneous vasculitis are β-lactam antibiotics, sulfonamides, NSAIDs, diuretics, and the thiouracils, although any drug may cause vasculitis. Anti-tumor necrosis factor agents, such as infliximab, have also been associated with cutaneous vasculitis. Some commonly associated medication triggers are ciprofloxacin, acetylsalicylic acid, and carbamazepine.

Once a diagnosis of cutaneous vasculitis is established, attempts should be made to identify an underlying cause. The differential diagnosis is broad and includes medication reaction, connective tissue disease, primary systemic vasculitis, infection, and malignancy. A diagnosis of idiopathic vasculitis may be made only after all other possibilities have been fully evaluated. A careful history and physical examination will often reveal clues to the specific systemic process, although most patients will also require laboratory tests to fully exclude disorders such as systemic lupus erythematosus (SLE), primary vasculitides, and infection.

Treatment of cutaneous vasculitis is directed toward the underlying cause. If the rash is suspected to be drug induced, removal of the offending agent generally results in rapid improvement over a period of 1 to 3 weeks. Occasionally, patients will require more aggressive therapy with systemic corticosteroids or other immunosuppressive agents, although this is usually necessary only in patients with an underlying systemic process such as a connective tissue disease.

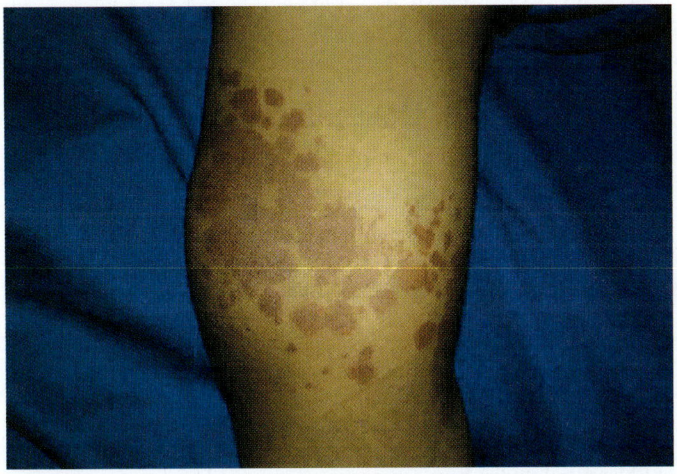

FIGURE 61-5. Drug-induced vasculitis with palpable purpura.

DIFFERENTIAL DIAGNOSIS AND DIAGNOSTIC EVALUATION

The diagnosis of a drug-induced eruption begins with a careful history and physical examination. The clinician should evaluate the timeline of medication(s) initiation as it relates to the development of the rash, especially in scenarios where there may be multiple offending agents that the patient may have been exposed to. Frequently, chronology is the most helpful factor in correctly diagnosing a drug reaction. Most reactions occur within 1 to 3 weeks of starting a new medication and resolve when the medication is fully excreted or metabolized. However, reactions may occur earlier if the patient is being re-exposed to the drug. An accurate description of the eruption is extremely important, including the morphology and distribution of the rash and, specifically, whether or not urticaria are present. Many drugs can induce acute urticaria. Antibiotics are commonly implicated, with penicillin being the most frequent. Other important agents include cephalosporins, sulfonamides, and tetracyclines. The urticaria caused by factors other than drug exposure is morphologically identical. Such factors include infection, autoimmune disease, temperature changes, pressure, sunlight, and exercise, among others.

In general, diagnostic tests are of limited value in the evaluation of drug eruptions. However, testing could be considered in select scenarios. For example, diagnostic tests may be helpful when evaluating rashes in the context of systemic reactions or a suspected immunologic process(es), if the offending agent has not been identified, if rashes occur repeatedly (i.e., two to three times in a year), in life-threatening presentations, and/or in cases where patients may be restricted from taking certain medications (e.g., specific antibiotic and/or anticonvulsant medication groups). Some tests that may be helpful in determining the etiology of drug rashes are antibody and/or immune-serology tests, serum chemistry to look for liver involvement in drug hypersensitivity syndrome, and targeted cultures if an infectious etiology is suspected. Skin biopsy may also be helpful in categorizing drug-associated rashes, and can assist with the diagnosis of urticaria, exanthema, erythema multiforme, toxic epidermal necrolysis, and other entities in the differential diagnosis, such as graft versus host disease if the cause remains unclear after other investigative studies; biopsies should be obtained in consultation with a dermatologist. Radioallergosorbent testing (RAST), skin testing, and patch testing are other useful investigative tools but may be limited to selected cases. Additionally, for a subset of patients with nonserious reactions, rechallenge with the medication may be appropriate, which may be accomplished in the outpatient setting.

CONSULTATION

Consultation needs should be considered and limited to when there is diagnostic uncertainty or a need for subspecialist support in regard to testing or procedural evaluations. The specific consultant needed would be determined based on specific concerns in individual cases.

Dermatology should be involved when there is diagnostic uncertainty, especially if considering the need for a skin biopsy, such as in the case of drug-induced vasculitis. These specialists can obtain specimens for histopathology and assist in the evaluation and management of complex or recalcitrant cases. Their input is especially useful for exfoliative conditions, where management of skin care is particularly challenging.

Involving rheumatology consultants can be helpful in drug-induced vasculitides, drug-induced lupus, and serum sickness, especially if the symptoms are severe, progressive, recurrent, or recalcitrant to initial therapy.

In patients with DRESS syndrome complicated with visceral involvement, consultations with multiple specialists are often indicated (e.g., dermatology, allergy/immunology, rheumatology).

DISCHARGE CRITERIA

Patients may be discharged after the following conditions have been met:

- Symptoms have stabilized, are improving, or are well controlled by therapy that is able to be continued after discharge.
- The underlying condition is well controlled despite discontinuation of medication.
- Adequate follow-up has been arranged with the primary care physician or, if needed, with subspecialists.

KEY POINTS

- Drug eruptions are common in hospitalized pediatric patients, and the majority are benign and self-limited. A subset of drug-associated rashes can be serious and even life threatening, including DRESS.
- Drug reactions result from both immunologic (e.g., IgE or T-cell mediated) and non-immunologic (e.g., cumulative toxicity, drug-drug interactions, or idiosyncrasy) mechanisms.
- The drug hypersensitivity syndrome (DRESS) is characterized by the triad of cutaneous eruption, fever, and multi-system internal organ dysfunction associated with exposure to a drug. There is a 10% mortality rate, with fulminant hepatic failure being the most common cause of death.
- Drug-induced vasculitis, drug-induced lupus, and serum sickness may present as rheumatologic conditions, but identification and discontinuation of the inciting agent are key to treatment.

SUGGESTED READINGS

Bigby M. Rates of cutaneous reactions to drugs. *Arch Dermatol.* 2001;137:765-770.

Bocquet H, Bagot M, Roujeau J. Drug-induced pseudolymphoma and drug hypersensitivity syndrome (drug rash with eosinophilia and systemic symptoms–DRESS). *Semin Cutan Med Surg.* 1996;15:250-257.

Bocquet H, Bagot M, Roujeau J. Drug-induced pseudolymphoma and drug hypersensitivity syndrome (drug rash with eosinophilia and systemic symptoms–DRESS). *Semin Cutan Med Surg.* 1996;15:250-257.

Crowson AN, Magro CM. Drug eruptions. In: Barnhill R, Crowson AN, Busam K, et al., eds. *Textbook of Dermatopathology*. New York: McGraw-Hill; 1998:257-270.

Crowson AN, Magro CM. Recent advances in the pathology of cutaneous drug eruptions. *Dermatol Clin.* 1999;17:537-560, viii.

Doyle MK, Cuellar ML. Drug-induced vasculitis. *Exp Opin Drug Saf.* 2003;2:401-409.

Drake LA, Dinehart SM, Farmer ER, et al. Guidelines of care for cutaneous adverse drug reactions; Guideline/Outcome Committee of the American Academy of Dermatology. *J Am Acad Dermatol.* 1996; 35(3 pt 1):458-461.

Husain Z, Reddy BY, Schwartz RA. DRESS syndrome: Part II. Management and therapeutics. *J Am Acad Dermatol.* 2013;68(5):709.e1-9.

Joint Task Force on Practice Parameters; American Academy of Allergy, Asthma and Immunology; American College of Allergy, Asthma and Immunology; Joint Council of Allergy, Asthma and Immunology. Drug allergy: an updated practice parameter. *Ann Allergy Asthma Immunol.* 2010;105(4):259-273.

Lawley TJ, Bielory L, Gascon P, et al. A prospective clinical and immunologic analysis of patients with serum sickness. *N Engl J Med.* 1984;311:1407-1413.

Leape LL, Brennan TA, Laird N, et al. The nature of adverse events in hospitalized patients: results of the Harvard Medical Practice Study. *N Engl J Med.* 1991;324:377-384.

Lowitt M, Shear N. Pharmacogenomics and dermatologic therapeutics. *Arch Dermatol.* 2001;137:1512-1514.

Mahboob A, Haroon TS. Drugs causing fixed eruptions: a study of 450 cases. *Int J Dermatol.* 1998;37:833-838.

Martinez-Mir I, Garcia-Lopez M, Palop V, et al. A prospective study of adverse drug reactions as a cause of admission to a pediatric hospital. *Br J Clin Pharmacol.* 1996;42:319-324.

Morelli JG, Yong-Kwang T, Rogers M, et al. Fixed drug eruptions in children: clinical and laboratory observations. *J Pediatr.* 1999;134:365-367.

Ozkaya-Bayazit E. Specific site involvement in fixed drug eruption. *J Am Acad Dermatol.* 2003;49:1003-1007.

Scheuerman O, Nofech-Moses Y, Rachmel A, Ashkenazi S. Successful treatment of antiepileptic drug hypersensitivity syndrome with IVIG. *Pediatrics.* 2001;107(1):E14.

Segal AR, Doherty KM, Leggott J, et al. Cutaneous reactions to drugs in children. *Pediatrics.* 2007;120(4):e1082-1096.

Tas S, Simonart T. Management of drug rash with eosinophilia and systemic symptoms (DRESS): an update. *Dermatology.* 2003;206:353-356.

Treat JR. Skin signs of severe systemic medication reactions. *Curr Probl Pediatr Adolesc Health Care.* 2012;42(8):193-197.

Volchek GW. Clinical evaluation and management of drug hypersensitivity. *Immunol Allergy Clin North Am.* 2004;24:357-371, v.

Williams EL, Gadola S, Edwards CJ. Anti-TNF-induced lupus. *Rheumatology.* 2009;48(7):716-720.

Zuberbier T, Greaves MW, Juhlin L, et al. Management of urticaria: a consensus report. *J Invest Dermatol Symp Proc.* 2001;6:128-131.

CHAPTER 62 Erythema Multiforme

Sarah Kitts, MD and Kalyani Marathe, MD, MPH

BACKGROUND

Erythema multiforme (EM) is an acute, self-limited, cutaneous and mucosal, immune-mediated hypersensitivity reaction that may be elicited by a variety of inciting agents. The disease is characterized by an abrupt onset of red papules that progress to form targetetoid, bullous, and necrotic lesions. EM can present at any age but frequently occurs in young adults (i.e., 20-30 years of age); 20% of cases occur in children and adolescents, with a small male preponderance. EM can occur in all seasons of the year; however, there is an increased incidence during the spring and fall.

Erythema multiforme is often separated into two forms: EM minor and EM major. EM minor refers to EM without or with only limited mucosal involvement, while EM major describes the more severe form with extensive mucosal involvement. EM major can occasionally be associated with systemic symptoms including fevers and arthralgias. EM major is less common than EM minor, but it does have a higher predilection for the pediatric population, especially adolescents. EM major can often be difficult to distinguish from Steven-Johnson Syndrome (SJS) and Toxic Epidermal Necrolysis (TEN), though these are two distinct diseases with differing pathologic triggers. SJS and TEN are discussed in Chapter 63.

PATHOPHYSIOLOGY

The exact pathophysiologic mechanism of EM is unknown, though many triggers have been linked to EM, including medications, vaccinations, autoimmune diseases and bacteria, fungi, and viruses. **Table 62-1** lists the commonly encountered potential triggers of EM in children. Approximately 90% of cases are associated with infections; viruses, particularly herpes simplex virus (HSV), and *Mycoplasma pneumoniae* are the most frequent infectious causes.

Most data assessing pathophysiology has come from studies investigating HSV-induced EM. EM is thought to be due to a cell-mediated immune response to cutaneous and mucosal antigens leading to local tissue damage, though it is unclear whether this mechanism occurs when other triggers cause EM. Genetic susceptibility may also play a role in the development of EM; several studies have demonstrated increased frequencies of certain HLA antigens, particularly HLA-DQB1*0301, in the development of EM.

TABLE 62-1 Potential Triggers of Erythema Multiforme in Children

Idiopathic
Viral
Herpes simplex virus (often implicated in recurrent bouts)
Enterovirus (e.g., coxsackievirus)
Epstein-Barr virus
Bacterial
Streptococcus (e.g., group A streptococcus, pneumococcus)
Mycoplasma pneumoniae (generally erythema multiforme major)
Drug induced
Nonsteroidal anti-inflammatory drugs
Antiepileptic medications
Antibiotics (e.g., sulfonamides, penicillins, cephalosporins)
Other
Vaccines (reported after varicella and COVID vaccination)
Progesterone (flares during luteal phase when serum progesterone levels peak)

CLINICAL PRESENTATION

EM typically begins with a red papule or plaque that evolves into a fixed, targetoid skin lesion. The target lesion is characterized by a central dusky area surrounded by a ring of pallor and a peripheral rim of erythema; collectively, it often appears as a ring-like shape. EM lesions may develop central vesiculation. The eruption is symmetric and may develop anywhere on the body, but often presents on the extensor surfaces of the extremities, gradually progressing proximally. Palms and soles are frequently involved. Once lesions appear, they remain fixed in the affected areas for at least a week or longer. The cutaneous lesions are typically asymptomatic but occasionally can be pruritic or painful. Images of EM are depicted in **Figures 62-1** through **62-4**.

Mucosal lesions of the oral, ocular, and genital mucosa are classically seen in EM major, though limited mucosal involvement may occur in EM minor. By definition, EM minor involves a single mucous membrane while in EM major at least two sites are involved. The oral mucosa is most frequently affected and presents with painful erythema and erosions. Some oral lesions are vesicular in character and others may appear ulcerated and/or blood crusted. The eyes may be injected or ulcerated and produce discharge. Inflammation of the genitourinary mucosa may cause dysuria, and gastrointestinal tract involvement may lead to dyschezia. Rarely, pulmonary mucosal surfaces are affected. Many patients with EM minor do not have prodromal or systemic symptoms; however, fever and myalgias can be seen in EM minor with mucosal involvement. Those with EM major often have a prodrome of symptoms such as headache, fever, and malaise that may present from a few days to 2 weeks before onset of the eruption. The nonspecific prodromal symptoms are followed by an abrupt and rapid onset of cutaneous and mucosal lesions. The skin may become red and tender and then rapidly progress to vesicles and ulcerations, with bullous lesions being much more common in EM major than EM minor. As EM progresses large areas of skin may be left with exposed, tender ulcers.

EM is generally a self-limited illness that typically lasts about 2 to 4 weeks. The lesions develop over the course of 3 to 5 days and often resolve without sequelae over the next 2 to 4 weeks. Occasionally, lesions may scar or resolve with postinflammatory hyperpigmentation. EM major can last somewhat longer, and resolution can take up to 6 weeks.

A subset of patients develops recurrent EM, which is usually related to underlying HSV. This can occur even without active symptoms of HSV.

DIFFERENTIAL DIAGNOSIS

The classic target lesion of EM is nearly diagnostic; however, these lesions may be difficult to identify, and several other disorders can present similarly to EM which may complicate diagnosis. The differential diagnosis should include urticaria multiforme, SJS/TEN, fixed drug eruption, Kawasaki Disease, and reactive infectious mucocutaneous eruption (RIME).

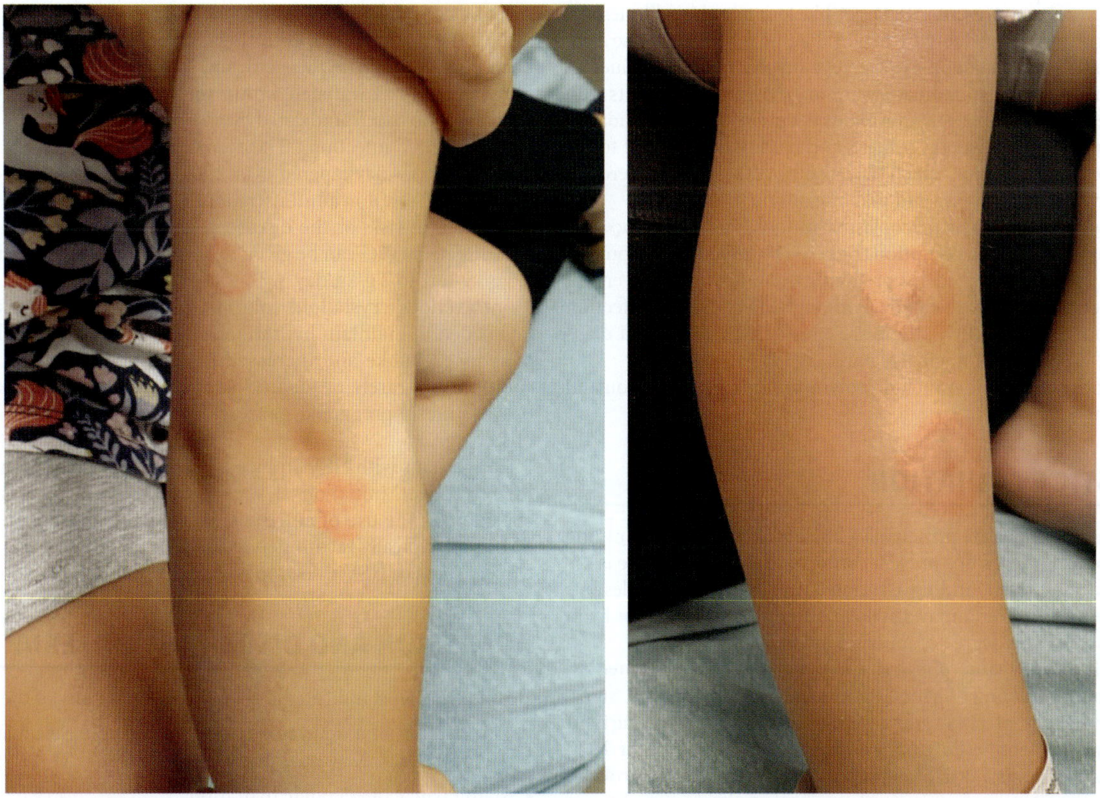

FIGURES 62-1 AND 62-2. Typical erythema multiforme lesions on the arm and leg of a young patient.

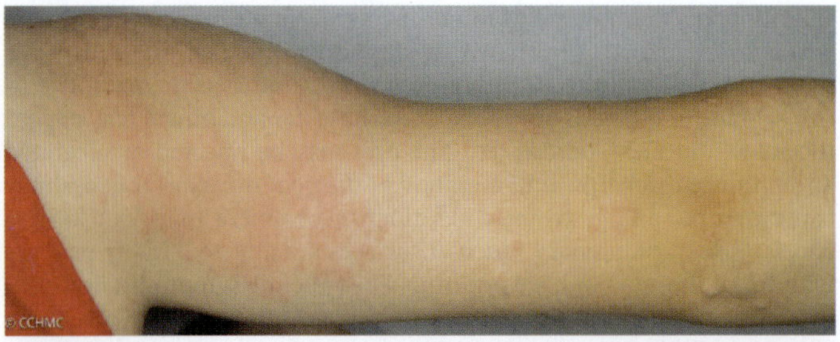

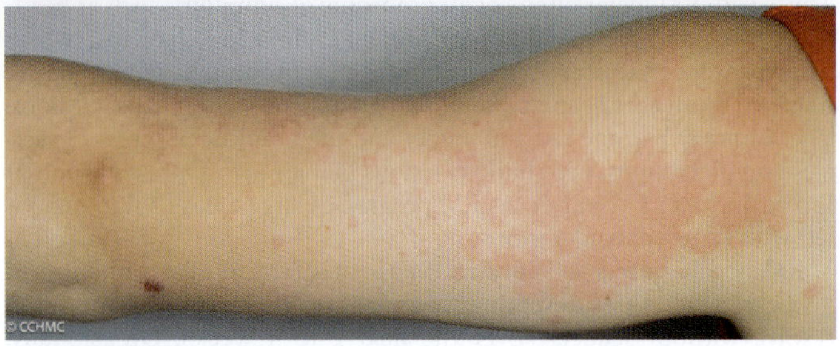

FIGURES 62-3 AND 62-4. Erythema multiforme lesions with a central dusky appearance and vesiculation.

Urticaria multiforme is commonly misdiagnosed as EM. In contrast to EM, lesions of urticaria multiforme are evanescent, with lesions resolving and appearing elsewhere within 24 hours. They frequently show central clearing which occurs due to vasoconstriction and are often pruritic. Brusing can occasionally be seen. On the contrary, lesions of EM show central duskiness and may be tender or painful but are less likely to be pruritic. **Figures 62-5** through **62-8** depict the appearance of urticaria multiforme.

SJS/TEN can also present with targetoid lesions and mucosal involvement, similarly to the presentation of EM major. However, the targetoid lesions of SJS tend to be macular, while the lesions of EM tend to be papular. Additionally, SJS is typically medication induced. Similarly, fixed drug eruptions are also more commonly medication induced. Although fixed drug eruptions can appear similarly to EM, the lesions of EM are more numerous and more widely distributed.

Kawasaki disease may present with target-like lesions or hive-like lesions and should be strongly considered when evaluating for EM because both conditions may be accompanied by fever, eye involvement, oral mucosal changes, and occasionally inflammatory urethritis. However, patients with Kawasaki disease may have a polymorphous eruption with nonexudative conjunctival injection, strawberry tongue, and red lips, as opposed to the targetoid lesions of EM major, which may also be associated with erosive mucosal involvement of the eyes and oral mucous membranes.

RIME, previously known as mycoplasma-induced rash and mucositis (MIRM), is a mucocutaneous eruption triggered by infection. In contrast to EM, RIME is characterized by predominant mucosal involvement with limited cutaneous involvement. Although mycoplasma infection can trigger both EM and RIME, these are considered two distinct diagnoses with different morphological features.

Other diagnoses to consider include polymorphous light eruption and viral exanthems.

DIAGNOSTIC EVALUATION

EM minor and EM major are principally clinical diagnoses. Determining that at least some of the lesions present conform to the target shape is the hallmark of the diagnosis. Finding associated mucous membrane lesions may aid in the diagnosis and may also help differentiate EM minor from EM major based on the degree of mucosal involvement.

A thorough history and physical exam should be performed to assess potential underlying triggers. Recent medication changes, signs, symptoms, or history of HSV, and respiratory symptoms are particularly important to identify. Polymerase chain reaction (PCR) for HSV can confirm the diagnosis of HSV-induced EM. Molecular or serologic testing for *M. pneumoniae* from nasopharyngeal or throat samples can be a useful tool in patients with respiratory symptoms. Additionally, performing PCR testing of lesions on the palms and soles may help identify enterovirus as a potential trigger for EM. Enterovirus causing systemic illness can also be identified in the blood and urine by PCR.

Laboratory tests are not typically indicated in order to diagnose EM minor, although they may provide support for an alternative diagnosis as well as identify complications of disease. Elevated inflammatory markers (i.e., erythrocyte sedimentation rate, C-reactive protein, ferritin), leukocytosis, and, if dehydrated, related electrolyte changes may be seen in EM major. Biopsy is not typically necessary but may help differentiate the condition from other dermatologic diagnoses, especially in patients with vesiculobullous eruptions.

MANAGEMENT

For all forms of EM, removal or treatment of the causative factor, if identified, may help to shorten disease duration. Most patients with EM minor can be managed as an outpatient; younger children often require hospitalization for intravenous fluids to treat severe dehydration and for intravenous medications to improve pain control. In mild forms of EM minor, treatment is supportive. Antihistamines and topical steroids can be used to help control itch. A medium potency topical steroid (group 4 or 5) can be used for the trunk and extremities, while a low potency steroid (group 6 or 7) can be used for the face and intertriginous sites. Diphenhydramine elixir with aluminum/magnesium hydroxide suspension (Maalox), and at times viscous lidocaine (the so-called magic mouthwash) may reduce oral discomfort and improve fluid intake. High potency topical steroids (group 1 or 2) can also be used for painful lesions of the mouth and genitals. Nonsteroidal anti-inflammatory medications may be used for arthralgias, but clinicians should remain cognizant that ibuprofen has been reported as a cause of EM. For patients with ocular involvement, ophthalmology should be consulted to assess and treat visual impairment and ocular scarring.

In contrast, EM major often warrants admission to manage localized, organ-specific, or systemic complications. Prompt discontinuation of any etiologic drug triggers and identification and treatment of underlying infections (such as *Mycoplasma* or HSV) may mitigate the duration of illness though this hypothesis has not been studied in randomized trials. In more advanced forms of EM, use of IVIG or systemic corticosteroids must be considered. This issue is still controversial, with support for and against the use of these medications, though no high-quality studies have been done to evaluate their efficacy. The use of systemic corticosteroids may be helpful if initiated within the first 24 to 72 hours of the eruption and if not contraindicated by an underlying infectious trigger for the EM (e.g., HSV infection). The recommended dose is 0.5 to 1 mg/kg of prednisone per day tapered over 2 to 4 weeks. Several studies have also suggested a role for administration of IVIG, particularly when ocular integrity is at risk, or the disease is severe with increased body surface area affected. IVIG can be given for 1 to 5 days with doses reported from 0.5 g/kg/day to 2 g/kg/day, with total doses ranging from 1 to 6 g/kg.

Intravenous crystalloid solution with electrolyte replacement may be needed to maintain hydration in severely affected children because of reduced intake and increased loss through damaged skin. Colloid solutions are rarely needed. Wound care with silicone-based dressing or Vaseline-impregnated gauze can be helpful in areas of erosion or blistering.

For patients with HSV-induced EM or recurrent EM without an identifiable trigger, initiation of suppressive antiviral treatment should be considered. The use of antivirals for an acute episode of HSV-induced EM is not typically recommended as EM develops several days after the clinical signs of HSV infection.

ADMISSION AND DISCHARGE CRITERIA

Hospitalization is indicated if there is a need for any of the following:

- Clarification of a definitive diagnosis, including evaluation for other diagnoses (e.g., Kawasaki disease, SJS/TEN)
- Maintenance of adequate hydration
- Correction of electrolyte abnormalities

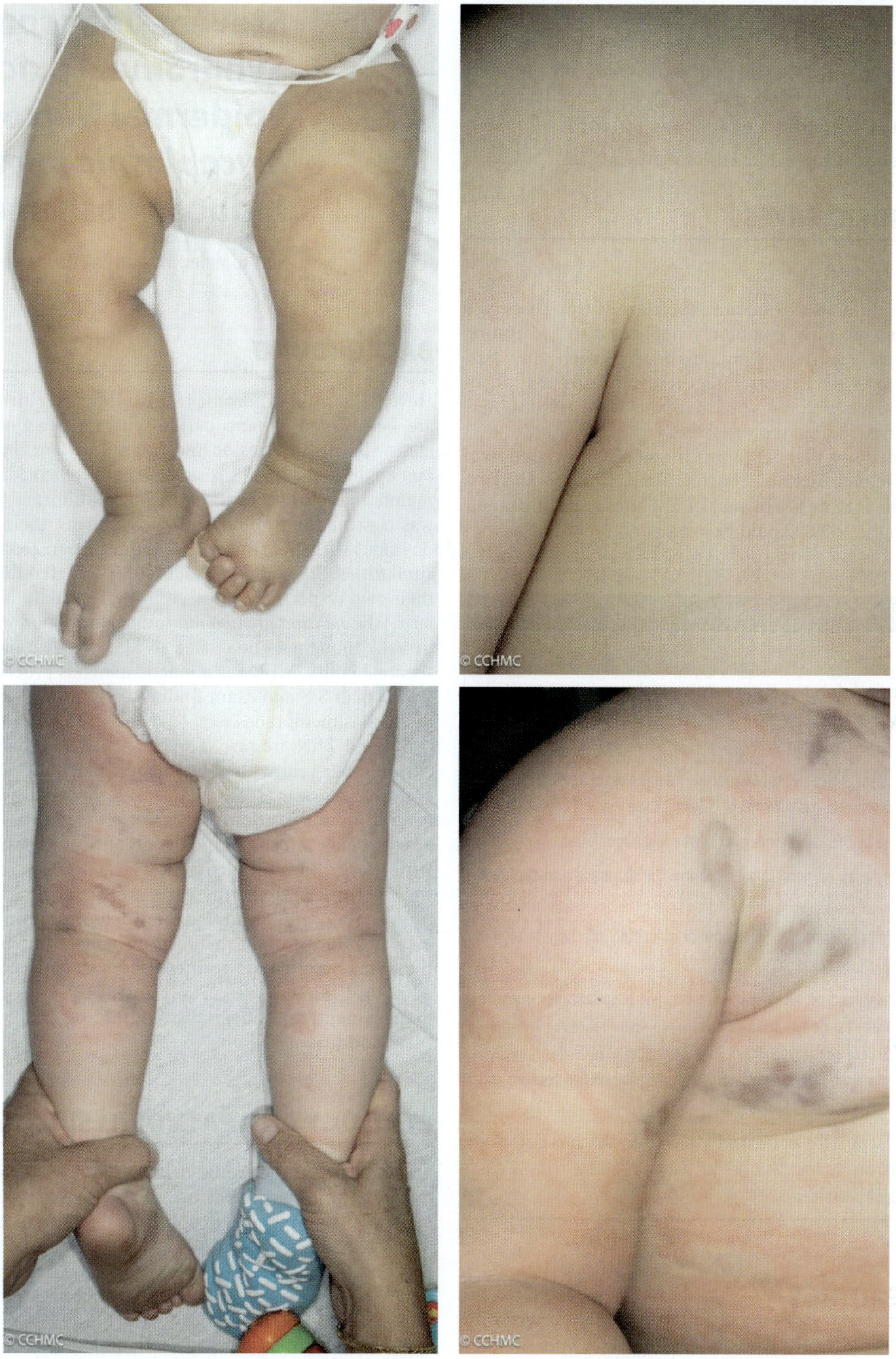

FIGURES 62-5, 62-6, 62-7, AND 62-8. Typical urticaria multiforme in a young child showing central pallor. Bruising can occasionally be seen.

- Wound management of large areas of denuded skin to decrease the risk for infection and/or dehydration
- Involvement of other organs requiring subspecialty involvement, ongoing observation, stabilization, or treatment

The following will be needed before discharge:

- Ability to maintain adequate oral/enteral hydration
- Resolution of symptoms to the point that the family can manage them at home
- Arrangement of follow-up to address all complications and remaining signs of illness

CONSULTATION

- Dermatology: For diagnosis, possible skin biopsy and management of severe mucosal and skin involvement
- Ophthalmology: Ocular involvement
- Infectious disease: Concern for alternative infectious processes, such as recurrent HSV as a cause of repeated episodes of EM minor and *Mycoplasma pneumoniae* as a cause of EM major
- Rheumatology: Progressive arthralgia, concern for other causes of arthralgia

- Plastic surgery: Extensive skin surface areas involvement as well as prevention of adhesions/strictures around mouth or eyes
- Critical care: Extensive blistering and body surface area involvement, significant electrolyte abnormalities, pulmonary involvement
- Urology: Treatment of urethral strictures if present
- Gynecology: Treatment of vaginal strictures if present

SPECIAL CONSIDERATIONS

PREVENTION

Prevention of EM is a difficult task because there are several suspected causes. Viral infections are most commonly implicated in EM minor, especially HSV. Because recurrent symptoms may be seen after outbreaks of HSV in an individual, controlling these outbreaks may theoretically lessen or eliminate symptoms of EM minor. These patients may benefit from suppressive antiviral prophylaxis.

Avoidance of medications that are more commonly associated with EM is difficult because the reaction is uncommon, and if it is the first episode, unpredictable. If there is a history of EM after a specific medication, other drugs in that class should be avoided.

KEY POINTS

Presentation

- EM minor: Symmetrically distributed, erythematous papules evolving into classic target lesions with involvement of the extremities, as well as the palms and soles. A single mucous membrane may be involved.
- EM major: More severe form with at least two mucous membranes involved by definition. Other organ systems may also be involved.
- EM is clinically diagnosed by the appearance of at least a few target lesions.
- Occasionally, skin biopsy may be necessary to confirm the diagnosis and facilitate treatment.
- Discontinuation of etiologic drug triggers or treatment of inciting infections is key for both the minor and major forms.
- EM minor is typically managed on an outpatient basis, but hospitalization may be required if there is concern for dehydration or electrolyte disturbances or for management of extensive severe skin involvement. Symptomatic relief is the mainstay of treatment with nonsteroidal anti-inflammatory drugs, topical corticosteroids, and pain-relieving mouthwashes.
- EM major is often managed in the inpatient setting for timely definitive diagnosis, supportive care, subspecialty involvement as needed, or consideration of systemic corticosteroid or immunoglobulin therapy.

SUGGESTED READINGS

Heinze A, Tollefson M, Holland KE, Chiu YE. Characteristics of pediatric recurrent erythema multiforme. *Pediatr Dermatol.* 2018; 35:97.

Hötzenecker W, Prins C, French LE. Erythema Multiforme, Stevens-Johnson Syndrome, and Toxic Epidermal Necrolysis. In Bolognia JL, Schaffer JV, Cerroni L *Dermatology*. 4th ed. Elsevier; 20: 332-347.

Huff JC, Weston WL, Tonnesen MG. Erythema multiforme: a critical review of characteristics, diagnostic criteria, and causes. *J Am Acad Dermatol.* 1983;8:763.

Zoghaib S, Kechichian E, Souaid K, et al. Triggers, clinical manifestations, and management of pediatric erythema multiforme: a systematic review. *J Am Acad Dermatol.* 2019; 81:813.

CHAPTER 63 Stevens-Johnson Syndrome, Toxic Epidermal Necrolysis, and *Mycoplasma pneumonia*-Induced Rash and Mucositis

Amy E. Miller, MD and Erik R. Hoefgen, MD

BACKGROUND

Stevens-Johnson syndrome (SJS) and toxic epidermal necrolysis (TEN) are both severe cutaneous idiosyncratic reactions commonly associated with medications or infections. They are characterized by cutaneous epidermal skin necrosis and involvement of at least two mucous membranes. In the past, erythema multiforme (EM, see Chapter 62) was classified into minor and major forms, the major form being synonymous with SJS. However, it is now recognized that, despite histologic similarities, SJS and EM should be considered distinct conditions with their own respective causes, clinical presentations, and outcomes. Similarly, *Mycoplasma pneumonia*-induced rash and mucositis (MIRM) was initially thought to be related to SJS; it is also now considered to be a separate entity. MIRM is a mucocutaneous process that is typically less severe than SJS and exam findings may be limited only to involvement of mucous membranes.

SJS and TEN are rare. The incidence of SJS is 5.3 cases per million children per year, while the incidence of TEN is 0.4 cases per million children per year. Regional differences in drug prescription patterns, genetic predisposition, cancer/other comorbidities, and radiotherapy use may affect the incidence of both conditions. Patients living with human immunodeficiency virus (HIV) are particularly susceptible with a 100-fold increase in annual incidence compared with the general population. Factors including immune dysregulation or exposure to multiple medications, including antiretroviral medications, may contribute to increased susceptibility of this population. Although relatively rare, SJS and TEN typically require inpatient management, and hospitalists should be able to recognize and treat these conditions.

ETIOLOGY AND PATHOPHYSIOLOGY

SJS and TEN appear to be delayed hypersensitivity reactions that culminate in epidermal detachment; reactions are characterized by T-cell–mediated keratinocyte apoptosis followed by epidermal necrolysis. Multiple pathways are thought to drive this process, including the Fas-FasL interaction, perforin/granzyme B, and granulysin; cytotoxic T lymphocytes (CTLs) and natural killer (NK) cells are also thought to play an important role. Histologic features of SJS and TEN include full-thickness epidermal necrosis with sparse inflammatory cells. The pathogenesis and histologic features of MIRM may be distinct from SJS/TEN, although more research in this area is required.

SJS can be caused by medications or infectious agents, but TEN is almost exclusively caused by medications, which is an important distinction. Although more than 100 drugs have been associated with SJS/TEN, most cases are attributable to a small group of medications including sulfonamides, other antibiotics, and antiepileptics. Drug dosage and/or duration of exposure appear to be related to risk of SJS/TEN. For example, allopurinol (a common inciting agent in adults, though not used widely in children) has been associated with SJS/TEN at higher doses (>200 mg). Drugs causing SJS/TEN after a relatively short duration of exposure include trimethoprim-sulfamethoxazole and other sulfonamides, aminopenicillins, cephalosporins, and quinolones. Conversely, lamotrigine, carbamazepine, oxcarbazepine, phenytoin, phenobarbital, valproic acid, nonsteroidal anti-inflammatory drugs (particularly of the oxicam type), and allopurinol are medications that typically cause SJS/TEN after exposures of longer duration. Generally, the first 2 months of treatment are a high-risk period for the development of SJS/TEN. Clinicians should also be aware that using drugs with similar molecular structures to an agent that caused SJS/TEN may provoke an additional reaction; if a patient developed SJS/TEN on carbamazepine, oxcarbazepine, phenytoin, and phenobarbital, they should not be prescribed another medication in this group of drugs.

Infections, underlying systemic diseases (e.g., inflammatory bowel disease), and immunizations may also be associated with SJS. However, these etiologies are less commonly identified as clear inciting factors, and direct associations are often difficult to prove. Of these etiologies, infections may be the most readily identifiable cause of SJS/TEN in hospitalized children. Herpes simplex virus (HSV), group A streptococci, hepatitis B, Epstein-Barr virus, and enteroviruses have been associated with SJS. HSV is also associated with EM. Underlying infections are also important considerations; immunocompromised patients, especially those who are HIV positive, are known to be at particular risk for the development of SJS/TEN.

Genetic predisposition is likely to be an important factor in some cases of SJS/TEN, particularly with regard to HLA alleles and families, and may play a role in pathogenesis. Specific alleles (e.g., HLA-B*1502) and HLA families (e.g., HLA-B75) have been implicated as risk factors for development of SJS/TEN susceptibility. HLA-B*1502 occurs more often in individuals of Asian descent and increases their risk of SJS/TEN particularly in association with carbamazepine. Notably, the FDA recommends testing for HLA-B*1502 in Asian patients prior to starting carbamazepine and to consider testing prior to using similar anticonvulsants such as oxcarbazepine. Other specific HLA-associated reactions have been identified in relation to abacavir, allopurinol, methazolamide, nevirapine, oxicams, and sulfonamides.

CLINICAL PRESENTATION

SJS/TEN is heralded by a prodrome of nonspecific constitutional symptoms that generally occurs 1 to 14 days prior to the development of necrotic mucosal or skin lesions. Children with SJS/TEN appear acutely ill. Fever and malaise are universal and are often accompanied by upper respiratory, gastrointestinal symptoms, or both. When due to drug exposure, SJS/TEN most commonly develops 2 to 8 weeks after drug initiation.

Skin lesions, which may begin simultaneously or after the onset of mucosal lesions, consist of tender, red to dusky macules that are often targetoid. Lesions generally appear first on the trunk and face and less commonly on the palms or soles. As the disease progresses, the face, neck, trunk, proximal ends of the extremities, and palms and soles may be involved, and rapid coalescence may occur (see **Figure 63-1**). Blistering, often heralded by the development of a central gray area within the skin lesions, may develop within hours or after several days. Blistering may be limited or consist of widespread epidermal detachment. In the latter case, large areas of raw, bleeding dermis may be seen. The frequent presence of overlapping clinical features in a given patient often makes definitive distinction between SJS and TEN difficult. According to a consensus definition for the classification of SJS and TEN, epidermal detachment (skin sloughing) of 10% or less of total body surface area is classified as SJS, greater than 30% is classified as TEN, and between 10% and 30% as on a spectrum between SJS and TEN. Large areas of skin sloughing, in the absence of mucosal involvement, are more characteristic of TEN.

Mucosal surfaces most commonly affected in SJS and TEN include the intraoral and ocular mucosa, but may also include the urethra, anus, vaginal vault, and upper aerodigestive tract. Classically, hemorrhagic crusts develop on the lips (Figure 63-1), and painful stomatitis leads to decreased oral intake. The conjunctivae also sloughs leading to a purulent conjunctivitis. As the denuded mucosa of the eye attempts to heal,

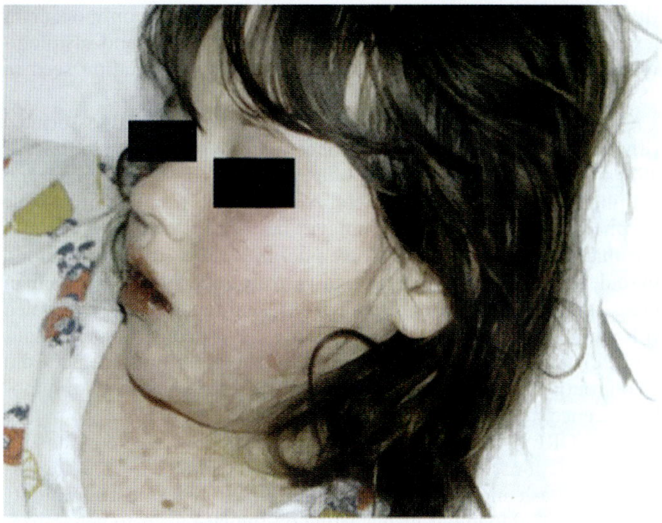

FIGURE 63-1. Oxcarbazepine-induced Stevens-Johnson syndrome. On the day of admission, hemorrhagic crusting of the lips and coalescing erythematous macules on the face and upper part of the trunk were apparent, along with early blister formation.

it can form synechiae and either cause the lids to adhere to each other or the palpebral conjunctivae to adhere to the bulbar conjunctiva, which can lead to blindness. Genital mucosal involvement is complicated by pain, bleeding, and possible scarring. Respiratory or gastrointestinal mucosal involvement and sloughing may also occur in more severe cases.

Potential systemic complications of SJS/TEN include generalized lymphadenopathy, hepatosplenomegaly, hepatitis, arthritis, and arthralgias. Less common findings are myocarditis, pancreatitis, pulmonary complications (especially pneumonia, pneumothorax, and bronchiolitis obliterans), and nephritis.

In MIRM, children will develop cough, fever, and malaise 1 week prior to the development of cutaneous and mucosal lesions. MIRM involves at least two mucous membranes, but commonly lacks the classic cutaneous lesions. Therefore, isolated and severe mucositis without cutaneous involvement should always prompt serologic or polymerase chain reaction testing for *M. pneumonia*, particularly if there is ocular involvement.

DIFFERENTIAL DIAGNOSIS

Differential diagnoses that should be considered when there is a high clinical concern for SJS/TEN or MIRM include Kawasaki disease (KD), staphylococcal scalded skin syndrome (SSSS), paraneoplastic pemphigus, drug reaction with eosinophilia and systemic syndrome (DRESS), EM, and graft-versus-host disease.

Kawasaki disease (KD) and SSSS are two childhood entities that may be difficult to distinguish from SJS/TEN or MIRM. In KD, mucosal involvement consists of chapped, red lips, without the erosions and hemorrhagic crusts typical of SJS. In addition, the conjunctival injection associated with KD lacks the purulent exudate of SJS. The skin lesions of KD are polymorphous and generally transient, without targetoid lesions or blistering, although superficial peeling of the fingertips and perineum is a characteristic finding seen later in the course of KD (see Chapter 148). SSSS, which usually occurs in infants and children younger than 2 years, is characterized by the onset of widespread, tender skin erythema (see Chapter 102). Crusting and superficial fissuring of the perioral and periocular skin is common, although mucous membrane involvement is universally absent. Staphylococcal exfoliative toxin selectively hydrolyzes desmoglein 1 (Dsg-1), which is found in all the strata of the skin. However, desmoglein 3 (Dsg-3), which is present in the deeper layers, compensates in these areas (hence the superficial skin involvement of SSSS). Since Dsg-3 is found in all the strata of mucous membranes, mucosal exfoliation does not occur in SSSS.

Although very superficial erosions, which most commonly occur in flexural areas, are a feature of SSSS, they are clinically and histologically distinct from the blistering and deeper skin separation seen in SJS/TEN.

Although rare, paraneoplastic pemphigus, which is usually associated with malignancy, can present with mucosal findings identical to those of SJS. Painful, severe oral erosions, often involving the lateral tongue and vermilion, tend to precede a generalized cutaneous eruption of variable morphology. Paraneoplastic pemphigus has a more subacute presentation than SJS and may also involve internal organs such as the lungs, thyroid, kidney, smooth muscle, and gastrointestinal tracts. Castleman disease and lymphoma are the malignancies most commonly associated with paraneoplastic pemphigus in children. Paraneoplastic pemphigus can be diagnosed with a skin biopsy, which shows features distinct from SJS on routine histology, and yields positive direct and indirect immunofluorescence studies.

While DRESS and SJS/TEN are both considered severe cutaneous adverse reactions, they can typically be differentiated by the appearance of the rash and associated lab findings. DRESS is most commonly a pruritic maculopapular rash starting on the face prior to generalization while SJS and TEN more commonly start on the trunk. Mucosal involvement in DRESS is rare. By definition, DRESS always has eosinophilia and is commonly associated with elevated liver enzymes and decreased renal function, all of which occur less commonly with SJS/TEN.

Grade IV acute graft-versus-host disease can also mimic TEN and should be considered in the appropriate clinical setting.

EM, which may also have infectious and drug-induced etiologies, was previously thought to be on a spectrum with SJS but is now differentiated as a separate entity. Although EM can present with painful acral targetoid papules and plaques that blister, as well as oral ulcerations, EM does not typically involve a second mucous membrane, which is characteristic of SJS. In addition, EM tends to have a much better prognosis.

MANAGEMENT

As soon as the diagnosis of SJS/TEN is suspected, any potential drug trigger should be immediately discontinued. Early withdrawal of the causative drug may reduce morbidity and mortality. Supportive therapy is the standard of care for SJS/TEN and includes close monitoring of fluid and electrolyte status, hydration, nutritional support, ophthalmologic care, wound care, and control of pain and infection. In MIRM, it is not clear whether antibiotic treatment of the underlying *Mycoplasma* infection leads to less severe mucosal injury or course of illness.

Insensible losses are increased as a result of fever and open skin lesions in SJS/TEN. Oral intake is often limited because of intraoral mucositis, making administration of parenteral fluids with careful monitoring of urine output and electrolytes even more essential. Nutritional support, preferably enteral, may be necessary when oral intake is inadequate for a prolonged period. A nasogastric (NG) tube may be appropriate, however, there are known complications of NG tube placement including risk of injury to the nasal and esophageal mucosa.

Attempts to limit ongoing skin loss should be instituted. Even minor manipulation of intact skin can cause sloughing. Maneuvers to protect fragile skin may include assistance with repositioning, devices to protect against friction and pressure, and assistance with activities of daily living. Use of a controlled-pressure, thermoregulated bed can also be beneficial.

Meticulous wound care is of utmost importance. Areas of skin sloughing and open wounds should be treated conservatively, without wide skin debridement unless the skin is entirely necrotic and becoming an infection risk. The blistered skin effectively serves as a natural dressing and may enhance re-epithelization. Areas with skin sloughing can be covered with petroleum gauze, non-adhesive biologic dressings, or silver-based dressings. Perioral erosions and hemorrhagic crusts should be gently cleansed daily and protected with petrolatum or a similar ointment. The mouth should be rinsed several times daily with a solution such as sterile isotonic saline. When the skin begins to heal, denuded areas will often adhere to each other inappropriately and then heal permanently. Care should also be taken to assure that any denuded areas of the oral mucosa, and genital mucosa of the labia, penis, and perianal areas do not fuse together; applying petrolatum multiple times per day may help prevent this. Care must also be taken if intubation is necessary, as more blisters may be induced, and the necrotic mucosa can be inadvertently pushed into the tracheobronchial tree. Transfer to an experienced burn unit or intensive care unit may be necessary to effectively manage wounds and monitor fluid and electrolyte status in patients with extensive surface area involvement.

Because sepsis is the principal cause of death, patients should be closely monitored for signs of secondary infection. Additional workup should be performed based on clinical concern for complications such as electrolyte abnormalities, sepsis, nephritis, hepatitis, and pulmonary complications.

The importance of early ophthalmologic consultation cannot be overemphasized because ocular complications, including blindness, are an important potential source of morbidity. The denuded areas of the conjunctiva will adhere to each other very rapidly and synechiae must be cleaved immediately by an experienced ophthalmologist to prevent permanent ocular damage. Amniotic membrane transplantation is a potential therapy that could be considered in cases of severe ocular inflammation.

There is currently no evidence-based, specific therapy accepted as the standard of care for pharmacologic management of SJS/TEN. Because of the rarity of such disorders and the frequent delay in diagnosis, large controlled studies are lacking. Treatment modalities are challenging to study as well due to the lack of in vitro cell cultures and appropriate animal models.

Intravenous immunoglobulin (IVIG) and corticosteroids are the most frequent immunomodulators used in the treatment of SJS/TEN in the pediatric population. Although commonly used, there is no definitive evidence that treatment with IVIG, corticosteroids, or a combination of corticosteroids/IVIG has beneficial effects on various outcomes in pediatric patients with SJS/TEN. In isolated pediatric cases, IVIG infusion has been associated with stopping the progression of skin blistering (**Figures 63-1** and **63-2**). Further investigation is needed on the efficacy of corticosteroids and/or IVIG in the management of pediatric patients with SJS/TEN.

Several other treatments, including plasmapheresis, cyclosporine, cyclophosphamide, TNF antagonists, calcineurin inhibitors,

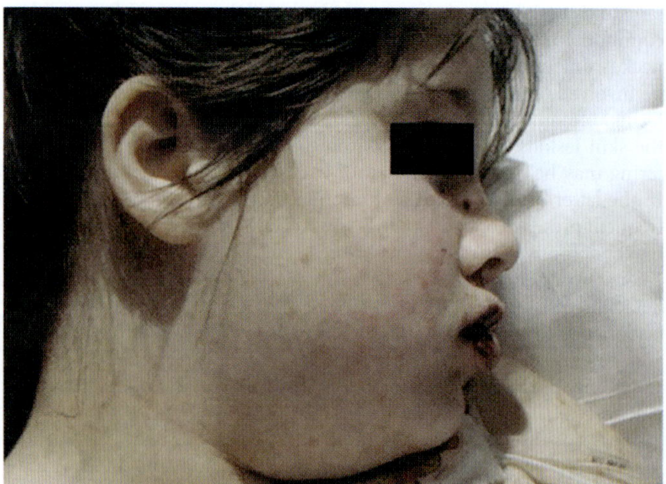

FIGURE 63-2. Clinical improvement (hospital day 5) of the patient in Figure 63-1 after four consecutive daily doses of intravenous immunoglobulin.

plasmapheresis, and *N*-acetylcysteine, have been reported with variable results.

CONSULTATION

- Dermatology: Can assist with diagnosis and wound management
- Ophthalmology: Due to the high risk of ocular involvement and long-term complications, ophthalmology consultation and long-term post-discharge follow-up are always recommended
- Plastic surgery: For wound management, acutely and long-term if needed
- Wound Service: If available, for wound management

ADMISSION CRITERIA

Patients are managed in the hospital setting because progression of the illness can be swift. Inpatient care centers on:

- Fluid and electrolyte management and nutritional support
- Meticulous care of areas of denuded skin and monitoring for secondary infection
- Close observation for multiorgan involvement, including respiratory compromise as a result of airway mucosal sloughing
- Coordination of subspecialty services

Transfer to a critical care setting is warranted in patients with cardiorespiratory instability, sepsis, or if the level of bedside care needed exceeds the capacity of non-intensive care unit staffing. Care in a burn center is often optimal for patients with extensive skin loss.

DISCHARGE CRITERIA

Care can be transitioned to the outpatient setting when:

- Progression of the illness has ceased, and the patient has stabilized
- Hydration and nutrition can be maintained
- Wound care can be managed in the home
- Appropriate outpatient follow-up is in place with subspecialists based on the morbidity and complications at time of discharge

PROGNOSIS

As expected, cases of TEN with the most extensive skin and mucosal sloughing, particularly respiratory and GI sloughing, are associated with the highest mortality rates. Cases of SJS/TEN triggered by drugs with a long half-life are more likely to result in a fatal outcome. In adults, mortality rates for TEN can reach as high as 30%, however in children mortality rates are lower, <1% in SJS and ~3% in TEN. Lower mortality rates in children may be associated with more rapid re-epithelization than in adults.

Ocular sequelae are the most common serious morbidity from SJS/TEN. Potential complications include pseudomembrane formation with immobility of the eyelids, symblepharon (adhesion of the palpebral conjunctivae to the bulbar conjunctivae), entropion (inward turning of eyelid margin), trichiasis (eyelashes misdirected toward globe surface secondary to entropion), corneal scarring, and permanent visual impairment. Lacrimal scarring with subsequent excessive tearing, anterior uveitis, and panophthalmitis may also occur.

Labial adhesions, esophageal and anal strictures, vaginal stenosis, urethral meatal stenosis, and phimosis can all occur as long-term complications. Late cutaneous complications of SJS/TEN include scarring, abnormal pigmentation, and fingernail loss and deformity. Large areas of scarring over joints may cause contractures, so physical therapy is an important prophylactic measure for patients at risk.

KEY POINTS

- Stevens-Johnson syndrome and toxic epidermal necrolysis are severe mucocutaneous disorders that occur secondary to idiosyncratic drug-related reactions that result in widespread skin breakdown and systemic toxicity.
- Upon recognition of SJS or TEN, any potential drug trigger should be immediately discontinued and admission to hospital advised to provide appropriate supportive care to limit morbidity and mortality.
- In the hospital setting, sepsis is the most common cause of mortality in patients with SJS and TEN. Patients should be closely monitored for signs of secondary infection.
- Common drugs causing these severe drug reactions include, but are not limited to, allopurinol, anticonvulsants, and antibiotics (particularly sulfonamides).
- Genetic susceptibility to SJS and TEN have been documented and patients of Asian descent receiving high-risk drugs (such as carbamazepine) should be screened for HLA susceptibilities prior to receiving these medications.
- Mycoplasma induced rash and mucositis (MIRM) is a mucocutaneous disorder associated with *Mycoplasma pneumoniae* infections. It is similar but distinct from SJS, predominately affects mucous membranes, and is less likely to result in skin involvement. Additional research is needed to better understand how this entity differs from SJS/TEN.

SUGGESTED READINGS

Antoon JW, Goldman JL, Lee B, Schwartz A. Incidence, outcomes, and resource use in children with Stevens-Johnson syndrome and toxic epidermal necrolysis. *Pediatr Dermatol.* 2018;35(2):182-187.

Antoon JW, Goldman JL, Shah SS, Lee B. A retrospective cohort study of the management and outcomes of children hospitalized with Stevens-Johnson syndrome or toxic epidermal necrolysis. *J Allergy Clin Immunol Pract.* 2019;7(1):244-250.e1.

Assier H, Bastuji-Garin S, Revuz J, Roujeau JC. Erythema multiforme with mucous membrane involvement and Stevens-Johnson syndrome are clinically different disorders with distinct causes. *Arch Dermatol.* 1995;131:539-543.

Bastuji-Garin S, Rzany B, Stern RS, et al. Clinical classification of cases of toxic epidermal necrolysis, Stevens-Johnson syndrome, and erythema multiforme. *Arch Dermatol.* 1993;129:92-96.

Brüggen MC, Le ST, Walsh S, et al. Supportive care in the acute phase of Stevens-Johnson syndrome and toxic epidermal necrolysis: an international, multidisciplinary Delphi-based consensus. *Br J Dermatol.* 2021;185(3):616-626.

Canavan TN, Mathes EF, Frieden I, Shinkai K. Mycoplasma pneumoniae-induced rash and mucositis as a syndrome distinct from Stevens-Johnson syndrome and erythema multiforme: a systematic review. *J Am Acad Dermatol.* 2015;72(2):239-245.

Chave TA, Mortimer NJ, Sladden MJ, et al. Toxic epidermal necrolysis: current evidence, practical management and future directions. *Br J Dermatol.* 2005;153:241-253.

Chen J, Wang B, Zeng Y, et al. High-dose intravenous immunoglobulins in the treatment of Stevens-Johnson syndrome and toxic epidermal necrolysis in Chinese patients: a retrospective study of 82 cases. *Eur J Dermatol.* 2010;20:743-747.

Chung W, Shuen-Iu H. Recent advances in the genetics and immunology of Steven-Johnson Syndrome and toxic epidermal necrolysis. *J Dermatol Sci.* 2012;66:190-196.

Garcia-Doval I, LeCleach L, Bocquet H, et al. Toxic epidermal necrolysis and Stevens-Johnson syndrome: does early withdrawal of causative drugs decrease the risk of death? *Arch Dermatol.* 2000;136:323-327.

Harr T, French L. Toxic epidermal necrolysis and Stevens-Johnson syndrome. *Orphanet J Rare Dis.* 2010;4:39.

Hsu DY, Brieva J, Silverberg NB, Paller AS, Silverberg JI. Pediatric Stevens-Johnson syndrome and toxic epidermal necrolysis in the United States. *J Am Acad Dermatol.* 2017;76(5):811-817.e4.

Hsu M, Jayaram A, Verner R, et al. Indications and outcomes of amniotic membrane transplantation in the management of acute Steven-Johnson Syndrome and toxic epidermal necrolysis: a case-control study. *Cornea*. 2012;31:1394-1402.

Koh MJ, Tay YK. Stevens-Johnson syndrome and toxic epidermal necrolysis in Asian children. *J Am Acad Dermatol*. 2010;62(1):54-60.

Li K, Haber R. Steven-Johnson syndrome without skin lesions (Fuchs syndrome): a literature review of adult cases with Mycoplasma cause. *Arch Dermatol*. 2012;148:963-964.

Lyell A. Toxic epidermal necrolysis: an eruption resembling scalding of the skin. *Br J Dermatol*. 1956;68:355-361.

Metry DW, Jung P, Levy ML. Use of intravenous immunoglobulin (IVIG) in children with Stevens-Johnson syndrome and toxic epidermal necrolysis: 7 cases and review of the literature. *Pediatrics*. 2003;112:1430-1436.

Pozzo-Magana BRD, Lazo-Langner A, Carleton B, et al. A systematic review of treatment of drug-induced Stevens-Johnson syndrome and toxic epidermal necrolysis in children. *J Popul Ther Clin Pharmacol*. 2011;18:e121-e133.

Prins C, Kerdel FA, Padilla RS, et al. Treatment of toxic epidermal necrolysis with high-dose intravenous immunoglobulins: multicenter retrospective analysis of 48 consecutive cases. *Arch Dermatol*. 2003;139(1):26-32.

Ravin KA, Rappaport LD, Zuckerbraun NS, et al. Mycoplasma pneumonia and atypical Stevens-Johnson syndrome: a case series. *Pediatrics*. 2007;119:e1002-1005.

Roujeau JC. The spectrum of Stevens-Johnson syndrome and toxic epidermal necrolysis: a clinical classification. *J Invest Dermatol*. 1994; 102:28S-30S.

Sekula P, Dunant A, Mockenhaupt M, et al. Comprehensive survival analysis of a cohort of patients with Stevens-Johnson syndrome and toxic epidermal necrolysis. *J Invest Dermatol*. 2013;133(5): 1197-204.

Stella M, Clemente A, Bollero D, et al. Toxic epidermal necrolysis (TEN) and Stevens-Johnson syndrome (SJS): experience with high-dose intravenous immunoglobulins and topical conservative approach, a retrospective analysis. *Burns*. 2007;33:452-459.

Sullivan JR, Shear NH. The drug hypersensitivity syndrome. What is the pathogenesis? *Arch Dermatol*. 2001;137:357-364.

CHAPTER 64 Skin Diseases in Immunocompromised Hosts

Maria C. Widmann, MD, FAAP and Megan E. Coe, MD, FAAP

BACKGROUND

Immunocompromised patients are at high risk for many serious and significant health complications. Cutaneous disorders are common in immunocompromised patients, and while they are often accompanied by other signs and symptoms of systemic disease, they may also be the first and only sign of illness or an underlying immunocompromised state. Many of the skin conditions seen in these patients are also commonly seen in the general immunocompetent population—newborn rashes, eczema, cutaneous bacterial and viral infections, mucocutaneous candidiasis, nevi, acne vulgaris, aphthous ulcers—thus, it is imperative that pediatric hospitalists recognize how these disorders may manifest differently in immunocompromised patients. Atypical features, unusual clinical courses, recurrent infections, and difficult-to-treat conditions should raise suspicion for cutaneous disease secondary to immunodeficiency or immunosuppression. Dermatologic conditions associated with immune dysregulation are generally a consequence of primary immunodeficiency, acquired immunodeficiency, or immunosuppressive medical therapy.

Although primary immunodeficiencies are rare, many have cutaneous manifestations. Some genetic conditions may be diagnosed via newborn screening, but many inherited immunodeficiencies are diagnosed in childhood after recurrent infections; other signs and symptoms of underlying immunodeficiency may or may not be present. Acquired immunodeficiencies, in contrast, are not inherited and are most commonly caused by human immunodeficiency virus (HIV), human T-lymphotropic virus 1 (HTLV-1), and oncologic processes such as leukemia and lymphoma. Immunosuppressive states often occur due to medications when patients are treated for autoimmune disorders, solid organ transplants, bone marrow transplants, stem cell transplants, and cancer. Immunosuppressants and chemotherapeutic agents may have short- and long-term sequelae. In this chapter, we will discuss the common skin manifestations seen in immunodeficient and immunosuppressed patients. **Table 64-1** highlights the various dermatologic conditions that can be seen in immunocompromised patients.

NONINFECTIOUS SKIN CONDITIONS

Although superficial and systemic infections are common in primary immunodeficiencies, non-specific cutaneous manifestations of disease are equally, if not more, common. Nearly half of all children with primary immunodeficiencies present with skin disease, and an additional third have early skin-related symptoms. Examples of primary immunodeficiencies with frequent cutaneous symptoms include severe combined immunodeficiency (SCID), Omenn syndrome, common variable immunodeficiency (CVID), Wiskott-Aldrich syndrome (WAS), ataxia-telangiectasia, hyper-IgE syndrome (Job syndrome), X-linked agammaglobulinemia (Bruton hypogammaglobulinemia), chronic granulomatous disease (CGD), and leukocyte adhesion deficiency. Common skin manifestations of primary immunodeficiencies include eczema, erythroderma, alopecia, noninfectious granulomas, and vasculitis (**Figure 64-1**).

Eczema is frequently seen in a variety of primary immunodeficiencies. Hyper-IgE syndrome is characterized by an eczematous rash secondary to increased circulating IgE levels. The rash often presents shortly after birth and is almost always apparent within the first month of life. Patients with immune dysregulation polyendocrinopathy enteropathy X-linked syndrome (IPEX) may have severe widespread eczema, erythroderma, or psoriasis. This syndrome occurs exclusively in males and is also associated with early-onset diarrhea, diabetes, and thyroid disease. Patients with WAS may have atopic dermatitis as well, though this condition often manifests with a more hemorrhagic-appearing rash. These patients will have associated neonatal thrombocytopenia and severe recurrent infections.

Cutaneous granulomas are also associated with multiple primary immunodeficiencies. Ataxia telangiectasia is characterized by ocular and cutaneous telangiectasias (dilated blood vessels) as well as with development of cutaneous granulomas. These granulomatous lesions are typically slow growing, well-defined, erythematous papules or plaques that may progress to central ulceration (**Figure 64-2**). Interestingly, noninfectious granulomas are also fairly common in patients with CVID, though they tend to occur more frequently in adults than in children (**Figure 64-3**).

Hospitalists should also be aware of other types of skin lesions. Papular pruritic eruptions are one of the most common cutaneous manifestations of HIV infection and often indicate waning immunity and decreasing CD4 count. These eruptions typically consist of excoriated reddish-brown papules on the extremities but may also include lesions on the face and trunk (**Figure 64-4**). Cutaneous vasculitis may also be seen in patients with HIV secondary to the infection itself, superimposed bacterial or viral infection, or drug reaction.

Graft versus host disease (GVHD) is a multisystem disorder that occurs as a complication of a solid organ transplant, bone marrow transplant, or a stem cell transplant. Interestingly, it can also occur in neonates with SCID who undergo maternal-fetal transfusion (maternal isoimmunization) during pregnancy. GVHD often presents with a nonspecific maculopapular rash and may be difficult to differentiate from other more benign skin disorders.

TABLE 64-1 Skin Diseases in Immunocompromised Hosts

Noninfectious	Medication side effects
Eczema	Corticosteroid side effects
Erythroderma	Skin thinning and atrophy
Alopecia	Hair thinning
Noninfectious granuloma	Striae
Vasculitis	Cushingoid facies
Papular pruritic eruption	Facial erythema
Graft versus host disease (GVHD)	Acne vulgaris or acneiform rash
Infectious	Hirsutism
Bacteria	Perioral dermatitis
Fungi	Ecchymosis
Viruses	Poor wound healing
Mycobacteria	Other side effects
Parasites	Acneiform rash
Neoplasms	Mucositis
Malignant	Stomatitis
Skin cancer	Xerosis
Squamous cell	Hypertrichosis
Basal cell	Gingival hyperplasia
Melanoma	Nonspecific maculopapular, eczematous, or psoriatic rashes
Post-transplant lymphoproliferative disorder	Pruritic morbilliform rash
Sarcoma	Inflammatory skin eruption
Kaposi sarcoma	Paronychia
Lymphoma	Edema
Carcinoma	Photosensitivity
Skin and lip	Hyperpigmentation
Genital (anal or vulvar)	Toxic erythema of chemotherapy
Benign	
Melanocytic nevus	
Pyogenic granuloma	

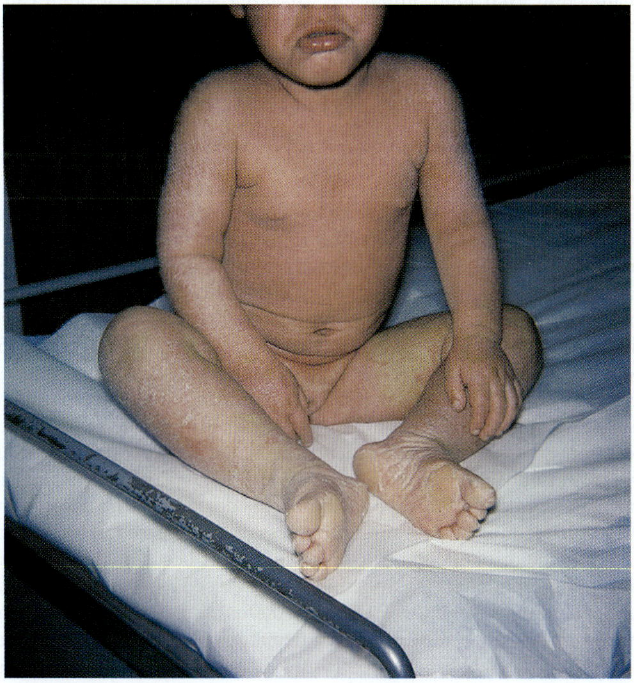

FIGURE 64-1. Generalized erythroderma in an infant with underlying atopic dermatitis. (From Shah BR, Mahajan P, Amodio J, Lucchesi M. *Atlas of Pediatric Emergency Medicine*. 3rd ed. New York: McGraw Hill; 2019, Figure 7.38. Reproduced with permission from photo contributor: Binita R. Shah, MD.)

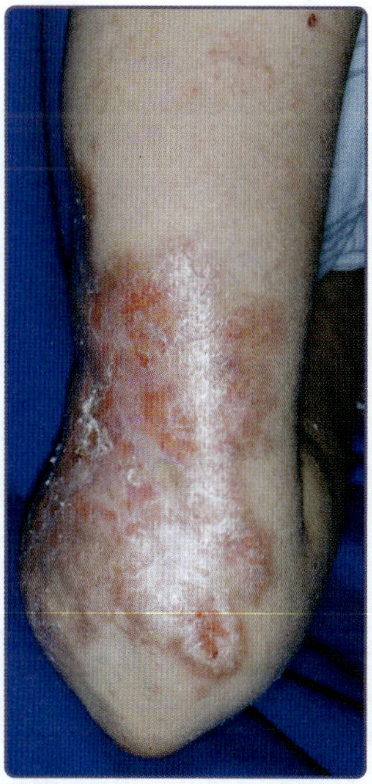

FIGURE 64-2. Noninfectious granulomatous dermatitis in a patient with ataxia telangiectasia. (Reproduced with permission from Kang S, Amagai M, Bruckner AL, et al, eds. *Fitzpatrick's Dermatology*. 9th ed. New York: McGraw Hill; 2019, Figure 132-12.)

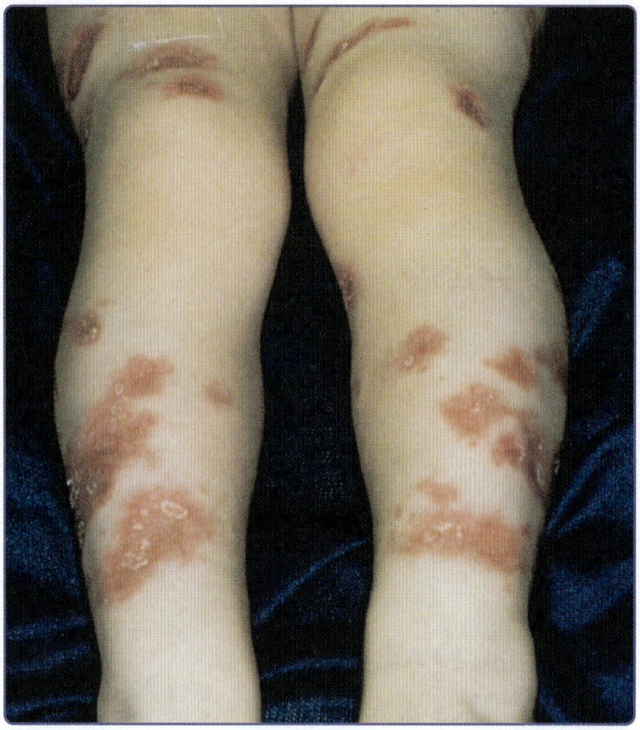

FIGURE 64-3. Multiple noncaseating granulomas in a child with CVID. (Reproduced with permission from Kang S, Amagai M, Bruckner AL, et al, eds. *Fitzpatrick's Dermatology*. 9th ed. New York: McGraw Hill; 2019, Figure 132-2.)

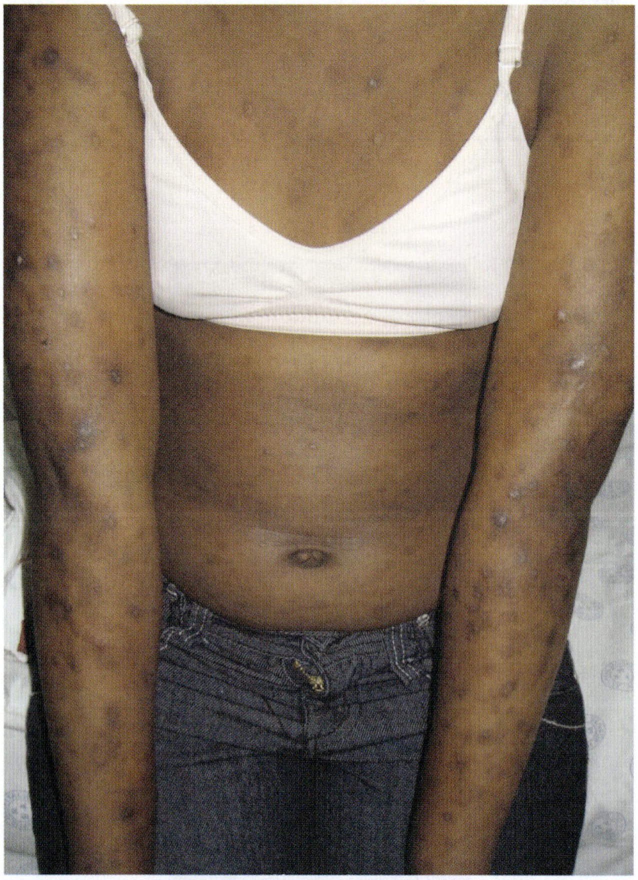

FIGURE 64-4. Papular pruritic eruption in a 23-year-old female with HIV. There are numerous excoriated papules on the bilateral arms and trunk. (From Wolff K, Johnson RA, Saavedra AP, Roh EK. *Fitzpatrick's Color Atlas and Synopsis of Clinical Dermatology*. 8th ed. New York: McGraw Hill; 2017, Figure 27-64. Reproduced with permission from Adam Lipworth, MD.)

INFECTIOUS SKIN CONDITIONS

Cutaneous bacterial, viral, and fungal infections are a common complication of immunodeficiency and immunosuppression. Hospitalists must be aware of the increased morbidity and mortality associated with cutaneous infections in the setting of a poorly functioning immune system. Even the most banal skin lesion can herald a life-threatening disease, thus a high index of suspicion, prompt evaluation, and urgent treatment of any cutaneous infection is essential to optimize outcomes. Cutaneous lesions in immunocompromised patients should be biopsied and sent for histology, special stains, and tissue culture as superficial skin cultures are often not sufficient to establish a diagnosis. Relatively minor but still problematic skin infections—tinea corporis, pityriasis (tinea) versicolor, and viral warts—may cause extensive disease in immunocompromised patients and must be evaluated and treated promptly.

BACTERIAL INFECTIONS

Common bacterial infections such as impetigo, folliculitis, and cellulitis may arise in immunocompromised patients. These infections may coincide with a known underlying systemic infection but may also occur as a result of occult disease. Typical pathogens such as *Staphylococcus aureus* and group A *Streptococcus* are also common in the immunocompromised patient population. More concerning, however, are the organisms that do not routinely cause infection in immunocompetent patients. *Pseudomonas aeruginosa* infections are a well-known cause of severe disease in debilitated, critically ill, and immunocompromised patients. Mortality associated with missed or delayed diagnosis may be up to 70%. A fairly benign and localized skin infection may quickly progress to necrotizing fasciitis or pyomyositis. Ecthyma gangrenosum, a necrotizing vasculitis, is one of the more severe manifestations of *Pseudomonas* sepsis. It begins as an erythematous or purpuric patch that evolves into a hemorrhagic bulla which progresses to a necrotic ulcer or eschar (**Figure 64-5**). This life-threatening infection is discussed in detail in Chapter 60. *Stenotrophomonas maltophilia* is another common cause of bacterial infection in immunocompromised patients, and cutaneous lesions may also progress to necrotizing fasciitis or ecthyma gangrenosum. Resistance to many common, broad-spectrum antibiotics is frequently encountered, making early suspicion and recognition of infection even more important. *Nocardia* species most often cause infection via direct inoculation of the skin secondary to trauma. In immunocompromised patients, however, cutaneous *Nocardia* infection (nonspecific erythematous papules and nodules) may represent disseminated infection from a pulmonary source.

FUNGAL INFECTIONS

Cutaneous fungal infections, such as seborrheic dermatitis, mucocutaneous candidiasis, folliculitis, intertrigo, and various tinea infections, occur commonly in both immunocompetent and immunocompromised patients. In immunocompromised patients, however, these generally minor infections can spread rapidly and have devastating consequences. Skin lesions may represent primary cutaneous infections that have the potential to disseminate to other organs, but they may also represent systemic dissemination of occult infection. Significant infections caused by yeasts and molds are most common in patients being treated with immunosuppressants or chemotherapeutic agents. They also tend to occur when immunosuppression is most severe. For transplant patients in particular, peak immunosuppression occurs during the first few months after transplant or when immunosuppression is increased to treat rejection. The majority of cutaneous mold infections occur in children with hematologic malignancies. Systemic disease caused by a variety of pathogens including *Aspergillus*, *Fusarium*, *Alternaria*, *Paecilomyces*, and the mucoromycetes may present as erythematous patches or nodules that evolve into ulcerated, necrotic plaques or multiple erythematous pustules and nodules (**Figure 64-6**).

As noted previously, *Candida* species can cause localized skin disease such as intertrigo and folliculitis. *Candida* sepsis, a much more severe and systemic infection, may present as erythematous papules or papulopustules, often on the trunk and extremities. Biopsy and culture of

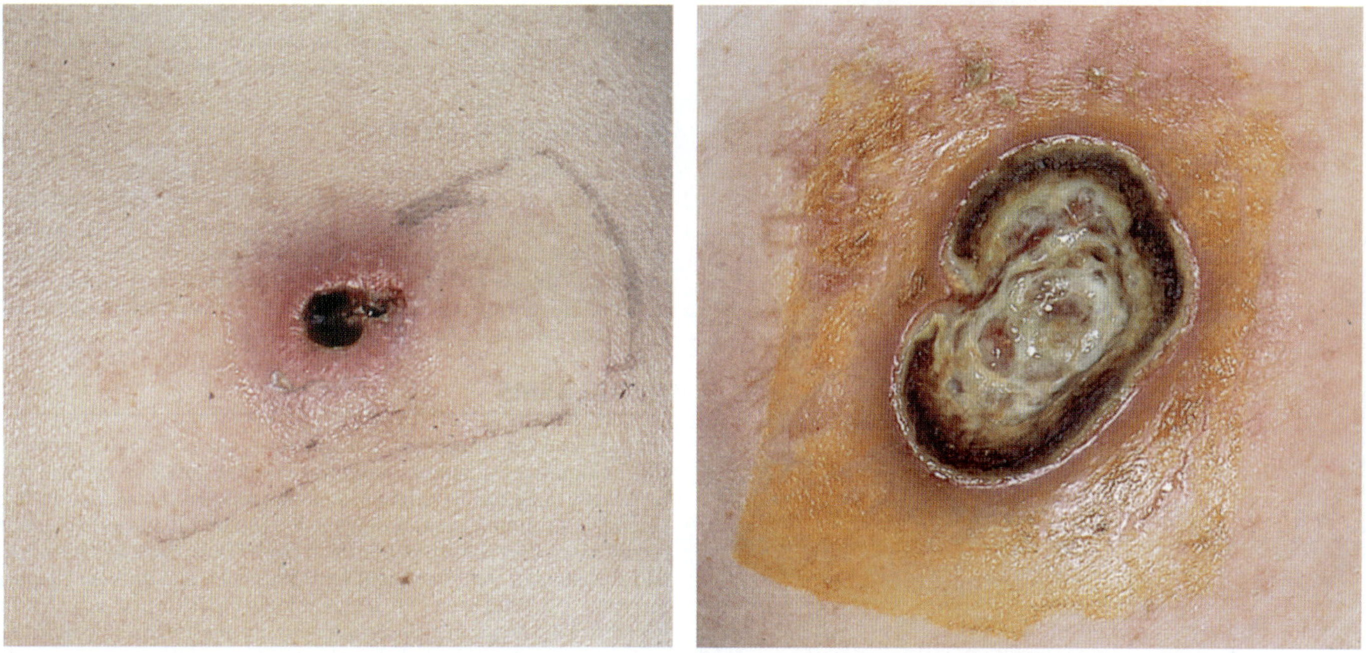

A B

FIGURE 64-5. Ecthyma gangrenosum of the buttock caused by *Pseudomonas aeruginosa* in a 30-year-old male with HIV. (A) Painful, infarcted lesion with surrounding erythema. (B) Progression of the same lesion to a large ulcer. (Reproduced with permission from Wolff K, Johnson RA, Saavedra AP, Roh EK. *Fitzpatrick's Color Atlas and Synopsis of Clinical Dermatology*. 8th ed. New York: McGraw Hill; 2017, Figure 25-32.)

lesions can aid in diagnosis of *Candida* sepsis as blood cultures are not always positive. Mucocutaneous candidiasis—in the forms of thrush, cheilitis, glossitis, papillary hyperplasia—is one of the most common presentations of *Candida* infection in immunocompromised individuals; infection may quickly spread beyond the mouth (**Figure 64-7**). Some studies suggest that in patients with HIV, thrush may be a marker of worsening disease and increased mortality.

Disseminated cryptococcosis primarily affects patients with acquired immunodeficiency. And like many other infections, nonspecific papules or cellulitic areas may be the first sign of systemic infection. Other cutaneous manifestations of cryptococcosis include abscesses, vesicles, ulcers, and granulomas. *Cryptococcus*, in particular, has a propensity for CNS spread in immunocompromised patients. Given this risk, cutaneous *Cryptococcus* lesions should prompt consideration of additional evaluation for systemic infection including lumbar puncture and CSF studies.

Dermatophytes cause widespread superficial skin infections such as tinea capitis, tinea pedis, and tinea corporis. These common infections are usually not life-threatening but may serve as a portal of entry for other pathogens that cause systemic disease. Severe onychomycosis of the fingernails and toenails is a common finding in patients with HIV. *Trichosporon* species, which most commonly cause innocuous superficial infections of the hair in immunocompetent hosts, are a known cause of systemic illness in immunocompromised patients. Again, a high index of suspicion is paramount in the diagnosis of life-threatening disseminated *Trichosporon* infections as cutaneous manifestations are often nonspecific.

VIRAL INFECTIONS

Patients with decreased or impaired immunity are at increased risk of primary and recurrent herpesvirus infections—herpes simplex virus

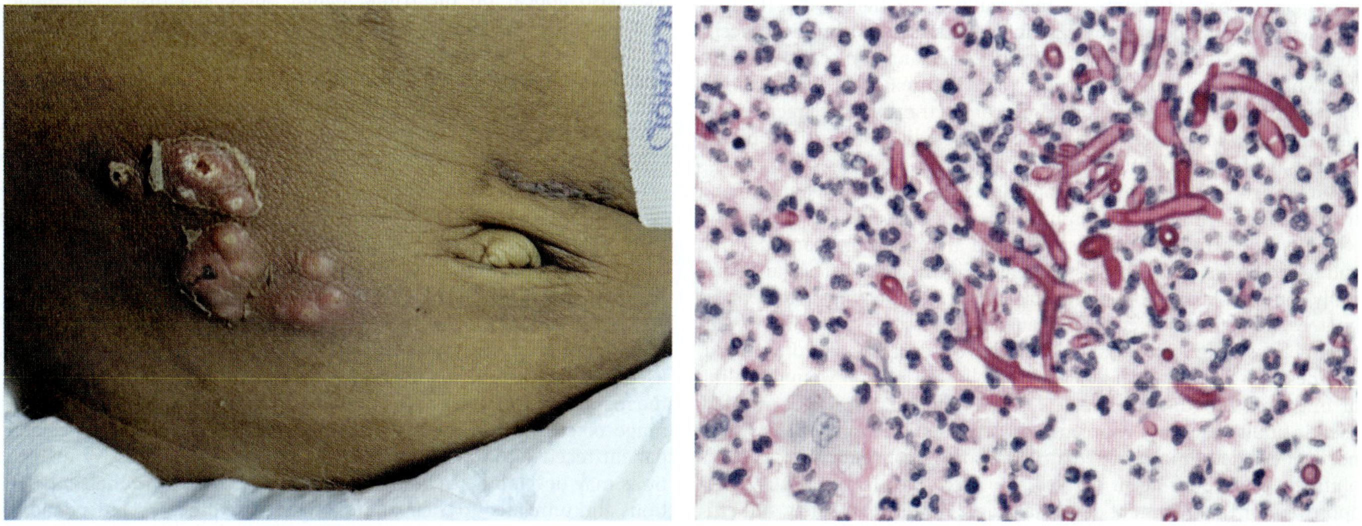

A B

FIGURE 64-6. (A) Collection of abscesses caused by *Rhizopus* in a neutropenic child. (B) PAS staining of *Rhizopus* species will demonstrate broad-based, ribbon-like nonseptate hyphae. (Images used with permission of Dr. Melinda Jen.)

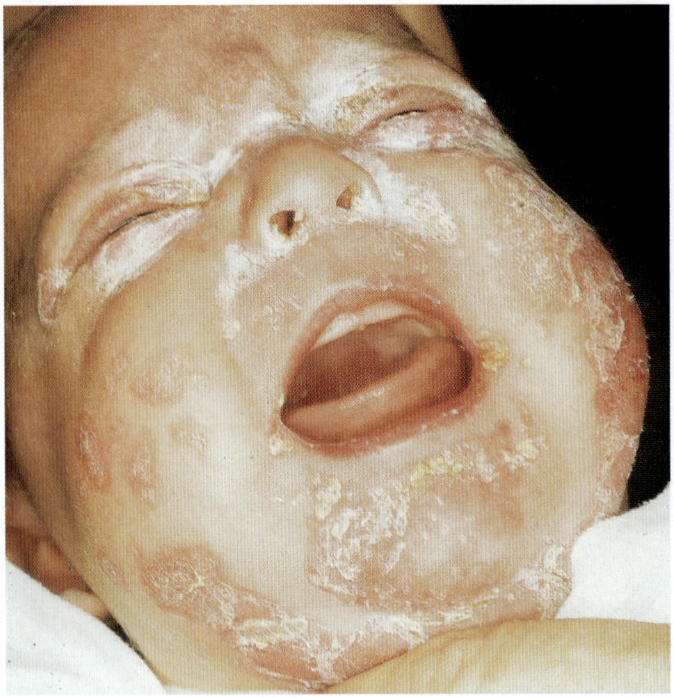

FIGURE 64-7. Persistent mucocutaneous candidiasis in an immunocompromised infant. There is diffuse scaling and crusting on the face as well as oropharyngeal candidiasis. (Reproduced with permission from Wolff K, Johnson RA, Saavedra AP, Roh EK. *Fitzpatrick's Color Atlas and Synopsis of Clinical Dermatology*. 8th ed. New York: McGraw Hill; 2017, Figure 26-12.)

(HSV), varicella zoster virus (VZV), cytomegalovirus (CMV). Cutaneous viral infections caused by HSV 1 and 2 may be more extensive in transplant recipients and may even cause lesions that mimic pressure ulcers. Lesions are most common in the periorificial and genital regions but may appear in other locations as well.

Reactivation of VZV commonly leads to herpes zoster in immunocompromised hosts. Unlike in immunocompetent patients, however, the presentation of herpes zoster may not follow a dermatomal distribution (**Figures 64-8** and **64-9**). Early initiation of antiviral therapy is imperative to decreasing the incidence of cutaneous and visceral dissemination which can result in life-threatening complications. Disseminated zoster infection is diagnosed when more than 20 skin lesions are present outside the affected dermatome or the immediately adjacent dermatomes (**Figure 64-10**). These patients are also at increased risk of post-herpetic neuralgia compared to immunocompetent peers. Patients with HIV may also develop a unique form of VZV infection known as chronic varicella zoster. This is characterized by recurrent vesicular and ulcerative lesions following a more standard VZV infection (**Figure 64-11**). CMV, a common cause of systemic infection in solid organ transplant recipients, may also cause a wide variety of skin lesions including periorificial ulcers, nodules, plaques, and diffuse exanthem.

Viral warts caused by human papillomavirus (HPV) are common and troublesome to immunocompromised patients. Lesions can occur anywhere on the skin or mucosal surface and are often numerous, painful, and felt to be unsightly by most patients (**Figure 64-12**). They are especially common in solid organ transplant patients, affecting up to approximately half of these patients. Spontaneous regression is uncommon, and treatment is often challenging. Destructive treatments are often used, but these can be painful and may be complicated by poor wound healing or infection. Imiquimod, a topical immunomodulator, has been safely used in adult transplant recipients; however, its safety and efficacy have not yet been determined in pediatric transplant recipients. Sinecatechins ointment is a newer agent derived from green tea leaves and is FDA-approved for the treatment of genital warts; however, its safety and efficacy have not been studied in immunocompromised adults or children.

Molluscum contagiosum occurs in approximately 7% of pediatric solid organ transplant recipients. Lesions arise in common locations—the face, trunk, extremities, and especially skin folds—but are often numerous and resistant to conventional treatments. They can also present atypically and in large numbers. Vesicular lesions, papules without typical umbilication, and giant nodules with ulceration have all been reported.

MYCOBACTERIAL INFECTIONS

Nontuberculous mycobacteria *(Mycobacterium kansasii, M. avium-intracellulare, M. fortuitum, M. marinum, M. abscessus*, and others) may present as subcutaneous nodules, abscesses, ulcerated lesions, or sinus tracts. These pathogens are most commonly known for causing chronic pulmonary infections, but they are a fairly common cause of skin infection in immunosuppressed patients, especially those who have undergone bone marrow or stem cell transplant.

NEOPLASMS

An increased risk of malignant neoplasms is one of the most concerning consequences of immunosuppressive medications. This elevated risk is thought to be due to reduced immune-mediated tumor surveillance secondary to chronic immunosuppression. An overall three- to fourfold increase in cancer risk is reported. Skin cancer (squamous cell, basal cell, and melanoma), post-transplant lymphoproliferative disorder, Kaposi sarcoma, and other sarcomas are commonly reported malignancies. In pediatric solid organ transplant recipients, the most frequently reported malignant neoplasms include lymphoma, skin and lip carcinoma, various sarcomas, and genital (anal or vulvar) carcinoma.

The incidence of skin cancer in solid organ transplant recipients increases with age, duration of immunosuppression, intensity of immunosuppression, infection with HPV, ultraviolet light exposure, and fair skin. Notably, pediatric solid organ transplant patients also have increased rates of skin cancer metastasis and mortality. Squamous cell carcinoma is the most common form of skin cancer diagnosed in solid organ transplant patients and often presents with multiple lesions at a younger age compared to the general population; the clinical course is often aggressive. Skin cancer risk is also increased in patients with hematologic malignancies, in bone marrow transplant and stem cell transplant recipients, and in patients who have received chemotherapy or immunosuppression for chronic autoimmune conditions. Cutaneous malignancies secondary to childhood cancer therapy are a consequence of disease-associated immunosuppression, chemotherapy-associated immunosuppression, immunosuppression associated with GVHD prophylaxis, and radiation therapy.

Kaposi sarcoma, an angioproliferative disorder, occurs in immunosuppressed patient populations after infection with human herpesvirus 8 (HHV-8). Tumors typically present as painless purple, red, or brown/black macules, plaques, or nodules on the extremities or face. Lesions may also appear on the trunk, palms, soles, and inside the mouth (**Figures 64-13** and **64-14**). In severe cases, lesions may also develop in the lungs or gastrointestinal tract. Kaposi sarcoma is seen in older males of Mediterranean or Middle Eastern descent, in people of all ages in sub-Saharan Africa, in transplant recipients on chronic immunosuppression, and in people with HIV. In HIV-positive individuals, development of Kaposi sarcoma indicates progression to acquired immunodeficiency syndrome (AIDS) and is considered an AIDS-defining illness. It occurs rarely in children. Lesions concerning for Kaposi sarcoma should always be biopsied as HIV status, especially in children, may not be known.

MEDICATION SIDE EFFECTS

Many immunosuppressive medications and immune-targeted therapies used to treat malignant and autoimmune conditions interrupt or affect the regulatory processes in the dermis and epidermis resulting in a wide range of cutaneous adverse effects. As such, a hospitalized pediatric patient receiving immune-modulating or immunosuppressive medications may develop dermatologic conditions secondary to their medications and unrelated to their underlying disease process. Understanding the more common dermatologic manifestations associated with these medications will help guide the diagnostic evaluation of immunosuppressed patients presenting with new skin lesions. The most frequently used immunosuppressive agents in pediatric patients are glucocorticoids;

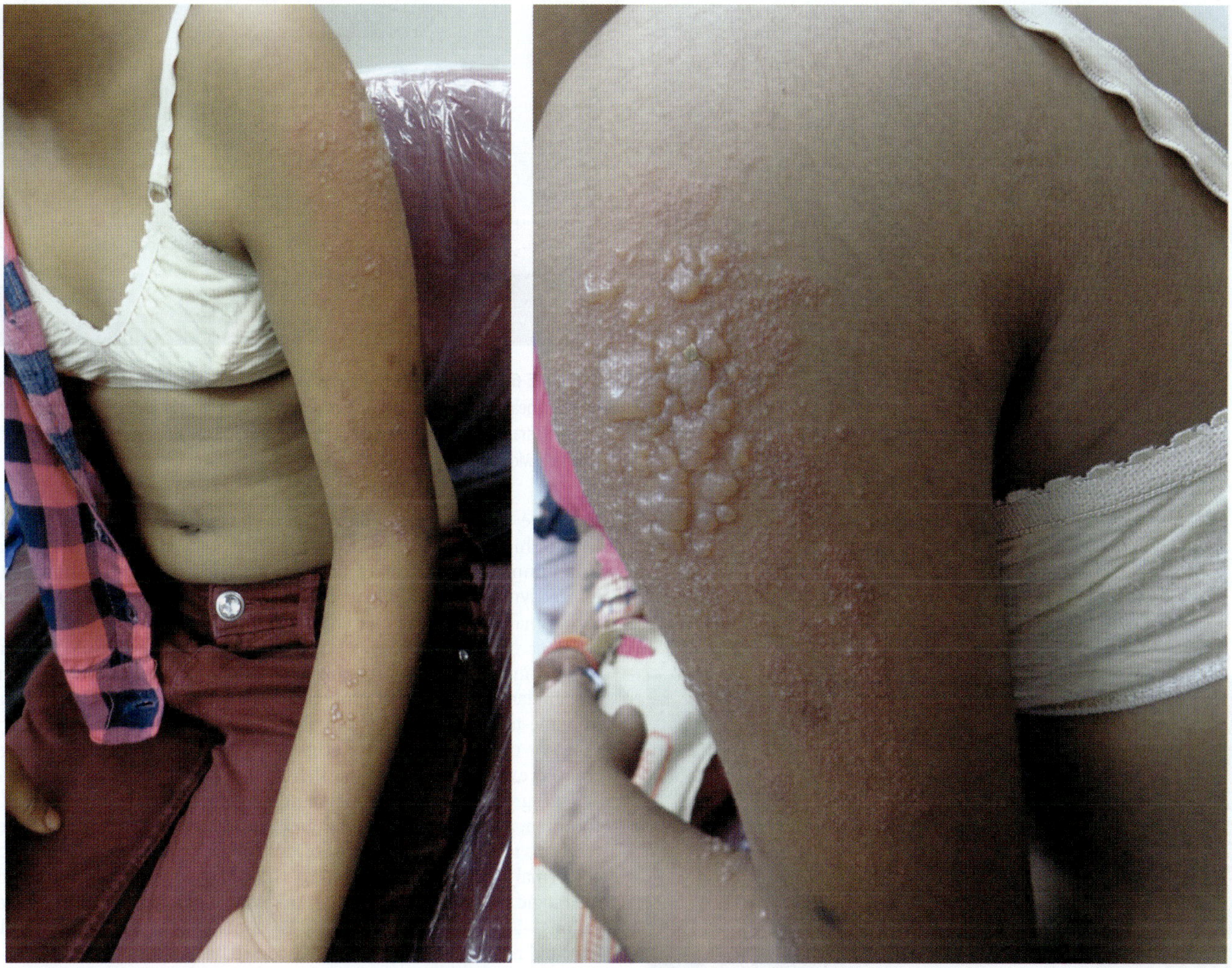

A B

FIGURE 64-8. Herpes zoster involving the C7 and C8 dermatomes of a 16-year-old female with steroid-resistant nephrotic syndrome on long-term mycophenolate. (From Shah BR, Mahajan P, Amodio J, Lucchesi M. *Atlas of Pediatric Emergency Medicine*. 3rd ed. New York: McGraw Hill; 2019, Figure 3.50. Reproduced with permission from photo contributor: Abhijeet Saha, MD.)

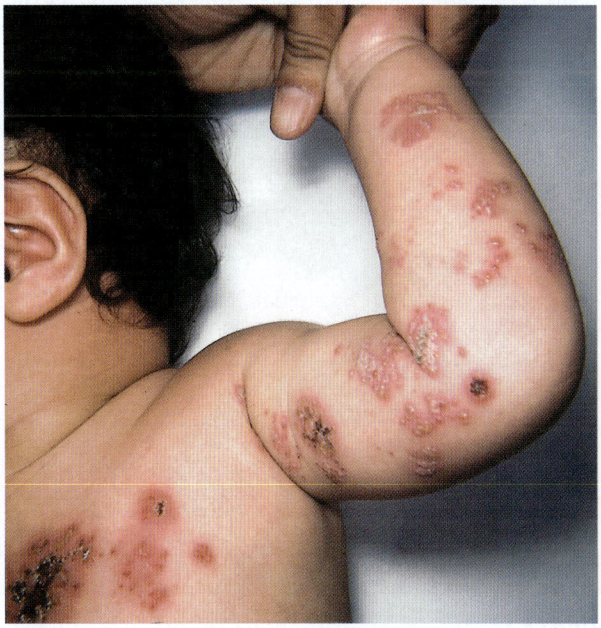

FIGURE 64-9. Herpes zoster involving the C5 and C6 dermatomes of an 8-month-old infant whose mother contracted VZV during pregnancy. (Reproduced with permission from Shah BR, Laude TL. *Atlas of Pediatric Clinical Diagnosis*. Philadelphia, PA: WB Saunders; 2000, p. 55.)

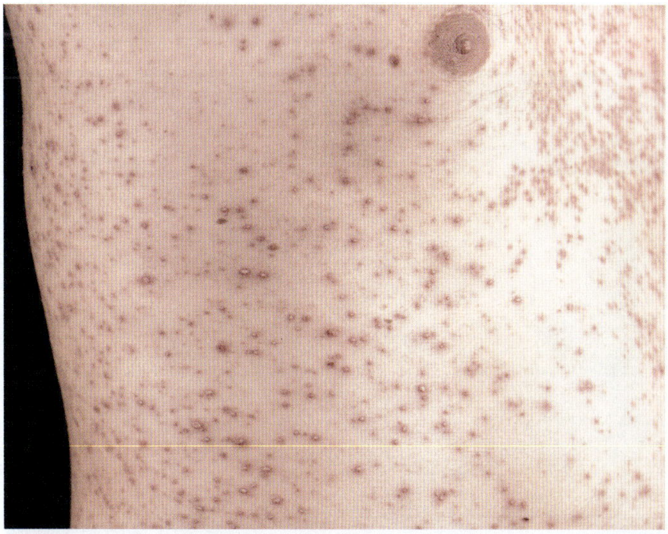

FIGURE 64-10. Disseminated cutaneous zoster in an immunocompromised patient with lymphoma. There are hundreds of vesicles and pustules on erythematous bases. The lesions are indistinguishable from VZV and disseminated HSV. (Reproduced with permission from Wolff K, Johnson RA, Saavedra AP, Roh EK. *Fitzpatrick's Color Atlas and Synopsis of Clinical Dermatology*. 8th ed. New York: McGraw Hill; 2017, Figure 27-57.)

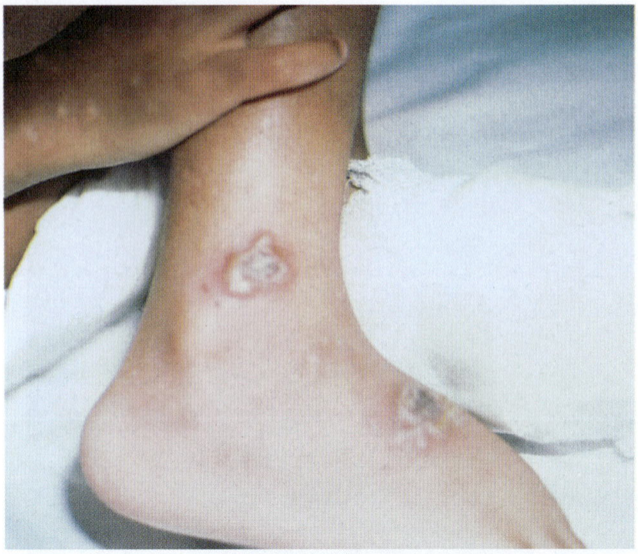

FIGURE 64-11. Chronic varicella zoster infection in a 6-year-old child. (Reproduced with permission from Prose NS, Kristal L. *Weinberg's Color Atlas of Pediatric Dermatology*. 5th ed. New York: McGraw Hill; 2017, Figure 18-1.)

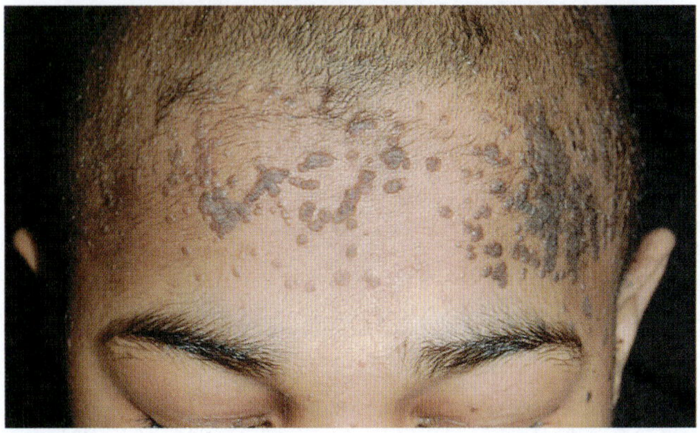

FIGURE 64-12. Numerous plane warts in a 12-year-old male kidney transplant recipient. (Reproduced with permission from Wolff K, Johnson RA, Saavedra AP, Roh EK. *Fitzpatrick's Color Atlas and Synopsis of Clinical Dermatology*. 8th ed. New York: McGraw Hill; 2017, Figure 27-17.)

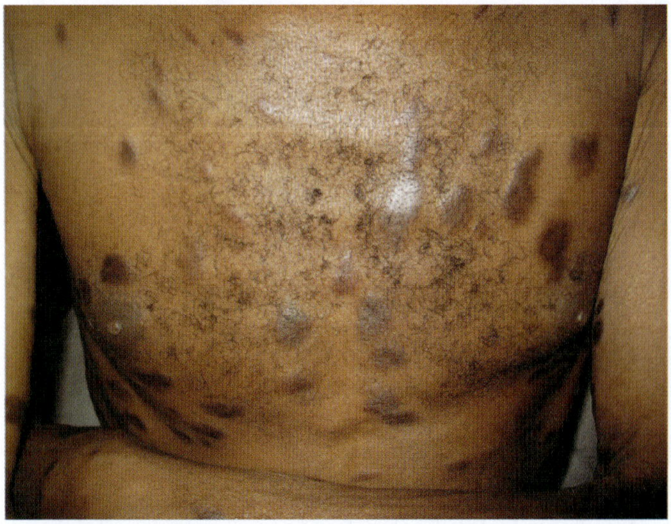

FIGURE 64-13. HIV-associated Kaposi sarcoma. (From Wolff K, Johnson RA, Saavedra AP, Roh EK. *Fitzpatrick's Color Atlas and Synopsis of Clinical Dermatology*. 8th ed. New York: McGraw Hill; 2017, Figure 21-20. Reproduced with permission from Adam Lipworth, MD.)

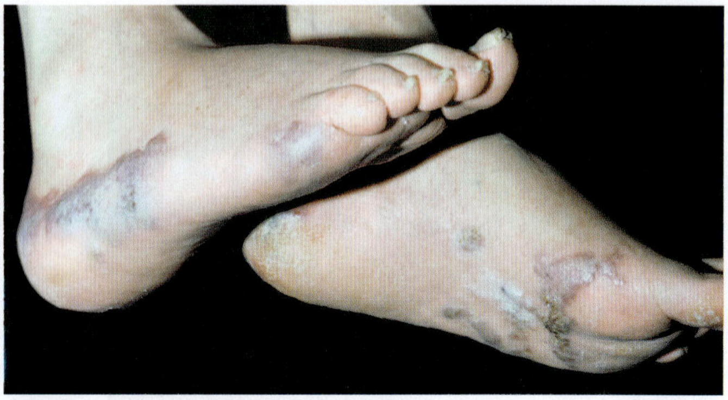

FIGURE 64-14. Classic Kaposi sarcoma of the feet. This is the form seen in older males of Mediterranean or Middle Eastern descent. (Reproduced with permission from Wolff K, Johnson RA, Saavedra AP, Roh EK. *Fitzpatrick's Color Atlas and Synopsis of Clinical Dermatology*. 8th ed. New York: McGraw Hill; 2017, Figure 21-18.)

there are many well-established dermatologic effects related to long-term or high-dose glucocorticoid use. These side effects include skin and hair thinning, skin atrophy, cushingoid facies, an increased propensity for ecchymosis, development of acne, mild hirsutism, facial erythema, abdominal striae, dermatitis, and generalized poor wound healing.

Other commonly encountered immunosuppressive, immune-modulating, or immune-targeting medications may cause nonspecific maculopapular, eczematous, or psoriatic rashes. Some immunosuppressive and immune-targeting therapies can also lead to pruritic, morbilliform eruptions, or other inflammatory eruptions—lichenoid reactions, acute generalized exanthematous pustulosis, small vessel vasculitis, erythroderma, and drug rash with eosinophilia and systemic symptoms (DRESS). Less common, but more concerning and life-threatening, cutaneous adverse reactions to be aware of include Stevens-Johnson syndrome (SJS) and toxic epidermal necrolysis (TEN). Some of the more frequently encountered dermatologic side effects of immunosuppressive and immune-targeting medications—acneiform rashes, mucositis, stomatitis, xerosis, and other skin, hair, and nail manifestations—are discussed further below.

ACNEIFORM RASH

Acneiform rash is the most commonly occurring cutaneous adverse effect and can be seen with glucocorticoids ("steroid acne"), azathioprine, sirolimus, cyclosporine, epidermal growth factor receptor (EGFR) inhibitors, and mitogen-activated protein kinase inhibitors (**Figure 64-15**).

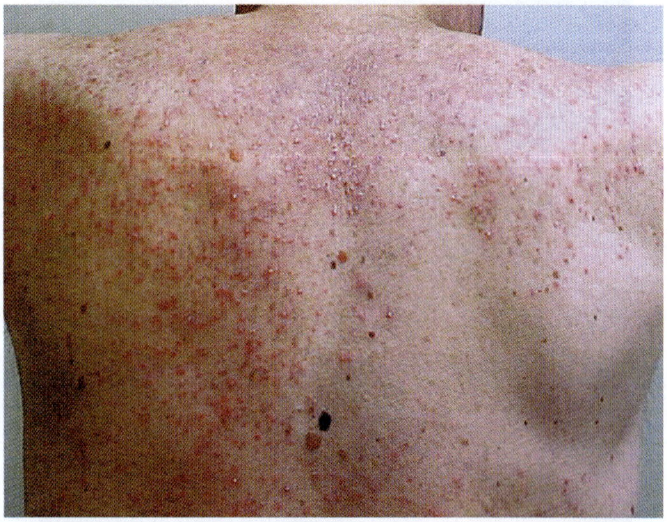

FIGURE 64-15. An acneiform eruption associated with epidermal growth factor receptor-targeted chemotherapy. (Reproduced with permission from DeWitt CA, Siroy AE, Stone SP. Acneiform eruptions associated with epidermal growth factor receptor-targeted chemotherapy. *J Am Acad Dermatol*. 2007;56(3):500-505.)

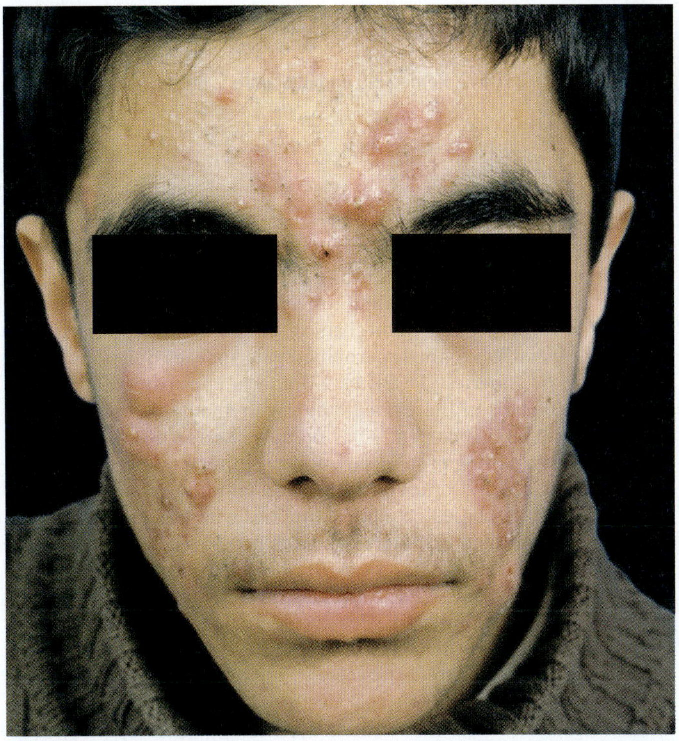

FIGURE 64-16. Nodulocystic acne on the face of a teenage boy. (Reproduced with permission from Wolff K, Johnson RA, Saavedra AP, Roh EK. *Fitzpatrick's Color Atlas and Synopsis of Clinical Dermatology*. 8th ed. New York: McGraw Hill; 2017, Figure 1-3.)

This rash is characterized by papules and pustules with surrounding areas of inflammation less than 5 mm in diameter. It occurs most often on the face and trunk. Pruritus, lack of comedones, and presence of monomorphic lesions in atypical locations (arms, back, and genitalia) help distinguish acneiform eruptions secondary to medication effect from acne vulgaris. Onset of this rash can be abrupt or more gradual and generally arises within 2 to 4 weeks of starting therapy. Less severe acneiform rashes typically do not require treatment and often improve with cessation of medications. If the rash is problematic for the patient—cosmetic appearance or pruritus—topical acne therapies such as benzoyl peroxide, topical antibiotics, or topical retinoids may be used.

Less commonly, a severe and often painful form of this rash can occur. This is better described as nodulocystic acne and is characterized by tender, draining nodules and cysts (**Figure 64-16**). This rash often leads to scarring or keloid formation and is susceptible to bacterial superinfection. Dermatology consultation should be considered to assist with management. Treatment consists of a combination of oral retinoids and antibiotics; topical treatments are ineffective. Severe or refractory cases may warrant dose adjustment or transition to an alternative agent.

MUCOSITIS

Mucositis is a well-known complication of most chemotherapy agents and radiation therapy, and it frequently arises in pediatric patients receiving oncologic treatments. General inflammation and irritation can occur anywhere in the gastrointestinal tract—from oral mucosa to anus—and can range from mild to severe in intensity. Mucositis often interferes with oral intake due to significant pain. A specific form of oral toxicity, stomatitis, may occur as a side effect of other immune-targeted therapies including EGFR inhibitors, HER inhibitors, and mTOR inhibitors like sirolimus. Stomatitis is distinct from the more general mucositis seen with chemotherapy and is characterized by superficial, painful, round, well-circumscribed aphthous ulcers. Treatment and prevention of both entities relies on early detection, good oral care regimens, topical anesthetics, use of localized NSAIDs like benzydamine, and monitoring for superinfection. Prophylactic antimicrobial rinses such as chlorhexidine are often used for children undergoing chemotherapy or radiation therapy. Knowledge of medication side effects can help pediatric hospitalists distinguish chemotherapy- and radiation-induced mucositis from the similar-appearing mucosal lesions seen with viral illnesses, Stevens-Johnson syndrome, toxic epidermal necrolysis, and inflammatory bowel disease.

XEROSIS

Xerosis, or moderate-to-severe dry skin or mucus membranes, is a common complication of certain medications such as EGFR inhibitors and MEK inhibitors. Breakdown of the epidermal layer can lead to cracking or fissuring of the skin which can result in pain, pruritus, and risk of secondary skin infections. Clinical appearance and presentation may be similar to the dry skin associated with atopic dermatitis and is treated in a similar fashion, primarily with topical skin emollients.

OTHER SKIN, HAIR, AND NAIL MANIFESTATIONS

Many other skin, hair, and nail manifestations may occur secondary to immunosuppressive, immune-targeting, or immune-modulating therapies. Gingival hyperplasia, which can lead to bone and tooth loss, is commonly seen with cyclosporine and less commonly with tacrolimus. Strict adherence to dental hygiene can help prevent gingival hyperplasia. Treatment includes tooth scaling and root planing to remove accumulated minerals (i.e., tartar); surgical treatments such as gingivectomy are occasionally required. Hypertrichosis, excessive hair growth throughout the body, can also be seen as a side effect of cyclosporine. Changes in hair quality and texture, including fine and brittle hair or total hair loss (alopecia), is commonly encountered with chemotherapeutic agents. Phototoxicity, photoaging, and photocarcinogenesis can be challenging side effects of the RAF inhibitors (used to treat melanoma) and of voriconazole (an antifungal often used as a prophylactic agent in immunosuppressed patients). Exaggerated sunburn response, cheilitis, exfoliative dermatitis, pseudoporphyria cutanea tarda, and lupus-like skin eruptions are some of the phototoxicities that may develop.

Nail changes secondary to immunosuppressive medications include paronychia and periungal pyogenic granulomas. They tend to occur more commonly with EGFR inhibitors, MEK inhibitors, and mTOR inhibitors and can develop slowly over weeks to months of therapy. Other common nail changes include brittle nails, onycholysis (separation of the nail from the nail bed), and slow nail growth. Extreme cases of nail damage or infection may require surgical removal of the nail plate.

KEY POINTS

- Cutaneous disorders are common in immunocompromised patients and may be the first and only sign of illness or an underlying immunocompromised state secondary to a primary immunodeficiency, acquired immunodeficiency, or immunosuppressive medical therapy.
- It is important for pediatric hospitalists to recognize that skin conditions which are common in the immunocompetent pediatric population may present differently in immunocompromised hosts.
- Atypical features, unusual clinical courses, recurrent infections, and difficult-to-treat conditions should raise suspicion for cutaneous disease secondary to immunodeficiency or immunosuppression.
- Cutaneous infectious are associated with significantly increased morbidity and mortality in patients with poorly functioning immune systems which necessitates a high index of suspicion, prompt evaluation, and urgent treatment in order to optimize patient outcomes.
- An increased risk of malignant neoplasm—skin cancer, post-transplant lymphoproliferative disorder, Kaposi sarcoma, other sarcomas—is one of the most concerning consequences of chronic immunosuppression and immunosuppressive medications.
- Many immunosuppressive medications and immune-targeted therapies used to treat malignant and autoimmune conditions interrupt or affect the regulatory processes in the dermis and epidermis resulting in a wide range of cutaneous adverse effects.
- Understanding the more common dermatologic manifestations associated with immunosuppressive medications and immune-targeted therapies will help guide the diagnostic evaluation of immunosuppressed patients presenting with new skin lesions.

SUGGESTED READINGS

Bhat T, Coughlin CC. Dermatologic considerations in pediatric transplant recipients. *Curr Opin Pediatr.* 2018 Aug;30(4):520-525.

Burke VE, Lopez FA. Approach to skin and soft tissue infections in non-HIV immunocompromised hosts. *Curr Opin Infect Dis.* 2017 Aug;30(4):354-363.

Chelidze K, Thomas C, Chang AY, Freeman EE. HIV-related skin disease in the era of antiretroviral therapy: recognition and management. *Am J Clin Dermatol.* 2019 Jun;20(3):423-442.

Cutaneous manifestations of HIV disease. In: Prose NS, Kristal L. eds. *Weinberg's Color Atlas of Pediatric Dermatology, 5e.* McGraw Hill; 2017.

Fogel AL, Miyar M, Teng JM. Cutaneous malignancies in pediatric solid organ transplant recipients. *Pediatr Dermatol.* 2016 Nov;33(6): 585-593.

Fuleihan RL, Paller AS. Genetic immunodeficiency diseases. In: Kang S, Amagai M, Bruckner AL, Enk AH, Margolis DJ, McMichael AJ, Orringer JS. eds. *Fitzpatricks' Dermatology.* 9th ed. McGraw Hill; 2019.

Jenkins S, Cotes M, Zwald F. Skin cancer in the organ transplant patient. In: Avram MR, Avram MM, Ratner D. eds. *Procedural Dermatology.* McGraw Hill; 2015.

Lacouture M, Sibaud V. Toxic side effects of targeted therapies and immunotherapies affecting the skin, oral mucosa, hair, and nails. *Am J Clin Dermatol.* 2018;19(Suppl 1):31-39.

Lewis DJ, Wu JH, Boyd M, Duvic M, Feldman SR. Cutaneous manifestations of genodermatoses and primary immunodeficiency. *Dermatol Online J.* 2019 Jun 15;25(6):13030/qt1gj1n07j.

Lipworth AD, Freeman EE, Saavedra AP. Cutaneous manifestations of HIV and human T-lymphotropic virus. In: Kang S, Amagai M, Bruckner AL, Enk AH, Margolis DJ, McMichael AJ, Orringer JS. eds. *Fitzpatricks' Dermatology.* 9th ed. McGraw Hill; 2019.

López-Quintero W, Cleves D, Gomez-Vasco JD, et al. Skin manifestations in pediatric patients with primary immunodeficiency diseases (PIDs) in a Tertiary Care Hospital in Colombia. *World Allergy Organ J.* 2021 Mar 1;14(3):100527.

Macdonald JB, Macdonald B, Golitz LE, LoRusso P, Sekulic A. Cutaneous adverse effects of targeted therapies: Part I: Inhibitors of the Cellular Membrane. *J Am Acad Dermatol.* 2015; 72(2): 203-220.

Macdonald JB, Macdonald B, Golitz LE, LoRusso P, Sekulic A. Cutaneous adverse effects of targeted therapies: Part II: Inhibitors of Intracellular Molecular Signaling Pathways. *J Am Acad Dermatol.* 2015; 72(2): 221-238.

Moffarah AS, Al Mohajer M, Hurwitz BL, Armstrong DG. Skin and soft tissue infections. *Microbiol Spectr.* 2016 Aug; 4(4).

Ng CY, Chen CB, Wu MY, et al. Anticancer drugs induced severe adverse cutaneous drug reactions: an updated review on the risks associated with anticancer targeted therapy or immunotherapies. *J Immunol Res.* 2018 Jan;2018:5376476.

Relan M, Lehman HK. Common dermatologic manifestations of primary immune deficiencies. *Curr Allergy Asthma Rep.* 2014 Dec;14(12): 480.

Sachdeva M, Lara-Corrales I, Pope E, et al. Outcomes of skin cancers in pediatric solid organ transplant patients: a systematic review. *Pediatr Transplant.* 2022 Feb;26(1):e14146.

Shah S, Shelburne S. Skin and soft tissue infections in non-human immunodeficiency virus immunocompromised hosts. *Infect Dis Clin N Am.* 2021 Mar;35(1):199-217.

Sillevis Smitt JH, Kuijpers TW. Cutaneous manifestations of primary immunodeficiency. *Curr Opin Pediatr.* 2013 Aug;25(4):492-497.

Yasir M, Goyal A, Bansal P, Sonthalia S. Corticosteroid adverse effects. In: StatPearls. StatPearls Publishing, Treasure Island (FL); 2021. PMID: 30285357.

CHAPTER 65

Epidermolysis Bullosa

Lisa M. Remer, MD and Benjamin S. Bolser, MD

BACKGROUND

Epidermolysis bullosa (EB) refers to a family of rare inherited genodermatoses with skin fragility leading to recurrent cutaneous and mucosal blistering; sites susceptible to mechanical trauma are especially prone to blistering. According to the Dystrophic Epidermolysis Bullosa Research Association of America (DEBRA), EB affects approximately 1 out of every 20,000 births in the United States with about 200 children born annually with EB. EB currently has no cure. Research into treatments and cures are exploring protein, cell, and gene therapies.

Historically, EB and other blistering skin conditions have been classified into subtypes based on clinical findings with nomenclature based on eponyms; multiple distinctive variants have been described in the literature. Efforts to streamline classification and incorporate underlying molecular differences led to the classification system most recently updated by Has et al in 2020. This system divides EB into four major types based on the ultrastructural level of blister formation (**Figure 65-1**): EB simplex (EBS; intraepidermal level), junctional EB (JEB; junctional level), dystrophic EB (DEB; dermal level), and Kindler EB (mixed levels). Future iterations of this classification system may divide types by causative genetic mutations.

Depending on where mutations occur on the chromosome and which protein is affected, the clinical manifestations of EB may range from dystrophic nails or minimal superficial blistering of the hands or feet to severe, widespread, disfiguring blistering and scarring. In general, more superficial cleavage planes (such as in EB simplex) are associated with less severe phenotypes and deeper cleavage planes (such as dystrophic EB) with more severe phenotypes. Damage to epithelial mucosa is not limited to the skin. The mouth, esophagus, and urethra are often prone to injury. Although all patients with EB are at risk of complications such as pain, intractable itching, infection, and scarring, those with more severe variants are also at risk for multiple chronic, systemic comorbidities. Some examples include nutritional deficiencies and failure to thrive, esophageal strictures, laryngeal complications such as granulation tissue in the airway, anemia and iron deficiency, severe scarring of extremities with resultant contractures, cardiomyopathy, renal insufficiency, depression and anxiety, and ocular complications that may lead to blindness. EB patients are also high risk for cutaneous squamous cell carcinoma, which may be fatal, in the second decade of life.

A multidisciplinary approach is key to comprehensive care for patients with EB given the variety of possible clinical sequelae. Basic care incorporates both lifestyle modifications and specialized skin care. Subspecialty care from a variety of medical and surgical specialties, nutrition experts, physical and occupational therapists, and behavioral health professionals is nearly always required to identify, prevent, and mitigate the sequelae of EB. Hospitalists may be involved in the care of patients with EB at diagnosis in the newborn period, or later in life, as several of the acute and chronic complications associated with EB require hospitalization and care coordination.

Inpatient management of a patient with EB requires a comprehensive understanding of the expected clinical features, severity, and common complications associated with the type of EB present. Interpreting clinical information in a patient-specific and compassionate context is essential for providing the highest level of care, especially in patients with more severe types of EB and multi-system involvement. When caring for a child with EB, it is important to remember that they are susceptible to common pediatric illnesses, though the presentation of illness may be influenced by the chronic conditions related to EB.

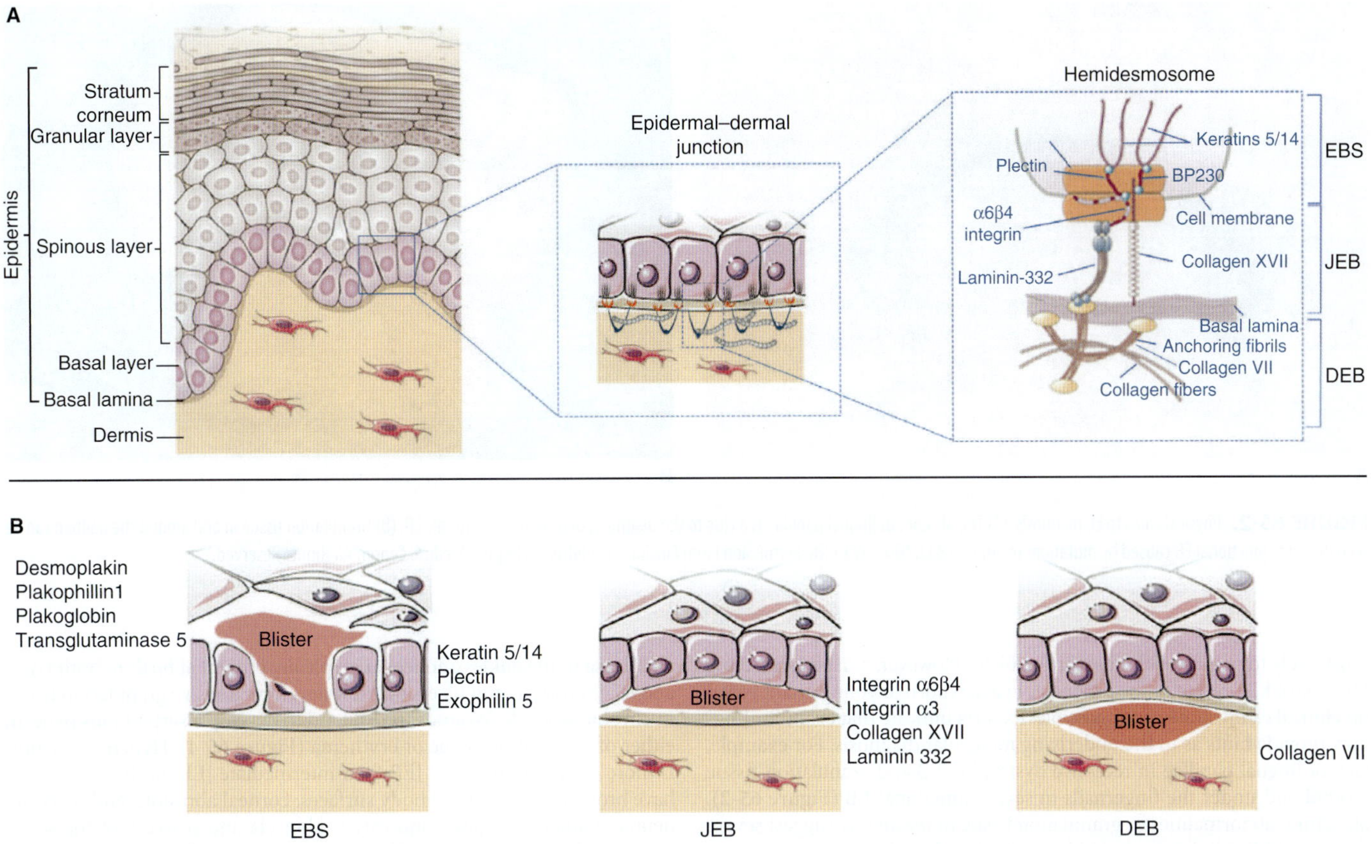

FIGURE 65-1. Schematic representation of human skin and epidermolysis bullosa (EB). (A) epidermal layers (*left*) and the epidermal-dermal junction (*middle*) are designated. The right panel denotes the hemidesmosome and its components, in relation to EB simplex (EBS), junctional EB (JEB), and dystrophic EB (DEB). (B) Proteins involved in the pathogenesis of EBS, JEB, and DEB and the site of blister formation. (Reproduced with permission from De Rosa L, et al. Toward combined cell and gene therapy for genodermatoses. *Cold Spring Harb Perspect Biol.* 2020;12(5):a035667.)

PATHOPHYSIOLOGY

EB results from mutations in genes for proteins that maintain the resilience of skin to mechanical stress. These genetic mutations may be inherited in an autosomal dominant or recessive manner and also occur as the result of de novo mutations. Further detail on genes affected in various subtypes of EB is available in **Table 65-1.**

CLINICAL PRESENTATION

NEWBORN PERIOD

Skin and mucosal blistering, the cardinal clinical features of EB, may be present at birth, may develop shortly after birth or in early infancy, or less commonly, may present later in life. The most severe subtypes of EB (severe RDEB, severe JEB, severe EBS, and EB with pyloric atresia) are

TABLE 65-1 Classification of Classic Types of EB

Level of Skin Cleavage	EB Type	Inheritance	Mutated Gene(s)	Targeted Protein(s)
Epidermis	EB simplex	Autosomal dominant	KRT5, KRT14	Keratin 5, Keratin 14
			PLEC	Plectin
			KLHL24	Kelch-like member 24
		Autosomal recessive	KRT5, KRT14	Keratin 5, Keratin 14
			DST	Bullous pemphigoid antigen 230/dystonin
			EXPH5/SLAC2B	Exophilin-5/synaptotagmin-like protein homolog lacking C2 domains b
			PLEC	Plectin
			CD151/TSPAN24	CD151 antigen/Tetraspanin 24
Basement Membrane	Junctional EB	Autosomal recessive	LAMA3, LAMB3, LAMC2	Laminin 332 (Lam A3, B3 and C2)
			COL17A1	Type XVII collagen
			ITGA6, ITGB4	Integrin α6 and β4
			ITGA3	Integrin α3 subunit
Dermis	Dystrophic EB	Autosomal dominant	COL7A1	Type VII collagen
		Autosomal recessive	COL7A1	Type VII collagen
Mixed	Kindler EB	Autosomal recessive	FERMT1/KIND1	Fermitin family homolog 1/kindlin-1

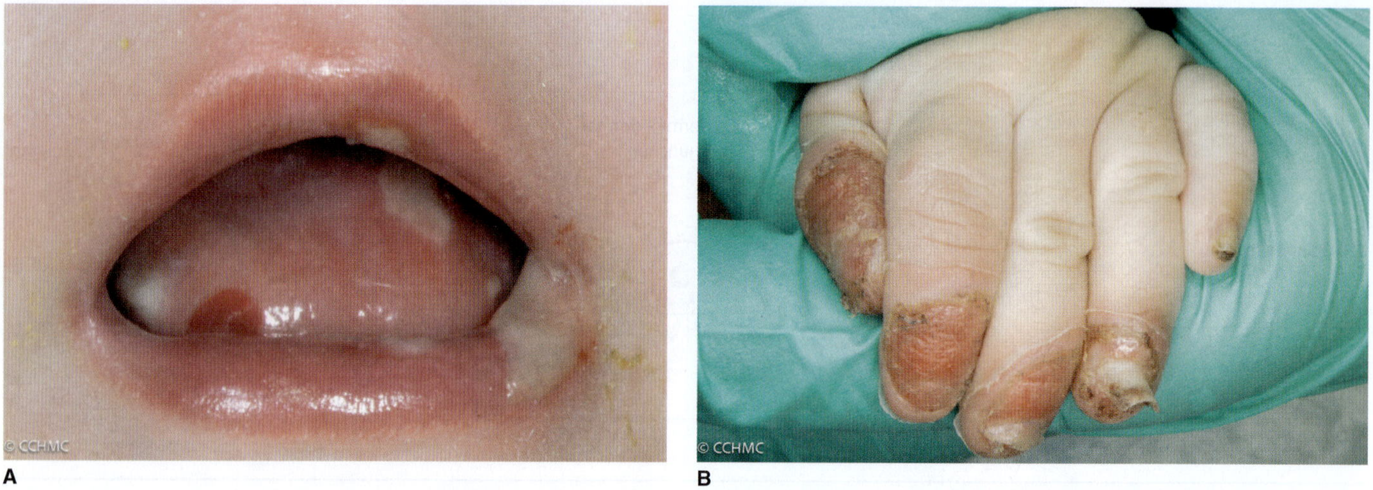

FIGURE 65-2. Physical clues to EB diagnosis. (A) The absence of lingual papillae is a clue to the diagnosis of recessive dystrophic EB. (B) Granulation tissue in and around the nailbed can be seen in severe junctional EB caused by mutations in laminin 332. (Used With The Permission From Cincinnati Children'S Hospital Medical Center. All Rights Reserved.)

most likely to present with blistering at birth. However, reliably predicting the type of EB present or the prognosis in a newborn or young infant based on clinical exam alone is not possible. Experts indicate that exam findings may provide hints as to the underlying molecular diagnosis. For example, lack of lingual papillae in recessive dystrophic EB and granulation tissue around and under the fingernails in severe junctional EB (**Figure 65-2**). Structural abnormalities or granulation tissue in the airway suggest severe junctional EB. Clinicians should have a high index of suspicion for severe junctional EB in infants with these findings as these children typically have a markedly shortened life expectancy due to risk of sepsis or airway compromise, especially if they also have extensive aplasia cutis congenita. Pyloric atresia can be associated with both plectin and ITGα6β4 mutations (classified as EBS and JEB, respectively). However, overlapping clinical findings and phenotypic heterogeneity in patients with similar genotypes preclude accurate prognostication based on clinical findings.

EB SIMPLEX

EB simplex (EBS), the most common type of EB, is divided into three subtypes: localized EBS, intermediate EBS, and severe EBS. Many mild cases are undiagnosed. Autosomal dominant EBS, the most common type of EBS, is due to keratin 5 and 14 mutations and characterized by disruption of the basal layer of the epidermis. This leads to superficial blisters that do not scar. Common findings in localized, intermediate, and severe EBS include blistering and milia that appear at birth or within the first few weeks of life, although in some cases blisters may not appear until childhood or early adulthood. Palmar and plantar keratoderma are also common, as are thick and dystrophic finger and toenails (**Figure 65-3**). Oral mucosal involvement may be extensive, occurring commonly in severe EBS; infants with oral mucosal involvement are at higher risk of gastroesophageal reflux, growth failure, constipation, and death in infancy. Blistering in EBS tends to diminish in adolescence and later in life. Rare forms of EBS may be associated with other conditions based on the gene affected, such as cardiomyopathy (KLHL24), pyloric atresia (plectin and integrin α6β4), muscular dystrophy (plectin), and nephropathy (CD151).

JUNCTIONAL EB

Junctional EB (JEB) is characterized by blistering with the plane of cleavage at the lamina lucida at the basement membrane zone and is subdivided into intermediate and severe (previously Herlitz) subtypes. The severity varies greatly between intermediate and severe types; patients with intermediate JEB improve slightly with age whereas patients with severe JEB typically have a life expectancy of 6 to 24 months. Most severe types of JEB are due to laminin A3, B3, and C2 mutations, and intermediate EB is often due to collagen 17 mutations. Blisters on the diaper area, lower extremities, and dorsa of the ankles and feet are typically present at birth in both types and leave erosions and ulcers that can develop extensive granulation tissue in chronic wounds. Wounds in JEB tend to develop a serpiginous pattern, either of granulation tissue or erythema (**Figure 65-4**). Hypergranulation is more common in severe JEB than intermediate JEB. Both types of JEB have broad involvement of body surfaces: corneal abrasions and scarring, dental enamel hypoplasia and caries, alopecia and scarring of the scalp, absent or dystrophic nails, and blistering and scarring of the genitourinary mucosa causing urethral strictures.

Within their first weeks of life, infants with severe JEB develop blistering on the buttocks, elbows, and around the nails; subsequently chronic wounds develop with hypergranulation on the face and extremities and severe, large wounds develop on the buttocks. Severe JEB is also associated with laryngeal mucosal involvement, leading to blistering, erosions, granulation tissue and scarring in the airway, causing obstruction, and manifesting as hoarse voice, stridor, or respiratory distress. Chronic severe JEB disease causes failure to thrive and anemia. Patients with severe JEB are at high risk of death from sepsis and airway compromise compared to patients with other types of EB. Intermediate JEB is associated with squamous cell carcinoma in teens and young adulthood. As with EBS, there are rare syndromes in which JEB occurs with other conditions such pyloric atresia, interstitial lung disease, and nephrotic syndrome.

DYSTROPHIC EB

Dystrophic EB (DEB) involves blister formation below the level of the basement membrane zone within the dermis; blisters then scar and cause a variety of complications. All types of DEB are due to mutations in collagen 7 which forms the anchoring fibrils that attach the basement membrane of the epidermis to the dermis. Inheritance may be autosomal dominant or recessive. In general, recessive dystrophic EB (RDEB) is more severe than dominant dystrophic EB (DDEB), though there is substantial phenotypic overlap. There are four main subtypes of DEB: localized DDEB, intermediate DDEB, intermediate RDEB, and severe RDEB. All forms of DEB present at birth or in early childhood, with severe RDEB having the most significant blistering very early in life. See **Figure 65-5** for findings in DEB.

Although a few rare and milder forms of DEB have been described, DEB generally has broad involvement of the oral mucosa and nails. With the exception of localized DDEB, patients with DEB are also prone to a variety of associated sequelae. Blistering and fissuring of the anal mucosa commonly occurs, setting off a cycle of chronic constipation in which associated pain leads to holding behavior and worsens constipation. Esophageal blistering may lead to strictures impeding oral intake (**Figure 65-6**). Failure to thrive may be multifactorial and is often associated with strictures, microstomia, dental caries, and high metabolic demands due to chronic wounds. Eye involvement is common. Joint

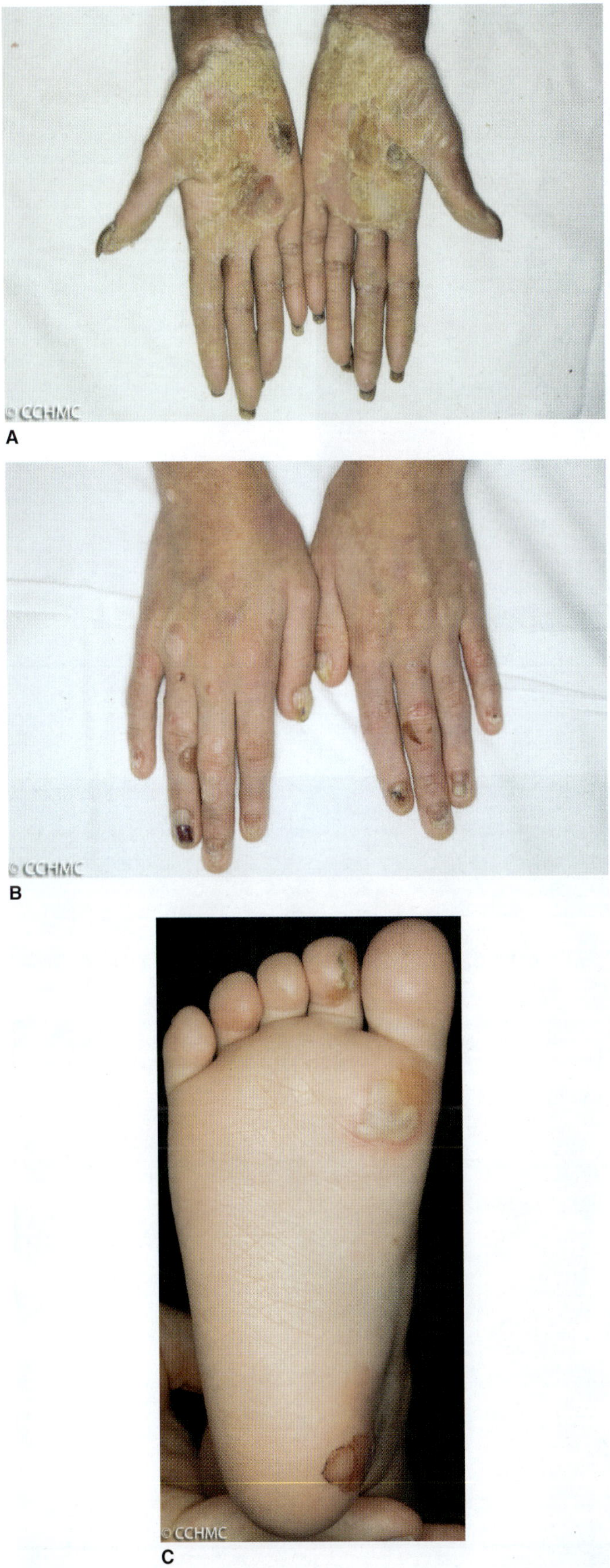

FIGURE 65-3. Findings in EB simplex: (A) Palmar keratoderma. (B) Dystrophic/thickened nails with characteristic blistering. (C) Typical blisters on foot.

contractures may occur due to scarring from recurrent wounds. Squamous cell carcinoma may develop later in life.

Severe RDEB is the most severe of the DEB subtypes and often includes: pseudosyndactyly ("mitten deformity") of the hands and feet due to scarring from recurrent wounds, flexion contractures, resorption of distal digits, severe failure to thrive, pubertal delay, osteoporosis and spinal stress fractures, multifactorial anemia (chronic blood loss, iron deficiency, and of chronic disease), renal impairment (IgA nephropathy, post-streptococcal glomerulonephritis, renal amyloidosis or acute kidney injury), and rarely cardiomyopathy (due to chronic anemia or micronutrient deficiencies such as selenium and carnitine). Patients with severe RDEB are also at highest risk of developing and dying of squamous cell carcinoma; up to 70% of cases become metastatic and life expectancy is on average five years after diagnosis.

KINDLER EB

Kindler EB is a very rare type of autosomal recessive EB primarily present in isolated or consanguineous populations. Blister formation can involve many skin layers and typically improves with age. Blistering is typically present at birth and generalized, though it is most consistently present on the extremities. Patients with Kindler EB develop cutaneous atrophy and poikiloderma (blotchy discoloration) of the dorsum of the hands and neck during childhood; this typically progresses to the rest of the body with age. Over time palmoplantar keratoderma (severe thickening of the palms and soles) occurs with loss of dermatoglyphs (ridges of the skin including fingerprints). Kindler EB can also result in corneal erosions, skin photosensitivity, esophageal strictures, urethral strictures, gingival hyperplasia, gingivitis, and colitis. Patients with Kindler EB have an increased risk of mucocutaneous squamous cell carcinoma.

DIFFERENTIAL DIAGNOSIS

The differential diagnosis of blistering disorders in neonates and infants is extensive and includes other inherited diseases characterized by skin blistering or erosions, infectious diseases, and immunobullous disorders (**Table 65-2**). Early consultation with the appropriate subspecialists based on history and exam is crucial.

DIAGNOSTIC EVALUATION

The diagnosis of EB is based on a combination of clinical features, family history, and laboratory findings. Clinical features alone are unreliable for diagnostic purposes. Relevant family history includes family members with known EB, or those with easy blistering or dystrophic nails who may have undiagnosed EB. Laboratory techniques include immunofluorescence mapping (IFM), transmission electron microscopy (TEM), and molecular genetic testing; genetic testing is now the preferred diagnostic tool. Where possible, evaluation of the neonate or infant with cutaneous blistering should be directed by a clinician with expertise in EB given the complexity of diagnosis and in order to make an accurate prognosis.

TREATMENT

GENERAL APPROACH

The majority of EB patients requiring hospital care are those with severe RDEB and severe JEB. Therefore, much of the following discussion pertains to this specific EB patient population. These conditions are debilitating and progressive, resulting in a perpetual inflammatory state that directly or indirectly affects every organ system. Frequent hospitalizations are often needed, especially in older children, adolescents, and young adults.

Hospitalists should approach patients and families with the understanding that they may have suffered traumatic healthcare encounters in the past and may be nervous or frightened while in the hospital. Often, iatrogenic complications occur as a result of healthcare providers that are not familiar with EB and the necessary precautions needed to avert harm

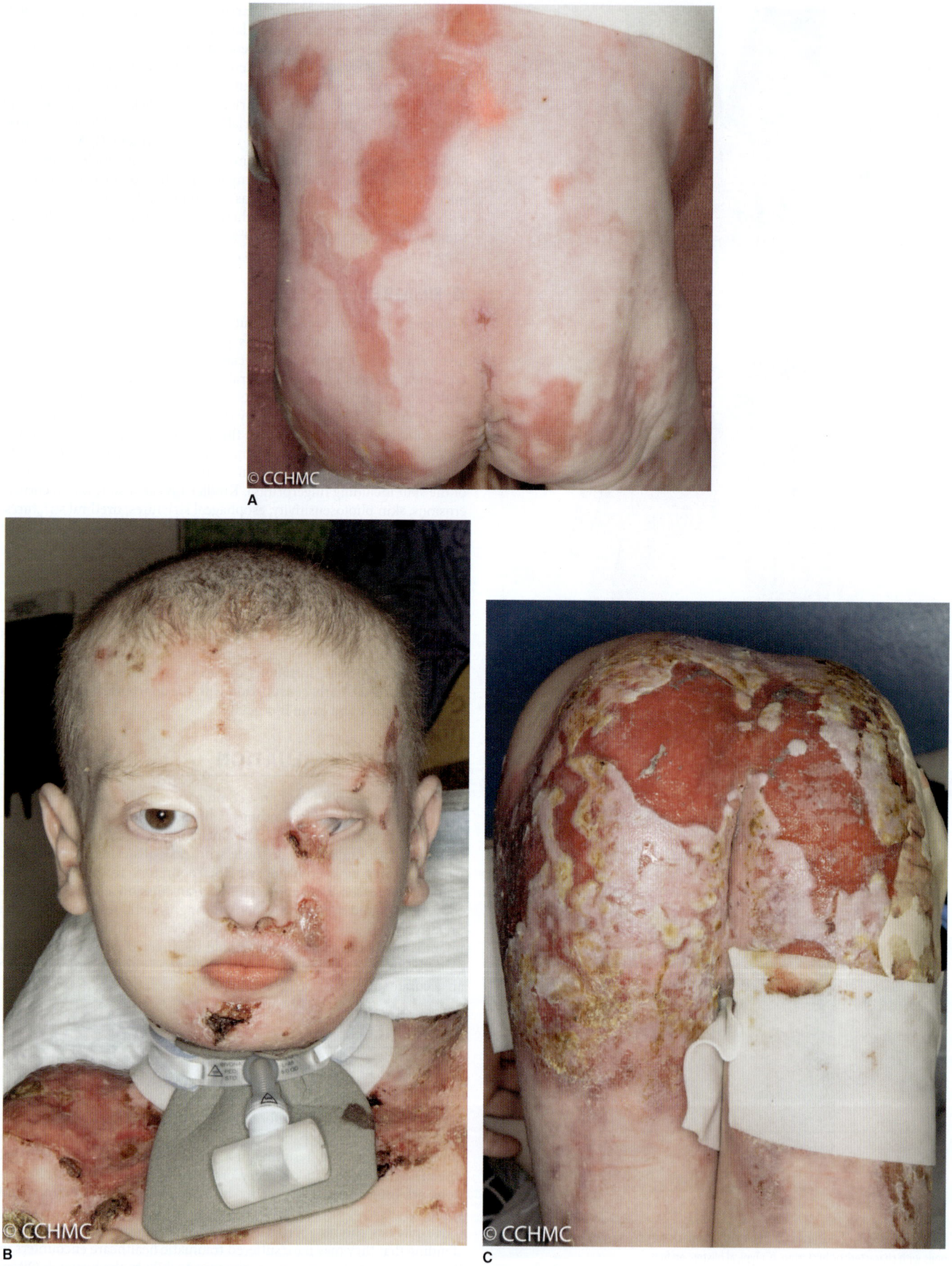

FIGURE 65-4. Findings in JEB: (A) Serpiginous erythema on infant's back. (B) Hypergranulation on face with eye involvement. (C) Large buttock wounds.

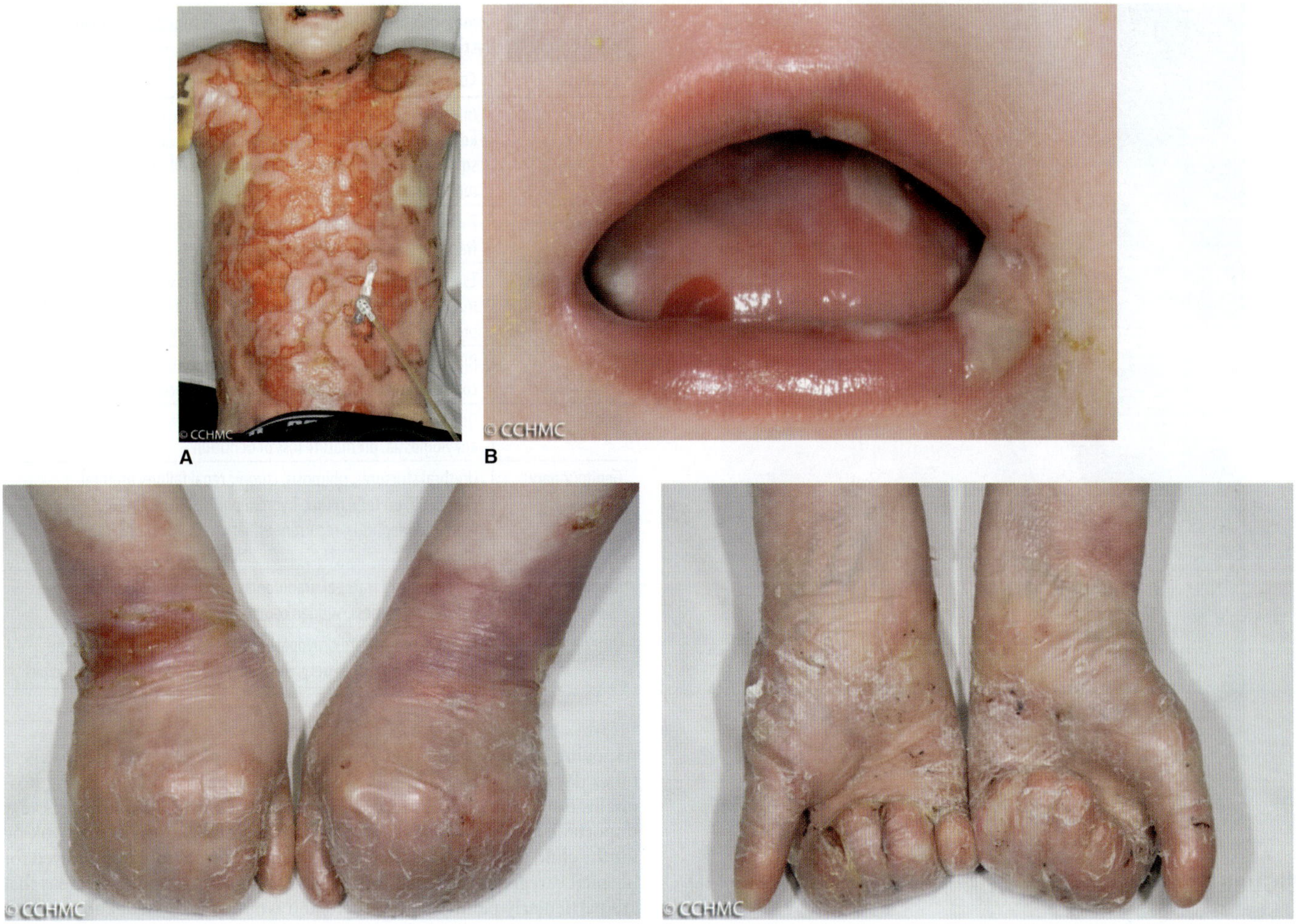

FIGURE 65-5. Findings in DEB. (A) Typical appearance of torso after blisters drained. (B) microstomia with oral and perioral blisters. (C and D) Pseudosyndactyly.

during hospitalization. For example, routine placement of pulse oximetry probes, EKG leads, or typical positioning for surgical procedures can easily lead to severe, painful skin wounds or blistering. Creative and strategic mitigation plans are often needed to avoid such harm; these are explored further later in the chapter. The astute hospitalist will gain trust and rapport by first acknowledging the family's extensive knowledge and lived experience as well as by reassuring the patient, especially if a younger child, that providers will not touch him/her without first explaining what to expect. It can be helpful to ask the patient or the caregiver how to touch, move, or manipulate the patient during an examination to minimize pain and discomfort. Finally, it is important to realize that the patient and caregivers *are* experts in managing the day-to-day dressing changes and skin care. Practicing these behaviors and modeling them to other providers will increase the chance that patients and families are comfortable, while lessening the chances of undesirable, traumatic experiences.

Unfortunately, there are no therapies that consistently reduce blister formation in patients with EB. Management of patients with EB focuses on the prevention and treatment of skin blistering and infections, pain control, and on careful monitoring for and treatment of EB-related complications, particularly in patients with JEB and RDEB (**Table 65-3**). Although children with EB may be hospitalized for a variety of EB-related complications, they may also be admitted for non-EB indications including typical childhood illnesses. The inpatient team should be aware of the myriad of complications and issues that may arise with EB patients, as well as with the general principles of skin and wound care for patients with EB. Additionally, it is important for providers to modify certain hospital interventions such as cardiorespiratory monitoring, EKG, intravenous (IV) catheter placement, intubation, severe constipation management, and bladder catheterization to prevent iatrogenic damage to the skin or other affected organs.

SKIN CARE

Bandaging regimens are often directed by dermatologists and aim to minimize disease severity and associated complications. General guidelines for skin care both at home and in the hospital are summarized in **Table 65-4**. In general, excessive friction, pressure, or rubbing of the skin is to be avoided where possible to minimize trauma that causes blistering. Vigilance for early detection and management of new blisters, and their potential complications such as infection, should be common practice. Providers should apply petrolatum or Aquaphor to fingertips of their gloves before contact with the skin. Overheating the patient or environment should be avoided, as it can exacerbate blistering and pruritus. Patients with poor mobility may require airbeds to reduce pressure on susceptible areas. Gentle handing by all caregivers is essential to minimize pain and risk of blistering. Soft coverings on infant highchairs and seats can help reduce skin friction. Use of adhesive tape on the skin is contraindicated. Use of a silicone-based foam dressing such as Mepilex or a silicon-based tape such as Mepitac, Adaptic touch, or Siltape may be helpful in securing percutaneous catheters and nasogastric feeding tubes (**Figure 65-7**). G-tube sites may develop local erosions, and placement of a layer of petrolatum gauze, a silicone-based foam dressing, such as Mepilex Transfer, or contact layer such as Mepitel may minimize local complications.

A thorough skin evaluation is an important component of the initial assessment of every child with EB who is hospitalized. This evaluation is best coordinated with a regular dressing change. Caregivers for older infants and children typically have an established routine for bathing,

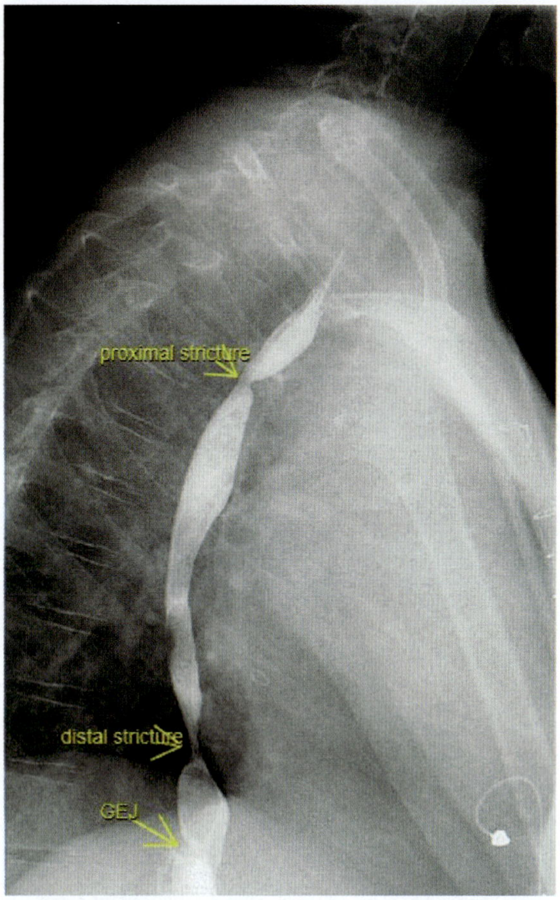

FIGURE 65-6. Esophagram showing distal and proximal esophageal strictures. GEJ, gastroesophageal junction.

TABLE 65-2 Differential Diagnosis of Blistering Disorders in the Neonate or Infant

Congenital Disorders:
- Epidermolytic hyperkeratosis
- Ichthyosis bullosa of Siemens
- Pachyonychia congenita
- Incontinentia pigmenti
- Aplasia cutis congenita
- Ankyloblepharon-ectodermal dysplasia-cleft lip syndrome

Immunobullous Disorders:
- Bullous pemphigoid
- Pemphigus vulgaris
- Chronic bullous dermatosis of childhood (linear IgA disease)
- Epidermolysis acquisita
- Neonatal lupus

Infectious Disorders:
- Staphylococcal scalded skin syndrome
- Bullous impetigo
- Herpes simplex
- Congenital syphilis
- Cutaneous candidiasis

Other:
- Bullous mastocytosis
- Sucking blisters
- Traumatic blisters
- Thermal or chemical burns

TABLE 65-3 Common Complications Associated With Junctional and Recessive Dystrophic Epidermolysis Bullosa

System	Complications
Skin, hair, nails	Infection, scarring, milia formation, excessive granulation tissue, keratoderma, alopecia, nail dystrophy, skin cancer (predominantly squamous cell carcinoma, although basal cell carcinoma and melanoma may also be seen)
Musculoskeletal	Pseudosyndactyly, contractures, osteoporosis, osteopenia, scoliosis, fractures
Gastrointestinal	Esophageal strictures, dysphagia, anal stenosis, constipation, malnutrition, failure to thrive, protein losing enteropathy, rectal prolapse, gastroesophageal reflux disease, liver disease
Ocular	Blepharoconjunctivitis, keratitis, pannus formation, symblepharon, corneal ulceration and scarring, ectropion, lacrimal duct obstruction
Oral	Oral erosions, dental enamel hypoplasia, severe caries, microstomia, ankyloglossia, premature loss of dentition
Genitourinary	Urethral strictures, phimosis, chronic renal failure, urethral diverticuli, ureteral reflux, hydronephrosis, hydroureter, glomerulonephritis, recurrent urinary tract infections, urinary retention
Respiratory	Laryngeal and tracheal granulomas/strictures, tracheal stenosis, stridor, hoarseness, sudden complete upper airway occlusion
Other	Anemia, sepsis, cardiomyopathy, otitis externa, occlusion of the nares, depression, anxiety, delayed puberty, developmental delays

removing bandages, and re-dressing wounds (typically every day or every other day), and preserving this routine should be prioritized during hospitalization. Providing appropriate pain control during wound care is very important, as dressing changes are typically painful and anxiety-provoking for the child as well as the caregivers. Adequate time should be allowed for hospital caregivers to visualize the entire skin surface, noting all areas that are particularly painful, and blisters and wounds with any exudate, odor, increased erythema, or poor healing. Alternatively, photos can be taken and shared later with medical providers. For infants and children with generalized blistering, this process may take 1 to 2 hours or more. The skin condition should be reassessed intermittently during the hospitalization, with more frequent evaluations if clinically indicated.

Detailed consensus recommendations for EB wound care are easily found online. Some general principles are as follows. Dressings should never be forcibly removed, but instead soaked off in a warm bath or with tap water or saline soaks if they are adherent. During or after removal, gentle bathing in warm water with a gentle non-soap cleanser such as Cetaphil is recommended. Bath additives may be beneficial about once or twice per week for patients prone to recurrent skin infections and may help reduce bacterial overgrowth; possible additives include bleach (1 capful of common household bleach per gallon of water; ⅛ to ¼ cup per 40-gallon bathtub of water), or acetic acid (white vinegar diluted 1:10 in bath water). For patients admitted with significant cutaneous blistering and/or crusting wounds, hydrotherapy can help clean and debride wounds, thus removing contaminated biofilm and dead skin. Sedation and monitoring with anesthesiology may be necessary for this. Intact blisters should always be immediately decompressed with a sterile needle to prevent them from enlarging. The roof of the blister should be left intact to provide a natural sterile dressing. Before new dressings are applied, all wounds should be evaluated for signs of infection and poor healing.

When applying new bandages, it is essential to use materials which will not adhere to the skin. Silicone-based specialty dressings are preferable and not likely to adhere to skin or wounds; these are available from a variety of manufacturers. Petrolatum gauze is another reasonable option. These dressings can be secured by wrapping with rolled gauze and/or a tubular dressing/elastic net dressing over the top. Use of emollients such as petrolatum before placing dressings also helps to reduce skin friction. The assistance of a wound care specialist such as a wound, ostomy, and continence nurse (WOCN) may also be helpful in managing acute and chronic wounds, especially if a specialized EB team is not available. Prolonged use of topical steroids is generally

TABLE 65-4 General Care for Infants and Children With Epidermolysis Bullosa

Type of Care	Recommendations
General skin care	Lift infants by supporting buttocks and head; avoid lifting from under the arms
	Provide a cool, air-conditioned environment; consider a room fan
	Avoid taking rectal temperatures
	Take blood pressure readings only when necessary; use soft gauze beneath the blood pressure cuff
	Use petrolatum gauze under pulse oximetry probes and a hydrogel dressing such as Duoderm under electrocardiogram electrodes, may secure with silicon tape (Mepitac®)
	Do not use tape to secure dressings or intravenous lines; use Mepitac®, gauze or tubular dressings
	Monitor for signs of skin infection
Bath care	Avoid rubbing the skin vigorously; pat the skin instead
	Cleanse skin gently with a mild nonsoap cleanser such as Dove or Cetaphil
	Apply an emollient such as petrolatum twice daily to decrease friction
	Give weekly baths using saline, dilute bleach, or dilute vinegar to help reduce bacterial skin colonization
Diet, nutrition, and oral care	For infants: Use soft or Haberman nipples on bottles
	For older infants and children: Provide soft, cool foods and teething gels Clean the mouth gently using a soft toothbrush and toothpaste Avoid suctioning the oropharynx Give multivitamins, stool softeners and supplements of nutrients tested to be deficient
Bedding and clothing	Use loose-fitting clothing and cloth diapers; avoid elastic
	Use protective foam or fleece padding on seatbelts and shoes and over elbows and knees
	Pad mattresses and cribs with foam or fleece
	For poorly mobile inpatients, use air-cushioned mattresses to help reduce blisters
Wound care and dressings	Clean erosions with saline-soaked gauze
	Decompress blisters by puncturing with a sterile needle; leave blister roof intact where possible as a natural sterile dressing
	Apply emollients to erosions; topical antimicrobials as indicated
	Apply petrolatum gauze or nonadherent dressing (e.g., Telfa, Mepilex Transfer, Mepitel)
	Use gauze wraps or tubular dressings; avoid tape and adhesive bandages
	Soak old dressings before removal if there is crusting or if the dressing sticks to the skin

contraindicated in patients with EB due to poor wound healing and risk of systemic absorption; they are used in some cases to control excess granulation tissue. Other medications to avoid due to risk of systemic absorption via the wounds are salicylic acid, prilocaine, lidocaine, or lactic acid-containing preparations. Finally, a cool environment can help minimize blistering and pruritis and improve overall comfort for most patients. In the inpatient setting many patients prefer to use a room fan.

CARE OF THE NEWBORN WITH EB

Newborns with skin blistering disorders and suspicion for EB require unique considerations. While most involve skin care, there are a few that should specifically be pointed out as they could be easily overlooked. Infants with suspected EB may be breastfed or fed with a Haberman bottle; infants with EB typically require more calories than the average newborn so most will require fortification of feeds. NG placement should be avoided to avoid nasopharyngeal and esophageal trauma. Pacifiers may be used for comfort if the infant tolerates them; if blistering occurs periorally, lubrication can be

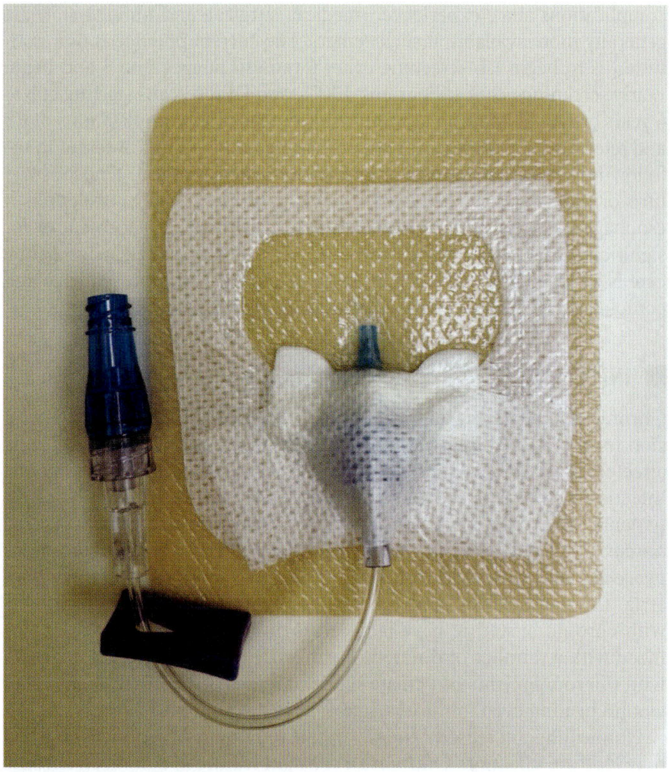

FIGURE 65-7. Securing lines in patients with EB. This photograph shows a secured central venous catheter on the chest of a neonate with severe junctional EB. (Provided courtesy of Beth Moeves, MSN, FNP-BC of Cincinnati Children's Hospital Epidermolysis Bullosa Center.)

placed around the ring. Reflux precautions should be initiated early with any spitting up or vomiting as many babies with EB develop GERD. A weak cry, hoarse cry, or stridor should be monitored closely as they may indicate granulation tissue in the airway, especially if an infant has granulation tissue at the finger or toenails. Suctioning should be done sparingly and then only with lubrication of the suction catheter. Infants typically require dressing changes every 2 to 3 days. They may be immersed in a bath as tolerated, or one body part dribbled with warm saline and rewrapped at a time. As with any patient with EB, all shearing forces and adhesives should be avoided, lubrication placed on gloves before the infant is touched, and blisters drained but not de-roofed as soon as they develop to avoid enlargement. Adhesives should be removed from EKG and cardiorespiratory monitor leads and replaced with Mepitac tape. Blood pressure cuffs should be cushioned with dressings underneath. Rectal temperatures should be avoided. Lubrication should be applied to diaper edges and any other areas of friction, such as the elbows or back of the head and heels may need dressings placed to avoid friction while lying on the bed. The diaper area should be cleansed with a patting motion using mineral oil and cotton balls. Elastic from diapers should be removed and the diaper lined with Mepilex transfer; the diaper edges should be folded over so as not to contact the skin. Even infants with EB experience pain with oral blisters, bandages that become stuck, or when air comes in contact with wounds; pain control can usually be achieved with acetaminophen or sucrose water. Parents should be encouraged to hold and dress their babies; we recommend breathable fabrics such as cotton for clothing. If there is concern for infection, wounds should be cultured and topical antibiotics such as bacitracin considered first line. As discussed above, genetic testing should be sent as soon as possible to inform discussions on diagnosis and possible prognosis.

MITIGATION OF SEQUELAE AND REFERRAL TO AN EB CENTER

Regular visits to an EB center every 6 to 12 months are strongly recommended to prevent and mitigate common complications of EB. EB centers are often better equipped to improve outcomes and minimize complications since experienced medical, surgical, and nursing staff are generally more available at such centers. The current practice at our institution is to begin lab screening every 6 months at ages 2 to 3 and begin yearly screening echocardiograms, EKGs, and DEXA scans starting at 5 to 6 years of age. In addition to monitoring for expected complications of EB and referrals for routine care, patients may benefit from an EB center in the following circumstances: when significant tracheolaryngeal stenosis, stricture, or occlusion have occurred, if a tracheostomy is being considered, if esophageal strictures require dilatation, for gastrostomy placement or for significant gastrostomy complications, and when comprehensive dental care is needed. The following subsections outline common sequelae and complications of EB as well as management approaches.

INFECTION

Chronic skin blistering and ulceration, combined with immune suppression from chronic disease and poor nutrition, predispose many severely affected EB patients to infection. Local wound infection and systemic infection account for a significant proportion of hospitalizations of EB patients. The most commonly isolated organisms are *Staphylococcus aureus* (consider MRSA), *Pseudomonas aeruginosa,* and *Streptococcus pyogenes*. Infections with other gram-negative bacteria, anaerobic bacteria, *Candida* species, and mixed flora can also occur. Most patients with chronic blistering have large areas of exposed skin that are colonized with a number of different organisms. Heavy wound colonization with microorganisms can create significant local inflammation and stall wound healing even in the absence of a true wound infection.

Nonhealing, increased exudate, friable red tissue, or wound sloughing may indicate infection. Odors are a constant feature of colonized chronic wounds, and therefore odor is not a reliable indicator of true infection. A suspect wound should be cultured and treated with a topical antimicrobial agent, while also considering use of an antimicrobial dressing or bath additive such as bleach or vinegar. Practitioners should consider asking patients and families directly which wounds they are concerned about and culturing those wounds in particular or allowing families to obtain cultures during dressing changes. Ideally, cultures are obtained from dressings saturated with exudate rather than from the wound bed itself; this practice will reduce unnecessary discomfort from swabbing skin directly. Commonly used topical antimicrobial agents are mupirocin, bacitracin/polymyxin B, gentamicin, ketoconazole, and medical grade honey. Neomycin is not recommended due to risk of developing contact allergic sensitization, and while silver sulfadiazine is also an effective antimicrobial, prolonged use can lead to argyria (skin discoloration). Newer dressings that contain nanocrystalline silver or polyhexamethylenebiguanide (PHMB) may be useful adjuncts.

Topical therapy is generally first line for patients that are not systemically ill and when infection appears superficial and nonsevere. The use of systemic therapy should be guided by the results of wound culture for bacterial and fungal organisms, when available. Otherwise, empiric antibiotic choice may be informed by the more common organisms as outlined above. In general, however, systemic therapy should be reserved for patients in whom there is evidence of more than superficial infection. The exception is when Group A streptococcus is isolated, in which case systemic antibiotic treatment is necessary because of the risk of complications such as sepsis, toxic shock, glomerulonephritis, or rheumatic heart disease. When Group A Streptococcus is identified, it is our practice to test a patient's family members and treat those who test positive in an effort to reduce the risk of reinfection from household contacts. In all other cases, judicious antibiotic use prevents the selection of multidrug-resistant organisms over the patient's lifetime. Clinical features that may indicate systemic antimicrobial therapy is needed are increasing size of the wound, increased temperature of the wound and surrounding skin, exposed bone, new areas of skin breakdown around the wound, erythema and/or edema of the surrounding skin, increasing exudate, and increasing odor or a change in odor. Fever and/or other signs and symptoms of more significant infection will guide inpatient management of suspected sepsis (**Figure 65-8**). Keep in mind that fevers should be evaluated in a manner similar to how non-EB patients are evaluated; other sources of fever should be considered before concluding that skin infection is the definite source.

Aside from skin infections, abscesses and osteomyelitis may also occur in patients with EB. The diagnostic process for these conditions is typically the same as for patients with and without EB; one potential exception is osteomyelitis (see musculoskeletal below). Inflammatory markers such as ESR, CRP, and ferritin levels are chronically elevated in patients with EB; therefore, high values should not be immediately interpreted as indicative of infection. Following the trends of these markers is more useful than individual values. Imaging results may also be impacted by the chronic inflammation of EB which is discussed further below.

ACUTE AND CHRONIC PAIN AND PRURITIS

Although all patients with EB experience pain with blistering, pain control is often a larger challenge in patients with more severe forms of EB, specifically RDEB and severe JEB. At some point in their lives, almost every severely affected EB patient will require daily use of opiates to address their chronic pain; acute pain exacerbations should also be anticipated with worsening skin or other complications, and medication regimens should be adjusted accordingly. Anxiety plays a substantial role in pain perception, so addition of an anxiolytic may be a useful therapeutic adjunct. Pain and anxiety create significant challenges during dressing changes, bathing, and skin care at home; in the hospital these issues are magnified by the stress of hospitalization. Pharmacologic options for pain management include topical preparations (e.g., morphine gel), traditional medications (e.g., acetaminophen, NSAIDs, opiates, gabapentin), and nontraditional agents (e.g., tricyclic antidepressants, cannabinoids). Hospitalists should strongly consider involving pain management experts in the care of EB patients, especially in cases where high doses of pain medications are needed or multiple agents are required; providers with expertise in pain management may be particularly helpful in tailoring pain medication regimens, addressing side effects, and troubleshooting drug interactions. Nonpharmacologic interventions such as relaxation and guided imagery have also been successfully used in EB patients.

Patients with EB also suffer from extreme and chronic pruritus which may be even more troublesome than pain. Chronic scratching can lead to open and nonhealing wounds. Antihistamines are first-line treatment, but for many the pruritus is recalcitrant to initial treatment with antihistamines such that other agents are needed (e.g., doxepin, ondansetron, gabapentin, aprepitant).

NUTRITION AND HYDRATION

A complete nutritional assessment should be performed in all patients with EB who are admitted to the hospital. Useful screening serum laboratory studies include electrolytes, albumin, prealbumin, blood urea nitrogen, liver transaminases, triglycerides, calcium, magnesium, and phosphate. Serum levels of specific vitamins and minerals may also be evaluated as indicated (e.g., iron, vitamin D, vitamin A, zinc, selenium, carnitine). Careful monitoring of growth parameters, especially BMI, in conjunction with dietary assessments are needed to ensure adequate calorie and protein intake; this is especially important when complications such as infection, oral blisters, or esophageal strictures predispose patients to poor oral intake and/or increase metabolic demand. In general, albumin is more helpful as a negative indicator of severity of disease than as a positive indicator of nutritional well-being, as it typically falls with increasing system-wide inflammation. Gastrostomy placement should be considered when the patient's BMI begins to drop despite other reasonable nutritional interventions. Poor nutrition and growth are associated with delayed puberty and osteopenia/osteoporosis.

Careful monitoring of fluid status in EB patients is very important, because patients with significant skin involvement and subsequent loss of skin barrier function can have significant transepidermal water loss and quickly become dehydrated. Patients that are febrile or unable to take in sufficient enteral fluids are at particularly high risk of dehydration.

GASTROINTESTINAL TRACT COMPLICATIONS

Gastrointestinal problems that may require hospitalization of the severe RDEB patient include pyloric atresia in the neonate, esophageal stricture,

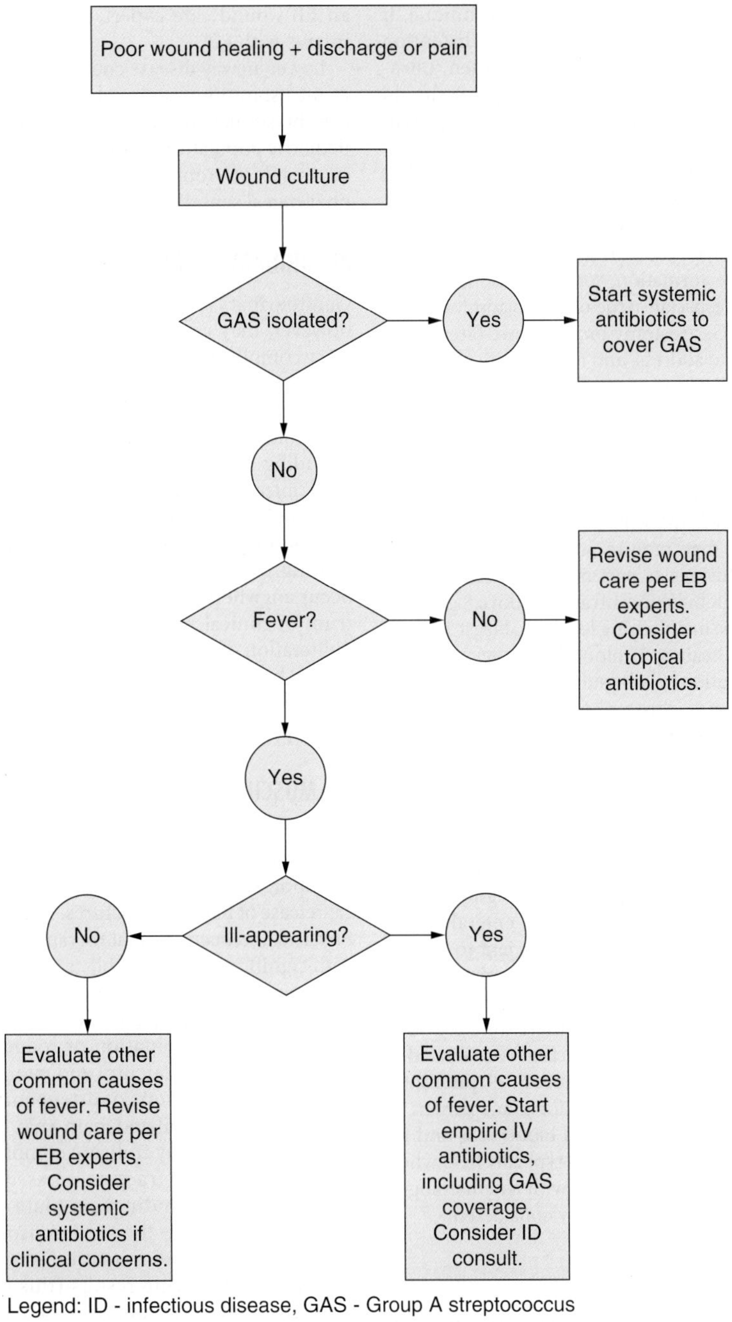

FIGURE 65-8. Approach to treatment of fever and suspected wound infection in patients with EB.

feeding intolerance, intestinal dysmotility, severe constipation/fecal impaction, and postoperative care after gastrostomy tube placement. All EB patients with dysphagia or odynophagia and infants who feed poorly should be evaluated for gastrointestinal dysfunction, notably esophageal stricture formation. A contrast study of the esophagus (barium swallow study or esophagram) is indicated to evaluate the anatomy and function of the esophagus. It is crucial to ask the radiologist to include the upper one-third of the esophagus in the images; this is the typical site of stricture formation and is not included in routine upper GI imaging. Esophageal stricture formation is directly related to mucosal blistering in RDEB and severe JEB; it is best treated with esophageal balloon dilatation by gastroenterology, general surgery, or interventional radiology. Overnight observation after dilatation may be required for pain control and/or diet advancement. Steroid use after dilation may be useful in some patients to prevent post-dilation swelling, and usage varies among providers and centers.

Dysmotility and constipation most often result from the necessary use of opiates for acute and chronic pain control; anal fissures may contribute to withholding stool as well. Hospital management of dysmotility should include gastroenterology consultation and diagnostic studies as they would be used to evaluate any patient with dysmotility; individualized treatment plans are essential. Constipation is a chronic problem; the home treatment regimen should be continued while in hospital. Severe constipation may require aggressive bowel cleanout and/or manual disimpaction by a surgeon under anesthesia. Important points to note regarding management of severe constipation include the following: (1) digital rectal exam should be avoided unless absolutely necessary, and then should be performed by an experienced provider with excess lubrication; (2) enemas should be avoided; (3) nasogastric tube placement, when needed for administration of electrolyte bowel prep solutions, should be performed carefully, with plenty of water-soluble lubricant, and secured with a non-adhesive, frictionless technique, if secure placement is necessary; (4) although gross abdominal distention is more commonly due to gaseous distention and stool burden, ultrasound imaging to rule out organomegaly (e.g., hepatomegaly) should be considered since physical examination is often limited by patient discomfort.

When gastrostomy is indicated for failure to thrive, an open surgical technique can be used, though minimally invasive techniques may result in less pain and fewer complications. A patient with a gastrostomy tube may require hospitalization to manage problems at the ostomy site such as skin erosions, granulation tissue formation, local infection, chronic leakage, or surgical revision. This is especially true of gastrostomies which have been in place for many years. Gastrostomy problems are often complex, may take long periods of time to address, and may require referral to larger centers with experienced medical and surgical practitioners.

HEMATOLOGIC COMPLICATIONS

Anemia is the predominant hematologic complication in patients with RDEB and JEB. The anemia associated with EB is multifactorial and often recalcitrant to treatment. Patients may require admission for IV iron preparations and/or red cell transfusions as part of therapy for anemia. Consensus views are to keep hemoglobin concentrations above 8 g/dL. In the setting of poorly healing wounds, maintaining levels of at least 10 g/dL has been shown to benefit wound healing. If blood iron levels are adequate, then enteral iron supplementation may be sufficient. However, iron levels are often low from chronic losses, chronic consumption, and poor absorption. It should be noted that simple iron and ferritin blood levels are respectively low and high in many EB patients; a true measurement of iron levels is best calculated by a ratio of soluble transferrin receptor (sTfR) to log of ferritin as a more accurate measurement in EB, with a value >1 indicating iron deficiency. Enteral iron supplementation is sometimes difficult as dyspepsia or constipation may limit tolerance; enteral replacement may also be insufficient to address substantial ongoing losses. An enteral iron absorption test may be useful to determine if enteral iron is beneficial. If enteral iron cannot be absorbed or is insufficient to meet a patient's needs, periodic IV iron infusion is preferred. The newest formulation of iron dextran is a safe and efficient way to deliver higher iron doses, and iron sucrose has also been used. Although there were previous concerns about high risk of anaphylactic or anaphylactoid reactions, this risk is minimized with current iron formulations. **Figure 65-9**, published by Simpson et al, can be used as a helpful reference for management of anemia in EB. Some patients receive both packed red blood cells and IV iron in the same hospital admission, though IV iron is typically held when there is concern for systemic infection. Consultation with a hematologist for chronic management of anemia should be strongly considered.

RESPIRATORY TRACT COMPLICATIONS

Airway and respiratory problems in EB patients that the hospitalist may encounter are few but significant and include tracheolaryngeal stenosis or stricture and airway occlusion. Patients with severe JEB can develop airway-threatening granulomas in the supra- and subglottic areas; this causes stenosis and laryngeal webbing. These most often present in infancy. Therefore, stridor and other signs or symptoms of upper airway obstruction must be viewed seriously in any patient with known EB or a neonate with suspicion of EB, especially JEB. The upper airway should be evaluated to rule out obstruction, starting with airway x-rays, and when necessary, direct visualization in the operating room by an otorhinolaryngologist. Acute airway obstruction can occur in the more severe types of EB if large enough pieces of oropharyngeal mucosa are sloughed and aspirated, such as may occur after trauma, instrumentation, forceful vomiting, or severe coughing. Treatment of upper airway obstruction is based on identification of the cause; if acute, urgent evaluation in the operating room is indicated. Granulation tissue can be cauterized and excised, but for recurrent obstruction, tracheostomy may eventually be needed. In EB patients that have a tracheostomy, maintaining it in place with tracheostomy ties without injuring the skin is fraught with difficulty. Skin complications associated with a tracheostomy should ideally be managed jointly by the caregiver, the hospitalist, an EB wound care expert, and an ENT surgeon with experience with infants with EB.

Lower airway disease could be related to acute and chronic aspiration. Acute aspiration events, which may lead to pneumonitis, are characterized by similar history and physical findings as are seen in the general pediatric population. Chronic silent aspiration can also be seen, typically as a result of oropharyngeal scarring, which can decrease epiglottic and pharyngeal sensation, causing chronic lung disease over time.

URINARY TRACT COMPLICATIONS

Genitourinary tract complications are associated more often with JEB; however, they can also be seen in patients with RDEB. Genitourinary tract complications typically include urethral stenosis and renal failure caused by glomerulonephritis. Hydronephrosis, obstruction of the ureteropelvic junction, and acquired dysfunctional voiding (from voluntary holding of urine) may also occur. Patients with urinary symptoms, including dysuria, hematuria, urinary retention, or recurrent urinary tract infections, may have a urethral stricture and should be seen by a urologist for a full evaluation of the genitourinary system; this may include imaging studies such as renal ultrasonography and possibly a voiding cystourethrogram. In boys with JEB, urethral strictures can occur anywhere along the length of the urethra and can result in a spectrum of clinical manifestations from mild meatal stenosis to complete obliteration of the urethra due to scarring. Surgical dilatation and repair should be attempted with caution, and ideally only by providers with EB experience. Some patients may require urinary diversion via placement of a suprapubic catheter or in extreme cases, nephrostomy.

MUSCULOSKELETAL COMPLICATIONS

Musculoskeletal complications are a major cause of morbidity in patients with RDEB, and include joint contractures, muscle atrophy, scoliosis, osteoporosis, and pseudosyndactyly. Hand surgeons can attempt surgical release of hand contractures, though there is a high rate of recurrence. Physical and occupational therapy evaluation are essential in all patients with significant pain and blistering to help maintain adequate function, conditioning, and range of motion, especially during hospitalization.

In RDEB, osteopenia and osteoporosis are not uncommon and result from a combination of reduced weight-bearing activity, poor nutrition with low calcium and vitamin D intake, and chronic inflammation. Complications of osteopenia and osteoporosis may manifest as bone pain. Localized pain may signify a fracture or microfracture. Spine pain may indicate compression fractures of the vertebrae. Diagnosis of spinal fracture is based on clinical findings in combination with typical findings on plain radiographs. Bone scans may be of limited use since they are nonspecific, and there are usually also multiple areas of inflammation in soft tissues that could lead to difficulty in interpreting results (this is also the case when looking for osteomyelitis). Generalized bone pain can result from osteopenia or osteoporosis in the absence of fracture. Lumbar dual-energy x-ray absorptiometry (DEXA) scans can be used to quantify low bone mineral density. Severely low scores have been used as markers for treating RDEB patients with IV bisphosphonates. In patients with delayed puberty, careful hormonal replacement, especially androgens in boys, may improve bone mineral density.

ENDOCRINOLOGIC COMPLICATIONS

In addition to abnormal vitamin D metabolism and poor bone health, other endocrinologic issues may also arise. Poor thyroid function also frequently occurs in the EB population. TSH and free T4 levels may be obtained to screen for thyroid dysfunction. Delayed puberty is also very common and may be managed with hormone replacement therapies. Consultation with a pediatric endocrinologist should be made for any patients that have such clinical concerns.

OPHTHALMOLOGIC COMPLICATIONS

Eye care for hospitalized EB patients is important, as ocular complications are common in almost all patients with EB. Erosions and blisters involving

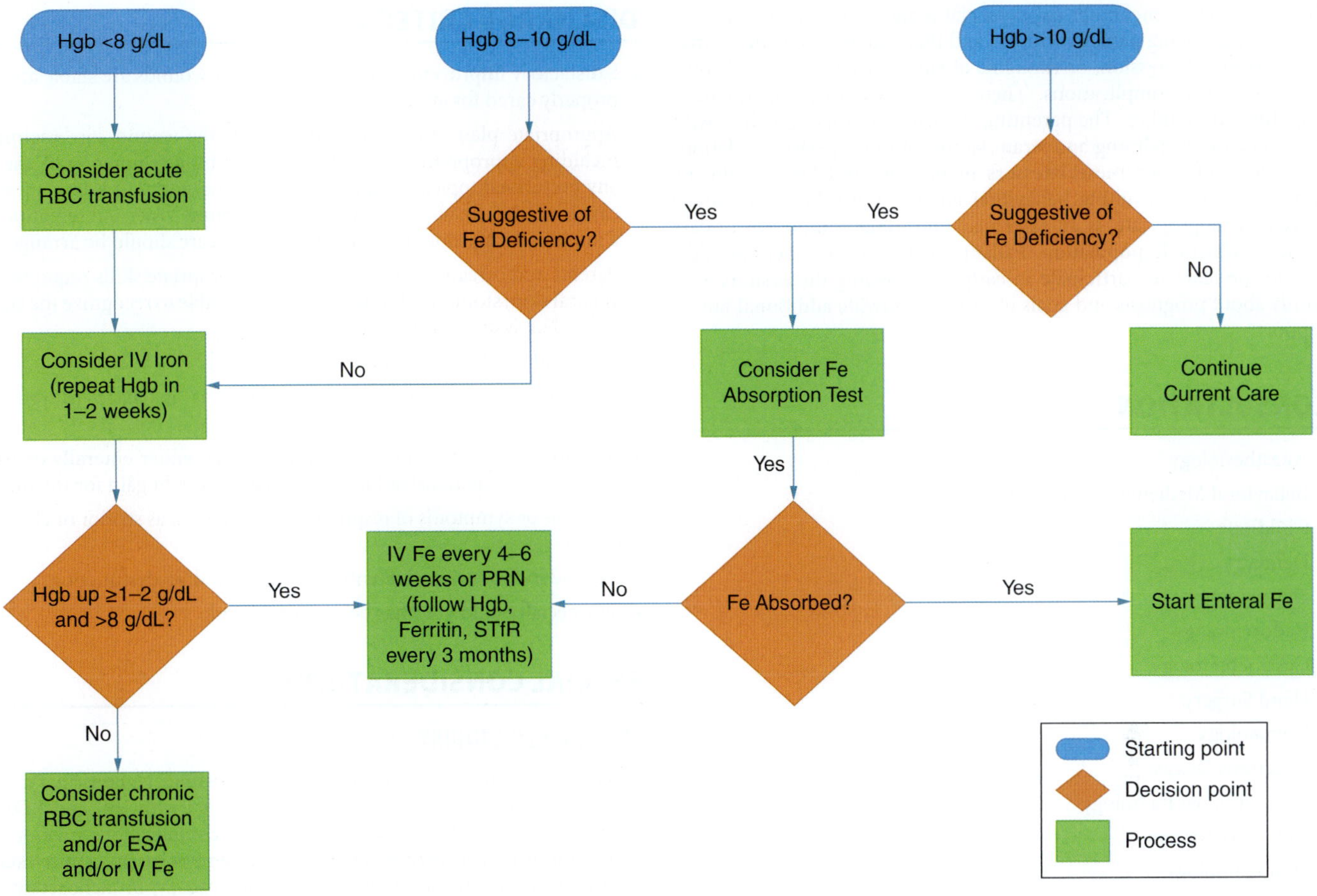

FIGURE 65-9. Epidermolysis bullosa anemia flow chart. Hgb, hemoglobin; Fe, iron; RBC, red blood cell; IV, intravenous; ESA, erythropoietin stimulating agent; sTfR, soluble transferrin receptor. (Reproduced with permission from Simpson B, Tarango C, Lucky AW. Clinical algorithm to manage anemia in epidermolysis bullosa. *Pediatr Dermatol.* 2018; 35(5):e319-e320.)

the bulbar conjunctiva and cornea are particularly common, as are chronic blepharitis, conjunctivitis, keratitis, and ectropion. Corneal scarring can result from repeated corneal abrasions and corneal ulceration, threatening vision. Because of this high risk of corneal abrasion, every consideration should be given to maintaining sufficient lubrication of the eyelids and corneas, especially during procedures requiring general anesthesia or sedation. Patients should not have their hospital beds placed directly under vents that may dry out the cornea. Ointments provide more protection and last longer than aqueous drops; use of these treatments can also be guided by patient and caregiver preference. Ocular antibiotics, analgesics, and cycloplegics may be required to treat corneal erosions and should be managed by ophthalmology. Recent evidence suggests that vitamin A deficiency contributes to corneal disease, and therefore now patients have vitamin A and retinol binding protein levels measured to determine whether vitamin A supplementation is indicated. Regular eye exams should be done every 6 to 12 months. Patients with eye pain, discharge, or blepharitis should undergo a full ophthalmologic examination.

CARDIAC COMPLICATIONS

Dilated cardiomyopathy is associated with RDEB and JEB and appears to be related to a complex interplay of several factors (i.e., chronic anemia, micronutrient deficiency, transfusion-associated iron overload, and/or viral myocarditis). The typical features noted on echocardiogram include dilated cardiomyopathy and aortic root dilatation. Presenting signs and symptoms such as fatigue, exercise intolerance, and malaise may be noted with many other disease processes; therefore, cardiomyopathy can easily go undetected. For this reason, it is recommended that all RDEB patients be evaluated by cardiology consultation with echocardiogram prior to any general anesthesia, and annually thereafter. Treatment of cardiomyopathy associated with RDEB ranges from active non-intervention to micronutrient supplementation with carnitine and selenium, to use of medications such as beta-receptor antagonists or angiotensin-converting enzyme inhibitors and should be managed by cardiology. Screening for a long QTc interval is also warranted in cases where medications, or combinations of medications (such as methadone and ondansetron) could prolong it further.

ONCOLOGIC COMPLICATIONS

Patients with JEB, RDEB, and Kindler EB are at high lifetime risk of squamous cell carcinoma, and in these patients, squamous cell carcinoma is a significant cause of mortality. There is no "typical" appearance of squamous cell carcinoma in EB, so skin biopsy should be obtained whenever it is suspected. Concerning hallmarks are chronically nonhealing wounds or wounds that feel different than a patient's normal EB wounds. Dermatology should be involved in diagnosis and an experienced oncology team should be involved in staging and treatment decisions, and orthopedic surgery and plastic surgery if amputation or wide excision is indicated.

DENTAL COMPLICATIONS

Dental hygiene is particularly difficult for patients with EB. Many patients have limited mouth opening which renders good oral care more challenging. Some patients may have pain with attempts to brush teeth and may be concerned about mucosal injury with oral care. Consequently, patients with EB are often susceptible to dental caries and may require exams under anesthesia for adequate evaluation or dental rehabilitation. Ideally, these procedures should be bundled with other procedures that require sedation.

PSYCHOSOCIAL COMPLICATIONS

In addition to the significant physical stressors and challenges of living with EB, particularly the more severe forms of disease, hospitalists should expect to encounter psychosocial issues given the broad array of challenges facing patients with EB and their caregivers. Patients may have anxiety, depression, or thoughts of suicide as a result of chronic pain and other complications. There are often devastating financial hardships for families. The parenting challenges of raising a child with EB can be overwhelming and strain family and interpersonal relationships. Screening for these stressors in patients and families during admission, and consulting behavioral medicine, psychiatry, or social services as appropriate, is an extremely important component of care for this vulnerable population. Palliative care can be a helpful addition to the team to participate in early and ongoing discussions with family about prognosis and goals of care and provide additional family support.

CONSULTATION

- Anesthesiology
- Behavioral Medicine/Clinical Psychology
- Child Life
- Dentistry
- Dermatology
- Endocrinology
- Gastroenterology
- Hand Surgery
- Hematology
- Infectious Disease
- Interventional Radiology
- Nutrition Therapy
- Ophthalmology
- Otolaryngology
- Pain Management
- Palliative Care
- Pediatric Surgery
- Physical Therapy/Occupational Therapy
- Plastic and/or Orthopedic Surgery
- Psychiatry
- Urology

ADMISSION CRITERIA

- Severe or extensive skin blistering not responsive to outpatient management
- Secondary infection, such as cellulitis, osteomyelitis, or sepsis
- Uncontrolled pain
- Severe malnutrition and failure to thrive
- Esophageal strictures that prevent adequate oral intake or cause aspiration
- Severe anemia requiring blood transfusion and monitoring for complications
- Respiratory compromise in more severe forms of EB (junctional or dystrophic)
- Acute urinary retention
- Perioperative care for surgical management of pseudosyndactyly with mitten-hand deformities or severe contractures that significantly impair function, including lower extremities
- Non-EB-related medical conditions (e.g., pneumonia, dehydration), or surgical conditions (e.g., appendectomy) for which admission is appropriate
- End-of-life palliative care related to metastatic squamous cell carcinoma or other lethal complications

DISCHARGE CRITERIA

- Satisfactory improvement in wounds and/or wounds are stable and be properly cared for at home.
- Appropriate plan of care regarding the home wound care regimen, including appropriate use of dressings, bathing regimen, and use of any prescribed topical medications. If the assistance of home nursing care is needed, an appropriate schedule of home visits and retention of a nurse with appropriate training in wound care should be arranged.
- Parents and caregivers demonstrate the appropriate skills required for general skin, stoma, and wound care and are able to recognize the signs of local or systemic infection.
- Pain is adequately controlled.
- Appropriate preventative bowel regimen is in place to prevent constipation.
- Able to receive adequate nutritional support, either enterally or parenterally with demonstration of appropriate weight gain for infants.
- No signs or symptoms of respiratory distress such as stridor or chronic cough.
- No evidence of urinary retention or other voiding dysfunction.
- Subspecialty follow-up has been coordinated.

SPECIAL CONSIDERATIONS

IATROGENIC INJURY

Mucosal blistering may occur in the gastrointestinal, genitourinary, and respiratory tracts, as well as the eyes in patients with JEB and RDEB. Hospitalists should be aware, therefore, that complications may occur as a result of routine care practices and more invasive procedures such as endotracheal intubation, endoscopy, colonoscopy, bronchoscopy, or urinary catheterization. Consequently, meticulous planning is needed to reduce the risk of iatrogenic harm, ideally with input from the patient or family. Modifications to routine procedures are often necessary, such as attachment of identification bracelets to clothing or gowns instead of around the wrist or ankle, where pressure and friction may result in skin damage. Adhesive cardiac monitor leads and EKG leads should not be used. Standard adhesive on leads should be removed and the leads should instead be attached with Mepitac. Adhesive pulse oximetry probes are contraindicated. If needed, probes with wrap-around hook-and-loop closure are preferable. A clip-on probe may be used on the earlobe. Bedside signs should indicate that tape should never be used. Hospitalists should also proactively discuss other routine precautions families use when hospitalized as families are experts in their child's care.

INTRAVENOUS ACCESS

IV catheter placement is often difficult in patients with RDEB and severe JEB due to extensive blistering and scarring and the frequency with which IV access is required. Only skilled practitioners should try to obtain IV access. A percutaneously inserted central catheter (PICC) is preferred if long-term IV access is required or anticipated, or if central access is not needed, a mid-line catheter may also be considered. Once IV access has been established, it should be secured in a manner that minimizes trauma to the surrounding skin. One technique that may be used to place and secure IV access involves a two-step process: (i) preparing skin at the site with a mild adhesive barrier such as 3M Cavilon No Sting Skin Barrier Spray and (ii) application of Mepiform (usually a 3 × 3 in dressing for a peripheral IV, larger for a PICC), with an opening in the center of the dressing to accommodate the catheter. The Mepiform is used as a "false skin" to which the line is secured using conventional methods. This technique facilitates safer removal of the dressing (Figure 65-7).

ANESTHESIA AND PERIOPERATIVE ISSUES

Preoperative assessment should include obtaining and securing IV access, screening for and treating severe anemia and electrolyte disturbances, examining mouth opening for potential difficulty with intubation and dental issues, and ensuring that a recent echocardiogram has been performed for all RDEB patients. All staff involved in handling and transporting EB patients should be completely briefed on skin fragility and coached on correct techniques for transferring patients to and from beds, examination tables, and wheelchairs. Correct techniques include the use of a slide sheet or allowing patients to move themselves to the operating table or other location. Use of a foam egg crate mattress pad or other soft covering is recommended if the patient will be positioned on a hard surface. Intraoperative measures to minimize iatrogenic trauma should be confirmed before the procedure begins and include placement of padding under the blood pressure cuff, application of a lubricating ophthalmic ointment to protect the corneas, and use of a foam dressing such as Mepilex or petrolatum gauze to protect the face and chin from device-related pressure or pressure due to prone positioning. Protective dressings must be placed—without tape on the eyelids and face to avoid denuding skin.

Anesthesiologists, pulmonologists, or otolaryngologists with experience treating EB patients with complicated airways should be consulted for assistance with endotracheal intubation. Their expertise is invaluable in preventing trauma to the upper airway that may result in blistering and scarring. Microstomia and jaw contractures, which are common in patients with RDEB, combined with fragile mucosa, make it very challenging for even the most skilled anesthesiologist to intubate with minimal trauma to the facial skin, eyes, airway, and oropharynx. Endoscopic-assisted intubation is generally recommended in these cases. Patients requiring esophageal dilatation may require retrograde dilation to avoid upper esophageal trauma.

DebRA: SUPPORT FOR FAMILIES AND CLINICIANS

The Dystrophic EB Research Association of America (DebRA) (https://www.debra.org) is a national, nonprofit organization dedicated to funding research and providing services and programs for those with EB. DebRA provides many programs and services for patients and clinicians, including educational and social support opportunities for families, information on the different types of EB and basics of care for patients with EB, a wound care product clearinghouse that can provide supplies for families in temporary need, a national physician referral service for families to find the EB Center of Excellence closest to them, and a family crisis fund. An EB nurse educator is also available to assist patients, families, and providers with EB-related questions or concerns. DebRA International (https://www.debra-international.org) is another excellent source of information and may be used to access the Clinical Practice Guidelines for EB care (in English); these guidelines are international consensus reports from multiple EB specialists. DebRA Chile (https://www.debrachile.cl) provides information about EB in Spanish.

BONE MARROW TRANSPLANTATION

Bone marrow transplantation (BMT), also referred to as hematopoietic stem cell transplantation, has been performed on a relatively small number of patients who have severe, generalized forms of EB, predominantly RDEB. Outcomes after BMT have been mixed and clinical benefits have varied. BMT is not considered the standard of care and is not routinely performed, though it is still available at select medical centers worldwide. Patients who undergo BMT are at significant risk of complications, including medication toxicity, susceptibility to infection, and other complications of immunosuppression, as well as graft-versus-host disease. BMT experts should be involved in the care of any hospitalized patient with EB who has undergone transplantation.

ROUTINE PEDIATRIC AND ADOLESCENT CARE WHILE HOSPITALIZED

Given the frequency with which some patients with EB are hospitalized, and the prolonged duration of some admissions, some patients and families may seek or require parts of routine pediatric or adolescent care during hospital admissions. Patients that require very frequent hospitalizations may not have a primary care provider they routinely follow with. Hospitalists may be asked to provide routine immunizations, and these may be provided at the discretion of the clinical team based on the clinical condition of the patient. Other patients may inquire about routine gynecologic or reproductive health. Given the medical complexity of these patients, it may be reasonable to involve gynecology during hospital admission if contraception decisions may be complicated by aspects of medical complexity.

TRANSITIONS OF CARE AND ADULT CARE

Patients with EB will continue to require multi-disciplinary care as they become adolescents and adults. Transitioning to adult-based care may be especially challenging as adult medical providers familiar with EB may be difficult to identify, and patients may find it logistically difficulty to identify and transition care to multiple adult-based subspecialists. Consequently, adult patients may continue to be hospitalized at pediatric centers given the expertise of their pediatric providers and established relationships with these providers. Hospitalists should be prepared to proactively contact adult care experts to provide input on management of hospitalized adult patients with EB. Some pediatric EB centers may have access to internal medicine physicians that are readily available for consultation or co-management. If this resource is not available, consulting with patients' adult-based primary care providers may be helpful. Adult care providers may offer insight into issues such as medication for smoking cessation, anticoagulation, managing risk of substance abuse, and other medical issues that pediatricians are less likely to routinely manage.

KEY POINTS

- EB, the prototype of skin fragility disorders, is a diverse group of inherited blistering diseases with no cure, some forms of which can result in severe, generalized cutaneous blistering with systemic involvement of extracutaneous mucosa. The morbidities associated with EB often require hospitalization.
- Four major subtypes of EB have been defined based on the level at which skin blistering occurs and commonality in genetic mutations: EB simplex, Junctional EB, dystrophic EB, and Kindler EB.
- JEB and RDEB are considered the most severe forms of EB and carry the highest risk for systemic complications. RDEB and JEB account for most EB patient admissions.
- Although patients with EB may be hospitalized for non-EB related disease, those with severe disease are frequently admitted for management of extensive blistering, poor wound healing, and/or infectious complications, or for management of systemic complications, in particular of the gastrointestinal, genitourinary, and respiratory tracts, many of which may require surgical intervention.
- Patients with RDEB are at high risk of squamous cell carcinoma which may be life limiting.
- Inpatient care of the patient with EB requires meticulous attention to skin and wound care and modification of routine patient care procedures to minimize blistering and iatrogenic complications.
- Caring for patients with EB requires a multidisciplinary approach involving pediatric hospital medicine, dermatology, pain management, ophthalmology, general surgery, plastic surgery, gastroenterology, clinical psychology, and nutrition experts.
- Suspected wound colonization or minor/ superficial infections should be cultured and initially treated with topical antibiotics rather than systemic antibiotics whenever possible. Use of systemic antibiotics should be reserved for deteriorating wounds, streptococcal infection of the skin, or when true cellulitis or systemic symptoms are present.
- Patients with EB commonly suffer significant psychosocial distress, chronic pain, and other comorbidities common to all patients with chronic, complex diseases.

ACKNOWLEDGMENTS

The authors gratefully acknowledge the assistance of Anne W. Lucky, MD, Beth Moeves, APRN, Nichole Halliburton, APRN, Sue Rowe, RN, Jean Whalen, RN, and Caitlin Treuting of the Epidermolysis Bullosa Center at Cincinnati Children's Hospital.

SUGGESTED READINGS

Augsburger BD, et al. Enteral iron absorption in patients with recessive dystrophic epidermolysis bullosa. *Pediatr Dermatol.* 2020;37:817-820.

Cohn HI, Teng JMC. Advances in management of epidermolysis bullosa. *Curr Opin Pediatr.* 2016;28(4):507-516.

De Rosa L, Latella MC, Seconetti AS, et al. Toward combined cell and gene therapy for genodermatoses. *Cold Spring Harb Perspect Biol.* 2020;12(5):a035667.

Fine JD, Mellerio JE. Extracutaneous manifestations and complications of inherited epidermolysis bullosa: part II. Other organs. *J Am Acad Dermatol.* 2009;61(3):387-404.

Fine JD, Mellerio JE. Extracutaneous manifestations and complications of inherited epidermolysis bullosa: part I. Epithelial associated tissues. *J Am Acad Dermatol.* 2009;61(3):367-386.

Goldschneider KR, Lucky AW. Pain management in epidermolysis bullosa. *Dermatol Clin.* 2010;28(2):273-282, ix.

Goldschneider K, et al. Perioperative care of patients with epidermolysis bullosa: proceedings of the 5th international symposium on epidermolysis bullosa, Santiago Chile, December 4-6, 2008. *Paediatr Anaesth.* 2010;20(9):797-804.

Has C, et al. Consensus reclassification of inherited epidermolysis bullosa and other disorders with skin fragility. *Br J Dermatol.* 2020;183: 614-627.

Has C, et al. Practical management of epidermolysis bullosa: consensus clinical position statement from the European Reference Network for Rare Skin Disease. *JEADV.* 2021;35:2349-2360.

Ida JB, Livshitz I, Azizkhan RG, et al. Upper airway complications of junctional epidermolysis bullosa. *J Pediatr.* 2012;160(4):657-661.e1.

Lara-Corrales I, Mellerio JE, Martinez AE, et al. Dilated cardiomyopathy in epidermolysis bullosa: a retrospective, multicenter study. *Pediatr Dermatol.* 2010;27(3):238-243.

Lucky AW, et al. Diagnosis and care of the newborn with epidermolysis bullosa. *Neoreviews.* 2021;22(7):e438-451.

Mellerio JE, et al. Emergency management in epidermolysis bullosa: consensus clinical recommendations from the European reference network for rare skin diseases. *Orphanet J Rare Dis.* 2020;15:142.

Mellerio JE, Uitto J. Meeting Report: The First Global Congress on Epidermolysis Bullosa, EB202 London: Toward a Treatment and Cure. *J Invest Dermatol.* 2020;140:1681-1687.

Simpson B, Tarango C, Lucky AW. Clinical algorithm to manage anemia in epidermolysis bullosa. *Pediatr Dermatol.* 2018;35:e319-e320.

Tarango C, Quinn CT, Augsburger B, Lucky AW. Iron status and burden of anemia in children with recessive dystrophic epidermolysis bullosa. *Pediatr Dermatol.* 2023;1-6.

Wasserman H, Dumenigo A, Hornung L, et al. Prevalence of delayed puberty and low bone density in patients with epidermolysis bullosa: insight from a large single center's experience. *Pediatr Dermatol.* 2023; 40(1):100-106.

SECTION F
Endocrinology

CHAPTER 66 Diabetes Mellitus and Hyperglycemia

Amanda Messer, MD and Amy Prudhomme, DO

BACKGROUND

Diabetes mellitus in the United States is a growing concern for pediatric patients. The incidence of both type 1 and type 2 diabetes has increased in recent decades. According to the SEARCH for Diabetes in Youth Study, the estimated prevalence of type 1 diabetes is 2.15 per 1000 youth. For type 2 diabetes, the prevalence is 0.67 cases per 1000 youth. These numbers represent an increase in prevalence during the last two decades. While diabetes is usually managed in an outpatient setting, initial presentations and complications often present to the pediatric hospitalist.

PATHOPHYSIOLOGY

Insulin is produced by beta cells in the islets of Langerhans in the pancreas. Insulin secretion is regulated by glucose influx into the beta cell, which is dependent on the serum glucose level. Insulin acts on target tissues including liver, fat, and muscle to stimulate glucose uptake and inhibit gluconeogenesis, glycogenolysis, lipolysis, and ketogenesis. Hyperglycemia results from abnormal insulin production, abnormal insulin action, or both.

TYPE 1 DIABETES MELLITUS (T1DM)

In T1DM, autoimmune destruction of beta cells results in an absolute insulin deficiency. Approximately 90% of patients with T1DM have measurable serum antibodies against islet cells, glutamic acid decarboxylase (GAD), or insulin. However, although autoimmunity is an essential component of the pathogenesis of T1DM, it alone is not sufficient; environmental factors including diet, prenatal influences, infectious exposures, stress, and genetic factors contribute to development of this disease. Younger age at presentation, a close relative with T1DM, and non-Hispanic white ethnicity is associated with increased likelihood of T1DM. Forty-five percent of children present before 10 years of age.

TYPE 2 DIABETES MELLITUS (T2DM)

T2DM is characterized by insulin resistance, often in relation to obesity, with resulting beta cell dysfunction and glucotoxicity that results in a relative insulin deficiency despite hyperinsulinemia. Although the etiology of T2DM is multifactorial, there is a stronger genetic component than for T1DM. Risk factors for T2DM include: family history, child of a mother with gestational diabetes, and concomitant conditions related to insulin resistance (including overweight, high blood pressure, high cholesterol, or polycystic ovarian syndrome).

MATURITY ONSET DIABETES OF THE YOUNG (MODY)

MODY is a relatively rare group of disorders of insulin secretion and glucose disposal. They vary in their severity and presentation, and management often differs from that of T1DM and T2DM. Each is caused by a single gene mutation and is inherited in an autosomal dominant pattern. Insulin resistance and obesity are not features of these disorders.

CLINICAL PRESENTATION

Patients with hyperglycemia often present with polyuria, polydipsia, polyphagia, nocturia, weight loss, and/or fatigue. Depending on the duration of illness and the underlying pathophysiology, the patient may or may not have ketosis or acidosis as a consequence of absolute or relative insulin deficiency. Acidosis is more commonly seen in T1DM, though ketosis and acidosis can also occur in T2DM.

Children with newly diagnosed diabetes may present to the hospital in advanced stages of metabolic decompensation if the initial symptoms of hyperglycemia were not recognized. Treatment of diabetic ketoacidosis (DKA) and Hyperglycemic Hyperosmolar Syndrome (HHS) in childhood requires admission for strict attention to fluid balance and neurologic status because of the increased risk of cerebral edema in the pediatric population. Early detection of diabetes can reduce these risks.

Obesity and acanthosis nigricans (thickening and darkening of the skin in flexural areas such as the axillae and posterior of the neck) should raise the possibility that a child has T2DM, even in the setting of ketoacidosis. These patients typically do not have antibodies against islet cells, GAD, or insulin. This form of diabetes was previously labeled as "adult-onset" diabetes; however, the incidence of T2DM in the pediatric population is increasing rapidly as childhood obesity has become more prevalent.

DIFFERENTIAL DIAGNOSIS

The cause of hyperglycemia is not always apparent at initial presentation. The differential diagnosis includes:

- T1DM
- T2DM
- MODY
- hyperglycemia secondary to stress, illness, or trauma
- pancreatitis and other pancreatic dysfunction (e.g., cystic fibrosis)
- drug effect (glucocorticoids, antipsychotics, etc.)

Less commonly, hyperglycemia may be seen in the setting of other endocrine disorders such as excess endogenous glucocorticoid, growth hormone, or catecholamine response. T1DM can also be a component of Autoimmune Polyendocrine Syndrome Type 2, which includes autoimmune primary adrenal insufficiency (Addison disease) and autoimmune thyroid disease (Hashimoto thyroiditis or Graves disease).

DIAGNOSTIC EVALUATION

Criteria for the diagnosis of diabetes includes:

- a random plasma glucose ≥200 mg/dL with symptoms of hyperglycemia OR
- hemoglobin A1c ≥ 6.5% OR
- fasting (at least 8 hours) plasma glucose ≥126 mg/dL on more than one occasion OR
- a 2-hour plasma glucose ≥200 mg/dL during an oral glucose tolerance test using a glucose load of 1.75 g/kg (up to 75 g).

If an asymptomatic patient is found to have a fasting plasma glucose ≥126 mg/dL or a random plasma glucose ≥200 mg/dL as part of screening labs, these should be repeated on a second day to confirm these results. However, if a patient with signs and symptoms of diabetes including polyuria, polydipsia, or weight loss is found to have a random glucose of ≥200 mg/dL, no further testing is needed for diagnosis.

HYPERGLYCEMIC STATES

Patients with diabetes can present in various hyperglycemic states, each with its own diagnostic criteria and management.

Hyperglycemia With Ketoacidosis DKA is defined by a glucose ≥200 mg/dL, venous pH <7.3 or HCO_3 <15 mEq/L, and ketonuria or ketonemia. Patients presenting with DKA should be admitted to an intensive care unit (ICU) or a medical unit that is prepared to handle a patient requiring close monitoring of vital signs and neurologic status, frequent blood glucose monitoring, and frequent lab draws.

Hyperglycemia With Ketosis and Without Acidosis Diabetic ketosis without acidosis is defined by a glucose ≥200 mg/dL, venous pH ≥7.3 or HCO_3 ≥15 mEq/L, and the presence of ketones in urine or blood. In the patient who has a history of diabetes, it is reasonable to consider emergency department management with a discharge to home if there is a good response to intravenous fluids and insulin.

Hyperglycemic Hyperosmolar Syndrome Hyperglycemic hyperosmolar syndrome (HHS), also known as hyperosmolar hyperglycemic nonketotic (HHNK) syndrome, is defined by a glucose >600 mg/dL, serum osmolality >330 mOsm, venous pH >7.3, HCO_3 >15 mEq/L, and absent to small ketonuria or ketonemia. It is often accompanied by hypernatremia, significant dehydration, and altered mental status. Admission to an ICU is indicated due to increased risk of cerebral edema and stroke in these patients even in comparison to DKA.

Mixed Hyperglycemic Hyperosmolar State and Ketoacidosis Mixed hyperglycemic hyperosmolar state and ketoacidosis, defined by glucose >600 mg/dL, serum osmolality >320 mOsm, venous pH <7.3, HCO_3 <15 mEq/L, and moderate or large ketonuria or ketonemia, often with hypernatremia, significant dehydration, and altered mental status. This presentation warrants admission to a critical care setting, particularly if there is evidence of altered mental status.

INITIAL ASSESSMENT

The initial assessment of a patient with hyperglycemia includes a physical exam that pays careful attention to vital signs, status of the respiratory, cardiovascular, and neurologic systems, and to hydration status. The patient's body mass index and the presence or absence of acanthosis nigricans may provide insight into the underlying pathophysiology.

The initial laboratory evaluation of newly diagnosed diabetes should include a venous or arterial blood gas, basic metabolic panel (to evaluate electrolytes, CO_2, BUN, and creatinine), phosphorus, magnesium, insulin, C-peptide, hemoglobin A1c, GAD-65 antibodies, islet cell antibodies, and insulin autoantibodies. Urine should be assessed for the presence of glucose and ketones. In patients with significant electrolyte abnormalities, an electrocardiogram (ECG) should be obtained. If the patient is experiencing altered mental status, evaluate for cerebral edema.

The history should include the duration of illness, precipitating factors (such as infection, trauma, stress, puberty, or pregnancy), the patient's previous weight, and any prescription or nonprescription drugs the patient may have taken. If diabetes has previously been diagnosed, it is helpful to know the current insulin regimen, time of the last insulin dose, and the patient's adherence with treatment. If this is the patient's first presentation with hyperglycemia, any family history of autoimmune disease, T1DM or T2DM, and gestational diabetes should be elicited. Patients with T1DM should have inappropriately low insulin and C-peptide levels. Most but not all patients with T1DM have positive antibodies. It is not uncommon for patients with T2DM to also have inappropriately low insulin and C-peptide levels given their blood glucose level, due to beta cell toxicity at the time of initial presentation; however, most patients with T2DM present with hyperinsulinemia indicative of insulin resistance (**Figure 66-1**).

MANAGEMENT

Rapid evaluation of the patient should be quickly followed by initiation of treatment. The aim is to reverse the metabolic disturbance and restore and maintain intravascular volume. However, fluid and insulin management must be titrated carefully because rapid changes in glucose and osmolality may contribute to the development of complications.

TREATMENT OF DIABETIC KETOACIDOSIS

This section is not intended as a rigid protocol but is offered as a guideline. DKA management is dynamic and each case should be assessed individually and reassessed frequently during the course of treatment.

Fluids Emergency fluid resuscitation is determined by assessment of the patient's hydration status (perfusion, heart rate, and blood pressure). A bolus of 10 to 20 mL/kg of normal saline (NS) over a 1-hour period is typically used in a mildly to moderately dehydrated patient (keep in mind that the degree of dehydration is often underestimated). Assess need for second 10 to 20 mL/kg bolus if needed. Clinical status and medical history will dictate whether a conservative or aggressive approach to fluid management is warranted. Following this acute management, the fluid deficit should be replaced evenly over a minimum of 48 hours, in addition to maintenance fluids. Evidence exists for providing fluids at 1.5 maintenance or 2.5 L/m^2/day not to exceed 4 L/m^2/day. The patient's ongoing losses must also be monitored, and if excessive, these losses may require replacement as well. Fluid management must be reassessed at a minimum of every 4 hours. Inadequate hydration will contribute to persistent acidosis. Prolonged administration of fluids with excess chloride can result in hyperchloremic metabolic acidosis. Normal saline can be used for fluid resuscitation at 1.5 maintenance rate when in DKA. The sodium content of the fluid may need to be adjusted, depending on the patient's age, serum osmolality, and serum electrolytes. The patient in DKA should remain without oral intake during the initial stabilization due to potential risk of decompensation.

Slower fluid replacement should be considered in a patient who is very young, has had a prolonged prodrome, has severe acidosis, has an elevated corrected sodium, or has significantly elevated serum osmolality (>300 mOsm).

$$\text{corrected sodium} = \text{measured sodium} + [1.6 \times (\text{serum glucose} - 100)/100]$$

If serum osmolality is <300 mOsm, aim to replace the deficit over a 48-hour period. If serum osmolality is ≥300 mOsm or dehydration is >10%, aim to replace the deficit over a 48-hour period or longer. NS should be used for replacement fluids. The volume of the initial resuscitation fluid should be subtracted from the total deficit when calculating the volume that should be replaced over the following 48 hours. Ongoing fluid losses are not generally replaced unless they are excessive (urine output >4 mL/kg/hr); such losses include urine, vomiting, and Kussmaul respirations.

Potassium Total body potassium is depleted in DKA and should be added to the intravenous fluids as soon as serum potassium is <6.0 mEq/L. EKG should be obtained if potassium is less than 2.5 mEq/L. Because potassium will be driven back into cells as the acidosis resolves, timely addition of potassium will help avoid the development of life-threatening arrhythmias that can occur if hypokalemia develops with correction of the acidosis. Potassium should be added to fluids in the form of potassium phosphate, potassium chloride, or potassium acetate.

Phosphorus Total body phosphorus is also depleted in patients who present with DKA. However, symptomatic hypophosphatemia is extremely rare, and intravenous replacement of phosphorus is not routinely recommended. Phosphate supplementation may be considered if there has been a prolonged period of illness or if an extended period of fasting is anticipated. Potassium phosphate can be used along with potassium chloride in this instance to provide both potassium and phosphorus intravenously. The major risk with phosphate administration is the development of hypocalcemia and arrhythmia. Calcium levels must be monitored carefully, and if hypocalcemia develops, the phosphate infusion should be discontinued immediately. Hypocalcemia may be challenging to correct in the unusual setting of concurrent untreated hypomagnesemia.

Bicarbonate Bicarbonate level will improve with administration of insulin and fluid resuscitation. DKA is the result of increased ketogenesis due to insulin deficiency and should reverse with insulin therapy.

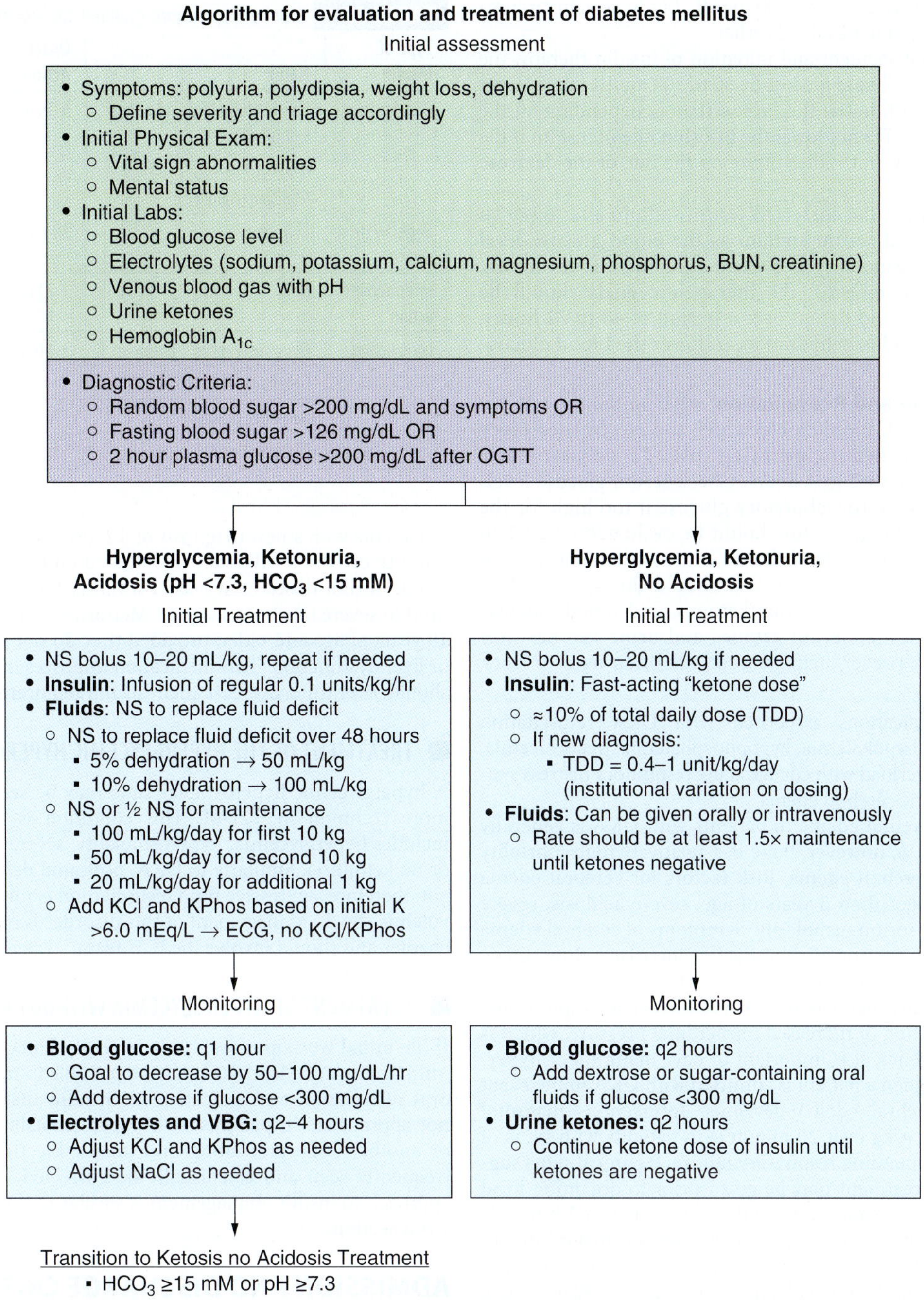

FIGURE 66-1. Algorithm for evaluation and treatment of diabetes mellitus. NS, normal saline; OGTT, oral glucose tolerance test; TDD, total daily dose.

Administration of bicarbonate is not recommended in the management of DKA and should be undertaken with extreme caution when being considered. Bicarbonate may be appropriate in certain situations, but it is important to consider that there is evidence that sudden correction of blood pH can paradoxically lower cerebrospinal fluid pH. Moreover, bicarbonate administration has been shown to be an independent risk factor for cerebral edema. It is important to recognize that endogenous production of bicarbonate will occur as ketones are metabolized once insulin is administered. As a result, the usual calculation used for the correction of acidosis will overestimate the bicarbonate required to correct acidosis in patients with DKA. The effect of bicarbonate administration on serum potassium must also be considered, and additional potassium administration may be required.

Insulin Although differentiating between T1DM and T2DM is important for long-term therapy and education, any patient with fasting hyperglycemia, ketosis, and metabolic abnormalities requires insulin therapy to reverse these derangements. Administration of insulin via an intravenous drip allows for rapid insulin action and dose adjustment. Ideally, an insulin infusion should be initiated within the first 2 hours of treatment of DKA. The initial insulin infusion rate should be 0.1 units/kg/hr. To ensure good flow of insulin into the patient, it is recommended to mix insulin with NS at a concentration of 0.1 units/mL (50 units of regular insulin in 500 mL of 0.9% NS). The insulin infusion must be regulated with a pump and should be included when calculating total fluids.

The response to insulin therapy is ultimately measured by resolution of ketosis and a rise in the serum bicarbonate level. The insulin infusion rate should be maintained until the ketosis and acidosis has markedly improved or resolved. Since insulin will lower blood sugar before resolution of the ketosis and acidosis, dextrose will need to be added to the intravenous fluids at some point to avoid a rapid decline in serum glucose or frank hypoglycemia, or both. Generally, dextrose is added to the fluids when serum glucose levels fall below 300 mg/dL, but in certain circumstances dextrose may need to be added earlier.

After initial fluid management and initiation of insulin therapy, the goal should be to decrease blood glucose by 50 to 100 mg/dL/hr. A larger decrease may be seen with initial fluid resuscitation, depending on the patient's hydration status. Do not lower the infusion rate of insulin if the glucose drops too quickly, but rather titrate up the rate of the dextrose containing fluids.

The goal is to maintain the corrected serum sodium and to see an increase in the measured serum sodium as the blood glucose level falls. If marked hyperosmolality is present (glucose >1200 mg/dL, serum osmolality >300 mOsm), the therapeutic goals should be adjusted to replace the fluid deficit over a period of 48 to 72 hours, and after an initial period of rehydration, to lower the blood glucose by 50 mg/dL/hr.

Continued Monitoring and Reevaluation After initial therapy for DKA has been instituted, monitor blood pH and electrolytes every 1 to 2 hours until the patient is improving (pH >7.3 or bicarbonate >15 mEq/L) and then every 2 to 4 hours. Check serum glucose levels every hour via finger stick (or laboratory glucose if too high for the glucose monitor). Neurologic status should be evaluated every 1 to 2 hours. Urine ketones and output should be recorded, and overall input and output reviewed frequently. One should closely track fluid balance, vital signs, electrolytes, urine ketones, and blood glucose. It is important to note that serum ketones and urine ketones may not exactly coincide; however, urine ketones are often used to track improvement in DKA.

Complications Complications associated with DKA resuscitation include hypoglycemia, hypokalemia, hypophosphatemia, hypocalcemia, hypernatremia, fluid overload with edema, acute respiratory distress syndrome, and symptomatic cerebral edema.

The incidence of cerebral edema in patients with DKA is generally reported as less than 1%; however, there is a relatively high mortality rate associated with cerebral edema. Risk factors for cerebral edema include: patients younger than 5 years of age, severe acidosis, severe dehydration, and high serum osmolarity. Symptoms of cerebral edema include any change in sensorium, headache, increased drowsiness, deepening coma, and cranial nerve abnormalities. Cushing's triad (increased blood pressure, decreased heart rate, irregular respirations) may be seen in the setting of increased intracranial pressure, which is a neurosurgical emergency. It is important to have mannitol or hypertonic saline available when a patient is admitted with DKA in the event that symptomatic cerebral edema develops. Intravenous mannitol should be given (0.5-1 g/kg over 20 minutes) in patients with signs of cerebral edema and impending respiratory failure. If clinical signs suggest cerebral edema, treatment may be given prior to obtaining head CT. If there is no initial response, it should be repeated in 2 hours. If there is concern for hypotension (and cerebral hypoperfusion) due to an osmotic diuresis that could be seen with mannitol administration or if mannitol is unavailable, 3% normal saline (5 mL/kg over 30 minutes), could be an alternative to mannitol. Intubation and ventilation may be necessary in severe DKA. Mild hypercapnea, however, should be tolerated, as aggressive hyperventilation has been associated with poor outcomes in DKA-related cerebral edema.

Transition to Subcutaneous Insulin The criteria for switching from an intravenous insulin infusion to subcutaneous insulin injections include the ability to tolerate oral intake, a normal mental status, and resolved acidosis (bicarbonate ≥15 mEq/L or pH ≥7.3). The first dose of long acting subcutaneous insulin should be given 60 minutes before stopping insulin infusion to allow sufficient time for absorption. A typical starting total daily dose of insulin for a patient with T1DM is between 0.4 and 1 units/kg/day. In general, approximately half of the total daily dose will be long acting and the other half will be short acting to cover meals. The dose and type of subcutaneous insulin varies by institution and should be taken into consideration when planning a regimen (**Table 66-1**). Treatment needs to be individualized for each patient and should be discussed with a pediatric endocrinologist. Patients with previously diagnosed diabetes can usually be started on their home insulin regimen.

TABLE 66-1 Insulin Preparations Available for Subcutaneous Therapy

Type of Insulin	Name	Onset of Action	Peak Action	Duration of Action
Rapid acting	Lispro (Humalog®, Admelog®, Lyumjev®) Aspart (NovoLog®, Fiasp®) Glulisine (Apidra®)	5-15 min	1-3 hrs	3-5 hrs
Regular/Short acting	Regular	30-60 min	2-4 hrs	5-8 hrs
Intermediate acting	NPH	1-2 hrs	4-12 hrs	10-12 hrs
Long acting	Glargine (Lantus®, Basaglar®)	3-4 hrs	None	up to 24 hrs
	Detemir (Levemir®)	1 hr	3-14 hrs	up to 24 hrs
	Degludec (Triseba®)	1 hr	None	up to 42 hrs
	Glargine U-300 (Toujeo®)	6 hrs	None	up to 36 hrs

Patients with a new diagnosis of T2DM who present with a hemoglobin A1c of ≥8.5% will likely be initiated on insulin therapy and require initial insulin doses of at least 1 unit/kg/day, as they will demonstrate mild to severe insulin resistance. Metformin can also be used in patients 10 years of age and older, provided they do not have significant kidney or liver dysfunction. This medication improves insulin sensitivity, which should, over time, decrease their insulin requirement.

TREATMENT OF THE HYPERGLYCEMIC HYPEROSMOLAR STATE

A hyperglycemic hyperosmolar state may be seen in T1DM, although more common in T2DM. This condition is rare and presentation includes hyperglycemia, hyperosmolality, severe dehydration, and little or no ketonuria. Similarly to DKA, profound dehydration is often present; therefore, aggressive fluid resuscitation is imperative to avoid hypovolemic shock. Management of this disorder is outside the scope of this chapter and should involve the ICU team.

TREATMENT OF HYPERGLYCEMIA WITHOUT ACIDOSIS

If the initial workup reveals only hyperglycemia or hyperglycemia with mild to moderate ketosis, it may be possible to manage the patient with oral rehydration and subcutaneous insulin therapy. This approach is not appropriate in patients with hyperosmolality, nausea or vomiting, or another issue precluding oral intake. Electrolyte imbalance is less frequently seen and can usually be corrected with oral therapy. The approach to insulin management is similar to that described in the previous section.

ADMISSION AND DISCHARGE CRITERIA

ADMISSION CRITERIA

- Hyperglycemia accompanied by ketosis and acidosis
- Altered mental status
- Any patient receiving insulin who is unable to tolerate sufficient oral intake to prevent hypoglycemia and dehydration
- Pediatric patients with newly diagnosed diabetes requiring initiation of insulin therapy if intensive education is not immediately available on an outpatient basis

DISCHARGE CRITERIA

- Normal electrolytes and hydration status
- Ability to tolerate oral intake
- It is not necessary to obtain perfect glucose control before discharge; insulin doses will require adjustments after discharge and on an ongoing basis.

- For a patient being discharged on insulin therapy, it is necessary to ensure that the family has been educated regarding the following:
  - Definition and pathophysiology of the different types of diabetes
  - Insulin action
  - Signs and symptoms of hypoglycemia
  - Treatment of hypoglycemia and use of glucagon
  - Proper technique in using the glucometer
  - Proper technique in drawing up and administering insulin
  - Consequences of poor glycemic control
- Follow-up should be arranged with a pediatric endocrinologist as an outpatient. Access to medications should be discussed with patients and their caregivers.

CONSULTATIONS

- Pediatric endocrinology
- Pediatric critical care, as needed
- Pediatric neurosurgery, as needed

SPECIAL CONSIDERATIONS

COMORBIDITIES

Patients with T1DM are at increased risk for other autoimmune disorders such as hypothyroidism and celiac disease. Patients with T2DM are at increased risk for nonalcoholic steatohepatitis and dyslipidemia. Patients with known diabetes should have screening for these comorbidities, in addition to annual urine microalbumin screen and dilated retinal exam to detect nephropathy and retinopathy respectively.

PREVENTION

Prevention of T1DM is currently being studied but there is no current knowledge to prevent development of T1DM. For patients with T1DM, the main focus is on prevention of complications from T1DM with tight glycemic control. Dietary recommendations include an energy distribution of 45% to 55% carbohydrate, 30% to 35% fat, and 15% to 20% protein. Some patients incorporate carbohydrate restrictive diets. There is theoretical concern for inadequate bone mineralization and poor linear growth thus close surveillance of growth patterns is vital in patients adhering to a low carbohydrate diet.

Prevention of T2DM involves lifestyle modifications such as dietary alterations and increased exercise to induce weight loss. Bariatric surgery can prevent progression of and reverse metabolic syndrome and T2DM, and has shown successful results in adolescents with severe obesity and type 2 diabetes.

NEW THERAPIES

Several newer drugs that were initially approved for use in adults with type 2 have proven beneficial to the pediatric population. Glucagon like peptide (GLP-1) medications increase insulin output as well as decrease appetite and delay gastric emptying. Weight loss is commonly reported. Sodium-glucose like co-transporter 2 inhibitors (SGLT2) are T2DM medications that block glucose reabsorption in the kidneys. Patients on these medications are at higher risk for genitourinary infections.

Hybrid closed loop insulin delivery systems utilize data from a patient's continuous glucose monitor to adjust basal insulin delivery from an insulin pump. This system has shown to be successful in children with reported improvement in quality of life by patients' parents and caregivers. Investigational therapies for type 1 diabetes include immunomodulators, improved islet transplantation techniques, and stem cell differentiation.

KEY POINTS

- Hyperglycemia can present in the inpatient setting and may be a result of type 1 (autoimmune) diabetes mellitus, type 2 diabetes mellitus, illness, sepsis, or drug effects.
- History should note presence of polyuria, polydipsia, polyphagia, and weight loss.
- The presence or absence of ketosis and acidosis at initial presentation does not necessarily differentiate type 1 from type 2 diabetes.
- Physical examination should focus on vital signs, neurologic status, and clinical signs of dehydration during initial evaluation of a patient with hyperglycemia.
- Management of patients with DKA is individualized and aimed at correcting the underlying insulin deficiency, ketosis, and acidosis, as well as replacing the fluid deficit over a 48-hour period or longer if clinically indicated.

SUGGESTED READINGS

Alemzadeh R, Ali O. Diabetes mellitus in children. In: Kliegman RM, Stanton BF, St. Gemel III JW, et al., eds. *Nelson Textbook of Pediatrics*. 19th ed. Philadelphia, PA: Elsevier Saunders; 2011: 1968-1997.

Copeland KC, Silverstein J, Moore KR, et al. Management of newly diagnosed type 2 diabetes mellitus (T2DM) in children and adolescents. *Pediatrics*. 2013;131(2):364-382.

Glaser N, Barnett P, McCaslin I, et al. Risk factors for cerebral edema in children with diabetic ketoacidosis. *N Engl J Med*. 2001;344(4): 264-269.

Inge T, et al. Comparison of surgical and medical therapy for type 2 diabetes in severely obese adolescents. *JAMA Pediatr*. 2018;172(5): 452-460.

Lawrence JM, et al; SEARCH for Diabetes in Youth Study Group. Trends in prevalence of type 1 and Type 2 diabetes in children and adolescents in the US, 2001-2017. *JAMA*. 2021 Aug 24;326(8): 717-727.

Majidi S, Maahs DM. Update on care of children with type 1 diabetes. *Adv Pediatr*. 2012;59(1):303-327.

Majidi S, Maahs DM. Update on care of children with type 1 diabetes. *Adv Pediatr*. 2012;59(1):303-327.

Prevent Type 2 Diabetes in Kids. Center for Disease Control and Prevention. August 10, 2021. https://www.cdc.gov/diabetes/prevent-type-2/type-2-kids.html.

Soto-Rivera CL, Asaro LA, Agus MS, DeCourcey DD. Suspected cerebral edema in diabetic ketoacidosis: is there still a role for head CT in treatment decisions? *Pediatr Crit Care Med*. 2017;18(3): 207-212.

Tamborlane W, et al. Liraglutide in children and adolescents with type 2 diabetes. *N Engl J Med*. 2019;381:637-646.

Tauschmann M, et al; KidsAP Consortium. Home use of day-and-night hybrid closed-loop insulin delivery in very young children: a multicenter, 3-week, randomized trial. *Diabetes Care*. 2019;42(4): 594-600.

Wolfsdorf J, Craig ME, Daneman D, et al. ISPAD clinical practice consensus guidelines 2009 compendium: diabetic ketoacidosis in children and adolescents with diabetes. *Pediatr Diabetes*. 2009; 10(Suppl 12):118-133.

Writing Group for the SEARCH for Diabetes in Youth Study Group. Incidence of diabetes in youth in the United States. *JAMA*. 2007; 297(24):2716-24.

Zeitler P, Haqq A, Rosenbloom A, Glaser N. Hyperglycemic hyperosmolar syndrome in children: pathophysiological considerations and suggested guidelines for treatment. *J Pediatr*. 2011;158(1):9-14.

CHAPTER 67

Disorders of Thyroid Hormone

Anuradha Pavuluri, MD and Lauren A. Wagner, DO

BACKGROUND

Thyroid hormone has many effects on the human body. It plays an essential role in growth and development; thermogenesis; oxygen consumption; and the metabolism of carbohydrates, lipids, and proteins. Although thyroid hormone is essential for the normal function of many tissues, thyroid dysfunction is frequently insidious and may be missed.

The hypothalamic-pituitary-thyroid axis is finely tuned to maintain stable levels of thyroid hormone. Thyrotropin-releasing hormone (TRH) is produced in the hypothalamus and stimulates the production and secretion of thyroid-stimulating hormone (TSH) by the anterior pituitary gland. Through binding of the thyroid-stimulating hormone receptor (TSHR), TSH leads to production and release of both thyroid hormones, thyroxine (T_4) and triiodothyroxine (T_3), as well as thyroid cell growth. Thyroid hormones feedback on the anterior pituitary and hypothalamus, decreasing secretion of TSH and TRH, respectively, allowing for tight regulation of thyroid hormone concentrations. The predominant form of hormone secreted by the thyroid is T_4, which is converted peripherally to the metabolically active hormone T_3, which exerts its effects by binding to nuclear receptors and influencing DNA transcription.

The majority of thyroid hormone circulates bound to thyroid-binding globulin (TBG) and other serum proteins. The unbound (free) hormones are the metabolically active forms.

The maturity level of the hypothalamic-pituitary-thyroid axis must be considered to correctly interpret thyroid function tests in newborns and children. At birth, an acute surge in TSH occurs in response to the cold extrauterine environment, followed by a rapid decline over 24 hours and slower decline over the next 5 days. This TSH surge causes a rise in T_4 and T_3 with a subsequent slower decline of T_4 and T_3 over the next 2 weeks. During childhood, there is a progressive decrease in TSH and thyroid hormone levels until adult levels are reached around 15 to 16 years (**Table 67-1**).

HYPOTHYROIDISM

CLINICAL PRESENTATION

Congenital Hypothyroidism The prevalence of congenital hypothyroidism is approximately 1 in 2000 newborns and is one of the leading causes of preventable intellectual disability. Most cases are due to abnormal formation of the thyroid gland (dysgenesis), while some are due to defective thyroid hormone synthesis (dyshormonogenesis). Placental transfer of maternal thyroid hormone protects the developing fetus. Despite the implementation of newborn screen in the 1970s, congenital hypothyroidism should remain as a differential diagnosis for any neonate presenting with symptoms of lethargy, difficulty feeding, constipation, hoarse cry, or prolonged jaundice. Physical exam may show protuberant abdomen, goiter, pallor, hypothermia, coarse facial features, hypotonia, edema (especially eyelids, hands, and feet), and macrosomia. Widely open anterior and posterior fontanelles at birth may be the first clues to recognizing congenital hypothyroidism.

Acquired Hypothyroidism Hashimoto thyroiditis (chronic lymphocytic thyroiditis or autoimmune thyroiditis) is the most common cause of acquired hypothyroidism in children. The child may be euthyroid, hypothyroid, or transiently hyperthyroid at initial presentation. Children may have neck swelling, dry skin, fatigue, constipation, cold intolerance, dyslipidemia, or menstrual irregularities. Seventy percent to 80% of children with hypothyroidism will present with a goiter, which is typically symmetric, firm, and nontender. Other exam findings include bradycardia, proximal muscle weakness, delayed deep tendon reflexes, and growth failure (**Figure 67-1**). Hypothyroidism produces poor linear growth with preservation of normal weight gain, leading children to be overweight for their height, however, hypothyroidism generally does not cause obesity.

Autoimmune hypothyroidism has a female predominance and 25% of patients will have a positive family history of autoimmune thyroid disease. It can be associated with other autoimmune disorders, including type 1 diabetes mellitus, autoimmune polyglandular syndromes, primary adrenal insufficiency (Addison disease), vitiligo, and celiac disease. Autoimmune thyroiditis is also more common in patients with certain chromosomal disorders, such as Down syndrome, Turner syndrome, and Klinefelter's syndrome.

DIFFERENTIAL DIAGNOSIS

Congenital Hypothyroidism Congenital hypothyroidism can be permanent or transient. It is classified as primary, when due to an inherent defect of the thyroid gland or thyroid hormone production or secretion; or secondary (central), when due to defects in the pituitary/hypothalamus. Eighty-five percent of primary congenital hypothyroidism is caused by thyroid gland dysgenesis. The gland may be ectopically located, hypoplastic, or absent. Iodine deficiency is an important cause of congenital hypothyroidism, however, is rare in developed countries. Isolated TSH deficiency is very rare and central congenital hypothyroidism occurs more commonly in the presence of other pituitary deficiencies.

Transient congenital hypothyroidism is rare and can be caused antithyroid medications taken by the mother during pregnancy that cross the placenta, inhibiting fetal thyroid hormone production. Generally, neonatal hypothyroidism induced by maternal medication resolves within 1 to 2 weeks. Other causes of transient congenital hypothyroidism include maternal iodine deficiency or excess, pre- or postnatal exposure to radioactive iodine, and maternal TSH receptor-blocking antibodies that cross the placenta and block thyroid hormone production in the fetus/neonate.

TABLE 67-1 Normal Values for Thyroid Function Tests

Age	TSH (μU/mL)	T_4 (μg/dL)	Free T_4 (ng/dL)	T_3 (ng/dL)	Reverse T_3 (ng/dL)
Premature infants (26-32 wk): 3-4 days of life	0.8-6.9 (2.3)	2.6-14.0 (6.4)	0.4-2.8 (1.5)	24-132 (65)	
Full-term infants: 1-3 days of life		8.2-20.0 (14.6)		89-405 (273)	90-250+
Full-term infants: 3-7 days of life	1.3-16.0 (4.9)	6.0-15.9 (12.0)	2.0-4.9 (3.5)	91-300 (190)	
1-12 mo of life	0.9-7.7 (2.9)	6.1-14.9 (9.8)	0.9-2.6 (1.6)	82-250 (175)	
Prepubertal	0.6-5.5 (1.9)	1-3 yr: 6.8-13.5 (9.3)	0.8-2.2 (1.6)	119-218 (168)	10-50
		3-10 yr: 5.5-12.8 (8.6)			
Pubertal	0.5-4.8 (1.6)	4.9-13.0 (8.0)	0.8-2.3 (1.5)	80-185 (116)	10-50

Source: Adapted with permission from Expected Values & S.I. Unit Conversion Tables. Laboratory Corporation of America Holdings; 2021.

TSH, thyroid-stimulating hormone; T_3, triiodothyronine; T_4, thyroxine.

*Range of values, with mean in parentheses.

†Levels decline to the adult range by 1 wk of life.

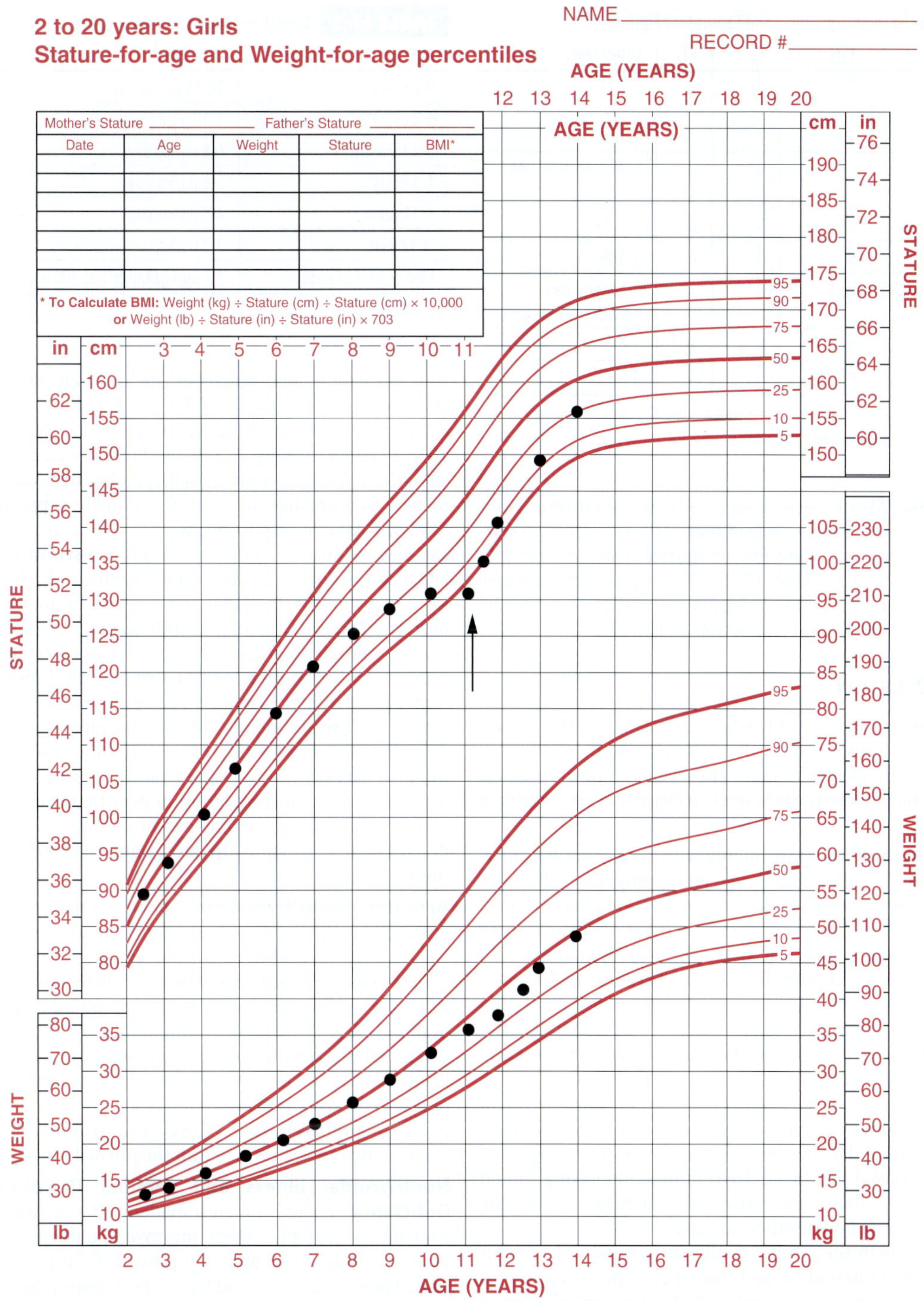

FIGURE 67-1. Growth chart demonstrating growth failure from undiagnosed hypothyroidism. Although weight remains relatively stable, linear growth slows significantly, and the girl eventually has declining height percentiles. Catch-up growth occurs with initiation of levothyroxine treatment (arrow). (Developed by the National Center for Health Statistics in collaboration with the National Center for Chronic Disease Prevention and Health Promotion; 2000. http://www.cdc.gov/growthcharts.)

Acquired Hypothyroidism Acquired hypothyroidism is also classified as primary or secondary. Hashimoto, or autoimmune, hypothyroidism, is the most common cause of primary acquired hypothyroidism. Other causes include radiation to the neck, and surgical resection of the thyroid gland for treatment of Graves disease or thyroid cancer. Certain medications can also induce hypothyroidism. Drugs that downregulate the release of TSH from the pituitary include glucocorticoids and dopamine. Glucocorticoids also inhibit the peripheral conversion of T_4 to T_3. Drugs that affect thyroid hormone synthesis and release include amiodarone (which contains iodine), iodine, and lithium. Although iodine is essential for proper thyroid function, it can block the release of preformed thyroid hormone and synthesis of new hormone. Lithium carbonate inhibits thyroid hormone release. Antiepileptic medications, particularly phenytoin, phenobarbitone, and carbamazepine, increase hepatic metabolism of thyroxine, which can result in low levels of total T_4 with normal TSH and T_3 levels.

Central hypothyroidism should be suspected in children with a history of central nervous system disease, such as hydrocephalus, hemorrhage, brain tumor, meningitis, head injury, traumatic delivery, or central nervous system malformations. In any patient with central hypothyroidism, it is important to investigate pituitary hormone deficiencies.

Thyroid-Binding Globulin Deficiency Thyroid-binding globulin deficiency is an X-linked condition that is characterized by low total T_4, normal TSH, and normal FT_4.

TABLE 67-2 Causes of Hypothyroidism and Laboratory Findings

	TSH	T_4	FT_4	Other tests
Primary hypothyroidism (e.g. dysgenesis, agenesis, dyshormonogenesis]	↑	↓	↓	
Autoimmune [Hashimoto] thyroiditis	↑	↓	↓	+ TPO-Ab +TBG-Ab
Subclinical hypothyroidism	slightly↑	N	N	
TBG deficiency	N	↓	N	↓TBG
Central hypothyroidism	N, ↓	↓	↓	Other pituitary hormone deficiencies
Sick euthyroid syndrome	N, ↓	N, ↓	N, ↓	↓T_3
Resistance to thyroid hormone	N, ↑	↑	↑	↑T_3

FT_4 = free thyroxine; T_3 = total triiodothyronine; T_4 = total thyroxine, TBG-Ab = thyroid-binding globulin antibodies, TPO-Ab = thyroid peroxidase antibodies.

Nonthyroidal Illness Also known as sick euthyroid syndrome, nonthyroidal illness (NTI) is seen in severely ill patients and in states of starvation. Patients will commonly have low or normal TSH, low total T_4 and T_3, and normal or high FT_4 **(Table 67-2).** Multiple mechanisms may give rise to these changes, including suppression of TSH secretion by cytokines and decreased peripheral conversion of T_4 to T_3.

DIAGNOSTIC EVALUATION

An elevated TSH in the presence of low T_4 is consistent with primary hypothyroidism. In subclinical primary hypothyroidism, there will be a mildly elevated TSH with normal T_4 levels. However, a child with central hypothyroidism can have a low, normal, or even elevated TSH combined with low T_4 levels.

Congenital Hypothyroidism Most infants with congenital hypothyroidism are identified through newborn screening programs. The newborn screen is based on the measurement of either T_4 or TSH (or both) between 2 and 5 days of life. There are advantages and disadvantages to either a T_4 or TSH screening approach. If T_4 is measured, infants with a T_4 level below a specific cutoff point have their TSH measured as well. This method can miss subclinical hypothyroidism (i.e., normal T_4 but elevated TSH levels). Primary screening with TSH has a higher false-positive rate owing to the early screening (before 2 days of life) and it also misses infants with central hypothyroidism.

When the newborn screen reports abnormal thyroid tests, the infant should be seen and examined immediately, and serum confirmatory testing should be obtained. The newborn screen should not be repeated as that can result in delayed treatment. Thyroid function testing should include TSH and FT_4. A pediatric endocrinologist can help to determine the utility of thyroid ultrasound or other imaging.

Low thyroid hormone in the setting of a low or normal TSH level is suggestive of central hypothyroidism and should prompt evaluation for hypopituitarism. It is important to identify if there is central adrenal insufficiency, and if detected, cortisol must be adequately replaced prior to initiating thyroid hormone replacement. Thyroid hormone supplementation increases cortisol clearance from the circulation and could precipitate adrenal crisis with cardiovascular collapse in patients with adrenal insufficiency.

Acquired Hypothyroidism Evaluation of older children with suspected acquired hypothyroidism should include a TSH and FT_4. Diagnosis of autoimmune hypothyroidism can be confirmed by identifying Thyroid peroxidase antibodies (TPO-Ab) and/or Thyroglobulin antibodies (Tg-Ab). Thyroid imaging in acquired hypothyroidism is not usually warranted unless a nodule is present.

MANAGEMENT

Congenital Hypothyroidism The goal of treatment for congenital hypothyroidism is to adequately replace thyroid hormone as early as possible to maximize the chances for normal neurologic development.

TABLE 67-3 Levothyroxine Dosing

Age	Oral Dose*
0-3 months	10-15 μg/kg/day
3-6 months	8-10 μg/kg/day
6-12 months	6-8 μg/kg/day
1-5 years	5-6 μg/kg/day
6-12 years	4-5 μg/kg/day
> 12 years	2-3 μg/kg/day
Post-pubertal/adult	1.7 μg/kg/day or 100-200 μg/day (average adult dose)

*Intravenous dose is 50% of oral dose.

Neurodevelopmental outcomes are inversely related to age at start of treatment. Levothyroxine (T_4) is the first line of treatment for all children with hypothyroidism. The starting dose for newborns is generally 10 to 15 μg/kg (usually 37.5-50 μg/day) once daily, however optimization should occur with pediatric endocrinologist guidance. The goal of treatment is to normalize the T_4 level as quickly as possible, recognizing that TSH will take longer to normalize. Overtreatment with levothyroxine can lead to advanced bone age and craniosynostosis. For infants with a late diagnosis of congenital hypothyroidism who have been hypothyroid for 2 to 3 months, it is advisable to work up to a full replacement dose over 1 to 2 weeks to avoid precipitating rapid mobilization of fluid.

Levothyroxine can be given as a crushed tablet in a small amount of formula, breast milk, or water or by liquid formulation. During the first 3 years of life, T_4 should be kept in the upper half of the reference range. AAP recommends clinical and biochemical monitoring at 2 to 4 weeks following levothyroxine initiation; every 1 to 2 months for 6 months; every 3 to 4 months from 6 months to 3 years; then every 6 to 12 months until completion of growth. Given the risk of neurologic damage, careful and ongoing parental counseling is essential to decrease nonadherence, which is the most common cause of elevated TSH during treatment.

Acquired Hypothyroidism The treatment for primary or central acquired hypothyroidism is also levothyroxine, which is dosed based on weight and age (**Table 67-3**). For younger children, liquid or crushed tablets may be given mixed with a small amount of liquid or food. Absorption of levothyroxine is greatest on an empty stomach, however higher doses can be used to compensate for any decrease in absorption due to taking it with a meal. Consistency of time of administration is key to identifying the optimal dose. Iron, calcium supplements, and soy products decrease the absorption of levothyroxine and should be administered at a different time. The goal of treatment is to keep TSH within age specific range and T_4 within the normal range.

Nonthyroidal Illness and Familial Thyroid-Binding Globulin Deficiency There is no clear evidence that treatment of NTI with thyroid hormone replacement improves outcomes. Consultation with a pediatric endocrinologist may prove helpful for any diagnostic confusion. These patients should have repeat thyroid function tests when they are well. Treatment is not indicated in familial thyroid-binding globulin deficiency.

HYPERTHYROIDISM

CLINICAL PRESENTATION

Neonatal Hyperthyroidism Neonatal thyrotoxicosis (neonatal Graves disease) is a rare disorder, occurring in approximately 1% to 10% of pregnancies affected by maternal Graves disease (autoimmune hyperthyroidism). It is caused by transplacental passage of TSH receptor-stimulating immunoglobulins (TSIs) leading to increased thyroid hormone production in the fetus. The hyperthyroid state persists until maternal antibodies are cleared from the infant's circulation in 3 to 12 weeks. Clinical symptoms in the neonate are variable and may not occur until several days after birth due to antithyroid medications taken by the mother during pregnancy. Neonates may present with low birth weight, heart failure, hypertension, irritability, tachycardia, jaundice, poor weight gain, poor sleep, diarrhea, frontal bossing, hepatosplenomegaly, goiter, and/or thrombocytopenia. Affected infants need to admission to an intensive care unit for close monitoring of vital signs and frequent thyroid labs, as neonatal hyperthyroidism can result in high-output cardiac failure and death. Long-term untreated hyperthyroidism can lead to craniosynostosis, developmental delay, hyperactivity, poor growth, and/or behavior issues.

Graves Disease The most common cause of hyperthyroidism in children is Graves disease (autoimmune hyperthyroidism), occurring in 1:10,000 children in the United States. There is a female predominance and peak incidence is during adolescence. In Graves disease, TSIs mimic TSH function which leads to the overproduction and secretion of thyroid hormone. The etiology is thought to be a combination of genetics, immunity, and environmental factors. Due to the symptoms being insidious and nonspecific combined with the rarity of the disorder often result in a delay in diagnosis. Children may present with fatigue, weight loss, palpitations, headache, mood disturbance, behavioral issues, hyperactivity, anxiety, increased bowel movements without diarrhea, irritability, and difficulty sleeping. Parents may report that their child has deteriorating school performance and decreased concentration. Increased growth may lead to bone age acceleration. In severe cases this can result in delayed puberty and menstruation changes. On examination, the thyroid is generally diffusely enlarged, smooth without nodules, and may have a thyroid bruit. The patient may have tachycardia, hypertension, hyperreflexia, or a fine tremor. Ophthalmopathy (thyroid eye disease) may occur in children, but less commonly than in adults and tends to remit more often when the patient becomes euthyroid.

Thyroid Storm This is an extremely rare medical emergency in children. It consists of acute hyperthermia, tachycardia, and encephalopathy in a patient with hyperthyroidism. Multiorgan failure including heart failure can result. It progresses rapidly and should be cared for in an intensive care unit. Thyroid storm may be precipitated by infection, surgery, nonadherence with antithyroid medications, radioactive iodine therapy, and/or acute illness.

DIFFERENTIAL DIAGNOSIS

Other causes of hyperthyroidism in childhood and adolescence include autonomously functioning thyroid nodules, infections of the thyroid, McCune–Albright syndrome, gain of function TSHR mutations, TSH secreting adenoma, and toxic multinodular goiters. Hashimoto thyroiditis may have a hyperthyroid phase during destruction of the thyroid gland resulting in release of pre-formed thyroid hormone and transient hyperthyroidism. Drugs that can cause hyperthyroidism include amiodarone, iodine, and ingestion of exogenous thyroid hormone.

DIAGNOSTIC EVALUATION

Neonatal Hyperthyroidism Laboratory evaluation shows low TSH, elevated T_4, FT_4, and T_3. Also seen are elevated TSIs which slowly resolve by 3 months of age. All infants born to mothers with Graves disease or history of Graves disease should be screened at delivery, 3 to 5 days of life, and 10 to 14 days of life.

Graves Disease Low TSH and elevated T_4 and T_3 levels are consistent with primary hyperthyroidism. The initial laboratory tests should include serum TSH, FT_4 or total T_4, and total T_3 levels. Measurements of TSIs should be obtained to confirm the diagnosis of Graves disease. A radionucleotide uptake scan may be necessary to distinguish Hashimoto thyroiditis from Graves. Exophthalmos is seen in Graves but not in Hashimoto's. Imaging, such as thyroid ultrasound, is generally not indicated unless there is a nodule present or asymmetric gland.

MANAGEMENT

Neonatal Hyperthyroidism Given the risk of cardiac failure and death, treatment for neonatal thyrotoxicosis should be initiated as soon as possible. Methimazole, an antithyroid medication that blocks the production of thyroid hormone is the first-line agent for treatment of neonatal hyperthyroidism. Propranolol should be administered to treat sympathetic hyperactivity. In severe cases, a saturated potassium iodide solution or Lugol iodide solution may be used to decrease thyroid hormone production more swiftly. If heart failure develops, Digoxin or glucocorticoids may be needed. Frequent monitoring of thyroid levels is essential. As the TSIs are cleared from the infant's circulation, the antithyroid medications and propranolol can be weaned and are typically discontinued after 3 months once the TSIs are no longer detectable.

Graves Disease The first-line treatment for Graves disease in children and adolescents is the antithyroid drug methimazole. Use of propylthiouracil (PTU) is avoided due to the association with acute liver failure. These medications inhibit thyroid hormone formation but not its release, so it may take several weeks until circulating thyroid hormone levels begin to decrease. A beta-blocker may be added to control tachycardia and ameliorate symptoms while the antithyroid medications take effect. Thyroid levels, including TSH, T_4, and T_3, should be checked 2 weeks after starting therapy, and monthly once on a stable dose and euthyroid. Severe side effects of methimazole include agranulocytosis, hepatitis, vasculitis, lupus-like syndrome, and liver failure. Children with ophthalmopathy should be referred to a pediatric ophthalmologist.

Remission rates for Graves disease are lower in children than in adults. Given the difficulty of maintaining compliance and the risk of side effects from antithyroid drug therapy, definitive therapy can be pursued if remission is not achieved within 12 to 24 months or sooner if methimazole cannot be tolerated. With the goal of inducing a permanent hypothyroid state, definitive therapy consists of either radioiodine ablation or surgical removal of the thyroid gland. Radioiodine ablation is a safe and effective treatment in children older than 5 years, with long-term studies showing no evidence of decreased fertility or increased malignancy rates. Thyroidectomy is generally recommended for younger children (<10 years), those with large glands, or those with severe eye disease.

Thyroid Storm Treatment of thyroid storm includes: glucocorticoids for reduction of conversion of T_4 to T_3, Lugo solution to decrease release of T_4, and beta blockade for tachycardia. Methimazole or PTU are also used for anti-thyroid hormone formation properties. Aggressive cooling and supportive measures will also be needed.

ADMISSION AND DISCHARGE CRITERIA

ADMISSION CRITERIA

- Neonatal thyrotoxicosis
- Thyroid storm
- Congenital hypothyroidism or severe hypothyroidism in an older child if there is concern for adherence to medication administration.

DISCHARGE CRITERIA

- Resolution of acute symptoms of neonatal thyrotoxicosis or thyroid storm and improving thyroid function tests on medication.
- Patient/family comprehension of proper dosing and administration of medication.

CONSULTATION

Most often, thyroid disorders are diagnosed and managed in the outpatient setting. Interpretation of thyroid function tests obtained on a hospitalized pediatric patient during period of illness can be challenging. A pediatric endocrinologist should always be consulted for patients with possible thyroid storm or infants with suspected neonatal thyrotoxicosis.

PREVENTION

Congenital hypothyroidism is the most common preventable cause of intellectual disability. Early recognition and initiation of treatment leads to better neurologic outcomes. Therefore, it is essential that newborn screens are promptly followed up, to confirm and initiate treatment of hypothyroidism.

KEY POINTS

- Congenital hypothyroidism is a preventable cause of intellectual disability, and early initiation of treatment with levothyroxine improves neurodevelopmental outcomes.
- Autoimmune hypothyroidism is the most common cause of acquired hypothyroidism.
- Neonatal hyperthyroidism is a rare but potentially fatal disorder which requires close monitoring and rapid initiation of treatment.
- Methimazole is the first-line agent for treating Graves disease. PTU is no longer recommended, given its association with severe liver failure.
- Illness may produce thyroid abnormalities, known as nonthyroidal illness; there is no evidence to support treating this condition in children.

SUGGESTED READINGS

Alarcon G, Figueredo V, Tarkoff J. Thyroid disorders. *Pediat Rev.* 2021;42(11):604-618.

Counts D, Varma SK. Hypothyroidism in children. *Pediat Rev.* 2009;30(7):251-258.

Diaz A, Lipman Diaz EG. Hypothyroidism. *Pediat Rev.* 2014;35(8):336–349.

Srinivasan S, Misra M. Hyperthyroidism in children. *Pediat Rev.* 2015; 36(6):239-248.

CHAPTER 68 Disorders of Pituitary Function

Emilee Colella Lewis, MD and Jennifer Fuchs, MD

BACKGROUND

The pituitary gland coordinates endocrine functions including growth, sexual development and function, thyroid function, stress response, and salt and water balance in the body. The pituitary gland is located in the sella turcica below the optic chiasm, just outside the brain dura, and is comprised of two parts with distinct embryologic origins. The hypothalamus sends signals to the pituitary gland, which then releases hormones that regulate endocrine target organs, such as the adrenal gland, ovary, testis, and thyroid gland. Disorders of the pituitary and hypothalamus result in disruption of these hypothalamic-pituitary-target organ axes. Dysfunction of the endocrine target organ itself is considered "primary," abnormalities in end-organ hormone release caused by pituitary dysfunction are considered "secondary," and those caused by a hypothalamic abnormality are considered "tertiary." Pituitary disorders may be genetic or acquired and in children commonly present as failure of growth and sexual maturation.

Pituitary function is dependent on the hypothalamus which secretes releasing factors that travel via the portal circulation to the anterior pituitary gland and include growth-hormone releasing hormone (GHRH), thyrotropin-releasing hormone (TRH), corticotropin-releasing hormone (CRH), and gonadotropin releasing hormone (GnRH). These factors stimulate or inhibit release of the six peptide hormones produced by the five distinct cell types of the anterior pituitary gland: (i) growth hormone (GH) from somatotropes, (ii) prolactin by lactotropes, (iii) thyroid-stimulating hormone (TSH) from the thyrotropes, (iv) adrenocorticotropic hormone (ACTH) via corticotropes, and (v) follicle-stimulating hormone (FSH), and (vi) luteinizing hormone (LH), secreted by gonadotropes.

The posterior pituitary gland releases arginine vasopressin, also known as antidiuretic hormone (ADH), and oxytocin. The neurons that produce vasopressin originate in the paraventricular and supraoptic nuclei of the hypothalamus. For this reason, diabetes insipidus (DI) can occur with hypothalamic disease, but may not always occur with pituitary disease, even if the stalk has been transected (depending on the level of transection). This chapter will review genetic and acquired causes of hypopituitarism, anterior pituitary dysfunction, central diabetes insipidus, and syndrome of inappropriate antidiuretic hormone secretion.

CLINICAL PRESENTATION

GENETIC CAUSES OF HYPOPITUITARISM

Hypopituitarism is defined as the decreased or absent secretion of pituitary hormones and can result from defects in the pituitary gland or the hypothalamus. There are several genetic causes of pituitary hormone deficiency including mutations integral to the embryonic development of the pituitary; however, these mutations account for less than 20% of hypopituitarism. Congenital malformations involving the midline of the central nervous system (CNS) are associated with pituitary deficiencies. Midline defects elsewhere may alert clinicians to screen for pituitary deficiency (e.g., single central incisor, cleft lip and palate, tracheo-esophageal fistula, omphalocele and gastroschisis, and exstrophy of the bladder). In the newborn, pituitary deficiency may present as fasting hypoglycemia (due to GH and/or ACTH deficiency), micropenis (combination of GH and gonadotropin deficiency), or unconjugated hyperbilirubinemia. Septo-optic-dysplasia, with optic nerve hypoplasia, is often associated with pituitary deficiencies as is holoprosencephaly and absence of the septum pellucidum. Findings on magnetic resonance imaging may include a small or absent anterior pituitary gland, an absent or ectopic posterior pituitary "bright spot," or a transected pituitary stalk.

ACQUIRED CAUSES OF HYPOPITUITARISM

Mass-occupying lesions in the hypothalamic area may result in disruption of pituitary function. Tumors such as craniopharyngiomas and, less commonly, germinomas and astrocytomas may first present during childhood with growth failure, DI, and/or visual complaints. Even in cases when the tumor does not cause loss of pituitary function, surgery or radiation may result in panhypopituitarism. Higher doses of radiation may precipitate precocious pubertal development. Hypothalamic hamartomas and pineal tumors are associated with precocious pubertal development during childhood. Pituitary adenomas are rare in childhood and may or may not actively produce peptide hormones. When active, they most often secrete prolactin (50%) or GH (20%).

Langerhans cell histiocytosis is a rare disorder that most often presents with DI, but it may also affect the production of other pituitary hormones. Inflammatory, postinfectious, and traumatic lesions of the CNS may cause hypopituitarism as well.

Clinical signs of pituitary deficiency in children include poor linear growth (GH deficiency), fatigue and malaise (TSH and ACTH deficiency), delayed pubertal development, amenorrhea, or sexual dysfunction (LH and FSH deficiency), hypotension or hypoglycemia (ACTH deficiency). Inability to regulate temperature, appetite, thirst, and vital signs may be seen in hypothalamic dysfunction. Signs of central nervous system lesions, including headaches, vision changes, and other neurological disturbances, may be seen.

ANTERIOR PITUITARY HORMONE DYSFUNCTION

DIAGNOSTIC EVALUATION

Diagnosis of anterior pituitary dysfunction typically requires a combination of random hormone measurements and stimulation tests with known secretagogues specific for the pituitary hormone in question.

TSH deficiency can be diagnosed by observing low thyroid hormone (T4) with low or inappropriately normal TSH levels (distinguished from primary hypothyroidism in which TSH is elevated). See chapter 67, Disorders of Thyroid Hormone, for more information.

Random GH measurements can be diagnostic in the newborn period prior to establishment of the diurnal and pulsatile secretion pattern at

2 to 4 weeks of life. Levels greater than 20 ng/mL are unequivocally sufficient. After this point, or when the diagnosis is not clear, stimulation tests must be performed. Commonly used secretagogues include arginine, clonidine, and glucagon; insulin-induced hypoglycemia was considered a gold standard but is rarely used due to safety concerns. Stimulated growth hormone peaks >10 ng/mL are normal.

Diagnosis of gonadotropin deficiency can be made in the first 6 months for males and before 2 to 3 years of life for females when the gonadotropin axis is active by measuring random LH and FSH.

Secondary or tertiary adrenal insufficiency is diagnosed by observing ACTH and cortisol rise after administration of CRH. See chapter 70, Disorders of the Adrenal Gland, for more information.

MANAGEMENT

Treatment of anterior pituitary deficiency consists of replacement of the pituitary or target gland hormone. Levothyroxine is used for thyroid hormone replacement, growth hormone for GH deficiency, and testosterone or estrogen (usually during puberty, though testosterone may be given in neonates to correct micropenis) for gonadotropin deficiency. In primary adrenal insufficiency, both glucocorticoids and mineralocorticoid replacement are required. However, in secondary or tertiary adrenal insufficiency, only cortisol replacement is required. For secondary adrenal insufficiency, maintenance doses of hydrocortisone may be used, though may not be required for all children. Mineralocorticoid replacement is not needed in secondary adrenal insufficiency, as ACTH does not control the zona glomerulosa where mineralocorticoid is produced. Cortisol replacement should be undertaken prior to thyroid hormone replacement, as this may precipitate adrenal crisis. See Chapter 70, Disorders of the Adrenal Gland, for more on maintenance and stress dosing of hydrocortisone. The stress dose should be continued until the patient is recovered from inciting illness, and daily dosage immediately resumed.

POSTERIOR PITUITARY DYSFUNCTION

Common presentations of posterior pituitary dysfunction include diabetes insipidus and syndrome of inappropriate antidiuretic hormone secretion.

DIABETES INSIPIDUS

Diabetes insipidus (DI) is defined as an inability to concentrate urine despite increasing serum osmolality due to inadequate secretion of ADH (central DI) or unresponsiveness of the kidney to ADH (nephrogenic DI). Patients present with excessive drinking (polydipsia) and excessive urine output (polyuria) in response to elevated serum sodium and osmolality. Polyuria may present as enuresis in a previously toilet-trained child. If thirst is intact and access to free water unrestricted, patients can compensate for urinary water loss with water intake and remain well hydrated and stable. However, when access to water is interrupted due to illness, fatigue, or lack of an intake thirst center, dehydration and hypernatremia will occur. Infants and patients with neurologic impairments are high risk to develop dehydration and electrolyte abnormalities. Additional symptoms at presentation may include feeding difficulty, poor growth, fever, constipation, irritability, headache, visual disturbances, vomiting, and/or seizures. Patients with combined anterior pituitary (ACTH or TSH) deficiency may not exhibit symptoms of DI due to increased ADH secretion secondary to cortisol deficiency or increased absorption of ADH in the renal tubule.

DIFFERENTIAL DIAGNOSIS

- diabetes mellitus (hyperglycemia with osmotic diuresis)
- hypercalcemia or hypokalemia (can cause ADH unresponsiveness)
- osmotic diuretics (mannitol, high glucose, intravenous contrast)
- psychogenic polydipsia (excess free water intake causing reduced renal responsiveness to ADH and decreased renal concentrating gradient)
- Nephrogenic DI which may be caused by: Renal tubular acidosis, Fanconi' syndrome, cystinosis, concentrating defect in chronic renal failure, structural malformations (post obstructive diuresis or post-acute tubular necrosis, drug toxicity (e.g., lithium, phenytoin, amphotericin)

DIAGNOSIS AND EVALUATION

To establish the diagnosis of DI, it is necessary to confirm that urinary osmolality remains inappropriately low during a period when serum osmolality has increased to an abnormally high level. Hypernatremia (>145 mEq/L) with urine specific gravity <1.010, urine osmolality of <300 mOsm/kg, and serum osmolality >300 mOsm/kg is highly suggestive of DI. It is important to remember that the administration of IV fluids prior to obtaining these labs will alter the interpretation of the results. Diagnosis may require fluid restriction and careful monitoring of the clinical status of the patient during a water deprivation test.

In consultation with a pediatric endocrinologist, a water deprivation test can be performed to confirm the diagnosis of DI. Fluid restriction should only occur in an age-appropriate patient in a setting where electrolytes can be closely monitored and corrected. Further differentiation between central and nephrogenic DI can be distinguished via a vasopressin stimulation test as plasma ADH will be low or absent in central DI and normal in nephrogenic DI.

Brain MRI is recommended for patients with central DI. For patients with a family history suggestive of DI or early onset idiopathic DI, genetic testing should be performed.

TREATMENT

The initial treatment of DI involves stabilization followed by electrolyte and fluid management. An accepted approach includes resuscitation with 0.9% normal saline, followed by slow correction of hypernatremia and remaining fluid deficit with 0.45% normal saline. Once the diagnosis of diabetes insipidus is established, fluids should be calculated to include the free water deficit (free water deficit (L) = ([0.6 × {wt in kg}] × [1-desired Na/actual Na]), maintenance fluid replacement and insensible losses (1/3 maintenance).

Mild forms of central DI may not require treatment if serum sodium is less than or equal to 145 mEq/L and serum osmolality is less than 195 mOsm. Significant polyuria and polydipsia are treated effectively with desmopressin in divided doses. Nasal spray or tablets are preferred due to ease of administration, though desmopressin can be administered parenterally. The dose should be titrated according to the patient's response to the initial dose with close monitoring of weight, intake/output, and electrolytes.

IMPORTANT CONSIDERATIONS

- DI may be transient, particularly after traumatic brain injury or surgery.
- Posttraumatic or postoperative DI may be followed by the syndrome of inappropriate ADH secretion (SIADH), which may be followed by recurrence of DI (triphasic pattern of DI/SIADH/DI).
- Avoid hyponatremia, which can exacerbate posttraumatic cerebral edema. Warning signs include nausea, vomiting, lethargy, headaches, confusion, seizures, and coma.
- In general, always start with the lowest recommended dose of desmopressin and adjust the dosage as necessary based on ongoing laboratory evaluations.

SYNDROME OF INAPPROPRIATE ANTIDIURETIC HORMONE SECRETION

Syndrome of inappropriate antidiuretic hormone secretion (SIADH) is an important consideration for patients with hyponatremia in the inpatient setting. When ADH is released, it stimulates water reabsorption in the renal tubule. This results in reduced urine volume and increased urine osmolality. SIADH should be considered when hyponatremia with

TABLE 68-1 Causes of Syndrome of Inappropriate Anti-Diuretic Hormone in Children

Conditions	Stress, nausea, pain
Pulmonary disease	Bronchiolitis, asthma, cystic fibrosis, pneumonia
Neurologic disease	Meningitis, encephalitis, tumor, trauma, hydrocephalus, brain abscess, stroke, Guillain-Barré syndrome/acute inflammatory demyelinating polyradiculopathy
Postsurgical	Neurosurgery including spinal surgery
Medications	Carbamazepine, vincristine, cyclophosphamide, opioids, non-steroidal anti-inflammatory drugs, Methylenedioxymethamphetamine (MDMA), tricyclic antidepressants, selective serotonin reuptake inhibitors, desmopressin, ciprofloxacin, amiodarone
Malignancy	Lymphoma, Ewing sarcoma, carcinoma

decreased urine output develops. By definition, the patient needs to be euvolemic for the secretion of ADH to be considered "inappropriate." Symptoms of acute hyponatremia may include nausea, vomiting, headache, lethargy, altered mental status, and/or seizures. See **Table 68-1** for Causes of SIADH in children.

DIFFERENTIAL DIAGNOSIS

- Hyponatremic dehydration
- Congestive heart failure
- Inadequate free water excretion secondary to ACTH/cortisol deficiency or thyroid hormone deficiency
- Hyperglycemia, hypertriglyceridemia (factitious)
- Other forms of salt loss (GI)
- Salt wasting via the kidney (should be accompanied by increased urine output)
- Cerebral salt wasting

DIAGNOSTIC EVALUATION

The diagnosis of SIADH should be considered when a patient has decreased urine output and low serum sodium. The evaluation should include strict measurement of input and output, measurement of serum sodium and osmolality, and measurement of urine sodium and osmolality. Typically, in isolated SIADH, the serum sodium and osmolality are low (<135 mEq/L and <280 mOsm/kg), the urine sodium is above 20 meq/L (except during sodium restriction), and the urine osmolality is inappropriately concentrated (>100 mOsm/kg). Findings should include the absence of dehydration on physical examination, and there should be evidence of intravascular volume expansion (low blood urea nitrogen, low hematocrit, low uric acid) on laboratory evaluation. Causes of factitious hyponatremia (hypertriglyceridemia, hyperglycemia) and other hormonal deficiencies that may interfere with free water excretion should be ruled out. Additionally, ensure renal, cardiac, hepatic, adrenal, and thyroid functions are normal.

TREATMENT

- Restriction of fluid to 400 to 600 mL/m^2/day (40% of maintenance) or less (not <25% of daily maintenance)
- Strict input and output; monitor urine specific gravity
- For symptomatic hyponatremia, raise serum sodium via administration of 3% saline 2 mL/kg bolus (max 100 mL).
- Frequent measurement of serum sodium levels. Correct <0.5 mEq/L per hour.
- In cases of chronic hyponatremia, correction should be even more gradual to avoid osmotic demyelination syndrome.

CONSULTATION

- Pediatric Endocrinologist
- Pediatric Neurosurgeon, as needed
- Pediatric Intensivist, as needed

ADMISSION AND DISCHARGE CRITERIA

ADMISSION CRITERIA

- Electrolyte imbalance
- Altered mental status
- Hemodynamic instability

DISCHARGE CRITERIA

- For DI and SIADH, input and output can be monitored at home and a caregiver can administer medication as needed.
- Patient is clinically stable with normalized vital signs and electrolytes.
- Regular follow-up for monitoring of serum electrolytes and the underlying disease is arranged.

KEY POINTS

- Anterior pituitary dysfunction may be congenital or acquired and result in hypothyroidism, adrenal insufficiency, growth failure, and/or lack of pubertal maturation.
- Patients with adrenal insufficiency require stress dose steroids during illness, injury, or procedures.
- If DI is secondary to surgery, it may be transient and part of the triphasic response of DI, followed by SIADH, followed by DI.
- DI is most often secondary to congenital abnormalities of the posterior pituitary or disturbance of the pituitary stalk in the setting of a CNS tumor, surgery, or both.
- Hyponatremia is often seen in the setting of dehydration, but can be from SIADH, which is associated with a number of conditions, as well as from surgery or stress state.

SUGGESTED READINGS

Bowden SA, Henry R. Pediatric adrenal insufficiency: diagnosis, management, and new therapies. *Int J Pediatr*. 2018;2018:1739831.

Di Iorgi N, Napoli F, Allegri AEM, et al. Diabetes insipidus—diagnosis and management. *Horm Res Paediatr*. 2012;(77):69-84.

Driano JE, Lteif AN, Creo AL. Vasopressin-dependent disorders: what is new in children? *Pediatrics*. 2021;147(5):e2020022848.

Jones DP. Syndrome of inappropriate secretion of antidiuretic hormone and hyponatremia. *Pediatr Rev*. January 2018;39(1):27-35.

Kirkgoz T, Guran T. Primary adrenal insufficiency in children: diagnosis and management. *Best Pract Res Clin Endocrinol Metab*. 2018;32(4):397-424.

Moritz ML. Syndrome of inappropriate antidiuresis. *Pediatr Clin North Am*. 2019;66(1):209-226.

Nisticò D, Bossini B, Benvenuto S, Pellegrin MC, Tornese G. Pediatric adrenal insufficiency: challenges and solutions. *Ther Clin Risk Manag*. 2022;18:47-60.

Patti G, Guzzeti C, Di Iorgi N, et al. Central adrenal insufficiency in children and adolescents. *Best Pract Res Clin Endocrinol Metab*. 2018;32(4):425-444.

Patti G, Napoli F, Fava D, Casalini E, Di Iorgi N, Maghnie M. Approach to the pediatric patient: central diabetes insipidus. *J Clin Endocrinol Metab*. 2022;107(5): 1407-1416.

CHAPTER 69

Disorders of Calcium Metabolism

Stephanie Berger, MD, Rebecca Cantu, MD, MPH, and Brian May, MD, MEd

BACKGROUND

Calcium, the most abundant mineral in the body, is required for proper functioning of numerous intracellular and extracellular processes, including muscle contraction, nerve conduction, hormone release, and blood coagulation. Calcium also plays a unique role in intracellular signaling and is involved in the regulation of enzyme activity. Maintenance of calcium homeostasis is therefore critical. Ionized calcium, which is responsible for the physiologic effects, is maintained under normal conditions within a narrow normal range.

The majority of total body calcium exists as bone mineral, with serum calcium representing less than 1% of total body calcium. Although total serum calcium levels are routinely measured, it is the ionized fraction that is biologically active. Total serum calcium levels include both ionized and bound calcium. The total serum calcium level reflects serum changes in albumin, pH, phosphate, magnesium, and bicarbonate. Ionized calcium may be reduced by exogenous factors such as citrate from transfused blood or free fatty acids from total parenteral nutrition. At physiologic pH, 40% of total serum calcium is bound to albumin, 10% can be bound to bicarbonate, phosphate, or citrate, and the remaining 50% exists in the ionized form.

Calcium absorption and regulation involves a complex interplay between multiple organ systems and regulatory hormones. Serum calcium levels are detected by calcium-sensing receptors located on the parathyroid glands and renal tubule cells resulting in regulation of parathyroid hormone (PTH) secretion and renal reabsorption of calcium, respectively. This tight regulation of circulating calcium is controlled through constant adjustment of PTH secretion, 1,25-dihydroxyvitamin D (1,25$(OH)_2$D) production, calcitonin, and renal handling of calcium.

CALCIUM REGULATION

The three major targets for calcium regulation (both to increase and decrease) include bone, intestine, and kidney. Ten percent of ingested calcium is absorbed in the intestines through passive, concentration-dependent absorption. The majority (60%-70%) of calcium is passively reabsorbed in the proximal tubule of the kidney that is driven by a gradient generated by sodium and water reabsorption. Individuals with normal kidney function have protection against calcium overload by virtue of their ability to increase renal excretion of calcium and reduce intestinal absorption of calcium by actions of PTH and 1,25$(OH)_2$D.

Endogenous Mechanisms to Increase Calcium In bone, PTH stimulates bone resorption, thereby increasing total serum calcium levels. In the kidney, PTH activates 1-α-hydroxylase leading to conversion of 25-hydroxyvitamin D (25(OH)D) to 1,25$(OH)_2$D, commonly known as the active form of vitamin D, allowing for increased intestinal absorption via vitamin D-dependent absorption. PTH also increases renal calcium reabsorption and phosphorus excretion.

Endogenous Mechanisms to Decrease Calcium Calcitonin, produced by the thyroid gland, inhibits osteoclasts, decreasing bone resorption, thereby decreasing total serum calcium. Calcitonin also decreases serum calcium levels by increasing renal excretion. Suppression of PTH is essential given effects of PTH as described above.

HYPOCALCEMIA

Hypocalcemia is generally defined as:

- Children and adolescents: less than 8.5 mg/dL (ionized calcium <4.6 mg/dL or <1.15 mmol/L)
- Term Neonates: less than 8 mg/dL (ionized calcium <4.4 mg/dL or 1.1 mmol/L)
- Preterm Neonates: less than 7 mg/dL (ionized calcium <3.2 mg/dL or 0.8 mmol/L)

If ionized calcium level is not available, calculate the corrected calcium by adding 0.8 mg/dL to the total calcium for every 1-mg decrease in the serum albumin below 4 mg/dL. Individual laboratory norms should be used when available.

CLINICAL PRESENTATION

Hypocalcemia is frequently observed in the inpatient setting, and incidentally noted biochemical hypocalcemia is often asymptomatic. Symptomatic hypocalcemia occurs in response to a rapid decrease in calcium concentration, as well as in response to the absolute calcium level. Symptoms tend to be more severe if hypocalcemia develops acutely.

The predominant clinical symptoms and signs in children and adolescents include perioral paresthesia, tingling of the fingers and toes, spontaneous or latent tetany, carpopedal spasms, and/or seizures. In neonates, manifestations of hypocalcemia are more nonspecific and include jitteriness, feeding intolerance, lethargy, apnea, and/or seizures. Physical examination may reveal hyperreflexia, a positive Chvostek sign (twitching of facial muscles after tapping the facial nerve anterior to the ear), or the Trousseau sign (carpopedal spasm after maintaining a blood pressure cuff above systolic blood pressure for 3 to 5 minutes). Less often seen features are cataracts, papilledema, rachitic deformities, and/or abnormal dental development.

DIFFERENTIAL DIAGNOSIS

The etiology of hypocalcemia in pediatrics can vary by the age of the child at presentation. **Table 69-1** highlights the clinically important categories of hypocalcemia and associated laboratory findings.

Early Neonatal Hypocalcemia In infants presenting with hypocalcemia within 48 to 72 hours of birth, the differential diagnosis includes prematurity, birth asphyxia, maternal diabetes, and maternal hyperparathyroidism. In preterm infants, hypocalcemia is essentially due to an insufficient increase in PTH secretion along with a relative resistance to 1,25$(OH)_2$D. In addition, premature infants have limited intake of milk, which contributes to hypocalcemia. In infants of diabetic mothers, magnesium deficiency may also play an important role in the development of early neonatal hypocalcemia. Whenever neonatal hypocalcemia occurs in the absence of these risk factors, the diagnosis of congenital hypoparathyroidism must be considered.

Late Neonatal Hypocalcemia Late neonatal hypocalcemia presents clinically at 5 to 10 days of life in healthy full-term infants. The three major causes of late neonatal hypocalcemia are phosphate loading, hypoparathyroidism, and magnesium deficiency. Other causes include vitamin D deficiency, PTH resistance, inborn errors of metabolism, and iatrogenic causes (e.g., diuretics, glucocorticoids, and citrated blood products). Phosphate-induced hypocalcemia should be differentiated from congenital hypoparathyroidism. While in both situations, serum calcium is low and serum phosphorus is high, the PTH is appropriately elevated in phosphate-induced neonatal hypocalcemia and the hypocalcemia resolves spontaneously when the neonate is placed on a low-phosphorus formula. In contrast, in congenital hypoparathyroidism, the PTH levels are low.

Childhood Hypocalcemia Causes of hypocalcemia in children include PTH deficiency, calcium-sensing receptor defects, vitamin D deficiency, and resistance to the biologic effects of these calcium-regulating hormones. The differential diagnosis includes vitamin D deficiency, vitamin D resistance, hypoparathyroidism, pseudohypoparathyroidism, metabolic bone disease, and drug effect. Abnormalities in vitamin D metabolism can be seen in both renal disease and liver disease. In patients with renal failure, 1α-hydroxylation of 25(OH)D is impaired, and therefore, the stored form of vitamin D (25(OH)D) cannot be converted to the biologically active form 1,25$(OH)_2$D. Hyperphosphatemia may further aggravate hypocalcemia in renal failure and lead to secondary hyperparathyroidism and renal osteodystrophy.

TABLE 69-1 Classification of Hypocalcemia in Childhood

Category	Phosphorus	25(OH)D	$1,25(OH)_2D$	PTH	Comments
Neonate					
Early hypocalcemia	N	N	N/ L	N/L	Prematurity, IUGR, birth asphyxia, diabetic mother
Late hypocalcemia	H	N	L	L	Low GFR, intake of high-phosphate milk
Older Child					
Congenital hypoparathyroidism	H	N	L	L	DiGeorge syndrome
Autoimmune hypoparathyroidism	H	N	L	L	Part of polyendocrinopathy syndrome, type 1
Pseudohypoparathyroidism	H	N	L	H	Peripheral resistance to PTH
Vitamin D deficiency	L/N/ H	L	L/N/ H	H	Exclusively breastfed with maternal vitamin D deficiency, sunlight avoidance, fat malabsorption
Vitamin D dependent	L	N	H	H	Caused by loss-of-function mutation of 1α -hydroxylase gene
Critical illness	N	N	N	L	PTH dysfunction and increase in cortisol
Magnesium deficiency	H	N	N/L	L	May be part of Bartter syndrome, malabsorption, renal disease
Renal disease	H	N	L	H	Abnormal renal function, metabolic acidosis

GFR, glomerular filtration rate; H, high; IUGR, intrauterine growth restriction; L, low; N, normal; 25(OH)D, 25-hydroxyvitamin D; $1,25(OH)_2D$, 1,25- dihydroxyvitamin D; PTH, parathyroid hormone.

Vitamin D Deficiency Vitamin D deficiency may be a primary nutritional deficiency or may be secondary to malabsorption. Nutritional deficiency is more common in infants 3 to 36 months of age, with dark skin or from northern latitudes, and in premature or exclusively breastfed infants. Conditions predisposing to malabsorption of vitamin D include celiac disease, cystic fibrosis, pancreatic insufficiency, intestinal bypass, and laxative abuse. Children on anti-seizure medication such as phenobarbital and phenytoin are at increased risk for vitamin D deficiency because of increased hepatic metabolism of vitamin D into inactive metabolites. Biochemical features of rickets are often seen with vitamin D deficiency, including secondary hyperparathyroidism, low serum phosphorus, phosphaturia, high serum alkaline phosphatase, and low 25(OH)D. Clinical features of vitamin D deficiency vary with severity, ranging from a normal exam to severe features seen with rickets including deformities of weight-bearing limbs, growth retardation, frontal bossing of the skull, rachitic rosary (string of beads appearance along the costochondral junctions), Harrison sulcus (indentation on the anterior chest roughly around the 6th rib), or delayed dentition. Radiographic evidence of rickets may also be present on radiographs if fusion of the epiphyses has not yet occurred.

To prevent vitamin D deficiency, the American Academy of Pediatrics (AAP) and the Institute of Medicine have established recommended daily intake guidelines for vitamin D. The current recommended daily intake for infants age 0 to 12 months is 400 international units (IU) daily and for children age 1 to 21 years is 600 IU daily. Any breastfeeding infant, regardless of amount of formula supplementation, should receive a daily supplement of 400 IU per day. If infants are exclusively formula-fed, they typically do not require vitamin supplementation, as they should receive their daily recommended dose of vitamin D in the formula.

Hypoparathyroidism Hypoparathyroidism may be secondary to surgery, polyglandular autoimmune disease, infiltrative disease, neck irradiation, or an idiopathic process. The diagnosis of hypoparathyroidism is suggested by low calcium levels, high phosphorus levels, an inappropriately low PTH level, and absence of bone disease on radiographs. Hypomagnesemia may be a causative factor in the development of hypoparathyroidism. Severe hypomagnesemia will suppress PTH secretion, and mild hypomagnesemia will interfere with PTH activity.

Autosomal Dominant Hypocalcemia Autosomal Dominant Hypocalcemia is due to a gain-of-function mutation in the calcium-sensing receptor on the parathyroid gland leading to a lowering of the calcium set-point and resulting in hypocalcemia with an inappropriately normal PTH.

Pseudohypoparathyroidism The diagnosis of pseudohypoparathyroidism (PHP) is characterized by hypocalcemia, hyperphosphatemia, and elevated PTH concentrations. PHP type 1 is a result of a dominantly inherited mutation in *GNAS1*. PHP type 1a is the result of an inactivating mutation in *GNAS1* on the maternal allele (either maternally inherited or de novo) resulting in characteristic biochemical findings and a phenotype known as Albright's hereditary osteodystrophy (AHO). The AHO phenotype includes short stature, round face, shortened fourth metacarpal bones, obesity, subcutaneous ossifications, and developmental delay. PHP type 1b has the biochemical findings of PHP but not the AHO phenotype. Elevated PTH levels, hypocalcemia, and hyperphosphatemia can also be seen in children with renal failure or those who have received treatment with phosphate enemas.

Other Causes Other conditions associated with hypocalcemia include renal failure, hungry bone syndrome, tumor lysis syndrome, rhabdomyolysis, acute illness, and certain medications (furosemide, calcitonin, bisphosphonates, and antineoplastic agents).

DIAGNOSTIC EVALUATION

The diagnosis of hypocalcemia is suspected based on the total serum calcium concentration corrected for albumin. However, this equation can be inaccurate, particularly, in the setting of significant albumin derangements. For this reason, the diagnosis should be confirmed with ionized calcium (if the appropriate tools are available for rapid processing). It is also important to note that ionized calcium itself can provide inaccurate results with acid/base derangements. The evaluation of calcium abnormalities should include total calcium, ionized calcium, phosphorus, magnesium, alkaline phosphatase, parathyroid hormone, 25(OH)D, $1,25(OH)_2D$, electrolytes, BUN, creatinine, and albumin. The phosphate level can greatly aid in narrowing the differential as a high phosphate concentration suggests a deficiency of PTH action, whereas a low phosphate concentration favors increased PTH effect. Urine studies including calcium, phosphorus, and creatinine are needed. An electrocardiogram should be performed to assess for QT prolongation. The algorithm shown in **Figure 69-1** (hypocalcemia) will assist in diagnosis.

MANAGEMENT

Although mild hypocalcemia may not require therapy, any neonate with a serum calcium less than 7.5 mg/dL or any older child with a serum calcium less than 8 to 8.5 mg/dL should be treated to prevent tetany and other symptoms. Oral therapy is preferable whenever possible.

In acute symptomatic hypocalcemia (tetany, seizures), intravenous (IV) therapy is required. For patients with acute life-threatening symptoms of hypocalcemia, IV calcium gluconate is the treatment of choice. Calcium gluconate 10% solution (9.4 mg elemental calcium/mL) can be given by slow intravenous push. Continuous cardiac monitoring must be in place as rapid injection can cause serious cardiac dysrhythmias. All

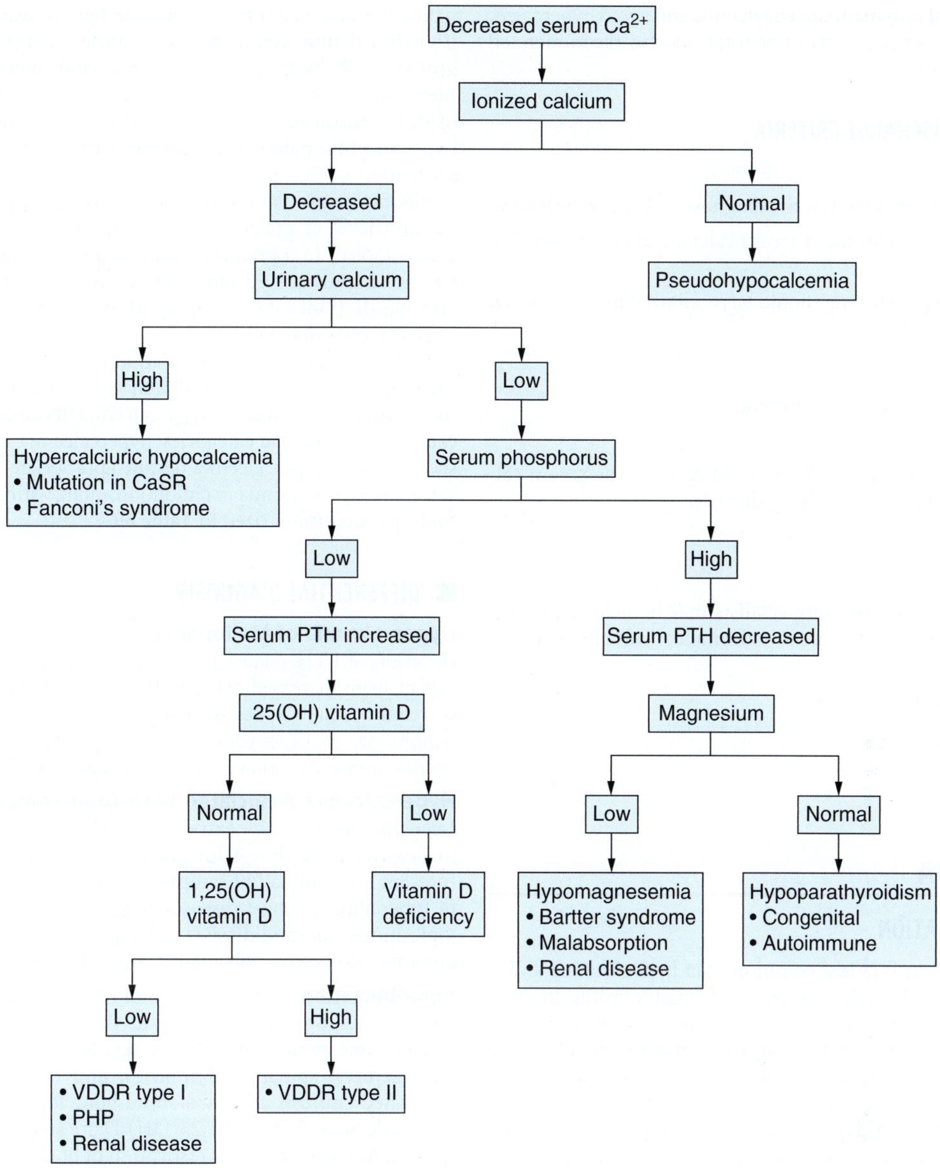

FIGURE 69-1. Flow chart for diagnosing the cause of hypocalcemia. CaSR, calcium-sensing receptor; PHP, pseudohypoparathyroidism; PTH, parathyroid hormone; VDDR, vitamin D-dependent rickets.

calcium salts are locally toxic and can lead to tissue damage if accidental extravasation occurs. A freely running intravenous line should be used to avoid extravasation. Calcium salts can also interfere with the administration of other IV medications. For this reason, multiple IVs may be needed. Calcium chloride is an alternative formulation used in shortages of IV calcium gluconate. However, it has higher risk of local reactions and IV complications rates.

In the absence of tetany or seizures, oral therapy will suffice. Calcium glubionate is the most suitable agent for infants and young children because it is dispensed as palatable syrup. Alternatively, chewable calcium carbonate is available. In older children, tablets of calcium gluconate, carbonate, or lactate can be given. A dosage of 50 mg elemental calcium/kg/day is generally prescribed, with a maximum adult dose of 2000 mg of elemental calcium per day.

When symptoms of hypocalcemia resolve, serial calcium determinations will determine the need for and route of further therapy. Because serum calcium levels may fall gradually after the initial infusion, ongoing treatment may be necessary.

If children are vitamin D-deficient, they will require vitamin D supplementation. Two preparations are currently available: vitamin D_2 (ergocalciferol) and vitamin D_3 (cholecalciferol). Supplementation recommendations from the AAP: 1000 IU per day for infants <1 month of age, 1000 to 5000 IU per day for children age 1 to 12 months, and >5000 IU per day for children 1 year of age and older. Guidelines for weekly vitamin D supplementation have been provided by the Endocrine Society, at a dose of 50,000 IU once per week for children ages 0 to 18 years. Treatment should continue for 6 weeks, at which time children should be continued on a maintenance dose of vitamin D based on recommended daily intake. Dose adjustment should be considered in children with malabsorptive disorders. Calcitriol may be used if the patient is unable to produce $1,25(OH)_2D$ because of renal disease or severe hypoparathyroidism. However, calcitriol bypasses the body's ability to regulate vitamin D activity and therefore carries the risk of hypercalcemia and hypercalciuria. It has a short half-life and persists in the body for only 1 to 2 days. Because calcitriol will not replenish vitamin D stores, 25(OH)D should be given as well if a true deficiency of vitamin D is suspected. The usual dosage of calcitriol is 0.25 μg/day but varies with body weight and the disorder for which it is being used. The dosage may be adjusted until calcium levels have improved. Children with significant malabsorption, 1-α hydroxylase deficiency, and vitamin D receptor defects may require high dose calcitriol and/or chronic intravenous calcium therapy.

Individualization of therapy is essential. It is crucial to monitor serum and urinary calcium and creatinine levels frequently to adjust the doses of medications. The goal is to maintain eucalcemia and avoid hypercalcemia and hypercalciuria. Annual renal sonography is also recommended to detect nephrocalcinosis.

ADMISSION AND DISCHARGE CRITERIA

Admission

- Symptomatic hypocalcemia (unless the diagnosis is hyperventilation)
- Severe hypocalcemia; specifically, a serum calcium level less than 7 to 7.5 mg/dL
- Any newborn with hypocalcemia should be monitored in the neonatal intensive care unit (NICU)

Discharge

- Asymptomatic and clinically stable patient
- Conversion to oral medications
- Arrangements made for regular follow-up to monitor the serum calcium concentration and the underlying disorder

CONSULTATION

Consultation from the following subspecialists may be helpful in diagnosis and/or management. Recommend tailoring consultants based on patient diagnosis.

- Pediatric Endocrinology
- Pediatric Nephrology
- Genetics
- Pediatric Cardiology

HYPERCALCEMIA

CLINICAL PRESENTATION

In childhood, hypercalcemia is less common than hypocalcemia and is frequently discovered incidentally on a routine chemistry profile. Because of the potential clinical significance of a slight elevation in serum calcium levels, it is important to obtain an accurate measure by taking the serum albumin concentration and acid-base status into account.

Symptoms of hypercalcemia vary little with age. Lethargy, weakness, inability to concentrate, and depression may develop. Many patients have nausea, vomiting, anorexia, constipation, and weight loss. Older children and adolescents may have psychiatric symptoms including hallucinations. Patients may become hypertensive with extreme elevations in calcium. Neonates may manifest symptoms of gastroesophageal reflux, lethargy, poor weight gain, and a decrease in linear growth. Elevations in extracellular calcium impair the ability of the distal tubule of the nephron to respond to antidiuretic hormone (ADH); therefore hypercalcemic patients may present with polyuria, dehydration, and azotemia.

The normative values for calcium are age dependent. A total serum calcium level of greater than 9.2 mg/dL (ionized Ca >5.8 mg/dL or 1.42 mmol/L) in a premature infant, greater than 10.4 mg/dL (ionized Ca >5.0 mg/dL or 1.22 mmol/L) in a full-term infant, and greater than 10.8 mg/dL (ionized Ca >5.0 mg/dL or 1.22 mmol/L) in a child or adolescent is considered elevated.

Because serum calcium regulation is dependent on PTH, vitamin D, calcium intake, and renal calcium excretion, derangements in any of these systems can produce hypercalcemia. It can be useful to separate the causes into two broad categories: hypercalcemia with *inappropriate* PTH secretion and hypercalcemia despite appropriate PTH suppression. The causes of hypercalcemia in childhood, along with associated biochemical findings, are summarized in **Table 69-2**.

DIFFERENTIAL DIAGNOSIS

Hypercalcemia of Malignancy Hypercalcemia may be caused by an elevation of PTH-related protein (PTH-rp) in patients with malignancies or from increased osteoclastic activity at the tumor site. PTH-rp is secreted by many types of malignant tumors, most notably leukemia, lymphoma, rhabdomyosarcoma, and Ewing sarcoma. Hypercalcemia results from activation of the PTH receptor by PTH-rp.

Hypercalcemia Associated With Granulomatous Disease Hypercalcemia from excessive extrarenal production of $1,25(OH)_2D$ may occur in diseases presenting with granulomas. It is common in sarcoidosis (present in about half of symptomatic cases) but has also been reported in tuberculosis, fungal diseases (e.g., berylliosis, coccidiomycosis, histoplasmosis, or candidiasis), inflammatory bowel disease, sarcoidosis, granulomatosis with polyangiitis, and cat-scratch disease.

Immobilization Hypercalcemia of immobilization occurs more commonly in children and adolescents than in adults because of a higher rate of bone remodeling at this age. It is seen most frequently after leg fractures, spinal cord injuries, and burns. Hypercalciuria with associated enuresis and substantial bone loss are more common than hypercalcemia. PTH and $1,25(OH)_2D$ are suppressed, and bone biopsy specimens show increased resorption of bone and decreased formation of bone.

TABLE 69-2 Classification of Hypercalcemia in Childhood

Type	Phosphorus	25(OH)D	$1,25(OH)_2D$	PTH	Urine Ca^+	Notes
Williams syndrome	N	N	N	N	H	Deletion in 17q11.23 Cognitive impairment, elfin facies, aortic stenosis
Primary hyperparathyroidism	L	N	H	H	H	Rare in children Part of MEN types I and II
Secondary hyperparathyroidism (secondary to renal insufficiency)	H	N	L	H	H	Can lead to tertiary autonomous hyperparathyroidism
Familial hypocalciuria	N	N	N	N	L	Loss-of-function mutation (generally heterozygous) in CaSR
Hypervitaminosis D	N/L	H	N/H	N	H	Overdose of vitamins, fad megavitamin diets
Increased 1α-hydroxylation of 25-hydroxyvitamin D	N	N	H	N	N	Granulomatous diseases, subcutaneous fat necrosis, neoplasm
Immobilization	N	N	L	L	H	Increased resorption and decreased bone formation
Malignancy	N	N	N	L	H	Release of bone-resorbing substances: PTH-rp
Adrenal insufficiency	N	N	N/L	L	N	Increased GI calcium absorption
Hyperthyroidism	N	N	N/L	L	N	Active bone turnover and enhanced resorption

CaSR, calcium-sensing receptor; GI, gastrointestinal; H, high; L, low; MEN, multiple endocrine neoplasia; N, normal; PTH, parathyroid hormone; PTH-rp, PTH-related protein.

Hyperparathyroidism Hyperparathyroidism is very rare in childhood. It is characterized by autonomous PTH secretion independent of the serum calcium level. Affected children are hypercalcemic as a result of increased calcium resorption from bone, increased renal reabsorption, and increased intestinal absorption. Serum phosphorus is usually reduced but may be normal. The skeletal erosion is most commonly observed in the phalanges and clavicles. Sporadic cases may result from either a parathyroid adenoma or hyperplasia of the parathyroid gland's chief cells.

Any child with hyperparathyroidism should be evaluated for multiple endocrine neoplasia (MEN) syndromes. Ninety percent of patients with MEN-I have parathyroid hyperplasia along with a pituitary adenoma and/or a pancreatic tumor. In MEN-IIA, medullary thyroid carcinoma and pheochromocytoma are the main features; chief cell hyperplasia (with resultant hyperparathyroidism) is sometimes associated.

Hypervitaminosis D Vitamin D intoxication is uncommon but can arise from chronic overdosage of vitamin D given for therapeutic purposes or self-administration of vitamin preparations. The resultant hypercalcemia can be severe and prolonged because of storage of vitamin D in fat. Specific therapy includes discontinuation of vitamin D and ingestion of a low-calcium diet.

Hypervitaminosis A Excessive intake of vitamins may result in vitamin A excess in addition to vitamin D excess. Excess amounts of the fat-soluble vitamin A also increase bone resorption, which may result in hypercalcemia.

Thiazide Diuretics Thiazides may cause hypercalcemia as a result of increased renal resorption of calcium and increased calcium binding protein levels.

Williams Syndrome Williams syndrome is the result of a large contiguous deletion on chromosome 7q11.23 involving approximately 28 different genes. Patients with Williams syndrome may have hypercalcemia in addition to characteristic features including elfin facies, congenital cardiovascular anomalies, and cognitive impairment. The cause of the hypercalcemia is not currently understood. The hypercalcemia may respond to a diet low in calcium and usually remits between 9 and 18 months of age. It is important to consider Williams syndrome in the setting of hypercalcemia in an infant because of the associated cardiac defects.

Idiopathic Hypercalcemia of Infancy Idiopathic hypercalcemia of infancy was initially described by Kenny et al. in 1963 in a report of an infant with asymptomatic hypercalcemia. The hypercalcemia improved when vitamin D intake was limited and would recur when given replacement doses of only 400 IU daily, suggesting a problem with the removal or deactivation of vitamin D. The *CYP24A1* gene encodes the 24-hydroxylase that breaks down vitamin D metabolites, and recently, loss-of-function mutations in the *CYP24A1* gene have been described in patients with idiopathic hypercalcemia of infancy, confirming that the mechanism of hypercalcemia is due to problems with deactivation of vitamin D.

Familial Hypocalciuric Hypercalcemia Familial hypocalciuric hypercalcemia (FHH) is a usually asymptomatic condition of parathyroid insensitivity to the normal suppressive effect of calcium on PTH secretion due to a loss-of-function mutation in the calcium-sensing receptor gene. This mutation results in an elevation in the normal calcium setpoint, leading to hypercalcemia with an inappropriately normal PTH. It is inherited in an autosomal dominant fashion. A homozygous calcium-sensing receptor gene mutation is characterized by severe and often lethal neonatal hyperparathyroidism.

Other Causes Other conditions associated with hypercalcemia include adrenal insufficiency, hyperthyroidism, subcutaneous fat necrosis, and high calcium intake.

DIAGNOSTIC EVALUATION

The evaluation of hypercalcemia should include initial laboratory evaluation similar to that recommended for hypocalcemia: total calcium, ionized calcium, phosphorus, magnesium, alkaline phosphatase, parathyroid hormone, 25(OH)D, $1,25(OH)_2D$, electrolytes, BUN, creatinine, albumin, and a urine calcium to creatinine ratio. Other laboratory tests to consider if warranted include PTHrp or *N*-terminal telopeptide, a marker of bone turnover. The algorithm shown in **Figure 69-2** (hypercalcemia) will assist in diagnosis. EKG may reveal short QT and prolonged PR interval.

MANAGEMENT

Appropriate management of a patient with hypercalcemia depends on the severity and cause of the hypercalcemia. When the calcium concentration is less than 12 mg/dL in an asymptomatic patient, treatment may be delayed until the cause of the hypercalcemia is known. If the total serum calcium concentration exceeds 12 mg/dL or the child is symptomatic, efforts to lower calcium levels should be instituted to prevent the adverse effects of hypercalcemia while awaiting the laboratory results. After initial stabilization, attention should turn to treatment of the underlying cause of the hypercalcemia.

Volume Repletion The mainstay of initial therapy for acute symptomatic hypercalcemia is vigorous hydration with normal saline. Twice the maintenance infusion rate is recommended initially, if tolerated. Urine output must be closely monitored, and any net fluid deficit should be replaced on an ongoing basis. The goal is to maintain an increased urinary rate and to have input exceed urinary output.

Pharmacotherapy • ***Calcitonin*** In cases of severe hypercalcemia, calcitonin (2-4 U/kg) via subcutaneous injection can be given every 6 to 12 hours as needed, but rapid tachyphylaxis to this medication is common and limits its utility.

Glucocorticoids Oral glucocorticoids decrease calcium, principally by decreasing absorption from the intestine by inhibiting synthesis of $1,25(OH)_2D$ from 25(OH)D. They also have a role in treating hypercalcemia that arises from granulomatous disease by treating the underlying disease. Caution should be exercised if an oncologic diagnosis has not been excluded given pretreatment can induce tumor lysis syndrome and complicate risk stratification.

Diuretics Once adequate hydration has been achieved, furosemide (1-2 mg/kg) may be administered intravenously to increase urinary calcium excretion if the serum calcium level is not improving. However, diuretics must be used with caution, as they may lead to fluid losses and worsening dehydration and can increase the risk of nephrocalcinosis with long-term use.

Phosphates Oral phosphate may be used to bind calcium in the intestine, but its efficacy is limited and its use may result in nausea, abdominal cramps, and diarrhea.

Bisphosphonates Bisphosphonate therapy should be reserved for refractory cases in which the underlying cause of hypercalcemia is not amenable to other therapies. These agents act via inhibition of osteoclastic bone resorption. Pamidronate (0.5-1 mg/kg per dose) may be given intravenously over a period of 4 to 5 hours. The peak effect will not be seen for 48 hours or longer and effects may last up to 24 weeks. Other electrolyte imbalances are frequently seen with bisphosphonate therapy, and patients must therefore be monitored for hypocalcemia, hypophosphatemia, hypomagnesemia, and hypokalemia. If renal failure coexists, bisphosphonate therapy may only be indicated in severe cases and at reduced doses. Renal dialysis may be necessary to decrease calcium levels in these patients (severe cases).

Hemodialysis Dialysis using a low-calcium dialysate is generally reserved for those patients with life-threatening hypercalcemia that is resistant to medical therapy.

Surgery Parathyroidectomy may be indicated for patients with primary hyperparathyroidism. Surgery should be performed by an experienced surgeon to avoid injury to recurrent laryngeal nerves and hypoparathyroidism. If malignancy-derived PTH-rp is the cause of hypercalcemia, treatment of the underlying malignancy is the treatment of choice.

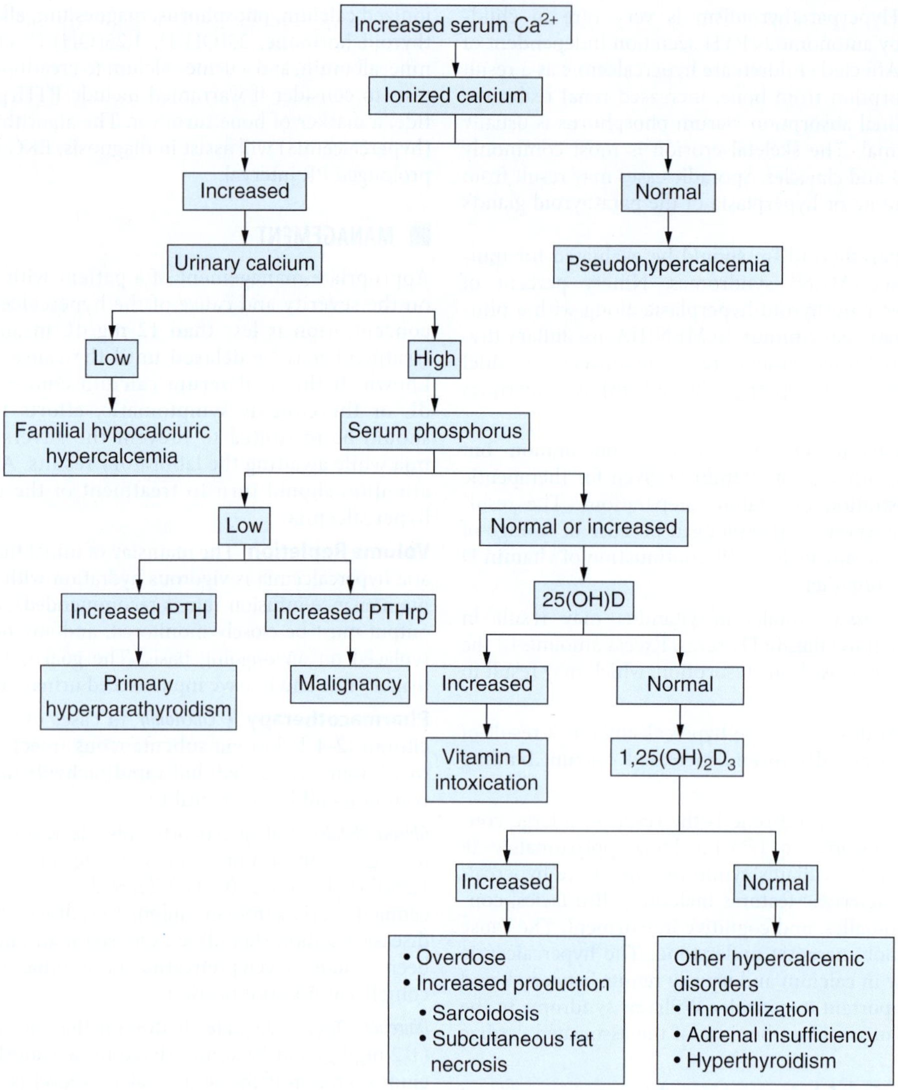

FIGURE 69-2. Flow chart for diagnosing the cause of hypercalcemia. PTH, parathyroid hormone; PTHrp, PTH-related protein.

ADMISSION AND DISCHARGE CRITERIA

Admission

- Symptomatic hypercalcemia
- Severe hypercalcemia, specifically, serum calcium greater than 12 mg/dL (except familial hypocalciuric hypercalcemia)
- Any newborn with hypercalcemia should be monitored in the NICU

Discharge

- Asymptomatic and clinically stable patient
- Arrangements made for regular follow-up to monitor the serum calcium concentration and the underlying disorder

CONSULTATION

Consultation from the following subspecialists may be helpful in diagnosis and/or management. Recommend tailoring consultants based on patient diagnosis.

- Pediatric Endocrinology
- Genetics
- Pediatric Cardiology
- Pediatric Rheumatology
- Pediatric Oncology

KEY POINTS

- The concentration of calcium in serum is modulated through a delicate interplay between PTH and vitamin D via their actions on target organs such as bone, kidney, and the gastrointestinal tract.
- Pediatric reference ranges should be used to interpret levels of total serum calcium, ionized calcium, and phosphorus because levels differ significantly with age.
- PTH and vitamin D levels should be checked before any intervention.
- Hypocalcemia may develop as a result of decreased calcium intake or absorption, excessive urinary loss of calcium, abnormal parathyroid gland development or destruction of the gland, synthesis of an abnormal form of PTH, impaired cellular responsiveness to PTH, restricted exposure to sunlight, or abnormal intake, absorption, or activity of vitamin D and its metabolites.
- Hypercalcemia in children can occur when there is increased resorption of calcium from bone, when the intestinal rate of calcium absorption exceeds renal excretory capacity, or when there is augmented renal tubular absorption of calcium.
- Treatment of hypocalcemia is mainly calcium replacement. Concurrent administration of vitamin D may be required, if vitamin D deficiency is found.
- Treatment of hypercalcemia typically begins with volume expansion to increase urinary calcium excretion. Correction of the underlying cause should be the next focus, but additional pharmacologic management strategies may be necessary depending on the severity of the hypercalcemia and response to volume expansion.

SUGGESTED READINGS

Auron A, Alon US. Hypercalcemia: a consultant's approach. *Pediatr Nephrol.* 2018;33(9):1475-1488.

Gorvin CM. Genetic causes of neonatal and infantile hypercalcaemia. *Pediatr Nephrol.* 2022;37(2):289-301.

Humphrey E, Clardy C. A framework for approaching refractory hypocalcemia in children. *Pediatr Ann.* 2019;48(5):e208-e211.

Kenny CM, Murphy CE, Boyce DS, Ashley DM, Jahanmir J. Things We Do for No Reason™: Calculating a "Corrected Calcium" Level. *J Hosp Med.* 2021;16:499-501.

Nadar R, Shaw N. Investigation and management of hypocalcaemia. *Arch Dis Child.* 2020;105:399-405.

Stokes VJ, Nielsen MF, Hannan FM, Thakker RV. Hypercalcemic disorders in children. *J Bone Miner Res.* 2017;32(11):2157-2170.

CHAPTER 70 Disorders of the Adrenal Gland

Hannah M. Gardner, MD, MSHQS and Jennifer A. Hoefert, MD

BACKGROUND

Adrenal glands are composed of two parts—the adrenal cortex, the outer region of the gland, and the adrenal medulla, located inside the adrenal cortex. The adrenal cortex is divided into three different zones, each of which produces a different type of steroid hormone—the outer zona glomerulosa produces aldosterone (mineralocorticoid), the middle zona fasciculata produces cortisol (glucocorticoid), and the inner zona reticularis produces the androgens dehydroepiandrosterone (DHEA) and dehydroepiandrosterone-sulfate (DHEA-S) which are converted into sex hormones. The adrenal medulla produces catecholamines which contribute to the body's response to stress.

Control of steroid hormone production and release occurs outside of the adrenal gland: aldosterone is primarily controlled by the renin-angiotensin system, and cortisol is regulated by adrenocorticotropic hormone (ACTH) which is stored in the anterior pituitary and is released in response to corticotropin-releasing hormone (CRH).

Each of the steroid hormones produced by the adrenal gland can be pathologically elevated or absent. Additional pathologies can be seen within the adrenal gland leading to the absence of one type of steroid and the overproduction of a precursor steroid (e.g., congenital adrenal hyperplasia), as well as an alteration in timing of steroid production and/or release (e.g., premature adrenarche).

HYPOTHALAMIC-PITUITARY-ADRENAL AXIS

CRH is secreted from the hypothalamus in response to serum cortisol level and stress and stimulates the release of ACTH from the anterior pituitary. ACTH, which regulates the secretion of glucocorticoids from the adrenals, is secreted in a pulsatile manner which varies based on the time of day, leading to a diurnal pattern of cortisol secretion. Cortisol secretion is highest in the early morning prior to waking, decreases in the afternoon and evening, and is lowest at midnight, or a few hours after sleep initiation. Cortisol provides negative feedback on the synthesis and secretion of ACTH and CRH. Interleukin-6 (IL-6), which regulates immune response and inflammatory reactions, also causes stimulation of the hypothalamic-pituitary-adrenal axis (HPA), leading to increased ACTH and cortisol secretion.

ADRENAL CORTEX

Mineralocorticoids, such as aldosterone, regulate sodium and potassium exchange in the distal tubule of the kidney, thereby maintaining electrolyte equilibrium, controlling fluid balance, and blood pressure. Glucocorticoids are responsible for multiple essential body functions: protein degradation, regulation of metabolic activity to increase and maintain serum glucose levels, stimulation of gluconeogenesis, and increasing central fat storage. Glucocorticoids play a role in the immunologic response with anti-inflammatory activity, as well as helping to regulate vascular tone through their action on endothelial and vascular smooth muscle cells. Androgens, which are synthesized in the gonads in addition to the adrenal glands, are responsible for initiation of puberty. DHEA is a precursor of both androgen and estrogen sex hormones.

RENIN-ANGIOTENSIN-ALDOSTERONE SYSTEM

The renin-angiotensin-aldosterone system helps to regulate blood volume and systemic vascular resistance through its effects on sodium and water reabsorption and vasoconstriction. The production and secretion of aldosterone is regulated by renin as well as serum potassium levels. Renin is produced in the juxtaglomerular apparatus of the kidney and leads to the production of angiotensin I. Angiotensin-converting enzyme converts angiotensin I to angiotensin II, which is cleaved to angiotensin III. Angiotensin II and III stimulate the synthesis and secretion of aldosterone from the adrenal cortex, leading to increased sodium reabsorption and potassium excretion. Renin production is stimulated in response to decreased sodium levels, decreased blood pressure, or reduced blood flow to the kidneys.

ADRENAL MEDULLA

The medulla and central nervous system produce catecholamines, including epinephrine, norepinephrine, and dopamine. Vanillylmandelic acid (VMA) and metanephrine are urinary metabolites of catecholamines and are typically elevated in patients with catecholamine-secreting tumors.

ADRENAL INSUFFICIENCY

PATHOPHYSIOLOGY

Adrenocortical deficiency typically refers to a deficiency in either aldosterone or cortisol. It can occur for a variety of reasons, either congenital or acquired, and may affect the adrenal cortex, the pituitary gland, or the hypothalamus. A deficiency in aldosterone leads to sodium wasting and hyperkalemia, while a deficiency in cortisol leads to hypotension and risk for hypoglycemia. Primary adrenal insufficiency refers to a problem within the adrenal gland. Secondary (or tertiary) adrenal insufficiency refers to a central problem with either the pituitary or the hypothalamus.

CLINICAL PRESENTATIONS

The clinical manifestations of an adrenal crisis will vary based on age, but may present with failure to thrive, vomiting, lethargy, anorexia, hypoglycemia, and/or shock. Because cortisol signaling is permissive for catecholamine action, hypotension is particularly challenging to manage as it often does not respond to catecholamines or fluid resuscitation, making it fatal. Other illnesses with similar presentations would include sepsis, colitis, inborn errors of metabolism, and hyperinsulinism. In the absence of crisis, adrenal insufficiency may present as decreased exercise tolerance or lethargy, particularly in the afternoon, and/or muscle aches or nonspecific complaints. Illnesses a hospitalist may consider with these symptom complaints would include hypothyroidism, myositis, neurologic or autoimmune etiologies, and depression. In disorders associated with excess ACTH, there can be hyperpigmentation of the skin and oral mucosa because of increased melanocyte-stimulating hormone (MSH) levels.

DIFFERENTIAL DIAGNOSIS

See **Table 70-1** for causes of adrenal insufficiency.

Congenital Adrenal Hyperplasia Congenital adrenal hyperplasia (CAH) is the most common cause of primary adrenal insufficiency in children and is due to an enzyme deficiency in adrenal steroidogenesis. This results in excess accumulation of steroid precursors and deficiencies

TABLE 70-1 Differential Diagnosis of Adrenal Insufficiency

Category	ACTH	Aldosterone	Comments
Congenital			
Congenital adrenal hyperplasia	↑	Normal or ↓	May see virilization in female neonates; may have salt wasting
Congenital adrenal hypoplasia	↑	Normal	Severe salt wasting always present
ACTH unresponsiveness	↑	Normal	May be associated with alacrimia and achalasia (triple A syndrome)
ACTH/CRH deficiency	↓	Normal	May occur with other pituitary hormone deficiencies
Adrenoleukodystrophy	↑	Normal or ↓	Patients have elevated levels of VLCFA
Wolman disease	Normal	Normal or ↓	Lysosomal storage disease
Aldosterone deficiency	Normal	↓	Deficiency of aldosterone synthase
Pseudohypoaldosterone		↑	Resistance to aldosterone action
Liddle Syndrome		↓	Hypertension and hypokalemia
Neonatal hemorrhage	↑	Normal	Often asymptomatic
Acquired			
Autoimmune/Addison disease	↑	Normal or ↓	May be associated with other autoimmune endocrinopathies
Trauma, hemorrhage, or surgery	↑	Normal or ↓	
Infiltrative	↑	Normal or ↓	Metastatic malignancies, hemochromatosis, sarcoidosis, amyloidosis
Infectious	↑	Normal or ↓	Tuberculosis, HIV, coccidioidomycosis, histoplasmosis, etc.
Acquired ACTH/CRH deficiency	↓	Normal	May be secondary to CNS tumor or trauma
Drugs directly interfering with steroid synthesis	↑	Normal or ↓	May be seen with ketoconazole, rifampin, phenobarbital, phenytoin, etc.
Drugs suppressing the HPA axis	↓	Normal	Steroids
Critical illness	↑	Normal	Likely an inability to keep up with production of steroid in the setting of continuous high demand

ACTH, adrenocorticotropic hormone; CNS, central nervous system; CRH, corticotropin-releasing hormone; HPA, hypothalamic-pituitary-adrenal; VLCFA, very long chain fatty acid.

of end products. Different forms of CAH exert their effects variably due to altered androgen and mineralocorticoid activity (**Figure 70-1**).

The majority of cases (95%) are due to 21-hydroxylase deficiency from a mutation in the CYP21A gene. This occurs in roughly 1 in 13,000 live births. This disease is classically characterized by salt-wasting with adrenal crisis around 2 weeks of age in its severe form. Female infants are virilized at birth, but newborn males have no physical exam findings, putting them at higher risk for delayed diagnosis until presentation in adrenal crisis. Most states have implemented universal screening with 17-hydroxyprogesterone levels for early detection. Some patients have late onset CAH due to mild enzyme deficiencies; they present with features of androgen excess with premature adrenarche and early initiation of puberty.

Addison Disease Addison disease is an acquired primary adrenal insufficiency due to autoimmune destruction of the adrenal cortex and sparing of the adrenal medulla. In older children, adrenal insufficiency caused by Addison disease presents gradually with muscle weakness, lassitude, anorexia, weight loss, wasting, hypotension, salt-craving, and abdominal pain. Elevated ACTH causes hyperpigmentation, either with a generalized tan or localized to the gums or creases in the palms.

Addison disease occurs with other endocrinopathies, such as autoimmune polyglandular syndrome (APS). APS type 1 is an autoimmune polyendocrinopathy which also presents with candidiasis and ectodermal dystrophy. Patients typically have mucocutaneous candidiasis, hypoparathyroidism, and Addison disease. Gonadal failure, alopecia, vitiligo, enamel hypoplasia, intestinal malabsorption, chronic acute hepatitis, and hypothyroidism can also occur in APS type 1. APS type 2 is characterized by Addison disease, autoimmune thyroid disease, and type 1 diabetes mellitus, but gonadal failure, vitiligo, alopecia, and atrophic gastritis can also commonly occur. APS type 2 is associated with HLA-DR3 and HLA-DR4 markers, affecting multiple generations.

Isolated Aldosterone Deficiencies Isolated deficiency of aldosterone is a rare autosomal recessive disorder. Pseudohypoaldosteronism occurs when there is target organ unresponsiveness to aldosterone. It can be limited to the kidney or may involve multiple target organs (sweat glands, salivary glands, and colon). Both autosomal dominant and autosomal recessive inheritance has been reported.

Other Other causes for adrenal insufficiency may involve pathologic or iatrogenic processes affecting the pituitary or hypothalamus. This can include hypopituitarism (Sheehan's syndrome from postpartum hemorrhage and pituitary necrosis), isolated ACTH defect, septo-optic dysplasia, or other midline cerebral defects such as craniopharyngioma, infiltrative pituitary or hypothalamic lesions (Langerhans cell histiocytosis, sarcoidosis), pituitary surgery, irradiation, and head trauma. Likewise, insults to the adrenals can cause corticosteroid deficiencies such as infections (TB, HIV, fungal, sepsis), adrenal hemorrhage, infarctions, or adrenal infiltration. Waterhouse-Friderichsen syndrome is hemorrhagic destruction of the adrenal glands in the context of systemic infection, most commonly by *Neisseria meningitidis*.

Certain medications can cause a state of steroid deficiency. Ketoconazole can inhibit adrenal enzymes. Rifampin, Phenytoin, and Phenobarbital can reduce the bioavailability and effectiveness of exogenously administered corticosteroids. Stopping pharmacologic doses of exogenous corticosteroids in someone with long-standing use of these agents can induce abrupt deficiency of glucocorticoids, which is one of the most common causes of secondary adrenal suppression seen clinically. These patients require a slow steroid taper as the HPA axis suppression may take up to 12 months to recover after chronic use.

DIAGNOSTIC EVALUATION

Obtaining the following labs is helpful for the diagnosis of adrenal insufficiency: sodium, potassium, bicarbonate, pH, glucose, AM cortisol, ACTH, renin, aldosterone, urine sodium, urine chloride, and urine potassium. Laboratory findings will vary based on the underlying etiology. See **Table 70-2**. ACTH will be elevated in primary adrenal insufficiency. In secondary or tertiary adrenal insufficiency, ACTH levels will be low. Mineralocorticoid activity is normal in secondary adrenal insufficiency; therefore, hyperkalemia is not present. Hyponatremia can still occur due to decreased water excretion from lack of glucocorticoid activity.

A morning cortisol level is the initial screening method for glucocorticoid deficiency. If this value is below 10 mcg/dL, a stimulation test should be performed. ACTH normally stimulates adrenal gland production of cortisol to greater than 18 mcg/dL. In primary adrenal insufficiency, there is minimal to no response to the standard/high ACTH dose of 250 mcg (125 mcg for infants) given IV, with cortisol measured at 0, 30, and 60 minutes. In secondary adrenal insufficiency, there may be some response until the adrenal glands atrophy over time, so a low ACTH dose (1 mcg) is used to prevent false positives. A CRH stimulation test is a preferred test for secondary adrenal insufficiency when CRH is available. To administer, give CRH 1 mcg/kg IV and measure ACTH and cortisol levels at 15, 30, 60, and 90 minutes.

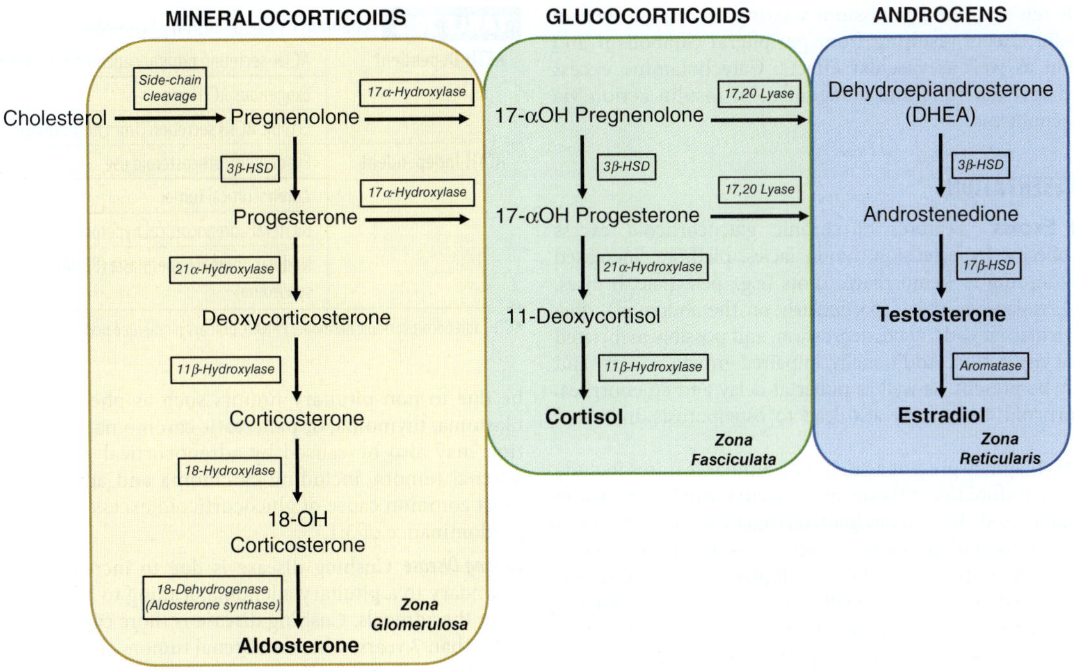

FIGURE 70-1. Adrenal cortical steroidogenic pathway including the mineralocorticoid, glucocorticoid, and androgen pathways.

Abdominal radiographs may show calcification of the adrenal gland secondary to infection or hemorrhage. Abdominal ultrasound may reveal enlarged adrenals bilaterally in CAH. Magnetic resonance imaging (MRI) of the brain/pituitary should be obtained in patients found to have secondary adrenal insufficiency to assess for central nervous system lesions.

In any patient presenting with symptoms of classic adrenal crisis, a serum ACTH and cortisol level should be drawn if possible prior to emergent treatment with stress-dose steroids. Because steroid administration is urgent in these cases, steroids should not be delayed pending the results of these tests. Elevation of both ACTH and cortisol levels can provide post-treatment reassurance of normal adrenal function.

MANAGEMENT

Treatment of adrenal insufficiency includes both acute and chronic therapy. Adrenal crisis requires immediate treatment with stress-dose steroids (100 mg/m^2 of hydrocortisone or glucocorticoid equivalent), dextrose, and normal saline to correct hypoglycemia and salt loss. For those with both glucocorticoid and mineralocorticoid deficiency, chronic treatment includes oral hydrocortisone two to three times daily (6-12 mg/m^2/day of hydrocortisone or glucocorticoid equivalent) and the mineralocorticoid fludrocortisone once daily. In some cases, sodium chloride supplementation may also be required. Plasma renin and serum sodium concentrations may be used to monitor the adequacy of mineralocorticoid replacement, and morning ACTH can be monitored to prevent overtreatment with glucocorticoid. Increased doses of hydrocortisone will need to be given during periods of stress (e.g., fever, illness, and/or surgery). Glucocorticoid therapy for CAH not only replaces the deficient cortisol but also suppresses the excessive ACTH secretion, resulting in a decrease in adrenal androgen secretion and thereby limiting virilization.

When patients with known adrenal insufficiency are admitted to the hospital with acute illness, they may have a relative insufficiency of steroids, and present with symptoms of adrenal insufficiency even when provided maintenance therapy. It is critical these children receive stress-dose steroids during acute illness.

ADMISSION AND DISCHARGE CRITERIA

Criteria for admission include:

- Electrolyte imbalance
- Hemodynamic instability
- Altered mental status
- Dehydration or inability to tolerate enteral steroids

Criteria for discharge include:

- Asymptomatic and clinically stable patient
- Regular follow-up arranged for monitoring serum electrolytes and/or blood pressure and the underlying disease
- Patient and/or patient's guardians/caretakers have received education on stress dosing, including IM injection if unable to take oral stress doses

CONSULTATION

- Pediatric endocrinologist
- Geneticist for patients with genetic forms of adrenal insufficiency
- Pediatric neurologist for patients with adrenoleukodystrophy

HYPERADRENAL STATES

PATHOPHYSIOLOGY

Similar to adrenal insufficiency, the pathophysiology of hyperadrenal states follows in a straightforward manner from the physiological effects of each of the adrenal hormones. Aldosterone excess leads

TABLE 70-2 Common Lab Values in Adrenal Insufficiency

	Na	K	HCO3	Glucose	AM cortisol	ACTH	Renin	Aldosterone
Primary Adrenal Insufficiency	↓	↑	↓	↓	↓	↑	↑	↓
Secondary Adrenal Insufficiency	↓ or normal	Normal	Normal	↓ or normal	↓	↓	Normal	Normal

ACTH, adrenocorticotropic hormone; HCO3, bicarbonate; K, Potassium; Na, Sodium.

to increased salt retention and potassium wasting. Excess of cortisol leads to metabolic effects resulting from peripheral catabolism and central anabolism as well as vascular effects. Catecholamine excess causes increased vascular tone and antagonism of insulin action via β-adrenergic mechanisms.

CLINICAL PRESENTATIONS

Glucocorticoid Excess Features of chronic glucocorticoid excess include central obesity, hypertension, moon facies, plethora, increased capillary fragility leading to hemorrhagic spots (e.g., petechiae, bruises, and hematomas), violaceous striae (particularly on the abdomen), dorsal and supraclavicular fat pads, acne, depression, and possibly associated signs of abnormal virilization. Additionally, impaired growth velocity and short stature may be present, as well as pubertal delay and amenorrhea. Chronic glucocorticoid excess may also lead to osteoporosis and renal stones.

Other problems that may present acutely with similar features include obesity and thyroid dysfunction. Obesity often occurs with hypertension and insulin resistance and also can be characterized by striae, as well as a buffalo hump distribution of fat. However, obesity is usually associated with increased growth as opposed to the growth plateau typically associated with glucocorticoid excess. Additionally, the degree of hypertension in glucocorticoid excess is generally higher than that observed with obesity. Hypothyroidism can lead to obesity, hypertension, and growth failure, but is usually not associated with striae or moon facies. Conversely, hyperthyroidism can lead to hypertension, but is more commonly associated with thin body habitus rather than central obesity.

Aldosterone Excess Patients with hyperaldosteronism may have moderate or severe hypertension, hypokalemia, weakness, tetany, growth failure, and intermittent paralysis. Some patients may be asymptomatic, and blood pressures can range from normotensive to severe or refractory hypertension.

Catecholamine Excess Symptoms of catecholamine excess may present differently in children than in adults. In children with pheochromocytoma, more than 90% of the hypertension is sustained instead of paroxysmal (as often observed in adults with pheochromocytoma). While the hypertension is often sustained, many of the most common complaints (headache, sweating, nausea, abdominal pain, and palpitations) may occur in a paroxysmal fashion. Sweating, visual changes, nausea and vomiting, weight loss, polyuria, and polydipsia are more common in children than adults. Pallor (and infrequently flushing), weight loss, weakness, and fatigue may also be noted. Symptoms may be precipitated by exercise, Valsalva maneuvers, alcohol ingestion, and intubation. If the catecholamine excess has been long standing, cardiac examination may reveal left ventricular hypertrophy or even cardiomyopathy, and there may be changes on fundoscopic examination. Elevated fasting plasma glucose levels and glycosuria may be present.

In patients with symptoms of catecholamine excess, acute ingestion of muscarinic antagonists should be considered, which appears very similar to catecholamine excess.

Patients with neuroblastoma may present with an abdominal mass, fever, weight loss, bone pain, periorbital ecchymosis/proptosis, anemia or pancytopenia, flushing, headache, and hypertension. Infants may present with nontender bluish subcutaneous nodules.

DIFFERENTIAL DIAGNOSIS

Glucocorticoid Excess

Cushing syndrome Cushing syndrome is a constellation of symptoms, including obesity, poor growth, and hypertension, which is secondary to chronic glucocorticoid excess. Cushing syndrome is seen with both exogenous use of corticosteroids and endogenous causes that lead to increased cortisol (see **Table 70-3**). The most common cause of Cushing syndrome is long-term administration of systemic glucocorticosteroids or ACTH. Following exogenous causes, the most common cause in older children is bilateral adrenal hyperplasia, which affects males and females equally. It may be due to hypersecretion of ACTH from a pituitary adenoma (Cushing disease) or ectopic ACTH secretion (may be due to non-pituitary tumors such as pheochromocytoma, neuroblastoma, thymoma, or pancreatic carcinoma). Excess cortisol production may also be caused by adrenocortical nodular hyperplasia and adrenal tumors, including carcinoma and adenoma. Tumors are the most common cause of glucocorticoid excess in infants, with a female predominance of 3:1.

TABLE 70-3 Common Causes of Cushing Syndrome

ACTH-Dependent	ACTH-secreting pituitary adenoma (Cushing disease)
	Exogenous ACTH use
	Ectopic ACTH secretion (from non-pituitary site)
ACTH-Independent	Exogenous corticosteroid use
	Adrenocortical tumor
	Bilateral adrenocortical hyperplasia
	Nodular adrenal hyperplasia (PPNAD, McCune-Albright syndrome)

ACTH, adrenocorticotropic hormone; PPNAD, primary pigmented nodular adrenocortical disease.

Cushing Disease Cushing disease is due to increased ACTH production secondary to a pituitary adenoma, leading to hypersecretion of cortisol from the adrenals. Cushing disease is more commonly seen in children older than 7 years, whereas adrenal tumors are more commonly seen in patients younger than 7 years.

Aldosterone Excess

Primary Hyperaldosteronism Primary hyperaldosteronism is uncommon in children and includes all disorders in which the increased production of aldosterone is independent of the renin-angiotensin system. Primary hyperaldosteronism can be due to an aldosterone-secreting adenoma, which is typically unilateral and mainly affects girls, or bilateral micronodular adrenocortical hyperplasia, which is typically seen in adolescents. An uncommon form of low-renin hypertension is an autosomal dominant disorder with increased ACTH secretion and subsequent hypersecretion of aldosterone.

Secondary Hyperaldosteronism Secondary hyperaldosteronism is due to an activated renin-angiotensin-aldosterone system (RAAS). Excess renin production leads to increased aldosterone release and can be seen in renal artery stenosis, Wilms tumor, and juxtaglomerular cell tumors. Renin production may also be increased due to sodium loss or volume depletion and in edematous states such as congestive heart failure, cirrhosis, and nephrotic syndrome. There are also genetic disorders leading to secondary hyperaldosteronism, including Bartter syndrome and Gitelman syndrome.

Catecholamine Excess Excess production of catecholamines occurs with tumors affecting the adrenal medulla, such as pheochromocytoma, paraganglioma, and neuroblastoma, but can additionally be seen with stress, alcohol ingestion, and use of certain medications (e.g., monoamine oxidase inhibitors, tricyclic antidepressants, adrenergic receptor agonists) and drugs (amphetamines, nicotine). Tumors of the adrenal medulla lead to increased catecholamine production.

Mercury toxicity is another cause of catecholamine excess, as elemental mercury interferes with catecholamine catabolism, resulting in elevated levels of catecholamines and clinical symptoms of tachycardia, hypertension, and sweating.

Pheochromocytoma Pheochromocytomas are rarely seen in childhood, but children with pheochromocytoma are more likely than adults to have bilateral tumors, multiple tumors, and tumors at extra-adrenal sites, usually within the abdominal cavity. Extra-adrenal pheochromocytomas are also called paragangliomas. The majority of cases in childhood occur between ages 6 and 14 years, with tumors varying in size and are more frequently found on the right side of the body. Pheochromocytomas can be seen with other disorders, including neurofibromatosis, von Hippel-Lindau disease, multiple endocrine neoplasia (MEN) type II, tuberous sclerosis, Sturge-Weber syndrome, and ataxia-telangiectasia.

Neuroblastoma Neuroblastoma is a malignant tumor and can be found anywhere along the sympathetic chain, including the adrenal medulla.

It is the most common extracranial solid tumor in children and is most commonly diagnosed in children <5 years old. It can spontaneously regress in infants younger than 6 months. Neuroblastomas typically are not associated with hypertension. Cervical tumors may present with Horner's syndrome (ptosis, miosis, anhidrosis), which is more frequently seen in infants. The most common sites of metastasis include regional lymph nodes, bone and bone marrow, liver, and skin; metastasis to the brain and lung are less frequently seen.

DIAGNOSTIC EVALUATION

Glucocorticoid Excess Initial screen for glucocorticoid excess is a nighttime salivary cortisol. If positive (greater than 1 mcg/dL at bedtime or > 0.27 mcg/dL at midnight), the next appropriate test is a 24-hour urinary free cortisol and midnight serum cortisol. In glucocorticoid excess, results should demonstrate elevated midnight serum cortisol (>2 mcg/dL) and 24-hour urinary free cortisol levels (>4 times the upper limit of normal). Complete blood count (CBC) may demonstrate polycythemia, lymphopenia, and decreased eosinophils. Serum electrolytes may also demonstrate hypokalemia and hyperglycemia. Further testing may reveal abnormal glucose tolerance or diabetes.

If the 24-hour urinary cortisol is positive or equivocal in the context of a high index of suspicion for glucocorticoid excess, an overnight dexamethasone suppression test can aid in diagnosis. In children without glucocorticoid excess, administration of dexamethasone 15 mcg/kg (maximum 1 mg) between 10 PM and 12 AM will usually suppress the following 8 AM cortisol level to less than 5 mcg/dL. In patients with pathologic excess of cortisol, cortisol levels will not be suppressed (>5 mcg/dL is diagnostic, normal is suppression to <1.8 mcg/dL) in response to an overnight dexamethasone suppression test. In this circumstance, a two-step (low-dose and high-dose) suppression test may be performed. In the low-dose test, 30 mcg/kg/day is administered in four divided doses for 2 days. The high-dose test consists of administration of 120 mcg/kg/day in four divided doses for 2 days. In patients with Cushing disease, cortisol levels will not be suppressed with low-dose but will be with high-dose dexamethasone.

Midnight ACTH level can be obtained for further evaluation; in causes with excess cortisol production (e.g., cortisol-secreting tumors), ACTH should be low, and in cases with excess ACTH production (e.g., ACTH-secreting tumors), ACTH is expected to be high, but could be normal with some pituitary adenomas.

MRI or CT of the abdomen can rule out an adrenal tumor and MRI of the head can help rule out an ACTH-secreting pituitary tumor.

In psychiatric diseases such as depression, the diurnal variation of cortisol production flattens out due to increased nighttime production of cortisol. This alteration can lead to false positives on screening midnight salivary cortisol but typically the overall cortisol production as measured by 24-hour urinary cortisol is normal. The increase in nighttime cortisol is not thought to be a primary defect.

Aldosterone Excess To diagnose primary hyperaldosteronism, renin, aldosterone, sodium, and potassium levels should be obtained simultaneously. Patients with primary hyperaldosteronism have hypokalemia, low renin, and increased blood and urinary aldosterone levels. Patients with secondary hyperaldosteronism are often normotensive and workup may reveal hypokalemic alkalosis and increased renin levels. In glucocorticoid-suppressible hyperaldosteronism, dexamethasone (0.25 mg every 6 hours) will suppress aldosterone and normalize blood pressures. In patients with clinical suspicion for a tumor, abdominal CT or MRI and adrenal vein catheterization can help localize the tumor.

Catecholamine Excess Dopamine is metabolized to homovanillic acid (HVA), norepinephrine to normetanephrine, and epinephrine to metanephrine. Metanephrine and normetanephrine are further metabolized by VMA. In individuals with catecholamine excess, the catecholamines or their metabolites may be elevated in the blood or urine. Episodic secretion of catecholamines by tumors can make it difficult to detect elevated levels. Furthermore, catecholamine levels may be falsely elevated by medication (e.g., calcium channel blockers, beta blockers, mood stabilizers, and stimulants) or in response to stressful stimuli. Evaluation of catecholamine metabolites is recommended, including plasma free metanephrines (metanephrine and normetanephrine) and 24-hour urinary fractionated metanephrines. As the production of plasma free metanephrines is constant and independent of the release of catecholamines, which are episodically secreted, these are the gold standard for diagnosis.

The degree of elevation of catecholamine metabolites should be assessed; values of greater than 4x the upper limit of normal are highly suggestive of a tumor. If urine or plasma metanephrines are only mildly to moderately elevated (greater than the upper limit of normal but less than 4x the upper limit of normal), this should be confirmed with a second 24-hour urine collection prior to obtaining imaging. Additionally, if there is a high index of suspicion for catecholamine excess secondary to tumor, the diagnosis should not be ruled out by a single normal 24-hour urine collection; repeat measurements may be required before an abnormality is observed.

If significant elevations of catecholamines or metabolites are identified, imaging for localization should be obtained with a CT or MRI of the abdomen and pelvis, as well as the head, neck, and chest. CT and MRI have similar diagnostic sensitivities (90%-100%), with specificities around 70% to 80%; MRI has higher sensitivity at locating extra-adrenal tumors and can better evaluate for involvement of major vessels or invasion into the spinal canal. If indicated, functional imaging via I-metaiodobenzylguanidine (I-MIBG) scintigraphy or positron emission tomography (PET) should be undertaken; these may be used to detect multifocal disease and malignancy, or if prior imaging was negative but there remains a high index of suspicion for catecholamine-secreting tumors.

If pheochromocytoma is identified, screening for genetic disorders such as MEN type IIA and IIB, von Hippel-Lindau disease, and neurofibromatosis should occur.

MANAGEMENT

Glucocorticoid Excess Treatment of glucocorticoid excess is based on its etiology. Cushing disease is treated with transsphenoidal adenomectomy. Adrenal adenomas, as well as ectopic ACTH-secreting tumors, are treated by surgical removal of the tumor; if the tumor is not resectable, adrenalectomy may be indicated. Nodular adrenal hyperplasia is treated with bilateral adrenalectomy. These patients require perioperative and postoperative glucocorticoid treatment until their HPA axis recovers (evaluated by ACTH-stimulation test). Surgery on or near the pituitary may lead to postoperative hypopituitarism.

Mineralocorticoid Excess Treatment of mineralocorticoid excess involves electrolyte correction (predominantly hypokalemia) as well as addressing the underlying renin and aldosterone abnormalities. Definitive therapy may include surgical resection if adenoma is present or adrenalectomy if unilateral disease is present; aldosterone antagonists (e.g., spironolactone, eplerenone) are used more frequently in bilateral hyperplasia. If elevated blood pressures persist despite treatment, blood pressure control is recommended for prevention of morbidity and mortality related to hypertension.

Catecholamine Excess Pheochromocytomas are treated with surgical resection and require lifelong follow-up. Pre-operative management includes blood pressure control with alpha- and beta-blocker medications, with beta-blockade not initiated until adequate alpha-blockade (typically with phenoxybenzamine) has been established. Beta-blockade in the absence of alpha-blockade can worsen hypertension and is generally used as adjunctive therapy in cases where alpha-blockade has induced severe tachycardia or tachyarrhythmias.

Treatment for neuroblastoma depends on the staging and if metastatic disease is present. Low-risk patients are typically treated with surgical resection alone, while patients with intermediate-risk disease are treated with a combination of surgery and chemotherapy, as well as radiation therapy if tumor debulking is indicated prior to surgery or if there is poor response to chemotherapy. Treatment for high-risk patients involves multimodal therapy involving surgical resection, chemotherapy, radiation therapy, and stem cell transplant and immunotherapy.

ADMISSION AND DISCHARGE CRITERIA

Criteria for admission include:

- Electrolyte imbalance
- Hemodynamic instability
- Altered mental status

Criteria for discharge include:

- Adequate control of symptoms and clinical stability
- Regular follow-up established for monitoring serum electrolytes and/or blood pressure as well as underlying disease

CONSULTATION

- Pediatric endocrinologist
- Pediatric surgeon (as needed)
- Pediatric oncologist (as needed)

KEY POINTS

- The pathophysiology of adrenal excess and insufficiency follow from the physiology of the hormone that is at altered concentration
- In suspected adrenal crisis, if possible, obtain a serum ACTH and cortisol prior to administering stress dose steroids
- The tests to determine adrenal deficit are different from adrenal excess
    - To evaluate for glucocorticoid insufficiency, screen with an AM serum cortisol
    - To evaluate for glucocorticoid excess, screen with midnight salivary cortisol or 24-hour urinary cortisol and midnight serum cortisol
- Hyperaldosteronism may present with hypertension and/or electrolyte derangements
- Catecholamine-secreting tumors in children may present with episodic symptoms but sustained hypertension
- Evaluate for catecholamine-secreting tumors with plasma free metanephrines and 24-hour urinary fractionated metanephrines

SUGGESTED READINGS

Auron, M, Raissouni, N. Adrenal insufficiency. *Pediatr Rev.* 2015;36(3):92-103.

Bholah R, Bunchman TE. Review of pediatric pheochromocytoma and paraganglioma. *Front Pediatr.* 2017;5:155.

Bowden SA, Henry R. Pediatric adrenal insufficiency: diagnosis, management, and new therapies. *Int J Pediatr.* 2018;2018:1739831.

Ferrigno R, Hasenmajer V, Caiulo S, et al. Paediatric Cushing's disease: epidemiology, pathogenesis, clinical management and outcome. *Rev Endocr Metab Disord.* 2021;22:817-835.

Konrad M, Nijenhuis T, Ariceta G, et al. Diagnosis and management of Bartter syndrome: executive summary of the consensus and recommendations from the European Rare Kidney Disease Reference Network Working Group for Tubular Disorders. *Kidney Int.* 2021;99(2):324-335.

Lodish MB, Keil MF, Stratakis CA. Cushing's syndrome in pediatrics: an update. *Endocrinol Metab Clin North Am.* 2018;47(2):451-462.

Nisticò D, Bossini B, Benvenuto S, Pellegrin MC, Tornese G. Pediatric adrenal insufficiency: challenges and solutions. *Ther Clin Risk Manag.* 2022;18:47-60.

Speiser PW, et al. Congenital adrenal hyperplasia due to steroid 21-hydroxylase deficiency: an endocrine society clinical practice guideline. *J Clin Endocrinol Metab.* 2018;103(11):4043-4088.

Witchel SF. Congenital adrenal hyperplasia. *J Pediatr Adolesc Gynecol.* 2017;30(5):520-534.

Young WF Jr. Diagnosis and treatment of primary aldosteronism: practical clinical perspectives. *J Intern Med.* 2018;285(2):126-148.

SECTION G
Gastroenterology and Nutrition

CHAPTER 71
Pediatric Biliary Disease

Anika Nelson, MD and Amethyst C. Kurbegov, MD, MPH

BACKGROUND

The biliary tree includes a series of ducts that drain bile from the liver, gallbladder, and pancreas into the duodenum. Biliary tract diseases can present at any age and have become increasingly recognized in pediatric practice as diagnostic tests have improved. While some diseases of the biliary system are associated with liver disease, others are specific to the biliary tract alone.

PATHOPHYSIOLOGY

Primary biliary tract diseases fall into two pathologic categories: obstructive and inflammatory. Obstruction of bile flow from the liver into the duodenum results in pressure in the biliary system (leading to pain, jaundice, and potentially pancreatitis), fat malabsorption (from poor micelle formation in the gut), and potential infection (from gut flora contamination of static biliary tree fluid). Obstruction is most often caused by gallstones but may be due to anatomic abnormalities, such as choledochal cysts. Inflammatory processes are most often autoimmune in nature but can be due to chronic infections or genetic diseases. These conditions often progress unrecognized until significant biliary damage has occurred, leading to bile duct scarring, obstruction, or malignancy. If biliary inflammation and obstruction are not relieved or treated, hepatic damage may result. Finally, gallbladder dysfunction in storing and/or evacuating bile can lead to the organ's distention and inflammation leading to subsequent chronic pain and dyspepsia.

CLINICAL PRESENTATIONS

Jaundice is typically the first sign of biliary disease that prompts medical evaluation. Complete or near-complete obstruction of bile flow can result in acholic stools that are light yellow to clay in color. For infants in diapers, stools may occasionally have a hint of pigment on the exterior surface due to sloughing of enteric cells or staining from bile-pigmented urine. Once this layer is removed, however, the clay-colored stool inside is apparent. Dark urine, associated with renal excretion of bilirubin, may also be found.

The clinical presentation of primary biliary tract disease varies by age. Approximately 60% of term and 80% of preterm infants develop jaundice without other signs of biliary disease, the vast majority of which is physiologic and resolves without intervention. However, this can lead to complacency by clinicians and delays in diagnosing more serious neonatal biliary and liver diseases. While older children with biliary disease also present with jaundice, they often have additional signs or symptoms indicating biliary obstruction or inflammation. These include right shoulder, epigastric, or upper quadrant pain (during inspiration, Murphy sign); postprandial pain or nausea (particularly with high-fat foods); vomiting; light-colored stools; or dark urine. Specifically, Charcot's Triad of fever, right upper quadrant abdominal pain, and jaundice points toward cholangitis. Bacterial cholangitis can progress to bacteremia and sepsis, particularly if obstruction is present. Systemic illnesses, such as scarlet fever, Kawasaki disease, and leptospirosis, can lead to acute gallbladder distension and poor contractility, known as hydrops, with findings of right upper quadrant pain, mass, and evidence of systemic disease.

Biliary disease also may present with poor weight gain due to inadequate bile salts in the intestinal lumen and fat malabsorption. In addition, symptoms or physical findings indicative of fat-soluble vitamin deficiencies may be found, including hemorrhage or hematoma (vitamin K deficiency), rickets (vitamin D deficiency), night blindness and corneal xerophthalmia (vitamin A deficiency), and peripheral neuropathy (vitamin E deficiency). Subacute biliary disease, such as acalculous cholangitis, can present more gradually with persistent or worsening right upper quadrant pain and nausea or vomiting with high-fat foods, but no fever or jaundice.

Hepatosplenomegaly is not typically associated with primary biliary tract conditions. However, the cholestasis of chronic biliary disease can result in hepatocellular injury, which may ultimately lead to liver fibrosis and portal hypertension.

DIFFERENTIAL DIAGNOSIS

The differential diagnosis of biliary disease in children is best categorized by age of presentation (**Table 71-1**). Metabolic, congenital endocrinologic, and genetic disorders are more likely to present in neonates and infants, while gallbladder dysfunction and cholelithiasis are more typically found in older children and adolescents. Anatomic abnormalities, such as biliary atresia, often present in infancy, but some conditions, such as choledochal cysts, can become apparent at any age.

DIAGNOSTIC EVALUATION

Although the evaluation for possible biliary tract disease should be tailored to the individual patient, the initial steps are usually similar (**Table 71-2**). First and foremost, serum fractionated bilirubin is required to determine if jaundice is due to conjugated ("direct") versus unconjugated ("indirect") hyperbilirubinemia, as cholestasis, or poor bile flow, is (by definition) associated with elevated conjugated bilirubin. Thereafter, studies should be selected based on clinical suspicion, feasibility, and invasiveness. Management of conditions detected during diagnostic evaluation is addressed in the discussions of each specific diagnosis.

An elevated conjugated bilirubin is associated with obstruction of bile flow through or from the liver due to either congenital or acquired lesions. Conditions of hepatic dysfunction can also be associated with elevated bilirubin, such as occurs in viral hepatitis or gram-negative rod sepsis, due to intracellular disruption of the bile flow. In contrast, an elevated unconjugated bilirubin is found in various hemolytic and abnormal liver conjugating conditions, such as breast milk jaundice and Crigler-Najjar syndrome and does not indicate diseases of bile flow.

It is particularly important to maintain a low threshold for obtaining a fractionated bilirubin in older neonates with persistent jaundice because timely intervention is required if biliary atresia is found. Biliary atresia is the most common cause of cholestasis in infants and must be treated early. The most recent American Academy of Pediatrics Guideline on the management of hyperbilirubinemia in newborns (2022) recommends measurement of fractionated serum bilirubin in any jaundiced infant at 2 weeks of age if formula fed and at 3-4 weeks of age if exclusively breast fed. In the presence of elevated total bilirubin, direct/conjugated bilirubin levels are considered abnormal when values are >1.0 mg/dL (17 μmol/L) regardless of the total bilirubin; this finding requires efficient and aggressive evaluation and management in any young infant.

In addition to a fractionated bilirubin, a broader laboratory assessment of liver inflammation and function should be pursued in all patients with suspected biliary disease. These include alanine transaminase (ALT), aspartate transaminase (AST), alkaline phosphatase, gamma-glutamyl transferase (GGT), total protein, and albumin levels and prothrombin time (PT)/INR. ALT and AST are markers of hepatocyte inflammation

TABLE 71-1 Differential Diagnosis of Biliary Tract Disease by Age

Infancy
Biliary atresia
Choledochal cyst
Gallstone, gallbladder sludge
Cystic fibrosis
Bile duct paucity
Syndromic (Alagille syndrome)
Nonsyndromic
Hypothyroidism
Panhypopituitarism
Congenital infection
Spontaneous perforation of common bile duct
Childhood
Gallstone
Choledochal cyst
Cholangitis
Acalculous cholecystitis
Hydrops of gallbladder
Biliary dyskinesia
Primary sclerosing cholangitis
Common bile duct stricture
Malignancy
Biliary helminthiasis
Graft-versus-host disease

and breakdown and may be elevated if biliary tract disease is severe enough to generate secondary inflammation in the liver. Alkaline phosphatase and GGT are more specific for the biliary tract and are usually elevated, possibly 10 times normal or more, with acute biliary tree obstruction or inflammation. Albumin and PT are indicators of liver synthetic function and are less likely to be abnormal in an acute biliary process. Although not common, liver failure can be seen with some biliary tract diseases, including biliary atresia and untreated common bile duct cholelithiasis. In patients with fever, a complete blood count and blood culture should be obtained given the possibility of cholangitis and subsequent bacteremia.

Ultrasonography is the most useful first imaging modality for assessing biliary tract disease. A carefully performed ultrasound can detect stones in the gallbladder, common bile duct, or elsewhere in the biliary tree. Dilatation of bile ducts, either intra- or extrahepatic, can indicate obstruction. Congenital malformations of the biliary tree, primarily choledochal cysts, are also typically detected by ultrasonography. Finally, abdominal ultrasonography allows the evaluation of other organs that can be affected by or associated with biliary disease, such as the pancreas, liver, and spleen.

TABLE 71-2 Evaluation of Suspected Biliary Tract Disease

All Patients
History and physical examination
Laboratory studies
Fractionated bilirubin
Aspartate transaminase, alanine transaminase, γ-glutamyl transferase, alkaline phosphatase
Albumin, prothrombin time/INR
Complete blood count, blood culture (in presence of fever)
Abdominal ultrasonography
Further Options
Hepatobiliary iminodiacetic acid scan (HIDA)
Liver biopsy
Sweat test
Magnetic resonance cholangiopancreatography (diagnostic)
Endoscopic retrograde cholangiopancreatography (therapeutic)
Genetic and metabolic testing
Thyroid function tests
Congenital infection tests (urine CMV PCR or culture, TORCH titers)

SPECIFIC DISEASES AND THEIR MANAGEMENT

This section discusses in greater depth the pathophysiology and management of those biliary diseases most likely to be encountered by the pediatric hospitalist. Biliary atresia and choledochal cysts are typically diagnosed in infancy, although the latter may rarely present in older children and adults. Cholelithiasis, cholangitis, acalculous cholecystitis, biliary dyskinesia, gallbladder hydrops, and primary sclerosing cholangitis are more likely to be found in older children and adolescents, although infants may develop cholelithiasis, particularly if treated with parenteral nutrition in the neonatal period. Biliary dyskinesia and primary sclerosing cholangitis are typically evaluated on an outpatient basis so will not be discussed.

BILIARY ATRESIA

Biliary atresia accounts for 40% to 50% of all cases of neonatal cholestasis and occurs in 1 in 8000 to 12,000 births. It is the leading indication for pediatric liver transplantation worldwide. In this condition, all or part of the extrahepatic bile ducts are destroyed or absent, leading to early cholestasis and rapidly progressive liver disease. While 15% to 20% of cases of biliary atresia are associated with congenital malformations (e.g., biliary atresia splenic malformation), the remaining cases result from acquired inflammatory processes. The etiology of this inflammation is still not fully understood, although several mechanisms have been implicated, such as viral triggers, environmental toxins, and immune dysregulation. Without surgical correction, death occurs in the first 2 years of life from liver failure; even with therapy, timing and surgical expertise are crucial to patient outcomes.

Biliary atresia typically presents with prolonged neonatal jaundice, acholic stools, and possibly malnutrition due to fat malabsorption. Since early surgical intervention is critical for patient outcomes, evaluation for biliary atresia must be pursued promptly. Laboratory studies reveal an elevated conjugated bilirubin and often only mildly elevated liver enzymes. The GGT and alkaline phosphatase are typically disproportionately high compared to the AST and ALT. Abdominal ultrasound findings may include an absent gallbladder and a "triangular cord" in the porta hepatis, but it is important to note that the presence of a gallbladder does not rule out biliary atresia. Radioisotope studies with technetium cholescintigraphy (also referred to as a "HIDA scan") can be helpful in distinguishing between biliary atresia and neonatal hepatitis. Classically, tracer is taken up well by the liver but is not excreted into the bowel in biliary atresia, whereas the opposite is true in neonatal hepatitis and other nonobstructive lesions. An abnormal study by itself is not diagnostic of biliary atresia, however, because other causes of chronic cholestasis, such as cystic fibrosis, Alagille syndrome, total parenteral nutrition (TPN)-cholestasis, and α-1-antitrypsin deficiency, may also have nonexcretion of tracer.

The definitive diagnosis of biliary atresia is made by liver biopsy and/or intraoperative cholangiogram. Liver biopsy shows proliferation of intrahepatic bile ductules, diffuse cholestasis, and often fibrosis. If the biopsy is suggestive of obstruction, an intraoperative cholangiogram should be performed to confirm the diagnosis and determine the degree of anatomic involvement. When suspicion of biliary atresia is high, particularly since time is of the essence in infants older than 6 weeks of age, proceeding directly to operative cholangiogram and open liver biopsy should be considered. These evaluations and interventions should take place at a tertiary pediatric hospital with a hepatology center.

A Kasai procedure (hepatoportoenterostomy) should follow cholangiogram if biliary atresia is confirmed. The goal of this surgery is to reestablish bile flow from the remaining patent ductules in the liver to a jejunal limb attached to the porta hepatis via a Roux-en-Y anastomosis. The timing of surgery is crucial, with correction before 60 days of life vastly improving outcomes. This procedure is successful in 80% to 90% of infants if it is performed during this time frame by an experienced surgeon in a center with significant numbers of biliary atresia patients. The success rate drops to <20% in patients 90 days of age or older at the time of surgery. Establishment of adequate bile flow immediately after surgery predicts a good outcome, but progressive liver disease and fibrosis usually still occur after surgery. Overall, following a Kasai procedure, approximately 50% of children require liver transplantation by 5 years of age and 70% by age 20. Transplantation is not pursued at the time of diagnosis due to neonatal size and the possibility of long-term success with hepatoportoenterostomy alone. Children's post-transplant survival and outcomes are greatly improved by successful Kasai procedures due to the gain of years of functional bile flow with subsequently enhanced growth and nutritional status.

CHOLEDOCHAL CYSTS

Choledochal cysts are congenital cystic dilations of the biliary tree; they may be extrahepatic, intrahepatic, or both. The incidence of cysts varies worldwide, occurring in about 1 in 13,000 to 15,000 births in Western countries but as frequently as 1 in 1000 births in Japan. There is a 4:1 female predominance. Choledochal cysts are typically present in infancy and are found in up to 2% of infants presenting with obstructive jaundice. Cysts may occasionally present as late as adulthood, and unrecognized malformations may lead to malignant cholangiocarcinoma in adults.

Patients with choledochal cysts most commonly present with jaundice, although vague right upper quadrant pain, cholangitis, and, rarely, recurrent pancreatitis may also be present. The classic triad of intermittent abdominal pain, jaundice, and right upper quadrant mass is found relatively infrequently. Jaundice is much more common in infants and young children, particularly those presenting under 2 years of age, while pain is the most common symptom in adults. Cholangitis (fever and biliary infection) may occur in a third of patients. Infants present similarly to those with biliary atresia, including jaundice and acholic stools. Diagnosis is usually made by ultrasonography showing abnormal biliary tree dilations in the absence of obstruction. Cross-sectional imaging with a computerized tomography (CT) scan or, ideally, magnetic resonance cholangiopancreatography (MRCP) is the next step to confirm presence of cyst(s), investigate for obstruction, examine for cyst communication with the biliary tree, and detect an abnormal pancreatobiliary junction (**Figure 71-1**). Once confirmed, both endoscopic retrograde cholangiopancreatography (ERCP) evaluation and surgical correction should be carried out at a tertiary care pediatric hospital with advanced endoscopy and hepatobiliary surgical expertise.

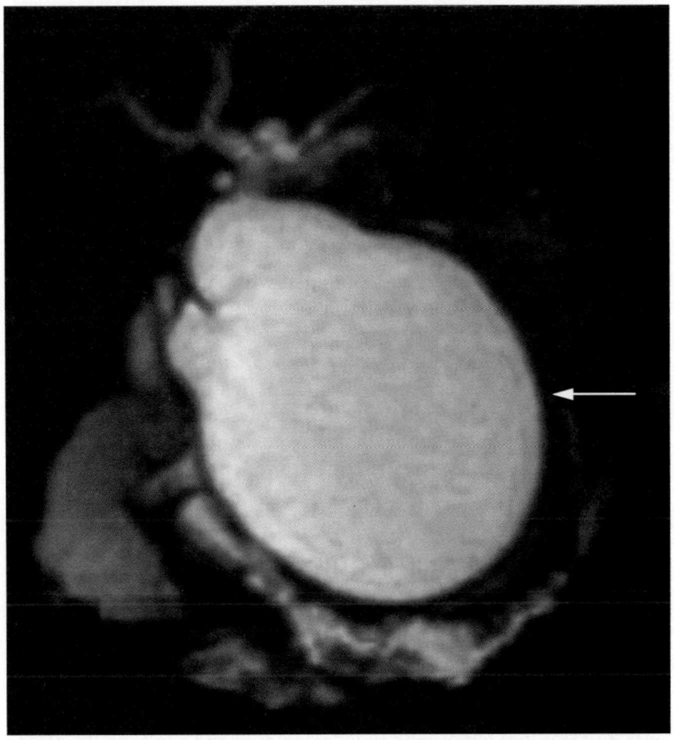

FIGURE 71-1. Type 1 choledochal cyst (arrow) in an 11-month-old girl. Magnetic resonance cholangiopancreatography maximum intensity projection reveals cystic dilation of the common bile duct without abnormality of the intrahepatic duct. (Image used with permission from the Children's Hospital Colorado Department of Radiology and reviewed by Christina J. White, DO and Laura Z. Fenton, MD.)

Treatment consists of complete surgical excision of the cyst and creation of a Roux-en-Y choledochojejunostomy proximal to the most distal lesion. The goals of surgery are adequate bile drainage and complete cyst removal to reduce the risk of future malignancy. Biliary adenocarcinoma rates are 20 times higher in patients with choledochal cysts than in the general population, and carcinoma rates are between 10% and 26% in patients left with residual cystic tissue after surgery. With successful radical excision of the cyst and Roux-en-Y formation, now often done laparoscopically, long-term outcomes are excellent. However, patients should be followed lifelong by gastroenterologists to monitor for recurrent cholangitis, pancreatitis, and malignancy.

CHOLELITHIASIS

Cholelithiasis, or stone formation in the gallbladder, occurs in up to 10% of the North American adult population. The prevalence is lower in children, 0.13% to 0.22%, but has risen over the last 30 years. Cholelithiasis in children is frequently associated with predisposing conditions such as obesity, hemolytic diseases, ileal disease, TPN, prolonged fasting, cephalosporin use, and pregnancy. Some studies show that up to half of infants and a quarter of older children with gallstones have no identifiable underlying condition. Children of Hispanic ethnicity have higher rates of gallstones than Caucasian or Black children, particularly if obesity is present. Pigmented stones are most common in children younger than 6 years and in patients with hemolytic processes, while cholesterol stones predominate in school-age children and adolescents.

Epigastric and right upper quadrant abdominal pain, vomiting, and jaundice are common presenting symptoms, and pancreatitis may be a complication of gallstone passage in 5% to 10% of patients. Laboratory studies may be normal in asymptomatic patients, but liver enzymes, GGT, alkaline phosphatase, and conjugated bilirubin may all be elevated in the presence of ductal obstruction from a dislodged stone or infection. Ultrasonography is the best initial study as it can identify both gallstones or sludge, a thickened gallbladder wall, and biliary tree dilation. If biliary obstruction with gallstones is suspected but not definitively seen on ultrasound, then additional imaging with MRCP (or CT if MRCP unavailable) should be pursued. Pediatric patients with hemolytic diseases are at particular risk for gallstone formation, with 30% to 60% of patients with sickle cell disease developing stones in the first 14 years of life. These patients may require ERCP to accurately identify common bile duct stones, and it is generally recommended they undergo cholecystectomy for gallstones even if asymptomatic due to high risk for obstruction, cholecystitis, and pancreatitis from stone passage. Of note, despite the benefits of cholecystectomy, patients with hemolytic disease, particularly sickle cell disease, may continue to form biliary tree stones several years after surgery, and these may cause clinically significant common bile duct obstruction.

Asymptomatic or "silent" stones found incidentally generally do not require therapy and will often resolve spontaneously. For children <2 years old, a single stone and small size of stone (< 5mm) are associated with spontaneous dissolution. For symptomatic gallstones, the definitive therapy is cholecystectomy, usually done laparoscopically. In acute cholecystitis, urgent or even emergent gallbladder removal may be warranted, but in those patients without infection or obstruction, surgery can usually be delayed for a few days to a month to allow for convenient timing. Laparoscopic cholecystectomy is the standard surgical approach to gallbladder removal. For uncomplicated cases, it can often be done with discharge in 24 hours or even as an outpatient day procedure.

Acute complications of cholelithiasis include cholecystitis, obstructive hepatitis, and/or pancreatitis (see Chapter 78, Pancreatitis). Cholecystitis is discussed later. Obstructive hepatitis typically resolves once the obstruction is relieved. Gallstone pancreatitis is an indication for cholecystectomy which should be performed during the initial hospitalization to avoid the development of further pancreatobiliary complications.

For stones obstructing the common bile duct (choledocholithiasis), therapeutic ERCP has become standard in both children and adolescents. The procedure is often combined with sphincterotomy of the sphincter of Oddi to allow balloon clearance of common bile duct stones. ERCP is safe in children and has been performed effectively by experienced practitioners for a variety of indications in children of all ages, even younger than 1 year. Complication rates are typically around 4% and can include post-ERCP pancreatitis, bleeding, infection, and biliary or duodenal hematoma or perforation. Following clearance of the acutely obstructing stone, cholecystectomy should be performed.

CHOLANGITIS AND CHOLECYSTITIS

Cholangitis is a bacterial infection of the biliary tree and cholecystitis is infection of the gallbladder alone. Patients with choledochal cysts, cholelithiasis, biliary atresia following a Kasai portoenterostomy, or strictures of the biliary tree (e.g., primary sclerosing cholangitis) are all at risk for cholangitis. Charcot's triad of right upper quadrant abdominal pain, fever, and jaundice is common in older children and adults while infants may present with fever and acholic stools as well as jaundice.

Therapy includes decompression of obstruction (if it exists), fluid resuscitation, and intravenous antibiotics. The timing of decompression depends on patient stability. Toxic patients often need emergent endoscopic or operative decompression, whereas most stable patients can be treated with antibiotics initially until they are afebrile for 24 to 48 hours before undergoing therapeutic interventions. Decompression usually involves ERCP with removal of a stone or stenting of a stricture. In patients with cholelithiasis, a cholecystectomy should be performed once the patient has recovered from the acute illness. Duration of antibiotic administration following ERCP and decompression has been debated. Several recent studies have shown good outcomes in adult patients treated with 3 days of intravenous antibiotics after relief of biliary obstruction, provided the patient was doing well and defervesced after surgery. The key criteria in these studies were resolution of fever before discontinuation of antibiotics and observation another 24 to 72 hours after antibiotics stopped to confirm no return of infection. Up to half of patients with bacterial cholangitis have positive blood cultures, and in those cases, cultures can help direct and narrow antibiotic choices. The most common bacteria identified on both blood and biliary fluid cultures are *Escherichia coli*, *Klebsiella* spp., *Bacteroides* spp., enterococci, *Enterobacter* spp., and *Pseudomonas* spp. Mixed infections with both aerobic and anaerobic bacteria commonly occur. Piperacillin-tazobactam may be used as a first-line single agent with meropenem or imipenem preferred in more severe cases.

ACALCULOUS CHOLECYSTITIS

Acalculous cholecystitis is acute gallbladder distention and inflammation resulting from gallbladder hypokinesis in the absence of gallstones. In severe cases, it can result in gallbladder necrosis or perforation. Anatomically, cystic duct narrowing due to a congenital anomaly, edema, or lymph node compression prevents gallbladder drainage and bile stasis and infection develop. It is typically associated with significant systemic infection or illness, prolonged fasting and TPN use, or episodic ischemia. The use of opiates in critically ill or postoperative patients may also contribute to its development. Several systemic illnesses have been associated with acalculous cholecystitis, including Epstein-Barr virus, streptococcal and gram-negative sepsis, leptospirosis, Rocky Mountain spotted fever, typhoid fever, ascariasis, and *Giardia lamblia* infection. Parasitic, candidal, and viral infections have been identified in immunocompromised patients.

Clinically, patients present with right upper quadrant abdominal pain, nausea, vomiting, and possibly fever, and may have a palpable gallbladder on examination. Diagnosis is typically made by ultrasound followed by HIDA scan. Increased gallbladder wall thickness on ultrasonography is an inconsistent finding, but progressive thickening of the wall in serial examinations may be suggestive. Other ultrasound findings include an absence of calculi, gallbladder distention, and poor contraction in response to cholecystokinin (CCK). A HIDA scan is sensitive for detecting the cystic duct obstruction suggestive of acalculous cholecystitis. Findings show good hepatic uptake and intestinal excretion of isotope *without* gallbladder filling. In the event of gallbladder perforation, tracer extrudes into the abdominal cavity. The HIDA scan has come to largely replace ultrasound as the most reliable way to confirm acalculous cholecystitis, but ultrasound is needed initially to confirm the absence of gallstones or mechanical obstruction.

Therapy for acalculous cholecystitis includes intravenous antibiotics, treatment of any underlying systemic illness, and possible cholecystectomy. Surgical consultation is appropriate to determine the need for cholecystectomy, which may be necessary to avoid gallbladder necrosis and possible perforation with bile peritonitis.

HYDROPS OF THE GALLBLADDER

Hydrops is acute gallbladder distention and poor contractility without concomitant inflammation, obstruction, or infection. The lack of gallstones, infection, or anatomic abnormality of the biliary system distinguishes this condition from several of those previously mentioned. It is associated with several systemic illnesses, including Kawasaki syndrome, in which it is found in up to 20% of patients. Other associated conditions include staphylococcal or streptococcal infection, leptospirosis, sepsis, TPN administration, mesenteric adenitis (often with a preceding viral syndrome) and several common viruses including Epstein-Barr virus.

Hydrops is a self-limited condition that usually does not require surgical intervention. Symptoms and signs often include right upper quadrant or epigastric abdominal pain, vomiting, and sometimes a palpable mass, in addition to those symptoms associated with the underlying disease. Ultrasonography reveals a markedly distended, acalculous, and unthickened gallbladder with no other biliary tree dilatation. HIDA scan showing good tracer uptake by the distended gallbladder points toward hydrops rather than acalculous cholecystitis. Serial examinations can confirm a return to normal gallbladder size and function. The need for surgery arises only if severe hydrops leads to insufficient gallbladder perfusion, with subsequent gangrene or perforation. Overall, most cases resolve without surgical intervention as the underlying systemic inflammatory disease resolves.

ADMISSION AND DISCHARGE CRITERIA

ADMISSION CRITERIA

- Infant with direct hyperbilirubinemia to evaluate for biliary atresia, choledochal cyst, or other causes of jaundice.
- Jaundice accompanied by fever to assess for underlying infection, provide intravenous antibiotics for treatment of cholangitis.
- Biliary tree anomaly in the presence of jaundice or fever for intravenous antibiotics and surgical correction of anomaly.
- Biliary tree obstruction for surgical or endoscopic relief of obstruction.

DISCHARGE CRITERIA

Patients may be discharged when the diagnosis has been established or when serious or life-threatening disorders are treated or no longer being considered. Further diagnostic evaluation and treatment may proceed after discharge, as appropriate, such as genetic, metabolic, or hemolytic evaluations, serial radiologic studies, completion of antibiotics, or scheduling outpatient surgery. Many biliary disorders will need follow-up by pediatric gastroenterology, pediatric surgery, or both.

CONSULTATION

Subspecialty consultation should be considered in the following circumstances:

- Biliary tree anomaly: Pediatric surgery and gastroenterology
- Jaundice with hepatosplenomegaly: Pediatric gastroenterology
- Jaundice with dysmorphism or associated congenital anomalies: Pediatric genetics and gastroenterology
- Obstructive cholelithiasis: Pediatric surgery and gastroenterology
- Gallstones with hemolysis: Pediatric hematology and surgery

KEY POINTS

- Diseases of the biliary tract range from those that need urgent surgical correction, such as biliary atresia, acute obstruction, or septic cholangitis, to genetic conditions that require lifelong subspecialist management.
- Jaundice, abdominal pain (often localized to the right upper quadrant), and fever are the most frequent presenting signs of biliary disease.
- A basic evaluation includes fractionated bilirubin, hepatic enzymes including GGT, liver function tests (PT/INR and albumin), a complete blood count, and abdominal ultrasonography. This evaluation typically indicates whether the disease is a primary liver disorder or biliary tract disease.
- Infants with suspected biliary atresia warrant transfer to a pediatric hepatology center for prompt evaluation and treatment of their jaundice, including performance of a Kasai procedure by an experienced pediatric surgeon.
- Biliary tract disease, particularly gallstones and gallbladder dysfunction, have increased with the rising incidence of obesity in children and adolescents in Western societies.
- Therapeutic ERCP has gained importance in the acute management of obstructive gallstones in the pediatric population, and children with obstructive gallstones often warrant ERCP followed by surgical cholecystectomy.
- Laparoscopic cholecystectomy has become a safe, frequently performed, and effective procedure in children for the treatment of gallstones, cholangitis, and acalculous cholangitis.

SUGGESTED READINGS

Badru F, Saxena S, Breeden R, et al. Optimal timing of cholecystectomy in children with gallstone pancreatitis. *J Surg Res*. 2017;215:225-230.

Dekonenko C, Holcomb GW. Laparoscopic Cholecystectomy in Children. *J Laparoendosc Adv Surg Tech A*. 2021;31(10):1180-1184.

Di Serafino M, Gioioso M, Severino R, et al. Ultrasound findings in paediatric cholestasis: how to image the patient and what to look for. *J Ultrasound*. 2020;23(1):1-12.

Fawaz R, Baumann U, Ekong U, et al. Guideline for the evaluation of cholestatic jaundice in infants: joint recommendations of the North American Society for Pediatric Gastroenterology, Hepatology, and Nutrition and the European Society for Pediatric Gastroenterology, Hepatology, and Nutrition. *J Pediatr Gastroenterol Nutr*. 2017; 64(1): 154-168.

Hull NC, Schooler GR, Lee EY. Hepatobiliary MR imaging in children: up-to-date imaging techniques and findings. *Magn Reson Imaging Clin N Am*. 2019;27(2):263-278.

Keil R, Drábek J, Lochmannová J, et al. ERCP in infants, children, and adolescents—different roles of the methods in different age groups. *PLoS One*. 2019;14(1):e0210805.

Kemper AR, Newman TB, Slaughter JL, et al. Clinical practice guideline revision: management of hyperbilirubinemia in the newborn infant 35 or more weeks of gestation. *Pediatrics*. 2022;e2022058859.

Lacaille F, Allali S, de Montalembert M. The liver in sickle cell disease. *J Pediatr Gastroenterol Nutr*. 2021;72(1):5-10.

Pakarinen MP, Johansen LS, Svensson JF, et al. Outcomes of biliary atresia in the Nordic countries—a multicenter study of 158 patients during 2005-2016. *J Pediatr Surg*. 2018;53(8):1509-1515.

Poddighe D, Sazonov V. Acute acalculous cholecystitis in children. *World J Gastroenterol*. 2018;24(43):4870-4879.

Tagawa M, Morita A, Imagawa K, Mizokami Y. Endoscopic retrograde cholangiopancreatography and endoscopic ultrasound in children. *Dig Endosc*. 2021;33(7):1045-1058.

Yakupovich A, Rajeswaran S, Green J, Donaldson JS. Role of interventional radiology in children with biliary and gallbladder diseases. *Semin Intervent Radiol*. 2021;38(3):356-363.

CHAPTER 72 Constipation

Michelle W. Parker, MD and Sean O'Brien, MD

BACKGROUND

Constipation is a common pediatric disorder, with a prevalence up to 30%. In special patient populations, such as children with complex chronic conditions or autism spectrum disorder, prevalence is even higher and increases with increasing number of complex chronic conditions. Because normal stooling patterns vary greatly among individuals and by age, constipation is generally defined as infrequent and difficult passage of hard stool, often associated with pain and straining. Average stooling frequencies at different ages have been defined (**Table 72-1**).

Constipation can occur at any age but is particularly common in toddlers and elementary school-age children. In most studies, no significant gender-specific prevalence difference has been reported.

PATHOPHYSIOLOGY

The causes of constipation can be divided into anatomic, physiologic, and functional (**Table 72-2**). Anatomic causes of constipation include Hirschsprung disease, imperforate anus, and bowel obstruction. Physiologic causes include several processes that alter bowel motility or fluid reabsorption, such as opioid administration, hypothyroidism, spinal cord defects, and other neuropathies, or celiac disease. Functional constipation, which results from voluntary stool withholding, is the most common cause of constipation (90%-97% of cases). It is often a self-perpetuating condition that starts with an episode of pain on defecation in the context of initiation of toilet training or other significant life change. Functional constipation may progress to encopresis, which is either voluntary or involuntary fecal incontinence in a child at least 4 years of age. It involves leakage of stool around a firm, distal fecal impaction and is thought to result from chronic constipation secondary to functional fecal retention.

The long-term complications of constipation are generally related to loss of normal colonic size and tone and the development of encopresis. In severe cases, chronic anorexia, and failure to thrive can result. Psychosocial functioning can also be severely affected in children with chronic constipation, leading to poor self-esteem, poor school performance, and family stress and conflict.

TABLE 72-1 Normal Stooling Patterns

Age Group	Average Frequency of Stools
0-3 months: breast-fed	2.9/day
0-3 months: formula fed	2.0/day
6-12 months	1.8/day
1-3 years	1.4/day
>3 years	1.0/day

TABLE 72-2 Differential Diagnosis of Constipation

Functional
Toilet phobia
Toilet training
School bathroom avoidance
Dietary change
Sexual abuse
Anatomic
Hirschsprung disease
Imperforate anus
Anal stenosis
Anteriorly displaced anus
Bowel obstruction, pseudo-obstruction
Tethered cord
Physiologic
Celiac disease
Hypothyroidism
Hypercalcemia
Diabetes mellitus
Cystic fibrosis
Bowel motility disorders
Spinal cord abnormalities
Neuropathic conditions
Drugs (opiates, anticholinergics, lead, iron, antidepressants)
Inadequate fluid or fiber intake
Depression
Connective tissue disorders (scleroderma, systemic lupus erythematosus, Ehlers-Danlos syndrome)
Infant botulism

CLINICAL PRESENTATIONS

Constipation does not always present with the obvious history of infrequent or hard stools. Children may have regular, even daily bowel movements but incomplete stool evacuation leading to progressive fecal retention that goes undetected by caregivers. The presenting complaint is often abdominal pain, which may be intermittently severe but is typically low grade and difficult for the child to describe. The location of the pain is usually periumbilical. On examination, there may be abdominal tenderness but usually no rebound or guarding. Other manifestations of constipation include diarrhea (encopresis), abdominal distention, anorexia, nausea, vomiting, flatulence, dyschezia, or blood-streaked stools. Constipation can even progress to bowel obstruction.

DIFFERENTIAL DIAGNOSIS

Constipation can be diagnosed with specificity by the presence of infrequent and hard stools. However, there is a large differential diagnosis of underlying disorders that can lead to constipation (see Table 72-2). Although functional constipation is the most common etiology, it is important to keep other disorders in mind, especially in children with new onset or refractory constipation or those with complex chronic conditions.

DIAGNOSTIC EVALUATION

The diagnosis and evaluation of constipation rests on a thorough history and physical examination. History alone may differentiate those children with an organic cause of constipation from those with functional constipation (**Table 72-3**). Besides stool consistency and frequency, the history should include time to passage of the first meconium stool, age at onset of symptoms, details of toilet training, urinary retention or incontinence, lower extremity weakness, and associated symptoms of rectal pain and bleeding, abdominal pain, and stool incontinence. An evaluation of other constitutional symptoms, such as fevers, weight loss, and nausea, should also be considered for those who have an acute or subacute onset of symptoms and those with severe enough symptoms to require hospitalization, as they may suggest an underlying organic disorder. A history of delayed passage of the first stool beyond 48 hours of life raises the suspicion of Hirschsprung disease, as would a longstanding family or personal history of constipation starting in infancy. A history of stool withholding or of constipation associated with toilet training or toilet phobia is strongly suggestive of functional constipation.

TABLE 72-3 Historical Factors of Importance in the Evaluation of Constipation

Historical Factor	Special Significance
Constipation history	
Timing of first stool in neonatal period	Delay >48 hours suggestive of Hirschsprung disease
Onset of symptoms	Onset <1 month suggestive of Hirschsprung disease
Quality of stool	Soft but infrequent stools may not indicate constipation
Frequency of stool	
Duration of symptoms	Sudden onset may indicate non-functional causes
Family history	Identify potentially inherited predisposition to constipation
Hirschsprung disease	
Other causes of constipation	
Other systemic disease (e.g. thyroid, cystic fibrosis, inflammatory bowel disease)	
Diet	May identify contributors to constipation or trigger suggestions for dietary modifications
Amount of fluid	
Amount of fiber	
General nutrition	
Significant dietary changes	
Social	Absence of these may raise concern for non-functional causes of constipation. Alternately, treatment of contributing behavioral concerns may be helpful achieving long-term therapeutic success
Toilet training	
Toilet phobia	
Change of school or childcare	
Family or social stressors	
History of withholding behavior	
Sexual abuse	
Medications, ingestions, or exposures	
Narcotic use or ingestion	May suggest medication-induced constipation
Any other ingestions	
Previous medication for constipation	
Lead exposure	Toxicity may lead to constipation
Associated symptoms	
Abdominal pain	
Nausea	
Vomiting	Suggestive of non-functional cause
Weight loss	May indicate encopresis; if bloody suggestive of non-functional cause
Diarrhea	
Pain with defecation	
Blood in stool	
Fever	Suggestive of non-functional cause
General medical history	Positive history may suggest underlying physiologic reason for constipation
Neuropathic disorder	
Cerebral palsy	
Spina bifida	

A careful and thorough physical examination can help identify underlying disorders. Children with constipation may or may not have abdominal distension or palpable stool. For children with functional constipation, a large rectal impaction may be found on digital rectal examination, but the remainder of the physical examination should be normal, including normoactive bowel sounds and no significant abdominal tenderness. Hirschsprung disease may be suggested by an empty, non-distended rectum or by expulsion of gas and stool following a digital rectal examination. Inspection of the anus may reveal anal stenosis, and fissures may be detected in those with a complaint of bloody stools. Bowel obstruction, which can be caused by constipation or can lead to constipation, would be associated with abdominal distension along with persistent vomiting and inability to tolerate food or liquids. Auscultation may reveal "tinkling" or hypoactive bowel sounds. On neurologic examination, deep tendon reflexes may be sluggish in hypercalcemia and hypothyroidism, or hyperreflexic in patients with spinal cord abnormalities. An abnormal gait, lower extremity weakness, and an absent anal wink are suggestive of a neurologic cause of constipation. Examination of the lumbosacral area of the spine may reveal a hairy patch, sinus tract, or other midline defect which could suggest spina bifida.

Laboratory studies or imaging are not recommended unless there is concern about an underlying organic cause of constipation based on the history or physical examination. Routine use of an abdominal radiograph should not be used to diagnose constipation but can be considered to diagnose fecal impaction when physical exam is not possible or is unreliable (**Figure 72-1**). For patients in whom an underlying organic cause is suspected, evaluation should be tailored to the diagnosis under consideration. A contrast enema or rectal biopsy to assess for an aganglionic colon performed in consultation with a pediatric gastroenterologist or surgeon may be considered for diagnosis of Hirschsprung disease or other motility disorders. Imaging may be needed to diagnose bowel obstruction and would necessitate the involvement of a pediatric surgeon. Laboratory studies may be obtained when concerns exist for underlying pathology, but their routine use for functional constipation is not recommended. Testing, if performed, should be judicious and may include thyroxine, thyroid-stimulating hormone, calcium, glucose, lead, anti-tissue transglutaminase antibodies, total serum IgA, and cow-milk protein allergy testing (by specific IgE or skin prick testing). If the patient presents with abdominal pain or urinary complaints, a urinalysis and urine culture may be indicated, because constipation increases the risk of a urinary tract infection as well as other urinary complaints. A sweat test to evaluate for cystic fibrosis may also be considered, especially in the presence of accompanying failure to thrive or pulmonary symptoms. Finally, spinal magnetic resonance imaging and colonic transit time may be warranted if there is concern for an occult spinal abnormality or neuropathy.

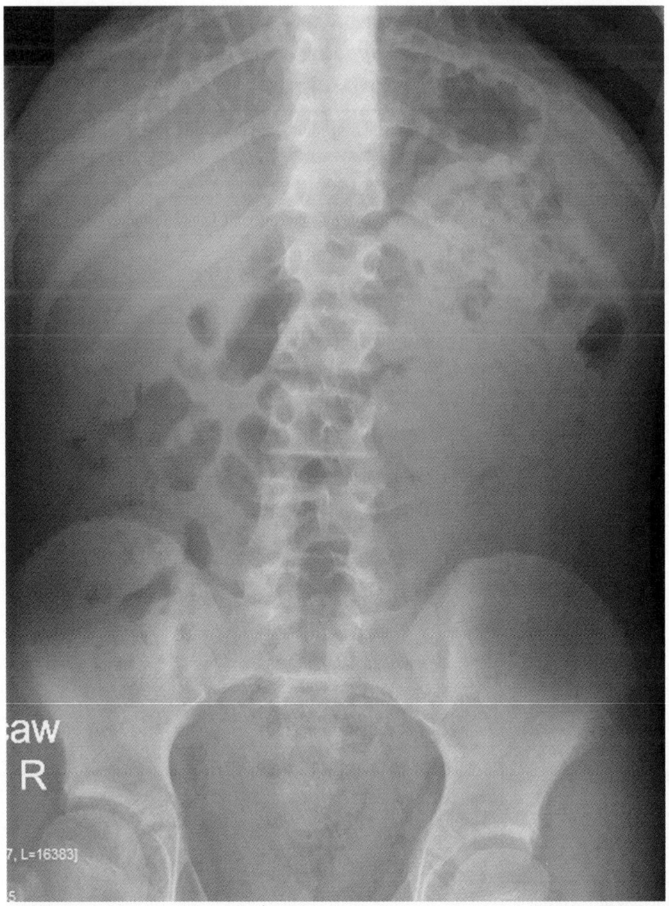

FIGURE 72-1. Abdominal radiograph showing stool burden with fecal impaction.

MANAGEMENT

Constipation is often a chronic problem that requires long-term management. Most patients with a clear diagnosis of functional constipation can be managed without hospitalization if close outpatient follow-up is available. After the initial diagnosis and initiation of therapy, reassessment of the frequency and character of stools and observation for new symptoms or findings are necessary. Patients should be followed at regular intervals until the child is having regular soft stools with no evidence of stool withholding or fecal soiling.

The successful treatment of functional constipation and encopresis requires a multipronged approach. The patient should be adequately hydrated prior to initiation of therapy to avoid sudden shifts in fluids and electrolytes. Acutely, the child may require disimpaction, which can be accomplished by either rectal enema, oral/nasogastric polyethylene glycol, or a combination of both (**Table 72-4**). For inpatients, disimpaction is often initiated by the administration of rectal enemas, which can be repeated as needed until no hard stool is present in defecation or rectal effluent. Stool may also be evacuated via oral or nasogastric polyethylene glycol with or without electrolytes at a dose of 25 to 40 mL/kg/hr until effluent is clear. Rarely, stool impaction is refractory to pharmacologic therapy. In this case, manual disimpaction should be considered and is often done in consultation with pediatric surgery and under anesthesia for young patients to maximize cooperation and minimize discomfort to the patient.

In the inpatient setting, acute impaction can often be relieved and the patient discharged home in 1 to 2 days; however, a maintenance plan for ongoing pharmacologic therapy must be established (**Table 72-5**). It should be continued for at least 2 months, with all symptoms of constipation resolved for at least 1 month prior to a gradual discontinuation of treatment. The goal is to keep stools soft and prevent reaccumulation of hard stool. Polyethylene glycol, an osmotic laxative, has been shown to be the most effective medication to treat constipation when compared with lactulose, milk of magnesia, mineral oil, or placebo. It is therefore recommended as the first-line therapy at a dose of 0.4 g/kg/day mixed in the indicated volume of fluid. Caregivers should be advised to adjust the dosage according to clinical response. Lactulose is the recommended second-line therapy and should be administered at a dose of 1 to 2 g/kg once or twice daily. Lubricants, such as mineral oil and other osmotic laxatives (e.g., magnesium hydroxide), have also been found to be effective and safe for long-term use. Stimulant laxatives, such as senna or bisacodyl, are best used only on a short-term or intermittent basis as "rescue" therapy to prevent ongoing or recurrent stool retention. Other classes of drugs, such as serotonin 5-HT4 receptor agonists, and intestinal fluid modulators, have demonstrated effectiveness in adults, but currently lack sufficient evidence to routinely recommend in pediatric populations.

Caregiver counseling and education should include promotion of adequate fluid intake and a healthy diet, which includes whole grains, fruits, and vegetables. If functional constipation is the diagnosis, behavioral factors must also be addressed. Families should be instructed to initiate regular toileting times and durations. On average, a child should be placed on the toilet for 5 to 10 minutes once or twice a day, ideally after meals. With younger or smaller children, the use of a footstool may

TABLE 72-4 Disimpaction Guidelines

Method	Dosage	Comments and Side Effects
Enemas		
Bisacodyl	2-10 y: 5 mg >10 y: 5-10 mg	Rare electrolyte abnormalities include metabolic acidosis or alkalosis, hypocalcemia
Docusate	2-<12 y: 283 mg/5 mL once	
	12+ y: 283/5 mL 1-3 times daily	
Sodium phosphate	1-18 y: 2.5 mL/kg, max 133 mL/dose	Not for use in patients with renal insufficiency, colitis or megacolon
Normal saline	>1 y: 6 mL/kg	
Mineral oil	2-11 y: 30-60 mL	
	>11 y: 60-150 mL	
Glycerin suppository	<6 y: 1 pediatric suppository (1 g)	Anal irritation
	≥6 y: 1 adult suppository (2 or 3 g)	
Oral/Nasogastric tube solutions		
Polyethylene glycol-electrolyte solution	Children ≥6 mo: Inpatient: 25-40 mL/kg/h for 4-10 hr or until rectal effluent is clear Outpatient: daily dosing x 3-6 days	Watch children younger than 2 y carefully for electrolyte abnormalities
	Adults: 240 mL (8 oz) every 10 min, until 4 L are consumed or rectal effluent is clear	Rapid drinking of each portion is preferred to drinking small amounts over a period of time

allow proper foot support to permit 90 degrees of hip and knee flexion. Importantly, children should not be punished if they fail to produce stool, but encouraged if they attempt to do so. The purpose of these postprandial toileting routines is to resensitize the body to the gastrocolic reflex. Parents should explicitly be told not to make this process a source of anxiety for the child, and encouraged to be patient as the process of resensitization may take time. Children with severe emotional disorders or avoidance of stool production may benefit from psychological evaluation and therapy.

Children younger than 1 year of age with functional constipation should be managed more conservatively. For this age group, emphasis is placed on adequate intake of fluids and only modest consumption

TABLE 72-5 Stool Softener and Laxative Guidelines

Method	Mechanism	Dosage	Comments and Side Effects
Mineral oil oral	Lubricant	>12 mo: 1-3 mL/kg/day	Do not use in children younger than 12 mo or in those at risk of aspiration Can cause anal leakage Long-term use (>1-2 y) can cause fat-soluble vitamin deficiency
Polyethylene glycol 3350	Osmotic laxative	0.8 g/kg/day of powder starting dose, adjusted to clinical response; each 17-g dose should be dissolved in 4-8 oz of liquid	First line maintenance medication
Magnesium hydroxide (milk of magnesia)	Osmotic laxative	<2 y: 0.5 mL/kg/dose	Can cause hypermagnesemia Use with caution in those with renal failure
		2-5 y: 1-3 tsp once a day	
		6-11 y: 1-2 tsp once a day	
		≥12 y: 2-4 tsp once a day	
Senna	Stimulant laxative	2-6 y: Start with ½ tablet, or 2.5 mL syrup daily	Forms: 8.6 mg tablet, 15 mg/5 mL granules, 8.8 mg/5 mL syrup Start as suggested, monitor effect, and increase dose as needed to maximum doses, as follows: 2-6 y: 1 tablet, or 3.75 mL syrup twice a day 7-12 y: 2 tablets, or 7.5 mL syrup twice a day ≥12 y: 4 tablets or 15 mL twice a day Can cause abdominal cramping
		7-12 y: Start with 1 tablet or 5 mL syrup once a day	
		>12 y: Start with 2 tablets or 10-15 mL	
Bisacodyl oral	Stimulant laxative	≤12 y: 5-10 mg daily	Do not use for more than 1 week Can cause abdominal cramping
		>12 y: 5-15 mg daily	
Bisacodyl rectal	Stimulant laxative	6 mo-2 y: 5 mg suppository daily	Do not use for more than 1 week Can cause abdominal cramping
		3-11 y: 5-10 mg suppository daily	
		≥12 y: 10 mg suppository daily	
Lactulose	Osmotic laxative	Children: 1-2 g/kg/day	Can cause abdominal cramping and flatulence
		Adults: 15-30 mL/day, increased to 60 mL/day in 1-2 divided doses if necessary	

of juices containing sorbitol (prune, pear, or apple). Pharmacologic treatment may include lactulose, which is approved for all ages. While enemas should generally be avoided, rectal glycerin suppositories may be helpful for disimpaction but should be used sparingly to avoid rectal irritation. Infants in this young age group should have careful consideration of possible underlying conditions contributing to constipation.

ADMISSION AND DISCHARGE CRITERIA

ADMISSION CRITERIA

- Unclear cause, with concern about potentially life-threatening conditions or those that require presumptive inpatient evaluation and treatment (e.g., cystic fibrosis, bowel obstruction).
- Persistent vomiting or inability to tolerate oral intake.
- Severe abdominal pain.
- Nasogastric electrolyte solution administration for bowel cleanout when oral and rectal routes have failed.
- Lack of appropriate outpatient support or follow-up.

DISCHARGE CRITERIA

- Successful evacuation of stool.
- Ability to tolerate oral or enteral fluids and nutrition.
- Stable or resolving signs and symptoms that the family can manage at home.
- Reliable outpatient follow-up with primary pediatrician and, if indicated, pediatric gastroenterologist or other specialist.

CONSULTATION

Subspecialty consultation should be considered if the workup raises concern for any of the following:

- Chronic or refractory constipation, possible bowel motility disorder, celiac disease: Pediatric gastroenterology
- Hirschsprung disease, bowel obstruction, acute abdomen: Pediatric general surgery
- Hypothyroidism: Pediatric endocrinology
- Spinal dysraphism, spina bifida, neuromuscular disorders: Pediatric neurology
- Severe toilet phobia: Pediatric clinical psychology

SPECIAL CONSIDERATIONS

Special consideration should be given to children with cerebral palsy, other neuromuscular disorders, autism spectrum disorder, or complex chronic conditions. These children are at greater risk for the development of constipation because of their relative inactivity, decreased muscle use and tone, and/or low-fiber diets. Therefore, efforts should be made to prevent constipation in these children by the routine use of stool softeners and other maintenance therapy. Clinicians should escalate therapy or begin disimpaction promptly if stools become more infrequent or hard.

PREVENTION

Eating a well-balanced diet with plenty of fruits, vegetables, and water can help prevent constipation, as can regular physical activity. Most importantly, hospitalization can usually be prevented by educating parents about the importance of appropriate toileting regimens. It is critical to address behavioral issues around toileting early, before severe constipation and encopresis result.

KEY POINTS

- Constipation is defined by the infrequent passage of hard stool and may present with a variety of signs and symptoms, including abdominal pain, abdominal distention, pain with defecation, nausea and even diarrhea (in the setting of encopresis).
- Treatment mainstays include initial disimpaction followed by long-term maintenance therapy, dietary changes, and behavioral modification.
- Indications for hospitalization include failure of outpatient management to resolve excessive stool burden or inability to maintain adequate intake due to associated vomiting or abdominal pain.
- Post-discharge follow-up is critical for preventing repeat episodes through dosage adjustments, rescue plans, and ongoing caregiver education.

SUGGESTED READINGS

McElhanon BO, McCracken C, Karpen S, Sharp WG. Gastrointestinal symptoms in autism spectrum disorder: a meta-analysis. *Pediatrics.* 2014;133(5):872-883.

Robin SG, Keller C, Zwiener R, et al. Prevalence of pediatric functional gastrointestinal disorders utilizing the Rome IV Criteria. *J Pediatr.* 2018;195:134-139.

Stephens JR, Steiner MJ, DeJong N, et al. Healthcare utilization and spending for constipation in children with versus without complex chronic conditions. *J Pediatr Gastroenterol Nutr.* 2017;64(1):31-36.

Tabbers MM, DiLorenzo C, Berger MY, et al. Evaluation and treatment of functional constipation in infants and children: evidence-based recommendations from ESPGHAN and NASPGHAN. *J Pediatr Gastroenterol Nutr.* 2014;58(2):258-274.

van Summeren JJGT, Holtman GA, van Ommeren SC, et al. Bladder symptoms in children with functional constipation: a systematic review. *J Pediatr Gastroenterol Nutr.* 2018;67(5):552-560.

CHAPTER 73 Dyspepsia

Laura P. Chen, MD and Daniel M. O'Connell, MD

BACKGROUND

Dyspepsia is defined as chronic or recurrent pain or discomfort in the abdomen above the umbilicus. Children often experience dyspepsia either as a presenting symptom or during hospitalization. The challenge to the hospitalist is to identify the cause or causes based on typically nonspecific symptoms (which vary widely based on age, cognitive and verbal ability), a wide differential, indirect examination of the affected area, and laboratory and radiographic evaluations that are rarely diagnostic.

CLINICAL PRESENTATIONS

Common presentations of dyspepsia include nausea, vomiting, regurgitation, fullness, early satiety, retching, postprandial abdominal bloating or distension, and excess gas with or without belching or flatulence. These symptoms typically exclude "heartburn" or a burning sensation in the retrosternal region, which is usually presumed to be gastroesophageal reflux disease (GERD). Dyspepsia symptoms overlap with those of other disorders, such as gastric ulceration, gastrointestinal (GI) bleed, failure to thrive, and feeding difficulties, which can make diagnosis challenging. The timing of symptoms can be helpful in determining the presence of underlying disease. For example, pain secondary to gastric ulceration often peaks when the stomach is empty, whereas pain associated with functional dyspepsia usually develops immediately after eating and may linger for hours.

DIFFERENTIAL DIAGNOSIS

Many disorders can cause dyspepsia, including functional, inflammatory/mucosal, and anatomic abnormalities of the stomach or extragastric GI system. In addition, disorders outside of the GI tract, such as genitourinary or psychiatric disorders, may have prominent dyspeptic symptoms (**Table 73-1**).

DIAGNOSTIC EVALUATION

The broad differential diagnosis and subjective nature of dyspepsia make it difficult to establish a standard diagnostic approach. Asking a patient or family to keep a symptom journal may be helpful. Initial questions should include symptom duration, degree of disability, antecedent infection or antibiotic use, medication history, and measures (both effective and ineffective) taken thus far to address the symptoms. An initial laboratory workup might include a complete blood count, inflammatory markers (erythrocyte sedimentation rate or C-reactive protein), chemistry profile (including liver and renal function tests), lipase, celiac screening, stool testing for Giardia, fecal calprotectin screening for inflammatory bowel disease, urinalysis, and *Helicobacter pylori (H. pylori)* testing.

Of the workup mentioned above, *H. pylori* screening is the diagnostic test most likely to yield a positive result. However, a positive *H. pylori* screen does not necessarily mean the source of dyspepsia has been identified given that most pediatric patients with *H. pylori* are asymptomatic. A hospitalized child with severe dyspepsia with a positive noninvasive *H. pylori* test (stool antigen or urea breath test) may benefit from upper endoscopy for direct visualization of possible ulcers and mucosal biopsy for definitive diagnosis. Patients should be off antibiotics for 4 weeks and off proton pump inhibitors for 2 weeks (when practical) prior to *H. pylori* testing to increase the sensitivity of the noninvasive tests.

Further evaluation should proceed in a stepwise fashion based on clinical suspicion and may include radiographic imaging or endoscopy. Ultrasonography, upper GI series, or computed tomography should be considered if there is suspicion for obstruction, pancreatitis, or liver, biliary or renal disease. Hydrogen breath tests may be a useful diagnostic tool for the evaluation of suspected bacterial overgrowth or carbohydrate malabsorption; however, these are rarely indicated in the inpatient setting. An upper endoscopy with possible colonoscopy should be strongly considered in patients with red-flag symptoms, such as dysphagia, odynophagia, persistent vomiting, GI bleeding, nocturnal diarrhea, arthritis, perianal disease, unintentional weight loss, delayed puberty, or unexplained fever. An upper endoscopy in the setting of dyspepsia is generally a low-yield diagnostic procedure, but negative findings may still be helpful in management.

Patients with severe chronic symptoms without identifiable disease may require motility testing using manometry or a nuclear medicine gastric emptying study. A psychosocial evaluation may also be warranted because children with chronic dyspeptic symptoms are at risk for depression and functional impairment.

TABLE 73-1 Differential Diagnosis for Dyspepsia

Functional disorders
Functional dyspepsia
Rumination syndrome
Aerophagia
Abdominal migraine
Post-viral gastroparesis
Inflammatory or mucosal disorders
GERD including acid mediated gastritis and esophagitis
Helicobacter pylori gastritis and ulcers
Peptic ulcer
NSAID-related ulcer
Eosinophilic GI diseases including esophagitis, gastritis, or enteritis
Infection: *Giardia, Blastocystis hominis, Dientamoeba fragilis*, and *Cytomegalovirus*
Bacterial overgrowth
Inflammatory bowel disease (Crohns disease)
Ménétrier disease
Celiac disease
Autoimmune gastritis
Collagenous gastritis
Lymphocytic gastritis
Lactose or other carbohydrate malabsorption or intolerance
Henoch-Schönlein purpura
Anatomic disorders
Malrotation with or without volvulus
Duodenal web
Psychiatric disorders
Psychogenic vomiting
Somatization related to underlying depression or anxiety
Panic disorders
Anorexia nervosa or other eating disorder
Other disorders
Chronic pancreatitis
Chronic hepatitis
Ureteropelvic junction obstruction
Biliary dyskinesia
Intestinal pseudo-obstruction
Lymphoma, carcinoma
Post-viral gastroparesis

GERD, gastroesophageal reflux disease; NSAID, nonsteroidal anti-inflammatory drug.

MANAGEMENT

Treatment for dyspepsia should be directed at the specific disorder if one is identified. For instance, in patients who test positive for *H. pylori*, antibiotic choice should be guided by local resistance patterns, if known. Empiric treatment with a 14-day course of amoxicillin, clarithromycin, and a proton pump inhibitor is a standard first-line treatment in most children. If antibiotic susceptibility profiles are not known, clinicians should treat with high dose triple therapy with amoxicillin, metronidazole, and a proton pump inhibitor or bismuth-based quadruple therapy.

Frequently no obvious cause is found. In this case, a diagnosis of functional dyspepsia is generally made, and empiric management is often warranted (**Table 73-2**).

TABLE 73-2 Management Options for Dyspepsia

Diet
Small, frequent low-fat meals
Solid vs. liquid diet, use of liquid nutritional supplements
Low FODMAP (Fermentable Oligo-, Di-, Monosaccharides and Polyols)
Pharmacology
H2 agonists (e.g., famotidine)
Proton pump inhibitors (e.g., omeprazole, esomeprazole, lansoprazole, pantoprazole)
Prokinetic agents (e.g., metoclopramide, erythromycin, azithromycin, prucalopride)
Neuromodulation (e.g., tricyclic antidepressants such as amitriptyline, cyproheptadine, mirtazapine)
Serotonin-1 agonists (e.g., sumatriptan, buspirone)
Supplements (e.g., ginger, Iberogast, probiotics)
Behavioral therapies directed at the Gut-Brain Axis
Cognitive-Behavioral Therapy
Hypnotherapy
Biofeedback

FUNCTIONAL DYSPEPSIA

Functional dyspepsia is diagnosed using the Rome IV criteria (2016) and must include 1 or more of the following bothersome symptoms at least 4 days per month and not fully attributed by another medical condition: postprandial fullness, early satiety, and epigastric pain or burning not associated with defecation. Functional dyspepsia can be further classified into two subtypes: postprandial distress syndrome and epigastric pain syndrome. In one study of children at a tertiary center evaluated for unexplained recurrent abdominal pain, 15.9% met criteria for functional dyspepsia. Functional dyspepsia fits under the larger umbrella of functional GI disorders, more accurately called disorders of gut brain interaction.

The most effective therapy is avoidance of dietary or medication-induced triggers when they can be identified. Conservative measures, such as dietary modifications (e.g., decreasing meal size, reducing fat, avoiding caffeine, carbonated beverages, and bedtime snacks) and avoiding nicotine (including cigarettes and vaping) may be helpful. Empiric acid blocking medication trials with proton pump inhibitors or H_2 receptor antagonists is typically first-line therapy for pain-predominant symptoms. Prokinetic agents, including erythromycin and azithromycin, may be considered in patients with predominant symptoms of fullness, bloating, or early satiety.

Similar to treatment of irritable bowel syndrome and other pain-predominant functional GI conditions, neuromodulation may have some benefits to decrease pain processing and visceral hypersensitivity in functional dyspepsia. Tricyclic antidepressants (e.g., amitriptyline), cyproheptadine, mirtazapine, and buspirone have been used, with amitriptyline often first line in children older than 5 years old. Cyproheptadine and mirtazapine can be particularly helpful if symptoms include concurrent chronic nausea, poor appetite, and weight loss. Auricular neurostimulation, a newer non-medication modality, is the only FDA-approved treatment for functional abdominal pain in children. Gastric electrical stimulation also shows some promise in pediatric populations refractory to medical treatment.

Adequate nutrition and hydration may be barriers to discharge in select patients. Emphasizing oral hydration strategies and calorie-dense liquid nutrition supplementation during acute and subacute illness should be a focus. Alternative enteral access with nasal or surgically placed feeding tubes or parenteral nutrition should be avoided and only considered within the context of a multidisciplinary team, which ideally includes pediatric gastroenterology, nutrition, pharmacy, social work, and a primary care provider.

ADMISSION AND DISCHARGE CRITERIA

ADMISSION CRITERIA

Persistent vomiting, severe abdominal pain, hematemesis, bilious emesis, dehydration, persistent weight loss, and significant hematochezia or melena all indicate the need for inpatient evaluation and management.

DISCHARGE CRITERIA

Once a patient can tolerate adequate oral intake, the remainder of the evaluation can usually be completed as an outpatient. It is important to ensure adequate follow-up, as these problems are often chronic and require long-term management.

CONSULTATION

Evaluation for chronic symptoms should initially occur in the outpatient setting, but when they are identified in the inpatient setting, consultation from a pediatric gastroenterologist may be helpful in providing management advice, performing endoscopy, addressing patient and parent concerns, and establishing outpatient follow-up. Further consultation should be tailored to the specific etiology of dyspepsia, if known.

KEY POINTS

- Dyspepsia is defined as chronic or recurrent upper abdominal pain or discomfort and can represent esophageal, gastric, intestinal, or non-GI disorders.
- Symptomatic treatment is often warranted and can be initiated before completion of the diagnostic evaluation.
- Upper endoscopy should be considered in dyspeptic patients presenting with red flag signs or symptoms, such as weight loss, recurrent vomiting, bleeding, anemia, dysphagia, or jaundice, patients taking NSAIDs, and patients with severe or persistent symptoms. Acid blockade, prokinetic agents, and diet modification are standard empirical therapy. Neuromodulation can be considered for refractory cases.

SUGGESTED READINGS

Hyams JS, Di Lorenzo C, Saps M, Shulman RJ, Staiano A, van Tilburg M. Functional disorders: children and adolescents. *Gastroenterology*. 2016;S0016-5085(16) 00181-5.

Jones NL, Koletzko S, Goodman K, et al. Joint ESPGHAN/NASPGHAN Guidelines for the management of *Helicobacter pylori* in children and adolescents (Update 2016). *J Pediatr Gastroenterol Nutr*. 2017;64(6):991-1003.

Rippel SW, Acra S, Correa H, Vaezi M, Di Lorenzo C, Walker LS. Pediatric patients with dyspepsia have chronic symptoms, anxiety, and lower quality of life as adolescents and adults. *Gastroenterology*. 2012;142(4):754-761.

Rodriguez L, Diaz J, Nurko S. Safety and efficacy of cyproheptadine for treating dyspeptic symptoms in children. *J Pediatr*. 2013; 163(1):261-267.

Romano C, Valenti S, Cardile S, Benninga MA. Functional dyspepsia: an enigma in a conundrum. *J Pediatr Gastroenterol Nutr*. 2016; 63(6):579-584.

Simren M, Barbara G, Flint HJ, et al. Intestinal microbiota in functional bowel disorders: a Rome foundation report. *Gut*. 2013;62(1):159-176.

Talley NJ, Ford AC. Functional dyspepsia. *N Engl J Med*. 2015;373(19): 1853-1863.

Tam YH, Chan KW, To KF, et al. Impact of pediatric Rome III criteria of functional dyspepsia on the diagnostic yield of upper endoscopy and predictors for a positive endoscopic finding. *J Pediatr Gastroenterol Nutr*. 2011;52(4):387-391.

Teich S, Mousa HM, Punati J, Di Lorenzo C. Efficacy of permanent gastric electrical stimulation for the treatment of gastroparesis and functional dyspepsia in children and adolescents. *J Pediatr Surg*. 2013;48(1):178-183.

Teitelbaum JE, Arora R. Long-term efficacy of low-dose tricyclic antidepressants for children with functional gastrointestinal disorders. *J Pediatr Gastroenterol Nutr*. 2011;53(3):260-264.

Zhou X, Su J, Xu G, Zhang G. Accuracy of stool antigen test for the diagnosis of *Helicobacter pylori* infection in children: a meta-analysis. *Clin Res Hepatol Gastroenterol*. 2014;38(5):629-638.

CHAPTER 74 Disorders of Gastric Emptying

Bianca N. Quiñones-Pérez, MD and Amy Turner, MD, MSHPEd

BACKGROUND

Passage of the food bolus from the stomach to the duodenum constitutes an important anatomical and functional transition point in the digestive process. The stomach functions as a reservoir for food and can accommodate changes in volume from the fasted to the postprandial state via receptive relaxation. Weak contractions propel the bolus toward the antrum, where stronger contractions are coordinated with the duodenum and result in progressive emptying of the stomach across the pylorus. This process is controlled by the intrinsic motor neurons of the gastric myenteric plexus. These, in turn, are modulated by the central nervous system via the vagus nerve, which can activate both inhibitory and excitatory post-ganglionic myenteric neurons. Activation of these neurons is essential for the propulsion of the food bolus, whereas inhibitory signals are necessary for fundic and pyloric relaxation. The rate of gastric emptying is influenced by the physical nature of the meal, with liquids emptying more rapidly than solids, and foods with lower caloric density emptying more rapidly than foods with higher caloric density.

PATHOPHYSIOLOGY

Abnormal gastric emptying includes disorders that cause delayed and accelerated emptying into the duodenum. Gastroparesis is defined as a delay in gastric emptying in the absence of a mechanical obstruction. In adults, this has been shown to be secondary to impaired gastric accommodation, postprandial antral hypomotility, pyloric dysfunction, duodenal dysmotility, dysfunction of the autonomic nervous system, and visceral hypersensitivity. On the contrary, accelerated emptying, or dumping, relates to the rapid passage of undigested, hyperosmolar food into the duodenum. This triggers a fluid shift from the intravascular to the extravascular space that results in depletion of intravascular volume, distension of the small intestine, and gastrointestinal peptide hormone release. Both conditions may result in symptoms that require hospitalization for supportive care, diagnostic evaluation, and therapeutic management. To simplify this review, the terms gastroparesis and dumping are utilized for delayed and accelerated gastric emptying, respectively.

CLINICAL PRESENTATIONS

Gastroparesis usually presents with vomiting, which is the most common symptom in infants, but it can also present with abdominal pain and nausea in older children. Other symptoms can be more vague and include postprandial fullness, early satiety, heartburn, bloating, belching, and weight loss in severe cases. Rapid gastric emptying can also result in nausea, abdominal pain, bloating, diarrhea, and early satiety. In a minority of patients, it may progress into the classic dumping syndrome. Early dumping syndrome, which occurs as early as 30 minutes after a meal, is characterized by vasomotor symptoms including tachycardia, hypotension, diaphoresis, or syncope. Symptoms of late dumping occur 1 to 3 hours after a meal and are mostly related to reactive hypoglycemia from persistently elevated insulin levels.

DIFFERENTIAL DIAGNOSIS

Before considering a diagnosis of gastroparesis, a mechanical gastric outlet obstruction must be ruled out, particularly in younger children who may have a congenital or acquired anatomical anomaly. The most common cause of gastric outlet obstruction in children is hypertrophic pyloric stenosis (HPS). Other causes may include antral and duodenal webs, ectopic pancreatic tissue, pyloric duplication cysts, polypoid tissue, bezoars, or intermittent intussusception (see Chapter 155, Gastrointestinal Obstruction: Pyloric Stenosis, Malrotation and Volvulus, and Intussusception). Other conditions that may present with similar symptoms to gastroparesis, but have normal gastric emptying include gastroesophageal reflux (see Chapter 79, Feeding Issues) and other causes of functional dyspepsia (see Chapter 73, Dyspepsia).

Over half of patients with gastroparesis have no identifiable underlying abnormality, termed idiopathic gastroparesis. When a cause can be identified, it is usually related to viral illnesses, medication side effects, post-surgical complications, mitochondrial diseases, metabolic problems, or other neuromuscular conditions (**Table 74-1**).

Post-viral or post-infectious gastroparesis, which has been described in up to 18% of pediatric patients with gastroparesis, is defined as having persistent symptoms for more than 1 month after the onset of a viral illness. Various medication classes commonly used in the hospital setting, such as opiates, anticholinergics (imipramine), and tricyclic antidepressants, can also have profound untoward effects on the ability of the stomach to empty promptly. Any history of intra-abdominal or thoracic operative procedures where vagal injury could have occurred, such as scoliosis surgery, may predispose a child to delayed or accelerated gastric emptying.

TABLE 74-1 Differential Diagnoses of Delayed and Accelerated Gastric Emptying

Delayed Gastric Emptying (Gastroparesis)	
Metabolic or electrolyte disturbance	Hypothyroidism
	Hypokalemia
	Acidosis
Medications	Opioids
	Anticholinergics
	Antidepressants
Neuromuscular dysfunction	Conditions of the central nervous system (e.g., Cerebral Palsy)
	Post-vagotomy
	Chronic idiopathic pseudoobstruction
	Autonomic dysfunction
	Visceral myopathy
	Systemic sclerosis
	Myotonic dystrophy
Malnutrition / Eating disorder	Anorexia nervosa
	Bulimia
Infectious disease	Viral
	Post-infectious
Other	Idiopathic
	Prematurity
	Post-surgical
Accelerated Gastric Emptying (Dumping Syndrome)	
Post-Surgical	Fundoplication
	Pyloric operative procedures
	Partial gastrectomy (proximal or distal)
	Vagotomy

Mitochondrial disorders may present with gastroparesis or dysmotility. Anorexia nervosa and bulimia are also frequently associated with a secondary gastroparesis that responds to improved nutrition and weight gain. Hypothyroidism decreases antroduodenal motility and resolves with treatment that restores the euthyroid state. Acid-base and electrolyte disturbances, present in conditions such as diabetes mellitus or renal insufficiency, may result in impaired motility and delayed gastric emptying. Diseases primarily affecting the neuromuscular components of the gastrointestinal tract can have a profound effect on gastric emptying. These might include primary central nervous system disease, vagotomy (planned or inadvertent), visceral myopathy, autonomic dysfunction, systemic sclerosis, myotonic dystrophy, or chronic idiopathic pseudoobstruction. Prematurity is also a known risk factor for gastroparesis, as normal gastric emptying mechanisms are not fully developed until 32 weeks of gestation.

Dumping syndrome is most commonly seen in post-surgical states where the normal proximal compliance or distal tone of the stomach has been affected. In children, the most likely procedure to result in dumping syndrome is fundoplication and it should always be considered in patients with feeding disorders who have had this procedure. Pyloroplasty is occasionally performed with a fundoplication and can result in even more severe dumping.

DIAGNOSTIC EVALUATION

The history should focus on evaluating the timing and nature of the symptoms, their relation to feeding and whether they occur when eating liquids, solids, or both. Physical examination should focus on determination of clinical hydration and general toxicity of the patient.

TABLE 74-2 Modalities Used to Diagnose Gastric Emptying Disorders

Laboratory studies	Electrolytes, blood urea nitrogen, glucose
	Complete blood count
	Liver aminotransferases
	Amylase, lipase
	Glucose tolerance tests
Radiographic studies	Upper gastrointestinal series
	Gastric emptying scintigraphy
Procedural Studies	Endoscopy
	Antroduodenal manometry

Evaluation for gastric emptying disorders can include laboratory, radiographic, and procedural studies (**Table 74-2**). Laboratory evaluation should address other potential etiologies of recurrent vomiting, if applicable. Electrolytes, glucose, and blood urea nitrogen are critical toward the diagnosis of metabolic disturbances that may either cause or be exacerbated by dysfunctional gastric emptying. Other laboratory evaluation may include liver aminotransferases, amylase, lipase, and a complete blood count. In cases where dumping is suspected, a glucose tolerance test may also be helpful.

Radiographic studies may be the most informative at differentiating gastroparesis from other structural causes of vomiting. An upper gastrointestinal series has been shown to be the most cost-effective study in infants presenting with vomiting and has the added benefit of diagnosing malrotation and small bowel obstruction, but it is not able to measure gastric motility. Although gastroparesis is often diagnosed based on clinical symptoms, delayed gastric emptying must be demonstrated to confirm the diagnosis. A gastric emptying scintigraphy is the standard method to assess for delayed gastric emptying. For this study, the patient ingests a radiolabeled meal and serial measurements of radioactivity in the stomach, correlating to the amount of meal remaining, are recorded. The test must be done after a prolonged period of fasting and after discontinuation of medications that may affect gastric motility. Studies of liquid emptying are performed in infants, whereas studies of liquid and solid emptying are more useful in older children and adults. Unfortunately, reference ranges are based on adult data and there are no established normative values for adequate gastric emptying times for children, which may vary based on age and size.

Finally, a contrast study via gastrostomy or nasogastric tube can quantify the volume of liquid the stomach will hold prior to emptying and may aid in the diagnosis of dumping syndrome.

Endoscopy can be performed to assess for other conditions that may present with similar symptoms. Furthermore, endoscopy can also be used to place catheters utilized for antroduodenal motility studies to diagnose primary motility disorders and for the injection of botulinum toxin into the pylorus.

MANAGEMENT

Clinical management for abnormal gastric emptying is mostly supportive and should focus on correcting fluid and electrolyte disturbances, optimizing nutrition, and, if able, identifying a cause to provide definitive treatment.

FLUID AND ELECTROLYTES

Both delayed and accelerated gastric emptying may result in marked alterations of fluid status and electrolytes that must be promptly identified and corrected. Recurrent vomiting can lead to the loss of sodium, potassium, and chloride resulting in a hypochloremic metabolic alkalosis. This is accentuated by paradoxical aciduria that results from renal retention of sodium and intravascular fluid.

Patients with severe dumping syndrome may require aggressive fluid resuscitation due to intravascular fluid depletion from rapid passage of hyperosmolar fluid into the small bowel, as well as glucose control, as these patients may present with initial hyperglycemia followed by hypoglycemia resulting from persistent elevated insulin levels.

NUTRITION

Nutritional management is typically the primary focus of gastroparesis treatment. If definitive treatment is not available or indicated, symptomatic improvement can often be achieved with use of small frequent meals, meals low in fat and non-digestible fiber, and/or with liquid supplementation, which may be better tolerated since liquids will empty faster than solids. If such modifications to intragastric feeding are not successful, the stomach may be bypassed with placement of a nasojejunal tube, surgical jejunostomy, or intravenous catheter. Lastly, patients with gastroparesis often develop micronutrient and vitamin deficiencies and require vitamin supplementation.

Treatment of dumping syndrome involves longer-term dietary changes with smaller, more frequent meals, eaten slowly and chewed well. Patients are also advised to eliminate rapidly absorbable carbohydrates and add foods rich in protein and fiber to their diet.

MEDICATIONS

Pharmacologic options for treatment of gastroparesis are relatively limited and inconsistent in their efficacy. Drugs that function as 5-HT4 receptor agonists (cisapride, tegaserod), dopamine-2 receptor antagonists (domperidone, metoclopramide), and motilin receptor agonists (erythromycin), have been considered as promotility agents. However, to date, these agents have had limited success due to low response rates and/or side effects. Agonism of 5-HT4 receptors in the digestive tract results in prokinetic effects beneficial in treating gastrointestinal motility problems; however, these receptors are also found in the cardiac atria where agonism may result in arrhythmia, perhaps due to QT interval prolongation. As a result, cisapride and tegaserod were both removed from the market due to concerns for cardiovascular effects. Dopamine antagonists have also had problems; domperidone has never been approved for use in the United States. Metoclopramide, while still available, carries a "black box label" warning of the potential for tardive dyskinesia and should not be used chronically. Motilin receptor agonist erythromycin is available and does not have safety issues; however, it may not have sustainable effects due to tachyphylaxis. The outcome of medical treatment appears to be inversely related to patient age, with a larger fraction of infants resolving their gastroparesis when compared to children and adolescents.

The gastric fundus is mainly used to accommodate food without significantly increasing gastric pressure. Early satiety, postprandial fullness, nausea, and abdominal pain symptoms can be associated with impaired gastric accommodation and/or increased gastric sensitivity to distention. Cyproheptadine is an antiallergic medication and an antagonist of serotonin receptors (5-HT2A, 5-HT2B, and 5-HT2C). The anti-serotoninergic effect of cyproheptadine is postulated to lead to improvement in gastric accommodation, so, although it is not a pro-motility agent, it can be used to help improve symptoms in patients with delayed gastric emptying.

Prucalopride is a selective 5-HT4 receptor agonist approved for treatment of constipation in adults. However, it is being used off label for upper gastrointestinal symptoms in both adults and children. In adult studies, prucalopride has been shown to improve gastric emptying and reduce gastroparesis symptoms in patients with and without delayed gastric emptying. A pediatric retrospective, open label study of patients with refractory upper gastrointestinal symptoms showed symptomatic improvement in 65% of patients after starting prucalopride.

Observationally, intrapyloric injection of botulinum toxin appears to reduce symptoms and accelerate gastric emptying in patients with gastroparesis. A randomized control trial in adults with gastroparesis did show improvement in gastric emptying after intrapyloric injection of botulinum toxin; however, 1 month after injection, there was no significant improvement in symptoms and the effect in gastric emptying was not superior to that of placebo.

The first-line treatment for dumping syndrome consists of dietary modifications, but when these are not effective, pharmacologic therapy may be considered. Acarbose, an alpha-glycosidase inhibitor that slows the release of monoglycerides from nutritional carbohydrates to the diet, can help reduce symptoms of dumping syndrome by improving glucose tolerance, reducing gastrointestinal hormone release, and reducing the incidence of hypoglycemia. In adults, somatostatin analogs, such as octreotide, have been shown to slow the rate of gastric emptying, slow small bowel transit time, inhibit insulin secretion, and inhibit postprandial vasodilation. However, there are no studies that have evaluated the efficacy of somatostatin analogs in pediatric patients with dumping syndrome.

ADMISSION AND DISCHARGE CRITERIA

ADMISSION CRITERIA

- Toxic appearance or signs of severe dehydration on physical examination
- Undernutrition based on height, weight, physical examination, and/or laboratory and micronutrient analysis
- Fluid and electrolyte disturbances

DISCHARGE CRITERIA

- No significant electrolyte disturbances
- Ability to tolerate feeds without excessive vomiting or diarrhea to maintain hydration and ensure weight stabilization
- Outpatient plan and follow-up in place

CONSULTATION

- Pediatric gastroenterology if endoscopy or long-term nutritional management are required
- Pediatric neurology, nephrology, endocrinology, or infectious diseases depending on the specific underlying diagnosis, if present

SPECIAL CONSIDERATIONS

PREVENTION

The most effective prevention for disorders of gastric emptying is careful consideration of operative procedures that may impair gastric function; most prominent among these is fundoplication. In some patients, a feeding jejunostomy may provide similar airway protection to a fundoplication with decreased morbidity. Knowledge of medication side effects that could play a role in a patient's symptoms is also of importance.

KEY POINTS

- Disorders of gastric emptying may present with severe symptoms that require hospitalization for supportive care, such as vomiting, abdominal pain, dehydration, and/or weight loss.
- The most common cause of gastroparesis is idiopathic, but the differential diagnosis includes multiple etiologies, including secondary to viral illnesses, medication side effects, post-surgical complications, mitochondrial diseases, metabolic problems, or other neuromuscular conditions.
- A gastric emptying scintigraphy is the standard method to assess for delayed gastric emptying, but this can be challenging due to a lack of standardized pediatric normative values.
- Management is directed at both supportive care and nutritional optimization.

SUGGESTED READINGS

Abell TL, Camilleri M, Donohoe K, et al. Consensus recommendations for gastric emptying scintigraphy: a joint report of the American Neurogastroenterology and Motility Society and the Society of Nuclear Medicine. *J Nucl Med Technol.* 2008;36(1).

Ambartsumyan L, Rodriguez L. Gastrointestinal motility disorders in children. *Gastroenterol Hepatol.* 2014;10(1):16-26.

Di Lorenzo C, Hyman PE. Gastrointestinal motility in neonatal and pediatric practice. *Gastrointest Motil Clin Pract.* 1996;25(1):203-224.

Friedenberg FK, Palit A, Parkman HP, Hanlon A, Nelson DB. Botulinum toxin A for the treatment of delayed gastric emptying. *Am J Gastroenterol.* 2008;103(2).

Hirsch S, Nurko S, Mitchell P, Rosen R. Prucalopride for treatment of upper gastrointestinal symptoms in children. *Pediatr Drugs.* 2022;24(1).

Kneepkens CMF, Fernandes J, Vonk RJ. Dumping syndrome in children. Diagnosis and effect of glucomannan on glucose tolerance and absorption. *Acta Paediatr Scand.* 1988;77(2).

Lu PL, Di Lorenzo C. Gastroparesis in the pediatric patient: children are not little adults. *Gastrointest Disord.* 2020;2(2):86-95.

Ogorek CP, Davidson L, Fisher RS, Krevsky B. Idiopathic gastroparesis is associated with a multiplicity of severe dietary deficiencies. *Am J Gastroenterol.* 1991;86(4).

Rodriguez L, Irani K, Jiang H, Goldstein AM. Clinical presentation, response to therapy, and outcome of gastroparesis in children. *J Pediatr Gastroenterol Nutr.* 2012;55(2):185-190.

Scarpellini E, Arts J, Karamanolis G, et al. International consensus on the diagnosis and management of dumping syndrome. *Nat Rev Endocrinol.* 2020;16(8).

Waseem S, Islam S, Kahn G, Moshiree B, Talley NJ. Spectrum of gastroparesis in children. *J Pediatr Gastroenterol Nutr.* 2012;55(2).

Wong GK, Shulman RJ, Chumpitazi BP. Gastric emptying scintigraphy results in children are affected by age, anthropometric factors, and study duration. *Neurogastroenterol Motil.* 2015;27(3).

CHAPTER 75

Liver Failure

Ellen Overson, MD and Scott A. Elisofon, MD

BACKGROUND

Liver failure, or hepatic failure, is a clinical condition that results from significant hepatocyte dysfunction or death. Criteria for acute liver failure differ between adults and children. The criteria for acute or fulminant liver failure in *adults* include encephalopathy, coagulopathy, and evidence of hepatic dysfunction without prior evidence of liver disease that occurs within 8 weeks of onset of illness. Because encephalopathy is uncommon and difficult to identify in infants and young children, the criteria for acute or fulminant liver failure in *children* include only uncorrectable coagulopathy and acute hepatic dysfunction occurring within 8 weeks of onset of illness. Coagulopathy, in this case, is defined as an International Normalized Ratio (INR) ≥ 2.0 without encephalopathy. If encephalopathy is present, an INR ≥ 1.5 is sufficient to diagnose acute liver failure.

Liver failure accounts for up to 15% of pediatric liver transplants in the United States each year. Thus, recognition of liver failure and its complications (**Table 75-1**) is crucial so that supportive therapy can be provided until recovery or transplantation. In this chapter, we will highlight the differing causes of both acute hepatitis and acute liver failure by age while reviewing key aspects of management.

PATHOPHYSIOLOGY

Hepatocytes perform many important functions, including the synthesis of many vital proteins and the clearance of ammonia and other metabolites from the body. When hepatocytes are inflamed or a small number are damaged or dying, this results in acute *hepatitis.* When a larger number of hepatocytes are dying and cannot recover, acute hepatitis leads to acute liver failure. Unlike in acute hepatitis, patients with acute liver failure must have coagulopathy (that is not correctable after parenteral vitamin K administration) with or without encephalopathy.

TABLE 75-1 Complications of Acute Hepatic Failure

Metabolic
Hypoglycemia
Hypokalemia
Hypophosphatemia
Hyponatremia
Neurologic
Encephalopathy
Cerebral edema
Intracranial hemorrhage
Acid-base imbalance
Respiratory alkalosis
Metabolic acidosis
Hematologic
Coagulopathy
Disseminated intravascular coagulation
Aplastic anemia
Multiorgan dysfunction
Gastrointestinal hemorrhage
Ascites
Pancreatitis
Renal failure (hepatorenal syndrome)
Shock
Sepsis
Respiratory failure
Pulmonary hemorrhage

Source: Reproduced with permission from Squires R. Liver failure. In: Rudolph CD, Rudolph AM, Hostetter MK, et al. eds. *Rudolph's Pediatrics.* 21st ed. New York: McGraw-Hill; 2002.

Hepatocyte death can be caused by different mechanisms, including infections, ischemia, drugs, inflammation, or metabolic/organelle dysfunction. Infections, especially viruses, can cause direct hepatocyte injury or can promote an inflammatory condition that injures hepatocytes. Ischemia causes direct hepatocyte injury and death from lack of blood flow. Drug-induced liver injury is thought to be either direct hepatocyte injury or the immunologic/inflammatory response to the drug or drug metabolite. Genetic diseases of organelle dysfunction, such as mitochondrial diseases, create an acute dysfunction of mitochondria in response to an infectious or stressful stimulus.

CLINICAL PRESENTATIONS

Many patients or families of patients with acute liver failure initially report a nonspecific prodrome of fever, nausea, vomiting, and abdominal discomfort and are then found to have some degree of abnormal liver testing (e.g., elevated bilirubin and/or transaminases) and an abnormal INR. The child may or may not have ascites, hepatosplenomegaly, or encephalopathy. Encephalopathy is characterized by mental status changes, such as reversal of the day-night sleep cycle, uncooperative behavior, delirium, stupor, or coma. The examination of a child with acute liver failure may also reveal clonus or asterixis.

The etiology and clinical presentation of liver failure can be categorized by age.

NEONATES AND INFANTS <3 MONTHS

There are a few entities which can present with acute liver failure already at birth or progress to acute liver failure shortly thereafter. These mainly include gestational alloimmune liver disease (GALD) or congenital infections (maternal infection with vertical transmission). GALD is caused by maternal immune attack of fetal liver tissue and characterized by iron overload in the liver and other organs, such as the pancreas, heart, and thyroid. Infants with GALD also may have intrauterine growth restriction. Congenital infections, such as enterovirus or adenovirus, present at birth and maternal symptoms of infection may be the only clue. Of note, the classic "TORCH" infections (e.g., cytomegalovirus, rubella, and syphilis) commonly cause signs of hepatitis but rarely present with acute liver failure.

Infants with hypoxic/ischemic injury due to liver hypoperfusion tend to present with acute liver failure in the first few days of life. This injury may be due to surgical or delivery complications (e.g., placental abruption, shoulder dystocia, emergent cesarean-section, maternal shock). Symptoms may be like those seen in neonatal sepsis, such as hypoglycemia, hypotension, poor perfusion (beyond acrocyanosis), lethargy, or acidosis. In these infants, direct bilirubin is generally more elevated than indirect bilirubin (a reverse pattern than that seen in breastfeeding or breast milk jaundice). Hypoxic/ischemic injury is one of two major causes of acute liver failure which result in transaminases in the tens of thousands (the other being drug-induced liver injury from acetaminophen).

Perinatally acquired infections (e.g., infant is infected in the first days to weeks after birth), such as herpes simplex virus (HSV) and enterovirus, can also cause an acute liver failure picture. These infants tend to present just prior to or soon after discharge from the newborn nursery.

At 1 to 2 months, infants with some metabolic disorders may present with worsening direct hyperbilirubinemia and liver failure. These include galactosemia, tyrosinemia, Niemann-Pick type C, mitochondrial hepatopathies, hereditary fructose intolerance, or urea cycle disorders.

OLDER INFANTS AND SCHOOL AGE CHILDREN

Viral infections and toxic ingestions are more common causes of acute liver injury in this age group. Hepatitis A, Epstein-Barr virus, and parvovirus B19 tend to be the most common culprits for acute hepatitis. In the developing world, hepatitis D and E make up a larger proportion of cases. While most of these viral illnesses are self-limited and hepatitis may go unrecognized, a small number of infected children go on to develop acute liver failure. Ingestion of medications, toxins, and accidental overdoses can occur in this age group. There is a long list of medications that have the potential to cause hepatitis (e.g., minocycline, sulfamethoxazole-trimethoprim, anti-epileptics, or anti-fungals), but very few progress to acute liver failure. Accidental overdoses of over-the-counter medications (e.g., acetaminophen or iron) occur more commonly in this age group due to the exploratory neurodevelopmental stage of these children.

ADOLESCENTS

Overdose of acetaminophen is the most common cause of acute liver failure in this age group. While accidental overdoses occur (typically due to co-ingesting multiple acetaminophen-containing medications), intentional ingestions in the setting of a suicide attempt are much more common. The acetaminophen level is very much dependent on timing of ingestion and presentation. A negative acetaminophen level does not rule out acetaminophen ingestion if the patient presents either very early relative to the ingestion or well after the ingestion. Ingestion of natural herbs, such as pennyroyal and kava, can also cause liver failure. Autoimmune hepatitis may progress to acute liver failure. Metabolic diseases, such as fatty acid oxidation defects, can present with high transaminase levels and hypoglycemia. Wilson disease would be more likely in an older child or teenager, especially if their presentation includes a Coombs-negative hemolytic anemia.

DIFFERENTIAL DIAGNOSIS

The causes of acute liver failure are almost identical to those of acute hepatitis (**Table 75-2**). They include infectious, metabolic, autoimmune, or toxic causes. Infectious hepatitis is most likely viral. Hepatitis B and C are uncommon causes of acute hepatitis or failure in children. It is important to recognize that 30% to 50% of all acute liver failure cases in children are determined as "indeterminate," with no cause identified.

In addition to those with acute liver injury, patients with underlying liver disease may present with increasing transaminases, jaundice, and coagulopathy, with or without encephalopathy. This is referred to as an acute decompensation of chronic liver disease or acute on chronic

TABLE 75-2 Causes of Acute Hepatic Failure in Children

Cause	Perinatal Period	Infants	Children and Adolescents
Infectious	Herpes simplex virus	Hepatitis A	Hepatitis A
	Enterovirus	Hepatitis B	Hepatitis B
	Adenovirus	Epstein-Barr virus	Hepatitis D
	Hepatitis B	Non-A-E hepatitis	Epstein-Barr virus
			Non-A-E hepatitis
Metabolic	Tyrosinemia	Tyrosinemia	Wilson disease
	Galactosemia	Hereditary fructose intolerance	
		Fatty acid oxidation defects	
		Mitochondrial disorders	
Immune	Gestational alloimmune liver disease	Autoimmune hepatitis	Autoimmune hepatitis
Toxic		Medications	Medications
		Herbs	Herbs
Miscellaneous	Congenital heart disease	Congenital heart disease	Ischemia
	Cardiac surgery	Cardiac surgery	Budd-Chiari syndrome
	Severe asphyxia	Severe asphyxia	Malignancy

liver failure. Diseases that involve significant liver fibrosis, such as α_1-antitrypsin deficiency, autoimmune hepatitis, primary sclerosing cholangitis, and Wilson disease, can present in this fashion. An acute exacerbation of chronic liver disease can have very similar clinical findings to acute liver failure. Evidence that a more chronic process is at play would be signs of portal hypertension (e.g., splenomegaly, ascites, or thrombocytopenia).

DIAGNOSTIC EVALUATION

A careful history is important to determine the cause and progression of liver failure. This should include the time course of symptoms, exposures (e.g., infections, chemicals, or drugs), and family history of liver disease. In the case of ill infants, questions should focus on maternal infections (hepatitis B, human immunodeficiency virus, herpes simplex virus, enterovirus) and a family history of genetic or metabolic diseases. Maternal human immunodeficiency virus does not cause acute liver failure, but it can increase risk of maternal co-infection with hepatitis B or hepatitis C. While vertical transmission of hepatitis B rarely causes acute liver failure in neonates, a child who is chronically infected with hepatitis B is more likely to develop cirrhosis and acute decompensation later in life.

The physical examination may direct the physician to further specific testing. Splenomegaly, ascites, or cutaneous spider angiomas suggest worsening of underlying chronic liver disease. Splenomegaly also may be present in acute processes, such as atypical viral infections or vascular events (e.g., hepatic vein thrombosis), but it is usually more suggestive of portal hypertension from chronic liver disease. Skin vesicles suggest systemic infection with agents such as herpes simplex virus. The liver may be enlarged, normal, or shrunken in acute liver failure; a shrunken liver indicates significant hepatic necrosis. If Wilson disease is suspected, the patient should undergo a slit-lamp ophthalmic examination to identify Kayser-Fleischer rings.

All patients should undergo careful monitoring of liver synthetic and metabolic function. Further workup should be tailored by findings on the history and physical exam (**Table 75-3**). Elevated transaminases, aspartate aminotransferase (AST) and alanine aminotransferase (ALT), are suggestive of hepatocyte injury and may be quite high. The ALT is more specific to liver tissue, while AST is found in other sites, such as red blood cells, cardiac muscle, skeletal muscle, and kidneys. Alkaline phosphatase (which can be tested in combination with gamma-glutamyl transpeptidase for more specificity) is generally elevated in cholestasis. Elevated bilirubin, particularly conjugated/direct, is indicative of hepatocyte or biliary tract disease. Albumin is synthesized by hepatocytes as are the blood clotting factors (except for Factor VIII). Patients with hepatic failure usually have a PT greater than 18 to 20 seconds (equivalent to INR >1.5 to 2). While ammonia elevation can be suggestive of liver dysfunction, it may not always correlate with actual encephalopathy.

TABLE 75-3 Laboratory Evaluation in Acute Hepatic Failure

Test	Description
Hematology	Complete blood count with platelets; differential; PT, PTT, INR
Chemistry	AST, ALT, bilirubin (total, direct), alkaline phosphatase, GGTP, total protein, albumin, glucose, blood urea nitrogen, creatinine, electrolytes, ammonia
Infectious evaluation	HAV, HBV, HCV, Epstein-Barr virus, Adenovirus
	Herpes simplex culture, fluorescent antibody of scraped vesicle or PCR (neonates)
	Enteroviral PCR (neonates)
	Maternal hepatitis B serologies (neonates)
Other studies	
Neonates and infants	Ferritin, lactate, pyruvate, plasma amino acids, urine succinylacetone (tyrosinemia), urine organic acids, urine ketones, urine-reducing substances (galactosemia)
Children and Adolescents	Antinuclear, anti-smooth muscle, anti-liver-kidney microsomal antibody; copper, ceruloplasmin, 24-hr urine copper, toxicology screen, acetaminophen level

ALT, Alanine transaminase; AST, Aspartate transaminase; GGTP, γ-glutamyl transpeptidase; HAV, Hepatitis A virus; HBV, Hepatitis B virus; HCV, Hepatitis C virus; INR, International normalized ratio; PT, Prothrombin time; PTT, Partial thromboplastin time; PCR, Polymerase chain reaction.

Ultrasonography of the abdomen with Doppler interrogation of the vessels can provide information about the size and consistency of the liver, patency of the biliary tree, presence of ascites, and patency of the hepatic veins to rule out hepatic vein thrombosis (Budd-Chiari syndrome).

MANAGEMENT

The most important first step when addressing suspected acute liver failure is confirmation that the patient indeed has coagulopathy (prolonged INR) and not just acute hepatitis. The next step is confirming that the prolonged INR is not secondary to vitamin K deficiency. This is done by empiric administration of parenteral (intramuscular, subcutaneous, or intravenous) vitamin K. Recommended dosing is 1 mg/y of age to a maximum dose of 10 mg. If this intervention does not improve the coagulopathy, acute liver failure is confirmed and close consultation with a pediatric gastroenterologist is recommended to initiate evaluation and transfer to a liver transplant center. Complications of liver failure are illustrated in Table 75-1 and management of the most common abnormalities delineated by system and prioritized by acuity are described below.

NEUROLOGIC

Frequent neurologic examinations are warranted to detect encephalopathy. Sedatives, such as benzodiazepines, should be avoided because they can alter the patient's mental status examination. Mental status changes, such as confusion or somnolence, should be taken quite seriously as the patient could rapidly progress to stupor or coma. Overall, advanced stages of encephalopathy are associated with higher mortality. Interestingly, however, children with early encephalopathy (within 7 days) after the first laboratory evidence of liver disease have a better prognosis than patients with late encephalopathy. Encephalopathy can be a prelude to cerebral edema and subsequent cerebral herniation—the most common cause of mortality in patients with acute liver failure. Enteral lactulose may be used if the child is euvolemic and electrolytes are normal.

CARDIOVASCULAR

If hypoxia or ischemia from cardiac surgery or insult is suspected, prompt support of perfusion and maintenance of normal blood pressure and oxygenation are crucial.

RENAL

Patients presenting with dehydration secondary to vomiting or poor oral intake should receive intravenous fluids to correct fluid balance. Once dehydration is corrected, fluids should be restricted to approximately 75% of maintenance requirements to avoid fluid overload and progression to cerebral edema. Renal function and urine output should be closely monitored.

METABOLIC

Hypoglycemia is frequently seen with acute liver failure due to hepatocyte failure of gluconeogenesis and mobilization of glucose. Many children require infusions of 10% dextrose to remain euglycemic. Hypokalemia, hypophosphatemia, or other metabolic abnormalities are also common and should be corrected in a timely manner to avoid cardiac arrhythmias. Infants with suspected galactosemia should have galactose-containing formulas withheld.

INFECTIOUS

Patients with hepatic failure are more susceptible to bacterial infections. If the patient develops fever or other clinical signs of infection (e.g., tachycardia or hypotension), a sepsis evaluation should be undertaken and there should be a low threshold to start empiric intravenous antibiotics. Any infant or child with suspected herpes simplex virus infection should receive intravenous acyclovir. Infection, either bacterial or fungal, is also a significant cause of mortality.

HEMATOLOGIC

Bleeding, especially gastrointestinal, is less common in children with acute liver failure than adults, unless there is underlying chronic liver disease with esophageal or gastric varices from portal hypertension. Transfusion of products to improve clotting (fresh frozen plasma, cryoprecipitate, or platelets) should be given only for significant bleeding or prevention of bleeding during invasive procedures. Excess blood product can contribute to fluid overload, and artificial correction of INR can make clinical assessment difficult. If the patient is having significant gastrointestinal bleeding and has evidence of portal hypertension (splenomegaly, ascites, and/or spider angiomas), octreotide should be considered.

Patients in acute liver failure should receive intravenous gastric acid suppressants to prevent gastrointestinal bleeding from gastritis or ulcers. Blood counts must be monitored closely because some children with acute liver failure develop aplastic anemia. Bone marrow failure may present at the onset of liver disease, develop as the liver is improving, or even after transplantation.

RESPIRATORY

Patients can have a respiratory alkalosis due to liver metabolite build-up affecting the respiratory centers of the brain. This tends to have little clinical significance other than how it affects the acid-base interpretation. In the more severe cases, actual respiratory failure can occur due to neurologic depression from encephalopathy.

OTHER CONSIDERATIONS

All noncritical medications and herbal supplements should be considered as possible causes or as aggravating factors and discontinued. Patients with known acetaminophen ingestion should receive *N*-acetylcysteine. Administration of *N*-acetylcysteine for non-acetaminophen-induced liver failure is not recommended, as studies in children have not shown the same benefit as in adults with liver failure. Some medications should be avoided, and others require dose adjustment in patients with significant liver injury. Consultation with a clinical pharmacist may be useful to determine appropriate medication dosages.

PROGNOSIS

The cause of liver failure is important in terms of prognosis. Patients with acetaminophen overdose, autoimmune hepatitis, or hepatitis A virus infection have a much higher survival rate than do those with hepatitis B or liver failure with an unknown cause. In some cases, with or without specific therapy, the INR and mental status begin to improve as transaminase values decrease. However, falling transaminases with a rising INR and bilirubin suggest worsening hepatic necrosis and may indicate the need for liver transplantation. Even with a known cause of liver failure, many cases are irreversible at the time of diagnosis. Treatment remains mostly supportive. The key concepts in management are correction of metabolic abnormalities and prevention of potentially lethal complications such as bleeding, sepsis, multiorgan failure, and cerebral edema.

ADMISSION AND DISCHARGE CRITERIA

ADMISSION CRITERIA

The following are reasons to consider hospitalization of a child with acute hepatitis:

- Dehydration or the inability to tolerate liquids by mouth
- Encephalopathy or any mental status changes
- Coagulopathy, with INR $\geq$ 1.5
- Bleeding complications, regardless of INR (most importantly, gastrointestinal bleeding)

DISCHARGE CRITERIA

A child with acute hepatitis or acute liver failure may be ready to go home when they have:

- A steadily improving INR
- Normal mental status
- Improving transaminases and bilirubin

CONSULTATION

If possible, children with acute hepatitis should be seen by a pediatric gastroenterologist or hepatologist. If the child subsequently develops acute liver failure, the child should be immediately transferred to a critical care unit, preferably at a tertiary referral center that has a liver transplant program.

SPECIAL CONSIDERATIONS

PREVENTION

There is no single strategy for prevention of acute hepatic failure. All infants should be immunized for hepatitis B, and all children older than 1 year of age should be immunized for hepatitis A. If a contagious virus is suspected, all caretakers should wear personal protective equipment for both contact, respiratory and droplets precautions. Any prescription or over-the-counter medication should be considered potentially hepatotoxic and discontinued promptly if evidence of significant hepatic dysfunction develops.

KEY POINTS

- Most cases of acute liver failure have no identifiable cause.
- Infants or children with liver failure present with abnormal transaminases, jaundice, uncorrectable coagulopathy, and possibly mental status changes or hypoglycemia.
- Management of liver failure is largely supportive, including correction of metabolic disturbances, attention to coagulopathy, and rapid referral to tertiary care center for further evaluation and treatment.
- At this time, *N*-acetylcysteine should only be used for acetaminophen-induced liver injury.

SUGGESTED READINGS

Centers for Disease and Control and Prevention. Surveillance for acute viral hepatitis—United States, 2007. *MMWR Morb Mortal Wkly Rep.* 2009;58(SS-3).

Lee WM, Hynan LS, Rossaro L, et al. Intravenous *N*-acetylcysteine improves transplant-free survival in early stage non-acetaminophen acute liver failure. *Gastroenterology*. 2009;137(3):856-864, 864 e851.

O'Grady JG, Schalm SW, Williams R. Acute liver failure: redefining the syndromes. *Lancet*. 1993;342(8866):273-275.7.

Squires JE, Alonso EM. Acute liver failure in children. In: Suchy FJ, Sokol RJ, Balistreri WF, eds. *Liver Disease in Children*. 5th ed. New York, NY: Cambridge University Press; 2021:36-57.

Squires JE, Alonso EM, Ibrahim SH, et al. North American Society for Pediatric Gastroenterology, Hepatology, and Nutrition position paper on the diagnosis and management of pediatric acute liver failure. *J Pediatr Gastroenterol Nutr*. 2022;74(1):138-158.

Squires RH Jr, Shneider BL, Bucuvalas J, et al. Acute liver failure in children: the first 348 patients in the pediatric acute liver failure study group. *J Pediatr*. 2006;148(5):652-658.

Squires RH, Dhawan A, Alonso E, et al. Intravenous *N*-acetylcysteine in pediatric patients with nonacetaminophen acute liver failure: a placebo-controlled clinical trial. *Hepatology*. 2013;57(4):1542-1549.

Taylor SA, Whitington PF. Neonatal acute liver failure. *Liver Transpl.* 2016;22(5):677-685.

CHAPTER 76 Inflammatory Bowel Disease

Elliott S. Gordon, MD, MSc and Elaine B. Barfield, MD

BACKGROUND

Inflammatory bowel disease (IBD) is the umbrella term used to describe Crohn's disease (CD) and ulcerative colitis (UC), two idiopathic chronic, inflammatory conditions of the gastrointestinal (GI) tract that can manifest during childhood and adolescence. Pediatric IBD is on the rise, with an incidence of approximately 15 per 100,000 children in North America. It is likely that a pediatrician will be faced with a diagnosis of IBD one to three times per year, while a busy hospital-based pediatric gastroenterology practice will diagnose one or more cases per week. Approximately 25% of children with CD and 10% with UC require surgical intervention within the first 2 years of their diagnosis. This epidemiologic data highlights both the significant impact of IBD on patients and their families, as well as the importance of knowledgeable pediatric hospitalists in the care and appropriate management of children with IBD.

PATHOPHYSIOLOGY

The etiopathogenesis of IBD has been linked to a combination of genetic, environmental, immunologic, and microbial factors, but the exact cause remains elusive. It is believed that patients with a genetic predisposition to IBD develop an immune-mediated response to an environmental trigger or intestinal microbial dysbiosis, which leads to chronic inflammatory dysregulation. The early discovery of several genes, including CARD15 and the OCTN cation transporter associated with CD, lends support to this hypothesis. Chronic inflammation in CD can involve any part of the GI tract (from mouth to anus) and is characterized by discontinuous inflammation with intervening areas of normal mucosa (so-called skip lesions). Transmural inflammation is also pathognomonic for CD and can result in fistulae, perforations, and strictures. Another hallmark of CD is noncaseating granulomas which may be noted on histologic examination of mucosal biopsies. In contrast, intestinal involvement in UC is limited to superficial mucosal inflammation within the colon. Inflammation typically begins distally in the rectum with sequential proximal extension that may end in the cecum but does not include the terminal ileum.

CLINICAL PRESENTATIONS

Patients with IBD may present with a diverse constellation of signs and symptoms. The clinical presentation of CD depends on the anatomic location(s) of involvement. In UC, the symptoms may be more predictable because intestinal involvement is limited to the colon. In both cases, the severity of inflammation may or may not correlate with the severity of clinical presentation. Recognition of the various clinical presentations of IBD can aid in early diagnosis and initiation of therapy.

Symptoms in patients presenting with IBD may include abdominal pain, hematochezia, diarrhea, anorexia, nausea, weight loss, fatigue, and oral ulcerations. Signs may include abdominal tenderness, perianal skin tags, fistulae, delayed puberty, iron deficiency anemia, hypoalbuminemia, and extra-intestinal complications, including joint pain, rashes, and uveitis (**Table 76-1**). Laboratory tests frequently reveal elevated Erythrocyte Sedimentation Rate (ESR), C-reactive protein (CRP) and hypoalbuminemia. Stool studies are often notable for elevated fecal calprotectin. Calprotectin is a calcium- and zinc-binding protein that reflects the quantity of neutrophils at a site of inflammation and correlates well with other measures of acute inflammation.

Up to 15% of patients may initially present with signs or symptoms which are not definitive for either CD or UC. These patients may be

TABLE 76-1 Extra-Intestinal Manifestations of IBD

Skin	**Blood**
Erythema nodosum	Iron deficiency anemia
Pyoderma gangrenosum	Anemia of chronic disease
Perianal disease	Thrombocytosis
Joints	Autoimmune hemolytic anemia
Arthralgia	**Vascular**
Arthritis	Vasculitis
Ankylosing spondylitis	Thrombosis
Eye	**Kidney**
Uveitis	Nephrolithiasis
Episcleritis	Obstructive hydronephrosis
Conjunctivitis	Enterovesical fistula
Liver	Urinary tract infection
Primary sclerosing cholangitis	Amyloidosis
Hepatitis	**Pancreas**
Cholelithiasis	Pancreatitis
Bone	**Lung**
Osteoporosis	Pulmonary vasculitis
Mouth	Fibrosing alveolitis
Cheilitis	**Growth**
Stomatitis	Delayed growth
Aphthous ulcerations	Delayed puberty

categorized as "inflammatory bowel disease–unspecified (IBD-U)" until the individual pattern of IBD behavior declares itself. A rapidly growing trend is the diagnosis of IBD in children under the age of 6 years known as very early-onset inflammatory bowel disease (VEO-IBD). These children present with severe, extensive, and aggressive disease patterns and are often found to have an underlying primary immunodeficiency.

DIFFERENTIAL DIAGNOSIS

Several enteric pathogens can also cause diarrhea and rectal bleeding that may mimic IBD, such as *Salmonella*, *Shigella*, *Campylobacter*, *Yersinia*, *Escherichia coli* 0157/H7, and *Clostridium difficile*. Other diagnostic considerations in adolescents with abdominal pain and rectal bleeding include intussusception and systemic vasculitis, such as Henoch-Schonlein purpura, Behçet's disease, and hemolytic–uremic syndrome. If an abdominal abscess is found during the investigation of abdominal pain, a perforated appendix, trauma, and gynecologic diseases must also be considered.

DIAGNOSTIC EVALUATION

The diagnosis of IBD is usually confirmed by a combination of clinical observations and laboratory, radiographic, endoscopic, and histological findings (**Table 76-2**). A detailed history and physical examination are critical first steps in the evaluation of a child with abdominal pain. The most appropriate initial diagnostic approach includes laboratory tests—complete blood count, ESR, CRP, albumin, and stool specimens evaluating for inflammation and the presence of protozoal pathogens.

Endoscopic evaluation with upper endoscopy and colonoscopy with biopsies is key to confirming the diagnosis (**Figure 76-1**). Since these procedures are unable to evaluate the small intestine, magnetic resonance enterography (MRE) has become the primary tool for evaluation of the jejunum and ileum given its low risk and lack of ionizing radiation. although small bowel follow through and more recently intestinal ultrasound are other options. In the hospitalized patient, however, a computerized tomography (CT) scan may be necessary to quickly rule out acute developing processes, such as appendicitis, infection with abscess formation, or colonic perforation. Small bowel imaging may also reveal signs suggestive of CD (e.g., "creeping fat" in the mesentery). Enteroclysis or WBC scanning have fallen out of favor for the evaluation of small bowel CD; instead, video capsule endoscopy has emerged as the most sensitive

TABLE 76-2 Diagnostic Evaluation of the Child With Suspected IBD
Laboratory studies
CBC with differential, reticulocyte count
Sedimentation rate
Total protein, albumin
Aminotransferases, alkaline phosphatase, bilirubin
Serum iron, ferritin
Vitamin levels (Vit D 25-OH, B12, folate)
Quantiferon Gold
Stool studies
GI Pathogen Panel (for bacteria, including *E. coli* 0157/H7, *C. difficile*)
Fecal calprotectin
Imaging
Abdominal and pelvic MRE scan (or CT scan if abscess is suspected or if patient cannot tolerate MRE)
Upper GI series with small bowel follow through
Endoscopy
Upper endoscopy, colonoscopy, ileoscopy, and biopsies
Video-capsule endoscopy (capsule enteroscopy, small bowel endoscopy, "Pillcam")

MRE, magnetic resonance enterography.

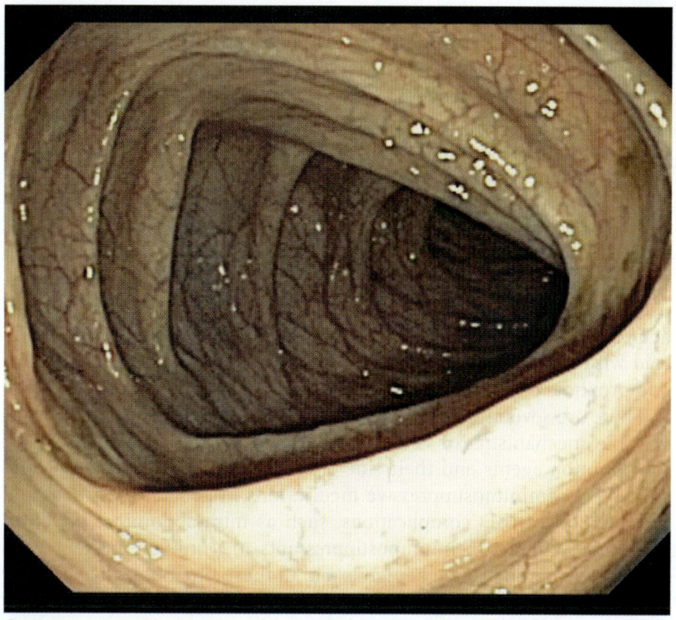

A

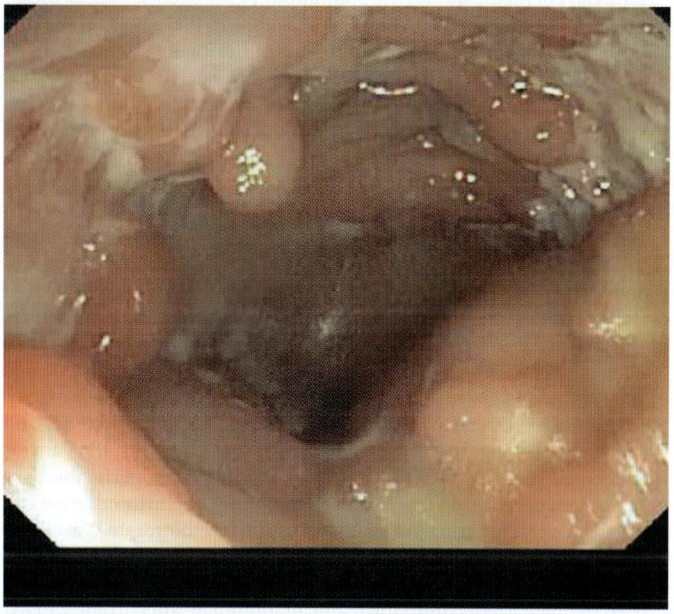

B

FIGURE 76-1. Photos from a colonoscopy showing (A) a normal appearing colon and (B) a colon from a patient with severe ulcerative colitis, which reveals serpiginous deep ulcerations along with pseudopolyps because of chronic inflammation.

means to assess the small intestine without radiation exposure. Capsule endoscopy is currently FDA approved in children aged 2 years and older; however, it has been used successfully in children as young as 8 months of age or 7.9 kg. The use of capsule endoscopy requires careful consideration and discussion with a pediatric gastroenterologist because there is a risk of capsule retention in patients with intestinal narrowing due to stenosing or stricturing disease. This is a particularly important issue to consider in the smaller child or children with severe, aggressive disease as a retained capsule would necessitate surgical intervention.

MANAGEMENT

Advances in medical therapy have revolutionized the management of IBD and reduced the need for hospitalization in many cases. As there is no known cure for IBD, the goal of therapy is to induce and maintain remission from disease activity. Nutritional therapy is the front-line therapy of choice in many Canadian and European IBD centers. Exclusive elemental or polymeric formula administrated via nasogastric tube as the primary source of nutrition has been shown to reduce inflammation and induce remission in many patients. As children tend to oppose the use of a fully liquid diet and nasogastric tube as an exclusive source of therapy, this treatment modality has not gained popularity in the United States.

Corticosteroids are sometimes used for short-term relief of symptoms and may be utilized as a bridge to disease control with more appropriate long-term treatment. Steroids are avoided for maintenance therapy, however, due to their side effect profile and lack of long-term efficacy. In the United States, IV corticosteroids (e.g., methylprednisolone) may be used to alleviate symptoms in the hospitalized patient presenting with an acute, severe IBD flare. Oral budesonide, a newer generation corticosteroid with fewer adverse effects, is effective in disease of the distal ileum and proximal colon because it specifically targets these areas.

There are several medications available in the treatment of IBD with variable mechanisms of action. **Table 76-3** provides a partial list of the common agents and their side effects. In addition to drug-specific side effects, immunosuppressive medications in general may mask the presentation of IBD complications, such as intra-abdominal infection or sepsis. Patients on immunosuppressants may initially present with minimal symptoms and a benign exam. In these situations, the clinician should maintain a low threshold for performing imaging and endoscopic evaluation and initiating empiric therapy.

One class of medication is the 5-aminosalicylate agents, such as mesalamine. These agents can be thought of as topical therapy for the colon and provide sustained remission in only a minority of patients, primarily those with mild to moderate UC. Antibiotics, such as metronidazole, ciprofloxacin, and piperacillin/tazobactam, are used as adjunct therapy in the case of abscess or infection but do not induce remission of IBD.

Immunomodulating agents, including thiopurines (azathioprine and 6-mercaptopurine), tacrolimus, cyclosporine, and methotrexate, were developed in the 1980s and initially used in the treatment of cancer. In lower doses, however, they were found to be effective for the treatment of IBD. The immunomodulators are slow acting and may take weeks to months to reach **maximum effect and achieve remission.** Tacrolimus and cyclosporine are used most as rescue or bridging therapies in the acutely ill hospitalized patient with colitis, often to avoid colectomy until more effective therapy with a biologic agent, for example, can be initiated. Side effects of thiopurines include bone marrow suppression, hepatotoxicity, pancreatitis, hypersensitivity, and an increased risk for infections and malignancy. Testing for thiopurine methyltransferase insufficiency is the accepted standard of practice prior to starting a thiopurine because patients with genetic polymorphisms in thiopurine methyltransferase can be at greater risk for bone marrow suppression. Methotrexate is available in oral and subcutaneous form and is a teratogen; counseling is required if it is used in the treatment of females with IBD who are of childbearing age.

Two biologic agents, infliximab and adalimumab, are currently FDA-approved for the management of moderate to severe pediatric IBD. Other biologics currently approved in the adult population, such as ustekinumab and vedolizumab, are sometimes used off label in pediatric patients who have experienced treatment failure or adverse reactions to infliximab and adalimumab. Risks of biologics include hypersensitivity reaction, hepatotoxicity, reactivation of tuberculosis and hepatitis B, and, rarely, hepatosplenic T-cell lymphoma. Newer therapies are aimed at either selectively blocking detrimental mucosal immune responses and/or decreasing the level of luminal antigens.

Careful attention to nutritional status is important in managing IBD in children. Quantifying caloric intake can help the clinician determine the best dietary intervention tailored to the patient's needs. Patients with upper intestinal CD may have secondary disaccharidase (e.g., lactase, sucrase) deficiency and require a low-carbohydrate, lactose-free diet. Patients with UC experiencing diarrhea need strict monitoring of fluid intake and losses and, in many cases, will require resuscitation either with oral rehydration or intravenous (IV) fluids. In patients with significant intestinal narrowing resulting from inflammation or stricture, a liquid diet may be better tolerated. Enteral nutrition is always preferable to parenteral nutrition and the route of administration is typically dictated by the degree of illness.

When hospitalization is required for patients with IBD, the 2011 ECCO/ESPGHAN (European Crohns and Colitis Organization and

TABLE 76-3 Common Side Effects/Adverse Reactions to IBD Drugs

Drug	Side effects/adverse reactions
5-Aminosalicylates	Allergic reactions Interstitial nephritis Colitis exacerbation Agranulocytosis
Corticosteroids	Adrenal suppression Cushingoid features Diabetes Hypertension Osteoporosis Cataracts Mood effects Growth retardation
Thiopurines (6-mercaptopurine, azathioprine)	Bone marrow suppression Hepatitis Pancreatitis Allergic reactions
Methotrexate	Bone marrow suppression Hepatitis Nausea
Anti-TNF, biologics Infliximab[a] Adalimumab[a] Certolizumab[b] Golimumab[b]	Injection site reaction Infusion reaction, anaphylaxis Autoantibody formation Antibodies against the medication Infections Reactivation of quiescent tuberculosis Neutropenia Lupus-like reaction CNS vasculitis Malignancy
Anti-IL 12/23 biologics Ustekinumab[b] (targets p40 subunit of both IL12 and IL23)	Injection site reaction Autoantibody formation Antibodies against the medication Infections (including nasopharyngitis) Malignancy
Anti-IL 23 biologics Mirikizumab (Omvoh)[b] (targets the p19 subunit of IL-23) Risankizumab (Skyrizi)[b] (targets the p19 subunit of IL-23)) Guselkumab (Tremfya)[b] (humanized monoclonal IgG4-variant antibody that selectively binds to the p19 subunit of human IL-23 cytokine and inhibits its interaction with the IL-23 receptor)	Injection site reaction Autoantibody formation Antibodies against the medication Infections (including nasopharyngitis) Malignancy
Humanized anti-alpha-4-beta-7 integrin monoclonal antibody Vedolizumab[b]	Autoantibody formation Antibodies against the medication Infections Reactivation of quiescent tuberculosis Progressive Multifocal Leukoencephalopathy (PML)
Sphingosine-1-phosphate (S1P receptor modulators) Ozanimod (Zeposia)[b] Etrasimod (Veltre)[b]	Infections Elevated liver enzymes Heart-related issues.
JAK inhibitors Tofacitinib (Xeljanz)[b] Upadacitinib (Rinvoq)[b]	Infections Hypercholesterolemia Venous thromboembolism Major adverse cardiovascular events Malignancy
Metronidazole	Neuropathy Yeast infections Coated tongue
Cyclosporine	Renal toxicity Anaphylaxis Seizures Hypertension Hirsutism Gum hyperplasia

[a]FDA approved in children and adolescents.
[b]FDA approved in patients 18 years and old.

European Society for Pediatric Gastroenterology, Hepatology, and Nutrition) guidelines outline the most appropriate inpatient treatment course. Initial management of the patient hospitalized with IBD must be tailored to the degree of illness while also attempting to relieve the patient's symptoms. Primary interventions should aim to stabilize the patient while the clinician determines if emergent surgical intervention is required. IV fluids and/or blood transfusions may be required if the patient presents with severe dehydration or anemia. Careful attention to hydration status is critical in the patient with significant hypoalbuminemia. If complications such as appendicitis, infection, abscess formation, or other surgical emergencies are suspected, it is prudent to withhold oral intake and administer IV broad-spectrum antibiotics that empirically cover intestinal flora (e.g., piperacillin-tazobactam). Once stabilized, oral intake may be permitted while evaluation and monitoring continue. If a patient presents with significant diarrhea followed by cessation of stooling, consider this an emergency as the patient may have developed toxic megacolon and could be at risk for impending intestinal perforation. In this case, a stat abdominal radiograph would be necessary to evaluate for signs of perforation including the presence of free air.

When a patient with severe UC is admitted to the hospital, the Pediatric Ulcerative Colitis Activity Index (PUCAI) should be calculated daily to assess disease activity. This six-item validated index includes elements such as stool consistency, number of stools in 24 hours, amount of rectal bleeding, activity level, and abdominal pain (**Table 76-4**). Calculating this index daily assists in monitoring the patient's response to therapy and can help direct management and next steps in care.

Surgical management remains an important consideration in the management of severe IBD with complications such as stricture, fistulae, and intestinal perforation. Colectomy must be considered in the patient who is steroid-dependent or unresponsive to medical management or in patients with longstanding colitic disease given increased risk of malignancy. Emergent colectomy may be necessary in patients who develop toxic megacolon or perforation. Though colectomy is often considered "curative" in UC, appropriate medical therapy may need to be continued in many cases and the rectal stump remaining after a subtotal colectomy must be surveyed at intervals for cancer screening. Surgical resection should not be a first-line therapy in CD as there is a high incidence of disease recurrence in other parts of the gastrointestinal tract since the location of disease can be unpredictable.

TABLE 76-4 Pediatric Ulcerative Colitis Disease Activity Index (PUCAI)

Abdominal pain	
No pain	0
Pain can be ignored	5
Pain cannot be ignored	10
Rectal bleeding	
None	0
Small amount only <50% of stools	10
Small amount with most stools	20
Large amount (>50% of stool content)	30
Consistency of most stools	
Formed	0
Partially formed	5
Completely unformed	10
Number of stools per 24 hours	
0-2	0
3-5	5
6-8	10
>8	15
Nocturnal bowel movements	
No	0
Yes	10
Activity level	
No limitation of activity	0
Occasional limitation	5
Severely restricted activity	10

RISK OF VENOUS THROMBOEMBOLISM

Adult guidelines recommend prophylaxis for venous thromboembolism (VTE) in patients hospitalized with severe colitis. The 2011 pediatric ECCO/ESPGHAN guidelines do not recommend prophylaxis in children, citing a lack of evidence demonstrating a favorable benefit-to-risk ratio. However, it has now been demonstrated that children with IBD do have an increased risk of thrombosis.

ADMISSION AND DISCHARGE CRITERIA

ADMISSION CRITERIA

- Persistent fever with worsening symptoms, such as abdominal pain or distention.
- Signs of intestinal obstruction or persistent and severe symptoms, which may necessitate IV antibiotics or surgical intervention.
- Active disease refractory to outpatient steroid, mesalamine, immunomodulator, or biologic therapy.
- Significant gastrointestinal blood loss leading to anemia with potential need for transfusion.
- Persistent diarrhea and inability to maintain hydration orally.

DISCHARGE CRITERIA

Discharge may considered when the child:

- Can tolerate an enteral (oral or nasogastric) diet and maintain hydration and a positive nutritional balance.
- Has stable or improving signs and symptoms of active disease (e.g., improved hemoglobin, stable stool output, improved pain).
- Has reliable outpatient follow-up and family has the ability to manage therapy and monitor recovery at home.

CONSULTATION

A pediatric gastroenterologist should be consulted for all patients with IBD. Surgical consultation may be necessary in patients with suspected abscesses or fistulae (penetrating disease), intestinal strictures, concern for toxic megacolon or intestinal perforation, or in those who are poorly responsive to medical management. Nutrition or dietary consultation is warranted in patients with poor weight gain or failure to thrive. Genetics evaluation may be merited in patients diagnosed with IBD under 6-years of age or in those with a strong family history (first-degree relative) also with IBD. Consultation with psychology or social work may also be beneficial for patients as they adjust to a new diagnosis of IBD.

KEY POINTS

- There is no known cause of Inflammatory Bowel Disease (IBD) though it is theorized that genetic, environmental, and microbial factors contribute to disease pathogenesis.
- The diagnosis of IBD should be considered in the pediatric patient presenting with abdominal pain, weight loss or failure to thrive, diarrhea, blood in stools, anemia, and/or fatigue.
- The definitive diagnosis of IBD requires mucosal specimens with histopathologic features suggestive of the disease. Elevated inflammatory markers, low iron, ferritin, and albumin may support a diagnosis.
- Treatment for IBD may include the use of biologic therapies, immunomodulators, corticosteroids, 5-ASA, and nutritional considerations.

SUGGESTED READINGS

Baldassano RN, Han PD, Jeshion WC, et al. Pediatric Crohn's disease: risk factors for postoperative recurrence. *Am J Gastroenterol.* 2001;96:2169-2176.

Escher JC, Taminiau JA, Nieuwenhuis EE, Buller HA, Grand RJ. Treatment of inflammatory bowel disease in childhood: best available evidence. *Inflamm Bowel Dis*. 2003;9:34-58.

Fiocchi C. Inflammatory bowel disease: etiology and pathogenesis. *Gastroenterology*. 1998;115:182-205.

Griffiths AM, Nguyen P, Smith C, MacMillan JH, Sherman PM. Growth and clinical course of children with Crohn's disease. *Gut*. 1993;34:939-943.

Griffiths, et al. Inflammatory bowel disease. In: Walker WA, et al., eds. *Pediatric Gastrointestinal Disease: Pathophysiology, Diagnosis, Management*. Hamilton, Ontario: B.C. Decker, 2000:613-651.

Heyman MB, Kirschner BS, Gold BD, et al. Children with early-onset inflammatory bowel disease (IBD): analysis of a pediatric IBD consortium registry. *J Pediatr*. 2005;146:35-40.

Kirschner BS. Safety of azathioprine and 6-mercaptopurine in pediatric patients with inflammatory bowel disease. *Gastroenterology*. 1998; 115:813-821.

Kugathasan S, Judd RH, Hoffmann RG, et al. Epidemiologic and clinical characteristics of children with newly diagnosed inflammatory bowel disease in Wisconsin: a statewide population-based study. *J Pediatr*. 2003;143:525-531.

Podolsky DK. Inflammatory bowel disease. *N Engl J Med*. 2002;347: 417-429.

Shashinder H, Integlia MJ, Grand RJ. *Clinical Manifestations of Pediatric Inflammatory Bowel Disease*. Sanders; 2000.

CHAPTER 77 Malnutrition

Diana L. Culbertson, PA-C, MMSc, MS and
Indi Trehan, MD, MPH, DTM&H

BACKGROUND

Malnutrition refers to disorders of nutritional status from either deficiencies or excess (i.e., imbalance) of energy, protein, and/or other nutrients that lead to adverse effects on tissue and body form and function as well as adverse clinical outcomes. Malnutrition includes undernutrition, overweight, and obesity; multiple forms of malnutrition may (and often do) exist within the same patient. Despite significant advances in prevention and treatment worldwide, malnutrition still contributes to nearly half of the deaths in children under five worldwide.

This chapter addresses ***undernutrition***, focusing on problems relating to inpatient care. The prevalence of undernutrition among hospitalized children in the United States varies by age and disease state and may be as high as 50%. The presence of undernutrition during hospitalization has been associated with an increased risk of adverse clinical events, prolonged length of stay, and increased hospital charges and costs.

PATHOPHYSIOLOGY

Pediatric undernutrition is defined as an imbalance between nutrient requirement and intake, resulting in cumulative deficits of energy, protein, or micronutrients that may negatively affect growth, development, and other outcomes. Undernutrition is often related to environmental, socioeconomic, or behavioral factors. Many hospitalized children have illness-related malnutrition, with one or more conditions directly resulting in a nutrient imbalance. This occurs because of decreased essential nutrient intake, altered utilization, excessive losses, or increased requirements not matched by nutrient intake. Furthermore, illness-related malnutrition is often associated with an inflammatory component, which increases nutrient requirements and promotes a nutrient-wasting catabolic state. The presence and severity of the inflammatory state may also impair the effectiveness of therapeutic nutrition interventions. Secondary complications of malnutrition include compromised immune function, impairments of gastrointestinal (GI) tract function, suboptimal response to medical or surgical therapy, bacterial and toxin translocation across the gut mucosa, and abnormal cognitive and behavioral development.

CLINICAL PRESENTATIONS

Physical examination findings in children with malnutrition are variable and related to the chronicity, severity, and type of nutrient imbalance. **Table 77-1** lists some findings associated with macro- and

TABLE 77-1 Physical Examination Findings Associated With Macro- and Micronutrient Deficiencies (Partial Listing)

Finding	Nutrient Deficiency
General	
Short stature	Multiple macronutrients and micronutrients
Decreased subcutaneous fat	Multiple macronutrients and micronutrients
Muscle wasting	Protein, calorie
Muscle tenderness	Thiamine, biotin
Edema, ascites	Protein, thiamine
Hepatosplenomegaly	Protein
Hair	
Alopecia or sparse hair	Protein, zinc, biotin, copper
Easy pluckability	Protein
Flag signs (bands of light and dark hair)	Protein
Skin	
Follicular hyperkeratosis	Vitamins A, C
Dermatitis	Niacin, zinc, biotin, vitamin B_6
Poor wound healing	Protein, zinc, vitamins A and C
Dry, xerosis	Essential fatty acids
Petechiae, purpura	Vitamins C, K
Nails	
Koilonychia (spoon shaped)	Iron
Transverse ridging	Protein
Dry, brittle	Essential fatty acids
Eyes	
Xerophthalmia, Bitot spots (conjunctival spots), night blindness	Vitamin A
Angular palpebritis	Riboflavin
Oropharynx	
Dental caries	Fluoride
Cheilosis	Riboflavin, niacin, vitamin B_6
Glossitis	Riboflavin, niacin, pyridoxine, folate, vitamin B_{12}
Angular stomatitis	Riboflavin, niacin, iron, vitamins B_6 and B_{12}
Hypogeusia (reduced ability to taste)	Zinc
Bleeding gums	Vitamin C
Bone	
Craniotabes, rachitic rosary, bowing of legs	Vitamin D
Bony tenderness	Vitamin C
Nervous system	
Neuropathy (weakness, paresthesias)	Niacin, thiamine, copper, vitamins B_6, B_{12}, E
Dementia	Niacin
Seizures	Vitamin B_6
Miscellaneous	
Goiter	Iodine

micronutrient deficiencies. Abnormal growth ultimately occurs in all patients with ongoing undernutrition, and, in some cases, it may be the only objective marker of poor nutritional status. Careful anthropometric measurements can assess growth cross-sectionally (e.g., triceps skinfold thickness) or longitudinally (length or height).

CLASSIFICATION

Historically, physical findings and anthropometry have been used to divide patients with acute malnutrition into two broad categories (which may overlap): marasmus and kwashiorkor. Marasmus generally develops after severe nutritional deprivation, resulting in weight loss and marked fat and muscle wasting. Children with marasmus appear emaciated, weak, or lethargic and may be irritable and difficult to console. Their skin is dry, loose, and wrinkled without a specific dermatosis. They may also have abnormal vital signs including bradycardia, hypotension, and hypothermia. Although both height and weight measurements are abnormally low, weight is often decreased out of proportion to height (reduced weight-for-height). Kwashiorkor develops more acutely, as a maladaptive response to starvation of protein and calories. The distinguishing clinical finding of kwashiorkor is the presence of bilateral pitting edema, without another medical cause, such as renal, cardiac, or hepatic insufficiency. Although some degree of growth failure is likely, weight may appear normal (or even elevated) for height due to fluid retention. Children with kwashiorkor may have various dermatoses including shiny, varnished-looking skin, dark erythematous macules, hypo- or hyperpigmentation, and areas of confluent hyperkeratosis which may split when stretched.

LONG-TERM CONSEQUENCES

There is growing recognition of the lifelong impairment of chronic or prolonged childhood malnutrition, which manifests physically as stunting (reduced height-for-age), but more profoundly as reduced cognitive capacity and an increased risk of nutrition-related chronic diseases in adulthood. Many children with acute malnutrition (kwashiorkor and/or marasmus) will also show evidence of stunting, especially in resource-limited settings. The prevention and reversal of stunting is unlikely beyond about the first 2 years of age.

DIAGNOSTIC EVALUATION

Several validated tools are available to screen hospitalized patients for malnutrition or at risk for malnutrition (**Table 77-2**). The presence of one or more of these risk factors should prompt a comprehensive evaluation including a thorough history, socioeconomic assessment, physical examination, anthropometry, and laboratory data to define nutritional status and develop a proper nutrition plan. The Subjective Global Nutrition Assessment (SGNA) is used to assess a child's current nutritional status, while the STRONGkids tool predicts risk of developing malnutrition during hospitalization. Both tools can help guide decisions about when to start nutritional interventions.

The medical history should include the use of any dietary supplements, a careful dietary history, and a detailed psychosocial history. Special emphasis should also be placed on conditions or medications that impair the ability to ingest and absorb food or that might result in high metabolic demands. The dietary history should focus on the type and preparation of food or formula and the amount, frequency and route of feedings. Prospectively, a 3 to 5-day diet diary can provide an objective and accurate method of assessing intake and may be an important part of discharge recommendations. Important psychosocial factors include adequacy of resources to purchase, store, and prepare food; level of parental knowledge and skills; drug and alcohol use or mental illness among caregivers; and potential child abuse or neglect.

TABLE 77-2 Risk Factors for Malnutrition

Risk Factors for Malnutrition
Recent unintentional weight loss of >10%
Weight 20% over or under ideal body weight
No oral intake for >7 days
Any medical condition resulting in the following:
Inadequate intake (e.g., oromotor or swallowing dysfunction, anorexia)
Malabsorption (e.g., cystic fibrosis, short gut syndrome)
Increased metabolic needs (e.g., congenital heart disease, bronchopulmonary dysplasia, trauma, burns, sepsis, severe or chronic infection)
Protracted nutrient losses (e.g., vomiting, diarrhea, skin wounds)
Medications with catabolic properties (e.g., steroids, chemotherapy)

A thorough physical examination and precise anthropometry provides essential and noninvasive evaluations of both acute and chronic nutritional status. Basic measurements include weight, height (for children aged 2 years or older) or recumbent length and head circumference (children younger than 2). Body mass index (BMI), normalized to age-based norms, is the best measure of adiposity (when balancing convenience and accuracy) and is commonly used to define underweight, overweight, and obesity in children older than 2 years. It is calculated by the following formula:

$$\text{BMI} = \frac{\text{Weight (kg)}}{[\text{height (m)}]^2}$$

Nutritional assessment with standardized anthropometric data is equally valid for children in both resource-replete and resource-constrained settings. The World Health Organization (WHO) has published universal growth standards for children under 5 years old. For those over 5, either the 2000 Centers for Disease Control and Prevention growth standards or the WHO's 2007 growth references may be used, depending on local practices. Reference values for children with special healthcare needs are also available. Expressing a child's growth in terms of *Z* scores, which express in standard deviation units how far a child's measurements are from the median of the population reference standard median, is preferred as this can most accurately quantify the degree of malnutrition. Acute malnutrition (or "wasting") is classified as moderate when the weight-for-height/length *Z* score is 2 to 3 standard deviations below the median and severe when more than 3 standard deviations below the median. Children with more long-standing undernutrition may present underweight (low weight-for-age) or stunted (low height-for-age).

Certain measurements of the arm can provide additional data and may be especially helpful when body weight and/or height measurements are difficult to obtain or are inaccurate (e.g., cerebral palsy, critical illness, limited resource settings). Measurements of the triceps and/or biceps skinfold thickness (TSF and BSF) using skin calipers or mid-upper arm circumference (MUAC) using a non-stretchable tape measure, can be used to estimate peripheral lean body mass. The WHO criteria for the diagnosis of acute malnutrition includes the use of MUAC measurements, with moderate malnutrition being a MUAC of 115 to 124 mm and severe malnutrition being a MUAC <115 mm for children between 6 and 59 months of age.

Several common blood tests can provide additional information about nutritional status (should there be diagnostic ambiguity) or help guide management. While not required, the initial evaluation may include:

- Electrolytes, including calcium, phosphorus, and magnesium
- Liver enzymes, prealbumin, albumin, prothrombin time, and bilirubin
- Complete blood count with differential and peripheral smear
- C-reactive protein (CRP) or erythrocyte sedimentation rate (ESR)

Depletion of electrolyte stores or metabolic bone disease may result in abnormal chemistry and mineral profiles. Several vitamin and mineral deficiencies can result in lymphopenia and thrombocytopenia, as well as hemolytic, microcytic, or megaloblastic anemia. Vitamin K deficiency often leads to a prolonged prothrombin time. CRP and ESR may indicate the degree of concomitant inflammation, although these provide no specific management guidance.

While serum protein levels often reflect the degree of malnutrition, they must be interpreted with caution. They can be influenced by the presence of systemic disease and the body's response to trauma, infection, and inflammation. Because albumin has a half-life of 14 to 20 days and undergoes shifts in body stores with changes in acute nutritional status, it may be more reflective of chronic malnutrition. Other proteins synthesized by the liver have shorter half-lives and more accurately reflect acute changes in protein stores and metabolism. These include

TABLE 77-3 WHO Criteria for the Diagnosis of Malnutrition for children aged 6-59 months

	Acute Malnutrition		Chronic Malnutrition	
	Severe	Moderate	Severe	Moderate
WHO z score	WLZ or WHZ < -3	WLZ or WHZ -2 to -3	LAZ or HAZ < -3	LAZ or HAZ -2 to -3
MUAC	< 115 mm	115-124 mm	N/A	N/A
Edema	+/–	–	+/–	+/–

WLZ: Weight-for-length, WHZ: Weight-for-height, LAZ: Length-for-age, HAZ: Height-for-Age.

+: Finding may be present, –: Finding is absent.

Source: World Health Organization (WHO), 2013.

transferrin (half-life 8 days), prealbumin (half-life approximately 2 days), and retinol-binding protein (half-life 12 hours). However, their utility beyond an effective clinical and historical assessment of the patient's condition is relatively limited.

If renal function is normal, urine studies can also provide additional information about total-body protein reserves and turnover. The creatinine-height index evaluates lean muscle mass by comparing the patient's 24-hour urinary creatinine excretion with the predicted urinary excretion for a child of similar height. Nitrogen balance compares 24-hour protein intake with 24-hour urinary urea nitrogen and reflects the rate of protein turnover. A positive nitrogen balance indicates an anabolic state, and a negative nitrogen balance indicates a catabolic state.

MANAGEMENT

Hospitalized patients who are malnourished or at risk for malnutrition need a formal plan that outlines their nutritional deficiencies, goals, and monitoring parameters. The plan should include the most appropriate route of administration of nutritional support and method of nutrition access, and the anticipated duration of therapy. An interdisciplinary approach is often necessary to ensure that the nutritional needs of the patient are adequately addressed and integrated into medical and surgical treatment plans. **Figure 77-1** presents an algorithm for determining the optimal route of nutritional support when oral intake is insufficient or not possible.

The nutrition plan should include an estimate of total caloric needs. Caloric needs can be impacted by several individual factors, such as activity level (e.g., bed rest vs. active), stress level (e.g., well vs. postoperative), and weight (e.g., obese vs. underweight). The starting point for computing basic caloric and protein needs are determined by the patient's age (**Table 77-4**) and adjusted for factors that may increase or decrease the need.

Daily caloric needs for infants and toddlers who need catch-up growth can be estimated using established guidelines, such as those from WHO. It is important to supplement energy and protein to optimize catch-up of both lean and fat mass (**Table 77-5**). It should be noted that these guidelines do not replace disease specific requirements that have been published on, for example, cardiac, renal, and cystic fibrosis energy and protein requirements.

ENTERAL NUTRITION

Enteral nutrition—the provision of nutrients by tube directly into the GI tract—is indicated when an individual is unable to ingest or absorb

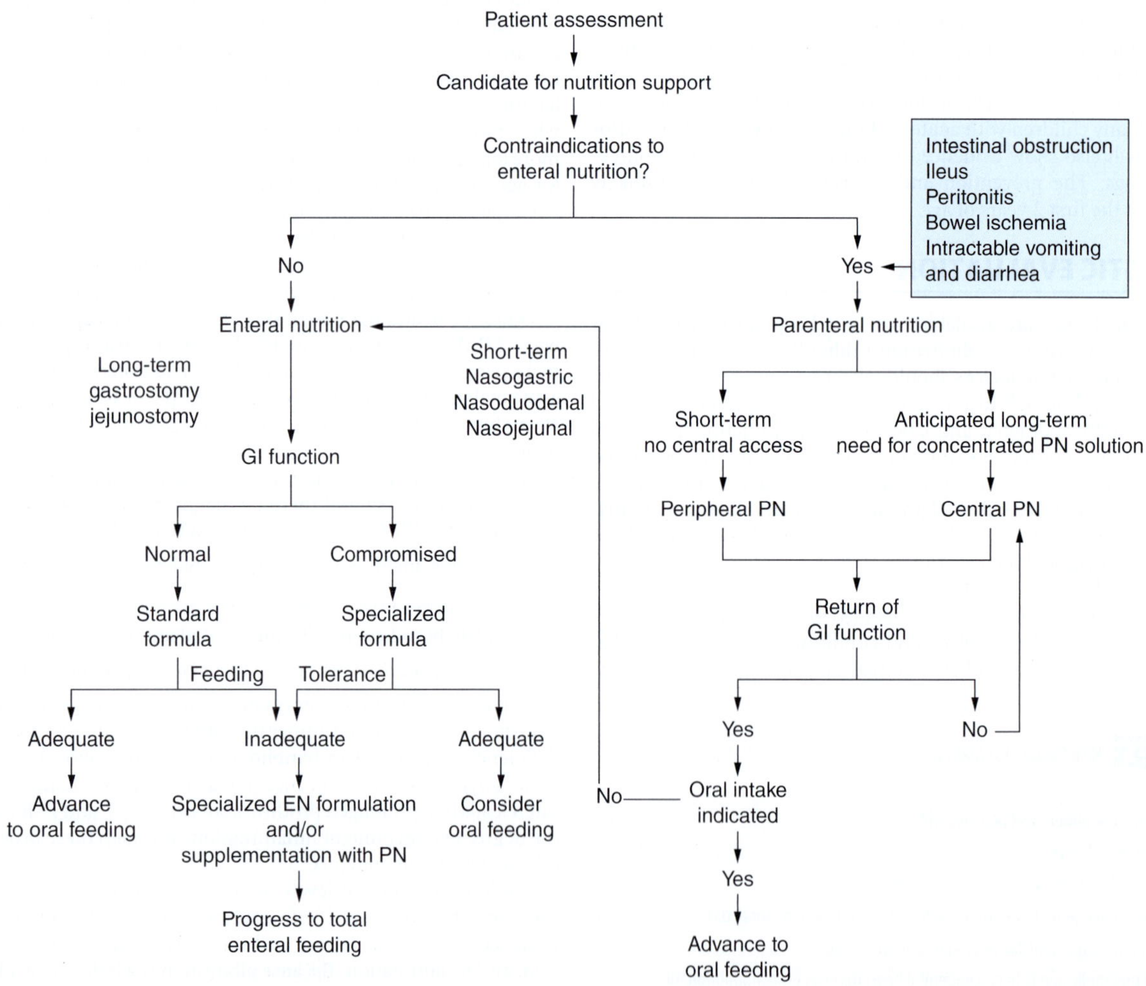

FIGURE 77-1. Route of administration of specialized nutrition support. GI, gastrointestinal; EN, enteral nutrition; PN, parenteral nutrition. (Modified with permission from Ukleja A, Freeman KL, Gilbert K, et al. Task Force on Standards for Nutrition Support: Adult Hospitalized Patients and the American Society for Parenteral and Enteral Nutrition Board of Directors. Standards for nutrition support: adult hospitalized patients. *Nutr Clin Pract.* 2010;25(4):403-414.)

TABLE 77-4 Recommended Daily Allowance for Calories and Protein by Age

Age	Calories (kcal/kg/day)	Protein (g/kg/day)
0-6 mo	108	1.5
7-12 mo	98	1.5
1-3 y	102	1.1
4-6 y	90	0.95
7-10 y	70	0.95
11-14 y		
Girls	47	0.95
Boys	55	0.95
15-18 y		
Girls	40	0.85
Boys	55	0.85

Source: Data from *Dietary Reference Intakes for Energy, Carbohydrates, Fiber, Fat, Fatty Acids, Cholesterol, Protein, and Amino Acids*. National Academy of Sciences, 2002-2005. http://nap.edu.

enough nutrition orally to meet requirements. Some specific indications for enteral nutrition are listed in **Table 77-6**. Bowel obstruction, paralytic ileus, intractable vomiting or diarrhea, and other disease processes that severely impair the function of the GI tract are contraindications to enteral nutrition. Therapy for oral-motor stimulation should be provided to patients throughout enteral nutritional support to help avoid the development of oral aversion and food refusal.

Selection of the appropriate delivery device and method of administration for enteral nutrition is dependent on the anticipated duration of nutrition support, GI tract anatomy and function, and associated medical conditions. Options include nasogastric (NG), nasoduodenal (ND), nasojejunal (NJ), gastrostomy (GT), and jejunosotomy (JT) tubes. Generally, nasoenteric tubes are used for short-term enteral nutrition (<3 months), and tube enterostomies are used for long-term enteral nutrition.

Gastric feedings are more physiologic and are preferred in children who require short-term nutritional support, have intact gag and cough reflexes, and have a normally functioning GI tract. Gastric feedings may exacerbate underlying gastroesophageal reflux or gastroparesis and increase the risk for aspiration. These patients, as well as those with known tracheal aspiration, gastric outlet obstruction, and congenital anomalies of the upper GI tract, usually require transpyloric feedings. See Chapter 182 on enteral tubes for more information.

The patient's age, nutritional requirements, and medical condition(s) determine the selection of formula. In most cases, enteral feedings are started at a continuous rate and advanced by increasing either the concentration or rate of infusion. A feeding pump can be used to control the feeding rate. Patients receiving transpyloric feedings or with impaired absorption typically remain on continuous feeding. Optimally, patients may advance to more physiologic bolus feedings once tolerance to full continuous feeding has been demonstrated (except those receiving transpyloric feeding). Feeding intolerance is manifested by nausea, pain, persistent regurgitation, malabsorption, dumping syndrome, and aspiration.

Compared with parenteral nutrition, enteral nutrition is better at maintaining the physiologic and immunologic integrity of the GI tract. The administration of enteral nutrition is easier, more economical, and results in fewer metabolic and infectious complications. Selected complications of enteral nutrition are listed in **Table 77-7**.

TABLE 77-5 WHO Guidelines for Energy and Protein Intake for Catch-up Growth

Rate of weight gain (g/kg/day)	Protein (g/kg/day)	Energy (kcal/kg/day)	Protein-Energy Ratio (PE%)
10	2.82	126	8.9
20	4.82	167	11.5

Source: WHO/FAO/UNU expert consultation, 2007.

TABLE 77-6 Selected Indications for Enteral Nutrition

Category	Example
Inadequate oral intake	Disorders of sucking or swallowing
	Congenital anomaly of upper airway or GI tract
Abnormal function of GI tract	Inflammatory bowel disease
	Gastroesophageal reflux
	Short bowel syndrome
	Hirschsprung disease
	Chronic liver disease
	Motility disorder
Increased metabolic demands	Cystic fibrosis
	Congenital heart disease
	Chronic pulmonary or renal disease
	Sepsis or severe infection
	Trauma or burns
Growth failure or chronic malnutrition	Anorexia nervosa
	Nonorganic failure to thrive

GI, gastrointestinal.

PARENTERAL NUTRITION

Parenteral nutrition—the provision of nutrients intravenously—is indicated when an individual is unable to meet ongoing nutritional needs with either oral or enteral nutrition. Selected indications for parenteral nutrition are listed in **Table 77-8**. Relative contraindications include short anticipated duration of nutritional support and probability of imminent death.

Parenteral nutrition can be administered peripherally via a standard intravenous catheter if the duration of nutritional support is short-term. However, peripheral veins are not tolerant of highly osmotic solutions, and it is often difficult to provide adequate calories, protein, and electrolytes in this manner. Central venous access, via either a peripherally inserted central catheter or a semipermanent catheter, allows for the provision of nutrients at a greater concentration.

The composition of a parenteral nutrition solution is determined by the patient's age, weight, and nutritional and medical needs. Solutions are typically infused over 24 hours in hospitalized patients, but may be cycled over shorter periods of time. Several resources exist for

TABLE 77-7 Selected Complications of Enteral Nutrition

Category	Complication
Feeding tube related	Clogging of tube
	Dislodgment/malposition of tube
	Nasopharyngeal ulceration or necrosis
	Hoarseness and vocal cord paralysis
	Bowel perforation
	Bowel obstruction
	Hemorrhage
	Stomal leakage
Infectious	Sinusitis and otitis media
	Aspiration pneumonia
	Cellulitis
Gastrointestinal	Vomiting
	Diarrhea
	Abdominal cramping or bloating
	Dumping syndrome
Metabolic	Electrolyte abnormalities

TABLE 77-8 Selected Indications for Parenteral Nutrition

Prematurity and low birth weight
Congenital gastrointestinal anomalies
Necrotizing enterocolitis
Short bowel syndrome
Intestinal obstruction
Gastrointestinal fistula
Severe motility disorders
Intractable diarrhea
Severe pancreatitis
Severe trauma or burns
Severe protein–energy malnutrition

determination of the normal requirements for energy, fluid and electrolytes, protein, carbohydrates, lipids, and micronutrients for children; early involvement of a clinical dietician and/or pharmacist is strongly recommended.

Selected complications of parenteral nutrition are listed in **Table 77-9**. Catheter-related infections can be reduced by limiting the frequency of manipulation/access and by adherence to the use of correct aseptic technique. Hepatic dysfunction is more likely to occur in young patients or neonates. The risk of hepatic dysfunction decreases with the early introduction of enteral feedings, which stimulate bile flow and GI hormones production. Transition back to oral or enteral feedings should begin when GI function returns.

MONITORING

A sample monitoring schedule to ensure the efficacy of supplemental nutritional support and to screen for complications is shown in **Table 77-10**. Aggressive monitoring is indicated for patients with severe protein-energy malnutrition and patients receiving parenteral nutrition.

REEDING SYNDROME

Refeeding syndrome refers to the metabolic and physiologic consequences of rapid electrolyte repletion, fluid resuscitation, and reintroduction of carbohydrates in a patient with chronic caloric deprivation and severe malnutrition. During prolonged starvation, glycogen stores are exhausted, protein is conserved for intracellular enzymatic and structural function, and fats become the predominant source of energy. In addition, both intracellular and extracellular ions are depleted over time. As carbohydrates are reintroduced, there is a rapid transition back to the use of glucose as the predominant fuel, with a resultant high demand to produce phosphorylated intermediates of glycolysis (i.e., adenosine triphosphate and 2,3-diphosphoglycerate). This can lead to the precipitous development of hypophosphatemia, which is the hallmark of refeeding syndrome. Other electrolyte, vitamin, and trace element imbalances may occur as well, such as hypomagnesemia, hypokalemia, hyperglycemia, and thiamine (vitamin B_1) deficiency. Electrolyte disturbances are exacerbated by insulin secretion in response to the carbohydrate load, which further shifts electrolytes such as potassium intracellularly.

TABLE 77-9 Selected Complications of Parenteral Nutrition

Category	Complication
Catheter related	Malposition of catheter
	Occlusion of catheter
	Pneumothorax, hemothorax, hydrothorax
	Cardiac arrhythmia
	Brachial plexus injuries
	Air or catheter embolus
	Vascular injury
	Thrombosis
	Thrombophlebitis
Infectious	Line infection
	Sepsis
Metabolic	Glucose abnormalities
	Electrolyte and mineral abnormalities
	Acid-base imbalance
	Hypertriglyceridemia
	Biliary and hepatic dysfunction
	Metabolic bone disease
	Refeeding syndrome

TABLE 77-10 Sample Monitoring Schedule for Hospitalized Patients Receiving Nutritional Support

	Frequency	
Parameter	Initiation Phase of Support	Maintenance Phase of Support
Weight	Daily	Weekly
Length and head circumference	Weekly	Weekly
Serum electrolytes	Daily, then 3 times/week	Weekly
Serum calcium, magnesium, phosphorus	Daily, then 3 times/week	Weekly
Serum glucose*		
Liver function tests	Weekly	Weekly
Albumin	Monthly	Monthly
Triglycerides	Daily until lipid dose is stable	Weekly
Copper, ceruloplasmin, manganese	Monthly	Monthly

*The frequency and duration of serum glucose monitoring are dependent on the occurrence of hyperglycemia or hypoglycemia and the individual clinical scenario.

The earliest indicators of impending refeeding syndrome can be picked up with close electrolyte monitoring, but clinical symptoms may be noticeable as well. Sudden fluid and sodium intake results in volume expansion and fluid retention. Cardiac decompensation can be precipitated by the stress of increased circulatory volume on an already depleted cardiac muscle. Hypokalemia and hypomagnesemia may result in electrocardiographic changes prior to clinical manifestations of arrhythmia or even cardiac arrest. Low levels of adenosine triphosphate in red blood cells may result in impaired oxygen delivery, and diaphragmatic weakness may result in respiratory failure. Neurologic changes, including paresthesias, weakness, mental status changes, or seizures, can occur when serum levels of phosphorus fall to less than 1 to 1.5 mg/dL. Delirium can occur in the second week of refeeding and may be related to hypophosphatemia, other electrolyte abnormalities, or thiamine deficiency.

The refeeding syndrome can occur in patients receiving all forms of specialized nutritional support and typically occurs within 5 days of treatment. Although refeeding syndrome is commonly associated with the administration of parenteral nutrition, the risk is more closely linked to the degree of malnutrition than the route of nutritional support. The risk of refeeding syndrome is associated with severe malnutrition, and with rapid weight loss or acute weight loss. To prevent refeeding syndrome, careful correction of circulatory volume and electrolyte derangements should precede refeeding. Nutritional support should be started at no more than 20% of the basal energy expenditure in calories and slowly advanced toward goal levels as tolerated. Frequent monitoring of laboratory parameters is imperative; this often involves checking electrolytes at least daily in the first week of carbohydrate supplementation. Repletion of electrolytes is the cornerstone of management of refeeding syndrome. It may also be necessary to severely limit the rate of glucose infusion until electrolytes have stabilized. Patients may initially require treatment in the intensive care unit because of the need for frequent electrolyte monitoring and possibly replacement.

ADMISSION AND DISCHARGE CRITERIA

ADMISSION CRITERIA

- Physical examination or anthropometric evidence of severe protein-energy malnutrition.
- Significant dehydration or electrolyte abnormalities.
- Inability to meet nutritional needs with a standard oral diet.
- Failure of outpatient management.
- Lack of safe or stable home environment or appropriate outpatient follow-up.

DISCHARGE CRITERIA

- Completion of inpatient treatment of any urgent or underlying conditions is completed.
- Demonstrated ability to ingest adequate oral nutrients or tolerate a discharge regimen of enteral or parenteral nutrition.
- Stabilized fluid and electrolyte status and other pertinent laboratory parameters.
- Documentation of adequate weight gain on the discharge nutrition regimen.
- Safe home environment and home medical assistance and follow-up have been arranged, as needed.

CONSULTATION

Dieticians can provide valuable guidance in the evaluation and management of malnourished children. Pediatric gastroenterologists can offer help during hospitalization and may be key to ongoing management after discharge. For patients with evidence of cardiac dysfunction, conduction abnormalities, arrhythmia, or hemodynamic instability, input from a pediatric cardiologists may be useful. Critical care consultation is appropriate if severe electrolyte abnormalities or circulatory instability are present, or when the level of monitoring or frequency of intervention needed exceeds the capacity of a non-critical care setting.

SPECIAL CONSIDERATIONS

PREVENTION

Early recognition of patients at risk for malnutrition, as well as those with existing disorders of nutritional status, is imperative. Prompt institution of nutritional support can prevent the development or progression of malnutrition and its sequelae.

KEY POINTS

- Malnutrition refers to any disorder of nutritional status and varies in severity and clinical presentation. Abnormal growth ultimately occurs in all patients with ongoing malnutrition.
- A detailed history and physical examination, with supportive laboratory evidence, are sufficient to make the diagnosis of malnutrition. Anthropometric measurements are useful for the classification of malnutrition and monitoring of response.
- Enteral or parenteral nutritional support is indicated until the patient can ingest adequate oral nutrients; enteral support is preferred whenever possible.
- Laboratory parameters and anthropometric measurements must be carefully monitored to assess the efficacy of treatment and screen for complications.
- Refeeding syndrome is a complication of malnutrition that can occur with the introduction of increased nutrition. Hypophosphatemia, hypokalemia, and hypomagnesemia are the typical electrolyte abnormalities seen. Cardiac, respiratory, and neurologic impairment can occur.

SUGGESTED READINGS

American Academy of Pediatrics, Committee on Nutrition. *Pediatric Nutrition Handbook*. 6th ed. Elk Grove Village, IL: American Academy of Pediatrics; 2009.

American Society for Parenteral and Enteral Nutrition. *The A.S.P.E.N. Nutrition Support Manual*. 2nd ed. Silver Spring, MD: American Society for Parenteral and Enteral Nutrition; 2005.

Bhutta ZA, Berkley JA, Bandsma RHJ, Kerac M, Trehan I, Briend A. Severe childhood malnutrition. *Nat Rev Dis Primers*. 2017;3:17067.

Centers for Disease Control and Prevention. CDC Growth Charts. http://www.cdc.gov/growthcharts/cdc_charts.htm.

Corkins MR, Griggs KC, Groh-Wargo S, et al. Standards for nutrition support: pediatric hospitalized patients. *Nutr Clin Pract*. 2013;28(2):263.

McCarthy A, Delvin E, Marcil V, et al. Prevalance of malnutrition in pediatric hospitals in developed and in-transition countries: the impact of hospital practices. *Nutrients*. 2019;11(2):236.

Mehta NM, Corkins MR, Lyman B, et al. Defining pediatric malnutrition: a paradigm shift toward etiology related definitions. *J Parenter Enteral Nutr*. 2013;37(4):460.

Secker DJ, Jeejeebhoy KN. How to perform Subjective Global Nutrition assessment in children. *J Acad Nutr Diet*. 2012;112-424.

United Nations Children's Fund, World Health Organization, International Bank for Reconstruction and Development, World Bank Group. Levels and trends in child malnutrition: Key findings of the 2021 edition of the joint child malnutrition estimates. Geneva: World Health Organization, 2021.

WHO/FAO/UNU Expert Consultation (2007). Protein and Amino Acid Requirements in Human Nutrition, vol. 935. WHO: Geneva.

World Health Organization. *Guideline: Update on the Management of Severe Malnutrition in Infants and Children*. Geneva, Switzerland: World Health Organization; 2013. http://apps.who.int/iris/bitstream/10665/95584/1/9789241506328_eng.pdf.

World Health Organization. The WHO Child Growth Standards. http://www.who.int/childgrowth/standards/en.

CHAPTER 78 Pancreatitis

Jillian Wall, MD, MPH and Jared Kusma, MD

BACKGROUND

The incidence of acute pediatric pancreatitis has significantly risen over the past two decades, affecting approximately 1 per 10,000 children annually. The increase in incidence is multifactorial and likely secondary to improved clinical awareness, referral bias, rising prevalence of childhood obesity, and greater medical complexity in children. In the United States, an estimated 11,000 children are diagnosed with acute pancreatitis each year, with hospitalizations costing more than $200 million annually. Although the overall mortality is low and most often caused by underlying co-morbid disease, growth in the number of children diagnosed with pancreatitis poses a significant burden on the healthcare system and impacts the quality of life among patients affected.

PATHOPHYSIOLOGY

Acute pancreatitis is a reversible process characterized by pancreatic injury followed by a local and systemic inflammatory response. Although the pathogenesis of acute pancreatitis is not fully understood, autodigestion is the currently accepted disease model. In pancreatic autodigestion, proenzymes are activated in the pancreas acinar cell instead of inside the intestinal lumen causing cellular injury and triggering further enzyme activation. The healthy pancreas is normally protected from autodigestion by several mechanisms. Digestive proenzymes, such as trypsinogen, are packaged in their inactive state and kept in an optimal pH range. Additionally, enzyme activity is tightly regulated by intracellular calcium signaling and the presence of both protease inhibitors and trypsin-degrading proteases.

Histopathology in adults suggests that pancreatitis evolves in distinct phases. In the *initial phase,* proenzymes are prematurely activated to proteases, notably trypsin, by abnormal calcium signals within acinar cells resulting in local cellular injury. In the *second phase,* inflammatory cells infiltrate the pancreas and produce proinflammatory mediators. These mediators increase intra and extrapancreatic inflammation and speed progression to the *final phase,* in which the ensuing inflammatory cascade leads to fulminant pancreatitis. The active enzymes digest cellular membranes leading to varying degrees of edema, hemorrhage, parenchymal and vascular injury, and necrosis. The production of cytokines leads to a systemic inflammatory response that can precipitate multi-organ failure and shock. While rare in children, progression to this final phase results in significant morbidity and mortality.

ETIOLOGY

There are many causes of acute pancreatitis in children (**Table 78-1**), but the mechanisms by which these conditions trigger pancreatic inflammation are not fully understood. While gallstones and alcohol consumption cause most cases in adults, the most common etiologies of acute pancreatitis in children are biliary tract disease, drugs, systemic illness, and trauma. Up to one-third of cases are idiopathic.

Biliary tract disease is found in 10% to 30% of children diagnosed with acute pancreatitis. One-third of these cases are attributed to sludge in the gallbladder, as opposed to formed gallstones. Congenital anomalies such as pancreatic divisum, abnormal junction of the common bile duct and main pancreatic duct (common channel syndrome), choledochal cysts, and annular pancreas increase the risk for pancreatitis and are present in 5% to 20% of children who carry the diagnosis.

Ten to 25% of cases of acute pancreatitis in children have been attributed to drugs (**Table 78-2**). The most common medications include valproic acid, L-asparaginase, corticosteroids, 5-ASA derivatives, and thiopurines. True causality is difficult to establish because many patients receive concomitant medications for systemic illnesses that may predispose them to developing pancreatitis.

Pancreatitis associated with multisystem disease accounts for approximately one-third of pediatric cases. The most common associated systemic diseases include sepsis, shock, hemolytic-uremic syndrome, inflammatory bowel disease, and systemic lupus erythematous. While rare, Kawasaki disease has also been reported as a cause.

Trauma, previously thought to be a leading cause of acute pancreatitis in children, is a precipitating factor in 10% to 40% of patients. Episodes of traumatic pancreatitis typically occur secondary to blunt abdominal injury related to motor vehicle collisions, sports injuries, accidental falls, and child abuse.

Less common causes of acute pancreatitis in children include infectious, metabolic, and hereditary sources. Viral illnesses, especially those caused by enteric viruses, tend to predominate infectious etiologies; however, causation by any specific pathogen can be difficult to prove (Table 78-1). The most commonly associated metabolic diseases include diabetic ketoacidosis, followed by hypertriglyceridemia and hypercalcemia. Having an inborn error of metabolism, specifically a branched chained amino aciduria, is a risk factor for developing acute pancreatitis. Genetic factors that interfere with the pancreas's protective mechanisms can increase the susceptibility to and the severity of pancreatitis and are typically related to control of trypsin activity within the acinar cell.

CLINICAL PRESENTATION

HISTORY

Abdominal pain is the most common presenting symptom in children with acute pancreatitis. Pain is typically localized to the epigastrium; however, 20% of patients report diffuse pain, and less than 10% describe the "classical" radiation to the back. Rarely, patients may present complaining only of back pain. The pain may be more intense after eating and when supine and relieved with trunk flexion. In nonverbal children, unusual irritability may be the only indication of discomfort. Nausea or vomiting is present in up to 80% of patients. Other findings can include abdominal distension, fever, or jaundice. Infants and toddlers may have subtle symptoms and are more likely to experience abdominal distension and fever compared to older children. In episodes of severe pancreatitis, patients can present with signs of multi-organ failure, shock, coagulopathy, acute respiratory distress syndrome, renal failure, and secondary infections.

PHYSICAL EXAM

On exam, patients with pancreatitis are frequently distressed and uncomfortable. Pain is sharp, boring, and localizes to the epigastrium or upper quadrants. The epigastrium is often tender to palpation. Abdominal distension and hypoactive bowel sounds due to ileus may be present. Patients can develop a chemical peritonitis that manifests as abdominal rigidity and guarding. Tachycardia is frequently present. Compensated and uncompensated shock can result from hypovolemic dehydration, third spacing of fluid into the retroperitoneal space, and increased vasodilation and vascular permeability. Jaundice may occur in biliary pancreatitis or can be secondary to edema of the pancreatic head compressing the common bile duct. Rarely, cutaneous manifestations, termed Grey-Turner's (ecchymoses in the flanks) or Cullen's sign (ecchymoses in the periumbilical area), arise due to hemorrhagic pancreatitis.

DIFFERENTIAL DIAGNOSIS

The differential diagnosis for abdominal pain in children is broad and age-specific (see Chapter 16, Abdominal Pain). Although rare in infants and toddlers, pancreatitis can present at any age. Findings may be subtle, and a high index of suspicion is often required to make the diagnosis. There should be a low threshold to obtain laboratory studies if the history or clinical presentation is compatible.

DIAGNOSTIC EVALUATION

LABORATORY DATA

After obtaining a history and performing a physical examination that is suggestive, the diagnosis of acute pancreatitis can be confirmed based on laboratory investigation. Serum amylase and/or lipase values threefold or more above normal are consistent with acute pancreatitis and have a sensitivity of 50% to 85% and 87% to 100%, respectively. Amylase values rise within 2 to 12 hours of symptom onset and stay elevated for 2 to 5 days. Since amylase levels can normalize quickly, its role in delayed presentations is limited. Rarely, an increased amylase level may be the only serum biomarker abnormality. Serum lipase levels rise within 6 hours of symptoms and may remain elevated for 7 to 14 days. While serum lipase is generally considered the preferred test due to its greater sensitivity and specificity, the combined sensitivity of both enzymes is higher than lipase alone. It should be noted that amylase and lipase elevation can be seen in non-pancreatic conditions, such as renal insufficiency, liver disease, and inflammatory illnesses (**Table 78-3**). In addition, infants and toddlers may have lower than expected amylase and lipase values due to decreased expression of pancreatic enzymes during the first few years of life.

Obtaining serum electrolytes, blood urea nitrogen, creatine, and a complete blood count is recommended to help assess electrolyte derangements, hydration status, infectious or inflammatory states, and renal function. A liver function panel, triglyceride level, and calcium level are indicated to investigate the etiology of pancreatitis. Increased liver enzymes, particularly elevated transaminases, gamma-glutamyl transferase, and bilirubin, should prompt evaluation for biliary causes. Nonspecific laboratory findings may include leukocytosis, hemoconcentration, decreased calcium and magnesium levels, hyperglycemia, and evidence of disseminated intravascular coagulation. Metabolic alkalosis can result secondary to vomiting and acidosis may be present in severe pancreatitis.

TABLE 78-1 Causes and Conditions Associated With Pancreatitis

Cause	Conditions
Biliary Tract Disease, Abnormalities, or Obstruction	Cholelithiasis Choledochal cyst Biliary Sludge Annular pancreas Biliary tract malformations Choledochal cyst Cholelithiasis and choledocholithiasis Duplication cyst Endoscopic retrograde cholangiopancreatography complication Pancreas divisum Pancreatic ductal abnormalities Pancreatic pseudocyst Perforated duodenal ulcer Sphincter of Oddi dysfunction Tumors
Medications and Toxins	See Table 78-2

Systemic Diseases	α_1-Antitrypsin deficiency
	Celiac disease
	Collagen vascular disorders (lupus, polyarteritis nodosa)
	Cystic fibrosis
	Diabetes mellitus
	Envenomation (scorpion, spider)
	Head trauma
	Hemochromatosis
	Henoch-Schönlein purpura
	Hemolytic uremic syndrome
	Hyperalimentation
	Hypercalcemia
	Hyperparathyroidism
	Hyperlipidemia (see Metabolic disorders/inborn errors of metabolism)
	Hypertriglyceridemia (see Metabolic disorders/inborn errors of metabolism)
	Inflammatory bowel disease
	Intracranial tumors
	Kawasaki disease
	Malnutrition (starvation, eating disorders)
	Metabolic disorders/inborn errors of metabolism
	  Acute intermittent porphyria
	  Apolipoprotein C-II deficiency
	  Apolipoprotein lipase deficiency
	  Branched-chain ketoaciduria (maple syrup urine disease)
	  Cystinuria
	  Familial hypertriglyceridemia and chylomicronemia
	  Glycogen storage disease
	  Hereditary lipoprotein lipase deficiency
	  Homocystinuria
	  Lysinuric protein intolerance
	  Organic aciduria (3-hydroxy-3-methyglutaryl-coenzyme A lyase deficiency)
	  Pyruvate kinase deficiency
	Renal failure
	Sarcoidosis
	Sepsis
	Shock (multiorgan dysfunction syndrome, systemic inflammatory response syndrome)
	Sickle cell disease (vaso-occlusive)
	Transplantation (bone marrow, heart, kidney, liver, pancreas)

Trauma	Accidental blunt trauma Burns Child abuse Endoscopic retrograde cholangiopancreatography Surgical trauma

Infections	Viral
	  Cytomegalovirus
	  Epstein-Barr virus
	  COVID-19
	  Enterovirus (Coxsackie)
	  Hepatitis A and B
	  Human immunodeficiency virus
	  Influenza A and B
	  Measles
	  Mumps
	  Rubella
	  Rubeola
	  Varicella
	Bacterial
	  Campylobacter
	  Escherichia coli
	  Leptospirosis
	  Mycoplasma
	  Yersinia
	Parasitic
	  Ascaris lumbricoides (obstructive)
	  Clonorchis sinensis (obstructive)
	  Malaria

Genetic/Hereditary	Calcium sensing receptor (CASR) Cationic trypsinogen (PRSS1) Anionic trypsinogen (PRSS2) Chymotrypsinogen C Cystic fibrosis transmembrane conductance regulator (CFTR) Serine protease inhibitor of Kazal 1 (SPINK1)
Autoimmune	Type 1 Autoimmune pancreatitis Type 2 Autoimmune pancreatitis

TABLE 78-2 Drugs Associated With Pancreatitis

Class	Drug
Analgesics/Antipyretics	Acetaminophen
	Salicylates
	Sulindac
Immunosuppressants/Chemotherapy	Azathioprine
	L-asparaginase
	Cisplatin
	Cyclophosphamide
	Isoniazid
	6-Mercaptopurine
	Methotrexate
	Vincristine
Psychiatric	Amphetamine
Drugs of Abuse	Alcohol
	Heroin
Hematologic	Anticoagulants
Antibiotics/Antiviral	Didanosine
	Erythromycin
	Lamivudine
	Metronidazole
	Nitrofurantoin
	Penicillin
	Pentamidine
	Rifampin
	Sulfonamides
Neurologic	Carbamazepine
	Valproic Acid
Antihistamines	Cimetidine
	Histamine
	Ranitidine
Cardiology/Nephrology/Nutrition	Cholestyramine
	Clonidine
	Enalapril
	Methyldopa
	Procainamide
	Furosemide
	Vitamin D
Steroids/Hormones/Anti-inflammatories	Corticosteroids
	Estrogen
	Mesalamine

TABLE 78-3 Pediatric Conditions Associated With Elevation of Amylase or Lipase Levels

Cause	Elevation in Amylase	Elevation in Lipase
Abdominal	Acute pancreatitis	Acute pancreatitis
	Biliary tract disease	Acute cholecystitis
	Intestinal obstruction/ischemia	Esophagitis
	Mesenteric infarction	Intestinal obstruction/ ischemia
	Peptic ulcer	Peptic ulcer
	Appendicitis	
	Ruptured ectopic pregnancy	
	Ovarian neoplasm	
Salivary gland	Trauma	
	Infection (i.e., mumps)	
	Sialolithiasis	
	Irradiation	
Thoracic	Pneumonia	
	Pulmonary embolism	
	Myocardial infarction	
	Cardiopulmonary bypass	
Infectious	Viral gastroenteritis	Human immunodeficiency virus infection
	Pelvic inflammatory disease	
Metabolic	Diabetic ketoacidosis	Diabetic ketoacidosis
	Pheochromocytoma	Hypertriglyceridemia
Neoplastic	Ovarian, lung, esophageal, or thymic tumors	
Drugs	Opiates	
Trauma	Cerebral trauma	
	Burns	
Renal	Renal insufficiency	Renal insufficiency
	Renal transplantation	
Inflammatory	Macroamylasemia	Macrolipasemia
	Celiac disease	Celiac disease
Miscellaneous	Cystic Fibrosis	
	Acute liver failure	
	Viral gastroenteritis	
	Pregnancy	
	Eating disorders: anorexia, bulimia	

RADIOGRAPHIC EVALUATION

Radiographic evaluation in pediatric pancreatitis is typically not required if the patient's exam and laboratory findings are consistent with the diagnosis. Diagnostic imaging is indicated in cases where the presentation is vague, to assess for complications, or when planning interventions. Imaging is also indicated in cases concerning for biliary causes (with elevation of transaminases and/or hyperbilirubinemia), such as cholelithiasis.

Ultrasound (US) is considered the gold standard for imaging in cases of acute pancreatitis due to its high sensitivity in detecting biliary causes of pancreatitis. US is widely available, does not utilize radiation, has a high safety profile, and is non-invasive. The diagnostic accuracy of US is limited, however, by several factors. It is more operator dependent than other modalities, and this can be an issue when young children are being seen outside of pediatric centers. US imaging of the pancreas can also be hindered by patient factors such as bowel gas or obesity. Diagnostic features at presentation on abdominal US include focal or diffuse pancreatic enlargement, increased echogenicity, ductal dilation, peripancreatic fluid collections, and/or the presence of gallstones.

In cases where the patient is unstable and needs quicker imaging, has a large body habitus, or gas-distended bowels, a computed tomography (CT) scan may be considered. CT imaging is more sensitive than US in the detection of acute pancreatitis and should be considered in cases of severe, persistent symptoms, clinical deterioration, or to assess for complications. Complications that CT can detect include masses, cysts, pseudocysts, abscesses, and necrosis. Early imaging may not visualize complications and/or underestimate the extent of disease, so it is generally advised to delay CT imaging until at least 96 hours after presentation. When considering a CT scan, it is important to specify abdominopelvic imaging for complete coverage of possible complications, and the use of intravenous (IV) contrast to distinguish areas of pancreatic necrosis. Disadvantages of CT include the use of radiation and poor biliary assessment.

Magnetic resonance imaging (MRI) may be used in cases with late complications or for patients with acute recurrent or chronic pancreatitis. It can detect areas of necrosis, with greater sensitivity than CT, and interstitial edema. The benefits of MRI include a lack of radiation and the ability to use alternative IV contrast for patients with renal dysfunction or contrast allergies. MRI is a more expensive procedure, however, and may require anesthesia in younger children.

Finally, magnetic resonance cholangiopancreatography (MRCP) is another imaging modality that may be used in rare scenarios. It is most frequently utilized in cases with high concern for biliary causes of pancreatitis. It allows for greater visualization of the pancreatic parenchyma and duct. When secretin is used it also allows for detailed visualization of the common bile duct to assess for strictures or stones. MRCP is best utilized after an episode of acute pancreatitis resolves due to edema potentially obscuring duct visualization.

DIAGNOSTIC CRITERIA AND SEVERITY CLASSIFICATION

Diagnosis of acute pancreatitis, defined by the International Study Group of Pediatric Pancreatitis: In Search for a Cure (INSPPIRE), requires 2 of the following 3 criteria: (i) Abdominal pain compatible with acute pancreatitis, (ii) serum amylase and/or lipase activity at least three times greater than the upper limit of normal (IU/L), and (iii) imaging findings characteristic of or compatible with acute pancreatitis.

Currently, no validated scoring model exists for predicting severity in pediatric acute pancreatitis. Traditional adult scoring systems, such as APACHE II and BISAP, do not have acceptable positive and negative predictive values in children. The etiology and clinical presentation of pancreatitis is influenced by age, with adults having a higher proportion related to biliary cause or alcohol usage. Also, the definition of organ dysfunction in children varies with age.

Recently, the North American Society of Pediatric Gastroenterology, Hepatology, and Nutrition (NASPGHAN) proposed a pancreatitis severity classification system with 3 tiers: mild, moderately severe, and severe. Mild acute pancreatitis is not associated with local or systemic complications and is without organ failure. Moderately severe pancreatitis is defined as having transient organ dysfunction lasting <48 hours and/or development of local (peri or pancreatic complications such as fluid collection or necrosis) or systemic complications (exacerbation of previously diagnosed co-morbid disease). Severe acute pancreatitis is defined as development of organ dysfunction that persists >48 hours. Importantly, organ dysfunction is based on the International Pediatric Sepsis Consensus which defines it as: presence of hypotension, lactic acidosis, metabolic acidosis, Glasgow coma score ≤11 or acute change in mental status, thrombocytopenia, disseminated intravascular coagulation, serum creatinine ≥2 times upper limit of normal for age, total bilirubin ≥4mg/dL, alanine transaminase ≥2 times upper limit of normal for age, need for >50% FiO_2, arterial oxygen tension/fraction of inspired oxygen <300, arterial carbon dioxide tension >65 torr, or arterial carbon dioxide tension 20 mmHg over baseline.

MANAGEMENT

Once the diagnosis has been confirmed, management of acute pancreatitis is largely supportive. The NASPGHAN Pancreas Committee published a guideline for the management of pediatric acute pancreatitis in 2018 that included recommendations for fluid resuscitation, pain control, and initiation of early enteral nutrition.

FLUID RESUSCITATION

Aggressive fluid administration improves outcomes and decreases the risk of complications in acute pancreatitis. If there are signs of hypovolemia or hemodynamic compromise on assessment, a 10 to 20 mL/kg bolus of isotonic crystalloid should be given. This may be repeated until the patient shows improvement in heart rate and blood pressure. If a patient continues to be hypotensive or tachycardic despite 60 mL/kg of IV fluid, intensive care unit (ICU) transfer or admission is warranted, as shock may be present or imminent. Although there is limited pediatric data regarding the ideal rate of fluid administration following initial resuscitation, the consensus guideline recommends giving dextrose containing isotonic fluids at 1.5 to 2 times maintenance rate for the first 24 to 48 hours. IV fluid should be discontinued once the patient is clinically improved, hemodynamically stable, and is able to maintain adequate enteral hydration.

Adult literature supports the use of lactated Ringer's over normal saline, but pediatric studies on the optimal fluid regimen are sparse. A recent study suggests that the exclusive use of lactated Ringer's in the first 48 hours of admission is associated with a shorter and less expensive hospital stay.

MONITORING

Cardiac, renal, and pulmonary complications of pancreatitis are typically seen in the first 48 hours of illness and should prompt close monitoring. The consensus guideline recommends obtaining vital signs every 4 hours with frequent assessment of fluid status and urine output. Patients presenting with shock, receiving aggressive fluid resuscitation, or with persistent emesis are at risk for electrolyte imbalances. The correction and repletion of any electrolyte abnormalities is important in the initial phase of management. Electrolytes and renal function should be checked frequently early in the course. Lipase and amylase levels do not necessarily correlate with disease severity or recovery and should not be trended to assess improvement.

NUTRITION

Historically patients presenting with pancreatitis were made nil per os with strict bowel rest to prevent pancreatic stimulation; however, studies have shown improved outcomes with early enteral feeding. In adults, the early initiation of enteral nutrition shortens length of stay (LOS) and decreases morbidity and mortality. Recent pediatric studies support that early enteral feeding is safe in mild to moderate pancreatitis and does not worsen abdominal pain. Furthermore, patients who start enteral nutrition within 48 hours of admission have a shorter LOS, less frequent transfers to the ICU, decreased progression to severe pancreatitis, and improved weight gain after discharge. Standard fat diets do not appear to increase pain. Feeding should be initiated with a regular diet within 48 to 72 hours of presentation unless there is a contraindication, such as an ileus or fistula. If a child is unable to tolerate oral feeding, nasogastric or nasojuejunal feeds should be started. Total parenteral nutrition is generally not recommended unless a patient proves intolerant to enteral feeding for more than 5 days.

PAIN CONTROL

Pain control is an essential piece of supportive care in pancreatitis. There are no randomized trials identifying a superior agent for pain management. Despite case reports of morphine causing sphincter of Oddi dysfunction, opioids are safe for use in pancreatitis and may be used if pain is not well controlled with acetaminophen or nonsteroidal anti-inflammatory drugs (NSAIDs). Many patients respond to high-dose NSAIDs such as ketorolac; however, its use must be weighed against the increased risk of bleeding, gastric ulceration, or renal injury. Refractory cases may benefit from consultation from a dedicated pain service when available.

OTHER THERAPIES

Debate exists on the utility of proton pump inhibitors in the acute treatment phase for acute pancreatitis. Although commonly prescribed, currently there are no data indicating that proton pump inhibitors favorably alter the course of acute pancreatitis. Use of prophylactic antibiotics, protease inhibitors, probiotics, or antioxidants is not recommended. Endoscopic retrograde cholangiopancreatography has an important role in the treatment of pancreatic and biliary disease in children and is indicated in cases of biliary pancreatitis due to choledocholithiasis or sludge, pancreatic ductal strictures or stones, or pancreatic duct leaks.

CLINICAL COURSE

In most cases of pediatric acute pancreatitis, the disease is self-limited and resolves spontaneously. The typical duration of hospitalization for children with pancreatitis is 3 to 7 days. More severe cases may require clinical stabilization in an ICU, multidisciplinary involvement, and admissions may well last longer than 7 days. The presence of systemic inflammatory response syndrome at admission, underlying chronic illness, the use of parenteral nutrition during hospitalization, and undergoing a therapeutic procedure has been associated with a prolonged LOS.

COMPLICATIONS

Complications of acute pancreatitis can be divided into early vs. late onset. Early onset complications primarily include multi-organ dysfunction or shock. Patients can also develop peripancreatic fluid collections which tend to resolve spontaneously. Late onset complications include pancreatic necrosis or pseudocyst. Pseudocysts are defined as an extrapancreatic homogenous collection of fluid rich in pancreatic enzymes and a small amount of debris that lacks an epithelial lining. They typically develop after 4 weeks and are asymptomatic, but they can cause abdominal pain, vomiting, and/or fever. They also can become infected. Signs of pseudocyst development may include a sudden rise or persistent elevation in pancreatic enzymes or persistence/worsening of symptoms. Pancreatic necrosis typically develops earlier in the course as an acute necrotic collection but can present later (around 4 weeks) as walled-off necrosis. Management for both walled-off necrosis and pancreatic pseudocysts is ultrasound-guided or surgical drainage.

ADMISSION AND DISCHARGE CRITERIA

ADMISSION CRITERIA

Pediatric patients with mild acute pancreatitis do not need to be admitted if they are hemodynamically stable, can maintain nutrition and hydration enterally, and pain is well controlled on oral medication. Pediatric patients with moderate to severe pancreatitis, those who require IV pain medication, or those who would benefit from IV fluids, should be admitted. Floor vs. ICU care should be determined based on the severity level of the episode. Severe acute pancreatitis or the presence of fluid refractory shock warrants ICU admission. Moderately severe cases level of care should be determined on a case-by-case basis.

DISCHARGE CRITERIA

When the child is tolerating adequate intake to sustain hydration and nutrition with manageable pain, discharge home may be considered. Patients should be discharged on a regular diet. Plans for follow-up, including any repeat imaging, should be in place prior to discharge.

CONSULTATION

Consultation with a pediatric gastroenterologist regarding the acute management and follow-up of patients with acute pancreatitis is warranted in severe cases and those with complications. Surgical consultation may be necessary in cases of confirmed or suspected trauma, pancreaticobiliary anomalies, or cholelithiasis. The interventional radiologist may also provide valuable guidance and assistance when radioimaging is being considered. The pain service, where available, may assist with pain management, particularly in the acute setting. A genetics evaluation or consultation should be considered in cases of recurrent pancreatitis or in a child with a strong family history of pancreatitis.

SPECIAL CONSIDERATIONS

RECURRENT PANCREATITIS

Following resolution of acute pancreatitis, approximately 15% to 35% of children will experience recurrence. Progression from acute to recurrent pancreatitis typically occurs within 5 months of the initial attack. Recurrent pancreatitis is more common in patients with biliary anomalies, metabolic disorders, (particularly hypertriglyceridemia) and in children with genetic or hereditary pancreatitis. As such, patients with recurrent pancreatitis should be evaluated for anatomic, metabolic, and genetic risk factors. The diagnosis of acute recurrent pancreatitis requires at least two distinct episodes of acute pancreatitis, along with (i) complete resolution of pain with a pain free interval of at least 1 month between occurrences or (ii) complete normalization of serum pancreatic enzyme levels before the subsequent episode of acute pancreatitis, along with complete resolution of pain symptoms, irrespective of a specific time interval between acute pancreatitis episodes.

CHRONIC PANCREATITIS

Of children with recurrent pancreatitis, 20% to 40% will progress to chronic pancreatitis within 2 years. Chronic pancreatitis is characterized by irreversible pancreatic damage. The destruction of the pancreas and replacement of the parenchyma by fibrosis can result in pancreatic duct stricture, chronic pain, exocrine pancreatic insufficiency, and diabetes mellitus. The diagnosis requires imaging findings characteristic of chronic pancreatitis with at least one of the following: (i) abdominal pain consistent with pancreatic origin, (ii) exocrine pancreatic insufficiency, or (iii) endocrine pancreatic insufficiency. A biopsy specimen demonstrating histological features of chronic pancreatitis alone is sufficient to make the diagnosis.

KEY POINTS

- The diagnosis of pancreatitis should be considered in the pediatric patient with epigastric abdominal pain and vomiting. Irritability may be the only presenting symptoms in infants, toddlers, and nonverbal children.
- The most common etiologies of acute pancreatitis in children are biliary tract disease, medications, systemic illness, and trauma, followed by infectious, metabolic, and hereditary causes. One third of cases are idiopathic.
- The diagnosis of acute pancreatitis requires 2 of the following 3 criteria: (i) Abdominal pain compatible with acute pancreatitis, (ii) serum amylase and/or lipase activity at least three times greater than the upper limit of normal, and (iii) imaging findings characteristic of or compatible with acute pancreatitis.
- Mild acute pancreatitis is not associated with local or systemic complications and is without organ failure. Moderately severe pancreatitis is defined as having transient organ dysfunction lasting <48 hours and/or development of local or systemic complications. Severe acute pancreatitis is defined as development of organ dysfunction that persists >48 hours.
- Fluid resuscitation should be initiated promptly based on the clinical assessment and followed by maintenance fluid for the first 24 to 48 hours.
- Enteral nutrition should be initiated within the 48 hours of presentation and is associated with improved outcomes. Nasogastric or jejunal feeds should be started if the child is unable to tolerate oral feeds.
- No optimal regimen for pain control has been identified. Opioids may be used for pain refractory to acetaminophen and NSAIDS.
- Patients with persistent vomiting, abdominal pain, or fever despite proper management should undergo imaging (ultrasound or computed tomography based on clinical stability) to assess for complications such as pancreatic pseudocyst or pancreatic necrosis.
- Although complete recovery is usual in children, recurrence suggests underlying pathology and mandates evaluation for an underlying metabolic, genetic, or anatomic cause.
- Patients with recurrent pancreatitis can progress to chronic pancreatitis which has a high morbidity due to associated pancreatic endocrine and exocrine insufficiency and the development of chronic pain.

SUGGESTED READINGS

Abu-El-Haija M, Kumar S, Quiros JA, et al. Management of acute pancreatitis in the pediatric population: a clinical report from the North American Society for Pediatric Gastroenterology, Hepatology and Nutrition Pancreas Committee. *J Pediatr Gastroenterol Nutr.* 2018;66(1):159-176.

Abu-El-Haija M, Kumar S, Szabo F, et al. Classification of acute pancreatitis in the pediatric population: clinical report from the NASPGHAN Pancreas Committee. *J Pediatr Gastroenterol Nutr.* 2017;64(6): 984-990.

Abu-El-Haija M, Uc A, Werlin SL, et al. Nutritional considerations in pediatric pancreatitis. *J Pediatr Gastroenterol Nutr.* 2018;67(1):131-143.

Bai HX, Lowe ME, Husain SZ. What have we learned about acute pancreatitis in children? *J Pediatr Gastroenterol Nutr.* 2011;52(3):262-270.

Banks PA, Freeman ML. Practice guidelines in acute pancreatitis. *Am J Gastroenterol.* 2006;101(10):2379-2400.

Conwell DL, Banks P, Greenberger NJ. Acute and chronic pancreatitis. In: Kasper D, Fauci A, Hauser S, Longo D, Jameson JL, Loscalzo J, eds. *Harrison's Principles of Internal Medicine.* 19th ed. McGraw-Hill Education; 2014.

Dike CR, Abu-El-Haija M. Nutrition management and pancreatitis in children: new insights. *Curr Opin Clin Nutr Metab Care.* 2022;25(5): 321-324.

Farrell PR, Farrell LM, Hornung L, Abu-El-Haija M. Use of lactated ringers solution compared with normal saline is associated with shorter length of stay in pediatric acute pancreatitis. *Pancreas.* 2020;49(3): 375-380.

Freeman AJ, Maqbool A, Bellin MD, et al. Medical management of chronic pancreatitis in children: a position paper by the North American Society for Pediatric Gastroenterology, Hepatology, and Nutrition Pancreas Committee. *J Pediatr Gastroenterol Nutr.* 2021;72(2):324-340.

Gay AC, Barreto NB, Schrager SM, Russell CJ. Factors associated with length of stay and 30-day revisits in pediatric acute pancreatitis. *J Pediatr Gastroenterol Nutr.* 2018;67(2):e30-e35.

Kandula L, Lowe ME. Etiology and outcome of acute pancreatitis in infants and toddlers. *J Pediatr.* 2008;152(1):106-110, 110.e1.

Kliegman R, St Geme J, Blum N, Shah S, Tasker R, Wilson K. Pancreatitis. In: Werlin S, Wilschanski M, eds. *Nelson Textbook of Pediatrics.* 21st ed. Elsevier; 2020:2074-2080.

Ledder O, Duvoisin G, Lekar M, et al. Early feeding in acute pancreatitis in children: a randomized controlled trial. *Pediatrics.* 2020;146(3).

Párniczky A, Abu-El-Haija M, Husain S, et al. EPC/HPSG Evidence-Based Guidelines for the management of pediatric pancreatitis. *Pancreatology.* 2018;18(2):146-160.

Saeed SA. Acute pancreatitis in children: updates in epidemiology, diagnosis and management. *Curr Probl Pediatr Adolesc Health Care.* 2020;50(8):100839.

Sellers ZM, Dike C, Zhang KY, Giefer MJ, Uc A, Abu-El-Haija M. A unified treatment algorithm and admission order set for pediatric acute pancreatitis. *J Pediatr Gastroenterol Nutr.* 2019;68(6):e109-e111.

Suchman K, Raphael KL, Liu Y, Wee D, Trindade AJ. Acute pancreatitis in children hospitalized with COVID-19. *Pancreatology.* 2021; 21(1):31-33.

Templeton K, Grover AS. Acute pancreatitis in children. *Curr Treat Options Pediatr.* 2021;7(2):46-59.

Trout AT, Anupindi SA, Freeman AJ, et al. North American Society for Pediatric Gastroenterology, Hepatology and Nutrition and the Society for Pediatric Radiology Joint Position Paper on noninvasive imaging of pediatric pancreatitis: literature summary and recommendations. *J Pediatr Gastroenterol Nutr.* 2021;72(1):151-167.

Trout AT, Ayyala RS, Murati MA, et al. Current state of imaging of pediatric pancreatitis: *AJR* expert panel narrative review. *Am J Roentgenol.* 2021;217(2):265-277.

Uc A, Husain SZ. Pancreatitis in children. *Gastroenterology.* 2019; 156(7):1969-1978.

Wu BU, Conwell DL. Acute pancreatitis part I: approach to early management. *Clin Gastroenterol Hepatol.* 2010;8(5):410-416.

CHAPTER 79

Feeding Issues

Stephanie S. Squires, MD and Kim Hoang, MD

BACKGROUND

Feeding difficulties are frequent comorbid conditions in hospitalized infants and children with acute and chronic illnesses. The ability of children to feed and grow relies on an appropriate food source, safe oromotor coordination, endurance while feeding, adequate caloric intake, and positive feedback during the feeding experience. In this chapter, we will review the clinical presentations, diagnostic evaluation, and management of common feeding-related issues seen in pediatric inpatients including oral aversion, dysphagia, and gastroesophageal reflux disease (GERD).

ORAL AVERSION

Oral aversion or food refusal is common in pediatrics and can be influenced by multiple factors, such as discomfort from chronic gastritis or esophagitis, chronic aspiration, abnormal gastrointestinal motility, sensory abnormalities, and behavioral issues. Feeding refusal may stem from visceral hyperalgesia as a result of previous painful experiences, such as multiple painful procedures. Stressed mealtime interactions and behaviors between child and feeder, such as force-feeding, can also influence and exacerbate food refusal. Severe oral aversion that requires inpatient evaluation and intervention commonly presents among children with chronic illnesses.

DIAGNOSTIC EVALUATION

Evaluation of oral aversion requires a thorough review of a child's feeding, growth, and developmental history as well as any underlying medical causes or issues that led up to food refusal. It is important to also identify experiences that may have contributed to traumatically acquired feeding disorders (e.g., enterostomy tube feeding, intubation, suctioning). Parental reports and direct or videotaped mealtime observation are also helpful to evaluate feeding behavior and to identify problems with feeder-child interactions. Feeding questionnaires and structured observation tools, such as the Infant Feeding Behaviors-Rater checklist, are available to assist in the evaluation of oral aversion. A psychological assessment can also be helpful to understand the child's feeding behaviors. Children with persistent oral aversion and failure to thrive may warrant further work up (e.g., blood work and imaging) based specific findings on history and physical examination.

MANAGEMENT

Management of oral aversion requires a comprehensive multidisciplinary approach that is multifaceted, dynamic, and tailored to the needs of the patient. The priority is to develop a feeding plan that promotes healthy nutrition and growth. Although some children with oral aversion may require tube feeding to maintain adequate nutrition, it can be quite difficult to wean off enterostomy tube feeding once it has been initiated. Other children may benefit from admission to the hospital to observe multiple meals and introduce specific behavioral feeding techniques. While inpatient behavioral therapy may be effective in helping reinstate hunger cues and reducing the fear of swallowing, it often requires prolonged hospitalization. One study of an outpatient behavioral intervention using extinction and nutritional counseling over a 7-week period led to successful exclusive oral feeding in 50% of children. Children who fail to make progress may benefit from an even more intensive inpatient behavioral treatment program.

DYSPHAGIA

Dysphagia, or difficulty swallowing, is the term often used to refer to a swallowing abnormality. Swallowing can be divided into three phases: oral, pharyngeal, and esophageal. Problems at any stage of swallowing can affect eating to some degree. During the oral phase, an infant creates suction with the lips, tongue, and palate and forms a bolus of food. The bolus is then moved to the posterior pharynx. Children older than 3 to 4 months of age can move food of different consistencies by chewing and more mature tongue movements. The oral phase relies on normal oral anatomy, sensation and sensory feedback, strong sucking (in infants), and normal oral muscular function (in children). The pharyngeal phase of swallowing is an involuntary action that is initiated when the food bolus touches the posterior pharyngeal wall. During this phase, respiration ceases as the vocal cords close, the larynx elevates, and the upper esophageal sphincter relaxes to allow the bolus to enter the esophagus. In children with poor oral muscular coordination, early entry of the bolus into the pharynx before vocal cord closure may lead to aspiration into the trachea. Similarly, delay in relaxation of the upper esophageal sphincter allows food to pool above or penetrate the larynx and increases the risk for aspiration when the vocal cords open again. Finally, in the last phase of swallowing, the esophageal phase, food moves involuntarily through the esophagus to the stomach. Esophageal mucosal inflammation, stricture, dysmotility, and obstruction can all contribute to dysphagia.

Swallowing abnormalities are most common in premature infants and children with neurologic abnormalities or airway anomalies, such as laryngeal clefts, vocal cord palsy, and tracheoesophageal fistula. The most common disorders of swallowing in infants relate to immature or inefficient sucking and difficulty coordinating the suck-swallow-breathe rhythm. Less commonly, incoordination of swallowing may be due to an anatomic or neuromuscular abnormality that impairs one or several swallowing phases. Swallowing incoordination may cause aspiration into the respiratory tract and lead to acute pneumonitis, pneumonia, or nonspecific airway inflammation.

Although most children who aspirate have neurodevelopmental delay or airway anomalies, aspiration can also occur as an isolated phenomenon in neurologically normal infants, which is defined as isolated dysphagia. For these neurologically normal children without risk factors for aspiration, the typical presentation of aspiration is chronic unexplained respiratory symptoms (e.g., recurrent wheezing, frequent lower respiratory tract infections) or failure to thrive. While symptoms are often initially treated as reflux or asthma, these children are eventually diagnosed with isolated dysphagia via videofluoroscopic swallow study (VFSS). The prognosis of isolated dysphagia is good with up to 53% of infants returning to normal feeding with exclusive oral feeding within 3 years.

CLINICAL PRESENTATIONS

The most common symptoms associated with dysphagia are coughing, choking, and "blue" spells with feeding. Blue spells may be actual hypoxic events caused by impaired minute ventilation or aspiration of oral contents into the airway. These spells may be more marked in children who already have underlying cardiorespiratory compromise (e.g., congenital heart disease, bronchopulmonary dysplasia). Parents or caregivers may also report stridor, wheezing, or vomiting. Symptoms may vary in severity and quality depending on the feeding position, feed consistency, and feeding apparatus. The symptoms may occur exclusively during feeding (e.g., blue spells, choking, or sputtering), linger after completion of feeding (e.g., cough, stridor), or persist between feedings (e.g., increased secretions, wheezing). Some children have a history of pneumonia or a previous diagnosis of reactive airways disease, which may really reflect a previous aspiration event or chronic aspiration. A chest radiograph may show a focal infiltrate or chronic changes.

A larger proportion of children aspirate silently without associated symptoms or evidence of protective cough. Premature infants with immature swallowing function and children with developmental or congenital disorders have increased risk for silent aspiration. Aspiration should be considered in children with slow feeding, an anatomic or neuromuscular disorder, chronic respiratory symptoms, or recurrent pneumonia.

Children with cleft palate or cardiorespiratory illnesses (e.g., chronic lung disease, congenital heart disease, acute infectious respiratory illnesses) may become tachypneic, cyanotic, or diaphoretic and may have difficulty coordinating the suck-swallow-breathe cycle. These infants may suffer a significant reduction in minute ventilation while swallowing which may lead to hypoxia. Infants with cleft palate need extra assistance with control of the flow of liquid into the pharynx to prevent aspiration and may have difficulty organizing the swallow at the end of the oral phase. Healthy, term infants with recent lower respiratory tract infections, such as bronchiolitis, may also have increased risk of aspiration due to acute alterations in sucking and swallowing mechanisms. Infants with underlying dysphagia may experience worsening of their swallowing dysfunction and a further increase in their aspiration risk.

DIFFERENTIAL DIAGNOSIS

The symptoms and signs that suggest dysphagia warrant consideration of the underlying abnormalities that may contribute to the disorder, including esophageal dysmotility, GERD, and anatomic, sensory, or motor abnormalities of the oropharynx.

DIAGNOSTIC EVALUATION

Evaluation should include bedside clinical assessment of feeding performed by an experienced speech-language pathologist or occupational therapist. This assessment involves observation and assessment of tone, feeding position, sucking, tongue and jaw movements, food bolus formation, and bolus manipulation. Observation of changes in respiratory status (e.g., coughing, choking, increased secretions, adventitious sounds on auscultation) is also important. In addition, assessment includes an evaluation with various food thicknesses and textures, depending on the age of the child. The evaluation of the caregiver-infant feeding relationship and feeding safety serves as a guide for the need for additional diagnostic testing (e.g., VFSS). Clinical assessment of swallowing of liquids and solids at the bedside has a sensitivity of 90% and a specificity of 56% for risk for aspiration and is therefore a useful screening test to determine the need for radiographic evaluation.

VFSS is the gold standard for assessment of feeding function. Radiographic contrast material is mixed with foodstuff of variable consistency to visualize its dynamic passage from the mouth to the stomach. The nature and severity of specific abnormalities of function can be identified, including inefficient food bolus formation, abnormal movement of the bolus to the posterior pharynx, pooling above the larynx, penetration of the bolus into the trachea, and direct aspiration into the lungs. There is a relationship between the severity of laryngeal penetration and aspiration risk, particularly with thin liquids. Eighty-five percent of children with evidence of deep laryngeal penetration on VFSS also aspirate thin liquids on VFSS. Swallowing appears to become more dysfunctional after multiple swallows in infants, thus suggesting that longer assessments with videofluoroscopy are most useful. VFSS is also an excellent tool to evaluate the effect of changes in posture and texture on the safety of feeds to devise an optimal feeding plan for a child with dysphagia.

Because VFSS requires radiation exposure, alternatives have been explored, including fiberoptic endoscopic evaluation of swallowing (FEES). This method allows direct visualization of baseline swallowing, as well as observation of swallowing with liquid or solid boluses. Several reproducibility studies have demonstrated similar accuracy in diagnosing dysphagia between FEES and VFSS and there is not yet expert consensus regarding which study has greater diagnostic accuracy. FEES has the added benefit of enabling assessment of baseline swallowing without requiring the introduction of oral liquids or solids in high-risk children.

Salivagrams and milk scans are both nuclear medicine tests that have been used to assess swallowing and aspiration. Drawbacks to nuclear scintigraphy include the inability to assess tracheal penetration, making these tests only situationally useful rather than first-line investigations of dysphagia. Similarly, bronchoscopy can detect lipid-laden macrophages, making aspiration of food contents into the airways highly likely, but it cannot distinguish between dysphagia and GER as a cause of aspiration.

MANAGEMENT

The goal of dysphagia management is to establish a safe feeding regimen that improves the efficiency and enjoyment of feeding. Children with oromotor incoordination may benefit from an ongoing oral stimulation therapeutic program led by a speech pathologist or occupational therapist. It is vital to maintain positive oral experiences and reassess the safety of oral feeding clinically and radiographically, particularly in infants and young children, because there is a potential for improvement and maturation of the swallow mechanism. Without ongoing oral stimulation, oral aversion may develop in children whose dysphagia improves.

Intervention for children who aspirate depends on which food consistency, if any, is found to be safe. Foods that are associated with aspiration are restricted. Children who are safe only with pureed consistencies often require another method of feeding to receive adequate fluids. Depending on the cause of dysphagia and the likelihood of improvement, nasogastric or gastrostomy tube feedings are indicated. Children who are found to aspirate all consistencies require admission to the hospital to establish tube feeding and to either teach parents how to administer nasogastric feeding or arrange for insertion of a gastrostomy tube.

GASTROESOPHAGEAL REFLUX AND GASTROESOPHAGEAL REFLUX DISEASE

Gastroesophageal reflux (GER) is a normal physiologic process whereby gastric contents involuntarily pass into the esophagus. Most episodes of GER in infants, children, and adults are asymptomatic. Regurgitation of gastric contents into the oral cavity is often a normal process in healthy thriving infants that resolves by the second year of life. Factors that influence the incidence of GER include lower esophageal sphincter pressure, angle of insertion of the esophagus into the stomach, gastric volume and emptying, intra-abdominal pressure, esophageal innervation, and motility.

GERD is a group of symptoms or complications of GER **(Table 79-1)**. Overt regurgitation of food is not always present. While GERD is more common in children with a history of prematurity, neurological conditions, and esophageal anomalies, it is often diagnosed in otherwise healthy infants and children. Although GER is quite common in premature infants, there is insufficient evidence to suggest GER is a cause of apnea in premature infants.

DIAGNOSTIC EVALUATION

The evaluation depends on child age and clinical presentation. In most infants with vomiting and older children with heartburn and regurgitation, a history and physical examination are usually sufficient to exclude other diagnoses, support the diagnosis of GER or GERD, and differentiate between them. Warning signs that suggest an alternative diagnosis include bilious vomiting, gastrointestinal bleeding, projectile vomiting, onset of vomiting after 6 months of age or persistence of symptoms beyond 12 months, failure to thrive (although this may occur as a consequence of severe GERD), diarrhea, constipation, fever, lethargy, hepatosplenomegaly, bulging fontanelle, macrocephaly or microcephaly, seizures, abdominal distention or tenderness, and genetic disorders known to be associated with other diagnoses that cause vomiting.

TABLE 79-1 Gastroesophageal Reflux Disease

Symptoms/Signs	Complications
Brief Resolved Unexplained Event	Anemia
Chronic cough	Apnea
Dysphagia	Aspiration pneumonia
Failure to thrive	Asthma
Feeding aversion	Barrett esophagus
Heartburn or chest pain	Bronchiectasis
Hematemesis	Dental erosion
Irritability	Esophageal stricture
Recurrent vomiting	Esophagitis
Sandifer syndrome	Laryngitis
Stridor or hoarseness	Sinusitis
Wheezing	Upper airway inflammation

The utility of various gastrointestinal studies is provided in **Table 79-2.** An upper gastrointestinal series (contrast fluoroscopic evaluation of the esophagus, stomach, and duodenum) is not a useful test to rule in or rule out GER because of its low sensitivity and specificity. It may, however, be helpful in detecting other anatomic abnormalities that may present with vomiting, such as malrotation, pyloric stenosis, duodenal web, and duplication.

Overall, there is not enough evidence to support the routine use of pH monitoring for the diagnosis of GERD in infants and children. Intraesophageal pH monitoring (pH probe) is useful for objective quantification of acid reflux and identification of associated symptoms, but it has limitations. It is easily affected by diet and posture changes, does not detect non-acid reflux, and results do not always correlate with symptom severity. Further, to complete pH monitoring, a child must be able to tolerate a catheter in their nose which can be difficult for some children (e.g., those with developmental delay or autism). One potential alternative for these children is the use of a wireless pH probe that is clipped to the esophagus during endoscopy. Studies suggest that wireless pH recording may be associated with improved reflux detection given the extended length of recording available (2-5 days). Another modality includes multiple intraluminal impedance monitoring which measures esophagus impedance changes and retrograde changes typical of reflux irrespective of acidity.

Endoscopy and biopsy are useful in evaluating children with warning symptoms (e.g., hematemesis), severe GERD (for detection of severe esophagitis or stricture), or predisposing conditions (i.e., hiatal hernia). Biopsy is also an important tool when other differential diagnoses are being considered, such as infectious or eosinophilic esophagitis. The risks associated with the procedures, which usually requires general anesthesia or deep sedation in children, must be weighed against the potential diagnostic benefit in each case.

MANAGEMENT

Management options can be categorized as nonpharmacologic, pharmacologic, and surgical. Nonpharmacologic interventions include positioning, lifestyle changes, formula change, and thickened feedings. Placing an infant in an infant seat after feeding to provide a more upright position or elevating the head of the bed has not shown benefit in systematic reviews. Prone positioning is associated with lower reflux scores but is not recommended because the risk for sudden infant death syndrome is greater than the potential benefits of prone sleeping. Because some infants with cow's milk protein intolerance may present with GERD, there is evidence to support a 2- to 4-week trial of a hydrolyzed hypoallergenic or amino acid-based formula in formula-fed infants. Breastfed infants with GERD may benefit from a trial of withdrawal of cows' milk and eggs from the maternal diet, but the evidence for this is not strong. Cessation of breastfeeding as a treatment of GERD is not recommended. Thickening feeds with rice cereal or using a prethickened formula does not improve reflux scores as measured by pH probe. However, both methods of thickening decrease the number of vomiting episodes. Smaller ingested volumes per feed have also been suggested as a mechanism to improve reflux. While no studies have found a relationship between feeding volume and regurgitation volume, it is still recommended to adjust feeding frequency and volume according to age-based recommendations.

Pharmacologic therapy for GERD includes histamine H_2 receptor antagonists (H_2 blockers), proton pump inhibitors (PPIs), and prokinetic agents. H_2 blockers are less effective than PPIs in treating severe esophagitis and are known to cause tachyphylaxis, thereby limiting utility for chronic use. A systematic review of PPI use in infants concluded that they are not effective in reducing GERD symptoms in this age group. Potential concerns of chronic long-term acid suppression from PPI use include increased risk for infection (e.g., necrotizing enterocolitis, pneumonia, upper respiratory infections, *Clostridium difficile* infections, sepsis) as acid plays a protective effect against some infections.

TABLE 79-2 Comparison of Gastrointestinal Studies for Vomiting

Study	Diagnostic Utility	Advantages	Disadvantages
Upper GI series*	Assesses for malrotation, presence of stenosis or stricture	Readily available	Not useful in diagnosing GERD
pH probe	Objective quantification of acid GER	Helps assess effectiveness of acid suppression therapy; may help correlate other symptoms (discomfort, apnea, arching) with GER	Cannot evaluate non-acid reflux; invasive
Combined pH probe and multiple intraluminal impedance (MII) monitoring	Objective quantification of acid and non-acid GER	May help correlate symptoms with GER, whether acid or non-acid	Invasive; absence of age-specific norms for MII
Milk scan/Scintigraphy	Able to detect aspiration into the lungs from GERD	Noninvasive	May not identify GERD in the absence of aspiration to the lungs
Abdominal ultrasound	Helps rule out other causes of vomiting; assesses the presence of pyloric stenosis in infants and other causes of obstruction in older children such as uretero-pelvic obstruction, gallstones, ovarian torsion	Noninvasive	Cannot evaluate GER/GERD
Gastric emptying scan	May be helpful in identifying children with delayed emptying who would benefit from motility agents or from pyloroplasty with fundoplication	Noninvasive	Cannot evaluate GER/GERD

*Contrast fluoroscopic evaluation of the esophagus, stomach, and duodenum.

GER, gastroesophageal reflux; GERD, GER disease; GI, gastrointestinal; PPI, proton pump inhibitor.

The 2018 joint recommendations of the North American Society of Pediatric Gastroenterology, Hepatology and Nutrition and European Society of Pediatric Gastroenterology, Hepatology and Nutrition no longer include H_2 blocker or PPI empiric therapy in otherwise healthy infants and young children unless GERD symptoms are not improved following trial of feeding changes including a 2 to 4 week trial of hydrolyzed formula or milk elimination in maternal diet for breastfed infants. In older children with typical symptoms of GERD (i.e., heartburn, retrosternal or epigastric pain), a (4-8-week) trial of a PPI may be considered as a diagnostic test for GERD.

Prokinetic agents, including cisapride, metoclopramide, and domperidone, have been used as a way of enhancing gastric emptying. However, there is no clear evidence that these agents are effective in the treatment of GERD. Metoclopramide may have some benefit in reducing symptoms in infants; however, caution should be exercised when using these medications because many believe that the risks outweigh the benefits.

Surgical therapeutic options may be considered in children with GERD who symptoms are refractory to maximal pharmacologic therapy (**Table 79-3**). Surgical approaches include fundoplication, gastrostomy, or gastrojejunostomy (GJ) tube insertion. Gastrostomy tube insertion has been used for children who cannot maintain adequate growth with oral feeding because of GERD. It is also commonly used in neurologically impaired children, who may have both oromotor difficulties and GERD. When a gastrostomy tube is inserted without fundoplication, GERD can worsen, particularly in neurologically impaired children. Although the mechanism is not understood, the incidence of new or worsening GERD in neurologically impaired children after gastrostomy tube insertion may be as high as 20% to 25%.

Fundoplication, which can be performed by open means or laparoscopically, may be accompanied by pyloroplasty for children with slow gastric emptying. In addition, it is often paired with gastrostomy tube insertion for children who also aspirate with oral feedings or who cannot feed enough orally to maintain hydration or maintain adequate weight. Outcomes of open versus laparoscopic fundoplication are comparable. The concerns about fundoplication revolve primarily around complication rates in neurologically impaired children. Major complications, such as wrap disruption, increased dysphagia, respiratory deterioration, gas bloating syndrome, intestinal obstruction, and death, are more common in these children.

GJ tubes may facilitate postpyloric feeds in the setting of GERD and be inserted percutaneously under fluoroscopic guidance with sedation (rather than general anesthesia). No randomized controlled trials have evaluated fundoplication with gastrostomy versus GJ tube insertion. Findings from a meta-analysis suggest that GJ tube use in neurologically impaired children may be associated with fewer major but more minor complications than fundoplication with G-tube. Another retrospective study showed that neither treatment is superior in preventing subsequent aspiration pneumonia. Late complications after GJ tube placement include tube breakage and blockage, superficial stoma infection, dislodgement, intussusception, and small bowel obstruction. These complications need to be carefully considered when a patient lives far from a regional center with an interventional radiologist.

TABLE 79-3 Indications for Surgical Intervention for Gastroesophageal Reflux Disease

Life-threatening complications
Recurrent aspiration
Laryngospasm
Apnea or BRUE*
Barrett esophagus
Failure of optimal medical therapeutic interventions
Non-compliance to medical therapy
Chronic conditions (i.e., neurologically impaired, cystic fibrosis) with a significant risk of GERD-related complications
Benefits of surgery outweigh the risks

*Brief Resolved Unexplained Event.

ADMISSION AND DISCHARGE CRITERIA

ADMISSION CRITERIA

- Dehydration or failure to thrive
- Risk of aspiration or dysphagia requiring initiation of nasogastric feeding and caregiver education on nasogastric tube feeding
- Admission for evaluation of feeding behavior and intensive behavioral intervention
- Cyanotic or apneic spells
- Moderate to severe aspiration pneumonia
- Failed outpatient therapies or social concerns

DISCHARGE CRITERIA

- Caloric and fluid intake goals are being met by a safe feeding regimen
- Respiratory symptoms, if present, are being treated and improving

- An outpatient therapeutic plan and key individuals (e.g., dietitian, speech language pathologist or otolaryngologist, primary physician, pediatric gastroenterologist) have been identified.

CONSULTATION

Frequently, reevaluation of swallowing and ongoing support for behavioral interventions are required. Consultation should be considered from a speech pathologist (or otolaryngologist if abnormal anatomy is suspected as a cause of dysphagia), psychologist or psychiatrist with experience in feeding behavior, or a clinical dietitian. Referral to a pediatric outpatient rehabilitation program may be helpful. Decisions regarding treatment of severe GERD are best approached by a multidisciplinary team. Inpatient pediatricians, gastroenterologists, pediatric surgeons, clinical dietitians, and the child's primary care physician may all participate in establishing the diagnosis, choosing appropriate investigations (if any), optimizing nutrition, and optimizing medical management while minimizing symptoms. For children who fail medical and nutritional intervention, surgical options should be assessed by the team and discussed with the family to weigh the risks of the procedure with its expected benefits.

KEY POINTS

- Feeding issues in children are common and multifaceted. Careful history taking, physical examination, and observation of feeding are crucial to making an accurate diagnosis, and a multidisciplinary approach will benefit the infant or child.
- Although appropriate assessment of growth and parental reassurance are often all that is required in the management of GER, any vomiting infant with irritability, feeding refusal, disturbed growth or sleep, apnea, or other respiratory symptoms warrants consideration of a broader differential diagnosis and appropriate diagnostic evaluation.
- Early diagnosis of dysphagia or GERD and institution of an appropriate intervention may help avoid secondary oral aversion.
- Admission to the hospital for recurrent respiratory illness, vomiting, or failure to thrive may not at first glance be related to feeding problems. Inpatient pediatricians have an opportunity to further explore feeding during admission to identify such problems.

SUGGESTED READINGS

Arts-Rodas D, Benoit D. Feeding problems in infancy and early childhood: identification and management. *Paediatr Child Health*. 1998;3(1):21-27.

Benoit D, Wang EE, Zlotkin SH. Discontinuation of enterostomy tube feeding by behavioral treatment in early childhood: a randomized controlled trial. *J Pediatr*. 2000;137(4):498-503.

Davidson G. The role of lower esophageal sphincter function and dysmotility in gastroesophageal reflux in premature infants and in the first year of life. *J Pediatr Gastroenterol Nutr*. 2003;37 Suppl 1:S17-22.

East L, Nettles K, Vansant A, Daniels SK. Evaluation of oropharyngeal dysphagia with the videofluoroscopic swallowing study. *J Radiol Nurs*. 2014;33(1):9-13.

Edwards S, Davis AM, Ernst L, et al. Interdisciplinary strategies for treating oral aversions in children. *JPEN J Parenter Enteral Nutr*. 2015;39(8):899-909.

Giraldo-Cadavid LF, Leal-Leaño LR, Leon-Basantes GA, et al. Accuracy of endoscopic and videofluoroscopic evaluations of swallowing for oropharyngeal dysphagia. *Laryngoscope*. 2017;127(9):2002-2010.

Horvath A, Dziechciarz P, Szajewska H. The effect of thickened-feed interventions on gastroesophageal reflux in infants: systematic review and meta-analysis of randomized, controlled trials. *Pediatrics*. 2008;122(6):e1268-1277.

Jacobson JC, Pandya SR. A narrative review of gastroesophageal reflux in the pediatric patient. *Transl Gastroenterol Hepatol*. 2021;6:34.

Livingston MH, Shawyer AC, Rosenbaum PL, Jones SA, Walton JM. Fundoplication and gastrostomy versus percutaneous gastrojejunostomy for gastroesophageal reflux in children with neurologic impairment: a systematic review and meta-analysis. *J Pediatr Surg*. 2015;50(5):707-714.

Maffey A, Moviglia T, Mirabello C, et al. Swallowing and respiratory distress in hospitalized patients with bronchiolitis. *Dysphagia*. 2013;28(4):582-587.

Rosen R, Vandenplas Y, Singendonk M, et al. Pediatric Gastroesophageal Reflux Clinical Practice Guidelines: Joint Recommendations of the North American Society for Pediatric Gastroenterology, Hepatology, and Nutrition and the European Society for Pediatric Gastroenterology, Hepatology, and Nutrition. *J Pediatr Gastroenterol Nutr*. 2018;66(3):516-554.

Shay EO, Meleca JB, Anne S, Hopkins B. Natural history of silent aspiration on modified barium swallow studies in the pediatric population. *Int J Pediatric Otorhinolaryngology*. 2019;125:116-121.

Silverman AH, Kirby M, Clifford LM, et al. Nutritional and psychosocial outcomes of gastrostomy tube-dependent children completing an intensive inpatient behavioral treatment program. *J Pediatr Gastroenterol Nutr*. 2013;57(5):668-672.

Trayer J, Gilmore C, Dallapè S, Cox DW. Infants without apparent risk factors with aspiration as a cause of respiratory symptoms—a retrospective study. *Ir J Med Sci*. 2021;190(1):217-223.

Trivić I, Hojsak I. Evaluation and treatment of malnutrition and associated gastrointestinal complications in children with cerebral palsy. *Pediatr Gastroenterol Hepatol Nutr*. 2019;22(2):122.

SECTION H
Genetics and Metabolism

CHAPTER 80 Genetic Syndromes

Sarah Schmidt, MD and Hayley Ron, MD

BACKGROUND

A genetic diagnosis provides a strong basis for disease management, treatments (when available) or screening guidelines, counseling, and prognosis. Advances in the field have made genetic testing for inherited conditions available as early as 10 weeks of gestation. Individuals may opt for carrier screening prior to conception to better understand their risk for and potentially avoid devastating disease. At birth, every newborn in the United States undergoes newborn screening for the most common, treatable genetic diseases. For a vast range of clinical indications that arise throughout childhood and adolescence—including congenital anomalies, differences in development, biochemical abnormalities, organ dysfunction, and cancer, for example—further genetic testing is often warranted.

Our understanding of how genetics influences human health is growing rapidly, but much is yet to be discovered. We know that genetic conditions and predispositions play a role in the way an individual responds to medical challenges such as infection, surgery, and hospitalization. Individuals with a genetic condition have increased morbidity and mortality compared with controls hospitalized with the same chief complaint. Early genetic diagnosis can be a powerful tool in preventing morbidity and mortality. Early detection of certain genetic conditions can lead to impactful interventions. In this chapter, we review genetic syndromes that are more commonly encountered in the inpatient pediatric setting, the initial medical workup, and preferred genetic testing modality is outlined for each syndrome.

CLINICAL PRESENTATION

The essential tools that the clinical geneticist uses to diagnose genetic disorders include the following: prenatal, birth, and medical histories; detailed pedigree analysis; careful clinical evaluation, including dysmorphology examination; comprehensive literature searches; and cytogenetic and molecular genetic laboratory analyses. Key features of the family history include ancestral origin, consanguinity, related signs and symptoms within the family, and pregnancy losses. The dysmorphology examination is intended to reveal and quantify abnormal development of organs or other parts of the body, as outlined in **Table 80-1**.

GENETIC TESTING

The DNA that makes up the human genome is packaged into 23 pairs of chromosomes—22 pairs of autosomes and 1 pair of sex chromosomes. The most common mechanisms leading to genetic disease are (i) chromosomal abnormalities that increase or decrease the number of chromosomes ("aneuploidy"); (ii) a duplication or deletion of a piece of a chromosome that may include multiple genes in a row; (iii) an error in the DNA sequence of a single gene (akin to a spelling error) which results in a dysfunctional or absent protein product when that sequence is translated ("pathogenic variant," previously called "mutation"); and (iv) epigenetic changes that alter gene expression (e.g., DNA methylation).

The advent of next-generation sequencing has allowed increased use of whole exome sequencing (WES) and whole genome sequencing (WGS) in the clinical setting. Due to decreasing costs and increasing diagnostic yield, these tests are increasingly becoming the preferred diagnostic modality for pediatric populations with suspected rare genetic disorders. However, while next-generation sequencing is becoming more routinely utilized to diagnose underlying genetic disorders, the previous mainstays of molecular and cytogenetic testing, including sanger sequencing, chromosomal microarray, karyotype, and fluorescent in-situ hybridization (FISH) all have important indications for clinical use either in lieu of or in addition to next-generation sequencing with advantages including but not limited to cost efficacy, high sensitivity for specific indications, and more rapid turn-around-time. These tests are summarized in **Table 80-2.**

In this chapter, we review the various types of genetic testing, their utilities and limitations, and how to determine which genetic testing modality is the most appropriate for the clinical scenario.

KARYOTYPING

Karyotyping, a cytogenetic technique that stains and visualizes whole chromosomes, detects major chromosomal structural abnormalities including whole extra or missing chromosomes (aneuploidies), copy number variants larger than a single gene (microdeletions or duplications), and structural variants (translocations, inversions). A karyotype would be the recommended test when a patient has clinical features concerning for a recognizable chromosomal disorder, such as Trisomy 21, 13, or 18, or Turner syndrome. Karyotope analysis may also be appropriate for determining sex chromosome status in children with differences in sexual differentiation (e.g., ambiguous genitalia). Even in these cases, chromosomal microarray may be a reasonable secondary analysis to detect possible mosaicism (**Figure 80-1**).

FLUORESCENT IN SITU HYBRIDIZATION (FISH)

FISH uses a fluorescent-labeled segment of synthetic DNA, which is allowed hybridize to its corresponding chromosomal locations to label regions of interest with a fluorophore for visibility under a fluorescence microscope. FISH is used to identify small chromosomal deletions or duplications or small structural rearrangements, such as balanced or unbalanced translocations, which would not be discerned on karyotype. FISH can only be used to identify recurrent chromosomal regions for which specific probes exist (e.g. 22q11.2) (**Figure 80-2**).

CHROMOSOMAL MICROARRAY

Chromosomal microarrays (CMAs) use millions of small probes across the genome to detect chromosome copy number changes, such as deletions and duplications, down to 100 kb in size. The most common type of CMA in the 2020s utilizes single-nucleotide polymorphisms (SNPs) to assess parent of origin for chromosome regions. SNP-CMAs can additionally detect regions of homozygosity due to either consanguinity or uniparental isodisomy. The resolution of CMA far exceeds that of a karyotype. CMA can detect very small deletions and duplications as small as 50,000 bp. However, CMA cannot detect balanced translocations. CMA also does not analyze the sequence of genes—it is a tool for looking for changes in copy number in genetic information. Therefore, single gene variants are not detected by CMA. CMA are the preferred testing modality when there are clinical features strongly overlapping with a specific deletion syndrome. CMA previously was the preferred first-line analysis for multiple congenital anomalies, as well as neurodevelopmental disorders (NDD), such as autism spectrum disorder and intellectual disability. However diagnostic yield for WES and WGS for congenital anomalies, developmental delays, and intellectual disabilities have consistently outperformed chromosomal microarray, leading to recommendations that WES/WGS be offered as first-line testing for congenital anomalies and NDD.

TABLE 80-1 Elements of the Dysmorphology Examination

Category	Subcategory	Examples of Abnormalities
General	Height	Overgrowth, short stature
	Weight	Small for gestational age, failure to thrive, obesity
	Head circumference	Microcephaly, macrocephaly
Head	Shape	Brachycephaly (disproportionately wide head), turricephaly (cone-shaped head), craniosynostosis (premature closure of one or more cranial sutures)
	Fontanelles	Large, small, accessory fontanelles
	Hair distribution	Scalp defects, high or low hairline, hair whorls, sparse, full
Eyes	Shape	Almond, proptotic, periorbital fullness
	Eyebrows	Synophrys (meeting at the midline), interruption, absent, full, arched
	Structures	Colobomas, iris irregularities, blue sclera
	Spacing	Hypertelorism, hypotelorism
	Palpebral fissures	Up-slanted, down-slanted, epicanthal folds, colobomas
Ears	Placement	Low set
	Rotation	Posteriorly rotated
	Length	Short or long
	Helices	Overfolded, simple, squared off
	Preauricular surface	Pits, tags
Nose	Shape of tip	Bulbous, pointed, prominent/fleshy
	Alae nasi (sides)	Hypoplastic
	Nares	Anteversion
	Columella	Long or short
	Choana patency	Choanal stenosis
Mouth	Lips	Thin, simple, pits, downturned, full, open-mouthed expression, tented
	Frenulum	Absent, duplicated
	Teeth	Natal, absent, single front incisor, widely spaced
	Tongue	Protuberant, lobulated, cleft
	Palate	Cleft, high arched, short
	Uvula	Bifid
Neck	Chin	Retrognathic, micrognathic, pointed, large mandible
	Folds	Excess nuchal folds, webbing
Chest	Cardiac	Murmurs
	Thorax	Pectus deformity, bell-shaped, absent clavicles, supernumerary ribs
	Size	Broad (increased internipple distance-chest ratio)
	Superficial findings	Supernumerary nipple
Back	Shape	Scoliosis, lordosis, kyphosis
	Sacrum	Dimple, myelomeningocele, hair tuft
Abdomen	Umbilicus	Two-vessel cord, umbilical hernia, omphalocele, diastasis recti
	Visceromegaly	Hepatosplenomegaly
Genitourinary	Phallus, clitoris	Hypospadias, chordee, clitoromegaly
	Labia, scrotum	Bifid scrotum, shawl scrotum, micropenis, ambiguous genitalia
	Testes	Undescended, hydrocele
Extremities	Limb length	Brachymelia (short limbs), rhizomelia (shortening of proximal limbs), mesomelia (small intermediate segments of long bones), acromelia (shortening of distal limb segments)
	Digit number	Polydactyly (pre- or postaxial), oligodactyly
	Digit formation	Syndactyly (digit fusion), broad thumbs, broad hallux, slender fingers, arachnodactyly (long fingers), brachydactyly (short fingers), contractures
	Position of digits	Proximally placed thumbs, clinodactyly, camptodactyly (bent position)
Skin	Pigmentation	Café au lait spots, ash-leaf spots, hyperpigmentation, hypopigmentation/albinism
	Vascular	Hemangioma, telangiectasia, nevus simplex
	Hair	Brittle, steely, absent, hypertrichosis
	Sweat	Absent, hyperhidrosis
Neurologic	Alertness	Lethargic, nonresponsive, hyperactive
	Tone	Hypertonia, hypotonia, head lag
	Feeding	Poor, hyperphagic
	Movements	Fasciculations, seizures, choreas, clonus, ataxia, hand/arm flapping, jerky movements
	Speech	Hypernasal, absent, unintelligible

SANGER SEQUENCING

Previously the mainstay of genetic sequencing, introduced in 1977 by Fredrick Sanger, this test sequences a gene of interest and will identify missense, frameshift, and small deletions or duplication within the specific gene or gene region. This method is most currently used for confirmation of known familial variants or variants identified using next-generation sequencing as well as sequencing of technically difficult regions. Sanger sequencing, or single gene sequencing is appropriate if there is a strong clinical suspicion for a genetic disorder associated with a single gene.

NEXT-GENERATION SEQUENCING

Next-generation sequencing has dramatically changed the landscape of genetic testing by significantly reducing time and cost of genetic sequencing. This test allows for massive parallel sequencing by fragmenting the genome, then simultaneously sequencing the millions of small fragments of DNA and aligning them.

Panel Sequencing applies next-generation sequencing to a selection of genes that are associated with a specific phenotype, for example "hypoglycemia panel" or "kidney disease panel." These range from small panels with as few as 3 genes to 100's of genes.

Whole Exome Sequencing (WES) sequences the entire protein-coding region of the genome (exons) and several hundred intronic nucleotides at the ends of exons. These regions are approximately 2% of the genome but contain approximately 85% of known disease causing variants.

Whole Genome Sequencing (WGS) sequences all exons and 90% of the genome. Meta-analysis of previous studies has not shown a significant difference in the diagnostic yield between WES and WGS. A more recent comparative retrospective analysis of 108 patients who underwent both clinical WES and WGS found an additional diagnostic rate of 3 cases (3%) for WGS. As testing costs for WGS are higher, WES remains the more common clinical default; that may change as testing cost decrease that may change. In the setting of a non-diagnostic WES in an individual highly suspected of having and underlying genetic disorder, WGS can be considered.

TABLE 80-2 Type of Genetic Testing

Test	Type of Genetic Change Detected	Indication	Limitations
Karyotype	• Whole chromosome deletion/duplication • Multi-gene deletion/duplication	• High suspicion of recognizable aneuploidy syndrome • Sex chromosome analysis • Analysis for suspected balanced rearrangement (parent of child with unbalanced rearrangement, recurrent miscarriage)	• Can only detect very large rearrangements • Not sensitive to mosaicism
FISH	• Multi-gene deletion/duplication	• Rapid testing for specific deletion/duplication systems • Determine if a deletion/duplication represents a translocation or other structural change	• Can only be utilized for specific regions for which probes exist
CMA	• Multi-gene deletion/duplication • Whole chromosome deletion/duplication	• Screening for congenital anomalies, intellectual disability/developmental delay with normal WES/WGS • Mosaicism evaluation for patients with aneuploidy	
Sanger Sequencing	• Errors in gene sequence		• Used for single genes
Next Generation Sequencing	• Errors in gene sequence	• First line testing for congenital anomalies, intellectual disability, developmental delay that do not match a known clinical syndrome	• Cannot detect repeat expansion disorders

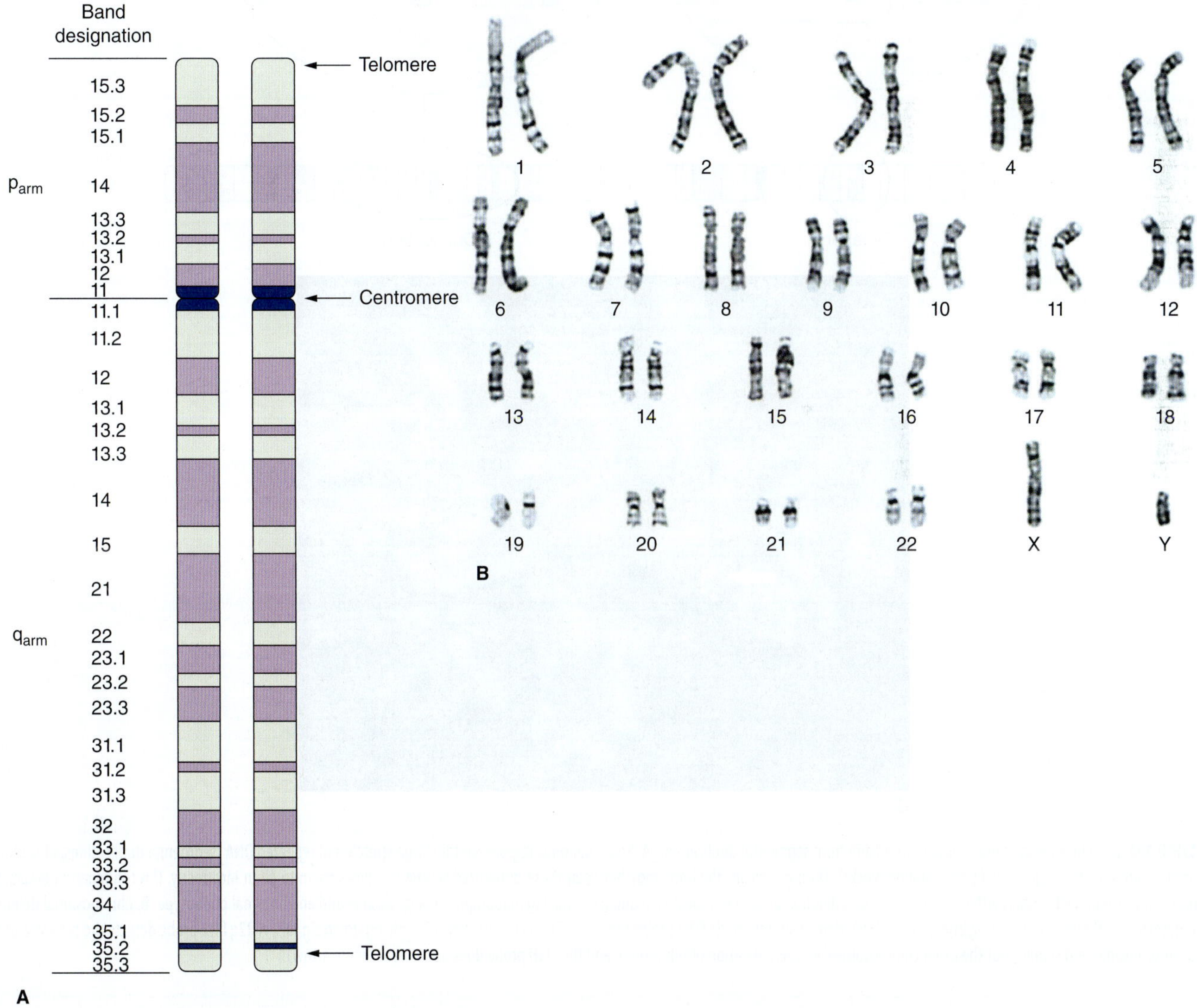

FIGURE 80-1. Chromosome structure and karyotyping. A. Structure of human chromosome: 5. Band designations for each arm start at the centromere and increase progressively toward the telomere. Therefore, band 5q21 and 5q34 are both on the long arm of chromosome 5, and 5q34 is closer to the telomere. B. Normal human male karyotype, showing 22 pairs of autosomes, one X chromosome, and one Y chromosome.

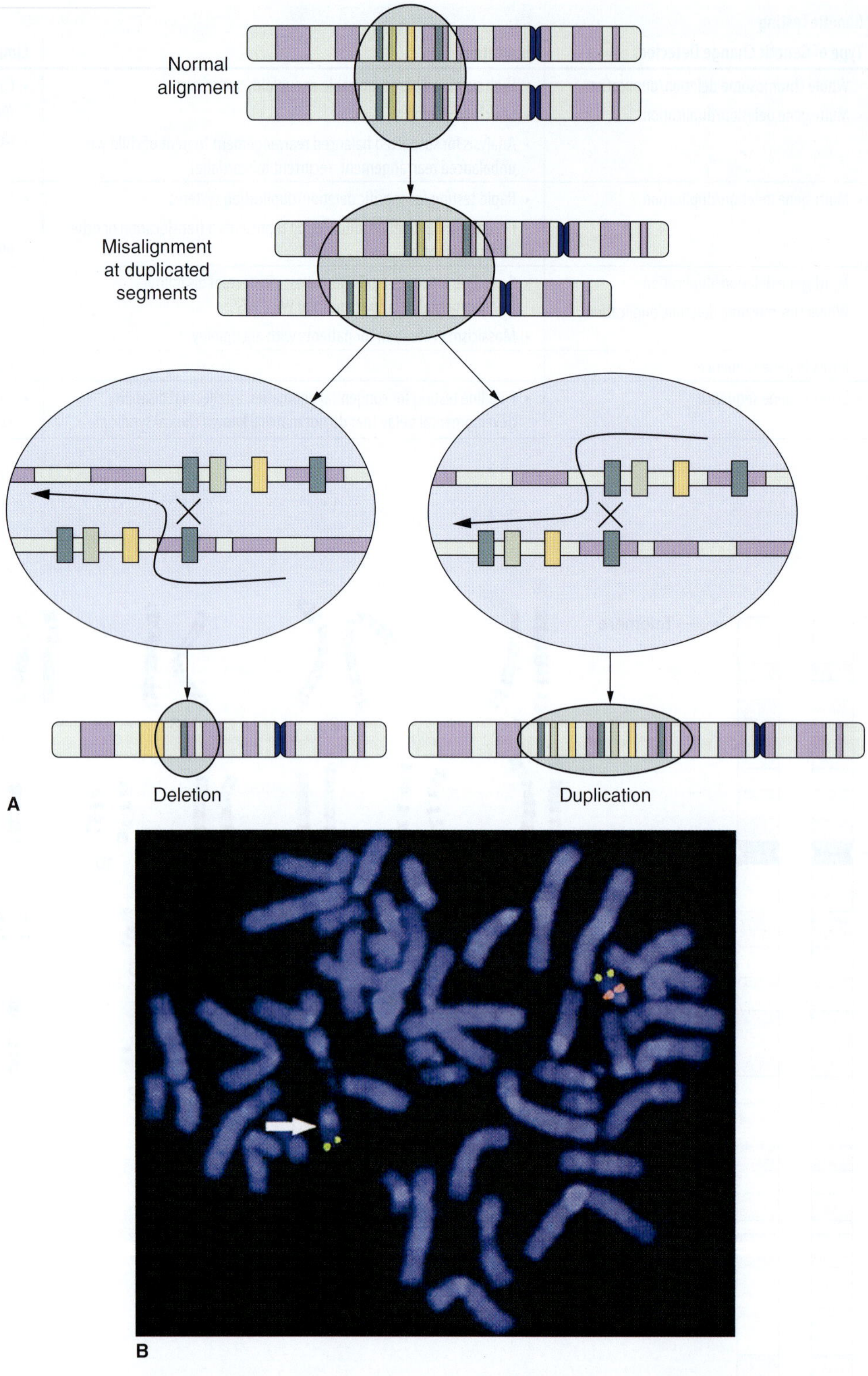

FIGURE 80-2. Chromosomal rearrangements arising from segmental duplications. A. Some genomic regions contain large stretches of repeated DNA (segmental duplications, blue blocks) surrounding nonrepeated sequences (green, orange blocks). During meiosis, the homology between these duplicated segments allows them to align incorrectly. If recombination occurs, the resulting chromosome will contain either a duplication or a deletion of the nonrepeated sequences, causing inappropriate gene dosage and an abnormal phenotype. B. Chromosomal deletions can be detected by fluorescent in situ hybridization (FISH). Here, a subtelomeric FISH probe anneals to both chromosomes 22, giving green signals. A 22q11.2 probe detects the presence of the normal chromosome (red signal), but the other chromosome contains a deletion of this region, and the FISH probe does not anneal (white arrow).

The diagnostic yield of WES/WGS is highest when performed in "trio:" samples from the "proband" or patient, and each parent. This allows better contextualization of rare variants aiding in the interpretation of the variant as pathogenic, benign, or of uncertain significance. The limitations of WES include that it typically cannot detect intronic variants, repeat expansion disorders (Fragile X, Huntington's, myotonic dystrophy, etc.), methylation abnormalities. WES also has historically been limited in the ability to detect copy-number variants. WGS overcomes all these limitations. The primary limitation of WGS is the inability to detect epigenetic changes. It is critical for pediatricians to understand that WES/WGS are dependent on bioinformatic algorithms that are informed by a patient's reported phenotype. The most important role of a pediatrician performing WES/WGS is carefully characterizing the patient's phenotype.

COMMON ANEUPLOIDY SYNDROMES

TRISOMY 21 (DOWN SYNDROME)

Trisomy 21 is the most common chromosomal disorder in humans. Non-invasive prenatal screening (NIPS) can detect trisomy 21 prenatally with high sensitivity and specificity and has reduced the need for invasive prenatal genetic testing. A confirmatory diagnosis of trisomy 21 can be obtained via amniocentesis after 15 weeks of gestation, by chorionic villus sampling (CVS) after 10 to 12 weeks, or after delivery. The clinical features of DS are summarized in **Table 80-3**. Postnatal clinical investigations should include a confirmatory karyotype, echocardiogram, screening for gastrointestinal anomalies such as duodenal atresia or Hirschsprung disease, serum thyrotropin level, and a complete blood count. The most immediately concerning malformation is congenital heart disease, which occurs in about half of infants with DS and may require surgical intervention. The complete blood count screens for various hematologic abnormalities associated with DS, including transient myeloproliferative disease in the newborn period and acute lymphoblastic leukemia later in life. Congenital hypothyroidism occurs in about 1% and should be evaluated for prior to birth hospital discharge. Guidelines for the ongoing care of children with Down syndrome have been published by the American Academy of Pediatrics.

Down syndrome can be due either to a full extra chromosome 21 ("free trisomy") or due to a translocation, where the extra chromosome 21 has become attached to another translocation. Free trisomy 21 is always spontaneous (not inherited). After having one child with trisomy 21, a mother's risk of having another affected child is approximately 1% point higher than her age-specific risk. The risk is higher if either parent carries a balanced translocation involving chromosome 21; therefore, if a karyotype shows that the proband has a translocation, parental karyotypes should be performed to determine if they are balanced translocation carriers. Since knowing the location of the extra genetical material is so important, if trisomy 21 is detected by microarray, secondary testing by either karyotype or FISH is needed to evaluate for translocation.

TRISOMY 18 (EDWARDS SYNDROME)

Trisomy 18 occurs is the second most common aneuploidy syndrome in live born infants. Diagnosis is usually made prenatally based on the presence of congenital anomalies, high risk NIPS, and/or confirmatory genetic testing through CVS or amniocentesis. There is a high rate of fetal loss. Of the live born infants, few survive to the age of 1 year. Prenatal and postnatal clinical features are listed in Table 80-3.

Trisomy 18 carries an extremely poor prognosis with death usually resulting from central apnea, infection, or congestive heart failure. The neonatal period is characterized by poor feeding and growth, and patients typically require tube feedings. Poor growth, profound intellectual disability, and lack of developmental progress beyond that of a 6-month-old infant have been universally documented. In the few cases attempted, cardiac surgery has not improved the outcome.

TRISOMY 13 (PATAU SYNDROME)

A small fraction of fetuses with trisomy 13 survive to birth. Diagnosis is usually made prenatally owing to a combination of abnormalities on ultrasound, high risk NIPS, and/or genetic testing through CVS or amniocentesis.

Classic features of trisomy 13 include congenital heart disease, cleft palate, holoprosencephaly, renal anomalies, and postaxial polydactyly. Additional findings are noted in Table 80-3. The prognosis for an infant born with trisomy 13 is extremely poor, with 80% mortality in the neonatal period and less than 5% survival at 6 months. Intellectual disability is profound, and many patients are blind and deaf.

SEX CHROMOSOME ABNORMALITIES

A male's sex chromosomes consist of an X and a Y chromosome. A female's sex chromosomes consist of two X chromosomes, one of which is inactivated, or lionized, to form a Barr body. Multiple syndromes originate from an abnormal number of sex chromosomes, including Turner syndrome and Klinefelter syndrome.

Turner Syndrome results from loss of an X chromosome in a female conceptus and occurs in approximately 1 in 2500 female newborns. The 45, XO karyotype, (loss of an entire X chromosome) accounts for roughly half of the cases. Deletions, translocations, and isochromosomes (i.e., a chromosome with two p arms or two q arms) of the x chromosome account for the remainder. The vast majority of 45, XO fetuses are spontaneously aborted. This underscores the requirement for both x chromosomes during early embryonic development.

Features of Turner syndrome that are recognizable at birth include short stature, webbed neck, craniofacial differences (epicanthal folds and high arched palate), shield chest, renal anomalies, lymphedema of the hands and feet, nail hypoplasia, and congenital heart disease. Typical cardiac defects include bicuspid aortic valve, coarctation of the aorta, hypoplastic left heart, valvular aortic stenosis, and mitral valve prolapse. Glucose levels should be monitored in the neonatal period due to the risk of hypoglycemia. Some affected individuals are diagnosed later during childhood and adolescence owing to growth issues, especially short stature. The remaining individuals are diagnosed due to primary ovarian failure caused by gonadal dysgenesis or streak gonads.

Additional features of Turner syndrome may include hypothyroidism, strabismus, cataracts, sensorineural hearing loss, structural renal malformations, and learning difficulties. Approximately 10% of Turner syndrome patients have substantial developmental delays requiring assistance in adult life (Sybert, VP).

A karyotype would detect most cases of classic 45, XO Turner syndrome. A subset of patients are mosaic for a population of cells with a Y chromosome, however, which confers an increased risk of gonadoblastoma and can be missed on a standard karyotype. A chromosomal microarray is therefore recommended to detect whether any Y chromosome material is present.

Klinefelter Syndrome occurs in a male who has two or more X chromosomes. The most common genotype is 47, XXY, but other possible genotypes include 48, XXXY and 49, XXXXY or mosaic 46, XY/47, XXY.

The neonate with Klinefelter syndrome may present with hypotonia and abnormal genitalia. Children may experience developmental delays and adolescents with Klinefelter syndrome come to attention with learning or behavioral difficulties, tall stature with decreased upper/lower segment ratio, small testicular size, and gynecomastia. There may be less facial or body hair than expected. Adults may experience infertility due to hyalinization and fibrosis of seminiferous tubules (Los et al 2021).

Management should focus on interventions such as speech and physical therapies as needed. In adolescence, testosterone therapy may help support virilization and reduce gynecomastia. Cryptorchidism or inguinal hernia should be referred to urology or pediatric surgery. Klinefelter syndrome can be diagnosed via karyotype or chromosomal microarray. NIPS can detect Klinefelter syndrome prenatally but has a high false positive rate. Therefore, confirmatory genetic testing is required to make a diagnosis.

DEVELOPMENTAL DELAY AND INTELLECTUAL DISABILITY

Genetic testing is an important component of the workup for developmental delay and intellectual disability—two common findings in the pediatric population. When the medical history and physical exam are not suggestive of a particular diagnosis, the AAP supports first-tier testing with a chromosomal microarray and Fragile X testing (Moeschler et al 2014). Metabolic testing should be considered when certain elements in the history are present (discussed below), as

TABLE 80-3 Common Autosomal Trisomies

Feature	Trisomy 21	Trisomy 18	Trisomy 13
Eponym	Down Syndrome	Edwards Syndrome	Patau Syndrome
Live-born incidence	1 in 800	1 in 6000	1 in 12,000
Prenatal	NIPS >99% sensitivity	NIPS 97%-98% sensitivity	NIPS: 93%-99% sensitivity
	Ultrasound: cardiac defects, duodenal atresia, shortened long bones, nuchal translucency, echogenic small bowel	Ultrasound: IUGR, oligohydramnios or polyhydramnios, microcephaly, Dandy-Walker malformation, cardiac defects, myelomeningocele, clenched fists, limb anomalies, single umbilical artery	Ultrasound: cardiac anomalies, omphalocele, renal anomalies, pyloric stenosis
Growth	Low-normal at birth (10%-25%), slow postnatal growth velocity	IUGR at birth (1500-2500 g); FTT due to poor feeding, requiring tube feedings	FTT due to feeding difficulties
Tone	Hypotonia	Hypertonia	Hypo- or hypertonia
Cranium, brain	Mild microcephaly, flat occiput, 3 fontanelles or confluence between anterior and posterior fontanelle	Microcephaly, narrow cranium, prominent occiput, open metopic suture	Microcephaly, anophthalmia, sloping forehead, split sutures, open fontanelles
Eyes	Up-slanting palpebral fissures, epicanthal folds, speckled iris, Brushfield spots (75%), strabismus, cataracts, myopia, glaucoma	Small palpebral fissures, corneal opacity, microphthalmia, coloboma, cataracts	Microphthalmia, hypotelorism, iris coloboma, retinal dysplasia, hamartomatous cartilage "islands", low-vision
Ears	Small, low-set, posteriorly rotated, overfolded upper helix; hearing loss (50%)	Low-set, posteriorly rotated, malformed	Low-set, malformed, sensorineural hearing loss
Nose, mouth	Holds mouth open; prominent tongue; large cheeks; low, flat nasal bridge	Small mouth, micrognathia, choanal atresia	Cleft lip and palate
Neck	Short neck with excess skin, atlantoaxial subluxation		
Skeletal	Brachyclinodactyly of 5th digit, gap between toes 1 and 2, excess nuchal skin, short stature, ligamentous laxity	Clenched hands, overlapping 2nd and 5th digits, absent 5th finger, distal crease, hypoplastic nails, short rocker-bottom feet, prominent heels, convex soles, clubfoot, vertebral anomalies, radial ray limb defects, dorsiflexed great toes	Postaxial Polydactyly; hypoconvex fingernails; flexed, overlapped fingers; camptodactyly; rocker-bottom feet
Cardiorespiratory	60% with CHD; AV canal, VSD, ASD, tetralogy of Fallot, PDA	90% with CHD; ASD, VSD, PDA, pulmonic stenosis, aortic coarctation, pulmonary hypoplasia; central apnea	80% with CHD; VSD, ASD, PDA, dextrocardia
Gastrointestinal	Duodenal atresia (2%-5%); Hirschsprung disease; esophageal atresia, fistulas, and webs	Omphalocele, malrotation, ileal atresia, hernias	Omphalocele, hernias
Genitourinary	Short labial folds	Polycystic kidneys, ureteral anomalies, unilateral renal agenesis, hypospadias, cryptorchidism	Genital anomalies, polycystic kidneys
Endocrine	Hypothyroidism (5%); men are almost always infertile, but some women have reproduced	Thyroid and adrenal hypoplasia	
Hematologic, oncologic	Neonatal thrombocytopenia, leukemoid reaction, acute nonlymphoblastic leukemia in first 3 yr, ALL	Thymic hypoplasia, increased incidence of hepatoblastoma and Wilms tumor	Increased nuclear projections in neutrophils ("drumstick" appearance), increased risk for malignancy, capillary hemangioma
Dermatoglyphics (skin)	Single palmar crease, plantar crease between 1st and 2nd toes, distal triradii	Excess arch pattern, hypoplastic nails	Occipital scalp defects (cutis aplasia, 50%); single palmar crease; hyperconvex, narrow nails
Neurologic	Seizures (5%-10%), early-onset Alzheimer neurodegeneration	Seizures	Holoprosencephaly (50%), seizures
Developmental	Language and motor delay, mean IQ 54 (range, 35-65), intensive early intervention critical	Severe delay (100%)	Severe delay
Survival	Long term; death typically related to heart disease, infection, malignancies	95% die within first year; 1% live to age 10 yr; death often due to apnea, cardiac disease, infection	80% die as neonates; death often related to cardiopulmonary arrest, CHD, pneumonia

AFP, α-fetoprotein; ALL, acute lymphoblastic leukemia; ASD, atrial septal defect; AV, atrioventricular; CHD, congenital heart disease; FTT, failure to thrive; HCG, human chorionic gonadotropin; IUGR, in utero growth retardation; NIPS: Non-invasive prenatal screening PDA, patent ductus arteriosus; VSD, ventricular septal defect.

Source: Data from Epstein CJ. Down syndrome (trisomy 21). In: Scriver CR, Sly WS, Childs B, et al., eds. *The Metabolic and Molecular Bases of Inherited Disease*. 8th ed. New York: McGraw-Hill; 2001:1223-1256; and Zackai EH, Anyane-Yeboa K, Bergoffen J, et al. Genetics. In: Polin RA, Ditmar MF, eds. *Pediatric Secrets*. 3rd ed. Philadelphia, PA: Hanley & Belfus; 2001:251.

universal testing has a low diagnostic yield. If the microarray does not reveal an etiology, whole exome and whole genome sequencing have a higher diagnostic yield, particularly if there are dysmorphic features, congenital anomalies, or involvement of another system (Manickam, 2021—ACMG Guidelines).

Features that increase suspicion for metabolic disease include, but are not limited to, recurrent vomiting, failure to thrive, hepatic dysfunction, developmental regression or loss of milestones (especially if the timing correlates with illness or fever), seizures, muscle weakness, and dietary preferences such as aversion to protein. If the infant was born outside of the United States, and therefore did not undergo newborn screening, metabolic testing should include plasma amino acids, acylcarnitine profile, total homocysteine, biotinidase activity, urine organic acids, and glycosaminoglycans.

This section details several syndromes that are commonly associated with developmental delays and intellectual disability (**Table 80-4**). It is important to note that within each syndrome the spectrum is vast and some patients may be mildly affected or seemingly unaffected, while others have more severe manifestations.

22Q11 DELETION SYNDROME

DiGeorge syndrome, velocardiofacial syndrome, Shprintzen syndrome, conotruncal anomaly face syndrome, Caylor cardiofacial syndrome, and autosomal dominant Opitz syndrome are all synonyms for the clinical spectrum of disorders caused by deletion of chromosome 22q11.2. Estimates indicate that the 22q11 deletion, which occurs in approximately 1 in 3000 live births, is the most common microdeletion syndrome in humans.

Common components of this syndrome include congenital heart disease, palatal anomalies, and aplasia or hypoplasia of the thymus and parathyroid glands. Even in children with structurally normal thymus glands, qualitative and quantitative lymphocyte defects can occur. Most patients diagnosed with a 22q11.2 deletion present as newborns or infants owing to cardiovascular malformations, including tetralogy of Fallot, ventricular septal defect, interrupted aortic arch type B, or truncus arteriosus, along with T-cell abnormalities and hypocalcemia. Facial dysmorphisms may include hooded eyelids, hypertelorism, overfolded ears, bulbous nasal tip, small mouth, and micrognathia.

Developmental delays and learning disabilities occur in 70% to 90% of patients with the 22q11.2 deletion. Severe cognitive disability is uncommon; if present, it may be due to a secondary insult. Most 22q11 deletions occur de novo, with less than 10% inherited from an affected parent. CMA will detect the presence and size the deletion. Some institutions use an alternate test, called multiplex ligation-dependent probe amplification (MPLA), which may have a faster turn-around-time than CMA.

PRADER-WILLI SYNDROME

Prader-Willi syndrome (PWS) results from the loss of activity of paternally inherited genes on the long arm of chromosome 15 (15q11). This can occur through deletion or disruption of this region on the paternally inherited chromosome or through the presence of two maternal and no paternal chromosomes (maternal uniparental disomy). Chromosome 15q11 contains both maternally and paternally imprinted genes, the significance of which is suppression or "silencing" of the imprinted gene. Children lacking paternal expression of this region have PWS, and those lacking maternal expression have Angelman syndrome (see below).

Newborns with PWS have pronounced central hypotonia, weak cry, and hyporeflexia. Consistent with hypotonia, breech presentation, and perinatal insults are more frequent than usual. Poor tone usually manifests as sucking and swallowing difficulties that lead to failure to thrive and the need for gavage feeding during infancy. Facial findings include bifrontal narrowing, almond-shaped eyes, and a small, downturned mouth. Genitalia are often hypoplastic, and cryptorchidism is common in boys. Small hands and feet are usually demonstrated in childhood.

The extreme hypotonia improves in the first year of life, as does motor development. Developmental delay is universal. Uncontrollable hyperphagia and subsequent obesity begin in the second year. This and other behavioral problems, including severe temper tantrums, are lifelong. Most patients have mild to moderate intellectual disability.

Methylation analysis is the first-tier test when PWS is suspected. It will detect most cases by determining if the region has maternally inherited genetic material only—whether due to a 15q11 deletion, maternal uniparental disomy or, infrequently, a methylation defect. Uniparental disomy as a cause of PWS is associated with advanced maternal. Microarray can detect 15q11 deletion or uniparentaly disomy, but cannot differentiate between PWS and Angelman, and cannot detect cases due to methylation defects.

ANGELMAN SYNDROME

Loss of the maternal copy of chromosome 15q11 is associated with Angelman syndrome. After an often normal prenatal and perinatal course, patients present with delayed milestones and acquired microcephaly. Seizures typically begin between 1 and 3 years of age. There is a significant delay in walking. Once children walk they have a jerky, ataxic gait. Facial features may include a protruding jaw, wide mouth, thin upper lip, and widely spaced teeth. Behavioral features include tongue thrusting, drooling, exaggerated bursts of laughter, sleep disturbance, hyperactivity, proclivity for water, and social-seeking personalities. Severe language impairment is common.

Methylation analysis is the best first test when Angelman syndrome is suspected. It most cases (about 80%) including those with a 15q11 deletion, UPD, or a methylation defect. A microarray alone would identify a 15q11 deletion or UPD but cannot differentiate Angelman from PWS and should be followed by methylation testing which determines the parental chromosome of origin of the deletion. Approximately 11% have a pathogenic variant in the *UBE3A* gene, which causes methylation defects and can be detected by sequence analysis of *UBE31*. Finally, approximately 10% of patients do not have an identifiable genetic change. Most cases are sporadic, but *UBE3A* variants may be inherited.

WAGR SYNDROME (11P13 DELETION SYNDROME)

Wilms tumor, Aniridia, Genital anomalies, Range of developmental delays (WAGR) syndrome results from a deletion involving chromosome 11p12-p14, which includes the *WT1* and *PAX6* genes. Pathogenic variants or deletions of *WT1* have been implicated in the pathogenesis of Wilms tumor. The risk of Wilms tumor in WAGR patients approaches 50%. The *WT1* gene has also been implicated in renal and genitourinary abnormalities, including uterine abnormalities, hypospadias, cryptorchidism, ambiguous genitalia, urethral strictures, fused kidneys, ureteric abnormalities, and gonadoblastoma.

Aniridia is characterized by bilateral aplasia or dysplasia of the iris and optic nerve hypoplasia, leading to visual impairment. Cataracts, glaucoma, and corneal opacification and vascularization can also be seen. These findings are caused by deletion of the *PAX6* gene. The cause of the mild intellectual disability seen in WAGR patients is unclear but is likely due to the role of *PAX6* in the developing forebrain.

Ongoing care of these patients includes frequent ophthalmic assessment, renal ultrasonography every 3 months until age 8 years, urologic, nephrologic, and endocrine management for gonadal abnormalities, and early cognitive assessment and intervention if developmental delay is noted.

Microarray allows for detection and sizing of this deletion. Most mutations are de novo. Transmission occurs in an autosomal dominant manner.

CHROMOSOME 1P36 DELETION SYNDROME

Deletion of the 1p36 region is estimated to occur in approximately 1 in 5000 births and has been associated with a constellation of clinical findings. The characteristic features include microbrachycephaly, large and late-closing anterior fontanelle, deep-set eyes, flattened midface, flat nose, pointed chin, short fifth finger, global developmental delay, hypotonia, oropharyngeal dysphagia, low-set ears, and hearing loss. Some are affected by orofacial clefting, hyperopia, seizures, brain anomalies, hypothyroidism, renal anomalies, dilated cardiomyopathy, and congenital heart defects. Intellectual disability is present in all affected individuals, ranging from moderate to severe, and speech delay is almost universal. Behavioral issues may include aggression and self-harm (e.g., headbanging and biting).

Most deletions arise de novo, but 5% are due to a balanced parental translocation. The size of the deletion varies from 1.5 to greater than 10.5 Mb, and there appears to be a correlation between the size of the deletion and the severity of clinical features. Chromosomal microarray will detect the presence and size of the deletion, but FISH or karyotype

TABLE 80-4 Syndromes Detectable by Chromosomal Microarray and Their Features

Syndrome	Locus	Mechanism	Features	Incidence
Monosomy 1q21	1q21.1	Deletion	Microcephaly, cardiovascular malformations, psychiatric illness, developmental delay	Unknown
Trisomy 1q21	1q21.1	Duplication	Macrocephaly, developmental delay	Unknown
Monosomy 1p	1p36	Deletion	Developmental delay, seizures, hypotonia, orofacial clefting, dysmorphia, deafness, cardiomyopathy	1 in 5000
Wolf-Hirschhorn	4p16	Deletion	Pre- and postnatal growth retardation, "Greek warrior helmet" facies, developmental delay, skeletal anomalies, cardiac septal defects, hearing loss, urinary tract abnormalities	1 in 50,000
Cri du chat	5p15	Deletion	Catlike cry, SGA, microcephaly, hypotonia, cardiac defects, intellectual disability	1 in 50,000
Russell-Silver	7p12	Maternal uniparental disomy (some cases)	Pre- and postnatal growth retardation with sparing of head; triangular facies; limb and facial asymmetry	1 in 100,000
Williams-Beuren	7q11.23	Deletion	"Jowly" facies, cardiac disease (supravalvular aortic stenosis), growth and developmental delay, overfriendliness, infantile hypocalcemia	1 in 25,000
Trisomy 7q11.2	7q11.23	Duplication	Developmental delay, speech delay, autism spectrum, hypotonia	Unknown
Trichorhinophalangeal, type I	8q24	Deletion	Sparse, thin hair; pear-shaped nose; short metacarpals; small, delayed teeth; infantile hypotonia	Unknown
Langer-Giedion	8q24.1	Deletion	Multiple exostoses; sparse, thin hair; pear-shaped nose; short metacarpals; small, delayed teeth; infantile hypotonia	Unknown
Potocki-Shaffer	11p11.2	Deletion	Multiple exostoses, skull defects, brachycephaly, developmental delay, genital anomalies	Unknown
WAGR	11p13	Deletion	Wilms tumor, aniridia, genitourinary and renal anomalies, intellectual disability	Unknown
Beckwith-Wiedemann	11p15.5	Paternal uniparental disomy, imprinting defect	Macrosomia, hemihypertrophy, abdominal wall defects, macroglossia, risk for Wilms tumor and hepatoblastoma	1 in 14,000
Prader-Willi	15q11-13	Paternal deletion, imprinting defect	Newborn hypotonia, hyporeflexia, cryptorchidism, failure to thrive that converts to hyperphagia, behavioral problems, intellectual disability	1 in 15,000
Angelman	15q11-13	Maternal deletion, imprinting defect, UBE3A pathogenic variant	Developmental delay, seizures, exaggerated laughter, repetitive hand movements, movement or balance disorder (ataxia and/or tremulousness)	1 in 15,000
Monosomy 15q13	15q13.3	Deletion	Intellectual disability, seizures, autism, neuropsychiatric disorders	Unknown
Monosomy 16p11	16p11.2	Deletion	Developmental delay, autism, seizures, abnormal muscle tone	Unknown
Smith-Magenis	17p11.2	Deletion	Brachycephaly, flat midface, hoarse voice, brachydactyly, intellectual disability, sleep disturbance, hyperactivity, self-destructive behavior	1 in 25,000
Duplication 17p11.2	17p11.2	Duplication	Short stature, mild intellectual disability, behavioral difficulties, dental crowding	Unknown
Hereditary neuropathy with pressure palsies	17p12	Deletion	Peripheral weakness and neuropathy from pressure on nerves	Unknown
Charcot-Marie-Tooth type 1A	17p12	Duplication	Distal limb muscle weakness, decreased motor nerve conduction velocities	Unknown
Miller-Dieker	17p13.3	Deletion	Lissencephaly; prominent forehead; bitemporal narrowing; short, upturned nose; protuberant upper lip; small jaw; profound intellectual disability	Unknown
Monosomy 17q11	17q11.2	Duplication	Potocki-Lupski syndrome: hypotonia, feeding difficulties, failure to thrive, congenital cardiovascular malformations, sleep apnea, developmental delay, verbal apraxia, autism hyperactivity, anxiety	1 in 25,000
Monosomy 17q21	17q21.31	Deletion	Intellectual disability, low birth weight, neonatal hypotonia, poor feeding, oral apraxia	1 in 16,000
Alagille	20p11.23	Deletion, JAG1 pathogenic variant	Chronic cholestasis, triangular facies, peripheral pulmonic stenosis, vertebral anomalies, posterior embryotoxin of eye	1 in 70,000
DiGeorge-velocardiofacial	22q11.2	Deletion	Cardiac conotruncal anomaly, parathyroid hypoplasia, hooded eyelids, bulbous nasal tip, developmental delay	1 in 4000
Cat-eye	22q11.2	Supernumerary marker chromosome	Iris coloboma, anal atresia, down-slanted eyes, ear tags or pits, cardiac or renal malformations	Unknown
Duchenne muscular dystrophy	Xp21	Deletion, pathogenic variant in *DMD1*	Muscular dystrophy	1 in 5000 males

TABLE 80-4 Syndromes Detectable by Chromosomal Microarray and Their Features

Syndrome	Locus	Mechanism	Features	Incidence
Complex glycerol kinase deficiency	Xp21	Deletion, pathogenic variant in *GK*	Glyceroluria, adrenal hypoplasia, ambiguous male genitalia, muscular dystrophy (if inherited as contiguous gene deletion)	Unknown
Adrenal hypoplasia congenita	Xp21	Deletion, pathogenic variant in *NROB1*	Adrenal hypoplasia, ambiguous genitalia	Unknown
Dosage-sensitive sex reversal	Xp21	Duplication associated with segmental duplication, pathogenic variant in *NROB1*	External genitalia appears consistent with typical female and abnormal gonadal development in XY males	Unknown
X-linked ichthyosis	Xp22.3	Deletion or pathogenic variant in *STS*	Dark, scaly skin; steryl-sulfatase deficiency	1 in 5000 males
Kallmann	Xp22.3	Deletion or pathogenic variant in *ANOS1* or *PROKR2*	Hypogonadotropic hypogonadism, anosmia	Unknown
Hemophilia A (severe)	Xq28	Inversion associated or pathogenic variant in *F8*	Bleeding diathesis, factor VIII deficiency	1 in 8000 males
Pelizaeus-Merzbacher	Xq22	Duplication or pathogenic variant in *PLP1*	Progressive neurodegeneration, microcephaly, hypotonia, rotary nystagmus, optic atrophy, head rolling	Unknown

SGA, small for gestational age.

Source: Data from Shaffer LG, Ledbetter DH, Lupski JR. Molecular cytogenetics of contiguous gene syndromes: mechanisms and consequences of gene dosage imbalance. In: Scriver CR, Sly WS, Childs B, et al, eds. *The Metabolic and Molecular Bases of Inherited Disease.* 8th ed. New York: McGraw-Hill; 2001:1291-1324; Emanuel BS, Shaikh TH. Segmental duplications: an "expanding" role in genomic instability and disease. *Nat Rev Genet.* 2001;2:791-800; Slavotinek A. Novel microdeletion syndromes detected by chromosome microarrays. *Hum Genet.* 2008;124:1-17; and Berg JS, Potocki L, Bacino CA. Common recurrent microduplication syndromes: diagnosis and management in clinical practice. *Am J Med Genet.* 2010;152A:1066-1078.

testing is necessary to rule out translocation for predicting recurrence risk.

At diagnosis, workup should include an echocardiogram and renal ultrasound; a brain MRI should be strongly considered to look for structural abnormalities. Owing to the presence of oropharyngeal dysfunction, swallow studies may be beneficial. Ongoing care of these patients includes yearly hearing and vision screening, monitoring for seizure activity, and thyroid function assessment.

CRI DU CHAT SYNDROME (5P DELETION SYNDROME)

Deletion of chromosome 5p is seen in approximately 1 in 37,000 live births. The hallmark clinical feature is a high-pitched, monotonous cry. Other features include low birth weight, microcephaly, hypotonia, dysmorphic facies, and heart defects. These infants tend to be irritable with failure to thrive and pronounced developmental delays. Survival into adulthood is possible, but often with severe intellectual disability.

Management is focused on therapies to ameliorate associated feeding difficulties, motor delays, and behavioral issues. Audiograms should be obtained on a regular basis as sensorineural deafness is a common complication. Mortality is 90% in the first year of life. The severity of the phenotype correlates with the size of the deletion, therefore genetic testing is an important predictor of prognosis.

CMA will detect and size the deletion. Approximately 85% of 5p deletions are *de novo*. The remaining deletions are inherited from a parent carrying a balanced translocation in a carrier parent, which is associated with a 10% to 15% risk of 5p deletion syndrome in a future liveborn child. Therefore, FISH and/or karyotype analysis of both parents is important for predicting risk of recurrence.

WOLF-HIRSCHHORN SYNDROME (4P DELETION SYNDROME)

Distal deletions of chromosome 4p cause Wolf-Hirschhorn syndrome (WHS), which is estimated to occur in 1 in 50,000 births. Infants with WHS demonstrate characteristic craniofacial features described as a "Greek warrior helmet" appearance: a high nasal bridge, that extends onto forehead. They also have microcephaly, hypertelorism with epicanthal folds, high forehead, prominent glabella, and high arched eyebrows. Prominent low-set ears with pits or tags are also seen.

The first signs of WHS are marked intrauterine growth restriction followed by failure to thrive with hypotonia and muscle underdevelopment. Developmental delay and intellectual disability of varying degrees are seen in all patients, and seizures occur in 50% to 100%. Other findings include skeletal anomalies, cleft lip and palate, hearing loss, cardiac septal defects, structural brain anomalies, and urinary tract malformations. Approximately 20% of WHS infants die in the first 2 years of life. Many patients, however, can live into adulthood with profound growth retardation and intellectual disability.

CMA detects WHS. More than 75% of 4p16 deletions arise *de novo*, with a minimal risk of recurrence. About 12% of patients have an unusual cytogenetic abnormality (such as ring chromosome 4), and about 13% are inherited from a parent carrying a balanced translocation. Therefore, patient and/or parental karyotypes are necessary to provide appropriate counseling regarding the recurrence risk.

OVERGROWTH SYNDROMES

BECKWITH-WIEDEMANN SYNDROME

Beckwith-Wiedemann syndrome (BWS) is a disorder of genomic imprinting that typically manifests as an overgrowth syndrome. Characteristic findings are macrosomia, macroglossia, visceromegaly, omphalocele, embryonal tumors, transient neonatal hypoglycemia, and ear creases or pits. Affected infants are large for gestational age, with proportionate weight and length. Advanced bone age, hemihypertrophy due to asymmetrical growth, and visceromegaly of various organs, including the spleen, kidneys, liver, pancreas, and adrenal glands, are often seen. There is an approximately 20% mortality rate in infants with BWS due to complications of omphalocele, macroglossia, neonatal hypoglycemia, and, rarely, cardiomyopathy.

Embryonal tumors seen with BWS include Wilms tumor, hepatoblastoma, neuroblastoma, and rhabdomyosarcoma. Cancer surveillance is important: serum alpha fetoprotein level and abdominal ultrasound should be done prior to birth hospital discharge and continued every 3 months until the fourth birthday. Renal ultrasounds should be performed every 3 months until the seventh birthday. The AFP trend is more informative than any single value. The values should be compared to the norms for BWS patients, which are higher than the general pediatric population.

A variety of genetic mechanisms underlie the known causes of BWS including uniparental disomy of chromosome 11p, loss (or gain) of methylation on the maternal 11p chromosome, paternal uniparental disomy of 11p, chromosomal alterations (translocation, inversion, duplication), or a pathogenic variant on the maternal allele of the *CDKNIC* gene. When BWS is suspected, genetic testing can be initiated with a CMA and methylation studies, followed by *CDKNIC* gene if the former is negative. In about 20% of cases, a genetic cause is not identified, which may be due to mosaicism (genetic change present in some, but not all tissues in the body).

CONNECTIVE TISSUE SYNDROMES

WILLIAMS-BEUREN SYNDROME (7Q11.2 DELETION SYNDROME)

Williams-Beuren syndrome is characterized by distinct facies, cardiovascular disease, growth and developmental delay, a "cocktail party" personality, and occasionally, infantile hypercalcemia. It is due to a deletion on chromosome 7 (7q11.2).

Neonates with this syndrome demonstrate intrauterine growth restriction and mild microcephaly. They may be small for gestational age and subsequently experience poor growth. Facial features include epicanthal folds with periorbital fullness, flat midface, anteverted nostrils, long philtrum, full lips, wide mouth, small jaw, and prominent earlobes. Children have full cheeks, small, widely spaced teeth, and stellate irises that may not be observed at birth. Adults typically have gaunt appearance caused by a long face and neck.

Most infants have a cardiovascular anomaly, most commonly supravalvular aortic stenosis (75%). Peripheral pulmonic stenosis is seen in infancy. Arterial narrowing, including pulmonary artery stenosis is also associated. Severe hypercalcemia occurs in a subset of infants. Other endocrine findings include hypercalciuria, hypothyroidism, and early (not precocious) puberty. Mild to moderate intellectual disability occurs in most patients. The characteristic personality of a patient with Williams-Beuren syndrome includes overfriendliness, excessive empathy, attention problems, and anxiety.

The elastin (*ELN*) gene falls within the deleted region in Williams syndrome. This gene codes the elastin protein, an important component of connective tissue that makes up many organs. This results in findings such as hoarseness, inguinal or umbilical hernia, joint limitation or laxity, and soft "doughy" skin.

The diagnosis is confirmed by CMA or MLPA. Most deletions arise *de novo* and are not inherited from a parent.

MARFAN SYNDROME

Marfan syndrome is an autosomal dominant condition caused by pathogenic variants in the *FBN1* gene, which encodes fibrillin-1, an important extracellular matrix protein. The salient features of this condition include aortic root disease, ectopia lentis, and skeletal deformities. Marfan syndrome commonly presents as a tall, slender individual with a pectal deformity or pneumothorax.

The physical exam in patients with Marfan syndrome may be notable for tall stature, with proportionally long arms and legs, long fingers, scoliosis, pectus deformities, hypermobile joints, and striae. The most common cardiac lesion is aortic root dilation, which puts the individual at high risk for an aortic dissection. Aortic root dilation typically only begins in adolescence. Aortic valve regurgitation, mitral valve prolapse, and mitral valve regurgitation also may occur. Common ophthalmologic complications include myopia, lens dislocation, presenile cataracts, and strabismus (secondary to unilateral dislocated lens).

The Ghent nosology are the consensus clinical criteria for establishing a diagnosis of Marfan Syndrome. The diagnosis is made in the presence of both of the cardinal features: ectopia lentis and dilated aortic root. If one or more of those are absent (which is typical in children with Marfan Syndrome), a pathogenic variant in *FBN1* mutation or positive systemic score is diagnostic. The systemic score includes features such as wrist and/or thumb sign, pneumothorax, anterior chest deformity, and myopia each of which holds a different weight in tabulating the score.

In patients with suspected Marfan Syndrome, an echocardiogram is essential to determine the risk of aortic dissection, which is proportional to the aortic diameter Z-score. Ophthalmologic emergencies include retinal detachment and glaucoma. Skeletal deformities of the chest that may require surgical repair include dyspnea secondary to diminished lung capacity, and compression of cardiac structures.

EHLERS-DANLOS SYNDROME

VASCULAR EDS (vEDS) is a connective tissue disorder caused by a pathogenic variant in *COL3A1*. It is characterized by fragility of skin, arteries, and hollow internal organs. There is a characteristic facial appearance (thin nose and lips, small chin, and prominent eyes). The major complications include arterial aneurysms, vessel dissection or rupture, intestinal rupture, and uterine rupture during pregnancy. Fatality is very high. A patient with any of these or a family history of vEDS should be evaluated for this diagnosis. vEDS is particularly challenging for the pediatrician, as the hallmark features typically do not occur until adulthood. Children more typically present joint hypermobility, easy bruising, thin skin, and/or talipes equinovarus. Neonates may present with hip dislocation, limb deficiencies, or amniotic banding. vEDS is inherited in an autosomal dominant manner, so it is important to screen the children of anyone with known vEDS. Any instance of sudden, severe pain in a patient with vEDS needs to be fully evaluated to rule out vessel or organ rupture. There are no guidelines for evaluation at the time of diagnosis, but visualization of the arterial tree may be beneficial.

Hypermobile EDS (hEDS) is a common non-monogenic clinical entity that spans many medical specialties. It is possibly a heritable condition, and some families demonstrate apparently autosomal dominant transmission and variable expressivity, but there is no known etiology (genetic or otherwise) for this diagnosis. There is a female predominance, like other chronic pain syndromes. Individuals present with complaints related to joint hypermobility or hyperflexibility, chronic pain, fatigue, dysautonomia, gastrointestinal issues, headaches, and neuropsychiatric complaints. Physical exam may reveal soft and hyperextensible skin. Wound healing may be impaired when compared to the general population, but much less so than in other types of EDS. No genetic testing is needed in a patient suspected to have hEDS as long as more serious connective tissue diseases are ruled out clinically. The mainstay of management is physical therapy and treatment should focus on alleviating disease manifestations acutely (e.g., dislocation) and chronically (e.g., pain and fatigue).

CRANIOFACIAL SYNDROMES

Orofacial clefts are one of the most common congenital anomalies. They fall into two distinct categories: cleft lip with or without cleft palate (CL/P) and cleft palate only (CP). CL/P occurs in 1/700 births and is usually unilateral (80%). It is nonsyndromic in about 70% of cases. Midline clefts are rare and may occur with orofaciodigital syndrome, and holoprosencephaly. Cleft palate is less common and entails a spectrum of defects ranging from isolated cleft uvula to complete clefing of the soft and hard palate. It is nonsyndromic in about 50% of cases. CL/P and/or CP are a feature in many genetic diseases.

VAN DER WOUDE SYNDROME

Van der Woude (VWS) is the most common syndromic cause of CL/P. VWS is inherited in an autosomal dominant manner. The syndrome can vary even within a single family from simple lip pits, usually on the inside of the lower lip, to "pseudo-cleft lip" (a congenital appearance of an area of hypotrophic skin along the lip, which looks similar to a surgically corrected cleft lip), CL/P or CP. In about 72% of cases that are clinically consistent with VWS, a pathogenic variant on *IRF6* is identified. All children with unexplained CL/P should be at least clinically evaluated for VWS (taking a careful family history and close physical exam of the proband and all first-degree relatives to look for lip pits and pseudo-cleft lip) because of the recurrence risk.

PIERRE ROBIN SEQUENCE

Pierre Robin Sequence (PRS) describes a developmental triad of mandibular hypoplasia, glossoptosis (downward displacement of the tongue) and upper airway obstruction. The term "sequence," rather than syndrome indicates that it describes a phenotype, rather than a specific cause. PRS is commonly associated with U-shaped cleft palate, which can lead to respiratory and feeding complications. PRS may be caused by a large number of genetic syndromes associated, such as Stickler syndrome (featuring myopia, hearing loss, short stature), Treacher Collins syndrome (featuring lower eyelid colobomas, abnormal ears, zygomatic dysplasia), Trisomy 18, and 22q11.2 deletion syndrome. The *SOX9* gene has been linked to nonsyndromic cases of PRS.

OTHER CAUSES OF CL/P AND CP

Other conditions to consider in association with CL/P or CP include Opitz G/BBB syndrome, Kabuki syndrome, Smith-Lemli Opitz syndrome, X-linked CP ankyloglossia, and ectrodactyly, ectodermal dysplasia and clefting syndrome. Genetics consultation is strongly recommended in an infant with CL/P or CP for diagnostic purposes and genetic counseling for the family.

CRANIOSYNOSTOSIS

Craniosynostosis is defined as premature fusion of one or more cranial sutures. This leads to abnormalities in the shape of the skull, development of the face, and, in some cases, increased intracranial pressure. A CT of the skull gives the most detail, but a skull x-ray is an acceptable first test.

Saggital synostosis is the most common type and causes elongation of the skull. Metopic synostosis occurs in about 15% and creates a triangular shape to the forehead with a noticeable ridge. Unilateral coronal synostosis occurs in about 10% to 15% and leads to asymmetry of the skull and face. Bicoronal synostosis occurs in 5% to 10% and is often related to a genetic syndrome, as is multiple suture involvement.

Syndromic causes of craniosynostosis usually occur *de novo*. When inherited, craniosynostosis is typically autosomal but there are exceptions. Pathogenic variants in the genes for FGF receptors (*FGFR1, FGFR2, FGFR3*, and *MSX2)* cause several known syndromic diagnoses. Although the same genes cause multiple syndromes (Apert, Crouzon, Muenke, and Pfeiffer syndrome), these can be differentiated from each other based on accompanying features. For example, Apert syndrome has a pathognomnic finding of complete syndactyly of the fingers and toes, resulting in a "mitten hand" appearance. Crouzon syndrome features a hooked nose and shallow orbits leading to a bulging appcarancc of the eyes. Muenke syndrome classically also causes brachydactyly and deafness, but the clinical spectrum is broad. In Pfeiffer syndrome pansynostosis of the sutures occurs, which in the most severe form causes a "clover leaf skull." Hand and foot anomalies are also seen in Pfeiffer syndrome.

When craniosynostosis is suspected, head imaging and neurosurgical consultation is of paramount importance given the risk of increased intracranial pressure and compression of brain structures. Expertise of neurosurgeons and plastic surgeons will typically guide any necessary corrective surgeries.

SUGGESTED READINGS

Alfares A, Aloraini T, Subaie LA, et al. Whole-genome sequencing offers additional but limited clinical utility compared with reanalysis of whole-exome sequencing. *Genet Med*. 2018;20(11):1328-1333.

Berg JS, Potocki L, Bacino CA. Common recurrent microduplication syndromes: diagnosis and management in clinical practice. *Am J Med Genet*. 2010;152A:1066-1078.

Botstein D, Risch N. Discovering genotypes underlying human phenotypes: past successes for mendelian disease, future approaches for complex disease. *Nat Genet*. 2003;33(3):228-237.

Bull MJ. Committee on Genetics Health supervision for children with Down syndrome. *Pediatrics*. 2011;128(2), 393–406.

Cassidy SB, Dykens E, Williams CA. Prader-Willi and Angelman syndromes: sister imprinted disorders. *Am J Med Genet*. 2000;97: 136-146.

Clark MM, Stark Z, Farnaes L, et al. Meta-analysis of the diagnostic and clinical utility of genome and exome sequencing and chromosomal microarray in children with suspected genetic diseases. *NPJ Genomic Med*. 2018;3:16.

Emanuel BS, McDonald-McGinn D, Saitta SC, Zackai EH. The 22q11.2 deletion syndrome. *Adv Pediatr*. 2001;48:39-73.

GeneTests. Medical Genetics Information Resource (online database). Seattle: University of Washington, 1993-2013. www.genetests.org.

Gjorgioski S, Halliday J, Riley M, Amor DJ, Delatycki MB, Bankier A. Genetics and pediatric hospital admissions, 1985 to 2017. *Genet Med*. 2020;22(11):1777-1785.

Hall JG, Froster-lskenius UG, Allanson JE. *Handbook of Normal Physical Measurements*. Oxford: Oxford University Press; 1989.

Hall JG, Powers EK, Mcllvaine RT, Ean VH. The frequency and financial burden of genetic disease in a pediatric hospital. *Am J Med Genet*. 1978;1(4):417-436. doi:10.1002/ajmg.1320010405

Heilstedt HA, Ballif BC, Howard LA, et al. Population data suggest that deletions of 1p36 are a relatively common chromosome abnormality. *Clin Genet*. 2003;64:310-316.

Higurashi M, Oda M, lijima S, et al. Livebirth prevalence and follow-up of malformation syndromes in 27,472 newborns. *Brain Dev*. 1990;12:770-773.

Jones KL. *Smith's Recognizable Patterns of Human Malformation*. 5th ed. Philadelphia, PA: WB Saunders; 1997.

Manickam K, McClain MR, Demmer LA, et al. Exome and genome sequencing for pediatric patients with congenital anomalies or intellectual disability: an evidence-based clinical guideline of the American College of Medical Genetics and Genomics (ACMG). *Genet Med*. 2021;23(11):2029-2037.

McCandless SE, Brunger JW, Cassidy SB. The burden of genetic disease on inpatient care in a children's hospital. *Am J Hum Genet*. 2004;74(1):121-127.

McDonald-McGinn D, Emanuel BS, Zackai EH. 22q11.2 deletion syndrome. Gene Reviews 2013. www.genetests.org.

McDonald-McGinn DM, LaRossa D, Goldmuntz E, et al. The 22q11.2 deletion: Screening, diagnostic workup, and outcome of results; report on 181 patients. *Genet Test*. 1997;1:99-108.

Milewicz DM, Braverman AC, De Backer J, et al. Marfan syndrome [published correction appears in Nat Rev Dis Primers. 2022;8(1):3]. *Nat Rev Dis Primers*. 2021;7(1):64.

Online Mendelian Inheritance in Man (OMIM). Baltimore: McKusick-Nathans Institute for Genetic Medicine, Johns Hopkins University, and National Center for Biotechnology Information, National Library of Medicine. 2013.

Scriver CR, Neal JL, Saginur R, Clow A. The frequency of genetic disease and congenital malformation among patients in a pediatric hospital. *Can Med Assoc J*. 1973;108(9):1111-1115.

Shaffer LG, Lupski JR. Molecular mechanisms for constitutional chromosomal rearrangements in humans. *Annu Rev Genet*. 2000;34: 297-329.

Shannon NL, Maltby EL, Rigby AS, Quarrell OW. An epidemiological study of Wolf-Hirschhorn syndrome: life expectancy and cause of mortality. *J Med Genet*. 2001;38:674-679.

Shuman C, Weksberg R. Beckwith-Wiedemann syndrome. Gene Reviews 2010. www.genetests.org.

Sybert VP, McCauley E. Turner's syndrome. *N Engl J Med*. 2004;351: 1227-1238.

Tinkle B, Castori M, Berglund B, et al. Hypermobile Ehlers-Danlos syndrome (a.k.a. Ehlers-Danlos syndrome Type III and Ehlers-Danlos syndrome hypermobility type): Clinical description and natural history. *Am J Med Genet C Semin Med Genet*. 2017;175(1): 48-69.

Yoon PW, Olney RS, Khoury MJ, Sappenfield WM, Chavez GF, Taylor D. Contribution of birth defects and genetic diseases to pediatric hospitalizations: a population-based study. *Arch Pediatr Adolesc Med*. 1997;151(11):1096-1103.

Zackai EH, Anyane-Yeboa K, Bergoffen J, et al. Genetics. In: Polin RA, Ditmar MF, eds. *Pediatric Secrets*. Philadelphia, PA: Hanley & Belfus; 2001:731.

CHAPTER 81

Hyperammonemia

Laura O'Neill, MD, MS, MEd and Karen L. Smith, MD, MEd

BACKGROUND

PATHOPHYSIOLOGY

Ammonia, the nitrogen-containing waste product of protein metabolism, is extremely toxic at high concentrations. Under normal circumstances, blood ammonia is cleared rapidly by the urea cycle, a biochemical pathway in hepatocytes that converts ammonia into water-soluble urea, which can then be excreted in urine (**Figure 81-1**). This system keeps ammonia levels under 100 μM/L in neonates and generally 20 to 60 μM/L in infants and older children. Elevated blood ammonia levels (hyperammonemia) trigger a variety of neurotoxic consequences that result in aberrant neurotransmitter levels and cerebral edema, causing severe and potentially irreversible injury to the central nervous system.

Hyperammonemia occurs during periods of "nitrogen imbalance," when nitrogen load exceeds the capacity for clearance. Nitrogen load is proportional to circulating amino acid levels, which are the result of both dietary protein intake and breakdown of endogenous protein (e.g., from muscle). Nitrogen clearance depends primarily on the ability of the liver to perform the urea cycle. Therefore, diseases that drastically increase nitrogen load or compromise liver function can result in hyperammonemia. Restoring nitrogen balance is the main goal in treating hyperammonemia. The urea cycle defects (UCDs) are an important category of diseases that present with severe hyperammonemia and are the main focus of this chapter.

CLINICAL PRESENTATION

Symptoms associated with hyperammonemia primarily reflect ammonia's neurotoxicity; therefore, hyperammonemia should be considered in patients with unexplained changes in mental status, encephalopathy, or signs of increased intracranial pressure (**Table 81-1**). A longitudinal study of children with UCDs revealed that children usually present with neurologic findings (80%) and/or gastrointestinal complaints (33%) such as vomiting and poor feeding. In addition, this study found that many patients with UCDs presented beyond the neonatal period.

The typical presentation of hyperammonemia in neonates with UCDs is an unremarkable term gestation newborn who is well for the first few days of life. However, normal increased protein intake leads to nitrogen imbalance and hyperammonemia in these infants, usually within the first week of life. A retrospective analysis of 74 infants with ornithine transcarbamoylase (OTC) deficiency, the most common UCD, demonstrated a mean onset of illness at 63 hours of life, with a range of 12 to 240 hours. In neonates, symptoms of hyperammonemia may be impossible to distinguish from those of sepsis: decreased activity, poor feeding, encephalopathy, and seizure. An important distinguishing characteristic is that neonates with hyperammonemia may have a primary respiratory alkalosis (average pH 7.5, with a PCO_2 of 24) because ammonia stimulates hyperventilation. Furthermore, these infants usually fail to improve after fluid resuscitation and antimicrobial therapy; instead, neurologic symptoms may progress to coma. In such cases, a UCD should be strongly suspected.

Although most presentations are neonatal, late-onset UCD may present throughout life. In older children, hyperammonemia may be even harder to identify because symptoms are either nonspecific (cyclic vomiting, headache, poor appetite) or easily confused with more common problems such as drug abuse or primary psychiatric disease (acute mental status changes, frank psychosis). A complete dietary history is important since children with UCD will often self-restrict protein intake by refusing or limiting high-protein foods such as meat and cheese.

Children with most types of UCDs have a lifetime risk of hyperammonemia episodes, which usually occur when a new nitrogen imbalance is introduced. This may be caused by dietary protein intake in excess of protein needs or catabolic stress-induced muscle protein turnover, which occurs during prolonged fasting, fever, or increased exercise. Protein needs change with age, linear growth rate and skeletal muscle mass; therefore, tolerated protein amounts may vary throughout an individual's life and vary between individuals. Blood ammonia levels can increase rapidly during these periods, and prompt treatment is critical. Similarly, children with mild forms of UCDs may not suffer an initial hyperammonemia crisis until an illness during infancy or even later in childhood or adolescence when nitrogen imbalance causes acute mental status changes or other signs of hyperammonemia.

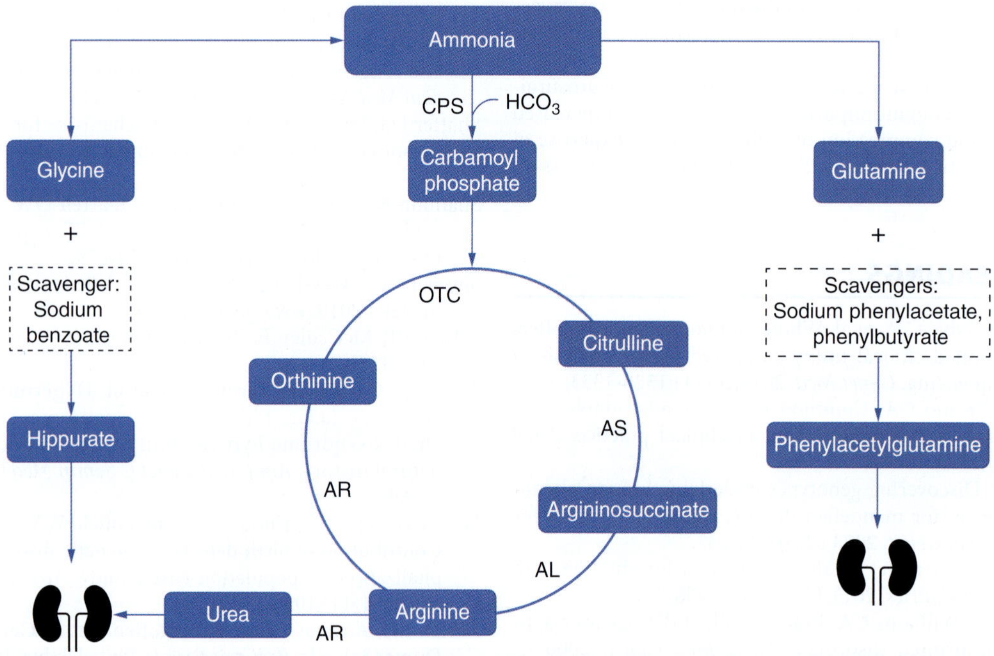

FIGURE 81-1. The urea cycle. The most common urea cycle defects are abbreviated as follows: AL, argininosuccinic acid lyase; AR, arginase; AS, argininosuccinic acid synthetase; CPS, carbamoyl phosphate synthetase; OTC, ornithine transcarbamoylase. Pharmacologic treatments used in the scavenger pathway are indicated by boxes with dotted lines.

In such patients, a thorough history may reveal the cause of the imbalance, such as a sudden increase in dietary protein intake or a dramatic increase in exercise.

DIFFERENTIAL DIAGNOSIS

Although numerous inborn errors of metabolism present in the neonatal period, it is important to remember that many cases of hyperammonemia are due to acquired problems (**Table 81-2**). Neonates with hyperammonemia should be carefully evaluated for treatable problems, especially infection with either bacterial pathogens or herpes simplex virus. In addition, liver function should be evaluated, because hyperammonemia is a complication of liver failure from a variety of causes. Transient hyperammonemia of the newborn (THAN), a phenomenon that generally occurs in premature infants with pulmonary disease, may present similar to UCDs, causing ammonia levels to rise high enough to induce coma. The precise biochemical defect responsible for THAN is not known, and symptoms tend to resolve after initial treatment, often without neurologic sequelae. These children do not have recurrences and tolerate normal amounts of dietary protein.

Metabolic causes of hyperammonemia include diseases that compromise the urea cycle either directly (e.g., UCDs) or indirectly through hepatic toxicity (Table 81-2). Although a definitive diagnosis of these disorders usually requires metabolic testing, a reasonable differential diagnosis can be established based on the results of common screening tests. For example, the presence of hypoglycemia is more consistent with fatty acid oxidation defects or defects in carbohydrate utilization (e.g., galactosemia, hereditary fructose intolerance) rather than UCD. Although hyperammonemia in UCD can be associated with respiratory alkalosis, the absence of respiratory alkalosis does not rule out UCD. Respiratory alkalosis may disappear as cerebral edema progresses; this normalization may be a sign of advanced ammonia intoxication. The presence of metabolic acidosis should raise suspicion for an organic acidemia or a primary lactic acidosis syndrome, such as pyruvate carboxylase deficiency. In nearly all states, newborn screening programs provide diagnostic information within the first week of life that can rule in or rule out many inborn errors associated with hyperammonemia; however, while specific, the newborn screen is not sensitive to distal UCDs. In these instances, a prompt call to the newborn screening laboratory may allow the physician to establish a tentative diagnosis and proceed with a logical round of confirmatory tests and presumptive treatment.

Collectively, the UCDs have an incidence of roughly 1 in 35,000, with OTC deficiency being the most common disease by far. The UCDs are autosomal recessive disorders, with the exception of OTC deficiency, which is X-linked. As a result, the classic presentation of OTC deficiency in an affected male is catastrophic neonatal hyperammonemia. In females, the severity is determined in large part by the pattern of hepatic X-inactivation; depending on the skewing, patients may be essentially asymptomatic or severely affected. In addition, as with most inborn errors of metabolism, the phenotype depends on the severity of the pathogenic variant and the amount of residual enzyme activity. Therefore, in both sexes, a less deleterious variant can leave a relatively high amount of residual enzyme activity and result in a milder phenotype.

Arginase deficiency differs from other UCDs in that its clinical course is characterized by chronic, progressive neurologic dysfunction rather than catastrophic hyperammonemia crises, although these episodes may occasionally occur as well. Symptoms include progressive spastic diplegia or quadriplegia, ataxia, and choreoathetosis.

TABLE 81-1 Symptoms Associated With Hyperammonemia

Neonates
Decreased activity
Poor feeding
Acid–base disturbance (classically respiratory alkalosis)
Clinical signs of increased intracranial pressure
Emesis
Seizures
May progress to coma if not corrected
Infants and Children
Decreased appetite
Emesis
Headache
Acute or progressive mental status disturbance
Mood lability
Aggression, combativeness
Psychosis
Neurologic deficits
May progress to coma if not corrected

TABLE 81-2 Differential Diagnosis of Hyperammonemia

Acquired Causes
Liver failure (various causes)
Infection
Sepsis
Hepatitis
Infection with urease-positive bacteria
Herpes simplex virus infection
Iatrogenic
Valproic acid
Asparaginase
Severe hypovolemia
Transient hyperammonemia of the newborn
Perinatal depression
Intrinsic Causes (Inborn Errors of Metabolism)
Urea cycle defects
Ornithine transcarbamoylase deficiency
Argininosuccinic acid synthetase deficiency (citrullinemia)
Argininosuccinic acid lyase deficiency
Carbamoyl phosphate synthetase deficiency
N-Acetyl glutamate synthetase deficiency
Arginase deficiency
Organic acidemias
Methylmalonicacidemia
Isovalericacidemia
Propionicacidemia
Multiple carboxylase deficiency
Others
Fatty acid oxidation defects
Long-chain fatty acid oxidation defects
Multiple acyl-CoA dehydrogenase deficiency
Hyperornithinemia-hyperammonemia-homocitrullinemia syndrome
Pyruvate carboxylase deficiency
Hyperammonemia-hyperinsulinemia syndrome
Galactosemia
Hereditary fructose intolerance

DIAGNOSTIC EVALUATION

Table 81-3 outlines the laboratory evaluation that should be considered in patients with hyperammonemia. A plasma ammonia level greater than 150 μM with a normal anion gap and normal glucose is particularly concerning for a UCD. Ammonia levels need to be

TABLE 81-3 Laboratory Studies for Hyperammonemic Children

Initial laboratory studies
- Electrolytes
- Blood glucose
- Liver enzymes
- Coagulation studies (for liver synthetic function)
- Blood gas (pH, PCO2, lactate)
- Plasma amino acids
- Urinalysis for ketones and reducing substances
- Urine for organic acids and orotic acid

Studies to consider
- Infectious workup if sepsis is a possibility
- Plasma acylcarnitine profile (for fatty acid oxidation defects)
- Lactate, pyruvate if elevated lactate on blood gas

obtained from free-flowing blood, transported immediately to the laboratory on ice, and processed within 15 minutes to ensure accuracy. In many cases, the initial workup rapidly narrows the differential diagnosis. This is especially true for UCDs, in which the combination of hyperammonemia and amino acid abnormalities is often suggestive of a particular disorder (**Table 81-4**). Emergent intervention to treat hyperammonemia must begin as soon as an elevated ammonia level is known; however, the ability to identify the specific UCD within a few hours allows ongoing treatment to be tailored accordingly.

If the initial workup uncovers metabolic abnormalities in addition to hyperammonemia (e.g., metabolic acidosis with a high anion gap, hypoglycemia), the child could have some other type of inborn error of metabolism. For example, both organic acidemias and fatty acid oxidation defects can present with hyperammonemia crises in neonates and can be diagnosed with additional metabolic tests.

Expanded newborn screening using tandem mass spectrometry can diagnose distal UCDs, including citrullinemia, argininemia, and argininosuccinic acid lyase deficiency. This may allow newborns to be placed on carefully tailored diets before suffering an initial episode of hyperammonemia. Unfortunately, the onset of illness may occur before the results of screening tests are received. If there is suspicion of a UCD in a symptomatic newborn, most laboratories can rush the processing and provide results in 1 to 2 days. The newborn screen is not sensitive for OTC deficiency, therefore a high index of suspicion for OTC should be maintained for a hyperammonemic patient even in the face of a normal newborn screen.

TABLE 81-4 Specific Amino Acid Abnormalities in Urea Cycle Defects

Deficiency	Amino Acid Abnormality	Orotic Acid
Ornithine transcarbamoylase	Elevated glutamine	Increased
	Decreased citrulline, arginine	
Argininosuccinic acid synthetase (citrullinemia)	Massively increased citrulline	Increased
	Decreased arginine	
Argininosuccinic acid lyase	Elevated citrulline, argininosuccinic acid (may not be detected in all laboratories)	Increased or normal
	Decreased arginine	
Arginase	Elevated arginine	Increased or normal
Carbamoyl phosphate synthetase	Elevated glutamine	Decreased or Normal
	Decreased citrulline, arginine	

Source: Data from Bachman C. Inherited hyperammonemias. In: Blau N, Duran M, Blaskovics ME, Gibson KM, eds. *Physician's Guide to the Laboratory Diagnosis of Metabolic Diseases*. 2nd ed. New York: Springer; 2003.

HOSPITAL MANAGEMENT

The treatment guidelines outlined in this section reflect the recommendations of the 2001 Consensus Conference for the Management of Patients with Urea Cycle Disorders. Because of the potential for rapid deterioration and mortality associated with UCDs and other inborn errors of metabolism, a metabolic specialist should be contacted immediately when one of these diseases is suspected. However, management can and should be initiated by the general practitioner. Immediate management of patients with UCD-related hyperammonemia should focus on supportive care of ABCs (airway, breathing, circulation), reversing the nitrogen imbalance by eliminating protein intake, initiating intravenous dextrose infusion to reverse catabolism (typically twice the maintenance rate with 10% dextrose; D10), and improving ammonia clearance.

Patients with hyperammonemia secondary to UCDs who present with mental status changes require rapid mobilization of resources and constant monitoring in an intensive care unit. Once the patient's respiratory and circulatory status has been stabilized, access should be obtained and intravenous infusion with a D10-based solution at twice the maintenance rate should be initiated. If intravenous nitrogen-scavenging agents are used, they should be given in D10W or D10/¼NS solutions. No amino acid–containing solutions should be used during this critical initial period (typically the first 24-48 hours). Intralipids may be useful to boost caloric intake and prevent catabolism.

AMMONIA CLEARANCE

Hemodialysis is the most efficient means of reducing blood ammonia levels in UCD patients. The decision to pursue hemodialysis should be made in conjunction with metabolic, nephrology, and intensive care specialists. The severity of hyperammonemia and clinical symptoms usually determine the need for hemodialysis. If hemodialysis is not available, hemofiltration or another method of dialysis can be used, but they are less effective. Some authors recommend continuing hemodialysis until the ammonia level falls below 200 μM.

In addition to dialysis, nitrogen scavengers sodium phenylacetate and sodium benzoate can help reduce blood ammonia via urinary excretion of alternate nitrogenous wastes. Central intravenous access is recommended for medication administration because of the potential for local tissue necrosis. Recommended doses for scavenging medications are given in **Table 81-5**. These medications are given as an initial loading dose in D10 over 90 minutes, followed by a continuous infusion of the same dose, but given over the next 24 hours. Repeating the loading dose is not recommended, even for patients on hemodialysis, because toxic levels of scavenger drugs can be lethal. Once the serum ammonia level is below 100 μM and stable, intravenous scavenger treatment can be converted to oral supplements by providing sodium benzoate and sodium phenylbutyrate, or glycerol phenylbutyrate. Depending on the type of UCD, other supplements should also be given, such as citrulline for OTC deficiency, and arginine for citrullinemia or argininosuccinic acid lyase deficiency to replete the urea cycle and provide essential amino acids.

LABORATORY MONITORING

In the most acute phase of treatment, while on hemodialysis, ammonia level should be checked every hour until the level is less than 300 μM. Other laboratory testing, such as blood gas, electrolytes, and glucose, should also be frequently monitored (every 4 hours). Once ammonia levels have stabilized, testing frequency can be reduced to every 4 to 6 hours. When patient is no longer on hemodialysis, ammonia levels should be checked every 12 to 24 hours. It is important for clinicians to remember to monitor sodium levels as both intravenous and oral scavenging medications can lead to sodium overload. Daily plasma amino acids are also useful for assessing the reversal of metabolic decompensation.

NUTRITION

Slow introduction of protein should begin in approximately 24 to 48 hours to provide essential amino acids and prevent ongoing protein

TABLE 81-5 Nitrogen Scavenger Therapy for Urea Cycle Defects

Deficiency	Sodium Phenylacetate	Sodium Benzoate	Arginine Hydrochloride*
Children			
Presumed UCD, undiagnosed type	250 mg/kg	250 mg/kg	600 mg/kg
CPS, OTC	250 mg/kg	250 mg/kg	200 mg/kg
AS, AL	250 mg/kg	250 mg/kg	600 mg/kg
Adolescents, adults			
CPS, OTC	5.5 g/m^2	5.5 g/m^2	4.0 g/m^2
AS, AL	5.5 g/m^2	5.5 g/m^2	12 g/m^2

*10% solution.

AL, argininosuceinic acid lyase deficiency; AS, argininosuccinic acid synthetase deficiency; CPS, carbamoyl phosphate synthetase deficiency; OTC, ornithine transcarbamoylase deficiency; UCD, urea cycle defect.

Source: Modified from Summar M. Current strategies for the management of neonatal urea cycle disorders. *J Pediatr.* 2001;138:S30-S34.

turnover. An initial amount of 1 to 1.5 g protein/kg per day is reasonable; this should be coordinated with a nutritionist to ensure that at least 50% of the essential amino acids are provided. Protein intake can be gradually increased toward baseline during the course of hospitalization. Enteral feeding should resume when gastrointestinal and mental status abnormalities have resolved. Enteral feeding may utilize medical foods that provide just essential amino acids ("incomplete protein") in addition to a source of complete protein (e.g., breast milk or traditional formula).

ADMISSION AND DISCHARGE CRITERIA

ADMISSION

It is crucial that patients with UCDs be admitted for intravenous nutrition with an adequate amount of carbohydrate (with or without lipids) to stop or prevent catabolism. A patient with a known or suspected UCD should be admitted for any of the following criteria:

- Inability to take adequate oral or enteral nutrition
- Persistent vomiting
- Elevated blood ammonia levels either above normal or above the baseline for a patient with a known UCD
- Admission to an intensive care unit is recommended for patients with altered mental status or hemodynamic compromise

DISCHARGE

A patient with a UCD is appropriate for discharge when the following criteria are met:

- Ammonia level has fallen and stabilized at normal or near-normal values.
- Toleration of a low-protein diet, and the parent is able to obtain the appropriate formula or diet.
- The parent is able to obtain the appropriate medications. (Even some large nationwide pharmacies do not carry these medications and may not be able to order them.)
- Appropriate follow-up has been arranged.

CONSULTATION

Metabolic specialists should be involved with the care of children with hyperammonemia or UCDs. They can offer guidance to confirm or refute a diagnosis, and they are essential for the ongoing management of these children, especially for the management of acute decompensation. Infants and children with UCDs are at risk for developmental disabilities and should be evaluated by the appropriate local county or state early intervention services.

SPECIAL CONSIDERATIONS

PROGNOSIS

Children with neonatal-onset of UCDs have the highest mortality (65%) compared to those with later onset UCD and those neonates who do survive will most likely suffer some degree of neurologic disability. Infants not treated early will be severely disabled, and many will not survive the initial presentation. One study of neonates with UCD found a 94% survival rate for neonates with a maximal ammonia level of 500 μM/L compared to a 38% survival rate with a maximal level of 1000 μM/L. Other studies have shown that neurologic outcome can be predicted based on the duration of encephalopathic coma with poor results for comas lasting longer than 48 hours. Presentation in late infancy or childhood usually results in a better outcome with a survival rate of 78% to 87%. Even children with mild disease are at risk for neurologic disability, although optimal management is associated with better developmental outcomes.

PREVENTION

Intensive parental and patient education on dietary limitations, the early signs of elevated ammonia, and situations likely to result in increased ammonia (e.g. illness with vomiting or poor oral intake) is essential to maximize the child's developmental potential. Parents should be given a written treatment protocol explaining the disease and the appropriate therapy. This document is especially useful when the pediatric patient requires treatment in an emergency room or other facility not familiar with UCDs. Healthcare providers may not be aware that aggressive management is necessary for what may appear to be a minor illness.

RECENT ADVANCEMENTS

Pharmaceutical In 2013, the Food and Drug Administration (FDA) approved a new medication, glycerol phenylbutyrate (GPB), for the chronic management of UCDs in children (2 years and older) and adults. The advantages of GPB over standard nitrogen scavengers, such as sodium benzoate and sodium phenylbutyrate, include improved tolerability with no taste and slow release of phenylbutyrate, resulting in more stable control of ammonia levels throughout a 24-hour period. GPB is an oil and the patient must have appropriate pancreas function. GPB can be prescribed by body surface area or per protein intake and urea synthesis capability.

Transplant In the past two decades, liver transplant has emerged as a potential curative treatment in some patients with UCDs and organic acidemias (OA). However, the benefits of liver transplant for resolution of hyperammonemia crises must be balanced with the morbidity and mortality risks of liver transplant and lifelong immunosuppression. From 2002 to 2020, the United Network of Organ Sharing (UNOS) reported 424 children with UCDs were listed for transplant and 403 were successfully transplanted. The UCD types receiving liver transplant included ornithine transcarbamylase deficiency (46.2%), citrullinemia (20.3%), and argininosuccinic aciduria (12.9%). The 1-, 3-, and 5-year graft survival rates were 90.4%, 86.3%, and 85.2%, respectively. The majority (59%) of liver transplants for UCDs were performed in children less than 2 years of age. Other studies have documented the 5-year patient survival was 88% for children less than 2 years old vs. 99% for children 2 years old or greater at the time of transplant. Even with a successful liver transplant, children with UCDs were more likely to have cognitive and motor delays compared to other children receiving a liver transplant. As experience and success with long-term transplant increases, this may become the treatment of choice for all children with moderate to severe UCDs.

KEY POINTS

- Respiratory alkalosis in a newborn with poor feeding and lethargy should prompt an immediate evaluation of ammonia levels and raise concern for a UCD.
- In older children, mental status changes out of proportion to the level of illness or frequent episodes of vomiting should raise suspicion of a UCD.
- Testing for inborn errors of metabolism should be done immediately on presentation, because abnormalities often resolve with appropriate IV fluids and therapy.
- If there is a concern for possible UCD, immediately stop protein consumption and start dextrose (D10) at twice maintenance rate (± lipids) to reverse the catabolic state.
- Decrease ammonia levels promptly with hemodialysis and the use of scavenger pathways.
- Catabolic states including fasting and fever should be avoided, and if a patient cannot tolerate oral nutrition, intravenous dextrose should be started immediately and ammonia level checked.
- A minor illness to a child with a metabolic disorder can be life-threatening. Prompt treatment and involvement of a metabolic specialist is essential.

SUGGESTED READINGS

Batshaw ML, Tuchman M, Summar M, et al. A longitudinal study of urea cycle disorders. *Mol Genet Metal.* 2014;113(0):127-130.

Brusilow SW. Hyperammonemic encephalopathy. *Medicine.* 2002;81: 240-249.

Burton BK. Inborn errors of metabolism in infancy: a guide to diagnosis. *Pediatrics.* 1998;102:E69.

Enns GM, Berry SA, Berry GT, et al. Survival after treatment with phenylacetate and benzoate for urea-cycle disorders. *N Engl J Med.* 2007;356:2282-2292.

Glycerol Phenylbutyrate (Ravicti) [Internet]. Ottawa (ON): Canadian Agency for Drugs and Technologies in Health; 2017 Apr. 1, INTRODUCTION. Available from: https://www.ncbi.nlm.nih.gov/books/NBK476305/.

Maestri NE, Clissold D, Brusilow SW. Neonatal onset ornithine transcarbamylase deficiency: a retrospective analysis. *J Pediatr.* 1999;134: 268-272.

Perito ER, Rhee S, Roberts JP, Rosenthal P. Pediatric liver transplantation for urea cycle disorders and organic acidemias: United Network for Organ Sharing data for 2002-2012. *Liver Transpl.* 2014; 20(1):89-99.

Summar M. Current strategies for the management of neonatal urea cycle disorders. *J Pediatr.* 2001;138:S30-S34.

Summar M, Dobbelaere D, Brusilow S, et al. Diagnosis, symptoms, frequency and mortality of 260 patients with urea cycle disorders from a 21-year, multicenter study of acute hyperammoniaemic episodes. *Acta Paed.* 2008;97:1420-1425.

Summar M, Tuchman M. Proceedings of a consensus conference for the management of patients with urea cycle disorders. *J Pediatr.* 2001;138:S6-S20.

Urea Cycle Disorders Conference Group. Consensus statement from a conference for the management of patients with urea cycle disorders. *J Pediatr.* 2001;138:S1-S5.

U.S. Department of Health and Human Services. (2011) Secretary's Advisory Committee on Heritable Disorders in Newborns and Children. www.hrsa.gov/advisorycommittees/mchbadvisory/heritabledisorders/recommendedpanel/index.html. Accessed July 1, 2022.

Ziogas IA, Wu WK, Matsuoka LK, et al. Liver transplantation in children with urea cycle disorders: the importance of minimizing waiting time. *Liver Transpl.* 2021;27(12):1799-1810.

CHAPTER 82 Hypoglycemia

Herodes Guzman, MD, MPH and Rebecca D. Ganetzky, MD

BACKGROUND

Hypoglycemia is the most common biochemical emergency in pediatric patients. Therefore, the ability to efficiently evaluate and treat this condition is essential for the pediatric hospitalist. Four broad categories of problems can cause hypoglycemia: loss of homeostatic control, inadequate caloric intake, intoxication with a substance that induces low blood sugar, and inborn errors in the utilization, production, or release of sugar. In normal physiology, there is a balance of supply and demand to maintain normal blood sugar (euglycemia) through a high variety of environmental conditions.

Euglycemia is maintained by balancing of glucose intake and production with glucose consumption. In the immediate postprandial period, there is a transient increase in the blood glucose level from glucose provided by digested food. However, this rapidly normalizes, primarily through the action of insulin, which promotes the consumption and storage of glucose. In all cells, glucose is consumed primarily through the glycolytic pathway, by which the breakdown of glucose produces energy in the form of adenosine triphosphate (ATP), as well as products that can be further used in the tricarboxylic acid cycle or for lipogenesis. Insulin also promotes the uptake of glucose into the liver, where it is stored in the form of glycogen.

By 3 hours after the last meal, glucose production is needed to maintain euglycemia. Initially, this is done by glycogenolysis—the fast release of free glucose via the breakdown of liver glycogen. However, after about 8 to 12 hours glycogen stores are exhausted and glucose is synthesized (gluconeogenesis) from amino acids and triglycerides. As fasting time lengthens into days, although euglycemia is maintained, the glucose level is lower. The maintenance of euglycemia in the face of fasting is coordinated by several hormones, including glucagon, cortisol, epinephrine, and norepinephrine.

Different organ systems have distinct roles in glucose homeostasis. Different organs also have different energy demands and different avidities for glucose as an energy source. The brain preferentially consumes glucose and is responsible for 15% to 18% of glucose consumption. The liver is the most important buffer for blood glucose, storing glucose as glycogen during times of excess and providing glucose from glycogenolysis and gluconeogenesis during times of fasting. Muscle produces glucose only for use within the myocyte and cannot release it into circulation. Adipose tissue provides energy in the form of fatty acids that can be used as a glucose-sparing fuel during fasting.

Ketogenesis is a key component of the normal physiological response to fasting. Ketones are produced by the breakdown of fatty acids. Ketones are a glucose-sparing energy source, as they can enter the tricarboxylic acid cycle to drive the production of ATP. Fatty acid oxidation is also critical to maintaining euglycemia, as in addition to producing ketones, fatty acid oxidation provides the necessary ATP for gluconeogenesis.

CLINICAL PRESENTATION

As hypoglycemia develops, catabolic hormones are released as a counterregulatory measure. Chief among these enzymes are epinephrine and norepinephrine. Therefore, the earliest manifestations of hypoglycemia are sympathetic symptoms, such as diaphoresis, pallor, and tachycardia. Because the brain is a major consumer of glucose, if hypoglycemia persists, neurologic symptoms are manifest, including fatigue, altered mental status, seizures, and ultimately coma. These symptoms are neither invariantly present nor specific to hypoglycemia. Therefore, clinicians should maintain a low threshold to suspect hypoglycemia, particularly in a child with neurologic manifestations.

Although hypoglycemia is common, controversy exists about laboratory cutoffs for hypoglycemia. Most sources agree that a blood glucose less than 50 mg/dL (40 mg/dL in neonates) warrants urgent correction. This level is chosen because of evidence that shows lower levels may produce long-term neurologic sequelae. Patients who have symptomatic hypoglycemia should be immediately corrected, regardless of the value of their blood glucose. Diagnostic workup of persistent or recurrent hypoglycemia should be pursued, even if it does not meet this threshold.

Newborns as a population are at special risk of hypoglycemia. There are several reasons for this: (i) Glucose is provided *in utero* through placental circulation. Within 2 hours of separation from placental circulation, blood glucose nadirs. Glucose does not stabilize until 4 to 6 hours postpartum. (ii) The brain is proportionally larger in newborns and therefore there is increased glucose demand per body weight as compared to different age groups. (iii) Newborns have small glycogen stores. (iv) Several biochemical pathways, including glycogenolysis, ketogenesis, and gluconeogenesis, are immature in the newborn, resulting in poor response to fasting.

In addition to these physiologic factors, several common conditions can lead to hypoglycemia in the newborn. In the normal newborn, primary factors include hypothermia, delayed feeding, or difficultly with breastfeeding. Infants of mothers with diabetes may have high insulin levels from placental circulation, predisposing them to hypoglycemia. Infants who have intrauterine growth restriction or who are small for gestational age may have an exaggerated physiologic nadir, with particularly low glycogen stores and particularly high brain to bodyweight ratios.

The symptoms of hypoglycemia may be subtle in newborns. Therefore, a low index of suspicion must be maintained and all infants with symptoms such as poor feeding, hypothermia, jitteriness, or lethargy should have a blood glucose checked. To help expedite diagnosis of hypoglycemia in the newborn period, nurseries should have a standard protocol for glucose monitoring that identifies infants at risk for hypoglycemia, including infants of mothers with diabetes, infants who are large for gestational age, and infants who are small for gestational age.

It is extremely important to note that hypoglycemia with neurologic symptoms may be the hallmark of other serious problems, including sepsis and inborn errors of metabolism. Neonates in distress who do not respond to or cannot tolerate oral or gavage feedings with breast milk or formula need rapid administration of intravenous dextrose and a full diagnostic evaluation that includes screening for sepsis, endocrinopathies, and inborn errors of metabolism.

DIFFERENTIAL DIAGNOSIS

EXTRINSIC CAUSES OF HYPOGLYCEMIA

Extrinsic causes are among the most frequent cause of hypoglycemia in the pediatric population; most common is ingestion of oral hypoglycemics. These medications affect glucose metabolism through several distinct mechanisms. Thiazolidinediones sensitize target cells to insulin so that glucose clearance from the bloodstream is increased, metformin interferes with glucose production by the liver, and sulfonylureas increase insulin secretion. All these medications may lead to hypoglycemia in a normal child, but the effects of sulfonylurea poisoning can be the most severe.

Insulin overdose should be suspected in patients with diabetes. Accidental overdose, insulin pump misuse, iatrogenic error, and factitious disorder imposed on self or another are all possible causes. Home glucagon kits are always provided to pediatric patients with insulin-dependent diabetes to correct insulin overdose.

Alcohol may also cause hypoglycemia. It leads to symptoms by blocking gluconeogenesis. The actual frequency of alcohol-induced hypoglycemia is quite low; however, the hypoglycemic effect of alcohol is an important factor in the care of all inebriated children, because they are often unwilling or unable to eat and may have had a prolonged fast by the time they reach medical attention.

INTRINSIC CAUSES OF HYPOGLYCEMIA

The intrinsic causes of hypoglycemia can be loosely grouped into the following subcategories: inborn errors of carbohydrate metabolism, inborn errors of fatty acid oxidation, glycogen storage disorders, deficiencies of counterregulatory hormones, and hyperinsulinism. Patients may also have hypoglycemic crises precipitated by attempted fasting, times of increased caloric need (such as illness), or ingestion of foods that cannot be properly metabolized.

Children with intrinsic metabolic defects tend to present with repeated bouts of hypoglycemia. One clue to the presence of an underlying metabolic defect is severity of hypoglycemia and symptoms out of proportion to the length of fasting. The history and physical examination in patients with suspected inborn errors of metabolism may reveal hepatomegaly due to hepatic steatosis or storage of glycogen, abnormal odors of sweat and/or urine, feeding aversions, events precipitated by specific foods, fasting or viral infections and/or unexplained episodes of acidosis during prior illnesses.

Hypoglycemia is endemic among children with inborn errors of metabolism, therefore this chapter will limit the discussion to those most commonly encountered by the pediatric hospitalist. However, it is important to refer hypoglycemic patients to an endocrinologist and/or biochemical geneticist for diagnosis and management. While such evaluation is pending, the principles of immediate treatment in patients with signs and symptoms of hypoglycemia is useful even when the underlying disorder is unknown. The following disease categories provide an overview of the most common and most severe of these disorders seen in children.

GLYCOGEN STORAGE DISEASES

The glycogen storage diseases are a family of syndromes caused by defects in glycogen synthesis, storage, degradation of glycogen into glucose, and/or release of glucose. The glycogen storage diseases have diverse manifestations, based on the different errors in the glycogen metabolism pathway. Indeed, not all patients with glycogen storage diseases are prone to hypoglycemia. The most common glycogen storage diseases are hepatic and feature hypoglycemia and hepatomegaly due to glycogen accumulation. However, rare but underdiagnosed glycogen storage diseases without hepatomegaly exist. Glycogen storage disease features low glucose with normal ketone response (high) and normal counterregulatory hormone levels (high). The most common glycogen storage disorder is glycogen storage disease type I, caused by deficiency of glucose-6-phosphatase, which is also key for gluconeogenesis. Loss of both pathways result in lactic acidemia and a characteristic rounded "cherubic" face due to triglyceride accumulation.

In children with glycogen storage diseases, hypoglycemia occurs when glycogenolysis is necessary to maintain blood glucose (approximately 3-8 hours post feeding). Therefore, the tempo of hypoglycemia is typically within a few hours after starting the last meal. Proper management of these patients requires that they avoid prolonged fasting, and for many patients, even sleeping through the night without caloric intake is impossible. The use of uncooked cornstarch or Glycosade for intermittent overnight feedings or nasogastric feedings is required for glycogen storage disease type I. There are many long-term complications with all these disorders, including hyperuricemia, hypertriglyceridemia, renal failure, and hepatic adenomas, which may be minimized by proper treatment.

Hereditary Fructose Intolerance Hereditary fructose intolerance is caused by inherited defects in fructose-1-phosphate aldolase, which is necessary to convert fructose into glucose. Children present with hypoglycemia and associated symptoms after ingestion of fructose. Hereditary fructose intolerance usually presents after the first fructose ingestion (e.g., fruit or juice), typically around 4 to 6 months of age. Sucrose is a disaccharide of fructose and glucose and also provokes symptoms. Unmetabolized fructose-1-phosphate is toxic, causing vomiting, lethargy, and hypoglycemia shortly after ingestion. The hypoglycemia may be severe but is often transient. Failure to detect this condition can lead to hepatitis, renal failure, and even death if the patient continues to be fed sucrose- or fructose-containing juices or foods. If the condition is not recognized in infancy, most children develop food aversions that limit or prevent toxic ingestion, but they continue to be at risk any time a novel food containing fructose or sucrose is given to them. Diagnosis requires an accurate dietary history. Targeted history should be obtained in any hypoglycemic child. Particular care is needed to make the diagnosis in young infants as many infant formulas may contain fructo-oligosaccharides or corn syrup solids; symptoms may also be provoked even by low volumes of sucrose-sweetened medication suspensions and sweet-ease® (sucrose). Ingestion of any of these substances can cause uncharacteristically young presentation.

Fatty Acid Oxidation Defects Fatty acid oxidation defects interfere with the ability to utilize fatty acids for oxidative metabolism and ketogenesis. Hypoglycemia occurs because patients are overly dependent on glucose as an energy source since they are unable to produce ketones as an alternate energy source. Gluconeogenesis is also impaired as it requires ATP, typically derived from ketolysis and fatty acid oxidation.

Although many such disorders exist, medium-chain acyl-CoA dehydrogenase (MCAD) deficiency is the most common, with an incidence of roughly 1 in 10,000. Children with MCAD deficiency are developmentally and physically normal and present to medical attention only when a significant illness prevents the intake of calories. The most remarkable presenting feature is inappropriately low urine and serum ketones in the face of hypoglycemia. Unfortunately, children can die at this initial presentation if the hypoglycemia is not quickly recognized and treated. Treatment with intravenous dextrose is life-saving. Hypoglycemia occurs with any sustained fast. Parental understanding and awareness are important aspects in the care of these children. Most fatty acid oxidation defects become less clinically significant with age as the glycogen reserve increases. Many of these defects, including MCAD deficiency, are now detectable on newborn metabolic screens. However, newborn screening may miss mild or intermittent cases, especially in children where the newborn screen is sent early, late or while the child is on intravenous fluids. Fatty acid oxidation defects are an easily treatable and potentially lethal cause of hypoglycemia, therefore they should be considered in any child with hypoketotic hypoglycemia, even if newborn screening was normal.

Hyperinsulinism Excessive release of insulin from pancreatic beta cells causes severe hypoglycemia that can be refractory to medical management. In these patients, insulin is continually and inappropriately released, causing the uptake of circulating glucose into the liver and muscle. This results in a unique clinical history of hypoglycemia that happens "constantly" or "frenetically" without any temporal relationship to last meal. Insulin also suppresses the endogenous synthesis of glucose by inhibiting glycogenolysis, gluconeogenesis, and ketosis, exacerbating the hypoglycemia. The most common form of hyperinsulinism is a transient form that is not inherited and is typically seen in small for gestational age infants. Several genetic defects causing hyperinsulinism have also been identified. Moreover, hyperinsulinism may occur secondary to other genetic conditions. For instance, patients with congenital disorders of glycosylation have dysregulated insulin release and may develop hyperinsulinemic hypoglycemia. Hyperinsulinism is also a notable feature of several well-recognized genetic syndromes, such as Turner syndrome, Beckwith-Wiedemann syndrome, and Kabuki syndrome.

Patients with primary hyperinsulinism often present shortly after birth with lethargy or seizure. Their hypoglycemia is refractory to enteral and parenteral calories. Management often requires very high intravenous glucose infusion rate and/or targeted medications to prevent insulin release. Clinical suspicion of hyperinsulinism and referral to a specialized center are required for the diagnosis and management of this condition. In older children with suspected hyperinsulinism, evaluation for insulinoma is critical.

Endocrine Deficiencies The counterregulatory hormones oppose insulin activity: glucagon, catecholamines, cortisol, and growth hormone. Generally, these hormones have metabolic effects that lead to increased conversion of glycogen to glucose and the breakdown of fats and protein for use in energy production. Thus, conditions limiting the production or secretion of the counterregulatory hormones, such as panhypopituitarism can lead to fasting hypoglycemia.

Ketotic Hypoglycemia Idiopathic ketotic hypoglycemia is a fairly common phenomenon characterized by reduced fasting tolerance in children who are otherwise healthy. Ketotic hypoglycemia is not a disease, *per se*, but rather reflects inadequate glycogen and fat stores to support the degree of fasting. In particular, many children with ketotic hypoglycemia have inefficient production or utilization (or both) of precursors for gluconeogenesis, particularly alanine. It is important to note that the ketosis is not pathologic *per se*; rather, it is protective in the setting of hypoglycemia. Ketotic hypoglycemia is a diagnosis of exclusion. The condition responds well to avoidance of fasting and typically resolves spontaneously by adolescence, if not sooner.

DIAGNOSTIC EVALUATION

The most important step in the evaluation of a child with hypoglycemia is a careful history. Key features of the history are the temporal relationship of the onset of hypoglycemia and the last meal, provocation by specific foods, the possibility of accidental drug ingestions, and any previous similar episodes.

The timing of symptoms alone is extremely powerful for narrowing the differential. Onset of hypoglycemia within 3 hours of a previous meal, or in a random temporal fashion occurs when dietary sugars are not utilized properly. This strongly implies an abnormal insulin response—either endogenous hyperinsulinism or exogenous insulin or oral hypoglycemic agents. Onset of hypoglycemia between 3 and 12 hours after the last meal suggests impaired glycogenolysis, including decreased glycogenolysis secondary to adrenal insufficiency. Finally, hypoglycemia that occurs more than 8 hours after the last meal is seen in disorders of gluconeogenesis.

Several strategies exist to further narrow the differential diagnosis of a patient with hypoglycemia. Included here is the scheme created by Saudubray and colleagues (**Figure 82-1**). In general, regardless of the algorithm used, key differentiating features include the presence of ketones, elevated lactate, and organomegaly. Once the differential has been narrowed down, additional labs are helpful in further differentiating the specific cause of hypoglycemia. Biochemical abnormalities often normalize when the hypoglycemia resolves; therefore, measuring "critical" tests during the symptomatic period is important. If possible, critical laboratory testing should be drawn prior to correcting the hypoglycemia. This may make more complex testing such as diagnostic fasting studies, unnecessary. Of course, testing should not delay administration of

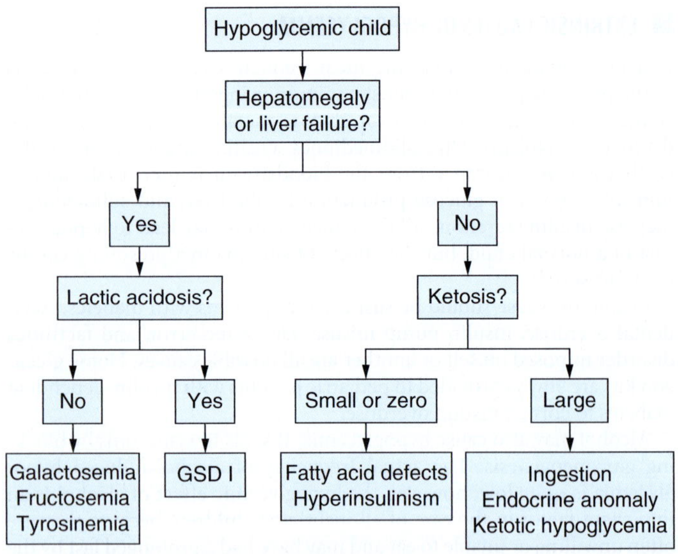

FIGURE 82-1. Evaluation of a child with hypoglycemia. GSD, glycogen storage disease.

TABLE 82-1 Laboratory Evaluation of a Hypoglycemic Child

Test	Analysis
Confirmatory glucose	Confirms presence of hypoglycemia
Insulin, C peptide	Elevated insulin can often (but not always) be documented in hyperinsulinism, but normal levels should not preclude consideration of this group of disorders; insulin level should be very low or undetectable in other types of hypoglycemia
	C-peptide testing determines whether the excess insulin is endogenous or exogenous in origin
Ketones	Hypoketotic hypoglycemia suggests hyperinsulinism or fatty acid oxidation defects
Free fatty acids	Falling insulin levels normally stimulate lipolysis; low fatty acids suggest hyperinsulinism
Cortisol, growth hormone	These hormones should increase during hypoglycemic episodes; inappropriately low levels suggest hormone deficiency and should be followed up with hormone stimulation testing
Lactate	Elevated lactate, especially with elevated fatty acids and uric acid, suggests impaired gluconeogenesis, most commonly type I glycogen storage disease. Lactate can also be elevated in fatty acid oxidation defects and some rarer metabolic causes of hypoglycemia
Acylcarnitine profile	Profile of fatty acid metabolites; primary method of diagnosing fatty acid oxidation defects; should be collected prior to performing a diagnostic fasting study as fasting children with fatty acid oxidation defects may be fatal.
Urinalysis	Useful screen for ketonuria
Urine reducing substances	Present in galactosemia, hereditary fructose intolerance; testing is sensitive, but not specific, as IV dextrose may result in positive reducing substances, especially in neonates
Urine organic acids	Quantitation is useful in identifying abnormal metabolites that arise in a variety of disorders, including fatty acid oxidation defects

IV dextrose in patients with life-threatening symptoms. **Table 82-1** provides a list of useful laboratory studies in an undiagnosed patient with hypoglycemia.

Establishing the presence or absence of ketones is essential both for evaluation and triaging of the patient. This can be done quickly and easily from a urine sample (sterility is not important). Ketosis is the physiologic response to hypoglycemia. Ketones are only absent if fatty acid oxidation is impaired, either in a primary fatty acid oxidation defect, or when fatty acid oxidation is inhibited by endogenous or exogenous insulin. A nonketotic or hypoketotic hypoglycemia is an absolute emergency.

FASTING STUDIES

When a definitive cause of hypoglycemia cannot be established, fasting studies may be considered. Fasting studies should only be performed in the inpatient setting in highly experienced centers so that the response to hypoglycemia can be evaluated safely. Fasting studies are not necessary in most cases of hypoglycemia, which can be established using the algorithm outlined above, but can be particularly useful for the diagnosis of abnormal hormonal regulation of glucose. "Safety fasts" can also be utilized to determine the length of fasting that a child can safely tolerate while well and ill. These tests are usually done in collaboration with a pediatric endocrinology service and significant nursing support, and specific protocols are followed that provide guidelines for laboratory testing (see **Table 82-2**), evaluation of hypoglycemia, and the administration of glucagon. Before pursuing fasting studies, conditions that make fasting dangerous, such as inborn errors of metabolism, must be ruled out to prevent harm.

GLUCAGON STIMULATION TESTING

Response to glucagon may also be helpful in differentiating among different causes of hypoglycemia. Glucagon stimulation testing may be done at the end of a fasting study if ketones are inappropriately low or absent or when there is high suspicion of hyperinsulinism. Serial glucose testing is done after the administration of glucagon to determine whether a response is observed. If no appreciable change in blood glucose is seen at 20 minutes, the patient should be allowed to eat or dextrose should be given. Glucagon stimulation testing is very dangerous in glycogen storage disease type 1, where it can exaggerate the metabolic acidosis. Therefore, similar to fasting studies, glucagon stimulation testing should only be performed in highly experienced inpatient settings with established algorithms and appropriate nursing support.

TREATMENT

In children who can take liquids by mouth, oral replenishment is preferred. However, if this is not possible, an intravenous solution of dextrose (the D-isomer of glucose that is nutritionally equivalent to glucose) is indicated. In general, a rapid intravenous infusion of 2 to 4 mL/kg of 10% dextrose (D10W) is administered. If hypoglycemia persists, a continuous infusion of dextrose is indicated. The continuous glucose infusion rate (GIR) should be initiated at 6 to 9 mg/kg of dextrose per minute, then titrated to maintain euglycemia. The GIR can be calculated by the following formula:

$$\text{GIR} = (\text{IVR} \times \%\ \text{Dextrose solution})/6 \times \text{Weight}$$

where the GIR is measured in mg/kg per minute, IVR is the intravenous infusion rate in mL/hour, and weight is expressed in kilograms.

To calculate the initial IVR, the formula can be rearranged as follows:

$$\text{IVR} = \text{GIR} \times 6 \times \text{Weight}/\%\ \text{Dextrose solution}$$

For simplicity, a typical GIR of 8 mg/kg/minute using D10W can be quickly calculated as:

$$\text{IVR} = 4.8 \times \text{Weight}$$

For example, a 10-kg child would receive D10W at 48 mL/hr to deliver 8 mg/kg glucose per minute. Using this simplified formula also conveniently provides maintenance fluid requirements for a child weighing less than 10 kg.

If the patient does not tolerate enteral glucose replenishment and intravenous access is unavailable, glucagon can be administered. It is important to note that this strategy will only work effectively and safely in those patients whose hypoglycemia is a result of hyperinsulinemia or insulin overdose. The dose of glucagon is 1 mg subcutaneously, regardless of patient size. Response to glucagon should be evaluated and noted within 10 minutes of administration, and blood sugar monitoring should be continued at least hourly until the patient returns to a safe, stable range. Rehydration and sugar replenishment usually lead to a rapid improvement in symptoms such as lethargy or jitteriness.

Management of overdose of oral hypoglycemics is largely supportive. Intravenous or oral glucose is often required until enough of the offending agent is cleared. Depending on the timing of the exposure and the release form of the medication, activated charcoal can be used to bind unabsorbed medications, especially some of the sustained-release formulations. Communication with poison control centers can provide information on drug half-life and appropriate techniques for detoxification. Octreotide, a long-acting somatostatin analog, has been used in some cases of sulfonylurea overdose.

Children with metabolic or endocrine abnormalities predisposing them to hypoglycemia require intervention to prevent recurrent crises. Although the particular therapies vary with the underlying disease, a few general guidelines are applicable to many disorders:

TABLE 82-2 Clinical Manifestations and Differential Diagnosis of Hypoglycemia

		URINE			SERUM		EFFECT OF 24–36 HR FAST ON PLASMA[4]					GLYCEMIC RESPONSE TO GLUCAGON		GLYCEMIC RESPONSE TO INFUSION OF	
Condition	Hypoglycemia	Ketones[2]	Reducing Sugars[3]	Hepatomegaly	Free fatty acids	Uric Acid	Glucose	Insulin	Ketones[2]	Alanine	Lactate	Fed	Fasted	Alanine	Glycerol
Hyperinsulinism	Severe with unpredictable timing	↓	–	–	Normal or Decreased ↑	Normal	↓↓	↑↑[5]	↓	↓	Normal	↑	↑	↑	↑
Ketotic hypoglycemia	Severe with missed meals/ illnesses	↑↑↑	–	–	Normal	Normal	↓↓	↓	↑↑↑	↓[6]	Normal	↑	–	↑	↑
Fatty acid oxidation disorders	Severe with fasting	↓	–	+/–; occasional abnormal liver function tests	↑	↑	↓↓↓	↓	↓	↓	Normal to ↑	↑	–	Not indicated	
Hypopituitarism	Moderate with missed meals	↑	–	–	Normal	Normal	↓↓	↓	↑	↓	Normal	↑	–	↑	↑
Adrenal insufficiency	Severe with missed meals	↑	–	–	Normal	Normal	↓↓	↓	↑	↓	Normal	↑	–	↑	↑
Enzyme deficiencies															
Glucose-6-phosphatase	Severe within hours of meal	↑↑	–	+++	↑↑	↑↑	↓↓	↓	↑↑	↑↑	↑↑	–[7]	–	–	–
Debrancher	Moderate with fasting	↑↑	–	++	Normal	Normal	↓↓	↓	↑↑	↓↓	Normal[8]	↑	–	↑	↑
Phosphorylase	Mild-moderate	↑↑	–	+	Normal	Normal	↓	↓	↑↑	↓↓	Normal	– to ↑	–	↑	↑
Fructose-1,6-bisphosphatase	Severe with fasting	↑↑	–	+++	↑↑	↑↑	↓↓	↓	↑↑	↑↑	↑↑	↑	–	↓	↓
Galactosemia[1]	After milk or milk products	↑	↑	+++	Normal	Normal	↓	↓	↑	↓	Normal	↑	–	↑	↑
Fructose intolerance	After fructose	↑	↑	+++	Normal	Normal	↓	↓	↑	↓	Normal	↑	–	↑	↑

1. Newborn screening in the United States is highly sensitive for galactosemia. A negative newborn screen makes galactosemia highly unlikely.

2. Ketones must be considered in the context of the severity of hypoglycemia. In this table ↓ ketones represents both negative ketones but may also include trace-small ketones in the face of extreme hypoglycemia. ↑ Represents the ketone response in a biochemically normal individual in response to the degree of hypoglycemia (such as provoked by fasting.) It is also important to remember that the ketone response is attenuated in neonates.

3. Reducing substances are sensitive, but poorly specific and false positives are common.

4. Intentional fasting should not be attempted until fatty acid oxidation disorders have been ruled out. Even in patients in whom fatty acid oxidation defects have been ruled out, the use of diagnostic fasting is controversial and should only be attempted by experienced endocrinologists.

5. This column represents the level of insulin in the context of the severity of hypoglycemia. Insulin may fall in hyperinsulinism during a fast; however, it will stay disproportionately high in comparison to the level of glucose.

6. Hypoalaninemia is a normal response to hypoglycemia. In this table ↓ represents a normal physiologic response to the degree of hypoglycemia. It was previously thought that there was exaggerated depletion of alanine in patients with ketotic hypoglycemia; however, the degree of hypoalaninemia is now believed to be proportional to hypoglycemia in these patients. See Wolsdorf JI, Sadeghi-Nejad A, Senior B. Hypoalaninemia and ketotic hypoglycemia: cause or consequence? *Eur J Ped.* 1982;138(1):28-31.

7. Glucagon is contraindicated in patients with known GSD I, in whom it can worsen metabolic acidosis.

8. Patients with GSD III (debrancher deficiency) experience a transient lacticemia after feeding, which can overlap the beginning of hypoglycemia; however, lactate normalizes during a fast. Therefore, if lactate is checked prior to a full fast (for instance, when a fast is terminated early for hypoglycemia), it may be elevated.

In children older than 2 years with early-morning hypoglycemia after an overnight fast, a pre-bedtime snack with complex carbohydrates often helps sustain adequate glucose levels overnight. Glucose is slowly released from the starch polymers, mimicking a glucose infusion. If starch snacks are inadequate, gastric feedings may be necessary. Even short periods of fasting pose a significant danger to children at risk for hypoglycemia. When an overnight fast is required (e.g., for anesthesia), the child should be admitted to the hospital and placed on intravenous dextrose during the fasting period.

Measures should be taken to reduce the risk of crisis during other times of stress. For example, febrile illnesses, especially when associated with emesis or diarrhea, often necessitate dextrose infusions. Consider prophylactic antipyretics in these children when they receive immunizations to curtail catabolic periods with increased metabolic demand.

Medical management of hyperinsulinism includes the use of diazoxide and octreotide (or lanreotide, a long-acting somatostatin analog), which interfere with the release of insulin from the beta cell, and glucagon infusion. Definitive treatment of hyperinsulinism may require partial or near-total pancreatectomy depending on the type of hyperinsulinism identified (focal versus diffuse forms). Frequently, these patients require background enteral dextrose infusions as a bridge to definitive therapy or during medication trials.

ADMISSION & DISCHARGE CRITERIA

ADMISSION

- Clinical evidence of lethargy, sweating, or pallor; neurologic symptoms such as syncope, seizure, or coma; unresponsiveness for unknown reasons.
- Persistent or recurrent serum glucose values less than 55 mg/dL.
- Known or suspected ingestion of medications or other toxins that can cause hypoglycemia.
- Known or suspected overdose of insulin.
- For neonates: listlessness, vomiting, poor suck, or serum glucose levels less than 36 mg/dL, particularly in infants of diabetic mothers or small- or large-for-gestational-age infants.

Admission or transfer to an intensive care unit is appropriate when an infant or child with hypoglycemia requires close observation, frequent laboratory studies requiring prompt reporting of results, and rapid adjustments in treatment based on laboratory results and changes in clinical status.

DISCHARGE

- Resolution of laboratory findings of hypoglycemia and the ability to maintain stable serum glucose levels without hospital-level support.
- A clinically stable patient with normal activity, adequate enteral intake, and established medical follow-up after discharge.
- Often, a "safety" fast is performed just prior to discharge to determine how long a patient can safely fast when well and ill on their current hypoglycemia treatment plan.

CONSULTATION

Consultation with specialists in endocrinology, metabolism, and/or neonatology can be helpful in patients with severe, recurrent, or prolonged hypoglycemia. These consultants can also guide the diagnostic evaluation, and when appropriate, follow patients after discharge.

Evaluation by a pediatric or neonatal intensivist is warranted when placement in an intensive care setting is being considered.

Involvement of a diabetes team is needed when a patient with diabetes presents with persistent or recurrent hypoglycemia. The team can evaluate the diet, the insulin regimen, and adherence, as well as provide ongoing education, support, and medical management for these patients.

KEY POINTS

- Hypoglycemia can present with a broad range of symptoms that are often nonspecific, including changes in mental status or seizure. Owing to the compensatory catecholamine release, findings of diaphoresis, tachycardia, and pallor are often present.
- Evaluation of an infant or child with new neurologic findings or a deteriorating neurologic status should routinely include a blood glucose analysis.
- Neonatal hypoglycemia is a common problem and is especially likely in small- or large-for-gestational-age babies and infants of mothers with diabetes.
- Patients with extrinsic causes of hypoglycemia have often been exposed to suspect medications, including oral hypoglycemics.
- Patients with intrinsic causes of hypoglycemia are more likely to have low blood sugar during illnesses and with fasts.
- Immediate treatment of hypoglycemia is far more important than determining the cause. However, blood samples should be obtained if this can be accomplished without delaying the necessary interventions.
- Treatment of hypoglycemia involves the delivery of glucose enterally or intravenously. Ongoing delivery may be needed if the hypoglycemia is severe, recurrent, or persistent.

SUGGESTED READINGS

Chen YT. Glycogen storage diseases. In: Scriver CR, Sly WS, Childs B, et al, eds. *The Molecular and Metabolic Bases of Inherited Disease.* 8th ed. New York: McGraw-Hill; 2001.

Cornblath M, Hawdon JM, Williams AF, et al. Controversies regarding definition of neonatal hypoglycemia: suggested operational thresholds. *Pediatrics.* 2000;105:1141-1145.

Kishnani PS, Austin SL, Abdenur JE, et al. Diagnosis and management of glycogen storage disease type I: a practice guideline of the American College of Medical Genetics and Genomics. *Genet Med.* 2014:16;e1.

McLaughlin SA, Crandall CS, McKinney PE. Octreotide: an antidote for sulfonylurea-induced hypoglycemia. *Ann Emerg Med.* 2000;36:133-138.

Saudubray JM, Ogier de Baulny H, Charpentier C. Clinical approach to inherited metabolic disease. In: Fernandes J, Saudubray JM, Tada K, eds. *Inborn Metabolic Diseases: Diagnosis and Treatment.* 3rd ed. Berlin: Springer-Verlag; 2000:3-41.

Stanley C, Thornton P, Finegold D, Sperling M. Hypoglycemia in infants. In: Sperling M, ed. *Pediatric Endocrinology.* 2nd ed. Philadelphia, PA: WB Saunders; 2002.

CHAPTER 83

Metabolic Acidosis

Jessica R. C. Priestley, MD, PhD

BACKGROUND

Metabolic acidemia is a common laboratory finding, usually the result of common ailments such as hypovolemia, systemic infection, or acute diarrhea. Rarely, it can result from a heritable or acquired disorder predisposing to acidemia. Specifically, many inborn errors of metabolic can present with severe metabolic acidemia. The challenge for the physician is to confirm that the acidemia has a presentation, history, and response to treatment consistent with a common, as opposed to a rare, etiology. This chapter presents a framework from which clinicians can recognize the signs and symptoms of severe metabolic acidemia, treat that acidemia if necessary, and broaden the differential diagnosis when an acidemia is not adequately explained by the clinical presentation and laboratory workup.

Acidemia, or "acid in the blood" denotes a state of acidic pH measured through blood gas analysis or serum bicarbonate level. *Acidosis* is reserved for cases of acidemia in which a specific acidic substance is suspected or has been identified in the blood (e.g., lactic acidosis, ketoacidosis). *Metabolic Acidemia* refers to acidemia when the serum bicarbonate level is low, in contrast to *respiratory acidemia* (associated with a high carbon dioxide level).

PATHOPHYSIOLOGY

Endogenous acid production can be generally categorized into volatile and nonvolatile components. The most significant volatile acid is carbon dioxide, which is eliminated through pulmonary ventilation. Nonvolatile acids are generated by dietary acid intake, amino acid catabolism, and fatty acid oxidation, productive of ketones and lactic acid. Elimination of nonvolatile acids occurs through renal mechanisms, including bicarbonate reclamation and ammoniagenesis. Acidemia of any type ultimately represents an imbalance between acid production and elimination.

Buffering systems play a critical role in the maintenance of acid-base homeostasis. In the blood, proteins such as albumin and hemoglobin form the largest quantitative reserve of immediate buffer and the bicarbonate-carbonic acid system has the largest capacity to alter its flux in response to an acid challenge. Modulation of renal bicarbonate reabsorption occurs more slowly, but also represents an important mechanism through which normal body pH is maintained. Impairment of any of these mechanisms can decrease the body's ability to respond to perturbations in acid-base status.

Because the bicarbonate buffering system plays such a critical role in the maintenance of acid-base homeostasis, metabolic acidemia can be the result of excessive loss of bicarbonate, rather than increased acid production. Acidemia secondary to bicarbonate loss is immediately differentiable by the presence of a compensatory increase in plasma chloride concentration and normal anion gap.

Bicarbonate losses may occur either via the gastrointestinal tract (e.g., acute diarrhea) or via the renal tubules (e.g., renal tubular acidosis). Injury to the proximal renal tubules can result in bicarbonate loss by presenting the reabsorption of small molecules, including bicarbonate, glucose, amino acids, phosphate, and urates. This pattern of renal metabolite losses is termed renal Fanconi syndrome. There are both acquired and inherited causes of renal Fanconi syndrome (**Table 83-1**). In these cases, metabolic acidemia may be accompanied by other signs of renal dysfunction (e.g., growth failure, osteopenia).

TABLE 83-1 Selected Causes of Fanconi Syndrome

Acquired	Inherited
Medications	Alport syndrome
Heavy metal toxicity	Classical galactosemia
Nephrotic syndrome	Cystinosis
Malignancy	Fanconi-Bickel syndrome
Vitamin D deficiency	Glycogen storage disease type I
	Glycogen storage disease type XI
	Hereditary fructose intolerance
	Lowe's syndrome
	Lysinuric protein intolerance
	Primary mitochondrial disorders
	Tyrosinemia type I
	Wilson's disease

CLINICAL PRESENTATION

Untreated metabolic acidemia causes malaise and a host of end-organ effects. Physiologic effects of acidemia include pulmonary vasoconstriction, decreased myocardial contractility, and a shift in the oxygen-hemoglobin dissociation curve resulting in decreased oxygen saturation. The typical breathing pattern is characterized by tachypnea and air hunger—hyperventilation ("Kussmaul respirations") is a physiologic mechanism for raising pH by carbon dioxide removal. Patients may be confused, lethargic, or ataxic. Nausea, vomiting, and abdominal pain are useful but nonspecific clues—vomiting is a physiologic mechanism for raising pH by proton removal. Myocardial suppression and cardiac conduction anomalies may result in chest pain or palpitations. Muscle weakness and bone pain can also be features.

Acute metabolic acidemia can occur from any process that reduces ventilation or perfusion. It is also the hallmark of specific inborn of metabolism. Episodes of metabolic acidemia due to inborn errors of metabolism can be triggered by an acquired illness, typically a viral infection, and progress rapidly from anorexia and lethargy to somnolence, coma, and death.

Chronic metabolic acidosis in children is associated with growth failure and developmental delays. Bone demineralization can result in osteopenia. Other signs and symptoms are largely determined by the underlying disease mechanism. Recognition of chronic acidosis should prompt subspecialty referral to a nephrologist, gastroenterologist, or biochemical geneticist, depending on the suspected mechanism.

DIFFERENTIAL DIAGNOSIS

The differential diagnoses and causes of metabolic acidosis are extensive and detailed in **Tables 83-2 to 83-4.**

DIAGNOSTIC EVALUATION

The following steps can guide the clinician toward an accurate diagnosis or referral point: (i) Confirm metabolic acidemia; (ii) Review standard laboratory data; (iii) Differentiate secondary metabolic acidemia due to common illnesses from cases requiring further evaluation; (iv) Differentiate acid accumulation from bicarbonate loss; (v) If acidic molecules are accumulating, determine the type if possible; and (vi) Consider specialized investigations if a rare cause of acidemia is suspected.

CONFIRMATION OF METABOLIC ACIDEMIA

The initial laboratory tests for a child with suspected unexplained metabolic acidemia include serum electrolytes (sodium, potassium, chloride, bicarbonate), renal function tests (creatinine and BUN), serum osmolality, glucose, blood gas analysis, and urinalysis. If a particular acid is suspected based on the presentation or a preexisting diagnosis, the initial studies should include measurement of that acid (e.g., ketones in a child

TABLE 83-2 Causes of Non-Anion Gap Metabolic Acidemia

Gastrointestinal Bicarbonate Loss	Renal Bicarbonate Loss	Chemicals That Alter Measured Acid	Other
Diarrhea	Renal tubular acidosis	HCl	Excessive chloride in intravenous fluids
Surgical drains distal to the pylorus	Renal compensation for chronic respiratory alkalosis	NH_4Cl	Carbonic anhydrase inhibitors
Cholestyramine	Renal Fanconi syndrome	Arginine	Dilution acidosis
		Lysine	

TABLE 83-3 Causes of Anion Gap Metabolic Acidosis

C	Carbon monoxide, cyanide
A	Aminoglycosides
T	Toluene, theophylline
M	Methanol
U	Uremia, renal failure
D	Diabetic ketoacidosis, ketoacidosis secondary to starvation
P	Paraldehyde
I	Iron, isoniazid, inborn errors of metabolism
L	Lactic acid
E	Ethanol, ethylene glycol, and other alcohols
S	Salicylates

with diabetes mellitus). Ketoacids and lactic acid have rapid measurements readily available in most pediatric chemistry labs and are good adjuvant laboratory tests.

REVIEW OF STANDARD LABORATORY DATA

Standard laboratory data should be reviewed prior to the consideration of specialized tests. Calculation of the anion gap is critical to interpreting the acid-base information provided by a standard electrolyte panel. The anion gap should be determined using the following formula:

$$\text{anion gap} = Na^+ - (Cl^- + HCO_3^-)$$

The anion gap calculation attempts to determine whether the measured cations and anions are present in proportionate amounts. A gap acidosis is present when the concentration of anions is lower than expected. The assumption is that some nonmeasured anion is present in an amount sufficient to satisfy electroneutrality. The anion gap's normal range (12 ± 2 mEq/L) assumes a normal amount of serum protein. Hypoalbuminemia may create a falsely normal anion gap in the presence of a significant amount of unmeasured anion.

Calculation of the osmolar gap can be useful to identify exogenous substances responsible for metabolic acidosis in the blood. It is calculated according to the following formula:

$$\text{osmol gap} = \text{measured serum osmolality} - \text{calculated osmolality}$$

where:

$$\text{calculated osmolarity} = (2 \times \text{Plasma } [Na^+] + [\text{Glucose}]/18 + \text{Blood urea nitrogen}/2.8)$$

The normal range is 10 to 15. An abnormal osmolar gap suggests the presence of bloodstream substances that are not accounted for in the osmolar equation such as methanol or ethylene glycol.

TABLE 83-4 Causes of Lactic Acidosis

Type A - Mismatch in O_2 delivery/consumption			Type B - No mismatch in O_2 delivery/consumption
States of increased metabolic activity		Toxins	Inborn errors of metabolism
	Strenuous exercise	Cyanide	Electron transport chain defects
	Seizures		Pyruvate dehydrogenase deficiency
	Respiratory distress		Glycogen storage disease type I
States of inadequate oxygen delivery to end organs			Pyruvate carboxylase deficiency
	Shock - cardiogenic, septic, hypovolemic, etc.		Biotinidase deficiency
	Anemia		Disorders of gluconeogenesis
	Hypoxemia		Others
	Ischemia		

Other diagnostic clues can also be gleaned from review of standard laboratory data. Blood gas and serum bicarbonate measurements may prompt further investigation based on the severity of the acidemia. Markedly abnormal serum pH (6.9-7.2) and serum bicarbonate levels (sometimes below the laboratory's limit of quantification) should raise suspicion for an inborn error of metabolism. Inappropriately alkalotic urine (pH > 7.0) in the setting of acidemia suggests renal tubular acidosis. Urine pH should be measured on a fresh sample, as prolonged exposure to air may alter urine pH. Creatinine and blood urea nitrogen should be scrutinized to rule out renal impairment. Hyperglycemia may indicate diabetes. Hypoglycemia is seen with disorders of gluconeogenesis, fatty acid oxidation disorders, and some organic acidemias and mitochondrial diseases.

DIFFERENTIATE ACIDEMIA DUE TO COMMON ILLNESSES FROM CASES REQUIRING FURTHER EVALUATION

An acidemia may not require further evaluation if it presents as the expected consequence of a common illness and is consistent in magnitude and response to treatment. Sepsis, diarrhea, and dehydration are the root causes of most cases of pediatric metabolic acidemia. Severity, chronicity, history, and context can all be helpful in determining how comprehensive the ensuing workup should be.

DIFFERENTIATE ACID ACUMMULATION FROM BICARBONATE LOSS

Acidosis may result from either increased acid production or loss of bicarbonate buffering capacity through the kidneys or gastrointestinal tract. Effective treatment depends on distinguishing between these two possibilities. The history, physical examination, and routine laboratory studies allow some acidemias to be sorted into the bicarbonate-losing category.

A typical bicarbonate-losing acidemia is associated with hyperchloremia and a normal anion gap. Causes of non-anion gap metabolic acidemia are listed in Table 83-2. Measurement of urine pH and serum potassium can support a diagnosis of renal tubular acidosis but should be interpreted with caution in the setting of gastrointestinal bicarbonate losses. Clues to the presence of Fanconi syndrome include hypophosphatemia, alkaline urine in the setting of acidemia, and the presence of urine-reducing substances, including glucose.

In contrast, typical acid-accumulation acidemia is associated with normochloremia and an anion gap (Table 83-3). Even with an equivocal gap, an unexplained acidemia may warrant additional workup to identify a possible accumulating anion.

DETERMINE THE TYPE OF ACCUMULATED ACID

Acid accumulation can be caused by normal stress physiology, toxic ingestion, and inborn errors of metabolism. Toxins may cause an acidosis by acting as an acid themselves or by causing secondary, acid-producing metabolic derangements. For example, methanol is metabolized to formic acid, which as an unmeasured anion increases the anion gap. Alternatively, cyanide is not a strong acid but causes a lactic acidosis by impairing mitochondrial energy metabolism. Other important toxins with the potential to cause acidosis include toluene, sulfur, iron, isoniazid, ethylene glycol, and salicylates. Similarly, inborn errors of metabolism can cause primary or secondary acidemia. Methylmalonic acidemia, an organic acidemia, causes a primary acidosis through the accumulation of several organic acids including propionic acid, methylmalonic acid, lactic acid, and ketone bodies. By contrast, some fatty acid oxidation disorders can cause cardiomyopathy, with a secondary lactic acidosis as the result of decreased tissue perfusion.

Among the types of nonvolatile acids associated with anion gap acidemia when produced in excess, three categories are particularly important in the pediatric population: lactic acid, ketone bodies, and other organic acids that accumulate in specific inborn errors of metabolism.

Lactic Acid Although pyruvate is the product of glycolysis, it exists in equilibrium with lactic acid in a molar ratio of approximately 10:1. Under conditions in which pyruvate accumulates (hypoxia, impairment of the mitochondrial respiratory chain or TCA cycle, impairment of gluconeogenesis), lactic acid also accumulates. Excess lactic acid is the most common cause of metabolic acidosis in the pediatric population. The differential diagnosis for lactic acidosis is broad. Categorization into type A, resulting from a mismatch in oxygen delivery and consumption, and type B, which occurs without evidence of tissue hypoperfusion, lactic acidosis can be helpful (Table 83-4). Because glycolysis is the primary metabolic pathway when oxygen is in short supply, most cases of lactic acidosis are type A and due to tissue hypoperfusion and hypoxia. Lactic acidosis may also be a clue to an inborn error of metabolism and can occur due to decreased utilization of pyruvate by downstream enzymes (Table 83-4). Lactic acid levels may be elevated without frank acidemia or an anion gap, which is an important consideration when ruling out inborn errors of metabolism associated with excess lactic acid.

A departure from the normal 10:1 ratio of lactate to pyruvate also helps narrow the differential diagnosis for lactic acidosis. For example, if a lactic acidosis is due to a respiratory chain defect, lactate and pyruvate usually have a ratio greater than 10:1. By contrast, pyruvate dehydrogenase deficiency is associated with increases in both lactate and pyruvate, yielding a normal ratio.

Whenever possible, a free-flowing venous or arterial sample should be collected for lactate and pyruvate measurements to prevent false metabolite elevations from sample handling. Pyruvate measurement is technically challenging and may not be available in all academic centers. Pyruvate measurement requires rapid cooling of the sample and preferably blood collection in a perchloric acid tube. Blood collected distal to the capillary bed may result in a falsely elevated lactate levels and lactate-pyruvate ratio. The use of a tourniquet can also cause false positive results.

Ketones The primary ketones, 3-hydroxybutyrate and acetoacetate, are the result of oxidation of fatty acids by the liver. Ketones are strong acids and can cause a significant elevation of the anion gap and depression in the blood pH when present in millimolar amounts (ketoacidosis), as commonly occurs in diabetes, certain organic acid disorders, and inborn errors of ketone metabolism. Specific ketone body concentrations can be measured to confirm that accumulation is contributing to measured academia. Total ketones are usually around 0.1 mM in the nonfasting state, but can increase to 2 mM with vigorous exercise or as high as 3 mM with a 24-hour fast. Ketone levels exceeding 3 mM or an elevation or depression in the setting of an incongruent history suggests a biochemical disorder. Additional, pathologic ketone species can be produced by genetic disorders in the metabolism of amino acids.

Other Organic Acids The organic acidemias are a group of relatively rare inborn errors of metabolism that share the common features of generating significant amounts of nonvolatile acidic metabolic intermediates called organic acids. These non-amino carbon-containing acids are usual derived from aberrant amino acid oxidation. Examples include methylmalonic acidemia, propionic acidemia, glutaric acidemia, and isovaleric acidemia. Many organic acidosis can be detected, or even definitively diagnosed, by urinary organic acid analysis. Presentations vary from acute to chronic acidemia, with correspondingly dramatic or indolent clinical courses. The presence of an organic acidosis is suggested by anion gap metabolic acidemia, an acidemia insufficiently explained by the clinical circumstances, and/or a profound ketoacidosis in an otherwise unexpected setting. During a metabolic decompensation, it is not uncommon to find serum bicarbonate concentrations less than 15 mEq/L and venous pH less than 7.2.

CONSIDERATION OF SPECIALIZED INVESTIGATIONS

The investigations used to work up rare causes of acidemia may benefit from subspecialist consultation, including a biochemical genetics (metabolism) specialist. Some tests require specific procedures and/or testing materials. Specimen collection may require "free-flowing" blood sample (ammonia, lactate, pyruvate) and/or rapid processing (plasma total homocysteine) to avoid spuriously elevated results. Attempting to perform testing without adequate procedures in place runs the risk of generating equivocal or misleading results.

Assuming that standard serum electrolytes and liver enzyme tests, urinalysis, and blood gas measurements have been performed and reviewed, additional tests for a patient with acidemia of an unclear etiology include those listed in **Table 83-5**. Of note, plasma amino acid and urinary organic acid analysis are particularly useful as they have the potential to detect a broad spectrum of specific hereditary diseases known to cause acidemia. Some toxic ingestions, such as with ethylene glycol, can also be diagnosed.

Additionally, the newborn screening results should be reviewed for every neonatal patient with a septic or catastrophic shock-like presentation. If an inborn error of metabolism is suspected and the newborn screening results are not yet available, the state or reference laboratory should be alerted and instructed to process the sample urgently. If a sample has not yet been obtained, it should be done immediately and always prior to blood product transfusion, including fresh frozen plasma.

TABLE 83-5 Specialized Investigations in Acidotic Children

Clinical Test	Utility
Acylcarnitine profile—plasma	Quantitative acylcarnitine patterns are essentially diagnostic for a variety of organic acidemias and fatty acid oxidation disorders
Amino acids—plasma	Patterns of abnormalities can suggest specific inborn errors of metabolism
Amino acids—urine	Global elevations in urinary amino acid excretion occur in renal Fanconi syndrome (N.B. newborns physiologically have elevated urinary amino acid excretion, making this test less helpful in the newborn period)
Ammonia	Hyperammonemia occurs in liver failure and in some inborn errors of metabolism; it can contribute to encephalopathy in acidotic patients
Free and total carnitine—plasma	Decreased carnitine occurs in a variety of organic acidemias and fatty acid oxidation disorders; carnitine replacement is important for such patients
Ketones—blood or urine	Verify ketoacidosis; note that plasma beta-hydroxybutyrate tests for only that ketoacid while urine ketones are more non-specific
Lactate, pyruvate—plasma	Used to identified disorders with primary or secondary lactate elevations; the ratio of lactate to pyruvate is sometimes useful in differentiating among lactic acidosis syndromes
Organic acids—urine	Patterns of metabolite excretion can aid in the diagnosis of many inborn errors of metabolism; excretion of ketones and lactate can also be documented and quantified
Various studies—CSF	Amino acids, lactate, pyruvate, and organic acidosis can be measured from cerebrospinal fluid specimens; if a patient with a suspected inborn error of metabolism has a lumbar puncture, consider saving a small amount of sample for metabolic studies

MANAGEMENT

Most metabolic acidemia encountered by the practicing pediatric hospitalist will be mild or moderate and caused by common illnesses resulting in bicarbonate loss or hypovolemia. In that setting, direct treatment of the underlying disease process generally reverses the acidosis. However, severe and/or unexplained acidemia should prompt consideration of both a broader differential diagnosis and direct treatment of the acidemia.

An algorithm for the treatment of a decompensated child with unexplained severe acidemia is presented in **Table 83-6**. The general approach is like that for any critically ill child: airway, breathing, and circulation are initial priorities. Laboratory testing as outlined above should be obtained to the extent practical. Subsequent steps serve to reverse the often-precipitous decline in homeostasis accompanying severe acidemia. Fluid resuscitation should be undertaken carefully with 5 to 10 mL/kg boluses of normal saline, followed by reassessment. Over-vigorous resuscitation may increase the risk for fluid shifts and cerebral edema. Many patients have coexisting volume losses, making sodium and potassium balance important.

Direct correction of acidemia using bicarbonate, citrate, or acetate have risks and benefits that depend on the underlying condition, which need to be carefully weighed. Buffering agents may correct a pH value, but they do not correct the underlying source of acidemia. Alkalinization may also help encourage excretion of organic acids. Risks of sodium bicarbonate therapy include volume overload, central nervous system

TABLE 83-6	Acute Correction Algorithm for Patients With Suspected Inborn Errors of Metabolism
1.	ABCs (airway, breathing circulation); anticipate circulatory impact of profound acidemia
2.	Cautious fluid resuscitation
3.	Dextrose infusion with appropriate electrolytes
4.	Calculate base deficit and consider correction if severe
5.	Consult Biochemical Genetics

acidosis, hypernatremia, hypokalemia, and hypercapnia. Citrate and acetate require a functional Krebs cycle in the liver in order to replenish bicarbonate, and therefore are avoided in children with Krebs cycle errors and respiratory chain defects. If supplemental bicarbonate is to be delivered, it is useful to calculate a base deficit using the following equation:

$$\text{base deficit (mEq)} = [\text{desired } HCO_3^- - \text{measured } HCO_3^-] \times \text{weight (in kg)} \times 0.4$$

As an initial approximation, many clinicians start by giving one-half deficit replacement and titrating additional therapy based on the change in acid-base status. Serum potassium levels must be followed closely while acidemia is being corrected.

In severe cases of exogenous intoxication or accumulation of organic acids due to an inborn error of metabolism, hemodialysis can be considered to acutely lower the presence of the offending agent. For endogenous diseases this works best as a temporary bridge to medical therapies. Medications that bind to organic acids and facilitate excretion may also be utilized.

When the result of an inborn error of metabolism, metabolic acidemia is often triggered by catabolism (e.g., fasting physiology). Thus, promotion of anabolism is a useful general principle. If an inborn error is suspected, dextrose is administered at a high concentration and rate. As a starting point, peripheral intravenous access permits infusion of a 12.5% dextrose solution with appropriate electrolytes at 1.5 times the maintenance rate. This provides a glucose infusion rate approximately equivalent to the basal glucose utilization rate of the liver. For critically ill children, central access should be obtained promptly. Insulin can be used to address hyperglycemia and promote anabolism. Additionally, children should receive adequate nutrition as soon as possible, especially those with inborn errors of metabolism, even if parenteral nutrition is necessary. This reverses catabolism and provides for the ongoing anabolic demands of growth and development.

ADMISSION AND DISCHARGE CRITERIA

ADMISSION CRITERIA

For patients with metabolic disorders known to cause rapid decompensation, there is a low threshold for hospitalization. Patients with unknown causes of acidemia should also be worked up aggressively. Criteria for admission include:

1. Symptomatic presentation including vomiting, lethargy, and/or rapid or labored breathing.
2. Young age, particularly neonates.
3. Lack of an obvious cause for the acidemia.
4. Anion gap acidosis.
5. Evidence of systemic decompensation (e.g., hemodynamic instability, altered perfusion, respiratory insufficiency).

DISCHARGE CRITERIA

1. Stabilization of acid-base balance.
2. Establishment of a diagnosis.
3. Initiation of appropriate medical and/or dietary therapy.
4. Confirmation of adequate feeding and weight gain.
5. Establishment of appropriate follow-up and family education.

CONSULTATION

Depending on the underlying cause of the metabolic acidemia, the following consultative services may be helpful:

1. Gastroenterology or Hepatology—for evaluation of patients with suspected primary hepatic disorders.
2. Genetics or Biochemical Genetics—for determination of a specific inborn error of metabolism and assistance in obtaining specialized laboratory tests, including genetic testing.
3. Nephrology—for evaluation of patients with suspected primary renal disorders.
4. Neurology—for evaluation of the variety of abnormal neurologic findings in patients with metabolic acidemia.
5. Nutrition—for assistance in obtaining specialized diets when indicated.

SUGGESTED READINGS

Berend K, de Vries APJ, Gans ROB. Physiological approach to assessment of acid-base disturbances. *N Engl J Med.* 2014;371(15):1434-1445.

Jaber S, Paugam C, Futier E, et al. Sodium bicarbonate therapy for patients with severe metabolic acidaemia in the intensive care unit (BICAR-ICU): a multicentre, open-label, randomised controlled, phase 3 trial. *Lancet.* 2018;392(10141):31-40.

Kappy MS, Morrow G III. A diagnostic approach to metabolic acidosis in children. *Pediatrics.* 1980;65(2):351-356.

Korang SK, Safi S, Feinberg J, Nielsen EE, Gluud C, Jakobsen JC. Bicarbonate for acute acidosis. *Cochrane Database Syst Rev.* 2021;2021(3):CD014371.

Kraut JA, Madias NE. Lactic acidosis. *N Engl J Med.* 2014;371(24):2309-2319.

Levy PA. Inborn errors of metabolism: Part 1: overview. *Pediatr Rev.* 2009;30(4):131-138.

Levy PA. Inborn errors of metabolism: Part 2: specific disorders. *Pediatr Rev.* 2009;30(4):e22-e28.

Nitu M, Montgomery G, Eigen H. Acid-base disorders. *Pediatr Rev.* 2011;32(6):240-251.

Vergano SAS. Inborn errors of metabolism: becoming ready for rare. *Pediatr Rev.* 2022;43(7):371-383.

SECTION I Hematology

CHAPTER 84 Anemia

Michael Contarino, MD and Adolfo Molina, MD, MSHQS

BACKGROUND

Anemia is a common pediatric condition. The World Health Organization reported a prevalence of 6.1% in 2019 in children 6 months to 59 months of age. Anemia requiring hospitalization accounts for approximately 1600 hospitalizations per year in the United States. Defined as insufficient red blood cell (RBC) mass for the age of the patient, anemia can develop acutely or insidiously. Mild anemia between 6 and 9 weeks of age is typically consistent with physiologic nadir, which is not considered pathologic. In children, anemia that develops gradually over several weeks to months may be profound but with few clinical signs and symptoms. However, if anemia develops acutely, the patient has no time to compensate for decreased oxygen carrying capacity, and symptoms of anemia (ranging from fatigue to cardiovascular collapse) can develop rapidly. Because anemia can result from many disease processes, it is helpful to divide anemia into three broad pathophysiologic categories: (i) decreased production of either hemoglobin or RBCs, (ii) premature RBC destruction, or (iii) blood loss. Fortunately, distinguishing among these processes usually requires only basic, widely available laboratory tests making the evaluation much less daunting. This chapter focuses primarily on children with newly recognized anemia during hospitalization.

CLINICAL PRESENTATION

Anemia is often discovered incidentally during laboratory screening for other indications in a child who otherwise exhibits no symptoms of anemia. Systematic evaluation of febrile hospitalized children demonstrated that a majority exhibit mild, clinically insignificant anemia. Alternatively, pallor and fatigue, the cardinal symptoms of anemia, may bring the patient to medical attention. Severe anemia, especially when there is a rapid onset, may present with weakness, obtundation, syncope, exertional dyspnea, congestive heart failure, or shock.

HISTORY

A directed history should thoroughly review the child's diet, including the amount and type of milk, red meat, fruits, and vegetables consumed daily, as well as a history of pica. Growth and development, blood loss (i.e., melena, hematemesis, hemoptysis, hematuria, menstruation, trauma), and recent illnesses are important areas of inquiry. History of systemic illness is also essential as acute and/or chronic inflammation are often underlying causes of anemia in hospitalized patients. Because many causes of anemia are inherited, the family history should include questions about transfusions, bleeding, splenectomy, cholelithiasis or cholecystectomy, and prior diagnoses of anemia among family members. In the case of trauma, consider blood loss from long bone fractures with major hematoma, hemothorax, or hemoperitoneum.

PHYSICAL EXAMINATION

The physical examination should focus on manifestations of anemia and diagnostic clues. Tachycardia, systolic murmur, and pallor suggest a moderate degree of anemia. Severe anemia can be accompanied by symptoms of congestive heart failure and tachypnea, despite children's typically profound and effective cardiovascular compensatory mechanisms. Jaundice or dark urine suggests intravascular hemolysis. Similarly, evaluation for hepatosplenomegaly is essential in an anemic patient, suggesting extramedullary hematopoiesis (as in chronic hemolytic anemias) or other diagnoses (e.g., storage diseases, bone marrow infiltration, infections, sequestration).

DIAGNOSTIC EVALUATION

The initial laboratory evaluation typically includes a basic panel of hematologic studies, followed by selected studies as directed by the presentation and the history. A complete blood count (CBC) with differential is central for initial classification. RBC indices included in the CBC provide additional clues to the pathophysiology of the anemia (**Table 84-1**). Comparing current RBC indices with those of previous blood examinations may provide important information, such as the rate and timing of onset of the anemia. It is critical to interpret both the hemoglobin and the mean corpuscular volume (MCV) based on the child's age, because normal RBC parameters change with age.

Secondary analysis commonly requires a reticulocyte count, Coombs testing, and examination of the peripheral blood smear, with particular attention to RBC morphology and evidence of hemolysis (**Table 84-2**). Some examples of RBC abnormalities that are seen on the peripheral smear are provided in **Figure 84-1**.

TABLE 84-1 Red Blood Cell Indices and Anemia-Related Laboratory Studies

Index	What It Measures	What It Tells Us
Hemoglobin	Concentration of hemoglobin in blood	Inclusive quantitation of red cell hemoglobin
Hematocrit	Volume of packed cells (may be calculated from red cell numbers/whole blood volume)	Red cell concentration in plasma
Mean corpuscular volume	Average volume (size) of red cells	Helpful in classifying pathophysiologic mechanisms of anemia
Mean corpuscular hemoglobin (MCH)	Average hemoglobin content per red cell	Low MCH suggests inefficient hemoglobin synthesis
Mean corpuscular hemoglobin concentration	Average concentration of hemoglobin per red cell volume	Elevated values suggest membranopathy or hemoglobinopathy
Red cell count	Direct quantitation of red cell number	Provides insight into red cell production somewhat independently of hemoglobin synthesis
Red blood cell distribution width	Measure of variability of red cell size	Indicates variation in red cell populations; often high in iron-deficiency anemia and low in thalassemias
Reticulocyte count	Quantitation of immature red cells	Increased number demonstrates active bone marrow red cell synthesis
Haptoglobin	Hemoglobin binding plasma protein	Depleted in conditions of intravascular hemolysis
Direct Coombs	Immunoglobulin or complement bound to erythrocytes	Detects the presence of bound autoreactive antibodies
Indirect Coombs	Serum immunoglobulin or complement capable of binding donor erythrocytes	Demonstrates alloantibody development or unbound autoantibodies

TABLE 84-2 Red Blood Cell Findings on Peripheral Blood Smear

Finding	Description	Commonly Associated Conditions	Comments
Microcytosis	Small erythrocytes	Iron deficiency Thalassemias Hemoglobinopathies	Interpret in context of age-dependent norms
Macrocytosis	Large erythrocytes	Folate deficiency Vitamin B_{12} deficiency Bone marrow failure	
Hypochromia	Decreased hemoglobin	Iron deficiency	
Spherocytosis	Erythrocytes without central pallor	Hereditary spherocytosis AIHA	Associated with loss of membrane
Schistocytosis (also referred to as burr or helmet cells)	Erythrocyte fragments	Hemolytic uremic syndrome Mechanical or vascular-mediated destruction Thrombotic thrombocytopenic purpura DIC	Microangiopathic hemolysis
Polychromasia	Variability in erythrocyte staining	Hemolytic anemias Recovery from anemia	Reflects mix of reticulocytes with older cells
Target cells	Erythrocytes with an island of hemoglobin within the area of central pallor	Hemoglobinopathies (especially hemoglobin C disease) Obstructive liver disease	
Basophilic stippling	Punctate pattern in erythrocytes	Lead poisoning Hemoglobinopathies Enzymopathies Infection	
Sickle cells	Crescent-shaped cells	Sickle cell anemia	
Reticulocytosis	Increased number of young erythrocytes	Hemolytic anemias	Can be seen in conditions of elevated red cell destruction or hemorrhage
Howell-Jolly bodies	Fragments of nuclei containing condensed DNA	Asplenia (anatomic or functional)	Associated with impaired splenic function
Acanthocytes	Red cells with multiple variable small protrusions	Hypothyroidism Liver disease Abetalipoproteinemia	
Heinz bodies	Accumulation of precipitated hemoglobin	Unstable hemoglobin Erythrocyte enzymopathy	Requires a special stain

AIHA, autoimmune hemolytic anemia; DIC, disseminated intravascular coagulation.

If there is concern for occult blood loss, a stool guaiac test may identify subclinical gastrointestinal bleeding. Subclinical hematuria usually involves only small amounts of blood in the urine and generally does not result in significant anemia in the absence of some other causative factor. However, blood detected by urinalysis is an important finding and requires attention to both the urine dipstick and microscopic analysis. Blood detected by dipstick without a significant number of RBCs on the microscopic examination indicates the presence of either hemoglobin (suggesting intravascular RBC hemolysis) or myoglobin (due to rhabdomyolysis). Serum concentrations of creatine kinase should help differentiate between myoglobinuria and hemoglobinuria.

Depending on the patient's age, history, and physical examination findings, and results from the initial workup, further evaluation can be tailored accordingly. For example, iron deficiency is the most common cause of microcytic anemia in children, so further evaluation of microcytic anemia includes a serum iron level, total iron binding capacity, and ferritin. Microcytic anemia with risk factors for plumbism should prompt the measurement of serum lead levels. In the special population of premature infants, intracranial hemorrhage can account for significant anemia, and consideration of cranial imaging may be indicated, especially in the presence of neurologic symptoms or signs.

Clinical concerns for endocrine, renal, or hepatic disease justify the assessment of hepatic transaminases and thyroid and renal function. Hematologic consultation is often useful if initial workup fails to yield a definitive diagnosis, especially those other than iron deficiency and inflammation-related anemia. Further laboratory studies such as hemoglobin electrophoresis (to investigate hemoglobinopathies) and osmotic fragility studies (to rule out spherocytosis) may be indicated. Bone marrow aspiration and biopsy may be useful in the diagnosis of anemias of unclear cause and to rule out diagnoses such as myelodysplastic syndrome, congenital dyserythropoietic anemias, aplastic anemia, and leukemia. Although occasionally presenting with isolated anemia, myelodysplastic syndrome and leukemia usually result in pancytopenia or the appearance of abnormal (e.g., dysplastic or immature) cells in the peripheral blood.

Whenever possible, specific laboratory studies should be obtained before blood product transfusion so that they reflect the patient's condition rather than that of the blood donor.

DIFFERENTIAL DIAGNOSIS

Anemia is associated with various pathophysiologic abnormalities; thus, functional classification simplifies the initial evaluation. One approach divides anemia into those with microcytic, normocytic, or macrocytic erythrocytes based on the MCV with careful attention to the possibility of blood loss or hemolysis. **Figure 84-2** diagrams a diagnostic approach to common anemias encountered by pediatric hospitalists. Multiple concurrent pathophysiologic processes often complicate even straightforward diagnoses. For example, it can be challenging to evaluate anemia in a patient with chronic renal failure and possible nutritional deficiencies who develops subclinical hemorrhage. Below we present a broad overview of common anemia types based on

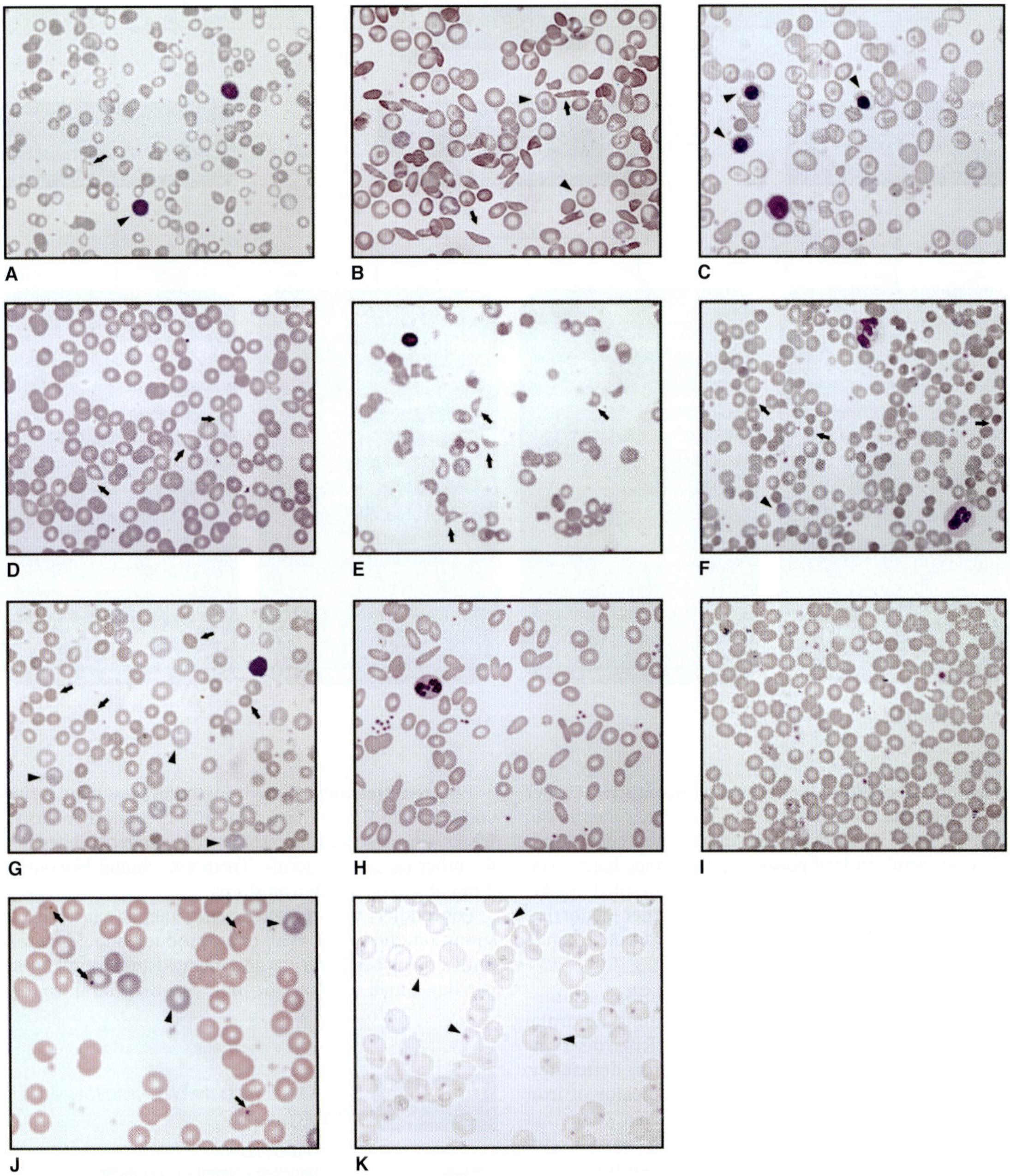

FIGURE 84-1. Erythrocyte morphologic abnormalities. A. Microcytosis and hypochromia associated with severe iron-deficiency anemia. Infrequent elliptocytes (pencil cells) can be seen (*arrow*). Note erythrocyte sizes relative to lymphocytes (*arrowhead*). B. Sickle (*arrows*) and target (*arrowheads*) erythrocytes associated with sickle cell anemia. C. Target erythrocytes associated with hemoglobinopathy or liver disease. Nucleated red blood cells (*arrowheads*) and polychromasia suggest increased red cell production. D. Teardrop-shaped cells (*arrows*) associated with marrow replacement (myelophthisis). Note the otherwise normal erythrocytes. E. Schistocytes (*arrows*) associated with microangiopathic hemolytic anemia. Note thrombocytopenia. F. Spherocytic erythrocytes (*arrows*) associated with hereditary spherocytosis. Note polychromasia, suggestive of reticulocytosis (*arrowheads*). G. Microspherocytes (*arrows*) and polychromasia from reticulocytosis (*arrowheads*) in autoimmune hemolytic anemia. H. Elliptocytes associated with hereditary elliptocytosis. Infrequent elliptocytes can also be seen in other anemias. I. Burr cells (echinocytes) may be associated with uremia. J. Howell-Jolly bodies (*arrows*) associated with impaired splenic function. Note polychromasia from reticulocytosis (*arrowheads*). K. Special stains detect Heinz bodies (*arrowheads*), which are associated with unstable hemoglobins and enzymopathies.

the aforementioned classification schemas, including clinical and historical features, diagnosis, and treatment.

CAUSES OF ANEMIA

DISORDERS OF RED CELL PRODUCTION: THE RETICULOCYTOPENIC ANEMIAS

This class of disorders is characterized by anemia, generally in the absence of other cytopenias, together with reduced or inappropriately normal reticulocyte counts, and a negative Coombs test, also known as the direct antiglobulin test (DAT).

Microcytic Anemia • *Iron-Deficiency Anemia* Iron deficiency is the most common cause of anemia in the pediatric population, displaying a bimodal age of distribution affecting mainly toddlers and female adolescents. Premature infants are at high risk because of their inability to accumulate sufficient iron stores during the third trimester. Although iron supplementation of infant formula and cereals has diminished its incidence, the absence of sufficient iron intake after the depletion of stores commonly results in anemia in older infants and toddlers. Inequitable access to iron-fortified infant formulas is an important contributor to the disparities seen in iron-deficiency anemia. Additionally, over consumption of cow's milk is a leading cause of iron-deficiency anemia in both infants and toddlers. Patients with iron-deficiency anemia may

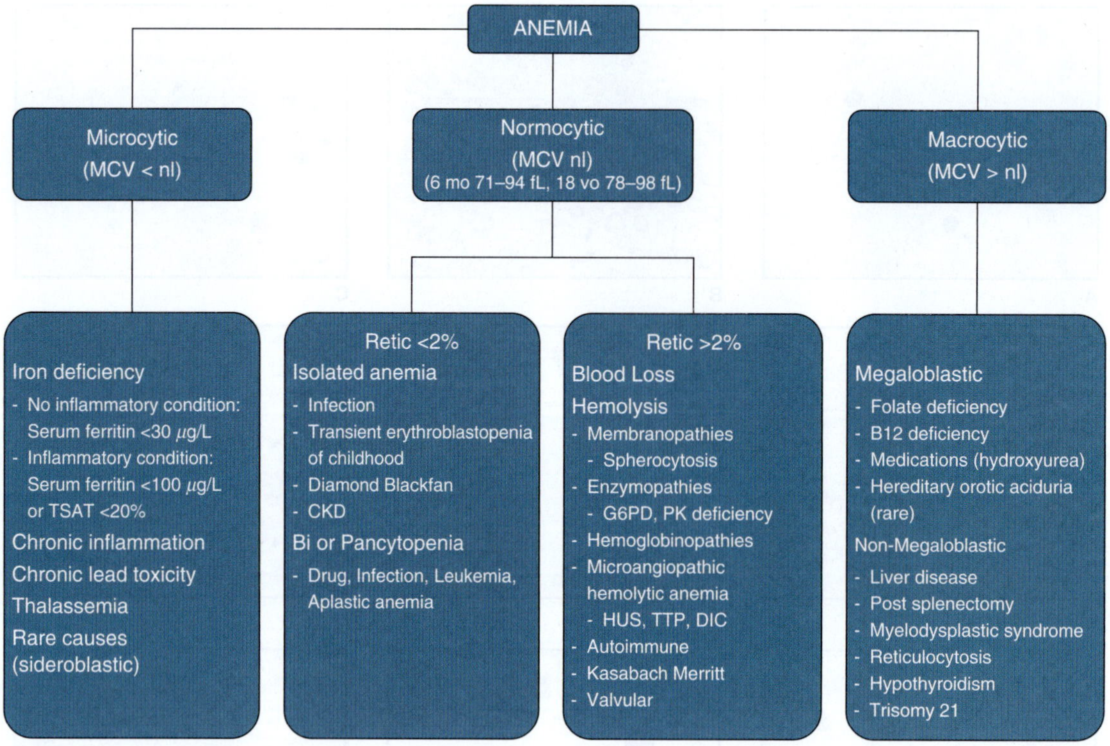

FIGURE 84-2. Anemia flowchart.

also exhibit microscopic stool blood loss from enterocolitis (e.g., cow's milk protein allergy in infants). In toddlers, iron-deficiency anemia can be accompanied by pica, the involuntary ingestion of inert compounds such as dirt, which can result in lead poisoning; this exacerbates iron-deficiency anemia because lead competes with iron for intestinal uptake. In young women, iron deficiency usually results from either menorrhagia or typical menstrual blood loss. Anemia in this context can be severe if associated with low dietary iron intake.

Diagnosis A nutritional history suggestive of excessive milk consumption or poor iron intake associated with microcytic anemia, a normal to slightly elevated reticulocyte count, an elevated RBC distribution width, and erythroid hypochromasia suggests iron deficiency. Reticulocyte hemoglobin content may be an early indicator of iron deficiency. Typical laboratory findings in iron-deficiency anemia are summarized in **Table 84-3**. Serum ferritin is the most useful laboratory test for evaluation of iron deficiency when an inflammatory condition is not present; ferritin is an acute phase reactant that may be falsely elevated with illness. Interpretation in the context of a C-reactive protein level increases utility, and evaluation of transferrin saturation (TSAT) is helpful. Concurrent causes of microcytic anemia such as α-thalassemia trait can be difficult to diagnose in the context of severe iron deficiency.

Treatment A therapeutic trial of oral iron is appropriate for iron-deficiency anemia before referral to a hematologist. Mild anemia can be treated with 3 mg elemental iron/kg per day, given once daily. Severe anemia may justify dosing up to 6 mg elemental iron/kg per day, given in divided doses. Although historically associated with the risk of significant side effects due to prior formulations, parenterally administered iron is generally safe, particularly when there is concern for limited absorption or oral intake is insufficient to replenish iron stores. Given the gradual development of iron-deficiency anemia, pediatric patients rarely exhibit significant physiologic consequences necessitating RBC transfusion, despite presenting with profoundly low hemoglobin levels and thus the American Association of Blood Banks (Choosing Wisely) does not recommend routine RBC transfusion for iron-deficiency anemia. However, diminishing physiologic compensation for severe anemia leading to hemodynamic instability is more commonly seen in hospitalized patients and may justify RBC transfusion.

Effective treatment with iron should result in a rising reticulocyte count within 2 to 3 days and an increasing hematocrit within a few weeks. The absence of a response to iron necessitates further evaluation for other causes of anemia. Treatment should be continued for at least 3 months to replenish iron stores.

For toddlers with iron-deficiency anemia caused by excess milk consumption, the intake of all dairy products should be initially restricted until a rising hematocrit is documented and overall limited to 16 ounces per day. Small amounts of milk can then be introduced with meals,

TABLE 84-3 Studies Pertinent to the Evaluation of Suspected Iron-Deficiency Anemia

Study	Finding in Iron-Deficiency Anemia	Comment
Plasma iron level	Low	Varies with recent iron intake
Serum ferritin level (No inflammatory condition present)	Low	Serum ferritin <30ug/L is both sensitive (92%) and specific (98%) for iron deficiency
Serum ferritin level (Inflammatory condition present)	Variable	Serum ferritin <100ug/L or TSAT <20% If ferritin is 100-300ug/L, a TSAT test should be used to confirm iron deficiency
Total iron binding capacity (TIBC)	Normal to elevated	A measure of plasma transferrin concentration
Mean corpuscular volume	Low	Reflects decreased hemoglobin production
Red blood cell distribution width	Increased	Reflects increased variability of cell size due to variable hemoglobin incorporation or increased numbers of reticulocytes
Reticulocyte count	Variable	Expect increase 2-3 days after starting effective iron therapy
Reticulocyte hemoglobin concentration	Low	Provides measure of heme synthesis in youngest erythrocytes and may indicate early iron deficiency

provided that allergic enterocolitis and occult gastrointestinal bleeding from milk protein allergy have been excluded as diagnostic possibilities.

Normocytic or Macrocytic Anemia • ***Anemia of Acute Inflammation*** Despite a paucity of literature, available data suggest that anemia associated with acute infection is common, particularly in very young children, with an incidence second only to iron-deficiency anemia. Anemia associated with acute infection/inflammation has been documented in acutely ill children in the outpatient setting, and at an even higher frequency in hospitalized patients, with two-thirds to three-quarters of children presenting with at least mild anemia. The anemia is normochromic and usually mild and other cytopenias are usually absent. Hemoglobin levels are about 1 to 1.5 grams lower than pre- and post-hospitalization values. The anemia typically resolves after the infection/inflammatory condition has been treated. Although the precise time course of resolution has not been well documented, it is unlikely to persist longer than 1 month after the resolution of the infection/inflammatory condition in an otherwise healthy child. The precise mechanism of the development of the anemia of acute infection/inflammation is not known. The cause is likely a combination of inhibition of response to endogenous erythropoietin, increased adhesion of red cells to endothelium (sequestration of red cells), and alteration of iron metabolism as shown by hypoferremia, low TIBC, and transferrin saturation with elevated ferritin—effects that are directly or indirectly cytokine mediated.

Extensive investigation of a mild to moderate normocytic anemia in a child without other cytopenias who has an uncomplicated infection is unwarranted. Although iron deficiency and anemia of acute infection can coexist, serum iron, transferrin, and ferritin may not accurately reflect iron status if measured during or soon after an infection. Definitive investigation of possible underlying iron deficiency, unless severe, should wait for at least 1 month after resolution of the infection.

Anemia of Chronic Inflammation Also called anemia of chronic disease or anemia of inflammation, anemia of chronic inflammation produces a mild to moderate normocytic to microcytic anemia. It is associated with infection, inflammatory disorders, and malignancy, and is common. For example, about 40% of children with inflammatory bowel disease have anemia of chronic inflammation. Anemia of chronic inflammation is due to ineffective hematopoiesis resulting from restricted iron availability along with decreased erythrocyte life span. Erythropoiesis is inhibited by TNF-α and interferons with a blunted response to endogenous erythropoietin. Hepcidin also has a role as an important mediator between immunity and erythropoiesis.

Anemia of chronic inflammation should be suspected by the presence of mild to moderate anemia with typically normocytic or slightly microcytic RBC in the setting of chronic inflammation, low serum iron, and elevated ferritin. Although bone marrow examination is not usually performed to make this diagnosis, when done it shows iron accumulation in macrophages, reflecting a block in the release of iron from the reticuloendothelial system. Although considered a diagnosis of exclusion, an extensive laboratory evaluation of an isolated anemia in a child with chronic inflammation may be of limited utility. However, a careful history may suggest concurrent iron or other nutritional deficiencies. Treatment of the underlying inflammatory condition is required to correct this anemia.

Transient Erythroblastopenia of Childhood Transient erythroblastopenia of childhood (TEC) is a relatively uncommon cause of normocytic anemia in young children (aged 6 months to 5 years). Most commonly presenting at age 2 years, TEC is probably an immune-mediated bone marrow suppression of RBC production that frequently follows mild viral infections (e.g., upper respiratory tract infections); tests of anti-red cell antibodies (e.g., Coombs tests) are negative as a rule. Hemolysis is not present in TEC; therefore, lactate dehydrogenase, bilirubin, haptoglobin, and urinary bilirubin and hemoglobin are within normal limits. TEC should be strongly suspected in the setting of moderate to severe normocytic anemia with an inappropriately low reticulocyte response, although it is worth noting that reticulocytosis may be present if TEC is detected during the recovery phase. TEC must be distinguished from Diamond-Blackfan anemia (pure red cell aplasia), an inherited bone marrow failure syndrome that usually presents in the first year of life. TEC resolves over a period of weeks to months, whereas Diamond-Blackfan anemia persists. Infectious causes of bone marrow suppression should also be considered (e.g., parvovirus B19, human herpesvirus 6, Epstein-Barr virus, cytomegalovirus, human immunodeficiency virus). Bone marrow examination may be warranted, especially if reticulocytopenia continues for more than a few weeks, repeated blood transfusions are required, or other hematopoietic lineages are affected. Complete recovery usually occurs in 4 to 8 weeks. Transfusion of RBCs may be indicated with clinical decompensation or severely low hemoglobin levels. Patients should be monitored with weekly blood and reticulocyte counts until they recover.

Inherited Bone Marrow Failure Syndromes If the anemia is chronic, is present from a young age, or is refractory to treatment, one must suspect an inherited cause, especially if the MCV is normal or slightly elevated. Frequently, inherited marrow failure syndromes are accompanied by physical abnormalities (birth defects), necessitating a careful examination for physical stigmata (e.g., short stature, limb abnormalities, cardiac defects, skin pigmentation changes). Some inherited causes of bone marrow suppression are specific to RBCs (e.g., Diamond-Blackfan anemia), whereas others (e.g., Fanconi anemia) affect multiple cell lines, resulting in pancytopenia. Careful attention must be paid to the remainder of the CBC when considering bone marrow failure syndromes. In general, hematologist consultation is recommended to diagnose and treat these rare diseases.

Megaloblastic Anemia Patients with anemia caused by dietary deficiencies of folic acid or cobalamin (vitamin B_{12}) present with reticulocytopenic macrocytic anemia. The MCV is generally quite elevated (often >100 fl). Other clues to the diagnosis may derive from examination of the peripheral blood smear, most notably hypersegmented neutrophils (>5 nuclear lobes). Folic acid is naturally found in fruits, vegetables, and cow's milk, and deficiency is normally limited to those patients with self-imposed dietary restrictions (e.g., consumption of only unfortified goat's milk or a diet devoid of fruits and vegetables).

Fortification of foods in the United States, aimed at preventing neural tube defects, has been successful. However, global access to folic acid containing foods may be limited. Serum or RBC folate levels can be assayed; the latter is less susceptible to short-term fluctuation and more reflective of tissue stores. Vitamin B_{12} is present in animal products, so a dietary basis for vitamin B_{12} deficiency is usually limited to strict vegans. Vitamin B_{12} and folate deficiencies can also result from malabsorption. In contrast to folate, however, vitamin B_{12} absorption depends on the activity of a gastric-derived cofactor (intrinsic factor); therefore, vitamin B_{12} deficiency can be due to a lack of intrinsic factor (e.g., pernicious anemia) rather than simple dietary deficiency or malabsorption. Prompt diagnosis of vitamin B_{12} as the cause of megaloblastic anemia is critical because of the risk of irreversible neuropathy that can accompany vitamin B_{12} deficiency.

DISORDERS OF RED CELL DESTRUCTION: THE HEMOLYTIC ANEMIAS

Hemolytic anemias result from the accelerated destruction of RBCs and should be suspected when there are signs of hemolysis such as jaundice, hyperbilirubinemia, organomegaly, dark urine, and reticulocytosis. RBCs survive approximately 120 days, so any cause of premature destruction can result in anemia, particularly when bone marrow production fails to keep pace with the destructive process. Hemolytic anemias result from factors either intrinsic or extrinsic to the RBC. In general, intrinsic defects are inherited, whereas extrinsic causes are usually acquired. Inherited hemolytic anemias can be caused by defects in the erythrocyte membrane (e.g., spherocytosis), defects in globin genes (e.g., sickle cell anemia, thalassemia, unstable hemoglobin), or defects in RBC metabolism (e.g., pyruvate kinase deficiency, glucose-6-phosphate dehydrogenase deficiency). A directed family history is critical in the workup of patients with hemolytic anemias since family members will often share a history of anemia or side effects of anemia. The primary causes of extrinsic destruction of RBC in children are immune mediated; these include autoimmune hemolytic anemia and alloimmune hemolytic anemia (hemolytic disease of the newborn). Microangiopathy can also result in significant hemolytic anemia; these include typical and atypical hemolytic uremic syndrome, thrombotic thrombocytopenic purpura, and disseminated intravascular coagulation.

Inherited Hemolytic Anemias • ***Hemoglobinopathies*** Many abnormal hemoglobin variants result in premature destruction of the RBC by relative insolubility and precipitation of hemoglobin in the red cell cytoplasm. Hemoglobin precipitation leads to less deformable RBC membranes, resulting in accelerated splenic clearance of the affected cells. Hemoglobin defects can result from either unbalanced expression of α- and β-globin genes (thalassemias) or mutations of the globin genes themselves (e.g., sickle cell, hemoglobin C, hemoglobin E, unstable hemoglobins). Although abnormal RBC morphology is a common finding in hemoglobinopathy, hemoglobin evaluation by electrophoresis, sequencing, and other tests, along with Heinz body testing (which detects hemoglobin precipitation in RBCs), is the more accurate method of diagnosing this group of hemolytic anemias. Early diagnosis is important to prevent disease morbidity highlighting the importance of improved newborn screening methodologies given challenges in detecting less common thalassemias. Children who did not receive newborn screening may present with undiagnosed sickle cell disease or thalassemia. Owing to its high incidence and special management considerations, sickle cell anemia is discussed separately in Chapter 85, Sickle Cell Disease.

Membranopathies The most common genetic RBC membrane abnormality is hereditary spherocytosis (HS), which is usually inherited in an autosomal dominant manner and results from defects in membrane proteins that bridge the actin cytoskeleton and the phospholipid bilayer. Defective membrane–protein interactions lead to the loss of small segments of the lipid membrane, resulting in spherocytic red cells that have lost their biconcave discoid shape and have an increased mean corpuscular hemoglobin concentration. Spherocytic cells are less deformable and are cleared rapidly by the spleen, resulting in a much-shortened life span. Patients with HS usually have mild chronic hyperbilirubinemia and splenomegaly. HS patients are normally well-compensated but are also susceptible to aplastic crises, worsening anemia with infection and gallstones. HS can be challenging to diagnosis, particularly in the neonate, as spherocytes can be produced naturally and infants may not be able to produce adequate marrow response necessitating transfusion. Classically diagnosed with osmotic fragility testing, however improved genetic testing has led to the recommendation for follow up gene panel studies typically performed with hematologist consultation. Other rarer membrane abnormalities associated with hemolysis include hereditary elliptocytosis, hereditary pyropoikilocytosis, and hereditary stomatocytosis.

Enzymopathies To survive normally, the RBC must be replete with the enzymes needed for adenosine triphosphate (ATP) generation and reduced nicotinamide adenine dinucleotide phosphate (NADPH) production. Defective enzymes of the hexose monophosphate shunt or Embden-Meyerhof pathway can result in anemia by limiting the RBCs energy or antioxidant capabilities, shortening their life span in the circulation. The most common enzymopathy is glucose-6-phosphate dehydrogenase (G6PD) deficiency. The enzyme G6PD protects the RBC from oxidative damage. Cells deficient in G6PD are susceptible to injury from oxidant drugs, infection, acidosis, and fava bean ingestion. The most likely presentation of this disorder to a hospitalist would be a child of Mediterranean or Asian descent who develops acute hemolysis marked by jaundice, dark urine, and anemia. G6PD deficiency should be suspected in the setting of prolonged jaundice in the neonatal period after alloimmune hemolysis has been ruled out by a normal Coombs test. G6PD testing can be performed, although the results may be falsely normal soon after a hemolytic event owing to selective hemolysis of cells with the lowest G6PD levels and increased G6PD levels in remaining reticulocytes. Inheritance of pyruvate kinase deficiency, the second most common enzymopathy, is autosomal recessive. Pyruvate kinase deficiency can result in severe anemia, with reticulocytosis and splenomegaly. In general, the management of patients with enzymopathies is supportive (chronic folic acid supplementation), with an emphasis on the avoidance of known oxidative stressors (e.g., medications, foods, environmental exposure).

Treatment of Inherited Hemolytic Anemias In general, treatment of inherited hemolytic anemias is dictated by the severity of the anemia, the nature of the defect, and its clinical consequences. Patients with mild anemia can be observed, whereas those with severe anemia may require chronic transfusions or splenectomy. In general, patients with chronic hemolytic anemias require only supportive care (e.g., folic acid supplementation) to facilitate chronic compensatory reticulocytosis. These children generally do well clinically unless an intercurrent illness slows bone marrow production of new RBCs. Parvovirus B19, the causative agent of erythema infectiosum (fifth disease), replicates in RBC precursors and can almost completely cease erythropoiesis for 1 to 2 weeks, leading to aplastic crisis in children with hemolytic anemias. Often, RBC transfusion is required to maintain homeostasis until erythropoiesis recovers from the infection (typically within 1 month). In general, it is recommended to involve hematology subspecialists in the diagnosis and long-term management of patients with inherited hemolytic anemias.

Acquired Hemolytic Anemias • ***Immune-Mediated Hemolytic Anemias*** Immune-mediated hemolytic anemias are common causes of acquired anemia in the pediatric population. By definition, antibody is produced against one or more antigens on the surface of RBCs, promoting premature destruction by opsonization and subsequent erythrocyte removal by the reticuloendothelial system or by complement-mediated lysis of RBCs in the bloodstream. Antibodies may come from the patient (in which case the process is known as autoimmune hemolytic anemia [AIHA]) or from another source (alloimmune hemolytic anemia), as occurs in hemolytic disease of the newborn. Unlike hemolytic disease of the newborn, which is invariably caused by transplacental maternal immunoglobulin (IgG) and is a problem only *in utero* and in the newborn period, AIHA can affect patients of any age and can be caused by either IgM or IgG.

Autoimmune Hemolytic Anemia Patients with AIHA often relate a history of previous viral or viral-like illness preceding the development of fatigue and pallor. The presentation of AIHA is usually sudden and may include symptoms of severe anemia. A history of dark urine suggests acute intravascular hemolysis and argues for complement-mediated red cell lysis (see later). Jaundiced sclerae or pruritus suggests hyperbilirubinemia. Mild splenomegaly is occasionally present.

AIHA can result in intravascular or extravascular hemolysis. Intravascular hemolysis is complement-mediated and caused by IgM or complement-fixing IgG directed against RBC antigens, resulting in lysis of RBCs directly in the plasma and leading to jaundice or hyperbilirubinemia, elevated lactate dehydrogenase, and low haptoglobin. In contrast, extravascular hemolysis is typically mediated by IgG without complement-fixing characteristics. Extravascular hemolysis may result in little or no increase in lactate dehydrogenase and bilirubin, presumably because RBCs are destroyed in the phagocytic cells of the reticuloendothelial system rather than in the plasma itself. Laboratory evaluation of AIHA reveals a moderate to severe anemia with a brisk reticulocytosis. However, it is important to note that the reticulocyte count may be unexpectedly low if the reactive antibody also results in clearance of young RBCs. Review of the peripheral blood smear may show spherocytosis, polychromasia, and RBC clumping. Urinalysis may show hemoglobinuria in the absence of hematuria. Direct Coombs testing (which tests for antibody bound to the patient's RBCs) is almost always positive in AIHA. Indirect Coombs testing, which tests for free anti-erythrocyte antibody in the patient's serum, usually detects alloantibodies but may be positive in AIHA when the antibody titer exceeds antigen binding; this can help define which isotype and RBC antigen are involved. If multiple cell lineages are depressed or Coombs testing is negative, examination of the bone marrow should be considered to rule out leukemia or aplastic anemia. Primary AIHA can be divided into three types based on the nature, thermal reactivity, and amplitude of the implicated antibody.

Warm-reactive autoimmune hemolytic anemia In warm-reactive AIHA, antibody (usually IgG) binds RBC antigens at 37°C, resulting in extravascular hemolysis. Warm-reactive IgG typically binds common RBC protein antigens, which explains why blood bank testing often demonstrates a pan-reactive pattern. Warm-reactive AIHA tends to behave in a more chronic fashion than cold agglutinin disease and may warrant a more long-term treatment approach.

Paroxysmal cold hemoglobinuria In paroxysmal cold hemoglobinuria (PCH), complement-fixing IgG autoantibody binds RBCs at low temperatures (usually in the extremities *in vivo*) and then causes complement-dependent intravascular hemolysis at warm temperatures (in central, warmer parts of the body). PCH sometimes follows infection with *Mycoplasma pneumoniae* or other atypical organisms. Testing for the cold-reactive (Donath-Landsteiner) antibody of PCH is performed by maintaining freshly drawn venous blood at 37°C until it is intentionally cooled in the laboratory, permitting antibody binding. Erythrocyte-antibody complexes are then warmed, inducing complement activation and hemolysis.

Cold agglutinin disease In cold agglutinin disease, antibody (usually IgM) binds erythrocyte antigens (typically red cell surface polysaccharides) and fixes complement at temperatures below 37°C. In this manner, IgM efficiently results in intravascular hemolysis. Because IgM inefficiently binds antigen at 37°C, unbound antibody can frequently be detected in the plasma. Cold agglutinin AIHA is usually a self-limited process and typically does not respond well to immunosuppressive therapy.

Alloimmune Hemolytic Anemia

Hemolytic disease of the newborn Although great progress has been made in reducing the incidence of erythroblastosis fetalis caused by Rh incompatibility between mother and infant, hemolytic disease of the newborn caused by ABO mismatch and mismatch related to minor red cell antigen systems still occurs, as does classic hemolytic disease of the newborn, particularly in the later pregnancies of sensitized women. Much of the initial management occurs prenatally or in the NICU—including intrauterine transfusions, and exchange transfusions for hyperbilirubinemia as well as administration of immunoglobulin to slow the immune-mediated destruction.

Despite perinatal management, these infants are susceptible to persistent anemia due to the persistence of maternally derived antibodies to their red cells in the infants' circulation. Hemolysis may continue for several months postnatally. The developing red cells in the bone marrow are also often subject to hemolysis. Typically, this process declines to a clinically insignificant level within a few weeks, but for some babies this can persist for up to 4 months of age. A careful history is one key to diagnosis, being sure to ask about mother's Rh status, administration of RhD immune globulin, the performance of prenatal procedures, and prior affected pregnancies. The anemia is normocytic, and some spherocytes can be seen on the smear. The direct antiglobulin test is positive. There may be reticulocytopenia. The decision to transfuse rests on the infant's physiologic response to the anemia, as well as the rate of fall of the hemoglobin and the reticulocyte count.

Microangiopathic hemolytic anemia The hallmark of microangiopathy is the finding of schistocytes (red cell fragments) on peripheral blood smear analysis. Infection, including recent recognition of COVID-19, can result in thrombotic microangiopathy through uncontrolled fibrinogenesis and consequent physical disruption of RBCs by shearing forces that occur when blood circulates through vessels clogged with fibrin strands. RBC destruction in this setting can be severe and may be accompanied by thrombocytopenia and coagulation factor consumption, resulting in disseminated intravascular coagulation (DIC). These patients are typically quite ill and often have multiorgan pathology in addition to hemolytic anemia.

Microangiopathic anemia also occurs with hemolytic uremic syndrome (HUS) and thrombotic thrombocytopenic purpura (TTP). HUS and TTP exist on a continuum and have decreased activity of von Willebrand protease (ADAMTS13) in common. HUS (covered in more detail in Chapter 111, Hemolytic Uremic Syndrome) is far more common in the pediatric population and typically results from infection with enteric bacteria, classically *Escherichia coli* 0157:H7, which expresses the Shiga toxin that directly interferes with ADAMTS13. Atypical HUS (aHUS) is due to one of several inherited or acquired disorders of the complement system. Guidelines on the management of aHUS recommend treatment with a combination of plasma exchange and complement-inactivating humanized monoclonal antibody (eculizumab). The clinical syndrome of HUS together with neurologic symptoms suggests TTP and justifies prompt consultation for possible multimodal treatment plan (i.e., plasma exchange, steroids, eculizumab, rituximab, etc.). Regardless of degree of thrombocytopenia, platelet transfusions are contraindicated. If HUS or TTP is suspected, prompt consultation with hematology and nephrology should be obtained.

Treatment of Acquired Hemolytic Anemias Treatment of hemolytic anemias due to extrinsic defects is normally directed toward the underlying problem resulting in hemolysis. Severe anemia may justify RBC transfusion, although the underlying pathophysiologic mechanism will likely destroy the newly transfused cells as well as the patient's own RBCs. Transfusion of other blood products may also be beneficial; however, platelet transfusion should be avoided when TTP is a consideration, given the increased risk of thrombosis.

The appropriate treatment of AIHA depends on the degree of hemolysis and resulting anemia. Children with mild anemia associated with postinfectious antibody development can usually be observed without transfusion. However, children with severe anemia or anemia with physiologic consequences should be promptly transfused with erythrocytes. Determination of the antigenic target of the autoantibody can be helpful in the selection of compatible blood for transfusion. If time permits, blood bank personnel should select the most compatible (or least incompatible) blood available, but emergent transfusion should not be delayed for this purpose. Transfusion in this challenging situation can be facilitated by direct clinician-blood bank interaction. Children with cold-reactive antibodies should avoid cold exposure, and blood should be administered with the use of a blood warmer. AIHA is often responsive to immunosuppression, and systemic corticosteroids are particularly effective for patients with warm-reactive IgG. Treatment may be initiated with combinations of steroids and other immunomodulatory agents and should be done in consultation with a hematology or immunology specialist.

ADMISSION CRITERIA

- Severe anemia complicated by physiologic changes.
- Ongoing hemolytic process that requires monitoring and possible transfusion.
- Anemia associated with severe neutropenia or thrombocytopenia.
- Lack of appropriate follow-up
- Need for expeditious workup.

DISCHARGE CRITERIA

- Absence of physiologic manifestations of anemia.
- No evidence of excessive ongoing hemolysis.
- Reliable outpatient follow-up with a pediatric practitioner to evaluate for a durable response to treatment and for recurrence of anemia. Communication of the inpatient treatment, laboratory values at the time of discharge, and pending laboratory studies is critical for appropriate post-hospital care.
- Follow-up with a hematology or oncology specialist is necessary for children with ongoing hemolysis, unclear diagnoses, bone marrow failure syndromes, or possible neoplastic processes.

CONSULTATION

Hematology or oncology consultation should be obtained in cases of unclear diagnoses, persistent or refractory anemia, requirement for bone marrow examination, concern about bone marrow failure syndromes, possible need for immunosuppressive therapy, or blast forms seen on the peripheral blood smear. Such specialists should also be consulted during the diagnostic workup before transfusion and for the long-term management of patients with chronic or refractory anemia.

Transfusion medicine specialists can be of assistance when there is a need for plasmapheresis or exchange transfusion, there are difficulties in blood crossmatching due to autoantibody production, or a determination of autoantibody specificity is required. They will typically work in conjunction with a pediatric hematologist.

KEY POINTS

- The clinical syndrome of anemia can have diverse causes and varied presentations including an asymptomatic state.
- Anemia of inflammation is common in hospitalized children and may coexist with other causes of anemia.
- The evaluation of anemia is best performed in a systematic and stepwise fashion (refer to Figure 84-2).
- Children with mild anemia are most appropriately evaluated in the outpatient setting. However, children with severe anemia, especially when the cause is uncertain, may require hospitalization for evaluation and treatment. Hospitalization allows the close monitoring of physiologic indicators (heart and respiratory rate) and blood counts, affording the ability to respond rapidly to changes.
- Severe anemia, especially with signs of cardiovascular compromise, should be treated with blood transfusion to enhance oxygen carrying capacity and reverse the associated physiologic changes. It is important to note that transfusion of blood products complicates subsequent laboratory testing by infusing donor cells and plasma. Thus, it is critical to collect samples for laboratory investigation before transfusion, which justifies consultation with a hematologist in unclear cases.

SUGGESTED READINGS

Afshar-Kharghan V. Atypical hemolytic uremic syndrome. Hematology 2014, the American Society of Hematology Education Program Book. 2016;2016(1):217-225.

Ball SE, Gordon-Smith EC. Failure of red cell production. In: Lilleyman J, Hann I, Blanchette V, eds. *Pediatric Hematology*. London: Churchill Livingstone; 1999:65-81.

Ballin A, Lotan A, Serour F, et al. Anemia of acute infection in hospitalized children-no evidence of hemolysis. *J Pediatr Hematol Oncol*. 2009;31:750-752.

Brugnara C, Oski F, Nathan DG. Diagnostic approach to the anemic patient. In: Orkin SH, Nathan DG, Ginsberg D, Look AT, Fisher DE, Lux SE, eds. *Nathan and Oski's Hematology of Infancy and Childhood*. Philadelphia: Saunders Elsevier; 2009:455-466.

Brugnara C, Oski FA, Nathan DG. Diagnostic approach to the anemic patient. In: Orkin SH, Nathan DG, Ginsberg D, Look AT, Fisher DE, Lux SE, eds. *Nathan and Oski's Hematology of Infancy and Childhood*. Philadelphia: Saunders Elsevier; 2009:455-466.

Cetinkaya F, Yildirmak Y, Kutluk G. Severe iron-deficiency anemia among hospitalized young children in an urban hospital. *Pediatr Hematol Oncol*. 2005;22:77-81.

Delaney M, Matthews DC. Hemolytic disease of the fetus and newborn: managing the mother, fetus, and newborn. Hematology 2014, the American Society of Hematology Education Program Book. 2015;2015(1):146-51.

Dignass A, Farrag K, Stein J. Limitations of serum ferritin in diagnosing iron deficiency in inflammatory conditions. *Int J Chronic Dis*. 2018;2018:9394060.

Grace RF, Lux SE. Disorders of the erythrocyte membrane. In: Orkin SH, Nathan DG, Ginsberg D, Look AT, Fisher DE, Lux SE, eds. *Nathan and Oski's Hematology of Infancy and Childhood*. Philadelphia: Saunders Elsevier; 2009:661-836.

Joly BS, Coppo P, Veyradier A. Thrombotic thrombocytopenic purpura. *Blood*. 2017;129(21):2836-2846.

Kalfa TA. Diagnosis and clinical management of red cell membrane disorders. *Hematology*. 2021;2021(1):331-340.

Kwiatkowski JL, West TB, Heidary N, et al. Severe iron deficiency anemia in young children. *J Pediatr*. 1999;135:514-516.

Means RT, Glader B. Anemia: General Considerations. In: Greer JP, Foerster J, Rodgers GM, et al, eds. *Wintrobe's Clinical Hematology*. 12th ed. Vol 1. Lippincott Williams and Wilkins, Philadelphia; 2009:784.

Traxler SG, Benjamin JT. The incidence, treatment, and follow-up of iron deficiency in a tertiary care pediatric clinic. *Clin Pediatr (Phila)*. 2005;44:333-337.

Ware RE. Autoimmune hemolytic anemia. In: Orkin SH, Nathan DG, Ginsberg D, Look AT, Fisher DE, Lux SE, eds. *Nathan and Oski's Hematology of Infancy and Childhood*. Philadelphia: Saunders Elsevier; 2009:613-658.

CHAPTER 85

Management of Sickle Cell Disease

Eric Choy, MD, MPH and Venée N. Tubman, MD, MMSc

BACKGROUND

Sickle cell disease (SCD) is an inherited hemolytic anemia that causes lifelong medical complications in most affected individuals. Complications include acute pain crises, stroke, and end-organ damage which can significantly reduce life expectancy. The most common causative mutations originated in Africa and India, where carrying a single gene mutation conferred an evolutionary advantage of protection against malaria. However, globalization and population migration has allowed SCD to distribute worldwide and the global burden of disease has continued to rise due to improved survival in resource poor countries and migration to higher income countries. It is estimated that globally over 300,000 children are born each year with SCD, including almost 3000 annually in the United States. SCD affects approximately 100,000 persons in the United States, mostly in the Black population, but millions worldwide. More than 500 children die every day due to lack of access to treatment. Complications of SCD can be divided into those that are acute and those that are the result of the chronic repetitive vaso-occlusion of target organ systems (**Table 85-1**). This chapter focuses on the acute complications that the hospitalist is likely to encounter.

PATHOPHYSIOLOGY

SCD refers to a group of hemolytic anemias in which the β^S- globin (HbS) is present in either a homozygous state (HbSS) or in a compound heterozygous state, as when combined with β^C-globin (HbSC), β^+-thalassemia (HbS-β^+thalassemia), or any other variant hemoglobin. The HbS mutation is the result of an amino acid substitution (valine is substituted for glutamic acid at position 6) in the β-globin protein of the hemoglobin heterotetramer. The mutation creates a hydrophobic region that in the deoxygenated state facilitates polymerization of HbS molecules into rigid strands. These HbS polymers damage the erythrocyte membrane, resulting in erythrocyte dehydration, hemolytic anemia, and vaso-occlusion. While sickling initiates a damaging cascade of events intracellularly, the physiology of SCD is driven by resultant activation of the innate immune system, damage to microvasculature, inflammation due to byproducts of hemolysis, and aberrant cellular adhesion.

CLINICAL PRESENTATION

The National Institutes of Health recommends that all infants be screened in the neonatal period for SCD; all 50 states and the District of Columbia perform universal screening for SCD. For this reason, most children born in the United States with SCD are identified early and medical management is initiated before the usual age of presentation. Because the sickle mutation affects β-globin, a component of adult hemoglobin ($\alpha 2\beta 2$) rather than fetal hemoglobin (HbF, $\alpha 2\gamma 2$), affected infants are usually asymptomatic for the first 6 months of life. Anemia and complications from SCD usually present toward the end of the first year of life, after the physiologic switch from fetal to adult hemoglobin.

TABLE 85-1 Medical Complications of Sickle Cell Disease

Acute	
Vaso-occlusive	Stroke/Cerebrovascular accident
	Acute chest syndrome
	Pain crises
	Splenic sequestration
	Priapism
	Dactylitis (hand foot syndrome)
Non–Vaso-occlusive	Aplastic Crisis
	Bacteremia
	Cholelithiasis/Cholecystitis
Chronic	
Constitutional	Decreased stamina
Cardiovascular	Pulmonary hypertension
	Cardiomegaly
Renal	Hyposthenuria
	Hematuria
	Nocturnal enuresis
Eyes	Proliferative retinopathy
Lungs	Chronic lung disease
Skin	Leg ulcers
Musculoskeletal	Osteonecrosis
	Avascular necrosis
Endocrine	Growth failure
	Delayed puberty
Neurologic	Learning disability
	Motor deficits
Psychiatric	Poor self-image
	Depression

Despite newborn screening and early identification, cases of previously undiagnosed SCD presenting with a medical complication do occur, especially in persons born outside of the United States. The clinician is advised to consider SCD in the differential of all patients with non-immune hemolytic anemia. Although affected patients typically have moderate or severe anemia with hemoglobin values ranging from 7 to 9 g/dL, they generally are not overtly symptomatic from the anemia (e.g., weakness, fatigue) given its chronicity that allows for physiologic compensation. As the result of a markedly shortened red cell survival time, bone marrow production of new erythrocytes is brisk, as indicated by chronically elevated reticulocyte counts (usually 10%-20% or absolute reticulocyte count >150). Patients will often be slightly icteric due to chronic hemolysis and may have splenomegaly and skull bone deformities due to extramedullary hematopoiesis.

HEALTH MAINTENANCE

Infants diagnosed by newborn screening should be referred to Pediatric Hematology for confirmation of the diagnosis with blood tests such as hemoglobin electrophoresis, parental education on SCD, genetic counseling, and long-term follow-up. Routine health maintenance visits with a Pediatric Hematologist are usually scheduled for every 3 months in the first 2 years of life, then every 6 months until 4 to 5 years of age, and annually thereafter. These "well visits" allow the hematologist to obtain baseline clinical, laboratory, and radiological data that is important in the event of an acute complication and also affords the opportunity for ongoing education and anticipatory guidance. More frequent visits may be required for patients with increased educational needs, accumulated complications, and need for therapeutic monitoring (e.g., hydroxyurea and/or chronic transfusion therapy).

COMPLICATIONS AND MANAGEMENT

Management of acute and chronic complications of SCD is crucial to reducing morbidity and mortality (Table 85-1). Although the hematologist manages conditions associated with chronic disease, the hospitalist may need to consider these complications and their impact when caring for children with SCD. The discussion below focuses on the acute complications.

FEVER

Children with SCD are at risk for invasive and overwhelming infections due to functional asplenia. Children with HbSS and HbS-β^0thalassemia develop impaired splenic function in the first year of life and are functionally asplenic by 2 years of age. Children with HbSC and HbS-β^+thalassemia may develop functional asplenia at older ages and with less profound effect. Despite the introduction of routine vaccination in many countries, life-threatening infections with encapsulated bacteria (e.g., *Streptococcus pneumoniae, Haemophilus influenzae, Neisseria meningitidis*) remain a significant threat in the functionally asplenic child. Antibiotic prophylaxis should be initiated when the diagnosis of SCD is made (**Table 85-2**). In addition to completing the routine immunization schedule, children with SCD should receive additional immunizations with a pneumococcal polysaccharide vaccine (i.e., PPSV23) and immunization against meningococcus (both quadrivalent meningococcus and meningococcus B) during infancy. Boosters are given at appropriate intervals. These additional vaccines and earlier timing provide broader protection against the most invasive bacterial serotypes to which immunosuppressed SCD patients are more susceptible. Influenza vaccine should be administered to all sickle cell patients annually and the COVID vaccination as per the CDC recommended schedule.

Even with antibiotic prophylaxis and complete immunizations, all persons with SCD should be considered high risk for bacteremia and overwhelming sepsis. Prompt evaluation and empiric treatment of fever in persons with SCD is necessary to reduce both mortality and morbidity of sepsis. The key to the proper management of febrile persons with SCD (or any person with asplenia) involves rapid triage and assessment with administration of empiric parenteral antibiotics within 1 hour of presentation. A focused history, physical examination, and laboratory evaluation, including blood cultures, should be done promptly. If the patient has a central line or implanted port, blood cultures must be drawn off this line. Additional peripherally obtained cultures are not necessary for those with central access. A chest radiograph is recommended for patients with tachypnea, cough, hypoxemia, or thoracic pain, and considered for patients with a history of asthma or recurrent acute chest syndrome (ACS). Urinalysis and urine culture are recommended for all males <6 months and females <2 years. Other cultures (e.g., throat, urine), respiratory viral panels, and other studies should be obtained as clinically indicated. Children with an obvious source of infection (e.g., otitis, gastroenteritis) presenting with fever should still receive full evaluation and empiric treatment until bacteremia has been excluded.

All febrile patients with SCD require empiric parenteral antibiotic coverage for at least 24 hours. A broad-spectrum agent such as ceftriaxone, given at 50 mg/kg IV/IM (maximum 2 grams/day), is the mainstay of empiric therapy. Other third-generation cephalosporins (e.g., ceftazidime) may be used depending upon institutional guidelines or formulary though these will require multiple doses in the first 24 hours.

TABLE 85-2 Antibiotic Prophylaxis

Age	Antibiotic Dose*
Birth-3 years	Penicillin VK 125 mg PO BID
3 years-5 years	Penicillin VK 250 mg PO BID
>5 years	Discontinue, except in the circumstance of previous surgical splenectomy or prior serious bacterial infection, after which antibiotic prophylaxis should be continued indefinitely.

*Erythromycin can be substituted in patients with penicillin allergies.

For patients allergic to cephalosporins, other broad-spectrum possibilities include clindamycin and quinolones (e.g., levofloxacin). Vancomycin is usually reserved for those with signs of meningitis, a history of pneumococcal sepsis, or toxic appearance. Vancomycin should also be considered in areas with high local prevalence of resistant organisms or if a central venous line is present. If a central venous line is present, antibiotics should be administered via this route. If a new infiltrate is identified on chest radiograph, a macrolide antibiotic should be added to the previously mentioned empiric antibiotics because of the high incidence of pneumonia caused by atypical organisms in the presence of fever.

Admission to hospital should be considered if there is any indication of possible complications or if high-risk features are present (**Figure 85-1**). If none of these features are present, one may consider discharge from the acute care setting if the patient is stable after receiving empiric antibiotics with 24-hour coverage such as ceftriaxone. Patients should be counseled to return immediately for persistent fever longer than 48 hours, or worsening symptoms—especially respiratory decline, dehydration, lethargy, or pain. Clear instructions should also be given for follow-up in 24 hours with primary care physician, emergency department, or by phone so that pending cultures will be tracked.

CEREBROVASCULAR ACCIDENT

Vaso-occlusive stroke represents one of the most important causes of disability in the sickle cell population. Sickle cell patients are at increased risk of stroke starting in the late school-age period. Without screening, primary stroke affects approximately 10% of patients with HbSS before the end of their second decade of life. Risk factors for primary stroke include previous transient ischemic attack, low baseline hemoglobin, preceding ACS, hypertension, and abnormal transcranial Doppler ultrasound (TCD) screen. TCD is a reliable screening test to identify patients with HbSS and HbS-β^0 thalassemia at highest risk of stroke. Abnormal TCD is defined by an increased velocity through the internal carotid or middle cerebral artery of >200 cm/s and predicts a 44-fold increased risk of stroke within 3 years. Higher velocities suggest vessel narrowing and poor blood flow. If the TCD is abnormal, these patients are prescribed chronic monthly transfusion therapy, with a goal of suppressing endogenous erythropoiesis and maintaining the HbS fraction at less than 30% as measured by hemoglobin electrophoresis. Chronic transfusion therapy has been demonstrated to reduce the risk of recurrent stroke and to reduce the risk of primary stroke in those children with elevated TCD velocities.

Any acute neurological findings such as weakness, altered consciousness, seizure, or language/speech disturbance must prompt immediate evaluation for cerebral ischemia. The majority of childhood stroke in SCD is caused by a nonhemorrhagic vaso-occlusion, although infection, tumor, intoxication, and thromboembolic disease should be considered. Obtaining or reviewing neuroimaging should not delay the initiation of transfusion therapy, especially if symptoms have persisted for more than 24 hours. Computerized tomography (CT) findings may be normal in early ischemia. Highly sensitive MRI diffusion and T2-weighted-Fluid-Attenuated Inversion Recovery (FLAIR)-weighted images remain abnormal for several days after significant cerebral ischemia.

Initial stabilization should include fluid hydration with crystalloid while samples for cross-matching are sent in preparation for red blood cell exchange transfusion. Correction of dehydration plus maintenance hydration alone may quickly reverse symptomatology, though should not be so aggressive as to risk the formation of cerebral edema. The goal of exchange transfusion is to reduce the proportion of sickle hemoglobin to below 30% while achieving a Hb 11 to 12 g/dL. Patients should be monitored for metabolic or electrolyte disturbances, such as hypocalcemia or hyperkalemia, arising from large transfusion, with prompt treatment, as necessary. Exchange transfusion may be achieved through manual exchange techniques, though automated exchange transfusion by erythrocytapheresis is the preferred method of treatment. Automated exchange transfusion requires specialized equipment, trained personnel, and central access in most children. Simple transfusion may be a temporizing measure until adequate cross-matched blood and personnel are present to perform the exchange. Consultation with a pediatric hematologist should be considered to assist in acute management.

Other symptoms or signs should also be investigated and treated, such as EEG and anti-epileptics for seizure activity, and antipyretics for fever. Treatments with tissue–plasminogen activator (tPA), antiplatelet agents, and hypothermia have not been studied adequately in childhood and are generally not indicated in the acute setting. If a central line is placed for exchange transfusion, consider prophylactic anticoagulation while the line is in place.

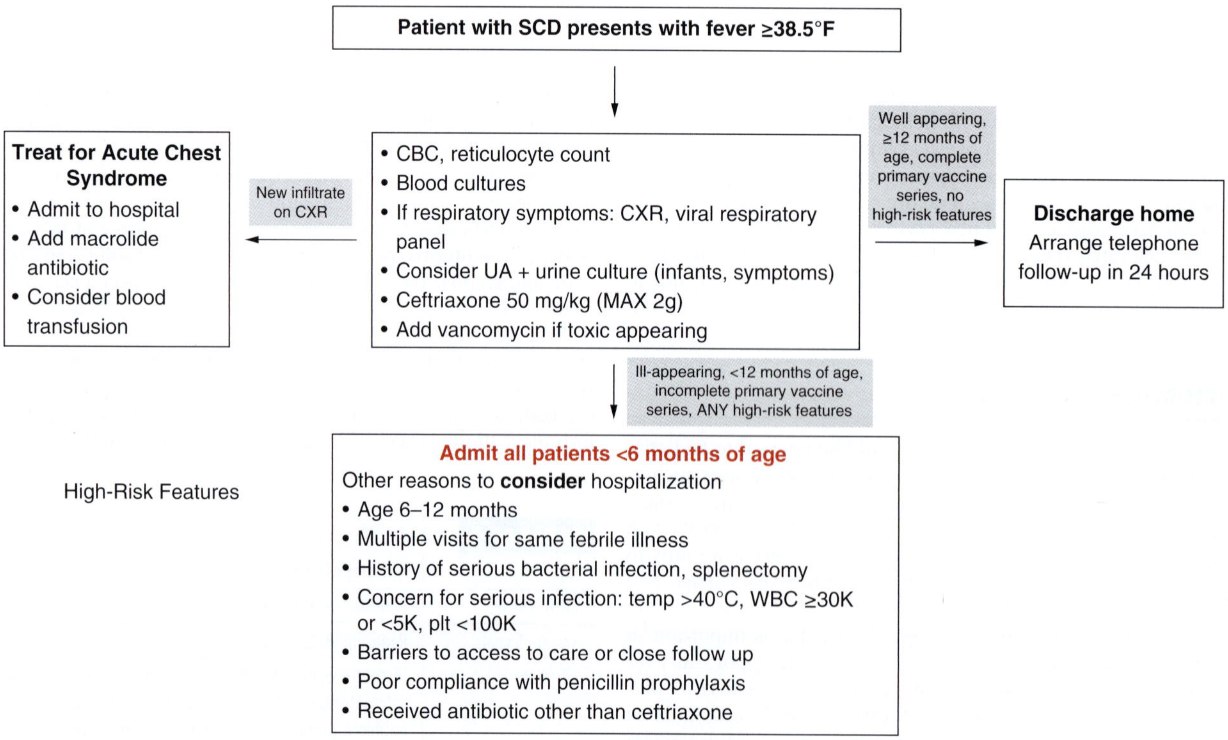

FIGURE 85-1. Algorithm for the management of fever in a child with sickle cell disease. (Reproduced with permission from Mary C Shapiro, MD. *The Handy Dandy: Sickle Cell Disease & Infection Figure, Texas Children's Cancer & Hematology Center Pediatric Hematology-Oncology-BMT Fellow's Handbook*. 2022-2023.)

Patients with recurrent neurological events should undergo further evaluation by MR Angiography for Moyamoya disease, a cerebrovascular disorder marked by progressive stenosis of cerebral arteries leading to development of a poorly defined network of fragile collateral vessels. Patients with significant cerebral vasculopathy have increased risk of recurrent stroke despite chronic transfusion therapy. Cohorts of patients with SCD and Moyamoya have been treated with pial synangiosis or encephalo-duro-arteriosynangiosis (EDAS) with demonstrated fivefold reduction of stroke risk.

ACUTE CHEST SYNDROME

ACS is a leading cause of morbidity and mortality in children with SCD. It is an acute illness characterized by fever, respiratory symptoms (one or more of tachypnea, cough, wheeze, or hypoxemia relative to baseline), and a new infiltrate on chest radiograph. Risk factors for the development of ACS include low HbF, elevated steady-state WBC counts, comorbid asthma, preceding vaso-occlusive pain crisis (VOC), and general anesthesia. The underlying pathophysiology is unclear, though infection, infarction, and pulmonary fat embolism have been implicated. Infectious agents most often identified are *Chlamydophila pneumoniae*, *Mycoplasma pneumoniae*, and viruses, with children showing a seasonal variation of presentation. Inadequately treated vaso-occlusive pain involving the sternum, ribs, trunk, or abdomen may lead to splinting respirations, decreased tidal volume, and the development of atelectasis, ventilation/perfusion mismatching, hypoxemia, and progression to ACS. Use of incentive spirometry has been shown to decrease incidence of ACS in patients hospitalized with vaso-occlusive crisis and should be used routinely in the care of all hospitalized sickle cell patients. ACS is the most common complication of surgery and anesthesia in patients with SCD, likely related to high risk of cold exposure, hypoxia, acidosis, atelectasis, and psychological stress in the perioperative period.

Initial treatment of patients with ACS should include supplemental oxygen if patients are hypoxemic (PaO_2 < 75 mmHg or oxygen saturation < 95%) or are below their known baseline. Control of chest pain with frequent incentive spirometry (5-10 times/hr) and avoidance of oversedation with analgesics are key to minimizing hypoventilation. Fever should be investigated with blood cultures prior to the administration of empiric broad-spectrum antibiotic (e.g., ceftriaxone), as well as a macrolide (e.g., azithromycin) for atypical bacterial pathogens. Judicious fluid replacement should correct deficits but should not exceed 100% maintenance as rapid or excessive hydration may contribute to pulmonary edema, effusions, and respiratory distress. Bronchodilators should be used aggressively in patients with history of asthma or clinical evidence of wheezing, and bear consideration in any patient if worsening clinically. Systemic corticosteroids have been shown to hasten recovery from ACS but are also associated with rehospitalization from "rebound" vaso-occlusive crisis and generally require a taper if used. Systemic corticosteroids should be strongly considered in the setting of comorbid asthma, as patients with asthma are more likely to require readmission without standard asthma therapies.

Red blood cell transfusion is the mainstay of therapy for ACS. While there are no randomized controlled trials comparing outcomes following transfusion versus supportive care, transfusion has been shown to reduce length of stay. Simple transfusion should be considered early in the presentation or progression in an attempt to abort progressive hypoxemia. Various triggers for simple transfusion have been suggested including >5% drop in SaO_2 from baseline or PaO_2 < 70 mmHg. There is no standard goal for transfusion to treat acute chest syndrome, however many will transfuse to a goal Hb 9 g/dL or until the patient begins to improve clinically. If simple transfusion is not effective in aborting the progression of respiratory symptoms, or if anemia is too mild to allow for simple transfusion, exchange transfusion must be considered. If mechanical ventilation is required, frequent therapeutic bronchoscopy with aggressive suction removal of tenacious plastic bronchial casts is often indicated, and inhaled mucolytics can be considered. A clinical respiratory score and clinical practice guideline have been used successfully in reducing the length of hospital admission in patients with ACS.

VASO-OCCLUSIVE PAIN

Acute vaso-occlusive [bone] pain crises (VOC) are the central clinical manifestation of SCD and are characterized by their recurrent, excruciating, and often unpredictable nature. As HbF wanes in the first year of life, the proportion of HbS increases, and patients with SCD become vulnerable to VOC pain episodes. The first manifestation of VOC pain seen in infants and young children is secondary to infarction of the small bones of the hands and feet leading to painful swelling referred to as dactylitis, or "hand-foot" syndrome. In older children, VOC pain of the long bones (humerus, tibia, and femur particularly), vertebrae, ribs, and sternum are more common. There may be associated warmth, swelling, and decreased range of motion of adjacent joints. Chronic or recurrent VOC may lead to osteonecrosis, with the femoral head and humeral head most commonly affected.

Acute VOC pain requires urgent attention. Episodes can be mild and transient or intense and of several weeks' duration. VOC pain is the leading cause of acute care visits and admissions to hospital for patients with SCD. Parental education and an effective outpatient pain management plan are critically important in the prevention and initial management of VOC pain. Rapid assessment and treatment can halt progression of VOC to life-threatening events such as ACS or stroke. Ineffective treatment is most often a result of inadequate provider knowledge of SCD, poor pain assessment skills, unfamiliarity, or discomfort with the use of opioid analgesics, and poor understanding of concepts of opioid tolerance, dependence, and addiction.

The assessment of sickle cell pain must include standardized assessment tools, such as visual analog scale or Wong-Baker Faces scale that facilitate frequent repeated subjective patient report of pain and may be useful for trending pain severity. Care must be taken during the assessment to look for comorbid processes that may complicate the pain (e.g., pneumonia, cholelithiasis, splenic sequestration, and appendicitis).

The mainstay of medical therapy for acute VOC pain is pharmacologic therapy. Treatment of mild/moderate pain begins with nonsteroidal anti-inflammatory (NSAID) agents either orally (e.g., ibuprofen) or parenterally (e.g., ketorolac). If these agents have been initiated at home and/or the pain is more severe, clinicians should not hesitate to use parenteral opioid medications. Reassessment of pain and level of sedation should be performed at the anticipated peak effect of the chosen opioid and frequently thereafter. If there is inadequate analgesic effect, repeated bolus opioid doses should be administered approximately every 30 to 60 minutes, with frequent reassessment until pain reduction to at least 50% of initial score is achieved without excessive sedation. If pain control is not achieved after three or more bolus doses, one should strongly consider patient-controlled anesthesia (PCA), which often plays an important role in pain management of the older child and adolescent. For young children that may not understand how to use PCA, the analgesia can be nurse-controlled (NCA).

In addition to diligent pharmacologic therapy, the initial management of pain crisis also includes attention to non-pharmacologic and psychosocial interventions. Important supportive measures include heating pads, massage, distraction with art or music by Child Life specialists, and ensuring adequate oral and/or parenteral hydration. Correction of fluid deficits with normal saline should be followed by continued intravenous or oral hydration not exceeding maintenance. Due to sickle-associated hyposthenuria, initial maintenance fluid choice should be relatively hypotonic (i.e., 5% dextrose + 1/2 normal saline + 20 mEq KCl/L) and adjusted for chemistry results. Based on age and cognitive-developmental stage, progressive muscle relaxation, meditation, guided imagery, or self-hypnosis may prove helpful. In addition, attention should be given to the elimination/diminution of psychosocial stressors that may potentiate pain perception (i.e., supporting and educating family members to avoid dysfunctional family interactions).

Discharge may be considered when consistent analgesia is achieved, and if needed, parenteral opioids can be converted to oral formulations. Optimal outpatient pain management often involves use of long-acting controlled-release opioids (e.g., morphine sulfate controlled-release capsules, methadone) with short-acting immediate-release preparations (e.g., morphine sulfate, oxycodone) for breakthrough pain.

ACUTE SPLENIC SEQUESTRATION

Acute splenic sequestration is a significant cause of mortality in children with SCD. With this event, the hypoxic environment of the spleen promotes acute sickling and trapping of erythrocytes leading to acute anemia and hypovolemia, manifested by weakness, pallor, tachycardia, tachypnea, and abdominal distention. This acute hypovolemic state can progress to shock. Peak incidence of splenic sequestration occurs between 6 months and 5 years of age, though has been described in early infancy and adulthood. Recurrent acute splenic sequestration occurs in approximately half of those who survive the first event, and subsequent mortality may be as high as 20%. Acute splenic sequestration occurs most commonly in homozygous SCD (HbSS) but also occurs in HbSC and HbS-β^0thalassemia, often at a later age. Acute splenic sequestrations occurring prior to age 1 year should be managed more aggressively than those occurring later, as younger age of onset predicts risk of recurrence.

The definition of acute splenic sequestration is a drop of 2 g/dL in steady-state hemoglobin, evidence of compensatory marrow response (i.e., reticulocytosis above baseline), and an acutely enlarging spleen. The splenomegaly may be massive such that the splenic tip may be found in the right lower quadrant. Parents should be educated in the technique of palpating the spleen in their infant and instructed to seek medical attention if it becomes enlarged.

Treatment of acute splenic sequestration is focused on the emergent correction of hypovolemia with crystalloid and/or erythrocyte transfusion. Improvement of circulating volume is often accompanied by release from the spleen of sequestered sickle erythrocytes leading to an increase in hemoglobin higher than predicted by the volume of transfused erythrocytes alone. This autotransfusion phenomenon can occur over several days after transfusion. One must take into account this phenomenon when planning the transfusion volume so as to not to risk hyperviscosity associated with hemoglobin > 10 g/dL. The rate of recurrent sequestration is high in children, and although observation may be recommended in adults, children 2 years or older should be considered for laparoscopic splenectomy once symptoms of the acute episode have waned. Laparoscopic splenectomy is the treatment of choice for the child requiring transfusion support during the acute episode, those with persistent hypersplenism (splenomegaly associated with premature/inappropriate clearance of blood elements from the circulation resulting in new or accentuated anemia, leukopenia, and/or thrombocytopenia), or for children who have suffered multiple episodes of sequestration. Polysaccharide vaccines should be given at least 4 weeks prior to splenectomy. Post-splenectomy antibiotic prophylaxis should continue indefinitely.

PRIAPISM

Priapism is defined as a sustained, painful, and unwanted erection usually unrelated to sexual activity. It should be treated as a medical emergency because of the subsequent high incidence of erectile dysfunction and impotence in affected males if not treated promptly. Priapism may be subclassified as prolonged or stuttering. Prolonged priapism refers to an episode lasting greater than 4 hours and stuttering refers to recurrent episodes lasting minutes to less than 3 hours duration, though may herald a prolonged event. Recurrent or prolonged priapism can result in corpus cavernosal fibrosis and erectile dysfunction, the incidence of which may be correlated to the duration of priapic events.

Priapism is reported to have affected as many as 75% to 89% of males with SCD by the time they reach 20 years of age. It may occur in patients as young as 3 years old. Triggers for priapism include prolonged sexual arousal/intercourse, fever, cold exposure, nocturnal tumescence (REM sleep), full bladder, dehydration, alcohol, and testosterone. Lack of awareness of this sickle-related complication and embarrassment to discuss an acute event represent significant hurdles to appropriate care.

The goals of management are pain relief, detumescence, and preservation of erectile function. Effective treatment of early priapism includes increased fluid intake, urination, oral pain medications, warm baths, gentle exercise, and oral pseudoephedrine. The patient should seek urgent medical attention if priapism is accompanied by inability to void, unusually severe pain, or no improvement with home treatment within 2 hours.

Emergency care should include prompt institution of supportive medical therapy (i.e., intravenous fluids, analgesia, oxygen) and catheterization if there is inability to void. Ice packs should never be used in SCD, despite their use in non-sickle priapism, because they may cause vasoconstriction and further impair blood flow. Urgent urology consultation is required for adjunctive corporeal aspiration with possible injection of vasoactive medications if medical therapy is ineffective in the first 3 to 4 hours of presentation. After conscious sedation and local anesthesia, the urologist can perform irrigation of the corpus cavernosa with a dilute epinephrine or phenylephrine solution while aspirating until detumescence is achieved. If this fails to produce consistent detumescence, exchange transfusion has been shown to be effective in small series. If sustained detumescence is not achieved, surgical shunting between the corpus cavernosa and draining veins may be indicated. Complications of priapism and its surgical treatment include infection, stricture, fistula, and high risk of impotence. Long-term management of patients with recurrent priapism requires collaboration between hematologists and urologists.

TRANSIENT APLASTIC CRISIS

In hemolytic anemias, due to the shortened erythrocyte lifespan, there is compensatory increased bone marrow erythropoietic rate and peripheral reticulocytosis. Transient suppression of the bone marrow response can lead to a rapid and severe decline in hemoglobin, the magnitude of which depends on the underlying rate of hemolysis and the duration of the suppression. Transient aplastic crises often have an infectious etiology, as evidenced by preceding viral symptoms. Other family members with an underlying hemolytic anemia may be affected within days of one another. Typical presentation includes symptoms of exacerbated anemia (e.g., fatigue, dyspnea, and tachycardia) and a relative reticulocytopenia and anemia compared to baseline values. Suppression of erythropoiesis is typically 7 to 10 days, and the convalescent phase is marked by a brisk reticulocytosis with gradual return to baseline hemoglobin levels.

The great majority of aplastic crises in SCD are related to infection with human parvovirus B19, though other viruses have been implicated. Parvovirus B19 has direct cytolytic effect on erythroid progenitors in the bone marrow, though it may affect several cell lines. Diagnostic elevated parvovirus B19 IgM titers usually occur within 1 to 2 weeks of the acute infection and are followed by seroconversion to IgG and the slapped-cheek appearance of erythema infectiosum, or fifth disease. Recurrent parvovirus B19 infection is rare in the immunocompetent host, suggesting exposure provides long-term immunity. Transient aplastic crisis often resolves spontaneously, although some patients may require hospitalization and erythrocyte transfusion to bridge their anemia until baseline erythropoiesis returns.

CHOLELITHIASIS AND CHOLECYSTITIS

Any patient with chronic hemolytic anemia is at risk of developing gallstones because of precipitation of excess bilirubin derived from the catabolism of heme released by prematurely senescent red blood cells. Approximately one-third of patients with SCD will develop cholelithiasis by adulthood. Cholelithiasis is responsible for considerable morbidity including recurrent abdominal pain mimicking vaso-occlusive painful events, cholecystitis, and choledocholithiasis with the possible complication of pancreatitis. To avoid these clinical consequences, elective cholecystectomy is often recommended even for those with asymptomatic cholelithiasis or biliary sludge; however, controversy exists for these indications, as a more conservative approach with serial ultrasound is advocated by some. Cholecystectomy has become the most common elective surgical procedure performed in the United States for patients with SCD, and the laparoscopic approach has become the favored method for children.

CHRONIC MANAGEMENT

Increasingly, SCD is understood to have a complex mechanism of action, whereby intracellular sickling initiates a cascade of events resulting in hemolysis, local inflammation, and vasculopathy. In response, existing and emerging treatments deploy a range of mechanisms. Optimal management of SCD may require using multiple disease-modifying agents and medications for control of symptoms (**Table 85-3**).

TABLE 85-3 Therapies for SCD

	Mechanism of Action	Laboratory Changes	Common Adverse Effects	Notes
Folic Acid	• RBC membrane component	None	None	Many foods in the United States are supplemented with folic acid; additional supplementation in the United States is often not necessary
Hydroxyurea	• Induces HbF • Lowers white blood cell count	• Increased HbF • Increased MCV	• Eczema • GI upset • Hyperpigmentation of nails	Mainstay of therapy
L-glutamine	• Reduce oxidative stress in RBC	None	• GI upset • Headache	
Voxelotor	• Impairs intracellular HbS polymerization	• Increased Hb	• GI upset • Headache • Rash	
Crizanlizumab	• Inhibits adherence to vascular endothelium by blocking p-selectin	None	• Allergic reaction • Arthralgia • GI upset	

Hydroxyurea is a ribonucleotide reductase inhibitor that has several beneficial effects in sickle cell disease. Treatment with hydroxyurea raises the level of HbF and therefore decreases the tendency for RBC sickling. Hydroxyurea also decreases the white blood cell count and reduces expression of selectins on the vascular endothelium, thereby decreasing blood viscosity and intravascular adhesion that can worsen vaso-occlusion. Clinically, it reduces the frequency of pain crises, ACS, and need for blood transfusions. In long-term studies, hydroxyurea has demonstrated an extension of life expectancy. It has become a mainstay of SCD therapy to prevent acute complications and provides therapeutic benefits for many patients, while being inexpensive, orally administered, and causing relatively few adverse effects.

Hematopoietic stem cell transplantation provides a tantalizing opportunity of cure, and continued improvements in outcome have been observed. However, widespread adoption of hematopoietic stem cell transplant has been hampered by donor availability, identification of the ideal stem cell source, attributes of the ideal recipient, and the toxicity of current conditioning regimens. Gene therapy techniques are under study and offer a promise of a more widely available curative therapy.

ADMISSION CRITERIA

Admission to hospital is required for many of the acute complications of SCD outlined (Table 85-1), especially if outpatient management is complex or follow-up is not assured. Fever with complicated or high-risk features, new neurological symptoms, and features of acute chest syndrome or VOC pain not controlled by an outpatient pain management plan are absolute indications for admission.

DISCHARGE CRITERIA

Discharge may be considered when the acute complication has been diagnosed and managed. Completion of treatment or transition to continued outpatient treatment should be in place. This would include institution of any preventative therapies or follow-up necessary for possible recurrence. Further details are provided in the subsections above.

KEY POINTS

- SCD is an inherited hemolytic anemia with wide phenotypic variation despite being a single gene disorder.
- Increased risk of serious bacterial infections, especially with encapsulated organisms, is related to functional asplenia. Empiric antibiotic therapy is indicated when patients develop fever. Immunizations and antibiotic prophylaxis are vital tools in reducing the risk of overwhelming bacterial infection.
- Clinical signs of stroke should be managed emergently. Provide simple or exchange transfusion as soon as possible. Do not delay transfusion for imaging.
- Acute chest syndrome is a common complication of SCD with high mortality. ACS should be treated with antibiotics, transfusion, and supportive care (e.g., supplemental oxygen, bronchodilators) as indicated clinically.
- Vaso-occlusion can lead to serious complications in virtually any organ system and is associated with significant morbidity and mortality. Euvolemia and aggressive use of analgesics are the key initial interventions for VOC pain. Transfusion plays a role primarily in the treatment and prevention of cerebrovascular accident and acute chest syndrome.
- Splenic sequestration can lead to hypovolemia that can progress to shock, along with significant splenomegaly. Initial treatment focuses on reestablishing intravascular volume with crystalloid or, if needed, transfusion.

SUGGESTED READINGS

Adams RJ, McKie VC, Hsu L, et al. Prevention of a first stroke by transfusions in children with sickle cell anemia and abnormal results on transcranial Doppler ultrasonography. *N Engl J Med.* 1998;339(1):5-11.

Bellet PS, Kalinyak KA, Shukla R, et al. Incentive spirometry to prevent acute pulmonary complications in sickle cell diseases. *N Engl J Med.* 1995;333(11):699-703.

Boyd JH, Macklin EA, Strunk RC, DeBaun MR. Asthma is associated with Increased mortality in individuals with sickle cell anemia. *Haematologica.* 2007;92(8):1115-1118.

Brandow AM, Carroll CP, Creary S, et al. American Society of Hematology 2020 guidelines for sickle cell disease: management of acute and chronic pain. *Blood Adv.* 2020;4(12):2656-2701.

Brousse V, Elie C, Benkerrou M, et al. Acute splenic sequestration crisis in sickle cell disease: cohort study of 190 paediatric patients. *Br J Haematol.* 2012;156(5):643-648.

Chou ST, Alsawas M, Fasano RM, et al. American Society of Hematology 2020 guidelines for sickle cell disease: transfusion support. *Blood Adv.* 2020;4(2): 327-355.

Consensus conference. Newborn screening for sickle cell disease and other hemoglobinopathies. *JAMA.* 1987;258(9):1205-1209.

Davies JM, Lewis MP, Wimperis J, et al. Review of guidelines for the prevention and treatment of infection in patients with an absent or dysfunctional spleen: prepared on behalf of the British Committee for Standards in Haematology by a working party of the Haemato-Oncology task force. *Br J Haematol.* 2011;155(3):308-317.

DeBaun MR, Jordan LC, King AA, et al. American Society of Hematology 2020 guidelines for sickle cell disease: prevention, diagnosis, and treatment of cerebrovascular disease in children and adults. *Blood Adv.* 2020;4(8):1554-1588.

Han H, Hensch L, Tubman VN. Indications for transfusion in the management of sickle cell disease. *Hematology Am Soc Hematol Educ Program.* 2021;2021(1):696-703.

Kanter J, Liem RI, Bernaudin F, et al. American Society of Hematology 2021 guidelines for sickle cell disease: stem cell transplantation. *Blood Adv.* 2021;5(18):3668-3689.

Kato GJ, Piel FB, Reid CD, et al. Sickle cell disease. *Nat Rev Dis Primers.* 2018;4(1):18010.

Serjeant BE, Hambleton IR, Kerr S, et al. Haematological response to parvovirus B19 infection in homozygous sickle-cell disease. *Lancet* 2001;358(9295):1779-1780.

Shah R, Taborda C, Chawla S. Acute and chronic hepatobiliary manifestations of sickle cell disease: a review. *World J Gastrointest Pathophysiol.* 2017;8(3):108-116.

Sobota A, Graham DA, Heeney MM, et al. Corticosteroids for acute chest syndrome in children with sickle cell disease: variation in use and association with length of stay and readmission. *Am J Hematol.* 2010;85(1):24-28.

Strouse JJ, Takemoto CM, Keefer JR, et al. Corticosteroids and increased risk of readmission after acute chest syndrome in children with sickle cell disease. *Pediatr Blood Cancer.* 2008;50(5):1006-1112.

US Department of Health and Human Services. Evidence-Based Management of Sickle Cell Disease. 2014.

van Beers EJ, van Tuijn CF, Nieuwkerk PT, et al. Patient-controlled analgesia versus continuous infusion of morphine during vaso-occlusive crisis in sickle cell disease, a randomized controlled trial. *Am J Hematol.* 2007;82(11):955-960.

Vichinsky E, Hurst D, Earles A, et al. Newborn screening for sickle cell disease: effect on mortality. *Pediatrics.* 1988;81(6):749-755.

Vichinsky EP, Haberkern CM, Neumayr L, et al. A comparison of conservative and aggressive transfusion regimens in the perioperative management of sickle cell disease. The Preoperative Transfusion in Sickle Cell Disease Study Group. *N Engl J Med.* 1995;333(4):206-213.

Vichinsky EP, Neumayr LD, Earles AN, et al. Causes and outcomes of the acute chest syndrome in sickle cell disease. National Acute Chest Syndrome Study Group. *N Engl J Med.* 2000;342(25):1855-1865.

Wang WC, Ware RE, Miller ST, et al. Hydroxycarbamide in very young children with sickle-cell anaemia: a multicentre, randomised, controlled trial (BABY HUG). *Lancet.* 2011;377(9778):1663-1672.

West TB, West DW, Ohene-Frempong K. The presentation, frequency, and outcome of bacteremia among children with sickle cell disease and fever. *Pediatr Emerg Care.* 1994;10(3):141-143.

Yee ME, Lai KW, Bakshi N, et al. Bloodstream Infections in Children With Sickle Cell Disease: 2010-2019. *Pediatrics.* 2022;149(1).

CHAPTER 86 Neutropenia and Bone Marrow Failure

Akshay Sharma, MBBS, John D'Orazio, MD, PhD, and Jill Azok, MD

BACKGROUND

Neutrophils are the cellular elements of the blood, which provide a large portion of anti-bacterial immunity to the body. Neutrophils phagocytize microorganisms opsonized by either immunoglobulin or complement and kill them by means of enzymatic and oxidative mechanisms. Neutropenia, defined by a low absolute neutrophil count (ANC), can be caused by a variety of conditions. The risk of sepsis, fungal infections, and mucositis correlate with the severity of neutropenia. Because neutrophils play such an important role in the killing of bacteria and fungi, neutropenic patients may succumb to severe infections caused by either. Immunity is generally preserved until absolute neutrophil counts (ANC) are profoundly decreased, usually below 500 neutrophils/μL.

As with red blood cells or platelets, the absolute number of circulating neutrophils depends on both the rate of production in the marrow and the circulating half-life. Therefore, ANC will be influenced by processes that affect production or maturation of neutrophils in the marrow as well as conditions that shorten neutrophil survival in the periphery. Since the life span of a circulating neutrophil is on the order of hours rather than days, ANC can be an early indication of impairment of hematopoietic activity in the marrow compartment. There are two distinct populations of neutrophils in the circulation—one free in the blood and the other associated with the endothelial surface of blood vessels. Glucocorticoids such as prednisone or dexamethasone have a demarginating effect on neutrophils to promote their entry into the bloodstream, resulting in higher ANCs in blood samples, especially in the first hours-to-days of taking such medications. Therefore, neutrophil counts can be influenced by the rate of demargination of endothelial-associated cells into the circulation.

ANC, determined by total white blood cell count in the complete blood count (CBC) and by the percentage of cells of the neutrophilic lineage in the differential, is calculated as follows:

$$\text{ANC} = \text{WBC} \times (\%\ \text{segmented neutrophils} + \%\ \text{band or earlier myeloid forms})/100$$

Normal neutrophil levels vary between individuals of different races and ages. Conventionally, neutropenia is classified by the absolute number of circulating neutrophils (i.e., the ANC) and may be classified as mild (1000-1500 cells/μL), moderate (500-1000 cells/μL), severe (<500 cells/μL), or very severe (<200 cells/μL). Generally, an ANC sustained below 1000 cells/μL is abnormal and warrants further investigation.

Neutropenia, whether isolated or as part of a broader clinical scenario, may be caused by many different underlying conditions (**Table 86-1**). The epidemiology, presenting symptoms, risk of infection, clinical course, and management differ depending on the etiology. The diagnostic approach to the neutropenic patient depends on clinical context and should be guided by whether neutropenia is accompanied by other hematologic imbalances.

ISOLATED NEUTROPENIA

"Isolated neutropenia" implies that every other aspect of the complete blood count (CBC) (differential, hemoglobin/hematocrit, mean corpuscular volume [MCV], and platelet count) is normal for age. Congenital forms of neutropenia such as Kostmann disease, cyclic neutropenia, and Shwachman-Diamond syndrome generally result in lifelong neutropenia with frequent, severe bacterial infections. Acquired causes of neutropenia may be acute or more chronic. In many cases, no identifiable diagnosis can be made at the onset, and the cause of neutropenia can only be made retrospectively or with the clarity of time.

PANCYTOPENIA

"Pancytopenia" refers to insufficiency of all three cell lines (white blood cells, red blood cells, and platelets), while "bicytopenia" more appropriately describes patients with two lines affected instead of three. However, as their differential diagnosis, workup, and management are similar, we will simply use the more inclusive and widely used term of pancytopenia to refer to conditions where more than one blood cell element is affected. Pancytopenia often reflects serious pathology in the bone marrow, and many patients who eventually develop pancytopenia first present either with a single cytopenia or bicytopenia. For this reason, patients with any cytopenia should be carefully followed over time and should be referred for hematology consultation if laboratory abnormalities persist, worsen, or are accompanied by worrisome clinical findings. Some cases of pancytopenia may resolve, particularly if associated with viral infection or autoimmunity; however, pancytopenia in many patients will persist and worsen over time. Presenting symptoms of marrow failure depend upon the cell line(s) affected. Pallor, lethargy, and easy fatigability are suspicious for anemia. Easy bruising and bleeding or the appearance of petechiae suggest thrombocytopenia. Neutropenia can present with infections, fevers, mouth ulcers, and skin abscesses.

It is important to determine if pancytopenia is caused by defective production or by peripheral destructive processes. Most of the time, destructive processes robust enough to cause pancytopenia will be clinically evident (e.g., severe sepsis, burns, thrombotic thrombocytopenic purpura [TTP], disseminated intravascular coagulation). Red cell indices can be especially useful in distinguishing between problems of

TABLE 86-1 Differential Diagnosis of Cytopenias in Children[a]

Disease Category	Examples
Bone marrow failure	• **Aplastic anemia** • Congenital dyserythropoeitic anemias (CDAs) • Diamond-Blackfan anemia • Dyskeratosis congenita • ELANE-related neutropenic diseases (severe congenital neutropenia [Kostmann syndrome], cyclic neutropenia) • Fanconi anemia • Myelodysplastic syndromes • Paroxysmal nocturnal hematuria • Reticular dysgenesis • Shwachman-Diamond syndrome
Immune-mediated	• Evans syndrome (concomitant ITP and autoimmune hemolytic anemia or neutropenia) • **Maternal autoimmune cytopenia with transplacental transfer of antibodies to infant** • Neonatal alloimmune cytopenias • Post-transfusion cytopenias • **Post-vaccination (especially MMR)** • Primary autoimmune cytopenias • **Secondary autoimmune cytopenias (e.g., in the setting of lupus or rheumatoid disorders)**
Infection-associated	• Congenital TORCH infection (especially rubella or CMV) • Histoplasmosis, toxoplasmosis • Rickettsial diseases (RMSF) • **Sepsis** • Toxic shock syndrome • Tuberculosis • **Viral infection (EBV, VZV, influenza, rubella, CMV, HIV, hepatitis viruses, others)**
Malignancy-associated	• Hemophagocytic lymphohistiocytosis (and other macrophage activation syndromes) • **Leukemias and lymphoproliferative disorders** • **Myelodysplastic syndromes (pre-leukemia)** • Myelophthisis (marrow infiltration) • Post-chemotherapy nadir • Post-stem cell transplantation (e.g., poor engraftment)
Medications, iatrogenic	• Drugs that cause marrow suppression by interfering with cell division **(Chemotherapy)** ∘ Alkylating agents (e.g., cyclophosphamide, ifosfamide, temozolomide, busulfan, melphalan) ∘ Anthracyclines (e.g., doxorubicin, daunorubicin) ∘ Antifolates (e.g., methotrexate) ∘ Antimitotics (e.g., vinblastine, colchicine) ∘ Nucleotide analogs (e.g., cytarabine, 6-mercaptopurine, 6-thioguanine) ∘ Topoisomerase inhibitors (etoposide, etc.) • Drugs that sometimes cause cytopenias, mechanisms may vary ∘ **Anti-epileptics (e.g., phenytoin, carbamazepine, valproate)** ∘ Antihistamines ∘ Antimalarials (chloroquine, quinidine, others) ∘ Chloramphenicol ("grey baby syndrome") ∘ NSAIDs (e.g., indomethacin) ∘ **Sulfa antibiotics (e.g., trimethoprim-sulfamethoxazole)** ∘ Thiazide diuretics ∘ Many others
Nutritional deficiency (Vitamin B_{12} or folate)	• **Inadequate dietary intake** • Crohn's disease • **Surgical resection of stomach or small bowel ("short gut syndrome")** • Pernicious anemia • Bacterial overgrowth
Environmental exposures	• Ionizing radiation • Benzene • Carbon tetrachloride • Heavy metals • Insecticides
Systemic diseases	• Sarcoidosis • Storage disease (e.g., Gaucher, Niemann-Pick) • Systemic lupus erythematosus, Sjögren syndrome • Hypersplenism

[a]This is a partial list focusing on the common causes, the most common causes are **bolded**. The reader is encouraged to seek further information about specific syndromes from current resources such as GeneReviews (http://www.ncbi.nlm.nih.gov/sites/GeneTests/review) or Online Mendelian Inheritance in Man (http://www.ncbi.nlm.nih.gov/omim).

CMV, cytomegalovirus; EBV, Epstein-Barr virus; HIV, human immunodeficiency virus; MMR, measles-mumps-rubella; RMSF, Rocky Mountain spotted fever; TORCH, toxoplasmosis, other agents, rubella, cytomegalovirus, herpes simplex; VZV, varicella zoster virus.

production versus destruction. Laboratory evidence of defective hematopoiesis includes a low reticulocyte count, low or normal markers of hemolysis (lactate dehydrogenase [LDH], free serum hemoglobin, bilirubin, and haptoglobin), and the absence of autoantibodies (e.g., negative Coombs testing).

Bone marrow failure syndromes due to injury to hematopoietic stem cells themselves or marrow abnormalities that interfere with normal hematopoiesis can be challenging to diagnose, as many share similar symptoms and signs such as pallor, petechiae, and purpura. The differential for marrow failure is extensive (Table 86-1), but it is critical to assess children accurately because of profound prognostic and management implications that accompany certain diagnoses. Though marrow failure can be due to inherited causes, most cases occur in previously well children without a recognizable genetic problem and are therefore acquired rather than inherited. Nonetheless, a detailed history including extended family medical history is imperative to rule out major causes of bone marrow failure. Replacement of the marrow by malignancy—either leukemia or metastatic solid tumor—can crowd out and suppress hematopoiesis, leading to marrow failure and cytopenias. Thus, physical examination should include attention to signs of malignancy, especially lymphadenopathy and organomegaly. Marrow failure can also occur in the context of genetic syndromes, and physical examination should note dysmorphic features, short stature, and pigmentary findings or congenital abnormalities. Certain environmental agents such as toxins, radiation, and chemicals are clearly associated with acquired bone marrow failure; however, etiologic agents are identified only in a handful of cases, and most cases of acquired bone marrow failure in children are idiopathic.

PATHOPHYSIOLOGY

Disorders of formed blood elements can be due to inherited genetic deficiencies or they can be acquired. In general, inherited causes are associated with progressive bone marrow failure, while acquired cases may be either temporary (e.g., drug- or virus-induced marrow suppression or immune-mediated cytopenias) or more permanent (e.g., aplastic anemia).

In fact, the underlying cause for many cases of pediatric cytopenia is often never identified, and the clinician must determine how aggressively patients should be managed based on symptoms, duration, and degree of cytopenia.

CLINICAL PRESENTATION

Neutropenia can present as a laboratory abnormality in an asymptomatic child, as part of a broader disease process, or with severe, unusual, or frequent bacterial infections. The severity of infections coincident with the abnormal ANC assists in identifying an etiology. In general, children with mild or moderate neutropenia have only a minimally increased risk of infection while those with severe neutropenia have a significantly increased risk of infection. Certain causes of neutropenia (e.g., benign neutropenia of childhood) can present with profound neutropenia yet have little clinical consequence, presumably because the patient can summon neutrophils if needed to fight off infection. The most common types of infections seen in neutropenic patients are otitis media, skin infections (cellulitis and abscesses), gingivitis, pneumonia, and bacteremia or sepsis. The bacteria most commonly isolated are *Staphylococcus aureus*, *Pseudomonas* species, *Escherichia coli*, other enteric species, *Streptococcus pyogenes*, and *Streptococcus pneumoniae*. Fungal infections such as candidiasis or aspergillosis occur particularly if duration of neutropenia is long (lasting more than 3-4 weeks) or in the setting of malignancy or concomitant corticosteroid or immunosuppressant use. Increased susceptibility to viral pathogens is not characteristic of neutropenia because antiviral immunity is mainly carried out by lymphocytes rather than neutrophils. In addition to infections, symptoms that suggest pathologic neutropenia include fever, oral ulcers or stomatitis, frequent paronychia, and delayed separation of the umbilical cord in infants.

For patients with other cytopenias, there may be important clues in the history. Isolated pallor or fatigue suggest anemia, which is usually nutritional in etiology in children (e.g., iron deficiency). Menorrhagia is also a common cause of anemia in adolescent and young adult women. Easy bruising and petechiae without pallor, fatigue, fever, or infections suggest childhood immune thrombocytopenic purpura (ITP), particularly if the platelet count is extremely low (< 20,000/μL). Constitutional symptoms such as weight loss or prolonged unexplained fevers along with pallor and bruising may be ominous signs indicating a hematologic malignancy. Finally, a history of exposure to medications, drugs, pesticides, or other toxic substances that could lead to cytopenias should be evaluated.

DIFFERENTIAL DIAGNOSIS

Cytopenias can result from a variety of causes (Table 86-1). We mention only the more common causes of neutropenia and pancytopenia and refer the reader to more comprehensive reviews on the topic.

BENIGN NEUTROPENIA OF CHILDHOOD

Benign neutropenia of childhood is characterized by neutropenia lasting at least 6 months without identifiable etiology and without apparent association of severe neutropenia-associated infection. The low infectious risk and self-resolving nature of benign neutropenia of childhood mimic that of primary autoimmune neutropenia. Once believed to be the most common cause of pediatric neutropenia, it is suspected that many prior cases of benign neutropenia of childhood may have been autoimmune in nature, with diagnoses confounded by the inadequate antineutrophil antibody testing. In fact, it is possible that unrecognized autoantibodies may still be responsible for many cases of "benign neutropenia of childhood." Not every child with clinical features of benign neutropenia will demonstrate (or even be tested for) the presence of antineutrophil antibodies. Benign neutropenia of childhood affects mainly toddlers and preschoolers, and rarely affects those under 1 year or older school-age children and adolescents. Definitive diagnosis of benign neutropenia of childhood implies resolution of the neutropenia over time; affected children should be carefully followed until ANC normalizes. Bone marrow examination is usually not indicated unless another CBC abnormality or worrying clinical feature (e.g., organomegaly, serious infection) develops. If tested, the marrow will usually demonstrate adequate cellularity and myeloid maturation with a reduction in the number of mature neutrophils. It is likely that because of adequate bone marrow reserves, children with benign neutropenia of childhood are usually able to resist serious infections that plague children with congenital neutropenias. Chronic benign neutropenia usually lasts no more than 2 to 3 years and has an excellent prognosis.

NEUTROPENIA SECONDARY TO INFECTION

Neutropenia occasionally accompanies some childhood infections (Table 86-1), often independent of the severity of infection. Mechanisms of neutropenia may include suppression of granulopoiesis, interference with neutrophil maturation, immune-mediated clearance, or premature destruction of mature neutrophils. Infections do not typically cause severe neutropenia. Viruses known to cause neutropenia include parvovirus B19, Epstein-Barr virus (EBV), human immunodeficiency virus (HIV), measles, human herpesvirus 6 (HHV-6), varicella, rubella, and hepatitis viruses. Bacterial infections associated with neutropenia include typhoid fever, tularemia, brucellosis, and, rarely, *Mycoplasma pneumoniae*. Sepsis, particularly in neonates, can result in neutropenia. Infection with the tick-born rickettsial organism that causes ehrlichiosis predictably causes leukopenia and neutropenia that is often associated with thrombocytopenia.

IMMUNE-MEDIATED NEUTROPENIA

Immune-mediated neutropenias, humorally mediated by antineutrophil antibodies, can be classified as primary, secondary, or alloimmune, depending on clinical context. Definitive diagnosis is made by the identification of antineutrophil antibodies. However, testing for such antibodies is challenging because repeated testing may be required for detection and the lack of positive antibody testing does not necessarily rule out the diagnosis. Immune-mediated neutropenia is most often due to premature destruction of mature granulocytes. Bone marrow biopsy, which is not a necessary part of the diagnostic evaluation if antibodies are identified, typically shows hypercellularity with normal neutrophil maturation but a decreased number of mature myeloid cells presumably due to antibody-mediated clearance of neutrophils.

Primary Autoimmune Neutropenia Primary autoimmune neutropenia, with an incidence of 1 in 100,000, usually occurs in young children between 5 and 15 months of age. To be diagnosed with autoimmune neutropenia, children must have neutropenia, evidence of antineutrophil antibodies, and not have an underlying autoimmune disease. ANC may decrease below 500 cells/μL but often increases during periods of infection. Risk of infection is moderate. In one large series of patients with primary autoimmune neutropenia, 12% developed severe bacterial infections such as sepsis, pneumonia, or meningitis; therefore, fevers should be evaluated conservatively in affected patients. Almost all patients with primary autoimmune neutropenia will undergo spontaneous remission within 7 to 24 months of diagnosis. Because neutropenia is transient, and the infection risk is only moderate, specific treatment of neutropenia is not required. When treatment of neutropenia is required, as for severe infection or surgery, granulocyte-colony stimulating factor (G-CSF), steroids, and intravenous immunoglobulin (IVIG) have all been used with moderate degrees of success. Prophylaxis with sulfamethoxazole and trimethoprim may decrease the frequency of infections without significant side effects.

Secondary Autoimmune Neutropenia Secondary autoimmune neutropenia can be seen in association with a number of chronic conditions and therefore can last longer than primary autoimmune neutropenia. Leading comorbid conditions include rheumatologic conditions such as systemic lupus erythematous, Sjögren syndrome, and scleroderma, malignancies, and certain immunodeficiency states (e.g., common variable immunodeficiency). The risk of opportunistic infections and their management generally depends on the duration of neutropenia and the underlying condition. If the neutropenia is prolonged (lasting weeks to months), antibiotic prophylaxis may be justified.

Alloimmune Neutropenia Alloimmune neutropenia occurs because of passive transfer of antineutrophil antibodies to the patient. It can occur following transfusions with blood products or from intrauterine transfer of maternal IgG directed against paternally derived neutrophil antigens to neonates (neonatal alloimmune neutropenia). Like Rh disease of the newborn, alloimmune neonatal neutropenia usually affects the infants of multiparous women, because maternal humoral response to paternal neutrophil antigens strengthens with each subsequent pregnancy. Neonatal neutropenia is typically severe and can last for several weeks. Fortunately, infections tend to be mild, with skin infections being the most common type. Specific treatment of neutropenia is usually not required, but, if necessary, ANC can be increased with administration of G-CSF, glucocorticoids, or IVIG.

DRUG-INDUCED NEUTROPENIA

Medications that inhibit cell division predictably cause cytopenias by stunting marrow hematopoiesis, which requires enormous proliferation of blood cell precursors. In fact, neutropenia is such an expected side effect of chemotherapy that many cancer patients are routinely placed on G-CSF to limit the duration and intensity of neutropenia. Other drugs, however, may cause neutropenia by alternative, sometimes ill-defined means. Certain medications are well known to cause neutropenia (Table 86-1). Drug-induced neutropenia typically occurs 1 to 2 weeks after initiation of an offending agent and is treated by removal of the drug. Once the responsible medication has been discontinued, neutrophil levels typically return to normal over the next 1 to 2 weeks. Children with drug-induced neutropenia are at high risk of infection. If the neutropenia is expected to last longer than a week, is profound, or if the offending drug cannot be discontinued, any fever in the patient should be treated with caution and empiric antibiotic coverage considered for febrile episodes. When treatment of neutropenia is required for severe infection or surgery, G-CSF, steroids, and IVIG have all been used with moderate success.

APLASTIC ANEMIA

"Aplastic anemia" is a descriptive term referring to pancytopenia resulting from a long-lasting, often permanent failure of hematopoiesis due to marrow pathology. The natural history of untreated aplastic anemia in most cases is an inexorable and progressive decline in marrow function, with patients succumbing to marrow failure and infection. "Idiopathic" aplastic anemia is the type most commonly diagnosed, in the absence of known exposure to marrow toxins ("secondary aplastic anemia") or genetic marrow failure syndromes ("inherited aplastic anemia") such as Fanconi anemia. In fact, identifying a cause for aplasia is quite unusual, and the great majority of pediatric cases are "idiopathic." It is critical to rule out inherited causes of aplastic anemia because of key medical and genetic implications that accompany their diagnoses. All children with aplastic anemia must be evaluated with a thorough medical history (including in-depth family medical and environmental exposure history), physical examination (especially focused on features suggestive of an inherited syndrome), and extensive laboratory evaluation including bone marrow examination and tests for known marrow failure syndromes. As a rule, the bone marrow will look too "empty" on biopsy, with normal hematopoietic elements replaced by fat.

Aplastic anemia occurs in roughly 1 in 500,000 children annually, roughly 25 times less frequent than acute leukemia. Prognosis and treatment are guided by the degree of pancytopenia. "Severe aplastic anemia" features at least two of the following: ANC < 500/μL, platelet count < 20,000/μL, and/or an absolute reticulocyte count of $\leq 40 \times 10^9$/L. If the ANC falls below 200/μL, then the patient is diagnosed with "very severe aplastic anemia." Milder forms of aplastic anemia exist with less profound cytopenias, and in general can be managed less intensively; however, pancytopenia may worsen over time. Prognosis for aplastic anemia has improved over the past several decades. Whereas less than 10% of patients survived before the 1960s, improved supportive care and advances in hematopoietic stem cell transplantation have resulted in current overall survival rates of over 70% for aplastic patients. Management includes judicious blood product support, infectious disease prophylaxis, and therapies aimed at restoring marrow hematopoiesis. If an appropriate HLA-matched donor can be identified, outcomes are best with timely hematopoietic stem cell transplantation. If transplantation must be delayed, most centers will offer immunosuppressive therapy incorporating antithymocyte globulin, cyclosporine, and corticosteroids. This approach benefits many patients and reduces their transfusion requirement, but relapses occur in many patients, and immunosuppressive therapy does little to curb risk for myelodysplastic syndrome (MDS) and leukemia in aplastic anemia patients over time. In general, because of the complexity of their medical issues, children with aplastic anemia should be managed by experienced pediatric hematology/oncology or bone marrow failure teams.

INHERITED NEUTROPENIA AND MARROW FAILURE SYNDROMES

There are inherited forms of neutropenia and marrow failure that are beyond the scope of this chapter. In general, these present with signs of hematopoietic deficiency, manifesting with easy bruising, anemia symptoms, or severe infections. Patients affected by these syndromes are best managed by hematology or marrow failure specialists. For more information, please refer to the many excellent reviews on this topic.

DIAGNOSTIC EVALUATION

HISTORY

When evaluating the patient with cytopenia, the history should include questions about a personal history of fevers, mouth sores, and infections, as well as a thorough family history focusing on blood disorders, transfusions, infections, or untimely childhood deaths. A family history of immunodeficiency, transfusion support, or hematologic malignancy may indicate inherited bone marrow failure syndromes. A family history of gallstones or cholecystectomy may suggest inherited hemolytic disorders which can present with isolated anemia. Consideration should be given to recent and remote medication and toxic exposure history.

PHYSICAL EXAM

Physical examination should pay particular attention to the presence of oral lesions, lymph nodes, organomegaly, height/weight, skin, teeth, nails, and subtle signs of infection. Certain findings on physical exam can offer clues for diagnostic workup. For instance, bruising from marrow failure or leukemia tends to "look" more chronic (i.e., petechiae/purpura in various stages of healing) rather than the "all-fresh" look of typical ITP. Aphthous ulcers, paronychia, enlarged lymph nodes, and skin abscesses suggest immunodeficiency syndromes, such as chronic neutropenia. Thumb/forearm abnormalities, short stature, pigmentary findings, nail dystrophy, and other deformities may indicate inherited conditions such as thrombocytopenia absent radii (TAR) syndrome, Diamond Blackfan anemia, or Fanconi anemia.

INITIAL LABORATORY EVALUATION

Manual review of the peripheral blood smear should be performed for every patient with cytopenias. Isolated profound thrombocytopenia (platelet count < 20,000/uL) in an otherwise well child points strongly to ITP. Manual review of the blood smear also helps to rule out spurious cytopenias that may occur due to cellular clumping or artifacts. Depending on clinical context, the finding of more than one abnormality in the CBC suggests either a global problem of destruction of mature blood elements (e.g., sepsis, TTP, Evans syndrome) or widespread hematopoietic suppression as might be observed in marrow failure or leukemia. Significant red cell macrocytosis may reflect megaloblastic anemias, stressed hematopoiesis (e.g., bone marrow failure), or reticulocytosis from recovering anemia.

One should always check a reticulocyte count when evaluating a patient with anemia or pancytopenia. The reticulocyte stain identifies red blood cells that emerged from the marrow in the preceding 24 to 48 hours and is therefore a helpful indication of marrow hematopoietic response. However, it is important to consider the reticulocyte count in the context of hemoglobin/hematocrit. A reticulocyte in the "normal range" may be inappropriately low in the setting of profound anemia. An absolute reticulocyte count is hence a better measure than a percentage of reticulocytes in the peripheral blood.

in infancy, history of mouth ulcers, and past infections

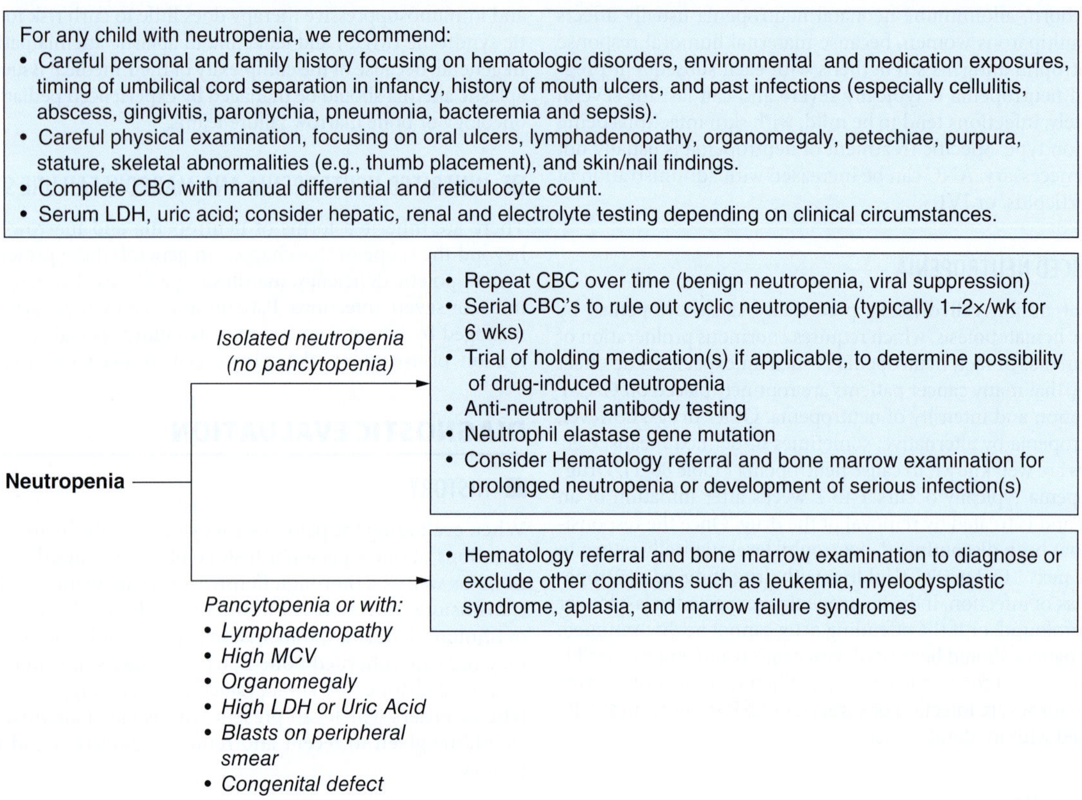

FIGURE 86-1. Recommended diagnostic approach to children with neutropenia.

FURTHER DIAGNOSTIC TESTING

Further laboratory evaluation will vary depending on the most likely etiology (**Figure 86-1**) based on the history and initial evaluation. Consultation with a pediatric hematologist is indicated whenever neutropenia is persistent or associated with additional abnormalities. Bone marrow examination should be considered if clinical or laboratory features suggest the possibility of bone marrow failure syndromes, myelodysplastic syndromes, and leukemias. A marrow biopsy and aspirate should be performed to evaluate cellularity as well as cytogenetics (looking for malignancy-associated chromosomal changes).

Depending on which cell lines are affected, searching for antibodies against that particular blood cell element can be quite helpful. For example, a positive direct or indirect antiglobulin (Coombs) test suggests the diagnosis of immune-mediated hemolytic anemia. Anti-neutrophil and antiplatelet antibodies may be responsible for destruction of neutrophils or platelets but may also be nonspecific. Hemoglobin identification by electrophoresis or high-performance liquid chromatography can be helpful at determining the cause of cytopenias. Fetal hemoglobin is often elevated in many cases of marrow failure syndromes (stressed hematopoiesis). Hemoglobin identification may reveal unstable hemoglobins (such as hemoglobin Köln or hemoglobin Zürich) which can cause hemolysis and isolated anemia. Anemia may also be the only presenting symptom of mild alpha or beta thalassemia trait or carriers. Serum LDH and uric acid may be elevated in proliferative conditions such as acute leukemia. Prolongation of coagulation tests and elevated creatinine may accompany TTP, hemolytic uremic syndrome (HUS), or disseminated intravascular coagulopathy (DIC). High serum bilirubin, low haptoglobin, and high free serum hemoglobin suggest hemolysis. Thrombocytopenia can be part of immunodeficiency syndromes such as common variable immunodeficiency (CVID), in which case assessment of quantitative immunoglobulins may be helpful. Macrocytosis of red blood cells, indicated by an elevated MCV, may indicate vitamin deficiency such as B12 or folate, or can reflect the stressed marrow of marrow failure. Peripheral blood flow cytometry can help detect clonal disorders such as leukemias or to rule out paroxysmal nocturnal hemoglobinuria (PNH, anti-CD55/59 testing). Urinalysis and testing of stool for occult blood are helpful to rule out occult blood loss. If urinalysis demonstrates hematuria or proteinuria, consider systemic lupus erythematosus (SLE) in the differential. Tests for exocrine pancreatic function such as 72-hour fecal fat, serum trypsinogen, and isoamylase may be helpful to evaluate for Schwachman-Diamond syndrome and Pearson syndrome. Chromosome breakage studies (diepoxybutane or mitomycin C testing) should be sent if there is clinical suspicion for Fanconi anemia, such as presence of skeletal abnormalities or family history of cancer and bone marrow failure. Telomere length determination should be done if there are other physical stigmata of dyskeratosis congenita such as dystrophic nail changes or skin/mucosal abnormalities. If neutropenia is associated with fevers, tests for infections known to be associated with neutropenia should be considered.

Finally, radiologic evaluation can be an important part of the evaluation for a patient with cytopenias. Findings such as lymphadenopathy, anterior mediastinal mass, or hepatosplenomegaly could indicate a solid tumor or a hematologic malignancy. Splenomegaly can also be seen in a sequestration crisis in patients with sickle cell disease leading to profound acute pancytopenia. Plain films of extremity bones can help evaluate TAR syndrome or Schwachman-Diamond syndrome. Similarly, an echocardiogram may be indicated to evaluate for cardiac structural defects that can accompany certain heritable marrow failure syndromes such as Diamond-Blackfan anemia and Fanconi anemia.

MANAGEMENT

Management of a child with neutropenia or pancytopenia is dictated by clinical circumstance, severity of cytopenias, and underlying pathology. In general, self-resolving cytopenias are managed supportively, whereas

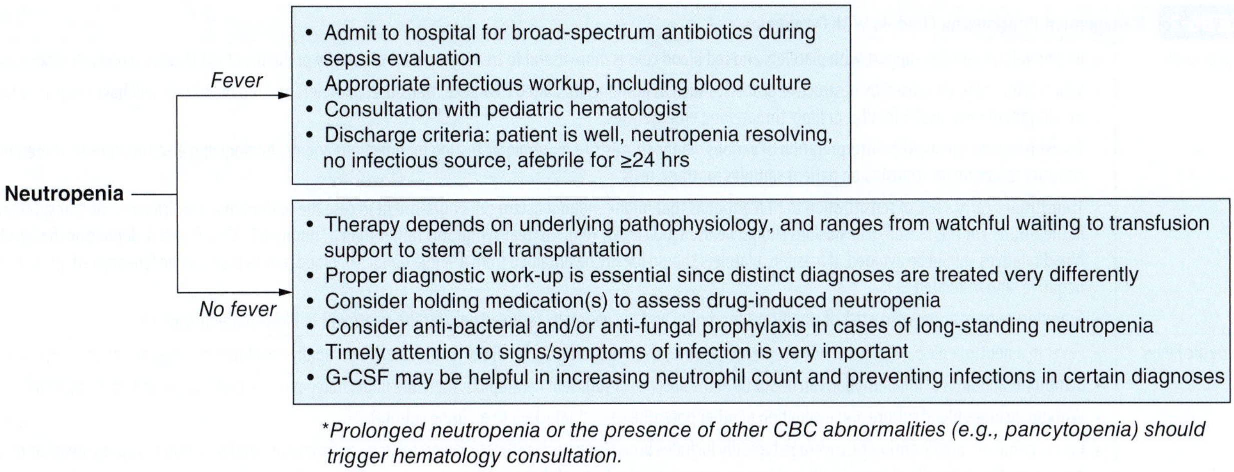

FIGURE 86-2. Treatment approach to children with cytopenias. G-CSF, granulocyte colony-stimulating factor.

marrow failure syndromes must be approached more aggressively. There are excellent reviews that cover treatment suggestions for most of the conditions listed in this chapter, thus we include a general overarching treatment approach relevant to the universal care of patients with cytopenias (**Figure 86-2**). Therapy is aimed at normalization of blood counts, antimicrobial prophylaxis for preventing infections, and monitoring for known complications.

If there is the possibility of a lymphoproliferative disorder such as acute leukemia, it is critical to rule out malignancy with a bone marrow examination prior to starting glucocorticoid medications given the risk of partially treating leukemia and contributing to eventual poorer outcome. Further, hematology consultation should be considered prior to blood product transfusions if feasible because transfusions may jeopardize interpretation of some diagnostic tests (e.g., serologic testing for infectious agents) and they carry a risk of sensitization to HLA antigens that might endanger stem cell engraftment if the patient requires stem cell transplantation in the future. In general, transfusions should be used judiciously (e.g., to treat symptoms rather than a "number"), and all blood products should be leukocyte-depleted, cytomegalovirus (CMV) negative, and irradiated (**Table 86-2**).

Digital rectal examination and any other manipulation of the rectum such as rectal temperatures and suppositories should be avoided in children with severe neutropenia because of the risk of translocating gut bacteria during the procedure and inadvertently raising infectious risk.

ADMISSION AND DISCHARGE CRITERIA

In general, neutropenic patients or patients with pancytopenia may be managed as outpatients provided, they are well-appearing (show no signs of infection) and afebrile. Fever in a neutropenic patient is a medical emergency since overwhelming bacterial sepsis and death can rapidly develop in the absence of adequate neutrophils. Therefore, it is standard to admit neutropenic patients who are febrile to obtain appropriate infectious workup (including a blood culture) and to administer broad-spectrum antibiotic coverage until cultures prove negative (typically 24-36 hours) and symptoms resolve (e.g., afebrile for 24 hours). In almost every case, patients with cytopenias should be followed closely upon discharge. Neutropenia in the absence of fever does not generally require admission to the hospital.

CONSULTATION

Formal hematologic consultation is recommended for children with any of the following:

- Prolonged cytopenias or cytopenias of unclear etiology
- Pancytopenia or severe level of single cytopenia
- Clinical features suggestive of marrow failure or lymphoproliferative syndromes (low reticulocyte count, immature cells on differential, high MCV, high LDH, high uric acid, splenomegaly, lymphadenopathy, weight loss, night sweats, fevers, etc.)
- Family history of cytopenias
- Before starting a child on steroids, immunosuppressive therapy, or hematopoietic growth factors (e.g., G-CSF)
- When marrow examination is being considered

PREVENTION

Most cases of neutropenia or pancytopenia in children occur in the absence of identifiable environmental or infectious risk factors. When using agents known to promote bone marrow suppression such as anti-epileptic drugs, blood cell count monitoring is recommended (Table 86-1).

KEY POINTS

- Neutropenia is defined as an ANC less that 1500 cells/µL. It is classified as mild (1000-1500 cells/ µL), moderate (500-1000 cells/ µL), or severe (<500 cells/ µL). Frequency and severity of infections in neutropenic patients depend on degree and duration of neutropenia.
- Most neutropenia-associated infections are bacterial, with the most common illnesses being otitis media, cellulitis, gingivitis, pneumonia, and bacteremia or sepsis.
- Congenital neutropenias present with lifelong neutropenia complicated by frequent and severe infections. In many congenital disorders, neutropenia can be ameliorated with G-CSF.
- The majority of cases of isolated neutropenias in childhood are transient and "benign" (e.g., primary autoimmune neutropenia, neutropenia secondary to infection).
- Any child with neutropenia and fever should be evaluated for occult infection, given intravenous broad-spectrum antibiotics, and admitted to the hospital.
- Clinical signs of infection (erythema, edema, tenderness, etc.) will as a rule be more subtle in a neutropenic child because neutrophils mediate many inflammatory processes.
- Pancytopenia suggests serious bone marrow pathology and usually warrants hematology consultation.
- Bone marrow failure can be inherited or acquired, idiopathic or secondary. Complete blood count and a thorough history and physical examination may help identify the cause.
- Packed red cell or platelet transfusions are standard therapies for bone marrow failure, but white blood cell transfusion remains risky. Consultation with a hematologist is recommended as evaluation of a cytopenia may be challenging once a patient has received a blood product transfusion.
- Many cases of bone marrow failure syndromes require hematopoietic stem cell transplant for definitive therapy; therefore, all transfused blood products should be CMV-negative, leukocyte reduced, and irradiated when possible.

TABLE 86-2 Management Principles for Children With Cytopenias

Blood products	• In general, transfusion support with platelets and red blood cells is more useful to treat cytopenias caused by problems of inadequate blood cell production. • When cytopenias are caused by destructive processes such as immune-mediated clearance, transfused platelets and red blood cells will have very short half-lives, making them most useful for life- or limb-threatening emergencies. • Transfusions may jeopardize interpretation of various diagnostic tests (e.g., serologic testing for infectious agents, hemoglobin electrophoresis), therefore consider reserving pre-transfusion patient samples for these tests. • Transfusions carry a risk of sensitization to HLA antigens that might endanger stem cell engraftment in case the patient may require stem cell transplantation in the future. For this reason, transfusions should be used judiciously (e.g., to treat symptoms rather than a "number"). Also, directed-donor transfusions from blood relatives should be avoided. If feasible, platelets should ideally be obtained from a single donor. All blood products should be leukocyte-depleted, CMV-negative, and irradiated. • Granulocyte transfusions carry risk of significant morbidity and are generally reserved only for the treatment of life-threatening infections.
Neutropenic Fever	• Fever in a neutropenic patient is a medical emergency since overwhelming bacterial sepsis and death can rapidly develop in the absence of adequate neutrophils. • Symptoms and signs of inflammation can be subtle in the absence of sufficient neutrophils, therefore understated physical findings can, in fact, be quite relevant. • Workup includes blood culture and evaluation of other potential sites of infection (e.g., urine culture). • Recommended empiric antibiotic coverage typically includes broad-spectrum antibiotic coverage (e.g., antipseudomonal β-lactam or carbapenem) until cultures prove negative (typically at least 24-48 hrs) and symptoms resolve (e.g., afebrile for 24 hrs). • Reserve addition of a second gram-negative directed antibiotic and/or vancomycin for clinical instability or in centers with high rates of resistant pathogens. • Consider the possibility of invasive fungal disease (e.g., Aspergillus, Candida) and adding antifungal therapy for persistent and high fevers.
Discontinue drugs that may suppress marrow function	• If drug-induced cytopenia is a possibility, then a trial off medication is generally recommended. Note that several days may be required for counts to normalize. • Exposure to any drugs, toxins, or radiation which impair marrow production of the cellular elements or impair the function-formed elements should be avoided.
Antimicrobial prophylaxis	• Antimicrobial prophylactic approaches include trimethoprim-sulfamethoxazole, pentamidine, fluconazole, neutropenic precautions, good personal hygiene, and avoidance of sick contacts.
Menstrual control	• Consider suppressing in thrombocytopenic women by the use of hormonal contraceptives. • Antifibrinolytic agents, such as aminocaproic acid, may be helpful to reduce non-urinary bleeding in thrombocytopenic patients.
Hematology consultation	• Prolonged cytopenias or cytopenias of unclear etiology. • Pancytopenia or particularly severe level of single cytopenia. • Clinical features suggestive of marrow failure or lymphoproliferative syndromes (low reticulocyte count, immature cells on differential, high MCV, high LDH, high uric acid, splenomegaly, lymphadenopathy, weight loss, night sweats, fevers, etc.). • Family history of cytopenias. • Before starting a child on steroids, immunosuppressive therapy, or hematopoietic growth factors (e.g., G-CSF). • When marrow examination is being considered.
Hematopoietic growth factors	• Cytokines such as G-CSF, GM-CSF, erythropoietin, thrombopoeitin, and androgens may be useful in raising blood counts in patients with marrow failure, but responses vary according to underlying pathology.
Immunosuppressive therapy	• Immunosuppressive therapy (e.g., ATG, cyclosporine, and corticosteroids) may be effective in PNH and aplastic anemia. • It is critical to rule out malignancy with a bone marrow examination prior to starting steroids. • Immunosuppressive agents carry an increased risk of infection, particularly in the setting of marrow failure syndromes and cytopenias.
Hematopoietic stem cell transplantation	• Generally reserved for treatment-refractory bone marrow failure syndromes, idiopathic aplastic anemia or conditions that carry substantial risk of myelodysplasia and leukemia. • Outcomes of HSCT have improved but vary with institutional experience. • In general, it is preferable for patients to go to transplant as early as possible to minimize neutropenia-related infections and HLA sensitization prior to transplant. • In general, the most favorable outcomes are realized with HLA-matched sibling transplants. • Reduced conditioning regimens have been developed and are especially important for underlying genomic instability disorders (e.g., Fanconi anemia).
Gene therapy	• Still investigational and not widely available.

ATG, antithymocyte globulin; CMV, cytomegalovirus; HLA, human leukocyte antigen; HSCT, hematopoietic stem cell transplant; LDH, lactate dehydrogenase; MCV, mean corpuscular volume; PNH, paroxysmal nocturnal hemoglobinuria.

SUGGESTED READINGS

Alter BP. Inherited bone marrow failure syndromes: considerations pre- and posttransplant. *Blood.* 2017;130(21):2257-2264.

Boxer LA. How to approach neutropenia. *Hematology Am Soc Hematol Educ Program.* 2012;2012:174-182.

Connelly JA, Walkovich K. Diagnosis and therapeutic decision-making for the neutropenic patient. *Hematology Am Soc Hematol Educ Program.* 2021;2021(1):492-503.

Dale DC, Bolyard AA, Shannon JA, et al. Outcomes for patients with severe chronic neutropenia treated with granulocyte colony-stimulating factor. *Blood Adv.* 2022;6(13):3861-3869.

Dale DC. How I diagnose and treat neutropenia. *Curr Opin Hematol.* 2016;23(1):1-4.

Newburger PE. Autoimmune and other acquired neutropenias. *Hematology Am Soc Hematol Educ Program.* 2016;2016(1):38-42.

Shimano KA, Narla A, Rose MJ, et al. Diagnostic work-up for severe aplastic anemia in children: Consensus of the North American Pediatric Aplastic Anemia Consortium. *Am J Hematol.* 2021;96(11):1491-1504.

Solomou EE, Salamaliki C, Lagadinou M. How to make the right diagnosis in neutropenia. *Clin Hematol Int.* 2021;3(2):41-46.

CHAPTER 87

Thrombocytopenia

Kathryn C. Hines, MD and Christina Bemrich-Stolz, MD

BACKGROUND

Thrombocytopenia, usually defined as an absolute platelet count less than 150,000/μL, is a common cause of bleeding in pediatric patients. The differential diagnosis is broad, and includes self-limited, relatively benign disease processes as well as chronic and life-threatening diagnoses. This chapter focuses on major causes of thrombocytopenia, and how a pediatric hospitalist might approach the evaluation and management of a child with thrombocytopenia.

PATHOPHYSIOLOGY

Platelets are small, anucleated blood cells that are vital in hemostasis and thrombosis. Derived from megakaryocytes in the bone marrow, platelets survive in circulation for 7 to 10 days prior to being cleared in the liver, spleen, or lungs. Details regarding the specific role of platelets in hemostasis and thrombus formation are found in Chapter 88. When considering the etiology of thrombocytopenia, it is helpful to consider possible pathophysiologic mechanisms including: (i) immune-mediated platelet destruction—platelets are targeted by autoantibodies; (ii) decreased platelet production; (iii) platelet consumption—platelets are depleted by ongoing activation of the coagulation cascade or destruction via microangiopathic processes; and (iv) sequestration—platelets are "trapped" in the spleen or a vascular tumor.

CLINICAL PRESENTATION

Formation of a platelet plug is vital to hemostasis. Regardless of the cause, when platelets are decreased, there can be petechiae, bruising, or bleeding. The bleeding is typically mucocutaneous and may include epistaxis, bleeding gums, gastrointestinal bleeding, and/or menorrhagia. The body has a remarkable capacity to maintain hemostasis despite low platelet numbers, so symptoms may not become evident until the platelet count is quite low—usually below 50,000/μL. Patients with moderately decreased platelet counts may be asymptomatic, with thrombocytopenia being noted incidentally.

DIFFERENTIAL DIAGNOSIS

A partial differential diagnosis for thrombocytopenia is included in **Table 87-1**. A thorough history and physical exam is most important in narrowing the differential diagnosis.

TABLE 87-1 Partial Differential Diagnosis for Thrombocytopenia

Immune-Mediated Platelet Destruction
Immune thrombocytopenia (ITP)
Evans syndrome (ITP with another immune-mediated cytopenia)
Neonatal ITP (secondary to maternal ITP)
Neonatal alloimmune thrombocytopenia (NAIT)
Heparin-induced thrombocytopenia (HIT)
Systemic lupus erythematosus (SLE)
Decreased Platelet Production
Viral infection
Drug induced
Malignancy/bone marrow failure (leukemia, bone marrow infiltration from other malignancies, aplastic anemia)
Genetic/inherited (Fanconi anemia, thrombocytopenia with absent radii)
Vitamin B_{12}/folate/iron deficiencies
Inborn errors of metabolism
Marrow infiltration
Storage diseases
Platelet Consumption/Sequestration
Disseminated Intravascular Coagulation (DIC)
Hemolytic uremic syndrome (HUS)
Thrombotic thrombocytopenic purpura (TTP)
Kasabach-Merritt phenomenon (KMP)
Hypersplenism
Von Willebrand Disease 2B

IMMUNE THROMBOCYTOPENIA

Immune thrombocytopenia (ITP), formerly known as immune or idiopathic thrombocytopenic purpura, is an acquired autoimmune condition caused by antiplatelet antibodies, resulting in peripheral platelet count <100,000/μL. Primary ITP occurs in the absence of medications or other conditions associated with immune-mediated thrombocytopenia, whereas secondary ITP refers to immune-mediated thrombocytopenia secondary to drug exposure or underlying disease. Commonly recognized precipitants of secondary ITP are listed in **Table 87-2**.

Clinical Presentation The annual incidence of ITP in children is about 50 per million; it most commonly affects children between 2 and 6 years of age. A common presentation of primary ITP is an otherwise healthy child with sudden onset of petechiae, bruising, and/or mucosal bleeding, often with an antecedent febrile illness. The age distribution and presenting symptoms of ITP can mimic acute leukemia, though the history, physical examination, and review of the complete blood count (CBC) parameters and peripheral blood smear typically differentiate ITP from other causes of thrombocytopenia including acute leukemia. **Table 87-3** highlights differentiating factors between ITP and acute leukemia specifically.

Diagnosis The diagnosis of ITP is one of exclusion. A CBC demonstrates a normal number of white blood cells and a relatively normal hematocrit. The platelet count is typically extremely low, often less than 10,000/μL. The peripheral blood film should be examined by an experienced hematologist or pathologist to ensure no blasts are present. Any aberrations in the history, physical examination, or laboratory findings warrant a bone marrow examination to rule out acute leukemia or aplastic anemia as a cause of thrombocytopenia. Investigation into concurrent infection or additional autoimmune process is not warranted unless history or physical exam suggests an additional process.

Treatment Recommendations regarding treatment of primary ITP have changed significantly since the American Society of Hematology (ASH) first published treatment guidelines in 1996. Based on the most recent guideline update in 2019, children with newly diagnosed ITP and only minor bleeding (skin manifestations) can be managed with observation alone, regardless of platelet count. There is less clear guidance regarding whether to treat patients with acute ITP and "moderate" bleeding (defined as mucosal bleeding that does not require immediate intervention, such as wet purpura, minor epistaxis, microscopic blood in gastrointestinal or urinary tracts). The decision to treat versus observe children with moderate bleeding should be a joint decision with the

TABLE 87-2 Potential Etiologies of Secondary ITP

Class	Examples
Drugs	Quinines, sulfonamides, alcohol
Infection	Parvovirus, HIV, rubella, infectious mononucleosis, VZV, CMV, H. pylori, Hepatitis C
Autoimmune	SLE, Antiphospholipid Syndrome, Evans syndrome, CVID
Other	Vaccinations (MMR most recognized), post-transplant

CMV, cytomegalovirus; CVID, combined variable immunodeficiency; HIV, human immunodeficiency virus; MMR, measles, mumps, and rubella combination vaccine; SLE, systemic lupus erythematosus; VZV, Varicella zoster virus.

TABLE 87-3 Differentiating Between Immune Thrombocytopenia (ITP) and Leukemia

	ITP	Leukemia
Review of systems	Otherwise healthy	History of fevers, swollen glands, bone or joint pain, other systemic complaints
Physical examination	Findings limited to petechiae, purpura, and epistaxis	Splenomegaly, hepatomegaly, lymphadenopathy
Complete blood count	Extremely low platelets with normal red and white cell count	Multiple cell lines may be decreased
Blood smear	Paucity of platelets, otherwise normal	Blast forms

patient and/or family, after counseling regarding the risks and benefits of both treatment and observation.

Historically, physicians have been inclined to treat primary ITP patients with very low platelet counts (<10,000/μL) who are accident-prone (such as toddlers, young children, and athletes), regardless of bleeding symptoms, in an effort to prevent significant bleeding. The most feared complication of ITP, intracranial hemorrhage (ICH), is rare, with reported incidence less than 1%. Risk factors associated with development of ICH in ITP patients include platelet count <10,000/μL, head trauma, mucous membrane bleeding, and hematuria. While ITP-directed therapies may raise the platelet count, there is not substantial evidence to suggest it shortens the duration of the disease state or prevents significant bleeding.

Treatment options for acute ITP include systemic corticosteroids, intravenous immunoglobulin (IVIG), and anti-Rh$_0$D therapy. Short courses of corticosteroids versus IVIG or anti-Rh$_0$D are favored for those patients with mild or moderate bleeding. For patients with severe bleeding, IVIG is typically the treatment of choice, as it has been shown to raise platelet count more quickly. In the face of any immune-mediated thrombocytopenia, platelet transfusions will raise the count only briefly at best and are reserved for children with acute life- or limb-threatening bleeding. A comparison of recommended treatment regimens for acute ITP is found in **Table 87-4**.

Hospitalization is not required for children with no or mild bleeding, regardless of platelet count. Although many families feel reassured by spending a night or two in the hospital, the artificial environment (e.g., high beds, hard floors) of the inpatient unit may actually predispose toddlers to falls or accidents. Those patients who are managed outpatient do require prompt outpatient follow-up, preferably with a pediatric hematologist, within 72 hours. Children with active bleeding, other comorbidities, a clinical picture not completely consistent with ITP, or those with complex social factors (inability to ensure proper follow up) should be admitted to the hospital for additional evaluation and/or education. Duration of hospitalization should be based on bleeding symptoms, confidence in the family's ability to observe the child at home, and availability of appropriate outpatient follow-up. Patients should not remain in the hospital simply for trending platelet count, as timing of platelet count recovery is highly variable.

ITP spontaneously resolves in 70% to 80% of children, regardless of treatment rendered. Some children will have relapses of declining platelet count and/or symptomatic bleeding after having initially responded

TABLE 87-4 Comparison of Treatment Options for ITP

Treatment	Dosage	Pros	Cons
First-Line Treatment Options			
Steroids	Prednisone 2-4 mg/kg/day, maximum 120 mg daily, for 5-7 days *Is preferred to* Dexamethasone 0.6 mg/kg/day, maximum 40 mg per day, for 4 days	Inexpensive Easy to administer Fairly rapid response (usually within a week) Does not (in and of itself) require hospitalization	Can cause mood changes acutely and serious side effects when used chronically Can induce temporary remission if given to child with acute lymphoblastic leukemia, compromising ultimate diagnosis and treatment
IVIG	1-2 g/kg IV	Quick response (usually days)	Expensive Likely requires hospitalization (8-12 hr infusion) Commonly causes side effects (headache, nausea, vomiting) that may result in additional imaging (head CT to evaluate for intracranial bleed) Is a blood product (risk of allergic reaction)
Anti-Rh$_0$D (WinRho)	50-100 μg/kg IV	Lower incidence of side effects compared to IVIG Less expensive than IVIG Fast infusion	More expensive than steroids Patient must be Rh-positive Must exclude concurrent hemolytic anemia (Evans Syndrome) with negative Coombs test Risk of hemolysis Not effective in patients who have had splenectomy
Second-Line Treatment Options			
TPO-RA	Eltrombopag Starting dose 25 or 50 mg oral daily, depending on age Romiplostim Starting dose 1 μg/kg subcutaneously weekly	Can be effective for chronic or refractory ITP	Both require ongoing lab monitoring for platelet response, as dose is adjusted based on platelet response Expensive Eltrombopag requires dietary restrictions with administration. Eltrombopag has been associated with hepatic toxicity and requires monitoring of liver function tests. Romiplostim frequently requires administration in physician's office due to difficulty obtaining prior authorization for home use
Rituximab (anti-CD20)	Typically a course of 4 weekly doses	Can be effective for chronic or refractory ITP Low side effect profile	Expensive Allergic reactions possible Profound depletion of B cells, often requiring subsequent IVIG for agammaglobulinemia
Splenectomy	N/A	Can be curative in chronic refractory patients	Risk for overwhelming sepsis with encapsulated organisms

IVIG, intravenous immunoglobulin; TPO-RA, thrombopoietin receptor agonists.

to treatment. The decision to repeat first-line therapy or pursue secondary therapies in these children should be informed by consultation with a pediatric hematologist. Chronic ITP (active disease 12 months after diagnosis) develops in 20% to 30% of cases. Treatment of refractory or chronic ITP is beyond the scope of the pediatric hospitalist. Several second-line treatment options exist (Table 87-4); these should be used under the direction of a pediatric hematologist.

The physician seeing a child with suspected ITP should seek consultation with a pediatric hematologist, even if the presentation is "classic," as the child will need follow-up with a hematologist, and establishing this relationship early is beneficial.

EVANS SYNDROME

Evans Syndrome is an autoimmune disorder characterized by ITP in combination with autoimmune hemolytic anemia (AIHA). Evans Syndrome might also occur in conjunction with autoimmune neutropenia, primary immunodeficiencies, and additional autoimmune diseases such as SLE and Autoimmune Lymphoproliferative Syndrome. It is not uncommon for isolated ITP or AIHA to be diagnosed initially, as development of additional symptoms and lab derangements may be delayed several years. Although patients with isolated ITP who have had a significant amount of bleeding can present with anemia, patients with moderate or severe anemia should have direct antiglobulin test (DAT) checked to rule-out concurrent AIHA. Additional evaluation for patients suspected of having Evans Syndrome may include immunodeficiency evaluation and genetic testing. This testing should be performed in consultation with experts in hematology/oncology, immunology, and/or genetics. Steroids and IVIG remain the mainstay of treatment for patients with ITP associated with Evans Syndrome. Given the increased risk of hemolysis, these patients should not be treated with anti-Rh_0D. Patients with Evans Syndrome are more likely to require second-line treatment, and the risk of mortality is 2.5 times greater in Evans Syndrome as compared to isolated ITP.

NEONATAL ALLOIMMUNE THROMBOCYTOPENIA

Neonatal alloimmune thrombocytopenia (NAIT) is characterized by hastened destruction of fetal platelets by maternal immunoglobulin G (IgG) against paternal antigens on fetal platelets. It is similar to Rh disease of the newborn, but unlike Rh disease, antigenic exposure can occur early in gestation and lead to an affected offspring with the first pregnancy. Generalized petechiae can develop within minutes of birth. Intracranial hemorrhage can occur, sometimes in utero with potential for fetal demise.

NAIT is different than neonatal ITP, which is characterized by maternal ITP and passage of antiplatelet antibodies to the fetus. Additional causes of neonatal thrombocytopenia include congenital infection (cytomegalovirus [CMV], toxoplasma, rubella), metabolic (e.g., organic acidemias), inherited (e.g., congenital amegakaryocytic thrombocytopenia), thrombocytopenia secondary to hypoxia, asphyxia, disseminated intravascular coagulation, or Group B streptococcus infection.

Unexplained severe thrombocytopenia in the first 48 hours of life has a high likelihood of being due to NAIT. Unlike neonatal ITP secondary to maternal ITP, the mother's platelet count should be normal in NAIT. Diagnosis can be confirmed by demonstrating serologically that the mother possesses antibodies to paternal human platelet antigens (HPA).

Thrombocytopenia associated with NAIT is usually self-limited. Therapy depends on the platelet count and neonate's clinical condition. Neonates with suspected NAIT should be evaluated by head ultrasound for intracranial hemorrhage (ICH) within 24 hours of delivery. Platelet transfusion is the mainstay of therapy for NAIT. Neonates with life-threatening bleeding (including ICH and gastrointestinal bleeding) should receive platelet transfusion to maintain platelets > 100,000/μL initially, and subsequently above 50,000/μL when more clinically stable. Infants without life-threatening bleeding should receive platelet transfusion when platelets fall below 30,000/μL. Transfusion with HPA negative platelets is preferred, and those infants diagnosed prenatally should have HPA-negative platelets available at delivery. If the infant has concern for life-threatening hemorrhage, random donor platelets can be used while obtaining HPA-negative platelets, as a temporary increase can be expected even with random platelets. IVIG can be considered as adjunct therapy in the case of life-threatening bleeding or if platelets are less than 30,000/μL and platelet transfusion is unavailable. Once an infant is diagnosed with NAIT, every effort should be made to determine the platelet genotypes of the mother and father, because this will be important for both verifying the diagnosis of NAIT and for genetic counseling and obstetric care in future pregnancies. All neonates with immune-mediated thrombocytopenia should be evaluated by a pediatric hematologist.

HEPARIN-INDUCED THROMBOCYTOPENIA

Heparin-induced thrombocytopenia (HIT) is a rare immune-mediated process that results in thrombocytopenia and increased risk of arterial and venous thrombosis following heparin exposure. The typical presentation is a significant fall in platelet count (frequently 50% or more) occurring 5 to 10 days after heparin exposure. However, a significant thrombotic event can precede the platelet drop. The vast majority of cases occur following exposure to unfractionated heparin, though cases following administration of therapeutic dosing of low molecular weight heparin (LMWH) have occurred. The diagnosis is confirmed with detection of HIT-antibodies. If HIT is confirmed or highly suspected, heparin should be discontinued, and anticoagulation should be achieved by alternate means.

BONE MARROW SUPPRESSION

A number of external factors including medications, infections, and nutritional deficiencies may result in decreased bone marrow production of platelets. Thrombocytopenia is a predictable iatrogenic consequence of treatment with cytotoxic drugs that suppress hematopoiesis of all bone marrow elements. In addition to chemotherapeutic agents, ibuprofen, ranitidine, vancomycin (and other antibiotics), and phenytoin can cause thrombocytopenia. Bone marrow suppression can be seen as a sequela of common childhood infections. Parvovirus B19 is known to cause a global aplastic process, especially in patients with shortened red cell life spans (such as sickle cell anemia and hereditary spherocytosis) but can also cause isolated thrombocytopenia. Other common infections that can result in bone marrow suppression of platelet production include EBV, CMV, HIV, rickettsia, and COVID-19; sepsis from any organism may also lead to bone marrow suppression. Deficiencies in B12, folate, iron, and vitamin C have also been associated with bone marrow failure or thrombocytopenia secondary to bone marrow suppression. Though iron deficiency can be associated with thrombocytosis, more severe deficiency can occasionally lead to thrombocytopenia.

BONE MARROW FAILURE SYNDROMES

Thrombocytopenia can also be a prominent feature of bone marrow failure syndromes such as Fanconi anemia, but generally more than one blood cell line will be affected in most of these syndromes. Thrombocytopenia–absent radii (TAR) syndrome presents with signs of thrombocytopenia in infants with upper limb abnormalities. Fortunately, patients with TAR syndrome need only supportive care in the first few years of life, including platelet transfusions, because thrombocytopenia frequently improves with age. Wiskott-Aldrich syndrome is an X-linked disorder consisting of the triad of atopic dermatitis, immune dysfunction, and thrombocytopenia. Effective treatment of Wiskott-Aldrich syndrome requires stem cell transplantation. Finally, there are rare types of bone marrow failure specific to platelet precursor stem cells, most notably amegakaryocytic thrombocytopenia, that also require stem cell transplantation. One clue to decreased bone marrow production in a child with a low platelet count is the presence of tiny platelets on the blood smear and low mean platelet volume on the complete blood count. One should also note the MCV in these patients as an elevated MCV may be present prior to other cytopenias in patients with bone marrow failure.

DISSEMINATED INTRAVASCULAR COAGULATION

DIC is generally a consequence of overwhelming sepsis or other systemic illness that results in an imbalance between the clot promotion and clot lysis systems in the body. Its presence always represents another underlying problem (e.g., infection, malignancy, major trauma). Activation of the coagulation system leads to a depletion of clotting factors, and platelets are consumed and activated by both thrombin and the underlying process. The prothrombin time (PT) and thromboplastin time (PTT) are usually high, and the platelet count and fibrinogen level are usually low. Treatment of DIC-induced thrombocytopenia is supportive while treating the underlying disease process. While replacement of clotting factors and platelets may be a temporizing measure in patients with active bleeding or need for surgery, the consumptive process will continue until the underlying problem is corrected.

HEMOLYTIC UREMIC SYNDROME

Hemolytic uremic syndrome is a thrombotic microangiopathy defined by presence of microangiopathic hemolytic anemia, thrombocytopenia, and acute kidney injury. Endothelial cell injury and inhibition of the ADAMST13 metalloproteinase result in a pro-thrombotic state. Platelets are inappropriately activated and subsequently trapped in small vessels, resulting in depletion from the circulation. Treatment is largely supportive with diligent fluid and electrolyte management, dialysis as indicated, and transfusion of blood products as indicated. While platelet transfusion was previously thought to perpetuate the disease process and contribute to worse outcomes, more recent studies do not support this. Platelet transfusion should be reserved for those patients with active bleeding. Further discussion of HUS can be found in Chapter 111.

THROMBOTIC THROMBOCYTOPENIC PURPURA

Clinical Presentation Thrombotic thrombocytopenic purpura (TTP) is another (less common) thrombotic microangiopathy characterized by hemolytic anemia and thrombocytopenia, with or without end-organ ischemia. TTP occurs because of hereditary deficiencies in, or more commonly, development of autoantibodies to ADAMTS13, which leads to platelet clumping, red blood cell destruction, and microvascular ischemia. Both hereditary and acquired TTP can have a relapsing/remitting course of variable severity. The brain is the organ most commonly affected by microischemia, thus neurologic symptoms (e.g., headache, confusion, seizure, weakness, coma) are common. The heart and kidney are less commonly affected.

Diagnosis The clinical presentation of TTP frequently overlaps with other disease entities (HUS, hematologic malignancies). This overlap, combined with the rarity of TTP in the pediatric population, results in initial misdiagnosis in almost one-third of patients with acquired TTP. A diagnosis of TTP is supported by findings of thrombocytopenia, hemolytic anemia, coagulopathy, and lab markers or imaging suggestive of end-organ damage. However, none of these are specific for TTP, and absolute diagnosis requires confirmation of significantly decreased (<10%) ADAMTS13 activity. This assay is limited to specialized laboratories, and thus turn-around-time may be delayed. TTP is life-threatening, and treatment should not be delayed while awaiting confirmatory testing. Once diagnosis is confirmed, ADAMTS13 autoantibodies and/or gene testing can be completed based on suspicion for acquired versus congenital TTP.

Treatment Treatment of TTP is aggressive daily exchange plasmapheresis, typically performed in an ICU setting. In cases of acquired TTP, steroids, rituximab, and other immunosuppressive agents have been used as adjunct therapy. Patients with congenital TTP are candidates for prophylactic plasmapheresis. As with HUS, platelet transfusion is generally avoided unless the patient is having life-threatening bleeding.

KASABACH-MERRITT PHENOMENON

Kassabach-Merritt Phenomenon (KMP) is a rare entity characterized by thrombocytopenia and consumptive coagulopathy associated with specific vascular tumors, namely Kaposiform hemangioendothelioma (KHE) and tufted angioma. KMP does not occur in conjunction with the more common infantile hemangiomas. Like infantile hemangiomas, KHE and tufted angioma typically present in infancy with an expanding violaceous or blue vascular mass. The majority have cutaneous features, though some are deep and not apparent with simple visual inspection. In contrast to infantile hemangiomas, KHE and TA are not expected to regress without intervention. In addition to KMP, complications can include musculoskeletal infiltration causing pain and deformity, lymphedema, and compression of vital structures. The development of KMP is evidenced by rapid growth and increasing purpura of the tumor and evolving thrombocytopenia and coagulopathy. The thrombocytopenia arises secondary to platelet trapping by the vascular endothelium that leads to platelet activation and subsequent consumption of clotting factors. Pathophysiology is similar to DIC, though in the case of KMP, the process is localized to the vascular lesion. The profound thrombocytopenia (sometimes less than 20,000/μL) along with the coagulopathy leads to a very high risk for devastating bleeding.

Therapeutic regimens for KHE with or without KMP have evolved in recent years. Despite expert consensus recommendations for first-line management of KMP with combination therapy of corticosteroids and vincristine, combination therapy of corticosteroids and sirolimus is more commonly used based on recent efficacy data and ability to administer sirolimus orally. Those patients with KHE or tufted angioma alone (without concurrent KMP) may require treatment as well due to symptoms associated with tumor growth. A prophylactic regimen with sirolimus has not been established for patients with asymptomatic KHE or tufted angioma, and close observation is recommended. Topical sirolimus and tacrolimus may be beneficial for uncomplicated, superficial tumors. While surgical resection can be curative, it is rarely possible for infiltrative tumors or patients with severe coagulopathy secondary to active KMP. Patients should be referred to a tertiary care center that can offer support from hematology, dermatology, and vascular surgery.

HYPERSPLENISM

Many conditions (e.g., liver disease, infection, malignancy) are associated with an enlarged spleen. As the spleen enlarges, there is greater opportunity for blood cells to be damaged and for platelets to be sequestered. This is purely a physical phenomenon, and splenectomy is often helpful in cases of protracted, chronic thrombocytopenia. Removing the spleen of a young patient carries a significant risk, especially infection with encapsulated organisms as well as increased risk of thrombosis. Therefore, splenectomy is only rarely offered as a primary treatment option.

MANAGEMENT

The management for thrombocytopenia varies based on the mechanism by which thrombocytopenia has occurred and specific diagnosis (if known). A more detailed discussion regarding management of specific disease processes is found in the preceding section.

In general, platelet transfusion is indicated for any life-threatening bleeding, regardless of cause. However, disorders of platelet destruction are not expected to have long-lasting response to platelet transfusion. For disorders of platelet production, platelets should be transfused for symptomatic bleeding. There is not a widely accepted threshold for which platelets should be transfused for patients without bleeding, though many experts would recommend platelet transfusion once platelets are less than 10,000/μL. This threshold may be increased for those patients with increased risk of severe bleeding.

ADMISSION AND DISCHARGE CRITERIA

Thrombocytopenia, in and of itself, is not an indication for hospital admission. The decision for admission (and discharge) is dependent upon many factors, including degree of thrombocytopenia, bleeding symptoms, confidence in diagnosis, need for additional diagnostic evaluation that requires inpatient admission, and ability to formulate a reliable follow-up plan.

CONSULTATION

Consultation with a hematologist is warranted for most cases of severe or persistent thrombocytopenia, with the exception being thrombocytopenia associated with bone marrow suppression.

SPECIAL CONSIDERATIONS

It has been typical practice for children with low platelets (<50,000/μL in the United States, though thresholds vary by country) to receive platelet transfusion prior to certain procedures, including lumbar puncture. The risk of spinal hematoma is exceedingly rare in general, and though the evidence is limited, studies suggest that this risk remains quite low even in children with severe thrombocytopenia. However, given the potential morbidity associated with spinal hematoma, national guidelines continue to recommend platelet transfusion to achieve a platelet count of at least 50,000/μL prior to lumbar puncture. This is also the platelet transfusion threshold for major surgery. A transfusion threshold of 20,000/μL is widely accepted for placement of a central venous line.

Children with platelet counts less than 50,000/μL should refrain from any high-impact activities, including contact sports and situations in which they are at risk for falls and injuries. The lower limit is controversial, but most physicians let their patients participate in sports once their platelet count reaches 75,000/μL and usually when it is above 100,000/μL.

KEY POINTS

- Thrombocytopenia can result from immune-mediated mechanisms (ITP, Evans Syndrome, NAIT, HIT), impaired platelet production (as occurs in marrow failure syndromes), or from consumption (DIC, HUS, TTP, KMP).
- ITP typically presents as an otherwise healthy child with isolated (often severe) thrombocytopenia and minor bleeding. The majority of cases resolve with or without medical therapy, and the risk of intracranial hemorrhage is low (<1%).
- HUS or TTP must be considered in any sick child with thrombocytopenia because failure to make the diagnosis quickly may have devastating consequences.
- Transfusion of platelets is indicated for any life-threatening bleeding, though will only have a sustained effect for thrombocytopenia secondary to decreased platelet production.
- Consultation with a hematologist is indicated in any case of persistent or severe thrombocytopenia, or if the diagnosis is not clear.

SUGGESTED READINGS

Audia S, Grienay N, Mounier M, et al. Evans' Syndrome: from diagnosis to treatment. *J Clinical Med.* 2020;9(12):3851.

Bennett CM, Neunert C, Grace RF, et al. Predictors of remission in children with newly diagnosed immune thrombocytopenia: data from the Intercontinental Cooperative ITP Study Group Registry II participants. *Pediatr Blood Cancer.* 2018;65(1).

Cines DB, Bussel JB, Liebman HA, et al. The ITP syndrome: pathogenic and clinical diversity. *Blood.* 2009;113(26):6511-6521.

Cody EM, Dixon BP. Hemolytic uremic syndrome. *Pediatr Clin N Am.* 2019;66(1):235-246.

Elalfy MS, Eltonbary KYEM, El Ghamry IR, et al. Intracranial hemorrhage in primary immune thrombocytopenia (ITP): 20 years' experience in pediatrics. *Eur J Pediatr.* 2021;180(5):1545-1552.

Estcourt LJ, Malouf R, Hopewell S, Doree C, Van Veen J. Use of platelet transfusions prior to lumbar punctures or epidural anaesthesia for the prevention of complications in people with thrombocytopenia. *Cochrane Database of Syst Rev.* 2018;4(4):CD011980.

Foerster MV, Pedrosa Fde P, da Fonseca TC, Couceiro TC, Lima LC. Lumbar punctures in thrombocytopenic children with cancer. *Paediatr Anaesth.* 2015;25(2):206-210.

Ji Y, Chen S, Yang K, Xia C, Li L. Kaposiform hemangioendothelioma: current knowledge and future perspectives. *Orphanet J Rare Dis.* 2020;15:39.

Joly BS, Coppo P, Veyradier A. Pediatric thrombotic thrombocytopenic purpura. *Eur J Haematol.* 2018; 101:425-434.

Kim TO, Despotovic J, Lambert, MP. Eltrombopag for use in children with immune thrombocytopenia. *Blood Adv.* 2018: 2(4): 454-461.

Lieberman L, Greinacher A, Murphy MF, et al. Fetal and neonatal alloimmune thrombocytopenia: recommendations for evidence-based practice, an international approach. *British J Hematol.* 2019;185: 549-562.

Neunert C, Terrel DR, Arnold DM, et al. American Society of Hematology 2019 guidelines for immune thrombocytopenia. *Blood Adv.* 2019; 3(23): 3829–3866.

Neunert CE, Rose MJ. Romiplostim for the management of pediatric immune thrombocytopenia: drug development and current practice. *Blood Adv.* 2019: 3(12); 1907-1915.

Risch L, Huber AR, Schmugge M. Diagnosis and treatment of heparin-induced thrombocytopenia in neonates and children. *Thromb Res.* 2006; 118: 123-135.

Rodeghiero F, Stasi R, Gernsheimer T, et al. Standardization of terminology, definitions and outcome criteria in immune thrombocytopenic purpura of adults and children: report from an international working group. *Blood.* 2009;113(11):2386-2393.

CHAPTER 88

Disorders of Coagulation and Thrombosis

Alicia Caldwell, MD and Stephanie Moss, MD

OVERVIEW

Under normal homeostatic conditions, the human body maintains a balance between clot formation and destruction. Physiologic hemostasis involves a complex interaction among platelets, the vascular endothelium, the coagulation cascade, and the fibrinolytic system. It is a dynamic system maintained by a balance of procoagulant and anticoagulant factors. Disruption of this equilibrium may lead to bleeding or thrombotic complications.

PATHOPHYSIOLOGY

The intact vascular endothelium provides a smooth surface that promotes blood flow and inhibits coagulation. When disrupted, blood comes in contact with the subendothelial matrix, which activates the hemostatic system. The first step in this process—formation of the platelet plug—consists of adherence of platelets to the margins of the injured vessel, followed by platelet activation and release of procoagulant substances. Here, von Willebrand factor (vWFct) acts as a bridging protein between platelets and the vascular wall. The next step is the coagulation cascade, a carefully regulated series of procoagulant events initiated by tissue factor released from the subendothelial matrix. Tissue factor along with factor VII activates factor X, which together with factor V forms the prothrombinase complex, subsequently activating factor II (prothrombin) to generate thrombin. Thrombin converts fibrinogen to fibrin. Fibrin crosslinks into polymers with the help of factor XIII to form a strong mesh that traps red cells, white cells, and more platelets to form the final clot. This pathway, known as the "extrinsic" pathway, feeds an auto-amplification loop to recruit the "intrinsic" pathway to further clot formation (**Figure 88-1**). Thrombin activates factors IX and VIII, which in turn activate factor X to further increase thrombin (and subsequently fibrin) production several thousand-fold. Once enough fibrin is generated, the coagulation cascade is terminated by natural anticoagulant factors. The fibrin clot will persist until the vascular wall is repaired; the clot is then broken down by the fibrinolytic system. The main fibrinolytic enzyme is plasmin, which is kept in check by the inhibitory action of antiplasmin.

DISORDERS OF COAGULATION

CLINICAL PRESENTATION

The main issues to consider in a patient with a suspected coagulation disorder are the severity of the bleeding episodes, the pattern of bleeding, and family members with similar manifestations.

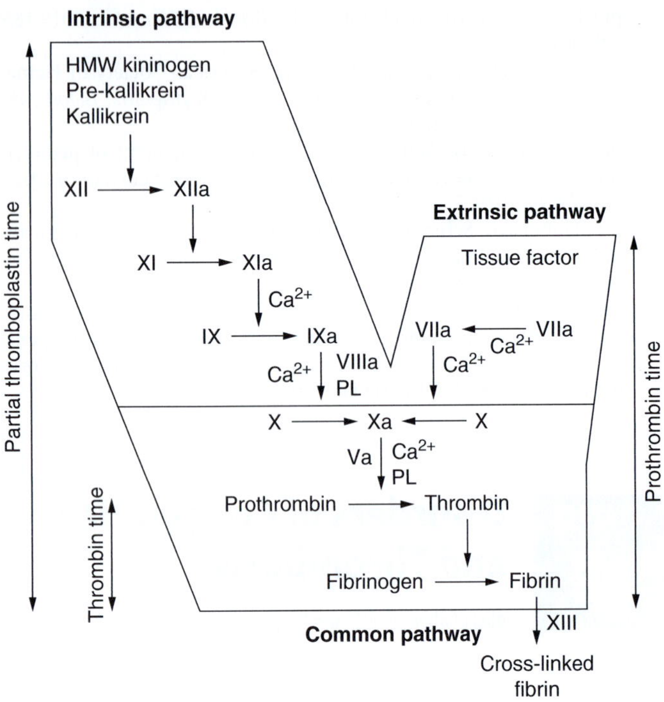

FIGURE 88-1. The coagulation cascade, showing the steps of the intrinsic pathway (measured by the PTT) and the extrinsic pathway (measured by the PT).

Magnitude of the Bleed in Relation to the Causative Factor Intense trauma will always cause vascular injury and bleeding. However, patients with coagulation disorders have bleeding that is spontaneous or disproportionate to the severity of the inciting event, lasts longer than expected, and/or recurs. Important hemostatic challenges include surgeries (including circumcision), dental extractions, traumatic events (including sports injuries), and menstruation.

Bleeding Pattern Mucocutaneous bleeds including purpura, epistaxis, gastrointestinal bleeding, and menorrhagia suggest a defect of primary hemostasis involving platelets (i.e., diminished number or function), vWFct, or the vessel wall (e.g., inflammation, collagen defect). Deep-seated bleeds, such as muscular hematomas or hemarthroses, suggest a coagulopathy, most commonly caused by a deficit of factor VIII, IX, or XI. Generalized bleeding combining the two patterns is encountered in consumptive coagulopathies such as disseminated intravascular coagulation (DIC), which is seen in patients who are critically ill.

Family History Most pediatric bleeding disorders are inherited. Hemophilia A (factor VIII deficiency) and B (factor IX deficiency) have an X-linked pattern of inheritance, while von Willebrand disease (vWD) most often has an autosomal dominant inheritance with variable expressivity and penetrance.

LABORATORY EVALUATION

For any patient with a history of abnormal bleeding, the evaluation should start with a complete blood count (CBC) and routine coagulation tests (prothrombin time and activated partial thromboplastin time) to help narrow the differential and direct further testing. An exception would be for the patient with a known family history of a specific disorder, in which case directed testing may be indicated without following the stepwise approach presented. A summary of laboratory findings for disorders of coagulation is present in **Table 88-1** and an algorithm for work up of abnormal coagulation tests is presented in **Figure 88-2**.

Complete Blood Count Only when the platelet count is less than 50,000 to 70,000/μL does bleeding tendency meaningfully increase. Severe thrombocytopenia, with platelet counts below 10,000 to 20,000/μL, puts the patient at risk for serious spontaneous bleeds. The approach to thrombocytopenia is discussed in Chapter 87.

Prothrombin Time (PT) PT is influenced by the activity of factors II, VII, IX, X, and fibrinogen, reflecting the function of the extrinsic and common coagulation pathways. It is commonly reported as the international normalized ratio (INR), allowing comparison of results across different laboratories. Isolated PT prolongation (i.e., prolonged PT and normal aPTT) is suggestive of factor VII deficiency, which may be inherited or secondary to liver failure.

Activated Partial Thromboplastin Time (aPTT) The aPTT evaluates the activities of coagulation factors of the intrinsic and common pathway: II, V, X, VIII, IX, XI, XII, prekallikrein, and bradykinin. In general, levels

TABLE 88-1 Laboratory Results for Disorders of Coagulation

	Platelets	PT/INR	aPTT	Mixing Study	Factor VIII	Factor IX	vWFct Antigen	vWFct Activity	vWFct Activity: Antigen Ratio	Platelet Aggregation Studies	D-dimer	Fibrinogen
Hemophilia A	Normal	Normal	High	Corrects unless inhibitor present	Low	Normal	Normal	Normal	n/a	Normal	Normal	Normal
Hemophilia B	Normal	Normal	High	Corrects unless inhibitor present	Normal	Low	Normal	Normal	n/a	Normal	Normal	Normal
VWD Type 1	Normal	Normal	Normal	n/a	Normal	Normal	Low	Low	>0.7	Normal	Normal	Normal
VWD Type 2	Normal or Low	Normal	Normal or High	Corrects	Normal or Low	Normal	Normal or Low	Low	<0.7	Normal	Normal	Normal
VWD Type 3	Normal	Normal	High	Corrects	Low	Normal	Absent or Low	Absent or Low	n/a	Normal	Normal	Normal
Bernard-Soulier	Decreased but large in size	Normal	Normal	n/a	Normal	Normal	Normal	Normal	n/a	Abnormal for ristocetin	Normal	Normal
Glanzmann Thrombasthenia	Normal, isolated platelets without clumping	Normal	Normal	n/a	Normal	Normal	Normal	Normal	n/a	Abnormal for ADP, collagen	Normal	Normal
DIC	Decreased	High	High	Does not correct	Normal	Normal	Normal	Normal	n/a	n/a	High	Low

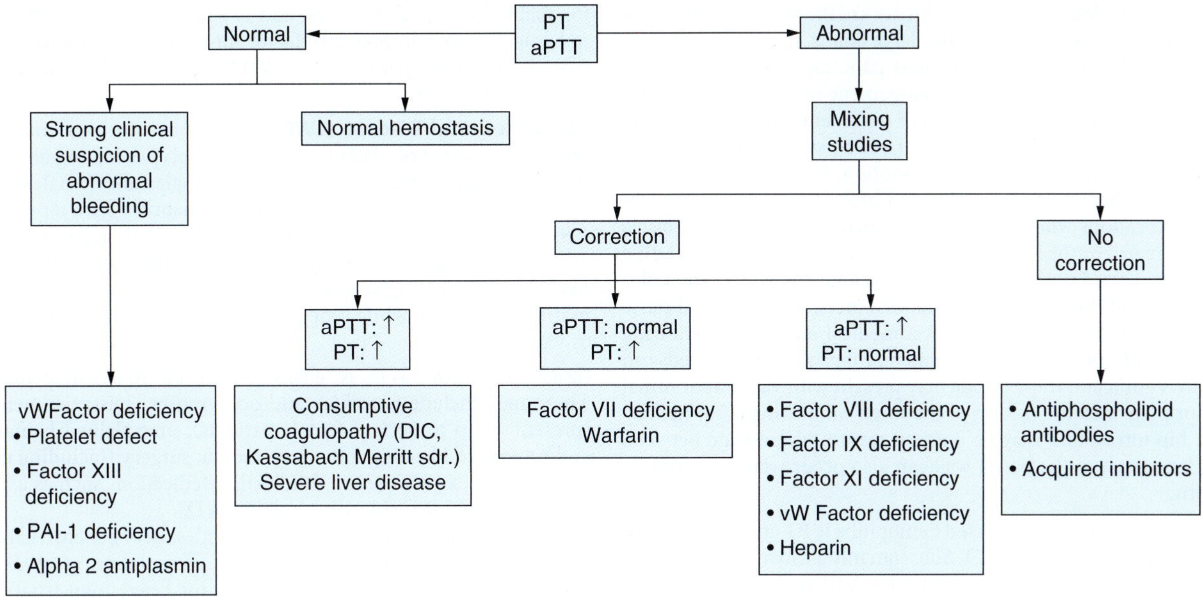

FIGURE 88-2. Algorithm of the laboratory evaluation for the patient with abnormal bleeding.

of any given factor must decrease below 40% before the aPTT is prolonged. aPTT is longer during infancy due to comparatively low levels of factor IX. Deficiency of factors VIII, IX, and XI result in bleeding disorders, whereas deficiencies of factor XII, bradikinin, or prekallikrein are not associated with bleeding despite prolonging the aPTT.

Mixing Studies Abnormal coagulation studies can be due to true deficiency of or acquired antibodies against one or more clotting factors. To distinguish between these possibilities, mixing studies can be helpful. Mixing studies involve combining the patient's plasma with normal plasma and determining the effect on the PT and aPTT. Correction of the patient's prolonged PT or aPTT after mixing suggests a clotting factor deficiency, while lack of correction suggests the presence of an inhibitor. Inhibitors can be specific for a particular clotting factor or more general such as lupus anticoagulant or antiphospholipid antibody. In children, inhibitors most commonly arise in response to factor replacement for known hemophilia. Not all inhibitors lead to clinical bleeding despite the effect on in vitro mixing studies. For example, lupus anticoagulants and antiphospholipid antibodies prolong the aPTT but are associated with thrombosis rather than bleeding.

Specific Factor Level Testing If mixing studies demonstrate correction of the PT and aPTT, further testing for specific factor deficiencies is indicated. An isolated prolonged PT that corrects with mixing study is indicative of factor VII deficiency. An isolated prolonged aPTT which corrects may indicate a deficiency in factor VIII, IX, or XI.

von Willebrand Factor (vWFct) Activity and Antigen Testing vWFct facilitates adherence of platelets to the injured endothelium. vWFct antigen is a quantitative measure of vWFct protein. Qualitative vWFct activity is measured by several different assays evaluating how well vWFct binds to cofactors, most commonly platelets, but also collagen and factor VIII. Historically the ristocetin cofactor assay was commonly used to assess the ability of vWFct to bind to platelets, but this test is limited by low reproducibility. Therefore, recent guidelines recommend newer assays to assess platelet binding. The ratio of vWFct activity to antigen, indicating concordance between function and amount, is helpful in distinguishing between VWD types.

Platelet Aggregation Studies These evaluate platelet clumping in response to various agonists (e.g., ADP, collagen, ristocetin), generally as a panel. It is time consuming and requires large quantities of blood, making it impractical for many pediatric patients. However, this testing can be used to distinguish between inherited platelet function disorders, such as Glantzmann thrombasthenia and Bernard Soulier syndrome.

D-dimer D-dimer is a product of degradation of cross-linked fibrin by plasmin and is elevated in the presence of ongoing coagulation and fibrinolysis. Fibrinolysis, and subsequently elevated D-dimer, is a hallmark of DIC, which presents with evidence of simultaneous clotting and bleeding. D-dimer is also used to screen for thrombosis. A normal D-dimer has a strong negative predictive value for venous thromboembolism in adults. In pediatrics, the negative predictive value of the D-dimer is weaker, as 13% to 40% of children with pulmonary embolization may have a normal D-dimer. D-dimer is elevated in other conditions of inflammation, including COVID-19.

Fibrinogen Fibrinogen is low in DIC due to consumption but can also be low in patients with liver disease as the liver is the sole site of production. Inherited causes of low or dysfunctional fibrinogen are very rare. Fibrinogen is an acute phase reactant and can be elevated in myriad inflammatory conditions.

INDIVIDUAL DISORDERS OF COAGULATION

Hemophilia The term hemophilia refers to a group of bleeding disorders characterized by deep-seated bleeds (hematomas, hemarthroses) due to congenital deficiencies in factors VIII (hemophilia A), IX (hemophilia B), or XI (hemophilia C). Factor XI deficiency is uncommon, and bleeding manifestations are generally milder.

The incidence of hemophilia is about 1:5000 males; about 85% have factor VIII deficiency and 15% have factor IX deficiency. Inheritance for both is X-linked recessive. Males are much more commonly affected; females are generally asymptomatic carriers or may have mild bleeding. About one-third of factor VIII mutations are spontaneous, thus there may be no family history of a bleeding disorder.

Clinical Presentation The clinical manifestations of hemophilia A and B correlate with their respective factor levels. Individuals with severe deficiency (<1%) may develop joint bleeds and hematomas during routine daily activities with no or minimal trauma. Severe disease occurs in approximately 60% of patients with hemophilia A and 30% to 40% of those with hemophilia B. Patients with moderate deficiency (1%-5%) may bleed with mild to moderate trauma and have significant bleeds with surgical or dental procedures. Both moderate and severe phenotypes typically have bleeding within the first year of life. Factor levels between 5% and 30% are associated with a milder clinical course.

Bleeding events in the newborn period have a distinct profile. The most common occurrence is post-circumcision, though the procedure can be safely performed with appropriate prophylaxis. Intracranial hemorrhage is another significant cause of bleeding, occurring in 3.5% to 4% of newborns with hemophilia with an estimated 20% mortality and long-term neurologic sequelae in 60% to 75% of cases. Instrumentation such as forceps or vacuum-assist increases the risk for intracranial hemorrhage.

In children and adolescents, hemarthroses are the most common type of hemorrhage, typically affecting the large joints (i.e., ankles, knees, elbows). The first sign of hemarthrosis is pain, especially with weight bearing or movement, followed by enlargement of the joint, warmth, and reduced range of motion. Repeated or persistent joint bleeds lead to chronic hemophilic arthropathy, characterized by synovial proliferation, damage of the cartilage, limited range of motion, and chronic pain.

Intramuscular hematomas are also common. Large muscle bleeds, occurring in locations where the muscle is surrounded by a tight fascia such as the forearm or the lower leg, can compromise blood flow leading to compartment syndrome. Clinical signs include changes in the color and temperature of the skin, paresthesia, weakness, and decreased pulse amplitude. Compartment syndrome is a medical emergency requiring fasciotomy in addition to factor replacement. Iliopsoas muscle bleeds can be clinically significant; these bleeds may present with vague abdominal pain and/or pain with the flexion of the thigh mimicking a hip hemarthrosis. A hip ultrasound may be a useful test to differentiate between the two. Hematoma in the bowel wall can also occur which can mimic appendicitis.

Diagnosis The initial test for suspected hemophilia is PT and aPTT, which will demonstrate a prolonged aPTT. Subsequently a mixing study should demonstrate correction of the aPTT. Factor VIII and factor IX levels should then be drawn to distinguish between hemophilia A and B.

Treatment Timely intervention is essential for the treatment of all acute bleeds in patients with hemophilia. Clotting factor replacement therapy should be given immediately, prior to any diagnostic testing to determine the location/extent of bleeding. A pediatric hematologist should be involved early.

Specific treatment of an acute hemarthrosis/hematoma includes:

- Correcting the coagulopathy with clotting factor replacement and antifibrinolytic therapy (aminocaproic acid and tranexamic acid)
- Decreasing the blood flow to the site of bleeding and reducing local inflammation through limb elevation, pressure, and ice packs
- Resting the affected joint or muscle until the pain subsides
- Managing pain
- Arthrocentesis is generally avoided unless there is suspicion for infection or for a tense effusion that has not improved despite factor replacement.

Clotting factor concentrates are either plasma derived or artificially produced by recombinant technology. The risk of transmitting a severe infection such as HIV or hepatitis through clotting factor concentrates is extremely low, with no documented transmissions for decades. Joint and muscle bleeds typically respond to treatment within 1 to 2 days. The dose of factor concentrate and length of therapy for any bleed are based on patient factors and bleed type. Recommendations for dosing are provided by the World Federation of Hemophilia (WFH) Guidelines.

The main treatment complication of using factor concentrates is the development of inhibitors, which are inactivating antibodies triggered by exposure to the factor. Inhibitors develop in approximately 30% of patients with hemophilia A and 2% to 3% of those with hemophilia B, mostly in patients with severe disease. The lower rate of inhibitors in hemophilia B is thought to relate to the lower incidence of severe disease in hemophilia B. If the inhibitor titer is low, the patient can be treated with larger amounts of factor to overwhelm the inhibitors. If, however, the inhibitor titer is high, giving the patient enough factor becomes impractical. In such cases, bleeding is best treated by administering an agent that bypasses factor VIII or IX in the coagulation cascade, such as activated factor VII (Novo-Seven) or the prothrombin complex concentrate (FEIBA). Long-term therapy for high titer inhibitors is immune tolerance induction, with the goal of eliminating the inhibitor by making the immune system tolerant to factor infusions. Of note, although development of inhibitors is less common in patients with hemophilia B, those patients do not respond as well to immune tolerance therapy as patients with hemophilia A, and are more prone to factor IV induced anaphylaxis, making it harder to treat these patients.

Prevention Bleed prevention is critically important in the management of hemophilia. Prophylactic therapy is superior to on-demand therapy for maintaining joint function and is associated with a 90% reduction in hemarthrosis rate. Standard factor infusions for prophylaxis are given two to three times per week. The WFH recommends initiating prophylaxis prior to age 3.

von Willebrand Disease (vWD) vWD is caused by a quantitative or qualitative defect of vWFct, with most subtypes having an autosomal dominant inheritance pattern affecting males and females equally. It is the most common inherited bleeding disorder with a prevalence of 1 in 1000. The most common form, type 1 vWD, accounts for 75% of cases and is characterized by low levels of functional vWFct. Type 2 vWD (encompassing several subtypes) is caused by functional abnormalities of vWFct, while type 3 vWD represents the complete absence of vWFct.

Clinical Presentation vWD is characterized by mucocutaneous bleeds. These may include petechiae and ecchymoses, epistaxis, menorrhagia (present in up to 90% of female patients), unexplained hematochezia, and prolonged bleeding following trauma, surgery (including circumcision), dental extractions, or childbirth. Medications such as aspirin and NSAIDs can increase bleeding risk in vWD.

In the absence of prior bleeding episodes, heavy menstrual bleeding at the onset of menarche is a common presentation of vWD. Among adolescents who require hospitalization for heavy menstrual bleeding, approximately one third will be diagnosed with a bleeding disorder, of which vWD is most common.

Type 3 vWD has the most severe phenotype and behaves similarly to hemophilia A as vWFct also serves as carrier for circulating factor VIII; Type 3 vWD may be associated with hemarthroses in addition to mucocutaneous bleeding. Type 2 vWD generally presents with moderate to severe mucocutaneous bleeding. Due to both incomplete penetrance and variable expressivity, type 1 vWD is the most variable ranging from asymptomatic to moderate mucocutaneous bleeding.

Diagnosis The initial tests used in the diagnosis of vWD include vWFct antigen level, platelet dependent vWFct activity, and factor VIII activity. Type 1 vWD is diagnosed by vWFct antigen level < 30 IU/dL or < 50 IU/dL with abnormal bleeding and is characterized by an activity: antigen ratio of > 0.7. Type 2 vWD patients have an activity level of < 30% or 30% to 50% with a bleeding history, and characteristically have an activity: antigen ratio < 0.7, or decreased activity out of proportion to vWFct level. The vWFct multimeric analysis or vWFct collagen binding are helpful in differentiating between the different type 2 subtypes; platelet level and factor VIII level can also be suggestive.

Among the general population, vWFct antigen may be increased by acute inflammation, exercise, pregnancy, or estrogen therapy. Conversely, levels may be falsely low if the blood was not rapidly processed. Blood type O individuals have physiologically low levels of vWFct.

Treatment The main goal of therapy is to elevate levels of vWFct at the time of bleeding or in preparation for a procedure. Desmopressin acetate (DDAVP) administered intranasally or intravenously stimulates the release of vWFct from the endothelial cell stores. DDAVP is usually effective in type 1 vWD, may be useful in certain subtypes of type 2 vWD, but is ineffective for type 3 vWD. The response is not always predictable, especially for the intranasal preparation. A trial of DDAVP should be performed in a nonbleeding state in order to ensure adequate response. Response to DDAVP decreases after 2 to 3 daily doses, as the endothelial reserves are depleted. DDAVP causes free water retention and may lead to hyponatremia; it should not be used in patients with seizure disorders. DDAVP is not indicated for patients under 2 years of age due to higher risk of side effects.

vWFct concentrates are used for treatment of type 3 vWD and severe bleeds in type 1 and 2 vWD, or perioperatively for a major surgery, (typically 20-60 U/kg every 8-24 hours depending on indication). For severe bleeding, the initial goal is to target a level of 100 IU/dL and maintain a level of 50 IU/dL. Some vWFct concentrates also contain factor VIII and others do not. Inhibitors can develop with vWFct concentrates though less commonly than in hemophilia patients, and most likely in patients with type 3 vWD.

Antifibrinolytic therapy with either aminocaproic acid or tranexamic acid may be useful for menorrhagia, gingivorhagia, and epistaxis. These agents are generally well-tolerated by patients.

Prevention The American Society of Hematology recommends prophylactic treatment with vWFct concentrate for patients with a history of severe bleeding. Prior to anticipated procedures, DDAVP and/or antifibrinolytics can be given. Other strategies include use of estrogen-containing oral contraceptive pills for women with menorrhagia and avoidance of medications with antiplatelet or anticoagulant effect.

Inherited Platelet Function Disorders Inherited platelet function disorders are uncommon and include Bernard Soulier and Glanzmann thrombasthenia. These two autosomal recessive disorders result from defects in membrane receptor glycoproteins. They present with mucocutaneous bleeding and prolonged bleeding with trauma and surgery.

Diagnosis Evaluation should begin with a CBC to evaluate platelet number, size (mean platelet volume), and appearance. Patients with Bernard Soulier syndrome have thrombocytopenia with large platelets. In Glanzmann thrombasthenia platelets are normal in appearance but there is absent clumping on a non-anticoagulated peripheral smear. Platelet aggregation studies offer functional information regarding response to different agonists that can distinguish between disorders.

Treatment Platelet transfusion should be used for severe bleeds; however, repeated transfusions may lead to the formation of antibodies against platelet-associated proteins and accelerated clearance of transfused platelets. Activated factor VII (Novo Seven) has been used off-label for such situations. DDAVP and antifibrinolytics may shorten bleeding time and reduce bleeding in certain cases.

Disseminated Intravascular Coagulation (DIC) DIC is not a primary disease process, but a secondary syndrome characterized clinically by both bleeding and clotting resulting from dysregulation of hemostasis. DIC can be triggered by myriad conditions including sepsis (classically meningococcemia), malignancy, trauma, liver disease, necrotizing enterocolitis, and respiratory distress syndrome. Tissue damage from the underlying condition leads to activation of the clotting cascade with fibrin deposition. This leads to fibrinolysis generating fibrin degradation products (thus resulting in elevated D-dimer and decreased fibrinogen) and a consumptive coagulopathy (i.e., decreased clotting factors and platelets). The combination of hemorrhage and microvascular thromboses in severe cases leads to life-threatening end-organ damage.

Diagnosis Laboratory abnormalities include thrombocytopenia, increased PT and aPTT, decreased fibrinogen, presence of schistocytes on peripheral blood smear, and elevation of D-dimer.

Treatment Treatment requires identification and management of the underlying cause and is otherwise supportive. This may include platelet transfusion for thrombocytopenia and/or fresh frozen plasma and cryoprecipitate for abnormal coagulation studies. The goal of transfusion support is to stop bleeding as laboratory tests may not normalize until the underlying condition is treated. Anticoagulation should only be pursued for life-threatening thrombosis in DIC due to bleeding risk.

DISORDERS OF THROMBOSIS

Venous thromboembolism (VTE) includes deep vein thrombosis (DVT), pulmonary embolism (PE), and clots in less common locations including cerebral venous sinus thrombosis (CVST), portal vein thrombosis, among others. Clots can cause significant morbidity and even associated mortality in pediatric and adult patients. The incidence of venous thromboembolism in children is low, especially when compared to the adult population, but has been increasing over the past several decades. Rates of VTE in children are >58 cases per 10,000 hospital admissions or 0.07 to 0.14 cases per 10,000 children. More than 90% of children who develop VTEs have at least one risk factor, making it a disease of mostly sick children.

RISK FACTORS

The mechanisms of venous thrombosis described in the nineteenth century by the German physician Rudolf Virchow are still valid today: venous stasis, endothelial damage, and hypercoagulability. Most risk factors for venous thromboembolism act through one of these mechanisms. The incidence of venous thromboembolism among children is highest in the first year of life, declines during childhood, and then increases again in adolescence. VTEs occurring in infancy are often related to use of central venous access devices (CVAD), congenital heart disease, and invasive procedures. In older children and adolescents, venous thromboembolism often occurs in the presence of traditional adult risk factors, including central venous lines, malignancy, recent procedures, and inherited hypercoagulable states.

TABLE 88-2 Venous Thromboembolism Risk Factors

Acquired Pediatric VTE Risk Factors	Inherited VTE Risk Factors
Central Venous Access Device	Antithrombin deficiency
Congenital Heart Disease	Protein S deficiency
Malignancy	Protein C deficiency
Chronic Inflammatory State	Prothrombin G20210A
Acute Infection	Factor V Leiden gene mutation
Surgery/Anesthesia	MTHFR gene mutation
Estrogen Use	History of VTE or inherited thrombophilia
Trauma (TBI, spinal cord, pelvic or long bone fracture)	Family history of thrombophilia
Altered Mobility	
Nephrotic Syndrome	
Obesity	

Acquired Risk Factors Many risk factors for developing a VTE are acquired either through medical comorbidities, medications, or indwelling devices (**Table 88-2**).

Special attention should be paid to CVAD-associated thrombosis, which has become more prevalent as indwelling central venous catheters for prolonged intravenous therapies have become more common. Presence of a CVAD can lead to endothelial injury and venous stasis; further, these are often placed in patients with underlying risk factors for thrombosis. Greater than 90% of neonatal and greater than 60% of pediatric VTEs are associated with CVAD. A clot may occur inside the lumen, around the catheter in a sleeve distribution, or it may attach to the vessel wall. Often the occlusion is gradual, allowing for development of collateral venous circulation that leads to catheter-associated thrombosis remaining clinically silent. It is important to review a patient's acquired VTE risk factors, as controlling underlying conditions and removing unnecessary medications or central lines can decrease their risk of thrombosis.

Inherited Risk Factors Inherited hypercoagulability traits may be separated into those that are uncommon but confer a high risk of thrombosis (i.e., protein C deficiency, protein S deficiency, antithrombin deficiency) and those that are relatively prevalent but increase risk of thrombosis only moderately (i.e., factor V Leiden, prothrombin gene mutation, hyperhomocystenemia, elevated factor VIII). Evaluation for inherited hypercoagulable risk factors is especially warranted in adolescents, patients with a prior personal or family history of VTE (including DVT, stroke, or myocardial infarction), or cases wherein the cause of the thrombotic event is not apparent. Identification of thrombophilic traits is critical to inform patients of their personal risk and to facilitate lifestyle choices to lower thrombotic risk (Table 88-2). With rare exceptions, the results do not influence the management of the acute thrombosis in the type or duration of therapy.

CLINICAL PRESENTATION

DVT can present with pain, edema, plethora, and manifestations related to the location of the thrombus. Thrombi occurring in the deep venous system, especially in the proximal veins of the extremities, may embolize in the pulmonary circulation. Clinical manifestations of PE include chest pain, shortness of breath, hypoxia, cough, hemoptysis, anxiety, and tachycardia. PE is a life-threatening complication of DVT and requires urgent treatment. VTE can occur in other locations as well, including renal vein, portal vein, and cerebral venous sinus. Symptoms vary based on the location, and may include renal failure, hematuria, ascites, liver dysfunction, and headache among other symptoms.

DIAGNOSIS AND EVALUATION

Compression duplex ultrasound is the test of choice in diagnosis of DVT. It is very sensitive for the DVT in the lower or upper extremity but is less useful for evaluation of intrathoracic and pelvic veins. The test of choice for diagnosing PE is CT pulmonary angiography. However, this test does expose the patient to radiation and IV contrast. Ventilation/perfusion (V/Q) scintigraphy is considered safe and sensitive, but specificity is lower when used in patients with congenital heart disease or those with right-to-left shunts, and can be difficult to obtain urgently. Magnetic resonance pulmonary angiography is an alternative that offers sensitive evaluation of the pulmonary circulation without exposing the patient to radiation, and it uses a contrast material (gadolinium) with fewer side effects than CT contrast. Though the sensitivity and specificity of MR pulmonary angiography are above 95%, the procedure is long and frequently requires anesthesia in young children. Echocardiogram is used in assessing right ventricular function and possible pulmonary hypertension as well as in visualization of intracardiac or large vessel thrombi. When renal vein thrombosis is suspected, doppler ultrasound is the initial recommended imaging to confirm diagnosis. Doppler ultrasound can also be used for initial evaluation of portal vein thrombosis but is often confirmed with cross sectional imaging. Cerebral venous sinus thrombosis can be diagnosed with CT or MRI depending on the urgency of evaluation and availability.

TREATMENT

The treatment of VTE includes medications (anticoagulants, thrombolytic agents) and vascular procedures (placement of inferior vena cava filters or surgical removal of the clot). A summary of anticoagulants and their general dosing and required monitoring is provided in **Table 88-3**. The reader is referred to the 2018 American Society of Hematology guidelines for detail regarding the specific treatment of pediatric thrombosis.

For CVAD associated VTE, treatment decisions are influenced by the presence of signs and symptoms of obstruction and the ongoing need for vascular access. If the line is no longer needed and or the patient is symptomatic, the catheter should be removed, preferably after 3 to 5 days of anticoagulation. If the line is needed one may consider anticoagulation at therapeutic levels for 3 months, followed by prophylactic doses until the line is removed.

Anticoagulants The goal of anticoagulation therapy is to prevent clot progression and embolization, to facilitate resolution of the thrombus, and to prevent recurrence. Prior to initiating anticoagulation, it is prudent to obtain a history of any clinical bleeding or risk factors for bleeding. CBC, PT, aPTT, should be obtained. In neonates, baseline head ultrasound is recommended prior to starting therapeutic anticoagulation. In general, patients with secondary or provoked thrombosis, where a causative factor can be identified and removed, should receive up to 3 months of anticoagulation. Idiopathic or unprovoked thrombosis is treated with anticoagulants for 6 months or more. If an unprovoked thrombosis recurs after the initial treatment or if the causative factor cannot be removed, there should be strong consideration for long-term, even lifelong, anticoagulation.

Currently there are no formal guidelines for the use of prophylactic anticoagulation in children at risk for VTE. However, most published literature on this subject recommends completing a risk assessment for hospitalized children by screening for known risk factors and categorizing them into low, moderate, or high risk. Based on the risk category, providers can consider early ambulation, sequential compression devices (SCD) or prophylactic doses of anticoagulants for VTE prevention. Primary prophylaxis with an anticoagulant may be considered for patients with inherited or acquired prothrombotic traits who have a transiently increased thrombotic risk (e.g., surgery, immobilization, pregnancy) until that risk factor is removed.

Unfractionated Heparin (UFH) Heparin binds to and activates antithrombin, thereby inhibiting thrombin activity and activated factor X among other clotting factors. Its main advantages are the rapid onset of action, the short half-life (1.5 hours), and the ability to reverse the anticoagulant effect with protamine. The disadvantages include the need for continuous intravenous infusion, unpredictable clinical response, and frequent monitoring. The risks are bleeding, heparin-induced thrombocytopenia, and potential risk of osteoporosis with prolonged use. Given the complexity in titrating UFH, the use of algorithms detailing changes based on lab monitoring is recommended. In the case of clinically significant bleeding, anticoagulant effect use can be reversed using protamine sulfate if risk of reversal does not outweigh risk of bleeding.

Low Molecular Weight Heparins (LMWH) The most commonly used LMWH in pediatrics is enoxaparin, and like UFH, its anticoagulant action depends on amplifying the activity of antithrombin. It differs from UFH, however, in that LMWH inhibits activated factor X more than it inhibits thrombin. Nonetheless, LMWH has become the heparin of choice for many

TABLE 88-3 Table Summarizing Anticoagulants, General Dosing, Monitoring Strategies, and Reversal Options

	Route (treatment)	General Treatment Dosing	FDA approved in children?	Monitoring/Goals*	Reversal
Heparin					
UFH	IV	Continuous	No	aPTT (goal 1.5-2.5 x baseline) vs anti Xa (goal 0.35-0.7 U/mL) Platelets	Protamine
LMWH (enoxaparin, dalteparin)	Subcutaneous	Daily to BID	Some (dalteparin in 2019)	Anti-Xa (treatment goal 0.5-1 IU/mL, prophylaxis goal 0.1-0.3 IU/mL) Creatinine Platelets	Protamine (partial)
Vitamin K Antagonist					
Warfarin	PO	Daily	No	INR (goal typically 2-3)	Vitamin K, Fresh Frozen Plasma
Direct Thrombin Inhibitors					
Argatroban	IV	Continuous	No	aPTT	None
Bivalirudin	IV	Continuous	No	Activating clotting time, aPTT	None
Dabigatran	PO	BID	Yes	None	Idarucizumab Activated PCC
Direct Factor Xa Inhibitors					
Apixaban	PO	BID	No	None	Andexanet alpha, PCC
Edoxaban	PO	Daily	No	None	Andexanet alpha (off label), PCC
Rivaroxaban	PO	Varies by weight	Yes	None	Andexanet alpha, PCC

*Treatment goal may vary based on indication for anticoagulation.

pediatric VTE patients because of its ease of use, including its ability to be utilized in the outpatient setting. The typical starting treatment dose is 1 mg/kg subcutaneously every 12 hours, with a larger dose in newborns and young infants. Anticoagulant activity is monitored by measuring anti-Xa activity. Other advantages of LMWH are its predictable response, less frequent monitoring, and lower risk of heparin-induced thrombocytopenia. Disadvantages of LMWH include its higher cost and only partial reversibility with protamine.

Vitamin K Antagonists Vitamin K plays an essential role in the activation of coagulation factors II, VII, IX, and X, as well as protein C and protein S. The vitamin K antagonist available in the United States is warfarin, and its anticoagulant activity is monitored by PT/INR. The INR therapeutic range is generally 2 to 3 (inferred from adult patients), though target INR can be higher for certain clinical circumstances. The typical starting dose of warfarin is 0.1 mg/kg (max 5 mg) administered orally; steady-state levels are achieved after 5 to 7 days. Importantly, the anticoagulant proteins C and S are also vitamin K-dependent factors. Thus, thrombotic risk is paradoxically increased when first starting warfarin due to the inhibition of protein C and S, often necessitating "bridging" with heparin until the appropriate INR is achieved. Warfarin is often avoided in newborns and young infants because of their decreased vitamin K dependent coagulation factors, variable vitamin K intake and absence of liquid formulation. The main adverse effect is bleeding. The activity of warfarin can be reversed with vitamin K, or in an emergent situation with fresh frozen plasma (FFP) or protein complex concentrates (PCC). Choice of reversal agent and route depends on the degree of INR elevation and clinically significant bleeding given that vitamin K is longer acting and FFP has a shorter duration.

Direct Thrombin Inhibitors (DTI) Unlike the heparins, which inhibit thrombin indirectly via their action on antithrombin, DTIs inhibit thrombin directly, thus producing more predictable pharmacokinetics and pharmacodynamics. Parenterally administered DTIs include lepirudin, desirudin, bivalirudin, and argatroban, while dabigatran is an orally administered DTI. The FDA-approved dabigatran for use in children as of 2021 based on pediatric trials rather than extrapolation of adult data. Routine coagulation studies are not required while using dabigatran. However, if the clinical situation necessitates, the preferred laboratory test for monitoring anticoagulation with DTIs is the thrombin time (TT) or the ecarin clotting time (ECT). However, neither the TT nor the ECT are readily available in many clinical labs. aPTT can be used to screen for the presence of DTI-induced anticoagulation; a normal aPTT excludes significant anticoagulation. However, the aPTT reaches a plateau with direct thrombin inhibitors. Thus, the degree of elevation in the aPTT does not correlate well with the degree of anticoagulation. Idarucizumab is used for reversal of dabigatran anticoagulant effects in the setting of clinically significant bleeding.

Factor Xa Inhibitors In addition to DTIs, factor Xa inhibitors have been used in adults for several years, with FDA approval of rivaroxaban in children in 2021 based on pediatric clinical trial data. Unlike traditional anticoagulants (heparin, LMWH, vitamin K antagonists), factor Xa inhibitors can be considered either direct inhibitors (e.g., rivaroxaban or apixaban), or indirect inhibitors (e.g., fondaparinux). Benefits of direct factor Xa inhibitors include oral administration, no recommended blood level monitoring, predictable pharmacokinetics, and decreased variability based on dietary intake. Andexanet alpha is a reversal agent that acts as a decoy factor Xa and binds direct factor Xa inhibitors with high affinity.

Other Treatment for VTE Thrombolytic therapy has been used more extensively in adults; pediatric experience is limited. The agent of choice in children is tissue–plasminogen activator (tPA). This intervention is reserved for limb- or life-threatening thrombosis, including cerebrovascular accidents and PE with hemodynamic compromise, and should only be performed under the supervision of a physician familiar with this therapy.

Inferior vena cava filters have been used in adults to reduce the risk of pulmonary embolization, but guidelines in pediatrics recommend against routine use. Recommended pediatric use is limited to special cases including patients with a DVT and absolute contraindication for anticoagulation, or those who have failed standard therapy.

Thrombectomy refers to mechanical removal of the clot, either through open surgical procedure or through percutaneous catheterization. It has been used mostly for life-threatening intracardiac or large vessel thrombosis leading to hemodynamic compromise.

SPECIAL CONSIDERATIONS

COVID-Related Thrombosis Adult patients with COVID-19 have developed acute thromboembolic complications raising questions about the merits of VTE prophylaxis. The American Society of Hematology released a guideline panel in 2021 with recommendations for VTE prophylaxis in patients hospitalized with COVID-19. The guidelines suggest prophylactic anticoagulation for patients admitted with COVID-19 rather than therapeutic anticoagulation, with specific dosing recommendations based on risk and benefit assessment for individual patients. The expert panel included pediatric hematologists; however, the guidelines do not specify differences in recommendations based on age. Recommendations may evolve as ongoing trials in this area are completed. The guidelines also discussed the need to prioritize research in pediatric patients with COVID, among other groups. While more specific pediatric VTE prophylactic guidelines are being developed, it is important to work within individual institutions to develop risk stratification tools and protocols for prophylaxis when indicated.

KEY POINTS

- The diagnosis of a bleeding disorder relies on:
  - Personal and family history of abnormal bleeding or clotting
  - Bleeding pattern
  - Appropriate screening laboratory tests which may include CBC, PT, aPTT, mixing study, specific factor levels, and vWFct testing
- Hemophilia is an X-linked congenital deficiency in the production of factor VIII (hemophilia A) or factor IX (hemophilia B). It is characterized by deep bleeds of joints or muscles. Hemophilia is treated with factor replacement, but inhibitors can complicate treatment. For acute hemarthrosis supportive therapy is also important: Rest, Ice, Compression, Elevation.
- von Willebrand disease is the most common coagulation disorder, with most commonly an autosomal dominant inheritance, resulting from decreased levels of, or dysfunctional, vWFct. DDAVP, vWFct concentrates, and antifibrinolytic drugs are the mainstays of treatment.
- The incidence of venous thromboembolism in children is on the rise as a result of more complex medical interventions, better imaging modalities, and increased awareness. Unfractionated heparin, LMWH, and warfarin have been the main treatment options for management of venous thromboembolism.
- New anticoagulants that directly inhibit thrombin (dabigatran) or activated factor X (rivaroxaban) have recently been approved and more commonly used in pediatrics.

SUGGESTED READINGS

Bawazir OA, Alharbi I. Circumcision in hemophilia: a multicenter experience. *J Pediatr Hematol Oncol.* 2021;43(1):e33-e36.

Connell NT, Flood VH, Brignardello-Petersen R, et al. ASH ISTH NHF WFH 2021 guidelines on the management of von Willebrand disease. *Blood Adv.* 2021;5(1):301-325.

Croteau SE. Hemophilia A/B. *Hematol Oncol Clin North Am.* 2022;36(4):797-812.

Cuker A, Tseng EK, Nieuwlaat R, et al. American Society of Hematology 2021 guidelines on the use of anticoagulation for thromboprophylaxis in patients with COVID-19. *Blood Adv.* 2021;5(3):872-888.

DiMichele D. Inhibitor development in haemophilia B: an orphan disease in need of attention. *Br J Haematol.* 2007;138(3):305-315.

Grainger JD, Thachil J, Will AM. How we treat the platelet glycoprotein defects; Glanzmann thrombasthenia and Bernard Soulier syndrome in children and adults. *Br J Haematol.* 2018;182(5):621-632.

Halton J, Brandão LR, Luciani M, et al. Dabigatran etexilate for the treatment of acute venous thromboembolism in children (DIVERSITY): a randomised, controlled, open-label, phase 2b/3, non-inferiority trial. *Lancet Haematol.* 2021;8(1):e22-e33.

James PD, Connell NT, Ameer B, et al. ASH ISTH NHF WFH 2021 guidelines on the diagnosis of von Willebrand disease. *Blood Adv.* 2021;5(1):280-300.

Kulkarni R, Soucie JM. Pediatric hemophilia: a review. *Semin Thromb Hemost.* 2011;37(7):737-744.

Male C, Lensing AWA, Palumbo JS, et al. Rivaroxaban compared with standard anticoagulants for the treatment of acute venous thromboembolism in children: a randomised, controlled, phase 3 trial. *Lancet Haematol.* 2020;7(1):e18-e27.

Meier KA, Tarango C. Treatment of Pediatric Venous Thromboembolism. *J Hosp Med.* 2019;14(8):497-498.

Monagle P, Cuello CA, Augustine C, et al. American Society of Hematology 2018 Guidelines for management of venous thromboembolism: treatment of pediatric venous thromboembolism. *Blood Adv.* 2018;2(22):3292-3316.

Monagle P, Newall F. Management of thrombosis in children and neonates: practical use of anticoagulants in children. *Hematology Am Soc Hematol Educ Program.* 2018; 2018 (1):399-404.

Papageorgiou C, Jourdi G, Adjambri E, et al. Disseminated intravascular coagulation: an update on pathogenesis, diagnosis, and therapeutic strategies. *Clin Appl Thromb Hemost.* 2018;24(9_suppl):8S-28S.

Puetz J, Soucie JM, Kempton CL, Monahan PE; Hemophilia Treatment Center Network (HTCN) Investigators. Prevalent inhibitors in haemophilia B subjects enrolled in the Universal Data Collection database. *Haemophilia.* 2014;20(1):25-31.

Ramiz S, Rajpurkar M. Pulmonary embolism in children. *Pediatr Clin North Am.* 2018;65(3):495-507.

Screening and Management of Bleeding Disorders in Adolescents with Heavy Menstrual Bleeding: ACOG COMMITTEE OPINION, Number 785. *Obstetrics & Gynecology.* 2019;134(3):e71-e83.

Srivastava A, Santagostino E, Dougall A, et al. WFH Guidelines for the Management of Hemophilia. 3rd ed. *Haemophilia.* 2020:26(Suppl 6): 1-158.

Witmer C, Raffini L. Treatment of venous thromboembolism in pediatric patients. *Blood.* 2020;135(5):335-343.

CHAPTER 89

Transfusion Medicine

HyoJeong Han, MD and Huay-ying Lo, MD

INTRODUCTION

Blood transfusions are one of the most common procedures performed in the United States, with >14 million units of blood transfused annually. Transfusion therapy is frequently utilized as a lifesaving intervention for a variety of medical conditions such as acute blood loss, anemia, and/or thrombocytopenia. Providing safe transfusion therapy is essential, and blood products undergo rigorous monitoring, screening, and testing from the time of blood donation until even after the product is transfused to the recipient. This chapter will review the processes involved in providing blood products to patients, indications for transfusion, and the symptoms and management of potential adverse events associated with transfusion therapy.

PRE-TRANSFUSION PROCESS AND BLOOD BANK TESTING

TYPE AND SCREEN

An updated "type and screen" (T&S) is required prior to issuing any blood products. This test identifies the individual's ABO status (type) and screens for any clinically significant red blood cell (RBC) alloantibodies besides ABO (screen). The T&S detects antibodies against RBC antigens to avoid issuing incompatible blood products.

Type RBCs have ABO antigen(s) on their cell surface. Individuals can express either A antigen (blood type A), B antigen (blood type B), both A and B antigens (blood type AB), or no antigens (blood type O). Based on which ABO antigen(s) an individual has on their RBC surface, they will also have naturally occurring antibodies against the antigen(s) absent from their RBCs. Typing an individual's blood involves determining what type of antigen is expressed on their RBC surface and whether the patient has correlating antibodies against antigens(s) absent from their RBCs. Even if an individual has never received blood products, antibodies against A or B antigens are present because the body naturally creates these antibodies from exposure to gut microbes, pollen particles, and other substances present in nature which are chemically similar to A or B antigens. Therefore, if the wrong ABO group is transfused, the patient's antibodies can cause rapid destruction of the donor RBC (also known as intravascular hemolysis), which can potentially result in death.

Screen In addition to ABO antigens, RBCs have multiple other antigens on their cell surface such as D antigen. The "screen" portion of a T&S identifies clinically significant alloantibodies that can target specific RBC antigens which are not present on the recipient's RBCs. Unlike anti-A or anti-B alloantibodies, these alloantibodies require prior exposure to the RBC antigen either via transfusion or pregnancy. The presence of these alloantibodies can decrease the survival of any RBCs that possess the target antigen. Therefore, both a type and screen are performed to ensure that compatible blood product is provided to the individual.

BLOOD COMPONENTS AND TRANSFUSION INDICATIONS

Whole blood can be divided into multiple blood components such as RBCs, platelets, plasma, and cryoprecipitate. These components can be further processed to make products like albumin, IVIG, or concentrated clotting factor. Children usually receive RBCs, platelet, plasma, and rarely cryoprecipitate. A description of each blood component and their transfusion indications are summarized in **Table 89-1**. Unfortunately, transfusion guidelines for children are limited, and most recommendations are extrapolated from adult studies. Therefore, a child's clinical status is important in determining the transfusion threshold.

RED BLOOD CELLS (RBCs)

RBCs are the most transfused blood product in pediatric patients. Over 400,000 units of RBCs are transfused annually in pediatric patients in the United States. RBC transfusions are considered in children with symptomatic anemia (tachycardia, tachypnea, dizziness, weakness, poor concentration, headache, decreased energy) or acute blood loss. Unfortunately, an ideal hemoglobin threshold to initiate RBC transfusion is not known. A large pediatric prospective randomized study found no significant difference in outcomes among children admitted to the pediatric intensive care unit when using a transfusion threshold of 7 versus 9.5 g/dL, and children in the first group received 44% fewer transfusions. Based on this and other studies, the Pediatric Critical Care Transfusion and Anemia Expertise Initiative recommends RBC transfusion threshold

TABLE 89-1 Blood Component and Brief Transfusion Indications

Blood Component	Transfusion Indication(s)
Red Blood Cells	• Symptomatic anemia • Acute blood loss
Platelets	• Low platelet count with bleeding • Low platelet count with planned invasive procedure/surgery • Platelet dysfunction
Plasma	• Coagulopathy • Warfarin reversal • Plasma exchange
Cryoprecipitate	• Low fibrinogen • Low Factor XIII

of 5 g/dL and does not recommend transfusion for children with hemoglobin ≥7 g/dL in hemodynamically stable patients. The American Society of Hematology Choosing Wisely Campaign also recommends transfusing enough RBCs to alleviate the symptoms of anemia or to reach a safe hemoglobin range, which is typically 7 to 8 g/dL in stable, noncardiac patients. Thus, RBC transfusion is generally indicated for symptomatic anemia or acute blood loss resulting in hemodynamic instability.

There are exceptions to the above recommendations. For children with malignancies or bone marrow failure syndromes, the median transfusion threshold used is frequently 7.0 g/dL. Children with transfusion-dependent thalassemias such as beta thalassemia major and alpha thalassemia major may receive chronic transfusions to promote growth and maintain hemoglobin trough levels of 9 to 10.5 g/dL to inhibit extramedullary hematopoiesis. Children with sickle cell disease (SCD) may require RBC transfusions for acute splenic sequestration, transient aplastic crisis, acute chest syndrome (ACS), or pre-operatively. Pre-operative RBC transfusion to hemoglobin goal of 10.0 g/dL in SCD patients has been shown to reduce the rate of post-op complications including ACS. Chronic transfusion therapy is indicated for stroke prevention in SCD patients with abnormal transcranial Doppler findings or prior history of strokes.

In a typical 70 kg adult, one unit of RBC is expected to increase the hemoglobin level by approximately 1 g/dL and hematocrit level by 3%. In children, 10 to 15 mL/kg of RBC will increase the hemoglobin by approximately 2 to 3 g/dL or hematocrit by approximately 6% to 9%. However, this increase will vary depending on the child's age and body mass. RBC are typically transfused over 2 to 4 hours, and lower volumes and/or slower transfusion rates are considered in children at risk of volume overload leading to cardiac failure.

PLATELETS

Platelets are essential for primary hemostasis or the formation of a "platelet plug." Therefore, platelet transfusion is usually indicated in children with bleeding associated with low platelet count or dysfunctional platelets, or children with thrombocytopenia undergoing invasive procedures. Like RBCs, the ideal platelet count threshold is not known. Several studies have shown no correlation between the degree of thrombocytopenia and the risk of bleeding. The largest prospective randomized platelet transfusion study that included pediatric patients found no difference in bleeding outcomes among children with hypoproliferative thrombocytopenia <10,000/μL who were randomized to receive low, medium, or high platelet doses. In adults, a transfusion threshold of 20,000/μL is typically recommended for minor invasive procedures such as central venous catheter (CVC) insertion, and a higher threshold of 50,000/μL is recommended for major, non-central nervous system surgery. For children not undergoing procedures, the threshold for prophylactic platelet transfusion to prevent bleeding is <10,000/μL, which is extrapolated from the American Society of Clinical Oncology recommendations. Generally, 10 to 15 mL/kg of apheresis platelets are transfused, but lower volumes may be considered in children at risk for volume overload.

PLASMA

Plasma is an acellular product which contains clotting factors. Plasma is used to treat multiple coagulation deficiencies, including liver failure, disseminated intravascular coagulopathy (DIC), massive transfusion, thrombotic thrombocytopenic purpura (TTP), and children with single factor (i.e., Factor V or XI) deficiencies where virus-safe fractionated product is unavailable. Plasma may also be given in cases of vitamin K deficiency or warfarin overdose; while these are typically treated with vitamin K, plasma transfusion may be indicated if there is active bleeding or urgent reversal is required for surgery.

Prophylactic plasma transfusion is not recommended for individuals with abnormal coagulation profiles like prolonged prothrombin time (PT), international normalized ratio (INR), or activated partial thromboplastin time (aPTT) to reduce the risk of bleeding. Coagulation studies are *in vitro* assays which have never been validated to predict the risk of bleeding, and plasma transfusions are associated with adverse events like allergic reactions, or transfusion-associated circulatory overload (TACO). In fact, expert consensus recommends against prophylactic plasma transfusion for correction of mild to moderate coagulopathies without active bleeding or planned invasive procedures. When plasma transfusion is indicated, usually 10 to 15 mL/kg of plasma is transfused.

CRYOPRECIPITATE

Cryoprecipitate contains clotting Factor VIII, Factor XIII, fibrinogen, von Willebrand factor (VWF), cryoglobulin, and fibronectin. It is prepared from frozen plasma that is thawed at 1°C to 6°C, which produces cold-insoluble clotting factor proteins also known as cryoprecipitate. Cryoprecipitate is extracted by centrifugation and removal of supernatant. Cryoprecipitate is recommended in the following clinical situations: Factor XIII deficiency, liver failure, DIC or massive transfusion, and afibrinogenemia, hypofibrinogenemia or dysfibrinogenemia complicated by bleeding or prophylaxis before invasive procedures.

Treatment of Factor XIII deficiency or hypofibrinogenemia may be supplemented with Factor XIII or fibrinogen concentrates, respectively. Of note, there is no ideal Factor XIII or fibrinogen threshold, but recommended fibrinogen levels range from 100 mg/dL to 200 mg/dL. Plasma also contains fibrinogen, but the volume needed to correct low fibrinogen is a lot less in cryoprecipitate than plasma (10-15 mL of cryoprecipitate vs. 200-260 mL of plasma). Even though cryoprecipitate also contains Factor VIII and VWF, it should not be used to treat Hemophilia A or von Willebrand disease because virus-inactivated or recombinant factor concentrates are available. Usually, 1 unit of cryoprecipitate per 10 kg of body weight is given to children.

BLOOD PRODUCT MODIFICATIONS AND PREPARATION

LEUKOREDUCTION OR LEUKOCYTE REDUCTION

This process involves the removal of white blood cells (WBCs) from blood or blood components prior to transfusion using special filters that trap WBCs but allow RBCs or apheresis platelets to flow through. After leukoreduction, blood products contain <5.0 x 10^6 residual WBC per RBC or apheresis platelet unit. Leukoreduction helps to reduce the rate of febrile non-hemolytic transfusion reactions, reduce alloimmunization to leukocyte antigens that may complicate transplantation or chronic transfusions, and protect against transmission of CMV. Therefore, the majority of centers practice universal leukoreduction for RBCs and platelets. For smaller centers where leukoreduction is not standard, leukoreduction is considered in individuals at high risk for above events like neonates and Hematology/Oncology patients.

IRRADIATION

Irradiation involves irradiating cellular components like RBCs and platelets using either gamma rays (cesium-137 or cobalt-50) or X-rays. Irradiation damages the nucleic acid of the donor T-lymphocytes resulting in inability to proliferate and cause transfusion-associated graft versus host disease (TA-GVHD). TA-GVHD occurs when donor T-lymphocytes escape destruction by the recipient's immune system due to inability to detect and destroy the foreign cells. TA-GVHD will be discussed further in detail in the Transfusion Reactions section. Irradiation is indicated in individuals at risk of TA-GVHD, including oncology patients (specifically Hodgkin lymphoma, leukemia), immunocompromised patients like hematopoietic stem cell transplant recipients, congenital immunodeficiencies, fetuses receiving intrauterine transfusion, and in patients receiving blood-related or human leukocyte antigen (HLA)-matched blood products.

VOLUME REDUCTION

Volume reduction involves centrifugation of cellular products (RBC or platelets) to remove the supernatant in which the cells are suspended. However, the process can lead to loss of cells resulting in about 85% recovery. Therefore, the expected incremental rise in hemoglobin or platelets will be less in volume reduced components when compared to unmodified components. Volume reduction is considered in individuals at risk of circulatory overload or history of severe allergic reaction or anaphylaxis with transfusion which cannot be managed with medication prior to transfusion.

WASHING

RBCs are stored in a mixture of an additive solution, small volume of residual plasma, and an anticoagulant. Platelets are stored in a mixture of donor plasma and an anticoagulant. Washing a product involves removing the extracellular solution and replacing it with normal saline. Washing is considered in patients who have severe allergic reactions to proteins found in plasma. However, the washing process further decreases the recovery rate compared to volume reduction, and platelet function may be reduced due to platelet adhesion and activation during the washing. Therefore, the washing process should only be considered in patients who experience anaphylaxis with transfusions and who cannot be effectively managed with medications prior to transfusion.

CMV NEGATIVE

Cytomegalovirus (CMV) can be carried in latent or infectious form in WBCs, and a small number of WBCs are present in cellular products such as RBCs or platelets. Transfusion of these virus-infected cells in cellular products can potentially transmit infection, especially to vulnerable populations like immunosuppressed patients. The risk of CMV infection can be reduced by transfusing leukocyte reduced blood products or using CMV antibody-negative blood.

CMV-negative blood is recommended in individuals who are CMV-negative and at risk for severe CMV infections including fetuses, low birth weight premature infants born to CMV-negative mothers, and CMV seronegative recipients of organ or stem cell transplants.

If CMV-negative product is not available, leukoreduced products can be used to reduce the risk of CMV infection transmission. In fact, past studies have shown no difference in CMV transmission rates when leukoreduced versus CMV-negative cellular products were given to stem cell transplant recipients. In some institutions, leukoreduced blood products are used in all recipients regardless of the CMV status.

TRANSFUSION REACTIONS

As one of the most commonly performed procedures, it is important for providers to be aware of potential transfusion reactions. Different types of transfusion reactions, their presenting symptoms, and recommended management are included in **Table 89-2**. Alternately, **Table 89-3** describes possible symptoms that may present in patients receiving transfusions, and which types of transfusion reactions to consider and recommended management. National databases with standardized case definitions have been created to monitor transfusion reactions and efficacy of current transfusion safety measures, as well as to develop strategies to reduce the risk of transfusion-related events.

In children, the most common transfusion reactions are allergic transfusion reactions, followed by febrile non-hemolytic transfusion reaction. Children experienced approximately 1.5-fold higher transfusion reactions than adults, with a higher incidence of transfusion reactions with platelet and RBC products.

TYPES OF TRANSFUSION REACTIONS AND THEIR MANAGEMENT

Acute Hemolytic Transfusion Reactions (AHTRs) AHTRs occur when incompatible blood product (ABO, Rh, or other RBC antigen group) is transfused, resulting in hemolysis or destruction of transfused RBCs within 24 hours of transfusion. AHTR typically occurs with

TABLE 89-2 Transfusion Reactions and Their Management

Transfusion Reaction	Symptoms	Management
Acute onset (usually occurs during or <24 hours after transfusion)		
Acute Hemolytic Transfusion Reaction (AHTR)	Fever, chills, pain (back pain, pain along infusion site), anxiety, hemoglobinuria, bleeding, oliguria, or anuria	• Stop transfusion & initiate transfusion reaction work up • IV fluids to maintain adequate urine output • Analgesics to manage pain • Plasma or factor replacements to manage bleeding (DIC)
Allergic Transfusion Reaction	Pruritus, hives, angioedema, nausea/vomiting, diarrhea, abdominal pain, wheezing, stridor, dyspnea, tachycardia, hypotension, shock	• Stop transfusion & initiate transfusion reaction work up • Diphenhydramine • Corticosteroids • Anaphylaxis: epinephrine, diphenhydramine, corticosteroids, IV fluids
Febrile Non-Hemolytic Transfusion Reaction (FNHTR)	Fever, chills, rigor, headache	• Stop transfusion & initiate transfusion reaction work up • Rule out hemolysis and infection • Antipyretics
Transfusion-Associated Circulatory Overload (TACO)	Dyspnea, orthopnea, cough, respiratory distress, tachycardia, hypertension	• Stop transfusion & initiate transfusion reaction work up • Upright posture • Supplemental oxygen • Diuretics
Transfusion-Related Acute Lung Injury (TRALI)	Acute respiratory distress/failure, hypoxemia, fever, tachycardia, hypotension	• Stop transfusion & initiate transfusion reaction work up • Supplemental oxygen or mechanical ventilation if needed • Supportive care until recovery
Delayed onset (usually occur >24 hours after transfusion)		
Delayed Hemolytic Transfusion Reaction (DHTR)	Fever, decreasing hemoglobin trend or inadequate rise in hemoglobin post-transfusion, jaundice	• Repeat type and screen • Direct antiglobulin test (DAT) • Hemolysis work up (LDH, haptoglobin, unconjugated bilirubin, plasma free hemoglobin, etc.) • Supportive care
Transfusion-Associated Graft Versus Host Disease (TA-GVHD)	Maculopapular rash, fever, diarrhea, hepatomegaly, pancytopenia	• Skin biopsy for diagnosis • Immune suppression • Prevent TA-GVHD by transfusing irradiated blood product to at risk individuals

TABLE 89-3 Transfusion Reaction Differentials Based on Clinical Presentation and Management

Clinical Presentation	Management	Transfusion Reaction Differentials
Fever	• Rule out hemolysis and infection • Consider blood culture and IV antibiotics if concern for TTI • Antipyretics	AHTR, FNHTR, TRALI, TTI
Hypotension	• IV fluids and/or pressors	AHTR, TRALI, TTI, ATR
Hypoxemia, respiratory distress	• Supplemental oxygen • Epinephrine if concern for anaphylaxis	AHTR, TRALI, TACO, TTI, ATR
Rash (hives, pruritis)	• Diphenhydramine	AHTR, ATR
Pain—headache, infusion site, abdomen, chest	Pain control	AHTR, TRALI, TACO, TTI
Hemoglobinuria, Jaundice	IV fluids	AHTR, DHTR
Oliguria or anuria	IV fluids	AHTR

incompatible RBC transfusion but can also occur with large amounts of plasma transfusion. AHTR happens because of clerical errors which may include misidentification of the patient or mislabeling of the blood sample. Between 2013 and 2018, approximately 0.6% of transfusion-associated adverse reactions were AHTR, and approximately 26.7% of those AHTR were classified as serious adverse events in the United States. Presenting symptoms of AHTR are variable and can include fever (most commonly), hemoglobinuria, chills/rigors, body pain, oliguria or anuria suggestive of acute kidney injury, bleeding associated with DIC, or hypotension/shock.

Management of AHTR is supportive care which includes early and aggressive IV fluid resuscitation and blood pressure management to prevent hypotension, AKI, and shock. Aggressive IV fluid hydration also reduces the possible complications from free hemoglobin including oliguria, anuria, and DIC.

Allergic Transfusion Reaction (ATR) ATR are one of the most common transfusion reactions, accounting for ~40% of reported transfusion reactions in the United States. ATR is most often associated with platelet transfusion because platelets are stored in plasma which contains proteins that can trigger allergic reactions. ATR can be classified as mild, moderate, or anaphylaxis. Mild to moderate reactions are usually limited to skin and gastrointestinal (GI) tract manifestations. Anaphylaxis involves oral and/or throat symptoms, more severe GI symptoms, respiratory complaints, and/or life-threatening reactions which may include hypotension and shock. ATR can present with mucocutaneous symptoms (urticaria, pruritus, lip/tongue/periorbital swelling), gastrointestinal symptoms (nausea, vomiting, abdominal pain, diarrhea), respiratory symptoms (throat tightness, wheezing, dyspnea), or cardiovascular symptoms (hypotension, tachycardia, shock).

In addition to stopping the transfusion and initiating transfusion reaction workup, providers should assess the patient and administer medications based upon symptoms, including diphenhydramine for mucocutaneous symptoms, bronchodilators for respiratory symptoms, glucocorticoids for moderate ATR, and epinephrine for anaphylaxis.

Volume reduction or washed products can be considered in individuals who experience anaphylaxis despite receiving medication prior to transfusion, but these types of special processing result in lower cell recovery rate. Of note, there is no evidence showing that administering diphenhydramine and/or glucocorticoids before transfusion will prevent ATR. Therefore, children should not receive prophylactic diphenhydramine and/or glucocorticoids unless they have history of ATR requiring premedications as recommended by the transfusion medicine service.

Febrile Non-Hemolytic Transfusion Reaction (FNHTR) FNHTR is another of the most commonly reported transfusion reactions. In the United States, ~40% of reported transfusion reactions were FNHTR. The cause of FNHTR is thought to be due to either accumulation of proinflammatory cytokines from residual WBCs present, or the patient's WBC antibodies reacting to donor HLA or other WBC antigens. Prestorage leukocyte reduction reduces the risk of FNHTR by approximately 50%.

FNHTR presents with fever, chills, and/or rigors. Unfortunately, AHTR, TRALI, TACO, and TTI can also present with identical symptoms. Therefore, FNHTR is a diagnosis of exclusion and other serious transfusion reactions must be ruled out. Fever can be managed with antipyretics like acetaminophen. Administering antipyretics prior to transfusion to prevent FNHTR is not recommended and may potentially mask a fever caused by other serious reasons.

Transfusion-Associated Circulatory Overload (TACO) TACO is caused by excessive blood transfusion volumes or rapid rates of transfusion resulting in circulatory overload, typically exhibited as acute respiratory distress from pulmonary edema. Individuals at risk for TACO are those unable to accommodate the volume of blood transfusion due to poor cardiac or renal function. Other risk factors include older age and pre-existing fluid overload. While TACO only accounts for about 5% of transfusion reactions reported in the United States, TACO and TRALI represented the leading causes of transfusion-associated death in 2019.

TACO presents during or within 6 hours after transfusion with acute respiratory distress with evidence of left heart failure, elevated central venous pressure, or positive fluid balance. Chest x-rays findings include pulmonary edema, and labs will reveal an elevated brain natriuretic peptide (BNP). Management of TACO includes keeping the patient upright and administering supplemental oxygen and diuretics. Patients who are at risk for TACO should receive the smallest possible volume of blood products administered slowly over 3 to 4 hours.

Transfusion-Related Acute Lung Injury (TRALI) TRALI is a rare transfusion-associated adverse event but represents one of the leading causes of transfusion-associated death in the United States. TRALI is proposed to be caused by the two-event model, with the first event being an underlying disorder or illness (i.e., pneumonia) that causes activation of the pulmonary endothelium, resulting in the sequestration of neutrophils in the lung. Then, a second event occurs at the time of blood product transfusion, which activates the neutrophils in the lungs causing endothelial damage and acute lung injury. Neutrophil activation can be due to donor anti-HLA or anti-human neutrophil antigen (HNA) antibodies or the presence of pro-inflammatory cytokines or proteins in the blood product.

The prevalence of anti-HLA or anti-HNA antibodies increases with the number of pregnancies, and there is a strong association between multiparous female donors and TRALI. The risk of TRALI can be reduced by selecting male or nulliparous female donors and/or screening for HLA- and HNA-antibodies in female donors with previous pregnancies.

TRALI presents with acute respiratory distress, fever, rigors, tachycardia, hypothermia, and/or hypotension. Chest X-rays reveal bilateral lung infiltrates which can be similar in appearance to TACO or other acute respiratory distress syndrome (ARDS). Because TRALI is rare, other causes of pulmonary edema should be ruled out. Individuals with TRALI are managed with supportive care including supplemental oxygen or mechanical ventilation for respiratory distress or failure.

Delayed Hemolytic Transfusion Reaction (DHTR) DHTR is one of the delayed transfusion reactions and can occur between 24 hours and 28 days after transfusion. DHTR occurs in individuals who have been alloimmunized to RBC antigens from prior transfusion and/or pregnancies, but whose antibodies are not detected during type and screen due to low or evanescent antibody titers. However, re-exposure to antigen-positive RBCs leads to an anamnestic response with rapid rise in antibody resulting in hemolysis. Of note, RBC alloantibodies can become undetectable over time after initial development. DHTR can also occur in individuals who received RBC antigen mismatched product for the first time resulting in development of antibody against the donor RBC antigen (alloimmunization).

Individuals with DHTR will show an inadequate rise in hemoglobin after transfusion, or even a drop in hemoglobin to pretransfusion levels. Individuals may also show signs and symptoms of hemolysis including low haptoglobin and elevated LDH, unconjugated bilirubin, and plasma-free hemoglobin. A peripheral smear will show spherocytes because DHTR leads to extravascular hemolysis. Additional workup will reveal positive direct antiglobulin test (DAT) with newly identified alloantibody. DHTR is managed with supportive care and avoidance of RBC transfusion if possible. Patients may require close monitoring of renal function, urine output, and hemoglobin, similar to in AHTR, in cases of significant hemolysis.

Transfusion-Associated Graft Versus Host Disease (TA-GVHD) TA-GVHD is one of the rarest transfusion reactions reported with a rate of <1 per 1,000,000 transfusions. Generally, TA-GVHD is fatal with overall mortality of approximately 90% following the onset of symptoms; no effective treatment is available. Therefore, the focus is on prevention of TA-GVHD. TA-GVHD occurs in individuals who are unable to mount an appropriate defense against the donor T-lymphocyte, resulting in T-lymphocyte proliferation followed by attack and destruction of the recipient's organs. Individuals at risk for TA-GVHD include immunocompromised patients (patients with cancer and primary immunodeficiency), fetuses and neonates, and individuals undergoing transplantation. Other at-risk individuals include those receiving HLA-matched products; the genetic similarities between donor and recipient allows donor T-lymphocytes to escape recipient immune defense.

TA-GVHD can occur anytime between 2 days and 6 weeks after transfusion, and the diagnosis is confirmed by skin biopsy which shows histological features including superficial perivascular lymphocytic infiltration, compact orthokeratosis, bullae formation, and the presence of necrotic keratinocytes. Signs and symptoms of TA-GVHD include fever, skin rashes (maculopapular rashes, erythroderma), gastrointestinal symptoms (diarrhea, hepatomegaly, elevated liver enzymes), and pancytopenia.

Patients can deteriorate rapidly, with high rates of death despite starting immunosuppression. Therefore, prevention is key by providing irradiated blood products which inactivate donor T-lymphocytes.

TRANSFUSION REACTION WORKUP

The purpose of a transfusion reaction workup is to identify possible AHTR. Signs and symptoms of AHTR vary and may include fever, hypoxemia, tachycardia, hypertension, hypotension, hematuria, vomiting, chills, rigors, pain, oliguria, and/or DIC. Presenting symptoms alone cannot rule out AHTR. If not recognized early, AHTR can be fatal; therefore, a transfusion reaction workup is recommended if there are any new symptoms or vital sign changes.

Each hospital has its own policy on when to notify the provider for suspected transfusion reactions. When transfusion reaction is suspected, the first step is to stop the transfusion if it is still running, followed by sending the appropriate specimens to the blood bank for investigation. In the blood bank, the following procedures are then performed:

1. Check for clerical errors—includes checking blood component bag label, paperwork, and the recipient's pretransfusion type and screen specimen
2. Repeat ABO testing on post-transfusion specimen
3. Check for hemolysis—visual inspection of the pre- and post-transfusion specimens for hemolysis
4. Perform DAT on post-transfusion specimen
5. Notify transfusion medicine physician on service who can order additional testing as needed
6. Notify primary provider if hemolysis, bacterial contamination, or other serious adverse event related to transfusion is suspected
7. Generate a transfusion reaction report including recommendations for future transfusions

TRANSFUSION-TRANSMITTED INFECTIONS

DONOR SCREENING AND INFECTION TESTING

Transfusion-transmitted infections (TTI) are infections transmitted from blood components to the recipient. To reduce the risk of TTI, blood donors must meet specific criteria and undergo a rigorous collection process. Accredited blood collection facilities must follow national regulations and recommendations for donor selection that are intended to protect both blood donors and recipients. The screening includes a blood donor history questionnaire that assesses potential risk factors for TTI such as recent piercings, tattoos, and travel history. If the donor passes the screening, the donation process includes additional measures to reduce the risk of TTI, as listed below:

- At least the first 10 mL of blood are collected into a special diversion pouch which captures skin debris, which reduces the bacterial contamination of collected blood
- Collected blood undergoes required serologic testing for hepatitis B (HBV), hepatitis C (HCV), human immunodeficiency virus (HIV), human T-cell lymphotropic virus (HTLV-I/II), syphilis, CMV, *Trypanosoma cruzi*, as well as nucleic acid testing (NAT) for HBV DNA, HIV-1 RNA, HCV RNA, West Nile virus (WNV) RNA, and Zika virus (ZIKV) RNA
- Babesia screening occurs in states with endemic Babesia
- Platelets also undergo bacterial screening which includes inspection for discoloration, culture, and point of care testing for bacterial proteins

RISK OF TRANSFUSION-TRANSMITTED INFECTIONS

Due to the above rigorous screening process and more sensitive assay development, the incidence of HIV, HBV, and HCV TTI has decreased. In the United States, the risk of HIV, HCV, and HBV transmission per unit is approximately 1 in 2 million.

However, there are many organisms that are not tested for and can be transmitted through blood. These organisms include Epstein-Barr virus (EBV), parvovirus B19, Dengue virus, malaria, and prion disease. The donor questionnaire helps to identify donors with risk of transmitting these infections. Between 2013 and 2018, fewer than 1% of TTI events were reported in the United States, and these infections were primarily from platelet and RBC transfusions.

In the United States, bacterial contamination of platelet products is the most common cause of transfusion-associated morbidity and mortality because platelets are stored at room temperature. Bacterial contamination may occur from donor skin, contaminated equipment, or introduced during processing and storage. Thus, venipuncture site disinfection, utilization of the diversion pouch to collect skin debris, and additional bacterial screening for platelets has been implemented.

Signs and symptoms of TTI include fever, chills, rigors, hypotension, tachycardia, nausea/vomiting, and may progress to septic shock and DIC. TTI can potentially be misdiagnosed as other transfusion reactions like AHTR, febrile non-hemolytic transfusion reaction (FNHTR), transfusion-related acute lung injury (TRALI), or allergic reactions. Therefore, one must have high index of suspicion for TTI so that appropriate management can be taken including obtaining blood cultures and starting antibiotics.

SUGGESTED READINGS

Abdallah R, Rai H, Panch SR. Transfusion reactions and adverse events. *Clin Lab Med*. 2021;41(4):669-696.

Ainley LI, Hewitt PE. Haematology patients and the risk of transfusion transmitted infection. *Br J Haematol*. 2018;180(4):473-483.

American Society of Hematology Choosing Wisely: Ten Things Physicians and Patients Should Question.; 2013. https://www.choosingwisely.org/societies/american-society-of-hematology/. Accessed September 2, 2022.

Center for Disease Control—Division of Healthcare Quality Promotion. National Healthcare Safety Network biovigilance component hemovigilance module surveillance Protocol. 2018;(March):1-30. https://www.cdc.gov/nhsn/pdfs/biovigilance/bv-hv-protocol-current.pdf.

Cohn CS, Delaney M, Johnson ST, Katz LM, eds. *Technical Manual*. 20th ed. AABB; 2020.

Delaney M, Wendel S, Bercovitz RS, et al. Transfusion reactions: prevention, diagnosis, and treatment. *Lancet*. 2016;388(10061):2825-2836.

FDA. Fatalities Reported to FDA Following Blood Collection and Transfusion: Annual Summary for Fiscal Year 2019. *Center for Biologics Evaluation and Research (CBER)*. Published online 2020:1-16.

Goel R, Tobian AAR, Shaz BH. Noninfectious transfusion-associated adverse events and their mitigation strategies. *Blood*. 2019;133(17): 1831-1839.

Harmening D. *Modern Blood Banking and Transfusion Practices*. 7th ed. F.A. Davis; 2019.

Kracalik I, Mowla S, Basavaraju SV, Sapiano MRP. Transfusion-related adverse reactions: Data from the National Healthcare Safety Network Hemovigilance Module — United States, 2013–2018. *Transfusion (Paris)*. 2021;61(5):1424-1434.

Lacroix J, Hébert PC, Hutchison JS, et al. Transfusion strategies for patients in pediatric intensive care units. *N Engl J Med*. 2007;356(16):1609-1619.

Mainou M, Alahdab F, Tobian AAR, et al. Reducing the risk of transfusion-transmitted cytomegalovirus infection: A systematic review and meta-analysis. *Transfusion (Paris)*. 2016;56(6):1569-1580.

McCormick M, Delaney M. Transfusion support: Considerations in pediatric populations. *Semin Hematol*. 2020;57(2):65-72.

Mo YD, Delaney M. Transfusion in Pediatric Patients: Review of Evidence-Based Guidelines. *Clin Lab Med*. 2021;41(1):1-14.

Mowla SJ, Sapiano MRP, Jones JM, Berger JJ, Basavaraju S v. Supplemental findings of the 2019 National Blood Collection and Utilization Survey. *Transfusion (Paris)*. 2021;61(S2):S11-S35.

Oakley FD, Woods M, Arnold S, Young PP. Transfusion reactions in pediatric compared with adult patients: A look at rate, reaction type, and associated products. *Transfusion (Paris)*. 2015;55(3):563-570.

Panch SR, Montemayor-Garcia C, Klein HG. Hemolytic Transfusion Reactions. *N Engl J Med*. 2019;381(2):150-162.

Parker RI. Transfusion in critically ill children: Indications, risks, and challenges. *Crit Care Med*. 2014;42(3):675-690.

Parker V, Tormey CA. The direct antiglobulin test: Indications, interpretation, and pitfalls. *Arch Pathol Lab Med*. 2017;141(2):305-310.

Schiffer CA, Bohlke K, Delaney M, et al. Platelet transfusion for patients with cancer: American society of clinical oncology clinical practice guideline update. *J Clin Oncol*. 2018;36(3):283-299.

Valentine SL, Bembea MM, Muszynski JA, et al. Consensus recommendations for rbc transfusion practice in critically Ill children from the pediatric critical care transfusion and Anemia expertise initiative. *Pediatr Crit Care Med*. 2018;19(9):884-898.

SECTION J

Infectious Diseases

CHAPTER 90 Empirical Treatment of Bacterial Infections

Talene A. Metjian, Pharm.D. and Jeffrey S. Gerber, MD, PhD

BACKGROUND

The initiation of antibiotic therapy is a common challenge for clinicians caring for hospitalized patients. Many factors influence the choice of whether to start antibiotics, when to start, and which agent or agents to employ. Often the decision to initiate antibiotics and to select appropriate antibiotic agents happens before confirmation of the presence of a treatable infection and before its precise location, severity, and the specific infectious cause is identified. Some of the factors to consider include the likelihood of a treatable infection actually being present, the risks of an untreated infection, and which pathogen might be involved. Other, antibiotic-related factors include the toxicity profile and the pharmacodynamic parameters of the drug.

This chapter provides guidance for antibiotic selection according to (i) common pediatric clinical syndromes (**Table 90-1**) and (ii) specific bacteria pathogens (**Table 90-2**). Antibiotic susceptibilities of organisms vary by region, by hospital, and in some cases, by units within a hospital. For proper treatment and appropriate use, the clinician must remain cognizant of these ever changing antibiotic susceptibility profiles by reviewing the current literature and local antibiograms. Importantly, if culture and sensitivity results become available, the clinician should modify antibiotic coverage to the narrowest spectrum that effectively treats the relevant pathogen(s) and adequately targets the site of infection.

TABLE 90-1 Empirical Treatment for Common Childhood Bacterial Infections*

		ANTIBIOTIC	
Bacterial Infection	**Common Pathogens**	**Primary**	**Alternative**
Bites	Dog/Cat: *Pasteurella* spp., *Streptococcus* spp., *Staphylococcus* spp., *Capnocytophaga* spp., *Moraxella* spps., anaerobes	Ampicillin-sulbactam **or** amoxicillin-clavulanate	Trimethoprim-sulfamethoxazole + clindamycin **or** ciprofloxacin + clindamycin
	Human: *Streptococcus* spp., *Staphylococcus* spp., corynebacterium, eikenella, anaerobes	Same as above	Same as above
Brain abscess	Polymicrobial	Vancomycin + metronidazole + Ceftriaxone/cefotaxime¶	Vancomycin + carbapenem
Cellulitis	*Streptococcus pyogenes* (nonpurulent) *Staphylococcus aureus* (purulent)	Cefazolin **or** cephalexin	Clindamycin **or** (for severe or refractory infection) vancomycin **or** linezolid
Deep soft tissue abscess	***S. aureus***, *Streptococcus* spp.	Cefazolin **or** cephalexin (if low MRSA prevalence)	Trimethoprim-sulfamethoxazole **or** clindamycin **or** (for severe or refractory infection) vancomycin **or** linezolid
Periorbital/preseptal	*Streptococcus pyogenes* (nonpurulent) *Staphylococcus aureus* (purulent)	Cefazolin **or** cephalexin (if low MRSA prevalence)	Clindamycin **or** (for severe or refractory infection) vancomycin **or** linezolid
Orbital	***S. aureus*** ***S. pneumoniae*** ***Anaerobes*** *S. anginosus* *H. influenzae* *M. catarrhalis* *S. pyogenes*	Ampicillin-sulbactam	Clindamycin **or** (for severe or refractory infection) Ampicillin-sulbactam + vancomycin **or** linezolid
Cervical adenitis, acute	*S. pyogenes*, *S. aureus*	Cefazolin **or** cephalexin (if low MRSA prevalence)	Clindamycin **or** (for severe or refractory infection) vancomycin **or** linezolid
Epiglottitis	*S. pyogenes*, *S. aureus*, *S. pneumoniae*, *H. inflenzae* (rare)	Ceftriaxone/cefotaxime + vancomycin	Levofloxacin† + clindamycin
Intra-abdominal infection	Polymicrobial (*Escherichia coli* and anaerobes)	ceftriaxone/cefotaxime + metronidazole	Piperacillin-tazobactam **or** ciprofloxacin† + metronidazole
Meningitis	Neonates: **GBS, *E. coli***, *L. monocytogenes*, HSV	Ampicillin + cefotaxime/ceftazidime	Vancomycin + cefotaxime/ceftazidime *Consider acyclovir
	Infants: *S. pneumoniae*, *N. meningitidis*, late-onset GBS	Vancomycin + cefotaxime/ ceftriaxone	Vancomycin + levofloxacin† **or** vancomycin + carbapenem
	Children and adolescents: *S. pneumoniae*, *N. meningitidis*	Same as above	Same as above

(Continued)

TABLE 90-1 Empirical Treatment for Common Childhood Bacterial Infections[*] *(Continued)*

Bacterial Infection	Common Pathogens	ANTIBIOTIC Primary	ANTIBIOTIC Alternative
Osteomyelitis	*S. aureus*, *S. pyogenes*, *K kingae*	Nafcillin/oxacillin **or** cefazolin if low MRSA prevalence	Clindamycin or Vancomycin **or** linezolid + nafcillin/oxacillin or cefazolin *K kingae* covered by amoxicillin, cefazolin or cephalexin
Otitis media, acute	*S. pneumoniae*, *H. influenzae*, *M. cattarrhalis*	Amoxicillin[‡]	Amoxicillin-clavulanate **or** ceftriaxone
Pelvic inflammatory disease	*N. gonorrhoeae*, *C. trachomatis*, anaerobes, Enterobacteriaceae, streptococci, *S. agalactiae*	Ceftriaxone + doxycycline (PO or IV)[§] +metronidazole (PO or IV)	Doxycycline (PO or IV)[§] + cefoxitin **or** clindamycin + gentamicin (IV or IM)
Pharyngitis (group A *Streptococcus*)		Penicillin V (PO) **or** benzathine penicillin G (IM) (can combine with procaine penicillin 3:1 ratio)	Amoxicillin **or** cephalexin **or** clindamycin **or** azithromycin
Pneumonia			
Mild/moderate	*S. pneumoniae*, *S. aureus*, *S. pyogenes*, *Mycoplasma pneumoniae*	Ampicillin **or** amoxicillin Consider azithromycin with atypical symptoms and > 5 years	Clindamycin **or** levofloxacin[†]
Complicated (empyema or necrotizing)	Same as above	Clindamycin + cefotaxime/ ceftriaxone	Clindamycin + levofloxacin[†]
Severe	Same as above	Vancomycin + cefotaxime/ ceftriaxone	Vancomycin + levofloxacin[†]
Retropharyngeal/ peritonsillar abscess	*S. pyogenes*, anaerobes, *H. influenzae*, *S. pneumoniae*, *S. aureus*	Ampicillin–sulbactam **or** amoxicillin-clavulanate	Clindamycin **or** ampicillin-sulbactam + vancomycin (severe infection)
Sepsis (immunocompetent)		Vancomycin + ceftriaxone/cefotaxime	Vancomycin + one of the following: cefepime, ciprofloxacin[†], **or** carbapenem
Septic Arthritis			
Typical, acute	*S. aureus*, *S. pneumoniae*, *S. pyogenes*	Nafcillin/oxacillin **or** cefazolin	Clindamycin or vancomycin + cefazolin **or** nafcillin/oxacillin (severe infection)
Hip or shoulder	*K. kingae* (3 months – 4 years of age)	Cefazolin	
Presumed Lyme	*B. burgdorferi*	Doxycycline[§] or amoxicillin or cefuroxime axetil	
Sexually active	Same as above and *N. gonorrhoeae*	Ceftriaxone/cefotaxime	
Sinusitis (acute)	*S. pneumoniae*, *H. influenzae*, *M. catarrhalis*	Amoxicillin[‡]	Clindamycin **or** amoxicillin-clavulanate **or** levofloxacin[†]
Urinary tract infection			
Outpatient	*E. coli*, *Klebsiella*, *Proteus*, *Enterococcus*, *S. saprophyticus*	Trimethoprim-sulfamethoxazole **or** cephalexin **or** cefixime	Cefuroxime **or** cefprozil **or** cephalexin
Inpatient		Ampicillin + gentamicin **or** cefazolin	Ceftriaxone/cefotaxime **or** ciprofloxacin[†]

MRSA, methicillin-resistant *Staphylococcus aureus*.

[*]Definitive therapy should be based on the availability of additional information, including culture results.

[†]Ciprofloxacin is approved for complicated urinary tract infections and pyelonephritis in children. Levofloxacin is approved only for patients >18 years of age; use off-label in children <18 years of age if no other alternatives are available.

[‡]If no antibiotics were administered in the prior month, use high-dose amoxicillin (80-90 mg/kg divided every 12 hours). If antibiotics were given previously or otitis–conjunctivitis syndrome consider amoxicillin-clavulanate (80-90 mg/kg amoxicillin component divided every 12 hours); if clavulanate component exceeds 10 mg/kg/day, use a preparation with a higher ratio of amoxicillin-to-clavulanate (e.g., 14:1 or higher ratio of amoxicillin-to-clavulanate).

[§]Doxycycline can be used in children less than < 8 years of age when clinically indicated for short courses.

[¶] Cefotaxime availability may be limited in some countries

TABLE 90-2 Empirical Treatment of Bacterial Infections by Organisms[*]

Organisms	First Choice	Others
Acinetobacter spp.	Ampicillin-sulbactam **or** carbapenem **or** cefepime	Trimethoprim-sulfamethoxazole **or** ciprofloxacin[‡]
Bacteroides fragilis group	Metronidazole	Ampicillin-sulbactam **or** amoxicillin-clavulanate **or** cefoxitin
Bordetella pertussis	Erythromycin **or** azithromycin	Trimethoprim-sulfamethoxazole **or** clarithromycin
Campylobacter jejuni	Erythromycin **or** azithromycin	Ciprofloxacin[‡] **or** doxycycline[†]
Chlamydia trachomatis	Infants and children < 45 kg: erythromycin or azithromycin ≥ 45 kg: azithromycin	Doxycycline[†] See Chapter 45, Sexually Transmitted Infections
Citrobacter spp.	Cefepime **or** carbapenem	Trimethoprim-sulfamethoxazole **or** ciprofloxacin[‡]

(Continued)

TABLE 90-2 Empirical Treatment of Bacterial Infections by Organisms[*] *(Continued)*

Organisms	First Choice	Others
Clostridium difficile	Metronidazole (PO)	Vancomycin (PO) **or** metronidazole (IV)
Enterobacter spp.	Cefepime **or** carbapenem	Trimethoprim-sulfamethoxazole **or** ciprofloxacin[‡]
Enterococcus faecalis		
Non-invasive	Ampicillin	vancomycin
Invasive (endocarditis or meningitis)	Ampicillin + gentamicin	Ampicillin +ceftriaxone or vancomycin or linezolid
Enterococcus faecium		
Non-invasive	Vancomycin	Linezolid
Invasive (endocarditis or meningitis)	Vancomycin + gentamicin	Linezolid
Escherichia coli	Ceftriaxone/cefotaxime	Aztreonam **or** carbapenem **or** trimethoprim-sulfamethoxazole **or** ciprofloxacin[‡]
Fusobacterium spp.	Metronidazole	Clindamycin **or** ampicillin-sulbactam **or** piperacillin-tazobactam
Haemophilus influenzae	Amoxicillin-clavulanate **or** ampicillin-sulbactam	Ceftriaxone/cefotaxime
Klebsiella spp. (excludes *Klebsiella aerogenes*)	Ceftriaxone/cefotaxime	Aztreonam **or** carbapenem **or** trimethoprim-sulfamethoxazole **or** ciprofloxacin[‡]
Listeria monocytogenes	Ampicillin	Trimethoprim-sulfamethoxazole
Moraxella catarrhalis	Amoxicillin-clavulanate or ampicillin-sulbactam	Ceftriaxone/cefotaxime
Mycoplasma pneumoniae	Azithromycin	Doxycycline[†] **or** erythromycin **or** clarithromycin **or** levofloxacin[‡]
Neisseria gonorrhoeae	Ceftriaxone	Gentamicin (IM) + azithromycin (PO) See pelvic inflammatory disease chapter; infectious diseases consultation if recent travel outside the United States
Neisseria meningitidis	Penicillin G	Ceftriaxone/cefotaxime
Pasteurella multocida	Penicillin **or** ampicillin **or** amoxicillin	Doxycycline[†] **or** cefuroxime **or** ceftriaxone/cefotaxime **or** amoxicillin-clavulanate
Proteus mirabilis	Ceftriaxone/cefotaxime	Cefuroxime **or** trimethoprim-sulfamethoxazole
Providencia and *Morganella* spp.	Ceftriaxone/cefotaxime	Ciprofloxacin[‡] **or** aztreonam
Pseudomonas aeruginosa	Cefepime **or** piperacillin-tazobactam	Ciprofloxacin[‡]
Prevotella spp.	Clindamycin	Metronidazole **or** ampicillin-sulbactam **or** cefoxitin
Salmonella (systemic)	Ceftriaxone/cefotaxime	Trimethoprim-sulfamethoxazole **or** ampicillin **or** ciprofloxacin[‡]
Serratia spp.	Cefepime **or** carbapenem	Trimethoprim-sulfamethoxazole **or** ciprofloxacin[‡]
Shigella, intestinal	Ceftriaxone/cefotaxime	Azithromycin **or** ciprofloxacin[‡] **or** ampicillin **or** trimethoprim-sulfamethoxazole
Staphylococcus aureus		
MSSA	Nafcillin/oxacillin	Cefazolin **or** ampicillin-sulbactam
MRSA, community acquired[§]	Clindamycin	Vancomycin **or** trimethoprim-sulfamethoxazole **or** doxycycline[†]
MRSA, hospital acquired or serious infection	Vancomycin	Linezolid
Staphylococcus epidermidis (and other coagulase-negative staphylococci in context of an indwelling device)	Vancomycin	Linezolid **or** nafcillin/oxacillin (if susceptible)
Streptococcus pneumoniae		
Meningitis or critically ill	Ceftriaxone/cefotaxime + vancomycin	Levofloxacin[‡] + vancomycin **or** carbapenem + vancomycin
Pneumonia	Ampicillin **or** ceftriaxone/cefotaxime	Levofloxacin[‡]
Streptococcus pyogenes (group A *Streptococcus*)	Penicillin	Amoxicillin **or** ampicillin **or** cefazolin **or** clindamycin **or** azithromycin
Streptococcus agalactiae (group B *Streptococcus*)	Penicillin ± gentamicin	Ceftriaxone/cefotaxime **or** vancomycin[¶]
Treponema pallidum	Penicillin	Erythromycin[¶] **or** tetracycline[+] **or** ceftriaxone
Yersinia enterocolitica (invasive)	Trimethoprim-sulfamethoxazole	Ceftriaxone/cefotaxime **or** ciprofloxacin[‡]

[*]Empirical treatment should be guided by local and hospital sensitivity patterns. After sensitivities are known, use the effective antibiotic with the narrowest spectrum.

[†]Patient age, 8 years or older.

[‡] Ciprofloxacin is approved for complicated urinary tract infections and pyelonephritis in children. Levofloxacin approved for patients >18 years of age; use off-label in children <18 years of age if no other alternatives are available.

[§]Clindamycin can be used if test for inducible resistance ("D-test") is negative; otherwise, use vancomycin.

[¶]Penicillin-allergic patient.

SUGGESTED READINGS

American Academy of Pediatrics. Committee on Infectious Diseases. *Red Book: 2021-2024 Report of the Committee on Infectious Diseases.* 32nd ed. Elk Grove Village, IL: American Academy of Pediatrics. Systems-based Treatment Table (990-1003).

American Academy of Pediatrics Subcommittee on Urinary Tract Infection, Steering Committee on Quality Improvement and Management, Urinary tract infection: clinical practice guidelines for the diagnosis and management of the initial UTI in febrile infants and children 2 to 24 months. *Pediatrics.* 2011;128(3):595-610.

Bradley JS, Byington CL, Shah SS, et al. The management of community-acquired pneumonia in infants and children older than 3 months of age: Clinical Practice Guidelines by the Pediatric Infectious Diseases Society and the Infectious Diseases Society of America. *Clin Infect Dis.* 2011;53(7):e25-e76.

Gerber JS, Jackson MA, Tamma PD, Zaoutis TE; AAP Committee on Infectious Diseases, Pediatric Infectious Diseases Society. Antibiotic stewardship in pediatrics. *Pediatrics.* 2021;147(1): e2020040295.

Lantos PM, Rumbaugh J, Bockenstedt LK, et al. Clinical practice guidelines by the Infectious Diseases Society of America (IDSA), American Academy of Neurology (AAN), and American College of Rheumatology (ACR): 2020 guidelines for the prevention, diagnosis, and treatment of lyme disease. *Clin Infect Dis.* 2021; 72(1): e1-e48.

Lieberthal AS, Carroll AE, Chonmaitree T, et al. Clinical practice guideline: the diagnosis and management of acute otitis media. *Pediatrics.* 2013;131:e964-e999.

McDonald LC, Gerding DN, Johnson S, et al. Clinical Practice Guidelines for Clostridium difficile Infection in Adults and Children: 2017 Update by the Infectious Diseases Society of America (IDSA) and Society for Healthcare Epidemiology of America (SHEA). *Clin Infect Dis.* 2018;66(7):e1-e48.

Pantell R H, Roberts K B, Adams W G, et al. Evaluation and management of well-appearing febrile infants 8 to 60 days old. *Pediatrics.* 2021;148(2):e2021052228.

Spellberg B. Principles of Antiinfective Therapy. In: Mandell, Douglas, Bennett's *Principles and Practice of Infectious Diseases.* 9th ed. Philadelphia, PA: Elsevier; 2020:211-221.e2.

Tamma PD, Aitken SL, Bonomo RA, et al. Infectious Diseases Society of America Antimicrobial-Resistant Treatment Guidance: Gram-Negative Bacterial Infections. Infectious Diseases Society of America 2022; Version 1.1. Available at https://www.idsociety.org/practice-guideline/amr-guidance/. Accessed July 8, 2022.

Tamma PD, Aitken SL, Bonomo RA, et al. Infectious Diseases Society of America Guidance on the Treatment of AmpC β-lactamase-Producing Enterobacterales, Carbapenem-Resistant Acinetobacter baumannii, and Stenotrophomonas maltophilia Infections. Infectious Diseases Society of America 2022; Version 2.0. Available at https://www.idsociety.org/practice-guideline/amr-guidance-2.0/. Accessed August 21, 2022.

Tamma PD, Turnbull AE, Harris AD, et al. Less is more: combination antibiotic therapy for the treatment of gram-negative bacteremia in pediatric patients. *JAMA Pediatrics.* 2013;167(10):903-910.

Woods CR, Bradley JS, Chatterjee A, et al. Clinical Practice Guideline by the Pediatric Infectious Diseases Society and the Infectious Diseases Society of America: 2021 Guideline on Diagnosis and Management of Acute Hematogenous Osteomyelitis in Pediatrics. *J Pediatric Infect Dis Soc.* 2021;10(8):801-844.

Workowski KA, Bachmann LH, Chan PA, et al. Sexually transmitted infections treatment guidelines, 2021. *MMWR Recomm Rep.* 2021;70(4):1-187.

CHAPTER 91

Fever

Paul L. Aronson, MD, MHS and Rachel R. Osborn, MD

BACKGROUND

Fever, a pyrogen-mediated increase in body temperature, may have a multitude of disparate causes, including infection, inflammation, or malignancy. Therefore, the most important goal when confronted with a febrile patient is to determine the underlying cause. Owing to a differential risk of disease, the cutoff point of abnormal temperature is determined by the age of the child and the presence of any underlying immunodeficiencies. Although there is some overlap, in this chapter the discussion of fever is divided into two age groups: (i) neonates and young infants and (ii) older infants and toddlers.

FEVER IN NEONATES AND YOUNG INFANTS

Fever frequently prompts the medical evaluation of neonates (28 days or younger) and young infants (aged 29-90 days). In this age group, fever is generally defined as a temperature greater than 38.0°C (100.4°F). Up to 15% of neonates and young infants with fever have a urinary tract infection (UTI) or invasive bacterial infection (IBI), that is, bacteremia and/or bacterial meningitis. These infections together were historically called serious bacterial infections, but this terminology has been replaced by UTI and IBI as the risk and potential outcomes of these infections are distinct. The risk of UTI and IBI appears to be lower in certain subgroups, such as those with normal laboratory studies or with bronchiolitis.

The most common bacterial infections in febrile infants are UTIs (5%-10%), bacteremia (2%-3%), and bacterial meningitis (0.5%-1%). Bacterial pneumonia, gastroenteritis, septic arthritis, osteomyelitis, cellulitis, omphalitis, and mastitis also occur. Infecting organisms vary by the site of infection (**Table 91-1**). *Escherichia coli*, the most common cause of UTIs, has replaced group B *Streptococcus* (GBS) as the most common etiologic organism for bacteremia in febrile infants due to perinatal prophylaxis against GBS (see Prevention below). UTIs caused by *Staphylococcus aureus* and *Citrobacter* species are often associated with urinary tract abnormalities and extrarenal sites of infection. Early-onset

TABLE 91-1 Bacterial Pathogens Causing Urinary Tract Infection, Bacteremia, and Bacterial Meningitis in Febrile Infants Younger than 90 Days

Frequency	Urinary Tract Infection	Bacteremia	Bacterial Meningitis
Common	*Escherichia coli*	*E. coli*	Group B *Streptococcus*
	Klebsiella species	Group B *Streptococcus*	*E. coli*
Less common	Group B *Streptococcus* *Enterococcus* species	*S. aureus* *Enterococcus* species	*Klebsiella* species* *Streptococcus pneumoniae**
	Pseudomonas aeruginosa	*Klebsiella* species *Enterobacter* species	*Listeria monocytogenes**
	Staphylococcus aureus *Citrobacter* species	*Salmonella* species$	
	Enterobacter species		Other gram-negative organisms† Other gram-positive organisms&

$Often associated with *Salmonella* gastroenteritis.

*More common in infants older than 1 month.

†Includes *Neisseria meningitidis*, *Citrobacter* species, *Enterobacter* species, *Haemophilus* species.

&Includes *Streptococcus gallolyticus*, *Streptococcus bovis*.

(age younger than 1 week) GBS infections are typically associated with bacteremia, pneumonia, and meningitis; late-onset (older than 1 week) infections include septic arthritis, osteomyelitis, cellulitis, and adenitis. *Streptococcus pneumoniae* is responsible for up to 5% of cases of meningitis in neonates and a slightly greater proportion in infants 1 to 3 months of age. Brain abscesses are more likely in cases of meningitis caused by *Citrobacter koseri*, *Enterobacter sakazakii*, *Bacteroides fragilis*, and *Serratia marcescens*. Bacteremia complicates *Salmonella* gastroenteritis in 5% to 10% of cases. In contrast to older children, young infants with *Salmonella* bacteremia rarely have other immunocompromising conditions. Omphalitis, an infection of the umbilical stump, affects 0.2% to 0.7% of newborn infants; it occurs most often among hospitalized preterm infants undergoing umbilical catheterization. Although *S. aureus* remains the most common pathogen in omphalitis, gram-negative organisms have emerged as an important cause of omphalitis since the introduction of antistaphylococcal cord care, particularly *E. coli*; anaerobes may also be a pathogen. *S. aureus* causes most cases of neonatal mastitis.

Herpes simplex virus (HSV) infection should also be considered in febrile and acutely ill infants younger than 1 month of age. HSV infections in neonates are caused by both HSV type 1 and type 2, and are rare in infants >28 days of age. Fetal scalp electrode use increases the risk of neonatal HSV infection. The higher infection rate after primary maternal genital HSV infection (compared with recurrent infection) may be related to the higher viral load, the longer duration of viral excretion, and the absence of transplacentally acquired protective antibodies in infants born to mothers with primary HSV infection. Although the onset is typically between 11 and 17 days, 9% of infants develop symptoms within the first 24 hours of life. Most infants with skin, eye, and mouth involvement or disseminated disease present between 10 and 14 days of life. In contrast, most infants with isolated central nervous system involvement present on days 18 to 21 of life.

CLINICAL PRESENTATION

Symptoms and signs of illness vary considerably. Up to two-thirds of infants younger than 2 months appear well and have a normal physical examination at the initial evaluation, despite the presence of UTI or IBI. Signs of sepsis or other systemic disease are often nonspecific and include disturbances of thermoregulation, such as fever (defined as temperature ≥38°C) or hypothermia (temperature <36°C), poor feeding, and evidence of organ dysfunction. Potential cardiovascular disturbances include tachycardia (pulse >180 beats per minute), bradycardia (pulse <95 beats per minute), hypotension (systolic blood pressure <60 mmHg in full-term infants), weak or bounding femoral pulses, mottled skin, and delayed capillary refill (>2-3 seconds). Respiratory abnormalities include apnea, tachypnea (respirations >60 breaths per minute), grunting, nasal flaring, intercostal or subcostal retractions, and hypoxemia. Signs of gastrointestinal tract disturbances include a rigid or distended abdomen, absent bowel sounds, diarrhea, or bloody stools. Cutaneous findings such as jaundice, petechiae, and cyanosis may be present. Neurologic abnormalities can occur with any serious infection and include irritability, lethargy, hypotonia, and hypertonia.

Signs of a specific disease process may also be detected. Infants with meningitis may have a tense or bulging fontanelle, and up to one-third may develop seizures. The presence of vesicles warrants consideration of HSV infection; vesicles are detected in two-thirds of children with either central nervous system or disseminated HSV infection. Erythema, edema, induration, and tenderness of the breast tissue herald mastitis. Although most cases of mastitis are mild, the infection can progress rapidly. Involvement may extend beyond the breast tissue to the subcutaneous tissue around the shoulder and the abdomen. Periumbilical erythema, ecchymosis, edema, induration, or crepitus suggests omphalitis. Extremity abnormalities may be more noticeable to the parents. Local signs of septic arthritis or osteomyelitis include swelling, erythema, warmth, exquisite tenderness, and diminished range of motion of the affected joint or extremity. These infants often demonstrate an unwillingness to move the extremity, a finding known as pseudoparalysis.

DIFFERENTIAL DIAGNOSIS

The management of febrile infants younger than 90 days poses a challenge because of the relatively high prevalence of UTI and IBI and the inability to easily distinguish those with bacterial infections or HSV from those with uncomplicated, common viral illnesses caused by respiratory syncytial virus (RSV), parainfluenza viruses, influenza viruses, adenovirus, human metapneumovirus, and enteroviruses.

EVALUATION

Febrile infants in the first week of life require comprehensive evaluation for UTI and IBI because of a high-risk of early onset GBS sepsis. This evaluation includes cultures of urine, blood, and cerebrospinal fluid (CSF) followed by hospitalization and empirical antibiotic administration. The diagnostic evaluation of young febrile infants 8 to 60 days old is guided by the 2021 American Academy of Pediatrics (AAP) clinical practice guideline (CPG) for the evaluation and management of well-appearing febrile infants. Because of a lower prevalence of IBI in febrile infants after the first three weeks of life, the AAP CPG provides separate management recommendations for three age groups: 8-21 days, 22-28 days, and 29-60 days of age. The AAP CPG applies to previously healthy, full term, well-appearing febrile infants without clinical bronchiolitis, focal bacterial infections, high suspicion of HSV, or immunizations within the past 48 hours. Infants with upper respiratory symptoms and those with positive respiratory viral tests without bronchiolitis should be managed as per the AAP CPG.

Infants 8 to 21 days of age are at highest risk of IBI, and therefore urinalysis (UA, with urine culture if the UA is positive i.e., the presence of any leukocyte esterase (LE) on dipstick, >5 WBCs per high-power field (hpf) in centrifuged urine, or >10 WBCs/mm^3 in uncentrifuged urine on microscopic urinalysis using a hemocytometer), blood and CSF cultures, hospitalization, and empirical antibiotic administration are recommended by the AAP CPG. For infants 22 to 28 days and 29 to 60 days of age, a UA (with urine culture if the UA is positive) and blood culture are recommended, but CSF testing, hospitalization, and empirical antimicrobial administration are based on risk stratification using combinations of inflammatory markers (**Table 91-2**). If inflammatory markers are normal in infants 22 to 28 days of age, even with a positive UA, shared decision-making about lumbar puncture is recommended, with hospitalization and empiric antimicrobial therapy dependent on whether a lumbar puncture was performed and the results. If inflammatory markers are abnormal in infants 22 to 28 days of age, lumbar puncture, hospitalization, and empiric antimicrobial therapy administration are recommended. In contrast, infants 29 to 60 days with normal inflammatory markers, regardless of UA result, should be discharged home without lumbar puncture, with or without antimicrobial therapy based on the UA result. The rationale for not obtaining a lumbar puncture on febrile infants 29 to 60 days of age with positive UAs but negative inflammatory markers is that multiple studies have shown no difference in the prevalence of bacterial meningitis among febrile infants with positive versus negative UAs, indicating that the prevalence of meningitis is independent of a positive UA. Additionally, two retrospective studies reported that infants with positive UAs treated with antimicrobial therapy without lumbar puncture did well with no adverse sequelae or delayed diagnosis of meningitis. A multicenter, ambispective study also found that infants older that 15 days with normal inflammatory markers (i.e., procalcitonin [PCT] and C-reactive protein [CRP]) had a low risk of IBI. Similarly, a 2022 multicenter, prospective study from the Pediatric Emergency Care Applied Research Network (PECARN) found no cases of IBI among 148 febrile infants age 60 days or younger with normal PCT (<0.5 ng/mL) and ANC (<4000 cells/mm^3). For infants 29 to 60 days of age with abnormal inflammatory markers, the decision to obtain a lumbar puncture, hospitalize the infant, and initiate empiric antimicrobial therapy is based on the clinician's and caregiver's risk tolerance and preferences, with an opportunity for shared decision-making. All infants discharged from the emergency department require follow-up within 24 hours and clear discharge instructions about return to care for clinical worsening.

For risk stratification of febrile infants 22 to 60 days age, use of PCT with absolute neutrophil count (ANC) plus/minus CRP is recommended,

TABLE 91-2 AAP CPG Recommended Evaluation and Management of Well Appearing Febrile Infants by Age Group

8-21 Days of Age

Urinalysis	Inflammatory Markers	Lumbar Puncture	Antibiotics	Disposition
Positive or Negative	Not Indicated	Perform LP	IV antibiotics	Admit^

22-28 Days of Age

Urinalysis	Inflammatory Markers	Lumbar Puncture	Antibiotics	Disposition
Negative	Negative	*LP may be obtained	LP **not** performed: option to admit off antibiotics	Observe in hospital^
			LP performed: *May give IV antibiotics (required if CSF (+))	*May discharge home if CSF (-) and Ceftriaxone x 1 given
Positive	Negative	*LP may be obtained	IV antibiotics	Admit^
Positive or Negative	**Positive**	Perform LP	IV antibiotics	Admit^

29-60 Days of Age

Urinalysis	Inflammatory Markers	Lumbar Puncture	Antibiotics	Disposition
Negative	Negative	No LP	No antibiotics	Observe closely at home, f/u in 24 hrs
Positive	Negative	No LP	Oral antibiotics	Observe closely at home, f/u in 24 hrs
Positive or negative	**Positive**	*May perform LP, then:		
		• If CSF is negative	IV or oral antibiotics (if UA (+))	*May observe in hospital or home
		• If CSF is **positive**	IV antibiotics	Admit^
		• If CSF is not obtained or uninterpretable	IV antibiotics	*May observe in hospital or home

^Discharge at 24-36 hours if cultures negative and clinically improving

* Opportunity for Shared Decision Making

ELEVATED INFLAMMATORY MARKERS (IM)
- Procalcitonin (PCT) > 0.5 ng/mL
- C-reactive protein (CRP) ≥ 20 mg/L (2.0 mg/dL)
- Absolute neutrophil count (ANC) > 4000-5200 cells/mm³
- Temperature > 38.5°C

When PCT **available**: Use PCT with ANC +/− CRP
When PCT **not** available: Use ANC + CRP + Max Temp

Source: Reproduced with permission from McDaniel CE, Kerns E, Jennings B, Magee S, Biondi E, Flores R, Aronson PL; AAP REVISE II QI Collaborative. Improving Guideline-Concordant Care for Febrile Infants Through a Quality Improvement Initiative. *Pediatrics*. 153(5):e2023063339; Copyright © 2024 by AAP.

using either the PECARN prediction rule or the Step-by-Step approach. The PECARN prediction rule has higher sensitivity and specificity for IBI (**Table 91-3**). If PCT is not available, the AAP CPG recommends a combination of height of temperature, ANC, and CRP for risk stratification. This combination of inflammatory markers has high sensitivity for UTI and IBI but lower specificity than the PECARN prediction rule.

Due to a paucity of evidence relative to infants 8 to 60 days of age, febrile infants 61 to 90 days of age are not included in the AAP CPG. Although the prevalence of IBI is lower in febrile infants 61 to 90 days of age (~1%), the prevalence of UTI remains 5% to 10%. Therefore, a UA (with urine culture if the UA is positive) is recommended, plus/minus blood culture and inflammatory markers based on the clinician's and caregiver's risk tolerance. The Step-by-Step approach was validated in infants up to 90 days of age and can be used for risk stratification in this age group. However, as the prevalence of bacterial meningitis is low in this age group, non-low-risk, well-appearing infants do not necessarily require lumbar puncture.

TABLE 91-3 Comparison of Risk Stratification Algorithms to Identify Previously Healthy, Full Term, Well-Appearing Febrile Infants at Low and Non-Low-Risk of IBI*

Variable	Step by Step	PECARN	Temperature + ANC + CRP
Low-Risk Criteria	Age <21 days Normal urine dipstick PCT <0.5 ng/mL CRP ≤20 mg/L ANC ≤10,000/mm⁴	Normal urinalysis PCT ≤0.5 ng/mL ANC ≤4000/uL	Max Temperature ≤38.5 °C CRP ≤20 mg/L ANC ≤5200/mm³
Sensitivity (95% CI)	92 (84.3-96)	96.7 (83.3-99.4)	100 (87-100)
Specificity (95% CI)	46.9 (44.8-49)	61.5 (59.2-63.9)	46 (43-50)
Negative predictive value (95% CI)	99.3 (98.5-99.7)	99.9 (99.4-100)	100 (99-100)

*Sensitivity, specificity, and negative predictive value are presented for IBI.

In summary, the AAP CPG guides the evaluation and management of previously healthy, well-appearing febrile infants 8 to 60 days of age. As stated throughout the AAP CPG, ultimately clinicians should weigh their own risk tolerance, practice setting (e.g., availability of 24-hour follow-up), and parents' values and preferences in weighing the pros and cons the various options in certain scenarios (e.g., an infant 29-60 days of age with abnormal inflammatory markers).

We now discuss in more detail the individual components of evaluation included in the management of febrile infants

Urinalysis Several rapid screening tests are available to identify UTI. The traditional UA involves a combination of urine dipstick (uncentrifuged urine) detection of leukocyte esterase or, nitrites, or microscopic (centrifuged urine) detection of >5 WBCs per high-power field. The enhanced UA uses a combination of hemocytometry to provide a WBC count per cubic millimeter and Gram stain for bacteria on uncentrifuged urine specimens. An abnormal enhanced UA (>10 WBCs/mm³ or bacteria identified on Gram stain) has a higher negative predictive value and sensitivity compared with the traditional UA but the positive predictive value (10%-17%) is substantially lower than that of urine dipstick tests (38%-54%). The traditional UA has a sensitivity of 94% (95% CI: 91%-97%) for detection of UTI and up to 100% (95% CI: 87%-100%) for bacteremic UTIs. Because of this high sensitivity of a positive UA, few "missed" infants with UTIs and negative UAs, and the likely possibility that the "missed" infants have asymptomatic bacteruria or contamination, the AAP CPG only recommends sending a urine culture for testing in the presence of a positive UA. A UA is most commonly obtained by catheterization, though suprapubic aspiration or, in infants 22 to 60 days of age, clean bag or stimulated void with clean catch are also acceptable methods of collection.

Complete Blood Count Because of inferior test characteristics when compared with other biomarkers, in particularly PCT and CRP, the total peripheral white blood cell (WBC) count is no longer recommended for risk stratification of febrile infants. However, ANC is recommended for risk stratification in combination with other inflammatory markers, as described previously.

Chest Radiograph Chest radiographs are not considered a routine part of most protocols. Several studies specifically evaluated the need for routine chest radiographs in febrile infants, but they are of limited value because they included any radiographic abnormality (e.g., peribronchial thickening) rather than the more clinically meaningful, but more difficult to define, finding of pneumonia. A reasonable approach is to limit the use of chest radiographs to infants with abnormal respiratory signs (e.g., cough, tachypnea, hypoxia, abnormal lung auscultation).

Urine Culture For infants with a positive UA, urine culture should be obtained by catheterization or, if needed, suprapubic aspiration. A positive urine culture is defined as growth >10,000 colony-forming units per high powered field of a pathogenic organism in the setting of a positive UA.

Blood Culture Several important variables affect the volume of blood necessary for culture. The magnitude of bacteremia affects blood culture yield, especially when small blood volumes are used. Although it is often difficult to obtain adequate blood samples in pediatric patients, the volume of blood in a single blood culture bottle matters more than the total number of blood cultures obtained. A single culture containing 1 to 2 mL of blood is sufficient for the detection of most clinically important bacteremias; a 0.5-mL blood sample, though not ideal, permits the detection of some clinically important bacteremias.

Lumbar Puncture CSF should routinely be sent for Gram stain and culture, glucose, protein, and cell count. An additional tube is occasionally collected and held in the microbiology or chemistry laboratory in case other studies are required. Interpretation of CSF values varies by age (**Table 91-4**). Bacteria are evident on CSF Gram stain in up to 72% of infants with bacterial meningitis; premature infants with bacterial meningitis are less likely to have organisms detected by Gram stain. Because of the relatively low concentration of organisms, infants with *Listeria monocytogenes* meningitis rarely have bacteria detectable by Gram stain.

Detection of bacterial antigens in the CSF by latex particle agglutination (*S. pneumoniae, Neisseria meningitidis, Haemophilus influenzae*) or counterimmunoelectrophoresis (*E. coli*) has been described. Moderate sensitivity (70%-80%), changing antibiotic susceptibility patterns, and the availability of broad-spectrum antimicrobial therapy limit the usefulness of these tests. Multiplex polymerase chain reaction (PCR) assays for *E. coli, S. pneumoniae, N. meningitidis*, and other bacteria result in higher sensitivity (90%-100%) and specificity (93%-98%) than do bacterial antigen detection tests, but additional research is required in febrile infants younger than 90 days of age.

Contamination of CSF with blood during a traumatic lumbar puncture (e.g., ≥10,000 RBCs/mm^3) confounds the accurate interpretation of results. Correcting the CSF WBCs for CSF RBCs may raise or lower the suspicion for bacterial meningitis. A corrected CSF WBC count can be calculated using the 1:1000 ratio of CSF WBCs:RBCs, as per the following formula:

$$\text{Corrected CSF WBCs} = \text{CSF RBCs}/1000$$

A multicenter, retrospective cohort study determined that the corrected CSF WBC using the 1:1000 CSF WBCs:RBCs ratio had a sensitivity of 85.7% (95% CI: 42.1%-99.6%) for bacterial meningitis in infants

TABLE 91-4 Range of Normal Values for Cerebrospinal Fluid Studies in Neonates and Young Infants*

Age (days)	Cell Count (per mm^3)	Protein (mg/dL)	Glucose (mg/dL)†
≤28	<19	16-131	>30
29-60	<10	6-106	>20

*Data from Pantell RH, Roberts KB, Adams WG, et al. Evaluation and Management of Well-Appearing Febrile Infants 8 to 60 Days Old [published correction appears in *Pediatrics*. 2021 Nov;148(5):]. *Pediatrics*. 2021;148(2):e2021052228; Thomson J, Sucharew H, Cruz AT, et al. Cerebrospinal Fluid Reference Values for Young Infants Undergoing Lumbar Puncture. *Pediatrics*. 2018;141(3):e20173405.

†Cerebrospinal fluid glucose values are typically >40 mg/dL, or one-half to two-thirds of serum values.

29 to 60 days of age, and lower when applied to all infants ≤60 days old (66.7%). Because of the lower sensitivity of corrected CSF WBC, the AAP CPG discourages correcting CSF WBC for CSF RBC and instead using uncorrected CSF WBC in clinical decision-making. Infants with traumatic, uninterpretable lumbar punctures are often hospitalized and receive empirical antibiotic therapy. In certain situations, a repeat lumbar puncture 12 to 24 hours later may clarify the ambiguity of the initial results.

Additional Studies Certain infants ≤28 days of age (particularly those ≤21 days) are at higher risk of having HSV: maternal HSV symptoms perinatally, a close contact with oral HSV, ill or toxic-appearing infant, seizures, hypothermia, vesicles, hepatitis, or lymphocytic predominant CSF pleocytosis outside of enteroviral season. When HSV is a concern based on these high-risk features, CSF, blood, and swabs from skin lesions and mucus membranes (i.e., conjunctivae, mouth, rectum) should be sent for PCR testing. CSF PCR has a sensitivity and specificity of 96% and 99%, respectively, compared with brain biopsy. Blood PCR will be positive in many infants with central nervous system or disseminated HSV infection and some infants with skin, eye, or mucosal infection; thus a positive blood HSV PCR does not necessarily indicate disseminated infection. In infants with skin, eye, or mucous membrane HSV disease, and in many with either central nervous system or disseminated disease, HSV can often be isolated from conjunctival, throat, and rectal swabs by PCR. HSV from these cutaneous sites can usually be detected by PCR within 24 hours. Although a negative PCR result cannot completely exclude HSV infection, most infants with HSV infection have positive PCR results from one of these sites. False negative PCR results are rare but may occur when CSF specimens are obtained very early in the course of HSV illness. In such cases, repeat testing 2 to 3 days later confirms the diagnosis. PCR testing of CSF remains reliable for up to 7 days after the initiation of acyclovir; 50% of specimens remain PCR-positive 8 to 14 days after the initiation of acyclovir. Infants with disseminated HSV may also have laboratory evidence of hepatitis, coagulopathy, and thrombocytopenia.

In addition, during local enteroviral season, CSF enterovirus PCR testing has been shown to decrease length of hospitalization and unnecessary antibiotic use in neonates and young febrile infants by permitting earlier discharge as concomitant bacterial infection in these infants is unlikely. Parechovirus may also be detected with CSF PCR seasonally (e.g., summer and fall); some neonates with parechovirus may have severe illness. Point-of-care RSV and influenza testing may also be informative, as febrile infants younger than 60 days with RSV or influenza have lower risk of IBI but still have substantial risk of UTI. Infants with other viruses also have lower but non-negligible risk of UTI and IBI compared with infants who test negative for viruses, though the risk appears higher in infants who test positive for rhinovirus. The prevalence of UTI and, in particular, IBI, are low amongst febrile infants 8 to 60 days old who test positive for SARS-CoV-2, though prospective study is needed to determine how SARS-CoV-2 testing impacts risk stratification.

OTHER CONSIDERATIONS

The prevalence of UTI and IBI may be lower among some febrile infants with clinical bronchiolitis, which is the rationale for excluding these infants from the AAP CPG. In a 2011 systematic review, 3.3% of young infants with bronchiolitis had UTI combined across studies, with no cases of bacteremia in 8 of 11 studies and no cases of meningitis in any study. Focusing on RSV with or without bronchiolitis, in a prospective, multicenter study from the Pediatric Emergency Medicine Collaborative Research Committee (PEM CRC), RSV-positive infants younger than 60 days were less likely to have a UTI or IBI than were RSV-negative infants (7% vs. 12.5%). However, the subanalysis found some differences by age. Infants 28 days or younger had an overall UTI or IBI prevalence of 13.3% regardless of RSV status. In contrast, RSV-positive infants 29 to 60 days of age had a lower risk of UTI or IBI than did RSV-negative infants (5.5% vs. 11.7%; relative risk: 0.5), and all infections in RSV-positive infants aged 29 to 60 days were UTIs. No RSV-positive patient in this age group had bacteremia or meningitis.

In summary, among infants 28 days and younger, the risk of UTI or IBI is substantial and is not altered by the presence of RSV bronchiolitis.

In following the AAP CPG recommendations for infants without bronchiolitis, we continue to perform a comprehensive evaluation, including urine, blood, and CSF studies, in infants ≤21 days of age. For infants 22 to 28 days of age, we recommend UAs (with urine culture if the urinalysis is positive) and obtaining inflammatory markers to risk stratify the infant, similar to the AAP CPG recommended evaluation of infants 22 to 28 days of age. RSV-positive infants 29 to 60 days of age have a clinically important prevalence of UTI, and because we cannot exclude UTI or IBI in any febrile infant in this age group without a thorough evaluation, blood and urine cultures are routinely performed. Although inflammatory markers may also be used in this age group to risk stratify well-appearing infants, the lumbar puncture is often deferred unless changes in the patient's condition warrant additional evaluation. In determining the extent of laboratory evaluation for infants discharged from the emergency department, clinicians should consider these data in combination with other factors, including the family's reliability to assess the infant's clinical deterioration, access to a telephone, proximity to medical care, and likelihood of follow-up evaluation within 24 hours after emergency department discharge or availability of 24-hour physician support for hospitalized patients.

Preliminary prospective study demonstrates that the host gene expression analysis, the response of the host RNA to infection, may be able to differentiate between viral and bacterial infections causing fever in neonates and young infants with high sensitivity (87% overall, and 94% for bacteremia) and specificity (89% and 95%, respectively). The concept is that differing infections cause differing host leukocyte response and RNA production that can be measured by microarray analysis. In the future, this or other novel technology may provide improved ability to identify patients at risk for SBI or IBI.

OFFICE-BASED STRATEGIES

The protocols summarized in Table 91-3 were developed for use in the emergency department setting. A large proportion of office-based physicians do not routinely follow any of these strategies, though the 2021 AAP CPG is intended to be applied in any practice setting. In an office-based study of 3066 febrile infants younger than 3 months, the overall prevalence of UTI and IBI was similar to the rates found in studies conducted in the emergency department: UTI (5.4%), bacteremia (2.4%), and meningitis (0.5%). Most cases of bacteremia or meningitis occurred during the first month of life in which 4.1% of infants were affected; in contrast, 1.9% and 0.7% of cases occurred during the second and third months of life, respectively. Practitioners in this study followed guidelines in 42% of cases; however, they correctly treated 61 of 63 cases of bacteremia or bacterial meningitis with empirical antibiotics during the initial visit. These findings suggest that if close follow-up care is attainable in an office-based setting (most infants in the study had more than one office visit and multiple telephone contacts), the management of selected cases by an experienced clinician may be more important than strict adherence to published recommendations. This strategy can reduce costs and complications associated with routine evaluation and hospitalization. This study, however, illustrated limitations that warrant consideration. Two infants with life-threatening infections did not receive antibiotics initially; both these infants would have been treated initially if they had been evaluated by at least one of the commonly used screening protocols. Given the relatively high prevalence of UTI and the wide availability of screening UA tests, practitioners should strongly consider routine UA in all young febrile infants. A secondary analysis of this study population also indicated that infants with clinical bronchiolitis evaluated in the office setting were less likely than other febrile infants to have laboratory studies, and were at lower risk of UTI and IBI. A more recent study from Kaiser Permanente Northern California similarly found that the proportion of febrile infants ≤90 days of age who had bacterial cultures obtained decreased by month of life.

ADMISSION CRITERIA

As outlined in the AAP CPG (see Table 91-2), criteria for hospitalization of previously healthy, well-appearing febrile infants vary by age. Hospitalization is recommended for all infants ≤21 days of age, for infants 22 to 28 days of age with positive inflammatory markers and based on shared decision-making for infants with negative inflammatory markers, and for infants 29 to 60 days of age with CSF results concerning for bacterial meningitis and based on clinician and caregiver risk tolerance and preferences for infants with positive inflammatory markers but without concern for meningitis. Any ill-appearing infant, regardless of laboratory test results, also requires hospitalization and empirical antimicrobial therapy.

TREATMENT

The antimicrobial therapy recommended by the AAP CPG varies by age and the suspected type of infection (see **Table 91-5**). For infants ≤21 days of age, ampicillin is recommended in combination with gentamicin (if meningitis is not suspected) or ceftazidime (because of a shortage of cefotaxime). Because of the rarity of *Listeria* monocyotogenes, particularly after the first month of life, plus the increasing rate of ampicillin-resistant organisms, ampicillin is only recommended for infants 22 to 28 days age in whom meningitis is suspected (in combination with ceftazidime) and otherwise ceftriaxone monotherapy is recommended. The recommendations for infants 29 to 60 days of age are similar except that oral cephalexin or cefixime is recommended for infants with suspected UTIs and negative inflammatory markers, and vancomycin is substituted for ampicillin with meningitis is suspected. Additional considerations including adding vancomycin in any age group for ill-appearing infants, those with CSF parameters suggestive of bacterial meningitis, or those with gram-positive cocci identified on CSF Gram stain until cultures have excluded drug-resistant *S. pneumoniae*. Additionally, infants with gram-negative meningitis should have an aminoglycoside added and a carbapenem can be used instead of a cephalosporin if a multi-drug resistant organism is suspected, while awaiting results of antibiotic susceptibility testing. Empiric acyclovir is indicated for febrile infants with risk factors or clinical findings concerning HSV (including ill appearance, vesicular rash, hepatitis, abnormal neurologic status, or seizures).

Duration of therapy is discussed in detail in Chapter 94, Central Nervous System Infections, Chapter 100, Urinary Tract Infections in Childhood, and Chapter 98, Lower Respiratory Tract Infections. In general, infants with UTI receive a total of 7 to 14 days of therapy. If there is associated bacteremia, early transition from parental to oral therapy has been increasingly common at many centers and is not associated with higher risk of treatment failure or readmission. Recommended duration of therapy for meningitis in young infants varies by organism and usually ranges from 14 (gram positive organisms) to 21 days (gram negative organisms).

TABLE 91-5 Antimicrobial Therapy for Febrile Young Infant

Age	Antimicrobial Therapy
1-21 days	Ampicillin/ceftazidime (or gentamicin if meningitis not suspected)/acyclovir*
22-28 days	Ceftriaxone or Ampicillin/ceftazidime (if meningitis suspected)
29-60 days	Ceftriaxone (add Vancomycin if meningitis suspected). Use oral cephalexin or cefixime for suspected UTI and negative inflammatory markers
Additional Considerations	
Ill appearing/+ CSF abnormality/Gram + organism on Gram stain in any age group	Consider adding vancomycin
Gram negative organism on Gram stain	Add an aminoglycoside. Use a carbapenem instead of a cephalosporin if a multidrug resistant organism is strongly suspected.
Risk factor for HSV (ill appearance, abnormal neurologic status, hepatitis, known exposure, maternal history)	Acyclovir

*Some institutions routinely send HSV testing and initiate acyclovir on all infants ≤21 days while other institutions use a more selective approach to testing and empiric acyclovir. The optimal strategy is not known.

Infants with suspected HSV infection should receive high-dose acyclovir (60 mg/kg per day). Infants with skin, eye, or mucous membrane disease receive 14 days of intravenous therapy. Infants with disseminated or central nervous system disease require at least 21 days of therapy. Many experts suggest repeating the lumbar puncture upon completion of the 21-day acyclovir course and extending the duration of acyclovir therapy if the CSF PCR remains positive for HSV. In such situations, consultation with a pediatric infectious disease specialist is recommended.

DISCHARGE CRITERIA

Emergency Department Discharge As delineated in Table 91-2, discharge from the ED is an option for infants 22 to 28 days of age with negative UAs and negative inflammatory markers in whom CSF testing is normal and shared decision-making is performed about disposition. For infants discharged from the ED in this age group, a dose of ceftriaxone is recommended prior to discharge. Infants 29 to 60 days of age with negative UAs and negative inflammatory markers should be discharged home without empiric antimicrobial therapy, while infants with positive UAs but negative inflammatory markers can be discharged with oral antimicrobial therapy for presumptive UTI. For infants with positive inflammatory markers in this age group, disposition is guided by clinician and caregiver risk tolerance and preferences. All infants discharged from the emergency department require follow-up within 24 hours and clear discharge instructions about return to care for clinical worsening.

Hospital Discharge Historically, infants were discharged if culture results had been negative for at least 48 hours. Multiple recent studies have demonstrated that 82% to 91% of pathogens will be detected in blood culture within 24 hours and 96% to 99% within 36 hours. Similarly, 82% to 88% of CSF pathogens will be detected in CSF culture within 24 hours and 86% to 95% within 36 hours. Earlier hospital discharge may therefore be indicated for many infants, and the AAP CPG recommends hospital discharge within 24 to 36 hours if the cultures are negative and the infant is clinically improving. Because of a very low but present risk of a delayed diagnosis of IBI in infants with negative cultures discharged at 24 to 36 hours, infants should have follow-up within 24 hours after hospital discharge. The patient's diagnosis (e.g., UTI, bacteremia, meningitis) and clinical response ultimately determine the duration of hospitalization for infants with positive urine, blood, or CSF cultures. Standardization of care through the use of evidence-based clinical pathways can decrease hospital length of stay, shorten antibiotic duration, and lower healthcare costs while improving patient outcomes.

PREVENTION

Group B Streptococcal Infection Antepartum screening for GBS is recommended weeks 36 to 37 of pregnancy, and maternal intrapartum chemoprophylaxis with at least two doses of penicillin or ampicillin reduces the vertical transmission of GBS from colonized mothers to their neonates. Pregnant patients who are allergic to penicillin without immediate-type hypersensitivity should receive cefazolin, and those with more severe allergies can receive clindamycin if susceptibility of the isolate has been performed. Over 40% of GBS isolates are clindamycin resistant, however, so this should not be used for prophylaxis without available susceptibility information. Vancomycin is another alternative with better resistance patterns, though in order to reach therapeutic levels high doses must be used in the antepartum period. Approximately 20% of pregnant patients require intrapartum chemoprophylaxis, based on current protocols. These strategies have dramatically decreased the incidence of early-onset GBS disease. However, because intrapartum penicillin administration does not reliably eradicate GBS from the colonized infant, its impact on late-onset disease is less significant. Some studies raised the concern that intrapartum ampicillin use led to an increase in neonatal infections with ampicillin-resistant pathogens. Antepartum testing is completed near delivery date to address the intermittent colonization of GBS in many vaginal flora. Even with this approach approximately 3% of women who test negative in the standard window will be GBS positive at time of delivery, so the absence of GBS on the antepartum screening does not rule out the possibility of early-onset GBS disease.

Herpes Simplex Virus Infection Mothers with active genital herpes at the time of delivery (including crusted lesions) or prodromal symptoms consistent with an early outbreak should undergo cesarean delivery as close as possible to the time of membrane rupture. C-section within 4 to 6 hours of rupture can reduce the risk of vertical transmission. However, three-fourths of mothers of infants with neonatal HSV infection are asymptomatic or have unrecognized infection, and neonatal infection can occur in an infant delivered by cesarean section in the presence of intact membranes. Chemoprophylaxis with acyclovir beginning at week 36 of pregnancy of women with history of HSV outbreak at any time during pregnancy has been associated with reduced viral shedding, reduced outbreaks at time of delivery and thus reduced need for cesarian delivery, but the impact of this approach on neonatal disease specifically is limited. For asymptomatic infants born to mothers with active genital HSV lesions, HSV cultures or PCR should be obtained at 24 to 48 hours of life from the conjunctiva, mouth, or nasopharynx and from the rectum or stool. Asymptomatic infants do not require any antiviral therapy while awaiting HSV culture results, although many experts suggest empirical acyclovir in those delivered vaginally.

FEVER IN OLDER INFANTS AND TODDLERS

Children between the ages of 3 and 36 months have increasing exposure to contagious illnesses and may experience multiple febrile illnesses each year. Differentiating serious illness from benign viral syndromes is the most important aspect of care of these febrile children. Although fever in older infants and toddlers (3-36 months) is still generally defined as body temperature greater than 38°C (100.4°F), fever of concern in this age group is generally defined as >39°C taken rectally without an identifiable source by history and exam. Healthy, well-appearing young children with fever but without an identifiable focal bacterial infection may have an occult infection, including occult bacteremia and UTI. UTI is discussed in detail in Chapter 100, but it is important to note that children with fever of concern have a ~7% risk of UTI, with the highest risk among girls younger than 12 months and uncircumcised male infants. Occult bacteremia is discussed in the following sections.

CLINICAL PRESENTATION

Occult bacteremia is defined as the presence of bacteria in the blood of a well-appearing child between the ages of 2 and or 36 months; fever is often the event that precipitates laboratory evaluation. By definition, these children have an intact immune system and lack an identifiable focal bacterial infection (e.g., abscess, cellulitis, pneumonia) or pathognomonic viral entity (e.g., herpes stomatitis, varicella).

Historically, occult bacteremia has overwhelmingly been due to *S. pneumoniae* and *H. influenzae* type B (HIB). Other causative organisms include *Salmonella* species, non-typeable *H. influenzae*, group A β-hemolytic streptococci, *Enterococcus* species, and *N. meningitidis*. In a 2022 multicenter study of febrile infants 2 to 6 months of age, 70% of bacteremia cases were caused by *E. coli* or GBS, and another 18% by *S. aureus* or *Salmomella* species. The overall risk of occult bacteremia among febrile infants and toddlers has been significantly reduced by administration of the HIB and heptavalent pneumococcal conjugate vaccines. Before the licensure of the HIB vaccine in 1987, the prevalence of occult bacteremia among febrile young children was between 3% and 11%. However, after widespread use of the HIB vaccine, the reported overall rate of occult bacteremia in immunized children became less than 2%. With the release of PCV7 in 2000, there was a nearly 70% decrease in the rate of invasive pneumococcal disease; in addition, the overall prevalence of occult bacteremia declined to less than 1%. In the aforementioned multicenter study of febrile infants 2 to 6 months of age, the prevalence of IBI was 0.48%, even lower (0.32%) in previously healthy, well-appearing infants without antibiotic pretreatment. The impact of vaccines has also benefitted unimmunized and underimmunized children through herd immunity. Although the risk of occult bacteremia in unimmunized and underimmunized children is thought to be elevated compared to their immunized peers, the prevalence of bacteremia is likely similarly low in these children.

The approach to diagnosis in older children with fever of concern is predominantly determined by immunization status. Occult bacteremia is a concern because of its possible progression to deep-seated focal infection, and in the pre-vaccine era approximately 5% of children with occult bacteremia developed severe invasive illness including possible meningitis. The risk of invasive disease due to occult bacteremia depends on the infecting organism. When HIB was a prominent causative organism, the risk of invasive disease with known occult HIB bacteremia was between 25% and 44%. However, occult pneumococcal bacteremia is associated with a significantly smaller risk (0.6%) of invasive disease. Because HIB is no longer a major concern in immunized populations, the risk of progression to meningitis or death is substantially reduced. Currently, the overall risk of meningitis or death in children with occult bacteremia is approximately 1.8%.

DIAGNOSIS

The diagnosis of occult bacteremia is dependent on a complete history and physical examination. Often subtle findings indicating a specific source are found on thorough examination including oral lesions or rash consistent with viral syndrome, musculoskeletal changes concerning for bone or joint infection, or tachypnea and nasal flaring concerning for possible occult pneumonia. If no identifiable source is located on exam, immunization status is often used as the primary branch point determining if additional testing is warranted.

Immunized children who are well-appearing presenting with a fever of concern generally do not require additional testing, excepting urine studies in patients as indicated by age and sex. There is very little data examining screening test characteristics in this population and because of the low overall prevalence of occult bacteremia in the post-vaccine era, these studies are limited in their positive predictive value. Studies completed prior to the introduction of the pneumococcal vaccine suggested a WBC count greater than 15,000/mm^3 as an indicator for occult bacteremia; though later data suggested an ANC cut-off of 10,000/mm^3 had improved sensitivity and specificity The positive predictive values for both of these cut-offs in the pre-vaccine era ranged from 5% to 8%, but multiple studies during the post-vaccine era the rate of occult bacteremia was lower than the rate of contaminated blood culture.

There are no clear consensus guidelines available, but some resources advocate that well-appearing, unimmunized children with fever of concern can have both a CBC with differential and a PCT drawn, along with a blood culture, though rates of occult bacteremia in this population have also fallen dramatically in the post-vaccine era. In some studies, the rates of true bacteremia in unimmunized or underimmunized children have been lower than the rates of contaminated blood cultures. Procalcitonin performs better than WBC count, ANC, band count, or CRP in identifying serious bacterial illnesses in febrile children less than 3 years of age, though the sensitivity of PCT alone is not sufficient to use PCT as the sole screening test for occult bacteremia. Given the slightly higher risk of occult bacteremia in the unimmunized population, the positive predictive value of procalcitonin may exceed the likelihood of blood culture contamination.

TREATMENT

As the incidence of occult bacteremia has decreased in the post-vaccine era, treatment approaches in the unimmunized child are also controversial. Owing to the difficulty of diagnosing occult bacteremia without waiting for test results, expectant antibiotic use in the unimmunized population has been advocated by some to decrease the risk of adverse outcomes such as meningitis or sepsis, though the efficacy of this approach was uncertain even in the pre-vaccine era. Practice variation exists, but unimmunized children with fever of concern may receive 50 mg/kg of IM ceftriaxone while their blood culture is monitored for 24 hours. If they have serious allergy to penicillin or cephalosporins and treatment is indicated, they can alternatively receive clindamycin dosing orally for 24 hours. As with the young infant, the overwhelming majority of true pathogens will have grown in this population by 24 hours.

DISCHARGE CRITERIA

When children with positive initial blood cultures warrant admission (i.e., their clinical appearance or laboratory studies are not reassuring), the repeat culture is followed closely for the first 24 hours. Several studies using continuously monitored carbon dioxide blood culture systems have documented that the great majority of pathogens from immunocompetent hosts are detected within 24 hours. Therefore well-appearing immunocompetent patients may be safely discharged home if their repeat blood cultures remain negative for at least 24 hours. Total length of treatment is determined by the presence or absence of any particular focal infection that may have developed and should be tailored to the identified infection.

PREVENTION

The HIB and conjugate pneumococcal vaccines are the most effective means of preventing occult bacteremia. The current conjugate pneumococcal vaccine is immunogenic for 13 of the 90 *S. pneumoniae* serotypes. Early data are promising with significant decreases in invasive pneumococcal disease. However, there is theoretical concern about serotype shift due to nonvaccine organisms, and close surveillance is necessary.

KEY POINTS

Fever in neonates and young infants

- Up to 15% of febrile infants younger than 90 days have a UTI or IBI.
- The 2021 AAP CPG provides evidence-based recommendations for the evaluation and management of previously healthy, well-appearing febrile infants in three age groups: 8 to 21 days, 22 to 28 days, and 29 to 60 days of age.
- For risk stratification of febrile infants 22 to 60 days of age, PCT in combination with ANC +/- CRP is recommended.
- Previously healthy, well-appearing febrile infants 29 to 60 days of age with negative inflammatory markers do not require a lumbar puncture or hospitalization, even if the UA is positive.
- Hospitalized febrile infants can be discharged at 24 to 36 hours if cultures are negative, the infant is clinically improving, and follow-up can be arranged.
- The prevalence of UTI and IBI are low in febrile infants who test positive for SARS-CoV-2.
- Intrapartum prophylaxis for GBS dramatically decreases the rate of early-onset group B streptococcal disease in neonates.

Fever in older infants and toddlers.

- Occult bacteremia is the presence of pathogenic bacteria in the blood of a well-appearing febrile child aged 2 to 36 months who lacks a focal bacterial infection.
- Occult bacteremia has the potential to progress to focal infection (including meningitis) or sepsis in 1% to 2% of cases.
- The overall prevalence of occult bacteremia in children after the introduction of the HIB and pneumoncoccal vaccination programs is less than 1%, and fully vaccinated well-appearing children with fever should not routinely undergo additional bloodwork.
- Procalcitonin is the test with the best test characteristics for identifying occult bacteremia and can be considered as a part of the diagnostic work up in unimmunized children with fever though further study is necessary.
- Expectant antibiotic treatment of patients with possible occult bacteremia has not been shown to definitively prevent subsequent focal or systemic infection and is not necessary in most cases of fever in the older age group.

SUGGESTED READINGS

Alpern ER, Alessandrini EA, Bell LM, et al. Occult bacteremia from a pediatric emergency department: current prevalence, time to detection, and outcome. *Pediatrics*. 2000;106:505-511.

Aronson PL, Louie JP, Kerns E et al. Prevalence of urinary tract infection, bacteremia, and meningitis among febrile infants aged 8 to 60 days with SARS-CoV-2. *JAMA Netw Open*. 2023;6(5):e2313354.

Aronson PL, Shabanova V, Shapiro ED, et al. A prediction model to identify febrile infants ≤60 days at low risk of invasive bacterial infection. *Pediatrics*. 2019;144(1):e20183604.

Aronson PL, Wang ME, Nigrovic LE, et al. Time to pathogen detection for non-ill versus ill-appearing infants ≤60 days old with bacteremia and meningitis. *Hosp Pediatr*. 2018;8(7):379-384

Biondi EA, Lee B, Ralston SL, Winikor JM, Lynn JF, Dixon A, McCulloh R. Prevalence of bacteremia and bacterial meningitis in febrile neonates and infants in the second month of life: a systematic review and meta-analysis. *JAMA Netw Open*. 2019;2(3):e190874.

Brower LH, Wilson PM, Murtagh Kurowski E, et al. Using quality improvement to implement a standardized approach to neonatal herpes simplex virus. *Pediatrics*. 2019;144:e20180262.

Bulloch B, Craig WR, Klassen TP. The use of antibiotics to prevent serious sequelae in children at risk for occult bacteremia: a meta-analysis. *Acad Emerg Med*. 1997;4:679-683.

Burstein B, Alathari N, Papenburg J. Guideline-based risk stratification for febrile young infants without procalcitonin measurement. *Pediatrics*. 2022;149(6):e2021056028

Burstein B, Sabhaney B, Bone JN, Doan Q, Mansouri FF, Meckler GD. Prevalence of bacterial meningitis among febrile infants aged 29-60 days with positive urinalysis results: a systematic review and meta-analysis. *JAMA Netw Open*. 4(5):e214544.

Carstairs KL, Tanen DA, Johnson AS, Kailes SB, Riffenburgh RH. Pneumococcal bacteremia in febrile infants presenting to the emergency department before and after the introduction of the heptavalent pneumococcal vaccine. *Ann Emerg Med*. 2007;49(6):772-777.

Corey L, Wald A. Maternal and neonatal herpes simplex virus infections. *N Engl J Med*. 2009;361:1376-1385.

Dunnick J, Taft M, Tisherman RT, Nowalk AJ, Hickey RW, Wilson PM. Association of bacteremia with vaccination status in children aged 2 to 36 months. *J Pediatr*. 2021;232:207-213.e2.

Green RS, Sartori LF, Lee BE, et al. Prevalence and management of invasive bacterial infections in febrile infants ages 2 to 6 months. *Ann Emerg Med*. 2022;80(6):499-506.

Hsiao AL, Chen L, Baker MD. Incidence and predictors of serious bacterial infections among 57- to 180-day-old infants. *Pediatrics*. 2006;117(5):1695-1701.

Kuppermann N, Dayan PS, Levine DA, et al. A clinical prediction rule to identify febrile infants 60 days and younger at low risk for serious bacterial infections. *JAMA Pediatr*. 2019;173(4):342-351.

Kyaw MH, Lynfield R, Schaffner W, et al. Active bacterial core surveillance of the Emerging Infections Program Network. Effect of introduction of the pneumococcal conjugate vaccine on drug-resistant Streptococcus pneumoniae. *N Engl J Med*. 2006;354(14):1455-1463.

Lee GM, Harper MB. Risk of bacteremia for febrile young children in the post-*Haemophilus influenzae* type B era. *Arch Pediatr Adolesc Med*. 1998;152:624-628.

Levine DA, Platt SL, Dayan PS, et al. Risk of serious bacterial infection in young febrile infants with respiratory syncytial virus infections. *Pediatrics*. 2004;113:1728-1734.

Mahajan P, Gryzbowski M. Procalcitonin as a marker of serious bacterial infectiojns in febrile children younger than 3 years old. *Acad Emerg Med*. 2014;21(2):171-179.

Mahajan P, VanBuren JM, Tzimenatos L, et al. Serious bacterial infectons in young febrile infants with positive urinalysis results. *Pediatrics*. 2022;150(4):e2021055633.

Pantell RH, Roberts KB, Adams WG, et al. Evaluation and management of well-appearing febrile infants 8 to 60 days old. *Pediatrics*. 2021;148(2):e2021052228.

Powell EC, Mahajan PV, Roosevelt G, et al. Epidemiology of bacteremia in febrile infants aged 60 days and younger. *Ann Emerg Med*. 2018;71(2):211-216.

Tzimenatos L, Mahajan P, Dayan PS, et al. Accuracy of the urinalysis for urinary tract infections in febrile infants 60 days and younger. *Pediatrics*. 2018;141(2):e20173068.

Woll C, Neuman MI, Pruitt CM, et al. Epidemiology and etiology of invasive bacterial infection in infants ≤60 day old treated in emergency departments. *J Pediatr*. 2018;200:210-217.e1.

CHAPTER 92

Fever of Unknown Origin

Danni Liang, MD and Nivedita Srinivas, MD

BACKGROUND

Fever is a common presentation of illness in children. Most causes are infectious, self-limited, and can be identified after obtaining a detailed history and physical exam. If fevers persist without distinguishing signs and symptoms, additional diagnostic approaches are often employed to delineate the etiology and appropriate management. The diagnosis of fever of unknown origin (FUO) is used to characterize this subset of children who present with prolonged fever duration requiring more extensive evaluation which may include hospitalization.

In 1961, Petersdorf and Beeson proposed their classic criteria for FUO in adults: (i) an illness of at least 3 weeks' duration, (ii) measured temperatures greater than 38.3°C on several occasions, and (iii) no etiologic diagnosis after 1 week of hospitalization, but FUO as an entity was not addressed in children until the 1970s. Since then, studies focusing on pediatric patients have used fever durations ranging from 1 to 3 weeks and temperatures ranging from 38.0°C to 38.3°C. A child with FUO remains a challenge for both the family and medical team, with many of these patients being admitted to the hospital for workup. Final diagnoses are determined in a number of ways (e.g., natural history, biopsy, imaging, serologic studies) and no single patient either receives or requires every diagnostic test. Therefore, FUO offers an opportunity to practice high-value care through stewardship in diagnostic testing and treatment.

CLINICAL PRESENTATION

In more recent pediatric literature, the accepted definition for FUO includes: (i) fever ≥ 8 days, (ii) temperature higher than 38.0°C (100.4°F), and (iii) no clear source. This is in contrast to fever without a source (FWS), defined as the occurrence of fever < 8 days without a clear etiology. Up to 50% of patients referred for evaluation of FUO have multiple unrelated and self-limited infections, parental misinterpretation of normal temperature variation, or complete absence of fever at the time of referral. Therefore, the initial history should include the method used to determine temperature (e.g., "felt warm" vs. actual measurement), the duration of thermometer insertion, location of insertion (tympanic membrane, oral, axillary, rectal), time of day, and confirmation by more than one person. Studies examining parents' ability to subjectively determine the presence of fever found a sensitivity of 74% to 84% and a specificity of 76% to 91% for tactile examination. Some studies of tactile examination reveal more accurate results for higher temperatures (>38.9°C) than for lower ones. The location of measurement also affects the accuracy of the reading. The oral temperature can be 0.3°C to 0.7°C lower than a simultaneous rectal measurement. Oral measurements are more easily influenced by other factors such as oral liquid intake and respiratory rate. Axillary and tympanic measurements are at least 0.5°C lower than simultaneous oral measurements. To compensate for such discrepancies, parents are sometimes instructed to add 0.5°C or 1°C to oral or axillary measurements to approximate the "real" temperature. Such corrections are often inaccurate, however, because the amount of underestimation varies from person to person and with the body temperature (differences are exacerbated at higher body temperatures); these corrections may further cloud the evaluation of a febrile child. The timing of measurement is also important because children's body temperature exhibits a daily variation; the normal temperature may be as high as 37.4°C (99.3°F) orally or 38.0°C (100.4°F) rectally in children older than 2 months and peaks in the early evening.

TABLE 92-1 Diagnoses in Pediatric Case Series of Prolonged Fever or Fever of Unknown Origin Including at Least 50 Patients[a]

	McClung (1972)	Pizzo et al (1975)	Lohr & Hendley (1977)	Steele et al (1991)	Jacobs & Schutze (1998)	Antoon (2018)	Szymanski (2020)	Total
No. of patients	99	100	54	109	146	102	110	819
No established diagnosis	32 (32)	12 (12)	10 (19)	73 (67)	62 (42)	6 (6)	42 (38)	257 (31)
Infection	29 (29)	52 (52)	18 (33)	24 (22)	64 (44)	42 (41)	41 (37)	366 (45)
Rheumatologic/ Auto-inflammatory	11 (11)	20 (20)	11 (20)	7 (6)	11 (8)	28 (27)	16 (15)	79 (10)
Malignancy	8 (8)	6 (6)	7 (13)	2 (2)	4 (3)	18 (17)	5 (5)	32 (4)
Other[b]	19 (19)	10 (10)	8 (15)	3 (3)	5 (3)	4 (4)	6 (5)	85 (10)

[a]Values listed are numbers of cases, with percentages in parentheses. Percentage values may not total 100 due to rounding.

[b]Includes drug fever, central nervous system fever, heavy metal poisoning, factitious fever, inflammatory bowel disease, hemophagocytic lymphohistiocytosis, macrophage activating syndrome, Kikuchi-Fujimoto disease, serum sickness, and other conditions.

DIFFERENTIAL DIAGNOSIS

New and more sensitive laboratory assays (e.g., multiplex polymerase chain reaction [PCR] panels to detect viruses and bacteria commonly implicated in childhood infections) and radiologic scanning procedures (e.g., magnetic resonance imaging) permit the earlier detection of many conditions. As a result, the differential diagnosis of FUO has evolved. In the 1970s only 10% to 25% of children presenting with FUO had fever resolution without determination of a cause. In more recent studies, the fever resolved in up to one-quarter of children without a specific discharge diagnosis. Infection remains the most common cause of FUO; rheumatologic diseases and malignancy are much less common (**Table 92-1**). A comprehensive list of causes is provided (**Table 92-2**). In most cases of FUO, the cause of the fever is a common pediatric infection with an uncommonly long-time course. In a series by Jacobs and Schutze, Epstein-Barr viral

TABLE 92-2 Causes of Fever of Unknown Origin in Previously Healthy Children

Infection	Hemophagocytic lymphohistiocytosis
Common infections	Macrophage activating syndrome
Respiratory infection	Hypothyroidism
Otitis media, mastoiditis	Serum sickness/serum sickness-like reaction
Sinusitis	*Less common and uncommon infections*
Cervical adenitis	Tuberculosis
Peritonsillar or retropharyngeal abscess	Infectious mononucleosis (Epstein-Barr virus, cytomegalovirus)
Pneumonia	Tick-borne diseases (e.g., Lyme disease, Rocky Mountain spotted fever, ehrlichiosis)
Systemic viral syndrome	Malaria
Urinary tract infection	Hepatitis
Central nervous system infection	Periodontal infection
Meningitis, meningoencephalitis	Endocarditis or endovascular infection
Intracranial abscess	Human immunodeficiency virus (HIV) infection
Bone or joint infection	Acute rheumatic fever
Osteomyelitis	Other zoonoses (brucellosis, leptospirosis, Q fever, tularemia)
Septic arthritis	Intra-abdominal abscess
Paravertebral abscess	Toxoplasmosis
Enteric infection (e.g., *Salmonella, Shigella*)	Syphilis
Cat-scratch disease	Parvovirus B19 infection
Rheumatologic/Auto-inflammatory	Rubella
Juvenile rheumatoid arthritis	Endemic mycoses (e.g., histoplasmosis, blastomycosis, coccidioidomycosis)
Systemic lupus erythematosus Dermatomyositis	Psittacosis
Scleroderma	Chronic meningococcemia
Sarcoidosis	**Drug Fever**[a]
Vasculitis (Granulomatosis with polyangiitis, polyarteritis nodosa, Behçet syndrome)	Penicillins
Malignancy[a]	Cephalosporins
Leukemia	Sulfonamides
Lymphoma	Phenytoin
Other Considerations	Methylphenidate
Central fever	Acetaminophen
Kikuchi-Fujimoto (histiocytic necrotizing lymphadenitis)	**Factitious Fever**
Kawasaki disease	Pseudofever
Inflammatory bowel disease	Factitious disorder by self or proxy

[a]Only common causes listed.

TABLE 92-3 Causes of Recurrent Fever

Regular Intervals
Cyclic neutropenia
Epstein-Barr virus infection[a]
Familial Mediterranean fever
Hyperimmunoglobulin D syndrome
Periodic fever with aphthous stomatitis, pharyngitis, and adenitis (PFAPA) syndrome
Relapsing fever (*Borrelia* species other than *burgdorferi*)[a]
Less Predictable Intervals
Behçet disease
Brucellosis
Central nervous system abnormalities (e.g., hypothalamic dysfunction)
Chronic meningococcemia
Familial dysautonomia (Riley-Day syndrome)
Inflammatory bowel disease
Lymphoma
Muckle-Wells syndrome
Nontuberculous mycobacteria
Parvovirus B19
Relapsing malaria (*Plasmodium vivax, Plasmodium ovale*)
Serial viral infections
Systemic-onset juvenile idiopathic arthritis
Tuberculosis
Tumor necrosis factor receptor-associated periodic fever syndrome (TRAPS)
Yersinia enterocolitica

[a]May also occur at less predictable intervals.

TABLE 92-4 Exposure History[a]

Animal	Travel
Pets (home, contacts, school) Occupational exposure to animals from household contacts Consumption of unpasteurized dairy, raw/uncooked meats Recreational activities (i.e., hunting) Insect or flea bites	Domestic travel or residence in certain areas of the US (endemic mycoses) Foreign travel Pre-travel immunizations Anti-malarial prophylaxis Measures taken to avoid contaminated food/water (*Salmonella typhi, Shigella* species, and others)
Medication Use	**Other considerations**
Antibiotics (β–lactams, sulfa- containing) Pain medications (acetaminophen, ibuprofen, aspirin) Antireflux agents (metoclopramide, cimetidine) Anticonvulsants Corticosteroids Methylphenidate	Antecedent illness Pica Family history including ethnicity: History of hemoglobinopathy, immune deficiency, autoimmune disease History of periodic fever syndromes

[a]Only common exposures listed.

infections (15%), osteomyelitis (10%), cat-scratch disease (5%), and urinary tract infection (4%) were the most frequent causes of FUO. Some infections caused by typical pathogens may be partially treated, blunting other manifestations of the disease. The causes of recurrent fevers differ from those of prolonged fever and FUO (**Table 92-3**). Recurrent fevers are not discussed in detail in this chapter.

A systematic review included 18 studies of FUO, 8 from developed countries and 10 from developing countries. The definitions of FUO varied widely, though most studies required at least 2 weeks of fever. The number of patients ranged from 10 to 221, with 1638 children included altogether. Infections accounted for 51% of all cases, with 9% of children having collagen vascular disease and 6% having malignancy. The most common infectious causes of FUO in developed countries were Epstein-Barr virus, osteomyelitis, and urinary tract infection/pyelonephritis. In developing countries, common infectious causes included brucellosis, tuberculosis, typhoid fever, malaria, leishmaniasis, toxoplasmosis, and parasitic infections, highlighting the importance of local epidemiologic considerations.

EVALUATION AND DIAGNOSIS

EVALUATION

A thorough history and physical examination are paramount in safely managing a child with FUO. In studies by Pizzo et al, McClung, and Lohr and Hendley, a careful history and physical examination yielded the ultimate diagnosis in more than two-thirds of patients, usually after repeated encounters. The pattern and duration of fever, response to antipyretic therapy, and presence of nonspecific complaints (e.g., anorexia, fatigue, weight loss) did not accurately predict the patient's diagnosis.

A number of specific questions in the history can contribute to making the diagnosis. The physician should attempt to clarify exposure to animals, travel history, medication use, family history, antecedent illnesses, and pica (**Table 92-4**). Animal exposure includes not only pets within the home but also contact with animals owned by others, animals encountered at school, or occupational exposures to farm animals or rodents from household contacts. The animal exposure history should also include questions regarding the consumption of unpasteurized dairy products and raw or undercooked meats, as well as participation in recreational activities such as hunting. Travel-related questions should elicit details about domestic and foreign travel or residence, appropriate pretravel immunizations and prophylaxis, and measures taken to avoid contaminated food and water. A family history of hemoglobinopathy, immune deficiency, and autoimmune disease can guide the evaluation. The patient's ethnicity may also suggest a cause, since some diseases are more prevalent among certain ethnic groups—for example, familial Mediterranean fever (Armenians, Arabs, Turkish, Sephardic Jews), hyperimmunoglobulin D syndrome (Dutch, French), and tumor necrosis factor receptor–associated periodic fever syndrome (Irish, Scottish).

Medications may also cause fever. Drug fever, defined as a febrile response to a drug in the absence of cutaneous manifestations, may be difficult to recognize because the presentation is often subtle. Drug fevers may occur any time after the initiation of therapy, but they frequently appear after 1 to 2 weeks of therapy. The patient usually appears remarkably well despite the presence of fever; however, rigors and other symptoms of systemic toxicity do not preclude a medication-related fever. Drug fever should be considered in a person receiving a potentially sensitizing medication with an otherwise unexplained fever. Medications implicated in drug fevers are extensive and include ß-lactam antibiotics, pain medications (acetaminophen, ibuprofen, aspirin), anti-reflux agents (metoclopramide, cimetidine), corticosteroids, methylphenidate, anticonvulsants, and sulfa-containing medications. Discontinuation of the offending agent results in resolution of the fever within 72 hours. Failure to recognize drug fever can lead to prolonged hospitalization, unnecessary diagnostic testing, and continuation or repeat administration of the sensitizing medication.

DIAGNOSIS

The approach to a child with FUO involves (i) documenting the fever, (ii) completing a thorough history and physical examination, (iii) creating a broad differential diagnosis, (iv) performing the initial laboratory evaluation (accounting for relevant findings on the history and physical examination) and tailoring it to the severity of the patient's illness, and (v) basing the subsequent evaluation on results of the initial laboratory studies and a repeated history and physical examination. Early in the diagnostic process, the child's caretaker should be urged to keep a fever diary or calendar documenting the temperature, time, and location of measurement, as well as timing of any antipyretics. Such documentation can clarify the presence or absence of a true fever, as well as determine whether the fever is prolonged or recurrent; this latter distinction has implications for the differential diagnosis (Table 92-3). Pizzo et al emphasized the importance of carefully reviewing laboratory data. Failure to correctly use existing data occurred in 50% of their cases and was the most important reason for failure to make the diagnosis before hospitalization.

A "shotgun" approach to the evaluation of FUO is seldom useful. Such an approach often creates misleading false positive results and additional unnecessary testing. The diagnostic benefit of each test should be considered carefully along with financial cost and physical/emotional distress to the patient. Steele et al evaluated the benefit of radiologic scanning procedures in children with FUO. Children with fever higher than 38.0°C, a fever duration of longer than 3 weeks, and a normal initial physical examination were included in the study. A specific diagnosis was determined in 36 of 109 children (33%). Abnormal results were detected in 8 of 43 (19%) abdominal ultrasound procedures, 5 of 11 (45%) indium scans, 1 of 4 (25%) gallium scans, 2 of 13 (15%) upper gastrointestinal barium studies with small bowel follow-through, 2 of 15 (13%) bone scans, and 1 of 16 (6%) bone marrow examinations. However, the abnormalities identified by these studies suggested a specific diagnosis in only seven children; in many of the other cases, the significance of the abnormalities evident on imaging was not known.

Routine echocardiography is also a low-yield procedure in the evaluation of a child with FUO. In one study examining the role of echocardiography in the diagnosis of endocarditis, persistent fever was the most common reason for performing an echocardiogram. Endocarditis was associated with at least two positive blood culture results, congestive heart failure, a new or changing heart murmur, and hematuria; no patient had fever as the sole manifestation of endocarditis. The Duke criteria may facilitate the evaluation for endocarditis (see Chapter 52, Infective Endocarditis).

Other tests listed in **Table 92-5** are performed even less often. Uveitis, detected by ophthalmic examination, suggests Behçet disease, Kawasaki syndrome, tuberculosis, syphilis, sarcoidosis, inflammatory bowel disease, or juvenile rheumatoid arthritis (polyarticular or pauciarticular, but not systemic). Bone marrow biopsy can detect some malignancies and some infections. Certain organisms that cause FUO readily grow in culture of bone marrow specimens (*Salmonella* species, mycobacteria, *Brucella*, and *Histoplasma capsulatum*) though bone marrow culture is rarely performed because the advent of sensitive and specific diagnostic test facilitates identification of these pathogens. Lumbar puncture occasionally sheds light on the cause of FUO in patients with chronic headache or other signs of central nervous system infection. Organisms and the appropriate tests to detect them include the following:

- Enterovirus: serum, urine, and cerebrospinal fluid (CSF) PCR
- Herpes simplex virus: blood and CSF PCR
- *Cryptococcus neoformans*: serum and CSF cryptococcal antigen and CSF culture
- *Mycobacterium tuberculosis*: CSF acid-fast smear and culture
- West Nile virus: serum antibodies and CSF PCR
- *Borrelia burgdorferi*: serum and CSF antibodies
- *Mycoplasma pneumoniae*: nasopharyngeal, throat, and CSF PCR

The increasing availability of rapid molecular testing and advanced imaging modalities has helped identify etiologies of FUO that previously went undiagnosed. Diagnostic stewardship and approaches which are patient- and family-centered should remain at the forefront as new technologies continue to emerge.

TABLE 92-5 Studies to Consider in the Initial and Subsequent Diagnostic Evaluations[a] of Children With Fever of Unknown Origin

Specimen	Initial Investigation	Subsequent Investigation
Blood	Blood culture Complete blood count Peripheral blood smear C-reactive protein Erythrocyte sedimentation rate Hepatic function panel Human immunodeficiency virus (HIV) antibodies Initial infectious disease serologic studies[c] Interferon-Gamma Release Assay (IGRA)[d]	Repeat blood culture (x3) Second-line infectious disease serologic studies[b] LDH Uric acid Ferritin Antinuclear antibody
Urine	Urinalysis Urine culture	Repeat urinalysis Repeat urine culture PCR for adenovirus or enterovirus
Stool	Hemoccult testing Culture (bacterial and viral) Ova and parasite examination (x3)[e]	*Clostridium difficile* toxins A and B
Radiologic	Chest radiograph	Sinus CT Upper GI barium study with small bowel follow-through Abdominal CT or ultrasonography MRI of pelvis, spine, or specific extremities Bone or gallium scan Echocardiogram
Other	Tuberculin skin test Nasal aspirate PCR for virus detection[f] Throat swab for rapid streptococcal antigen testing and culture	Ophthalmic examination Lumbar puncture Bone marrow biopsy Evaluation for primary immune deficiency

[a]Findings on the history, physical examination, and initial laboratory evaluation should direct the subsequent evaluation. A patient usually does not require all the tests listed.

[b]If relevant exposures can be documented, consider serologic testing for hepatitis A, B, and C; tularemia; brucellosis; leptospirosis; Rocky Mountain spotted fever; ehrlichiosis; Q fever; dengue fever; or leptospirosis.

[c]Potential serologic studies include Epstein-Barr virus, cytomegalovirus, *Bartonella henselae* (cat-scratch disease), *Borrelia burgdorferi* (Lyme disease), antistreptolysin-O and anti-DNase B (group A ß-hemolytic streptococci).

[d]IGRA may be considered as an alternative to tuberculin skin testing in children ≥2 years of age, though tuberculin skin testing is preferred in children under 2 years.

[e]Antigen testing is available for some organisms, including *Giardia lamblia*, *Cryptosporidium parvum*, and *Entamoeba histolytica*.

[f]Polymerase chain reaction tests widely available for respiratory syncytial virus, influenza viruses A and B, parainfluenza viruses types 1 to 3, human metapneumovirus, rhinovirus, human coronaviruses, and adenovirus. Polymerase chain reaction–based assays also provide a highly sensitive method of detecting adenovirus from nasopharyngeal aspirates, sputum, and conjunctival swabs. Rapid antigen detection by immunofluorescence is less sensitive but available for respiratory syncytial virus, influenza viruses A and B, parainfluenza viruses types 1 to 3, and adenovirus.

CT, computed tomography; GI, gastrointestinal; MRI, magnetic resonance imaging.

TREATMENT

Treatment depends on the diagnosis and the utility of empirical therapy, such as antibiotics, antituberculosis agents, or corticosteroids, has not been studied in FUO. Empirical therapy can obscure the diagnosis and exacerbate the underlying etiology and should therefore be avoided in children who otherwise appear well.

ADMISSION AND DISCHARGE CRITERIA

ADMISSION CRITERIA

Ill-appearing children require hospitalization. There are no firm criteria for the hospitalization of well-appearing patients with FUO. Generally, all the initial investigations (see Table 92-4) can be performed in the outpatient setting. Hospitalization should be considered for children requiring extensive subspecialist consultation or invasive procedures (e.g., lumbar puncture) to allow for better coordination of care.

DISCHARGE CRITERIA

The diagnosis determines the appropriate time for discharge. For patients in whom a diagnosis cannot be ascertained, outpatient follow-up is appropriate. Talano and Katz described the long-term outcome in children with FUO in whom no diagnosis was established after inpatient evaluation. Among the 19 patients studied, 16 had resolution of fever without recurrence, 2 were diagnosed with juvenile rheumatoid arthritis, and 1 patient had recurrent intussusception. Follow-up information was available for 63 of 73 patients studied by Steele et al for whom no diagnosis could be established. Most of these children recovered uneventfully; nine of them had continuation or recurrence of fever for brief periods, with ultimate resolution and no specific diagnosis. Nine additional patients were initially diagnosed with juvenile rheumatoid arthritis; on follow-up, five had resolution of fever without further recurrence and four had infections: Lyme disease, psittacosis, toxoplasmosis, and cat-scratch disease.

CONSULTATION

Subspecialty consultation can assist with diagnostic evaluation or, once the diagnosis has been made, treatment. Relevant subspecialties to consider include infectious diseases, rheumatology, and oncology. Other subspecialties may warrant consultation based on the results of historical features, physical examination findings or laboratory results.

KEY POINTS

- The definition for pediatric FUO is a fever ≥8 days with temperature higher than 38.0°C (100.4°F) without a clear source.
- The evaluation of FUO should include confirmation of fever, a thorough history and physical examination, and a tiered diagnostic approach guided by the patient's signs and symptoms.
- Advances in diagnostic testing reflect a changing landscape in FUO. Many FUO cases resolve without determination of a specific cause, and infections continue to be the most common identifiable cause of FUO.

SUGGESTED READINGS

Antoon JW, Potisek NM, Lohr JA. Pediatric Fever of Unknown Origin. *Pediatr Rev.* 2015;36(9):380-391.

Antoon JW, Peritz DC, Parsons MR, Skinner AC, Lohr JA. Etiology and resource use of fever of unknown origin in hospitalized children. *Hosp Pediatr.* 2018;8(3):135-140.

Calello DP, Shah SS. The child with fever of unknown origin. *Pediatr Case Rev.* 2002;2:226-239.

Chow A, Robinson JL. Fever of unknown origin in children: a systematic review. *World J Pediatr.* 2011;7:5-10.

Jacobs RF, Schutze GE. *Bartonella henselae* as a cause of prolonged fever and fever of unknown origin in children. *Clin Infect Dis.* 1998;26:80-84.

Lohr JA, Hendley JO. Prolonged fever of unknown origin: a record of experiences with 54 childhood patients. *Clin Pediatr.* 1977;16:768-773.

McClung HJ. Prolonged fever of unknown origin in children. *Am J Dis Child.* 1972;124:544-550.

Palazzi DL. Fever without source and fever of unknown origin. *Feigin and Cherry's Textbook of Pediatric Infectious Diseases.* 8:11.

Petersdorf RG, Beeson PB. Fever of unexplained origin: report on 100 cases. *Medicine.* 1961;40:1-30.

Pizzo PA, Lovejoy Jr FH, Smith DH. Prolonged fever in children: review of 100 cases. *Pediatrics.* 1975;55:468-473.

Shah SS, Ludwig S. *Pediatric Complaints and Diagnostic Dilemmas: A Case-Based Approach.* Philadelphia, PA: Lippincott Williams & Wilkins; 2004.

Statler VA, Marshall GS. Evaluation of prolonged and recurrent unexplained fevers. *Pediatr Ann.* 2018;47(9):e347-e353.

Steele RW, Jones SM, Lowe BA, Glasier CM. Usefulness of scanning procedures for diagnosis of fever of unknown origin in children. *J Pediatr.* 1991;119:526-530.

Szymanski AM, Clifford H, Ronis T. Fever of unknown origin: a retrospective review of pediatric patients from an urban, tertiary care center in Washington, DC. *World J Pediatr.* 2020;16(2):177-184.

Talano JA, Katz BZ. Long-term follow-up of children with fever of unknown origin. *Clin Pediatr.* 2000;39:715-717.

CHAPTER 93

Fever and Rash

Jodi Ehrmann, MD and Carolyn E. Beck, MD, MSc

INTRODUCTION

Fever, a common presenting complaint in the acute care setting, may be associated with rash. The disorders that present with fever and rash range from benign and self-limited to rapidly progressive and life-threatening. The entire clinical picture must be considered in a child presenting with fever and rash to facilitate timely diagnosis and treatment.

Fever and rash can be categorized into the most common etiologies which include infectious, inflammatory/autoimmune, or oncologic/immunosuppressive. The following chapter will be discussing only infectious etiologies. Additional etiologies will be discussed in other chapters.

The character of the rash combined with other signs and symptoms often suggests a specific cause of the illness. Based on this characterization, common clinical syndromes with the hallmark of fever and rash are as follows: (i) Viral exanthems; (ii) Meningococcal diseases; (iii) Group A Streptococcal diseases; and (iv) Rickettsial diseases.

VIRAL EXANTHEMS

The term exanthem refers to a rash that is abrupt and can affect several areas of the skin simultaneously. Viral exanthems in childhood are frequent and the appearance can range from macular, maculopapular, papular, urticarial, morbilliform, or vesicular. They are commonly associated with a prodrome of fever, malaise, rhinorrhea, and/or cough. The majority of viral exanthems are self-limited and with no identifiable specific virus, thus these rashes are often referred to as nonspecific viral exanthems. Nevertheless, a thorough history is important as viral exanthems can mimic other etiologies including drug eruptions (Chapter 61) and Kawasaki's Disease (Chapter 148). In other cases, a thorough history and exam can help point to a specific infectious etiology.

Measles and rubella are classic infections (**Table 93-1**) representing a morbilliform rash that presents 3 to 5 days after an influenza-like prodrome. The rash appears as a generalized erythematous to pink maculopapular rash that blanches with pressure. While widespread vaccination makes these diagnoses less likely, recent clusters of cases, particularly in unimmunized communities, should prompt consideration of these infections. Among immunized pediatric patients with fever and morbilliform rash, studies show viruses other than measles or rubella to be the cause, specifically parvovirus, human herpesvirus 6, enteroviruses, and group A *Streptococcus*. The most common of these is Parvovirus, also known as fifth disease and erythema infectiosum. Parvovirus typically begins with a 7 to 10 days prodrome of low-grade temperatures, myalgias, and headache followed by a facial rash. The rash is often described as a "slapped cheek" appearance with circumoral sparing. The rash can progress over 1 to 4 days to include the trunk and extremities which may last for 1 to 3 weeks. In pregnant women, parvovirus can cross the placenta and lead to severe fetal infection. Parvovirus is generally not contagious after the onset of rash.

TABLE 93-1 Key Features of Classic Childhood Exanthems

Disease	Cause	Rash	Clinical Findings	Complications
Measles (Rubeola)	Measles virus	Morbilliform rash, spreads from head to feet	Koplik spots, fever, cough, coryza, conjunctivitis	Bronchopneumonia, encephalitis, otitis media, myocarditis, encephalomyelitis, subacute sclerosing panencephalitis
Rubella (German measles)	Rubella virus	Discrete papular rash, spreads from head to feet	Exanthema, rhinorrhea, tender adenopathy (postauricular, posterior cervical, postoccipital), low-grade fever	Congenital rubella syndrome, arthritis, neuritis, encephalitis
Chickenpox	Varicella virus	Generalized, vesicular rash; "dewdrops on a rose petal"	Fever, malaise, myalgias, pruritus	Bacterial skin infection, pneumonia, hepatitis, encephalitis, cerebellar ataxia, other postinfectious neurologic syndromes
Erythema infectiosum (Fifth disease)	Parvovirus B19	Erythematous, lacy, reticular rash on trunk and extremities; "slapped cheek" appearance	Mild symptoms: headache, coryza, myalgia, arthralgia	Aplastic crisis in patients with chronic hemolysis, chronic anemia in those with immunodeficiency, arthritis
Exanthema subitum (Roseola)	Human herpesvirus 6	Centrally located, pink macular rash; onset as fever dissipates	Often asymptomatic; fever, mild rhinorrhea occasionally	Febrile seizures
Scarlet fever	*Streptococcus pyogenes* (group A *Streptococcus*)	Tiny, papular "sandpaper" rash; predilection for skin folds	Exudative pharyngitis, fever, "strawberry" tongue, late desquamation	Postinfectious sequelae (rheumatic fever, glomerulonephritis)

Certain viruses present with a characteristic vesicular or bullous rash and fever. A generalized pattern of vesicles on an erythematous base ("dewdrops on a rose petal") in various stages of eruption is characteristic of chicken pox, caused by the varicella-zoster virus. A dermatomal distribution of a painful rash suggests shingles, caused by the reactivation of varicella-zoster. This is possible in patients with a past history of varicella infection or vaccination. Vesicular lesions distributed on the palms and soles associated with mouth ulcers, most commonly in the posterior oropharynx, suggest hand-foot-and-mouth disease secondary to enterovirus infection, most commonly caused by coxsackievirus A16. Herpes simplex virus (HSV) causes localized vesicular lesions such as gingivostomatitis, herpes labialis and other genital infections, herpetic whitlow, and keratoconjunctivitis, typically with periocular skin involvement. A vesicular eruption in the neonatal period, with or without fever, raises suspicion for neonatal HSV infection. Bullae associated with erythema multiforme and mucosal involvement are characteristic of Stevens-Johnson syndrome (**Figure 93-1**), which will be further discussed in Chapter 65. Staphylococcal scalded skin syndrome results in bullae with significant skin peeling, which can look similar to toxic epidermal necrolysis, further discussed in Chapter 65.

Other types of rashes associated with fever should raise your concern for bacterial etiology. Petechiae are small red or purple lesions that do not blanch with pressure. Purpura are larger, non-blanching, purple or brown lesions; these may be raised, or palpable. Fever associated with petechiae or purpura may herald life-threatening conditions (e.g., rickettsiae, *Neisseria meningitidis*).

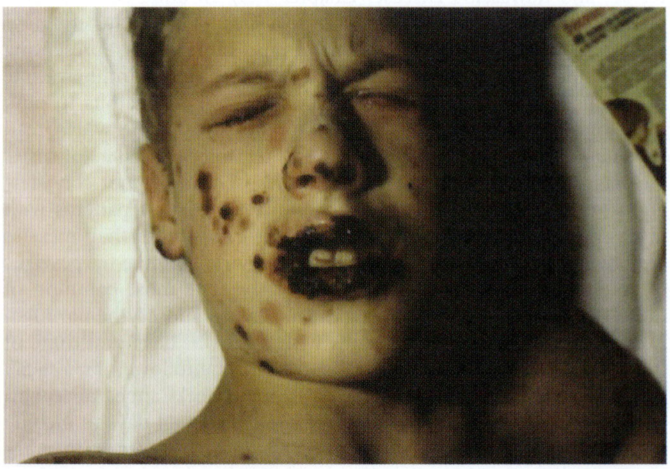

FIGURE 93-1. Stevens-Johnson syndrome with hemorrhagic crusting of the oral mucosa.

MENINGOCOCCAL INFECTIONS

Meningococcal infections are caused by the gram-negative diplococcus *N. meningitidis*. The peak incidence of these infections is during the first year of life after passive maternal antibody protection begins to wane; 40% of cases occur in children younger than 5 years. A smaller peak occurs during adolescence and young adulthood, with military recruits and first-year college students living in crowded dormitories at higher risk. Asplenia, complement deficiencies, immunoglobulin deficiencies, and infection with the human immunodeficiency virus (HIV) are risk factors for the development of severe meningococcal infections.

N. meningitidis is classified into serotypes based on the immunologic response to polysaccharides in the capsule. Further subclassification is based on outer membrane proteins and genetic sequencing of the bacteria. Historically, serotypes B and C accounted for the majority of meningococcal infections in the United States and the rest of the industrialized world. However, since vaccination for serotypes ACWY

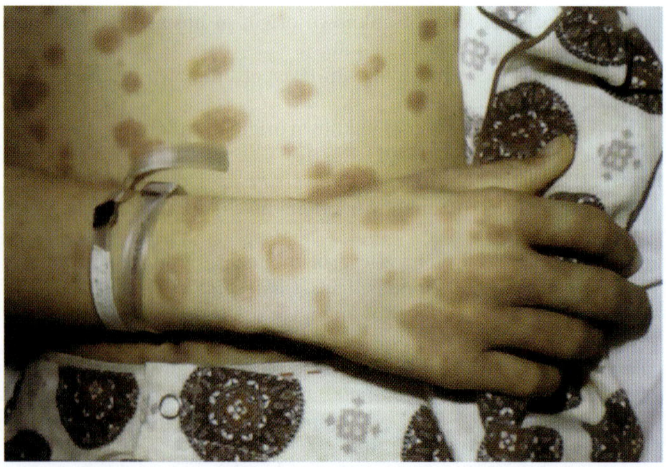

FIGURE 93-2. Erythema multiforme rash in an 8-year-old boy demonstrating discrete target lesions on the trunk and extremity, with confluence distally. Central bullae are seen in the lesion of the dorsal wrist. This patient also has substantial post-inflammatory hyperpigmentation.

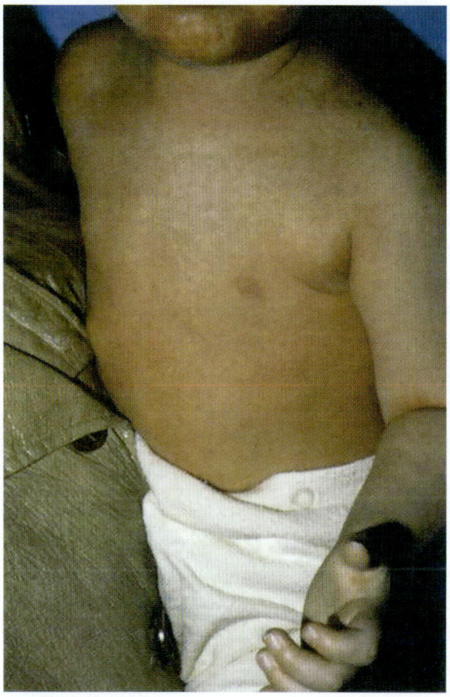

FIGURE 93-3. Scarlatina in an 18-month-old child with group A streptococcal infection.

became routine in the United States, serotype B is now the predominant cause of outbreaks. Serotype A is responsible for meningococcal epidemics, particularly in sub-Saharan Africa, the so-called meningitis belt.

Humans are the only reservoir for *N. meningitidis,* and the bacteria reside in the nasopharynx. In non-endemic areas, 5% to 10% of individuals are asymptomatic carriers. Transmission is from person to person through respiratory droplets or direct contact with secretions through activities such as kissing or sharing of drinking glasses. Disease develops when a pathogenic strain of *N. meningitidis* translocates across the mucosal barrier, with subsequent bacteremia. Exposure to cigarette smoke and concurrent upper respiratory infection are risk factors for this process.

PATHOPHYSIOLOGY

Once the bacteria enter the bloodstream, the release of lipopolysaccharides and other bacterial factors results in the release of cytokines and tumor necrosis factor, activation of the complement system, and

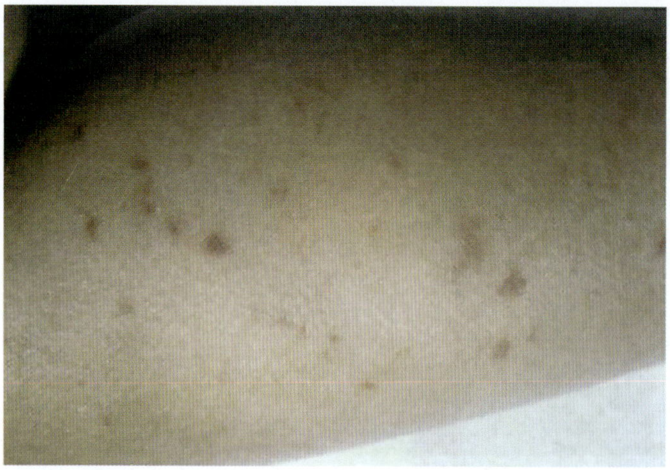

FIGURE 93-5. Maculopapular rash early in the course of meningococcemia.

subsequent development of the systemic inflammatory response. This response, in conjunction with a bacteria-induced procoagulant state, results in the clinical features seen in meningococcemia. In systemic disease, petechiae and purpura can develop as a result of vasculitis and thrombosis in the blood vessels of the skin. Meningococcal meningitis is secondary to bacterial seeding of the meninges subsequent to bacteremia.

CLINICAL PRESENTATION

Meningitis is the most common clinical presentation, accounting for approximately 50% of invasive meningococcal disease, with symptoms common to other forms of bacterial meningitis including fever, headache, neck stiffness, nausea, vomiting, altered mental status, and photophobia. Meningococcal septicemia accounts for about 40% of cases. The classic presentation of meningococcemia (septicemia) is the acute onset of fever in association with petechiae or purpura. Headache, myalgia, nausea, and vomiting may be present. Tachycardia, hypotension, and poor perfusion are evidence of septic shock. Early in the course of the disease, the rash can appear as a nonspecific, erythematous, maculopapular rash that blanches (**Figure 93-5**), followed by rapid progression to petechiae and purpura (**Figure 93-6**).

Rapid progression to multiorgan failure can occur; complications include shock, acute respiratory distress syndrome, seizures, increased intracranial pressure, electrolyte abnormalities, renal failure, adrenal hemorrhage, anemia, thrombocytopenia, coagulopathy, pancreatitis, myocardial dysfunction, and compartment syndrome. Purpura fulminans

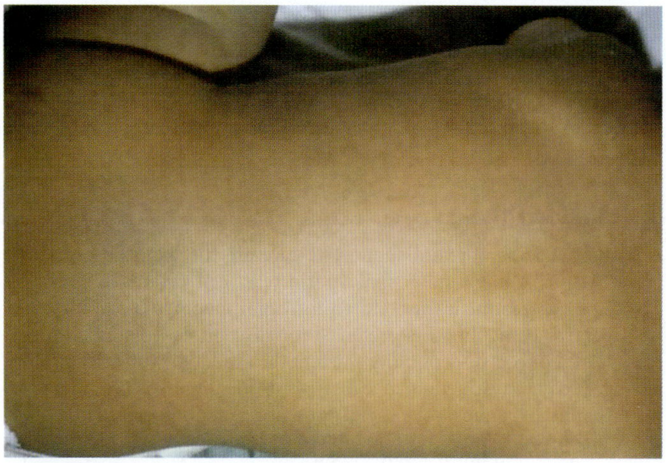

FIGURE 93-4. Erythroderma in a child with toxic shock syndrome.

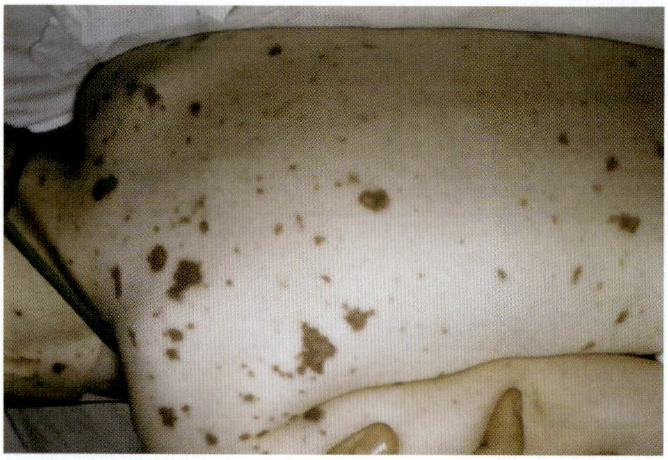

FIGURE 93-6. Purpuric rash in a 3-year-old with meningococcemia.

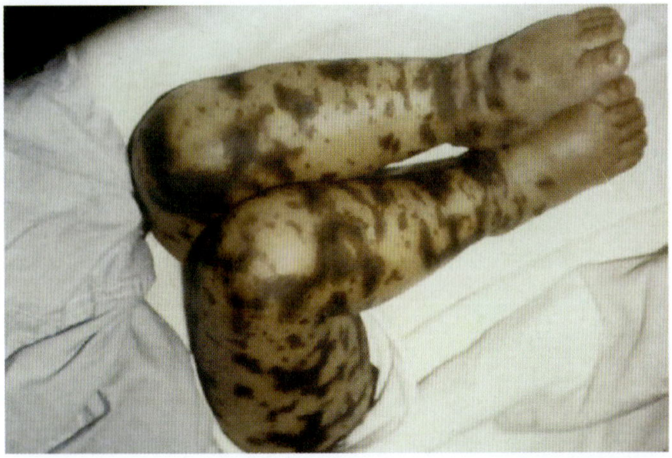

FIGURE 93-7. Purpura fulminans in an 11-month-old with meningococcemia.

(**Figure 93-7**), with necrosis of the skin and extremities (**Figure 93-8**), can develop.

The overall case fatality rate for meningococcal infections is 9% to 12%, with meningococcemia resulting in a higher mortality rate (up to 40%) compared with meningitis. The lower mortality rate seen in patients with meningitis is explained by the belief that patients who survive the initial bacteremia long enough to develop meningitis have a less pathogenic strain of meningococcus. Among survivors, permanent sequelae occur in 20% of people, with sensorineural deafness being the most common deficit. Other sequelae include neurologic damage and extremity or skin necrosis requiring amputation or skin grafting.

DIFFERENTIAL DIAGNOSIS

Current incidence rates of meningococcal disease in patients presenting with fever and petechial rash are not well defined. Past studies of patients presenting to the emergency department with fever and petechiae show that the incidence of invasive bacterial infections ranges from 2% to 8%, and the incidence of meningococcal infections may be as high as 7%. In pediatric patients hospitalized for fever and petechiae, the incidence of meningococcal infections may be as high as 15%. Invasive infections other than *N. meningitidis* causing fever and petechiae include *Staphylococcal aureus*, group A *Streptococcus*, *Streptococcus pneumoniae*, *Escherichia coli*, *Rickettsia rickettsii*, and *Ehrlichia chaffeensis*. *Haemophilus influenzae* type B should also be considered in an unimmunized population. Noninvasive causes of petechiae are listed in **Table 93-2**.

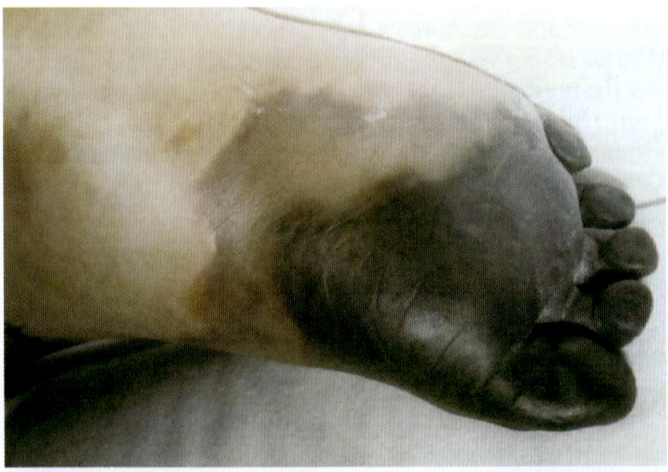

FIGURE 93-8. Necrosis and early gangrene in the toes and distal foot of a 14-month-old with meningococcemia.

TABLE 93-2 Commonly Described Causes of Petechiae

- Infectious
  - Group A streptococcal pharyngitis
  - Enterovirus infections
  - Rotavirus
  - Respiratory syncytial virus
  - Mycoplasma pneumoniae
  - Adenovirus
  - Influenza
  - Epstein-Barr virus
  - Cytomegalovirus
  - Neisseria *meningitidis*
- Mechanical
  - Vomiting
  - Cough
  - Blood pressure cuff
  - Tourniquet
- Other
  - Henoch-Schönlein purpura
  - Idiopathic thrombocytopenic purpura
  - Leukemia
  - Drug rash
  - Scurvy (Vitamin C deficiency)
- Immunization reaction (measles-mumps-rubella vaccine)

DIAGNOSTIC EVALUATION

Laboratory abnormalities often include leukocytosis, anemia, acidosis, electrolyte abnormalities, and uremia. Thrombocytopenia, prolonged prothrombin time and partial thromboplastin time, elevated fibrin degradation products, and depressed fibrinogen levels are characteristic of the disseminated intravascular coagulopathy associated with bacterial sepsis. In patients with meningitis, cerebrospinal fluid analysis may show an elevated white blood cell (WBC) count with high protein and low glucose levels, and gram-negative diplococci may be seen on Gram stain.

A number of studies have evaluated clinical and laboratory features in an attempt to exclude meningococcal infection at presentation. Petechiae limited to the distribution of the superior vena cava (superior to the nipple line), particularly if associated with coughing or vomiting, make meningococcal infection unlikely. Worrisome findings include ill appearance, evidence of shock, the presence of purpura, WBC count less than 5000 cells/dL or greater than 15,000 cells/dL, and C-reactive protein level greater than 5 mg/L. A few studies have found superior test accuracy of procalcitonin at detecting bacterial meningitis compared to WBC, ANC, and CRP.

Positive culture results of blood or spinal fluid confirm the diagnosis. Gram stain and culture of skin lesions may be helpful, particularly when antibiotics are given before the collection of samples. Frequently these cultures are sterile, however, and the diagnosis is made on clinical grounds. Antigen testing is unreliable; PCR testing is available in some areas.

MANAGEMENT

Antimicrobial therapy and supportive care are the mainstays of treatment. A third-generation cephalosporin (e.g., ceftriaxone) is the standard empiric treatment for children in whom meningococcal infection is suspected. Penicillin G is preferred for susceptible isolates, although reports of reduced susceptibility warrant the availability of susceptibility testing. Frequently, pneumococcal sepsis or meningitis is considered in the differential diagnosis of patients presenting meningococcal infection, and vancomycin is initially added to the third-generation cephalosporin to cover the possibility of resistant pneumococcus. Vancomycin can be discontinued when meningococcal infection is confirmed. Meropenem or chloramphenicol are alternatives in patients with anaphylaxis to penicillin and ceftriaxone. A 5 to 7 days course of antibiotics is an effective therapy for both meningococcemia and meningococcal meningitis. Additionally, all patients with meningitis should have a proper audiology evaluation and follow-up plan.

Supportive care includes fluid resuscitation and medications as appropriate based on patient symptoms. Of note, the need for pharmacologic vasoconstrictors (pressors) should be weighed carefully against the risk of extremity necrosis. Fasciotomy, amputation, and skin grafts are sometimes required.

ADMISSION AND DISCHARGE CRITERIA

All patients in whom meningococcal infection is suspected should be admitted to the hospital for prompt intravenous antibiotic therapy and monitoring of clinical status. Those with evidence of cardiovascular instability or multiorgan failure should be admitted to a pediatric critical care unit.

Patients may be discharged from the hospital after completion of an appropriate course of antibiotics, provided that any complications are stable and amenable to outpatient management.

CONSULTATION

Consultation with infectious diseases experts may be warranted in complicated meningococcal infections or when the diagnosis is in question.

PREVENTION

Droplet precautions are recommended for the first 24 hours of antibiotic therapy initiation, in addition to standard precautions, to prevent the spread of disease to other hospitalized patients and staff.

Chemoprophylaxis is recommended for (i) the index case (if treated only with penicillin); (ii) all intimate, household, or daycare contacts who have been exposed to the index case within 10 days of onset; and (iii) any individual with direct contact with the patient's secretions (e.g., mouth-to-mouth resuscitation), regardless of immunization status. Chemoprophylaxis of other contacts is recommended only during outbreaks or clusters of cases. Rifampin (2 days), ceftriaxone (one intramuscular dose), ciprofloxacin (single dose), and azithromycin are efficacious.

Polysaccharide vaccines that protect against serotypes A, B, C, Y, and W-135 are all available. A national update on meningococcal vaccine recommendations was published in 2020. Recommendations in the United States include routine immunization of 11- to 12-year-olds with a booster at 16 years of age. Since 2015 there has been a meningitis B vaccine approved for children 10 years or older with the recommended age of administration 16 to 18 years. Young children at higher risk of meningococcal infection because of anatomic or functional asplenia (including patients with sickle cell disease), terminal complement deficiencies or adolescents with HIV disease should also be vaccinated routinely with a two-dose primary series given 2 months apart and boosters administered in subsequent 5-year intervals based upon underlying diagnosis. Of note, Menactra is contraindicated for patients with functional asplenia or HIV below the age of 2 years as it is thought to interact with the pneumococcal vaccine. Instead, it is recommended that these patients receive Menveo.

GROUP A STREPTOCOCCUS AND RELATED DISEASES

Scarlatina, or Scarlet fever, is a diffuse, fine papular rash with a "sandpaper" texture, and it is associated with group A Streptococcus infection (**Figure 93-3**). A characteristic of this rash is exaggeration in the antecubital, axillary, and inguinal folds known as Pastia lines. Erythroderma is a diffuse erythema of the skin that is similar in appearance to a sunburn (**Figure 93-4**). Typically, erythroderma features extensive skin involvement that does not follow the pattern of sun exposure seen with sunburn. Scarlatina and erythroderma also raise the possibility of bacterial toxin production and toxic shock syndrome (TSS).

TSS is a life-threatening condition characterized by rash, fever, multiorgan failure, and shock. *Staphylococcus aureus* and *Streptococcus pyogenes* are the most common causative agents, and each organism results in a distinct clinical syndrome.

Menstruation-related staphylococcal TSS was first described in the 1970s, and an association with tampon use was noted in the 1980s. Subsequently, cases of TSS both with and without a link to menstruation have been reported, now with nearly equal frequency. Staphylococcal TSS results from the toxin produced by a strain of *S. aureus*. Streptococcal TSS became known in the 1990s with a resurgence of invasive group A streptococcal infections. It is associated with soft tissue infections such as pyomyositis and necrotizing fasciitis. Preceding skin lesions or infections, particularly varicella, and the use of nonsteroidal anti-inflammatory drugs are risk factors.

PATHOPHYSIOLOGY

Toxic shock syndrome toxin-1 (TSST-1) accounts for nearly all cases of menstruation-related TSS. Menstruation-related TSS typically occurs within 2 to 3 days of the onset of menses. TSST-1 production is enhanced by the neutral pH and high protein levels associated with menstruation. Tampon insertion contributes by elevating oxygen levels in a normally anaerobic environment. Elevation of intravaginal carbon dioxide levels with prolonged tampon insertion also contributes, especially with high-absorbency, rayon tampons. Unlike some of the other staphylococcal toxins, TSST-1 can easily cross the mucosal barrier, enter the bloodstream, and cause systemic manifestations. Non-menstruation-related TSS is caused by TSST-1 and staphylococcal enterotoxin serotypes B and C; it occurs in association with surgery, influenza infections, skin lesions and infections, foreign bodies, burns, and sometimes with no obvious focus of infection (e.g., sinusitis).

Streptococcal pyogenic exotoxin serotypes A and C are most commonly associated with severe disease. In addition, M typing appears to play an important role in the evasion of the host immune response, with M types 1 and 3 being the most common. These toxins can stimulate massive T-cell proliferation. Traditional antigens require recognition at multiple sites on the antigen-presenting cell, whereas these toxins require recognition at only one β-chain variable region. More than 20% of all T cells can be stimulated by these toxins, compared with less than 1% of T cells stimulated by traditional antigens. This ability has led these toxins to be called "superantigens." Massive cytokine release results, which can lead to capillary leak, hypotension, shock, multiorgan failure, and death.

CLINICAL PRESENTATION

Staphylococcal TSS begins with a 2- to 3-day prodromal phase characterized by malaise, myalgia, fever, and chills. Mental status changes, including lightheadedness, lethargy, and confusion, frequently bring the patient to medical attention. Diarrhea is common. Tachycardia and hypotension are usually evident at presentation. Generalized or patchy erythroderma is observed in many patients.

Streptococcal TSS has two major presentations. Some patients present with the acute onset of severe pain and fever. The pain is usually in an extremity, is out of proportion to the physical findings, and results from an underlying soft tissue infection such as necrotizing fasciitis. Alternatively, patients can present with an influenza-like syndrome characterized by fever, chills, myalgias, headache, nausea, vomiting, and diarrhea. Mental status changes ranging from confusion to coma occur in more than 50% of cases. Sore throat is unusual. The heart rate should be assessed carefully, because tachycardia out of proportion to the degree of fever may be the only evidence of impending cardiovascular collapse. Many patients are hypotensive on presentation, but commonly, blood pressure is initially normal and deteriorates rapidly within 4 hours. The typical rash seen in toxic shock syndrome, while only seen in a minority of patients, is erythroderma. Careful examination of the musculoskeletal system is important, because signs of soft tissue infection may not be obvious. When signs are present, they can range from local swelling to violaceous bullae suggestive of tissue necrosis. Diffuse edema from capillary leak may be evident in either form of TSS.

DIFFERENTIAL DIAGNOSIS

The differential diagnosis of fever and shock is broad. Presence of the typical rash should make TSS a strong consideration, but its absence should not exclude the possibility. In addition to TSS, gram-negative sepsis should be considered. Other non-infectious etiologies like heatstroke present similarly with hyperthermia and renal dysfunction and may have erythroderma. Meningococcal infections and Rocky Mountain spotted fever present with fever and shock, but the rash, when present, is petechial in nature. Pyomyositis and necrotizing fasciitis can occur without the shock or organ dysfunction associated with TSS. Kawasaki disease may present with fever, mucous membrane involvement, and scarlatina or erythroderma, but shock occurs in only a small percentage of patients. Kawasaki disease also has a younger age distribution than does TSS. Purulent conjunctivitis and the absence of shock differentiate viral infections, such as adenovirus and measles, from TSS. Normal heart rate and blood pressure in association with a scarlatiniform rash and exudative pharyngitis support the diagnosis of uncomplicated scarlet fever.

DIAGNOSTIC EVALUATION

The diagnosis of TSS is based on the clinical criteria outlined in **Table 93-3**. WBC counts are elevated in staphylococcal TSS, with an elevation of immature neutrophils. In streptococcal TSS, WBC counts are frequently normal to mildly elevated, with immature neutrophils accounting for as much as 50% to 60% of the total. Thrombocytopenia with an abnormal coagulation panel suggests the consumptive coagulopathy known to complicate these illnesses. Isolated thrombocytopenia is common with staphylococcal disease. Elevated blood urea nitrogen and serum creatinine are often evident at presentation and can occur before the onset of hypotension in streptococcal TSS.

TABLE 93-3 Clinical Criteria for Toxic Shock Syndrome
Streptococcal Toxic Shock Syndrome
Hypotension
Clinical or laboratory evidence of multisystem organ involvement (≥2 of the following):
Renal impairment
Coagulopathy
Liver abnormalities
Acute respiratory distress syndrome
Extensive tissue necrosis
Erythematous rash
Definite case: above criteria plus isolation of group A β-hemolytic streptococcus from sterile site
Probable case: above criteria plus isolation of group A β-hemolytic streptococcus from nonsterile site
Staphylococcal Toxic Shock Syndrome
Major criteria (3 of 3):
Acute fever ≥38.8°C
Hypotension
Characteristic rash
Minor criteria (3 of 7):
Mucous membrane involvement (conjunctival, oropharyngeal erythema)
Gastrointestinal abnormalities (vomiting, diarrhea)
Muscle abnormalities (myalgia, elevated creatine phosphokinase)
Central nervous system abnormalities (coma, obtundation)
Hepatic abnormalities
Renal abnormalities (pyuria, uremia)
Thrombocytopenia
Exclusionary criteria
Another explanation
Positive blood culture for an organism other than *Staphylococcus aureus*

Elevated serum transaminases, bilirubin, and prothrombin time are evidence of liver involvement. Direct hyperbilirubinemia out of proportion to other abnormalities in liver enzymes suggests hydrops of the gallbladder. Hypoalbuminemia can be secondary to capillary leak and liver dysfunction. Hypocalcemia can be significant. Creatine phosphokinase levels are elevated in both types of TSS and correlate with the degree of myositis in streptococcal TSS. Blood cultures are positive in 60% of those with streptococcal TSS but in only a minority of those with staphylococcal disease. *S. aureus* can be isolated from cultures of the anterior nares, rectum, and vagina, and throat culture can identify *S. pyogenes*. Cultures of wounds may be helpful in isolating either organism.

MANAGEMENT

Early recognition of TSS is paramount in appropriately managing this disease. Staphylococcal TSS can progress to shock and multiorgan failure, however appropriate intravenous antibiotics in combination with aggressive supportive care may decrease mortality to less than 5% of patients. Supportive therapy includes aggressive fluid resuscitation and the potential use of vasopressors to maintain hemodynamic stability. Use of a semisynthetic penicillin such as nafcillin generally provides good bactericidal coverage against *S. aureus* and *S. pyogenes*. In geographic areas demonstrating a significant presence of community-acquired methicillin-resistant *S. aureus*, vancomycin should be used instead. Adequate coverage for gram-negative organisms should be added when these organisms are being considered in the differential diagnosis. A third-generation cephalosporin such as ceftriaxone is appropriate. Additionally, administration of antimicrobial agents capable of suppressing toxin production, specifically clindamycin or linezolid, is important in treating TSS. Intravenous immunoglobulin can also be considered as it has the potential to neutralize the superantigen and may mitigate subsequent tissue damage.

The outcome of streptococcal TSS is worse than staphylococcal TSS. Despite appropriate treatment, shock and renal dysfunction are nearly universal and often progress over 48 to 72 hours. More than 50% of patients develop acute respiratory distress syndrome, with the majority requiring some degree of respiratory support. Mortality ranges from 30% to 70%. Those with deep soft tissue infections fare the worst. Renal dysfunction often persists for 4 to 6 weeks in survivors.

Animal models of streptococcal TSS demonstrate improved survival in clindamycin-treated mice versus those treated with penicillin. The decreased efficacy of penicillin is explained by the high inoculum of *S. pyogenes* in these infections, resulting in a static growth phase and decreased demonstration of penicillin-binding proteins. In addition, clindamycin inhibits bacterial protein synthesis and thus decreases the production of toxin and antiphagocytic M proteins. Last, clindamycin may modulate the host immune response by inhibiting tumor necrosis factor production by monocytes. Thus, an antibiotic regimen of a beta lactam antibiotic with clindamycin is superior than a beta lactam antibiotic alone. The benefits of clindamycin as an adjunct agent probably do not continue once the patient is stable and soft tissue collections have been adequately drained. A total course of 10 to 14 days of antibiotics is commonly prescribed. Transition to oral antibiotics at the time of discharge to complete this course is appropriate. The role of intravenous immune globulin (IVIG) is controversial. Larger observational studies have not demonstrated reduced mortality in children with streptococcal toxic shock syndrome. Therefore, IVIG should not routinely be used but may be considered in severe cases.

ADMISSION AND DISCHARGE CRITERIA

All patients with suspected TSS should be hospitalized for intravenous antibiotics and careful monitoring, rapid clinical deterioration is common, and further cardiovascular support may be necessary. Any indication of cardiovascular instability or acute respiratory distress syndrome warrants transfer to a critical care setting.

Patients can be discharged to home when:

- They are afebrile.
- They have negative blood culture results.

- They are hemodynamically stable.
- Complications are stable and manageable on an outpatient basis.

CONSULTATION

Consultation with infectious diseases experts may be warranted in complicated TSS cases or when the diagnosis is in question.

PREVENTION

Judicious use of tampons is an important measure to prevent staphylococcal TSS. Recommendations include using tampons of minimal absorbency, avoiding prolonged insertion of tampons (<4-8 hours), and alternating tampon and pad use. Patients with staphylococcal TSS who survive are at higher risk of recurrence and should be instructed not to use tampons. There are no preventive measures for streptococcal TSS. Vaccinations are not available for either entity.

DISEASES CAUSED BY RICKETTSIA, EHRLICHIA, AND ANAPLASMA

A dramatic petechial rash is frequently cited as the hallmark of Rocky Mountain spotted fever (RMSF), a potentially severe disease. However, the rash in RMSF, as with other rickettsial diseases and similar zoonoses, is a late clinical phenomenon. A delay in diagnosis is common, and few of these diseases are diagnosed at the first presentation of the illness. In addition, the empirical antimicrobial agents frequently prescribed for suspected systemic bacterial infections (e.g., β-lactams) are ineffective against these organisms. Because morbidity and mortality are significant, clinicians must consider empirical therapy for these diseases based on epidemiologic, clinical, and laboratory features.

ROCKY MOUNTAIN SPOTTED FEVER

Rickettsia rickettsii is a gram-negative coccobacillus that is an obligate intracellular pathogen; it cannot be cultured on routine microbiologic media. Ticks are the vector by which *R. rickettsii* is transmitted. *Dermacentor variabilis* (American dog tick) and *Dermacentor andersonii* (Rocky Mountain wood tick) are the vectors in the eastern and western United States, respectively.

The incidence of RMSF has increased over the past several years to over 13.5 cases per million people. Although RMSF has been described in most of the continental United States, 60% of cases occur in the southeastern and south-central states, with highly endemic areas in Oklahoma, North Carolina, Arkansas, Tennessee, and Missouri. A significant number of cases occur in children, with a slight peak in incidence in the 5- to 9-year-old age group; a male predominance is seen. As would be expected with a tick-borne illness, the majority of cases occur in rural areas, and there is usually a history suggesting significant tick exposure; however, many patients do not recall a tick bite. Most infections occur between April and September, correlating with outdoor recreation and tick activity. Case fatality has decreased over recent years and has the highest incidence in very young children and older adults.

Pathophysiology The primary targets of the organisms are the endothelial cells of small blood vessels of all major tissues and organs. This vasculitis accounts for the clinical manifestations of RMSF, including the rash, and the significant morbidity and mortality of the illness.

Clinical Presentation The classic triad of fever, headache, and rash is found in the minority of patients when they first present for medical care. Most of the initial symptoms are nonspecific. After an incubation of 2 to 14 days, patients often present with high fever exceeding 38.9°C, which is usually the earliest sign. Fever may be accompanied by severe myalgias and malaise. Headache is commonly frontal in location and is likely secondary to inflammation and increased intracranial pressure related to vasculitis; young children may present with fussiness. Abdominal pain may be severe enough to suggest an acute surgical abdomen and can be associated with vomiting or diarrhea.

Findings on physical examination may include hepatosplenomegaly, conjunctival injection, and periorbital or peripheral edema. Central nervous system findings may include neck stiffness, mental status changes, and focal neurologic deficits that may present a confusing clinical picture. The characteristic centripetally spreading rash, present in about 95% of children, usually occurs earlier in children than in adults but may not appear until the third or fourth day of illness. Diagnosis of RMSF should not await the appearance of a rash, because a delay in initiating therapy is associated with increased mortality. The rash frequently begins as macular or maculopapular lesions on the wrists and ankles and spreads to the palms and soles and centrally to the trunk. Because RMSF is a vasculitis, it is not surprising that the lesions often become petechial and occasionally purpuric later in the course of illness.

The course of illness includes progression of vasculitis and intravascular volume depletion secondary to vascular leak, which can lead to multiorgan involvement. Renal complications and hypotension are common, and cardiovascular collapse and myocarditis may occur in severe disease. Neurologic complications include headache, seizures, coma, cerebral edema, and intracranial hemorrhage. Pulmonary edema, hemorrhage, and respiratory failure are rare.

Differential Diagnosis The differential diagnosis may initially include nonspecific viral illness. As symptoms progress, the differential is broadened to include bacterial sepsis, especially meningococcemia. The clinical picture of ehrlichiosis may be quite similar (see later). Enteroviral infections may be associated with a petechial rash, headache, and myalgias, but clinical manifestations are usually not as severe as with RMSF. It is important to strongly consider RMSF in the differential diagnosis early in the disease course; delay in treatment is often related to lack of recognition, rather than patients not presenting early for medical care.

Diagnostic Evaluation The peripheral WBC count is frequently normal, especially early in the illness. Later evaluations may show either an increase or a decrease in the WBC count, making this test less useful for diagnosis. Thrombocytopenia, with values below 100,000/mm^3, is relatively common. This may be secondary to the vasculitis and endothelial expression of platelet-binding substances produced by *R. rickettsii.* A helpful diagnostic clue is that thrombocytopenia may be found in the absence of evidence of a consumptive coagulopathy. Hyponatremia is also common and is likely a result of disrupted vascular integrity and capillary leakage. Cerebrospinal fluid analysis may reveal a mild pleocytosis (polymorphonuclear or mononuclear) and may have elevated protein. Serum transaminase, blood urea nitrogen, and creatinine levels are frequently elevated and represent end-organ injury from vasculitis. Evidence of renal insufficiency may signal a poor prognosis.

Unfortunately, there are no generally available tests for rapid diagnosis during the acute illness. Serologic evaluation by the immunofluorescent antibody test can establish a diagnosis 10 to 14 days after the onset of illness with 90% sensitivity and is available at most state health departments and some commercial laboratories. Most tests measure both IgM and IgG, which often are not detectable in the first 7 days of illness. The use of paired acute and convalescent sera demonstrating a fourfold rise in titers against *R. rickettsii* is diagnostic. *R. rickettsii* may also be identified in skin biopsy specimens by direct immunofluorescent microscopy or immunoperoxidase staining, but this is not widely available.

Management As noted earlier, treatment targeting RMSF should be started promptly upon considering the diagnosis. Antibiotics used for typical bacterial agents (e.g. β-lactams) have no activity against *R. rickettsii.* The drug of choice, even in children, is doxycycline, which can be administered intravenously or orally, depending upon severity of disease. The consequences of RMSF far outweigh the small risk of dental staining from the use of tetracyclines (usually associated with repeated and prolonged courses). The dose of doxycycline is 2.2 mg/kg (maximum 100 mg/dose) every 12 hours. Chloramphenicol is an inferior agent that may be considered in rare cases, such as severe doxycycline allergy or in the treatment of pregnant women; it is no longer available in oral formulation in the United States. Antibiotics should be continued until the patient has been afebrile for 3 days with clinical improvement, generally resulting in 7 to 10 days of treatment. Although therapy for hospitalized patients is often completed intravenously, rapid improvement may allow completion of therapy with oral doxycycline.

Supportive care is indicated depending upon severity of progression of illness. Care may include the need for fluid resuscitation, blood products, vasoactive infusion support, or mechanical ventilation.

Admission and Discharge Criteria Oral outpatient therapy may be used for patients with normal vital signs, absence of end-organ damage, tolerance of oral therapy, and assurance of excellent follow-up. Abnormal vital signs (other than fever) and evidence of end-organ damage (e.g., mental status changes or renal dysfunction) are clear indications for hospital admission and may warrant admission to the pediatric critical care unit.

Patients may be discharged from the hospital when they show clinical improvement in admission symptoms, including recovery of organ function. Antibiotic regimen, if oral therapy continuation is indicated, should be tolerated and close follow-up assured.

Consultation Consultation with infectious diseases experts may be warranted in complicated RMSF cases or when the diagnosis is in question.

Prevention Standard precautions are recommended for the hospitalized patient.

Avoidance of ticks should be attempted in tick-endemic areas. This can be accomplished by avoiding bushy areas, wearing long sleeves and pants, and using effective insect repellents. Careful inspection of the body and household pets for ticks during the summer months may also decrease the risk of exposure. Prophylactic antibiotics after a tick bite are not recommended. No vaccine is available.

EHRLICHIOSIS AND ANAPLASMOSIS

Other zoonoses whose epidemiologic, clinical, and laboratory features mimic RMSF may in fact be more common. They are represented predominantly by the ehrlichioses. Like RMSF, ehrlichiosis and anaplasmosis represent a diagnostic challenge, and therapy is similar.

Ehrlichia chaffeensis, E. ewingii, and *E. muris* like agents cause human ehrlichiosis in the United States, while *Anaplasma phagocytophila* (formerly *E. phagocytophila*) causes a similar disease called anaplasmosis. The agents of these diseases are obligate intracellular bacteria with tick vectors and mammalian hosts. Target cells are mononuclear phagocytic cells for the ehrlichioses and neutrophils for *A. phagocytophila*. The clinical syndromes, human monocytic ehrlichiosis (HME) and human granulocytic anaplasmosis (HGA), correlate with these target cells.

Although HME has been reported in most of the continental United States, the highest incidence is in the southeastern and south-central states. The vectors are *Amblyomma americanum* (Lone Star tick) and *Dermacentor variabilis* (American dog tick). Deer are the natural reservoir.

The distribution of HGA is predominantly in the northeastern and upper midwestern United States. The vector is *Ixodes scapularis* (*I. pacificus* in California), with deer and white-footed mice serving as reservoirs. The zoonotic cycle is similar to that of *Borrelia burgdorferi*, the agent of Lyme disease. Co-infection with *B. burgdorferi* can occur, but it is unclear how frequently. HGA infection may be underrecognized. As the ticks are small, the bite itself is often difficult to appreciate. Both ehrlichiosis and anaplasmosis cases are on the rise in the United States. The incidence is highest in the summer months and in rural and suburban areas, and both have a more pronounced male predominance in comparison to RMSF; only a minority of cases occur in children. Incubation period for both diseases is typically 5 to 10 days.

Clinical Presentation The disease ranges from subclinical or asymptomatic cases to severe, life-threatening, and fatal illnesses. Initial symptoms are nonspecific and include fever, chills, severe headache, myalgias, arthralgias, abdominal pain, and weight loss. Central nervous system symptoms can include ataxia, vertigo, and delirium. Lymphadenopathy, which is uncommon with RMSF, may be noted. Organomegaly may result from granulomatous infiltration. Rash is less common than seen with RMSF, noted in about 60% of children with ehrlichiosis and only 10% with anaplasmosis. The rash involves the trunk and extremities and may be macular, maculopapular, or petechial.

Complications of ehrlichiosis include coagulopathy, hypotension, acute respiratory distress syndrome, and renal failure. Mortality can result from gastrointestinal or pulmonary hemorrhage, with case fatality rates of approximately 1% to 2%. Complications of anaplasmosis can include acute respiratory distress syndrome and neuropathy. The illness tends to be less severe than ehrlichiosis, with less frequent central nervous system involvement, organomegaly, and mortality. Mortality rates are also lower at about 0.5%.

Differential Diagnosis The differential diagnosis of ehrlichiosis and anaplasmosis is similar to that of RMSF. Most of the entities discussed in the previous sections of this chapter are given greater consideration than ehrlichiosis in patients with fever and rash; however, in patients with tick exposure in endemic areas and suspicious laboratory findings, ehrlichiosis or anaplasmosis should be considered.

Diagnostic Evaluation Laboratory features of ehrlichiosis or anaplasmosis are nonspecific but may provide helpful clues to the diagnosis. Abnormalities, particularly hematologic ones, are more common in children. Leukopenia, with WBC counts in the range of 1 to 4000, is often present early in the illness, along with lymphopenia or neutropenia. During the second week of illness these counts may be elevated; therefore, the timing of laboratory studies relative to the duration of the illness should be considered when interpreting these values. Leukopenia is likely due to peripheral destruction, margination, and sequestration of WBCs rather than bone marrow suppression. Other common lab abnormalities include thrombocytopenia and elevated transaminase levels in over 90% of patients, as well as hypoalbuminemia and hyponatremia in the majority of patients.

Serologic evaluation (immunoglobulin G and immunoglobulin M) for *E. chaffeensis* and *A. phagocytophilum* are available by indirect immunofluorescence. The gold standard for diagnosis is a fourfold increase in IgG titers in samples 2 to 4 weeks apart. Single elevated titers indicate probable infection, but levels can remain high after prior infection, so comparing two samples over time is best.

Management The initial treatment is frequently empirical, given the difficulty of obtaining timely confirmation of the diagnosis. Therapy should not await serologic confirmation. As with RMSF, doxycycline is the drug of choice in a dose of 2.2 mg/kg (maximum 100 mg/dose) every 12 hours. Therapy should be continued for at least 3 days beyond defervescence, with a total course between 7 and 14 days. As co-infection with *B. burgdorferi* and *A. phagocytophila* has been reported, it is essential to recognize that empirical therapy for Lyme disease with β-lactams (e.g., the treatment of young children with amoxicillin) is not adequate for anaplasmosis.

Supportive care is also indicated depending upon the severity of the progression of the illness and may include fluid resuscitation, vasoconstrictor (pressor) support, or mechanical ventilation.

Admission and Discharge Criteria Many cases of ehrlichiosis are unrecognized, but most patients who present to a hospital setting are admitted due to diagnostic confusion or severe symptoms. In general, admission should be prompted by central nervous system or cardiovascular dysfunction, hematologic abnormalities, or electrolyte disturbances; in severe cases, pediatric critical care unit admission may be necessary.

Patients may be discharged from the hospital when they show clinical improvement in admission symptoms, including resolution of neurologic or cardiovascular abnormalities. Antibiotic regimen, if oral therapy continuation is indicated, should be tolerated and close follow-up assured.

Consultation Consultation with infectious diseases experts may be warranted in complicated cases or when the diagnoses are in question.

Prevention Prevention is similar to that for RMSF (see above).

KEY POINTS

- The combination of fever and rash is a common clinical scenario. Careful characterization of the rash in conjunction with consideration for other clinical features, can provide clues to the cause of the illness.
- The characteristic rash may be absent in all the severe infections discussed.
- Although the presence of fever and petechiae raises concern for meningococcemia, other infections should be considered. Noninvasive etiologies account for the majority of these illnesses.
- In patients with fever and erythroderma or scarlatina, TSS should be considered in the differential diagnosis.
- TSS may present initially without apparent signs of shock, and tachycardia out of proportion to the fever may be an early sign of cardiovascular instability.
- Epidemiology, including a history concerning for tick exposure, is critical when considering the diagnoses of RMSF and ehrlichiosis.
- Thrombocytopenia and hyponatremia may be helpful clues to diagnosing RMSF and ehrlichiosis.
- Early and aggressive therapy improves the outcomes for meningococcemia, TSS, and rickettsial diseases. Therapy should be initiated at the first suspicion of these entities rather than waiting for confirmation.
- Antibiotics commonly used for the empirical treatment of serious bacterial infections are ineffective against RMSF, ehrlichiosis, and anaplasmosis. Doxycycline is the drug of choice.

SUGGESTED READINGS

Atkinson W, CDC. *Epidemiology and Prevention of Vaccine-Preventable Diseases*. 12th ed. The Public Health Foundation; 2012.

Brogan PA, Raffles A. The management of fever and petechiae: making sense of rash decisions. *Arch Dis Child*. 2000;83(6):506-507.

Buckingham SC, Marshall GS, Schutze GE, et al. Clinical and laboratory features, hospital course, and outcome of Rocky Mountain spotted fever Rocky Mountain spotted fever in children. *J Pediatr*. 2007;150(2):180-184, 184 e181.

Centers for Disease Control and Prevention (CDC). Rickettsial Diseases (Including Spotted Fever & Typhus Fever Rickettsioses, Scrub Typhus, Anaplasmosis, and Ehrlichioses) https://wwwnc.cdc.gov/travel/yellowbook/2020/travel-related-infectious-diseases/rickettsial-including-spotted-fever-and-typhus-fever-rickettsioses-scrub-typhus-anaplasmosis-and-ehr (Accessed September 23, 2022).

Chuang YY, Huang YC, Lin TY. Toxic shock syndrome in children: epidemiology, pathogenesis, and management. *Paediatr Drugs*. 2005;7(1): 11-25.

Conlon PJ, Procop GW, Fowler V, Eloubeidi MA, Smith SR, Sexton DJ. Predictors of prognosis and risk of acute renal failure in Rocky Mountain spotted fever patients. *Am J Med*. 1996;101(6):621-626.

Davidkin I, Valle M, Peltola H, et al. Etiology of measles- and rubella-like illnesses in measles, mumps, and rubella-vaccinated children. *J Infect Dis*. 1998;178(6):1567-1570.

Haj-Hassan TA, Thompson MJ, Mayon-White RT, et al. Which early 'red flag' symptoms identify children with meningococcal disease in primary care? *British J Gen Pract*. 2011;61(584):e97-104.

Jay R, Armstrong PA. Clinical characteristics of Rocky Mountain spotted fever in the United States: a literature review. *J Vector Borne Dis*. 2020;57(2):114-120.

Lappin E, Ferguson AJ. Gram-positive toxic shock syndromes. *Lancet Infect Dis*. 2009;9(5):281-290.

Leaute-Labreze C, Lamireau T, Chawki D, Maleville J, Taieb A. Diagnosis, classification, and management of erythema multiforme and Stevens-Johnson syndrome. *Arch Dis Child*. 2000;83(4):347-352.

Nielsen HE, Andersen EA, Andersen J, et al. Diagnostic assessment of hemorrhagic rash and fever. *Arch Dis Child*. 2001;85(2):160-165.

Mandl KD, Stack AM, Fleisher GR. Incidence of bacteremia in infants and children with fever and petechiae. *J Pediatr*. 1997;131(3):398-404.

Mbaeyi SA, Bozio CH, Duffy J, et al. Meningococcal vaccination: recommendations of the Advisory Committee on Immunization Practices, United States, 2020. *MMWR Recomm Rep*. 2020;69 (9): 1-41.

Ramsay M, Reacher M, O'Flynn C, et al. Causes of morbilliform rash in a highly immunized English population. *Arch Dis Child*. 2002;87(3):202-206.

Schutze GE, Buckingham SC, Marshall GS, et al. Human monocytic ehrlichiosis in children. *Pediatr Infect Dis J*. 2007;26(6):475-479.

Shah KN, Honig PJ, Yan AC. "Urticaria multiforme": a case series and review of acute annular urticarial hypersensitivity syndromes in children. *Pediatrics*. 2007;119(5):e1177-1183.

Stevens DL. Streptococcal toxic-shock syndrome: spectrum of disease, pathogenesis, and new concepts in treatment. *Emerg Infect Dis*. 1995;1:69-78.

Wells LC, Smith JC, Weston VC, Collier J, Rutter N. The child with a non-blanching rash: how likely is meningococcal disease? *Arch Dis Child*. 2001;85(3):218-222.

CHAPTER 94

Central Nervous System Infections

Lauren B. Nassetta, MD and Robert F. Pass, MD

INTRODUCTION

This chapter will cover bacterial and viral central nervous system (CNS) infections in children, focusing on meningitis, focal bacterial infections, and encephalitis/meningoencephalitis. Central nervous system infections are a common reason for hospitalization in children because they cause severe discomfort, altered consciousness, and neurologic abnormalities, and they are associated with risk of disabling sequelae and even death. Almost all children who present to the hospital with evidence of an acute CNS infection are hospitalized; the vast majority are later discharged home, **Table 94-1**.

BACTERIAL MENINGITIS

Meningitis is inflammation of the membranes surrounding the brain and spinal cord. Infectious causes include viruses, bacteria, fungi, protozoa, and helminths. Viruses and bacteria cause almost all meningitis cases in immunocompetent children in the community. Distinguishing

TABLE 94-1 Age Distribution and Hospitalization Rates for US Children With Meningitis or Encephalitis

	Age Group, years			
Variable	**<1**	**1-2**	**3-9**	**10-17**
% Of study population	45.5	4.43	21.9	28.2
Hospitalization rate, %	91.1	86.8	79.0	72.7
Admit from emergency department, %	76.2	76.6	83.4	80.8
Disposition, % discharges				
Home	94.3	88.8	94.6	93.8
Nursing home/rehab/hospice	3.9	7.6	3.8	4.5
Expired	0.6	0.8	0.7	0.6

Source: Adapted from Hasbun R, Wootton SH, Rosenthal N, et al. Epidemiology of Meningitis and Encephalitis in Infants and Children in the United States, 2011-2014. *Pediatr Infect Dis J*. 2019; 38(1):37-41.

bacterial from viral meningitis is a priority in caring for hospitalized children with meningitis.

EPIDEMIOLOGY

Bacterial meningitis is a relatively uncommon cause of hospitalization in children, though precise current data providing a population-based incidence in the United States are not available. Review of epidemiologic and administrative database studies allows for an approximation of about 1000 to 2000 cases of bacterial meningitis in children in the United States annually. Incidence rates vary by age. A meta-analysis by Nigrovic et al reports incidence rates in 2007 as 81, 6.9, 0.56, and 0.43 (cases per 100,000) respectively for ages < 2 months, 2 to 23 months, 2 to 10 years, and 11 to 17 years. *Haemophilus influenzae* type *b*, historically a leading cause of bacterial meningitis in children, became a rare cause in the 1990s after licensure and wide use of conjugate *H. influenzae b* vaccines in infants in the United States. The incidence of bacterial meningitis continued to decline over the past 20 years, based largely on the success of conjugate vaccines for *Streptococcus pneumoniae* and *Neisseria meningitidis.* In recent years, the decrease has been most dramatic in younger children with a higher proportion of cases in older children and adolescents. Children with bacterial meningitis are disproportionately male, from low-income families, and have chronic conditions that increase risk of infection. Chronic conditions associated with increased risk of bacterial meningitis include congenital and acquired immunodeficiency [disorders of complement, agammaglobulinemia, human immunodeficiency virus (HIV) infection, and asplenia], immunosuppression related to transplantation or cancer chemotherapy, anatomic defects (CSF leak and dermal sinus tract), and premature birth. Overall mortality of bacterial meningitis in children is around 3% in the United States. Mortality rates vary with age and are higher in developing countries and with pneumococcal infection.

ETIOLOGY

Table 94-2 lists the leading etiologies and associated exposures for bacterial meningitis in children and in newborn infants. Exposure to respiratory droplets from a colonized human is the primary mechanism for transmission of *S. pneumoniae, N. meningitides,* and *H. influenzae.*

TABLE 94-2 Key Exposures for the Most Common Causes of Bacterial Meningitis in Children

Pathogen	Usual Source of Infection	Risk Factor or Exposure
Streptococcus pneumoniae	Human contact, respiratory droplet	Incomplete pneumococcal conjugate vaccine series Crowded living conditions Antibody or complement deficiency
Neisseria meningitidis	Human contact, respiratory droplet	Incomplete Men A, C, W, Y vaccine series No Men B vaccine Household contact with a case of meningococcal disease Crowded living conditions, college dorm or military barracks Complement deficiency, asplenia
Hemophilus influenzae	Human contact, respiratory droplet	Incomplete *H flu b* vaccine series Crowded living conditions Day care center
Streptococcus agalactiae	Maternal	Newborn Infant < 3 months of age
Escherichia coli	Maternal or environment	Premature newborn Young infant
Listeria monocytogenes	Mother perinatal (newborn) Contaminated food	Maternal perinatal *Listeria* illness or colonization Contaminated food (dairy, vegetables, fruits, meats)

Outbreaks of meningococcal meningitis in the United States have occurred in college and military dormitories. Daycare center outbreaks of *H. influenzae b* invasive disease and meningitis occurred in the pre-vaccine era. *H. influenzae b* disease is still common in countries that have not achieved high rates of coverage with *H. influenzae b* vaccines. According to Tsang et al, in the United States, non-typeable *H. influenzae* strains now cause more invasive disease than the *b* serotype, and prevalence of serotype *a* is increasing. Strains of *N. meningitidis* and *S. pneumoniae* not covered by their conjugate vaccines have become more prevalent in nasopharyngeal colonization. Although meningitis incidence has steadily decreased in the post-conjugate-vaccine era, invasive disease due to serotypes of *S. pneumoniae* not covered by the licensed vaccines increased.

Meningitis due to *Mycobacterium tuberculosis* in children is both much less common than pneumococcal or meningococcal meningitis and significantly more likely to lead to death or disability. In 2020, there were 7174 tuberculosis infections in the United States, with 634 (8.8%) pediatric cases, which the Centers for Disease Control and Prevention (CDC) and international authorities define as including those in patients up to age 14 years. Although meningitis occurs in <1% of *M. tuberculosis* cases in adults, young children are more likely to have extrapulmonary disease, including meningitis, with recent *M. tuberculosis* infection. The CDC reports that in 2017, the proportions of pediatric *M. tuberculosis* cases complicated by meningitis by age group were: 11.2% (<1 year), 6.4% (1-4 years), 2.9% (5-9 years), and 2.6% (10-14 years). Incidence rates for *M. tuberculosis* in the United States by race/ethnicity data in 2020 show that the highest rates (cases/100,000 population) occurred in Native Hawaiians/other Pacific Islanders (18.7) and Asians (13.3), with notably lower rates among the Hispanic/Latino population (3.5), Black/African Americans (3.4), American Indian/Alaska Natives (3.2), multiple races/ethnicities (0.7), and whites (0.4). Demographic data also show that most *M. tuberculosis* cases in the United States are in persons not born in the United States. Although exposure to an adult with *M. tuberculosis* is the likely source of infection for children, medical history does not reveal a specific exposure in 30% to 50% of pediatric tuberculous (TB) meningitis cases. The rate of adverse outcomes (developmental, motor, or cognitive disability) in survivors is 40% or higher regardless of treatment. Mortality for TB meningitis in children is high, with around 10% in the United States and Western Europe and 20% or higher in developing countries.

Streptococcus agalactiae [group B *Streptococcus* (GBS)] and *Escherichia coli* are the major causes of meningitis in newborn infants. Although maternal screening for GBS colonization at 35 to 37 weeks gestation and intrapartum prophylactic treatment with antibiotics reduced the occurrence of early onset GBS disease (<7 days from birth) in the newborn by around 85%, it has not affected rates of late onset disease. The CDC Active Bacterial Core Surveillance program data for 2006 to 2015 reported that meningitis was part of GBS disease in 9.5% and 31.4% of early onset and late onset cases, respectively. GBS is the leading cause of bacterial meningitis in community dwelling infants up to 90 days of age, and approximately 10% of GBS meningitis cases occur in infants or children older than 3 months. *E.coli* is the second leading cause of meningitis in newborns and infants up to 90 days of age and the leading cause of meningitis in premature newborns. For infants who require prolonged hospitalization because of prematurity, surgical procedures, or other morbidities, a wider range of etiologies for sepsis and meningitis are seen, including *Enterobacter, Proteus, Klebsiella, Staphylococcus* species, and *Candida* species. *Listeria* is an uncommon cause of meningitis in the United States, but it can be a prominent cause of neonatal meningitis when community outbreaks of *Listeria* infection involve pregnant women. Almost all *Listeria* infections in young infants occur within the first postnatal month.

PATHOGENESIS

Acute Bacterial Meningitis The most common causes of childhood meningitis (*S. pneumoniae, N. meningitides,* and *H. influenzae*) colonize the nasopharynx. Specific bacterial cell surface molecules interact with host respiratory tract epithelial cells to facilitate host invasion. Differences in bacterial cell wall features can account for invasiveness and persistence in the nasopharynx. Similar mechanisms are involved in bacteria entering the bloodstream through capillary endothelial cells. Pattern-recognition molecules, phagocytic cells, complement and other elements of the innate immune system are the first line of host defense against invading bacteria. Specific antibody is also important but will not be present for several days unless the patient has previous experience with the pathogen, has maternal antibodies received prenatally or has been immunized. *S. pneumoniae, N. meningitides,* and *H. influenzae* have polysaccharide capsules which protect them from host immune responses and facilitate survival in the bloodstream long enough to reach the blood-brain barrier. Interaction between bacterial surface molecules and vascular endothelium allows the bacteria to pass through or around the endothelial cells, crossing into the subarachnoid space and escaping antibody and other host defense mechanisms in the bloodstream. Although astrocytes and microglial cells that are present at the blood-brain barrier have the ability to engulf and kill bacteria, high-level bacteremia will overcome that defense. Adaptive immune responses within the CNS take days to reach protective levels. Phagocytic cells (predominantly neutrophils) move to the subarachnoid space in response to astrocytic signaling and breaks in the blood-brain barrier. Escalating activation of systemic and local immune responses leads to cytokine release, intense inflammation, and thrombosis, the results of which can be focal areas of ischemia, cerebral edema, increased intracranial pressure (ICP), and obstructive hydrocephalus. Ischemia and activation of apoptotic pathways by cytokines lead to neuronal cell injury and death. In experimental models, inflammatory processes continue for days after elimination of bacteria. More detailed reviews of the pathogenesis of bacterial meningitis are available for the interested reader (see Suggested Readings).

Post-mortem findings provide insight into the damage wrought by infection and inflammation. Prominent macroscopic findings include brain swelling, exudate over cerebral hemispheres, compressed ventricular spaces, purulent fluid in ventricles, thrombosis of penetrating arteries, and infarcts. Microscopic findings reveal exudate extending into cortical surfaces of brain, perivascular inflammation, necrosis of blood vessels in periventricular white matter and infarcts in meninges and cortex.

Tuberculous Meningitis Airborne transmission of *M. tuberculosis* causes initial infection in the lung. The pathogenesis of TB meningitis is different from that of the more common acute bacterial meningitides in that it does not depend on acute bacteremia or the ability of bacilli to cross the blood-brain barrier. Wilkinson et al describes that during primary *M. tuberculosis* infection, bacilli from the site of infection in the respiratory tract spread through lymphoid tissue and blood vessels to establish foci of infection in other tissues, including the leptomeninges and brain. TB meningitis occurs when a focal lesion ruptures, releasing bacilli into the subarachnoid space or ventricles. Although the quantity of *M. tuberculosis* in CSF is low, and cultures are usually negative, the inflammatory reaction to infection is intense, especially at the base of the brain. There is marked perivascular inflammation and edema with obstruction of flow, focal infarction, and resulting cerebral edema. Obstructive hydrocephalus is present at the time of presentation in the majority of cases of TB meningitis in children. TB meningitis is also associated with pituitary dysfunction, low serum cortisol levels, cerebral salt wasting, and hypothyroidism. There is evidence that variations in strains of *M. tuberculosis* and in host innate immunity contribute significantly to development of TB meningitis.

CLINICAL PRESENTATION

Acute Bacterial Meningitis The clinical signs of acute bacterial meningitis vary with patient age and condition at the time of presentation. In newborns, initial signs and symptoms are nonspecific and indistinguishable from those expected with any serious bacterial infection: fever, fussiness, diminished oral intake, vomiting, and unwell appearance. Signs of meningeal irritation are not reliably elicited in newborns. More severely affected newborns will have a septic appearance, hypothermia, bulging fontanel, seizures, and altered level of consciousness. Older infants are usually febrile, fretful, unhappy, and difficult to console. Vomiting is common and infants sometimes stroke their heads as a sign of headache. A full fontanelle is notable, but dehydration from vomiting and decreased feeding can lead to a sunken fontanel.

In older children, initial signs and symptoms include fever, headache, malaise, and vomiting, any of which could be present for days. Children with mild or moderate symptoms may have meningismus. Examination in the supine position in children is not sensitive for detection of nuchal rigidity. A more sensitive means is to have the child seated in a chair, then attempt neck flexion with the child's legs extended. Kernig's or Brudzinski's signs could be present with more significant meningismus; however, evidenced-based guidelines of the European Society for Clinical Microbiology and Infectious Diseases in 2016 declared presence or absence of Kernig's and Brudzinski's signs "do not contribute to the diagnosis of bacterial meningitis." Delay in treatment or more rapid progression of disease is associated with seizures, altered level of consciousness, and even coma. Septic shock accompanies bacterial meningitis in around 10% of cases, and initial patient evaluation must consider this possibility with prompt administration of intravenous (IV) antibiotics and support of circulatory volume and tissue perfusion.

TABLE 94-3 British Research Council Severity Grading System for Tuberculous Meningitis

Severity	Clinical Status at Presentation	Estimated Rate death or disability
Grade I	GCS 15; no focal neurological signs	15%
Grade II	GCS 11-14 or 15 with focal neurological signs	30%
Grade III	GCS ≤10	50%

GCS, Glasgow Coma Score.

Source: Adapted with permission from Wilkinson RJ, Rohlwink U, Misra UK, et al. Tuberculous Meningitis. *Nat Rev Neurol.* 2017; 13(10):581-598.

Tuberculous Meningitis The symptom development in TB meningitis tends to be subacute compared with the more common acute bacterial causes. The onset can be insidious with weeks of nonspecific symptoms (loss of appetite, weight loss, low-grade fever, irritability, decreased activity, and increased sleeping) prior to the development of more disturbing symptoms that lead to medical evaluation. At the time of presentation, most patients will have some combination of fever, lethargy, persistent headache, vomiting, meningismus, seizures, altered mental status, obstructive hydrocephalus, and focal neurological abnormalities involving cranial nerves or extremities. Most cases of TB meningitis in the United States and Western Europe occur in preschool-aged children. Young children with TB meningitis often have a history of contact with an adult case of *M. tuberculosis* infection and have evidence of pulmonary or other extra-pulmonary involvement. The British Medical Research Council system for categorizing severity of TB meningitis based on findings at presentation is useful clinically because severity grade is a strong predictor of outcome, **Table 94-3**.

CLINICAL EVALUATION

Medical History and Physical Examination A careful and complete medical history is essential. **Table 94-4** provides a list of information from medical history that is necessary in order to determine whether the patient is at increased risk because of comorbidities, medications, inadequate immunization, specific exposures, or rate of progression of the current illness. The medical history can be completed shortly after the patient is stabilized and initial orders are placed.

Physical examination must focus on identifying signs of meningitis, neurological findings, and alterations in homeostasis that require immediate attention. It is important to determine whether the patient needs supportive care for shock and whether there is evidence of increased ICP. Examination with an ophthalmoscope can identify changes that occur early with increased ICP. Retinal veins become engorged when they are under increased pressure and are thus more easily seen. With increasing pressure, venous pulsations are lost, and optic disk margins become indistinct due to swelling of optic nerve axons. Although papilledema

TABLE 94-4 Key Elements of Medical History for Patient With Possible Meningitis

- Present illness
  - ✓ First day of symptoms, last day patient was well
  - ✓ Effect of illness on ability to perform usual daily activities
  - ✓ Changes in mental status
  - ✓ Presence or absence of fever, headache, neck stiffness, vomiting
  - ✓ Abnormal movements or seizures
  - ✓ Focal weakness or paralysis
  - ✓ Recent hospitalization or surgical procedures
  - ✓ Exposure to others with similar symptoms or acute febrile illnesses
  - ✓ Medications received for this illness
- Past medical history
  - ✓ Immunizations – documented if possible
  - ✓ Allergy to antibiotics
  - ✓ Infections requiring hospitalization
  - ✓ CNS surgery—shunts, implants
  - ✓ Head injury
  - ✓ Congenital heart disease or endocarditis
  - ✓ Daily immunosuppressive medications or antibiotics
- Family history
- Current or past meningitis
- Problems with serious or life threatening infections
- Social history
  - ✓ Group living arrangement: dormitory, homeless shelter
  - ✓ Day care, school attendance
  - ✓ Environmental exposures, freshwater recreation, camping
  - ✓ Travel history

is uncommon in bacterial meningitis, early diagnosis of increased ICP makes it possible to prevent complications. Other physical findings that are important to document are vital signs (heart rate, blood pressure, respiratory rate, temperature), evidence of head trauma, level of consciousness (pediatric Glasgow Coma Score), cranial nerve function (especially III and VI), focal neurological deficits, any focus of infection, cardiac abnormalities, petechiae, purpura, and skin rash. In most cases of possible meningitis, the medical history and physical examination are sufficient to reach a clinical diagnosis of meningitis.

Laboratory Evaluation Laboratory evaluation must include a complete blood count with differential and platelet count; blood culture; lumbar puncture to obtain CSF for gram stain, culture, white blood cell count (WBC) with differential, and glucose and protein concentrations. Other laboratory tests that can be useful in learning more about the disease process include a chemistry profile (hepatic and renal function, electrolytes), C-reactive protein, and procalcitonin. If tuberculous, fungal or parasitic meningitis are possible based on the CSF results, clinical presentation, or exposures, it is important to notify the laboratory and obtain organism-specific testing of CSF and blood. Viral testing of CSF can be helpful if a viral etiology is suspected or the gram stain is negative.

When TB meningitis is being considered, consultation with a specialist in pediatric infectious diseases is recommended. The CSF in TB meningitis will usually have fewer than 500 WBC/mm^3 (often predominantly monocytes), elevated protein (often more than 1 g/dL), and low glucose (10-40 g/dL). Cultures and stains for *M. tuberculosis* in CSF are positive in only around one-third of cases. Diagnostic evaluation will include a chest radiograph and either an interferon-γ release assay (IGRA) (preferred for all ages), which measure host cellular immunity to *M. tuberculosis* antigens, or a tuberculin skin test. Evaluation should also attempt to detect *M. tuberculosis* in gastric washings, urine, lower respiratory tract, and from any accessible extra-pulmonary sites of disease such as skin lesion or enlarged lymph nodes. Interferon-γ release assays measure host cellular immunity to *M. tuberculosis* antigens and can provide evidence of infection. New methods based on detection of *M. tuberculosis* nucleic acids or antigens in CSF will improve the ability to confirm the diagnosis of TB meningitis.

MANAGEMENT

Bacterial Versus Viral Meningitis CSF findings in viral meningitis are typically different from those in bacterial meningitis: no bacteria appear on gram stain; the glucose is ≥50% of serum glucose; the protein is not elevated to more than twice the upper limit of normal; the WBC is in the low hundreds rather than thousands, and there is not a neutrophil predominance. However, there is considerable overlap between viral and bacterial meningitis in CSF leukocyte counts, protein and glucose concentrations, and gram stain results are sometimes incorrect or negative due to prior antibiotic treatment. Although it is imperative to promptly identify and treat all cases of bacterial meningitis, antibiotics are of no benefit in viral meningitis, and their unnecessary use exposes patients to adverse effects and prolongs hospitalization. Results of CSF culture are not available when making initial decisions about antibiotics, so scoring systems are useful in helping to distinguish patients with bacterial meningitis from those who are more likely to have viral meningitis. A meta-analysis by Nigrovic et al establishes the Bacterial Meningitis Score (BMS) as an accurate scoring system to identify patients with CSF pleocytosis with very low risk of bacterial meningitis, **Table 94-5**.

Patients with none of the predictors listed in Table 94-5 are considered "very low risk" of having bacterial meningitis, while children with one or more predictors are considered "not low risk." A meta-analysis found this dichotomous scoring system had a sensitivity of 99.3% for bacterial meningitis. In the analysis, patients were excluded if they had any of the following: critical illness, purpura, CSF shunt, recent neurosurgery, immunosuppression, other bacterial infections that require inpatient antibiotic treatment, active Lyme disease, or receipt of antibiotics (oral or parenteral) within 72 hours prior to lumbar puncture. This scoring system makes it possible to identify patients who could possibly be followed as outpatients, potentially after administering a long-acting parenteral antibiotic. Thus, application of the score could reduce unnecessary hospitalizations, with the safety net of antibiotic coverage while awaiting culture results. However even with the score, some patients with viral meningitis will be considered "not low risk" prompting use of empiric antibiotics and hospitalization.

A multi-site study by Mintegi et al based on previously healthy children with CSF pleocytosis seen in emergency departments in Spanish hospitals incorporated results for CRP and procalcitonin into a scoring system (named the Meningitis Score for Emergencies, MSE) for identifying patients with bacterial meningitis. Points are assigned as follows: 3 points for serum procalcitonin >1.20 ng/mL, 2 points for CSF protein >80 mg/dL, 1 point for serum CRP >40 mg/L, and 1 point for CSF ANC >1000/μL. A score of 1 or greater is 100% sensitive for predicting bacterial meningitis (95% CI: 89.0%-100%), with a specificity of 77.4% (95% CI: 70.3%-83.2%). The exclusions for the MSE study were similar to those listed for the Bacterial Meningitis Score validation study. These scoring systems can be helpful in distinguishing patients who are unlikely to have bacterial meningitis from those in whom it is likely, but they are not a replacement for clinical judgment and cannot be used for patients who meet exclusion criteria for the validation studies. Before using these

TABLE 94-5 Components of the Bacterial Meningitis Score for Establishing Risk of Bacterial Meningitis

Score Predictors	Criteria
CSF Gram stain	Positive
CSF ANC	≥ 1000 cells/mm^3
CSF protein	≥ 80 mg/dl
Peripheral blood ANC	≥ 10,000 cells/mm^3
Seizure	Onset at or prior to presentation

Note: Patients who lack all five of the listed features have very low risk for bacterial meningitis (Nigrovic, 2012). This scoring system should not be used for patients who meet exclusion criteria used in the validation study; see text for details.

scoring systems in patient management, reading the publications that validate their accuracy is recommended.

Empiric Antibiotics Ampicillin and ceftazidime are the empiric antibiotics for community dwelling newborns up to a month of age to cover GBS, *E. coli* and *Listeria*. Perinatal *Listeria* transmission results in newborn infection during the first month of life. Empiric ampicillin is generally not needed for older infants unless exposure history or CSF findings suggest the possibility of *Listeria* infection. Up to 90 days of age, GBS and *E. coli* continue to be important causes of bacterial meningitis, especially for infants born prematurely. The combination of vancomycin and ceftriaxone will provide coverage for GBS and *E. coli* as well as *S. pneumoniae, N. meningitidis,* and *H. influenzae*. In communities in which *S. pneumoniae* resistance to ceftriaxone is rare, some clinicians do not include vancomycin in empiric regimens. Meropenem is used in place of ceftriaxone when there is concern for *E. coli* with extended-spectrum beta-lactamase (ESBL) resistance or for other gram negatives with resistance to cephalosporins. Antibiotic dosage recommendations are available in the *Red Book*, published by the American Academy of Pediatrics.

Empiric antibiotics for community acquired bacterial meningitis in patients older than 90 days primarily target *S. pneumoniae, N. meningitides,* and *H. influenzae,* though GBS meningitis is occasionally seen in infants older than 90 days. The combination of vancomycin and ceftriaxone is recommended. Similar to considerations for infants from 30 to 90 days of age, knowledge of antibiotic resistance patterns might justify use of ceftriaxone alone. Practitioners could add ampicillin if exposure history or CSF findings suggest the possibility of *Listeria* and substitute meropenem for ceftriaxone for patients allergic to cephalosporins.

Recommended empiric antibiotics are used for 48 to 72 hours with the expectation that bacterial culture results and organism specific antibiotic sensitivity will be available within that time interval. If there is no bacterial growth in blood or CSF, and the patient did not receive intravenous or oral antibiotics prior to lumbar puncture, antibiotics can usually be discontinued at that time.

Antibiotic Treatment of Bacterial Meningitis **Table 94-6** lists recommended treatment regimens for common causes of bacterial meningitis. Antibiotic dosages are provided in the *Red Book*. Initiation of pathogen specific treatment is based on laboratory identification of pathogen and available antibiotic sensitivity. Resistance or intermediate sensitivity to penicillin G, ampicillin, and third-generation cephalosporins are key factors in antibiotic selection. If *S. pneumoniae* is resistant

TABLE 94-6 Antibiotics for Treatment of Common of Bacterial Causes of Meningitis in Infants and Children

Microorganism	Antibiotic	Duration
S. agalactiae	Newborn: ampicillin or penicillin G plus gentamicin Infants/children: ampicillin or penicillin G. If allergic, ceftriaxone, or linezolid	14-21 days
E. coli	Ampicillin if sensitive	at least 21 days
	Ceftriaxone if resistant to ampicillin	
	meropenem if resistant to both	
N. meningitidis	Penicillin G or ampicillin	7 days
	ceftriaxone if resistant to penicillin G	
S. pneumoniae	Penicillin G or ampicillin	10-14 days
	Ceftriaxone if resistant to penicillin G	
	Meropenem if resistant to both	
H. influenzae	β-lactamase negative: ampicillin β-lactamase positive: ceftriaxone β-lactamase negative, ampicillin resistant: meropenem	7-10 days
L. monocytogenes	Ampicillin or penicillin G	At least 21 days

Source: Adapted from Kimberlin D, Barnett ED, Lynfield R, Sawyer MH, eds. *Red Book, 2021-2024 Report of the Committee on Infectious Diseases*. 32nd ed. Itasca, IL: American Academy of Pediatrics; 2021.

or of intermediate sensitivity to both penicillin G and ceftriaxone, continuing vancomycin is recommended. This will require close monitoring of renal function as well as pharmacokinetic monitoring of serum vancomycin concentrations. Vancomycin should not be used alone to treat meningitis because of difficulty in achieving effective levels in CSF. The addition of cefepime or preferably (authors' opinion), meropenem is recommended if there is resistance to ceftriaxone. Similar considerations apply if there is a history of allergy to penicillin or ampicillin with anaphylaxis. In this situation, ceftriaxone can be used with attention to the possibility of concurrent allergy to cephalosporins. Penicillin G or ampicillin are the drugs of choice for treatment of meningitis due to GBS, *S. pneumoniae* and *N. meningitidis*. If a patient has a history of penicillin allergy, properly supervised desensitization is recommended.

Patient receipt of oral or intravenous antibiotics prior to lumbar puncture causes around 10% to 50% of CSF cultures to be negative, making treatment decisions difficult. Greater length of prior treatment results in lower chance of growing the causative agent. When no pathogen is cultured from CSF, other laboratory results are helpful. Blood cultures are positive in approximately 50% to 90% of cases of bacterial meningitis when obtained prior to antibiotic exposure and sometimes even after antibiotics have been given. Blood culture that reveals a pathogen will provide antibiotic sensitivity results. When performed by an experienced technician, gram stain can accurately identify the most common bacterial causes of meningitis. Latex agglutination tests on CSF or other body fluids lack sensitivity and specificity and should not be used. Polymerase chain reaction (PCR) in some cases can identify the bacterial etiology; it is conceivable that in the near future PCR will provide both pathogen identification and presence of genes associated with antibiotic resistance. Availability of PCR testing for bacteria in CSF is variable and data on positive and negative prediction values is limited. A positive result from CSF PCR can be helpful, but a negative PCR might not rule out bacterial infection. If there is laboratory identification of the presumptive infecting agent (gram stain or PCR), but no cultured bacterium for antibiotic susceptibility testing, then antibiotic choice is based on knowledge of local and regional rates of antibiotic resistance. In cases of prior antibiotic treatment with all tests for pathogens negative, it could be helpful to examine the scoring systems (BMS and MSE). These are based on laboratory results that are available on all cases in which it was possible to obtain CSF. Applying these scoring systems could lead one to stop antibiotics and observe the patient carefully or proceed with treatment for bacterial meningitis.

Antimicrobial Treatment for Tuberculous Meningitis Initiation of empiric treatment for TB meningitis is recommended in any child with meningitis and evidence of basilar brain inflammation with hydrocephalus or cranial nerve involvement and no evidence for another cause. Treatment consists of antimicrobials with glucocorticoids for every patient, and neurosurgical intervention may be necessary for patients with hydrocephalus. A four-drug antituberculous regimen is recommended: isoniazid, rifampin, pyrazinamide, and ethambutol or an aminoglycoside. Glucocorticoids used for TB are dexamethasone or prednisone/prednisolone, and the WHO recommends six to eight weeks of treatment for suspected or confirmed TB meningitis. Pediatric hospitalists should consult pediatric infectious disease physicians at the time empiric treatment for TB meningitis is started.

Problems in Management of Bacterial Meningitis

Failed Lumbar Puncture If clinical assessment is compatible with bacterial meningitis, no CSF was obtained, and no pathogen identified by blood culture, continuing the empiric antibiotic regimen for a treatment course is recommended. In most cases like this, ceftriaxone alone is suitable in children with no comorbidities associated with immune system impairment, assuming the patient continues to improve.

Contraindications for Lumbar Puncture If there is evidence of increased intracranial pressure or an intracranial space-occupying lesion, it is reasonable to question the safety of removal of CSF by lumbar puncture. **Table 94-7** demonstrates factors associated with high risk of LP in adults, and Brouwer et al suggests that if none of the listed risk factors are present, brain imaging prior to LP in adults is not needed. This list could be helpful in management of children with possible meningitis; however, thrombocytopenia, coagulopathy due to disease or medication, septic shock and respiratory failure also need to be addressed before performing an LP in

TABLE 94-7 Possible Contraindications to LP Based Largely on Studies in Adults

- New onset seizures
- Immunocompromised state (HIV, organ transplantation, immunosuppressive medications)
- History of CNS lesion (mass lesion, stroke, focal infection)
- Signs of space occupying lesion (papilledema, focal neurological deficits, signs of brain shift)
- Moderate to severe impairment of consciousness
- Thrombocytopenia or coagulopathy
- Septic shock
- Respiratory failure

Source: Data from Brouwer MC, Thwaites GE, Tunkel AR, van de Beek D. Dilemmas in the diagnosis of acute community-acquired bacterial meningitis. *Lancet*. 2012; 380(9854):1684-1692.

children. When factors that increase the risk to the patient are present, it is reasonable to consider delaying LP until results of brain imaging are available and presumed risk factors for herniation are resolved. Brain herniation can occur in bacterial meningitis due to edema and brain swelling resulting from infection and inflammation even if no LP is performed. A goal of management of bacterial meningitis is administration of IV antibiotics within the first hour of care. If LP is delayed, antibiotic administration must not be delayed. It is important to obtain a blood culture prior to initiating antibiotics.

Steroids Adjunctive treatment with dexamethasone for children with nontuberculous bacterial meningitis remains controversial. Evidence of benefit of giving steroids after the etiology is identified or in meningitis due to bacterial causes other than *H. influenzae b* is lacking. Guidelines published in 2004 from the Infectious Disease Society of America (IDSA) recommend adjunctive treatment with dexamethasone for all adults with pneumococcal meningitis. For infants and children 6 weeks and older with pneumococcal meningitis, the American Academy of Pediatrics in 2021 suggests considering adjunctive therapy with dexamethasone. The dexamethasone should ideally be given before or concurrently with the first dose of antibiotic, but consensus from the European Society for Clinical Microbiology and Infectious Diseases states that "in the absence of scientific evidence," adjunctive dexamethasone could be started up to 4 hours after initiation of antibiotics. A 2013 systematic review by Brouwer et al of randomized clinical trials of corticosteroids in bacterial meningitis did not find evidence of benefit of corticosteroid use to prevent severe hearing loss in children with meningitis due to bacteria other than *H. influenzae b*. The same study did not find evidence of benefit in mortality or short-term neurological sequelae for *H. influenzae b* or other etiologies. Considering the goal of rapid initiation of antimicrobial therapy for children with bacterial meningitis, the rarity of *H. influenzae b* as a cause in the United States, and the fact that knowledge of the etiology is unlikely to be known within 4 hours of antibiotic administration, it is understandable that there is not a firm recommendation on use of adjunctive steroids for bacterial meningitis in children.

FOCAL BACTERIAL CNS INFECTIONS

Focal CNS bacterial infections include parenchymal abscesses, subdural empyema, epidural abscess, and septic venous thrombophlebitis. Abscess in the CNS is an enclosed collection of purulent material. Empyema is a collection of purulent material that is not enclosed and able to spread within an anatomical boundary. In otherwise healthy hosts, abscess and empyema are caused by bacteria and are rarely due to other microorganisms. Abscesses can be located anywhere within the CNS, including the brain or spinal cord parenchyma and epidural and subdural spaces. Empyemas are usually in the epidural or subdural space.

EPIDEMIOLOGY AND ETIOLOGY

CNS Abscess Bacterial brain parenchymal abscesses are reported by Weinberg et al to be as common as 0.3 to 1.3 per 100,000 persons per year. Almost one-quarter of all brain abscesses occur in children, mostly between 4 and 7 years of age. The majority of cases are associated with a predisposing factor, congenital heart disease, lung infection, meningitis or extension from infections in middle ear, mastoid, sinuses, or intracranial epidural abscess. Meningitis and postoperative surgical infections are rare causes of brain abscess. Epidural abscesses usually arise by extension of infection from contiguous sites: sinuses, middle ear, or orbit. Spinal epidural abscesses occur most frequently in children around age 7 to 8 years, while spinal subdural abscesses occur most commonly in infants and toddlers. Intramedullary spinal cord abscesses are extremely rare. The most common source of spinal epidural abscess is vertebral osteomyelitis, though it can also arise from hematogenous spread, contamination of surgical sites or needle sticks (including LP), or dermal sinus tracts. In younger children, subdural empyemas can occur as a complication of meningitis, and at any age from extension from infections in middle ear, sinuses, or osteomyelitis of the skull. Intracranial septic venous thrombophlebitis usually results from extension of infection from sphenoid or ethmoid sinuses, middle ear, or teeth.

These abscesses, particularly when resulting from extension of infection from the mastoids or sinuses, may be polymicrobial. The most commonly involved microorganisms in the etiology of intracranial infections in children are aerobic and anaerobic streptococci (60%-70%), gram-negative anaerobic bacilli (20%-40%), *Enterobacteriaceae* (20%-30%), *Staphylococcus aureus* (10%-15%), and fungi (1%-5%). Neonates and infants are more likely to have infections with gram-negative organisms than *S. pneumoniae*. Children with shunts, penetrating traumatic injuries, or nosocomial infections are more likely to have infections with methicillin resistant *S. aureus* (MRSA). Approximately one-third of brain abscesses are polymicrobial, including both aerobic and anaerobic organisms. No organism is identified in about half of case. Abscesses form equally as commonly in the right and left hemispheres, and approximately 80% are found in the frontal, parietal, or temporal lobes; while the remaining 20% are in the occipital lobe, brain stem, or cerebellum.

Septic Intracranial Venous Sinus Thrombosis Cerebral sinovenous thrombosis in children is rare. A Canadian study by deVeber et al estimated the incidence to be 0.67 cases per 100,000 children under 18 years of age per year; approximately 25% of these were due to infection. In neonates, the triggering infection is usually a systemic bacterial or fungal infection or meningitis. In older children, local suppurative infections—mastoiditis, otitis media, and sinusitis—are the leading causes. The bacterial etiologies are primarily those that cause the triggering infection: GBS, *E. coli*, *Staphylococcal* species, and *Candida* in newborns; and in older children aerobic and anaerobic streptococci, *S. aureus* and, occasionally, gram-negative anaerobic rods.

PATHOGENESIS

Brain parenchymal abscesses are thought to begin as a focal area of cerebritis that develop over days to weeks into an encapsulated collection of necrotic tissue and pus. Bacteremia increases risk of intracranial infection in patients with venous to arterial shunting (from uncorrected intracardiac shunts, arteriovenous malformations, hereditary hemorrhagic telangiectasia, hepatopulmonary syndrome, pulmonary arteriovenous malformation, or other conditions). Brain abscesses from hematogenous spread of bacteria are often multiple and in the distribution of the middle cerebral artery. In contrast, intracranial spread of infection from a contiguous site typically leads to a single abscess. Trauma that penetrates the dura will introduce bacteria from the skin and other contaminated sites into the CNS. Surgery or other invasive procedures (LP, medication injection, or epidural anesthesia) can introduce bacteria from the skin into the CNS and initiate cerebritis and abscess formation.

Most epidural and subdural abscesses develop by spread of infection from contiguous sites including acute otitis media, mastoiditis, sinusitis, facial infections, vertebral or cranial osteomyelitis (Pott puffy tumor), and facial or odontogenic infections. Sinusitis pathogens spread through vasculature to the dura, leading to abscess formation in the temporal and frontal lobes. Once the bacteria are in the subdural space, they can spread across the surface of brain and spinal cord. Neonates and young infants develop subdural empyema in about 2% to 10% of bacterial meningitis cases. Spinal epidural abscesses are more common in children with underlying disease including immunocompromise, tuberculosis, and vertebral osteomyelitis. Up to one-quarter of patients with spinal epidural abscess have a history of trauma with hematoma. By contrast, spinal abscesses in the subdural or intramedullary spaces are usually associated with midline congenital dermal sinus tracts. Other risk factors include spinal cord tumors, trauma, and bacterial meningitis.

CLINICAL PRESENTATION

Intracranial Abscess Signs and symptoms of brain parenchymal abscess can be subtle or nonspecific early in the illness, potentially leading to a delay in diagnosis. Oral antibiotics, if given, may provide temporary improvement and thus contribute to delayed diagnosis. Early in the illness, patients often have low-grade fever, headache, and malaise. Severity of illness can progress rapidly or gradually over a week or longer. As the illness progresses, headache is the most common symptom, occurring in about 70% of patients; pain is usually localized to the area of the abscess. Fever and vomiting occur in 40% to 60% of patients. Focal neurological findings and altered mental status occur in 30% to 50% of children. Seizures, meningeal signs, and hemiparesis occur less frequently. The classic triad of fever, headache, and focal neurologic deficits occurs in fewer than 30% of all cases. Lethargy, stupor, and coma are more likely late in the course of illness.

Intracranial epidural abscesses and subdural empyemas cause symptoms very similar to those of brain parenchymal abscesses. Patients with CNS empyemas tend to be sicker. They are consistently febrile and are more likely to have mental status changes, seizures, and hemiparesis. The size and location of abscesses as well as immune status of the child influence the clinical presentation.

Spinal Epidural and Subdural Abscesses Back or flank pain is often the initial symptom of spinal abscess, and movement, especially spinal rotation, worsens this pain. Nerve root compression produces localized pain or paresthesia that may help in localizing the abscess. Focal neurologic deficits are initially subtle but progress to weakness and alterations in sensation. Paraparesis can develop within 1 week from the onset of back pain, about 4 days from the onset of nerve root pain. Patients may experience bowel or bladder dysfunction and changes in mental status. Early intervention is essential to prevent permanent paralysis.

Septic Intracranial Venous Sinus Thrombosis Common presenting manifestations of septic intracranial sinovenous thrombosis are fever, headache, and vomiting. Neurological findings vary depending on the original site of infection, the involved venous sinus and the extent of thrombosis. Ethmoid and sphenoid sinusitis are associated with cavernous sinus thrombosis. Diplopia, blurred vision, chemosis, weakness of lateral gaze, and periorbital edema suggest cavernous sinus thrombosis. Otitis media and mastoiditis are the common infectious causes of lateral and superior sinus thrombosis. Patients with lateral sinus thrombosis are likely to complain of otalgia and have evidence of otitis media or mastoiditis. Cranial nerve VI palsy also occurs with lateral sinus thrombosis, and patients may complain of retro-orbital or facial pain due to cranial nerve V inflammation. Superior sagittal sinus thrombosis as a complication of meningitis tends to present with signs and symptoms of CNS involvement including mental status changes, seizures, meningismus, and papilledema.

CLINICAL EVALUATION

Medical History and Physical Examination A thorough medical history, particularly in search of risk factors for CNS infection and subtle changes in behavior, mobility, strength, mental status, focal pain, paresthesia, bowel and bladder control and ability to pursue usual daily activities is essential. In addition to a general physical exam, patients should have a thorough neurological exam documenting mental status, cranial nerve function, sensation, limb strength, and reflexes.

Laboratory Evaluation Routine blood tests for patients with possible focal CNS bacterial infections are the same as those recommended for patients with meningitis. Blood cultures should be obtained prior to starting antibiotics. Laboratory results will not allow one to accurately distinguish bacterial meningitis, brain or spinal parenchymal abscess, epidural or subdural abscess. It is important to identify a pathogen. Blood cultures are positive in only around 10% of patients. In patients with CNS infection related to otitis or mastoiditis, culture of fluid from middle ear could be helpful. Imaging guided needle aspiration will provide material for culture (aerobic and anaerobic bacteria and fungi) and abscess drainage. Neuroimaging rather than CSF analysis remains the diagnostic study of choice for establishing the diagnosis (**Figure 94-1**).

Neuroimaging CNS imaging is a critical step in evaluation of patients with suspected focal bacterial CNS infection and should be performed as rapidly as possible. Magnetic resonance imaging (MRI) with contrast is preferred. MRI is more sensitive in detecting early cerebritis, necrosis, edema, and satellite lesions and allows better visualization of the brain stem and posterior fossa. If spine or paraspinous infections are the concern, MRI is superior in identifying coinciding diskitis, osteomyelitis, and paraspinal abscesses. For suspected septic sinovenous thrombosis, MRI venography improves ability to identify and define the extent of a thrombus. If MRI is not available, or there will be a delay due to sedation needs of young children, high resolution CT scan with and without contrast and CT venography is acceptable

Differential Diagnosis The differential diagnosis of focal bacterial CNS infections includes many other infectious and noninfectious processes. In immunocompromised patients, the range of infectious causes includes bacterial species not mentioned here and a variety of fungi. Other space-occupying lesions include hemorrhage, cysticercosis, and primary and metastasized cancer. The majority of sinovenous thromboses are not caused by infection but arise from a variety of acute illnesses (including stroke, gastroenteritis, dehydration, and sepsis) and chronic conditions (including prothrombotic disorders, inflammatory bowel disease, lupus, diabetes, nephrotic syndrome, and hemoglobinopathies). For spinal cord and paraspinous abscess, other diagnoses to consider include diskitis, tuberculosis of the vertebrae or spine, vertebral osteomyelitis (particularly from *Bartonella henselae*), transverse myelitis, spinal cord tumor, lymphoma, vascular malformation, and hematoma in the spine or epidural or subdural spaces.

TREATMENT

Intracranial Abscess Neurosurgical consultation is recommended for all intracranial abscesses. Medical treatment alone may be successful in neurologically intact children who have no signs of increased ICP, and in whom the abscess is smaller than 3 cm in diameter. For most intracranial abscesses, image-guided needle aspiration for drainage in combination with antimicrobial therapy remains the treatment of choice. Subdural infections often require surgical intervention for drainage. In patients with intracranial empyema or abscess, antimicrobial therapy should be started immediately after sampling of the infection and blood cultures are obtained. Empirical treatment should cover likely pathogens for most infections: streptococci, staphylococci (including MRSA), anaerobes, and *Enterobacteriaceae.* A combination of vancomycin, a third-generation cephalosporin (e.g., ceftriaxone, cefotaxime, or ceftazidime) plus metronidazole is recommended. For brain abscesses that arise as a complication of meningitis, empiric antibiotics should be aimed at the known or likely cause of meningitis. The decision to narrow antibiotic coverage based on cultures remains controversial because many infections are polymicrobial, and there is a risk of failure to identify additional pathogens, especially anaerobic bacteria. If culture is negative for *S. aureus* and *Enterococcus*, then vancomycin can usually be discontinued. Unless a source of infection caused by a specific bacterium is known (as in endocarditis or meningitis), anaerobic coverage is usually continued at least until substantial clinical improvement has been achieved. In general, IV therapy is continued for 4 to 8 weeks. Some authorities recommend an additional 2 to 3 months of oral antibiotics. Response to therapy should be monitored with neuroimaging techniques. Even with therapy, mortality from brain abscess and empyema remains relatively high, and a third of survivors have neurologic sequelae. Poor prognostic indicators include age younger than 1 year, rapid neurologic impairment, multiple foci, and coma at the time of diagnosis.

Spinal Abscess In contrast to intracranial abscesses that may be treated without open surgical drainage, a space-occupying lesion of the spinal cord often requires urgent surgical intervention to relieve pressure

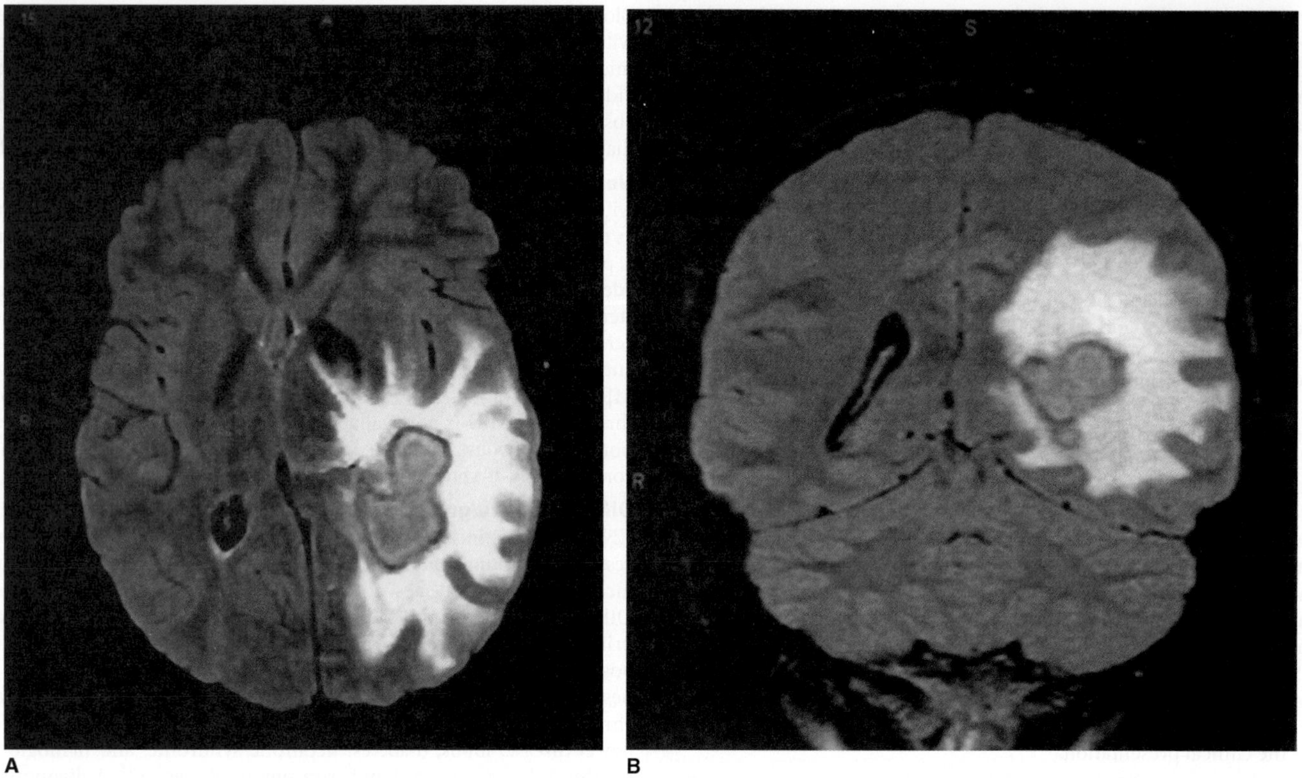

FIGURE 94-1. Brain magnetic resonance imaging in a 12-year-old girl demonstrates a multiloculated abscess in the left temporoparietal region. Thick rim enhancement (appears dark on these T2 images) is seen on both the axial (A) and coronal (B) views. Large amounts of vasogenic edema (appears bright white) is seen extending into the left cerebral hemisphere.

on nerves and stop the progression of permanent neurological deficits. Patients who have no signs of cord or nerve root compression for at least 3 days may be treated with antibiotics alone, but this requires frequent repeat MRI imaging and serial neurological exams. As in intracranial infections, selection of an antibiotic regimen will be guided by the most likely cause of infection. Antibiotic penetration of the CNS is essential for subdural abscesses but less so for infections limited to the epidural space.

DEVICE-RELATED CNS INFECTIONS

Chapter 103, Device-Related Infections, covers CSF shunt-related infections.

INFECTIONS ASSOCIATED WITH COCHLEAR IMPLANTS

Cochlear implants are used to facilitate hearing in children and adults with severe to profound sensorineural hearing loss. A cochlear implant is a complex device that receives auditory input from the environment, organizes these signals, and converts them to electrical impulses that are transmitted via a wire to electrodes arranged in the cochlea to stimulate hair cells. Placement of a cochlear implant results in an indwelling device installed below the skin surface on the skull near the ear and wires and electrodes that remain in the inner ear. Infection risk is related to the surgical procedure itself, an indwelling device, the opening of the cochlea, and the anatomical communication between the inner ear and the subarachnoid space. The presence of a cochlear implant makes it possible for many children to hear and achieve use of expressive and receptive spoken language, but it does carry increased risk of bacterial meningitis.

Epidemiology and Etiology Rates of cochlear implant–related infections over the past 3 decades range from 1% to 13% of patients, and are mostly soft tissue infections. Meningitis is much less common but remains more frequent in recipients of cochlear implants than in the general population. In the early years of use, implants had an additional internal connection through a positioner that was associated with an estimated meningitis risk 450 times that of the general population. That device is no longer used, and estimates that are more recent indicate the increased risk to be 2 to 10 times that of the general population. Risk factors for cochlear implant infections are young age (<5 years), previous meningitis, CSF shunt, cochlear trauma or failure to seal opening, and longer duration of surgical procedure.

Pathogenesis Understanding of the mechanisms that account for the increased risk of meningitis in cochlear implants is limited. A persistent opening in the cochlea allowing communication with the middle ear is a possibility. In children, frequent purulent otitis media is associated with implant infection. Lack of full immunization against *S. pneumoniae* is a key risk factor for pneumococcal meningitis in these patients.

Diagnosis and Management The possibility of cochlear implant infection and meningitis must be considered for any child admitted to the hospital with fever or evidence of inflammation at the site of the implant. The signs of implant device infection overlap significantly with skin infection. These include tenderness and swelling of soft tissue, erythema, and exudate at the surgical wound. Distinct tenderness at the external portion of the implant is more suggestive of infection of the device. Important details of medical history include: when and where cochlear implant was placed, the type of device, history of otitis media, known CSF leak, meningitis, and immunization status. It is essential to involve otolaryngology in the initial evaluation of any child with a cochlear implant who is hospitalized with an acute febrile illness or possible infection. The otolaryngologist will be able to provide information on risk factors for infection related to surgery or the specific device as well as the history of otitis media. In addition, the otolaryngologist will likely have experience evaluating children with possible implant infections.

Laboratory evaluation is essentially the same as for a patient with possible bacterial meningitis. A lumbar puncture must be performed unless the hospitalist and the otolaryngologist are confident that meningitis is not present. Blood culture and cultures at the site of infection can be very helpful. MRI cannot be used for cochlear implant patients without surgical removal of the magnets in the device, though there may be some exceptions. It is unclear whether CT imaging is helpful in identifying early meningitis in these patients. Antibiotic treatment will focus on the most common causes of implant infections: *S. pneumoniae, H. influenzae, S. aureus* (MRSA and MSSA), and *Streptococcus pyogenes*. *Pseudomonas* is less frequent overall but is more common in older children and those with a history of chronic, draining otitis media. A reasonable empiric choice for cochlear implant infection and possible meningitis is vancomycin and ceftriaxone, substituting ceftazidime or cefepime if *Pseudomonas* is a concern. Treatment of meningitis will be based on results of cultures of CSF and blood. Once bacterial meningitis has been ruled out, antibiotics can be adjusted appropriately for the situation. In the absence of meningitis, the goal of antibiotic treatment is to preserve the implant, which is successful in around 50% of patients.

VIRAL CNS INFECTIONS

Viral infections are the most common cause of hospitalization of children with acute onset of CNS symptoms not due to trauma or medication overdose. Viral CNS infections can generally be considered in two broad categories based on clinical presentation: meningitis and encephalitis, though there is considerable overlap in signs, symptoms, and viral etiologies. In addition to meningitis and encephalitis, viral infections of the CNS can also cause focal signs of motor nerve damage or peripheral neuropathy. *Herpes simplex virus* (HSV) is the only common cause of viral CNS infections for which there is effective antiviral treatment, and rapid initiation of empiric treatment for HSV is essential for any patient with concern for encephalitis until etiology is established.

EPIDEMIOLOGY

Exposure to an infected person is the most common source of viral infections associated with CNS disease in the United States. Humans are the source for almost all viruses. Lymphocytic choriomeningitis virus (LCMV) and arboviruses, of all the viruses listed in **Table 94-8,** are the exceptions.

Many people infected with viruses are asymptomatic or only mildly ill (sometimes without fever), making identifying the source of infection difficult. The CDC uses the following definition for surveillance of viral or aseptic meningitis: acute illness with fever and meningeal signs with CSF pleocytosis with neither culture nor serological evidence of bacterial or fungal infection. Viruses cause most meningitis in children. Among hospitalized children with meningitis, viruses are implicated in around threefold more cases than bacteria. Precise incidence rates are difficult to ascertain as patients who have received antibiotics prior to presentation are often assumed to have bacterial meningitis. In addition, the improvements in knowledge and available laboratory methods for establishing viral etiology of CNS infection make older data less relevant. Enteroviruses (EV) cause most cases of viral meningitis, usually with seasonal increases in infection rates between July and October in North America. EVs spread through various routes: fecal-oral, respiratory secretions, and vertically from mother to fetus. Sporadic enterovirus outbreaks in closed populations can involve any age, including hospitalized newborns. Mortality rates with viral meningitis are very low. Rudolph et al reports an estimated mortality rate of 0.03%, a calculation from WHO data not limited to hospitalized patients or children.

A study by Vora et al of hospital discharge data from 1998 to 2010 provided a US population-based estimate of 20,258 hospitalizations annually for encephalitis with 3648 cases per year in children (≤19 years). Annual incidence rates per 100,000 (95% confidence interval) for encephalitis hospitalization for children by age were 11.1 (10.1-12.1) for <1 year, 4.7 (4.3-5.1) for 1 to 4 years, and 4.0 (3.7-4.2) for 5 to 19 years. In only about half of encephalitis-associated hospitalizations was an etiology specified. A study by Bagdure et al based on hospital discharge diagnosis codes from 44 freestanding children's hospitals, for the 10-year interval, 2004 to 2013, identified 7298 admissions for encephalitis. The median age of patients was 9 years, and 51% were male. The median length of hospital stay was 16 days, and the overall mortality rate was 3.2%. Information on etiology of encephalitis was not included. More recent studies focused on hospital-based convenience samples and using molecular methods for diagnosis identified a viral etiology for the majority of children hospitalized with aseptic meningitis or encephalitis.

TABLE 94-8 Viral Etiologies of CNS Infection

Common Etiologies	Less Common and Rare Etiologies
Enteroviruses	Arboviruses
Coxsackievirus	California serogroup
Echovirus	La Crosse virus
Enterovirus	Jamestown Canyon virus
	California encephalitis virus
Parechoviruses	Chikungunya virus
Herpes simplex viruses 1 & 2	Dengue virus
	Eastern equine encephalitis virus
	Japanese encephalitis virus
	Powassan virus
	St. Louis encephalitis virus
	Tick-born encephalitis virus
	West Nile virus
	Western equine encephalitis virus
	Zika virus
	Herpesviruses
	Varicella Zoster Virus
	Epstein Barr Virus
	Cytomegalovirus
	Human herpes viruses 6 & 7
	Lymphocytic choriomeningitis virus
	Measles virus
	Mumps virus
	Polio Virus
	SARS-CoV-2 virus

ETIOLOGY

Table 94-8 lists common and uncommon viral etiologies of CNS infection. Virus names and groupings listed are those prevalent in clinically oriented literature and in viral diagnostic reports. While some viruses are listed as uncommon or rare, they can be common in an endemic area (like Dengue and Japanese encephalitis virus), during outbreaks (including arboviruses, mumps, and poliovirus), in areas with low levels of childhood vaccine coverage (for measles and mumps), or in a specific population (including newborns and cases of HSV encephalitis). Prior to widespread use of mumps vaccine in the United States, mumps was a common cause of meningitis.

Enteroviruses

Enteroviruses are the most common viral causes of CNS infections in children in the United States. For simplicity, common names for members of the enterovirus (EV) family (enterovirus, coxsackievirus, echovirus) are used in Table 94-8. There are 10 EV species, designated by letters A through J. Human pathogens are found almost entirely among A, B, and C species with two notable exceptions: EV D68 and EV D70. Parechoviruses were previously included as Echoviruses but are now recognized as a separate species. Enteroviruses and parechoviruses are prominent causes of acute febrile illnesses, viral exanthems, and "fever without source" in newborns and young infants. The development of molecular testing of CSF for viral etiologies has revealed the prominent role of enteroviruses and parechoviruses and provided evidence that aseptic meningitis in children is usually viral. Enteroviruses are also implicated as a cause of a variety of neurological disorders including cerebellar ataxia, meningoencephalitis, acute flaccid myelitis, brainstem encephalitis, and Guillain-Barré syndrome.

Arboviruses

An insect vector (most often a mosquito) transmits viruses identified as arboviruses. Arboviruses include viruses from different virus families. Most human arboviral infections result in subclinical disease or febrile syndromes that do not involve the CNS, but cases of arboviral CNS disease can involve meningoencephalitis with severe and concerning encephalitis. ArboNET, the US national arboviral surveillance system collects data on arbovirus infections and associated encephalitis. According to the CDC in 2022, La Cross encephalitis occurs sporadically in the United States with 5 to 150 cases reported each year. In 2020, there were 88 cases, and 83 (94%) of these were in children. Historically, cases of La Crosse encephalitis are more likely to occur in West Virginia and northern Midwestern states, but recently more cases are in mid-Atlantic and southeastern states.

West Nile virus (WNV) is the etiologic agent of West Nile fever and West Nile neuroinvasive syndromes. Transmission occurs through *Culex* mosquitos with seasonal (July-September) increases in cases during times mosquito activity and human outdoor exposure coincide. WNV is the leading cause of arboviral CNS disease in adults in the United States and is an important cause in children. According to Soto with the CDC, only 16/731 (2%) of reported WNV infections were in children < 18 years in 2020. However, WNV cases that year were around half what is typical. Herring reports that over the past two decades, around 4% of WNV neuroinvasive disease was children, and around 25% to 30% of reported pediatric cases have involved neuroinvasive disease.

St. Louis encephalitis virus is a flavivirus relative of WNV. Infections with this virus are much less common, with only 16 reported US cases in 2020, none of them in children. Eastern equine encephalitis and Powassan virus encephalitis cases are reported mostly in the Northeast, with 13 and 21 cases, three each in children, reported in 2020. Almost all cases of both involved neuroinvasive disease.

Herpes Viruses

HSV CNS infection at any age can be devastating. Neonatal HSV encephalitis occurs in the first weeks of life, and the incidence of neonatal herpes is reported by Whitley in 2018 to be 5.24 per 10,000 live births. Transmission usually occurs from mother to child during birth and rarely occurs prenatally. Infections can also occur after birth through contact with a person (usually a caregiver) with HSV infection. In the past, genital herpes and neonatal herpes were linked almost exclusively to the type 2 virus. It is now clear that both HSV 1 and 2 are responsible for adult genital herpes and neonatal HSV infection.

HSV encephalitis in older children and adults results from primary or recurrent HSV infection and is estimated to occur in approximately 1 in 100,000 to 150,000 individuals per year in the United States. Fewer than 10% of these cases are attributable to HSV type 2. In healthy children, the other members of the herpesvirus family (varicella-zoster virus [VZV], human herpesvirus 6 [HHV6], cytomegalovirus, and Epstein-Barr virus) rarely cause meningitis or encephalitis. Although VZV is a significant cause of CNS disease in older adults, routine childhood vaccination has made it rare in children. Cerebellar ataxia is the most common neurologic complication after primary VZV infection, occurring in approximately one in 4000 patients.

Other Viruses

Severe acute respiratory syndrome virus-2 (SARS-CoV-2), LCMV, measles, mumps, rubella, rabies, and polio are rare causes of CNS disease in the United States. With SARS-CoV-2, it is unclear whether the encephalopathy that has occurred in some severe cases in children is due to direct viral infection of the CNS or the result of severe systemic inflammation triggered by the infection.

Routine childhood immunization has made encephalitis due to measles, mumps, rubella virus, and polioviruses rare in the United States. However, recent outbreaks of measles and polio in communities affected by vaccine hesitancy show that infections and CNS disease will return if high immunization rates are not maintained.

Rabies virus infection results in a deadly encephalitis. Rabies virus infections are acquired from contact with secretions of infected wild and domestic animals. Vaccination of pets against rabies, animal control efforts, and availability of post-exposure prophylaxis have reduced rabies cases in the United States to fewer than three per year.

LCMV infection is present in around 5% of *Mus musculus*, the common house mouse. Human LCMV infection is acquired by contact with urine, droppings, saliva, or nesting materials of mice, other wild rodents, or less often, laboratory animals or pets. Infection is facilitated by breaks in the skin or rodent bites. Hamsters and other domestic rodents acquire infection from contact with wild rodents and can expose humans. LCMV infection can be transmitted transplacentally during pregnancy, with severe consequences for the fetus, including hydrocephalus, severe cognitive deficits and chorioretinitis. Population based data on incidence of human infection is not available, and most infections go unrecognized. Seroprevalence studies report antibodies to LCMV in from 2% to 5% of urban dwellers. Human to human transmission does not occur except in the setting of organ transplantation.

PATHOGENESIS

The pathogenesis of viral CNS infection likely follows the following steps: host entry; viremia; initial replication at permissive sites; secondary viremia; dissemination; penetration of blood-brain-barrier; and then infection of leptomeninges, glial cells, and neurons. For viruses transmitted by the fecal-oral route, the site of entry is likely intestinal lymphoid tissue. Respiratory-transmitted viruses enter through the nasopharyngeal epithelium. Among enteroviruses, it is likely that both fecal-oral and respiratory spread occur. Mosquito or tick vectors inject arboviruses directly into the blood stream. Regional lymphoid tissue and vascular endothelial cells are initial sites of replication common to different sites of entry. Initial replication rapidly (within hours) leads to a primary viremia allowing infection to spread through the body. Tropism determines which tissues are infected, based largely on the ability of viral surface molecules to bind to host cell receptors and facilitate entry into host cells. A secondary, higher level of viremia follows ongoing viral replication at multiple sites and is associated with initial symptoms like lethargy, malaise, fever and rash. Viruses get past the blood-brain barrier via a hematogenous route or by retrograde transport via neuronal axons (as for some enteroviruses, rabies virus, and herpesviruses). The precise mechanisms are not well defined. Within the CNS, viral infection can lead to death of infected glial and neuronal cells. Host immune and inflammatory responses also contribute to tissue damage and affect symptoms and outcomes.

An intact mucosal barrier and surface antibodies are the first lines of defense. Host innate immunity (including pattern recognition molecules, type 1 interferon, and natural killer cells) slow viral replication and spread, providing time for the adaptive immune responses to generate neutralizing antibodies and cytotoxic T lymphocytes. The importance of adaptive immunity is demonstrated by the near-elimination of polio and varicella zoster virus CNS disease in US children with vaccines.

CLINICAL PRESENTATION

Viral CNS infections present with fever and meningeal signs or signs of brain infection (including confusion, seizures, delirium, impaired consciousness, focal neurological signs, paresis or paralysis, new onset seizures, dysautonomia, or coma). Patients hospitalized with signs of encephalitis often have meningoencephalitis with clinical evidence of meningitis. Patients who have viral meningitis without clinical evidence of encephalitis typically present with fever, malaise, headache, vomiting and nuchal rigidity. Studies aimed at identifying features that help distinguish bacterial meningitis from viral meningitis have not identified any clinical features (exclusive of laboratory results) that reliably distinguish bacterial meningitis from viral meningitis. Although seizures, petechiae or purpura, and hemodynamic instability at the time of presentation occur more frequently in bacterial meningitis, they can also occur with viral meningitis. Most patients with viral meningitis for whom bacterial meningitidis excluded can be managed as outpatients if they do not have signs of encephalitis and do not require inpatient supportive care.

Clinical features in patients with viral CNS infection can sometimes suggest a specific etiology. In HSV encephalitis, seizures and neurological signs may relate to the temporal lobes. Unusual findings in HSV encephalitis include Bell's palsy, atypical pain syndromes, trigeminal neuralgia, myelitis, and recurrent or chronic inflammation of the meninges. Neonatal encephalitis from perinatal HSV infection has a typical clinical course starting with nonspecific symptoms like fussiness and difficulty with feeds as early as postnatal days 7 to 10, progressing by day 10 to 21 to worsening fussiness, vomiting, refusal to feed, lethargy, obtundation, and focal seizures. Enteroviral encephalitis can be associated with a biphasic fever pattern: the first fever with associated generalized symptoms, and the second with CNS symptoms. Enteroviral and parechovirus infections may be accompanied by exanthema.

Arboviruses characteristically have a prodrome of systemic illness that may also be accompanied by nausea and vomiting. VZV is associated with two distinct neurological illnesses: acute encephalitis and cerebellar ataxia. Cerebellar ataxia is associated with vomiting, nystagmus, headache, and can be associated with nuchal rigidity. Acute flaccid myelitis is a distinct, dangerous condition seen in previously healthy children with enterovirus infections, notably EV D68 and EV A71. It is characterized by acute onset of flaccid limb weakness and specific MRI findings of gray matter changes in the spinal cord. Up to 25% of involved patients require ventilatory support. A number of other viruses have been associated with acute onset of limb paralysis, including polio, LCMV, tick born encephalitis virus, and Japanese encephalitis virus.

MANAGEMENT

All patients with signs of encephalitis require hospital admission for diagnostic evaluation, antiviral treatment, and management of complications that impair homeostasis. A detailed medical history is essential to identify exposures and risk factors (Table 94-4). In addition to all elements of an age-appropriate physical examination, a thorough neurological examination is required. Ophthalmological examination and hearing testing can help define the extent of neurological involvement and contribute to diagnosis.

MRI with and without contrast is required for every patient hospitalized with encephalitis unless it is contraindicated. If there are physical findings compatible with spinal cord involvement, MRI should include brain and spinal cord. MRI is more sensitive than computed tomography for identifying changes early in disease associated with specific causes of encephalitis. Most notably, HSV encephalitis causes high-intensity T2-weighted lesions in bilateral temporal lobes. EEG may demonstrate abnormalities in the early stages of encephalitis and reveal changes that affect management such as status epilepticus or focal temporal lobe discharges suggestive of HSV encephalitis.

Laboratory Evaluation Encephalitis is often associated with signs of multi-system illness, and laboratory evaluation can contribute to understanding the extent of disease. In addition to tests focusing on the CNS, the hospitalist should obtain a complete blood count, electrolytes, renal and liver function tests, urine analysis, and acute phase reactants (CRP and procalcitonin). It is essential to obtain a blood culture prior to the first dose of any antibiotics that may be given. Every patient with encephalitis needs a lumbar puncture. Neurology consultation should be considered prior to lumbar puncture because they may aid in directing specialized testing of CSF for autoimmune encephalitis. LP can be deferred until imaging is performed, as MRI can relieve concerns for mass lesions, cerebral edema, increased intracranial pressure, and shifts in the brain. Routine CSF studies for cell count, gram stain, glucose, protein, and culture (for bacteria, fungi, and mycobacteria), HSV PCR and multiplex viral panel are necessary. CSF cell counts and chemistries are nonspecific in terms of identifying a virus and can occasionally be normal early in infection. Typically, cell counts range from 10 to a few hundred mostly lymphocytic cells; glucose is usually normal; and protein is often increased. Samples of serum and CSF should be retained for specific antibody testing if needed. For some viral causes of encephalitis, it is not possible to find the virus in CSF. Although serum immunoglobulins do not cross the blood-brain barrier in significant quantities, there are resident B-lymphocytes in the CNS that produce antibody in response to infection. In acute CNS infections due to enteroviruses, WNV and other arboviruses, detection of IgM antibody in CSF has established etiologic diagnosis when virus culture or PCR were negative. Antibody testing of serum and CSF can usually be arranged through reference laboratories or communicable disease services of state health departments and the CDC.

Differential Diagnosis Except during viral outbreaks, around half of encephalitis in hospitalized children is due to causes other than viral infection. Autoimmune encephalitides, medication (overdoses or side effects), trauma, and non-viral infections produce similar symptoms. Careful history, physical examination, and laboratory testing can identify CNS symptoms due to trauma or medication. Autoimmune encephalitis occurs in association with systemic rheumatologic disorders, paraneoplastic syndromes, and appears to be triggered by viral (usually HSV) encephalitis. The importance of early recognition of autoimmune encephalitis is demonstrated in cases of anti *N*-methyl-D-aspartate receptor (anti-NMDAR) encephalitis; early diagnosis and treatment is clearly associated with better outcome.

Nonviral infectious agents that cause encephalitis include bacteria, fungi, protozoa, and helminths. In depth discussion of these infections is beyond the scope of this text, but a few deserve mention. Bacteria found to cause encephalitis include *Treponema pallidum*, *Mycoplasma*, *Campylobacter*, *Bartonella*, *Leptospira*, *Borrelia burdorferi* (Lyme disease), and *Rickettsia*. The most common acquired fungal causes of encephalitis in immunocompetent children in the United States are *Blastomyces dermatitidis* and *Cryptococcus gattii*; both cause meningoencephalitis and are difficult to treat. Although fungal CNS infection is much more common in immunocompromised patients, both infections are also seen in healthy hosts. *C. gattii* infection is becoming more frequent in some geographic areas, perhaps related to climate change. Encephalitis due to helminths is rarely seen in US children. It can be due to a variety of tissue nematodes, notably *Toxocara canis*, *T. cati*, and *Baylisascaris procyonis*; tape worms, especially *T. solium* and protozoa. *T. solium* is the cause of neurocysticercosis, probably the most common parasitic CNS infection in the United States. It often presents with new onset focal seizures and has characteristic cystic lesions on brain imaging. Encephalitis due to ingestion of eggs of *Baylisascaris procyonis*, a roundworm that infects raccoons, is particularly concerning because this parasite can continue to grow in human tissues (including the brain), and mortality of infection is high. A rare protozoal infection that seems to be increasing in prevalence in the United States is encephalitis due to *Naegleria fowleri*, an amoebic species common in fresh water in warm climates. Amebic encephalitis due to this organism progresses rapidly and is almost uniformly fatal; any chance at successful treatment requires a high index of suspicion and rapid initiation of treatment.

Treatment of Viral Encephalitis For most pediatric patients with viral CNS infection, there is no antiviral treatment available. HSV encephalitis is the notable exception. It is a necrotizing brain infection that will quickly cause irreversible brain damage. Prior to effective antiviral treatment, the outcome of neonatal HSV encephalitis was death or severe neurological sequelae. With acyclovir treatment in neonates, mortality is reduced to 5% and neurological sequelae to 30%. The availability of antiviral treatment led to similar dramatic improvements in HSV encephalitis in older children and adults. Unless another etiology is confirmed, all children hospitalized with encephalitis should receive IV acyclovir as soon as possible and continue it until HSV infection is ruled out. Regimens for treatment of HSV encephalitis in newborns, infants and older children and for VZV infections are available in the *Red Book*. In newborns, induction treatment of at least 21 days of acyclovir is followed by 6 months of suppressive treatment. Neutropenia and impaired renal function are common adverse events during acyclovir treatment, especially at higher doses, so intermittent laboratory monitoring is required. Dosage adjustment is required if renal function is impaired and should occur regularly to accommodate for patient growth.

Studies by Antoon et al and Frankl et al show that CNS symptoms compatible with encephalitis occur in around 7% to 10% percent of children hospitalized with influenza. Evidence of direct infection of the CNS is lacking, and infection-related inflammation seems to be the likely cause. Treatment with oseltamivir is recommended for all children hospitalized with influenza. For those with CNS symptoms, 10 days of oseltamivir is recommended. At the time of publication of this chapter, baloxavir is currently approved for use in some children with influenza but not for those who are hospitalized.

Supportive Care for Viral Encephalitis Hospital care of patients with encephalitis is challenging. Admission to a critical care unit should be considered initially because these patients can experience rapid clinical deterioration. Complications including seizures, agitation, autonomic instability, dysphagia, respiratory insufficiency or failure, fluid and electrolyte problems, and hemodynamic instability can appear suddenly. Management often requires input from subspecialists (see Consultation section below). In the recovery period, patients often need supportive care for nutrition and temporary or persistent disabilities including weakness or paralysis, confusion, aphasia, dysphagia, and inability to perform activities of daily living. The length of hospital stay for acute viral encephalitis patients often ranges from 2 to 4 weeks.

OTHER CONSIDERATIONS

CONSULTATION

Pediatric hospitalists are expected to be able to diagnose and manage newborns, infants, and children with bacterial meningitis due to the causes listed in **Table 94-2**. For patients with chronic illnesses associated with impaired host defenses such as leukemia, cancer chemotherapy, organ or hematopoietic stem cell transplantation, HIV infection, or congenital immunodeficiency, it is important to coordinate care with the subspecialists who follow them. These patients have increased risk of meningitis due to fungi or parasites. Subspecialists will have experience with infections in their patients, and they will be able to guide modifications to immunosuppressive medication regimens that may help the patient overcome the infection. Consultation with a pharmacist is very helpful when antibiotic monitoring is required (as in vancomycin or aminoglycosides) or renal or hepatic insufficiency necessitates dosing adjustment. Consultation with a pediatric infectious disease specialist is recommended for all cases of meningitis or focal bacterial infections due to *M. tuberculosis*, fungi, protozoa, helminths, or bacteria that are resistant to commonly used β-lactam antibiotics, including ESBL and carbapenem-resistant organisms. Consultation with the infectious diseases service should also be considered in all patients with HSV or VZV CNS infections for assistance with antiviral management and follow-up after inpatient treatment is completed.

Patients with bacterial meningitis and shock require immediate fluid resuscitation to maintain adequate tissue perfusion. Patients with shock are best served by initial placement in a pediatric critical care unit. Initial placement in a critical care unit is also strongly recommended for all patients with possible CNS infections with evolving focal neurological signs, inability to respond to verbal stimuli, evidence of increased ICP, concerning abnormalities in heart rate, blood pressure or respirations, or new onset of seizures. If critical care placement is not available, the hospitalist should request consultation.

Neurosurgeons, and in some cases, otolaryngologists, should be consulted for CNS infections involving abscesses, empyema or surgical procedures, or trauma. A neurosurgeon will aid in determining the necessity of surgical drainage of the abscess or empyema and may be helpful in drainage and culture of the site prior to antibiotic administration. Neurosurgical consultation is also required for any patient with concern for infection of their CSF shunt. Consultation with otolaryngology is necessary for patients with abscess related to sinusitis, otitis, or mastoiditis and for all patients with concern for infections related to cochlear implants. When symptoms and signs suggest spinal cord involvement, involvement of both neurosurgery and orthopedics is recommended.

Patients with encephalitis or possible infectious sino-venous thrombophlebitis often require a multi-disciplinary team to finalize diagnosis and manage hospital care and complications. This team could include pediatric hospitalists working with specialists in critical care, neurology, neurosurgery, infectious diseases, and neuroradiology.

PREVENTION

Pediatric hospitalists can make a significant contribution to primary prevention of CNS infections by participating in ensuring necessary immunization of their patients. Vaccines for *H. influenzae b, S. pneumoniae, N. meningitidis*, measles, mumps, rubella, VZV, and polio have dramatically decreased CNS infections. Immunization status should be documented on all patients during hospitalization. When a patient is incompletely immunized, a plan for catching-up should be implemented during hospitalization and communicated to the primary care provider.

Chemoprophylaxis is essential in decreasing spread of *N. meningitidis* and *H. influenzae*. Thus, it is necessary to quickly identify people who have had significant contact with patients infected with these bacteria. Because it is necessary to provide chemoprophylaxis as soon as possible, the pediatric hospitalist should prescribe prophylactic antibiotics and instructions for family members and household contacts of the index case. In cases when contacts live outside of the patient's household, it is necessary to involve public health authorities. Recommendations for post-exposure chemoprophylaxis of contacts with a case of invasive meningococcal disease take into consideration the risk based primarily on closeness of contact, the age of the exposed person, antibiotic choices, and possible need for post-exposure meningococcal vaccine. Similar recommendations are provided for household and childcare contacts of children with invasive *H. influenzae* disease. With the exception of pregnant women, prophylaxis for both is with rifampin.

ADMISSION CRITERIA

With the exception of patients with established viral meningitis who do not require hospital level supportive care and for whom there is no concern for evolving meningoencephalitis or bacterial meningitis, all children with suspected or proven CNS infection require hospitalization for diagnosis and management.

DISCHARGE PLANNING

In children with bacterial CNS infection or HSV encephalitis, discharge may be considered once the patient has completed antimicrobial therapy and no longer requires inpatient supportive care. Some patients with bacterial infections may be candidates for parenteral outpatient therapy. Most patients hospitalized with CNS infections will require post-hospitalization follow-up to confirm continued improvement, identify signs of persistent impairments, and in some cases, complete treatment (outpatient antibiotics or oral suppressive acyclovir for neonatal HSV infection, or anticoagulants for sino-venous thrombosis). In addition, at the time of hospital discharge, some patients will have cognitive, sensory or motor impairments. The hospital medicine service must see that those services that are involved in post-hospital care are involved in discharge planning. This will include the primary care provider for all patients and could include specialists in infectious diseases, neurology, neurosurgery, otolaryngology, orthopedics, hematology, and rehabilitation medicine

SUGGESTED READINGS

Antoon JW, Hall M, Herndon A, et al. Prevalence, risk factors, and outcomes of influenza-associated neurologic complications in children. *J Pediatr*. 2021;239:32-38.

Bagdure D, Custer JW, Rao S, et al. Hospitalized children with encephalitis in the United States: A Pediatric Health Information System Database Study. *Pediatr Neurol*. 2016;61:58-62.

Brouwer MC, Thwaites GE, Tunkel AR, van de Beek D. Dilemmas in the diagnosis of acute community-acquired bacterial meningitis. *Lancet*. 2012;380(9854):1684-1692.

Brouwer MC, McIntyre P, Prasad K, van de Beek D. Corticosteroids for acute bacterial meningitis. *Cochrane Database Syst Rev*. 2013;(6):CD004405.

deVeber G, Andrew M, Adams C, et al. Cerebral sinovenous thrombosis in children. *N Engl J Med*. 2001; 345(6):417-423.

Frankl S, Coffin SE, Harrison JB, Swami SK, McGuire JL. Influenza-associated neurologic complications in hospitalized children. *J Pediatr*. 2021;239:24-31.

Harrison CJ, Berkovich R. Focal suppurative infections of the nervous system. In: Long SS; Prober CG; Fischer M; Kimberlin DW, Ed. *Principles and Practice of Pediatric Infectious Diseases, 6th ed*. Philadelphia, PA: Elsevier; 2022.

Hasbun R, Wootton SH, Rosenthal N, et al. Epidemiology of meningitis and encephalitis in infants and children in the United States, 2011-2014. *Pediatr Infect Dis J*. 2019;38(1):37-41.

Bennett JE, Dolin R, Blaser MJ, eds. *Mandell, Douglas and Bennett's Principles and Practice of Infectious Diseases*. 9th ed. Philadelphia, PA: Elsevier; 2020. Two sections: Hasbun R, van de Beek D, Brouwer M, Tunkel AR. Acute Meningitis:1183-1219; and Tunkel AR. Subdural empyema, epidural abscess and supurative intracranial thbrombophlebitis:1262-1271.

Herring R, Desai N, Parnes M, Jarjour I. Pediatric West Nile virus-associated neuroinvasive disease: a review of the literature. *Pediatr Neurol*. 2019;92:16-25.

Holmquist L, Russo A, Elixhauser A. Meningitis-related hospitalizations in the United States, 2006. In: Services HaH, ed. *Statistical Brief #57*. Rockville, MD: Agency for Healthcare Research and Quality 2008.

Kim KS. Bacterial meningitis beyond the neonatal period. In: Cherry JD, Harrison GJ, Kaplan S, Steinbach WJ, Hotez PJ, eds. *Feigin and Cherry's Textbook of Pediatric Infectious Diseases*. 8th ed. Philadelphia, PA: Elsevier; 2019:309-336.

Kimberlin D, Barnett ED, Lynfield R, Sawyer MH, eds. *Red Book, 2021-2024 Report of the Committee on Infectious Diseases*. 32nd ed. Itasca, IL: American Academy of Pediatrics; 2021.

Mintegi S, García S, Martín MJ, et al. Clinical prediction rule for distinguishing bacterial from aseptic Meningitis. *Pediatrics*. 2020;146(3):e20201126.

Nigrovic LE, Malley R, Kuppermann N. Meta-analysis of Bacterial Meningitis Score validation studies. *Arch Dis Child*. 2012;97(9):799-805.

Rudolph H, Schroten H, Tenenbaum T. Enterovirus infections of the central nervous system in children: an update. *Pediatr Infect Dis J*. 2016;35(5):567-569.

Shachor-Meyouhas Y, Bar-Joseph G, Guilburd JN, Lorber A, Hadash A, Kassis I. Brain abscess in children—epidemiology, predisposing factors and management in the modern medicine era. *Acta Paediatr*. 2010;99(8):1163-1167.

Soto RA, Hughes ML, Staples JE, Lindsey NP. West Nile virus and other domestic nationally notifiable arboviral diseases—United States, 2020. *MMWR Morb Mortal Wkly Rep*. 2022;71:628-632.

Tsang RS. A narrative review of the molecular epidemiology and laboratory surveillance of vaccine preventable bacterial meningitis agents: *Streptococcus pneumoniae, Neisseria meningitidis, Haemophilus influenzae* and *Streptococcus agalactiae*. *Microorganisms*. 2021;9:449.

Tunkel AR, Hartman BJ, Kaplan SL, Kaufman BA, Roos KL, Scheld WM, Whitley RJ. Practice guidelines for the management of bacterial meningitis. *Clin Infect Dis*. 2004;39:1267-1284.

Tyagi R. Spinal infections in children: a review. *J Orthop*. 2016;13:254-258.

van de Beek D. European Society for Clinical Microbiology and Infectious Diseases (ESCMID) Guideline: diagnosis and treatment of acute bacterial meningitis. *Clin Microbiol Infect*. 2016;22:S37-62.

Vora NM, Holman RC, Mehal JM, Steiner CA, Blanton J, Sejvar J. Burden of encephalitis-associated hospitalizations in the United States, 1998-2010. *Neurology*. 2014; 82(5):443-451.

Weinberg GA. Brain abscess. *Pediatr Rev*. 2018;39:270-272.

Whitley R, Baines J. Clinical management of Herpes Simplex Virus Infections: past, present, and future. *F1000Res*. 2018; 7:F1000 Faculty Rev-1726.

Wilkinson RJ, Rohlwink U, Misra UK, et al. Tuberculous meningitis. *Nat Rev Neurol*. 2017;13(10):581-598.

CHAPTER 95 Complications of Acute Otitis Media and Sinusitis

Peter J. Gill, MD, DPhil and Karen E. Jerardi, MD, MEd

BACKGROUND

Uncomplicated acute otitis media (AOM) and sinusitis are generally managed in the outpatient setting with excellent outcomes. Occasionally, complications from these infections arise, and a subset of these complications requires immediate intervention and hospitalization (**Table 95-1**). Children with AOM and sinusitis are predisposed to infectious and inflammatory complications because of their close proximity to orbital and parameningeal structures. The separation between these structures and the middle ear or sinuses may be breached by two main mechanisms: (i) direct extension via communication between the middle ear and the mastoid airspace and thin bony walls separating the sinuses from intraorbital area, and (ii) hematogenous spread via penetrating veins from infected sinuses or mastoid spaces to the intracranial region.

TABLE 95-1 Complications of Acute Otitis Media and Sinusitis

Complications of Acute Otitis Media
Surrounding Bone
Mastoiditis
Petrositis
Middle/inner ear
Hearing loss
Cholesteatoma
Labyrinthitis
Facial nerve palsy
Intracranial
Meningitis
Epidural or intracranial abscess
Lateral sinus thrombosis
Complications of Acute Sinusitis
Extracranial
Periorbital cellulitis
Orbital cellulitis
Pott's puffy tumor
Intracranial
Meningitis
Epidural, subdural, or intracranial abscess
Venous sinus thrombosis

ACUTE OTITIS MEDIA AND COMPLICATIONS

AOM is defined as inflammation of the mucoperiosteal lining of the middle ear. An upper respiratory tract infection (URI) precedes most episodes of AOM and causes edema and obstruction of the Eustachian tube, which then impedes drainage of middle ear fluid. One-third of all URIs are complicated by AOM. Children under 3 years of age have a combination of narrower and more horizontal positioning of the Eustachian tubes and a relatively immature immune system, thus making them more susceptible to infection. Most episodes of AOM are treated with oral antibiotics in the outpatient setting. For treatment with parenteral antibiotics, a single dose of ceftriaxone eradicates AOM caused by *Haemophilus influenzae* and penicillin-susceptible *Streptococcus pneumoniae*. However, three intramuscular or intravenous doses are required to eradicate non-penicillin susceptible *S. pneumoniae*. In practice, given the lack of knowledge of the underlying causative agents in most children, three doses of parenteral antibiotics are recommended.

In the postantibiotic era, complications from AOM have decreased significantly, and are estimated to occur in 0.04% to 0.4% of cases. However, recent population based-studies suggest an increase in complications over the past decade. The sites of these complications include the surrounding bone, middle/inner ear, and intracranial spaces (**Table 95-1**).

MASTOIDITIS

Background and Pathophysiology The mastoid is the inferior posterior portion of the temporal bone and consists of air cells separated by bony septa. Although present at birth, the air cells are not fully pneumatized until 2 to 3 years of age. The mastoid air cells are adjacent to the middle ear, and the two are connected via a narrow opening called the aditus ad antrum. The middle ear and the mastoid share a continuous mucoperiosteum, so the mastoid air cells often become inflamed with middle ear infection. In cases of acute mastoiditis, the aditus ad antrum becomes obstructed and the inflammation within the mastoid air cells progresses to suppuration and necrosis.

Clinical Presentation The age-related incidence of mastoiditis mirrors that of otitis media. Some controversy exists regarding whether infants, whose mastoids are not fully formed, can truly have mastoiditis. However, inflammation and suppuration of the mastoid or antrum, or both, have been observed in this age group.

Children with mastoiditis may present with postauricular erythema, edema, and tenderness in association with fever and ear pain. Symptoms typically develop several days to weeks after an episode of treated or untreated AOM. The tympanic membrane appears abnormal in approximately 90% of cases. The examiner should look for the presence of a cholesteatoma, because it is frequently associated with subperiosteal abscesses in older children. If a subperiosteal abscess is present, the area posterior to the ear may be fluctuant and tender. In children younger than 1 year, the fluctuance is typically superior and posterior to the ear with the pinna displaced downward and outward. In children older than 1 year, the fluctuance is most commonly posterior and inferior to the ear with the pinna displaced upward and outward.

Differential Diagnosis The differential diagnosis of mastoiditis includes lymphadenopathy, parotitis, lateral sinus thrombosis, mastoid tumors, and branchial cleft cysts.

Evaluation and Diagnosis While the diagnosis can be made clinically, computed tomography (CT) of the mastoid/temporal bone with contrast enhancement should be obtained to evaluate for intratemporal or intracranial complications. On CT, children with early mastoiditis will demonstrate clouding or opacification of the mastoid air cells. Destruction of the bony septa and empyema formation indicate mastoiditis with osteitis. Subperiosteal abscess is also readily visualized by CT (**Figure 95-1A**).

An elevated C-reactive protein (CRP), erythrocyte sedimentation rate (ESR), and white blood cell count, with a predominance of neutrophils or band forms, may be observed with mastoiditis; however, these tests are neither sensitive nor specific. A blood culture should be obtained. Middle ear fluid samples collected after tympanocentesis or placement of a myringotomy tube should be sent for aerobic and anaerobic culture. Culture of fluid in the canal is less reliable than culture of the middle ear or the mastoid because of possible contamination with ear canal flora. Additionally, a lumbar puncture should be considered for patients with findings concerning for meningitis.

Course of Illness Acute mastoiditis is defined as the presence of symptoms for less than a month. Although most cases of mastoiditis are isolated, a small percentage may be complicated by extension of the infection. The possibility of extension of the mastoiditis necessitates frequent assessment of the patient's neurologic status and neck examination.

A subperiosteal abscess may occur if the infection extends to and penetrates the external cortex of the mastoid. A Bezold abscess occurs if the infection progresses inferiorly and extends into the deep tissues of the neck. It results in a collection beneath the sternocleidomastoid with swelling and tenderness. The facial nerve courses through the middle ear, thus making it susceptible to both direct infectious injury and mechanical compression from surrounding structures. Facial nerve palsy is usually unilateral, and paresis of the lower part of the face, as well as the forehead, would be seen, as expected with this peripheral neuritis. CT can identify the bony erosions and is important to assess for the possibility of cholesteatoma or other middle ear tumor. The facial nerve palsy generally improves as the infection is treated, usually with intravenous antibiotics and surgical drainage with placement of myringotomy tubes. If the infection extends into the petrous portion of the temporal bone (petrositis), Gradenigo syndrome, a triad of pain behind the eye, ear discharge, and abducens nerve palsy, may develop.

Intracranial complications occur either by hematogenous spread or by bony erosion leading to direct extension. Children with these complications frequently present with headache, fevers, and vomiting and may or may not demonstrate neurologic impairment. If intracranial complications are suspected, CT with contrast or magnetic resonance imaging (MRI) of the brain should be performed immediately, and neurosurgical consultation should be sought.

Lateral sinus thrombosis is a rare but well-described intracranial complication of AOM. While more often described in areas of the world with limited healthcare access, cases still occur in developed countries despite effective antibiotic therapy for AOM. Sinus wall inflammation resulting from middle ear infection can result in thrombosis, most typically in the sigmoid sinus given its position within the mastoid bone (**Figure 95-1B**). Children with lateral sinus thrombosis may present with spiking fevers (often called "picket fence" fevers), neck pain, headache, emesis, neurologic signs and symptoms, or any combination of these findings. They may also demonstrate evidence of distant septic thromboemboli. Case series have described signs and symptoms of elevated intracranial pressure (ICP) and cranial neuropathies (specifically

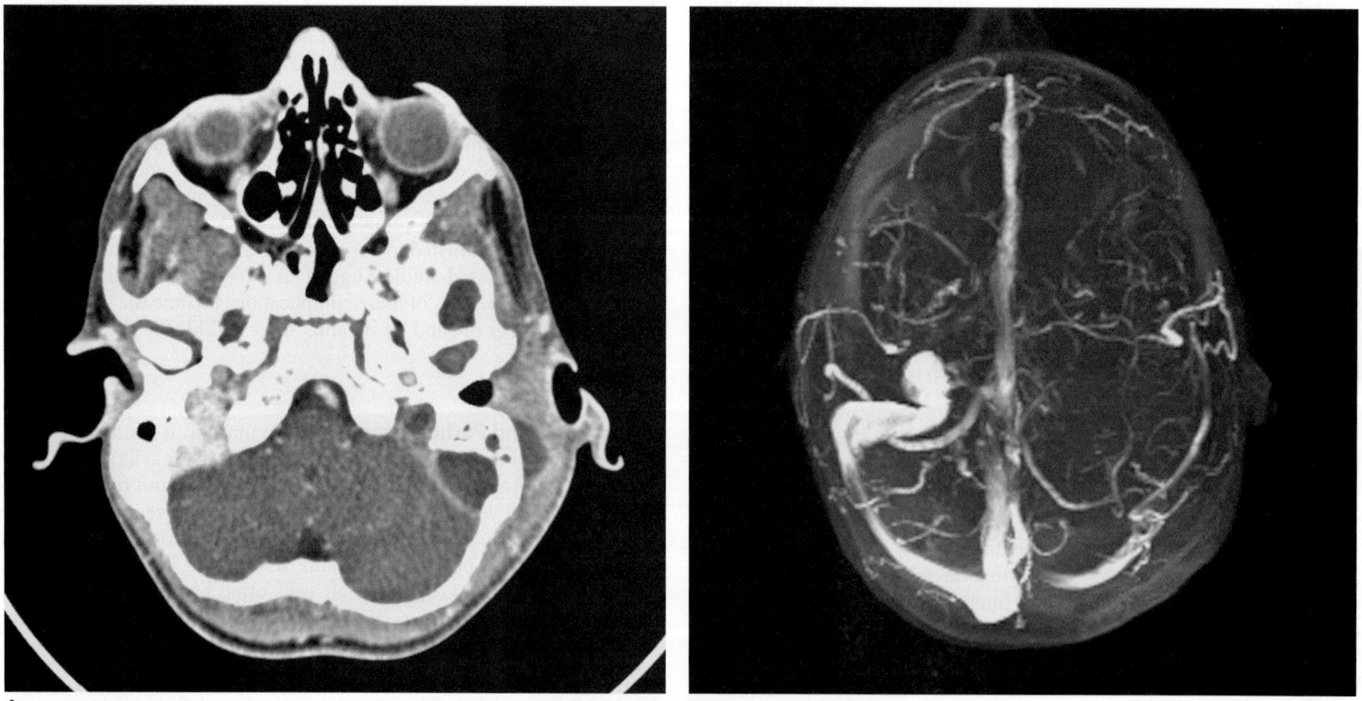

A B

FIGURE 95-1. A 12-year-old boy with acute left-sided mastoiditis complicated by epidural abscess and sigmoid sinus thrombosis. (A) Head CT in coronal view reveals a large rim-enhancing fluid collection along the left petrous bone that is consistent with a subdural abscess. (B) MRI with MR venography reveals venous thrombosis in the left sigmoid sinus to the proximal internal jugular vein.

6th and 7th nerve palsies) as being more often reported than symptoms of otalgia and fevers, despite most patients having recent AOM. Thrombosis may also occur in the mastoid emissary vein as a complication of AOM or mastoiditis. This results in edema or bogginess over the posterior mastoid, known as Griesinger sign.

Treatment • ***Medical management*** Antibiotic coverage should target the most common pathogens with cognizance of local resistance patterns. The microbiology of mastoiditis and AOM differs to some degree. As in AOM, *S. pneumoniae* is the most common pathogen. However, whereas *Moraxella catarrhalis* and nontypeable *Haemophilus influenzae* are the second and third most common organisms responsible for AOM, *Staphylococcus aureus* and group A β-hemolytic *Streptococcus* (GABHS; *Streptococcus pyogenes*) are the next most common bacteria found in mastoiditis. Anaerobes are isolated in up to 10% of cases. *Pseudomonas aeruginosa* (usually with chronic mastoiditis), and *Proteus* species, in addition to *M. catarrhalis* and nontypeable *H. influenzae*, also have been implicated.

Empirical antibiotic regimens typically include a third-generation cephalosporin or ampicillin-sulbactam. Patients should also receive clindamycin or vancomycin if they are seriously ill or methicillin-resistant *S. aureus* (MRSA) covered is desired. Patients with intracranial involvement should receive a third-generation cephalosporin with vancomycin and metronidazole. Antibiotic therapy can be modified based on intraoperative culture results if available. Most children require 4 weeks of antibiotics, though children with severe illness or intracranial complications may require 6 or more weeks of antibiotic therapy. Patients with mastoiditis with or without mastoidectomy can receive oral antibiotic therapy at discharge; patients with intracranial complications should receive parenteral antibiotics for the entire treatment course. The role of adjunctive corticosteroids is currently under investigation but they are not routinely recommended.

Surgical management Consultation from otolaryngology should be sought in the management of children with mastoiditis. Neurosurgical involvement should be considered if intracranial complications exist.

Tympanocentesis (with middle ear fluid culture) should be performed, preferably with tympanostomy tube placement. Indications for mastoidectomy include (i) osteitis or subperiosteal abscess, (ii) poor response to medical therapy within 48 hours, or (iii) evidence of intracranial complications. Treatment of petrositis involves intravenous antibiotics, placement of myringotomy tubes, and surgical drainage of the petrous portion of the temporal bone. Surgical decompression of the facial nerve is considered in some cases of facial nerve palsy associated with AOM/mastoiditis. Surgical drainage may also be indicated for a Bezold abscess that does not respond to antibiotic therapy.

Other Considerations For lateral sinus thrombosis, diagnosis is made with MRI with angiography/venography. Treatment should involve culture-directed antibiotic therapy and otolaryngology consultation for consideration of myringotomy tube placement and mastoidectomy. Additionally, if deemed safe after head imaging, lumbar puncture with measurement of opening pressure may be both diagnostic and therapeutic for otic hydrocephalus (benign increased ICP secondary to infectious process of the inner ear, not related to brain abscess or meningitis); repeat lumbar puncture may be necessary to manage increased ICP, and acetazolamide may be helpful by reducing production of cerebrospinal fluid. Anticoagulation should be considered, especially for patients with high risk for thrombus, clot extending beyond the sigmoid sinus, or neurologic changes. Consultation from hematology and neurosurgery is also warranted.

On completion of therapy, an audiogram should be considered for all children with mastoiditis.

Admission and Discharge Criteria Children with suspected mastoiditis, with or without evidence of further complications, should be hospitalized for intravenous antibiotics, definitive diagnosis, and, if needed, surgical management.

Discharge criteria include:

- Afebrile for 48 hours with an improving overall clinical picture
- No evidence of further complications (normal or improving neurologic findings)
- Ability to tolerate oral nutrition
- Compliance with oral antibiotic regimen or home parenteral therapy, if necessary
- Reliable follow-up with a generalist and otolaryngologist

Prevention The extent to which antibiotic therapy for AOM prevents complications of AOM, such as mastoiditis, is controversial. Up to 80% of children with untreated AOM will have resolution of symptoms within 7 to 14 days. A 2015 Cochrane review concluded that 20 children with AOM would need to receive antibiotic treatment to improve the clinical outcome (pain at 2-7 days) in one of the children. This evidence has led to the wait-and-see approach that asks caregivers to start the antibiotic if the patient is not improved in 48 hours; in these circumstances, the family receives a prescription for the antibiotic but does not obtain the medication unless symptoms have not improved. This approach significantly decreases antibiotic use and is not associated with differences in subsequent fever or ear pain at follow-up. Additionally, a systematic review concluded that if 100 children were treated with immediate antibiotic therapy for AOM, 12 more would improve than if none had received antibiotics, but up to 10 would develop a rash and 10 would develop diarrhea.

In the 2013 American Academy of Pediatrics clinical guideline, Lieberthal et al concluded that a "watch and see" approach to antibiotic use did not increase the risk for mastoiditis, and concluded that this approach is acceptable for children older than 2 years with a definite diagnosis of AOM but without severe illness (moderate to severe otalgia, otalgia lasting >48 hours, or fever >39°C) or in children between 6 months and 2 years of age without severe illness and without a certain diagnosis of bilateral AOM. This age-stratified recommendation was based on evidence indicating higher risk for severe illness and poor outcomes in children younger than 2 years of age. Further, a study in the United Kingdom examined records of over 2 million children and found risk of mastoiditis was halved by use of antibiotics but that almost 5000 episodes of AOM would need to be treated to prevent one case of mastoiditis, which was felt to preclude the use of antibiotic treatment of AOM as a method of preventing mastoiditis.

ACUTE SINUSITIS AND COMPLICATIONS

Sinusitis develops in 6% to 8% of episodes of URI, and typical cases can be diagnosed clinically. The peak incidence is in children age 2 to 6 years; by 3 years of age, 10% of children will have had sinusitis. Sinusitis is diagnosed when patients present with: (i) persistent symptoms or cough for >10 days without resolution; (ii) worsening course after initial improvement; or (iii) severe symptoms with purulent rhinorrhea, and fever >38.5°C for at least 3 to 4 days. URIs facilitate the development of sinusitis by causing mucosal edema with subsequent obstruction of the ostia and by impairing ciliary clearance of bacteria.

Whereas adults possess well-developed bilateral frontal, ethmoid, sphenoid, and maxillary sinuses (**Figure 95-2**), the presence of these sinuses in children depends on age. The maxillary and ethmoid sinuses begin to develop during the third month of gestation and are therefore present at the time of birth. In contrast, the frontal and sphenoid sinuses do not pneumatize until a child is approximately 5 years of age and are not completely developed until late adolescence. Extracranial complications from acute sinusitis include periorbital cellulitis, orbital cellulitis, and Pott's puffy tumor (subperiosteal abscess of the frontal bone); intracranial complications include meningitis, subdural empyema, epidural or intracranial abscess, and venous sinus thrombosis.

PERIORBITAL CELLULITIS AND ORBITAL CELLULITIS

Background and Pathophysiology • ***Periorbital Cellulitis*** Periorbital cellulitis involves inflammation anterior to the orbital septum, and is also referred to as preseptal cellulitis. The orbital septum, which extends from the periosteum of the inferior and superior orbital rims to the tarsal plates of the eyelids, provides a protective barrier for the deeper orbital structures as well as structural support for the lids.

Infections in deeper orbital structures are referred to as orbital cellulitis. Periorbital cellulitis may result from inoculation of bacteria into the skin surrounding the eye, such as from abrasions, lacerations, or insect bites or stings, known as traumatic periorbital cellulitis. Less commonly, conjunctivitis may cause inflammation of the periorbital skin, which may allow cellulitis to develop. Periorbital swelling may accompany underlying sinusitis but is thought to be sympathetic inflammation caused by poor venous drainage. Uncommonly, sinus infection may extend to the periorbital tissue and result in nontraumatic periorbital cellulitis. Occasionally, periorbital cellulitis may develop secondary to hematogenous spread of bacteria.

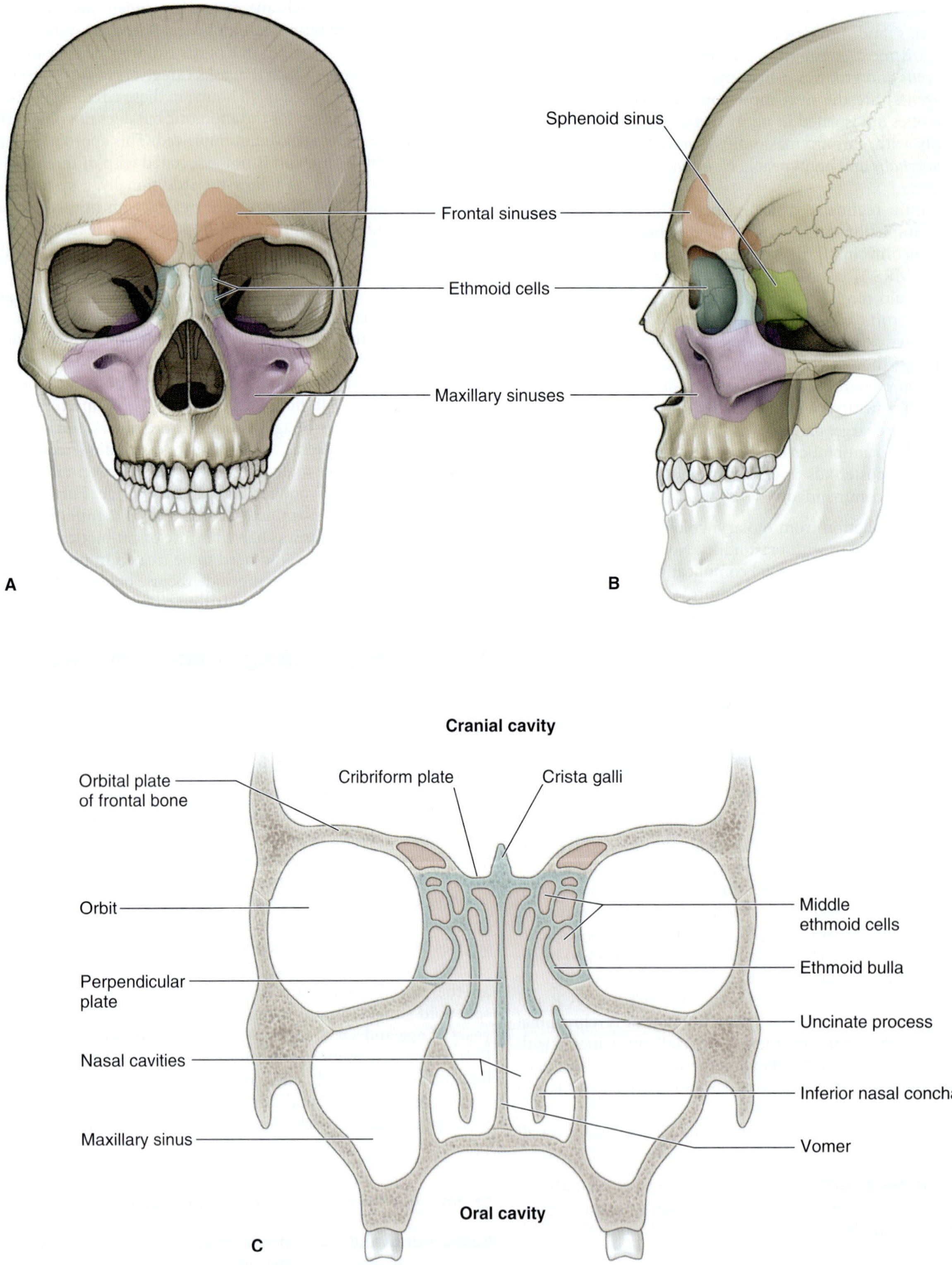

FIGURE 95-2. Anatomy of the sinuses. (Original Legend: "Anterior (A) and lateral (B) views of the paranasal sinuses. C. Coronal section of the skull revealing the cranial, orbital, and nasal cavities and their relationships to the paranasal sinuses.") (Reproduced with permission from Morton DA, Foreman KB, Albertine KH eds. The Big Picture: Gross Anatomy. McGraw-Hill Education; 2011.)

Orbital Cellulitis In orbital cellulitis, the infection is deep to the orbital septum and involves the bony orbit or the intraorbital structures. Most commonly, orbital cellulitis results from extension of sinusitis (usually ethmoid), but it can also occur as a result of direct inoculation from penetrating trauma to the intraorbital or postseptal areas or hematogenous spread. Multiple factors facilitate direct extension of sinusitis into the orbits. First, the orbit is surrounded by and in close proximity to the paranasal sinuses. Second, the bony walls that separate the paranasal sinuses from the orbit are thin, thereby providing a permeable barrier. For example, the lamina papyracea is a paper-thin bone that separates the ethmoid sinus from the medial aspect of the intraorbital structures. Extension of infection from this sinus is the most common route by which orbital cellulitis develops. Finally, the orbital veins that drain the sinuses are valveless, which allows both anterograde and retrograde spread of infections. With progression, orbital cellulitis may lead to a subperiosteal or orbital abscess and/or cavernous sinus thrombosis.

Clinical Presentation • *Periorbital Cellulitis* Periorbital cellulitis occurs most commonly in children younger than 5 years. Hallmarks of the clinical presentation include unilateral eyelid erythema, edema, and tenderness (**Figure 95-3**). The skin may display evidence of recent trauma, insect bite, or a break in the skin. The contralateral eye may appear mildly edematous secondary to associated compression of the superior and inferior ophthalmic veins. Proptosis, chemosis, pain with extraocular movements, limitation of extraocular movements, and diminished visual acuity are not consistent with a periorbital process and suggest orbital involvement. Constitutional features such as fever or a toxic appearance are uncommon. Purulent drainage and pronounced conjunctival injection occur if concomitant conjunctivitis is present.

Differentiating preseptal swelling from proptosis by physical examination is challenging because protrusion of the lid is present with both. Furthermore, retracting the lid is often difficult because of soft tissue swelling, tenderness, and poor cooperation from young children, which makes evaluation of the appearance and function of the globe especially problematic.

Orbital Cellulitis In contrast to periorbital cellulitis, orbital cellulitis occurs most commonly in older children. Similar to children with periorbital cellulitis, those with orbital cellulitis present with edema and erythema around the eye. However, children with orbital cellulitis may also have painful, limited extraocular movement and proptosis. Fever is less common in periorbital cellulitis, and children with orbital cellulitis are often more ill-appearing than those with periorbital cellulitis. Factors associated with severe orbital infection and need for surgical intervention include proptosis, elevated WBC of 12-20,000/μL, ANC >10,000/mm, elevated CRP >120 mg/L, absence of conjunctivitis, edema beyond the eyelid on exam, and age >9 years. Pupillary function and visual acuity should be carefully assessed because optic dysfunction is a vision-threatening complication.

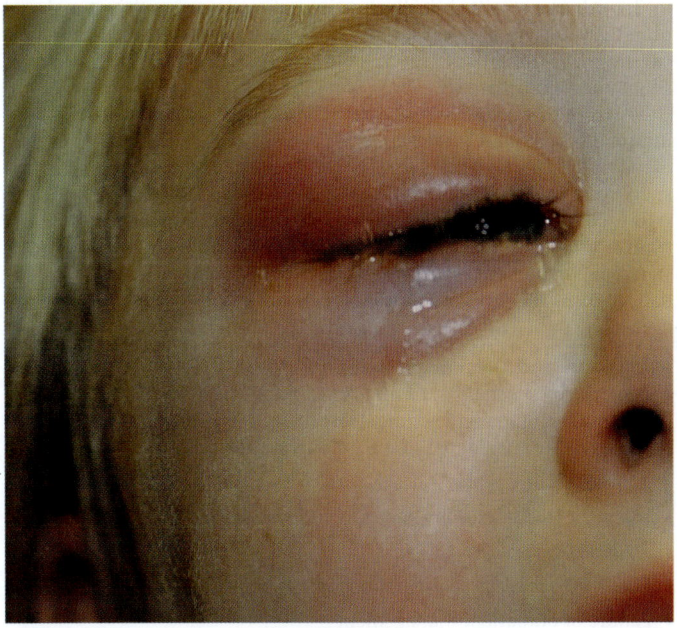

FIGURE 95-3. Child with periorbital cellulitis.

Differential Diagnosis The clinician must distinguish between periorbital cellulitis and orbital cellulitis. Other diagnoses to consider in the differential for periorbital cellulitis include allergic reaction, chemical irritation, trauma (especially nasal and zygomatic fractures), hordeolum or chalazion, dacryocystitis, and conjunctivitis. The differential diagnosis of orbital cellulitis is similar to that for periorbital cellulitis. Orbital pseudotumor and intraocular masses/tumors, including retinoblastoma, lymphoma, and rhabdomyosarcoma, must also be considered.

Evaluation and Diagnosis Visual acuity should always be assessed, with glasses worn by patients who require them. Contrast CT of the brain and orbits should be performed if orbital involvement is a consideration and sinus disease is the suspected etiology (**Figure 95-4**). CT will delineate the extent of the infection and provide information about the presence or absence of an orbital or subperiosteal abscess. If there are no red flag features, consider deferring a CT scan for patients who fail to improve from medical therapy at 36-48 hours. Consider MRI in patients with suspected complications.

In the post-Hib vaccination era, concurrent bacteremia decreased from reported rates of 30% to close to 0% of cases. Rates of bacteremia in orbital cellulitis have remained low after the addition of 7-valent pneumococcal conjugate vaccine (PCV 7). Regardless, a blood culture should be considered as it may be useful in targeted antibiotic selection. Leukocytosis and an elevated CRP are common but, as with mastoiditis, are neither sensitive nor specific. Culture of the eye discharge is rarely diagnostic or useful, and is not routinely recommended. A lumbar puncture should be considered in children with significant irritability, altered mental status, focal neurologic deficits, or other findings suggestive of concomitant bacterial meningitis.

Course of Illness • *Periorbital cellulitis* Periorbital cellulitis typically improves within 24 hours of initiation of antibiotic therapy. Additionally, it is uncommon for true periorbital cellulitis to progress to orbital cellulitis but as the initial diagnosis may be difficult, especially in young children, care should be taken to ensure close follow-up to monitor for clinical improvement, and appropriate education provided to caregivers about when to seek care.

Orbital cellulitis Although most cases of orbital cellulitis resolve with proper therapy, rare but serious sequelae include loss of vision and central nervous system (CNS) infection. Visual loss is most frequently due to traction on the optic nerve with progressive proptosis or compression of the optic nerve from adjacent abscess or foraminal impingement. The resultant nerve injury is not always reversible.

Treatment • *Periorbital Cellulitis* For traumatic periorbital cellulitis, the most common organisms are *S. aureus* and group A beta-hemolytic *Streptococcus* (GABHS; *S. pyogenes*); anaerobic bacteria are occasionally isolated. For nontraumatic periorbital cellultis associated with sinusitis, the practitioner should base treatment on common sinusitis pathogens. Before widespread immunization against *H. influenzae* type B, bacteremia from this organism was a common, virulent cause of periorbital cellulitis. Today, *S. pneumoniae* is most often implicated in periorbital infection by this route followed by *M. catarrhalis* and nontypeable *H. influenzae*. Of note, adenovirus is a causative agent that can mimic bacterial infection. With adenoviral conjunctivitis, the eye and surrounding tissues are edematous, the conjunctiva is hyperemic, and copious mucopurulent discharge is present. The periorbital inflammation may allow invasion of bacteria and progression to secondary periorbital cellulitis. Additionally, immunocompromised patients are more at risk for sinusitis caused by *Pseudomonas aeruginosa*, anaerobes, or molds, particularly *Aspergillus* species.

The choice of antibiotic should be guided by the most frequent pathogens. In traumatic periorbital cellulitis, cephalexin or cloxacillin provides adequate coverage for *S. aureus* and GABHS. In nontraumatic periorbital cellulitis, amoxicillin-clavulanate or cefuroxime

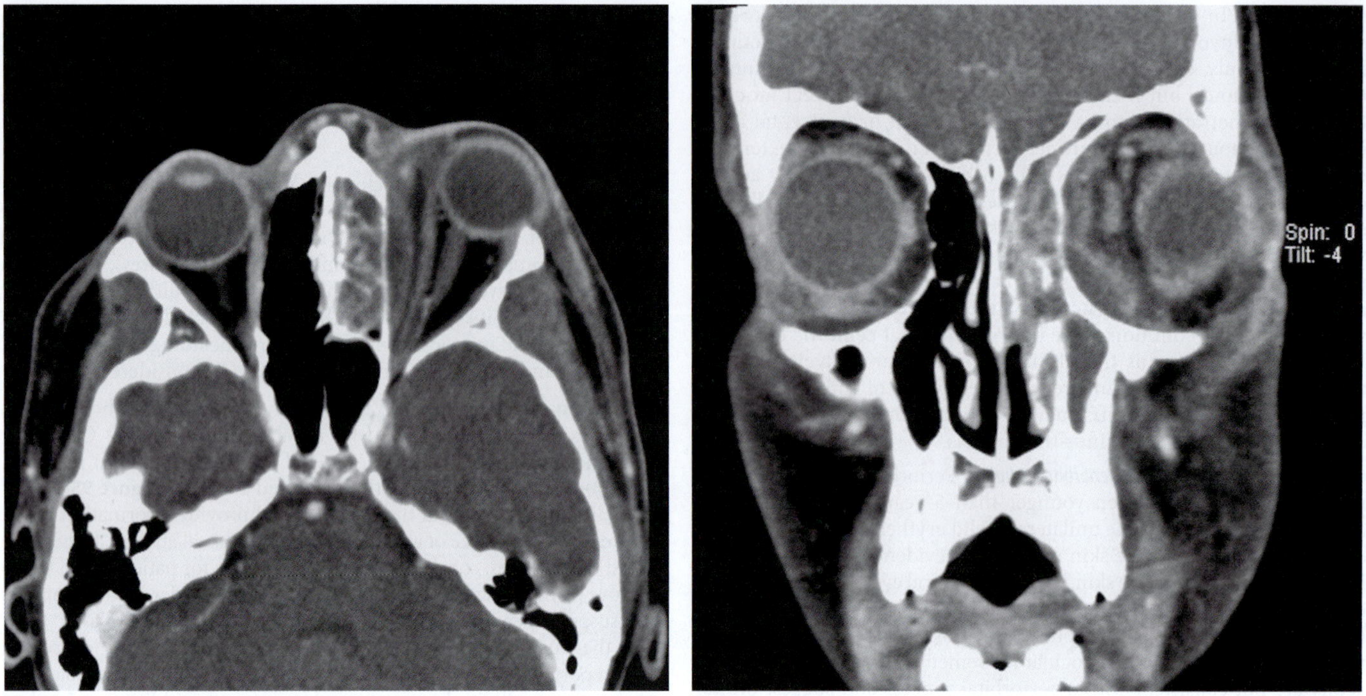

A B

FIGURE 95-4. CT scan of a 13-year-old boy with left-sided orbital cellulitis. (A) Axial and (B) coronal views reveal left proptosis with post-septal inflammation and a subperiosteal abscess in the medial aspect of the orbit. The left ethomoid sinus demonstrates near total opacification.

are appropriate antibiotics. Because of the increasing prevalence of community-acquired MRSA in many areas, clindamycin is an appropriate alternative. If a patient is treated as an outpatient for periorbital cellulitis, close monitoring by a pediatrician is recommended, and the patient should be advised to return to the hospital in the event of any photophobia, decreased vision, pain with eye movement, or diplopia.

Children who are hospitalized for management of periorbital cellulitis should receive intravenous antibiotics. Consider adding clindamycin if there is concern for MRSA. Patients with periorbital cellulitis can be transitioned to oral antibiotic therapy at discharge to complete a 7- to 10-day course of antibiotic.

Orbital Cellulitis For orbital cellulitis, the most common organisms are those associated with sinusitis and include *S. pneumoniae*, nontypeable *H. influenzae*, *M. catarrhalis*, and facultative anaerobes such as *Streptococcus milleri* group bacteria. Additionally, orbital cellulitis may be caused by *S. aureus* and *S. pyogenes*. Ampicillin-sulbactam or a third-generation cephalosporin (e.g., ceftriaxone) is a reasonable choice for empirical intravenous therapy. Although MRSA is uncommonly present in sinusitis, and therefore less often the causative organism in orbital cellulitis compared with periorbital cellulitis, empiric coverage for MRSA should be considered given the high risk of untreated MRSA infection in certain jurisdictions based on the changing epidemiology. Recent studies have indicated that in the post-PCV 7 vaccination era, *S. pneumoniae* is a decreasing and *S. aureus* is an increasing causative organism. Antibiotic therapy can then be narrowed as appropriate based on culture results and clinical response. Transition to oral therapy at discharge is reasonable if there is a comparable oral antibiotic available, the patient is willing and able to take oral antibiotics, and there are no conditions that would preclude adequate drug absorption (e.g., diarrhea). Oral antibiotic options include amoxicillin-clavulanate, clindamycin in combination with an oral second- or third- generation cephalosporin (e.g., cefuroxime), or respiratory fluoroquinolones (e.g., levofloxacin). The total duration of antibiotic therapy is 14 to 21 days.

Ideally, children with orbital cellulitis should be managed in consultation with ophthalmology and otolaryngology. The physical examination should be monitored closely because progression of the infectious process is usually heralded by clinical deterioration. If a child does not demonstrate improvement with intravenous antibiotics in 24 to 48 hours, repeat imaging is warranted to check for the development of an abscess.

The need for prompt surgical drainage of an intraorbital or subperiosteal abscess is controversial. Medical management may be appropriate for a small subperiosteal abscess that does not impair vision or cause excessive pain. A large subperiosteal abscess or an intraorbital abscess that results in impaired vision, often because of optic nerve or retinal compromise, requires prompt surgical drainage. If the surgeons elect to not drain a subperiosteal abscess immediately, the patient's clinical status should be assessed frequently for any changes. Several studies have attempted to determine subperiostal abscess volumes that require surgical compared with medical care, with volumes ranging from 0.5 to 3.4 mL as cut-offs, but diagnostic performance is sub-optimal and none have been externally validated. If there is worsening or no clinical improvement after 48 hours of antibiotic therapy, surgical drainage should be reconsidered.

The role of systemic corticosteroids in reducing complications and improving outcomes is unclear, and routine use is not currently recommended. Despite the lack of evidence, there is wide variation of corticosteroid use in hospitalized children. Similarly, intranasal agents, such as saline, corticosteroids, decongestants, are often suggested, extrapolating from studies in adult patients with bacterial sinusitis. In the 2013 AAP statement on pediatric sinusitis, Wald et al did not provide a recommendation given the weak underlying evidence base supporting intranasal agents.

Admission and Discharge Criteria • ***Periorbital Cellulitis*** Most patients with periorbital cellulitis are managed successfully with oral antibiotic therapy in the outpatient setting. Hospitalization and intravenous antibiotics should be considered in the following situations:

- Younger than 1 year
- Incomplete vaccination against *H. influenzae* type B (Hib)
- Toxic appearance
- Inability to tolerate oral/enteral feedings or antibiotics
- Failure of outpatient management
- Concern for orbital involvement

Discharge criteria for patients with periorbital cellulitis include:

- Improving clinical findings, including downtrending fever curve
- Ability to tolerate oral nutrition and oral antibiotics
- Reliable outpatient follow-up

Orbital Cellulitis Children with suspected or confirmed orbital cellulitis or abscess should be admitted for intravenous antibiotics, subspecialty consultation, definitive diagnosis, and possible surgical drainage.

Discharge criteria for patients with orbital cellulitis or abscess include:

- Improving physical examination findings/resolving symptoms
- Afebrile for 24 to 48 hours
- Ability to tolerate oral nutrition
- Compliance with oral antibiotic regimen or home parenteral therapy, if necessary
- Appropriate outpatient follow-up with a generalist, an ophthalmologist, and if appropriate, an otolaryngologist.

Prevention Periorbital cellulitis secondary to Hib bacteremia has been nearly eradicated in immunized children. Because minor trauma, insect bites, and conjunctivitis are the most common preceding events that lead to periorbital cellulitis, a prevention strategy is difficult.

Orbital cellulitis is most commonly a sequela of sinusitis, and prevention focuses on treatment of paranasal sinusitis. Timely and accurate recognition as well as appropriate treatment of sinusitis is important. However, in view of the impressive frequency of childhood sinusitis, the high rate of spontaneous resolution, the small proportion that progress to complications, and the conflicting data available in the literature, diagnosis and treatment remain a challenge for primary care clinicians.

INTRACRANIAL COMPLICATIONS

Background and Pathophysiology Perhaps the most serious complication of sinusitis involves extension of infection into the intracranial space and progression to meningitis, epidural abscess, subdural abscess, or intraparenchymal abscess. These complications are reported to occur in 3% to 4% of pediatric patients admitted for management of rhinosinusitis. Although these complications are rare, morbidity and mortality are significant although only reported in small case series.

Most commonly, intracranial complications result from frontal or ethmoid disease either from direct extension from the sinuses or from hematogenous spread via thrombophlebitis of the valveless diploic veins that connect the sinuses to the dura. Frontal sinusitis resulting in osteomyelitis of the frontal bone may lead to intracranial extension, but extension anteriorly is also seen. When the infection progresses in this direction, a subperiosteal abscess known as a Pott's puffy tumor develops. Intracranial extension may coexist with this condition, and evaluation for intracranial involvement is recommended.

Sagittal venous sinus thrombosis is a rare complication of sinusitis in children. Most cases result from thrombophlebitis of the valveless diploic veins that drain from the sinuses into the superior sagittal venous sinus.

Clinical Presentation Intracranial complications of sinusitis are more common in older age children. The increased rate of intracranial infection in adolescents is due to the peak growth of their frontal sinus, with resultant increased vascularity. The most common presenting signs and symptoms of the suppurative intracranial complications of sinusitis include headache, vomiting, and fever. Neurologic symptoms are present in only one-third to one-half of patients at presentation. Case series have differing views about the frequency of upper respiratory tract symptoms at the time of presentation, with reports varying from approximately 20% to 75% of patients.

A Pott's puffy tumor presents as a painful, tender, erythematous, and often fluctuant mass adjacent to the glabella (**Figure 95-5**). The patient complains of headache, fever, and concomitant or recent symptoms of sinusitis. Clinical signs of coexisting intracranial involvement may be present.

Differential Diagnosis The differential diagnosis includes other CNS infections, CNS tumor, intracranial hemorrhage, and if altered mentation is present, toxin ingestion.

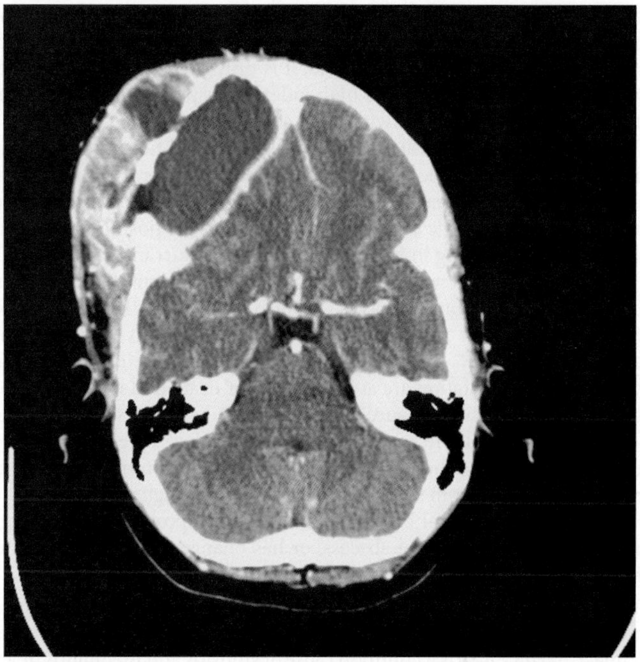

FIGURE 95-5. CT of an 11-year-old boy with Pott's puffy tumor who presented with headache, emesis, and scalp swelling. The CT reveals extensive right scalp subcutaneous swelling with multiple small subcutaneous abscesses overlying the right portion of the frontal bone. There is also marked destruction of the right portion of the frontal bone with a ring-enhancing 6 cm × 3 cm epidural abscess.

Evaluation and Diagnosis Rapid diagnosis is essential to prevention of long-term sequelae. Imaging with both CT and MRI should be considered (**Figure 95-6**). While CT can provide more rapid results, occult intracranial infections may be missed in up to 50% of cases.

Course of Illness Intracranial abscesses complicating sinusitis often present with vomiting, headache, confusion, or behavioral changes, which indicate increased ICP. Other neurologic signs are related to the

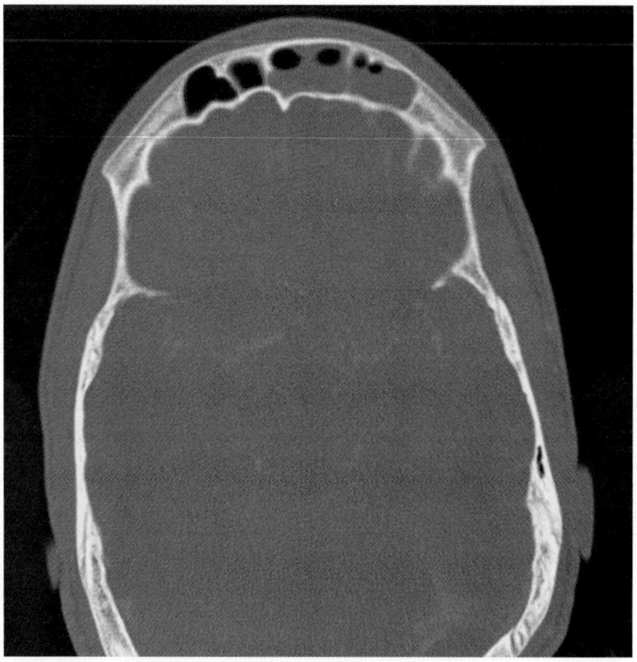

FIGURE 95-6. CT scan of a 14-year-old boy receiving antibiotics for treatment of sinusitis who presented with altered mentation. He had near-total opacification of the left frontal and ethmoid sinuses with intracranial extension. The CT reveals a large subdural empyema containing fluid and air.

location of the infection, and often these signs occur late in the clinical course. While the triad of fever, headache, and neurological deficit is worrisome for intracranial abscess, it is only present in 30% of cases, which indicates the need for a high index of suspicion in patients with atypical findings associated with acute sinusitis.

For most abscesses, drainage of the lesion in addition to appropriate antibiotic therapy will lead to improvement and reversal of previously present neurologic signs and symptoms as the ICP normalizes. Careful and frequent neurologic exams should be part of the postoperative evaluation. Repeat imaging in follow-up may also be warranted.

Epidural abscesses without intracranial involvement have excellent prognosis. For intracranial abscesses, approximately two-thirds of patients will recover without significant sequelae, and mortality rates are now reported between 2% and 15%. Those with more acute onset or severe symptoms at presentation are at higher risk for death and long-term neurologic deficits such as seizure, hydrocephalus, hemiparesis, and cranial nerve palsy. Abscesses in the frontal or temporal lobes are more likely to result in seizures, and these may present years after the initial infection has resolved. Mortality from septic thrombosis remains high at 35%.

A patient with orbital cellulitis who fails to improve, requires surgical intervention for orbital abscess, or has change in neurologic status should be evaluated for concurrent intracranial complication.

Treatment • ***Medical Management*** Case reports of bacterial isolates in intracranial abscesses report a polymicrobial culture in 30% to 50% of cases. While *S. pneumoniae* is a common cause of sinusitis and meningitis, it less commonly implicated as a cause of intracranial abscesses. The *S. milleri* group bacteria are most commonly isolated, followed by *S. aureus* and anaerobic bacteria. Empiric treatment should include broad-spectrum antibiotic therapy directed at most likely pathogens with adequate CNS penetration; a combination of vancomycin, a third-generation cephalosporin, and metronidazole provides reasonable coverage of expected organisms. If MRSA or other resistant gram-positive bacteria are not identified in operative cultures, vancomycin may be discontinued unless other patient factors warrant continuation. Obviously, treatment should be modified as necessary based on culture results and the patient's clinical status. There is no consensus on duration of therapy; typical courses are 4 to 6 weeks of antibiotics administered intravenously.

Surgical Management Neurosurgical and/or otolaryngology consultation is also warranted. Surgical intervention is likely required, especially for subdural or cerebral collections as well as Pott's puffy tumor. Surgical management includes both direct sinus drainage and drainage of the infectious fluid collection.

Admission and Discharge Criteria Children with suspected or confirmed intracranial complications of sinusitis should be admitted for intravenous antibiotics, subspecialty consultation, definitive diagnosis, and possible surgical drainage.

Discharge criteria include:

- Improving physical examination findings/resolving symptoms
- Afebrile for 24 to 48 hours
- Ability to tolerate oral nutrition
- Completion of intravenous antibiotic therapy or the ability to complete this treatment at home
- Outpatient follow-up with a generalist, a neurosurgeon, and an otolaryngologist.

Prevention Similar to prevention of orbital cellulitis, prevention of intracranial complications consists of appropriate management of acute sinusitis and timely recognition of treatment failure.

SUGGESTED READINGS

Bair-Merritt MH, Shah SS, Zaoutis TE, Bell LM, Feudtner C. Suppurative intracranial complications of sinusitis in previously healthy children. *Pediatr Infect Dis J*. 2005;24(4):384-386.

Burek AG, Melamed S, Liljestrom T, et al. Evaluation and medical management of the pediatric patient with orbital cellulitis/abscess: a systematic review. *J Hosp Med*. 2021;16(11):680-687.

Cassano P, Ciprandi G, Passali D. Acute mastoiditis in children. *Acta Biomed*. 2020;91(1-S):54-59.

Chow AW, Benninger MS, Brook I, et al. IDSA clinical practice guideline for acute bacterial rhinosinusitis in children and adults. *Clin Infect Dis*. 2012;54(8):e72-e112.

Coker TR, Chan LS, Newberry SJ, et al. Diagnosis, microbial epidemiology, and antibiotic treatment of acute otitis media in children: a systematic review. *JAMA*. 2010;304(19):2161-2169.

Corticosteroids as an Additional Treatment for Mastoiditis in Children—Full Text View—Clinicaltrials.gov. Accessed July 25, 2022. https://clinicaltrials.gov/ct2/show/NCT04828525

Crosbie RA, Nairn J, Kubba H. Management of paediatric periorbital cellulitis: Our experience of 243 children managed according to a standardised protocol 2012-2015. *Int J Pediatr Otorhinolaryngol*. 2016;87:134-138.

DeMuri GP, Wald ER. Clinical practice. Acute bacterial sinusitis in children. *N Engl J Med*. 2012;367(12):1128-1134.

Feigin RD, Cherry JD. *Textbook of Pediatric Infectious Diseases*. 4th ed. W B Saunders; 1997.

Garcia C, Salgueiro AB, Luís C, Correia P, Brito MJ. Acute mastoiditis in children: middle ear cultures may help in reducing use of broad spectrum antibiotics. *Int J Pediatr Otorhinolaryngol*. 2017;92:32-37.

Gill PJ, Drouin O, Pound C, et al. Factors associated with surgery and imaging characteristics in severe orbital infections. *J Pediatr*. 2022; 248:66-73.e7.

Gill PJ, Mahant S, Hall M, et al. Association between corticosteroids and outcomes in children hospitalized with orbital cellulitis. *Hosp Pediatr*. 2022;12(1):70-89.

Hauser A, Fogarasi S. Periorbital and orbital cellulitis. *Pediatr Rev*. 2010;31(6):242-249.

Kornelsen E, Mahant S, Parkin P, et al. Corticosteroids for periorbital and orbital cellulitis. *Cochrane Database Syst Rev*. 2021;4: CD013535.

Krueger C, Mahant S, Begum N, et al. Changes in the management of severe orbital infections over seventeen years. *Hosp Pediatr*. 2021;11(6):613-621.

Leibovitz E, Piglansky L, Raiz S, Press J, Leiberman A, Dagan R. Bacteriologic and clinical efficacy of one day vs. three day intramuscular ceftriaxone for treatment of nonresponsive acute otitis media in children. *Pediatr Infect Dis J*. 2000;19(11):1040-1045.

Lieberthal AS, Carroll AE, Chonmaitree T, et al. The diagnosis and management of acute otitis media. *Pediatrics*. 2013;131(3):e964-99.

Loh R, Phua M, Shaw CKL. Management of paediatric acute mastoiditis: systematic review. *J Laryngol Otol*. 2018;132(2):96-104.

Long SS, Prober CG, Fischer M, Kimberlin D, eds. Principles and Practice of Pediatric Infectious Diseases. 6th ed. Elsevier—Health Sciences Division; 2022.

McKerlie MF, Wolter NE, Mahant S, et al. Periorbital and Orbital Cellulitis (POC); Multicentre Study Group and Canadian Pediatric Inpatient Research Network (PIRN). Abscess volume as a predictor of surgical intervention in children hospitalized with orbital cellulitis: A multicentre cohort study. *Int J Pediatr Otorhinolaryngol*. 2023;171:111629. doi: 10.1016/j.ijporl.2023.111629. Epub 2023 Jul 8. PMID: 37437497.

Peña MT, Preciado D, Orestes M, Choi S. Orbital complications of acute sinusitis: changes in the post-pneumococcal vaccine era. *JAMA Otolaryngol Head Neck Surg*. 2013;139(3):223-227.

Ren Y, Sethi RKV, Stankovic KM. Acute otitis media and associated complications in United States Emergency Departments. *Otol Neurotol*. 2018;39(8):1005-1011.

Reviews C. Nelson Textbook of Pediatrics: Medicine, Pediatrics. 15th ed. Cram101; 2016.

Rudloe TF, Harper MB, Prabhu SP, Rahbar R, Vanderveen D, Kimia AA. Acute periorbital infections: who needs emergent imaging? *Pediatrics*. 2010;125(4):e719-26.

Venekamp RP, Sanders SL, Glasziou PP, Del Mar CB, Rovers MM. Antibiotics for acute otitis media in children. *Cochrane Database Syst Rev*. 2015;(6):CD000219.

Wald ER, Applegate KE, Bordley C, et al. Clinical practice guideline for the diagnosis and management of acute bacterial sinusitis in children aged 1 to 18 years. *Pediatrics*. 2013;132(1):e262-80.

Wong SJ, Levi J. Management of pediatric orbital cellulitis: a systematic review. *Int J Pediatr Otorhinolaryngol*. 2018;110:123-129.

CHAPTER 96

Neck and Oral Cavity Infections

Jessica L. Markham, MD, MSc and
Katherine M. Richardson, MD

BACKGROUND

Children with complaints of mouth and/or throat pain may have infections that range from mild and self-limited in nature to severe and life threatening. With the advent of childhood immunizations and the increased availability of effective antimicrobials, we have seen improved outcomes and decreased incidence of many serious, life-threatening infections. Yet infections of the oral cavity and neck remain an important cause of pediatric hospital admission and childhood morbidity. This chapter focuses on common oral cavity and neck infections that result in hospitalization or have potential for serious complications.

STOMATITIS

BACKGROUND

The term stomatitis describes inflammatory lesions of the oral mucosa, usually presenting as small, shallow, painful ulcerations. Stomatitis is caused by both infectious and noninfectious etiologies. The location of lesions and accompanying historical and physical exam findings can help to identify the underlying cause and guide further management. Most cases of stomatitis are isolated occurrences and self-limited, and can be managed in the outpatient setting. However, stomatitis can be a sign of an underlying systemic condition and some children may develop severe pain or dehydration that necessitates inpatient management.

CLINICAL PRESENTATION

The most common causes of stomatitis in children are recurrent aphthous ulcers, herpangina, hand, foot, and mouth disease (HFMD), and herpetic gingivostomatitis.

Recurrent Aphthous Ulcers Commonly referred to as "canker sores," recurrent aphthous ulcers are the most common cause of inflammatory ulcerations of the oral mucosa. They typically present as small (<5 mm), round, painful ulcerations with clearly defined erythematous borders on the mucosal surface of the inner lip or buccal mucosa. Small lesions heal spontaneously within 4 to 7 days of onset without any scarring, but recurrence is common. Familial tendencies have been noted, but the cause remains unknown. There are hypotheses that there may be a relation to alterations in local cell-mediated immunity, trauma, emotional stress, and possibly nutritional deficiencies. Other systemic symptoms, such as fever, are usually absent.

Herpangina and Oral Manifestations of Hand, Foot, and Mouth Disease Herpangina is a self-limited clinical syndrome, usually caused by group A coxsackieviruses, found in young children during the summer and early fall. Children with herpangina typically present with sore throat, mouth pain with mucosal lesions, and fever. Mucosal involvement characteristically includes clusters of small papules that vesiculate and progress to shallow yellow/gray ulcerations with hyperemic borders involving the anterior faucial pillars and soft palate. Lesions are occasionally observed on the hard palate, tongue, or buccal mucosa.

HFMD, another manifestation of group A coxsackieviruses, is characterized by mouth/throat pain, oral lesions, and a viral exanthem. As with herpangina, oral lesions typically occur anterior to the faucial pillars; however, involvement of the tongue and buccal mucosa occurs more frequently. Children with HFMD present with non-pruritic macular, maculopapular, or vesicular exanthems in addition to oral changes. Exanthems characteristically involve the hands and feet, with lesions frequently observed on the dorsum and lateral aspects of fingers and toes with nail changes also reported (**Figure 96-1**). Lesions may also appear in other areas, particularly the buttocks and knees, though less commonly appear on the face and trunk. While these lesions typically will heal spontaneously over 3 to 5 days, oral intake can be markedly decreased during the illness due to severe odynophagia and lead to dehydration.

Herpetic Gingivostomatitis Gingivostomatitis is the most common manifestation of herpes simplex virus (HSV) infection in childhood, with primary herpetic gingivostomatitis typically occurring between 6 months and 5 years of age. It is primarily due to HSV type 1, resulting from direct exposure to oral secretions or lesions present in close contacts. Symptoms typically begin with a viral prodrome of low-grade fevers, malaise, and decreased appetite. Lesions begin as small vesicles clustered on the gingiva that subsequently rupture and coalesce to form large, painful ulcerations. The gingiva becomes very red, edematous, bleeds easily, and may become covered with a thick, black crust. Most lesions are anterior and involve the lips and gingiva, although lesions on the tongue, hard palate, and pharynx can occur (see **Figure 96-2**). Healing may take up to 3 weeks in those with severe involvement. Spread of the infection beyond the oral mucous membranes is sometimes seen with spread to the perioral skin, fingers (herpetic whitlow), or eyes (HSV keratitis).

DIFFERENTIAL DIAGNOSIS

In addition to HSV and coxsackieviruses described above, other viruses such as varicella, human immunodeficiency virus (HIV), SARS-CoV-2 virus, and other enteroviruses can cause stomatitis. Infections with *Candida albicans* are common in infants and older patients who are immunocompromised and can cause erythematous and painful oral lesions, but are accompanied by white plaques. Lesions can also be seen in *Mycoplasma pneumoniae*-induced rash and mucositis. Patients receiving certain chemotherapy regimens are at high risk for severe mucositis, requiring immediate recognition and supportive care. Traumatic ulcers can be due to mechanical, chemical, or thermal injuries. Some systemic illnesses can present with oral ulcerations in association with other systemic signs and symptoms, including Crohn's disease, Behçet's disease, systemic lupus erythematosus, and reactive arthritis. Cyclical occurrences of stomatitis can be seen in children with cyclic neutropenia or PFAPA (periodic fever with aphthous stomatitis, pharyngitis, and adenitis). In toxic-appearing patients with hemorrhagic oral lesions and discoloration of oral mucosa, Stevens-Johnson syndrome should be considered.

DIAGNOSTIC EVALUATION

Diagnosis can usually be made on historical and clinical grounds alone. Further testing is only necessary when the cause is unclear or thought to be due to systemic illness. When necessary, HSV and many other viruses can be identified using viral polymerase chain reaction (PCR) (preferred), culture, serology, or immunofluorescence. For patients with reduced oral intake and possible dehydration, consideration should be given to checking serum electrolytes. If patients are ill-appearing or secondary bacterial infections are suspected, blood cultures and complete blood count (CBC) should also be considered.

MANAGEMENT

Pain control and hydration are the primary focus when managing patients with stomatitis. Pain is often well controlled with acetaminophen or ibuprofen. Other supportive management options include the use of topical medications such as benzocaine (e.g., Orabase®), sucralfate, or "magic mouthwash" and in some rare instances the use of systemic agents such as colchicine. One common "magic mouthwash" preparation includes equal-parts mixture of Maalox®, 2% viscous lidocaine, and diphenhydramine. Due to concern for toxicity due to systemic absorption, lidocaine use should be avoided in younger patients. In patients with HSV gingivostomatitis, if given within 3 to 4 days of disease onset, acyclovir may be able to decrease the duration of pain, fever, and viral shedding.

ADMISSION CRITERIA

Most patients with stomatitis can be managed in an outpatient setting. Admission should be considered for patients with severe pain despite

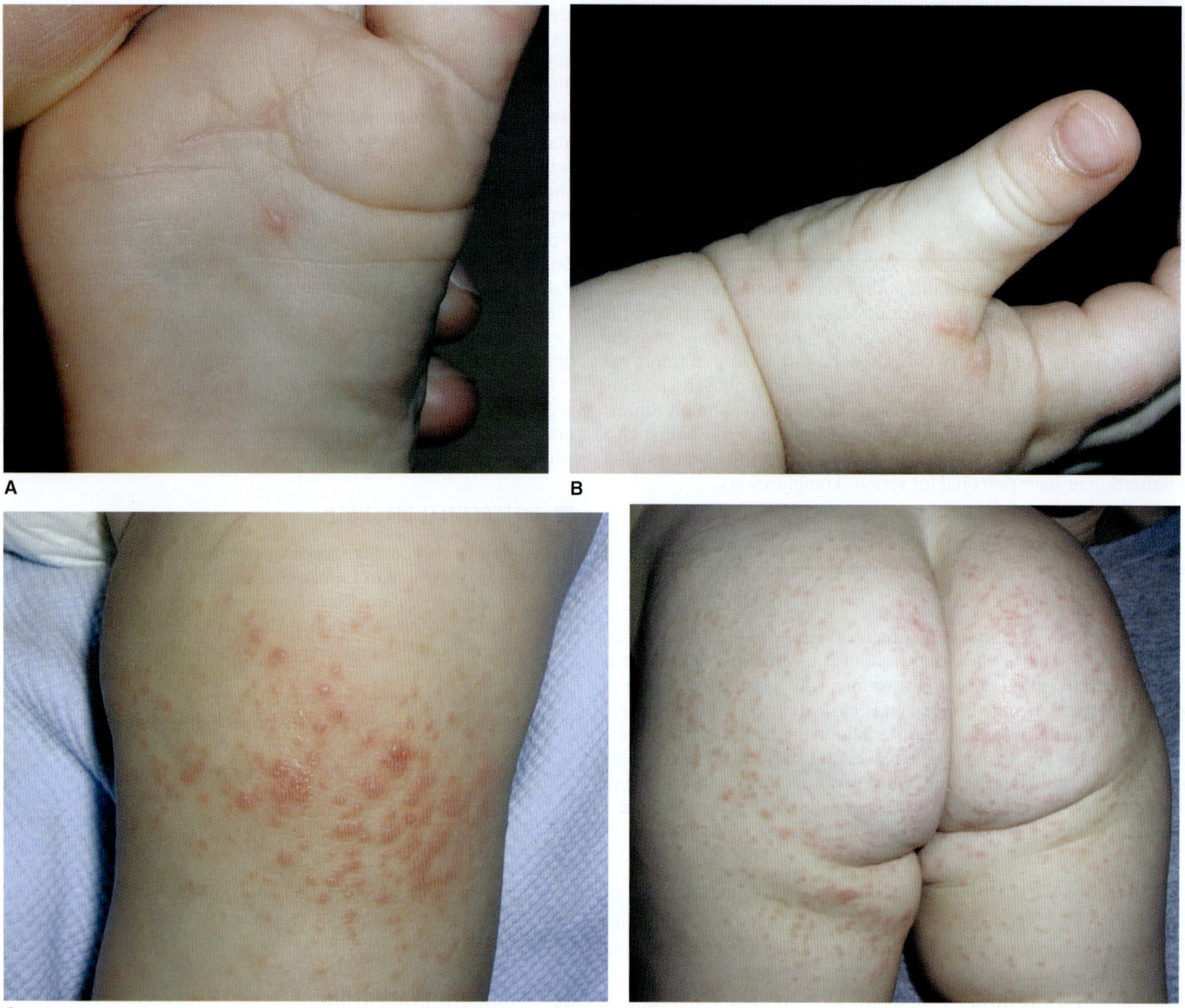

A B C D

FIGURE 96-1. Typical cutaneous manifestations of hand, foot, and mouth disease on a toddler. (A) Inflammatory vesicles on the foot; (B) inflammatory vesicle on the hand; (C, D) numerous small erythematous papules and vesicles on the knees and buttocks. (Reproduced with permission from Shah KN. Case 9-6. In: Shah SS, Ludwig S eds. *Symptom-based Diagnosis in Pediatrics.* New York: McGraw-Hill Medical; 2014:254, Figure 9-6.)

oral medications, dehydration, or concern for secondary bacterial infection or other serious conditions such as Stevens-Johnson syndrome. In addition, immunocompromised patients and children with mucositis related to chemotherapy often require admission for supportive care and close monitoring.

PREVENTION

When infectious causes are suspected, patients and families should reduce contact with oral secretions and be encouraged to practice good hand hygiene to minimize the spread of infection from oral secretions and stool. Hospitalized patients can be placed in isolation according to the standards of the admission facility.

PHARYNGITIS

BACKGROUND

With an estimated 15 million visits to healthcare providers annually in the United States, sore throat is one of the most common presenting complaints in children. Pharyngitis in children is most frequently caused by viral infections. However, bacterial causes are not uncommon, with group A β-hemolytic streptococcus (GABHS) comprising 15% to 30% of all cases of pediatric pharyngitis. Clinicians are often challenged with deciding which children have benign, self-limited conditions and which require further evaluation to prevent serious complications and spread of infection.

CLINICAL PRESENTATION

Nearly every child with pharyngitis will present with pharyngeal erythema and a history of sore throat. However, distinguishing the underlying cause (i.e., viral from bacterial etiologies) can be challenging based on history and exam findings alone though findings such as rhinitis, cough, stridor, conjunctivitis, hoarseness, oral ulcerations, or diarrhea are more suggestive of a viral etiology. Exudative pharyngitis can be seen in both bacterial and viral infections. Findings often associated with GABHS infection include palatal petechiae, sandpaper-like rash, and anterior cervical lymphadenopathy, but these are nonspecific findings. GABHS infections peak between 5 and 11 years of age, with symptoms typically lasting 3 to 5 days. Pharyngitis in infants and children are most likely to be due to viral infections, and symptoms may be slightly more prolonged, lasting >5 days. Both GABHS and viral pharyngitis are common in the colder months between the winter and early spring.

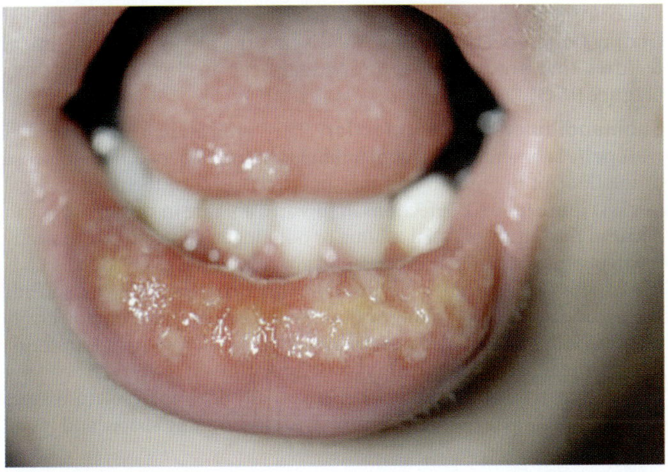

FIGURE 96-2. Stomatitis caused by herpes simplex virus. (From Knoop K, Stack L, Storrow A, Thurman RJ. *Atlas of Emergency Medicine*. 4th ed. New York: McGraw-Hill; 2016, Figure 6.44. Reproduced with permission from photo contributor: Lawrence B. Stack, MD.)

Arcanobacterium haemolyticum is another important cause of pharyngitis that is often overlooked due to the time required to grow on culture. *A. haemolyticum* classically causes pharyngitis and rash in adolescents. The rash typically appears several days after the onset of pharyngitis and starts on the extensor surfaces of the extremities and moves centrally. It can appear urticarial, maculopapular, or scarlatiniform.

DIFFERENTIAL DIAGNOSIS

Viral infections are the most common etiology of pharyngitis in children. However, aside from GABHS, there are several other bacterial causes to consider as well. Noninfectious causes of pharyngitis are less common, but should also be considered in the proper context. **Table 96-1** lists the various causes of pharyngitis in children. The presenting history and physical exam are critical to help determine the most likely cause in each individual patient.

DIAGNOSTIC EVALUATION

The goal of diagnosis is to identify treatable causes of pharyngitis and to prevent complications and transmission of illness to others. If symptoms are consistent with uncomplicated viral pharyngitis, monitoring the patient without further workup may be reasonable. However, if GABHS is suspected, further testing is needed. Evaluation for GABHS infection should begin with a throat swab sent for a rapid antigen detection test (RADT). Testing is not indicated if there are overt signs of viral infection present (e.g., rhinorrhea, conjunctival infection) and should generally be avoided in children under 3 years of age unless other risk factors are present. Because RADTs are highly specific but have a sensitivity of approximately 70% to 90%, children with positive tests should be treated as having a GABHS infection, but negative RADT tests warrant culture for confirmation. Care must be taken to distinguish a positive test for GABHS in patients with an acute infection versus those who have viral pharyngitis but are colonized with GABHS. Some estimates have placed the colonization rate as high as 20%. Pharyngeal swabs can also be sent for culture of bacteria other than GABHS, such as *Neisseria gonorrhoeae*, *Arcanobacterium haemolyticum*, or *Fusobacterium necrophorum*. In order to ensure proper collection, test selection and performance, communication with laboratory personnel is recommended.

Rapid diagnostic tests are also available for various viral pathogens, including respiratory syncytial virus (RSV), influenza A and B, and heterophile antibody spot (Monospot) tests for Epstein-Barr virus (EBV). However, unless management will change, these tests may not be necessary. Serologic tests can be ordered but are generally not indicated.

TABLE 96-1 Causes of Pharyngitis in Children and Adolescents

Viral	Bacterial	Non-infectious
Adenovirus	*Arcanobacterium haemolyticum*	Allergic rhinitis
Coronavirus (including SARS-CoV-2)	*Chlamydophila pneumoniae*	Caustic ingestions
Cytomegalovirus	*Chlamydia trachomatis*	Chronic cough
Enterovirus	*Corynebacterium diphtheriae*	Foreign body
Epstein-Barr virus	*Francisella tularensis*	Gastroesophageal reflux
Herpes simplex virus	*Fusobacterium necrophorum*	Inhaled irritants
Human immunodeficiency virus	Group A *Streptococci*	Malignancy
Influenza	Group C and G *Streptococci*	Multisystem inflammatory syndrome in children (MIS-C)
Parainfluenza	*Mycoplasma pneumoniae*	Postnasal drip
Respiratory syncytial virus	*Neisseria gonorrhoeae*	Rheumatologic condition
Rhinovirus	*Yersinia* spp.	

MANAGEMENT

Supportive care alone is usually all that is required for patients with viral pharyngitis. Acetaminophen and ibuprofen can be used to treat throat pain or fevers. In addition, there are several over-the-counter lozenges and throat sprays that patients can use for pain relief. Patients with EBV infections and splenomegaly are at risk for splenic rupture and should be instructed to refrain from all contact sports until the patient's symptoms and splenomegaly are resolved.

Systemic corticosteroids have been used in patients with pharyngitis, but their use remains controversial. Studies in both adults and children have shown modest but statistically significant reductions in duration of pain when systemic corticosteroids are added to standard antimicrobial regimens. However, there continue to be concerns about adverse outcomes associated with steroid use in these patients, particularly as it relates to patients with pharyngitis or adenitis and undiagnosed malignancy.

For patients with confirmed GABHS infection, first-line therapy includes either a single dose of IM penicillin G, or oral penicillin V or oral amoxicillin for 10 days. Antibiotic options for patients with an allergy to penicillin include cephalexin for children with nonsevere penicillin allergy or clindamycin for severe penicillin allergy for 10 days or azithromycin for 5 days. Of note, macrolide resistance has been reported in some areas of the United States, and local resistance patterns should be consulted when selecting empiric therapy.

Pharyngitis caused by *A. haemolyticum* can resolve in the absence of treatment. Antibiotics may shorten the duration of symptoms though rigorous controlled trials have not been conducted. When antibiotics are indicated, *A. haemolyticum* is virtually always susceptible to macrolides and clindamycin, and is usually susceptible to penicillin, though penicillin treatment failures have been reported.

ADMISSION CRITERIA

Most patients with pharyngitis can be managed in an outpatient setting. Admission should be considered for patients with severe pain that is not adequately controlled with oral medications, those with dehydration who are unable to tolerate oral medications, or if there are signs of worsening infection and possible airway compromise. Suppurative complications of pharyngitis such as peritonsillar abscess, parapharyngeal abscess, mastoiditis, or other invasive infections may also necessitate admission to the hospital.

DEEP NECK SPACE INFECTIONS

BACKGROUND

The neck anatomy includes a complex fascial system that divides the neck into different spaces that communicate with each other and serve as potential areas for the contiguous spread of infection. Infections that develop in these spaces, termed deep neck space infections, remain a relatively common reason for hospital admission in the pediatric population. Early recognition and treatment are essential to avoid significant morbidity and mortality associated with these conditions. Deep neck space infections are generally polymicrobial in nature, involving a combination of oral anaerobes, *Staphylococcus aureus*, and various streptococcal species. Below we review the most common and clinically relevant infections involving the submandibular, peritonsillar, retropharyngeal, and parapharyngeal spaces.

ANATOMY AND CLINICAL PRESENTATION OF SPECIFIC DEEP NECK SPACE INFECTIONS

Patients with deep neck space infections commonly present with fever, malaise, drooling, mouth pain, and dysphagia/odynophagia. Trismus, pain with neck movement, stridor, and "hot potato" voice are other classic features that may be present. While clinical findings often overlap, below we discuss the anatomic and clinical features that are unique to individual deep neck space infections (**Figure 96-3**).

Submandibular Space Infection The submandibular space lies within the submental and submandibular triangles between the mucosa of the floor of the mouth and the superficial layer of the deep cervical fascia (**Figure 96-3A**). Infections in this area are rare in children, but can occur in the setting of facial trauma or odontogenic infections classically involving the mandibular molars, and are commonly referred to as Ludwig's angina. The infection begins in the floor of the mouth and spreads rapidly and aggressively along both sides of the floor of the mouth, creating a "woody" cellulitis. On exam there may be elevation and posterior displacement of the tongue.

Infection in the submandibular space usually does not result in abscess formation, though contingous spread to surrounding spaces and fascia is observed.

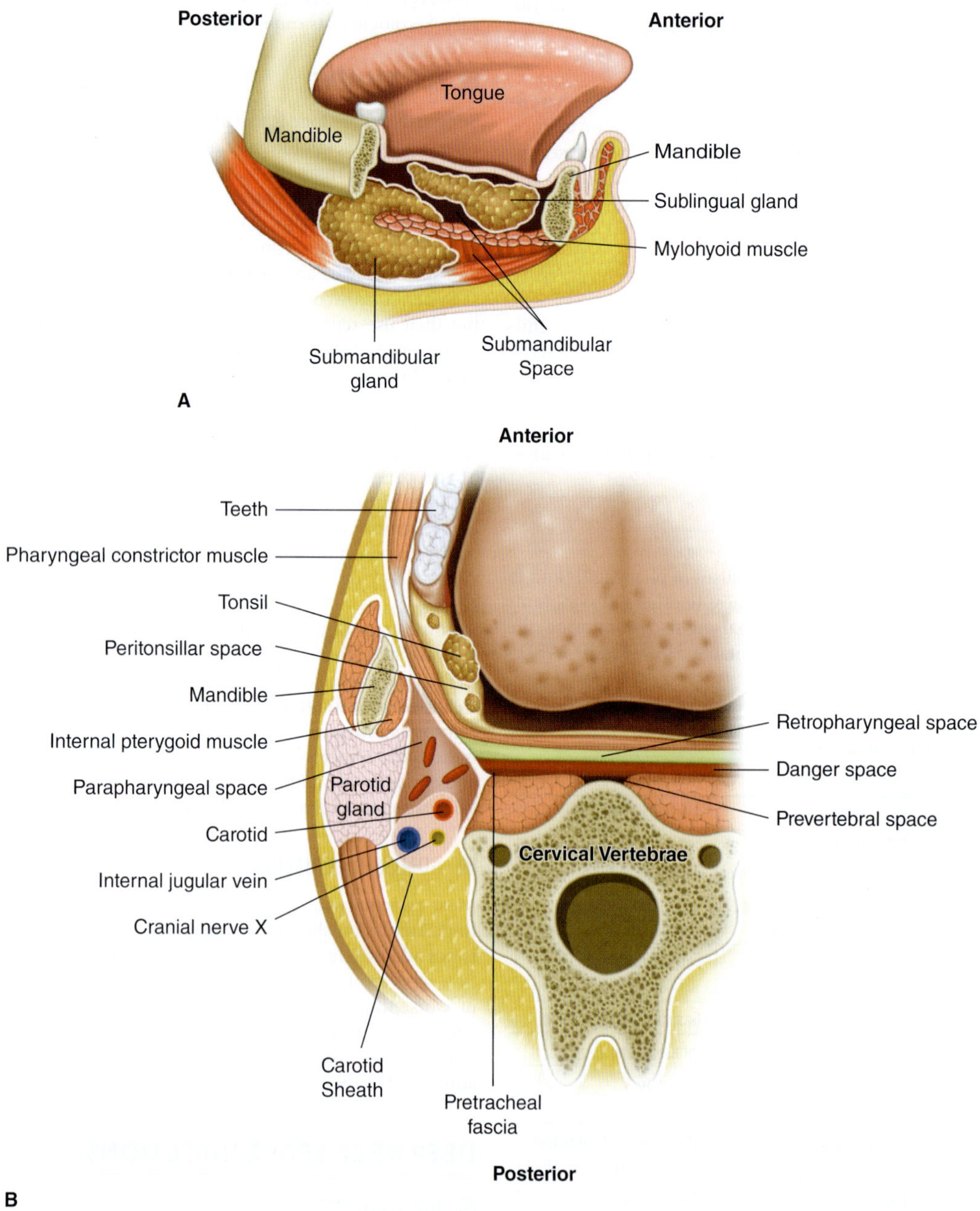

FIGURE 96-3. Anatomy of the deep neck spaces. A. Submandibular space and surrounding structures. B. Parapharyngeal, peritonsillar, and retropharyngeal spaces and their surrounding structures.

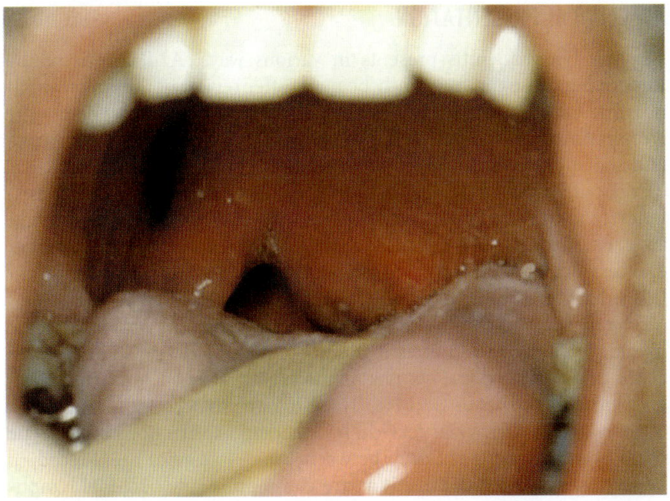

FIGURE 96-4. Peritonsillar abscess with marked deviation of the uvula. (From Knoop K, Stack L, Storrow A, Thurman RJ. *Atlas of Emergency Medicine*. 3rd ed. New York: McGraw-Hill; 2010, Figure 5.43. Reproduced with permission from photo contributor: Kevin J. Knoop, MD, MS.)

Peritonsillar Abscess The peritonsillar space is found in the peritonsillar fossa, between the tonsillar capsule medially and the superior constrictor muscle laterally (**Figure 96-3B**). Peritonsillar abscess (PTA) is the most common infection arising in this space and is the result of a purulent fluid collection in this area, often resulting from direct extension of local pharyngitis or tonsillitis. PTA occurs most commonly in older children and adolescents. On exam, the affected tonsil is enlarged and displaced anteriorly and medially by the abscess, causing deviation in the uvula to the contralateral side (see **Figure 96-4**).

Retropharyngeal Abscess The retropharyngeal space is a potential space that lies between the constrictor muscles of the neck anteriorly and the deep cervical fascia posteriorly and communicates with the parapharyngeal spaces laterally (Figure 96-3B). A pair of lymph node chains runs through this space and drains the nasopharynx, adenoids, and paranasal sinuses. Infections of the retropharyngeal space frequently arise due to suppurative infection involving these lymph nodes, but may also occur following trauma or foreign body ingestion. Retropharyngeal abscesses are seen most commonly in children less than 6 years of age. Involution of the lymph nodes in the retropharyngeal space usually takes place in early childhood, which may explain, in part, the decreasing likelihood of retropharyngeal abscess in older children.

Parapharyngeal Abscess The parapharyngeal spaces are located in the lateral aspect of the neck bilaterally and shaped like inverted cones, extending from the base of the skull to the hyoid bone (Figure 96-3B). Infections in this area have the potential to be life-threatening due to the close proximity of vital structures, including the internal jugular vein, the internal carotid artery, the cervical sympathetic trunk, and cranial nerves IX, X, and XII. Infections of the parapharyngeal space usually occur secondary to spread from other sites, such as odontogenic, peritonsillar, and retropharyngeal infections and symptoms may be overshadowed by these other infections contributing to delays in diagnosis. On exam there may be induration below the angle of the mandible and medial bulging of the pharyngeal wall. It is important to recognize complications of parapharyngeal deep neck space infections which include bacteremia/septic shock, septic emboli, and cavernous venous thrombosis. Horner syndrome (decreased pupil size, drooping eyelid, and decreased sweating on the affected side of the face) and changes to the voice can be seen when parapharyngeal deep neck space infections involve neurologic structures. In addition, extension of infection to the carotid artery can produce varying effects ranging from direct compression to arteritis, aneurysm formation, and even rupture. Extension to the jugular vein can cause septic thrombophlebitis (i.e., Lemierre syndrome), a finding commonly observed in association with *Fusobacterium necrophorum*.

DIAGNOSTIC EVALUATION

Laboratory evaluation can help support a diagnosis of deep neck space infection, though testing is nonspecific. White blood counts and inflammatory markers are frequently elevated. Blood cultures rarely identify a causative organism, though aerobic and anaerobic cultures obtained from aspirated fluid are most helpful in this regard. Throat swabs can be helpful in rapidly assessing for GABHS and sent for culture if negative.

Diagnostic imaging is helpful to determine the location, severity, and extent of an infection for most deep neck space infections and can be especially useful when the exam is limited due to trismus. In patients with peritonsillar abscess that can be diagnosed clinically based on direct visualization during physical exam, or those without severe symptoms, imaging may not always be necessary. Currently, neck computed tomography (CT) with contrast has become the imaging modality of choice for assessing most deep neck space infections and offers the advantages of better localization of abscesses, identifying the extent of spread of infection, and better differentiation between true abscesses and cellulitis (**Figure 96-5**). Ultrasonography can be considered cases involving infection of superficial structures, but deep neck spaces are rarely discernible using ultrasound.

MANAGEMENT

If a deep neck space infections is suspected, initial attention should focus on airway evaluation and maintaining a patent airway. Most patients will require admission to the hospital for ongoing evaluation and initiation of therapy. In otherwise healthy children requiring hospitalization, empiric parenteral antibiotics effective against both anaerobic and the most common gram-positive bacteria involved in these infections should be initiated. A penicillin in combination with a β-lactamase inhibitor, such as ampicillin-sulbactam, or clindamycin would be a good initial choice. In patients who are not improving or have a life-threatening infection, the addition of vancomycin should be considered. If an organism is identified from culture, antibiotic therapy can be narrowed. Duration of treatment varies based on location and severity of the infection. Most patients require treatment for at least 2 weeks, but treatment may be extended for more complicated, undrained infections, or specific organisms. For patients with peritonsillar, retropharyngeal, or parapharyngeal abscesses, a transition to oral antibiotics can be considered after patients are showing clinical improvement.

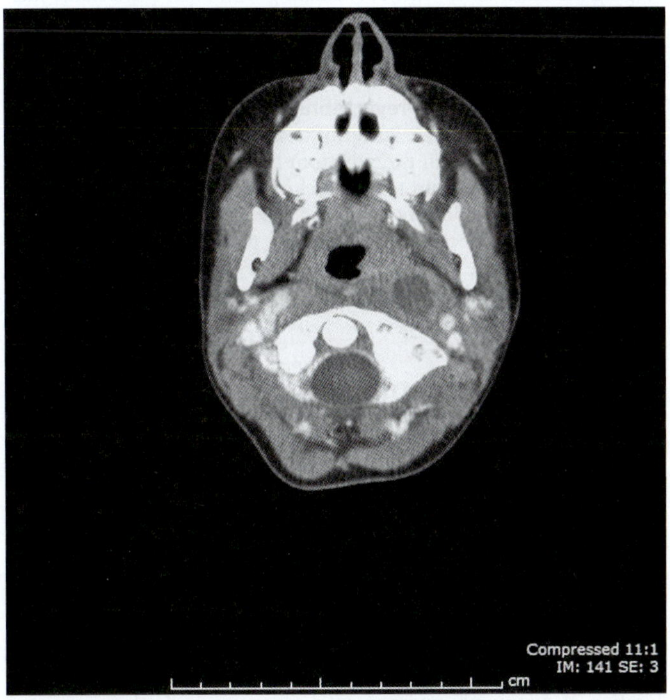

FIGURE 96-5. Neck CT showing a large, left-sided parapharyngeal abscess.

In addition to antibiotics, steroids may be of benefit in deep neck space infections with some studies showing decreased need for surgery and more rapid clinical improvement, though administration may not decrease symptom duration or length of hospitalization. Many children, recover with medical management alone, however surgical drainage is still recommended for patients who present with evidence of airway compromise, have large abscesses (>2 cm), fail to respond to parenteral antibiotics within 24 to 48 hours, or have other life-threatening complications. In patients with Ludwig's angina, surgery is usually performed if decompression is necessary or if abscess formation occurs later in the course of the illness.

ADMISSION AND DISCHARGE CRITERIA

Nearly all children with deep neck space infections are admitted for antibiotics and airway monitoring; however, patients with peritonsillar abscess can be successfully managed in the outpatient setting. Discharge for the remainder of patients can be considered after there has been clear improvement in symptoms, resolution of any airway compromise, and demonstration of the ability to maintain hydration and tolerate oral antibiotics.

CONSULTATION

Early consultation with an otolaryngologist is appropriate for most cases of suspected deep neck space infections to assist with management and planning for possible surgical intervention, particularly if children fail to respond to initial empiric antibiotic therapy.

SPECIAL CONSIDERATIONS

Epiglottitis Although epiglottitis is rarely seen in industrialized countries with widespread immunization especially against *Haemophilus influenza* type B (Hib), it still deserves special consideration due to the potential for life-threatening airway obstruction associated with this acute infection. Its classic presentation includes sore throat, drooling, respiratory distress, "tripod" posture, and a toxic appearance. The diagnosis should be considered in any child with these symptoms, particularly if there is a history of incomplete or lack of immunization against Hib, as historically this was the most common cause, though serotype non-type b *H. influenzae* is the more prevalent organism isolated in invasive infections. Immediate interventions should focus on keeping the child calm while coordinating with other physicians, such as otolaryngology, anesthesia, and the intensive care service, to examine the child in a setting where the airway can be secured immediately if necessary.

The Danger Space and Prevertebral Space These two spaces are also of clinical significance. Posterior to the retropharyngeal space lies the "danger space," which extends from the base of the skull through the posterior mediastinum to the level of the diaphragm. The danger space provides an important anatomic route for contiguous spread of infection from the neck to the chest. The prevertebral space extends from the base of the skull to the coccyx (**Figure 96-3B**). This space similarly provides a direct route for passage of organisms distally from the neck to the psoas muscles.

CERVICAL LYMPHADENITIS

BACKGROUND

Enlargement of cervical lymph nodes occurs frequently in the pediatric population and happens for a variety of reasons, ranging from benign and self-limited inflammatory responses to potentially serious infections and malignancy. The lymph nodes of the neck serve as the major drainage system for the head and neck area and commonly become inflamed in response to upper respiratory infections or other local inflammatory processes. The key to accurate diagnosis and management of children with cervical lymphadenitis relies on a thorough history focused on duration of symptoms, environmental exposures, and other associated symptoms.

CLINICAL PRESENTATION

Cervical lymphadenitis presents in various ways. A diagnosis of the underlying cause can frequently be made after review of the course of illness and exposure history. Distinction should be made as to whether the lymphadenopathy is acute versus chronic, disseminated versus localized, and unilateral versus bilateral. When examining the patient, particular care should be taken to include the number, location, size, shape, consistency, tenderness, mobility, and color of the lymph nodes involved. Once assessed, most patients fall into one of three categories: (i) acute unilateral cervical lymphadenitis, (ii) acute bilateral cervical lymphadenitis, or (iii) subacute/chronic cervical lymphadenitis.

The majority of children with cervical lymphadenitis present as acute infections that develop over a period of several days. Children with acute, unilateral cervical lymphadenitis usually have bacterial infections with either *S. aureus* or GABHS. These organisms account for over 80% of cases of acute bacterial cervical lymphadenitis. Infections of this type often occur in young children between 1 and 4 years of age. Preceding upper respiratory tract infections are common. Acute bacterial lymphadenitis can also occur as a complication of other infections such as pharyngitis, dental abscess, or facial impetigo. Nodes vary greatly in size, measuring from 1.5 cm to >6 cm, and are often accompanied by tenderness, erythema, and fever.

On the other hand, children with acute bilateral cervical lymphadenitis usually have self-limited, systemic viral infections caused by viruses such as EBV and cytomegalovirus. Inflammatory changes such as tenderness and erythema associated with these infections are typically mild when compared to cases of lymphadenitis caused by bacteria. Therefore, the term lymphadenopathy is sometimes used in these situations instead of lymphadenitis, indicating a simple, reactive enlargement of the lymph node in response to regional infection or inflammation. Fever and other associated viral symptoms such as sore throat, rash, hepatomegaly, or splenomegaly may be present and aid in diagnosis. These infections are more typical of patients in the preschool to adolescent age range.

Subacute or chronic lymphadenitis usually has a more indolent course, worsening over a period of several weeks. Presentation varies depending on the inciting agent, with *Bartonella henselae* and mycobacterial organisms being two of the most common infectious causes. Infection with *B. henselae*, also known as cat-scratch disease, causes tender lymphadenopathy measuring over 4 cm, usually in a regional distribution and often involving nodes in the axilla or cervical areas. Symptoms begin anywhere from 5 days to 2 months after inoculation, classically after being scratched by cats or kittens. Sometimes a papule or pustule can be seen at the site of inoculation. Lymphadenopathy persists for several weeks, but usually will diminish in size by 6 weeks unless suppurative complications occur. Associated symptoms of fever, malaise, and headache often occur, but typically resolve prior to the onset of lymphadenitis.

Mycobacterial causes of chronic lymphadenitis can be due either to *Mycobacterium tuberculosis* or nontuberculous mycobacterium (NTM). NTM infections usually occur in young children and typically result from environmental exposure, as organisms are ubiquitous in soil. Such infections are typically localized to a unilateral lymph node and have an insidious onset with gradual increase in size over several weeks. The majority of involved nodes are under 3 cm in size and other symptoms such as pain, fever, and erythema are less common. Overlying skin may change from pink to a violaceous discoloration. Untreated cases may resolve, but there is a risk of spontaneous drainage with sinus tract formation. Clinical signs of NTM lymphadenitis are often very similar to those of *M. tuberculosis*.

DIFFERENTIAL DIAGNOSIS

The differential for possible causes of enlarged cervical lymph nodes is quite broad, with other infectious etiologies often to blame. In addition to the common etiologies discussed above, there are many other infectious agents to consider when evaluating children with enlarged lymph nodes. A comprehensive listing can be found in **Table 96-2**. While infiltration of inflammatory cells is a major cause of enlarged lymph nodes, infiltration by neoplastic cells is also possible and is an important diagnosis to consider. In these cases, enlarged nodes are often painless, firm, and fixed to adjacent tissues. While not specific to neoplastic disease,

TABLE 96-2 Infectious Causes of Cervical Lymphadenitis

Bacteria	Viral	Other
Anaerobes	Adenovirus	*Aspergillus* spp.
Actinomyces israelii	Cytomegalovirus	*Candida* spp.
Bartonella henselae	Enterovirus	*Coccidioides* spp.
Brucella spp.	Epstein-Barr virus	*Cryptococcus* spp.
Corynebacterium diphtheriae	Human herpesvirus 6, 7, or 8	*Histoplasma* spp.
Francisella tularensis	Human immunodeficiency virus	*Leptospira* spp.
Group A *Streptococci*	Herpes simplex virus	*Toxoplasma* spp.
Group B *Streptococci*	Influenza	*Treponema pallidum*
Mycobacterium tuberculosis	Parvovirus B19	
Mycoplasma pneumoniae	Rhinovirus	
Nocardia spp.	Rubella virus	
Nontuberculous mycobacterium		
Pasturella multocida		
Staphylococcus aureus		
Yersinia spp.		

lymphadenopathy related to malignancy may be found in the posterior cervical or supraclavicular areas. Additionally, some congenital malformations in the neck can be mistaken for lymphadenitis, particularly if they become secondarily infected. These lesions include thyroglossal duct cysts (midline defect), branchial cleft cysts (anterior along the cervical chain), and cystic hygromas (located posteriorly, above the clavicles). Other causes include medications (phenytoin or carbamazepine) and systemic illnesses such as Kawasaki disease, histiocytosis, Castleman disease, Kikuchi-Fujimoto disease, sarcoidosis, Kimura disease, and PFAPA.

DIAGNOSTIC EVALUATION

The evaluation of cervical lymphadenitis should be guided by the initial presenting history and exam findings. As discussed previously, attention to pertinent exposure history and determination of whether the onset of lymphadenitis has been acute or chronic, and unilateral or bilateral, will help limit the likely causes and focus the diagnostic evaluation.

An acutely inflamed solitary nodule in an otherwise well-appearing child may not require any further workup, as the most likely cause would be a localized bacterial infection with either *S. aureus* or GABHS. If fluctuance of the affected node is appreciated on exam, needle aspiration can be not only therapeutic, but also helpful in identifying an etiology. Though aspiration should be avoided in the case of suspected NTM infection due to risk of fistula formation. Aspirated fluid can be sent for bacterial (aerobic and anaerobic), fungal, and mycobacterial culture. Blood culture is not indicated routinely, but should be obtained if the child is febrile and ill-appearing. *B. henselae* can be detected by serologic studies. Lymph node tissue specimens can be sent for *B. henselae* PCR, but the PCR is not helpful when performed from blood. For children with persistent or severe symptoms, further workup can be considered including complete blood count, erythrocyte sedimentation rate (ESR), C-reactive protein (CRP), hepatic function panel, tuberculin skin test (TST), interferon gamma release assay (IGRA), and other serologic testing for specific pathogens as indicated by history and exam. In children with NTM infections the TST may be positive but the patient will have negative IGRA.

Imaging of the neck with either ultrasound or CT can be useful in guiding surgical management, detecting the extent of infection, and identifying the presence of a drainable fluid collection. If the diagnosis continues to remain in question and symptoms are persistent or worsening, an excisional lymph node biopsy can be done to help evaluate further for malignancy or other infectious causes.

MANAGEMENT

Management of cervical lymphadenitis depends on what is deemed as the most likely underlying etiology. Patients with uncomplicated bilateral lymphadenitis that is thought to be secondary to a viral infection require supportive care and observation only. Children who have acute onset of unilateral lymphadenitis and are thought to have a bacterial etiology will require treatment with antibiotics.

Recommendations for initial antibiotic coverage may vary based on local resistance patterns. Empiric therapy should include coverage for *S. aureus* and GABHS; however, empiric coverage for methicillin-resistant *S. aureus* (MRSA) depends on regional susceptibilities. In patient's with low risk of MRSA based on history or local resistance patterns, cefazolin, oxacillin, or nafcillin may be utilized. When MRSA coverage is desired, clindamycin is a reasonable empiric option, but is unlikely to cover all MSSA and MRSA. Linezolid or vancomycin cover MRSA, but consultation with an infectious disease specialist is advised. If the patient's symptoms are associated with periodontal disease, the addition of anaerobic coverage should be considered and treatment begun with either amoxicillin-clavulanic acid, ampicillin-sulbactam, or clindamycin. Symptomatic improvement is usually seen within 48 to 72 hours after starting treatment, but it may take up to 6 weeks for the enlarged node to completely resolve depending on etiology.

When an abscess is seen on imaging or palpable on exam, treatment with either incision and drainage or needle aspiration can be therapeutic. For *B. henselae*, surgical drainage is rarely necessary, and some argue that no treatment is necessary at all due to the self-limited course of the infection. If treatment is desired, azithromycin, rifampin, or trimethoprim-sulfamethoxazole can be used. In patients with NTM infection, excisional biopsy is the most effective therapy, but is often accompanied or preceded by antimicrobial therapy as there can be risk for facial nerve injury with full excision.

ADMISSION AND DISCHARGE CRITERIA

Nontoxic and well-hydrated children should be managed in the outpatient setting. Admission is appropriate for patients who are ill-appearing, dehydrated, or have failed outpatient therapy with oral antibiotics. Discharge from the hospital should be considered when patients have shown symptomatic improvement and are able to be transitioned to an oral antibiotic.

CONSULTATION

Surgeons, usually otolaryngologists, should be consulted when considering incision and drainage or excisional biopsies of infected nodes. Infectious diseases specialists may be needed for atypical cases or those in which a patient is not responding to initial therapy. If there is concern for an oncologic process, consultation with a hematology/oncology specialist is warranted to help guide further evaluation.

SUGGESTED READINGS

Bridwell R, Gottlieb M, Koyfman A, Long B. Diagnosis and management of Ludwig's angina: an evidence-based review. *Am J Emerg Med.* 2021;41:1-5.

Cui RZ, Bruce AJ, Rogers RS. Recurrent aphthous stomatitis. *Clin Dermatol.* 2016;34(4):475-481.

Dudas R, Serwint JR. In brief: retropharyngeal abscess. *Pediatr Rev.* 2006;27(6):e45-e46.

Gereige R, Cunill-De Sautu B. Throat infections. *Pediatr Rev.* 2011; 32(11):459-468; quiz 469.

Hoffmann C, Pierrot S, Contencin P, Morisseau-Durand MP, Manach Y, Couloigner V. Retropharyngeal infections in children. Treatment strategies and outcomes. *Int J Pediatr Otorhinolaryngol.* 2011;75(9):1099-1103.

Krol DM, Keels MA. Oral conditions. *Pediatr Rev.* 2007;28(1):15-22.

Lipsett SC, Porter JJ, Monuteaux MC, Watters K, Hudgins JD. Variation in the management of children with deep neck infections. *Hosp Pediatr.* 2021;11(3):277-283.

Neff L, Newland JG, Sykes KJ, Selvarangan R, Wei JL. Microbiology and antimicrobial treatment of pediatric cervical lymphadenitis requiring surgical intervention. *Int J Pediatr Otorhinolaryngol.* 2013; 77(5):817-820.

Peters TR, Edwards KM. Cervical lymphadenopathy and adenitis. *Pediatr Rev*. 2000;21(12):399-405.

Shulman ST, Bisno AL, Clegg HW, et al. Clinical Practice Guideline for the diagnosis and management of Group A Streptococcal Pharyngitis: 2012 Update by the Infectious Diseases Society of America. *Clin Infect Dis*. 2012;55(10):e86-e102.

Vieira F, Allen SM, Stocks RMS, Thompson JW. Deep neck infection. *Otolaryngol Clin North Am*. 2008;41(3):459-483, vii.

CHAPTER 97

Middle Respiratory Tract Infections and Bronchiolitis

Julia A. Marlow, MD, MS and Todd A. Florin, MD, MSCE

BRONCHIOLITIS

Acute bronchiolitis is the most frequent cause of infant hospitalization in the United States. Both bronchiolitis and laryngotracheobronchitis (croup) are common and lead to significant morbidity. Epiglottitis, although rare since introduction of the *Haemophilus influenzae* type B (Hib) vaccine, warrants inclusion because of its life-threatening nature.

PATHOPHYSIOLOGY

Bronchiolitis, a common communicable respiratory illness, is characterized by signs and symptoms of both upper and lower respiratory tract infection. Most episodes occur in otherwise healthy children younger than 2 years. Children younger than 3 months are at high risk for severe disease. Other groups at risk for serious illness secondary to bronchiolitis include young infants less than 37 weeks gestation with and without chronic lung disease, children with hemodynamically significant congenital heart disease, and those with severe immune deficiency such as hematopoietic stem cell transplantation, solid organ transplantation, and cellular immune deficiencies (e.g., 22q11.2 chromosome deletions).

Respiratory syncytial virus (RSV), a single-stranded RNA paramyxovirus, and Rhinovirus, a single-stranded RNA picornavirus, accounts for 50% to 80% of cases of bronchiolitis. Less common causes of bronchiolitis include parainfluenza virus types 1, 2, and 3, influenza viruses A and B, coronavirus (including SARS-CoV-2), adenovirus, human metapneumovirus, other enteroviruses and human bocavirus (**Table 97-1**). Rare bacterial causes of bronchiolitis include *Mycoplasma pneumoniae and Bordetella pertussis*.

Overall, bronchiolitis is most prevalent between October and May, although sporadic cases occur throughout the year. Epidemic RSV bronchiolitis displays remarkable seasonality, with a peak occurrence between December and April and virtually no occurrence between June and October. Peak activity of hMPV occurs in March and April, just as RSV activity begins to wane. The typical seasonal prevalence of specific pathogens is shown in **Figure 97-1**. The COVID-19 pandemic has altered the typical seasonal cycle of RSV and other viral pathogens, though it is expected that as SARS-CoV-2 becomes endemic, the typical seasonality will return. In the United States, 1% to 3% of affected infants require hospital care; most hospital admissions for bronchiolitis occur between December and March. Although the clinical manifestations of bronchiolitis and asthma overlap to some extent, the pathogenesis of the two conditions differs, a fact that has important therapeutic implications. In bronchiolitis, progressive infection of the respiratory mucosa induces desquamation of ciliated respiratory epithelial cells and lymphocytic infiltration of peribronchial epithelial cells. These changes lead to small-airway obstruction as intraluminal cellular debris accumulates and mucosal edema worsens. The concomitant increase in mucus production and, in some children, enhanced airway smooth muscle reactivity compounds the small airway obstruction that characterizes bronchiolitis. The relatively small caliber of their distal airways predisposes young infants to more severe obstructive symptoms.

TABLE 97-1 Prevalence of Detected Respiratory Pathogens in Infants With Severe Bronchiolitis

Detected Pathogen	Prevalence Detected (%)
RSV	77.1
Rhinovirus	23.8
Coronavirus	6.9
Adenovirus	6.4
Human metapneumovirus	6.0
Parainfluenza viruses	2.5
Enterovirus	2.3
Bocavirus	1.8
Influenza virus	1.4
Mycoplasma pneumoniae	1.0
Bordetella pertussis	0.2

CLINICAL PRESENTATION

Symptoms appear 5 to 7 days after exposure, although the incubation period is often shorter for parainfluenza (2-4 days) and influenza (1-7 days) viruses. The initial symptoms include nasal congestion, rhinorrhea, and cough. Poor feeding, posttussive emesis, and irritability may accompany these symptoms. Fever develops in half to three-fourths of patients. These findings persist for several days, and then lower respiratory tract involvement develops precipitously. Dyspnea and audible wheezing are common. In younger infants, especially those younger than 2 months, apnea may develop as the initial manifestation of bronchiolitis.

Tachypnea, tachycardia, and mild to moderate hypoxemia are often present during the physical examination. The infant may appear barrel-chested because of air trapping. Labored breathing, with flaring of the alae nasi, grunting, abdominal breathing, and suprasternal, intercostal, subcostal, and supraclavicular retractions, may be observed. On auscultation, harsh rhonchi, expiratory wheezing, and rales are heard diffusely throughout the chest. As the illness progresses, wheezing is often heard without the aid of a stethoscope. In children with severe lower airway obstruction, wheezing may not be readily appreciated because of poor aeration. Although not common in a tachypneic young infant, marked prolongation of the expiratory respiratory phase occurs with more severe lower airway obstruction.

Other findings in children with bronchiolitis can include conjunctivitis, otitis media (up to 50% of cases), and pharyngitis. The liver and spleen may be palpable because of air trapping and flattening of the diaphragm. Signs of dehydration may be noted in children with decreased fluid intake due to cough or respiratory distress and in those with significant posttussive vomiting.

In older children and adults, infections caused by RSV and hMPV usually cause symptoms of upper respiratory tract involvement such as rhinorrhea, cough, coryza, and pharyngitis. Any of the agents that cause bronchiolitis in younger children can exacerbate asthma or other chronic lung diseases in older children and adults.

DIFFERENTIAL DIAGNOSIS

In young infants early in the course of illness, the cough is occasionally staccato in nature, which makes it difficult to differentiate clinically from infection with *Bordetella pertussis* or *Chlamydia trachomatis*. Asthma, as well as other conditions that cause wheezing (see Chapter 142), must also be considered in the differential diagnosis.

DIAGNOSIS

The diagnosis of bronchiolitis can generally be made by the history and physical examination findings alone. No tests are routinely required.

In the hospital setting, an etiologic diagnosis may facilitate the implementation of strategies to limit nosocomial transmission of respiratory viruses (e.g., type of precautions, patient cohorting). However, institution of these interventions can be based on the clinical diagnosis (e.g., bronchiolitis) rather than the specific infectious agent.

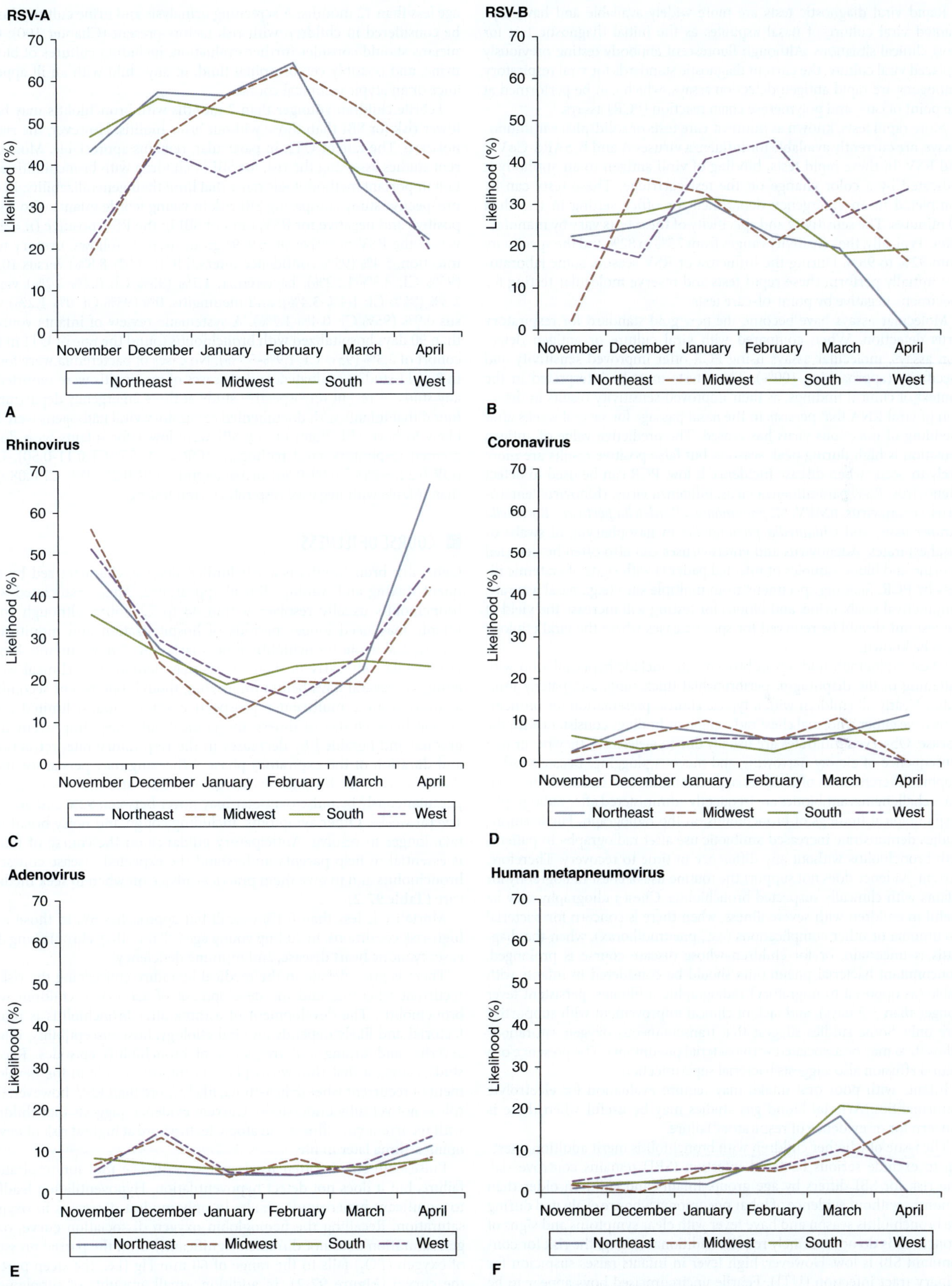

FIGURE 97-1. Temporal change in the likelihood of having each of five most common pathogens in infants with severe bronchiolitis, by U.S. census region. Respiratory syncytial virus (A) (RSV)-A, (B) RSV-B, (C) rhinovirus, (D) coronavirus, (E) adenovirus, and (F) human metapneumovirus (hMPV). (Reproduced with permission from Hasegawa K, Goto T, Hirayama A, et al. Respiratory virus epidemiology among US infants with severe bronchiolitis: analysis of 2 multicenter, multiyear cohort studies. *Pediatr Infect Dis J*. 2019;38(8):e180-e183.)

Rapid viral diagnostic tests are more widely available and have supplanted viral culture of nasal aspirates as the initial diagnostic test for most clinical situations. Although fluorescent antibody testing previously replaced viral culture, the current diagnostic standards for viral respiratory pathogens are rapid antigen detection assays, which can be performed at the point of care, and polymerase chain reaction (PCR) assays.

More rapid tests, known as point-of-care tests or solid-phase immunoassays, are currently available for influenza viruses A and B, SARS-CoV-2 and RSV. In these rapid tests, binding of viral antigen to an antibody is indicated by a color change on the test cartridge. These tests can be completed in an emergency department or office setting in less than 30 minutes. The sensitivity and specificity of these tests vary by manufacturer. Typically, the sensitivity ranges from 75% to 82% and the specificity from 92% to 98%. During the influenza or RSV season, some laboratories initially perform these rapid tests and reserve molecular testing for specimens negative by point-of-care tests.

Molecular assays have become the new gold standard for respiratory virus detection. When compared with viral culture or antigen detection assays, molecular assays using PCR offer improved sensitivity and specificity (approaching 100%). These tests must be interpreted in the context of clinical findings, as their improved sensitivity results in detection of viral RNA that persists in the nasal passage for several weeks after shedding of infectious virus has ceased. The predictive value of antigen detection is high during peak seasons, but false positive results are more likely to occur when disease incidence is low. PCR can be used to detect adenovirus, RSV, parainfluenza virus, influenza virus, rhinovirus/enterovirus, coronavirus, hMPV, *M. pneumoniae*, *Bordetella pertussis*, *Bordetella parapertussis*, and *Chlamydia pneumoniae* in nasopharyngeal swabs or nasal aspirates. Adenovirus and enteroviruses can also often be detected in urine and blood samples of infected patients with signs of systemic illness by PCR. Sending specimens from multiple sites (e.g., nasal aspirate, conjunctival swab, urine, and blood) for testing will increase the yield of the test but should be reserved for specific cases where the viral etiology must be known.

Chest radiograph findings in bronchiolitis include hyperinflation with flattening of the diaphragm, peribronchial thickening, and patchy infiltrates. Nearly all children with a typical clinical presentation for bronchiolitis have either a normal chest radiograph or findings consistent with the disease. Observed infiltrates are usually due to atelectasis; they occur as a consequence of airway narrowing and mucous plugging. Because radiographic differentiation of atelectasis, pneumonitis, and bacterial pneumonia is challenging, antibiotics are frequently administered after radiography despite typical findings of bronchiolitis on the radiograph. Furthermore, studies demonstrate increased antibiotic use after radiography in patients with bronchiolitis without any difference in time to recovery. Therefore, current evidence does not support the routine use of chest radiography for infants with clinically suspected bronchiolitis. Chest radiography may be useful in children with severe illness, when there is concern for bacterial pneumonia or other complications (e.g., pneumothorax), when the diagnosis is uncertain, or for children whose disease course is prolonged. Concomitant bacterial pneumonia should be considered in infants with stable (as opposed to migratory) radiographic infiltrates, persistent fever (longer than 3-5 days), and lack of clinical improvement with supportive care only. Some studies suggest that transcutaneous oxygen saturations below 92% may be associated with bacterial pneumonia. The presence of a pleural effusion also suggests bacterial superinfection.

Infants with poor oral intake may require evaluation for electrolyte abnormalities. Arterial blood gas studies may be useful when there is concern for or evidence of respiratory failure.

The issue of whether children with bronchiolitis merit additional testing to exclude serious bacterial infection (SBI) remains controversial. The risk for SBI differs by age group. Infants and children older than 2 months without evidence of lobar pneumonia who are evaluated during the bronchiolitis season and have fever with clear symptoms and signs of bronchiolitis do not routinely require additional testing; the risk for concomitant SBI is low. However, high fever in infants raises suspicion for urinary tract infection (UTI). Febrile uncircumcised boys appear to be at particularly high risk. Risk factors for UTI in infant boys include temperature ≥39°C, fever lasting more than 24 hours, and absence of another infectious source. Infant girls are at risk for UTI with temperature ≥39°C, fever lasting 2 days or more, absence of another infectious source, and age less than 12 months. A screening urinalysis and urine culture should be considered in children with risk factors present (Chapter 100). Clinicians should consider further evaluation, including cultures of blood, urine, and possibly cerebrospinal fluid, in any child with an ill appearance or an atypical clinical course.

Febrile children younger than 2 months with bronchiolitis may be at lower risk for SBI than those without bronchiolitis. However, the risk is not zero. The rate of UTI, in particular, remains appreciable. Most current studies assessing the risk for SBI in children with bronchiolitis contain important methodologic flaws that limit their generalizability. In one prospective study comparing SBI risk in young febrile infants who tested positive and negative for RSV, rates of SBI in the RSV-positive ($n = 269$) versus the RSV-negative ($n = 979$) group were as follows: urinary tract infection, 5.4% (95% confidence interval [CI]: 3.0%-8.8%) versus 10.1% (95% CI: 8.3%-12.2%); bacteremia, 1.1% (95% CI: 0.2%-3.2%) versus 2.3% (95% CI: 1.4%-3.4%); and meningitis, 0% (95% CI: 0%-1.2%) versus 0.9% (95% CI: 0.4%-1.7%). A systematic review of infants younger than 90 days hospitalized with bronchiolitis found the rate of UTI in this cohort of 3.3% (95% CI: 1.9%-5.7%). No cases of bacteremia were found in 8 of 11 studies evaluated, and no cases of meningitis were reported in any study. A recent retrospective study at three emergency departments found that infants with documented respiratory viral pathogens were less likely to have SBI. Rates of any SBI were lower for infants with documented respiratory viral pathogens (OR 0.23, 95%CI 0.11-0.50), UTI (OR 0.22, 95%CI 0.09-0.56) or bacteremia (OR 0.27, 95% CI 0.08-0.9) than infants with negative respiratory viral testing.

COURSE OF ILLNESS

Generally, bronchiolitis is a self-limited disease, characterized by frequent waxing and waning clinical appearance. Apnea associated with bronchiolitis usually resolves within 48 to 72 hours, although some infants may need longer periods of hospitalization and monitoring. The typical acute bronchiolitis illness lasts 3 to 7 days. Infants hospitalized relatively early in their illness may demonstrate clinical worsening for several days before improving, though one recent secondary analysis from 2 multicenter prospective studies found limited association between day of illness and clinical outcomes. Improvement is gradual and heralded by decreases in the respiratory rate, retractions, and duration of the expiratory phase. Wheezing may persist for more than a week after hospital discharge. Oxygen saturation as measured percutaneously by pulse oximeter may hover between 92% and 96% for several weeks. Other symptoms, including cough and noisy breathing, take longer to resolve. Anticipatory guidance on the course of illness is essential to help parents understand the expected disease course of bronchiolitis and to give them practical advice on when to seek medical care (**Table 97-2**).

Mortality is less than 0.1% overall but approaches 5% in those with high-risk conditions, including young age (<2 months), chronic lung disease, cyanotic heart disease, and immune deficiency.

There is great debate in the medical literature concerning the risk of recurrent wheezing and the development of asthma in children with bronchiolitis. The development of asthma after bronchiolitis is multifactorial and likely depends on viral etiology, host susceptibility, illness severity, and timing and frequency of bronchiolitis episodes. Recent studies suggest that rhinovirus plays an important role in the development of recurrent wheeze in asthma, likely more than RSV; however, this role is not yet fully understood. Current evidence suggests that children with recurrent viral illness and atopic features are at highest risk of developing asthma later in life.

Pulse oximetry is often used as a surveillance tool for respiratory failure, but it does not detect hypoventilation. Hypoventilation leading to significant hypercapnia results in only modest decreases in oxygen saturation. Recalling the hemoglobin-oxygen dissociation curve, oxygen saturation does not diminish significantly until the partial pressure of oxygen (PO_2) falls to the range of 60 mm Hg (i.e., the steep part of the curve) (**Figure 97-2**). In addition, small amounts of supplemental oxygen will restore PO_2, thereby normalizing oxygen saturation, which would allow unrecognized inadequate ventilation to progress without further derangements in pulse oximeter readings. Respiratory acidosis ensues with increasing hypercapnia. Bedside evaluation of an

TABLE 97-2 Anticipatory Guidance for Bronchiolitis

Clinical Course: Bronchiolitis typically starts with upper respiratory tract symptoms, progressing to lower respiratory tract symptoms after 2-3 days. Disease symptoms vary, but often peak during days 4-6. Resolution of symptoms may take 1-2 weeks, with approximately 10% of patients having persistent symptoms at 4 weeks.

Transient Nature: Symptoms in bronchiolitis can change frequently. Children with bronchiolitis may look to have only mild symptoms at one moment, which can be promptly followed by significant distress. When the child appears in moderate-to-severe distress, attempt to calm the child, provide supportive treatment measures, and if significant distress persists, contact the child's physician.

Treatment at Home:

- Nasal suctioning and saline drops*
  - Nasal suctioning may be helpful before feeding, before sleeping, or if the baby appears to have trouble breathing due to nasal congestion. Avoid suctioning after feeding, as this may cause the baby to vomit.
  - Saline drops or sprays can be purchased at most pharmacies or can be made at home by mixing ¼ teaspoon of salt to 8 ounces of warm water, stirring to dissolve the salt, and storing in a clean, covered jar for no more than 1 week.
  - After washing your hands, with the baby on their back drop 3-4 drops of saline into one nostril and keep baby in this position for 1 minute.
  - Push all of the air out of the bulb suction with your thumb, hold in place and carefully place the tip of the bulb into the nostril until the nostril is sealed
  - Slowly release thumb letting air back into the bulb, which will suction mucus out of the baby's nose.
  - Remove the bulb from the baby's nose and squeeze out the mucus from the bulb.
  - Repeat this procedure on the other nostril. This may need to be done several times to fully clear the mucus.
  - Gently wipe the baby's nose and clean the bulb syringe with warm, soapy water.
- Maintaining adequate hydration: Babies with bronchiolitis often have trouble eating and drinking due to nasal congestion or respiratory distress. Attempt small feedings at more frequent intervals than the baby's usual schedule, with a goal of attaining at least 70–80% of the baby's usual intake when healthy over a 24-hour period. For example, instead of taking 4 ounces of fluid every 4 hours, the baby may need to take 1 ounce of fluid every hour. Urine output should be monitored, with a goal of at least 3 wet diapers each day.
- Use a cool-mist humidifier in the baby's room.
- Fever may be treated with over-the-counter medicines, such as acetaminophen. AVOID cough suppressants and decongestants in children with bronchiolitis.
- The baby's physician may prescribe additional therapies, such as albuterol, if they have been found to be helpful for your child. These therapies do not work in most children with bronchiolitis.

Indications to return to medical care: apnea (pause in breathing for more than 15 seconds), cyanosis, not able to maintain hydration or poor feeding, fever, increased respiratory rate (more than 60 breaths per minute that persists for more than 15–30 minutes), increased work of breathing (grunting, flaring, retractions)

Prevention:

- Hand washing with soap and water or an alcohol-based hand sanitizer is essential to minimize spread of infection.
- Avoid exposing the baby to cigarette smoke.
  - If smoking outside, wear a "smoking jacket" that is removed before entering the home.
- Avoid contact with other individuals with respiratory infections.
- Parents and children should receive the flu shot each year.

*Adapted from http://www.cincinnatichildrens.org/health/s/suction.

infant with respiratory failure would reveal somnolence and tachypnea with shallow respirations, which can progress to bradypnea or apnea. Expected derangements in arterial blood gas results would progress from hypocapnia associated with tachypnea and hyperventilation to the normal-range partial pressure of carbon dioxide (PCO_2). This "normal" PCO_2 would be inappropriate in the setting of hyperventilation and should be considered a harbinger of respiratory insufficiency. Progression to respiratory failure would be confirmed by worsening hypercapnia and respiratory acidosis (i.e., falling blood pH on an arterial blood gas specimen).

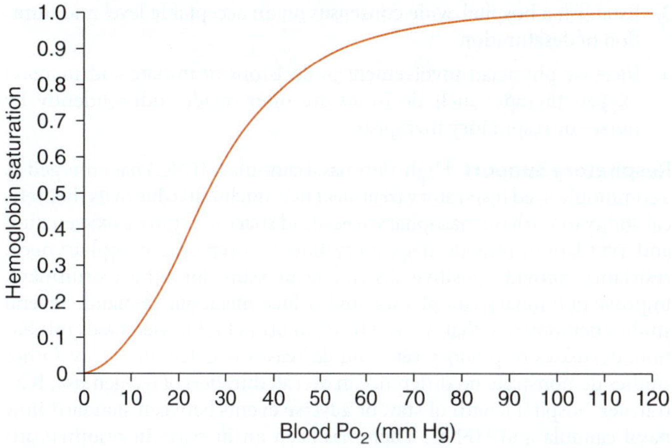

FIGURE 97-2. Hemoglobin-oxygen dissociation curve. (Reproduced with permission from Gutierrez G, Bismar H. Oxygen transport and utilization. In: Dantzker DR [ed]. *Cardiopulmonary Critical Care.* 2nd ed. Philadelphia: WB Saunders;1991.)

TREATMENT

The primary care physician manages most infants and children with bronchiolitis in the outpatient setting. Certain high-risk children and children with severe symptoms require closer monitoring and often hospitalization. Factors associated with a more severe disease course where hospitalization should be considered include age less than 3 months, prematurity (gestational age <34 weeks), significant retractions, tachypnea, tachycardia, and hypoxia (oxygen saturation ≤94%).

Oxygen Therapy The mainstay of treatment in infants and children with bronchiolitis is supportive. Infants and children admitted with bronchiolitis and hypoxia require supplemental oxygen. The appropriate lower limits for oxygen saturation in children with bronchiolitis are not known, but various guidelines suggest values ranging from 90% to 94%. However, no guideline specifies the acceptable duration of desaturation below these thresholds. Furthermore, normal transient desaturation and measurement error because of poor pulse pressure and motion artifact occur frequently. Considerable uncertainty remains over when to begin, increase, or discontinue supplemental oxygen therapy. As a consequence, abnormalities in pulse oximetry readings alone often unnecessarily prolong hospitalization in children with bronchiolitis as a result of the perceived requirement for supplemental oxygen. Healthy infants with bronchiolitis who have oxygen saturations at or above 90% while breathing room air benefit little from increasing PaO_2 with supplemental oxygen (Figure 97-2), particularly in the absence of significant respiratory distress and feeding difficulties. Thus, the American Academy of Pediatrics Bronchiolitis Clinical Practice Guidelines recommend that supplemental oxygen should be initiated in previously healthy infants only if oxygen saturation values fall persistently below 90%, and should be discontinued if oxygen saturation is greater than 90% while feeding well with minimal respiratory distress. Fever, acidosis, and hemoglobinopathies shift the oxyhemoglobin dissociation curve to the right; a higher oxygen saturation should be maintained in patients with these factors. Data are lacking as to safe upper saturations to support discontinuation of supplemental oxygen. Evidence in neonatal literature demonstrates harm secondary to hyperoxemia; similar evidence is growing in pediatric and adult critical care literature, yet data are needed in pediatric respiratory illnesses including bronchiolitis. Careful consideration is necessary to prevent potential harm secondary to hyperoxemia. The following strategies can help to limit overreliance on pulse oximetry:

1. Discontinue the use of pulse oximetry or transition to intermittent pulse oximetry during the convalescent stage of illness. Recent research has demonstrated continued focus on desaturations and overreliance on pulse oximetry. Innovative methods to deimplement the pulse oximeter, including a multi-center RCT, are currently underway.
2. Initiate or increase supplemental oxygen therapy only in children with increasing respiratory distress or when other maneuvers such as stimulation, suctioning, or repositioning fail to improve oxygenation.

3. Establish a hospital-wide consensus on an acceptable level and duration of desaturation.
4. Increase physician involvement in decisions to initiate and increase oxygen therapy; such decisions are often made independently by nurses or respiratory therapists.

Respiratory Support High-flow nasal cannula (HFNC) has emerged as a commonly used respiratory treatment in bronchiolitis due to its theoretical ability to wash out nasopharyngeal dead space to improve oxygenation and ventilation, provide inspiratory flow to overcome nasopharyngeal resistance, provide positive distending pressure for lung recruitment, improve pulmonary compliance, and reduce metabolic demand. Several studies demonstrate that use of HFNC in bronchiolitis decreases intubation, decreases respiratory rate, and decreases ICU length of stay. Other studies demonstrate no difference in overall duration of oxygen use, ICU transfer, hospital length of stay, or adverse events between standard flow nasal cannula and HFNC. There has been an increase in resource utilization and cost with the implementation of HFNC. One retrospective study found a 13-fold increase in HFNC use over a 6-year period, but no changes in rates of hospital or ICU admission. Less than 30% of children initiated on HFNC were hypoxic. It remains unclear if HFNC has a role as a rescue therapy to minimize the need for intensive therapies. Several single center, retrospective studies have explored feeding while on HFNC and report low rates of adverse events (e.g., aspiration pneumonia) at various ranges of high flow support. The most beneficial and cost-effective methods of using HFNC have yet to be determined. Further prospective studies are necessary to define objective clinical criteria for initiating HFNC therapy as well as efficient weaning protocols.

Other potential respiratory support interventions include heliox therapy, nasal continuous positive airway pressure (CPAP), and endotracheal intubation with mechanical ventilation. Administration of heliox (70% helium, 30% oxygen) through a non-rebreather (reservoir) facemask may improve respiratory effort by preserving laminar airflow at higher flow rates. While heliox has been shown to reduce respiratory distress in infants with bronchiolitis within the first hour of initiation, it has not been shown to reduce either the rate of endotracheal intubation or length of ICU stay. In several small studies, CPAP has been shown to reduce pCO_2 and improve clinical respiratory scores. A small international randomized controlled trial compared CPAP to HFNC for infants with severe bronchiolitis and found CPAP was better at preventing treatment failure than HFNC. A recent meta-analysis comparing 5 randomized controlled trials found higher failure rates with HFNC, no difference in PICU length of stay and no difference in need for intubation (latter 2 only had data from 4/5 trials). A European RCT found no difference in pCO_2, respiratory rate, treatment failure or length of stay alluding to the benefit of HFNC being better tolerated. Mechanical ventilation should be considered for infants with signs of respiratory failure, shock, or persistent apnea.

Medications Several meta-analyses have systematically reviewed the efficacy of β-agonists in the treatment of bronchiolitis. In a systematic review of 13 trials consisting of 956 patients, most of the studies compared nebulized albuterol with nebulized saline, unspecified placebo, or no treatment, while four studies also compared nebulized albuterol with nebulized ipratropium bromide. Nine of the 13 trials showed no difference in various clinical measures (e.g., oxygen saturation, respiratory rate) between children treated with and without β-agonist therapy, three demonstrated short-term improvement in various clinical measures, and one demonstrated a worsening of these parameters. There were no significant differences between the groups in need for or length of hospitalization. Another meta-analysis of 48 trials including 4897 patients revealed that β-agonist use was not associated with lower hospitalization rates at 1 and 7 days after presentation to the emergency department or with a shorter hospital length of stay. A third meta-analysis of 28 trials (1912 infants) found that β-agonists do not improve oxygen saturation, reduce hospitalizations, shorten the duration of hospitalization, or reduce time to resolution of illness. The average improvement in clinical score with β-agonists vs placebo, though statistically significant, was of small magnitude, limiting its clinical significance (standardized mean difference: −0.37; 95% CI: −0.62 to −0.13). In summary, although some trials of β-agonist therapy demonstrated mild improvement in some clinical features of bronchiolitis, β-agonist use must be weighed carefully against potential adverse effects and cost of these therapies. In addition, β-agonists appear to have no effect on other clinically important factors, such as oxygen saturation, need for hospitalization, duration of illness, and hospital length of stay.

In addition to bronchodilating effects, nebulized racemic epinephrine adds β-agonist properties that are thought to reduce airway edema and mucus production by inducing vasoconstriction of the bronchial vasculature. Compared to placebo, epinephrine showed a significant reduction in hospitalization at one day after presentation in outpatients (risk ratio [RR]: 0.67; 95% CI: 0.5-0.89), but no difference at 7 days, in a meta-analysis of 19 trials (2256 patients). There was no difference in admission rates when epinephrine was compared to β-agonists. For inpatients, there was no difference in hospital length of stay when comparing epinephrine to placebo, although the mean length of stay was 0.28 (95% CI: 0.46-0.09) days less in those receiving epinephrine compared to β-agonists. This analysis also found a statistically significant, though clinically modest, improvement in clinical score at 1 hour after treatment when comparing epinephrine to placebo in outpatients (standardized mean difference: −0.40; 95% CI: −0.58 to −0.23) with no differences in oxygen saturation or respiratory rate. When compared to β-agonists, epinephrine appears to have modest benefits in short-term clinical outcomes in the first 24 hours of care, such as clinical score and respiratory rate.

Although the benefit of administering bronchodilators has not been established, they are often used in clinical practice, as clinical experience suggests that bronchodilators improve the clinical condition in selected infants. There is currently no evidence-based means of determining which infants may benefit from bronchodilators. Bronchodilators may be considered in patients with severe respiratory distress, hypoxia, or impending respiratory failure. Attempting a trial of nebulized bronchodilator and evaluating clinical response may be considered in patients with moderate to severe bronchiolitis. It is critical to evaluate response to therapy with objective scores before and after the bronchodilator trial. If no significant improvement occurs within 60 minutes of administration, treatment should be discontinued. Although studies suggest that racemic epinephrine may be superior to β-agonists in the emergency department and for hospitalized patients, it is not typically prescribed in the outpatient setting due to potential adverse effects.

Systemic corticosteroids are not indicated in the routine management of bronchiolitis. Studies have typically used 3- to 5-day courses of either dexamethasone (0.6 mg/kg to a maximum of 15 mg orally once daily) or prednisolone (1-2 mg/kg/day to a maximum of 60 mg orally divided twice daily). One of the largest clinical trials examining corticosteroids in bronchiolitis enrolled 600 infants 2 to 12 months of age with moderate to severe bronchiolitis across 20 pediatric emergency departments in the United States. This study demonstrated that a single 1 mg/kg dose of oral dexamethasone did not change hospitalization rate, respiratory state at 4 hours after treatment, or longer-term outcomes compared to placebo. A meta-analysis of six placebo-controlled studies (347 patients) of corticosteroid therapy demonstrated a small but statistically significant reduction in the length of hospital stay; the mean duration of hospitalization was 0.43 day (95% CI: 0.05-0.81) shorter in the corticosteroid group than in the placebo group. When the studies that included patients with a history of wheezing were omitted from the analysis, this difference was no longer significant, a finding that supports the notion that certain subgroups with bronchiolitis may benefit from corticosteroid treatment. A subsequent meta-analysis of 17 trials including 2596 patients found that corticosteroids did not reduce hospitalization rates or inpatient length of stay.

Several studies have examined the synergistic effects of corticosteroids and inhaled epinephrine. Unadjusted results from a single multicenter study examining nebulized epinephrine and dexamethasone (1 mg/kg initially, followed by 5 days of 0.6 mg/kg/day) found that only those infants who received both treatments (as opposed to epinephrine and placebo, dexamethasone and placebo, or two placebos) had reduced hospital admissions at 7 days after treatment (RR: 0.65; 95% CI: 0.45-0.95). After adjustment, this effect was not significant, making these results exploratory. In another trial of children with severe bronchiolitis requiring positive-pressure ventilatory support, the duration of respiratory support was reduced in the combination corticosteroids-epinephrine group versus standard care. These results require confirmation in future research, and it remains unclear whether a combination of corticosteroids and inhaled epinephrine should be used and, if so, which infants are most likely to benefit.

Overall, the risks and benefits of corticosteroid administration must be weighed. Because bronchiolitis is generally self-limited and corticosteroid use prolongs viral shedding in RSV bronchiolitis, many clinicians do not favor their routine use in the treatment of children with bronchiolitis. However, subgroups that may benefit from corticosteroid administration include those with recurrent wheezing in the context of a strong family history of atopy and asthma (provided that evaluation for other causes of recurrent wheezing has been undertaken) and those with severe illness or respiratory failure. In summary, current evidence suggests that corticosteroids should not be routinely administered to infants with bronchiolitis. Future studies may demonstrate benefit in combination with certain medications or in certain populations.

Nebulized hypertonic saline is believed to increase mucociliary clearance of pulmonary secretions through its ability to lower the viscosity of mucus, stimulate cilial beat, and reduce airway edema by absorbing water from the mucosa. Although initial trials found that 3% saline reduced hospital length of stay by more than 1 day compared with 0.9% saline, these studies occurred in hospitals with long mean lengths of stay. More recent trials with lengths of stay <72 hours, more consistent with most US hospitals, demonstrate no difference in length of stay between 3% and 0.9% saline. Recent systematic reviews have shown either an attenuated effect of 3% saline compared with prior reviews or no effect on length of stay. There have been concerns about bronchospasm related to hypertonic saline administration. AAP bronchiolitis guidelines therefore do not recommend hypertonic saline use for infants with bronchiolitis. A systematic review and meta-analysis of 29 studies and 1583 patients challenges the placebo status of nebulized normal saline. The review showed statistically significant improvement in respiratory rate and respiratory score without change in oxygen saturation. It did not explore other relevant outcomes, such as overall disease course or hospital length of stay.

Ribavirin, a synthetic purine nucleoside analogue, exerts its effect by lethally mutating the viral RNA genome. Although initially thought to be a promising treatment in bronchiolitis, a recent systematic review of 10 trials of ribavirin in severe RSV bronchiolitis found no evidence that its use results in consistent improvements in clinical outcomes. Its cumbersome delivery requirements, potential health risks for caregivers (anemia, hemolysis, bone marrow suppression, conjunctival irritation, transient worsening of pulmonary function), and high cost have led the AAP to recommend against routine use of ribavirin in bronchiolitis. Ribavirin may be considered in highly selected situations in patients with severe illness where the potential benefit in reducing duration of mechanical ventilation outweighs the above risks.

Additional therapies evaluated in bronchiolitis include leukotriene receptor antagonists (e.g., montelukast), inhaled corticosteroids, steam inhalation or mist therapy, nasal phenylephrine, nebulized deoxyribonuclease, and surfactant (for critically ill patients). None of these therapies have been shown to be effective and are not currently recommended in the treatment of bronchiolitis.

Hydration & Supportive Care Maintaining hydration with intravenous fluids may be necessary, but nasogastric feeding is an alternative. One open randomized trial found that both intravenous and nasogastric fluids were appropriate hydration methods for infants with bronchiolitis, but nasogastric insertion may require fewer attempts and have higher insertion success rates than intravenous access. Infusing nasogastric feeding slowly tends to minimize gastric distention and vomiting. Daily weights and careful documentation of intake and output are helpful in assessing and tracking fluid status.

Mechanical airway clearance involves improving symptoms of bronchiolitis through mobilizing and eliminating respiratory secretions. Chest physiotherapy through chest percussion and postural drainage has been proposed as a physical mechanism to help clear bronchial secretions. A meta-analysis of nine trials involving 891 patients found no differences between chest physiotherapy and no intervention in disease severity, respiratory parameters, oxygen requirements, or length of stay. Chest physiotherapy should therefore not be routinely used in infants with bronchiolitis. Suctioning may provide temporary relief and improve the ability to sleep and feed. Deep suctioning has been shown to be associated with increased hospital length of stay, likely due to airway trauma and resultant edema. There is no evidence to support deep suctioning of the lower pharynx, larynx, or trachea, and such techniques may be potentially harmful.

CONSULTATION

- Pediatric critical care for an infant or child with respiratory distress requiring intensive monitoring and mechanical ventilation.
- Pediatric infectious diseases for a child with concern over an alternative infectious process or for a child at risk for severe disease in whom ribavirin is being considered.
- Pediatric pulmonology for an infant or child with severe or persistent symptoms requiring further evaluation or follow-up.

ADMISSION CRITERIA

Hospitalization may be considered for the following reasons:

- Respiratory distress or respiratory difficulties requiring close monitoring, especially in young infants early in the course of their illness
- Persistent tachypnea or tachycardia
- Hypoxia (percutaneous oxygen saturation <90%)
- Evidence of respiratory insufficiency by clinical evaluation or arterial blood gas findings of hypercapnia or respiratory acidosis
- Dehydration or inability to maintain oral intake
- Apnea or cyanosis
- Infant with risk factors for severe disease
- Lack of outpatient support and follow-up

DISCHARGE CRITERIA

- Resolution of respiratory distress with stable or improving respiratory status that is well tolerated
- Respiratory rate consistently less than 60 to 70 breaths per minute with no more than modest increase in respiratory effort
- Percutaneous oxygen saturation >90% on room air or eligible for home oxygen therapy
- Resolution of apnea
- Ability to maintain adequate hydration
- Ability of a caregiver to provide adequate support at home
- Appropriate outpatient follow-up (requires thoughtful attention to which patients benefit from follow up and if recommended, is ideally scheduled prior to discharge)

PREVENTION

The goals of prevention are to minimize nosocomial transmission of the viruses that cause bronchiolitis and reduce the risk for RSV infection in high-risk infants by providing immunoprophylaxis.

INFECTION CONTROL MEASURES

RSV is the leading cause of nosocomial respiratory illness. Several factors contribute to the frequency of nosocomial RSV infection:

- RSV can spread by large-particle droplets or by contaminated secretions carried on infected patients, healthcare workers, and fomites.
- Transmission to 45% of contacts may occur in the absence of infection control measures.
- Repeat infections may be acquired by both adults and children, because RSV infection does not induce long-term immunity.

Control measures that have been shown to reduce rates of nosocomial infection and save money include:

- Recognizing patients with respiratory symptoms early and implementing infection control precautions
- Establishing cohorts of patients and nursing staff
- Instituting gown, glove, and mask barrier precautions
- Monitoring and education of staff

IMMUNOPROPHYLAXIS

For many years, palivizumab (Synagis) was the only licensed product currently available to provide passive immunity for infants at high risk for a poor outcome if infected with RSV (**Table 97-3**). RSV-IGIV, a polyclonal hyperimmune globulin prepared from donors with high serum titers of RSV-neutralizing antibody, was used for RSV prophylaxis but is no longer available. Palivizumab, a genetically engineered humanized murine monoclonal antibody to RSV, is given at monthly intervals (15 mg/kg intramuscularly) during the RSV season. Several randomized, multicenter placebo-controlled trials have demonstrated the safety and efficacy of palivizumab in children. The IMpact-RSV trial enrolled 1502 patients. Prophylaxis decreased RSV-related hospitalization rates from 10.6% to 4.8% in the placebo versus palivizumab recipients, respectively. This study also demonstrated decreases in the duration of hospitalization, requirement for supplemental oxygen, and need for intensive care unit admission in the palivizumab versus the placebo group. Among 1287 infants with hemodynamically significant congenital heart disease, palivizumab recipients had lower hospitalization rates than placebo recipients did (5.3% vs. 9.7%). No serious adverse events were attributed to palivizumab. Advantages of palivizumab include its safety in children with cyanotic congenital heart disease, ease of intramuscular versus intravenous administration, and low complication rate. Moreover, immunizations do not need to be delayed after palivizumab administration.

Palivizumab is expensive and uses a significant amount of healthcare resources. Therefore, its use is restricted to groups that would most benefit from passive immunization (Table 97-3). Hospitalized infants who qualify for prophylaxis during the RSV season should receive their first dose of palivizumab 2 to 3 days before discharge or soon after discharge. The families of all high-risk infants should receive counseling regarding smoking cessation and influenza vaccination for all family members, including infants older than 6 months.

A second monoclonal antibody against severe RSV recently entered the market in 2023. For infants less than 8 months of age, pooled efficacy from phase 2 and 3 trials of nirsevimab (Beyfortus) demonstrated an efficacy of 80.6% in preventing RSV-associated LRTI hospitalization and 90% in preventing RSV-associated LRTI intensive care unit (ICU) admission. It is administered in a single dose and has broader inclusion criteria (**Table 97-3**).

Advances in vaccine development—including mRNA vaccines—in the setting of the COVID-19 pandemic have led to the recent development of an RSV vaccine. RSVpreF is a recombinant protein vaccine for adults that entered the market in 2023. There are two forms (GSK Arexvy and Pfizer Abrysvo). Abrysvo received approval for use in pregnant women (target administration at 32-36 weeks gestation) in 2023. Research is underway for both vaccines; preliminary evidence indicates acceptable tolerability, safety, and immunogenicity in older adults and pregnant women. Further research is necessary in the pediatric population.

TABLE 97-3 Indications for Prophylaxis against Respiratory Syncytial Virus

Palivizumab

Administer palivizumab (maximum of 5 doses)* in the first 12 months of life if:

- Premature infants born *before* 29 weeks, 0 days' gestation if younger than 12 months at the start of the RSV season
- Infants with chronic lung disease of prematurity (birth at <32 weeks, 0 days' gestation AND a requirement of >21% oxygen for at least 28 days after birth)
- Infants with hemodynamically significant cyanotic or acyanotic congenital heart disease (those most likely to benefit include those receiving medication to control congestive heart failure, moderate-to-severe pulmonary hypertension, cyanotic heart disease)†

Consider palivizumab for:

- Infants in the first 12 months of life with pulmonary abnormalities or neuromuscular disease that impairs the ability to clear secretions from the upper airways
- Children <2 years of age with profound immunocompromised during RSV season

Palivizumab prophylaxis *not* recommended in the second year of life *except* in:

- Children who required at least 28 days of supplemental oxygen after birth and continue to require medical interventions (e.g. supplemental oxygen, diuretics, chronic corticosteroids)

If an infant receiving monthly prophylaxis experiences a breakthrough RSV hospitalization, monthly prophylaxis should be discontinued due to extremely low likelihood of second RSV hospitalization in the same season (<0.5%).

Nirsevimab

Administer 1 dose of nirsevimab (50 mg for infants <5 kg and 100 mg for infants ≥5 kg) to infants < 8 months of age if the mother did not receive the RSV vaccine during pregnancy, has unknown RSV vaccination status, or the infant is born within 14 days of maternal RSV vaccination.

For infants < 8 months of age born shortly before or during the RSV season:

- Administer nirsevimab in the first week of life. The dose can be administered either in the birth hospital or outpatient clinic. For infants with prolonged hospitalization (e.g., preterm infants), immunize shortly before or promptly after discharge. Nirsevimab administration should be offered during the season to those who have not received a dose.

For infants < 8 months of age born outside the RSV season:

- Administer a single dose of nirsevimab (50 mg for infants <5 kg and 100 mg for infants ≥5 kg) shortly before the start of their first RSV season.

For children ages 8 through 19 months who are at increased risk of severe RSV disease:

- Administer a single dose of nirsevimab (200 mg) shortly before the start of their second RSV season.

*Once a child qualifies for initiation of prophylaxis at the start of the RSV season, administration should continue throughout the season and not stop when an infant reaches either 6 or 12 months of age.

†The following conditions generally do *not* require prophylaxis: lesions adequately corrected by surgery do not require prophylaxis unless infants continue to need medication for congestive heart failure, hemodynamically insignificant disease (eg, secundum atrial septal defect, small ventricular septal defects, uncomplicated aortic stenosis, pulmonic stenosis, mild coarctation of the aorta, and patent ductus arteriosus), mild cardiomyopathy not requiring medical therapy, children in the 2nd year of life.

Summarized from AAP Policy Statement: updated guidance for palivizumab prophylaxis among infants and young children at increased risk of hospitalization for respiratory syncytial virus infections. *Pediatrics*. 2014;134:415-420.

CROUP

Croup, or laryngotracheobronchitis, is a common acute respiratory tract infection in children. Children between the ages of 6 months and 6 years are most affected, and the highest incidence of disease occurs during a child's second year of life. Each year up to 6 cases per 100 children are evaluated in primary care offices and emergency departments. The seasonal predilection of croup is the fall and early winter, but cases occur throughout the year.

Parainfluenza viruses type 1 to 3, members of the Paramyxoviridae family, account for almost three-quarters of all cases of croup. Type 1 is most commonly isolated, followed by type 3 and then type 2. Other viral causes of croup include RSV, influenza A and B, adenovirus, hMPV, and coronavirus HCoV-NL63. Rare causes of croup include *M. pneumoniae*, and in unimmunized children, measles, and diphtheria. SARS-CoV-2 has been associated with croup in children, most notably with the omicron variant. Further research is needed to characterize the condition.

Croup results from an infection of the upper and middle respiratory tract and is manifested as inflammation and edema of the larynx, trachea, and bronchi. The inflammation and edema lead to narrowing of the airway and increased resistance to airflow. In young children this becomes problematic because of the funnel-like anatomy of their airway. The increased resistance causes the classic "croupy" or barky cough and inspiratory stridor. In severe cases, respiratory distress or respiratory failure can occur.

CLINICAL PRESENTATION

Croup is an illness characterized by a bark-like cough, hoarseness, inspiratory stridor, and potentially respiratory distress. Commonly, a child initially experiences nasal congestion and cough. After 12 to 48 hours the cough progressively worsens and becomes barky in nature, and hoarseness and intermittent inspiratory stridor arise. For reasons that are unclear, the cough and stridor are more severe during the night. Mild pharyngeal erythema, coryza, and fever are common. The symptoms of croup often progress along a spectrum classically divided into mild, moderate, and severe based on the level of respiratory distress. In mild croup, physical examination reveals a comfortable patient who is mildly tachypneic with a hoarse voice. Stridor is generally absent or observed only when the child is agitated. In moderate croup, the child appears uncomfortable, is tachypneic, and has a pronounced cough. Inspiratory stridor is present at rest and suprasternal and intercostal retractions may be present. Children with severe croup have significant respiratory distress with tachypnea, nasal flaring, and retractions and may appear agitated or lethargic. Stridor occurs at rest, and with increasing airway narrowing, may be present with inspiration and expiration. Tachycardia, and in some cases pulsus paradoxus, are observed.

DIFFERENTIAL DIAGNOSIS

The differential diagnosis for croup should focus on the potential causes of stridor. Stridor is defined as a medium-pitched respiratory sound, usually with inspiration, that represents resistance to airflow through the airway. The level of resistance determines the timing of the stridor. During inspiration, negative pressure is transmitted to the intraluminal space of the extrathoracic airway and leads to narrowing of the upper airway and partial obstruction, and thus inspiratory stridor is produced. Within the chest cavity, the downward excursion of the diaphragm with inspiration produces negative pressure in the pleural space, thereby allowing expansion of the intrathoracic airways. This increased airway diameter would reduce or relieve partial obstruction of these airways.

Conversely, on expiration, positive pressure is created within the extrathoracic (upper) airway and expands its luminal diameter. With expiration, there is a relative positive pressure in the intrapleural space in comparison to the intraluminal space of the intrathoracic airways. This would lead to narrowing of these airways and worsening of any partial obstruction, thus producing expiratory stridor.

Biphasic stridor represents a fixed obstruction that is unaltered by changes in intraluminal diameter or a combination of upper and lower airway involvement. The differential diagnosis for stridor is presented in **Table 97-4**. Although children with classic signs and symptoms of croup will only very rarely have an alternative diagnosis, vigilance for other diseases presenting with stridor and respiratory distress is essential in atypical presentations. For example, bacterial tracheitis is a rare but life-threatening bacterial infection that typically presents with acutely worsening symptoms after 2 to 7 days of mild to moderate illness. Bacterial tracheitis should be considered in children with stridor who are febrile, appear toxic, and typically do not respond to treatment with nebulized epinephrine. Epiglottitis is a rare, life-threatening infection presenting with high fever, drooling, dysphagia, anxiety, and preference to sit forward with the head extended. Other considerations in atypical presentations include foreign body aspiration, retropharyngeal or peritonsillar abscess, angioneurotic edema, and allergic reaction.

DIAGNOSIS AND EVALUATION

Croup is a clinical diagnosis that can safely be made without the use of diagnostic tests. Performing diagnostic tests has the potential to agitate the patient and further worsen the respiratory distress.

TABLE 97-4 Differential Diagnosis of Stridor

Quality of Stridor	Inspiratory	Biphasic	Expiratory
Location of Pathology	Supraglottic	Glottic	Subglottic
Condition	Croup	Croup	Bacterial tracheitis
	Epiglottitis	Bacterial tracheitis	Foreign body
	Peritonsillar abscess	Foreign body	Tracheomalacia
	Retropharyngeal abscess	Laryngomalacia	Hemangioma
	Foreign body	Laryngeal web	Subglottic stenosis
	Laryngomalacia	Vascular ring	Pulmonary sling
	Hemangioma	Hemangioma	
	Supraglottic web	Vocal cord paralysis	

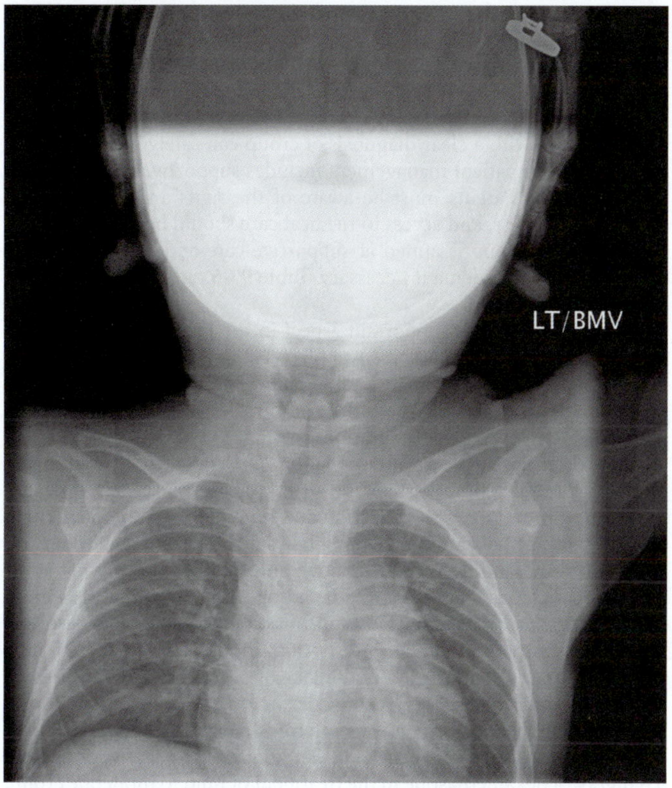

FIGURE 97-3. Airway radiograph demonstrating "steeple sign" of croup.

In most instances, radiographic studies are not necessary. However, anteroposterior and lateral neck radiographs may confirm typical changes in the contour of the airway seen in croup. These films are particularly useful if there is concern for an airway foreign body. In the anteroposterior view the "steeple sign," the classic finding in croup, reveals narrowing of the subglottic air column (**Figure 97-3**). Widening of the hypopharynx is observed in the lateral view. This finding is not present in all children with croup and can be found in some healthy children, depending on the phase of inspiration and positioning of the child when the radiographs are obtained.

In the outpatient setting, routine laboratory testing in children with croup is not needed. However, patients sufficiently ill to warrant hospitalization may require additional laboratory evaluation. Pulse oximetry is a useful tool for detecting oxygen desaturation. In patients with severe respiratory distress, arterial blood gas analysis could be helpful in evaluation of the potential respiratory insufficiency or failure. Electrolytes may be appropriate in patients with significant dehydration. Concurrent bacterial infections in the setting of croup are rare. However, patients with high spiking fevers who continue to worsen despite proper treatment should be evaluated for a secondary bacterial infection. Studies to consider include chest radiography as well as blood and urine cultures.

Children with uncomplicated croup do not require routine direct visualization of the airway by laryngoscopy. This test should be considered in children with noisy breathing or a hoarse cry between croup illnesses, frequent or progressively worsening episodes of croup, a severe episode requiring intubation, and a history of intubation in the neonatal period. Children with an episode of choking or gagging at the onset of the illness should be evaluated for foreign body aspiration.

COURSE OF ILLNESS

Croup is a self-limited disease. Symptoms typically worsen during the first 2 to 3 days of the illness and then remit over the next 3 to 7 days. A decrease in oral intake can occur as a result of a sore throat or respiratory distress. Hospitalization occurs in less than 2% of children with croup. Of those hospitalized, less than 1.5% require endotracheal intubation. Long-term sequelae and death are rare. Bacterial tracheitis is a potentially severe complication of croup. There are also sporadic reports of tracheitis caused by *Candida* species after prolonged corticosteroid administration for recurrent stridor.

TREATMENT

Most children with a clear diagnosis of croup can safely be managed as outpatients. Outpatient management includes supportive care and often corticosteroids. Parents must be aware of the signs and symptoms of respiratory distress, and access to medical care should be ensured.

Therapy for croup is aimed at supportive care and reducing airway inflammation and edema if necessary. **Table 97-5** outlines management for a child with croup.

Supportive care is an important aspect in the management of croup. Adequate hydration should be ensured; consider administering intravenous isotonic saline in those not taking fluids well by mouth. Although hypoxemia is rare, oxygen should be administered in cases associated with persistent low oxygen saturations.

Corticosteroids decrease inflammation and edema of the laryngeal mucosa. Multiple clinical trials and meta-analyses have demonstrated their utility in reducing the duration and severity of symptoms, return office visits, hospitalization rates, length of stay in the emergency department and ward, and need for intubation and reintubation. Recent studies have concluded that oral dexamethasone is the optimal treatment modality because of its ease of administration, low cost, and widespread availability. Intramuscular administration should be considered in a child with difficulty tolerating oral intake or severe respiratory distress, and has equivalent efficacy to oral dexamethasone. Investigations of the smallest effective dose of corticosteroids have been conducted. One study demonstrated that a dose of 0.15 mg/kg was as effective as 0.3 and 0.6 mg/kg of dexamethasone in the treatment of mild to moderate croup; however, a meta-analysis of six studies indicates that a higher dose may be more effective in children with severe disease. Adverse events from the use of corticosteroids for croup have been rare. Corticosteroids should not be administered to patients with tuberculosis unless they are receiving appropriate antituberculosis treatment or to patients with varicella.

Nebulized epinephrine is well established as an effective treatment for children with moderate to severe croup. Epinephrine improves croup symptoms by its α-adrenergic properties. It is composed of an equal mixture of the *d*- and *l*-isomer of epinephrine. The *l*-isomer binds the α-receptors on the precapillary arterioles and causes fluid resorption and a decrease in laryngeal edema. The dose of racemic epinephrine is 0.25 to 0.75 mL of a 2.25% solution. Racemic epinephrine was initially used because it was thought to be associated with less tachycardia and hypertension. It has been shown that *l*-epinephrine is as effective and the cardiovascular effects are similar to those of racemic epinephrine. Nebulized epinephrine has an onset of action of 10 minutes and lasts approximately 2 hours. Some children return to their pretreatment state once the effect of the medication dissipates. This return of symptoms has historically been referred to as the "rebound phenomenon." Initially, it was believed that all children receiving racemic epinephrine required hospitalization. In one study evaluating the safety of sending children treated with epinephrine home, patients with severe respiratory distress after 20 minutes of mist therapy were administered 0.5 mL of 2.25% racemic epinephrine and 0.6 mg/kg of oral dexamethasone. After 2 to 3 hours if a child had a sustained response without return of symptoms, the child was discharged home. Of the patients discharged, none had a return of their respiratory distress. Subsequent studies have found similar results. One retrospective study did not find differences in return rates in those discharged after fewer than 2 hours after receiving inhaled epinephrine. Therefore, children receiving racemic epinephrine in the emergency department should receive corticosteroids and be monitored for approximately 2 hours after the racemic epinephrine. If they remain stable and have a lack of stridor at rest and a normal level of consciousness, discharge can be considered.

Heliox is believed to reduce severe respiratory distress by increasing laminar flow (and thus decreasing turbulent flow) through the narrowed airway. When compared to racemic epinephrine, patients treated with heliox had similar improvements in croup score over time. As it has not been shown to be superior to standard therapies and requires skilled personnel to administer, there is currently insufficient evidence to recommend the general use of heliox in severe croup. Additionally, heliox may provide insufficient supplemental oxygen in a child with severe hypoxia.

If respiratory failure or complete airway obstruction is imminent, the airway should be secured by tracheal intubation or tracheostomy. In children who require intubation, the endotracheal tube should be 0.5 to 1 mm smaller than the predicted size for age. Extubation is recommended when a positive pressure of 25 cm H_2O causes a significant air leak.

Older therapies thought to be beneficial to croup patients included steam and cool night air. These two treatments are still recommended for patients at home with evidence of mild croup. Use of humidified air via mist tents in the emergency department or hospital setting has been shown to be ineffective and is not without its adverse effects. Nebulized saline may precipitate bronchospasm in children with underlying airway hyperreactivity and is not recommended. Problems exist with the use of mist tents in the hospital setting. First, mist therapy can worsen bronchospasm in children with wheezing. Second, it separates children from their parents, which may cause anxiety and potentially worsen a child's respiratory status. Third, mist tents have been reported to disperse fungus and molds into the environment if not properly cleaned. Finally, the cumbersome tent precludes frequent reevaluation, an important aspect of croup management. Therefore, the use of mist tents in the hospital is no longer recommended.

TABLE 97-5 Treatment of Croup

Severity of Symptoms	Management
Mild	Anticipatory guidance
	Ensure appropriate follow-up and access to medical services
	Consider dexamethasone, 0.15-0.6 mg/kg orally × 1 dose
Moderate	Dexamethasone, 0.15-0.6 mg/kg orally × 1 dose; consider IM or IV if unable to take PO
	Racemic epinephrine, 0.25-0.75 mL of a 2.25% solution with 2.5 mL normal saline via nebulizer
	Consider hospital admission if repeated doses of racemic epinephrine are needed or if patient has one or more criteria for admission
Severe	Secure the airway if necessary
	Racemic epinephrine, 0.25-0.75 mL of a 2.25% solution with 2.5 mL normal saline via nebulizer
	Dexamethasone, 0.6 mg/kg IV or IM
	Consider heliox (70%-80% helium) via face mask
	Close observation for possible respiratory decompensation
	Admit to the hospital; consider admission to the intensive care unit

CONSULTATION

- Critical care: Children with respiratory distress requiring intensive monitoring and the possibility of endotracheal intubation or tracheostomy
- Otolaryngology or pulmonology: Children with unusual or persistent symptoms for which laryngoscopy or bronchoscopy may be warranted
- Infectious diseases: Children with suspected alternative infectious processes (e.g., epiglottitis, bacterial tracheitis)

ADMISSION CRITERIA

Hospitalization may be considered for any of the following reasons:

- Persistent moderate to severe symptoms despite outpatient therapy (corticosteroids and aerosolized epinephrine)
- Respiratory distress
- Hypoxemia
- Young infant; for example, younger than 4 to 6 months
- Dehydration or inability to tolerate feeding
- Inability to manage at home or ensure follow-up
- Uncertain diagnosis in which further evaluation and treatment are necessary

DISCHARGE CRITERIA

- Resolution of respiratory distress
- Resolution of hypoxemia
- Tolerating sufficient fluids
- Ability of caregivers to provide appropriate support at home and to understand the signs of a worsening clinical condition
- Establishment of appropriate outpatient follow-up

PREVENTION

Prudent hand washing is the mainstay of prevention for exposed individuals. Adherence to the immunization guidelines will prevent the rare cases caused by measles and diphtheria.

EPIGLOTTITIS

Acute epiglottitis, an illness characterized by fever, dysphagia, and dysphonia, rapidly progresses to upper airway obstruction secondary to edema of the epiglottis and aryepiglottic folds. In the past it was predominantly a disease of otherwise healthy children. More recent reports emphasize the development of epiglottitis in immunocompromised patients. After the 1988 introduction of the conjugate Hib vaccine and the 1991 recommendation to routinely immunize all infants starting at 2 months of age, invasive Hib disease, including epiglottitis, declined by more than 99%. Affected children are now also older than in the pre-Hib vaccine licensure period; the typical age presently ranges from 5 to 12 years rather than 3 to 6 years. In the pre-vaccination era, Hib accounted for up to 90% of cases. Currently, Hib is responsible for approximately 25% of cases of epiglottitis; other bacteria, viruses, and noninfectious agents now cause most cases. Responsible organisms include group A β-hemolytic streptococcus; *Staphylococcus aureus*; nontypable and type A *H. influenzae*; group B, C, and G streptococci; viridans group streptococci; *Streptococcus pneumoniae*; and *Candida* species. Among immunosuppressed patients *S. pneumoniae* and *Candida* species have been reported more commonly than other organisms. Bacterial superinfection causing epiglottitis may follow viral respiratory infections, particularly herpes simplex virus, varicella-zoster virus, Epstein-Barr virus, and parainfluenza viruses. Noninfectious causes include thermal injuries, trauma, and post-transplant lymphoproliferative disorder.

CLINICAL PRESENTATION

A child with acute bacterial epiglottitis initially has a fever and dysphagia. Antecedent cough and upper respiratory tract infection are uncommon. The illness evolves rapidly over a 12- to 24-hour period with the development of drooling, dysphonia (usually a muffled or "thick-sounding" voice), and progressive irritability, restlessness, and anxiety. Hoarseness of the voice is uncommon. On physical examination the child appears extremely toxic. The child may sit in the tripod position (sitting up and leaning forward with the neck hyperextended and the mouth open) to maximize airway diameter. Often there is drooling. In contrast to croup, stridor in epiglottitis is rarely severe. However, its presence indicates impending complete airway obstruction. Hypoxia, hypercapnia, and acidosis worsen with the progressive deterioration in air exchange.

DIFFERENTIAL DIAGNOSIS

The differential diagnosis for epiglottitis is that of edema and inflammation of the upper airway. An aspirated foreign body can present with a sudden onset of respiratory distress and may be accompanied by drooling. It should be considered in a child with a history of a choking episode that precedes the development of respiratory distress. Laryngotracheobronchitis, or croup, can present with stridor and respiratory distress and should be considered, especially if the child has the associated barky cough and hoarse voice. Cough is more likely to be associated with croup while drooling, refusal to swallow, and dysphagia or odynophagia were more likely to be associated with epiglottitis. Bacterial tracheitis can present with respiratory distress in a toxic-appearing child and should be considered in a child with a more slowly evolving course. Peritonsillar abscess and retropharyngeal abscess should be considered. Angioneurotic edema that involves the epiglottis resembles epiglottitis; however, fever is noticeably absent. Isolated uvulitis can cause dysphonia. Although usually viral in origin, cases of bacterial uvulitis with concomitant epiglottitis have been described.

DIAGNOSIS AND TREATMENT

Management of epiglottitis involves securing the airway and then administering appropriate antibiotics. Most epiglottitis-related deaths occur en route to the hospital or within the first few hours of evaluation. Epiglottitis represents an airway emergency; delays of even a few hours may prove fatal. In cases in which suspicion of epiglottitis is high, radiographic confirmation of the diagnosis causes unnecessary delay and should not be considered until airway patency has been established.

Care should be taken to keep the child calm and comfortable. Anxiety-provoking maneuvers such as phlebotomy, intraoral examination, or removal of the child from the comfort of a caregiver's arms should be avoided. Agitation of the child can lead to obstruction of the airway and decompensation. A clinician with experience in pediatric airway management should perform a diagnostic evaluation by direct laryngoscopy with endotracheal intubation, and tracheostomy equipment should be available at bedside. This evaluation should take place in the operating suite whenever possible, but the emergency department and pediatric critical care unit are other good options. Direct visualization of the epiglottis provides the definitive diagnosis. The epiglottis and aryepiglottic folds appear inflamed, often described as a "cherry red" epiglottis. An abscess on the lingual surface of the epiglottis may obscure some landmarks.

A child with epiglottitis requires endotracheal intubation, with nasotracheal placement preferred. Age-appropriate endotracheal tubes as well as several smaller tubes should be readily available. Supplies should also be available to perform a tracheostomy if required. In a true emergency, experienced personnel can insert a 13- or 15-gauge needle through the cricothyroid membrane. This needle thoracostomy can provide temporary means of oxygenation while more definitive methods to secure the airway are being established. Culture specimens from the surface of the epiglottis and from blood should be obtained after establishment of an artificial airway. Cultures are particularly important given the diversity of organisms causing epiglottitis.

Once the airway has been secured, the child should be examined for secondary sites of infection, which are present more than half the time and include otitis media, pneumonia, meningitis, and cellulitis.

Culture of blood or epiglottis may identify the causative organism. Blood cultures were positive in approximately 75% of patients in the pre-Hib vaccine era. Limited data suggest that the yield of positive blood cultures in the post-Hib era ranges from 40% to 60%. A complete blood count may reveal leukocytosis with a predominance of neutrophils and band forms. Additional diagnostic evaluation is unnecessary except for studies pertaining to evaluation of respiratory status and to assessment of end-organ damage (e.g., liver, kidneys, brain) as required.

In patients with a high likelihood of epiglottitis, radiography should be deferred until after endotracheal intubation. In stable patients in whom clinical suspicion is low, a lateral radiograph of the neck should be obtained and examined to determine whether it suggests epiglottitis or other pathology. Positioning for radiographs should not compromise the patient's comfort, so flexion of the neck to a neutral position or supine positioning may need to be avoided. On a lateral soft tissue radiograph, the epiglottis appears rounded and thickened (thumb sign) with loss of the vallecular airspace (**Figure 97-4**). The aryepiglottic folds may be thickened, and the hypopharynx distended. Anteroposterior views of the neck reveal a normal-caliber subglottic space. A clinician skilled in airway management should accompany the child if radiographic studies are performed, and whenever possible, obtaining portable (bedside) films is preferred.

Ceftriaxone and ampicillin-sulbactam are reasonable options for empirical therapy in a child with suspected epiglottitis. Alternative choices in patients with hypersensitivity reactions to β-lactam antibiotics include carbapenem-class (e.g., imipenem, meropenem) and fluoroquinolone-class (e.g., levofloxacin) antibiotics. Therapy should be continued

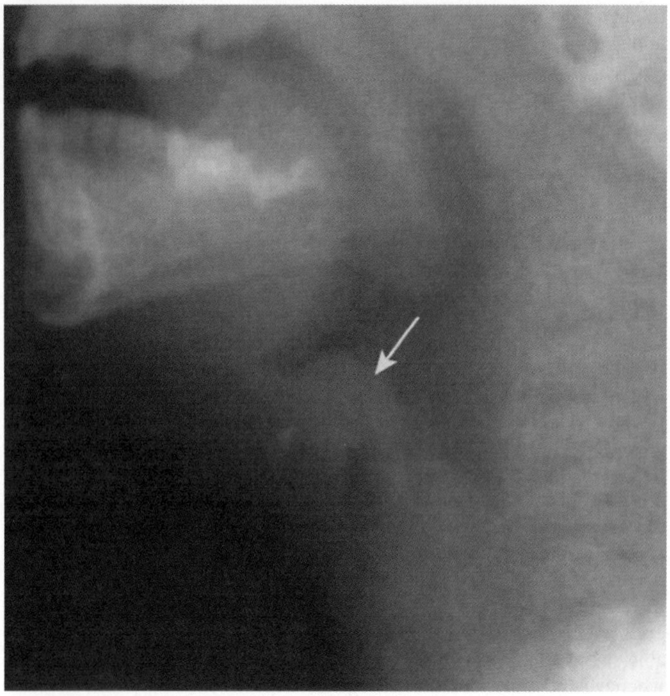

FIGURE 97-4. Lateral neck radiograph demonstrating epiglottis with the "thumb sign."

for 7 to 10 days. The therapeutic agent should be altered according to the results of culture and antimicrobial susceptibility testing.

COURSE OF ILLNESS

Epiglottitis is a life-threatening illness. Mortality in various studies has ranged from less than 1% to 30%. Early and aggressive airway management increases survival. Complications include post obstructive pulmonary edema after insertion of the endotracheal tube to relieve laryngeal obstruction, and metastatic foci of infection. In the Hib era, epiglottitis was often associated with pneumonia, cervical adenitis, and otitis media and rarely with meningitis, septic arthritis, and cellulitis. Other complications occur as a consequence of initial hypoxia or subsequent mechanical ventilation.

CONSULTATION

- Pediatric critical care: Airway and ventilator management and treatment of hemodynamic complications.
- Pediatric anesthesiology, otolaryngology: Assistance with airway management. Emergency tracheostomy, if needed, may require the assistance of general surgeons.
- Pediatric infectious disease: Antibiotic selection.

ADMISSION CRITERIA

- All children with suspected epiglottitis require hospitalization for diagnostic evaluation. Those with proven epiglottitis require hospitalization in an intensive care setting for intravenous antibiotics, endotracheal intubation, and monitoring.

DISCHARGE CRITERIA

- No airway compromise is present.
- Completed antibiotic therapy or appropriate oral antibiotics are available.
- Parents/caregivers understand the disease course, treatment, and follow-up.

PREVENTION

The mainstay of prevention of epiglottitis secondary to Hib is adherence to the immunization guidelines. Secondary disease may occur in contacts of patients with Hib disease. Although the rate of secondary illness after cases of Hib-related epiglottitis is less than that after other invasive Hib infections, prophylaxis of contacts is still recommended as follows: Rifampin prophylaxis (20 mg/kg/day once daily, maximum of 600 mg/dose), when prescribed, should continue for 4 days. In households with one or more infants younger than 12 months, the index case and all household contacts should receive rifampin prophylaxis. The same applies in households with children younger than 4 years who are incompletely vaccinated and in families with a fully vaccinated but immunocompromised child. For school or childcare contacts, chemoprophylaxis is not indicated unless there is more than one case of invasive Hib disease. Local public health officials as well as hospital infection control personnel can assist in identification of individuals requiring prophylaxis.

KEY POINTS

Bronchiolitis

- Clinical presentation: viral infection of the middle and lower respiratory tract with cough, wheezing, or crackles and varying degrees of respiratory distress most often caused by RSV.
- Diagnosis: Diagnosis is clinical.
- Treatment: Hospitalized patients require supportive care, usually for inadequate oral intake, respiratory distress, or hypoxemia.
- Bronchodilators are used often but have not been proven to be effective.
- Steroids should not be routinely used in children with bronchiolitis but may be of benefit to children with a personal or family history of asthma or atopy.
- Prophylaxis is indicated during the RSV season for children at high risk for significant morbidity or mortality.
- Prevention: Development of an RSV vaccine could provide active immunity, in contrast to the passive immunity provided by palivizumab.
- Research: Further research is needed to understand the role of RSV infection in recurrent wheezing.
- It remains unclear if corticosteroids or bronchodilators are beneficial for a sub-population of patients with bronchiolitis.

Croup

- Clinical presentation: A short nonspecific upper airway illness followed by a barking cough, hoarse voice, and stridor.
- Diagnosis: Diagnosis is clinical. Neck radiographs, viral testing, and laryngoscopy are reserved for patients with atypical presentations or severe symptoms.
- Treatment: Often managed on an outpatient basis. Corticosteroids are beneficial in mild, moderate, and severe cases. Aerosolized epinephrine can improve airway edema acutely if stridor present at rest or with moderate-to-severe respiratory distress. Mist is ineffective.
- Research: The optimal dosing, frequency, and route of administration of steroids needs to be further delineated. The role of adjunctive supportive therapies needs to be further investigated.
- The potential role of heliox in moderate-to-severe croup needs to be further explored.

Epiglottitis

- Clinical presentation: Epiglottitis is an airway emergency characterized by fever, dysphagia, and dyspnea. The child is often drooling and sitting in the tripod position with a toxic appearance.
- Diagnosis: A child with suspected epiglottitis should be cared for by the person most skilled in pediatric airway management and intubated in a controlled setting. Laryngoscopy will support the diagnosis by revealing a "cherry red" swollen epiglottis.
- Since the development of the *H. influenzae* (Hib) vaccine, the incidence of epiglottitis has decreased significantly.
- In fully vaccinated patients, a diversity of organisms may cause epiglottitis.
- Treatment: Treatment involves securing the airway and systemic antibiotics.

SUGGESTED READINGS

American Academy of Pediatrics Committee on Infectious Diseases, American Academy of Pediatrics Bronchiolitis Guidelines Committee. Updated guidance for palivizumab prophylaxis among infants and young children at increased risk of hospitalization for respiratory syncytial virus infection. *Pediatrics*. 2014;134(2):e620-e638.

Bjornson C, Russell K, Vandermeer B, Klassen TP, Johnson DW. Nebulized epinephrine for croup in children. *Cochrane Database Syst Rev*. 2013;(10):CD006619.

Bordley WC, Viswanathan M, King VJ, et al. Diagnosis and testing in bronchiolitis: a systematic review. *Arch Pediatr Adolesc Med*. 2004;158(2):119-126.

Corneli HM, Zorc JJ, Mahajan P, et al. A Multicenter, Randomized, Controlled Trial of Dexamethasone for Bronchiolitis. *N Engl J Med*. 2007;357(4):331-339.

Dafydd C, Saunders BJ, Kotecha SJ, Edwards MO. Efficacy and safety of high flow nasal oxygen for children with bronchiolitis: systematic review and meta-analysis. *BMJ Open Respir Res*. 2021;8(1):e000844.

Fernandes RM, Bialy LM, Vandermeer B, et al. Glucocorticoids for acute viral bronchiolitis in infants and young children. *Cochrane Database Syst Rev*. 2013;(6):CD004878.

Franklin D, Babl FE, Schlapbach LJ, et al. A Randomized Trial of High-Flow Oxygen Therapy in Infants with Bronchiolitis. *N Engl J Med*. 2018;378(12):1121-1131.

Gadomski AM, Scribani MB. Bronchodilators for bronchiolitis. *Cochrane Database Syst Rev*. 2014;(6):CD001266.

Gates A, Gates M, Vandermeer B, et al. Glucocorticoids for croup in children. *Cochrane Database Syst Rev*. 2018;8:CD001955.

Greenfield BW, Lowery BM, Starke HE, et al. Frequency of serious bacterial infections in young infants with and without viral respiratory infections. *Am J Emerg Med*. 2021;50:744-747.

Hartling L, Bialy LM, Vandermeer B, et al. Epinephrine for bronchiolitis. *Cochrane Database Syst Rev*. 2011;(6):CD003123.

Hasegawa K, Goto T, Hirayama A, et al. Respiratory virus epidemiology among US infants with severe bronchiolitis: analysis of 2 multicenter, multiyear cohort studies. *Pediatr Infect Dis J*. 2019;38(8):e180-e183.

Jones JM, Fleming-Dutra KE, Prill MM et al. Use of Nirsevimab for the Prevention of Respiratory Syncytial Virtus Disease Among Infants and Young Children: Recommendations of the Advisory Committee on Immunization Practices - United Stats, 2023. *MMWR Morb Mortal Wkly Rep*. 2023;72:920.

Kepreotes E, Whitehead B, Attia J, et al. High-flow warm humidified oxygen versus standard low-flow nasal cannula oxygen for moderate bronchiolitis (HFWHO RCT): an open, phase 4, randomised controlled trial. *Lancet*. 2017;389(10072):930-939.

Levine DA, Platt SL, Dayan PS, et al. Risk of serious bacterial infection in young febrile infants with respiratory syncytial virus infections. *Pediatrics*. 2004;113(6):1728-1734.

Luo J, Duke T, Chisti MJ, Kepreotes E, Kalinowski V, Li J. Efficacy of High-Flow Nasal Cannula vs Standard Oxygen Therapy or Nasal Continuous Positive Airway Pressure in Children with Respiratory Distress: A Meta-Analysis. *J Pediatr*. 2019;215:199-208.e8.

Mahajan P, Browne LR, Levine DA, et al. Risk of Bacterial Coinfections in Febrile Infants 60 Days Old and Younger with Documented Viral Infections. *J Pediatr*. 2018;203:86-91.e2.

Milési C, Essouri S, Pouyau R, et al. High flow nasal cannula (HFNC) versus nasal continuous positive airway pressure (nCPAP) for the initial respiratory management of acute viral bronchiolitis in young infants: a multicenter randomized controlled trial (TRAMONTANE study). *Intensive Care Med*. 2017;43(2):209-216.

Mussman GM, Parker MW, Statile A, Sucharew H, Brady PW. Suctioning and Length of Stay in Infants Hospitalized With Bronchiolitis. *JAMA Pediatr*. 2013;167(5):414-421.

Plint AC, Johnson DW, Patel H, et al. Epinephrine and Dexamethasone in Children with Bronchiolitis. *N Engl J Med*. 2009;360(20):2079-2089.

Ralston S, Hill V, Waters A. Occult serious bacterial infection in infants younger than 60 to 90 days with bronchiolitis: a systematic review. *Arch Pediatr Adolesc Med*. 2011;165(10):951-956.

Ralston SL, Lieberthal AS, Meissner HC, et al. Clinical Practice Guideline: The diagnosis, management, and prevention of bronchiolitis. *Pediatrics*. 2014;134(5):e1474-e1502.

Schondelmeyer AC, Simmons JM, Statile AM, et al. Using quality improvement to reduce continuous pulse oximetry use in children with wheezing. *Pediatrics*. 2015;135(4):e1044-e1051.

Schroeder AR, Destino LA, Ip W, et al. Day of illness and outcomes in bronchiolitis hospitalizations. *Pediatrics*. 2020;146(5):e20201537.

Schroeder AR, Marlow JA, Bonafide CP. Improving value in bronchiolitis care. *JAMA Netw Open*. 2021;4(2):e210157.

Schroeder AR, Marmor AK, Pantell RH, Newman TB. Impact of pulse oximetry and oxygen therapy on length of stay in bronchiolitis hospitalizations. *Arch Pediatr Adolesc Med*. 2004;158(6):527.

Schuh S, Lalani A, Allen U, et al. Evaluation of the utility of radiography in acute bronchiolitis. *J Pediatr*. 2007;150(4):429-433.

Zhang L, Mendoza-Sassi RA, Wainwright C, Klassen TP. Nebulised hypertonic saline solution for acute bronchiolitis in infants. *Cochrane Database Syst Rev*. 2017;12:CD006458.

Zhong Z, Zhao L, Zhao Y, Xia S. Comparison of high flow nasal cannula and non-invasive positive pressure ventilation in children with bronchiolitis: A meta-analysis of randomized controlled trials. *Front Pediatr*. 2022;10:947667.

CHAPTER 98 Lower Respiratory Tract Infections

Meghan E. Hofto, MD, MPH

PNEUMONIA

BACKGROUND

Epidemiology Pneumonia is the leading cause of death of children worldwide, with nearly 1 million deaths annually among children less than 5 years of age. Mortality is exceedingly rare in the developed world, occurring in less than 1% of hospitalized pneumonia cases. While hospitalization rates have decreased with the advent of the 13-valent pneumococcal conjugate vaccine, morbidity remains substantial with estimated hospitalization rates of 88.4 to 665.5 per 100,000 children in the United States, with the highest rates in those less than 5 years old. This translates to over 100,000 hospitalizations per year in the United States, making childhood pneumonia one of the most common conditions encountered in the hospital setting and also one of the most costly, with aggregate hospitalization costs approaching $1 billion annually.

ETIOLOGY

Viruses Respiratory viruses lead to pneumonia by direct extension from the upper respiratory tract and progressive invasion of the respiratory epithelium, which may lead to diffuse lymphocytic proliferation and interstitial pneumonitis and/or alveolar destruction depending on the specific etiology. Viruses are detected in 60% to 80% of children with pneumonia in both ambulatory and hospitalized settings (**Table 98-1**). Viral pathogens represent the predominant cause of pneumonia in children under 5 years of age, either alone or in combination with bacteria. Respiratory syncytial virus (RSV), parainfluenza viruses, influenza viruses, and adenovirus have long been considered causative pneumonia pathogens; human metapneumovirus and novel coronaviruses, including SARS-CoV-2, are more recently discovered etiologies of potentially severe disease. Human bocavirus and rhinoviruses have also been implicated.

Bacteria Bacteria causing pneumonia often colonize the nasopharynx and access the lower respiratory tract directly by inhalation, although this alone is not sufficient to cause disease as it likely happens frequently. Only when bacteria overcome the typical pulmonary host defenses does pneumonia develop. Often this occurs in the setting of a viral upper

TABLE 98-1 Common Causes of Pneumonia by Age

Age	Pathogen
1-3 mo	*Chlamydia trachomatis*
	Respiratory syncytial virus
	Parainfluenza viruses
	Metapneumovirus
	Streptococcus pneumoniae
	Bordetella pertussis
	Staphylococcus aureus
3 mo-5 yr	Respiratory syncytial virus
	Parainfluenza viruses
	Metapneumovirus
	Influenza viruses
	Adenoviruses
	Streptococcus pneumoniae
	Mycoplasma pneumoniae
	Haemophilus influenzae, nontypable*
	Staphylococcus aureus
	Streptococcus pyogenes
	Bordetella pertussis
5-15 yr	*Mycoplasma pneumoniae*
	Chlamydophila pneumoniae
	Streptococcus pneumoniae
	Staphylococcus aureus

*Rarely seen in immunocompetent children in developed nations.

respiratory tract infection or other period of impaired immunity. Bacterial replication in the lower airways leads to alveolar fluid accumulation and neutrophilic inflammation with rapid involvement of contiguous alveoli progressing to lobar consolidation. Occasionally, pneumonia develops by hematogenous dissemination, either from a distant site of infection (e.g. osteomyelitis) or from primary bacteremia.

A number of different bacteria may cause pneumonia (Table 98-1); however, *Streptococcus pneumoniae* is considered the major pathogen, implicated in up to 50% of pneumonia cases in clinical and epidemiologic studies. Following the introduction of the 7-valent pneumococcal conjugate vaccine, rates of all-cause and pneumococcal pneumonia declined substantially, as did rates of pneumococcal penicillin resistance. However, non-vaccine serotypes quickly emerged, and despite reductions in pneumonia hospitalizations and systemic complications, disease complicated by parapneumonic effusion and empyema increased substantially.

Non-vaccine serotype 19A, often multidrug-resistant and associated with severe disease, was responsible for the majority of culture-positive pneumococcal cases reported following the introduction of the heptavalent pneumococcal conjugate vaccine and is likely partially responsible for increases in rates of complicated pneumonia. Overall disease rates, however, have yet to approach pre-conjugate vaccine era levels, and the licensure of the 13-valent pneumococcal conjugate vaccine in 2010, targeting six additional clinically important serotypes including 19A, has led to further declines in both hospitalizations and complications such as empyema.

Other bacteria-causing pneumonia include the atypical pathogens *Mycoplasma pneumoniae* and *Chlamydophila pneumoniae*, as well as *Staphylococcus aureus*, *Streptococcus pyogenes*, *Haemophilus influenzae*, and *Moraxella catarrhalis*. Atypical pathogens, particularly *M. pneumoniae*, are common causes of pneumonia, especially in school-age children and outpatients. However, asymptomatic carriage of *M. pneumoniae* has been detected, raising questions on overall burden of disease. Both *S. aureus* and *S. pyogenes* are notable for causing rapidly progressive disease that is often severe and associated with frequent complications. *S. aureus*, especially community-associated methicillin-resistant *S. aureus* (CA-MRSA), has become an increasingly important consideration in the United States. The CA-MRSA epidemic also parallels the rise of local pneumonia complications. In contrast, *H. influenzae* is no longer a major pneumonia pathogen due to widespread use of conjugate vaccines targeting *H. influenzae* type B. Non-type B *H. influenzae*, along with *M. catarrhalis*, are frequent colonizers of the upper respiratory tract, but only occasionally cause pneumonia.

Viral-Bacterial Coinfection The influenza pandemic of 1918 killed more than 600,000 US children and adults, but it is believed most deaths resulted from bacterial coinfection. Thus, viral-bacterial coinfections are well recognized, particularly the association of influenza with bacterial pneumonia caused by either *S. pneumoniae* or *S. aureus*. Other viruses have also been implicated as co-pathogens in bacterial pneumonia (20%-35%). Viral infections often precede the development of bacterial pneumonia, although it is not always clear if the infection is purely a "secondary" bacterial pneumonia or if the virus and bacterium coinfect the lower airways simultaneously. However, in vitro and animal studies demonstrate that the virulence of both bacteria and viruses is enhanced in coinfections, and clinical studies of pediatric pneumonia indicate worse outcomes among coinfected children compared with those without viral coinfection.

Occasional Pathogens and Disease Occurring in Specific Populations Several other pathogens, including viruses, bacteria, and fungi, may occasionally cause pneumonia. Often these occur in neonates, children with congenital or acquired immunodeficiency, those with specific animal or environmental exposures, and in children at risk for aspiration pneumonia. Key animal exposures for bacterial and viral pneumonia include wild and domesticated animals such as cattle, sheep, and goats (*Coxiella burnetii*, *Bacillus anthracis*, *Brucella abortus*), rodents (*Yersinia pestis*, lymphocytis choriomeningitis virus), pigeons or pet birds (*Chlamydia psittaci*), and rabbits (*Francisella tularensis*). Key exposures for endemic fungi include bird droppings (*Histoplasma capsulatum*, *Cryptococcus neoformans*) and geographic location: Midwestern United States (*H. capsulatum*, *Blastomyces dermatiditis*), Southeast (*B. dermatiditis*), Southwest (*Coccidioides immitis*), and Eastern and Central (*H. capsulatum*). *Mycobacterium tuberculosis* should also be suspected in children with chronic cough.

CLINICAL PRESENTATION

Signs and Symptoms Children with pneumonia typically present with one or more of the following clinical signs and symptoms: fever, cough, tachypnea, increased respiratory effort (retractions, nasal flaring, grunting), hypoxemia, and asymmetric or decreased breath sounds and crackles on auscultation. Retractions and respiratory rate have acceptable interrater reliability. Fever and abdominal pain suggestive of an acute abdomen may occur, particularly in the presence of a parapneumonic effusion or lobar consolidation adjacent to the diaphragm. Tachypnea is considered the most sensitive marker for pneumonia, present in up to 80% of radiographic-confirmed cases, but tachypnea alone is relatively nonspecific. Further, defining appropriate age-based reference ranges for respiratory rate and other vital signs has proven difficult, especially among hospitalized children. The World Health Organization (WHO) case definition of pneumonia, applicable to children less than 5 years of age, includes cough or difficulty breathing and tachypnea at rest, and is widely used in the developing world. A Brazilian study demonstrated sensitivity of 84% for the WHO case definition but specificity of only 19%, although the addition of fever improved specificity to 42% without reducing sensitivity. In contrast, a study conducted among US children with clinical suspicion of pneumonia demonstrated poor sensitivity for the WHO case definition (34%) compared with the reference standard of radiograph-confirmed pneumonia.

Presentation According to Microbiologic Etiology The clinical presentation may also provide etiologic clues. Viral pneumonia typically evolves gradually over several days and includes both upper and lower respiratory tract symptoms, such as cough, coryza, post-tussive emesis, and generalized malaise. Fever is typical but may not be present. Upper respiratory tract rhonchi and bilateral wheezes or rales may be appreciated on auscultation. In contrast, bacterial pneumonia often presents rapidly with high fever and ill or toxic appearance. In a child with preceding viral illness, this typically occurs several days after the initial illness and represents an abrupt and significant change in clinical status. Auscultation may reveal focal abnormality (e.g., rales, whispered pectoriloquy, egophony) indicative of parenchymal consolidation; such focal findings are more challenging to appreciate in young children. The presentation of atypical pneumonia is more insidious and is difficult to distinguish from viral pneumonia; persistent cough is typical. Respiratory symptoms may be preceded by pharyngitis. Wheezing is also frequently present in children with atypical pneumonia, and like some viral pathogens, atypical pneumonia has been implicated as a trigger of recurrent wheezing and asthma.

COMPLICATIONS AND SPECIAL CONSIDERATIONS

Parapneumonic Effusion and Empyema Parapneumonic effusion and empyema represent the most common complications, occurring in up to 25% of children hospitalized with pneumonia. Parapneumonic effusion is not always apparent at presentation and may develop and evolve despite adequate antimicrobial therapy. Persistent fever, worsening respiratory distress, painful respirations, or pain referred to the back, shoulder, or abdomen may herald the development of a significant parapneumonic effusion. Physical examination may reveal dullness to percussion, decreased breath sounds, or egophany; tracheal deviation is also possible. Most effusions are small and resolve following treatment of the underlying pneumonia; about 5% of hospitalized children develop large and/or persistent complicated effusions that necessitate intervention and are associated with significant morbidity. Large effusions are most indicative of typical bacterial disease; however, small effusions, either unilateral or bilateral, are occasionally encountered in children with *M. pneumoniae* and viral pneumonia.

Necrotizing Pneumonia and Lung Abscess Other local complications include necrotizing pneumonia (**Figure 98-1**) and lung abscess. These complications are rare due to routine and prompt antimicrobial therapy. The same organisms that cause complicated parapneumonic effusions are also implicated in necrotizing pneumonia, specifically *S. pneumoniae*, *S. aureus*, or *S. pyogenes*, and may also lead to abscess formation as well as bronchopleural fistula. Lung abscess may also be the primary source of infection and is often associated with aspiration; anaerobes and polymicrobial infections are frequently implicated. Prolonged fever and poor response to therapy are usually cardinal features of both necrotizing pneumonia and lung abscess; cough productive of purulent sputum and/or blood may also be noted.

Systemic and Metastatic Complications

Systemic Complications Systemic complications, including respiratory failure and severe sepsis/shock, occur in approximately 5% to 10% of hospitalized children, and are highest in very young children. Respiratory failure is the most common systemic complication, and may progress to acute respiratory distress syndrome (ARDS) in a small minority of children. For these children, extracorporeal membrane oxygenation (ECMO) can be lifesaving. *S. pneumoniae*-associated hemolytic uremic syndrome is also a rare but severe complication of pneumococcal disease that is most often associated with empyema.

Metastatic Complications Metastatic complications include distant sites of infection (e.g., meningitis, endocarditis, osteomyelitis) and occur as a result of hematogenous seeding; however, these complications are exceedingly rare.

Aspiration Pneumonia Children who lack adequate airway protection (e.g., seizure disorders, neuromuscular disease, or other neurologic impairment) may aspirate oral or gastric contents, leading to chemical pneumonitis and/or infectious pneumonia. Aspiration is a frequent reason for hospitalization among these children, although distinguishing between pneumonitis and pneumonia is difficult. Sterile chemical pneumonitis results from the aspiration of sterile stomach contents with symptoms beginning immediately following or within hours of a witnessed aspiration event, whereas infectious pneumonia typically follows aspiration of oropharyngeal contents and becomes symptomatic many hours to days following an aspiration event. In the case of pneumonia, although typical community-acquired pneumonia pathogens are a consideration, anaerobes and gram-negative bacilli may be more prevalent. Typically, radiographic infiltrates develop in dependent areas of the lungs, such as the posterior upper lobes or apical lower lobes, in children who aspirate while lying down, or basilar lower lobes in those who aspirate while upright; the right lung is also more often implicated in aspiration.

DIFFERENTIAL DIAGNOSIS

The clinical presentation of pneumonia may mimic other infectious and non-infectious conditions. Lack of fever, historical features or associated

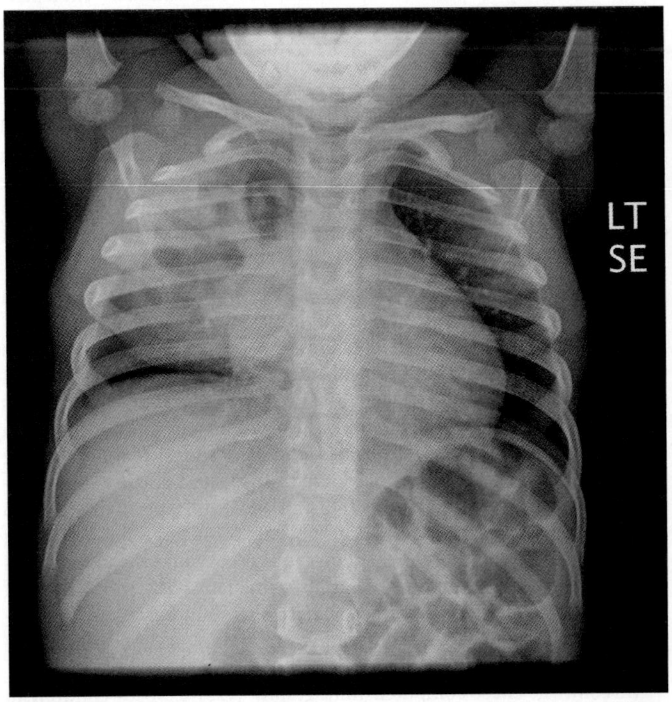

A

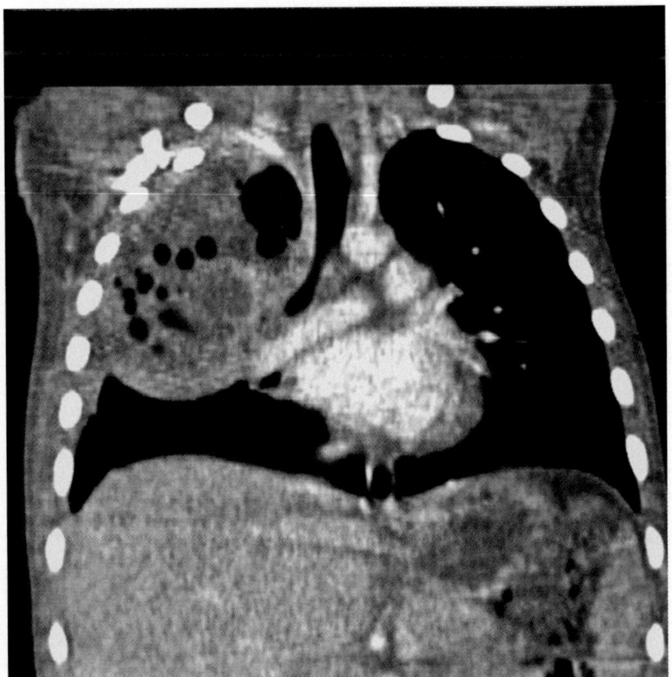

B

FIGURE 98-1. (A) Chest radiograph reveals a complex air space opacity in the right upper lobe with central lucency consistent with cavitating pneumonia. (B) Computed tomography demonstrates a large cavity with central necrosis containing multiple air fluid levels and a thick peripheral irregular rim of enhancement encompassing and replacing much of the right upper lobe. There is also a compressive mass effect, which displaces the minor fissure inferiorly and slightly displaces the trachea to the left.

signs or symptoms, and poor response to therapy should prompt consideration of alternative diagnoses. Children with asthma or bronchiolitis may have opacities on chest radiograph that represent alveolar consolidation of viral origin or atelectasis.

DIAGNOSTIC EVALUATION

Imaging

Chest Radiographs Chest radiographs are typically recommended for children suspected of having pneumonia who require hospitalization, as they help to distinguish among other possible diagnoses and can reveal complications and provide valuable prognostic and diagnostic clues. Both frontal and lateral views are recommended. Infiltrate patterns may be classified as alveolar (e.g., lobar consolidation) (**Figure 98-2**), interstitial (bilateral patchy or linear densities), or mixed. Chest radiographs are subject to variability in interpretation, although standardizing radiographic assessments for pneumonia in children has been a recent focus. Alveolar infiltrate has high inter-observer agreement (κ = 0.58-0.73 across studies), indicating good reliability, whereas inter-observer agreement for interstitial infiltrates is poor.

Radiographs also reveal the presence of complications. Opacification of the pleural space and blunting of the costophrenic angle indicative of parapneumonic effusion can be seen on upright chest radiographs; larger effusions may opacify an entire lung or demonstrate mediastinal shift to the unaffected lung (**Figure 98-3**). A lateral decubitus film may also be helpful for discerning effusion size and organization, although ultrasound is superior in this regard. Cavitation with air-fluid levels usually indicate lung abscess and/or pneumatocele formation with necrotizing pneumonia and may also be seen with any of the above described infiltrate patterns.

Although not absolute, radiographic patterns may offer clues to microbiologic etiology. Alveolar infiltrates are more suggestive of typical bacterial pathogens. Interstitial infiltrates are more often associated with viral and atypical bacterial pathogens; however, typical bacterial pathogens may also produce a similar pattern. The presence of large parapneumonic effusions and empyema (**Figure 98-4**) are strongly indicative of infection caused by *S. pneumoniae*, *S. aureus*, or *S. pyogenes*, whereas small effusions may indicate a typical or atypical bacterial or viral cause. Pneumatoceles are more commonly reported following

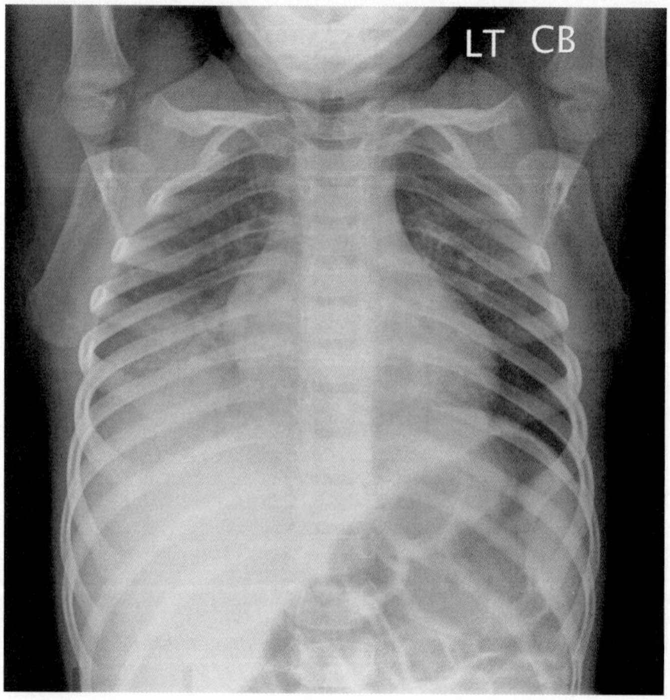

FIGURE 98-2. Chest radiograph of a 2-year-old child reveals right lower lobe consolidation with obliteration of the right hemidiaphragm.

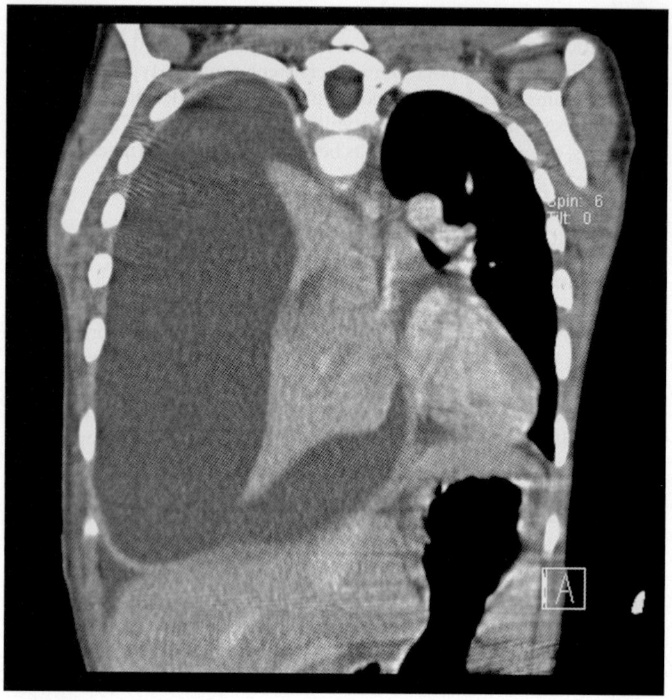

FIGURE 98-3. Computed tomography reveals a massive right pleural effusion with associated pleural enhancement with associated complete collapse of the right lung and leftward cardio-mediastinal shift.

pneumonia caused by *S. aureus*, gram-negative bacteria, and occasionally *S. pneumoniae*. The presence of round infiltrates ("round pneumonia") suggests *S. pneumoniae*. Prominent hilar adenopathy is commonly associated with *H. capsulatum* and other endemic fungi, *M. tuberculosis*, and occasionally *M. pneumoniae*, but may also indicate a noninfectious process such as malignancy.

Follow-up Chest Radiographs Once the diagnosis of pneumonia is confirmed by chest radiograph, follow-up studies are not routinely indicated. Radiographic findings may progress for several days despite clinical improvement and may remain abnormal for months. Repeat chest radiographs are suggested for children not responding or worsening after 48 to 72 hours of appropriate antimicrobial therapy to evaluate for development of complications. Radiographic resolution of severe or complicated pneumonia generally takes weeks to months, and pleural thickening months after the illness is not uncommon. A prior study found that 25% of children had clinical, radiographic, and/or pulmonary function abnormalities at 1 month, but few children had persistent morbidity at 12 months.

Chest Ultrasound and Computed Tomography Chest ultrasound provides an accurate estimate of effusion size and location and can detect the presence of stranding and degree of loculation, which are important factors for assessing the need for surgical intervention. More recently, chest ultrasound has been investigated as a means for the primary diagnosis of pneumonia, performing as well as or better than chest radiograph for detecting pulmonary infiltrates and was superior for detecting effusion. In a study among children with suspected pneumonia, ultrasonography demonstrated sensitivity of 86% and specificity of 89% for detection of lung consolidation and air bronchograms indicating pneumonia. This study is of particular interest because the ultrasounds were performed at the point of care by clinicians with only 1 hour of focused ultrasonography training. Chest ultrasound also has the benefit of non-exposure to ionizing radiation, making it especially attractive for use in children.

In contrast, chest computed tomography (CT) exposes children to high levels of ionizing radiation and should not be used routinely to diagnose pneumonia. The benefit of chest CT is that it offers a highly detailed view of the lung parenchyma, bronchial tree, and pleura. Thus, CT may be useful in instances of severe or complicated disease, especially

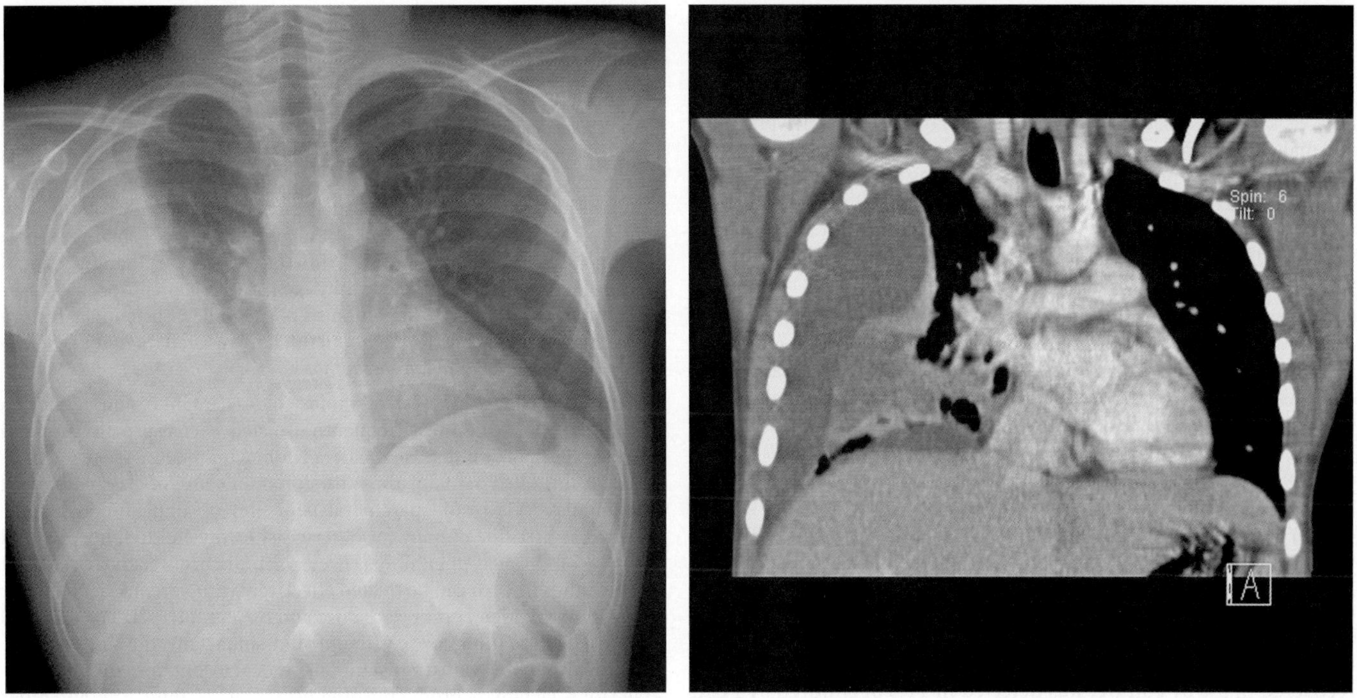

A B

FIGURE 98-4. (A) Chest radiograph reveals a large right-sided parapneumonic effusion. Computed tomography demonstrates a large right-sided parapneumonic effusion with significant compression of the lung. The lung has several areas of early cavitation. There is a smaller loculated collection in the medial right mid-thoracic area.

if surgical intervention is planned, and in children with recurrent or non-responding pneumonia to evaluate for underlying pathology.

Laboratory Diagnostics for Microbiologic Etiology

Culture-Based Methods

Blood. Blood cultures are positive in about 3% children with pneumonia who have blood cultures obtained. Blood cultures are positive in up to 10% to 13% of children with parapneumonic effusion. Because *S. pneumoniae* is most commonly isolated and few isolates are penicillin non-susceptible, blood cultures may be reserved for children hospitalized with more severe illness, including empyema.

Sputum and tracheal aspirates. Culture of sputum often aids in the diagnosis of bacterial pneumonia in adults; however, obtaining high quality sputum in children is hindered by the young age of most children hospitalized with pneumonia. Sputum cultures could contribute to the diagnosis of bacterial pneumonia in school-age children provided a high quality specimen is obtained (less than 10-25 epithelial cells and/or greater than 25 polymorphonuclear cells per low power field and culture isolation of a predominant organism at a concentration of 10^6/mL). Hypertonic saline may be helpful to induce sputum in younger children, although the yield of this approach is uncertain. Culture of tracheal aspirates among intubated children is similarly hampered by concerns regarding upper airway contamination as well as rapid colonization of tracheal tubing, making interpretation problematic unless samples are obtained at the time of intubation (or under direct laryngoscopy) and qualitative assessments similar to sputa are employed.

Pleural fluid and other lower respiratory tract samples. Among children with pneumonia complicated by parapneumonic effusion, culture of pleural fluid is positive in up to 25% of cases. With the exception of pleural drainage, sampling directly from the lower respiratory tract (e.g., bronchoalveolar lavage) is rarely indicated except in instances of non-responding or very severe pneumonia.

Antigen Detection Antigen testing by immunofluorescence from nasal or nasopharyngeal samples can be performed rapidly and is helpful for the detection of viruses. A positive test is usually highly specific; however, sensitivity is variable, particularly for influenza (sensitivity 19%-71%) and adenovirus, and is likely influenced by virus type and strain, viral load, and the test itself. Urinary antigen testing is available for both *Streptococcus pneumoniae* and *Legionella pneumophilia*, and both are useful tests in adults; however, in immunocompetent children, *L. pneumophilia* is rare except in localized outbreaks, and although test sensitivity for *S. pneumoniae* is generally excellent, frequent false positives due to nasopharyngeal colonization limit the clinical utility of urinary antigen detection. However, the pneumococcal urinary antigen tests could be useful for the detection of pneumococcus from normally sterile sites (e.g. blood, pleural fluid) with much less concern regarding test specificity. Studies have demonstrated sensitivities of >95% among children with documented pneumococcal bacteremia (from urine) and/or empyema (from pleural fluid), although test sensitivity is ultimately dependent on organism density within the fluid tested.

Serology Serologic testing is available for several different viral and bacterial pathogens and is used widely in epidemiologic studies. However, this method is hindered by the need for convalescent titers, making serologic testing impractical in most clinical scenarios. Testing for cold agglutinins to detect *M. pneumoniae* is no longer recommended due to poor test specificity since many conditions, including viral infections, may elevate cold agglutinin titers.

Molecular Diagnostics

Nasopharynx. Highly sensitive molecular diagnostics (e.g. polymerase chain reaction [PCR]) are available for a wide range of viral and bacterial respiratory pathogens. Viruses are readily detected from nasopharyngeal samples, and testing is highly specific; a positive test may also persuade one to withhold antimicrobial therapy for a child or to start antivirals for influenza. However, these tests are often expensive and not rapidly available at the point of care, barriers that must be overcome to increase their clinical utility. Frequent bacterial colonization of the upper respiratory tract makes detection of bacterial pathogens from nasopharyngeal samples problematic and is not advised, although quantitative PCR to assess bacterial load may prove useful for differentiating carriage from causal pathogen as well as predicting disease severity. There is debate over whether *M. pneumoniae* is a colonizer of the upper respiratory tract, but specificity of nasopharyngeal PCR is high (>95%) while test sensitivity is variable (9%-93%).

Blood. PCR testing of blood or pleural fluid for bacterial pathogens is less likely to produce false positive results and does not require viable organisms for detection, presumably reducing the influence of antimicrobial therapy on test performance compared to culture-based methods. However, lack of a well-defined reference standard for bacterial pneumonia makes interpreting clinical test characteristics problematic. Using culture-confirmed pneumococcal bacteremia as the reference standard, clinical sensitivity of whole-blood pneumococcal PCR ranges from 40% to 100%; however, sensitivity decreases to 26% to 32% in adult studies, which consider a broader reference standard (positive blood culture, sputum culture, or urinary antigen test).

Pleural fluid. PCR of pleural fluid samples is more likely to reveal a causative pathogen compared to whole-blood PCR for the same reasons pleural fluid culture is superior to blood culture. Several studies demonstrate the substantial improvement in diagnostic yield using both broad-range (16S ribosomal RNA) and species-specific PCR (69%-100%) compared with pleural fluid culture (19%-58%). Reliance on culture alone may also bias our understanding of the importance of individual pathogens, particularly resistant phenotypes. In a study of 63 children with pneumonia complicated by empyema, the etiologic yield increased from 35% with culture alone to 84% using pleural fluid PCR for specific bacteria. The typically drug-resistant pneumococcal serotype 19A and staphylococcal pneumonias accounted for 23% and 18% of culture positive cases, respectively, but only 2% each of culture negative cases. In contrast, *S. pyogenes*, recovered in 5% by culture, was detected in 11% of children by PCR. Overall, detection of *S. pneumoniae* doubled from 35% by culture alone to 71% using PCR and was largely due to increased yield of nonresistant serotypes.

Other Laboratory Testing Peripheral white blood cell count, C-reactive protein, erythrocyte sedimentation rate, and other acute-phase reactants are often abnormal in children with pneumonia, although the magnitude of abnormality is variable and likely affected by other factors including host characteristics, timing of illness, and infecting organism. Bacteria can induce a robust immune response with substantially elevated acute phase reactants, leading many to associate elevated inflammatory markers with bacterial infection. However, studies have failed to demonstrate adequate test sensitivity or specificity to reliably distinguish bacterial from viral etiologies limiting their clinical utility. As a result, these studies are not routinely recommended; however, in children with severe pneumonia, serial measurements may be helpful to assess response to therapy.

Biomarker discovery and the burgeoning "omics" fields are areas of intense research focus with implications for a wide range of disease states, including childhood pneumonia. A precursor to calcitonin, serum procalcitonin levels often rise substantially in response to serious bacterial infections and do not increase appreciably in the setting of viral infections or noninfectious inflammatory states. Specific to pneumonia, procalcitonin levels are typically higher among children with pneumonia caused by typical bacterial pathogens compared to viral or atypical bacterial pathogens. A randomized trial among children hospitalized with pneumonia demonstrated reduced antimicrobial prescribing (85% vs. 100%, $p < 0.05$) and duration of antibiotic exposure (5 vs. 11 days, $p < 0.05$) when procalcitonin (cutoff 0.25 ng/mL) was used to inform treatment decisions compared to usual care. In an observational study of 532 children with typical community acquired pneumonia, a procalcitonin level less than 0.25 ng/mL was found to have a 96% negative predictive value (95% confidence interval [CI], 93-99), 85% sensitivity (95% CI, 76-95), and 45% specificity (95% CI, 40-50) in identifying children without typical bacterial CAP who would not benefit from antibiotic treatment. A review of 14 randomized trials among adults with respiratory tract infections and sepsis reported consistent reductions in antimicrobial prescribing and duration of therapy when procalcitonin-based algorithms were used to guide treatment decisions compared to usual care. Pathogen and disease-specific biosignatures are also under development using whole-blood gene expression patterns and urinary metabolite profiles; whether or not this area of research translates to improved care and outcomes at the bedside remains to be determined.

MANAGEMENT

Antimicrobial Therapy

Bacterial Pneumonia (Table 98-2)

Neonates and Young Infants. Treatment for neonatal pneumonia should include coverage for both gram-positive and gram-negative bacteria commonly encountered in neonates (e.g., group B *Streptococcus*, *E. coli*, *Listeria monocytogenes*). This is usually accomplished with combination therapy consisting of parenteral aminopenicillin plus gentamicin or a third-generation cephalosporin. Anti-staphylococcal therapy should be considered in select cases. A third-generation cephalosporin is usually sufficient for infants 1 to 3 months of age, unless the clinical history raises suspicion for infection with methicillin-resistant *S. aureus*, *Bordetella pertussis*, or *Chlamydia trachomatis*.

Children 3 months to 17 years. Among older infants and children, *S. pneumoniae* is the most frequently isolated bacterial pathogen, and despite reductions in disease incidence following pneumococcal conjugate vaccine, likely remains the most common cause of classic bacterial pneumonia. As a result, parenteral penicillin or ampicillin is recommended as first-line therapy for otherwise healthy children hospitalized with uncomplicated pneumonia. Even pneumococci relatively resistant to penicillins in vitro can be treated effectively with parental penicillin or ampicillin provided appropriate dose and dosing interval. The addition of a β-lactamase inhibitor (e.g., ampicillin-sulbactam) does not provide additional activity against resistant pneumococci, but does improve coverage for β-lactamase producing organisms (e.g., *H. influenzae* and other gram-negative bacilli). Parenteral third-generation cephalosporins, such as ceftriaxone, are appropriate alternatives, particularly for children with severe or complicated disease. For children with severe penicillin allergy, alternatives include clindamycin and levofloxacin, although pneumococcal resistance to clindamycin is high in some areas. In addition, anti-staphylococcal therapy (including clindamycin or vancomycin in MRSA prevalent regions) is recommended for children with severe or rapidly progressive disease and in those with poor treatment response after 48 to 72 hours of therapy.

Antimicrobial therapy for children with significant parapneumonic effusion and/or necrotizing pneumonia should include coverage for *S. pneumoniae*, *S. aureus*, and *S. pyogenes*. A third-generation cephalosporin in combination with either an anti-staphylococcal penicillin or clindamycin/vancomycin (depending on regional MRSA prevalence) is recommended. In pleural fluid culture-negative cases, ampicillin is reasonable, as *S. pneumoniae* is the predominant pathogen detected by PCR in culture-negative cases. For lung abscess, treatment should also include coverage for oral anaerobes.

Coverage for Atypical Pathogens Consideration of atypical coverage (e.g., macrolide) is warranted in school-age children. However, differentiating atypical from viral or even typical bacterial pneumonia based on clinical or radiographic features is infeasible. Many children each year who are infected with *M. pneumoniae* recover uneventfully without specific antimicrobial therapy, and prior Cochrane reviews have demonstrated insufficient evidence to draw conclusions on antibiotic use for *M. pneumoniae* lower respiratory tract infections. However, macrolide therapy might be beneficial for hospitalized children with atypical pneumonia. A large retrospective study among more than 20,000 children hospitalized with pneumonia comparing β-lactam monotherapy to combination therapy with a macrolide demonstrated a 20% shorter average length of stay among the combination therapy group; the magnitude of effect increased with increasing age and was not significant among children less than 6 years of age. In the outpatient setting, children 6 to 18 years who received β-lactam/macrolide combination therapy had lower odds of treatment failure compared with those who received β-lactam monotherapy; this retrospective study was limited by the absence of confirmation of *M. pneumoniae* in study participants. Few studies have prospectively evaluated this treatment strategy, and studies among children with proven atypical disease are needed. Macrolide monotherapy is not typically recommended, as this strategy does not provide adequate pneumococcal coverage due to frequent resistance. Further, development of regional penicillin- and multidrug-resistant pneumococci has also been linked to frequent use of broad-spectrum antimicrobials, including macrolides.

TABLE 98-2 Empiric Antimicrobial Strategies for Pediatric Community-Acquired Pneumonia*

Population		Bacterial Pneumonia	Atypical Pneumonia
Outpatient			
Neonates-3 months			
Preschool (<5 years)	Preferred	Amoxicillin	Azithromycin
	Alternative(s)	Amoxicillin/clavulanate	Clarithromycin or erythromycin
5-17 years	Preferred	Amoxicillin	Azithromycin
	Alternative(s)	Amoxicillin/clavulanate	Clarithromycin or erythromycin Doxycycline if >7 years of age
Inpatient			
Neonates	Preferred	Ampicillin + gentamicin	N/A
	Alternative(s)	Ampicillin + third-generation cephalosporin	
1-3 months	Preferred	Third generation cephalosporin	N/A
	Alternative(s)	Azithromycin if suspect *C. trachomatis* or *B. pertussis*	
3 months-17 years, fully immunized, local epidemiology indicates low prevalence of penicillin non-susceptible *S. pneumoniae*	Preferred	Ampicillin or Penicillin G	Azithromycin
	Alternative(s)	Ceftriaxone Anti-staphylococcal coverage for suspected *S. aureus*, including clindamycin or vancomycin in MRSA prevalent regions	Clarithromycin or erythromycin Doxycycline Levofloxacin for those who have reached skeletal maturity
3 months-17 years, not fully immunized, or local epidemiology indicates moderate to high prevalence of penicillin nonsusceptible *S. pneumoniae*	Preferred	Ceftriaxone	Azithromycin
	Alternative(s)	Levofloxacin Anti-staphylococcal coverage for suspected *S. aureus*, including clindamycin or vancomycin in MRSA prevalent regions	Clarithromycin or erythromycin Doxycycline Levofloxacin for those who have reached skeletal maturity

MRSA, methicillin-resistant *Staphylococcus aureus*; N/A, not applicable.

Source: Adapted from Bradley JS, Byington CL, Shah SS, et al. Empiric therapy for pediatric community-acquired pneumonia (CAP). The management of community-acquired pneumonia in infants and children older than 3 months of age: clinical practice guidelines by the Pediatric Infectious Diseases Society and the Infectious Diseases Society of America. *Clin Infect Dis*. 2011;53:e34, Table 7.

Transition to Oral Therapy and Treatment Duration Transition to oral therapy should be accomplished early in the hospital course and as soon as a child demonstrates clinical improvement. With few exceptions, prolonged or outpatient parenteral therapy is usually not required, as oral equivalents are generally available that are similar in spectrum and efficacy to commonly used parenteral agents. Treatment for uncomplicated bacterial pneumonia generally includes antimicrobial therapy for 7 to 10 days; shorter treatment durations may also be effective. Recent randomized controlled trials have demonstrated that for young children in the outpatient setting, 5 days of antibiotics of antibiotics is noninferior and may be superior to 10 days; this has not yet been well studied in the hospitalized population, although one study did show that 3 days was noninferior to 7 in a small sample of children hospitalized for less than 48 hours. Optimal treatment duration for significant parapneumonic effusion or empyema, necrotizing pneumonia, and/or lung abscess is not well studied but likely depends on the infecting organism and extent of disease as well as the effectiveness of drainage if performed. The typical duration of therapy is 2 to 3 weeks. Other special circumstances (e.g., severe staphylococcal pneumonia or metastatic complications) may also require prolonged antimicrobial therapy.

Influenza-Associated Pneumonia Antivirals (i.e., neuraminidase inhibitors) are recommended for children hospitalized with influenza. Treatment is likely most beneficial early during the course of illness, but neuraminidase inhibitors such as osteltamivir should not be withheld for high-risk children presenting to the hospital more than 48 hours after symptom onset, as clinical benefit has been demonstrated. The role of antiviral therapy for otherwise healthy children with influenza is evolving. Osteltamivir modestly reduces time to alleviation of symptoms by 12 to 48 hours; however, adverse effects include vomiting (10% vs. <2% of placebo recipients), headaches, and renal and psychiatric syndromes (number needed to harm = 94). Zanamivir also reduces time to first alleviation of symptoms and total symptom duration. Available data should prompt greater consideration of benefits and harms when making decisions for neuraminidase treatment for influenza in patients at low risk of complications. Randomized trials of neuraminidase inhibitors for hospitalized and severely ill patients are needed to inform clinical practice. Recommendations for treatment of influenza vary by season; the Centers for Disease Control and Prevention (CDC) provides annual recommendations at www.cdc.gov/flu.

Other Viral Pneumonia The majority of pneumonia in children under 5 years old is caused by viruses and so would not need antibiotic treatment. While children managed outpatient do not routinely require antibiotics, the current recommendation is to empirically treat inpatients with pneumonia. Recent studies in the outpatient and emergency department setting have indicated that antibiotics are not always beneficial, but there is little evidence in the inpatient setting. Further research needs to be done to identify children who do not require antibiotics in the inpatient setting, particularly as unnecessary antibiotic use can lead to developing antimicrobial resistance and other adverse events.

Adjunctive Therapies Adjunctive therapies for children with uncomplicated pneumonia primarily focus on respiratory support, minimizing discomfort, and optimizing nutrition. Oxygen therapy should be instituted to maintain oxygen saturation >90%. Incentive spirometry or bubble therapy may be helpful for children with poor inspiratory effort and/or atelectasis. Inadequate analgesia may also contribute to poor respiratory effort. Nutrition promotes healing and recovery and should not be overlooked; if oral intake remains poor after 48 to 72 hours of therapy, consideration of nasogastric feedings or other means of nutrition should be considered.

Corticosteroid therapy has been suggested and may be beneficial among adults with severe pneumonia. Although not well studied, corticosteroid therapy among children hospitalized with pneumonia has not demonstrated benefit, except among children with suspected reactive airways disease or concomitant asthma exacerbation. In the outpatient setting, adjunct corticosteroid therapy was associated with treatment failure among children diagnosed with CAP who did not have underlying asthma. Chest physiotherapy is likely not beneficial, may prolong symptoms and cause discomfort, and is not recommended except possibly for children with neurologic impairment or other conditions associated with poor airway clearance.

Drainage for Parapneumonic Effusion and Empyema The decision to perform a therapeutic drainage is informed by the effusion size and character, as well as the degree of respiratory compromise. Diagnostic thoracentesis may also be helpful if noninfectious effusion is suspected. Small effusions (arbitrarily defined as <10 mm on decubitus films or occupying less than 25% of the hemithorax on upright films) are likely to resolve with treatment of the underlying pneumonia and typically do not require additional intervention. Children with moderate (25%-50% of hemithorax opacified) to large (>50% opacified) effusions are more likely to develop respiratory compromise, and drainage should be considered. Early drainage is preferred, as delayed drainage may result in the need for more invasive or repeated interventions as well as increased morbidity and prolonged hospitalization. Drainage also offers the potential for identifying a causative organism. Choice of drainage procedure is informed by the degree of organization of the fluid collection and may also be influenced by local expertise. A child with a moderately sized free-flowing effusion may improve with the placement of a simple thoracostomy tube. More complicated (loculated) effusions typically require chemical (fibrinolysis) or mechanical (video-assisted thoracoscopic surgery [VATS]) intervention. The decision to pursue thoracostomy tube placement with instillation of fibrinolytics (tissue plasminogen activator, urokinase) or VATS is dictated by local expertise. It is unclear whether one strategy is superior to the other for the initial management of complicated effusion; several small randomized trials demonstrated equivalent patient outcomes. Thoracostomy tube placement occasionally fails, necessitating definitive therapy with VATS. Open thoracotomy and decortication is associated with significant morbidity and is rarely indicated.

When a drainage procedure is performed, fluid Gram stain and culture should be performed. If available, bacterial PCR or antigen detection should also be performed, as these tests improve diagnostic yield over culture. Cell counts and differential analysis may be helpful if the diagnosis is in question. Additional fluid analysis (pH, glucose, protein) is rarely helpful. **Table 98-3** provides interpretation of pleural fluid studies. Criteria for thoracostomy tube removal include decreased output (<1 mL/kg/24 hour measured over a 12-hour period or 25-60 mL in a 24-hour period) and absence of an air leak.

TABLE 98-3 Pleural Fluid Studies in Complicated Pneumonia

Study	Comments
Routine	
Cell count and differential	Usually >10,000 U/mL in parapneumonic effusion
	PMN predominance in bacterial PPE
	Lymphocytes and mononuclear cells predominate in TB, lymphoma, chylothorax
Glucose	Low glucose (<40 mg/dL) more likely to require intervention
pH	Low pH (<7.20) more likely to require intervention
LDH	If high (>1000 U/mL) or pleural fluid–plasma ratio >0.6, more likely to be exudative effusion and require intervention
Gram stain	If positive, more likely to require intervention
Acid fast stain	May be positive with *Mycobacterium tuberculosis* or *Nocardia*
Cultures*	Insensitive in setting of prior antibiotic therapy
Additional studies to consider	
Mycoplasma PCR	Also obtain PCR of nasal aspirate
Viral antigen immunofluorescence	Also obtain immunofluorescence of nasal aspirate; consider PCR testing for adenovirus
Viral culture	May be positive with negative immunofluorescence
Total protein	Indicative of exudates if >3 g/dL and pleural–serum ratio >0.5
Amylase	If concern for pancreatic disease or esophageal rupture
Cholesterol	If >60 mg/dL and pleural fluid–cholesterol ratio >0.3, indicative of exudate
Cytology	To exclude malignancy
Chylomicrons, triglycerides	Along with cholesterol if chylothorax suspected

*Aerobic and anaerobic; consider mycobacterial and fungal.

LDH, lactate dehydrogenase; PCR, polymerase chain reaction; PMN, polymorphonuclear neutrophils; PPE, parapneumonic effusion; TB, tuberculosis.

ADMISSION AND DISCHARGE CRITERIA

Although the majority of children with community-acquired pneumonia are successfully managed in the outpatient setting, pneumonia remains one of the most common indications for pediatric hospitalization in the United States. A tool to predict severe pneumonia outcomes was recently developed which may inform site of care and other management decisions but requires further validation prior to implementation. Ill appearance, moderate to severe respiratory distress with or without hypoxia, and inability to eat are common reasons necessitating hospitalization for children with pneumonia. Potential barriers to effective home care should also be considered. Children with severe respiratory distress and impending respiratory failure or hemodynamic instability require admission to a pediatric critical care unit. Children may be discharged once responding appropriately to therapeutic interventions, typically within 1 to 3 days.

CONSULTATION

Most children hospitalized with pneumonia improve quickly with appropriate antimicrobial therapy and supportive care under the direction of a pediatric care team that includes nursing, pharmacy, and respiratory care staff, and a generalist physician. Access to pediatric critical care services is paramount. When available, ancillary support services such as social work and child life can be an excellent resource. Subspecialty consultation may be beneficial for children with selected comorbidities, significant complications, or disease that is not responding to typical therapies, or in children with recurrent infections. Infectious disease specialists may assist with antimicrobial management or evaluation for underlying immunodeficiency in a child with non-responding pneumonia or frequent infections; pulmonary specialists can help with the evaluation of recurrent pneumonia in a single location indicative of an underlying structural or functional abnormality, those with significant respiratory comorbidity, or in children who require bronchoscopy, such as a child with non-responding pneumonia; general surgery or interventional radiology consultation is appropriate for children requiring intervention for local complications such as parapneumonic effusion or empyema.

PERTUSSIS

BACKGROUND

Epidemiology Pertussis is an acute infectious disease caused by the bacterium *Bordetella pertussis*. Outbreaks of pertussis were described as early as the 15th century, but the causative bacterium was not isolated until 1906. Pertussis is also called whooping cough, which is descriptive of the high-pitched inspiratory noise ("whoop") made by infected children.

Pertussis was one of the most common childhood diseases in the 20th century and a major cause of childhood mortality in the United States. There were more than 200,000 cases of pertussis reported annually before pertussis vaccine became available in the 1940s. With the advent of widespread vaccination in the United States, the incidence had decreased more than 80% compared with the pre-vaccine era; fewer than 2000 cases were reported in 1975. However, increasing rates of non-medical or personal belief vaccine exemptions to school immunization requirements, as well as decreased efficacy of DTaP vaccine, have contributed to increasing rates of pertussis through frequent outbreaks.

The incidence of pertussis most recently peaked in 2012 around 48,000 cases and has since improved somewhat, with around 18,000 cases in 2019. Secondary attack rates among unvaccinated people range from 50% to 100%, depending on proximity to the infected person. In a study of pediatric pertussis hospitalizations, family members were the source in nearly 75% of cases; daycare contacts accounted for 3% of cases. The highest case rates and mortality occur in infants <6 months of age. Pertussis remains a major health problem among children in developing countries, however, with an estimated 24.1 million cases of the disease worldwide in 2014 as well as >160,000 deaths, despite >80% coverage of the world by the vaccine.

Pathophysiology Pertussis is primarily a toxin-mediated disease. *B. pertussis*, a gram-negative nonmotile coccobacillus, is only infectious in humans. It is acquired by contact with aerosolized droplets from infected patients, and infection is limited to the ciliated epithelium of the respiratory tract. The bacteria attach to the respiratory cilia and produce toxins that paralyze the cilia, cause inflammation of the respiratory tract, and impair clearance of pulmonary secretions.

A variety of pertussis components and their contribution to disease have been studied. The antigenic and biologically active components currently thought to be responsible for the clinical features of pertussis disease include pertussis toxin, filamentous hemagglutinin, agglutinogens, adenylate cyclase, pertactin, and tracheal cytotoxin. The pertussis toxin is the major virulence protein and is expressed only by *B. pertussis*. It aids attachment of the bacteria to respiratory epithelium and has multiple systemic effects, including enhancement of insulin secretion, inhibition of leukocyte phagocytic function, and induction of lymphocytosis by inhibition of migration from the bloodstream. Filamentous hemagglutinin, pertactin, and agglutinogens play a role in the attachment to respiratory epithelium. Adenylate cyclase contributes to impairing the phagocytic function of lymphocytes, and tracheal toxin has a role in ciliary stasis. An immune response to one or more of these components produces immunity to subsequent clinical illness, although that immunity is not permanent.

CLINICAL PRESENTATION

B. pertussis disease presents with a wide clinical spectrum, and several clinical case definitions for pertussis exist. Pertussis is defined by the WHO as a case diagnosed as pertussis by a physician in a person with a cough lasting at least 2 weeks with at least one of the following symptoms: paroxysms of coughing, inspiratory whooping, and post-tussive vomiting without other apparent cause. The incubation period is commonly 7 to 10 days, with a range of 4 to 21 days. The clinical course of the illness is typically divided into three stages: catarrhal, paroxysmal, and convalescent.

The first stage, the catarrhal stage, is characterized by nonspecific symptoms such as rhinorrhea, sneezing, low-grade fever, and a mild cough. Caregivers often do not seek medical attention for these common symptoms, especially in infants and young children, and the nondistinctive symptoms rarely prompt investigation even if patients are brought to medical attention. Over the subsequent 1 to 2 weeks the cough gradually becomes more severe and the second stage, the paroxysmal stage, begins. Fever is usually minimal through the course of illness.

During the paroxysmal stage of classic pertussis disease, the patient has bursts of numerous, rapid coughs, and at the end of the paroxysm, a long inspiratory effort is usually accompanied by a characteristic high-pitched crowing or whoop as air is inspired across an inflamed partially closed glottis. Patients younger than 6 months of age may not have the strength to have a whoop, but they will have paroxysms of coughing and may also have choking, gasping, or apnea. Thick, clear mucus may be discharged with the coughing spells. Children and young infants often appear ill and distressed during the attack. A range of color changes may be seen, including cyanosis or pallor, and some children may develop a plethoric appearance to the face during coughing spells. Post-tussive emesis and exhaustion commonly follow the event. The patient's appearance is usually normal after recovery from the coughing paroxysm. During the first 1 or 2 weeks of the paroxysmal stage, the coughing spells typically increase in frequency, then remain at the same level for 2 to 3 weeks, and then will gradually decrease. Paroxysms may occur more frequently at night. The paroxysmal stage usually lasts 1 to 6 weeks but may persist for up to 10 weeks before entering the third stage.

In the third stage, the convalescent stage, the cough becomes less paroxysmal and gradually disappears over several weeks. Paroxysms often recur, especially with subsequent respiratory infections, for many months after the onset of pertussis. This is not due to reactivation or reinfection with *B. pertussis*.

Adolescents, adults, and those partially protected by vaccination may still become infected with *B. pertussis*. Their clinical course will typically be mild, ranging from few symptoms to mild cough with intermittent laryngospasm to classic pertussis, with persistent cough lasting more than several months. Inspiratory whoop is uncommon in this population. They usually do not demonstrate three distinct stages of disease.

DIFFERENTIAL DIAGNOSIS

Pertussis is uncommon in children with acute viral respiratory infections; however, infants <6 months of age with pertussis commonly have viruses concomitantly detected. Thus, identification of a virus does not exclude the possibility of pertussis. Prolonged cough may also be seen with adenovirus, parainfluenza, influenza, RSV, or *M. pneumoniae* infection and may be difficult to distinguish from pertussis. Adenovirus may present with pharyngitis and conjunctivitis not typical of pertussis. Mycoplasma may also present with fever, headache, and lung examination findings, such as rales, with patchy infiltrates on chest radiograph that are not common with pertussis. Pneumonia due to *Chlamydia trachomatis* or *pneumoniae* classically presents with a staccato cough, which implies a breath with each cough. Tachypnea, rales, and wheezes are often present. Patients with RSV infection often have prominent rhinorrhea with bronchiolitis symptoms that accompany or closely follow the nasal symptoms. *B. parapertussis* causes a similar although milder disease and is seen predominantly in Europe. Infection with *B. bronchiseptica* is more commonly an animal infection, although there are case reports of human infection.

Foreign body aspiration, gastroesophageal reflux, aspiration pneumonia, and asthma/reactive airways disease are non-infectious processes that may also present with intractable or prolonged cough.

DIAGNOSIS

The gold standard for diagnosis of pertussis is isolation of *B. pertussis* by culture. The fastidious nature of this organism results in the need for careful collection and culture methods. Isolation of *B. pertussis* using direct plating is most successful during the first 2 weeks of infection, in the catarrhal stage. Specimens should be obtained from the posterior nasopharynx, not from the throat. Cotton swabs should not be used because they will inhibit the growth of *B. pertussis*. Samples should be obtained using Dacron or calcium alginate swabs or by aspiration and should be plated directly onto the selective media. A holding broth or transport medium should be used if plating is not performed immediately. The cultures are grown for 10 to 14 days. Success in isolating the organism declines if the patient had prior antibiotic therapy effective against *B. pertussis*, if specimen collection is delayed beyond the first 2 weeks of illness, or if the patient has been vaccinated.

PCR testing of nasopharyngeal swabs or aspirates is an increasingly available rapid, sensitive, and specific method of diagnosing pertussis; throat and anterior nasal swabs have poor sensitivity and should not be used. Collection swabs may be Dacron, rayon, or nylon-flocked; cotton-tipped and calcium alginate swabs inhibit PCR and therefore should not be used for PCR testing. PCR tests from nasopharyngeal swab specimens are optimal for those who present relatively early in the course of illness (i.e., within 3-4 weeks from cough onset). The yield from PCR is less likely to be affected by prior antibiotic therapy than the yield from culture. Direct fluorescent antibody (DFA) testing of nasopharyngeal specimens is no longer recommended.

An elevated IgG titer to pertussis toxin is suggestive of recent infection in an individual who has not received immunization within 2 years. However, there are currently no commercially available serologic tests that are approved by the FDA, and diagnostic levels have not been established. Serologic tests are most useful for those who present later (i.e., 2-8 weeks after symptom onset) in the course of illness, a time when PCR and culture are typically negative; serology may be performed on specimens collected up to 12 weeks after cough onset. Serologic tests cannot reliably distinguish infection from vaccine response in those who have received the vaccine.

Leukocytosis (peripheral white blood cell count >16,000/mm^3) with lymphocyte predominance occurs in the late catarrhal and paroxysmal stages. Lymphocyte counts above the mean are seen in more than 75% of unimmunized patients with pertussis; patients with mild or modified cases of pertussis and adolescents may not present with lymphocytosis. White blood cell counts ≥30,000/mm^3 may portend worse outcomes among infants ≤90 days with pertussis.

COMPLICATIONS

Complications of pertussis may include pneumonia, middle ear infection, anorexia, dehydration, failure to thrive, apneic episodes, seizures, rectal prolapse, encephalopathy, pulmonary hypertension, and death. Eighty percent of deaths from pertussis occur in children under age 1 year. The most common complication, as well as the cause of most pertussis-related deaths, is secondary bacterial pneumonia. Neurologic complications such as seizures and encephalopathy may occur due to hypoxia from coughing, or possibly from toxin. Neurologic complications of pertussis are more common among infants. Complications resulting from pressure effects of severe paroxysms include pneumothorax, epistaxis, hernias, and rectal prolapse. Adolescents and adults may also develop complications of pertussis such as difficulty sleeping, urinary incontinence, and pneumonia.

TREATMENT/MANAGEMENT

The single most effective control measure is maintaining the highest possible level of immunization in the community. Anyone who comes into close contact with a person who has pertussis should receive antibiotics to prevent spread of the disease, as patients with pertussis are infectious from the onset of symptoms through the third week of illness. People who have or may have pertussis should stay away from young children and infants until properly treated. Treatment during the catarrhal stage may lead to resolution of the infection or may alleviate symptoms. Treatment during the paroxysmal or convalescent phases will have limited effect on symptoms but is recommended to limit the spread of disease to others. Infants under 1 year of age should be treated within the first 6 weeks of symptoms; everyone else should be treated within the first 3 weeks of suspected illness. Prophylaxis is recommended for household contacts.

Macrolide agents are the first-line treatment choices. According to the 2005 CDC guidelines, for patients older than 1 month, azithromycin, clarithromycin, or erythromycin is preferred for treatment. For infants less than 1 month of age, azithromycin is the drug of choice, and clarithromycin and erythromycin are not recommended; the risk of severe disease is greater than the risk of potentially developing infantile hypertrophic pyloric stenosis. In infants older than 2 months of age, trimethoprim-sulfamethoxazole is the recommended alternative agent. These recommendations from the CDC are provided even though the FDA has not licensed any macrolide for use in infants less than 6 months of age. Specific dosing recommendations are provided in **Table 98-4**.

Postexposure prophylaxis is recommended for household contacts and those in close contact with an infectious patient. Dosing is the same as for treatment (see Table 98-4).

ADMISSION CRITERIA

Indications for admission include severe paroxysms of cough, cyanosis, or apnea with or without cough, extreme fatigue or apnea after cough, obstruction after cough (from mucous plugs), inability to feed, and seizures. Children may also need to be hospitalized for pneumonia, the most common complication of pertussis. Infants younger than 6 months commonly require hospitalization for management of apnea, hypoxia, and feeding difficulties. Intensive care may be required for infants with severe respiratory failure, pulmonary hypertension, or severe apnea and hypoxia requiring ventilator support.

Supportive care is the mainstay of management. Environmental stimulation should be limited, a detailed cough record should be maintained, and oral intake with daily weights should be recorded. Electronic monitoring for heart rate, respiratory rate, and oxygen saturation is also indicated. Patients should be placed on standard and droplet precautions for the first 5 days on effective treatment or for 21 days after the onset of symptoms if untreated.

DISCHARGE CRITERIA

- Infant can tolerate adequate oral or enteral fluids and nutrition to maintain hydration and gain weight.
- Infant does not become hypoxic or bradycardic with coughing episodes.
- Caretakers are reliable and comfortable with infant's condition.
- Reliable outpatient follow-up has been established.

CONSULTATION

The need for cardiorespiratory support warrants involvement with intensivists. Subspecialty consultation is usually prompted by the development of specific complications (e.g., if seizures or encephalopathy develop, input from pediatric neurologists may be appropriate).

TABLE 98-4 Recommended Antimicrobial Treatment and Postexposure Prophylaxis for Pertussis, by Age Group

	PRIMARY AGENTS			ALTERNATE AGENT
Age Group	*Azithromycin*[*]	*Erythromycin*[†]	*Clarithromycin*	*TMP-SMZ*[‡]
<1 month	Recommended agent; 10 mg/kg per day in a single dose for 5 days (only limited safety data available)	Not preferred; 40-50 mg/kg per day in 4 divided doses for 14 days	Not recommended (safety data unavailable)	Contraindicated for infants aged <2 months (risk for kernicterus)
1-5 months	10 mg/kg per day in a single dose for 5 days	40-50 mg/kg per day in 4 divided doses for 14 days	15 mg/kg per day in 2 divided doses for 7 days	Contraindicated at age <2 months; for infants aged ≥2 months, TMP 8 mg/kg per day, SMZ 40 mg/kg per day in 2 divided doses for 14 days
Infants (aged ≥6 months) and children	10 mg/kg in a single dose on day 1 then 5 mg/kg per day (maximum: 500 mg) on days 2-5	40-50 mg/kg per day (maximum: 2 g per day) in 4 divided doses for 14 days	15 mg/kg per day in 2 divided doses (maximum: 1 g per day) for 7 days	TMP 8 mg/kg per day, SMZ 40 mg/kg per day in 2 divided doses for 14 days
Adults	500 mg in a single dose on day 1 then 250 mg per day on days 2-5	2 g per day in 4 divided doses for 7-14 days	1 g per day in 2 divided doses for 7 days	TMP 320 mg per day, SMZ 1600 mg per day in 2 divided doses for 14 days

[*]Use azithromycin with caution in persons with prolonged QT interval and other conditions predisposing to arrhythmia.

[†]Erythromycin is associated with infantile pyloric stenosis; use if azithromycin is unavailable or contraindicated.

[‡]Trimethoprim sulfamethoxazole (TMP-SMZ) can be used as an alternative agent to macrolides in patients aged ≥2 months who are allergic to macrolides, who cannot tolerate macrolides, or who are infected with a rare macrolide-resistant strain of *Bordetella pertussis*.

Source: From Centers for Disease Control and Prevention. Recommended antimicrobial agents for the treatment and postexposure prophylaxis of pertussis: 2005 CDC guidelines. *MMWR*. 2005;54(No. RR-14):1-16.

PREVENTION

The incidence of pertussis has markedly decreased worldwide with the advent of effective vaccinations. Major epidemics have been mostly eliminated, but there are still episodic spikes every 3 to 5 years in pertussis cases. Studies suggest that vaccine-induced cellular and humoral immunity lasts 3 to 5 years. Booster vaccination induces another 7 to 8 years of immunity. Natural infection with *B. pertussis* seems to confer a similar length of immunity as vaccination with whole-cell pertussis (5-8 years).

Children who have recovered from documented pertussis do not immediately need additional doses of pertussis vaccine. Satisfactory documentation includes recovery of *B. pertussis* on culture or typical symptoms and clinical course when these are epidemiologically linked to a culture-confirmed case. If confirmation of pertussis infection is lacking, vaccination should be completed.

In 2005, the FDA licensed two new Tdap (tetanus toxoid, reduced diphtheria toxoid, and acellular pertussis) vaccines for adolescents and adults. The CDC recommends that everyone 11 years or older receive a Tdap vaccine every 10 years. Pregnant women should be given a pertussis vaccine with every pregnancy during the third trimester to protect the infant.

SUGGESTED READINGS

Ambroggio L, Taylor JA, Tabb LP, Newschaffer CJ, Evans AA, Shah SS. Comparative effectiveness of empiric beta-lactam monotherapy and beta-lactam-macrolide combination therapy in children hospitalized with community-acquired pneumonia. *J Pediatr.* 2012;161(6):1097-1103.

Ambroggio L, Test M, Metlay JP, et al. Beta-lactam versus beta- lactam/macrolide therapy in pediatric outpatient pneumonia. *Pediatr Pulmonol.* 2016;51(5):541-548.

Andrews AL, Simpson AN, Heine D, Teufel RJ 2nd. A Cost-Effectiveness Analysis of Obtaining Blood Cultures in Children Hospitalized for Community-Acquired Pneumonia. *J Pediatr.* 2015;167(6):1280-1286.

Bielicki JA, Stöhr W, Barratt S, et al. Effect of amoxicillin dose and treatment duration on the need for antibiotic re-treatment in children with community-acquired pneumonia: The CAP-IT randomized clinical trial. *JAMA.* 2021;326(17):1713-1724.

Blaschke AJ, Heyrend C, Byington CL, et al. Molecular analysis improves pathogen identification and epidemiologic study of pediatric parapneumonic empyema. *Pediatr Infect Dis J.* 2011;30(4):289-294.

Bradley JS, Byington CL, Shah SS, et al. The management of community-acquired pneumonia in infants and children older than 3 months of age: clinical practice guidelines by the Pediatric Infectious Diseases Society and the Infectious Diseases Society of America. *Clin Infect Dis.* 2011;53(7):e25-76.

Centers for Disease Control and Prevention. 2019. Pertussis (whooping cough); clinicians. Centers for Disease Control and Prevention, Atlanta, GA. https://www.cdc.gov/pertussis/clinical/index.html.

Cherry JD. Epidemic pertussis in 2012–the resurgence of a vaccine-preventable disease. *N Engl J Med.* 2012;367(9):785-7.

Daniels HL, Sabella C. Bordetella pertussis (Pertussis). *Pediatr Rev.* 2018; 39(5): 247–257.

Gardiner SJ, Gavranich JB, Chang AB. Antibiotics for community-acquired lower respiratory tract infections secondary to Mycoplasma pneumoniae in children. *Cochrane Database Syst Rev.* 2015;1: CD004875.

Hofto ME, Samuy N, Pass RF. Antibiotic use and outcomes in young children hospitalized with uncomplicated community-acquired pneumonia. *Open Forum Infect Dis.* 2022;9(4):ofac123.

Jain S, Williams DJ, Arnold SR, et al. Community-acquired pneumonia requiring hospitalization among U.S. children. *N Engl J Med.* 2015; 372(9):835-845.

Lipshaw MJ, Eckerle M, Florin TA, et al. Antibiotic use and outcomes in children in the emergency department with suspected pneumonia. *Pediatrics.* 2020;145:e20193138.

Pernica JM, Harman S, Kam AJ, et al. Short-Course antimicrobial therapy for pediatric community-acquired pneumonia: The SAFER randomized clinical trial. *JAMA Pediatr.* 2021 May 1;175(5):475-482.

Shah SS, Hall M, Newland JG, et al. Comparative effectiveness of pleural drainage procedures for the treatment of complicated pneumonia in childhood. *J Hosp Med.* 2011;6(5):256-263.

Shah SS, Srivastava R, Wu S, et al. Intravenous versus oral antibiotics for postdischarge treatment of complicated pneumonia. *Pediatrics.* 2016; 138(6):e20161692.

Shah VP, Tunik MG, Tsung JW. Prospective Evaluation of Point-of-Care Ultrasonography for the Diagnosis of Pneumonia in Children and Young Adults. *JAMA Pediatr.* 2013;167(2):119–125.

Stockmann C, Ampofo K, Killpack J, et al. Procalcitonin accurately identifies hospitalized children with low risk of bacterial community-acquired pneumonia. *J Pediatric Infect Dis Soc.* 2018;7(1):46-53.

Tiwari T, Murphy TV, Moran J; National Immunization Program, CDC. Recommended antimicrobial agents for the treatment and post-exposure prophylaxis of pertussis: 2005 CDC Guidelines. *MMWR Recomm Rep.* 2005;54(RR-14):1-16.

Williams DJ, Creech CB, Walter EB, et al. Short- vs standard-course outpatient antibiotic therapy for community-acquired pneumonia in children: The SCOUT-CAP randomized clinical trial. *JAMA Pediatr.* 2022;176(3):253-261.

Williams DJ, Shah SS. Community-acquired pneumonia in the conjugate vaccine era. *J Pediatric Infect Dis Soc.* 2012;1(4):320.

CHAPTER 99 Gastrointestinal Infections

Aleisha Nabower, MD and Gwenn Skar, MD

ACUTE GASTROENTERITIS

BACKGROUND

Acute gastroenteritis (AGE) (often termed "diarrheal disease" when the global burden is discussed) is characterized by the sudden onset of diarrhea with or without vomiting. It results from inflammation of the epithelial lining of the gastrointestinal (GI) tract involving any region from the stomach to the colon, most often as a result of infection. The epidemiology, pathogenesis, clinical features, diagnosis, management, and prevention of the major pathogens causing AGE in children are reviewed in this chapter.

An estimated 500,000 children under 5 years old die due to diarrheal illness each year with morbidity and mortality disproportionately found in low-income countries. Diarrheal diseases also remain ubiquitous in middle- and high-income countries, although the severe consequences have become uncommon.

Viruses cause >60% of pediatrics cases of AGE, followed by bacteria and parasites, with rotavirus being the most common organism worldwide. There was a dramatic shift in the epidemiology of pediatric AGE after two rotavirus vaccines were recommended for routine immunization of all infants by the World Health Organization in 2006 to 2008 and the advent of molecular methods for identifying pathogens. Vaccine introduction has resulted in substantial reductions in rotavirus-associated and all-cause AGE hospitalizations in both vaccinated (direct protection) and unvaccinated individuals (indirect, or herd protection) living in high- and middle-income countries. Norovirus is now the most common enteropathogen identified in children hospitalized with AGE in the United States. Globally, however, rotavirus remains the most common detected organism in hospitalized children although the overall proportion of cases due to it have decreased, with norovirus being the next most common, followed by *Cryptosporidium, Shigella/enteroinvasive E. coli* (EIEC), heat-labile enterotoxin-producing *Escheria coli* (ST-ETEC), *and* adenovirus.

In addition, substantial declines in less severe disease are demonstrated by reductions in office visits for rotavirus AGE. Together, these changes translate into large savings of healthcare costs. Moreover, in Mexico and Brazil, reductions in all-cause AGE deaths have been observed. Because programmatic uptake is lagging in low-resource settings where most severe disease and death occurs, international efforts are focused on accelerated introduction in low-income countries. Vaccine efficacy has shown to be lower and wane more rapidly in lower income countries; however, these countries also see the majority of infections prior to 2 years of age so with broad coverage, the life-saving potential of vaccination is predicted to be substantial.

EPIDEMIOLOGY

Viruses, bacteria, and protozoa may all cause AGE in children (**Table 99-1**).

Viral Many viruses can be identified in the GI tract, but only a handful have been associated with AGE in humans. The most common viruses found to cause gastroenteritis seen by a medical provider in the United States includes norovirus, rotavirus, adenovirus, sapovirus, and astrovirus. However, it is important to note that almost 1 in 5 healthy patients had a virus detected by PCR. Among the more than 50 serotypes of adenovirus, types 40 and 41 are most often associated with diarrhea, whereas the remaining serotypes are more commonly found in asymptomatic patients. Astroviruses that cause disease in humans belong to the *Mamastrovirus* genera (types 1-8).

Seasonality provides an epidemiologic clue to implicate specific pathogens, although patterns may differ in tropical and temperate climates. Rotavirus peaks in the cool months, as do norovirus and astrovirus. Enteric adenovirus infections are seen throughout the year, with some increase in summer.

Bacterial The major bacterial enteropathogens responsible for AGE are *Shigella*, nontyphoidal *Salmonella*, *Campylobacter*, and *Yersinia*. Four species of *Shigella* cause human disease: *S. sonnei* (the major cause of shigellosis in industrialized and transitional countries), *S. flexneri* (the major cause of shigellosis in low resource countries), and less commonly *S. boydii* and *S. dysenteriae*. Endemic shigellosis peaks in 1- to 4-year-olds. Human *Salmonella* are classically divided into the human-restricted typhoidal *Salmonella* (*S. typhi* and *S. paratyphi* A and B) which cause enteric fever, and nontyphoidal *Salmonella*, which contains the majority of other serovars causing human AGE and are transmitted mostly from zoonotic reservoirs (asymptomatic young birds, amphibians, and reptiles). *S. typhimurium* and *S. enteritidis* are the most common human nontyphoidal *Salmonella* serovars globally.

Two species of *Campylobacter* traditionally were thought to affect humans: *C. jejuni* and *C. coli* with greatest incidence in infants and young adults. However, recent data suggests other strains may be a key contributor to severe diarrhea and dysentery in children in low-income countries, although it also can be seen in asymptomatic infections. Only two of the 11 species of *Yersinia* cause diarrhea in humans (*Y. enterocolitica* and *Y. pseudotuberculosis*). *Salmonella*, *Shigella*, and *Campylobacter* peak in the warm season, while the ability of *Yersinia* to tolerate cold likely influences its winter seasonality, higher prevalence in northern regions of Europe and Canada, and ability to survive in contaminated blood products during refrigeration.

Five pathotypes of *Escherichia coli* infect humans: enterotoxigenic (ETEC), enteropathogenic (EPEC), Shiga toxin-producing (also known as enterohemorrhagic) (STEC), enteroinvasive (EIEC), and enteroaggregative (EAEC). Pathogenic *E. coli* are identified according to genotypic or phenotypic features that indicate the serologic or antigenic type or the virulence factors that they produce. There are >200 serogroups of *V. cholerae* but only two (O1 or O139) have been associated with epidemic cholera and cause nearly all sporadic cases. The O1 serogroup can be further classified by serotype (e.g., Ogawa and Inaba) and biotype (El Tor or classical) which produces high attack rates and mortality in all age groups, and often affect displaced persons in emergency settings.

TABLE 99-1 Common Pathogens Causing Gastrointestinal Disease

Agent	Clinically Relevant Typing Scheme	Most Relevant Strains for Humans	Available in Most Clinical Labs
Bacteria			
Campylobacter spp.	Speciation	*C. jejuni* (90%-95%) and *C. coli*	Yes
Clostridioides difficile	Virulence factors	Toxigenic *C. difficile*	Yes
		Hypervirulent strain NAP1/B1/02 7(outbreaks since 2000)	No
Enterotoxigenic *E. coli*	Virulence factors	Toxin: Heat labile toxin (LT), heat stable toxin (ST), or LT and ST	Yes
		Colonization factor antigens (CFA/I, CFA/II, or CFA/IV)	No
Enterohemorrhagic *E. coli*	Serotyping	*E. coli* that produce the potent Shiga toxin	Yes
		Most are serotype 0157:H7 (50%-70% in the United States)	
		Other serotypes: 026, 0111, 0105, 0121, 045, 0145, and 0104:H4	
Salmonella	Serogroup	*S. enteritidis,*, *S. typhimurium*, *S. newport*, *S. Heidelberg*, *S. choleraesuis*,	No
	Serotype	*S. paratyphi* A-C, *S. typhi S. dublin*	
Shigella species	Serogroup	*S. sonnei* (endemic diarrhea in middle-high income countries)	Yes
		S. flexneri (endemic diarrhea in developing countries)	Yes
		S. boydii (uncommon)	Yes
		S. dysenteriae (uncommon)	Yes
Vibrio cholerae 01, 0139	Serogroup	98% of diarrheagenic strains are O type 1 or 139, the only two that cause epidemic disease.	Yes
Yersinia enterocolitica	Speciation	*Y. enterocolitica* and *Y. pseudotuberculosis*	Yes
Viruses			
Rotavirus	G and P genotypes	G1P[8], G2P[4], G3P[8], G4P[8], and G9P[8]	Yes
Calicivirus	Genera	Norovirus, sapovirus	Yes
	Genogroup	Norovirus: GI and GII; sapovirus: GI, GII, GIV, GV	Yes
	Genotype	Many	No
Adenovirus	Serotype	Enteric serotypes are 40 and 41	Yes
Astrovirus	Serotyping	1-8	Yes
Protozoa			
Cryptosporidium	Speciation	*C. hominus* (most common), *C. parvum*	Yes

Foodborne diseases are an important public health problem in the United States, causing an estimated 4562 hospitalizations and 68 deaths annually. Children <5 years old have the highest incidence of disease, while the elderly experience the highest frequency of hospitalization and death. The most common foodborne causes of AGE are norovirus, nontyphoidal *Salmonella*, *C. perfringens*, *Campylobacter*, and *S. aureus*, while nontyphoidal *Salmonella* is the leading cause of hospitalization and death.

The epidemiology of zoonotic infections is influenced by the organism's behavior in the animal host. Nontyphoidal *Salmonella*'s capability of transovarian passage in hens can result in large outbreaks related to intact grade A pasteurized eggs. Although *Campylobacter* is prevalent in poultry, it has lower outbreak potential, at least in part because it is incapable of transovarian spread in hens and has stringent growth requirements, which limit its ability to replicate in foods. On the other hand, because of its extensive reservoir in domestic and wild animals, *Campylobacter* has emerged as the most common cause of sporadic bacterial foodborne disease in many industrialized countries, usually from consumption of contaminated chicken, beef, and milk. The ubiquitous animal reservoir has resulted in widespread contamination of surface waters with *Campylobacter*, and as a result, diarrhea in hikers who drink untreated surface water in wilderness areas is often due to *Campylobacter*, exceeding *Giardia*. The predilection for STEC to asymptomatically colonize the intestines of ruminant animals explains why unpasteurized dairy products, fruits harvested from fields where cattle graze, and undercooked hamburger are common vehicles. The major animal reservoir for *Yersinia* is pigs, so ingestion of raw or undercooked pork products is an important risk factor.

Clostridiodes difficile (formerly *Clostridium difficile*) that produce toxin are pathogenic for humans over 1 year of age. Hospitalization and antibiotic therapies contribute to the risk of toxigenic *Clostridiodes difficile*, with rates of pediatric infection ranging from 2-420/10,000 day for inpatients and 14-80/100,000 for outpatients, peaking around 4 years of age. However, community-acquired C. *difficile* disease is becoming more common, accounting for up to 41% of cases. While a hypervirulent strain (NAP/027/BI) has been detected in outbreaks among adults, it accounts for <20% of the isolates in kids, with the most common strain identified being 014. There is little doubt that children develop severe *C. difficile* disease, but it appears to be uncommon, and occurs mostly among older children. Children with cancer have an increased risk for severe disease, while *C. difficile* infection exacerbates inflammatory bowel disease. There is a high frequency (up to 70%) of asymptomatic colonization among healthy newborns that gradually falls to adult levels as the microbiota of the lower intestine becomes established by about 2 years of age, rendering the significance of identifying the organism in an individual child <2 years of age uncertain.

Protozoal *Cryptosporidium* is an oocyst-forming coccidian protozoa. At least 13 of the more than 60 species have been found to cause human disease, but *C. hominus*, and to a lesser extent *C. parvum*, account for the vast majority (~90%) of human infections. Water treatment systems and recreational swimming facilities have provided vehicles for massive outbreaks of the chlorine-resistant *Cryptosporidium*. These outbreaks are sustained by the ability of *Cryptosporidium* to spread person-to-person via a small inoculum. *Cyclospora cayetanesis* is another coccidian protozoa. The genus *Entamoeba* includes six species that colonize humans; *E. histolytica* is thought to be the sole pathogen causing intestinal illness. *Giardia intestinalis* (formerly *G. lamblia* and *G. duodenalis*) is a flagellate protozoan that infects the small intestine and biliary tract.

The epidemiologic features of the major AGE pathogens are listed according to pathogen in **Table 99-2** and according to risk factor in **Table 99-3**.

PATHOPHYSIOLOGY

Viral In viral AGE, cytolytic infection of the small intestinal villus tips leads to decreased absorption of water, disaccharide malabsorption

TABLE 99-2 Vehicles, Epidemiology, and Routes of Transmission Favored by Major Enteropathogens

Agent	Principal Vehicles/Transmission	Peak Age	Setting	Season	Estimated Annual No. Cases in the United States, All Age Groups (Deaths)*	Risk Factors
Bacteria						
Campylobacter spp.	Wild and domestic animals and animal products, including pets	Young children, young adults	Global	Warm/late summer and autumn in temperate zones	1.5 million (119)[1]	Ingestion of raw or undercooked poultry, untreated water, unpasteurized milk; improper food handling; animal contact; travel to developing country, backpackers, hikers, and campers who drink untreated, unfiltered water
Clostridioides difficile	Person-to-person (fecal-oral) mostly within inpatient healthcare facilities; source of community-acquired infection unknown	Elderly	IC	None	223,900 healthcare-associated cases of infection (12,800)	Immunosuppression, intestinal surgery, inflammatory bowel disease, Hirschsprung disease, prolonged hospitalization, antibiotic usage
Enterotoxigenic *E. coli* (ETEC)	Food and water contaminated with human feces	Infants, young children	LDC	Warm, wet seasons	79,420 (0)	Infants and young children in endemic areas, travel to LDC
Shiga toxin-producing *E. coli* (STEC)	Food and water contaminated with feces from cattle or other ruminants; person-to-person or animal-to-person (fecal-oral), predominantly in industrialized countries	All, with most severe illness in very young and elderly	IC	None	16,939 (30)	Ingestion of undercooked ground beef, unpasteurized dairy products or juices, untreated water; petting zoos, recreational swimming; day care centers; risk of HUS increased with use of antidiarrheal agents and antibiotics
Nontyphoidal *Salmonella*	Food from infected animals (eggs, poultry, beef, milk) that is either eaten or that cross-contaminates other foods; pet reptiles or amphibians and birds	Infants, young children 0-4 years of age	Global	Warm/late summer and autumn in temperate zones	58,371 million (400)	Ingestion of raw or undercooked food, improper food handling, travelers, immunosuppression, antibiotics, hemolytic anemia, achlorhydria, contact with infected animal

(*Continued*)

TABLE 99-2 Vehicles, Epidemiology, and Routes of Transmission Favored by Major Enteropathogens (*Continued*)

Agent	Principal Vehicles/Transmission	Peak Age	Setting	Season	Estimated Annual No. Cases in the United States, All Age Groups (Deaths)*	Risk Factors
Shigella spp.	Person-to-person by fecal oral route, also food or water contaminated with human feces	Toddlers 2-4 years of age	Global	Warm/late summer and autumn in temperate zones	18,574 (10)[1]	Travelers, day care, prisoners, MSM, poor hygiene and/or sanitation
Vibrio cholerae	Food and water contaminated with human feces, shellfish, food from street vendors	Children (all ages in naïve populations)	LDC	Warm seasons/ before and after monsoons	14 (0)[1]	Travelers to endemic or epidemic settings, blood group O, vitamin A deficiency
Yersinia enterocolitica	Pig is major human reservoir and food is major source (most cases are sporadic with occasional outbreaks, occasional animal-to-human, waterborne, bloodborne; can multiply during refrigeration	Young children	IC (especially Europe and Canada)	Cool	117,000(35)	Undercooked pork, improper food handling, unpasteurized milk, transfusion from a bacteremic person, cirrhosis, chelation therapy
Bacillus cereus	Soil and water	All ages	IC[£]	All	63,000 (0)	Cooked rice, meats (emetic toxin) Meats, stews, gravies, vanilla sauce (diarrhea toxin)
Clostridium perfringens	Environment, intestines of humans and animals	All ages	IC[£]	All	965,958 (26)	Beef, poultry, gravies, dried or precooked foods subject to poor temperature control, usually produced in commercial kitchens
Staphylococcus aureus toxin	Contamination during food preparation from bird, mammal, or environmental sources, direct contamination of ruminant animal dairy products	All ages	IC[£]	All	240,000 (0)	Sliced meat, puddings, pastries, sandwiches, dairy products, and salads subject to poor temperature control
Viruses						
Rotavirus Astrovirus Enteric adenovirus	Person-to-person (fecal-oral), fomites	Infants	Global	Cool	593,007 (37)[2 *]	Infants and young children worldwide
Norovirus	Person-to-person (fecal-oral and aerosolized vomit), and fomites, food, or water contaminated with human feces	All	Global	Year-round with peak in cool season	20 million (900)	Very contagious (chlorine and heat resistant), producing large outbreaks in closed settings such as cruise ships
Protozoa						
Entamoeba histolytica	Person-to-person (fecal-oral), and fomites, food, and water contaminated with human feces	Unknown	LDC	Unknown	Unknown (unknown)	Travelers to LDC, institutionalized persons, MSM
Cryptosporidium	Person-to-person and animal-to-person (fecal-oral), food or water (including contaminated municipal water and recreational water) contaminated with human or animal feces	Infants	Global	Warm/ warm rainy seasons	13,975 (4)	Child care settings, swimmers, backpackers, hikers, and campers who drink untreated, unfiltered water, untreated water from unprotected, shallow wells, cowhands, MSM, recreational water venues, malnutrition, immunodeficiency
Giardia	Waterborne from lakes or streams, person-to-person or animal-to-person	Bimodal in IC, unclear in DC	Global	Warm	14,860 (2)[1]	Hikers drinking unfiltered, untreated water, travelers to endemic settings, animal contact, MSM, IgA deficiency
Cyclospora	Fresh produce, contaminated water	All	LDC	Varies	4,703 (0)[1]	Travelers, fresh produce imported from endemic areas

HUS, hemolytic uremic syndrome; IC, industrialized country; LDC, less developed country; MSM, men who have sex with men.

*Unless otherwise specified, data are derived from http://www.cdc.gov/az/c.html.

1. Geissler AL, Carrillo FB, Swanson K, et al. Increasing campylobacter infections, outbreaks, and antimicrobial resistance in the United States, 2004–2012. *Clin Infect Dis*. 2017;65(10):1624-1631.

2. Troeger C, Khalil IA, Rao PC, et al. Rotavirus vaccination and the global burden of rotavirus diarrhea among children younger than 5 years. *JAMA Pediatr*. 2018;172(10):958–965. *Rates per children < 5 years not entire population.

TABLE 99-3 Exposures Associated With Specific Pathogens That Cause Diarrhea

Travel to developing countries	Enterotoxigenic *E. coli* (ETEC), *Shigella*, nontyphoidal *Salmonella*, *Campylobacter*, *Entamoeba*
Swimming in or drinking contaminated water	*Campylobacter*, *Cryptosporidium*, *Giardia*
Swimming in recreational facility	*Cryptosporidium*
Institutional exposure, healthcare setting, or day care	*Shigella*, *Cryptosporidium*, *Giardia*, Shiga toxin-producing *E. coli*, norovirus, rotavirus, *C. difficile*
Antibiotic therapy	*Clostridioides difficile*
Foodborne outbreak in hotel, cruise ship, resort, restaurant, catered event	Norovirus, nontyphoidal *Salmonella*, *C. perfringens*, *B.* cereus, *S. aureus*, *Campylobacter* spp.
Unpasteurized milk	*Salmonella*, *Campylobacter*, *Yersinia*, *Staphylococcus aureus* toxin
Consumption of raw or undercooked meat	Shiga toxin-producing *E. coli* (hamburger), *Salmonella* (poultry), *Campylobacter* (poultry), *Yersinia* (pork, chitterlings), *Vibrio* (shellfish)
Consumption of fruits or unpasteurized fruit juices harvested from fields where cattle graze	Shiga toxin-producing *E. coli*
Exposure to animals	Puppies and kittens with diarrhea (*Campylobacter*, *Yersinia*), asymptomatic chicks and reptiles (non-typhoidal *Salmonella*), petting zoos (Shiga toxin-producing *E. coli*)
Hemochromatosis	*Yersinia*
Underlying immunocompromising condition	Nontyphoidal *Salmonella*, protozoa, *Cryptosporidium*, *Campylobacter*, *Shigella*, *Yersinia*

(occurs in 10%-20%, but is transient and subclinical in most instances), mononuclear cell infiltration in the lamina propria, and cytokine activation. Rotavirus also produces an enterotoxin that opens cellular calcium channels, causing secretory diarrhea. Additionally, rotavirus activates the enteric nervous system causing decreased gastric emptying and increased intestinal motility. A unique feature of norovirus infection is that susceptibility is mediated by histo-blood group antigens on the epithelial cell surface and in mucous secretions, in particular those controlled by the fucosyltransferase 2 gene.

Bacterial *Shigella*, nontyphoidal *Salmonella*, *Campylobacter*, and *Yersinia* share the ability to invade the intestinal epithelium, evoke an inflammatory response, and evade the host immune system but have evolved different mechanisms to achieve this. *Shigella* and EIEC invade and destroy the colonic epithelial cells and produce an intense inflammatory response characterized by infiltration with neutrophils, leading to loss of epithelial cell barrier function, diarrhea, and formation of mucosal micro-abscesses and ulcerations. One serotype of *Shigella* (*S. dysenteriae* type 1) also produces a potent cytotoxin called Shiga toxin that irreversibly inhibits protein synthesis, manifests enterotoxic and neurotoxic features, and is associated with hemolytic uremic syndrome (HUS). STEC produces a biologically similar toxin that induces bloody diarrhea and also is associated with HUS.

Nontyphoidal *Salmonella* invade the mucosal epithelium of the small intestine and colon and are engulfed by dendritic cells in intestinal lymphoid tissue, evoking an inflammatory response dominated by neutrophils, with mucosal edema and crypt abscesses. While the neutrophil response helps to prevent NTS from disseminating to the bloodstream, it may nonetheless contribute to the development of diarrhea by causing epithelial cell disruption and increased vascular permeability. *Salmonella* that spread systemically pass to the reticuloendothelial system via the mesenteric lymph nodes and/or invade the bloodstream and depending on the virulence of the organism and host factors, may disseminate to contiguous or distant sites. The invasive phenotype is also a feature of *Campylobacter* and *Yersinia* infections, although it is mediated by a distinct array of virulence factors which are less well-characterized compared to *Shigella* and nontyphoidal *Salmonella*. Flagellar-mediated motility and cytolethal distending toxin are putative virulence factors contributing to the invasiveness and immunomodulary properties of *C. jejuni*, while production of a heat-stable enterotoxin is thought to contribute to the pathogenesis of *Yersinia*. The association of *Campylobacter* infection with Guillain Barré syndrome arises from immunologic cross-reactivity between the lipooligosaccharide antigens of specific serogroups and gangliosides present in neural myelin.

Pathogenic *V. cholerae* attach to the small intestinal epithelium via the toxin-coregulated pilus and elaborate an enterotoxin that produces secretory diarrhea by activating adenylate cyclase and raising intracellular cAMP. Similarly, ETEC causes secretory diarrhea by adhering to the small intestine via colonizing fimbrial antigens (CFAs) and elaborating heat-labile toxin (LT), which is nearly identical to cholera toxin, and/or heat-stable enterotoxin (ST) which increases secretion of water and electrolytes by activating cGMP. ETEC that produce either ST alone or ST plus LT are pathogenic, while many of those producing only LT are not. EPEC undergo *eae*-encoded intimin-mediated attachment to the intestinal epithelium to form a pedestal-like lesion. So-called typical EPEC also possess *bfpA*, which encodes localized adherence on cultured epithelial cells. Like EPEC, STEC produce a pedestal malformation at the intestinal attachment site and do not invade; the mechanism of local and systemic illness involves elaboration of toxins, including two potent cytotoxins, Shiga-like toxins 1 and 2 that are involved in the pathogenesis of bloody diarrhea and HUS.

The diarrheagenic phenotype of *C. difficile* is attributed to production of toxin B (all strains) and toxin A (most strains). After entry into the colonic epithelial cells, the toxins glucosylate and inactivate host GTPases, leading to alterations in the cytoskeletal structure, disruption of barrier function, and apoptosis. They also evoke an inflammatory response. Both toxins have enterotoxic properties, but toxin B is considered the major cytotoxin. The epidemic NAP1 strain is also produces a binary toxin, which may enhance colonization and augment the capacity to produce toxins A and B. NAP1 is resistant to fluoroquinolones in vitro. The pathogenicity of *C. difficile* among infants and young children is a subject of controversy, as asymptomatic colonization with toxigenic strains is frequently seen, attributed to diminished toxin A receptor sites along the intestinal epithelium.

Staphylococcal food poisoning results from ingestion of food contaminated with preformed *S. aureus* ST enterotoxin. Enterotoxin types A to E cause enteric disease. *B. cereus* is an aerobic gram-positive spore-forming bacillus that produces two distinct forms of GI illnesses. One syndrome resembles *S. aureus* food poisoning and is caused by a preformed emetic toxin that survives high temperatures, exposure to trypsin, and pH extremes. The other is caused by a group of three enterotoxins formed in vivo that are sensitive to high temperatures, proteolytic enzymes, and acids. After ingestion of the anaerobic gram-positive bacillus *Clostridium perfringens*, in vivo sporulation occurs in the small intestine with release of a heat-labile, single-polypeptide enterotoxin.

Protozoal After excystation in the lumen, *E. histolytica* trophozoites that are pathogenic attach to the colonic epithelium via a surface lectin and create channel-forming peptides called amebophores, which cause cell lysis resulting in bloody diarrhea. Organisms reaching the lamina propria trigger an inflammatory cascade. Armed with the ability to resist complement-mediated lysis and to kill host inflammatory cells, trophozoites can disseminate via the portal vein to the liver and other viscera.

Cryptosporidium sporozoites released from ingested oocysts penetrate small intestinal epithelial cells and develop into trophozoites within vacuoles in the intracellular, but extracytoplasmic, apical space. After undergoing asexual multiplication and sexual development, they are released as either infectious oocysts that enter the feces or thin-walled sporulated oocysts capable of autoinfection. Host factors, particularly T cell function and nutritional status, play a critical role in disease severity.

In contrast to *Cryptosporidium*, *Cyclospora* oocysts are not infectious in freshly passed stools and therefore direct fecal-oral transmission is not seen. Sporulation occurs after 1 to 2 weeks in the environment, and the infectious oocysts are ingested in contaminated fresh produce and water. The pathophysiologic mechanisms of this human pathogen are likely similar to *Cryptosporidium*.

CLINICAL PRESENTATION

Diarrhea is usually defined as the passage of three or more loose or liquid stools per day (or more frequent passage than is normal for the individual). Frequent passage of formed stools is not diarrhea, nor is the passing of loose, "pasty" stools by breastfed babies. Three clinical syndromes are often described because they have different (albeit overlapping) etiologies, outcomes, and treatments: acute (non-bloody) diarrhea, bloody diarrhea or frank dysentery (the frequent passage of scant stools containing blood and mucus, often accompanied by fever, lower abdominal cramps, and rectal tenesmus), and persistent diarrhea (lasting more than 14 days).

In the initial evaluation of all patients with AGE, the physician should focus on the patient's hydration status and electrolyte balance as well as evidence of sepsis or invasive bacterial infection, which could complicate bacterial AGE. Important elements of the medical history include the duration of diarrhea and a description of stools (frequency, amount, presence of blood or mucus), fever (duration, magnitude), vomiting (onset, amount and frequency), and the amount and type of solid and liquid oral intake. Additionally, the past medical history should identify comorbidities that might increase the risk or severity of AGE.

Vital signs and weight should be measured. Certain physical signs are best assessed before approaching the child directly so he/she remains calm, including general appearance (activity, response to stimulation) and respiratory patterns. Hyperpnea (deep, rapid breathing) suggests acidosis secondary to dehydration, while respiratory distress (tachypnea, grunting, nasal flaring, head bobbing, and retractions) suggests pneumonia. Skin turgor is assessed by pinching a small skin fold on the lateral abdominal wall at the level of the umbilicus. If the fold does not promptly return to normal after release, the recoil time is quantified as delayed slightly or ≥2 seconds. Note that excess subcutaneous tissue and hypernatremia may result in a false negative test and malnutrition can prolong the recoil time. Capillary refill time is assessed by gradually pressing the palmar surface of the child's distal fingertip, with the child's arm at heart level, until blanching occurs. When dehydration is present, the time elapsed until normal color is restored after release usually exceeds 2 seconds. Ambient temperature and autonomic dysfunction are among the factors that can modify the results.

In the past, many guidelines divided patients into subgroups for mild (3%-5%), moderate (6%-9%), and severe (≥10%) dehydration. While multiple severity prediction scales have been developed, none have shown sufficient reliability to be widely adapted. Additionally, it is difficult to distinguish between mild and moderate dehydration based on clinical signs alone. Therefore most current guidelines combine mild and moderate dehydration and simply use none, some, and severe dehydration. Symptoms of dehydration that should be evaluated are urine output (number of wet diapers per day and time since the last urination), whether eyes appear sunken, whether the child is active, whether the child drinks vigorously, and the date and value of the most recent weight measurement. Documented weight loss can be used to calculate the fluid deficit.

The three individual signs that best predict dehydration are prolonged capillary refill time, abnormal skin turgor, and hyperpnea (**Table 99-4**). As the number of signs increases, so does the likelihood of dehydration. For example, one study found that the presence of two or more of the following findings had a sensitivity of 79% and specificity of 87% in predicting dehydration: capillary refill >2 seconds, dry mucous membranes, absent tears, and general appearance (including activity level and thirst).

Once the patient is stabilized, the history and physical examination can focus on detecting risk factors and exposures, as well as the clinical features (**Table 99-5**) that may suggest specific etiologic agents. Although there is considerable overlap, high fever >40°C, overt fecal blood, abdominal pain, no vomiting before diarrhea onset, and high stool frequency (>10 per day) are more common with bacterial pathogens. Although high fever and overt fecal blood are often absent in bacterial enteritis, when present there is a high probability of a bacterial etiology.

Viral Symptoms of rotavirus AGE usually begin 2 to 4 days after exposure with the onset of vomiting followed by frequent passage of watery non-bloody stools, associated with fever in about half the cases.

TABLE 99-4 Management of Dehydration According to Severity Classification in Children With Diarrhea

Severe Dehydration	Management[1,2]
Two or more of the following signs[1]: • Lethargy/unconsciousness • Sunken eyes, more than usual • Unable to drink or drinks poorly • Skin pinch goes back very slowly >2 seconds) Other signs and symptoms that may be present[2,3]: • Respirations deep and rapid • Hypotension • Rapid, weak radial pulse • Extremities cool and mottled • Urine output ≪1 mL/kg/hr • Very sunken anterior fontanelle • Absent tears • Parched oral mucosa	Isotonic intravenous fluids • 20-30 mL/kg over 30-60 minutes (repeat if necessary) until pulse, perfusion, and mental status normalize • Then provide maintenance fluids and replace the remaining deficit either intravenously, or enterally as described below if the child is awake, has no risk factors for aspiration, and no evidence of ileus
Some Dehydration	**Management[1,2]**
Two or more of the following signs[1]: • Restlessness, irritability • Sunken eyes, more than usual • Drinks eagerly, thirsty • Skin pinch goes back slowly but <2 seconds Other signs and symptoms that may be present[2,3]: • Fatigue • Respirations normal to rapid • Normal to increased • Mildly delayed capillary refill • Urine output decreased or <1 mL/kg/hr • Sunken anterior fontanelle • Decreased tears • Dry oral mucosa	Replace deficit: • Give 50-100 mL/kg of oral rehydration solution (ORS) over 2-4 hr; if the child wants more to drink, give more • Provide frequent, small amounts of ORS by spoon or syringe (≤5 mL) to avoid triggering vomiting; increase volume as tolerated • Administer as continuous nasogastric infusion for patients with persistent vomiting or refusal to drink • Keep child in healthcare setting until rehydrated Replace ongoing losses • 1 mL ORS for each 1 g of stool or vomitus, if known • Alternatively, Provide nutrition • Continue breastfeeding • When rehydrated, resume age-appropriate, unrestricted diet

References

1. World Health Organization. Pocket book of Hospital Care for Children: Guideline for the Management of Common Illnesses with Limited Resources. 2005. http://whqlibdoc.who.int/publications/2005/9241546700.pdf. Accessed December 11, 2013.

2. King CK, Glass R, Bresee JS, Duggan C. Managing acute gastroenteritis among children: oral rehydration, maintenance, and nutritional therapy. *MMWR Recomm Rep*. 2003;52:1-16.

3. Steiner MJ, DeWalt DA, Byerley JS. Is this child dehydrated† *JAMA*. 2004;291:2746-2754.

The diarrhea lacks fecal leukocytes, but stools from 20% of cases contain mucus. Recovery with complete resolution of symptoms generally occurs within 7 days. Although disaccharide malabsorption is found in 10% to 20% of episodes, it is rarely clinically significant.

Other viral agents elicit similar symptoms and cannot be distinguished from rotavirus based on clinical findings. In an outbreak setting, the pattern of a brief incubation period (12-48 hours), short duration of illness, and clustering of cases is shared by caliciviruses and preformed bacterial toxin. However, unlike preformed toxins, calciviruses cause secondary infections, which confirm the contagious nature of the outbreak. Diarrheal illnesses caused by enteric adenovirus infections tend to be more prolonged than rotavirus (7-10 days), while astroviruses cause a shorter course (~5 days), usually without significant vomiting.

TABLE 99-5 Typical Clinical Features of Illness with Major Enteropathogens

Causative Agent	Usual Incubation Period	Usual Duration of Illness	CLINICAL ILLNESS Fever	Diarrhea	Vomiting	Bloody Stools	Other Features*
Staphylococcus aureus enterotoxin *Bacillus cereus* emetic toxin	1-6 hours	1-3 days	+	++	++++	Absent	–
Clostridium perfringens enterotoxin *B. cereus* enterotoxin	8-16 hours	1-2 days†	+	++++	++	Absent	–
Clostridioides difficile toxin	Unknown**	Variable	++	++++	+	++	Mild-moderate watery diarrhea may progress to severe, pseudomembranous colitis with systemic toxicity
Shigella	1-5 days (up to 8 days for *S. dysenteriae* 1)	5-7 days	+++	++++	+	+++	Dysentery (frequent scant bloody stools, often with tenesmus); *S. dysenteriae* type 1 associated with high case-fatality
Non-typhoidal *Salmonella* *Campylobacter* *Yersinia*	1-5 days	5-7 days, occasionally >10 days	++	++++	++	++	Relapsing or prolonged diarrhea (10%-20%) dysentery; bacteremia, extra-intestinal infections; severe disease in immunocompromised persons
Vibrio cholerae O1 and O139 Enterotoxigenic *E. coli* (ETEC)	1-5 days (can be as short as 2 hours)	3-7 days	++	++++	++	Absent	Cholera gravis in 5%-10% (profuse watery diarrhea – "rice water stools," vomiting, leg cramps), can lead to hypovolemic shock and death within hours
Rotavirus Enteric adenovirus Astrovirus	2-4 days	3-8 days	++	++++	+++	Absent	Illness often begins with vomiting
Norovirus	12-48 hours	1-3 days	++	++++	++++	Absent	Headache, myalgia
Shiga toxin-producing *E. coli* (STEC)	1-9 days (usually 3–4 days)	4-7 days	++ (low grade)	++++	+++	+++	Watery diarrhea becomes bloody in 1-4 days in ~40% of infections; in contrast to bacillary dysentery, bloody stools are large volume and fever/toxicity is minimal
Cryptosporidium parvum *Cyclospora cayetanensis*	1-11 days	1-2 weeks	+	++++	++	Absent	Frequent, sometimes explosive stools, bloating, flatulence, weight loss, fatigue; symptoms may wax and wane. In persons with AIDS or malnutrition, *Cryptosporidium* can cause prolonged diarrhea, malabsorption, and death
Giardia lamblia	1-4 weeks	2-4 weeks	+	++++	++	Absent	Steatorrhea, borborygmi, flatulence, weight loss; symptoms may wax and wane
Entamoeba histolytica	2-4 weeks	Variable	+ (8–38%)	++++	+	+++	Gradual onset over 1-3 weeks; typically there is dysentery, can become chronic

*All etiologies are associated with abdominal cramps, which are typically most severe with dysentery.

**Symptoms may begin during antibiotic therapy and as long as 10 weeks after its cessation.

†Occasionally *C. perfringens* causes prolonged illnesses for up to 2 weeks.

Bacterial The signs and symptoms of bacterial AGE overlap considerably with those of other causes. Below is a description of the presentations of classical bacterial agents, the *E. coli* pathotypes, and other bacterial agents.

Classical Bacterial Agents In general, the classical agents, nontyphoidal *Salmonella*, *Shigella*, *Campylobacter*, and *Yersinia*, present with one of five syndromes.

1. *Acute diarrhea*, the most common presentation, may be accompanied by fever and vomiting. Clinically silent bacteremia accompanying uncomplicated nontyphoidal *Salmonella* AGE can be seen among otherwise healthy children younger than 2 years living in industrialized countries.
2. *Bloody diarrhea or frank dysentery*. *Shigella* is the classical cause of bacillary dysentery. Watery diarrhea (small bowel disease) typically precedes dysentery and is often the sole clinical manifestation of mild infection. Progression to dysentery indicates colitis and may occur within hours to days. Patients with severe infection may pass more than 20 dysenteric stools in one day. Dysenteric illnesses due to *Campylobacter* have been confused with inflammatory bowel disease.
3. *Invasive, non-focal disease (enteric fever)* is a febrile illness associated with bacteremia without localized infection. Diarrhea may be minimal or absent. Although classically the result of *S.* Typhi or Paratyphi A and B, enteric fever can result from systemic spread of the classical bacterial enteropathogens. Whereas enteric fever caused by *S.* Typhi or Paratyphi A and B primarily affect preschool and school-age children in endemic countries, other bacterial enteropathogens most often cause disease in infants (particularly <3 months), the immunocompromised, and children with malnutrition. Additional risk factors include hemolytic anemia and intravascular lesions for nontyphoidal *Salmonella*, and iron overload, cirrhosis, and chelation therapy for *Yersinia* sepsis. The distinct clones of nontyphoidal *Salmonella* that have arisen in sub-Saharan Africa are causing enteric-fever type illnesses often in the absence of AGE. *Shigella* sepsis is rare, and is seen most often in malnourished and immunocompromised hosts.
4. *Localized extraintestinal invasive infections* can result from either local invasion or bacteremic spread. Local invasion may result in mesenteric adenitis, appendicitis, and rarely cholecystitis, mesenteric venous thrombosis, pancreatitis, hepatic or splenic abscess.

Bacteremic spread may result in abscesses or local infections such as pneumonia, osteomyelitis, or meningitis (three conditions seen most commonly with nontyphoidal *Salmonella*), cellulitis, septic arthritis, and endocarditis. *Shigella* also can cause noninvasive contiguous infections such as vaginitis and urinary tract infections.

5. *Perinatal infection* can result from vertical transmission of *Shigella*, nontyphoidal *Salmonella*, and *Campylobacter*, resulting in a spectrum of illness from isolated diarrhea or hematochezia to fulminant neonatal sepsis. One species of *Campylobacter*, *C. fetus*, is particularly virulent in pregnant women and can result in chorioamnionitis, abortion, and neonatal sepsis and meningitis.

Diarrheagenic E. coli *E. coli* pathotypes cause a variety of diarrheal diseases. Illness with STEC typically follows 3 to 4 days after ingestion of as few as 100 organisms. Crampy abdominal pain and non-bloody diarrhea are the first symptoms, sometimes with vomiting. By the second or third day of illness, diarrhea becomes bloody in approximately 90% of cases and abdominal pain worsens. Bloody diarrhea lasts between 1 and 22 days (median 4 days). In contrast to dysentery, the stools associated with STEC hemorrhagic colitis are large volume, and signs of high fever and toxicity are usually absent. ETEC produce a secretory watery diarrhea that affects infants and young children in low-income countries; in addition, ETEC is the major causative agent of traveler's diarrhea, accounting for about half of all episodes in some studies. In its most severe form, ETEC can cause cholera-like purging, even in adults. Although previously a cause of summertime non-bloody diarrhea in infants in the United States, EPEC has become extremely uncommon in industrialized countries, but remains a leading cause of persistent diarrhea (14 days or longer) associated with malnutrition among infants and young children from low-income countries. EIEC is genetically, biochemically, and clinically nearly identical to *Shigella*. It causes rare foodborne outbreaks in industrialized countries. EAEC has been associated with persistent diarrhea in immunocompromised persons and sporadic diarrhea in infants in countries with varying levels of economic development; however, some studies have not found an association with disease. It is likely that further elucidation of the mechanisms that define pathogenic infection will allow studies to better discern the disease-producing strains.

C. difficile is associated with several clinical syndromes. The most common is mild to moderate watery diarrhea, low-grade fever, and mild abdominal pain. Occasionally the illness will progress to full-blown pseudomembranous colitis characterized by diarrhea, abdominal cramps, and fever. The colonic mucosa contains 2- to 5-mm raised, yellowish plaques. Fatal cases are associated with systemic toxicity and multisystem organ failure, possibly related to systemic absorption of toxin. The illness associated with *S. aureus* and *B. cereus* emetic toxin is dominated by vomiting, while diarrhea is the major manifestation of *C. perfringens* and *B. cereus* enterotoxin.

Protozoal Parasitic protozoa such as *Giardia*, *Cryptosporidium*, *Cyclospora*, and *E. histolytica* are the most common parasites that cause diarrhea in the United States. These illnesses tend to be more prolonged, sometimes for 2 weeks or more, but are usually self-limited in the otherwise healthy host. A protozoal etiology should be suspected when there is a prolonged diarrheal illness characterized by episodes of sometimes-explosive diarrhea with nausea, abdominal cramps, and abdominal bloating. The stools are usually watery, but can be greasy and foul smelling due to concomitant malabsorption of fats, which is more likely to occur if the parasite load is high. Occasionally diarrhea may alternate with constipation.

In low-income countries, *Cryptosporidium* is a cause of moderate-to-severe diarrhea in infants, leading to increased risk of growth faltering and death. In general, the duration and severity of diarrhea is strongly influenced by the immune and nutritional status of the host.

Although infection with *E. histolytica* causes the typical syndrome of protozoal diarrhea (known as intestinal amebiasis), a range of other syndromes may occur, including amebic dysentery and hepatic amebiasis. Amebic dysentery is characterized by bloody or mucoid diarrhea, which may be profuse and lead to dehydration or electrolyte imbalances. Hepatic amebiasis is limited to abscess formation in the liver, which may occur with or without intestinal disease.

DIFFERENTIAL DIAGNOSIS

The infectious causes of bloody diarrhea or dysentery include *Shigella*, nontyphoidal *Salmonella*, *Campylobacter*, *Yersinia*, and STEC. If the exposure history is suggestive, *C. difficile* and *E. histolytica* should also be entertained. The physician should also consider noninfectious diseases that can present with bright red blood per rectum (hematochezia). In an infant or young child without systemic symptoms, the differential diagnosis includes anal fissures, intermittent intussusception, juvenile polyps, arteriovenous malformations and Meckel's diverticulum. Necrotizing enterocolitis can cause lower GI bleeding in infants, especially premature neonates. Inflammatory bowel disease should be considered in older children, particularly those experiencing systemic signs and symptoms. The most likely diagnosis in an infant or child who presents with watery diarrhea is viral AGE; however, infection with any enteropathogen can produce watery diarrhea. If the watery diarrhea is persistent, noninfectious causes can be considered, although these are rare. Examples include congenital secretory diarrheas, endocrine disorders (hyperthyroidism), neoplasms, food intolerance, and medications (particularly antibiotics). Chronic or relapsing diarrhea with or without malabsorption should trigger a search for intestinal protozoa; noninfectious causes that should be considered include cystic fibrosis, celiac disease, milk protein intolerance, and congenital or acquired disaccharidase deficiency. Significant abdominal pain should raise suspicion of other infectious processes in the abdomen such as apendicitis and pelvic inflammatory disease. Prominent vomiting with or without abdominal pain can be a manifestation of pyloric stenosis, intestinal obstruction, pancreatitis, appendicitis, and cholecystitis.

DIAGNOSTIC EVALUATION

Most cases of AGE do not require diagnostic laboratory testing. Suspicion of a causative agent that might require specific therapy, cohorting of patients to limit the spread of infection, or that has been linked to a possible outbreak, may necessitate laboratory investigation. Stool can be examined for mucus, blood, and leukocytes; however, the use of stool leukocytes or fecal lactoferrin are not recommended in the diagnostic evaluation of acute gastroenteritis.

When microbiologic diagnosis is sought, a stool sample must be evaluated. Timely submission of a fresh or well-preserved stool is of paramount importance to maximize identification of pathogens and best inform treatment choices. If the child has not passed a stool, a rectal swab can be collected promptly. After dipping the cotton tip into the medium that will be used for transport, it is gently inserted into the child's rectum and rotated 360°. A properly collected rectal swab is stained or covered with fecal material. A stool sample should still be sent for studies when available given the conflicting yield of rectal swabs.

The advent of multiplex nucleic acid amplification testing has drastically changed the ability to receive rapid pathogen identification from stool. These tests however are costly, with most isolates having limited impact on clinical management. They should be reserved for cases of blood or mucoid stools, severe pain, signs of sepsis, immunocompromised patients, or when testing occurs in the setting of a suspected outbreak. A positive result does not necessarily predict actual disease, with almost 1/3 of asymptomatic patients testing positive for an organism. Unlike stool cultures, PCR testing is not impacted by antibiotic or bismuth use. Specific organisms targeted in the assay vary between panels. Especially in immunocompromised hosts, it is important to recognize that many opportunistic pathogens are not included in the panel. Additionally, these panels do not provide information on isolate or antimicrobial susceptibility so culture should be obtained as well in those cases. Similar to stool cultures, the diagnostic yield of stool PCR >3 days after admission is low and should not routinely be obtained.

For children older than 2 years who have recently received antibiotics or have other risk factors, evaluation for *C. difficile* infection may be appropriate. The cytotoxin assay detects toxin B, but testing for toxin A is also available in some laboratories. Several tests are commercially available to detect toxin-producing *C. difficile* in stool, including enzyme immunoassays for toxins A and B, cell culture cytotoxicity assay, and polymerase chain reaction (PCR). The sensitivity of cell culture and PCR are superior to that of immunoassay and only require one sample; however confirmatory testing for toxin production should be obtained to confirm PCR results. Testing for *C. difficile* toxin in children younger than 2 years is discouraged because the organism and its toxins are commonly detected in asymptomatic infants.

Evaluation for intestinal protozoa that cause diarrhea is usually indicated in patients who recently traveled to an endemic area, have contact with untreated water, or manifest suggestive symptoms. The advent of PCR testing allows for more sensitive and rapid detection of *Giardia, Enatmoeba, Cyclospora*, and *Cryptosporidium* compared to direct microscopy of stool for cysts and trophozoites, modified acid fast staining, or antigen testing. Additional testing for organisms such as *D. fragilis and B. hominis* is available in expanded panels, although the pathogenicity of these organisms remains unclear. In addition, enzyme immunoassays are available for *Cryptosporidium, Giardia*, and *Entamoeba* that are more sensitive and specific than direct microscopy and provide a useful diagnostic tool.

Most episodes of diarrheal dehydration are isonatremic and do not warrant serum electrolyte measurements. These should be reserved for children with severe dehydration, or children with lesser dehydration whose clinical picture raises a concern, for example when the skin pinch feels doughy without delayed recoil, which suggests hypernatremia, or when inappropriate rehydration fluids have been administered at home. A complete blood count and blood culture should be obtained if there is concern for systemic bacterial infection. This includes infants <3 months of age and high-risk children (e.g., immunocompromised, underlying hemolytic anemia) with fever and/or blood in the stool. A suspicion for HUS prompts a complete blood count with review of the peripheral smear, serum electrolytes, and renal function tests. If diarrhea persists with no cause identified, endoscopic evaluation may be indicated. Biopsy specimens help in diagnosing inflammatory bowel disease or identifying infecting agents that may mimic it. A sweat test is warranted if cystic fibrosis is suspected.

MANAGEMENT

Six principles guide the management of AGE: (i) rapid rehydration (over 4 hours) with an oral rehydration solution (ORS); (ii) continued breastfeeding; (iii) additional ORS for ongoing diarrheal losses; (iv) refeeding with an age-appropriate, unrestricted diet as soon as dehydration is corrected—complex carbohydrates, fresh fruits, lean meats, yogurt, and vegetables are recommended; (v) if normal diet includes infant formula, it should not be diluted or changed to a lactose-free preparation unless lactose malabsorption is evident; and (vi) no unnecessary laboratory tests or medications.

Hydration ORS is the method of choice for some dehydration regardless of age, causative agent, presence of vomiting, or initial serum sodium value (Table 99-4). Children with some dehydration can be managed successfully with ORS in over 80% of cases at a lower cost and complication rate compared to intravenous rehydration; despite this fact, ORS is underused in the United States. The principle guiding ORS is that the sodium-coupled co-transport with organic solutes such as glucose remains intact during AGE. To be effective, equimolar concentrations of glucose and sodium are required. Some prepared ORS fluids available in the United States are CeraLyte, Enfalyte, Pedialyte, and Redhydralyte. WHO-ORS packets that require reconstitution with water are an inexpensive alternative. Traditionally, guidelines have suggested avoiding fluids with high glucose concentrations (e.g., fruit juices and soda beverages) or high sodium (e.g., chicken broth) as they were thought to exacerbate diarrheal losses. However, recent studies have demonstrated that giving diluted apple juice followed by the child's preferred fluid for minimal dehydration in high resource countries has better outcomes than the use of ORS. Intravenous fluids are appropriate for children who are severely dehydrated, are moderately dehydrated with persistent vomiting, failed oral rehydration, have altered mental status with concern for aspiration, ileus, a malabsorption syndrome, or have an underlying condition that can be exacerbated by dehydration. Continued breastfeeding and resumption of normal diet as soon as rehydration is complete have been shown to decrease the duration of diarrhea when compared with oral or intravenous hydration alone. Most children can be managed in the emergency department or outpatient setting. Hospitalization is recommended when there is severe dehydration, when there are concerns about the ability of families to provide adequate care at home or return promptly to a medical setting if symptoms worsen, when ORS administered orally or enterally is not retained, when the child does not improve or has large ongoing fluid losses, when the child has comorbidities such as prematurity or undernutrition that could interfere with recovery, and so forth.

Pharmacologic Therapy for Symptom Relief Numerous medications are available aimed to alleviate the symptoms of gastroenteritis using a variety of mechanisms.

Agents in the following categories are not recommended for use in children

1. **Antimotility agents**: opiates, e.g., loperamide (Imodium) and difenoxylate and atropine (Lomotil). These agents do not prevent dehydration or improve nutritional status and have dangerous, sometimes fatal, side effects.
2. **Antisecretory agents**: e.g., bismuth subsalicylate (Pepto-Bismol).
3. **Agents designed to adsorb toxins and water**: e.g., kaolin and pectin (Kaodene NN).

Agents in the following categories have benefits in selected situations

1. **Anti-emetics**: Over the years multiple studies have been done to assess various antiemetics efficacy in allowing for oral rehydration in the setting of gastroenteritis presenting to an emergency department. Thus far, the strongest support is for ondansetron, (Zofran), an oral and parenteral serotonin (5-HT_3) receptor antagonist, is used in children to prevent and treat nausea and vomiting during chemotherapy, radiation therapy, and surgery. A meta-analysis found ondansetron to be superior to other antiemetics and placebo with regards to cessation of vomiting, need for IV hydration, and hospitalization with mixed data on if it prevents revisits. Although generally safe, with rates of side effects and diarrhea similar to placebo in the metanalysis there is some risk of inducing dose-dependent QT-prolongation and torsades de pointes, although this appears to be a minimal risk at least in single doses. However, the efficacy of ondansetron outside of the emergency department remains unclear, with limited studies.
2. **Micronutrients**: Zinc supplementation results in clinically significant reductions in the duration and severity of AGE when given to children in low-income countries as an adjunct to ORS. Although there are no apparent safety issues, similar efficacy has not been shown among children in developed countries. Therefore zinc is not recommended, except perhaps if malnutrition is present.

Probiotics While initial studies on the effectiveness of probiotics, specifically *Lactobacillus Rhamnosus, Lactobacillus reuteri, and Saccharomyces boulardii* were promising, with recommendations for their use being added to some guidelines, multiple recent randomized control trials call the effectiveness of lactobacillus into question. Meanwhile, a recent meta-analysis on *Saccharomyces* found a 1.1 day reduction in hospitalization when used, and reduced duration of diarrhea; however, the evidence is low quality.

Antibiotics Judicious use of antibiotics for suspected or proven bacterial AGE is recommended for specific indications (**Table 99-6**). Several factors justify limited use. For one, most episodes of AGE are self-limited among otherwise healthy children. Second, the increasing prevalence of antibiotic resistance has prompted restrictions in promiscuous use of these drugs. Third, antibiotics may actually worsen outcome, as some studies have shown that antibiotic therapy of STEC infection increases the risk of Hemolytic Uremic Syndrome (HUS). Therefore antibiotics are used primarily to treat severe infections to decrease the duration and severity of symptoms, to treat or prevent complications in high-risk hosts, or to limit the spread of infection. Microbiologic confirmation of the etiology should be sought prior to treatment if possible.

Special Considerations

C. difficile The most important intervention for *C. difficile* infection is removal of the offending antibiotic, if possible. Antibiotic therapy

TABLE 99-6 Therapy for Bacterial Pathogens That Cause Acute Gastroenteritis

Pathogen Recovered From Stool Culture	Indication for Therapy	Empiric Antibiotic Choices	Route	Duration
Clostridioides difficile	Mild-moderate colitis	Metronidazole	Oral	10 days
	Severe colitis	Vancomycin, or	Oral	10 days
		Vancomycin plus	Enema	10 days
		Metronidazole	IV	
Campylobacter	Dysentery, gastroenteritis (effective if treated within 3 days of onset in the illness), to reduce transmission (e.g., daycare attendee)	Erythromycin or Azithromycin	Oral	3-5 days
Enterotoxigenic *Escherichia coli* (ETEC)	Watery diarrhea in a traveler returning from an endemic area	Azithromycin, Fluoroquinolone,† or TMP-SMX*	Oral	5 days
E. coli, Shiga-toxin producing (STEC)	Gastroenteritis, hemorrhagic colitis, hemolytic-uremic syndrome	Avoid administration of antimicrobials	–	–
Salmonella, nontyphoidal (NTS)	Gastroenteritis in normal host	None (ineffective, may prolong excretion)		
	Gastroenteritis in special host without bacteremia (Infants <3 months, chronic gastrointestinal disease, immunocompromise, hemolytic anemia, malignancy, HIV)	Azithromycin, Fluoroquinolone,† Amoxicillin,* or TMP-SMX*	Oral	5-7 days
	Bacteremia (proven or until blood culture results are available in a high-risk host)	Ceftriaxone or Ampicillin*	IV then oral	10-14 days
Salmonella enterica Typhi or Paratyphi	History of international travel presenting with bacteremia, constitutional symptoms, or gastroenteritis. Oral antibiotic therapy is indicated for asymptomatic contacts of a positive case.	Ceftriaxone Azithromycin Additional antibiotic options depend on organism susceptibilities	IV then oral	7-10 days
Shigella	Severe disease, dysentery, underlying immunosuppression, to reduce transmission (e.g., daycare attendee)	Azithromycin,	IV or oral	3 days
		Ceftriaxone, or	IV	3-5 days
		Fluoroquinolone†	IV or oral	3-5 days
Yersinia	Gastroenteritis	Self-limited and clinical benefits of treatment not established	–	–
Vibrio cholerae	Gastroenteritis, moderate to severe	Azithromycin, Erythromycin, Doxycycline (for children ≥8 years), or Fluoroquinolones (for resistant strains)	Oral	3 days
Other: *Staphylococcus aureus*, *C. perfringens*, or *Bacillus cereus*	Gastroenteritis (food poisoning)	Antibiotics are not indicated	–	–

TMP-SMX denotes trimethoprim-sulfamethoxazole.

*Indicates high rates of resistance reported. Consider other options if possible until the susceptibility pattern is known.

† Not approved <18 years of age.

directed against *C. difficile* should be instituted if the symptoms are severe or persistent (**Table 99-7**). Oral vancomycin and metronidazole for 7 to 14 days (first line agents) displayed equivalent efficacy in a prospective randomized trial; however, metronidazole is preferred because of lower cost and decreased potential for inducing vancomycin-resistant enterococci. Recurrences of *C. difficile* infection in children is slightly less than rates in adults, at an estimated 20%. There are no pediatric studies on optimal treatment for recurrences, but in adults, tapering and/or pulsed regimen of oral vancomycin over a 4- to 6-week period has shown some benefit. In the absence of ongoing symptoms, a test of cure is not necessary. Early limited data suggest probiotics may have a role in preventing antibiotic associated C. *difficle*, with *S. boulardii* having the most data.

Traveler's Diarrhea Empirical antibiotics are generally recommended to treat traveler's diarrhea when the traveler is still abroad. According to the Foodborne Diseases Active Surveillance Network (foodNet), the pathogens identified most commonly in travelers in the United States were *Campylobacter* (42%), nontyphoidal *Salmonella* (32%), and *Shigella* (13%). Children younger than 2 years are at higher risk for traveler's diarrhea as well as more severe disease. Azithromycin is a reasonable choice for empiric treatment of children. In older children and adults, a fluoroquinolone is recommended. If the patient has returned home with diarrhea, a microbiologic evaluation can be obtained before initiating antibiotic therapy. Prolonged diarrhea should prompt further investigation into possible parasitic infections. Prophylactic antibiotics for travelers are not recommended.

Antimicrobial therapy for parasitic infections is listed in Table 99-7.

Complications The major complications of diarrhea from any cause are dehydration and electrolyte abnormalities (**Table 99-8**). Viral AGE illnesses are usually self-limited and resolve after several days. Supportive care with either oral, enteral, or intravenous hydration prevents most common complications related to dehydration, electrolyte abnormalities, or acid-base derangements. Rarely, intussusception may be triggered by lymphoid hyperplasia associated with viral AGE. Ensuring continued nutritional support is also important, as prolonged limitation of the diet may extend diarrheal symptoms. Reestablishing a normal diet generally restores villous anatomy and function with resolution of loose stools.

Bacterial AGE has been associated with a variety of intestinal and extraintestinal complications due to either end-organ damage that results directly from the infectious process and its extension to other sites, unusual manifestations of infection, or post-infectious immune-mediated events. *C. difficile* toxin can induce some of these same

TABLE 99-7 First-Line Oral Therapies for Intestinal Protozoa That Cause Acute Gastroenteritis

Giardia lamblia (when symptoms are severe or persistent)	Tinidazole single dose (for children ≥3 years old) Nitazoxanide for 3 days (for children ≥1 year old) Metronidazole for 5-10 days
	Alternatives: Paromomycin for 5-10 days, Furazolidone for 7-10 days, OR Quinacrine for 5 days
*Cryptosporidium**	Nitazoxanide for 3 days if ≥1 year old (dosed by age)
Cyclospora	TMP-SMX for 7-10 days†
	Alternative; Ciprofloxaxin for 7 days§
Entamoeba histolytica Asymptomatic cyst excreters Mild to moderate intestinal disease, and Severe intestinal or extraintestinal disease (including liver abscess)	Iodoquinol for 20 days, Paromomycin for 7 days, or Diloxanide furoate for 10 days Metronidazole for 7-10 days, or Tinidazole (for children ≥3 years old) for 3 days if mild to moderate intestinal disease, or 5 days for severe intestinal or extraintestinal disease **Either followed by (to prevent relapse):** Iodoquinol for 20 days, or Paromomycin for 7 days

*Although no anti-parasite therapy is effective for patients with advanced AIDS, improvement in CD4+ T-lymphocyte counts using antiretroviral therapy can lead to symptom resolution and cessation of oocyte shedding. High-dose nitazoxanide or combination of paramomycin and azithromycin may be tried; expert consultation is advised.

§ Not approved <18 years of age.

†Maintenance therapy may be needed for immunocompromised individuals.

Source: Data from Drugs for parasitic infections. *Treat Guidel Med Lett*. 2013;11:e1. New Rochelle, NY: The Medical Letter, Inc.

TABLE 99-8 Unique Intestinal and Extra-Intestinal Manifestations of Enteric Infections

Intestinal complications	Major causes
Toxic megacolon	*Shigella, C. difficile, E. histolytica*
Intestinal perforation	*Shigella, Yersinia, C. difficile, E. histolytica*
Rectal prolapse	*Shigella*, STEC, *C. difficile*
Persistent diarrhea	All causes
Recurrent diarrhea (usually immunocompromised persons)	*Salmonella, Shigella, Yersinia, Campylobacter, C. difficile*
Enteritis necroticans—jejunal hemorrhagic necrosis	*Clostridium perfringens* type C beta toxin
Extra-intestinal complications	
Dehydration and metabolic disturbances, malnutrition, micronutrient deficiency	All causes
Bacteremia with distant infectious foci	*Salmonella, Shigella, Yersinia, Campylobacter, C. difficile*
Pseudoappendicitis (older children and adolescents)	*Yersinia* (rarely *Campylobacter*)
Exudative pharyngitis, cervical lymphadenopathy	*Yersinia*
Rhabdomyolysis and hepatic necrosis	*Bacillus cereus* emetic toxin
Postinfectious complications	
Glomerulonephritis, myocarditis, pericarditis	*Campylobacter*
Guillain-Barré (polyneuritis with ascending paralysis and autonomic dysfunction) or Miller Fisher syndrome (ophthalmoplegia, areflexia, ataxia)	*Campylobacter*
Hemolytic uremic syndrome	STEC, *Shigella dysenteriae* type 1
Seizure or encephalopathy	*Shigella* spp.
Erythema nodosum or other rash	*Yersinia, Campylobacter, Salmonella*

STEC, Shiga toxin-producing *E. coli*.

complications (toxic megacolon, intestinal perforation, rectal prolapse, systemic disease). However, the most dreaded complication of pediatric diarrhea in the United States is HUS, the leading cause of acquired renal failure in children. HUS develops in 5% to 15% of patients infected with STEC, with *E. coli* O157:H7 being the predominant cause. Approximately half of the children with HUS need kidney replacement therapy, and 20% to 25% develop chronic kidney disease. It is usually diagnosed 2 to 14 days after the onset of diarrhea. HUS is unlikely to occur once diarrhea has remained resolved for 2 or 3 days with no evidence of hemolysis. Risk factors include under 3 years of age, bloody diarrhea, the presence of Shiga toxin 2a, elevated leukocyte count, and treatment with anti-motility agents. Two-thirds of patients no longer excrete the organism at the time they develop HUS.

So-called "pseudo-appendicitis" secondary to mesenteric adenitis is a notable complication of *Yersinia*, and sometimes *Campylobacter*. Usually seen in older children and adolescents, it typically presents with fever and abdominal pain, with tenderness localized to the right lower quadrant, with or without diarrhea, which can be confused with appendicitis. CT scan may be helpful to distinguish true appendicitis from *Yersinia* infection.

Immune-mediated complications that are thought to result from immunologic cross-reactivity between bacterial antigens and host tissues are more often seen in adults than children. These include reactive arthritis following infection with the classical bacterial enteropathogens and Guillain-Barré syndrome following *Campylobacter* infection.

Protozoan illnesses, when persistent, can lead to poor weight gain in the young and immunocompromised individuals, malnutrition, or vitamin deficiencies. Infection with *Entamoeba* can cause severe ulcerating colitis, colonic dilation, and perforation. The parasite may spread systemically, most commonly causing liver abscesses. It is critical to exclude *Entamoeba* infection and tuberculosis before initiating corticosteroids for presumed ulcerative colitis.

ADMISSION CRITERIA

- Severe dehydration or moderate dehydration with continuing losses via diarrhea or vomiting.
- Suspected bacteremia, sepsis, or metastatic bacterial infection.
- Suspected HUS.
- Suspected intra-abdominal complication (e.g., intussusception, perforation, toxic megacolon).

DISCHARGE CRITERIA

- Able to maintain adequate oral/enteral hydration.
- If a bacterial infection is identified and the patient requires therapy, the patient can be discharged if treatment is complete, if an appropriate oral antibiotic is available, or if intravenous therapy can be administered at home.

CONSULTATION

- Gastroenterology to evaluate persistent diarrhea, significant GI bleeding, or suspected inflammatory bowel disease.
- Nephrology for HUS.
- Surgery for evaluation of acute abdomen or suspected intestinal perforation.
- Intensive care for severe dehydration, refractory hypotension or tachycardia, or complications such as suspected sepsis and GI bleeding.

PREVENTION

Insufficient access to adequate hygiene, sanitation, and clean drinking water are the major risk factors for the heavy burden of diarrheal diseases in low-income countries. At the same time, there are many examples of how food production and water treatment in industrialized countries poses risks for transmission of enteric agents. For instance, the ability to mass produce and widely distribute products enables large, multistate outbreaks of foodborne agents. The increasing prevalence of antibiotic-resistant enteric bacterial infections has been linked to use of antibiotics as growth promoters in feed given to animals bred for food. Globalization has cultivated a market for tropical fruits and vegetables, creating a mechanism for importation of novel foodborne pathogens, while those who travel to less-developed regions can acquire these infections abroad. Semi-closed settings where catered food is served to large groups, such as hotels, resorts, and cruise ships, are conducive to large outbreaks, as are institutions where hygiene is compromised, such as daycare centers, prisons, and nursing homes.

With this in mind, transmission of enteric infections via the fecal-oral route can be interrupted by vigilant hand hygiene, especially in centers that provide care for children in diapers. Attention to food preparation and adequate cooking of meat can prevent many foodborne infections, coupled with public health initiatives such as microbiological surveillance can further decrease the risk of food-borne illnesses. Maintenance of a clean water supply is a most important intervention to prevent bacterial and parasitic infections worldwide.

A rotavirus vaccine was licensed in 2006. It is an oral vaccine composed of five reassorted viruses from human and bovine rotavirus strains. The vaccine is administered during infancy at 2, 4, and 6 months in the United States. For travelers, two forms of typhoid fever vaccine are available: a polysaccharide vaccine delivered intramuscularly that can be administered to children older than 2 years and an oral, live attenuated vaccine that can be administered to children over 6 years of age. An effective cholera vaccine is not yet available in the United States.

PERITONITIS

Peritonitis refers to inflammation of any aspect of the peritoneum. Infectious peritonitis can be considered as a primary or secondary disease. Bacterial infection of the peritoneum that arises from the bloodstream or lymphatics is termed primary, or spontaneous, peritonitis. It is much more frequently found in patients with ascites secondary to nephrotic syndrome or cirrhosis. Secondary peritonitis develops from contamination of the peritoneal cavity by contents of the GI tract or by indwelling devices such as peritoneal dialysis catheters or ventriculoperitoneal shunts.

CLINICAL PRESENTATION

Children with peritonitis are ill appearing and febrile. They complain of abdominal pain and distention and often have vomiting as a result of ileus. The abdomen is usually distended, and with severe disease, the overlying skin may appear shiny and erythematous. On auscultation, bowel sounds are absent or decreased. The abdomen may be rigid, rebound tenderness or tenderness with percussion may be elicited.

DIAGNOSIS AND EVALUATION

An obstruction series may reveal an air-fluid level indicative of bowel obstruction, free air found with perforation, or a ground-glass appearance suggesting the presence of intraperitoneal fluid. Ultrasound may demonstrate intraperitoneal fluid as well as bowel wall inflammation, masses, and organomegaly. The most sensitive study is computed tomography with contrast enhancement to delineate the extent of the disease and identify causes of secondary peritonitis such as a ruptured viscus or abscess.

Because ascites may be present in many conditions and may be a baseline finding in some patients being evaluated for peritonitis, direct examination of the fluid is essential. More than 50 white blood cells/mm^3 is abnormal; however, the white blood cell count in peritoneal fluid in patients with peritonitis generally reaches 5000 to 10,000 cells/mm^3. Cultures for bacteria, fungi, and mycobacteria should be obtained, and specific stains for these organisms should be performed on fresh specimens. Multiple organisms or the presence of anaerobes should raise concern for secondary peritonitis. If tuberculous peritonitis is suspected, Interferon Gamma Release Assay (IGRA), direct visualization of the abdomen, and peritoneal biopsy aid in the diagnosis.

Children with a catheter in place for peritoneal dialysis are at high risk for the development of peritonitis, with the potential loss of peritoneal membrane transport capacity. Peritonitis is generally suspected when fever with abdominal pain and tenderness develops. The effluent appears cloudy and demonstrates an elevated leukocyte count (>100 cells/mm^3) with greater than 50% polymorphonuclear leukocytes. When infection is suspected, peritoneal fluid should be obtained for analysis and culture as described earlier.

Blood cultures are frequently positive in children with primary peritonitis but generally negative in children with secondary peritonitis.

DIFFERENTIAL DIAGNOSIS

When children initially have a peritoneal catheter placed for dialysis, an eosinophilic peritonitis often develops but is usually self-limited. A mild to moderate elevation in the peritoneal leukocyte concentration has been attributed to chemical peritonitis in these patients as well.

Intra-abdominal infections such as hepatitis, cholecystitis, or early appendicitis may cause fever and inflammation of the visceral peritoneum without frank infection of the peritoneal space. Symptoms tend to be more localized, but rebound tenderness may be present. Girls or young women with pelvic infections or ovarian torsion may present similarly.

Bowel obstruction or severe ileus may also produce abdominal distention and tenderness. Fever is usually absent, and significant ascites is not common (unless the ileus is occurring secondary to infected intraperitoneal fluid).

Children with a ventriculoperitoneal shunt generally have a low level of peritoneal inflammation at baseline with increased amounts of fluid in the abdomen. However, when the fluid becomes infected, clinical signs of peritonitis or central nervous system infection generally develop.

TREATMENT

In children with a previously normal peritoneum and those with ascites but without indwelling catheters, *Streptococcus pneumoniae* is the most common cause of primary bacterial peritonitis. Empiric therapy with parenteral third-generation cephalosporins should be administered to treat possible penicillin-resistant *S. pneumoniae* until culture and susceptibility results are known. Children with ascites are also at risk for peritonitis with gram-negative organisms, even in the absence of intestinal pathology. If the patient does not clinically improve after 1 to 2 days, repeat paracentesis should be performed. In children without any complicating factors, systemic antibiotics alone are sufficient to treat primary peritonitis, without drainage of the infected fluid. Treatment for 14 days is usually adequate. In patients with nephrotic syndrome or cirrhosis, data are insufficient to determine whether drainage of the infected fluid improves outcomes. Management of any underlying disease is often needed to achieve a clinical cure.

In children who have peritoneal dialysis catheters in place, gram-positive cocci (coagulase-negative *Staphylococcus* and *S. aureus*) from the skin are the most common organisms that cause peritonitis. Gram-negative rods, including *Pseudomonas*, can also cause peritonitis in this population. Antimicrobial therapy directed toward these bacteria should be started promptly because of the risk for loss of functional membrane. Intraperitoneal antibiotic administration of antimicrobial agents is preferred route of administration if the catheter remains in place as peritonitis associated with a peritoneal catheter is considered a localized infection, and adequate levels of antimicrobial agents to treat peritonitis can be achieved by intraperitoneal administration. Moreover, for most currently used antibiotics, the doses recommended by intraperitoneal administration to achieve adequate blood levels have been established in pharmacokinetic studies. Continuous dosing is preferred to intermittent dosing to ensure constant therapeutic concentrations of antibiotic locally. Most dosing regimens include an initial extended-dwell cycle with a higher antibiotic concentration followed by maintenance dosing. Detailed guidelines for both continuous and intermittent antibiotic administration and monitoring of drug levels are available from the International Society for Peritoneal Dialysis. Empiric antibiotic therapy should be guided by local susceptibility patterns and the individual patient's history of resistant infections. However, cefepime monotherapy is typically recommended as the drug of choice for empiric treatment as it provides coverage for methicillin susceptible *S. aureus* and gram-negative organisms including *Pseudomonas*. If cefepime is not available, intraperitoneal cefazolin plus either ceftazidime or an aminoglycoside is recommended. Aminoglycosides can also be administered into the peritoneum but are often avoided to preserve any remaining kidney function. In centers where >10% of *S. aureus* are resistant to oxacillin, or when the patient has a history of methicillin-resistant *S. aureus* (MRSA), addition of vancomycin to cefepime, or replacement of cefazolin with vancomycin is recommended. In addition, these guidelines suggest that vancomycin replace the first-generation cephalosporin if the patient is younger than 2 years or has severe symptoms. Antibiotics should be modified when the offending organism has been identified based on the results of susceptibility testing.

The duration of intraperitoneal treatment of peritonitis in children with peritoneal catheters in place is usually 2 weeks for coagulase-negative staphylococci and 3 weeks for *S. aureus*, *Enterococcus*, and gram-negative infection. Catheter removal should be considered if the patient fails to clinically improve or the infection fails to clear after 5 days on appropriate antibiotic therapy. Fungi have been associated with peritonitis in this population, although it has not been well studied. Amphotericin B (intravenously) or fluconazole (orally or intravenously) is recommended for the treatment of *Candida* peritonitis. If a peritoneal catheter is present, removal of the catheter as soon as possible to help clear the fungus is essential. If no organism is identified but evaluation of peritoneal fluid supports the diagnosis of peritonitis, the initial empirical therapy should be continued.

Patients who fail to improve may require a change in antibiotic therapy or catheter removal. Experts generally recommend that once removed, the catheter can be replaced after 2 to 3 weeks, although there have been some reports of success with simultaneous removal of the infected catheter and replacement with a new catheter.

CONSULTATION

- Nephrology for patients maintained on peritoneal dialysis to ascertain that the membrane is functioning properly and for management of intraperitoneal antibiotic therapy.
- Surgery for patients with possible secondary peritonitis or if removal of the peritoneal catheter may be necessary.
- Infectious diseases to assist with antibiotic selection and duration especially in resistant infections or immunocompromised patients.

ADMISSION CRITERIA

- Children with suspected bacterial or fungal peritonitis require inpatient evaluation.

DISCHARGE CRITERIA

- Defervescence and overall clinical improvement
- Ability to complete the antibiotic regimen after discharge
- Stability or improvement of any underlying medical condition
- Appropriate follow-up with primary care or subspecialists, or both

HEPATITIS

Hepatitis is a final common pathway of hepatocyte injury by both infectious and noninfectious causes. Infectious causes of hepatitis include hepatotropic and systemic viral infections as well as bacterial, parasitic, and fungal pathogens. This section focuses on the infectious etiologies. The infecting agents that cause primary hepatitis include hepatitis A virus (HAV), hepatitis B virus (HBV), hepatitis C virus (HCV), hepatitis D virus (HDV), and hepatitis E virus (HEV), which was previously referred to as non-A, non-B hepatitis.

EPIDEMIOLOGY AND TRANSMISSION

Hepatitis A The incidence of HAV infection has diminished in the United States from about 12 cases per 100,000 in 1995 to 0.4 cases per 100,000 in 2015. Children under 10 years of age had the highest rates in 2000 and the lowest rates in 2011. This decline has been attributed to the introduction of vaccination for high-risk persons in 1996 and subsequently for all infants in 2006. Nonetheless, HAV remains a common infection worldwide. This 27-nm single-stranded nonenveloped RNA virus of the *Picornaviridae* family is acquired through fecal-oral spread during close personal contact. In daycare settings, particularly those with children in diapers, spread usually takes place to adult caretakers and family members in the community before the index case (usually an asymptomatic child) has been recognized. Outbreaks due to contaminated food or water are also described. Adult international travelers, international adoptees, men who have sex with men, and illicit drug users (both injecting and non-injecting) are also at increased risk. When a case is found, an epidemiologic investigation is necessary to identify individuals in need of post-exposure prophylaxis and vaccination.

Hepatitis B HBV is a highly infectious 42-nm enveloped virus with a partly double-stranded, relaxed circular DNA genome belonging to the *Hepadnaviridae* family. A single HBV particle is sufficient to establish infection. Since introduction of effective HBV vaccine strategies in 1990, the incidence among children <19 years has decreased from 13.8 to 1.1 cases per 100,000 population in 2015. It is estimated that 700,000 to 1.4 million people living in the United States are chronically HBV infected, about half of whom are persons born in Asia and Asian-Americans who were born to HBV-infected mothers in the United States.

HBV is transmitted through activities that involve percutaneous or mucosal contact with infected blood or body fluids, including sex, drug injection, birth, human bites, contact with blood or open sores, needle sticks, and sharing items such as razors and toothbrushes. HBV can survive at room temperature in the environment for up to 7 days; concentrations of 10^2 to 105 virions/mL can be present on surfaces without any visible blood and still cause transmission. Both percutaneous and non-percutaneous transmission of HBV is highly efficient, which should be kept in mind when evaluating likelihood of infection. Injection drug use is the most common risk factor reported (18.3%). The risk of secondary spread to susceptible household contacts of persons with chronic infection is 14% to 60%. Without post-exposure prophylaxis, the risk of perinatal transmission is 70% to 90% by 6 months of age if the mother is positive for both hepatitis B surface antigen (HBsAg) and hepatitis B e antigen (HBeAg), but <10% if the mother is only HBsAg-positive. Travelers to countries with high HBV prevalence are also at risk. HBV is not spread through food or water or breastfeeding.

Hepatitis C Routine HBV vaccination of infants in the United States has left HCV as the most common cause of chronic viral hepatitis in children and adults. HCV is a positive sense, single-stranded RNA virus in the *Flaviviridae* family. The number of reported cases of acute HCV infection in the United States was 0.8 cases per 100,000 in 2015. For all age groups the incidence of Hepatitis C infection declined rapidly and reached its lowest incidence from 2006 to 2010. This increase has been attributed to accelerated transmission among adolescents and young adults living in non-urban areas of eastern and midwestern states who have a history of injecting and other illicit drug use. Nonetheless, the incidence among children <19 years is low and has remained constant at about 0.1 cases per 100,000 population. An estimated 3.5 million US residents suffer from chronic HCV infection, with the highest prevalence among adults born from 1945 to 1965.

HCV is transmitted primarily through contact with infected blood. In contrast to HBV, non-percutaneous transmission of HCV is uncommon. Household transmission without a direct blood exposure is very unlikely, and sexual contact and perinatal transmission rates are low.

The overall adjusted rate of perinatal transmission is estimated at 1.7%, but can be as high as 20% in the presence of HIV coinfection. Despite the low rates, perinatal transmission is the most common source of infection in children, accounting for about 750 new cases annually in the United States. Adolescents may be exposed through high-risk behaviors such as current or prior injecting drug use and shared tattoo equipment. Other risk groups include recipients of blood and blood products and solid-organ transplantation prior to systematic screening in the early 1990s, and chronic hemodialysis patients, persons with HIV/AIDS, and victims of needle sticks. Currently the risk related to blood transfusion is considered to be less than 1 per 2 million units transferred.

Hepatitis D HDV, also known as delta agent, is a defective RNA virus. It is the only virus in the genus Deltaviridae, and is capable of encoding only one antigen. It transmitted through blood products, sexual contact, and tattooing or drug use with contaminated needles. Although HDV can replicate autonomously, the simultaneous presence of HBV is required for complete virion assembly and secretion. Therefore, it can cause infection only in patients with active HBV co-infection. Worldwide, the prevalence of HDV does not mirror that of HBV. Endemic areas for HDV include the Mediterranean basin and the Far East. HDV is uncommon in the United States, except in injecting drug users and hemophiliacs.

Hepatitis E HEV infection is a 27- to 34-nm nonenveloped, single-stranded RNA virus of the family *Hepeviridae.* Like HAV, it is acquired by the fecal-oral route, and epidemics have occurred from contaminated water sources. In endemic areas, transmission by blood transfusion has also been reported. Zoonotic transmission may occur via consumption of insufficiently cooked game meat and pork products, and exposure to rats. Clinical infection is rare in the United States and most developed countries even though many people are seropositive. Endemic areas include South Asia, North Africa, the Middle East, and Central America. In North Africa and the Middle East, it is the most common cause of sporadic hepatitis.

CLINICAL PRESENTATION AND COURSE OF ILLNESS

The clinical presentation of hepatitis is often nonspecific, and because the symptoms can be insidious, identifying the onset of the disease can be challenging. In addition to jaundice, scleral icterus, right upper quadrant tenderness, and hepatomegaly, constitutional symptoms of poor oral intake, lethargy, vomiting, fever, arthralgia, rash, or pruritus may be reported. There may be ascites, arthritis, or manifestations of more systemic illness in which liver involvement is not the primary process.

Hepatitis A The clinical manifestations of HAV infection are age dependent. Children younger than 2 years are generally asymptomatic. Before 6 years of age, children are usually anicteric and only 30% have symptoms, whereas infection is typically symptomatic in older children and adults, of whom 70% have jaundice. Symptomatic infections are typically biphasic, with acute onset after an incubation period of 15 to 50 days (average 28 days). The prodromal phase consists of fever and diarrhea and usually lasts 1 to 7 days. The icteric phase follows accompanied by nonspecific symptoms such as fever, malaise, poor appetite, nausea, vomiting, abdominal discomfort, diarrhea, clay-colored (acholic) stools, and dark urine, lasting 2 to 10 weeks. Fulminant hepatitis is rare, but patients with chronic liver disease and HCV co-infection are at risk for more severe infection. Occasionally illness is prolonged, with cholestasis lasting more than 12 weeks, or relapsing, but chronic HAV infection does not occur. The highest concentrations of virus in stool occur during the incubation period (before the onset of jaundice). Shedding in children is longer than in adults, sometimes lasting 10 weeks or longer. Liver enzymes rise during the icteric phase. Viremia begins soon after infection and persists through the period of transaminase elevation.

Hepatitis B The average incubation period is 90 days (range 60-150 days) from exposure to onset of jaundice and 60 days (range 40-90 days) from exposure to elevation of ALT levels. HBV infection produces a wide range of manifestations, including asymptomatic infection, a self-limited moderate illness with features typical of clinical hepatitis, a rare fulminant lethal hepatitis, and chronic disease. Usually, symptomatic illness begins with the insidious onset of constitutional symptoms such as malaise, anorexia, nausea, vomiting, and abdominal pain, which may be accompanied by extrahepatic complaints of arthralgia or rash. The icteric phase follows and may last for weeks, after which convalescence occurs over weeks to months. HBV has been associated with Gianotti-Crosti syndrome, also known as papular acrodermatitis, which is a symmetric papular eruption with an acral distribution (cheeks, buttocks, and extensor surfaces of forearms and legs) of several weeks duration, seen primarily among children younger than 5 years.

Although neonates who are infected during the perinatal period are at highest risk for development of chronic infection with HBV, their infection is generally clinically silent. Chronic infection occurs in approximately 90% of infants with perinatal infection, whereas the risk for young children who become infected is 25% to 50%, and that for older children is 6% to 10%. Immunosuppression, for example, secondary to hemodialysis and HIV/AIDS, increases the risk of chronicity. Chronically infected people serve as the major reservoir for continued transmission.

Chronic HBV infection may be associated with normal physical examination and liver function test results or only subtle signs of liver disease. Approximately 25% of those who become chronically infected during childhood die prematurely from cirrhosis or hepatocellular carcinoma (HCC). Patients with chronic infection, especially those with cirrhosis or a family history of HCC, should be monitored for the development of HCC.

Hepatitis C Acute infection is often mild and insidious, most infections are asymptomtic with jaundice occurring in less than 20% of patients. Spontaneous clearance of perinatal infection has been reported in about 20% of cases. The remainder develop chronic infection which usually remains asymptomatic with normal or nearly normal liver function tests; 10% have hepatomegaly. Clearance is less likely in children who remain PCR positive beyond infancy and those who are persistently PCR positive during the first year of life. Hepatitis C progresses slowly. Over decades, mild, stable hepatic inflammation, severe progression to cirrhosis or fibrosis without cirrhosis, and infrequently, HCC develops. Severe liver disease occurs in a small percentage of children during childhood. Prior HCV infection does not protect against later infection with the same or different genotypes of the virus.

Hepatitis D HDV can only cause infection in individuals with underlying acute or chronic HBV infection. After an incubation period of 3 to 7 weeks, nonspecific symptoms appear for 3 to 7 days, followed by an icteric phase. Simultaneous HDV and HBV infection (co-infection) usually results in acute, self-limited hepatitis, which rarely becomes chronic. In contrast, HDV superinfection of a chronic HBsAg carrier usually causes severe acute hepatitis and chronic HDV infection. Chronic HDV infection is associated with annual rates of development of cirrhosis and HCC of 4% and 2.8%, respectively.

Hepatitis E HEV produces a clinical illness similar to HAV after an incubation period of 15 to 60 days. The clinical picture of HEV infection is similar to that of HAV, and most children have a self-limited infection lasting 4 to 6 weeks with no long-term complications. However, HEV infection is associated with significant mortality in pregnant women. For unclear reasons, fulminant hepatic failure occurs more often during pregnancy, resulting in a mortality rate of 15% to 25%, primarily during the third trimester. More severe disease has also been reported in immunosuppression, including transplant recipients.

DIFFERENTIAL DIAGNOSIS

A wide range of infectious and noninfectious processes can lead to hepatic inflammation and damage. Infections that can cause hepatitis, usually as part of a generalized illness, include Epstein-Barr virus, cytomegalovirus, varicella-zoster virus, herpes simplex virus, yellow fever, measles, mumps, rubella, rubeola, enterovirus, adenovirus, HIV, syphilis, and toxoplasmosis. Noninfectious causes of hepatitis that should be considered include cystic fibrosis, metabolic disorders, Wilson disease, α_1-antitrypsin deficiency, and autoimmune hepatitis. Toxins, including medications such as acetaminophen, accidental ingestions, and selected complementary and alternative medicines, can cause hepatic injury.

In newborns, hepatic injury is frequently due to congenital anatomic abnormalities such as biliary atresia and choledochal cysts.

DIAGNOSIS AND EVALUATION

To explore the possible cause of liver injury, the physician should ask about the progression of symptoms; potential exposure to toxins, medications, infected contacts; associated medical problems or symptoms; and travel and family history. Patients should be specifically questioned about a history of blood transfusion, and in older children and adolescents, sexual activity and the use of intravenous drugs. The physical examination should focus on physical findings associated with liver disease as well as signs of extrahepatic disease.

The initial laboratory evaluation aims to identify the extent of liver injury (**Table 99-9**). Elevated serum alanine and aspartate transaminase levels indicate hepatocellular injury, the primary pathologic feature in hepatitis. In general, levels exceeding 10,000 IU/mL are found in patients with toxin- or ischemia-mediated hepatitis, whereas levels of 1000 to 3000 IU/mL are more typical of acute viral hepatitis. Lower degrees of elevation are seen in chronic viral infection and metabolic disorders. Bilirubin is often elevated as well, but the result should be further fractionated into direct and indirect components and measured in conjunction with alkaline phosphatase and γ-glutamyltransferase (GGT), to assess hepatic excretory function. Serum albumin, prothrombin time, and ammonia are measures of the liver's synthetic function. Once the diagnosis of hepatitis has been made, the cause should be identified if possible. In infants and young children with jaundice, imaging of the liver is important because anatomic abnormalities are a leading cause of hepatitis. Ultrasound of the liver is often the first imaging study obtained. It can demonstrate its size, uniformity of composition, and blood flow and can identify most anatomic abnormalities. Although sedation may be required in younger children, computed tomography or magnetic resonance imaging may more accurately detect small tumors or abscesses. In some cases, liver biopsy may be necessary to determine the cause of the hepatitis, assess the extent of liver injury, and determine the need for therapy.

Hepatitis A The initial evaluation for infectious causes should include studies for HAV, HBV, and HCV. The gold standard for diagnosis of HAV is serum IgM antibody to capsid proteins, which become detectable 5 to 10 days before the onset of symptoms and disappears within 6 months. IgG anti-HAV appears early and persists, providing lifelong protection against disease.

Hepatitis B To evaluate for acute or chronic hepatitis B, studies should be sent for HBsAg as well as antibodies against hepatitis B core antigen (anti-HBc) and surface antigen (anti-HBs), as detailed in **Table 99-10**. Detection of HBeAg in serum indicates that the virus is replicating and abundant; it portends a high risk for chronic infection. Patients who have detectable HBsAg are infectious, and those with HBeAg, without antibody formation, are at highest risk for transmission. When HBsAg clears and anti-HBs appears, the infection is considered resolved, although it may reactivate with immunosuppression. Vaccination also evokes

TABLE 99-9 Recommended Evaluation of Patients With Hepatitis

Laboratory Test	Utility of Test
Bilirubin-total and direct	• Indirect hyperbilirubinemia (direct <20%) ∘ Overproduction (e.g. hemolysis, extravasation of blood into tissues) ∘ Impaired uptake or conjugation (e.g., neonates, Wilson disease, Gilbert disease, Crigler Najjar syndrome, drugs such as rifampin, viral hepatitis) • Direct hyperbilirubinemi ∘ Intrahepatic cholestasis (decreased excretion in bile ductules or leakage from hepatocytes into serum (e.g., viral hepatitis, sepsis and hypoperfusion states, total parenteral nutrition; Dubin-Johnson syndrome and Rotor syndrome cause mild direct hyperbilirubinemia in the absence of other enzyme abnormalities) • Elevated in nearly equal proportions in viral hepatitis
Alanine transaminase (ALT, formerly SGPT) and aspartate transaminase (AST, formerly SGOT)	• Indicate hepatocellular damage • ALT is more specific to the liver than AST • >25-fold elevations suggest acute viral hepatitis • >50-fold elevations suggest ischemic hepatitis (in addition, the lactate dehydrogenase if often markedly elevated) • Chronic viral or metabolic disease elevation usually <10-fold • In hepatitis, level of elevation is disproportionately higher than that of alkaline phosphatase
Alkaline phosphatase	• Levels >4 times normal indicate cholestasis (intrahepatic, or extrahepatic) • Found in liver, bone predominantly (can be fractionated, but usually a liver source can be confirmed by simultaneous elevation of other measures of cholestasis) • Levels generally much higher in growing children than in adults • In cholestasis, level of elevation is disproportionately higher than that of serum aminotransferases
γ-Glutamyl transpeptidase (GGT)	• Found in hepatocytes and biliary epithelial cells and elevated in cholestasis, but lacks specificity with elevations in a variety of conditions • >300 IU/mL in cases of biliary atresia and α_1-antitrypsin deficiency
Albumin	• Reduced levels indicate longstanding liver dysfunction or malnutrition
Prothrombin	• Factors I, II, V, VII, and X are synthesized in the liver • If fails to correct with vitamin K, suggests severe hepatocellular dysfunction
Ammonia	• Elevated in hepatic encephalopathy

TABLE 99-10 Serologic Diagnosis of Hepatitis B Virus (HBV) Infection

HBsAg	Total anti-HBc	Anti-HBs	IgM anti-HBc*	Interpretation
–	–	–	–	Naïve/susceptible to infection
–	–	+	–	Vaccine-induced immunity (immune if >10 IU/mL), recent HBIG
+	–	–	–	Early acute infection or <3 weeks post-vaccination
+	+	–	+	Acute infection
–	+	–	+	Resolving acute infection
–	+	+	–	Recovered from acute infection and immune
+	+	–	–	Chronic infection
–	+	–	+/–	False positive (i.e., susceptible); low-level chronic infection; resolving acute infection; passive transfer of maternal antibody from HbSAg-positive mother (total anti-HBc only)

anti-HBc, antibody-to-core antigen; anti-HBs, antibody-to-surface antigen; HBc, hepatitis B core antigen; HBIG, hepatitis B immune globulin; HBsAg, hepatitis B surface antigen.

TABLE 99-11 Children Who Should Be Tested for Hepatitis C Virus (HCV) Infection

- Born to mothers who are HCV-positive or have a history of injecting drug use (to avoid detecting maternal antibody, screen serologically after 18 months of age or perform HCV RNA assay at 4 months of age)
- International adoptees or refugees
- Victims of sexual abuse or a history of multiple sex partners
- Injected illegal drugs, even once
- Recipient of chronic hemodialysis
- Received blood or organs from a donor who later tested HCV-positive
- Infected with HIV

Consultation:

- Gastroenterologist or hepatologist for unexplained, persistent LFT elevations ≥1.5- to 2-fold above the upper limit of normal

anti-HBs. Anti-HBc appears at the onset of symptoms and persists for life, so it is not helpful in distinguishing the stage of infection. However, IgM anti-HBc appears at the onset of HBV infection and persists for up to 6 months if disease resolves, making it a good marker for recent infection. In chronic infection, IgM anti-HBc can rise during viral replication, but it has low predictive value in asymptomatic patients and should not be performed unless there is hepatitis or an epidemiologic link to a case. The diagnosis of chronic HBV infection is made when HBsAg is present for more than 6 months.

Hepatitis C Because antiviral treatment is intended for persons with current HCV infection, these individuals need to be distinguished from those who cleared their infection. Children in whom screening for HCV should be performed are shown in **Table 99-11**. The initial step in screening is recommended is an assay to detect IgG anti-HCV antibody either the recently licensed rapid test (OraQuick HCV Rapid Antibody Test) or another FDA-approved antibody test. Antibodies may not develop for 6 weeks after exposure. Persons with positive HCV antibody, or those whose exposure was recent, or infants younger than 18 months of age, should undergo a nucleic acid test for HCV RNA in blood, which indicates current infection. A negative HCV RNA test suggests either past, resolved infection or a false positive antibody assay. Once it has been present for 3 months, the virus is unlikely to be cleared. The diagnosis of chronic disease is established by the presence of HCV RNA with elevated alanine transaminase, positive serology for 6 months, or positive HCV RNA with liver biopsy–proven chronic hepatitis.

Hepatitis D Because HDV infection occurs solely with acute or chronic hepatitis B, testing for antibody against HDV is considered only if HBsAg is present. Assays for anti-HDV IgM and IgG antibodies and RT-PCR are available in reference laboratories. All of these markers disappear within months of recovery but persist in chronic infection.

Hepatitis E HEV infection is exceedingly rare in developed countries but should be considered if there is a history of recent travel to the Indian subcontinent, Asia, Africa, or Mexico. IgM antibody testing in serum or assay for HEV RNA in serum or feces collected during the acute phase is performed only at reference laboratories.

TREATMENT

Most cases of infectious hepatitis are managed successfully on an outpatient basis with supportive care and serial office visits to monitor the course of the illness. Acute hepatitis with inadequate oral/enteral intake may require intravenous hydration. Cases of hepatic failure with impaired synthetic function require inpatient management. Coagulopathies with or without active bleeding may necessitate replacement of clotting factors or parenteral administration of vitamin K, or both.

Ascites may develop in patients with severe or chronic liver involvement. Dietary salt restriction and diuretics are often helpful. Spontaneous bacterial peritonitis is a known complication and is discussed in detail in the later section on peritonitis.

If mental status changes occur, consider the complication of hyperammonemia due to liver failure. Deterioration of renal function as evidenced by oliguria, azotemia, acidosis, or hyperkalemia indicates hepatorenal syndrome. These conditions are usually managed in intensive care units. Progressive, irreversible liver failure with or without renal involvement warrants prompt referral for possible liver transplantation.

Treatment of HAV and HEV infection is supportive. Case reports have suggested a benefit from ribavirin with or without interferon-alpha or immunosuppression for HEV, but more data are needed.

Hepatitis B Indications for treatment of HBV include evidence of ongoing viral replication as indicated by the presence for longer than 6 months of serum HBV DNA >20,000 IU/mL without HBeAb positivity, >2000 IU/mL with HBeAg positivity, and ALT concentrations two times higher than the upper limit of normal for longer than 6 months or evidence of chronic hepatitis on liver biopsy. Numerous nucleos(t)ide analogues and two interferon-alfa (IFNα) drugs are approved by the FDA for use in adults. Of these, FDA licensure for use in children is as follows: interferon alfa-2b, ≥1 year of age; peginterferon alpha-2a, ≥3 years of age; lamivudine, ≥3 years of age; adefovir, ≥12 years of age; tenofovir disoproxil fumarate, ≥12 years of age and entecavir, ≥16 years of age. The American Association for the Study of Liver Diseases Web site (www.aasld.org) contains information on treatment options. The optimal agent and duration of therapy for chronic HBV infection in children remain unclear, as there are few randomized controlled trials for guidance. Virologic responses have been observed in children treated with IFNα, and some practitioners consider it to be first-line therapy in children without an underlying autoimmune disorder, organ transplant, or serious psychiatric disease. Children with perinatal infection, those with a prolonged immune tolerant phase of infection, and those infected with HBV genotype C are associated with reduced response to IFNα. Lamivudine or adefovir can be used as second-line therapy; however, these drugs are most efficacious in advanced liver disease. Enrolling a child in an ongoing clinical trial involving agents shown to be more efficacious with lower rates of resistance in adults is sometimes a preferable option. Consultation with healthcare professionals experienced in treating chronic HBV in children is recommended.

Hepatitis C Recently significant advancements in the treatment of HCV infection with direct acting antivirals (DAA) have been made and information regarding treatment options is available on The American Association for the Study of Liver Diseases Web site (www.aasld.org). Research has demonstrated that treatment of HCV infection during early childhood is cost effective and has the potential to decrease the lifetime risk of complications. For treatment-naïve children and adolescents that are ≥3 years of age three separate treatment regimens are available depending on viral genotype. For children and adolescents that are DAA experienced additional regimens are recommended depending on viral genotype and patient's previous treatment history.

Hepatitis D Effective treatments have been sought for patients with chronic HDV infection and active liver disease demonstrated as elevated ALT levels or chronic hepatitis on liver biopsy because of the poor outcome. Treatment of HDV is the same as that for HBV, there are no approved therapies specifically for HDV. Some data suggests treatment including IFNα and lamivudine is beneficial. IFNα confers a modest benefit in suppressing viral activity and hepatocellular injury in some patients, but benefits are not sustained.

CONSULTATION

- Gastroenterology if liver biopsy may be needed and for further evaluation and treatment recommendations for patients with hepatitis C; hepatitis B with persistently elevated transaminases, increased α-fetoprotein concentration, or abnormal ultrasound findings; active GI bleeding; and hepatitis that does not resolve.
- Rheumatology for evaluation of autoimmune hepatitis.
- Hematology for management of coagulopathy.
- Infectious diseases for guidance regarding diagnosis, therapy, isolation, and prophylaxis.
- Intensive care for evidence of acute hepatic failure with or without renal insufficiency/failure and severe GI bleeding.

ADMISSION CRITERIA

- Inadequate oral/enteral intake
- Worsening liver function (coagulopathy, encephalopathy)
- Renal dysfunction
- Severe ascites or pleural effusion
- Need for further evaluation, including liver biopsy

DISCHARGE CRITERIA

- Stable liver function
- Control of coagulopathy, active bleeding, and encephalopathy
- Appropriate primary care and subspecialty follow-up

PREVENTION

Hepatitis A All susceptible people traveling internationally to countries with an intermediate or high HAV endemnicity should be immunized or receive immune globulin before departure. Immune globulin is given as pre-exposure prophylaxis for travelers younger than 6 months and should be repeated every 2 months for long-term travelers. Children 6 months of age or older should receive HAV vaccine as pre-exposure prophylaxis. Any doses of HAV vaccine given to children 6 to 11 months of age do not count towards the routine vaccine series and a two-dose series should be completed per the typical vaccination schedule. For travelers for whom vaccine is contraindicated or who choose not to receive vaccine, immune globulin should be used as pre-exposure prophylaxis.

HAV vaccine is safe and highly immunogenic. Three inactivated vaccines containing HAV antigen are currently licensed in the United States Vaqta (≥6 months), Havrix (≥6 months), and Twinrix (≥18 years). All children should receive vaccine at age 1 year (12–23 months) with a second dose 6 to 12 months later (Havrix) or 6 to 18 months later (Vaqta). Individuals traveling to endemic countries, children living in US communities with high rates of hepatitis A, and patients with chronic liver disease and clotting factor disorders, and illicit drug users (injecting and non-injecting) should also be vaccinated.

After identification of an index case of HAV infection, post-exposure prophylaxis is indicated in all unimmunized household members, sexual contacts, and child care contacts. Although perinatal transmission is rare and infants usually have few symptoms, administration of immune globulin to newborn infants of HAV-infected mothers should be considered if the mother's symptoms began between 2 weeks before and 1 week after delivery. Immune globulin should be administered within 2 weeks of exposure to those who are less than 1 year old, adults who are >40 years, immunocompromised persons, and those with chronic liver disease. HAV vaccine is preferred as post-exposure prophylaxis for most people between 1 and 40 years of age.

Hepatitis B HBV vaccine is recommended for all infants, for children and adolescents who were not vaccinated in infancy, and for individuals at risk for occupational exposure. The vaccine elicits a protective immune response in more than 95% of infants and 90% of adults. Patients who are seronegative despite vaccination should be revaccinated. Pooled hepatitis B immune globulin (HBIG) is available for exposure of non-immune individuals. Patients with chronic hepatitis B should be vaccinated against HAV if they are not immune.

Full-term and preterm infants born to mothers with HBV infection should receive the initial dose of HBV vaccine within 12 hours of birth. HBIG should be administered at the same time, but at a different site. If the mother's hepatitis B status is unknown, the infant should receive the vaccine within the first 12 hours. If the mother is found to be HBV-positive, HBIG should be administered as soon as possible, but within the first 7 days of life. For infants weighing <2000 grams at birth this first dose of HBV vaccine in noncountable and the routine series should be initiated at 1 month of age in medically stable preterm infants.

Children with chronic HBV infection should undergo periodic screening for disease progression and development of HCC. Screening should include serum transaminase levels, α-fetoprotein concentration, and abdominal ultrasound.

Hepatitis C Patients with HCV infection should be vaccinated against HAV and HBV. The rate of vertical transmission of HCV from mother to child is increased from 5% to 12% if the mother is positive for human immunodeficiency virus (HIV). There is no clear evidence that cesarean section prevents mother-to-child transmission of HCV. At this time the risk for transmission of HCV through breast milk is considered negligible. Anti-HCV antibodies can cross the placenta, so exposed infants should not undergo antibody testing until 18 months of age. FDA-licensed diagnostic NAATs for qualitative detection of HCV RNA are available. HCV RNA can be detected in serum or plasma within 1 to 2 weeks after exposure to the virus and weeks before onset of liver enzyme abnormalities or appearance of anti-HCV. Assays for detection of HCV RNA are used commonly in clinical practice to identify anti-HCV-positive patients who have HCV infection, for identifying infection in infants early in life (i.e., perinatal transmission), and for monitoring patients receiving antiviral therapy. However, false positive and false negative results can occur.

Hepatitis D Prevention of HBV infection with the licensed vaccine is the best means for preventing HDV infection.

Hepatitis E An effective vaccine has been developed but is not yet commercially available.

KEY POINTS

Acute Viral Gastroenteritis

- Clinical presentation: Viral gastroenteritis generally presents with vomiting and diarrhea without blood or mucus, whereas bacterial infections may present with bloody or mucoid stools.
- Diagnosis: Pursue a bacterial or parasitic diagnosis if blood or mucus is present in stool or if there is high fever, a history of travel, or prolonged illness.
- Treatment: Rehydration is the most important intervention with enteral repletion being first line. Antimicrobial therapy should be judiciously used depending on the organism.
- Antibiotic-associated diarrhea: Antibiotics should be discontinued if possible.
- Vaccines against important enteric bacterial and viral infections are gradually changing the epidemiology of gastroenteritis worldwide.

Peritonitis

- Clinical presentation: Fever, abdominal pain, and tenderness, especially in children with ascites, or indwelling peritoneal catheters or ventriculoperitoneal shunts.
- Diagnosis: Paracentesis, except when the peritonitis is secondary to gastrointestinal perforation.
- Treatment: Intravenous or intraperitoneal antibiotics or laparotomy if a ruptured viscus is suspected or confirmed.

Hepatitis

- Clinical presentation: Clinical findings include jaundice and hepatomegaly but can otherwise be nonspecific. Infections with hepatotropic viruses are often asymptomatic in children.
- Diagnosis: Laboratory tests to assess the extent of hepatocyte damage, excretory function, synthetic function, and cause.
- Treatment: Supportive care is usually sufficient for uncomplicated cases. Complications often warrant subspecialty input and transfer to an intensive care unit. Hepatic failure may necessitate liver transplantation.
- Prophylaxis: Both primary prophylaxis and postexposure prophylaxis are important, and recommendations vary according to the specific infecting agent.
- Genotyping of HBV and HCV aid in prognosis and the choice of therapy.
- Updated HBV and HCV treatment guidelines are available from The American Association for the Study of Liver Diseases (www.aasld.org).

SUGGESTED READINGS

Barnett E, Kimberlin D, Sawyer M, et al. *Red Book 2021-2024 Report of the Committee on Infectious Diseases*. 32nd ed. Itasca, IL: American Academy of Pediatrics; 2021. http://www.r2library.com/resource/title/9781610025218.

Clark A, van Zandvoort K, Flasche S, et al. Efficacy of live oral rotavirus vaccines by duration of follow-up: A meta-regression of randomised controlled trials. *Lancet Infect Dis*. 2019;19(7):717-727.

Freedman SB, Williamson-Urquhart S, Farion KJ, et al. Multicenter trial of a combination probiotic for children with gastroenteritis. *N Engl J Med*. 2018;379(21):2015-2026.

Hitchcock MM, Gomez CA, Banaei N. Low yield of FilmArray GI panel in hospitalized patients with diarrhea: an opportunity for diagnostic stewardship intervention. *J Clin Microbiol*. 2018;56(3).

Li PK, Chow KM, Cho Y, et al. ISPD peritonitis guideline recommendations: 2022 update on prevention and treatment. *Perit Dial Int*. 2022;42(2):110-153.

Liu J, Platts-Mills J, Juma J, et al. Use of quantitative molecular diagnostic methods to identify causes of diarrhoea in children: a reanalysis of the GEMS case-control study. *Lancet*. 2016;388(10051):1291-1301.

McFarland LV, Ozen M, Dinleyici EC, Goh S. Comparison of pediatric and adult antibiotic-associated diarrhea and clostridium difficile infections. *World J Gastroenterol*. 2016;22(11):3078-3104.

Nelson NP, Weng MK, Hofmeister MG, et al. Prevention of hepatitis A virus infection in the united states: Recommendations of the advisory committee on immunization practices, 2020. *MMWR*. 2020;69(5):1-38.

Niño-Serna L,F., Acosta-Reyes J, Veroniki A, Florez ID. Antiemetics in children with acute gastroenteritis: a meta-analysis. *Pediatrics*. 2020;145(4).

Operario DJ, Platts-Mills J, Nadan S, et al. Etiology of severe acute watery diarrhea in children in the global rotavirus surveillance network using quantitative polymerase chain reaction. *J Infect Dis*. 2017;216(2):220-227.

Schnadower D, O'Connell KJ, VanBuren JM, et al. Association between diarrhea duration and severity and probiotic efficacy in children with acute gastroenteritis. *Am J Gastroenterol*. 2021;116(7):1523-1532.

Shane AL, Mody RK, Crump JA, et al. 2017 infectious diseases society of america clinical practice guidelines for the diagnosis and management of infectious diarrhea. *Clin Infect Dis*. 2017;65(12):e45-e80.

Stinco M, Rubino C, Trapani S, Indolfi G. Treatment of hepatitis B virus infection in children and adolescents. *World J Gastroenterol*. 2021;27(36):6053-6063.

Tilmanne A, Martiny D, Quach C, et al. Enteropathogens in paediatric gastroenteritis: Comparison of routine diagnostic and molecular methods. *Clin Microbiol Infect*. 2019;25(12):1519-1524.

Ylinen E, Salmenlinna S, Halkilahti J, et al. Hemolytic uremic syndrome caused by shiga toxin-producing escherichia coli in children: incidence, risk factors, and clinical outcome. *Pediatr Nephrol*. 2020;35(9):1749-1759.

CHAPTER 100 Urinary Tract Infections in Childhood

Catherine S. Forster, MD, MSc and Nader Shaikh, MD, MPH

INTRODUCTION

Urinary tract infections (UTIs) are a common and important clinical problem in childhood. In the short term, UTIs may lead to systemic illness. Repeated infections can be associated with renal scarring, hypertension, and end-stage renal dysfunction.

TABLE 100-1 UTI Prevalence by Demographic Group

	Female	Male	
		Uncircumcised Male	*Circumcised Male*
>3 months and febrile	7.5% (5.1-10.0)	2.4% (1.4-3.5)	20.1% (16.8-23.4)
3-6 months and febrile	5.7% (2.3-9.4)	3.3% (1.3-5.3)	
6-12 months and febrile	8.3% (3.9-12.7)	1.7 (0.5-2.9)	
12-24 months and febrile	2.1% (1.2-3.6)	<1%	

Data from Shaikh N, Morone NE, Bost JE, Farrell MH. Prevalence of urinary tract infection in childhood: a meta-analysis. *Pediatr Infect Dis J*. 2008;27(4):302-308.

The overall prevalence of UTI is estimated at 7% in febrile infants but varies widely by gender. The highest prevalence rates of childhood UTI occur in uncircumcised male infants under 3 months of age (prevalence ~20%), and among females (prevalence ~8%). Circumcised older male children have the lowest prevalence of UTI (~1%) (**Table 100-1**). The probability of UTI in a given patient can be estimated using an online calculator (https://uticalc.pitt.edu/); this may help select patients who may benefit from catheterization to assess for UTI.

PATHOPHYSIOLOGY

Most UTIs beyond the newborn period represent an ascending infection. The first step in the pathogenesis of UTI is colonization of the periurethral area by uropathogenic enteric organisms. *Escherichia coli*, which accounts for about 90% of UTIs in children, is the most common causative pathogen. Other bacteria include both gram-negative species (*Klebsiella*, *Proteus*, *Enterobacter*, and *Citrobacter*) and gram-positive species (*Staphylococcus saprophyticus* and *Enterococcus*).

There are both bacterial and host factors that predispose to UTIs. With regard to bacterial factors, uropathogens have specific virulence mechanisms to facilitate infection of the urinary tract. Attachment of bacteria to uroepithelial cells is an active process mediated by specific bacterial adhesions and specific receptor sites on the epithelial cells. This process allows bacteria to ascend into the kidney, even in children without vesicoureteral reflux (VUR). In the kidney, the bacterial inoculum can produce an infection with an intense inflammatory response that may ultimately lead to renal scarring.

Host factors that increase risk of UTI include genetic factors, genitourinary anatomy and function, instrumentation (including the need for urinary catheterization for bladder management), presence of kidney or bladder stones, and sexual activity. Specific factors that increase the risk of UTI include uncircumcised males, bladder and bowel dysfunction, VUR, obstructive lesions, alterations in the periurethral flora, and use of urinary catheterization for bladder management.

Uncircumcised febrile male infants have a four- to tenfold higher prevalence of UTIs than circumcised males do. Although uncircumcised males are at increased risk for the development of a UTI, it is important to point out that UTIs do not develop in most uncircumcised boys. It is estimated that 195 circumcisions would be needed to prevent one hospital admission for UTI in the first year of life. The most recent AAP policy statement on circumcision suggests that the benefits of circumcision with regards to UTI is likely greater in those boys who are already at increased risk of UTI due other factors.

Bowel and bladder dysfunction, previously known as dysfunctional elimination syndrome or voiding dysfunction, is a functional disorder of unknown etiology characterized by the features delineated in **Table 100-2**. Bowel and bladder dysfunction usually appears in healthy school-aged children and may persist for months to years. Although it is a relatively common condition in the pediatric population, with a prevalence estimated at 15%, it is often underdiagnosed and undertreated by primary care physicians. Bowel and bladder dysfunction is a known risk factor for UTI, with a hypothesized causative relationship. Data suggests that the rectal distension seen in bowel and bladder dysfunction can compress the bladder neck, leading to incomplete bladder emptying, which is associated with UTI. Indeed, symptoms of bowel and bladder dysfunction were reported in approximately 40% of toilet-trained children with their first UTI and 80% of children with recurrent UTI.

TABLE 100-2 Bowel and Bladder Dysfunction

Clinical Triad	Symptoms
Abnormal elimination pattern	• Frequent voiding (>10 times/day) • Infrequent voiding • Urgency (often runs to the bathroom) • Infrequent painful stools (ask the child, not the parent)
Incontinence	• Bladder (ask about damp underwear) • Bowel (ask about streaks of stool in underwear)
Withholding maneuvers	• "Pee dance" • Kneeling with the perineum on the heel (Vincent's curtsy)

In a study of 141 girls older than 3 years with more than three UTIs, 108 had bowel and bladder dysfunction. In addition to its association with UTI, bowel and bladder dysfunction is also a risk factor for persistence of VUR and for renal scarring. The presence of VUR potentiates the risk of UTI in bowel and bladder dysfunction: As shown by Keren et al, the 2-year risk of UTI seen with any grade of VUR in combination with bowel and bladder dysfunction is 56%.

VUR is the most common urologic abnormality in children, with an overall prevalence of 1% and a prevalence of 40% in young children with febrile UTIs. A strong genetic predisposition for VUR exists and has been identified in up to 40% of siblings of children with VUR. VUR is graded according to the international classification from grade I to grade V (**Figure 100-1**). Hoberman et al found that in children presenting with their first UTI to a primary care physician, 95% of cases of VUR have been found to be grades I to III. Most VUR improves or resolves as the child ages, with resolution occurring more frequently in children with low-grade and unilateral disease. The likelihood of resolution of VUR, 5 years after detection, as derived from a large meta-analysis, is summarized in **Figure 100-2**.

Current evidence suggests that isolated VUR is neither necessary nor sufficient to cause renal scarring. Nevertheless, the risk of renal scarring increases in children with VUR compared with children without VUR (41% vs. 17% in a systematic review) and increases with increasing grades of VUR.

Children with obstructive abnormalities, whether anatomic (e.g., posterior urethral valves, ureteropelvic junction obstruction, constipation), neurologic (e.g., myelomeningocele with neurogenic bladder), or functional (e.g., bowel and bladder dysfunction), are at increased risk for the development of UTIs. Stagnant urine is an excellent culture medium for most uropathogens. However, obstructive anatomic abnormalities in children presenting with their first UTI are infrequent (1%-4%) in nonsyndromic children. Obstruction should be suspected in a child with UTI when there is a family history of urologic abnormalities, when dysmorphic features are detected on physical examination, or when symptoms do not respond to appropriate therapy.

Emerging evidence suggests that the microbiome may play a role in development of UTI. The vast majority of children have identifiable microbiomes in the bladder, urethra, perineum, and vagina. Decreased diversity of the urinary microbiome, as measured by the Shannon Diversity Index, been found in children with acute UTI compared to those without UTI. Further, there is indirect evidence that alteration of the normal periurethral flora in females (*Lactobacillus* and *Corynebacterium* spp.) promotes attachment of pathogenic bacteria to the urothelium. Sexual activity is also associated with UTI in women. In a prospective study of young sexually active women, recent intercourse was independently associated with the development of UTIs. The use of spermicidal condoms and spermicidal jelly with diaphragms has been independently associated with *E. coli* bacteriuria, thus suggesting that these agents predispose to UTI by altering the vaginal flora. Finally, in adult women with recurrent UTIs, there is an association between specific patterns of symptoms and urobiomes that are predominated by specific bacteria.

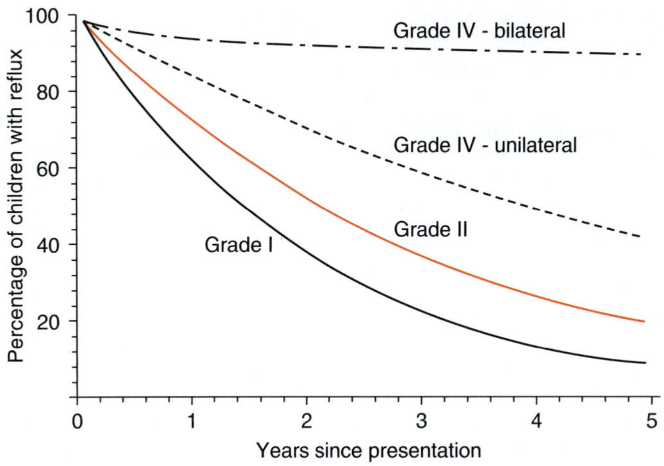

FIGURE 100-2. Persistence of vesicoureteral reflux in young children.

Urinary catheterization, whether used acutely during a hospitalization or as part of a chronic bladder management routine, is a known risk factor for UTI. Children with spina bifida who use clean intermittent catheterization have an average of 1.5 UTIs a year. In terms of urinary catheterization for acute needs, a 7-year retrospective study found that nosocomial UTIs were the fifth most common infection in hospitalized children. However, only 50% of children with nosocomial UTIs were catheterized, and nosocomial UTIs occurred with a disproportionately high rate in newborns.

CLINICAL PRESENTATION

In general, the younger the child, the less specific the presenting signs and symptoms of UTI; many infants with UTI are described as "well appearing."

Several prospective studies have shown that infants and young children can present with fever as the sole manifestation of UTI. Furthermore, the presence of another potential source for fever (upper respiratory tract infection, acute otitis media, acute gastroenteritis, etc.) does not rule out the possibility of UTI. In one study, the prevalence of UTI in infants and young girls with fever was 6% if no other potential source of fever was

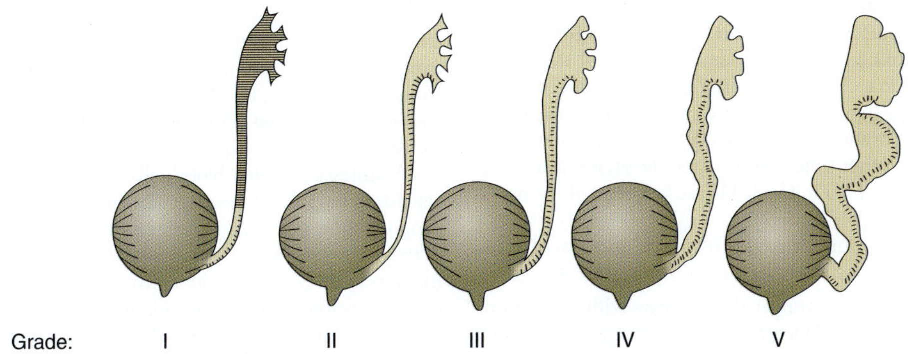

FIGURE 100-1. Grading of vesicoureteral reflux.

identified, but the prevalence was 3% even if another potential source of fever was identified. This finding highlights the importance of considering urine cultures in all febrile infants.

DIFFERENTIAL DIAGNOSIS

The differential diagnosis of a well-appearing infant or young child with "fever without a definite source" is extensive but most commonly includes UTI, occult bacteremia, and viral infections. In children vaccinated against *Haemophilus influenzae* type b and *Streptococcus pneumoniae*, the odds of UTI are much higher than the odds of occult bacteremia. The differential diagnosis of an older child presenting with urinary symptoms and bacteriuria includes nonspecific vulvovaginitis, an abdominal process such as appendicitis, urinary calculi, urethritis secondary to sexually transmitted disease, and a vaginal foreign body. Patients with group A streptococcal infection, appendicitis, and Kawasaki disease may also present with fever, abdominal pain, and pyuria.

DIAGNOSIS AND EVALUATION

Particular elements of the history of present illness should include the height and duration of fever and the presence of both urinary symptoms (e.g., hematuria, dysuria, vomiting) and nonurinary symptoms (e.g., rash, rhinorrhea, and cough), genitourinary instrumentation, sexual activity, and method of contraception. The past medical history should include any history of chronic constipation or chronic urinary symptoms (incontinence, lack of proper stream, frequency, urgency, withholding maneuvers) that may suggest an underlying diagnosis of bowel and bladder dysfunction, previous UTIs, VUR, and previous undiagnosed febrile illnesses. Relevant family history would include frequent UTIs, VUR, and other genitourinary abnormalities in close relatives.

Key elements of the physical examination include blood pressure and temperature, assessment of suprapubic and costovertebral tenderness, and if febrile, a search for signs of other sources of fever. The external genitalia should be examined for signs of vulvovaginitis, labial fusions, vaginal foreign body, sexually transmitted diseases, and anatomic abnormalities.

Given that the signs and symptoms of UTI in children are nonspecific, diagnosis of UTI requires laboratory confirmation. A clean-catch specimen and a catheterized specimen are the preferred methods of urine collection in a toilet-trained and a diapered child, respectively. Suprapubic aspiration may also be used to collect a specimen in young children. The use of a sterile bag is not generally recommended because up to 85% of positive cultures from bag urine specimens will represent false positive results; therefore, results are useful only if negative. Some institutions use a two-step approach in which a bagged specimen is used to obtain urine for a screening urinalysis, with urethral catheterization performed for culture in patients whose urinalysis results are suggestive of UTI. Regardless of the collection method, specimens should be examined soon after collection as a delay of even a few hours substantially increases both false positive and false negative rates.

The decision to obtain a urine sample for culture is best made on a case-by-case basis, taking into consideration the child's age, gender, circumcision status, and the presenting signs and symptoms (**Figure 100-3**). UTICalc (https://uticalc.pitt.edu/) aids in the estimation of the pretest probability of UTI based on a child's presenting symptoms and may help identify children who may benefit from urine culture. This tool, which includes age, height and duration of fever, history of UTI, gender, presence of circumcision, and other potential source of fever, has a sensitivity of 96% for the outcome of UTI. The UTICalc is intended for use in children 2 to 23 months of age.

In general, urine samples for urinalysis (dipstick and microscopic examination) and culture are indicated in the following patients:

- Girls and uncircumcised boys younger than 2 years with at least one risk factor for UTI (history of UTI, temperature >39°C, fever without apparent source [particularly if the child will be treated with antibiotics], ill appearance, suprapubic tenderness, or fever >24 hours).
- Circumcised boys younger than 2 years with suprapubic tenderness or at least two risk factors for UTI (history of UTI, temperature >39°C, fever without apparent source [particularly if the child will be treated with antibiotics], ill appearance, suprapubic tenderness, or fever >24 hours).
- Girls and uncircumcised boys older than 2 years with any of the following urinary symptoms: abdominal pain, back pain, dysuria, frequency, high fever, or new-onset incontinence.
- Circumcised boys older than 2 years with multiple urinary symptoms (abdominal pain, back pain, dysuria, frequency, high fever, or new-onset incontinence).
- Febrile infants and children with abnormalities of the urinary tract or family history of urinary tract disease.

The accuracy of the various diagnostic tests for UTI has been the subject of two meta-analyses. The sensitivity, specificity, and likelihood ratios of bedside tests available to diagnose UTIs in children are summarized in **Table 100-3**.

Dipstick tests are convenient and inexpensive and require little training for proper use, but they may miss some children with UTI (88% sensitivity at best). Furthermore, a positive leukocyte esterase test does not always confirm the diagnosis of UTI, which is why microscopic examination for urine white blood cells is used. Microscopic examination requires more equipment and training than dipstick tests do. Traditionally, a centrifuged sample of unstained urine is examined for the presence of bacteria and white cells. The accuracy of microscopic analysis is improved by using (i) an uncentrifuged specimen, (ii) a Gram-stained smear, and (iii) a hemocytometer (results reported as white blood cells/mm^3). Examination of urine with these three techniques has been termed "enhanced urinalysis." In young children, in whom prompt diagnosis and treatment are paramount, the enhanced urinalysis offers the best combination of sensitivity and specificity. A child with neither pyuria nor bacteriuria on the enhanced urinalysis is very unlikely to have a UTI, whereas a child with both pyuria and bacteriuria is very likely to have a UTI.

UTI is best defined as significant bacteriuria on urine culture in a patient with signs of urinary tract inflammation. Determination of "significant" bacteriuria by culture depends on the method of collection. Historically, >100,000 CFUs/mL indicated a UTI. These data were derived from morning collections of urine from adult women, with comparison of specimens from women without symptoms and women considered clinically to have pyelonephritis. The transition range at which the proportion of women with pyelonephritis exceeded the proportion of women without symptoms was 10,000 to 100,000 CFUs/mL. In children a threshold of 50,000 CFU/mL has been the accepted standard for some tome; however, some experts have supported the use of 10,000 CFU/mL as the cutoff to use for febrile infants undergoing bladder catheterization.

The American Academy of Pediatrics (AAP) criteria for UTI required evidence of inflammation in addition to positive culture results. Although true UTI without pyuria is unusual, the absence of pyuria in the presence of significant bacteriuria may occur early in the course of UTI (before the local inflammatory response develops), in colonization of the urinary tract (i.e., asymptomatic bacteriuria), as a result of contamination of the culture, or with certain organisms other than *E. coli*. In children who are suspected of having UTI but in whom pyuria is not detected on dipstick or microscopic analysis, repeating the urinalysis and urine culture can help to distinguish between early infection, colonization of the urinary tract, and contamination. Given that pyuria has been absent in at least 10% of children with bacteriuria plus symptoms of a UTI in a few studies, some experts have suggested that the requirement for pyuria should be removed from the definition of UTI in febrile children undergoing bladder catheterization for presumed UTI, particularly because the prevalence of asymptomatic bacteriuria in this population is very low (approximately 1/500).

Obtaining a complete blood cell count, a C-reactive protein level, or procalcitonin level is not necessary because, as of yet, no evidence exists that supports different management strategies for children based on the levels of these markers. Indeed, a meta-analysis that looked at the utility of these markers in diagnosing pyelonephritis reported the cumulative evidence as low to very low quality. Determination of serum creatinine is appropriate in a child with multiple UTIs and suspected renal involvement to assess for associated chronic kidney disease. Although 8% to 10% of young infants with UTI are bacteremic, and although fever in bacteremic infants with

UTI may persist on average 1 day longer than in nonbacteremic children, the organisms isolated from blood and urine are identical, as is the prognosis. For these reasons, routine performance of a blood culture in children older than 2 months with a UTI is not necessary because it does not alter management in the vast majority of children. Children younger than 1 month with high fever and abnormal urinalysis results should undergo lumbar puncture as part of the initial evaluation as some neonates (0.5%-1%) with UTI may also have bacterial meningitis.

COURSE OF ILLNESS

Two large studies have documented the details of the hospital course in children with UTI. Mean time to defervescence was approximately 24 hours. Approximately 90% of children were afebrile by 48 hours, and only 5% of children remained febrile for longer than 72 hours. None of the follow-up urine cultures, including cultures from children with fever that lasted longer than 48 hours, were positive. No renal abscesses were found. Since the incidence of renal abscess formation is very low (about 4% of all children hospitalized for UTI in one, single-center study), children who are clinically improving do not routinely need a repeat urine culture or a renal ultrasound despite persistent fever. A renal ultrasound is indicated in children who are clinically deteriorating or whose symptoms do not resolve in the time periods above.

MANAGEMENT

Treatment of children with presumed UTI depends on a number of factors, including age, severity of illness, presence of vomiting, duration of fever, degree of underlying medical complexity, availability of outpatient follow-up, and antimicrobial resistance patterns in the community.

The probable organisms and local resistance patterns should guide the practitioner in the choice of initial antimicrobial agent. Gram-staining of urine, if readily available, provides additional guidance for this choice. *E. coli* is the most common causative uropathogen, which can guide empiric antibiotic choices. However, antibiotic resistance to many previously used first-line agents is increasing. One paper found that resistance to amoxicillin in community-acquired UTIs due to *E. coli* increased from 47% to 89% in a 5-year period. Therefore, these agents cannot be recommended routinely for the empiric treatment of a young child with UTI. First-generation cephalosporins, amoxicillin-clavulanate or ampicillin-sulbactam, and trimethoprim-sulfamethoxazole can all be considered, but local antibiotic resistance patterns should be used to guide choice of

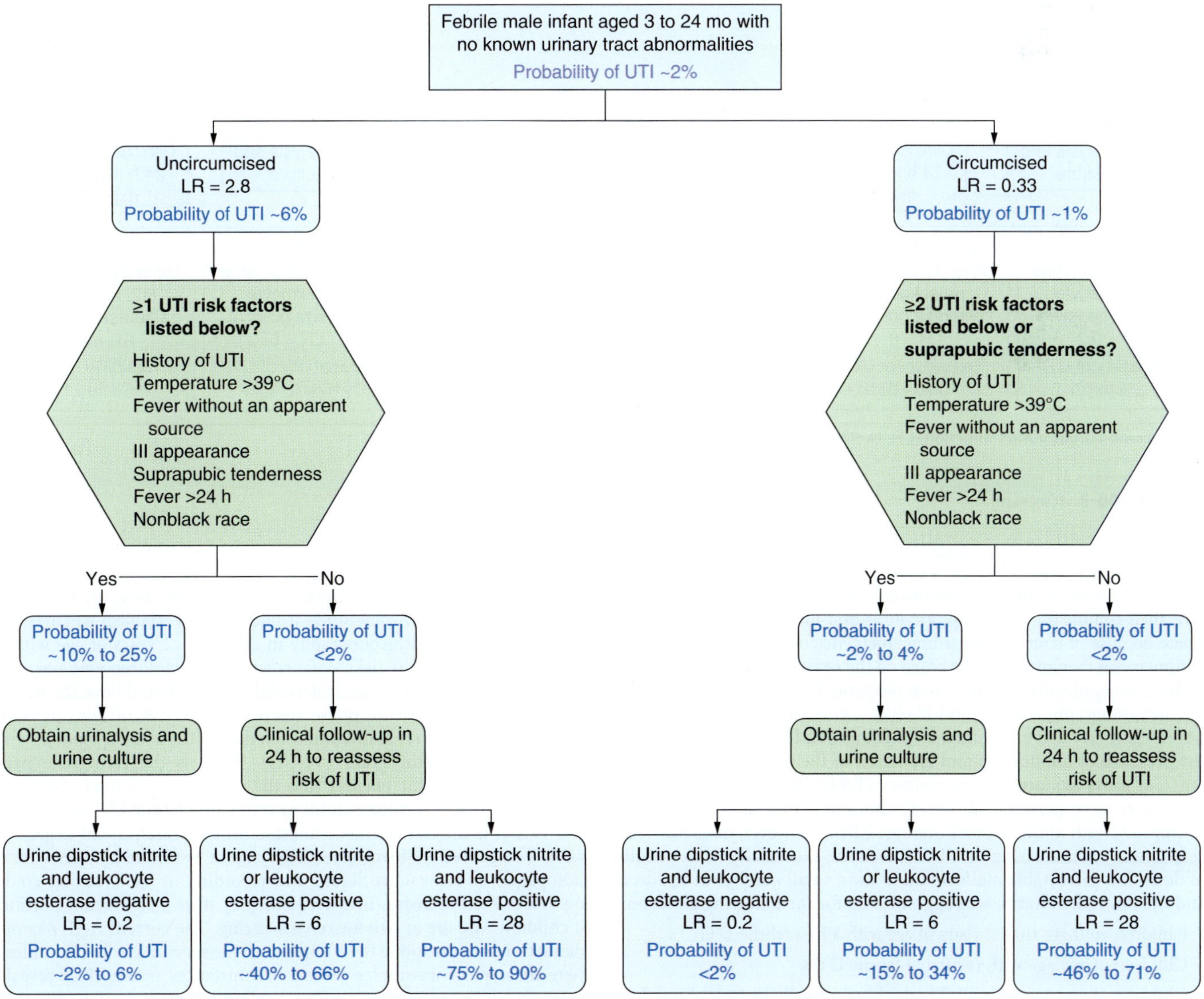

UTI indicates urinary tract infection; LR, likelihood ratio.

A

FIGURE 100-3. Diagnostic algorithm for verbal children older than 24 months with urinary or abdominal symptoms.

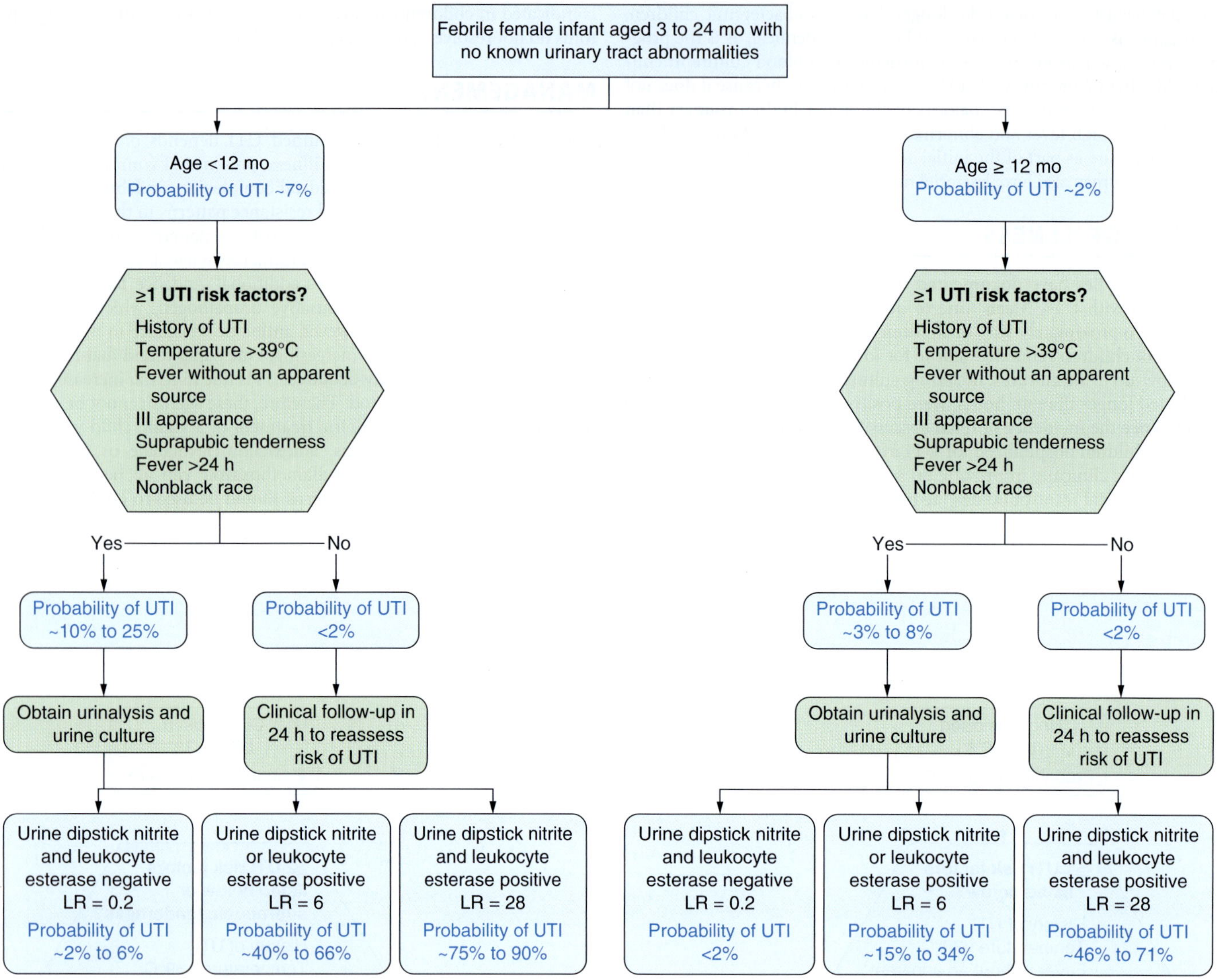

UTI indicates urinary tract infection; LR, likelihood ratio.

B

FIGURE 100-3. *(Continued)*

empiric antibiotics. Although quinolones are effective and resistance is rare, their routine use is not appropriate as first-line therapy is not appropriate because of concerns regarding emergence of resistance. Definitive antimicrobial therapy should be based on the resistance pattern of isolates within the organism(s) cultured from the patient's urine.

Ultrasonography—Renal and bladder ultrasonography (RBUS) is a noninvasive test that can demonstrate the size and shape of the kidneys, the presence of duplication and dilatation of the ureters, and the existence of gross anatomic abnormalities (**Table 100-4**). RBUS can also identify renal or perirenal abscess in children with acute UTI who fail to improve with antimicrobial therapy. RBUS, however, does not reliably detect renal scarring or VUR. Given the potentially large benefit of detecting correctable malformations for a small number of children and the low risk of harm, we suggest RBUS for the following children:

- Children younger than 2 years of age with a first febrile UTI
- Children of any age with recurrent febrile UTIs
- Children of any age with a UTI who have a family history of renal or urologic disease, poor growth, or hypertension
- Children who do not respond as expected to appropriate antimicrobial therapy (to identify complications; e.g., renal or perirenal abscess, pyonephrosis).

It is important to note that the recommendations above are not based on empiric evidence. A new study is underway to establish whether the benefits of routine ultrasonography in children <2 years of age with a febrile UTI outweigh its risks. Infants and young children who respond as expected to appropriate antimicrobial therapy should have the RBUS performed after the acute phase (to reduce the risk of false positive results secondary to renal inflammation during the acute episode).

Voiding cystourethrogram (VCUG)—VUR is the retrograde passage of urine from the bladder into the upper urinary tract. Approximately 40% to 50% of young children with a first febrile UTI have VUR. The VCUG is the test of choice to establish the presence and degree of VUR. The procedure involves catheterization to fill the bladder with a radiopaque or radioactive liquid and recording of VUR during voiding. VCUG is expensive, invasive, and may miss a significant portion of children who are at risk for renal scarring. The current AAP recommendation is to postpone the VCUG until the second febrile UTI unless there are atypical or complex clinical circumstances, or the RBUS reveals hydronephrosis, scarring, or other findings suggestive of high-grade (IV or V) VUR or obstructive uropathy. According to the guideline, the benefit of avoiding radiation exposure and discomfort in the majority of patients outweighs delayed detection of a small number of cases of high-grade reflux or surgically correctible abnormalities. One study found

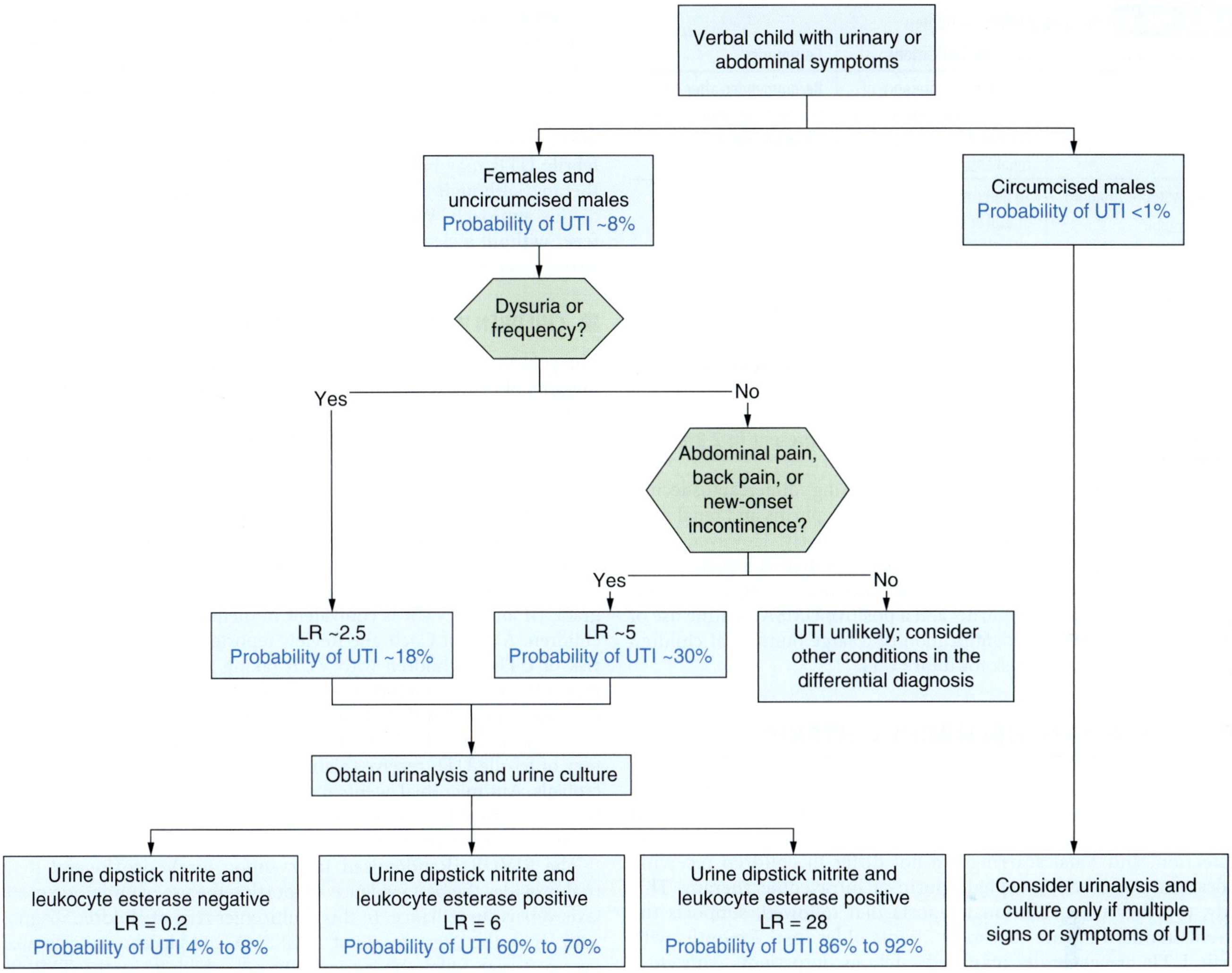

UTI indicates urinary tract infection; LR, likelihood ratio.

C

FIGURE 100-3. (*Continued*)

TABLE 100-3 Diagnostic Accuracy of Bedside Tests Available to Diagnose UTI

	Sensitivity	Specificity	Positive Likelihood Ratio	1/Negative Likelihood Ratio
Dipstick				
Leukocyte esterase (LE)	84%	78%	4	5
Nitrite	50%	98%	25	2
Nitrite or LE	88%	93%	13	8
Nitrite and LE	72%	96%	18	3
Microscopy				
Uncentrifuged				
Pyuria (≥10/mm³) (all ages)	77%	89%	7	4
Pyuria (>10/mm³) (<2 yr)*	90%	95%	18	10
Bacteriuria (Gram stained)	93%	95%	19	14
Overall (P+B) = enhanced	85%	99.9%	85	7
Overall (P or B)	95%	89%	9	17
Centrifuged				
Pyuria (>5/hpf)	67%	79%	3	0.4
Bacteriuria	81%	83%	5	0.2
Overall (P+B)*	66%	99%	7	0.4

*Indicates data from: Gorelick MH, Shaw KN. Screening tests for urinary tract infection in children: a meta-analysis. *Pediatrics*. 1999;104(5):e54.

Source: Data taken from Huicho L, Campos-Sanchez M, Alamo C. Metaanalysis of urine screening tests for determining the risk of urinary tract infection in children. *Pediatr Infect Dis J.* 2002;21(1):1-11, 88 unless otherwise specified.

TABLE 100-4 Imaging Studies in Children

Diagnostic Study	Purpose/Indications	Comments
Renal ultrasound	To determine presence of anatomic abnormalities, or complication of UTI such as renal abscess.	Recommended after 1st UTI; best performed after the acute phase
Voiding cystourethrogram Radiographic Nuclear	To determine the presence of VUR or obstruction. May also identify adequacy of bladder emptying.	Recommended after 2nd UTI
Renal scintigraphy (DMSA scan)	To determine presence or extent of renal scarring.	Not routinely performed

DMSA, 99m technetium-dimercaptosuccinic acid; UTI, urinary tract infection; VUR, vesicoureteral reflux.

high-grade reflux (defined as grade IV or V) was present in 2.8% of all patients who underwent VCUG following UTI.

Renal scintigraphy—Renal scintigraphy using dimercaptosuccinic acid (DMSA) can be used to detect acute pyelonephritis and renal scarring in the acute and chronic settings, respectively. However, using DMSA as the initial test to identify high-risk children is expensive and involves radiation exposure. Furthermore, since most young febrile children with UTI have pyelonephritis and a positive DMSA, routine use of DMSA scans may lead to identification of a large number of children who may or may not be at risk for future UTI.

ADMISSION AND DISCHARGE CRITERIA

Traditionally, young children with febrile UTIs were managed as inpatients. In a double-blind randomized controlled trial of 306 children 1 to 24 months of age with a febrile UTI, rates of symptom resolution, reinfection, and renal scarring did not differ in children receiving an oral third-generation cephalosporin or intravenous therapy. This study, together with additional reports that followed, supports the current standard of care that most infants older than 2 months with febrile UTIs are generally managed safely as outpatients with close follow-up. Indeed, the 2021 AAP febrile infant guidelines recommend that well-appearing infants with a negative urinalysis (a positive urinalysis is any leukocyte esterase, >5 urine white blood cells per high-powered field OR >10 white blood cells per mm^3) and negative inflammatory markers (abnormal inflammatory markers include procalcitonin >0.5mg/mL, CRP >20mg/L, absolute neutrophil count >4000 or >5200) can be safely monitored at home with close outpatient follow-up. The following subgroups of children, however, should be hospitalized:

- Those with vomiting who cannot tolerate oral medications or cannot maintain adequate hydration
- Those that have significant underlying medical disorders that may complicate management of the underlying illness or the UTI
- Those with inadequate outpatient support or availability of close follow-up
- Those who have responded inadequately to outpatient therapy

Children with bacteremic UTIs have traditionally been treated with longer courses of IV antibiotics. However, several studies have not shown differences in outcomes for infants with bacteremic UTIs who are treated with short versus long-course IV antibiotics. Children who are clinically improving and who are tolerating oral fluids may be discharged from the hospital on a regimen of oral antibiotics. Follow-up studies (e.g., RBUS and VCUG) are generally scheduled on an outpatient basis.

POSTDISCHARGE CONSIDERATIONS

CHILDREN WITH RECURRENT URINARY TRACT SYMPTOMS

Approximately 8% to 30% of children with UTI experience one or more symptomatic reinfections, usually within the first 6 months after the initial UTI. Prompt recognition and treatment of UTIs may be the most important factor in the prevention of renal scarring, as delay in antibiotic initiation is associated with the development of new renal scarring. Routine surveillance of asymptomatic children with monthly urine studies has not been shown to be associated with a better prognosis and is therefore not recommended. Children with recurrent febrile UTIs may be candidates for low-dose long-term antimicrobial therapy, although there is no evidence demonstrating the efficacy of this approach. When children with a history of UTI present with fever without a clear focus of infection, evaluation for possible UTI is strongly recommended.

CHILDREN WITH VESICOURETERAL REFLUX

The goal of treating VUR is to prevent progressive renal damage. The majority of young children with VUR will have low-grade VUR (grades I to III), which will often resolve spontaneously as the child ages. Children with grades IV and V VUR and older children are less likely to experience spontaneous resolution. Children with VUR have traditionally been treated either medically with low-dose long-term antimicrobials to prevent recurrent infection, or surgically. Surgical treatment involves reimplantation of the ureter or ureters into the bladder and creation of a longer mucosal tunnel. Several large prospective studies have demonstrated that the incidence of renal scarring in children with persistent grade III and IV VUR is equivalent in medically and surgically treated children. A recent Cochrane Review reported a modest decrease in the risk of UTIs in children with VUR taking antibiotic prophylaxis (risk ratio of 0.65, 95% confidence interval of 0.39-1.07). Therefore, it has been recommended that children less than 1 year of age with VUR and a history of febrile UTI, or children with grade III-V VUR and no history of febrile UTI, receive treatment with low-dose long-term antimicrobials. Antimicrobial agents most appropriate for prophylaxis include trimethoprim-sulfamethoxazole and nitrofurantoin in half the usual therapeutic doses given once daily.

The RIVUR (Randomized Intervention for VesicoUreteral Reflux) trial provides the best evidence supporting the use of antibiotic prophylaxis versus surveillance. In this multicenter trial of children diagnosed with VUR, the effectiveness of TMP-SMX and placebo were compared over a 2-year follow-up period. Overall, children in the TMP-SMX group were less likely to have recurrent febrile or symptomatic UTI than those in the placebo group (13 vs. 24%) (HR 0.50, 95% CI 0.34-0.74). In subgroup analysis, antibiotic prophylaxis was most effective in children with bowel and bladder dysfunction (HR 0.21, 95% CI 0.08-0.58) and in children whose first UTI was febrile (HR 0.41, 95% CI 0.26-0.64). The occurrence of renal scarring did not differ significantly between the prophylaxis and placebo groups. A meta-analysis similarly did not find a difference in renal scarring between children who did and did not receive antibiotic prophylaxis. However, the RIVUR trial also found that children who received antibiotic prophylaxis had higher rates of subsequent infections with organisms resistant to the antibiotic used for prophylaxis.

CONSULTATION

Subspeciality consultation should be considered for outpatient management of children with anatomic anomalies of the kidney and urinary tract, VUR, or chronic kidney disease.

SPECIAL CONSIDERATIONS

Children with neurogenic bladders, which are most commonly due to spina bifida, are a unique population. Notably, the AAP guidelines on diagnosis and management of UTIs are specifically designed for children with normal genitourinary anatomy and function. However, there are no widely accepted guidelines for the diagnosis or management of UTIs in children with neurogenic bladder: thus, many clinicians apply the AAP guidelines to this population. It is important to note that children with neurogenic bladders frequently have bacteriuria and pyuria in the absence of symptoms. Treatment of asymptomatic bacteriuria in children with neurogenic bladder is not recommended as asymptomatic bacteriuria in this population is not associated with the development of renal scars. Further, the rate of resistance to third-generation cephalosporins in bacteria cultured from urine from children who use clean intermittent catheterization is increasingly rapidly, underscoring the critical need for antibiotic stewardship.

SUGGESTED READINGS

Bocquet N, Sergent Alaoui A, Jais JP, et al. Randomized trial of oral versus sequential IV/oral antibiotic for acute pyelonephritis in children. *Pediatrics.* 2012;129(2):e269-275.

Desai S, Aronson PL, Shabanova V, et al. Parenteral antibiotic therapy duration in young infants with bacteremic urinary tract infections. *Pediatrics.* 2019;144(3).

Finnell SM, Carroll AE, Downs SM, et al. Technical report—diagnosis and management of an initial UTI in febrile infants and young children. *Pediatrics.* 2011;128(3):e749-e770.

Gorelick MH, Shaw KN. Screening tests for urinary tract infection in children: a meta-analysis. *Pediatrics.* 1999;104(5):e54.

Hewitt IK, Pennesi M, Morello W, Ronfani L, Montini G. Antibiotic prophylaxis for urinary tract infection-related renal scarring: a systematic review. *Pediatrics.* 2017;139(5).

Hoberman A, Wald ER, Hickey RW, et al. Oral versus initial intravenous therapy for urinary tract infections in young febrile children. *Pediatrics.* 1999;106:79-86.

Hoberman A, Charron M, Hickey RW, Baskin M, Kearney DH, Wald ER. Imaging studies after a first febrile urinary tract infection in young children. *N Engl J Med.* 2003;348(3):195-202.

Hoberman A, Wald ER, Penchansky L, Reynolds EA, Young S. Enhanced urinalysis as a screening test for urinary tract infection. *Pediatrics.* 1993;91(6):1196-1199.

Hoberman A, Wald ER, Hickey RW, et al. Oral versus initial intravenous therapy for urinary tract infections in young febrile children. *Pediatrics.* 1999;104(1 Pt 1):79-86.

Hoberman A, Chesney RW, Investigators RT. Antimicrobial prophylaxis for children with vesicoureteral reflux. *N Engl J Med.* 2014;371(11):1072-1073.

Huicho L, Campos-Sanchez M, Alamo C. Metaanalysis of urine screening tests for determining the risk of urinary tract infection in children. *Pediatr Infect Dis J.* 2002;21(1):1-11, 88.

Keren R, Shaikh N, Pohl H, et al. Risk factors for recurrent urinary tract infection and renal scarring. *Pediatrics.* 2015;136(1):e13-21.

Koff SA, Wagner TT, Jayanthi VR. The relationship among dysfunctional elimination syndromes, primary vesicoureteral reflux and urinary tract infections in children. *J Urol.* 1998;160(3 Pt 2):1019-1022.

Lavelle JM, Blackstone MM, Funari MK, et al. Two-step process for ED UTI screening in febrile young children: reducing catheterization rates. *Pediatrics.* 2016;138(1).

Montini G, Toffolo A, Zucchetta P, et al. Antibiotic treatment for pyelonephritis in children: multicentre randomised controlled non-inferiority trial. *BMJ.* 2007;335(7616):386.

Naseer SR, Steinhardt GF. New renal scars in children with urinary tract infections, vesicoureteral reflux and voiding dysfunction: a prospective evaluation. *J Urol.* 1997;158(2):566-568.

Nelson CP, Johnson EK, Logvinenko T, Chow JS. Ultrasound as a screening test for genitourinary anomalies in children with UTI. *Pediatrics.* 2014;133(3):e394-403.

Pantell RH, Roberts KB, Adams WG, et al. Evaluation and Management of Well-Appearing Febrile Infants 8 to 60 Days Old. *Pediatrics.* 2021;148(2):e2021052228.

Shaikh N, Ewing AL, Bhatnagar S, Hoberman A. Risk of renal scarring in children with a first urinary tract infection: a systematic review. *Pediatrics.* 2010;126(6):1084-1091.

Shaikh N, Hoberman A, Keren R, et al. Recurrent urinary tract infections in children with bladder and bowel dysfunction. *Pediatrics.* 2016;137(1).

Shaikh N, Mattoo TK, Keren R, et al. Early antibiotic treatment for pediatric febrile urinary tract infection and renal scarring. *JAMA Pediatr.* 2016;170(9):848-854.

Shaikh N, Osio VA, Wessel CB, Jeong JH. Prevalence of asymptomatic bacteriuria in children: a meta-analysis. *J Pediatr.* 2020;217:110-117 e114.

Shaikh N, Lee MC, Stokes LR, et al. Reassessment of the role of race in calculating the risk for urinary tract infection: a systematic review and meta-analysis. *JAMA Pediatr.* 2022;176(6):569-575.

Shaikh N, Morone NE, Bost JE, Farrell MH. Prevalence of urinary tract infection in childhood: a meta-analysis. *Pediatr Infect Dis J.* 2008;27(4):302-308.

Shaikh N, Morone NE, Lopez J, et al. Does this child have a urinary tract infection? *JAMA.* 2007;298(24):2895-904.

Storm DW, Copp HL, Halverson TM, Du J, Juhr D, Wolfe AJ. A Child's urine is not sterile: a pilot study evaluating the Pediatric Urinary Microbiome. *J Pediatr Urol.* 2022;18(3):383-392.

Subcommittee on Urinary Tract Infection SCoQI, Management, Roberts KB. Urinary tract infection: clinical practice guideline for the diagnosis and management of the initial UTI in febrile infants and children 2 to 24 months. *Pediatrics.* 2011;128(3):595-610.

Tamminen-Mobius T, Brunier E, Ebel KD, et al. Cessation of vesicoureteral reflux for 5 years in infants and children allocated to medical treatment. The International Reflux Study in Children. *J Urol.* 1992;148(5 Pt 2):1662-1666.

Thomson J, Cruz AT, Nigrovic LE, et al. Concomitant bacterial meningitis in infants with urinary tract infection. *Pediatr Infect Dis J.* 2017;36(9):908-910.

Weiss R, Duckett J, Spitzer A. Results of a randomized clinical trial of medical versus surgical management of infants and children with grades III and IV primary vesicoureteral reflux (United States). The International Reflux Study in Children. *J Urol.* 1992;148(5 Pt 2):1667-1673.

Williams G, Craig JC. Long-term antibiotics for preventing recurrent urinary tract infection in children. *Cochrane Database Syst Rev.* 2019;4:CD001534.

CHAPTER 101 Bone and Joint Infections

Brandon Palmer, MD and Matthew P. Kronman, MD, MSCE

OSTEOMYELITIS

BACKGROUND

Osteomyelitis is an inflammatory process of the bone and bone marrow that is most commonly due to an acute bacterial infection. The most common form in childhood is acute hematogenous osteomyelitis (AHO); 50% of cases occur in children younger than 5 years. The incidence of AHO is approximately 1 in 10,000 children, and boys are about twice as likely to be affected as girls. The majority of cases are limited to a single site and occur in long bones, with the femur and tibia accounting for almost half of all cases.

Staphylococcus aureus is the most commonly identified organism, accounting for 78.2% of cases of AHO. Group A Beta-hemolytic streptococci and *Haemophilus influenzae* were commonly encountered in the past, but effective immunization has decreased the incidence dramatically. *Kingella kingae* is an important pathogen to consider in young children (<4 years) following an upper respiratory tract infection or stomatitis. Group B *Streptococcus* and enteric gram-negative organisms such as *Escherichia coli* may be identified in neonates with osteomyelitis but are rare in older children. *Salmonella* species are commonly identified in patients with sickle cell disease, and *Pseudomonas aeruginosa* is often identified in cases of osteochondritis following puncture wounds of the feet. Mycobacteria and fungi are rare causes of osteomyelitis. *Bartonella henselae*, a less typical cause of osteomyelitis, occurs in patients with cat scratch disease.

PATHOPHYSIOLOGY

While the exact pathogenesis of osteomyelitis is not known, several routes of infection are hypothesized. In children, most cases result from hematogenous spread after a transient episode of bacteremia. About one-third of patients report a history of blunt trauma, which increases the likelihood of seeding an infection during an episode of bacteremia (due to disruptions in the microcirculation in the medullary bone). Direct inoculation of bacteria into bone, occurring as a result of penetrating trauma or surgery, is a less common cause of osteomyelitis in children.

Osteomyelitis most commonly begins in the highly vascular metaphysis of long bones. Certain bacteria such as *S. aureus* adhere to bone by expressing receptors (adhesins) for a component of the bone matrix. Growing colonies of bacteria surround themselves with a protective glycocalyx, shielding them from circulating white blood cells. As infection advances, cortical bone is destroyed, and infection and inflammation may extend into the subperiosteal space.

The periosteum in young infants is thin and is not tightly adherent to the underlying bone. As a result, the periosteum is more likely to perforate, spreading infection into the surrounding tissues. In young infants, blood vessels extend into the epiphyses, which increase the likelihood of growth plate damage as well as septic arthritis. The hips and shoulders are common sites of epiphyseal infection.

TABLE 101-1 Common Etiologic Agents in Pediatric Bone and Joint Infections

Organisms	Typical Age Range	Recommended Antibiotics*
Group B strep	Neonate-2 months	Ampicillin 200 mg/kg/day
S. aureus (MSSA)	Any	Oxacillin 200 mg/kg/day**
S. aureus (MRSA)	Any	Vancomycin 60 mg/kg/day*** Target trough level: 15-20
Group A strep	Infant-adolescent	Ampicillin or cephalosporin
Kingella kingae	Infant-4 years	Ampicillin or cephalosporin
Salmonella spp.	Any (sickle cell disease)	Ceftriaxone 100 mg/kg/day (base on susceptibilities)
N. gonorrhoeae	Adolescent	Ceftriaxone 100 mg/kg/day
Pseudomonas	Older child/Adolescent	Cefepime 150 mg/kg/day or Piperacillin/Tazobactam 300 mg/kg/day

*See standard references for neonatal and adult maximum doses.

**Nafcillin 200 mg/kg/day and cefazolin 100 mg/kg/day are alternatives.

***Clindamycin may be used if organism susceptible and patient not bacteremic.

CLINICAL PRESENTATIONS

Patients often present after experiencing symptoms for days, most commonly complaining of fever and pain at the affected site. Infants and toddlers may present with irritability, limp, or refusal to bear weight on an extremity. Neonates with osteomyelitis may present with pseudoparalysis (refusal to move) of the affected extremity. Erythema, warmth, and swelling of the affected site may be noted. The lower extremities account for most cases, followed by the humerus and pelvis. A subacute presentation, often for weeks or months, can be associated with a Brodie abscess. Due to improved diagnosis and earlier treatment, chronic osteomyelitis is now uncommon. If not properly treated, the effects of inflammation or tissue destruction of the growth plate can cause persistent symptoms for life.

DIFFERENTIAL DIAGNOSIS

The differential diagnosis for osteomyelitis includes other skin and soft tissue infections such as cellulitis, septic arthritis, and toxic synovitis. Cancers such as leukemia, osteosarcoma, and Ewing sarcoma are important causes of bone pain that should be considered in the differential diagnosis of osteomyelitis. Thrombophlebitis, trauma, fracture, rheumatologic diseases such as juvenile rheumatoid arthritis, vitamin deficiencies (such as scurvy in patients with extremely limited diets), and pain crisis in sickle cell disease should also be considered.

DIAGNOSTIC EVALUATION

Noninvasive Evaluation There are no specific biomarkers of osteomyelitis. A microbiological diagnosis in AHO is of high value, as it leads to optimization of spectrum and duration of antimicrobial therapy. A blood culture should always be performed as part of the initial evaluation *before* initiating antibiotics. Blood cultures have a positivity rate of about 31%, and pathogen yield on blood culture may decrease the need for more invasive testing. Per the 2021 national guidelines by Woods et al, C-reactive protein (CRP) is the test of choice to assess response of osteomyelitis to therapy, and therefore is recommended to obtain at time of presentation and to trend throughout illness course. CRP has a sensitivity of 80.5% for diagnosing AHO. CRP usually peaks in the first 2 to 4 days of treatment and normalizes in 9 to 12 days. While there is not a definitive CRP numeric cutoff value for diagnosis, higher peak CRPs are associated with complications such as subperiosteal abscesses and multifocal disease. Other inflammatory markers such as the erythrocyte sedimentation rate (ESR) and procalcitonin may be elevated at time of presentation, but are not recommended to obtain or trend, as CRP has been shown to have superior sensitivity. A complete blood count may be important to help rule out leukemia, and is likely to reveal a leukocytosis with a left shift, as well as reactive thrombocytosis.

Invasive Evaluation Given the high value of microbiological diagnosis, invasive diagnostic procedures such as bone aspirate or bone biopsy should be done in non-critically ill children per Woods et al. The addition of bone/tissue culture to blood cultures increases pathogen yield from 32.9% to 55.4%, and can lead to more targeted antimicrobial therapy in up to 85% of cases. For the most part, culture-negative cases behave similarly to cases in which a pathogen is identified. Open procedures involving metaphyseal drilling may enhance the yield and can also be therapeutic. **Table 101-1** lists the most common causes of osteomyelitis by age.

Imaging The advantages and disadvantages of various imaging techniques are summarized in **Table 101-2**. Plain radiographs are low cost, readily available and can help rule out other causes of bone pain such as fracture or neoplasm. However, plain radiographs have low sensitivity (16%-37%) (**Figure 101-1**) and are dependent on the duration of active disease. In the first 3 days, these films may reveal soft tissue swelling; by days 3 to 7, swelling of the surrounding muscle leads to obliteration of the normally translucent fat planes. Osteolytic lesions are generally not apparent until days 10 to 21, at which point there has been greater than 50% loss of bone density. In contrast, patients presenting with discitis may show narrowing of the disc space early on, with involvement of the vertebral bodies later.

TABLE 101-2 Advantages and Disadvantages of Imaging Modalities for the Diagnosis of Osteomyelitis

Modality	Advantages	Disadvantages
Plain radiographs	Inexpensive Quick Easy	Insensitive in early disease
Computed tomography	Improved sensitivity Relatively quick	Radiation exposure May require sedation
Magnetic resonance imaging	Very sensitive, even in early disease May reveal pus collections or extension into adjacent joint or soft tissue	Long study Often requires sedation Expensive
Three-phase nuclear bone scan (technetium 99m methylene diphosphonate)	Very sensitive Identifies multifocal disease May reveal unsuspected sites in preverbal children	Long study Often requires sedation Expensive Radiation exposure

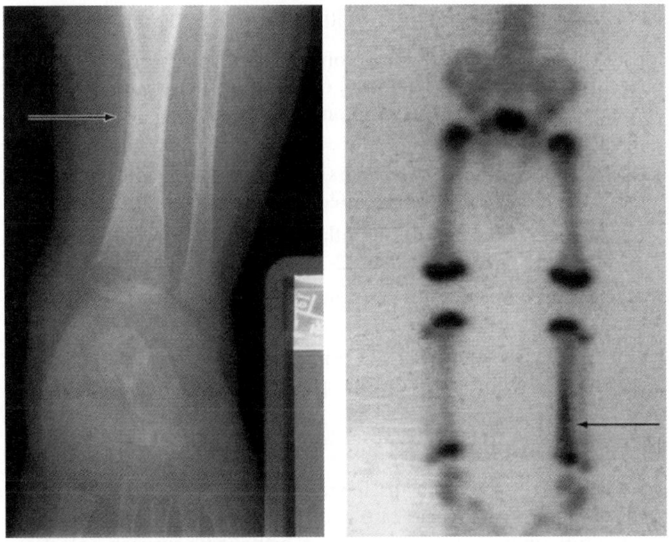

A B

FIGURE 101-1. A. Anteroposterior radiograph of the leg in a 6-month-old infant reveals periosteal new bone formation along the tibial diaphysis (*arrow*). B. Anterior bone scan of the same patient reveals increased uptake along the distal tibial diaphysis extending into the metaphysis (*arrow*). These images are consistent with osteomyelitis. (Used with permission of Lisa States, MD.)

When clinical findings and radiographs are sufficiently suggestive of AHO, advanced imaging is not required. However, when advanced imaging is required, MRI has superior sensitivity (81%-100%) and specificity (67%-94%) compared to computerized tomography (CT), ultrasound, or nuclear scintigraphy (bone scan). Edema and exudate of the medullary space may be noted in early osteomyelitis (**Figure 101-2**) on MRI. Coronal or sagittal images are especially useful for planning surgical procedures and assessing the growth plates and epiphyses. Gadolinium enhancement is recommended. While MRI is typically a time-consuming procedure that requires sedation for young children in order to obtain optimal images, newer "fast" MRI techniques are being developed that may avoid these problems.

Nuclear scintigraphy (bone scan) can be helpful in young patients who are unable to verbalize the location of their pain, when multiple sites are suspected, or in differentiating osteomyelitis from cellulitis (see Figure 101-1). Technetium-99m methylene diphosphonate has increased uptake in areas of osteoblastic activity, and the three-phase bone scan is the study of choice. The technetium scan is not specific for infection and may be abnormal with fractures, tumors, and other bone pathology. Tagged leukocyte scans (e.g., indium 111 or technetium-99m) are more specific for infection but are laborious, time consuming, and may yield false positive results.

CT allows a cross-sectional assessment and can reveal areas of cortical bone destruction, periosteal reaction, sequestration, and soft tissue abscesses. Images should be obtained with and without enhancement. CT involves significant radiation exposure and is not necessary in most cases of pediatric osteomyelitis.

MANAGEMENT

Empiric Therapy Antimicrobial therapy should be started immediately for ill-appearing children, but according to Woods et al, antibiotics can be withheld for up to 48 to 72 hours in well-appearing children in whom an invasive diagnostic procedure is planned to increase the likelihood of pathogen identification. Empirical therapy should be active against *S. aureus,* and guided by local *S. aureus* resistance susceptibilities, rates of community-acquired MRSA (CA-MRSA), and clindamycin resistance. In regions with CA-MRSA rates less than 10% to 20%, cefazolin, oxacillin, or nafcillin are appropriate first-line choices for stable children. If the CA-MRSA rates are >20% and clindamycin resistance rates are less than 10% to 20%, clindamycin is preferred over vancomycin as it is associated with less toxicity and there is no requirement to measure levels. If vancomycin is used to treat osteomyelitis, a potentially severe infection, trough concentrations between 15 and 20 mg/mL have historically been targeted in order to ensure adequate bacterial killing, though many centers are moving to area under the curve (AUC) to minimum inhibitory concentration (MIC) ratios, which can provide a measure of treatment efficacy while generally avoiding the toxicities associated with higher vancomycin levels.

Targeted Therapy Among children 4 years and younger, *Kingella kingae* is an important cause of bone and joint infection. Lower extremity involvement, subacute presentation, and preceding URI symptoms

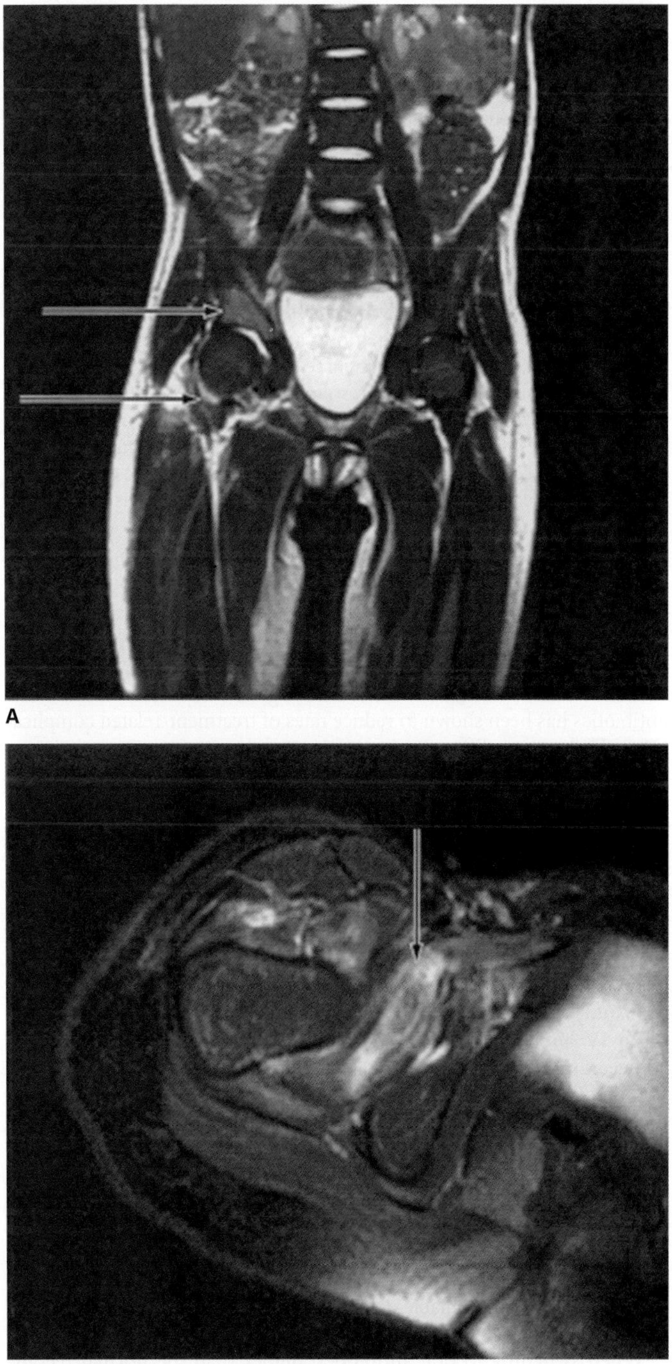

A

B

FIGURE 101-2. A. T2-weighted coronal MRI scan in a 4-year-old girl demonstrates increased signal in the right ischium due to marrow edema, consistent with osteomyelitis (*upper arrow*). Also noted is increased signal in the joint space, consistent with a small joint effusion (*lower arrow*). B. T2-weighted axial image in the same patient reveals increased signal in the deep muscles of the pelvis, consistent with myositis. (Used with permission of Lisa States, MD.)

or oral ulcers are features of this infection. The initial indolent features, including normal or mildly elevated CRP values at presentation, contribute to delays in diagnosis. The organism can be difficult to grow (inoculating a blood culture bottle with the clinical specimen enhances yield) and grows late. Neither vancomycin nor clindamycin is active, but penicillin, ampicillin, and cephalosporins are effective against *K. kingae*. Using cefazolin as initial empiric therapy is appropriate for the young child when *S. aureus*, GABHS, and *K. kingae* are all considerations. If MRSA is strongly considered, initial empiric therapy can include combining cefazolin with either clindamycin or vancomycin depending on resistance patterns, though a treatment goal should be to work toward antibiotic monotherapy if possible.

Neonates with osteomyelitis often have a history of a preceding infection, and about half have involvement of multiple sites. Rapid screening tests can help identify the newborn colonized with MRSA and the results can influence antibiotic choice. Empirical therapy should cover group B streptococci and enteric gram-negative rods in addition to the pathogens common in older infants and children. An intravenous third-generation cephalosporin such as ceftriaxone or ceftazidime (based on the age of the neonate) may be used for empirical therapy, and coverage can be narrowed once culture results and sensitivities are available. If MRSA is considered likely based on local epidemiology, screening results, or initial Gram stain and culture results, vancomycin should be added.

Monitoring Response Treatment response should be monitored through serial clinical examinations and serial CRP measurements. Signs of clinical improvement include improvement in pain, mobility and range of motions, as well as resolution of fever. Persistently elevated CRP with slower than expected clinical improvement may be a sign of failure to respond to therapy and prompt re-evaluation. Additional imaging should be considered, as well as further diagnostic or therapeutic surgical intervention. A reconsideration of the diagnosis is also warranted if clinical and lab response is not as expected.

Treatment Duration and Oral Therapy Once an organism has been identified, coverage can be narrowed according to the results of susceptibility testing. The minimum recommended length of treatment is 20 days, with a recommended total length of treatment of 3 to 4 weeks per the IDSA guidelines by Woods et al. Children should be transitioned to oral antibiotics if feasible at time of discharge or earlier. Transition to oral antibiotics has been shown to reduce rates of treatment-related complications. There is no difference in treatment failure rates in completion of treatment with oral antibiotics compared to parenteral therapy, and studies have shown a very low failure rate in children transitioned to oral antibiotics when they were clinically improving and their CRP was <3 mg/dL. Children with *S. aureus* detected on bacterial culture without concerns of endocarditis can also be transitioned to oral antibiotic therapy based on clinical course and response to treatment. A longer antibiotic course (e.g. 6 weeks, or occasionally longer) may be considered in especially complicated cases. If long-term intravenous antibiotics will be administered, placement of a peripherally inserted central catheter (PICC) should be considered.

A study by Peltola et al in 2010 described good results using 2 to 4 days of an IV antibiotic, followed by oral antibiotics to complete a 20-day course. It should be noted that no patients in that study had MRSA infection and the population may have been less ill than is often described in the United States, so the results may not be generalizable. Additionally, the response of MRSA to vancomycin is slower than the response of MSSA to a beta-lactam antibiotic. Recent studies by Zaoutis et al and Keren et al showed equivalent failure rates among children who were transitioned to oral antibiotics early compared with those who received more prolonged IV treatment. Catheter-related complications were more common in the latter group. Caution should be used in interpreting these findings because of the limitations of available database information (e.g. less sick patients may have been more likely to have early transition to oral therapy).

When switching to oral antibiotics, higher than the normal recommended doses are often used. Typical dosing for cephalexin would be 100 to 150 mg/kg/day, for dicloxacillin 100 mg/kg/day, and for clindamycin 40 mg/kg/day. For neonatal osteomyelitis, many experts would favor the use of IV antibiotics for the entire course given concerns about enteral antibiotic absorption and the limited knowledge of the pharmacokinetics of these agents in very young or premature neonates.

ADMISSION AND DISCHARGE CRITERIA

Most children will require admission for the treatment of osteomyelitis, to identify the causative pathogen, optimize the antimicrobial therapy, and demonstrate improving symptoms.

Discharge criteria include:

- Afebrile for at least 24 to 48 hours, general clinical improvement, and improvement of the localized osteomyelitis symptoms.
- Substantive improvement in inflammatory markers such as CRP; some studies have used a CRP <2-3 mg/dL as one discharge criterion.
- Ability to complete antibiotic therapy (oral or intravenous) as an outpatient.
- Comprehensive follow-up with primary care provider and/or subspecialists such as infectious disease specialist or orthopedic surgeon.

CONSULTATION

A collaborative and multi-disciplinary approach in the treatment of AHO promotes high-value care and optimizes outcomes. Oftentimes the multidisciplinary team includes an orthopedic surgeon, infectious disease specialist, physical therapist, and the hospital medicine team. It is especially important to consult an orthopedist if imaging reveals subperiosteal or soft tissue abscesses, sequestra, intramedullary purulence, or involvement of the growth plate. The surgeon's role may include performing the diagnostic procedure, decompression and drainage (when necessary), and long-term follow-up in complicated cases. In some institutions, interventional radiology (IR) may be consulted to perform the invasive diagnostic testing.

SPECIAL CONSIDERATIONS

Chronic Osteomyelitis Two to 5% of patients with AHO develop a chronic, suppurative course with intermittent acute exacerbations, which may develop after an open fracture or if initial therapy was quite delayed. Treatment consists of long-term antibiotics (intravenous followed by oral therapy for up to 6-12 months) and often requires surgical debridement of necrotic or poorly vascularized tissue or reconstructive surgery. The relative merits of prolonged intravenous therapy compared with short-course intravenous therapy followed by prolonged oral therapy have not been studied rigorously.

Chronic Nonbacterial Osteomyelitis Chronic nonbacterial osteomyelitis (CNO) is a noninfectious entity characterized by bony inflammation and pain, with or without fever. Some patients experience recurrent episodes with periodic exacerbations and remissions, for which the term "chronic recurrent multifocal osteomyelitis (CRMO)" was first used, but not all patients experience these symptoms, so the broader term CNO is preferred to encompass more presentations. CNO occurs in approximately 0.4 to 2 per 100,000 children, is more common in girls, and its pathogenesis is likely driven by both genetic and cytokine dysregulation components. If cultures are obtained, they are negative, and antibiotics do not alter the course of the disease. CNO is associated with Sweet syndrome, psoriasis, and pustulosis palmaris et plantaris; some authors consider CNO the pediatric form of SAPHO (synovitis, acne, pustulosis, hyperostosis, osteitis/osteomyelitis). Plain radiographs or technetium bone scan may demonstrate multiple areas of osteolysis and sclerosis, especially in the long bones, vertebral bodies, and clavicles. Treatment generally involves nonsteroidal anti-inflammatory drugs (NSAIDs). Other reported therapies include corticosteroids, methotrexate, sulfasalazine, tumor necrosis factor inhibitors, and bisphosphonates.

Brodie Abscess A Brodie abscess is a subacute form of osteomyelitis resulting in a collection of necrotic bone and pus in a fibrous capsule. It occurs most commonly in the long bones of adolescents and may be seen on plain radiographs. Management typically involves surgical drainage followed by antibiotic therapy.

Osteomyelitis in Patients With Sickle Hemoglobinopathies Osteomyelitis may be difficult to differentiate from vaso-occlusive crises in patients with sickle cell disease, because both syndromes can present with fever, bone pain, and tenderness. Spiking fevers above 39°C, chills, toxic appearance, and leukocytosis are more indicative of osteomyelitis in this population. Infection can be difficult to differentiate from infarction on imaging studies, and needle aspiration or biopsy of the affected site may be required. In the United States, *Salmonella* spp. are the most common pathogens, while in African patients, *Staphylococcus aureus* is more common. Prolonged parenteral therapy is sometimes required.

Pelvic Osteomyelitis Osteomyelitis of the pelvis or spine should be considered in children presenting with fever and gait abnormalities. Pain is often localized to the hip, groin, or buttocks, but may be poorly localized. Patients may also present with abdominal pain mimicking appendicitis. Point tenderness may be elicited over the affected bone, and rocking of the pelvis is often painful. As with other forms of osteomyelitis, *S. aureus* is the most commonly identified organism. Surgical drainage is often required, and pelvic venous thrombosis can be a complication.

***Pseudomonas* Osteochondritis** *Pseudomonas aeruginosa* infection of the bones and cartilage in the feet complicates up to 2% of puncture wounds. *P. aeruginosa* can be found in the linings of sneakers, although infection may occur after puncture wounds through other types of shoes or even bare feet. Management generally involves surgery to remove necrotic cartilage and to obtain a specimen for culture. Traditionally, an intravenous antibiotic with coverage for *Pseudomonas* as well as the more common pathogens (e.g., cefepime or piperacillin-tazobactam) was used for 7 to 14 days. However, adult studies indicate that oral ciprofloxacin for 7 to 14 days is usually adequate.

Spinal Osteomyelitis Osteomyelitis of the spine occurs along a spectrum including discitis, vertebral osteomyelitis, or spondylodiscitis; these presentations can occur in isolation or in combination. Discitis is an inflammatory process, usually of a lumbar disk, and is most common in children younger than 5 years. Discitis generally results from a low-grade bacterial infection, although some authors believe that it can be noninfectious (e.g., following trauma to the spine). Patients may present with a limp, backache, a lordotic gait, or refusal to walk. Fever is generally absent or low grade. Plain radiographs may demonstrate narrowing of the disk space. Empiric antibiotic therapy should cover *S. aureus* and GABHS. Clinical course and inflammatory markers should guide treatment duration as described above; some children with discitis appear to respond to a relatively short course of IV and total antibiotic therapy.

Vertebral osteomyelitis occurs in 1% to 3% of cases of osteomyelitis and is more common in boys. It may result from hematologic seeding of the vertebrae or through extension of a local infection such as discitis. *S. aureus* is the most common organism, but *B. henselae* (cat-scratch disease), *K. kingae*, and others have been reported. In some areas of the world, tuberculosis of the spine (Pott's disease) is not uncommon. Patients may manifest neurologic deficits or loss of normal spinal curvature, and surgery may be required urgently if there is evidence of spinal cord compression or large epidural abscess. Diagnosis is often based on MRI of the spine. Antibiotics should be administered for at least 4 weeks.

PREVENTION

No specific measures can be taken to prevent osteomyelitis. Cleaning of minor scrapes and wounds may reduce the chance of the transient bacteremia hypothesized to be part of the pathophysiology of this infection.

SEPTIC ARTHRITIS

BACKGROUND

Septic arthritis refers to bacterial invasion of the joint space by viable bacteria. Septic arthritis is commonly a childhood condition, with approximately half of all cases occurring in patients younger than 20 years. The peak incidence is in children younger than 3 years, and boys are affected approximately twice as often as girls.

PATHOPHYSIOLOGY

The synovium is a highly vascular layer of connective tissue that lacks a limiting basement membrane, which allows bacteria to enter the joint space more readily. Septic arthritis may occur after hematogenous seeding of the synovium during a transient episode of bacteremia, contiguous spread of an adjacent infection such as osteomyelitis, or direct inoculation during surgery or as a result of penetrating trauma. In response to bacterial endotoxin, cytokines such as tumor necrosis factor and interleukin-1 are released, which in turn stimulate the release of proteolytic enzymes and increase leukocyte migration. This combination of factors leads to destruction of the synovium and cartilage matrix. When the hip is involved, increased pressure within the joint can interrupt blood flow, leading to avascular necrosis of the femoral head; a similar process can occur in the shoulder joint. Although septic arthritis is rarely fatal since the introduction of antibiotics, destruction of the joint space can lead to long-term sequelae and prompt recognition and aggressive management are therefore critical.

S. aureus is the most common organism identified in patients with septic arthritis. Other frequently identified organisms include GABHS and *S. pneumoniae*. Now an unusual cause of septic arthritis, *H. influenzae* type B was commonly identified before the introduction of effective vaccines. *K. kingae* may be identified in toddlers with a preceding history of an upper respiratory tract infection and has been implicated in preschool outbreaks. In addition to *S. aureus*, neonates are also at risk for group B streptococci and gram-negative enteric bacilli. Neonates and sexually active adolescents are at risk for infection by *Neisseria gonorrhoeae*. In addition to the usual organisms, patients with sickle cell disease are at risk for bone and joint infections caused by *Salmonella* species. *Neisseria meningitidis* is a rare cause of septic arthritis, but a reactive arthritis is not uncommon following bacteremia or meningitis secondary to this organism.

CLINICAL PRESENTATIONS

Septic arthritis usually presents with systemic symptoms such as fever, malaise, and poor appetite. Local findings at the infected joint include edema, erythema, and tenderness, and patients tend to keep the affected joint in a position that maximizes intracapsular volume and therefore comfort. Knees are held moderately flexed, and hips are kept flexed, abducted, and externally rotated. Refusal to move an affected joint or extremity is referred to as pseudoparalysis, and even small passive movements may be extremely painful.

Approximately 75% to 80% of cases involve joints of the lower extremities, with the knees and hips most commonly affected. Other commonly affected joints include the ankles, wrists, elbows, and shoulders. Small, distal joints are less likely to be involved.

DIFFERENTIAL DIAGNOSIS

Multiple entities can be confused with septic arthritis, including trauma, bursitis, transient synovitis, reactive arthritis, Lyme arthritis, juvenile idiopathic arthritis, acute rheumatic fever, osteomyelitis, tumor, slipped capital femoral epiphysis, and Legg-Calvé-Perthes disease, among others. In particular, transient synovitis (also known as toxic synovitis) often mimics septic arthritis. Transient synovitis is presumed to be a postviral phenomenon, often affecting the hip in boys between the ages of 3 and 10 years; a number of clinical prediction rules have been developed to differentiate septic arthritis from transient synovitis, the most widely used of which is that by Kocher et al. The arthritis that occurs with Lyme disease is also a great imitator of septic arthritis and must be considered in endemic areas. Classically, it is a monoarticular or oligoarticular arthritis, involving the knee in 90% of cases, followed by ankle, elbow, and shoulder. The joint effusions in Lyme arthritis are typically larger than the effusions seen in septic arthritis, and usually the child is weight bearing with some active range of motion of the affected joint. A serum C6 peptide enzyme immunoassay has been shown to have good ability to discriminate between Lyme arthritis and septic arthritis, and other diagnostic criteria that include serum inflammatory markers and synovial white blood cell (WBC) count have been proposed (Lyme arthritis management is discussed further in Chapter 153, Infection-Associated Arthritis). In addition, multiple bacteria, including *N. meningitidis*, *Streptococcus* species, *Salmonella* species, and *Mycoplasma pneumoniae*, are associated with postinfectious reactive arthritides that may be difficult to differentiate from septic arthritis. In cases of suspected septic arthritis, concomitant osteomyelitis of an adjacent bone should also be suspected, especially in neonates and infants.

DIAGNOSTIC EVALUATION

In general, the WBC count, CRP, and ESR are elevated in patients with septic arthritis. Blood cultures are positive in about one-third of cases, and they occasionally yield the pathogen even when culture of the synovial fluid is negative.

For both osteomyelitis and septic arthritis it should be emphasized that, when possible, administration of antibiotics should be delayed until cultures can be obtained. The cornerstone of diagnosis is the evaluation of aspirated joint fluid. Synovial fluid should be aspirated into a heparinized syringe. If *K. kingae* is a concern, synovial fluid should be inoculated directly into a blood culture bottle to increase the chance of recovering this organism; PCR for *K. kingae* is now commercially available for synovial fluid specimens as well. Joint fluid should be sent for Gram stain, aerobic and anaerobic culture, and cell count with differential. Typical findings of aspirated synovial fluid are presented in **Table 101-3.** Note that Lyme arthritis can have WBC counts in the septic range, but the Gram stain and bacterial culture are invariably negative.

Plain radiographs may demonstrate a widened joint space in a patient with a septic hip, but they are most useful for eliminating other conditions such as fractures, Legg-Calvé-Perthes disease, and slipped capital femoral epiphysis. Ultrasonography is useful for identifying and quantifying a joint effusion, especially in deeper joints such as the hips, and it may be used to guide needle aspiration of these joints. MRI is often performed and may play a critical role in diagnosing concomitant osteomyelitis. However, imaging studies should not delay joint aspiration or prompt surgical and antibiotic management when septic arthritis is suspected.

MANAGEMENT

Antibiotic therapy should be initiated immediately after blood and synovial fluid cultures have been obtained. The Gram stain can help guide the initial antibiotic choice; however, antibiotic therapy should not be delayed if these specimens cannot be obtained promptly. If gram-positive cocci are seen, or if the patient is severely ill, coverage for community-acquired MRSA should be considered, using clindamycin, vancomycin, linezolid, or others based on the local antibiogram. If gram-negative organisms are found, a third-generation cephalosporin will cover most gram-positive organisms (except MRSA), as well as *K. kingae*, *Salmonella* species, and *H. influenzae*. If no organisms are seen on Gram stain, empiric antibiotics should target *S. aureus* based on local susceptibility patterns (using cefazolin, clindamycin, vancomycin, or other agents). In sexually active adolescents, ceftriaxone may be used to cover *N. gonorrhoeae*. Neonates are often treated with ceftazidime or ceftriaxone, which cover the most likely causative agents. However, if there is concern for MRSA, appropriate coverage should be added as above. Coverage can be narrowed once identification of the organism and susceptibilities are available. Table 101-1 lists the common bacterial etiologies and recommended antibiotics.

Most authors agree that septic arthritis of the hip is a medical emergency requiring immediate surgical drainage; septic arthritis of the shoulder is often treated similarly. When other joints are affected, some authors advocate repeated daily arthrocentesis, which proved to be superior to surgical drainage in an adult study. However, if there is a large amount of fibrin or debris, the infection is loculated, or there is a lack of improvement within 3 days, formal surgical drainage with arthroscopy or arthrotomy is recommended. Physical therapy may be beneficial as adjunctive management in some cases, especially when the child is reluctant to use the joint.

In uncomplicated cases, a prospective randomized trial by Peltola et al in 2009 demonstrated that 10 days of therapy is as effective as 3 weeks of therapy, provided that a good clinical response has been achieved and the CRP has decreased below 2mg/dL. One critique of this study is that it did not include patients with MRSA or the USA300 clone of *S. aureus*, based on being conducted before their widespread prominence. Current guidance from the AAP Committee on Infectious Diseases recommends a total duration of therapy of 2 to 3 weeks, often with initial antibiotics given intravenously until the patient has demonstrated clear clinical improvement and inflammatory markers are improved. In the modern era, serious sequelae of septic arthritis are uncommon, but close follow-up in all patients and physical therapy in selected patients are nonetheless essential to monitor for any loss of joint function, growth plate damage and growth arrest, and avascular necrosis.

TABLE 101-3 Typical Synovial Fluid Findings

Finding	Septic Arthritis	Transient Synovitis	Normal Joint
Color	Serosanguineous	Yellow	Yellow
Clarity	Turbid	Generally clear, but depends on number of white blood cells	Clear
White blood cells	>50,000-100,000/mm^3	5000-15,000/mm^3	<200/mm^3
Neutrophils (%)	>75	<25	<25
Culture	Positive in 70%-80%	Negative	Negative
Glucose	<40 mg/dL	Equal to serum	Equal to serum

ADMISSION AND DISCHARGE CRITERIA

As with osteomyelitis, most children will require admission for the treatment of septic arthritis, to identify the causative pathogen, optimize the antimicrobial therapy, and demonstrate improving symptoms.

Discharge criteria include:

- Clinical improvement with resolution of fever and improved range of motion of the affected joint, along with decreased inflammatory markers.
- Ability to complete intravenous or oral antibiotic therapy (oral or intravenous) as an outpatient.
- Reliable outpatient follow-up with orthopedics and potentially with physical therapy.

CONSULTATION

Involvement of Orthopedic surgeons and Infectious Diseases specialists is important both in the acute surgical and medical management of septic arthritis, and to provide longer-term follow up after hospitalization to monitor for late complications.

PREVENTION

As with osteomyelitis, no specific measures can be taken to prevent septic arthritis. Cleaning of minor scrapes and wounds may reduce the chance of the transient bacteremia hypothesized to be part of the pathophysiology of this infection.

KEY POINTS

- Pediatric bone and joint infections are serious conditions requiring prompt, aggressive evaluation, and management.
- Various imaging modalities play an important role in diagnosis; MRI has generally become the preferred modality.
- If at all possible, perform blood and bone/joint fluid cultures *before* initiating antibiotic therapy. If a patient is septic or not stable, begin antibiotics after blood culture is obtained.
- Orthopedic (or interventional radiology) consultation is critical for obtaining proper specimens. The orthopedist may need to do additional procedures in complicated cases.
- Empiric antibiotic therapy may need to include coverage for MRSA based on your local *S. aureus* epidemiology—consult your local hospital antibiogram. When microbiology laboratory results are available, antibiotics can be adjusted to provide optimal therapy.
- Most patients should be able to transition to oral antibiotic therapy, guided by clinical response and the use of inflammatory markers, unless the causative organism has no oral therapy options. Appropriate follow-up is required.

SUGGESTED READINGS

Benvenuti MA, An TJ, Mignemi ME, Martus JE, Thomsen IP, Schoenecker JG. Effects of antibiotic timing on culture results and clinical outcomes in pediatric musculoskeletal infection. *J Pediatr Orthop*. 2016;22:22.

Cruz AI Jr, Anari JB, Ramirez JM, Sankar WN, Baldwin KD. Distinguishing pediatric Lyme arthritis of the hip from transient synovitis and acute bacterial septic arthritis: a systematic review and meta-analysis. *Cureus*. 2018;10(1):e2112.

Dartnell J, Ramachandran M, Katchburian M. Haematogenous acute and subacute paediatric osteomyelitis: a systematic review of the literature. *J Bone Joint Surg Br*. 2012;94(5):584-595.

Dich VQ, Nelson JD, Haltalin KC. Osteomyelitis in infants and children. *Am J Dis Child*. 1975;129:1273-1275.

Donaldson N, Sanders J, Child J, Parker S. Acute hematogenous bacterial osteoarticular infections in children. *Pediatr Rev*. 2020;41(3):120-136.

Ferri I, Ristori G, Lisi C, Galli L, Chiappini E. Characteristics, management and outcomes of spondylodiscitis in children: a systematic review. *Antibiotics (Basel)*. 2020;10(1):30.

Grant DS, Neville DN, Levas M, et al. Validation of septic knee monoarthritis prediction rule in a Lyme disease endemic area. *Pediatr Emerg Care*. 2022;38(2):e881-e885.

Jaramillo D, Dormans JP, Delgado J, et al. Hematogenous osteomyelitis in infants and children: imaging of a changing disease. *Radiology*. 2017; 283:629-643.

Karen R, Shah SS, Srivastava R, et al.; Pediatric Research in Inpatient Settings Network. Comparative effectiveness of intravenous vs oral antibiotics for postdischarge treatment of acute osteomyelitis in children. *JAMA Pediatr*. 2015; 169:120–128.

Kocher MS, Zurakowski D, Kasser JR. Differentiating between septic arthritis and transient synovitis of the hip in children: an evidence-based clinical prediction algorithm. *J Bone Joint Surg Am*. 1999;81(12):1662-1670.

Kocher MS, Mandiga R, Zurakowski D, Barnewolt C, Kasser JR. Validation of a clinical prediction rule for the differentiation between septic arthritis and transient synovitis of the hip in children. *J Bone Joint Surg Am*. 2004;86(8):1629-1635.

Manz N, Krieg AH, Heininger U, Ritz N. Evaluation of the current use of imaging modalities and pathogen detection in children with acute osteomyelitis and septic arthritis. *Eur J Pediatr*. 2018; 177:1071–80.

McNeil JC, Forbes AR, Vallejo JG, et al. Role of operative or interventional radiology-guided cultures for osteomyelitis. *Pediatrics*. 2016; 137(5):e20154616.

McNeil JC, Vallejo JG, Kok EY, et al. Clinical and microbiologic variables predictive of orthopedic complications following Staphylococcus aureus acute hematogenous osteoarticular infections in children. *Clin Infect Dis*. 2019;69:195.

Nigrovic LE, Bennett JE, Balamuth F, et al. Diagnostic performance of C6 enzyme immunoassay for Lyme arthritis. *Pediatrics*. 2020;145(1): e20190593.

Nuruzzaman F, Zhao Y, Ferguson PJ. Chronic nonbacterial osteomyelitis: insights into pathogenesis, assessment, and treatment. *Rheum Dis Clin North Am*. 2021;47(4):691-705.

Pääkkönen M, Kallio MJ, Kallio PE, Peltola H. Sensitivity of erythrocyte sedimentation rate and C-reactive protein in childhood bone and joint infections. *Clin Orthop Relat Res*. 2010;468(3): 861-866.

Pääkkönen M, Kallio MTJ, Kallio PE, Peltola H. Significance of negative cultures in the treatment of acute hematogenous bone and joint infections in children. *J Pediatr Infect Dis Soc*. 2013;2:119-125.

Palmer B, Wang ME. Clinical guideline highlights for the hospitalist: diagnosis and management of acute hematogenous osteomyelitis in children. *J Hosp Med*. 2022;17:114-116.

Peltola H, Pääkkönen M, Kallio P, Kallio MJ; Osteomyelitis-Septic Arthritis (OM-SA) Study Group. Prospective, randomized trial of 10 days versus 30 days of antimicrobial treatment, including a short-term course of parenteral therapy, for childhood septic arthritis. *Clin Infect Dis*. 2009;48(9):1201-1210.

Peltola H, Pääkkönen M, Kallio P, Kallio MJT. Short- vs long-term antimicrobial treatment for acute hematogenous osteomyelitis of childhood: prospective, randomized trial on 131 culture positive cases. *Pediatr Infect Dis J*. 2010;29(12):1123-1128.

Russell CD, Ramaesh R, Kalima P, Murray A, Gaston MS. Microbiological characteristics of acute osteoarticular infections in children. *J Med Microbiol*. 2015;64(Pt 4):446-453.

Samara E, Spyropoulou V, Tabard-Fougere A, et al. Kingella kingae and osteoarticular infections. *Pediatrics*. 2019;144(6):e20191509.

Shaikh N, Umscheid J, Rizvi S, et al. National trends of acute osteomyelitis and peripherally inserted central catheters in children. *Hosp Pediatr*. 2021;11(7):662-670.

Tetzlaff TR, McCracken GH Jr, Nelson JD. Oral antibiotic therapy for skeletal infections of children. II. Therapy of osteomyelitis and suppurative arthritis. *J Pediatr*. 1978;92(3):485-490.

van der Merwe M, Rooks K, Crawford H, et al. The effect of antibiotic timing on culture yield in paediatric osteoarticular infection. *J Child Orthop*. 2019;13:114-119.

Woods CR, Bradley JS, Chatterjee A, et al. Clinical Practice Guideline by the Pediatric Infectious Diseases Society and the Infectious Diseases Society of America: 2021 Guideline on Diagnosis and Management of Acute Hematogenous Osteomyelitis in Pediatrics. *J Pediatric Infect Dis Soc*. 2021;10(8):801-844.

Yagupsky P, El Houmami N, Fluss R. Outbreaks of *Kingella kingae* infections in daycare centers suggest tissue tropism of the causative strains. *J Pediatric Infect Dis Soc*. 2020;9(6):695-700.

Zaoutis T, Localio AR, Leckerman K, Saddlemire S, Bertoch D, Keren R. Prolonged intravenous therapy versus early transition to oral antimicrobial therapy for acute osteomyelitis in children. *Pediatrics*. 2009;123:636-642.

Zhao Y, Wu EY, Oliver MS, et al. Consensus treatment plans for chronic nonbacterial osteomyelitis refractory to nonsteroidal antiinflammatory drugs and/or with active spinal lesions. *Arthritis Care Res (Hoboken)*. 2018;70(8):1228-1237.

CHAPTER 102 Skin and Soft Tissue Infections

Andrew Haynes, MD and Kimberly O'Hara, MD

INTRODUCTION

Intact skin serves as an effective mechanical barrier to prevent infection, and constant desquamation continually removes potentially invasive bacteria. When skin integrity is compromised by injury or disease, patients are at increased risk for skin and other soft tissue infections, including staphylococcal scalded skin syndrome, cellulitis, erysipelas, pyomyositis, and necrotizing skin infections, among others. A patient's age, comorbidities, immunocompetency, immunization status, as well as community prevalence of methicillin-resistant *Staphylococcus aureus* (MRSA), and other exposures impact the type, progression, and treatment of the infection. Hospitalists should know when a patient may need to be admitted to the hospital, if consultation with sub-specialists or surgical intervention is required, appropriate treatment options, expected clinical course, and discharge criteria for children presenting with skin and soft tissues infections.

STAPHYLOCOCCAL SCALDED SKIN SYNDROME

BACKGROUND

Staphylococcal scalded skin syndrome (SSSS), alternatively known as Ritter's disease, is a toxin-mediated exfoliative dermatitis caused by toxigenic strains of *S. aureus*, characterized by skin tenderness and erythema, flaccid bullae, and eventual skin sloughing. The disease occurs most commonly in children with slight male predominance; 98% being younger than the age of 6 years, 62% under the age of 2 years, and neonates being especially susceptible. SSSS can lead to serious complications, such as pneumonia, hypothermia, dehydration, and secondary infections, particularly in newborns and immunocompromised adults in whom these complications can be lethal.

PATHOPHYSIOLOGY

SSSS generally begins with colonization of the conjunctivae, naris, perioral region, perineum, or umbilical stump by specific strains of *S. aureus* capable of producing the exfoliative toxins A (ETA) or B (ETB). ETA accounts for an estimated 89% of cases. Both exfoliative toxins cause intraepidermal splitting at the zona granulosa by cleaving desmoglein 1 complex, an important desmosomal protein, leading to fragile, flaccid bullae and eventual detachment of the superficial epidermis. Of note, desmoglein 3 is more prominent than desmoglein 1 in mucous membranes, and since the exfoliative toxins only target desmoglein 1, mucous membranes are characteristically spared in SSSS. Subsequent hematogenous spread of the toxin results in other areas of skin involvement and constitutional symptoms in SSSS. While the toxin spreads hematogenously, the toxin-producing *S. aureus* population remains localized to the colonized area (generally the perioral region), so the blood and diffuse skin lesions are typically sterile. The exfoliative toxins, unlike the toxin involved in staphylococcal toxic shock syndrome, are not known to produce direct hemodynamic compromise. Neonates are thought to be particularly vulnerable to SSSS due to their immature immunity and decreased renal excretion of the toxin.

CLINICAL PRESENTATION

The clinical presentation of SSSS depends on age; neonates tend to present with generalized exfoliation, while older children develop a tender scarlatiniform eruption and localized bullous impetigo; older infants and toddlers present with a combination of these with desquamation of their skin. A local skin infection may be the first sign of SSSS, with impetigo-associated crusting around the nares and perioral skin among the most common. Other possible sources include a purulent circumcision site or umbilical stump, or rarely, as a complication of measles or varicella though the source of infection may not be apparent. A prodrome of fever, irritability, malaise, and coryza is common, especially in neonates and young children. Following an incubation period of 1 to 10 days after initial skin infection, patients develop diffuse, tender, blanchable erythroderma usually beginning around the mouth. Flaccid, thin-walled bullae then appear within 1 to 2 days of the erythroderma and can demonstrate a positive Nikolsky sign, where applying lateral pressure to the border of a blister leads to dislodgment of the normal epidermis and extension of the blister. The bullae typically rupture within hours, followed by sloughing of the superficial epidermis in large sheets (**Figure 102-1**). Perioral radial fissures may also be present; however, other mucus membranes are spared (**Figure 102-2**). Within 1 to 3 days of the initial skin detachment, a second flaky desquamation of the denuded skin occurs. Due to the denuded skin, dehydration from fluid loss, temperature instability, and secondary infections may occur. The dermis is not typically involved, and scarring is not expected as the skin gradually heals over the following 1 to 2 weeks.

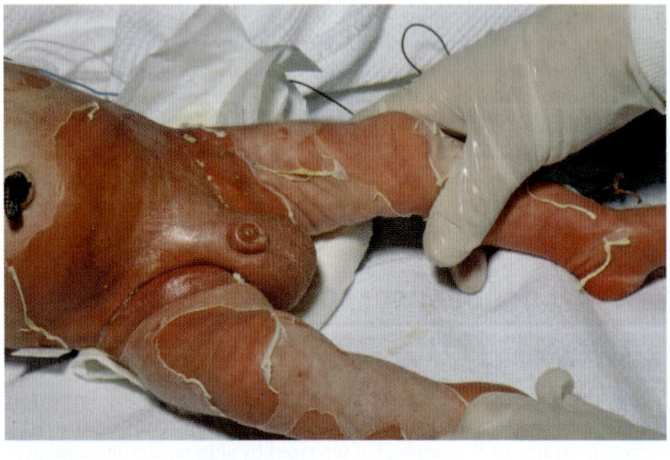

FIGURE 102-1. Staphylococcal scalded skin syndrome of a neonate with sloughing of superficial epidermis and denuded, glistening cutaneous surfaces.

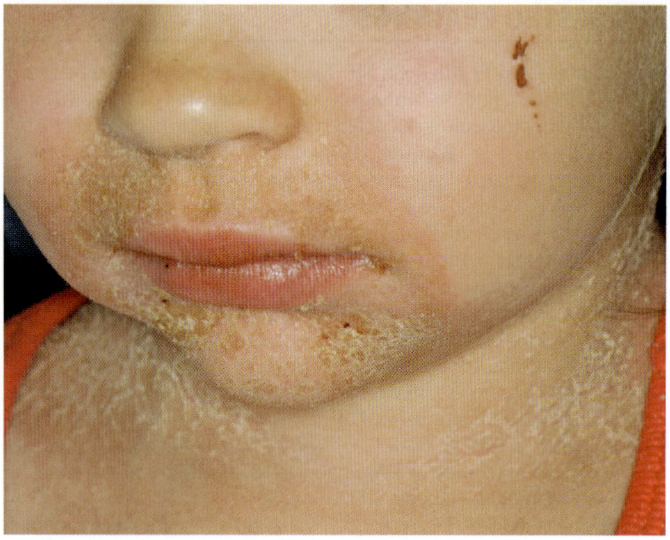

FIGURE 102-2. Staphylococcal scalded skin syndrome of an older child highlighting perioral radial fissures.

DIFFERENTIAL DIAGNOSIS

The main differential diagnosis to consider for SSSS is toxic epidermal necrolysis (TEN), a severe exfoliative dermatitis that is usually drug induced and has a high mortality rate. Mucosal membranes are typically spared in SSSS, which helps to distinguish it from TEN. SSSS may also mimic Kawasaki Disease (KD), as both can present with erythematous exanthema. Additional laboratory testing, mucosal involvement (among the other clinical criteria of KD), and development of a Nikolsky sign can all help differentiate between these two disease processes. Other diagnoses to consider are Stevens-Johnson syndrome, scarlet fever, bullous impetigo, burn injury, epidermolysis bullosa, graft-versus-host disease, erythrodermic psoriasis, pemphigus, and methylmalonic acidemia.

DIAGNOSTIC EVALUATION

The diagnosis of SSSS can usually be made on clinical presentation alone. The fluid within intact bullae is generally sterile, and swabs should be directed toward more typical areas of carriage or sites that appear purulent. However, wound cultures and swabs of the nasopharynx, eyes, axillae, groin, and any other suspected foci of infection, such as the umbilicus in neonates, can also help identify the likely causal pathogen (typically methicillin-sensitive *S. aureus* or MSSA and rarely MRSA) and guide antibiotic selection. Because SSSS is generally a clinical diagnosis and improves with supportive care and anti-staphylococcal antibiotics, most workup beyond surface cultures (e.g., blood and urine cultures, complete blood count, inflammatory markers, and other labs) rarely changes the outcome (such as length of stay, cost, readmission rates, and return rates to the emergency department) in children as found by Neubauer et al. in 2018. Blood cultures are usually negative, but should be considered in neonates or those who are critically ill or with hemodynamic compromise.

If the diagnosis is in question, particularly if TEN cannot be excluded, microscopic examination of a blister roof or a skin biopsy could be performed; SSSS will demonstrate cleavage at the level of the granular epidermis and TEN usually below the dermal-epidermal junction.

MANAGEMENT

Adequate analgesia and minimizing skin manipulation are the mainstays of treatment. Although there are minimal data guiding antibiotic use, and it is possible that some patients could improve with supportive care only, anti-staphylococcal antibiotics are almost universally used. Cefazolin (or alternatively a penicillinase-resistant penicillin, such as nafcillin or oxacillin) is recommended because most cases are due to MSSA. Addition of clindamycin may be considered for additional MRSA coverage depending on regional MRSA prevalence, but clindamycin monotherapy is generally not recommended because of staphylococcal resistance. Vancomycin or linezolid could also be considered in areas with a high prevalence of community-acquired MRSA or in those who have failed to respond to anti-MSSA therapy; however, SSSS from MRSA is much less common and is more frequently reported in those with risk factors, such as recent healthcare exposure. Clindamycin has also been considered in those with severe illness to inhibit bacterial ribosomal exotoxin production, but there are no data showing a clear benefit from adding clindamycin. Patients with severe allergy to penicillin may receive cefazolin or vancomycin. If *S. aureus* is isolated from culture, antibiotic susceptibilities can guide therapy.

Even when antibiotics are started early in the disease process, SSSS can continue to progress though most patients will see some clinical improvement within 2 to 3 days. Continued symptoms for multiple days after antibiotics are started can still occur on appropriate therapy and does not necessarily indicate staphylococcal resistance. Patients can be transitioned from IV to oral antibiotics once clinically improved. The optimal duration of total antibiotic therapy is not definitively known, but a total course of 7 to 10 days is generally sufficient.

Corticosteroids should not be given, and topical antibiotics have not been shown to be effective. Intravenous (IV) immunoglobulin had also been proposed to treat SSSS, but there is no definitive evidence of benefit and its use has been linked to longer hospitalizations.

Supportive skin care, including application of thick emollients along with semi-occlusive, nonadherent dressings (similar to how burns are treated), should be provided. Minimizing skin manipulation is important, and adherent stickers (such as for cardiac monitoring, unless necessary) should be avoided. Hydration status and electrolytes should be monitored closely. Depending on the severity of skin involvement, admission to the intensive care unit (ICU) or a burn unit may be necessary. Serious complications can develop, such as hypothermia, electrolyte derangements, dehydration, renal failure, and secondary infections even with optimal therapy. Recurrence is rare and not expected due to the development of neutralizing antibodies, but this has been reported in the context of immature immune systems or immunosuppression.

ADMISSION CRITERIA

Patients with suspected SSSS should be admitted for monitoring, microbial cultures, intravenous antibiotics, analgesia, and supportive skin care. Outpatient therapy may be an option for older children as their disease tends to be milder or more similar to bullous impetigo. ICU or burn unit transfer may be required for fluid and electrolytes management, if temperature control becomes difficult, if the patient becomes critically ill, or if extensive time is needed to provide supportive skin care.

DISCHARGE CRITERIA

Patients may be discharged once hemodynamically stable, maintaining adequate hydration and nutrition orally, and if pain is well controlled. Antibiotics can be transitioned to an oral formulation at discharge. Caregivers should be able to provide all necessary supportive skin care though home nursing services may be an option for some families.

CONSULTATION

Dermatology can assist with diagnosis, specifically if a skin biopsy is indicated to exclude TEN. Infectious diseases consultation can guide diagnosis and initial and ongoing antibiotic recommendations. Wound care specialists can advise and assist with emollients and dressing needs if needed. Critical care may be needed if any complications develop. Infection control services should be involved if an outbreak is suspected.

SPECIAL CONSIDERATIONS

Adults possess the neutralizing antibodies against the exotoxins and have increased renal clearance of the exotoxins so it is rare for healthy adults to acquire SSSS. Adults who are immunocompromised or have an underlying comorbidity are more likely to develop SSSS, unlike children with SSSS who are typically otherwise healthy. SSSS preferentially impacts neonates and children due to their lack of antitoxin antibodies and decreased renal excretion of the toxin. The prognosis in children is excellent, while the prognosis in adults varies, with mortality rates as high as 60% reported.

PREVENTION

Close attention to hand hygiene and institution of contact precautions are paramount to prevent the development of outbreaks, which have been reported in multiple nurseries. Patients admitted to the hospital with SSSS should remain on contact precautions for the duration of their hospitalization.

KEY POINTS

- Staphylococcal scalded skin syndrome is an exfoliative dermatitis caused by toxigenic strains of *S. aureus* and is predominantly a disease of young children or the immunocompromised.
- Following an initial local infection and prodrome of fever, irritability, and coryza, a tender erythroderma ensues, with eventual development of flaccid, thin-walled bullae demonstrating a positive Nikolsky sign, with sparing of the mucous membranes.
- Prior to initiating antibiotics, sites that appear purulent as well as common areas of carriage should be cultured to provide antibiotic susceptibility data.
- Treatment involves prompt initiation of intravenous antibiotics, supportive skin care, analgesia, and close attention to hydration, electrolytes, and temperature.

CELLULITIS AND ERYSIPELAS

BACKGROUND

Cellulitis and erysipelas, referring to skin infections that develop as a result of bacterial entry by breeches in the skin barrier, manifest as areas of skin erythema, edema, and warmth. They are distinguished from one another in several important aspects, primarily by the depth of infection. Specifically, cellulitis is an acute, noncontagious infection of the skin and subcutaneous tissue. Erysipelas is a superficial infection, affecting the upper dermis with prominent lymphatic involvement. Raised edges and well-demarcated edges of affected skin are seen in erysipelas and may help differentiate it from cellulitis as well as other skin infections. Both conditions require prompt diagnosis and antibiotic therapy. The majority of children can be managed safely and effectively in the outpatient setting, but hospital admission may be prudent in some cases. It is important to note that there has been an increasing burden on Emergency Departments from children presenting with cellulitis or erysipelas, possibly due to disparities in healthcare access, and that the mean costs of children presenting with these conditions has recently tripled.

PATHOPHYSIOLOGY

The most common causative organisms of cellulitis are *Streptococcus pyogenes* (group A beta-hemolytic streptococcus, GABHS) and *S. aureus*, but other gram-positive bacteria such as *Streptococcus pneumoniae* and group C or G streptococci may be involved. GABHS is by far the most common causative organism of erysipelas, although groups B, C, D, and G streptococci, and uncommonly, *S. aureus*, *Klebsiella pneumoniae*, and *Yersinia enterocolitica* may be involved. Although not reliable distinguishing features, infection with *S. aureus* tends to be more localized and suppurative, whereas *S. pyogenes* tends to spread more rapidly with associated lymphangitis.

The skin barrier may be compromised by trauma, pre-existing skin infections, such as impetigo, eczema, fungal infections, ulceration, or fissured toe webs. Breaks in the skin may be clinically inapparent. Venous and lymphatic damage from past surgeries, trauma, thromboses, or congenital vascular malformations may result in chronic limb edema and serve as significant predisposing factors for cellulitis.

CLINICAL PRESENTATION

Cellulitis presents as ill-defined erythema, warmth, edema, and/or tenderness of the affected skin in a patient who may also have systemic symptoms of fever, malaise, and fatigue. Although a leading edge of the erythema can sometimes be determined, this edge is not raised or sharply demarcated from the adjacent normal skin (**Figure 102-3**).

Periorbital (preseptal) cellulitis deserves mention due to its potential confusion with the more concerning diagnosis of orbital cellulitis. Periorbital cellulitis is limited to the periorbital tissues, and while often due to skin trauma, it can also occur via spread of *Haemophilus influenzae* type b (among the unimmunized) or *S. pneumoniae* from the paranasal sinuses or bloodstream. If the infection crosses the orbital septum, it may result in orbital cellulitis, which is concerning for its potential to cause orbital abscesses as well as cavernous sinus thrombosis. Patients with orbital cellulitis may present with proptosis, ophthalmoplegia, and decreased visual acuity, in which case computed tomography (CT) imaging and ophthalmology consultation are indicated.

Perianal streptococcal dermatitis (sometimes referred to as cellulitis), presenting with sharply circumscribed perianal erythema, is also a distinct clinical entity that is important to recognize. It may be associated with rectal itching, painful defecation, constipation, and blood-streaked stools. Fever is rare, but a concomitant streptococcal pharyngitis is sometimes present.

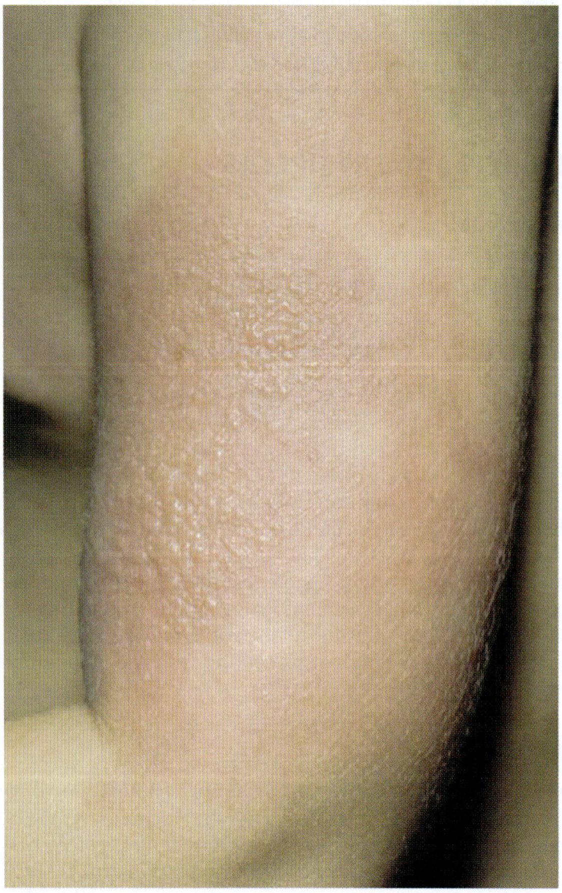

FIGURE 102-3. Cellulitis, presenting as ill-defined erythema, warmth, edema, pain, and in this case multiple overlying vesicles.

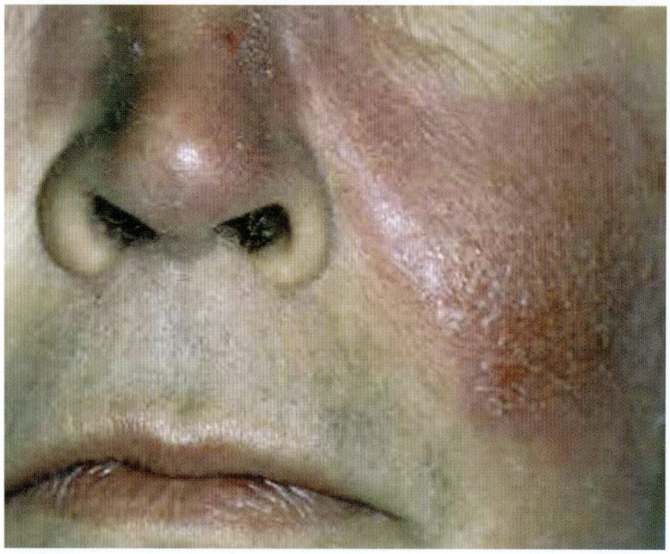

FIGURE 102-4. Erysipelas, characterized by a bright red, confluent, indurated, tender plaque with elevated, sharply defined margins.

Erysipelas is characterized by the abrupt onset of fever, chills, and malaise, followed by the development of a warm, shiny, bright red, tender plaque with elevated, sharply defined margins (**Figure 102-4**). Due to the tender, "firey" rash or skin involvement, erysipelas is also known as "St. Anthony's Fire." It classically presents with better-defined borders and develops more quickly, while cellulitis has ill-defined borders and develops more slowly. In erysipelas, superficial cutaneous edema surrounding hair follicles and lymphatic involvement can lead to a "peau d'orange" (orange peel) appearance of the skin. The face, scalp, and hands are most commonly involved in pediatrics. Involvement of the ear (Milian's ear sign) indicates erysipelas and not cellulitis, as the pinna does not contain deep dermal and subcutaneous tissue.

Distinct clinical settings or presentations may suggest alternative infectious agents. In neonates, group B *Streptococcus* (GBS) should be suspected, and a full sepsis evaluation initiated. Buccal cellulitis, a facial cellulitis with red-blue discoloration of the cheek, suggests infection with *H. influenzae* type b, but this is rarely seen since routine childhood Hib immunization. Infections following cat or dog bites may be due to *Pasteurella multocida* or *Capnocytophaga canimorsus*. Infection after contact with fresh or salt water should raise the possibility of *Aeromonas hydrophila* or *Vibrio vulnificus*, respectively, as well as *Pseudomonas* species. *Pseudomonas* should also be suspected in diabetic patients, particularly if they have foot ulcers. Circumstances, such as frequent subcutaneous injection of medications (e.g. insulin) or recreational drugs, as well as iatrogenic or congenital immunosuppression necessitate a wider differential diagnosis (including a large array of bacterial, fungal, and mycobacterial organisms) and greater scrutiny in terms of diagnosis and management.

With early diagnosis and treatment, the prognosis is excellent. However, complications of cellulitis include abscess formation, bacteremia, osteomyelitis, septic arthritis, necrotizing soft tissue infections, and streptococcus-associated nephritis. Recurrent bouts of cellulitis may occur after successful treatment as each episode of cellulitis causes lymphatic inflammation and damage, which may lead to lymphedema and that predisposes to cellulitis formation.

DIFFERENTIAL DIAGNOSIS

There are several noninfectious causes of swollen, warm, red skin that must be considered in the differential diagnosis of cellulitis and erysipelas. Most can be distinguished by the history and the lack of systemic symptoms, but in some cases, a skin biopsy may be needed to make the correct diagnosis. With insect bite hypersensitivity reaction or allergic contact dermatitis, itch is usually the predominant symptom, and the history may provide a clue to the cause. These hypersensitivity reactions tend to be more acute than cellulitis. Injection sites from vaccines administered intramuscularly may also present with local reactions, but these rarely become infected. It is important to distinguish between cellulitis and abscesses, as well-defined fluid collections often require surgical incision and drainage. Necrotizing soft tissue infections, septic arthritis, and deep venous thrombosis may also present with some similar findings. Toxic shock syndrome may include skin erythema and warmth though hemodynamic compromise would not be expected in most cases of cellulitis.

DIAGNOSTIC EVALUATION

Cellulitis and erysipelas can usually be diagnosed by their typical clinical presentation, and diagnostic studies, including blood cultures and cutaneous aspirates, biopsies or swabs, are not routinely needed. Interestingly, GABHS can be readily isolated from perianal swabs in perianal streptococcal dermatitis, but in most other cellulitic settings, wound swabs are typically unhelpful. Punch biopsies may be helpful when the diagnosis is in question, the response to therapy has been poor, or more unusual organisms are suspected (for example, in an immunocompromised patient or with unusual exposures). Blood cultures are not typically useful in managing immunocompetent patients hospitalized with uncomplicated superficial skin and soft tissues infections.

Radiologic studies are not helpful in managing cellulitis but should be obtained if symptoms suggest an associated osteomyelitis, orbital cellulitis, or other infection that may require surgical intervention.

MANAGEMENT

Antibiotic management should be guided by the likely causal pathogens. In most cases of cellultis, treatment should cover GABHS and MSSA. In patients able to receive oral therapy, a first-generation cephalosporin (such as cephalexin) is typically recommended. Erysipelas can be difficult to distinguish from cellulitis though patients with mild erysipelas may be treated with oral penicillin or amoxicillin.

Coverage of methicillin-resistant *S. aureus* (MRSA) is prudent in regions with high MRSA prevalence or if patients have associated purulent drainage/abscess or have certain risk factors (e.g., critically ill, history of MRSA infection, evidence of MRSA infection elsewhere, nasal MRSA colonization, and cellulitis associated with penetrating trauma or injection drug use). For suspected MRSA infections, clindamycin, trimethoprim sulfamethoxazole (TMP-SMX), linezolid, or doxycycline (durations <21 days are considered safe in children regardless of age) can be considered. Doxycycline does not have good antistreptococcal activity, so it is generally combined with amoxicillin or cephalexin if the causal pathogen is unknown. The other listed anti-MRSA agents are likely sufficient as monotherapy even if GABHS is possible.

For those who require hospitalization or who are unable to tolerate oral medications, antibiotics should be administered intravenously. If there is a low likelihood of MRSA, cefazolin (or an antistaphylococcal penicillin) is a reasonable option to reliably treat both GABHS and MSSA. IV options that expand coverage to MRSA include vancomycin, daptomycin, ceftaroline, or linezolid.

It is typical for cellulitis to continue progressing while on appropriate therapy in the first 24 to 48 hours. Extension beyond the initial borders of cellulitis after starting antibiotic therapy does not necessarily warrant a change in antibiotic. The total duration of antibiotic therapy in most cases should be 5 days but must be gauged by the health of the patient and duration extended (sometimes up to 10-14 days) for severe infections or if symptoms are not improved during this time period. Management should also include elevation of the affected area and treatment of any underlying conditions, such as lymphedema, ulcers, poorly controlled diabetes mellitus, and eczema, which can lead to skin breakdown or edema.

When the presentation or clinical setting increases the concern for uncommon pathogens, antibiotic coverage should be broadened appropriately. Empiric therapy is initiated based on the presentation, particular exposures (such as water, soil, etc.), and the appearance of the involved skin. For example, in children with facial or periorbital cellulitis, the possibility of *S. pneumoniae* and *H. influenzae* should be considered in the context of the patient's age and immunization status, with antibiotics chosen accordingly. If the pathogen is identified and antibiotic susceptibilities are available, coverage can be adjusted.

ADMISSION CRITERIA

Most children with cellulitis or erysipelas can be treated as outpatients, but admission should be considered in the following situations: most neonates due to the need for initial parenteral antibiotics, if the child appears ill or is immunocompromised, concern for necrotizing infection, if there is clinical worsening despite appropriate outpatient therapy, if the patient is unable to tolerate oral medications, or poor adherence with treatment.

DISCHARGE CRITERIA

If a patient does require admission, several criteria should be met prior to discharge home. The patient must be able to take adequate oral fluids as well as oral medications, with improving clinical symptoms, such as decreased erythema and tenderness at the infected site and a downtrending fever curve or no fever.

CONSULTATION

While not typically required, dermatology consultation can be obtained when the diagnosis is in question or if punch biopsies are needed to identify unusual organisms. Pediatric infectious disease consultation can be obtained in the context of unusual suspected organisms or failed treatment response. Ophthalmology consultation is indicated if there is concern for orbital cellulitis.

SPECIAL CONSIDERATIONS

In neonates who are systemically well and not febrile, cefazolin monotherapy is reasonable in areas with low MRSA rates. If a neonate is febrile, ill-appearing, or being an admitted after a larger workup (e.g., blood, urine, and CSF cultures were obtained), empiric therapy should include coverage for common neonatal pathogens.

In nondiabetic adult patients, systemic corticosteroids could be considered to complement antibiotic treatment of cellulitis, but this is not the case for pediatric patients.

Children diagnosed with GABHS skin infections should not return to child care settings or school until they are well-appearing and have been taking appropriate antibiotics for at least 12 hours.

PREVENTION

Treatment of underlying predisposing factors is the principle means of preventing cellulitis and erysipelas and includes management of obesity, eczema, venous insufficiency, any interdigital maceration, scaling or fissuring, and reduction of any underlying edema. The efficacy of prophylactic antibiotics for recurrent cellulitis is unclear, but such antibiotics are sometimes used in adults with >3-4 episodes of cellulitis per year despite attempts to treat predisposing factors. When considering skin and soft tissue infections due to MRSA, decreased recurrence has been associated with decolonization protocols though results widely vary.

KEY POINTS

- Cellulitis and erysipelas are typically clinical diagnoses. Fever, chills, and malaise accompanied by ill-defined soft tissue erythema, warmth, and edema indicate cellulitis; raised, sharply defined margins that develop more quickly suggest erysipelas.
- Blood cultures are not usually useful in immunocompetent children hospitalized with skin and soft tissue infections.
- Typically, oral or IV antibiotics effective against *S. aureus* and *S. pyogenes* are needed for 5 days; however, the patient's response to therapy must be assessed and distinct clinical settings or presentations may suggest alternative or atypical infectious agents or the need for longer therapy.

PYOMYOSITIS

BACKGROUND

Pyomyositis is a bacterial infection of skeletal muscle that arises from hematogenous spread and typically results in local abscess formation. It is a disease endemic to the tropics though it has become increasingly more prevalent in temperate regions. In tropical areas, 33% to 40% of all cases of pyomyositis are seen in children, with the peak incidence between the ages of 2 and 5; males appear to be more commonly affected, and most patients are otherwise healthy prior to infection. Older children and adults are more often diagnosed in temperate regions, with a peak age of 5 to 9 years in the United States. Pyomyositis is more frequent in the West and South than the Midwest or Northeast of the United States, presumably due to climate differences.

PATHOPHYSIOLOGY

S. aureus, both MSSA and MRSA, is the most common pathogen identified in pyomyositis, causing 90% of cases in most regions. GABHS is the second most common pathogen, followed by non-group A streptococci, *S. pneumoniae*, gram-negative enteric bacilli (especially in patients with hematologic malignancy where *E. coli* and *Pseudomonas aeruginosa* are more prevalent), and rarely, mycobacteria. The strongest risk factors for pyomyositis are immunodeficiency, including HIV, hematologic malignancy, and organ transplantation. Other risk factors include diabetes mellitus, malnutrition, chronic kidney disease, and obesity. Intravenous drug use has been implicated in multiple cases of pyomyositis, not just for its association with HIV transmission, but also as a direct means of seeding the bloodstream with bacteria. Trauma or even minor muscle damage due to vigorous exercise has also been strongly linked with pyomyositis, associated with 25% to 50% of cases.

CLINICAL PRESENTATION

Pyomyositis presents with fever along with pain and cramping localized to a single muscle group. The majority of cases occur in the thigh, calf, or buttocks, but any muscle group has the potential for involvement. Multifocal infection is not uncommon, observed in 15% to 43% of cases. The course of clinical pyomyositis has classically been divided into three stages. Stage I, also known as the invasive stage, is characterized by low-grade fever, malaise, and the insidious onset of dull muscle pain and cramps as the infected muscle becomes inflamed. At this stage, the overlying skin usually appears normal, without fluctuance or erythema, but a "woody" texture may be appreciated on deep palpation of the affected muscle. Presentation at Stage I is rare, thought to occur in only 2% of patients. Stage II, also referred to as the suppurative phase, occurs 10 to 21 days after the onset of initial symptoms and is characterized by the formation of a local abscess. Muscle tenderness is usually exquisite, and there often is overlying erythema and edema. Most patients present in Stage II. Stage III, known alternatively as the late phase, is notable for systemic toxicity and fluctuance in the muscle. Metastatic abscesses, rhabdomyolysis, renal failure, septic arthritis, endocarditis, and septic shock have all been reported to occur in this stage.

DIFFERENTIAL DIAGNOSIS

The differential diagnosis of pyomyositis is broad; it includes infectious, inflammatory, neoplastic, and mechanical syndromes, and distinguishing these diagnoses often requires imaging and laboratory studies. Infectious processes include septic arthritis, cellulitis, osteomyelitis, various necrotizing soft-tissue infections, and non-bacterial forms of myositis, such as viral (e.g., influenza), fungal, and parasitic. Inflammatory conditions that may mimic pyomyositis include gout, deep venous thrombosis, thrombophlebitis, and polymyositis. Neoplastic diagnoses depend on the site affected but include sarcomas, Langerhans cell histiocytosis, and leukemia. Mechanical causes, such as muscle strain, contusion, hematoma, and muscle infarction, can also present similarly to pyomyositis.

DIAGNOSTIC EVALUATION

Identification of pyomyositis is often delayed because of its vague presentation, with an average of 10 days between the onset of symptoms and the correct diagnosis. Pyomyositis should be considered in children with fever and acute muscle pain, with or without recent trauma, especially in areas with high temperatures and humidity. Pelvic pyomyositis, a common location, may present with referred pain to the hip and may be difficult for the patient to localize, making diagnosis more difficult. Imaging is ultimately how most pyomyositis is diagnosed. Plain films can be used to rule out osteomyelitis but are otherwise of little diagnostic value. CT is helpful for detecting muscle edema and abscesses and can also be used for radiographic-guided drainage. While CT is more definitive, ultrasound is a reasonable first step given that is non-invasive, inexpensive, and does not use radiation. MRI provides the most definitive diagnosis, offering the most soft tissue contrast and the earliest detection of abscesses. Compared to imaging, laboratory tests tend to be nonspecific. Interestingly, creatine kinase levels are almost always normal. Cultures collected from abscesses can guide antibiotic therapy. Because pyomyositis is a hematogenously spread infection, and can be complicated by metastatic seeding of infection, all patients should have blood cultures obtained, which are positive in up to 30% of patients.

MANAGEMENT

Treatment is dictated by the stage of the disease at presentation. In most patients with Stage I pyomyositis, antibiotics alone are effective therapy. However, because most patients present in either Stage II or Stage III, typical treatment consists of antibiotics along with surgical or percutaneous incision and drainage. For immunocompetent individuals, empiric IV antibiotics should be directed against *S. aureus* and streptococci. In areas with relatively low prevalence of MRSA, initial therapy with cefazolin (or alternatively oxacillin or nafcillin) is reasonable. If there is a high local prevalence of MRSA, vancomycin (often combined with cefazolin for improved killing of MSSA and GABHS), daptomycin, ceftaroline, or linezolid could be considered. In clinically stable patients, clindamycin (possibly in combination with cefazolin) may be considered though the prevalence of clindamycin-resistant *S. aureus* may limit the effectiveness of this approach. In immunocompromised hosts, coverage should be expanded to include gram-negative and anaerobic organisms, with either vancomycin (or other anti-MRSA agent) plus a beta-lactam/beta-lactamase inhibitor, an extended-spectrum cephalosporin plus metronidazole, a fluoroquinolone plus metronidazole, or a carbapenem, depending on the clinical scenario. The length of therapy should be dictated by clinical improvement, but 2 to 3 weeks is sufficient in most cases. In the absence of a specific complication that requires prolonged IV therapy (e.g., endocarditis), patients should be transitioned to oral therapy once clinically improved. Oral options include cephalexin (for MSSA); amoxicillin (for GABHS); clindamycin (susceptible MRSA); linezolid, doxycycline, or TMP-SMX (for clindamycin-resistant MRSA); or matching the spectrum of their empiric therapy if no organism is isolated. Recurrent infection is rare but has been reported in immunocompromised individuals. The prognosis for most patients with pyomyositis is generally favorable and most recover without further sequelae. However, with delays in treatment, complications can include osteomyelitis, muscle scarring, residual weakness, functional impairment, and a mortality rate as high as 10%.

ADMISSION CRITERIA

Inpatient admission is generally required as these patients will require both parenteral antibiotics and surgical or percutaneous incision and drainage. Stage III patients are also at risk for significant complications, such as renal failure or septic shock, which warrant close monitoring of hemodynamics and electrolytes, and urgent need for intensive care if these develop.

DISCHARGE CRITERIA

Prior to discharge, a patient admitted for pyomyositis should demonstrate clinical improvement, exhibit hemodynamic and electrolyte stability, remain afebrile for 24 hours, and have an established plan to complete the appropriate course of antibiotics as an outpatient.

CONSULTATION

General surgery or interventional radiology consultation will be required for drainage of all but the most superficial soft tissue abscesses. Infectious disease consultation should be considered. Critical care would be required if a patient develops signs of systemic toxicity.

SPECIAL CONSIDERATIONS

Immunocompromised patients warrant additional coverage for gram-negative and anaerobic organisms. Patients with extensive, multifocal disease may warrant longer courses of antibiotics, as would patients found to have endocarditis, osteomyelitis, or other sequelae of bacteremia.

PREVENTION

While certain immunodeficiencies may be nonmodifiable, avoidance of all other risk factors, such as trauma, obesity, diabetes, intravenous drug use, tropical travel, and malnutrition will limit the likelihood of pyomyositis development.

KEY POINTS

- Classically, pyomyositis is an infection of the tropics though it is becoming increasingly prevalent in temperate zones.
- *S. aureus* is responsible for ~90% of pyomyositis cases, followed by GABHS.
- Pyomyositis typically progresses through three stages of development: invasion, suppuration, and systemic toxicity.
- Ultrasonography may quickly and inexpensively diagnose pyomyositis though CT and MRI have a higher sensitivity of detection.
- Antibiotics targeting *S. aureus* and GABHS are indicated in most patients, along with incision and drainage for all those who demonstrate abscess formation.

NECROTIZING SOFT-TISSUE INFECTIONS

BACKGROUND

Necrotizing soft tissue infections (NSTIs) are rapidly progressive and potentially fatal infections involving soft tissue, with tissue involvement ranging from epidermis to deep musculature. They are characterized by fulminant tissue destruction and systemic toxicity and have high rates of mortality. NSTIs collectively refer to various pathophysiologically distinct clinical entities, but each are similar necrotizing processes that have overlapping clinical risk factors, presenting symptoms, and treatments. Type I (polymicrobial) and Type II (monomicrobial) necrotizing fasciitis refer to the subsets in which infection specifically spreads along the plane between the superficial muscle fascia and the overlying subcutaneous tissue. In addition to necrotizing fasciitis, NSTIs include clostridial myonecrosis (also termed gas gangrene) and streptococcal myonecrosis (generally non-gas forming), among others.

NSTIs can occur after penetrating trauma, surgery, or other minor skin insults (e.g., eczema, primary varicella infection), but up to a quarter of cases occur without any identified initial skin lesion. Though rare overall, NSTIs are more common in adults, with an annual incidence ranging from 0.3 up to 16 cases per 100,000 persons; in children, the incidence is as low as 0.08 to 0.13 per 100,000. Prompt surgical intervention is critical for survival as antibiotic therapy alone, while necessary, is insufficient to stop the spread of infection.

PATHOPHYSIOLOGY

Necrotizing fasciitis is divided into two distinct bacteriologic entities: type I (polymicrobial) and type II (monomicrobial, usually due to group A streptococcus). Type I infections are more common in adults, typically due to a combination of aerobic (e.g., enteric gram-negative bacilli, *S. aureus*, streptococci, *Enterococcus*) and anaerobic (e.g., *Clostridium* species, *Bacteroides* species). Type I infections are often associated with penetrating trauma, gastrointestinal or genitourinary/gynecologic surgery, decubitus ulcers, and patient-specific risk factors, such as neutropenia, diabetes, peripheral vascular disease, and injection drug use.

In type II necrotizing fasciitis, GABHS is the most common pathogen though monobacterial infections due to *S. aureus* or clostridial species can be seen. It can occur among healthy individuals and in any age group. Predisposing factors include a history of skin injury, such as abrasions, burns, eczema, insect bites, lacerations, childbirth, primary varicella infection, and even minor non-penetrating trauma. Up to 20% of patients have no visible skin lesion, and these infections likely arise from hematogenous spread of GABHS to sometimes undetectable sites of blunt trauma or muscle injury. GABHS can also cause a necrotizing myositis (also termed streptococcal myonecrosis), which is sometimes classified as a distinct entity. Monomicrobial infections can also be seen due to *Aeromonas hydrophila* and *Vibrio vulnificus* (occurring after injuries associated with freshwater and saltwater, respectively), and some authors classify these infections as type III necrotizing fasciitis.

Across all NSTIs, the possible association with nonsteroidal anti-inflammatory drug (NSAID) use has been raised. Speculated mechanisms have included inhibition of neutrophil function, augmentation of cytokine release, and masking of usual signs of inflammation, delaying diagnosis. Some clinical and experimental data suggest a causal relationship with NSAIDs; however, the association may be secondary to the use of NSAIDs for pain and fever following the onset of infection without a true cause-effect relationship.

CLINICAL PRESENTATION

Most NSTIs begin with an inciting skin trauma, with extension of infection from the initial skin lesion. However, diagnosis can be difficult, especially in children, because the initial symptoms may be non-specific; fever and erythema may not initially be present, and there may not be apparent trauma or skin breakdown. In cases with an associated trauma, an area of ill-defined erythema, warmth, swelling, and exquisite tenderness will develop within 1 to 4 days of the initial injury. Such exam findings may be otherwise indistinguishable from a cellulitis. The affected area may progress rapidly or more indolently (**Figure 102-5**). The pain is often noted as being out of proportion to the cutaneous signs of infection.

Within 24 hours, swelling, induration, and a distinguishing wooden-hard feel are generally appreciated. Erythema is usually but not always present. Specific to pediatrics, infants and toddlers at this stage may be merely fussy or irritable without an obvious localizing infection; toddlers and young children may present with limp or refusal to bear weight on an affected lower extremity. In these cases, careful physical exam is important to identify severe pain with movement/palpation out of proportion to the skin's superficial appearance. Patients with NSTI due to GABHS may present with concomitant toxic shock syndrome, with associated systemic symptoms of vomiting, diarrhea, diffuse myalgias, respiratory distress, along with laboratory evidence of multiorgan dysfunction (elevated creatinine, transaminases). Over the next several days, the overlying skin color may change to red-purple and patches of blue-gray, sometimes with blistering. The infection and inflammation will continue to extend deeper through the fascial planes, which emphasizes the importance of rapid diagnosis and ultimately surgical dissection. As the infection progresses, signs of systemic toxicity with high fevers will appear. After 3 to 5 days of onset, skin breakdown typically occurs, with bullae containing pink/purple fluid, frank gangrene, and in type I, often subcutaneous gas. By this point, the affected area has usually become anesthetic.

DIFFERENTIAL DIAGNOSIS

The main differential diagnoses for NSTI are the other forms of soft tissue infections. NSTI may appear clinically similar to cellulitis and erysipelas early in the course of infection; however, the presence of systemic signs,

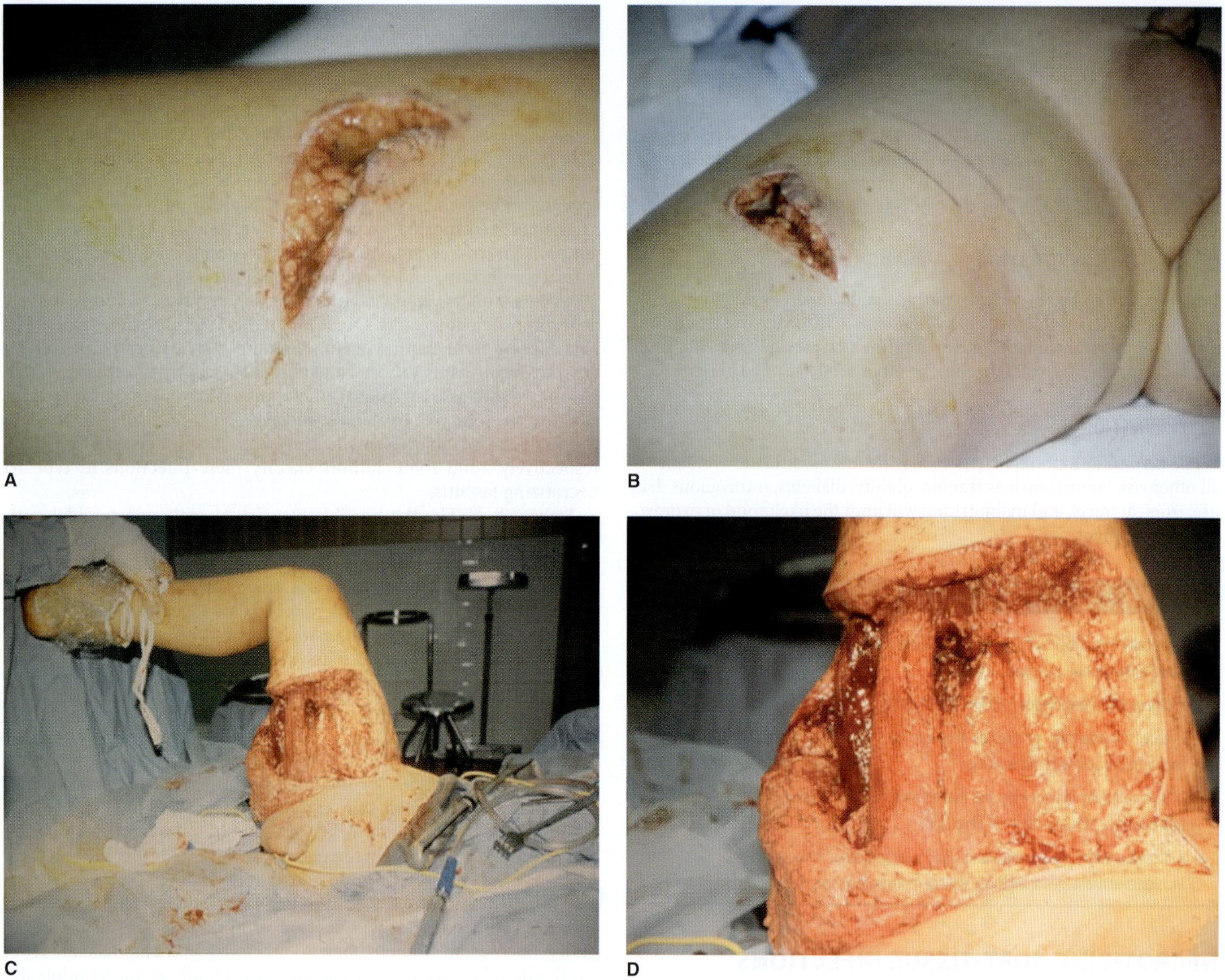

FIGURE 102-5. Necrotizing fasciitis. Note the size of the initial trauma and the extent of the surgical debridement ultimately required. (Photographs used with permission of Michael Ryan, DO, FAAP, FACOP.)

character of induration, loss of fascial plane and muscle group differentiation (in necrotizing fasciitis), lack of response to antibiotic therapy, and a more fulminant nature distinguish NSTIs from these superficial infections. Pyomyositis may have a similar "wooden-like" texture of induration, but it is characterized by abscess formation instead of gangrenous necrosis and is generally associated with less systemic toxicity. Streptococcal toxic shock syndrome may be caused by the same toxigenic bacteria that cause type II necrotizing fasciitis and should be considered in all cases. The systemic and GI symptoms of toxic shock syndrome can be wrongly diagnosed as food poisoning or viral gastroenteritis. Some symptoms of NSTI can overlap with osteoarticular infections. Non-infectious differential diagnoses include musculoskeletal injury, deep venous thrombosis, warfarin-induced skin necrosis, and brown recluse spider bites. Severe pain is sometimes attributed to the prior injury or surgery instead of the necrotizing infection.

DIAGNOSTIC EVALUATION

Early diagnosis of NSTIs is essential to facilitate urgent surgical intervention. NSTIs should be considered in any patient with a combination of fever, systemic toxicity, and soft tissue symptoms, such as swelling, erythema, and pain out of proportion to visible skin findings. While diagnostic imaging may be useful in some settings, time-consuming diagnostic testing should not delay surgical exploration when there is a high index of suspicion. Radiographic imaging is rarely diagnostically helpful beyond the physical exam though it can demonstrate gas in the fascial plane, a highly specific finding. Non-contrast CT, the initial imaging of choice, is the most expedient approach to assess for the extent of soft tissue involvement and/or gas in the fascial planes, but early surgical exploration is frequently preferrable to obtaining any imaging, unless there is a low index of suspicion. MRI may show thicking and T2 hyperintensity of intramuscular fascia, but its role in NSTIs is unclear due to the time required for these scans. Marked swelling and edema may produce a compartment syndrome. Measurement of intracompartmental pressure may aid in evaluation early in the course of infection if significant pain and swelling are present without associated skin changes.

Initial laboratory studies may include a complete blood count (CBC), serum electrolytes, C-reactive protein (CRP), creatine kinase (CK), and aerobic as well as anaerobic blood cultures. The white blood cell (WBC) count may be elevated or normal, frequently with immature granulocytes and bands, and thrombocytopenia may be seen. Patients may have evidence of coagulopathy, renal failure, acidosis, hyperglycemia, and/or myocardial dysfunction. Blood cultures are more likely to be positive in infections due to GABHS but are otherwise positive in the minority of patients. Aspiration of skin or bullae for Gram stain and culture may be useful and provide an early clue to therapy though these are not as reliable as deep tissue cultures obtained during surgery.

The Laboratory Risk Indicator for Necrotizing Fasciitis (LRINEC) scoring system has been used to help distinguish necrotizing fasciitis from other soft-tissue infections. It incorporates CBC parameters, electrolytes, creatinine, and CRP values. High LRINEC scores have been associated with high positive and negative predictive values for necrotizing fasciitis; however, the diagnostic value of this scoring system has been questioned in more recent studies. Of note, this system was developed and validated in adult populations, and children with necrotizing fasciitis often have lower LRINEC scores on average than adults, so its role in the evaluation of children with suspected NSTIs is unclear.

Surgical exploration is the only way to definitively establish the diagnosis of NSTIs and facilitates necessary debridement of affected tissue. If an open wound is present, probing the edges with a blunt instrument will demonstrate ready dissection of the superficial fascial plane well beyond the wound margins. Upon direct inspection, the fascia will appear swollen and dull gray, with stringy areas of necrosis. Intraoperative frozen section biopsy has been used diagnostically in the past but is now rarely used due to low accuracy.

MANAGEMENT

Early surgical intervention is the primary treatment modality for NSTIs, as without appropriate exploration and debridement, these cases are almost universally fatal. In addition to rapid surgical intervention, antibiotics, fluid and electrolyte management, pain control, and management of organ failure are also essential. The goal of operative management is both therapeutic, to debride all areas of necrosis, and diagnostic, to assess the extent of infection and obtain specimens for Gram stain and culture. Patients should be taken to surgery as soon as possible, ideally within 24 hours of presentation though surgery within 6 hours of presentation may yield even better outcomes. Most patients will require multiple surgeries, generally daily, until the surgical team finds no need for further debridement. Negative-pressure devices are commonly used to improve wound healing. If recognized early and treated aggressively, some patients will be able to avoid highly morbid surgical resections, but the need for amputations, allografting, and reconstructive surgery is unfortunately common.

Antibiotic therapy consists of immediate broad-spectrum antimicrobials, including activity against gram positive (including MRSA), gram negative, and anaerobic organisms. Common therapies include a primary regimen of piperacillin-tazobactam, meropenem, or an extended-spectrum cephalosporin plus metronidazole, with additional MRSA coverage (e.g., vancomycin, daptomycin, or linezolid) and a protein-synthesis inhibitor to suppress toxin and/or M protein synthesis (e.g., clindamycin or linezolid). A regimen that includes linezolid is an appealing option to provide both MRSA coverage and toxin inhibition. Less typical organisms, such as *A. hydrophila* or *V. vulnificans*, may require additional agents, such as doxycycline. Antibiotic therapy can then be tailored to the tissue culture and susceptibility results. Both GABHS and clostridial species are optimally treated with penicillin plus clindamycin, for example. The optimal duration of antibiotic treatment has not been well-studied, but most experts recommend continuation until operative procedures are no longer needed, obvious clinical improvement has been demonstrated, and a lack of fever for 48 to 72 hours. Invasive GABHS infections are generally treated for 10 to 14 days total, and the course can be completed with oral antibiotics once the patient is stable. The use of intravenous immunoglobulin for its activity against bacterial toxins is controversial. It may have limited benefit in severe cases of GABHS infections, particularly those associated with streptococcal toxic shock syndrome, but it is not routinely recommended. Hyperbaric oxygen has been considered as a possible adjunctive therapy, but the evidence is weak and controversial. It should not be routinely used due to inadequate evidence of benefit.

ADMISSION CRITERIA

All patients with NSTIs will require admission, typically in an intensive care setting, for extensive surgical debridement, close attention to fluid volume status, pain control, and potential management of multiorgan failure.

DISCHARGE CRITERIA

Discharge of a patient with a NSTI may be considered after all of the following conditions have been demonstrated. There should be no evidence of systemic toxicity, specifically absence of fever and hypotension for 48 to 72 hours, complete surgical debridement of all necrotic tissue has been accomplished, and surgical wounds should exhibit appropriate healing. If indicated, a plan to complete outpatient antibiotics, generally with oral therapy, should be in place.

CONSULTATION

Early surgical consultation is essential, often with general/pediatric surgery and/or orthopedic surgery. Plastic surgery consultation may be needed in some cases for allografting or tissue reconstruction. Infectious disease consultation is generally warranted to guide initial and definitive therapy as well as treatment duration.

SPECIAL CONSIDERATIONS

In type I (polymicrobial) necrotizing fasciitis, several unique presentations should be kept in mind. Bacterial penetration through the fascial components of the head and neck can result in Ludwig angina, a rapidly expanding inflammation in the submandibular and sublingual regions, which may be life-threatening due to the potential for airway obstruction. Necrotizing infection of the male perineum is known as Fournier gangrene and can result from breaches in the gastrointestinal or urethral mucosa, with rapid extension from the perineum to the anterior abdominal wall, buttocks, and genitalia. It can occur in any age group but is seen most commonly in elderly men. In neonates, necrotizing fasciitis can be a complication of omphalitis, balanitis, circumcision, and fetal scalp monitoring.

PREVENTION

In cases of invasive GABHS infection, prophylaxis of close contacts is considered though the risk of developing a secondary case of necrotizing fasciitis or toxic shock syndrome is still very low. Varicella vaccination decreases the incidence of necrotizing fasciitis, generally due to GABHS, and is one of the main reasons universal childhood varicella vaccination has been implemented in the United States.

KEY POINTS

- Necrotizing soft tissue infections, including necrotizing fasciitis and other related processes, are rapidly progressive and potentially fatal soft tissue infections characterized by fulminant tissue destruction and systemic toxicity.
- Necrotizing fasciitis is typically divided into the categories of type I (polymicrobial) and type II (group A streptococcal) due to their similar but still distinct clinical presentations.
- The main differential diagnoses for necrotizing soft tissue infections are less invasive forms of soft tissue infections.
- Radiographic imaging and laboratory work may guide treatment, but necrotizing soft tissue infections remain a surgical diagnosis, for which surgical intervention should not be delayed by other studies.
- Optimal treatment consists of early and aggressive surgical debridement, broad-spectrum empiric antibiotic therapy, and hemodynamic support.

SUGGESTED READINGS

Assadian A, Assadian O, Simon A, Kramer A. Infection control consequences—early staphylococcal scalded skin syndrome or Kawasaki syndrome?. *GMS Krankenhhyg Interdiszip*. 2009;4(2):Doc05.

Barnett E, Kimberlin D, Sawyer M, et al. *Red Book 2021-2024 Report of the Committee on Infectious Diseases*. 32nd ed. Itasca, IL: American Academy of Pediatrics; 2021. http://online.statref.com/document/wjranW4si1KCK_3E0AU5QD.

Dalal A, Eskin-Schwartz M, Mimouni D, et al. Interventions for the prevention of recurrent erysipelas and cellulitis. *Cochrane Database Syst Rev*. 2017;6(6):CD009758.

Eckmann C, Montravers P. Current management of necrotizing soft-tissue infections. *Curr Opin Infect Dis*. 2021;34(2):89-95.

Gupta A, Jacobs N. Visual diagnosis: 2-week-old has a red, peeling rash. *Pediatr Rev*. 2013;34(3):e9-e12.

James WD, Elston DM, Treat JR, Rosenbach MA, Neuhaus IM. Bacterial infections. In: James WD, Elston DM, Treat JR, Rosenbach MA, Neuhaus IM. *Andrews' Diseases of the Skin: Clinical Dermatology*. 13th ed. Elsevier; 2020: 252-290.e4.

Liy-Wong C, Pope E, Weinstein M, Lara-Corrales I. Staphylococcal scalded skin syndrome: an epidemiological and clinical review of 84 cases. *Pediatr Dermatol*. 2021;38(1):149-153.

Maravelas R, Melgar TA, Vos D, Lima N, Sadarangani S. Pyomyositis in the United States 2002-2014. *J Infect*. 2020;80(5):497-503.

Mishra AK, Yadav P, Mishra A. A Systemic review on staphylococcal scalded skin syndrome (SSSS): a rare and critical disease of neonates. *Open Microbiol J*. 2016;10:150-159.

Mitsionis GI, Manoudis GN, Lykissas MG, et al. Pyomyositis in children: early diagnosis and treatment. *J Pediatr Surg*. 2009;44(11):2173-2178.

Neubauer HC, Hall M, Lopez MA, et al. Antibiotic regimens and associated outcomes in children hospitalized with staphylococcal scalded skin syndrome. *J Hosp Med*. 2021;16(3):149-155.

Neubauer HC, Hall M, Wallace SS, et al. Variation in diagnostic test use and associated outcomes in staphylococcal scalded skin syndrome at Children's Hospitals. *Hosp Pediatr*. 2018;8(9):530-537.

Noor A, Krilov LR. Necrotizing fasciitis. *Pediatr Rev*. 2021;42(10):573-575.

Paller AS, Mancini AJ. Bacterial, mycobacterial, and protozoal infections of the skin. In: Paller AS, Mancini AJ, eds. *Hurwitz Clinical Pediatric Dermatology: A Textbook of Skin Disorders of Childhood and Adolescence—Expert Consult*. New York, NY: Saunders; 2011:321-347.

Stevens DL, Bisno AL, Chambers HF, et al. Practice guidelines for the diagnosis and management of skin and soft tissue infections: 2014 update by the Infectious Diseases Society of America [published correction appears in Clin Infect Dis. 2015;60(9):1448.

Stevens DL, Bryant AE, Goldstein EJ. Necrotizing soft tissue infections. *Infect Dis Clin North Am*. 2021;35(1):135-155.

Stevens DL, Bryant AE. Necrotizing soft-tissue infections. *N Engl J Med*. 2017;377(23):2253-2265.

VanderMeulen H, Pernica JM, Roy M, Kam AJ. A 10-year review of necrotizing fasciitis in the pediatric population: delays to diagnosis and management. *Clin Pediatr (Phila)*. 2017;56(7):627-633.

Verma S. Pyomyositis in children. *Curr Infect Dis Rep*. 2016;18(4):12.

CHAPTER 103 Device-Related Infections

Katherine MacKrell, MD and Russell McCulloh, MD

INTRODUCTION

Invasive medical devices are commonly used in hospitalized children. They result in more than 250,000 infections each year in the United States. A catheter-related bloodstream infection (CRBSI) is defined as bacteremia or fungemia in a patient with an intravascular catheter that is the presumed source of infection. This definition belies the challenges a clinician faces in accurately diagnosing CRBSI in children, including difficulties in diagnostic testing and variability in epidemiology based on age, intravascular device used, infusate being given, and underlying clinical condition. Additionally, central venous catheters (CVCs) pose other infectious complications aside from CRBSI, including local infection at exit sites, and they can become secondarily infected through seeding of bacteria due to bacteremia originating from infection at a distant site. With varying pathogens, patients present with a variety of time to onset and manifestations of symptoms—often including proliferations of the bacteria to cause local damage (wound dehiscence, etc) and systemic manifestations such as fever and sepsis.

Nationwide approximately 4700 children are hospitalized for initial placement of cerebrospinal fluid (CSF) shunts annually, with more than 2400 children hospitalized for shunt-related infections at a cost of over $250 million. The most common CNS shunt placed in children is the ventriculoperitoneal (VP) shunt. These devices breach natural barriers to infection and provide access for bacteria to enter and proliferate in a site relatively sequestered from the immune system and rich in nutrients. Diagnosis and management of these infections usually involves invasive procedures and prolonged hospitalization, with marked burdens on children and their families, including prolonged hospital stays, potential morbidity, and significant healthcare costs.

Pediatric hospitalists care for a population of children that is increasingly medically complex, often including children in the neonatal intensive care unit (NICU) and/or pediatric intensive care unit (PICU), both sites of care where intravascular and CNS catheters are commonly used. Knowledge of optimal diagnostic and treatment strategies for device-related infections is a vital skill for hospitalists. This chapter will help provide information clinicians can use to help develop expertise in the management of infectious complications from these devices.

CENTRAL VENOUS CATHETER-RELATED INFECTIONS

BACKGROUND

Pediatric bloodstream infections account for approximately 13.5% of all nosocomial bloodstream infections, at per-episode cost of approximately $39,000 per episode in PICU patients and catheter-related bloodstream infections have an associated mortality rate of 12% to 25% each year. The majority of nosocomial bacteremias present in the setting of a central venous catheter and divergence from care recommendations in both ICU and non-ICU settings is often a factor in these infections. Poorly intact dressings and incorrectly placed catheter caps and taps are seen as major breeches in care and can directly contribute to infection risk. Risk of infection is present both for CVCs inserted directly into a central vein as well as peripherally inserted central venous catheters (PICCs), which are more commonly used outside of the intensive care unit.

Multiple factors influence the risk of infection, including patient age, medical comorbidities, site of device placement, types of infusate being administered, frequency of times the device is accessed, duration the CVC is in place, and the device type. **Table 103-1** lists the most commonly used CVC types in pediatrics. In general, tunneled catheters are a lower long-term risk for infection than non-tunneled catheters, with implanted venous access devices (ports) having the lowest rates of infection. Although tunneled catheters are associated with fewer infections, ultimately the decision between using a tunneled catheter, a fully implanted catheter, or a PICC should be based on duration of treatment,

TABLE 103-1 Commonly Used Central Venous Catheters

Catheter Type	Description
Peripherally inserted central catheter	Inserted via a peripheral vein (usually basilic, cephalic, or brachial) into the superior vena cava
Non-tunneled CVC	Inserted directly into a central vein (usually subclavian, internal jugular, or femoral) through a skin incision
Tunneled CVC	Inserted through a subcutaneous tunnel on the chest wall before entering the superior vena cava (e.g. Broviac, Hickman, Groshong, Quinton catheters); a Dacron cuff located at the tunnel exit site contributes to long-term catheter stability by stimulating tissue growth around the tunneled portion of the catheter
Totally implanted venous access device ("port")	Subcutaneous port or reservoir with self-sealing septum accessed by a needle through intact skin; the catheter tip is located in the subclavian or internal jugular vein

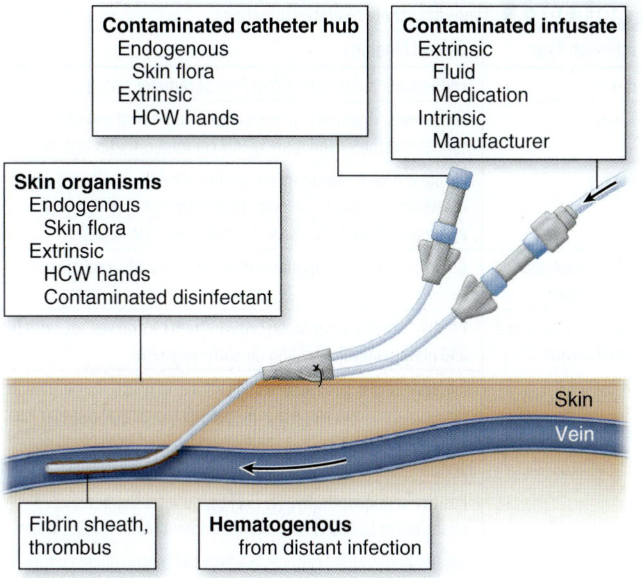

FIGURE 103-1. Routes of microorganism entry for colonization/infection of vascular catheters. HCW, healthcare worker.

level of care, the patient's dexterity/mobility, and the underlying medical condition necessitating vascular access.

PATHOPHYSIOLOGY

Central venous catheters provide multiple avenues for microbial colonization and infection (**Figure 103-1**). First, CVCs have at least one access port/hub which can become colonized with organisms from environmental exposure or from accessing/de-accessing the device. Cutaneous flora may also translocate through the barrier defect provided by the CVC or from contaminated healthcare worker hands during dressing changes or device manipulation, which can result in exit site infections or infection of the subcutaneous length of the catheter in the case of tunneled devices. Fibrin sheaths and thrombi can develop along the intravascular portions of the catheter, an ideal site for colonization by organisms during episodes of transient bacteremia or from bacteremia due to infection at a distant site. Finally, materials being infused through the catheter may be contaminated with organisms, resulting in direct inoculation of both the device and the bloodstream. Thus, infection can be local, systemic, or secondary to another infectious process.

Table 103-2 summarizes the pathogens most commonly associated with catheter-related bloodstream infections. Coagulase-negative staphylococci (CONS) account for approximately 40% of children diagnosed with nosocomial bloodstream infections; this increases to 50% in neonates. Gram-negative aerobic bacilli account for approximately 25% of CRBSI, followed by enterococci (11%-15%), and *Candida* species. Among gram-negative bacilli isolated, the most common pathogens include *Enterobacter* species, *Pseudomonas aeruginosa*, *Klebsiella pneumonia*, *Escherichia coli*, *Serratia marcescens*, *Acinetobacter* species, and *Citrobacter* species. Children with CVCs managed mostly in home healthcare settings may be at higher risk for non-endogenous gram-negative pathogens from water or environmental sources such as *Pseudomonas*, *Acinetobacter*, and *Agrobacterium* species, especially during the summer. Fungal infections remain an uncommon cause of bloodstream infections associated with an indwelling catheter, with *Candida spp.* being the most common pathogens isolated.

Available data are biased toward PICUs, NICUs, and oncology units, as surveillance for bloodstream infection is usually performed in these high-risk patient populations. It is likely that a similar spectrum of organisms cause CRBSI in children in non-ICU inpatient settings, but there is limited information to support this. One study of outpatient parenteral therapy in children with osteoarticular infections found that the rate of infectious complications associated with the catheter was 6.3 per 1000 catheter days and occurred in approximately 10% of patients. The average time to development of infectious complications was 24.5 days.

CLINICAL PRESENTATION

Children with local site infections and tunnel infections may present with focal erythema, induration, tenderness, warmth, a fluctuant mass, and/or purulent or foul-smelling discharge. For tunnel infections these

TABLE 103-2 Most Common Pathogens Reported for Pediatric Central Line-Associated Bloodstream Infection (CLABSI) Pathogens, by Location Type 2015-2017

	NICUs[b]		Pediatric ICUs[a]		Pediatric Oncology Units[a]		Pediatric Wards[a,b]	
Pathogen	No. (%) Pathogens	Rank	No. (%) Pathogens	Rank	No. (%) Pathogens	Rank	No. (%) Pathogens	Rank
Staphylococcus aureus	1,381 (25.2)	1	420 (12.6)	2	266 (7.7)	5	313 (12.4)	2
Coagulase-negative staphylococci	1,145 (20.9)	2	345 (10.4)	4	316 (9.1)	4	289 (11.4)	3
Escherichia coli	596 (10.9)	3	151 (4.5)	9	429 (12.4)	2	205 (8.1)	5
Enterococcus faecalis[c]	483 (8.8)	4	492 (14.8)	1	179 (5.2)	7	264 (10.4)	4
Selected *Klebsiella* spp	408 (7.5)	5	368 (11.0)	3	374 (10.8)	3	375 (14.8)	1
Candida albicans[c]	243 (4.4)	6	130 (3.9)	10	41 (1.2)	14	94 (3.7)	9
Enterobacter spp	229 (4.2)	7	278 (8.3)	5	218 (6.3)	6	191 (7.5)	6
Pseudomonas aeruginosa	156 (2.8)	8	167 (5.0)	7	173 (5.0)	8	78 (3.1)	10
Serratia spp	150 (2.7)	9	166 (5.0)	8	20 (0.6)	20	66 (2.6)	11
Other *Candida* spp[c,d,e]	141 (2.6)	10	207 (6.2)	6	138 (4.0)	9	120 (4.7)	7
Streptococcus agalactiae (GBS)	130 (2.4)	11	8 (0.2)	24	7 (0.2)	35	6 (0.2)	23
Acinetobacter spp	47 (0.9)	12	43 (1.3)	13	24 (0.7)	18	29 (1.1)	14
Other *Enterococcus* spp[c,d]	46 (0.8)	13	38 (1.1)	14	60 (1.7)	11	36 (1.4)	13
Candida glabrata[c]	36 (0.7)	14	32 (1.0)	15	21 (0.6)	19	23 (0.9)	16
Citrobacter spp	27 (0.5)	15	19 (0.6)	18	25 (0.7)	17	23 (0.9)	16
Other	256 (4.7)		468 (14.0)		1,177 (33.9)		418 (16.5)	
Total	5,474 (100.0)		3,332 (100.0)		3,468 (100.0)		2,530 (100.0)	

Source: Reproduced with permission from Winer-Lastinger L, et al. Antimicrobial-resistant pathogens associated with pediatric healthcare-associated infections: Summary of data reported to the National Healthcare Safety Network, 2015-2017. *Infect Control Hosp Epidemiol.* 2020;41(1):19-30, Table 5.

symptoms can extend along the length of the subcutaneous portion of the catheter. Site infections may extend deep into subcutaneous tissues, including fat, muscle, fascia, or bone. Additionally, these localized infections can still be associated with bloodstream infection.

Catheter-related bloodstream infections are difficult to diagnose clinically. The most common symptom in children with CRBSI is fever, but this has poor specificity as most febrile children with a CVC in place do not have bloodstream infection. For example, among febrile cancer patients with intravascular catheters, only 10% and 24% of all febrile episodes were associated with bacteremia in non-neutropenic and neutropenic patients, respectively. Episodic symptoms of fever and/or hypotension associated with infusion times may be an indicator of introduction of bacteria into the bloodstream through either an infected catheter hub or lumen or from the infusate. Complications of bacteremia may also be the presenting symptoms, which could include sepsis, or disseminated infection to multiple end organs (including the eyes, heart, bones, skin, or visceral organs) which can manifest as embolic phenomena, multifocal abscesses, or immune complex disease such as nephritis. Finally, catheter malfunction, such as inability to infuse fluids or aspirate blood from the catheter, may indicate infection. Such malfunction is often due to fibrin or thrombus deposition which can readily become colonized or infected, but can also arise due to deep venous thrombosis.

Despite the variety of potential clinical features of CRBSI, in many cases, a positive blood culture alone may be the presenting feature, especially among patients transferred from outside facilities or seen for inpatient consultation. A positive blood culture—with or without associated symptoms—can be difficult to interpret as representative of a true infection versus contaminant. Below we discuss several approaches to help make this distinction.

TABLE 103-3 Types of Catheter-Related Infections

Infection Type	Clinical Findings
Exit site	Erythema or induration within 2 cm of catheter exit site
Tunnel	Tenderness, erythema, or induration along subcutaneous tract of tunneled catheter and more than 2 cm from catheter exit site
Pocket	Purulent fluid in subcutaneous pocket of totally implanted venous access device; may be accompanied by overlying tenderness, erythema, induration, visible drainage, and skin necrosis
Infusate-related bloodstream	Growth of the same organism from infusate and bloodstream
Catheter-associated bloodstream	Positive simultaneous blood cultures from central venous catheter and peripheral vein yielding the same organism
	Simultaneous quantitative blood cultures in which the number of CFUs isolated from blood drawn through the central catheter is at least fivefold greater than the number isolated from blood drawn peripherally
	Positive semiquantitative (≥15 CFUs/catheter segment) or quantitative (≥100 CFUs/catheter segment) catheter tip cultures
	Simultaneous blood cultures in which the central blood culture grows ≥2 hr earlier than the peripheral blood culture
	Simultaneous quantitative blood cultures drawn from separate lumens of a multiple-lumen catheter in which the number of CFUs isolated from blood drawn through one lumen is at least threefold greater than the number isolated from blood drawn from the other lumen

DIFFERENTIAL DIAGNOSIS

Given that children presenting with fever in the setting of indwelling CVC usually do not have CRBSI, the differential diagnosis can be quite broad. Often children with CVCs have significant chronic medical conditions, including immune-compromised states, previously diagnosed infection at a different site, or systemic illnesses requiring parenteral medications or nutrition. Among children with long-term CVCs in place, catheter malfunction is a common occurrence; secondary infection of a malfunctioning catheter may occur concomitantly. In all these cases, a thoughtful evaluation that includes blood cultures from the CVC and, when possible, peripheral sites are important for accurate diagnosis.

DIAGNOSIS

Local Infection Local infections associated with a central venous catheter (including exit site, tunnel, and pocket infections) are readily recognizable by physical examination (**Table 103-3**). Ultrasonography of the area to assess deep fluid collection/abscess can aid in establishing the extent of infection and identify areas that may require drainage after catheter removal.

Catheter-Related Bloodstream Infections Accurate diagnosis of CRBSI in children can be challenging. Although pediatric-specific data are lacking, in adults, rates of confirmed catheter infection from removed CVCs in bacteremic patients are only 15%. Current methods available for increasing accuracy of diagnosing CRBSI in children include quantitative blood cultures obtained through the catheter and a peripheral vein, semiquantitative cultures of a catheter segment, and differential time to positivity of cultures (Table 103-3). Additionally, organism type remains an important factor in diagnosing CRBSI, as it can differentiate a true pathogen from a contaminant.

Diagnosis of CRBSI can be made by comparing quantitative differences in colony counts of a pathogen isolated from blood cultures from a CVC versus a peripheral culture. A fivefold or greater difference in number of colonies from the CVC culture versus the peripheral culture establishes the diagnosis. In practice, this technique is rarely used due to cost and logistic limitations of most microbiology laboratories.

Differential time to positivity of blood cultures drawn from two different sites may also be used to establish the diagnosis. Time to positivity is defined as the duration of time necessary for the blood culture to grow the causative organism. This can only be used reliably when identical blood volumes are drawn from each site, due to the influence of blood volume on time to positivity (see below). This testing method is most commonly performed by obtaining a blood culture from the catheter and a separate culture via peripheral venipuncture. Positive blood culture from the catheter in at least 2 hours less than peripheral culture positivity has a sensitivity of 93% and a specificity of 75% for catheters in place for greater than 30 days, and a sensitivity of 81% and a specificity of 92% for catheters in place for less than 30 days. Alternatively, in patients with a dual-lumen catheter, observing a difference in time to positivity between cultures drawn from each hub of ≥180 minutes was associated with a sensitivity of 61% and a specificity of 94%. This latter approach may be helpful in cases where obtaining a peripheral culture is not feasible.

In cases where the catheter is removed, the tip may be sent for culture via quantitative or semiquantitative methods. In the first case, a catheter segment including the tip is flushed with broth or vortexed in broth, followed by culture of the broth on agar plates. Semiquantitative, or roll-plate methods, involve rolling a sliced segment of the removed catheter across the surface of an agar plate; colony-forming units are counted after overnight incubation.

Timing of Blood Cultures Optimal timing of blood cultures has not been studied extensively. In CRBSI, unlike other infections causing bacteremia, patients are only intermittently subjected to bacteremia due to the fact that bacteria residing in the catheter lumen are not continuously exposed to the intravascular space. Prior evidence suggests that bacteremia may precede fever onset, which may mean that, in children with CRBSI, by the time fever is noted and blood cultures are drawn, the transient bacteremia has cleared. There is some evidence to suggest that this could be overcome by taking multiple blood cultures in a 24-hour period.

For critically ill patients with hemodynamic instability, two sets of blood cultures from two separate sites should be drawn promptly before the patient receives initial empiric antibiotic therapy, but this should not delay initiation of antibiotics in a septic patient. For more stable patients, multiple sets of blood cultures can be obtained in a 24-hour period to improve yield. For patients already on antibiotics, obtaining blood cultures right before the next scheduled dose (when drug levels in the body are lowest) theoretically improve blood culture yield; alternatively, "isolator" culture bottles—culture bottles with resins or chemical beads designed to remove antibiotics from sampled blood—could be used in these patients, although data are lacking on the effectiveness of these strategies.

Volume of Blood for Culture The sensitivity of blood cultures for detecting a pathogen can vary by the magnitude of bacteremia, the sensitivity of the blood culture detection system, and the volume of blood aspirated into the bottle. Smaller blood volumes (<0.5 mL) used for culture can prolong time to positivity and reduce the overall likelihood of organism growth, particularly when bacterial concentrations are low in the obtained blood. Volume of blood obtained per culture bottle is more important than number of blood cultures obtained. For example, one study found that positive yield for one large-volume (6 mL) blood culture was 72% versus only 47% for two separate smaller-volume (2 mL) blood cultures. Similar results are found in adult data as well, with standard adult-volume cultures (mean 8.7 mL) having a 92% pathogen recovery rate versus only 69% for low-volume (mean 2.7 mL) blood cultures. In adults, blood culture yield is increased approximately 3% per mL of blood cultured. In part this may be due to inadequate nutrients present in blood necessary for bacterial growth (as in the case of *Haemophilus influenzae*) after dilution in culture broth.

Conversely, overfilling blood culture bottles may also reduce yield. Broth dilution of blood, and the phagocytic cells, complement proteins, and antibodies present therein, may enhance blood culture yield. Given these constraints, each blood culture system has an optimal blood volume:broth ratio, which is usually in the range of 1:5 to 1:10. Clinicians should become familiar with the blood culture system used at their own institutions and the optimal blood volumes that should be obtained. Finally, despite the lower yield of low-volume blood cultures, it is important to note that modern culture systems supplement the broth with other materials that may increase their yield. Thus, in pediatric blood cultures, even low-volume cultures (e.g., 0.5 mL) may detect significant bacteremias, although 1 to 5 mL of blood is preferred.

Primary Bloodstream Infection Versus Contaminated Culture The most important predictor of true pathogen vs culture contamination is organism type. Expert consensus and prior data support the assertion that *Staphylococcus aureus*, *Streptococcus pneumoniae*, *Escherichia coli*, *Pseudomonas aeruginosa*, *Candida* species, and *Enterobacteriaceae* should always be thought of as true pathogens. However, given that skin flora—especially coagulase-negative staphylococci (CONS)—are commonly identified in catheter-related bloodstream infections, differentiating contaminated blood cultures from true infections can pose a challenge. Multiple cultures prior to antibiotic administration can help clarify the issue; a single blood culture contaminated with CONS, *Micrococcus*, or *Bacillus* species may represent contamination, whereas isolation of the organism from multiple cultures is more concerning for infection. Prior studies estimating the positive predictive value of a single blood culture positive for CONS in patients with central venous lines found a positive predictive value as high as 55% if it was the only culture obtained, 20% if two cultures were performed, and only 5% if three total were performed. Conversely, if two of two cultures were positive, the positive predictive value was 98% if both samples were obtained from a peripheral vein, 96% if one was obtained through a CVC and the other through a peripheral vein, and 50% if both samples were from a CVC. Differences in antibiotic susceptibility patterns between isolates of CONS obtained from multiple blood cultures may also help differentiate true infection from contamination, as differing susceptibility patterns between isolated organisms could suggest the presence of multiple contaminated blood cultures. Multiple positive cultures with a pathogenic organism are typically used in clinical practice to confirm the diagnosis of CRBSI and most labs nationwide report using this method.

Age of the child and underlying medical condition also influences the likelihood of a blood culture positive for skin flora being positive for a true pathogen. Neonates more frequently have CRBSI caused by coagulase-negative staphylococci, but it remains the predominant organism identified in children in PICUs as well. The identification of CONS in blood culture often results in administration of antibiotics, particularly vancomycin, with such overuse likely being a contributing factor to increasing vancomycin resistance among gram-positive organisms. Current recommendations from the American Academy of Pediatrics (AAP) and the Centers for Disease Control and Prevention (CDC) provide a highly sensitive method for detecting primary bloodstream infections, although from a clinician's perspective these definitions may overestimate the true incidence of bloodstream infection.

Future Detection Methods It is important to note that, although marked strides have been made in blood culture technology, the basic techniques for growing bacteria from blood samples remain relatively unchanged. Future molecular-based methods for detection of bacterial genetic material are being developed and evaluated and have proven fairly accurate in determining if two isolates come from the same strain of bacteria—thus making them more likely to represent persistent bacteremia and a true pathogen. While the technology for molecular-based methods is currently helpful for research models, it remains largely impractical for clinical purposes and nothing to date has replaced blood cultures as the gold standard for detecting bacteremia.

TREATMENT

Treatment guidelines for catheter-related bloodstream infections in children are based on limited data; most recommendations are derived from data from adult populations. Even adult data are limited, as there are no randomized control trials that address the optimal management of CRBSI.

Empiric therapy in children with suspected CRBSI should include an antibiotic with gram-positive activity such as nafcillin, oxacillin, or vancomycin, and an anti-pseudomonal gram-negative agent such as cefepime or piperacillin-tazobactam in cases where the patient is at increased risk for *Pseudomonas* such as in immunocompromised populations or in those children with underlying GI disease, etc. In cases where infection with multidrug-resistant gram-negative bacteria is suspected, use of an aminoglycoside in addition to an anti-pseudomonal β-lactam may be appropriate. More recent data exists supporting the use of beta-lactam/beta-lactamase inhibitors in the treatment of multidrug-resistant gram-negative bacteria. Vancomycin should be used in children with current or recent prolonged hospitalizations or in institutions where methicillin-resistant *Staphylococcus aureus* is common. Fluoroquinolones are rarely utilized in children as empiric treatment of a suspected CRBSI.

Clinicians should refine antibiotic therapy to target the isolated pathogen(s) based on organism morphology (e.g. coccus or bacillus, gram-positive or -negative, fungal elements) and antimicrobial susceptibility data as they become available. Pathogen identification and antibiotic susceptibility data is becoming available earlier from the time of culture positivity with molecular rapid diagnostic tests (RDTs). Use of these RDTs reduces time to definitive therapy and length of stay but are so far not associated with decreased mortality.

One of the most important issues to address in treating CRBSI is that of catheter removal (**Table 103-4**). For adults, most non-tunneled CVCs should be removed in cases of CRBSI. Adult patients whose central line is removed may experience up to a 10-fold reduction mortality rate. Removal may not always be feasible in children given lack of alternative vascular access sites or potential complications associated with reinsertion or replacement. Thus, treatment of the infection with retention of the infected catheter is often attempted. Tunneled catheters or catheters with subcutaneous access ports where there is associated tunnel or port site infection present an additional complicating issue; cure of the tunnel or site infection is rarely achieved without removal of the catheter. Successful treatment of CRBSI with retention of the catheter has been reported, however. Regardless, successful treatment of catheter-associated infection should be tailored to the device-type and organism identified.

Optimal duration of therapy for catheter-related infection is another issue of debate, and depends in part on pathogen isolated, catheter device involved, whether the device is removed, type of infection (local or systemic), and whether there are complications related to the infection, such as septic thrombosis, endocarditis, or metastatic foci of infection. In the case of complications, duration is tailored to address the most serious

TABLE 103-4 Catheter Management in Patients With Central Venous Catheter-Related Infection

Infection Type	Catheter Management
Exit site	Remove CVC if:
	No longer required
	Alternative site exists
	Patient is critically ill (e.g., hypotension)
	Infection is due to *Pseudomonas aeruginosa* or *fungi*
Tunnel	Remove CVC
Pocket	Remove CVC
Catheter-related bloodstream	Remove CVC if:
	No longer required
	Infection is due to *Staphylococcus aureus*, *Candida* species, or mycobacteria
	Patient is critically ill
	Bacteremia fails to clear in 48-72 hr
	Symptoms of bloodstream infection persist beyond 48-72 hr
	Patient has any of the following:
	Noninfectious valvular heart disease (increased risk of endocarditis)
	Endocarditis
	Metastatic infection
	Septic thrombophlebitis

complications (e.g. a patient with CRBSI and endocarditis would receive antibiotics for the duration necessary to treat endocarditis). Route of antibiotic administration is also not well-studied, although in cases of resistant organisms parenteral therapy may be the only available option. While there are very little published data to support the exact timing of transition to oral therapy and with which infections transition to oral antibiotics may/should occur, the IDSA and majority of practicing ID physicians use the following as criteria for considering transition to an alternative antibiotic with excellent oral bioavailability: (i) the catheter has been removed; (ii) the bacteremia has cleared; (iii) there are no contraindicating infectious complications; (iv) adherence to therapy is assured; (v) there are no significant barriers to medication absorption; and (vi) the patient is clinically improved. Following are some pathogen-specific recommendations.

Coagulase-Negative Staphylococci Coagulase-negative staphylococci (CONS) are considered less virulent than other pathogens causing CRBSI. Infections caused by CONS are often associated with isolated fever or local infection/inflammation at the exit site. Severe systemic illness is rare, although it is more common in neonates. Removal of the catheter without antimicrobial therapy may be sufficient treatment for CONS bacteremia, although repeat blood cultures should be obtained after catheter removal to document clearance, and most experts recommend at least a short course (e.g., 3-5 days) of antibiotic therapy after catheter removal. Treatment of infection when the catheter is retained should last 10 to 14 days after negative blood cultures. Neonates with CONS infection can be treated with retention of the catheter, but if three separate repeat blood cultures remain positive after initiation of adequate antibiotic therapy, the catheter should be removed to minimize the risk of end-organ damage. Relapse rates of CONS bacteremia from adult data in cases of retained catheters are 20% versus 3% when the catheter is removed.

Staphylococcus aureus Infections caused by *Staphylococcus aureus* can be quite severe, resulting in significant complications and risk of mortality. Although adults with CRBSI from *S. aureus* are at significant risk for bacterial endocarditis, the risk appears to be much lower in children. Regardless, echocardiography to evaluate for infective endocarditis should be performed in cases of persistent bacteremia despite adequate antibiotic therapy, or if a new murmur is identified on physical exam. In a prospective study of 51 children with *S. aureus* bacteremia, definite or possible endocarditis was diagnosed in 52% of patients with congenital heart disease, but in only 3% of patients with structurally normal hearts. Neonates are particularly susceptible to complications from *S. aureus* bloodstream infections. In cases of neonatal CRBSI from *S. aureus*, some researchers suggest removing the catheter promptly to improve patient outcomes. A minimum of 2 weeks of antimicrobial therapy is recommended for uncomplicated *S. aureus* CRBSI, and, especially in cases of methicillin-resistant *S. aureus*, should be extended in cases of complications or prolonged bacteremia, to as long as 4 to 6 weeks.

Gram-Negative Bacilli Aside from neonatal data, there is a dearth of research to guide whether intravascular catheters should be removed in patients with CRBSI caused by gram-negative bacteria. Although CRBSIs caused by certain gram-negative bacteria have been successfully treated without catheter removal, catheter removal is beneficial in treating infection cause by *Pseudomonas* species, *Burkholderia cepacia*, *Acinetobacter baumanni*, and *Stenotrophomonas* species. A study in adults reported reduced relapse rates in patients who underwent catheter removal as part of their treatment. In general, antibiotic therapy should be given for 10 to 14 days.

Fungemia Treatment of fungal CRBSI without catheter removal is associated with generally poor outcomes, although these studies were confounded by illness severity (i.e., sicker patients often required catheter retention and were the most likely patients to die). Retaining catheters infected with *Candida* species may prolong fungemia, which can increase the risk for disseminated infection. Metastatic infection from candidemia to end organs (lung, liver, spleen, eye, brain, heart) is reportedly 17%, and the crude mortality rate in children with candidemia is 26%. In general, catheters should be removed in children with candidemia whenever possible, and therapy with an appropriate antifungal therapy should be continued for 2 weeks from negative culture. All children diagnosed with candidemia should have an ophthalmologic examination to evaluate for endophthalmitis, preferably after the infection appears to be controlled and further dissemination is unlikely. Abdominal and renal ultrasounds and echocardiogram should be considered in the following situations: (i) neonatal age group; (ii) older children with prolonged candidemia; and (iii) any child with concern for disseminated infection.

Antibiotic Lock Therapy Instillation of antimicrobial solutions intended to dwell in the catheter lumen can increase the likelihood of successful treatment of CRBSI in cases where catheter retention is necessary. So-called antibiotic lock therapy utilizes solutions that often achieve concentrations of antimicrobial agents 40 to 120 times serum concentrations while imposing minimal risk of systemic toxicity to the patient. Researchers have reported use of several antimicrobial agents in lock therapy, with variable success (**Table 103-5**). Lock therapy can be used in conjunction with systemic antibiotic therapy, although clinicians should maximize the time lock solutions dwell in the catheter lumen undisturbed (usually 12-24 hrs/dwell). Lock therapy should not be attempted in patients with complicated infections, *Candida* species infection, or in cases of tunnel, exit site, or port site infections.

CONSULTATION

Involvement of the team that prescribed the central catheter is appropriate, such as gastroenterology if the catheter was placed for parenteral

TABLE 103-5 Recommended Concentrations of Antimicrobial Agents Used in Lock Therapy*

Agent	Concentration (mg/mL)
Vancomycin	1-5
Gentamicin	1-2
Amikacin	1-2
Cefazolin	5
Ceftazidime	0.5
Ethanol	25%-50% solution

*Solutions made with heparin 50-100 UOR 0.9% sodium chloride solution to volume of 2-5 mL.

nutrition, orthopedics for treatment of osteomyelitis, and oncology for chemotherapy. Infectious disease specialist consultation can be helpful, especially if outpatient antibiotic therapy services are desired or if there is clinical uncertainty about when or if transition to parenteral antibiotics is appropriate. Including the clinical service that initially inserted the catheter may also be necessary, especially in cases where replacement of the line will likely be necessary.

ADMISSION AND DISCHARGE CRITERIA

Most patients with CRBSI are initially evaluated and treated as inpatients. Children with associated sepsis with hemodynamic instability require intensive management in a critical care setting.

Discharge criteria for children with catheter-related bloodstream infection include:

- Resolution of bacteremia
- Ability to safely provide ongoing antibiotic therapy in the outpatient setting if required
- Institution of an appropriate plan to continue therapy for the underlying condition that initially warranted catheter placement

PREVENTION

Current practices associated with a reduced risk of catheter-related infections include the following:

- Use of maximal barriers during catheter placement
- Use of chlorhexidine-isopropyl alcohol solution to prepare the skin prior to catheter placement and during routine catheter care/dressing changes
- Prompt removal of catheters as soon as they are no longer required
- Strict adherence to appropriate hand hygiene practices
- Scrubbing the catheter hub with chlorhexidine-isopropyl alcohol solution prior to every access/entry into the catheter hub
- Using the most peripheral insertion site possible
- Application of topical antibiotics to skin surrounding the catheter with dressings

A systematic review of the use of antibiotic impregnated central lines for the prevention of bloodstream infections found a modest benefit to the use of such catheters. Finally, monitoring/oversight systems should be employed to ensure compliance with multiple risk reduction interventions (bundled interventions).

CEREBROSPINAL FLUID (CSF) SHUNTS

BACKGROUND

Infection is one of the most common complications of cerebrospinal fluid (CSF) shunts with 11% to 25% of VP shunts placed in children and neonates developing infection within the first year. Shunt infections account for 2200 to 2400 admissions and 49,000 to 59,000 hospital days in the United States yearly. CSF shunt infections are associated with increased risk of seizure disorder, intellectual impairment, and long-term mortality.

PATHOPHYSIOLOGY

Shunt obstruction is the most common reason for shunt revision, but shunt infection follows as a close second, leading to many costly admissions including ICU stays and need for prolonged IV antibiotics. **Table 103-6** summarizes the organisms most commonly found in CSF shunt infections. Accounting for two-thirds of shunt infections, *Staphylococcus* species are by far the most common species identified with coagulase-negative staphylococci as the most prevalent organism. Various gram-negative organisms, including *Escherichia coli*, *Klebsiella pneumonia*, and *Pseudomonas aeruginosa*, can also be responsible for shunt infections. Anaerobic bacteria, especially *Cutibacterium* (formerly *Propionibacterium*) *acnes*, cause low-grade, indolent shunt infections. They have historically been implicated in culture-negative infections, and they can be difficult to grow, especially if CSF is not sent for anaerobic culture. Shunt infections with fungi, predominantly *Candida* species, have been reported in premature neonates as well as patients who are immune compromised or receiving parental nutrition.

Shunt infections caused by skin organisms are thought to occur with introduction of the bacteria at time of shunt placement or shortly following shunt placement with wound breakdown. Up to 85% of shunt infections that occur within the first 15 days after surgery are caused by the common skin flora staphylococci. By contrast, *S. aureus* rarely causes infection in shunts placed more than 9 months prior to infection.

Shunt infections caused by gram-negative organisms are thought to arise from ascending infection of enteric organisms that colonize the distal portion of the shunt, as the catheter often terminates in the abdomen. These infections typically occur a longer time after the initial surgery, with 64% of gram-negative infections occurring more than 15 days following surgery. Ventriculoatrial (VA) shunts in particular are at increased risk of infection from hematogenous spread of pathogens due to their interface with the vascular system.

Many studies have attempted to define factors that predispose children to shunt infection. Several retrospective studies have identified increased risk of infection with younger patient age, insertion of shunt into a premature neonate, more frequent shunt revisions, insertion following infection, and neuroendoscope use for shunt insertion. Infection risk is higher among younger patients. Premature infants have a nearly fivefold increase in risk of infection.

Infection is up to fourfold higher in cases of reinsertion following treatment of initial infection. A retrospective multicenter cohort study of 675 patients with first CSF shunt infection found an overall 6-month reinfection rate of 14.8%. There were no differences between those with and without reinfection in age or number of shunt revisions at first infection, but those with reinfection did have less time between their shunt placement and initial infection. Children who experience a second shunt

TABLE 103-6 Pathogens Commonly Found in Shunt Infections

	NUMBER OF PATIENTS (%)						
Organism	McGirt et al, 2003 ($n = 92$)	Odio et al, 1960 ($n = 59$)	Ronan et al, 1995 ($n = 41$)	Mancao et al, 1998 ($n = 29$)	Kontny et al, 1993 ($n = 28$)	Enger et al, 2003 ($n = 9$)	Total ($n = 258$)
Staphylococcus epidermidis	49 (53)	27 (46%)	7 (17)	14 (48)	16 (57)	7 (78%)	120 (47)
Staphylococcus aureus	24 (26)	17 (29)	12 (30)	7 (24)	1 (4)	1 (11%)	62 (24)
Gram negatives	8 (9)	15 (25)	10 (24)	3 (10)	2 (7)	–	38 (15)
Viridans streptococcus	–	6 (10)	–	–	–	–	6 (2)
Enterococcus	4 (4)	3 (5)	2 (5)	–	–	–	9 (3)
Mixed	–	–	–	3 (10)	5 (18)	–	8 (3)
Other*	4 (4)	–	–	2 (7)	4 (14)	2 (22)	12 (5)

*Other culture results include *Candida* species ($n = 2$; Enger), no growth ($n = 4$; Kontny), *Corynebacterium* ($n = 1$) and group B *Streptococcus* ($n = 1$; Mancao), and *Propionibacterium* ($n = 4$; McGirf).

TABLE 103-7 Percentage of Patients With Clinical Findings of Possible Shunt Infection

Presentation	Odio et al, 1960 ($n = 59$)	Rogers et al, 2012 ($n = 58$)	Ronan et al, 1995 ($n = 41$)	Mancao et al, 1998 ($n = 29$)	Kontny et al, 1993 ($n = 28$)	Total ($n = 215$)
Fever	87	59	72	62	96	74
Irritability	81	26	27	69*	25	47
Vomiting	39	48	24	–	–	28
Abdominal pain	22	16	15	17†	36	20
Shunt malfunction	–	–	36	–	50	13
Cellulitis	19	–	15	24	–	11
Headache	–	28	5	–	–	10
Lethargy	–	24	12	–	–	8
Meningismus	–	–	20	–	21	6
Seizure	–	3	7	–	–	1

*This percentage represents patients with "neurologic signs," which included vomiting, irritability, bulging fontanelle, or meningismus.

†This percentage represents patients with "abdominal signs," which included abdominal pain, ileus, or diarrhea.

infection are at substantially higher risk for further repeated infections with 60% developing a third infection and 47% developing a fourth infection in one study. Up to two-thirds of recurrent infections are caused by the same organism as the initial infection.

CLINICAL PRESENTATION

While fever and shunt malfunction are common presenting symptoms of shunt infection, early diagnosis is difficult due to the lack of reliable predictive factors to distinguish shunt infection from other causes of fever and shunt malfunction. For example, shunt infection is the cause of malfunction in only 3% to 8% of shunt malfunctions.

The clinical manifestations of shunt infections can be quite varied (**Table 103-7**), owing to the existence of different locations along the shunt track that are prone to infection. These include the lumen of the shunt itself, the extraluminal ventricles, and the cranial and distal surgical sites of insertion. While proximal shunt malfunctions and infections may present with neurologic features of increased intracranial pressure (including headache, vomiting, lethargy, and/or seizures), distal shunt malfunction, and infections commonly present with abdominal pain.

Pseudocysts, inflammatory reactions around the distal catheter tip that result in the collection of CSF, may be the direct consequence of a shunt infection or may develop in the absence of infection and become secondarily infected. If an infected pseudocyst leaks into the abdominal cavity, patients often present with frank peritonitis. If leakage does not occur, abdominal symptoms may be more indolent.

Patients with wound infections present with incisional erythema and purulence, with or without local collections of CSF. Although physical exam findings suggestive of wound infection should prompt evaluation for shunt infection, they are rarely present.

DIFFERENTIAL DIAGNOSIS

Most children with CSF shunts who present with fever do not have shunt infections. While the full spectrum of causes of fever should be considered, it will be tailored by other presenting symptoms. For instance, in a child with fever and altered mental status, the differential diagnosis should include meningoencephalitis.

In children presenting with symptoms of shunt malfunction without fever, mechanical obstruction of CSF flow should be considered. Obstruction may occur proximally, at the intake portion of the device (e.g., clogging, blockage from adjacent tissue), at any point along the tubing (e.g., kinking), or at the point of fluid exit. If the tubing becomes disconnected, flow may cease.

DIAGNOSIS

Diagnosis of a shunt infection necessitates the isolation of a bacterial pathogen from ventricular fluid, lumbar CSF, or blood, with or without CSF pleocytosis (>50 white blood cells/mm^3) and at least one symptom of CSF shunt infection (fever, shunt malfunction, neurologic symptoms, or abdominal pain).

Ventricular fluid should be obtained under sterile conditions via percutaneous aspiration by a practitioner with experience in the procedure. In a patient with more than one shunt, it is important to obtain cultures of each shunt as the collections of CSF drained by separate shunts may not be in communication. Once obtained CSF should be sent for cell count, glucose, protein, Gram stain, and aerobic and anaerobic cultures. Fungal cultures should be considered in patients at high risk for fungal infections.

Positive blood cultures are frequently seen with VA shunt infections as infected CSF drains directly into the bloodstream. However, bacteremia is a relatively uncommon finding in VP shunt infections as many patients who require CSF shunts have underlying impairment or absence of CSF reabsorption into the venous blood system limiting passage of bacteria into the bloodstream. Additionally, negative cultures from lumbar CSF should be interpreted with caution. Lumbar CSF culture may not always reflect the CSF in the ventricles as the ventricles have little or no communication with lumbar spinal fluid when a shunt is in place. Thus, while cultures of blood and lumbar CSF can be helpful in diagnosis, culture of the ventricular fluid is the mainstay of diagnosis.

In analysis of ventricular CSF, pleocytosis is a helpful marker, but is not diagnostic of infection alone. CSF white blood cell (WBC) count of >100/mm^3 has a specificity of 96% for shunt infection (i.e., of those without shunt infection, 96% will have 100 or fewer white blood cells/mm^3); the sensitivity of that finding is only 60%. This modest sensitivity may reflect inflammation that can occur following shunt placement. However, as many shunt infections occur shortly after placement it is important to have a high index of suspicion for infection when CSF pleocytosis is seen. In addition, shunt infections caused by indolent organisms (e.g., *Cutibacterium acnes* and coagulase-negative staphylococci) may not have a reactive CSF pleocytosis. CSF neutrophilia (neutrophils >10% of CSF white blood cells) is a more sensitive marker of infection, with sensitivity of 90% and a specificity of 90%.

When considered in association with other clinical markers, the CSF white blood cell count and differential is of greater diagnostic value. In a meta-analysis of 49 studies on pediatric shunt infections, when fever was combined with CSF pleocytosis, diagnosis of shunt infection was made with sensitivity of 82% and specificity of 99%. The combination of fever with ventricular fluid neutrophilia (>10%) has been shown to have a specificity of 99% and positive and negative predictive values of 93% and 95%, respectively, for identifying or excluding shunt-related infection. While pleocytosis, elevated CSF lactate or procalcitonin, and other markers of inflammation and infection are often used as a supporting factor, CSF culture is still the gold standard—often along with patient symptomatology—in diagnosing shunt infection.

A "shunt series" (x-ray of the skull, neck, chest, and abdomen) as well as head computed tomography (CT) should be obtained to evaluate for signs of shunt malfunction. Additional imaging is dependent on the type of shunt in place—for example, abdominal ultrasound or abdominal CT to evaluate for pseudocyst formation in the child with a VP shunt presenting with abdominal pain.

TREATMENT

It is generally accepted that optimal management of a shunt infection includes treatment with antibiotics in combination with and shunt removal or externalization with delayed replacement until the CSF is sterile. In retrospective studies, this approach has been clearly associated with better outcomes than other approaches including intravenous antibiotics without shunt removal, intravenous and intraventricular antibiotics without shunt removal, and intravenous antibiotics with shunt removal and immediate shunt replacement. In a prospective cohort study of shunt infections treatment the authors found no difference in outcomes between those patients who underwent shunt removal and those treated with externalization. An analysis of the treatment options for shunt infection, including 17 studies published over 30 years, revealed that antibiotics in combination with shunt removal (either complete removal or externalization with delayed replacement until CSF sterility) successfully treated 88% of 244 infections. In contrast, antibiotic therapy alone was successful in only 33% of 230 infections.

Empirical antibiotic therapy should include broad-spectrum antibiotics that cover the major pathogens associated with shunt-related infections. Vancomycin is recommended for gram-positive coverage of staphylococcal species, including the common *Staphylococcus epidermidis* and the increasingly prevalent methicillin-resistant *S. aureus*. Addition of cefepime or meropenem is recommended for coverage of gram-negative organisms including *P. aeruginosa*. *C. acnes* is generally susceptible to penicillin and ceftriaxone; vancomycin is an alternate option. Therapy should be tailored based on the identification and susceptibility of the causative organism identified on culture. The addition of oral rifampin is often recommended, despite a lack of strong evidence, for gram-positive infections that fail to clear with vancomycin monotherapy.

If appropriate systemic therapy fails to eradicate the infection, neuroimaging should be obtained to detect possible intracranial abscess. The presence of an intracranial abscess might lead to surgical drainage and/or prolonged antibiotic therapy. In the case of continued infection and negative neuroimaging, the addition of intrathecal antibiotics or assessment of antibiotic therapy should be considered. While not approved by the Food and Drug Administration for intraventricular use, vancomycin and aminoglycosides have been commonly used. Trough ventricular antibiotic concentration or ventricular fluid bactericidal titers may be used in consultation with infectious disease specialists to determine the adequacy of antibiotic therapy.

Duration of antibiotic therapy varies widely, largely dependent on the pathogen involved, time to CSF sterilization, clinical response, and the surgical approach. The duration of therapy recommended is largely consensus based as there is no good evidence surrounding treatment time and clinical outcomes.

See **Figure 103-2** for an algorithm of management of suspected CSF shunt infection.

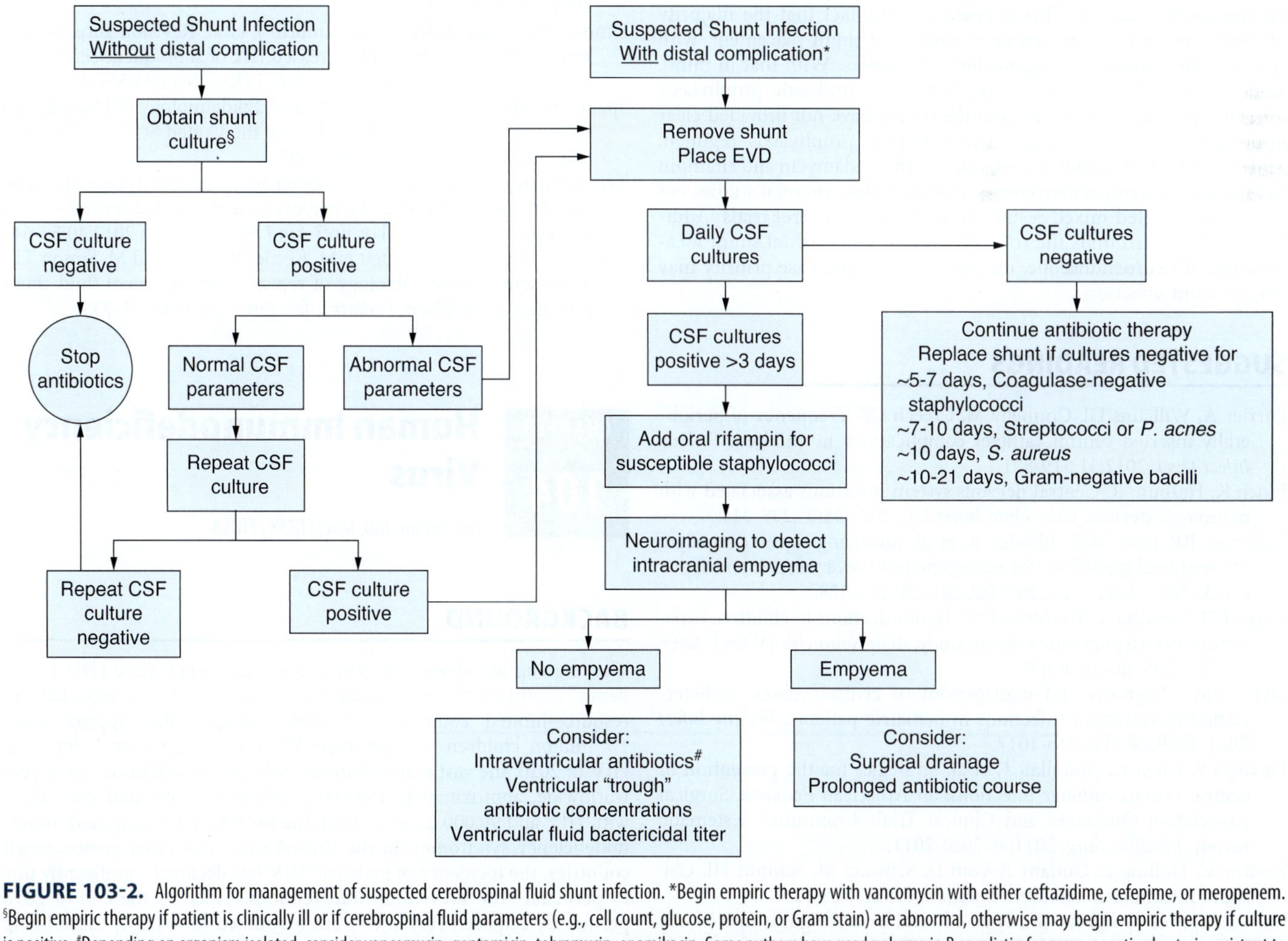

FIGURE 103-2. Algorithm for management of suspected cerebrospinal fluid shunt infection. *Begin empiric therapy with vancomycin with either ceftazidime, cefepime, or meropenem. §Begin empiric therapy if patient is clinically ill or if cerebrospinal fluid parameters (e.g., cell count, glucose, protein, or Gram stain) are abnormal, otherwise may begin empiric therapy if culture is positive. #Depending on organism isolated, consider vancomycin, gentamicin, tobramycin, or amikacin. Some authors have used polymyxin B or colistin for gram-negative bacteria resistant to commonly used antibiotic agents.[103-105] Intraventricular administration is not a Food and Drug Administration-approved indication for any of the listed antibiotics. (Reproduced with permission from Hart JK, Shah SS. Cerebrospinal fluid shunt infections. In: Shaw SS, ed. *Pediatric Practice: Infectious Diseases*. New York, NY: McGraw-Hill Medical; 2009.)

CONSULTATION

Neurosurgery and infectious disease consultants should be involved in the care of a child with a CSF shunt infection. Neurosurgeons are routinely involved with the evaluation of infections and are responsible for surgical management of CSF shunt infections. Infectious disease specialists can provide guidance on empiric therapy, need for further evaluation, and antibiotic management decisions. Critical care involvement varies with the patient's condition and the particular institution, though most centers require at least some time in the ICU following shunt revision surgery.

ADMISSION AND DISCHARGE CRITERIA

The majority of patients with shunt infections require hospitalization owing to the complexity of care, including parenteral antibiotic therapy and externalization of the shunt. Frequent assessments of the neurologic and overall clinical status of the patient are required. Additionally, externalized shunts require close attention to the rate of drainage, as adjustments may be needed to remain within satisfactory parameters. Transfer to a critical care setting may be appropriate, depending on the clinical status of the patient and the ability to provide close medical support in a non-intensive care environment.

Discharge can be considered when the infection has resolved, and a stable CSF drainage management system is in place. Close outpatient follow-up is needed to watch for reinfection, malfunction, and signs of raised intracranial pressure.

PREVENTION

Despite aseptic technique in the operating room with skin cleansing and site preparation (with hair clipping and shampoo), surgical contamination still occurs. This is evident in the fact that the majority of shunt infections occur within 6 months of shunt placement, with approximately half occurring in the first 2 weeks. With that in mind, several studies have examined the benefit of antibiotic prophylaxis for shunt placement surgeries, but the results have not provided clear information on the most effective antibiotic prophylaxis regimen. More recently, CSF shunts impregnated with clindamycin and rifampin have demonstrated positive effects in several observational studies but have demonstrated mixed results in randomized control trials. Additional debate surrounds the role that type of shunt, distal shunt location, use of neuroendoscope, duration of case, and case priority may play in shunt infection.

SUGGESTED READINGS

Barrier A, Williams DJ, Connelly M, Creech CB. Frequency of peripherally inserted central catheter complications in children. *Pediatr Infect Dis J.* 2012;31:519-521.

Bloch K, Hasbun, R. Central nervous system infections associated with neurologic devices. *Curr Opin Infect Dis.* 2021;34(3):238-244.

Dellinger RP, Levy MM, Rhodes A, et al. Surviving sepsis campaign: international guidelines for management of severe sepsis and septic shock, 2012. *Intensive Care Med.* 2013;39:165-228.

Enger PO, Svendsen F, Wester K. CSF shunt infections in children: experiences from a population-based study. *Acta Neurochir (Wien).* 2003; 145:243-248; discussion 8.

Flynn PM. Diagnosis and management of central venous catheter-related bloodstream infections in pediatric patients. *Pediatr Infect Dis J.* 2009;28(11):1016-1017.

Huang EY, Chen C, Abdullah F, et al. Strategies for the prevention of central venous catheter infections: an American Pediatric Surgical Association Outcomes and Clinical Trials Committee systematic review. *J Pediatr Surg.* 2011;46:2000-2011.

Kontny U, Hofling B, Gutjahr P, Voth D, Schwarz M, Schmitt HJ. CSF shunt infections in children. *Infection.* 1993;21:89-92.

Liu C, Bayer A, Cosgrove SE, et al. Clinical practice guidelines by the Infectious Diseases Society of America for the treatment of methicillin-resistant *Staphylococcus aureus* infections in adults and children. *Clin Infect Dis.* 2011;52:e18-e55.

Mancao M, Miller C, Cochrane B, Hoff C, Sauter K, Weber E. Cerebrospinal fluid shunt infections in infants and children in Mobile, Alabama. *Acta Paediatrica* (Oslo, Norway: 1992). 1998;87:667-670.

McGirt MJ, Zaas A, Fuchs HE, George TM, Kaye K, Sexton DJ. Risk factors for pediatric ventriculoperitoneal shunt infection and predictors of infectious pathogens. *Clin Infect Dis.* 2003;36:858-862.

Megged O, Shalit I, Yaniv I, et al. Outcome of antibiotic lock technique for persistent central venous catheter-associated coagulase-negative Staphylococcus bacteremia in children. *Eur J Clin Microbiol Infect Dis.* 2010;29:157-161.

Mermel LA, Allon M, Bouza E, et al. Clinical practice guidelines for the diagnosis and management of intravascular catheter-related infection: 2009 Update by the Infectious Diseases Society of America. *Clin Infect Dis.* 2009;49(1):1-45. Erratum in: *Clin Infect Dis.* 2010; 50(7):1079. Dosage error in article text. Erratum in: *Clin Infect Dis.* 2010;50(3):457.

Odio C, McCracken GH Jr, Nelson JD. CSF shunt infections in pediatrics. A seven-year experience. *Am J Dis Child* (1960). 1984;138:1103-1108.

Paff, M. Alexandru-Abrams, D. et al. Ventriculoperitoneal shunt complications: a review. *Interdisciplinary Neurosurg.* 2018;13:66-70.

Rinke ML, Heo M, Saiman L, Bundy DG, et al. Pediatric ambulatory central line-associated bloodstream infections. *Pediatrics.* 2021;147(1): e20200524.

Rogers EA, Kimia A, Madsen JR, Nigrovic LE, Neuman MI. Predictors of ventricular shunt infection among children presenting to a pediatric emergency department. *Pediatr Emerg Care.* 2012;28:405-409.

Ronan A, Hogg GG, Klug GL. Cerebrospinal fluid shunt infections in children. *Pediatr Infect Dis J.* 1995;14:782-786.

Selby LM, Rupp ME, Cawcutt KA. Prevention of central-line associated bloodstream infections: 2021 update. *Infect Dis Clin North Am.* 2021;35(4):841-856.

Simon TD, Whitlock KB, Riva-Cambrin J, et al. Revision surgeries are associated with significant increased risk of subsequent cerebrospinal fluid shunt infection. *Pediatr Infect Dis J.* 2012;31:551-556.

Spaulding AB, Watson D, Dreyfus J, et al. Epidemiology of bloodstream infections in hospitalized children in the United States, 2009-2016. *Clin Infect Dis.* 2019;69(6):995-1002.

Tsai MH, Hsu JF, Lien R, et al. Catheter management in neonates with bloodstream infection and a percutaneously inserted central venous catheter in situ: removal or not? *Am J Infect Control.* 2012;40:59-64.

Tuan TJ, Thorell EA, Hamblett NM, Kestle JR, Rosenfeld M, Simon TD. Treatment and microbiology of repeated cerebrospinal fluid shunt infections in children. *Pediatr Infect Dis J.* 2011;30:731-735.

CHAPTER 104 Human Immunodeficiency Virus

Ari Bitnun, MD, MSc, FRCPC, FIDSA

BACKGROUND

The ongoing world-wide human immunodeficiency virus (HIV) pandemic continues to exact a dramatic toll on children, especially in resource-limited countries. UNAIDS estimates that approximately 1.7 million children younger than 15 years of age were living with HIV in 2020, the vast majority in sub-Saharan Africa. In the same year worldwide, approximately 150,000 children were infected perinatally with HIV and 99,000 children died due to HIV/AIDS (acquired immunodeficiency syndrome). In the United States and other resource-rich countries, the incidence of pediatric HIV has declined significantly due to perinatal HIV prevention interventions. Thus, by the end of 2018 perinatally acquired HIV infections accounted for <1% of those living with HIV in the United States. Youth aged 13 to 24 years, who most often acquire infection sexually or via injection drug use, accounted for approximately 20% of new HIV infections in the United States in 2020.

Prior to the availability of preventive interventions, vertical HIV transmission occurred at rates of 15% to 40%. Sixty percent to 75% of infections occurred during the process of delivery, while 10% to 20% occurred in utero and 10% to 15% as a consequence of breastfeeding. With the routine implementation of preventive interventions including routine prenatal counseling and testing for HIV, antenatal antiretroviral therapy (ART) for pregnant women and zidovudine (ZDV, also known as AZT) prophylaxis for newborns, and where appropriate, elective cesarean delivery and ZDV infusion during labor, the vertical transmission rate has been reduced to about 1% of infants born in the developed world. Ongoing challenges include primary prevention of infection in girls and young women, incomplete testing during pregnancy, and failure to implement preventive interventions once the diagnosis is established. Substance abuse, psychiatric illness, and socioeconomic issues such as poverty, limited access to medical care, and inadequate housing are associated with HIV infection and vertical HIV transmission.

The pediatric hospitalist needs to be familiar with the care of HIV-exposed newborns and newborns of mothers with unknown HIV status as these mothers can be at elevated risk of having undiagnosed HIV infection. It is also important for pediatric hospitalists to know when to consider HIV infection in children hospitalized with undifferentiated symptoms and be familiar with the management of infectious and non-infectious complications of HIV infection as well as the management of occupational and non-occupational HIV exposures.

CLINICAL PRESENTATION

Most infants infected vertically with HIV acquire the infection intrapartum and are asymptomatic as newborns. Rates of prematurity and low birth weight are higher in HIV-infected than in uninfected infants, but there are usually no physical examination findings that would specifically implicate HIV as the cause. Consequently, any newborn whose mother's HIV status is unknown should be considered at risk.

The natural history of HIV infection in vertically infected children is one of rapid progression when compared to adolescents and adults infected horizontally, likely due to immunologic immaturity at the time of infection. In developed countries, approximately 20% develop profound immunosuppression and AIDS-defining conditions during the first year of life. Without treatment, these "rapid progressors" typically succumb to the disease by 2 years of age. Of the remaining 80%, onset of disease is more gradual with 4% to 8% progressing to AIDS each year. In the absence of treatment, only 2% remain completely asymptomatic and have preserved immune function, as measured by CD4 count, at 10 years of age.

The most common AIDS-defining conditions in children are *Pneumocystis jirovecii* pneumonia (PJP), lymphoid interstitial pneumonitis (LIP), multiple or recurrent invasive bacterial infections, HIV wasting syndrome, HIV encephalopathy, esophageal candidiasis, cytomegalovirus (CMV) disease, and disseminated infection with *Mycobacterium avium-intracellulare* complex. However, clues to the diagnosis are evident prior to development of AIDS in most children. Recurrent sinopulmonary infections, prolonged or atypical course of common childhood infections, impaired growth, or delayed attainment of developmental milestones may be evident. Nonspecific findings on physical examination, such as generalized lymphadenopathy, parotitis, hepatosplenomegaly, or dermatitis and laboratory abnormalities, such as anemia, neutropenia, thrombocytopenia, or hypergammaglobulinemia may be seen. Youth with acute HIV infection, most often acquired sexually or through injection drug use, can present with an acute retroviral syndrome that resembles infectious mononucleosis with fever, headache, pharyngitis, fatigue, rash, generalized lymphadenopathy, myalgia, arthralgia, and other non-specific symptoms.

The clinical and immunologic classification of HIV/AIDS can be helpful in assessing how advance HIV disease is at baseline, how well a person living with HIV is doing while on treatment and as a guide to when antimicrobial prophylaxis is warranted. The need for antimicrobial prophylaxis is primarily determined by immunologic status, as defined by CD4 count or CD4%. Both CD4 count and CD4% decline with age until about 6 years of age when they stabilize at adult levels. The stages of HIV infection progression is depicted in **Figure 104-1**, the World Health Organization (WHO) clinical staging of HIV/AIDS for children

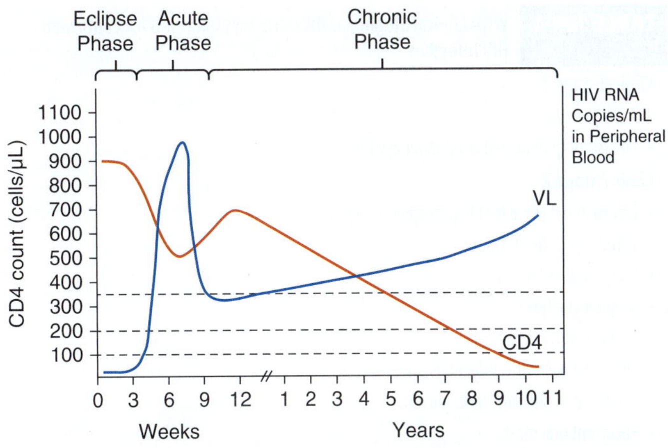

FIGURE 104-1. Disease progression following horizontally acquired HIV infection in the absence of antiretroviral treatment. In the absence of treatment, HIV infection can be broadly divided into three phases: eclipse, acute, and chronic phases. The eclipse phase reflects initial HIV infection of immune cells in the mucosa at the site of infection, systemic spread of the virus via local lymph nodes, absence of detectable virus in peripheral blood and non-reactive HIV serology. The acute phase is characterized by detection of the virus in blood, a decline in CD4 cell count, initial cytotoxic T cell response, and seroconversion to HIV, and in some cases a non-specific febrile illness (acute retroviral syndrome). The chronic phase, which is variable in length but can last for many years, can be roughly divided into an initial asymptomatic period and a subsequent symptomatic period. During the asymptomatic period viral load stabilizes at a level that varies widely between patients ("viral set point") with CD4 count partially recovering from its nadir during the acute phase and stabilizing at a level below its pre-infection level. The symptomatic period reflects declining immune function with CD4 counts dropping below 350 cell/μL and a gradual viral load rise in peripheral blood. Opportunistic infections and other AIDS-defining complications characteristically occur when CD4 count declines to less than 200 cells/μL. VL, viral load.

in **Table 104-1** and the immunologic classification for established HIV infection in **Table 104-2**.

DIAGNOSIS

Diagnosis of HIV infection during early infancy relies on detection of the virus in serum using DNA or RNA polymerase chain reaction (PCR); serology is of little utility due to transplacental passage of maternal antibodies. Cord blood samples should not be used for testing because maternal blood may contaminate the sample. HIV PCR should be performed within 48 hours of birth, at 1 to 2 months, and at 4 to 6 months of age. A positive result within 48 hours of birth is indicative of in utero transmission while a reactive PCR at or beyond 1 month of age, subsequent to a negative birth to 48 hour test, reflects infection acquired during the birthing process or via breast milk. Exclusion of HIV infection in non-breastfed infants requires either: (i) two negative HIV DNA or RNA virologic test results from separate specimens obtained at 1 month of age or later, one of which was obtained at 4 months of age or later; or (ii) two or more negative HIV antibody tests taken at 6 months of age or later. In children 24 months of age or older, HIV infection is confirmed by a two step process, an initial antigen/antibody combination immunoassay that detects antibodies to HIV-1 and HIV-2 and HIV p24 antigen, followed by a supplemental immunoassay that differentiates HIV-1 from HIV-2 antibodies. Two important caveats to HIV diagnostic tests are that perinatally exposed children aged 18 to 24 months can occasionally have residual maternal antibody in their blood and that HIV-1 PCR primers have reduced sensitivity for HIV-2.

MANAGEMENT

MANAGEMENT OF THE HIV-EXPOSED NEWBORN INFANT (TABLE 104-3)

The initial evaluation of an HIV-exposed neonate begins with a detailed prenatal history. In addition to the typical elements (e.g., prenatal

TABLE 104-1 WHO Clinical Staging of HIV/AIDS for Children With Confirmed HIV Infection

Clinical stage 1
- Asymptomatic
- Persistent generalized lymphadenopathy

Clinical stage 2
- Unexplained persistent hepatosplenomegaly
- Papular pruritic eruptions
- Fungal nail infections
- Angular cheilitis
- Linear gingival erythema
- Extensive wart virus infections
- Extensive molluscum contagiosum
- Recurrent oral ulcers
- Unexplained persistent parotid enlargement
- Herpes zoster
- Recurrent or chronic upper respiratory tract infections (otitis media, otorrhea, sinusitis, tonsillitis)

Clinical stage 3
- Unexplained moderate malnutrition or wasting not adequately responding to standard therapy
- Unexplained persistent diarrhea (14 days or more)
- Unexplained persistent fever (above 37.5°C intermittent or constant; longer than 1 month)
- Persistent oral candidiasis (after first 6-8 weeks of life)
- Oral hairy leukoplakia
- Acute necrotizing ulcerative gingivitis or periodontitis
- Lymph node tuberculosis
- Pulmonary tuberculosis

Severe recurrent bacterial pneumonia
- Symptomatic lymphoid interstitial pneumonitis
- Chronic HIV-associated lung disease including bronchiectasis
- Unexplained anemia (<8 g/L), neutropenia ($<0.5 \times 10^6$/L), or chronic thrombocytopenia ($< 50 \times 10^9$/L)

Clinical stage 4[§]
- Unexplained severe wasting, stunting or severe malnutrition not responding to standard therapy
- *Pneumocystis jirovecii* pneumonia
- Recurrent severe bacterial infections (such as empyema, pyomyositis, bone or joint infection or meningitis but excluding pneumonia)
- Chronic herpes simplex infection (orolabial or cutaneous of more than one month's duration or visceral at any site)
- Esophageal candidiasis (or candidiasis of trachea, bronchi or lungs)
- Extrapulmonary tuberculosis
- Kaposi sarcoma
- Cytomegalovirus infection: retinitis or cytomegalovirus infection affecting another organ, with onset at age older than one month
- Central nervous system toxoplasmosis (after one month of life)
- Extrapulmonary cryptococcosis (including meningitis)
- HIV encephalopathy
- Disseminated endemic mycosis (coccidiomycosis or histoplasmosis)
- Disseminated non-tuberculous mycobacterial infection
- Chronic cryptosporidiosis (with diarrhea)
- Chronic isosporiasis
- Cerebral or B-cell non-Hodgkin lymphoma
- Progressive multifocal leukoencephlopathy
- Symptomatic HIV-associated nephropathy or HIV-associated cardiomyopathy

[§]Some additional specific conditions can also be included in regional classifications (such as reactivation of American trypanosomiasis [meningoencephalitis and/or myocarditis] in the WHO Region of the Americas, disseminated penicilliosis in Asia and HIV-associated rectovaginal fistula in Africa).

Source: Reproduced with permission from World Health Organization; 2007. Available at: https://apps.who.int/iris/bitstream/handle/10665/43699/9789241595629_eng.pdf?sequence=1&isAllowed=y.

TABLE 104-2 WHO Immunological Classification for Established HIV Infection

	Age			
HIV-Associated Immunodeficiency	<11 months (CD4%)	12-35 months (CD4%)	36-59 months (CD4%)	>5 years (CD4 count or CD4%)
None or not significant	>35	>30	>25	>500
Mild	30-35	25-30	20-25	350-499
Moderate	25-29	20-24	15-19	200-349
Severe	<25	<20	<15	<200 or <15%

CD4 count—absolute number per mm^3.

Source: Reproduced with permission from World Health Organization; 2007. Available at: https://apps.who.int/iris/bitstream/handle/10665/43699/9789241595629_eng.pdf?sequence=1&isAllowed=y.

TABLE 104-3 Key Elements of Maternal History and Infant Management in the Immediate Post-Partum Period

Antenatal maternal history
- Timing of HIV diagnosis
- Prenatal antiretiviral regimen(s)
- Timing of antiretroviral treatment initiation
- Antiretroviral medication adherence
- Viral loads during pregnancy
- CD4 counts during pregnancy

Intrapartum history
- Intravenous zidovudine administration (yes/no)*
- Mode of delivery; if Cesarean section reason (related to HIV)

Infant feeding plan
- Exclusive formula feeding is the preferred recommendation in resource rich settings
- Women who indicate an intention to breastfeed should receive urgent counseling by a pediatric HIV expert[||]

Infant investigations[||]
- Bloodwork in the newborn period not routinely required for term infants receiving a shortened (2 week) course of zidovudine
- Complete blood count and differential at baseline for infants receiving 4-6 weeks of zidovudine or pre-emptive antiretroviral treatment
- HIV PCR within 48 hours of birth for infants receiving 4-6 weeks of zidovudine or pre-emptive antiretroviral treatment

Infant antiretroviral medications[||]
- Zidovudine monotherapy for 2-6 weeks for infants at lower risk of HIV infection[‡¥]
- Pre-emptive treatment with zidovudine, lamivudine and nevirapine, or raltegravir for 2-6 weeks for infants at high risk of HIV infection[§]

*Intravenous intrapartum zidovudine is not required for women who are receiving antiretroviral therapy, are adherent to treatment and have an undetectable viral load.

[||]For infants who are being breastfed, their management, including bloodwork and antiretroviral treatment, should be directed by a pediatric HIV expert.

[‡]Zidovudine for 2 weeks is appropriate for term infants if the mother received at least 10 weeks of antiretroviral therapy by time of delivery, achieved and maintained an undetectable viral load and did not have acute HIV infection during the current pregnancy.

[¥]For infants born prematurely and for term infants who do not fulfill the above criteria but whose mothers achieved an undetectable viral load at or after 36 weeks, zidovudine for 4-6 weeks is recommended.

[§]Warranted for situation where the mother received no antenatal antiretroviral therapy, received only intrapartum antiretroviral medications, received antenatal antiretroviral medications but did not achieve an undetectable viral load within 4 weeks of delivery.

laboratory studies, medical complications of pregnancy, alcohol or illicit drug use, mode of delivery [elective cesarean section recommended when maternal viral load is >1000 copies/mL]), the nursery clinician should determine the following aspects of the prenatal history: when the mother was diagnosed with HIV; the prenatal antiretroviral regimen, if any; the most recent maternal viral load and CD4 count; and whether the mother received intravenous ZDV during labor (recommended when maternal viral load is >1000 copies/mL and selectively when maternal viral load is detectable, but ≤1000 copies/mL).

The appropriate ART regimen for the infant is determined primarily by timing of maternal ART initiation and maternal viral load at or near the time of delivery. For infants whose mothers received at least 10 consecutive weeks of ART during pregnancy and achieved and maintained virologic suppression (viral load < 50 copies/mL) prior to delivery, ZDV monotherapy for 2 to 6 weeks is recommended (depending on gestational age). Pre-emptive treatment with ZDV, lamivudine and nevirapine or raltegravir is recommended for infants of mothers who did not receive antepartum ART, did not have virologic suppression despite antenatal ART or who had acute or primary HIV infection in pregnancy.

Routine bloodwork is not required for most term newborns at low risk of HIV infection who are prescribed a shortened (2 week) course of zidovudine. For those who are going to receive 4 to 6 weeks of zidovudine or pre-emptive antiretroviral treatment (combination antiretroviral therapy at treatment doses) due to elevated risk of HIV infection, a baseline complete blood count (CBC) with differential should be performed due to elevated risk of anemia and neutropenia. HIV PCR should also be done within 48 hours of birth in those at elevated risk of HIV infection.

Exclusive formula feeding is recommended for infants of mothers living with HIV in the United States and other resource-rich countries because vertical transmission may occur despite a fully suppressed maternal viral load in serum. However, because the risk of vertical transmission via breastmilk is less than 1% when the mother is receiving ART with good adherence and sustained virologic suppression, some have advocated for a more nuanced approach to infant feeding in the HIV context. Healthcare providers caring for newborns whose mothers indicate an interest in breastfeeding should consult with a pediatric HIV expert so that timely comprehensive counseling of the mother can be done and a management plan for the mother and infant put in place. Specific guidance regarding infant feeding in the HIV context is available.

MANAGEMENT OF THE NEWBORN INFANT OF A MOTHER WITH UNKNOWN HIV STATUS

The evaluation of a newborn infant whose mother received incomplete or no prenatal care should include evaluation of the adequacy of routine prenatal infectious diseases workup, any treatments administered for specific infections and the timing of these treatments (gestational age), and an assessment of ongoing risk of exposure to infectious diseases during the pregnancy. Routine prenatal testing varies by jurisdiction, but in most includes testing for HIV, hepatitis B virus, hepatitis C virus, syphilis, *Neisseria gonorrhoeae*, *Chlamydia trachomatis*, group B streptococcus, and rubella. Intrapartum maternal testing for these infections is warranted in all women if not performed antenatally and repeat testing for HIV, hepatitis B virus, hepatitis C virus, syphilis, *Neisseria gonorrhoeae,* and *Chlamydia trachomatis* selectively for women previously tested but deemed to be at significant ongoing risk. HIV antigen/antibody testing as well as hepatitis B surface antigen and syphilis serology should be expedited as positive results impact immediate management of the infant. If the mother is not available for testing, HIV antigen/antibody and syphilis serologic testing of the infant can serve as a surrogate for maternal status. A clear plan, with assured follow-up, is essential for infants discharged from hospital when the maternal HIV, hepatitis B, or syphilis status has not been finalized.

If intrapartum maternal HIV antigen/antibody testing is reactive in a previously undiagnosed or untreated woman, consultation with a pediatric HIV expert is advised as urgent initiation of pre-emptive HIV treatment with ZDV, lamivudine and nevirapine or raltegravir is warranted for the infant. As outlined in the diagnosis section above, HIV PCR should be done on such infants within 48 hours of birth. The management of infants born to mothers who are chronic hepatitis B carriers or inadequately treated for syphilis in pregnancy is outlined in Chapters 99 and 128.

TREATMENT OF HIV INFECTION

Combination antiretroviral therapy has dramatically improved the health and life expectancy of children living with HIV and is recommended for all such children regardless of clinical status, immunologic status (CD4 count), or viral load. The immediate goals of therapy are to achieve and maintain an undetectable viral load and to restore normal CD4 count while minimizing adverse effects of the medications. Ensuring retention in care and adherence to ART and appropriate management of comorbidities and complications are essential in optimizing outcomes.

Five classes of antiretroviral agents are available for treatment of HIV infection: (i) entry inhibitors (including CCR5 antagonists and fusion inhibitors); (ii) nucleoside reverse transcriptase inhibitors (NRTIs); (iii) non-nucleoside reverse transcriptase inhibitors (NNRTIs); (iv) integrase strand transfer inhibitors (INSTIs); and (v) protease inhibitors (PIs). Combination ART comprises at least three agents from at least two classes of medication. Up-to-date guidelines for the use of antiretroviral medications, published by the US Department of Health and Human Services, are available online. Currently, the recommended first-line ART regimens consist of a dual-NRTI "backbone" in combination with either an INSTI, NNRTI, or a PI.

Adjunctive therapies, used for children with poorly controlled or advanced HIV, include intravenous immunoglobulin infusions every 3 to 4 weeks and antimicrobial prophylaxis. Commonly used prophylactic agents include trimethoprim-sulfamethoxazole and azithromycin for the prevention of *P. jiroveci* pneumonia and disseminated *Mycobacterium avium-intracellulare* complex infection, respectively. Specific recommendations for the prevention of opportunistic infections and use of prophylactic medications by the US Department of Health and Human Services are available online.

INFECTIOUS COMPLICATIONS IN HIV INFECTED CHILDREN

When evaluating a child living with HIV for infection, it is crucial to determine the child's most recent viral load, CD4 count (and CD4%), ART regimen, and their adherence to the ART regimen. CD4 count (and CD4%) must be interpreted according to age-specific ranges.

In children with normal immunologic function, as determined by CD4 count or CD4%, the infectious agents are usually similar to those seen in children without HIV. However, they are at higher risk of invasive bacterial infection and therefore, a lower threshold for obtaining blood culture, urinalysis, urine culture, stool culture, chest radiograph, and lumbar puncture may be appropriate, on a case-by-case basis. The need for antimicrobial therapy should be determined in a manner similar to children without HIV.

In children with CD4 counts or CD4% in the severe immunodeficiency range, the risk of opportunistic infection increases dramatically. Multiple concurrent infections are not uncommon. Such children should be admitted for investigation. Broad-spectrum empirical antimicrobial therapy may be warranted and should be chosen in consultation with an infectious disease specialist. Treatment guidelines for opportunistic infections in HIV-infected children by the US Department of Health and Human Services are available online. Key management aspects for HIV-infected children presenting with fever and symptoms indicative of central nervous system, respiratory tract, and gastrointestinal tract are provided later.

Fever Acute onset of fever is a common reason for an HIV-infected child to be brought to medical attention. As with all children, the majority of febrile illnesses are due to common, self-limited infections, such as a viral upper respiratory infection. However, children with HIV have a higher incidence of bacteremia and invasive bacterial disease than does the general population, regardless of CD4 count (or CD4%). *Streptococcus pneumoniae* is the most common cause of invasive bacterial infection, but rates of disease due to other pathogens, including *Staphylococcus aureus*, *Haemophilus influenzae* type B, *Escherichia coli*, non-typhi *Salmonella* species, and other gram positive and negative pathogens, are also higher than in HIV-negative children.

The absence of localizing signs in a child with a fever and a low CD4 count (or CD4%) dictates a broader, more intensive diagnostic evaluation because of the breadth of potential infectious causes. The compromised immunity caused by advanced HIV disease may obscure the focus of infection, including infection within the central nervous system (CNS). A child whose CD4 count (or CD4%) is in the severe immunodeficiency range may have an infection caused by either typical pathogens or opportunistic pathogens. The scope and tempo of the evaluation are dictated by the child's immunologic status and the acuity of presentation. A partial list of causes of undifferentiated fever in HIV-infected children is provided in **Table 104-4**.

Central Nervous System In children living with HIV who are on ART with sustained virologic suppression and CD4 counts (or CD4%) in the normal range, CNS infections are usually caused by the same pathogens as in HIV-uninfected children. They are however, at slightly increased risk for bacterial meningitis compared with children without HIV. Empiric antibiotic therapy for meningitis in children older than 2 to 3 months of age should target *S. pneumoniae* and *Neisseria meningitidis*, and in the unimmunized, *Haemophilus influenzae* type B.

Children with untreated or inadequately treated HIV infection and severe immunodeficiency are at increased risk for infectious as well as non-infectious complications involving the CNS. Opportunistic infections that can involve the CNS include CMV and other herpes group viruses, *Mycobacterium tuberculosis*, *Cryptococcus neoformans*, *Toxoplasma gondii*, and human polyoma virus-2 (JC virus). CMV is the most common opportunistic infection of the CNS in children, typically presenting as subacute or chronic meningoencephalitis. Cryptococcal meningitis, the most common opportunistic fungal infection of the CNS, presents insidiously with a gradual onset of fever, headache, malaise, and emesis. Frank signs of meningismus are often absent; a lymphocytic pleocytosis is characteristic, but the cerebrospinal fluid findings may be completely normal. Progressive multifocal leukoencephalopathy, due to reactivation of latent JC virus, presents with slowly progressive confusion, personality changes, and focal neurologic findings. Noninfectious conditions, which often present with focal neurologic deficits, include stroke secondary to cerebrovascular disease and primary CNS lymphoma.

TABLE 104-4 Selected Causes of Undifferentiated Fever in Children Living With HIV[§]

Infectious
Focal bacterial infection (with symptoms and signs obscured)
Bacteremia without a focus (e.g., *S aureus*, *S pneumoniae*)
Salmonellosis
Bartonellosis (e.g., *Bartonella henselae*, *Bartonella quintana*)
Mycobacterium tuberculosis
Atypical mycobacteria (e.g., *Mycobacterium avium intracellulare*)
Cryptococcus neoformans
Dimorphic fungi (e.g., *Blastomyces dermatitidis*, *Histoplasma capsulatum*)
Pneumocystis jirovecii
Toxoplasma gondii
Herpes virus infections (CMV, EBV, HSV and VZV)
Hepatitis viruses (hepatitis A mainly)
Parvovirus B19
Non infectious
Malignancy (primarily lymphoma)
Drug fever
Autoimmune disorders

[§]The specific causes to be considered will depend on many factors including the epidemiologic history (where the child lives, travel, exposures etc.), degree of immune compromise and associated symptoms and signs.

Abbreviations: CMV = cytomegalovirus, EBV = Epstein Barr virus; HSV = herpes simplex virus; VZV = varicella zoster virus.

Respiratory Tract Bacterial pneumonia is common in children living with HIV regardless of their immunologic status and is more prevalent than in otherwise healthy uninfected children. *Streptococcus pneumoniae* is the most common pathogen. Other causative agents include *Staphylococcus aureus*, *Streptococcus pyogenes*, non-typeable *Haemophilus influenzae*, *Klebsiella pneumoniae*, *Pseudomonas aeruginosa*, non-typhi *Salmonella* species, and *Mycobacterium tuberculosis*. In children with suspected bacterial pneumonia and normal immunologic function, empiric antibiotic therapy should target the same pathogens as in otherwise healthy uninfected children.

Pneumocystis jiroveci pneumonia (PJP) is the most common AIDS-defining condition in children living with HIV. The peak incidence is between 3 and 6 months of age. In young infants, co-infection with CMV is common. Beyond the first year of life, PJP is seen almost exclusively in children with a CD4 count (or CD4%) in the severe immunodeficiency range. The classic presentation consists of fever, tachypnea, dyspnea, and non-productive cough. The degree of hypoxemia and respiratory distress is usually out of proportion to the relatively nontoxic appearance of the child. The most common radiographic findings are bilateral perihilar interstitial infiltrates (butterfly pattern); however, PJP is renowned for its multiplicity of radiographic presentations, including lobar infiltrates, pneumothorax, and pneumatoceles. Diagnosis is most often established by demonstrating the organism in sputum, bronchoalveolar lavage material, or lung biopsy specimen by various staining techniques and more recently PCR. The treatment of choice is trimethoprim-sulfamethoxazole for 21 days. Corticosteroids may be of benefit in children with significant hypoxemia.

A common noninfectious cause of chronic cough in HIV-infected children is lymphocytic interstitial pneumonitis (LIP). LIP has an insidious onset and an indolent course, which can mimic PJP, CMV pneumonitis, and miliary tuberculosis. Initial symptoms typically include mild cough, fatigue, dyspnea, and tachypnea. Generalized lymphadenopathy, hepatomegaly, parotid gland enlargement, and clubbing may be present. A typical reticulonodular pattern may be seen on chest radiographs, with or without hilar lymphadenopathy. LIP often resolves with effective control of HIV using ART. Corticosteroids may be of benefit in severe cases.

Gastrointestinal System The clinical presentation and course of gastrointestinal disorders in HIV-infected children with preserved immunologic function are similar to those in otherwise healthy children. Causes of non-bloody diarrhea include rotavirus, adenovirus, enterotoxigenic *Escherichia coli*, and *Giardia lamblia*. Bloody, dysentery-like diarrheal disease, may be caused by *Salmonella* species, *Shigella* species, *Campylobacter jejuni*, enteroinvasive *E. coli*, or *Entamoeba histolytica*. The need for and choice of antimicrobial therapy in this context is similar to otherwise healthy children.

Persistent diarrhea is common in children with advanced HIV infection. The differential diagnosis is broad and includes infections with common or opportunistic pathogens, noninfectious conditions, and side effects of antiretroviral medications. Opportunistic pathogens that can cause chronic diarrhea include CMV, *Mycobacterium avium-intracellulare* complex, *Cryptosporidium* spp., *Microsporidia* spp., and *Isospora belli*. Pathogen-specific treatment recommendations by the US Department of Health and Human Services are available online. Failure to detect a secondary infection in a child with persistent diarrhea, malabsorption, and failure to thrive is suggestive of HIV-associated enteropathy; ART is the treatment of choice for this condition. Chronic diarrhea due to antiretroviral medications sometimes necessitates a change in the ART regimen.

Common abnormalities of the oral cavity in advanced HIV disease include persistent oral thrush, stomatitis secondary to HSV or CMV, hairy leukoplakia, periodontal disease, and oral ulcers associated with neutropenia. Esophagitis is most often due to *Candida*, but can also be caused by HSV or CMV; dysphagia and odynophagia are the most common clinical manifestations, but fever or irritability may occasionally be the only presenting signs.

Other Organ Systems Any organ system can be affected by HIV or its complications. Common dermatologic disorders that can be persistent and more severe in HIV-infected children with moderate or severe immune compromise include atopic dermatitis, warts, molluscum contagiosum, scabies, HSV, herpes zoster, and dermatophytic infections of the skin and nails. CMV and toxoplasmosis are important, albeit uncommon, causes of chorioretinitis in children with advanced HIV disease. Neutropenia and immune thrombocytopenia are common hematologic abnormalities. HIV-associated cardiomyopathy and nephropathy are well-recognized entities.

IMMUNE RECONSTITUTION INFLAMMATORY SYNDROME

The HIV-associated immune reconstitution inflammatory syndrome (IRIS) is characterized by paradoxical worsening of symptoms of a known opportunistic infection (or condition) or unmasking of a previously "silent" opportunistic infection (or condition), caused by a heightened inflammatory response associated with immunologic recovery following the initiation of ART. In some cases, multiple concurrent opportunistic infections can be unmasked. As such, newly diagnosed patients with advanced HIV require a thorough workup to detect asymptomatic infections that could manifest once ART is initiated. IRIS develops in approximately 20% of newly diagnosed HIV-infected children. Risk factors for IRIS include profound immune suppression (CD4 count often <50 cells/mm^3) at the time of ART initiation as well as rapid recovery of CD4 count and rapid decline in viral load subsequent to ART initiation. Any child with advanced HIV who has new or worsening symptoms within 2 months of ART initiation should be evaluated for possible IRIS.

The most common infections associated with IRIS include tuberculosis, atypical mycobacterial infections, cryptococcal meningitis, herpesvirus infections (CMV, HSV, and VZV), hepatitis B and C, molluscum contagiosum, and progressive multifocal leukoencephalopathy. Autoimmune conditions and malignancies can also present with IRIS. Infections involving the CNS are of particular concern due to the risk of increased intracranial pressure secondary to exacerbation of the inflammatory process; a mortality rate of approximately 20% has been noted among adult patients with cryptococcal meningitis-associated IRIS.

Prevention and treatment of IRIS depends on the specific pathogen as well as organ system involvement. Overall, early initiation of ART lowers the rate of AIDS-defining events and mortality at the cost of increasing the risk of IRIS. Consequently, for most opportunistic infections outside the CNS, early initiation of ART is recommended. For infections involving the CNS, the risk of increased intracranial pressure in the presence of CNS infections is a major concern. Delaying the initiation of ART until 2 to 6 weeks after starting treatment for cryptococcal meningitis has been associated with reduced mortality. The optimal timing of ART initiation in CNS tuberculosis is unknown. Corticosteroids are recommended for IRIS due to CNS tuberculosis and are likely of benefit in cryptococcal meningitis and progressive multifocal leukoencephalopathy-associated IRIS. Corticosteroids may reduce the duration and severity of symptoms in non-CNS IRIS; in some, nonsteroidal anti-inflammatory agents may suffice.

ADVERSE EFFECTS OF ANTIRETROVIRAL MEDICATIONS

Potentially life-threatening adverse effects of antiretroviral medications, though rare, should always be considered in HIV-infected children presenting to the emergency department with fever, rash, or gastrointestinal or respiratory symptoms. The most serious of these reactions are due to NRTIs and NNRTIs. If such a reaction is suspected, the medication should be discontinued and an HIV expert consulted.

Lactic acidosis and hepatic steatosis leading to liver failure is a rare but potentially fatal complication of stavudine and didanosine, and to a lesser extent other NRTIs. Symptoms are nonspecific and include fatigue, persistent nausea and vomiting, abdominal pain, and compensatory hyperventilation. A serum lactate greater than 5 mmol/L and moderate elevation in liver enzyme levels is helpful diagnostically. Mortality is extremely high if the offending agent is not discontinued in a timely manner. Abacavir hypersensitivity is characterized by fever, malaise, rash (which is often minimal), abdominal pain, nausea, vomiting, diarrhea, and cough that develop within 1 to 2 months of treatment initiation. Symptoms resolve once the medication is stopped. The incidence of abacavir hypersensitivity reactions has been dramatically reduced through pretreatment screening for the abacavir hypersensitivity locus (HLA B*5701) and avoidance of its use in those testing positive.

Nevirapine and to a lesser extent other NNRTIs can cause idiosyncratic hypersensitivity reactions, usually within 4 to 6 weeks of treatment initiation. The spectrum of clinical manifestations ranges from acute hepatitis with fulminant liver failure to skin rashes with mild elevation of liver enzymes. Risk factors include female sex and high CD4 count at treatment initiation.

CONSULTATION

Consultation with an infectious disease specialist is appropriate when managing newborn infants at elevated risk of perinatal HIV infection; when the diagnosis of HIV is being considered; when opportunistic infections or other AIDS-defining conditions are suspected or identified; when HIV-infected patients present with fever, especially when no source is identified; and for long-term management. Whenever possible, contact with the physicians involved in the ongoing management of an HIV-infected child is desirable.

If specific organ systems are affected by HIV-related complications, involvement of the appropriate subspecialists is recommended. Their involvement may be necessary for a single event (e.g., biopsy) or for long-term management.

ADMISSION CRITERIA

Febrile children living with HIV with normal CD4 counts (or CD4%) should be admitted according to the same criteria used for HIV-uninfected children. A more thorough evaluation in the emergency department for invasive bacterial infection should be considered, however. Most children with normal CD4 counts (or CD4%) can be discharged while appropriate cultures are incubating in the clinical microbiology laboratory.

All febrile children living with HIV who have CD4 counts (or CD4%) indicative of severe immunodeficiency should be admitted for investigation. Because of their immunologic compromise, they may not localize infections well, including those involving the CNS. Additionally, such children are at risk for rapid decompensation of clinical status. The need to admit children with moderate immune compromise, based on CD4 count (or CD4%), depends on their past history and clinical status. The threshold to admit should be lower for children with a history of recurrent bacterial infections or AIDS defining conditions.

Children with HIV infection and CNS symptoms and signs (usually with the exception of mild headaches) should be admitted for evaluation. The cause of CNS findings may be infectious, neoplastic, or vasculitic and may present irrespective of CD4 count (or CD4%). Progressive, worsening headache should be evaluated more intensively than in a child without HIV.

Children with advanced HIV disease in whom ART was initiated during the preceding 2 months who present with worsening or new symptoms potentially related to an opportunistic infection should be admitted and evaluated for possible IRIS. This is of particular importance with respect to neurologic symptoms as IRIS related to CNS infections can be rapidly fatal.

PREVENTION OF OCCUPATIONAL AND NON-OCCUPATIONAL TRANSMISSION OF HIV

MANAGEMENT OF OCCUPATIONAL HIV EXPOSURE

Transmission of HIV to healthcare personnel due to occupational exposure has been reported since the beginning of the AIDS epidemic. The US Public Health Service guidelines for the management of occupational exposure to HIV were most recently updated in 2018 and are available online. Healthcare personnel are defined as all paid and unpaid personnel who work in a healthcare setting and have the potential for exposure to HIV-infected body fluids or contaminated material. An occupational exposure is defined as any percutaneous injury (e.g., needle stick) or contact of a mucous membrane or nonintact skin with a potentially infectious fluid or substance, including blood and bloody bodily fluids. The risk of transmission from the following fluids has not been studied epidemiologically, but they should be considered infectious: cerebrospinal, pericardial, pleural, ascitic, vaginal, seminal, and amniotic fluids. Other fluids, such as tears and saliva, should not be considered infectious unless they are visibly contaminated with blood.

The risk for acquisition of HIV due to a percutaneous injury with a visibly contaminated sharp object from a source patient known to be HIV positive is approximately 0.3% (95% confidence interval [CI], 0.2-0.5). The risk resulting from a mucous membrane exposure with blood is approximately 0.09% (95% CI, 0.006-0.5). Factors associated with an increased risk for transmission of HIV to healthcare personnel include a sharp object visibly contaminated with blood, a procedure involving the placement of an intravascular device, a deep injury, and a source patient with end-stage AIDS. Although the risk of HIV transmission from a patient with an undetectable viral load is likely significantly reduced, it is not zero, and therefore percutaneous and other significant body fluid exposures to such patients should still be considered a risk to healthcare personnel.

The current US Public Health Services guidelines recommend HIV-post exposure prophylaxis (HIV-PEP) when the source patient is known to be HIV-infected or is at high risk of being HIV-infected. The preferred regimen consists of raltegravir or dolutegravir combined with tenofovir disoproxil fumarate and emtricitabine (Truvada®). HIV-PEP should be initiated as soon as possible after exposure, preferably within 1 hour of exposure. HIV-PEP is not recommended if the exposure occurred more than 72 hours before presentation, if the exposed person refuses HIV-PEP, or if the exposed person is unwilling or unable to commit to 28 days of therapy and appropriate follow-up.

Rapid testing for HIV with Food and Drug Administration (FDA)-approved kits should also be performed on healthcare workers to determine their baseline status. HIV-PEP should be discontinued if the source patient is determined to be HIV-negative. Institutions should have personnel responsible for responding to occupational exposure to HIV, available 24 hours a day as well as procedures for HIV testing and HIV-PEP administration. The National Clinical Consultation Center provides online guidance and consultation services pertaining to occupational exposures (PEPLine at 888-448-4911).

MANAGEMENT OF NON-OCCUPATIONAL EXPOSURE

Updated guidelines for HIV-PEP following non-occupational exposure to HIV were published by the US Department of Health and Human Services in 2016 and are available online. Unprotected sex, whether consensual or following sexual assault, and percutaneous exposure due to use of nonsterilized needles (needle sharing) are reasons adolescents may seek HIV-PEP. Potential HIV exposures unique to young children include sexual abuse, percutaneous exposure to discarded syringes, human bites, and ingestion of human breast milk.

The general principles of assessment, including the characteristics of the exposure source and the type and extent of exposure are similar to those for occupational exposure. HIV-PEP should be considered if: (i) the source is known to be HIV positive; (ii) the exposure is deemed to be associated with a substantial risk of infection; and (iii) the exposed individual seeks care within 72 hours of the exposure. In general, HIV-PEP is not routinely recommended following percutaneous exposure to discarded syringes or human bites in the absence of blood in the saliva and blood in the bite wound. HIV-PEP is also likely not warranted following a single exposure to breast milk from an HIV-infected woman as the risk of transmission is exceeding low (1-4 per 100,000). For any case deemed to have potential risk of HIV acquisition the child and caregiver's preference should also be taken into account in making the decision regarding HIV-PEP.

The decision to prescribe HIV-PEP should be made in consultation with a clinician who has experience in the management of HIV infection. A three drug regimen consisting of raltegravir or dolutegravir combined with tenofovir disoproxil fumarate and emtricitabine (Truvada®) is preferred for adolescents 13 years of age and older. For children 3 to 12 years of age the same three medications, dosed according to age and weight, are recommended. In children 2 years of age or younger, the combination of zidovudine, lamivudine, and raltegravir is preferred.

KEY POINTS

- In children younger than 18-24 months of age the diagnosis of HIV infection is established by detection of the virus using molecular detection methods (HIV DNA or RNA PCR).
- In children older than 24 months, HIV infection is confirmed by an initial combination immunoassay that detects antibodies to HIV-1 and HIV-2 and HIV-1 p24 antigen, followed by a supplemental immunoassay that differentiates HIV-1 from HIV-2 antibodies.
- The ART regimen administered to newborn infants depends on the level of risk of perinatal transmission. Zidovudine monotherapy for 4 weeks is indicated for newborns whose mothers received antenatal ART and had an undetectable viral load prior to delivery. Pre-emptive treatment with combination ART is warranted for neonates born to mothers who did not receive antenatal ART or who did not have virologic suppression prior to delivery despite ART.
- Acute retroviral syndrome should be considered in youth with a febrile mononucleosis-like syndrome who have risk factors for HIV infection including a history of being sexually active or injecting drugs.
- Children living with HIV who have a normal CD4 count and CD4% are not at increased risk for opportunistic infections; however, their risk for invasive bacterial infection is higher than in a child without HIV infection.
- Children living with HIV who have severe immune compromise as determined by CD4 count or CD4% are at risk for opportunistic infections and other AIDS-defining conditions.
- Immune reconstitution inflammatory syndrome is a potentially life-threatening complication observed in children with advanced HIV within weeks or months of initiation of effective ART.
- Potentially life-threatening complication of antiretroviral medications includes NRTI-induced lactic acidosis with hepatic steatosis, abacavir hypersensitivity, and NNRTI-induced liver toxicity.
- Although the risk for HIV transmission through occupational and non-occupational exposure is low, it does occur. Timely initiation of HIV-PEP needs to be considered and extra care must be taken to monitor for medication toxicity.

SUGGESTED READINGS

American Academy of Pediatrics. Human Immunodeficiency virus. In: Kimberlin DW, Barnett ED, Lynfield R, Sawyer MH, eds. *Red Book 2021 Report of the Committee on Infectious Diseases*. Elk Grove Village, IL. American Academy of Pediatrics; 2021:427-440.

Armstrong WS. The immune reconstitution inflammatory syndrome: a clinical update. *Curr Infect Dis Rep*. 2013;15(1):39-45.

Centers for Disease Control and Prevention. HIV and Pregnant Women, Infants, and Children. Page last reviewed: June 28, 2022. Available at: https://www.cdc.gov/hiv/group/gender/pregnantwomen/index.html.

Centers for Disease Control and Prevention, US Department of Health and Human Services. Updated U.S. Public Health Service Guidelines for the Management of Occupational Exposures to HIV and Recommendations for Postexposure Prophylaxis Update (May 23, 2018). Available at: https://stacks.cdc.gov/view/cdc/20711.

Centers for Disease Control and Prevention, US Department of Health and Human Services. Updated guidelines for antiretroviral postexposure prophylaxis after sexual, injection drug use, or other nonoccupational exposure to HIV—United States, 2016 (Update May 23, 2018). Available at https://stacks.cdc.gov/view/cdc/38856.

Centers for Disease C, Prevention. Revised surveillance case definition for HIV infection—United States, 2014. *MMWR Recomm Rep*. 2014;63(RR-03):1-10.

Muller M, Wandel S, Colebunders R, Attia S, Furrer H, Egger M. Immune reconstitution inflammatory syndrome in patients starting antiretroviral therapy for HIV infection: a systematic review and meta-analysis. *Lancet Infect Dis*. 2010;10(4):251-261.

Panel on Treatment of HIV During Pregnancy and Prevention of Perinatal Transmission. Recommendations for Use of Antiretroviral Drugs During Pregnancy and Interventions to Reduce Perinatal HIV Transmission in the United States. Department of Health and Human Services. Available at https://clinicalinfo.hiv.gov/en/guidelines.

Panel on Antiretroviral Therapy and Medical Management of Children Living with HIV. Guidelines for the Use of Antiretroviral Agents in Pediatric HIV Infection. Department of Health and Human Services. Available at https://clinicalinfo.hiv.gov/en/guidelines.

Panel on Opportunistic Infections in HIV-Exposed and HIV-Infected Children. Guidelines for the Prevention and Treatment of Opportunistic Infections in HIV-Exposed and HIV-Infected Children. Department of Health and Human Services. Available at https://clinicalinfo.hiv.gov/en/guidelines.

Panel on Guidelines for the Prevention and Treatment of Opportunistic Infections in Adults and Adolescents with HIV. Guidelines for the Prevention and Treatment of Opportunistic Infections in Adults and Adolescents with HIV. National Institutes of Health, Centers for Disease Control and Prevention, the HIV Medicine Association, and the Infectious Disease Society of America. Available at https://clinicalinfo.hiv.gov/en/guidelines.

World Health Organization. WHO case definitions of HIV for surveillance and revised clinical and immunological classification of HIV-related disease in adults and children, 2007. Available at: https://apps.who.int/iris/bitstream/handle/10665/43699/9789241595629_eng.pdf?sequence=1&isAllowed=y.

CHAPTER 105

Infections in Special Hosts

Mark Murphy, DO and Grant Paulsen, MD

BACKGROUND

The definition of immune compromise is characterized by an impairment of a host's ability to effectively handle infectious challenges. As new therapeutic options for previously untreatable illnesses become available, a growing number of children fall into this category. This chapter focuses primarily on the infection-related issues among children who are immunocompromised owing to solid organ or hematopoietic cell transplantation; splenic dysfunction will also be addressed. These special hosts may present for the evaluation of unexplained fever, or with focal signs of infection, and often require a different approach than pursued in an otherwise healthy child. The goal of this chapter is to provide the pediatric hospitalist with a framework for infectious disease evaluation in these children. Infectious complications related to chemotherapy for malignancy are discussed in Chapter 133.

PATHOPHYSIOLOGY

Solid organ transplantation (SOT) was revolutionized in the early 1980s with the introduction of the immunosuppressant cyclosporine. Heart, kidney, liver, lung, and small bowel transplants have become acceptable therapies for end-organ disease. Although these procedures allow improved survival, infectious complications are among the leading causes of morbidity and mortality in the SOT population. While the surgical procedure itself carries risk of infection following SOT, the immunosuppressive medications used to avoid graft rejection pose significantly higher and more prolonged infectious risks for transplant recipients. The underlying medical conditions necessitating SOT also carry infectious risks that need to be considered. Patients with cystic fibrosis, for example, are colonized with pathogens in their sinuses and upper respiratory tracts which are not impacted by lung transplant. Patients with renal or liver failure, meanwhile, may be predisposed to infection prior to transplant owing to end-organ dysfunction.

Hematopoietic cell transplantation (HCT), which includes transplantation of marrow- or blood-derived stem cells derived from peripheral blood, umbilical cord blood, or bone marrow, treat certain malignancies, metabolic disorders, and immune dysfunctions. Advances in immunosuppression have dramatically improved survival in HCT, but have led to an increased risk of infectious complications. Despite preventive antimicrobial therapies, infection is a leading cause of morbidity and mortality in both autologous and allogeneic HCT recipients.

CLINICAL PRESENTATION

There are several important variables when evaluating transplant recipients with suspected infection: the type of transplant (type of organ; allogeneic vs autologous HCT), the amount of time since transplantation (state of immunosuppression), the underlying disease (indication for transplantation), and the environment of the recipient. In SOT, the type of organ transplanted confers different technical challenges. Understanding the basic anatomical considerations of organ transplantation facilitates diagnosis and guides empiric antimicrobial therapy during postoperative infections. In HCT, autologous transplants (cells derived from the patient) affords lower risk of infection than use of allogeneic, or donor-derived, cells. As will be discussed later under Differential Diagnosis, the time since transplantation is a critical component to assessing the risk of infection in transplant recipients. The degree of immunosuppression varies over time and with it the risk for reactivation of old and acquisition of new infections. HCT patients also deserve particular attention with regard to the stages of engraftment and recent or current graft versus host disease (GVHD). Neutropenia, defects in cell-mediated immunity and altered antibody-mediated immunity occur at predictable times in HCT patients. Finally, it is important to consider the physical setting of the transplant recipient when assessing for infection. The management will differ according to the risk for community- and hospital-acquired infections based on the environment of the patient prior to evaluation. Each institution carries its own set of nosocomial pathogens, and knowledge of local antibiograms is crucial when determining appropriate empiric antimicrobial therapy in immunocompromised hosts. Meanwhile, transplant recipients who have been home are at risk for community-acquired infections, making it important to be aware of seasonal infections and community outbreaks. Further, regional infections (e.g., histoplasmosis, blastomycosis, coccidioidomycosis, strongyloides) should be considered; a detailed travel history should be obtained.

Other considerations include the patient's age, preoperative risk factors such as malnutrition, donor and recipient serostatus for Epstein-Barr virus (EBV) and cytomegalovirus (CMV), intraoperative complications, and the specific postoperative immunosuppressive regimen.

DIFFERENTIAL DIAGNOSIS

The time from transplantation is a key factor that influences infection risk following transplant. For both HCT and SOT recipients, the time period between transplantation and evaluation influences the differential diagnosis for suspected infection. Prior to implementation of prophylactic and preventive antimicrobials, certain infections in the posttransplant period followed a predictable pattern that allowed for prioritized evaluation and empiric treatment. **Figure 105-1** depicts the classic timetable for the development of infections after SOT and HCT. Some of the listed infections, such as CMV and HSV, have shifted their timeframes to develop later after transplant due to common use of prophylaxis or preventive antimicrobials.

EARLY POSTTRANSPLANT PERIOD

Solid Organ Transplantation (0–30 Days) Immediately after transplantation, bacterial pathogens predominate as the cause of infection. In SOT recipients, the source of bacterial infection is typically related

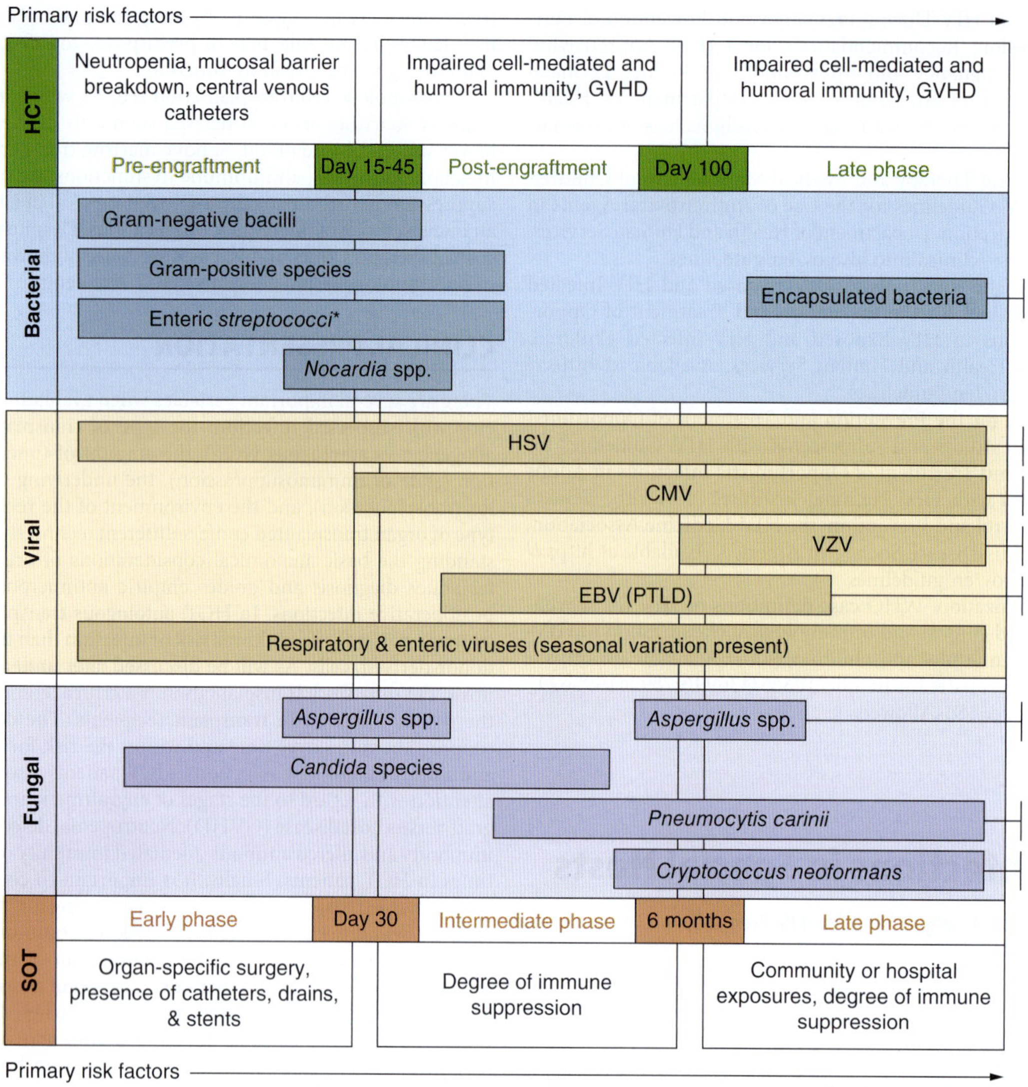

FIGURE 105-1. Timetable of infection following solid organ and hematopoietic cell transplantation. Solid lines and end brackets indicate that risk of infection may extend beyond period shown depending on degree of ongoing immunosuppression and underlying disease. HSV, herpes simplex virus; CMV, cytomegalovirus; VZV, varicella zoster virus; EBV, Epstein-Barr virus; PTLD, posttransplant lymphoproliferative disorder. *Enteric *Streptococci* include *Enterococcus* spp. and viridans group streptococci. (Reproduced with permission from Tomblyn M, Chiller T, Einsele H, Gress R, et al. Guidelines for preventing infectious complications among hematopoietic cell transplantation recipients: a global perspective. *Biol Blood Marrow Transplant.* 2009;15(10):1143-1238.)

to the surgical procedure performed or the presence of an indwelling device (e.g., catheter, drain, stent). Although immunosuppression is implemented during this period, most infections are directly related to surgery and peri- and postoperative care. For example, peritonitis is the principal postoperative infection in liver transplant recipients, whereas urinary tract infections are common following renal transplantation. Infection can also be conveyed with the allograft (donor-derived infections) or reactivation of an infection present at surgery can resurface, although these occur less frequently.

Fungal infections, predominantly caused by *Candida* species, also occur early after SOT. Factors predisposing to fungal infection include disruption of anatomic barriers by surgery, fungal colonization enhanced by broad-spectrum antibiotic therapy, and presence of indwelling catheters. The incidence varies by type of organ transplanted; lung and liver transplants involve a higher incidence of fungal infection than do kidney transplants. Particularly problematic is fungal pneumonia after lung transplantation, because colonization is frequent and difficult to distinguish from infection. Infections caused by *Aspergillus* species, although less common than *Candida* spp, infections are associated with high mortality.

Hematopoietic Cell Transplantation—Preengraftment (First 15-45 Days) For HCT recipients, the preengraftment period begins with conditioning therapy that eradicates or reduces the patient's burden of abnormal or malignant cells to below detectable levels and suppresses the patient's immunity to prevent the rejection of donor cells. This period, which extends until approximately 5 to 15 days after transplantation, is complicated by neutropenia, lymphopenia, and mucositis. Patients react similarly to those with neutropenia from other forms of chemotherapy. Bacterial and fungal infections commonly can gain entry through indwelling venous catheters or through mucosal breakdown along the gastrointestinal tract. If initial conditioning therapy includes agents directed at T cells, the patient is predisposed to an earlier onset of viral infection, particularly EBV, CMV, adenovirus, and BK virus. Reactivation of herpes simplex virus (HSV) may also occur, making antiviral prophylaxis part of standard therapy during the preengraftment period.

INTERMEDIATE POSTTRANSPLANT PERIOD

Solid Organ Transplantation (1–6 Months) Between 30 and 180 days posttransplantation, viral causes of infection predominate. During this time, opportunistic infections and posttransplant lymphoproliferative disorder (PTLD) must also be considered. The type of organ transplanted influences the risk of specific infections. For example, bacterial and fungal pneumonia are common in lung transplant patients and recurrent bacterial cholangitis occurs in liver transplant patients with biliary strictures and drains. However, CMV, EBV, adenovirus, varicella-zoster virus (VZV), and the childhood respiratory viruses must be considered in all SOT patients with fever during this period.

Opportunistic infections are relatively rare following pediatric SOT. Because trimethoprim-sulfamethoxazole prophylaxis has been incorporated into treatment regimens, early infection with *Pneumocystis jirovecii* (previously *Pneumocystis carinii)* has been almost eliminated. *Toxoplasma gondii* infection should be considered in seronegative heart transplant recipients, especially if the donor is seropositive.

Hematopoietic Cell Transplantation—Postengraftment (Marrow Recovery—100 Days) In HCT patients, the postengraftment period begins with marrow recovery and extends to 100 days after transplantation, when functional lymphocyte recovery is apparent. This is a time of impaired cellular immunity. GVHD and the use of calcineurin inhibitors, which blunt T-lymphocyte reconstitution via their inhibitory effect on interleukin-2, also play a role in risk for infection. CMV, EBV, and VZV are frequent causes of infection during this time. Bacterial infections from indwelling catheters and fungal infections, both *Candida* and *Aspergillus* species, continue to be a problem as well. Other opportunistic infections, such as *P. jirovecii*, and reactivation of *T. gondii* may occur during this period.

LATE POSTTRANSPLANT PERIOD

Solid Organ Transplantation (>6 Months) Late infections, typically occurring 180 days or longer after transplantation, include many of the same viral illnesses that occur in the immunocompetent population (e.g., gastroenteritis, viral respiratory infection). Particular attention should be paid to varicella, influenza, and adenovirus infection because these can be particularly severe in transplant recipients. EBV-associated posttransplant lymphoproliferative disorders (PTLDs) can also occur during this period. In lung transplant patients, bacterial (including gram-negative bacilli) and fungal pneumonia remains a concern. Additionally, with routine use of ganciclovir and valganciclovir for CMV prophylaxis, late-onset CMV disease (after discontinuation of prophylaxis) is also an important consideration during this period.

Hematopoietic Cell Transplantation—Late Phase (>100 Days) The late phase begins 101 days after transplantation. Impaired cellular immunity persists and GVHD can become a chronic problem. The risk of infection during this period is directly related to underlying disease state and the need for ongoing immunosuppression. The use of prophylactic antimicrobials may shift reactivation of certain infections, such as CMV, VZV, and HSV, to this period. The presence of chronic GVHD predisposes to EBV-related complications as well as to late-onset infections with encapsulated organisms, particularly pneumococci. The risk for community-acquired infections is greatest during this period as patients' care is transitioned to the outpatient setting.

SPECIFIC INFECTIONS FOLLOWING TRANSPLANTATION

Bacterial Infections Infections are common immediately after liver transplantation, and most are associated with either central venous line or abdominal infections. Factors predisposing to infection include previous abdominal surgery, known multidrug-resistant bacteria carrier, prolonged operating time, elevated tacrolimus level, hepatic artery thrombosis, and biliary strictures. Prolonged operating time and repeated surgical procedures increase the risk for bowel perforation and subsequent infection with *Enterococcus* species or gram-negative bacilli. Biliary strictures and hepatic artery thrombosis predispose to cholangitis and hepatic abscesses with similar organisms. Postoperative cholangitis is particularly difficult to differentiate from acute cellular rejection, and a biopsy is often warranted to help choose the appropriate therapy.

Postoperative bacterial infections in renal transplant patients are similar to those of any postoperative patient and include pneumonia, wound infection, central venous catheter infection, and urinary tract infection (UTI). However, uncomplicated urinary tract infection, pyelonephritis, and urosepsis all occur with increased frequency in this population. Historically, one-third of renal transplant patients developed recurrent urinary tract infections in the first 6 months after transplantation, but this number is now lower with increased use of prophylactic antibiotics with fewer than 20% having a febrile UTI in the first year.

Blood and pulmonary infections are the most common bacterial infections in pediatric heart transplant recipients. *Staphylococcus aureus* is the organism most likely to cause mediastinitis and colonization with methicillin-resistant *S.aureus* is a risk factor. Surgical reexploration of the wound is critical for successful treatment. Infants younger than 6 months of age appear to have a higher risk of bacterial infection than older pediatric heart transplant recipients.

Bacterial pneumonias following lung transplantation occur in the majority of patients and infections in the first 30 days after transplant are common. Cystic fibrosis patients have a challenging microbial ecosystem which is not eliminated by transplantation. Gram-negative bacilli, *Staphylococcus aureus*, and atypical mycobacterial pathogens are common following lung transplant in cystic fibrosis patients and multidrug resistance should be expected. Pre-transplant colonization with *Burkholderia cepacia* complex (*B. cenocepacia*) portends a lower survival following transplant. Bloodstream infections are also frequent following lung transplantation, primarily due to the presence of central venous catheters, and complicate more than a quarter of postoperative lung transplantation courses.

Bacteremia and serious bacterial infections caused by gram-positive organisms are common after HCT. Mucositis and indwelling catheters in the preengraftment period and chronic GVHD in the late phase predispose to such infections. Mucositis and indwelling catheters predispose to infections with *Staphylococcus epidermidis*, *Staphylococcus aureus*, *Streptococcus pneumoniae*, viridans group *Streptococci (VGS)*, *Streptococcus pyogenes*, *Enterococcus* as well as gram-negative bacteria such as *E.coli* and *Klebsiella*. *VGS* is particularly important, being isolated from approximately 15% of adult transplant patients with mucositis and neutropenia in the weeks following transplant. In pediatric HCT it can present with fever alone or with overwhelming sepsis. Viridans group streptococci usually gain access to the bloodstream via mucositis and can cause a sepsis syndrome with multiorgan dysfunction in the early preengraftment period. Infection with *S. pneumoniae* continues to be a problem in patients with chronic GVHD despite the use of prophylactic penicillin or trimethoprim-sulfamethoxazole in many centers. Gram-negative organisms can present with a more fulminant, devastating course.

Clostridioides difficile (formerly *Clostridium difficile*) infection (CDI) should be considered in any transplant patient with diarrhea, especially if prolonged or severe. Exposure to antibiotics and immunosuppressives following transplantation increases the likelihood of disease and complications. While peak onset in adults is in the first 1 to 2 weeks following SOT, pediatric SOT can have CDI years after transplant and recurrent infections are common. In HCT recipients, *C. difficile* may also predispose patients to GHVD, and severe infection is associated with decreased overall survival.

Viral Infections Unlike bacterial infections, viral infections tend to have lower organ specificity because they are usually related to immunosuppression. Transmission can occur through reactivation of a latent virus, transmission via the transplanted organ, or person-to-person spread. The herpesviruses are a major source of posttransplant morbidity and mortality, especially CMV, EBV, HSV, and VZV. Other important viral infections in solid organ transplant patients include adenovirus, parvovirus, influenza virus, parainfluenza virus, and respiratory syncytial virus (RSV).

Cytomegalovirus (CMV) Despite various preventive regimens with antiviral agents and CMV-specific immune globulin, CMV remains a common cause of morbidity in the transplant population. Primary infection after SOT, whereby a CMV-naïve (seronegative, R-) recipient receives an organ or blood products from a CMV-infected (seropositive, D+) donor, is the most severe. Primary infection can also occur in a D-/R- patient due to nosocomial or community exposures. HCT recipients can acquire CMV through receipt of blood products, including stem cells, from CMV-seropositive donors or via hospital or community exposures. The use of CMV-safe blood products is recommended. HCT recipients at risk for CMV disease include those who are CMV-seropositive prior to transplant and all who are CMV-seronegative and have a CMV-seropositive donor.

Primary infection occurs more frequently in children than in adults because a greater proportion of children are CMV naïve at the time of transplant. Secondary infection, or reactivation of a previously acquired (latent) CMV infection usually results in less severe disease. In addition to CMV naïveté, high doses of immune suppression (especially antilymphocyte therapy used for rejection) and EBV coinfection (due to the immune-modulating effects of EBV) increase the risk for CMV disease.

CMV infection can present as asymptomatic viremia, a nonspecific viral syndrome, termed CMV syndrome, or it can present as CMV disease with end-organ involvement. CMV syndrome usually involves several of the following symptoms: fever, malaise, weakness, myalgia, and arthralgia. There is often an accompanying myelosuppression. End-organ CMV disease often affects the transplanted organ, with hepatitis in liver transplant patients and pneumonitis in lung transplant patients being the most common associations. The gastrointestinal tract can be affected regardless of the organ transplanted, and lower gastrointestinal bleeding in a transplant patient should raise the suspicion of CMV colitis. Tissue-invasive CMV disease can also compartmentalize in specific organs (e.g., liver or colon) without associated CMV viremia.

CMV is a significant cause of morbidity and mortality in HCT recipients as well. Pretransplant exposure with documented CMV IgG levels is a risk factor for recurrence after transplantation due to reactivation of latent disease. End-organ disease from CMV can include pneumonitis, hepatitis, enteritis, and retinitis. As in solid organ transplants, the immune-modulating properties of CMV link it to graft rejection. More unique to HCT, however, is its occurrence in conjunction with GVHD.

Diagnosis of CMV disease has changed in the past decade. CMV serology still plays an important role in risk stratification prior to transplantation in both SOT and HCT but does not have a role in diagnosis of active infection. Quantitative real-time polymerase chain reaction assay (QRT-PCR) is now the most frequently implemented tool for diagnosis and surveillance posttransplantation.

Diagnosis of CMV infection and disease must take current prevention strategies into account for a given patient. Preemptive antiviral therapy, which involves initiation of therapy when infection meets a predefined threshold based on elevated CMV DNA viral loads, is utilized by many centers for low-risk patients. This differs from prophylaxis, which consists of empiric therapy and aims to prevent development or spread of infection. For both prevention and treatment, the drugs of choice for CMV are intravenous ganciclovir and oral valganciclovir, which inhibit CMV DNA polymerase.

Epstein-Barr Virus (EBV) Primary infection from an infected donor to a naïve recipient represents the most common and severe form of EBV infection in SOT recipients. Children are particularly prone to infection owing to the relatively high incidence of EBV-naïve recipients. Clinical manifestations of primary infection include enteritis, hepatitis, encephalitis, and mononucleosis-like symptoms including fever, hepatosplenomegaly, and lymphadenopathy. EBV disease in HCT is most often from reactivation of endogenous infection or transmission due to receipt of a graft from an EBV-seropositive donor. Primary infection due to community contact with an individual with EBV disease is also possible.

Following primary infection, EBV, like other herpesviruses, persists for the lifetime of the host despite the presence of a strong humoral and cell-mediated immune response. Ongoing low-grade viral replication normally occurs in the oropharynx simultaneously with a predominantly latent infection of B cells in the peripheral blood and lymphoid tissues. In cases of severe immunosuppression (e.g., following hematopoietic stem cell or SOT), the equilibrium is disrupted in favor of the virus. The uncontrolled proliferation of EBV-infected B cells that occurs in this context may result in a spectrum of PTLD, ranging from self-limited polyclonal proliferation to true malignancies containing clonal chromosomal abnormalities.

Factors associated with increased risk for PTLD include younger patient age, EBV seronegative recipient, intestinal or multivisceral transplants, more intense immune suppression, and coinfection with other pathogens. T-cell lymphopenia is a strong predictor of PTLD in HCT recipients. The specificity of calcineurin inhibitors and antilymphocyte antibodies for the T-cell limb of the immune response may explain in part the higher frequency of PTLD associated with the use of these agents. Coinfection with other herpesviruses such as CMV and human herpesvirus-8 also increases the risk of PTLD.

The clinical presentation of PTLD can be variable, ranging from a benign illness with self-limited lymphoproliferation to fulminant disease that presents with localized nodules, multifocal disease, or a sepsis-like picture. The most common presentation in children is similar to that of mononucleosis, with vague constitutional symptoms of fever, fatigue, and myalgias accompanied by a sore throat, cervical lymph node hypertrophy, and tonsillar enlargement. Gastrointestinal involvement can present with bleeding, weight loss, constipation, diarrhea, hypoalbuminemia, or intussusception. Pulmonary involvement can present with respiratory distress or lung nodules on the chest radiograph.

Diagnosis is best made by taking a tissue sample of the affected lymph node or tissue. Similar to CMV, nucleic acid PCR for EBV is an invaluable diagnostic tool. Elevated levels can prompt the early adjustment of immune suppression, which may impact development of PTLD.

Reduction in immune suppression is the recommended first treatment step and alone is often successful in treating PTLD limited to the allograft. If reduction of immune suppression is ineffective, or if the patient presents with advanced disease, there are other treatment options. Treatment with rituximab, a monoclonal antibody to CD20-positive B cells, can be added. Other chemotherapeutic agents, such as cyclophosphamide and infusions of donor-derived EBV-specific cytotoxic T lymphocytes also have a role in individual cases.

Varicella-Zoster Virus (VZV) Most children are either exposed to varicella before adolescence or immunized at 1 year of age. Children who receive organs before being either exposed or immunized are at risk for severe varicella infection, although herd immunity and the relatively low incidence of varicella lessen that risk somewhat.

VZV can cause illness as a primary infection or after reactivation of latent virus. Reactivation is much more common and typically occurs several months after transplantation. Patients may have typical painful vesicular lesions in a dermatomal distribution, or the lesions may be atypical with a less obvious pattern. The lesions may also be present for a prolonged period despite appropriate antiviral treatment. Dissemination can occur with primary infection (rarely with reactivation) and can result in significant end-organ disease, including hepatitis and pneumonitis; visceral dissemination does not have to be accompanied by rash.

The most effective means of preventing severe VZV disease is pretransplant vaccination. Although studies have shown live-attenuated VZV vaccine to be safe and effective following SOT, it is not routinely recommended outside of a research setting or following detailed patient evaluation and risk stratification. Recombinant zoster vaccine is a non-live VZV vaccine approved for immunocompromised adults aged 18 years and older. It has been shown to elicit an immune response in SOT recipients and is an option for that age group. If a VZV-seronegative, immunosuppressed transplant patient has a significant contact with a VZV-infected person (>5 minutes face-to-face contact, intimate contact, or contact with an immune-compromised individual with VZV), VZV-specific immune globulin (Varizig) should be administered within 96 hours of the exposure. Intravenous immunoglobulin (IVIG) can be used as an alternative if Varizig is unavailable. If clinical disease develops, either primary infection or reactivation (herpes zoster), patients should receive intravenous acyclovir in the hospital.

Herpes Simplex Virus (HSV) HSV is the most common viral infection following HCT and often occurs fairly early in the preengraftment or conditioning phase. HSV usually presents with oral or perianal vesicular or ulcerative lesions but occasionally progresses to systemic disease with hepatitis or encephalitis. Marked reduction in the incidence of HSV has been achieved with the use of prophylactic acyclovir.

HSV reactivation appears to be more common in HCT than in solid organ transplant recipients and has led to the universal use of prophylactic acyclovir for all seropositive patients. If oral vesicles occur, diagnosis is achieved when HSV is detected by PCR. Viral culture of the vesicle is typically only done as the initial step to test for acyclovir resistance. Dissemination can occur with primary infection and, less commonly, with reactivation and can result in significant end-organ disease, including hepatitis and pneumonitis.

Patients with suspected HSV infection should receive intravenous acyclovir empirically while awaiting diagnostic confirmation.

Adenovirus Adenovirus is a common cause of infection in all transplant recipients and clinical manifestations can vary from asymptomatic to severe, disseminated disease. As in solid organ transplant recipients, adenovirus can cause significant disease in HCT recipients but seems to be more common in patients with GVHD. Clinical manifestations include hemorrhagic cystitis, pneumonitis, nephritis, gastroenteritis, and hepatitis.

Risk factors for severe infection are similar to those for other viruses and include extremes of age, infection within 1 month of transplantation, and high levels of immunosuppression. Different adenovirus serotypes have a propensity to infect different organs, leading to specific clinical manifestations. For example, liver transplant recipients tend to develop hepatitis or gastroenteritis from serotypes 1, 2, and 5. In contrast, lung transplant recipients develop pneumonitis and obliterative bronchiolitis, and renal transplant recipients often develop hemorrhagic cystitis or prolonged urinary tract infections caused by serotypes 11, 34, and 35.

Detection of adenovirus by PCR suggests infection only in the context of compatible clinical symptoms. Diagnosis of disease can be challenging to distinguish from shedding because immunocompromised patients may shed adenovirus asymptomatically for prolonged periods.

While primary management consists of supportive care and judicious reduction in immunosuppression, the role of antiviral agents is unclear and there are currently no FDA-approved treatments. Most centers consider cidofovir as standard antiviral treatment for severe or disseminated disease, with reports of success in severe infections. Adoptive viral-specifc T-cell (VST) therapy, also known as cytotoxic T lymphocyte (CTL) therapy is a potentially promising option, but currently, there are minimal data on efficacy and availability is limited. Antibody preparations, such as IVIG, have also been used in some cases with unclear benefit. Patients with severe hypogammaglobulinemia (IgG <350 mg/dL) may benefit from supplementation.

Parvovirus Parvovirus B19 was first recognized as a cause of red cell aplasia in sickle cell patients. It has also been identified as a cause of aplastic anemia and, to a lesser extent, pancytopenia in the transplant population. The aplasia can occur with or without systemic signs of fatigue, malaise, fever, and arthralgias. In HCT patients, Parvovirus B19 has also rarely been associated with graft failure. Parvovirus DNA can be detected by PCR and low-level viremia may persist for several months following initial infection. Testing is indicated in the setting of chronic anemia and treatment is with IVIG, although adjustment in immunosuppression may also be needed and recurrences have been reported.

Influenza Virus Influenza virus has significant morbidity and mortality in both immunocompetent and immunocompromised populations. Morbidity in transplant patients increases with lung transplantation, extremes of age, high levels of immunosuppression, and occurrence of infection immediately posttransplant. The Centers for Disease Control and Prevention (CDC) has long recommended vaccination before influenza season and chemoprophylaxis during outbreaks for immunocompromised patients. If a transplant patient presents with signs and symptoms compatible with influenza, early diagnosis with a rapid antigen assay and empiric treatment with oral antiviral therapy are warranted. Oral oseltamivir is often used owing to its efficacy against both influenza A and B with peramivir as an intravenous option. Baloxavir is a small molecule inhibitor of influenza mRNA synthesis that is approved for children >12 years old and appears to be as effective as oseltamivir. Baloxavir has not yet been well studied in immunocompromised patients and due to the risk of treatment emergent resistance it is not currently routinely recommended in immunocompromised patients. Chemoprophylaxis should be offered to all transplant recipients who come in close contact with an individual with suspected or confirmed influenza infection. The CDC maintains the latest information on seasonal influenza activity and sensitivities, providing up-to-date guidance on optimal antiviral treatments (http://www.cdc.gov/flu/professionals/index.htm).

Respiratory Syncytial Virus (RSV) RSV causes a wide range of symptoms in transplant patients, although upper and lower respiratory tract infections are most common. The risk factors for severe disease are similar to those for influenza: lung transplantation, extremes of age, greater immune suppression, and infection early after transplantation. Unlike influenza, however, there is no proven therapy. Inhaled, IV or oral ribavirin could be considered in severe cases. There are insufficient data to determine whether palivizumab is effective in treating RSV pneumonia in solid organ recipients.

Other Viruses Human herpesvirus-6 (HHV6) is a common infection following transplantation owing to a high rate of reactivation. Although the vast majority of patients (99%) are asymptomatic, this virus has been associated with development of numerous clinical symptoms including fever, rash, hepatitis, pneumonitis, graft dysfunction, and encephalitis. Diagnosis is most often made by PCR, but the significance of detection of HHV6 DNA is challenging given the frequency of asymptomatic reactivation. When treatment is indicated, foscarnet or ganciclovir typically have activity and are recommended first-line agents.

Parainfluenza viruses (PIV) are common respiratory viruses. Infections generally begin as mild upper respiratory symptoms but may progress to severe lower respiratory tract infections including giant cell pneumonia. Risk of lower tract disease appears to relate to use of corticosteroids, lymphopenia, and coinfections with other respiratory pathogens. The efficacy of ribavirin has not been established in PIV. DAS181, a novel sialidase fusion protein, has shown promise in prevention and treatment of PIV disease but is available for investigational use only.

BK virus causes infections predominantly in renal transplant and HCT recipients. Although adult patients are affected more commonly, pediatric kidney transplant recipients may develop BK nephropathy due to reactivation or primary infection which may lead to graft loss. In HCT recipients, BK virus may cause hemorrhagic cystitis, generally after the first few weeks posttransplant. In any HCT patient with hematuria, BK virus infection should be suspected. Cidofovir is the primary treatment for both BK nephropathy and hemorrhagic cystitis.

Fungal Infections In SOT recipients, the risk of fungal infection varies depending on the organ that is transplanted. *Candida* species infections are more common in heart, liver, small bowel, and kidney transplants. Meanwhile, *Aspergillus* species predominate in lung transplant recipients, most often due to pretransplant colonization and a direct connection between the graft and the environment. Although the use of prophylactic fluconazole has decreased the overall incidence of fungal infections, it remains a relatively common cause of morbidity due to the emergence of resistant strains of *Candida* species and the presence of *Aspergillus* species.

Risk factors in HCT recipients include mucositis, neutropenia, GVHD, the need for corticosteroid therapy, and potentially CMV infection due to the immunosuppressive effects of the infection. Given the antibacterial and immunosuppressive therapies given to transplant patients, fungal infection should always be included in the differential diagnosis of fever in a transplant recipient. Mucormycoses, which include *Mucor*, *Rhizopus*, *Rhizomucor*, and other species, cause devastating invasive disease in immunocompromised patients. Rhinocerebral and pulmonary infections are most common and have a high mortality; aggressive surgical debridement as well as antifungal treatment is paramount. Diagnosis is made with peripheral blood cultures and cultures of any suspicious lesions, particularly those seen on computed tomography (CT) of the chest.

DIAGNOSTIC EVALUATION

The evaluation of a transplant patient with fever or any concerns for infection should begin with a thorough history and physical examination, attempting to localize the symptoms to a specific location or organ system. **Table 105-1** lists common diagnostic tests that should be considered based on the presenting symptoms. For HCT recipients, the phase of engraftment should also be considered when beginning this assessment.

Diagnosis of viral infections in transplant recipients may be difficult. PCR has largely replaced other diagnostic tools for detection and quantification of viral infections. PCR is the most commonly used method of detection of viral DNA for CMV, EBV, VZV, HSV, adenovirus, and respiratory viruses. While clinical availability of specific viral PCRs may vary between institutions, they are generally highly sensitive and specific tests. PCRs can be performed on blood/serum, cerebrospinal fluid (CSF), urine, stool, bronchoalveolar lavage fluid, and tissue. While the

TABLE 105-1 Diagnostic Considerations for Infection in Transplant Recipients

PRESENTATION AND DIAGNOSTIC CONSIDERATIONS			COMMON ORGANISMS		
Clinical presentation	*Disease processes*	*Diagnostic tests*	*Bacteria*	*Viruses*	*Fungi & Parasites*
Fever without localizing symptoms	Occult bacteremia (if neutropenic) CVC-associated bloodstream infection Viral infection or reactivation PTLD	Blood cultures (central line & peripheral) Urine culture (especially young age) Respiratory Viral PCR Panel CMV quantitative PCR EBV quantitative PCR Adenovirus quantitative PCR	*Staphylococcus* species Gram-negative bacilli	CMV EBV Adenovirus COVID-19	Candida species (early posttransplant)
Headache Meningismus Neurologic changes Altered mental status	Meningitis Encephalitis Cerebral abscess	CSF cell counts and cultures (bacterial, fungal) CSF PCR: enterovirus, HSV, VZV, EBV, CMV, LCMV, HHV6, mycoplasma, *Toxoplasma* Arbovirus serology (seasonal) Cryptococcal antigen (CSF & serum) CNS imaging (head CT with contrast if intracranial abscess suspected)	*Streptococcus* spp. *Listeria monocytogenes* *Salmonella* spp. *Pseudomonas aeruginosa* *Escherichia coli* *Nocardia* spp.	Enterovirus HSV VZV EBV CMV HHV6 JC virus	*Cryptococcus neoformans* *Aspergillus* spp. *Candida* spp. Mucormycoses *Toxoplasma gondii*
Oral ulcers	Stomatitis Mucositis	HSV PCR/DFA Enterovirus PCR swab/serum/stool		HSV Enterovirus	
Tonsillar hypertrophy Cervical lymphadenopathy	PTLD Lymphadenitis	EBV PCR (blood) Lymph node biopsy/incision and drainage (ultrasound guidance may be needed)	*Staphylococcus aureus* Oral anaerobes (if cervical adenopathy) Atypical mycobacteria *Actinomyces* spp.	EBV Adenovirus CMV	
Sinus pain or tenderness Tooth pain	Sinusitis	Head/sinus CT with contrast Sinus aspirate and culture (in refractory or severe cases, or when fungal infection suspected)	*Staphylococcus aureus* *Streptococcus pneumoniae* *Haemophilus influenza* *Moraxella catarrhalis* *Pseudomonas aeruginosa* (CF patients) Oral Anaerobes		Mucormycoses *Aspergillus* spp.
Nasal congestion Rhinorrhea Cough	Upper respiratory tract infection Sinusitis	Respiratory Viral PCR Panel Enzyme immunoassays (EIA) or DFA for viral pathogens Rapid influenza/RSV diagnostic tests	(see above)	Influenza Parainfluenza RSV Rhinovirus Enterovirus Adenovirus Coronavirus Human metapneumovirus	
Cough Tachypnea Respiratory distress	Pneumonia Pneumonitis	Chest x-ray Chest CT scan Bronchoscopy: GMS stain and/or PCR for PJP, bacterial and fungal cultures, respiratory viral PCRs, legionella antigen or PCR, AFB stain and cultures Lung biopsy with histology and cultures	*S. pneumoniae* *Staphylococcus aureus* *Haemophilus influenzae* *Legionella* *Pseudomonas* *Acinetobacter* *Burkholderia* (cystic fibrosis patients) *Bordetella pertussis*	Influenza Parainfluenza RSV CMV Rhinovirus Human metapneumovirus HSV (pneumonitis)	*Aspergillus* spp. *Candida* spp. *Pneumocystis jirovecii* *Histoplasmosis capsulatum* *Coccidioides* spp. *Blastomycosis dermatitidis* *Cryptococcus neoformans*
Dysphagia Odynophagia	Esophagitis	Esophagogastroduodenoscopy: HSV PCR, CMV PCR, fungal culture		CMV HSV	*Candida* spp.

(*Continued*)

TABLE 105-1 Diagnostic Considerations for Infection in Transplant Recipients (*Continued*)

PRESENTATION AND DIAGNOSTIC CONSIDERATIONS			COMMON ORGANISMS		
Clinical presentation	*Disease processes*	*Diagnostic tests*	*Bacteria*	*Viruses*	*Fungi & Parasites*
Diarrhea Abdominal pain	Gastroenteritis Colitis/enteritis	Stool multiplex PCR *Clostridium difficile* toxin EIA or PCR Rotavirus antigen EIA Norovirus PCR CMV PCR (blood) Giardia/cryptosporidium antigen Ova and parasite testing Colonoscopy with biopsy	*Clostridium difficile* *Salmonella* *Shigella* *Campylobacter* *E. coli*	Rotavirus Norovirus CMV Adenovirus Hepatitis A	*Giardia lamblia* *Cryptosporidium* *Strongyloides stercoralis*
Right upper quadrant abdominal pain Vomiting Hepatomegaly Jaundice	Hepatitis Cholangitis/liver abscess	Liver function tests/enzymes Liver ultrasound Abdominal CT scan Blood culture Liver biopsy	Enteric gram-negative bacilli *Enterococcus* spp. Anaerobes	CMV HSV VZV EBV HHV6 Hepatitis A, B, C Adenovirus	*Candida* spp. *Aspergillus* spp.
Erythematous rash	Cellulitis Folliculitis	Bacterial culture from incision and drainage (if warranted)	*Staphylococcus aureus* *Streptococcus pyogenes*		*Candida* spp.
Vesicular rash	Chickenpox/zoster	VZV and HSV PCR of scraping of base of unroofed vesicle		VZV HSV	
Nonspecific rash	Viral exanthem	PCRs from blood Respiratory viral PCR panel		EBV CMV VZV HHV6 Parvovirus Adenovirus Enterovirus	

Abbreviations: CMV, cytomegalovirus; CT, computed tomography; EBV, Epstein-Barr virus; HHV6, human herpesvirus-6; HSV, herpes simplex virus; LCMV, lymphocytic choriomeningitis virus; PCR, polymerase chain reaction; RSV, respiratory syncytial virus; VZV, varicella zoster virus.

presence of viral DNA in blood/serum and CSF is generally indicative of active infection, interpretation may be needed to determine the clinical significance of viral DNA in other sites due to prolonged shedding and asymptomatic carriage. Rapid enzyme immunoassays (EIAs) may also be offered for RSV and influenza at some institutions.

Candidal infections are diagnosed using site-specific cultures, such as blood cultures from indwelling intravascular catheters, urinary cultures, and peritoneal cultures. *Candida* identified from tracheal or bronchial cultures usually represents colonization rather than true infection. Patients with candidemia should undergo evaluation for disseminated candidiasis. Ophthalmic evaluation of the retina should be performed; abdominal ultrasonography is useful to demonstrate candidal lesions in the liver, spleen, or kidney; and echocardiography can reveal fungal endocarditis. Infection with *Aspergillus* species is diagnosed by culturing these organisms from a sterile body site (e.g., cerebrospinal fluid) or biopsy specimen (e.g., lung tissue). The identification of *Aspergillus* from nonsterile body fluids (e.g., sputum) must be interpreted with caution, because colonization may occur among transplant patients. Novel testing assays including fungal PCRs (blood and bronchial fluid) and free-cell DNA (blood) testing are becoming more commercially available, but their positive and negative predictive values remain uncertain.

MANAGEMENT

PREVENTION AND PROPHYLAXIS

There are a number of preventive strategies used to reduce infectious diseases and their complications in transplant recipients including the use of isolation precautions, vaccination, preemptive antimicrobial treatment, and prophylaxis for specific infections. The use of preemptive treatment, which entails initiation of therapy when infection meets a predefined threshold (i.e., level of viremia), differs from prophylaxis, which aims to prevent development or spread of infection. The decision to use preemptive antimicrobials versus prophylaxis varies from institution to institution and depends largely on the underlying risk of disease versus side effects of the medication in the transplant recipient.

Understanding prophylaxis strategies is important when evaluating a transplant patient with suspected infection. Knowing which patients should be on prophylaxis and whether they have received it helps to stratify risk and shape the diagnostic approach. Intravenous immunoglobulin (IVIG) is often given to HCT recipients with hypogammaglobulinemia to prevent bacterial infections. Other infections, such as HSV, CMV, EBV, *Pneumocystis jirovecii*, and fungal infections, may require prophylactic strategies depending on the type of transplant, time since transplantation, and the donor/recipient status. Specific prophylactic and preventive treatments are summarized in **Table 105-2**. However, approaches to prophylaxis may vary widely from one center to another and providers should be familiar with their local practices.

TREATMENT

Bacterial Infections Empirical antimicrobial coverage for SOT patients varies depending on the organ transplanted. In liver and intestinal transplant recipients with suspected bowel perforations, antibiotics should include coverage for *Streptococcus* species, gram-negative rods, anaerobes, and *Candida* species. Therapeutic options include the combination of piperacillin-tazobactam and fluconazole, or the combination of antipseudomonal cephalosporin, metronidazole, and fluconazole.

In renal transplant recipients, infections with gram-negative bacilli predominate. Antibacterial coverage should include an antipseudomonal

TABLE 105-2 Therapies Used for Prevention and Prophylaxis of Specific Pathogens in Transplant Recipients

PATHOGEN	PREVENTATIVE THERAPY AND PROPHYLAXIS	
Viruses	**Solid Organ Transplant (SOT)**	**Hematopoietic Cell Transplant (HCT)**
Cytomegalovirus (CMV)	Primary: ganciclovir/valganciclovir Alternative(s): foscarnet, cidofovir, letermovir *Highest-risk patients are CMV-seronegative recipients of organs from CMV-seropositive donors (D+/R-); prophylaxis generally given for 3-6 months following transplant in all high-risk (D+/R-) SOT patients and 3 months in lower-risk (D+ or D-/R+) patients*	Primary: ganciclovir/ valganciclovir Alternative(s): foscarnet, cidofovir, letermovir *Pre-emptive or prophylactic strategies used for at-risk allogeneic HCT recipients from engraftment to day 100 post-HCT. Dose and frequency of administration will vary depending on underlying risk. Valganciclovir used for pre-emptive therapy >100 days post-HCT in low-risk patients.*
Epstein Barr virus (EBV)	*Routine prophylaxis not recommended; serial monitoring of EBV viral load is often implemented in high-risk patients*	Primary prevention of EBV-related PTLD: rituximab *Used in high-risk patients only (EBV viremia in context of T-cell depletion)*
Herpes simplex virus (HSV)	Primary: acyclovir, valacyclovir Alternative(s): ganciclovir, foscarnet *Prophylaxis offered to all seropositive SOT recipients during early posttransplant period to prevent reactivation of disease, typically for 3 months; patients receiving ganciclovir for CMV do not need additional HSV prophylaxis with acyclovir*	Primary: acyclovir, valacyclovir Alternative(s): ganciclovir, foscarnet *Offered to all seropositive allogeneic HCT recipients during early posttransplant period; continue until engraftment occurs*
Varicella zoster virus (VZV)	*Routine prophylaxis of VZV is not recommended; VZV immunoglobulin (Varizig) and acyclovir are given in cases of VZV exposure, particularly in seronegative patients*	Primary: acyclovir, valacyclovir Alternative(s): varizig, foscarnet *Offered for the first year after HCT in seropositive patients; may require longer therapy if chronic GVHD or chronic immunosuppression. Post-exposure prophylaxis with Varizig.*
BK virus (BKV)	*Routine prophylaxis of BKV is not recommended; serial screening with BKV DNA PCR recommended in renal transplant patients*	*Routine prophylaxis of BKV hemorrhagic cystitis is not recommended in HCT recipients*
Fungi	**Solid Organ Transplant (SOT)**	**Hematopoietic Cell Transplant (HCT)**
Invasive candidiasis	Primary: fluconazole Alternative(s): oral nystatin, echinocandins, amphotericin B *Generally offered to all SOT recipients; Recipients of lung, small bowel, and pancreas considered high-risk; no uniform approach to prophylaxis; therapy typically 4 weeks*	Primary: fluconazole Alternative(s): echinocandins *Offered to 1) all allogeneic HCT recipients or, 2) autologous HCT recipients with underlying hematologic malignancies, prolonged neutropenia and mucosal damage; given from conditioning through engraftment; prophylaxis with echinocandins may be needed in patients with a history of known azole-resistant fungal pathogens*
Moulds (Aspergillus spp., etc.)	Primary: azole agents with activity against *Aspergillus* sp. (voriconazole, posaconazole, isavuconazole) Alternative(s): amphotericin B *Lung transplant recipients at highest risk for Aspergillus; liver transplant recipients at high risk for Aspergillus may also receive prophylaxis; treatment typically 4-6 months*	Primary: voriconazole, posaconazole, isavuconazole Alternative(s): amphotericin B *Prophylaxis is increasing across the US; may be offered to patients at high-risk for mould infection (prolonged neutropenia or severe GVHD) or with prior history of invasive mould infection*
Pneumocystis jirovecii	Primary: trimethoprim-sulfamethoxazole (TMP-SMX) Alternative(s): pentamidine, dapsone, atovaquone *Recommended for all SOT recipients for 6-12 months post-transplant; lifelong prophylaxis indicated for lung and small bowel recipients, or anyone with prior PJP infection or chronic CMV disease; lifelong prophylaxis may also be indicated in heart and liver recipients depending on underlying risk and immunosuppression*	Primary: trimethoprim-sulfamethoxazole (TMP-SMX) Alternative(s): pentamidine, dapsone, atovaquone *Used in all allogeneic transplant recipients from engraftment to >6 months post-transplant; offered to autologous HCT recipients requiring significant immunosuppression*
Other	**Solid Organ Transplant (SOT)**	**Hematopoietic Cell Transplant (HCT)**
Toxoplasma gondii	Primary: trimethoprim-sulfamethoxazole (TMP-SMX) Alternative(s): pyrimethamine plus sulfadiazine *Cardiac transplant recipients most likely to receive prophylaxis; TMP-SMX typically used in R+ patients; pyrimethamine/sulfadiazine may be offered to high-risk (D+/R-) recipients; prophylaxis usually for 6 months*	Primary: trimethoprim-sulfamethoxazole (TMP-SMX) Alternative(s): not well-established *May be offered to seropositive allogeneic HCT recipients; used from engraftment through end of immunosuppression*

penicillin or cephalosporin, especially in the first month after transplantation.

Bacteremia from gram-positive and gram-negative organisms occurs in the HCT population for a variety of reasons, including immune suppression, mucosal breakdown, and frequent central venous catheterization. In SOT recipients, the most common sources of bacterial infection are surgery and indwelling catheters. Resistant organisms are being seen with increasing frequency in transplant populations and knowledge of local antibiograms is critical.

For HCT recipients with suspected infection, typical empirical broad-spectrum antibiotic coverage should include an antipseudomonal agent such as cefepime, piperacillin-tazobactam, or a carbapenem. Vancomycin is often added for the following indications: (1) HCT patients with mucositis and neutropenia; (2) hypotension or other evidence of cardiovascular dysfunction, particularly in the presence of a central venous catheter; (3) known colonization with an organism resistant to penicillins and cephalosporins (e.g., methicillin-resistant *S. aureus*, some *Enterococcus* species); (4) growth of a gram-positive organism from the blood with pending susceptibilities; and (5) recent parenteral antibiotic use. Caution should be employed when using empiric vancomycin therapy in other situations given the increasing prevalence of vancomycin-resistant enterococci in pediatric transplant populations. Increasing use of alternative agents for resistant gram-positive infections include daptomycin and ceftaroline to mitigate nephrotoxicity risk that is associated with vancomycin.

Viral Infections Therapies used to treat various viral infections are discussed under each specific virus in the Differential Diagnosis section. **Table 105-3** provides a summary of common therapeutics used against the most common viral infections in transplant recipients.

TABLE 105-3 Treatment Strategies for Select Viral Infections in Transplant Recipients

Pathogen	Primary Agent	Alternative(s)
Cytomegalovirus (CMV)	Primary: IV ganciclovir (5 mg/kg/dose every 12 hours) *dosing may vary depending on severity of disease and underlying renal function; optimal length of therapy determined by reduction in viral loads and clinical response, generally until complete resolution of viremia for at least two weeks; response typically seen within 5-7 days; longer therapy may be needed if evidence of severe disease or tissue invasion; early transition to oral therapy (valganciclovir) possible according to clinical response*	Alternative(s): Valganciclovir (dose based on age and creatinine clearance)—*oral drug used in cases of nonsevere disease with low-level viremia or following demonstrable response to IV therapy* Foscarnet (60 mg/kg/dose)—*dose adjustments needed for renal dysfunction; used in cases of ganciclovir resistance or intolerance; electrolyte abnormalities common* Cidofovir (5 mg/kg/dose/wk or 1 mg/kg/dose 3 times weekly)—*in cases of ganciclovir resistance; nephrotoxicity common* Maribavir (>12 y/o; 400 mg twice a day)—*in cases of multidrug resistance or intolerance*
Epstein-Barr Virus (EBV)	Primary: No recommended treatment. For EBV-related PTLD, initial options include: Rituximab (375 mg/m^2 weekly)—*anti-CD20 monoclonal antibody used in PTLD and EBV disease; may require several doses to achieve reduction in EBV viral load* Reduction in immunosuppression—*critical in treatment of EBV disease and PTLD*	Alternative(s): EBV donor-derived or third-party adoptive cytotoxic T lymphocytes (CTL)—*may have a role in select cases; risk of GVHD following CTL therapy* Infusion of donor lymphocytes—*used to restore T cell function* Chemotherapy—*may have a role in select cases*
Herpes simplex virus (HSV)	Primary: IV acyclovir (10 mg/kg/dose every 8 hours)—*therapy of choice for systemic or severe mucocutaneous disease; prolonged therapy (14-21) days needed for CNS disease*	Alternative(s): Oral acyclovir (1000 mg/day divided 3-5 times daily not to exceed 80 mg/kg/day), valacyclovir (15-30 mg/kg/dose 3 times daily)—*could be considered in less serious cases* Foscarnet (40-60 mg/kg/dose)—*dose adjustments needed for renal dysfunction; used in cases of acyclovir-resistant disease* Cidofovir (dose not established for this indication)—*for acyclovir-resistant disease*
Varicella zoster virus (VZV)	Primary: IV acyclovir (10 mg/kg/dose every 8 hours)—*key drug used to stop viral replication and prevent progression of disease* Varicella immunoglobulin (Varizig; 125 units/10 kg)— *should be offered within 96 hours of exposure in seronegative patients*	Alternative(s): Oral acyclovir (20 mg/kg/dose 4 times daily)—*could be considered in mild cases of mucocutaneous disease* Oral valacyclovir 20 mg/kg/dose 2-3 times daily Foscarnet (40-60 mg/kg/dose)—*dose adjustments needed for renal dysfunction; higher doses may be needed in older children; used in cases of acyclovir-resistant disease* Cidofovir (dose not established for this indication)—*for acyclovir-resistant disease*
Influenza	Primary: Neuraminidase inhibitors: oseltamivir (dose varies by weight), peramivir (12 mg/kg one-time dose) *activity against both influenza A and B; prompt initiation of therapy is key; attention should be paid to viral resistance patterns*	Alternative(s): Baloxavir <80 kg: 40 mg one time dose >80 kg: 80 mg one-time dose
Parainfluenza virus	Primary: Supportive care—*no proven effective treatments*	Alternative(s): Intravenous immunoglobulin (400 mg/kg/dose)—*efficacy is unclear*
Respiratory syncytial virus (RSV)	Primary: Ribavirin (aerosolized, intravenous, oral; dose varies by route of administration)—*used in high-risk patients (HCT, lung transplant) with evidence of lower respiratory tract infection; some centers may use in upper respiratory tract infection; efficacy is unclear*	Alternative(s): Intravenous immunoglobulin (400 mg/kg/dose)—*use varies by center; role and efficacy not clearly established*
Adenovirus	Primary: Cidofovir (5 mg/kg/dose/wk or 1mg/kg/dose 3 times weekly)—*specific regimens may vary; early initiation of therapy may prevent dissemination and end-organ disease*	Alternative(s): Cytotoxic T lymphocytes—*donor-derived or third party if available.*
Human herpesvirus-6 (HHV-6)	Primary: Treatment not indicated in asymptomatic reactivation or during coinfection with CMV	Alternative(s): Ganciclovir (5 mg/kg/dose), foscarnet (40-60 mg/kg/dose), cidofovir (dose not established)—*can be used in setting of HHV-6 encephalitis or other severe disease; HHV-6A has variable resistance to ganciclovir*
BK virus	Primary: Reduction in immunosuppressant medications is important, if possible Cidofovir (dosing regimens vary)—*may be beneficial in both hemorrhagic cystitis (HCT recipients) and BK nephropathy (renal transplant recipients); should be used with close monitoring given nephrotoxicity* Adequate hydration essential for hemorrhagic cystitis	Alternative(s): Cytotoxic T lymphocytes Leflunomide (pediatric dose not established)—*used for BK virus allograft nephropathy; no controlled trials to demonstrate efficacy*

Fungal Infections Routine prophylaxis with fluconazole has led to an overall decrease in the number of fungal infections; however, there appears to be an increase in the number of fluconazole-resistant *Candida* species and continued concern about *Aspergillus*. Antifungal coverage with amphotericin is often added for HCT patients with fever for longer than 3 to 5 days with no identifiable source; if *Aspergillus* infection is a possibility, based on an identifiable site of infection (sinusitis, pneumonia); or in high-risk patients, such as those with GVHD.

First-line antifungal agents for invasive candidal infections are the echinocandins (caspofungin, micafungin, anidulafungin) which typically have good activity against all *Candida* species. Alternatively, amphotericin and fluconazole can be used as second-line agents, but lessor favored due to susceptibility patterns and side effect profiles. Removal of infected hardware (central venous catheters, peritoneal catheters, etc.) is critical and treatment without removal of infected devices should be avoided when possible.

The drugs of choice for the treatment of invasive aspergillosis are the later-generation azoles, voriconazole, posaconazole, and isavuconazole. Alternative agents include amphotericin B products but have inferior outcomes and higher rates of adverse effects. Other molds, including mucormycoses, should be treated with lipid formulations of amphotericin B. In patients with renal dysfunction, posaconazole can be considered as an alternative agent. Susceptibility testing should be performed on all fungal isolates as resistance cannot be predicted merely by organism identification. Aggressive surgical debridement often plays a crucial role in successful treatment of invasive mold infections as medical therapy alone is frequently ineffective.

Treatment for *PJP* pneumonia is with trimethoprim-sulfamethoxazole (TMP-SMX). Steroids are used concomitantly in severe disease cases where hypoxia is present. In patients who are allergic to TMP-SMX or do not respond to therapy, intravenous pentamidine or clindamycin plus primaquine could be used. Atovaquone is an option for mild cases.

Numerous antimicrobials require close monitoring in transplant recipients due to their side effect profile or drug-drug interactions with immunosuppressants. Aminoglycosides, vancomycin, extended-spectrum penicillins with β-lactamase inhibitors (piperacillin-tazobactam, ticarcillin-clavulanate), and amphotericin may potentiate nephrotoxicity of several immune-suppressant drugs resulting in acute kidney injury. Patients receiving calcineurin inhibitors in conjunction with azoles require frequent monitoring of the serum levels of calcineurin inhibitor because azoles inhibit hepatic P450 metabolism and can cause a patient's calcineurin inhibitor level to rise. Rifampin upregulates P450 enzymes and affects drug levels as well. Macrolides inhibit tacrolimus metabolism and concomitant use should be avoided, although azithromycin may have less of an effect than other drugs in this class.

ADMISSION AND DISCHARGE CRITERIA

In most instances, when infection is suspected in a transplant recipient, hospital admission is warranted. No specific guidelines exist regarding admission or discharge criteria. But, the majority of centers will approach immunocompromised individuals, including transplant recipients, more conservatively than others. In cases when discharge is contemplated prior to establishing a diagnosis or before completing treatment for an established infection, close follow-up needs to be arranged.

CONSULTATION

Depending on the institution, pediatric hospitalists may be the first to evaluate, stabilize, perform diagnostic tests, and initiate empiric antimicrobial treatment in transplant recipients with suspected infections. Due to the vulnerable and complex nature of this patient population, consultation with an infectious diseases specialist is recommended when managing transplant recipients with suspected or documented infections. Additional consultation with surgeons, in the setting of SOT, and organ-specific transplant specialists (hepatologists, nephrologists, pulmonologists, cardiologists, oncologists) is also warranted. While pediatric hospitalists may be required to provide care for transplant recipients, assistance from trained subspecialists is advised. If these services are unavailable, consideration could be given to transfer of the patient as needed.

SPECIAL CONSIDERATIONS

ACQUIRED AND FUNCTIONAL ASPLENIA

The spleen is an important organ in the defense against infection. It produces antibodies, and macrophages within the spleen engulf bacteria and eliminate them from the circulation. Patients who are asplenic or have functional asplenia are at risk for a variety of severe infections, particularly with encapsulated bacterial organisms: *S. pneumoniae*, *Neisseria meningitidis*, and *Haemophilus influenzae*. *Salmonella*, although not an encapsulated organism, is also a common cause of infection, particularly in patients with sickle cell disease. Intracellular organisms that cause babesiosis and malaria also cause disease in asplenic patients. Although the risk of bacterial infection with asplenia is highest in the first several years after the spleen is removed (or functionally absent), the risk of infection is lifelong. To reduce the risk of infection, antibiotic prophylaxis with penicillin, amoxicillin, amoxicillin-clavulanate, trimethoprim-sulfamethoxazole, or cefuroxime is standard therapy for the first several years after splenectomy, although the optimal duration of prophylaxis is not known. Asplenic patients with suspected bacterial infection should be admitted to the hospital and placed on broad-spectrum antibiotic therapy, typically with a third-generation cephalosporin pending blood culture results.

PREVENTION

VACCINATIONS FOR PATIENTS POSTTRANSPLANTATION

Vaccination of patients following transplantation is important to protect individuals who may be more prone to illness and complications from vaccine-preventable illnesses. However, special consideration needs to be given to the safety and timing of vaccine administration. Transplant recipients may be at higher risk for complications from vaccines, some of which may be contraindicated depending on the degree of ongoing immunosuppression. Additionally, patients may generate suboptimal immunologic responses to immunizations both due to underlying disease and the use of immunosuppressive medications. For all transplant recipients, long-lasting immunity from vaccines given posttransplant has not been well established and reevaluation for booster doses may be needed.

In general, all age-appropriate vaccines should be encouraged prior to SOT and an accelerated schedule should be pursued in anticipation of transplantation. Live virus vaccines are contraindicated within 4 weeks prior to transplant and while can be given in specific settings following transplant, they are not routinely recommended outside of a research setting or following detailed patient evaluation and risk stratification. For transplant recipients unable to get live vaccines, antibody (IgG) levels to live vaccine components (measles, mumps, rubella, varicella) can be measured pretransplant and 1 year following transplantation to determine if a patient should require passive immunization if exposed to disease. Inactivated vaccines can be resumed 3 to 6 months following transplantation, although timing may vary by center and depending on the degree of ongoing immunosuppression. Influenza vaccine should be given annually and vaccination during the early transplant period appears to be safe, although immunogenicity may be impaired.

Hematopoietic cell transplant (HCT) recipients should be routinely re-vaccinated with inactivated vaccines following transplant, typically 6 to 12 months following transplantation. Influenza vaccine could be given as early as 4 months after transplant, but a second dose may need to be given. MMR and varicella vaccines can be administered ≥24 months following HCT, if the patient is no longer immunocompromised and has not had recent episodes of GVHD. Specific guidelines for immunization practices in HCT recipients have been published by the American Society for Blood and Marrow Transplantion (Tomblyn 2009).

Household and close contacts of transplant recipients should be strongly encouraged to receive all age-appropriate vaccines as this is an important way to provide added protection for the vulnerable patient in the immediate posttransplant period. With the exception of the smallpox vaccine, live vaccines are not contraindicated for close contacts of transplant recipients and should be administered when indicated. Live attenuated influenza vaccine (LAIV) should be avoided if possible for contacts of a profoundly immunosuppressed patient (i.e., requires strict contact precautions), although transmission of LAIV has not been reported. Individuals who receive varicella virus-containing vaccines and develop skin lesions should avoid contact with a transplant recipient. Good hand hygiene practices are important for contacts whose children have received rotavirus vaccine.

VACCINATIONS IN ASPLENIC PATIENTS

All patients should receive immunization with meningococcal, pneumococcal, and *H. influenzae* type B vaccine, preferably before the onset of asplenia. Pneumococcal conjugate vaccine (PCV) should be given to all asplenic children; the number of administrations depend on prior receipt of the vaccine. Following completion of the full PCV series, a 23-valent pneumococcal polysaccharide vaccine (PPSV23) should be administered at >24 months of age, as soon as 8 weeks after the last PCV13, and then again 5 years later. The *H. influenzae* type B conjugate vaccine should be administered immediately to any unvaccinated or undervaccinated child. For children 2 to 24 months of age, MenACWY-CRM should be administered in a 2 to 4-dose series depending on age of child at dose 1. Patients older than 2 years of age who have not received MenACWY-CRM should receive 2 doses of meningococcal conjugate vaccine (MenACWY-D4 or MenACWY-CRM). MenACWY-D must be administered at least 4 weeks after completion of all PCV doses. Serogroup B meningococcal vaccines MenB-FHbp and MenB-4C are recommended at age 10 years and older. Of note these vaccine series are not interchangeable and the same product should be used to complete the entire series.

KEY POINTS

- Transplant recipients represent a special population with unique risks for infectious complications.
- The risk of infection in solid organ transplant recipients is dependent upon the type of organ transplanted, the time since transplantation, the amount of ongoing immunosuppression, the physical environment of the patient, and infectious diseases history of the organ donor and recipient.
- The level of infection risk in hematopoietic cell transplant recipients depends on the stage of engraftment, indication for HCT, degree of immunosuppression (and presence of graft-versus-host disease), and infectious diseases history.
- A careful history and physical examination are critical to determine the appropriate evaluation for transplant recipients with concerns of infection, which is often more thorough than is implemented in an immune-competent individual.
- Signs of infection in transplant recipients may be subtle and atypical features of common infections may be present in transplant recipients.
- Viral infections may be associated with significant morbidity and mortality in transplant recipients and numerous preventive strategies have been implemented to decrease the incidence and severity of these infections in transplant patients.
- Consultation with infectious diseases and/or transplant specialists is recommended to assist with diagnostic and therapeutic approaches in transplant recipients.

SUGGESTED READINGS

Allen U, Green M. Prevention and treatment of infectious complications after solid organ transplantation in children. *Pediatr Clin North Am.* 2010;57(2):459-479.

Fishman JA. Infection in organ transplantation. *Am J Transplant.* 2017; 17(4):856-879.

Danzinger-Isakov L, Kumar D; AST Infectious Diseases Community of Practice. Vaccination of solid organ transplant candidates and recipients: Guidelines from the American society of transplantation infectious diseases community of practice. *Clin Transplant.* 2019;33(9): e13563.

Styczynski J, Reusser P, Einsele H, et al. Management of HSV, VZV and EBV infections in patients with hematological malignancies and after SCT: guidelines from the Second European Conference on Infections in Leukemia. *Bone Marrow Transplant.* 2009;43(10):757-770.

Tomblyn M, Chiller T, Einsele H, et al. Guidelines for preventing infectious complications among hematopoietic cell transplantation recipients: a global perspective. *Biol Blood Marrow Transplant.* 2009; 15(10):1143-1238.

Cornely OA, Alastruey-Izquierdo A, Arenz D, et al. Global guideline for the diagnosis and management of mucormycosis: an initiative of the European Confederation of Medical Mycology in cooperation with the Mycoses Study Group Education and Research Consortium. *Lancet Infect Dis.* 2019;19(12):e405-e421.

Dutta A, Flores R. Infection prevention in pediatric oncology and hematopoietic stem cell transplant recipients. *Healthcare-Associated Infections in Children.* 2018:281-299.

Freifeld AG, Bow EJ, Sepkowitz KA, et al. Clinical practice guideline for the use of antimicrobial agents in neutropenic patients with cancer: 2010 update by the Infectious Diseases Society of America. *Clin Infect Dis.* 2011;52(4):e56-93.

Kotton CN, Kumar D, Caliendo AM, et al. The Third International Consensus Guidelines on the Management of Cytomegalovirus in Solid-organ Transplantation. *Transplantation.* 2018;102(6):900-931.

Lehrnbecher T, Fisher BT, Phillips B, et al. Guideline for Antibacterial Prophylaxis Administration in Pediatric Cancer and Hematopoietic Stem Cell Transplantation. *Clin Infect Dis.* 2020;71(1):226-236.

So M, Hand J, Forrest G, et al. White paper on antimicrobial stewardship in solid organ transplant recipients. *Am J Transplant.* 2022;22(1): 96-112.

CHAPTER 106 Coronavirus Disease 2019 (COVID-19)

Hayden T. Schwenk, MD, MPH and Roshni Mathew, MD

BACKGROUND

Coronavirus disease 2019 (COVID-19) is caused by severe acute respiratory syndrome coronavirus 2 (SARS-CoV-2) and was initially identified in Wuhan, China in December 2019 before rapidly spreading worldwide. SARS-CoV-2 is an enveloped, single-stranded ribonucleic acid (RNA) virus that belongs to the family *Coronaviridae* which includes human coronaviruses that cause the common cold as well as SARS-CoV and Middle East respiratory syndrome coronavirus. The viral envelope is coated with a club-shaped spike (S) glycoprotein that mediates host cell binding and entry and has been an important target for vaccine and drug development. SARS-CoV-2 has continually evolved over the course of the pandemic with accumulated mutations resulting in variants of the original virus. The World Health Organization has designated specific variants as "variants of concern" based on different factors (e.g., transmissibility, virulence) and named them using letters of the Greek alphabet. These definitions and nomenclature have been incorporated by the Centers for Disease Control and Prevention (CDC) with Alpha, Beta, and Gamma designated variants of concern in December 2020, Delta in June 2021, and Omicron in November 2021. Some of these variants have been associated with evasion of vaccine- or infection-associated immunity and reduced response to therapeutics.

PATHOPHYSIOLOGY

SARS-CoV-2 enters the host cell via binding of the receptor binding domain of the S protein to the angiotensin-converting enzyme 2 receptor of nasal and bronchial epithelial cells. Within the host cell, the virus undergoes RNA replication, transcription, translation, and assembly before being released to propagate infection of the next host cell. SARS-CoV-2 infection elicits both innate and adaptive immune responses. Proinflammatory chemokines and cytokines such as tumor necrosis factor alpha, interleukin-1, interleukin-6, and interferons help control the infection; however, a dysregulated immune response may result in more severe COVID-19 disease. This aberrant inflammatory response results in acute respiratory distress syndrome and is more common among adults than children. Endothelial barrier disruption and impaired oxygen diffusion capacity are characteristic features associated with critical COVID-19. Severe COVID-19 is also characterized by coagulopathy and disseminated intravascular coagulation. Severely inflamed tissues can result in microthrombi formation with resultant thrombotic arterial complications and pulmonary embolism. The adaptive immune response is mediated by CD4 and CD8 T-lymphocytes that are activated by viral peptides. The B-lymphocytes generate antibodies against the S and other viral proteins. Viral antigens, either through natural infection or vaccination, generate immunologic memory through T- and B-lymphocyte memory cells and neutralizing antibodies that protect the host, although the duration of protective immunity remains poorly understood.

CLINICAL PRESENTATION

Much of our knowledge about the clinical features of COVID-19 in children comes from reports published when the majority of infections were due to the original SARS-CoV-2 strain. Initial accounts suggested that most children with COVID-19 were either asymptomatic or had mild-moderate disease, characterized by cough and fever. Subsequent systematic reviews of publications during the first several months of the pandemic confirmed that severe disease requiring oxygen supplementation was rare in children. Various classification schemas, most of which were designed for adult patients, have been proposed to describe the clinical spectrum of SARS-CoV-2 infection (**Table 106-1**).

The clinical spectrum of disease is influenced by several factors, including the patient's age and underlying medical conditions, as well as the infecting SARS-CoV-2 variant. The median duration of illness is 5 to 6 days, with older children tending to experience a more prolonged illness. Contemporary data suggest that the majority of children with COVID-19 are asymptomatic or have a mild illness characterized by fevers and chills, cough, sore throat, nasal congestion, and headache. Unlike adults, children with COVID-19 may not present with the classic symptoms of fever, cough, shortness of breath, and olfactory dysfunction. Hoarse voice, sore throat, croup, and other upper respiratory tract symptoms appear to have been more common when the Omicron variant was the predominant circulating strain, while fever, loss of smell, and persistent cough were more common during the Delta period.

A variety of gastrointestinal symptoms including nausea, vomiting, diarrhea, and abdominal pain have been reported in children. Vomiting and poor feeding may be particularly common among neonates. Although cholestasis appears to be less common in children than adults with COVID-19, liver enzyme elevations are not uncommon. Dermatologic manifestations, including chilblain-like lesions of the extremities or "COVID toes," erythema multiforme-like lesions, and a varicella-like papulovesicular eruption have been reported in ~8% of children. A variety of neurologic symptoms, ranging from headache and fatigue to encephalopathy and seizures, have also been described. Although cardiac complications, including myocarditis and pericarditis, have been reported following both COVID-19 infection and messenger RNA (mRNA) COVID-19 vaccination, the incidence is significantly higher after COVID-19 infection than following receipt of an mRNA COVID-19 vaccine.

TABLE 106-1 Classification Schemas for the Clinical Spectrum of COVID-19

	Classification Schema		
Illness severity	**NIH**	**PIDS**	**WHO**
Asymptomatic or Presymptomatic Infection	Individuals who test positive for SARS-CoV-2 using a virologic test (i.e., a nucleic acid amplification test [NAAT] or an antigen test) but who have no symptoms that are consistent with COVID-19.	Individuals who test positive for SARS-CoV-2, but who have no symptoms consistent with COVID-19.	N/A
Mild Illness	Individuals who have any of the various signs and symptoms of COVID-19 (e.g., fever, cough, sore throat, malaise, headache, muscle pain, nausea, vomiting, diarrhea, loss of taste and smell) but who do not have shortness of breath, dyspnea, or abnormal chest imaging.	No new or increased supplemental oxygen requirement, with symptoms limited to the upper respiratory tract.	N/A
Moderate Illness	Individuals who show evidence of lower respiratory disease during clinical assessment or imaging and who have an oxygen saturation (SpO_2) ≥94% on room air at sea level.	No new or increased supplemental oxygen requirement, with symptoms involving the lower respiratory tract, or radiographic findings on chest x-ray.	N/A
Severe Illness	Individuals who have SpO_2 <94% on room air at sea level, a ratio of arterial partial pressure of oxygen to fraction of inspired oxygen (PaO_2/FiO_2) <300 mm Hg, a respiratory rate >30 breaths/min, or lung infiltrates >50%.	New or increase from baseline supplemental oxygen requirement without need for new or increase in baseline noninvasive/invasive mechanical ventilation.	Oxygen saturation <90% on room air, signs of pneumonia, or signs of severe respiratory distress (in adults, accessory muscle use, inability to complete full sentences, respiratory rate >30 breaths per minute; and, in children, very severe chest wall in-drawing, grunting, central cyanosis, or presence of any other general danger signs including inability to breastfeed or drink, lethargy, convulsions or reduced level of consciousness).
Critical Illness	Individuals who have respiratory failure, septic shock, and/or multiple organ dysfunction.	New or increased requirement for invasive or noninvasive mechanical ventilation, sepsis, or multiorgan failure OR rapidly worsening clinical trajectory that does not yet meet these criteria	Individuals with acute respiratory distress syndrome (ARDS), sepsis, septic shock, or other conditions that would normally require the provision of life-sustaining therapies (e.g., mechanical ventilation or vasopressor therapy).

References: COVID-19 Treatment Guidelines Panel. Coronavirus Disease 2019 (COVID-19) Treatment Guidelines. Available at https://www.covid19treatmentguidelines.nih.gov/. Accessed July 20, 2022; Chiotos K, Hayes M, Kimberlin DW, et al. Multicenter Interim Guidance on Use of Antivirals for Children With Coronavirus Disease 2019/Severe Acute Respiratory Syndrome Coronavirus 2. *J Pediatric Infect Dis Soc*. 2021;10(1): 34-48; and, World Health Organization. Therapeutics and COVID-19: living guideline. Available at https://app.magicapp.org/#/guideline/nBkO1E. Accessed September 28, 2022.

It is estimated that ~6% of children with COVID-19 require hospitalization. Reassuringly, the need for invasive mechanical ventilation and the incidence of in-hospital death among infants and children have remained rare. Surveillance data from the CDC found that although there were more infections, hospitalizations, and intensive care unit (ICU) admissions among children <12 years of age during the period of time when Omicron was the predominant circulating variant in the United States, the proportion of children with SARS-CoV-2 infection who required hospitalization or ICU admission was higher during the Delta period. Another study found no difference in COVID-19 severity across a period when the Alpha variant, Delta variant, and subsequently, Omicron variant, were the dominant strains.

Risk factors for severe and critical COVID-19 in children remain poorly understood. The need for hospitalization and risk for severe disease is similar between male and female children, while non-Hispanic Black and Hispanic children have higher rates of hospitalization compared to non-Hispanic White children. Young age has been inconsistently linked to a greater risk for severe disease, with some studies suggesting that infants may be at increased risk for severe illness, and others finding no difference in length of stay, ICU admission, and/or need for respiratory support. Prematurity may be a risk factor for severe disease among children ≤1 year of age. Compared to younger children, disease may also be severe in adolescents and young adults. Since the advent of effective vaccines, the majority of children hospitalized with COVID-19 have been unvaccinated.

Data during the period of Omicron predominance suggest roughly one-third of children 0 to 4 years of age and two-thirds of children aged 5 to 11 years of age hospitalized with COVID-19 had an underlying medical condition. A variety of comorbidities have been variably associated with hospitalization and/or severe COVID-19 in children including obesity, diabetes, sickle cell disease, asthma, gastrointestinal disease, neurological comorbidities, and underlying cardiac disorders. Immunocompromising conditions have not been consistently associated with worse outcomes in children with COVID-19. Laboratory and radiographic abnormalities potentially associated with severe disease include elevated inflammatory markers, elevated white blood cell count, thrombocytopenia, lymphopenia, and bilateral infiltrates on chest x-ray. Examination findings associated with hospitalization and worse outcomes include fever, shortness of breath, vomiting, and hypoxia.

DIFFERENTIAL DIAGNOSIS

Symptoms and radiographic findings of COVID-19 infection are relatively nonspecific and overlap with other viral illnesses common during childhood. A report from early during the pandemic found a combination of anosmia/ageusia, nausea/vomiting, and headache with fever to be most strongly associated with a positive SARS-CoV-2 result in children. Common viral (e.g., respiratory syncytial virus, influenza virus, human metapneumovirus) and bacterial (e.g., *Mycoplasma pneumoniae*, *Streptococcus pneumoniae*, *Streptococcus pyogenes*) pathogens are all considerations when patients present with upper or lower respiratory tract illness symptoms potentially consistent with COVID-19.

DIAGNOSTIC EVALUATION

There are several diagnostic testing options for SARS-CoV-2. Nucleic acid amplification tests (NAATs), such as the reverse transcription polymerase chain reaction (RT-PCR), are considered most sensitive to diagnose symptomatic or asymptomatic infection. The Infectious Diseases Society of America (IDSA) Guidelines on the Diagnosis of COVID-19: Molecular Diagnostic Testing recommends NAATs be performed on one of the following samples: nasopharyngeal (NP), mid-turbinate, anterior nares, combination of anterior nares and oropharyngeal, or saliva. While NP sampling has been heralded as the "gold standard" due to possible loss of sensitivity when other sites are used, the advantage of being less invasive makes alternate sampling sites attractive. Lower respiratory tract NAAT has higher sensitivity for viral detection but is generally reserved for critically ill patients in the intensive care setting. RT-PCR testing results are reported qualitatively as "detected" or "not detected"; however, there has been an interest in using the cycle threshold value of the RT-PCR as a surrogate for viral load.

SARS-CoV-2 antigen testing has become widely available and is used as point-of-care testing in clinical settings as well as for in-home testing. Antigen tests are less sensitive compared to NAAT, with highest sensitivity in symptomatic individuals tested within the first 7 days of symptom onset. Antigen tests have excellent specificity and do not typically require confirmatory testing if positive. The IDSA Guidelines on the Diagnosis of COVID-19: Antigen Testing recommends the use of NAAT over antigen testing when missing the diagnosis of SARS-CoV-2 has significant downstream implications, such as in hospitalized patients. In other settings, the quick turnaround time and lower cost make it an attractive testing option.

Serological testing for SARS-CoV-2 measures the host's humoral response to current or past infection or vaccination. While a vaccinated, uninfected individual would only develop antibodies against the S protein of SARS-CoV-2, additional antibodies, such as anti-nucleocapsid antibody, would be generated following infection. Anti-SARS-CoV-2 antibodies are detectable more than 2 weeks after the onset of the illness. Serological testing is not used for diagnosis of acute COVID-19, but can be used in scenarios where there is high clinical suspicion and a NAAT is repeatedly negative. It is also used as additional laboratory data for patients suspected of having postinfectious manifestations such as multisystem inflammatory syndrome in children (MIS-C) and post-acute sequelae of SARS-CoV-2 or post-COVID syndrome. Assays have also been developed that can detect the cell-mediated immune response to SARS-CoV-2.

MANAGEMENT

The limited evidence evaluating currently available therapies, exclusion of infants and children from most clinical trials, and generally favorable outcomes in pediatric patients make it difficult to provide definitive recommendations for the management of children with COVID-19. Factors that should be considered when determining whether and what treatment is most appropriate for a child include their illness trajectory, illness severity, potential risk factors for a poor outcome, patient and caregiver preferences, and the strength and applicability of available evidence. Given the rapidly evolving nature of the COVID-19 pandemic, we refer the reader to treatment guidelines and recommendations published by the IDSA, National Institutes of Health, and American Academy of Pediatrics for the most up-to-date information.

For children in the early stages of COVID-19 infection and those with mild-moderate disease, the mainstay of treatment remains supportive care. Bacterial coinfection in infants and children with COVID-19 appears to be relatively uncommon. If broad-spectrum antibiotics are started, the need for continued use should be re-evaluated daily. Antithrombotic therapy may be appropriate for some patients (see Chapter 88, Disorders of Coagulation and Thrombosis). Despite theoretical concerns, nonsteroidal anti-inflammatory drugs are not associated with worse outcomes in patients with COVID-19 and can be used when indicated.

Most children with asymptomatic or mild-moderate illness are expected to recover; however, a minority of children will progress to severe disease. While specific risk factors for worse outcomes have not been completely elucidated in children, anti-SARS-CoV-2 monoclonal antibodies, ritonavir-boosted nirmatrelvir, molnupiravir, and remdesivir have all been shown to reduce the risk for hospitalization and/or death in high-risk adults in the ambulatory setting. A number of factors, including product availability, the feasibility of medication administration, potential drug-drug interactions, and the regional prevalence of circulating SARS-CoV-2 variants and subvariants, affect the selection of the best treatment option for a specific patient. Since there are no data to support safety and efficacy in pediatric patients, these medications are not routinely recommended for use in outpatients <18 years of age.

Treatment options for patients with severe COVID-19 infection include remdesivir, corticosteroids, and immunomodulatory agents.

Remdesivir is approved for the treatment of COVID-19 in adults and pediatric patients (28 days of age and older and weighing at least 3 kg) with positive results of SARS-CoV-2 viral testing who require hospitalization. Published data suggest that patients who require minimal oxygen supplementation (e.g., nasal canula) are most likely to benefit from receipt of remdesivir. There are limited pediatric data to support the routine administration of remdesivir to children hospitalized with COVID-19, although a recent multicenter guidance document on the use of antivirals for children with COVID-19 suggests its use for children with severe disease. Pediatric-specific studies are ongoing to help determine the role of remdesivir in the management of infants and children with COVID-19 infection. When used, remdesivir should be continued for 5 days or until discharge, whichever comes first. The duration can be extended up to 10 days if the patient does not demonstrate clinical improvement and for children requiring invasive mechanical ventilation and/or extracorporeal membrane oxygenation (ECMO).

The disease process in patients who require oxygen through a high-flow device or require noninvasive or mechanical ventilation is likely related, at least in part, to a hyperinflammatory host response, and these patients have not been found to consistently benefit from remdesivir administration. Dexamethasone has been associated with reduced mortality in patients who require oxygen supplementation or invasive mechanical ventilation and is recommended for hospitalized adults who require supplemental oxygen, noninvasive ventilation, mechanical ventilation, or ECMO. Although there are limited data to support the use of dexamethasone for COVID-19 treatment in pediatric patients, there is extensive experience with the use of corticosteroids in children. Dexamethasone is recommended for pediatric patients who require high-flow oxygen, noninvasive ventilation, mechanical ventilation, or ECMO and should be considered for any patient with a new or increase from their baseline oxygen requirement. If dexamethasone is not available, an equivalent dose of another corticosteroid may be used. The addition of other immunomodulators (e.g., anti-interleukin-6 receptor monoclonal antibodies, Janus kinase inhibitors) may be appropriate for children with rapidly escalating oxygen requirements and systemic inflammation or with critical illness requiring mechanical ventilation and/or ECMO. Given the extremely limited data to support their use and potential for significant immunosuppression, it is recommended that these agents be administered under expert guidance and, preferably, as part of a clinical trial. Medications not recommended for the treatment of COVID-19 infection include hydroxychloroquine, azithromycin, ivermectin, and lopinavir/ritonavir.

ADMISSION AND DISCHARGE CRITERIA

As described above, to date, most children with COVID-19 infection have not required inpatient hospitalization. Children with dehydration or poor feeding may require admission. Children with severe COVID-19 (i.e., new or increased from baseline oxygen requirement) and those with respiratory distress should be admitted to the hospital. Patients with severe or critical COVID-19 may require intensive care. Patients with underlying comorbidities may require admission due to the risk of serious infection or because of chronic disease-related complications potentially triggered by COVID-19 infection. Patients are generally safe for discharge to home when able to maintain adequate hydration and once any hypoxia and respiratory distress have resolved. The American Academy of Pediatrics recommends that infants with positive SARS-CoV-2 testing and without signs of COVID-19 can be discharged per usual practice with close outpatient follow-up for the first 14 days of life.

CONSULTATION

Given the rapid pace at which our understanding of COVID-19 infection and putative therapeutics are evolving, consultation with infectious diseases should be considered for patients requiring hospitalization. Consultation with subspecialists with experience in the management of immunosuppressive medications (e.g., rheumatology) is recommended if the receipt of secondary immunomodulatory therapy is being considered. Hematology consultation may be necessary for patients who require therapeutic anticoagulation.

PREVENTION

Like other respiratory viruses, SARS-CoV-2 is primarily transmitted through respiratory droplets from an infected person that land on the mucous membranes of a susceptible host. Transmission through suspended smaller droplets or aerosols can occur in poorly ventilated spaces. Close and prolonged duration of contact is associated with a higher risk of transmission. The use of a well-fitting face mask has been one of the nonpharmaceutical interventions applied to reduce the transmission of COVID-19. Other nonpharmaceutical interventions include physical distancing, adherence to hand hygiene, environmental cleaning, and observing isolation if symptomatic. COVID-19 acquisition in healthcare settings, either by patients or healthcare personnel, has been lower than acquisition from community settings and can be attributed to use of appropriate personal protective equipment, air changes that allow for adequate ventilation in the healthcare setting, and stringent screening protocols.

The risk of infectiousness is highest during the presymptomatic phase (i.e., 2 days prior to onset of symptoms) through the initial days of symptoms. With improved symptoms, the risk of infectiousness rapidly declines. For immune competent hosts, viable virus has not been recovered through cultures beyond 10 days after the onset of illness. For immunocompromised hosts or individuals with severe or critical illness, the duration of infectiousness can be longer. Guidance on the duration of isolation for different patient populations has been recommended based on the evidence gathered. Although the role of children in the spread of COVID-19 was unclear at the beginning of the pandemic, we now know they can transmit infection similar to adults.

In addition to nonpharmaceutical interventions, vaccination remains an important public health strategy to protect against serious disease and reduce stress on the healthcare system. As of July 2024, two categories of COVID-19 vaccines are currently approved or authorized under an Emergency Use Authorization by the U.S. Food and Drug Administration—mRNA, protein subunit. The protein subunit vaccine (Novavax) is authorized for use as a two-dose series in children 12 years of age and older while two different mRNA vaccines (Pfizer-BioNTech and Moderna) are available for children 6 months of age and older. There is no preferential recommendation for the use of one COVID-19 vaccine over another when more than one recommended age-appropriate vaccine is available. The reader is encouraged to consult the Advisory Committee on Immunization Practices COVID-19 Recommendations and the CDC Interim Clinical Considerations for the Use of COVID-19 Vaccines Currently Approved or Authorized in the United States for the latest COVID-19 vaccine guidance.

SUGGESTED READINGS

Advisory Committee on Immunization Practices. COVID-19 ACIP Vaccine Recommendations. Available at https://www.cdc.gov/vaccines/hcp/acip-recs/vacc-specific/covid-19.html. Accessed 29 September 2022.

American Academy of Pediatrics. Critical Updates on COVID-19. Available at https://www.aap.org/en/pages/2019-novel-coronavirus-covid-19-infections/. Accessed 29 September 2022.

Bhimraj A, Shumaker A, Lavergne V, et al. IDSA Guidelines on the Treatment and Management of Patients with COVID-19. Available at https://www.idsociety.org/practice-guideline/covid-19-guideline-treatment-and-management/#. Accessed 20 July 2022.

Beigel JH, Tomashek KM, Dodd LE, et al. Remdesivir for the Treatment of Covid-19 - Final Report. *N Engl J Med*. Nov 5 2020;383(19):1813-1826. doi:10.1056/NEJMoa2007764

Block JP, Boehmer TK, Forrest CB, et al. Cardiac complications after SARS-CoV-2 infection and mRNA COVID-19 vaccination - PCORnet, United States, January 2021-January 2022. *MMWR Morb Mortal Wkly Rep*. Apr 8 2022;71(14):517-523. doi:10.15585/mmwr.mm7114e1.

Centers for Disease Control and Prevention. Ending Isolation and Precautions for People with COVID-19: Interim Guidance. Available at: https://www.cdc.gov/coronavirus/2019-ncov/hcp/infection-control-recommendations.html.

Cevik M, Kuppalli K, Kindrachuk J, Peiris M. Virology, transmission, and pathogenesis of SARS-CoV-2. *BMJ*. 2020;371:m3862.

Chiotos K, Hayes M, Kimberlin DW, et al. Multicenter interim guidance on use of antivirals for children with coronavirus disease 2019/severe acute respiratory syndrome Coronavirus 2. *J Pediatric Infect Dis Soc*. Feb 13 2021;10(1):34-48. doi:10.1093/jpids/piaa115

COVID-19 Treatment Guidelines Panel. Coronavirus Disease 2019 (COVID-19) Treatment Guidelines. Available at https://www.covid19treatmentguidelines.nih.gov/. Accessed 20 July 2022.

Dulek DE, Fuhlbrigge RC, Tribble AC, et al. Multidisciplinary guidance regarding the use of immunomodulatory therapies for acute coronavirus disease 2019 in pediatric patients. *J Pediatric Infect Dis Soc*. Dec 31 2020;9(6):716-737. doi:10.1093/jpids/piaa098

Goldman DL, Aldrich ML, Hagmann SHF, et al. Compassionate use of remdesivir in children with severe COVID-19. *Pediatrics*. May 1 2021;147(5):e2020047803.

Gottlieb RL, Vaca CE, Paredes R, et al. Early remdesivir to prevent progression to severe Covid-19 in outpatients. *N Engl J Med*. Jan 27 2022;386(4):305-315. doi:10.1056/NEJMoa2116846

Group RC, Horby P, Lim WS, et al. Dexamethasone in hospitalized patients with Covid-19. *N Engl J Med*. Feb 25 2021;384(8):693-704. doi:10.1056/NEJMoa2021436

Gruell H, Vanshylla K, Weber T, Barnes CO, Kreer C, Klein F. Antibody-mediated neutralization of SARS-CoV-2. *Immunity* 2022;55:925-944.

Hammond J, Leister-Tebbe H, Gardner A, et al. Oral nirmatrelvir for high-risk, nonhospitalized adults with COVID-19. *N Engl J Med*. Apr 14 2022;386(15):1397-1408. doi:10.1056/NEJMoa2118542

Hanson KE, Caliendo AM, Arias CA, et al. Infectious Diseases Society of America Guidelines on the Diagnosis of COVID-19: Molecular Diagnostic Testing. Infectious Diseases Society of America. Available at https://www.idsociety.org/practice-guideline/covid-19-guideline-diagnostics/. Accessed 28 September 2022.

Henderson LA, Canna SW, Friedman KG, et al. American College of Rheumatology Clinical Guidance for Multisystem Inflammatory Syndrome in Children Associated With SARS-CoV-2 and Hyperinflammation in Pediatric COVID-19: Version 3. *Arthritis Rheumatol*. Apr 2022;74(4):e1-e20. doi:10.1002/art.42062

Jimenez-García R, Nogueira J, Retuerta-Oliva A, et al. Pneumonia in hospitalized children during SARS-CoV-2 pandemic. Is it all COVID-19? Comparison between COVID and non-COVID pneumonia. *Pediatr Infect Dis J*. 2021;40:e111-e113.

Lu X, Zhang L, Du H, et al. SARS-CoV-2 Infection in children. *N Engl J Med*. Apr 23 2020;382(17):1663-1665. doi:10.1056/NEJMc2005073

Parcha V, Booker KS, Kalra R, et al. A retrospective cohort study of 12,306 pediatric COVID-19 patients in the United States. *Sci Rep*. May 13 2021;11(1):10231. doi:10.1038/s41598-021-89553-1.

Wiersinga WJ, Rhodes A, Cheng AC, Peacock SJ, Prescott HC. Pathophysiology, transmission, diagnosis, and treatment of coronavirus disease 2019 (COVID-19): a review. *JAMA*. 2020;324:782-793.

Wolf J, Abzug MJ, Anosike BI, et al. Updated guidance on use and prioritization of monoclonal antibody therapy for treatment of COVID-19 in adolescents. *J Pediatric Infect Dis Soc*. May 30 2022;11(5):177-185. doi:10.1093/jpids/piab124.

World Health Organization. Therapeutics and COVID-19: living guideline. Available at https://app.magicapp.org/#/guideline/nBkO1E. Accessed 28 September 2022.

Zachariah P, Johnson CL, Halabi KC, et al. Epidemiology, clinical features, and disease severity in patients with coronavirus disease 2019 (COVID-19) in a children's hospital in New York City, New York. *JAMA Pediatr*. Oct 1 2020;174(10):e202430. doi:10.1001/jamapediatrics.2020.2430.

CHAPTER 107

Multisystem Inflammatory Syndrome in Children (MIS-C)

Beth D. Gamulka, MDCM, FRCPC and
Rae S. M. Yeung, MD, PhD, FRCPC

BACKGROUND

During the first few months of the SARS-CoV-2 pandemic in 2020, pediatric specialists in SARS-CoV-2 epicenters in the United Kingdom, Italy, and New York City identified a severe systemic inflammatory syndrome associated with features similar to Kawasaki disease and toxic shock syndrome. The initial alert from the United Kingdom in April 2020 described a novel Paediatric Inflammatory Multisystem Syndrome Temporally Associated with COVID-19 (PIMS-TS) at a time when the country was experiencing a high incidence of acute SARS-CoV-2 infection. Several weeks later the World Health Organization (WHO) coined the term Multisystem Inflammatory Syndrome in Children and Adolescents temporally associated with COVID-19 (MIS) and the Centers for Disease Control (CDC) adapted the same term, defining the pediatric syndrome as MIS-C to distinguish it from a similar yet distinct syndrome in adults (MIS-A). Aside from differences in nomenclature, many expert bodies have distinct definitions. For instance, the Royal College of Pediatrics and Child Health in the United Kingdom, the WHO, the CDC, and the Canadian Paediatric Society all have slight variations in their case definitions, making comparative research of an emerging syndrome challenging.

EPIDEMIOLOGY

Irrespective of the definition used, MIS-C is a rare but serious postinfectious complication of SARS-CoV-2 in children and can occur after symptomatic or asymptomatic SARS-CoV-2 infection. Given that many acute cases of infection have been underreported, the true incidence of MIS-C in children is difficult to estimate and varies by ethnicity, race, age, geographic area, and potentially SARS-CoV-2 subvariant wave. The estimation of MIS-C incidence during the first wave of the pandemic was also affected by initial delays in the identification, surveillance, and reporting of cases. Epidemiological estimates are also dependent on the case definition used since some definitions rely on evidence of a temporal association with a recent SARS-CoV-2 infection and others do not. The peak incidence of cases of MIS-C in a geographic area occurs 2 to 6 weeks (median 4 weeks) after each wave's infection peak in that region.

The overall incidence of MIS-C in one study using the CDC definition for MIS-C was 5.1 per 1 000 000 person-months. The overall incidence of MIS-C in Black and Hispanic/Latino populations was 9-fold higher than in White populations, corresponding to the burden of illness in communities of color during the initial waves of the pandemic. Similarly, the overall incidence in Asian or Pacific Islander populations was 3-fold higher than in White populations. Of note, affected populations have changed in accord with the ethnicities affected by MIS-C in the community. The median age of affected children is 8 years, with higher incidence noted in both the ≤5 years and the 6 to 10-year age category. As the pandemic has progressed and all population groups have been affected more equally by SARS-CoV-2, there is less of a racial disparity among patients with MIS-C.

PATHOPHYSIOLOGY

The hallmark of MIS-C is the presence of fever and hyperinflammation occurring between 2 and 12 weeks after acute infection with SARS-CoV-2. The degree of inflammation may differ from that seen with acute SARS-CoV-2 infection and from pre-pandemic cohorts of patients with Kawasaki disease. As part of the hyperinflammatory immune state, cytokine storm is a notable feature of MIS-C. End-organ involvement in MIS-C varies slightly from classic Kawasaki disease and may reflect different parts of the hyperinflammatory disease spectrum. Research focusing on genetic susceptibility to the development of hyperinflammation after SARS-CoV-2 infection is ongoing.

CLINICAL PRESENTATION

Patients with MIS-C all have unremitting fever as well as the involvement of at least two organ systems (**Table 107-1**). Most present 2 to 6 weeks from an initial acute SARS-CoV-2 infection (range 2-12 weeks) but asymptomatic infection, household infections, or presentation in a region with a high burden of acute infection may be sufficient to suspect an epidemiologic link to SARS-CoV-2.

There are several phenotypes observed in patients with MIS-C, with the most recognizable being Kawasaki-like disease, shock, and isolated fever with hyperinflammation. While some children present with Kawasaki disease-like features (meeting the criteria for complete or incomplete Kawasaki disease), others present with suspected septic shock, significant neurologic signs and symptoms, evidence of macrophage activation system on laboratory investigations, or with a clinical picture of peritonitis. Some children have one feature of Kawasaki disease and one other organ system involved. MIS-C, when untreated, can progress to involve more organ systems, therefore any child with suspicion of MIS-C should be appropriately screened, thoroughly assessed, and have a clear follow-up plan if not admitted to hospital for observation or treatment.

DIAGNOSTIC EVALUATION

Patients presenting with shock or cardiac dysfunction during periods during or within 12 weeks of local acute SARS-CoV-2 infection peaks should have expanded investigations for MIS-C along with investigations usually undertaken for critically ill children.

For children seeking care with fever who are not critically ill, the diagnostic approach is often stepwise. During the pandemic, many centers adopted a two-tiered approach to screening patients with unremitting fever who presented to care without clinical concern for shock or cardiorespiratory compromise. Access to some of the investigations suggested in the diagnostic evaluation of children suspected of having MIS-C is influenced by cost and local laboratory resources and may not be available in all settings.

SCREENING INVESTIGATIONS

For children with fever without focus and no clinical concern for shock or cardiorespiratory compromise, who also have at least two clinical features suggestive of MIS-C (see Table 107-1), several initial investigations are useful as a way of screening for hyperinflammation, and biochemical abnormalities that have been associated with MIS-C (**Table 107-2**). While screening tests may be more inclusive in some institutions, at a minimum, a CBC and differential, C-reactive protein (CRP), erythrocyte sedimentation rate (ESR), sodium, albumin, blood culture, urine analysis and urine culture, and nasopharyngeal SARS-CoV-2 PCR should be collected. Expanded investigations are performed on any patient with an elevated CRP or ESR, and at least one of the following: significant neutrophilia, lymphopenia, hypoalbuminemia, hyponatremia, or thrombocytopenia.

TABLE 107-1 Clinical Presentation

- **Fever**
- **Evidence of hyperinflammation on lab investigations**
- **Evidence of or suspected past SARS-CoV-2 exposure**
- **AND at least two of:**
  - Nonvesicular rash
  - Bilateral nonpurulent conjunctivitis
  - Oral mucosal changes (red or cracked lips, strawberry tongue, oropharyngeal erythema)
  - Erythema or edema of hands or feet
  - Cervical lymphadenopathy ≥ 1.5 cm
  - Gastrointestinal symptoms (abdominal pain, vomiting, diarrhea)
  - Neurologic symptoms (headache, seizures, altered mental status, encephalopathy, papilledema, meningismus, focal neurologic deficits)
  - Cardiac involvement (signs of shock or heart failure)

TABLE 107-2 Two-tiered Approach to Investigation of Children With Fever Without Shock and Features of MIS-C

Screening Investigations	Expanded Investigations
CBC/differential	AST/ALT
CRP and or ESR	Troponin I
Urine analysis and urine culture	Creatinine
Blood culture	Electrolytes
Sodium	Ferritin
Albumin	Triglycerides
Nasopharyngeal PCR swab for SARS-CoV-2	NT-proBNP
	INR/PTT
	LDH
	SARS-CoV-2 serology
	Von Willebrand factor
	IL-1β and IL-6
	D-Dimer
	Echocardiogram
	EKG

EXPANDED INVESTIGATIONS

Children with MIS-C all have evidence of hyperinflammation and fever. Expanded investigations are used to show evidence of end-organ involvement, macrophage activation syndrome, elevated cytokines and to confirm past exposure to acute SARS-CoV-2 if not yet known (see Table 107-2).

SEROLOGIC TESTING

While evidence of past infection using either viral PCR or SARS-CoV-2 serology along with a strong epidemiological link to SARS-CoV-2 infection (such as positive household contacts within the previous 12 weeks) has been used in most case definitions, it is unclear how future interpretation of serologic testing will change as the target population is vaccinated and more individuals recover from acute infection. Timely serologic testing varies across regions such that its use in clinical decision-making and diagnosis may be limited. The ability of serologic tests to distinguish between wild-type infection and immunity from vaccination may also vary among commercially available tests. Since remote SARS-CoV-2 infections may confer evidence of immunity on serologic testing, past case definitions relying on antibody positivity to the virus may need revision. Alternatively, serologic testing will need to be refined to successfully distinguish recent from remote infection to remain clinically useful in attributing symptoms of MIS-C to a recent SARS-CoV-2 infection.

DIFFERENTIAL DIAGNOSIS

Depending on the organ systems involved, children may present with serious bacterial infections, non-SARS-CoV-2 viral myocarditis, or new hematologic disorders. The presence of a recent SARS-CoV-2 infection, whether documented or suspected, does not preclude the possibility of other diagnoses, even during periods of high acute SARS-CoV-2 burden within a particular community. It is imperative that healthcare providers maintain a broad differential diagnosis during the initial assessment to reduce the likelihood of anchoring bias and premature closure.

It is important to maintain a high index of suspicion for serious bacterial infection and other diagnoses, including but not limited to severe acute SARS-CoV-2 infection, sepsis/septic shock (especially from toxin-producing bacteria), perforated appendicitis/peritonitis, pyelonephritis, bacterial pneumonia, osteomyelitis, intraabdominal abscess, retropharyngeal abscess, cervical adenitis, and meningitis in ill children presenting with fever and hyperinflammation depending on the organ systems involved. For children presenting with signs of macrophage activation syndrome (MAS), including pancytopenia, consideration must be given to other conditions associated with MAS, such as systemic juvenile inflammatory arthritis (sJIA) as well as to primary or secondary bone marrow disorders such as hemophagocytic lymphohistiocytosis, aplastic anemia, profound viral suppression, and hematologic malignancies.

MANAGEMENT

Empiric antibiotic therapy is recommended if the index of suspicion for serious bacterial infection is high or infection has not been excluded.

The American College of Rheumatology Guidelines for the treatment of MIS-C were based on limited evidence reports with consensus built through a modified Delphi process. These guidelines aim to reduce the inflammatory response, provide cardiorespiratory support, reduce the risk of coronary artery aneurysm, and provide antiplatelet therapy +/– thromboprophylaxis. The mainstays of treatment for MIS-C are rooted in proven therapies for Kawasaki disease, including intravenous immunoglobulin (IVIG), low-dose acetylsalicylic acid (ASA), and systemic glucocorticoids at moderate doses. Compared to traditional protocols for Kawasaki disease; however, protocols for MIS-C treatment only use a single dose of IVIG. Steroid dosing is weaned slowly over 2 to 3 weeks. Severe cases of MIS-C unresponsive to initial therapy and all patients with cardiac dysfunction or shock should receive high-dose pulse intravenous glucocorticoids. Refractory cases of MIS-C can be treated with biologic immunomodulators such as anakinra, an interleukin-1 receptor antagonist or infliximab, a TNF-alpha inhibitor. Infliximab should not be used in patients with MIS-C and features of MAS.

Patients presenting in shock or with evidence of reduced cardiac function require monitoring in an intensive care setting, inotropic support, and in some cases, respiratory support.

Stratification for thrombosis risk and the need for anticoagulation should be done in conjunction with pediatric intensivists and pediatric hematologists. In some patients, there is a role for prophylactic anticoagulation to reduce the risk of thrombosis. This includes patients who develop coronary artery aneurysms.

Patients receiving IVIG are at risk for acute anaphylactic reactions during the infusion, fluid overload because of the volume infused, and post-IVIG hemolysis. Patients receiving systemic glucocorticoids together with ASA should receive gastric protection and may need transient treatment for hypertension or hyperglycemia.

CONSULTATION

Children with MIS-C benefit from collaborative care between pediatric hospitalists and pediatric cardiologists and rheumatologists. For children requiring inotropic support and those with severely reduced cardiac function, consultation with pediatric intensivists is recommended. Prophylactic anticoagulation protocols may vary from institution to institution and consultation with pediatric hematologists or thrombosis specialists should be considered for patients with risk factors for thrombosis, such as the presence of a central venous catheter, markedly reduced cardiac function, significantly elevated D-dimers and immobility. In some centers, pediatric infectious disease specialists are involved with the care of all patients admitted with postinfectious complications, including MIS-C.

ADMISSION CRITERIA

Any child presenting in shock or with features consistent with complete or incomplete Kawasaki disease should be admitted and treated for MIS-C. Patients with fever, evidence of hyperinflammation, and any evidence of cardiac dysfunction, ECG abnormalities, or elevation of cardiac biomarkers require admission and treatment for MIS-C. Patients with fever and hyperinflammation and normal cardiac assessment should be admitted and treated if at least two abnormalities are found on expanded investigations or if there is laboratory evidence of MAS. Admission is also recommended for patients with fever and hyperinflammation with neurologic, cardiac, or respiratory compromise.

Many children with fever for 3 to 5 days without focus who have normal screening and/or expanded investigations should have reliable timely clinical reassessment in 24 to 48 hours. Some children with fever and isolated hyperinflammation who are not admitted for treatment would benefit from repeat expanded investigations at that time if fever persists.

TABLE 107-3 Discharge Criteria

- Resolution of fever
- Improving inflammatory markers
- Discharge treatment plan established
- Discharge medication teaching completed
- Discharge counseling completed (return of fever, effect of IVIG on vaccination scheduling, COVID vaccination recommendations for patients with MIS-C)
- Follow-up referrals and investigations arranged

DISCHARGE CRITERIA

Children with MIS-C are usually ready for discharge when they show clinical improvement, including resolution of fever, improving markers of inflammation and cardiac function, and are tolerating oral medications. Discharge teaching should include patient education regarding medications, including instructions about steroid weaning, delayed administration of live vaccination post-IVIG for 11 months, as well as recommendations regarding future SARS-CoV-2 vaccination (**Table 107-3**). While SARS-CoV-2 vaccination is recommended for children after diagnosis of MIS-C, the timing of dose administration should occur after the return to normal cardiac function and for at least 90 days after diagnosis.

OUTCOME AND FOLLOW-UP

Children who recover from MIS-C benefit from standardized follow-up including repeat cardiac echocardiogram and bloodwork to confirm the resolution of inflammation and derangements in renal, hematologic, and hepatic function. In most pediatric centers, children are re-evaluated by a pediatric cardiologist or by a multidisciplinary team comprised of pediatric cardiologists, rheumatologists, and in some cases thrombosis specialists.

While signs and symptoms of MIS-C are generally responsive to steroid initiation, fever and other clinical features of MIS-C can recur as steroid dosing is weaned. Follow-up is usually arranged to ensure clinical assessment occurs prior to steroid discontinuation. Subsequent long-term evaluation of children with MIS-C varies but may be useful as the medical community learns more about the long-term outcomes of MIS-C. Research into the long-term cardiac outcomes of children with MIS-C is currently underway.

SUGGESTED READINGS

Berard RA, Tam H, Scuccimarri R, et al. Paediatric inflammatory multisystem syndrome temporally associated with COVID-19. *Canadian Paediatric Society*. May 2021. https://cps.ca/documents/position/pims.

Consiglio CR, Cotugno N, Sardh F, et al. The immunology of multisystem inflammatory syndrome in children with COVID-19. *Cell*. 2020;183(4):968-981.

Dufort EM, Koumans EH, Chow EJ, et al. Multisystem inflammatory syndrome in children in New York State. *N Engl J Med.* 2020;383(4):347-358.

Feldstein LR, Rose EB, Horwitz SM, et al. Multisystem inflammatory syndrome in U.S. children and adolescents. *N Engl J Med.* 2020;383(4):334-346.

Henderson LA, Canna SW, Friedman KG, et al. American College of Rheumatology clinical guidance for pediatric patients with multisystem inflammatory syndrome in children (MIS-C) associated with SARS-CoV-2 and hyperinflammation in COVID-19. Version 3. *Arthritis Rheumatol.* 2022;74(4):e1-20.

Payne AB, Gilani Z, Godfred-Cato S, et al. Incidence of multisystem inflammatory syndrome in children among US persons infected with SARS-CoV-2. *JAMA Netw Open.* 2021;4(6):e2116420.

Riphagen S, Gomez X, Gonzalez-Martinez C, Wilkinson N, Theocharis P. Hyperinflammatory shock in children during COVID-19 pandemic. *Lancet.* 2020;395:1607-1608.

Verdoni L, Mazza A, Gervasoni A, et al. An outbreak of severe Kawasaki-like disease at the Italian epicentre of the SARS-CoV-2 epidemic: an observational cohort study. *Lancet.* 2020;395:1771-1778.

SECTION K
Nephrology

CHAPTER 108 Acute Kidney Injury

Laura O'Neill, MD, MS, MEd and Yi Shi, MD, PharmD

BACKGROUND

Acute kidney injury (AKI) is a sudden decline in renal function that results in an increase in metabolic waste products in the blood and dysregulation of extracellular electrolytes and volumes. AKI is usually marked by elevations in serum creatinine and may be associated with increased, normal, or decreased urine output. The terms polyuria, oliguria, and anuria sometimes are used to characterize the type of failure. The term AKI has replaced acute renal failure (ARF) in the literature to better characterize the spectrum of impairment in renal function before complete failure.

Two classification systems are currently used to standardize assessment of AKI for clinical and research purposes. Both use creatinine and urine output criteria to stratify acute renal injury from stage 1 to stage 3 based on severity (**Table 108-1**).

The pediatric risk, injury, failure, loss, end-stage renal disease (pRIFLE) criteria were developed by modifying existing adult RIFLE criteria. The Kidney Disease: Improving Global Outcomes (KDIGO) criteria were developed by unifying previously existing definitions and are applicable to both children and adults. The use of the KDIGO criteria has been found to detect more patients with AKI compared to the pRIFLE criteria.

Traditionally, elevated serum creatinine is used to make the diagnosis of AKI. Reliance solely on an increase in creatinine is problematic for several reasons. Serum creatinine is an isolated measurement and does not accurately reflect ongoing changes in renal function. Creatinine takes time to accumulate so an early normal value may not reflect ongoing and potentially severe injury. In children, the baseline creatinine level for a patient often is not known and a rise from the baseline may still fall within the "normal" range for lab values. Additionally, once dialysis is started, creatinine is no longer helpful in assessing renal function.

Given the limitations of creatinine measurement in accurately diagnosing early renal injury and the improved outcomes when renal injury is treated early, much research is now focused on biomarkers. The most promising biomarkers of renal injury in urine and blood are neutrophil gelatinase-associated lipocalin (NGAL), cystatin C, kidney injury molecule-1 (KIM-1), liver-type fatty acid binding protein (L-FABP), and interleukin-18 (IL-18). Compared to creatinine, NGAL has been shown to be a potentially superior early marker of kidney injury and correlates with severity and length of ICU stay. Unlike creatinine, cystatin C is not affected by weight or muscle mass. It has increasingly shown usefulness in diagnosing AKI, and it has been used more commonly in an outpatient setting for evaluation of renal function. Continued work in this area may provide clinically useful assays that result in earlier diagnosis and treatment of renal injury.

TABLE 108-1 Criteria for Diagnosis of Acute Kidney Injury

	KDIGO	pRIFLE
Stage 1	Cr increase 1.5-1.9 times baseline Absolute Cr increase ≥0.3 mg/dL UOP <0.5 mL/kg/hr for 6-12 hours	eGFR decrease by 25%* UOP <0.5 mL/kg/hr for 8 hours
Stage 2	Cr increase 2.0-2.9 times baseline UOP <0.5 ml/kg/hr for 12-24 hours	eGFR decrease by 50% UOP <0.5 mL/kg/hr for 16 hours
Stage 3	Cr increase ≥3 times baseline or Cr ≥4 mg/dL or eGFR <35 mL/min/1.73m^2 UOP <0.3 mL/kg/hr for ≥24 hours or anuria for 12 hours Received renal replacement therapy	eGFR decrease by 75% or eGFR <35 mL/min/1.73 m^2 UOP <0.3 mL/kg/hr for 24 hours or anuria for 12 hours

*If no baseline then use 100 mL/min per 1.73m^2 for baseline value.

Cr, serum creatinine; eGFR, estimated glomerular filtration rate; KDIGO, Kidney disease: Improving Global Outcomes; pRIFLE, pediatric risk, injury, failure, loss, end-stage renal disease.

Sources: Data from Khwaja A. KDIGO clinical practice guidelines for acute kidney injury. *Nephron Clin Pract*. 2012;120(4):c179-184; Akcan-Arikan A, Zappitelli M, Loftis LL, et al. Modified RIFLE criteria in critically ill children with acute kidney injury. *Kidney Int*. 2007;71:1028-1235.

PATHOPHYSIOLOGY

Impairment in renal function can occur for a variety of reasons and is often multifactorial in hospitalized children. Kidney damage can result from impairment in blood flow, direct damage to the filtration system itself, or by increased pressure on the filtration system by impaired output. The classic names for these categories are prerenal, intrinsic, and postrenal (**Table 108-2**).

Prerenal causes all result in decreased renal perfusion leading to decreased glomerular perfusion and filtration with subsequent elevation of blood urea nitrogen and creatinine. Intrinsic causes are a larger and more varied group as any cause of direct damage to the filtration function of the kidney is included. These include vascular, tubular, interstitial, and glomerular processes. Acute tubular necrosis, nephrotoxins, hemolytic uremic syndrome (HUS), and primary renal diseases are included as they result in direct damage to the glomeruli or renal tubule. Iatrogenic administration of nephrotoxic medications is the fastest-growing cause of renal injury in hospitalized children. Postrenal causes, also called obstructive, include examples such as posterior urethral valves and bladder catheter obstruction. It is also important to recognize that one type of injury can progress to another. Untreated hypoperfusion, for instance, may eventually result in intrinsic damage in the form of acute tubular necrosis. A patient with dehydration who is given ibuprofen may have components of both prerenal and intrinsic renal injury.

CLINICAL PRESENTATION

HISTORY

The clinical presentation of AKI varies depending on the underlying cause. The history and physical examination provide clues to guide the workup. On history, urine changes should be assessed—color, volume, and frequency. Intake and output history will give information to assess volume status, and other elements of the history may provide clues to possible diagnosis. For example, history of bloody diarrhea will raise concern for HUS. A thorough medication history is necessary and should include prescriptions, over-the-counter medications, supplements, and all other possible nephrotoxic substances. Systemic complaints such as fever, joint pain, and rash could indicate a postinfectious or rheumatologic condition. Edema raises suspicion for intrinsic renal disease.

TABLE 108-2 Differential for Causes of Acute Kidney Injury

Prerenal

Decreased intravascular volume
- Dehydration
- Hemorrhage
- Burns
- Diuretics

Decreased cardiac output
- Heart failure
- Arrhythmias

Vascular changes (peripheral vasodilation and/or renal vasoconstriction)
- Sepsis
- Anaphylaxis
- Antihypertensives
- Nonsteroidal anti-inflammatories

Intrinsic

Tubular injury/Acute tubular necrosis
- Hypotension
- Prolonged ischemia

Sepsis

Nephrotoxins
- Drugs: aminoglycosides, acyclovir, radiocontrast medium, cyclosporine, amphotericin B, cisplatin
- Toxins: ethylene glycol, heavy metals
- Pigments: hemolysis, rhabdomyolysis

Interstitial disease
- Acute interstitial nephritis
- Infection
- Malignant infiltrations

Vascular disease
- Hemolytic uremic syndrome
- Vasculitides (e.g., granulomatosis with polyangiitis, antiglomerular basement membrane (GBM) disease)
- Thrombosis

Glomerulonephritis
- Postinfectious glomerulonephritis
- Systemic lupus erythematosus
- Membranoproliferative glomerulonephritis
- IgA nephropathy
- IgA vasculitis

Postrenal (Obstructive)

Bladder calculi

Posterior urethral valves

Bladder catheter obstruction

Neurogenic bladder

PHYSICAL EXAMINATION

Physical examination should focus on assessment of volume status. Careful attention should be given to heart rate, blood pressure (high or low), weight (change from "dry weight"), mucus membranes, and skin turgor. Assessment for areas of edema should be performed—lower extremity for ambulatory children, sacral for nonambulatory and acutely ill children, and facial/periorbital in all. Growth parameter abnormalities can indicate the presentation of a chronic disease rather than an isolated acute process. The skin and musculoskeletal examination may provide clues to rheumatologic conditions. The abdominal examination may reveal enlarged bladder or palpable kidneys, both concerning signs for obstructive conditions.

DIFFERENTIAL DIAGNOSIS

The differential for AKI is broad, and classically divided into prerenal, intrinsic, and postrenal categories (Table 108-2).

DIAGNOSTIC EVALUATION

Initial diagnosis of AKI is generally made by elevations in serum creatinine—either isolated elevation or increases over time. Serum creatinine is an indirect reflection of glomerular filtration rate (GFR). Equations are available to estimate GFR, though an exact value is not always necessary to diagnose AKI and will not provide information about etiology. In pediatrics, the chronic kidney disease in Children Under 25 (CKiD U25) equation was recently developed based on data from the Chronic Kidney Disease in Children study and has greater internal validity compared to previous published equations for measuring eGFR. However, the bedside Schwartz equation is still commonly used to quickly estimate eGFR.

In addition to measurement of serum creatinine, serum electrolytes, urinalysis, and renal ultrasound may be useful in determining the cause of the AKI. Electrolyte assessment should include sodium, potassium, bicarbonate, blood urea nitrogen (BUN), calcium, and phosphorous. These electrolytes can be significantly abnormal and may prompt preemptive treatment in often asymptomatic patients. Elevated BUN/creatinine ratio over 20 can be a clue that the kidney injury is prerenal. Urinalysis with microscopy looking for cells and casts can provide indications of an intrinsic renal process. Renal ultrasound should be performed to evaluate structural changes in the kidneys and urinary tract. Swollen echogenic kidneys suggest an acute process, whereas small kidneys suggest chronic renal disease. A Doppler study can evaluate the renal vasculature.

Initial history, examination, and imaging should identify postrenal causes of AKI. It is often more difficult to differentiate prerenal from intrinsic renal injury. Plasma and urine sodium and creatinine measurements should be obtained to help differentiate the two (**Table 108-3**).

Fractional excretion of sodium (FENa) is the most often used measurement to differentiate prerenal disease from intrinsic due to acute tubular necrosis (ATN). Due to impaired sodium reabsorption, neonates have different expected values. Additionally, FENa calculations are not helpful if patients have received diuretics as these medications affect sodium reabsorption.

If the initial workup suggests an intrinsic cause for renal injury, then further studies may be indicated. Often complete blood count and complement studies will be done. Additional studies such as streptococcal serologies may be done based on history, examination, and initial laboratory findings. If renal function does not improve, then a renal biopsy may be necessary to find a specific diagnosis.

TABLE 108-3 Laboratory Characteristics of Prerenal Versus Intrinsic Acute Kidney Injury

	Prerenal	Intrinsic
Urine specific gravity	>1.020	<1.010
Plasma BUN/Cr ratio	>20	<20
FENa*	<1%	>2%
	<2% (neonate)	>2.5% (neonate)
Urine Na (mEq/L)	<20	>40
Urine osmolality (mOsm)	>500	<350
	>400 (neonate)	<400 (neonate)

*Fractional excretion of sodium $(FE_{Na}) = (U_{Na}/P_{Na}) \times (P_{creat}/U_{creat}) \times 100$.

BUN, blood urea nitrogen; Cr, creatinine; FENa, fractional excretion of sodium.

TABLE 108-4	Principles of Management of Acute Kidney Injury (FFENA)
Find	Find and treat underlying cause
Fluids	Achieve and maintain euvolemia
Electrolytes	Monitor for and treat electrolyte abnormalities Na, K, HCO_3, Ca, Phos
Nutrition	Adequate caloric and protein intake to minimize catabolism
Avoid	Avoid further harm by careful attention to medications.

MANAGEMENT

There are five principles to the management of AKI: Find, Fluids, Electrolytes, Nutrition, and Avoid (**Table 108-4**).

FIND

Finding and treating the underlying cause of kidney injury, if possible, is the first principle of management. The approach explained in the diagnostic evaluation section should help narrow the differential.

FLUIDS

The goal of fluid management in patients with AKI is achieving and maintaining euvolemia. Assessment of fluid status is essential so frequent physical examinations (heart rate, blood pressure, mucus membranes), strict intake/output measurements, and weights are necessary. If a patient is found to be hypovolemic then initial treatment is to bolus with normal saline until intravascular volume is restored. For patients with prerenal disease, adequate hydration may be sufficient to restore renal function. Studies have not supported the routine use of dopamine in the management of AKI and dopamine use is associated with negative respiratory, fluid, electrolyte, and hemodynamic changes. For patients with signs of hypervolemia, such as hypertension, pulmonary edema, or heart failure, fluid restriction is indicated. Fluid removal with diuretics is only indicated if the fluid overload is clinically concerning. Pulmonary edema resulting in hypoxemia and the need for increased respiratory support would necessitate fluid removal while isolated peripheral edema may not. Diuretics may pull off excess fluid in the short term but will not significantly change outcomes in patients with AKI. Excessive use of diuretics can result in additional renal injury in the setting of hypovolemia or intravascular depletion. In a symptomatic hypervolemic patient, a trial of furosemide may be performed with close monitoring of response. If responsive, additional doses may be given until euvolemia is achieved. If no increase in urine output is achieved within 2 hours, diuretics should be discontinued immediately. Persistent hypertension unresponsive to diuretics may not be due to hypervolemia alone. Other therapies may be indicated and should be chosen with the consultation of a nephrologist.

Once euvolemia is achieved, total fluid volume should be calculated and administered to maintain that fluid balance. Insensible losses should be replaced with 300 to 500 mL/m^2 per day of fluids. Urine and gastrointestinal losses should be monitored and replaced. It is important to account for nutrition and medications when calculating total fluid volume. Total fluid volume should be adjusted frequently to maintain euvolemia.

ELECTROLYTES

Electrolyte abnormalities are common in patients with AKI and are usually asymptomatic. Most frequent issues arise with potassium, sodium, bicarbonate, phosphorous, and calcium. As a result, electrolytes should be monitored frequently, and a few precautions should be taken. In general, patients with AKI should not receive potassium or phosphorous and should be restricted to 2 to 3 mEq/kg per day of sodium. Patients with polyuric kidney injury are at increased risk for electrolyte losses and may need even closer monitoring and frequent replacement of electrolytes.

Hyperkalemia is an acute life-threatening complication of renal injury as it can result in cardiac arrhythmia. Assessment of a patient with hyperkalemia should include an electrocardiogram. Treatment for hyperkalemia depends on the level and rate of rise. Urgent treatment focuses on stabilizing the cardiac membrane with calcium and decreasing the serum potassium level quickly, albeit transiently, by shifting potassium into cells to decrease risk of cardiac arrhythmia. Additional treatment is needed to remove and decrease total body potassium. Urgent treatment includes intravenous calcium, intravenous glucose and insulin, intravenous sodium bicarbonate, and may also include inhaled a beta-agonist such as albuterol. Sodium polystyrene sulfonate should be given orally or rectally to remove potassium from the body by ion exchange. Potassium intake should be avoided in all forms—nutrition and medication. If these measures are unsuccessful in critical hyperkalemia, then dialysis is indicated.

Hyponatremia can result from fluid retention, hypotonic fluid administration, and excessive sodium losses. Once euvolemia has been achieved, volume restriction is required. Hypertonic saline administration is generally limited to patients with severe hyponatremia and seizure. Severe hyponatremia may require dialysis.

In AKI, renal excretion of acid and reabsorption of bicarbonate is impaired, resulting in an anion gap metabolic acidosis. This acidosis may also be worsened by the underlying cause of renal injury such as shock or heart failure. Treatment of these underlying causes may help limit and eventually improve the degree of acidosis. Compensatory respiratory alkalosis may help correct the acidosis and prevent exacerbation of additional electrolyte abnormalities. Sodium bicarbonate treatment is controversial but may be indicated in severe situations such as worsening hyperkalemia.

Elevated phosphorous is mostly due to impaired renal excretion but may be coupled with overproduction such as in rhabdomyolysis. Elevated phosphorous can contribute to hypocalcemia. Management must include assessment and treatment of both electrolytes. Phosphorous intake is restricted and oral phosphate binders such as calcium carbonate or calcium acetate can be administered.

NUTRITION

Nutrition is a key part of management of AKI as it is associated with a catabolic state—specifically protein catabolism and abnormal amino acid synthesis. In addition to overall increased caloric needs, patients also need increased protein intake. Goal caloric intake should be approximately 150% of maintenance needs. Protein intake needs to be balanced with the goal of preventing catabolism yet limited to avoid uremia. Usual range is 1 to 1.5 g/kg/day but may be higher than 3 g/kg/day in a critically ill patient or potentially higher in patients on renal replacement therapy. Nutrition should be initiated either enterally or parenterally as early as possible with careful attention to total fluid volume. Dialysis may be indicated if the patient is unable to tolerate adequate nutrition due to volume restriction.

AVOIDANCE OF HARM

Avoidance of further harm is the last principle in management of AKI. Careful attention to all medications is needed. Potentially nephrotoxic medications should be discontinued. Dosages for all medications should be frequently reviewed and adjusted for current renal function. As function changes or dialysis is initiated, dosages will need to be readjusted to avoid toxicity but also ensure therapeutic dosing.

Dialysis, also known as acute renal replacement therapy, is indicated for fluid overload, electrolyte abnormalities, uremia, and hypertension not responsive to the above measures. There are many modalities for renal replacement therapy; all of which require the expertise of a nephrologist and fall outside the scope of this chapter.

ADMISSION CRITERIA

- Unknown etiology or rapidly progressing kidney injury
- Oliguria (e.g., < 0.5 mL/kg/hr urine output) or anuria
- Increase in serum creatinine >/= 0.3 mg/dL in past 48 hours or increase by 1.5 above the normal or baseline value
- Severe or potentially dangerous fluid (e.g., hypo- or hypervolemia) or electrolyte (e.g., hyperkalemia, hyponatremia) abnormalities
- Need for urgent renal biopsy

DISCHARGE CRITERIA

- Electrolyte abnormalities corrected and/or well-controlled on medical therapy
- Renal function normal or clearly improving
- Suspected intrinsic causes known and appropriate therapies initiated
- Urine output normal or patient is stable on appropriate renal replacement therapy

CONSULTATION

Nephrology consultation should be obtained for any child with suspected intrinsic kidney injury. Early consultation for suspected intrinsic problems is indicated as long-term prognosis improves dramatically with rapid identification and treatment of the primary disorder. Nephrologist and/or intensivist consultation is indicated for management of patients with AKI associated with diuretic refractory hypertension or electrolyte abnormalities that are progressive or severe as they may indicate a need for renal replacement therapy. Pharmacist consultation may be helpful in adjusting medication dosing and nutritionists may help achieve the right nutritional balance in acutely ill patients.

SPECIAL CONSIDERATIONS

PREVENTION

As treatment of AKI is supportive and new evidence shows that even mild injury poses an increased risk of chronic renal dysfunction, special attention to prevention of renal injury is crucial. All hospitalized patients should be considered at risk so administration of potentially nephrotoxic medications should be limited. Routine use of nonsteroidal anti-inflammatories should be discouraged, especially in potentially hypovolemic patients. Protocol orders should be reviewed for indications, appropriate dose and frequency information, and exclusion criteria. Patients with multiple risk factors (e.g., sepsis, hypotension, nephrotoxic drug use) should have close monitoring of intake and output, weight, and overall fluid balance to assist in early recognition of renal dysfunction. Drug levels are available for many nephrotoxic medications such as vancomycin and tacrolimus and should be closely monitored.

KEY POINTS

- Treatment of acute kidney injury is supportive, and prevention is crucial.
- Etiology of acute kidney injury in hospitalized patients is usually multifactorial.
- Key principle of management of all cases of kidney injury is avoiding further harm.
- Early involvement of pediatric nephrologist in suspected intrinsic renal injury can result in improved outcomes with early initiation of treatment of the primary disease.

SUGGESTED READINGS

Akcan-Arikan A, Zappitelli M, Loftis LL, et al. Modified RIFLE criteria in critically ill children with acute kidney injury. *Kidney Int.* 2007;71:1028-1235.

Andreoli SP. Acute kidney injury in children. *Pediatr Nephrol.* 2009;24(2):253-263.

Andreoli SP. Management of acute kidney injury in children: a guide for pediatricians. *Paediatr Drugs.* 2008;10(6):379-390.

Askenazi D. Evaluation and management of critically ill children with acute kidney injury. *Curr Opin Pediatr.* 2011;23(2):201-207.

Basu RK, Devarajan P, Wong H, Wheeler DS. An update and review of acute kidney injury in pediatrics. *Pediatr Crit Care Med.* 2011;12(3):339-347.

Bellomo R, Kellum JA, Ronco C. Acute kidney injury. *Lancet.* 2012;380(9843):756-766.

Bennett M, Dent CL, Ma Q, et al. Urine NGAL predicts severity of acute kidney injury after cardiac surgery: a prospective study. *Clin J Am Soc Nephrol.* 2008;3(3):665-673.

Devarajan P. Biomarkers for the early detection of acute kidney injury. *Curr Opin Pediatr.* 2011;23(2):194-200.

Goldstein SL, Devarajan P. Acute kidney injury in childhood: should we be worried about progression to CKD? *Pediatr Nephrol.* 2011;26(4):509-522.

Hsu CW, Symons JM. Acute kidney injury: can we improve prognosis? *Pediatr Nephrol.* 2010;25(12):2401-2412.

Khwaja A. KDIGO clinical practice guidelines for acute kidney injury. *Nephron Clin Pract.* 2012;120(4):c179-184.

Koeze J, Keus F, Dieperink W, van der Horst ICC, Zijlstra JG, van Meurs M. Incidence, timing and outcome of AKI in critically ill patients varies with the definition used and the addition of urine output criteria. *BMC Nephrol.* 2017;18(1):70.

Krawczeski CD, Goldstein SL, Woo JG, et al. Temporal relationship and predictive value of urinary acute kidney injury biomarkers after pediatric cardiopulmonary bypass. *J Am Coll Cardiol.* 2011;58(22):2301-2309.

Mak RH. Acute kidney injury in children: the dawn of a new era. *Pediatr Nephrol.* 2008;23(12):2147-2149.

Nakhjavan-Shahraki B, Yousefifard M, Ataei N, et al. Accuracy of cystatin C in prediction of acute kidney injury in children; serum or urine levels: which one works better? A systematic review and meta-analysis. *BMC Nephrol.* 2017;18(1):120.

Patzer L. Nephrotoxicity as a cause of AKI in children. *Pediatr Nephrol.* 2008;23(12):2159-2173.

Schwartz GM, Brion LP, Spitzer A. The use of plasma creatinine concentration for estimating glomerular filtration rate in infants, children, and adolescents. *Pediatr Clin North Am.* 1987;34:571-590.

Slater MB, Anand V, Uleryk EM, Parshuram CS. A systematic review of RIFLE criteria in children, and its application and association with measures of mortality and morbidity. *Kidney Int.* 2012;81(8):791-798.

Sutherland SM, Kwiatkowski DM. Acute kidney injury in children. *Adv Chronic Kidney Dis.* 2017;24(6):380-387.

Twombley K, Baum M, Gattineni K. Accidental and iatrogenic causes of acute kidney injury. *Curr Opin Pediatr.* 2011;23(2):208-214.

CHAPTER 109 Chronic Renal Failure

Celina Brunson, MD and Elizabeth W. Pingree, MD

BACKGROUND

Chronic renal failure (CRF) is an irreversible reduction in renal function, or glomerular filtration rate (GFR), with accompanying derangements in biochemical homeostasis. The term *chronic kidney disease* (CKD) incorporates CRF and chronic renal insufficiency, which are considered part of the spectrum of CKD. End-stage renal disease (ESRD) is defined as CRF so severe that a form of renal replacement therapy (such as peritoneal dialysis) is required. The National Kidney Foundation define CKD as being present in any patient who meets one of two criteria: (1) there is evidence of kidney damage for 3 months or more, as defined by structural abnormalities of the kidney with or without decreased GFR, as evidenced by abnormalities in the composition of blood or urine, abnormalities in imaging tests, or abnormalities on kidney biopsy; (2) the GFR is less than 60 mL/minute per 1.73 m^2 for 3 months or more, with or without any structural changes. GFR is not adequately determined using serum creatinine alone; it should be

TABLE 109-1 Estimating Creatinine Clearance

kL/P_{Cr} = Estimated creatinine clearance
k = Age-dependent constant:
k = 0.33 for low-birth-weight infants during first year of life
k = 0.45 for term infants during first year of life
k = 0.55 for children and adolescent girls
k = 0.7 for adolescent boys
L = Height (cm)
P_{Cr} = Serum creatinine

Source: From Schwartz GM, Brion LP, Spitzer A: The use of plasma creatinine concentration for estimating glomerular filtration rate in infants, children, and adolescents. *Pediatr Clin North Am.* 1987;34:571-590.

estimated using a prediction equation such as the Schwartz equation (**Table 109-1**).

The incidence of CRF in children is low, and the incidence of ESRD is 11 children per 1 million of the age-related population. Unlike adults with CRF, in which the renal disease is secondary to diseases such as diabetes and hypertension, the overwhelming majority of children with CRF have primary renal disease, usually of a congenital origin including congenital anomalies of the kidney and urinary tract (CAKUT). This means that the care of children with CRF can deviate dramatically from that of adults.

There have been remarkable improvements in the treatment of children with CRF and ESRD, with a subsequent increase in the prevalence of CRF in the pediatric population. Children with CAKUT disorders such as renal dysplasia or obstructive uropathy are more likely to have polyuria and salt wasting, complicating their care as compared to adults with CRF. Additionally, they have the requirement for growth and development. Normalization of these parameters is the key to successful treatment. These factors, along with the psychosocial issues specific to childhood, make the treatment of children with CRF challenging, but with meticulous care and attention to detail, these children can reach adulthood with minimal associated morbidity.

PATHOPHYSIOLOGY

There is a wide spectrum of causes of childhood CRF. Regardless of the underlying cause, the basic pathophysiology is the same. Damage to the nephron can be direct or as the result of adaptive hyperfiltration in which other areas try to compensate for the loss of nephrons from the initial injury. The increased filtration leads to increased glomerular pressure which over time causes inflammation and damage. Both pathways lead to glomerular scarring, tubular atrophy, and interstitial fibrosis, with an ultimate reduction in normal renal function. The consequences of decreased function are usually not evident until renal function is less than 30% to 50%. These consequences can include acidosis, hyper- or (more rarely) hypokalemia, anemia, deranged calcium-phosphorus balance (hyperphosphatemia and hypocalcemia), abnormal bone metabolism, hypertension, short stature, hyponatremia, and disrupted water homeostasis.

CLINICAL PRESENTATION

The clinical presentation of children with CRF varies tremendously due to both the wide range of causes and the different stages of disease at which a child may present. Stage 1 and Stage 2 patients are generally asymptomatic. Polyuria is often an early sign of many congenital anomalies and diseases that impair urine concentrating ability before GFR decreases. The most universal finding in children presenting with undiagnosed CRF is growth failure. Fatigue, anorexia, malaise, and worsening school performance are also common findings in patients with Stage 3 and above. Renal osteodystrophy can be seen, regardless of the cause of CRF. Signs and symptoms may include bone pain, refusal to walk, valgus deformities of the lower extremities, frontal bossing, and a rachitic rosary. Children with congenital uropathies or nephropathies are likely to present with the symptoms of polyuria and salt wasting: dehydration, emesis, acidosis, hyperkalemia, and either hyper- or hyponatremia, depending on the salt and water balance of the individual patient. This subset of patients rarely has hypertension. Children with juvenile nephronophthisis (chronic, progressive tubulointerstitial nephritis) can also present with signs and symptoms of polyuria, but they often have accompanying hypertension and ocular abnormalities. Children with reflux nephropathy may present initially with signs and symptoms of pyelonephritis and develop hypertension as the nephropathy progresses. Edema and hypertension are typically found in children with CRF due to a glomerulopathy. Polycystic renal disease and renal tumors may present with abdominal pain, hypertension, and an abdominal mass.

CRF should be suspected in children with marked nonhemolytic anemia, hyperparathyroidism, small kidneys on renal ultrasonography, or physical findings consistent with rickets.

DIFFERENTIAL DIAGNOSIS

There is a wide spectrum of causes of childhood CRF (**Table 109-2**). In developed countries, approximately two-thirds of children with CRF have congenital conditions such as posterior urethral valves or renal dysplasia.

TABLE 109-2 Causes of Chronic Renal Failure in Children

Congenital urinary tract malformations
Renal dysplasia
Renal hypoplasia
Obstructive uropathies
Posterior urethral valves
Ureteropelvic junction obstruction
Megaureter
Glomerulopathies
Focal segmental glomerulosclerosis
Rapidly progressive glomerulonephritis
Membranoproliferative glomerulonephritis
Membranous nephropathy
IgA nephropathy
Hereditary diseases
Polycystic kidney disease
Alport syndrome
Cystinosis
Oxalosis
Nephronophthisis
Systemic diseases
Systemic lupus erythematosus
Goodpasture disease
Wegener granulomatosis
Polyarteritis nodosa
Vascular diseases
Hypertension
Diabetes mellitus
Miscellaneous causes
Denys-Drash syndrome
Wilms tumor
Neuroblastoma

DIAGNOSTIC EVALUATION

Once a patient has had impaired kidney function with associated metabolic derangements for 3 months or more, he or she is considered to have CRF. A patient with suspected CRF presenting to the hospital for the first time may not meet the time criterion but should be evaluated as if CRF were present as the early identification of CRF can improve a patient's long-term outcome.

The evaluation of a patient with suspected CRF should be directed toward determining the cause of kidney disease, its severity, comorbid conditions such as hypertension and dyslipidemia, complications such as renal osteodystrophy, and the risk for further loss of renal function. The initial evaluation to determine the cause of kidney disease should be done with the guidance of a pediatric nephrologist. Important historical information includes previous kidney disease, hypertension, diabetes, abnormal prenatal ultrasonography, fetal drug exposures, or oligohydramnios. Practitioners should have elevated concern for patients with polyuria, dysuria, or gross hematuria and systemic complaints such as anorexia, fatigue, malaise, fever, or arthralgias. Deteriorating school performance and a family history of renal disease are also important indicators. Pertinent findings of the physical examination may include short stature, elevated blood pressure, edema, rashes, joint effusions or arthritis, ascites, or evidence of rickets.

Initial laboratory studies should include a complete urinalysis, serum electrolytes (including calcium and phosphorus), albumin, complete blood count, parathyroid hormone, and renal ultrasonography. Children with proteinuria on the initial urinalysis should have a 24-hour urine collection for protein and creatinine or a spot urine protein-creatinine ratio (normal is <0.18) on a first-morning void if 24-hour urine collection is not feasible. Daily weights and accurate monitoring of urine output are also important.

MANAGEMENT

The focus of management in CRF is fourfold: monitoring and correcting biochemical disturbances, managing and preventing comorbidities, avoiding further damage and renal replacement therapy (e.g., hemodialysis) for ESRD. Additionally, for some patients with acquired causes of CRF, treatment of the primary disease is required.

BIOCHEMICAL DISTURBANCES

Biochemical disturbances associated with CRF include hyperkalemia, metabolic acidosis, hyperphosphatemia, hypocalcemia, and sodium derangement. Hyperkalemia results from increased catabolism associated with uremia, coupled with diminished excretion due to both decreased GFR and tubular dysfunction. Acidosis can worsen hyperkalemia by inducing the extracellular shift of intracellular potassium. Hyperkalemia is a potentially life-threatening condition owing to its effect on cardiac conductivity. At levels greater than 7 mEq/L, electrocardiographic abnormalities can be seen, including potentially life-threatening arrhythmias. Acute hyperkalemia can be treated by administering sodium bicarbonate, Kayexalate cation-exchange resins, loop diuretics, beta-agonists, or dialysis. For acute hyperkalemia with electrocardiographic changes, cardiac stabilization with calcium infusion or intravenous insulin and glucose is also required. However, in CRF, the goal is to prevent the need for acute interventions, and central to preventing hyperkalemia is dietary control of potassium intake. In patients with moderate CRF, chronic loop diuretics can be used to increase potassium excretion.

Metabolic acidosis is another common abnormality seen in CRF, resulting from the inadequate excretion of ammonium by the kidney. Chronic acidosis results in impaired growth through both inadequate caloric intake (due to the accompanying anorexia and nausea) and abnormal bone formation (due to hydrogen ion deposition in bone, which acts as a buffer to maintain normal body pH). Acidosis also induces hyperpnea, which is a compensatory mechanism to remove excess acid via increased ventilation. Acidosis is treated by the administration of alkali, usually in the form of sodium bicarbonate or sodium citrate, to maintain serum bicarbonate levels above 22 mEq/L.

Hyperphosphatemia results from diminished phosphate excretion. As serum phosphate levels increase, serum calcium levels drop; this stimulates parathyroid hormone excretion, leading to secondary hyperparathyroidism. Hyperphosphatemia also has a direct stimulatory effect on the parathyroid gland. Chronic hyperphosphatemia can be associated with an elevated serum calcium-phosphorus product, leading to metastatic calcifications and increased atherosclerosis. There are two treatments for hyperphosphatemia, both of which are usually necessary: (1) dietary restriction of phosphorus intake, usually 800 to 1200 mg/day, depending on the age of the child; and (2) administration of phosphate binders with meals to prevent the intestinal absorption of ingested phosphorus. These phosphate binders include calcium salts, such as calcium carbonate and calcium acetate, as well as synthetic polymers, such as sevelamer hydrochloride and lanthanum carbonate. Aluminum salts were once widely used as phosphate binders but are no longer used because of their association with bone deposition and dementia due to aluminum toxicity.

Hypocalcemia occurs as a physiologic response to hyperphosphatemia and as a result of the diminished levels of activated vitamin D that occur with reduced renal function. Activation of vitamin D to calcitriol (1,25-dihydroxyvitamin D) normally takes place in the proximal nephron, but with CRF, inadequate production of this active hormone leads to diminished intestinal calcium absorption, diminished release of calcium from bone, and diminished renal tubular calcium reabsorption, all of which contribute to hypocalcemia. Although extreme hypocalcemia may require treatment with calcium supplements, the majority of patients respond to the administration of activated vitamin D metabolites such as calcitriol or dihydrotachysterol.

Sodium derangement can result from both sodium retention and sodium wasting. Glomerular diseases are often associated with impaired sodium excretion, and patients can develop edema and hypertension if they are not placed on a sodium-restricted diet. CRF caused by CAKUT, in contrast, is frequently associated with polyuria and renal salt wasting due to impaired urinary concentrating ability. These patients may present with normal serum sodium levels because of simultaneous intravascular volume depletion, or they may have hyponatremia. In both scenarios, there is often decreased circulating plasma volume with subsequent renal hypoperfusion. These children frequently need sodium and fluid supplementation.

COMORBIDITIES

Anemia frequently occurs in patients with CRF once the GFR falls to less than 30 mL/minute per 1.73 m^2, mainly due to inadequate erythropoietin production by the kidneys. Although chronic blood transfusions were once a mainstay of treatment, the development of recombinant human erythropoietin means that, for most CRF patients, transfusions can be avoided. Additionally, iron supplementation is required; current recommendations are for a target hemoglobin between 11 and 12 g/dL.

Renal osteodystrophy results from secondary hyperparathyroidism, which is a result of hypocalcemia and hyperphosphatemia. Additionally, skeletal resistance to parathyroid hormone is present in those with uremia, further contributing to the development of renal osteodystrophy. Treatment is aggressive control of hyperphosphatemia by dietary restriction and the administration of oral phosphate binders and activated vitamin D metabolites. In rare cases, some patients with severe hyperparathyroidism who are nonresponsive to these measures may require a parathyroidectomy. Oversuppression of the parathyroid hormone is associated with aplastic bone disease, so the goal is not complete normalization of intact parathyroid hormone levels but rather a target level between 150 and 300 pg/mL.

Growth failure is frequently associated with CRF once the GFR has fallen to less than 30 mL/minute per 1.73 m^2, although it may occur earlier. Although acidosis and renal osteodystrophy contribute to the poor growth seen in children with CRF, the major cause of growth failure in those older than 2 years is growth hormone resistance due to decreased tissue expression of insulin-like growth factor (IGF) and increased IGF-binding proteins. The use of recombinant human growth hormone is effective in maintaining normal growth. In contrast, in infants with CRF, poor growth is likely due to inadequate nutrition. These babies benefit from aggressive nutritional management; in those with congenital renal disease, high-volume gavage feedings with sodium supplements may normalize growth.

Cardiac dysfunction is frequently seen in individuals with CRF. Hypertension is frequently associated with CRF and can result in left ventricular hypertrophy. Severe hypertension can result in congestive heart failure. Patients with oliguria may also develop congestive heart failure due to hypervolemia. With marked uremia, pericarditis and pericardial effusions can occur. Appropriate blood pressure control and close cardiovascular monitoring are key to decreasing morbidity and mortality for CRF patients.

Uremic patients may have increased bleeding due to platelet dysfunction. This can be an especially important issue for menstruating girls or patients requiring surgery. Patients with CRF and uremic bleeding have normal prothrombin times and partial thromboplastin times but an elevated platelet function assay or skin bleeding time. Desmopressin, administered intravenously, subcutaneously, or intranasally, can be used acutely to treat uremic bleeding, although it is ineffective for the control of prolonged bleeding due to tachyphylaxis. Cryoprecipitate can be used in patients with prolonged bleeding or in those who are unresponsive to desmopressin. Antifibrinolytic agents such as ε-aminocaproic acid are also effective in treating acute hemorrhage. Patients who require prolonged therapy can be treated with conjugated estrogens, although these compounds are not effective in the acute setting.

RENAL REPLACEMENT THERAPY

Some method of renal replacement, either dialysis or transplantation, is needed once the GFR has decreased to less than 15 mL/minute per 1.73 m^2. Some patients may require intervention earlier owing to uncontrolled metabolic complications. There are also relative indications for initiating dialysis including symptoms such as fatigue, decreased school performance, depression, anorexia, etc. which can all be secondary to uremia. Although hemodialysis is the primary modality used in adult patients with ESRD, peritoneal dialysis plays a more predominant role in children. Continuous cycling peritoneal dialysis, in which the child is dialyzed overnight through a peritoneal catheter using an automated cycler, has several advantages. It can be done at home by the child's caregiver, with minimal interference with the patient's schooling. Peritoneal dialysis also allows increased sodium and fluid intake, which makes compliance with dietary restrictions easier. Peritoneal dialysis is frequently complicated by peritonitis and catheter site infection, however. Recurrent infections can result in scarring of the peritoneum, making it unusable for dialysis.

Hemodialysis is an option for patients who do not have an intact peritoneum, those whose caregivers are not capable of performing peritoneal dialysis, or those for whom the presence of a peritoneal dialysis catheter is unacceptable. Chronic hemodialysis is usually performed three times a week in an outpatient setting, although some patients require more frequent dialysis. Dialysis access is a problem in children on hemodialysis, especially in very small children in whom placement of a dialysis fistula or shunt is impractical. The intermittent nature of hemodialysis also requires more severe dietary and fluid restrictions, especially for children with oliguria.

Renal transplantation is the renal replacement modality of choice for children with ESRD. Children receiving kidney transplants from living, related donors have excellent long-term survival rates, and the average half-life of a renal allograft is now 13 years or more. Suspected allograft rejection is one of the most common causes of hospitalization in transplant patients following the initial surgery. Infectious complications, especially viral, are other common reasons for the hospitalization of children with kidney transplants. The immunosuppressive agents used in transplant patients may have significant interactions with a variety of drugs, and great care must be used in prescribing additional medications in this patient population.

SPECIAL DOSING OF MEDICATIONS

Because the kidneys are responsible for the elimination of many drugs, once renal function drops to less than 50%, many medications require adjustments in dosage, dosing interval, or both. All patients with CRF should have their renal function calculated and their medication lists reviewed often to determine whether alterations in drug dosing are indicated.

ADMISSION AND DISCHARGE CRITERIA

ADMISSION CRITERIA

- Initial diagnosis and stabilization
- Life-threatening electrolyte disturbance
- Congestive heart failure
- Severe anemia requiring blood transfusion
- Malignant hypertension
- Infection associated with hemodynamic compromise
- Dialysis access complication
- Suspected allograft rejection

DISCHARGE CRITERIA

Children hospitalized for suspected CRF can be discharged once the diagnosis has been confirmed, the cause established, and any electrolyte or volume derangements normalized. Other children with CRF who require hospitalization can be discharged once the condition leading to their hospitalization (e.g., severe hyperkalemia, peritonitis, suspected rejection) has been corrected.

CONSULTATION

Any child admitted for suspected CRF requires a pediatric nephrology consultation. Similarly, any dialysis or renal transplant patient who requires hospitalization needs to be followed by a pediatric nephrologist. Other patients with CRF who are hospitalized for reasons unrelated to their kidney disease do not necessarily require nephrology consultation, although it may be helpful, especially when adjustments in medications are necessary to account for abnormal renal function.

SPECIAL CONSIDERATIONS

PREVENTION

CRF is usually a progressive disease with an orderly sequence of deterioration. Interventions that can slow the progression of renal failure include meticulous blood pressure control, proper dietary management, control of proteinuria, reduction of glomerular hyperfiltration, and control of dyslipidemia. In patients with CRF, the goal of antihypertensive therapy should be maintenance of blood pressure below the 90th percentile for age and height. Protein restriction is not as clearly indicated in children as it is in adults, because children have the additional burden of growth; in general, however, infants and toddlers should have a protein intake of 2 g/kg per day, and older children should have 1 to 1.5 g/kg per day. Angiotensin-converting enzyme inhibitors and angiotensin II receptor inhibitors are both effective in reducing intraglomerular pressure, even without associated systemic hypertension, and their use can slow the progression of CRF. Both drugs can be useful in controlling proteinuria as well. Providers should avoid further renal injury by appropriately dosing and/or avoiding certain medications such as nonsteroidal anti-inflammatories and antibiotics.

KEY POINTS

- Congenital anomalies of the kidney and urinary tract are the most common cause of CRF in children and, unlike other types of CRF, can be associated with polyuria and salt wasting.
- The evaluation of a patient with suspected CRF should be directed toward determining the cause and severity of kidney disease, identifying comorbid conditions and complications, and assessing the risk for further loss of renal function.
- Comorbidities of CRF include anemia, osteodystrophy, growth failure, cardiac dysfunction, and abnormal bleeding.
- Estimates of GFR can be made using the patient's height and plasma creatinine concentration.
- Many medications require dosage adjustments when administered to children with diminished GFR.
- Slowing the progression of CKD is an important goal of therapy, and effective interventions include control of blood pressure, proteinuria, dyslipidemia, and reduction of glomerular hyperfiltration.

SUGGESTED READINGS

Chan JCM, Williams DM, Roth KS. Kidney failure in infants and children. *Pediatr Rev*. 2002;23:47-60.

Fadrowski JJ, Rees L. The demographics of dialysis in children. In: Warady, BA, Alexander SA, Schaefer F, ed. *Pediatric Dialysis*. 3rd ed. Cham, Switzerland: Springer; 2021:35-46.

Harambat J, Van Stralen KJ, Kim JJ, et al. Epidemiology of chronic kidney disease in children. *Pediatr Nephrol*. 2012;27(3):363-373.

Harmon WE. Treatment of children with chronic renal failure. *Kidney Int*. 1995;47:951-961.

Hogg RJ, Furth S, Lemley KV, et al. National Kidney Foundation's Kidney Disease Outcomes Quality Initiative: clinical practice guidelines for chronic kidney disease in children and adolescents: evaluation, classification and stratification. *Pediatrics*. 2003;111:1416-1421.

Salman S. Uremic bleeding: pathophysiology, diagnosis, and management. *Hosp Physician*. 2001;76:45-50.

Schwartz GM, Brion LP, Spitzer A. The use of plasma creatinine concentration for estimating glomerular filtration rate in infants, children, and adolescents. *Pediatr Clin North Am*. 1987;34:571-590.

United States Renal Data System. 2021 USRDS Annual Data Report: Epidemiology of kidney disease in the United States. National Institutes of Health, National Institute of Diabetes and Digestive and Kidney Diseases, Bethesda, MD, 2021.

Wuhl E, Schaefer F. Therapeutic strategies to slow chronic kidney disease progression. *Pediatr Nephrol*. 2008;23(5):705-716.

Zahr RS, Greenbaum LA, Schaefer F. The decision to initiate dialysis in children and adolescents. In: Warady, BA, Alexander SA, Schaefer F, ed. *Pediatric Dialysis*. 3rd rd. Cham, Switzerland: Springer; 2021:115-130.

CHAPTER 110 Glomerulonephritis

Bakri J. Alzarka, MD, MS and
Stephanie R. Davis-Rodriguez*, MD, MS

BACKGROUND

Glomerulonephritis (GN) is not a specific disease, but rather an inflammatory state within the renal glomerulus. This inflammation causes glomerular injury and results in impaired glomerular filtration with subsequent abnormal urinary sediment and possibly decreased kidney function. It is often associated with edema and hypertension. Clinically, GN spans a wide spectrum of disease from a benign, self-limited condition to an aggressive systemic disease that can lead to rapid loss of kidney function and end-stage kidney disease (ESKD). This chapter focuses on the four common presentations of GN that are most likely to be found in hospitalized patients: asymptomatic hematuria, acute GN, rapidly progressive GN (RPGN), and chronic GN.

PATHOGENESIS

Major advances toward understanding the mechanism of GN have been made recently. However, the pathogenesis of GN is not completely understood. Autoimmunity and genetic predisposition play a major role. Evidence suggests environmental insults including infections as the trigger for many forms of GN. This immune response is mediated by antibodies, T-cells, and likely complement dysregulation as well.

CLINICAL PRESENTATION

ASYMPTOMATIC HEMATURIA

Asymptomatic hematuria can be either microscopic or gross and is not associated with hypertension, impaired kidney function, edema, or proteinuria. It is important to distinguish hematuria from other sources of discolored urine. Aside from hematuria, changes in urine color can be seen in patients taking certain medications (e.g., rifampin, Senna, and pyridium) or in the presence of heme (e.g., myoglobinuria or hemoglobinuria). Myoglobinuria or hemoglobinuria will present as positive urinary dipstick for blood and can be discriminated by the absence of red blood cells on microscopic examination. Asymptomatic isolated microscopic hematuria is commonly seen in hospitalized patients and is usually transient. It can be the result of many different conditions such as febrile illness, urinary tract infection (UTI), and trauma to the kidney or urinary tract including bladder catheterization. In cases of asymptomatic isolated microscopic hematuria, experts recommend at least two of three urinalyses show microhematuria over 2 to 3 weeks before further evaluation is performed. Outpatient follow-up is appropriate in these patients unless also associated with proteinuria. The combination of hematuria, either microscopic or gross, associated with proteinuria or hypertension is concerning for possible GN, and diagnostic evaluation is therefore indicated.

ACUTE GLOMERULONEPHRITIS

Acute GN is characterized by an abrupt onset of hematuria (gross or microscopic), proteinuria, decrease in glomerular filtration rate (GFR), and water and sodium retention leading to hypertension and edema. Proteinuria is rarely within the nephrotic range (nephrotic range is >40 mg urinary protein/m^2/hr or a urinary protein/creatinine ratio >2.0 mg/mg).

Poststreptococcal glomerulonephritis (PSGN) is the most common form of acute GN in children, typically affecting children aged 4 to 12 years old and rarely seen in children less than 2 years or more than 18 years old. It is caused by specific nephritogenic strains of Group A Streptococcus (GAS) promoting a glomerular immune complex disease. In its classic form, there is a sudden onset of painless gross hematuria (often described as "tea or coke colored") 1 to 3 weeks after GAS pharyngitis and 3 to 6 weeks after GAS skin infection. Hematuria is nearly always present, but only one-third of patients will report gross hematuria. Physical examination often reveals edema and hypertension. The latter is the most common reason for hospitalization and can be severe enough to cause hypertensive encephalopathy and seizures. PSGN is a self-limited disease. Edema and hypertension improve within 7 to 10 days and kidney function returns to baseline within three to four weeks. Proteinuria and hematuria may last for months. There are other forms of postinfectious GN caused by various microorganisms. It is important to note that several etiologies of chronic GN can present as acute GN. The initial course can be very similar, requiring careful evaluation and follow up.

RAPIDLY PROGRESSIVE GLOMERULONEPHRITIS (RPGN)

RPGN is a clinical syndrome characterized by the signs of GN (microscopic or gross hematuria and proteinuria), and loss of kidney function

TABLE 110-1 Clinical Presentation Concerning for Rapidly Progressive Glomerulonephritis

Prodrome of vague systemic symptoms such as fatigue and malaise before the development of glomerulonephritis
Acute onset of hematuria, edema, hypertension, and rapid deterioration in kidney function
Associated systemic symptoms such as upper or lower airway, pulmonary hemorrhage, musculoskeletal, skin, or central nervous system symptoms concurrent with glomerulonephritis

TABLE 110-2 Glomerulonephritis Classification

Primary GN	Secondary GN
Membranoproliferative glomerulonephritis (MPGN)	Poststreptococcal GN (PSGN)
Immunoglobulin A (IgA) nephropathy	IgA vasculitis
Anti-glomerular basement membrane (GBM) disease	Systemic lupus erythematosus nephritis
Idiopathic crescentic GN	ANCA-associated vasculitis

over a relatively short period of time (**Table 110-1**). Systemic complaints are common, including fever, malaise, and anorexia. On kidney biopsy, cellular crescent formation is the pathologic hallmark of RPGN. Unlike PSGN, RPGN can result in ESKD in a significant portion of afflicted children.

RPGN is due to one of three glomerular injury mechanisms: anti-GBM antibody disease, immune complex-mediated disease, or pauci-immune GN. Anti-GBM disease is a small vessel vasculitis related to circulating antibodies affecting glomerular and alveolar basement membranes. In addition to RPGN, anti-GBM disease also presents with pulmonary hemorrhage.

Immune complex-mediated GN consists of a variety of renal diseases characterized by immune complex deposition within the glomeruli, including systemic lupus erythematosus (SLE), membranoproliferative glomerulonephritis (MPGN), IgA vasculitis, and IgA nephropathy. Extrarenal manifestations, serologies, and histologic findings are used to distinguish the etiology. SLE GN presents with systemic signs and symptoms consistent with lupus including arthralgias, joint effusions, fatigue, malaise, leukopenia, anemia, and thrombocytopenia. IgA vasculitis usually manifests with palpable purpura, arthralgias, and abdominal pain in addition to the kidney disease. MPGN and IgA nephropathy manifestations tend to be isolated to the kidney.

Pauci-immune glomerulonephritides have few or no immune complex deposition, are often antineutrophile cytoplasmic antibody (ANCA) positive, and cause necrotizing crescentic GN. ANCA-associated vasculitides include microscopic polyangiitis (MPA) and granulomatosis with polyangiitis (GPA). Both conditions can affect small vessels in any organ; however, they most commonly involve the kidneys and upper and lower respiratory tract. Nonspecific symptoms can include fever, weight loss, myalgias, and arthralgia. Pauci-immune GN also includes eosinophilic granulomatosis with polyangiitis (EGPA), previously called Churg-Strauss. EGPA is a small and medium-size vessel vasculitis affecting multiple organs including the kidneys, lung, heart, gastrointestinal tract, and central nervous system. It presents most commonly with difficult-to-treat asthma, chronic rhinosinusitis, and peripheral neuropathy. A distinguishing feature is eosinophilia.

CHRONIC GLOMERULONEPHRITIS

Chronic GN can present acutely, but more commonly presents as persistent hematuria and proteinuria, with or without hypertension or decrease in kidney function. Chronic GN can manifest as isolated renal disease, as is seen with IgA nephropathy and MPGN, or as part of a systemic disease, such as SLE or IgA vasculitis. Hospitalization for chronic GN is unusual, although children may be hospitalized after kidney biopsy.

DIFFERENTIAL DIAGNOSIS

Hematuria has a broad differential, but the presence of proteinuria in addition to hematuria, particularly in the setting of other findings such as hypertension, edema, and decreased kidney function should prompt the clinician to suspect GN. In the absence of these findings, the initial evaluation of hospitalized patients with hematuria should focus on causes other than GN, including infection, trauma, nephrolithiasis, papillary necrosis, acute interstitial nephritis, and obstruction. Asymptomatic isolated microscopic hematuria in an otherwise healthy individual may be followed closely in the outpatient setting.

DIAGNOSTIC EVALUATION

Glomerulonephritides can be divided into primary GN, a disease isolated to the kidney, and secondary GN as a manifestation of a systemic disease (**Table 110-2**).

All patients with suspected GN should undergo urine microscopic evaluation. The presence of red blood cell (RBC) casts or dysmorphic RBCs suggest a glomerular source of hematuria. The evaluation should also include a complete blood count, a comprehensive electrolyte panel including serum albumin, phosphorus, and magnesium, and C3 and C4 complement levels. Proteinuria should be quantified with a urine protein-to-creatinine ratio. Other tests can be considered based on history and physical examination.

Given the latency period between GAS infection and PSGN manifestation, rapid streptococcal antigen testing and throat culture will often be negative at the time of nephritic symptoms; however, elevated titers of streptococcal antibodies can provide evidence of recent GAS infection. Multiple streptococcal antibodies are available including antistreptolysin (ASO), anti-DNase B, antihyaluronidase (AHase), and antistreptokinase (ASKase). ASO titers are the most commonly used, and the clinician should be aware of their limitations. ASO titers peak 2 to 4 weeks after acute infection and remain elevated for up to 6 months. Therefore, serial ASO titers demonstrating a rise over time are more diagnostic than one isolated measurement that may be too early in the PSGN course or may reflect a more remote GAS infection. Lastly, ASO titers are often negative in patients with skin infections. Obtaining additional GAS antigen titers in combination increases the sensitivity and specificity when compared to a single antigen test.

Serum complement measurement provides helpful information in the classification of GN. It is usually low in PSGN and immune-complex mediated GN. The exception is IgA nephropathy which is usually associated with normal complement levels. Serum complement levels are typically normal in anti-GBM and pauci-immune GN as well (**Table 110-3**).

Isolated asymptomatic microscopic hematuria and PSGN do not usually require a kidney biopsy. In the case of PSGN, a kidney biopsy may be warranted in patients with persistent symptoms or low C3 levels beyond 8 weeks. For other types of suspected GN or if there is evidence of progressive disease including sustained decreased kidney function or hypertension, a kidney biopsy is often necessary for diagnosis. Nephrotic-range proteinuria should also prompt a kidney biopsy.

TABLE 110-3 Complement Levels in Glomerulonephritis

	C3	C4	Other Diagnostic Tests
PSGN	Low	Normal	Streptococcal antigen titers
MPGN	Low	Low or normal	
IgA nephropathy	Normal	Normal	
GBM disease	Normal	Normal	Anti-GBM antibodies
IgA vasculitis	Normal	Normal	
SLE nephritis	Low	Low	ANA, dsDNA
ANCA-associated vasculitis	Normal	Normal	ANCA

Source: Made de novo (new) by the authors.

MANAGEMENT

Management of GN is guided by the underlying cause; however, the initial approach is similar. Initial treatment focuses on stabilization of blood pressure and strict fluid management. Nephrology consultation is warranted for patients with suspected GN associated with refractory hypertension and fluid overload or decrease in kidney function to provide dialysis and perform kidney biopsy if needed. Dialysis is indicated in patients with uncontrollable hyperkalemia, life-threatening fluid overload (pulmonary edema, heart failure, hypertensive encephalopathy) refractory to medical therapy, or rapidly increasing BUN/severe uremia.

Blood pressure control is the most important initial concern in patients with GN. The etiology of hypertension in GN is excess salt and water retention. Therefore, initial management should include restricted fluid and sodium intake and diuresis. Both thiazide and loop diuretics can be used for mild edema and hypertension. If hypertension is not well controlled with diuretic therapy, other antihypertensives can be added such as a calcium channel blocker. Angiotensin-converting enzyme inhibitors (ACEIs) should be used with caution in acute GN due to the risk of further worsening glomerular filtration and hyperkalemia. Children with symptomatic hypertension (i.e., headache, mental status changes including irritability, symptoms of congestive heart failure, or papilledema) should be treated as hypertensive emergencies. Potential parenteral therapies include nicardipine (calcium channel blocker) and labetalol (β-blocker).

RPGN is a medical emergency, and the long-term prognosis improves dramatically with early initiation of treatment. Pulse corticosteroid therapy is the initial treatment of all forms of RPGN. Treatment should not be withheld in a patient with suspected RPGN because of difficulty obtaining a renal biopsy or in patients requiring dialysis. Additional management depends on the type of GN but may include cytotoxic agents such as cyclophosphamide and plasma exchange.

POST-BIOPSY PATIENTS

Care of patients after kidney biopsy focuses on pain control and preventive measures to decrease the risk of postprocedural hemorrhage. Expert consensus recommends strict bed rest while lying on the back for 6 to 12 hours after the procedure along with frequent vital signs for 6 to 8 hours. Gross hematuria is common after biopsy occurring in up to 30% of patients and usually resolves within one or two voids. Microscopic hematuria can persist for several days. Persistent gross hematuria, presence of clots, or severe suprapubic or flank pain should prompt urgent nephrology consultation. Acetaminophen is typically adequate pain control postprocedure. Ibuprofen and other nonsteroidal anti-inflammatory drugs (NSAIDs) should be avoided due to the risk of bleeding and potential nephrotoxicity. Some patients may experience severe pain after kidney biopsy, presumably from subcapsular hematoma. If unaccompanied by tachycardia, these patients may be treated symptomatically with narcotics. Pain unrelieved by narcotics or associated with persistent tachycardia requires Nephrology consultation and further investigation for hemorrhage.

ADMISSION CRITERIA

Most pediatric patients with acute GN require hospitalization. Suggested admission criteria include:

- Moderate to severe edema and/or hypertension
- Moderate to severe acute kidney injury
- Suspected RPGN
- Presentation of GN in patients younger than 2 years or older than 12 years

DISCHARGE CRITERIA

- Stabilization of kidney function
- Adequate blood pressure control
- Completion of therapies that require close monitoring or inpatient level of support (e.g., pulse steroids)
- Establishment of appropriate referrals and follow-up

CONSULTATION

Consultation with pediatric Nephrologists can assist with diagnostic evaluation and management of patients with GN. RPGN should be considered a nephrologic emergency, and rapid consultation with a Nephrologist is essential. Consultation is warranted in patients with acute GN who do not demonstrate resolution over time, those with recurrent disease, or patients with symptoms that are difficult to control. Methylprednisolone or cyclophosphamide for GN should be administered under the guidance of a Nephrologist.

SPECIAL CONSIDERATIONS/PREVENTION

At this time there are no good preventive strategies to avoid the development of GN. Early detection plus intervention is the best option presently available. Excellent blood pressure control and avoidance of further renal injury through careful fluid and electrolyte control, along with nutritional management, will decrease the morbidity associated with GN.

KEY POINTS

- GN spans a wide spectrum of disease from self-limited conditions such as PSGN to aggressive systemic disease.
- There are three common presentations of GN: acute GN, RPGN, and chronic GN.
- All patients with suspected GN need a complete blood count, a comprehensive electrolyte panel, serum C3 and C4 complement levels, and urinalysis with urine microscopy.
- Acute management is directed at controlling blood pressure, achieving fluid and electrolyte balance, and providing adequate nutrition.
- Early Nephrology consultation should be considered in complex cases, especially if there is evidence of progressive deterioration in renal function, recurrence, or symptoms that are difficult to control.

SUGGESTED READINGS

Cameron JS, Vick RM, Ogg CS, Seymour WM, Chantler C, Turner DR. Plasma C3 and C4 concentrations in management of glomerulonephritis. *Br Med J*. 1973;3(5882):668-672.

A clinico-pathologic study of crescentic glomerulonephritis in 50 children. A report of the Southwest Pediatric Nephrology Study Group. *Kidney Int*. 1985;27:450-458.

Couser WG. Pathogenesis and treatment of glomerulonephritis-an update. *J Bras Nephrol*. 2016;38(1):107-122.

Couser WG, Johnson RJ. The etiology of glomerulonephritis: roles of infection and autoimmunity. *Kidney Int*. 2014;86(5):905-914.

Eison TM, Ault BH, Jones DP, Chesney RW, Wyatt RJ. Post-streptococcal acute glomerulonephritis in children: clinical features and pathogenesis. *Pediatr Nephrol*. 2011;26(2):165-180.

Kaartinen K, Safa A, Kotha S, Ratti G, Meri S. Complement dysregulation in glomerulonephritis. *Semin Immunol*. 2019;45:101331.

Kambham N. Postinfectious glomerulonephritis. *Adv Anatom Pathol*. 2012;19:338-347.

Mayer U, Schmitz J, Bräsen JH, Pape L. Crescentic glomerulonephritis in children. *Pediatr Nephrol*. 2020;35(5):829-842.

Meyers KE. Evaluation of hematuria in children. *Urol Clin North Am*. 2004;31:559-573, x.

Rianthavorn P, Chacranon M. Long-term renal outcome in pediatric glomerulonephritis associated with crescent formation. *Clin Exp Nephrol*. 2018;22(3):661-667.

Rodríguez-Iturbe B, Batsford S. Pathogenesis of poststreptococcal glomerulonephritis a century after Clemens von Pirquet. *Kidney Int*. 2007;71(11):1094-1104.

Twilt M, Benseler S, Cabral D. Granulomatosis with polyangiitis in childhood. *Curr Rheum Rep*. 2012;14:107-115.

CHAPTER 111 Hemolytic Uremic Syndrome

Samar A. Hussein, MD, FAAP

BACKGROUND

Hemolytic uremic syndrome (HUS) was first described in 1955. It is one of the most frequent causes of acute renal failure in children and is defined by a triad of microangiopathic hemolytic anemia, thrombocytopenia, and acute kidney injury. The incidence of HUS is 2.7 cases per million people per year in the United States. HUS can occur at any age but most often presents between 2 months and 8 years of age. It has a seasonal peak in the summer and early fall. HUS is divided into two main categories, typical diarrhea-associated (D+ HUS) and atypical non-diarrhea associated HUS (aHUS). The most common form is D+ HUS, which is caused by Shiga toxin-producing bacteria and accounts for 90% of cases. Atypical HUS (aHUS), sometimes called D-HUS, accounts for the remaining cases (**Table 111-1**). Recently, it has become recognized that the two categories of HUS are not mutually exclusive. Some cases of HUS are multifactorial, with as many as 25% of patients with D+ HUS having mutations in complement system gene sequences.

PATHOPHYSIOLOGY

Typical D+ HUS Shiga toxin-producing *Escherichia coli* (0157:H7 and other strains) are found in the gastrointestinal (GI) tract of beef cattle and can be isolated from inadequately cooked ground beef. Shiga toxin can also be produced by *Shigella dysenteriae* and may be present in contaminated water. Other reported vehicles of transmission include deer jerky, salami, unpasteurized milk, unpasteurized apple cider, salmon, and lettuce or radish sprouts. After an exposure to contaminated water or food, the average incubation period is 3 days prior to the development of diarrhea. Shiga toxin targets microvascular endothelial cells. This damaging effect on the vascular endothelium triggers multiple cellular and vascular phenomena leading to thrombus formation (a.k.a. thrombotic microangiopathy). Of note, urinary tract infections caused by Shiga toxin-producing *E. coli* have also been reported prior to the development of HUS.

Atypical HUS In contrast to typical D+ HUS, aHUS is seen in individuals with a genetic predisposition to complement dysregulation. Genetic mutations decrease the activity of complement regulatory proteins, and thus when exposed to an inciting trigger, these individuals may have an uncontrolled complement response leading to endothelial damage and thrombosis. Environmental triggers such as infection, drugs such as immunosuppressants and oral contraceptives, and pregnancy can all trigger aHUS. Infectious diseases account for the trigger in 50% to 80% of patients, and Shiga toxin-induced diarrhea triggers aHUS in 30% of cases.

TABLE 111-1 Causes of Atypical Hemolytic Uremic Syndrome (aHUS)

Drug related
Oral contraceptives
Post-transplant immunosuppressants (cyclosporine, tacrolimus)
Chemotherapy (mitomycin, cisplatin, bleomycin)
Idiopathic
Infections
*Streptococcus pneumoniae**
Human immunodeficiency virus (HIV)
Genetic
Complement regulatory protein mutations (C3, Factor H, B, I, CD46)
Methylmalonic acidemia†

*The most common cause of aHUS.

†Usually a neonatal presentation of aHUS.

Five percent of aHUS cases in children are caused by *Streptococcus pneumoniae* strains. This bacteria produces the enzyme neuraminidase, which exposes cryptoantigen in the T cell surface, producing thrombotic microangiopathy. HUS triggered by *S. pneumoniae* is usually associated with severe invasive infection such as sepsis, meningitis, or complicated pneumonia.

CLINICAL PRESENTATION

Typical D+ HUS Classic D+ HUS presents 2 days to 2 weeks after a prodrome of diarrheal illness. Typically, the diarrhea is nonbloody for 1 to 3 days before becoming bloody and is associated with abdominal pain and vomiting. Just as the child's symptoms of colitis seem to be resolving, he or she presents with pallor, irritability, and sometimes oligoanuria. Patients commonly have petechiae, edema, dehydration, hypertension, and electrolyte abnormalities. Some patients may appear fluid-overloaded despite intravascular depletion. Third spacing of fluid to extravascular tissues can result from the combined effects of hypoalbuminemia, vascular injury, and hyponatremia. Patients may develop pulmonary edema and effusions due to third spacing.

Neurologic findings such as irritability and lethargy often occur and most commonly may be related to dehydration, fatigue, or direct neuronal effects of Shiga toxin. However, practitioners must carefully evaluate patients with neurologic symptoms since thrombotic microangiopathy can also occur in the brain, causing 10% of children to develop seizures, coma, or stroke. Neurologic complications of HUS have been associated with higher rates of morbidity and mortality. Endothelial damage of blood vessels can also occur elsewhere in the body, leading to pancreatitis, hepatitis, GI bleeding, intussusception, and myocarditis.

Atypical HUS aHUS predominantly affects the renal vessels, but due to the diffuse thrombotic microangiopathy, other organ systems (brain, heart, intestines, pancreas, and lungs) are more commonly affected than with D+ HUS. The most frequent extrarenal symptoms are neurological (48%), which can include irritability, somnolence, confusion, convulsions, encephalopathy, cerebrovascular accidents, hemiparesis, hemiplegia, and coma. Myocardial infarction has been described in 3% of patients with aHUS and can cause sudden death. Cardiomyopathy, heart failure, and peripheral ischemic heart disease have also been described, in addition to diarrhea (30%), vomiting, and abdominal pain. Variability in presentation makes aHUS more difficult to diagnose, and in some cases difficult to distinguish from D+ HUS.

HOSPITAL COURSE

The course of HUS can be variable in severity and duration, but there is a general pattern to the illness. Patients are diagnosed following the usual clinical course of resolving colitis and the onset of anemia, thrombocytopenia, and renal dysfunction. Over the next hours to days of illness, the patient's general clinical picture worsens, with further decreases in hemoglobin, platelets, and urine output and increasing blood urea nitrogen and creatinine. Thirty percent to 50% of patients may progress to renal failure with anuria, requiring dialysis, while others follow a milder course of illness. After this period of decline, there is usually a plateau that lasts for several days or even weeks. The child may remain on dialysis and be transfusion dependent during this time. Eventually, most patients recover, heralded by an increase in platelets. Recovery of other systems follows slowly. Most children survive the acute phase; however, there is a mortality rate of 2% to 5%. The mortality rate has decreased in recent years, and this has been attributed to increased transfer of patients to institutions with pediatric nephrologists and improvement in the use of dialysis in pediatric patients.

PROGNOSIS

Although the majority of children with D+ HUS are thought to have complete recovery, up to 30% of patients may have long-term sequelae including renal impairment, hypertension, or central nervous system manifestations. Studies show that mild chronic renal sequelae such as hypertension, proteinuria, or low creatinine clearance may persist in 10% to 50% of patients, depending on the population. End-stage renal disease (ESRD) occurs in 3% to 6% of patients. In a 20-year longitudinal study in Utah, 11% of patients with D+ HUS had a negative outcome, defined as either death, ESRD, or stroke.

Predictors of poor prognosis include severe prodromal illness, increased white blood cell count at presentation (>20 K), increasing number of days of anuria, multisystem involvement (especially CNS), and age <2 years. Severe dehydration at the time of initial diarrheal illness with resultant acute tubular injury may increase the chance of developing oligoanuric HUS and chronic renal sequelae.

In contrast to typical HUS, aHUS is a chronic condition due to its genetic origins and has a poorer prognosis. More than 50% of patients with aHUS die from the illness, require dialysis, or develop permanent kidney damage during the year following diagnosis. Morbidity and mortality remains high despite the use of monoclonal antibodies for treatment. aHUS triggered by *S. pneumoniae* is also associated with severe illness, with higher long-term morbidity compared to D+ HUS.

DIFFERENTIAL DIAGNOSIS

When present, the constellation of findings in HUS is generally easily recognized. Early in the course, however, diagnosis can be more difficult. Other causes of enterocolitis, such as *Salmonella*, *Campylobacter*, *Yersinia*, *Clostridium difficile*, and *amebiasis* may cause dehydration and acute kidney injury but usually do not cause thrombocytopenia or hemolytic anemia. Diseases that cause acute renal failure, such as the glomerulonephritides and vasculitides may mimic HUS. Other considerations are early ulcerative colitis, bilateral renal vein thrombosis, systemic lupus erythematosus, and malignant hypertension.

Diseases that cause thrombotic microangiopathy can also be confused with HUS. Disseminated intravascular coagulation (DIC) as seen in sepsis may be confused with HUS due to presence of thrombocytopenia and anemia. However, coagulation profiles will be normal in HUS. Thrombotic thrombocytopenic purpura (TTP) has a similar presentation to HUS. However, TTP involves the central nervous system much more often than HUS. Also, patients with TTP have a deficiency of ADAMSTS13, which is a von Willebrand factor–cleaving protease that regulates thrombus formation, while patients with HUS have normal ADAMSTS13 levels.

DIAGNOSTIC EVALUATION

The diagnosis of HUS depends on history, physical examination, and laboratory findings. Stool cultures obtained during the acute diarrheal phase may reveal *E. coli* O157:H7 and therefore heighten the suspicion for HUS. However, stool cultures obtained after the acute diarrheal phase are not as useful since the yield of positive cultures decreases dramatically after the sixth day of illness. Some centers perform both stool culture and Shiga toxin testing simultaneously from a single stool sample.

Laboratory evaluation usually reveals thrombocytopenia as the first sign of HUS followed by the development of anemia with hemoglobin levels in the range of 5 to 9 g/dL. Red blood cells have the morphology of schistocytes and helmet-shaped forms due to the microangiopathic hemolysis caused by cell trauma from the renal microvasculature. Fibrin degradation products are elevated, but coagulation studies are normal. White blood cell counts are often increased, and the reticulocyte count may be increased as the marrow attempts to replace hemolyzed red blood cells. Laboratory criteria to diagnose HUS are hemoglobin level <10 g/dL with signs of fragmented erythrocytes on peripheral smear, thrombocytopenia with a platelet count <150, and acute renal impairment with glomerular filtration rate (GFR) <90 mL/min/1.73 m^2.

A broad range of electrolyte abnormalities can be seen related to the renal dysfunction; most often patients have hyperkalemia, hypocalcemia, and either hypo- or hypernatremia. Both blood urea nitrogen and creatinine are variably elevated, based on the degree of renal involvement. Urine samples are usually not considered helpful since they are often contaminated as diarrhea is subsiding, but if obtained, may reveal microscopic hematuria, proteinuria, and casts. Amylase, lipase, and liver enzymes may be elevated. Renal ultrasonography is generally not useful as it typically reveals nonspecific findings. Echocardiography should be considered in the face of myocarditis or other cardiac dysfunction. Electrocardiography may be considered to evaluate for the effects of hyperkalemia or if myocardial ischemia is suspected. Computed tomography or magnetic resonance imaging of the brain should be considered when neurologic complications arise. Air or contrast enema can be helpful when GI complications such as intussusception, perforation, stricture, or toxic megacolon are suspected.

MANAGEMENT

The mainstay of therapy is management of renal dysfunction. Urine output and electrolytes should be monitored closely, and fluids adjusted as necessary. Fluid balance is a challenging issue in HUS since renal perfusion must be maintained while avoiding fluid overload. Daily weights and strict intake and output should be recorded during hospitalization to monitor fluid status. Anuric patients should have fluid intake limited to insensible losses (about one-third maintenance) plus output. Diuretics should be avoided in absence of severe fluid overload since they may decrease intravascular volume and perfusion to the kidneys. Dialysis is a most effective mode of management for severe fluid overload. Other indications for dialysis include hyperkalemia, severe metabolic acidosis (persistent bicarbonate <10 mmol/L), severe uremia (BUN >36 mmol/L), or signs and symptoms of volume overload.

Nutritional support is imperative for recovery. Enteral feeding is preferred if permitted by the patient's clinical status. If this is not possible, parenteral nutrition should be initiated. Diarrhea should be managed with supportive care with the avoidance of antimotility agents and nephrotoxic agents such as NSAIDs. Narcotics should also be avoided since they can cause seizures in children with renal failure. Avoidance of antibiotics during the acute phase of diarrheal illness continues to be a controversial topic. A 2002 meta-analysis that concluded that antibiotic therapy may not be harmful has been widely discredited due to the inclusion of one large study that showed beneficial effect of Fosfomycin administration. Fosfomycin was compared to other antibiotics in this study and not placebo. A recent prospective cohort study showed that antibiotic exposure significantly increased the odds of developing oliguric and nonoliguric HUS. Currently, antibiotics should be avoided since it seems that risks outweigh any potential benefits.

Hypertension is initially controlled through the careful stabilization of volume status. If hypertension persists, medical management can be initiated. Calcium channel blockers such as nifedipine are frequently used as first-line agents. In cases of long-term renal sequelae, such as hypertension and proteinuria, ongoing surveillance and close follow-up are indicated.

Patients who develop neurologic symptoms, such as irritability, lethargy, confusion, seizures, or abnormal neurologic examination require urgent brain imaging to evaluate for stroke. These patients should be transferred to an intensive care unit for closer monitoring. Neurologic complications are known to be important determinants of morbidity and mortality.

Patients can become profoundly and rapidly anemic and may require transfusion if they develop any cardiovascular or respiratory compromise. Eighty percent of patients with HUS need erythrocyte transfusions. Blood products should be volume-reduced and given slowly to prevent the chance of worsening hypertension. Leukocyte depletion of packed red blood cells is recommended to reduce alloimmunization in case renal transplantation is required in the future. Platelets should be given only in the face of active bleeding or the need for an invasive procedure (e.g., dialysis catheter placement, central venous line placement). More liberal use of platelets can actually increase thrombus formation in the renal microvasculature and cause clinical deterioration.

In aHUS, plasma exchange was traditionally used early in the illness to decrease toxin load. Most recently experts are recommending the use of Eculizumab, if available, instead of plasma exchange. Eculizumab is an IgG-humanized monoclonal antibody that binds to complement proteins with great affinity and blocks excision of complements that lead to the formation of membrane attack complexes and ensuing damage. Positive clinical responses to eculizumab have been reported. If Eculizumab is not available, plasma exchange should be done early. Although the evidence is sparse, some practitioners also use Eculizumab and plasma exchange for severe D+ HUS accompanied by neurologic complications. This approach makes sense given the severity of illness, poor prognosis, and possibility of multifactorial disease (underlying genetic predisposition). Practitioners should be aware that patients receiving eculizumab have increased susceptibility to encapsulated bacterium, such as meningococcus, pneumococcus, and *Haemophilus influenzae* type b, due to the suppression of complement activity. Patients should receive vaccinations against these organisms as a preventive measure.

ADMISSION CRITERIA

Any child with suspected or confirmed HUS should be admitted for close monitoring and evaluation.

Patients with neurologic symptoms, hypertensive emergency, and/or the need for urgent dialysis (severe volume overload, electrolyte derangements, severe acidosis, severe uremia) require admission to an intensive care unit.

DISCHARGE CRITERIA

- Renal function improving and electrolytes stable
- Platelet count rising
- Hemoglobin stable or increasing
- Ability to maintain adequate oral intake for fluid and nutritional needs
- Hypertension resolved or controlled with medication

CONSULTATION

Specific consultation services should be based on the severity of illness and the organ systems involved. Examples include the following:

- Nephrology evaluation for significant renal dysfunction and management of hypertension.
- Cardiology consultation if carditis is present.
- Hematology evaluation for management of hemolytic anemia and indications for transfusion.
- Gastroenterology or surgical evaluation for complications of colitis.

SPECIAL CONSIDERATIONS

EARLY IDENTIFICATION

Since HUS is a rare but serious complication of a common presenting condition, it may be helpful to identify clinical or laboratory predictors for children at risk for development of HUS. Many children with severe diarrhea may be briefly hospitalized due to dehydration and then discharged prior to development of HUS symptoms, and stool culture results may not be available at the time of discharge. Anticipatory guidance and follow-up can be tailored for a high-risk group. Several recent prospective studies have sought to identify predictors for development of HUS in children with Shiga toxin-associated diarrhea. One prospective cohort study reported that higher leukocyte count, vomiting, and exposure to antibiotics during the acute phase of illness among children with *E. coli* 0157:H7 may predict the development of HUS. Higher white blood cell count with neutrophilic predominance on admission was also associated with development of HUS in children in a prospective epidemiologic surveillance study in Argentina. Further studies are needed to assess cost-benefit and patient outcomes with the use of screening white blood cell counts in patients hospitalized with bloody diarrhea. Interestingly, the study in Argentina also identified high serum Shiga toxin levels at the beginning of a diarrheal illness in patients who later developed HUS. A screening strategy using serum Shiga toxin levels at the time of hospital admission for patients with suspected bacterial gastroenteritis also warrants further study.

Early identification may also be useful because early management decisions during the diarrheal phase may modify HUS outcomes. Generous administration of intravenous fluids during the first 4 days of gastroenteritis and use of isotonic fluids may reduce the risk for development of oligoanuric HUS, which is usually associated with a more complicated hospital course and long-term renal sequelae. No studies have identified methods to prevent the development of HUS at this time.

PREVENTION

Because many cases of HUS follow a GI illness, prevention of the inciting illness may lead to the prevention of HUS. This is relevant in the case of infection with *E. coli* 0157:H7, because about 13% of infected pediatric patients develop HUS. Reduction in *E. coli* infection can be accomplished by avoiding raw or undercooked ground beef and unpasteurized milk, cheese, or cider. Decreasing levels of 0157:H7 in cattle, thereby reducing the risk of humans acquiring the disease, can be accomplished by modification of the animals' diet before slaughter, and by irradiation of meat.

Infection can be associated with exposure to farm and zoologic animals (e.g., petting zoos, farm tours) because many animals shed this organism. Person-to-person transmission is also a concern, especially in places such as daycare centers, where outbreaks might occur. Hand hygiene is an effective tool to reduce transmission, although compliance can be a challenge. In the hospital setting, contact precautions are indicated to limit the risk of transmission.

Routine antibiotic treatment of *E. coli* 0157:H7 is not recommended, because antimicrobial therapy of the diarrheal illness may increase and certainly does not decrease the risk of developing HUS.

KEY POINTS

- HUS is defined by a clinical triad of microangiopathic hemolytic anemia, thrombocytopenia, and varying degrees of acute kidney injury.
- Ninety percent of cases are preceded by Shiga toxin-induced enteritis.
- A small percentage of atypical cases follow an invasive *S. pneumoniae* infection or occur in genetically predisposed hosts.
- Multisystem extrarenal involvement can occur in severe cases, with involvement of the brain, heart, lungs, pancreas, liver, and intestines.
- Diagnosis is made clinically and by laboratory findings.
- Management for typical D+ HUS involves meticulous fluid balance, judicious red cell transfusions, nutritional support, antihypertensive medication, and dialysis when indicated.
- Patients with aHUS and/or neurologic symptoms may benefit from Eculizumab and plasma exchange therapy.

ACKNOWLEDGMENT

The author wishes to acknowledge the work of Dr. Sowdhamini Wallace on the prior version of this chapter.

SUGGESTED READINGS

Ake JA, Jelacic S, Ciol MA, et al. Relative nephroprotection during Escherichia coli 0157:H7 infections: association with intravenous volume expansion. *Pediatrics*. 2005;115(6):e673-e679.

Campistol JM, Arias M, Ariceta G, et al. An update for atypical haemolytic uraemic syndrome: diagnosis and treatment. A consensus document. *Nefrologia*. 2013;33(1):27-45.

Gianviti A, Tozzi A, DePetris L, et al. Risk factors for poor renal prognosis in children with hemolytic uremic syndrome. *Pediatr Nephrol*. 2003;18:1229-1235.

Hogan MC, Gloor JM, Uhl JR, et al. Two cases of non-0157H7 Escherichia coli hemolytic uremic syndrome caused by urinary tract infection. *Am J Kid Dis*. 2001;38:E22.

Kazumoto I, Kamioka I, Nozu K. Management of diarrhea-associated hemolytic uremic syndrome in children. *Clin Exp Nephrol*. 2008;12:16-19.

Lopez EL, Contrini MM, Glatstein E, et al. An epidemiologic surveillance of Shiga-like toxin-producing Escherichia coli infection in Argentinean children. Risk factors and serum Shiga-like toxin 2 values. *Pediatr Infect Dis J*. 2012;31(1):20-24.

Miller DP, Kaye JA, Shea K, et al. Incidence of thrombotic thrombocytopenic purpura/hemolytic uremic syndrome. *Epidemiology*. 2004;15:208-215.

National Association of State Public Health Veterinarians, Inc. Compendium of measures to prevent disease associated with animals in public settings, 2005. *MMWR Recomm Rep*. 2005;54:1-12.

Safdar N, Said A, Gangnon RE, Maki DG. Risk of hemolytic uremic syndrome after antibiotic treatment of *Escherichia coli* 0157:H7 enteritis: a meta-analysis. *JAMA*. 2002;288:996-1001.

Scheiring J, Rosales A, Zimmerhackl LB. Today's understanding of the haemolytic uraemic syndrome. *Eur J Pediatr*. 2010;169:7-13.

Serna A, Boedeker EC. Pathogenesis and treatment of Shiga toxin-producing Escherichia coli infections. *Curr Opin Gastroenterol*. 2008;24(1):38-47.

Siegler RL, Pavia AT, Christofferson RD, Milligan MK. A 20-year population-based study of postdiarrheal hemolytic uremic syndrome in Utah. *Pediatrics*. 1994;94:35-40.

Spizzirri FD, Rahman RC, Bibiloni N, et al. Childhood hemolytic uremic syndrome in Argentina: long term follow-up and prognostic features. *Pediatr Nephrol*. 1997;11:156-160.

Tarr PI, Gordon CA, Chandler WL. Shiga-toxin producing Escherichia coli and haemolytic uraemic syndrome. *Lancet*. 2005;365:1073-1086.

Wong, CS, Mooney JC, Brandt JR, et al. Risk factors for the hemolytic uremic syndrome in children infected with Escherichia coli 0157:H7: a multivariable analysis. *Clin Infect Dis*. 2012;55(1):33-41.

CHAPTER 112 Interstitial Nephritis

Samar A. Hussein, MD, FAAP

BACKGROUND

Interstitial nephritis was first described histologically in 1898 in the kidneys of patients who died from diphtheria and scarlet fever. Interstitial nephritis is characterized by histologic changes due to infiltration of the renal interstitium and tubular cells by inflammatory cells accompanied by interstitial edema or fibrosis and varying degrees of tubular atrophy. These inflammatory changes usually spare the glomeruli and renal vasculature. Therefore, interstitial nephritis is now termed tubulointerstitial nephritis (TIN). Acute TIN refers to acute renal dysfunction and is usually reversible. Common types of acute TIN include drug induced, infectious, immune mediated, and idiopathic.

Chronic TIN describes a more insidious decline in renal function. Chronic TIN in children is far less common than acute TIN and is most often seen in the setting of obstructive uropathy, progressive renal disorders, and metabolic and hereditary disorders. In chronic TIN the tubular epithelial cell damage is similar to that seen in acute TIN, but with eventual progression to interstitial fibrosis and tubular atrophy. Tubulointerstitial nephritis with uveitis (TINU) syndrome is a rare form of TIN in which the renal findings are associated with uveal inflammation. Uveitis may recur and persist even when renal symptoms resolve.

The true prevalence of TIN in the pediatric population is difficult to determine. The diagnosis of acute TIN is often made when there is clinical improvement or, as is the case of drug-induced acute TIN, after empiric removal of the likely trigger. According to the 2008 annual report from the North American Pediatric Renal Transplant Cooperative Study, TIN and pyelonephritis account for approximately 1.8% of all identified causes of chronic kidney disease and 1.7% of all causes of end-stage renal disease in the United States. Published data between 1983 and 2009 show that acute TIN has been diagnosed by percutaneous kidney biopsy in 3% to 7% of children and adolescents with acute kidney injury. The incidence of TINU has been reported anywhere from 10% up to 25% in some case series. This incidence is higher than previously reported in the literature.

PATHOPHYSIOLOGY

The exact pathophysiologic mechanism for TIN in humans is not completely understood. The most widely accepted hypothesis is that of cell-mediated immunity via T-lymphocyte infiltration in response to endogenous antigens (Tamm-Horsfall proteins, megalin, cumulin), or to exogenous antigens internalized and processed by tubular membrane cells. After internalization and processing, MHC class I molecules then present potential antigens to CD8+ cytotoxic T-cells leading to tubular cell damage. Delayed or type IV hypersensitivity reactions are also thought to play a role in the pathogenesis of drug-induced TIN with a mixture of CD8+ and CD4+ T-cells, B-cells, macrophages, and natural killer cells. Immunohistochemical staining of kidney tissue in TIN occasionally demonstrates the presence of antibodies, antibody-antigen complexes, and complement proteins, suggesting a role for antibody-mediated immunity and the complement cascade. Antigens of drug origin or microbial origin can mimic tubular basement membrane (TBM) antigens or renal interstitial antigens and induce an immune response against the TBM or renal interstitium. Alternatively, drugs or drug components can bind to the renal interstitial cells and act as haptens, stimulating the production of anti-TBM antibodies. One additional mechanism described is direct binding of antigens to the TBM or deposition of antigen-antibody complexes into the renal interstitium. This can lead to MHC class II processing of antigens by renal tubular epithelial cells and presentation to CD4+ T-cells. Activation of cytokines leads to amplification of renal injury.

CLINICAL PRESENTATION

The clinical presentation of TIN is quite variable. Fever, abdominal pain, nausea, vomiting, arthralgia, myalgia, and rash are some of the common presenting symptoms in children. Complaints of malaise, weight loss, and asthenia have also been reported in some case series. Often there are no specific signs or symptoms that point to a renal etiology unless some degree of renal failure is already present. If hematuria is present, it is usually microscopic, while oliguria is not a common finding on presentation. Nocturia, polyuria, and polydipsia may be present in some patients as a sign of tubular dysfunction and defective sodium reabsorption. Patients with chronic TIN may exhibit symptoms of anorexia, weight loss, poor growth, and hypertension.

Due to the nonspecific nature of many presenting signs and symptoms, clinicians must have a high index of suspicion in cases of acute TIN. History of exposure to medications and the temporal relationship to such exposure as well as knowledge of any concurrent conditions known to cause TIN have significant diagnostic importance. The onset of symptoms can occur as late as 7 to 10 days after drug exposure in acute TIN. It is also important to note that drug-induced acute TIN is not a dose-dependent phenomenon, but symptoms can reoccur if a patient is exposed to the offending drug again. A classic hypersensitivity triad of fever, rash, and eosinophilia was frequently reported in early literature. More recent evidence suggests that only about 15% of patients present with this constellation of symptoms. In children, the most common medications known to cause acute TIN are antibiotics and nonsteroidal anti-inflammatory drugs (NSAIDs). A common clinical scenario in the inpatient setting is one of an already hospitalized patient with an otherwise unexplained acute rise in serum creatinine or blood urea nitrogen levels. A listing of some specific etiologic agents and disorders is provided in **Table 112–1**.

Patients with TINU may present with blurred vision, photophobia, and eye redness and pain. However, in up to 50% of reported cases of TINU, patients had no ophthalmologic complaints at presentation.

DIFFERENTIAL DIAGNOSIS

The differential diagnosis for acute TIN can be quite broad initially since symptoms are often vague and nonspecific. Viral syndromes, urinary tract infection, trauma, renal calculi, renal vein thrombosis, and hemorrhagic cystitis are some of the renal and nonrenal disorders to consider. In the setting of acute renal failure, intrinsic renal causes should be considered such as the glomerulonephritides and the vasculitides (see Chapters 108 and 109 on acute and chronic renal failure, respectively).

DIAGNOSTIC EVALUATION

Percutaneous kidney biopsy is the only definitive way to diagnose TIN, but it is not routinely recommended. Kidney biopsy should be reserved for those patients who do not respond to standard treatment or in whom

TABLE 112-1 Causes of Tubulointerstitial Nephritis

Infections	Drugs	Immune Mediated	Other
Bacterial	**Antibiotics**	**Anti-TBM antibodies**	**Metabolic**
β-Hemolytic streptococci	Penicillins	Primary anti-TBM nephritis	Oxalate nephropathy
Corynebacterium	Cephalosporins	Secondary anti-TBM nephritis	Hypercalcemic nephropathy
Brucella sp.	Sulfonamides	Anti-GBM disease	Urate nephropathy
Legionella pneumophila	Rifampin	Membranous nephropathy	Cystine nephropathy
Campylobacter jejuni	Ethambutol	Immune complex deposits	
Mycoplasma spp.	Azithromycin	Primary immune complex nephritis	**Heavy metal**
Salmonella spp.	Ciprofloxacin	Secondary immune complex nephritis	Lead
Yersinia pseudotuberculosis	Tetracycline	Lupus nephritis	Cadmium
	Vancomycin	Sjögren syndrome	Mercury
Viruses	Erythromycin	MPGN	
Measles	Aminoglycosides	Membranous nephropathy	**Hereditary**
Epstein-Barr virus		Mixed cryoglobulinemia	Alport syndrome
HIV	**Anti-inflammatory drugs**		Nephrolithiasis-medullary cystic kidney
Hepatitis viruses	Ibuprofen	**T cell–mediated**	
Cytomegalovirus	Indomethacin	Tubulointerstitial nephritis with uveitis syndrome	
Polyomavirus (BK)			**Miscellaneous**
Hantavirus		**Sarcoidosis**	Chinese herb nephropathy
Adenovirus	**Diuretics**	Granulomatous tubulointerstitial nephritis	Radiation nephritis
	Furosemide		Ischemic nephropathy
Fungi	Thiazides		Balkan endemic nephropathy
Candida spp.			
Aspergillus spp.	**Other medications**		
Cryptococcus neoformans	Cimetidine		
Histoplasma capsulatum	Omeprazole		
Coccidioides immitis	Captopril		
Blastomyces dermatitidis	Carbamazepine		
Mucormycosis	Phenobarbital		
	Cyclosporine		
Parasites	Lithium		
Plasmodium spp.	Gold		
Schistosoma spp.	Aspirin		
Filariasis	Azathioprine		

GBM, glomerular basement membrane; HIV, human immunodeficiency virus; MPGN, membranoproliferative glomerulonephritis; TBM, tubular basement membrane.

the diagnosis of acute TIN is in question. Noninvasive serum and urine tests can be useful tools along with clinical information in establishing the diagnosis. The most common laboratory abnormality in TIN is elevated serum creatinine with a decreased calculated or measured glomerular filtration anywhere in the range from mild azotemia to acute renal failure. Microscopic proteinuria is a prominent finding, but often less than that found in nephrotic syndrome. As noted earlier, microscopic hematuria is sometimes also present, and sterile pyuria has also been reported. TIN can affect all parts of the nephron, and laboratory findings of renal dysfunction may be evident depending on which parts of the nephron are involved. Evidence of Fanconi syndrome and impaired glucose, sodium bicarbonate, phosphorous, and amino acid reabsorption may be present if proximal tubules are damaged. Renal tubular acidosis may reflect injury to the distal convoluted tubule. Other nonspecific laboratory findings include anemia, leukocytosis with eosinophilia, and elevated erythrocyte sedimentation rate. Eosinophiliuria has low specificity for TIN but it may be helpful in making the diagnosis, as it is found in up to 25% of patients with acute TIN. **Table 112-2** summarizes some of the laboratory findings seen in acute TIN, and **Table 112-3** provides comparisons of laboratory findings in acute glomerulonephritis, acute renal failure, and TIN.

There are no indications for routine diagnostic use of imaging in acute TIN. Renal ultrasonography may prove helpful in cases of acute renal failure when the diagnosis is in question and TIN is in the differential. On ultrasound, the kidneys often appear larger in width, depth, and length in patients with acute TIN than in normal, age-matched pediatric patients. In addition to nephromegaly, the kidneys may appear diffusely echogenic in comparison to the liver and spleen, with increased echogenicity occurring particularly in the renal cortices. In contrast, chronic TIN is characterized ultrasonographically by small renal size and diffusely increased echogenicity.

TABLE 112-2 Laboratory Abnormalities in Tubulointerstitial Nephritis

CBC	Chemistry	Immunology	Urinalysis
Anemia	Acute renal failure	Elevated ESR	FENA >2%
Leukocytosis	Hypoalbuminemia	Elevated IgG	Proteinuria
Eosinophilia		Hypocomplementemia	Hematuria
			Leukocyturia
			Glycosuria
			Granular casts

CBC, complete blood count; ESR, erythrocyte sedimentation rate; FENA, fractional excretion of sodium.

TABLE 112-3 Key Laboratory Findings in Acute Renal Failure, Acute Glomerulonephritis, and Tubulointerstitial Nephritis

	Prerenal Acute Renal Failure	Acute Glomerulonephritis	Tubulointerstitial Nephritis
Serum creatinine	↑	↔ or ↑	↑
Serum potassium	↑	↔ or ↑	↓
Serum HCO_3^-	↓	↓ or ↔ or ↑	↓
Proteinuria	None	>2 g/24 hr (Upr/Ucr >2.0)	<1 g/24 hr (Upr/Ucr <1.0)
Hematuria	None	↔ or ↑	↔ or ↑
Pyuria	None	↔ or ↑	↔ or ↑
Urine sediment	Hyaline casts	RBC, WBC, granular or hyaline casts	Granular, hyaline, or WBC casts
FENA	<1%	<2%	>2%

↓, Decreased; ↔, normal; ↑, increased; FE_{NA}, fractional excretion of sodium; RBC, red blood cell; Upr/Ucr, urine protein-to-urine creatinine ratio; WBC, white blood cell.

MANAGEMENT

Symptomatic and supportive care is the primary focus of treatment in acute TIN. Correction of any electrolyte abnormalities and monitoring for improvement in renal function is important. If drug-induced acute TIN is suspected, identification and prompt removal of the offending medication is essential. If a medication is necessary for treatment of an underlying disorder and an appropriate substitute agent is available, replacement of the suspected medication is justified. If an infectious cause is suspected, prompt medical treatment with appropriate antibiotics, antifungals, or antiviral medications should be initiated. For patients presenting with acute renal failure and indications for dialytic therapy, renal replacement therapy (e.g., hemodialysis) should be provided until the patient's renal function recovers.

The routine use of corticosteroids for acute TIN in children is not recommended. There are no large, randomized controlled prospective studies that compare supportive care versus corticosteroids in acute TIN in children. A small prospective nonrandomized study reported that patients who were treated early with corticosteroids returned to baseline renal function sooner than those patients who received only supportive care; however, no significant difference was found in creatinine levels, GFR, or low-molecular-weight proteinuria at 6-month follow-up between those patients treated with corticosteroids or supportive care alone. The current accepted recommendation for treatment is to reserve the use of corticosteroids in acute TIN for patients in whom renal function does not improve after removal of the suspected inciting agent. If a patient does not respond to symptomatic or supportive care, consultation with a pediatric nephrologist is recommended to discuss treatment with corticosteroids and whether percutaneous kidney biopsy should be done prior to initiating the treatment. When corticosteroids are necessary, published treatment regimens recommend prescribing prednisone at a dose of 1 to 2 mg/kg/day (maximum of 60 mg/day) as a single dose or in divided doses for approximately 1 to 3 months, followed by a taper. Total duration of treatment will depend on the patient's response. A recent prospective study demonstrated no statistically significant difference in the rate of occurrence of uveitis in patients with TIN in steroid-treated patients versus those treated with supportive care alone. There are currently no high-quality studies that support the use of cyclophosphamide or cyclosporine in the treatment of corticosteroid-resistant acute TIN.

The overall prognosis of acute TIN in children is rather good, in contrast to that reported for TIN in adults. Several studies have shown that most patients have complete recovery of renal function after supportive therapy alone in a matter of weeks. A recent study suggests that patients who require treatment with corticosteroids or cytotoxic agents have eventual normalization of renal function as soon as 6 months after treatment. Prognosis for renal recovery in children with TINU has a similarly good long-term prognosis, but uveitis can be persistent.

ADMISSION CRITERIA

- Acute renal failure
- Progressive decrease in renal function as measured by serum creatinine or urine output, or both
- Failure to respond to supportive care (i.e., those requiring steroid initiation with or without biopsy)
- Age younger than 2 years or older than 12 years
- Nephrotic-range proteinuria
- Recurrent episodes of acute TIN

DISCHARGE CRITERIA

- Stabilization of renal function
- Establishment of appropriate referrals and follow-up

CONSULTATION

- Nephrology: Consultation should be considered when acute TIN is a diagnostic consideration. Consultation is absolutely recommended when symptoms persist despite discontinuation of the suspected inciting agent, renal function is compromised, corticosteroid therapy is being considered, and/or recurrent disease is present.
- Ophthalmology: Inpatient or prompt outpatient consultation with an ophthalmologist is recommended to rule out uveitis.

SPECIAL CONSIDERATIONS

PREVENTION

Prevention of acute TIN is probably difficult, especially during the initial episode. It may be preventable by careful consideration of medications prescribed to pediatric patients. Early recognition of systemic symptoms and discontinuation of the potential offending medication may circumvent the development of acute TIN.

KEY POINTS

- TIN is inflammation of the renal interstitium and tubular cells that can be accompanied by interstitial edema, fibrosis, or tubular atrophy.
- Medication-induced acute TIN is a common type of TIN. Removal of the offending medication is key to management of this disorder.
- The clinical presentation of TIN may consist of constitutional symptoms, including rash, fever, abdominal pain, nausea, vomiting, anorexia, weight loss, polydipsia, polyuria, hypertension, and headaches.
- Laboratory findings include anemia, leukocytosis, eosinophilia, elevated erythrocyte sedimentation rate, elevated fractional excretion of sodium, sterile pyuria, proteinuria, hematuria, and evidence of acute renal failure.
- The prognosis in children is good, with recovery of renal function occurring in most patients with proper treatment.
- Treatment involves support of renal function and removal of an inciting medication or treatment of a causative infection when such triggers can be identified. In some cases, corticosteroid therapy may be indicated.

SUGGESTED READINGS

Alon US. Tubulointerstitial nephritis. In: Avner ED, Harmon WE, Niaudet P eds. *Pediatric Nephrology*. Philadelphia: Lippincott, Williams & Wilkins; 2004:817-831.

Cavallo T. Tubulointerstitial nephritis. In: Jennette JC, Olson LL, Schwartz MM, Silva FG eds. *Heptinstall's Pathology of the Kidney*. 5th ed. Philadelphia: Lippincott-Raven; 1998:667-723.

Clarkson MR, Giblin L, O'Connell FP, et al. Acute interstitial nephritis: clinical features and response to corticosteroid therapy. *Nephrol Dial Transplant*. 2004;19(11):2778-2783.

Councilman WT. Acute interstitial nephritis. *J Exp Med*. 1898;(4-5): 393-420.

Dell KM, Kaplan BS, Meyers CM. Tubulointerstitial nephritis. In: Barratt TM, Avner ED, Harmon WE eds. *Pediatric Nephrology*. 4th ed. Baltimore: Lippincott Williams & Wilkins; 1999:823-834.

Ellis D, Fried WA, Yunis EJ, Blau EB. Acute interstitial nephritis in children: a report of 13 cases and review of the literature. *Pediatric Nephrol*. 1981;862-870.

Goda C, Kotake S, Ichiisi A, Namba K, Kitaichi N, Ohno S. Clinical features in tubulointerstitial nephritis and uveitis (TINU) syndrome. *Am J Ophthalmol*. 2005;140(4):637-641.

Gonzalez E, Gutierrez E, Galeano C, et al. Early steroid treatment improves the recovery of renal function patients in drug-induced acute interstitial nephritis. *Kidney Int*. 2008;73(8):940-946.

Greising J, Trachtman H, Gauthier B, Valderrama E. Acute interstitial nephritis in adolescents and young adults. *Child Nephrol Urol*. 1990;10(4):189-195.

Hiraoka M, Hori C, Tsuchida S, et al. Ultrasonographic findings of acute tubulointerstitial nephritis. *Am J Nephrol*. 1996;16:154-158.

Jahnukainen T, Ala-Houhala M, Karikoski R, et al. Clinical outcome and occurrence of uveitis in children with idiopathic tubulointerstitial nephritis. *Pediatr Nephrol*. 2011;26 (2):291-299.

Lanewala A, Mubarak M, Akhter F, Aziz S, Bhatti S, Kazi JI. Pattern of pediatric renal disease observed in native renal biopsies in Pakistan. *J Nephrol*. 2009;22(6):739-746.

North American Pediatric Renal Transplant Cooperative Study. The North American Pediatric Renal Transplant Cooperative Study (NAPRTCS) 2008.

Perazella MA, Markowitz GS. Drug-induced acute interstitial nephritis. *Nat Rev Nephrol*. 2010;6(8):461-470.

Praga M, Gonzalez E. Acute interstitial nephritis. *Kidney Int*. 2010;77(11):956-961.

Ruffing KA, Hoppes P, Blend D, Cugino A, Jarjoura D, Whittier FC. Eosinophils in urine revisited. *Clin Nephrol*. 1994;41(3):163-166.

Saarela V, Nuutinen M, Ala-Houhala M, Arikoski P, Ronnholm K, Jahnukainen T. Tubulointerstitial nephritis and uveitis syndrome in children: a prospective multicenter study. *Ophthalmology*. 2013;120(7):1476-1481.

Thomassen VH, Ring T, Thaarup J, Baggesen K. Tubulointerstitial nephritis and uveitis (TINU) syndrome: a case report and review of the literature. *Acta Ophthalmol*. 2009;87(6):676-679.

Ulinski T, Sellier-Leclerc AL, Tudorache E, Bensman A, Aoun B. Acute tubulointerstitial nephritis. *Pediatr Nephrol*. 2012;27(7):1051-1057.

Winkler P, Altrogge H. Sonographic signs of nephritis in children: a comparison of renal echography with clinical evaluation, laboratory data and biopsy. *Pediatr Radiol*. 1985;15(4):231-237.

CHAPTER 113 Nephrotic Syndrome

Deborah R. Stein, MD

BACKGROUND

Nephrotic syndrome is one of the most common renal diseases in childhood. In recent estimates, the most common type, idiopathic nephrotic syndrome, occurs in about 2 to 3 per 100,000 children per year. Nephrotic syndrome is caused by abnormalities of the selective permeability of the glomerular filtration system. It includes four key clinical features: proteinuria, hypoalbuminemia, edema, and hyperlipidemia. The most common types of childhood nephrotic syndrome are responsive to steroids. The majority of patients with nephrotic syndrome have a relapsing course.

TABLE 113-1 Classification of Nephrotic Syndrome*

- Idiopathic (primary) nephrotic syndrome
  - Minimal change disease (MCD)
  - Focal segmental glomerulosclerosis (FSGS)
  - Membranous nephropathy
- Secondary nephrotic syndrome = systemic disease
  - Membranous nephropathy
  - Systemic lupus erythematosus
  - Diabetes mellitus
  - Amyloidosis
  - Vasculitis (IgA vasculitis, ANCA vasculitis)
  - Membranoproliferative glomerulonephritis
  - Nephritis (post-infectious glomerulonephritis, thrombotic microangiopathy)
  - Alport syndrome
  - Infection (HIV, Hepatitis B, Hepatitis C, CMV, Parvovirus)
  - Preeclampsia
- Congenital/infantile nephrotic syndrome = classified based on gene mutations
  - Finnish type
    - Mutation of NPHS1, which encodes nephrin
    - Mutation of NPHS2, which encodes podocin
  - Denys-Drash syndrome: mutation of WT1, which encodes transcription tumor suppressor
  - Pierson syndrome: mutation of LAMB2, which encodes laminin β1
  - Diffuse mesangial sclerosis: mutation of PLCE1, which encodes phospholipase C epsilon
  - Others

*This list is not exhaustive.

PATHOPHYSIOLOGY

Nephrotic syndrome may be classified in several ways, including histopathology, inclusion/exclusion of systemic disease, and responsiveness to steroids. The disease can be divided into three major categories—primary or idiopathic nephrotic syndrome, secondary nephrotic syndrome, and congenital/infantile nephrotic syndrome. The most common form in childhood is idiopathic nephrotic syndrome (**Table 113-1**). In secondary nephrotic syndrome, the disease may demonstrate histology similar to that of primary forms; however, the disease stems from a systemic, rather than nephrologic, illness, such as lymphoma or HIV.

In all forms of nephrotic syndrome, there is abnormal selectivity of the permeable barrier, which leads to pathologic protein loss across the glomerular basement membrane (GBM) (**Figure 113-1**). Typically this barrier exhibits both charge and size selectivity. Charge selectivity arises from the normally negatively charged endothelial cells on the GBM, which serve as a barrier to large anions such as albumin crossing into the urine. Size selectivity arises from podocyte foot processes that form an intricate layer with interposition that further inhibits protein loss.

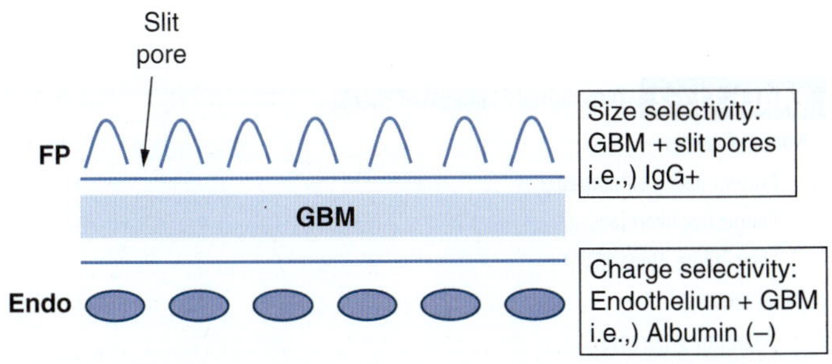

FIGURE 113-1. Pathogenesis of nephrotic syndrome. FP: foot processes; GBM: glomerular basement membrane; Endo: endothelium

Minimal change disease (MCD), the most common type of idiopathic nephrotic syndrome, is caused by a loss of the negative charge secondary to structural damage to the epithelium. As a result, albumin and other proteins are lost in the urine. In addition, the foot processes and slit pores on the Bowman's capsule side of the GBM that typically serve as a size barrier are effaced and thus contribute to protein loss. In patients with nephrotic syndrome, large neutral proteins such as IgG also cross these barriers into urine, often leading to a state of hypogammaglobulinemia. Additional proteins such as thyroid-binding globulin, coagulation factors, and others are lost in the urine during a period of active nephrotic syndrome.

CLINICAL PRESENTATION

Patients with nephrotic syndrome present with edema, often periorbital, sometimes following an upper respiratory illness or other viral illness. This may be diagnosed initially as an allergic reaction, but edema eventually becomes more generalized and severe. The edema is gravity dependent, may be more prominent in the lower extremities, back/sacral area, and genital area, and may progress to ascites and anasarca. Many believe the edema is caused by hypoalbuminemia and subsequent low intravascular oncotic pressure, which allows third spacing of fluid, as well as sodium and water retention due to increased aldosterone as the kidneys sense reduced effective circulating volume.

DIFFERENTIAL DIAGNOSIS

The differential diagnosis for edema includes nonrenal disease (such as protein-losing enteropathy and congestive heart failure) and primary and secondary nephrotic syndrome (**Table 113-2** and **Figure 113-2**). The causes of edema can be categorized based on changes in pressure. If there is increased capillary hydrostatic pressure, decreased capillary oncotic pressure, increased interstitial hydrostatic pressure, or increased capillary permeability, edema may develop.

DIAGNOSTIC EVALUATION

In addition to edema, three key laboratory features define nephrotic syndrome: nephrotic-range proteinuria, hypoalbuminemia, and hyperlipidemia. Nephrotic range proteinuria is urine protein excretion >50 mg/kg/day (or 40 mg/m^2/hr) or alternatively, a spot urine sample that is >300 mg protein/mmol of creatinine (or 3 mg protein/mg creatinine) or urine protein to creatinine ratio greater than 2. Urine protein to creatinine ratios on spot samples (ideally first morning) are preferred over 24-hour collections due to inaccuracies in 24-hour collection and the cumbersome nature of the 24-hour collection procedure. Serum albumin <2.5 g/Dl (25 g/L) is a second key feature. Finally, although not diagnostic, hyperlipidemia is often seen in patients with nephrotic syndrome—specifically, elevated serum total cholesterol, triglycerides, and lipids. Additional recommended laboratory evaluation includes the following:

- Urinalysis
- First morning urine protein/creatinine ratio (normal is ≤0.2 mg/mg in children older than 2 years of age and normal is <0.5 in children younger than 2 years of age. Urine protein creatinine ratio values above these numbers and below 2 are considered non-nephrotic range proteinuria).

TABLE 113-2 Differential Diagnosis of Edema

Nonrenal causes
Protein-losing enteropathy
Congestive heart failure
Liver failure, Hepatitis
Renal causes
Nephrotic syndrome
Nephritic syndrome
Renal failure (acute or chronic)

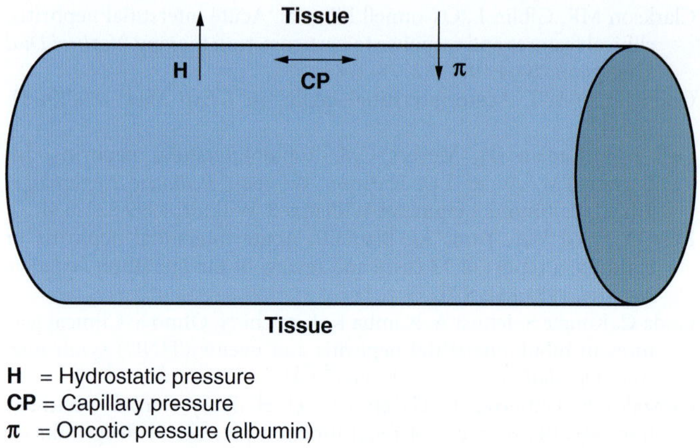

FIGURE 113-2. Pathophysiology of edema in nephrotic syndrome. H: hydrostatic pressure; CP: capillary pressure; π: oncotic pressure (albumin).

- Blood tests: electrolytes, urea nitrogen, creatinine, glucose; cholesterol; albumin; C3 if hematuria present; ANA for children ≥10 years of age or with signs/symptoms of systemic lupus erythematosus (SLE); hepatitis B antigen, hepatitis C, and HIV.
- Assessment for tuberculosis, given anticipated therapy with steroids, either by skin test or blood test.
- Renal biopsy; the age at which a renal biopsy is conducted prior to any therapy will vary depending on the region, prevalence of steroid-responsive nephrotic syndrome, and other patient-specific factors.

MANAGEMENT

Children with nephrotic syndrome should be managed by a pediatric nephrologist. The management of childhood nephrotic syndrome depends on the suspected disease. Management includes both symptomatic relief as well as treatment of the underlying condition.

In general, the use of 25% albumin with a loop diuretic such as furosemide may be considered when there are signs/symptoms of intravascular hypovolemia and total body fluid overload that is causing distress or discomfort. Of note, therapy with albumin and diuretics does not address the underlying nephrosis, and fluid restriction and salt restriction must be implemented as well. Infants with nephrotic syndrome are at high risk for infection and should be treated aggressively if infection is suspected or confirmed.

If MCD is suspected, steroid therapy may be initiated without a renal biopsy. In addition to normal renal function and a negative workup for the chronic diseases above, a classic study by the International Study of Kidney Disease in Children proposes the following findings suggest a diagnosis of MCD:

- Age >1 and <10 years
- Absence of hematuria, though up to 20% of children with MCD may have microscopic hematuria
- Absence of hypertension and gross hematuria
- Normal complement levels
- Normal renal function
- Absence of systemic symptoms such as malar rash, purpura, or joint pain

A set of guidelines from the 2012 Kidney Disease Improving Global Outcomes (KDIGO) recommends the following treatment for an initial episode: prednisone 60 mg/m^2/day (2 mg/kg/day) × 4 to 6 weeks, followed by a taper over the subsequent 4 to 6 weeks. Remission of nephrotic syndrome is defined by the absence of proteinuria. In most practices, families monitor the child's first morning urine at home by dipstick, and thus both remission and subsequent relapses may be detected without formal laboratory assessment. In patients who relapse frequently and/or are steroid dependent, steroid-sparing agents such as mycophenolate and rituximab are considered. In those who are steroid-resistant, several therapies may be considered, including tacrolimus, cyclophosphamide, cyclosporine, and levamisole. Cyclosporine has fallen out of favor, as other calcineurin inhibitors with less toxicity and better tolerability are now available (tacrolimus). For patients with steroid-resistant nephrotic syndrome or those who have signs or symptoms concerning more complex renal or systemic disease, renal biopsy is recommended, as therapy will be tailored based on renal histopathology.

In children younger than 1 year of age with nephrotic syndrome, congenital/genetic disorders are more likely, and steroid therapy should not be initiated as first-line therapy. In these cases, symptoms are managed, often with diuresis, and intensive monitoring for infection and thrombosis is critical. Genetic testing may confirm the underlying cause of nephrotic syndrome. The vast majority of infants with congenital nephrotic syndrome progress to have end-stage renal disease and require dialysis and transplant.

Additional therapies are targeted to specific consequences of nephrotic syndrome. A no-added salt diet is recommended along with fluid restriction to decrease the edema. ACE inhibitors and/or angiotensin II receptor blockers (ARBs) may be used for hypertension as these also serve to decrease proteinuria. Lipid-lowering medications are employed if hyperlipidemia is longstanding.

COMPLICATIONS

Complications may arise from both the disease itself and from the treatment of childhood nephrotic syndrome (**Table 113-3**). Children with nephrotic syndrome are at increased risk for infection. Impaired complement-dependent opsonization of encapsulated bacteria (i.e., *Streptococcus pneumoniae*, *Neisseria meningitidis*, and *Haemophilus influenza*) can lead to severe infections including pneumonia, cellulitis, bacteremia, peritonitis, and sepsis. In addition, hypogammaglobulinemia leads to an increased risk of infection from encapsulated organisms and *Candida* species. The risk of infection may be increased further by factors such as immunosuppressive therapy, and stagnant fluid in the setting of edema and ascites.

Patients with active nephrotic syndrome are hypercoagulable due to loss of protein C and S in the urine, and abnormalities in hemostasis activation, such as fibrinogen, and thrombocytosis. The risk of thrombosis is compounded by relative intravascular depletion. While renal vein thrombosis is rare in patients with nephrotic syndrome, there must be a high index of suspicion for deep vein thrombosis, especially if there is asymmetric swelling or pain in a lower extremity. Patients with nephrotic syndrome have also been reported with pulmonary embolism, cerebral venous thrombosis, and arterial thrombosis. Renal vein thrombosis is most common in infants, in the absence of nephrotic syndrome. In such cases, consultation with hematology as well as pediatric surgery are in order. In many cases, surgical intervention is not warranted but may be considered if there is a thrombus extending to the inferior vena cava, or bilateral disease with renal failure. The decision to provide anticoagulation is case dependent and varies based on risk factors and the clinical status of the child.

ADMISSION CRITERIA

Some patients with childhood nephrotic syndrome may be managed as outpatients following the initial diagnosis. Infection and thromboembolism require hospitalization when suspected.

TABLE 113-3 Complications of Nephrotic Syndrome

- Edema
- Hypertension
- Hyperlipidemia
- Obesity
- Growth impairment
- Infection
- Thromboembolism

Indications for admission include the following:

- Patients <1 year of age
- Systemic symptoms including fever
- Abdominal pain concerning for peritonitis
- Signs/symptoms of acute renal failure (i.e., oliguria, elevated creatinine)
- Uncontrolled hypertension
- Severe edema causing patient discomfort
- Infection
- Concern for/presence of thromboembolism
- Concern for fluid overload causing organ dysfunction (pulmonary edema, congestive heart failure)
- Lack of appropriate outpatient education, support, or follow-up

DISCHARGE CRITERIA

Indications for discharge include the following:

- Adequate treatment of underlying condition requiring hospitalization
- Appropriate patient and family education
- Established treatment plan and follow-up

CONSULTATION

Indications for nephrology consult include:

- All cases of suspected or confirmed nephrotic syndrome
- Patients <1 year of age in whom congenital/infantile nephrotic syndrome is suspected

All children with nephrotic syndrome would benefit from dietary or nutrition consultation to aid in appropriate interventions including salt restriction. Children with a history of thrombosis require an evaluation with a pediatric hematologist. Those who are unvaccinated or under vaccinated may benefit from evaluation with infectious diseases, given the risk for infections that are rarely seen in current hospital settings (such as primary varicella). All children treated with steroids should undergo an annual dilated ophthalmologic exam.

SPECIAL CONSIDERATIONS

PREVENTION

There is no way to prevent a patient from developing nephrotic syndrome. After the diagnosis is established, key components in prevention of major complications include close monitoring, appropriate diet, adherence to therapy, adherence to fluid restriction when necessary, and vaccinations. Patients should be instructed to call the medical team with fevers, especially while undergoing immunosuppression.

Parameters to monitor include weight, height, body mass index (BMI), and blood pressure. Laboratories such as creatinine, electrolytes, glucose, CBC, UA, lipid profile, and liver function should also be monitored periodically. Patients who require ongoing steroid therapy should have an annual eye examination to evaluate for steroid side effects.

The following are recommendations for vaccination:

- Pneumococcus: immunize with 23-valent and heptavalent conjugated vaccines
- Influenza: immunize all actively nephrotic patients, immunosuppressed patients, and household contacts with inactivated influenza vaccine early
- COVID-19: immunize all actively nephrotic patients, immunosuppressed patients, and household contacts
- Defer live vaccines
  - Until prednisone dose is <2 mg/kg/day
  - Until 3 months after completion of therapy with cytotoxic agents
  - Until 1 month after completion of other daily immunosuppression

- For all patients receiving mycophenolate
- Consider IV acyclovir for immunosuppressed patients with onset of varicella lesions

- If vaccination status is unclear, consider assessing titers to determine the need for re-vaccination.

KEY POINTS

- Childhood nephrotic syndrome is diagnosed by four key clinical features: nephrotic range proteinuria, hypoalbuminemia, edema, and hyperlipidemia.
- The most common type of childhood nephrotic syndrome—idiopathic nephrotic syndrome, specifically minimal change disease—is often treatable with steroids without the need for renal biopsy.
- Consultation with a nephrologist is required for all suspected cases of nephrotic syndrome. Hospitalization is recommended for the majority of newly diagnosed patients, to address fluid overload, monitor for signs of complications, and provide education regarding the disease.
- After diagnosis is made, prevention of treatment failure and complications is centered around close monitoring, detection of relapses, and vaccine administration.

SUGGESTED READINGS

Hahn D, Samuel SM, Willis NS, et al. Corticosteroid therapy for nephrotic syndrome in children. *Cochrane Database Syst Rev*. 2015:CD001533

Hodson EM, Willis NS, Craig JC. Interventions for idiopathic steroid-resistant nephrotic syndrome in children (review). *The Cochrane Library*. 2010;11.

Hodson EM, Willis NS, Craig JC. Non-corticosteroid treatment for nephrotic syndrome in children (review). *The Cochrane Library*. 2010;4.

Kidney Disease: Improving Global Outcomes (KDIGO) Glomerular Diseases Work Group (2021) KDIGO 2021 clinical practice guideline for the management of glomerular diseases. *Kidney Int*. 100:S1-S276.

Lombel RM, Gipson DS, Hodson EM. Treatment of steroid-sensitive nephrotic syndrome: new guidelines from KDIGO. *Pediatr Nephrol*. 2013;28:415-426.

Nephrotic syndrome in children: prediction of histopathology from clinical and laboratory characteristics at time of diagnosis. A report of the International Study of Kidney Disease in Children. *Kidney Int*. 1978;13:159-165.

Trautmann A, Vivarelli M, Samuel S, et al; International Pediatric Nephrology Association. IPNA clinical practice recommendations for the diagnosis and management of children with steroid-resistant nephrotic syndrome. *Pediatr Nephrol*. 2020;35:1529-1561.

Veltkamp F, Rensma LR, Bouts AHM. Incidence and relapse of idiopathic nephrotic syndrome: meta-analysis, LEARNS consortium. *Pediatrics*. 2021;148(1):Epub 2021 Jun 30.

CHAPTER 114 Renal Tubular Acidosis

Nirupama Gupta, MD and Amina Khan, MD, MPH

BACKGROUND

Renal tubular acidosis (RTA) occurs when the kidneys are unable to maintain normal acid-base homeostasis because of renal transport defects in bicarbonate reabsorption, acid excretion, or both, resulting in a hyperchloremic, non-anion gap metabolic acidosis. RTA can be an isolated disorder or a feature of a more complex disease or syndrome. Because RTA can present with nonspecific symptoms such as failure to thrive, vomiting, and myalgia, recognizing, diagnosing, and managing these disorders is important for inpatient providers.

RTA is categorized into four types, depending on the location of the tubular dysfunction. Distal RTA (Type I) is characterized by impairment of the urinary acidification process in the distal tubule. Proximal RTA (Type II) refers to disorders involving bicarbonate reabsorption at the proximal tubule. Type III RTA is rare and has features of both type I and II RTA. Type IV RTA is characterized by hyperkalemic acidosis, due to aldosterone deficiency or resistance in the distal tubule.

PATHOPHYSIOLOGY

A normal functioning kidney maintains acid-base homeostasis by two main processes: reabsorption of filtered bicarbonate (HCO_3^-) at the proximal tubule and excretion of hydrogen ion (H^+) as ammonium (NH_4^+) at the distal nephron. Under normal circumstances, the kidney excretes acid at the same rate that metabolic processes generate acid. Metabolic acidosis is defined as an excess in nonvolatile acid load that results in a primary decrease in plasma HCO_3^- leading to a low plasma pH. RTA is characterized by hyperchloremic normal anion gap metabolic acidosis, and it occurs when the kidneys are unable to reclaim the filtered HCO_3^- or secrete sufficient H^+.

Mechanism for Proximal HCO3⁻ Reabsorption Most tubular reabsorption of bicarbonate occurs in the proximal tubule of the nephron. It is indirectly driven by H^+ secretion at the luminal membrane (cell membranes of the proximal tubular cells that face the tubular lumen) via Na^+/H^+ exchanger (NHE-3) and H^+-ATPase pump (not pictured in **Figure 114-1**). The intraluminal and intracellular carbonic anhydrases (CAII and CAIV) also facilitate bicarbonate reclamation. The HCO_3^- that is reclaimed/formed within the proximal tubular cells exits via the Na^+-HCO_3^- cotransporter (NBC-1) on the basolateral membrane (cell membrane that faces the blood) and is absorbed in the blood. Additionally, some HCO_3^- is also reabsorbed along the spaces in between the proximal tubular cells.

Mechanism for Distal Urinary Acidification Urinary acidification at the distal collecting tubule of the nephron is characterized by three related processes:

a. Reclamation of the remaining HCO_3^- that escapes reabsorption in the proximal tubule
b. Titration of divalent basic phosphate (HPO_4^-) to monovalent acid form ($H_2PO_4^-$), or titratable acid
c. Pairing intraluminal ammonia (NH_3) with secreted H^+ to make non-diffusible ammonium (NH_4^+)

In the distal tubule, H^+ ion secretion is mediated by the H^+-ATPase and H^+/K^+-ATPase pumps on the luminal aspect of the distal tubular cells (**Figure 114-2**). After H^+ enters the lumen, it is quickly buffered by ammonia (NH_3) and monohydrogen phosphate (HPO_4^{2-}) to form ammonium (NH_4^+) and titratable acid ($H_2PO_4^-$). The HCO_3^- formed within the cell (due to carbonic anhydrase CA II) exits via the Cl^-/HCO_3^- exchanger on the basolateral membrane.

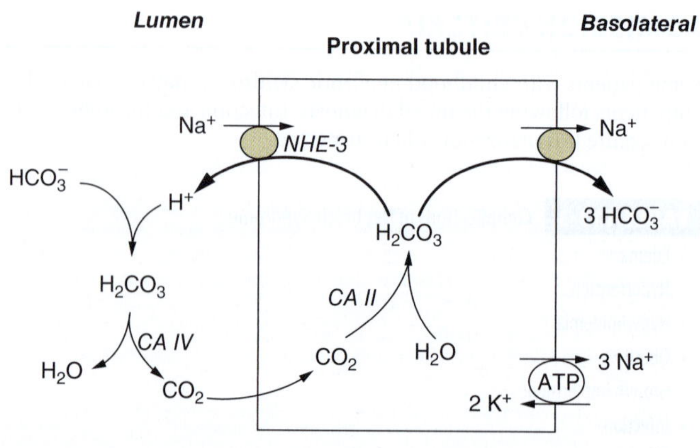

FIGURE 114-1. Bicarbonate reabsorption in the proximal tubule.

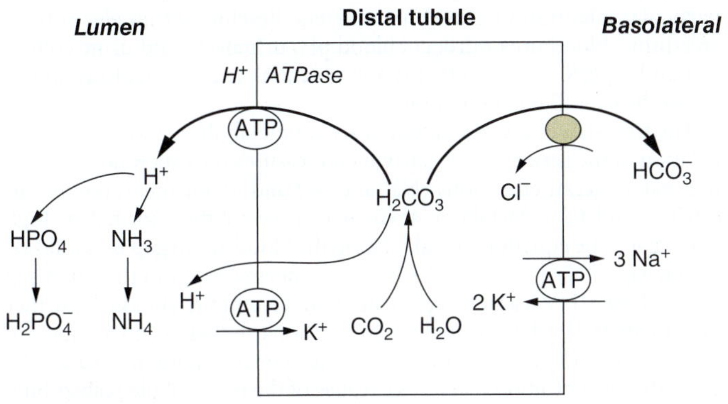

FIGURE 114-2. Distal urinary acidification.

Aldosterone also influences distal urinary acidification in following ways:

a. Enhancing Na^+ transport in the distal nephron, which favors H^+ and K^+ secretion
b. Specific localization of sodium channels (ENaC) in the apical membrane of the collecting tubular cells
c. Enhancing H^+-ATPase activity in the distal collecting tubules
d. Increasing NH_3 synthesis

In hyperkalemic, or type IV, RTA, there is a defect in the hormonal message initiating this distal acid excretion—that is, aldosterone is not sent or received correctly.

Proximal Renal Tubular Acidosis (Type II RTA) Proximal RTA is caused by a defect in HCO_3^- reabsorption in the proximal convoluted tubule, which presents as non-anion gap metabolic acidosis due to HCO_3^- wastage. There is a set point or threshold of serum bicarb concentration that regulates the amount of bicarbonate that is absorbed in the blood from the renal tubules. In older children/adults normally this setpoint keeps serum bicarbonate concentration around 22 mEq/L and 26 mEq/L, respectively. In proximal RTA, the threshold serum concentration for HCO_3^- reabsorption is reduced (to around 15 mEq/L), which leads to the delivery of excess filtered HCO_3^- to the distal nephron and urinary HCO_3^- wastage. When the lower new threshold is reached, a new steady state is achieved, and the proximal tubule begins reabsorbing bicarbonate again. The distal acidification continues to remain intact. Therefore, due to excess HCO_3^- waste in the urine, the urine remains alkaline (urine pH >5.5). Patients with proximal RTA often have hypokalemia because the increased loss of bicarbonate and sodium in the urine along with intravascular volume depletion results in increased aldosterone-mediated potassium excretion.

Distal Renal Tubular Acidosis (Type I RTA) Distal RTA can occur from an impaired H^+ secretion through decreased net activity of H^+-ATPase or H^+/K^+-ATPase pumps (secretory defect) or increased H^+ permeability of the luminal membrane (gradient defect). As a result, a lesser amount of ammonium and titratable acids are excreted, and there is a net acidosis due to the accumulation of H^+ ions. Unlike proximal RTA, the urine cannot be acidified to pH < 6.5, even in the face of severe systemic acidosis. Hypokalemia is also seen in distal RTA.

Hyperkalemic Renal Tubular Acidosis (Type IV RTA) Type IV RTA is characterized by impaired ammoniagenesis, mainly caused by aldosterone deficiency or resistance to aldosterone in the collecting ducts. Aldosterone normally promotes retention of sodium and the excretion of potassium. Aldosterone also stimulates acid excretion in two ways: a) induces the H^+-ATPase pump that secretes H^+ in the distal tubule, and b) generates the ammonia that buffers the H^+ in the collecting duct. Hypoaldosteronism causes reduced Na^+ reabsorption, which diminishes H^+ and K^+ excretion. Hyperkalemia inhibits NH_3 synthesis in the proximal tubule, further reducing renal acid excretion. Unlike type I RTA, type IV RTA maintains the ability to lower urinary pH in response to systemic acidosis. Reductions in urine NH_3 can be detected by a positive urine anion gap and a failure to increase the urine osmolal gap.

TABLE 114-1 Causes of Proximal RTA (Type II RTA)

I. Primary RTA
1. Genetic
a. Autosomal dominant
b. Autosomal recessive
2. Sporadic (usually transient)
II. Secondary RTA
1. Fanconi syndrome (phosphaturia, glycosuria, aminoaciduria, uricosuria, and proteinuria)
2. Drugs (ifosfamide, 6-mercaptopurine, valproic acid, carbonic anhydrase inhibitors, outdated tetracycline)
3. Other disease (Wilson disease, amyloidosis, hyperparathyroidism, vitamin D deficiency, tetralogy of Fallot, osteopetrosis)

CLINICAL PRESENTATION

Proximal RTA (Type II RTA) Proximal RTA can be primary (inherited) or secondary (acquired). The primary form can be either sporadic or genetically inherited in an autosomal dominant or autosomal recessive manner. The diagnosis of isolated proximal RTA is rare and typically suspected with the following clinical presentations: hypokalemia, normal anion gap metabolic acidosis, and acidic urine (pH <5.5). Proximal RTA is more often associated with Fanconi syndrome, which is characterized by urinary wastage of solutes and presents with hypophosphatemia, hypouricemia, euglycemic glycosuria, aminoaciduria, and proteinuria. The secondary forms of proximal RTA are numerous and include a variety of diseases, but most commonly proximal RTA is induced by drugs and toxins (**Table 114-1**). The prognosis of secondary proximal RTA depends on the underlying condition.

Hereditary forms of proximal RTA usually present in childhood. Autosomal recessive proximal RTA is associated with severe growth restriction leading to short stature, intellectual disability, and ocular abnormalities such as glaucoma or cataracts. The rarer autosomal dominant proximal RTA includes reduced bone density and mild growth restriction. Faltering growth, vomiting, and dehydration are prominent clinical features. Rickets and osteomalacia are observed if there is a presence of hypophosphatemia, as in Fanconi syndrome. Nephrocalcinosis and hypercalciuria are infrequent. Other manifestations, which are related to untreated hypokalemia, include polyuria, polydipsia, dehydration, vomiting, anorexia, constipation, and muscle weakness.

Distal RTA (Type I RTA) Distal RTA can also be classified as primary or acquired (i.e., secondary). In children, distal RTA is commonly a primary entity. The most common primary distal RTA among children is caused by autosomal recessive mutations in the subunit genes of H^+-ATPase and is mostly diagnosed in the infantile period of life or early childhood. Autosomal dominant primary distal RTA can be caused by mutation in the *AE1* gene encoding the basolateral Cl^-/HCO_3^- exchanger protein and presents in adolescence or adulthood. Secondary distal RTA often develops in association with systemic diseases or as a drug side effect (**Table 114-2**).

Clinical manifestations in children with distal RTA include stunted growth and polyuria, with laboratory findings of hypokalemia, hyperchloremic metabolic acidosis with normal anion gap, and hypercalciuria. Nephrolithiasis, nephrocalcinosis, and metabolic bone disease occur secondary to H^+ retention, which leads to decreased renal calcium reabsorption and increased calcium release from the bones, leading to hypercalciuria. Increased citrate reabsorption in the proximal tubules leads to hypocitraturia. Hence, hypercalciuria, hypocitraturia, and alkaline urinary pH all promote calcium phosphate precipitation (kidney stones). Clinical manifestations secondary to hypokalemia are also present. Some with the genetic form of distal RTA may also present with sensorineural deafness.

Hyperkalemic RTA (Type IV RTA) Type IV RTA is usually an acquired defect of aldosterone deficiency or relative aldosterone resistance. Children with type IV RTA are often asymptomatic but can present with muscle weakness and potentially life-threatening cardiac arrhythmias

TABLE 114-2 Causes of Distal RTA (Type I RTA)

I. Primary RTA
   1. Persistent
      a. Genetic (autosomal dominant or autosomal recessive)
      b. Sporadic
   2. Transient (in infancy)
   3. Incomplete RTA
II. Secondary RTA
   4. Genetic diseases (osteopetrosis, sickle-cell disease, Ehlers-Danlos syndrome, hereditary ovalocytosis, Wilson disease, hereditary fructose intolerance with nephrocalcinosis, primary hyperoxaluria type 1, carnitine palmitoyltransferase-1 deficiency, X-linked hypophosphatemia, congenital adrenal hyperplasia)
   5. Drugs (amphotericin B, lithium, analgesic abuse, toluene, amiloride, trimethoprim, pentamidine, vanadium)
   6. Renal disease (transplantation, tubulointerstitial disease, obstructive uropathy, pyelonephritis, nephrotic syndrome)
   7. Other disease (hyperparathyroidism, congenital adrenal hyperplasia, hypothyroidism, amyloidosis, hyperparathyroidism, vitamin D deficiency, tetralogy of Fallot)

due to hyperkalemia. In contrast to those with distal RTA, the urine in patients with type IV RTA can be acidified to less than pH 6.5 in the setting of systemic acidosis. Type IV RTA patients do not have nephrocalcinosis, nephrolithiasis, or metabolic bone disease.

Causes of type IV RTA are various, including genetic, syndromic, and medication related (**Table 114-3**). Serum levels of aldosterone and renin are the key to distinguishing among these different types.

DIFFERENTIAL DIAGNOSIS

When faced with a patient with a nongap metabolic acidosis, one must consider diarrheal illness, exogenous acid administration (e.g., hyperalimentation), ureterosigmoidostomy, and extensive pancreatic fluid drainage in addition to RTA. If there is concern about acidosis caused by metabolic compensation for primary respiratory alkalosis, arterial blood gas analysis can clarify the diagnosis. Patients with a *Proteus* urinary tract infection can appear to have RTA because their urine is alkaline secondary to the bacteria's capacity to split urea.

DIAGNOSTIC EVALUATION

The diagnosis of RTA should be considered in patients with persistent hyperchloremic metabolic acidosis with a normal anion gap. Evaluation should begin with a complete history and physical examination, paying particular attention to growth parameters. Baseline serum electrolytes, creatinine, blood urea nitrogen, blood pH, urinalysis, and urine culture should be performed to identify the potential cause of acidosis and to assess the overall renal function.

The first step in the evaluation of serum metabolic acidosis is the calculation of the serum anion gap, which measures the difference between the major measured cations (Na^+ and K^+) and major measured anions (HCO^{3-} and Cl^-). Metabolic acidosis can have either normal or high anion gap. The equation for calculating the blood anion gap is as follows: Anion gap = $[Na^+] - [HCO_3^-] + [Cl^-]$. The normal range of the anion gap is 12 ± 4 mEq/L. An anion gap greater than 18 mmol/L should be further investigated. RTA has normal anion gap because there is no addition of unmeasured anion. When the bicarbonate concentration decreases, the chloride concentration increases because of the renal tubule reabsorbing chloride to balance electrical neutrality when it absorbs sodium.

To assess the integrity of the distal urinary acidification, begin by checking the patient's urinary pH with a formal urinalysis. If the urine pH is 5.5 or higher in the presence of metabolic acidosis, the patient most likely has distal RTA (Type I RTA). A high urine pH may be secondary to urinary infection with urea-splitting organisms, which convert urea to ammonia and bicarbonate, therefore, a urinalysis and urine culture should be done, if warranted. If the urine pH <5.5, the patient could have either proximal or type IV RTA (**Figure 114-3**).

To distinguish between proximal RTA and type IV RTA, the urinary anion gap (UAG) should be calculated. UAG is an indirect index of urinary NH_4^+ concentration, and it is calculated as follows:

$$\text{Urinary anion gap} = [\text{Urinary Na}^+ + \text{Urinary K}^+] - \text{Urinary Cl}^-$$

In a state of acidosis, a normal response to bicarbonate losses is the production of ammonium in the distal tubule. Since ammonium (an unmeasured cation) accompanies chloride, any increase in $NH4^+$ excretion parallels an increase in Cl^- excretion. Thus, the UAG becomes progressively more negative as NH_4^+ excretion increases. Both distal and type IV RTA have impaired ammonium excretion in the distal tubule; therefore, they will have a positive UAG. Proximal RTA is most likely if UAG is negative. Patients with proximal RTA should also be evaluated for Fanconi syndrome with serum and urine measurements looking for renal glycosuria, phosphaturia, aminoaciduria, hypocitraturia, and hypophosphatemia. Renal ultrasonography can be used to identify nephrocalcinosis. **Table 114-4** presents the distinguishing characteristics of the different types of RTA.

MANAGEMENT

Successful treatment of RTA improves the growth of affected children and prevents the progression of nephrocalcinosis and chronic renal failure.

Acute Phase Treatment The first phase of treatment is fluid resuscitation and correction of any electrolyte abnormalities. Potassium should be normalized before alkali therapy is initiated. Replace bicarbonate over 1 to 2 days using the following formula to calculate the deficit:

$$\text{Bicarbonate deficit} = 0.5 \times \text{Body weight in kg} \times [\text{Desired HCO}_3 - \text{Measured HCO}_3]$$

Chronic Phase Treatment The treatment is typically lifelong alkali supplementation. The alkali supplementation is titrated to maintain normal serum bicarbonate levels, which usually begins with oral bicarbonate replacement at 1 to 2 mEq/kg/day of sodium bicarbonate or potassium citrate. In distal RTA, alkali therapy is often about 4 to 8 mEq/kg/day. Of all the types, proximal RTA usually requires the most alkali for successful treatment, often doses greater than 10 mEq/kg/day, due to marked bicarbonate diuresis. Occasionally, hydrochlorothiazide can be added to the regimen to decrease the alkali dose, because it enhances proximal tubule bicarbonate reabsorption. Alkali therapy also increases urinary potassium losses secondary to the increased sodium and water delivery to the distal tubule, which stimulate potassium secretion.

TABLE 114-3 Causes of Hyperkalemic RTA (Type IV RTA)

I. Primary hyperkalemic RTA
   1. Early childhood hyperkalemia (transient)
II. Secondary hyperkalemic RTA
   1. Mineralocorticoid deficiency
      a. In absence of renal disease (Addison disease, congenital adrenal hyperplasia)
      b. Hyporeninemic hypoaldosteronism in patients with chronic nephropathies (diabetic nephropathy, systemic lupus erythematosus)
      c. Hyporeninemic hypoaldosteronism in patients with acute glomerulonephritis
   2. Mineralocorticoid resistance
      a. In genetic diseases (primary pseudohypoaldosteronism type 1)
      b. In chronic interstitial nephropathies (obstructive uropathy, drug-induced interstitial nephritis)
   3. Drug-induced hyperkalemia
      a. Inhibitors of renal K^+ secretion (potassium-retaining diuretics, trimethoprim)
      b. Altered K^+ distribution (insulin antagonists, beta-adrenergic antagonists, alpha-adrenergic agonists)

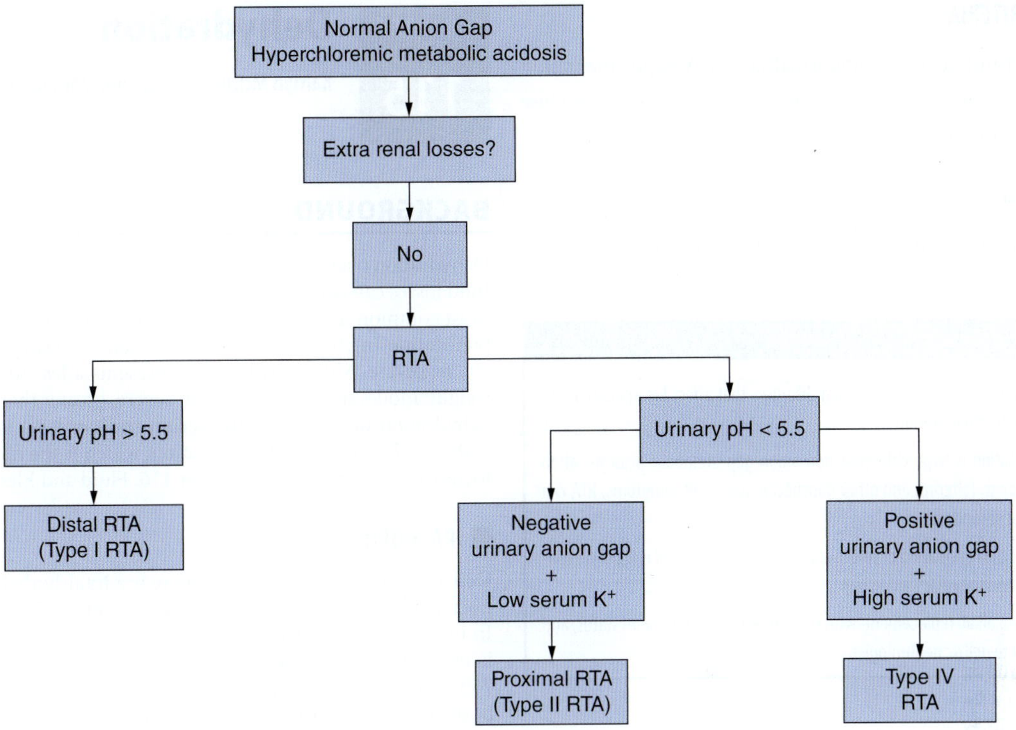

FIGURE 114-3. Flowchart for diagnostic evaluation of RTA.

Thus, potassium levels must be monitored, and potassium supplementation should be administered as needed. With appropriate therapy, the symptoms can resolve (including resolution of nephrolithiasis), and growth can improve, if treated early. The urinary calcium-to-creatinine ratio and urinary citrate-to-creatinine ratio should be followed to assess for hypercalciuria and to target the appropriate amount of alkali supplementation.

Treatment of type IV RTA is slightly different. Like other RTAs, its treatment consists of alkali therapy. However, due to hyperkalemia, treatment also involves removal of excess dietary potassium. Volume contraction should be treated, and sodium supplementation should be considered. In cases of hypoaldosteronism, mineralocorticoid therapy can be useful. For severe hyperkalemia, furosemide or potassium resins may be helpful.

ADMISSION CRITERIA

- Severe metabolic acidosis
- Severe electrolyte abnormalities
- Growth faltering with failure of outpatient management

TABLE 114-4 Summary of Distinguishing Features of RTA Types and Treatment Options

	Distal RTA (Type I)	Proximal RTA (Type II)	Hyperkalemic RTA (Type IV)
Primary defect	Decreased distal tubule acid excretion or increased H^+ membrane permeability	Decreased proximal reabsorption of HCO_3^-	Reduced excretion of acid and K^+ in the collecting duct
Symptoms	Polydipsia, polyuria, muscle weakness, nephrolithiasis, nephrocalcinosis, growth retardation, faltering growth restriction, rickets	Muscle weakness or paralysis (if severely hypokalemic), growth retardation in early childhood	Often asymptomatic, occasional muscle weakness or cardiac arrhythmia
Serum anion gap	Normal	Normal	Normal
Serum potassium	Low (<3.5 mmol/L)*	Low (<3.5 mmol/L)	High (5.5-6.5 mmol/L)
Urinary pH	>5.5	<5.5	<5.5
Urinary anion gap	Positive	Negative	Positive
Urinary ammonium	Decreased	Normal	Decreased
Nephrolithiasis	Yes	No	No
Diagnostic tests	Positive urinary anion gap after NH_4^+ loading test	pH > 7.5 after HCO_3^- loading test Glycosuria, hypophosphatemia, and hypouricemia indicate Fanconi syndrome	Urinary K^+ <40 mmol/L, abnormal serum aldosterone with near-normal renal function
Treatment			
Diet and lifestyle modifications	Increased citrus fruit and fluid intake, restricted intake of Na^+, oxalate, fructose, and animal protein	Limit acidic foods (animal protein), increase alkaline foods (fruits and vegetables)	Dietary K^+ restriction, increase alkaline foods, limit acidic foods
Pharmacotherapy	Bicarbonate supplementation, Potassium supplementation for severe hypokalemia	Alkali therapy, fluids, electrolytes, vitamin D, phosphate, hydrochlorothiazide	Low-dose fludrocortisone, loop diuretics, oral NaHCO3 for low serum HCO_3^-, K^+ binders

DISCHARGE CRITERIA

- Correction of pH and electrolyte abnormalities off IV supplementation
- Availability of correct forms and dosages of medications for outpatient use
- Assured close nephrology follow-up

CONSULTATION

A nephrologist is routinely involved in the initial evaluation, treatment decisions, and long-term follow-up.

KEY POINTS

- RTA encompasses a collection of renal tubular disorders that affect bicarbonate reabsorption and/or renal acid excretion.
- The typical presentation is hyperchloremic non-anion gap metabolic acidosis, often associated with growth faltering and other nonspecific signs and symptoms. RTA can be either primary or secondary.
- Diagnosis is based on an evaluation of serum and urinary pH levels and electrolyte concentrations in addition to urinary anion gap.
- Treatment consists of alkali replacement, with close attention to potassium status, and consultation with a pediatric nephrologist.

SUGGESTED READINGS

1. Quigley R. Chapter 39: Renal tubular acidosis. In: Avner ED, Harmon WE, Niaudet P eds. *Pediatric Nephrology*. 6th ed. Berlin: Springer; 2009:979-1002.
2. Palmer BF, Kelepouris E, Clegg DJ. Renal tubular acidosis and management strategies: A narrative review. *Adv Ther*. 2021;38: 949-968.
3. Kurtz, I. Renal tubular acidosis: H^+/Base and ammonia transport abnormalities and clinical syndromes. *Adv Chronic Kidney Dis*. 2018;25(4):334-350.
4. Soriano JR. Chapter 31: Renal tubular acidosis: The clinical entity. *J Am Soc Nephrol*. 2002;13:2160-2170.
5. Gowrishankar M, Pinsk M. Renal tubular acidosis. In: Geary DF, Schaefer F. *Comprehensive Pediatric Nephrology*. 1st ed. Philadelphia: Mosby/Elsevier; 2008:477-488.
6. Johnson V, Perelsteine E. Tubular diseases. In: Trachtman H, Gauthier B eds. *Pediatric Nephrology*. Amsterdam: Henwood Academic Publishers; 1998:231-239.
7. Zelikovic I. Chapter 18: Hereditary tubulopathies. In: Oh W, Guignard JP, Baumgart S eds. *Nephrology and Fluid/Electrolyte Physiology, Neonatology Questions and Controversies*. 2nd ed. Saunders/Elsevier; 2012:305-334.
8. Gil-Pena, H, Mejia N, Santos Fernando. Renal tubular acidosis. *J Pediatr*. 2014;691-698.
9. Bianchetti, MG, Bettinelli A. Chapter 27: Differential diagnosis and management of fluid, electrolyte, and acid-base disorder. In: Geary DF, Schaefer F. *Comprehensive Pediatric Nephrology*. 1st ed Mosby/ Elsevier; 2008:395-431.
10. Mustaqeem R, Arif A. Renal tubular acidosis. In: StatPearls [Internet]. Treasure Island (FL): StatPearls Publishing; 2022 Jan.
11. Haque SK, Ariceta G, Batlle D. Proximal renal tubular acidosis: a not so rare disorder of multiple etiologies. *Nephrol Dial Transplant*. 2012 Dec;27(12):4273-4287. doi: 10.1093/ndt/gfs493. PMID: 23235953; PMCID: PMC3616759.

CHAPTER 115 Dehydration

Kaitlyn McQuistion, MD and Margaret Rush, MD

BACKGROUND

Dehydration occurs when there is fluid loss in excess of intake. Although fluid losses can occur for different reasons, gastrointestinal losses are the most common. Dehydration is one of the most frequent reasons for hospitalization in children. Dehydration can be classified as mild, moderate, or severe. Mild dehydration represents a less than 5% loss of body weight; moderate, 5% to 10%; and severe, greater than 10%. Isonatremic dehydration occurs when the serum sodium level is between 130 and 150 mEq/L. This type of dehydration, which is the most common, is the focus of this chapter. (See Chapter 116: Fluid and Electrolyte Therapy.)

PATHOPHYSIOLOGY

Dehydration is a state in which there is a total-body fluid deficit. Under normal physiologic conditions, water constitutes 70% of lean body mass. In infants, the proportion is approximately 75%. Two-thirds of the fluid is intracellular, and one-third is extracellular. Of the extracellular fluid, 75% is interstitial and 25% is intravascular. Fluid that is lost from the body often has an electrolyte composition similar to that of plasma. Most of the fluid deficit during the early stages of dehydration is from the extracellular space, but over time, the fluid losses equilibrate, and fluid leaves the intracellular space. During the recovery phase, fluid administered to the patient is located in the extracellular space and needs time to equilibrate with the intracellular space.

CLINICAL PRESENTATIONS

INITIAL STABILIZATION

Careful attention to CABs (circulation, airway, breathing) is required for appropriate stabilization in any emergent situation. However, with dehydration, circulatory derangements are most common. In particular, it is important to identify signs of shock, which include poor peripheral perfusion, obtundation, severe tachycardia, and blood pressure changes—either narrowed pulse pressure or frank hypotension. Blood pressure changes in the pediatric population are a late sign of dehydration and often signal impending circulatory failure. Any dehydrated patient in shock should receive large amounts of isotonic fluid administered via large-bore intravenous (IV) lines in 20 mL/kg boluses. Recently published pediatric sepsis guidelines recommend 40 to 60mL/kg of fluid boluses administered over the first hour with intensive care availability. Frequent reassessment of the patient's vital signs, urine output, and physical findings can assist in determining the appropriate therapy. Even in initially stable-appearing patients, paying careful attention to early indicators of shock can avoid a precipitous deterioration in their condition.

HISTORY AND PHYSICAL EXAMINATION

Because treatment may depend on an estimation of degree of dehydration, it is important to be as accurate as possible in the history and physical examination. In the setting of acute illness (<5 days of symptoms), acute weight loss is the best indicator of the fluid deficit; each 1 kg of weight loss indicates a fluid deficit of 1 L. Unfortunately, a recent "well" weight is rarely known in children being treated for dehydration; thus, an estimate of the deficit must be made on clinical evaluation.

The history is perhaps most helpful in determining the cause of dehydration, particularly the symptoms, their duration, and what therapies have been implemented (**Table 115-1**). Of specific interest are the presence, quality, and quantity of both vomiting and diarrhea. Determining whether there has been a reduction in urine output is helpful; while decreased urination has a low positive predictive value for dehydration, a history of normal urine output is reassuring.

TABLE 115-1 Focused History

Description of the illness
- How many days has the child been sick?
- Does the child have vomiting, and if so, how many times per day?
- Does the child have diarrhea, and if so, how many times per day?
- Did the abdominal pain start before the vomiting?
- What has the urine output been?
- Who else has been ill?
- Does the child have fever?
- How has the child been eating and drinking?

Description of treatment administered
- What has been tried at home?
- How is the infant formula made?
- What other health care providers have been involved?

Past medical history
- Does the child have any cardiac, renal, gastrointestinal, endocrine or metabolic disorders?
- If yes, is the child on fluid restriction?
- Any other relevant past medical or surgical history?

Other history
- Does the family use well water?
- Was there any recent travel?
- Was there any recent antibiotic use?

Because dehydration is such a ubiquitous problem in ill children, an overall assessment of hydration status should be part of the routine physical assessment of all patients. Mild dehydration is typically not detected on physical examination. Potential markers of moderate to severe dehydration include ill appearance, prolonged capillary refill (>2 seconds), absent tears, dry mucus membranes, decreased skin elasticity, abnormal respirations, sunken eyes, sunken fontanelle, abnormal radial pulse, tachycardia, widened pulse pressures, and ultimately hypotension. Several tools exist to attempt to improve the assessment of dehydration including the Clinical Dehydration Scale (CDS), the WHO Scale, and the Gorelick Scale. Attempts to validate these tools have revealed significant limitations; however, the most support is for the CDS, which is presented in **Table 115-2**. The CDS involves assessing four clinical features (general appearance, eyes, mucous membranes, and tears) each on a 0 to 2-point scale. A score of 0 represents no dehydration, a score of 1 to 4 represents mild dehydration, and a score of 5 to 8 represents moderate to severe dehydration. Systematic review and metanalysis of the CDS performed by Falszewska et al. and Freedman et al. indicate that the CDS is helpful in identifying moderate to severe dehydration in high-resource healthcare settings.

Children with hyponatremia have a greater relative loss of extracellular fluid and may manifest more marked clinical findings for a given degree of dehydration; conversely, hypernatremia leads to relative preservation of the extracellular fluid compartment and the consequent amelioration of clinical signs.

TABLE 115-2 Clinical Dehydration Scale (CDS)

Characteristic	0	1	2
General appearance	Normal	Thirsty, restless, or lethargic but irritable when touched	Drowsy, limp, cold, sweaty +/− comatose
Eyes	Normal	Slightly sunken	Very sunken
Mucous membranes (tongue)	Moist	"Sticky"	Dry
Tears	Tears	Decreased tears	Absent tears

Clinical Dehydration Scale: score of 0 = no dehydration; score of 1-4 = mild dehydration; score of 5-8 = moderate to severe dehydration.

Source: Modified with permission from Friedman JN, Goldman RD, Srivastava R, Parkin PC. Development of a clinical dehydration scale for use in children between 1 and 36 months of age. *J Pediatr.* 2004; 145(2):201-207.

DIFFERENTIAL DIAGNOSIS

Dehydration is not a disease but rather a symptom or consequence of another process. It can be thought of as a common final pathway. The clinician must search for the cause of dehydration, which can be due to decreased intake, increased losses, or a combination of the two (**Table 115-3**). Among the myriad causes of dehydration, a few stand out. The most common cause that brings patients to medical attention is acute gastroenteritis. Decreased intake secondary to stomatitis, pharyngitis, or viral respiratory disease are also common. Although gastroenteritis is the most common cause of dehydration, it is important to remember that numerous diseases can present similarly, and the clinician will need to obtain a thorough history and examination to rule out alternative causes. Common diseases occasionally misdiagnosed as gastroenteritis include pyelonephritis, pancreatitis, lower lobe pneumonia, intussusception, and appendicitis. Vomiting without diarrhea in the correct clinical context may warrant consideration of increased intracranial pressure.

DIAGNOSTIC EVALUATION

The majority of children with uncomplicated dehydration do not require laboratory testing. A decreased serum bicarbonate concentration is often associated with dehydration; however, this usually reflects the ketoacidosis that accompanies fasting, and by itself does not determine the need for hospitalization. Measurement of serum electrolytes is indicated for children with severe dehydration or those with risk factors for hypo- or

TABLE 115-3 Causes of Dehydration

Increased Losses	Decreased Intake
Gastroenteritis* (viral or bacterial)	Gingivostomatitis*
Vomiting	Pharyngitis*
Pyloric stenosis	Febrile episode*
Pyelonephritis	Altered mental status
Increased intracranial pressure	Systemic illness (malignancy, heart failure, etc.)
Abdominal obstruction	Dependence on caregiver
Appendicitis	Restrictive eating disorder
Pancreatitis	Respiratory distress
Hepatitis	
Cholecystitis/biliary disease	
Pregnancy/Hyperemesis gravidarum	
Pelvic inflammatory disease	
Nephrolithiasis	
Cyclic vomiting syndrome	
Cannabis hyperemesis syndrome	
Purging eating disorder	
Diarrhea	
Carbohydrate or other malabsorption	
Milk/food protein allergy	
Inflammatory bowel disease	
Increased insensible losses (fever, tachypnea)	
Burns	
Diabetes insipidus	
Diabetic ketoacidosis	
Cystic fibrosis	

*The most common causes.

hypernatremia (see Chapter 116). A substantial percentage of moderate to severely dehydrated patients are also hypoglycemic, making it important to consider checking a glucose level. Bedside ultrasound evaluation of IVC:aorta ratio and urinalysis evaluation of specific gravity and/or ketones have also been explored as methods to assess dehydration severity, but current evidence does not support their routine use.

MANAGEMENT

ORAL REHYDRATION THERAPY

Oral rehydration therapy (ORT) is recommended by the American Academy of Pediatrics (AAP) and the World Health Organization (WHO) as the treatment of choice for mildly and moderately dehydrated patients. Contraindications to ORT include shock or suspected acute abdomen. Vomiting itself is not a contraindication to a trial of ORT. Because ORT can be instituted rapidly and treatment failure is typically apparent early on, it is reasonable to start with ORT and if it is unsuccessful, progress to IV fluids (**Figure 115-1**).

ORT uses the sodium-glucose cotransport mechanism to passively absorb water across the intestinal mucosa. Hence, the oral rehydration solution (ORS) should have the correct sodium-to-glucose ratio, which is optimally 1:1. Commonly used solutions include the WHO ORS packets (1:1 ratio), Rehydralyte (1:2 ratio), and Pedialyte (1:3 ratio). The proper procedure for administering ORT is shown in Figure 115-1. The aim is to replace fluid losses over 4 to 6 hours. When vomiting is a prominent part of the clinical picture, administration of small, frequent aliquots is necessary. ORT failure is defined as progression of signs of dehydration, failure to replace the deficit over 8 hours, or the presence of intractable vomiting. In a Cochrane review, Hartling et al. found that for approximately every 25 children treated with ORT, one will fail and go on to require IV fluid therapy.

Breastfed infants should continue breastfeeding during periods of mild to moderate dehydration. Once older patients are better able to tolerate oral intake, a normal diet can be reintroduced. If the gastroenteritis is severe, the brush border of the small bowel may be injured, causing a temporary secondary lactase deficiency. Lactose-free milk may be recommended for 48 hours to 1 week, depending on the severity of diarrhea, but lactose restriction is not a routine recommendation in most children.

Despite the recommendations and evidence that ORT is as effective as IV fluids for mild and moderate dehydration, in North America, especially the United States, ORT is underused in cases for which it is indicated. Work by Creedon et al. suggests that adoption of an evidence-based care pathway may improve ORT implementation, and decrease the need for IV therapy, ED length of stay, and healthcare costs.

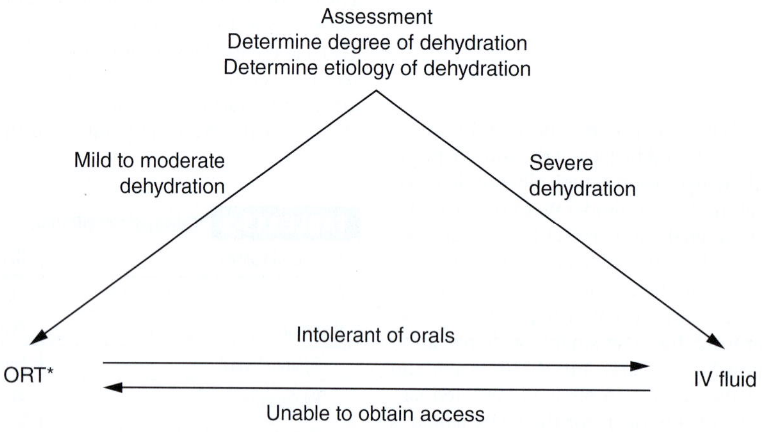

* If intolerant of orals, a nasogastric tube may be used to administer appropriate electrolyte solutions.

ORT medical personnel directions:
- ORT works via the sodium glucose cotransport mechanism.
- Utilizing the correct electrolyte solution is critical for its success.
- Choose appropriate solution:
  - Maintenance electrolyte solution (e.g., Pedialyte) as first line
  - May use 1/2.strength sports beverage (e.g., Gatorade) with saltine crackers in older patients.

Caution: Do not add juice to the Pedialyte as it alters the sodium-to-glucose concentration, which is important for fluid absorption across the GI tract.
- Calculate total volume to be administered over 4-hr rehydration phase.
  - Mild dehydration: 50 mL/kg
  - Moderate dehydration: 100 mL/kg
  - Severe dehydration: 150 mL/kg
- Calculate 5-min aliquot volume
  - (Total volume) ÷ 4 ÷ 12, i.e., 4-hr rehydration period and 12 five-min blocks in an hour
- Administer the aliquot over the 5-min period.
- Increase volume as tolerated.

ORT family directions:
- ORT is a specific treatment technique for dehydrated patients.
- A small amount of liquid is administered every few minutes with a syringe—although the child may want more, the stomach needs a chance to digest the liquid before the next syringe feed.
- If the child has been vomiting, he or she may continue to vomit.
- Please try to collect the vomit in a bucket so we can measure it.
- If it is only a small amount of vomit, we will continue.
- If it is a large amount of vomit, we may need to stop and place on IV.
- You should watch the clock and every 5 min give the syringe.
- It may be hard at first, but with a few feeds it gets much easier and the child begins to take the feeds.
- If your child refuses the feeds, then we may need to place an IV as well.
- This is a treatment that you are able to do at home to continue treating this illness as well as any future cases of dehydration that may occur.

FIGURE 115-1. Algorithm for the treatment of dehydration. GI, gastrointestinal; IV, intravenous line; ORT, oral rehydration therapy.

NASOGASTRIC FLUID THERAPY

Fluids may also be administered in children via a nasogastric (NG) tube. This is especially helpful in infants and younger children who may voluntarily withhold from drinking in the setting of illness. In children with mild to moderate dehydration, ORS may be administered via NG tube as a continuous bolus of 50 to 100 mL/kg over a 4-hour period. Maintenance fluids may also be provided via NG tube at similar rates to expected IV fluid administration. Rapid NG hydration has been found to be equally effective and to have fewer complications than rapid IV hydration in children with mild to moderate dehydration.

INTRAVENOUS FLUID THERAPY

IV fluid therapy is needed when ORT fails or is contraindicated. The WHO recommends rapid administration of 70 to 100 mL/kg of isotonic fluid over 3 to 6 hours for severe dehydration. However, others have cautioned about the risk of aggressive fluid expansion. A systematic review and metanalysis by Iro et al. found that when volumes of 20 to 60 mL/kg were administered over 1 to 2 hours versus 2 to 4 hours, there were no significant differences in outcomes. Therefore, a reasonable approach is to administer a 20 mL/kg bolus of isotonic fluid (e.g., normal saline) over 20 to 60 minutes, followed by frequent reexamination to determine the need for additional bolus administration up to a total of 60 mL/kg. At that point, additional support, such as vasopressors, should be considered for persistent hemodynamic instability.

After initial resuscitation has been achieved, isotonic fluid containing adequate dextrose and potassium concentrations can be administered at a maintenance IV fluid rate as outlined by the AAP Clinical Practice Guideline on maintenance IV fluid administration (see Chapter 116). In general, for children older than 28 days of age requiring maintenance IV fluids, 5% dextrose with normal saline and potassium chloride as clinically appropriate is the fluid of choice. Additional fluid administration should be considered to account for ongoing copious losses, either in the form of an increased rate of fluid administration (1.5-2 times maintenance) or as intermittent fluid boluses for replacement. Intermittent replacement plans should attempt to replicate the electrolyte content of the ongoing losses. IV fluids may be discontinued when clinical signs are improving, and the patient is able to take sufficient oral fluids to meet maintenance needs and ongoing losses.

SUBCUTANEOUS REHYDRATION THERAPY

A renewed interest in subcutaneous rehydration has recently come about due to the advent of a recombinant human hyaluronidase enzyme. The hyaluronidase enzyme is administered under the skin and allows fluids to be administered and rapidly absorbed into the vascular system through the capillary beds. Although this method is not common practice now, there are years of experience with the use of subcutaneous hydration in children in the era prior to IV rehydration therapy. There are a few recent industry-sponsored clinical trials by Spandorfer and Allen et al. that show ease of use and safety of the subcutaneous method with recombinant hyaluronidase. Subcutaneous therapy may be an option for mildly and moderately dehydrated children who fail ORT and need short-term isotonic fluids. It has also been found clinically to be useful as a bridge for providing fluids to a patient who will ultimately need an IV line but has poor access due to dehydration.

ANTIEMETICS

Traditionally, the routine use of antiemetics was discouraged in pediatric patients owing to the side effects of the commonly used drugs (i.e., promethazine, prochlorperazine, etc.). However, ondansetron, which selectively blocks serotonin 5-HT_3 receptors, has an acceptable side effect profile. Approximately 80% of these receptors are located in the emetic center in the brain. Ondansetron can be administered either orally or intravenously, with the orally disintegrating tablet being particularly easy to administer to children. Several studies, including those by Freedman et al. and Danewa et al., have shown that when given prior to ORT, ondansetron reduces emesis and increases the likelihood of ORT success in patients with viral gastroenteritis. Although a majority of patients stop vomiting with routine rehydration measures alone, these studies found that 20% to 30% more patients stop vomiting after ondansetron administration. Cost analysis by Freedman et al. demonstrated that administration of ondansetron early in the course is cost effective.

ADMISSION CRITERIA

- Inability to tolerate ORT due to persistent vomiting, high stool output, or inability to cooperate, requiring ongoing IV fluid therapy.
- Signs or symptoms of severe dehydration (>10% loss of body weight).
- Significant electrolyte abnormalities (see Chapter 116).

DISCHARGE CRITERIA

- Ability to maintain hydration status orally.
- Correction of abnormal electrolyte status.

CONSULTATION

Most cases of dehydration are managed solely by the pediatric hospital medicine physician. ICU consultation may be considered for patients with evidence of shock or severe electrolyte derangements.

SPECIAL CONSIDERATIONS

PREVENTION

Hand hygiene, infection control measures, food safety practices, and sanitation infrastructure are all crucial to preventing underlying infectious illnesses that often result in dehydration. Universal infant rotavirus vaccination has significantly reduced hospitalizations for gastroenteritis. Typhoid and cholera vaccines are also available for high-risk groups.

KEY POINTS

- Dehydration is one of the most common reasons for hospitalization in children.
- ORT is the treatment of choice for mildly and moderately dehydrated patients.
- Intravenous fluid therapy is needed when ORT fails or is contraindicated.
- Ondansetron reduces emesis and improves ORT success in patients with viral gastroenteritis.

SUGGESTED READINGS

Allen CH, Etzwiler LS, Miller MK, et al. Recombinant human hyaluronidase-enabled subcutaneous pediatric rehydration. *Pediatrics.* 2009;124(5):e858-e867.

American Academy of Pediatrics, Provisional Committee on Quality Improvement, Subcommittee on Acute Gastroenteritis. Practice parameter: the management of acute gastroenteritis in young children. *Pediatrics.* 1996;97:424.

Centers for Disease Control and Prevention. Managing acute gastroenteritis among children: oral rehydration, maintenance, and nutritional therapy. *MMWR.* 2003;52:1-16.

Creedon JK, Eisenberg M, Monuteaux MC, Samnaliev M, Levy J. Reduction in resources and cost for gastroenteritis through implementation of dehydration pathway. *Pediatrics.* 2020;146(1):e20191553.

Danewa AS, Shah D, Batra P, Bhattacharya SK, Gupta P. Oral ondansetron in management of dehydrating diarrhea with vomiting in children aged 3 months to 5 years: a randomized controlled trial. *J Pediatr.* 2016;169:105-9.e3.

Falszewska A, Szajewska H, Dziechciarz P. Diagnostic accuracy of three clinical dehydration scales: a systematic review. *Arch Dis Child.* 2018;103(4):383-388.

Feld LG, Neuspiel DR, Foster BA, et al. Clinical Practice Guideline: Maintenance intravenous fluids in children. *Pediatrics.* 2018;142(6):e20183083.

Fonseca BK, Holdgate A, Craig JC. Enteral vs intravenous rehydration therapy for children with gastroenteritis, a meta-analysis of randomized controlled trials. *Arch Pediatr Adolesc Med.* 2004;158: 483-490.

Freedman SB, Adler M, Seshadri R, Powell EC. Oral ondansetron for gastroenteritis in a pediatric emergency department. *N Engl J Med.* 2006;354:1698-1705.

Freedman SB, Steiner MJ, Chan KJ. Oral ondansetron administration in emergency departments to children with gastroenteritis: an economic analysis. *PLoS Med.* 2010;7(10):e1000350.

Freedman SB, Vandermeer B, Milne A, Hartling L; Pediatric Emergency Research Canada Gastroenteritis Study Group. Diagnosing clinically significant dehydration in children with acute gastroenteritis using noninvasive methods: a meta-analysis. *J Pediatr.* 2015;166(4): 908-16.e166.

Friedman JN, Goldman RD, Srivastava R, Parkin PC. Development of a clinical dehydration scale for use in children between 1 and 36 months of age. *J Pediatr.* 2004;145(2):201-207.

Gorelick MH, Shaw KN, Murphy KO. Validity and reliability of clinical signs in the diagnosis of dehydration in children. *Pediatrics.* 1997;99:e6.

Hartling L, Bellemare S, Wiebe N, Russell K, Klassen TP, Craig W. Oral versus intravenous rehydration for treating dehydration due to gastroenteritis in children. *Cochrane Database Syst Rev.* 2006; 2006(3):CD004390.

Houston KA, Gibb J, Olupot-Olupot, et al. Gastroenteritis aggressive versus slow treatment for rehydration (GASTRO): a phase II rehydration trial for severe dehydration: WHO plan C versus slow rehydration. *BMC Medicine.* 2019;17(1):122.

Iro MA, Sell T, Brown N, Maitland K. Rapid intravenous rehydration of children with acute gastroenteritis and dehydration: a systematic review and meta-analysis. *BMC Pediatr.* 2018;18(1):44.

Maitland K, Kiguli S, Opoka RO, et al. Mortality after fluid bolus in African children with severe infection. *N Engl J Med.* 2011;364(26):2483-2495.

Nager AL, Wang VJ. Comparison of nasogastric and intravenous methods of rehydration in pediatric patients with acute dehydration. *Pediatrics.* 2002;109(4):566-572.

Poonai N, Powell EC, Schnadower D, et al. Variables associated with intravenous rehydration and hospitalization in children with acute gastroenteritis: a secondary analysis of 2 randomized clinical trials [published correction appears in JAMA Netw Open. 2021;4(6):e2116800]. *JAMA Netw Open.* 2021;4(4):e216433.

Shane AL, Mody RK, Crump JA, et al. 2017 Infectious Diseases Society of America Clinical Practice Guidelines for the Diagnosis and Management of Infectious Diarrhea. *Clin Infect Dis.* 2017;65(12): 1963-1973.

Spandorfer PR. Subcutaneous hydration: updating a traditional technique. *Pediatr Emerg Care.* 2011;27(3):230-236.

Spandorfer PR, Alessandrini EA, Joffe M, et al. Oral vs intravenous rehydration of moderately dehydrated children: a randomized controlled trial. *Pediatrics.* 2005;115:295-301.

Steiner MJ, DeWalt DA, Byerley JS. Is this child dehydrated? *JAMA.* 2004;291:2746-2754.

Wathen JE, MacKenzie T, Bothner JP. Usefulness of the serum electrolyte panel in the management of pediatric dehydration treated with intravenously administered fluids. *Pediatrics.* 2004;114: 1227-1234.

World Health Organization. *The treatment of diarrhoea: a manual for physicians and other senior health workers.* 4th ed. Geneva: World Health Organization; 2005. https://apps.who.int/iris/handle/10665/43209.

World Health Organization. *Updated guideline: Paediatric emergency triage, assessment and treatment.* Geneva: World Health Organization; 2016. https://www.ncbi.nlm.nih.gov/books/NBK350528/.

CHAPTER 116

Fluid and Electrolyte Therapy

Yuliya Oumarbaeva-Malone, MD and Lana Ismail, MD

PHYSIOLOGY OF WATER AND ELECTROLYTE REGULATION

DISTRIBUTION OF WATER, CATIONS, AND ANIONS

Total body water (TBW) is distributed as follows: two-thirds in the intracellular space (ICF) and one-third in the extracellular space (ECF). Seventy-five percent of the water of the ECF is located interstitially, and 25% is located intravascularly. Sodium is the primary cation in the ECF, while chloride and bicarbonate are the primary anions. In intracellular fluid (ICF), potassium is the primary cation, while phosphate is the primary anion.

TONICITY, OSMOLALITY, AND SODIUM CONCENTRATION

Tonicity refers to the osmotic pressure gradient, while osmolarity is a measurement of the concentration of solute particles per kilogram. The body tightly regulates tonicity within an osmolality range of 275 to 290 mOsm/kg. Serum osmolality may be measured using the following formula:

$$\text{Osmolality} = 2\,[\text{Na}^+] + \text{BUN (mg/dL)}/2.8 + \text{glucose (mg/dL)}/18$$

Sodium concentration is the dominant factor in serum osmolality as it is the primary cation in ECF. In most cases the tonicity and osmolality closely align and will be used interchangeably throughout this chapter. The few notable instances when they do not align are in cases of measured high osmolality due to for example, urea, ethanol, methanol or ethylene glycol that do not translate to high tonicity. These substances freely cross the cell membrane and do not cause water shifts, and therefore they do not cause cell volume changes. In these instances, high osmolality would not translate to high tonicity.

REGULATORY MECHANISMS

The two principal regulatory factors that maintain osmolality (and indirectly, the sodium concentration) are antidiuretic hormone (ADH) and thirst.

Antidiuretic Hormone ADH is the main driver of free water excretion. It is synthesized in the supraoptic and paraventricular nuclei of the hypothalamus and stored in the posterior pituitary. Hypertonicity is the main trigger of its release, causing resorption of water by the kidney's collecting tubules. ADH is also released to a lesser extent when hypovolemia is sensed by carotid sinuses' receptors. ADH can also be released inappropriately, in a condition called the syndrome of inappropriate antidiuretic hormone (SIADH), which can be caused by stress, pain, postoperative state, malignancies, and CNS disorders. When ADH is present, urine osmolality generally ranges from 300 to 1200 mOsm/kg, and urine specific gravity is >1.010. When ADH is absent, urine osmolality ranges from 50 to 80 mOsm/kg, and urine specific gravity is <1.005. However, as specific gravity reflects the weight of particles in the urine, rather than just their number, it is not always an accurate measure of ADH action. For example, proteinuria may lead to a high urine specific gravity but a low urine osmolality.

Thirst A small rise in ECF tonicity stimulates thirst. Consequent decreased water excretion and increased water intake restore body fluid tonicity. High serum sodium and osmolality stimulate thirst and the intake of hypotonic fluids, while low serum sodium and osmolality suppress thirst.

Renin/Angiotensin/Aldosterone The renin/angiotensin system also regulates ECF volume, especially in cases of hypovolemia. Renin is produced by the juxtaglomerular cells of the kidney when they are hypoperfused. Renin stimulates angiotensin I production, which is then converted to angiotensin II by angiotensin-converting enzyme produced by the pulmonary and renal endothelium. Angiotensin II increases blood pressure by constricting the blood vessels and stimulating aldosterone secretion. Aldosterone is secreted by the adrenal cortex and acts on the distal tubules and collecting ducts to increase sodium and water resorption and potassium excretion.

Bottom-Line Summary The body has multiple mechanisms to regulate tonicity, osmolality, and indirectly, sodium concentrations. Thirst drives the body to add free water (lowering tonicity), ADH signals the kidneys to hold on to more free water (also lowering tonicity), and aldosterone signals the kidneys to retain sodium, which pulls in water with it (increasing total volume without changing tonicity).

FLUID THERAPY

PHYSIOLOGIC APPROACH TO FLUID DECISIONS

MAINTENANCE WATER REQUIREMENTS (HOLLIDAY-SEGAR METHOD)

"Maintenance" fluids are the volume required to achieve homeostasis of fluid balance on an ongoing basis. The most common approach to calculation of maintenance water requirements is the Holliday-Segar Method. This calculation is based on the basal metabolic rates and total energy requirements of healthy children. A rough estimate is 1 mL of water is needed for each kilocalorie of energy expended. Younger infants and children have higher metabolic rates and therefore require more fluids per unit of body weight than adolescents and adults. The Holliday-Segar method can be simplified and used to calculate fluids on a daily or hourly basis (**Table 116-1**). The hourly calculation is often referred to as the "4-2-1" rule. An important caveat to the Holliday-Segar Method is that it assumes the patient is healthy. Therefore, it does not account for clinical conditions that alter insensible losses (respiratory distress, prematurity, burns, other dermatologic impairment, etc.), urinary output (SIADH, diuresis, etc.), or metabolic demand (fever, paralysis, neuroleptic malignant syndrome, etc.). In such cases, fluid rates may require adjustment beyond empiric "maintenance."

MAINTENANCE SODIUM AND POTASSIUM REQUIREMENTS

The Holliday-Segar method refers only to water requirements and does not take into consideration electrolyte losses and needs. In healthy children, most electrolyte loss is through urine. An average of 3 mEq of Na^+ and 2 mEq of K^+ is lost for every 100 kcal of energy expended or 100 mL of maintenance fluid required per 24 hours. Identifying the underlying etiology of the patient's hospitalization can help guide the need for electrolyte measurement and/or replacement.

FLUID DEFICITS

The fluid deficit is the volume of fluids needed for a hypovolemic patient to become euvolemic.

The fluid deficit calculation is as follows:

Well weight – ill weight = kg of fluid lost
(remember that 1 kg = 1 L of fluid lost)

TABLE 116-1 Fluid Requirements Based on the Holliday-Segar Formula

Patient Weight	24-Hour Calculation	Hourly Calculation
3–10 kg	100 mL/kg	4 mL/kg
>10 but <20 kg	1000 mL + 50 mL/kg*	40 mL + 2 mL/kg
>20 kg	1500 mL + 20 mL/kg†	60 mL + 1 mL/kg

*This additional amount for the weight >10 kg only.

†This additional amount for the weight >20 kg only.

Source: This table has been updated according to the latest clinical practice guidelines 2018 from Feld LG, Neuspiel DR, Foster BA, et al. Clinical Practice Guideline: Maintenance Intravenous Fluids in Children. *Pediatrics.* 2018;142(6):e20183083.

If a well weight is not available, please refer to Chapter 115 which discusses how to use clinical signs to estimate a patient's level of dehydration.

ELECTROLYTE DEFICITS

Sodium deficit calculation:

$$[\text{Liters of fluid lost}] \times [\text{Percent from extracellular fluid}^*] \times [\text{measured Na}^+] = \text{Sodium deficit}$$

*In cases of acute dehydration, use 0.8. In cases of chronic dehydration, use 0.6. In acute dehydration (3 days or less), most of the fluid loss is from the ECF (80% extracellular, 20% intracellular). In chronic dehydration (longer than a 3-day period), there is greater intracellular fluid loss (60% extracellular, 40% intracellular). Intracellular fluid will move into the ECF, particularly the interstitial space, to make up for the loss of fluid in that space. Osmotic shifts start to occur, making rapid fluid replacement more dangerous. In this case, fluid replacement should be slower and more controlled.

SUMMARY OF THE PHYSIOLOGIC APPROACH

Combine the fluid deficit and electrolyte deficits with the maintenance requirements to determine the total amount of fluid and electrolytes that need to be replaced in 24 hours. Using that total volume and the total amounts of sodium and potassium needed, calculate the concentration of sodium and potassium for the patient's intravenous fluids. Then, calculate the hourly rate to administer that total volume over 24 hours. See **Table 116-2** for an example that uses this approach to calculate a patient's fluid needs. In addition, replace ongoing fluid losses 1:1 with the appropriate solution (**Table 116-3**).

EMPIRIC APPROACH TO FLUID DECISIONS

ENTERAL FLUID THERAPY

Oral rehydration is the best first therapy in uncomplicated mild and moderate dehydration (see Chapter 115). For mild dehydration, the American Academy of Pediatrics (AAP) and World Health Organization (WHO) recommend the use of oral rehydration therapy (ORT) first line, and studies have shown it is as effective as IV therapy for mild to moderate dehydration. Some studies have shown parental preference for IV therapy over nasogastric hydration, and when possible shared decision-making with the caregiver should be done.

INTRAVENOUS RESUSCITATION OF ACUTE HYPOVOLEMIA

Upon evaluation of a patient, one should first determine the degree of dehydration or hypovolemia by clinical history and physical examination to help guide rate of correction, as described in Chapter 115. It is important to identify signs of clinical shock such as hypotension and decreased organ perfusion as initial resuscitation efforts should be begun rapidly. Recent pediatric sepsis guidelines recommend that in a setting with intensive care availability, 40 to 60 mL/kg of fluid boluses should be administered over the first hour. It is important to note that after each bolus of 10 to 20 mL/kg of fluid, a focused physical examination should be performed to assess for signs of fluid overload such as development of crackles or hepatomegaly. While this may be difficult to ascertain in young children, other clinical markers such as respiratory distress or radiographic findings can help determine fluid overload and guide the need for further fluid administration.

HYPOTONIC VERSUS ISOTONIC INTRAVENOUS FLUIDS

In the past, hypotonic solutions such as 0.2 normal saline (NS) or 0.45 NS were often used as maintenance IV fluid therapy. However, over the past several years, multiple studies have highlighted the increased rates of iatrogenic hyponatremia in hospitalized patients due to such practice. As most children who are acutely ill and hospitalized display a degree of

TABLE 116-2 Example: Isonatremic Dehydration

A 7-year-old boy is admitted with a 2-day history of vomiting and diarrhea. He is estimated to be 7% dehydrated and vomited all attempts at oral rehydration in the emergency department. He was given a 20-mL/kg bolus of IV normal saline prior to transfer to the inpatient unit. His weight is 23 kg and his serum sodium level is 139 mEq/L.

	Water		Sodium	
	Calculation	Result	Calculation	Result
Maintenance				
1st 10 kg = 100 mL/kg	**10 kg** × 100 mL/kg = 1000 mL	**1560 mL**	**1560 mL** × 3 mEq/100 mL	**47 mEq**
2nd 10 kg = 50 mL/kg	**10 kg** × 50 mL/kg = 500 mL			
>20 kg = 20 mL/kg	**3 kg** × 20 mL/kg = 30 mL			
Total Fluid Deficit				
= weight × % dehydration × 1000 mL/kg or = (normal wt – dehydrated wt) × 1000 mL/kg	**23 kg** × **0.07** × 1000 mL/kg	**1610 mL**	—	—
ECF Na⁺ Deficit				
= 0.6 × total fluid deficit × 140 mEq/L	—	—	**1.61 L** × 0.6 × 140 mEq/L	**135 mEq**
Correction for Sodium Derangement				
No sodium derangement	—	—	—	—
Total Requirements	—	**3170 mL**	—	**182 mEq**
Previous Replacement	**23 kg** × **20 mL/kg**	**–460 mL**	**0.46 L** × 154 mEq/L	**–71 mEq**
Balance of Requirements	**3170 mL – 460 mL**	**2710 mL**	**182 mEq – 71 mEq**	**111 mEq**
Concentration of Saline Solution	**111 mEq ÷ 2.71 L**	**41 mEq/L**		

Note: Numbers that are in bold are specific for the patient data provided in the example.

Maintenance: This boy's maintenance water needs for the first 24 hours are 100 mL/kg for his first 10 kg of body weight (1000 mL) plus 50 mL/kg for the second 10 kg of body weight (500 mL) plus 20 mL/kg for the last 3 kg of body weight, which yields a total of 1560 mL. Only a current weight is available for this child but provides a sufficiently close approximation of his normal body weight to be used in these calculations. His daily maintenance sodium needs are 3 mEq for each 100 mL of water, or 47 mEq.

Total Fluid Deficit: This child's weight loss is used to approximate his total fluid loss. Since he is estimated to be 7% dehydrated, the weight loss can be calculated by multiplying his body weight by the estimated percent of dehydration (23 kg × 0.07). Since each kilogram of weight loss is equivalent to 1000 mL, the total fluid loss would be 1610 mL.

ECF Sodium Deficit: The sodium content of this total fluid deficit is based on the proportion of the fluid that is made up by the extracellular fluid (ECF), which is 60% of the total. The sodium concentration is normally 140 mEq/L; therefore, the sodium content in the total fluid deficit is found by multiplying this concentration by the volume of ECF deficit: (140mEq/L x 1.61 L × 0.6), which yields 135 mEq.

Correction for Sodium Derangement: Since this child is isonatremic, no additional water or sodium deficits beyond that already approximated above are expected.

Total Requirements: The total water requirements are equal to the sum of the maintenance (1560 mL) and volume of the total fluid deficit (1610 mL), which is 3170 mL. The total sodium requirements are the maintenance sodium needs (47 mEq) plus the amount of sodium in the ECF deficit volume (135 mEq), which is 182 mEq.

Previous Replacement/Balance of Requirements: This boy received a bolus of 20 mL/kg of normal saline, which provided some portion of his total water and sodium needs. The total volume of water in this saline bolus is equal to the total volume (23 kg × 20 mL/kg = 460 mL = 0.46 L). Since the concentration of normal saline solution is 154 mEq/L, the amount of sodium in that volume is 71 mEq (= 0.46 L × 154 mEq/L). These amounts of water and sodium are subtracted from the total requirements, which leaves the balances of 2710 mL of water and 111 mEq of sodium.

Concentration of Saline Solution: An appropriate concentration of intravenous saline would be 111 mEq of sodium in 2710 mL (2.71 L) of water, or 41 mEq/L. Since normal saline is 154 mEq/L, this would be proportional to approximately ¼ normal saline solution (41 mEq/L ÷ 154 mEq/L = 0.27 ≈ ¼.)

Concentration of Potassium Solution: The potassium needs are estimated by multiplying the daily maintenance potassium needs (2 mEq/100 mL) by the maintenance daily fluid requirements (1560 mL), which would be 31 mEq. This amount should be added to the balance of fluids that he will receive in the first day (2710 mL, or 2.71 L), which is equivalent to 11 mEq/L (31 mEq ÷ 2.71 L). A standard or "stock" solution that contains 10 or 20 mEq/L KCl can be used. Potassium should not be added routinely to an intravenous solution if renal failure is suspected.

Calculate the Hourly Rate and Add Glucose: The hourly rate at which the fluids should be delivered is calculated by dividing the balance of the fluids needed in the first day (2710 mL) by 24 hours, or 113 mL/hour for the first 24 hours. To provide some caloric support and to deliver a more isotonic fluid through the vein, the saline is provided in a 5% dextrose solution.

Answer: D5/¼ NS + 20 mEq/L KCl at 113 mL/hour (or D5/¼ NS + 10 mEq/L KCl at 113 mL/hour).

****NOTE: This is a calculation only, however, after the 2018 AAP Clinical Practice Guideline: Maintenance Intravenous Fluids in Children, isotonic fluid is recommended for children >28 days of age. Therefore, the ideal fluid for this child would instead be D5NS + 20 mEq/L KCl.**

Source: This table has been updated according to the latest clinical practice guidelines 2018 from Feld LG, Neuspiel DR, Foster BA, et al. Clinical Practice Guideline: Maintenance Intravenous Fluids in Children. *Pediatrics*. 2018;142(6):e20183083.

TABLE 116-3 Electrolyte Content of Various Fluids

Site	Na^+ (mEq/L)	K^+ (mEq/L)	Cl^- (mEq/L)	HCO_3^- (mEq/L)
Gastric	20–80	5–30	100–140	0
Small intestine	100–140	5–25	90–135	0
Ileostomy	45–135	3–15	20–115	110
Diarrhea	50–100	5–80	10–110	15–50

Source: This table has been updated according to the latest clinical practice guidelines 2018 from Feld LG, Neuspiel DR, Foster BA, et al. Clinical Practice Guideline: Maintenance Intravenous Fluids in Children. *Pediatrics*. 2018;142(6):e20183083.

SIADH which stops free water excretion, hypotonic solutions may further exacerbate developing hyponatremia.

In 2018, the American Academy of Pediatrics released new clinical practice guidelines recommending the use of isotonic fluids with appropriate dextrose and potassium chloride for hospitalized patients aged 28 days to 18 years for maintenance fluid use. This recommendation aims to decrease the risk of iatrogenic hyponatremia, which when unrecognized can lead to potentially devastating consequences of hyponatremic encephalopathy. Critics of the guideline note the risk of inducing hypernatremia and hyperchloremic metabolic acidosis; however, studies do not show this trend broadly. Most studies to date have shown that the adverse effect of hyperchloremia from NS is primarily seen in patients with acute shock who develop acute kidney injury.

During the establishment of the new maintenance fluid guidelines, studies reviewed primarily included those using normal saline (0.9% NaCl (NS)) or PlasmaLyte. New data especially for patients with acute sepsis have recommended the use of lactated ringer's (LR) solution as it is isotonic but with a more balanced chloride concentration (109 mEq/L Cl^- in LR vs 154 mEq/L Cl^- in NS). However, its use as maintenance therapy in the general pediatric population has yet to be established. In addition, due to calcium content in LR, it is often incompatible with various medications, requiring dual access or pause of IV hydration therapy.

VALUE OF INITIAL CHEMISTRY PANEL WHEN TREATING DEHYDRATION WITH INTRAVENOUS FLUIDS

One investigation of the utility of obtaining a chemistry panel found that 10% of these results altered clinical management in the emergency department setting (due to hypoglycemia, hypokalemia, hypernatremia, or severe acidosis). This investigation also found the treating physicians did not reliably predict which children would have clinically significant electrolyte abnormalities (58% sensitivity). Therefore, the decision to obtain initial chemistry panel should rely on a thorough physical examination and critical history taking.

BOTTOMLINE SUMMARY

The degree and method of rehydration should be guided by the degree of dehydration and physical examination findings. If signs of shock or sepsis are identified, it is important to aggressively resuscitate with 40 to 60 mL/kg of isotonic fluids within the first hour with multiple repeat exams to monitor for fluid overload. When choosing maintenance fluid therapy, current clinical guidelines recommend that isotonic fluids be used to avoid iatrogenic hyponatremia. IV fluid therapy is not benign and should be discontinued once fluid balance is restored and the patient can be transitioned to oral fluid hydration.

ELECTROLYTE DISORDERS

HYPONATREMIA (TOO MUCH WATER, COMPARED WITH SODIUM)

Background Hyponatremia is defined as serum sodium less than 135 mEq/L. Hyponatremia is usually caused by sodium loss in excess of free water loss. It is important to note that the serum sodium concentration does not accurately reflect total body sodium; rather, hyponatremia reflects a relative excess of free water. To determine the cause and treatment of hyponatremia, three factors are most important: the patient's volume status, urine sodium, and urine osmolality.

Before beginning therapy, it is important to determine whether true (hypotonic) hyponatremia is present. Pseudohyponatremia exists when serum is either isotonic (as in severe hyperlipidemia or hyperproteinemia) or hypertonic (as in hyperglycemia). In isotonic pseudohyponatremia caused by hyperlipidemia or hyperproteinemia, the volume of lipid or protein displaces plasma water so that a smaller volume of sodium-containing plasma is measured. In hypertonic or "dilutional" hyponatremia, hyperglycemia causes fluid to shift into the vascular space such that a decrease in serum Na^+ of 1.6 mEq/L occurs for every 100 mg/dL elevation in serum glucose (e.g., a serum glucose concentration of 800 results in a sodium concentration of 124: $800 - 100 = 700$, $1.6 \times 7 = 11$, $135 - 11 = 124$).

True hyponatremia (Na^+ <130 mEq/L) occurs when serum is hypotonic. True hyponatremia may be associated with changes in TBW and categorized as hypovolemic, euvolemic, or edematous.

Hypovolemic hyponatremia (or dehydration) occurs in the face of sodium and total fluid loss such as from diarrhea, excessive sweating, renal salt wasting, or excessive diuretics. The body responds with increased ADH secretion leading to increased free water retention, thereby dropping the sodium concentration. This is the most common cause of hyponatremia in children.

Euvolemic hyponatremia results from SIADH, psychogenic polydipsia, or inadequate sodium intake. Hyponatremia associated with euvolemia is most commonly seen in SIADH secretion, which may be due to glucocorticoid deficiency, hypothyroidism, stress (especially pain in the postoperative period), drugs (including selective serotonin reuptake inhibitors, antineoplastic agents, and anticonvulsants), or positive-pressure ventilation. Further, some of the most common pediatric diagnoses resulting in hospitalization, such as bronchiolitis, pneumonia, meningitis, and various febrile inflammatory states, have a degree of inappropriate ADH release during the acute stress period.

Hyponatremia with edema exists when renal mechanisms inappropriately conserve excessive sodium and water, such as in congestive heart failure or nephrotic syndrome. This may be due to acute or chronic renal failure, or due to decreased effective circulating blood volume because of decreased cardiac output (congestive heart failure) or decreased oncotic pressure (cirrhosis or nephrotic syndrome).

Clinical Presentation Patients with mild hyponatremia (serum Na^+ 134-130mEq/L) are generally asymptomatic. Those with moderate hyponatremia (serum Na^+ 129-120mEq/L) can experience muscular weakness, headaches, lethargy, ataxia, and psychosis due to fluid shifts from hypotonicity. Severe hyponatremia (serum Na^+ <120mEq/L) leads to increased intracranial pressure from cerebral edema presenting with nausea, vomiting, and sometimes seizures, coma, tentorial herniation, respiratory depression, and death.

Diagnostic Evaluation Volume status is diagnosed from either known weight change or clinical criteria, as discussed above. In determining the cause of hyponatremia, supportive lab data include the urine osmolarity and urine sodium concentration.

Hypovolemic hyponatremia is characterized by urine osmolality greater than 100 mOsm/kg (threshold between maximally dilute and concentrated urine). If urine Na^+ is less than 20 mEq/L, hyponatremia is due to extrarenal losses such as vomiting and diarrhea. If urine Na^+ is greater than 20 mEq/L, renal losses may occur as a result of diuretics, mineralocorticoid deficiency, salt-losing nephropathy, bicarbonaturia, ketonuria, or osmotic diuresis.

In **euvolemic hyponatremia** due to SIADH, urine osmolality is greater than 100 mOsm/kg and urine Na^+ is greater than 20 mEq/L. Euvolemic hyponatremia with urine osmolality less than 100 mOsm/kg is due to water intoxication.

When there is **hyponatremia with edema**, urine osmolality is greater than 100 mOsm/kg. In renal failure, urinary sodium is >20 mEq/L. In cases of decreased cardiac output (congestive heart failure) or decreased oncotic pressure (cirrhosis or nephrotic syndrome), the urinary sodium is <20 mEq/L.

Management • *Emergency Treatment of Hyponatremia* Patients with severe acute hyponatremia (Na^+ usually <120 mEq/L) can present with generalized seizure activity or coma. In such instances, raising Na^+ by 5 mEq/L (over 6 hours) or increasing the serum sodium level above 125 mEq/L will typically improve symptoms. Note that this rate of rapid correction of sodium is reserved only for patients presenting with seizure activity or coma. The initial treatment of symptomatic severe acute hyponatremia is hypertonic (3%) saline, which has 513 mEq/L of sodium. In general, administration of 1 mL/kg of hypertonic (3%) saline raises serum Na^+ by approximately 1 mEq/L. The initial dose of hypertonic saline is 2 to 5 mL/kg administered over 20 minutes to treat hyponatremic seizures. This dose can be repeated up to twice more as needed to stop the hyponatremic seizure, with a goal correction of 4 to 6 mEq/L Na^+ over the first 1 to 4 hours of symptoms.

Importantly, the duration of hyponatremia plays a large role in the possible sequelae from rapid sodium correction. Chronic hyponatremia (>48 hours) has a much higher risk of osmotic demyelination syndrome when sodium is corrected too rapidly, and therefore the goal sodium correction has been listed anywhere from <8 mEq/L/24 hours for chronic hyponatremia and up to 10 to 12 mEq/L/24 hours for acute hyponatremia. Osmotic demyelination syndrome (which encompasses central pontine myelinolysis and extrapontine myelinolysis) occurs due to osmotic stress to the brainstem and is characterized by encephalopathy sometimes accompanied by seizures, dysphagia, ataxia, spastic quadriparesis, and in severe cases, a persistent "locked in" neurologic state. It often presents anywhere from one day to two weeks after sodium is corrected. Once hyponatremic seizures are controlled, treatment should transition from rapid correction to slow correction of sodium.

Hyponatremia With Hypovolemia Treatment should always be guided by the attempt to correct the underlying condition (diarrhea, vomiting, osmotic diuresis) and administration of isotonic fluid until the intravascular volume is normalized. This clinical scenario is caused by increased ADH that was triggered by hypovolemia. Since ADH has a short half-life (about 10-15 min), volume repletion with isotonic fluid rapidly corrects the sodium level in this setting, and water restriction is not necessary.

In hyponatremic dehydration, aside from the sodium and water deficit that would be expected with isonatremic dehydration, an additional amount of sodium must be given to correct the sodium deficit. The following formula is used to calculate the additional sodium deficit that occurs:

$$0.6 \times \text{Wt} \times (\text{Desired Na}^+ - \text{Current Na}^+)$$

The "desired" sodium should be no more than 12 to 14 mEq/L above the current sodium level so that a rapid shift in fluid does not ensue. Electrolytes should be monitored closely until serum sodium is in the 130 mEq/L range.

Example: See **Table 116-4** for an example of fluid calculations for hyponatremic hypovolemia.

Hyponatremia With Euvolemia Treatment should be focused on the underlying disease. Fluid restriction and administration of NS and a loop diuretic may be indicated.

Fluid Restriction Due to insensible losses and obligatory excretion of water in the urine, the serum sodium will increase if the amount of water ingested is less than the amount of water excreted.

Loop Diuretics Loop diuretics (furosemide, bumetanide, torsemide) increase urinary free water excretion. They need to be used along with water restriction, because they indirectly increase ADH release and thirst. If patients are allowed free access to water, the sodium level will not improve. Loop diuretics should not be administered to patients with volume depletion.

ADH-Antagonists These include demeclocycline and lithium carbonate. Clinical data on their effectiveness in management of pediatric hyponatremia are limited. Tolvaptan and conivaptan are expensive, do not improve mortality in adults with hyponatremia, and pediatric drug safety data are limited.

Hyponatremia With Edema In addition to treating the underlying disorder, hyponatremia is treated by sodium and fluid restriction and possibly the use of a loop diuretic or an angiotensin-converting enzyme inhibitor.

HYPERNATREMIA (NOT ENOUGH WATER, COMPARED WITH SODIUM)

Background and Pathophysiology Hypernatremia is defined as serum sodium more than 150 mEq/L. It may result from excessive free water loss with low total body sodium, from water loss with normal total body sodium, or from increased TBW and sodium. Hypernatremic (or hypertonic) dehydration occurs when sodium and water are lost but there is excess loss of free water, or when volume losses are replaced with inadequate free water. Young infants and cognitively impaired children who are unable to obtain free water in response to thirst stimulus are at particular risk. Breastfeeding failure has been associated with hypernatremic dehydration in the newborn. Hypernatremia secondary to water loss with normal total body sodium is due to inadequate secretion of ADH by the posterior pituitary gland (central diabetes insipidus) or inappropriate response to ADH by the renal collecting tubule to reabsorb water (nephrogenic diabetes insipidus). Central diabetes insipidus occurs more commonly and is idiopathic or autoimmune in at least 30% of cases. It can also be due to injury or destruction of the hypothalamus or posterior pituitary from meningitis or tumor (craniopharyngioma, histiocytosis X) and less commonly due to cerebral midline defects or to genetic defects in ADH synthesis and release. Nephrogenic diabetes insipidus may be due to a genetic defect in the membrane receptor protein. It may also be acquired as a result of an illness or insult that damages the renal medulla, such as from medication, obstructive uropathy, or electrolyte disturbances, including hypokalemia and hypercalcemia. Infants with nephrogenic diabetes insipidus are polyuric and also may have unexplained fever, irritability, vomiting, or lethargy in association with hypernatremic dehydration. Hypernatremia with edema means that there is increased total body sodium and an increase in TBW. The cause is usually iatrogenic and due to excessive administration of hypertonic dialysis fluid, $NaHCO_3$ or NaCl, or saline for therapeutic abortion. Primary hyperaldosteronism and Cushing syndrome are rare causes of edema and hypernatremia in childhood.

Clinical Presentation Hypernatremia generally equates with hypertonicity, causing water to move out of cells, leading them to shrink. When brain cells shrink, serious neurologic complications can occur, such as seizure, coma, cerebrovascular hemorrhage, and death. Cerebrovascular hemorrhage can occur secondary to ischemia from blood vessel sludging or from tension on bridging vessels from the shrinking brain. Less severe clinical signs of hypernatremia include hyperpnea, muscle weakness, restlessness, a high-pitched cry, and lethargy. If the increased tonicity occurs less acutely (over days or weeks), neurologic complications from the hypertonicity are much less likely. Brain cells adapt by taking up "osmolytes," causing water to move back into cells and restoring cell volume.

In hypernatremic dehydration the skin may feel "doughy." In addition, in contrast to patients with hyponatremic dehydration, patients with hypernatremic dehydration may have less prominent signs and symptoms of dehydration because circulating blood volume is preserved.

Diagnostic Evaluation As with hyponatremia, the first step is to determine the patient's volume status. The cause of hypernatremic dehydration can be narrowed down by examining the urine sodium concentration. Renal losses from osmotic diuresis (such as from glucose, mannitol, or urea) result in urine Na^+ more than 20 mEq/L. Extrarenal losses caused by vomiting and diarrhea, excessive sweating, or breastfeeding failure result in urine Na^+ less than 20 mEq/L. The diagnosis of diabetes insipidus is made by finding an inappropriately low urine osmolality (specific gravity <1.005, urine osmolarity of 50-200) with a low serum ADH level in the face of increased serum osmolality after a period of water deprivation. Diabetes insipidus can also result in hyperosmolar dehydration if the patient is unable to drink enough to compensate for deficient levels of ADH. Hypernatremia with edema is marked by urine Na^+ greater than 20 mEq/L.

Management • ***Hypernatremic Dehydration*** The goal of treatment is to avoid cerebral edema or herniation by decreasing serum sodium slowly, by a maximum rate of 0.5 mEq/L/h. While in the past, acute hypernatremia (< 24 hours) was corrected with a higher sodium correction goal of up to 1 mEq/L/hr, now this is less commonly practiced given more studies showing higher rates of cerebral edema or seizures in these cases. Patients with chronic onset of hypernatremia especially need slower correction because they are particularly vulnerable to the risk of cerebral edema and herniation (due to the presence of brain cells' adaptive osmolytes). Patients with a serum sodium concentration higher than 170 mEq/L should be managed in an intensive care unit (ICU) setting for close monitoring of electrolytes and cardiovascular and neurologic status.

Management of hypernatremic dehydration involves determination of hydration status, correction of free water deficit in addition to solute fluid deficit, and providing hydration to cover maintenance needs and ongoing losses. The free water deficit is calculated as follows:

$$(\text{Current Na}^+ - \text{Desired Na}^+) \times 4 \text{ mL/kg} \times \text{Patient weight (in kg)}$$

In this formula, it is estimated that it takes 4 mL/kg of free water to decrease serum Na^+ by 1 mEq/L, and the desired sodium is generally 145 mEq/L to prevent overly rapid correction.

Example: See **Table 116-5** for an example of fluid calculations for hypernatremic hypovolemia.

Generally, half of the free water deficit, along with all the maintenance and solute deficit, is administered in the first 24 hours. Although the formula for calculating the free water deficit is a good general starting point, the rate of decrease in serum sodium is not predictable. No formula can replace frequent reassessment of the patient's sodium level and mental status. It is important to check electrolytes frequently (every 2-4 hours initially) to be sure that the sodium level does not drop too quickly (a rate of decrease no greater than 0.5 mEq/L per hour).

TABLE 116-4 Example: Hypovolemic Hyponatremia

A 10 month-old girl is admitted with a 5-day history of vomiting, diarrhea, and now mild encephalopathy. Her weight is 1 kg less than baseline, currently at 8 kg, and she vomited all attempts at oral rehydration in the emergency department. She was given a 20-mL/kg bolus of IV normal saline prior to transfer to the inpatient unit. Her serum sodium level is 122 mEq/L.

	Water		Sodium	
	Calculation	**Result**	**Calculation**	**Result**
Maintenance 1st 10 kg = 100 mL/kg 2nd 10 kg = 50 mL/kg >20 kg = 20 mL/kg	**9 kg** × 100 mL/kg	**900 mL**	**900 mL** × 3 mEq/100 mL	**27 mEq**
Total Fluid Deficit = weight × % dehydration × 1000 mL/kg or = (normal wt – dehydrated wt) × 1000 mL/kg	**(9 kg – 8 kg)** × 1000 mL/kg	**1000 mL**	—	—
ECF Na⁺ Deficit = 0.6 × total fluid deficit × 140 mEq/L	—	—	**1 L** × 0.6 × 140 mEq/L	**84 mEq**
Correction for Sodium Derangement Sodium deficit: = (desired Na⁺ – current Na⁺) × wt × 0.6	—	—	**(134 – 122)** × **9 kg** × 0.6	**65 mEq**
Total Requirements	—	**1900 mL**	—	**176 mEq**
Previous Replacement	**9 kg** × **20 mL/kg**	**–180 mL**	**0.18 L** × 154 mEq/L	**–28 mEq**
Balance of Requirements	**1900 mL – 180 mL**	**1720 mL**	**183 mEq – 28 mEq**	**148 mEq**
Concentration of Saline Solution	**148 mEq ÷ 1.72 L**	**86 mEq/L**		

Note: Numbers that are in bold are specific for the patient data provided in the example.

Maintenance: This child's maintenance water needs for the first 24 hours are 100 mL/kg for each of her 9 kg of body weight, or 900 mL. Her maintenance sodium needs for this time period are 3 mEq for each 100 mL of water, or 27 mEq.

Total Fluid Deficit: Her total fluid deficit is calculated by the difference between her pre-illness weight (9 kg) and her weight at the time she presented with dehydration (8 kg), which is 1 kg. This indicates that she is 11% dehydrated, i.e., 1 kg is 11% of her pre-illness weight (9 kg). If a pre-illness weight were not available, estimates of degree of dehydration would be made based on physical findings (see Chapter 57). Since each 1000 mL weighs 1 kg, her total fluid deficit is 1000 mL.

ECF Sodium Deficit: The sodium content of this total fluid deficit is based on the proportion made up by her extracellular fluid (ECF) compartment, which is 60% of the total fluid deficit. The sodium concentration in the ECF is normally 140 mEq/L; therefore, this little girl's estimated sodium deficit is the product of her ECF deficit (expressed in liters) and the normal sodium concentration, or 84 mEq.

Correction for Sodium Derangement: However, this child is hyponatremic; therefore, she has an additional sodium deficit, beyond that already approximated above. The additional sodium deficit is estimated by the difference between her current serum sodium level and her desired serum sodium level for her whole body ECF compartment. The whole body ECF volume is 60% of the total body weight. Rather than target a complete correction of her serum sodium level, a desired sodium level 12 mEq/L higher than her current level, or 134 mEq/L, is used. Therefore, the sodium deficit is calculated by multiplying her ECF volume (body weight × 0.6) by the difference between her desired and current serum sodium level. For this example, the sodium deficit would be 65 mEq.

Total Requirements: The maintenance water (900 mL) and total fluid deficit (1000 mL) are added to determine the total water requirements for the first 24 hours (1900 mL). The total sodium requirements are the sum of the maintenance sodium needs (27 mEq), the amount of sodium in the ECF deficit (84 mEq), and the additional sodium deficit due to her hyponatremia (65 mEq), which is 176 mEq.

Previous Replacement/Balance of Requirements: However, her initial resuscitation included 20 mL/kg of normal saline. This provided her with 180 mL of water and 28 mEq of sodium, which are subtracted from the total needs. This leaves the balances of water and sodium needed in the first 24 hours of 1720 mL and 148 mEq, respectively.

Concentration of Saline Solution: If a saline solution containing the proportions of salt and water from the balance of requirements were prepared, it would yield a saline concentration of 79 mEq/L. Since normal saline is 154 mEq/L, this would be approximately equivalent to a ½ normal saline solution.

Concentration of Potassium Solution: The potassium needs are approximated by multiplying the daily maintenance potassium needs (2 mEq/100 mL each day) by the maintenance fluid requirements (900 mL), which yields 18 mEq/day. This amount should be added to the balance of fluids that she will receive in the first 24 hours (1720 mL, or 1.72 L), which is equivalent to 10 mEq/L (18 mEq ÷ 1.72 L = 10 mEq/L). Potassium should not be added routinely to intravenous solutions if renal failure is suspected.

Calculate the Hourly Rate and Add Glucose: To provide some caloric support, the saline is provided in a 5% dextrose solution. The total volume should be delivered over 24 hours, so one would divide 1720 mL by 24 hours to provide a rate of 72 mL/hour.

Answer: D5/½ NS + 10 mEq/L KCl to run at 72 mL/hour. For patients with hyponatremia secondary to excessive renal sodium loss, the underlying disorder should be corrected if possible. Mineralocorticoid supplementation should be given for deficient states such as congenital adrenal hyperplasia. Long-term oral sodium supplementation is often needed if the underlying defects cannot be completely corrected.

****NOTE: This is a calculation only, however, after the 2018 AAP Clinical Practice Guideline: Maintenance Intravenous Fluids in Children, isotonic fluid is recommended for children >28 days of age. Therefore, the ideal fluid for this child would instead be D5NS + 20 mEq/L KCl.**

Source: This table has been updated according to the latest clinical practice guidelines 2018 from Feld LG, Neuspiel DR, Foster BA, et al. Clinical Practice Guideline: Maintenance Intravenous Fluids in Children. *Pediatrics*. 2018;142(6):e20183083.

Diabetes Insipidus Primary treatment is to administer free water. Inadequate endogenous ADH may be treated by replacement with desmopressin (DDAVP), a synthetic analogue. DDAVP is given as a nasal spray, orally, or intravenously/subcutaneously as replacement therapy for central diabetes insipidus. Patients with nephrogenic diabetes insipidus may benefit from the addition of a thiazide diuretic in combination with a potassium-sparing diuretic. Typical agents used are hydrochlorothiazide plus amiloride. NSAIDs have also been used to inhibit the prostaglandin effect of ADH antagonism. Children with non-hereditary nephrogenic DI sometimes have partial resistance to desmopressin and thus desmopressin may also be administered. Patients without a thirst mechanism must be monitored extremely carefully, as they will be unable to alert the provider to an imbalance of water intake and urinary losses.

TABLE 116-5 Example: Hypernatremic Dehydration

An 8-month-old boy is admitted with a 4-day history of vomiting and diarrhea. He is currently 6.2 kg, down from his baseline of 7 kg, and he vomited all attempts at oral rehydration in the emergency department. He was given a 20-mL/kg bolus of IV normal saline prior to transfer to the inpatient unit. His serum sodium level is 155 mEq/L.

	Water		Sodium	
	Calculation	Result	Calculation	Result
Maintenance 1st 10 kg = 100 mL/kg 2nd 10 kg = 50 mL/kg >20 kg = 20 mL/kg	**7 kg** × 100 mL/kg	**700 mL**	**700 mL** × 3 mEq/100 mL	**21 mEq**
Total Fluid Deficit = weight × % dehydration × 1000 mL/kg or = (normal wt – dehydrated wt) × 1000 mL/kg	**(7 kg – 6.2 kg)** × 1000 mL/kg	**800 mL**	—	—
ECF Na⁺ Deficit = total fluid deficit × 0.6 × 140 mEq/L		—	**0.8 L** × 0.6 × 140 mEq/L	**67 mEq**
Correction for Sodium Derangement Free water deficit = (current Na⁺ – desired Na⁺) × wt × 4 mL/kg	**(155** – 145) × **7 kg** × 4 mL/kg (Divide this number by 2 for the amount of free water deficit to be corrected in the first 24 hours)	**140 mL**	—	—
Total Requirements		**1640 mL**		**88 mEq**
Previous Replacement		**0**		**0**
Balance of Requirements		**1640 mL**		**88 mEq**
Concentration of Saline Solution	**88 mEq** ÷ **1640 L**	**54 mEq/L**		

Note: Numbers that are in bold are specific for the patient data provided in the example.

Maintenance: For this 7-kg boy, his maintenance water needs are 10 mL/kg for each of his 7 kg of body weight, or 700 mL each day. His maintenance sodium needs for this time period are 3 mEq for each 100 mL of water, or 27 mEq/day.

Total Fluid Deficit: The difference between his pre-illness weight (7.0 kg) and his weight at the time of presentation (6.2 kg) indicates the total fluid deficit, which is 0.8 kg, or equivalent to 800 mL.

ECF Sodium Deficit: Despite the fact that this child is hypernatremic, he still has a sodium deficit due to fluid losses from the ECF, which makes up 60% of the total fluid deficit. The sodium content of this total fluid deficit is calculated by multiplying the ECF proportion of the total fluid deficit (0.6 × 800 mL) by the sodium concentration of the ECF (approximately 140 mEq/L), which yields 67 mEq/L.

Correction for Sodium Derangement: However, this boy's hypernatremia is caused by an additional loss of free water, which needs to be replaced. The amount of free water is calculated based on the difference between the current serum sodium level and the desired serum sodium (155 – 145), which is multiplied by a factor of 4 mL/kg and the patient's weight. Since corrections of hypernatremia should proceed more slowly, only half of the estimated free water deficit is replaced in the first 24 hours, which yields a result of 140 mL.

Total Requirements: The water and sodium requirements are totaled, which indicated that this patient should receive 1640 mL of water and 88 mEq of sodium in the first 24 hours.

Previous Replacement/Balance of Requirements: In this example, the patient did not receive a normal saline bolus or any other replacement therapy, so the balance of water and sodium requirements are the same as for the total requirements.

Concentration of Saline Solution: If the sodium requirements were mixed in the amount of water required, it would yield a saline solution containing 54 mEq/L, which is equivalent to ⅓ normal saline solution. To avoid the risk of correcting the serum sodium level too quickly, i.e., more than 0.5 mEq/L per hour, most clinicians would select a stock solution of ½ normal saline for this patient.

Concentration of Potassium Solution: As previously calculated, the potassium needs are estimated by multiplying the daily maintenance potassium needs (2 mEq/100 mL each day) by the maintenance fluid requirements (700 mL), which yields 14 mEq/day. This amount should be added to the total fluids that this boy will receive in the first 24 hours (1640 mL), which is equivalent to 9 mEq/L (14 mEq ÷ 1640 mL = 8.5 mEq/L). A standard solution that contains 10 mEq/L of KCl can be used. Potassium should not be added routinely to intravenous solutions if renal failure is suspected.

Calculate the Hourly Rate and Add Glucose: To provide some caloric support, the saline solution is provided with 5% dextrose solution. The total volume should be delivered over 24 hours, so one would divide 1640 mL by 24 hours to provide a rate of 68 mL/hour.

Answer: D5/½ NS + 10 mEq/L KCl to run at 68 mL/hour.

Subsequent Therapy: The entire deficit of ECF, along with half of the additional free water deficit, is replaced during the first 24 hours. The remaining free water deficit is then replaced over the next 24 hours. For this period, the maintenance needs remain the same: 700 mL of water, 21 mEq of sodium, and 14 mEq of potassium per day. Adding the 140 mL of free water yields a total of 840 mL of water with 21 mEq of sodium, or 25 mEq/L, which is equivalent to ¼ normal saline with 17 mEq/L of potassium. A stock solution of D5¼ normal saline with 10 or 20 mEq/L of KCl may be used at a rate of 35 mL/h (840 mL ÷ 24 hours).

Source: This table has been updated according to the latest clinical practice guidelines 2018 from Feld LG, Neuspiel DR, Foster BA, et al. Clinical Practice Guideline: Maintenance Intravenous Fluids in Children. *Pediatrics*. 2018;142(6):e20183083.

Hypernatremia with Edema Treatment is a loop diuretic along with administration of free water.

DISORDERS OF POTASSIUM

Background and Pathophysiology Ninety-five percent of total body potassium is intracellular, mostly in muscle cells, in a concentration of 150 mEq/L. Most (90%) potassium is excreted in urine under normal conditions. Renal excretion of potassium is very efficient, but unlike sodium, conservation is not efficient, and occurs only in states of extreme deprivation. Aldosterone plays a critical role in potassium secretion in the distal tubule in exchange for sodium or hydrogen ions, or both. Delivery of sodium to the distal tubule for resorption is necessary for normal potassium excretion.

Most conditions resulting in dehydration cause depletion of total body potassium and sodium. Because potassium is an intracellular cation, serum potassium represents only 2% of total body potassium. A general principle regarding potassium therapy is to avoid instituting K^+ repletion until a patient has established urine output. Also, ideally one would not exceed 4 mEq/kg/day of K^+ repletion. The potassium requirement for maintenance fluid in a patient with normal body potassium is approximately 2 mEq/100 kcal or per 100 mL of fluid. In practice, giving a patient 10 to 20 mEq/L of fluid provides adequate maintenance potassium.

HYPERKALEMIA

Definition Hyperkalemia is defined as serum K^+ greater than 5.5 mEq/L. Moderate to severe hyperkalemia (K^+ >6.1 to 6.9 mEq/L) is potentially life threatening because high serum potassium disrupts the normal cellular conduction system. True hyperkalemia (**Table 116-6**) most commonly results from a decrease in potassium excretion in the kidney or redistribution of potassium from the intracellular to the ECF. Shifts in potassium from the intracellular to the ECF, as in metabolic acidosis or with nonselective beta-blockers, can lead to an increase in serum potassium, although total body potassium is normal. Extreme and rapid cellular destruction can overwhelm the kidney's ability to excrete the increased potassium load.

Pseudohyperkalemia, or falsely elevated potassium level, is usually due to inappropriate specimen collection, such as squeezing a digit too strenuously when obtaining a finger-stick blood draw, which causes the blood collected to be hemolyzed and release potassium from red blood cells. Severe leukocytosis greater than 70,000/cm^3 or thrombocytosis greater than 1,000,000/cm^3 may also result in pseudohyperkalemia.

Clinical Presentation Within the muscular system, hyperkalemia causes skeletal muscle weakness, and smooth muscle inhibition can cause respiratory depression. Most seriously, disruption of the cardiac conduction system can lead to cardiac arrhythmias and ultimately to cardiac arrest. Electrocardiographic manifestations include peaked T waves, prolongation of the PR interval, and widening of the QRS complex.

TABLE 116-6 Causes of Hyperkalemia

Decrease in K^+ Excretion
Acute or chronic kidney disease
Aldosterone deficiency: Addison disease or congenital adrenal hyperplasia
Drugs
Potassium-sparing agents
Angiotensin-converting enzyme inhibitors
Nonsteroidal anti-inflammatory drugs
Miscellaneous (trimethoprim-sulfamethoxazole, heparin, pentamidine, alpha- and beta-blockers)
Increase in K^+ Load: Cellular Destruction
Ingestion of a K^+-rich diet
Tumor lysis syndrome
Rhabdomyolysis
Trauma
Intravascular hemolysis
Transfusion of stored red blood cells
Catabolic states
Redistribution of K^+
Metabolic acidosis
Infusion of hypertonic solution
Hyperkalemic periodic paralysis
Nonselective beta-blockers
Tubular Unresponsiveness to Aldosterone
Sickle cell anemia
Systemic lupus erythematosus
Amyloidosis
Renal transplantation

Source: This table has been updated according to the latest clinical practice guidelines 2018 from Feld LG, Neuspiel DR, Foster BA, et al. Clinical Practice Guideline: Maintenance Intravenous Fluids in Children. *Pediatrics*. 2018;142(6):e20183083.

Diagnostic Evaluation If the patient has none of the above causes of hyperkalemia and the serum potassium level is reported as high, it is often prudent to recheck the potassium from a venous, easy-flowing blood draw and minimize the use of a tourniquet to avoid pseudohyperkalemia from a hemolyzed blood specimen. In metabolic acidosis from bicarbonate losses in diarrhea or from diabetic ketoacidosis, buffering occurs at the cellular level as potassium shifts from the intracellular to the ECF while hydrogen ion shifts to the ICF. Correction of acidosis will usually correct hyperkalemia.

If repeat testing reveals true hyperkalemia, an electrocardiogram should be obtained to evaluate for prolongation of the PR or QRS intervals and for peaked T waves.

Management For potassium levels ≥6.5 mg/dL, or in the setting of significant arrhythmia or widened QRS, the patient should have an electrocardiogram (ECG) obtained, be placed on a cardiorespiratory monitor, and transferred to an ICU setting. All potassium intake should be discontinued. Further management in order of priority is as follows:

1. Stabilize the myocardium: Cardiac membrane excitability can be decreased by infusing 10% calcium gluconate, 0.5 to 1 mL/kg (60–100 mg/kg per dose, maximum 2000 mg/dose) by peripheral IV/IO; or calcium chloride, 20 mg/kg (20 mg/kg per dose, maximum 2000 mg) through a central venous line, not to exceed 100 mg/min. Follow infusion with a flush. Calcium infusion may be repeated as needed for persistent ECG abnormalities or arrhythmia.
2. Shift potassium intracellularly:
   a. Infuse Sodium bicarbonate ($NaHCO_3$), 1 to 2 mEq/kg per dose IV over 5 to 10 minutes. This works best in the presence of metabolic acidosis. **Note: Calcium gluconate and calcium chloride are not compatible with $NaHCO_3$ as it will precipitate to form chalk ($CaCO_3$). Therefore, flush lines between infusions or use a different IV site.
   b. Infuse 0.1 U/kg of insulin with 0.5 g/kg dextrose (e.g., 2 mL/kg of 25% dextrose or 5mL/kg of 10% dextrose) infused in separate bags simultaneously over 30 minutes.
3. Remove excess potassium from the body:
   a. Administer sodium polystyrene sulfonate (Kayexalate) at 1g/kg every 4 hours orally or by retention enema. Sodium polystyrene sulfonate works as a cation exchange, removing potassium in lieu of sodium. It can cause constipation and may be given with polyethylene glycol. Per the 2009 FDA report, avoid use with sorbitol due to reported colonic necrosis.
   b. Use a loop or thiazide diuretic if the patient is not hypovolemic and has normal renal function. Often furosemide 1mg/kg/dose IV is used in combination with a 10 to 20 mL/kg NS bolus. If effective, furosemide can be repeated every 6 hours as needed. Hemodialysis or peritoneal dialysis can also be used in patients with renal failure or severe poisoning.

HYPOKALEMIA

Definition Hypokalemia is defined as a serum potassium concentration less than 3.5 mEq/L. Severe hypokalemia exists when serum K^+ is less than 2.5 mEq/L. Causes of hypokalemia (**Table 116-7**) can be divided into increased potassium losses in urine or stool or shift of potassium into the ICF. Stool losses occur as a result of diarrhea or laxative abuse.

Clinical Presentation The most common clinical signs and symptoms of hypokalemia are caused by disordered electrical conduction in cardiac, skeletal, and smooth muscle. Electrocardiographic changes include U waves, depressed ST segments, prolonged QTc, and many other arrhythmias. Skeletal muscle effects include generalized (sometimes severe) muscle weakness, rhabdomyolysis, paralytic ileus, and impaired respiration. In addition, hypokalemia impairs the ability of the kidneys to reabsorb hydrogen ion, thereby promoting metabolic alkalosis and renal medullary dysfunction with an inability to dilute or concentrate the urine.

TABLE 116-7 Causes of Hypokalemia

Increase in Renal K$^+$ Excretion
Metabolic alkalosis
Chloride responsive
Volume contraction
Chloride unresponsive
Primary hyperaldosteronism
Hypertension
Liddle syndrome
11β-Hydroxysteroid dehydrogenase deficiency
No hypertension
Bartter syndrome
Gitelman syndrome
Metabolic acidosis
Type I and II renal tubular acidosis
Drugs
Diuretics
Fluorinated steroids
Penicillins
Transcellular K$^+$ Shift
β-Adrenergic agonists
Insulin administration
Theophylline and caffeine
Verapamil and chloroquine ingestion
Hyperthyroidism
Familial hypokalemic paralysis
Excessive K$^+$ Loss in Stool
Laxative abuse
Diarrheal illness
Miscellaneous
Mg^{2+} depletion

Source: This table has been updated according to the latest clinical practice guidelines 2018 from Feld LG, Neuspiel DR, Foster BA, et al. Clinical Practice Guideline: Maintenance Intravenous Fluids in Children. *Pediatrics*. 2018;142(6):e20183083.

All of the tables are sourced from the previous version of the book. They have been edited to be updated according to the latest clinical practice guidelines 2018 from Feld LG, Neuspiel DR, Foster BA, et al. Clinical Practice Guideline: Maintenance Intravenous Fluids in Children. *Pediatrics*. 2018;142(6):e20183083.

Diagnostic Evaluation If the cause of the hypokalemia is not clear, a urine potassium level higher than 10 mEq/L indicates excess urine loss. In the face of volume contraction, as seen in chloride-responsive metabolic alkalosis, urine Cl$^-$ is less than 25 mEq/L and the renin/angiotensin system is activated by the low circulating blood volume, which leads to increased aldosterone secretion to retain sodium and chloride and results in continued potassium excretion by the kidney. Chloride-unresponsive metabolic alkalosis, as occurs with mineralocorticoid excess, is characterized by urine Cl$^-$ >40 mEq/L.

Management The treatment of hypokalemia is potassium repletion. For symptomatic, severe hypokalemia, use 0.25 to 0.5 mEq/kg/dose (maximum dose: 40 mEq) to infuse at 0.25 mEq/kg/hour (maximum dose/rate: 1 mEq/kg/hour). If infusions of >40 mEq/L are needed, patients should be monitored in an ICU setting and a central line should be used for administration. The concentration should not exceed 0.1 mEq/mL in a peripheral line and 0.2 mEq/mL in a central line. Generally, for patients who are asymptomatic, enteral potassium replacement therapy is preferred (oral or via nasogastric tube). Dosing and duration of therapy should be driven by the underlying cause or monitored if the reason for hypokalemia is short-lived such as in the case of exposure to beta adrenergic in asthma. In cases where expected intracellular shifts occur, addition of potassium to maintenance IV fluids is likely to be sufficient and hypokalemia will usually resolve when the patient can tolerate a regular diet. For hypokalemia in the face of metabolic acidosis, potassium may be given as phosphate or acetate, whereas with metabolic alkalosis it is given as KCl. For patients with ongoing and severe potassium losses, such as patients with Bartter syndrome, repletion doses may need to be increased.

ADMISSION AND DISCHARGE CRITERIA

- Any patient with a significant electrolyte abnormality should be hospitalized, especially if the cause of the abnormality is unclear. Placement on an acute care floor versus the intensive care unit admission will be institution-dependent based on how frequently labs or symptom monitoring is required.
- Discharge is contingent upon correction of the abnormal electrolyte status, presence of a treatment plan to maintain normal electrolyte status, and appropriate follow up after discharge.

CONSULTATION

Given the myriad of disease states that can lead to electrolyte disturbances, the hospitalist may consult with several specialists, including renal, endocrine, or critical care colleagues, to assist in the management of these patients, especially if the electrolyte derangements are severe.

SUGGESTED READINGS

Bruno J, Canada N, Canada T, Tucker AM, Ybarra JV, eds. *ASPEN Fluids, Electrolytes*, and *Acid-Base Disorders Handbook*. 2nd Ed. Silver Spring: MD: American Society of Parenteral and Enteral Nutrition, 2020.

Feld LG, Neuspiel DR, Foster BA, et al. Clinical Practice Guidelines: Maintenance Intravenous Fluids in Children. *Pediatrics*. 2018;142(6): e20183083.

Holliday MA, Segar WE. The maintenance need for water in parenteral fluid therapy. *Pediatrics*. 1957;19(5):823-832.

Roberts KB. Fluid and electrolytes: parenteral fluid therapy. *Pediatrics Review*. 2001;22(11):380-387.

Singh TD, Fugate JE, Rabinstein AA. Central pontine and extrapontine myelinolysis: a systematic review. Eur J Neurol. 2014;21(12): 1443-1450.

Spandorfer PR, Alessandrini EA, Joffe MD, Localio R, Shaw KN. Oral versus intravenous rehydration of moderately dehydrated children: a randomized, controlled trial. *Pediatrics*. 2005;115(2):295-301.

Weiss SL, Peters MJ, Alhazzani W, et al. Surviving Sepsis Campaign International Guidelines for the Management of Septic Shock and Sepsis-Associated Organ Dysfunction in Children. *Pediatric Crit Care Med*. 2020;21(2):e52-e106.

CHAPTER 117

Hypertension

Rasheda Z. Amin, MBBS, MSHS

BACKGROUND

Cardiovascular disease is the leading cause of mortality in the United States; hypertension is a well-documented risk factor for cardiovascular disease in both the adult and pediatric populations. The population prevalence of hypertension is estimated to be 4.2% based on analysis of data from 12,004 participants aged 12 to 19 years in the 2001 to 2016 National Health and Nutrition Examination Survey (NHANES). Prevalence of elevated blood pressure and hypertension in children has been linked to obesity, high salt food intake, and a sedentary lifestyle.

When only considering overweight or obese children, the estimated proportion of children afflicted with hypertension is much greater, ranging from 20% to 47%. Hypertension in children is thus increasingly recognized as one of the most important pediatric preventable diseases and is especially important in view of the observation that pediatric hypertension correlates to hypertension in adulthood.

Regardless of etiology, depending on the degree of elevation and the duration of onset, hypertension can lead to both acute and chronic organ dysfunction. In ambulatory settings, otherwise healthy hypertensive children have been found to be more likely to have left ventricular hypertrophy, accelerated atherosclerosis, proteinuria, and decreased cognitive function. In hospitalized children, hypertension may complicate the management of coexisting clinical conditions, and there is the additional burden of determining whether the high blood pressure is a primary problem or whether it stems from an ongoing condition or its treatment.

Accordingly, a child who presents with hypertension may require treatment while the diagnostic evaluation is ongoing. The approach to the evaluation and treatment of hypertension is often both more directed and more intensive in a hospitalized child than in an ambulatory setting. The extent of the blood pressure elevation and the degree of clinical concern for immediate harm to the child from the hypertension also guides the tempo of diagnostic evaluation and therapeutic intervention.

DEFINITION

The latest clinical practice guidelines for diagnosis and management of elevated blood pressure and hypertension were published in 2017 and contain several modifications to the previous guidelines. Normative reference data and blood pressure tables were revised to be based on normal body weight (body mass index <85th percentile), resulting in blood pressure values several mm Hg lower compared to previous normative data which included overweight and obese children. A simplified table listing systolic and diastolic blood pressure levels at the 90th percentile by age and sex was provided for screening purposes to facilitate detection of abnormal blood pressure levels in clinical practices. The term "prehypertension" was replaced by the term "elevated blood pressure."

The revised definitions of categories and stages of blood pressure are as follows:

For Children between the ages 1 and 13 years:

Normal Blood Pressure (BP): Less than the 90th percentile.

Elevated BP: Equal to or greater than the 90th percentile to less than the 95th percentile or 120/80 mm Hg to less than the 95th percentile (whichever is lower).

Stage 1 Hypertension: Equal to or greater than the 95th percentile to less than the 95th percentile + 12 mm Hg, or 130/80 to 139/89 mm Hg (whichever is lower).

Stage 2 Hypertension: Equal to or greater than the 95th percentile + 12 mm Hg, or equal to or greater than 140/90 mm Hg (whichever is lower).

For Children Ages 13 years or older:

Normal BP: Less than 120/80 mm Hg.

Elevated BP: 120/80 to less than 129/80 mm Hg.

Stage 1 HTN: 130/80 to 139/89 mm Hg.

Stage 2 HTN: Equal to or greater than 140/90 mm Hg.

The revised staging criteria for stage 1 and stage 2 hypertension for the adolescent age group are aligned with the new definitions of abnormal blood pressure in the guidelines for hypertension in adults developed by the American Heart Association and the American College of Cardiology

MEASUREMENT OF BLOOD PRESSURE

Performing a proper blood pressure measurement is essential for accurate diagnosis of hypertension in children. A misdiagnosis of hypertension is often made if the proper sized cuff, for example, is not used. The patient should have rested for 3 to 5 minutes before the blood pressure measurement and should be sitting in an upright position, with back supported, feet flat on the floor with the cubital fossa at the heart level. Younger children may be lying down. Since blood pressure readings from the leg are usually 10 to 20 mm Hg higher than those from the arm, blood pressures should ideally be taken from the arm; right arm is preferable unless the child has abnormal anatomy of the aortic arch such as coarctation. The width of the cuff bladder should be at least 40% of the mid-arm circumference and the bladder length should wrap around at least 80% or two-thirds of the upper arm circumference.

Oscillometric devices (such as Dynamap) or mercury or aneroid sphygmomanometers can be used to measure the blood pressure. When using the auscultatory method, the stethoscope should be placed over the brachial artery below the bottom edge of the cuff and just above the medial cubital fossa. The systolic blood pressure is measured on the first Korotkoff sound (K1) and the diastolic blood pressure at the fifth Korotkoff sound (K5), or when the Korotkoff sound completely disappears. In some children where the K5 is close to 0, the diastolic blood pressure can be measured at K4 (muffling of sounds). Most automated blood pressure machines use the oscillometric technique, which determines the mean arterial pressure by measuring the peak amplitude of oscillation of the arterial wall as the blood pressure cuff deflates. The machine then calculates the systolic and diastolic blood pressures from this mean arterial pressure. The oscillometric systolic blood pressures tend to be 10 mm Hg higher than the auscultatory systolic blood pressures, while the diastolic blood pressures tend to be 5 mm Hg higher for the oscillometric technique compared to the auscultatory technique.

If the initial blood pressure is elevated (≥90th percentile), two additional auscultatory blood pressure measurements should be obtained at the same visit and the mean obtained to determine the blood pressure category.

AMBULATORY BLOOD PRESSURE MONITORING

An ambulatory blood pressure monitor (ABPM) comprises of a blood pressure cuff attached to a small monitor (slightly larger than a cellphone) which is programmed to record blood pressure every 20 to 30 minutes, usually for a 24-hour period. ABPM has been demonstrated as being more accurate for diagnosis of hypertension, correlates better with cardiovascular target organ damage such as left ventricular hypertrophy, and allows evaluation of nocturnal blood pressure. Nocturnal blood pressure readings are usually 10% lower than daytime readings, a phenomenon known as nocturnal dipping. The 2017 pediatric hypertension guidelines recommend ABPM for confirmation of abnormal blood pressure status in several clinical situations, including confirmation of the diagnosis of hypertension in patients with concern for elevated blood pressure, identification of white coat hypertension, detection of masked hypertension, and evaluation of treatment effectiveness in patients receiving antihypertensive therapy. White coat hypertension refers to elevated blood pressure in the office or clinical setting and normal blood pressure in other settings. In contrast, masked hypertension is normal blood pressure reading in clinical setting but elevated blood pressure in other settings. The incidence of masked hypertension is higher in patients with chronic kidney disease, heart and kidney transplant recipients, and children with history of coarctation of aorta. ABPM procedures are usually done by a nephrology or cardiology subspecialist.

PATHOGENESIS

Hypertension can be largely classified into essential or primary hypertension and secondary hypertension. The mechanism for essential hypertension is not entirely clear; however, it has been linked to various genetic and environmental factors, and is strongly associated with obesity. Obese children are three times more likely to be hypertensive compared to nonobese children, and the prevalence of systolic hypertension rises with increasing body mass index (BMI). Insulin resistance is also prevalent in overweight children, and the metabolic syndrome, a constellation of clinical findings including obesity, hyperinsulinemia, hypertension, and hyperlipidemia, is becoming a major health concern worldwide, especially in the pediatric population. Essential hypertension associated with obesity may be a result of various factors including dysfunctional autonomic regulation, abnormal vascular structure and function, and insulin resistance. Secondary hypertension is more common in younger children and can be a result of renal and renovascular disease, cardiac abnormalities, hormonal excess, genetic conditions, low birth weight and prematurity, or medication related (**Table 117-1**). Sleep-disordered breathing, often associated with obesity, can also increase the risk of developing hypertension.

CLINICAL PRESENTATION

Most patients with essential hypertension are asymptomatic, but some may present with headaches, blurry vision, dizziness, epistaxis, or fatigue. Often, patients with secondary hypertension are found to have elevated blood pressures during evaluation for the underlying disease and usually present with symptoms related to that disease. For example, patients with pheochromocytoma and hyperthyroidism may present with symptoms such as tachycardia and diaphoresis. The presence of rashes, joint swelling, or gross hematuria may indicate an autoimmune-mediated glomerulonephritis. Delayed puberty might be a clue to congenital adrenal hyperplasia, while muscle cramps and constipation could be signs of hypokalemia from hyperaldosteronism.

In cases of severe hypertension, mental status changes can occur. Posterior reversible encephalopathy syndrome, a syndrome that manifests as headaches, seizures, encephalopathy, or loss in vision can be caused by hypertension and is a result of vasogenic edema typically in the occipital and parietal lobes.

TABLE 117-1 Etiology of Secondary Hypertension

Vascular	Coarctation of the aorta
	Renal artery stenosis
	Renal artery thrombus
	Umbilical artery catheterization (leading to renal artery stenosis)
Neurologic	Increased intracranial pressure
	Seizures
	Familial dysautonomia
	Guillain-Barre syndrome
Endocrine	Pheochromocytoma
	Neuroblastoma
	Cushing syndrome
	Congenital adrenal hyperplasia
	Aldosterone-secreting tumors
	Thyroid disorders
Pulmonary	Obstructive sleep apnea
	Bronchopulmonary dysplasia
	Pneumothorax
Renal or genitourinary	Glomerulonephritis, acute and chronic
	Polycystic kidney disease
	Chronic kidney disease
	Renal scars
	Obstructive uropathy
Monogenic	Liddle's syndrome, Type 1 pseudohypoaldosteronism, Type 2 pseudohypoaldosteronism, or Gordon syndrome
Drugs	Steroids
	Calcineurin inhibitors
	Epinephrine
	Amphetamines
	Cocaine
	Oral contraceptive drugs
	Pseudoephedrine

EVALUATION

Once hypertension is confirmed, further evaluation should include a detailed history, physical examination, laboratory testing, and imaging studies. An algorithm for the diagnostic evaluation of hypertension in hospitalized children is provided in **Figure 117-1**.

HISTORY

The clinician should focus on disorders or conditions that predispose to hypertension and, in a hospitalized patient, should begin with the history of present illness leading to the child's admission. For instance, in a postoperative patient who is otherwise healthy, pain or anxiety may play a role in hypertension. In a child hospitalized with severe reactive airway disease, steroid therapy or frequent administration of β-agonists may be the cause of hypertension.

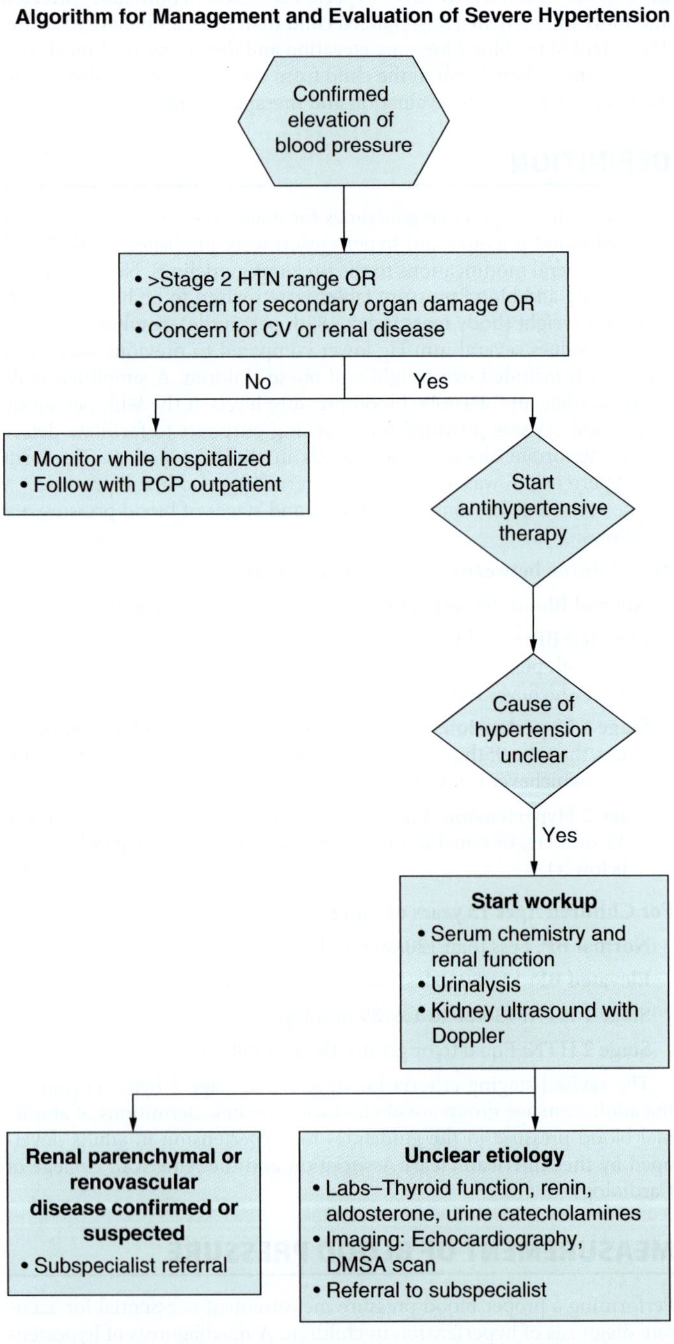

FIGURE 117-1. Algorithm for management and evaluation of severe hypertension. (Courtesy of Rasheda Amin MBBS, MSHS.)

In the absence of an obvious precipitating factor related to an acute illness or medical condition, the history should begin with the perinatal period. Prematurity is a risk factor for hypertension, because premature babies are born with fewer nephrons, have a reduced renal reserve, and may be more prone to hyperfiltration injury and glomerulosclerosis as both a child and adult. In addition, placement of umbilical catheters in the nursery or periods of hypotension early in life can mediate renal injury by thrombosis or hypoperfusion with increased risk for subsequent renal scarring.

Especially in preschool children, febrile urinary tract infections commonly leave renal parenchymal scars that can then lead to hyperreninemic hypertension over time. These infections may have been misdiagnosed or even gone unappreciated, so any history of unexplained recurrent febrile illness should be elicited.

Glomerulonephritis can present with edema, hematuria, and hypertension and may be isolated to the kidney or associated with systemic disorders such as systemic lupus erythematosus. Relevant extrarenal findings include joint symptoms, rashes, and recurrent unexplained fevers or constitutional symptoms. A recent history of pharyngitis or skin infection is suggestive of postinfectious glomerulonephritis and may be associated with gross hematuria or tea-colored urine in addition to high blood pressure.

The family history focuses on relatives with pediatric or early-onset hypertension and inherited diseases that affect the kidneys, such as the polycystic kidney disease complexes, tuberous sclerosis, and neurofibromatosis. A strong family history of cardiovascular disease, such as coronary artery disease, stroke, and hyperlipidemia, can be suggestive of essential hypertension, especially in older children.

Certain medications are known to cause hypertension, including oral contraceptives, corticosteroids, stimulants, decongestants, and calcineurin inhibitors (cyclosporine, tacrolimus). Recreational drugs with stimulant effects, such as cocaine, nicotine, and ephedra, can also raise blood pressure, as can withdrawal from the effects of central nervous system depressants such as ethanol or narcotic analgesics.

The review of systems should evaluate for symptoms such as headache, chest pain, visual changes, or mental status changes, because these may be related to severe hypertension or end-organ damage. Sweating, palpitations, and flushing are associated with states of catecholamine excess such as occurs with a pheochromocytoma.

PHYSICAL EXAMINATION

The most essential part of the physical assessment of a child with suspected hypertension is accurate measurement of the blood pressure. Blood pressure should be measured in all four extremities. When measured at the same encounter with the same equipment, the blood pressure in the lower extremities is typically 10 to 20 mm Hg higher than in the right arm. If lower extremity blood pressure is not higher, this suggests a coarctation or other narrowing of the aorta and is often associated with diminished femoral pulses.

Height, weight, and BMI should be measured to assess for growth anomalies or to document obesity. The physical examination should look for signs of end-organ damage from hypertension. This involves fundoscopy and cardiovascular, pulmonary, and neurologic examinations. Although the finding is uncommon, the abdomen should be auscultated for abdominal bruits, which can be seen in renovascular hypertension.

The physical examination should also look for findings of genetic syndromes that may explain the elevated blood pressure. These include neurofibromatosis (café au lait spots, axillary freckling, Lisch nodules), tuberous sclerosis (ash-leaf macules, shagreen patches, adenoma sebaceum, peri- or subungual fibromas, retinal hamartomas), Turner syndrome (short stature, shield chest, upturned mouth, webbed neck), and Williams syndrome (overfriendly personality, cognitive impairment, prominent ears).

LABORATORY AND RADIOLOGIC STUDIES

A urinalysis should be performed on a freshly voided urine sample, and if the dipstick is positive for blood or protein, microscopy should be performed. Initial screening blood work should include electrolytes, blood urea nitrogen, and creatinine. This effectively evaluates renal function and screens for states of mineralocorticoid excess that lead to hypokalemia and alkalosis. The presence of hematuria or proteinuria can be detected with a urinalysis. In patients where specific symptoms such as tachycardia or diaphoresis are present, thyroid function tests or urine catecholamines can be sent.

The 2017 AAP high BP guidelines recommend a kidney ultrasound initially for children presenting with hypertension at age <6 years and those with laboratory findings concerning for kidney disease (e.g., abnormal kidney function tests or urinalysis). An ultrasound study will uncover solitary kidney, differential renal size, hydronephrosis, changes in parenchymal echogenicity, or diffuse cystic changes. More extensive areas of renal scarring will often be appreciated on ultrasound as thinning of the renal cortex or loss of parenchyma. Subtler scarring may not be seen on ultrasonography, but a size discrepancy of greater than 1 cm between the two kidneys is unusual and may reflect scarring in the smaller kidney.

Since there is low yield in routinely doing other laboratory work or imaging studies with initial screening, each individual's history and physical examination findings should guide further evaluation. For example, tachycardia suggests hyperthyroidism or high-catecholamine states and should trigger blood thyroid function tests and quantification of catecholamines. A history of urinary tract infections with unexplained fevers or positive urine cultures should prompt evaluation with a dimercaptosuccinic acid (DMSA) scan to determine the presence of cortical scars.

The diagnosis of renal artery stenosis continues to be challenging in children. The gold standard study for diagnosis remains angiography. It allows for both diagnostic and therapeutic interventions, although the invasive nature of angiography limits its use as first-line approach. Doppler studies of renal vasculature can show changes in flow rates through areas of measurement and may suggest the presence of renovascular hypertension. A normal Doppler study does not, however, rule out renal artery stenosis, especially stenosis in the smaller segmental arteries that are not well visualized by Doppler. Computed tomographic angiography (CTA) and magnetic resonance angiography (MRA) have been studied as alternate imaging modalities. MRA lacks the spatial resolution of CTA but avoids the radiation exposure that comes with CT. When compared with renal angiography, one study that included both pediatric and adult patients showed that the sensitivity and specificity for the detection of renal artery stenosis was 94% and 93% for CTA and 90% and 94% for MRA, respectively. Consultation with a pediatric radiologist is recommended to decide which imaging study may be best, always considering that angiography may ultimately still be necessary if there is a high level of suspicion for renal artery stenosis.

Echocardiography is necessary in any child suspected of having a structural lesion causing hypertension. In addition, echocardiography may be a sensitive tool to measure cardiac changes such as left ventricular hypertrophy that accompanies sustained hypertension and can be used over time to assess the impact of antihypertensive therapy on end-organ damage.

Similarly, in some children with hypertension, formal ophthalmology examinations may provide initial information about the chronicity of a child's hypertensive state and help document amelioration of vascular changes with therapy.

Plasma renin activity and serum aldosterone level should also be sent to screen for renal and mineralocorticoid disorders. Plasma renin activity and aldosterone levels are helpful only if the results are unequivocally low or very high. They are most useful when a diagnosis of mineralocorticoid excess is suspected because plasma renin activity is typically suppressed. Aldosterone levels may be low or high, depending on the specific cause of the mineralocorticoid excess.

TARGET ORGAN DAMAGE

Although long-term complications of hypertension such as cardiovascular, cerebrovascular, renal, and retinal disease usually manifest in adulthood, there is growing evidence of their presence in pediatric patients. The markers for cardiovascular target organ damage are left ventricular mass index, elevated carotid intima media thickness (cIMT), higher pulse wave velocity (PWV), and diastolic dysfunction. The most common cardiovascular complication is left ventricular hypertrophy and its prevalence has been reported to be 5% to 50% in pediatric patients with primary hypertension.

Cerebrovascular accidents, the more common manifestation of hypertension in adults, are relatively uncommon in the pediatric population; however, there is also a growing body of evidence showing an association between primary hypertension and cognitive function decline and learning disabilities. Changes from hypertensive retinopathy characterized by arteriolar narrowing have been identified in the pediatric population.

TREATMENT OF PEDIATRIC HYPERTENSION

ACUTE MANAGEMENT

Since hospitalization is an anxiety-provoking experience for most children, transient elevation in blood pressure below the Stage 2 hypertension threshold can be monitored with frequent readings to document the trend of measurements. As the child recovers and acclimates to the hospital, blood pressure often falls to normal ranges. If there is concern that the blood pressure may adversely affect a clinical condition or is directly related to a primary disease process (e.g., glomerulonephritis), more immediate measures may be necessary. If blood pressure readings are still consistently elevated by the time of discharge, it is judicious to arrange follow-up with the child's primary care provider and further evaluation as an outpatient.

In a child with sustained blood pressure exceeding the Stage 2 hypertension threshold, diagnostic evaluation and therapy must be carefully considered (see Figure 117-1). The timing and urgency of the intervention are guided by the individual child's clinical presentation and course.

Children with sustained blood pressure readings more than 30 mm Hg above the 95th percentile are at particular risk of developing acute sequelae; even if they are asymptomatic, blood pressure control must begin immediately to prevent progression to a hypertensive urgency (severely elevated blood pressure that is potentially harmful but without evidence of secondary/target organ damage or dysfunction) or emergency (severely elevated blood pressure associated with evidence of secondary/target organ dysfunction). A sequential approach to management of severe acute hypertension is outlined in **Figure 117-2**.

Severe acute hypertension requires immediate treatment with short-acting antihypertensive medications. Treatment can be initiated with oral agents if tolerated and if there is no concern for severe secondary end-organ dysfunction, otherwise intravenous therapy is indicated. Intravenous drips allow for more controlled blood pressure reduction in conditions that warrant it, such as congestive heart failure. The blood pressure should be lowered by 25% in the first 8 hours and once the blood pressure falls into a range that is not acutely dangerous for the patient, it should be lowered more gradually over the remaining 24 hours, aiming eventually for pressures around 95th percentile for a patient's age, gender, and height. The medications most commonly used in a hypertensive crisis are outlined in **Table 117-2**.

Hydralazine is a commonly used vasodilator with a rapid onset that can often be titrated to achieve good blood pressure control. It is well tolerated and can be given readily in a nonintensive care unit setting. Nifedipine is another short-acting agent and has the advantage of oral administration. Its use in adults is rare owing to reports of myocardial infarction. The use of short-acting nifedipine in children is safe, although a higher incidence of adverse events was seen in patients with preexisting central nervous system disease. The sublingual route is somewhat controversial because accurate dosing is problematic since it requires aspiration of liquid from within a capsule, moreover, its absorption is erratic. Nicardipine and isradipine can be used for vasodilation as intravenous calcium channel blockers in cases where oral nifedipine or intravenous hydralazine cannot be considered. Labetalol and esmolol can also be used as intermittent intravenous medications if necessary.

Severe hypertension refractory to intermittent therapy may require continuous infusions to reduce blood pressure to safe levels. Ideally, the setting for such continuous infusions should be an intensive care unit. Historically, nitroprusside and labetalol have been used most in children. Both agents are shorter-acting than hydralazine, and continuous infusions may be titrated to achieve specific target blood pressures.

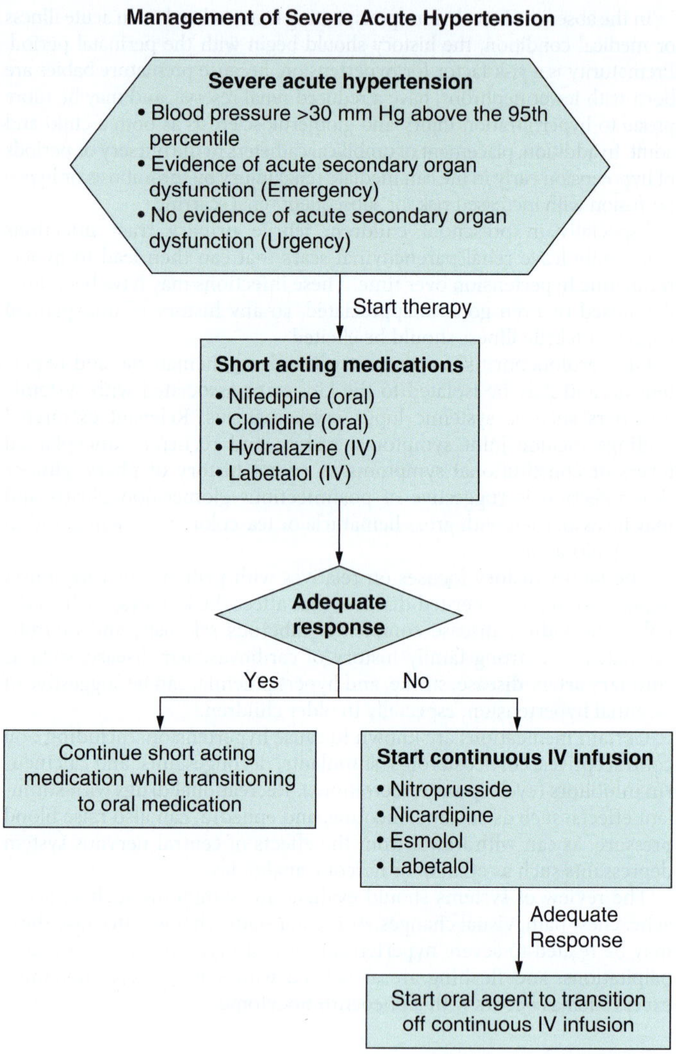

FIGURE 117-2. Algorithm for management of severe acute hypertension. (Courtesy of Rasheda Amin, MBBS, MSHS.)

Labetalol can be administered via both continuous infusion and scheduled intravenous dosing. It is the only drug that is both an alpha- and beta-adrenergic blocker. Nitroprusside is a vasodilator with a wide dosage range. The drug is photosensitive and must be protected from light. Its use is limited by the toxicity of its metabolites; nitroprusside is converted to cyanide by tissue sulfhydryl groups, and cyanide is converted to thiocyanate in the liver. In patients with liver disease, cyanide levels

TABLE 117-2 Short-acting Antihypertensive Agents for Severe Hypertension

Drug	Dose	Onset	Duration
Hydralazine	IV: 0.1-0.4 mg/kg to max dose of 20 mg	5-15 min	3-8 h
Labetalol	Initial IV bolus: 0.25 mg/kg; repeat q15min at increasing doses up to 1 mg/kg until effective or to total dose of 4 mg/kg	5 min	2-6 h
	Maintenance IV drip: 1-3 mg/kg/hr		
Nitroprusside	IV: start at 0.5 µg/kg/min	1-2 min	3-5 min
Nifedipine	PO: 0.25-0.5 mg/kg	10-20 min	3-6 h
Nicardipine	IV: 0.5-5 µg/kg/min	10 min	2-6 h
Esmolol	Loading dose: 500 µg/kg over 2 min	Seconds	10–20 min
	Maintenance IV drip: 50-250 g/kg/min		
Enalaprilat	IV: 5-10 µg/kg q 8-24 h	0.5-4 h	6 h

should be followed. Thiocyanate levels should be monitored in patients on nitroprusside for more than 72 hours and in patients with renal insufficiency. Thiocyanate toxicity manifests primarily as neurotoxicity and includes psychosis, blurred vision, confusion, weakness, tinnitus, and seizures. An early sign of cyanide toxicity includes metabolic acidosis; other signs of toxicity include tachycardia, pink skin, decreased pulse, decreased reflexes, altered consciousness, coma, almond smell on breath, methemoglobinemia, and dilated pupils.

Continuous infusions of the calcium-channel blocker nicardipine or the beta-blocker esmolol have also been used in hypertensive children. In most children who require continuous infusions for a limited time, there is no specific advantage to using any of these therapies versus older therapies.

LONG-TERM MANAGEMENT

Antihypertensive medication should be started in children who have symptomatic hypertension, stage 2 hypertension without a modifiable etiology, have other risk factors such as chronic kidney disease, or have failed lifestyle modifications. Therapy should be initiated with a single agent at the starting dose and titrated to achieve good blood pressure control. The goal of therapy is to reduce blood pressure to < 90th percentile. The first-line medications are angiotensin-converting enzyme inhibitors (ACEIs) and angiotensin receptor blockers (ARBs), calcium channel blockers, and thiazide diuretics (**Table 117-3**). ACE inhibitors and ARBs block the action of angiotensin II, a hormone that induces

TABLE 117-3 Long-acting Antihypertensive Medications in Children

Class	Drug	Dose	Dosing Interval	Formulations
Angiotensin-onverting enzyme (ACE) inhibitors	• Common side effects: cough, headache, dizziness • Serious side effects: Angioedema, teratogenicity, azotemia, hyperkalemia • Contraindications: pregnancy and angioedema			
	Captopril	Initial: Infants: 0.05 mg/kg/dose Children:0.3-0.5 mg/kg/dose Maximum: 6 mg/kg per day	Daily to 4 times a day	Tablet: 12.5, 25, 50, 100 mg Compounded liquid: 1 mg/mL
	Enalapril	Child ≥1 month*: Initial: 0.08 mg/kg per day up to 5 mg/d Maximum: 0.6 mg/kg per day up to 40 mg/d	Once or twice a day	Tablet: 2.5, 5, 10, 20 mg Solution: 1 mg/mL
	Lisinopril	Child ≥6 y/o*: Initial: 0.07 mg/kg per day up to 5 mg/day Maximum: 0.6 mg/kg per d up to 40 mg/d	Once a day	Tablet: 2.5, 5, 10, 20, 30, 40 mg Solution: 1 mg/mL
Angiotensin-receptor blocker	• Common side effects: cough, headache, dizziness • Serious side effects: Angioedema, teratogenicity, azotemia, hyperkalemia • Contraindications: pregnancy			
	Losartan	Child ≥6 y/o*: Initial: 0.7 mg/kg per d up to 50 mg/d Maximum: 1.4 mg/kg per d up to 100 mg/d	Daily	Tablet: 25, 50, 100 mg Compounded liquid: liquid: 2.5 mg/mL
	Valsartan	Child≥6 y/o*: Initial: 1.3 mg/kg (up to 40 mg) Maximum: 2.7 mg/kg (up to 160 mg)	Daily	Tablet: 40, 80, 160, 320 mg Compounded liquid: 4 mg/mL
Calcium channel blockers	• Common side effects: headache, flushing, peripheral edema, tachycardia • Serious side effects: angioedema • Contraindications: hypersensitivity to calcium channel blockers			
	Amlodipine	Child 1 < 6y/o: Initial: 0.1 mg/kg per day Maximum: 0.6 mg/kg per day up to 5 mg Child≥6 y/o*: Initial: 2.5 mg Maximum: 10 mg	Daily	Tablet: 2.5, 5,10 mg Compounded liquid: 1 mg/mL
	Nifedipine (ER-Extended release)	Initial: 0.2-0.5 mg/kg per day Maximum: 3 mg/kg/d (up to 120 mg per day)	Daily or twice a day	Tablet (ER): 30, 60, 90 mg
Thiazide Diuretics	• Common side effects: dizziness, hypokalemia • Serious side effects: cardiac dysrhythmias, cholestatic jaundice, new-onset diabetes mellitus, pancreatitis • Monitoring: electrolytes should be periodically • Contraindications: anuric state			
	Hydrochlorothiazide (HCTZ)	Child*: Initial dose: 1 mg/kg per day Maximum dose: 2 mg/kg per day (up to 37.5 mg)	Daily or twice a day	Tablet: 12.5, 25, 50 mg
	Chlorothiazide	Child*: Initial dose: 10 mg/kg per day Maximum dose: 20 mg/kg per day (up to 375 mg)	Daily or twice a day	Tablet: 250, 500 mg Suspension: 250/5 mL Compounded liquid: 1 mg/mL

(Continued)

TABLE 117-3 Long-acting Antihypertensive Medications in Children (*Continued*)

Class	Drug	Dose	Dosing Interval	Formulations
Potassium-sparing diuretics†	• Common side effects: • Serious side effects: hyperkalemia • Contraindications: hyperkalemia, Addison disease			
	Spironolactone	Initial: 1 mg/kg per day Maximum: 3.3 mg/kg per day (up to 100 mg)	Daily or twice a day	Tablet: 25, 50, 100 mg Suspension: 25 mg/5 mL
α- and β-Blocker[b]	• Common side effects: bradycardia, fatigue, sleep changes, sexual dysfunction, weight gain. • Serious side effects: bronchospasm (nonselective beta-blockers) • Contraindications: Asthma, (nonselective beta-blockers should not be used), Raynaud phenomenon.			
α- and β-Blocker	Labetalol	Initial: 1-3 mg/kg per day Maximum: 10-12 mg/kg/day up to 1200 mg/day	Twice a day	Tablet: 100, 200, 300 mg
β-Blocker	Atenolol	Initial: 0.5-1 mg/kg per day Maximum: 2 mg/kg per day up to 100 mg/d	Once to twice a day	Tablet: 25, 50, 100 mg
	Metoprolol	Initial: 0.5-1 mg/kg per day Maximum: 6 mg/kg per day or 200 mg/day (whichever is less)	Twice a day Once a day (XL: extended release)	Tablet: 25, 50, 75, 100 mg Tablet XL: 25, 50, 100, 200 mg
	Propranolol	Initial: 1-2 mg/kg per day Maximum: 4 mg/kg per day or 640 mg/day (whichever is less)	Two to four times a day	Tablet: 10, 20, 40, 60, 80 mg Solution: 20 mg/5mL
Vasodilator†	• Common side effects: tachycardia, fluid retention; hypertrichosis (minoxidil) • Serious side effects: can cause lupus-like syndrome (hydralazine); pericardial effusion (minoxidil) • Contraindications: hypersensitivity			
	Hydralazine	Initial: 0.75 mg/kg per day Maximum: 7.5 not to exceed 200 mg/day	Two to four times a day	Tablet: 10, 25, 50, 100 mg
	Minoxidil	Children <12 years: Initial: 0.2 mg/kg per day Maximum: 50 mg/day Children ≥12 years: Initial: 5 mg/day Maximum: 100 mg/day	One to three times a day	Tablet: 2.5, 10 mg
Central α-agonist†	• Common side effects: xerostomia, sedation • Serious side effects: severe rebound hypertension if stopped suddenly, angioedema, AV block, depression. • Contraindications: hypersensitivity			
	Clonidine	Children ≥12 years: Initial: 0.2 mg/d Maximum: 2.4 mg/d	Oral: Twice a day Patch: Once a week	Tablet: 0.1, 0.2, 0.3 mg Transdermal patch: 0.1, 0.2, 0.3 mg/24 hr

*FDA pediatric labeling.

†Not recommended as first-line agents for pediatric hypertension.

Source: Adapted and Modified from National High Blood Pressure Education Program Working Group on High Blood Pressure in Children and Adolescents; The Fourth Report on the Diagnosis, Evaluation, and Treatment of High Blood Pressure in Children and Adolescents. Pediatrics August 2004; 114 (Supplement_2): 555-576, Table 9.

vasoconstriction, increases sympathetic activity, and reduces renal sodium excretion. These drugs also possess additional beneficial effects of decreasing proteinuria and delaying the progression of kidney damage in glomerular hypertension. Some side effects include hyperkalemia, acute renal failure, angioedema, teratogenic effects, and dry cough. Another commonly used first line of drug is the calcium-channel blocker (CCB). Some side effects of CCBs include peripheral edema, facial flushing, and headaches. Diuretics reduce blood pressure by increasing renal sodium excretion. Care should be taken to restrict sodium in patients taking diuretics since a high sodium intake will reduce the effect of the diuretic. Diuretics should be avoided in athletes. Side effects include electrolyte abnormalities and dehydration.

Beta-blockers, alpha-1 adrenergic receptor antagonists, vasodilators, and centrally acting alpha-2 agonists are not recommended as first-line drugs for management of pediatric hypertension and should be reserved for refractory hypertension. Beta-blockers decrease sympathetic activity, cardiac output, and renin and aldosterone release. Alpha-1 adrenergic receptor antagonists, including doxazosin, prazosin, and terazosin, act peripherally to reduce arteriolar resistance. They are often used in conditions wherein the sympathetic system is activated, such as in pheochromocytoma, metabolic syndrome, and in cases of severe and resistant hypertension. Vasodilators reduce blood pressure by lowering peripheral vascular resistance. The use of vasodilators is generally reserved for refractory hypertension. Clonidine, a centrally acting alpha-2 agonist. Clonidine lowers blood pressure and heart rate by relaxing the arteries and increasing the blood supply to the heart. It has a sedative effect, and thus may be used in children with hyperactivity disorder.

NONPHARMACOLOGIC TREATMENT

Children with elevated blood pressure and no end-organ target damage can be treated with lifestyle modifications that include weight reduction and dietary changes. Exercise leads to a decrease in abdominal fat, arterial stiffness, and therefore blood pressure in prepubertal obese children. Children should devote at least 30 to 60 minutes daily to exercise and reduce their sedentary activities. Physical activity has also been linked to dietary habits. For example, television viewing has been associated with poor diet quality, including higher intake of fast food and lower intake of fruits and vegetables.

Dietary modifications include salt restriction. Current recommendations include restricting sodium to less than 1.2 g/day for 4- to 8-year-old children and 1.5 g/day for children older than 9 years. Other dietary recommendations include adopting the DASH (Dietary Approaches to Stop Hypertension) diet, a diet rich in vegetables, fruits, and low-fat dairy foods which has been shown to reduce blood pressure in hypertensive patients. The DASH diet provides a rich source of calcium, potassium, and magnesium elements that have been associated with decreased blood pressures.

SUBSPECIALTY CONSULTATION

Most hospitalized children with mild to moderate hypertension requiring admission can be managed effectively by the pediatric clinician without referral to a sub-specialist, especially when the high blood pressure is transient and linked to anxiety or an acute self-limited illness. Certain clinical situations may require specialty input. These include the following:

- Hypertension requiring continuous infusions of antihypertensive medications for blood pressure management
- Hypertension requiring more than one agent for effective control
- Hypertension accompanied by renal insufficiency or other evidence of end-organ damage such as left ventricular hypertrophy, retinal vessel changes, or seizures
- Hypertension accompanied by any urinary abnormalities, or urinary tract or renal parenchymal abnormalities on imaging
- High index of clinical suspicion for renovascular hypertension
- Suspected coarctation of the aorta
- Hypertension accompanied by finding of high catecholamine levels

KEY POINTS

- The prevalence of high blood pressure in children in both the hospital and ambulatory settings is estimated to be about 4% and much higher in obese or overweight children.
- There is strong evidence linking pediatric hypertension to hypertension during adulthood.
- Blood pressure should be obtained using proper technique and an elevated reading should be confirmed by repeated measurements.
- There have been several changes to the definition, evaluation approach, and treatment of hypertension in the updated clinical practice guideline for screening and management of high blood pressure in children and adolescents published in 2017.
- The evaluation for secondary causes should focus primarily on renal parenchymal disease, with other causes suspected mainly from the history and physical examination.
- Symptomatic hypertension or sustained hypertension >95th percentile +12 mm Hg should be treated while an evaluation is ongoing.
- The first line of medications to be used for long-term management of hypertension is calcium channel blockers, ACE inhibitors, angiotensin receptor blockers, or a thiazide diuretic.
- Subspecialty referral should be initiated if an intensive care setting is required because of the hypertension, if end-organ damage is discovered, or if management or diagnostic evaluation becomes complicated.

SUGGESTED READINGS

Berenson GS, Srinivasan SR, Hunter SM, et al. Risk factors in early life as predictors of adult heart disease: The bogalusa heart study. *Am J Med Sci.* 1989;298(3):141-151.

Flynn J. The changing face of pediatric hypertension in the era of the childhood obesity epidemic. *Pediatric Nephrology.* 2013;28(7):1059-1066.

Flynn JT, Kaelber DC, Baker-Smith CM, et al. Clinical practice guideline for screening and management of high blood pressure in children and adolescents. *Pediatrics.* 2017;140(3).

Foster BJ, Khoury PR, Kimball TR, Mackie AS, Mitsnefes M. New reference centiles for left ventricular mass relative to lean body mass in children. *J Am Soc Echocardiogr.* 2016;29(5):441-447.e2.

Fugate JE, Rabinstein AA. Posterior reversible encephalopathy syndrome: Clinical and radiological manifestations, pathophysiology, and outstanding questions. *Lancet Neurology.* 2015;14(9):914-925.

Gadde KM, Martin CK, Berthoud H, Heymsfield SB. Obesity: Pathophysiology and management. *J Am Coll Cardiol.* 2018;71(1):69-84.

Jackson SL, Zhang Z, Wiltz JL, et al. Hypertension among youths—United States, 2001–2016. *Am J Transplant.* 2018;18(9):2356-2360.

Jacobs DR, Woo JG, Sinaiko AR, et al. Childhood cardiovascular risk factors and adult cardiovascular events. *N Engl J Med.* 2022;386(20):1877-1888.

Juonala M, Magnussen CG, Berenson GS, et al. Childhood adiposity, adult adiposity, and cardiovascular risk factors. *N Engl J Med.* 2011;365:1876-1885.

Koechli S, Endes K, Infanger D, Zahner L, Hanssen H. Obesity, blood pressure, and retinal vessels: a meta-analysis. *Pediatrics.* 2018;141(6).

Konecny T, Kara T, Somers VK. Obstructive sleep apnea and hypertension: an update. *Hypertension.* 2014;63(2):203-209.

Lande MB, Kupferman JC. Blood pressure and cognitive function in children and adolescents. *Hypertension.* 2019;73(3):532-540.

Leyvraz M, Chatelan A, da Costa BR, et al. Sodium intake and blood pressure in children and adolescents: A systematic review and meta-analysis of experimental and observational studies. *Int J Epidemiol.* 2018;47(6):1796-1810.

Parker ED, Sinaiko AR, Kharbanda EO, et al. Change in weight status and development of hypertension. *Pediatrics.* 2016;137(3).

Roth GA, Johnson CO, Abate KH, et al. The burden of cardiovascular diseases among US states, 1990-2016. *JAMA Cardiology.* 2018;3(5):375-389.

Rountas C, Vlychou M, Vassiou K, et al. Imaging modalities for renal artery stenosis in suspected renovascular hypertension: Prospective intraindividual comparison of color doppler US, CT angiography, GD-enhanced MR angiography, and digital substraction angiography. *Ren Fail.* 2007;29(3):295-302.

Sharma AK, Metzger DL, Rodd CJ. Prevalence and severity of high blood pressure among children based on the 2017 American Academy of Pediatrics guidelines. *JAMA Pediatrics.* 2018;172(6):557-565.

Whelton PK, Carey RM, Aronow WS, et al. 2017 ACC/AHA/AAPA/ABC/ACPM/AGS/APhA/ASH/ASPC/NMA/PCNA guideline for the prevention, detection, evaluation, and management of high blood pressure in adults: a report of the American College of Cardiology/American Heart Association Task Force on Clinical Practice Guidelines. *J Am Coll Cardiol.* 2018;71(19):e127-e248.

Woroniecki RP, Kahnauth A, Panesar LE, Supe-Markovina K. Left ventricular hypertrophy in pediatric hypertension: a mini review. *Front Pediatr.* 2017;5:101.

SECTION L
Neurology

CHAPTER 118 Seizures

Paul E. Manicone, MD and Marina M. Eskandar, MD

BACKGROUND

Approximately 4% to 10% of children will have at least one seizure before the age of 16 years. A seizure is the manifestation of abnormally synchronized electrical activity in the brain. The initial approach to a patient with a seizure should focus on stabilizing the patient and evaluating for potentially reversible seizure causes. While most unprovoked seizures are brief and resolve spontaneously, seizures secondary to metabolic disturbances, infections, or intracranial hemorrhage may be more prolonged. Timely evaluation and treatment are essential in preventing or minimizing the complications of a prolonged seizure, including hypoventilation, tissue hypoxia, and cerebral edema.

Most children who experience a single seizure, which is often provoked by fever or acute illness, do not go on to develop epilepsy. Epilepsy is diagnosed by the presence of recurrent unprovoked seizures and has a prevalence in childhood of approximately 0.5%.

EPILEPTIC SEIZURES

CLINICAL PRESENTATION

The presentation and seizure semiology (symptoms during a seizure) depends on the region of brain involved as well as the underlying etiology. Epilepsy classification systems are clinically useful frameworks and provide diagnostic and therapeutic criteria.

Previous classification systems (e.g., the 1981 International Classification of Epileptic Seizures and the 1989 International Classification of Epilepsies, Epileptic Syndromes, and Related Disorders), although widely accepted, were based primarily on the phenomenology of the seizure and concepts that predate the era of neuroimaging, genetic technologies, and modern molecular biology. Since 2001, the International League Against Epilepsy (ILAE) has moved toward a classification that allows for neuroscientific advances to be incorporated into clinical practice.

According to the 2017 ILAE revised terminology, seizures have been classified as either generalized onset or focal onset (**Table 118-1**). Generalized seizures are defined as originating anywhere within, and rapidly involving bilateral hemispheres. This produces a loss or impairment of consciousness and may present as bilateral tonic activity (stiffening), clonic activity (rhythmic jerking), tonic-clonic activity (stiffening followed by or alternating with rhythmic jerking), atonic activity (loss of tone), myoclonic activity (sudden contraction of muscles), or absence seizures (typically with staring, blinking, and automatisms).

Focal seizures originate from networks limited to one hemisphere. Simple partial and complex partial terms, now less used in clinical practice, have been replaced by different focal seizure descriptors according to the degree of impairment during seizures (**Table 118-2**). For example, a focal seizure beginning in or rapidly spreading to the left motor strip (left frontal cortex) would likely involve clonic movements of the right arm, leg, or face without impairment of consciousness. A focal seizure arising from the temporal lobe might result in an abnormal psychic experience, such as déjà vu. A focal seizure can spread to involve the entire cortex and produce generalized seizure activity, but the emphasis is on the unilateral onset.

If a seizure's onset was unobserved (either because the patient was alone or because the observers did not notice the presence of focal features due to distraction at the manifestation of the seizure itself), it is deemed unknown onset. A seizure should also remain unclassified until further information is collected if the nature of the seizure does not allow it to fit into the previous categories.

The stereotypical presentations of focal and generalized seizures are as described earlier, but any change in consciousness or unexplained loss of consciousness can be due to electrical seizure activity without other outward signs. Therefore seizure—particularly nonconvulsive status epilepticus—must be included in the differential diagnosis of any patient with an altered mental status or altered level of consciousness (see Chapter 18, "Altered Mental Status").

The ILAE classification also formalized the term *electroclinical syndrome,* defined as a constellation of clinical and EEG features often with similar age-dependent features and comorbidities. It frequently

TABLE 118-1 Classification of Seizures

Generalized-onset seizures
Tonic-clonic
Clonic
Tonic
Myoclonic
Myoclonic-atonic
Myoclonic-tonic-clonic
Atonic
Epileptic spasms
Absence (typical, atypical, special features such as myoclonic absence or eyelid myoclonia)
Focal-onset seizures
Automatisms
Atonic
Clonic
Epileptic spasms
Hyperkinetic
Myoclonic
Tonic
Autonomic
Behavior arrest
Cognitive
Emotional
Sensory
Unknown onset
Tonic-clonic
Epileptic spasms
Behavior arrest

TABLE 118-2 Descriptors of Focal Seizures According to Degree of Impairment During Seizure

Without impairment of consciousness or awareness
With motor or autonomic symptoms (corresponds to "simple partial seizure")
With subjective sensory or psychic symptoms (corresponds to "aura")
With impairment of consciousness or awareness (corresponds to "complex partial seizures")
Evolving to a bilateral, convulsive seizure (corresponds to "secondarily generalized seizure")

has associated implications for etiology, prognosis, and treatment (**Table 118-3**).

Approximately one-third of children have epilepsy due to a specific electroclinical syndrome, but the majority of epilepsies are related to other causes such as structural abnormalities in the cortex (including tumor, stroke, or congenital malformations), genetic, metabolic, infectious, or immune conditions.

Status epilepticus, or a continuous seizure, was formerly defined as any single seizure lasting 30 minutes or recurrent seizures over a period longer than 30 minutes without intervening return to baseline mental status. In 2015 the ILAE revised the definition for generalized convulsive status epilepticus to be "≥5 minutes of continuous seizure or two or more discrete seizures between which there is incomplete recovery of consciousness." Status epilepticus for a focal seizure with impaired awareness is defined as ≥10 minutes of continuous seizure or multiple discrete seizures between which there is incomplete recovery of consciousness.

TABLE 118-3 Electroclinical Syndromes Arranged by Age at Onset

Neonatal-infant period
Self-limited (familial) neonatal epilepsy
Early infantile developmental and epileptic encephalopathy (includes Ohtahara syndrome and early myoclonic encephalopathy)
Epilepsy in infancy with migrating focal seizures
Infantile Epileptic Spasm Syndrome (includes West syndrome)
Myoclonic epilepsy in infancy (MEI)
Self-limited (familial) infantile epilepsy
Self-limited familial neonatal and infantile epilepsy
Dravet syndrome
Gelastic seizures with hypothalamic hamartoma
Etiology-specific developmental epileptic encephalopathies (e.g., KCNQ2, pyridoxine-dependent and pyridoxamine 5′ phosphate deficiency, CDKL5, PCDH19, GLUT1 transporter deficiency, Sturge Weber Syndrome)
Childhood
Genetic epilepsy with febrile seizures plus (GEFS+) (can start in infancy)
Self-limited epilepsy with autonomic seizures (e.g., Panayiotopoulos syndrome)
Epilepsy with myoclonic atonic seizures
Self-limited (Childhood) epilepsy with centrotemporal spikes (SeLECTS)
Childhood occipital visual epilepsy (Gastaut type epilepsy)
Photosensitive occipital lobe epilepsy
Epilepsy with myoclonic absences
Epilepsy with eyelid myoclonia
Lennox-Gastaut syndrome
Developmental and/or epileptic encephalopathy with Spike-Wave Activation in sleep (DEE-SWAS)
Childhood absence epilepsy (CAE)
Febrile infection-related epilepsy syndrome
Hemiconvulsion-hemiplegia-epilepsy
Adolescence-Adult
Juvenile absence epilepsy (JAE)
Juvenile myoclonic epilepsy (JME)
Epilepsy with generalized tonic-clonic seizures alone
Variable age
Familial focal epilepsy with variable foci
Epilepsy with reading-induced seizures
Sleep-related hypermotor (Hyperkinetic) epilepsy (Autosomal-dominant nocturnal frontal lobe epilepsy)
Epilepsy with auditory features
Familial Mesial Temporal Lobe Epilepsy
Progressive myoclonic epilepsy (PME)
Mesial temporal lobe epilepsy with hippocampal sclerosis
Rasmussen syndrome

TABLE 118-4 Differential Diagnosis of Seizures

Syncope (in which anoxia may also precipitate a provoked seizure)
Cardiac arrhythmia with collapse
Breath-holding spell
Tics
Myoclonus (including benign neonatal sleep myoclonus, benign myoclonus of early infancy)
Migraine variant (complicated migraine)
Other paroxysmal disorders of childhood (e.g., movement disorders, paroxysmal tonic upgaze, shuddering attacks, benign paroxysmal vertigo, etc.)
Gastroesophageal reflux disease (including Sandifer syndrome)
Behavioral event (e.g., nonepileptic staring, self-gratification disorder, stereotypies)
Sleep-related condition
Psychogenic nonepileptic seizure

DIFFERENTIAL DIAGNOSIS

The differential diagnosis of seizure includes a variety of neurologic and non-neurologic conditions (**Table 118-4**). In a previously normal child, the evaluation of a first seizure should include a careful review of the event itself to determine whether or not it was in fact a seizure and its possible precipitating factors. In most cases, a description of the event by the parent or caretaker, or possibly from the child, must suffice in arriving at a working clinical diagnosis.

DIAGNOSTIC EVALUATION

The causes of a new seizure in a previously healthy child or an increase in seizure frequency in a child with known seizures should always be investigated. Although an otherwise healthy child is unlikely to have an occult abnormality, it is important to distinguish an unprovoked seizure from an acute symptomatic (or provoked) seizure if this is the child's first presentation. An unprovoked seizure occurs in the absence of an apparent precipitating illness or condition. Two unprovoked seizures taking place at least 24 hours apart or a high risk of recurrence (as defined by an expert) after one unprovoked seizure constitutes a diagnosis of epilepsy. Meanwhile, a symptomatic seizure is due to a temporarily lowered seizure threshold in the setting of an acute central nervous system (CNS) insult such as a metabolic, toxic, structural, infectious, or inflammatory etiology. The seizure is "not expected to recur once the precipitating factor or condition has been removed or reversed."

Children with known epilepsy may have an underlying infection, such as a urinary tract infection, or other systemic disturbance that tends to decrease the seizure threshold. Factors that can provoke seizures are listed in **Table 118-5**. The likelihood of each must be judged based on the entire clinical picture. The same precipitating factors apply to children with epilepsy who are taking antiepileptic medication, along with the additional considerations listed in **Table 118-6**.

The pace and extent of the diagnostic evaluation depend on the clinical setting. A detailed history and physical examination—with immediate assessment of airway, breathing, circulation, and glucose, followed by a comprehensive general and neurologic examination—should guide the evaluation. **Table 118-7** presents several approaches to the diagnostic evaluation of a child with seizures, based on the clinical history and state of the patient.

In a stable, well-appearing, otherwise healthy child who presents with a brief new-onset seizure, extensive laboratory evaluation is of little diagnostic value. In the emergency department, a typical evaluation includes measurement of glucose, serum electrolytes, and calcium. There is evidence that even this limited screen for abnormalities is not necessary in patients older than 6 months with no concern for dehydration or gastrointestinal losses who have returned to baseline mental status. The history and clinical judgment must be used to decide whether other tests, such as urine toxicology screening, are needed. A previously healthy child with a new unprovoked seizure should have neurologic follow-up within 1 to 2 weeks for a comprehensive evaluation. Additional workup may include an electroencephalogram (EEG) or outpatient magnetic

TABLE 118-5 Factors That May Precipitate Seizures

Fever
Infection
Meningitis (bacterial; viral, including herpes simplex virus)
Encephalitis (infectious; autoimmune)
Sepsis (especially in neonates)
Minor afebrile infection (commonly diarrheal illness)
COVID-19
Hypoxia or ischemia
Head trauma-producing concussion or intracranial hemorrhage
Cerebral venous thrombosis
Posterior reversible encephalopathy syndrome
Metabolic disturbance
Low or high glucose
Low or high sodium
Low calcium
Low magnesium
Hyperammonemia
Uremia and renal failure
Hyperthyroidism
Pregnancy or toxemia (usually second or third trimester)
Inborn error of metabolism
Medication (e.g., imipenem, meperidine, cyclosporine)
Medication withdrawal (e.g., benzodiazepines)
Toxin or illicit substance (e.g., cocaine)

resonance imaging (MRI). Outpatient MRI should be performed after a first-time seizure for children younger than 1 year of age, and children with a history of focal seizures or convulsive seizures for which the onset may have been focal, even if not directly observed. In addition, children with an abnormal neurologic history or examination (e.g., significant cognitive or motor impairment of unknown etiology) or with EEG abnormalities that do not fall into the category of a primary generalized or benign epilepsy syndrome (e.g., childhood absence epilepsy) should have an outpatient MRI. Both EEG and MRI can be helpful in assessing the risk of seizure recurrence.

Ill-appearing children warrant a more extensive initial evaluation. In the presence of fever and findings that suggest the possibility of meningitis or encephalitis, computed tomography (CT) of the head should be followed by lumbar puncture. These tests should not delay the administration of broad-spectrum antibiotics or acyclovir in an ill-appearing febrile child who has had a seizure. If a patient does not return to a normal baseline neurologic status, an EEG is required to evaluate for nonconvulsive status epilepticus, and the patient should be admitted to a unit with appropriate monitoring capability.

TABLE 118-6 Additional Factors That May Precipitate Seizures in Patients with Epilepsy

Systemic infection (with or without fever)
Urinary tract infection
Upper or lower respiratory tract infection
Sinusitis
Bacteremia
Other systemic disturbance
Dehydration
Subtherapeutic antiepileptic medication
Illness causing decreased intake or absorption of antiepileptic medication
Concurrent use of other medications that lower antiepileptic medication levels
Noncompliance
Toxic level of antiepileptic medication (e.g., phenytoin, valproic acid)

TABLE 118-7 Diagnostic Evaluation of a Patient With Seizure

Basic Evaluation
Vital signs, history, and physical examination
Electrocardiogram
Blood glucose level
Serum electrolytes, magnesium, and calcium levels*
Urine toxicology screen*
Urine pregnancy screen in age-appropriate girls*
If febrile, evaluation for source of fever (e.g., CBC, viral PCR testing, blood culture, urine culture, chest radiograph)
Additional Studies
In well-appearing, previously normal patients who return to baseline after a first seizure
Outpatient neurologic consultation with EEG
Possible outpatient MRI
In a patient with recent head trauma, persistent headache, acute focal neurological deficit, ventricular shunt, signs of increased intracranial pressure, or history of malignancy, immunocompromise, anticoagulation, or bleeding diathesis
CT of the head, consider CT or MR venogram
In a patient with meningitic features (i.e., fever, photophobia, neck stiffness)
CT of the head
Lumbar puncture following CT
If the patient has altered consciousness
Liver transaminases
Consider blood ammonia level, thyroid studies, and screening tests for other inborn errors of metabolism
Consider arterial blood gas
CT of the head
Consider lumbar puncture after CT when patient is stable
EEG if patient does not return to baseline or nonconvulsive status epilepticus is suspected
In patients with persistent focal neurological abnormality following a focal seizure
CT of the head with consideration of CT or MR venogram
If patient has transient or no focal deficits following a focal seizure and is back to baseline, may perform expedited MRI of the brain
In patients with neuropsychiatric and cognitive symptoms or dyskinesias
Thyroid studies
Consider ESR and screening tests for rheumatologic disease if additional systemic signs such as rash, arthralgia, etc. MRI brain with and without contrast
Lumbar puncture to evaluate for autoimmune encephalitis in consultation with a neurologist
In patients with a prior history of seizures
Liver transaminases and blood urea nitrogen level
Serum ammonia level if taking valproic acid or if comatose
Consider other screens for inborn errors of metabolism if cause of patient's seizures is not well established
Consider arterial blood gas
Appropriate anticonvulsant levels
CBC with platelets
CT of the head in those with a ventricular shunt, history of recent head trauma, coma, or focal neurologic abnormality
EEG if patient does not return to baseline or nonconvulsive status epilepticus is suspected

CBC, complete blood count; CT, computed tomography; EEG, electroencephalogram; ESR, erythrocyte sedimentation rate; MRI, magnetic resonance imaging.

*Depending on history, at clinician's discretion.

Children with epilepsy might have the same seizure precipitants as children without prior seizures, therefore particular attention should be given to a history of recent infection, head trauma, or toxin ingestion. A change in the medication regimen, lack of adherence to medication plan, or conditions causing malabsorption can lead to increased seizure frequency. Anticonvulsant levels must be obtained and interpreted with regard to the timing of last administered dose, and, when possible, those levels should be compared to the patient's prior levels.

The clinical course of a patient with seizures depends on the cause of the seizures. An otherwise well child with a provoked seizure in the setting of a mild self-limited illness, a toxic exposure, or an electrolyte abnormality does not have a significantly increased risk of seizure recurrence, whereas a child with acute symptomatic seizures caused by structural brain pathology is at increased risk for developing epilepsy later in life as a sequela of the prior injury. A previously healthy child with a first-time unprovoked seizure has a 50% chance of seizure recurrence within 3 years (further increased risk if they have a focal seizure, epileptiform discharges on EEG, or family history of epilepsy). A child with a known chronic encephalopathy with seizures has an even higher likelihood of seizure recurrence.

Most individual seizures are brief and cause no damage to the brain. A fall during a seizure might result in head trauma, and aspiration of gastrointestinal contents or excessive saliva could result in pneumonia, but these are uncommon events. The development of status epilepticus can result in respiratory or cardiovascular complications, which necessitate respiratory support in an intensive care setting. Status epilepticus that persists for 30 minutes or longer may cause long-term consequences such as neuronal death or alteration of neuronal networks.

MANAGEMENT

Seizure treatment generally consists of two main elements: acute seizure management and seizure prevention in patients with a risk of recurrence. Because most seizures are self-limited, initial management consists of stabilization of the airway, breathing, and circulation, and prompt evaluation of underlying causes of the seizure. Proper monitoring should be established, including cardiorespiratory monitoring and pulse oximetry. Supplemental oxygen should be administered as needed and whenever possible, intravenous access should be obtained. Reversible causes of the seizure should be appropriately corrected. Hypoglycemia requires rapid correction, and disturbances in sodium balance require judicious, slow correction. Broad-spectrum antibiotics with good CNS penetration should be given at doses appropriate to treat meningitis until CNS or other infection has been excluded in any child with signs of CNS infection; acyclovir should be added if CNS herpetic infection is suspected.

Intervention for a child with continuous or recurrent seizures (whether provoked or unprovoked), should begin by 5 minutes into the seizure (per definition of status epilepticus) because a seizure of that length is unlikely to self-terminate and may become more resistant to antiseizure medications. Pharmacologic treatment should be initiated sooner than 5 minutes in these high-risk settings: a child at increased risk of intracranial pathology (such as increased intracranial pressure or brain edema), a child with a severe known epileptic syndrome who has a seizure lasting longer than their typical seizure, or a child with multiorgan failure who is unlikely to tolerate the sympathetic activity generated by a seizure. These children should all be considered to have incipient status epilepticus and treated immediately.

Treatment of the seizure should not be delayed during the process of cardiorespiratory stabilization and workup for reversible causes. Pharmacologic management to stop the seizure activity should be initiated at 5 minutes regardless of the patient's stability or the cause of the seizure. Medications used in the acute treatment of seizures are outlined in **Table 118-8**. If intravenous (IV) access cannot be established within the first 5 minutes, a benzodiazepine should be administered via other routes such as intramuscular, rectal, buccal, or nasal. Vigilant monitoring of oxygenation, ventilation, and circulatory status is essential during the administration of these medications because of their sedative and potential respiratory and cardiovascular effects. If the medications listed in Table 118-8 are not effective, further therapy with agents such as pentobarbital, midazolam (by continuous IV infusion), or general anesthesia

TABLE 118-8 Medications for the Acute Treatment of Seizures

After 5 minutes, or sooner if warranted by the clinical situation:
Intravenous lorazepam 0.1 mg/kg/dose (maximum 4 mg/dose), may repeat dose once in 5 minutes OR
Intramuscular midazolam 10 mg for >40 kg, 5 mg for 13-40 kg, single dose. If no IV access may give buccal 0.5 mg/kg or intranasal 0.2 mg/kg (maximum for both 10 mg/dose)
Intravenous diazepam 0.15-0.2 mg/kg/dose (maximum: 10 mg/dose), may repeat dose once in 5 minutes. If no IV access may give rectal diazepam 0.2-0.5 mg/kg up to 20 mg in children older than 2 years.
If seizures persist after 10 minutes, proceed to:
Intravenous fosphenytoin 20 mg phenytoin equivalents/kg (maximum 1500 mg PE/dose), single dose OR
Intravenous valproic acid 40 mg/kg (max 3000 mg/dose), single dose* OR
Intravenous levetiracetam 60 mg/kg (max 4500 mg/dose), single dose OR
Intravenous phenobarbital 15-20 mg/kg, single dose

Source: Adapted from: Glauser T, Shinnar S, Gloss D, et al. Evidence-based guideline: treatment of convulsive status epilepticus in children and adults: report of the guideline committee of the American Epilepsy Society. *Epilepsy Curr*. 2016;16(1):48-61.

*Use valproic acid if child is older than 2 years and there is no suspicion of metabolic disease or liver dysfunction; higher doses should be used in children also on enzyme-inducing agents.

should be administered in an intensive care setting, ideally with continuous EEG monitoring.

The initial treatment of a child with a new diagnosis of epilepsy requires an accurate diagnosis of the particular seizure disorder as well as an understanding of the wide range of available antiseizure medications (**Table 118-9**). There are limited studies of antiseizure medications in children, and some are not yet approved by the Food and Drug Administration for specific indications. **Table 118-10** provides the generic and select trade names of antiseizure medications used in children with epilepsy and a limited list of their adverse reactions.

ADMISSION AND DISCHARGE CRITERIA

Admission Criteria

Acute care unit

- First-time unprovoked seizure in a child <1 year of age
- Increased or prolonged seizures compared to baseline in a child with known history of seizures (but able to be controlled without IV infusions of antiseizure medications)
- High caregiver anxiety following the seizure
- Treatment of the underlying cause of the seizure, such as infection or metabolic abnormality
- Patient does not return to baseline mental status >1 hour after the seizure
- Inability to identify the underlying cause of the seizure in an ill-appearing child, or a child with an abnormal examination

Intensive care unit

- Patient is in status epilepticus
- Close neurological monitoring is required due to increased intracranial pressure, intracranial hemorrhage, ischemic stroke, correction of severe metabolic abnormalities, or need for cardiorespiratory support.

Discharge Criteria

- The patient is medically stable, and seizure control is adequate for outpatient management.
- The patient's caretakers are trained in basic cardiopulmonary resuscitation and first aid during seizures. Some caretakers can be instructed in the use of diazepam rectal gel for the initial management of a prolonged seizure.
- Patients who are started on antiepileptic medications are able to take them orally and do not have significant side effects, such as excessive drowsiness, severe nausea, or ataxia.

TABLE 118-9 Antiseizure Medications for Pediatric Seizures and Epileptic Syndromes

Seizure Disorder	Drugs of Choice
Generalized tonic-clonic seizures	Topiramate
	Valproic acid
	Lamotrigine
	Carbamazepine
	Levetiracetam
Generalized absence seizures	Ethosuximide
	Valproic acid
	Lamotrigine
Focal seizures	Carbamazepine
	Oxcarbazepine
	Lamotrigine
	Topiramate
	Lacosamide
Self-limited Epilepsy with Centrotemporal Spikes (SeLECTs), formerly known as benign rolandic epilepsy	Carbamazepine
	Oxcarbazepine
	Levetiracetam
Juvenile myoclonic epilepsy	Valproic acid
	Lamotrigine
	Levetiracetam
	Topiramate
Neonatal seizures	Phenobarbital
	Phenytoin
	Levetiracetam
	Topiramate
Infantile spasms	ACTH
	Prednisolone
	Vigabatrin
	Topiramate
Lennox-Gastaut syndrome	Clobazam
	Rufinamide
	Lamotrigine
	Valproic acid
	Topiramate
	Felbamate

ACTH, adrenocorticotropic hormone.

CONSULTATION

Consultation with a neurologist is advised for new-onset seizures, especially in the case of a focal neurologic deficit, and for seizures that are not self-limited. Neurology consultation is also advised when initiating and adjusting antiseizure medications in patients with a diagnosis of epilepsy.

Critical care consultation is required when the patient's cardiorespiratory status is unstable, for intractable status epilepticus that requires cardiorespiratory support (e.g., intravenous infusion sedatives or general anesthesia), or if the cause of the seizure warrants close neurologic monitoring (e.g., increased intracranial pressure, ischemic injury, intracranial hemorrhage).

FEBRILE SEIZURES

BACKGROUND

Febrile seizures are the most common seizures seen in children younger than 5 years. The 1993 ILAE guidelines defined a febrile seizure as an epileptic seizure occurring in children older than 1 month and associated with a febrile illness, excluding those with prior unprovoked or neonatal seizures, acute CNS infection, or electrolyte imbalance, and not meeting criteria for other acute symptomatic seizures. According to the American Academy of Pediatrics (AAP) 2011 guidelines on febrile seizures, a febrile seizure is defined as a seizure accompanied by a fever (temperature greater than 100.4°F or 38.0°C by any method) without CNS infection that occurs in infants and children 6 through 60 months of age.

Febrile seizures are classified as simple or complex. Simple febrile seizures, which constitute 85% of all febrile seizures, last for less than 15 minutes, are generalized with no evidence of focality and do not occur more than once in 24 hours. Febrile seizures that last for more than 15 minutes, have focal features (at any time), or recur within 24 hours are considered complex. Most febrile seizures are self-limited and last only a few minutes.

Febrile seizures occur in 2% to 5% of all children. The peak age of onset is 14 to 18 months. A strong family history of febrile seizures in siblings and parents suggests a genetic predisposition. Twenty-five percent to 40% of patients have an immediate family member with a history of febrile seizures. If one parent has a history of febrile seizures, a child's risk of having a febrile seizure is greater than four times that of the general population. If both parents have a history of febrile seizures, the risk increases to 20 times that of the general population. Siblings of a child with febrile seizures have a risk 3.6 times greater than that of the general population. Even the concordance rate in monozygotic twins is higher than that in dizygotic twins.

PATHOPHYSIOLOGY

The underlying pathophysiology of febrile seizures is unknown. Viral infections are frequently associated with febrile seizures, particularly human herpesviruses and influenza A and B. It is estimated that human herpesvirus 6 accounts for one-third of first-time febrile seizures in children younger than 2 years, and human herpesvirus 7 is increasingly being recognized as a causative agent as well. Severe Acute Respiratory Syndrome Coronavirus 2 (SARS-CoV-2) has also been associated with febrile seizures in infants and children less than 5 years of age during the COVID-19 pandemic. The rates of serious bacterial infection in patients with febrile seizures are similar to the rates in age-matched febrile children without seizures.

CLINICAL PRESENTATION

Children with simple febrile seizures are neurologically and developmentally normal before and after the seizure. Simple febrile seizures often occur with the initial temperature elevation at the onset of illness. The seizure may be the first indication that the child is ill.

The history should address the details of the event to characterize the seizure as simple or complex. Additional information should focus on the fever's duration, exposures, and associated symptoms. Medications given at home should also be checked, especially antibiotics. The possibility of partially treated meningitis in an infant or child with recent or current antibiotic use should be considered.

The physical examination should concentrate on identifying the underlying fever source, assessing the likelihood of meningitis or encephalitis, and identifying generalized or focal neurologic abnormalities. The child should have a normal neurologic examination or, if presenting in the postictal period, should be observed until the examination returns to normal. Any prolonged alteration in the child's general appearance or mental status or any finding suggestive of a focal deficit signifies the need for a more aggressive evaluation, such as neuroimaging and lumbar puncture.

DIFFERENTIAL DIAGNOSIS

A broad range of entities can present with a febrile seizure, seizure-like activity, or altered mental status (**Table 118-11**). Convulsive behavior may be a consequence of the fever itself or of the condition that caused the fever.

TABLE 118-10 Antiseizure Medications and Prominent Adverse Effects

Generic Name	Trade Name	Side Effects*
ACTH	Acthar Gel	Irritability, Cushingoid features, hypertension, hyperglycemia, electrolyte imbalance, immunosuppression
Carbamazepine	Tegretol, Carbatrol	Cardiac arrhythmia and conduction delays, sedation, dizziness, GI symptoms, SJS, bone marrow suppression, hepatitis, SIADH
Clobazam	Onfi, Sympazan	Sedation, dry mouth, decreased appetite, constipation, aggressive outbursts
Ethosuximide	Zarontin	Sedation, headache, GI symptoms, SJS, hiccups, dyskinesia, granulocytopenia, behavioral disturbances
Felbamate	Felbatol	GI symptoms, dizziness, insomnia, aplastic anemia, hepatotoxicity, diplopia
Gabapentin	Neurontin	Sedation, ataxia, diplopia, agitation, GI symptoms, increased appetite, pancreatitis
Lacosamide	Vimpat	Dizziness, headache, nystagmus, GI symptoms, PR interval prolongation (avoid in second or third-degree heart block or other cardiac conduction problems). If cardiac history unknown, obtain EKG prior to initiating
Lamotrigine	Lamictal	Rash, dizziness, sedation, SJS, GI symptoms, increased risk of cardiac arrhythmia
Levetiracetam	Keppra	Somnolence, ataxia, behavioral symptoms (agitation, oppositional behavior, anxiety, emotional lability, depression)
Oxcarbazepine	Trileptal, Oxtellar XR	Somnolence, dizziness, GI symptoms, hyponatremia, rash
Phenobarbital	Luminal	Sedation, hyperactivity/irritability in some children, cognitive impairment, decreased bone mineral density, SJS, megaloblastic anemia, respiratory depression, may reduce serum levels of a wide variety of drugs
Phenytoin	Dilantin, Phenytek	Ataxia, lethargy, nystagmus, GI symptoms, hepatotoxicity, folic acid depletion, SJS, hirsutism, gingival hyperplasia, decreased bone mineral density, increased risk of SI, may reduce serum levels of a wide variety of drugs
Rufinamide	Banzel	Dizziness, somnolence, GI symptoms, hypersensitivity syndrome, decreases QTc interval
Topiramate	Topamax, Trokendi XR	Cognitive slowing, psychomotor slowing, ataxia, metabolic acidosis, hypohydrosis, paresthesias, GI symptoms, decreased appetite, weight loss, nystagmus, nephrolithiasis
Valproic acid	Depakene, Depakote, Epival	Ataxia, irritability, alopecia, thrombocytopenia, GI symptoms, hepatotoxicity (particularly under age 2), hyperammonemia, carnitine depletion, decreased bone mineral density, pancreatitis, weight gain, teratogenicity
Vigabatrin	Sabril, Vigadrone	Ataxia, rash, visual field defects, nystagmus, GI symptoms, weight gain, reversible changes on MRI of the brain, may increase seizures in patients with myoclonic or absence seizures
Zonisamide	Zonegran	Drowsiness, Ataxia, psychomotor slowing, behavioral symptoms, anorexia, metabolic acidosis, hypohydrosis, rash, SJS, nephrolithiasis, paresthesias, weight loss

ACTH, adrenocorticotropic hormone; GI, gastrointestinal; MRI, magnetic resonance imaging; SI, suicidal ideation; SIADH, syndrome of inappropriate antidiuretic hormone; SJS, Stevens-Johnson syndrome.

*This is only a partial list. Prescribers should consult pharmaceutical references for complete information.

DIAGNOSTIC EVALUATION

When a child presents with a febrile seizure, the evaluation should involve the seizure component as well as the febrile illness. This discussion will focus on the neurodiagnostic evaluation.

Routine laboratory studies are usually not indicated for patients with simple febrile seizures, with the exception of serum glucose. Laboratory studies should be driven by the nature of the underlying illness rather than the presentation of a febrile seizure. For example, patients with dehydration may warrant an electrolyte panel to evaluate for hyponatremia, which can cause convulsions.

Many physicians are faced with the decision of whether to perform a lumbar puncture to rule out meningitis in a patient with a febrile seizure. According to the AAP 2011 practice guidelines for children with a first simple febrile seizure, a lumbar puncture should be performed in any child presenting with a febrile seizure and who has meningeal signs and symptoms. The guidelines for infants younger than 6 months are not part of this practice guideline, as by definition, these children do not fit the age category of febrile seizures. A lumbar puncture, however, should be performed in that age group. In infants between 6 and 12 months of age, the AAP 2011 practice guidelines deem a lumbar puncture optional since the widespread immunization for *Haemophilus influenzae* type B and *Streptococcus pneumoniae*, two of the most common causes of bacterial meningitis in this age group. A recent analysis of the evaluation and management of simple febrile seizure from before and after the AAP 2011 guidelines showed a decrease in lumbar puncture from 11.6% in 2005 to 0.6% in 2019, as well as significant reductions in head CT, complete blood counts, hospital admissions and cost, without a significant change in delay of diagnosis of bacterial meningitis.

Patients with simple febrile seizures have the same risk for bacterial illnesses, including meningitis, as those who present with similar febrile illnesses without seizures. The indications for lumbar puncture in **Table 118-12** reflect the recommendations for a similarly aged patient with fever but no seizure.

The 2011 AAP practice guideline does not recommend neuroimaging (CT or MRI) for the routine evaluation of children with first simple febrile seizures. There are currently no guidelines for complex febrile seizures; however, studies have demonstrated that the risk of intracranial pathology requiring emergency neurosurgical or medical intervention is low in children with first complex febrile seizures. This suggests that routine imaging in patients with complex febrile seizures may be unnecessary as well. Neuroimaging should be considered in the following situations: uncertain diagnosis, inability to exclude increased intracranial

TABLE 118-11 Differential Diagnosis of Febrile Seizure

Seizures
- Epilepsy (decreased seizure threshold secondary to fever)
- Acute disseminated encephalomyelitis
- Intracranial infection (e.g., meningitis, encephalitis, brain abscess, epidural or subdural infections)

Seizure-like symptoms
- Shivering or rigors
- Febrile myoclonus
- Febrile delirium
- Drug-induced hyperthermia

TABLE 118-12 Indications to Perform Lumbar Puncture in a Child Younger Than 18 Months With a Febrile Seizure

- History of irritability, poor feeding, or lethargy
- Abnormal mental status beyond the postictal period
- Physical signs of meningitis, such as bulging fontanelle, Kernig or Brudzinski sign, photophobia, or inconsolable crying
- Pretreatment with antibiotics

pressure by physical examination, status epilepticus, persistent focal features, evidence of trauma, or presence of ventriculoperitoneal shunt.

The AAP practice guideline does not recommend an EEG for a neurologically healthy child with a first simple febrile seizure. The EEG does not reliably predict which patients will have recurrent febrile seizures or subsequently develop epilepsy. An EEG might be indicated in patients with evidence of developmental delay or underlying neurologic abnormalities, but this study is rarely needed on an urgent basis in the emergency room or inpatient setting.

MANAGEMENT

Several approaches have been investigated for the management and prevention of febrile seizures. These strategies include continuous or intermittent anticonvulsant therapy, prophylactic benzodiazepine therapy, and prophylactic antipyretic therapy.

Based on a risk-benefit analysis, neither long term nor intermittent anticonvulsant therapy is indicated for children who have experienced one or more simple febrile seizures. Phenobarbital is effective in preventing febrile seizures but has serious adverse effects, such as hyperactivity, hypersensitivity reactions, and a risk of cognitive impairment. Valproic acid is similarly effective in preventing febrile seizures but is associated with hepatotoxicity, thrombocytopenia, weight changes, gastrointestinal disturbances, and pancreatitis.

Oral diazepam given at the first sign of a febrile illness is effective in preventing febrile seizures; however, the adverse effects include lethargy, drowsiness, and ataxia. In addition, oral diazepam could mask the evolving signs of a CNS infection. In the rare instances where preventing subsequent febrile seizures is essential, diazepam is considered the treatment of choice.

Antipyretic agents are not effective in preventing recurrent febrile seizures. Although the routine use of prophylactic medications for simple febrile seizures is not indicated, there is insufficient evidence regarding their role in the treatment of complex febrile seizures.

Abortive therapy for future febrile seizures is another important consideration because approximately one in three children with a first febrile seizure will experience at least one recurrence with future febrile illnesses. Rectal diazepam gel (Diastat) has been approved by the Food and Drug Administration for home administration by trained nonprofessional caregivers and is effective in terminating febrile seizures. Because most febrile seizures are brief, abortive therapy is often not necessary. Those children with a history of prolonged seizure activity or multiple seizures, those who live far from medical care, or those with overly anxious caregivers may benefit from this medication. Proper training in use of the drug should occur before the child is discharged from the hospital. Abortive therapy for children who are actively seizing in the hospital setting is similar to the therapy for ongoing nonfebrile seizure activity. Intravenous or rectal diazepam is a good first choice.

The prognosis for children with febrile seizures is excellent. One-third of all children will experience a recurrent febrile seizure with a subsequent febrile illness. Children younger than 12 months at the time of their first simple febrile seizure have a 50% probability of recurrence. After 12 months, the risk decreases to 30%. Several risk factors for recurrence have been identified and are listed in **Table 118-13**.

The development of epilepsy and cognitive impairments are the two most important long-term outcomes that concern physicians and caregivers. In the general population, the risk of developing epilepsy by age 7 years is approximately 1%. Children younger than 12 months at the time of a first simple febrile seizure or those who have had multiple simple febrile seizures have a 2.4% risk of developing epilepsy. The risk is higher in patients with one or more complex febrile seizures. There is no evidence that children with simple febrile seizures develop any cognitive impairment. The long-term cognitive outcome for children with complex febrile seizures has not been well studied.

TABLE 118-13 Risk Factors for Recurrence of Febrile Seizure

Age younger than 18 months
Family history of febrile seizures or epilepsy
Lower peak fever (<40°C or <104°F) with prior febrile seizure
Shorter duration of fever with prior febrile seizure
Initial complex febrile seizure

ADMISSION AND DISCHARGE CRITERIA

Admission Criteria Hospitalization is generally not necessary for the evaluation or management of a febrile seizure in a child who meets the criteria for a simple febrile seizure, has a normal neurologic examination, is well hydrated, and has access to appropriate follow-up. The following are indications for hospitalization:

- Prolonged or persistent alteration of mental status.
- Clinical or laboratory evidence of meningitis or encephalitis.
- Multiple complex features requiring further monitoring or workup.
- Inadequate enteral hydration or nutrition due to underlying source of infection.
- Inadequate follow-up or lack of family reliability.
- Fever source requiring inpatient treatment.

Discharge Criteria

- Normal neurologic examination.
- Reassuring results of cerebrospinal fluid tests if performed.
- Neuroimaging not consistent with any evolving neurosurgical condition (e.g., space-occupying lesion, increased intracranial pressure) or infectious process (e.g., brain abscess) if performed.
- Demonstration of adequate oral hydration and nutrition.

CONSULTATION

Input from a neurologist may be warranted, especially if the diagnosis is in question, there are multiple complex features, or outpatient neurologic evaluation or management is needed.

KEY POINTS

- Most spontaneous or unprovoked seizures are self-limited. Children with underlying metabolic abnormalities, intracranial infection, or trauma are more likely to have prolonged seizures.
- The evaluation of children with seizures is guided by clinical assessment, including well versus ill appearance and first seizure versus history of previous seizures.
- Nonconvulsive status epilepticus may present as an altered mental status or an altered level of consciousness.
- Initial management includes cardiorespiratory stabilization, correction of metabolic disturbances, treatment of underlying localized or systemic infection, and, if there is ongoing seizure activity, pharmacologic therapy to abort the process.
- Children with known seizure disorders (with or without anticonvulsant therapy) may have a lower seizure threshold in the face of fever, metabolic abnormalities, or infection. When these patients show an increase in their baseline seizure activity, they require the same evaluation as patients without a history of seizures.
- Consultation with a neurologist is recommended when seizure activity is not self-limited, is difficult to control, includes focal neurologic deficits, when starting or adjusting antiseizure medications, or if the patient does not return to baseline neurologic status.
- Adherence to the 2011 AAP practice guideline on the evaluation of simple febrile seizures has resulted in fewer lumbar punctures, neuroimaging, laboratory studies, admissions, and a reduction in cost without a significant change in delay in diagnosis of bacterial meningitis
- Current and future studies will focus on complex febrile seizures: their evaluation and management and the associated risks. A practice guideline for complex febrile seizures will help reduce the wide variation in how this condition is evaluated and managed.
- Ongoing research in the area of genetic mapping will enhance our understanding of the genetic predispositions to febrile seizures.

ACKNOWLEDGMENTS

The authors would like to acknowledge the oversight of Dr. Claudine Sinsioco in assisting with revisions to this chapter.

SUGGESTED READINGS

American Academy of Pediatrics. Febrile seizures: guideline for the neurodiagnostic evaluation of the child with a simple febrile seizure. *Pediatrics*. 2011;127:389-394.

Bauman RJ, Duffner PK, Schneider S. Practice parameter: long-term treatment of the child with simple febrile seizures. American Academy of Pediatrics, Committee on Quality Improvement, Subcommittee on Febrile Seizures. *Pediatrics*. 1999;103:1307-1309.

Baumer JH. Evidence based guideline for post-seizure management in children presenting acutely to secondary care. *Arch Dis Child*. 2004;89(3):278-280.

Cadet K, Boegner J, Ceneviva G, et al. Evaluation of febrile seizure diagnosis associated with COVID-19. *J. Child Neurol*. 2022:27(5):410-415.

Camfield P, Camfield C. Incidence, prevalence and aetiology of seizures and epilepsy in children. *Epileptic Disorders*. 2015;17(2):117-123.

Engel J Jr. A proposed diagnostic scheme for people with epileptic seizures and with epilepsy: report of the ILAE task force on classification and terminology. *Epilepsia*. 2001;42(6):796-803.

Fisher RS, Cross JH, French JA, et al. Operational classification of seizure types by the International League against Epilepsy: position paper of the ILAE commission for classification and terminology. *Epilepsia*. 2017;58(4):522-530.

Friedman MJ, Sharieff GQ. Seizures in children. *Pediat Clin North Am*. 2006;53(2):257-277.

Glauser T, Shinnar S, Gloss D, et al. Evidence-based guideline: treatment of convulsive status epilepticus in children and adults: report of the guideline committee of the American Epilepsy Society. *Epilepsy Curr*. 2016;16(1):48-61.

Gogou M, Cross JH. Seizures and epilepsy in childhood. *CONTINUUM: Lifelong Learning in Neurology*. 2022;28(2):428-456.

Hirtz D, Ashwal S, Berg A, et al. Practice parameter: evaluating a first nonfebrile seizure in children: report of the quality standards subcommittee of the American Academy of Neurology, the Child Neurology Society, and the American Epilepsy Society. *Neurology*. 2000;55(5):616-623.

Mauritz M, Hirsch LJ, Camfield P, et al. Acute symptomatic seizures: an educational, evidence-based review. *Epileptic Disord*. 2022;24(1):26-49.

McLauchlan DJ, Powell R. Acute symptomatic seizures. *Pract Neurol*. 2012;12:154-165.

Mula M, Coleman H, Wilson SJ. Neuropsychiatric and cognitive comorbidities in epilepsy. *CONTINUUM: Lifelong Learning in Neurology*. 2022;28(2):457-482.

Pellino G, Faggioli R, Madrassi L, Falsaperla R, Suppiej A. Operational diagnosis of epilepsy in children at undetermined risk: a meta-analysis of prognostic factors for seizure recurrence. *Epilepsy Behav*. 2022;127:108498.

Ragahavan V, Porter J, Neuman M. et al. Trends in management of simple febrile seizures at US children's hospitals. *Pediatrics* 2021;148(5):e2021051517.

Takasaki K, Diaz Stransky A, Miller G. Psychogenic nonepileptic seizures: diagnosis, management, and bioethics. *Pediatr Neurol*. 2016;62:3-8.

Trinka E, Cock H, Hesdorffer D, et al. A definition and classification of status epilepticus - Report of the ILAE Task Force on Classification of Status Epilepticus. *Epilepsia*. 2015;56(10):1515-1523.

Wirrell EC, Nabbout R, Scheffer IE, et al. Methodology for classification and definition of epilepsy syndromes with list of syndromes: Report of the ILAE Task Force on Nosology and Definitions. *Epilepsia*. 2022;63(6):1333-1348.

Zerr DM, Blume HK, Berg AT, et al. Nonfebrile illness seizures: a unique seizure category? *Epilepsia*. 2005;46(6):952-955.

Zuccarelli BD, Hall AS. Utility of obtaining a serum basic metabolic panel in the setting of a first-time nonfebrile seizure. *Clin Pediatr (Phila)*. 2016;55(7):650-653.

CHAPTER 119 Headache

Dana M. Foradori, MD, MEd and Gary Hsich, MD

BACKGROUND

Headache is a common condition in children and adolescents. Patients may be hospitalized for headaches or develop headaches during hospitalization. In either situation, it is important to determine whether the headache represents a primary headache disorder, such as migraine or tension headache, or a secondary disorder resulting from potentially serious intracranial or systemic processes (**Table 119-1**).

Epidemiologic studies in large cohorts of American children reveal an estimated 1-year prevalence rates of frequent or severe headaches of 17%. In general, postpubertal girls have the highest prevalence rates of both migraine and tension headache. The most recent classification criteria established by the International Headache Society (IHS) in 2018 provide a detailed classification of headaches in children.

CLINICAL PRESENTATION

Head pain (cephalgia) is a symptom, and the diagnosis of a primary headache disorder, such as migraine, is a diagnosis of exclusion. Evaluation of headache consists chiefly of a detailed history and thorough physical examination. Efficient history-taking is focused on any symptoms or signs of altered intracranial pressure (ICP) (**Table 119-2**), risk factors for increased ICP, or focal deficits. A more expanded history should assess possible contributing stress and mood disorders.

Any abnormalities on neurologic examination in a previously healthy child or changes from neurologic baseline in a child with previous abnormalities warrant expeditious evaluation. The absence of worrisome symptoms and abnormalities in the physical (including neurologic)

TABLE 119-1 International Headache Society Classification of Headache Disorders

Primary headaches
Migraine
Tension-type headache
Cluster headache and other trigeminal autonomic cephalgias
Other primary headaches
Secondary headaches associated with one of the following:
Head and/or neck trauma
Cranial or cervical vascular disorders
Examples: stroke, hematoma, subarachnoid hemorrhage, unruptured vascular malformation, arteritis, carotid/vertebral artery pain, hypertension, other vascular disorder
Nonvascular intracranial disorders
Examples: idiopathic intracranial hypertension, low cerebrospinal fluid pressure, intracranial infection, inflammatory condition such as neurosarcoidosis, intracranial neoplasm, intrathecal injection, ictal or post-ictal state
Substances or withdrawal
Examples: analgesic overuse; cocaine, alcohol use; opiate, caffeine withdrawal
Intracranial or systemic infection
Disorders of homeostasis
Examples: hypoxia, hypercapnia, hypertension, fasting, dialysis, lead
Disorders of the cranium, neck, eyes, ears, nose, sinuses, teeth, mouth, or other facial or cranial structure
Somatization or psychotic disorders
Cranial neuralgias, central and primary facial pain, and other disorders

Source: Data from Headache Classification Committee of the International Headache Society (HIS). *International Classification of Headache Disorders*, 3rd ed. Cephalalgia. 2018;38(1):1-211.

TABLE 119-2 Concerning Symptoms and Signs Suggesting Headache From Increased Intracranial Pressure

Symptoms of Increased Intracranial Pressure
"First or worst" headache
Chronic and progressively worsening headache
Sudden "thunderclap" headache
Early morning headache or headache worse in the morning
Headache worse in the supine position
Change from mental status baseline (including irritability)
Associated loss of vision or other neurologic deficit
Associated vomiting, especially upon awakening
Transiently worsens with cough or Valsalva maneuver
Other Historical Details
Presence of a ventriculoperitoneal shunt
Recent head trauma or neurosurgery
Signs of Increased Intracranial Pressure
Depressed or abnormal mental status
Papilledema
Cranial nerve abnormalities, particularly 3rd nerve palsy (including "blown pupil") and 6th nerve palsy (impaired abduction)
Asymmetry in the motor examination
In infants: bulging fontanelle, split sutures, setting sun sign (impaired upward gaze), macrocephaly, failure to thrive, shrill cry

examination is reassuring against serious pathology in majority of headaches. The physician should consider the following key questions during the evaluation:

- Are there warning signs or symptoms suggesting increased ICP or focal neurologic abnormalities?
- Are there any predisposing factors to secondary headaches, such as a ventriculoperitoneal (VP) shunt?
- Do the symptoms fit into the pattern of a typical headache syndrome?

Although less common than primary headaches, secondary headaches are of greater immediate clinical concern, especially for the physician evaluating a child in the emergency department or the inpatient hospital setting. The typical presentations of headaches caused by increased ICP, other secondary headaches, and common primary headache disorders will be reviewed. Familiarity with the particular symptoms for each of these categories guides differential diagnoses.

HEADACHES ASSOCIATED WITH INCREASED INTRACRANIAL PRESSURE

Symptoms and signs that should alert the physician to the possibility of a headache secondary to increased ICP are reviewed in Table 119-2.

A "first or worst" headache warrants immediate evaluation for the possibility of a mass lesion causing increased ICP, but additional historical details tailor the degree of suspicion.

A sudden "thunderclap" headache or the report of the "worst headache of my life" may suggest an acute intracranial hemorrhage. These can be caused by either spontaneous aneurysmal rupture (rare) or arterial-venous malformation (more common). A severe headache in the setting of recent head trauma or in a patient with a bleeding diathesis may suggest acute or subacute hemorrhage into the epidural, subarachnoid, or subdural space.

Headaches caused by mass lesions and slowly increasing ICP are often worse in the morning or after a period of lying supine. Headaches may be associated with emesis, visual disturbance (e.g., blurring or enlargement of the blind spot caused by optic nerve swelling), or other complaints reflecting focal neurologic deficits. Children with posterior fossa tumors, which account for a small minority of children with headache, may present with ataxia and other symptoms referable to the brainstem, such as diplopia and dysphagia. A child with such symptoms will also most likely have corresponding abnormalities on neurologic examination. The presence of all three features of the Cushing triad (hypertension, bradycardia, and irregular respirations) is a late sign of increased ICP that indicates brainstem compression and represents impending coma or a comatose state.

Headaches from increased ICP should also be considered in several special circumstances. These circumstances include a known bleeding diathesis or disseminated intravascular coagulation. Patients with a clotting tendency are also at risk of developing cerebral venous sinus thrombosis. Predispositions include factor V Leiden, antithrombin III deficiency, malignancy, inflammatory bowel disease, or secondary coagulopathies as a result of rheumatologic disease (e.g., systemic lupus erythematosus associated with lupus anticoagulant). Hypertension, chemotherapeutic agents, and immunosuppressants are associated with a posterior leukoencephalopathy syndrome presenting with headache, seizures, cortical blindness, and hallucinations.

Another important historical detail is the presence of a VP shunt. Not every headache in a child with a VP shunt represents a neurosurgical emergency, but one must be suspicious of shunt malfunction and increasing ICP. This is particularly true if the headache is severe, is a first or new type of headache for the child, or additional symptoms or signs suggest increased ICP. Of note, early in the process of VP shunt obstruction, accompanying abnormalities may include subtle mood changes or decreased energy. Papilledema and other signs of increased ICP may not be present early in their presentation. For all these reasons, headache in a patient with a VP shunt should be considered secondary to shunt obstruction until proven otherwise, unless it is a typical headache for a given child and there are no other worrisome features in the history or physical examination to suggest otherwise.

OTHER SECONDARY HEADACHE PRESENTATIONS

The history and physical examination assist in identifying secondary headaches not associated with increased ICP. For example, headache may be a presenting feature of meningitis, but there are typically other features, such as fever and meningismus, to suggest this diagnosis.

Headache with or without neck pain in the setting of head or neck trauma, even relatively trivial trauma, can be caused by dissection of the carotid or vertebral arteries. Although less common in children than adults, this entity deserves consideration due to the risk of embolic stroke from the clot that forms in response to the dissection.

Secondary headaches may herald otherwise occult head and neck conditions, such as dental abscess, otitis media, or sinusitis. Pain may not be well localized in these conditions.

Other causes of secondary headaches, particularly in the inpatient setting, include metabolic disturbances (listed in Table 119-1 as disorders of homeostasis), intracranial hypotension (or a "low-pressure" or "post-lumbar puncture" headache) caused by a cerebrospinal fluid (CSF) leak after lumbar puncture (LP), and opiate withdrawal in patients receiving analgesia for other conditions or for headache itself.

Benign idiopathic intracranial hypertension (IIH), or pseudotumor cerebri, is considered a secondary headache, although the underlying cause is often not determined. Patients with this condition have symptoms suggesting increased ICP. They may also report transient visual obscurations, a large blind spot, or diplopia. Typical examination findings include papilledema and enlargement of the blind spot on visual fields examination. Occasionally, IIH may cause pressure on the sixth cranial nerves, resulting in weakness of the lateral rectus muscle and decreased eye abduction. Findings on computed tomography (CT) can be normal, and CSF opening pressure at LP is >280 mm H_2O. Often the patient experiences relief of symptoms transiently after LP. Although not a life-threatening condition, untreated IIH can lead to permanent loss of vision if not treated expeditiously.

COMMON PRIMARY HEADACHE DISORDER PRESENTATIONS—MIGRAINE OR TENSION HEADACHES

Migraines and tension headaches account for the vast majority of all pediatric headaches and may be challenging to distinguish due to overlapping clinical features. The pathophysiology of these headaches is incompletely understood and likely includes a multifactorial interplay of

TABLE 119-3 Common Features of Migraine (Not All Required)
Unilateral or bilateral, especially in younger children
Pulsating or throbbing quality
Nausea, vomiting
Photophobia, phonophobia
Visual aura (e.g,. scintillating scotoma)
Desire for sleep
Family history of migraine

vascular, neurotransmitter-mediated, electrophysiologic, inflammatory, stress, and mood components. Migraines and tension headaches are frequently triggered by stress, exercise, head trauma, decreasing estrogen levels prior to menstruation, and many other environmental factors.

Migraine may occur without or with an aura, which typically precedes the headache onset by less than 60 minutes. Auras are most frequently visual but may also cause sensory, motor, retinal, or brainstem symptomatology (see below). Visual auras are frequently "scintillating scotomas," or shining, brightly colored regions of the visual field with transient visual obscuration in the affected area. The nausea associated with a migraine may be profound. Notably, a headache reaching maximal severity at onset merits consideration of alternative diagnoses. The typical constellation of symptoms associated with migraine headaches is listed in **Table 119-3,** but not all patients with migraine experience all features.

Tension-type headaches are characterized by bilateral pain with a pressing or tightening quality, as well as tenderness of pericranial and neck musculature. Patients with both tension-type headaches and migraine may have concurrent photophobia and phonophobia, which may be expressed by a preference to remain in a dark, quiet room during the episode.

Children with headaches often express the desire to sleep, and most patients with tension and migraine headaches report that their headaches are relieved by sleep. Typical migraine duration is 2 to 6 hours; however, longer durations are not uncommon, which may prompt patients to seek medical attention and result in hospitalization. Status migrainosus is defined as a debilitating migraine or associated symptoms lasting >72 hours. Emesis and fatigue frequently occur near the end of the migraine, with symptom resolution upon awakening.

Migraine equivalent syndromes, also known as complicated migraines, present with transient neurological deficits and mimic stroke, hemorrhage, or other intracranial processes. In many cases, neurological symptoms precede headache onset. Migraine equivalent syndromes warrant emergent evaluation, especially with the initial episode of symptoms. For example, migraines with brainstem aura, also known as basilar artery migraines, include combinations of dysarthria, paresthesias, tinnitus, vertigo, diplopia, vision loss, ataxia, and depressed consciousness. Hemiplegic migraines include reversible motor weakness and may be familial or sporadic in origin. Retinal migraines may cause unilateral visual disturbances, sometimes including unilateral blindness. Ophthalmoplegic migraines (also known as ophthalmoplegic neuropathy) are characterized by ocular nerve palsies, resulting in ptosis, ophthalmoplegia, and pupillary defects. Acute confusional migraines present with impaired mentation, and transient global amnesia is characterized by inability to form new memories. Complicated migraines are diagnoses of exclusion; urgent brain MRI is usually necessary to rule out a worrisome intracranial process. Fortunately, in the pediatric population, complicated migraines are often more likely than worrisome neurological disorders, and the neurological deficits seen in complicated migraines typically resolve within 24 hours.

Migraine variants are more common during childhood and consist mainly of syndromes that appear in children with a family history of migraines. These include cyclic vomiting syndrome (CVS), abdominal migraine, benign paroxysmal torticollis, and benign paroxysmal vertigo. While headache is not the primary presenting symptom of these syndromes, it is important to note that they are considered part of a continuum of paroxysmal disorders that fall under the broad category of migraine. CVS consists of vomiting attacks that are typically self-limited, with or without headaches. Abdominal migraines are characterized by attacks of abdominal pain with less prominent vomiting than with CVS. Paroxysmal vertigo is typically sudden and consists of unexplained fear of falling and refusal to stand; it is most common among infants and young children. Paroxysmal torticollis is characterized by recurrent episodes of head tilting. Both paroxysmal vertigo and paroxysmal torticollis can be accompanied by vomiting. Other medical conditions must be ruled out before diagnosing a migraine variant.

DIFFERENTIAL DIAGNOSIS

The IHS classification system presented in Table 119-1 offers a general framework for considering the differential diagnosis of headache. The chief distinction lies between primary and secondary headaches, with the latter typically requiring more urgent medical attention. A more comprehensive differential diagnosis is included in **Table 119-4**. This table is organized to depict the most likely diagnoses for patients with headache and normal neurologic findings versus headache with signs of increased ICP or focal neurologic abnormalities.

DIAGNOSTIC EVALUATION

The history and physical examination form the basis for evaluation of patients with headache. Physicians evaluating patients with headache must perform a careful neurologic examination, including mental status, fundoscopic evaluation, horizontal eye movements, and motor symmetry. Further evaluation of a secondary headache may be warranted, as dictated by specific circumstances. For example, a patient with symptoms and signs of sinusitis and normal neurologic findings might receive empiric antibiotic therapy and symptomatic pain relief with outpatient follow-up and no further diagnostic testing. In contrast, a child with headache, fever, and meningeal signs warrants an LP. **Table 119-5** provides an overview of the general principles of headache diagnosis.

The role of neuroimaging in the evaluation of a child with headache requires clinical judgment. Not every headache warrants a head CT or magnetic resonance imaging (MRI), but prudent and judicious use of these modalities clearly has a place in the evaluation of headache. The likelihood of identifying a significant abnormality in a patient with headache and normal neurologic findings is extremely low, especially in a patient with recurrent episodic headache suggestive of a primary headache disorder. While it is difficult to generalize, a well-appearing child without worrisome features and with a normal neurological examination can often be observed without neuroimaging.

Any patient with focal neurological signs or "red flag" signs and symptoms of increased ICP (see Table 119-2) should undergo an emergency CT scan. It is usually more convenient and expeditious to perform a CT scan than MRI; this factor, as well as the fact that CT scans are more sensitive in the evaluation of acute hemorrhage, makes CT the first line of neuroimaging for an acute headache and for most headaches that warrant neuroimaging. A limitation of CT scans is their decreased ability to evaluate the posterior fossa, and MRI is warranted as a first-line study if there is high suspicion of a brain tumor or other posterior fossa lesions. In addition, although the ionizing radiation associated with repeat CT scans must be considered, the dose of radiation per scan should be based on the size of the patient in any center that routinely performs these studies in children; fear of ionizing radiation should not preclude the performance of a clinically warranted scan in an acutely ill patient who may require emergency intervention.

Lumbar puncture is indicated for the diagnosis of meningitis or encephalitis, subarachnoid hemorrhage, or pseudotumor cerebri. When increased ICP is caused by a mass lesion, such as an abscess or tumor, the pressure differential created by LP can lead to catastrophic herniation of the brainstem (see Chapter 187 Lumbar Puncture). A CT scan should be obtained before LP if there is suspicion of such a space-occupying lesion. Although LP is a safe procedure in the majority of cases, there is a minute risk of herniation following an LP and therefore should be performed when believed to be safe and useful for diagnosis and/or treatment.

TABLE 119-4 Differential Diagnosis of Headache

Patients with Normal Neurologic Examination and No Concern for Increased Intracranial Pressure
Migraine, tension headache, or other primary headache disorder
Head and neck problems
Orbital disease
Sinusitis
Otitis
Dental infection
Temporomandibular joint pain
Recurrent facial pain syndromes (e.g., trigeminal neuralgia)
Visual refractive error
Metabolic disturbance
Hypoglycemia
Hypoxia
Hypercapnia
Dialysis headache
Carbon monoxide poisoning
Intracranial hypotension ("post-lumbar puncture" headache)
Ingestions from food—monosodium glutamate, nitrites, individual food triggers
Marijuana
Oral contraceptives
Substance withdrawal
Analgesics (including those used for headache treatment)
Opiates
Caffeine
Infections
Group A Strep pharyngitis
Viral meningitis
Patients with Abnormal Neurologic Examination or Concern for Increased Intracranial Pressure
Central nervous system infection
Meningitis
Encephalitis
Brain abscess
Intracranial hemorrhage
Subarachnoid hemorrhage (presents with "worst headache of my life")
Epidural hemorrhage, often after trauma and associated with skull fracture
Subdural hemorrhage, often associated with trauma
Posttraumatic headache
Cerebral venous sinus thrombosis
Stroke
Complicated migraine, in which stroke must be suspected and ruled out, especially at first presentation
Hypertensive encephalopathy
Carotid or vertebral artery dissection
Ventriculoperitoneal shunt obstruction
Inflammatory disease with central nervous system involvement (e.g., vasculitis)
Brain tumor
Pseudotumor cerebri/Benign idiopathic intracranial hypertension
Ictal or postictal headache, possibly after an unwitnessed seizure
Functional Neurological Symptom Disorder—diagnosis of exclusion

The platelet concentration should be at least 50×10^9/L to minimize the risk for epidural hemorrhage.

Electroencephalograms are not routinely indicated in the evaluation of headache unless there is a high degree of suspicion for seizure or postictal state as its etiology. Similarly, laboratory evaluation is not routinely indicated for children with headaches.

TABLE 119-5 Diagnostic Evaluation of Headache

History
With attention to worrisome features, as outlined in Table 119-2
Physical Examination
Focus should be on identifying secondary causes of headache, particularly worrisome causes requiring hospitalization and close observation:
General examination: temperature, blood pressure
Head, ears, eyes, nose, and throat examination: palpation of the head and face, sinus percussion, eyes for papilledema, ears and tympanic membranes, neck for tenderness, mouth, throat, teeth
Neurologic examination
Mental status
Cranial nerves
Motor
Cerebellar
Computed Tomography (CT) of the Head
To evaluate for hemorrhage if headache is first or worst, if mental status is abnormal, or if findings on neurologic examination are focal
To evaluate for a mass lesion causing hydrocephalus and increased intracranial pressure (Table 119-2)
Magnetic Resonance Imaging of the Brain with Gadolinium Enhancement
If stroke is suspected, MRI with diffusion-weighted images
If venous sinus thrombosis is suspected, MRI and MR venography
If posterior fossa tumor is suspected
Lumbar Puncture (LP)
Prior to LP, ensure that platelet concentration >$50 \times 10 \times 10^9$/L. For any suspicion for increased ICP, obtain a head CT prior to LP.
If infection is likely (after CT is performed, if there is any concern for increased intracranial pressure)
To measure opening pressure to evaluate for pseudotumor cerebri/idiopathic intracranial hypertension (after CT)
If inflammatory disease is suspected.
If subarachnoid hemorrhage is suspected. LP evaluates for elevated opening pressure, xanthochromia, and persistent red blood cells (no clearance demonstrated between tubes 1 and 4). Head CT may be insufficient to rule out early subarachnoid hemorrhage.
Laboratory Studies
Glucose, others on a case-by-case basis
Urine human chorionic gonadotropin in girls
Electroencephalography
Only if transient focal neurologic symptoms and signs are present

MANAGEMENT

Management of the pain of a secondary headache depends on the underlying cause of the headache. Narcotics and nonsteroidal anti-inflammatory drugs (NSAIDs) should be avoided during the initial phase of evaluation. Narcotics might interfere with accurate monitoring of changes in mental status and NSAIDs can worsen intracranial hemorrhage. Acetaminophen is an appropriate alternative that can be given orally, per rectum, or intravenously. Once the patient is deemed stable and the risk for hemorrhage low, NSAIDs may provide additional symptomatic relief while underlying causes are under investigation.

Increased ICP warrants urgent neurosurgical consultation. Pending surgical intervention, multiple interventions should be employed. Elevation of the head of the bed to 30 to 45 degrees may lower ICP. To prevent worsening, efforts should be made to maintain normal sodium levels, blood glucose, oxygenation, ventilation, and blood pressure. Fevers, seizures, pain, and agitation should be treated promptly to avoid increasing cerebral metabolic demand. In consultation with intensivists, consider hyperventilation and provision of corticosteroids, osmolar diuretics, or hypertonic saline.

In the acute management of a migraine, ensuring adequate hydration is important, especially if the migraine has been protracted and has led to decreased oral intake or vomiting. If home medications at appropriate doses have been ineffective or if oral therapy is not tolerated, intravenous fluids and medications should be considered. Due the the high placebo response rate, there is no proven or single accepted medication treatment for acute migraines. Options may include NSAIDs (including ketorolac), triptans, or dihydroergotamine. Associated nausea and emesis can be treated with ondansetron, prochlorperazine, metoclopramide, or promethazine. While narcotics often provide rapid pain relief and may help the patient achieve sleep, they should be avoided in the treatment of chronic headache exacerbations due to concern for potential addiction or drug-seeking behavior, as well as rebound headache. Procedural interventions, such as nerve blocks, botulinum toxin injections, transcutaneous electrical nerve stimulation, should be reserved for medication-refractory headaches.

Although the majority of headaches in children do not represent life-threatening emergencies, the pain experienced by the child and the ensuing anxiety of the family can be great. Once a patient with headache is deemed stable and relevant secondary causes have been considered and ruled out, the focus should shift to providing reassurance

The addition of complementary and alternative medicine is likely to have a growing role in the management of chronic headache.[8] When patients are admitted for exacerbations of chronic headache conditions, it is important to incorporate aspects of nonpharmacologic treatment in keeping with their outpatient treatment strategies. Lifestyle modifications should be discussed. These include adequate hydration, sleep hygiene, regular meals, exercise, and avoidance of medication overuse. Patients should be screened for stress, anxiety, and depression, with referrals for psychological or psychiatric services, as indicated. Headache diaries may help the patient and family to gain insight into triggers, especially related to lifestyle factors. Additional complementary therapies for headache include biofeedback, relaxation therapy, acupuncture, massage, craniosacral therapy, and vitamin supplementation.

COURSE OF ILLNESS

The course of the headache will depend on its cause. Secondary headaches usually respond to treatment of the causative condition. Primary headache disorders in children, as in adults, are typically recurrent and may require prophylactic management depending on their frequency and severity.

ADMISSION AND DISCHARGE CRITERIA

ADMISSION CRITERIA

- Suspected or identified underlying cause that requires prompt investigation, ongoing observation, or intervention (e.g., increased ICP, intracranial mass or hemorrhage, bacterial meningitis)
- Severe pain that cannot be managed with outpatient medications

DISCHARGE CRITERIA

- Completion of urgent diagnostic studies
- Definitive treatment or initiation of therapy for an underlying process
- Pain management regimen that can be continued after discharge
- Appropriate outpatient follow-up with a primary care clinician and, if needed, a subspecialist

CONSULTATION

Consider subspecialty consultation for any of the following reasons:

- Neurosurgical consultation for patients with increased ICP, intracranial hemorrhage, and VP shunt
- Neurologic consultation for patients with abnormal neurologic examination, for suspected intracranial etiology of headache, and for patients with known primary headache disorders that have become refractory to standard management
- Ophthalmologic consultation for patients with pseudotumor cerebri to assess and monitor the visual fields

KEY POINTS

- The history and physical examination form the cornerstone of evaluation of headache in the hospital setting.
- A careful neurologic examination must include evaluation of mental status, optic fundi, horizontal eye movements, and motor symmetry.
- Distinction between primary and secondary headache is important in determining the likelihood of an acute intracranial process that may require emergent or urgent intervention.
- Patients with a history or physical examination findings suggesting increased ICP should undergo emergency neuroimaging, in most cases with CT. This category includes patients with a VP shunt.
- Patients with signs and symptoms suggesting increased ICP from a posterior fossa lesion should undergo CT acutely and MRI for detailed posterior fossa evaluation.
- Most patients with a history of headache but without "red flag" features worrisome for increased ICP and without abnormalities on neurologic examination do not have serious intracranial pathology. In these cases, headache should be managed symptomatically.
- Headache management depends upon the suspected underlying cause.
- Exacerbations of chronic headache conditions require a multipronged approach, including medical management of pain, nausea, and hydration, as well as consideration of lifestyle factors, stressors, underlying mood disorders, and nonpharmacologic therapies.
- As the underlying mechanisms of headache are more completely understood, more specific treatment strategies may be available.

SUGGESTED READINGS

Alehan FK. Value of neuroimaging in the evaluation of neurologically normal children with recurrent headache. *J Child Neurol.* 2002;17:807-809.

Headache Classification Committee of the International Headache Society. The International Classification of Headache Disorders. 3rd ed. Cephalalgia. 2018;38(1):1-211.

Joffe AR. Lumbar puncture and brain herniation in acute bacterial meningitis: a review. *J Intensive Care Med.* 2007;22(4):194-207.

Kline J, Kock T. Headache in children. *Pediatr Rev.* 2020;41(4).

Lateef TM, Merikangas KR, He J. Headache in a national sample of American children: prevalence and comorbidity. *J Clin Neuro.* 2009;24(5):536-543.

Lewis DW, Ashwal S, Dahl G, et al. Quality Standards Subcommittee of the American Academy of Neurology; Practice Committee of the Child Neurology Society. Practice parameter: evaluation of children and adolescents with recurrent headaches: report of the Quality Standards Subcommittee of the American Academy of Neurology and the Practice Committee of the Child Neurology Society. *Neurology.* 2002;59(4):490-498.

Maytal J, Bienkowski RS, Patel M, Eviatar L. The value of brain imaging in children with headaches. Pediatrics. 1995;96:413-416.

Medina LS, Kuntz KM, Pomeroy S. Children with headache suspected of having a brain tumor: a cost-effectiveness analysis of diagnostic strategies. *Pediatrics.* 2001;108:255-263.

Medina LS, Pinter JD, Zurakowski D, Davis R, Kuban K, Barnes PD. Children with headache: clinical predictors of the surgical space-occupying lesions and the role of neuroimaging. *Radiology.* 1997;202: 819-824.

Piña-Garza JE, James KC. *Fenichel's Clinical Pediatric Neurology: A Signs and Symptoms Approach*. 8th ed. Elsevier; 2019.
Silberstein SD, Lipton RB, Goadsby PJ. *Headache in Clinical Practice*. London: Martin Dunitz; 2002.
Swaiman KF, Ashwal S eds. *Pediatric Neurology, Principles and Practice*. 6th ed. Elsevier; 2017.
Van Crevel H, Hijdra A, De Gans J. Lumbar puncture and the risk of herniation: when should we first perform CT? *J Neurol*. 2002;249:129-137.

CHAPTER 120

Hypotonia and Weakness

Joy L. Solano, MD, MHPE and Ashley N. Lepse, MD

BACKGROUND

Hypotonia and weakness may indicate a variety of systemic, neurologic, neuromuscular, and muscular disorders (**Table 120-1**). Evaluation of hypotonia and weakness can be challenging as the list of possible diagnoses is extensive and includes many rare conditions. After considering systemic causes, a logical next step in the evaluation is to localize the lesion to the central nervous system (CNS) or the peripheral nervous system (PNS), which frequently can be accomplished by detailed birth and medical history, along with thorough general and neurological examination. It should be noted that not all conditions fit perfectly in the CNS or PNS categories, and there is often overlap. Pediatric hospitalists should know and be able to teach a general approach to patients presenting with hypotonia or weakness and have a basic understanding of the diagnostic possibilities and their clinical presentations, pathophysiology, diagnostic strategies, comorbid conditions, and management.

TABLE 120-1 Differential Diagnosis of Hypotonia and Weakness

Systemic Causes

- Severe illness (e.g., sepsis), medication toxicity, malnutrition

Central Causes

- Brain: hypoxic ischemic injury, static encephalopathy, trauma, infection, malformations, genetic conditions (e.g., Trisomy 21, Prader-Willi syndrome [PWS], etc.), metabolic conditions (e.g., hypothyroidism, Zellweger syndrome, neonatal adrenoleukodystrophy, biotinidase deficiency, mitochondrial diseases, aminoacidopathies, organic acidurias, urea cycle disorders, etc.), autoimmune/inflammatory diseases, functional neurologic disorders, malignancy
- Spinal cord: trauma, infection, autoimmune/inflammatory diseases, malignancy

Peripheral Causes

- Anterior horn cell disease: spinal muscular atrophy (SMA), infantile neuroaxonal dystrophy, poliomyelitis, polio-like illnesses
- Peripheral neuropathy: Riley-Day syndrome, Charcot-Marie-Tooth disease, autoimmune inflammatory demyelinating neuropathy (AIDP), chronic inflammatory demyelinating neuropathy (CIDP)
- Neuromuscular junction defect: transient neonatal myasthenia gravis, congenital myasthenic syndrome, infant botulism, juvenile myasthenia gravis
- Muscle
  - Muscular dystrophy: congenital myotonic dystrophy, congenital muscular dystrophy
  - Metabolic myopathies: glycogen storage disease type II (Pompe), mitochondrial cytopathy
  - Congenital myopathy: nemaline myopathy, myotubular myopathy, central nuclear myopathy, central core myopathy, congenital fiber type disproportion, and others
  - Infectious or autoimmune myositis

CLINICAL PRESENTATIONS

HISTORY

An infant or child presenting with hypotonia or weakness requires a thorough history and comprehensive physical and neurological examination. Presentation can vary based on age. During the neonatal period and infancy, patients frequently present with poor tone (e.g., "floppy") or with delay in achieving developmental milestones. Poor tone can be manifested in both resting posture and in inability to feed effectively. In older children, the most common complaints relate to weakness and include an unusual gait, frequent falls, inability to run or climb stairs, inability to keep up with peers, inability to lift heavy objects, and clumsiness with fine motor functions, such as writing and manipulating small objects. It is important to clarify with careful questioning and examination whether these signs reflect problems of strength or coordination.

Information about the time course of symptom development (acute/subacute/chronic and static/progressive) is an important element in sorting the diagnostic possibilities. When hypotonia or weakness occurs acutely in an otherwise healthy infant or child, they are most commonly the result of severe infection, fluid or electrolyte derangements, toxic ingestion, immune-mediated processes, trauma, or mass lesion(s). If present at birth, they may be the result of perinatal injury to the nervous system, brain malformation, or genetic diseases. Progressive hypotonia and weakness may herald the onset of several neurodegenerative diseases. This may manifest as delay in achieving or regression of developmental milestones.

Birth and pregnancy history are also of critical importance, especially in young patients. Infants with hypoxic-ischemic encephalopathy may have a history of prenatal or perinatal complications, anoxia/hypoxia, low cord pH, and low Apgar scores. A history of infection during pregnancy, especially during the first trimester, raises a concern for in-utero infection or exposure to systemic inflammation, potentially exacerbating hypoxic injury. Decreased fetal movements, polyhydramnios, or breech presentation may be reported in infants with neuromuscular disorders. A maternal history of multiple late spontaneous abortions suggests an inherited condition.

Finally, a detailed review of systems along with complete past medical histories is also pertinent. A history of seizures and cognitive impairment support a CNS etiology. Syndromic features, such as facial dysmorphisms or other congenital malformations, offer support for a genetic or metabolic etiology. Fevers, rashes, malaise, and weight loss can suggest an infectious, rheumatologic, or other systemic etiology. For older children, medication use by them or those in the household in case of accidental or purposeful ingestion should be noted. A full family history should be taken to specifically note anyone with underlying neurological (at any level) disorders, multiple miscarriages, rheumatological diseases, or a history of sudden death in a child. Finally, a thorough social history is important. This should include risk factors for possible nonaccidental trauma or ingestion along with assessment of family supports should a diagnosis that requires lifelong medical care be made.

PHYSICAL EXAMINATION

As with any child presenting with a neurologic complaint, a complete general examination should not be neglected. Vital signs should be obtained with particular attention to respiratory effort. If there is concern for inadequate respiratory effort, bedside tests such as vital capacity (VC) and negative inspiratory force (NIF) should be obtained. The results must be interpreted within the context of the patient's developmental abilities (e.g., ability to generate an adequate seal). If the results of VC and NIF are concerning, consideration should be given to transfer to the intensive care unit for impending respiratory failure. It is critical to remember that patients with neuromuscular weakness will not develop increased work of breathing so close monitoring of respiratory parameters is vital. With the general examination, particular attention should be paid to head circumference and growth curves. Assessment for organomegaly, lymphadenopathy, joint swelling, and skin changes may point toward systemic infection or rheumatological disorders rather than primary neurological disorders. Small stature and dysmorphic features may indicate genetic or metabolic disorders.

The neurologic examination should be conducted in the standard way with additional focus on tone, strength, and reflexes (**Table 120-2**). Assessment of mental status may reveal encephalopathy, which can be seen with chronic static encephalopathy, genetic or metabolic disorders, and acute illness, among others. Funduscopic examination is important as retinal pigmentary degeneration or optic atrophy is frequently seen in certain metabolic disorders and cherry-red spot of the macula may be present in some lysosomal disorders. Weakness of extraocular eye muscles or the face can be seen with neuromuscular junction disorders, such as myasthenia gravis, or with some neuropathies. Hearing loss can be seen with some genetic or metabolic disorders. Tongue fasciculations can be seen with spinal muscular atrophy. In infants and young children, most of the examination will need to be done by careful observation, such as watching the child track objects, watching spontaneous facial expressions, listening to strength of spontaneous vocalizations and cries, a quick look inside the mouth to note tongue and palate positioning if the patient cries, watching for spontaneous movement, and evaluating resistance to examiner's evaluation.

Muscle tone and strength should be evaluated when the infant or child is awake and comfortable. It should be noted that evaluation of strength and tone can be influenced by illness, malnutrition, psychological stress, and medication use. The provider must distinguish hypotonia (reduced resistance to passive range of motion) from muscle weakness (reduced maximum power generated). For example, weak infants are often hypotonic, but hypotonic infants are not necessarily weak.

Tone in an infant or a child is assessed by passive and active maneuvers. The overall resting posture of a hypotonic infant shows decreased flexion in the arms, with legs flexed at the hips and externally rotated ("frog leg" posture). Passive maneuvers require only gravity to stretch the muscles. A hypotonic infant supported beneath the axillae (vertical suspension) will slip through the hands of the examiner unless lateral pressure is exerted. An inverted "U" curvature of the spine is observed (with abnormal lack of extension of the head and legs) while the infant is held prone in one hand of the examiner (Landau maneuver). Poor head control and head lag are seen on "pull to sit." Active maneuvers are those in which the examiner actively stretches the muscle, such as those used to assess immaturity on the Dubowitz scale (heel-to-ear or scarf sign). Ligament laxity, which may occur in connective tissue disorders or marked hyperextensibility as a normal variant, may be mistaken for hypotonia.

TABLE 120-2 Comprehensive Neurological Examination

Mental status
Speech
Cranial Nerves
II: Symmetry of pupils, reactivity to light, funduscopic, visual acuity
III, IV, VI: Extraocular movements
V: Facial sensation, muscles of mastication
VII: Facial movements, taste on anterior one-third of tongue
VIII: Hearing, vestibular system (passively assessed with coordination during the Romberg test)
IX/X: Palate elevation, cough, gag reflex
XI: Head turning (sternocleidomastoid muscle function)
XII: Tongue strength
Motor
Tone and bulk
Strength
Sensory
Anterolateral tracts (pain/temperature)
Dorsal columns (vibration/proprioception)
Reflexes
Upper extremity: brachial, brachioradialis
Lower extremity: patellar, Achilles, plantar (Babinski)
Coordination
Finger to nose
Heel to shin
Romberg test
Gait
Baseline (ask to walk across the room)
Toe walk
Heel walk
Tandem gait

TABLE 120-3 Medical Research Council (MRC) Scale for Muscle Strength

Grade	Muscle Activity
0	No contraction
1	Flicker/trace contraction
2	Active movement with gravity eliminated
3	Active movement against gravity but not against resistance
4	Active movement against gravity and resistance
5	Normal strength

The central component of motor examination in a weak patient is strength testing. Strength may be difficult to assess in an infant. Hypotonic infants frequently have paucity of spontaneous movement. With stimulation, hypotonic infants without muscle weakness usually demonstrate antigravity limb movements, whereas hypotonic, weak infants frequently do not. Other signs of weakness can be inferred by a weak cry, paradoxical breathing pattern ("belly breathing"), swallowing difficulty manifesting as poor suck, slow feeding, oropharyngeal pooling of secretions or food, and choking.

Muscle strength in older and cooperative children can be graded with the Medical Research Council (MRC) grading scale (**Table 120-3**). In younger children, formal muscle strength testing often cannot be performed due to lack of cooperation or lack of understanding of the testing; thus, functional testing is necessary. Functional testing includes watching the child walk, run, stand up from a supine position, and climb stairs. The Gowers sign is when a child rises from a supine position on the floor by turning to the prone position, using hands to first push off the floor and then to "climb" up his/her legs (**Figure 120-1**). Difficulty with ascending stairs suggests hip extensor weakness and difficulty with descending stairs suggests quadriceps (flexor) weakness. Push-ups are a good test of muscle strength in arms. A child with shoulder girdle or upper arm muscle weakness has difficulty with the "wheelbarrow walk" (walking on hands while someone holds their legs up).

Once assessment of overall tone and weakness has been completed, evaluation of the pattern of any motor deficits can help localize the lesion. Weakness with upper motor neuron (UMN) signs may present with hemiparesis, quadriparesis, or paraparesis (lower extremities) (**Table 120-4**). Oculomotor dysfunction and cranial nerve dysfunction may indicate brainstem involvement. Hemiparesis typically localizes the lesion to the brain contralateral to the paretic side due to decussation of the corticospinal tracts at the level of the medulla. Quadriparesis can be the result of bilateral brain disease, brainstem lesions, or a cervical spinal cord process. Paraparesis with sparing of the arms raises a concern for spinal cord disease in the thoracic or lumbosacral region. These lesions are also typically accompanied by sensory deficits and possible bowel/bladder incontinence. In an acute setting, this is a neurologic emergency. Focal weakness with lower motor neuron (LMN) signs localizes the lesion to the anterior horn cells, spinal nerve roots, the brachial (upper extremity) or lumbosacral (lower extremity) plexus, nerves, neuromuscular junction, or muscles (see Table 120-4). Finally, it should be noted that in infants younger than 18 months, both UMN and LMN lesions may present initially as hypotonia due to incomplete myelination of the corticospinal tracts. Many patients with central hypotonia may evolve to have increased tone (spasticity/dystonia) in the extremities while retaining axial hypotonia as they get older. For example, an infant with kernicterus due to hyperbilirubinemia is initially hypotonic but frequently develops spasticity and/or dystonia over time.

To complete the neurologic examination, sensation, reflexes, coordination, and gait should be assessed. Sensory testing should include

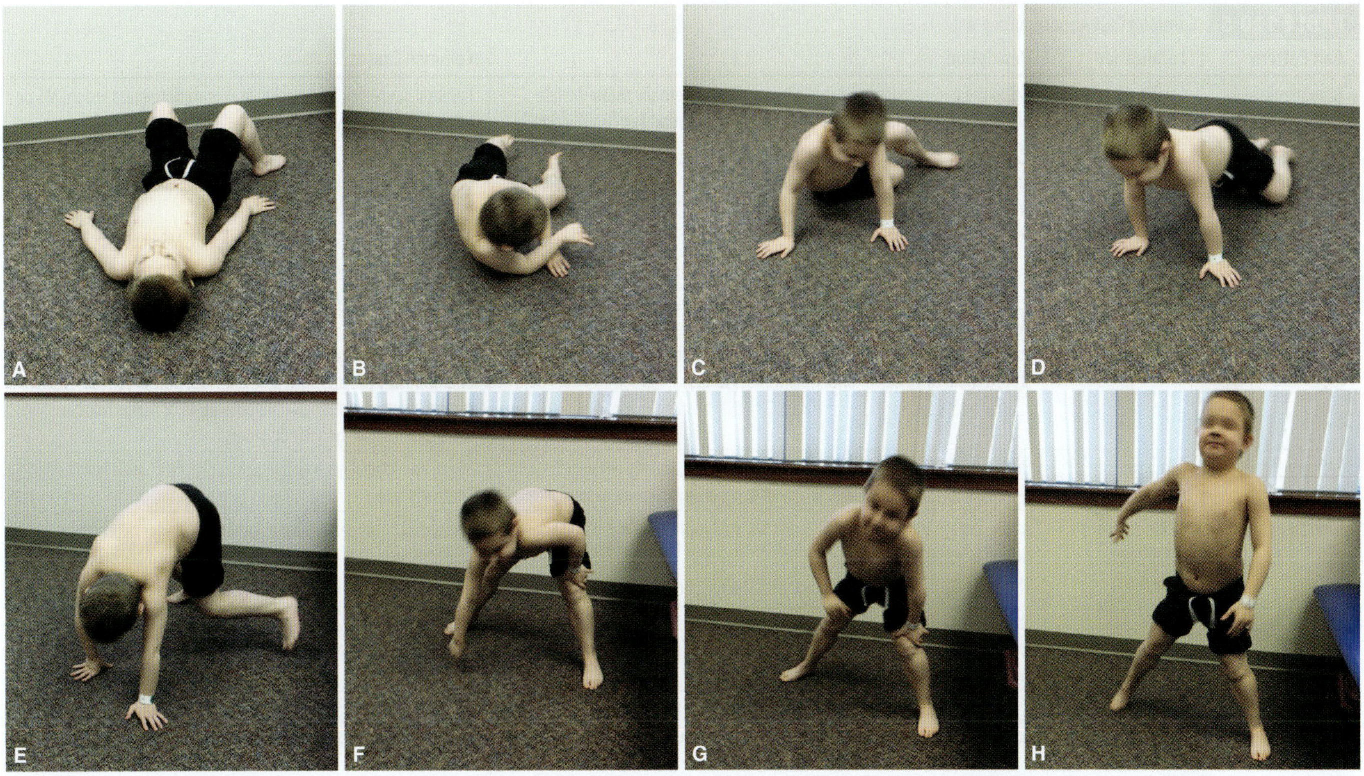

FIGURE 120-1. A boy with Duchenne muscular dystrophy demonstrates the sequence of maneuvers that constitutes the Gowers sign while getting up from the floor because of marked weakness of the hip extensors. (A) begins the exam with the child lying supine (B-C) the child starts by rolling over to the side, turning around to get on four extremities to prepare to get up (D-E), then moves his hands close to his feet, moves one hand on the thigh, then moves another hand to another thigh to push up to erect position.

assessment of sensory domains that involve both the anterolateral tract (pain/temperature) and the dorsal columns (vibration/proprioception). Testing should be completed in both upper and lower extremities. Reflexes should be obtained in all extremities. Upper extremity reflexes should include brachial and brachiocephalic. Lower extremity reflexes should include patellar and Achilles. The plantar reflex should also be assessed as an extensor (upgoing) response is a key UMN finding. Coordination should be assessed with tasks such as finger-nose-finger and heel-to-shin testing in children who are able to follow commands. In younger children, this can be assessed by having them give a "high-five," reach out for a toy, or touch the nose of a stuffed animal. Lower extremity coordination can be assessed by asking them to kick a target. The assessment of coordination can be limited by weakness. If the patient does not have at least 3/5 strength, coordination may not be able to be accurately assessed.

Gait is assessed with watching the child walk normally followed by toe-walking, heel walking, and tandem gait (heel to toe). There are several types of abnormal gaits (**Table 120-5**). A spastic hemiparetic gait is characterized by circumduction of the affected leg, and frequently accompanied by arm adduction (held close to the body) and elbow flexion with hand pronation, often with cortical thumb (thumb held under the fingers or "palmed") on the same side. With mild hemiparesis, loss of normal arm swing and slight circumduction of the leg may be the only abnormalities. Scissoring gait, frequently accompanied by crouching at the knees and toe walking, is seen in spastic diplegia due to tightness of hip adductors, hamstrings, and calf muscles. With proximal weakness, the pelvis is not stable and waddles from side to side as the child walks (Trendelenburg sign). Running is particularly difficult or impossible and accentuates the waddling. With distal leg weakness, the child has difficulty with heel-walking due to weakness of the anterior compartment muscles (shin) of the legs. Difficulty with toe-walking suggests weakness of gastrocnemius muscles (calf). Children with foot drop tend to raise their knee high in air so the toes can clear the ground, and then the weak leg comes down with a slapping motion (high steppage gait).

TABLE 120-4 Upper Motor Neuron Versus Lower Motor Neuron Signs

Signs	Upper Motor Neurons	Lower Motor Neurons
Muscle tone	Increased/spastic*	Decreased/flaccid
Muscle atrophy	No†	Yes
Weakness	No/Yes	Yes
Fasciculations	None	Present
Reflexes	Increased††	Decreased/absent
Babinski sign	Present	Absent

*With acute spinal cord lesion/injury, tone and reflexes can be decreased initially.

†Mild atrophy may develop due to disuse.

††With acute spinal cord lesion/injury, tone and reflexes can be decreased initially.

LESION-BASED DIFFERENTIAL DIAGNOSIS

A myriad of conditions can cause hypotonia and weakness in infants and children admitted to the hospital. The differential includes systemic conditions, stroke, genetic diseases, and acquired diseases (e.g., perinatal hypoxic ischemic events, infection, autoimmune, trauma, oncologic). The underlying cause of the hypotonia and weakness can often be linked to lesions in the brain, spinal cord, nerves, neuromuscular junction, muscles, or a combination of the above. The diseases presented below most often cause symptoms within the location they are listed in but may not be exclusive to that location. Within each section, certain diseases are highlighted based on conditions a hospitalist is likely to see or conditions that hospitalists may need to quickly review when considering the differential diagnosis of patients presenting with hypotonia and weakness.

SYSTEMIC CONSIDERATIONS

Changes in tone or strength in a hospitalized patient may be due to conditions that are not caused by a primary neurological disorder, and these should be considered early on as treatment of these conditions may lead to resolution of symptoms. Severe illness of any variety (i.e., infection,

TABLE 120-5 Common Gait Abnormalities

Gait Pattern	Localization	Description	Common Causes
Hemiplegic	Corticospinal tract contralateral to the paretic side	Holds the paralyzed arm flexed, adducted and internally rotated while walking, with hip hike, plantar flexion of the foot and circumduction (swing around) of the leg	Cerebral causes include stroke, malformation, mass lesion, MS or other inflammatory process
Spastic diplegic	Bilateral corticospinal tracts	Scissoring gait, frequently accompanied by crouching at the knees and toe walking	Cerebral causes include cerebral palsy due to PVL, cerebral midline lesion, brain stem lesion/mass Spinal cord causes include mass, trauma, MS or other inflammatory lesions, myelopathy due vitamin B_{12} or vitamin E deficiency, hereditary spastic paraparesis
Cerebellar ataxia	Cerebellum	Wide-base, lateral instability of trunk, erratic foot placement and staggering, difficulty maintaining balance when making turn or sudden stop, unable to perform tandem gait (heel to toe)	Toxins, such as alcohol, or medications such as benzodiazepine, carbamazepine, diphenhydramine, infarct; mass lesion; inflammatory process such as ADEM, MS, postinfectious cerebellar ataxia; cerebellar degeneration or malformation; certain metabolic/genetic disorders
Sensory ataxia	Large sensory nerve fibers	Unsteady gait especially with eyes closed or in dark, usually not wide based, tends to look down at the feet when walking, positive Romberg sign	Sensory peripheral neuropathy such as GBS, CIDP, and Charcot-Marie-Tooth disease
High steppage	Ankle and toe dorsiflexor weakness	A gait pattern in which the feet and toes are lifted through hip and knee flexion to excessive heights. The foot will slap at initial contact with the ground secondary to decreased control	Peripheral neuropathy such as peroneal/fibular neuropathy, sciatic neuropathy, L5 radiculopathy, Charcot-Marie-Tooth disease, CIDP, GBS; distal myopathy or some forms of muscular dystrophy; spina bifida; cauda equina syndrome
Trendelenburg (or waddling)	Weakness of hip girdle muscles	Exaggerated pelvic swing, with abnormal drop of pelvis on the side of swing leg and weight shifting over the stance leg	Myopathy, muscular dystrophy, spinal muscular atrophy
Antalgic	Pain from disorders of various tissues	A protective gait pattern where the involved step length is decreased in order to avoid weight bearing on the involved side, usually secondary to pain	Pain from fracture, ankle sprain; hip dislocation/subluxation; osteomyelitis; transient synovitis
Astasia-abasia (psychogenic gait)	Psychogenic	Inability to stand or walk in the absence of other neurologic abnormalities; Dramatic fluctuation of gait; Often the patient sways wildly and nearly falls, but recovers at the last moment	Functional neurological disorders

ADEM, acute disseminated encephalomyelitis; CIDP, chronic inflammatory demyelinating neuropathy; GBS, Guillain-Barré syndrome; MS, multiple sclerosis; PVL, periventricular leukomalacia.

significant electrolyte abnormalities, intestinal ischemia, all types of shock, etc.) may lead to hypotonia due to a relative brain energy crisis in the setting of high energy demands. Additionally, acute and chronic malnutrition affects the body's ability to use energy both centrally and peripherally, and neurological symptoms may be reversible with adequate nutrition and physical and occupational therapies. Encephalopathy of any etiology may interfere with a patient's ability to participate in strength testing. Intoxication, intentional or accidental, should be considered in all patients, no matter their age, especially in patients with a sudden onset of symptoms. Hospitalists often manage patients with baclofen pumps and worsening hypotonia in these patients may be due to baclofen overdose. Early recognition and appropriate subspecialty consultation is imperative to appropriately treat these patients. In all of these cases, if symptoms persist after appropriate treatment for the presumed underlying cause, alternative diagnoses must be considered.

BRAIN

Most intracranial pathology in newborns and infants presents with hypotonia. A variety of perinatal events can damage UMN structures and result in congenital hypotonia, including congenital infections (classically TORCH - **t**oxoplasmosis, **o**ther [congenital syphilis and viruses], **r**ubella, **c**ytomegalovirus, and **he**rpes simplex virus), toxin exposure, trauma, intracranial bleeding, and hypoxic-ischemic injury. Other causes of central hypotonia include brain malformations, chromosomal/genetic syndromes (such as trisomy 21, Prader-Willi syndrome [PWS], Zellweger syndrome, and neonatal adrenoleukodystrophy), and metabolic disorders. Certain medical emergencies, such as stroke, need to be considered early on.

Stroke While rare in children and typically identified prior to admission to a pediatric hospitalist service, strokes are a "can't miss" diagnosis. Risk factors include recent viral illness in young children leading to focal cerebral arteriopathy, sickle-cell disease, congenital heart disease, and other disorders associated with hypercoagulability (e.g., lupus, malignancy). See Chapter 121 for more on Stroke.

Cerebral Palsy (CP) Chronic static encephalopathy (CSE) of infancy and childhood is a term used by neurologists to refer to chronic, permanent, and nonprogressive brain disorders, with resultant cognitive and motor impairment. This terminology does not imply specific etiology. The symptoms and effect on development depend on the part(s) of the brain involved and the severity of the injury. CSE can be due to acquired conditions, such as hypoxic ischemic brain injury, trauma, or infection; in-utero toxin exposure, such as in fetal alcohol syndrome; or congenital brain malformation.

CP, a type of CSE, is a broad term used to describe a heterogeneous group of disorders affecting motor control and posture due to damage to the immature and developing brain, especially the corticospinal tract or the cerebral white matter. CP is typically present early in life and is not caused by a degenerative disorder. CP is the most common childhood physical disability, with an overall prevalence at 2 to 3.5 cases per 1000 live births. The prevalence has increased among very small premature infants as more have survived. Identification of causal relationships in CP has been challenging. Seventy to 80% of CP cases are acquired prenatally and from largely unknown causes. In about 10% of patients, CP is acquired postnatally, mainly due to brain damage from bacterial meningitis, viral encephalitis, hyperbilirubinemia, motor vehicle accident, or accidental or nonaccidental head trauma.

Clinical Features Common manifestations of CP include hypotonia, spasticity, or both; global developmental delay or developmental arrest in very severe cases; epilepsy; visual and hearing impairment; and feeding difficulty due to cortical and/or bulbar dysfunction. For patients with CP, the initial presentation may be hypotonia at birth or during infancy that subsequently evolves to increased tone (spasticity/dystonia). Some patients may present later in life with motor developmental delay or an abnormal gait. Traditionally, CP has been classified based on the pattern of motor impairment: the spastic (diplegia, quadriplegia, or hemiplegia) type accounts for

TABLE 120-6 Gross Motor Function Classification System (GMFCS)

Level 1	Walks and climbs stairs without support and can run and jump, though moves with slower speed and with decreased balance and coordination
Level 2	Walks and climbs stairs with support (e.g., railing), struggles in areas with inclines or uneven surfaces, decreased ability to run and jump
Level 3	Walks with assistance (e.g., mobility device), may climb stairs with railing, may be able to push self in manual wheelchair
Level 4	Has significant difficulty walking even with assistance, usually dependent on wheelchair, though may be able to power their own power wheelchair
Level 5	Has significant difficulty voluntarily controlling their movement and holding head and neck in upright position, cannot sit, stand, or walk independently

Source: From Palisano R, Rosenbaum P, Walter S, Russell D, Galuppi B. Development and reliability of a system to classify gross motor function in children with cerebral palsy. *Dev Med Child Neurol.* 1997;39(4):214-223.

85% to 91% of cases. Other types include athetoid/dyskinetic and ataxic types. Mixed type is used for patients with a combination of symptoms. The effect of CP on functional abilities varies greatly. Some patients are ambulatory with only mild motor deficit, while others are not able to walk. The degree of functional ability can be described using the Gross Motor Function Classification System (GMFCS) (**Table 120-6**).

Although CP is defined as a motor disability, other neurological disabilities frequently co-occur. Intellectual disability occurs in around 50% of individuals with CP. It is more common among those with spastic quadriplegia than in those with other types of CP. About 35% of pediatric patients have seizures. Children with both CP and epilepsy are more likely to have intellectual disability. Speech and language disorders are present in more than one-third of individuals with CP. Growth problems are common, as well as other neurological deficits such as visual and hearing impairment and abnormal sensation.

By definition, CSE and CP are nonprogressive, but progressive joint contractures can cause deterioration of motor function. Poorly controlled epilepsy resulting from the brain injury can cause regression of motor and cognitive function. It is also important to note that many slowly progressive conditions can be misdiagnosed as CSE or CP.

Diagnosis Laboratory tests are not necessary to confirm the diagnosis of CSE or CP, as it is based on the history and examination. Historically, diagnosis was thought to be inaccurate if attempted before 12 to 24 months of age, but newer tools have been identified with high predictive validity for use before 6 months of age, including standardized motor assessment and neuroimaging. Infants >6 months of age who are not sitting independently by 9 months of age, have hand function asymmetry, or are unable to put weight on the entirety of their foot (heel and forefoot) should have standardized neurological assessment, neuroimaging, and standardized motor assessment performed. This testing should occur in conjunction with Neurology consultation.

Management Optimal management of individuals with CSE or CP requires CP-specific early intervention to maximize neuroplasticity and optimize motor, cognitive, and communication outcomes. Treatment requires a multidisciplinary approach involving neurologists, physiatrists, orthopedics, neurosurgery, and therapists (i.e., occupational, physical, speech, etc.). Physical therapy and occupational therapy complemented by daily home stretching exercises are essential for prevention of joint contractures and promotion of improved motor function.

Clear objectives and goals should be set before initiation of pharmacological and surgical intervention. Some individuals with more diffuse spasticity may benefit from pharmacological therapy with medications such as baclofen or benzodiazepines. Most of these medications used are off-label for age and indication, and thus should be used only by experienced physicians, such as neurologists or physiatrists. CNS depressant side effects may limit the use of these medications. Intrathecal baclofen administration with a surgically implanted pump may improve the effectiveness of the medication with reduced side effects. The baclofen dose can be adjusted with an external handheld programmer. However, there are neurological emergencies associated with baclofen withdrawal from pump malfunction or an empty reservoir. Infection is another potential complication. Botulinum toxin (Botox) type A may reduce spasticity in injected muscles, but the injection needs to be repeated every 3 to 6 months to maintain the beneficial effects. Phenol intramuscular neurolysis can be considered for spasticity involving large muscles or several muscles, but sedation or anesthesia is required due to severe pain at the injection site.

Scoliosis and hip dislocation are the most common conditions requiring surgery. Tendon lengthening or transfer can improve passive range motion and reduce deformity. Selective dorsal rhizotomy, a procedure involving laminectomy and then surgical ablation of 70% to 90% of the dorsal or sensory nerve roots, may be beneficial for select patients, but it may potentially worsen lumbar lordosis a few years later and can worsen dystonia in patients with mixed spasticity and dystonia.

Genetic/Metabolic Diseases Genetic and metabolic causes of hypotonia and weakness comprise a very large, heterogenous group of conditions. Hypotonia is a common symptom in all these disorders. An overview of PWS, leukodystrophies, lysosomal storage disorders (LSDs), and congenital disorders of glycosylation (CDGs) is provided but does not exhaust the list of genetic or metabolic causes of hypotonia and weakness in infants and children. When suspected, the differential should be broadened in conjunction with expert consultation.

Prader-Willi Syndrome PWS is a complex genetic condition and the most common genetic cause of life-threatening obesity. It is a paternally inherited condition that arises due to lack of expression of genes imprinted on chromosome 15.

Clinical Features Prenatally, patients often have reduced fetal activity and are breech. At birth, the following features are usually present: profound hypotonia, poor suck, and hypogonadism. The profound hypotonia can be easily mistaken for a presentation of spinal muscular atrophy but is differentiated by the presence of deep tendon reflexes. The profound hypotonia improves with age, though affected children often remain hypotonic. Craniofacial differences include dolichocephaly, narrow forehead, strabismus, almond-shaped eyes, enamel hypoplasia, and short upturned nose. Beginning in early childhood, affected individuals develop an insatiable appetite, which leads to chronic overeating and morbid obesity. Patients typically have mild to moderate intellectual impairment and learning disabilities. Behavioral problems are common. Puberty is delayed or incomplete, and most affected individuals are infertile.

Diagnosis Testing should begin with DNA methylation analysis; if abnormal, further genetic testing should be performed. Chromosome analysis via fluorescence in situ hybridization will identify typical gene deletions on chromosome 15 suggestive of PWS, but microarray will better identify the size of the deletion and assess for other PWS subtypes.

Management Treatment is targeted toward the multiple comorbidities patients with PWS develop. In infancy, enteral tube feeding may be needed to assure adequate nutrition. In childhood, strict supervision of daily food intake is essential to limit weight gain. Hormone replacement at puberty may help to produce adequate secondary sexual characteristics. Scoliosis is present in about 40% of patients and should be closely monitored. Behavioral management can be challenging and comanagement with Psychiatry and Psychology is often helpful. Finally, individuals with PWS are also at increased risk of epilepsy, so there should be a low threshold for referral to Neurology with episodes of altered awareness or abnormal movements concerning for seizure.

Leukodystrophies Leukodystrophies are a large group of rare, heterogenous genetic disorders predominantly affecting CNS white matter. They are caused by defects in myelin, astrocytes, microglia, and small blood vessels. The list of defined genetic leukodystrophies is extensive but includes lysosomal disorders (e.g., metachromatic leukodystrophy and Krabbe disease) and peroxisomal disorders (e.g., Zellweger [cerebrohepatorenal] syndrome, neonatal adrenoleukodystrophy, and X-linked adrenoleukodystrophy), mitochondrial disorders, metabolic disorders, and DNA repair defects.

Clinical Features Most patients with leukodystrophies present with motor symptoms, in contrast to primary neuronal disorders (or gray matter diseases) which frequently present with cognitive decline and seizures. CNS defects lead to severe hypotonia during infancy that frequently evolves to axial hypotonia and appendicular spasticity and/or dystonia over time. Some may present with delayed acquisition of motor milestones, developmental arrest, or regression of motor function. In older children, the presenting symptoms may be frequent falls, clumsy gait, or decline in sporting skills or other functional skills. Some patients may develop dystonia or movement disorders when deep gray matter is involved, and ataxia when cerebellum is involved. Peripheral neuropathy is seen in Krabbe disease, metachromatic leukodystrophy, adrenoleukodystrophy, and peroxisomal disorders. Problems with vision are also common in leukodystrophies. These can be due to intraocular pathology (cataract, retinitis pigmentosa, retinal cherry-red spots, optic atrophy, nystagmus) or problems with the cortical visual pathways. Cortical visual impairment can be a late manifestation of many types of leukodystrophies due to involvement of the cortical visual pathway. In late stages, cognitive decline and seizures may occur.

Typically, these diseases involve organ systems beyond the nervous system. The precise constellation of organ systems involved can help determine the diagnosis. Patients with Zellweger syndrome have characteristic dysmorphic features (e.g., high forehead, enlarged fontanelle, and shallow orbits), profound hypotonia, and organomegaly. Adrenal insufficiency is seen in X-linked adrenoleukodystrophy and peroxisome biogenesis disorders. Patients with 4H leukodystrophy have associated hypogonadotropic hypogonadism, growth hormone deficiency, and hypothyroidism. Hypothyroidism can also be seen in Aicardi-Goutières syndrome.

Diagnosis The hallmark of leukodystrophy is abnormal white matter on brain MRI. If MRI shows patterns consistent with a specific leukodystrophy, targeted metabolic and genetic testing should be pursued. If MRI findings are unclear, nontargeted genetic testing or generalized metabolic screening should be pursued. Whole exome sequencing has helped decrease the number of leukodystrophy cases without an identifiable genetic cause significantly over the last several years.

Management Some leukodystrophies have disease-specific therapies available; for example, patients with Addison disease in X-linked adrenoleukodystrophy may require hydrocortisone supplementation. Patients with metachromatic leukodystrophy may require cholecystectomy due to gallbladder dysfunction. Hematopoietic stem cell transplantation (HSCT) or bone marrow transplantation (BMT) may be used in a few specific cases (e.g., X-linked adrenoleukodystrophy, metachromatic leukodystrophy, Krabbe). Generally, patients may require treatment for spasticity, malnutrition, bowel and bladder dysfunction, hip dislocation, scoliosis, epilepsy, and other comorbidities.

Lysosomal Storage Diseases LSDs are a group of rare, inherited, and progressive metabolic disorders that result from lysosomal dysfunction, usually as a consequence of deficiency of a vital single enzyme required for the metabolism of lipids, glycoproteins, or mucopolysaccharides. The accumulation of macromolecules results in cellular and tissue dysfunction and symptom development and progression. Traditionally, LSD is classified based on the nature of the accumulating storage material—as in sphingolipidoses (e.g., Gaucher disease, Fabry disease, Niemann-Pick diseases, Tay-Sachs disease, Krabbe disease, etc.), mucopolysaccharidosis (e.g., Hurler syndrome, Hunter syndrome, etc.), and oligosaccharidoses (e.g., Pompe disease, which is discussed in the metabolic myopathy section later in this chapter, gangliosidoses, etc.). Some lysosomal storage diseases are also considered leukodystrophies based on their primary CNS involvement and include Fabry disease, Krabbe disease, and GM1 gangliosidosis.

Clinical Features The signs and symptoms of LSDs vary depending on disease type, age of onset, and other factors. Signs and symptoms often include dysmorphic features (coarse facies, macroglossia), visual loss and ophthalmologic findings (corneal clouding or macular cherry-red spot), bony abnormalities (dysostosis multiplex), cardiac involvement (arrhythmia or cardiomegaly), hepatosplenomegaly, and progressive neurological symptoms (intellectual disability, developmental delay or development regression, epilepsy, ataxia, hypotonia and/or spasticity, peripheral neuropathy).

Diagnosis Diagnosis of LSD can be made by demonstrating lysosomal enzyme deficiency in peripheral white blood cells, or fibroblasts. Urine can be screened for excretion of substrates. The diagnosis of specific types of LSD is confirmed by genetic testing.

Management Some LSDs can be efficiently treated by substrate reduction therapies or enzyme replacement therapy (ERT). Unfortunately, however ERT has been largely unsuccessful in improving CNS symptoms in neuronopathic forms of lysosomal diseases, likely due to difficulty in getting the enzymes to penetrate the blood-brain barrier. Increasing data suggest that HSCT might be effective in preventing progression of neurological symptoms in individuals with asymptomatic Krabbe disease and may have some efficacy in patients with mucopolysaccharidoses. Multiple subspecialists need to be involved to provide holistic care to these patients.

Congenital Disorders of Glycosylation CDGs are a fast-growing group of inherited metabolic disorders characterized by defective activity of enzymes involved in glycosylation—the process of adding complex sugar chains to proteins and lipids. More than 140 genetic disorders of glycosylation have been discovered. The most common type of protein glycosylation disorder is N-glycosylation disorders, but others have been described (e.g., disorders of O-glycosylation). Abnormal glycosylation of proteins disrupts their function thereby disrupting the function of organs and tissues. CDGs are multisystem disorders but neurological symptoms often predominate.

Clinical Features Clinical presentation and course are highly variable, ranging from death in the first year of life to mildly affected adults. As with other genetic and metabolic disorders discussed in this chapter, CDGs can present with hypotonia in infancy and early childhood. Additional signs and symptoms may include developmental delay, intellectual disability, feeding problems, inadequate weight gain, abnormal liver function, coagulopathy, hypothyroidism, hypogonadism, pericardial effusion or cardiomyopathy, abnormal fat deposits (subcutaneous fat pad) and inverted nipples, microcephaly, seizures, stroke-like episodes, and ataxia due to cerebellar hypoplasia/atrophy.

Diagnosis Brain MRI may show a variety of changes related to CDGs including polymicrogyria, lissencephaly, pontocerebellar atrophy, cerebellar atrophy, and many other changes. Evaluation of plasma transferrin isoforms remains the diagnostic standard but is now used in conjunction with brain imaging and genetic testing. Genetic testing is especially important in identifying the CDG subtype.

Management Current treatment for CDG is supportive based on associated comorbidities. Some subtypes may respond to treatment with galactose, mannose, or fructose.

Autoimmune/Neuroinflammatory Diseases There are multiple autoimmune/neuroinflammatory disorders that can present with weakness. These include multiple sclerosis (MS), neuromyelitis optica (NMO), acute demyelinating encephalomyelitis (ADEM), and myelin oligodendrocyte glycoprotein antibody disease (MOGAD). See Chapter 122 "Demyelinating Diseases" for a discussion of these diseases.

Functional Neurologic Disorder (FND) FND, according to the National Institute of Health, describes a group of common neurological movement disorders caused by an abnormality in how the brain functions that is not associated with structural abnormalities or another disorder. It can manifest with various symptoms including psychogenic nonepileptic events, functional tics and tremor, functional gait abnormalities, and functional weakness. It is important to recognize that FND is no longer a diagnosis of exclusion. There are key observances and physical examination findings that can help rule out this diagnosis. A working knowledge of the nervous system is also critical to identify inconsistencies between a patient's signs and symptoms and known neuroanatomical pathways or neuropathologic findings.

Clinical Features Patients can present with sudden or gradual onset of weakness. There is frequently a preceding minor injury or trauma. Additionally, paresthesias are commonly associated with the weakness. Key findings are incongruity and inconsistency. Incongruity describes weakness that cannot be explained by a peripheral nerve, plexus, nerve root, spinal cord, or intracranial pathology. Inconsistency describes variable strength with different modes of strength testing. For example, a patient with functional weakness may have significant weakness (1 or 2 out of 5) with formal testing but when passively observed maneuvering in bed or completing minor tasks, such as taking off shoes or using a phone, they are noted to have at least anti-gravity strength. Frequently, there are psychiatric comorbidities.

Diagnosis Diagnosis is clinical. The Diagnostic and Statistical Manual of Mental Disorders, version 5 lists four criteria for diagnosis: 1) one or more symptoms of altered voluntary motor or sensory function, 2) clinical findings provide evidence of incompatibility between the symptom and recognized neurological or medical conditions, 3) the symptom or deficit is not better explained by another medical or mental disorder, and 4) the symptom or deficit causes clinically significant distress or impairment in social, occupational, or other important areas of functioning or warrants medical evaluation. With a careful history and physical examination, the physician should be able to identify findings that rule in the diagnosis of FND. Thus, neuroimaging or further diagnostic studies are not necessary.

Management Delivering the diagnosis is the first and most critical step in management for patients with FND. It is critical to acknowledge that the disorder is not voluntary or "made up." The patient and their family should be provided with a detailed explanation of findings that rule in the diagnosis of FND. Resources should then be given to provide further understanding of the disease. Referrals should be made for cognitive behavioral therapy or other forms of psychotherapy and physical therapy. If there is concern for comorbid psychiatric conditions, a referral to a Child and Adolescent Psychiatrist should be made as well.

SPINAL CORD

Patients with spinal cord disease (myelopathy) usually present with bilateral weakness involving both arms and legs in a cervical spinal cord lesion (quadriparesis) or legs only in thoracic or lumbar lesions (diplegia). Sensory level deficits, incontinence, and hyperreflexia are classic findings seen with spinal cord disease. Depending on the exact location of the lesion, findings can be symmetric or asymmetric (e.g., hemi-cord or Brown-Sequard syndrome). As with intracranial lesions, the differential of potential etiologies for spinal cord pathology causing weakness is extensive and includes ischemia, inflammatory/demyelinating diseases, vasculitis, malignancy, trauma, and infection. Highlighted below are a few of the most common pathologies that lead to myelopathy, which the pediatric hospitalist should be familiar with.

Structural There are several congenital and acquired structural abnormalities of the spine that can result in weakness. Examples of congenital etiologies include spina bifida or myelomeningocele and tethered cord. Examples of acquired structural abnormalities include injury from trauma and compression from infection or malignancy. It is critical to know that a patient presenting with signs of acute spinal cord pathology, such as sudden onset weakness or a sensory level defect with bowel or bladder incontinence should be treated as having a neurologic emergency. Neurosurgical consultation should be considered. Depending on the pathology of the acute lesion, steroids may be considered, however should not be initiated without expert consultation.

Transverse myelitis Transverse myelitis is an immune-mediated demyelinating lesion of the spinal cord. The potential etiologies include those discussed above with intracranial demyelinating lesions (e.g., MS, NMO, ADEM, MOGAD) along with potential infectious etiologies (e.g., viral, Mycoplasma, Bartonella) and systemic autoimmune diseases (e.g., sarcoidosis, lupus), among others. See Chapter 122 "Demyelinating Diseases."

Acute Flaccid Myelitis (AFM) AFM is a predominantly childhood polio-like illness resulting in acute flaccid weakness in one or more limbs and occurs most commonly in young children. There is often a febrile prodrome with associated respiratory symptoms in the days prior to onset of weakness. Thus far, enterovirus D68 is strongly implicated as a primary cause of AFM although other viruses have been reported. The pathophysiological mechanism by which these viruses lead to AFM is unclear. See Chapter 122, "Demyelinating Diseases."

NERVE

Peripheral neuropathies are disorders in which the primary pathological process affects the axons of motor and/or sensory neurons or their myelin sheath and associated Schwann cells. Although acquired neuropathies such as Guillain-Barré syndrome (GBS) and the extremely rare chronic inflammatory demyelinating neuropathy occur in children, most chronic polyneuropathies in children are genetically determined. The largest group is the hereditary motor and sensory neuropathies such as Charcot-Marie-Tooth disease.

Complex syndromes associated with inborn errors of metabolism or neurodegenerative disorders may have polyneuropathy as one of their features. Different from adults, the incidence of toxic neuropathy or neuropathy secondary to systemic diseases such as diabetes, cancer, and collagen vascular diseases is low. In addition to polyneuropathy, focal or compressive neuropathy such as carpal tunnel syndrome (median neuropathy at wrist), ulnar neuropathy, or peroneal neuropathy can occur but are uncommon in children.

Acute Demyelinating Inflammatory Polyneuropathy (Guillain-Barré Syndrome [GBS]) GBS is an immune-mediated rapidly progressive disorder of peripheral nerves and nerve roots; see Chapter 122 "Demyelinating Diseases" for a full discussion.

Spinal Muscular Atrophy (SMA) SMA is characterized by progressive muscle weakness resulting from degeneration and loss of anterior horn cells in the spinal cord and the brainstem nuclei. The incidence of SMA varies from 1 in 6000 to 1 in 10,000 in different populations. Age of onset varies from birth to adulthood. Some forms are degenerative/progressive disorders while others have a more static process. The most common form of SMA is an autosomal recessive disorder resulting from mutations in the survival motor neuron (*SMN*) 1 gene. In humans, most functional SMN protein is produced from the *SMN1* gene, with a small amount produced from the *SMN2* gene. The severity of the disease is modified by the copy numbers of the *SMN2* gene.

Clinical Features Patients present with hypotonia and symmetric weakness. Weakness affects proximal muscles more than distal, and legs more than arms. Intercostal muscles may also be affected, but there is relative sparing of the diaphragm, which creates a "bell-shaped" chest. Poor weight gain, pneumonia, nocturnal hypoventilation, respiratory insufficiency/failure, scoliosis, and joint contractures are common complications of SMA. Cardiac function is typically not affected. Based on the age of onset of symptoms and maximum function achieved, SMA is clinically classified into types 0 to IV:

- SMA type 0 (prenatal) has prenatal onset of the disease. Patients are born with multiple joint contractures (arthrogryposis), facial weakness, lack of movement, and respiratory failure requiring immediate mechanical ventilation. Decreased fetal movement, polyhydramnios, and breech presentation are common. Death usually occurs from respiratory failure before age 1 month.
- SMA type I (also called Werdnig-Hoffman disease) is the most common inherited cause of death in infancy, with onset of weakness before 6 months but frequently presenting as a neonate. It presents with progressive weakness causing paradoxical respiration and impaired swallowing. Patients may have a history of reduced fetal movements and polyhydramnios. Affected individuals do not acquire the ability to sit unsupported. Characteristic findings include hypotonia, weakness, tongue fasciculations, absent reflexes, and a coarse tremor sometimes called minipolymyoclonus. Patients frequently have an alert and very interactive appearance as their facial muscles are spared.
- SMA type II has onset between 6 and 12 months. Patients can sit unsupported but do not stand or walk. Affected individuals typically lose the ability to sit unsupported by the mid-teen years.
- SMA type III (also called Kugelberg-Welander disease or juvenile type) has a milder phenotype with variable severity of weakness and clinical course. Patients typically develop weakness after 1 year of age, though it may not develop until late childhood and adolescence. Patients achieve the ability to walk unsupported at least 25 m. The clinical course is variable. Typically, patients never climb stairs without holding a rail and lose the ability to walk independently by the mid-teens. Those who acquired normal walking before onset of weakness, however, can remain ambulatory independently until the third and fourth decade of life.
- SMA type IV has adult-onset of disease, typically after 25 years of age, with proximal weakness. There can be associated tremor and respiratory insufficiency.

Diagnosis SMA is diagnosed with molecular genetic testing. Eighteen states have SMA testing on the newborn screen. About 96% of patients are homozygous for deletion of the *SMN1* gene. Generally, the presence of three or more copies of *SMN2* correlates with milder phenotypes. Muscle biopsy and electromyography (EMG) are not usually needed to make a diagnosis.

Management Treatment should be guided based on the most recent consensus guidelines, which were originally published in 2007 and updated in 2018. Patients are best managed in a multidisciplinary setting where nutritional status, respiratory function, and orthopedic issues can be evaluated and managed. Nusinersen was the first drug to be approved to treat SMA by increasing *SMN2* production. Several other drugs have since been developed, and common among them is their startling cost ($125,000 per injection for nusinersen). The use of these medications should be guided by the appropriate subspecialists. Proper genetic counseling and parental testing for carrier status is also an important part of SMA management.

Charcot-Marie-Tooth Disease (CMT) Hereditary motor and sensory neuropathies are a clinically and genetically heterogeneous group of diseases that are often collectively referred to as CMT. CMT is commonly divided into demyelinating and axonal forms. The demyelinating form is the most common form and is caused by defects in myelin-forming Schwann cells. The less common axonal form is caused by defects in the nerve axon or its interaction with Schwann cells. More than 80 causative genes have been identified, making an accurate genetic diagnosis of CMT increasingly possible.

Clinical Features The longest nerves in the body are affected first and most severely as CMT neuropathy is length dependent. Patients frequently present within the first decade of life with toe walking, progressive pes cavus, frequent trips and falls due to distal weakness and gait instability, high steppage gait, and difficulty running. Hand weakness leads to difficulty with buttoning, opening bottles, writing, or using utensils. A small percentage of patients present early during the neonatal period and infancy with hypotonia, profound weakness, areflexia, and other problems, which in rare cases can be life-threatening. However, in most affected individuals, CMT does not affect life expectancy.

Diagnosis Current diagnostic strategy of CMT is based on clinical and electrophysiologic features. NCS results and pattern of inheritance help divide CMT into the autosomal dominantly inherited demyelinating form (CMT1) and the axonal form (CMT2). For patients with CMT1 (based on significant slowing of conduction on NCS and a family history of a dominant pattern of inheritance), it is most cost-effective to start with testing for *PMP22* duplication, as it accounts for up to 70% of CMT1. The unique features of other types of CMT may also allow for more targeted genetic testing. If no unique features are identified however, the next-generation sequencing technology has become a robust and powerful tool that can deliver increased diagnostic yield at a relatively low cost.

Management There is no cure for CMT at the present time. Medical interventions focus on enhancing physical mobility and preventing complications and contractures. Physical therapy, braces, heel cord, and foot joint surgery are used to correct foot deformities and contractures, to improve the quality of gait or prolong walking. Adaptive utensils, writing tools, and devices help to increase efficiency and performance of daily tasks. Scoliosis surgery is performed in patients with severe spinal curvature. It is important to avoid neurotoxic medications, especially vincristine, which can cause paralysis in patients with CMT1.

NEUROMUSCULAR JUNCTION

Neuromuscular junction transmission defects are classified into immune-mediated, toxic or metabolic, and congenital syndromes. These disorders are typically pure motor syndromes preferentially affecting extraocular, bulbar, and proximal limb muscles, and are characterized by fluctuating weakness that classically worsens after repeated or sustained muscle activity and improves with rest, though there are some exceptions. Specific symptoms and signs include fluctuating and frequently asymmetrical or unilateral ptosis, diplopia due to oculomotor dysfunction, dysarthria or hypophonia, dysphagia, dyspnea, and systemic weakness affecting proximal greater than distal muscles. These disorders can be mistaken as myopathy. It should also be noted that certain medications that impair neuromuscular transmission may cause neonatal hypotonia when administered to mothers in labor or to newborn infants. For example, magnesium used to treat pre-eclampsia and preterm labor may cause apnea, respiratory depression, lethargy, hypotonia, and poor sucking in the newborn.

Infantile Botulism Infant botulism is a toxin-mediated disease of the neuromuscular junction that commonly strikes between 6 weeks and 6 months of age. It is the most common form of human botulism in the United States, with between 80 and 110 cases recognized annually. The disease is caused by ingestion of the spores of *Clostridium botulinum*, which germinate in the sterile intestines of infants and produce the botulinum neurotoxin that irreversibly blocks presynaptic release of acetylcholine at both somatic and autonomic synapses. This causes flaccid paralysis. There is a strong geographic clustering of cases in regions of eastern Pennsylvania, New Jersey, Delaware, Utah, and California.

Clinical Features Constipation is often one of the early but frequently overlooked symptoms, followed by difficulty feeding (sucking and swallowing) and progressive bulbar and muscle weakness in a descending pattern, manifested as weak cry, diminished facial expression due to facial weakness, ptosis, ophthalmoplegia, hypotonia with poor head control, and decreased spontaneous movement. Deep tendon reflexes can be normal or depressed/absent. About 50% of patients may develop hypoventilation and require mechanical ventilation as the weakness progresses. Signs of autonomic dysfunction including sluggish pupillary reaction, tachycardia, and hypotension are frequently found. The disease typically progresses for about 1 to 2 weeks, followed by gradual improvement over the next few weeks.

Diagnosis A high degree of clinical suspicion is needed to make a prompt diagnosis of infant botulism. The diagnosis is made on clinical grounds and is confirmed by identification of the neurotoxin or the *C. botulinum* organisms in the stool, but it may take a few days to get the result. NCS and EMG can provide rapid bedside substantiation of the clinical diagnosis but are rarely indicated.

Management Urgent treatment with BabyBIG, Botulism Immune Globulin Intravenous (BIG-IV), is the current standard of treatment and should not be delayed for confirmatory testing. BIG-IV is derived from pooled plasma of immunized adult volunteers; it neutralizes free toxin. To be most effective, BIG-IV should be administered as early as possible. Infants receiving this treatment have shorter hospital stays and less severe illness. If antibiotics are needed to treat infections that arise, aminoglycosides should be avoided as they decrease acetylcholine release from diaphragmatic nerves and can potentiate respiratory compromise. Proper nutritional and respiratory support are essential. In the absence of complications, patients recover completely from the disease.

Myasthenia Gravis (MG) Three forms of myasthenia gravis occur in childhood: (1) transient neonatal myasthenia, occurring in the newborn secondary to transplacental transmission of maternal antibodies from a mother with MG; (2) the immune-mediated form of MG (also known as juvenile MG) associated with antibodies directed against components of the neuromuscular junction (acetylcholine receptor [AChR] or muscle-specific kinase [MuSK]); and (3) congenital myasthenic syndrome (CMS) due to various genetic defects in the structure and function of proteins in the neuromuscular junction.

Transient Neonatal Myasthenia Transient neonatal myasthenia complicates pregnancy in as many as 5% to 30% of mothers with MG. Most mothers of affected infants have active clinical disease, but some may be in remission or have no evidence of MG. Neonates present with hypotonia, weak cry, poor suck, respiratory distress, and weakness in extraocular muscles. The severity of symptoms in the newborn may be profound, depending on the timing (early vs. late gestation) and severity of exposure. Both AChR and MuSK antibodies cross the placenta. The illness is usually mild and self-limiting, but neostigmine and plasmapheresis have been used with success.

Juvenile Myasthenia Gravis In older children and adolescents, MG is an autoimmune disease in which antibodies are directed against the postsynaptic membrane of the neuromuscular junction, resulting in muscle weakness and fatigability. The majority of cases of MG are caused by antibodies against the nicotinic AChR (binding, blocking, modulating). Antibodies to MuSK have been reported in some patients who are seronegative for AChR antibodies. Antibodies against the low-density lipoprotein receptor-related protein 4 (LRP-4) and other potential immune targets at the muscle endplate have been recently identified.

Clinical Features Juvenile MG shares the symptoms and signs of the later-onset adult autoimmune disease. The first symptoms occur after age 10 in most pediatric patients but may appear as early as infancy. Unilateral or bilateral ptosis, which is often asymmetric and fluctuating (i.e., worse at the end of the day or after school, better after a nap), is the most common presentation. Unilateral or asymmetric ophthalmoplegia can be a particular concern in children as it may cause amblyopia. Individual patients can have different patterns and severity of weakness. Weakness may remain in the ocular muscles (ocular MG) or spread to the facial, bulbar, and respiratory muscles (bulbar MG) or also involve the limbs (generalized MG). Patients may complain of hypophonia and dysphagia. Patients with MG are at risk for choking and respiratory failure, which can be life-threatening. MuSK antibody-positive patients may present with symptoms indistinguishable from AchR-positive MG patients, but some patients have unique features presenting with prominent faciopharyngeal weakness with sparing of ocular muscles, or with relatively isolated neck extensor and respiratory muscle weakness.

Diagnosis Diagnosis is typically suggested by a thorough history and examination. At the bedside, the clinician can perform the ice-pack test and assess for improvement in ptosis. Ice is held over the eye for 2 minutes and an increase in eye opening of 2 mm is considered a positive result. The ice decreases the rate of acetylcholine breakdown at the neuromuscular junction allowing increasing acetylcholine available for binding to the motor endplate. Confirmation of the diagnosis can be achieved by serologic testing showing elevated anti-AChR or anti-MuSK antibodies. In patients who are negative for tested antibodies but clinical suspicion remains, EMG and NCS can be performed. EMG will classically show decrement with repetitive nerve stimulation and excessive "jitter" on single-fiber EMG. Diagnosing autoimmune MG in young children can be complicated by the need to differentiate from CMS, as anti-AChR or anti-MuSK antibodies are frequently undetected in younger children. Chest CT scan may detect thymic abnormalities (thymic hyperplasia vs. thymoma) and should always be completed, although thymoma is rare in children.

Management Treatment commonly includes oral acetylcholine esterase (AChE) inhibitors (e.g., pyridostigmine) for symptomatic treatment and/or immunomodulating therapy with corticosteroids or steroid-sparing agents. Plasmapheresis and IVIG are the mainstays in the treatment of myasthenic crisis or for preparing a myasthenic patient for surgery or other stressful procedure. Thymectomy is absolutely indicated in patients with thymoma. Thymectomy is also recommended in nonthymomatous AChR-positive MG with severe symptoms. There are a few important differences in the treatment of MuSK MG. Patients with MuSK MG often do not respond or may actually worsen with oral anticholinesterase drugs. There is often a remarkable response to plasmapheresis, while the response to IVIG may be more modest. The role of thymectomy in MuSK MG is not clear.

Congenital Myasthenic Syndromes (CMS) CMS is a growing family of genetic disorders that affect specific components of the neuromuscular junction. They are not autoimmune diseases. CMS is classified according to the affected anatomy of the neuromuscular junction—presynaptic, synaptic basal lamina-associated, or post-synaptic. The most common cause of CMS is an alteration in the structure, presence, or function of AChR. Most are autosomal recessive, although at least one condition is autosomal dominant. A full discussion is beyond the scope of this chapter.

MUSCLE

Disorders affecting the muscles primarily are referred to as myopathies and can be either inherited or acquired conditions. Inherited conditions include congenital myopathies, muscular dystrophies, metabolic myopathies, mitochondrial cytopathy, channelopathies, and myotonic syndromes. Acquired conditions include inflammatory/infectious myopathies, endocrine myopathies, toxic myopathies, and critical illness myopathy.

Congenital Myopathies Congenital myopathies are a heterogeneous group of genetic myopathies defined by their characteristic structural findings on muscle biopsy. Autosomal dominant, autosomal recessive, and X-linked inheritance patterns have been recognized.

Clinical Features Congenital myopathies usually manifest at birth with profound hypotonia, hyporeflexia, facial and generalized weakness, motor developmental delay, feeding difficulty, and in severe cases, respiratory insufficiency/failure. Patients presenting later in infancy or early childhood may have more mild symptoms. Associated findings can include features such as dolichocephaly (i.e., abnormally long and narrow head), a long, narrow face, a high-arched palate, and pectus excavatum. Ophthalmoplegia, frequently associated with ptosis, is a consistent finding in X-linked *MTM1*-related myotubular myopathy and recessive *RYR1*-related myopathies. Orthopedic complications may include kyphoscoliosis or rigid spine, hip dislocation, and progressive contracture. A history of malignant hyperthermia or rhabdomyolysis associated with generalized anesthesia strongly suggests *RYR1*-related myopathies. Cardiomyopathy is not a typical feature except in *TTN*- and *MYH7*-related myopathies. Respiratory insufficiency disproportional to the severity of muscle weakness, along with early development of scoliosis or rigid spine, should prompt consideration of *SEPN1*- or *LMNA*-related myopathies. Unlike muscular dystrophies, the clinical course of many congenital myopathies may be relatively static, and many individuals show some improvement after the neonatal period. On the other hand, cases with facial, ocular, and respiratory muscle involvement may be lethal in infancy.

Diagnosis The creatine kinase (CK) level is typically normal or only mildly elevated. CK elevation more than 5 times normal should prompt consideration of muscular dystrophies. It should be noted that serum CK level is frequently elevated even in normal neonates during the first week of life. EMG usually shows myopathic features but can be normal in mild cases. The diagnosis is made by demonstrating characteristic structures on muscle biopsy with special stains and electron microscopy. At least seven distinctive subtypes have been recognized, and these include central core disease, nemaline myopathy, centronuclear/myotubular myopathy, centronuclear myopathy, multicore disease, congenital fiber-type disproportion, and hyaline body myopathy. Muscle ultrasound and muscle MRI have increasingly been used to differentiate between different forms of congenital myopathy by identifying selective muscle involvement patterns that are associated with specific gene defects. Features on clinical examination, investigations, imaging studies, and pathological findings provide guidance in prioritization of genetic testing. Rapid advances in sequencing technology have allowed genetic confirmation of congenital myopathy in many patients in recent years.

Management Supportive treatment may involve orthopedic treatments, as well as physical, occupational, or speech therapy. Nutritional support and assisted breathing may be needed. Children with central core disease due to *RYR1* mutations may have life-threatening reaction to general anesthesia, and malignant hyperthermia protocols should be used.

Muscular Dystrophies Muscular dystrophies (MDs) are a group of more than 30 different genetic disorders featuring progressive muscular weakness along with wasting and degeneration of skeletal muscles. MD is classified based on the distribution and severity of muscle involvement, age of onset, rate of progression, and pattern of inheritance. Some forms become evident at birth, infancy, and early childhood; others may not manifest symptoms until adolescence or adulthood. The pattern of inheritance can be autosomal recessive, autosomal dominant, or X-linked. Duchenne muscular dystrophy (DMD) and Becker muscular dystrophy (BMD) are X-linked conditions and are the most prevalent forms of MD. There are several other forms of MD including congenital muscular dystrophy (CMD), facioscapulohumeral muscular dystrophy (FSHD), myotonic dystrophy (DM1 and DM2), limb-girdle muscular dystrophies (LGMD), Emery-Dreifuss muscular dystrophy (EDMD) and collagen VI disease (Ulrich muscular dystrophy and Bethlem myopathy) (**Table 120-7**).

TABLE 120-7 Muscular Dystrophies

Type	Inheri-tance	Defective Gene	Onset Age	Clinical Features	Other Organ/System Involvement	Treatment
DMD	XR	Dystrophin	3-5 years	Progressive proximal > distal weakness, loss of independent ambulation at 12 years, respiratory failure during 2nd or 3rd decade	Cardiomyopathy Learning disabilities	Corticosteroids Supportive
BMD	XR	Dystrophin	Early childhood to adult	Progressive proximal > distal weakness with variable course, Some with hyper-CK only	Cardiomyopathy	Supportive
Limb-girdle	AD/AR	Many different genes	Early childhood to adult	Progressive limb girdle weakness	± Cardiomyopathy ± Learning disabilities	Supportive
EMDB	XR/AD	Emerin, lamin A/C	Childhood	Progressive joint contracture disproportional to weakness Humeral and peroneal weakness	Cardiomyopathy	Supportive
Congenital	AR	Many different genes	At birth or infancy	Hypotonia, diffuse weakness	CNS abnormalities ± Eye abnormalities	Supportive
Ullrich	AR/AD	COL6	Birth or infancy to adulthood	Distal hyperlaxity and progressive joint contracture, progressive weakness	Rigid spine	Supportive
FSHD	AD	DUX4 SMCHD1	Childhood to adult	Slowly progressive weakness facial and shoulder girdle and foot dorsiflexors, Scapular winging	Deafness Coat's disease	Supportive
Oculo-pharyngeal	AD/AR	Expansion of GCN trinucleotide repeat of the *PABPN1*	5th to 6th decade	Ptosis, slowly progressive facial, bulbar, and limb muscles		Supportive
Myotonic	AD	DM1: Expansion of a CTG trinucleotide repeat DM2: expansion of CCTG repeat	Infancy to adult	Hypotonia, weakness, feeding difficulty, and respiratory compromise in congenital form, Myotonia, distal weakness in classical and mild forms	Cognitive impairment in congenital form Cardiac conduction defect and cardiomyopathy Cataract, hypothyroidism, hyperglycemia and diabetes, hypogonadism, infertility	Supportive

AD, autosomal dominant; AR, autosomal recessive; CK, creatine kinase; CNS, central nervous system; XR, X-linked recessive.

Dystrophinopathies Dystrophinopathies are the most common forms of MD during childhood and are X-linked recessive disorders. They are caused by mutations in the *DMD* gene (encodes dystrophin) that lead to either severe DMD or a milder form of the disease called Becker muscular dystrophy (BMD). Most mutations causing DMD and BMD are deletions. Dystrophin deficiency leads to sarcolemma weakening, functional ischemia, free-radical damage, calcium overloading, and regeneration failure leading to muscle degeneration. The damaged cells are cleared by the inflammatory system and later are replaced by fatty and fibrotic tissue.

Clinical Features Symptoms of DMD become clinically evident in the preschool years when male children present with delayed milestones or a gait disorder. The mean age of walking is 18 months (ranging from 12 to 24 months). Pelvic girdle muscle weakness causes a waddling and lordotic gait and difficulty climbing stairs, running, jumping, and standing up from a squatting position. These patients use the Gowers maneuver to get up from a supine position (see Figure 120-1). Progressive calf muscle hypertrophy is almost always present. The untreated natural history of DMD shows a predictable clinical course. Weakness and contractures progress such that patients lose independent ambulation at a mean age of 9 years. There is also development of clinically significant scoliosis in up to 90% of boys, respiratory insufficiency, and cardiomyopathy. The incidence of cardiomyopathy steadily increases in the second decade of life, with all individuals affected after 18 years of age, although many boys remain asymptomatic until left ventricular ejection fraction is decreased from 10% to 15%. Death typically occurs in the late teens or early twenties as a result of respiratory or cardiac failure. Despite improvement in survival with advanced pulmonary care, early treatment of cardiomyopathy, scoliosis surgery, and nutritional support, survival beyond age 30 years is still uncommon. Most patients have normal cognitive function throughout the course of their disease, but some patients have nonprogressive cognitive impairment, with the average IQ left-shifted in the DMD population. Some also have attention or behavioral issues.

BMD is characterized by later onset of skeletal muscle weakness, with a much more variable clinical course. Individuals with BMD typically lose independent ambulation by 16 years of age, but some may remain ambulatory up to 20 years of age or older. It is increasingly recognized that some patients with BMD may have a much milder spectrum of disease, presenting with elevated creatinine kinase, myalgia, muscle cramps, and exertional myoglobinuria without muscle weakness or with only subclinical weakness. Despite the milder skeletal muscle involvement, heart failure from dilated cardiomyopathy (DCM) is a common cause of morbidity and the most common cause of death. The development of DCM is disproportional to the degree of skeletal muscle weakness. Mean age at cardiomyopathy diagnosis is 14 years, similar to that in DMD.

Diagnosis Serum CK levels are massively elevated with levels greater than 20,000 U/L not uncommon. EMG demonstrates myopathic features but is not needed to make a diagnosis in the setting of markedly elevated CK level. The characteristic findings on muscle biopsy in the dystrophies include fiber splitting and necrosis, variation in fiber size, and progressive replacement of muscle tissue by fat and connective tissue. Genetic testing has largely replaced invasive muscle biopsies in patients with classical presentations. Genetic confirmation of the disease should be performed even in those with the diagnosis established by muscle biopsy, as the genetic testing result is essential for proper genetic counseling, prenatal diagnosis, and consideration for future mutation-specific therapies.

Management Although there is no curative therapy, advances in medical management and multidisciplinary approaches, in conjunction with steroid therapy, have altered the natural history of DMD and improved survival into adulthood. Glucocorticoids have been shown to significantly slow progression of muscle weakness, prolong independent ambulation, and delay loss of pulmonary function. They should be initiated after age 2, most often around age 4 or 5. However, significant long-term side effects of chronic steroid therapy have limited their use in some patients. New therapies are currently being researched and consultation with Neurology should occur when considering these medications. The child should be cared for by a multidisciplinary team including Neurology, Pulmonology, Cardiology, Orthopedics, Genetics, physical therapy, occupational therapy, nutrition, and social work. The sub-specialists will be able to help treat comorbidities such as hypoventilation, DCM, contractures, and scoliosis.

Congenital Myotonic Dystrophy Myotonic dystrophy type 1 is an autosomal-dominant, multisystem disorder that affects skeletal and smooth muscle, as well as the eye, heart, endocrine system, and CNS. It is caused by the expansion of a CTG trinucleotide repeat in the noncoding region of the *DMPK* gene. Subsequent generations may have a greater number of repeats and earlier and more severe expression of the disease (anticipation). Genetic counseling is thus an important aspect of care of the child and family.

Clinical Features Congenital myotonic dystrophy type 1 may present prenatally with spontaneous abortions, decreased fetal movements, or polyhydramnios. Characteristic presenting symptoms and signs in live born neonates include profound hypotonia, feeding difficulties, severe generalized weakness, club foot, and respiratory insufficiency/failure requiring mechanical ventilation. Infants requiring ventilation for longer than 3 months have around a 30% mortality rate in the first year of life. Other common signs and symptoms include eyelid ptosis, developmental delay, constipation or diarrhea, scoliosis, behavior problems, and arrhythmias. Later in childhood, myotonia gradually develops and some patients may complain about muscle cramps/pain and frequent falls, often at initiation of walking after resting because legs are "stuck" due to myotonia.

Diagnosis Affected infants are typically born to mothers (rarely to fathers) with myotonic dystrophy type 1. It is essential to examine parents for signs of grip and percussion myotonia (i.e., delayed relaxation of muscles after contraction). The affected infant's mother may or may not have obvious signs or symptoms of the disease. Characteristic facies and inability of the mother to release her handshake (grip myotonia) may be the only clue that she is affected. The diagnosis is confirmed by molecular genetic testing of the *DMPK* gene. CTG repeat length exceeding 50 establishes the diagnosis of myotonic dystrophy type 1.

Management Treatment is primarily aimed at supporting the weak respiratory musculature; many babies need mechanical ventilation and assisted feeding. Patients are best cared for in a multidisciplinary setting. Patients are at risk for nocturnal hypoventilation or obstructive sleep apnea and need to be monitored by a pulmonary specialist. Regular cardiac evaluation to monitor for development of cardiac conduction defects and cardiomyopathy is essential. Orthopedic evaluation is needed for management of clubfoot, joint contracture, and scoliosis. Anticipatory developmental support and optimization of the educational environment is important. Extensive genetic counseling should be provided.

Metabolic Myopathies Metabolic myopathies comprise a heterogeneous group of genetic disorders characterized by abnormalities in skeletal muscle energy production due to defects in glycogen catabolism (i.e., glycogenolysis and glycolysis), fatty acid oxidation, Krebs cycle, or mitochondrial respiratory chain and oxidative phosphorylation. The main categories include glycogen storage diseases, fatty acid oxidation defects, disorders of purine metabolism, and mitochondrial myopathies.

Clinical Features The clinical presentation of metabolic myopathy is variable. Generally, patients may present with exercise-related symptoms and signs (e.g., exercise intolerance, exercise-induced muscle cramp, myalgia, or exercise-induced elevated CK level or myoglobinuria) with normal examination between the attacks or fixed or progressive skeletal muscle weakness frequently associated with other systemic symptoms (such as cardiomyopathy, respiratory insufficiency, encephalopathy, endocrine dysfunction). Short-burst intense exercise (such as sprinting)-induced symptoms suggest glycogen metabolism defects as seen in myophosphorylase deficiency (e.g., McArdle disease, glycogenosis type V), whereas prolonged exercise (such as hiking or playing football or soccer)-triggered symptoms suggest defects of fatty acid oxidation, as seen in carnitine palmitoyltransferase II deficiency. A typical and unique feature of McArdle disease is a spontaneous "second wind," which is marked improvement of exercise tolerance and exercise-induced tachycardia after about 8 to 10 minutes into aerobic exercise involving large muscles.

Pompe disease, also referred to as acid maltase deficiency or glycogen storage disease type II (GSDII), is an autosomal recessive disorder caused by a deficiency of the lysosomal enzyme acid-glucosidase (GAA). The incidence is approximately 1 in 40,000. Glycogen accumulates in lysosomes in many tissues with skeletal, cardiac, and smooth muscles and anterior horn cells most prominently affected. Pompe disease is a continuum of disease spectrum varying by age of onset, organ involvement, and the severity of the myopathy. Classic infantile-onset Pompe disease presents shortly after birth with profound muscle weakness, hypotonia, and hypertrophic cardiomyopathy. Macroglossia, mild hepatomegaly, and feeding difficulty are also typical symptoms and signs. It is rapidly progressive and fatal before 1 year of age due to respiratory and cardiac failure. The less severe late-onset form of Pompe disease can present from childhood to adulthood, often as a limb-girdle dystrophy with early-onset respiratory insufficiency, but typically without cardiomyopathy. Many such patients are ultimately wheelchair dependent and require artificial ventilation if not treated.

Diagnosis CK is generally elevated in metabolic myopathies but is frequently normal between attacks for those presenting with exercise-induced symptoms. Definitive diagnosis requires an assay of acid maltase and genetic testing for Pompe disease, and genetic testing is now available for many different types of metabolic myopathies. Some patients with late-onset Pompe disease may still have up to 10% residual enzyme activity. Prenatal testing is available on chorionic villous cells once genetic diagnosis is established.

Management Treatment for metabolic myopathies is primarily supportive. Glucose intake before and during exercise may decrease symptoms in McArdle disease but may exacerbate muscle symptoms (out-of-wind phenomenon) in phosphofructokinase (PFK) deficiency. It is important to avoid fasting and high fat intake in patients with fatty acid oxidation defects. ERT with recombinant human alglucosidase alfa has proven life-saving when instituted early in Pompe disease. ERT has prolonged overall survival and ventilator-free survival in infantile-onset Pompe disease. Motor function was maintained when infants with classic infantile-onset Pompe disease were diagnosed through newborn screening and received very early treatment with ERT. ERT for late-onset Pompe disease has been associated with improved motor capability and stabilized pulmonary function. Supportive therapy includes respiratory support, management of cardiomyopathy and renal failure, nutritional support, and physical therapy.

Mitochondrial Myopathies Mitochondrial myopathies are genetic disorders that arise from mitochondrial dysfunction affecting predominantly the skeletal muscle. Mutation of genes encoded by either nuclear DNA (patients typically present in infancy or early childhood) or mitochondrial DNA (mtDNA; patients can present at any age). Mitochondrial diseases often have multisystem involvement with involvement of organs/tissues highly dependent on oxidative aerobic metabolism such as brain, retina, heart, and skeletal muscles preferentially affected. Recognized clinical syndromes include Leber hereditary optic neuropathy (LHON), Kearns-Sayre syndrome (KSS), Pearson syndrome, Leigh syndrome (subacute necrotizing encephalomyelopathy), mitochondrial encephalomyopathy with lactic acidosis and stroke-like episodes (MELAS), mitochondrial neurogastrointestinal encephalopathy (MNGIE), and myoclonic epilepsy with ragged red fibers (MERRF).

Clinical Features Infants and children frequently present with hypotonia, weakness, developmental delay or regression, and difficulty feeding. Older children demonstrate delayed motor milestones and exercise intolerance. These symptoms combined with hearing loss, optic atrophy, peripheral neuropathy, seizures, ataxia, stroke-like episodes, cardiomyopathy, nephropathy, and diabetes should raise suspicion for a mitochondrial disease. The clinical course may range from an acute life-threatening metabolic derangement or episodic crises (frequently in the setting of illness) with partial recovery to a more gradual progressive neurodevelopmental regression.

Leigh syndrome is a severe and progressive neurometabolic disorder resulting from defects in oxidative phosphorylation or additional steps relating to energy production secondary to mutations in mitochondrial or nuclear DNA. More than 75 different genes have been identified, and the metabolic defects cause spongy degeneration and necrosis of the basal ganglia and cerebellum. Typically, psychomotor regression develops in an otherwise normal infant in the first year of life, often following a viral illness. Rarely, it occurs in older children and adults. Initial symptoms may be nonspecific, such as failure to thrive and persistent vomiting. Neurological features include hypotonia, feeding and swallowing difficulties, seizures, spasticity, movement disorders, ataxia, ophthalmoplegia, nystagmus, and peripheral neuropathy. Extraneurological manifestations include hypertrophic cardiomyopathy. About 50% of affected individuals die by 3 years of age, often due to respiratory or cardiac failure.

Diagnosis The diagnosis of mitochondrial myopathies is supported by the findings of elevated plasma and/or CSF lactate level. However, spurious elevation of plasma lactate can occur due to poor collection or handling methods or due to secondary mitochondrial dysfunction, while a normal lactate level does not exclude the presence of mitochondrial diseases. Quantitative plasma amino acids analysis may show elevated alanine level. Serum ammonia is frequently normal. On brain MRI, nonspecific delayed myelination pattern can be seen in early disease, stroke-like lesions (in a nonvascular distribution, which resolve with minimal atrophy) are suggestive of MELAS, and cerebral and/or cerebellar atrophy with bilateral deep gray lesions are frequently seen in mitochondrial DNA-deletion disorders. Bilateral symmetric hypodensities in the basal ganglia on head CT or bilateral symmetric hyperintense signal abnormality in the dorsal brainstem (periaqueductal gray matter) and/or basal ganglia (specifically the putamen and caudate) on T_2-weighted imaging on MRI of the brain are characteristic features of Leigh syndrome. Magnetic resonance spectroscopy (MRS) may be used to detect an elevated lactate level in the brain, which is a nonspecific marker for cellular injury. Molecular genetic testing for mtDNA or nuclear gene mutations is needed. Many patients may not have the diagnosis confirmed by molecular genetic testing from blood and require further investigation with muscle biopsy for respiratory chain function, analysis for mtDNA depletion, mtDNA mutation, and duplication/deletion to establish the diagnosis. The classic hallmark of mitochondrial diseases is subsarcolemmal and intermyofibrillar accumulation of mitochondria visualized on Gomori trichrome stain, termed "ragged red fibers." Genetic testing from leukocytes has replaced biopsy for many of these patients.

Management Treatment of mitochondrial diseases is primarily supportive, with particular attention to management of feeding and the airway and ventilation. Therapies to treat specific symptoms and signs of mitochondrial diseases are very important. Seizures are common in patients with CNS involvement and should be treated aggressively to achieve good seizure control. However, it is very important to avoid valproic acid (i.e., Depakote or Depakene) because of the significant risk of precipitating and/or accelerating liver disease or other diseases in patients with mitochondrial diseases. Insulin and other standard treatments are effective for diabetes mellitus. Vitamins and respiratory chain cofactors (such as succinate, riboflavin, thiamine, and coenzyme Q10) supplements are often recommended for patients with mitochondrial diseases, although much of the evidence comes from case reports and small open-label studies. Supplementation is most useful in patients with specific deficiencies. For example, coenzyme Q10 (CoQ10) supplementation is particularly effective in patients with CoQ10 deficiencies, and individuals with complex I and/or complex II deficiency may benefit from oral administration of riboflavin.

DIAGNOSTIC EVALUATION

As with all patients, the patient presenting with hypotonia and weakness should first be evaluated with a detailed history and physical examination as discussed above. With this information, the physician should then be able to localize the lesion to involve the UMNs or LMNs, noting this distinction can be particularly challenging in neonates. If there is uncertainty, expert consultation should be obtained. After localizing to the UMNs or LMNs, further testing can be obtained to narrow the differential (see Table 120-1).

DIAGNOSTIC TESTING

If there is concern for an UMN lesion, MRI of the brain and/or spinal cord should be obtained. Weakness and UMN signs involving all four extremities suggest a lesion at the cervical cord or above. Lesions involving only the lower extremities suggest a lesion below the cervical cord. Knowledge of sensory levels (dermatomes) and muscle groups supplied by each level of the cord (myotomes) can be helpful in further localization.

With concern for a lesion distal to the UMN (lower motor neuron, neuromuscular junction, muscle), multiple studies can be considered to aid in diagnosis, including EMG and nerve conduction studies (NCS), imaging, biopsy, and laboratory evaluation. EMG/NCS can be ordered to further localize lesions of the peripheral nervous system. Nerve conduction velocities are normal or mildly slowed in axonal peripheral neuropathies but markedly slowed in demyelinating peripheral neuropathies. Significant decremental responses on repetitive stimulation testing are seen in disorders of neuromuscular junction transmission, such as myasthenia gravis. EMG can distinguish a neurogenic process from a myopathic process. The muscle action potentials in myopathies have polyphasic morphology, reduced duration and amplitude, and increased recruitment, in contrast to the prolonged-duration, polyphasic, high-amplitude potentials and reduced recruitment seen in chronic denervation. Abnormal spontaneous activities including fasciculation and fibrillation on EMG indicate ongoing denervation. Myotonic discharge is seen in myotonic syndromes such as myotonic dystrophy and myotonia congenita.

Muscle imaging is gaining traction in the clinical setting. Ultrasound of muscles is a useful noninvasive, convenient technique for visualizing normal and pathological skeletal muscle. It can be done at the bedside without sedation but requires significant training for interpretation. In neuromuscular diseases, the increased fatty tissues, fibrosis, and inflammation result in increased echogenicity of muscles. A myopathic process frequently shows homogeneous fine granular echogenicity, whereas a neurogenic process typically shows streak-like, inhomogeneous echogenicity within muscles. Additionally, fasciculations can be observed in many cases of neurogenic diseases. MRI of muscles is growing in its clinical use with improved ability to distinguish between various types of myopathies. Distinct imaging patterns have been identified for a number of diseases.

Muscle biopsy with histologic examination, specific immunostaining techniques, and electron microscopy is essential for morphologic diagnosis. It remains quite helpful in diagnosing specific forms of congenital myopathies even with the recent advances in genetic testing, inflammatory myositis, and rare forms of muscular dystrophies. Nerve biopsy is rarely helpful in diagnosing CMT but may be performed on occasion when chronic inflammatory demyelinating neuropathy is suspected, especially in patients with atypical features and poor response to standard therapies.

Regardless of localization, genetic and metabolic testing should be considered and guided by clinical evaluation. Targeted studies are preferred. The availability of next-generation sequencing (i.e., high-throughput sequencing technologies that parallelize the sequencing process, producing thousands or millions of sequences concurrently) and whole-exome sequencing (i.e., selectively sequencing the coding regions of the genome) has allowed identification of gene mutations that cause many undiagnosed childhood neuromuscular and neurological diseases. However, it has added much more complexity and ethical issues. There is growing concern that complete sequencing data may lead to weakly justified claims of association between genetic variants and disease. Furthermore, certain genetic mechanism such as trinucleotide repeats, deletion, or duplication will not be detected by whole-exome sequencing. Proper genetic counseling must be provided before and after the testing, and the ordering physician should be prepared to interpret the results, especially variants that have not been previously reported (or variants of unknown clinical significance), and to deal with unexpected and unrelated findings.

Serum CK is a nonspecific marker of leaky muscle membranes. CK isoforms occur in the brain (BB), heart (MB), and skeletal muscle (MM). It is markedly elevated in muscular dystrophy, especially in Duchenne and Becker muscular dystrophy, certain LGMDs, and inflammatory myositis such as dermatomyositis and polymyositis. Patients with congenital myopathies typically have a normal CK level. Some neurogenic disorders such as type III SMA may also have elevated CK, but to a much lesser extent.

Metabolic studies may be indicated on samples of serum, urine, or CSF. Such studies include blood glucose, potassium, CO_2, ammonia, lactate, pyruvate, carnitine, coenzyme Q_{10}, acylcarnitines, amino acids, enzyme study for CDG, and urine organic acids. CSF lactate and pyruvate are more sensitive as screening for mitochondrial diseases. Characteristic findings may suggest oxidative phosphorylation defects, glycolytic disorders, and amino and organic acid disorders.

ADMISSION AND DISCHARGE CRITERIA

ADMISSION CRITERIA

Patients should be considered for inpatient admission if they:

- Are unable to protect their airway due to altered mental status or weakness
- Are unable to maintain fluid or nutritional needs, especially if accompanied by poor growth and signs of aspiration with feeds
- Have evidence of inadequate ventilation or oxygenation
- Have evidence of cardiac compromise including heart failure and uncontrolled arrhythmia
- Report rapid deterioration in their ability to perform activities of daily living
- Require urgent work-up to determine acute treatment
- Are unsafe at home, especially if caregivers report difficulty meeting their needs

DISCHARGE CRITERIA

Patients may be considered for discharge if they:

- Have a safe airway in place
- Can adequately ventilate and oxygenate on their own or with assistance from supplemental oxygen, noninvasive ventilation, and/or tracheostomy
- Can maintain adequate nutrition and fluid needs whether it be fully by mouth or via gastrostomy tube or parenteral nutrition
- Have sufficient medical support personnel (i.e., home nursing, home health aides, etc.) and equipment (i.e., walkers, wheelchairs, assistive devices, etc.) in the home environment
- Have long-term follow-up with appropriate specialists in place

CONSULTATION

Neurology can offer guidance in clinical evaluation, diagnostic testing, and short- and long-term management.

Consider the following indications for consulting other subspecialists:

- Pulmonology: Need for home oxygen or noninvasive ventilation
- Cardiology: Presence of cardiomyopathy or dysrhythmias
- Gastroenterology: Feeding difficulties not responsive to basic interventions
- General surgery: Gastrostomy tube placement, if needed
- Genetics: Patient has dysmorphic features, signs of metabolic disease, or strong family history of certain diseases
- Physical medicine and rehabilitation: Assessment and management of physical disabilities

KEY POINTS

- The differential for hypotonia and weakness is very broad but a thorough history and physical examination can narrow the possibilities significantly.
- Evaluation of negative inspiratory force can help assess infants and children at risk for respiratory failure.
- Pediatric hospitalists should be aware of the variable time periods for progression of disease as some diseases progress rapidly and early recognition of subsequent respiratory failure is imperative.
- Neurology can offer guidance in clinical evaluation, diagnostic testing, and short- and long-term management.

SUGGESTED READINGS

Abicht A, Müller JS, Lochmüller H. Congenital Myasthenic Syndromes Overview. *GeneReviews®[Internet]*.2021.

Bakare AB, Lesnefsky EJ, Iyer S. Leigh syndrome: a tale of two genomes. *Front Physiol.* 2021;12.

Brenton JN. Pediatric Acquired Demyelinating Disorders. *Continuum.* 2022;28(4):1104-1130.

Butler MG, Miller JL, Forster JL. Prader-Willi syndrome-clinical genetics, diagnosis and treatment approaches: an update. *Curr Pediatr Rev.* 2019;15(4):207-244.

Colver A, Fairhurst C, Pharoah POD. Cerebral Palsy. *Lancet.* 2014; 383(9924):1240.

Duan D, Goemans N, Takeda SI, Mercuri E, Aartsma-Rus A. Duchenne muscular dystrophy. *Nat Rev Dis Primers.* 2021;7(1):1-9.

Ferriero DM, Fullerton HJ, Bernard TJ, et al. Management of stroke in neonates and children: a scientific statement from the American Heart Association/American Stroke Association. *Stroke.* 2019; 50(3):e51-e96.

Finkel RS, Mercuri E, Meyer OH, et al. Diagnosis and management of spinal muscular atrophy: Part 2: Pulmonary and acute care; medications, supplements and immunizations; other organ systems; and ethics. *Neuromuscul Disord.* 2018;28(3):197-207.

Gomez-Andres D, Oulihissane A, Quijano-Roy S. Two decades of advances in muscle imaging in children: from pattern recognition of muscle diseases to quantification and machine learning approaches. *Neuromuscul Disord.* 2021;31(10):1038-1050.

Johnson NE, Aldana EZ, Angeard N, et al. Consensus-based care recommendations for congenital and childhood-onset myotonic dystrophy type 1. *Neurol Clin Pract.* 2019;9(5):443-454.

Korinthenberg R, Trollmann R, Felderhoff-Müser U, et al. Diagnosis and treatment of Guillain-Barré Syndrome in childhood and adolescence: an evidence-and consensus-based guideline. *Eur J Paediatr Neurol.* 2020;25:5-16.

Lilleker JB, Keh YS, Roncaroli F, Sharma R, Roberts M. Metabolic myopathies: a practical approach. *Pract Neurol.* 2018;18(1):14-26.

Mercuri E, Finkel RS, Muntoni F, et al. Diagnosis and management of spinal muscular atrophy: Part 1: Recommendations for diagnosis, rehabilitation, orthopedic and nutritional care. *Neuromuscul Disord.* 2018;28(2):103-115.

Murphy OC, Messacar K, Benson L, et al. Acute flaccid myelitis: cause, diagnosis, and management. *Lancet.* 2021;397(10271):334-346.

O'Connell K, Ramdas S, Palace J. Management of juvenile myasthenia gravis. *Front Neurol.* 2020;11:743.

Olimpio C, Tiet MY, Horvath R. Primary mitochondrial myopathies in childhood. *Neuromuscul Disord.* 2021;31(10):978-987.

Paprocka J, Jezela-Stanek A, Tylki-Szymańska A, Grunewald S. Congenital disorders of glycosylation from a neurological perspective. *Brain Sci.* 2021;11(1):88.

Peragallo JH. Pediatric Myasthenia Gravis. *Semin Pediatr Neurol.* 2017; 24(2):116-121.

Roscow LK, Strober JB. Infant botulism: review and clinical update. *Pediatric Neurol.* 2015;52(5):487-492.

Schorling DC, Pechmann A, Kirschner J. Advances in treatment of spinal muscular atrophy–new phenotypes, new challenges, new implications for care. Journal of neuromuscular diseases. 2020;7(1):1-3.

Stone J, Carson A. Functional Neurologic Disorders. *Continuum.* 2015; 21(3):818-837.

Sun A. Lysosomal storage disease overview. *Ann Transl Med.* 2018;6(24).

van der Knaap MS, Schiffmann R, Mochel F, Wolf NI. Diagnosis, prognosis, and treatment of leukodystrophies. *Lancet Neurol.* 2019;18(10):962-972.

West E, Shah U. Diagnosis of functional weakness and functional gait disorders in children and adolescents. *Semin Pediatr Neurol.* 2022;41:100955.

CHAPTER 121 Cerebrovascular Disease

Melissa Cossey, MD and Louisa Keith, MD

BACKGROUND

Stroke is a major cause of acquired brain injury in children and can be associated with significant morbidity and mortality. The presentation, etiology, and management of stroke in pediatric patients differs from those of older patients. The prompt recognition of stroke by clinicians is essential to implementing early treatment strategies and preventing recurrence.

In simple terms, stroke is an acute neurologic injury related to infarction or hemorrhage within the central nervous system. The term stroke is generally limited to focal or multifocal lesions and excludes the diffuse infarction resulting from global anoxia. Stroke in pediatric patients can be classified in several ways. When characterized by age, stroke can be divided into perinatal and childhood stroke, with perinatal stroke occurring from 28 weeks of gestation to 28 postnatal days of age, and childhood stroke occurring from 29 postnatal days of age up to 18 years. Perinatal stroke involves different clinical presentations and risk factors than childhood stroke and will not be addressed in detail in this chapter.

Subtypes of childhood stroke are hemorrhagic stroke and ischemic stroke. Hemorrhagic stroke is defined as brain injury that is attributable to the nontraumatic extravasation of blood from a ruptured or damaged blood vessel. Hemorrhagic stroke can be caused by intracerebral hemorrhage (ICH), intraventricular hemorrhage (IVH), or subarachnoid hemorrhage (SAH).

Ischemic stroke is an acute focal infarction of central nervous system tissue resulting from lack of tissue perfusion, and infarction is defined as cell death attributable to ischemia. Ischemic stroke is divided into arterial ischemic stroke (AIS), in which injury occurs in a discrete arterial distribution, and venous infarction, which is most often caused by cerebral sinovenous thrombosis (CSVT). The size and location of infarction largely determines the clinical manifestations of the stroke, although smaller lesions can remain asymptomatic. A transient ischemic attack (TIA) is a temporary episode of neurologic dysfunction caused by focal ischemia of the brain, spinal cord, or retina without an acute infarction. A TIA is traditionally defined as an ischemic deficit lasting less than 24 hours; however, the typical duration is less than 1 to 2 hours, and longer-lasting episodes are often associated with infarction, even in individuals with complete resolution of their symptoms.

EPIDEMIOLOGY

Globally, the incidence of stroke in children appears to be increasing, although this may reflect improved diagnosis rather than a true increase in incidence. In developed countries, current estimates place the incidence of childhood ischemic stroke at 1 to 2 per 100,000. The incidence is higher in infants, children younger than 5 years of age, Black and Asian children, children with cardiac disease, and boys. The annual incidence of AIS in patients with cardiac disease is as high as 132 per 100,000, but the frequency is far greater in children with complex congenital heart lesions than among children with a relatively uncomplicated septal defect. For patients with sickle cell disease (SCD), the annual incidence of childhood stroke is increased by more than 200-fold. If an individual with SCD experiences an ischemic stroke, the likelihood of this person having another stroke within the following year increases dramatically. Hemorrhagic stroke in children has a similar incidence to ischemic stroke at approximately 1 to 1.7 cases per 100,000 annually, making up approximately half of stroke cases in children. CSVT is much less common, with an estimated annual incidence that is four times lower than AIS. In pediatric CSVT, approximately half of cases occur in children under 1 year of age.

Stroke is among the top 10 causes of death for US and Canadian children. Case fatality rates are estimated at 4% to 10% for AIS, up to 23% for CSVT, and 4% for hemorrhagic stroke. Some deaths, however, may be due to the comorbid conditions that lead to stroke (e.g., meningitis or congenital heart disease) rather than the stroke itself. Among survivors, two-thirds or more may have permanent neurological deficits, cognitive impairment, or epilepsy.

PATHOPHYSIOLOGY

Arterial Ischemic Stroke AIS is defined as focal brain ischemia conforming to the distribution of one or more cerebral arteries (**Figure 121-1**) and results when arterial blood flow is focally obstructed or diminished (**Figures 121-2** and **121-3**). This obstruction may be caused by multiple mechanisms: a thromboembolism that begins at a local or distant site, inflammatory or noninflammatory steno-occlusive disease intrinsic to the arterial wall (arteriopathy or vasculopathy), or an extrinsic process that results in vessel wall compression (e.g., mass lesion, trauma, or cerebral edema). Unlike adults, atherosclerosis is seldom a cause of AIS in children.

Ischemia deprives neurons of their two primary substrates, oxygen and glucose, triggering a cascade of molecular and cellular events that culminate in cell death and coagulation necrosis. This process begins within minutes, creating a window of therapeutic opportunity during the time between occlusion and the point at which the injury is irreversible. The extent of ischemic injury is influenced by several factors. The size of the occluded artery determines the size of the ischemic injury and, consequently, the potential for recovery of function. Other factors include the duration of vessel occlusion, the degree of collateral circulation, the maturational status of the brain, concurrent disease processes, and the basal metabolic rate of affected cerebral tissue.

After a substantial ischemic injury, there is a core of infarcted cerebral tissue which is encompassed by a concentric penumbra of potentially salvageable tissue. The penumbra is tissue with decreased perfusion that is likely to perish unless adequate blood flow is quickly restored. Restoration of blood flow to the penumbra is the goal of neuroprotective and thrombolytic strategies, which will be outlined in later sections. It is important to note that AIS can be complicated by the development of hemorrhagic transformation, resulting either from the ischemic stroke itself or from antithrombotic therapies.

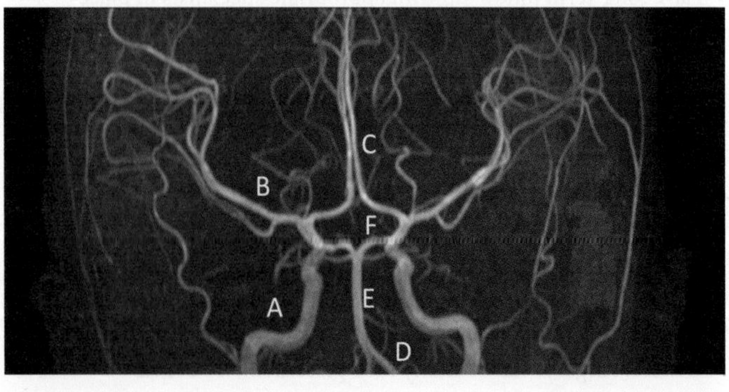

FIGURE 121-1. MRA showing normal arterial anatomy. A. Right internal carotid artery. B. Right middle cerebral artery. C. Left anterior cerebral artery. D. Left vertebral artery. E. Basilar artery. F. Left posterior cerebral artery. Anterior and posterior communicating arteries are not easily visible.

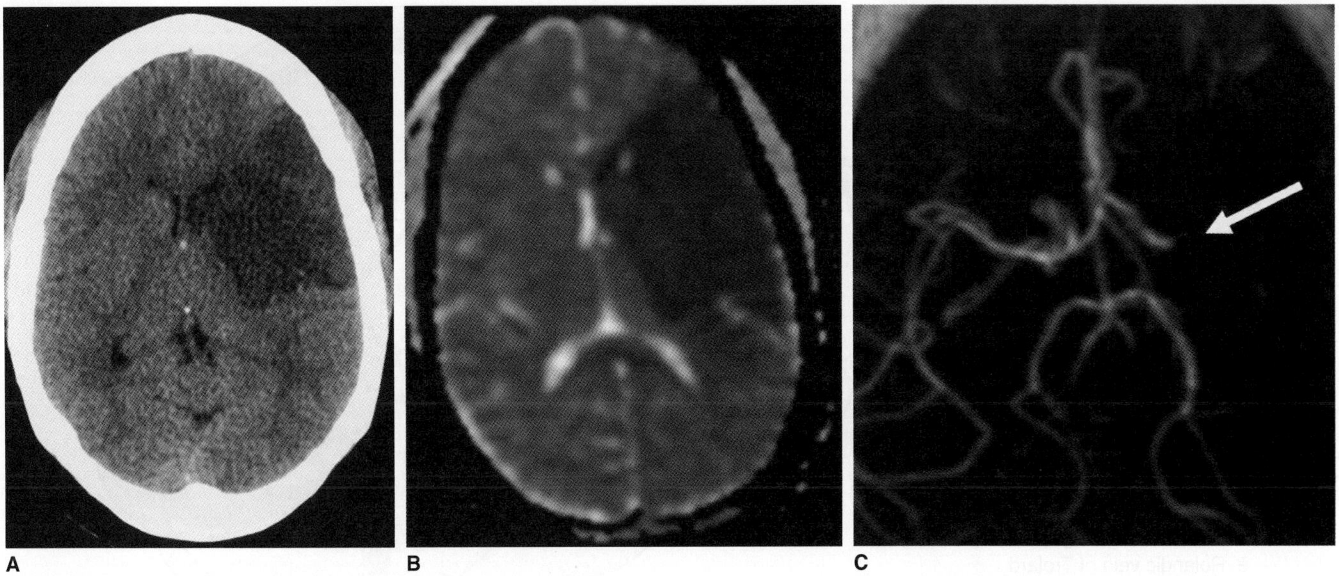

FIGURE 121-2. Left middle cerebral artery stroke in a previously healthy 16-year-old girl. A. Axial head CT demonstrates large hypodensity in region of left middle cerebral artery. B. Axial apparent diffusion coefficient (ADC) map MRI confirming stroke in the left middle cerebral artery territory. C. Axial MRA demonstrates abrupt cutoff in left middle cerebral artery (clot) with absent flow to distal branches of left middle cerebral artery.

Cerebral Sinovenous Thrombosis CSVT involves partial or complete occlusion of any of the venous sinuses or veins of the deep and/or superficial drainage system of the brain. In the central nervous system, blood is drained from the brain into the internal jugular veins by a system of superficial and deep venous sinuses and veins lying within the dura and subarachnoid space (**Figure 121-4**).

Superficial drainage occurs mainly by way of cortical veins, which drain into the superior sagittal sinus, which in turn drains via the torcula (or confluence of sinuses—the joining of the superior sagittal, straight, and transverse sinuses) into the right and left transverse sinuses. Some superficial drainage flows into the right and left cavernous sinuses, through which the internal carotid artery and several cranial nerves pass; cavernous sinus thrombosis, although rare, can therefore be life-threatening. Deep venous drainage occurs via the internal (deep) cerebral veins and basal veins of Rosenthal, which drain into the great cerebral vein (of Galen) and from there into the straight sinus, then via the torcula into the bilateral transverse sinuses. The transverse sinuses, carrying drainage from both superficial and deep systems, become the sigmoid sinuses, which exit the skull to become the bilateral internal jugular veins. The right transverse sinus is dominant in the majority of individuals and may appear visibly larger than the left transverse sinus on venography. This may confound neuroimaging interpretation and make it difficult to differentiate a congenitally narrow left transverse sinus from one that is narrowed by thrombus.

CSVT most frequently involves the major superficial sinuses (i.e., the superior sagittal sinus and transverse sinuses). An imaging example

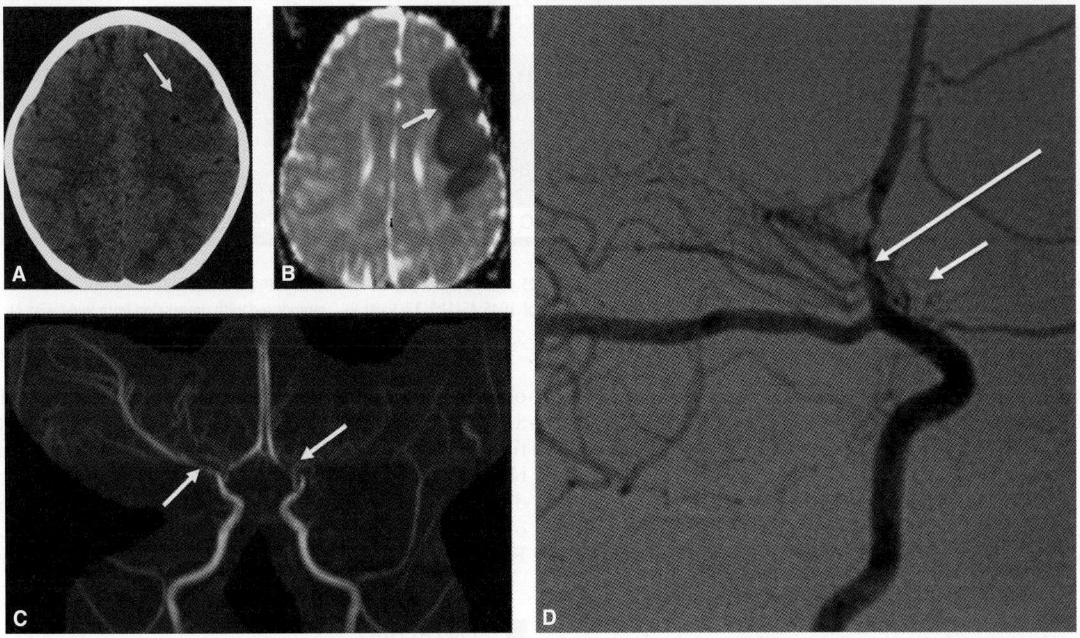

FIGURE 121-3. Moyamoya disease in a 2-year-old who presented with complex partial seizures. A. Axial head CT with hypodensity (arrow) in the region of the left middle cerebral artery. B. Axial apparent diffusion coefficient (ADC) map confirming left MCA stroke (arrow). C. Coronal MRA demonstrates occlusion of the internal carotid arteries bilaterally (arrows). D. Conventional catheter angiogram shows occlusion of the internal carotid artery (long arrow) with "puff of smoke" appearance (short arrow) of compensatory collaterals.

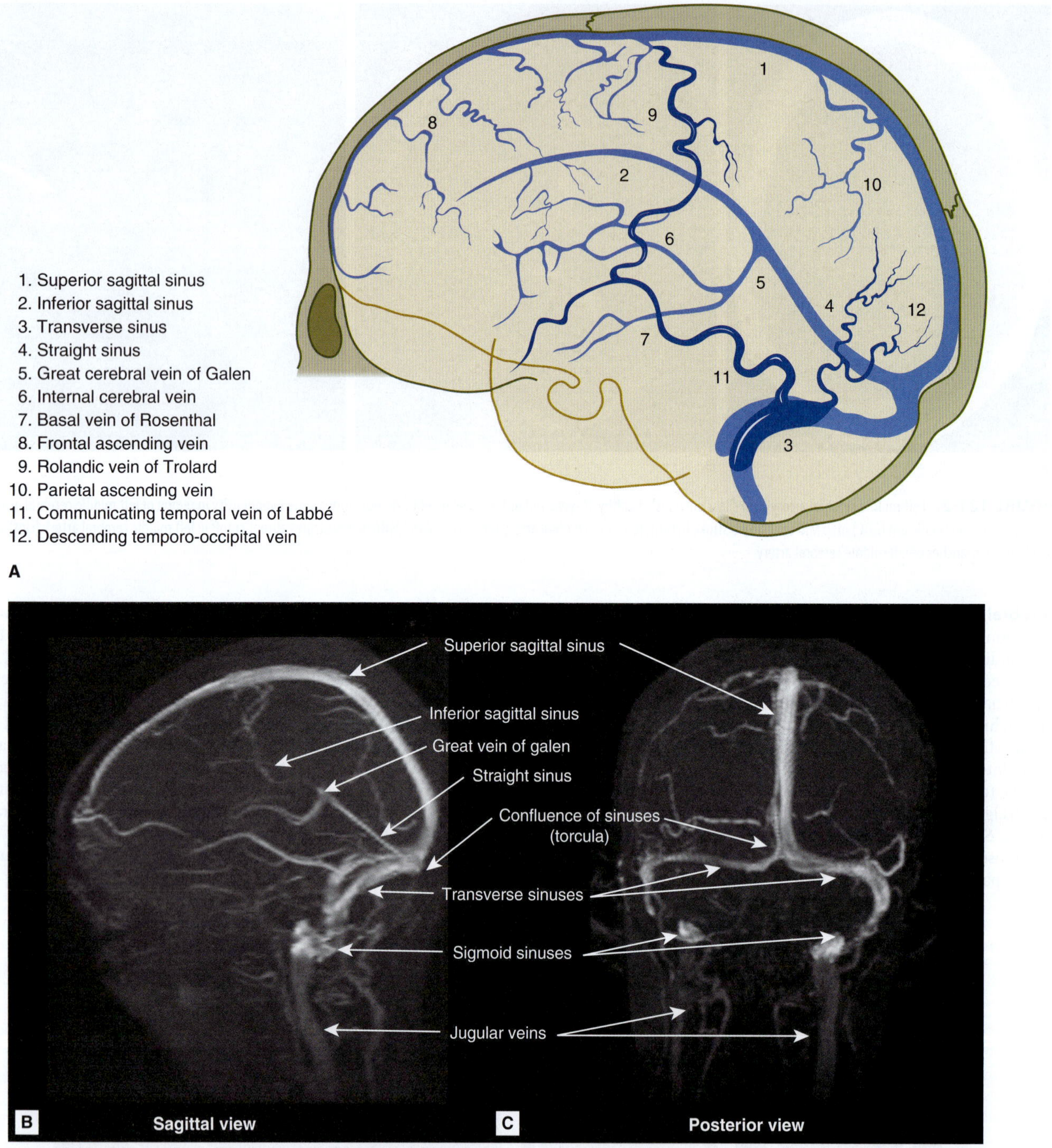

FIGURE 121-4. Cerebral venous sinuses. A: Schematic lateral view of cerebral venous sinuses. B–C: Magnetic resonance venogram (MRV) in lateral view (B) and posterior coronal view (C). (Part A reproduced with permission from List CF, Burge CH, Hodges FJ: Intracranial angiography. *Radiol.* 1945;45(1):1-14. Parts B–C reproduced with permission from Berkowitz AL. *Clinical Neurology & Neuroanatomy: A Localization-Based Approach*. 2nd ed. New York, NY: McGraw Hill; 2022, Figure 3–5.)

involving the straight sinus is seen in **Figure 121-5**. Both occlusive and nonocclusive sinovenous clots may occur.

If collateral venous channels are unable to sufficiently drain blood around a thrombus, intracranial pressure will increase and ischemia can occur when capillary hydrostatic pressure exceeds arterial pressure. A persistent increase in hydrostatic pressure can also cause leakage of red blood cells, resulting in hemorrhage.

Hemorrhagic Stroke The mechanisms underlying hemorrhage-induced brain injury include chemical irritation of neurons via red blood cell lysis, thrombin formation, iron toxicity, and edema formation. In both ICH and SAH, intraventricular and subarachnoid blood can cause irritation to the ependymal lining of the ventricle and obstruction of arachnoid granulations (or villi), resulting in secondary obstructive or communicating hydrocephalus. Children with ICH or SAH may suffer from secondary arterial ischemic or watershed infarction due to compression of adjacent arteries, vasospasm, or decreased blood flow resulting from increased intracranial pressure (ICP) with decreased cerebral perfusion pressure. An imaging example of hemorrhagic stroke from an arteriovenous malformation can be seen in **Figure 121-6**.

RISK FACTORS

As demonstrated in **Table 121-1**, risk factors for childhood stroke vary according to the stroke category, and the identification of risk factors depends greatly on the extensiveness of the evaluation. The most

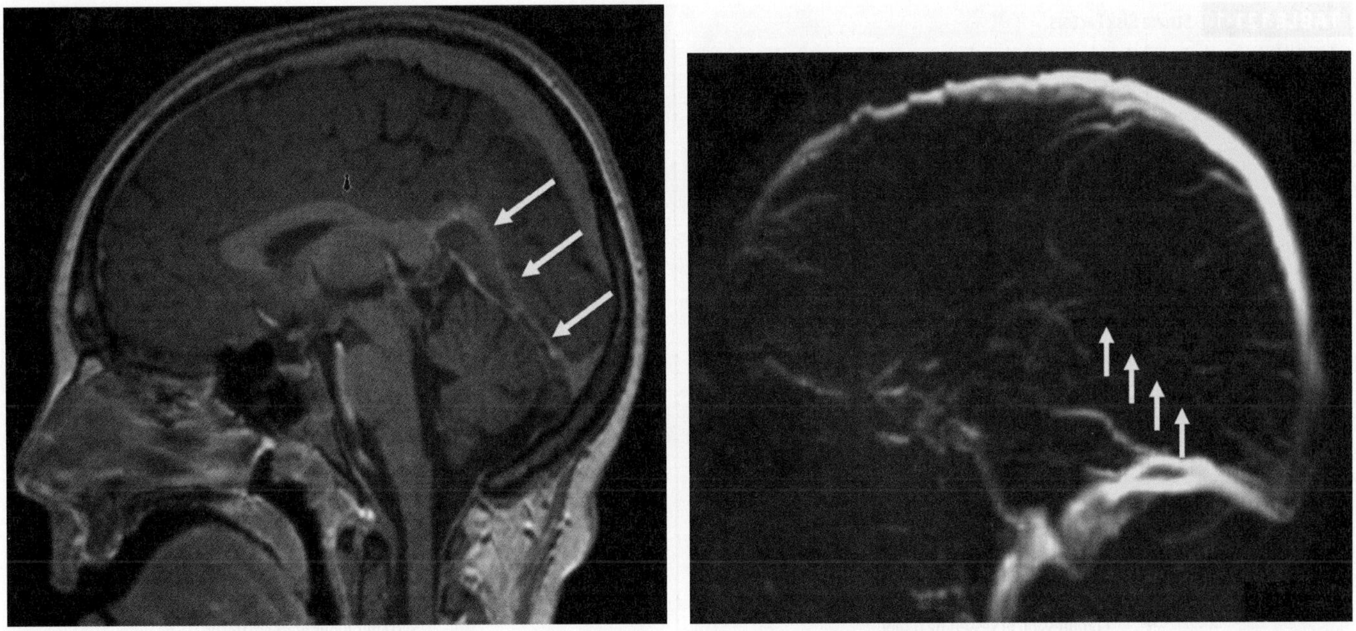

A B

FIGURE 121-5. Cerebral sinovenous thrombosis. A. Sagittal T1-weighted post-contrast MRI demonstrates dark clot (arrow) within the straight sinus. Bright contrast surrounds the clot. B. Sagittal MRV with arrows in the typical position of the straight sinus. No flow is evident.

common risk factors for ischemic stroke include cardiac disease, intra- and extracranial arteriopathies, hematologic and prothrombotic disorders, inflammatory states, vascular malformations, and infection. For many patients, particularly with CSVT, multiple risk factors are present. In at least 10% of childhood stroke, no risk factors are identified and the underlying etiology is unknown.

An important group of children at high risk of stroke are those with congenital and acquired cardiac disease. These children have a high rate of cardioembolic stroke, although hemorrhagic stroke may also occur. Risk in this population is highest for children with cyanotic and complex congenital heart disease, particularly those with single-ventricle physiology and right-to-left shunts, endocarditis, cardiomyopathy, Fontan physiology, recent cardiac catheterization, and with use of extracorporeal membrane oxygenation (ECMO) and ventricular assist devices (VADs).

Arteriopathies are genetic or acquired abnormalities in the cervical, vertebral, or cerebral arteries and are found in nearly half of all children with stroke. Arteriopathies can lead to dissection or stenosis of the artery, and the presence of arteriopathy increases the risk of both primary and recurrent stroke. Moyamoya and focal cerebral arteriopathy are two of the most common arteriopathies of childhood. Moyamoya is characterized by progressive stenosis and occlusion of the distal internal carotid arteries with dilated collateral channels in the brain distal to the occlusion. It can be either idiopathic or associated with other underlying conditions or genetic syndromes. Focal cerebral arteriopathy (FCA) describes a limited area of stenosis or vessel wall irregularity in one of the large intracranial arteries of the anterior circulation. While typically transient in nature, FCA is associated with a high 1-year risk of stroke recurrence. This abnormal area may result from inflammation (i.e., a focal vasculitis) or from a limited area of intracranial dissection, which can be caused by trauma. Most inflammatory cases of FCA are thought to relate to recent infection, with post-varicella FCA being particularly well described.

Children with SCD (either hemoglobin SS disease or hemoglobin Sβ^0 thalassemia) have a significantly increased risk of childhood stroke, not only for AIS but also for CSVT and hemorrhagic stroke. Cerebral arteriopathy is present in approximately 25% of patients with SCD, further increasing the risk of stroke. Stroke, including silent infarcts, contributes to a large amount of morbidity in SCD. In recent years, stroke prevalence has been decreased by use of transcranial Doppler and regular red blood cell transfusions for those at heightened risk.

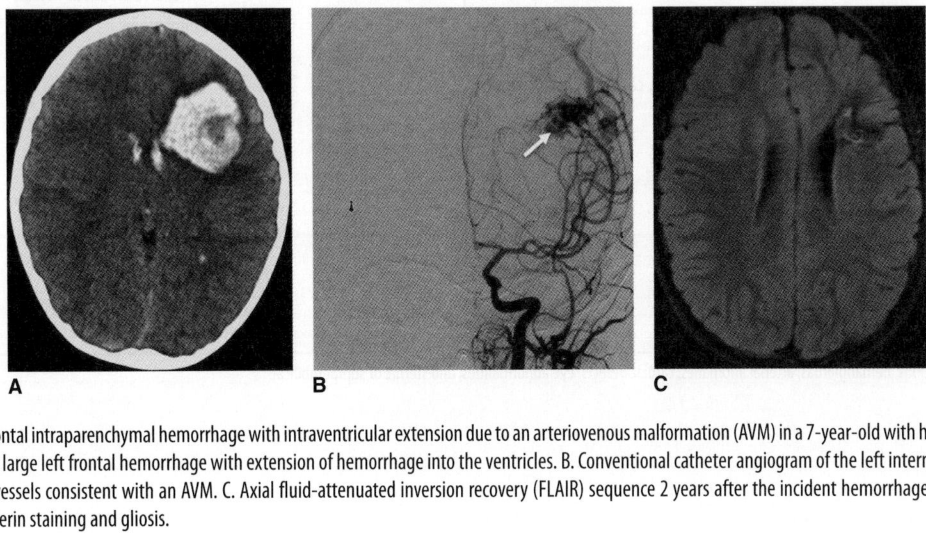

A B C

FIGURE 121-6. Left frontal intraparenchymal hemorrhage with intraventricular extension due to an arteriovenous malformation (AVM) in a 7-year-old with hereditary hemorrhagic telangiectasia. A. Axial head CT with large left frontal hemorrhage with extension of hemorrhage into the ventricles. B. Conventional catheter angiogram of the left internal carotid artery demonstrates a tangle of abnormal blood vessels consistent with an AVM. C. Axial fluid-attenuated inversion recovery (FLAIR) sequence 2 years after the incident hemorrhage demonstrates reabsorption of the hematoma with hemosiderin staining and gliosis.

TABLE 121-1 Stroke Risk Factors

Stroke type	Risk factors
Arterial ischemic stroke	Intracranial Arteriopathy
	Focal cerebral arteriopathy of childhood
	Dissection type (most commonly related to trauma)
	Inflammation type (e.g., post-varicella arteriopathy or transient cerebral arteriopathy)
	Moyamoya disease (idiopathic)
	Moyamoya syndrome (associated with)
	Type 1 diabetes mellitus
	Sickle cell disease
	Trisomy 21
	Neurofibromatosis type 1
	Williams syndrome
	Alagille syndrome
	Noonan syndrome
	Vasculitis (primary or secondary)
	Fibromuscular dysplasia
	Post-radiation arteriopathy
	Genetic/syndromic arteriopathy (e.g., PHACES)
	Compression of vessels by tumor
	Vasospasm related to tumor or tumor resection
	Extracranial arteriopathy
	Craniocervical dissection
	Head or neck trauma
	Bow hunter syndrome
	Connective tissue disorder
	Hematologic
	Inherited or acquired prothrombotic disorders
	Sickle cell disease
	Iron deficiency anemia
	Disseminated intravascular coagulation
	Thrombotic thrombocytopenic purpura
	Malignancy
	Cardiac
	Ventricular assist device
	Extracorporeal membranous oxygenation
	Congenital heart disease with right-to-left shunts
	Fontan
	Valve abnormalities
	Intracardiac septal defect
	Intracardiac tumors
	Intracardiac thrombus
	Cardiomyopathy
	Arrhythmia
	Periprocedural including surgery, catheterization, and line placement
	Infectious
	Meningitis
	Endocarditis
	Human immunodeficiency virus
	Rheumatologic
	Anticardiolipin antibody syndrome
	Systemic lupus erythematosus
	Childhood primary angiitis of the central nervous system (cPACNS)
	Polyarteritis nodosa
	Takayasu arteritis
	Other
	Hereditary hemorrhagic telangiectasia
	Connective tissue disorder
	Drug abuse, especially cocaine and amphetamines
Cerebral sinovenous thrombosis	Head and neck infections
	Mastoiditis
	Otitis media
	Orbital cellulitis
	Sinusitis
	Meningoencephalitis
	Severe dehydration
	Chronic conditions
	Inflammatory bowel disease
	Bechet syndrome
	Systemic lupus erythematosus
	Homocystinuria
	Protein-losing enteropathy
	Liver failure
	Congenital heart disease
	Nephrotic syndrome
	Thyrotoxicosis
	Malignancy
	Hematologic
	Inherited or acquired prothrombotic disorders
	Iron deficiency anemia
	Recent head injury or surgery
	Pregnancy
	Mass effect with venous compression from CNS tumor
	Medications
	L-asparaginase
	Oral contraceptives
	Systemic corticosteroids
Hemorrhagic stroke	Vascular malformations
	Arteriovenous malformations
	Cavernous angiomas
	Aneurysms
	Dural arteriovenous fistulas
	Coagulopathies
	Hemophilia A or B
	von Willebrand disease
	Clotting factor deficiencies
	Thrombocytopenia
	Anticoagulation use
	Tumors
	Hypertension
	Drug abuse

PHACES, posterior fossa malformations, hemangiomas, arterial anomalies, cardiac defects, eye abnormalities, and sternal or supraumbilical.

In children and adolescents, the most common cause of nontraumatic hemorrhagic stroke is vascular malformations, most commonly an arteriovenous malformation (AVM). Less commonly, hemorrhagic stroke is related to other structural abnormalities, such as a cavernous malformation, an arteriovenous fistula (AVF), or an aneurysm. Most AVMs are isolated developmental lesions, although some known genetic conditions predispose individuals to multiple AVMs. AVFs may be congenital or acquired, such as with venous sinus hypertension or following CSVT. AVFs are at particularly high risk of rupture and neuronal injury because of their high flow.

Cavernous malformations (CM) are low-flow lesions and are composed of sinusoidal vessels. Dysfunctional endothelial vessels contribute to the leaking of blood into surrounding tissues. CMs can occur sporadically as single lesions or as an inherited trait resulting in multiple lesions. CMs can also be acquired following radiation therapy.

Nontraumatic SAH is most commonly caused by ruptured aneurysms, although many aneurysms in children are discovered prior to acute rupture. Aneurysms can be categorized as either saccular or dissecting, based on their appearance on imaging. Mycotic aneurysms are infections of the vessel wall and can result from conditions such as endocarditis.

Examples of genetic disorders associated with vascular malformations include hereditary hemorrhagic telangiectasia, CLOVES syndrome, PHACE syndrome, polycystic kidney disease, fibromuscular dysplasia, and connective tissue disorders, such as Ehlers-Danlos type IV, Marfan syndrome, and Loeys-Dietz syndrome. A smaller proportion of hemorrhagic stroke is attributed to hematologic abnormalities such as primary or secondary coagulopathies, platelet dysfunction, brain tumors, and SCD. Hypertension and drug-related hemorrhage are rare in the pediatric population.

CLINICAL PRESENTATION

Any acute onset of focal neurologic deficit in a child should prompt consideration of stroke. While adult stroke symptoms are commonly recognized by even the lay population, signs and symptoms of acute stroke in infants and children can be subtle and nonspecific, making stroke diagnosis easy to miss for even experienced medical professionals. Rapid identification and diagnosis of pediatric stroke therefore depends on a familiarity with both stroke risk factors and the range of possible presenting signs and symptoms, which can vary by patient age as well as size and location of the lesion. As a further challenge to diagnosis, perinatal strokes may be clinically silent, with symptoms manifesting months to years later when motor asymmetry emerges as the child develops voluntary movements.

TABLE 121-2 Presentation
Cortex and subcortical white matter
Cognitive and behavioral abnormalities:
Irritability, hyperactivity, lethargy
Coma (malignant cerebral edema)
Contralateral monoparesis or lower facial weakness
Contralateral hemiparesis (face and arm > leg)
Contralateral hemisensory loss
Visual field loss, hemianopsia
Gaze preference (conjugate gaze paresis) toward side of stroke
Contralateral gaze palsy
Dysarthria (from facial paresis)
Receptive and/or expressive aphasia (if dominant hemisphere affected)
Sensory extinction or neglect (if nondominant hemisphere affected)
Subcortical (basal ganglia, thalamus)
Contralateral sensory loss
Contralateral hemiparesis
Pain
Choreoathetosis (rare in children)
Tremor
Brainstem
Pure motor hemiparesis without cortical deficits
Nystagmus
Diplopia
Gaze palsy
Vertigo
Dysarthria
Dysphagia
Nausea, vomiting
Horner syndrome
Coma
Cerebellum
Limb and/or truncal ataxia
Nystagmus
Vertigo
Dysarthria
Dysphagia
Nausea, vomiting

ARTERIAL ISCHEMIC STROKE

Arterial ischemic stroke (AIS) in children may present with nonlocalizing symptoms, such as headache, altered mental status, or seizure. Seizure, typically with focal onset, is the presenting symptom in more than 70% of neonates and up to 25% of older infants and children, particularly those under the age of 6 years.

In older infants and children, AIS presents similarly to adult stroke, with the symptom pattern based on the size and location of the infarct. **Table 121-2** lists possible neurological deficits based on stroke location. Up to 90% of children with AIS present with acute unilateral weakness of the face or extremities. Other common symptoms include speech or language disturbance, vision disturbance, or ataxia. Large infarctions of the middle cerebral artery territory with accompanying malignant edema, large cerebellar strokes with edema and herniation, or brainstem strokes are relatively rare but can lead to rapidly progressive encephalopathy or coma. Age and developmental stage of an infant or young child can make clinical localization of symptoms challenging.

CEREBRAL SINOVENOUS THROMBOSIS

Symptoms of CSVT in children may be acute in onset; however, unlike in AIS, they also may progress gradually over days. Most commonly, symptoms of ICP predominate, including headache, nausea and vomiting, lethargy, or diplopia resulting from sixth nerve palsy. Focal symptoms and signs of seizures may occur when there is an ischemic or hemorrhagic injury to surrounding brain parenchyma.

HEMORRHAGIC STROKE

In childhood, sudden-onset of severe headache is a typical presenting symptom, along with other signs and symptoms of acutely increased ICP (e.g., emesis, altered mental status, seizure). The description of "worst headache of [their] life" should always call to mind SAH, but may also occur with other forms of ICH; neck pain or nuchal rigidity may also be present as symptoms of blood causing meningeal irritation.

DIFFERENTIAL DIAGNOSIS

Stroke must be differentiated from diagnoses that can mimic stroke (**Table 121-3**). The most common mimics are migraine with aura, new-onset seizure (particularly with associated postictal Todd's paralysis), Bell's palsy, and functional neurological disorders. The term "complex migraine" was previously used to describe migraine associated with focal neurological deficits; current headache classification guidelines

TABLE 121-3 Stroke Mimics

Stroke Mimics
Migraine aura (+/− headache at presentation)
• *Unilateral sensory loss*
• *Unilateral weakness*
• *Vision deficits*
Seizure, +/− Todd's paralysis
Bell's palsy
Functional neurological symptoms
Demyelinating disease
• *Transverse myelitis*
• *Multiple sclerosis*
• *Acute disseminated encephalomyelitis (ADEM)*
Posterior reversible encephalopathy syndrome (PRES)
Intracranial infection
• *Abscess*
• *Meningitis*
• *Encephalitis*
Post-infectious process
• *Cerebellitis*
• *Acute cerebellar ataxia*
Brain tumor
Chemotherapeutic neurotoxicity
• *Methotrexate*
Metabolic condition
• *Hypo- or hyperglycemia*
• *Inborn errors of metabolism*
• *Mitochondrial disease (e.g., mitochondrial encephalomyelopathy, lactic acidosis, and stroke-like episodes [MELAS])*
Traumatic brain injury
Musculoskeletal injury

identify these deficits as variations of migraine aura, and the term "complex migraine" is no longer preferred (see Chapter 119). Other mimics include brain tumors, methotrexate and other chemotherapeutic agent neurotoxicity, intracranial infection, demyelinating disease, posterior reversible encephalopathy syndrome, metabolic derangements such as hypoglycemia, neurological manifestations of metabolic or mitochondrial disorders, and musculoskeletal abnormalities. Rapidity of onset of the neurological deficit can be helpful in differentiating the clinical syndrome: stroke symptoms typically evolve over seconds to minutes and are maximal at onset, and deficits associated with other disorders often develop more slowly. However, TIA or stroke due to vasculopathy may follow a more stuttering, gradually evolving course. Given that clinical symptomatology alone is not adequate to differentiate stroke from its mimics, or to distinguish between stroke subtypes (e.g., ischemic vs. hemorrhagic), neuroimaging is required for acute diagnosis.

DIAGNOSTIC EVALUATION

Diagnostic delay is common for children with stroke, delaying or preventing the hyperacute or acute interventions that are critical to optimizing perfusion of at-risk brain tissue. These delays occur both for patients presenting to the emergency department with new onset of symptoms and for acute stroke occurring in hospitalized patients; contributing factors include after-hours presentation, as well as delayed consideration of stroke among frontline providers and delays in accessing MRI imaging. Over the past decade, pediatric acute stroke pathways or response protocols have been developed and increasingly implemented in medical centers where the expertise of multiple subspecialists (i.e., neurologists, interventional neuroradiologists, neurosurgeons, anesthesiologists, neuroradiologists) is available. These ideally include guidelines for rapid assessment, an order set, and imaging protocol. Variability exists in the specifics of each center's protocol, but initial outcomes data has been favorable regarding time to diagnosis and treatment for eligible patients.

HISTORY AND PHYSICAL

Time is of the essence when evaluating an infant or child with suspected stroke. A careful history and both general and neurological examinations must be performed as soon as concern is identified. The history should include the time course and evolution of neurological symptoms: time of onset or time last seen well, whether symptoms were maximal at onset or progressive, and whether they are worsening, stable, or improving with time. A complete history should also elicit the presence of headache, associated signs of ICP, potential risk factors for stroke, and prior personal history of stroke. Family history of stroke at an early age, hematologic disorders, or vascular malformations should also be elicited. The general examination should focus on signs of trauma or underlying cardiac, inflammatory, hematologic, genetic, or infectious disease. While a detailed neurological examination is ideal and should be completed eventually, an initial abbreviated assessment can be helpful in quantifying the extent of neurological deficit and stratifying potential severity of symptoms. The Pediatric National Institutes of Health Stroke Scale (PedNIHSS), which has been validated for use in children and infants, is used in many institutional stroke pathways and provides a semiquantitative assessment of clinical stroke severity that has demonstrated good interrater reliability among pediatric neurologists.

NEUROIMAGING

Arterial Ischemic Stroke Evaluation of suspected AIS in children necessitates rapid access to neuroimaging. MRI brain with diffusion-weighted sequences is the gold standard and preferred initial modality of imaging for the diagnosis of AIS in children. It is highly sensitive for acute ischemia and able to delineate parenchymal abnormalities, including nonischemic lesions that clinically mimic AIS. Unlike computed tomography (CT), it does not involve exposure to ionizing radiation. Vessel imaging with MR angiography (MRA) of the brain and neck should be obtained simultaneously, if possible, to evaluate for arteriopathy or dissection, as identification of these contributors to stroke pathogenesis can impact immediate and long-term management. Barriers to use of MRI as first-line imaging modality include clinical instability of a patient, lack of MRI availability in some hospitals, and need for anesthesia for many (particularly younger) children. Many institutions have developed abbreviated MRI protocols that incorporate critical diagnostic sequences only (including diffusion-weighted imaging [DWI] with apparent diffusion coefficient [ADC] maps to confirm presence of ischemia and susceptibility-weighted imaging [SWI] or gradient echo [GRE] to identify hemorrhage) and can be completed in 15 to 20 minutes. If stroke is present on a rapid MRI study, a full protocol MRI with vessel imaging, if not already completed, can be performed later in the hospitalization. Clinicians should note that orthodontic braces can obscure MR imaging and should be removed prior to MR whenever possible.

In an unstable child, a child with contraindications to MRI (e.g., the presence of an implanted cardiac device), in settings where MRI is not readily available, or when the need for anesthesia will significantly delay the MRI, a noncontrast head CT can be performed as an initial assessment. Advantages of CT include the short duration of imaging, a lower cost, and the ability to rapidly identify or exclude hemorrhage. On head CT, acute AIS can show up as a wedge-shaped area of hypodensity involving cortex and subcortical white matter. Disadvantages of CT imaging include exposure to ionizing radiation and lower sensitivity for ischemia, especially within the first several hours and for small lesions; therefore, a normal CT head does not definitively make or rule out the diagnosis of AIS. If CT imaging is obtained, a contrast-enhanced CT angiogram (CTA) of the head and neck should also be performed to evaluate the intracranial vasculature.

Conventional catheter angiogram of the bilateral carotid and vertebral arteries, with careful delineation of anterior and posterior circulations, may be undertaken when MRA or CTA of the brain or neck is inconclusive and care would be altered with a definitive diagnosis of arterial dissection, vasculitis, or other intracranial vasculopathy. Almost all patients with Moyamoya vasculopathy will require a catheter angiogram of the intracranial and extracranial vasculature for evaluation of arterial collaterals prior to revascularization surgery, but this is not necessarily performed in the acute setting. Catheter angiography is invasive and involves fluoroscopic radiation, so the benefit of the potential additional information gained must be carefully weighed against any potential risk. It should be noted that there is a risk of stroke associated with the angiogram procedure itself, though this risk is low and is dependent on the experience of the interventional radiologist. Perceived risk and availability of angiography will therefore vary from center to center. Finally, the appropriate imaging modality and sequences to be obtained should be reviewed with a local neuroradiologist, preferably one with pediatric experience, as well as an interventional neuroradiologist when conventional catheter angiography is considered.

Cerebral Sinovenous Thrombosis MRI with MR venography (MRV) is the most sensitive modality to evaluate for both thrombosis of the cerebral venous drainage system and associated hemorrhagic or ischemic infarction. While MR imaging without contrast is often adequate to confirm diagnosis, addition of gadolinium contrast maximizes sensitivity for detecting lack of flow in the affected vessels. CT head and contrast-enhanced CT venography (CTV) may be considered if there is lack of availability of or contraindication to MRI (e.g., presence of implanted device not compatible with MRI or contraindication to sedation for younger children). Compared to MRI, CT venography offers comparable sensitivity and specificity for detecting thrombi, but sensitivity for parenchymal injury is much lower. Focal parenchymal changes may be identified in up to half of patients, with hemorrhagic infarct occurring most commonly. Depending on identified risk factors of the patient with CSVT, CT head may be needed to evaluate for mastoiditis or sinusitis. If there is concern for meningitis as a precipitating factor for CSVT, lumbar puncture with routine and infectious studies should be considered.

Hemorrhagic Stroke For detection of intracranial hemorrhage, head CT carries the advantages of rapid access and availability in the emergency setting and easily identifying blood (appears bright white). It is therefore typically the first study obtained when hemorrhagic stroke is suspected. Intraparenchymal hemorrhages are readily apparent; however, SAH may be more subtle and appear as hyperdensities following the cortical surface into the sulci and cisterns. Further neuroimaging is often required after the initial, emergent management to delineate an underlying vascular abnormality (e.g., AVM, AVF, or aneurysm) in preparation for definitive surgical management. For a stable and cooperative child, MRI can be considered first-line imaging as it has the ability to identify blood on SWI or GRE sequences and offers an improved image of the brain parenchyma. MRI can be combined with MRA to diagnose a vascular malformation and assess the etiology and extent of brain injury with more certainty.

In a child who is deteriorating, comatose, or who is suspected to have isolated SAH, an emergency CTA or conventional angiogram should be considered since these modalities are more sensitive for small aneurysms and can define the AVM for definitive endovascular or surgical treatment. AVMs that have an aneurysmal component may be at higher risk for acute rebleeding and therefore may need definitive treatment more urgently.

If a vascular malformation is suspected in the acute setting but is not found, follow-up vascular imaging should be performed weeks to months later because some malformations can be obscured or compressed by large hemorrhages and edema in the acute period. Patients who have a vascular malformation generally require follow-up imaging at regular intervals, the timing of which depends on both the type of malformation and its treatment status.

ADDITIONAL LAB TESTING AND STUDIES

All children with AIS diagnosed on neuroimaging should undergo an electrocardiogram to evaluate for arrhythmia and a transthoracic echocardiogram (TTE) with a bubble study (agitated saline) to evaluate for intra- and extracardiac shunts or thrombus and to assess ventricular function. Continuous cardiac monitoring to assess for arrhythmia is also recommended. If the bubble study indicates the presence of a right to left cardiac shunt, a four-extremity Doppler study should be considered to assess for deep vein thrombosis which might lead to paradoxical embolus. While previously undiagnosed severe congenital heart disease is rare in otherwise healthy children, a patent foramen ovale, atrial septal defect, valvular abnormality, fibroelastoma, or pulmonary AVM associated with hereditary hemorrhagic telangiectasia may be uncovered. A pediatric cardiologist can help to interpret EKG and ECHO abnormalities, their potential contribution to an AIS, and the need for additional investigations and treatment.

If a clear alternative cause has not been identified (e.g., known traumatic dissection or Moyamoya), all children with AIS or CSVT should undergo a complete prothrombotic workup, as well as initial evaluation for inflammatory pathology (**Table 121-4**). This should include a complete blood count (CBC) with differential to evaluate for infection and anemia and coagulation studies to evaluate for evidence of acquired or inherited thrombophilia. Importantly, pediatric normal values for many of these studies can vary with age, and in some instances, abnormalities

TABLE 121-4 Stroke Investigations*

Initial Diagnostic Imaging	
Suspected AIS	MRI brain with MRA head and neck
Suspected CSVT	MRI brain with MRV head
Suspected HS *Or if history of head trauma*	Consider initial CT head, followed by MRI with MRA
Investigation for Common Causes	
Follow-up Neuroimaging	Consider catheter angiography, if: • Strongly suspect arteriopathy or dissection and MRA is negative • Moyamoya disease on MRI/MRA • Suspect vascular malformation and MRA nondiagnostic (e.g., obscured by hemorrhage)
Cardiac Evaluation	Transthoracic echocardiogram with bubble study Electrocardiogram and inpatient telemetry Consider 4-extremity Doppler ultrasound if positive bubble study
Laboratory Investigations	
Thrombophilia (AIS, CSVT)	CBC Protein C Protein S Lupus anticoagulant Lipoprotein (a) Anticardiolipin antibody (IgG/IgM) Anti-β2 glycoprotein antibody (IgG/IgM) Homocysteine Specific gene mutation testing: • Prothrombin • Factor V Leiden • Antithrombin • Methylene tetrahydrofolate reductase (MTHFR)
Inflammatory (AIS)	ESR, CRP, ANA
Infectious (AIS, CVST)	*If infection suspected* • Lumbar puncture with CSF studies: glucose, protein, cell count, CSF culture; consider HSV PCR, VZV PCR, VZV antibodies (IgM/IgG)
Coagulopathy (HS)	CBC with differential PT, PTT, INR Factor VIII, IX, and XIII levels

*AIS, arterial ischemic stroke; ANA, antinuclear antibody; CBC, complete blood count; CSF, cerebrospinal fluid; CRP, C-reactive protein; CSVT, cerebral sinovenous thrombosis; CT, computed tomography; ESR, erythrocyte sedimentation rate; HS, hemorrhagic stroke; HSV, herpes simplex virus; IgG, immunoglobulin G; IgM, immunoglobulin M; INR, international normalized ratio; MRA, magnetic resonance angiography; MRI, magnetic resonance imaging; MRV, magnetic resonance venography; PT, prothrombin tine; PTT, partial thromboplastic time; VZV, varicella zoster virus.

appear to resolve with repeat testing, suggesting a transient process or epiphenomenon. Abnormalities uncovered during thrombophilia testing should be discussed with a pediatric hematologist. Initial laboratory evaluation in these patients should also include evaluation of inflammatory markers such as erythrocyte sedimentation rate, C-reactive protein, and antinuclear antibody.

Children with fever or symptoms of infection should be evaluated for infection. If meningitis is suspected, a lumbar puncture should be performed if there is no concern that this will precipitate herniation. FCA may also warrant evaluation for underlying infectious (e.g., herpes simplex virus or varicella-zoster virus) or rheumatological pathology. Finally, it should be noted that while atherosclerotic risk factors (e.g., obesity, hypertension, hyperlipidemia, diabetes, and smoking) are uncommon in children with AIS, their contribution to stroke risk increases in young adulthood; therefore, identifying these features in children and adolescents allows the clinician to counsel around mitigation of these risk factors for secondary stroke prevention.

In children with hemorrhagic stroke, basic laboratory studies, including CBC and coagulation studies (PT, PTT, INR), should be performed urgently. Any abnormalities in these studies should be corrected acutely as part of initial management steps, which are discussed in further detail below. If brain and vascular imaging do not demonstrate a vascular malformation, more hematological studies may be pursued, ideally with guidance from a pediatric hematologist.

Additional testing to consider includes evaluation for metabolic or mitochondrial disorder in a child with infarcts not fitting a classic vascular distribution, especially symmetric lesions affecting deep gray matter structures or occipital lobes. For example, individuals with mitochondrial myopathy, encephalopathy, lactic acidosis, and stroke-like episodes (MELAS) syndrome can have episodes of focal neurological deficits with imaging findings similar to ischemic infarction; suggestive clinical history includes short stature, seizures, and migraine headaches. POLG1 spectrum disorder, associated with often severe episodes of status epilepticus and hepatic dysfunction, can lead to infarctions of the occipital lobes. Evaluation may include initial screening with plasma lactate, pyruvate, ammonia, acylcarnitine profile, plasma amino acids, and urine organic acids; ultimately, genetic testing with mitochondrial analysis is often useful for definitive diagnosis.

Clinical features or family history of connective tissue disorder in a child with craniocervical arterial dissection should prompt further evaluation for connective tissue disorder, which may involve a genetic panel. In general, genetic testing and counseling play a growing role in the evaluation of pediatric stroke patients when there is clinical suspicion of an inherited disorder. Examples in which hereditary disorders should also be considered include patients with Moyamoya disease or other intracranial vasculopathies, those with multiple cavernous angiomas, or those vascular abnormalities and associated skin or mucosal vascular lesions to suggest hereditary hemorrhagic telangiectasia.

MANAGEMENT

Over the past decade, dedicated pediatric stroke centers have evolved at many institutions. The goal of these centers is to improve patient outcomes by delivering comprehensive stroke care via multidisciplinary pediatric stroke teams comprised of pediatric neurologists, vascular neurologists, neurocritical care intensivists, hematologists, neurosurgeons, neuroradiologists, interventional neuroradiologists, and experts in neurorehabilitation. Care strategies at such centers encompass best practices in acute interventions including tissue plasminogen activator (tPA), antiplatelet and anticoagulation therapy, neuroprotective and supportive care, prevention of stroke complications and recurrence, rehabilitation efforts, and neuropsychological and educational endeavors. Many of these institutions have established acute stroke protocols, provide advice to outside referring centers, and accept regional transfers of care. All individuals caring for children with stroke are encouraged to seek out their closest pediatric stroke center for support and guidance.

Many aspects of stroke management in children are derived from adult data and further study is needed to confirm or refute the efficacy and safety in children. Updated national guidelines for neonatal and childhood stroke were released by the American Heart Association (AHA) in 2019 and currently serve as the best practice guidelines for the management of stroke in children. The development of institutional guidelines for the management of pediatric stroke is associated with more timely recognition of stroke and improved time to initiation of management.

ARTERIAL ISCHEMIC STROKE

The goals of AIS care are focused on restoring and/or maintaining perfusion to injured brain, limiting the area of infarction, salvaging the surrounding healthy tissue or penumbra, promoting recovery and neuronal plasticity, monitoring for and preventing complications, and preventing stroke recurrence. Elements of care include arterial recanalization therapy, when applicable, and employing neuroprotective measures to limit neuronal metabolic demand and optimize penumbral perfusion and substrate delivery.

Neuroprotective Care and Monitoring In general, patients with childhood stroke should be admitted to the intensive care unit for close monitoring and implementation of neuroprotective measures. Although objective evidence of effectiveness is relatively limited, examples of neuroprotective measures include treating fevers, maintaining blood pressure within certain parameters, treating and preventing seizures, and treating hypo- or hyperglycemia. Hypertension should be treated cautiously to avoid cerebral hypoperfusion. Hypotension should be avoided. Administration of intravenous fluids at the child's maintenance rate may help by increasing the circulating blood volume and protecting against hypotension. If clinically feasible, clinicians may also consider keeping the head of the bed flat to avoid postural perfusion fluctuations. Cardiorespiratory monitoring should be initiated, and supplemental oxygen should be considered for any child with Moyamoya vasculopathy, SCD, or whose oxygen saturation is below 95%. Anticonvulsant medications should be started for children who present with seizures. As is the case for all pediatric stroke subtypes, the duration of anticonvulsant therapy for acute symptomatic seizures in the setting of AIS is unknown. Evaluation with routine or continuous EEG should be considered in all children with seizures at stroke diagnosis, particularly if there is persistent altered mental status, as subclinical, or nonconvulsive, seizures may be detected.

Recanalization Therapy For adult patients presenting within hours of AIS symptom onset, arterial recanalization through hyperacute stroke therapies, which includes thrombolysis or endovascular thrombectomy, is the standard of care based on a substantial body of scientific literature and best-practice guidelines published by the AHA. Trials in adults demonstrated the safety and efficacy of intravenous tPA within 4.5 hours of stroke onset and intra-arterial tPA within 6 hours of stroke onset. Thrombectomy can be utilized up to 24 hours after stroke onset in some cases. Although age-specific data supporting the use of these procedures in children is less robust, hyperacute stroke therapies can be considered in childhood AIS for patients who present to care within hours of symptom onset. Use of these therapies beyond this time frame may increase the risk of hemorrhagic transformation, reperfusion injury, or other complications. Since pediatric data about the efficacy and safety of these interventions is limited, decisions on the use of hyperacute stroke therapies should be made on a case-by-case basis in conjunction with a neurologist who is experienced in treating pediatric stroke. In general, since stroke mimics in children are common, these therapies should only be employed after an arterial obstruction is confirmed on imaging.

Sickle Cell Disease In patients with SCD who present with a focal neurologic deficit, early consultation with a hematologist is important. Blood transfusion is generally indicated even before the results of imaging studies are known. Intravenous thrombolysis is not recommended for children with SCD.

Neurosurgical Intervention Hemicraniectomy can be lifesaving for some children with a large supratentorial stroke. A neurosurgeon should be consulted early for any child with a large volume infarct, evidence of midline shift, or significant cerebral edema. For these patients, if early prophylactic hemicraniectomy is not performed, the patient should undergo frequent neurological examinations and serial imaging for the first 72 hours to assess the need for surgical intervention. Worsening headache, combativeness, and late signs such as Cushing's triad (i.e., hypertension, bradycardia, and irregular breathing), should prompt immediate neuroimaging with a noncontrast head CT. Neurosurgical consultation can also be helpful for placement of an intracranial pressure monitor or in the setting of hemorrhagic transformation if the hemorrhage is large and compressive.

Secondary Stroke Prevention While investigations into the etiology of a child's AIS are underway, and in the absence of known hemorrhagic transformation, the majority of children with childhood AIS are started on antiplatelet or anticoagulation therapy to prevent stroke recurrence. The most common empiric prevention therapy used in children is aspirin; however, other options include low molecular weight heparin (LMWH) and unfractionated heparin (UFH), among others. Consultation with a pediatric hematologist with experience in stroke management is important as these decisions should be individualized. Stroke prevention is discussed in more detail later in this chapter.

CEREBRAL SINOVENOUS THROMBOSIS

The goals of CSVT care are focused on prevention of clot propagation, promotion of recanalization, and prevention of new or worse venous infarction or hemorrhagic transformation. Admission to an intensive care unit and use of a multidisciplinary treatment team including neurology, hematology, neurosurgery, intensive care, and otolaryngology is needed. When the CSVT is accompanied by ischemia and/or hemorrhage, supportive care for the patient's symptoms, such as nausea, headache, seizures, and focal deficits, is critical. Correction of anemia, dehydration, or hypovolemia with isotonic IV fluids is important in children in whom this is found. Anticonvulsants should be used for the treatment of seizures. Intravenous antibiotics are needed when systemic or local head and neck infections (e.g., meningitis, otitis media, or mastoiditis) have contributed to the CSVT. Surgical interventions, such as mastoidectomy, myringotomy, and tympanostomy tube placement for otitis media and/or mastoiditis-related CSVT are usually needed.

Monitoring for ICP is important and can be accomplished by regular use of fundoscopy and visual field testing. Surgical management of ICP must be balanced by the increased risk of bleeding related to anticoagulation, so medical management of ICP with carbonic anhydrase inhibitors can be beneficial.

Anticoagulation therapy with UFH, LMWH, or warfarin is the mainstay of treatment for pediatric CSVT. If there is concern for hemorrhage or patient-specific bleeding risk factors, some pediatric stroke experts prefer to start UFH initially so that it can be reversed quickly when needed. Transition to LMWH can occur later when hemorrhage has been ruled out or is stable on subsequent neuroimaging. Anticoagulation therapy needs to be carefully monitored with activated partial thromboplastin time (aPTT) for heparin, anti-Xa levels for LMWH, and international normalized ratio (INR) for warfarin. Newer anticoagulants such as dabigatran have not been tested in children in the setting of CSVT. Thrombus extension may be seen in up to one-third of children who are not treated with anticoagulation, and clot propagation may result in new venous infarcts and worse outcomes in up to 40%. Thrombolysis or thrombectomy should be considered in rare situations in which there is a high risk of deterioration or death despite anticoagulation. Examples include when there is extensive, deep multifocal, or diffuse sinovenous involvement.

Treatment regimens vary from center to center, but most pediatric stroke experts and hematologists recommend completion of at least 3 to 6 months of anticoagulation therapy. Anticoagulation may be discontinued earlier if complete vessel recanalization is observed on follow-up neuroimaging. Therapy may also be prolonged in certain high-risk children.

HEMORRHAGIC STROKE

The management of hemorrhagic stroke focuses on stabilizing the child and preventing additional neurologic injury. When the diagnosis is suspected or definitively made, a neurosurgeon should be consulted immediately. The head of the bed should be elevated to at least 30° to promote venous drainage, thereby reducing ICP. If the patient is obtunded, comatose, or has a deteriorating mental status, the child should be intubated for airway protection. Hypertension can occur after hemorrhage, and the management of each case should be individualized to balance concern for rebleeding with that of maintaining cerebral perfusion pressure. As with all stroke types, normothermia and normoglycemia should be maintained. Anticonvulsants are commonly given following hemorrhagic stroke to prevent seizures.

Monitoring for elevated ICP is critical. An external ventricular drain can be used to both monitor and manage intracranial pressure. If an intraventricular catheter is not needed but pressure monitoring is required, a subdural bolt can be placed. For management of increased ICP, hyperventilation can be used acutely but should not be maintained for a prolonged period. Mannitol or hypertonic saline are additional useful temporizing measures, and serum osmoles and sodium must be monitored closely. Surgical evacuation of a parenchymal hematoma may be necessary to control intracranial pressure and/or mass effect and is sometimes performed concomitantly with resection of a vascular malformation, even in a stable patient. Finally, decompressive craniectomy can be life-saving and function-sparing in cases of increased ICP or mass effect that are refractory to medical intervention. In the case of cerebellar hematomas, a suboccipital craniectomy may be needed to prevent brainstem compression and death. It is important to monitor the child's neurological examination at least hourly for signs of neurological worsening and herniation syndromes. An urgent head CT should be performed for any neurological deterioration or change or for worsening headache.

Endovascular and/or surgical management of vascular malformations may be needed in the acute setting, depending on the type of malformation and the condition of the child. In general, aneurysms are addressed acutely due to their high rate of acute rebleeding.

Treatment of any known bleeding diathesis is another important component of care. In a child with low or abnormal platelets, a platelet transfusion may be needed. Specific treatments such as intravenous immunoglobulin are required for diseases such as idiopathic thrombocytopenic purpura. Coagulopathy may be corrected with intravenous vitamin K and fresh frozen plasma, depending on the underlying cause. Children with factor VIII or IX deficiency and hemorrhagic stroke typically require urgent factor replacement. Any child with hemorrhage on anticoagulation should have their anticoagulation held or reversed.

Children with hemorrhagic stroke often have severe headache. While pain should be treated, nonsteroidal anti-inflammatory drugs should be avoided because they can theoretically worsen bleeding through their action on platelet function. Additionally, narcotics should be used with caution since they can cause altered mental status that can be difficult to differentiate from true neurological worsening. Acetaminophen, topiramate, and gabapentin can be used safely and with good effect in these children.

REHABILITATION AND SCHOOL TRANSITION

All children with a confirmed diagnosis of stroke should be comprehensively assessed by physical, occupational, and speech therapists as early in their hospitalization as possible. Splints and braces as well as stretching exercises are often necessary, even in the acute hospitalization. Many children will require inpatient rehabilitation before they may be discharged home safely. Disposition planning should begin soon after the stroke diagnosis is made so that candidacy for inpatient or outpatient rehabilitation regimens can be determined and insurance coverage for necessary therapy verified. Psychology assessment after the neurologic injury and ongoing assessments in the future can be an important component of determining cognitive deficits and assisting with any mental health or behavioral concerns that have developed. Likewise, most school-age children with stroke should have formal neuropsychological testing performed to gauge cognitive and behavioral strengths and weaknesses that may affect school programming. The knowledge gained from these therapeutic assessments can help with planning for school reentry. Many children are fatigued after a stroke and may need to return to school on a half-time or modified basis. Some children will require school accommodations or the development of an individualized education program. A school liaison may be necessary to provide stroke education and to outline physical activity restrictions when relevant.

ADMISSION AND DISCHARGE CRITERIA

All children with acute AIS, CSVT, and HS should be hospitalized. The first hospital days are usually in the pediatric intensive care unit so that appropriate monitoring can be provided. The child with stroke may be safely discharged from the hospital when the child is neurologically and medically stable, his/her investigations for underlying etiologies and ongoing risk factors are complete, and antiplatelet or anticoagulation treatment has been initiated, when appropriate. Many children with stroke must be discharged to an inpatient rehabilitation facility to maximize their recovery. For those who are discharged home, outpatient rehabilitation including varying degrees of physical therapy, occupational therapy, and speech therapy, are usually needed. Prior to discharge, follow-up with neurology and any other specialists should be scheduled. Additionally, accommodations in the home or at school may be needed.

CONSULTATION

- **Neurology:** A neurologist should be consulted on any case of suspected or confirmed pediatric stroke, regardless of subtype.
- **Neurosurgery:** Neurosurgery should be consulted for children with a large ischemic stroke with potential for cerebral edema swelling and herniation, for children with CSVT and rapidly evolving encephalopathy or with an associated large venous hemorrhagic infarction, and for most children with hemorrhagic stroke. Even if the child is initially stable, a consultation is reasonable.
- **Hematology:** A hematologist is often helpful when evaluating children with AIS or CSVT who may have thrombophilia or when anticoagulation is being considered. A hematology consult is also useful for children with ICH or SAH who are suspected to have a platelet abnormality or coagulopathy. Hematology should also be involved in the care of children with SCD and suspected or confirmed stroke.
- **Cardiology:** A cardiologist should be consulted for children with suspected congenital heart disease or an abnormal echocardiogram. A bubble study indicating flow from the right to the left side of the heart can suggest a patent foramen ovale, atrial septal defect, or pulmonary AVM.
- **Neuroradiology:** When available, consultation with a neuroradiologist for imaging interpretation can be useful. A neuroradiologist can also assist with choosing the most appropriate imaging modalities for a particular patient.
- **Interventional neuroradiology:** Interventional neuroradiologists often have a role in the management of pediatric stroke patients. Though rarely used, intra-arterial tPA is always administered by an interventional neuroradiologist. Occasionally, an interventional radiologist may be needed for a child with CSVT for clot removal. The most common role for an interventional neuroradiologist is with children with AVMs or aneurysms. AVMs can be embolized, most often prior to surgical resection. Aneurysms can be embolized or coiled.
- **Rheumatology:** A child with suspected rheumatologic disease or inflammatory process may benefit from a pediatric rheumatology consultation.
- **Metabolism and genetics:** Children with a suspected metabolic disease, mitochondrial disease, or genetic syndrome should be evaluated by a specialist.
- **Infectious disease:** Some children with endocarditis, meningitis, encephalitis, or a brain abscess benefit from an infectious disease consultation.
- **Radiation oncology:** Some AVMs are best treated with gamma knife or proton beam therapy. If the neurosurgeon suggests that a lesion would be difficult to treat surgically or by an endovascular approach, radiation may be a consideration.
- **Physical medicine and rehabilitation:** During the acute hospitalization, a physical therapist, occupational therapist, and speech therapist should evaluate the child. Additionally, a physical medicine and rehabilitation expert should be consulted to help inform a rehabilitation program and to determine whether the child requires an inpatient rehabilitation program or an outpatient program.

SPECIAL CONSIDERATIONS

PROGNOSIS

Arterial Ischemic Stroke The literature has reported a range of outcomes following AIS in childhood, largely owing to variability in follow-up intervals and outcome definitions and measures. Mortality due to AIS specifically is likely in the range of 4% to 5%. Long-term sequelae include hemiparesis, speech/language deficits, cognitive impairment, and behavioral problems. A significant number also develop epilepsy, particularly those with acute symptomatic seizures at presentation. Neurological impairments have been reported in up two-thirds of children leaving the hospital, with moderate or greater functional deficits persisting at 1 year in up to 50%. While the plasticity of the developing brain may confer some advantages in recovery from injury, outcomes vary widely, with long-term follow-up studies indicating more nuanced interactions between age at injury, size of lesion, and location of lesion in influencing outcome.

The Pediatric Stroke Outcome Measure (PSOM) is a quantitative, validated measure of outcome following pediatric stroke. A longitudinal prospective cohort found that PSOM score at 1 month following AIS was predictive of motor and adaptive behavior outcomes at 1 year. The PSOM was also used in the Felling et al 2020 publication of a follow-up of 413 childhood and 174 neonatal International Pediatric Stroke Study (IPSS) study participants at 2 years from discharge, which is the largest study to date evaluating longitudinal outcomes using a standardized pediatric stroke-specific outcome measure. Overall, outcomes were favorable in most patients. At 2 years, moderate to severe neurological impairment was present in 24.7% of childhood AIS patients. Sensorimotor problems were more common than language or cognitive/behavioral problems. The most severe outcomes were seen in young infants who experienced AIS at ages 1 month to 1 year, compared to both younger and older age groups. Poor outcome was predicted by age between 1 month and 1 year, underlying chronic disorder, and involvement of both small and large vascular territories.

Cerebral Sinovenous Thrombosis Reports of long-term outcomes and recurrence risk for patients with CSVT are limited by small sample size. Mortality has been reported up to 25%, although in reality may be lower as the primary cause of death is not consistently identified in studies reporting outcomes. Reported morbidity also varies, but up to two-thirds may have long-term neurological sequelae. Early diagnosis, older age, and treatment with anticoagulation have been associated with lower mortality and more favorable outcomes. Decreased levels of consciousness and focal parenchymal lesions on imaging have been associated with less favorable outcomes. Reported rates of remote symptomatic seizures and epilepsy range from 10% to 25%.

Hemorrhagic Stroke Mortality reported after ICH is typically less than 10% but varies widely by cause of hemorrhage. More than one-third may have significant disability at 2 years. Predictors of mortality and poor outcomes include coagulopathy, decreased mental status at presentation, aneurysmal cause of hemorrhage, and increased volume of hemorrhage. Long-term risk of epilepsy increases with time, and more than 10% of survivors may develop seizures by 2 years after hemorrhage.

RECURRENCE RISK

Stroke recurrence is influenced heavily by underlying risk factors. Secondary prevention strategies for all stroke subtypes hinge upon accurate characterization of underlying pathogenesis and risk factors, of which there are often more than one, and, when possible, treatment or mitigation of those risk factors and presumed etiologies.

Arterial Ischemic Stroke Stroke recurrence is identified in a significant minority of children with AIS, and short- and long-term rates of recurrence are dependent upon the primary etiology for the stroke and associated risk factors, keeping in mind that many children with AIS have multiple risk factors contributing to their initial stroke. The risk of recurrence of AIS is highest within the first year of the index stroke. In their 2016 publication, Fullerton et al found recurrence rate globally to be 12% at 1 year. Recurrence risk is also highest for children with arteriopathy, in whom up to 1 in 3 will have recurrent stroke within 1 year, and higher for posterior circulation as compared to anterior circulation strokes. More than 25% of children with congenital heart disease have recurrence within 10 years.

Cerebral Sinovenous Thrombosis Overall recurrence rate of CSVT is less than 10%, and recurrent thrombosis may be cerebral or noncerebral. A 2007 publication by Kenet et al evaluating risk factors for recurrence, found recurrence risk to be highest in first 6 months, with risk factors including age >2 years at time of onset, non-use of anticoagulation, persistent venous occlusion at short-term follow-up imaging, and presence of *G20210A* mutation in factor II (prothrombin). Early clot propagation portends potential for worse outcome; however, once the clot stabilizes, persistence of thrombosis at 6 months after diagnosis is presumed to have low risk of further extension. Complete recanalization may not occur, but this does not necessarily impact prognosis or risk of recurrence. Therefore, while there are no clinical trials to support dose or duration of anticoagulation therapy following CSVT, most pediatric stroke experts and hematologists recommend 3 to 6 months of therapy, or longer for patients with ongoing systemic risk factors that cannot be mitigated.

Hemorrhagic Stroke The risk of recurrent hemorrhagic stroke has been estimated at 10% at 5 years, with most recurrences occurring within the first 6 months. Children with structural lesions (vascular malformations or tumors) and with medical etiologies are at highest risk of recurrence. Prevention of recurrent hemorrhage is thus in part dependent upon correcting any underlying vascular malformation or hematologic abnormality. Follow-up vascular imaging at least annually for the first 5 years is recommended for most vascular malformations, even following successful treatment, as lesions may recur or new lesions develop over time.

PREVENTION

Arterial Ischemic Stroke Except in certain circumstances, the primary prevention of childhood AIS is challenging, since for many patients, their stroke risk factors may not be identified until after the first stroke. Examples in which primary prevention can be accomplished include SCD, certain cardiac conditions, known thrombophilia, known arteriopathy, and known thrombus. Following the first episode of AIS, prevention of recurrent stroke, referred to as secondary prevention, is an important component of care.

Because of the complexities of decisions surrounding secondary stroke prevention through use of antithrombotic therapy, these decisions are best made at pediatric centers with on-site expertise. Except in the cases of SCD or in cases of concomitant coagulopathy, most children with AIS require an antithrombotic medication to prevent stroke recurrence. The choice of an antiplatelet agent (most commonly aspirin) or an anticoagulant (standard UFH, LMWH, or warfarin) for secondary stroke prevention is controversial and lacks evidence from pediatric clinical trials. Antithrombotic choice is based on the underlying mechanism or risk factor(s) for stroke and should be made in conjunction with a neurologist and hematologist, particularly when thrombophilia has been identified.

Most commonly, children with stroke of unknown etiology continue antithrombotic therapy for 2 years. Children with FCA and Moyamoya are typically treated with aspirin indefinitely unless a contraindication arises. Children with AIS in the setting of prior thrombosis, extracranial dissection, or known pro-thrombotic disorder are often treated with anticoagulation for 3 months or longer.

Prevention of stroke recurrence in Moyamoya is accomplished through surgical revascularization procedures. Surgery is done as soon as medically feasible but is typically planned several weeks after a stroke or series of TIAs to reduce the risk of perioperative complications. Evidence shows that surgical revascularization can reverse prior white matter changes and reduces the risk of future TIA, ischemic stroke, and hemorrhagic stroke. Because of suspected familial inheritance, clinicians should recommend that first-degree relatives of a child with Moyamoya disease receive routine screening with an MRI brain.

Children with heart disease and AIS deserve special consideration due to the complex nature of their care and shifting hemodynamics over time. Consultation with cardiology, hematology, and neurology is often necessary to choose the appropriate antithrombotic agent for the patient's clinical circumstances. Patients with known cardiac thromboembolism are typically anticoagulated with LMWH or warfarin for 3 to 6 months to prevent stroke recurrence. Some children are treated with life-long antithrombotic therapy. The role of patent foramen ovale closure in reduction of primary or recurrent stroke risk is uncertain.

Primary and secondary prevention of stroke in children with SCD is a vital component of SCD care. National guidelines by the American Hematology Society recommend that children with SCD be screened yearly with transcranial Doppler ultrasound. Additionally, early school-aged children with SCD should be screened for silent infarction with an MRI brain without sedation. Children found to have abnormal transcranial Doppler ultrasound are known to have a markedly reduced risk of stroke with chronic transfusion therapy. Patients with SCD with prior stroke and those with steno-occlusive vasculopathy suspicious for Moyamoya disease should be managed with chronic transfusion protocols. Patients with SCD and known Moyamoya vasculopathy should also undergo surgical revascularization procedures for risk reduction.

Cerebral Sinovenous Thrombosis Primary prevention of CSVT is generally limited to patients with known thrombophilia. To prevent recurrence of CSVT after a first episode, children with underlying risk factors may be candidates for ongoing anticoagulation therapy. These patients may include those who are receiving chemotherapy with prothrombotic agents or those who are found to have prothrombotic abnormalities that carry a high rate of recurrent venous thromboembolism (e.g., homozygous for Factor V Leiden or prothrombin gene mutations). Additionally, patients who are at high risk of nephrotic syndrome relapse or with active inflammatory bowel disease may be candidates for continued anticoagulation. Modifiable hypercoagulable risk factors, such as use of systemic corticosteroids or exogenous estrogen, should also be addressed when possible.

Hemorrhagic Stroke For patients with a known AVM, the primary or secondary prevention of hemorrhagic stroke can often be achieved through surgical resection, embolization, and/or stereotactic radiosurgery. In some cases, such as large AVMs or for those within certain regions of the brain, the risks of AVM treatment may outweigh the risks of observation, and serial imaging is performed instead.

High flow or symptomatic AVFs should be considered for treatment, particularly those determined to have a greater risk of hemorrhage. Lower flow asymptomatic lesions may be candidates for observation. When indicated, the treatment of AVFs is aimed toward closure of the fistulous connection which is most commonly achieved via endovascular or microsurgical techniques. Likewise, high-risk cavernous malformations (such as those with prior hemorrhage, symptomatic lesions, or posterior fossa location) may be candidates for surgical resection or other treatment modalities.

Decisions about the treatment of aneurysms is complex and best made by a multidisciplinary team. Similar to other CNS vascular abnormalities, decisions about treatment are partly based on the size and location of the lesion. At times, monitoring of an asymptomatic aneurysm for signs of enlargement or the development of symptoms may be preferred. Treatment options may include open surgery and/or endovascular techniques.

Prevention of hemorrhagic stroke in patients with a known coagulopathy should be guided by a pediatric hematologist. Avoidance of head injuries is important, and the use of blood products, clotting factors, or antifibrinolytic agents may be needed.

KEY POINTS

Clinical presentation

- Pediatric stroke presentation can include nonspecific symptoms such as headache, altered mental status, and seizure. Clinicians should maintain a high index of suspicion for stroke in children with known risk factors.
- Arterial ischemic strokes present with acute, focal neurologic deficits, most often including hemiparesis.
- Cerebral venous sinus thrombosis most often presents with headache, emesis, diplopia, and/or altered mental status. Focal deficits can occur.
- Hemorrhagic stroke typically presents with severe headache, emesis, and altered mental status. Focal neurologic deficits are common, and neck stiffness is common with subarachnoid hemorrhage.

Diagnosis

- Head CT is the most common first-line imaging study obtained. It is sensitive to all types of hemorrhage, but is less sensitive for cerebral sinovenous thrombosis and insensitive for acute arterial ischemic stroke.
- MRI and angiography and/or venography are the gold standard for diagnosis of stroke and for evaluation of the underlying cause.

Treatment

- Antiplatelet agents and anticoagulation are the most common treatments for pediatric arterial ischemic stroke.
- In consultation with a neurologist, alteplase (tPA) and mechanical clot thrombectomy can be considered for pediatric patients with stroke.
- Most pediatric cerebral sinovenous thrombosis, even with concomitant hemorrhage, is treated with anticoagulation.
- Neurosurgical intervention is often required in patients with hemorrhagic stroke.
- All pediatric acute stroke subtypes require admission to the pediatric intensive care unit and systematic evaluation for the underlying cause.
- Physical, occupational, and speech therapy, as well as inpatient rehabilitation, are important for recovery following stroke.
- Childhood stroke outcomes may be improved by stroke identification pathways and comprehensive care teams within dedicated pediatric stroke centers.

ACKNOWLEDGMENTS

The authors would like to thank Lauren A. Beslow and Lori Billinghurst for their prior contributions to this chapter and E. Steve Roach for his suggestions and edits.

SUGGESTED READINGS

Berkowitz AL. Overview of the anatomy of the nervous system. In: Berkowitz AL. *Clinical Neurology & Neuroanatomy: A Localization-Based Approach*. 2nd ed. New York, NY: McGraw Hill; 2022. https://accessmedicine-mhmedical-com.ezproxy.lib.utexas.edu/content.aspx?bookid=3206&sectionid=267213261. Accessed August 27, 2022.

Bernson-Leung ME, Rivkin MJ. Stroke in neonates and children. *Pediatr Rev*. 2016;37(11):463-477.

Billinghurst LL, Beslow LA, Abend NS, et al. Incidence and predictors of epilepsy after pediatric arterial ischemic stroke. *Neurol*. 2017;88(7):630-637.

Cornelius LP, Elango N, Jeyaram VK. Clinico-etiological factors, neuroimaging characteristics and outcome in pediatric cerebral venous sinus thrombosis. *Annals Ind Acad Neurol*. 2021;24(6):901-907.

DeBaun MR, Jordan LC, King AA, et al. American Society of Hematology 2020 guidelines for sickle cell disease: prevention, diagnosis, and treatment of cerebrovascular disease in children and adults. *Blood Adv*. 2020;4(8):1554-1588.

DeLaroche AM, Sivaswamy L, Farooqi A, Kannikeswaran N. Pediatric stroke and its mimics: limitations of a pediatric stroke clinical pathway. *Pediatr Neurol*. 2018;80:35-41.

Dlamini N, Billinghurst L, Kirkham FJ. Cerebral venous sinus (sinovenous) thrombosis in children. *Neurosurg Clin N Am*. 2010;21(3):511-527.

Felling RJ, Rafay MF, Bernard TJ, et al. Predicting recovery and outcome after pediatric stroke: results from the International Pediatric Stroke Study. *Ann Neurol*. 2020;87(6):840-852.

Ferriero DM, Fullerton HJ, Bernard TJ, et al. Management of stroke in neonates and children: a scientific statement from the American Heart Association/American Stroke Association. *Stroke*. 2019;50(3):e51-e96.

Harrar DB, Salussolia CL, Kapur K, et al. A Stroke alert protocol decreases the time to diagnosis of brain attack symptoms in a pediatric emergency department. *J Pediatr*. 2020;216:136-141 e136.

Hutchinson ML, Beslow LA. Hemorrhagic transformation of arterial ischemic and venous stroke in children. *Pediatr Neurol*. 2019;95:26-33.

Ichord RN. Cerebral sinovenous thrombosis. *Front Pediatr*. 2017;5:163.

Ichord RN, Bastian R, Abraham L, et al. Interrater reliability of the Pediatric National Institutes of Health Stroke Scale (PedNIHSS) in a multicenter study. *Stroke*. 2011;42(3):613-617.

Kenet G, Kirkham F, Niederstadt T, et al. Risk factors for recurrent venous thromboembolism in the European collaborative paediatric database on cerebral venous thrombosis: a multicentre cohort study. *Lancet Neurol*. 2007;6(7):595-603.

Malone LA, Felling RJ. Pediatric stroke: unique implications of the immature brain on injury and recovery. *Pediatr Neurol*. 2020;102:3-9.

Mirsky DM, Beslow LA, Amlie-Lefond C, et al. Pathways for neuroimaging of childhood stroke. *Pediat Neurol*. 2017;69:11-23.

Porcari GS, Beslow LA, Ichord RN, Licht DJ, Kleinman JT, Jordan LC. Neurologic outcome predictors in pediatric intracerebral hemorrhage: a prospective study. *Stroke*. 2018;49(7):1755-1758.

Roach ES, Bernard T, deVeber G. Defining a pediatric stroke center. *Pediatr Neurol*. 2020;112:11-13.

Statistics Canada. Table 13-10-0392-01. Deaths and age-specific mortality rates, by selected grouped causes. https://www150.statcan.gc.ca/t1/tbl1/en/tv.action?pid=1310039201. Accessed July 1, 2022.

Swaiman KF, Ashwal S, Ferriero DM, et al, eds. *Swaiman's Pediatric Neurology*. 6th ed. Elsevier; 2018.

CHAPTER 122 Central Nervous System Demyelinating Disease

Brooke Surran, MD and Jeremy Yardley, MD, FAAP

BACKGROUND

Acquired demyelinating syndromes (ADS) encompass both acute and chronic immune-mediated disorders of the central nervous system (CNS) and include acute disseminated encephalomyelitis (ADEM), optic neuritis (ON), transverse myelitis (TM), multiple sclerosis (MS), myelin-oligodendrocyte glycoprotein associated disease (MOGAD), and neuromyelitis optica (NMO). These disorders are all characterized by CNS inflammation. Although these syndromes overlap in their neurologic symptoms, the clinical severity, radiologic features, response to treatment, and prognosis for neurologic recovery vary between the disorders. In recent decades, the recognition of disease entities characterized by the presence of circulating antibodies directed toward CNS antigens (i.e., AQP4 and MOG) has led to a shift in diagnosis, understanding of prognosis, and directed therapies.

Given the complexity of ADS, pediatric providers must have a high index of suspicion for these disorders. Subtle neurologic symptoms and signs may be difficult to identify in young children. For example, sensory and visual symptoms are often difficult for young children to describe and may not be brought to the attention of a care provider or parent unless they are severe or impacting activities of daily living.

Patients with symptoms concerning for an acute or chronic demyelinating disorder require prompt evaluation so that a diagnosis can be confirmed and treatment initiated. This chapter reviews clinical features, differential diagnosis, and management of demyelinating disorders in the inpatient setting and then describes the prototypical ADS in greater detail, highlighting the unique features of the disorders.

The global incidence of pediatric ADS is estimated to be 0.87 per 100,000 children per year. Approximately 20% of children with ADS are ultimately diagnosed with MS though, pediatric-onset MS represents less than 5% of all patients with a diagnosis of MS. In a North American pediatric cohort, 71% with incidental ADS had monophasic disease and relapses were rare in patients who did not meet criteria for MS and were seronegative for anti-MOG and anti-AQP4 antibodies.

CLINICAL PRESENTATIONS

ADS cause various symptoms that localize to the CNS. Common symptoms include vision loss or visual disturbance (such as blurry or double vision), sensory abnormalities (including numbness or tingling), weakness, balance difficulties, gait abnormalities, and bowel and bladder dysfunction. Neurologic symptoms may localize to one particular area of the CNS (termed monofocal); however, symptoms and signs can affect various regions (polyfocal) and reflect the presence of diffuse inflammation throughout the CNS.

DIFFERENTIAL DIAGNOSIS OF DEMYELINATING DISORDERS IN CHILDREN

The differential diagnosis for an acute or subacute neurologic event in a previously well child is extensive and must be tailored to the individual's clinical history and examination findings. ADS are diagnosed based on clinical criteria, with accompanying supportive laboratory and radiographic features. The prototypical demyelinating disorders are listed in **Table 122-1** and discussed in greater detail later in the chapter. However, diagnosis of a demyelinating syndrome is often difficult at presentation, and other etiologies, such as infection, rheumatologic processes, genetic/metabolic disorders, and malignancy, must be carefully considered prior to making the diagnosis. **Table 122-2** provides a differential diagnosis that may be considered in the appropriate clinical context as well as supportive laboratory and imaging features to determine whether an alternative diagnosis exists.

DIAGNOSTIC EVALUATION

The evaluation of a child with acute neurologic symptoms begins with a detailed history that includes information about the timing and duration of symptoms. Although a thorough neurologic examination should be performed to help localize neurologic dysfunction, asymptomatic inflammation (i.e., lesions that do not cause symptoms or findings on examination) is also common in these disorders. Similarly, a normal sensory or ophthalmologic examination does not preclude the possibility of CNS demyelinating lesions. Therefore, extensive imaging (i.e., brain, cervical, and thoracic spine) is often indicated, even without symptoms or examination findings that specifically localize to these areas of the CNS. Though magnetic resonance imaging (MRI) is required to determine the extent of CNS inflammation, computed tomography (CT) of the brain may be performed acutely if there are signs of elevated intracranial pressure, altered mental status, or new focal neurologic deficits. Due to the inflammatory nature of ADS, MRI should be completed both with and without gadolinium.

In all children with suspected CNS inflammation, cerebrospinal fluid (CSF) analysis should be considered. In addition to obtaining CSF cell count, protein, glucose, Gram stain and culture, and other clinically indicated tests (i.e., for infectious etiologies), an evaluation for immunoglobulin synthesis within the CNS should be performed. The intrathecal synthesis of immunoglobulins is a hallmark of CNS inflammation but not specific to demyelinating diseases. To interpret these studies, CSF and blood should be drawn at the same time and sent for an oligoclonal band profile, which includes a qualitative test to visualize the oligoclonal bands through isoelectric focusing, as well as quantitative measures of these immunoglobulins through an immunoglobulin G (IgG) index and IgG synthesis rate. Children presenting with first ADS should be evaluated with serology directed at anti-AQP4 and anti-MOG IgG as seropositivity may alter the diagnosis and treatment regimen (see disorder-specific discussion below).

TABLE 122-1 Characteristic Features of Pediatric Acquired Demyelinating Syndromes

Diagnosis	Clinical Features	Radiographic Features	CSF and Other Labs	Demographics
Acute disseminated encephalomyelitis (ADEM)	Acute encephalopathy with polyfocal neurologic symptoms Seizures, fever, headache can occur Typically monophasic	Lesions are asymmetric, large, and often have poorly defined borders Visible lesions in the deep gray matter are common	Oligoclonal bands are rarely positive	Common in children and young adults Male predominance in few pediatric cohorts
Multiple Sclerosis (MS)	Neurologic features are variable; encephalopathy and seizures are rare Typically a relapsing course	Periaqueductal, corpus callosum, and periventricular white matter often involved T1 hypointense lesions present commonly at onset	Oligoclonal bands are typically positive (>95% in post-pubertal patients)	Commonly presents in adolescence and young adulthood Female predominance (1.8:1.0 female to male)
Myelin Oligodendrocyte Glycoprotein antibody-associated disease (MOGAD	Neurologic features are variable with frequent optic neuritis, transverse myelitis, and ADEM phenotypes	Large cerebral lesions, longitudinally extensive optic nerve and/or spinal cord lesions	CSF pleocytosis common. Serum anti-MOG antibodies always positive.	Frequent onset before 10 years
Optic neuritis (ON)	Vision loss Pain with eye movement Change in color vision	Increased T2 signal, swelling, or Gd enhancement of the optic nerves	Can see elevated CSF WBC, CSF protein/glucose is typically normal	Can occur at any age Bilateral ON is more common in younger children (<10 years of age)
Transverse myelitis (TM)	Weakness Paresthesias Bowel/bladder dysfunction	Increased T2 signal, swelling, or Gd enhancement of the spinal cord	CSF pleocytosis and/or elevated protein seen in at least half of cases	Can occur at any age
Neuromyelitis optica (NMO)	Must have ON and TM	Spinal cord and optic nerve lesions longitudinally extensive. Brain lesions, if present, tend to occur in the hypothalamic region or midbrain	Positive NMO IgG in serum and/or CSF CSF WBC often very elevated (can be >100 cells)	Females predominantly affected (4.0:1.0 female to male) More commonly reported in African-American children

CSF, cerebrospinal fluid; Gd, gadolinium; IgG, immunoglobulin; WBC, white blood cells

TABLE 122-2 Differential Diagnosis of Demyelinating Disease

Diagnostic Category	Characteristic Clinical Features	Additional Investigations
Infectious/peri-infectious Bacterial, viral, fungal, or parasitic infections, such as: Herpes virus (HSV, VZV, CMV) EBV Mycoplasma Enterovirus Neuroborreliosis HIV Neurosyphilis Tuberculosis (TB) JC virus HTLV-1 Hepatitis A, B, and C Cryptococcus	Fever Meningsmus Rash (such as petechiae in bacterial meningitis or vesicles in herpes viruses) Systemic evidence of infection Alteration in mental status Acute, asymmetric flaccid myelitis	Blood and CSF cell counts and cultures PCR testing for infection in CSF TB testing Fungal culture
Rheumatologic Primary CNS angiitis Sarcoidosis Sjogren syndrome System lupus erythematosus Bechet syndrome Anticardiolipin or antiphospholipid antibody syndrome	Persistent and prominent headache Systemic evidence of vasculitis (not required) *Note:* Clinical, laboratory, and radiographic evidence of systemic disease may be absent in CNS vasculitis	ESR, ANA profile ACE level Antiphospholipid and anticardiolipin antibodies MRA of head Cerebral angiography Brain biopsy
Malignancy CNS lymphoma Glioma	History of prior malignancy and/or chemotherapy Systemic symptoms (weight loss, night sweats, fever) *Note:* With CNS lymphoma, symptoms may improve with administration of steroids	Blood smear CSF cytology Brain biopsy
Neuroimmune disorders Autoimmune encephalitis (such as NMDA-R encephalitis)	Encephalopathy Vital sign instability Movement abnormalities Psychiatric symptoms	Anti-NMDA receptor antibody from CSF and blood Abdominal ultrasound in females; testicular ultrasound in males (evaluate for teratoma) Consider other paraneoplastic antibody testing (based on clinical symptomatology)
Macrophage activation syndromes	History of similarly affected sibling Systemic signs of liver, skin, renal, or bone marrow involvement Persistent fever	Serum ferritin and triglycerides Soluble IL-2 receptor level Blood, CSF, and bone marrow evaluation for hemophagocytosis
Metabolic, Genetic, or mitochondrial disease Leukodystrophies MELAS	Symptomatic worsening with fever Pre-existing progressive neurologic deterioration, developmental delay, or cognitive dysfunction	Serum and CSF lactate/pyruvate MR spectroscopy Consider plasma amino acids, urine organic acids, ammonia, acylcarnitine profile
Vascular Cerebral Autosomal Dominant Arteriopathy with Subcortical Infracts and Leukoencephalopathy (CADASIL) Anterior spinal artery infarction	Prominent headaches Cognitive and psychiatric symptoms are common Family history of migraines, early onset dementia, and strokes	NOTCH3 genetic testing

Source: Data from Banwell B. Acute disseminated encephalomyelitis. In: Lisak R, Truong D, Carroll W, Bhidayasiri R, eds. *International Neurology*. Wiley-Blackwell; 2009:381-385; and Waldman AT, Shumski MJ, Tennekoon GI. Acquired demyelinating syndromes of the central nervous system. In: Abend NS, Helfaer MA, eds. *Pediatric Critical Care*. Demos Medical; 2012.

MANAGEMENT

In severe cases, acute demyelination may be life threatening and can impair respiration, especially if upper cervical cord or brainstem lesions are present. As a result, assessment of vital signs is a key part of the initial management of any patient with acute demyelination. Airway, breathing, and circulation should be assessed, and respiratory support should be quickly obtained if needed.

It is not always possible at the onset of CNS inflammation to determine the diagnosis. For example, inflammation of the optic nerves causing visual loss (i.e., ON, described below) may occur without any other clinical or radiographic neurologic findings (termed a clinically isolated syndrome) or may be a feature of ADEM, MS, MOGAD, or NMO. Therefore, acute therapy, targeting the CNS inflammation, is similar at presentation regardless of diagnosis. Most clinicians initiate a short course of corticosteroids intended to rapidly decrease inflammation and promote symptom recovery. Other therapies include intravenous immunoglobulin (IVIG) or plasma exchange in severe or refractory cases.

The care of children with ADS requires complex and multidisciplinary care teams, including practitioners experienced in the care of neuroimmune disorders, social workers, neuropsychologists, psychologists/psychiatrists, and physical, occupational, and speech therapists. Additional factors that impact outcomes in children with ADS include healthy weight, vitamin-D supplementation, avoidance of exposure to cigarette smoke, and physical activity.

CORTICOSTEROIDS

Though the optimal dose has not been established for pediatric patients, most clinicians prescribe 20 to 30 mg/kg/day (with a maximum of 1000 mg/day) of intravenous methylprednisolone for 3 to 5 days for initial treatment of an ADS requiring hospitalization. The use of a subsequent steroid taper is physician-dependent. If symptoms have markedly improved after intravenous treatment, additional treatment with oral prednisone may not be required and is controversial. For children with partial improvement but ongoing deficits, oral prednisone, starting at a dose of 1 mg/kg/day (max of 60 mg), can subsequently be administered and tapered over a few weeks.

Often treatment with corticosteroids is delayed due to concern for infection. Of note, corticosteroids are often used to treat patients with *Haemophilus influenzae* type b and pneumococcal meningitis and have been safely given in severe cases of herpes encephalitis. Therefore delaying treatment with corticosteroids due to concern for infection may not be necessary and is under further investigation. While steroids may be safe even in the presence of a viral or bacterial CNS infection, corticosteroids are contraindicated in fungal infections.

When administering high-dose corticosteroids, it is important to remember to also treat with an H_2 blocker or a proton pump inhibitor for gastrointestinal prophylaxis. Other less common side effects of corticosteroids to consider include hyperglycemia, hypertension, psychiatric symptoms (e.g., anxiety, psychosis), insomnia, and weight gain. Avascular necrosis can also occur and has been reported in a patient treated with corticosteroids for less than 1 month.

INTRAVENOUS IMMUNOGLOBULIN

IVIG has been reported to be effective in some children with ADS who do not respond to corticosteroids, or in some patients who experience recurrence of neurological deficits upon corticosteroid withdrawal. The typical dose administered is 2 g/kg divided over 2 to 5 days, though faster infusions can be safely used.

PLASMA EXCHANGE

For patients with ADS and severe neurologic deficits who fail to demonstrate clinical improvement by the third to fifth day of corticosteroid treatment or children with life-threatening demyelination or paralysis at onset, plasma exchange (PE) is the preferred second-line treatment modality. A typical PE regimen consists of 5 to 7 exchanges over a 2-week period. Notably, PE may impact interpretation of antibody assays for MOGAD and NMO and, when possible, laboratory testing should be undertaken prior to initiation of plasma exchange.

REHABILITATION

Physiatrists and physical, occupational, and speech therapists play a major role in the recovery of patients with CNS inflammation and should be consulted as early as appropriate during an admission. Some children will require transfer to a rehabilitation facility after discharge from the acute care setting, depending upon their clinical recovery.

CHRONIC IMMUNOMODULATION

Consideration of chronic immunomodulatory therapies, often referred to as disease-modifying therapies, should be entertained early in the disease course for cases of pediatric MS, relapsing MOGAD, and NMOSD. In particular, the treatment of pediatric MS focuses on preventing relapses and reducing the risk for secondary disease progression. There are well-established therapeutic strategies for pediatric MS and NMOSD and emerging consensus on similar chronic therapies for relapsing MOGAD. These therapies should be guided by subspecialty consultation.

In summary, ADS occur in children and often require hospitalization at symptom onset to fully evaluate the CNS and exclude alternative diagnoses. Treatment of CNS inflammation is often initiated before all of the diagnostic studies are obtained in the inpatient setting. The prototypical ADS are described in more detail below.

DEMYELINATING SYNDROMES

ACUTE DISSEMINATED ENCEPHALOMYELITIS

Approximately 25% of all children with an ADS will manifest with ADEM, which is defined by the International Pediatric Multiple Sclerosis Study Group (IPMSSG) as a clinical CNS event with a presumed inflammatory cause characterized by polyfocal neurologic deficits and encephalopathy not explained by fever or systemic illness. Though ADEM is typically a monophasic (i.e., isolated illness followed by recovery and no recurrence) pediatric disorder, multiphasic forms have been reported. ADEM-like initial attack can be the first presentation of a chronic demyelinating disorder, such as MS, MOGAD, or NMO.

Clinical Presentation To meet consensus criteria for ADEM, a patient must present with encephalopathy, which can be manifested by behavioral change, profound irritability, altered consciousness (including coma), and polyfocal neurologic deficits. Prodromal systemic symptoms such as fever, headache, and malaise can occur in the days prior to the onset of neurologic symptoms. The initial symptoms of ADEM may occur spontaneously without antecedent illness, but more typically begin within days to weeks of a febrile illness of presumed viral etiology. Upper respiratory tract infections are the most commonly reported preceding illnesses, followed by gastrointestinal infection, and then nonspecific febrile illnesses. Once neurologic symptoms begin, the clinical course progresses quickly and patients typically develop maximal symptoms over the following 3 to 5 days.

Neurologic symptoms in ADEM can vary and correspond to the sites of CNS inflammation in a particular patient. The most common neurologic features other than encephalopathy in ADEM include upper motor neuron symptoms, such as weakness, increased tone, and hyperreflexia, followed by ataxia and cranial nerve palsies.

DIFFERENTIAL DIAGNOSIS

In a patient with encephalopathy and neurologic symptoms, with or without a recent fever or illness, investigations are initially directed toward excluding active CNS infections and evaluating for recent viral exposures. The presence of fever, meningismus, rash, or systemic illness should raise suspicion for an infectious process rather than ADEM, although it may often be difficult to differentiate infections from postinfectious disorders if the neurologic symptoms coincide with the fever and systemic illness. Other symptoms and signs are particularly relevant, such as pain over a dermatome (with or without vesicular lesions), which may be caused by herpes infections. Adenopathy is present in cat-scratch disease and other infections. A patient presenting with encephalopathy and psychiatric symptoms or a movement disorder should raise concern for autoimmune encephalitis.

Diagnostic Evaluation • ***CSF Analysis*** A lymphocytic CSF pleocytosis (>10 cell/μL) and/or elevation of CSF protein is present in more than half of cases of ADEM. Oligoclonal bands detected in CSF but not detected in concurrent serum are rare but have been reported to be present acutely in up to 19% of patients with ADEM. Presence of CSF oligoclonal bands in this population is nonspecific, as intrathecal immunoglobulins can also be seen with CNS infection, but it is still recommended as part of the diagnostic evaluation in patients presenting with ADEM. Serologic evaluation for anti-MOG antibodies is recommended in patients who present with an ADEM phenotype.

MRI Features Radiologically, ADEM is typically characterized by multifocal T2/FLAIR hyperintense lesions in both the white and gray matter of the brain and spinal cord. Lesions are typically large with poorly demarcated margins. Visible lesions in the deep gray matter (i.e., thalamus and basal ganglia) are frequently noted. Typical radiologic features of ADEM are demonstrated in **Figure 122-1**. Though ADEM is thought to be an acute disorder, it is rare for all lesions to enhance with gadolinium, and some patients have no enhancing lesions. Meningeal enhancement, the presence of completely ring-enhanced lesions, and lesions that are

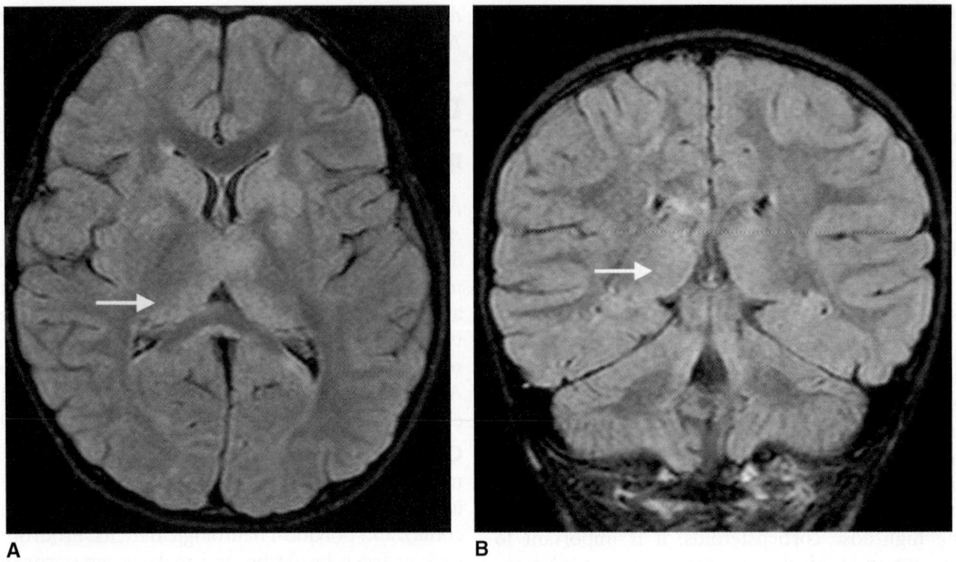

FIGURE 122-1. Common radiologic features of acute demyelinating encephalomyelitis: (A) axial and (B) coronal fluid-attenuated inversion recovery (FLAIR) images demonstrating typical radiologic features of ADEM. Lesions are typically large, asymmetric, and have poorly demarcated borders. Deep gray lesions are often visualized (arrow).

persistently T1 hypointense are uncommon in ADEM and suggest alternative diagnoses.

Management Treatment is based on the severity of neurologic symptoms. If the encephalopathy and polyfocal symptoms have resolved by the time of medical evaluation, acute treatment may not be necessary. For children with neurologic deficits, intravenous corticosteroids should be initiated. Typically, intravenous methylprednisolone is given for 3 to 5 days, during which time clinical improvement often occurs. An oral prednisone taper may be used subsequently if there is partial improvement but significant persistent neurologic deficits remain.

If the symptoms do not improve with intravenous steroids or children have life-threatening demyelination at onset, plasma exchange should be considered. IVIg has been reported to be effective in some children with ADEM who do not respond fully to corticosteroids, or in some patients who seem to experience recurrence of neurological deficits upon corticosteroid withdrawal. Additional details can be found in the Management section.

Although rare, some children with ADEM experience fulminant, life-threatening cerebral edema refractory to conventional medical management. In these cases, decompressive craniectomy may lead to rapid improvement and an improved outcome. Survival has been reported with combination treatment using corticosteroids, early plasma exchange, and decompressive craniectomy, if needed, in such cases.

Prognosis While the acute phase of ADEM can be severe and children are often ill-appearing, the prognosis of ADEM is generally favorable and the majority patients with ADEM recover fully. The average time to complete recovery ranges between 1 and 6 months, though patients typically show some improvement within a few days of starting treatment. Despite the favorable prognosis, minor residual deficits have been reported in up to 20% to 30% of children. Residual deficits depend on the clinical sites involved, with the most common residual deficits including motor dysfunction, visual and cognitive impairment, behavioral problems, and seizures.

Although ADEM is typically monophasic, a child may rarely experience a second ADEM-like attack. According to the most recent IPMSSG consensus criteria, multiphasic ADEM can be diagnosed if a patient experiences two attacks consistent with ADEM separated by at least 3 months. The second attack may be characterized by new symptoms or recurrence of prior symptoms. Should a patient have a third event, the diagnosis is no longer consistent with ADEM, and investigations into a more chronic inflammatory disorder should be pursued.

CLINICALLY ISOLATED SYNDROMES

As defined by the IPMSSG, clinically isolated syndrome (CIS) represents an initial event of CNS inflammation characterized by either monofocal or polyfocal neurologic dysfunction. In contrast to ADEM, encephalopathy is not a clinical feature in CIS and should not be present unless the brainstem is involved. CIS is a heterogeneous clinical syndrome and symptoms reflect the involved areas in the CNS. The two most common clinically isolated syndromes, ON and TM, are described below. Visual disturbances and spinal cord disease can also be seen in ADEM, MS, MOGAD, and NMO; therefore, it is important to determine whether the patient meets criteria for these alternate diagnoses. This often requires comprehensive imaging of the brain and spine for asymptomatic lesions. In other words, a patient presenting with a first clinical attack may actually have MS if the 2010 McDonald criteria are fulfilled (see MS section below).

Optic Neuritis ON is an acute inflammatory demyelinating event in which the anterior visual pathway (i.e., the optic nerve and/or chiasm) is affected. ON can be either unilateral or bilateral. Additionally, ON can occur either in insolation, or in the context of diffuse demyelination (e.g., as part of an attack of ADEM, MS, or NMO).

Clinical Presentation ON is typically associated with a disturbance in vision or decreased visual acuity, reduced color vision, decreased depth perception, and sometimes visual field defects. See **Table 122-3** for a summary of the ophthalmologic findings in ON. Eye pain is also typically reported with ON, and generally worsens with eye movement. Disc swelling can occur in ON, but it is not a required feature since its visualization depends on the site of optic nerve inflammation. If the inflammation occurs at the junction between the retina and optic nerve, disc swelling may be seen on funduscopic examination. However, if the inflammation affects the posterior optic nerve, disc swelling is not typically visible, and the term retrobulbar ON is preferred.

Differential Diagnosis ON can occur as an isolated inflammatory event but can also manifest as part of other inflammatory disorders, such as MS, MOGAD, NMO, ADEM, or chronic relapsing inflammatory optic neuropathy (CRION). Presence of other clinical features (e.g., myelopathy, encephalopathy, relapsing course, or poor response to therapy) can help to differentiate these entities.

Neuroretinitis, characterized by vision loss, optic disc swelling, and macular exudate, often occurs in the setting of infection and must be considered in the differential of inflammatory ON. Cat-scratch disease, caused by *Bartonella henselae*, is a common cause of neuroretinitis. Another common cause of optic neuropathy in the pediatric population is Lyme disease, caused by *Borrelia burgdorferi*, which should be investigated in the appropriate clinical context.

TABLE 122-3 Ophthalmologic Findings in Optic Neuritis

Test	Method		Findings
	Bedside Tests	Ophthalmologic Tests	
Visual acuity	Near card	Snellen or equivalent distance eye charts	Decreased visual acuity ranging from subtle deficits (such as 20/40) to severe visual loss (no light perception).
Color vision	Red desaturation	Ishihara color plates	Dyschromatopsia (difficulty with color vision).
Visual fields	Confrontational testing	Perimetry testing	Visual field defect (especially central scotoma).
Afferent pupillary defect	Swinging flashlight test: the examiner swings a light back and forth from one pupil to the other, and observes the size of the pupils as the patient gazes straight ahead	Swinging flashlight test	Normally, both the illuminated and nonilluminated pupil will constrict. In cases of optic neuritis, when light is moved away from the unaffected eye and toward the affected eye, the non-illuminated pupil will dilate from its prior constricted state.
Funduscopic examination	Undilated exam with an ophthalmoscope	Dilated examination with indirect and direct visualization of the optic nerve	Normal in retrobulbar optic neuritis, or disc edema is present in papillitis.

Leber hereditary optic neuropathy is a mitochondrial disorder that should be considered in patients presenting with bilateral subacute, painless vision loss. Vision loss typically progresses over weeks to months, and final visual acuity is less than 20/200 in both eyes. This disorder is most commonly diagnosed in males between the ages of 15 and 35 years.

Diagnostic Evaluation

CSF Analysis CSF analysis is not always obtained in cases of isolated ON. When done acutely, a lymphocytic pleocytosis has been reported in about 33% to 50% of patients, and CSF protein and glucose are usually normal. The presence of oligoclonal bands has been reported in patients with ON and can be predictive of a diagnosis of MS, especially when seen in conjunction with an abnormal brain MRI.

Imaging MRI of the orbits may be obtained to confirm a diagnosis of ON, and typically reveals optic nerve swelling, T2/FLAIR hyperintensity, and/or contrast enhancement of the optic nerve (**Figure 122-2**). In a study of 36 children with ON followed prospectively, neuroimaging of the optic nerve was found to be abnormal in 55% of the cohort.

In cases of ON, a brain MRI can lead to the confirmation of an MS diagnosis if asymptomatic brain lesions are present, thereby demonstrating dissemination in time and space (see Prognosis section below). Inflammation of the optic chiasm seen on a brain or orbit MRI should also raise suspicion for NMO or MOGAD. Similarly, an MRI of the cervical and thoracic spine can also be helpful, as they may reveal lesions suspicious for MS, MOGAD, or NMO.

Management In adults, the Optic Neuritis Treatment Trial has shown that treatment does not affect the long-term recovery of visual function (acuity) in ON. In this trial, the visual acuity at the conclusion of the study was favorable regardless of whether a subject received IV methylprednisolone, oral prednisone, or placebo. However, treatment with IV steroids has been shown to increase the rate of visual recovery in patients with ON. In addition, the use of oral steroids (specifically prednisone 1 mg/kg/day) in adults was associated with an increased risk of ON relapse. Therefore, many neurologists and ophthalmologists still administer IV methylprednisolone for 3 days, often followed by a taper of oral prednisone over 1 to 2 weeks.

Prognosis In pediatric patients with monophasic ON, visual recovery is typically excellent. The majority (76%-80%) of patients regain visual acuity of better than 20/40 in the affected eye. Of note, many children in these studies received IV methylprednisolone.

Though ON can be isolated and monophasic, it can also be the initial presentation of a chronic demyelinating disorder, such as MS, MOGAD, or NMO. Studies have shown that the presence of one of more clinically silent white matter lesions (outside the optic nerve) on brain imaging is strongly associated with a subsequent MS diagnosis. Children without additional clinically silent white matter lesions at onset are at very low risk for MS. ON is also a major criterion for NMO (discussed below). The visual deficits in NMO may not recover as readily as seen in monophasic ON. Finally, isolated ON (without brain or spinal cord lesions) can also rarely recur and is termed either sequential or recurrent ON depending on the affected eye and timing of relapse.

Transverse Myelitis TM is an inflammatory demyelinating disorder characterized by acute or subacute motor, sensory, and/or autonomic spinal cord dysfunction. Diagnostic criteria established by the Transverse Myelitis Consortium Working Group in 2002 require the presence of spinal cord inflammation, as evidenced by CSF pleocytosis, elevated IgG index, or gadolinium enhancement on spine MRI, with the exclusion

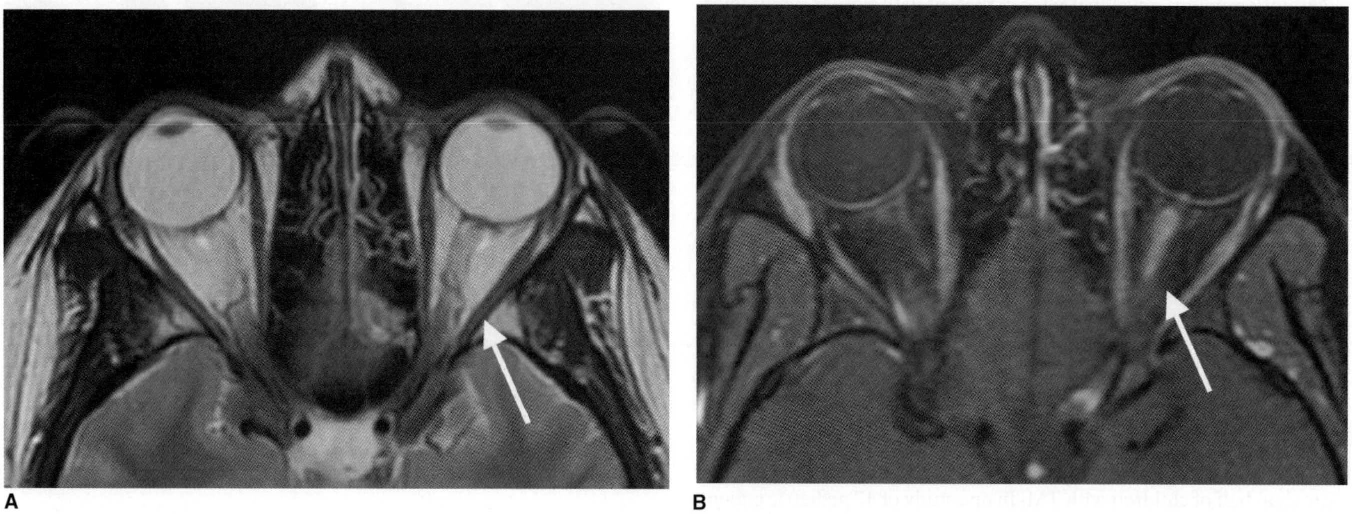

FIGURE 122-2. Typical radiologic features of optic neuritis: axial T2 weighted image (A) showing enlargement and increased signal (arrow). Axial T1 post-contrast image (B) demonstrating enhancement of the intraorbital left optic nerve (arrow).

of CNS infection, compressive myelopathy, or another underlying disease process that may account for symptoms (such as connective tissue disease or vascular malformations). Like ON, transverse myelitis can occur as a clinically isolated syndrome in which only spinal cord signs and symptoms occur, or can occur in the context of another demyelinating disease in which there may be brain and/or optic nerve involvement as well.

Clinical Presentation Symptoms that suggest spinal cord inflammation include acute respiratory failure, bowel or bladder dysfunction, weakness involving the legs and/or arms, and a Lhermitte sign (i.e., an electrical sensation that extends down the spine and is often elicited by forward flexion of the neck) with the absence of cortical signs (e.g., visual field deficits, aphasia, or neglect). In addition, positive sensory symptoms (e.g., tingling, burning) or sensory loss/numbness are common in patients with TM. Symptoms typically progress over days, and most patients reach their clinical nadir between 2 and 10 days after their first clinical symptom. In terms of motor dysfunction, while flaccidity and depressed reflexes are typically present initially, this evolves into spasticity and hyperreflexia over the course of about 1 week.

In patients with inflammatory TM, a sensory level (i.e., rostral border of sensory loss) may be detected on neurologic examination. In one case series, the sensory level was detected most commonly at a thoracic level. Additional findings on examination may include extremity weakness, sensory dysfunction (e.g., vibration, light touch, or temperature discrimination), and abnormal reflexes (may be depressed acutely or brisk if few days into the course).

Differential Diagnosis When a patient presents with suspected spinal cord pathology, a careful history and examination are urgently needed to determine the extent of neurologic injury, risk factors, and time course. First, a compressive lesion must be excluded. This is considered a neurologic emergency for which prompt imaging is required (see below). Compressive lesions can be caused by herniated discs, neoplasms, and other causes. A history of trauma or malignancy raises concern for a herniated disc or metastasis, respectively. Pathologic vertebral fractures or spondylolisthesis have also caused compressive lesions.

Guillain-Barré syndrome (GBS), an acute polyneuropathy, is another important entity to consider in the differential of TM and can sometimes be differentiated by a history of ascending weakness and lower extremity pain. Reflexes are often absent or depressed with GBS. CSF sampling, looking for elevated protein without an accompanying pleocytosis, and electromyography can help to confirm this diagnosis.

Acute flaccid myelitis (AFM) is a disorder seen with biennial outbreaks associated with enterovirus infection. AFM is a consideration in patients presenting with acute flaccid limb weakness. Contrary to TM, the motor involvement in AFM is often significantly asymmetric or unilateral. MRI of the spine shows predominantly gray matter lesions of the spinal cord in contrast to the white matter lesions typical of TM.

Noninflammatory myelopathies can present with similar symptoms to TM. These disorders include vascular, metabolic/nutritional, and neoplastic myelopathies. Vascular myelopathies should be considered particularly in patients with vascular territory lesions of the anterior spinal artery. Historical risk factors should prompt consideration of nutritional myelopathies related to vitamin B12, vitamin E, or copper deficiencies. Neoplastic myelopathies can occur as a result of primary spinal malignancies as well as CNS and intravascular lymphomas.

The timing of symptoms should also be noted and can help to differentiate TM from other disorders. As described above, symptoms in inflammatory TM progress over days, typically 2 to 10 days. In contrast, an ischemic process nadirs over several hours. The presence of fever, rash, meningismus, adenopathy, and active systemic infections are worrisome for an infectious etiology rather than an inflammatory process. The differential for infectious etiologies affecting the CNS is similar to other disorders and outlined in Table 122-2.

Diagnostic Evaluation

CSF Analysis A CSF pleocytosis or abnormal CSF protein is reported in more than half of children with TM. In one study of 47 pediatric patients with TM, the mean CSF WBC was 137 ± 67 cells/mm^3 and the mean CSF protein was 173 ± 75 mg/dL. In cases of isolated TM, it is uncommon for oligoclonal bands to be present in the CSF, which has been reported in less than 5% of cases. In fact, the presence of CSF oligoclonal bands should raise suspicion for another process such as MS, and further investigation should be pursued.

Imaging An MRI of the spine is typically notable for T2 signal abnormality in either the thoracic or cervical levels of the spinal cord in TM. Lesions can be small or longitudinally extensive (≥3 spinal segments) and there may be more than one lesion present (See **Figure 122-3**). One case series reported that the average number of spinal cord segments spanned for an acute TM lesion was six. Of note, longitudinally extensive cord lesions are also sometimes seen in cases of ADEM or NMO. Gadolinium enhancement of spinal cord lesions is also common in TM and has been reported in up to 74% of cases.

Rarely, the spine MRI in TM can be normal. In these cases, clinical symptoms and CSF findings are used to make the diagnosis.

Management When the diagnosis of TM is suspected, prompt treatment with corticosteroids should be initiated (see Management section above). If symptoms are severe or do not improve with steroids, early initiation of plasma exchange should be considered. In severe cases unresponsive to steroids and plasma exchange, immunosuppressive therapies such as cyclophosphamide can be used.

Prognosis The prognosis for acute TM is variable, and many children require intensive rehabilitation and ongoing support for activities of daily living. Studies have reported that up to 40% of children surviving TM remain wheelchair-dependent, 80% are left with residual bladder symptoms (30% of whom remain catheter dependent), and 27% require assistance for tasks of daily living. Pain and sensory symptoms may also persist. Depending on the severity of symptoms, evaluation by pain management specialists may be necessary.

Clinical factors that have been associated with better functional outcomes include shorter time to diagnosis, absence of complete paraplegia, and a lower sensory level found on examination. Young age at onset, requirement of respiratory support during the acute illness, and higher CSF WBC counts have all been shown to predict worse functional outcomes. In terms of prognostic radiologic features, the presence of T1 hypointensity at onset may correlate with worse ambulation outcomes.

Although TM is most commonly isolated and monophasic, it can also be the first presentation of a more chronic process such as MS or NMO. A number of studies have shown that with a normal brain MRI, likelihood of an MS diagnosis after the initial attack of TM is low. Longitudinally extensive cord lesions should prompt consideration of NMO or

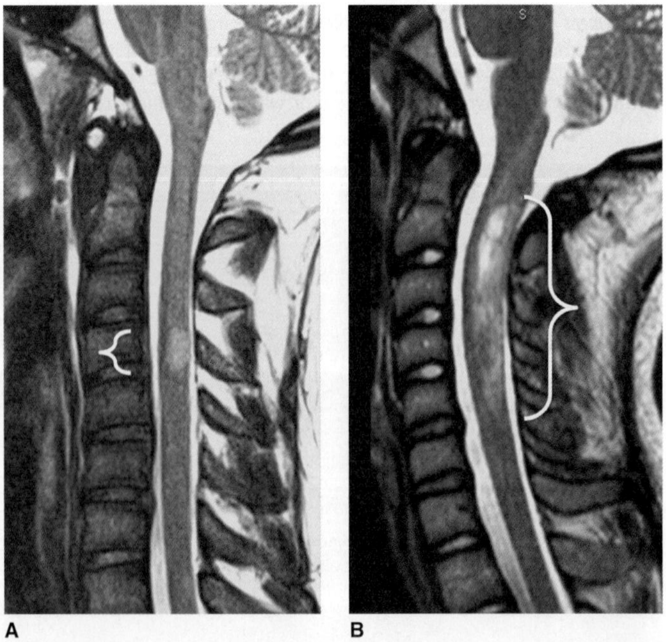

FIGURE 122-3. Common radiologic features of transverse myelitis: Sagittal T2 weighted images demonstrating short segment versus (left, small bracket) longitudinally extensive (right, large bracket) myelitis.

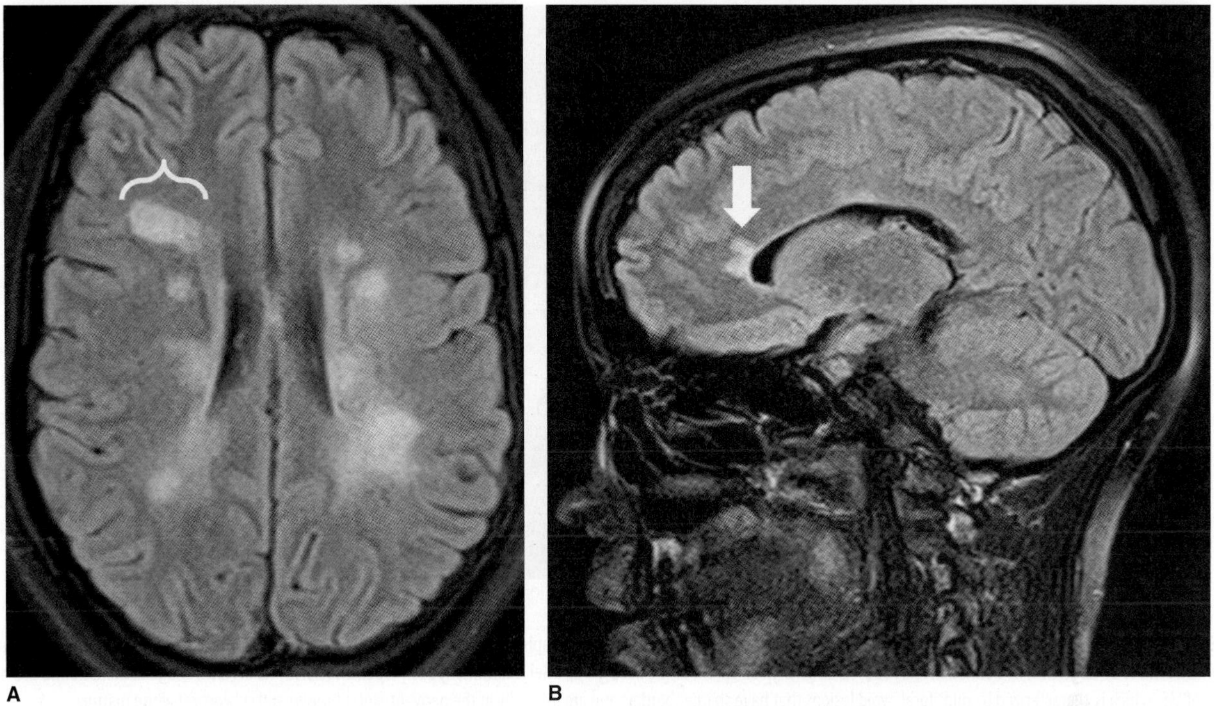

FIGURE 122-4. "Dawson's fingers"—A common radiologic feature of multiple sclerosis: (A) axial FLAIR image illustrating typical periventricular sharply demarcated ovoid lesions, (B) sagittal FLAIR image depicting Dawson's fingers extending from the corpus callosum, arranged at right angles to the ventricle.

MOGAD, especially if there is optic nerve or brainstem/hypothalamic involvement on MRI.

MULTIPLE SCLEROSIS

MS is a chronic demyelinating disease resulting in multiple areas of CNS inflammation in both children and adults. Using the 2010 revised McDonald criteria, a diagnosis of MS is confirmed after at least two clinical "MS-like" (i.e., nonencephalopathic) events separated by at least 30 days and involving different areas of the CNS (known as dissemination in time and space). Alternatively, a diagnosis of MS can be made at the time of a first clinical demyelinating "MS-like" event if a patient's MRI shows radiographic evidence of lesions that are disseminated in time and space using specific criteria.

As other diseases may clinically or radiologically mimic MS, it is imperative that an appropriate diagnostic workup be initiated to exclude these disorders in the correct clinical context (see differential diagnosis section and Table 122-1).

Clinical Presentation MS is characterized by transient neurologic symptoms, lasting days to weeks, due to areas of focal inflammatory demyelination in the CNS. Presenting manifestations are heterogeneous, reflecting the regions of the CNS that are involved. While ON and sensory symptoms are the most common initial presentations, other symptoms such as weakness or hemiparesis, ataxia, diplopia (secondary to an isolated intranuclear ophthalmoplegia or other cranial nerve palsy), and bladder or bowel dysfunction can also herald onset of this disease.

Differential Diagnosis In children, MS is almost exclusively relapsing-remitting, defined as attacks of neurologic dysfunction followed by periods in which symptoms either partially or completely improve without accrual of disability. Therefore the diagnosis should be questioned in any patient who presents with progressive neurologic symptoms from onset. Additionally, seizures and encephalopathy (in the absence of a brainstem lesion) are uncommon in pediatric MS.

Diagnostic Evaluation • ***CSF Analysis*** A lymphocytic pleocytosis has been reported in about 50% of children with MS, though a CSF WBC count greater than 50 is uncommon. CSF protein may be elevated, but this is not a requirement. Oligoclonal bands, which are a key diagnostic feature in adult MS, are less commonly seen in young children with MS. Studies have reported positive oligoclonal bands in approximately 80% of pediatric patients, with some variability explained by different methodologies of oligoclonal band detection.

Imaging MS lesions are hyperintense on T2-weighted or FLAIR sequences and are most commonly found in the periventricular white matter, corpus callosum, junctions of the gray–white matter (i.e., juxtacortical areas), and the spinal cord. "Dawson fingers" are a radiographic feature depicting demyelinating plaques through the corpus callosum, arranged at right angles to the ventricle, along medullary veins (i.e., callososeptal location) (**Figure 122-4**). Lesions that are chronically hypointense on T1 sequences are termed "black holes" and are associated with areas of severe white matter destruction and axonal loss.

When trying to radiologically distinguish MS from ADEM, features such as T1 hypointense lesions, periventricular lesion location, and absence of bilateral diffuse lesions have been found to be more consistent and predictive of MS. **Figure 122-5** compares and contrasts radiologic features of MS and ADEM.

Management Similar to the other ADS, intravenous corticosteroids are typically used to treat moderate to severe neurologic symptoms. Acute treatment is thought to hasten clinical recovery of neurologic symptoms but has not been shown to impact disease course or prognosis in adults. Therefore, not all attacks require acute therapy. Instead, the decision to initiate inpatient treatment is based on the severity of symptoms.

After the diagnosis of MS is confirmed, a patient will be started on disease-modifying therapy; typically interferon-beta (e.g., Avonex, Betaseron, Extavia, and Rebif) and glatiramer acetate (Copaxone) in the outpatient setting. These medications are given by injection (intramuscular for Avonex, all others are subcutaneous) and are not on hospital formularies. For established MS patients who are hospitalized for an MS flare, they must bring their own medication from home. Natalizumab (Tysabri) has also been used in the pediatric population and is given intravenously every 28 days. There are significant risks with this medication, namely progressive multifocal leukoencephalopathy (PML). PML has been reported in adults receiving natalizumab, especially those with exposure to natalizumab over 2 years, John Cunningham (JC) virus (a polyomavirus) positivity, and a history of immunosuppression.

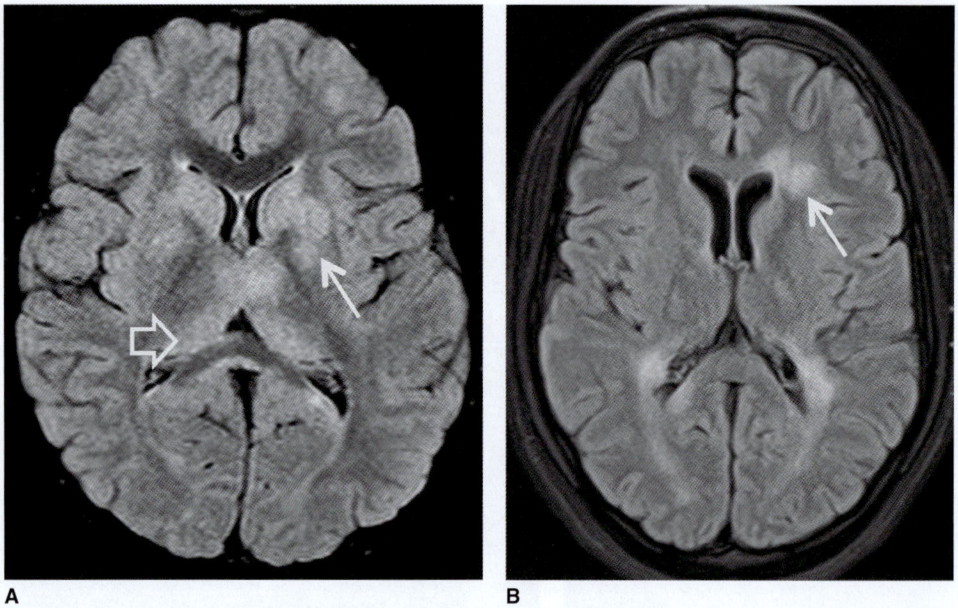

FIGURE 122-5. Acute demyelinating encephalomyelitis vs multiple sclerosis— contrasting radiographic features of ADEM and MS: (A) Axial FLAIR image demonstrating typical brain lesions in ADEM, which tend to be large with ill-defined borders (closed arrow). Involvement of the deep gray nuclei is commonly seen (open arrow). (B) Axial FLAIR image demonstrating the typical MRI appearance of MS, which is characterized by multifocal ovoid lesions that have sharper borders and are primarily in the periventricular (arrow) and subcortical white matter.

Given the risk of PML, natalizumab can only be given through certified centers familiar with the infusion protocol.

Prognosis Neurologic recovery after MS flares is typically more complete in children than in adults. As compared with adult patients, the relapse rate in children with MS is higher (1.12-2.76 in children vs 0.3-1.78 in adults), and 98% pediatric and adolescent patients have a relapsing-remitting course. Children typically accrue physical disability more slowly; however, children tend to have more relapses in the first 4 years after clinical onset and a larger number of and volume of new T2 lesions on brain MRI. One longitudinal study reported the median time from initial attack to secondary progression was 28 years, which is about 10 years longer than the average time reported for time to irreversible disability in adult MS patients.

NEUROMYELITIS OPTICA (NMO) AND NEUROMYELITIS OPTICA SPECTRUM DISORDERS (NMOSD)

NMO is a demyelinating disorder that is most commonly characterized by repeated attacks on the spinal cord and optic nerves. According to the most recent consensus criteria, a diagnosis of NMO requires at least one episode of ON and one episode of acute myelitis as major criteria, and either a longitudinally extensive cord lesion (≥3 spinal segments) or anti-aquaporin-4 antibody (NMO-IgG) seropositive status (discussed below). Of note, patients who are found to have a positive anti-aquaporin-4 antibody but do not meet all of the clinical criteria for NMO are considered to have an NMO-spectrum disorder.

Clinical Presentation ON occurs at disease onset in about half of pediatric patients with NMO, and about 15% of patients present with bilateral ON. Isolated TM, which often is longitudinally extensive, is the presenting episode in about one-quarter of patients with NMO, and simultaneous ON and TM is found in about 9% of patients at onset. In NMO, attacks are usually severe and can result in permanent motor and visual dysfunction.

Additionally, symptoms such as hiccups, nausea, and vomiting are often reported in patients with NMO and are usually referable to lesions involving the periaqueductal gray, an area rich in aquaporin-4. Coexisting autoimmune disorders are common in patients with NMO.

Differential Diagnosis Similar to the other acute demyelinating syndromes, infectious, metabolic, and systemic rheumatologic diseases must be considered (Table 122-2). Though recovery from clinical exacerbations may not be as complete or rapid in NMO as in MS, the diagnosis of NMO should still be questioned in any patient who presents with progressive neurologic symptoms from onset.

Diagnostic Evaluation • ***NMO-IgG*** NMO-IgG is considered a pathogenic autoantibody and biomarker for NMO that selectively binds aquaporin-4, a protein that is highly expressed in the astrocytic foot processes that forms a component of the blood-brain barrier. The antibody can be identified in both serum and CSF of NMO patients but is not currently required for diagnosis if the clinical criteria for NMO are met. In one study of a cohort of pediatric patients with clinically diagnosed NMO, 78% of children with relapsing NMO were found to be seropositive and only 12.5% of patients with monophasic NMO were found to have the NMO autoantibody. Serological testing for NMO-IgG has high specificity and has become more sensitive in recent years. Tests using recombinant aquaporin-4 antigen–based assays are preferred over tissue-based immunofluorescence.

CSF Analysis A CSF lymphocytic or neutrophil-predominant leukocytosis and/or elevated CSF protein are present in more than 70% of patients with NMO. In addition, it is not uncommon to have a CSF pleocytosis of more than 50 WBC per mm^3 in NMO. In fact, the CSF WBC may be several hundred or even reach 1000. Unlike with MS, oligoclonal bands are rare and are only reported in about 10% of cases.

Imaging In NMO, spine MRI commonly shows longitudinally extensive lesions spanning multiple cord segments often with cord edema. Brain imaging can vary from being normal without evidence of demyelination to showing large tumefactive supratentorial lesions. Most commonly, brain lesions in NMO tend to involve the brainstem and hypothalamic regions adjacent to the third and fourth ventricles. Acutely, MRI of the optic nerve in NMO patients may show longitudinally extensive, bilateral nerve swelling with enhancement that can include the optic chiasm. These lesions may later evolve to optic nerve atrophy.

Management To date, there have been few trials for the acute or chronic treatment of pediatric NMO. As a result, treatment recommendations are based on expert consensus and observational reports, although comprehensive reviews have become available in recent years. Management of an acute NMO attack is similar to treatment of any acute demyelinating flare (see Management section above) and begins with administration of high-dose intravenous corticosteroids. In contrast to the other disorders, early plasma exchange is recommended in patients with longitudinally extensive spinal cord lesions or those with significant brainstem involvement as it has been shown to improve clinical outcomes.

For long-term treatment, given the high rates of relapse in NMO, chronic immunosuppression is strongly considered to prevent ongoing attacks and disability accrual. A number of long-term treatments have been used for NMO including daily low-dose prednisone, mycophenolate mofetil, azathioprine, and rituximab, a monoclonal antibody to the CD20 antigen found on B cells, with variable success. Comprehensive reviews of therapeutic strategies are available for NMOSD; however, these therapies should be guided by subspecialty consultation.

Prognosis While NMO can be monophasic (i.e., a single event of simultaneous ON and TM without recurrent episodes of demyelination), >80% of patients have a relapsing course, with the diagnosis being confirmed at a time after the initial attack of isolated TM or ON. As compared with MS flares, recovery from NMO attacks is poor and patients can accrue permanent disability from each attack. Similar to MS, adults and children with NMO have been reported to have long-term cognitive sequelae that include memory, processing, and language dysfunction.

MYELIN-OLIGODENDROCYTE GLYCOPROTEIN ANTIBODY-ASSOCIATED DISEASE (MOGAD)

In recent decades, the recognition of ADS characterized by the presence of circulating antibodies toward myelin-oligodendrocyte glycoprotein (MOG) has led to a shift in diagnosis. While this disorder shares neuroimmune biology and may present with similar acute neurologic symptomatology as other ADS, such as MS and NMO, the underlying fundamental biological underpinnings and optimal treatments differ. MOG is a protein on the surface of oligodendrocytes that serves as a minor component of myelin with potential roles in cell adhesion. It is felt to be highly immunogenic and has been identified as a target of autoimmune antigens, particularly in children with ADS. MOGAD pathology has shown coexisting peri-venous and confluent demyelination with frequent presence of cortical and intracortical demyelinating lesions. CD4-positive T-cell inflammatory reaction with granulocytic inflammation is typical and differs from MS in which a CD8-positive predominant infiltrate is observed. The overall incidence is estimated between 1.6 and 3.4 per 1,000,000 person-years, with children accounting for up to half of reported cases. MOGAD is frequently diagnosed in younger children (age 10 and younger), as compared to MS and NMO, with a nearly equal male-to-female ratio.

Clinical Presentation While none of the clinical features of MOGAD are disease-specific, some are highly characteristic, including unilateral or bilateral ON, ADEM-phenotype, and TM. MOGAD is most often monophasic; however, relapsing courses can occur. The characteristic that distinguishes this disorder from other ADS (such as NMO, MS, and isolated ADEM, ON, and TM) is the presence of anti-MOG antibodies. The initial symptoms of MOGAD may occur spontaneously without antecedent illness, but more typically begin within days to weeks of a febrile illness of presumed viral etiology.

Differential Diagnosis The most common differential considerations include other ADS, such as NMOSD and MS. As with other ADS, additional differential considerations include genetic, infectious, inflammatory/autoimmune, neoplastic, toxic/metabolic, rheumatologic, and vascular disorders (Table 122-2).

Diagnostic Evaluation • ***MOG-IgG*** The antibody can be identified in both serum and CSF of MOGAD patients, although serum should be the specimen of choice given its greater sensitivity compared with CSF. Rarely, anti-MOG antibodies can be detected exclusively in the CSF. Antibody serology should be undertaken as close to a clinical episode as possible, as anti-MOG antibody titers decrease to below threshold levels within months. Anti-MOG-IgG seropositivity is considered necessary for the diagnosis of MOGAD. Serological testing for anti-MOG-IgG has high specificity and has become more sensitive and commercially available in recent years. Tests using cell-based assays are preferred. Low titers of anti-MOG antibodies have been occasionally detected in pediatric patients with typical MS, whereas detection of high anti-MOG antibody titers refutes a diagnosis of MS.

CSF Analysis A CSF lymphocytic or neutrophil-predominant leukocytosis is present in more than 70% of patients with MOGAD. Unlike with MS, oligoclonal bands are rare and are only reported in about 10% of cases.

MRI Features Often the MRI features of MOGAD have significant overlap with other ADS. Young children frequently present with ADEM phenotype with MRI revealing large, ill-defined lesions of the grey and white matter. These often show substantial improvement or resolution on follow-up imaging. White matter lesions can have a leukodystrophy-like pattern of involvement. In some cases, prominent cortical involvement can be present. MOGAD patients with optic nerve involvement often have longitudinally extensive and bilateral lesions. Similarly, spinal cord lesions in MOGAD can be longitudinally extensive and involve the conus.

Management For children with neurologic deficits, intravenous corticosteroids should be initiated. Typically, intravenous methylprednisolone is given for 3 to 5 days, during which time clinical improvement often occurs. An oral prednisone taper may be used subsequently if there is partial improvement, but significant persistent neurologic deficits remain.

If the symptoms do not improve with intravenous steroids or children have life-threatening demyelination at onset, addition of IVIg or plasma exchange should be considered. Plasma exchange is favored in children with severe or life-threatening demyelination. IVIg has been reported to be effective in some children with MOGAD who do not respond fully to corticosteroids, or in some patients who seem to experience recurrence of neurological deficits upon corticosteroid withdrawal. Additional details can be found in the Treatment section.

As a large portion of children with anti-MOG antibodies will remain monophasic, initiation of disease-modifying chronic immunomodulatory therapy may not be necessary after initial presentation. Consideration of chronic immunomodulatory therapy should be considered after a second event that signifies a relapse.

Prognosis Studies have indicated that many children with MOGAD will only have a single demyelinating event. A greater likelihood of having a monophasic disease course is associated with younger age of presentation, a presenting phenotype of ADEM, and conversion to seronegativity. In patients who do experience relapse, the time to second clinical event is typically between 5 and 12 months. In a prospective observational study, the majority (67%) of children who were positive for anti-MOG antibodies at initial presentation had complete neurologic recovery, 18% had marked improvement but did not return to entirely healthy neurologic function, 14% were left with moderate to severe neurologic deficits, and 1% died.

DEMYELINATING DISEASE WORKUP: KEY POINTS

- Brain MRI is always necessary in an acquired demyelinating syndrome as it delineates the extent of inflammation and can help prognosticate risk for MS diagnosis in CIS (especially cases of ON or TM).
- If clinical symptoms are referable to the spinal cord, spine MRI is warranted. Typically, the entire cord can be visualized with just a cervical and thoracic spine MRI.
- If CSF analysis is performed, oligoclonal bands should always be sent when considering a demyelinating etiology. A paired serum sample, which should ideally be collected at the same time, must also be sent within 48 hours.
- Screening labs for other systemic inflammatory diseases (see Table 122-2) should be considered and sent in the appropriate clinical context (i.e., other systemic symptoms present).
- Patients with demyelination may rarely have normal imaging and CSF studies at presentation. If the clinical level of suspicion remains high for demyelination, these studies should be repeated in 5 to 7 days, as the inflammation detected by these tests may lag behind the clinical symptoms.

ADMISSION CRITERIA

- Patient has persistent neurologic symptoms with or without clear etiology. Diagnostic workup should be tailored based on patient history and presenting symptoms.
- Intravenous therapy is required acutely due to the severity of symptoms.

DISCHARGE CRITERIA

- The patient is medically stable and has started to experience improvement of symptoms.
- No further IV therapy is required.
- The severity of neurologic symptoms does not warrant an inpatient admission for rehabilitation and the clinical course is improving without the need for escalating therapy.

CONSULTATION

Input from a neurologist is generally warranted to advise on diagnostic testing and appropriate treatment of all patients admitted with a demyelinating disease. Outpatient neurologic follow-up will be required whether the disease is monophasic or chronic. If a patient is diagnosed with MS or NMO, the patient will need to be started on immunomodulatory therapy by a neurologist, which is often done in the outpatient setting after discharge from the hospital. If a patient presents with visual dysfunction, an evaluation by an ophthalmologist or a neuro-ophthalmologist is also likely indicated.

KEY POINTS

- Visual or sensory disturbances are often the initial presenting symptoms of demyelination in the pediatric population. Therefore, practitioners should have a high index of suspicion when evaluating children with blurry or altered vision or paresthesias.
- The neurologic examination may be normal in children with isolated sensory or visual symptoms, and diagnostic imaging may still be warranted.
- When considering a demyelinating etiology based on symptoms, MRI of the brain, optic nerves, and cervical and thoracic spine may reveal pathology. Imaging should primarily be directed by presumed localization of symptomatology.
- Corticosteroids are first-line therapy for demyelination and their initiation should not be delayed unless there is a high suspicion for underlying CNS infection (especially fungal).
- Early referral to neurology can help guide evaluation and management of demyelinating disorders.

SUGGESTED READINGS

Banwell, B. Acute disseminated encephalomyelitis. In: Lisak R, Truong D, Carroll W, Bhidayasiri R, eds. *International Neurology*. Wiley-Blackwell; 2009:381-385.

Chitnis T. Pediatric central nervous system demyelinating diseases. *Continuum*. 2019;(3):793-814.

Defresne P, Hollenberg H, Husson B, et al. Acute transverse myelitis in children: clinical course and prognostic factors. *J Child Neurol*. 2003;18(6):401-406.

Lotze TE, Northrop JL, Hutton GJ, et al. Spectrum of pediatric neuromyelitis optica. *Pediatrics*. 2008;122(5):e1039-1047.

Murthy SN, Faden HS, Cohen ME, Bakshi R. Acute disseminated encephalomyelitis in children. *Pediatrics*. 2002;110 (2 Pt 1):e21.

Ness JM, Chabas D, Sadovnick AD, et al. International Pediatric MS Study Group. Clinical features of children and adolescents with multiple sclerosis. *Neurol*. 2007;68(16 Suppl 2):S37-45.

Polman CH, Reingold SC, Banwell B, et al. Diagnostic criteria for multiple sclerosis: 2010 revisions to the McDonald Criteria. *Ann Neurol*. 2011;69(2):292-302.

Waldman AT, Gorman MP, Rensel MR. Management of pediatric central nervous system demyelinating disorders: consensus of United States neurologists. *J Child Neurol*. 2011;26(6):675-682.

Waldman AT, Shumski MJ, Tennekoon GI. Acquired demyelinating syndromes of the central nervous system. In: Abend NS, Helfaer MA, eds. *Pediatric Critical Care*. Demos Medical; 2012.

Waldman AT, Stull LB, Galetta SL, et al. Pediatric optic neuritis and risk of multiple sclerosis: meta-analysis of observational studies. *J AAPOS*. 2011;15(5):441-446.

SECTION M
Newborn Medicine

CHAPTER 123 Delivery Room Medicine

Amy Rule, MD, MPH

BACKGROUND

A complicated and well-orchestrated sequence of physiologic cardiovascular and pulmonary changes must transpire in order for a normal transition from fetal to newborn physiology to occur. While most newborns transition from fetal to postnatal oxygenation and circulation without significant difficulty, ~10% require some degree of resuscitation in the delivery room and ~1% require significant resuscitation. Globally, perinatal events (e.g., birth asphyxia) account for almost one-third of the 2.4 million newborn deaths per year. Delays in establishing effective cardiorespiratory function may increase the risk for hypoxic-ischemic cerebral injury, pulmonary hypertension, and systemic organ dysfunction. Some of these injuries may be preventable with prompt and appropriate resuscitation. However, some of these outcomes are related to events or exposures that precede delivery, such as prenatal injuries, abnormal development, and insults to the intrauterine environment.

PATHOPHYSIOLOGY

The adaptation from intrauterine life to extrauterine life starts during the process of labor. Labor not only increases oxygen consumption in the transitioning fetus but also causes brief periods of asphyxia during contractions as umbilical venous blood flow is briefly interrupted. The fetus tolerates this interruption in blood flow because fetal tissue beds have greater resistance to acidosis than adult tissue beds. The fetus responds to bradycardia with the "diving reflex" whereby blood preferentially flows to the brain, heart, and adrenal glands. Finally, the fetus can switch to anaerobic sugar production when liver glycogen stores are adequate.

During labor and delivery, catecholamine levels surge and increase lung fluid resorption, release of surfactant, and stimulation of gluconeogenesis. This surge also helps direct blood flow to vital organs such as the heart and brain. With clamping of the umbilical cord, the low-resistance placental circuit is removed from the newborn's circulation. Systemic blood pressure increases, and transition to the postnatal circulation begins.

As a newborn takes the first few breaths, negative intrathoracic pressure is generated, which helps the lungs expand and become filled with air. Alveolar oxygenation increases as air replaces the fetal lung fluid. The negative intrathoracic pressure, however, is countered by lung compliance, lung fluid viscosity, and surface tension forces. Because these factors need to be overcome to establish adequate alveolar expansion, the newborn must take deep enough breaths to create the large transpulmonary pressure initially required after birth. Surfactant, a phospholipid-protein complex that is produced by type II pneumocytes and is deposited along the alveolar surfaces, also helps counteract alveolar surface tension and promote alveolar stability. As a result of the increasing effect of surfactant, less trans-pulmonary pressure is needed for subsequent breaths, and functional residual capacity is soon established. Pulmonary blood flow increases as the lungs expand, and pulmonary vascular resistance declines under the influence of oxygen-mediated relaxation of the pulmonary arterioles. This increase in pulmonary blood flow in turn allows the patent foramen ovale and the patent ductus arteriosus to functionally close, thereby allowing further blood flow to the lungs. The postnatal circulation is now that of a low-resistance pulmonary circuit and high-resistance systemic circuit, and the lungs assume the responsibility of gas exchange and oxygenation.

Asphyxia is defined as failure of gas exchange leading to a combination of hypoxemia, hypercapnia, and metabolic acidemia. If adequate ventilation and pulmonary perfusion are not rapidly established, a progressive cycle of worsening hypoxemia, hypercapnia, and metabolic acidemia ensues. Initially, blood flow to the brain and heart is preserved, whereas blood flow to the intestines, kidneys, muscles, and skin is sacrificed. However, maintenance of blood flow, even to vital organs, cannot be sustained endlessly. Ultimately, ongoing ischemia, hypoxia, and acidosis result in myocardial dysfunction and impaired cardiac output. Inadequate blood flow, perfusion, and tissue oxygenation may result in brain injury, multiorgan injury, and even death.

CLINICAL PRESENTATION

Clinical signs and symptoms of disrupted fetal-to-newborn transition include persistent cyanosis, bradycardia, hypotension, decreased peripheral perfusion, depressed respiratory drive, and poor muscle tone. Apgar scoring is an objective method of quantifying the newborn's status and to convey information about response to resuscitation, depicted in **Table 123-1**. The newborn is assessed at 1 and 5 minutes, and if the 5-minute score remains less than 7, additional scores should be assigned every 5 minutes for up to 20 minutes. Because resuscitation must be initiated before a 1-minute score is assigned, Apgar scores should not be used to determine need for resuscitation or to guide steps of resuscitation.

DIFFERENTIAL DIAGNOSIS

Multiple maternal, placental, mechanical, and fetal problems may occur at any point during pregnancy, labor, or delivery and can jeopardize a smooth fetus-to-newborn transition. During pregnancy, fetoplacental circulation can be compromised for a variety of reasons, including but not limited to maternal hypotension or hypertension, placental abnormalities (e.g., placenta previa, placental abruption) or maternal clotting or autoimmune disorders. During or around labor, a fetus with intrauterine growth restriction (IUGR) may be intolerant of even brief and intermittent interruptions of umbilical blood flow during contractions. Issues such as cord compression and shoulder dystocia during labor can also compromise blood flow to the newborn. After delivery, causes of newborn respiratory depression are numerous and can include respiratory

TABLE 123-1 Apgar Scoring

	Score of 0	Score of 1	Score of 2
Skin color/ Complexion	Blue or pale all over	Blue at extremities Pink body (acrocyanosis)	No cyanosis Body and extremities pink
Pulse rate	Absent	<100	≥100
Reflex irritability	No response to stimulation	Grimace/Feeble cry when stimulated	Cry or pull away when stimulated
Muscle tone	None	Some flexion	Flexed arms and legs that resist extension
Breathing	Absent	Weak, irregular, gasping	Strong, lusty cry

Source: Data from Weiner G, Zaichkin J, eds. *Textbook of Neonatal Resuscitation*. 8th ed. Elk Grove Village, IL: American Academy of Pediatrics and American Heart Association; 2021.

distress syndrome (lack of mature lung tissue for gas exchange), maternal narcotic administration or anesthesia, and airway obstruction from material such as meconium or blood.

The end result of any of these situations is inadequate alveolar oxygenation, which may lead to the development of persistent pulmonary hypertension of the newborn (PPHN). In this condition, also known as persistent fetal circulation, the pulmonary arterioles remain constricted, thereby preventing adequate blood flow to the lungs and resulting in hypoxia and acidosis. Hypoxia and acidosis mediate sustained constriction of the pulmonary arterioles, and a vicious cycle ensues as progressively deoxygenated blood circulates. Transitional physiology does not occur normally, and unoxygenated blood is shunted away from the high-pressure lung circuit. Systemic organ dysfunction and, more importantly, long-term neurologic compromise may result.

MANAGEMENT

OPTIMIZING DELIVERY ROOM RESUSCITATION

Anticipation, adequate preparation, accurate evaluation, and prompt initiation of support are critical for successful neonatal resuscitation. Well-trained personnel must be immediately available in any setting in which a newborn might be delivered. Every birth should be attended by at least one person whose primary responsibility is the newborn and who is able to initiate resuscitation if needed. Resuscitation equipment should be readily available for each and every birth and lists exist to help this preparation. Personnel attending deliveries should be familiar with the organization of the equipment so that resuscitation can be promptly initiated and support provided. Equipment should be checked at regular intervals and immediately before any delivery. Expiration dates of medications should be monitored regularly.

When preparing for delivery, trained neonatal providers should collaborate with obstetric providers and ask four questions in preparation for birth: (i) Gestational age?; (ii) Amniotic fluid color?; (iii) Additional maternal or fetal risk factors?; and (iv) Umbilical cord management plan? Significant maternal medical history, gestational age, prenatal complications, medications, illicit drug use, and prenatal laboratory values should be discussed. Risk factors for sepsis, including group B streptococcus carrier status, length of rupture of membranes, maternal fever, evidence of chorioamnionitis, and use of intrapartum antibiotics, should be assessed. Specific indicators of fetal condition such as heart rate monitoring, lung maturity, presence of meconium-stained fluids and antenatal ultrasound findings should be communicated. If a high-risk delivery is anticipated in which significant resuscitative intervention may be necessary, a prenatal consultation by the pediatric team should be performed if time permits, and additional skilled personnel should be present at delivery.

The final question is to discuss an umbilical cord management plan with the obstetrics team. Delayed umbilical cord clamping for 1 to 3 minutes is the standard of care for stable term and preterm newborns after either a vaginal and Cesarean delivery. This intervention been shown to raise hemoglobin levels after birth and increase iron stores up to 6 months of age, without increasing risk of hyperbilirubinemia or polycythemia. For preterm newborns, delayed cord clamping may be associated with decreased risk of interventricular hemorrhage and necrotizing enterocolitis. However, delayed cord clamping is contraindicated in the presence of a complication and/or a congenital anomaly requiring immediate attention.

INITIAL STEPS OF DELIVERY ROOM RESUSCITATION

At each birth, three primary questions about the newborn well-being should be asked when assessing need for intervention after birth: (i) Is the newborn at term gestational age?; (ii) Is there breathing or crying?; and (iii) Does the newborn have good tone? If the answer to any of these questions is "No," further resuscitation should be initiated. Newborns who are breathing/crying with good tone and at least 35 weeks can have delayed cord clamping and can stay skin-to-skin on their parent's chest and receive routine care. Providers can help parents consider early initiation of breastfeeding while continuing to monitor during the first hour of life.

For newborns in distress and/or who are preterm, warmth under a pre-heated radiant warmer or skin to skin with parent should be provided. Providers should initiate rapid drying and stimulating with prepared warm blankets. Newborns delivered preterm or term newborns who continue to show signs of distress after initial steps of warming and drying should be moved to a pre-warmed warmer for further evaluation if not already there.

At the warmer, the newborn's head should be positioned in a neutral or "sniffing" position, which allows alignment of the posterior pharynx, larynx, and trachea for maximal airway patency. Providers should evaluate if the newborn has visible secretions including but not limited to meconium in their mouth or nares. It is no longer recommended to suction all newborns. If secretions are visualized, a bulb suction should be used to clear the airway of any potential obstructions. The mouth should be suctioned first because suctioning the nose and nasopharynx may cause gagging and aspiration of oral secretions. Catheter suction should be reserved for significant airway obstruction with failure of improvement after bulb suction. Vigorous suctioning of the posterior pharynx should be avoided as it can delay positive pressure ventilation and can delay transitioning due to nasal or airway edema.

In addition to drying and airway clearance, respirations can be further encouraged by briefly providing tactile stimulation to the newborn with gentle yet vigorous rubbing of the trunk, back and extremities. These initial steps of newborn resuscitation should take less than 30 seconds, at which point respirations, presence of chest rise, and heart rate should be evaluated. Heart rate can be evaluated by auscultating the chest or palpating the umbilical pulse. The clinician checking the heart rate should verbalized to the team if the heart rate is less than or above a 100 beats per minute (bpm).

VENTILATION ASSISTANCE

The goal of resuscitation is for every newborn to either be breathing spontaneously or receiving effective positive pressure ventilation with consistent, symmetrical chest rise by 60 seconds of life. This is referred to as the "golden minute." If a newborn of any gestation is breathing spontaneously at 60 seconds and has a heart rate greater than 100 bpm, but demonstrates persistent respiratory distress or cyanosis, clinicians should administer continuous positive airway pressure (CPAP) starting at a positive end expiratory pressure (PEEP) of 5 cm H_2O. CPAP maintains pressure within the lungs of a breathing newborn, which can help to keep surfactant-deficient alveoli from collapsing and improve aeration and ventilation.

If the newborn is apneic, gasping or in severe distress, or if the heart rate is below 100 bpm, positive pressure ventilation (PPV) should be initiated at a rate of 40 to 60 breaths per minute. Initial peak inspiratory pressure should start at 20 mm Hg or with a self-inflating bag enough to obtain gentle chest rise. After 15 seconds of PPV, the newborn should be reevaluated to ensure ventilation is adequate. After 15 seconds of starting PPV the heart rate should be increasing and by 30 seconds should be greater than 100 beats per minutes. If heart rate is not improving, assure the chest is moving. For term and late preterm newborns, clinicians should be able to visualize the gentle rise and fall of chest rise with each breath. If the chest is moving, continue with an additional 30 seconds of PPV. If not moving, initiate corrective steps to improve ventilation.

If ventilation is inadequate without chest rise and/or no increase in heart rate after 15 seconds, corrective steps should be taken to improve chest rise and heart rate. It is helpful to remember the corrective steps through the acronym: MRSOPA: **M**ask adjustment, **R**eposition the head and neck, **S**uction the mouth and nose, **O**pen the mouth, **P**ressure increase, and **A**lternative airway (**Table 123-2**). With the initiation of either CPAP or PPV, a pulse oximeter should be applied to the right wrist and cardiac monitors should be initiated. In addition, when using of CPAP or PPV for longer than 30 to 60 seconds, clinicians should consider inserting an orogastric tube to decrease gastric distension.

ASSESSMENT OF SUPPLEMENTAL OXYGEN REQUIREMENT

Central cyanosis caused by low oxygen will appear as a blue hue to the lips, tongue, and torso. However, studies have shown that clinical assessment of skin color is not very reliable. Therefore, an oximeter probe should be placed in a preductal location (right wrist or right palm) to confirm perception of central cyanosis and to determine need for supplemental

TABLE 123-2 "MRSOPA" Acronym for Steps to Improve Response to Positive Pressure Ventilation

Step	Interventions
Mask Reposition	Check the seal of the mask; air leak most commonly occurs around the nasal bridge and more downward pressure may be required.
	Check the position of the mask on the face and consider different size if needed.
	Reposition the head to a sniffing position, assure no fingers are obstructing the airway externally
Suction	Suction the mouth then the nares to assure secretions and/or meconium are not obstructing the airway
Open Mouth/ Airway	In order to suction you will need to open the mouth. Assure that hand position around the mask is not preventing the mouth from opening.
Pressure Increase	Gently increase the pressure by small increments watching for gentle chest rise. It is important to do this gradually to decrease risk of barotrauma.
Alternative Airway	If all steps have been completed and chest rise cannot be achieved and/or the heart rate is not improving, consider endotracheal intubation or laryngeal mask airway placement.

oxygen whenever PPV or CPAP is initiated along with cardiac monitors. For newborns > 35 weeks, resuscitation should be initiated using room air (21%) and then be guided by oximetry to titrate supplemental oxygen to achieve saturations that approximate normal transitioning from in utero to extrauterine values. For newborns < 35 weeks, oxygen titration can start between 21% and 30%. **Table 123-3** demonstrates the time course for targeted oxygen saturation values after birth, which range from approximately 60% at 1 minute of life to approximately 90% at 10 minutes of life. If considering endotracheal intubation and/or chest compressions, the newborn should be given a 100% oxygen until the heart rate is at least 60 bpm.

BAG-MASK VENTILATION

The first breath must be large enough to ensure alveolar expansion such that functional residual capacity is established. This sometimes requires initial breaths with a pressure of 20 to 25 cm H_2O. Once functional residual capacity is established, less pressure is likely to be necessary. Care should be taken to prevent overdistention and hyperventilation during resuscitation. Over-distention from bag-mask ventilation using high airway pressure—and therefore applying large tidal volumes—may impair venous return to the heart and may also lead to air leak syndromes. The goal of positive-pressure ventilation is to provide just enough pressure to inflate and aerate the lungs and avoid injury.

Masks with air-filled cushions help maintain a tight seal without inflicting facial or ocular injury. The mask should rest on or just below the nasal bridge and the chin (not below the chin). Multiple mask sizes should be available at every birth. Infant masks are cushioned and come in two shapes (i) anatomically shaped triangle and (ii) round. The point of the anatomical mask goes over the nose. It is important to test a mask seal on your hand prior to delivery when checking equipment. A good seal is necessary to achieve effective positive pressure ventilation to inflate the newborn's lungs. For both administering PPV and CPAP, the mask should be held by cupping the chin with the thumb and index finger (a "C" shape of the clinician's hand). Additional fingers should be placed along the bony angle of the jaw and can aid in gently lifting the jaw upward and helping to maintain the sniffing position. Once in position, gentle pressure can be applied downward to achieve a good seal. Preterm or growth-restricted newborns may need a smaller mask than expected and this may lead to challenge in achieving a good seal. It may also be difficult to get a good seal if the mask is not sufficiently inflated. Corrective steps should be taken to achieve a good seal.

Three types of devices are available for PPV of the newborn. A self-inflating bag (Ambu) inflates automatically without a compressed gas source, and should be available as a backup wherever resuscitation may be needed, in case of other equipment failure. CPAP cannot be delivered reliably with this device, and maximal oxygen delivery is only 40% unless an oxygen reservoir is attached. A flow-inflating or "anesthesia" bag inflates only when there is continual flow from a compressed gas source and when the outlet of the bag is sufficiently occluded with a tight mask seal against the face. CPAP can be delivered with a flow-inflating bag. For both the self-inflating bag and the flow-inflating bag, the use of a pressure-gauge is recommended to monitor peak inspiratory pressure and to help maintain consistency of each assisted breath. Finally, a T-piece resuscitator (Neopuff™) provides flow-controlled and pressure-limited breaths using gas from a compressed source (see **Figure 123-2**).

ENDOTRACHEAL INTUBATION

Endotracheal intubation is required when adequate ventilation is not achieved using bag mask ventilation indicated by persistent heart rate under 100 bpm after at least 60 seconds of effective PPV or unsuccessful PPV after corrective steps. Endotracheal intubation as a step should be prioritized over chest compressions or medications in the setting of a heart rate under 60 bpm. The procedure for endotracheal intubation is detailed in Chapter 194 and gives specifics regarding correct endotracheal tube (ETT) sizes and insertion depth based on gestational age and weight. A CO_2 detector will assist in confirming tracheal placement of an ETT along with a rapidly, rising heart rate. However, a CO_2 detector may not change color if adequate circulation has not been established despite proper ETT placement, such as in the case of a patient in cardiopulmonary arrest. Moreover, a CO_2 detector will not indicate whether an ETT is in the correct position along the trachea. Therefore, it is recommended that a CO_2 detector be used during initial intubation but that the ETT position ultimately should be confirmed with chest radiograph. If intubation is not feasible or successful after several attempts, an alternative for newborns >2 kilograms (kg) is the use of a laryngeal mask (LMA). LMAs can provide a better seal than a face mask alone and may help improve ventilation. They are particularly helpful in newborns with craniofacial anomalies.

CIRCULATORY SUPPORT

Chest compressions are indicated if the heart rate is absent or remains less than 60 bpm after at least 30 seconds of effective ventilation, ideally through a properly inserted endotracheal tube or laryngeal mask. Inaccurate evaluation of heart rate can lead to unnecessary chest compressions, cardiac monitors should be used to full assess heart rate once PPV starts. Lack of circulation may make a pulse oximeter reading difficult in this setting, all newborns receiving chest compressions should be administered 100% oxygen.

The two thumb-encircling method is now the preferred technique to administer compressions, because it results in optimal peak systolic and coronary perfusion pressure. However, care should be taken to avoid limiting chest expansion during ventilation with this method. Chest compressions are performed on the lower third of the sternum immediately above the xiphoid process to a depth of one-third the anteroposterior diameter of the chest, with the goal of generating a palpable pulse. Chest compressions are performed in coordination with ventilations at a 3:1 ratio such that 90 compressions and 30 ventilations occur in 1 minute. As depicted in **Figure 123-1**, the newborn should be reassessed

TABLE 123-3 Target Ranges of Pre-Ductal Oximetry Values During First 10 Minutes of Life for Uncomplicated Term Newborns

	Target Oximetry Values
1 minute	60%-65%
2 minutes	65%-70%
3 minutes	70%-75%
4 minutes	75%-80%
5 minutes	80%-85%
10 minutes	85%-95%

Source: Data from Weiner G, Zaichkin J, eds. *Textbook of Neonatal Resuscitation*. 8th ed. Elk Grove Village, IL: American Academy of Pediatrics and American Heart Association; 2021.

60 seconds after initiation of chest compressions and coordinated ventilation to determine next steps in the resuscitation algorithm. If heart rate is >60 bpm, clinicians should continue PPV and adjust oxygen. If less than 60 bpm, clinicians should continue coordinated compressions with ventilation and consider medications.

VASCULAR ACCESS

If the newborn's response to resuscitative measures continues to be poor, vascular access should be obtained for administration of medications and volume expansion as needed. Peripheral intravenous access can be difficult and time consuming, especially if hypoxia or acidosis is present. Emergency vascular access can be achieved via the umbilical vein as described in Chapter 192. If the umbilical vein cannot be cannulated and peripheral access is unsuccessful, intraosseous access, described in Chapter 191, can be used as an alternative route for medications or volume expansion.

MEDICATIONS

Drugs are rarely but sometimes necessary in newborn resuscitation. Epinephrine is indicated when the heart rate remains lower than 60 bpm

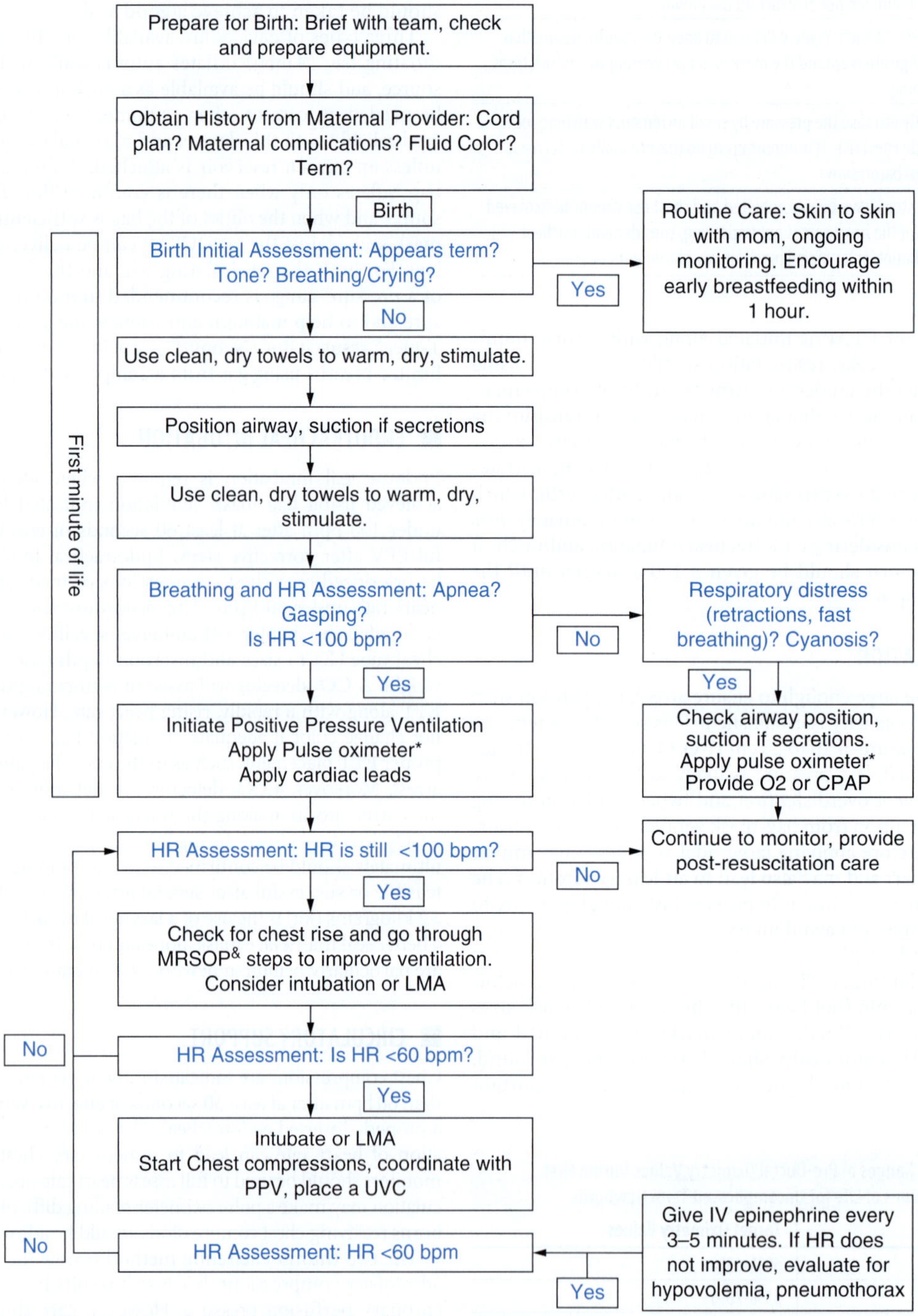

*Target oxygen saturations are as follows: 60–65% at 1 minute of life, 65–70% at 2 minutes, 70–75% at 3 minutes, 75–80% at 4 minutes, 80–85% at 5 minutes, and 85–95% at 10 minutes.

&MRSOP: adjust Mask to improve seal, Reposition head and airway, Suction, Open mouth and airway, increase Pressure

FIGURE 123-1. Algorithm for newborn resuscitation. (From Weiner G, Zaichkin J, eds. *Textbook of Neonatal Resuscitation*. 8th ed. Elk Grove Village, IL: American Academy of Pediatrics and American Heart Association; 2021. Copyright © 2022 American Academy of Pediatrics. All rights reserved.)

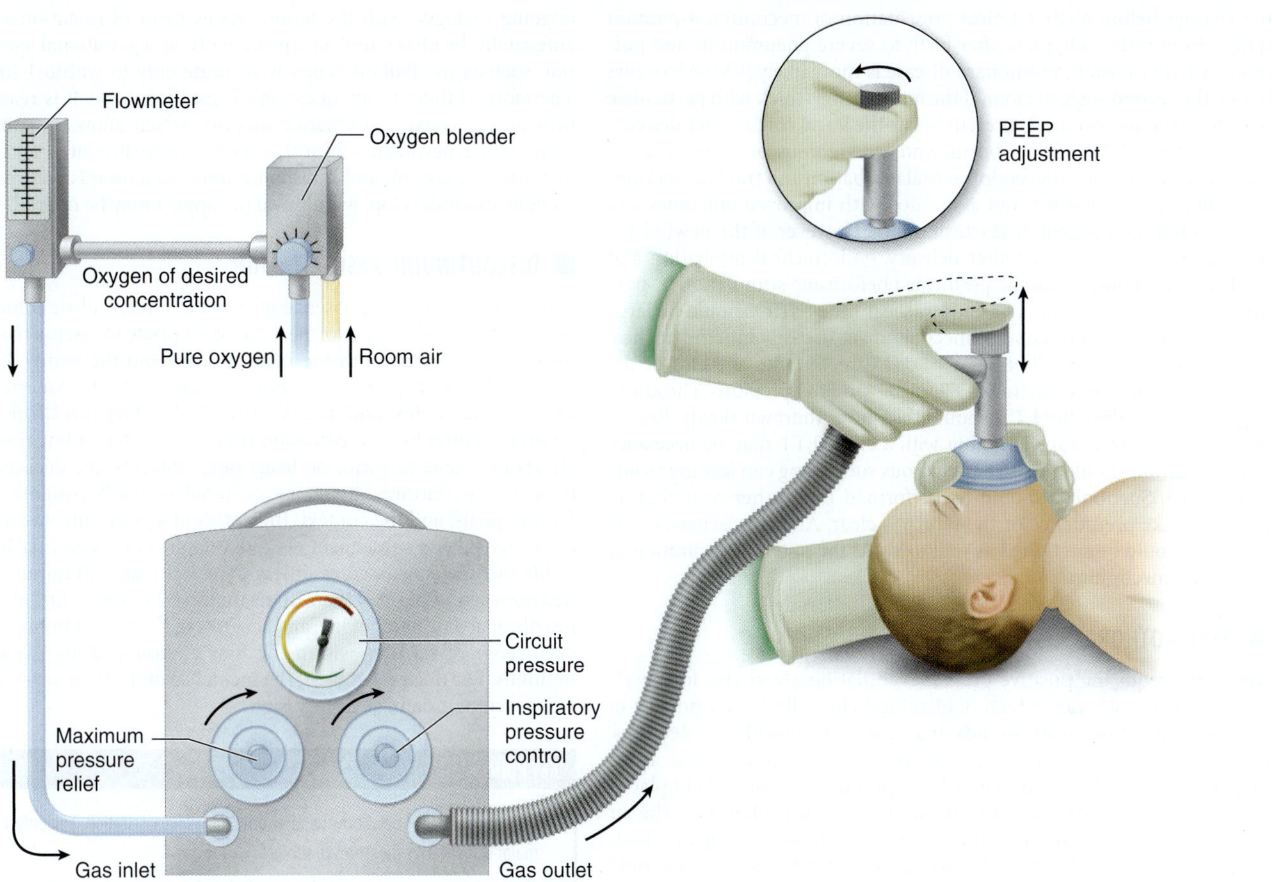

FIGURE 123-2. T-Piece resuscitator to provide continuous positive airway pressure, positive pressure ventilation, and blow-by oxygen. (Redrawn from Kattwinkel J, ed. *Textbook of Neonatal Resuscitation*. 6th ed. Elk Grove Village, IL: American Academy of Pediatrics and American Heart Association; 2011.)

after 30 seconds of effective ventilation and 60 seconds of coordinated PPV with 100% oxygen and cardiac compressions. Epinephrine is not indicated if the clinician has not established ventilation that inflates the lungs and moves the chest. The α-vasoconstrictive properties and the positive cardiac chronotropic effects of epinephrine aid in improving spontaneous circulation. The epinephrine concentration should be 0.1 mg/mL = 1 mg/10 mL for all newborns. If given intravenous/intraosseous a 1 mL syringe should be drawn up and labeled Epinephrine-IV. The IV/IO dose is 0.02 mg/kg (equal to 0.2 mL/kg) may be given rapidly every 3 to 5 minutes with a 3 mL saline flush. Epinephrine may be administered intratracheally; however, the intravenous route is preferred. If administered via the endotracheal tube, a 3 to 5 mL syringe should be prepared and labeled ET ONLY. The endotracheal dose is 0.1 mg/kg (1 mL/kg). The dose should be administered rapidly and can be repeated every 3 to 5 minutes as needed.

Naloxone administration is indicated for severe respiratory depression that persists despite a normal heart rate and color after delivery of positive-pressure ventilation in the setting of maternal narcotic administration within 4 hours of delivery. Naloxone has a rapid onset of action within 1 to 2 minutes, but it also has a short duration of action; repeated doses may therefore be needed. The dosage of naloxone is 0.1 mg/kg, and it can be administered via the endotracheal tube, subcutaneously, intramuscularly, or intravenously. If given to a newborn with chronic intrauterine opioid exposure, naloxone may precipitate acute withdrawal, including severe seizures and long-term sequelae, and it is therefore contraindicated in this scenario. Naloxone is ineffective for respiratory depression due to magnesium sulfate exposure.

Volume expansion should be considered in situations in which hypovolemia progresses to hypovolemic shock. This may occur as a result of inadequate supply, as with umbilical cord compression, or increased loss of blood. Significant hemorrhage may be due to placenta previa or placental abruption, fetomaternal bleeding, internal hemorrhage, or twin-twin transfusion syndrome. Recommended options for volume resuscitation include normal saline or type O-Rh-negative packed red blood cells. Any of these solutions should be administered slowly and in increments of 10 mL/kg, as cardiac function may be compromised during shock and may be exacerbated by an acutely expanded preload volume. Intracranial hemorrhage is a potential consequence of rapid volume expansion, especially in preterm newborns. Reassessment, including blood pressure, perfusion, and oxygenation, is essential before additional doses.

ADMISSION CRITERIA AND CONSULTATION

Transfer from the delivery room to a neonatal intensive care unit or consultation with a neonatologist (or both) is recommended in the following circumstances:

- Existence of or suspicion of a significant fetal anomaly, including Down syndrome, ambiguous genitalia, or cardiac or gastrointestinal malformation
- Persistent respiratory distress/tachypnea
- Newborns requiring respiratory or cardiac support
- Prolonged resuscitation or delivery requiring cardiac compressions

Of note, many newborns with minor concerns can remain in a mother's room to facilitate family bonding. Simple anomalies such as supernumerary digits, hypospadias, or a cleft lip or palate may not require admission to the neonatal intensive care unit.

SPECIAL CIRCUMSTANCES

MECONIUM-STAINED AMNIOTIC FLUID

Meconium-stained amniotic fluid (MSAF) is caused by a reaction to fetal hypoxemia, acidemia, stress, or any combination of these precipitants. If in utero stress is significant, the meconium may be aspirated into the airways before birth. Clinical presentation of meconium aspiration ranges from mild tachypnea after birth to severe pneumonitis and pulmonary hypertension. Pulmonary disease is more likely if MSAF occurs before the second stage of labor, if the meconium is thick with particulate material, or if meconium is present below the vocal cords. After delivery in the setting of MSAF, newborns who are vigorous or crying require routine resuscitation only; endotracheal intubation and tracheal suctioning is not indicated as it is not associated with improved outcomes and may result in esophageal or tracheal injury. However, if the newborn is non-vigorous or depressed after delivery, endotracheal intubation and tracheal suctioning should be performed before any stimulation or positive-pressure ventilation. The endotracheal tube (ETT) should be large enough to remove thick copious meconium yet fit easily into the trachea. A meconium aspirator should be placed directly onto the end of the ETT and connected to suction at 80 to 100 cm H_2O pressure. The entire apparatus, including the ETT, should then be withdrawn slowly. Repeat intubation and tracheal suctioning with a clean ETT may be necessary though caution should be used as vigorous suctioning can leading to airway edema. Suctioning should be performed until other resuscitation priorities take precedence or the return is clear. After resuscitation, the stomach should be suctioned as well to avoid the potential aspiration of swallowed meconium.

PNEUMOTHORAX

Newborns requiring positive pressure ventilation are at risk for developing a pneumothorax, which is identified clinically by asymmetry of chest movement or breath sounds. If a tension pneumothorax develops, venous return and cardiac output are compromised and cardiac arrest may occur. Transillumination may be helpful in diagnosis; a light placed next to the newborn's chest on the affected side will illuminate the air pocket of the pneumothorax more brightly compared with the unaffected side. A chest radiograph is diagnostic, but thoracentesis should be considered in life-threatening cases, even before a radiograph is available. This procedure is described in Chapter 195.

MULTIPLE GESTATIONS

Separate teams of skilled personnel are required for each newborn of a multiple gestation delivery. Multiple gestations are associated with an increased incidence of preterm labor and delivery, as well as an increased risk for IUGR in at least one fetus. Postnatally, there is a risk of higher sensitivity to asphyxia, hypoglycemia, or polycythemia in each newborn. Monozygotic twins are especially at high risk not only because of the potential for twin-twin transfusion syndrome, possibly with hydrops in either twin, but also because of the increased incidence of congenital anomalies.

PRETERM NEWBORNS

The incidence of perinatal depression is markedly increased before 37 weeks gestation due to physiologic and anatomic differences. Risk factors for this population include lungs deficient in surfactant, which can make ventilation difficult, immature brain development and weak respiratory muscles, which can decrease respiratory effort, thin skin and low fat stores, contributing to rapid heat loss, and fragile cerebral blood vessels that are more prone to bleeding under stress. Additional resources required at a preterm delivery include additional personnel to perform complex resuscitation. The temperature in the delivery room should be increased and the radiant warmer pre-heated. If the newborn is anticipated to be very preterm, that is less than 32 weeks gestation, a reclose-able, food-grade polyethylene bag, and a chemically activated warming pad should be used. An oxygen blender, an oximeter, and a transport incubator should always be available for preterm births. CPAP should be used when the newborn is breathing spontaneously and the HR is greater than 100 bpm to decrease risk of lung injury from mechanical ventilation. To further decrease neurological injury avoid rapid intravenous fluids, high PPV or CPAP pressures, and use a pulse oximeter and blood gases to adjust oxygen concentration to minimize toxicity.

For deliveries at the threshold of viability (22-23 weeks), it is especially important to provide antenatal counseling, as well as maintain an ongoing dialogue with the family. Assessment of gestational age both antenatally, by ultrasound, and postnatally, by a gestational age examination such as the Ballard Score, is accurate only to within 1 to 2 weeks. Therefore, if there is any question of gestational age, it is reasonable to provide aggressive resuscitative support, which allows ongoing assessment of the newborn. Clinical response to treatment is an important factor in assessment, and if response to resuscitation is poor or if severe complications develop, withdrawal of support may be offered.

DISCONTINUING RESUSCITATION

If there is a confirmed absence of heart rate after all standard steps of resuscitation has been performed, it is appropriate to discuss the cessation of resuscitation care with the medical team and the family. Guidelines differ by hospital systems and should be clarified. The American Academy of Pediatrics and the World Health Organization consider 20 minutes after birth a reasonable time to consider ending resuscitation efforts in a newborn with no heart rate. However, the decision to continue or discontinue should be centered on each patient's situation, family's goals, and the context. Indicators of a poor outcome in terms of both survival and subsequent neurodevelopment beyond first 20 minutes of life include Apgar scores of less than 3 at 5 and 10 minutes, cord or newborn blood pH less than 7.0 in the first 2 hours of life, absence of a heartbeat at 5 minutes of life, and seizures in the first 24 hours of life. The occurrence of seizures within the first 12 hours of life is particularly ominous. For these newborns, the incidence of death or severe, irreversible neurologic damage is very high.

KEY POINTS

- Only about 10% of newborns require some form of resuscitation, and only 1% require major resuscitative measures to survive.
- The most important and critical action during delivery room resuscitation is to assist with ventilation.
- Antepartum and intrapartum risk factors can be used to anticipate newborns who are more likely to require neonatal resuscitation.
- All newborns should be initially assessed at birth to determine whether resuscitative efforts are needed, and every birth should be attended by at least one person capable of initiating resuscitation.
- Personnel should be fully prepared for resuscitation at every delivery even if no risk factors are known.
- The initial steps of resuscitation are to provide warmth, position the head and clear the airway, provide tactile stimulation, and evaluate respirations, heart rate, and oxygenation.
- If further intervention is required after initial steps of resuscitation, positive pressure ventilation should be provided and pulse oximetry should be used to guide supplemental oxygen titration.
- Chest compressions are indicated if the heart rate is less than 60 breaths per minute after 30 seconds of effective assisted ventilation.
- A very small number of newborns will still have a heart rate less than 60 breaths per minute despite adequate positive pressure ventilation and chest compressions, requiring epinephrine.

SUGGESTED READINGS

Aziz K, Lee CHC, Escobedo MB, et al. Part 5: Neonatal Resuscitation 2020 American Heart Association Guidelines for Cardiopulmonary Resuscitation and Emergency Cardiovascular Care. *Pediatrics.* 2021;147(Suppl 1):e2020038505E.

Chen X, Li X, Chang Y, Li W, Cui H. Effect and safety of timing of cord clamping on neonatal hematocrit values and clinical outcomes in term infants: a randomized controlled trial. *J Perinatol.* 2018;38(3): 251-257.

Foster JP, Dawson JA, Davis PG, Dahlen HG. Routine oro/nasopharyngeal suction versus no suction at birth. *Cochrane Database Syst Rev.* 2017;4(4):CD010332.

Talati AJ, Scott TA, Barker B, Grubb PH; Tennessee Initiative for Perinatal Quality Care Golden Hour Project Team. Improving neonatal resuscitation in Tennessee: a large-scale, quality improvement project. *J Perinatol.* 2019;39(12):1676-1683.

Weiner G, Zaichkin J, eds. *Textbook of Neonatal Resuscitation.* 8th ed. Elk Grove Village, IL: American Academy of Pediatrics and American Heart Association; 2021.

Wyckoff MH, Wyllie J, Aziz K, et al. Neonatal Life Support: 2020 International Consensus on Cardiopulmonary Resuscitation and Emergency Cardiovascular Care Science with Treatment Recommendations. *Circulation.* 2020;142(16_suppl_1):S185-S221.

CHAPTER 124

The Well Newborn

Hayato Unno, MD and Neera Goyal, MD, MSc

BACKGROUND

The newborn birth hospital stay, though typically brief, is a multidimensional process with complex physiologic transitions for both the newborn and birthing parent. It is also a time when clinical decisions shape the basics of early parenthood—the fundamentals of feeding, caring for, and bringing home a new baby. Each of these early milestones provides an opportunity for parental self-affirmation and family bonding. For the newborn clinician, responsibilities are numerous and include: reviewing and interpreting perinatal and other historical data, identifying issues or risk factors that necessitate further evaluation, clinical assessment and management of the infant, and supporting families with anticipatory guidance and resources. The newborn hospital stay should be long enough for each of these tasks to be addressed, to ensure adequate outpatient follow-up, and to minimize the risk of a serious adverse outcome after discharge.

PATHOPHYSIOLOGY

Newborn physiology is fundamentally different from fetal physiology, and the transition from intra- to extrauterine life involves a rapid, complex cascade of structural and functional changes. Key physiologic changes include:

- an increase in systemic vascular resistance after clamping of the umbilical cord
- closure of the foramen ovale and ductus arteriosus
- lowering of pulmonary vascular resistance
- clearance of fluid from the airways and changes in airway pressure
- increased catecholamine levels to support higher blood pressure

In addition to these circulatory and respiratory changes, the immediate hours and days after birth are accompanied by significant metabolic and thermal adaptations, including changes in body water content and fluid homeostasis, gluconeogenesis, and temperature regulation. Transition to enteric nutrition also involves multiple steps including suck-swallow coordination, changes in gastric compliance, and establishing intestinal motility. While most newborns successfully transition as expected, delays or failure to undergo these physiological changes warrants prompt evaluation and management.

CLINICAL PRESENTATION

Assessment of the newborn begins with review of the maternal and family history, the pregnancy, and the delivery (**Table 124-1**). A physician must perform a thorough head-to-toe examination of the newborn infant within 24 hours of birth and daily while the infant is in the hospital. Every examination should start with a review of the vital signs, oral intake, and urinary and stool output; the range of normal values and patterns for newborns is provided in **Tables 124-2** and **124-3**. The initial examination should also include measurements of birth weight, length, and head circumference. These are plotted on standard growth curves (e.g., the World Health Organization curves) to determine whether they are proportional and appropriate for the gestational age.

The infant should be completely undressed and observed for any signs of distress, dysmorphology, asymmetry, or abnormal color. Pertinent

TABLE 124-1 Perinatal History Assessment

Maternal and Family	Fetus	Labor
Illnesses (current and past)	Prenatal ultrasonography (first trimester: dating, nuchal translucency. Second trimester: anatomy scan)	Gestational age at delivery Plurality
Medications	Triple or Quad screen (for chromosomal abnormalities and neural tube defects) NIPT	Progression of labor (e.g., duration of rupture of membranes, precipitous, arrest of descent)
Drug, alcohol, or tobacco use	CVS or amniocentesis	Delivery (vaginal: spontaneous, induced, forceps or vacuum assisted. Cesarean: elective, emergent. Fetal presentation)
Prenatal care (onset, sufficiency, use of fertility treatment, gravidity and parity)	Growth (e.g., IUGR, macrosomia)	Medications (analgesia, antibiotics)
Prenatal testing (HBsAg, HIV, RPR, other STIs, GBS, PPD, ABO, and Rh blood type)	Position (e.g., breech presentation in the third trimester)	Fetal distress (abnormal fetal heart rate monitoring) Meconium-stained amniotic fluid Evidence of chorioamnionitis
Complications of this pregnancy (e.g., diabetes, HTN, preeclampsia, multiple gestation, infection, premature labor, bleeding)	In utero interventions (e.g., surgery, infusions, selective reductions)	Resuscitation (per NRP)
Complications of previous pregnancies		Apgar scores
Disorders in other children or family members		Complications (e.g., shoulder dystocia, trauma)

CVS, chorionic villus sampling; GBS, group B streptococci; HBsAg, Hepatitis B surface antigen; HIV, human immunodeficiency virus; HTN, hypertension; IUGR, intrauterine growth restriction; NIPT, noninvasive prenatal screening; NRP, neonatal resuscitation algorithm; PPD, purified protein derivative (for tuberculosis); RPR, rapid plasma reagin (for syphilis); STI, sexually transmitted infection.

TABLE 124-2 Vital Signs in Full-Term Newborns

Vital Sign	Normal Range
Temperature	Axillary: 36.5°C to 37.5°C* Rectal: 36.5°C to 38°C
Heart rate	120-160 beats/min (can be as low as 85 beats/min while asleep)
Respiratory rate†	30-60 breaths/min

*While in an open crib.

†The respiratory rate should be obtained by counting breaths for 60 seconds, because newborns often exhibit periodic breathing.

TABLE 124-3 Expected Intake and Output

Intake	Output
Breastfeeding: Nurse on demand, until infant satisfied, every 1 to 3 hours (at least 8 to 12 times every 24 hours).	**Urine:** At least one void in the first 24 hours. Gradual increase to 6 or more voids per day by 5-7 days.
Formula: Between ¼ and 1 oz (approximately 7.5 and 30 mL) per feeding, every 3-4 hours, in the first 24 hours. 2-3 oz (60-90 mL) every 3-4 hours by days 3-4.	**Stool:** At least one bowel movement (i.e. meconium) in the first 48 hours. 1-2 stools per day (that begin to appear greenish to yellow and seedy) on days 3 and 4. 3-4 stools per day by 5-7 days.

findings of the newborn examination are summarized in **Table 124-4**. Abnormalities, including vital signs outside the normal range, often require further investigation or follow-up.

MANAGEMENT

Management of the newborn during birth hospitalization involves observation for expected physiologic transitions, screening for underlying pathology, and anticipatory guidance for families on newborn safety and health. Given the typically brief length of hospitalization for well-appearing newborns, discharge counseling and coordination should begin soon after birth to ensure a smooth transition to outpatient care.

FEEDING

One of the most important milestones for newborns and families after birth is establishment of oral feedings. The American Academy of Pediatrics (AAP) recommends exclusive breastfeeding for the first 6 months of life, with continuation of breastfeeding for 2 years or longer as mutually desired. Hospital practices to encourage and support the initiation of exclusive breastfeeding should be based on the AAP-endorsed "Ten Steps to Successful Breastfeeding" and have been demonstrated to increase breastfeeding success and duration. These practices include breastfeeding within the first hour after birth, continuous rooming-in to facilitate around-the-clock, on-demand feeding, and avoidance of non-medically indicated formula. Families should be counselled on the newborn and maternal health benefits of exclusive breastfeeding, educated on lactogenesis, and provided support with positioning, latch, and expression of colostrum. Given that the second stage of lactogenesis, onset of copious milk secretion, typically occurs on or after postpartum day two, mothers should be provided contact information for breastfeeding support after discharge from hospital. Given the myriad of factors, including socioeconomic barriers and personal experiences, that influence a family's plan for newborn feeding, providers should remain sensitive to family feeding preferences that do not involve exclusive breastfeeding. Undue pressure to exclusively breastfeed from the newborn provider could cause or exacerbate parental feelings of shame and guilt.

Medical contraindications to breastfeeding in the United States are rare and include infant galactosemia, maternal human immunodeficiency virus (HIV) infection, and certain drugs, including hazardous substance use (i.e., illicit opioids, cocaine, and phencyclidine), cytotoxic agents, and radioactive compounds. Medications taken while breastfeeding should be reviewed to ensure that their transfer via breast milk will not adversely affect the newborn. The Drugs and Lactation Database (LactMed), published by the National Library of Medicine and National Institutes of Health, is the most comprehensive source of information regarding the safety of maternal medications during lactation and is available online.

For newborns requiring formula due to family preference or medical indications, most can be offered any 20 kcal/oz cows-milk based formula that meets nutritional standards and provides adequate nutrients for term infants. Iron-fortified, 20 kcal/oz soy formula may be used for families seeking an option that is free of animal products; soy formula

TABLE 124-4 Newborn Examination

Site or System	Pertinent Findings
General	Vital signs, anthropomorphic measurements (weight, length, head circumference) Evidence of distress Symmetry of movements Dysmorphic or asymmetric features
Head	Skull shape (molding, overriding sutures) Fontanelles (size, bulging or sunken) Swelling (cephalohematoma, caput succedaneum, subgaleal hemorrhage) Scalp bruise, abrasion
Eyes	Shape, position, size, spontaneous opening Red reflex Scleral icterus, subconjunctival hemorrhage Conjugate gaze Conjunctival injection, eyelid edema, discharge
Ears	Shape and position Patency of external canals Preauricular pits or tags
Nose	Shape Patency of nares
Mouth	Keratin cysts, natal teeth Cleft lip, palate Ankyloglossia ("tongue-tie")
Neck	Range of motion (e.g., torticollis) Masses, sinuses, pits
Chest	Shape, symmetry of motion Breast tissue, supernumerary nipples Clavicular crepitus/fracture
Lungs	Symmetry of air entry Retractions, tachypnea, grunting, adventitial sounds
Cardiovascular	Heart rate, rhythm, sounds, murmurs, point of maximum impulse Pulses, capillary refill Cyanosis, acrocyanosis
Abdomen	Distention Bowel sounds Organomegaly, masses Umbilical stump (number of vessels) Hernia
Genitourinary	Females: size of clitoris and labia, presence of vaginal opening and hymenal tissue, discharge Males: presence and location of both testes, presence of epi- or hypospadias, chordee, penile torsion, hydrocele, inguinal hernia Ambiguous genitalia: (clitoromegaly, absent testes bilaterally)
Extremities	Symmetry and range of motion Hips: symmetry of thigh and gluteal folds, symmetry of abduction, Barlow and Ortolani maneuvers Extranumerary digits, metatarsus adductus, clubfeet
Neurologic	Tone Reflexes: Moro, suck, palmar, plantar, deep tendon
Back	Asymmetry (including gluteal cleft) Midline lesions (tufts of hair, pits, masses, skin tags) Position and patency of anus
Skin	Birthmarks (dermal melanosis, nevus simplex, nevus flammeus, hemangiomas) Rashes (erythema toxicum, pustular melanosis, milia, sebaceous hyperplasia) Jaundice Lanugo, vernix Abrasions, lacerations, contusions

can also be medically indicated in cases of newborn galactosemia or congenital lactase deficiency. Feeding difficulties in the first 48 hours can be caused by both maternal and newborn factors and can range in severity. Normal contents of emesis or spit-ups include breastmilk, formula, retained amniotic fluid, or swallowed maternal blood (usually bright red, in small amounts, and self-resolving). Parents should be counseled on the benign nature of gastroesophageal reflux, which occurs due to small gastric volumes, the intermittent relaxation of the esophageal sphincter in the newborn period, and their predominately recumbent positioning. Concerning features suggestive of pathology include bilious or coffee ground emesis, which may be accompanied by abdominal distension, firmness, or tenderness.

WEIGHT AND ELIMINATION

In the immediate newborn period, weight loss due to newborn diuresis and relatively low enteral intake is expected. The extent of newborn weight loss may be influenced by several factors, including delivery method, intrapartum fluids, and feeding status after birth. Most newborns tolerate this initial transition period of weight loss without event, begin gaining weight at 48 to 72 hours of age, and have regained back to their birth weight by 10 to 14 days of life. However, excessive weight loss, defined as ≥10% loss from birthweight, is associated with increased risk of hyperbilirubinemia and hypernatremic dehydration. Among exclusively breastfed newborns, almost 5% of vaginally delivered newborns and 10% of those delivered by cesarean can be expected to experience early excessive weight loss. Prior to discharge, newborns should be serially weighed with close monitoring for concerns of feeding inadequacy. Comparison to normative age-based nomograms of newborn early weight loss may be helpful for counselling and/or discharge planning.

Newborns with less frequent urination than expected for age should be evaluated for feeding difficulty or otherwise inadequate oral intake. Anatomic or functional abnormalities such as renal dysplasia or posterior urethral valves (in males) should also be considered, prompting careful review of prenatal ultrasounds for any abnormalities of the fetal urinary system or amniotic fluid index. Parents may be alarmed by urate crystals (a pinkish-orange, chalky stain) in the diapers but should be reassured that their appearance is normal in the first week after birth. While most cases of oliguria in the newborn period are due to inadequate oral intake, laboratory and imaging (i.e., renal and bladder ultrasound) evaluation could be considered if there is no improvement in urine output even after the initiation of supplemental feedings or the patient exhibits concerning clinical changes (e.g., abdominal distension).

Most newborns pass meconium (thick, sticky, black stool with a "tarry" appearance) in the first 24 hours of life, then transition to yellow, seedy stools in the first 48 hours of life. A delay in the passage of meconium may be a variant of normal or may signal a problem such as meconium plugging, Hirschsprung disease, or inadequate oral intake. When addressing a lack of stool production, it should be noted whether there was meconium staining of the amniotic fluid. An infant who has not produced a stool in 48 hours should undergo investigation for an underlying pathology (e.g., cystic fibrosis, Hirschsprung disease, imperforate anus, anorectal malformations, small left colon syndrome).

VITAMIN SUPPLEMENTATION

After delivery, all infants should receive prophylaxis against vitamin K deficiency bleeding (VKDB), which was formerly known as hemorrhagic disease of the newborn, with the intramuscular (IM) administration of 0.5 to 1.0 mg of vitamin K_1 (phytonadione). Infants are born with low levels of vitamin K because of poor transplacental transfer and because their intestines have not yet been colonized with bacteria that synthesize it. VKDB can occur anytime in the first 6 months of life, and the late-onset form of the disease presents with intracranial hemorrhage in 30% to 60% of cases. In a 2022 policy statement, the AAP acknowledged a recent rise in the incidence of VKDB and attributed it to increasing parental refusal of prophylaxis. The statement also stressed that oral vitamin K is not recommended because the oral dose is variably absorbed and is significantly less effective than the parenteral dose at preventing late-onset VKDB.

To prevent vitamin D deficiency and rickets, all exclusively breastfed infants and infants consuming less than 28 ounces of commercial infant formula per day should routinely receive an oral supplement of vitamin D, 400 IU per day, beginning at hospital discharge. Alternatively, a mother who breastfeeds can take 6400 IU of vitamin D to provide her infant with adequate supplementation.

OCULAR PROPHYLAXIS

Prophylaxis against ophthalmia neonatorum with topical antimicrobial application to the eyes is recommended immediately after birth for all newborns and is required by law in most of the United States. Today, the most commonly used treatment is 0.5% erythromycin ointment. If erythromycin ointment is unavailable, azithromycin ophthalmic solution 1% is an acceptable substitute. In the past, silver nitrate solution and tetracycline ointment were used, but these agents are no longer readily available in the United States. Silver nitrate is also associated with a transient chemical conjunctivitis. Although topical antimicrobial agents are highly effective in preventing ophthalmia neonatorum secondary to *Neisseria gonorrhoeae*, their effectiveness against *Chlamydia trachomatis* has not been established.

UMBILICAL CORD AND SKIN CARE

Newborn skin is covered in vernix and commensal bacteria after delivery, and aids in both immunologic protection and temperature homeostasis. Delaying the newborn bath for at least 12 hours has been shown to reduce risk of hypothermia and hypoglycemia, and to increase rates of breastfeeding. The application of antiseptics such as chlorhexidine or alcohol to the umbilical cord stump is not recommended, and families should be counseled that if left to dry naturally it should fall off within 2 weeks. Although omphalitis is uncommon and usually presents after hospital discharge, families should be counselled on indications to seek medical evaluation including erythema, induration around the umbilical stump, and foul-smelling discharge. Families can also be counselled that early application of emollients to the newborn's skin may reduce risk of early childhood atopic dermatitis.

MALE CIRCUMCISION

Whether to circumcise a newborn male is a personal choice, and many parents base their decision on religious or cultural factors. The current position of the AAP is that the health benefits are not great enough to recommend routine circumcision; however, the benefits are sufficient to justify access to this procedure for families choosing it. Potential benefits include decreased risk of urinary tract infection in the first year of life, decreased risk of penile cancer, and decreased risk of acquisition of syphilis, HIV, and other sexually transmitted infections. The risks of circumcision are minor but include bleeding, infection, poor cosmetic result, surgical trauma, meatal stenosis, skin bridges, and inclusion cysts. All infants undergoing circumcision should receive proper analgesia, either with topical anesthetic application, dorsal penile nerve block, or subcutaneous ring block, along with sucrose on a pacifier and proper positioning during the procedure. Potential but rare complications of analgesia include methemoglobinemia and hematoma. Prior to circumcision, the occurrence of at least one urinary void should be confirmed. It is also recommended that the infant receive the routine IM dose of vitamin K prior to the procedure. Congenital penile anomalies such as hypospadias, epispadias, chordee, webbed or buried penis, and penile torsion (raphe torsion of >60 degrees) are contraindications to newborn circumcision and should be referred to pediatric urology.

After circumcision, lubricant (e.g., petroleum ointment) should be applied to the newly exposed glans to prevent adherence to the diaper and repeated trauma to the healing tissue. This should be continued until the area is well healed, usually by the fifth day. The area can then be cleansed with water as needed. The infant should remain in the hospital for at least 2 hours after the circumcision to allow monitoring for any excessive bleeding from the site; any ongoing bleeding should be immediately addressed and investigated. For newborns who are not circumcised, families should be warned against retracting the foreskin, which is unnecessary, painful, and can lead to scarring and permanent adhesion.

HEPATITIS B VACCINE

Hepatitis B vaccine administration is recommended for all newborns prior to discharge to prevent perinatal or vertical transmission of hepatitis B virus. Exposure to hepatitis B virus places newborns at risk of congenital infection, which is associated with high rates of chronic carrier status, morbidity, and mortality due to complications of hepatitis, cirrhosis, and/or hepatocellular carcinoma.

Upon admission, careful review of prenatal labs and maternal infection history should focus on maternal hepatitis B surface antigen (HBsAg) status. If maternal HBsAg status is positive, the newborn should receive both hepatitis B immune globulin (HBIG) and the first dose of the hepatitis B vaccine administered as soon as possible within the first 12 hours of life, in opposite thighs. The vaccine alone is 70% to 95% effective, and the combination of hepatitis B vaccine and HBIG is 85% to 95% effective in preventing congenital infection. Newborns with a positive maternal HBsAg screen should also be bathed shortly after birth, prior to receiving any injections.

If maternal HBsAg status is unknown, newborns weighing > 2000 grams should receive the hepatitis B vaccine as soon as possible within the first 12 hours of life, and maternal HBsAg should be tested. If the test comes back positive, HBIG should be administered as soon as possible, with peak effectiveness before 7 days of age. If the results of the HBsAg test are still unavailable at 7 days, some experts recommend that the newborn receive HBIG. Infants of mothers with positive or unknown HBsAg results should be tested at 9 to 18 months of age for evidence of hepatitis B infection or immunity, after completing the hepatitis B vaccine series with the second and third doses administered at 1 month and 6 months, respectively.

SCREENING FOR HYPERBILIRUBINEMIA

All newborns should be clinically assessed for jaundice prior to discharge, with initial bilirubin measurement occurring at 24 hours of life or earlier if pathological jaundice is suspected; see Chapter 130 for specifics on screening and management of newborn hyperbilirubinemia.

SCREENING FOR CONGENITAL HEART DISEASE

Congenital heart disease (CHD) is the most common congenital anomaly in newborns. Although many newborns with critical CHD, defined as requiring surgery or catheter-based intervention in the first year of life, are symptomatic and identified soon after birth, others are not diagnosed until after discharge from the birth hospital. For those with a critical cardiac lesion, the risk of morbidity and mortality increases with any delay in diagnosis and referral to a tertiary care center. Refer to Chapter 51 for further details on pathophysiology and clinical presentation of CHD.

To improve identification of patients with critical CHD, pulse oximetry should be performed routinely in all newborns, using the right hand and either foot after 24 hours of life or as late as possible if discharge before 24 hours is planned. An abnormal screening result is defined as (i) any oxygen saturation measurement <90%; (ii) oxygen saturation 90% to 95% in both upper and lower extremities on three measurements, each separated by 1 hour; or (iii) a difference in oxygen saturation >3% between the upper and lower extremities on three measurements, each separated by 1 hour. Each birth hospital should establish procedures to ensure timely evaluation for newborns with an abnormal screening result, including echocardiography and interpretation by a clinician with expertise in CHD. Among infants with a normal pulse oximetry screen, an estimated 40% or more may provide false results, particularly in cases of aortic coarctation, Tetralogy of Fallot, and Ebstein anomaly. Careful and thorough physical examination both during hospitalization and after discharge is essential to CHD detection for all newborns, regardless of pulse oximetry screening results.

HEARING SCREENING

Before discharge from the hospital, all newborns should undergo screening for congenital hearing loss, which is estimated to affect between 1 and 3 per 1000 healthy newborns. Early detection and intervention for this diagnosis are critical to ensuring age-appropriate language development. Until universal hearing screening was implemented, most children with congenital hearing loss were not identified until 14 to 30 months of age.

There are two accepted and commonly used methods for screening hearing in newborns: the otoacoustic emissions (OAE) test and the auditory brainstem response (ABR) test. The OAE test measures sound waves generated by hair cells in the inner ear in response to clicks emitted and recorded by microphones in the outer ear canal. It detects sensory or inner ear hearing loss but not neural hearing loss. The ABR test measures neural impulses from the cochlea, auditory nerve, and auditory brainstem pathways. Three electrodes placed on the infant's scalp measure waves generated in response to clicks emitted in the ear canal. Both methods are quick and easy to perform but require a quiet infant and environment. False failures can occur if there is debris or fluid in the ear canal. A newborn who fails the initial hearing test should have a second test before discharge. A newborn who fails the second test should be referred prior to discharge from the nursery for outpatient screening within a 1 month of age. For rescreening, a complete screening on both ears is recommended, even if only one ear failed the initial screening. A referral for full audiologic evaluation is warranted for infants who fail this series of tests, and this referral should take place before the infant reaches 3 months of age.

There is compelling evidence for screening for congenital cytomegalovirus (CMV) infection in newborns who fail the newborn hearing screen, and several states have recently passed legislation mandating a hearing targeted approach to early CMV screening. Congenital CMV infection, which may not cause noticeable symptoms at birth, is a leading cause of non-genetic sensorineural hearing loss (SNHL) that is permanent and often progressive. Testing for congenital CMV must be performed before the age of 3 weeks because a later positive result may reflect postnatal infection, which is not associated with SNHL.

RED REFLEX SCREENING

All newborns should undergo retinal red reflex examination prior to hospital discharge and subsequently at all well child care visits. Red reflex examination screens for vision- and potentially life-threatening abnormalities such as cataracts, glaucoma, retinoblastoma, and retinal abnormalities, systemic diseases with ocular abnormalities, and high refractive errors. The exam is performed with an ophthalmoscope held close to the examiner's eye and with the light projected onto the eyes from approximately 18 inches, ideally in a darkened room. Normally, the red reflex is symmetric. The presence of dark spots, a markedly diminished reflex, a white reflex, or asymmetric findings are indications for referral to pediatric Ophthalmology. Additionally, any infant with a family history of retinoblastoma, (congenital, infantile, or juvenile) cataracts, glaucoma, or retinal abnormalities should be referred to Ophthalmology regardless of the red reflex exam.

METABOLIC SCREENING

Newborn screening for certain metabolic and genetic disorders began in the 1960s when Robert Guthrie devised a test that screened for phenylketonuria (PKU). He also developed a simple and inexpensive way of collecting blood samples from the heel of newborns on filter paper. Since then, screening for other disorders has become possible. The goal of newborn screening is to detect certain disorders early and provide treatment to prevent their clinical manifestations and subsequent morbidity and mortality. Today, all 50 states test for PKU and hypothyroidism; however, because there is no federal law regulating newborn screening programs, there is state-to-state variation in the testing for other disorders. Many states test for medium-chain acyl-CoA dehydrogenase deficiency, congenital adrenal hyperplasia, biotinidase deficiency, cystic fibrosis, maple syrup disease, galactosemia, homocystinuria, and sickle cell anemia. Clinicians must be familiar with the tests performed in the states where they practice and counsel parents appropriately about these conditions. It is important to ensure that the specimen is collected at least 24 hours after birth, because many of the disorders are based on abnormal protein metabolism. Some state laboratories may require specimen collection 24 hours after initiation of feedings.

PARENTAL SUPPORT AND EDUCATION

Parental bonding and caregiving skills should be assessed during the hospitalization. It is recommended that every mother be assessed with a screening tool such as the Edinburgh Postnatal Depression Scale prior to discharge. For any family with psychosocial concerns including barriers to healthcare access, prenatal substance use disorder, maternal mental illness, family violence, or lack of resources, professional guidance and family support should be instituted in the hospital and continued after discharge. Anticipatory guidance on newborn care should include counselling about normal newborn crying and sleep patterns, temperature measurement (as any fever in the first three months of life requires immediate attention), how to recognize jaundice, the need for a car seat (installed in the back seat and in the rear-facing position) when transporting the newborn in a vehicle, safe newborn sleep positioning, and when to call the physician. Parents should be provided with a telephone number where they can reach a medical professional if questions arise.

ADMISSION AND DISCHARGE CRITERIA

The American Academy of Pediatrics (AAP) recommends that routine newborn hospitalization should be long enough to allow identification of problems and to ensure safety of the newborn after discharge. Many newborn complications, including hyperbilirubinemia, CHD, and gastrointestinal obstruction require detection by skilled healthcare professional and may not present until well after 24 hours of life. Given the severe and potentially fatal consequences of these conditions, and in response to safety concerns related to rapid newborn discharge from hospitals after delivery, the US Congress passed the federal Newborns' and Mothers' Health Protection Act in 1996. This legislation mandated insurers to cover hospitalization for at least 2 days after vaginal birth and 4 days after cesarean birth.

Infants with feeding issues, significant weight loss, temperature instability, significant jaundice, or social concerns are not candidates for early discharge before 48 hours of life. Vital signs should be within normal ranges and stable for the 12 hours preceding discharge. At least two successful feedings should have occurred, and the infant should have voided and passed at least one stool spontaneously. All newborns should have a designated physician for follow-up care. For those being discharged before 48 hours of life, outpatient follow-up should occur preferably within 48 hours, and no later than 72 hours in most cases.

CONSULTATION

Consultation of neonatology is indicated for newborns with signs of impaired adaptation to extrauterine life, including persistent tachypnea, hypothermia, hypoglycemia, or difficulty feeding. Based on circumstances, consultation with pediatric subspecialists may be indicated, including but not limited to Infectious Disease (e.g., maternal HIV infection), Cardiology (e.g., abnormal cardiac exam), Urology (e.g., antenatal pylectasis), Hematology (e.g., family history of bleeding disorder), Genetics (e.g., concern for dysmorphic features), and Orthopedics (e.g., concern for femur or humeral fracture).

SPECIAL CONSIDERATIONS

DEVELOPMENTAL DYSPLASIA OF THE HIP

Developmental dysplasia of the hip (DDH—defined as an abnormal relationship of the femoral head to the acetabulum—includes frank dislocation (luxation), partial dislocation (subluxation), femoral head instability, and any malformation of the acetabulum. While the true incidence of DDH is unknown, it is estimated that 1 in 100 newborns has hip instability and 1 to 1.5 per 1000 has dislocation. The left hip is involved three times more often than the right hip. Risk factors for DDH include female gender, breech position, positive family history, and incorrect lower-extremity swaddling. Screening for DDH should start after birth and continue at each scheduled well-child visit until age 18 months.

Hip examination should be conducted while the newborn is quiet and relaxed. Although no physical examination signs are pathognomonic for a dislocated hip, suspicious findings include asymmetry of thigh or gluteal folds, apparent limb length discrepancy, and restricted mobility of the hip, especially abduction. The Barlow, Ortolani, and Galeazzi tests are physical maneuvers that suggest hip dislocation and should prompt further evaluation. It is not unusual for hip "clicks" to be elicited during the initial newborn examination; these usually represent ligamentous laxity. For newborns with a hip click or other suspicious finding (e.g., unequal gluteal folds) that persist by 2 weeks of age without evidence of true hip dislocation, further referral and evaluation may be warranted. Hip "clunk" on newborn examination is never normal and warrants prompt orthopedic evaluation after discharge (no need to confirm dislocation by radiographic studies). **Table 124-5** summarizes the evaluation and management of DDH. Double and triple diapering of newborns with suspected DDH is not recommended.

TABLE 124-5 Approach to Developmental Dysplasia of the Hip (DDH)

DDH Examination	Risk Factors	Recommended Action
Positive	–	Refer to orthopedist
Equivocal at birth	–	Repeat at 2 weeks
Equivocal at 2 weeks	–	Refer to orthopedist or perform ultrasonography at 3-4 weeks, determine risk factors
Negative	Girl or boy with breech presentation in third trimester	Recommend hip ultrasonography between 6 weeks and 6 months
Negative	Girl or boy with family history of DDH	Recommend hip ultrasonography between 6 weeks and 6 months
Negative	No risk factors	Reevaluate at well-child visits

SUPERNUMERARY DIGITS

Polydactyly is a common congenital deformity that in most affected newborns involves the border digits of the ulnar (postaxial) aspect of the hand. Ulnar supernumerary digits can range from rudimentary skin tags to well-developed, functional digits. Management is based on the degree to which the supernumerary digit is formed, and if osseous structures are felt on examination, radiographs of the hand should be obtained. Traditionally, soft-tissue–only postaxial polydactyly has been managed by a general pediatrician with suture ligation, which involves tying a silk suture at the digit base to occlude vascular inflow. Advantages of this approach are simplicity and safety of performing soon after birth, and convenience for the family. The disadvantage of suture ligation is the potential for complications: persistent dry gangrenous digit (i.e., does not fall off), symptomatic neuroma formation, cyst formation, aesthetically unacceptable residual stump, and infection. Orthopedic referral for surgical ligation may result in improved aesthetics and fewer complications, however the age of surgery is controversial. Of note, multiple genetic syndromes have been associated with postaxial polydactyly, including orofaciodigital syndrome and Smith–Lemhi–Optiz syndrome. In the absence of a strong family history, outpatient referral to a geneticist should be considered.

KEY POINTS

- Early screening and detection of certain clinical conditions in the newborn period may prevent long-term morbidity or even death.
- Assessment of every newborn should include a head-to-toe physical examination, evaluation of vital signs, and review of the maternal medical and social history.
- Hospital policies and procedures that promote exclusive breastfeeding after birth are important to successful initiation and longer duration of breastfeeding.
- All newborns should be assessed for jaundice and undergo a hearing screen, pulse oximetry screening, and newborn metabolic screening before discharge from the hospital.
- Evaluation of readiness for discharge should incorporate assessment of parental resources, access to timely follow-up care, and family risk factors.

SUGGESTED READINGS

American Academy of Pediatrics. Hepatitis B. In: Kimberlin DW, Barnett ED, Lynfield R, Sawyer MH, eds. *Red Book: 2021 Report of the Committee on Infectious Diseases*. Itasca, IL: American Academy of Pediatrics: 2021:381-399.

American Academy of Pediatrics Joint Committee on Infant Hearing. Year 2007 position statement: principles and guidelines for early hearing detection and intervention programs. *Pediatrics*. 2007; 120(4):898-921.

American Academy of Pediatrics. Neonatal Ophthalmia. In: Kimberlin DW, Barnett ED, Lynfield R, Sawyer MH, eds. *Red Book: 2021 Report of the Committee on Infectious Diseases*. Itasca, IL: American Academy of Pediatrics: 2021:1023-1026.

American Academy of Pediatrics; Section on Ophthalmology; American Association for Pediatric Ophthalmology And Strabismus; American Academy of Ophthalmology; American Association of Certified Orthoptists. Red reflex examination in neonates, infants, and children. *Pediatrics*. 2008;122(6):1401-1404.

American Academy of Pediatrics Task Force on Circumcision; Circumcision policy statement. *Pediatrics*. 2012;130(3):585-586.

Benitz WE; Committee on Fetus and Newborn, American Academy of Pediatrics. Hospital stay for healthy term newborn infants. *Pediatrics*. 2015;135(5):948-953.

Bhatia J, Greer F. Use of soy protein-based formulas in infant feeding. *Pediatrics*. 2008;121(5):1062-1068.

Centers for Disease Control and Prevention. Hepatitis B. In: Hall E, Wodi AP, Hamborsky J, et al, eds. *Epidemiology and Prevention of Vaccine-Preventable Diseases: The Pink Book*. 14th ed. Washington, DC: Public Health Foundation; 2021:143-164.

Comer GC, Potter M, Ladd AL. Polydactyly of the Hand. *J Am Acad Orthop Surg*. 2018;26(3):75-82.

Drugs and Lactation Database (LactMed). US National Library of Medicine. Available at: https://www.ncbi.nlm.nih.gov/books/NBK501922/.

Flaherman VJ, Schaefer EW, Kuzniewicz MW, Li SX, Walsh EM, Paul IM. Early weight loss nomograms for exclusively breastfed newborns. *Pediatrics*. 2015;135(1):e16-23.

Grosse SD, Ross DS, Dollard SC. Congenital cytomegalovirus (CMV) infection as a cause of permanent bilateral hearing loss: a quantitative assessment. *J Clin Virol*. 2008;41(2):57-62.

Hand I, Noble L, Abrams SA; American Academy of Pediatrics Committee on Fetus and Newborn, Section on Breastfeeding, Committee on Nutrition. Vitamin k and the newborn infant. *Pediatrics*. 2022; 149(3):e2021056036.

Martin GR, Ewer AK, Gaviglio A, et al. Updated strategies for pulse oximetry screening for critical congenital heart disease. *Pediatrics*. 2020;146(1):e20191650.

Meek JY, Noble L; Section on Breastfeeding. Policy Statement: Breastfeeding and the use of human milk. *Pediatrics*. 2022;150(1):e2022057988.

Morton SU, Brodsky D. Fetal physiology and the transition to extrauterine life. *Clin Perinatol*. 2016;43(3):395-407.

Shaw BA, Segal LS, American Academy Section on Orthopedics. Evaluation and referral for developmental dysplasia of the hip in infants. *Pediatrics*. 2016;138(6):e20163107.

Stewart D, Benitz W, American Academy of Pediatrics Committee on Fetus and Newborn. Umbilical cord care in the newborn infant. *Pediatrics*. 2016;138(3):e20162149.

Wisniewski JA, Phillipi CA, Goyal N, et al. Variation in newborn skincare policies across United States Maternity Hospitals. *Hosp Pediatr*. 2021;11(9):1010-1019.

Zangen S, Di Lorenzo C, Zangen T, Mertz H, Schwankovsky L, Hyman PE. Rapid maturation of gastric relaxation in newborn infants. *Pediatr Res*. 2001;50(5):629-632.

CHAPTER 125 Birth Injury

Mark D. Hormann, MD

INTRODUCTION

Birth injuries are an uncommon complication of vaginal and cesarean delivery. Injuries range from those that are minor and require no further diagnostic evaluation or treatment to those that are life threatening or associated with long-term morbidity. Risk factors for injury include macrosomia, precipitous or prolonged delivery, breech presentation, cephalopelvic disproportion, shoulder dystocia, and the use of forceps or vacuum to assist extraction. However, birth injuries also occur in infants with no identifiable risk factors, making prediction difficult.

FRACTURES

BACKGROUND

Fractures as complications of the delivery process most commonly occur in the clavicle, humerus, and femur. Skull fractures are also reported, usually in association with forceps delivery. Long bone fractures generally require evaluation by an orthopedic specialist, whereas skull fractures are usually simple linear fractures that do not require intervention. Infants rarely have more than one fracture; for those with multiple fractures, diagnoses such as osteogenesis imperfecta should be considered.

Pathophysiology Clavicle fractures occur as a complication of the delivery process in approximately 0.5% to 1.7% of all live births. Historically, clavicle fractures were thought to be a result of obstetric mismanagement. Recent studies, however, have shown that little can be done to prevent this complication. Clavicle fractures are most commonly reported with vaginal deliveries, but they are also reported with cesarean sections. Risk factors include fetal macrosomia, instrumented delivery, and a prolonged second stage of labor, but predictive models based on these factors have a high false-positive rate and have not been clinically useful.

The humerus is occasionally fractured during the delivery process, typically with a difficult vertex delivery of the shoulder or a breech delivery. The fracture may result from direct pressure or traction. A greenstick fracture is most common, but displaced fractures may also occur. Breech deliveries may also result in a femur fracture; most are complete fractures that result in obvious deformity.

CLINICAL PRESENTATION

Clavicular fractures are sometimes overlooked, particularly in the case of a nondisplaced fracture. Acutely, the examiner may feel crepitus, and irritability may be noted with pressure over the bone. In displaced fractures, a bony ledge may be palpated. The infant may have decreased movement of the ipsilateral arm with an asymmetric Moro response. This pseudoparalysis is typically related to pain but may also be the result of associated nerve damage. The diagnosis of a nondisplaced clavicular fracture is sometimes delayed for several weeks until normal healing occurs and the callus forms a visible or palpable mass.

Humerus fractures may present clinically with swelling and pain; in the case of a displaced fracture an obvious deformity will be noted. The infant may refuse to move the affected arm, thereby resulting in an asymmetric Moro reflex and pseudoparalysis; however, nerve involvement may also occur. Most femur fractures will present as an obvious deformity.

DIAGNOSTIC EVALUATION

The diagnosis of neonatal clavicle fracture may be made clinically either at the time of delivery or in the first month of life. A single anteroposterior radiograph of the chest is sufficient to confirm the fracture if the diagnosis is in question. Plain films are also usually sufficient to confirm the diagnosis of humerus or femur fractures.

MANAGEMENT

Clavicular fractures usually heal without sequelae or deformity. Management is conservative and involves keeping the infant off the affected side; immobilization of the arm may help to decrease pain. Healing should occur within 2 weeks, and callus formation may be seen radiographically in several weeks. Parents may complain of a bony irregularity as the clavicle heals, but this will become less prominent as the child grows.

Treatment of humerus fractures is generally limited to immobilization for 2 to 4 weeks in the adducted position, and the prognosis is excellent. Treatment of femur fractures is 3 to 4 weeks of traction and suspension of both lower extremities. Immobilization with a Pavlik harness may also be effective in treating femur fractures. The prognosis is excellent.

ADMISSION AND DISCHARGE CRITERIA

Admission to the neonatal intensive care unit for management and consultation with a pediatric orthopedic surgeon is indicated for infants with concerns for humerus or femur fracture, including focal pain, edema, erythema, or deformity. Infants with clavicular fracture can generally be managed in the routine well newborn nursery. Discharge criteria include adequate pain control and nutritional intake as well as timely access to primary care and orthopedics follow-up if indicated.

PERIPHERAL NERVE INJURIES

BACKGROUND

Nerve damage is an infrequent, but important complication of the birthing process. In some cases, injury may be traced to traction on the neck and thus on the brachial plexus during delivery. Severity can range from mild nerve stretching to nerve root avulsion. In the United States, brachial plexus injury is currently estimated to affect 1 in 1000 live vaginal births, and up to 0.2% of all live births. Risk of brachial plexus injury increases with higher birthweight, with an incidence as high as 3.6% among vaginally delivered newborns weighing over 4500 g. In addition to macrosomia, risk factors include shoulder dystocia, breech presentation, and instrumented delivery. However, because many cases of brachial plexus injury occur without these risk factors, an effective predictive model has not been established.

CLINICAL PRESENTATION

Clinical presentation is variable, depending on the location and extent of nerve injury. Injury to the fifth and sixth cervical (C5 and C6) nerve roots is the most common nerve injury (**Figure 125-1**) and results in partial paralysis of the upper extremity, known as Erb-Duchenne paralysis or Erb palsy. Affected infants have unilateral arm weakness and an asymmetric Moro response. The hypotonic extremity is adducted, internally rotated, and pronated at the forearm. Additional involvement of

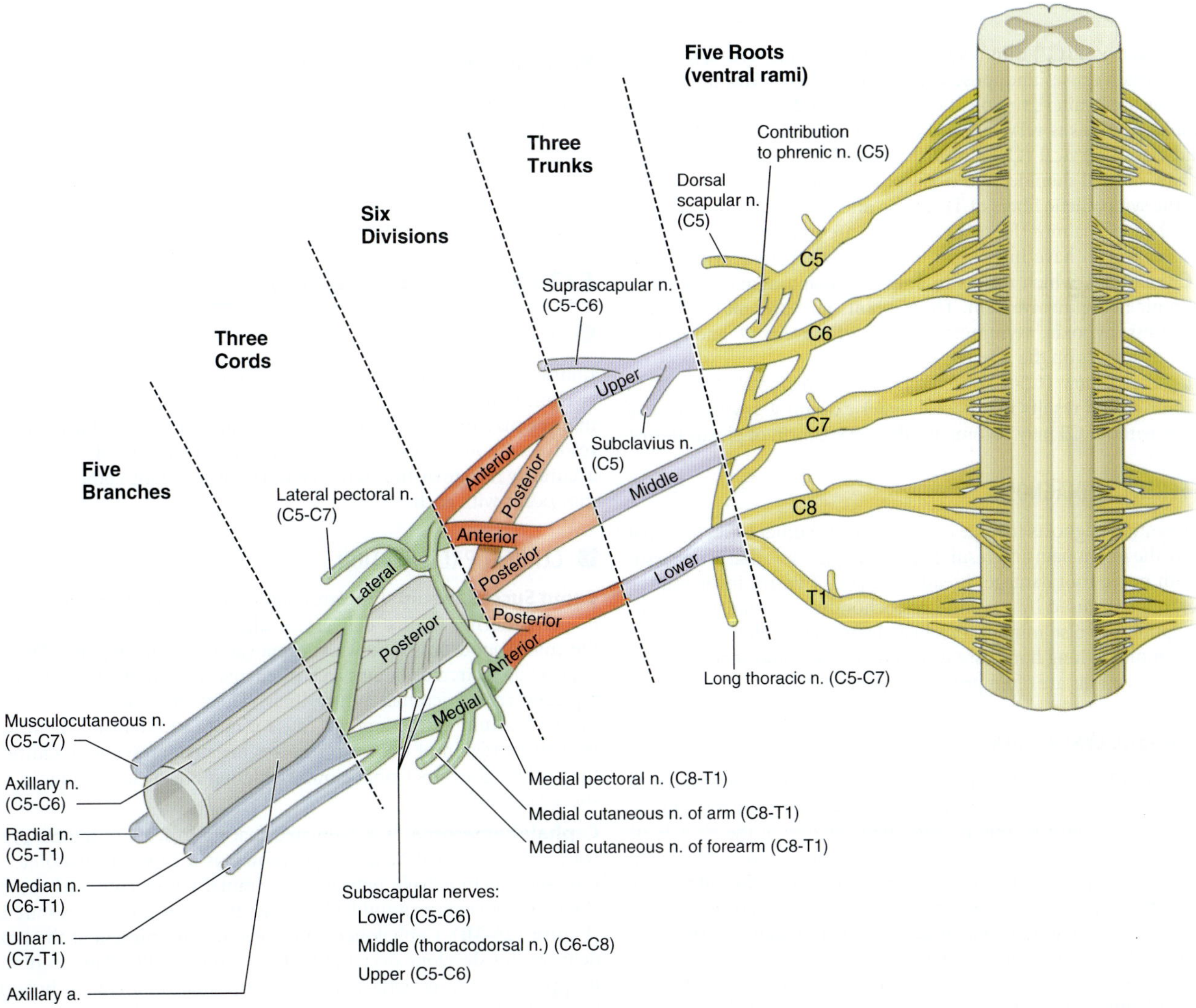

FIGURE 125-1. Schematic of the brachial nerve plexus. (Reproduced with permission from Morton DA, Foreman KB, Albertine KH. *The Big Picture: Gross Anatomy*. 2nd ed. New York: McGraw Hill; 2019, Figure 29-4.)

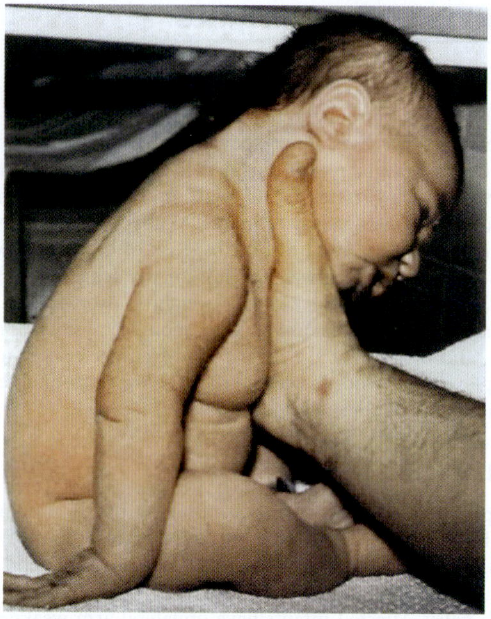

FIGURE 125-2. Waiter's tip position of Erb palsy. (Reproduced with permission from Balest AL, Riley MM, O'Donnell B and Zarit JS: Neonatology. In Zitelli BJ, Davis HW, eds. *Atlas of Pediatric Physical Diagnosis*. 8th ed. Philadelphia: CV Mosby; 2023. Copyright © Elsevier.)

the seventh cervical (C7) root results in paralysis of the wrist and finger extensors, which causes unopposed flexion of the hand. Together, this is described as the "waiter's tip" position (**Figure 125-2**).

Klumpke paralysis is very rare and involves isolated injury to the seventh and eighth cervical (C8) and first thoracic (Tl) nerve roots. These infants have normal shoulder and elbow position but a weak or paralyzed hand. If the sympathetic fibers of Tl are also affected, miosis, ptosis, anhidrosis, and enophthalmos (Horner syndrome) are additional findings.

Infants may also have injury to the third and fourth cervical nerve roots (C3 and C4), which results in unilateral diaphragmatic paralysis from phrenic nerve involvement. These infants may present with respiratory distress, hypoxia, asymmetric chest wall movement, and diminished breath sounds on the affected side.

Total plexus injury (C5-T1) accounts for approximately 20% of all plexus injuries and results in a flaccid upper extremity. Involvement of C4 with or without C3 may accompany this severe form of plexus injury.

DIFFERENTIAL DIAGNOSIS

The differential diagnosis includes a clavicular or humeral fracture that may cause the infant pain and result in a pseudoparalysis that is not associated with nerve root damage. Pseudoparalysis of Parrot involving the upper extremity caused by a painful osteochondritis secondary to congenital syphilis can also mimic a brachial plexus injury. However, in this condition multiple long bones are generally involved and other features of congenital syphilis are often present (Chapter 128).

DIAGNOSTIC EVALUATION

The diagnosis of nerve root injury is usually made clinically and based on the finding of an upper extremity with abnormal tone and movement. Plain radiography can rule out an associated fracture of the clavicle or humerus. Electromyography and nerve conduction studies may help clarify the injury in anticipation of surgical repair, but they are rarely necessary otherwise. These studies are typically performed several weeks after birth. When required, magnetic resonance imaging (MRI) can define the anatomy and extent of injury.

The diagnosis of diaphragmatic paralysis is made by demonstrating an elevated hemidiaphragm on the same side as the affected arm on an inspiratory radiograph. Real-time visualization with ultrasound or fluoroscopy will reveal paradoxical movement.

MANAGEMENT

Once fracture has been ruled out, initial management is rapid initiation of physical therapy. Therapy needs to include range-of-motion, stretching, and strengthening exercises. The therapist also needs to educate the parents of the infant in appropriate exercises at home. These exercises decrease the risk for contractures. Additionally, early involvement of an occupational therapist may be helpful.

There is some debate about how many infants have complete resolution of their injury without surgical intervention. Reported rates of spontaneous recovery after brachial plexus injury vary widely between 50% and 90%, with most studies suggesting a recovery rate of 66% to 75%. Those infants without complete recovery demonstrate varying degrees of residual weakness. Infants with upper arm paralysis do better than those with lower arm involvement. Other features associated with a less favorable outcome include diaphragmatic paralysis and Horner syndrome. Early signs of recovery, which may be noted by 2 weeks of age, favor complete resolution. Permanent weakness is likely if significant weakness is still present at 4 to 6 months.

CONSULTATION

Physical or occupational therapy should be consulted either during the initial hospitalization or shortly after discharge. Nerve reconstruction is an emerging technique that has shown promise in improving function in certain patients. The best timing for the procedure is still not clear, but several studies suggest that early repair may have a better long-term outcome. If the infant has persistent weakness of the biceps by 2 months, surgical consultation is indicated.

ADMISSION AND DISCHARGE CRITERIA

Admission to a neonatal intensive care unit is indicated for infants presenting with respiratory symptoms concerning for C3 and C4 nerve root injury. All infants with brachial plexus injury must have timely and serial follow-up with their physician to assess muscle function and recovery. Referral to a team or center specializing in brachial plexus injury care should occur by 2 months if there is persistent weakness.

EXTRACRANIAL INJURIES

BACKGROUND

Injuries to the scalp, subcutaneous tissue, and skull usually result in swelling that is apparent at birth or shortly thereafter. These extracranial injuries may occur from soft tissue swelling or hemorrhage and often resolve without treatment. However, the clinician needs to be able to accurately recognize these entities and be aware of the complications that may occur with each.

CLINICAL PRESENTATION

Caput Succedaneum Pressure applied to the scalp by the uterus, cervix, or pelvis during vaginal delivery results in a localized swelling outside the cranial aponeurosis known as caput succedaneum (**Figure 125-3A**). It appears as a circular boggy area of edema with indistinct borders that typically crosses cranial suture lines. There may be overlying ecchymosis. Vacuum extraction can cause a more pronounced caput as the presenting region of the scalp receives negative pressure in addition to the positive pressure from below. A chignon is a vacuum-induced caput succedaneum.

Cephalohematoma It is estimated that up to 2.5% of infants present with a subperiosteal hemorrhage known as a cephalohematoma. This represents hemorrhage between the cranial periosteum and the bony skull and presents as a fluid-filled mass that does not cross suture lines (**Figure 125-3B**). Cephalohematoma is often not present at the time of delivery but develops over the first few hours of life. Most commonly it appears in the parietal bone, but more than one cranial bone may be involved. Risk factors for cephalohematoma include a primiparous mother, forceps- or vacuum-assisted delivery, and prolonged labor. In one study, 90% of infants with cephalohematoma had an occiput

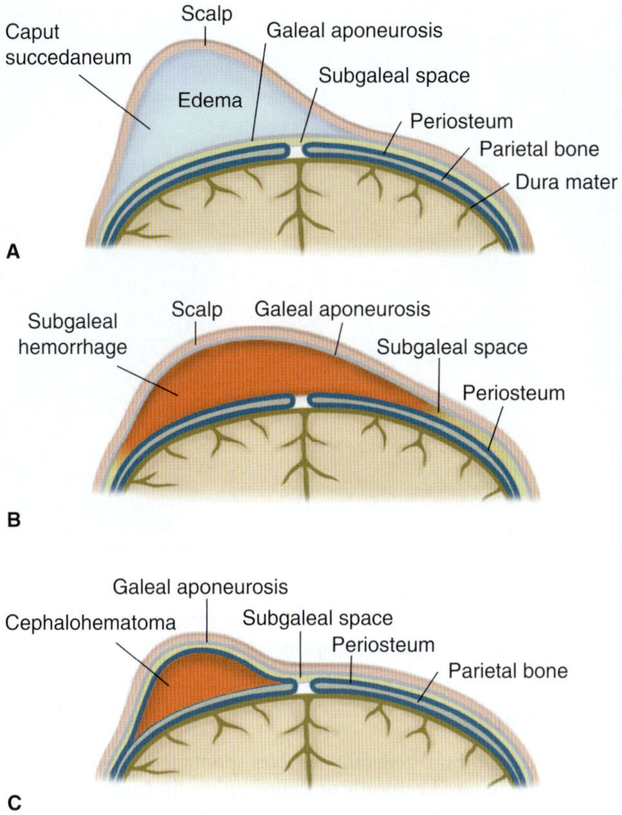

FIGURE 125-3. Drawing of caput succedaneum (A), subgaleal hemorrhage (B), and cephalohematoma (C). (Reproduced with permission from Cunningham FG, Leveno KJ, Dashe JS, et al, eds. *Williams Obstetrics*. 26th ed. New York: McGraw Hill; 2022, Figure 33-2.)

anterior presentation. In the same study, 7% of cephalohematomas were associated with an underlying skull fracture, with all these injuries being related to the use of forceps.

Subgaleal Hemorrhage Bleeding that occurs beneath the aponeurosis of the scalp but outside the cranial periosteum is termed a subgaleal or subaponeurotic hemorrhage. Similar to a cephalohematoma, a subgaleal hemorrhage is fluctuant because of the fluid collection that is present, but it extends over suture lines (**Figure 125-3C**). Unlike a cephalohematoma, the bleeding into the subgaleal space is not restricted by the boundaries of the sutures. Extensive bleeding may occur and the infant may present with signs of hypovolemic shock.

DIFFERENTIAL DIAGNOSIS

Other entities to consider in the differential of extrancranial hemorrhage are subarachnoid cyst, meningocele, or leptomeningeal cyst.

DIAGNOSTIC EVALUATION

The diagnosis is based on the feel and location of the scalp swelling. Ultrasonography is helpful when the clinical examination is not definitive. Because fractures are only occasionally associated with cephalohematoma and the majority of these fractures are benign linear skull fractures, routine skull radiographs are not generally necessary.

MANAGEMENT

Caput succedaneum resolves spontaneously over a period of several days; no management is needed other than parental reassurance. Cranial molding and prominent bony ridges as a result of overriding sutures may become more apparent as the soft tissue swelling improves. Parents can be reassured that these bony changes will improve over the next few weeks.

Cephalohematoma takes weeks to months to resolve. As resorption proceeds, the additional red cell destruction may cause or contribute to indirect hyperbilirubinemia. As the hematoma resolves, a firm calcified ring may form around the hematoma and cause the illusion of a depressed skull fracture. As previously noted, cephalohematomas are uncommonly associated with skull fractures, and they are almost always linear skull fractures that require no specific management.

Subgaleal hemorrhage requires prompt recognition because it is a much more serious entity with mortality estimated at up to 20%. Rapid bleeding can occur and may lead to hypovolemic shock. Serial hemoglobin and bilirubin levels as well as coagulation studies are indicated. Volume replacement or red cell transfusion may be needed. Surgical management is rarely indicated because the source of bleeding is typically not identifiable.

Aspiration of these fluid collections is discouraged because the procedure is rarely therapeutic or diagnostic. Imaging studies can determine the anatomic level of the bleeding and do not have the attendant risk of introducing infection.

Infection of the fluid collection can occur, especially when there is an overlying laceration or puncture secondary to forceps, scalp probes, or aspiration attempts. The area becomes erythematous and warm, and fever often develops. When infection is present, aspiration for Gram stain and bacterial culture and sensitivity studies is warranted while empirical antibiotic therapy is initiated. Coverage of skin flora and newborn pathogens is recommended.

ADMISSION AND DISCHARGE CRITERIA

Admission to the neonatal intensive care unit is indicated for infants with cephalohematoma who develop significant hyperbilirubinemia requiring exchange transfusion. Infants with subgaleal hemorrhage also may warrant admission to the neonatal intensive care unit for close vital sign monitoring, serial laboratory studies, and volume replacement or red cell transfusion as needed. Routine postnatal care and discharge can be anticipated for infants with caput succedaneum and for most infants with cephalohematoma.

INTRACRANIAL HEMORRHAGE

BACKGROUND

With advances in obstetric practices, hemorrhage within the bony skull is an increasingly uncommon occurrence in term newborns. Risk factors are similar to those for other birth injuries, including macrosomia and precipitous or instrument-assisted deliveries. Intraventricular hemorrhage is a significant consideration in preterm infants (<37 weeks gestation).

CLINICAL PRESENTATION

Subdural Hemorrhage Although often associated with vacuum-assisted deliveries, subdural hemorrhage is now known to occur in spontaneous vaginal deliveries as well as in utero before delivery. Clinical manifestations range from asymptomatic infants with no long-term sequelae to serious neurologic injury. The location of the hemorrhage can alter the presentation, but the most common locations are infra- and supra-tentorial, and intrahemispheric. Apnea or cyanotic episodes are the most common initial symptoms, although seizure, focal neurologic deficits, lethargy, or other global nonspecific findings may be the presenting early symptoms. Commonly, infants become symptomatic on the first day of life, but sometimes the findings are not apparent until several days after birth.

Epidural Hemorrhage Bleeding into the epidural space is the least common form of intracranial hemorrhage. The cause is injury to the middle meningeal artery, which is almost uniformly associated with an overlying fracture of the temporal bone and cephalohematoma. Focal or generalized neurologic symptoms are present shortly after birth, and evidence of raised intracranial pressure may be demonstrated by a bulging fontanelle.

Subarachnoid Hemorrhage In older children and adults, subarachnoid hemorrhage is most often due to aneurysms or arteriovenous malformations. By contrast, subarachnoid hemorrhage in newborns is due to rupture of small bridging veins of the subarachnoid space and is more common with vacuum- or forceps-assisted deliveries than with vaginal deliveries. The typical presentation in newborns with subarachnoid bleeding is seizure activity that starts on the second day of life, with normal neurologic findings between seizures. The prognosis is very good, with complete resolution of the hemorrhage and no neurologic sequelae, although children with asphyxia or underlying cortical injury are at risk for permanent deficits. Posthemorrhagic hydrocephalus may develop in the first few weeks of life and can be detected by routine monitoring of head circumference.

DIAGNOSTIC EVALUATION

For subdural, epidural, and subarachnoid hemorrhages, computed tomography (CT) of the head is the diagnostic tool of choice. This may also demonstrate any associated skull fracture in the case of epidural hemorrhage. For infants with subdural hemorrhage, MRI may be needed to clearly visualize bleeding in the posterior fossa. Because of the possibility of an underlying coagulopathy with subdural hemorrhage, a prothrombin time and partial thromboplastin time should also be obtained.

MANAGEMENT

In the case of subdural hemorrhage, surgical intervention is usually reserved for infants with evidence of brainstem compression. Surgical drainage for epidural hemorrhage is necessary for most newborns. Most infants with subarachnoid hemorrhage do not require surgical intervention unless the hemorrhage is very extensive.

ADMISSION AND DISCHARGE CRITERIA

Admission to the neonatal intensive care unit is indicated for infants presenting with neurologic symptoms consistent with intracranial hemorrhage, including apnea or cyanotic seizure, focal deficits, and lethargy. Discharge criteria should be determined in consultation with a neonatologist; consider consultation with a neurologist or neurosurgeon as well.

PNEUMOTHORAX

BACKGROUND

Spontaneous pneumothorax in term newborns has a reported incidence of 1% to 2%, although many are asymptomatic. It is thought to be the result of the intrathoracic pressure created by the infant during the first few attempts at respiration. Pneumothorax may also be seen in infants with meconium aspiration or pneumonia and in those with a history of receiving positive-pressure ventilation at delivery.

CLINICAL PRESENTATION

Most cases of spontaneous pneumothorax in newborns are not clinically apparent. However, if the volume of air in the pleural space is large or under pressure (tension pneumothorax), the infant will display signs of respiratory distress, including grunting, flaring, and retracting, with decreased breath sounds on the involved side. A tension pneumothorax may cause a shift in location of the point of maximal impulse of the heart, deviation of the trachea, or a distended hemithorax.

DIAGNOSTIC EVALUATION

If the diagnosis of pneumothorax is suspected and the infant is not clinically stable, intervention should not be delayed to obtain a chest radiograph. Initially, needle thoracostomy may be performed until a definitive chest tube can be inserted (see Treatment). An audible release of air under pressure along with an associated improvement in the patient's clinical status confirms the diagnosis.

If the diagnosis is in question and the infant is clinically stable, a chest radiograph is appropriate to confirm the presence and severity of the pneumothorax. Pneumothorax appears as a dark (radiolucent) area in the chest, without overlying lung markings (**Figure 125-4**). A radiograph of an infant with tension pneumothorax also displays a shift of the mediastinum and airway away from the affected side.

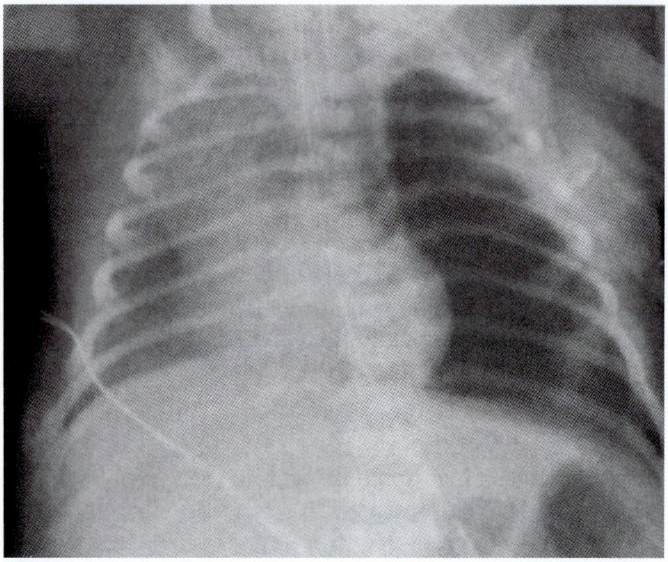

FIGURE 125-4. Radiograph of a newborn with a large left-sided pneumothorax displacing the mediastinal structures to the right. The mass effect from the pneumothorax is also causing compressive atelectasis in the right upper lung field.

MANAGEMENT

A small pneumothorax generally resolves spontaneously in a few days and may be monitored clinically or radiographically. Large pneumothoraces and those under pressure require evacuation of the air and continued drainage with a chest tube and negative pressure. When the air leak has stopped, the tube may be clamped. Without further evidence of reaccumulation, the chest tube may be removed (see Chapter 164 for further details on chest tube insertion).

ADMISSION AND DISCHARGE CRITERIA

Infants with large or symptomatic pneumothoraces should be admitted to the neonatal intensive care unit. Criteria for discharge include resolution of tachypnea, tachycardia, hypoxia, and other vital sign disturbances.

KEY POINTS

- While macrosomia, shoulder dystocia, and instrumented delivery increase the risk of birth injury, injury may be identified in newborns with no known risk factors.
- The clavicle is the most commonly broken bone in newborns.
- Most scalp injuries are benign and self-limited; however, a subgaleal hemorrhage must be recognized promptly, as these infants are at risk for hypovolemic shock.
- Pneumothorax and brachial plexus injury with diaphragmatic paralysis should be considered in the differential diagnosis for an infant with respiratory distress.

SUGGESTED READINGS

Beall MH, Ross MG. Clavicle fracture in labor: risk factors and associated morbidities. *J Perinatol.* 2001;21:513-515.

Chauhan SP, Rose CH, Gherman RB, Magann EF, Holland MW, Morrison JC. Brachial plexus injury: a 23-year experience from a tertiary center. *Am J Obstet Gynecol.* 2005;192:1795-1800.

Corsini I, Dani C. Pneumomediastinum in term and late preterm newborns: what is the proper clinical approach? *J Matern Fetal Neonatal Med.* 2015;28:1332-1335.

Demissie K, Rhoads GG, Smulian JC, et al. Operative vaginal delivery and neonatal and infant adverse outcomes: population based retrospective analysis. *BMJ.* 2004;329(7456):24-29. Erratum in: *BMJ.* 2004;329(7465):547.

Dodds SD, Wolfe SW. Perinatal brachial plexus palsy. *Curr Opin Pediatr.* 2000;12:40-47.

Koshinski JL, Russo SA, Zlotolow DA. Brachial plexus birth injury: a review of neurology literature assessing variability and current recommendations. *Pediatr Neurol.* 2022;136:35-42.

Noetzel MJ, Park TS, Robinson S, Kaufman B. Prospective study of recovery following neonatal brachial plexus injury. *J Child Neurol.* 2001;16:488-492.

Raio L, Ghezzi F, Di Naro E, et al. Perinatal outcome of fetuses with a birth weight greater than 4500 g: an analysis of 3356 cases. *Eur J Obstet Gynecol Reprod Biol.* 2003;109:160-165.

Sandberg DI, Lamberti-Pasculli M, Drake JM, Humphreys RP, Rutka JT. Spontaneous intraparenchymal hemorrhage in full-term neonates. *Neurosurgery.* 2001;48(5):1042-1048; discussion 1048-9.

Steele RW, Metz JR, Bass JW, DuBois JJ. Pneumothorax and pneumomediastinum in the newborn. *Radiology.* 1971;98:629-632.

Tasunaga S, Rivera R. Cephalohematoma in the newborn. *Clin Pediatr (Philadelphia).* 1974;13:256-260.

Werner EF, Janevic TM, Illuzzi J, Funai EF, Savitz DA, Lipkind HS. Mode of delivery in nulliparous women and neonatal intracranial injury. *Obstet Gynecol.* 2011;118(6):1239-1246.

CHAPTER 126

Care of the Late Preterm Infant

Kelly E. Wood, MD

BACKGROUND

DEFINITION

Late preterm (LPT) infants are premature infants born between 34 0/7 and 36 6/7 weeks of gestation. Formerly known as "near term," the term "late preterm" arose from a workshop held in 2005 by the National Institute of Child Health and Human Development. The change was driven by the recognition that these infants are not fully mature, and the final weeks of gestation are important for growth and development. The phrase "near term" may mislead some to think of these infants as "almost term," and subsequently fail to recognize their increased risk of complications compared with term infants and need for closer monitoring and follow-up. In 2007, the American Academy of Pediatrics (AAP) published a clinical report on LPT infants endorsing the terminology.

INCIDENCE AND EPIDEMIOLOGY

In the United States (US), LPT infants comprise 7% of all live births, and account for more than 70% of all preterm births. Disparities in LPT birth have persisted, with non-Hispanic black individuals disproportionately affected. LPT birth is also more common among individuals who conceived using assisted reproductive technology, in part because many procedures involve transferring multiple embryos resulting in multiple gestation pregnancies.

ETIOLOGY AND PATHOGENESIS

The etiology of LPT birth is multifactorial and can generally be categorized as spontaneous, elective without medical indication, or medically indicated. Most LPT births result from spontaneous preterm labor and/or preterm rupture of placental membranes, with identified risk factors including prior preterm delivery, infection, short cervix, multiple gestations, and smoking during pregnancy. Elective late preterm births without medical indication, though historically more common, are now infrequent due to recommendations from federal agencies (Centers for Disease Control and Prevention), professional societies (AAP, American College of Obstetricians and Gynecology [ACOG]), and national organizations (March of Dimes) to avoid elective deliveries before 39 weeks of gestation.

Medically indicated LPT birth results from pregnant person, placental, or fetal complications necessitating early delivery. Examples of pregnancy related medical conditions include poorly controlled chronic hypertension, gestational hypertension with severe range blood pressures, preeclampsia with severe features, intrahepatic cholestasis of pregnancy, and poorly controlled gestational diabetes. Placental indications include placenta previa; suspected accrete, increta, or percreta; vasa previa; prior classical cesarean section; and/or prior uterine rupture. Examples of fetal conditions include oligohydramnios, abnormal umbilical artery with absence of end-diastolic flow, and those related to multiple gestations such as triplet and higher order multiples and monochronic placentation.

CLINICAL PRESENTATION

LPT infants resemble term infants, and macrosomia may mask prematurity. Careful history taking is important, and includes details about the pregnancy, delivery including reasons for preterm delivery, and resuscitation. Carefully review prenatal test results to determine if the infant requires additional postnatal testing and/or treatment. Group B streptococcus (GBS) status of the pregnant person may be unknown as testing is recommended between 36 0/7 and 37 6/7 weeks of gestation. If GBS status is unknown, preterm prolonged rupture of membranes and premature labor are indications for intrapartum antibiotic prophylaxis.

ASSESSMENT OF GESTATIONAL AGE

Prenatally, gestational age and due date can be estimated using the date of last menstrual period and/or prenatal ultrasound. The most accurate method to determine and confirm gestational age is a first trimester (at or before 13 6/7 weeks gestation) ultrasound. During the ultrasound, the fetal crown-rump length is measured, and has an accuracy of ± 5 to 7 days. Dating is considered suboptimal if an ultrasound is not performed by 22 0/7 weeks gestation to confirm or revise the estimated due date.

Methods of postnatal assessment of gestational age include the Dubowitz method, new Ballard score, and eye exam evaluating vascularity of the lens capsule. Such assessments may be useful if pregnancy dating is unknown or suboptimal, but first trimester ultrasound is superior. The new Ballard score is a common method that uses physical and neurologic exam characteristics to estimate gestational age (**Table 126-1**). Each criterion is scored from −1 to 5 and then tallied to give a corresponding gestational age between 20 and 44 weeks. Accuracy increases with each week of gestational age, and performs best for infants over 38 weeks of gestation and up to 96 hours old. Illness, medications, neuromuscular disorders, and breech positioning may affect the neurologic exam.

GROWTH ASSESSMENT

Weight, length, and head circumference should be measured after birth, and plotted on a preterm growth chart to determine size classification. Currently, there is no agreed upon postnatal growth assessment tool for preterm infants. Typically, local practice and preference determines the growth chart used. Intrauterine curves also called size-at-birth charts, such as the Olsen and Fenton growth curves, use size at birth as a proxy for the healthy fetus size at the same post-menstrual age. The assumption that extrauterine growth of the infant should match intrauterine growth of a healthy fetus has been questioned. In 2015, the INTERGROWTH-21st preterm postnatal growth standards were developed. Conceptually similar to the World Health Organization (WHO) growth standards, the INTERGROWTH-21st compares the postnatal growth of preterm infants to that of other healthy preterm infants, not fetuses or term infants.

After discharge, growth should be monitored closely as growth failure is associated with poor neurodevelopmental outcomes and overnutrition may increase future cardiometabolic risk. It is important to correct for gestational age to avoid mislabeling an infant as having suboptimal growth, but there is no consensus for how long to correct. Eventually, all LPT infants should be transitioned to the WHO growth curve used for term infants.

TABLE 126-1 New Ballard Score—Common Findings for Late Preterm and Term Infants

	Late Preterm	Term
Physical characteristics		
Skin	Smooth, pink, veins visible	Peeling, cracking, rare or no veins
Lanugo	Abundant or thinning	Bald areas or mostly bald
Plantar surface (creases on sole)	Faint, anterior transverse crease only	Creases cover 2/3 to entire sole
Breast	Flat areola, no or small bud (1-2 mm)	Raised or full areola, progressively larger bud (3-10 mm)
Eye/Ear	Soft pinna, slow to ready recoil	Formed firm pinna, instant recoil
Genitalia (male)	Testes descending, few rugae	Testes descended, good to deep rugae
Genitalia (female)	Prominent clitoris, majora and minora equally prominent	Majora larger or cover minora and clitoris
Neurologic characteristics		
Posture	Extremities slightly flexed	Extremities fully flexed
Square window—*angle formed when wrist flexed*	45° or greater	30° or less
Arm recoil—*angle at elbow when extend supinated arm recoils toward shoulder*	110° to 140°	<90°-110°
Popliteal angle—*angle formed when knee extended*	120° or greater	100° or less
Scarf Sign—*pulling flexed elbow across the chest*	To or past midline of chest	Less than midline
Heel to Ear—*distance between when leg extended at hip and knee*	Able to extend heel to face or chest (above umbilicus)	Unable to extend heel past umbilicus

Abbreviations: mm, millimeter

TABLE 126-2 Common Complications After Birth for Late Preterm Infants

Complication	Etiology
Respiratory conditions	Surfactant deficiency Decreased fetal lung clearance Delayed postnatal transition Immature respiratory drive
Hypothermia	Large body surface area relative to weight Immature thermogenesis Decreased insulation
Hypoglycemia	Decreased glycogen stores Immature gluconeogenesis and glycogenolysis Ineffective adipose tissue lipolysis Poor feeding
Feeding difficulties	Neurologic immaturity Suck-swallow-breathe incoordination Low oromotor tone Fatigue with feeds
Infection	Invasive procedures Intraamnionic infection (chorioamnionitis) causing preterm labor Reduced barrier function of skin Immature immune system
Hyperbilirubinemia	Reduced hepatic uptake and conjugation of bilirubin Increased enterohepatic circulation Gastrointestinal immaturity Feeding difficulties Dehydration

MANAGEMENT

As shown in **Table 126-2**, LPT infants are at increased risk of complications related to their physiologic immaturity. The likelihood of complications decreases as gestational age at birth increases. Overall, most LPT infants do well without significant complications.

DELIVERY ROOM

LPT infants are more likely to require resuscitation after delivery. The increased risk is highest for those born at 34 weeks and decreases with each advancing week of gestation. Delivery rooms should be kept temperature neutral as LPT infants are at risk for hypothermia. Delayed cord clamping (DCC), greater than or equal to 60 seconds, is recommended for late preterm infants just like term infants, as long as they are vigorous and/or do not require immediate resuscitation after birth. Although DCC increases hemoglobin and hematocrit concentration after birth and improves iron status in early infancy, it has not been shown to prevent iron deficiency anemia or improve neurodevelopmental outcomes in this population.

RESPIRATORY

LPT infants are born during the transition from the terminal saccular to alveolar phase of lung development, therefore, they may be deficient in surfactant, have decreased ability to absorb lung fluid, and inefficient gas exchange. They are at increased risk for various respiratory complications including respiratory distress syndrome, transient tachypnea of the newborn (TTN), pneumonia, pulmonary hypertension, and apnea. They are at higher risk for respiratory failure requiring supplemental oxygen and assisted ventilation both mechanical and continuous positive airway pressure (CPAP). Delivery by cesarean section before the onset of labor greatly increases the odds of respiratory complications. The likelihood of respiratory complications and need for assisted ventilation decreases with each advancing week of gestation until 38 weeks and likely reflects lung maturation.

HYPOTHERMIA

Hypothermia is defined as a core temperature less than 36.5°C. In premature infants, hypothermia increases morbidity and mortality. Hypothermia may be environmental or a sign of a serious underlying condition such as sepsis.

In LPT infants, the risk of hypothermia is multifactorial including increased heat loss, decreased insulation, and impaired thermogenesis. LPT infants have increased body-surface area relative to body weight, thin skin, and decreased subcutaneous white fat for insulation which increases the risk of heat loss. Evaporative heat loss occurs after delivery, and can be prevented by drying the infant. Conductive heat loss occurs when the infant is placed in contact with a cold surface such as a scale. Unlike term infants who can generate heat by breaking down brown adipose tissue, LPT infants have less brown fat and the hormones needed to breakdown it down. Immaturity of the central nervous system, specifically the hypothalamus, results in impaired response to hypothermia with impaired release of thermogenic hormones such as thyroxine and norepinephrine. All increase the LPT infant's susceptibility to hypothermia. Cold stress increases the metabolic demand and oxygen consumption which can lead to delayed respiratory transition and exacerbate hypoglycemia.

Preventing hypothermia starts in the delivery room. To minimize heat loss in the delivery room, provide a warm environment, dry the infant after birth, and initiate early skin to skin contact with the birth parent or other caregiver. Outside of the delivery room provide a thermoneutral environment, postpone routine bathing, ensure proper dressing, and promote kangaroo care. Kangaroo care (early, prolonged skin to skin contact between the caregiver and infant) has been shown to be effective at preventing hypothermia.

HYPOGLYCEMIA

At delivery, all newborns must rapidly adapt to prevent hypoglycemia due to the abrupt loss of the placental glucose supply. The incidence of hypoglycemia is inversely proportional to gestational age. LPT infants are significantly more likely to develop hypoglycemia than term infants, and more likely to require an intravenous glucose infusion during the birth hospitalization. Decreased glycogen stores and immature hepatic gluconeogenesis and glycogenolysis, and adipose tissue lipolysis increases their susceptibility to developing hypoglycemia. Factors such as cold stress, sepsis, and poor feeding may exacerbate hypoglycemia. Clinical manifestations of hypoglycemia are similar to that seen in term infants and may include hypothermia, irritability, jitteriness, tachypnea, apnea, lethargy, hypotonia, and seizures. Hypoglycemia can be asymptomatic; therefore, the AAP recommends all LPT infants be screened prior to each feed during the first 24 hours of life. To prevent hypoglycemia, LPT infants should be fed every 2 to 3 hours, paying close attention for feeding difficulties.

FEEDING DIFFICULTIES

Feeding difficulties are more common in LPT infants, and one of the most common reasons for readmission. Feeding difficulties may lead to prolonged hospitalization, poor weight gain, and increase the risk of hyperbilirubinemia, hypoglycemia, and dehydration. Difficulties may be secondary to neurologic immaturity, suck-swallow-breathe incoordination, low oromotor tone, and fatigue with feeds. Feeding during the birth hospitalization may be successful but not sustained after discharge. To identify feeding problems, weight loss, stooling habits, and urine output should be closely monitored. Failure to recognize difficulties during the birth hospitalization may relate to shorter hospital stays and small initial volume of feedings.

LPT infants are at increased risk for breast/chest feeding difficulties, with lower reported rates of breast/chest feeding initiation and exclusive breast/chest feeding. Readmission rates for breast/chest fed LPT infants are almost twice as common as rates for breast/chest fed term or non-breast/chest fed LPT infants. Supportive practices such as rooming-in, latch assistance, and skin-to-skin care have been shown to improve breast/chest feeding outcomes in this population.

INFECTION

LPT infants have higher rates of sepsis and culture-positive infections than term infants. Their increased susceptibility is likely multifactorial including invasive procedures, intraamniotic infection (chorioamnionitis) as the cause of preterm labor, immunologic immaturity, and decreased protective barriers due to thin, immature skin. During the birth hospitalization, they are four times more likely to be evaluated for sepsis and receive antibiotics than term infants. Common conditions related to prematurity such as TTN, hypothermia, and hypoglycemia may be interpreted as signs of infection leading to evaluation and treatment for suspected sepsis.

Although LPT infants are at increased risk for early onset sepsis (EOS), empiric evaluation and treatment with antibiotics is not universally indicated. National guidelines for risk assessment and management of suspected EOS for well appearing LPT infants are divided by gestational age into ≤ 34 6/7 weeks and ≥ 35 weeks. Approaches to risk assessment for EOS in this population is described further in Chapter 128. Regardless of gestational age, any LPT infant with clinical signs of infection should have a blood culture obtained and started on empiric antibiotics.

HYPERBILIRUBINEMIA

Hyperbilirubinemia is more common and has a more prolonged course in LPT infants. They have a higher rate of bilirubin production, decreased hepatic conjugation, and impaired elimination. Their liver is immature and has decreased uridine diphosphate glucuronyl transferase enzyme activity resulting in decrease uptake and conjugation of bilirubin. Enterohepatic circulation is increased due to their immature gastrointestinal function and motility compounded by feeding difficulties and dehydration. The risk of developing high total serum bilirubin (TSB) levels (>20 mg/dL) is higher compared to term infants. Among LPT infants, identified risk factors for severe hyperbilirubinemia requiring treatment include large for gestational age (LGA), lower gestational age, birth trauma, and a previous sibling with severe hyperbilirubinemia.

The AAP recommends treatment with phototherapy and exchange transfusion at a lower TSB for LPT infants especially for those with risk factors (Chapter 136). There is data to suggest these infants are at greater risk for developing neurotoxicity at lower bilirubin levels and earlier postnatal age. LPT infants, especially those LGA, were overrepresented in the U.S. Pilot Kernicterus Registry, a database of voluntarily reported cases. In these cases, providers failed to recognize and act upon late prematurity as a risk factor for severe hyperbilirubinemia. It is vital that all LPT infants be assessed for hyperbilirubinemia prior to discharge, have close follow-up, and prompt initiation of treatment when indicated.

READMISSION

Readmission rates are 1.5 to 3 times higher for LPT infants compared to term infants. The most common reason for readmission is hyperbilirubinemia, followed by feeding difficulties, and infection/sepsis evaluation. The majority of readmissions occur within the first 5 days after discharge which is consistent with hyperbilirubinemia being the primary driver of readmission. Breast/chest feeding at discharge is a prominent risk factor for readmission, though the majority of breast/chest fed LPT infants do not require readmission.

NEURODEVELOPMENTAL OUTCOMES AND LONG-TERM SEQULAE

LPT infants are at risk for developmental delays, learning difficulties, poorer academic performance, and cognitive deficits compared to term infants. Problems with attention are also more likely. Interruption of in utero brain maturation during a critical period is felt to be the main reason for long-term neurodevelopmental outcomes. Additionally, they may be more likely to develop respiratory problems such as wheezing and asthma later in childhood.

ADMISSION CRITERIA

Compared to term infants, LPT infants are more frequently admitted to neonatal intensive care units (NICU). Yet, many LPT infants are admitted to well newborn nurseries (Level I) despite their increased risk of morbidity. For well appearing LPT infants, standardized admission criteria for the well newborn nursery have not been created leaving institutions to develop their own practice guideline. Gestational age and birth weight cutoffs are likely key decision factors. The medical needs of the infant and unit capabilities are important factors to consider when determining if the infant may remain with the caregiver(s) in the well nursery or requires admission to a higher level of care such as a NICU (Level III and IV) or special care nursery (Level II).

DISCHARGE CRITERIA

The AAP has established minimum discharge criteria for LPT infants many of which overlap with that recommended for term infants. Discharge criteria include vital sign stability for 12 hours prior to discharge; 24 hours of successful feeding; completion of standard screenings and assessments including for hyperbilirubinemia; passed a car seat tolerance screening; caregiver education completed; medical, family and social needs addressed; and follow-up 24 to 48 hours after discharge arranged. The AAP recommends that discharge timing should be individualized, but notes that LPT infants are not expected to meet all necessary discharge requirements before 48 hours of age. As LPT infants are at increased risk for readmission, providers must ensure infants and caregivers are ready for discharge, and that follow-up is timely.

CAR SEAT TOLERANCE TESTING

Preterm infants are at risk for proximal airway obstruction and cardiopulmonary events while in their car seats. As such, the AAP recommends car seat tolerance screening for all infants < 37 weeks gestation prior to discharge. Suggested length of screening is a minimum of 90 to 120 minutes or the duration of travel, whichever is longer.

KEY POINTS

- Late preterm infants are premature infants born between 34 0/7 and 36 6/7 weeks of gestation.
- Late preterm infants have increased morbidity and mortality compared to term infants, and are at increased risk for respiratory conditions, hypothermia, hypoglycemia, feeding difficulties, infection, and hyperbilirubinemia.
- Late preterm infants are at increased risk for readmission especially during the first week after discharge. Hyperbilirubinemia is the most common reason for readmission.
- The American Academy of Pediatrics has outlined minimal discharge criteria for late preterm infants to help clinicians assess discharge readiness.

SUGGESTED READINGS

Adamkin DH. Postnatal glucose homeostasis in late-preterm and term infants. *Pediatrics.* 2011;127(3):575-579.

Ballard JL, Khoury JC, Wedig K, Wang L, Eilers-Walsman BL, Lipp R. New Ballard Score, expanded to include extremely premature infants. *J Pediatr.* 1991;119(3):417-423.

Bhutani VK, Johnson L. Kernicterus in late preterm infants cared for as term healthy infants. *Semin Perinatol.* 2006;30(2):89-97.

Bull MJ, Engle WA. Safe transportation of preterm and low birth weight infants at hospital discharge. *Pediatrics.* 2009;123(5): 1424-1429.

Cordova EG, Belfort MB. Updates on assessment and monitoring of the postnatal growth of preterm infants. *Neoreviews.* 2020;21(2): e98-e108.

Goyal NK, Attanasio LB, Kozhimannil KB. Hospital care and early breastfeeding outcomes among late preterm, early-term, and term infants. *Birth.* 2014;41(4):330-338.

Kemper AR, Newman TB, Slaughter JL, et al. Clinical practice guideline revision: management of hyperbilirubinemia in the newborn infant 35 or more weeks of gestation. *Pediatrics.* 2022;150(3).

Martin JA, Hamilton BE, Osterman MJK. Births in the United States, 2020. *NCHS data brief; no 418.* 09/27/2021ed: National Center for Health Statistics (U.S.) National Vital Statistics System; 2021.

Natarajan G, Shankaran S. Short- and long-term outcomes of moderate and late preterm infants. *Am J Perinatol.* 2016;33(3):305-317.

Puopolo KM, Benitz WE, Zaoutis TE, Committee On F, Newborn, Committee On Infectious D, et al. Management of neonates born at ≥35 0/7 weeks' gestation with suspected or proven early-onset bacterial sepsis. *Pediatrics.* 2018;142(6):e20182894.

Raju TN, Higgins RD, Stark AR, Leveno KJ. Optimizing care and outcome for late-preterm (near-term) infants: a summary of the workshop sponsored by the National Institute of Child Health and Human Development. *Pediatrics.* 2006;118(3):1207-1214.

Shapiro-Mendoza CK, Tomashek KM, Kotelchuck M, Barfield W, Weiss J, Evans S. Risk factors for neonatal morbidity and mortality among "healthy," late preterm newborns. *Semin Perinatol.* 2006;30(2):54-60.

Stewart DL, Barfield WD, AAP Committee on Fetus and Newborn. Updates on an at-risk population: late-preterm and early-term infants. *Pediatrics.* 2019;144(5).

CHAPTER 127 Respiratory Distress and Transient Tachypnea of the Newborn

Ebony Beaudoin, MD

BACKGROUND

Respiratory distress occurs frequently in newborns and can be a presenting symptom of both benign and life-threatening diseases. Failure of any of a complex series of cardiovascular and pulmonary modifications that help the neonate transition to extrauterine life can manifest as neonatal respiratory distress. Clinical features of a newborn in respiratory distress include tachypnea of more than 60 breaths per minute; cyanosis; expiratory grunting; intercostal, subcostal, or supraclavicular retractions; and nasal flaring. Although the causes of respiratory distress are numerous, this chapter focuses on a relatively common cause of respiratory distress known as transient tachypnea of the newborn (TTN).

TTN is a benign, self-limited disorder that occurs during the transition from uterine to extrauterine life and results from the delayed clearance of excess lung fluid. It is the most common cause of respiratory distress in infants term (≥37 weeks' gestation) and late preterm (34-36 weeks gestation). TTN was first described in 1966 when it was observed that a subset of newborns exhibited respiratory distress, consisting primarily of tachypnea, at or shortly after birth. Although the tachypnea persisted for several days, it subsequently resolved completely without sequelae.

PATHOPHYSIOLOGY

At approximately 6 weeks of gestation, the fetal lung begins secreting alveolar fluid. Sodium and subsequently water are transported into the alveolar cells via aquaporin, a channel protein. Fetal lung volume is maintained by the larynx, which serves as a one-way valve for outflow. Late in gestation and culminating at the onset of labor, catecholamine release, and hormonal changes trigger the lungs to prepare for delivery and begin resorption of sodium and liquids into the neonatal pulmonary circulation and lymphatics.

TTN results from inadequate or delayed clearance of fetal lung fluid, which fills the alveolar space, then moves into the extra-alveolar space subsequently surrounding the perivascular tissue and lung fissures. This results in decreased compliance of the neonatal lung, ineffective gas exchange, and respiratory distress. Risk factors for TTN include delivery before completion of 39 weeks gestation, cesarean section without labor, gestational diabetes, and maternal asthma. The risk of TTN after cesarean section is significantly decreased if the mother undergoes a trial of labor. Additional known risk factors for TTN include male sex, perinatal asphyxia, prematurity, small for gestational age, and large for gestational age infants.

CLINICAL PRESENTATION

TTN presents within the first few minutes to hours of life with respiratory rates greater than 60 breaths per minute. Infants typically have shallow respirations, which may be accompanied by mild cyanosis. Increased work of breathing, including subcostal and intercostal retractions, expiratory grunting, and nasal flaring may also be present. Auscultation of the chest generally reveals clear breath sounds without rales, rhonchi, or crackles. Most infants do not require high levels of exogenous oxygen to ensure adequate oxygenation. Although symptoms usually resolve within the first 24 hours, TTN can persist for as long as 72 hours.

DIFFERENTIAL DIAGNOSIS

TTN is a diagnosis of exclusion, and the differential for this benign, self-limited condition is extensive (**Table 127-1**). Infants with TTN do not typically require high levels of oxygen (>60%) or respiratory support such as mechanical ventilation. Any newborn exhibiting prolonged

TABLE 127-1 Causes of Respiratory Distress in the Newborn

Structural and anatomic
Diaphragmatic hernia
Cystic adenomatoid malformation
Choanal atresia
Tracheomalacia
Laryngomalacia
Tracheoesophageal fistula
Vocal cord paralysis
Pulmonary
Transient tachypnea of the newborn
Respiratory distress syndrome
Meconium aspiration syndrome
Persistent pulmonary hypertension of the newborn
Pulmonary hypoplasia
Pneumothorax
Neonatal pneumonia
Pulmonary cysts
Infectious
Neonatal pneumonia
Sepsis
Systemic
Metabolic acidosis
Hypothermia
Encephalopathy
Cardiac
Congenital heart disease

respiratory distress, or who requires a high level of respiratory support, or who presents with respiratory distress after the first few hours of life, should undergo diagnostic evaluation.

DIAGNOSTIC EVALUATION

All newborns presenting with respiratory distress should be evaluated promptly. Initial general assessment should include physical exam to assess for respiratory rate, apnea, color, cyanosis, and cardiac murmur. Pulse oximetry should be monitored continuously, with supplemental oxygen provided for oxygen levels below 90%. Blood glucose is typically necessary to assess for hypoglycemia as a cause of respiratory distress. Additional evaluation including blood gas, complete blood count (CBC), and a chest radiograph may be indicated based on physical exam findings, severity of symptoms, and duration.

On chest radiograph, classic findings of TTN include prominent central markings suggestive of vascular engorgement, hyperinflation, and edema of the interlobar septae or fluid in the fissures (**Figure 127-1**). However, TTN can also be diagnosed in the presence of normal chest radiograph findings. Unless the infant's clinical symptoms suggest more serious disease, other studies are usually not necessary to confirm suspected TTN. If obtained, arterial blood gas evaluation in TTN should reveal a mild respiratory acidosis due to mild hypoxemia and hypercapnia, and a normal complete blood count and C-reactive protein.

PPHN may present initially with symptoms that overlap those of TTN, however PPHN can progress rapidly to cyanosis, systemic hypotension, and severe respiratory distress. With PPHN, insufficient or delayed decrease in pulmonary vascular resistance results in right-to-left shunting through the ductus arteriosus or foramen ovale and severe hypoxemia. Pre- and post-ductal oximetry may be significantly discordant to these infants. Echocardiography is typically used to confirm a diagnosis of PPHN. Similarly, significant cardiac malformations must be differentiated from TTN and other causes of respiratory distress, with diagnostic evaluation that should include chest radiography to assess for cardiomegaly or vascular congestion, pre- and post-ductal pulse oximetry, and echocardiography. Measurements of upper and lower extremity blood pressures may reveal a difference between the two readings and is suggestive of aortic coarctation.

If there are clinical features (e.g., temperature instability, lethargy) or risk factors for infection (e.g., maternal fever, chorioamnionitis, untreated, or incompletely treated maternal group B streptococcal colonization), appropriate cultures should also be obtained (see Chapter 134 for more information). Measurement of C-reactive protein (CRP) levels may be unreliable when obtained shortly after birth if there has been insufficient time for an inflammatory response to occur. Evaluation for hypoglycemia, metabolic acidosis, and hyperammonemia should occur for infants with suspected inborn errors of metabolism.

MANAGEMENT

Management of respiratory distress in newborns requires a systematic approach, with every effort to identify and address the underlying cause of symptoms. All newborns with respiratory distress should be monitored closely for hydration status and be maintained in a proper thermal environment. For those diagnosed with TTN, management is supportive. Newborns with mild tachypnea can typically be observed in the routine postpartum care unit, however pulse oximetry should be monitored and frequent assessments should be performed for signs of worsening distress or fatigue.

If mild hypoxia is associated with the TTN, supplemental oxygen may be administered via oxy-hood or nasal canula. Oxygen should be titrated to maintain oxygen saturation levels between 90% and 95%. Noninvasive support such as nasal CPAP (continuous positive airway pressure) should be considered in infants who require more than 40% FiO_2 and for those exhibiting persistent and significant work of breathing. Significant tachypnea (>60-80 bpm) prevents oral feeding and necessitates transfer to a higher level of care for initiation of intravenous fluids and monitoring. In selected situations, an orogastric or nasogastric tube can be

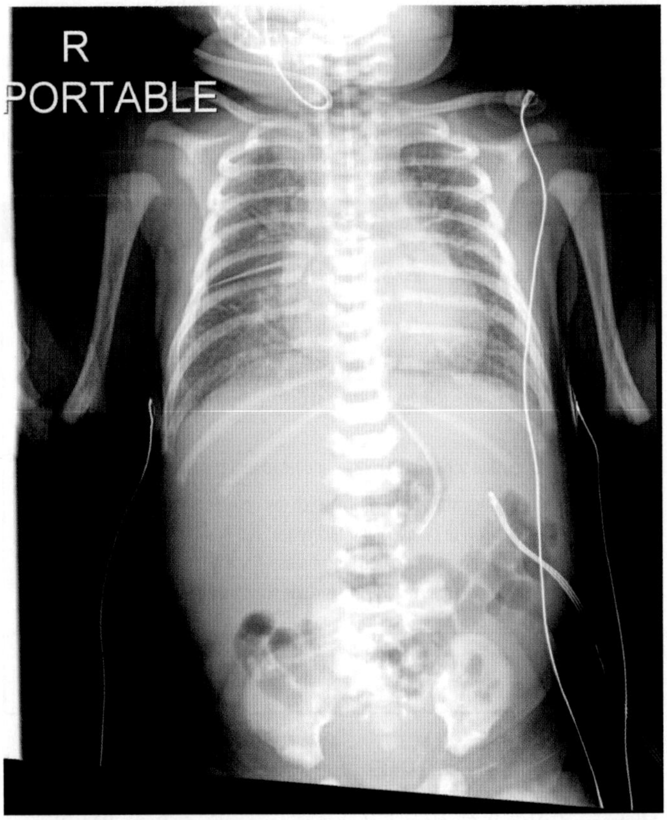

FIGURE 127-1. Chest radiograph of infant with TTN, which demonstrates interstitial edema and a right-sided linear mark consistent with fissural fluid.

placed for assistance with feeding, but only after determining that the infant is unlikely to require ventilatory support. Because of concerns about gastroesophageal reflux and aspiration, newborns with respiratory rates greater than 90 to 100 breaths per minute should not receive oral or gastric feedings. However, placement of an orogastric or nasogastric tube for stomach decompression may be helpful to maximize lung volume expansion.

ADMISSION AND DISCHARGE CRITERIA

Criteria for transfer to a neonatal intensive care unit include:

- Suspected or proven PPHN
- Respiratory distress requiring supplemental oxygen
- Significant tachypnea (>60-80 bpm) that requires frequent reassessment or precludes oral feeding
- Prolonged tachypnea (>4-6 hours)
- Respiratory distress that may require the administration of continuous positive airway pressure or other ventilatory support
- Suspected or proven infection
- Suspected or proven cardiac disease
- Respiratory distress for which there is an unclear diagnosis

Criteria for discharge in the setting of newborn tachypnea include:

- Resolved respiratory distress, defined as respiratory rate less 60 without grunting or retractions
- No supplemental oxygen requirement for at least 12-24 hours
- Able to feed adequately by mouth
- Blood culture negative (if obtained)
- Reliable outpatient follow-up

CONSULTATION

Consultation with a neonatologist should be sought for any newborn requiring escalation of care, including supplemental oxygen requirement, intravenous fluids, or orogastric feedings. Consultation with a pediatric cardiologist in indicated for concerns related to PPHN or congenital heart disease. Pediatric surgery should be consulted if there is suspicion of underlying pulmonary malformation, such as congenital diaphragmatic hernia or cystic adenomatoid malformation.

KEY POINTS

- TTN is a common cause of neonatal respiratory distress that usually presents in the first few hours of life with tachypnea, mild cyanosis, and mildly increased work of breathing.
- TTN is a clinical diagnosis but may require diagnostic tests to exclude other causes of respiratory distress, based on a history of risk factors and typical findings on chest radiographs.
- TTN has a benign and self-limited course, and treatment is supportive.
- TTN should be distinguished from PPHN, which can occur in term or near-term infants and presents with severe cyanosis and tachypnea. The findings on chest radiographs depend on the presence of associated lung disease. For any infant suspected of having PPHN, an echocardiogram is required to exclude structural heart defects as the cause of hypoxemia.
- PPHN is a life-threatening condition that requires management in an intensive care setting.

SUGGESTED READING

Alhassen Z, Vali P, Guglani L, Lakshminrusimha S, Ryan RM. Recent advances in pathophysiology and management of transient tachypnea of newborn. *J Perinatol.* 2021;41(1):6-16.

Avery ME, Gatewood OB, Brumley G. Transient tachypnea of newborn. *Am J Dis Child.* 1966;111:380-385.

Bruschettini M, Hassan KO, Romantsik O, Banzi R, Calevo MG, Moresco L. Interventions for the management of transient tachypnoea of the newborn—an overview of systematic reviews. *Cochrane Database Syst Rev.* 2022; 2(2):CD013563.

Jain L. Alveolar fluid clearance in developing lungs and its role in neonatal transition. *Clin Perinatol.* 1999;26:585-599.

Kim SS, Zhu Y, Grantz KL, et al. Obstetric and neonatal risks among obese women without chronic disease. *Obstet Gynecol.* 2016;128(1): 104-112.

Mc Gillick EV, Lock MC, Orgeig S, Morrison JL. Maternal obesity mediated predisposition to respiratory complication at birth and later in life: understanding the implications of the obesogenic intrauterine environment. *Paediatr Respir Rev.* 2017:21:11.

Tita AT, Landon MB, Spong CY, et al. Timing of elective repeat cesarean delivery at term and neonatal outcomes. *N Engl J Med.* 2009;360:111.

CHAPTER 128 Congenital and Perinatal Infections

Neha Shirish Joshi, MD, MS

CONGENITAL INFECTIONS

BACKGROUND

Congenital infections acquired in utero are a significant cause of neonatal mortality and childhood morbidity. The original concept of the TORCH acronym was to group five infections with similar presentations: toxoplasmosis, "other" (traditionally referring to syphilis), rubella, cytomegalovirus (CMV), and herpesvirus. However, recent additions have expanded the scope of this term to include infections such as human immunodeficiency virus (HIV), enteroviruses, parvovirus B19, and varicella. The incidence of TORCH infections in the United States is variable, ranging from 1 in 200 infants for CMV, the most common congenital viral infection, to ≤1 in 10,000 for rare infections such as rubella and toxoplasmosis. A high index of suspicion for congenital infection and awareness of the prominent features of the most common etiologies will help to facilitate early diagnosis and management.

Pathophysiology Transplacental spread and invasion of the bloodstream after maternal infection is the primary route for intrauterine infection, though it is also possible for the fetus to be infected by extension from adjacent infections of the peritoneum and the genitalia during the birth process or during invasive procedures such as fetal monitoring and intrauterine transfusion.

The placenta serves as a protective barrier that shields the fetus from maternal humoral and cell-mediated immune activity. The fetus is particularly vulnerable during the first trimester of pregnancy, when the most complex events in embryogenesis occur, including development of sensory organs such as the eyes and ears.

The outcome of fetal infection depends on several factors, including gestational age at the time of infection, organism virulence, degree of associated placental damage, and maternal disease severity. Primary infection is also likely to have more significant effects on the fetus than recurrent infection as existing maternal immunity is postulated to allow for efficient clearance of microbes before fetus can be infected. Infection during the first few weeks of gestation may cause embryonal death and resorption, sometimes prior to recognition of pregnancy. Spontaneous abortion and stillbirth are among the earliest recognizable effects of fetal infection after 6 to 8 weeks of pregnancy. In infants who are liveborn, effects of fetal infection may present as preterm birth, intrauterine growth restriction (IUGR), congenital anomalies, or local or systemic signs of infection. Alternatively, fetal infection may present in liveborn infants as the complete absence of any clinical signs of disease, with abnormalities becoming obvious only as the child develops and fails to reach appropriate physiologic or developmental milestones.

CLINICAL PRESENTATION

Intrauterine infection may present in the neonatal period with signs of widely disseminated disease caused by microbial invasion and proliferation over weeks or months prior to delivery. In such infants, it can be difficult to determine whether infection was acquired in utero, intrapartum, or postpartum. However, if the onset of clinical symptoms after birth occurs within the minimal incubation period for the disease, it is likely that infection was acquired before delivery.

Cytomegalovirus (CMV) Congenital CMV infection is the most common cause of sensorineural hearing loss. It may present at birth as small for gestational age, with generalized petechiae, direct hyperbilirubinemia, hepatosplenomegaly, purpuric rash, microcephaly, seizures, focal or general neurologic deficits, retinitis, and intracranial calcifications (usually periventricular) (**Figure 128-1A**). However, 90% of infants with congenital CMV infection are asymptomatic at birth, and therefore infection is often not recognized during the birth hospitalization. Increasingly in the United States, hospital-based and/or statewide initiatives have been implemented to promote targeted or universal screening for congenital CMV. Infants who are symptomatic at birth are at highest risk of long-term neurological sequelae including sensorineural hearing loss (30%-40%), intellectual disability, cerebral palsy, and vision impairment. Infected asymptomatic infants can also experience later, long-term adverse neurological outcomes such as hearing loss (as many as 5%-10% of infected, asymptomatic infants).

Herpes Simplex Virus (HSV) Intrauterine HSV transmission, though occurring uncommonly, is mostly likely during the first 20 weeks of pregnancy and can result in abortion, stillbirth, and, among infants who survive, congenital anomalies. Perinatal mortality is high, and infected infants usually have clinical abnormalities identified at birth. Typical presentation is a triad of clinical findings: cutaneous manifestations (i.e., scarring, active lesions, hypo- and hyperpigmentation, aplasia cutis, and/or an erythematous macular exanthem), ophthalmologic findings (i.e., micro-opthalmia, retinal dysplasia, optic atrophy, and/or chorioretinitis), and neurologic involvement (i.e., microcephaly, encephalomalacia, hydranencephaly, and/or intracranial calcification).

Most HSV infections result from peripartum exposure. Clinical presentation for infants infected with HSV during delivery can be divided into three categories, isolated skin, eye, and mucosal infection, central nervous system infection (CNS; with or without SEM manifestations), or disseminated infection (with or without CNS infection). These three manifestations are associated with different outcomes.

Neonates with infection confined to the skin, eyes, and mucosa (SEM) most often present with cutaneous or mucosal vesicular lesions. By definition, infants in this category have no central nervous system (CNS) or visceral organ involvement, although systemic therapy is required to prevent further disease progression. Infants with CNS disease usually present in the first 2 weeks of life, but can present as late as 6 weeks old. The second category is HSV infection with CNS involvement. CNS disease can present with lethargy, poor feeding, seizures, with or without cutaneous lesions. Infants with CNS disease usually present in the second or third week of life, but can present as late as 6 weeks old. Morbidity with CNS involvement is higher with HSV-2 than HSV-1 infection, with potential long-term sequelae including developmental delay, epilepsy, blindness, and cognitive disabilities. Relapses of CNS infection may also occur during childhood, further increasing morbidity. Disseminated HSV infection is the third category. Mortality risk is highest for these infants, as it is associated with multiorgan dysfunction. Clinical presentation can be indistinguishable from bacterial sepsis, and usually occurs in the first week of life.

A 2001 review summarized the effectiveness of high-dose acyclovir (60 mg/kg/day administered intravenously in three divided doses), and its significant reduction on both morbidity and mortality across all HSV infection types. With high-dose acyclovir treatment, the mortality is 29% for disseminated disease and 4% for CNS disease. Eighty-three percent of infants with disseminated disease who survive have normal development at 12 months of age, compared to 31% of infants with CNS disease. No infants treated with high-dose acyclovir for SEM HSV disease had neurological sequelae at 12 months of age.

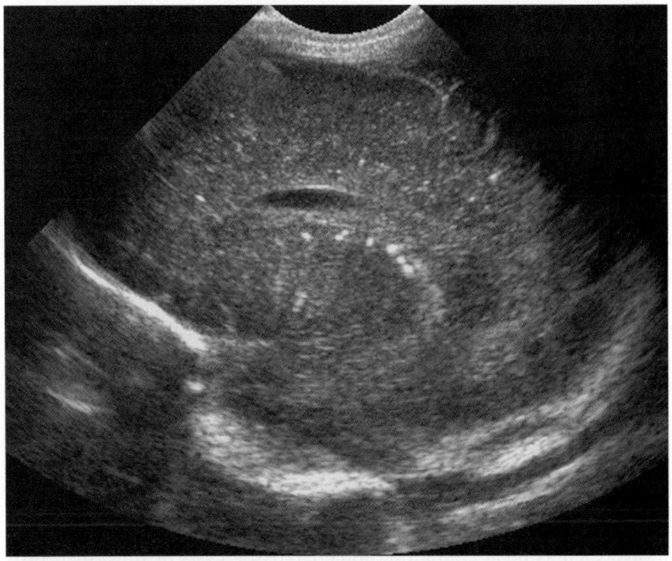

A

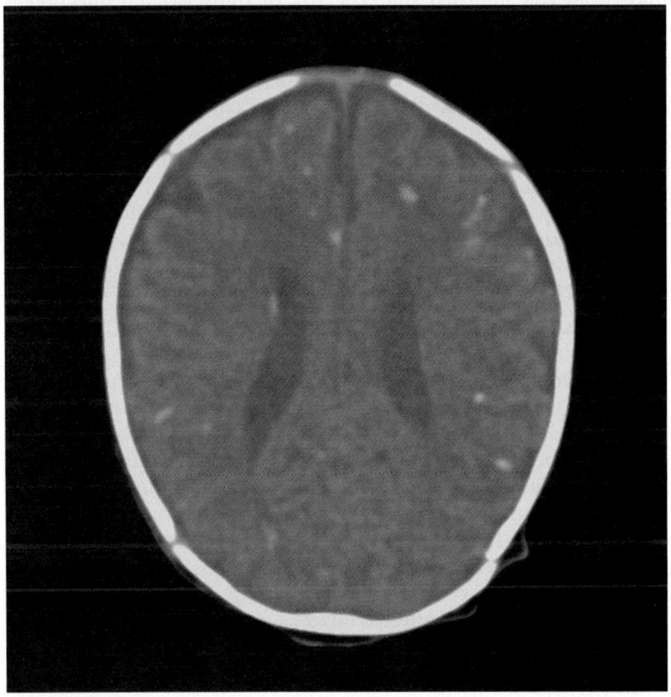

B

FIGURE 128-1. Intracranial calcifications in infants with congenital infection. A. Head ultrasound of an infant with congenital cytomegalovirus infection, note periventricular distribution. B. Head computed tomography in an infant with congenital toxoplasma infection, note scattered or generalized distribution. (Reproduced with permission from Shah SS, Ludwig S. *Symptom-Based Diagnosis in Pediatrics*. New York: McGraw-Hill Education; 2014:153, Figure 6-2; 477, Figure 19-3.)

Syphilis Congenital syphilis results from fetal infection with the spirochete *Treponema pallidum* via transplacental transmission. In recent years, the rate of congenital syphilis in the United States has more than tripled, and reflect rising infection rates in the general community. The Centers for Disease Control and Prevention recommend reporting cases of congenital syphilis to local or state health departments within 24 hours of diagnosis; more than 2000 cases were reported in 2020. Infected liveborn infants are often asymptomatic, with only severe cases clinically apparent at birth.

Early presentation of congenital syphilis, manifesting within the first 2 years of life, can include hepatosplenomegaly, jaundice, lymphadenopathy, meningoencephalitis, chorioretinitis, and mucocutaneous findings such as maculopapular erythema, bullae, and desquamation. Infants may present with failure to thrive and have a characteristic mucopurulent or blood-stained nasal discharge causing "snuffles." Osteochondritis of the long bones and ribs may cause pseudoparalysis of the limbs with characteristic radiologic changes. Late presentation of congenital syphilis, manifesting after the first two years of life, can include gummatous ulcers of the nose, septum, or hard palate; periosteal lesions resulting in saber shins and frontal and parietal bossing; juvenile paresis and tabes secondary to neurosyphilis; optic atrophy and interstitial keratitis; and progressive sensorineural deafness. Dental abnormalities include Hutchinson incisors (small, widely spaced, peg-shaped, notched upper incisors with thin discolored enamel), hypoplastic enamel, and mulberry molars. "Hutchinson triad" is a pathognomonic constellation of findings that consist of interstitial keratitis, Hutchinson teeth, and sensorineural hearing loss.

Toxoplasmosis *Toxoplasma gondii* is a protozoan parasite transmittable through contact with cat feces or consumption of contaminated foods, such as meat containing infective tissue cysts or unwashed produce from contaminated soil. The risk of transplacental infection is lower (10%-25%) when maternal infection occurs in the first trimester compared with the third trimester (60%-90%). However, severe sequelae, including stillbirth and neonatal death, are more likely when infection is acquired in the first trimester. Overall risk of congenital infection from acute prenatal infection ranges from approximately 20% to 50%. Most neonates with congenital toxoplasmosis are asymptomatic; however, clinical presentation can include hepatosplenomegaly, lymphadenopathy, maculopapular rash, jaundice, anemia, and thrombocytopenia. A classic triad of clinical findings associated with this disease is chorioretinitis with intracranial calcifications (typically generalized) (**Figure 128-1B**) and hydrocephalus.

Enteroviruses Enteroviruses are small, single-stranded RNA viruses belonging to the Picornaviridae family. Congenital enterovirus infection often presents with a maternal history of viral illness including fever, respiratory concerns, or abdominal symptoms preceding or immediately following delivery. There may also be a history of viral symptoms in other family members. Signs of infection in neonates may include temperature instability, irritability, lethargy, jaundice, emesis, abdominal distension, diarrhea, respiratory distress, and macular or maculopapular rash. Most affected neonates have mild disease; however, a small percentage develops severe sequelae including meningoencephalitis, myocarditis, pneumonia, hepatitis, and coagulopathy. Myocarditis, in particular, confers a high risk for mortality in affected infants.

Rubella Since licensure of live attenuated rubella vaccines in the late 1960s, the number of reported US cases of congenital rubella infection has declined dramatically to <1 case per year. Risk of infection and associated defects is highest during the first 12 weeks of gestation. Severe sequelae including spontaneous abortion and stillbirth are possible outcomes of infection early in pregnancy. Infection in the first trimester is considered to be uniformly teratogenic, while birth defects are rare among infants infected after 20 weeks of gestation. Common congenital manifestations include cataracts, congenital heart disease (most commonly patent ductus arteriosus or peripheral pulmonary artery stenosis), hearing impairment, and developmental delay. Eye findings including glaucoma, chorioretinitis, retinopathy, and cataracts. In some cases, congenital rubella may only be identified years after birth due to isolated hearing defects.

Human Immunodeficiency Virus (HIV) Although the transmission rate of HIV from an untreated mother to the fetus is estimated to be about 25%, this risk can be reduced to <2% with use of antiretroviral regimens and obstetrical intervention (i.e., zidovudine or nevirapine and elective cesarean section at 38 weeks of pregnancy), and by avoiding breastfeeding. Infants with congenital HIV infection are usually asymptomatic at birth and through the first few months of life. The median age of onset for clinical signs is approximately 3 years, but many children remain asymptomatic for more than 5 years. Clinical presentation of congenital HIV infection can include failure to thrive, persistent diarrhea, recurrent suppurative infections, and opportunistic infections that occur weeks to months or years after birth.

Varicella Varicella-zoster virus (VZV) is one of eight herpes viruses known to cause human infection; primary infection during pregnancy carries significant implications for both maternal and fetal health. Congenital varicella syndrome due to transplacental infection is rare and mostly occurs with infection between 8 and 20 weeks gestation. Characteristic findings in affected infants may include low birth weight; cutaneous scars in a dermatomal distribution; eye findings of cataracts, chorioretinitis, microphthalmos, or nystagmus; hypoplastic limbs; gastrointestinal abnormalities including bowel stenosis; and neurological findings of cortical atrophy or seizures. Varicella is not generally associated with spontaneous fetal loss, preterm birth, or stillbirth.

Parvovirus B19 Parvovirus B19 is a single-stranded, DNA virus that preferentially infects rapidly dividing cells and is cytotoxic for erythroid progenitor cells. The risk for transplacental transmission from an infected mother to the fetus is between 10% and 35%, and is highest in the first and second trimesters of pregnancy. Infection prior to 20 weeks gestation is associated with a higher fetal mortality rate (14.8%) compared with infection after 20 weeks (2.3%). Presentation is typically related to severe anemia, high-output cardiac failure, and extramedullary hematopoiesis, resulting in nonimmune hydrops fetalis, ascites, pleural effusion, and pericardial effusions. Persistent anemia due to hematopoietic suppression can also persist for months after birth.

Zika Virus Congenital Zika virus infection can occur infants whose mothers were infected with Zika virus during the first trimester. While the complete manifestations and incidence of congenital Zika syndrome are still not entirely understood, infants can present with microcephaly (notably with facial disproportion), seizures, abnormal ophthalmologic exam, sensorineural hearing loss, hypertonia, and abnormalities on neurological imaging such as ventriculomegaly and intracranial calcifications.

DIFFERENTIAL DIAGNOSIS

Clinical presentations for infections acquired in utero share many features, including but not limited to IUGR, microcephaly, cataracts, hearing loss, hepatosplenomegaly, cutaneous findings, and thrombocytopenia. Consequently, in the absence of maternal history or prenatal laboratory results that suggest a specific infection (e.g., positive syphilis serology), the differential diagnosis for each TORCH infection includes all of the other TORCH or TORCH-like infections. It is also important to note that neonates with suspected or confirmed congenital HIV or syphilis infection should also be considered at risk for other sexually transmitted infections including gonorrhea and *Chlamydia trachomatis*. Noninfectious diseases in the differential include genetic disorders (e.g., pseudo-TORCH syndrome), inborn errors of metabolism, ABO or Rh incompatibility, neoplastic disorders, and prenatal teratogen exposure.

DIAGNOSTIC EVALUATION

Initial evaluation of a neonate with suspected intrauterine infection should begin with a thorough review of maternal history (including routine prenatal laboratory studies, history of HSV, HIV, and other diseases), and potential exposures including contact with cats and persons infected with VZV (**Table 128-1**). A head-to-toe assessment should be performed to identify physical findings that may be more prominent features of a particular congenital infection. Additional helpful studies for initial evaluation are a complete blood count (CBC) with differential, liver function tests, long bone radiography, ophthalmologic and audiologic evaluation, neuroimaging, and lumbar puncture. Based on initial results, further tailored evaluation for a specific infection or group of infections may follow.

MANAGEMENT

Management of all infants with suspected or proven congenital infections should be done in consultation with an infectious diseases specialist, and other specialists (ophthalmology, neurology, audiology) as needed.

TABLE 128-1 Evaluation of the Infant With a Suspected Congenital Infection

Cerebrospinal fluid
CSF cell count, protein, glucose
CSF PCR (enterovirus, HSV)
CSF VDRL (syphilis)
Blood
IgG (specify *Toxoplasma* or rubella; if positive, send IgM)
RPR (syphilis)
Hepatitis B surface antigen
PCR (enteroviruses, HIV)
Skin lesions
Dark-field examination (syphilis)
PCR (HSV, varicella)
Direct fluorescent antibody (HSV, varicella)[a]
Tzanck smear (HSV)[a]
Culture (HSV)[a]
Urine
PCR (CMV, enteroviruses)
Culture (CMV)[b]
Mucosa
Conjunctiva culture (HSV)
Mouth or nasopharynx culture (HSV, enterovirus)[c]
Rectum culture (enterovirus, HSV)†
Other studies
Audiologic evaluation (CMV, rubella, toxoplasmosis)
Head CT (CMV, toxoplasmosis)
Ophthalmologic examination (toxoplasmosis, rubella, CMV, HSV, varicella, syphilis)
Radiograph of long bones (rubella, syphilis)

[a]PCR testing is typically used for diagnosis. Some centers may perform viral culture rather than PCR for HSV. Tzanck smear and direct fluorescent antibody are now rarely used. Culture may not be necessary if PCR is performed.

[b]CMV urine shell vial culture has been replaced by CMV PCR at most centers. Urine CMV shell vial culture is not necessary if CMV PCR is performed.

[c]Enteroviral cultures rarely performed given the high sensitivity of enteroviral PCR for detection of enterovirus in blood, urine, and stool specimens.

CMV, cytomegalovirus; CSF, cerebrospinal fluid; CT, computed tomography; HSV, herpes simplex virus; PCR, polymerase chain reaction; RPR, rapid plasma reagin; VDRL, Venereal Disease Research Laboratory.

Source: Reproduced with permission from Shah SS, Kemper A, Ratner AJ. *Pediatric Infectious Diseases: Essentials for Practice*. 2nd ed. New York: McGraw-Hill; 2019.

For many congenital infections, including Enterovirus, Rubella, Parvovirus, and Zika virus, there is no specific treatment other than supportive care.

CMV Symptomatic infants with one or more end-organ involvement secondary to congenital CMV are recommended treatment with antivirals (ganciclovir, valganciclovir) to improve long-term neurodevelopmental, including auditory, outcomes. Infants receiving antiviral therapy should receive close laboratory monitoring for side effects of the medications. Treatment with antivirals is not currently recommended for asymptomatic infants. There is no current consensus regarding whether the benefits of antivirals outweigh the risks for infants with isolated hearing loss from congenital CMV without other symptoms.

HSV Management of infants at highest risk for HSV infection varies significantly based on the maternal history of HSV (primary vs. recurrent illness) and whether active lesions are present at the time of delivery. For infants with known maternal recurrent genital HSV infection but no genital lesions at delivery, close observation without contact isolation or surface cultures is indicated. Parents or caregivers should be educated about the signs and symptoms of neonatal HSV infection at discharge.

For infants born to mothers with known prior HSV and now with active genital HSV lesions at delivery, surface cultures should be obtained at 12 to 24 hours of life from the nasopharynx, mouth, urine, and stool or rectum. Blood cultures should additionally be sent for HSV PCR. Cultures obtained prior to 12 hours may reflect contamination during birth rather than true infection. Positives cultures should be treated with a full antiviral course of acyclovir. Infants in this category do not necessarily need empiric antiviral treatment; however if other risk factors for infection are also present (preterm gestation, fetal scalp electrode, skin lacerations, rupture of membranes longer than 4-6 hours), empiric acyclovir treatment may be considered while awaiting PCR and culture results.

Infants born to mothers without a prior history of HSV but active lesions noted at the time of delivery (primary infection) have a high risk of HSV transmission. For these infants, empiric treatment with acyclovir is recommended. Infant testing at 24 hours after birth should include surface cultures for HSV, blood HSV PCR, cerebrospinal fluid testing, liver function tests, and a CBC with differential. Maternal testing should be completed to identify serotype of HSV.

Any neonate with a vesicular rash should be evaluated for HSV. Disseminated HSV infection should also be considered in neonates with signs of sepsis, particularly those with negative bacteriologic culture results and/or liver dysfunction. For infants with suspected or confirmed HSV infection, parenteral acyclovir is the treatment of choice regardless of manifestations and clinical findings. Treatment for infants with CNS involvement or disseminated disease is a minimum of 21 days. Use of oral acyclovir for 6 months following treatment of acute disease has been shown to improve neurodevelopmental outcomes and to prevent skin recurrences. In addition to parental acyclovir, infants with ocular involvement should also receive topical ophthalmic medication (1% trifluridine, 0.1% iododeoxyuridine, or 3% vidarabine).

Syphilis Parenteral penicillin remains the standard treatment for congenital syphilis. Factors to consider in treatment include adequacy of maternal treatment and response to treatment, infant serologic titers compared with maternal titers, and physical exam findings and other laboratory studies. The approach to diagnosis, evaluation, and treatment of infants with potential congenital syphilis is summarized in the syphilis figure, given in the AAP Redbook (https://publications.aap.org/redbook).

Toxoplasmosis For congenital toxoplasmosis infections, initial therapy for symptomatic infections is pyrimethamine combined with sulfadiazine (supplemented with folinic acid). Dosage and duration of therapy, and decision for empiric therapy pending confirmatory testing in asymptomatic infants should be determined in consultation with an infectious disease specialist.

HIV Because treatment recommendations change over time, consultation with a pediatric HIV expert is recommended in the care of HIV-exposed and infected infants. Care of the HIV-exposed infant is addressed in Chapter 104. Current treatment recommendations are available online at https://clinicalinfo.hiv.gov/en/guidelines. The National Perinatal HIV Hotline (1-888-448-8765) also provides free clinical consultation for providers.

Currently, post exposure prophylaxis is recommended in all infants born to mothers with HIV with the specifics determined by the virologic status of the mother. All infants should initiate treatment within the first 6-12 hours after birth. Infants born to mothers with a low/undetectable viral load (less than 50 copies/mL) in the 4 weeks prior to delivery need to be empirically treated with zidovudine for a minimum of 4 weeks. Infants at higher risk for perinatal HIV (mothers with unknown or ≥ 50 copies/mL viral levels, adherence challenges with antepartum antiretroviral therapy, acute/primary HIV infection during pregnancy) should receive empiric therapy with zidovudine plus lamivudine plus either nevirapine or raltegravir for at least 6 weeks.

It is recommended that for HIV-exposed infants, virologic testing should be performed within the first 2 to 3 weeks of life, at 1 to 2 months, and at 4 to 6 months of age. Virologic testing at birth is indicated for high-risk exposures, for example detectable maternal viral load near the time of delivery.

Because of the risk of HIV transmission through breast milk and alternative safe options available for infant feeding, infants born to mothers with HIV in the United States should not breastfeed. This includes infants born to mothers with undetectable viral loads prior to delivery as an undetectable viral load does not entirely eliminate the risk of HIV transmitted through breastmilk.

If the infant's virologic testing is positive at any time, chemoprophylaxis should be replaced with combination antiretroviral therapy at the recommendation of a pediatric HIV specialist.

Varicella Post exposure prophylaxis with varicella-zoster immunoglobulin may be recommended for certain infants with exposure to varicella infection in the peripartum period; this decision should be made with an infectious diseases specialist. Infants with severe symptomatic varicella infection may additionally be treated with acyclovir to reduce incidence of morbidity and mortality.

ADMISSION AND DISCHARGE CRITERIA

Admission to a neonatal intensive care unit can be considered for newborns with

- Severe IUGR or prematurity
- Respiratory compromise, including apnea, cyanosis, or requirement for supplemental oxygen or ventilator support
- Hemodynamic instability
- Concern for CNS involvement
- Gastrointestinal symptoms, including feeding difficulty or concern for intestinal anomalies
- Physical exam or laboratory findings concerning for disseminated infection

Discharge home is appropriate when

- Infant is clinically stable
- Any necessary diagnostic and hospital-based treatment regimens are complete
- Appropriate primary care and specialty follow-up appointments have been arranged

CONSULTATION

With suspected congenital infections, consultation with a pediatric infectious disease specialist may be warranted to help guide diagnostic workup, interpretation of laboratory results, and treatment. Ophthalmology and audiology referrals may also be required. Consultation with an expert in pediatric HIV infection is recommended in the care of HIV-exposed neonates.

SPECIAL CONSIDERATIONS

Prevention All women should be screened serologically for syphilis early in pregnancy with a nontreponemal test (e.g., RPR or VDRL) and preferably again at delivery. HIV screening is also recommended as part of standard prenatal care. Routine serological screening for herpes simplex virus (HSV) in asymptomatic pregnant women is not recommended, as it has not been shown to reduce transmission of HSV to newborns. Pregnant women identified as rubella nonimmune should be immunized in the immediate postpartum period to protect future pregnancies, however, immunization is contraindicated during pregnancy and in the 3 months before conception.

Awareness of congenital viral infections, their potential risks, and appropriate hand hygiene measures to minimize acquired infection are important for pregnant women and women of childbearing age. Serologic testing for varicella should be considered only for pregnant women who do not have evidence of immunity (reliable history of chickenpox or documented vaccination). There is no single recommendation for monitoring for parvovirus B19 in pregnancy, but serological testing may be indicated when there are potential exposures. Pregnant women whose serostatus for *T. gondii* is negative or unknown should avoid activities that potentially expose them to cat feces (such as changing litter boxes, gardening, and landscaping), or they should wear gloves and wash their hands if such activities are unavoidable.

PERINATALLY ACQUIRED INFECTION

BACKGROUND

In addition to congenital infections acquired in utero, infections acquired during birth from the maternal genital tract can present as systemic infection in the neonate. As a result of prevention efforts, including improved antenatal screening for Group B *Streptococcus* (GBS) and antibiotic prophylaxis for mothers with GBS positivity or chorioamnionitis, the incidence of early onset sepsis has declined dramatically over the past 15 years, from 1.7 cases per 1000 live births in the early 1990s to 0.34-0.37 cases per 1000 live births recently. Updated clinical practice guidelines from the American Academy of Pediatrics' Committee on Fetus and Newborn (AAP COFN) were released in 2018, with differing recommendations for infants born at <35 weeks' completed gestational age and infants born at ≥35 weeks' completed gestational age. These guidelines allow for stratification of infants deemed at lower risk for early onset sepsis, and therefore decrease overall empiric antibiotic usage. In infants born at ≥ 35 weeks' completed gestational age who are well appearing, early onset sepsis is especially rare. Additionally, nearly half of infants with early onset sepsis have no known risk factors for disease. The importance of close serial monitoring in all infants is especially critical knowing that infected late preterm and term infants nearly always display clinical signs of illness, and that maternal risk factors are seen in only half of infected infants.

Pathophysiology Early onset sepsis is usually defined as a bacterial infection of the newborn within the first 72 hours after birth, evidenced by a positive blood or cerebrospinal fluid culture growing a pathogenic organism. Some definitions of early onset sepsis can extend the timeframe to the first week after birth. Infections occurring one week after birth are classified as late onset sepsis. Although maternal antepartum risk factors (GBS positivity, prolonged rupture of membranes, intraamniotic infection or chorioamnionitis, preterm labor/delivery) are linked to early onset sepsis, they do not appear to be associated with late onset sepsis. In term infants, GBS remains the most common pathogenic organism causing early onset sepsis. *Escherichia coli* (*E. coli*) is the most common pathogenic organism causing early onset sepsis in preterm infants.

CLINICAL PRESENTATION

Infants with early onset sepsis generally present with respiratory distress, apnea, or other signs of sepsis (including temperature instability, tachycardia, lethargy, irritability, abdominal distention, and poor feeding) within the first 24 to 48 hours of life.

DIFFERENTIAL DIAGNOSIS

The differential diagnosis for symptoms of early onset sepsis is broad. Critical congenital heart disease should be considered, as many ductal-dependent anatomic lesions and tachyarrhythmias manifest early with features that can overlap with sepsis (i.e., tachypnea, tachycardia, and poor perfusion). Hypovolemia resulting from acute perinatal blood loss may also present with nonspecific signs including tachycardia, pallor, and hypotension. Additional conditions include transient tachypnea of the newborn, pneumothorax, pulmonary hypertension, respiratory distress syndrome, congenital anatomic lesions (e.g., congenital diaphragmatic hernia, choanal atresia), neonatal abstinence syndrome, polycythemia, and endocrine and metabolic abnormalities.

DIAGNOSTIC EVALUATION AND MANAGEMENT

Detection of early onset disease can be challenging, as clinical symptoms may be non-specific and overall incidence of early onset sepsis is low. Laboratory tests (such as a complete blood count and C-reactive protein) have limited specificity and sensitivity in the diagnosis of early onset sepsis, and should not be used on their own to guide the decision to initiate empiric antibiotics. The American Academy of Pediatrics' Committee on Fetus and Newborn Guidelines, released in December 2019, provide different recommendations for infants < 35 weeks' completed gestational age and infants born at ≥35 weeks' completed gestational age.

Preterm infants < 35 weeks' completed gestational age can be stratified by reasons behind the preterm delivery to determine risk levels for early onset sepsis. Low-risk infants include those who meet all the following criteria: delivered due to maternal indications (non-infectious), no labor or attempts to induce labor, and rupture of membranes at the time of delivery. For this lower risk set of infants, the risks and benefits of antibiotic treatment at the time of birth can be individually evaluated. Higher risk infants include those with spontaneous preterm labor, premature rupture of membranes, intraamniotic infection or chorioamnionitis, or non-reassuring fetal status. In these higher risk infants, initiation of empiric antibiotics and obtaining blood cultures are recommended. The American Academy of Pediatrics Committee on Fetus and Newborn's Clinical Practice Guidelines for infants born at < 35 weeks can be found at https://publications.aap.org/pediatrics/article/142/6/e20182896/37519/Management-of-Neonates-Born-at-34-6-7-Weeks.

As recommended by the American Academy of Pediatrics' Committee on Fetus and Newborn Clinical Practice Guidelines (https://publications.aap.org/pediatrics/article-pdf/142/6/e20182894/1075508/peds_20182894.pdf), one of three approaches can be used to evaluate risk for early onset sepsis for infants born at ≥ 35 weeks completed gestational age. The Categorical Risk Assessment (A) is based on the 2010 Centers for Disease Control guidelines and recommends initiation of empiric antibiotics in all infants born to mothers with fever during labor. The Neonatal Sepsis Calculator (B) approach [https://neonatalsepsiscalculator.kaiserpermanente.org] uses a multivariable risk assessment along with clinical status of infant to determine need for blood culture and/or antibiotics. The Enhanced Clinical Examination (C) approach relies on serial examinations of infants to identify those with signs of illness for the initiation of antibiotics.

ADMISSION AND DISCHARGE CRITERIA

Admission to a neonatal intensive care unit is indicated for any newborn with signs of sepsis. Well-appearing infants undergoing limited evaluation and empiric antibiotic treatment pending results may be appropriate for care in the routine mother-baby unit, depending on institution policies and procedures.

CONSULTATION

Consultation with a neonatologist should be considered for infants with symptoms of sepsis, including temperature instability, feeding difficulty, lethargy, abdominal distension, poor tone, respiratory distress, and hemodynamic instability.

SPECIAL CONSIDERATIONS

Prevention Prevention strategies have substantially reduced the burden of early-onset GBS disease. The 2010 CDC guidelines recommend universal screening of all pregnant women for vaginal and rectal colonization between 35 and 37 weeks gestation. Any woman with a positive screen, a history of GBS bacteriuria during pregnancy, or previous delivery of an infant with invasive GBS disease requires antibiotic prophylaxis at the time of labor onset or membrane rupture; a planned cesarean delivery obviates the need for antibiotics if labor has not begun and membranes have not ruptured. For women with an unknown GBS status, amniotic membrane rupture ≥18 hours, intrapartum temperature ≥100.4°F, preterm delivery (<37 weeks), or intrapartum testing positive for GBS are indications for intrapartum antibiotic prophylaxis.

Newborn providers should be aware of current recommendations for appropriate intrapartum prophylaxis regimens. As penicillin is the first-line agent for antibiotic prophylaxis, with ampicillin as an acceptable alternative. Penicillin-allergic women without a history of anaphylaxis or other severe allergic reactions should receive cefazolin. For penicillin-allergic women at high risk for anaphylaxis, susceptibility testing should be performed on antenatal GBS cultures. In such cases, clindamycin should be used if the GBS isolate is susceptible. If the isolate is resistant to clindamycin or demonstrates inducible resistance, penicillin-allergic women should receive vancomycin. Erythromycin should not be used as an alternative for GBS prophylaxis.

COVID-19 Infants born to mothers testing positive for SARS-CoV-2 are at risk of COVID-19 infection in the newborn period, with infants born at a premature gestational age and those with mothers positive during the birth hospitalization at highest risk for infection. Infants should be monitored for signs of illness, and should have nasopharyngeal testing completed prior to discharge home. No separation of the mother-infant dyad is required, and mothers should be encouraged to continue breastfeeding. Appropriate hand hygiene and mask wearing may reduce likelihood of infection transmission to the infant. For infected infants, supportive care is recommended. For further information, see Chapter 106.

KEY POINTS

- Current conceptualization of TORCH infections has expanded to include HIV, enterovirus, parvovirus B19, Zika, and varicella.
- Clinical presentation for intrauterine infections is dependent on several factors, including gestational age at infection, organism virulence, and maternal disease severity.
- Maternal history, prenatal laboratory results, physical exam findings, and initial laboratory studies should guide the approach to further diagnostic evaluation and management of congenital infections.
- Many infants with congenital infections are asymptomatic at birth, necessitating a thorough review of antenatal laboratory screening results and maternal exposure history.
- GBS remains the most common causative organism for early onset sepsis in term infants, while *E coli* is the most common causative organism in preterm infants.
- Newer stratification approaches exist for infants born at <35 weeks' completed gestational age and those born at ≥35 weeks' completed gestational age in the evaluation for early onset sepsis.

SUGGESTED READINGS

American Academy of Pediatrics. Herpes Simplex. In: Kimberlin DW, Barnett ED, Lynfield R, Sawyer MH, eds. *Red Book: 2021-2024 Report of the Committee on Infectious Diseases*. 32nd ed. Elk Grove Village, IL: American Academy of Pediatrics; 2021:407-417.

American Academy of Pediatrics. Syphilis. In: Kimberlin DW, Barnett ED, Lynfield R, Sawyer MH, eds. *Red Book: 2021-2024 Report of the Committee on Infectious Diseases*. 32nd ed. Elk Grove Village, IL: American Academy of Pediatrics; 2021:729-744.

Committee Opinion No. 712. Intrapartum management of intraamniotic infection. *Obstet Gynecol*. 2017;130:e95-101.

Kimberlin DW. Advances in the treatment of neonatal herpes simplex infections. *Rev Med Virol*. 2001 May-Jun;11(3):157-163.

Nicloux M, Peterman L, Parodi M, Magny JF. Outcome and management of newborns with congenital cytomegalovirus infection. *Arch Pediatr*. 2020;27(3):160-165.

Penner J, Hernstadt H, Burns JE, Randell P, Lyall H. Stop, think SCORTCH: rethinking the traditional 'TORCH' screen in an era of re-emerging syphilis. *Arch Dis Child*. 2021;106(2):117-124.

Puopolo KM, Benitz WE, Zaoutis TE. AAP Committee on Fetus and Newborn, AAP Committee on fetus and newborn. management of neonates born at ≤34 6/7 weeks' gestation with suspected or proven early-onset bacterial sepsis. *Pediatrics*. 2018;142:e20182896.

Puopolo KM, Benitz WE, Zaoutis TE. AAP Committee on Fetus and Newborn, AAP Committee on Infectious Disease. Management of neonates born at ≥35 0/7 weeks' gestation with suspected or proven early-enset bacterial sepsis. *Pediatrics*. 2018;142:e20182894.

Samies NL, James SH, Kimberlin DW. Neonatal herpes simplex virus disease: updates and continued challenges. *Clin Perinatol*. 2021;48(2):263-274.

Seedat F, Marshall J. Re: Universal screening versus risk-based protocols for antibiotic prophylaxis during childbirth to prevent early-onset group B streptococcal disease: a systematic review and meta-analysis. *BJOG: Int J Obstet Gynaecol*. 2020;127:1038-1039.

Verani JR, McGee L, Schrag SJ. Prevention of perinatal group B streptococcal disease—revised guidelines from CDC. *MMWR Recomm Rep*. 2010;59(RR-10):1-36.

Villar J, Ariff S, Gunier RB, et al. Maternal and Neonatal Morbidity and Mortality Among Pregnant Women With and Without COVID-19 Infection: The INTERCOVID Multinational Cohort Study. *JAMA Pediatr*. 2021; 175(8):817-826.

CHAPTER 129

Hypoglycemia and Infants of Diabetic Mothers

Terry Wall, MD, MPH

HYPOGLYCEMIA

BACKGROUND

Glucose is the preferred oxidative energy source for the central nervous system. At birth, the sudden loss of a continuous maternal glucose supply requires a response in newborn metabolism to maintain adequate serum glucose levels throughout the early feeding and fasting periods. The newborn's plasma glucose level drops quickly after delivery and generally reaches a nadir by 2 hours of age. It has been estimated that 5% to 15% of otherwise healthy newborns will develop persistent hypoglycemia; and that number increases to as high as 50% in high-risk newborns. If severe, newborn hypoglycemia may result in systemic effects and have potential neurological sequelae.

Pathophysiology Adaptive changes in hormonal regulation at birth conspire to maintain the newborn's plasma glucose concentration, reserve glucose for the central nervous system, and avoid hypoglycemia. Counterregulatory hormones, including glucagon, growth hormone, cortisol, and epinephrine, act together to increase blood glucose via glycogenolysis, gluconeogenesis, ketogenesis, and inhibition of peripheral glucose uptake and insulin release. These regulatory mechanisms support the transition from a continuous transplacental glucose source to an intermittent supply via feeding. The failure of one or several parts of this process can result in hypoglycemia.

Newborns at higher risk for hypoglycemia are those with diminished hepatic glucose production, increased metabolic need versus substrate availability, or increased insulin production (**Table 129-1**). Additional metabolic challenges such as immaturity, low glycogen reserves, and thermal stress may also render the newborn more susceptible to hypoglycemia. Hypoglycemia occurs in roughly half of newborns with known risk factors; up to 20% may have multiple episodes of hypoglycemia, and 20% may experience severe hypoglycemia.

CLINICAL PRESENTATION

In healthy adults, a decrease in blood glucose concentration inhibits the production of insulin and stimulates the production of glucagon. This prevents the blood glucose from dropping to less than 60 mg/dL, thus avoiding the development of typical symptoms of hypoglycemia such as diaphoresis, headache, and dizziness. In newborns, there is a weaker clinical correlation between blood glucose concentrations and symptoms of hypoglycemia. Although some newborns may display nonspecific signs and symptoms of hypoglycemia (**Table 129-2**), others may appear completely asymptomatic despite low blood and cerebral glucose levels.

Studying long-term outcomes of newborn hypoglycemia has proven to be difficult for several reasons: (i) variation in definition of hypoglycemia, (ii) presence of co-morbidities which may independently impact outcomes, and (iii) having varying etiologies of hypoglycemia which may themselves impact outcomes. However, some studies have suggested an increased risk of neurologic impairment, such as in measures of executive functioning, when newborn hypoglycemia is severe or prolonged. An association has also been shown between transient newborn hypoglycemia and lower achievement test scores at 10 years of age. The long-term neurologic effects of transient hypoglycemia in the newborn may vary depending on which age is examined.

Differential Diagnosis The presence of hypoglycemia is most often the result of a healthy newborn's inability to respond quickly and adequately to the dramatic loss of maternal sources of glucose. However, hypoglycemia may also be a signal of other stresses, including sepsis, inborn errors of metabolism, hyperinsulinism, polycythemia, and congenital hypopituitarism (see Table 129-1). Symptoms of hypoglycemia are nonspecific and overlap with other systemic conditions (e.g., neonatal abstinence syndrome). In addition, hypoglycemia may be one feature of a syndrome or multifaceted disorder (e.g., Beckwith-Wiedemann syndrome).

DIAGNOSTIC EVALUATION

There is no specific glucose value that defines significant hypoglycemia or that predicts neurologic injury in the newborn. Consequently, there is no consensus or numerical definition for newborn hypoglycemia. Uncertainty exists about where the appropriate lower limit of normal is for newborns, and there are limitations to a single cutoff value. In general, to avoid the systemic effects and potential neurologic sequelae of hypoglycemia, a conservative threshold for defining hypoglycemia is useful. An "operational threshold" has been suggested that takes into consideration the unstable relationship between plasma glucose levels and clinical signs of hypoglycemia. The operational threshold has been defined as "that concentration of plasma or whole blood glucose at which clinicians should consider intervention." The American Academy of Pediatrics (AAP) notes that the generally adopted level for an operational threshold for newborn hypoglycemia is less than 47 mg/dL and suggests a target glucose of ≥45 mg/dL prior to feeds. The 2011 AAP clinical report provides a strategy that accounts for infant risk factors, symptoms, and age in hours. Screening is recommended in preterm infants, small and large-for-gestational-age infants, and infants of diabetic mothers. Healthy term newborns who are delivered without complications after a normal pregnancy do not require routine glucose monitoring. Regardless of risk factors, any newborn with clinical signs consistent with hypoglycemia requires evaluation (see Table 129-2).

TABLE 129-1 Infants at Risk for Hypoglycemia*

Risk Due to Diminished Hepatic Glucose Production	Risk Due to Increased Glucose Utilization (Increased Metabolic Demand)	Risk Due to Excessive Transient Pancreatic Insulin Production (Hyperinsulinism)	Risk Due to Excessive and Persistent Pancreatic Insulin Production (Hyperinsulinism)	Other
SGA infant / IUGR	Perinatal stress / Hypoxia	Infant of diabetic mother	Congenital hyperinsulinism	Endocrine disorders¶
Prematurity	Thermal stress	LGA infant	Beckwith-Wiedemann syndrome	Delayed feeding
Post-term gestation	Polycythemia-hyperviscosity	Severe Rh incompatibility (erythroblastosis fetalis)	Pancreatic islet cell adenoma	Iatrogenic
Maternal beta-blockers	Congenital heart disease	Iatrogenic (maternal drugs)†	Adenomatosis	
Inborn errors of metabolism§	CNS abnormalities	High umbilical artery catheter		
	Sepsis	Exchange transfusion		

*Infants with hypoglycemia due to a lack of available glucose generally have ketones in the urine; infants with hypoglycemia due to excess insulin do not.

†Chlorpropamide, diazoxide, diuretics, salicyclates, alcohol, terbutaline, ritodrine.

§ Glycogen storage disease, galactosemia, tyrosinemia, hereditary fructose intolerance, α_1-Antitrypsin deficiency.

¶ Adrenal insufficiency (CAH), congenital hypopituitarism, hypothyroidism.

CAH, congenital adrenal hyperplasia; CNS, central nervous system; IUGR, intrauterine growth retardation; LGA, large for gestational age; SGA, small for gestational age.

TABLE 129-2 Symptoms of Hypoglycemia in Neonates

Irritability
Abnormal or high-pitched cry
Tremors
Jitteriness
Lethargy
Hypotonia
Poor suck reflex, poor feeding
Apnea
Tachypnea
Cyanosis
Seizures
Hypothermia
Vasomotor instability
Temperature instability
Cardiac arrest

The optimal timing of screening is not known. Hypoglycemia in newborns generally appears at 2 to 6 hours of life. As shown in **Figure 129-1**, the AAP recommends that infants at risk for hypoglycemia be screened within the first 1 to 2 hours after birth, with surveillance continuing before feedings for 12 to 24 hours of life.

Point-of-care glucometers are often used as a screening method to evaluate blood glucose; however, since point-of-care methods tend to measure whole blood glucose levels, their results may vary from plasma glucose levels by as much as 10 to 20 mL/dL. Therefore, laboratory confirmation of plasma glucose levels is necessary when point-of-care results are low.

MANAGEMENT

Because of the potential risk to the central nervous system, newborn hypoglycemia is treated aggressively with the early institution of oral feedings. However, hypoglycemia may still occur despite prompt feeding.

For asymptomatic newborns with hypoglycemia, intrabuccal dextrose gel (0.5mL/kg of 40% dextrose gel) can be administered in conjunction with a feeding. Although evidence for the effects of dextrose gel on long-term neurodevelopmental outcomes is inconclusive, dextrose gel has been shown to be safe and to possibly improve short-term outcomes, including improved glucose concentrations, improved breastfeeding rates, reduced admissions to intensive care settings, and reduced need for formula supplementation in breastfed newborns. Dextrose gel administration should be followed by a blood glucose check 30 minutes later.

In symptomatic newborns with significant hypoglycemia, or in newborns who are unable to feed, an intravenous bolus of 2 mL/kg of 10% dextrose (D10W) should be administered, followed by a maintenance infusion of 80 to 100 mL/kg per day of D10W (Figure 129-1). Refractory hypoglycemia may require an increase in the volume of fluid or the concentration of glucose. Newborns requiring greater than 100 mL/kg per day of D10W to maintain adequate serum glucose levels can be treated with D12.5W via a peripheral intravenous line. However, concentrations greater than this require central venous access. Once glucose levels have stabilized, infusions can be decreased by approximately 2 mL/hr while providing oral feedings. Glucose levels should be assessed before each oral feeding while the intravenous infusion is being decreased.

ADMISSION AND DISCHARGE CRITERIA

Admission or transfer to a neonatal intensive care unit is appropriate in the following circumstances:

- Persistent hypoglycemia despite adequate oral or gavage feeding
- Inability to tolerate an oral or gavage glucose load
- Presence of nonspecific signs of hypoglycemia (see Table 129-2) despite normalized serum glucose

Discharge criteria include:

- Clinically asymptomatic newborn with the ability to take breastmilk or infant formula by mouth at age-appropriate intervals
- Stable preprandial glucose level greater than 50 mg/dL

CONSULTATION

Subspecialty evaluation by a neonatologist or pediatric endocrinologist should be considered in infants with prolonged hypoglycemia, or when persistently high rates of glucose infusion are required to maintain normal glucose levels. Other situations in which to consider consultation include severe hypoglycemia associated with seizures in an otherwise healthy newborn, or those with physical exam findings consistent with underlying etiologies, such as hypotonia, hepatomegaly, omphalocele, or macroglossia.

SPECIAL CONSIDERATIONS

Prevention Newborn hypoglycemia may be prevented with the early initiation of feeds, at frequent intervals of every 2 to 3 hours. Cold stress in the newborn should be avoided by maintaining a neutral thermal environment.

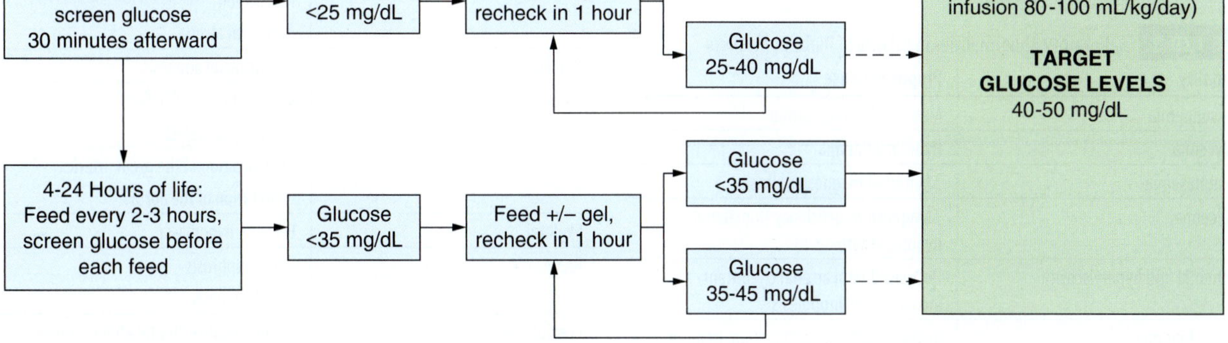

FIGURE 129-1. Screening and management of infants at risk for neonatal hypoglycemia.

This may be facilitated by early skin to skin contact with the mother. Newborns at high risk for hypoglycemia should undergo hypoglycemia screening, with close monitoring for symptoms.

INFANTS OF DIABETIC MOTHERS

BACKGROUND

Diabetes is a condition that is seen with increasing frequency worldwide and is one of the most common complications of pregnancy. It is estimated that gestational diabetes occurs in more than 8% of pregnancies, whereas pre-gestational diabetes is present in about 1% of women. Diabetes during pregnancy increases the risk of both fetal and neonatal morbidity and mortality.

Pathophysiology A unique metabolic consequence of pregnancy is a blunting of the effects of insulin in the mother. The normal clearance of glucose is delayed, which helps maintain a consistent level of maternal glucose for the fetus. Pre-gestational maternal diabetes potentiates these anti-insulin effects and causes an additional increase in glucose in the fetal environment. Fetal hyperglycemia induces fetal pancreatic islet hypertrophy and beta cell hyperplasia. This results in an elevation in fetal, and later, neonatal plasma insulin concentrations which can lead to neonatal hypoglycemia, occurring in up to 50% of infants of diabetic mothers (IDMs). In addition, the normal shift in energy metabolism that allows the newborn to use fat and amino acids may be hampered by hyperinsulinemia and may result in other metabolic abnormalities such as hypocalcemia and hypomagnesemia (**Table 129-3**). Furthermore, insulin acts as an anabolic growth hormone. In the presence of elevated fetal insulin levels, increased growth of insulin-sensitive tissues occurs, resulting in macrosomia and organomegaly. Chronic fetal hyperinsulinemia may also lead to fetal hypoxemia and placental insufficiency, resulting in higher fetal erythropoietin levels and polycythemia.

CLINICAL PRESENTATION

In addition to newborn hypoglycemia, IDMs may present with a variety of newborn complications, including excessive growth, respiratory distress, and cardiac disorders. The risk of complications for IDMs is related to the timing and intensity of maternal hyperglycemia (i.e., pre-gestational vs. gestational diabetes), and to the level of glycemic control during pregnancy.

Macrosomia Macrosomia, typically defined as a birth weight > 4000 grams, affects up to 40% of IDMs due to increased body fat, visceral organ hypertrophy, and increased skeletal growth. Owing to their large size, IDMs are more likely to be delivered by cesarean section and to experience complications of delivery, such as shoulder dystocia and brachial and facial nerve palsies (see Chapter 125). Preterm IDMs may have a birth weight that is below the cutoff for macrosomia, but still measure large for gestational age (LGA), defined as >90th percentile on adjusted growth curves, and have increased adiposity on physical exam. Excessive birth weight is the most common growth abnormality for IDMs and is associated with all types of maternal diabetes. However, intrauterine growth restriction (IUGR) can also occur in the presence of advanced vascular disease and hypertension in the mother. IUGR can lead to significantly reduced hepatic glycogen stores, making IDMs particularly vulnerable and dependent on an exogenous glucose supply. Macrosomic IDMs have adequate glycogen and lipid stores but cannot use them efficiently owing to the antagonistic effects of high insulin levels on glycogenolysis, gluconeogenesis, ketogenesis, and lipolysis.

TABLE 129-3 Laboratory Abnormalities in Infants of Diabetic Mothers

Abnormality	Proposed Cause
Hyperinsulinemia	Maternal hyperglycemia
Hypoglycemia	Hyperinsulinemia
Hypomagnesemia	? Maternal magnesium losses
Hypocalcemia	? Magnesium deficiency (functional hypoparathyroidism)
Polycythemia and hyperviscosity	Decreased fetal arterial O_2 content, increased erythropoiesis
Hyperbilirubinemia	Increased bilirubin production, impaired hepatic function, polycythemia

Congenital Malformations High maternal blood glucose is considered a teratogen and can have severe adverse effects on fetal development and organogenesis. Particularly for women with pre-gestational diabetes, the incidence of major congenital malformations is estimated to be 5% to 10%. Even strict glycemic control during pregnancy, including during the period of organogenesis, does not appear to completely eliminate excess risk of congenital malformations for IDMs. For women with gestational diabetes and type 2 non-insulin-dependent diabetes mellitus, the association with congenital anomalies is less well established, however greater glucose intolerance and poor first trimester glycemic control seems to increase the risk. Various congenital malformations associated with maternal diabetes are listed in **Table 129-4**.

Cardiac Hypertrophy In additional to structural cardiac malformations, IDMs can develop transient hypertrophic cardiomyopathy as a manifestation of visceromegaly. Most infants are asymptomatic, and the septal wall hypertrophy spontaneously resolves over several months. However, depending on the severity and extent of myocardial involvement, this can sometimes lead to severe morbidity and mortality.

Respiratory Distress Rates of respiratory distress syndrome and transient tachypnea of the newborn are increased in IDMs. Maternal diabetes is also associated with increased risk of persistent pulmonary hypertension, although this may be mediated by associated risk factors like macrosomia and increased rate of caesarean deliveries in this population.

Jaundice and Polycythemia IDMs are at increased risk of significant hyperbilirubinemia, likely due to associated polycythemia but also secondary to other factors such as preterm birth and/or impaired hepatic conjugation. Polycythemia, defined as a hematocrit > 65%, may present as a ruddy appearance to the skin, and poses an increased risk of hyperviscosity. Early symptoms may be nonspecific and include feeding problems, acrocyanosis, lethargy, hypotonia, respiratory distress, and irritability. Severe complications of hyperviscosity can include cerebral infarct, necrotizing enterocolitis, and deep vessel thrombosis.

DIFFERENTIAL DIAGNOSIS

The differential for macrosomia includes post-term pregnancy (>42 weeks gestational age), excessive maternal weight gain, multigravidity, and familial genetic factors (large parental size). Based on the presence of other findings, genetic syndromes associated with excessive fetal growth should also be considered including Beckwith-Wiedemann, Pallister-Killian, and Sotos syndrome.

TABLE 129-4 Congenital Malformations in Infants of Diabetic Mothers

System Affected	Defect
Neural tube	Caudal regression syndromes Holoprosencephaly
Gastrointestinal	Duodenal atresia Microcolon Anorectal atresia
Vertebral	Lumbosacral agenesis
Cardiac	Ventricular septal defect Atrial septal defect Transposition of the great arteries Coarctation of the aorta
Skeletal	Femoral hypoplasia
Renal	Hydronephrosis Renal agenesis
Craniofacial	Oculoauriculovertebral abnormalities Hemifacial microsomia

DIAGNOSTIC EVALUATION

IDMs are considered high-risk deliveries and are more likely to require resuscitation following delivery. Cardiorespiratory status should be assessed, and major anomalies should be identified. If stable, they should receive routine well newborn care and remain with their mother for skin to skin contact and early initiation of breastfeeding. As described in the section above, IDMs should be screened for hypoglycemia.

MANAGEMENT

See Figure 129-1 for the assessment and treatment of hypoglycemia in IDMs. Hyperviscosity requires treatment with intravenous hydration, and in severe cases partial exchange transfusion.

ADMISSION AND DISCHARGE CRITERIA

Admission or transfer to a neonatal intensive care unit is appropriate in the following circumstances:

- Persistent hypoglycemia despite adequate oral or gavage feedings, with or without dextrose gel
- Inability to tolerate enteral glucose load
- Presence of anomalies which necessitate higher level of care
- Respiratory compromise
- Hyperbilirubinemia or other complications of polycythemia requiring intensive intervention

Discharge criteria include:

- Clinically asymptomatic newborn with the ability to take breast milk or infant formula by mouth at age-appropriate intervals while maintaining stable glucose levels greater than 50 mg/dL
- Cardiorespiratory stability
- Resolution of significant hyperbilirubinemia

CONSULTATION

Consultation with a neonatologist should be considered in IDMs that have refractory or severe hypoglycemia or significant respiratory distress. Subspecialty evaluation by a cardiologist may be warranted for suspicion of cardiac anomalies or symptomatic hypertrophic cardiomyopathy. An evaluation by a geneticist may be indicated if there are multiple congenital anomalies.

SPECIAL CONSIDERATIONS

Prevention Pre-pregnancy care and counseling may influence pregestational glycemic control, which may lower the teratogenic effects of maternal metabolic derangements. Prenatal screening and ultrasounds may detect malformations and influence delivery site and plan. Close surveillance of the pregnancy is warranted to ensure fetal well-being. Careful management of maternal glycemic control, with nutritional support and attention to appropriate weight targets may minimize the risk of newborn hypoglycemia and other complications.

KEY POINTS

- Newborn hypoglycemia may present with typical signs and symptoms of hypoglycemia or be completely asymptomatic.
- Screening glucose monitoring is recommended for newborns with risk factors for hypoglycemia and for symptomatic newborns.
- Initial management depends on the degree of hypoglycemia and the infant's ability to maintain safe blood glucose levels (>45 mg/dL).
- Infants of diabetic mothers are at risk for hypoglycemia as well as other abnormalities, such as macrosomia, electrolyte abnormalities, organomegaly, congenital anomalies, respiratory distress syndrome, and hyperbilirubinemia.

SUGGESTED READINGS

American Academy of Pediatrics Committee on Fetus and Newborn. Clinical report—Postnatal glucose homeostasis in late-preterm and term infants. *Pediatrics*. 2011;127:575-579.

Cornblath M, Hawdon JM, Williams AF, et al. Controversies regarding definition of neonatal hypoglycemia: suggested operational thresholds. *Pediatrics*. 2000;105:1141-1145.

Coors SM, Cousin JJ, Hagan JL, Kaiser JR. Prophylactic dextrose gel does not prevent neonatal hypoglycemia: a quasi-experimental pilot study. *J Pediatr*. 2018;198:156-161.

Correa A, Gilboa SM, Besser LM, et al. Diabetes mellitus and birth defects. *Am J Obstet Gynecol*. 2008;199:237e1-e9.

Harris DL, Alsweiler JM, Ansell JM, et al. Outcome at 2 years after dextrose gel treatment for neonatal hypoglycemia: follow-up of a randomized trial. *J Pediatr*. 2016;170:54-9.e1-2.

Harris DL, Weston PJ, Harding JE. Incidence of neonatal hypoglycemia in babies identified as at risk. *J Pediatr*. 2012;161:787-791.

Harris DL, Weston PJ, Signal M, et al. Dextrose gel for neonatal hypoglycaemia (the Sugar Babies Study): a randomised, double-blind, placebo-controlled trial. *Lancet*. 2013;382:2077-2083.

Kaiser JR, Bai S, Gibson N, et al. Association between transient newborn hypoglycemia and fourth-grade achievement test proficiency: a population-based study. *JAMA Pediatr*. 2015;169:913-921.

McKinlay CJD, Alsweiler JM, Anstice NS, et al. Association of neonatal glycemia with neurodevelopmental outcomes at 4.5 years. *JAMA Pediatr*. 2017; 171:972-983.

Peters S, Andrews C, Sen S. Care of infants born to women with diabetes. *Curr Diab Rep*. 2020;20:39.

Thompson-Branch A, Havranek T. Neonatal hypoglycemia. *Pediatr Rev*. 2017;38:147-157.

Wight NE; Academy of Breastfeeding Medicine. ABM Clinical Protocol #1: Guidelines for glucose monitoring and treatment of hypoglycemia in term and late preterm neonates, Revised 2021. *Breastfeed Med*. 2021;16:353-365.

CHAPTER 130 Neonatal Hyperbilirubinemia

Pearl W. Chang, MD* and Thomas B. Newman, MD, MPH

BACKGROUND

Untreated severe hyperbilirubinemia can lead to kernicterus, or chronic bilirubin encephalopathy, a permanent and devastating condition associated with significant morbidity and mortality. A systematic approach to the detection and management of hyperbilirubinemia in newborns is therefore critical for prevention. While kernicterus in high-resource countries is a rare condition, with an estimated incidence of 0.4-1.3 per 100,000 full-term newborns, hyperbilirubinemia is one of the most common neonatal conditions requiring extension of the newborn hospital stay or readmission to the hospital after newborn discharge.

PATHOPHYSIOLOGY

Bilirubin is a breakdown product of heme, which is contained primarily in hemoglobin. Microsomal heme oxygenase catabolizes heme to biliverdin, which is then reduced to bilirubin by biliverdin reductase. The resulting unconjugated bilirubin is a lipid-soluble molecule that is transported to the liver bound to albumin in plasma. In the liver, bilirubin uridine diphosphate glucuronosyltransferase (UDPGT) conjugates bilirubin with glucuronic acid. Conjugated bilirubin is a water-soluble molecule that is excreted from the hepatocyte to the bile canaliculi, through the biliary tree, and into the duodenum. In the intestines, β-glucuronidase from breast milk or bacteria can convert conjugated bilirubin back to unconjugated bilirubin, which may be absorbed and returned to the liver (enterohepatic circulation). The rest may be converted by intestinal bacteria to urobilinogen, which may be reabsorbed and found in urine, and stercobilin and other substances excreted in the feces.

Hyperbilirubinemia is classified as either conjugated or unconjugated (also known as direct or indirect, referring to the van den Bergh reaction used to measure bilirubin). Unconjugated hyperbilirubinemia is caused by increased production, decreased hepatic uptake or metabolism, or increased enterohepatic circulation of bilirubin. Newborn infants are particularly susceptible to unconjugated hyperbilirubinemia because, compared with adults, they have more red blood cells with a higher turnover and shorter life span, and a limited ability to conjugate bilirubin. Newborn bilirubin levels typically peak at 3 to 5 days of age and then decrease over the next few weeks to adult levels. Unconjugated bilirubin that exceeds the binding capacity of albumin (maximum of 8.2 mg bilirubin per gram of albumin) may enter the brain and damage neurons primarily in the basal ganglia, hippocampus, cerebellum, and brainstem nuclei for oculomotor function and hearing. Factors that increase the risk of bilirubin neurotoxicity include the concentration of bilirubin and the duration of exposure to it, albumin levels, and conditions that decrease albumin binding or increase blood-brain barrier permeability (e.g., medications, such as sulfonamides, that displace bilirubin from albumin, infection, acidosis, hyperoxia, sepsis, prematurity, hyperosmolarity).

CLINICAL PRESENTATION

Jaundice, the yellow discoloration of the skin and conjunctivae, may rarely be present at birth but most often appears on the second or third day after birth. It generally starts on the face and spreads down the body in a cephalocaudal progression as the bilirubin rises. The extent of cephalocaudal jaundice progression can be used to estimate the bilirubin level, though differences as high as 13 to 15 mg/dL between visual estimation and the actual bilirubin level have been observed. More reassuringly, complete absence of jaundice in infants >3 days of age is helpful in predicting which infants will not develop significant hyperbilirubinemia. Unconjugated bilirubin in the skin appears bright yellow or orange, whereas conjugated bilirubin appears more greenish or muddy yellow. Infants with unconjugated hyperbilirubinemia secondary to suboptimal milk intake may also present with an ineffective latch or suck, a sunken fontanelle, and/or increased sleepiness, while infants with conjugated hyperbilirubinemia may also present with pale stools, dark urine, and/or hepatomegaly.

Acute bilirubin encephalopathy generally progresses through three stages: early, intermediate, and advanced. Progression through these stages depends on peak bilirubin level, duration of hyperbilirubinemia, host susceptibility, and presence of comorbidities. In the early phase of acute bilirubin encephalopathy, infants display lethargy, hypotonia, and poor ability to suck. In the intermediate phase, infants have stupor, irritability, and hypertonia (retrocollis-opisthotonos) alternating with drowsiness and hypotonia. They may also develop a fever and high-pitched cry. The advanced phase of acute bilirubin encephalopathy is associated with a high mortality rate—approximately 10%—and can be characterized by cessation of feeding, bicycling movements, inconsolable irritability and crying, seizures, fever, and coma. Survivors of this advanced stage are likely to develop chronic bilirubin encephalopathy, even after intensive treatment.

Chronic bilirubin encephalopathy (kernicterus) refers to permanent, chronic, and lifelong sequalae that become apparent within the first year of life, and may include extrapyramidal movement disorders (dystonia and athetosis), gaze abnormalities (especially upward gaze), auditory disturbances (especially sensorineural hearing loss with central processing disorders or auditory neuropathy), and enamel dysplasia of the deciduous teeth.

DIFFERENTIAL DIAGNOSIS

The most common contributors to significant hyperbilirubinemia in the first week after birth are lower gestational age, suboptimal breastmilk intake, cephalohematomas or excessive bruising, and isoimmune hemolytic disease (i.e., positive direct antiglobulin test [DAT]), due to ABO, Rh, or minor blood group incompatibility. Exclusive breastfeeding is strongly associated with hyperbilirubinemia. In particular, suboptimal milk intake contributes to decreased stool output and increased enterohepatic circulation of bilirubin. This is commonly referred to as "breastfeeding jaundice," though more accurately should be termed *suboptimal intake jaundice*. There may also be some increased β-glucuronidase activity in breast milk after birth, though results are conflicting. With the availability of Rh(D) immunoglobulin for mothers with Rh negative blood types, isoimmune hemolytic disease due to Rh incompatibility, once a leading cause of severe hyperbilirubinemia, is uncommon in resource-rich countries. Instead, ABO hemolytic disease, which occurs primarily in infants of blood group A or B born to group O mothers, is the most common cause of isoimmune hemolytic disease in resource-rich countries. Isoimmune hemolytic disease due to minor blood group antigens, such as C, c, E, e, and Kell, is a less common cause of hyperbilirubinemia, but may be more severe; the risk for hemolytic disease due to antibodies to these antigens should be identified on the mother's prenatal antibody screen.

Heritable causes of hemolysis are a less common cause of neonatal hyperbilirubinemia, but important to consider especially for infants with severe hyperbilirubinemia or atypical development of hyperbilirubinemia. Glucose-6-phosphate dehydrogenase (G6PD) deficiency, an X-linked recessive red blood cell enzyme deficiency, is the one of the most important causes of bilirubin encephalopathy in the United States. Other causes of hemolysis are listed in **Table 130-1**.

In approximately 20% of breastfed infants, jaundice persists beyond the first week after birth in what is termed *breast milk jaundice*, which in contrast to *suboptimal intake jaundice* (breastfeeding jaundice), occurs in infants with adequate breast milk intake and weight gain. With breast milk jaundice, bilirubin levels can peak as high as 10 to 25 mg/dL in the second to third week, and jaundice may persist for up to 10 weeks. Breast

TABLE 130-1 Differential Diagnosis of Neonatal Hyperbilirubinemia

Finding	Diagnosis
Unconjugated hyperbilirubinemia	
Increased production	Isoimmune hemolysis (ABO, Rh, other) Cephalohematoma Bruising Sepsis Polycythemia Congenital hemolytic anemias (spherocytosis, elliptocytosis, pyknocytosis) Erythrocyte enzyme defects (G6PD, pyruvate kinase, hexokinase)
Decreased uptake, storage, or metabolism	Prematurity Sepsis Gilbert syndrome Crigler-Najjar syndrome (Type I or II) Hypothyroidism Hypopituitarism Lucey-Driscoll syndrome
Increased enterohepatic circulation	Suboptimal intake jaundice Breast milk jaundice Intestinal obstruction (ileal atresia, Hirschsprung disease, meconium ileus)
Conjugated hyperbilirubinemia	
	Sepsis Extrahepatic biliary atresia Intrahepatic cholestasis Metabolic disorders Congenital viral infections

G6PD, glucose-6-phosphate dehydrogenase.

milk jaundice is not associated with conjugated or direct hyperbilirubinemia. Discontinuation of breastfeeding and substitution of formula for 1 to 2 days results in a rapid and sustained decline in serum bilirubin, but this is generally not recommended unless bilirubin levels approach treatment thresholds. The cause of breast milk jaundice is not known with certainty, although β-glucuronidase (resulting in deconjugation of bilirubin and increased enterohepatic circulation) and other factors in breast milk that might interfere with bilirubin conjugation (e.g., pregnanediol and free fatty acids) have been implicated as potential causes.

For breastfed infants who are still jaundiced at 3 to 4 weeks of age and for formula-fed infants who are still jaundiced at 2 weeks of age, the American Academy of Pediatrics (AAP) recommends that a conjugated or direct bilirubin be checked to rule out possible pathologic cholestasis. Causes of conjugated hyperbilirubinemia include extrahepatic biliary atresia, intrahepatic cholestasis, metabolic disorders, urinary tract infections, and congenital viral infections (see Chapter 71).

DIAGNOSTIC EVALUATION

RISK ASSESSMENT AND SCREENING

The 2022 AAP Clinical Practice Guideline recommends that all newborn infants ≥35 weeks' gestation have a transcutaneous bilirubin (TcB) or total serum bilirubin (TSB) measured at 24-48 hours after birth, or prior to birth hospitalization discharge if that occurs earlier. In addition to universal predischarge screening, bilirubin measurements should be obtained for infants who are jaundiced in the first 24 hours after birth and for those who appear excessively jaundiced for their age at any point. A high bilirubin rate of rise of ≥0.3 mg/dL/hr in the first 24 hours after birth or ≥0.2 mg/dL/hr thereafter suggests possible hemolysis, as do TSB levels that rise or fail to decline despite intensive phototherapy.

TRANSCUTANEOUS VERSUS TOTAL SERUM BILIRUBIN MEASUREMENT

TSB measured in a clinical laboratory is considered the gold standard for bilirubin measurement; however, there is still a disturbing level of interlaboratory variability in this measurement depending on the method used, and even intralaboratory variability when instruments are recalibrated. Clinicians should be aware of the method of testing used by their clinical laboratory; the Vitros method results in higher bilirubin values compared with traditional methods. The Vitros method will generally report total, conjugated and unconjugated bilirubin levels, while traditional methods measure and report total, direct, and indirect bilirubin levels.

TcB instruments do not directly measure bilirubin levels, but TcB measurements are a valid screening test to identify which infants require a TSB measurement. Transcutaneous bilirubinometers operate by transmitting light that penetrates the blanched skin and transilluminates the subcutaneous tissues. The yellowness of the reflected light is measured in a spectrophotometric module and converted into an estimate of the TSB concentration. Measurements should be taken on the forehead or sternum. Values generally correlate within 2 to 3 mg/dL of TSB values, although there is some evidence that transcutaneous instruments are less accurate at higher bilirubin levels (>15 mg/dL) or for darker-skinned infants. In addition, there may be inconsistencies in performances across instruments, and quality control is essential to ensure proper function and accuracy.

Therefore, if the TcB level is within 3 mg/dL of the phototherapy threshold or ≥15 mg/dL, the AAP recommends confirmation with a TSB measurement. TSB values should also be measured once infants begin phototherapy, as TcB measurements may underestimate the total bilirubin in this setting. If it has been at least 24 hours since phototherapy was stopped, or the area of skin used for testing was covered by an opaque patch during phototherapy, then use of TcB may be an option.

ADDITIONAL LABORATORY STUDIES

As part of routine prenatal care, maternal blood type and anti-erythrocyte antibody screening should be obtained; if the mother has not had prenatal antibody screening or is Rh-negative, the infant's cord or peripheral blood should be obtained for blood typing and a DAT as soon as possible after birth. Infant blood typing and DAT when the maternal blood is group O, Rh-positive is an option but not routinely recommended, as long as appropriate surveillance and follow-up for hyperbilirubinemia are performed. While knowing the DAT status is important for risk stratification, only ~25% of infants with ABO incompatibility who are DAT-positive develop significant hyperbilirubinemia.

Infants whose TSB levels require phototherapy should have fractionated (conjugated and unconjugated or direct and indirect) bilirubin levels checked, as well as blood type and DAT (if O positive mother), and at least a hemoglobin or hematocrit. If the DAT is negative and there remains concern for hemolysis, additional studies for inherited disorders such as spherocytosis and G6PD deficiency should be considered if the TSB does not decline promptly with phototherapy. Infants who are jaundiced beyond 2 weeks of age if formula-fed and beyond 3 weeks of age if breastfed should have total and conjugated (or direct) bilirubin levels measured and undergo evaluation for the cause of cholestasis if the conjugated or direct bilirubin level is elevated. The results of the newborn screen can be used to evaluate for congenital hypothyroidism and galactosemia as causes of jaundice.

MANAGEMENT

PHOTOTHERAPY

The primary goal of phototherapy is to prevent the TSB from rising to levels that may require an exchange transfusion. Hour-specific bilirubin thresholds for initiating phototherapy and exchange transfusion for infants ≥35 weeks gestational age have been recommended by the AAP based on expert opinion (see Figures 2, 3 and Figures 5, 6, respectively in https://publications.aap.org/pediatrics/article/150/3/e2022058859/188726/Clinical-Practice-Guideline-Revision-Management-of). The hour-specific thresholds, first established in 2004, were raised slightly in 2022 to decrease phototherapy overtreatment, given that there is no evidence of bilirubin toxicity at levels < 5 mg/dL above the previous 2004 AAP exchange transfusion thresholds. Clinicians should use the TSB, not the unconjugated (or indirect) fraction, in applying these treatment guidelines. Treatment thresholds depend on the infant's gestational age and other neurotoxicity risk factors, including albumin <3.0 g/dL, hemolysis (e.g., isoimmune hemolytic disease, G6PD deficiency), sepsis, or significant clinical instability in the previous 24 hours.

Phototherapy achieves reduction of hyperbilirubinemia by three mechanisms: (i) reversible photoisomerization of the nonpolar native unconjugated *4Z,15Z*-bilirubin into the polar configurational isomer *4Z,15E*-bilirubin, which is excreted in the bile without need for conjugation; (ii) irreversible conversion of native unconjugated bilirubin into the structural isomer lumirubin, which is excreted by both the liver and the kidneys; and (iii) photooxidation to various colorless compounds excreted in the urine. Phototherapy must contain light in the blue range (460-490 nm) and be of sufficient intensity to efficiently reduce hyperbilirubinemia. The AAP recommends that hospitals use intensive phototherapy light of at least 30 $\mu W/cm^2/nm$ measured by a radiometer at the infant's skin directly below the center of the unit. Depending on the intensity of the light and surface area exposed, intensive phototherapy can be expected to decrease the initial bilirubin level by 30% to 50% in the first 24 hours. Intermittent phototherapy, with interruptions for feeding and other infant care, has been shown to be as effective as continuous phototherapy. Feeding should be continued during phototherapy to avoid dehydration and promote bilirubin excretion. Brief supplementation with formula may lead to a more rapid TSB decline and reduce the risk of readmission for phototherapy, with possibly similar benefits with expressed or donor breast milk supplementation. Intravenous fluids are not necessary unless there is dehydration that cannot be corrected enterally or the TSB meets escalation of care threshold (see further).

For infants who have been discharged from the nursery, home phototherapy may be an alternative to hospital readmission for those who need treatment. Home phototherapy may be less costly than hospital phototherapy and less disruptive to infant breastfeeding and bonding.

However, the quality of home phototherapy equipment and the ability of parents to use the device influence the effectiveness of home treatment. The AAP recommends that home phototherapy be used only for infants of ≥38 weeks' gestation who are ≥48 hours old and clinically well, have no neurotoxicity risk factors, no history of phototherapy treatment, with a TSB level no more than 1 mg/dL above the phototherapy treatment threshold. For breastfed infants with excessive weight loss consistent with suboptimal intake hyperbilirubinemia and no concern for hemolysis, the use of supplemental formula, expressed or donor breast milk may be an alternative to phototherapy for a bilirubin level approaching or at treatment threshold.

The decision to discontinue phototherapy should balance the potential harms of a longer phototherapy course with the risk of rebound hyperbilirubinemia, defined as a TSB level that reaches treatment threshold for the infant's age within 4 days of phototherapy discontinuation. Lower gestational age, hemolytic disease, younger age at phototherapy initiation, and a TSB closer to the phototherapy threshold at the time of phototherapy termination are risk factors for rebound hyperbilirubinemia; risk prediction tools are available that can estimate the risk of rebound. For infants who start phototherapy at <48 hours of age or have a positive DAT or other known or suspected hemolytic disease, a rebound TSB measurement at 6 to 12 hours after phototherapy discontinuation should be considered, plus another follow-up TSB the day after. All other infants treated with phototherapy are at lower risk for rebound hyperbilirubinemia and should get either a repeat TSB or clinical follow-up in 1 to 2 days, depending on an infant's rebound and hyperbilirubinemia risk factors.

ESCALATION OF CARE AND EXCHANGE TRANSFUSION

If an infant reaches or exceeds the TSB level that is 2 mg/dL below their hour- and gestational-age specific exchange transfusion threshold ("escalation of care" threshold), the AAP recommends that care be escalated to prevent the need for an exchange transfusion. This includes additional laboratory tests (CBC, G6PD activity, serum albumin, serum chemistries, type and crossmatch), intensive phototherapy, intravenous hydration, and TSB monitoring every 2 hours until the TSB is lower than the escalation of care threshold. Intravenous immune globulin is an option for infants with isoimmune hemolytic disease whose bilirubin is approaching exchange levels despite phototherapy, especially in settings where timely exchange transfusion may not be available. In addition, there should be an urgent consultation with a neonatologist to discuss transfer to a neonatal intensive care unit.

Exchange transfusion should be performed for infants who reach the exchange transfusion threshold, unless the TSB declines with intensive phototherapy during preparations for the exchange transfusion and the infant has no signs of acute bilirubin encephalopathy. The bilirubin-to-albumin ratio can also be used, together with TSB level, as an additional consideration in determining the need for exchange transfusion (**Table 130-2**).

TABLE 130-2 Bilirubin: Albumin Ratio as an Additional Risk Factor When Considering Exchange Transfusion

Risk Category	Total Serum Bilirubin (mg/dl)-to-Albumin (g/dL) Ratio that suggests an exchange transfusion may be warranted
Gestational age ≥38 weeks with no neurotoxicity risk factors	≥8.0
Gestational age ≥38 weeks plus ≥1 neurotoxicity risk factor, or Gestational age 35-37 weeks with no neurotoxicity risk factors	≥7.2
Gestational age 35-37 weeks plus ≥1 neurotoxicity risk factor	≥6.8

Source: Adapted from Kemper AR, Newman TB, Slaughter JL, et al. Clinical practice guideline revision: management of hyperbilirubinemia in the newborn infant 35 or more weeks of gestation. *Pediatrics.* 2022;150(3):e2022058859.

FOLLOW-UP

Appropriate and timely follow-up should always be provided, as even for infants with a low predischarge TSB or TcB level the risk of subsequent hyperbilirubinemia is not zero. The AAP recommends using the difference between the bilirubin level and the phototherapy threshold at the age of bilirubin measurement to determine the timing of follow-up (https://publications.aap.org/pediatrics/article/150/3/e2022058859/188726/Clinical-Practice-Guideline-Revision-Management-of, Figure 7). Earlier or more frequent follow-up may be needed for infants who have hyperbilirubinemia risk factors or feeding and weight loss concerns. If follow-up cannot be assured, a clinician may opt to delay discharge until the bilirubin trajectory is elucidated and a decision can be made about the need for phototherapy or discharge home.

SPECIAL CONSIDERATIONS

POTENTIAL HARMS OF PHOTOTHERAPY

Decisions about whether to start phototherapy below treatment threshold or to continue phototherapy for a longer duration should weigh the benefits of phototherapy treatment against its potential harms. In addition to costs, separation of mother and baby in some hospital settings, and parental stress, there may be a small increased risk of childhood epilepsy after phototherapy treatment (about 2.4 per 1000 children over 10 years). Previous studies with concern for associations between phototherapy and melanocytic nevi have not been replicated in newer studies, and while some studies have reported associations between phototherapy and childhood cancer (particularly hematologic malignancies), the only studies that controlled for bilirubin levels did not find a significant independent association between phototherapy and cancer.

PREVENTION

A hospital-based approach to primary prevention of severe hyperbilirubinemia includes the establishment of standing protocols for nurses' assessment of jaundice, including measurement of TcB and TSB levels, without requiring a physician's order (similar to the protocols in place for measuring serum glucose levels). Checklists or reminders should prompt providers to consider risk factors and age at discharge, as well as laboratory test results that guide appropriate follow-up. Support for breastfeeding mothers and close monitoring of infant feeding are critical. Educational materials concerning the identification of jaundice and information about pre-discharge bilirubin levels and follow-up instructions should be provided to parents.

KEY POINTS

- Universal bilirubin screening, when combined with clinical risk assessment and targeted follow-up, is the most effective method of identifying infants at high or low risk for development of severe hyperbilirubinemia.
- Gestational age as a clinical risk factor has a strong impact on prediction of severe hyperbilirubinemia and bilirubin neurotoxicity, with risk decreasing continuously with each additional week of maturity.
- TSB or TcB measurement and interpretation compared with the hour-specific phototherapy threshold provides an immediate and quantitative method to assess current degree and future risk of hyperbilirubinemia and the need for additional surveillance and testing.
- Initiation of phototherapy or exchange transfusion should be guided using TSB levels, gestational age, and the AAP hour-specific treatment thresholds according to whether neurotoxicity risk factors are present.
- Timely follow-up to ensure hyperbilirubinemia surveillance should be provided for all newborns discharged at <72 hours of age, including those with a low predischarge TSB or TcB level.

SUGGESTED READINGS

Alkén J, Håkansson S, Ekéus C, Gustafson P, Norman M. Rates of extreme neonatal hyperbilirubinemia and kernicterus in children and adherence to national guidelines for screening, diagnosis, and treatment in Sweden. *JAMA Netw Open*. 2019;2(3):e190858.

Chang PW, Newman TB. A simpler prediction rule for rebound hyperbilirubinemia. *Pediatrics*. 2019 Jul;144(1).

Christensen RD, Baer VL, MacQueen BC, O'Brien EA, Ilstrup SJ. ABO hemolytic disease of the fetus and newborn: thirteen years of data after implementing a universal bilirubin screening and management program. *J Perinatol*. 2018;38(5):517-525.

Digitale JC, Kim MO, Kuzniewicz MW, Newman TB. Update on phototherapy and childhood cancer in a Northern California Cohort. *Pediatrics*. 2021;148(5).

Ebbesen F, Bjerre JV, Vandborg PK. Relation between serum bilirubin levels ≥450 μmol/L and bilirubin encephalopathy; a Danish population-based study. *Acta Paediatr*. 2012;101(4):384-9.

Flaherman VJ, Maisels MJ, Medicine AoB. ABM Clinical Protocol #22: Guidelines for management of jaundice in the breastfeeding infant 35 weeks or more of gestation-revised 2017. *Breastfeed Med*. 2017 June;12(5):250-257.

Gotink MJ, Benders MJ, Lavrijsen SW, Rodrigues Pereira R, Hulzebos CV, Dijk PH. Severe neonatal hyperbilirubinemia in the Netherlands. *Neonatology*. 2013;104(2):137-142.

Gourley GR, Li Z, Kreamer BL, Kosorok MR. A controlled, randomized, double-blind trial of prophylaxis against jaundice among breastfed newborns. *Pediatrics*. 2005;116(2):385-391.

Hansen TWR, Wong RJ, Stevenson DK. Molecular physiology and pathophysiology of bilirubin handling by the blood, liver, intestine, and brain in the newborn. *Physiol Rev*. 2020;100(3):1291-1346.

Hemati Z, Keikha M, Khoshhali M, Kelishadi R. Phototherapy and risk of childhood cancer: a systematic review and meta-analysis. *J Neonatal Nurs*. 2022;28:219-228.

Kemper AR, Newman TB, Slaughter JL, et al. Clinical practice guideline revision: management of hyperbilirubinemia in the newborn infant 35 or more weeks of gestation. *Pediatrics*. 2022;150(3): e2022058859.

Kuzniewicz MW, Greene DN, Walsh EM, McCulloch CE, Newman TB. Association between laboratory calibration of a serum bilirubin assay, neonatal bilirubin levels, and phototherapy use. *JAMA Pediatr*. 2016;170(6):557-561.

Kuzniewicz MW, Wickremasinghe AC, Wu YW, et al. Incidence, etiology, and outcomes of hazardous hyperbilirubinemia in newborns. *Pediatrics*. 2014;134(3):504-509.

Lai YC, Yew YW. Neonatal blue light phototherapy and melanocytic nevus count in children: a systematic review and meta-analysis of observational studies. *Pediatr Dermatol*. 2016 Jan-Feb;33(1):62-68.

Newman TB, Wu YW, Kuzniewicz MW, Grimes BA, McCulloch CE. Childhood seizures after phototherapy. *Pediatrics*. 2018;142(4).

Slaughter JL, Kemper AR, Newman TB. Technical report: diagnosis and management of hyperbilirubinemia in the newborn infant 35 or more weeks of gestation. *Pediatrics*. 2022 Sep 1;150(3):e2022058865.

Vandborg PK, Hansen BM, Greisen G, Ebbesen F. Dose-response relationship of phototherapy for hyperbilirubinemia. *Pediatrics*. Aug 2012; 130(2):e352-7.

Wickremasinghe AC, Kuzniewicz MW, McCulloch CE, Newman TB. Efficacy of subthreshold newborn phototherapy during the birth hospitalization in preventing readmission for phototherapy. *JAMA Pediatr*. 2018;172(4):378-385.

Wickremasinghe AC, Risley RJ, Kuzniewicz MW, et al. Risk of sensorineural hearing loss and bilirubin exchange transfusion thresholds. *Pediatrics*. 2015;129(3):505-512.

Wu YW, Kuzniewicz MW, Wickremasinghe AC, et al. Risk for cerebral palsy in infants with total serum bilirubin levels at or above the exchange transfusion threshold: a population-based study. *JAMA Pediatr*. 2015;169(3):239-246.

Yiğit S, Ciliv G, Aygün C, Erdem G. Breast milk beta-glucuronidase levels in hyperbilirubinemia. *Turk J Pediatr*. 2001 Apr-Jun;43(2):118-120.

Young PC, Korgenski K, Buchi KF. Early readmission of newborns in a large health care system. *Pediatrics*. May 2013;131(5):e1538-1544.

CHAPTER 131 Neonatal Opioid Withdrawal Syndrome

Jennifer McAllister, MD, IBCLC

BACKGROUND

Neonatal abstinence syndrome (NAS) refers to a constellation of symptoms that occur in newborns after the cessation of placental transfer of opioids and other substances after birth. In the United States, the number of pregnant people with opioid use disorder (OUD) has increased significantly with rates of maternal opioid-related diagnoses affecting 4.6 per 1000 birth hospitalizations and rates of NAS at 7.3 per 1000 birth hospitalizations. Recently, the terminology, neonatal opioid withdrawal syndrome (NOWS), has been more commonly used to distinguish neonatal withdrawal specific to opioids and is considered a subset of NAS. In utero opioid exposure can have both short- and long-term consequences for infants and children; prompt identification, diagnosis, management, and appropriate follow-up care will promote optimal health outcomes in this population.

PATHOPHYSIOLOGY

The terms opiates and opioids are often used interchangeably. However, opiates refer to natural occurring compounds such as heroin, morphine, and codeine whereas the broader category of opioids refers to all natural, semi-synthetic, and synthetic opioids including prescription pain medications and medications for opioid use disorder (MOUD). In general, opioids have low molecular weights, are water soluble, and are lipophilic, allowing for easy transfer through passive diffusion across the placenta. Synthetic opioids including buprenorphine, fentanyl, and methadone cross the placenta more easily than semi-synthetic compounds like oxycodone, but any opioids in the maternal blood stream can transfer into fetal circulation. As gestational age increases, the placental transfer of opioids also increases, resulting in a higher cumulative exposure for newborns delivered at term (≥ 37 weeks gestation). Compared with preterm infants (<37 weeks gestation), term newborns also have increased morphine clearance, another likely contributor to their increased risk of experiencing NOWS symptoms.

A variety of factors contribute to the symptoms experienced by newborns with NOWS. Opioid receptors are distributed across the central nervous system, peripheral nervous systems, and the gastrointestinal system. After birth, the lack of opioids in a previously chronically stimulated state leads to an increase in opioid receptor activity, resulting in the altered production of various neurotransmitters. Surges of norepinephrine, noradrenaline, corticotrophin, and acetylcholine, as well as decreases in serotonin and dopamine, all contribute to the multitude of NOWS symptoms.

CLINICAL PRESENTATION

Newborns with NOWS are often born small for gestational age and with reduced growth parameters. Most newborns with chronic in utero opioid exposure will experience some symptoms of NOWS affecting the neurologic, autonomic, and gastrointestinal (GI) systems (**Table 131-1**). Symptoms range from mild to severe, which may require pharmacologic intervention and often prolonged hospital stays. The most common signs of NOWS include excessive crying, fragmented sleep, tremors, hypertonia, and feeding difficulties. Timing of onset of symptoms is determined by the type of opioid exposure, half-life of the opioid, duration of exposure, and other pharmacologic properties or co-current substance exposures; however dose of maternal opioid use does not seem to affect the risk of symptom severity. Newborns exposed to immediate-release or short-acting opioids like fentanyl, heroin, and prescription pain medications may exhibit symptoms within hours up to a few days after birth whereas the onset of symptoms for infants exposed to

TABLE 131-1 Clinical Symptoms of NOWS

Neurologic Symptoms	Autonomic Symptoms	Gastrointestinal Symptoms
Excessive crying	Tachypnea	Loose, frequent stools
Fragmented sleep	Tachycardia	Hyperphagia
Tremors	Nasal stuffiness	Vomiting
Hypertonia	Sweating	Regurgitation
Irritability	Elevated temperature/fever	Poor feeding
Exaggerated moro reflex	Sneezing	Excessive weight loss
Excessive sucking	Mottling	
Myoclonic jerks	Frequent yawning	

longer-acting opioids often prescribed for MOUD including buprenorphine and methadone may be several days after birth. The duration of NOWS symptoms can also be variable, with some newborns experiencing symptoms for several months.

DIFFERENTIAL DIAGNOSIS

Withdrawal from other in utero exposures including nicotine, caffeine, antidepressants, and benzodiazepines may present similarly to NOWS and should be considered in the differential diagnosis. It is important to determine history of prenatal opioid exposure or other possible exposures when diagnosing NOWS, especially if the newborn requires pharmacologic treatment for symptoms. Medical conditions including electrolyte abnormalities and hypoglycemia, in utero central nervous system injuries, and congenital GI issues should also be assessed in newborns with NOWS-like symptoms.

DIAGNOSTIC EVALUATION

IDENTIFICATION OF IN UTERO EXPOSURE

A thorough prenatal history is required to help recognize mothers with OUD and infants with in utero opioid exposure. Validated screening questionnaires including the "4Ps" (parents, partners, past, and pregnancy), "CRAFFT" tool (car, relax, alone, forget, friends, trouble), and the National Institute on Drug Abuse quick screen should be administered during prenatal visits to help identify mothers with substance use or OUD. Toxicology testing can be performed for both the mother and newborn to identify and confirm prenatal exposures. Universal maternal toxicology testing can improve identification of newborns at risk for NOWS, however this approach should consider access to treatment and resources for mothers with a positive toxicology test, potential legal and mandatory reporting ramifications, and processes to minimize false positives. For all maternal toxicology testing, consent should be obtained.

Newborn Toxicology Testing Toxicology testing of the newborn can be performed using either an antibody-based immunoassay or specific drug identification test (mass spectroscopy). Immunoassay tests have the advantage of broad testing for multiple types of substances and can be quickly processed. However, they are more prone to false positive results due to cross-reactivity. Mass spectroscopy is superior for definitive testing and can also quantitate results, however this approach is more costly and time consuming. The most common method of newborn toxicology testing is urine immunoassay testing. However, the window of detection in urine is limited to the last several days prior to delivery and should be collected soon after birth as many substances are rapidly metabolized and eliminated (see **Table 131-2**). Meconium testing via mass spectroscopy is considered the gold standard and can detect exposures from the last 20 weeks of gestation providing information on chronic exposure, but it is cumbersome to collect and can also take several days to obtain results. Recently, umbilical cord testing via mass spectroscopy has become a common method of testing as cords are easy to obtain and may yield quicker results, with a window of detection that has been reported through the third trimester. However, studies comparing umbilical cord testing with meconium have demonstrated mixed results with some reporting discordance. As methods of umbilical cord testing improve, this may become a more popular method of testing for in utero substance exposure.

ASSESSMENT OF NOWS SYMPTOMS

All newborns with chronic in utero exposure to short-acting or long-acting opioids should be monitored for the development of NOWS symptoms. There is wide variation in hospital practices related to observation periods for NOWS, however, the American Academy of Pediatrics recommends observing newborns exposed to immediate-release opioids for at least 3 days, infants exposed to buprenorphine or sustained-release opioids for 4 to 7 days, and infants exposed to methadone for 5 to 7 days. Monitoring for NOWS symptoms is routinely performed in the postpartum or well-baby unit, and keeping the mother-infant dyad together is the preferred model of care.

Finnegan Score The most widely used assessment tool to evaluate NOWS symptoms is the Finnegan Neonatal Abstinence Scoring System (FNASS) or the Modified FNASS which assigns numbers or a score based on perceived severity of 21 clinical signs. Typically, a consecutive score of 8 to 12 or 2 scores of 13 or greater within 24 hours on the modified FNASS suggests that the infant is experiencing significant withdrawal and may require pharmacologic treatment. Scores should be obtained every 3 to 4 hours after feeding when the infant is awake, and scores should reflect the status of the infant at the time of assessment and during the previous time period. Despite its widespread usage there

TABLE 131-2 Common Opioids, Their Metabolites, and Approximate Urinary Detection Times

		Half-life	Other Metabolites	Urine Detection Time
SHORT-ACTING OPIOIDS	Heroin (diacetylmorphine)	2-6 minutes	6-acetylmorphine	2-8 hours
			morphine	1-2 days
	Morphine	2-3 hours	(<3%) hydromorphone	1-2 days
	Hydromorphone	2-3 hours		1-2 days
	Fentanyl	3-4 hours	Norfentanyl, despropionylfentanyl	1-3 days
	Codeine	3 hours	Morphine	2-3 days
	Hydrocodone	2-3 hours	Hydromorphone, norhydrocodone, dihydrocodeine	2-3 days
	Oxycodone	2-3 hours	Oxymorphone Noroxymorphone	2-3 days
	Tramadol	6 hours	O-desmethyltramadol	2-4 days
LONG-ACTING OPIOIDS	Buprenorphine	24-48 hours	Norbuprenorphine	1-7 days
	Methadone	12-60 hours	3-diphenylpyrrolidine (EDDP)	1-14 days

are potential limitations of the FNASS, including lack of validation to support pharmacologic treatment cutoffs, and questionable clinical relevance of scoring for certain symptoms.

Eat, Sleep, Console Approach The scoring assessment system called "Eat, Sleep, Console" (ESC) evaluates the key functions of a newborn; rather than characterizing all signs of withdrawal, it instead focuses on ability to eat at least 1 oz or breastfeed well, sleep undisturbed for at least 1 hour, and be consoled within 10 minutes. If a newborn is unable to meet these criteria, the care team meets to determine the need for further intervention or pharmacotherapy. Multiple published reports on ESC implementation have demonstrated shorter lengths of stay and less need for newborn pharmacotherapy with this approach, and it may also reduce the experience of stigma among mothers with OUD. Rigorous research comparing outcomes of ESC with FNASS in a randomized, control trial setting is currently ongoing.

MANAGEMENT

NONPHARMACOLOGIC INTERVENTION

The primary management strategy for all infants undergoing assessment for NOWS is nonpharmacologic care. These interventions should be initiated after birth and include providing a low-stimulus environment, allowing for on-demand feeding, minimizing interventions, and maximizing caregiver interactions through kangaroo care and skin to skin contact (**Figure 131-1**). Breastfeeding is safe and recommended for mothers who are stable in their treatment and without recurrence of substance use, and methadone and buprenorphine are found in low levels in human milk. Breastfeeding is also associated with reduced maternal stress, increased confidence and bonding, decreased risk of NOWS, and need for pharmacologic treatment. If newborns are not able to receive breastmilk, higher calorie formula, which has been associated with a shorter length of hospital stay, can be considered. Gavage feeding may be required in those with poor or uncoordinated feeding skills. Mothers and caregiver presence and rooming-in with their newborn have been shown to decrease the need for pharmacologic therapy and severity of withdrawal. Nonpharmacologic care should be individualized and tailored to the signs the symptoms the infant is exhibiting as well as support the needs of the caregiver.

PHARMACOLOGIC TREATMENT

For infants with severe NOWS symptoms not able to be controlled through supportive therapy, the use of medication in addition to continued nonpharmacologic interventions may be necessary (Figure 131-1). Opioids should be used as the first-line agent for treatment. Morphine is the most widely used medication and is prescribed every 3 to 4 hours or as needed for symptoms. Longer-acting opioids including methadone and buprenorphine are also used and have the benefit of less frequent dosing with some studies reporting shorter lengths of stay and opioid treatment days. If infants continue to experience significant symptoms of withdrawal despite maximized opioid dosing or if there is polysubstance exposure, adjunct therapy is often utilized. Phenobarbital, a nonspecific central nervous system depressant, is commonly given but has been associated with adverse developmental outcomes. Clonidine is a centrally acting α-2-adrenergic receptor agonist with a more specific mechanism for treating opioid withdrawal and has been used in combination with opioids with some success. Adjunct therapy is added with the goal of weaning the primary opioid. Clonidine is typically weaned during the hospitalization; however, phenobarbital can be continued and weaned after hospital discharge. Regardless of the primary opioid and adjunct therapy used, a standard treatment and weaning protocol can reduce length of hospital stay and outcomes.

ADMISSION AND DISCHARGE CRITERIA

ADMISSION CRITERIA

All newborns chronically exposed to opioids in utero should be monitored for signs and symptoms of NOWS in the hospital for a minimum of 72 hours or longer depending on the category of opioid exposure. Infants without known prenatal opioid exposure exhibiting clinical signs consistent with NOWS should also be monitored while a thorough evaluation for the cause of their symptoms is performed. If infants experience severe withdrawal requiring pharmacologic intervention, consideration should be given regarding the safest location for provision of medication therapy and the ability to be monitored for possible side effects which could include a Neonatal Intensive Care Unit, Special Care Nursery, or pediatric inpatient floor.

DISCHARGE CRITERIA

Newborns with NOWS are generally considered safe for discharge when they are without withdrawal symptoms that prevent them from adequately growing and thriving. In general, they should demonstrate ability to adequately eat with appropriate weight loss or weight gain for age, sleep well, and have NOWS symptoms that are manageable by a caregiver. If they received pharmacologic treatment for NOWS, they should have stable or improving symptoms of withdrawal without opioid therapy for a minimum of 48 hours. For those who required adjunct therapy that will be weaned as an outpatient, caregivers should demonstrate ability to administer this medication. In addition to normal newborn anticipatory guidance, caregivers of infants with NOWS should be educated on ongoing symptoms of NOWS, ways to support the infant through challenging times of irritability, sleeping, or feeding, and knowledge of when to seek care if signs of withdrawal are unmanageable or worsening.

READMISSION CONSIDERATIONS

It is possible for infants to experience worsening symptoms of withdrawal beyond the initial monitoring and treatment period during

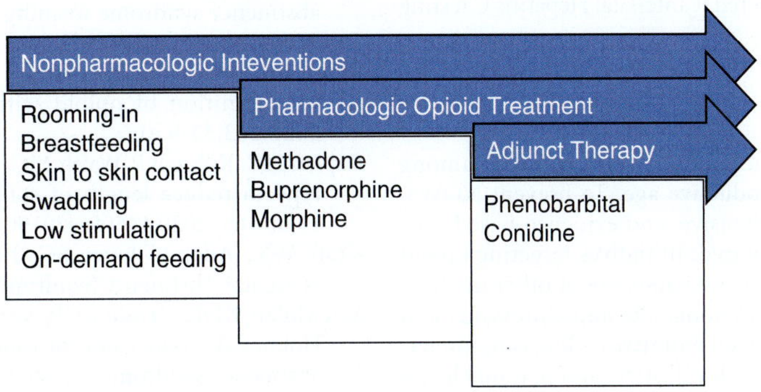

FIGURE 131-1. Treatment management for NOWS. Nonpharmacologic interventions should be initiated after birth and maintained through hospitalization. If required, primary pharmacologic management should be with a primary opioid and adjunct medications may be added.

birth hospitalization after they are discharged home. If severe withdrawal symptoms are present that are not able to be handled at home or infants have failure to thrive, further evaluation and treatment including hospitalization should be considered as infants with NOWS are at higher risk for hospital readmission compared to healthy term infants.

CONSULTATION

Support for the maternal and infant dyad affected by prenatal opioid exposure should be multidisciplinary including neonatal, pediatric and OB providers, nurses, social workers, and case managers. Consultation with occupational or physical therapists can support the sensory and neuromotor difficulties infants with NOWS may experience during hospitalization. The immediate postpartum period is a time of high risk for maternal relapse and overdose death. Referrals should be provided as needed to postpartum psychiatry or behavioral health services, OUD treatment and relapse-prevention programs, child welfare services, and harm reduction services (e.g., naloxone training). In addition to the healthcare team, other community members can be enlisted to serve as a trusted, consistent and non-judgmental support during the hospitalization; examples may include a peer support (another mother with OUD), an OUD program caseworker, or a doula. Plans of Safe Care should be developed to ensure wrap-around support services for all mothers with OUD and their newborns, as these often face economic and social hardships.

SPECIAL CONSIDERATIONS

Mothers with OUD face issues of stigma and criminality related to their substance use and often experience guilt, shame, and fear regarding their newborns with NOWS. Efforts should be made to provide nonjudgmental, trauma informed care to increase maternal confidence, develop rapport, and engage families in the care of their infants. The use of medically accurate, person-first, and non-stigmatizing terminology should be used in interactions with patients and families. Specifically, infants who experience neonatal withdrawal are not "born addicted," as infants cannot exhibit maladaptive behaviors associated with physiologic dependence to a substance, and use of this language is highly stigmatizing. Keeping families intact improves outcomes for parents and infants and should be prioritized if there are no concerns for child safety.

Follow-up care with a primary care physician knowledgeable about long-term considerations regarding potential adverse neurodevelopmental outcomes, behavior problems, and ophthalmologic issues specific to this population is important. Additionally, infants with NOWS should be referred to their local Early Intervention programs as these children often automatically qualify for these in-home developmental services. Finally, given the increased risk of Hepatitis C and HIV associated with OUD, subsequent testing for infectious diseases in infants with NOWS should be coordinated as appropriate. Nucleic acid testing at 2–3 months for Hepatitis C should be performed in the case of confirmed perinatal exposure, and considered if antenatal Hepatitis C testing was not done.

PREVENTION

The incidence of NOWS reflects the increase rates of OUD among pregnant people and people of reproductive age. To prevent NOWS, equitable access to effective, comprehensive, and evidence-based substance use treatment programs is required. Initiatives targeting opioid overprescribing practices as well as the judicious use of other medications that may exacerbate NOWS symptoms like antidepressants and benzodiazepines are also beneficial. Collaboratives addressing prenatal, hospital, and follow-up practices at local, state, and national levels have been shown to improve outcomes of infants with prenatal opioid exposure and should be continued to advance the health of this population.

KEY POINTS

- Rates of NOWS have increased over the last several decades as a consequence of the opioid epidemic.
- Hospitals should develop standardized protocols that address identification, assessment, and treatment for infants with NOWS.
- Nonpharmacologic, caregiver-based interventions should be emphasized, and if required, pharmacologic treatment should consist of a primary opioid agent.
- Care for infants affected by NOWS should be provided through nonjudgmental and trauma informed approaches to help engage families and build trust.
- A multidisciplinary team is important in addressing and supporting the physical, social, and emotional needs of the mother infant dyad.
- Plans of safe care should be developed to promote ongoing support for infants with NOWS.
- Infants with NOWS may be at risk for ongoing medical and developmental problems and should receive specific follow up screening targeted at these issues.

SUGGESTED READINGS

ACOG Committee on Obstetric Practice; American Society of Addiction Medicine. ACOG Committee Opinion No 711: opioid use and opioid use disorder in pregnancy. *Obstet Gynecol.* 2017;130: e81-e94.

Alinsky RH, Hadland SE, Quigley J, Patrick SW; Committee on Substance Use and Prevention. Recommended terminology for substance use disorders in the care of children, adolescents, young adults, and families. *Pediatrics.* 2022;149(6):e2022057529.

Bogen DL, Whalen BL, Kair LR, Vining M, King BA. Wide variation found in care of opioid-exposed newborns. *Acad Pediatr.* 2017;17:374-380.

Colby JM, Adams BC, Morad A, Presley LD, Patrick SW. Umbilical cord tissue and meconium may not be equivalent for confirming in utero substance exposure. *J Pediatr.* 2019;205:277-280.

Davis JM, Shenberger J, Terrin N, et al. Comparison of safety and efficacy of methadone vs morphine for treatment of neonatal abstinence syndrome: a randomized clinical trial. *JAMA Pediatr.* 2018;172:741-748.

Finnegan LP, Connaughton JF Jr, Kron RE, Emich JP. Neonatal abstinence syndrome: assessment and management. *Addict Dis.* 1975;2:141-158.

Goyal NK, McAllister J. Hospital care of opioid-exposed newborns: clinical and psychosocial challenges. *J Hosp Med.* 2020;15(10): 613-618.

Hall ES, Wexelblatt SL, Crowley M, et al. Implementation of a neonatal abstinence syndrome weaning protocol: a multicenter cohort study. *Pediatrics.* 2015;136:e803-10.

Jilani SM, Jones HE, Grossman M, et al. Standardizing the clinical definition of opioid withdrawal in the neonate. *J Pediatr.* 2022;243:33-9 e1.

Kaplan HC, Kuhnell P, Walsh MC, et al. Orchestrated testing of formula type to reduce length of stay in neonatal abstinence syndrome. *Pediatrics.* 2020;146(4):e20190914.

Kraft WK, Adeniyi-Jones SC, Ehrlich ME. Buprenorphine for the Neonatal Abstinence Syndrome. *N Engl J Med.* 2017;377:997-998.

MacMillan KDL, Rendon CP, Verma K, Riblet N, Washer DB, Volpe Holmes A. Association of rooming-in with outcomes for neonatal abstinence syndrome: a systematic review and meta-analysis. *JAMA Pediatr.* 2018;172:345-351.

Patrick SW, Barfield WD, Poindexter BB; Committee on Fetus and Newborn, Committee on Substance Use and Prevention. Neonatal opioid withdrawal syndrome. *Pediatrics.* 2020;146(5):e2020029074.

Reece-Stremtan S, Marinelli KA. ABM clinical protocol #21: guidelines for breastfeeding and substance use or substance use disorder, revised 2015. *Breastfeed Med.* 2015;10:135-141.

Schiff DM, Grossman MR. Beyond the Finnegan scoring system: novel assessment and diagnostic techniques for the opioid-exposed infant. *Semin Fetal Neonatal Med.* 2019; 24:115-120.

Young LW, Ounpraseuth ST, Merhar SL, et al. Eat, sleep, console approach or usual care for neonatal opioid withdrawal. *N Engl J Med.* 2023 Jun 22; 388(25):2326-2337.

van Hoogdalem MW, Wexelblatt SL, Akinbi HT, Vinks AA, Mizuno T. A review of pregnancy-induced changes in opioid pharmacokinetics, placental transfer, and fetal exposure: towards fetomaternal physiologically-based pharmacokinetic modeling to improve the treatment of neonatal opioid withdrawal syndrome. *Pharmacol Ther.* 2022;234:108045.

SECTION N
ONCOLOGY

CHAPTER 132 Childhood Cancer

Marni Shear, DO

BACKGROUND

Childhood cancer is rare, with nearly 16,000 new cases diagnosed each year in the United States. Nonetheless, cancer is the leading cause of disease-related mortality in children younger than 20 years of age. Pediatricians and general practitioners commonly encounter children with symptoms that could signal an undiagnosed cancer. The challenge is to identify those children who warrant an evaluation for malignancy. This chapter reviews the typical presentations of the most common pediatric hematologic malignancies and solid tumors and provides guidelines for the initial diagnostic evaluation. A review of current therapies and expected outcomes is beyond the scope of this chapter. However, it can be broadly stated that most children diagnosed with cancer can be cured of their disease with currently available treatment.

Cancer results from the uncontrolled proliferation of a clonal cell population, and can arise in essentially any cell type or organ. In general, children with cancer present with symptoms related to the location and extent of the tumor. Cancers cause symptoms by invading or obstructing tissues locally or by spreading to distant sites, leading to pain, organ dysfunction, or both. During childhood, the incidence of specific malignancies varies dramatically with age. The most common types of cancer in children are hematologic malignancies (i.e., leukemias, lymphomas), brain tumors, and extracranial solid tumors, including sarcomas and embryonal tumors.

CAUSES

Because childhood cancer is rare and heterogeneous, the elucidation of its causes is extremely challenging. Certain factors are associated with an increased risk of some types of childhood cancer. For example, in utero exposure to ionizing radiation leads to about a 1.5-fold increased risk of lymphoblastic leukemia. External beam radiation, sometimes used to treat patients with solid tumors, is associated with an increased risk of osteosarcoma within the radiation field. Chemotherapy with alkylating agents or etoposide may also increase risk of future malignancies, including leukemia and myelodysplastic syndrome. Patients with Down syndrome have a 10- to 20-fold increased risk of developing leukemia. Several other genetic syndromes are also associated with an increased risk of developing cancer, including neurofibromatosis, Beckwith-Wiedemann syndrome, and Li-Fraumeni syndrome (**Table 132-1**). However, in the vast majority of children with cancer, no predisposing factors are identified.

INCIDENCE

The incidence of childhood cancer is highest in the first year of life, declines until about age 9 years, and then gradually increases into adulthood. The peak rates of specific childhood malignancies occur at different ages. In a child with suspected cancer, the age at presentation has a major impact on the differential diagnosis.

Leukemia accounts for approximately one-third of cancers diagnosed in childhood. In contrast to adults, acute lymphoblastic leukemia (ALL) occurs relatively more commonly than acute myeloid leukemia (AML). ALL is the most common specific childhood malignancy, representing approximately 28% of cancers diagnosed in children younger than 15 years. The peak age at diagnosis of childhood ALL is 2 to 3 years. White children are about two times more likely than Black children to be diagnosed with ALL, with the highest incidence noted in Hispanic populations, and boys are affected slightly more commonly than girls. Precursor B-cell ALL accounts for the majority of cases of ALL. In contrast, the incidence of AML peaks in the first year of life, subsequently decreases, and then gradually increases late in childhood and throughout adulthood. Chronic leukemias are distinctly uncommon in childhood. Chronic myeloid leukemia accounts for only about 3% to 5% of childhood leukemia cases, and chronic lymphoid leukemia does not typically occur in children. Non-Hodgkin lymphoma (NHL) accounts for 6% of cancers diagnosed in children, and Hodgkin lymphoma accounts for about 3%.

Brain tumors are a diverse group of malignant neoplasms that, taken together, account for approximately 30% of childhood cancers. Among pediatric solid tumors that originate outside the central nervous system, neuroblastoma is the most common, representing 6% of childhood cancers, primarily affecting children younger than 5 years. Wilms tumor accounts for 6% of childhood cancers and also occurs primarily in those younger than 5 years. The bone sarcomas, including osteosarcoma and Ewing sarcoma, together represent 4% of childhood cancers. These tumors generally affect older children, with the highest incidence in adolescence and young adulthood.

HEMATOLOGIC MALIGNANCIES

LEUKEMIA

Clinical Presentation and Differential Diagnosis ALL arises as a consequence of malignant transformation of lymphocyte precursors in the bone marrow or lymphoid organs. AML is an analogous process

TABLE 132-1 Common Childhood Genetic Syndromes and Associated Malignancies

Genetic Syndrome	Associated Malignancy
Trisomy 21 (Down syndrome)	ALL, AML
Ataxia-telangiectasia	ALL, lymphoma
Familial monosomy 7	AML
Neurofibromatosis type 1	ALL, AML, optic glioma, rhabdomyosarcoma
Tuberous sclerosis	Brain tumors
Beckwith-Wiedemann syndrome	Wilms tumor, hepatoblastoma
Li-Fraumeni syndrome	Osteosarcoma, soft tissue sarcoma, brain tumor, adrenocortical carcinoma, ALL, AML
Nevoid basal cell carcinoma syndrome	Basal cell carcinoma, medulloblastoma, rhabdomyosarcoma

ALL, acute lymphoblastic leukemia; AML, acute myeloid leukemia.

TABLE 132-2 Differential Diagnosis of Childhood Transient Abnormal Myelopoiesis of Down Syndrome

Noncancer diagnoses
Infectious mononucleosis
Juvenile idiopathic arthritis
Systemic lupus erythematosus
Pertussis
Immune thrombocytopenic purpura
Aplastic anemia
Malignant diagnoses*
Neuroblastoma
Retinoblastoma
Rhabdomyosarcoma
Ewing sarcoma

*With small, round, blue cell morphology similar to acute lymphoblastic leukemia.

involving malignant transformation of myeloid progenitors. The presentation of new-onset leukemia may be dramatic, insidious, or rarely, even asymptomatic, with an incidental finding of leukemia blasts on peripheral blood smear. Often, the differential diagnosis includes benign conditions, such as acute viral infection (e.g., Epstein-Barr virus), aplastic anemia, hemophagocytic syndrome, and other rare congenital disorders (**Table 132-2**).

Children with new-onset acute leukemia usually present with symptoms caused by the impaired production of normal blood cells, owing to the proliferation of leukemia cells in the bone marrow. Fatigue, pallor, weight loss, and fever are common presenting symptoms. Decreased numbers of normal white blood cells lead to an increased risk of serious infection. Bruising and petechiae may be present due to thrombocytopenia. Concomitant coagulopathy may magnify the risk of serious bleeding, especially in certain leukemia subtypes, though serious bleeding as a presenting symptom is rare. Patients may complain of bone pain, back pain, or present with limp or refusal to walk related to bone marrow infiltration and expansion. Leukemia cells may infiltrate organs such as the lymph nodes, liver, or spleen, resulting in lymphadenopathy or hepatosplenomegaly. Leukemia cells may form solid masses, such as in the anterior mediastinum, leading to tracheal or vascular compression. Uncommonly, new-onset leukemia involves the central nervous system, testes, skin, gingivae, and eyes. CNS disease is higher risk in T-cell ALL, and may present as headache, seizure, visual changes, altered mental status, or cranial nerve deficits. Children with very large numbers of circulating malignant cells (white blood cell counts >100,000/μL) may experience symptoms of hyperleukocytosis with ocular, neurologic, or respiratory symptoms (see Chapter 133). Hyperleukocytosis occurs in patients with AML at relatively lower white blood cell counts than in ALL given the larger MCV of AML blasts.

Diagnostic Evaluation and Management When leukemia is suspected, immediate evaluation is warranted, beginning with a complete blood count. The white blood cell count may be low, normal, or elevated. Leukemia blasts may be seen in the peripheral blood smear. Anemia with reticulocytopenia and thrombocytopenia are usually present but of variable severity. When leukemia is strongly suspected, it is important to assess renal function and serum electrolytes, including calcium, phosphate, and uric acid. Patients with a large, rapidly proliferating leukemia burden may present with features of acute tumor lysis syndrome (see Chapter 133) even before the initiation of cytotoxic therapy. Marked elevation of lactate dehydrogenase may also be present. Liver function tests should also be performed because leukemic infiltration of the liver has been described, leading to coagulation abnormalities and hyperbilirubinemia. Coagulation studies should be obtained, and coagulation abnormalities should be corrected before high-risk invasive procedures are attempted, including lumbar puncture and central line placement. Blood cultures should be obtained from patients presenting with fever, and empiric antibiotics should be strongly considered, especially if the neutrophil count is low. A blood

TABLE 132-3 Initial Diagnostic Evaluation when Leukemia is Suspected

Study	Common Findings/Considerations
Complete blood count with differential	• Involvement of more than 1 cell line should raise suspicion for leukemia
White blood cell (WBC) count	◦ Elevated, but may also be low or normal; neutropenia is common; hyperleukocytosis commonly defined as WBC count >100k cell/mm^3
Hemoglobin	◦ Often low
Platelets	◦ Often low
Reticulocyte Count	• Usually low
Peripheral blood smear	• Blasts may be evident
Basic Metabolic Panel	
Potassium	◦ Elevated in tumor lysis syndrome
Calcium	◦ Low in tumor lysis syndrome secondary to precipitation of calcium phosphate in the microvasculature; elevation may suggest paraneoplastic syndrome
Creatinine	◦ Elevated in tumor lysis syndrome secondary to precipitation of uric acid and calcium phosphate crystals in the kidneys
Phosphate	• Elevated in tumor lysis syndrome
Uric Acid	• Elevated in tumor lysis syndrome
Lactate dehydrogenase	• Usually elevated at presentation
Hepatic Panel	
AST ALT	◦ Often normal, may be elevated; liver involvement is rarely attributable to leukemic infiltrate; consider possibility of infectious etiology, drug toxicity
Albumin	◦ Commonly low, but may be normal or elevated if dehydrated at presentation
PT/INR PTT	◦ Often normal, rarely elevated; if abnormal, coagulation abnormalities should be corrected before high-risk invasive procedures
Total bilirubin Direct bilirubin	◦ Jaundice is a rare presenting symptom of ALL; when present, most often conjugated secondary to leukemic infiltration of liver
Blood culture	Obtain if febrile at presentation
Urine culture	Obtain without catherization if febrile at presentation
Type and screen	Send in anticipation of possible transfusion needs
Chest radiograph	Screening for mediastinal mass

sample should be sent to the blood bank in preparation for red blood cell or platelet transfusion. A screening chest radiograph is also recommended. Intravenous access should be established and the patient should be hospitalized for completion of the diagnostic evaluation and initiation of therapy (**Table 132-3**).

Further diagnostic workup should then be performed under the direction of a hematologist/oncologist. Expert evaluation of the peripheral blood smear is often informative. When circulating blasts are present, flow cytometry of peripheral blood may establish the diagnosis. A bone marrow aspirate is needed to analyze morphology, and perform flow cytometry, cytogenetic studies, and molecular analysis. These studies have become increasingly important for risk stratification in patients with ALL and AML. In most cases, assessment of the cerebrospinal fluid by lumbar puncture is performed to document the presence or absence of leukemic involvement. At the time of the initial staging lumbar puncture, chemotherapy should be instilled directly into the spinal fluid. Diagnostic lumbar puncture without intrathecal chemotherapy is strongly discouraged.

NON-HODGKIN LYMPHOMA

Clinical Presentation and Differential Diagnosis Several different subtypes of Non-Hodgkin Lymphoma (NHL) occur in childhood, the most frequently encountered types demonstrating high-grade histology and aggressive behavior. Lymphoblastic lymphoma is a malignant

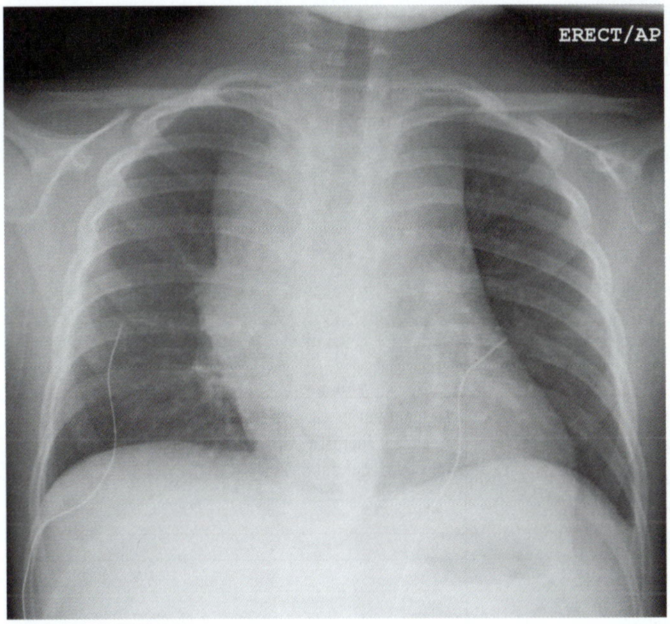

FIGURE 132-1. Chest X-ray demonstrating a mediastinal mass in a patient with lymphoblastic lymphoma.

lymphoma that is indistinguishable from ALL except that the extent of bone marrow involvement is, by definition, less than 25%. Most cases of lymphoblastic lymphoma are of precursor T-cell origin. Children with lymphoblastic lymphoma often present with an anterior mediastinal mass (**Figure 132-1**). Compression of the airway or vascular structures at or below the thoracic inlet can lead to dyspnea, stridor, dysphagia, orthopnea, or superior vena cava (SVC) syndrome. Patients may present with other manifestations of mass effect such as spinal cord compression, hepatosplenomegaly, testicular mass, or localized or diffuse lymphadenopathy. Diagnosis is made by means of biopsy of involved tissue. When a mass is present in the anterior mediastinum, biopsy requires extreme caution owing to the high risk of anesthesia in the setting of tracheal compression.

Burkitt lymphoma is a high-grade malignancy of mature B-cell origin. In the United States, the disease occurs in a sporadic form, with the majority of tumors presenting in the abdomen. Bone marrow or central nervous system involvement is relatively uncommon and is associated with a less favorable prognosis. Because of the extremely rapid growth rate of this tumor, patients are at high risk for the development of hyperuricemia and acute tumor lysis syndrome at presentation and after initiation of treatment. Patients with abdominal masses may present with symptoms that range from abdominal pain to intussusception, intestinal obstruction, or intestinal perforation.

Large-cell lymphomas may be of B-cell, T-cell, or null-cell origin. These tumors arise most commonly in the lymph nodes of the mediastinum and abdomen but may arise in or spread to skin, bone, and soft tissues.

Diagnostic Evaluation and Management The same laboratory assessment described above for leukemia, including measurement of electrolytes, creatinine, and uric acid, is recommended for all patients with suspected or confirmed NHL. Diagnosis depends on histopathologic examination of tumor tissue. Sufficient biopsy material should be obtained so that specialized flow cytometric and molecular studies can be performed. These studies may demonstrate specific molecular characteristics that define certain tumor types, such as rearrangement of the *MYC* oncogene in Burkitt lymphoma. Computed tomography (CT) of the chest, abdomen, and pelvis, fluorodeoxyglucose positron emission tomography (FDG-PET) scan and examination of the bone marrow and cerebrospinal fluid are usually performed to determine the stage of the disease. Because systemic therapy with chemotherapy and sometimes immunotherapy is necessary in nearly all cases of lymphoma, attempt at complete surgical resection is only warranted in some cases of localized disease.

HODGKIN LYMPHOMA

Clinical Presentation and Differential Diagnosis Hodgkin lymphoma is a relatively indolent malignancy that most commonly arises in the neck and is characterized by slowly progressive nodal enlargement and spread of tumor to contiguous lymph node groups over time. Involved lymph nodes are usually nontender and may have a firm, rubbery, or matted texture on physical examination. At initial presentation, the differential includes bacterial lymphadenitis, typical and atypical mycobacterial infections, EBV, bartonella, and other infectious and non-infectious etiologies that cause reactive hyperplasia of lymph nodes. Mediastinal involvement is common and may be demonstrated on chest radiographs. Uncommonly, bulky tumors in the mediastinum may be associated with vascular compression and symptoms of superior vena cava syndrome. Widespread nodal involvement, as well as extranodal spread of tumor to the liver, lung, cortical bone, and bone marrow, occurs in advanced stages of the disease. Some patients, especially those with extensive disease, may experience systemic symptoms, termed "B" symptoms, such as fevers, night sweats, and weight loss. For unclear reasons, some patients present with generalized pruritus. Nonspecific markers of inflammation, including the erythrocyte sedimentation rate and C-reactive protein, are often elevated at diagnosis, and current studies are exploring the prognostic utility of CRP in early stage disease.

Diagnostic Evaluation and Management Under most circumstances, the diagnostic evaluation of a patient with suspected Hodgkin lymphoma may be safely completed in the outpatient setting once respiratory insufficiency, hemodynamic instability, and metabolic derangement have been ruled out. Many children are referred for excisional node biopsy after a course of oral antibiotics for presumed lymphadenitis is ineffective. Once the diagnosis of Hodgkin lymphoma is established by biopsy of involved tissue, a staging evaluation is performed under the direction of the treating oncologist. Radiographic studies, including CT scan of the neck through pelvis and FDG-PET scan are usually obtained. Bone marrow aspiration/biopsy for staging is reserved for patients with B symptoms or advanced-stage disease.

SOLID TUMORS

BRAIN TUMORS

Central nervous system tumors are a diverse group of neoplasms that occur in the brain, brainstem, spinal cord, or ependymal lining of the ventricles. They are the second most common malignancy in the pediatric age group, after leukemia, and the number one cause of mortality secondary to cancer. Most brain tumors in children are primary tumors, whereas brain metastases of extra-axial tumors occur more commonly in adults. Pediatric brain tumors can be broadly classified as tumors of glial origin and those of primitive neuroectodermal cell origin. Tumors of glial origin can arise anywhere within the craniospinal axis and are of variable grade. Specific diagnoses in this group range from low-grade astrocytomas to high-grade glioblastoma multiforme and ependymoma. The neuroectodermal tumors presumably arise from primitive undifferentiated cells in the central nervous system. Tumors with this histology that arise in the cerebellum are called medulloblastomas.

Clinical Presentation and Differential Diagnosis Depending on their location, pediatric brain tumors come to medical attention because of signs and symptoms of increased intracranial pressure or because of the development of focal neurologic signs. Infratentorial tumors account for more than half of all pediatric brain tumors. Commonly, infratentorial tumors obstruct the flow of cerebrospinal fluid, leading to headache and vomiting (characteristically without nausea, especially in the morning). As symptoms of elevated intracranial pressure progress, patients may experience severe headache, intractable emesis, visual disturbances, abnormal eye movements, and eventually altered mental status. Infants may demonstrate bulging of the anterior fontanelle. Children with cerebellar tumors may demonstrate nystagmus and ataxia. Supratentorial tumors sometimes cause symptoms of

TABLE 132-4 Tumors Affecting the Central Nervous System

Location	Specific Tumor Types	Presenting Signs and Symptoms	Comments
Supratentorial hemispheric	Low-grade gliomas • Pilocytic • Fibrillary High-grade glioma Mixed neuronal-glial • Neoplasms • Ganglioglioma Ependymoma Choroid plexus tumors Primitive Neuroectodermal Tumor	Varies with site • Hemiparesis • Hemisensory deficits • Seizure • Hemianopsia	Mainstay of treatment is gross total resection, with adjuvant chemotherapy and/or radiation indicated in some types of cancer
Supratentorial midline	Chiasmatic/hypothalamic glioma Craniopharyngioma Germinoma/malignant germ cell tumors Pineoblastoma Primitive neuroectodermal tumor	Vision deficits Diencephalic syndrome Neuroendocrine symptoms Hydrocephalus Parinaud syndrome	Location and appearance on imaging guides diagnostic and treatment approach, with biopsy sometimes indicated to maximize adjuvant therapy
Infratentorial	Medulloblastoma Cerebellar astrocytoma Ependymoma Diffuse malignant brainstem glioma Benign focal brainstem glioma	Cranial nerve palsies Cerebellar signs • Ataxia • Dysmetria Brainstem signs • Weakness • Unsteady gait Increased intracranial pressure	

increased intracranial pressure but more commonly come to medical attention because of focal seizures, hemiparesis, or visual changes. Vague personality changes, ranging from lethargy to irritability, may be noted (**Table 132-4**).

For the general practitioner, a broad differential should be considered when evaluating neurologic symptoms. Patients who present with headache and emesis may have an infectious condition, such as a viral gastroenteritis or viral meningitis. They may also have a more serious infection, such as encephalitis or bacterial meningitis. Focal neurologic deficits or extremity weakness may occur with a wide range of diagnoses, as well, from seizure disorder to stroke to subacute combined degeneration of the spinal cord.

Diagnostic Evaluation and Management Imaging of the brain is usually the first step in the evaluation of a patient with a suspected brain tumor. A CT scan may be obtained emergently to look for a mass or associated findings such as hydrocephalus or cerebral edema. However, magnetic resonance imaging (MRI) is the preferred study for the diagnosis and follow-up of pediatric brain tumors because it is more sensitive than CT and does not expose the child to ionizing radiation. In the setting of increased intracranial pressure, lumbar puncture should not be performed because it may precipitate fatal herniation of the cerebellar tonsils.

When a brain tumor is suspected, the patient should be urgently referred to a pediatric neurosurgeon, preferably one who collaborates with an experienced multidisciplinary team that includes a pediatric oncologist, neurologist, and radiation oncologist. Depending on the size, appearance, and location of the tumor, biopsy, subtotal resection, or complete resection may be undertaken. Sometimes biopsy is not recommended because the radiographic appearance of the tumor is characteristic or because its location makes biopsy extremely risky. Patients with optic pathway gliomas (especially those known to have neurofibromatosis) and diffuse intrinsic pontine gliomas are usually not subjected to biopsy. Beyond surgery, therapeutic options for many types of brain tumors include chemotherapy, radiation, or both, depending on the tumor grade and histology. With advances in the molecular profiling of pediatric tumors, immunotherapy is also emerging as a promising treatment option, including adoptive cellular therapies, checkpoint blockade, vaccines, and viral therapies. Alternatively, some low-grade tumors may not require therapy if they are not causing symptoms and are stable in size.

EXTRACRANIAL SOLID TUMORS

Clinical Presentation and Differential Diagnosis Children with solid tumors may present with a range of signs and symptoms, depending on the size, location, and site of origin of the tumor. In children, malignant solid tumors most often arise in the abdomen, and less commonly in the thorax, extremities, and head and neck. In adolescents, extracranial germ cell tumors account for the majority of extracranial malignant solid tumors, followed by bone and soft tissue sarcomas, thyroid cancer, and melanoma.

Abdominal tumors come to medical attention because of abdominal pain, distention, vomiting, or change in bowel or bladder habits. An abdominal mass may be detected incidentally during routine child care or may come to medical attention when an individual without daily contact with the child notices abdominal distention. Abdominal masses may be difficult to palpate, especially in toddlers. Because most abdominal masses in children represent malignant disease, expedited evaluation is warranted. In most cases, abdominal ultrasonography is the first study performed to confirm the presence of the mass and to begin to formulate a differential diagnosis. Masses should not be palpated deeply, as a Wilm's tumors can rupture and result in upstage of disease. Once a mass is confirmed, the child should be referred to a pediatric oncologist or pediatric surgeon for further evaluation (**Table 132-5**).

Thoracic tumors can emanate from the chest wall or originate in any compartment of the mediastinum. Patients may complain of pain or show signs of respiratory compromise with coughing, stridor, wheezing, shortness of breath, or SVC syndrome. Apical lung or mediastinal tumors may lead to Horner syndrome (unilateral ptosis, miosis, and anhidrosis). A chest radiograph is the initial study of choice.

Extremity tumors are usually accompanied by pain. Soft tissue swelling with or without a palpable mass may be present. A history of trauma

TABLE 132-5 Benign and Malignant Abdominal/Pelvic Masses

Location	Benign	Malignant
Hepatic	Adenoma Hemangioma Storage disease Hamartoma Infectious	Hepatoblastoma Hepatocellular carcinoma Sarcoma Metastatic disease Leukemia
Kidney/Adrenal	Hydronephrosis Cysts Renal vein thrombosis Adrenal hemorrhage	Wilms tumor Renal cell carcinoma Rhabdoid tumor Neuroblastoma Pheochromocytoma
Gastrointestinal	Torsion/duplication Feces (constipation) Hernia Abscess Appendicitis	Gastrointestinal stromal tumor Lymphoma
Pancreas	Trauma Pseudocyst	Pancreaticoblastoma
Ovary	Torsion Cyst Mature teratoma	Lymphoma Germ cell tumor Sex cord/stromal tumor Carcinoma Immature teratoma
Bladder/Prostate	Duplication Cyst	Rhabdomyosarcoma

or athletic injury to the extremity is frequently reported. Again, plain films are obtained initially. Additional studies such as ultrasonography, CT, or MRI can help narrow the differential diagnosis and direct further diagnostic evaluation.

NEUROBLASTOMA

Clinical Presentation and Differential Diagnosis Neuroblastoma is the most common extracranial solid tumor in children and the most common cancer in children under one year of age. It is a diverse disease, ranging from a localized tumor with benign behavior to disseminated disease with extremely aggressive features. Neuroblastoma arises from primitive neural crest elements that make up the sympathetic ganglia and the adrenal medulla and can arise anywhere along the sympathetic nervous system. Most tumors arise in the abdomen, especially in the adrenal gland (**Figure 132-2**), though thoracic tumors also occur. Rarely, neck and brain tumors can occur. Abdominal neuroblastoma often presents with a firm, fixed, and non-tender abdominal mass but may be associated with abdominal pain or constipation. Infants with thoracic tumors may present with incidental findings on chest radiographs or with respiratory distress, wheezing, or facial swelling. Thoracic and retroperitoneal tumors may extend into the spinal canal and lead to spinal cord compression. These children may present with pain, numbness, limb weakness, bowel or bladder changes, or loss of reflexes. This represents a neurosurgical emergency, and diagnostic evaluation and initiation of treatment must be expedited to minimize the risk of irreversible spinal cord injury.

Fifty percent of children with neuroblastoma present with metastatic disease. Neuroblastoma may disseminate to regional distant lymph nodes, cortical bone, bone marrow, liver, or skin (cutaneous involvement is characteristic of infants with metastatic disease). Patients with disseminated disease experience bone pain, irritability, fatigue, pallor, bruising, and fevers. Spread of neuroblastoma to the orbital bones may lead to proptosis and orbital discoloration, a characteristic sign referred to as "raccoon eyes." Infants may also present with respiratory distress that results from hepatomegaly in the setting of metastatic tumor burden, and these patients require prompt admission to an inpatient pediatric setting under the care of a pediatric oncologist.

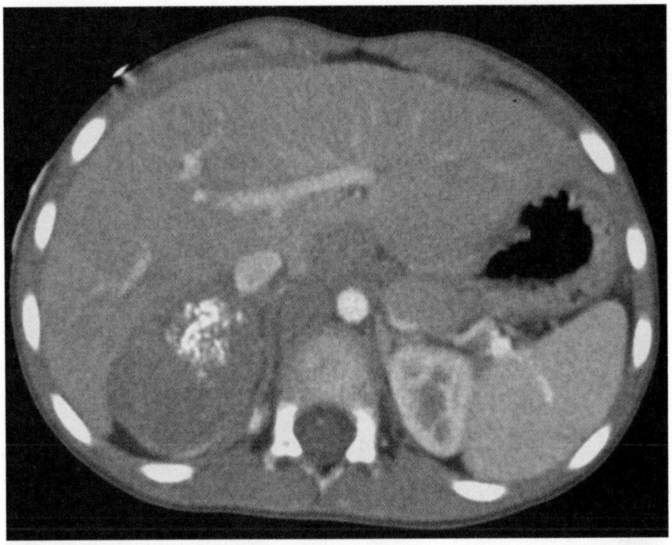

FIGURE 132-2. CT scan of a patient with a retroperitoneal mass demonstrating the typical calcifications seen in neuroblastoma.

Occasionally, neuroblastoma is associated with paraneoplastic syndromes. Secretion of vasoactive intestinal peptide (VIP) and catecholamines by the tumor may lead to secretory diarrhea and hypertension, respectively. Up to 5% of children with neuroblastoma develop opsoclonus-myoclonus syndrome ("dancing eyes, dancing feet") secondary to autoantibodies against neural tissue.

Diagnostic Evaluation and Management Blood tests in children with disseminated neuroblastoma may demonstrate cytopenias as a consequence of bone marrow infiltration. The peripheral blood may show myelophthisic features, including "teardrop" forms. Blood levels of lactate dehydrogenase and ferritin may be elevated. Elevated levels of the catecholamines vanillylmandelic acid and homovanillic acid are detectable in the urine in the majority of cases and support the diagnosis of neuroblastoma. Histopathologic examination of the primary tumor or of a metastatic focus is necessary to establish the diagnosis. When neuroblastoma is suspected, sufficient biopsy tissue should be obtained for analysis of *MYC-N*, ploidy, and cytogenetics, if possible. Evaluation for metastatic disease with CT, bone scan, I-131 metaiodobenzylguanidine (MIBG) imaging, and bone marrow aspirates and biopsies is usually indicated. If there is intraspinal extension of tumor, spinal MRI may be recommended to assess the risk to the spinal cord. Treatment varies significantly based on individual patient risk factors. Some patients require no intervention, while others may undergo surgical resection, chemotherapy, radiation, immunotherapy, or stem cell transplant. Prognosis is extremely variable, with spontaneous regression without intervention in the lowest risk populations to a survival rate of 5% in the highest risk patients.

RENAL TUMORS

Clinical Presentation and Differential Diagnosis The majority of primary renal tumors in children are Wilms tumor; however, several other histologic types do occur. Nearly 10% of Wilms tumors occur in children with congenital anomalies. An asymptomatic abdominal mass or abdominal distention without other symptoms is the most common presenting features. Abdominal pain may result from stretching of the renal capsule. Occasionally, patients come to medical attention because of rapid abdominal enlargement and signs of anemia due to intratumoral hemorrhage or tumor rupture. In extreme cases, sudden hemorrhagic shock can occur. While tumor rupture will upstage the disease, most ruptures do not result in a medical or surgical emergency, but are more often asymptomatic or

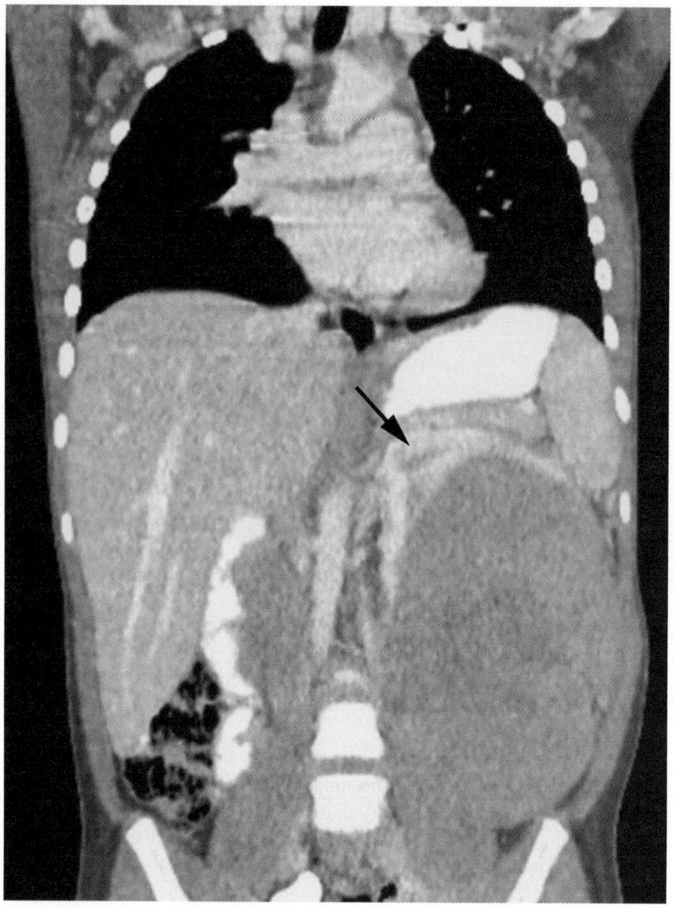

FIGURE 132-3. CT scan of a patient with a Wilms tumor demonstrating the characteristic "claw sign" of preserved renal parenchyma (arrow).

involve self-limited bleeding. As such, children with hemodynamically stable tumor ruptures should be referred to a pediatric oncology center rather than undergoing emergent surgical intervention. Between 1% and 8% of children with Wilms tumors may also develop von Willebrand disease. Gross or microscopic hematuria may be present, and moderate to severe hypertension is commonly seen.

Diagnostic Evaluation and Management Abdominal ultrasonography is useful to confirm the presence of a renal mass and may suggest renal origin of the tumor. CT with contrast may demonstrate the characteristic "claw sign" of preserved renal parenchyma adjacent to the tumor (**Figure 132-3**). The contralateral kidney should also be evaluated, because bilateral tumors do occur, with nearly 5% of children with Wilms tumors presenting bilaterally. Wilms tumor characteristically metastasizes via the renal vein into the inferior vena cava and to the lungs. Doppler ultrasonography of the venous system and a chest radiograph (or chest CT scan) are important for staging the tumor and planning therapy. When feasible, up-front nephrectomy is recommended for unilateral tumors that do not extend into the renal vein. However, in some circumstances preoperative chemotherapy is preferred. Biopsy of a renal mass is not recommended, however, as this may result in upstaging of the tumor. Patients with concern for a renal tumor should instead be referred to a pediatric oncology center. Among children who develop von Willebrand disease in the setting of a Wilms tumor, surgical excision of the tumor will resolve this bleeding disorder.

BONE TUMORS

Clinical Presentation and Differential Diagnosis Osteosarcoma is the most common primary malignant bone tumor in children and adolescents, followed by Ewing sarcoma. Children older than 10 years

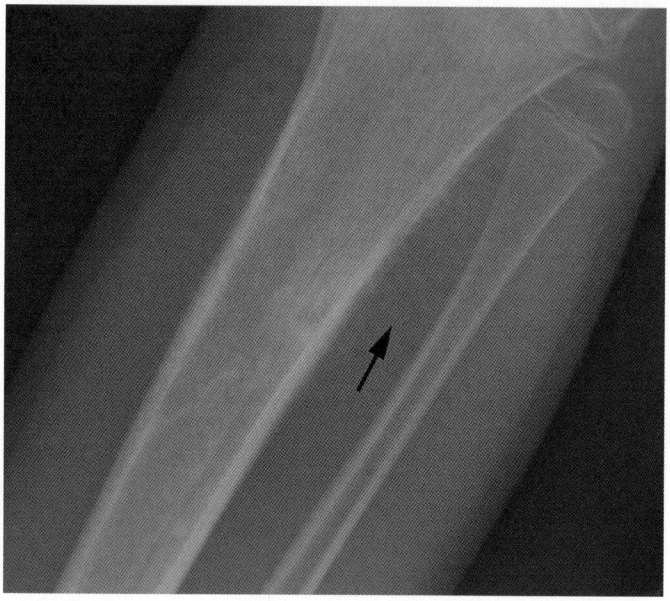

FIGURE 132-4. X-ray of a tibia demonstrating an osteosarcoma with a classic "sunburst" pattern (arrow).

are affected more frequently than are younger children. Both types of tumors can arise in any bone, but osteosarcoma is most likely to occur in the metaphysis of the distal femur or proximal tibia, while Ewing sarcoma is more likely to involve the diaphysis of the long bones, with up to 20% occurring extraosseously in soft tissue. A hallmark of bone malignancy is "deep," persistent, unrelenting pain that occurs at night and is poorly controlled with analgesics. Typically, these tumors grow relatively slowly, and the pain is chronic and progressive. Pain, swelling, and limitation of range of motion associated with the tumor may be attributed to a sports injury or to trauma for some time before medical attention is sought. Pathologic fracture may precipitate the diagnosis. X-ray typically demonstrates a destructive bone lesion (**Figure 132-4**). In patients with disseminated Ewing sarcoma, systemic symptoms such as fever, malaise, and weight loss sometimes occur, however, systemic symptoms are unlikely in osteosarcoma.

Diagnostic Evaluation and Management Plain radiograph remains the most common method for initial diagnosis of bone tumors, with periosteal reaction resulting in the classic sunburst appearance and codman triangle seen in osteosarcoma, and a moth-eaten appearance and onion skin periosteal reaction seen in Ewing sarcoma. Blood work is usually normal in patients with bone tumors, but alkaline phosphatase or lactate dehydrogenase may be elevated in some cases. Metastatic disease to the lungs and other bones may be present at diagnosis or may develop later. Unlike osteosarcoma, Ewing sarcoma may metastasize to the bone marrow, as well. If a primary bone tumor is suspected, referral to an orthopedic surgeon with experience in the surgical management of bone malignancies is strongly encouraged. In most cases, percutaneous biopsy is performed by interventional radiologists to establish the diagnosis. Surgical resection, or in some cases radiation therapy to the primary tumor, is often delayed until a course of systemic chemotherapy has been administered.

OTHER EMBRYONAL TUMORS

A variety of other solid tumors of embryonal origin occur in children, including rhabdomyosarcoma, hepatoblastoma, retinoblastoma, and germ cell tumors. The clinical manifestations correspond to the location and extent of the tumor.

Rhabdomyosarcoma is a soft tissue sarcoma with histologic features of primitive muscle development. It can arise anywhere in the body, but the most common sites are the head and neck, genitourinary tract, and extremities; chest wall tumors also occur. In advanced stages, rhabdomyosarcoma can spread to the lungs, bones, and bone marrow.

Hepatoblastoma is a primary tumor of the liver that occurs almost exclusively in children younger than 3 years. Abdominal distention is the most common presenting symptom. In most cases, serum levels of α-fetoprotein are elevated. Children with a history of low birth weight and those with Beckwith-Wiedemann syndrome are at increased risk for the development of this tumor, but the majority of cases are sporadic.

Retinoblastoma is an uncommon tumor of retinal origin that occurs in young children. Retinoblastoma was the first cancer to be linked to a specific genetic defect—namely, mutation of the *RB* gene on chromosome 13. Individuals with inherited or acquired constitutional mutations involving this genetic locus are at high risk of developing multiple and bilateral tumors. Unilateral (i.e., non-germline) retinoblastoma accounts for about 60% of cases and is associated with a slightly older median age at diagnosis. The most common presenting sign of retinoblastoma is leukocoria, or loss of the normal red retinal reflex. If the tumor is large enough, it may manifest as a painful red eye, decreased vision, strabismus, or proptosis.

Germ cell tumors (GCTs) are a heterogeneous group of malignant tumors of several different histologic types that, taken together, account for only about 1% of cancers in children, but 15% of extracranial solid tumors in adolescence. These tumors develop from primordial germ cells that migrate during embryogenesis from the yolk sac to the gonads. Therefore, these tumors may arise in gonadal or extragonadal (usually midline) sites. A mass in the abdomen or pelvis or in the male testis is the usual presenting complaint. Adolescent boys may be reluctant to complain about painless testicular enlargement, and some patients present with surprisingly large tumors discovered during a thorough physical examination. Ovarian GCTs may present as progressive abdominal distention. Several serum markers may be elevated in patients with germ cell tumors, including α-fetoprotein, β-human chorionic gonadotropin, lactate dehydrogenase, and placental alkaline phosphatase. When serum markers are elevated at diagnosis, they may be useful for following response to therapy and identifying disease recurrence.

SHORT TERM RISK OF CHEMOTHERAPEUTIC AGENTS

In caring for children that are receiving chemotherapeutic agents under the supervision of a pediatric oncologist, it is helpful to be aware of the most common side effects of the agents being used. While induction chemotherapeutic regimens for ALL include drugs that may place patients at risk for peripheral neuropathy, hypertension, hyperglycemia, constipation, poor wound healing, pancreatitis, myelosuppression, cardiomyopathy, thrombosis, and neurotoxicity, interim maintenance regimens may contribute to mucositis or renal insufficiency, in addition to myelosuppression, constipation, peripheral neuropathy, and neurotoxicity. As such, in addition to exploring specific drug side effects for each drug administered by the prescribing oncologist, it is important to ensure close communication around monitoring expectations and discharge criteria for each individual patient. While some patients may be safe to discharge with close outpatient follow-up after completion of an inpatient chemotherapeutic regimen, others may require close inpatient monitoring until cell counts recover to a sufficient level, while offering supportive care through blood product administration.

LONG-TERM SEQUELAE OF ONCOLOGIC TREATMENT

Pediatric cancer patients who receive care in pediatric oncology centers during their initial treatment are often followed by programs dedicated to survivorship. For some children who live far from such centers or lose insurance coverage after recovery from childhood cancer, future hospital admissions may reflect a new point of access to the healthcare system. As such, it is of critical importance to understand the ways in which early exposure to varied treatment modalities in pediatric cancer may place patients at risk for future sequelae, from neurologic toxicity such as peripheral neuropathy to development of secondary malignancies. A history obtained from childhood cancer survivors should include a detailed history of their diagnosis and treatment, including chemotherapeutic agents administered, location and duration of radiation, and duration of steroid use.

Chronic pain, sleep problems, fatigue, post-traumatic stress disorder, anxiety, depression, and suicidal ideation are common among pediatric cancer survivors. Children exposed to chemotherapy may also develop dental problems, including enamel dysplasia, microdontia, dental caries, root agenesis or shortening, or ectopic molar eruption. While long-term cardiotoxicity is low among patients with ALL, patients with AML receive larger doses of anthracyclines, increasing their risk of developing cardiomyopathy or heart failure. For many individuals that receive chemotherapy or radiation in childhood, hypothalamic-pituitary dysfunction may develop, with risk of impaired growth and delayed pubertal development, as well gonadal damage with the risk of fertility challenges, as well as subsequent thyroid dysfunction. An understanding of long-term risk factors for childhood cancer survivors is critical to ensuring patients receive appropriate long-term follow-up well beyond their time of diagnosis.

CONSULTATION, ADMISSION, AND DISCHARGE CRITERIA

- All patients with newly diagnosed leukemia should be admitted to a hospital experienced in the management of children with cancer.
- Patients with a new diagnosis of a solid tumor can be evaluated on an outpatient basis as long as pain is controlled and there is no evidence of superior vena cava syndrome, spinal cord compression, respiratory distress, bleeding, or metabolic derangement.
- The initial management of all childhood cancers is directed by a pediatric hematology-oncology team, with the consultation of other appropriate specialists.
- The primary care provider's support and involvement are needed for the optimal care of the patient and his or her family.
- Multidisciplinary care teams that include physician specialists from multiple subspecialties, nurses, social workers, psychologists, and other ancillary support staff are critical to ensuring the needs of each patient are met.
- Discharge criteria are determined by the type of cancer and by the recommendations of the hematology-oncology team and involved subspecialists.
- Long-term follow-up is extremely important in childhood cancer survivors, given both the risk of chronic sequelae secondary to treatment regimens received, as well as to ensure the unique psychosocial needs of this vulnerable population are appropriately addressed.

SUGGESTED READINGS

Allen-Rhoades W, Whittle, SB, Rainusso N. Pediatric solid tumors in children and adolescents: an overview. *Pediatr Rev.* 2018;39(9):444-453.

American Academy of Pediatrics Section on Hematology/Oncology Children's Oncology Group. Long-term follow-up care for pediatric cancer survivors. *Pediatrics.* 2009;123(3):906-915.

Butler E, Ludwig K, Pacenta HL, et al. Recent progress in the treatment of cancer in children. *CA Cancer J Clin.* 2021;71(4):315-332.

Cairo MS, Pinkerton R. Childhood, adolescent and young adult non-Hodgkin lymphoma: state of the science. *Br J Haematol.* 2016; 173(4):507-530.

Castle JT, Levy BE, Rodeberg DA. Abdominal tumors: wilms, neuroblastoma, rhabdomyosarcoma, and hepatoblastoma. *Surg Clin North Am.* 2022;102(5):715-737.

Corrigan JJ, Feig SA. Guidelines for pediatric cancer centers. *Pediatrics.* 2004;113(6):1833-1835. https://doi.org/10.1542/peds.113.6.1833

Creutzig U, van den Heuvel-Eibrink, MM, Gibson B, et al. Diagnosis and management of acute myeloid leukemia in children and adolescents: recommendations from an international expert panel. *Blood.* 2012;120(16):3187-3205.

Hunger SP, Mullighan CG. Acute lymphoblastic leukemia in children. *N Engl J Med.* 2015;373(16):1541-1552.

Kaplan JA. Leukemia in children. *Pediatr Rev.* 2019;40(7):319-331.

Lee P, Bhansali R, Izraeli S, et al. The biology, pathogenesis and clinical aspects of acute lymphoblastic leukemia in children with Down syndrome. *Leukemia.* 2016;30(9):1816-1823.

Olson TA, Murray MJ, Rodriguez-Galindo C, et al. Pediatric and adolescent extracranial germ cell tumors: the road to collaboration. *J Clin Oncol.* 2015;33(27):3018-3028.

Plant-Fox AS, O'Halloran K, Goldman S. Pediatric brain tumors: the era of molecular diagnostics, targeted and immune-based therapeutics, and a focus on long term neurologic sequelae. *Curr Probl Cancer.* 2021;45(4):100777.

Rao AA, Naheedy JH, Chen JY, et al. A clinical update and radiologic review of pediatric orbital and ocular tumors. *J Oncol.* 2013;2013:975908.

Siegel RL, Miller KD, Fuchs HE, et al. Cancer statistics, 2022. *CA Cancer J Clin.* 2022;72(1):7-33.

Zahnreich S, Schmidberger H. Childhood cancer: occurrence, treatment and risk of second primary malignancies. *Cancers (Basel).* 2021;13(11):2607.

CHAPTER 133

Oncologic Emergencies

Kelsey Johnson, MD

INTRODUCTION

Early recognition, prevention, and treatment of oncological emergencies improve clinical outcomes. Both at initial presentation and during treatment, pediatric cancer patients can develop acute, severe, and life-threatening conditions (**Table 133-1**). This chapter reviews the presentation and management of the most commonly encountered emergent conditions seen in pediatric cancer patients. The pediatric hospitalist should be able to identify at-risk patients, adopt preventive strategies, recognize clinical deterioration, and initiate prompt treatment of these emergencies.

When a new diagnosis of cancer or an oncologic emergency is suspected, a pediatric oncologist should be consulted to aid in the initial diagnostic evaluation and therapeutic management. Pediatric cancer patients benefit from rapid referral to a tertiary care center with a subspecialty pediatric oncology program. Ideal treatment of some oncologic emergencies will involve the initiation of chemotherapy or radiation therapy, which must be done at a facility experienced in the administration of these modalities in children and adolescents.

METABOLIC EMERGENCIES

TUMOR LYSIS SYNDROME

The rapid release of the intracellular contents of tumor cells into the plasma can cause significant metabolic derangements that can progress to multiorgan failure and death. The laboratory abnormalities most often associated with this tumor lysis syndrome (TLS) include hyperuricemia, hyperphosphatemia, hyperkalemia, and hypocalcemia. While there are no strict criteria defining TLS, the Cairo-Bishop definition proposed in 2004 and further modified by Howard et al in 2011 has been widely accepted. This classification system categorizes TLS into "laboratory" and "clinical" entities, the former being defined by simultaneous presence of two or more electrolyte abnormalities within 3 days before or up to 7 days after the initiation of chemotherapy and the latter by "laboratory" TLS plus the presence of at least one of the following clinical features: renal dysfunction, seizures, cardiac dysrhythmia, multiorgan system failure, or death (**Table 133-2**).

TLS is most commonly encountered shortly after initiation of therapy for malignancies with high tumor burden. TLS can also be identified prior to the initiation of therapy, especially in tumors with high cellular proliferation such as acute lymphoblastic leukemia (ALL) or Burkitt lymphoma. TLS prophylaxis recommendations are based on risk stratification. High-risk clinical features include diagnoses of acute myelogenous leukemia (AML), ALL and advanced-stage non-Hodgkin lymphoma (NHL), WBC count greater than 100,000 cells/mm^3, elevated

TABLE 133-1 Pediatric Oncologic Emergencies

Metabolic emergencies
Tumor lysis syndrome
Hyperuricemia
Hyperkalemia
Hyperphosphatemia/hypocalcemia
Syndrome of inappropriate antidiuretic hormone secretion (SIADH)
Hematologic emergencies
Hyperleukocytosis, leukostasis
Hemorrhage and disseminated intravascular coagulation (DIC)
Thrombosis
Infectious and inflammatory emergencies
Febrile neutropenia
Septicemia, shock
Neutropenic enterocolitis
Pancreatitis
Mechanical emergencies
Superior vena cava syndrome, superior mediastinal syndrome
Pleural and pericardial effusions
Cardiac tamponade
Neurologic emergencies
Spinal cord compression
Increased intracranial pressure
Pain
Altered mental status
Malignant hypertension
Seizure

TABLE 133-2 Classification of Laboratory and Clinical Tumor Lysis Syndrome

Laboratory TLS (≥ 2 abnormalities)*
Hyperuricemia: > the upper limits of normal for age
Hyperkalemia: > 6.0 mmol/L
Hyperphosphatemia: >6.5mg/dL (>2.1 mmol/L)
Hypocalcemia: <7.0 mg/dL (< 1.75 mmol/L) corrected calcium *or* <4.5 mg/dL (1.12 mmol/L) ionized calcium
Clinical TLS (≥ 1 abnormality plus laboratory TLS)
Acute Kidney Injury: serum creatinine > 1.5x the ULN for age
Cardiac arrhythmia or sudden death
Seizure
Multiorgan system failure (including neuromuscular instability, heart failure)

*Electrolyte abnormalities must be present in the same 24-hour period and within 3 days before or up to 7 days after initiating chemotherapy.

TLS, tumor lysis syndrome; ULN, upper limit of normal.

Source: Adapted from Howard SC, Jones DP, Pui CH. The tumor lysis syndrome. *N Engl J Med.* 2011;364(19):1844-1854.

TABLE 133-3 TLS: Risk-Stratified Prophylaxis Strategies

	Low Risk*	Intermediate Risk**	High Risk
AML	WBC <25 K *and* LDH <2 X ULN	WBC 25-100 K *or* WBC <25 K *and* LDH ≥2 X ULN	WBC ≥100 K
ALL		WBC <100 K *and* LDH <2 X ULN	WBC ≥100 K *or* LDH >2 X ULN
Hodgkin lymphoma	All stages		
Burkitt lymphoma		Stage I/II *and* LDH <2 X ULN	Stage III/IV *or* LDH ≥2 X ULN
Lymphoblastic lymphoma		Stage I/II *and* LDH <2 X ULN	Stage III/IV *or* LDH ≥2 X ULN
Anaplastic large cell lymphoma	Stage I/II	Stage III/IV	
Other NHL	Stage I/II	Stage III/IV *and* LDH <2 X ULN	Stage III/IV *and* LDH ≥2 X ULN
Solid tumors	Most	Few***	
TLS prophylaxis recommendation			
	Normal hydration +/– Allopurinol	Hyperhydration Allopurinol	Hyperhydration Rasburicase****

ALL, acute lymphoblastic leukemia; AML, acute myeloid leukemia; K, 10^3 cells/mm^3; LDH, lactate dehydrogenase; NHL, non-Hodgkin lymphoma; ST, solid tumors; ULN, upper limit of normal; WBC, white blood cell.

*Patients with lymphoma/leukemia initially stratified with LRD should be upstaged to IR if presenting with renal dysfunction and/or renal involvement.

**Patients initially stratified with IRD should be upstaged to HRD if presenting with renal dysfunction, renal involvement or increased serum uric acid, potassium or phosphate.

***Neuroblastoma, germ cell tumors and others with bulky or advanced stage disease may be classified as IRD.

****Contraindicated in patients with a history consistent with glucose-6 phosphate dehydrogenase deficiency. In these patients, rasburicase should be substituted with allopurinol.

Source: Adapted from Cairo MS, Coiffier B, Reiter A, Younes A. Recommendations for the evaluation of risk and prophylaxis of tumour lysis syndrome (TLS) in adults and children with malignant diseases: an expert TLS panel consensus. *Br J Haematol*. 2010;149(4):578-586.

lactate dehydrogenase (LDH), presence of renal dysfunction, or multiple electrolyte abnormalities (**Table 133-3**). Rapid identification of at-risk patients should expedite the initiation of prophylactic strategies to avoid complications of TLS (**Table 133-4**). TLS management requires close clinical and laboratory monitoring, including aggressive volume repletion/expansion to optimize kidney function. Since acute kidney injury (AKI) is a serious complication of TLS, patients with oliguria or suspected AKI should have prompt involvement of a pediatric nephrologist to undergo a full evaluation for the presence of AKI and guide management, including the role of diuretics or renal replacement therapy.

TABLE 133-4 Tumor Lysis: General Guidelines for Prevention and Treatment

Hydration 2500-3000 ml/m^2/day of D5 ½ NS or D5 NS to maintain urine output >100 mL/m^2/hr and specific gravity <1.010
May use furosemide (1-2 mg/kg) or mannitol (0.5 g/kg) to increase urine output if necessary; avoid in hypovolemic or hypotensive patients
Consider initiating uric acid–reducing therapy—allopurinol or rasburicase (see Tables 133-3 and 133-5)*
Monitor strict intake and output; measure weight bid
Take vital signs at least q4h; place on cardiovascular-respiratory monitor if any significant metabolic abnormalities
Monitor lysis laboratory studies based on risk (HR q4-6h, IR q8-12h, LR q12-24h, or more frequently if indicated): electrolytes, blood urea nitrogen, creatinine, uric acid, ionized calcium, magnesium, phosphorus, lactate dehydrogenase
Avoid nephrotoxic medications or IV contrast material
Avoid supplemental potassium or phosphorus intake even when potassium and phosphorus levels are not elevated
Monitor for associated hyperkalemia, hyperphosphatemia, and hypocalcemia and treat as clinically indicated (see Table 133-6)
For severe metabolic abnormalities, persistent oliguria, or renal failure, hemofiltration or dialysis may be warranted

*Rasburicase should not be used in patients with known or suspected glucose-6-phosphate dehydrogenase deficiency because severe hemolysis can occur, further increasing the likelihood of renal impairment.

HR, high risk; IR, intermediate risk; LR, low risk.

Hyperuricemia Hyperuricemia results from the breakdown of the purine components of DNA that are released in the circulation when tumor cells lyse. As shown in **Figure 133-1**, the purine metabolites hypoxanthine and xanthine are converted by xanthine oxidase to uric acid. In the acidic environment of the urine, uric acid precipitates and deposits in renal tubules causing uric acid nephropathy, which can lead to renal failure. The key strategies in both the prevention and management of hyperuricemia are to increase uric acid elimination and decrease uric acid production.

Hyperhydration is the most common strategy used to eliminate uric acid. Most pediatric patients can tolerate 3000 mL/m^2/day of IV fluid administration. The rare patient who does not respond to this therapy with copious urine output can be treated with diuretics. In settings where hyperhydration must be used with caution (pulmonary/pericardial effusions, preexisting heart dysfunction, large anterior mediastinal masses), maintaining a minimum urine output of at least 2 mL/kg/hr with a lower rate of IV fluid administration may suffice.

The classic teaching is that excretion of purine metabolites can be improved by alkalinization of the urine, which is most commonly achieved by addition of sodium bicarbonate to IV fluids. However, alkalinization can promote calcium-phosphate crystal formation and deposition in the renal tubules. Furthermore, the use of alkalinized fluids is falling out of favor owing to decreased availability of sodium bicarbonate, lack of evidence of clinical benefit, and increased use of alternative therapies (i.e., rasburicase).

Allopurinol has been the mainstay of the prevention and treatment of hyperuricemia for decades. Allopurinol inhibits xanthine oxidase and prevents the formation of uric acid. However, allopurinol does not aid in the elimination of previously formed uric acid and may also increase the concentrations of upstream purine metabolites, such as hypoxanthine and xanthine, which can also lead to renal dysfunction.

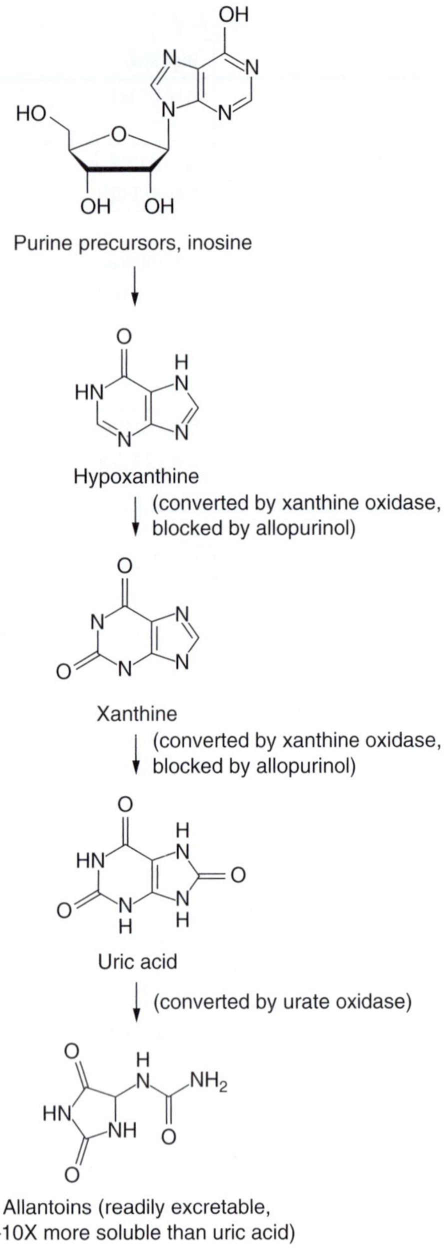

FIGURE 133-1. Uric acid metabolism.

The use and availability of recombinant urate oxidase (rasburicase) has significantly changed the landscape of TLS management in children. As an enzyme, rasburicase directly breaks down uric acid into highly soluble metabolites (allantoins) that are easily excreted by the kidney. Rasburicase not only eliminates uric acid but also promotes the elimination of upstream purine precursors. Rasburicase is approved for use in children for management of hyperuricemia associated with malignancy. It has been proven to be a safe alternative to allopurinol, while demonstrating increased efficacy. Unfortunately, rasburicase is much more expensive than allopurinol and thus should be reserved for a select population of patients. Strong consideration of rasburicase should be given to patients with elevated uric acid levels in combination with other predictive markers of severe TLS. Guidelines for administration of allopurinol and rasburicase are presented in **Tables** 133-4 and **133-5**. Of note, when obtaining uric acid levels after the administration of rasburicase, blood samples should be delivered to the clinical laboratory on ice in order to inhibit the continued enzymatic breakdown of uric acid in the test tube. G6PD deficiency is an absolute contraindication to rasburicase administration.

TABLE 133-5 Tumor Lysis Syndrome: Guidelines for Administration of Allopurinol and Rasburicase
Allopurinol
Begin 24-48 hours before start of cytoreductive chemotherapy
Administer IV or PO; children often have difficulty with oral administration
Allopurinol PO 10 mg/kg/day divided TID (maximum dose 800 mg/day)
Allopurinol IV 200 mg/m^2/day in 1-3 divided doses
Rasburicase
Recommended dose: 0.1-0.2 mg/kg daily for up to 5 days
Urine should not be alkalinized
Do not administer to G6PD-deficient patients; if G6PD deficiency is suspected, status should be confirmed before administration

G6PD, glucose-6-phosphate dehydrogenase.

Additional Electrolyte Abnormalities Associated With Tumor Lysis Syndrome Hyperkalemia is the most life-threatening complication of TLS, as it can cause sudden cardiac death. Avoiding exogenous potassium sources and implementing hyperhydration are usually adequate to avoid clinically significant hyperkalemia. While avoidance of potassium-containing fluids is often encouraged, some patients receiving hyperhydration can develop hypokalemia secondary to profuse urinary output ("solvent drag"). In these patients, supplemental potassium can be cautiously administered (preferably internally) with frequent laboratory assessment. It is important to review a patient's medication list closely for medications that may contribute to hyperkalemia, such as non-steroidal anti-inflammatory drugs, potassium-sparing diuretics, angiotensin-converting enzymes, angiotensin-receptor blockers, and others, which can impair the tubular secretion of potassium. In cases of severe hyperkalemia, additional modalities should be considered. Hyperphosphatemia can develop as a consequence of tumor lysis and lead to the development of calcium-phosphate crystals that can precipitate in the renal tubule and contribute to renal dysfunction. These calcium-phosphate complexes can also result in hypocalcemia. Treatment of hypocalcemia is usually reserved only for patients presenting with clinical signs such as positive Trousseau or Chvostek signs or tetany. Calcium supplementation in asymptomatic patients should be avoided, as this may enhance calcium-phosphate deposition. The clinical symptoms of the metabolic derangements seen in TLS and specific management guidelines are presented in **Table 133-6**.

SYNDROME OF INAPPROPRIATE ANTIDIURETIC HORMONE SECRETION

Syndrome of inappropriate antidiuretic hormone secretion (SIADH) can develop as a side effect of certain chemotherapeutics or can be associated with intracranial malignancies, and infections such as pneumonia. Common chemotherapeutic drugs associated with SIADH in children include vincristine, cyclophosphamide, ifosfamide, cisplatin, and melphalan. The resulting hyponatremia can be clinically significant and require intervention. While fluid restriction is the mainstay of therapy, this can compromise the hydration strategies utilized around certain chemotherapy regimens or clinical scenarios. For instance, in patients receiving hyperhydration for prevention of TLS or to aid clearance of methotrexate, fluid restriction may be contraindicated. Consultation with a pediatric oncologist is recommended in these cases.

HEMATOLOGIC EMERGENCIES

HYPERLEUKOCYTOSIS

The initial presentation of childhood ALL or AML can be complicated by the presence of a very elevated circulating blast count. Hyperleukocytosis is defined as a WBC greater than 100,000 cells/mm^3 and can

TABLE 133-6 Tumor Lysis Syndrome: Treatment of Metabolic Abnormalities

Disorder	Clinical Features	Treatment
Hyperkalemia	ECG abnormalities: peaked T waves, lengthening of P-R interval, widened QRS complex Arrhythmias and cardiac arrest Paresthesias, muscle cramps, paralysis	Avoid potassium administration Avoid medications that contribute to hyperkalemia Oral potassium-binding resin (sodium polystyrene sulfonate) 1 g/kg q6h IV furosemide 0.5-1 mg/kg/dose IV dextrose and insulin: 1 g/kg dextrose with 0.25 unit/kg regular insulin Beta-adrenergic agonist (ex: albuterol); should be used concomitantly with other modalities, not as sole agent IV sodium bicarbonate 1-2 mEq/kg IV calcium gluconate 60-100 mg/kg slow bolus; use only for severe life-threatening arrhythmias; may cause calcium phosphate precipitation
Hyperphosphatemia	Nausea, vomiting, diarrhea, lethargy, seizures Can lead to hypocalcemia	Avoid phosphate administration/ dietary restriction Oral phosphate binder: aluminum hydroxide 150 mg/kg/day divided every 4-6 hours; calcium acetate or sevelamer (dose varies by BSA/age) Forced diuresis (hydration, furosemide, mannitol) IV glucose and insulin (see hyperkalemia above) Dialysis or hemofiltration
Hypocalcemia	Positive Trousseau or Chvostek sign, tetany, seizure, laryngospasm, wheezing associated with bronchospasm, carpopedal spasm Prolonged Q-T interval on ECG	Control hyperphosphatemia Implement seizure precautions If severely symptomatic, treat with IV 10% calcium gluconate 30-50 mg/kg slow bolus; must monitor for bradycardia; may cause calcium phosphate precipitation
Hyperuricemia	Clinical symptoms usually associated with levels >10 mg/dL and include lethargy, nausea, vomiting, uric acid calculi, hematuria, oliguria, anuria	Hyperhydration Allopurinol or rasburicase (see Table 133-5)

ECG, electrocardiogram.

be seen in both ALL and AML. Hyperleukocytosis is more commonly seen in ALL, but clinical evidence of vascular obstruction by blasts (leukostasis) is more commonly encountered in patients with AML.

Hyperleukocytosis increases blood viscosity, which can ultimately result in leukostasis, small vessel obstruction, and decreased perfusion. The circulatory anatomy of the brain and lungs puts these organs at particular risk of developing life-threatening complications. Classic presenting symptoms of pulmonary leukocytosis include hypoxia, tachypnea, and respiratory distress. Chest x-rays are generally not indicated for the diagnosis of leukostasis, but when they are performed, may demonstrate bilateral "whiteout" of the lung fields, sometimes prompting an incorrect diagnosis of pneumonia. Central nervous system (CNS) manifestations of cerebral leukostasis may be subtle, so a thorough neurologic exam is essential. Common signs or symptoms include headache or somnolence, but altered metal status, seizure, or comas are also possible. Less common presentations of leukostasis include renal dysfunction, cardiac ischemia, priapism, and dactylitis. Leukocytosis may induce disseminated intravascular coagulopathy and hemorrhage. Close monitoring of patients presenting with hyperleukocytosis is important, as leukostasis is diagnosed clinically rather than by laboratory or imaging assessment.

Critical goals in the initial management of a patient with hyperleukocytosis include reduction of blood viscosity and initiation of TLS prevention. Administration of intravenous fluids aids both of these goals and should be promptly initiated. While patients with leukemia can present with exceptional anemia, red cell transfusions should be avoided if possible, because increasing the hematocrit will directly increase blood viscosity. Transfusion of platelets has less effect on viscosity, therefore may be used when indicated. Early consultation with a pediatric oncologist is critical, as initiation of hydroxyurea or induction chemotherapy should be started as soon as possible.

Cytoreduction by leukapheresis or exchange transfusion, though controversial, can be considered as an alternative method to decrease blood viscosity. Generally, these procedures are considered when peripheral blood WBC count is greater than 100,000 cells/mm^3 in AML or greater than 300 to 500,000 cells/mm^3 in ALL. However, these are typically offered only to patients whose chemotherapy is delayed and who are symptomatic of leukostasis. There are no studies comparing the use of leukapheresis to initiation of chemotherapy in pediatric patients with hyperleukocytosis or leukostasis. In addition, in cases where hyperleukocytosis is accompanied by coagulopathy (see later) or septic shock, leukapheresis may be unsafe. As a result, there are no uniformly accepted criteria supporting the use of leukapheresis or exchange transfusion in children with hyperleukocytosis. Leukapheresis should be initiated on a case-by-case basis after consultation with a pediatric oncologist. Considering the complexities of preparing for leukapheresis (e.g., catheter placement, blood product administration, and critical care support), the local blood bank and/or apheresis team should be quickly notified of any patient being considered for this procedure.

HEMORRHAGE AND DISSEMINATED INTRAVASCULAR COAGULATION

Severe thrombocytopenia is commonly seen in pediatric oncology patients, either as a result of direct invasion of the bone marrow by cancer cells or as a consequence of cancer therapy. Abnormal bleeding associated with thrombocytopenia typically presents with either petechiae or spontaneous mucosal bleeding, such as epistaxis. Less commonly, more severe bleeding such as intracranial hemorrhage or gastrointestinal bleeding can occur. Transfusing asymptomatic patients when their platelet count is below a specific threshold can prevent thrombocytopenia-related bleeding. Typically, this platelet count threshold is between 10,000 and 30,000 platelets/mm^3, but is variable among different centers and in certain clinical situations.

Hemorrhage in cancer patients can also occur because of acquired coagulation factor deficiency that occurs as a result of disseminated intravascular coagulation (DIC) or secondary to specific chemotherapeutics such as asparaginase, which blocks production of numerous coagulation factors. DIC in oncology patients is most commonly encountered when these patients are experiencing overwhelming infections, such as sepsis. However, certain subtypes of childhood AML, especially acute promyelocytic leukemia (APML), can present with life-threatening DIC prior to or immediately after initiation of therapy. The management of DIC in the setting of sepsis in the oncology patient is similar to non-oncology patients, with emphasis on fibrinogen and coagulation factor replacement through the administration of cryoprecipitate and fresh frozen plasma (FFP), respectively. In the case of APML-associated DIC, initiation of appropriate chemotherapy should be expedited, in addition to supportive administration of FFP and cryoprecipitate.

L-Asparaginase, a chemotherapeutic commonly used in the treatment of childhood ALL and AML, depletes asparagine, which starves tumor cells of this essential amino acid. Unfortunately, asparagine depletion also reduces the production of numerous coagulation factors, predisposing these patients to both hemorrhage and thrombosis.

TABLE 133-7 Transfusions in the Oncology Patient

Blood Product and Indication	Transfusion Threshold
Platelets	
Major surgery*	>40-50 K/mm^3
Active bleeding	>100 K/mm^3
Minor Procedures, such as bone marrow aspirations/biopsies, insertion/removal of central venous catheters*	>20 K/mm^3
Lumbar Puncture*	>50 K/mm^3
Mild Mucosal bleeding	>20-30 K/mm^3
Prevention of spontaneous bleeding	>10 K/mm^3
Red cells	
Prophylaxis against symptomatic anemia	>7 g/dL
Mildly symptomatic anemia**	>7 g/dL
Severe illness or sepsis	>9 g/dL
Radiation therapy	>10 g/dL

Product Guidelines	Platelet	Red Cells	Comment
Type and Cross	Yes	Yes	Type not required for platelet transfusion if prior type available in Blood bank
ABO matched	Preferred	Yes	
Rh matched	Preferred	Yes	If Rh+ platelets given to Rh- donor, must administer anti-D product within 72 hours
Irradiated	Yes	Yes	For prevention of graft-versus-host-disease
Leukoreduced	Yes	Yes	Reduces risk of transfusion reactions, alloimmunization, and CMV transmission
CMV negative	No	No	Leukoreduction is sufficient
HLA matched	Rarely	No	Only in platelet refractory patients
Single donor	Preferred	No	
Premedications	Possible	Possible	Acetaminophen if history of fevers Diphenhydramine if history of allergic reaction Hydrocortisone if history of allergic reaction despite administration of diphenhydramine or history of severe allergic reaction
Amount	1 unit/10 kg	~ 10-15 mL/kg (2 units for pts >50 kg)	Many institutional standards exist

*For platelet administration prior to a procedure, post-transfusion platelet counts should be obtained to confirm desired platelet count has been reached. Platelet transfusions should be on hold for a procedure in the event of peri-operative bleeding.

**For mildly symptomatic anemia related to bone marrow suppression, recovery can be aided with recombinant erythropoietin.

A detailed explanation of the management of blood product support in cases of severe hemorrhage and DIC is outside the scope of this chapter. However, the pediatric hospitalist should be knowledgeable about transfusion management strategies that are particular to the pediatric oncology patient. In general, transfusions of blood products should be minimized as much as possible to avoid the development of alloimmunization, transfusion reactions, infections, and iron overload. The transfusion thresholds for platelets and red blood cells vary by center and diagnosis but should always be tailored to the particular clinical scenario (**Table 133-7**).

It is common for family members of a newly diagnosed pediatric oncology patient to request direct donation of blood products for their loved one. This practice should be discouraged for two reasons. First, directly donated blood products have not been shown to be safer than anonymously donated blood products. Second, oncology patients may at some point need an allogeneic hematopoietic stem cell transplant, and exposure to familial human lymphocyte antigens may increase the risk of graft rejection and poor outcome.

THROMBOSIS

Risk of thrombosis is increased in pediatric cancer patients for numerous reasons. The most common risk factor in children is the presence of an indwelling central venous catheter. As mentioned earlier, certain medications, such as L-asparaginase, increase the risk of thrombosis through depletion of the coagulation factors like antithrombin III (ATIII), plasminogen, protein C, and protein S. Mechanical compression of large veins by tumors can also result in thrombosis. Other risk factors for thrombosis in the cancer setting include sepsis, prolonged immobility, and the underlying inflammatory state intrinsic to malignancy.

Presenting symptoms of thrombosis are related to location and may include extremity or facial swelling. When occurring in the cerebral venous sinuses, patients can present with headache, seizures, or other neurological manifestations. Central venous line (CVL)-associated thrombosis can present with line malfunction. Pulmonary embolism should be considered in patients with respiratory distress, chest pain, hypoxia, syncope, or with sustained tachycardia of unclear etiology. Once identified by appropriate imaging, the management of venous thrombosis must be tailored with consideration of thrombus location (superficial vs. deep vein thrombosis), provocative triggers (CVL vs. mass), type/duration of chemotherapy, and age of the child (ambulating vs. toddling), as these factors will influence the type and duration of anticoagulation as well as supportive care. For instance, during periods of chemotherapy-induced severe thrombocytopenia, anticoagulation may be reduced or discontinued. Furthermore, patients receiving anticoagulation with enoxaparin may need frequent repletion of ATIII in order to achieve therapeutic levels of enoxaparin; this is especially relevant if they are receiving L-asparaginase, which is known to inhibit ATIII synthesis.

While thrombosis in pediatric oncology patients is not uncommon, it is rarely associated with an underlying hypercoagulability syndrome (e.g., Factor V Leiden). The involvement of a pediatric hematologist is encouraged to help guide therapy and to determine the need for a hypercoagulability evaluation.

FEVER AND NEUTROPENIA

BACKGROUND

Neutropenia is a common side effect of chemotherapy administered to children, particularly alkylating agents, anthracyclines, and cytarabine. In contrast to thrombocytopenia and anemia, which can be treated with the transfusion of blood products, neutropenia resolves only after recovery of bone marrow function. While the transfusion of donor granulocytes is possible, this practice is controversial without clear clinical benefit. Severe neutropenia is commonly encountered in pediatric oncology patients and can lead to the development of life-threatening bacterial and fungal infections. The febrile and neutropenic patient is a true emergency, as overwhelming sepsis and death can occur in a matter of hours if appropriate interventions are not emergently implemented.

Fever and neutropenia guidelines have been published by the Infectious Diseases Society of America and the International Pediatric Fever and Neutropenia Guideline Panel. Common definitions used in these guidelines are presented in **Table 133-8**. The guidelines stress the importance of utilizing risk stratification in determining treatment strategies. However, there are still no universally accepted pediatric criteria to categorize neutropenic patients at low or high risk of developing severe infections. As a result, many institutions adopt specific algorithms that differentiate risk based on neutrophil count, clinical status, malignancy, and chemotherapy most recently given. What follows are general approaches to the neutropenic patient at high risk for serious infections.

PATHOGENS

The pediatric hospitalist should understand the microbiology of neutropenia-associated infections in order to optimize initial therapy. The most common pathogens encountered in neutropenic patients comprise gram-negative organisms, including *Escherichia coli*, *Klebsiella*, and *Pseudomonas* species, and gram-positive bacteria such as *Staphylococcus aureus*, *Enterococci*, *viridans* group *Streptococci*, and *Streptococcus pneumoniae*. Historically, gram-negative infections were the most commonly encountered organisms. However, over the last few decades, gram-positive organisms have accounted for the majority of documented infections in neutropenic patients. The use of prophylactic antibiotics, increased colonization of drug-resistant organisms, and use of indwelling catheters have been identified as contributing factors to this change.

Fungal infections are less commonly encountered, but can result in deep-seated infections that may require prolonged antifungal treatment and/or surgery. The likelihood of fungal infection increases with prolonged neutropenia and in neutropenic patients with prolonged fever despite administration of empiric antibiotics. The most common fungal pathogens are *Candida* and *Aspergillus* species.

TABLE 133-8 Fever and Neutropenia: Definitions and Initial Laboratory Assessment

Clinical Feature	Definition
Fever	• Single temperature greater than 38.3°C, *or* • Temperature greater than 38°C lasting more than 1 hour, or obtained twice within 12-24 hours
Neutropenia	ANC <500 cells/mm³ or with expected nadir <500 cells/mm³ within the next 48 hours
Absolute neutrophil count (ANC)	(% Granulocytes + % Bands) × WBC
Initial laboratory assessment	Blood culture from each lumen of indwelling catheter and consider obtaining peripheral cultures Urine analysis/culture if patients able to obtain clean catch specimen (no catheterizations) CBC with differential Chemistries including creatinine Liver panel (AST, ALT, direct and indirect bilirubin) *If abdominal pain:* Amylase and lipase

APPROACH TO PATIENT WITH FEVER AND NEUTROPENIA

A detailed history and physical examination must be obtained from each patient presenting with febrile neutropenia. Details of the expected duration of neutropenia, type and timing of chemotherapy administered, past infectious history, and presence or absence of indwelling catheter will help guide empiric therapy. Often, localizing symptoms of infection are absent, but localized pain or redness can guide initial antibiotic selection and appropriate ancillary testing (**Table 133-9**). The physical examination of the febrile neutropenic patient must be efficient but thorough, and include an examination of the perianal area, even in well-appearing patients. Rectal measurement of temperature should be avoided. The laboratory evaluation should include aerobic and anaerobic blood cultures from each lumen of any indwelling catheter. A peripheral culture should be considered as it increases the identification of true bacteremia. The laboratory assessment of every febrile oncology patient with suspected neutropenia should include a CBC with differential, liver function tests, and full chemistry panel, including creatinine. Obtaining a C-reactive protein can be considered to help risk stratify patients. In addition, urine analysis and culture can be considered in patients who can provide a clean catch sample, especially young patients. Neutropenic patients should not be routinely catheterized and should never have a digital rectal exam performed. A lumbar puncture to assess for meningitis is not indicated unless the patient presents with clinical signs or symptoms of meningitis or encephalitis. Patients presenting with abdominal pain should also have amylase or lipase obtained, particularly if they have recently received L-asparaginase, which is a known risk factor for pancreatitis (Tables 133-8 and 133-9).

CONSIDERATIONS IN INITIAL ANTIBIOTIC SELECTION

Prompt administration of antibiotics is paramount and should be considered a top priority. Standard goal times to antibiotic administration at pediatric emergency departments are generally considered less than 60 minutes. For ill-appearing patients, antibiotics should be administered emergently, even prior to obtaining a blood culture. The ideal antibiotic regimen will have broad-spectrum coverage of gram-positive and gram-negative organisms, including *Pseudomonas* species. Several monotherapy regimens are widely utilized including a fourth-generation cephalosporin, a carbapenem, or piperacillin/tazobactam (**Table 133-10**). The addition of vancomycin may also be considered, especially in patients with a history of methicillin-resistant *Staphylococcus aureus* infections or those with vital sign instability. For patients with a cephalosporin allergy, a combination of aztreonam (for gram-negative coverage) and vancomycin (for gram-positive coverage) or ciprofloxacin and clindamycin should be considered. Certain other clinical situations may warrant an alternative antibiotic choice (Table 133-9). For instance, the patient presenting with abdominal or perianal pain should have additional anaerobic coverage. These are general guidelines for empiric coverage, and individual institutions may have different algorithms based on the local prevalence of drug-resistant organisms. Antibiotic selection should be tailored further if a microbe is isolated from any culture. Isolation of certain organisms also warrants urgent removal of the indwelling CVL.

Initial or step-down outpatient management, as well as oral antibiotics, can be considered in patients with low-risk fever and neutropenia, if the infrastructure is in place to ensure careful follow-up and monitoring.

CONSIDERATIONS IN EMPIRIC ANTIFUNGAL THERAPY

Risk criteria have been developed to classify patients with persistent fever and neutropenia as low or high risk of invasive fungal disease. Patients with AML, high-risk ALL, relapsed acute leukemia, and allogeneic HSCT recipients are classified as high risk. Additionally, patients receiving high-dose corticosteroids and those with prolonged neutropenia are at high risk of invasive fungal disease. All other patients

TABLE 133-9 Fever and Neutropenia: Guidelines for Modifying Treatment

Clinical Finding	Action
Well-appearing child, non-focal exam	Standard empiric antibiotic plan.
Abdominal pain	Add anaerobic coverage. Consider abdominal imaging. Obtain amylase and lipase (pancreatitis).
Perianal pain or redness	Add anaerobic coverage (metronidazole) if not already receiving adequate anaerobic coverage (eg, piperacillin-tazobactam, meropenem).
Cough, dyspnea, or hypoxia	Obtain CXR, consider testing for respiratory viruses (eg, Influenza, RSV).
CVL-site infection	Add vancomycin.
Diarrhea	Test for *C. difficile –consider adding metronidazole (for non-severe episodes) or oral vancomycin (for non-severe, severe, or recurrent episodes), or oral fidaxomicin (for recurrent episodes)*. Consider testing of SSYCE organisms, rotavirus.
History of drug-resistant organism	Choose broad-spectrum antibiotic that covers particular organism or add additional agent.
Dysuria	Obtain UA and urine culture. Consider renal imaging.
Meningismus	*All patients*: Switch to meningitic dosing of a broad-spectrum BBB-penetrant antibiotic. Obtain lumbar puncture (platelets should be greater than 50,000/mm^3). *Patients with VP shunt or Ommaya reservoir:* Consider CNS imaging and neurosurgical consult prior to obtaining CSF
Periodontal infection	Add anaerobic coverage
Pulmonary infiltrates by CXR	*Diffuse/interstitial*: consider coverage for atypical microorganisms (macrolide antibiotic). *Localized*: Consider adding antifungal coverage and advanced imaging (CT) if persistently febrile.
Vital sign instability	Add vancomycin, consider removal of CVL, consult infectious disease and critical care expert.
Vesicular or ulcerative lesions	Test and culture for herpes simplex and varicella.
Positive Blood Cultures	
Bacillus species	Add vancomycin or meropenem and remove CVL. Consider solid-organ and CNS imaging after ANC recovery.
Candida species	Remove CVL, add antifungal agent. Consider solid-organ imaging at baseline and after ANC recovery.
Methicillin-resistant *S. aureus*	Add vancomycin, remove CVL.
Vancomycin-resistant *enterococcus*	Remove CVL, discuss antibiotic plan with infectious disease consultant.
Failure to clear positive blood culture by 48 hours	Remove CVL.
Persistent Fevers	
Febrile and neutropenic for ≥4-7 days	Add empiric antifungal therapy in those at high risk of invasive fungal disease: amphotericin B or echinocandins (e.g., caspofungin), or triazole derivatives (e.g., voriconazole, Posaconazole). Obtain fungal cultures. Consult infectious disease expert.

ANC, absolute neutrophil count; BBB, blood–brain barrier; CNS, central nervous system; CVL, central venous line; CXR, chest x-ray; RSV, respiratory syncytial virus; SSYCE, *Shigella, Salmonella, Yersinia, Campylobacter, enterohemorrhagic Escherichia coli*; VP, ventriculoperitoneal shunt.

should be considered low risk of invasive fungal disease. Empiric antifungal therapy should be initiated for the high-risk persistently febrile and neutropenic patient, who has not defervesced after several days of empiric therapy with broad-spectrum antibiotics. In patients at low risk of invasive fungal disease, who have been febrile and neutropenic and have not defervesced after 4 days despite broad-spectrum antibiotics, withholding empirical antifungal therapy should be considered. While

TABLE 133-10 Fever and Neutropenia: Guidelines for Initial Antibiotic Selection

Clinical Feature	Antibiotic
No antibiotic allergy	Cefepime 50 mg/kg (max. 2 g) IV Q8 hr; *or* Meropenem 20 mg/kg IV Q8 hr; *or* Piperacillin/tazobactam (varies by age)
Cephalosporin allergy	Aztreonam 30 mg/kg (max. 2 g) IV Q6 hr + vancomycin; *or* Ciprofloxacin + clindamycin; *or* Meropenem 20 mg/kg IV Q8hr

regimens may vary among institutions, most guidelines recommend the initiation of caspofungin or liposomal amphotericin B for empiric antifungal coverage. In regard to fungal markers to guide empirical antifungal management, in patients at high risk of invasive fungal disease, the most recent guidelines recommend considering not obtaining serum galactomannan, and recommend against using beta-D-glucan and fungal polymerase chain reaction. In patients with prolonged fever and neutropenia at high risk of invasive fungal disease, imaging may be needed. In these high-risk patients, CT of the lungs should be performed. Imaging of the abdomen can be considered in those without localizing signs or symptoms. Finally, CT of the sinuses should only be considered in patients with localizing signs or symptoms. Consultation with a pediatric oncologist or infectious disease expert should be considered in these cases.

WHEN TO STOP THERAPY

Most institutions discontinue antimicrobial therapy once the patient has been afebrile for 24 hours, ANC is greater than 500 cells/mm^3 (or is greater than 200 cells/mm^3 and rising), and blood cultures have been negative for at least 48 hours. For patients with low-risk febrile neutropenia, discontinuation of empiric antimicrobials can be considered at 72 hours, if blood cultures have remained negative and they have been afebrile for 24 hours, irrespective of ANC count, as long as close follow-up can be ensured. For patients receiving antifungal therapy, imaging of the lungs and abdominal viscera should be considered as aforementioned.

CARDIOPULMONARY EMERGENCIES

ANTERIOR MEDIASTINAL MASS

Large intrathoracic masses can lead to life-threatening cardiac and pulmonary complications. The management of anterior mediastinal masses (AMM) can be very challenging, because in addition to potentially devastating effects on ventilation and cardiac output, they can significantly delay or compromise the diagnosis of a new malignancy. The most common diagnoses presenting with an AMM are Hodgkin and non-Hodgkin lymphomas. In addition, AMM can present as an extramedullary complication of leukemia; this is most commonly seen in patients diagnosed with T-cell ALL. Solid tumors that can present with large anterior mediastinal masses include thymomas, thyroid cancers, germ cell tumors, neuroblastoma, Ewing sarcoma, and rhabdomyosarcoma. The compression of vital mediastinal structures causes two main clinical phenomena: tracheal compression and superior vena cava (SVC) syndrome. In superior mediastinum syndrome, these complications occur simultaneously.

Compression of the trachea or main stem bronchi can present with cough, wheeze, dyspnea (at rest or on exertion), orthopnea, chest pain, and syncope. These clinical manifestations can occur gradually over time or suddenly, depending on the location and proliferative capacity of the mass. Occasionally patients may be asymptomatic from the mass, or may only have symptoms that present with particular positions, such as laying supine. Patients will sometimes assume positions of comfort, such as "tripoding," which shift the mass away from the airways, alleviating the obstruction. The patient with a suspected mediastinal mass should be maintained in an upright or prone position during initial evaluation.

The workup of a patient with a suspected mediastinal mass should start with a chest x-ray (PA and lateral views) which can assess the size of the mass and identify tracheal deviation or compression. Once AMM is identified, the patient should be maintained in an upright position pending further evaluations. Subsequent diagnostic evaluations, including advanced imaging (CT, MRI) and biopsies, need to be carefully planned to avoid precipitating sudden cardiopulmonary arrest with improper positioning or sedation. An echocardiogram should be considered to assess cardiac compromise.

Ideally, the biopsy should be attempted through the least invasive method. For patients with suspected leukemia, peripheral blood blast analysis may lead to a diagnosis without the need for invasive procedures or sedation. Alternatively, an unsedated bone marrow or peripheral lymph node biopsy using local anesthesia can be considered. Additional sources of diagnostic material include pleural and pericardial effusions, though tapping these fluid collections would be contraindicated in the uncooperative, non-sedated child. Presence of specific tumor biomarkers, such as elevated urinary catecholamines (in neuroblastoma) or αFP/βHCG (in some germ cell tumors), may be of diagnostic assistance.

If sedation is required for biopsy, airway risk should be assessed with consultation from a multidisciplinary team that might include a pediatric oncologist, otolaryngologist, intensivist, or anesthesiologist depending on institutional practices. It is critical to recognize that endotracheal intubation may not maintain or secure the airway in these patients, especially patients whose obstruction is at or below the level of the tip of the endotracheal tube (carina). In addition, sedation of these patients during attempted intubation, imaging, or biopsy can lead to sudden cardiopulmonary arrest and death.

The presence of orthopnea has been associated with a high risk of respiratory collapse. The best radiologic evaluation of the trachea is with lateral films and CT scan, which may need to be obtained in the prone position. Risk of anesthesia can be assessed by measurement of the cross-sectional diameter of the trachea on CT as well as pulmonary function tests (PFTs)—in particular, peak expiratory flow rates (PEFRs). Patients with a >50% tracheal cross-section and PEFRs of >50% have been shown to tolerate anesthesia well. It should be noted that the benefits of obtaining PFTs is still being investigated. PFTs have the limitation of reliability given the dependence on effort and ability to cooperate. It also remains unclear whether obtaining PFTs in addition to history, physical examination, and imaging adds significant benefit.

In extreme circumstances, such as impending respiratory failure, implementation of empiric antineoplastic therapy must be considered prior to obtaining tissue for diagnosis. Strategies employed in this scenario include initiation of steroids, chemotherapy, or radiation therapy. In these situations, a pediatric oncologist should always be involved. Some malignancies, such as lymphoma, may have an exceptional response to empiric therapy with rapid resolution of both AMM size and symptoms. Such a response may make biopsy more challenging or infeasible, thus jeopardizing the ability to make an accurate pathological diagnosis.

SUPERIOR VENA CAVA SYNDROME/SUPERIOR MEDIASTINAL SYNDROME

SVC syndrome classically presents with upper extremity swelling and/or facial plethora resulting from decreased venous return from the head and upper extremities. Rarely, SVC syndrome is associated with cardiogenic shock or signs of increased intracranial pressure. SVC syndrome can also be caused by an occlusive thrombus resulting from the placement of an indwelling catheter into venous structures already narrowed by the mediastinal mass. Central venous catheter associated SVC syndrome may be treated by removing the central line, anticoagulation, or stenting when needed. One must also be careful with fluid administration in patients presenting with significant vascular compromise from anterior mediastinal masses. The increased intrathoracic pressure or direct compression of the right atrium from the tumor may make these patients particularly pre-load sensitive; hypovolemia in these patients may precipitate cardiopulmonary arrest secondary to poor cardiac output. On the other hand, hyperhydration may worsen symptoms of SVC syndrome, increasing upper extremity and facial swelling. As in the case of severe tracheal compression, antineoplastic therapy should be urgently initiated.

NEUROLOGIC EMERGENCIES

SPINAL CORD COMPRESSION

Rapid identification of spinal cord compression in the pediatric oncology patient is necessary in order to avoid permanent neurological disability. Spinal cord compression is most commonly encountered in solid tumors such as neuroblastoma, Ewing sarcoma, rhabdomyosarcoma, osteosarcoma, metastatic CNS tumors, lymphoma, and AML-related chloromas. Spinal cord compression can be associated with both advanced stage metastatic disease or at initial presentation. The presenting signs are dependent upon the location and severity of cord compression, but can include back pain, weakness, loss of bladder/bowel function, and changes in sensation. Clinicians must remain vigilant and be on the lookout for spinal cord compression lest the diagnosis be missed. In patients who are very young, for whom the neurologic exam is difficult to interpret, or for patients who are otherwise very ill, new findings consistent with spinal cord compression may be overlooked.

The workup of suspected spinal cord compression should be expedited as a medical emergency requiring a multidisciplinary approach, beginning with an efficient, thorough neurological examination followed by MRI of the spine. If cord compression is strongly suspected based on known areas of disease or clinical presentation, IV dexamethasone (1-2 mg/kg) may be administered prior to imaging. If imaging confirms cord compression, an emergent consultation with neurosurgery, radiation oncology, and pediatric oncology should be obtained in order to decide whether surgery, chemotherapy, or radiation therapy should be emergently initiated.

INCREASED INTRACRANIAL PRESSURE

The presence of an expanding intracranial mass or hydrocephalus can result in increased intracranial pressure (ICP) that can progress to uncal herniation. Intracranial malignancies can cause increased ICP by means of either mass effect or an obstructive hydrocephalus, depending on location. Increased ICP can also be caused by thrombosis, infarction, infection, or hemorrhage. Finally, malfunction of an indwelling ventriculoperitoneal (VP) shunt can cause elevated ICP.

Presenting symptoms of increased ICP include headache, nausea, emesis, and visual complaints. On physical examination, cranial nerve abnormalities (including papilledema), deficits in strength and sensation, and altered mental status may be encountered. Cushing's triad of bradycardia, hypertension, and respiratory irregularities must be recognized immediately, as they herald impending herniation.

A rapid evaluation of the patient with suspected increased ICP must occur concurrently with consideration of starting therapy. Imaging of the brain is most rapidly obtained with a CT scan. CT is able to identify the presence of increased ICP, impending cerebral herniation, and hemorrhage. MRI has the advantage of obtaining superior anatomical detail compared to CT, especially in the posterior fossa, and can be used initially if available, or after initial evaluation with CT. Patients with an indwelling ventricular shunt or Ommaya reservoir should have a radiographic shunt series performed and be referred for emergency neurosurgical consultation.

For emergent therapy, IV mannitol can be administered as a 25% solution at a dose of 0.25 to 1 g/kg. IV dexamethasone may also be indicated, and can be administered at a dose of 1 to 2 mg/kg IV. Once intubated, hyperventilation with a goal PCO_2 of 30-35 mmHg can be effective in the management of increased ICP. Early discussion with neurosurgery and critical care consultants will help optimize patient care.

PAIN EMERGENCIES

Despite favorable long-term outcomes in many forms of pediatric cancer, pain, whether acute or chronic, remains a significant clinical challenge. Patients can experience pain as a presenting symptom at time of diagnosis (e.g., bone pain with osteosarcoma), as a side effect of therapy (e.g. mucositis pain) or as a sign of tumor progression (e.g., gastrointestinal obstruction). Controlling pain in patients with advanced-stage disease or at end of life is particularly challenging. Unfortunately, there is evidence that pain and other discomfort at the end of life is often undertreated; however, recent studies indicate that patterns of end-of-life care are improving. A full discussion of palliative care can be found elsewhere in this text, but the pediatric hospitalist should be familiar with strategies to control pain in patients with advanced-stage disease or those approaching end of life. Severe pain in these patients is a medical emergency and should be approached with urgency.

In general, severe pain should be treated with a multidisciplinary approach, including pharmacologic interventions as well as nonpharmacologic integrative therapies. Management should begin with a developmentally appropriate pain assessment, characterization of type of pain, and identification of pathologic and psychosocial conditions contributing to pain. Initial interventions need to be closely monitored so as to capture pain control as quickly as possible. Advanced-stage oncology patients are likely to require rapid escalation of opioids or doses of opioids that are significantly larger than typically administered to opioid-naïve patients. Adequate pain control is determined by the amount of relief or comfort acceptable to the patient, not by the cumulative dosages of analgesics. The pediatric hospitalist should become familiar with institution-specific algorithms and policies around rapid escalation of opioids. In addition to opioids, non-opioid analgesics (e.g. acetaminophen) and integrative approaches (e.g., massage, music therapy, biofeedback) should be maximized. Not uncommonly, patients may require adjuvant therapies (e.g., anticonvulsants, benzodiazepines, dissociative agents) or more invasive approaches such as placement of epidural catheters or nerve blocks. Palliative care expertise is invaluable in these settings and can assist the pediatric hospitalist in optimizing comfort at end of life. Pediatric hospitalists should become familiar with interdisciplinary members available at their institution, including oncologists, oncology nurses, psychologists, pain specialists, occupational or physical therapists, and the palliative care team.

TABLE 133-11 Etiologies of Altered Mental Status in the Oncology Patient

Tumor	**Cytotoxic chemotherapy**
Primary CNS tumor	Methotrexate
Metastatic CNS tumor	Cytarabine
Leukemic or carcinomatous meningitis	Ifosphamide
Hyperleukocytosis	**Supportive care medications**
CNS infection	Opioids
Meningitis	Benzodiazepines
Viral encephalitis	Gabapentin
Brain abscess	Anticonvulsants
Cerebrovascular accident	Antidepressants
Ischemic or hemorrhagic stroke	Antihistamines
Sagittal venous sinus thrombosis	Dronabinol
Metabolic derangements	**Psychiatric conditions**
Hyponatremia	Adjustment disorders
Hypo/hyperglycemia	Depression
Hypomagnesemia	Anxiety
Uremia	Delerium
Hypo/hyperthyroidism	"ICU psychosis"
Increased intracranial pressure	**Cardiopulmonary insufficiency**
Tumor	Hypoxia
All-trans-retinoic acid	Hypercarbia
	Hypotension
	Seizure/postictal state

ALTERED MENTAL STATUS

Altered mental status in an oncology patient has a broad differential ranging from relatively benign causes to etiologies that are truly life threatening. The hospitalist should be familiar with this differential, as it will help guide a rapid assessment (**Table 133-11**).

SUGGESTED READINGS

Azizkhan RG, Dudgeon DL, Buck JR, et al. Life-threatening airway obstruction as a complication to the management of mediastinal masses in children. *J Pediatr Surg.* 1985;20(6):816-822.

Cairo MS, Bishop M. Tumour lysis syndrome: new therapeutic strategies and classification. *Br J Haematol.* 2004;127(1):3-11.

Cairo MS, Coiffier B, Reiter A, Younes A. Recommendations for the evaluation of risk and prophylaxis of tumour lysis syndrome (TLS) in adults and children with malignant diseases: an expert TLS panel consensus. *Br J Haematol.* 2010;149(4):578-586.

Fisher MJ, Rheingold SR. Oncologic emergencies. In: Pizzo P, Poplack D eds. *Principles and Practice of Pediatric Oncology.* 6th ed. Philadelphia, PA: Wolters Kluwer/Lippincott Williams & Wilkins Health; 2011:1125-1151.

Freifeld AG, Bow EJ, Sepkowitz KA, et al. Clinical practice guideline for the use of antimicrobial agents in neutropenic patients with cancer: 2010 update by the Infectious Diseases Society of America. *Clin Infect Dis.* 2011;52(4):e56-93.

Friedrichsdorf SJ. Pain management in children with advanced cancer and during end-of-life care. *Pediatr Hematol Oncol.* 2010;27(4): 257-261.

Goldman SC, Holcenberg JS, Finklestein JZ, et al. A randomized comparison between rasburicase and allopurinol in children with lymphoma or leukemia at high risk for tumor lysis. *Blood.* 2001;97(10): 2998-3003.

Hammer GB. Anaesthetic management for the child with a mediastinal mass. *Paediatr Anaesth.* 2004;14(1):95-97.

Holdsworth MT, Nguyen P. Role of i.v. allopurinol and rasburicase in tumor lysis syndrome. *AJHP.* 2003;60(21):2213-2222; quiz 2223-2214.

Howard SC, Jones DP, Pui CH. The tumor lysis syndrome. *N Engl J Med.* 2011;364(19):1844-1854.

Lehrnbecher T, Robinson P, Fisher B, et al. Guideline for the management of fever and neutropenia in children with cancer and hematopoietic stem-cell transplantation recipients: 2017 update. *J Clin Oncol.* 2017;35(18):2082-2094.

Lewis DW, Packer RJ, Raney B, Rak IW, Belasco J, Lange B. Incidence, presentation, and outcome of spinal cord disease in children with systemic cancer. *Pediatrics.* 1986;78(3):438-443.

Mullen E, Whangbo J, Vrooman L. Oncologic emergencies. In: Orkin S, Fisher D, Look A, eds. *Oncology of Infancy and Childhood.* 1st ed. Philadelphia, PA: Elsevier; 2009:1121-1143.

Pearson JK, Tan GM. Pediatric anterior mediastinal mass: a review article. *Semin Cardiothorac Vasc Anesth.* 2015;19(3):248-254.

Perger L, Lee EY, Shamberger RC. Management of children and adolescents with a critical airway due to compression by an anterior mediastinal mass. *J Pediatr Surg.* 2008;43(11):1990-1997.

Pollono D, Tomarchia S, Drut R, Ibanez O, Ferreyra M, Cedola J. Spinal cord compression: a review of 70 pediatric patients. *Pediatr Hematol Oncol.* 2003;20(6):457-466.

Pui CH, Mahmoud HH, Wiley JM, et al. Recombinant urate oxidase for the prophylaxis or treatment of hyperuricemia in patients with leukemia or lymphoma. *J Clin Oncol.* 2001;19(3):697-704.

Shamberger RC, Holzman RS, Griscom NT, Tarbell NJ, Weinstein HJ. CT quantitation of tracheal cross-sectional area as a guide to the surgical and anesthetic management of children with anterior mediastinal masses. *J Pediatr Surg.* 1991;26(2):138-142.

Shamberger RC. Preanesthetic evaluation of children with anterior mediastinal masses. *Semin Pediatr Surg.* 1999;8(2):61-68.

Snaman JM, Baker JN, Ehrentraut JH, Anghelescu DL. Pediatric oncology: managing pain at the end of life. *Paediatr Drugs.* 2016;18(3): 161-180.

Ullrich C, Berde C, Billett A. Symptom management in children with cancer. In: Orkin S, Fisher D, Look A, eds. *Oncology of Infancy and Childhood*. 1st ed. Philadelphia, PA: Elsevier; 2009:1204-1220.

Wolfe J, Grier HE, Klar N, et al. Symptoms and suffering at the end of life in children with cancer. *N Engl J Med*. 2000;342(5):326-333.

Wolfe J, Hammel JF, Edwards KE, et al. Easing of suffering in children with cancer at the end of life: is care changing? *J Clin Oncol*. 2008;26(10):1717-1723.

CHAPTER 134 Hematopoietic Stem Cell Transplant and Cellular Therapies

Malika Kapadia, MD and Christine N. Duncan, MD

INTRODUCTION

Over the years, there has been increasing use of cellular directed therapies including hematopoietic stem cell transplants (HSCT) and chimeric antigen receptor (CAR) T cell therapy. Thousands of transplants (HSCT) are performed in children and adolescents annually in the United States. HSCT is being used to treat a growing number of indications, including malignancies, nonmalignant hematologic diseases, immunologic disorders, inborn errors of metabolism, and autoimmune disorders (**Table 134-1**). HSCT is not the first line of therapy for many of these diseases but is reserved for patients for whom first-line therapy is not sufficient or is ineffective.

CAR T cell therapies are newly evolving, immune-directed, potentially less toxic, curative approaches for hematologic malignancies. Like HSCT, CAR T cells are not first-line therapies but are reserved for aggressive, relapsed, and/or refractory malignancies. Most of the experience in pediatrics has been with B cell malignancies, that is, B lymphoblastic leukemia (BALL). CAR T cells however are also used for Non-Hodgkin lymphoma (NHL), Chronic Lymphoblastic lymphoma (CLL) and newer trials directed toward CD19 negative B ALL, T cell malignancies, and solid tumor are emerging.

TABLE 134-1 Examples of Pediatric Diseases Treated With Stem Cell Transplant

High-Risk Hematologic Malignancies	Solid Tumors
Acute myelogenous leukemia	Neuroblastoma
Acute lymphoblastic leukemia	Burkitt lymphoma
Chronic myelogenous leukemia	Wilms tumor
Juvenile myelomonocytic leukemia	Certain brain tumors
Hodgkin and non-Hodgkin lymphoma	
Myelodysplastic syndrome (MDS)	
Bone Marrow Failure Syndromes	**Immunodeficiencies**
Aplastic anemia	Severe combined immunodeficiency
Shwachman-Diamond syndrome	Chronic granulomatous disease
Fanconi anemia	Wiskott-Aldrich syndrome
Diamond-Blackfan anemia	X-linked lymphoproliferative disease
	Primary immune regulatory disorders (PIRD)
Hematologic Disorders	**Metabolic and Inherited Disorders**
Sickle cell anemia	Lysosomal storage diseases
Thalassemia major	Osteopetrosis
Hemophagocytic lymphohistiocytosis	Niemann-Pick disease
	Adrenoleukodystrophy

While most pediatric transplants and CAR T-cell-directed therapies are performed at tertiary care centers, patients receive a portion of their care in community hospitals and local oncologists' offices. It is important for the pediatric hospitalist to have a general understanding of the medical issues facing HSCT and post CAR T cell patients who may present to their emergency departments or get admitted to inpatient units.

HEMATOPOIETIC STEM CELL TRANSPLANT

BACKGROUND

HSCT is the process of replacing diseased or dysfunctional bone marrow with stem cells capable of restoring normal hematopoietic function and immune reconstitution. The three main types of HSCT are autologous, allogeneic, and syngeneic. In autologous HSCT, stem cells are collected from the patient and stored until the time of infusion. *Autologous* transplant has the advantages of being readily available for current and future transplants if needed, eliminating the risk of graft-versus-host disease (GVHD), more rapid immune reconstitution, and lower short-term mortality rates. High-dose chemotherapy followed by autologous stem cell infusion (often called rescue) is used to treat children with some high-stage or relapsed solid tumors, and is employed in gene therapy transplants.

In *allogeneic* HSCT, stem cells are collected from another person and infused into the patient following conditioning with chemotherapy and/or radiation. A *syngeneic* HSCT is a transplant using the patient's identical twin sibling as a donor. The benefits of allogeneic transplants are that there is no risk of residual tumor cells in the graft, the stem cells have not been potentially damaged by prior therapy, and the cells may exhibit a graft-versus-leukemia effect. Disadvantages include the risk of GVHD, less flexible timing of donation, the need for immunosuppression following engraftment, slower immune reconstitution with increased risk of infection, and greater overall morbidity and mortality.

Human leukocyte antigen (HLA) typing is performed to determine the suitability of potential allogeneic donors. HLAs are genetic markers found on the surface of white blood cells. The genetic composition of these antigens, located on the short arm of chromosome six, is determined from a blood test or buccal swab of the recipient and potential donors. HLAs are inherited, making siblings more likely than unrelated donors or parents to have similar typing. There is an approximate 25% chance of two siblings having matching HLA typing. The closer the HLA match between the donor and the recipient, the lower the risk of GVHD, graft rejection, and better overall survival.

Allogeneic donors may be related to the patient or found through an unrelated donor search. Related donors have the advantages of being more closely HLA-matched, are typically readily available for donation, have lower risk of GVHD or graft failure and have higher survival rates. Unfortunately, only 30% of individuals needing an allogeneic HSCT have a suitably matched sibling, hence most HSCT are performed using unrelated donors. Unrelated allogeneic donors may be less readily available compared to related donors, may be unavailable for potential future transplants or cellular infusions, that is, donor specific lymphocytes (DLI), and may be less well-matched. Higher HLA disparity is associated with increased risk of both GVHD and graft failure.

The National Marrow Donation Program (NMDP) is a nonprofit organization in the United States that anonymously matches unrelated stem cell transplant recipients and donors. Using the NMDP and similar organizations, a suitable stem cell source can be found for approximately 80% of White patients with a transplantable disorder. However, Black, Hispanic, Asian, and Pacific Islander patients, as well as patients with more than one race, have a less than 50% chance of finding a well-matched, unrelated bone marrow or peripheral blood stem cell (PBSC) donor. Alternative donor sources, including umbilical cord blood and haploidentical transplants, are needed for many of these patients.

Sources of stem cells include bone marrow, peripheral blood, and umbilical cord blood (UCB). Bone marrow and umbilical cord blood are rich in stem cells and are the most commonly used stem cell sources for pediatric HSCT. Bone marrow is typically collected under anesthesia and requires no physical pre-donation preparation of the donor. Bone marrow donors undergo confirmatory HLA typing, health assessment, and infectious screening prior to being approved to donate. The process of identifying and clearing a bone marrow donor takes weeks to months.

UCB is removed via cannulation or drainage following delivery of the infant. The blood is stored frozen in public banks as an anonymous donation or in private banks for use by the family. The risk of GVHD is lower with UCB compared with bone marrow or PBSCs. UCB stem cells are naïve compared to bone marrow and PBSCs, hence higher HLA disparity/mismatch at HLA loci is more tolerable with equivalent GVHD risk compared to the other stem cell sources. This has increased the ability to find a suitable stem cell source for patients for whom fully matched unrelated bone marrow or PBSC donors are not found/available in international registries. Another advantage is the rapid availability of the stem cell product. Clinical challenges with the use of UCB is that the stem cell yield is limited to what is collected at birth, a single unit may not be adequate for adults or large children, there may be lack of complete medical follow-up on the child who donated the UCB, and immune reconstitution is slower compared to other stem cell sources.

Peripheral blood has a low concentration of circulating stem cells. Chemotherapy or stimulating factors are used to mobilize stem cells from the bone marrow into the peripheral circulation. Chemotherapy with or without stimulating factors is commonly given to autologous donors prior to PBSC collection as part of treatment of their underlying disease. Granulocyte colony stimulating factor (G-CSF) or granulocyte-macrophage colony-stimulating factor (GM-CSF) are given to allogeneic PBSC donors to release the stem cells from their niche and into the peripheral blood prior to collection. PBSCs are removed via apheresis through large peripheral intravenous access or central venous line. Advantages of using PBSCs are more rapid neutrophil and immune recovery, potentially greater graft-versus-leukemia effect, and less invasive collection procedure for the donor without the need for anesthesia. The primary disadvantage of using PBSC is the greater risk of chronic GVHD. In pediatrics the use of PBSC is associated with greater risk of chronic GVHD, increased mortality, without reducing relapse rate. As a result, it is a less favored stem cell source in pediatrics.

TRANSPLANT PROCEDURE

Prior to receiving stem cells, patients receive a conditioning regimen consisting of chemotherapy or chemotherapy with radiation. Patients are admitted to the hospital prior to conditioning and typically remain hospitalized until neutrophil engraftment, though some centers allow discharge prior to engraftment following autologous stem cell infusion. The duration of admission varies depending on the type of transplant, graft source, and possible complications. The purposes of conditioning are to create marrow space for the transplanted cells, eliminate diseased marrow cells when applicable, and remove host lymphocytes capable of rejecting the transplanted cells. The specific conditioning protocol used depends on the disease being treated and the practices of the transplanting institution. Commonly used myeloablative conditioning regimens include one or more of the following: cyclophosphamide, total body irradiation (TBI), busulfan, treosulfan, carboplatin, melphalan, etoposide, and carmustine. Toxicities common to many conditioning regimens are myelosuppression, nausea, emesis, mucositis (inflammation, irritation, and ulceration of oral and gastrointestinal mucosal cells), alopecia, increased risk of infection, organ dysfunction, and infertility. A detailed discussion of specific conditioning agents and their toxicities is beyond the scope of this chapter.

Patients receive supportive care in the forms of blood product transfusions, anti-emetics, analgesia, nutritional supplementation, antimicrobial agents, and other therapies targeted at individual toxicities. Select groups of patients receive growth factors (G-CSF or GM-CSF) following the stem cell infusion, again depending on the underlying disease, type of transplant, and the graft source.

Once conditioning is completed, stem cells are infused through a central venous line. This can be done by manual injection or by a pump similar to a blood transfusion. The day that the stem cells are infused is called "day zero." The days prior to day zero are referred to as "minus" days and the days following the transplant are referred to as "plus" days. For example, the day prior to stem cell infusion is considered day minus one, and the day following transplant is day plus one. This sets the stage and allows providers to anticipate complications that may arise, as many of the expected post-transplant toxicities can be caught early if watched for. The time from stem cell infusion to engraftment (defined as an absolute neutrophil count of 500/mm^3 for three consecutive days) can be a medically complex period. Patients are at risk for significant complications in addition to the expected toxicities of the conditioning and GVHD prevention regimen. Patients are profoundly immunosuppressed and at risk for severe, potentially life-threatening infections. They commonly experience mucositis requiring narcotic analgesia and the need for supplemental nutrition as the immense pain reduces their ability to take anything by mouth. Nausea and emesis remain a significant problem during this period, exacerbated by mucositis and the paralytic effects of narcotics on the gastrointestinal tract. Other less common, but important medical issues during this period are veno-occlusive disease (VOD) of the liver, transplant associated thrombotic microangiopathy (TA-TMA), GVHD organ dysfunction and failure, noninfectious pulmonary complications, and life-threatening bleeding.

Discharge criteria vary across institutions. However, discharge typically occurs following engraftment, once all acute medical issues resolve and the child tolerates enteral medications and is able to maintain an adequate hydration status at home. After hospital discharge, patients require close monitoring and are seen frequently in an outpatient HSCT clinic. The frequency of visits is dictated by the patient's condition and decreases as their clinical status improves. Patients are followed annually for an indefinite period to monitor for post-HSCT late effects.

GRAFT-VERSUS-HOST DISEASE

GVHD is a significant cause of morbidity and mortality in HSCT patients. It can present with either subtle or fulminant symptoms at any time following transplant. It is important that the pediatric hospitalist caring for HSCT patients has an understanding of the disease and its varied presentations. GVHD is a T-cell-mediated immunoreactive process in which donor cells react against recipient cells resulting in end organ and tissue damage. Tissue damage is caused by direct cytolysis and by the effects of inflammatory cytokines such as TNF-α, IL-6, and IL-10. Acute GVHD is an inflammatory process and commonly occurs in the first 100 days after transplant. While chronic GVHD may have elements of inflammation, it is also characterized by scarring and fibrosis. Chronic GVHD typically occurs after day (+)100. Risk factors for both acute and chronic GVHD are HLA mismatch between the host and the donor, the type of GVHD prophylaxis used, the use of PBSC as the stem cell source, increased age of donor and recipient, parity in female donors, and the presence of T-lymphocytes in the stem cell infusion. Additional risk factors described for chronic GVHD are previous acute GVHD, female donors, and the use of total body irradiation during conditioning.

Acute and chronic GVHD differ not only in time of onset, but also in presentation. The skin and gastrointestinal system are frequently affected in both acute and chronic GCHD. The rash seen in acute GVHD can have many different appearances. Acute skin GVHD often first appears as tender, erythematous patches on the palms, soles, occiput, posterior neck, or face. The patient may develop diffuse erythroderma. Severe skin GVHD can blister, ulcerate, and desquamate. Chronic skin GVHD commonly involves larger areas and presents with a dry, pruritic rash, which can progress to sclerodermatous changes. Extensive sclerodermatous GVHD may impair joint mobility and adversely affect quality of life and survival.

Oral changes are also seen in both acute and chronic GVHD. Oral changes may include ulcerative lesions, lichenoid patches, mucoceles, and fibrotic bands. Patients with chronic oral GVHD may develop sicca syndrome with severely dry mouth with the potential for salivary gland atrophy. The presence of GVHD is associated with increased risk of secondary malignancies, and patients should be followed by an oral medicine specialist familiar with oral cancers.

Acute gastrointestinal (GI) GVHD can affect any portion of the GI tract as well as the liver. The gold standard diagnostic tool is biopsy revealing cellular necrosis, glandular dropout, and apoptosis. However, the condition is often diagnosed clinically. Anorexia, nausea, emesis, weight loss, and abdominal pain are symptoms of upper GI GVHD. Lower GI GVHD presents with profuse, watery or bloody diarrhea, abdominal cramping, and anorexia. Severe lower tract GI GVHD may present with ileus. Abnormalities of cholestasis are the hallmarks of hepatic acute

TABLE 134-2 Signs and Symptoms of Graft-Versus-Host Disease

Acute
Erythematous rash on palms, soles, occiput, face and posterior neck
Bullous skin eruption with peeling skin
Oral ulceration and inflammation
Nausea, vomiting
Anorexia, weight loss
Profuse diarrhea, may be bloody
Liver function abnormalities
Jaundice
Chronic
Dry, pruritic diffuse rash
Sclerodermatous skin changes with contractures
Sicca syndrome (dry skin, dry eyes) with possible tooth decay and corneal ulceration
Dysphagia
Abdominal pain
Hyperbilirubinemia or transaminitis
Premature graying of hair
Patchy alopecia
Immune dysfunction
Bronchiolitis obliterans with organizing pneumonia
Genital or urinary stricture

and chronic GVHD, though transaminitis may be observed. Chronic GI GVHD is less common than acute. It presents with similar symptoms as acute (diarrhea, abdominal pain, nausea, emesis, weight loss, dysphagia, and early satiety). Histologically, chronic GVHD appears more fibrotic with crypt distortion. Other signs and symptoms of acute and chronic GVHD are listed in **Table 134-2**.

All patients undergoing allogeneic stem cell transplant receive GVHD prophylaxis. Immune modulation may include T-cell depletion of the stem cell product or the use of immunosuppressive medications. Methotrexate, calcineurin inhibitors, mycophenylate mofetil, rapamycin, and corticosteroids are commonly used prophylactic agents. The regimen used depends on the patient's risk factors for GVHD, type of transplant, graft source, and the practices of the transplanting institution. Allogenic stem cell transplant patients remain on immunosuppressive drug therapy for months following HSCT, even with no evidence of acute or chronic GVHD. Immunosuppressive drugs are tapered off over a period of weeks to months determined by the clinical situation. Patients post HSCT do not typically require life-long immune suppression.

Corticosteroid therapy is first-line treatment for acute and chronic GVHD. Additional and second-line therapies are directed at specific symptoms, and practices differ between institutions, however recently ruxolitinib, a selected Janus Kinase inhibitor, received FDA approval as a second-line agent. Patients with evidence of GVHD may remain on immunosuppressive therapy for years. In these cases, the clinician attempts to maintain the patient on the lowest dose of therapy that controls the patient's disease. In addition to immunosuppressive therapy, these patients receive prophylactic antiviral, antifungal, and antibacterial prophylaxis, to prevent opportunistic infections while on immune suppression. All patients with chronic GVHD should be considered functionally asplenic and receive appropriate therapy when febrile and as prophylaxis. Additionally, the patient should receive regular screening for long-term complications of immunosuppression and of GVHD. This should include routine evaluation by oral medicine and dermatologic specialists familiar with GVHD and secondary cancers. In addition, patients should undergo screening for skeletal, endocrinologic, cardiac, pulmonary, ophthalmologic, and reproductive health.

FEVER AND INFECTIONS

Infection is a significant cause of morbidity and mortality in HSCT patients. Profound immunosuppression, breakdown of the mucosal barriers, indwelling central lines, and disruption of skin integrity contribute to the infectious risk for patients during the acute transplant hospitalization. During the HSCT hospitalization, patients are placed on infectious prophylaxis and are isolated either in a hospital room or on the transplant floor, depending on air filtration and hospital policy. Bacterial, fungal, and viral prophylaxis are commonly given, and specific agents used differ between institutions. Trimethoprim-sulfamethoxazole or other agent for pneumocystis coverage is mandatory for all patients.

Fever and symptoms of potential infection during the inpatient hospitalization and post-transplant period are very common and warrant evaluation. Patients presenting to an emergency department should be moved to a private examination room as soon as possible. Patients should not spend time in a waiting room due to the risk of acquiring infections through exposure to patients in the waiting room. "Reverse" precautions should be observed (i.e., care provider wears a mask, protective gown, and gloves). All febrile HSCT patients require a meticulous physical exam. Special attention should be given to the skin, perirectal tissue, neurologic exam, and CVL site, when applicable. Rectal temperatures and rectal examinations **should not** be performed because of the risk of introducing infection. Blood cultures should be drawn from all central venous lines, or peripherally if lines are no longer present. Lumbar puncture in not routinely indicated for febrile HSCT patients unless specific signs or symptoms consistent with meningitis or encephalitis are present. A chest radiograph is recommended for any patient with respiratory symptoms. Broad-spectrum antibiotics should be started as soon as possible, with a goal of within 60 minutes of presentation. The start of antimicrobial therapy should not be delayed for diagnostic procedures including blood culture or lumbar puncture if there is difficulty obtaining the sample. Hospital admission for febrile HSCT patients depends on the time since transplant, degree of immunosuppression, central line in place, and the presence of post-transplant complications. Most allogeneic transplant recipients within a year of their transplant will need to be admitted for any episode of fever, particularly if remaining on immunosuppressive drugs. Hospitalization and the choice of antimicrobial therapy should be discussed with the HSCT team.

CAR T CELL THERAPY

BACKGROUND

The first experience reported using CAR T cells against B ALL was in 2013. T cells are collected from the patient, then genetically engineered to display receptor proteins to target specific antigens, such as CD19 for B ALL. Once collected the T cell are expanded and then transduced with CAR using either a retroviral or lentiviral vector. These receptors can both bind to antigen and activate the T cell.

Once engineered, which can take several weeks, patients undergo lymphodepletion chemo-therapy prior to CAR T cell infusion. This gives the engineered CAR T cells an advantage to expand and upregulate cytokines without competition from other lymphocytes. These cells can then migrate and target B cells anywhere including extramedullary sites such as central nervous system (CNS) and testes.

CYTOKINE RELEASE SYNDROME (CRS)

CAR T cell expansion can result in systemic inflammation with the rise of cytokines known as cytokine release syndrome (CRS) with or without neurologic manifestation known as immune effector cell associated neurotoxicity syndrome (ICANS). Evolving CRS can present similar to sepsis and should be treated with broad spectrum antibiotics. To establish a diagnosis of CRS, patient must have a fever of >38.0°C, along with other criteria listed in **Table 134-3**.

The American Society for Transplantation and Cell Therapy (ASTCT) defines CRS as a "supraphysiologic response following any immune therapy that results in the activation or engagement of endogenous or infused T cell and/or other immune effector cells. Symptoms can be progressive, must include fever at the onset and may include hypotension, capillary leak and end organ dysfunction." High disease burden and high CAR T Cell dose are associated with increased risk of CRS and ICANS. Increased T cell expansion leads to a rise in cytokines such as interferon gamma (IFNγ), interleukin-6 (IL-6),

TABLE 134-3 Signs and Symptoms of CRS and ICANS

CRS
Fever (required for diagnosis), fatigue, myalgia, malaise
Tachycardia, hypotension
Increased work of breathing, hypoxia
Diarrhea, nausea, abdominal pain
Transaminitis, hyperbilirubinemia, abnormal coagulation (Clotting or bleeding)
Acute kidney injury (AKI)
ICANS
Headaches (HA)
Increased lethargy, somnolence
Altered mental status
Memory loss
Tremors, weakness, seizures
Aphasia, intracranial bleeding, coma

granulocyte-macrophage colony-stimulating factor (GM-CSF), tumor necrosis factor (TNF), and interleukin-10 (IL-10), leading to exponential systemic inflammation.

CRS, unlike ICANS, can be treated. Tocilizumab, an IL-6 receptor antagonist, binds to IL-6 receptors and prevents IL-6 from binding to the reception site and promoting further cytokine release and inflammation. Other treatments targeting different pathways contributing to CRS are seen in **Figure 134-1**. If possible, systemic steroids should be avoided, as that would render the infused engineered T cells unable to function. One of the more readily available and least invasive markers to test the presence of CAR T cells and possible sign of continued remission is the presence of B cell aplasia. The use of CAR T-cell-targeted therapies have opened new doors to opportunities that showcase promising results for the future.

VACCINATION

Autologous and allogeneic HSCT recipients lose immunologic memory responses to most vaccinations. Thus, patients need to be revaccinated after transplant. The timing of revaccination differs among transplant institutions, though there are international recommendations from multiple organizations. Clinicians evaluating HSCT transplant patients should be aware of the patient's vaccination status and remain alert for unusual infections. Live vaccines should be avoided in any patient receiving immunosuppression and for a minimum of 2 years after transplant.

MEDICATION CONSIDERATIONS

HSCT patients are frequently on multiple medications which may interact with other drugs, including immunosuppressants, antimicrobials, and antiepileptics. Because of the potential for drug-drug interaction it is important to review medication lists with a pharmacist or other knowledgeable source before adding a new agent. This is also important when considering a dose change of a medication a patient is already taking. In addition to interacting with other drugs, some common medications are known to cause decreased blood counts due to either marrow suppression or peripheral destruction. These drugs should be avoided if possible. The primary transplant team can provide assistance in choosing appropriate medications for these patients.

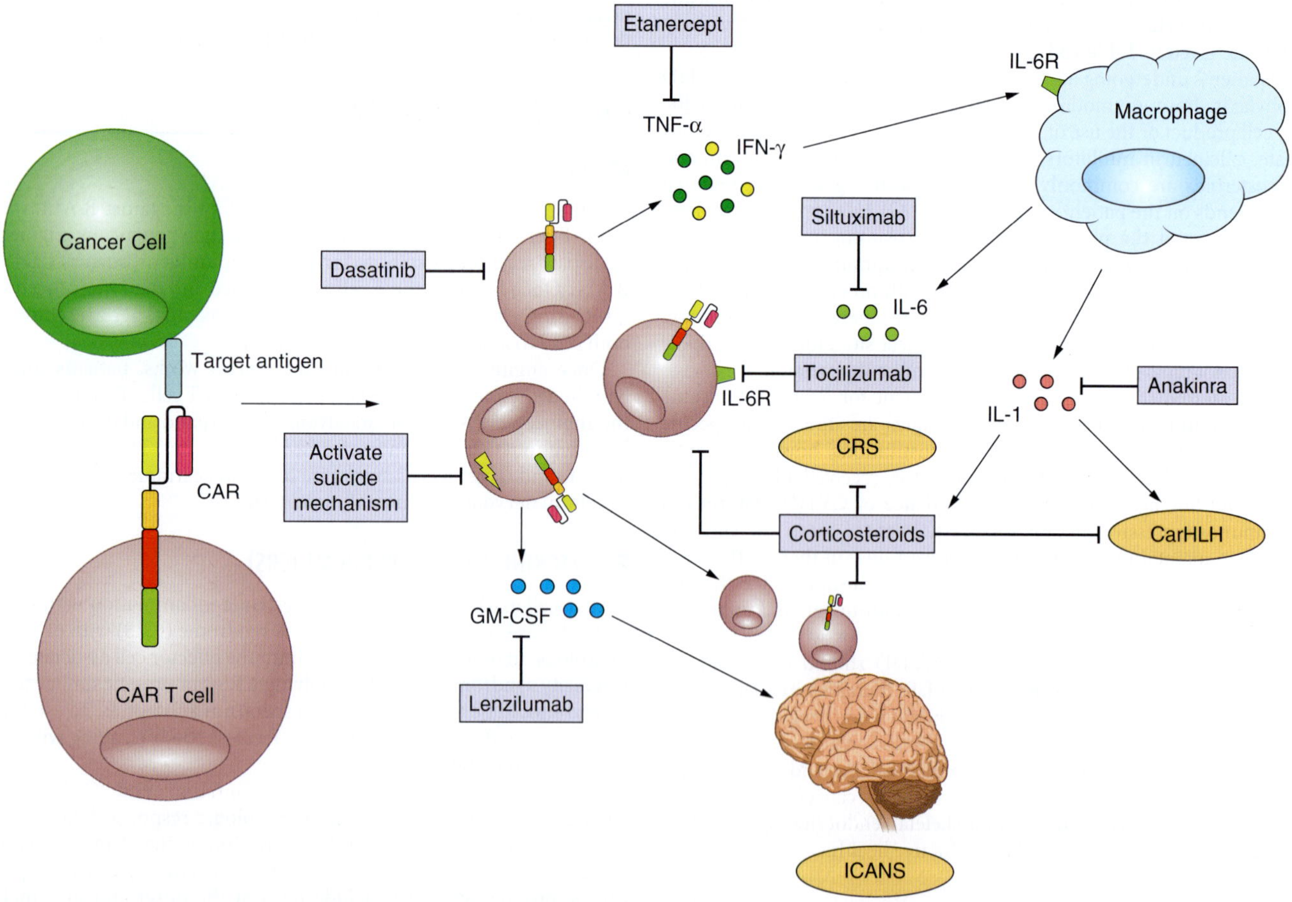

FIGURE 134-1. Mechanisms of toxicty and pathways for interventions. CAR T cells proliferate and expand resulting in pro-inflammatory cytokine production and activation of other immune cells. The penetration of these Inflammatory cytokines and CAR T cells into the central nervous system can promote ICANS or other neurologic sequle. There are multple pathways (pink boxes) which can be targeted to block further inflammation and progression of CRS. (Reproduced from Baumeister SHC, Mohan GS, Eihaddad A, Lehmann L. Cytokine Release Syndrome and Associated acute toxicities in pediatric patients undergoing immune effector cell therapy or hematopoietic cell transplantation. *Front Oncol.* 2022;12:841117.)

CONCLUSION

Patients who have undergone stem cell transplantation often are cared for in local community settings after their transplant. Pediatric hospitalists may be involved in the evaluation and treatment of these patients for both routine and acute post-transplant issues. Therefore, it is essential to have insight into the particular risks of this group of patients. This group of patients is at heightened risk for common and uncommon infections, and always require prompt and thorough evaluation and initiation of treatment. Communication with the patient's transplant center is crucial. The hospitalist needs to be informed of the patient's often complex history, and pediatric hospitalists should discuss management decisions with the primary transplant center.

HSCT is a rapidly changing field. The focus of much clinical development is on reducing the toxicity of the transplant process. This includes but is not limited to developing and improving non-ablative transplants, creating less immunosuppressive treatment strategies for GVHD, and decreasing the length of hospitalization. These and other developments would enable transplants to be extended to more diverse patient populations.

SUGGESTED READINGS

Arai S, Klingemann HG. Hematopoietic stem cell transplantation: bone marrow vs. mobilized peripheral blood. *Arch Med Res.* 2003;34: 545-553.

Baumeister, S.H.C, Mohan, G S., Eihaddad, A, et al. Cytokine release syndrome and associated acute toxicities in pediatric patients undergoing immune effector cell therapy or hematopoietic cell transplantation. *Front Oncol.* 2022;12:841117

Blazar BR, Murphy WJ. Bone marrow transplantation and approaches to avoid graft-versus-host disease (GVHD). *Philos Trans R Soc Lond B Biol Sci.* 2005;360:1747-1767.

Busca A, Amoroso A, Miniero R. Bone marrow transplantation from unrelated volunteer donors. An overview. *Panminerva Med.* 1997;39:71-77.

Cutler C, Ballen KK. Improving outcomes in umbilical cord blood transplantation: state of the art. *Blood Rev.* 2012;26:241-246.

Eapen M, Horowitz MM, Klein JP, et al. Higher mortality after allogeneic peripheral-blood transplantation compared with bone marrow in children and adolescents: the Histocompatibility and Alternate Stem Cell Source Working Committee of the International Bone Marrow Transplant Registry. *J Clin Oncol.* 2004;22:4872-4880.

Ferrara JL, Yanik G. Acute graft versus host disease: pathophysiology, risk factors, and prevention strategies. *Clin Adv Hematol Oncol.* 2005;3:415-419, 28.

Hilgendorf I, Freund M, Jilg W, et al. Vaccination of allogeneic haematopoietic stem cell transplant recipients: report from the international consensus conference on clinical practice in chronic GVHD. *Vaccine.* 2011;29:2825-2833.

Johns A. Overview of bone marrow and stem cell transplantation. *J Intraven Nurs.* 1998;21:356-360.

Lee DW, Gardner R, Porter DL, et al. Current concepts in the diagnosis and management of cytokine release syndrome. *Blood.* 2014;124(2): 188-95.

Lee DW, Santomasso BD, Locke FL, et al. ASTCT Consensus Grading for cytokine release syndrome and neurologic toxicity associated with immune effector cells. *Biol Blood Marrow Transplant.* 2019;25(4): 625-638.

Martin PJ, Carpenter PA, Sanders JE, Flowers ME. Diagnosis and clinical management of chronic graft-versus-host disease. *Int J Hematol.* 2004;79:221-228.

McCluskey J, Peh CA. The human leucocyte antigens and clinical medicine: an overview. *Rev Immunogenet.* 1999;1:3-20.

Neelapu SS, Tummala S, Kebriaei P, et al. Chimeric antigen receptor T-cell therapy-assessment and management of toxicities. *Nat Rev Clin Oncol.* 2018;15(1):47-62.

Pidala J, Kim J, Schell M, et al. Race/ethnicity affects the probability of finding an HLA-A, -B, -C and DRB1 allele-matched unrelated donor and likelihood of subsequent transplant utilization. *Bone Marrow Transplant.* 2013;48:346-350.

Saba N, Abraham R, Keating A. Overview of autologous stem cell transplantation. *Crit Rev Oncol Hematol.* 2000;36:27-48.

SECTION O
Psychiatry

CHAPTER 135 Mood and Anxiety Disorders

Katherine S. Spencer, PsyD, HSP and
Alison C. Herndon, MD, MSPH

BACKGROUND

The number of children and adolescents diagnosed with mental health disorders has increased dramatically in recent years with a rising volume presenting to children's hospitals. This trend has been exacerbated by the COVID-19 pandemic and led to a joint declaration of a national emergency in pediatric mental health by the American Academy of Pediatrics (AAP), American Academy of Child and Adolescent Psychiatry (AACAP), and Children's Hospital Association (CHA) in October 2021. The landscape of practice has changed such that pediatric hospitalists must recognize and feel comfortable managing children and adolescents with mental health disorders, whether their patients are admitted for primary physical illnesses or for primary mental health concerns.

Children and adolescents hospitalized for any reason may have feelings of sadness, frustration, irritability, or anxiety that represent a normal response to their experience. Children experience disruption of daily routine, separation from family and peers, uncertainty regarding diagnosis and/or prognosis, pain and discomfort related to the illness or its treatment, and fear of the illness or its sequelae. Children with chronic illness have increased risk of psychosocial challenges, depression, and anxiety. There is even greater vulnerability for children with preexisting mental health or developmental disorders or who have parents with mental illness. Hospitalized children may also experience exacerbation of preexisting mental health symptoms. The hospitalist must feel comfortable distinguishing normal feelings from underlying mental health disorders and also managing patients requiring admission for a primary mental health crisis. The purpose of this chapter is to provide the pediatric hospitalist with a framework for understanding the diagnosis and treatment of common mood and anxiety disorders.

CLINICAL PRESENTATION

In the acute medical setting, mood and anxiety disorders can interfere with hospital course, exacerbate medical symptoms (e.g., pain, gastrointestinal discomfort, sleep problems), and at times contribute to difficulty with medical adherence. Children and adolescents with mood or anxiety disorders have greater risk of poor future health, higher levels of pain, decline in physical, social, and general developmental functioning, poor adherence to treatment regimens, reduced immune function, increased disease severity, and risk of suicide attempts. There also appears to be a bidirectional relationship between biological and psychological factors in medical conditions, such as irritable bowel syndrome and pain.

ANXIETY DISORDERS

Anxiety disorders are the most common psychiatric illnesses affecting children and adolescents. These include disorders with common features of excessive fear, anxiety, and related behavioral disturbances, and differ from one another based on the source of threat and associated thoughts and behaviors (**Table 135-1**). Symptoms of anxiety disorder include surges of autonomic arousal and cautious or avoidant behaviors. Caregivers often refer to their anxious children as "sensitive," "self-conscious," "shy," "rigid," "homesick," or "perfectionistic."

Restlessness, stomachaches, palpitations, muscle tension, sweating, shaking, tingling, chest pain, insomnia, and hot flashes or chills are common somatic complaints. Children may have somatic symptoms before or during a feared situation (i.e., medical procedure, school) but may not complain about these same symptoms at other times (i.e., when playing a game or when on a vacation). When children have anxiety and are unable to avoid fears, they may escalate and appear agitated or become aggressive.

TABLE 135-1 General Overview of Anxiety and Related Disorders

Disorder	Description
Anxiety Disorders	
Generalized anxiety disorder	Excessive and difficult to control worry and general feeling of dread with uncontrollability of a number of events. Children constantly seek reassurance, have disrupted sleep, fatigue, restlessness, poor focus due to worries.
Panic disorder	Fear of panic attacks and their consequences, avoids places or activities related to panic attacks sensations. Panic attacks are an unexpected, abrupt surge of intense fear or discomfort, including physical symptoms (e.g., palpitations, sweating, shortness of breath, dizziness) and cognitive symptoms (i.e., fear of losing control or dying)
Separation anxiety	Excessive fear or worry about losing major attachment figures or untoward events that will cause separation. Co-sleeps, follows caregiver around home, avoids activities that cause separation (i.e., school, camp).
Agoraphobia	Fear of places where immediate escape may be embarrassing or difficult. Marked fear or anxiety outside of the home, in public spaces, in lines, crowds, in enclosed or open spaces.
Social phobia	Fear of humiliation, scrutiny, or embarrassment by peers. Anxiety about 1 or more social situations in which the individual is exposed to possible scrutiny by peers. Avoids eye contact, struggles to initiate conversation.
Specific phobia	Marked fear and avoidance of a specific object or situation (e.g., insects, heights, needles, weather, loud sounds). Children may express this by tantrums, freezing, or clinging.
Obsessive-Compulsive Disorders*	
	Presence of obsessions or compulsions. Obsessions are recurrent persistent thoughts, urges, or images that are experienced as intrusive and unwanted. Compulsions are repetitive behaviors or mental acts that an individual is driven to perform, often in response to an obsession or rigidly applied rules.
Trauma and Stress-Related Disorders*	
	Posttraumatic stress disorder (PTSD). Development of characteristic symptoms following exposure to an actual or threatened death, serious injury, or sexual violence.

*Both obsessive compulsive and related disorders and posttraumatic stress disorder were removed from the anxiety disorders chapter in the DSM-5.

Source: Derived from American Psychiatric Association. *Diagnostic and Statistical Manual of Mental Disorders*. 5th ed. Arlington, VA: American Psychiatric Association; 2013.

TABLE 135-2 Mood Disorders

Depressive Disorders	Bipolar and Related Disorders
Disruptive mood dysregulation disorder	Bipolar I disorder
Major depressive disorder	Bipolar II disorder
Persistent depressive disorder (Dysthymia)	Cyclothymic disorder
Premenstrual dysphoric disorder	Substance/medical induced bipolar disorder
Substance/medical induced depressive disorder	Bipolar disorder and related disorder due to another medical condition
Depressive disorder due to another medical condition	

Source: Derived from American Psychiatric Association. *Diagnostic and Statistical Manual of Mental Disorders*. 5th ed. Arlington, VA: American Psychiatric Association; 2013.

MOOD DISORDERS

Mood disorders include depressive disorders and bipolar and related disorders (see **Table 135-2**). Depressive disorders differ in terms of duration, timing, and presumed etiology. Bipolar and related disorders differ in terms of type of most recent mood episode, severity of manic or hypomanic symptoms, and frequency of mood shifts.

Psychological symptoms of depression in children and adolescents include dysphoric mood, irritability, anhedonia, feelings of helplessness or hopelessness, feelings of guilt or worthlessness, loss of self-esteem, decreased ability to concentrate, and thoughts of suicide. Somatic symptoms of depression include fatigue, sleep disturbance (insomnia or hypersomnia), appetite changes (decrease or increase), and motor restlessness or retardation.

The presentation of mood disorders depends largely on the child's developmental level. Signs of depression in young children (or with developmental delay) may include sad mood, depressed affect, somatic complaints (most commonly stomachaches and headaches), separation anxiety, low self-esteem, social withdrawal, academic decline, sleep or appetite disturbances, decreased concentration, and suicidal thoughts. In adolescents, depression frequently presents with an irritable rather than a depressed mood. Adolescents commonly experience motor hyperactivity, feelings of being unloved or misunderstood, self-deprecation, tearfulness, hopelessness, low self-esteem, hypersomnia, lethargy, anhedonia, weight gain, decreased concentration, declining school performance, psychomotor retardation, and suicidal ideation. Adolescents frequently do not recognize their symptoms as being part of a depressive disorder and may not report them unless specifically asked.

Primary symptoms of bipolar and related disorders include recurrent and cycling depression and mania or hypomania that often emerge in adolescence and early adulthood. Bipolar and related disorders vary in polarity, cyclicity, frequency, and status between episodes. Primary symptoms include at least 1 week of abnormally and persistently elevated, expansive, or irritable mood and abnormally and persistently increased goal-directed activity or energy, with symptoms of inflated self-esteem, decreased need for sleep, more talkative or pressured speech, flight of ideas or racing thoughts, distractibility, psychomotor agitation or increased goal-directed activity, and excessive involvement in activities with potentially painful consequences. Bipolar disorders can be diagnostically complex due to a significant number of initial mood episodes being depressive. Manic episodes often emerge in adolescence and are less commonly seen in young children. A full manic episode that emerges during antidepressant treatment may indicate a diagnosis of bipolar I disorder.

DIFFERENTIAL DIAGNOSIS

When assessing for a possible diagnosis of a mood or anxiety disorder in the hospitalized child, the provider must first consider the expected developmental response to the situation and/or illness. Hospitalized children and adolescents frequently appear sad, tearful, unmotivated, fearful, and overwhelmed. Acute-onset depressive or worry symptoms may resolve when the stressor is removed (or shortly after) and the patient is able to resume his or her usual routine following discharge from the hospital. Adjustment disorders are often included in differential diagnosis for anxiety and mood disorder. Assessment of timeline of onset of mood or anxiety symptoms (acute or chronic), duration or frequency of symptoms, severity, and interference in overall functioning can often help differentiate the two.

Differential diagnosis of mood and anxiety disorders is complex, and commonly hospitalists rely on their mental health specialist colleagues for specific diagnosis. In addition to comparison between disorder categories (e.g., mood versus anxiety disorder), comparisons are made within diagnostic categories (e.g., generalized versus social anxiety disorder). Attention-deficit hyperactivity disorder (ADHD) is often included in the differential with anxiety and mood disorders due to shared symptoms of distractibility and low frustration tolerance. Other considerations include trauma-related disorders such as posttraumatic stress disorder (see Chapter 140), psychotic disorders, and personality disorders.

When evaluating symptoms of bipolar and related disorders, it is very important to consider family psychiatric history. A child of a parent with bipolar disorder has over 10 times higher risk of this disorder. Differential diagnosis of bipolar disorders involves consideration of last mood episode, frequency, and severity. Individuals with past manic episodes can meet criteria for major depressive disorder, and major depressive episode with prominent irritable mood may be difficult to distinguish from manic or mixed mood episodes. When considering diagnosis of bipolar disorder, also consider ruling out anxiety disorders, stress and trauma-related disorders, substance/medication-induced symptoms, ADHD, personality disorders, and other disorders with significant irritability.

Additional diagnoses for depressive disorders, bipolar disorders, and anxiety disorders include substance/medication-induced disorder and disorder due to another medical condition. For more specific information and diagnosis criteria for mental health disorders, please refer to the Diagnostic and Statistical Manual of Mental Health disorders Fifth Edition (DSM-5). Differentiating a primary psychiatric disorder from one related to a general medical condition or substance requires close consideration of the temporal relationship between the onset, exacerbation, or remission of the mood disturbance and the medical disorder; medication; or drug of abuse. Certain medical conditions, medications, and drugs of abuse may be associated with depressive or anxiety symptoms and should be considered in the differential diagnosis (**Table 135-3**).

DIAGNOSTIC EVALUATION

When the hospitalist suspects a mood or anxiety disorder, consultation by a psychiatrist or psychologist should be obtained if available. If unavailable, the hospitalist can further assess a child's history and symptoms to clarify diagnosis and then support a treatment plan. A strong assessment of a child or adolescent with mood or anxiety disorder includes a thorough chart review, a mental status examination, a HEEADSSS examination, and assessment of the psychological and somatic symptoms of the mood and anxiety disorder. The mental status examination should include appearance, affect, mood, behavior (engagement with others, vocalization/verbalization, social interaction, any odd behaviors), suicidal or homicidal ideation, presence of auditory or visual hallucinations, and thought disorder (e.g., hallucinations, delusions). The HEEADSSS examination includes a series of questions about Home, Education/employment, Eating, Activities, Drugs, Sexuality, Suicidality, and Safety to help providers assess risk-taking behaviors. The hospitalist should also inquire about past individual and family psychiatric histories, social/peer relationships, family relationships, current or past history of trauma, and other psychosocial stressors. History of coping with prior hospitalization, illness, or injury may also be helpful information to obtain.

While not always possible, it can be particularly beneficial to meet with the patient and his or her parents or guardians both separately and together. Unique to the hospital setting, the hospitalist can also obtain details and observations from bedside staff related to current identified concerns.

It is important to assess for past and current suicidal ideation as suicidal ideation and suicide attempts may be tragic consequences of depression and anxiety. If there is any concern about suicide, a risk

TABLE 135-3 Common Medical and Pharmacologic Causes of Anxiety and Depression Symptoms

ANXIETY				
Endocrine	**Infectious**	**Neurologic**	**Medications**	**Other**
Hyperthyroidism	Encephalitis	Migraine	Stimulants	Illicit drugs: cocaine, lysergic acid diethylamide (LSD), methamphetamine, phencyclidine (PCP)
Hyperparathyroidism	HIV/AIDS	Post-concussive syndrome	Formulations that include caffeine	Alcohol
Diabetes mellitus	Hepatitis C	Traumatic brain injury	Short-acting beta agonists	Withdrawal (alcohol, benzodiazepines)
Pheochromocytoma	Cytomegalovirus	Encephalopathy	Corticosteroids	Asthma
Cushing disease	Varicella-zoster virus	Guillain-Barre	Levothyroxine	Inflammatory bowel disease
Hypoglycemia	Group A Strep		Antiepileptics	Cardiac dysrhythmia
	Respiratory infections causing SOB		Decongestants (pseudoephedrine)	SLE
	MIS-C		Antihistamines	Electrolyte disturbance
			Antidepressants (bupropion)	Sleep apnea
			Nicotine	
DEPRESSION				
Endocrine	**Infectious**	**Neurologic**	**Medications**	**Other**
Diabetes mellitus	Encephalitis	Epilepsy	Benzodiazepines	Drug abuse and withdrawal (cocaine, amphetamines, opiates)
Cushing disease	Hepatitis	Multiple sclerosis	Corticosteroids	Alcohol abuse
Hypothyroidism	Pneumonia	TBI	Oral contraceptives	Electrolyte abnormalities
Addison disease	Mononucleosis	Sleep apnea	Anticonvulsants	Anemia
Hypopituitarism	AIDS	Cerebrovascular accident	Antihypertensives	Failure to thrive
Parathyroid disorders (hyper- and hypo-)	Chronic fatigue syndrome	Huntington disease	Aminophylline	Lupus erythematosus
	Neurosyphilis	Hydrocephalus	Clonidine	Wilson disease
	MIS-C	Migraine	Ibuprofen	Uremia
		Neoplasm	Ampicillin	Porphyria
			Tetracycline	
			Sulfonamides	
			C-Asparaginase	
			Azathioprine	
			Bleomycin	
			Vincristine	
			Cimetidine	
			Interferon	

Sources: Wise MG, Rundell JR. *Concise Guide to Consultation Psychiatry*. Washington, DC: American Psychiatric Press; 1988; Martin A, Volkmar FR, Block MH. *Lewis's Child and Adolescent Psychiatry: A Comprehensive Textbook*. Wolters Kluwer, 2017; Skuse, D. et al. Child Psychology and Psychiatry: Frameworks for Clinical Training and Practice. John Wiley & Sons, Incorporated, 2017; Lexicomp Online, Pediatric and Neonatal Lexi-Drugs Online. Waltham, MA; UpToDate, Inc.; various websites including https://reference.medscape.com, https://www.uptodate.com.

assessment should be conducted to determine the history of previous suicide attempts, family history of suicide, exposure to family violence or abuse, level of impulsivity, access to lethal means, and presence of comorbid psychiatric disorders. For patients deemed at risk for suicide, one-to-one observation should be implemented to monitor the patient at all times until the patient is no longer at high risk of suicide or is transferred to a psychiatric hospital (see Chapter 136, Assessment and Management of the Suicidal Patient).

Diagnostic clarity is important for developing a robust treatment plan and appropriate mental health referrals. Hospitalists may also encounter children with longstanding histories of unrecognized anxiety or mood disorders who are learning of these diagnoses for the first time when symptoms are exacerbated in an acute care setting. Early identification and treatment of mental illness can have a positive impact on child health outcomes.

MANAGEMENT

The management of mood and anxiety disorders in hospitalized children and adolescents requires both an acute intervention in the hospital and a plan for follow-up after discharge, if necessary. If available, a mental health consultant, such as a psychologist or psychiatrist can be helpful to assess, clarify diagnosis, and create treatment recommendations. Bedside staff and family may support implementation of a treatment plan. If available, consultation with social workers, child life specialists, integrative health (e.g., aromatherapy, reiki), and creative arts or movement therapy (i.e., music, art, yoga) may also help. Sadness, irritability, and fear in hospitalized children may be due to unexpressed feelings related to hospitalization, disruption in routine, and loss of control. A combination of psychosocial and behavioral interventions can often help alleviate symptoms without the need for psychotropic medications.

The goal of psychosocial interventions implemented in the hospital setting is to help the patient and family better understand the medical condition and its treatment, and to facilitate coping with the illness and hospitalization. The mental health consultant can help explain medical issues and treatments to children in a developmentally appropriate manner to encourage feelings of mastery and control. Supportive therapy may include engaging younger children in therapeutic play with medical toys and dolls or having older patients create a scrapbook or a mood journal to cope with their feelings related to the illness and hospitalization. Validating a child's emotional experience is a vital component of supportive therapy. Parents should be encouraged to bring special items from home (e.g., favorite blanket, toys, pictures) to help the child feel more comfortable. If possible, the parents can inform the child's teacher to help facilitate contact with friends at school and develop a school plan. Contact with other patients can provide peer support and help the child understand that he or she is not alone; however, this may be limited due to infection prevention and related safety concerns.

Most common evidence-based therapeutic interventions for children and adolescents presenting with anxiety or mood disorders include cognitive behavioral therapy (CBT), dialectical behavioral therapy (DBT), and acceptance and commitment therapy (ACT). These are all skill-focused interventions that can be applied to treatment of individuals, groups, and families. CBT has robust research evidence in pediatric medical conditions, and there is growing evidence for DBT and ACT. Mental health providers can individualize and tailor treatment to the child's developmental level, symptoms, and family context. A psychologist may provide brief consultation services in a hospital or outpatient clinic, or 8 to 12 sessions of treatment outpatient. Duration and format of treatment varies. A growing number of mental health professionals are offering telehealth therapy options; preliminary research suggests similar effectiveness of both telehealth and in-person treatment.

CBT includes a range of techniques that promote identifying, challenging, and modifying maladaptive or negative thoughts and behaviors that interfere with adjustment to and management of the child's medical condition. CBT treatment in a medical setting often involves development of active coping strategies to increase positively reinforcing patterns of behavior (behavioral activation) and creating a daily routine to increase predictability and control in an often stressful environment. The CBT provider can help support engagement in distraction and pleasurable activities, in the form of movies, games, and crafts projects, to help alleviate depressive symptoms. CBT is an effective treatment for mental health conditions including anxiety and mood disorders and medical conditions such as chronic pain, irritable bowel disease, diabetes, chronic fatigue syndrome, headache, and others. Other behavioral techniques such as hypnosis, relaxation, and guided imagery can be helpful adjuncts in the management of somatic symptoms, acute and chronic pain. The Handbook of Cognitive Behavioral Therapy for Pediatric Medical Conditions (2019) offers descriptions of evidence-based practices.

DBT for Chronic Medical Illness (DBT-CMI) has shown preliminary efficacy in children with chronic illness, with significant improvements found in both depression and adherence. DBT is also the therapy of choice for children and teens with treatment-resistant depression, chronic suicidality and self-injury, and other high-risk behaviors.

Acceptance and Commitment Therapy (ACT) has similar efficacy to CBT for teens with anxiety and mood disorders. The main premise of ACT is to reduce rigid thought patterns and avoidance, increase psychological flexibility, be present, and purposefully change behavior in ways consistent with self-defined valued living.

Pharmacology While it is common for hospitalists to encounter children with mood disorders and anxiety in the acute medical setting, we caution against initiating chronic psychotropic medications without special consideration and specific plans for outpatient management. It is important to note that studies are limited regarding the use of psychotropic medications in children or adolescents. As most psychotropic medications take weeks to reach maximal efficacy, the formation of a treatment alliance with the patient and parents is crucial. It is imperative to inform the patient and parents about side effects, dosage schedule, lag in therapeutic efficacy, and danger of overdose for each agent prescribed. Following discharge from the hospital, the parents should be responsible for storing and administering these medications to minimize the risk of overdose. In addition, it is important to establish outpatient psychiatric follow-up to assess efficacy and monitor side effects of new medications. Families and caregivers should be advised of the need for close observation and communication with the prescriber.

Medications such as diphenhydramine or olanzapine are often used for acute anxiety or irritable depression in hospitalized patients. It is generally unnecessary to continue antianxiety medications after discharge. Patients with severe symptoms of depression may warrant a trial of an antidepressant medication and many pediatricians feel comfortable prescribing commonly used antidepressants (i.e., selective serotonin reuptake inhibitors [SSRIs]), although it is recommended to consult psychiatry when considering alternative (non-SSRI) treatments in youth or when considering treatment in youth who have failed first-line agents. Of note, the FDA issued a public health advisory requiring that antidepressant labels carry a black box warning informing patients of an increased risk of suicidal thoughts and behaviors among children and adolescents taking these medications. These potential risks should be discussed with patients and their families as part of the informed consent process and balanced against clinical need. Patients who are started on therapy should be observed closely for clinical worsening, suicidality, or unusual changes in behavior.

ADMISSION AND DISCHARGE CRITERIA

Most hospitalized children who are experiencing mood or anxiety symptoms are admitted for medical reasons; therefore, in most cases, discharge criteria will depend upon sufficient stabilization or improvement in the medical condition that prompted admission. Psychiatric admission criteria are an imminent danger to self or others, often due to suicidal or homicidal ideation or due to severe behavioral dysregulation likely to result in harm to self or others. Such determinations are best made via a psychiatric consultation. Discharge criteria will highly depend upon availability of appropriate psychiatric care and if the child meets criteria for outpatient, intensive outpatient, partial hospital, inpatient hospital, or residential treatment. When available, a mental health professional can be helpful in evaluating and securing appropriate psychiatric disposition.

A comprehensive follow-up treatment plan should be developed for the patient and family before discharge. This may include referrals to mental health providers for outpatient psychotherapy, psychiatry, family therapy, or group therapy. For children and adolescents with severe depression or suicidal ideation, transfer to an inpatient psychiatric unit or enrollment in a partial hospital program may be warranted. If available, at this stage of treatment, a mental health professional should be involved to assist in assessment and disposition planning.

PREVENTION

Pediatric anxiety and mood disorders are burdensome for affected children and families as well as the healthcare system, particularly given the association with chronic illness and future health outcomes. Given the changing landscape of pediatric practice, hospitalists must recognize and feel comfortable managing children and adolescents with mental health disorders, recognize risks related to comorbidity with medical conditions, and if necessary, help connect children and families with resources for evidence-based treatment.

KEY POINTS

- Mood and anxiety disorders are increasingly common comorbidities for children with medical and surgical illness.
- The hospitalist has an important role in both recognizing common mental health symptoms and connecting children to hospital-based and community support.
- Common therapy interventions for youth include CBT, DBT, and ACT. These treatments are evidence based for mood and anxiety disorders and are well studied in several illness groups.
- When prescribing psychotropic medications in an acute medical setting, it is important to also consider nonpharmacological interventions and short-term medication options to address situational concerns.
- If prescribing longer-term psychotropic medication in the hospital setting, take special caution to make specific plans for outpatient management after discharge.

SUGGESTED READINGS

Bitsko RH, Claussen AH, Lichstein J, et al. Mental health surveillance among children - United States, 2013-2019. *MMWR Suppl.* 2022;71(2):1-42.

Chiu A, Falk A, Walkup JT. Anxiety disorders among children and adolescents. *Focus Am Psychiatr Pub.* 2016;14(1):26-33.

Clark MS, Jansen KL, Cloy JA. Treatment of childhood and adolescent depression. *Am Fam Physician.* 2012;86(5):442-448.

Data and statistics on children's mental health. https://www.cdc.gov/childrensmentalhealth/data.html.
Davydow DS, Richardson LP, Zatzick DF, Katon WJ. Psychiatric morbidity in pediatric critical illness survivors: a comprehensive review of the literature. *Arch Pediatr Adolesc Med*. 2010;164(4):377-385.
Evidence Based Practice Resources for Pediatric Conditions: https://pedpsych.org/ebp_resources/.
Evidence Based Therapy Descriptions https://effectivechildtherapy.org/.
Fang S, Ding D. A meta-analysis of the efficacy of acceptance and commitment therapy for children. *J Contextual Behav Sci*. 2020;15:225-234.
Friedberg RD, Paternostro JK, SpringerLink (Online service). Handbook of Cognitive Behavioral Therapy for Pediatric Medical Conditions. 1st ed.:1 online resource (XVII, 466 p.) 24 illus., 11 illus. in color. https://yale.idm.oclc.org/login?URL=https://doi.org/10.1007/978-3-030-21683-2.
Kendall PC. *Child and Adolescent Therapy: Cognitive-Behavioral Procedures*. 4th ed. Guilford Press; 2012:xiv, 538.
Martin As, Scahill L, Kratochvil C. *Pediatric Psychopharmacology: Principles and Practice*. 2nd ed. Oxford University Press; 2011:xxvi, 810.
McCauley E, Berk MS, Asarnow JR, et al. Efficacy of dialectical behavior therapy for adolescents at high risk for suicide: a randomized clinical trial. *JAMA Psychiatry*. 2018;75(8):777-785.
Mehlum L, Ramberg M, Tormoen AJ, et al. Dialectical behavior therapy compared with enhanced usual care for adolescents with repeated suicidal and self-harming behavior: outcomes over a one-year follow-up. *J Am Acad Child Adolesc Psychiatry*. 2016;55(4):295-300.
Mojtabai R, Olfson M, Han B. National trends in the prevalence and treatment of depression in adolescents and young adults. *Pediatrics*. 2016;138(6):e20161878.
Palermo TM. Cognitive-behavioral therapy for chronic pain in children and adolescents. Oxford University Press; 2012:xii, 223.
Plemmons G, Hall M, Doupnik S, et al. Hospitalization for suicide ideation or attempt: 2008-2015. *Pediatrics*. 2018;141(6): e20172426.
Tran L, Mulligan K. A systematic review of self-management interventions for children and adolescents with inflammatory bowel disease. *Inflamm Bowel Dis*. 2019;25(4):685-698.
Trivedi HK, Kershner JD. Practical child and adolescent psychiatry for pediatrics and primary care. Hogrefe; 2009.

CHAPTER 136 Suicide Risk and Prevention

Jennifer Lee, MD, Jennifer L. McLaren, MD, and JoAnna K. Leyenaar, MD, PhD, MPH

BACKGROUND

Suicide is the second leading cause of death in children and adolescents aged 10 to 14 years and the third leading cause of death among individuals aged 15 to 24 years in 2020 (CDC WISQARS data accessed December 2, 2022), with rates increasing over time. In 2019, according to the Youth Risk Behavior Survey, 18.8% of high school-aged youths seriously considered attempting suicide and 15.7% made a plan about how they would attempt suicide. Additionally, 8.9% attempted suicide and 2.5% had a suicide attempt that resulted in an injury, poisoning, or overdose that required medical care. Suicide affects all populations but there are disparities in suicide rates, risk, and care across gender, race, sexual orientation, and socioeconomic status. Boys are more likely than girls to die by suicide but girls have higher rates of suicidal ideation and attempts. Emerging research demonstrates that rates of suicide are high across race and ethnicity, though data regarding multiracial youth are limited. Adolescents who identify as sexual minorities are more likely to attempt suicide compared to heterosexual adolescents.

The COVID-19 pandemic and subsequent disruptions were associated with increases in the proportion of mental health-related emergency department visits among adolescents aged 12 to 17 years, particularly among girls. In this context, global rates of depression and anxiety in children and adolescents have doubled. Several US states saw a rise in adolescent suicides when comparing data from 2015-2019 to 2020. The rising prevalence of mental health concerns led the American Academy of Pediatrics (AAP), the American Academy of Child and Adolescent Psychiatry and the Children's Hospital Association to jointly declare a National State of Emergency in Children's Mental Health in 2021.

With this rapidly shifting landscape, pediatricians should expect to care for patients at risk for suicide in hospital settings. This chapter describes an approach to assessing and managing patients at risk for suicide in the hospital setting.

PATHOPHYSIOLOGY

Suicide is complex and influenced by a combination of genetic, neurobiological, environmental, and psychologic/behavioral factors. Adolescents and children are a unique population with characteristics that may put them at increased risk.

There are a number of risk factors that are associated with suicide, but may not be directly causative. These factors can be classified as individual, relationship, community, and societal level risks. Individual risk factors for suicide include mental illness such as depression, feelings of worthlessness and low self-esteem, prior suicide attempts, self-injurious thoughts and behaviors, social isolation, impulsive or aggressive tendencies, chronic illnesses, and substance use disorder. Self-injurious thoughts and behaviors (SITB), including nonsuicidal self-injury (NSSI), confer risk for future suicidal thoughts and behaviors. While SITB are more prevalent in adolescents compared to younger children, rates of SITB are as high as 15% among preadolescents. Adolescents are prone to impulsivity, which may increase chances of acting on short-lived urges to commit suicide. Neurodevelopmental disabilities, including autism spectrum disorder, may increase risk of suicide in children, which may be under recognized by caregivers of this population.

Relationship risk factors for suicide include adverse childhood experiences such as child abuse and neglect, bullying, family history of suicide, relationship problems such as break-up or loss, and personal history of or exposure to physical, sexual, and emotional violence or assault. Discrimination is associated with suicidal ideation in children and adolescents and the impact of racism on mental health problems in children and adolescents may intersect with other factors to increase suicide risk for certain youth populations. Bullying involvement of any kind, as a victim, perpetrator, or bully-victim, is associated with suicidal ideation and behavior, though the relationship between bullying and suicide is complicated and not directly causative. Bullying via electronic communication, or cyberbullying, is also a risk factor for suicide. Cyberbullying differs from traditional bullying in anonymity of the perpetrator, proximity of relationships between victims and perpetrators, and potential for accumulation of communication that can occur any time of day. Children and youth with special healthcare needs are a particularly vulnerable population as they experience more adverse childhood experiences, are at increased risk for physical, emotional, and sexual abuse and neglect, and may be more likely to experience bullying. Their concurrent chronic physical and mental health conditions increase their risk for attempted suicide beyond what would be expected based on their chronic mental health condition alone.

Community risk factors include lack of access to mental healthcare and suicide clusters in communities. Adolescents in rural communities have higher rates of suicide than in urban communities, which may be explained in part by limited access to mental health resources in these areas. Societal risk factors include stigma associated with mental illness or help seeking, easy access to lethal means among people at risk (e.g., firearms, medication), and exposure to reports of suicides in the news or fictional portrayals of suicide. Increased screen time is associated with depressive symptoms among children and adolescents and exposure to suicide on the Internet may increase suicidal ideation by sensationalizing the use of suicide to solve problems and attract attention. However, this effect may be offset by online support groups that reinforce positive behaviors.

Biological processes, such as certain brain circuits and molecules, have been correlated with suicidal behavior in children and adolescents. Structurally different from adults, the developing brain in younger people likely contributes to differences in how the above risk factors play a role in suicidal behavior in children and adolescents. Recent studies suggest that several key brain circuits may differ in adolescents who have attempted suicide compared to adolescents who have not attempted suicide, including the hippocampus, dorsolateral prefrontal cortex, and the default mode network. Most neurochemical evidence implicates alterations of the serotonergic system in suicidal behavior. Additional molecules that may be correlated with suicide risk include proinflammatory markers such as tumor necrosis factor, interleukin-1 beta, and brain-derived neurotrophic factor, a protein involved in neuronal growth. It is possible that the correlation between these molecules and suicide are mediated by their relationship with chronic stress. Though data in pediatric populations are limited, these studies may be a starting point for identifying practical targets for interventions.

CLINICAL PRESENTATIONS

Pediatric hospitalists may provide care to children and adolescents with suicidality following a suicide attempt or following assessment in another healthcare setting where they were determined to have suicidal ideation and be unsafe for discharge to home. Additionally, children and adolescents admitted to a hospital medicine service for other reasons may screen positive for suicidality and require additional management during their hospital stay.

Following medical stabilization and treatment, some youth will need inpatient psychiatric hospitalization, which can occur on a voluntary or involuntary basis. Given a national shortage of inpatient pediatric psychiatric beds, some patients for whom inpatient psychiatric care is recommended may need to wait in the emergency department or be transferred to an inpatient medical unit to continue the wait. This practice is called "boarding," defined by The Joint Commission as "the practice of holding patients in the emergency department or another temporary location after the decision to admit or transfer has been made." There is variation in this practice regarding where patients may board, but a recent study demonstrated that pediatric hospitalists are frequently the attending physicians responsible for the care of youth during boarding. Children and youth with special healthcare needs may experience particularly long boarding times due to challenges in finding resources to meet both mental and physical health needs.

SCREENING

Suicidality can present with preceding stressors or behaviors that serve as warning signs, such as recent self harm, accessing mental health services, or expressing suicidal ideation. However, suicidality may not be preceded by these warning signs, and not all children and adolescents may volunteer this information. When parents are aware of suicidal thoughts, they can help children access mental health services. However, parents are often unaware of or underreport their children's suicidal thoughts. For these reasons, screening plays a crucial role in identifying children and adolescents at risk for suicide.

Screening for suicide can occur in all healthcare settings including outpatient clinics, emergency departments, and inpatient units. The AAP and Bright Futures recommend universal screening of patients ages 12 and older in any of these settings. Benefits of universal screening include identifying patients who may not disclose suicide risk, identifying patients who may not have typical risk factors, reducing stigma around mental health, reducing perceived isolation, and promoting equity by ensuring that all youth are screened. The AAP further recommends that youth ages 8 to 11 be screened when they are presenting with behavioral health complaints, if the patient or parent raises a concern, if there is reported history of suicidal ideation or behavior, or if the patient displays warning signs. Screening is not currently recommended for children under age 8, but assessing for suicidal thoughts and behaviors is needed if there are warning signs, or if a parent reports suicidal behaviors. Warning signs in this age group can include talking about wanting to die, actions such as placing their hands in the shape of a gun pointed toward their head, engaging in self-harming behaviors, acting with impulsive aggression, or giving away treasured toys or possessions.

The Joint Commission has approved a number of validated tools for screening in all ages and in all settings including inpatient medical/surgical settings. These tools are available publicly and in multiple languages.

> The Ask Suicide Screening Questions (ASQ), developed by the National Institute of Mental Health, consists of four questions that take about 20 seconds to administer. Initially validated in the emergency department, it has now also been shown to have high sensitivity and negative predictive value in inpatient medical-surgical units.
>
> The Columbia Suicide Severity Rating Scale (C-SSRS) consists of a short series of questions that can be asked by anyone in any setting and is recommended by multiple organizations. These questions seek to identify who is at risk for suicide and assess the severity and immediacy of that risk to guide the appropriate level of support.

Clinical pathways for youth suicide risk screening sponsored by the American Academy of Child and Adolescent Psychiatry and the National Institute of Mental Health have been published and offer a guide that can be adapted based on resources available at hospitals to implement universal screening in an inpatient medical setting. This pathway utilizes the ASQ as the first step, followed by the Brief Suicide Assessment Screening (BSSA) for patients who screen positive, and finally, if indicated by the BSSA, a full suicide safety assessment is conducted by a mental health professional.

DIFFERENTIAL DIAGNOSIS

A comprehensive mental health evaluation may be beneficial to help determine the underlying etiologic diagnosis associated with suicidal ideation (e.g., depression, anxiety, substance abuse, trauma). A mental health consultation should be conducted on youth who are screened at an intermediate/high or imminent risk. Youth may fall into the intermediate/high-risk categories if they have experienced active suicidal ideation with a plan in the past month. Youth who have had a suicide attempt, interrupted attempt, or preparatory acts in the past 3 months are also considered high risk and should have a mental health consultation. If these youth are having active suicidal thoughts, they are then considered an imminent risk and require safety precautions and an urgent mental health evaluation.

MANAGEMENT

ASSESSMENT

Patients who disclose suicidal ideation or behaviors on screening, or who present to the emergency department following suicide attempt or with suicidal ideation require assessment by a mental health professional to determine next steps. **Figure 136-1** summarizes features, warning signs, and risk factors that characterize various levels of risk and outlines appropriate next steps based on that risk. Evidence-based suicide assessment tools are used to determine the level of risk. These assessments focus on recent symptoms, stressors, current suicidal ideation, current and past suicide attempts and plans, risk factors, and protective factors. It is important to obtain information from the patient and caregivers and to consider additional collateral sources such as schools, other medical and mental health providers, and medical records.

The assessment determines risk and informs the treatment plan. For example, disposition recommendations may include referral for further mental health evaluation, or concern for imminent risk and need for urgent full mental health evaluation. It is important to keep the patient under direct observation until the assessment is complete. The Joint Commission recommends that this risk be explicitly documented in the medical record including the plan to decrease the risk. Furthermore, while in the hospital, children and adolescents should regularly be reassessed, as their symptoms and risk of suicide may change.

ACUTE Therapeutic Risk Management – *Risk Stratification Table*

ROCKY MOUNTAIN MIRECC

HIGH ACUTE RISK

Essential Features

- **Suicidal ideation with intent to die by suicide**
- **Inability to maintain safety independent external support/help**

Common Warning Signs

- A plan for suicide
- Recent attempt and/or ongoing preparatory behaviors
- Acute major mental illness (e.g., MDD episode, acute mania, acute psychosis, recent/current drug relapse)
- Exacerbation of personality disorder (e.g., increased borderline symptomatology)

Common Risk Factors

- Access to means
- Acute psychosocial stressors (e.g., job loss, relationship dissolution, relapse on alcohol)

Action

Typically requires psychiatric hospitalization to maintain safety and aggressively target modifiable factors.

These individuals need to be directly observed until on a secure unit and kept in an environment with limited access to lethal means (e.g., keep away from sharps, cords/tubing, toxic substances).

During hospitalization co-occurring psychiatric symptoms should also be addressed.

INTERMEDIATE ACUTE RISK

Essential Features

- **Suicidal ideation to die by suicide**
- **Ability to maintain safety, independent of external support/help**

These individuals may present similarly to those at high acute risk, sharing many of the features. The only difference may be lack of intent, based upon an identified reason for living (e.g. children), and ability to abide by a safety plan and maintain their own safety. Preparatory behaviors are likely to be absent.

Action

Consider psychiatric hospitalization, if related factors driving risk are responsive to inpatient treatment (e.g., acute psychosis).

Outpatient management of suicidal thoughts and/or behaviors should be intensive and include:

- frequent contact,
- regular re-assessment of risk, and
- a well-articulated safety plan

Mental health treatment should also address co-occurring psychiatric symptoms.

LOW ACUTE RISK

Essential Features

- **No current suicidal intent AND**
- **No specific and current suicidal plan AND**
- **No preparatory behaviors AND**
- **Collective high confidence** (e.g., patient, care provider, family member) in the ability of the patient to independently maintain safety

Individuals may have suicidal ideation, but it will be **with little or no intent or specific current plan**. If a plan is present, the plan is general and/or vague, and without any associated preparatory behaviors (e.g., "I'd shoot myself if things got bad enough, but I don't have a gun"). These patients will be capable of engaging appropriate coping strategies, and willing and able to utilize a safety plan in a crisis situation.

Action

Can be managed in primary care.

Outpatient mental health treatment may also be indicated, particularly if suicidal ideation and psychiatric symptoms are co-occurring.

*Overall level of individual risk may be increased or decreased based upon warning signs, risk factors and **protective factors**

FIGURE 136-1. Therapeutic risk management features of varying levels of risk and appropriate actions. (From Rocky Mountain Mental Illness Research Education and Clinical Center (MIRECC) for Suicide Prevention. Available at: https://www.va.gov/HOMELESS/nchav/resources/docs/prevention/Suicide/ACUTE-Therapeutic-Risk-Management-Risk-Stratification-Table.pdf.)

CHRONIC Therapeutic Risk Management – *Risk Stratification Table*

ROCKY MOUNTAIN MIRECC

HIGH CHRONIC RISK

Essential Features	Action
Common Warning Sign • Chronic suicidal ideation Common Risk Factors • Chronic major mental illness and/or personality disorder • History of prior suicide attempt(s) • History of substance abuse/dependence • Chronic pain • Chronic medical condition • Limited coping skills • Unstable or turbulent psychosocial status (e.g. unstable housing, erratic relationships, marginal employment) • Limited ability to identify reasons for living	These individuals are considered to be at chronic risk for becoming acutely suicidal, often in the context of unpredictable situational contingencies (e.g., job loss, loss of relationships, and relapse on drugs). These individuals typically require: • routine mental health follow-up • a well-articulated safety plan, including means safety (e.g., no access to guns, limited medication supply) • routine suicide risk screening • coping skills building • management of co-occurring psychiatric symptoms

INTERMEDIATE CHRONIC RISK

Essential Features	Action
These individuals may feature similar chronicity as those at high chronic risk with respect to psychiatric, substance abuse, medical and painful conditions. Protective factors, coping skills, reasons for living, and relative psychosocial stability suggest enhanced ability to endure future crisis without resorting to self-directed violence.	These individuals typically require: • routine mental health care to optimize psychiatric condition and maintain/enhance coping skills and protective factors. • a well articulated safety plan, including means safety (e.g., no access to guns, limited medication supply) • management of co-occurring psychiatric symptoms

LOW CHRONIC RISK

Essential Features	Action
These individuals may range from persons with no or little in the way of mental health or substance abuse problems, to persons with significant mental illness that is associated with relatively abundant strengths/resources. Stressors historically have typically been endured absent suicidal ideation. The following factors will generally be missing • history of self-directed violence • chronic suicidal ideation • tendency towards being highly impulsive • risky behaviors • marginal psychosocial functioning	Appropriate for mental health care on an as needed basis, some may be managed in primary care settings. Others may require mental health follow-up to continue successful treatments.

FIGURE 136-1. *(Continued)*

COMMUNICATION

At all stages in evaluation, optimizing communication with adolescents and their families is crucial. When possible, adolescents should be interviewed separately from the parent. If the child cannot be interviewed alone, the evaluation should continue with the understanding that the patient may not be as forthcoming during the evaluation. Minors should be informed of their rights to access and consent to mental health services on their own, though variations in practice exist across states. The limits of confidentiality and the duty to maintain safety should be disclosed to patients. Though preserving confidentiality is crucial in caring for adolescents, if the adolescent discloses risk of harm to themselves or others, the pediatrician has a responsibility to inform others, which can include parents or other medical providers. When speaking with adolescents, it is important to avoid trying to "fix it" and instead focus on listening and asking questions. Applying principles of trauma-informed care, such as ensuring the physical and psychological safety of the youth, recognizing the signs and symptoms of traumatic stress, and acknowledging the individual's strengths and resilience can help engage patients and create a safe setting when addressing suicide with adolescents and their families.

INITIAL STABILIZATION

Often, patients are screened for suicidal ideation in an emergency department or they may be referred to an emergency department following a positive screen, reported suicidal ideation, or a suicide attempt. In this setting, medical stabilization to address physical injuries, toxidromes in settings of overdose, or medical conditions unrelated to suicidal ideation and attempt may be necessary. Stabilization of any agitation may also be necessary, which can include verbal, chemical, and physical restraint guided by the following four principles: (1) maximizing the safety of the patient and treating staff; (2) assisting the patient in managing his or her emotions and maintaining or regaining control of his or her behavior; (3) using the least restrictive, age-appropriate methods of restraint possible; and (4) minimizing coercive interventions that may exacerbate agitation.

MEDICAL CLEARANCE

Following initial stabilization, medical clearance may be needed to determine whether the patient's suicidal thoughts and behaviors are caused or exacerbated by an underlying medical condition. Laboratory and radiographic testing should be informed by history and physical examination.

SAFE ENVIRONMENT

For patients who disclose suicidal ideation, it is necessary to address safety in all settings. Not every patient who has suicidal thoughts will need full safety precautions. Full safety precautions may vary across settings and can include changing into a hospital gown, removing personal belongings including cell phones, and placing the patient under 1:1 observation. Utilizing full safety precautions for patients who are not at imminent risk can be punitive or traumatizing, overtax the health system unnecessarily, and threaten the therapeutic alliance between patient and treatment team.

Securing the environment in inpatient medical settings has been shown to decrease risk. While individual hospital policies may vary, The Joint Commission currently recommends that nonpsychiatric units in general hospitals conduct an environmental risk assessment, which includes (1) an evaluation to identify self-harm issues before a patient is placed into the room, (2) a plan to identify someone to remove objects that cause potential self harm, and (3) resources to guide staff in this process. One of the most common environmental risks is ligature, which are objects used for tying or binding. While acute care hospital settings are not required to be entirely free of such items, they are expected to make routine assessments for potential environmental hazards and take action to protect individuals from potential risks. The Joint Commission supports a three-step approach to mitigate ligature risks provided by the American Society for Health Care Engineering. These three steps include (1) identifying patients who are at risk for harm to themselves or others, (2) providing 1:1 monitoring of patients performed by an individual who is able to intervene immediately, and (3) removing or mitigating all environmental risks when continuous observation is not possible, including in settings that require privacy such as bathrooms. The assessment is dynamic, as patients move to different settings throughout the hospital and visitors may bring objects into a patient's room that should be assessed.

DISCHARGE CRITERIA

The disposition of children or adolescents with suicidality depends on risk of suicide balanced against protective factors and available resources. A psychiatric hospitalization is recommended when a youth is at acute high risk for suicide or at acute intermediate risk with symptoms or risk factors that are anticipated to benefit from inpatient psychiatric treatment. Other patients may require acute residential treatment program, partial hospitalization, or can be safely discharged with outpatient follow up which may include intensive outpatient care/wraparound services.

When discharging someone with suicide risk from an inpatient to an outpatient setting, several best practices have been proposed: (1) developing protocols for safety and rapid referrals to outpatient care, (2) involving family members and other natural supports, (3) collaboratively developing a safety plan, (4) connecting with the outpatient provider, and (5) following up with the patient and outpatient provider (e.g., reviewing discharge paperwork, sending records, etc.)

For patients who are ready for discharge, The Joint Commission recommends safety planning and follow-up care upon discharge. Safety planning has been shown to reduce subsequent suicidal behavior and increase follow up, and involves collaboration between patients, families, and the treatment team to develop a personalized plan to help get through feelings of suicide should they occur in the future. The key elements of a safety plan include (1) recognizing the warning signs of a crisis; (2) identifying coping skills; (3) naming people who can support and distract; (4) identifying close friends/adults who can potentially help resolve a crisis; (5) knowing mental health professionals or agencies to contact; (6) ensuring a safe environment; and (7) having a positive focus to leverage.

Lethal means counseling is another evidence-based intervention supported by The Joint Commission. Lethal means reduction, which is the practice of limiting access to dangerous items that can be used in suicides such as firearms and medications, prevents death by suicide. Mental health professionals and others who work with patients with suicidality have access to an effective online training course that is publicly available through Zero Suicide. Firearms are important to discuss with patients and families as having a gun in the home is associated with increased risk for suicide among adolescents, and firearms are the most lethal means of suicide. The safest measure is to ensure there are no guns in the home. If this is not possible, the practice of keeping a gun locked, unloaded, storing ammunition locked and in a separate location without giving the adolescent access to the key or location reduces rates of firearm injuries including suicide in adolescents.

Similarly, restricting access to other dangerous items, such as medications, including prescription and over the counter, alcohol, and household cleaners, is important. Medications that are not needed or expired should be removed from the home. Obtaining medications in blister packs may mitigate risks during a crisis by slowing down the rate at which large quantities of medication may be ingested.

Follow-up is important to establishing safe disposition. Follow-up plans should include a patient's medical home when possible, as primary care clinicians play an essential role in ongoing care. A team-based approach, which supports partnership between children, families, medical providers, and other team members across settings including school and community partners, should be applied in discharge planning.

After discharge, following up with a "caring contact", or periodic, personalized text-based communications that express concern without demanding reciprocation, can prevent future suicide attempts. Examples of postcards that serve as "caring contacts" are provided to the public by Zero Suicide.

SPECIAL CONSIDERATIONS

PREVENTION

There are multiple different stakeholders to involve and strategies to utilize to prevent suicide. The World Health Organization recommends the following evidence-based interventions: limiting access to lethal means, encouraging the media to responsibly report on suicide, encouraging positive coping skills in youth, and monitoring of those affected by suicide. The Centers for Disease and Control and Prevention has noted several additional strategies to prevent suicide: strengthening economic supports, strengthening access to and delivery of suicide care, creating protective environments, promoting connectedness, teaching coping and problem-solving skills, and identifying and supporting people at risk.

SUGGESTED READINGS

Ahmedani BK, Simon GE, Stewart C, et al. Health care contacts in the year before suicide death. *J Gen Intern Med.* 2014;29(6):870-877.

Alderman EM, Breuner CC. Unique needs of the adolescent. *Pediatrics.* 2019;144(6).

American Academy of Pediatrics. AAP-AACAP-CHA Declaration of a National Emergency in Child and Adolescent Mental health. [updated 2021 Oct 19; cited 2022 Dec 2]. Available from: https://www.aap.org/en/advocacy/child-and-adolescent-healthy-mental-development/aap-aacap-cha-declaration-of-a-national-emergency-in-child-and-adolescent-mental-health.

American Academy of Pediatrics. Suicide: Blueprint for Youth Suicide Prevention [Internet]. [cited 2022]. Available from: https://www.aap.org/en/patient-care/blueprint-for-youth-suicide-prevention/.

Benton TD. Suicide and Suicidal Behaviors Among Minoritized Youth. *Child Adolesc Psychiatr Clin N Am [Internet]*. 2022;31(2):211-221. Available from: https://doi.org/10.1016/j.chc.2022.01.002.

Bitsko RH. Mental Health Surveillance Among Children—United States, 2013-2019. 2022;71(2):2013-2019. Available from: https://www.cdc.gov/mmwr/preview/mmwrhtml/su6202a1.htm%0Ahttp://files/1225/su6202a1.html.

Brahmbhatt K, Kurtz BP, Afzal KI, et al. Suicide risk screening in pediatric hospitals: clinical pathways to address a global health crisis. *Psychosomatics [Internet]*. 2019;60(1):1-9. Available from: https://doi.org/10.1016/j.psym.2018.09.003.

Bridge JA, Horowitz LM, Fontanella CA, et al. Age-related racial disparity in suicide rates among us youths from 2001 through 2015. *JAMA Pediatr*. 2018;172(7):696-697.

Cha CB, Franz PJ, Guzman EM, Glenn CR, Kleiman EM, Nock MK. Annual Research Review: Suicide among youth–epidemiology, (potential) etiology, and treatment. *J Child Psychol Psychiatr*. 2018;59(4):460-482.

Chitavi S, Paul S, Wells E, et al. Suicide Prevention Resources to support joint Commission Accredited organizations implementation of NPSG 15.01.01, revised July, 2020 [Internet]. The Joint Commission; 2020 [updated 2020; cited 2022]. Available from: https://www.jointcommission.org/-/media/tjc/documents/resources/patient-safety-topics/suicide-prevention/suicide_prevention_compendium_5_11_20_updated-july2020.pdf.

Chun TH, Mace SE, Katz ER. Evaluation and management of children and adolescents with acute mental health or behavioral problems. Part I: Common clinical challenges of patients with mental health and/or behavioral emergencies. 2016;138(3).

Curtin SC, Heron M. Death rates due to suicide and homicide among persons aged 10-24: United States, 2000-2017. *NCHS Data Brief.* 2019;(352):1-8.

Cwik M, Jay S, Ryan TC, et al. Lowering the age limit in suicide risk screening: clinical differences and screening form predictive ability. *J Am Acad Child Adolesc Psychiatry*. 2021;60(5):537-540.

Doupnik SK, Rudd B, Schmutte T, et al. Association of suicide prevention interventions with subsequent suicide attempts, linkage to follow-up care, and depression symptoms for acute care settings a systematic review and meta-analysis. 2022;19146(10):1021-1030.

Horowitz LM, Wharff EA, Mournet AM, et al. Validation and feasibility of the ASQ among pediatric medical and surgical inpatients. *Hosp Pediatr*. 2020;10:750-757.

Ivey-Stephenson AZ, Demissie Z, Crosby AE, et al. Suicidal ideation and behaviors among high school students - Youth Risk Behavior Survey, United States, 2019. *MMWR Suppl*. 2020;69(1):47-55.

Leyenaar JK, Freyleue SD, Bordogna A, Wong C, Penwill N, Bode R. Frequency and duration of boarding for pediatric mental health conditions at acute care hospitals in the US. *JAMA* 2021;326:2326-2328.

Liu RT, Walsh RFL, Sheehan AE, Cheek SM, Sanzari CM. Prevalence and correlates of suicide and nonsuicidal self-injury in children: a systematic review and meta-analysis. *JAMA psychiatry [Internet]*. 2022;02114:1-9. Available from: http://www.ncbi.nlm.nih.gov/pubmed/35612875.

Mangione CM. Screening for Depression and Suicide Risk in Children and Adolescents US Preventive Services Task Force Recommendation Statement. *JAMA*. 2022;1-9.

Maslow GR, Dunlap K, Chung RJ. Depression and suicide in children and adolescents. *Pediatr Rev*. 2015;36:299-310.

Mattson G, Kuo DZ. Psychosocial factors in children and youth with special health care needs and their families. *Pediatrics*. 2019;143(1).

National Action Alliance for Suicide Prevention. Best Practices in Care Transitions for individuals with Suicide Risk: Inpatient care to outpatient care [Internet]. [cited 2022]. Available from: https://www.samhsa.gov/sites/default/files/suicide-risk-practices-in-care-transitions-11192019.pdf.

Olfson M, Wall M, Wang S, et al. Suicide after deliberate self-harm in adolescents and young adults. *Pediatrics*. 2018;141(4).

Plemmons G, Hall M, Doupnik S, et al. Hospitalization for suicide ideation or attempt: 2008–2015. *Pediatrics*. 2018;141(6):2008-2015.

Posner K, Brown GK, Stanley B, et al. The Columbia–Suicide Severity Rating Scale: Initial validity and internal consistency findings from three multisite studies with adolescents and adults. *Am J Psychiatry*. 2011;168(12):1266-1277.

Racine N, McArthur BA, Cooke JE, Eirich R, Zhu J, Madigan S. Global prevalence of depressive and anxiety symptoms in children and adolescents during COVID-19: a meta-analysis. *JAMA Pediatr*. 2021;175(11):1142-1150.

Raifman J, Charlton BM, Arrington-Sanders R, et al. Sexual orientation and suicide attempt disparities among US adolescents: *Pediatrics*. 2020;145(3):2009-2017.

Rodway C, Tham SG, Turnbull P, Kapur N, Appleby L. Suicide in children and young people: can it happen without warning? *J Affect Disord [Internet]*. 2020;275(April):307-310. Available from: https://doi.org/10.1016/j.jad.2020.06.069.

Shaffer D, Pfeffer CR, the Work Group on Quality Issues. Practice Parameter for the Assessment and Treatment of Children and Adolescents With Suicidal Behavior. *J Am Acad Child Adolesc Psychiatry [Internet]*. 2001;40(7):24S-51S. Available from: http://dx.doi.org/10.1097/00004583-200107001-00003.

Shain B. Suicide and suicide attempts in adolescents. *Pediatrics*. 2016;138(1):1-11.

Skopp NA, Smolenski DJ, Bush NE, et al. Caring contacts for suicide prevention: a systematic review and meta-analysis. *Psychol Serv*. 2023;20(1):74-83.

Stanley B, Brown GK, Brenner LA, et al. Comparison of the safety planning intervention with follow-up vs usual care of suicidal patients treated in the emergency department. *JAMA Psychiatry*. 2018;75(9):894-900.

Trent M, Dooley DG, Dougé J. The impact of racism on child and adolescent health. *Pediatrics*. 2019;144(2).

Yard E, Radhakrishnan L, Ballesteros MF, et al. Emergency department visits for suspected suicide attempts among persons aged 12-25 years before and during the COVID-19 pandemic—United States, January 2019-May 2021. *MMWR Recomm Reports*. 2021;70(24):888-894.

Zalsman G, Hawton K, Wasserman D, et al. Suicide prevention strategies revisited: 10-year systematic. *Lancet Psychiatry*. 2016;3(July):646-659.

CHAPTER 137

Somatic Symptom and Related Disorders

Kimberly K. Monroe, MD, MS and Leah Rappaport, MD

BACKGROUND

The assessment and management of children and adolescents who present with medically unexplained symptoms or symptoms in excess of what would be expected for a particular medical illness can be a difficult task. According to the *Diagnostic and Statistical Manual of Mental Disorders*, 5th ed. (DSM-5), illnesses previously referred to as somatoform disorders are now defined as somatic symptoms and related disorders. Somatic symptoms and related disorders (SSRDs) include a number of diagnoses. Given the breadth of this diagnostic category, this chapter will focus on the two most common categories of SSRDs: somatic symptom disorder and conversion disorder (also known as functional neurological symptom disorder).

SSRDs are classified based on distressing somatic symptoms and excessive thoughts, feelings, or behaviors in relation to these symptoms. They are thought to result from the interaction of psychological and biological processes that exceed a person's coping abilities, resulting in significant distress and impairment. SSRDs can present with symptoms that range from pain to disabling neurological symptoms. The physical symptoms are not explained better by another mental illness, are spontaneous in nature, and are not contrived by the child or adolescent. In addition, a medical condition, if present, does not fully account for the level of impairment the child is displaying. Inability to identify and verbally express emotions and feelings, difficulty adjusting to and recognizing stress, and impactful life events can perpetuate or predispose children to SSRDs.

In early childhood, the most common symptoms of SSRDs are recurrent abdominal pain (RAP) and headaches, while older children also tend to experience symptoms of insomnia, pain, and fatigue. The symptoms of SSRDs can be severe, recurrent, impairing, and involve more than one body system. Impairment often involves withdrawal from activities and social relationships and avoidance of everyday responsibilities and stresses.

Patients with somatic symptoms disproportionately consume health resources by utilizing the emergency department, inpatient, and consultation services, and families may present to multiple health providers and have unnecessary testing in pursuit of a medical explanation for symptoms. Patients hospitalized with SSRDs generally have more significant and impairing symptoms as well as an increased risk of continued iatrogenic intervention and injury which can perpetuate the cycle of disability.

SOMATIC SYMPTOM DISORDER

Somatic symptom disorder (SSD) is characterized by somatic symptoms that are distressing or result in significant disruption of daily life. It is important to note that the individual's suffering is genuine. SSD may occur concurrently with other medical diagnoses. The following are diagnostic criteria per DSM-5 for somatic symptom disorder:

A. One or more somatic symptoms that are distressing or result in significant disruption of daily life

B. Excessive thoughts, feelings, or behaviors related to the somatic symptoms or associated health concerns as manifested by at least one of the following:

1. Disproportionate and persistent thoughts about the seriousness of one's symptoms
2. Persistently high level of anxiety about health or symptoms
3. Excessive time and energy devoted to these symptoms or health concerns

C. Although any one somatic symptom may not be continuously present, the state of being symptomatic is persistent (typically more than 6 months).

SSD with predominant pain should be suspected when there are excessive thoughts, feelings, or behaviors in relation to pain symptoms, an intense preoccupation with the pain, and resultant disruption of daily life. Severity (mild, moderate, or severe) is also specified. If the symptoms are severe and there is marked impairment with duration more than 6 months, the specifier "persistent" is added.

BIOLOGICAL FACTORS

The reactivity and recovery of the nervous system during times of stress can influence the experience of pain. Children with SSD likely exhibit a lower threshold to internal and external cues of painful stimuli. When there is a strong expectation of pain, the anterior insular cortex is activated in proportion to this expectation. Thus, the preactivation will predict the subjective intensity of subsequent pain stimulus. Studies of long-term pain suggest progressive loss of gray matter density in brain structures involved in registering pain, and in those involving inhibition of the pain signal.

PSYCHOLOGICAL FACTORS

Psychological factors related to pain include temperament, attention biases toward system-related stimuli, and use of coping strategies. Subjective representations of pain can occur as a result of emotional states, thoughts, beliefs, intentions, suggestions, injuries to social or attachment relationships, memories of past injuries, and the emotional state of others. Negative emotions such as sadness, fear, or anger can significantly influence how the brain processes pain and can increase the degree of pain felt by the child.

A meta-analysis shows that internalizing symptoms (e.g., depressed mood, anxious thoughts, negative self-talk) are approximately six times more likely to occur in children with RAP than in matched healthy controls. Thus, insecure attachment is a risk factor for the adjustment to pain, and patients with this attachment type have poor outcomes from a range of treatment interventions.

Somatization is thought to be a learned behavior that may begin because the experience of having a somatic complaint is more acceptable or more noticed in some households than the expression of strong emotions such as anxiety, fear, or anger. In such an environment, a child may repeatedly garner minimal attention for emotional distress, but obtain more attention and sympathy for physical symptoms that can accompany a disturbed emotional state. Pain behaviors may also be reinforced by inactivity or pain medication, or from the surrounding environment in the form of increased concern or interest from a family member or a highly regarded physician.

Somatic complaints and anxiety disorders commonly coexist. Evidence suggests that RAP and anxiety disorders share common risk factors or are different manifestations of a common causal process.

SOCIAL FACTORS

Social factors that can predispose to SSD include environmental stressors, especially chronic stress and parental functioning. Children with chronic pain symptoms often live with family members who complain of similar physical symptoms, and a parent's response to a child's pain and stressors can modulate pain symptoms. Additional predisposing for somatic symptoms include increased medical diagnoses, hospitalizations, being female, having problems in school, and having a parent who is stressed about their own pain.

CLINICAL PRESENTATION

The clinical presentation of SSD includes one or more distressing physical symptoms, such as pain, fatigue, or gastrointestinal complaints, that significantly impact daily functioning.

Pain is the presenting symptom in up to 70% of patients with physical complaints that cannot be fully explained by any physical health condition, and occurs in 4% to 15% of adolescents. Frequent complaints include headache, chest pain, and abdominal pain.

RAP is defined as intermittent pain with full recovery between episodes, lasting more than 3 months, and it is the most common recurrent pain complaint of childhood. RAP affects 8% to 25% of children ages 9 to 12 years. The prevalence of RAP increases with age into adolescence, with an equal gender ratio in early childhood and symptom reporting by girls predominating by late childhood. RAP is strongly associated with depressive symptoms, other pain syndromes such as headache, limb pain, and chest pain, as well as other somatic symptoms such as fatigue, dizziness, weakness, and numbness.

Complex regional pain syndrome is defined as pain that spreads along a dermatomal pattern beyond the location of the initial injury and is usually accompanied by autonomic dysfunction, movement deficits, dystrophy, and edema. Children with this syndrome have been shown to have an elevated risk of somatic symptoms and emotional distress, particularly anxiety.

DIFFERENTIAL DIAGNOSIS

When assessing a child with pain symptoms, it is important to evaluate any potential physical illnesses that may contribute to the pain. The differential diagnosis of physical conditions that could explain a child's symptoms will vary depending on a child's presenting symptoms. Evaluating for mental health conditions that may explain pain symptoms or coexist with SSD can help in diagnosis and management. For example, mood and anxiety disorders may also present with pain symptoms. Younger children may be affected by factious disorder imposed on another (formerly called "Munchhausen's disorder by proxy"). Although factitious disorders or malingering are less common in the pediatric age group, it is important to keep these diagnoses on the differential, particularly for older adolescents who may have secondary gain from somatic symptoms.

DIAGNOSTIC EVALUATION

The cornerstones of diagnostic evaluation in SSD are a thorough history and physical examination. Focused, limited medical testing can offer reassurance against physical pathology.

The medical history should include a, detailed assessment of the child's symptoms. Clinicians can obtain a current pain or symptom history using the mnemonic OPQRST (onset, provocation/palliation, quality, region/radiation, severity, and timing), along with developmentally appropriate structured pain assessment tools, and/or a pain diary. Past medical history of prior episodes of pain or other symptoms, psychiatric history, and family medical and mental health history should also be included in the assessment. The social history should include a careful assessment of the child's social and academic functioning, coping strategies, family functioning, and any stressors. Importantly, identification of a stressor is not required for diagnosis of SSD, but understanding stressors can help inform the treatment plan.

The physical examination may find that the child's symptoms are anatomically inconsistent or in excess of what would be expected from any physical health condition that is present. Patients may have changes on physical examination, which can be the result of immobilization or activity limitation (e.g., decreased muscle bulk or skin changes).

Many children with SSD endure potentially risky and unnecessary hospitalizations, tests, and procedures. Unnecessary testing increases the risk of iatrogenic injury and can reinforce a family's belief that symptoms may have a physical explanation. Nevertheless, for some families, limited medical testing can offer reassurance and reduce anxiety about possible missed diagnoses. In these situations, we recommend noninvasive testing within reason. For example, for a patient presenting with RAP, abdominal radiograph, urinalysis, and ultrasound might all be reasonable. In the absence of specific findings that warrant invasive testing, the diagnostic yield is low.

CONVERSION DISORDER (ALSO KNOWN AS FUNCTIONAL NEUROLOGICAL SYMPTOM DISORDER)

According to the DSM-5, conversion disorder, also known as functional neurological symptom disorder, is characterized by clinically significant distress leading to impairment in functioning due to a deficit affecting voluntary motor and sensory functioning. In conversion disorder, the symptoms cannot be better accounted for by another medical condition or mental illness. One specific subtype of conversion disorder that we will discuss in more detail is psychogenic nonepileptic seizures (PNES).

BIOLOGICAL FACTORS

Hyperactivity of the anterior cingulate cortex has been found in patients with conversion disorder, along with either increased or decreased activity of the dorsolateral prefrontal cortex. Patients with nonepileptic seizures have increased activity of neurobiological stress systems with lower heart rate variability at baseline and during recovery from an induced stress condition. Decreased heart rate variability is associated with increased arousal and poor emotion regulation. Patients with conversion disorders also have increased diurnal cortisol levels when compared to controls.

PSYCHOLOGICAL AND SOCIAL FACTORS

Psychological factors that can contribute to the etiology of conversion disorder include attachment, environmental stress, family discord, trauma, and culture. Many children have a parent or family member who models conversion symptoms. In some cases, the patient may be their own symptom model; a common example of this is children with epilepsy who also have PNES. Recent family stress, unresolved grief reactions, and family psychopathology occur at a higher frequency in children with conversion symptoms.

External environmental factors such as school stress or change in family situation, and internal factors such as coping deficits or poor behavioral self-control, are common in children presenting with conversion disorder. Common school stressors in this patient population include bullying, fear of exams, extracurricular activities, and beginning the new school year. A transition within the family system such as death of a family member, birth of a sibling, parental divorce, physical punishment by parents, and an increase in the number of arguments between parents have all been linked to conversion symptoms. Conversion symptoms may not immediately follow a specific stressor but instead can occur months or years later.

Conversion disorder presents differently in various cultures. The use of nonverbal body language as a way of communication or expression of self in response to interpersonal conflicts may represent a culturally determined and socially learned behavior. Emerging literature indicates the risk of conversion disorder may be higher in adolescents who have anxiety related to sexual behaviors, sexual orientation, or gender identity. The adolescent may struggle with communicating their internal turmoil due to fear of parental rejection, peer isolation, stigmatization, and victimization.

CLINICAL PRESENTATION

Clinical presentation can be variable and typically involves loss of function or ability to do activities of daily living in the absence of objective physical exam findings. The most frequently reported symptoms of conversion disorder in childhood are episodic loss of consciousness, typically syncope or PNES, and motor functioning, typically abnormal gait or the inability to walk. Early diagnosis can prevent symptom fixation and the performance of expensive and sometimes painful invasive procedures.

DIFFERENTIAL DIAGNOSIS

When evaluating a child with conversion symptoms it is important to keep in mind other medical causes that may lead to the same presentation. Thus, it is important to consider temporal lobe epilepsy, tumors of the central nervous system, multiple sclerosis, electrolyte abnormalities, drug use or exposure and myopathies. The pediatrician should keep in mind that the presence of a conversion disorder does not exclude the possibility of a physical condition in the same patient.

Apart from conversion disorder, other psychiatric disorders such as depression, anxiety, factitious disorder, and malingering may cause similar presentations. Factitious disorder and malingering are generally described in adults, although some cases are reported in older children and adolescents. Acute stress disorder and symptoms of posttraumatic stress disorder can present (and coexist) with symptoms similar to that of conversion disorder. Conversion symptoms can occur within other somatic symptom disorders with a combination of pain and gastrointestinal, sexual, and pseudoneurologic symptoms.

DIAGNOSTIC EVALUTION

Early diagnosis is important to avoid unnecessary hospitalization and investigations. Video-EEG monitoring remains the gold standard in diagnosing PNES, and the visualization can be helpful for caregivers. The use of provocative testing to confirm a diagnosis of nonepileptic seizures is not recommended.

Other neuroimaging studies and lumbar puncture with cerebrospinal fluid analysis may be indicated in certain types of conversion disorders to exclude specific CNS pathologies, although avoiding invasive procedures when possible is preferred. A psychiatric evaluation should be conducted to assess for biopsychosocial contributing and risk factors that would inform the diagnosis and treatment plan. Psychiatric evaluation can also help assess for feigned, falsified, and induced disorders. Maintaining an alert, transparent, empathic approach can help the patient shed the pretense of disease.

MANAGEMENT OF SSRDS

Although SSRDs are a diverse set of disorders and have a large range of clinical manifestations, management and treatment remain consistent across presentations.

PSYCHOEDUCATION

Psychoeducation and the management of children with somatic symptoms and their caregivers can be challenging. The hospitalist must convey an understanding that the patient's pain and symptoms are real. Psychoeducation is directed at understanding and adhering to a treatment regimen, clarifying when to worry about symptoms, enhancing communication and collaboration with treating professionals and using problem-solving coping techniques. As part of discussing the mind-body connection, it is helpful to use examples that allow the child and caregiver to better understand the connection between emotions and the body. For common example, the sensation of "butterflies in their stomach," can be related to anxiety. Showing respect for a patient's own perception of illness and allocating ample time for communicating the diagnosis are critical for successful treatment.

Families often worry about abandonment by the physician after a diagnosis of an SSRD; scheduled follow-up visits with the primary care provider and specialists are essential. Even if they disagree with their physicians, many families can accept treatment recommendations if they are assured regularly scheduled follow-up visits with their pediatrician. However, it is ideal to strive for full parental acceptance of the diagnosis as this may lead to an increased chance of functional recovery for the patient.

REHABILITATION MODEL

Based on a growing body of evidence, the main approach to treatment is based on the rehabilitation model. Goals are to reduce symptoms, improve normal functioning, enhance coping, and prevent secondary disabilities. It is helpful to establish realistic goals that emphasize improvements in functioning rather than the expectation that symptoms can be completely resolved. The implementation of interventions that simultaneously target "body and mind" can facilitate the family's acceptance of the psychological aspect of the treatment. The child actively participates in incentive-based intensive physical and occupational therapy to help restore their functioning. Parents should be encouraged to view their child's progress as evidence that they are capable and strong. Furthermore, parents should ignore or reduce attention to sick role behavior, use problem-solving coping techniques when the child struggles, and participate in family counseling to enhance parental competence to resolve family crises. A gradual return to school with a structured plan to address obstacles and support can be effective.

COGNITIVE BEHAVIORAL THERAPY

Cognitive behavioral therapy (CBT) techniques have demonstrated effectiveness in treating SSRDs. Providers encourage patients to participate in routine activities through gradual exposure and explore the links between physical and psychological pain.

ADDITIONAL TECHNIQUES

Programs that incorporate mindfulness meditation, yoga exercises, and group support have shown improvements in patients' pain, physical function, psychological health, and a reduction in perceived stress. In addition, techniques such as hypnosis and biofeedback have been helpful in treating SSRDs. There is some evidence in adults that hypnosis, alone or in the form of self-hypnosis using relaxation techniques has resulted in improvement in symptoms such as back pain, headache, and emotional arousal. Virtual reality modalities have shown evidence of improvements in patients with chronic pain and distraction for painful procedures. While the exact mechanism is not yet understood, it is thought that by processing virtual reality experiences, the nervous system undergoes remodeling resulting in less perceived pain.

PHARMACOLOGIC MANAGEMENT

There is a paucity of randomized, controlled trials investigating the use of psychotropic medication in the management of somatic symptoms in the pediatric population. A child who does not respond to intensive treatment should be evaluated for the possibility of comorbid disorders such as a mood disorder, anxiety disorder, and substance use disorder. Traditional pain medications like opioids and analgesics are not effective for treating SSRDs; nevertheless, many patients are prescribed opioids. Attempts should be made to decrease the use of opioids in these patients unless pain is postsurgical or from a traumatic injury, such as a fractured bone. Antidepressant medications are proven to be more beneficial for treatment of pain and comorbid psychiatric issues.

A small body of evidence from the 1950s to 1970s shows improvement in SSRD symptoms when patients are treated with psychedelics; however, additional research has not been conducted due to restrictions in licensing of psychedelics. Further study is needed into whether psychedelics can be a safe and effective treatment.

ADMISSION AND DISCHARGE CRITERIA

Ideally, medical hospitalization is avoided for patients with SSRDs. Nevertheless, patients may be referred for inpatient medical hospitalization if outpatient clinicians perceive a need to pursue an expedited medical workup to rule out an alternative medical explanation. Once any necessary medical workup has been completed, or if medical workup can be avoided based on reassuring history and physical examination, inpatient medical admission should be kept as short as possible while partnering with the patient, family, and outpatient team to make an ongoing plan of outpatient care, to avoid reinforcing the sick role. Medical hospital discharge criteria include that a patient is eating and drinking well enough to maintain nutrition and hydration, and can do activities of daily living with a level of support/supervision that is feasible for the patient's family.

Studies have suggested that the treatment of patients with SSRDs on medical-psychiatric units leads to a decrease in healthcare utilization and an appropriate increase in psychiatric interventions. If the frequency and duration of SSRD symptom episodes are unchanged or if symptoms escalate, psychiatric admission may be indicated for further evaluation of psychiatric comorbidities and continued acute intervention.

CONSULTATION

If SSRDs are suspected, psychology and psychiatric consultation should be included early in the evaluation process. The psychologist and/or psychiatrist should start seeing the child shortly after their medical admission, in parallel with the medical workup. It is helpful for the pediatrician to frame the consultation as a routine part of a comprehensive assessment for patients presenting in said manner. Interdisciplinary management may include the child psychologist, child psychiatrist, pediatric neurologist, pain specialist, physical therapist, social worker, occupational therapist, child life/activity therapist, and school personnel. It is important for physical and occupational therapy to be involved, to avoid chronic sequelae of contractures or decreased mobility.

PREVENTION

Given the chronicity of symptoms in some children, early identification of risk factors and prevention of further impairment and more disabling symptoms can be critical to the overall course of their illness. Early intervention and recognition have been reported to be associated with a good prognosis. The longer the duration of presenting symptoms, the more likely the child will have a relapse of symptoms. Short-term treatment goals are to stop or significantly decrease the frequency and duration of symptoms, limit medical interventions, and return the child to normal daily activities. It is imperative to involve and educate school personnel to help the school create a safe environment for the child's optimal functioning.

KEY POINTS

- Somatic symptom and related disorders are common in hospitalized children.
- We recommend using the American Academy of Child and Adolescent Psychiatry Pathways in Clinical Care Workgroup Consensus Pathway on SSRD Evaluation and Management, to help standardize care, promote patient recovery, and optimize cost-effectiveness.
- Include biological, psychological, developmental, and social factors when assessing a child with somatic symptoms to inform the treatment plan.
- A mental health specialist (psychologist or psychiatrist) should start evaluating the child shortly after admission in conjunction with the medical workup to limit over-medicalization and promote high-value care.
- An interdisciplinary team approach is integral to providing patients with comprehensive care: involve social work, child life, nursing, physical therapy, and occupational therapy.
- Emphasize the rehabilitation model with a focus on the connection between the mind and body.

SUGGESTED READINGS

Bakvis P, Spinhoven P, Giltay EJ, et al. Basal hypercortisolism and trauma in patients with psychogenic nonepileptic seizures. *Epilepsia*. 2009;51:752-759.

Borkum JM. Chronic headaches and the neurobiology of somatization. *Curr Pain Headache Rep*. 2010;14:55-61.

Bujoreanu IS, Ibeziako PI, DeMaso DR. Psychiatric concerns in pediatric epilepsy. *Child Adolesc Psychiatr Clin N Am*. 2010;371-386.

Bursch B. Pediatric pain. In: Shaw RH, DeMaso DR eds. *Textbook of Pediatric Psychosomatic Medicine: Mental Health Consultation with Physically Ill Children*. Washington DC: American Psychiatric Press; 2010:141-154.

Campo JV, Bridge J, Ehmann M, et al. Recurrent abdominal pain, anxiety, and depression in primary care. *Pediatrics*. 2004;113:817-824.

Chinta SS, Malhi P, Singhi P, Prabhakar S. Clinical and psychosocial characteristics of children with nonepileptic seizures. *Ann Indian Acad Neurol*. 2008;11(3):159-163.

Cloninger CR, Dokucu, ME. Somatoform and dissociative disorders. In: Fatemi SH, Clayton PJ eds. *The Medical Basis of Psychiatry*. 3rd ed. Humana Press; 2008:190-191.

Cruz N, O'Reilly J, Slomine BS, Salorio CF. Emotional and neuropsychological profiles of children with complex regional pain syndrome type-I in an inpatient rehabilitation setting. *Clin J Pain*. 2011;27(1):27-34.

Gates JR. Provocative testing should not be used for nonepileptic seizures. *Arch Neurol*. 2001;58(12):2065-2066.

Griffin A, Christie D. Taking the psycho out of psychosomatic: using systemic approaches in a pediatric setting for the treatment of adolescents with unexplained psychical symptoms. *Clin Child Psychol Psychiatry*. 2008;13:531-542.

Ibeziako PI, Bujoreanu S. Approach to psychosomatic illness in adolescents. *Curr Opin Pediatr*. 2011;4:384-389.

Ibeziako PI, DeMaso DR. The somatoform disorders. In: Klykylo WM, Kay JL, eds. *Clinical Child Psychiatry*. 3rd ed. West Sussex, England: Wiley. 2012;26:458-474.

Johnson KB, Harris C, Forstein M, Joffe A. Adolescent conversion disorder and the importance of competence discussing sexual orientation. *Clin Pediatr*. 2010;49:491-494.

Kanaan RA, Armstrong D, Wessely SC. Neurologists' understanding and management of conversion disorder. *J Neurol Neurosurg Psychiatry*. 2011;82:961-966.

Karterud HN, Knizek BL, Nakken KO. Changing the diagnosis from epilepsy to PNES: patients' experiences and understanding of their new diagnosis. *Seizure*. 2010;19:40-46.

Kozlowska K, Rose D, Khan R, MA, Kram S, Lane L, Collins J. A conceptual model and practice framework for managing chronic pain in children and adolescents. *Harvard Rev Psychiatry*. 2008;16: 136-150.

LaFrance WC Jr, Miller IW, Ryan CE, et al. Cognitive behavioral therapy for psychogenic non-epileptic seizures. *Epilepsy Behav*. 2009;14(4):591-596.

Leue C, Driessen G, Strik JJ, et al. Managing complex patients on a medical psychiatric unit: an observational study of university hospital costs associated with medical service use, length of stay and psychiatric intervention. *J Psychosomat Res*. 2010;68:295-302.

Libow J. Beyond collusion: active illness falsification. *Child Abuse Neglect*. 2002;26:525-536.

Meredith PJ, Ownsworth T, Strong J. A review of the evidence linking adult attachment theory and chronic pain: presenting a conceptual model. *Clin Psychol Rev*. 2008;28:407-409.

Nickel R, Ademmer K, Egle UT. Manualized psychodynamic interactional group therapy for the treatment of somatoform pain disorders. *Bull Menninger Clin*. 2010;74:219-237.

Plioplys S, Asato MR, Bursch B, et al. Multidisciplinary management of pediatric nonepileptic seizures. *J Am Acad Child Adolesc Psychiatry*. 2007;46(11):1491-1495.

Schroder A, Rehfeld E, Ornbol E, Sharpe M, et al. Cognitive-behavioural group treatment for a range of functional somatic syndromes: randomised trial. *Br J Psychiatry*. 2012;200(6):499-507.

Seshia SS, Phillips DF, von Baeyer CL. Childhood chronic daily headache: a biopsychosocial perspective. *Devel Med Child Neurol*. 2008;50:541-545.

Shaw R. Somatoform Disorder. In: Shaw RH, DeMaso DR eds. *Textbook of Pediatric Psychosomatic Medicine: Mental Health Consultation with Physically Ill Children*. Washington DC: American Psychiatric Press; 2010:121-139.

Siket MS, Merchant RC. Psychogenic seizures: a review and description of pitfalls in their acute diagnosis and management in the emergency department. *Emerg Med Clin N Am*. 2011;29:73-81.

Silber TJ. Somatization disorders: diagnosis, treatment and prognosis. *Pediatr Rev*. 2011;32:56-64.

Spratt EG, Thomas SG. Pediatric case study and review: is it a conversion disorder? *Int J Psychiatry Med*. 2008;38:185-193.

Stiles TC, Wright D. Cognitive behavioral treatment of chronic pain conditions. *Nordic J Psychiatry*. 2008;62(Suppl 47):30-36.

Sumathipala A, Siribaddana S, Hewege S, et al. Understanding the explanatory model of the patient on their medically unexplained symptoms and its implications on treatment development research: a Sri Lanka Study. *BMC Psychiatry*. 2008;8:54.

CHAPTER 138 Agitation

Evan Dalton, MD, MSHP and Roger K. Nicome, MD

BACKGROUND

Children with mental health conditions may become acutely agitated during their admission to a medical hospital. Medical hospitals work to keep these children, their families, and hospital staff safe during episodes of agitation. Clinicians can respond to these mental health emergencies by using a variety of interventions including verbal de-escalation, distraction, as-needed (PRN) psychotropic medications, and physical restraint—both through manual physical holds and mechanical devices. However, the environment of these pediatric medical units is typically not designed to care for children with mental health conditions and the staff on medical units often lack specialized training on the care of the agitated child. Consequently, agitation episodes can have a high risk of staff injuries.

Pediatric hospitalists have the opportunity to lead the treatment team in providing integrated, multi-disciplinary care to children experiencing agitation during their hospitalization. Hospitalists should foster partnerships with available experts in the field of pediatric mental health at their own institution to form this treatment team, including child and adolescent psychiatrists, psychologists, specialized nurses, therapists, social workers, and child-life specialists. This chapter reviews best practices in identifying, managing, treating, and preventing acute agitation in children with mental health conditions who are admitted to a medical hospital.

PATHOPHYSIOLOGY

Agitation in children exists across a spectrum, ranging from verbal outbursts to physical violence. Pediatric agitation can be driven by a variety of biopsychosocial factors. Since agitation is not a marker for a specific underlying diagnosis, the pediatric hospitalist's evaluation of an agitated child requires a thorough investigation that is best done in collaboration with the child's family members or caregivers. Factors that commonly contribute to agitation can be categorized into four groups: physiologic, mental, environmental, and historical **(Table 138-1)**. Children are often agitated by a combination of these factors, and each type of agitation driver has its own distinct method of diagnosis and treatment.

TABLE 138-1 Common Underlying Factors Contributing to Pediatric Agitation

Factors
Physiologic Factors
• Delirium (e.g., secondary to insomnia, sepsis)
• CNS (e.g., headache, trauma, meningoencephalitis, epilepsy)
• Metabolic (e.g., hypoxia, hypercarbia)
• Endocrine (e.g., hyperglycemia, hyperthyroidism)
• Pain (e.g., constipation, dental pain)
• Infection (e.g., acute otitis media, dental infection)
• Medication side effects (e.g., steroids, psychotropic medications)
• Catatonia
• Intoxication secondary to substance use
Mental & Behavioral Health Factors
• Attention deficit hyperactivity disorder (ADHD)
• Posttraumatic stress disorder (PTSD)
• Bipolar disorder
• Autism spectrum disorder (ASD)
• Disruptive mood dysregulation disorder (DMDD)
• Psychosis
• Anxiety
Environmental Factors
• Overstimulation from bright lights, noises of alarms and monitors, and unfamiliar smell
• Lack of physical space in hospital room
• Unfamiliar medical personnel
• Restriction of preferred activities
• Lack or restriction of limited food or drink preferences
Historical Factors
• Recent psychosocial stressors at home or school
• History of restraint or seclusion
• History of trauma including witnessed violence or victim of violence
• History of physical or sexual abuse
• Recent or remote history of agitation or physical aggression
• History of intellectual or cognitive disability

The multifactorial drivers of pediatric agitation can be demonstrated through the following case example. A nonverbal, male teenager with autism spectrum disorder presents to a pediatric medical hospital due to increasingly aggressive behaviors at home and at school, including head banging and property destruction. He has been admitted to this hospital multiple times before and was discharged to a local inpatient psychiatric facility following each admission. On obtaining a history, clinicians learn that he has chronic constipation and has not stooled in 7 days. His parents state that he has refused to take his home psychotropic medications for the past 3 days due to his abdominal discomfort. During his initial evaluation in the hospital's emergency department, he begins to become anxious. He vocalizes loudly and begins to scratch himself and his parents. He rocks back and forth, crying and screaming. As staff and security approach his room to verbally de-escalate, he jumps out of his bed and elopes into the hallway, pushing frantically past his parents and the treatment team before injuring a nurse. He is physically escorted back to his room by hospital staff in a manual hold, placed in four-point mechanical limb restraints and given an intramuscular psychotropic medication.

This vignette depicts the complex interplay among factors that contribute to agitation in children and adolescents. This patient had physical pain caused by constipation, leading to an inability to tolerate oral medications. Unable to receive his standing psychotropic medications, his frustration tolerance decreased, and his anxiety increased. He communicated his mental distress through escalating physical behaviors due to his lack of verbal communication skills. His anxiety worsened upon presentation to the medical hospital, likely due to past traumatic experiences in hospitals and sensory overload in a busy emergency department. He exhibited physical signs of agitation that escalated to physical aggression. Overwhelmed by the hospital environment, he tried to escape his room. Since he did not respond to verbal redirection and injured a staff member, he was placed in physical restraints and given an intramuscular medication, which will likely lead to a subsequent period of calm or sleep. However, he may awaken in a state of confusion from the side effects of the medication or the mental and physical trauma of the event, leading to the potential for recurrent agitation.

Adverse childhood experiences (ACEs) have a tremendous impact on the development of children's neurobiological systems and permanently alter their response to future stressors. The toxic stress of ACEs has been implicated in biological alterations to the limbic system and hypothalamic-pituitary axis, resulting in an enhanced and prolonged stress response. These changes enhance traumatic memories in the hippocampus and impair the child's ability to discriminate between safe and unsafe stimuli. Children with histories of trauma may experience an exaggerated response to stress and react with sudden outbursts before using their prefrontal cortex to assess or plan their response to the perceived threat. Since trauma is quite common and children and families may not always disclose trauma, pediatric hospitalists should treat all children as though they have had prior traumatic experiences and incorporate principles of trauma-informed care into their behavior plan. In cases where a specific prior trauma is known, such as physical or sexual abuse, loss of a primary caregiver, peer victimization or bullying, pediatric hospital teams should avoid recreating aspects of prior adverse experiences so the child is not re-traumatized during their hospitalization.

CLINICAL PRESENTATION

Agitation presents clinically as the outward manifestation of underlying mental distress. The pediatric hospitalist should recognize that the external physical symptoms of an agitated child are driven by the child's internal psychological state. Agitation can manifest across a spectrum as the child escalates through stages of agitation ranging from restlessness to physical violence.

The stages of agitation are commonly categorized within a paradigm of mild, moderate, or severe agitation **(Figure 138-1)**. Mild agitation is driven predominantly by underlying anxiety. Children with mild agitation may exhibit an increase in behaviors such as rocking, crying, pacing, posturing, fidgeting, restlessness, and excessive worrying. Mildly agitated children may be confused but should respond to instructions and verbal redirection. As the child progresses to a level of moderate agitation, they begin to challenge authority and refuse initial attempts at redirection. Moderately agitated children can be loud, boisterous, or irritable. They may use inappropriate language or verbal threats when communicating with others. They may show physical signs of escalation, such as scratching themselves, lightly head banging, or throwing objects. However, children at a moderate level of agitation have not yet endangered the safety of themselves or others. Severely agitated children exhibit physically aggressive behavior intended to hurt or damage themselves, others, or property.

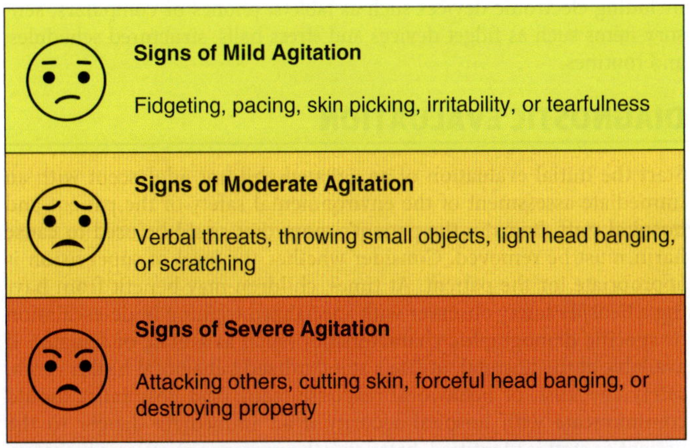

FIGURE 138-1. Signs of mild, moderate, and severe agitation.

Multiple validated scales such as the Brøset Violence Checklist (BVC), Brief Rating of Aggression by Children and Adolescents (BRACHA), and the Behavioral Activity Rating Scale (BARS) have been used in medical hospitals to score the clinical signs of agitation in both children and adults. These scales can be performed quickly, and their results are easily interpretable by staff. Pediatric hospitalists can utilize these scales to assess their patients' agitation severity and match their treatment interventions to the patient's level of agitation. Clinical protocols for treating agitation can be helpful in coordinating and scaling the response to agitation at pediatric medical hospitals. Optimal protocols target early identification and de-escalation of agitation through least restrictive means before the child reaches a severe level of agitation.

DIFFERENTIAL DIAGNOSIS

Agitation, like pain, is a symptom with many potential etiologies. Agitation can be treated like a vital sign for children, an indication of the child's distress that requires urgent evaluation and management. Pediatric hospitalists should assess agitated children with a broad differential, including broad considerations if the child has developmental or cognitive disabilities.

Physical diseases can contribute to pediatric agitation through underlying pain, irritation, or alteration of the patient's sensorium. Central nervous system disorders such as brain injury, epilepsy, encephalitis, brain tumors, and systemic conditions with neurologic manifestations such as sepsis, hyperthyroidism, delirium, medication side effects, and intoxication can agitate children. Common mental health conditions like anxiety and depression can predispose children to low frustration tolerance, depressed mood, panic, and other internal states that can predispose children to agitation. Less common mental health conditions such as psychosis or mania can cause cognitive and perceptual disturbances that predispose children to agitation. Chronic substance use can predispose children to substance withdrawal which can present with agitation.

Children with limited verbal communication, such as those with autism spectrum disorder or developmental delay, require additional clinical investigation when presenting with agitation. It is critical that the pediatric hospitalist acknowledge that conditions like autism are not a cause of agitation alone. Children with autism and developmental disabilities are more likely to have certain physical conditions, including constipation, gastrointestinal issues, epilepsy and insomnia, and mental health conditions, such as ADHD, anxiety, schizophrenia, bipolar disorder, and obsessive-compulsive disorder. These conditions can trigger agitation or aggression in children with autism or developmental delay. Common triggers for agitation include transitions between tasks, sensory overstimulation, overwhelming demands, the inability to engage in their preferred behaviors, and difficulty communicating their wants and needs to others. For children with autism and developmental disabilities, understanding unique interests, home routines, and medical comorbidities can help maintain a broad and appropriate differential diagnosis. The unique interests and triggers of these children should be explored, communicated among team members, and utilized in the child's treatment plan. For example, offer items that are soothing to children with autism including electronic devices such as tablets, phones or computers, sensory items such as fidget devices and stress balls, structured schedules, and routines.

DIAGNOSTIC EVALUATION

Start the initial evaluation of an agitated child or adolescent with an immediate assessment of the environmental safety of the patient and hospital staff. Items in the patient's room that could be used to cause harm must be removed. Consider whether the level of supervision is appropriate for the patient. At times, children may benefit from having a bedside safety observer with specialized training in de-escalation or specific demographic characteristics (such as a male or female). If available at the hospital, utilize a standardized behavioral health room, safety checklist, or behavioral response team. The hospitalist should communicate with hospital security if an immediate danger to the patient or staff is identified, balancing the presence of officers for safety with the potential that the child may become further escalated by their presence.

The next step in the evaluation of the agitated child is to assess the etiology and severity of the child's agitation. Obtain a focused history and physical examination as tolerated by the child. Then, investigate the child's medical, psychiatric, trauma, and developmental histories. Interview family members regarding their perception of the child's behavior, the child's interests and triggers, and any antecedents to the child's current behavior. In addition, ask about recent external stressors in the child's home and school environments. Consider using scales such as the modified overt aggression scale to help assess and monitor the frequency, severity, change, and character of the child's recent agitation episodes. We recommend evaluating for physical discomfort and pain using history, physical examination, and limited diagnostic studies as tolerated. Laboratory and imaging studies should be considered, if necessary, weighing the benefits of additional clinical information against the difficulty of performing these studies on an acutely agitated child.

The acutely agitated child may have difficulty participating in the examination, and their response to verbal redirection can assist the clinician in identifying their level of agitation. If the child responds to prompts and follows directions, they should be considered mildly agitated rather than moderately or severely agitated. If the underlying etiology of the child's agitation cannot be immediately identified, symptomatic management should be initiated via nonpharmacologic and, if necessary, pharmacologic measures. The child's response to this management should then be monitored and used to tailor the treatment plan.

Depending on the resources available, hospitalists should engage providers from other disciplines at this stage of the assessment. Child and adolescent psychiatrists, child-life specialists, social workers, nurses, and 1:1 observers can play critical roles in the assessment and treatment of agitated children. Consult these providers as early as possible in the patient's hospital course, so that a collaborative treatment plan can be established, and the appropriate disposition destination identified and facilitated.

MANAGEMENT

The management of an acutely agitated child can be structured through the following stepwise approach that is detailed further in **Figure 138-2.**

SECURING THE ENVIRONMENT

The initial step in the management of pediatric agitation is to immediately identify and mitigate risks to the safety of the patient or staff. Safety risks in the patient's room include unsecured objects (e.g., medical equipment, TV remote, chairs, trash cans, utensils) and people who may further escalate the patient. Consider which of the hospital staff need to be in the patient room and remove extraneous staff. In some cases, visitors or family members contribute to a patient's agitation. Once the room is as safe as possible, the hospitalist can assess the severity and etiologies of the patient's agitation.

NONPHARMACOLOGIC INTERVENTIONS

The next step is to engage the patient in nonpharmacologic measures of de-escalation. Use nonpharmacologic interventions proactively for all agitated children, regardless of their level of agitation to help prevent further escalation. When initiating an encounter with an agitated child, hospitalists should introduce themselves and emphasize that they are there to help the child. Speak to the patient clearly and slowly and at their level of understanding using simple phrases and commands that can be repeated as needed. State the goals for the encounter, such as improving the child's distress and ensuring safety for all parties, while showing empathy to the patient's condition. It is critical to remain cognizant of nonverbal communication when addressing an agitated child and avoid a threatening stance as much as possible, leaving arms uncrossed and knees slightly bent. Additionally, ensure that there is a clear line of sight to the door for both the child and the physician. If the child is nonverbal, it may be helpful to use images, storyboards, or even basic sign language

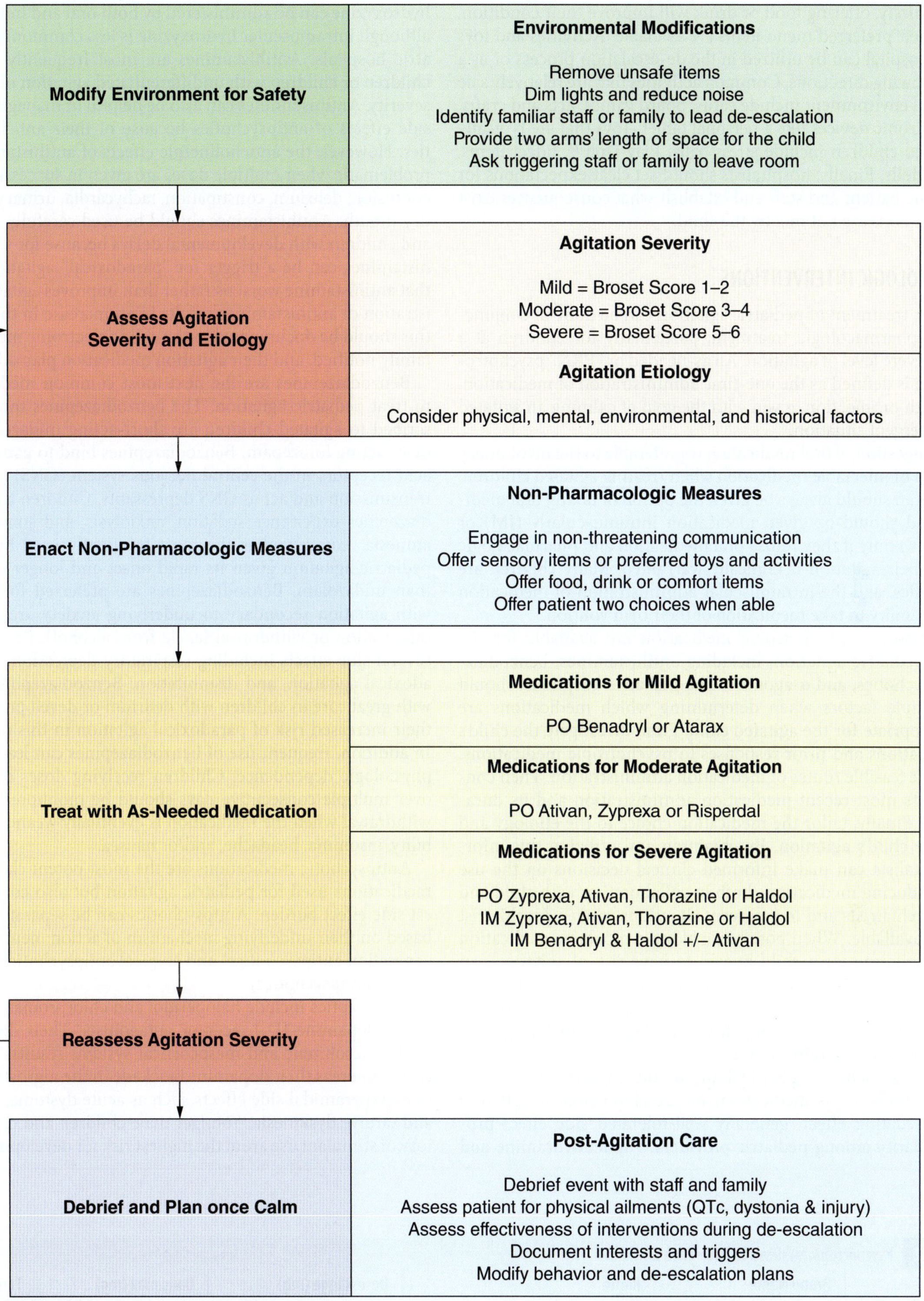

FIGURE 138-2. Management of hospitalized pediatric patients with acute agitation. (Adapted from Hoffmann JA, Pergjika A, Konicek CE, Reynolds SL. Pharmacologic management of acute agitation in youth in the emergency department. *Pediatr Emerg Care.* 2021;37(8):417-422.)

for communication. Quite often, the agitated child is reluctant to comply with instructions or procedures because they feel overwhelmed and powerless. In these circumstances, offering them simple binary options ("Can you sit on the bed or the couch?" or "Would you like me to take your blood pressure on your left arm or your right?") and encouraging them to choose can help them regain a sense of control and diffuse the interaction.

Additional nonpharmacologic management of agitation can be accomplished through modifications to the hospital environment, and the provision of toys and activities. Children may be overwhelmed by the sensory stimulation of the hospital. If the child appears to be triggered by noises, it is helpful to identify and play music that calms the child or provide noise-blocking headphones. The lights of the hospital room should be dimmed, and window blinds closed to lower the brightness. If the child is hungry or thirsty, offering food or drink will improve their condition, especially if their preferred menu items are available. Activities and toys found in the hospital can be utilized in the de-escalation process or as a reward for following directions. Common activities that are relatively safe for the hospital environment include cards, board games, arts and crafts, and some electronic devices like a personal tablet. Toys that are typically safe for agitated children include stress balls, Play Doh™, fidget items, blankets, and dolls. Finally, hospitalists should set clear expectations for the safety of the patient and staff and establish what consequences exist if these expectations are not met by the child.

PHARMACOLOGIC INTERVENTIONS

Pharmacologic treatment of pediatric agitation can be done in conjunction with nonpharmacologic treatment, particularly for children at a moderate or severe level of agitation. An as-needed or "PRN" psychotropic medication is defined as the one-time administration of medication, either by mouth or injection, given with the goal of calming an agitated child in an emergent situation.

Voluntary ingestion of oral medication is preferable to the involuntary administration of injectable medication when treating agitated children. Agitated children should always be given the option of taking oral medication first and should be given medication intramuscularly (IM) or intravenous (IV) only if they refuse oral medication and pharmacologic treatment of their agitation is clinically warranted. Many children are fearful of needles, and the intramuscular administration of medication removes their ability to take medication of their own volition.

Multiple classes of psychotropic medication are available for the treatment of pediatric agitation, including antihistamines, benzodiazepines, antipsychotics, and α-agonists. The pediatric hospitalist should consider multiple factors when determining which medications are the most appropriate for the agitated child. First, investigate the child's current medications and prior responses to psychotropic medications. Next, assess the feasible routes of medication administration. Then consider the child's most recent medication administration and its duration of action. Finally, tailor the medication choice to the etiology and severity of the child's agitation. By obtaining and utilizing this information, hospitalists can make informed clinical decisions on the use of agitation-reducing medications both in collaboration with child and adolescent psychiatrists and in emergent situations when a psychiatrist is not readily available. When possible, making a proactive medication plan to treat agitation for a child known to have risk of agitation can help providers offer medication for voluntary oral administration earlier and reduce polypharmacy. Additional reference information on the dosing and timing of as-needed psychotropic medications for agitated children can be found in **Table 138-2**.

Antihistamines such as diphenhydramine and hydroxyzine are the most utilized psychotropic medications for treating pediatric agitation due to their sedating effect, generally well-tolerated side effect profile, and familiarity among pediatric providers. Diphenhydramine and hydroxyzine can be administered by both oral and intramuscular routes, although intramuscular hydroxyzine is less commonly available in pediatric hospitals. Antihistamines are most frequently used for younger children or children with undifferentiated agitation of mild to moderate severity. Antihistamines can also be helpful in managing extrapyramidal side effects of antipsychotics because of their anticholinergic properties. However, the anticholinergic effects of antihistamines can become problematic when multiple doses are given in succession and may cause confusion, delirium, constipation, tachycardia, urinary retention, and/or dry mouth. Antihistamines should be used carefully in young children and children with developmental delays because for some children antihistamines can be a trigger for "paradoxical" agitation, paradoxical in that antihistamine worsens rather than improves agitation. If the administration of antihistamines results in an increase in the child's agitation, this should be documented in the child's electronic medical record, their family notified, and their agitation medication plan adjusted.

Benzodiazepines are the next most common medication class used to treat pediatric agitation. The benzodiazepines most frequently prescribed to agitated children are short-acting midazolam and intermediate-acting lorazepam. Benzodiazepines bind to gamma-aminobutyric acid receptors in the central nervous system (CNS) and inhibit neurotransmission and act as CNS depressants. Children treated with benzodiazepines experience sedation, anxiolysis, and some may experience amnesia. Lorazepam is the most frequently used benzodiazepine for pediatric agitation given its rapid onset and longer duration of action than midazolam. Benzodiazepines are preferred for treating children with agitation secondary to underlying anxiety, trauma, or substance intoxication or withdrawal (aside from alcohol). Benzodiazepines have several side effects including respiratory depression, hypotension, paradoxical agitation, and disinhibition. Benzodiazepines should be used with great care in children with delirium or developmental delay due to their increased risk of paradoxical agitation in this patient population. In addition, frequent use of benzodiazepines can lead to tolerance and physiologic dependence. Children receiving doses of benzodiazepines over multiple consecutive days should be monitored for symptoms of withdrawal when the medication is eventually weaned, including irritability, insomnia, headache, and/or nausea.

Antipsychotic medications are the most potent class of psychotropic medications used for pediatric agitation but also come with the greatest side effect burden. Antipsychotics can be separated into two classes based on their underlying mechanism of action: neuroleptics (i.e., first-generation antipsychotics) and atypical antipsychotics (i.e., second-generation antipsychotics).

Neuroleptics include haloperidol and chlorpromazine, both of which act as dopamine (D_2) receptor antagonists. Their dopamine blockade in the mesolimbic and mesocortical systems results in their treatment effect, whereas their dopamine blockade in the nigrostriatal system leads to extrapyramidal side effects such as acute dystonia, akathisia, tremor, and tardive dyskinesia. Younger male children and children with a history of stimulant use are at the highest risk for developing extrapyramidal

TABLE 138-2 Psychotropic Medication Reference Guide

Medication	Brand Name	Route	Dose Range (mg)	Daily max (mg)	Time until Peak (PO)
Diphenhydramine	Benadryl	PO, IM, IV	12.5-50	100-200	2 hours
Hydroxyzine	Atarax or Vistaril	PO	12.5-50	50-100	2 hours
Midazolam	Versed	PO, IM, IV, intranasal, buccal	0.5-2	6-10	30 minutes
Lorazepam	Ativan	PO, IM, IV	0.5-2	4-8	1-2 hours
Chlorpromazine	Thorazine	PO, IM	12.5-50	40-75	30-60 minutes
Haloperidol	Haldol	PO, IM, IV	1-5	6-15	2 hours
Olanzapine	Zyprexa	PO, IM, ODT	1.25-5	10-20	5 hours
Risperidone	Risperdal	PO, ODT	0.25-1	1 - 3	1 hour
Quetiapine	Seroquel	PO	12.5-100	400-800	1-2 hours
Clonidine	Catapres	PO	0.05-0.1	0.2-0.4	2-4 hours

symptoms when receiving antipsychotics for agitation. Acute dystonia is a movement disorder characterized by sustained muscle contractions that leads to abnormal postures, most commonly involving muscles of the face and neck. Acute dystonia is seen most often with haloperidol use and can be treated with intramuscular diphenhydramine or benztropine. Neuroleptics can also cause cardiac adverse effects including prolonged QTc interval, hypotension, and neuroleptic malignant syndrome. Neuroleptic malignant syndrome is a significant adverse reaction that includes symptoms of fever, altered mental status and muscle rigidity, and can be treated with discontinuation of the antipsychotic, supportive care, intravenous fluids, and bromocriptine or dantrolene.

Atypical antipsychotics used to treat pediatric agitation include olanzapine, risperidone, and quetiapine. Atypical antipsychotics work mechanistically through the blockage of both dopamine and serotonin receptors. Their affinity for dopamine receptors is less than that of neuroleptics, which reduces their risk of causing extrapyramidal symptoms. Atypical antipsychotics are commonly given as a tablet by mouth, but olanzapine can be given intramuscularly or as an oral dissolving tablet. Atypical antipsychotics have a similar side effect profile to typical antipsychotics, including extrapyramidal symptoms, respiratory depression, and hypotension. Intramuscular olanzapine should not be coadministered with intramuscular lorazepam due to the risk of cardiorespiratory collapse.

Antipsychotics can work well for calming agitated children with developmental delay, psychosis, or mania. They can be coadministered along with an anticholinergic medication such as diphenhydramine or benztropine to reduce their risk causing of extrapyramidal symptoms. Antipsychotics are often the preferred medication for treating children with severe agitation but should be used cautiously given their side effects.

Alpha-2 agonists like clonidine and guanfacine are the least commonly used class of psychotropic medication for treating pediatric agitation. Clonidine works by decreasing norepinephrine release in the central and peripheral nervous system and causes sedation in addition to side effects such as hypotension, dizziness, and dry mouth. The onset of these medications is relatively slow and their level of sedation is mild in comparison to other classes of psychotropic medications used for pediatric agitation. Alpha-2 agonists may be used as treatment of agitation for children who are already prescribed this class of medication and may benefit from an additional as needed dose for treatment.

PHARMACOLOGIC RESTRAINT

Pharmacologic or chemical restraint is different than PRN medication administration for treatment of agitation. A pharmacologic restraint is defined by the Code of Federal Regulations as a medication used to control behavior or to restrict the participant's freedom of movement and is not a standard treatment for the participant's medical or psychiatric condition. Pharmacologic restraint is a deviation from the patient's existing treatment plan and can be administered without the patient's consent. This is typically achieved through the coadministration of multiple intramuscular psychotropic medications and is designed for rapid-onset sedation of the patient. The definition of pharmacologic restraint includes the use of higher than necessary doses of mediations to treat agitation and unnecessary use of multiple medications. Pharmacologic restraint should be avoided in pediatric hospitals with the goal of using standard treatment doses for the appropriate medical management of agitation.

PHYSICAL RESTRAINT

Manual physical restraint is a last resort intervention for the management of pediatric agitation and is only indicated to prevent clear, imminent harm to the patient and others when all other interventions have failed. The Joint Commission (TJC), recognizing the severity of this type of restraint, has detailed standards that hospitals must follow when restraining patients. The use of manual restraint involves the restriction of the child's body using physical hold or mechanical limb devices, the latter being the more common in pediatric medical hospitals. Mechanical restraints are typically "four-point," meaning they fix each of the child's four limbs to the bedframe to restrict the child's movement. Physical restraints are used for safety purposes, but their application is a high-risk procedure that can result in patient and staff injury. In addition, restraint use can cause psychological trauma to patients and staff alike with lasting consequences on children's well-being. Unfortunately, racial and ethnic disparities in restraint use have been shown to exist at pediatric hospitals, with Black children more likely to be restrained than White children. While data on the frequency of physical restraint at pediatric hospitals in the United States are limited, published rates of restraint use range between 0.1% and 16% of patients across different medical units, reflecting variability in the threshold at which staff determine restraint use is necessary. Pediatric hospitalists should work to ensure that TJC standards are adhered to and minimize restraint use for agitated children through prevention efforts. If restraints are absolutely indicated, the hospitalist should examine the child during restraint and work with the team to minimize the child's time spent in restraints. If a child must be restrained, their physiologic state should be closely monitored, especially for signs of respiratory depression or restriction of freedom of movement of the chest and neck.

POST AGITATION CARE

The final step in the management of pediatric agitation is the initiation of postagitation care. An episode of agitation has resolved when the child demonstrates a decrease in physical and emotional energy and has regained rational control. The child may apologize, cry, sleep, or become engaged in an alternative activity. The child should be able to communicate and respond to redirection at this stage.

Following an episode of acute agitation, assess the child for physical ailments secondary to the medications or restraints used in the de-escalation. For medications, this includes calculation of the total medication dosage administered and monitoring for medication side effects such as extrapyramidal symptoms or arrythmias and injuries secondary to physical intervention including restraint. If a child requires physical restraints, they should be thoroughly assessed for injuries resulting from restraint application or use, including joint, skin, and soft tissue injury.

The hospitalist should then assist with leading a thorough debrief of the child's treatment team through a clinical event debriefing. A clinical event debriefing is a facilitated discussion with unit staff that occurs immediately following a significant clinical event and is meant to foster rapid-cycle improvement. The priority of the debrief is to ensure the physical safety of staff involved, assess for injuries, and confirm the unit can return to regular operations. Then, the debriefing team should review the child's history and antecedent triggers for their agitation, reflect on the strengths and opportunities for improvement of the team's response, identify system issues impacting the child and treatment team, and implement strategies to prevent recurrence of the child's agitation. A revised treatment plan should reflect identified triggers, future pharmacological and behavioral interventions, and preventative measures gathered from the event debriefing.

PEARLS AND PITFALLS

- Hospitals with the resources to support behavioral response teams have been successful in implementing processes for psychiatric "codes" which are designed to alert specialized staff of an ongoing psychiatric emergency. A group of clinicians (ideally mental health specialists) familiar with the management of acute agitation should be the designated behavioral response team, or "psychiatric code team." When an episode of acute agitation occurs on a medical floor or emergency department, this behavioral response team can be immediately notified and respond promptly and effectively to the psychiatric crisis.
- Children experiencing acute agitation may be more willing to take oral medications if they are in liquid form. Liquid formulations exist for multiple psychotropic medications including lorazepam, risperidone, haloperidol, and clonidine.
- Oral medications typically have an onset of action within 30 minutes of administration, whereas intramuscular medications may have onset as quickly as 5 to 10 minutes after administration. Hospitalists should be cognizant of the delayed onset of oral medications and use caution when administering multiple oral medications within short succession.

Hospitalists should also consider using medication when patients have mild to moderate agitation to allow time for the medication to take effect and avoid severe agitation.

KEY POINTS

Acute agitation in children and adolescents frequently occurs in pediatric acute care medical hospitals. Pediatric agitation is an emergency and should be assessed and managed immediately by pediatric hospitalists in collaboration with the available members of the child's treatment team and family. Nonpharmacologic interventions including environmental modifications, toys, and activities can help manage and prevent episodes of pediatric agitation. Various medication options are available for treatment of agitation in the pediatric population and guidelines exist to support the pediatric hospitalist in selecting the most appropriate medication for treatment. A multi-disciplinary approach to the management of pediatric agitation in the medical hospital setting can help ensure safety for the patient and staff through protocolized de-escalation and debriefing.

SUGGESTED READINGS

AAP, AACAP, CHA Declare National Emergency in Children's Mental Health. American Academy of Pediatrics https://publications.aap.org/aapnews/news/17718?autologincheck=redirected.

Dalton EM, Herndon AC, Cundiff A, et al. Decreasing the use of restraints on children admitted for behavioral health conditions. *Pediatrics*. 2021;148(1):e2020003939.

Galligan MM, DeBrocco D, Friedlaender E. Debriefing during a mental health crisis. *J Hosp Med*. 2021;16(7):440-442.

Gerson R, Malas N, Feuer V, Silver GH, Prasad R, Mroczkowski MM. Best practices for evaluation and treatment of agitated children and adolescents (BETA) in the emergency department: Consensus Statement of the American Association for Emergency Psychiatry. *West J Emerg Med*. 2019;20(2):409-418.

Goddard A. Adverse childhood experiences and trauma-informed care. *J Pediatr Health Care*. 2021;35(2):145-155.

Hoffmann JA, Pergjika A, Konicek CE, Reynolds SL. Pharmacologic management of acute agitation in youth in the emergency department. *Pediatr Emerg Care*. 2021;37(8):417-422.

Leyenaar JK, Freyleue SD, Bordogna A, Wong C, Penwill N, Bode R. Frequency and duration of boarding for pediatric mental health conditions at acute care hospitals in the US. *JAMA*. 2021;326(22):2326-2328.

Lo CB, Bridge JA, Shi J, Ludwig L, Stanley RM. Children's mental health emergency department visits: 2007–2016. *Pediatrics*. 2020;145(6):e20191536.

McMillan JA, Land M, Leslie LK. Pediatric residency education and the behavioral and mental health crisis: a call to action. *Pediatrics*. 2017;139(1):e20162141.

Nash KA, Tolliver DG, Taylor RA, et al. Racial and ethnic disparities in physical restraint use for pediatric patients in the emergency department. *JAMA Pediatr*. 2021;175(12):1283-1285.

Nicome R, Lo HY, Gupta S, et al. Utilizing a behavioral health bundle to improve patient and clinician safety for hospitalized children. *Pediatr Qual Saf*. 2021;6(2):e393.

Noah A, Andrade G, DeBrocco D, et al. Patient risk factors for violent restraint use in a children's hospital medical unit. *Hosp Pediatr*. 2021;11(8):833-840.

Plemmons G, Hall M, Doupnik S, et al. Hospitalization for suicide ideation or attempt: 2008–2015. *Pediatrics*. 2018;141(6):e20172426.

Poolman I. *Workforce Maps by State*. The American Academy of Child and Adolescent Psychiatry https://www.aacap.org/aacap/Advocacy/Federal_and_State_Initiatives/Workforce_Maps/Home.aspx.

Wong AH, Ray JM, Rosenberg A, et al. Experiences of individuals who were physically restrained in the emergency department. *JAMA Netw Open*. 2020;3(1):e1919381.

Worsley D, Barrios E, Shuter M, Pettit AR, Doupnik SK. Adolescents' experiences during "boarding" hospitalization while awaiting inpatient psychiatric treatment following suicidal ideation or suicide attempt. *Hosp Pediatr*. 2019;9(11):827-833.

CHAPTER 139 New-Onset Psychosis

Patricia A. Stoeck, MD and Charles R. Wulff, MD

BACKGROUND

Psychosis is a syndrome, the symptoms of which reflect a disruption and distortion of an individual's ability to effectively process their own thoughts and the world around them. Psychotic symptoms include hallucinations, delusions, or disorganization of thoughts and behavior. Children, adolescents, and adults can present with these symptoms in the context of psychiatric conditions such as depression, bipolar disorder, schizophrenia, substance use/abuse, and posttraumatic stress disorder, as well as medical conditions, including neurologic causes, metabolic disturbances, and infections.

Few studies have examined hallucination and delusion phenomenology in children, thereby making diagnosis and prevalence difficult to assess. Schizophrenia is estimated to impact 1% of the population, with a peak onset in late adolescence. Early-onset schizophrenia—before 18 years of age—is rare, occurring in less than 0.04% of children, and has a poor prognosis. Psychotic symptoms can also be present in other mood disorders in children and adolescents. For example, it is estimated that 40% of pediatric patients diagnosed with bipolar type I will have symptoms of psychosis during a mood episode. Regardless of the psychiatric diagnosis, hallucinations and delusions are present within the general population and appear to be associated with worse health function, higher incidence of depression, and higher likelihood of diagnosis and treatment for a psychiatric disorder.

CLINICAL PRESENTATION

Children with psychosis may present with cognitive abnormalities, emotional difficulties, and changes in social functioning. Studies indicate that premorbid social and emotional function is lower in patients who later develop schizophrenia or schizoaffective disorder, as opposed to mood disorders with psychotic features. In children and adolescents there is often a prodromal period, during which there is a decline in social, emotional, and academic function that precedes the onset of psychosis by a period of weeks to months. Changes in social functioning due to new-onset psychosis may present with disruptive behaviors, social withdrawal, or difficulties with peer relationships.

Cognitive manifestations of psychosis include distortions of thoughts to the extent of hallucinations or delusions (**Table 139-1**). Hallucinations are false sensory perceptions in the absence of stimuli; this is distinct from illusions, which are misinterpretations of actual stimuli, such as mistaking a jacket in the corner as a person. In children, hallucinations are most frequently auditory in nature. Delusions represent distorted or fixed beliefs that are not substantiated by evidence. Delusions can be impacted by the patient's interpretation of their environment, as well as their cultural and religious beliefs.

Patients presenting with new-onset psychosis can also present with alterations in their mood. Children can present as irritable, angry, or elevated (e.g., mania with psychosis). Negative symptoms may be present such as apathy, flat/blunted affect, and paucity of speech. Mood symptoms may change rapidly for patients and manifest in mood-congruent or -incongruent hallucinations or delusions. For example, a patient with a depressed mood may have mood-congruent hallucinations of voices speaking in a derogatory way about them, while having delusions of persecution by peers.

Speech and language may also be impacted by this altered cognitive state. In addition to hallucinations and delusions, patients with psychosis may respond to questions in a disorganized or nonsensical fashion. At times their dialogue may include perseveration on topics, creating new words/phrases (neologisms), or stereotypies (see Table 139-1). Behaviors may be congruent with the thought processes and patients may exhibit a regression of behaviors, bizarre behaviors, or other motoric disturbances.

TABLE 139-1 Symptoms Associated With Psychosis

Symptom	Clinical Presentation
Delusions	Fixed false belief without supporting evidence and inconsistent with patient's culture, social, or religious background. Types of delusions include: • Erotomanic: Individual believes another is in love with them • Grandiose: Belief one has exceptional, sometimes supernatural, abilities, fame, purpose, and/or insights • Persecutory: Belief an individual/organization/group is seeking to harm the individual in some manner • Jealous: Belief that a significant other is unfaithful • Referential: Belief that general elements of the environment and actions of others are specifically directed at the individual or carry content intended specifically for them; for example, an individual believing that a news broadcast is directly communicating to them • Somatic: belief about one's bodily functions or sensations; for example, believing one has a foul odor or that there are parasites under one's skin *Note*: Bizarre delusions are those with no clear grounding within reality. For example, a belief one is being monitored by the FBI through surveillance technology would not itself be bizarre, but the belief that the FBI surveillance is achieved using psychic powers would be considered bizarre.
Hallucinations	Sensory perception in the absence of a stimulus *Note*: auditory is the most common; other sensory perceptions (e.g., visual, tactile, olfactory, gustatory) are more concerning for underlying medical etiologies
Disorganized Thinking/Speech	• Looseness of associations: Speech content lacks clear tracking from one topic to another. This can range from tangential to flight of ideas to completely disorganized/loose associations • Though Blocking: Thought process abruptly stopped without clear conclusion, with no recall of train of thought • Incoherence: speech disorganized such that it appears as a "word salad," and can appear similar to receptive aphasia • Clanging: Word choice determined by similarity of sound, rather than means to convey content • Echolalia: Meaningless repetition of words/phrases patient has heard • Neologisms: Creation of new words, or use of words in new manner which is independent from its typical use
Disorganized/Catatonic Behavior	• Motor disturbances • Bizarre postures • Stereotypies: persistent, repetition of an action with no obvious purpose • Stupor: not actively relating to the environment • Extreme rigidity • Waxy flexibility: limbs retain the position into which another has placed them
Negative Symptoms	• Alogia: Limited/diminished speech • Avolition: Decrease in motivated, self-initiated, purposeful activities • Affective flattening: Diminished emotional expression • Anhedonia: Reduction in ability to experience pleasure • Asociality: Lack of interest in social engagement, social withdrawal

Source: Adapted from Schizophrenia Spectrum and Other Psychotic Disorders. In: *Diagnostic and Statistical Manual of Mental Disorders.* 5th ed,. Text Revision. American Psychiatric Association; 2022.

Catatonia represents the most extreme presentation of negative symptoms, including mutism, immobility, and avolition. Classical catatonia demonstrates severe bradykinesia with unusual properties such as waxy flexibility and stereotypies of the hand or other body parts. Conversely, excited catatonia can present with extreme psychomotor agitation without purposeful actions.

DIFFERENTIAL DIAGNOSIS

Given that clinical presentation may vary widely based on the underlying etiology, timing of presentation to care, and patient's developmental stage, a comprehensive medical history and physical examination is crucial for establishing the primary diagnosis leading to the onset of psychosis.

Determining whether psychotic symptoms are present in a child is challenging for several reasons. First, hallucinations are reported frequently in the pediatric population even in the absence of an underlying diagnosis. Second, identifying hallucinations or reactions to internal stimuli can be challenging depending on the child's developmental age, as they may respond with hyperactivity, aggression, tearfulness, or behavioral regression. Third, children with impaired receptive/expressive language or social capacity can present with disruptive and/or bizarre behavior in an effort to express their wishes. These behaviors can easily be misinterpreted as signs of a psychotic disorder. Finally, anxiety disorders can also mask or exacerbate behaviors in a way that appears psychotic when reviewed in isolation. For these reasons, a careful assessment should include comorbid psychiatric diagnoses, developmental stage, language capacity, and social/emotional development.

Further characterization of symptom onset is also necessary in diagnosing the underlying cause of new-onset psychosis. Acute onset of symptoms may indicate a possible physical insult to the body, including the central nervous system (CNS). Concurrent physiologic findings (e.g., fever, hypertension) also raise concern for underlying medical etiologies. By contrast, a more insidious onset of symptoms may be more consistent with a psychiatric diagnosis. For example, schizophrenia is associated with a prodromal period characterized by a reduction in functioning across social domains, while preceding or concurrent mood symptoms may help differentiate mood disorders with psychotic features from schizophrenia.

Regardless of presenting signs and symptoms, all patients who meet clinical criteria for new-onset psychosis should undergo a thoughtful diagnostic evaluation that is appropriately tailored to their clinical presentation. When psychotic symptoms manifest in very young children, clinical suspicion for medical conditions is much higher and more extensive diagnostic evaluation is likely warranted. See **Table 139-2**.

Children and adolescents should be evaluated for seizures, particularly when presenting with motor features such as alternating tonic-clonic movements or myoclonus. Furthermore, nonauditory hallucinations, such as visual, olfactory, and tactile hallucinations are less common in psychiatric conditions associated with psychosis and raise concern for seizure activity. Seizures may be the result of underlying epilepsy or other

TABLE 139-2 Medical Causes of New-Onset Psychosis: Clinical Features and Proposed Actions

	Clinical Features	Medical Condition	Actions
Autoimmune/ Rheumatologic/ Endocrine	Seizures, movement disorder, language regression, autonomic instability	Anti-NMDA receptor encephalitis	EEG, brain MRI, and LP; serum and CSF autoimmune encephalopathy panels *Note*: serum is 85% sensitive compared to 100% for CSF
	Malar rash, joint pain, fatigue, cytopenias	Systemic Lupus Erythematosus	Consult rheumatology; ESR, CRP, ANA, C3, C4, IgG
	Auditory or visual hallucinations, delusions of "impostors" (either of the patient or significant others), paranoia, few cognitive deficits, lethargy, normal level of consciousness	• Hashimoto thyroiditis • Hyperthyroidism	TSH/free T4, anti-thyroid antibodies
	Bruising, glucose intolerance, hyperlipidemia, hypertension, moon facies, truncal obesity, bitemporal hemianopsia or other visual impairment	• Cushing syndrome • Exogenous steroid use • Steroid-producing tumors (e.g., pituitary adenoma)	Consult endocrinology; prolactin, IGF-1, 24-hour urinary free cortisol, MRI
	Abnormal glucose metabolism, blurry vision, fatigue	Diabetes mellitus	Hemoglobin A1c, urinalysis
	Abdominal discomfort, bone disorders, kidney stones, confusion, depression, fatigue, hallucinations, paranoia	Parathyroid disease	Consult endocrinology; calcium, PTH, Vitamin D
Infectious	Fever, sore throat, lymphadenopathy, fatigue	Infectious mononucleosis	EBV titers
	Fever, cough, altered mental status	*Mycoplasma pneumoniae* Infection	Mycoplasma titers
	Target lesion, tick exposure	Lyme disease	*Borrelia burgdorferi* titers/tick-borne illness testing
	Cachexia, cognitive changes, delusions	HIV	Consult infectious disease; HIV testing
	Abnormal gait, cognitive deficits, headache, incontinence, seizures, visual disturbances	Neurosyphilis	Consult infectious disease; fluorescent treponemal antibody absorption test
Metabolic/Nutritional Deficiencies/Toxins	Tremors, muscle spasticity, abnormal liver function testing	Wilson disease	Ceruloplasmin; 24-hour urinary copper; consult ophthalmology
	Altered mental status, gaze palsy, unsteady gait/ataxia, progressive neurologic deterioration, cognitive decline, peripheral neuropathy, paresthesias, dystonia, hepatosplenomegaly, jaundice	Metabolic conditions: • Tay-Sachs disease • Niemann-Pick disease • Fabry's disease • Juvenile metachromatic leukodystrophy	Consult genetics/metabolism; ammonia level
	Regression, ataxia, visual hallucinations, post-surgery	Homocysteinemia	Consult metabolism; homocysteine
	Nausea/vomiting, encephalopathy, post-partum	Urea cycle disorders	Consult genetics/metabolism; ammonia level
	Nystagmus, ophthalmoplegia, confusion, gait ataxia, confabulation, poor diet, history of chronic alcohol dependence	Nutritional deficiencies	Consult nutrition; Thiamine (vitamin B1) testing
	Hallucinations, delusions, dermatitis, diarrhea, poor diet, history of chronic alcohol dependence or restrictive eating disorder		Consult nutrition; niacin (vitamin B3) testing
	Redness/swelling of the mouth and tongue, diarrhea, rash, poor diet, history of treatment for TB (INH)		Consult nutrition; pyridoxine (vitamin B6) testing
	Psychotic symptoms, poor diet, history of restrictive eating disorder		Consult nutrition; cobalamin (vitamin B12) testing
	Headache, fatigue, altered mental status, abdominal pain, bleeding gums, exposure concerns	Heavy metal toxicity	Depending on institutional availability, consult Environmental Health or Toxicology services; if not available, call the Poison Control Center or local health department; lead/mercury levels

*This table has also been included as part of the Boston Children's Hospital "New Onset Psychosis" clinical pathway. Accessed on November 21, 2023.

neurologic conditions such as CNS masses or infections. Encephalitis, which may also present with seizures, as well as unusual hallucinations or delusions, is characterized by decreased levels of consciousness and often accompanied by other symptoms of inflammation such as fever, headache, and nausea/vomiting. Infectious causes, such as viral etiologies, and inflammatory causes, such as autoimmune encephalitis, should be considered in this clinical context.

Delirium is another clinical entity that is often confused with psychosis and should be considered in patients presenting with hallucinations or delusions. In contrast to psychosis, it is often denoted by the presence of *waxing and waning* symptoms, particularly consciousness and cognition. However, delirium can also present with social and emotional regression, withdrawal, disordered mood, hallucinations, delusions, and sensory misperceptions in children. These patients often have accompanying risk factors, such as recent infection, surgery, intensive care unit (ICU) hospitalization, or medication changes. Further complicating this presentation is the phenomenon of behavioral health boarding, whereby patients evaluated for emergent crisis intervention are held in the ED or another temporary location for prolonged periods while awaiting inpatient psychiatric placement, often in rooms without windows or in the absence of regular daily routines, thereby placing them at greater risk for developing delirium.

DIAGNOSTIC EVALUATION

Since there is no definitive diagnostic test or laboratory analysis for psychosis, all patients presenting with new-onset psychosis should undergo a diagnostic evaluation that begins with a complete medical history, psychiatric evaluation, and physical examination.

Past medical history should be carefully reviewed for any risk factors that would increase susceptibility to schizophrenia. In addition to family history of psychiatric disorders, several environmental exposures have been identified as risk factors for the development of schizophrenia. A patient's prenatal and perinatal history should be reviewed carefully, as obstetric complications (e.g., maternal hypertension, prenatal exposure to analgesics, or maternal-fetal blood incompatibility), prenatal nutrition, and prenatal maternal stress have been shown to increase the odds of developing schizophrenia.

Patients with premorbid neurological disorders should be assessed carefully, as they may be at an increased risk for schizophrenia. In one meta-analysis of patients with schizophrenia, the prevalence rate of epilepsy was 1.3%. Traumatic brain injury has also been identified as a risk factor for the development of psychotic disorders. Autistic patients may have symptoms of social withdrawal (e.g., isolation, mutism), seizures, disorganized thinking or behavior, and increased risk for catatonia, all of which may place them at higher risk for the development of schizophrenia.

Childhood adversity and trauma have also been identified as possible factors in the development of schizophrenia. It is therefore essential to assess for trauma, including sexual, physical, and emotional trauma or abuse (including bullying), neglect, or exposure to intimate partner violence. These factors appear to act synergistically in increasing the risk for schizophrenia.

In assessing adolescents with new-onset psychosis, it is imperative to review their substance use history. In fact, cannabis users have a 2 to 5-fold increased risk of developing schizophrenia. Cannabis use confers a vulnerability to the development of schizophrenia that is mediated by both the duration and the amount used by the individual.

Any medication changes should be reviewed for their possible contribution to the patient's presentation. The examination should include a neurologic assessment, and ideally, neurology consultation to further evaluate for neurologic conditions. Based on these and other physical examination findings, additional laboratory and other diagnostic testing may be indicated to further assess for possible medical causes of psychotic symptoms.

Urine toxicology screening is crucial for the assessment of any intentional or accidental ingestion of a toxic substance. As some substances are often not included in standard toxicology screens, additional toxicology testing should be ordered when other substance use is suspected (e.g., amphetamine salt compounds, inhalants, synthetic marijuana, prescription opioids, hallucinogens, etc.). Additional screening medical testing should also include complete blood counts, electrolytes, renal, liver, and thyroid function testing, C-reactive protein, erythrocyte sedimentation rate, antinuclear antibodies, and urine pregnancy testing, as these are easy to obtain, relatively low cost, and screen for a variety of medical conditions. All patients should also undergo electrocardiogram to assess for underlying cardiac disease or rhythm disturbances, particularly prior to initiation of antipsychotic medications due to the risk of prolongation of the QTc interval.

Although there have been advances in our understanding of the genetic underpinnings of psychiatric disease, including schizophrenia, there is limited benefit to performing genetic testing to assist with the diagnosis of psychosis, unless there is concern for a specific genetic disorder with psychotic features (e.g., Huntington disease). Clinicians should assess the rationale for genetic studies on a case-by-case basis.

Given the poor diagnostic utility of universal screening for underlying medical conditions with more advanced testing, a tiered approach may be both evidence-based and cost-effective. Electroencephalogram (EEG) is most useful for identifying seizure activity and encephalitis, including autoimmune encephalitis. In the absence of witnessed seizure activity or with insufficient evidence of encephalitis, a history of characteristic abnormal movements, nonauditory hallucinations, or fixed and repetitive hallucinations may serve as relative indications for EEG monitoring; otherwise, EEG is likely not necessary.

Neuroimaging, particularly magnetic resonance imaging (MRI), may be useful to rule out any intracranial tumors or other lesions and should be performed for patients with new-onset focal neurologic deficits on examination, signs of increased intracranial pressure, or abnormal focal EEG findings; temporally related history of significant head trauma and other headache morphologies may also warrant cross-sectional imaging. In the absence of such indications, the vast majority of imaging findings are incidental and have no association with the patient's psychotic symptoms.

Finally, lumbar puncture (LP) may be indicated to assess for signs of infection or changes in cerebrospinal fluid (CSF) pressure for patients with relevant symptoms. Symptoms of fever or neck stiffness, evidence of abnormalities on EEG, or meningeal enhancement on MRI, are strong indications for pursuing LP (see Chapter 94). Clinical concern for autoimmune encephalitis, including reduced level of consciousness, concern for new-onset movement disorder, headache, or elevated inflammatory markers, should also prompt discussion of the value of CSF sampling. In the absence of such clinical findings suggestive of infection or changes in CSF pressure, diagnostic yield of LP is low. If LP is indicated based on clinical considerations, clinicians should consider obtaining CSF cell counts, total protein, glucose, gram stain, bacterial culture, opening pressure, oligoclonal bands, neopterin, and autoimmune encephalitis panel. If clinical suspicion for autoimmune encephalitis is high, concurrent serum anti-thyroperoxidase antibody, anti-thyroglobulin antibody, oligoclonal bands, and autoimmune encephalitis panel should be sent as well.

MANAGEMENT

Psychosis is a rare and complex disorder. Patients presenting with symptoms of psychosis in a medical setting are often experiencing extreme positive or negative symptoms. Urgent management is required when patients are experiencing significant positive symptoms such as auditory hallucinations, delusions, or disorganization.

The decision to initiate medication is based on the risk-versus-benefit assessment of the clinician. Patients at an imminent risk of harming themselves or others without intention should be considered for acute medication management. Patients who appear to be worsening or progressing in terms of their cognitive decline may also be considered for initiating treatment.

In addition to the medical and psychiatric factors listed above, providers should take into consideration the route of administration of medications. Patients who are acutely agitated and will not take tablets by mouth may require an injectable medication. Many first-generation (typical) and a smaller number of second-generation (atypical) medications come in the injectable form. Of the first-generation antipsychotics, haloperidol is the most commonly available. Olanzapine and ziprasidone are the only second-generation medications available in the intramuscular (IM) formulation, though studies have identified ziprasidone to be ineffective in a double-blind, placebo-controlled trial in children with schizophrenia. Ziprasidone may also be a less favorable option due to the finding of prolonged QTc interval in several trials. Risperidone and olanzapine are both available in an orally disintegrating tablet that can be used when a patient is able to cooperate with medication administration.

COMPLICATIONS AND CONSIDERATIONS

Medication Adverse Effects Initiating psychotropic medication should take into account multiple factors, including the patient's past medical history, allergies to medications, prior trials of psychotropic medications (including antihistamines and benzodiazepines), and other risk factors for side effects. Antipsychotics are the first line of medications for the treatment of schizophrenia in children (**Table 139-3**). Patients should be carefully assessed for cardiac conditions or movement disorders prior to initiation of these medications.

TABLE 139-3 Select First- and Second-Generation Antipsychotics for New-Onset Psychosis in Children and Adolescents

		First-Generation Antipsychotics			Second-Generation Antipsychotics			
	Medication	**Chlorpromazine (Thorazine)**	**Haloperidol (Haldol)**	**Fluphenazine (Modecate)**	**Aripiprazole (Abilify)**	**Olanzapine (Zyprexa, Zydis)**	**Quetiapine (Seroquel)**	**Risperidone (Risperdal)**
Basic Information	Formulations	PO, IM	PO, IM, LAI, IV*	PO, IM, LAI	PO, LAI	PO, IM, LAI	PO	PO, LAI
	Initial Dose	25 mg	0.5-1 mg BID or TID	1.5-2.5	2 mg	2.5-5 mg	25 BID	0.25 mg BID
	Typical Treatment Range (TDD)	150-375 mg	1-10 mg	1.5-10 mg	10-20 mg	10-20 mg	300-800 mg	1-4 mg
Relative Adverse Effects**	Abnormal Glucose	Sometimes	Seldom	Seldom	Seldom	Often	Sometimes	Sometimes
	Akathisia	Sometimes	Often	Often	Sometimes	Sometimes	Seldom	Sometimes
	Anticholinergic	Often	Seldom	Seldom	Seldom	Sometimes	Sometimes	Seldom
	Dystonia	Sometimes	Often	Often	Seldom	Seldom	Seldom	Sometimes
	Hyperlipidemia	Seldom	Seldom	Seldom	Seldom	Often	Often	Seldom
	Hyperprolactinemia	Seldom	Often	Often	Seldom	Sometimes	Seldom	Often
	Orthostasis	Often	Often	Often	Seldom	Sometimes	Sometimes	Sometimes
	Parkinsonism	Sometimes	Often	Often	Seldom	Sometimes	Seldom	Sometimes
	QT prolongation	Often	Sometimes	Sometimes	Seldom	Sometimes	Sometimes	Sometimes
	Tardive Dyskinesia	Often	Often	Often	Seldom	Seldom	Seldom	Sometimes
	Sedation	Often	Seldom	Seldom	Seldom	Often	Often	Sometimes
	Seizures	Sometimes	Seldom	Seldom	Seldom	Sometimes	Seldom	Seldom
	Weight gain	Sometimes	Sometimes	Sometimes	Seldom	Often	Sometimes	Sometimes

Note: While a number of antipsychotic agents are available, many are not readily available in inpatient medical settings, are not considered first-line agents for acute psychosis, have not been approved in children of any age, and/or can only be initiated by specifically trained individuals (e.g., Clozapine).

LAI: long acting, or Depot injection; not to be administered without psychiatric evaluation.

*IV haloperidol is not typically recommended due to high risk of QTc prolongation.

**Based on oral formulations/administration.

Source: The American Psychiatric Association Practice Guideline for the Treatment of Patients With Schizophrenia. Psychiatry Online, American Psychiatric Association, 31 Aug. 2020.

Patients should be carefully monitored for the development of side effects and treated appropriately (**Table 139-4**). Some of the most acute side effects are those related to the extrapyramidal system. In the acute phase, patients can present with acute dystonia, torticollis, or oculogyric crisis. Sub-acutely, patients can present with akathisia, restlessness, or bradykinesia. Chronic use of antipsychotics can cause tardive dyskinesias: involuntary repetitive movements usually involving the small muscles of the face. Neuroleptic malignant syndrome (NMS) can also occur in rare instances and presents with fever, autonomic dysregulation, and muscle rigidity after administration of an antipsychotic. Benztropine or diphenhydramine should be administered concurrently with antipsychotics to reduce the risk of extrapyramidal symptoms.

Furthermore, antipsychotic medications are associated with prolongation of the QTc interval and impairment in ventricular repolarization, which can place a patient at risk for torsades de pointes. The risk of QTc prolongation is related to the specific antipsychotic drug chosen, the route of administration, and the dose. Oral administration is associated with lower risk of QTc prolongation than intramuscular or intravenous administration, and lower doses are also associated with lower risk. When possible, patients should be assessed for any history of syncope, cardiac disease, family history of cardiac disease, and family history of sudden cardiac death, and they should have a baseline electrocardiogram performed prior to initiation of antipsychotic medication. After initiation, QTc should be monitored, with consideration for concurrent medical factors that could contribute to QTc prolongation.

Additional common side effects of antipsychotics include sedation, insomnia, orthostatic hypotension, rash, and sialorrhea. Although metabolic abnormalities associated with second-generation antipsychotics generally take some time to manifest, it is important to consider this side effect profile if initiating an agent from this medication class. Thus, baseline fasting glucose and lipids, hemoglobin A1c, LFTs, weight, and waist circumference should be obtained to establish a baseline prior to the initiation of a second-generation antipsychotic. Finally, some antipsychotics can induce neutropenia and agranulocytosis (with second-generation antipsychotics having a higher risk than first generation); thus a baseline CBC with differential is indicated prior to initiation of these medications. Patients should also be monitored for blood dyscrasias and hepatic injury, especially if initiated on clozapine.

Catatonia Similar to psychosis, catatonia is a neuropsychiatric syndrome. While historically associated with schizophrenia, this condition more commonly occurs with bipolar disorder and can be associated with a number of neurodevelopmental, psychiatric, and medical conditions. Furthermore, the treatment of psychosis with antipsychotics can induce the development of catatonia, and raises the risk of developing NMS, a life-threatening adverse reaction to antipsychotics. Finally, catatonia itself can be associated with autonomic instability requiring ICU support. Thus, while less common in pediatric populations, recognition of catatonia when it occurs is vital.

Catatonia can be complex and varied in its presentation, and the diagnosis is made by clinical history and exam identifying the presence of at least 3 of 12 symptoms (**Table 139-5**).

To assist in diagnosis and rating of symptom severity, screening and rating scales such as the Bush-Francis Catatonia Rating Scale and Pediatric Catatonia Rating Scale have been developed. In addition to dividing catatonia by the underlying condition giving rise to it, there are three primary categories of catatonia: akinetic, excited, and malignant. The more commonly occurring manifestation is akinetic catatonia, which is marked by psychomotor retardation and typically associated with mutism, stupor, and withdrawal. Excited catatonia, by contrast, is marked by psychomotor agitation, including excessive, yet purposeless, movement. The development of autonomic instability, delirium, or rigidity is concerning for malignant catatonia, a lethal manifestation which can arise either spontaneously or in the setting of excited or akinetic catatonia. Malignant catatonia indicates a need for even more emergent intervention and escalation of treatment due to high risk of mortality.

The use of benzodiazepines is considered the gold standard of catatonia management. High-dose IV lorazepam can both lead to rapid

TABLE 139-4 Significant Side Effects Associated With Antipsychotic Use

Side Effect	Clinical Presentation	Treatment and Management
Extrapyramidal side effects	Dystonia: Uncontrolled, painful muscle spasms; medical emergency if involving tongue, oropharynx, or muscles around eyes	Antihistamines (Diphenhydramine, benztropine)
	Akathesia: Combined feeling of restlessness and need to move in some manner	Propranolol, Benzodiazepines
	Tardive dyskinesia: Involuntary, painless, repetitive movements, including smacking of lips, tongue protrusion, and limb movements	Switching from first to second generation (especially clozapine) VMAT inhibitors (deutetrabenazine, valbenazine)
	Bradykinesia/drug-induced Parkinsonism	Switch to lower potency agent Anticholinergics Amantadine
Neuroleptic malignant syndrome	Muscle rigidity Autonomic dysregulation Fever Mental status changes Elevated creatine phosphokinase (CPK)	Symptom management (cooling blankets, antipyretics, fluids) Medications (dantrolene, amantadine, bromocriptine, benzodiazepines) Electroconvulsive therapy
Cardiac abnormalities	QTc prolongation* Torsades de pointes	Discontinuation/or reduction of antipsychotic
Metabolic syndrome	Obesity Glucose metabolism impairment Dyslipidemia	Weight loss/management Metformin Discontinuation or switching antipsychotics

*Black box warning for sudden cardiac death.

Source: The American Psychiatric Association Practice Guideline for the Treatment of Patients With Schizophrenia. Psychiatry Online, American Psychiatric Association, 31 Aug. 2020.

TABLE 139-5 Catatonia Associated With Another Mental Disorder (Catatonia Specifier)

(F06.1)

A. The clinical picture is dominated by three (or more) of the following symptoms:
1. Stupor (i.e., no psychomotor activity; not actively relating to environment).
2. Catalepsy (i.e., passive induction of a posture held against gravity).
3. Waxy flexibility (i.e., slight, even resistance to positioning by examiner).
4. Mutism (i.e., no, or very little, verbal response [exclude if known aphasia]).
5. Negativism (i.e., opposition or no response to instructions or external stimuli).
6. Posturing (i.e., spontaneous and active maintenance of a posture against gravity).
7. Mannerism (i.e., odd, circumstantial caricature of normal actions).
8. Stereotypy (i.e., repetitive, abnormally frequent, non-goal-directed movements).
9. Agitation, not influenced by external stimuli.
10. Grimacing.
11. Echolalia (i.e., mimicking another's speech).
12. Echopraxia (i.e., mimicking another's movements).

Coding note: Indicate the name of the associated mental disorder when recording the name of the condition (i.e., F06.1 catatonia associated with major depressive disorder). Code first the associated mental disorder (e.g., neurodevelopmental disorder, brief psychotic disorder, schizophreniform disorder, schizophrenia, schizoaffective disorder, bipolar disorder, major depressive disorder, or other mental disorder) (e.g., F25.1 schizoaffective disorder, depressive type; F06.1 catatonia associated with schizoaffective disorder).

Source: Reprinted with permission from the Diagnostic and Statistical Manual of Mental Disorders, Fifth Edition, Text Revision (Copyright © 2022). *American Psychiatric Association.* All Rights Reserved.

improvement of symptoms (in as little as 5 minutes), as well as serving as a diagnostic trial for confirming the diagnosis. However, some individuals have limited or no response to treatment, or there is acute need for intervention due to medical instability (such as in the case of malignant catatonia). In these settings, electroconvulsive therapy is indicated. Furthermore, treatment of the underlying condition which precipitated the catatonia is essential for recovery. Therapeutic strategies become challenging when the suspected underlying condition is a primary psychotic disorder, given the potential for antipsychotics to precipitate catatonia, as well as the increased risk for NMS when antipsychotics are used in the setting of catatonia.

Aggression and Risk for Self-Harm As their ability to effectively and appropriately interpret reality is by definition impaired in individuals with psychosis, they are at risk for abnormal cognition and behaviors which may put themselves and others at risk, even if this is not their intent. For example, an individual who is suffering a delusion where they believe others have been replaced by an identical appearing entity may react violently against the perceived imposter. An individual with the grandiose delusion they are able to fly may attempt to do so from the top of a tall building. Furthermore, the distress caused by their symptoms can precipitate suicidal or aggressive behaviors, such as when an individual suffering command auditory hallucinations to kill themselves feels overwhelmed and becomes suicidal. As such, management of agitation, as well as ensuring the patient remains safe and monitored to prevent potential self-harm, is indicated (see Chapters 136 and 138.)

Functional Impairment The presence of psychotic symptoms can lead to functional impairment which is not always acutely dangerous but can result in significant decline in health and capacity. This can occur indirectly due to the disruption of their normal organization and attention, or may occur directly as the patient's symptoms directly cause lack of engagement, such as a delusional belief that they no longer need to eat or a command auditory hallucination telling them not to shower. Depending on the nature of the deficit, consultation with a dietician, physical therapist, or occupational therapist may be clinically indicated. For patients presenting with acute food refusal, if oral intake is severely restricted, enteral tube feedings may be medically necessary, even if the patient requires a medical restraint to undergo tube placement (see Chapters 40 and 79).

ADMISSION CRITERIA

In patients for whom there is concern for new-onset psychosis, an initial medical hospitalization is often most appropriate to facilitate relevant diagnostic testing and to evaluate for medical or toxic causes of mental status changes. However, depending on the workflow of the institution, this evaluation may also be feasibly performed in the emergency department. Patients should be observed carefully during this time for any changes due to a general medical condition or intoxication. Some patients may require initial medical hospitalization for complications of psychosis, such as malnutrition, dehydration, or rhabdomyolysis.

Once a complete medical evaluation has been completed, the patient's mental status should be re-evaluated. If there is high suspicion for an ongoing psychiatric process, inpatient psychiatric hospitalization should be considered. Appropriate reasons for inpatient hospitalization include further diagnostic assessment and clarification, initiation of behavioral treatment, initiation or adjustment of psychotropic medication, assistance with activities of daily living such as maintenance of personal hygiene and adequate oral intake, or safety planning if at risk for harm to self or others.

DISCHARGE CRITERIA

Stable patients may be medically cleared for discharge to further psychiatric care. If there is concern about the patient's ability to care for themselves due to poor safety awareness, nutritional status, or other medical concerns, they may require transfer to a facility with both medical and psychiatric capabilities.

Patients who do not have ongoing medical needs, but are impaired significantly and require more intensive psychiatric treatments may be referred for inpatient psychiatric care. Patients who are functioning close to their baseline, but require intensive daily psychiatric treatment may be referred to a partial hospitalization program. This requires that the family be comfortable with the patient returning home for part of the day, including to sleep at night. If over the course of the patient's medical hospitalization the patient is close to or at their baseline mental status, clinicians may consider discharge to home with supports. This would most likely be feasible in a patient with a longstanding history of psychiatric treatment who already has a therapist and psychiatrist in the community. Providers may also coordinate additional in-home supports, family therapy, and school-based treatments that may allow the patient to return safely to the community. Clinical programs specifically designed to support individuals with psychosis exist in some regions, and when feasible, referral to such programs can benefit patients.

CONSULTATION

When feasible, all patients admitted to a medical facility with new-onset or ongoing psychiatric disorder should be referred for a psychiatric consultation. Ideally, the patient should be seen by a provider with a background in pediatric psychology/psychiatry.

The consultation team can assist in the diagnostic assessment of the patient by clarifying the patient's premorbid psychological and social functioning as well as current level of functioning. Consultants can assist with management if the patient is at risk of harm to themselves or others due to their level of disorganization or psychosis. This may include acute psychotropic management of agitation using antipsychotics, benzodiazepines, or antihistamines. Consultants can provide support and guidance to the medical staff, nurses, and child-life specialist caring for the patient. Recommendations made for the patient may include a structured day with a schedule of activities, 1:1 supervision for safety or observation, physical therapy for assistance with resolving dystonias or catatonia, and teaching distraction or relaxation techniques.

In the instance of new-onset psychosis, the consultation team may provide valuable psychoeducation for the family and patient. This could include information about diagnostic impressions, types of behavioral and medication treatment, and levels of care (e.g., outpatient, partial hospitalization, and inpatient hospitalization). The consultant can provide referrals for the required levels of psychiatric care. Depending on the structure of the institution, consulting teams may collaborate with social work to provide ongoing social and emotional support for the family throughout this process.

SUGGESTED READINGS

Beach SR, Celano CM, Sugrue AM, et al. QT prolongation, torsades de pointes, and psychotropic medications: a 5-year update. *Psychosomatics*. 2018;59(2):105-122.

Benarous X, Raffin M, Ferrafiat V, Consoli A, Cohen D. Catatonia in children and adolescents: new perspectives. *Schizophrenia Research*. 2018;200:56-67.

Bridgwater MA, Horton LE, Haas GL. Premorbid adjustment in childhood is associated with later emotion management in first-episode schizophrenia. *Schizophrenia Research*. 2022;240(June 2020):233-238.

Cardno AG, Selzam S, Freeman D, Ronald A. Psychotic-like experiences in adolescence occurring in combination or isolation: associations with schizophrenia risk factors. *Psychiatr Res Clin Pract*. 2021;3(2):67-75.

Carlisle LL, McClellan J. Psychopharmacology of schizophrenia in children and adolescents. *Pediatr Clin North Am*. 2011;58(1):205-218.

Cellucci T, van Mater H, Graus F, et al. Clinical approach to the diagnosis of autoimmune encephalitis in the pediatric patient. *Neurol (R) Neuroimmunol Neuroinflamm*. 2020;7(2).

Cirone C, Secci I, Favole I, et al. What do we know about the long-term course of early onset bipolar disorder? A review of the current evidence. *Brain Sciences*. 2021;11(3):1-16.

Clarke MC, Kelleher I, Clancy M, Cannon M. Predicting risk and the emergence of schizophrenia. *Psychiatr Clin N Am*. 2012;35(3): 585-612.

Coentre R, Silva-dos-Santos A, Talina MC. Retrospective study on structural neuroimaging in first-episode psychosis. *PeerJ*. 2016;2016(26):1-10.

Driver DI, Thomas S, Gogtay N, Rapoport JL. Childhood-onset schizophrenia and early-onset schizophrenia spectrum disorders: an update. *Child Adolesc Psychiatr Clin N Am*. 2020;29(1):71-90.

Edinoff AN, Kaufman SE, Hollier JW, et al. Catatonia: Clinical overview of the diagnosis, treatment, and clinical challenges. *Neurology International*. 2021;13(4):570-586.

Gadow KD. Association of schizophrenia spectrum and autism spectrum disorder (ASD) symptoms in children with ASD and clinic controls. *Res Dev Disabil*. 2013;34(4):1289-1299.

Garcia G, Logan GE, Gonzalez-Heydrich J. Management of psychotropic medication side effects in children and adolescents. *Child Adolesc Psychiatr Clin N Am*. 2012;21(4):713-738.

Guasp M, Giné-Servén E, Maudes E, et al. Clinical, neuroimmunologic, and CSF investigations in first episode psychosis. *Neurology*. 2021;97(1):e61-e75.

Hua LL, Alderman EM, Chung RJ, et al. Collaborative care in the identification and management of psychosis in adolescents and young adults. *Pediatrics*. 2021;147(6).

Kaar SJ, Natesan S, McCutcheon R, Howes OD. Antipsychotics: mechanisms underlying clinical response and side-effects and novel treatment approaches based on pathophysiology. *Neuropharmacology*. 2020;172:107704.

Kendall T, Hollis C, Stafford M, Taylor C. Recognition and management of psychosis and schizophrenia in children and young people: Summary of NICE guidance. *BMJ (Online)*. 2013;346(7892):1-5.

Lieberman JA, First MB. Psychotic disorders. *N Eng J Medicine*. 2018;379(3):270-280.

Luttrull MD, Boulter DJ, Kirsch CFE, et al. ACR Appropriateness Criteria® Acute Mental Status Change, Delirium, and New Onset Psychosis. *J Am Coll Radiol*. 2019;16(5):S26-S37.

Matheson SL, Shepherd AM, Pinchbeck RM, Laurens KR, Carr VJ. Childhood adversity in schizophrenia: a systematic meta-analysis. *Psychol Med*. 2013;43(2):225-238.

McCarthy-Jones S, Smailes D, Corvin A, et al. Occurrence and co-occurrence of hallucinations by modality in schizophrenia-spectrum disorders. *Psychiatry Research*. 2017;252(December 2016):154-160.

McClellan J. Psychosis in children and adolescents. *J Am Acad Child Adolesc Psychiatry*. 2018;57(5):308-312.

McCutcheon RA, Reis Marques T, Howes OD. Schizophrenia - an overview. *JAMA Psychiatry*. 2020;77(2):201-210.

Pientka LJ, Schulz SC, Lim KO, Jasberg SG. The clinical impact of neuroimaging in first-episode psychosis. *Clin Schizophr Relat Psychoses*. 2017;(aop).

Raybould JE, Alfers C, won Cho Y, et al. EEG screening for temporal lobe epilepsy in patients with acute psychosis. *J Neuropsychiatry Clin Neurosci*. 2012;24(4):452-457.

Robert Williams S, Yukio Koyanagi C, Shigemi Hishinuma E. On the usefulness of structural brain imaging for young first episode inpatients with psychosis. *Psychiatry Res - Neuroimaging*. 2014;224(2):104-106.

Santosh PJ, Bell L, Fiori F, Singh J. Pediatric antipsychotic use and outcomes monitoring. *J Child Adolesc Psychopharmacol*. 2017; 27(6):546-554.

Schizophrenia Spectrum and Other Psychotic Disorders. In: *Diagnostic and Statistical Manual of Mental Disorders*. 5th ed. Text Revision. American Psychiatric Association; 2022. doi:10.1176/appi.books.9780890425787.x02_Schizophrenia_Spectrum.

Sideli L, Murray RM, Schimmenti A, et al. Childhood adversity and psychosis: a systematic review of bio-psycho-social mediators and moderators. *Psycholo Med*. 2020;50(11):1761-1782.

Skikic M, Arriola JA. First episode psychosis medical workup: evidence-informed recommendations and introduction to a clinically guided approach. *Child Adolesc Psychiatr Clin N Am*. 2020;29(1):15-28.

Sommer IE, de Kort GAP, Meijering AL, et al. How frequent are radiological abnormalities in patients with psychosis? A review of 1379 MRI scans. *Schizophr Bull*. 2013;39(4):815-819.

Sood S. Neutropenia with multiple antipsychotics including dose dependent neutropenia with lurasidone. *Clin Psychopharmacol Neurosci*. 2017;15(4):413-415.

Starzer MSK, Nordentoft M, Hjorthøj C. Rates and predictors of conversion to schizophrenia or bipolar disorder following substance-induced psychosis. *Am J Psychiatry*. 2018;175(4):343-350.

Stoeck PA, Petersen E, Pereira-View K, et al. *Clinical Pathway for Evaluation and Management of New Onset Psychosis*. Boston Children's Hospital, 2021. Accessed: November 21, 2023.

CHAPTER 140

Trauma and Trauma-Informed Care

Heather Kreth, PsyD and Merranda D. Holmes, MD

BACKGROUND AND ETIOLOGY

Psychological trauma can generally be thought of as an event that causes extreme stress which overwhelms a person's ability to cope. The Substance Abuse and Mental Health Services Administration defines trauma as "an event, series of events, or set of circumstances that is experienced by an individual as physically or emotionally harmful or life-threatening and that has lasting adverse effects on the individual's functioning and mental, physical, social, emotional, or spiritual well-being." Others have defined trauma as an event or experience that overwhelms a person's capacity to depend on or protect themselves. Several types of trauma are particularly important for pediatric hospital medicine clinicians to be aware of medical trauma, child abuse and neglect, and adverse childhood experiences. Providers will also encounter individuals who have been exposed to traumatic experiences on larger population scales such as war, famine, forced displacement, immigration, and human trafficking.

Medical trauma can have lasting psychological impacts on children and their parents. Medical traumatic stress typically involves psychological and physiological responses to required painful procedures, critical illness, or frightening therapies to treat a known medical condition. Children's responses to medical trauma are often more related to their subjective experience of the medical event, rather than its objective severity. Nevertheless, pediatric hospital teams can be aware that certain types of medical experiences are particularly associated with medical trauma: repeat hospitalization, chemotherapy, intensive care unit (ICU) stays with sedation/intubation, uncontrolled pain, and dismissive medical treatment.

Children may require hospital care due to sequelae of child abuse or neglect, and hospital teams may encounter children who have experienced abuse or neglect and require hospitalization for other reasons. In 2020, over 3.1 million children in the United States received an investigation or alternative response from their local Child Protective Services (CPS) agency due to concern for abuse or neglect. Of these, 618,000 children were identified as having experienced abuse and neglect. While states have varying definitions of maltreatment, the experience of trauma extends beyond confirmed or substantiated cases of abuse and or neglect. In many families, multiple family members experience the same trauma; for example, in cases where violence occurs in the home. Families may also perpetuate generational trauma based on personal risk factors and social situations. Much child abuse and neglect remains unrecognized or unreported, but many traumatic experiences can be prevented with increased awareness and social support.

Adverse Childhood Experiences are potentially traumatic events that occur in childhood. The 1998 landmark Adverse Childhood Experiences (ACE) study examined three categories of abuse (psychological, physical, and sexual) and four categories of exposure to household dysfunction (mental illness, substance use, violence toward mother/stepmother, and criminal behavior). Other events in childhood like divorce or witnessing community violence also can be traumatic. About two in three adults have had at least one ACE, and nearly one in four have had at least three ACEs (**Table 140-1**).

TABLE 140-1 Examples of Adverse Childhood Experiences

Physical abuse	Emotional abuse
Sexual abuse	Physical and emotional neglect
Parental mental illness	Substance use within the household
Parental incarceration	Parental divorce/separation
Witnessing domestic violence	Witnessing community violence

Both psychosocial and medical trauma can interplay with acute medical illness and hospitalization. The inpatient provider must understand this linkage to support the child and family and prevent traumatic experiences when possible.

PATHOPHYSIOLOGY

The effects of trauma on the developing brain can be lasting and profound, and the impact varies with genetic predisposure and timing of traumatic events at different ages. The limbic-hypothalamic-pituitary-adrenal (LPHA) axis plays a central role in regulating the body's response to stress. When a person encounters a stressful situation, the sympathetic nervous system is acutely triggered, and signals from the locus coeruleus in the hypothalamus stimulate the adrenal medulla to release catecholamines—epinephrine and norepinephrine. Catecholamines are responsible for the "fight or flight" response and produce tachycardia, hypertension, increased alertness, and hyperglycemia. They can lead to shortness of breath, flushing, tingling of fingertips, chest pain, nausea, or difficulty focusing. In children, this experience can lead to fear and crying. With prolonged stress, the limbic system simultaneously triggers the hypothalamus to produce corticotropin-releasing hormone, which causes the release of adrenocorticotropin-releasing hormone (ACTH) from the anterior pituitary. ACTH then stimulates the production of cortisol by the adrenal cortex. Cortisol acts by stimulating receptors across the brain and body to regulate metabolism, immune function, glucose and protein homeostasis, stress responses and behaviors, cognitive development, and storage of memory.

Normally, a stress response serves an appropriate, protective function. When stressful amygdala triggers are ongoing, the typical negative feedback of cortisol on the hypothalamus is blunted, resulting in continued overproduction of cortisol, ongoing catecholamine release, and difficulty returning to homeostasis.

Patients who have experienced traumatic stress and have overstimulated these neurological pathways experience a "priming" of these chronic compensatory pathways. When a minor stressor occurs, the resultant acute stimulation of the stress response escalates quickly, having a much greater physiologic impact on the child, and can result in a response that is objectively out of proportion to the stressor. The child may find it difficult to filter between a perceived threat ("someone stole my pencil") and an actual threat ("someone is trying to physically harm me"), resulting in varying levels of behavioral dysregulation and ability to cope, even when the stressor is no longer present.

The long-term physiologic effects of childhood trauma are still being studied. The ACE study in adults has shown very strong correlations between these dysregulated neurobiological pathways and propensity to develop coronary artery disease, chronic obstructive pulmonary disease, asthma, depression and anxiety, substance abuse, and premature death, among others. One in six adults has experienced four or more ACEs, and at least five of the top 10 leading causes of death are associated with ACEs.

CLINICAL PRESENTATION

In an acute care hospital setting, children with complex trauma may present with low distress tolerance, emotional lability, behavioral dysregulation, difficulty tolerating limits, increased anxiety, or aggression. Responses to trauma are unique to the individual and can differ based on the age of the child (**Table 140-2**).

TABLE 140-2 Common Reactions to Trauma/Traumatic Experiences by Age

Age	Common Reactions
Early childhood	Change in appetite Behavioral regression and increased tantrums Toileting regression Increased separation anxiety Sleep or appetite disturbances
Elementary age	Mood lability: increased whining, aggression, acting out Separation anxiety New onset anxieties or phobias Sleep or appetite disturbances Withdrawal from peers or family/isolation Somatic symptoms such as headaches or stomachaches
Middle/High school age	Mood lability including agitation or depression New-onset anxieties or phobias Sleep or appetite disturbances Withdrawal from peers or family/isolation Loss of interest in activities Somatic symptoms such as headaches or stomachaches Difficulty completing activities of daily living

While some children may be exposed to a single traumatic event, studies such as the ACEs study have highlighted the reality that exposure to multiple events or types of trauma is common. Exposure to multiple, pervasive, sequential, and often highly interpersonal traumatic events, particularly in early childhood, is defined as complex trauma and is associated with increased complexity and severity of symptoms. Complex trauma has been proposed to lead to derailment of typical child development and to have profound and lasting impacts on children's beliefs about themselves, the world, and the safety of relationships.

For individuals exposed to sustained or repeated traumas, behaviors that may develop in response to the initial trauma are often in the service of coping with day-to-day threats to survival. Later, when the acute danger has passed, these behaviors may remain as lasting reminders of brilliant survival strategies that no longer work. Complex trauma can have profound, lasting impacts on multiple domains of functioning (**Table 140-3**).

TABLE 140-3 Complex Trauma and Associated Effects

Attachment and relationships	Safe, healthy relationships with caregivers teach us that we can trust others and the world around us. Repeated interactions with caregivers during times of distress teach emotion regulation skills. In the absence of a healthy or safe relationship with a primary caregiver, these basic skills are not developed or can be maladaptive. It is not unusual for children and adults with trauma histories to have difficulty developing healthy and trusting relationships.
Physical health	Physiological responses that might be adaptive when faced with a significant threat, can become overworked when children grow up in a constant state of stress or fear. Over activation of the sympathetic nervous system, or "fight-or-flight" response, can lead to responses that are out of proportion in the context of normal stress.
Emotional regulation	Children who have experienced trauma can have difficulty identifying, expressing, and managing emotions in adaptive and healthy ways. Reminders of traumatic events can be everywhere, and it is not unusual for those with trauma histories to struggle to identify triggers, cope-ahead for potential triggers, and manage their response when these triggers occur. Healthy and adaptive management of emotion is learned in the context of safe and healthy interpersonal relationships. In the absence of these kinds of relationships, children do not learn the skills to manage their feelings, and this can leave children with trauma histories appearing as though the "volume" has been turned up on their emotions.
Dissociation	When we encounter a terrifying experience, we may dissociate or mentally check out of our bodies as a means of surviving the experience. Repeated experiences of dissociation make it more likely for a child to dissociate again when presented with stress or a dangerous situation. This can have profound impacts on the child's ability to meaningfully engage in relationships, social situations, and learning.
Cognition	Cognitive energy is directed toward survival and not academic gains when a child is repeatedly exposed to traumatic events. Difficulties with attention, abstract reasoning, and problem solving are common.
Self-concept and future orientation	It is common for children to blame themselves for the abuse they have sustained. This can lead to feelings of worthlessness, shame, guilt, and a damaged sense of self. They can feel hopeless or powerless. Children who have experienced complex trauma may also later put themselves in dangerous situations or unhealthy relationships because they do not feel they deserve something better.

DIFFERENTIAL DIAGNOSIS

When a patient appears easily agitated, tearful, combative, or withdrawn in the inpatient setting, evaluation for medical triggers of the stress response including pain, infection, environmental change, and appropriateness of natural response for stage of development should be considered. Concurrently, the provider should be aware of the potential dysregulated stress response due to history of trauma. Often, a timeline of reported behavioral changes, social history, and traumatic events including at home (death, threatened death, serious injury, or sexual violence) and in the hospital (frequent or prolonged admissions with serious illness) will help lead the clinician to a comorbid psychological diagnosis. Children might react to traumatic events that they experienced, that they witnessed, or that a loved one experienced. When there is concern for a trauma-related illness, the provider in the acute setting must first focus on the methods of trauma-informed care. Second, providers must work with subspecialists to determine whether the patient meets criteria for Diagnostic and Statistical Manual of Mental Disorders: Fifth Addition (DSM-V) diagnosis of a trauma and stressor-related illness versus overlapping diagnoses such as major depressive disorder, generalized anxiety disorder, oppositional defiant disorder, intermittent explosive disorder, conduct disorder, attention deficit hyperactivity disorder, and obsessive-compulsive disorder. Clarifying the diagnosis may take time and may not occur during the hospitalization. However, an initial evaluation with a working differential diagnosis can inform appropriate management in the hospital and support a child in ongoing treatment after returning to the community. Often, a DSM-V diagnosis may not be made until further evaluation is conducted by outpatient clinicians. Below are specific trauma and stress-related disorders that are particularly relevant to pediatric hospital medicine:

- **Acute Stress Disorder:** Development of the stress response begins immediately, but these pervasive features (below) must last at least 3 days up to 1 month after a traumatic event for an acute stress disorder diagnosis.
- **Post-Traumatic Stress Disorder (PTSD):** Three groups of symptoms comprise PTSD: re-experiencing the traumatic event, avoidance of stimuli that serve as reminders of the event, and negative alterations in mood/cognition.
- **Complex PTSD:** Although the DSM-V does not currently include this diagnosis, the 11th revision of the International Classification of Diseases (ICD-11) has recognized the difference between PTSD and Complex PTSD (CPTSD). Diagnosis of CPTSD includes criteria of PTSD, with the addition of disturbances in self-organization like affect dysregulation, negative self-concept, and disturbances in relationships.

While a particular trauma can trigger any of the above diagnoses, CPTSD is most often attributed to recurrent trauma, whether it be the same trauma chronically, or multiple types of trauma during childhood (particularly highly interpersonal sexual and physical trauma). Some studies in adults and adolescents have shown that certain protective

TABLE 140-4 Criteria for Posttraumatic Stress Disorder and Complex Posttraumatic Stress Disorder

	DSM - 5	ICD - 11
PTSD	Exposure to traumatic events; intrusion symptoms; persistent avoidance of stimuli; negative alterations in cognitions and mood (dissociation, persistent negative beliefs of oneself, others or the world, distorted cognitions about the traumatic event, persistent negative emotional state, detachment from others, diminished interest or participation in previously enjoyed activities, etc.); alterations in arousal and reactivity; aggressive verbal and/or physical behavior, reckless or self-destructive behavior; depersonalization or derealization; significant impairment in all areas of functioning	Exposure to an extremely threatening or horrific event or series of events; vivid intrusive memories, flashbacks, or nightmares, which are typically accompanied by strong and overwhelming emotions; avoidance of thoughts and memories, events, people, activities, situations reminiscent of the event(s); persistent perceptions of heightened current threat, hypervigilance or an enhanced startle reaction. Significant impairment in personal, family, social, educational, occupational, or other important areas of functioning
Complex PTSD	Not included as a diagnostic entity	Exposure to an event(s) of an extremely threatening or horrific nature, most commonly prolonged or repetitive, from which escape is difficult or impossible; All diagnostic requirements for PTSD and additionally: severe and pervasive affect dysregulation; persistent negative beliefs about oneself; deep-rooted feelings of shame, guilt or failure; persistent difficulties in sustaining relationships and in feeling close to others. Significant impairment in all areas of functioning.

Source: Reproduced with permission from Giourou E, Skokou M, Andrew SP, et al. Complex posttraumatic stress disorder: the need to consolidate a distinct clinical syndrome or to reevaluate features of psychiatric disorders following interpersonal trauma? *World J Psychiatry*. 2018;8(1):12-19, Table 1.

factors such as family and school support have lessened the development of and duration of CPTSD (**Table 140-4**).

SCREENING

For all patient encounters, it is important to assess any threats to the child's safety or well-being. Pediatric clinicians can be alert to direct disclosures when a child or adolescent reports or describes threats to their safety and well-being. In other cases, clinicians may recognize the behavior symptoms outlined above, which can be suggestive of prior traumatic experience. Further evaluation, including trauma screening as described below can help clinicians understand what prior traumatic experiences might be contributing to a patient's behaviors and symptoms. Collaboration with social work or mental health service providers can be helpful in assessing trauma history, need for more robust or tailored screening, and identification of potential areas for intervention.

If a child or adolescent discloses current abuse or neglect, those concerns should be immediately reported to the appropriate local authorities. Even in the absence of current concerns for abuse or neglect, hospital clinicians can screen for history of trauma with developmentally appropriate questions or standardized measures. Standardized measures for assessment of current trauma-associated symptoms or risk for development of trauma-associated symptoms are widely available and include the Child Trauma Screen (10-item questionnaire available in English and Spanish) and the Trauma Symptom Checklist for Children.

Providers should be aware that while any child of any socioeconomic class, race, or religion is susceptible to ACEs, certain populations are at higher risk. In a study of self-reported ACE data, individuals who were identified as multiracial, Black, Hispanic, lesbian, gay, bisexual, transgender, or gender nonbinary had significantly more exposure to ACEs. Lack of a college degree and lower household incomes (particularly households experiencing poverty) were also associated with higher rates of experiencing ACEs. Individuals identifying as female reported sexual abuse more often than males. For all ACEs, including sexual abuse, perceived stigma may contribute to under-reporting.

INTERVENTION

In a systematic review of evidence-based treatments for trauma-related psychopathology, multiple studies confirmed the efficacy of Trauma-Focused Cognitive Behavioral Therapy (TF-CBT) and other forms of Cognitive Behavioral Therapy (CBT). Less well-known or well-investigated forms of treatment showed promise or merited further research. For all evidence-based trauma treatment, approaches are generally phase-based in nature, with focus on first ensuring safety and then building necessary skills for adaptive coping. For professionals working with individuals who have experienced trauma, it is imperative to remember that trauma processing work cannot be done in the absence of a foundation based on ensuring safety.

Many evidence-based interventions also involve caregivers in treatment and intervention when the caregiver was not the perpetrator of child abuse or neglect. Focus on providing psychoeducation, strengthening resources and support, and enhancing affect regulation skills in the caregivers are considered key to successful trauma treatment in the child. Interventions further focus on supporting coregulation opportunities, strengthening affect identification and regulation skills, and building resiliency.

TRAUMA-INFORMED CARE

Because trauma is so common and has important impacts on physical and mental health and well-being, healthcare organizations are increasingly incorporating trauma-informed practices into routine care. According to the Substance Abuse and Mental Health Services Administration, "a program, organization, or system that is trauma-informed realizes the widespread impact of trauma and understands potential paths for recovery; recognizes the signs and symptoms of trauma in clients, families, staff, and others involved with the system; and responds by fully integrating knowledge about trauma into policies, procedures, and practices and seeks to actively resist re-traumatization." In other words, a trauma-informed medical system involves organizational and clinical practices that recognize the impact of both preexisting trauma and new traumatic experiences related to medical care, and how these experiences affect patients, families, and staff. Organizations that are trauma-informed seek to actively resist re-traumatization of patients, families, and staff through policies and procedures that support (1) physical and psychological safety, (2) patient empowerment, (3) transparency and trustworthiness, (4) peer support, (5) collaboration, and (6) awareness of cultural, historical, and gender issues.

In an acute care medical setting, agitation can be a symptom of a child's current experience of medical trauma or a symptom of prior trauma. To prevent and manage agitation among hospitalized children, trauma-informed clinical practices prioritize environmental strategies, offering a child control over their environment and treatment to the extent that is possible, and behavior support strategies such as distraction and redirection. When agitation or escalation does occur, trauma-informed practice prioritizes early recognition and verbal de-escalation in an effort to avoid imposing further trauma if physical restraint or intramuscular medication injection is required to maintain patient and staff physical safety. The ability of adults (providers, staff, and family) to regulate their own affect in the face of a child's dysregulation can have a direct impact on the success of de-escalation attempts. A calm, neutral response with reassurances of safety is critical for helping children to access the affect regulation skills necessary to effectively cope with perceived stress or threats.

TABLE 140-5	Escalation Prevention and De-Escalation Strategies
Environmental Modifications	• Dim lights • Play low music • A favorite TV show • Minimize noise and unnecessary activity, people in the room
Psychological Interventions	• Provide one-to-one verbal support • Involve or limit family visitation as appropriate • Implement/explain • Ask eliciting questions and make uninterrupted time to listen to the patient • Remain neutral and calm
Behavioral Interventions	• Child life • Use simple age-appropriate directions and explanations • Verbal redirection • Distraction techniques • Set reasonable limits • Explain consequences of behavior in simple concrete terms
Nursing Interventions	• Assess for any physical/medical causes for behavior • Assess need for PRN medication • Consult MD for medication alternatives • Initiate a safety observation level, ask MD for order • Explain safety and support aspects of observation level

Source: Adapted from https://www.chop.edu/clinical-pathway/behavioral-health-issues-clinical-pathway-alternatives-restraints.

Confinement, boredom, and lack of access to healthy, adaptive coping mechanisms and other means of distraction can lead to agitation in adolescents and children. Often, parents have experienced similar traumas as their children, and clinicians may notice that the parent has similar difficulty regulating. In these cases, teams can recognize the importance of treating the parent from a trauma-informed lens as well (**Table 140-5**).

Early and proactive engagement of child life and consult-liaison psychiatry and other mental health specialist (psychology, clinical social work, behavior analyst) teams has been shown to have several positive effects ranging from improved staff satisfaction, to improvements in patient and family-centered care. A multidisciplinary team approach can also lead to the development of trauma-informed policies and procedures. Such teams often consist of existing key stakeholders, such as nursing administration, child life, social work, case management, and security services, and can examine safety protocols, develop a crisis response team, better coordinate care and communication, and provide education to staff on best practice in de-escalation and management of the distressed patient.

KEY POINTS

- Childhood trauma impacts physiology and neurocognitive development and can lead to maladaptive behavior and poor coping mechanisms, societal dysfunction, and chronic medical disease.
- Certain populations of children and families are at higher risk of Adverse Childhood Experiences (ACEs). Those who experience more than four ACEs are more likely to experience chronic disease and poor coping mechanisms as adults.
- Approaching all patient and family interactions from a trauma-informed lens is beneficial, regardless of known trauma history.
- Trauma-informed clinical interventions actively avoid re-traumatization and prioritize empowerment of the patient along with respect for their lived experience and ability to make the right decisions for themselves.
- Any clinician can practice trauma-informed care, and the best approach to avoiding re-traumatization is to build a trauma-informed health system by systematically integrating trauma-informed practices into clinical care.

SUGGESTED READINGS

Blaustein M, Kinniburgh K. *Treating Traumatic Stress in Children and Adolescents: How to Foster Resilience Through Attachment, Self-Regulation, and Competency*. 2nd ed. New York: Guilford Press; 2018.

Briere J, Kaltman S, Green BL. Accumulated childhood trauma and symptom complexity. *J Trauma Stress*. 2008;21:223-226.

Briere J. Trauma Symptom Checklist for Children. https://www.parinc.com/Products/Pkey/461.

CDC Fast Facts: Preventing Adverse Childhood Experiences. https://www.cdc.gov/violenceprevention/aces/fastfact.html.

Child Trauma Screen: https://www.chdi.org/our-work/trauma-informed-initiatives/ct-trauma-screen-cts/.

Cloitre M, Stolbach BC, Herman JL, et al. A developmental approach to complex PTSD: childhood and adult cumulative trauma as predictors of symptom complexity. *J Traumat Stress*. 2009;22:399-408.

Daniunaite I, Cloitre M, Karatzias T, et al. PTSD and complex PTSD in adolescence: discriminating factors in a population-based cross-sectional study. *Eur J Psychotraumatol*. 2021;12(1):1890937.

De Bellis MD, Zisk A. The biological effects of childhood trauma. *Child Adolesc Psychiatr Clin N Am*. 2014;23(2):185-222.

Felitti VJ, Andra RF, Nordenberg D, et al. Relationship of childhood abuse and household dysfunction to many of the leading causes of death in adults. the adverse childhood experiences (ACE) Study. *Am J Prev Med*. 1998;14(4):245-258.

Giano Z, Wheeler DL, Hubach RD. The frequencies and disparities of adverse childhood experiences in the U.S. *BMC Public Health*. 2020;20:1327.

Leenarts LE, Diehle J, Doreleijers TA, Jansma EP, Lindauer RJ. Evidence-based treatments for children with trauma-related psychopathology as a result of childhood maltreatment: a systematic review. *Eur Child Adolesc Psychiatry*. 2013;22(5):269-283.

Nicome R, Lo HY, Gupta S, et al. Utilizing a behavioral health bundle to improve patient and clinician safety for hospitalized children. *Pediatr Qual Saf*. 2021;6(2):e393.

Oldham MA, Walsh P, Maeng DD, et al. Integration of a proactive, multidisciplinary mental health team on hospital medicine improves provider and nursing satisfaction. *J Psychosom Res*. 2020;134:110112.

Sachser C, Keller F, Goldbeck, L. Complex PTSD as proposed for ICD-11: validation of a new disorder in children and adolescents and their response to trauma-focused cognitive behavioral therapy. *J Child Psychol Psychiatry*. 2017;58:160-168.

SAMHSA's Concept of Trauma and Guidance for a Trauma Informed Approach. SAMHSA's Trauma and Justice Strategic Initiative. https://ncsacw.acf.hhs.gov/userfiles/files/SAMHSA_Trauma.pdf.

Substance Abuse and Mental Health Services Administration. https://www.samhsa.gov https://www.samhsa.gov.

Thakur A, Creedon J, Zeanah CH. Trauma- and stressor-related disorders among children and adolescents. *Focus*. 2016;14(1):34-45.

Trauma and Stressor Related Disorders. American Psychiatric Association. *Diagnostic and Statistical Manual of Mental Health Disorders*: 5th ed. American Psychiatric Press: Washington D.C.

U.S Department of Health and Human Services, Administration for Children and Families, Child Maltreatment 2020. https://www.acf.hhs.gov/cb/report/child-maltreatment-2020.

Van der Kolk BA. Developmental trauma disorder: toward a rational diagnosis for children with complex trauma histories. *Psychiatric Annals*. 2005;35:401-408.

SECTION P
Pulmonology

CHAPTER 141 Obstructive Sleep Apnea and Central Sleep Apnea in Childhood

Marie-Hélène Bourassa, MD and
Evelyn Constantin, MD, CM, MSc(Epi), FRCPC

BACKGROUND

Children are often brought for urgent or emergent medical assessment due to abnormal breathing patterns or worrisome respiratory episodes during sleep. Children with preexisting or previously undiagnosed sleep apnea may also be referred for admission with symptoms of acute airway obstruction or significant apneas. Sleep-disordered breathing may also occur in the sedation suite or in a hospitalized patient admitted for an unrelated problem when severe snoring, labored breathing, or gas exchange abnormalities become evident during sleep. This is more common in a postoperative patient or a patient recently extubated from endotracheal intubation. Often these episodes resolve and do not recur. However, some children with respiratory episodes during sleep have significant underlying medical conditions or even life-threatening events. Some children will require hospitalization for monitoring, diagnostic testing, and management despite a stable appearance at presentation, while others are able to be managed as outpatients. This chapter addresses sleep apnea in childhood.

PATHOPHYSIOLOGY

Pathologic apnea is defined as an event associated with physiologic compromise, as indicated by changes in oxygenation, color, muscle tone, or bradycardia. Apneic events may be obstructive, central, or mixed. Obstructive apnea is associated with respiratory effort throughout the event (out of phase or paradoxical breathing) and is considered abnormal even if it is of brief duration. As per the American Academy of Sleep Medicine (AASM) guidelines, the duration of an obstructive apnea event during sleep is scored if it is a minimum duration of two typical breaths. Central respiratory pauses are generally considered abnormal when they last 20 seconds or longer Shorter central apneic episodes (minimum duration of two typical breaths) are considered abnormal when they are accompanied by physiologic compromise (oxygen desaturation or arousal). Mixed apnea combines the features of central and obstructive episodes in the same respiratory event. A mixed apnea therefore presents with and without respiratory effort during the event.

During sleep, polysomnography (PSG) is the gold standard method of diagnosing sleep apnea. As per AASM guidelines, an apnea requires a drop of at least 90% of previous respiratory excursion during PSG; a hypopnea only requires a drop of at least 30% and this drop must last for the duration of at least two breaths and be associated with an oxygen desaturation of ≥ 3% or an arousal. The hypopnea is considered obstructive if there is snoring, increased inspiratory flattening of the nasal pressure compared to baseline breathing or thoracoabdominal paradox during the event, whereas the hypopnea is considered central if none of these criteria are met.

Central sleep apnea (CSA) can result from the lack of brainstem-mediated respiratory effort, as can be seen in premature infants and many other etiologies. Obstructive sleep apnea (OSA) results from attempts to breathe against a blocked airway, as can be seen in laryngomalacia or, most commonly, in adenotonsillar hypertrophy. Other common causes of OSA include craniofacial abnormalities, neuromuscular diseases, and obesity. Just like in CSA, the events tend to be more significant in rapid eye movement (REM) sleep likely in context of increased hypotonia during that sleep stage.

A correlation between the physiopathology of central and obstructive sleep apnea has been suggested by studies showing improvement of CSA after OSA management likely secondary to better control of breathing and less postobstructive central apneas. Furthermore, some underlying medical conditions, such as Trisomy 21 and Arnold-Chiari malformations can cause both central and obstructive sleep apnea.

CENTRAL SLEEP APNEA

Central sleep apnea is defined as the absence of respiratory effort due to either a lack of brain output from the central respiratory centers or neuromuscular insufficiency. In CSA, chest and abdominal wall movement are decreased or absent, and no breath sounds are evident on auscultation of the chest. Significant central apnea is generally defined as cessation of inspiratory effort for at least 20 seconds; shorter events of at least the duration of two typical breaths are considered significant if they are associated with arousal, oxygen desaturation of a minimum of 3%, or bradycardia for infants. Pathologic apnea is associated with physiologic compromise. Sometimes, brief central pauses associated with movement arousals can be considered normal during sleep and these tend to decrease in frequency with age.

PERIODIC BREATHING

Periodic breathing is a breathing pattern that can be common during infancy and is defined as three or more respiratory pauses of greater than 3 seconds duration with less than 20 seconds of normal breathing between pauses. Periodic breathing is mostly seen between 2 and 4 weeks of age and usually resolves by 3 to 6 months of age. It can be considered normal in that age group, especially in preterm infants. However, if periodic breathing is associated with bradycardia, cyanosis, or desaturations, it is considered a pathologic breathing pattern and warrants evaluation for an underlying cause. In some cases, respiratory stimulants such as caffeine may be indicated for infants with prolonged cardiorespiratory immaturity.

APNEA OF PREMATURITY

A frequent cause of central, and more commonly mixed apneas, is apnea of prematurity. It is believed to be secondary to the immature breathing regulation of preterm infants and usually resolves by 37 weeks postconceptional age. However, in rare cases, it may persist beyond term, particularly in infants born at less than 28 weeks gestation. There is strong evidence that methylxanthines are effective in reducing the number of apneic events and the need for mechanical ventilation in preterm infants. Caffeine was identified as the methylxanthine associated with the least toxicity. When pathologic apnea occurs for the first time in an infant beyond 37 weeks postconceptional age, it is called apnea of infancy. In term infants, the efficacy of caffeine in the prevention of clinically significant apnea lacks convincing data.

CENTRAL SLEEP APNEA RELATED TO UNDERLYING MEDICAL CONDITIONS

CSA is mostly seen in children with underlying medical conditions such as neurological conditions, Arnold-Chiari malformation, brain

TABLE 141-1 Conditions Associated With Central Sleep Apnea

Prematurity
Arnold-Chiari malformations
Foramen magnum stenosis
Prader-Willi syndrome
Trisomy 21
Seizure disorder
Hypoventilation syndromes
Obesity
Central nervous system infection, hemorrhage, or tumor

TABLE 141-2 Symptoms and Physical Findings Associated With Obstructive Sleep Apnea

Symptoms	Findings
Snoring	Tonsillar hypertrophy
Restless sleep	Crowded oropharynx
Increased work of breathing	Nasal obstruction/swollen nasal turbinates
Breathing pauses during sleep	Macroglossia
Mouth breathing	Midface hypoplasia
Secondary enuresis	Micro/retrognathia
Neurobehavioral changes	Large neck

masses/tumors, seizure disorders, brainstem malformations, and hypoventilation syndromes (secondary CSA). Congenital central hypoventilation syndrome (CCHS) is a ventilatory control disorder that often presents with CSA in the neonatal period. It is frequently caused by a mutation of the *PHOX2B* gene which is also responsible for other hypoventilation syndromes that may present later in childhood and even in adulthood. Another hypoventilation syndrome is the rapid-onset obesity with hypothalamic dysfunction, hypoventilation, and autonomic dysfunction (ROHHAD). ROHHAD often presents in early childhood and after a rapid weight gain. The central hypoventilation typically presents after the endocrinologic disorders and these patients are more at risk for neuroendocrine tumor (ROHHAD-NET) (**Table 141-1**).

DIAGNOSIS AND MANAGEMENT

The gold standard for diagnosis of CSA is laboratory PSG, and a central apnea/hypopnea index of more than 1 per hour is abnormal. Neurology assessment including neuroimaging (brain +/− spine MRI) and electroencephalography (EEG) should be considered as a first step after confirmed CSA on PSG in an otherwise healthy child. Other investigations and consultations should be undertaken based on clinical symptoms and evolution. The management of CSA is specific to the patient's underlying medical conditions and underlying diagnosis. Treatment may include neurologic or neurosurgical interventions, as well as noninvasive ventilation, and often requires admission to hospital and often intensive care unit for noninvasive ventilation and close monitoring (**Table 141-1**).

OBSTRUCTIVE SLEEP APNEA

Obstructive sleep apnea is generally defined as the absence of airflow at the nose or mouth despite continued respiratory efforts during sleep. OSA has been defined as a disorder of sleep consisting of prolonged partial upper airway obstruction or episodic obstructive apneas that affects gas exchange or sleep architecture and quality.

CLINICAL PRESENTATION

OSA occurs in 1.2% to 5.7% of children. The peak incidence is between 2 and 8 years in context of increased relative size of adenoids and tonsils in the pre-school age. In children with obesity, midfacial hypoplasia, and micrognathia (commonly seen in craniofacial syndromes), and disorders associated with abnormal muscle tone, the risk of OSA is even greater with a prevalence of up to 76% for children with Trisomy 21 and of up to 60% for children with obesity.

As its name implies, OSA occurs only during sleep. Respiration during wakefulness may be completely normal, although mouth breathing, adenoidal facies, nasal obstruction, and chronic congestion may be evident. Gas exchange should be normal during wakefulness, even in patients who have significant OSA and severe gas exchange abnormalities during sleep. Most patients with OSA have a history of snoring and restless fragmented sleep. Labored breathing with respiratory pauses may be noticed by the healthcare team in the hospital setting or by the parents at home or in the hospital setting at the bedside. Children may experience daytime sleepiness or have behavioral or attention problems. Secondary enuresis may also be associated with OSA (**Table 141-2**).

In the absence of an underlying craniofacial skeletal dysplasia or neuromuscular syndrome, the physical examination may reveal adenotonsillar hypertrophy or possibly rhinosinusitis but is often within normal limits. Pectus excavatum in a young child may suggest prolonged and severe upper airway obstruction. Despite the association with adenotonsillar hypertrophy, the absolute size of the tonsils and adenoid does not correlate with the severity of OSA. The Mallampati score, which is often used by anesthesiologists prior to intubation, can also be used in children with suspected OSA to classify the oropharynx findings. A grade 1 is defined by a full visualization of the soft palate whereas a grade 4 is an absent visualization of the soft palate. Rarely, in severe cases of OSA, failure to thrive or even cor pulmonale may be evident. Obesity is an increasingly common comorbidity when screening for OSA. Anatomical findings that may be suggestive of underlying conditions include macroglossia, mid-face hypoplasia and micro/retrognathia.

RISK FACTORS

Allergic rhinitis has a high prevalence in children with OSA and is also considered a risk factor, although the association is likely bidirectional. Obesity is an increasingly frequent cause of OSA in older children. The correlation between obesity and OSA is multifactorial with adenotonsillar hypertrophy remaining the most common etiology. Inflammation, altered tone, and excess load on the chest wall's respiratory efforts are other contributing factors that have been suggested to explain the physiopathology for this population.

Children with underlying craniofacial syndromes or neuromuscular disorders are more at risk of OSA. Often, these children are cared for by the hospital medicine service and thus it is important to be aware of an increased risk of OSA even if these children are admitted for a different reason. Children with sickle cell disease also have an increased prevalence of OSA compared to the general population. The risk of OSA, as well as opioid-induced central apneas should be considered when these patients with sickle cell disease are hospitalized for a vaso-occlusive crisis (**Table 141-3**). Family history of OSA can also be considered a risk factor for pediatric OSA and can be asked during clinical evaluation.

DIAGNOSTIC EVALUATION

Although the diagnosis and management of pediatric OSA are generally performed on an outpatient basis, the hospitalist should be aware of specific circumstances where admissions are warranted. Simple bedside observation of snoring and obstructed breathing, with or without

TABLE 141-3 Conditions Associated With Obstructive Sleep Apnea

Adenotonsillar hypertrophy
Allergic rhinitis
Obesity
Prader-Willi syndrome
Trisomy 21
Sickle cell disease
Skeletal dysplasia syndromes
Craniosynostosis syndromes (Crouzon, Apert)
Neuromuscular disorders

oxyhemoglobin desaturation, can be highly suggestive of OSA and may prompt the need for definitive testing. However, it is not possible to make the diagnosis of OSA based on history alone, and the gold standard for diagnosis is PSG. All children with suspected OSA should either undergo a PSG or be referred to a specialist for further evaluation, including sleep medicine specialists, respirologists, and otolaryngologists. Nocturnal oximetry can also be used as part of the screening assessment for OSA to help detect children with OSA and oxygen desaturations. We have elaborated on these evaluations below.

PSG is often performed in an inpatient facility, and a patient who becomes unstable during the study may come to the attention of the hospitalist. PSG monitors multiple cardiorespiratory and neurological parameters to assess the central and/or obstructive breathing pauses. The PSG criteria for OSA are one or more obstructive respiratory events per hour of sleep OR obstructive hypoventilation for > 25% total of sleep time with hypercapnia (> 50 mm Hg) associated with either snoring, flattening of the nasal pressure waveform, or paradoxical respiratory events. Although PSG is considered the most accurate test for diagnosis of OSA, not all children will have access because of its high cost, technical complexity, and accessibility to pediatric sleep laboratories.

Overnight oximetry is an alternative abbreviated testing modality that requires less equipment and is frequently done in the pediatric inpatient setting. It measures pulse rate and oxygen levels and is useful to diagnose children with severe OSA, but may not be helpful for children with OSA who do not desaturate with sleep. The McGill Oximetry Score (MOS) is used widely and considers all the desaturation clusters and the saturations below 90%. This score has been shown to help children with adenotonsillar hypertrophy get diagnosed and treated for OSA faster. Other alternative sleep diagnostic tests include nap PSG, home PSG, and video/audio recording.

Tests that might be indicated to assess for the etiology and complications of OSA include anteroposterior and lateral neck radiographs looking for adenotonsillar hypertrophy, anteroposterior and lateral chest radiographs to assess cardiac silhouette, and electrocardiogram (EKG). Electrocardiographic findings indicative of cor pulmonale include right atrial and right ventricular hypertrophy. Blood work is usually unremarkable, although hypercapnia due to severe OSA could theoretically result in elevated CO_2 and serum bicarbonate. Elevated inflammatory markers may be seen as there is a clear association between OSA and inflammation. Children with evidence of severe OSA should be evaluated by a sleep medicine specialist, respirologist and pulmonologist, and otolaryngologist and should be assessed for underlying causes of OSA (including adenotonsillar hypertrophy). Bedside laryngoscopy by otolaryngology could be done in the hospital setting to examine upper airway. Hospitalists could also assess for possible cardiac sequelae for severe OSA, including chest X-ray and EKG. If the EKG is abnormal or if the hospitalist has clinical concern for possible cor pulmonale, including low baseline oxygen saturation, cardiology consultation should be obtained for consideration for echocardiography. Assessment for hypercapnia via blood gas and/or transcutaneous or end-tidal CO_2 measurements should also be considered in children with severe OSA.

More complex testing may be considered to assess the airway of children with persistent OSA such as a drug-induced sleep endoscopy or a cine magnetic reasonance imaging (MRI), which is a type of dynamic MRI that helps evaluate sites of airway obstruction during sleep. magnetic resonance imaging. These tests may be difficult to access as they require sedation and the involvement of specialized teams.

MANAGEMENT

When witnessing an apneic event in a child during sleep, stimulation/arousal and repositioning are key to help resolve the apneic event and ensure no further desaturations. Children who demonstrate recurrent events need further investigations and close monitoring, especially if they require stimulation, supplemental oxygen, or ventilatory assistance. This may best be accomplished in an intensive care setting. In some cases, ventilatory support with either noninvasive methods or endotracheal intubation may be necessary until the child stabilizes.

The management of pediatric OSA includes support of gas exchange and airway function during sleep and treatment of the underlying condition. Tonsillectomy +/− adenoidectomy (T+/−A) is usually curative in an otherwise healthy child and is considered a first-line treatment for those with adenotonsillar hypertrophy. PSG prior to T+/−A is the gold standard diagnostic tool for OSA, especially for children with comorbidities and for children with no obvious adenotonsillar hypertrophy on physical examination. Some centers use nocturnal oximetry testing as part of their investigations and screening for desaturations in children with suspected OSA on history and clinical examination, especially in centers where patients do not have access to PSG or sleep laboratories. T+/−A is the most common treatment in children with OSA and hypertrophy of the tonsils and/or adenoids. Children younger than 3 years of age and those with severe OSA are at risk of postoperative respiratory compromise and should be monitored overnight in an inpatient setting after the procedure. This may warrant monitoring in an intensive care setting, especially in children with preoperative diagnosis of severe OSA or if patient has significant comorbidities that may place them at risk of perioperative complications (e.g., patients with Trisomy 21 or neurologic or genetic conditions). Continuous or bilevel positive airway pressure most commonly administered via a nasal mask can be used acutely or chronically for specific patients. A challenge that hospitalists and parents may face with positive pressure therapy is the tolerance of the child to the mask during sleep.

Recent trials have demonstrated some efficacy of intranasal steroids and montelukast in mild OSA for children with nasal obstruction secondary to adenoidal hypertrophy. Furthermore, for children with obesity, weight loss is critical. Hospitalists can consider medical therapy for OSA, including nasal steroids, montelukast, and weight management, as part of inpatient treatment for OSA as well as for discharge planning.

ADMISSION CRITERIA

- Any ill-appearing patient
- Evidence of sequelae of untreated and long-standing symptoms (e.g., failure to thrive, cardiac implications)
- Inability to ensure patient safety, parental comfort, or adequate medical follow-up in a timely manner
- Need for inpatient diagnostic testing and investigations
- Initiation of noninvasive ventilation therapy
- Postadenotonsillectomy monitoring for patients with severe OSA and/or younger than 3 years of age and/or with comorbidities and/or with unanticipated perioperative complications

DISCHARGE CRITERIA

- Documented medical and airway stability
- Adequate initiation of therapy for any treatable underlying disorder identified
- Adequate parental education and training in airway management and safe infant sleep
- Plan in place for medical follow-up

CONSULTATION

Subspecialty consultation should be considered on a case-by-case basis for children with suspected sleep apnea with technology dependence or evidence of a serious underlying condition. This often facilitates additional testing (e.g., PSG), allows the initiation of medical therapy, or results in an evaluation for possible surgical intervention. Subspecialty consultants include neonatologists, pulmonologists, otolaryngologists, cardiologists, or sleep medicine specialists depending on the individual patient's clinical situation. The early involvement of a multidisciplinary team is important for children at risk of OSA, such as children with complex genetic syndromes. Consulting allied health groups such as nurses, respiratory therapists, speech therapists, and occupational therapists can also be beneficial for some patients. Referral patterns vary according to regional practice and availability of subspecialty support. A referral to anesthesiology is warranted for patients with suspected or confirmed sleep apnea prior to general anesthesia because of the increased risk of severe apneas while under sedation as well as to ascertain best and safe practices perioperatively.

SPECIAL CONSIDERATIONS

Children with sleep apnea are heavy consumers of the healthcare system, even in the years prior to their diagnosis. In children with severe cases of sleep apnea, home monitoring, noninvasive ventilation, or even tracheostomy may be required.. These children therefore become technology-dependent and the involvement of the respiratory medicine, sleep medicine, and/or complex care team is often warranted. The initiation of respiratory technology in the pediatric inpatient units may lead to a complex discharge, as such requires more involved discharge planning. Equipment availability and caregiver teaching should be part of the discharge planning. A child with respiratory technology will also require close follow-up of his respiratory status and equipment.

PREVENTION

Left untreated, sleep apnea can lead to serious health consequences. As a hospitalist, it is important to take the opportunity to screen for sleep apnea, especially in the high-risk populations and in those who do not have a primary care physician. Counseling parents and ensuring an appropriate follow-up for these children is essential prior to discharge.

KEY POINTS

- In central sleep apnea (CSA), chest and abdominal wall movement are decreased or absent secondary to a lack of output from the central respiratory centers or neuromuscular insufficiency.
- CSA is most commonly seen in children with underlying medical conditions.
- OSA is a sleep disorder consisting of obstructive apnea or prolonged partial upper airway obstruction that affects gas exchange and sleep quality or architecture.
- Adenotonsillar hypertrophy, obesity, and diminished neuromuscular tone are common underlying conditions in OSA.
- Some pediatric populations that are well-known to hospitalists, such as children with Trisomy 21, are more at risk of CSA and/or OSA.
- Polysomnography (PSG) is the gold standard for the diagnosis of CSA and OSA.
- When PSG is not available, an overnight sleep oximetry test is an alternative test that is often performed on the pediatric wards.
- Tonsillectomy +/− adenoidectomy is a first-line treatment of OSA for children with adenotonsillar hypertrophy and adequate postoperative care needs to be established on a case-by-case basis.
- Untreated sleep apnea can lead to long-term health-related consequences, such as impacts on growth, development, behavior, and cardiovascular health.

SUGGESTED READINGS

American Academy of Sleep Medicine. International Classification of Sleep Disorders. 3rd ed. American Academy of Sleep Medicine; 2014.

Arens R, Sin S, Nandalike K, et al. Upper airway structure and body fat composition in obese children with obstructive sleep apnea syndrome. *Am J Resp Crit Care Med*. 2011;183(6):782-787.

Baldassari CM, Kepchar J, Bryant L, Beydoun H,Choi S. Changes in central apnea index following pediatric adenotonsillectomy.*Otolaryngol Head Neck Surg*. 2012;146(3):487-490.

Baldassari CM, Lam DJ, Ishman SL, et al. Expert consensus statement: pediatric drug-induced sleep endoscopy. *Otolaryngol Head Neck Surg*. 2021;165(4):578-591.

Berry RB, Quand SF, Abreu AR, et al; for the American Academy of Sleep Medicine. The AASM Manual for the Scoring of Sleep and Associated Events: Rules, Terminology and Technical Specifications: American Academy of Sleep Medicine; 2020; Version 2.6: 64-69.

Brouillette RT, Morielli A, Leimanis A, et al. Nocturnal pulse oximetry as an abbreviated testing modality for pediatric obstructive sleep apnea. *Pediatrics*. 2000;105:405-412.

Cao Y, Wu S, Zhang L, Yang Y, Cao S, Li Q. Association of allergic rhinitis with obstructive sleep apnea: a meta-analysis. *Medicine* (Baltimore). 2018;97(51):e13783.

Chiang J, Amin R. Respiratory care considerations for children with medical complexity. *Children* (Basel, Switzerland). 2017;4(5):41.

Constantin E, Brouillette RT. Congenital central hypoventilation syndrome and other causes of sleep-related hypoventilation in children. In: UpToDate. 2022.

Erenberg A, Leff RD, Haack DG, et al. Caffeine citrate for the treatment of apnea of prematurity: a double-blind, placebo-controlled study. *Pharmacotherapy*. 2000;20:644-652.

Goldbart AD, Greenberg-Dotan S, Tal A. Montelukast for children with obstructive sleep apnea: a double-blind, placebo-controlled study. *Pediatrics*. 2012;130(3):575-580.

Hasuneh MM, Toubasi AA, Khraisat B, Aldabbas H, Al-Iede M. Risk factors of obstructive sleep apnea (OSA) in pediatric patients: a systematic review and meta-analysis. *J Pediatr Health Care*. 2024 Sep-Oct;38(5):717–726.

Horwood L, Brouillette RT, McGregor CD, Manoukian JJ, Constantin E. Testing for pediatric obstructive sleep apnea when health care resources are rationed. *JAMA Otolaryngol Head Neck Surg*. 2014;140(7):616-623.

Kheirandish-Gozal L, Gozal D. Intranasal budesonide treatment for children with mild obstructive sleep apnea syndrome. *Pediatrics*. 2008;122(1):149-155.

Lee CF, Lee CH, Hsueh WY, Lin MT, Kang KT. Prevalence of obstructive sleep apnea in children with Down syndrome: a meta-analysis. *J Clin Sleep Med*. 2018;14(5):867-875.

Mitchell RB, Archer SM, Ishman SL, et al. Clinical Practice Guideline: Tonsillectomy in Children (Update). *Otolaryngol Head Neck Surg*. 2019;160(1_suppl):S1-S42.

Narang I, Mathew JL. Childhood obesity and obstructive sleep apnea. *J Nutr Metab*. 2012;134202.

Oros M, Baranga L, Plaiasu V, et al. Obstructing sleep apnea in children with genetic disorders—a special need for early multidisciplinary diagnosis and treatment. *J Clin Med*. 2021;10(10):2156.

Reuveni H, Simon T, Tal A, Elhayany A, Tarasiuk A. Health care services utilization in children with obstructive sleep apnea syndrome. *Pediatrics*. 2022;110(1 Pt 1):68-72.

Schechter MS. Technical report: diagnosis and management of childhood obstructive sleep apnea syndrome. *Pediatrics*. 2022;109(4):69.

CHAPTER 142

Asthma

Katherine Pumphrey, MD, MHA, MSHP and Chén C. Kenyon, MD, MSHP

BACKGROUND

Over 4 million children in the United States have asthma and it is a leading cause of hospital admission in children. Each year, asthma results in approximately 10 million school absences, 800,000 emergency department (ED) visits, and 65,000 hospitalizations, and in 2020, 204 deaths of children under 18 years. Appropriate asthma treatment prevents ED visits and hospital admissions, reduces the risk of death, and improves the quality of life for children with asthma. The hospitalist is ideally situated to have a major impact on asthma by treating its acute manifestations, appropriately identifying and intervening upon comorbid conditions and modifiable environmental triggers, and adjusting long-term therapy commensurate with the child's impairment and risk.

Asthma is considered an "ambulatory-sensitive condition," meaning that effective outpatient treatment should prevent ED visits and hospitalization. Despite this, hospitalization rates for children with asthma remain high in many metropolitan areas. Disparities for asthma prevalence, morbidity, and mortality are well documented in the United States. Racial and socioeconomic disparities include African-American children experiencing higher rates of asthma diagnosis, as well as hospitalization and death, and children from low socioeconomic households more likely to have persistent asthma. Of particular note are persistent racial disparities. For instance, of the 204 children under 18 who died due to asthma in 2020, 119 (58%) were African American, while only 19% of children with asthma were African American. The causes of these disparities are multifactorial; yet hospitalists must ensure they address gaps in the implementation of evidence-based and guideline-consistent care for at-risk populations, as they perpetuate asthma disparities.

DEFINITION AND PATHOPHYSIOLOGY OF ASTHMA

Asthma was defined by the Global Initiative for Asthma (GINA) in 2022 as "a heterogeneous disease, usually characterized by chronic airway inflammation. It is defined by a history of respiratory symptoms, such as wheeze, shortness of breath, chest tightness or cough, that vary over time and intensity, together with variable expiratory airflow limitation." A similar working definition is used by the U.S. National Heart Lung and Blood Institute (NHLBI) in their 2007 guidelines. Early in the course of the disease, airway inflammation, bronchial hyperreactivity, and loss of lung function are often evident. Atopy and a family history of asthma are strongly correlated with childhood asthma. In children with atopic phenotypes, exposure to allergens activates mast cells and promotes inflammation and airway infiltration with neutrophils, eosinophils, and lymphocytes. The inflammation results in airway hyperresponsiveness, which causes bronchoconstriction, edema, and mucus plugging, all of which contribute to bronchial obstruction. Chronically, collagen deposition below the epithelial basement membrane results in narrowing of the airway due to remodeling.

ASTHMA EXACERBATIONS

Asthma exacerbations are acute or subacute episodes of progressively worsening shortness of breath, cough, wheezing, and chest tightness, or some combination of these symptoms. Exacerbations are characterized by decreases in expiratory airflow that can be documented and quantified by measurement of lung function. Status asthmaticus is continued or progressive airway obstruction despite bronchodilator therapy resulting in sustained or worsening respiratory distress.

Acute asthma exacerbations can be triggered by many exposures, including infectious respiratory illness, environmental allergen or irritant exposure, exercise, cold air, or combinations of these. An asthma exacerbation may involve either a slow onset of symptoms or a rapid decline in respiratory status. Persistent or acute allergen or irritant exposure promotes inflammation, bronchoconstriction, and airway hyperresponsiveness on an ongoing basis.

Viral infections cause asthma symptoms by promoting eosinophilic or neutrophilic airway inflammation. Viral-induced asthma exacerbations are common in children and most acute asthma admissions are associated with viral infections, especially rhinovirus. The risk of an asthma exacerbation can be modified by a patient's underlying inflammatory state and level of airway hyperreactivity. A patient with reduced airway inflammation due to adequate controller therapy is less likely to have a severe asthma flare when exposed to offending agents.

CLINICAL PRESENTATION

The presentation of an acute asthma exacerbation may vary, but all patients experience worsening airflow obstruction leading to various degrees of respiratory distress. Patients often complain of shortness of breath, chest tightness, and wheezing. Some patients describe chest pain, cough, or fatigue. Caregivers may report observations of breathlessness, trouble speaking, decreased activity, retractions, rapid breathing, wheezing noises, or relentless cough.

On physical examination, tachypnea is present, often accompanied by tachycardia. Pulse oximetry may reveal decreased oxygen saturation. There is often evidence of increased respiratory effort, such as subcostal, intercostal, and supraclavicular retractions. The paradoxical motion of the thoracoabdominal wall (e.g., expansion of the abdominal girth with inspiration), often referred to as "belly breathing," is another useful sign of increased work of breathing in younger children. Auscultation of the chest often reveals polyphonic wheezing—secondary to turbulent air flow through bronchioles of different diameter—and a prolonged expiratory phase. Rales or crackles are often heard and may shift in location over minutes to hours ("migratory atelectasis"). An assessment of air movement is determined by the loudness of breath sounds, often characterized as good, fair, or poor, in various areas of the chest and may vary over time. Patients with poor air movement may have minimal wheezing since the passage of air through the airway is what generates wheezing sounds. As air exchange improves, polyphonic wheezing may become more pronounced. Conversely, patients with a deteriorating clinical course may have diminishing wheezing, indicative of worsening air movement and poor ventilation. Agitation or somnolence are worrisome signs and may indicate hypercarbia or hypoxemia with impending respiratory failure.

DIFFERENTIAL DIAGNOSIS

Many conditions result in acute or chronic respiratory symptoms that mimic an asthma syndrome. Anatomical abnormalities should be considered in young children with frequent episodes of cough or wheeze. Inhaled foreign bodies are most common in toddler-aged children (see Chapter 146). These problems may present with cough, stridor, and/or monophonic wheeze—indicating turbulent airflow at a single area of airway obstruction. In all age groups, gastroesophageal reflux can contribute to underlying asthma. Cystic fibrosis is a genetic disorder that can also present with chronic cough or recurrent episodes of wheezing (see Chapter 145).

Viral infections often cause wheezing in childhood and may or may not be coincident with the underlying chronic inflammation and reversible airway obstruction of asthma. Respiratory syncytial virus (RSV) is the most common cause of bronchiolitis, but other respiratory viruses such as rhinovirus, parainfluenza virus, coronavirus (including SARS-CoV-2), adenovirus, and influenza viruses are other common infectious agents. Viral bronchiolitis classically presents in children less than 2 years of age and is associated with small airway edema, increased mucus production, and wheezing (see Chapter 97). Thus, in young children with a history of wheezing, it may be difficult to determine if a wheezing episode represents bronchiolitis or an asthma exacerbation triggered by the respiratory illness. In this circumstance, the Asthma Predictive Index, which assesses the frequency of wheezing in the past year, as well as personal and family history of atopy and asthma, may provide additional diagnostic utility. Atypical respiratory infections with agents such as *Mycoplasma*, *Chlamydia pneumoniae*, *Bordetella pertussis*, or *parapertussis* can present with chronic cough.

Functional disorders can coexist with or mimic asthma and include vocal cord dysfunction (VCD) and psychogenic cough. VCD usually presents in adolescence, with upper airway (laryngeal) inspiratory and/or expiratory stridor, which may be difficult to distinguish from lower airway wheezing. The diagnosis of VCD is confirmed by laryngoscopy demonstrating paradoxical adduction of the vocal cords seen during inspiration. Psychogenic cough is a habitual cough that can also persist for months, often occurring after an acute respiratory illness. A key feature of VCD and psychogenic cough is the lack of response to asthma therapy. In addition, they are not associated with hypoxia.

DIAGNOSTIC EVALUATION

In the United States, the 2007 NHLBI *Guidelines for the Diagnosis and Management of Asthma* (EPR-3) are available to guide clinicians through the diagnosis and management of chronic asthma. These guidelines are complementary to the material presented in this chapter. More recently, the NHLBI published the 2020 Focused Updates to the Asthma Management Guidelines, which include an updated stepwise approach to management of asthma. GINA, the International Asthma Guideline

TABLE 142-1 Questions to Ask Patients Who Present With Concern for Asthma Exacerbation

Types of Symptoms (Impairment)	Cough Wheeze Shortness of breath Chest tightness Sputum production
Frequency of Symptoms (Impairment)	Prior to this current illness, how many nights/month do they awaken with cough? Prior to this current illness, how many days/week does asthma interfere with their activity? Prior to this current illness, how many days/week do they use their albuterol? *If a patient has asthma and the answer is 3 or more for any of these questions, the asthma is not well controlled.*
Severity of Symptoms (Risk)	How many times in the last year have they used oral steroids? How many emergency room visits for asthma? How many visits to the hospital for asthma? Have they ever needed help with breathing (positive airway pressure, intubation) in an ICU?

Committee, has slightly different stepwise recommendations for asthma treatment that are more pragmatic and intended to apply more broadly to lower-resourced healthcare settings than the United States.

The initial evaluation of a patient presenting with an asthma exacerbation should include the assessment of the acute respiratory symptoms, signs, or symptoms of coexisting or precipitating conditions, and treatments initiated prior to presentation. History should be obtained regarding the characteristics of the patient's asthma symptoms, the pattern and frequency of the symptoms, any precipitating or aggravating factors as well as features indicative of the severity and level of control of their asthma (**Tables 142-1**).

The physical examination provides clues to the severity of the current illness as well as the presence of comorbidities. Important physical parameters include respiratory rate, work of breathing, air entry, wheezing, and oxygen saturation. Work of breathing refers to the use of accessory muscles of respiration and includes parameters such as nasal flaring, abdominal retractions, and depth of respiration.

During an asthma exacerbation, physical findings may vary and evolve with treatment or progression of the acute condition. A quiet or silent chest is a worrisome sign as poor movement of air can be associated with respiratory insufficiency or failure. Asymmetry of auscultatory findings may indicate other conditions. Unequal breath sounds can be found with pneumonia, effusion (especially in dependent regions of the lung), or atelectasis. Unilateral breath sounds may indicate an aspirated foreign body or a pneumothorax on the side with diminished breath sounds, and may be accompanied by hyperresonance on that side, especially if there is significant air trapping. Chest radiographs are typically not needed for patients who present with an asthma exacerbation; however, when obtained, typical radiographic findings include hyperinflation, peribronchial thickening, and atelectasis (**Figure 142-1**). **Chest radiographs** may be considered if concerned for additional etiologies of increased work of breathing such as foreign body or pneumothorax.

A classification system for the severity of an asthma exacerbation is provided in **Table 142-2**. Respiratory scoring algorithms may be used to assess the severity of an acute asthma exacerbation. Multiple algorithms are available and include the Pediatric Asthma Severity Score (PASS) and Pediatric Respiratory Assessment Measure (PRAM). PASS and PRAM both produce a score based on an assessment of the patient's wheezing, work of breathing, and prolongation of expiration, among other clinical factors. Validation studies of these scoring systems were performed in the ED; however, scoring algorithms are often used in the inpatient setting to complement the more subjective assessments of response to therapy provided by individual providers.

Patients in mild distress typically have slightly increased respiratory rates, may not use accessory muscles of respiration, and have end-expiratory wheezes with good air entry. Patients in severe distress are working hard to breathe, with inspiratory and expiratory wheezes, and are often hypoxemic. For infants and children under 2 years of age, clues to breathlessness include difficulty or reluctance to feed and changes in crying pattern (e.g., softer or shorter). Changes in vital signs in younger patients should be interpreted in the context of normal values for age. Interestingly, paradoxical thoracoabdominal movement, a sign associated with severe respiratory distress in older children, may be seen in young children and infants even in states of mild or moderate respiratory distress.

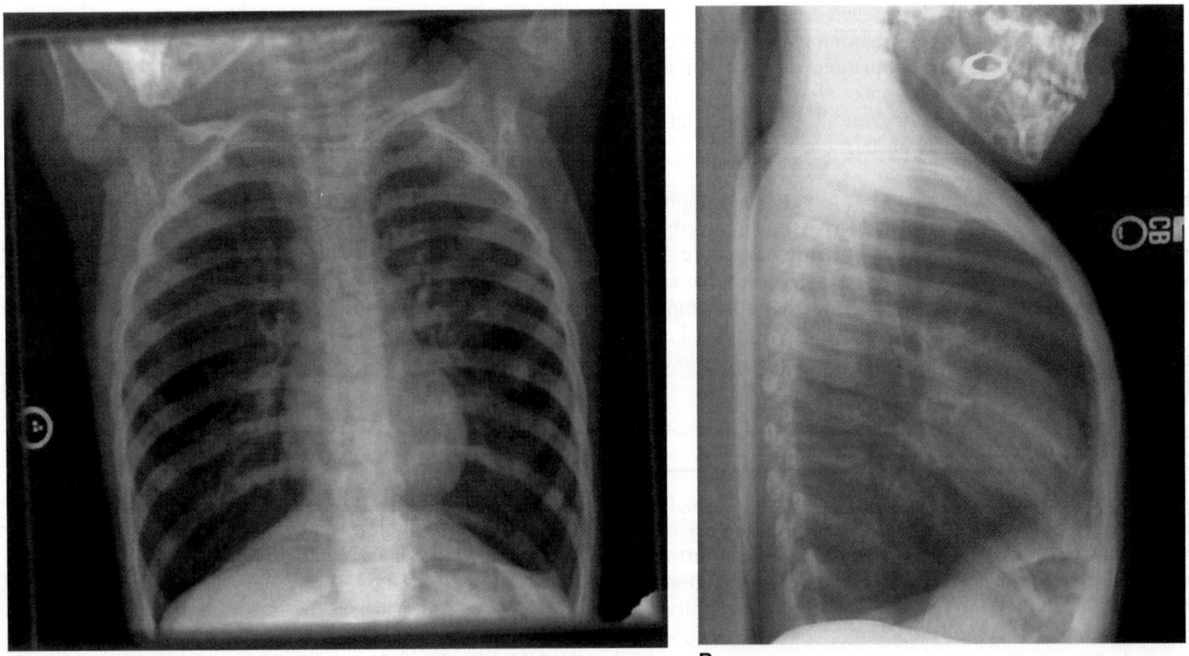

A B

FIGURE 142-1. Typical radiographic findings in a patient with an acute asthma exacerbation.

TABLE 142-2 Clinical Classification of Severity for Asthma Exacerbation in Patients ≥5 Years of Age

Exacerbation Severity	Mild	Moderate	Severe	Subset: Respiratory Arrest Imminent
Symptoms				
Breathlessness	While walking	While talking (infants: softer, shorter cry; difficulty feeding)	While at rest (infants: stop feeding)	
Positioning	Can lie down	Prefers sitting	Sits upright	Inability to lie supine
Speaks in	Sentences	Phrases	Words	Inability to speak
Alertness	May be agitated	Usually agitated	Usually agitated	Deteriorating mental status, lethargy, or agitation
Signs				
Respiratory rate	Increased	Increased	Often >30/min	
Use of accessory muscles, suprasternal retractions	Usually not	Commonly	Usually	Paradoxical thoracoabdominal movement
Wheeze	Moderate, often only end expiratory	Loud; throughout exhalation	Usually loud, throughout inhalation and exhalation	Poor air movement or silent chest in combination with increased respiratory effort, bradypnea, or disorganized breathing pattern
Pulse/min	<100	100-120	>120	Tachycardia or bradycardia
Pulsus paradoxus	Absent (<10 mm Hg)	May be present (10-25 mm Hg)	Often present (>25 mm Hg for an adult, 20-40 mm Hg for a child)	Increasing pulsus paradoxus or decreasing pulsus paradoxus in an exhausted patient
Functional Assessment				
PEF % predicted or % personal best	>70%	40% to 69% or response lasts <2 hours	<40% predicted or personal best	<25% Note: PEF test may not be needed for severe attacks
PaO_2 (on room air)	Normal (test not usually necessary)	>60 mm Hg (test not usually necessary)	<60 mm Hg, possible cyanosis	
And/or $PaCO_2$	<42 mm Hg	<42 mm Hg	>42 mm Hg, possible respiratory failure	PCO_2 >42 mm Hg
SaO_2 % (on room air) at sea level	>95%	90% to 95%	<90%	

Source: Modified from National Asthma Education and Prevention Program: Full Report of the Expert Panel: Guidelines for the Diagnosis and Management of Asthma (EPR-3). Bethesda, MD, National Heart, Lung, and Blood Institute, National Institutes of Health, 2007.

An exacerbation usually includes several parameters, but not necessarily all. These parameters serve only as general guidelines because many have not been systemically studied.

Objective measures of acute asthma exacerbation include pulse oximetry, venous and arterial blood gases, and, less frequently, pulmonary function testing. Patients with asthma exacerbations are at risk for hypoxemia. As a result, patients require frequent monitoring to ensure adequate oxygenation. During initial treatment of a severe exacerbation, continuous pulse oximetry is recommended, whereas intermittent oximetry is appropriate as the clinical course improves. Of note, however, pulse oximetry tends to underrepresent oxygen saturation by 3% to 4% compared to direct measurement with co-oximetry.

Venous blood gases are often obtained in the emergency department or inpatient setting and often reveal respiratory alkalosis with hypocapnia due to hyperventilation early in the course. Arterial blood gases are typically performed in critically ill patients and those with clinical deterioration or signs of respiratory insufficiency or failure and may also reveal hypoxemia due to ventilation-perfusion mismatch. A normal or elevated partial pressure of carbon dioxide on either venous or arterial blood gas may signal progression from respiratory distress to respiratory insufficiency or failure and may be associated with a decreased blood pH due to respiratory acidosis. In addition, lactic acidosis is a particularly concerning finding in status asthmaticus as patients with lactic acidosis are at high risk of respiratory failure.

Pulmonary function tests can be used to assess lung function even during an asthma exacerbation. Spirometric indices such as the measurement of the forced expiratory volume at 1 second (FEV_1), or peak expiratory flow rate (PEFR) have been recommended by the NHLBI consensus guidelines to assess the severity of asthma **(Figure 142-2)**. In patients presenting to an emergency room with an asthma exacerbation, the FEV_1 is typically 30% to 35% of normal, and the PEFR is less than 50% of normal. However, since spirometry is often not readily available and practicable in the emergency and inpatient settings and PEFR is effort- and technique-dependent, and thus unreliable, they are not frequently used in practice.

MANAGEMENT

Asthma exacerbations are treated with a combination of supportive therapy and pharmacological interventions. Treatment is tailored to the severity of the symptoms and adjusted based on response to therapy. Adequate hydration should be established and maintained either orally or with intravenous fluids. Physiologic monitoring should include vital signs and pulse oximetry. Oxygen supplementation is provided to maintain oxygen saturations in a safe range. Most agree that levels more than 90% are safe.

MEDICATIONS

Adrenergic Agonists This class of medications works by stimulating the β_2-adrenergic receptor causing activation of adenylate cyclase, which increases the production of cyclic 3′5-adenosine monophosphate (cAMP). This increase in cAMP depending on the site of stimulation results in bronchial smooth relaxation, skeletal muscle and cardiac muscle stimulation, and inhibition of the release of inflammatory mediators via stabilization of the mast cell membrane. Adrenergic agonists, such as albuterol, are used as first-line agents for acute asthma exacerbation due to their ability to open the airways rapidly and reliably. Albuterol can be administered by metered-dose inhaler (MDI) with a spacer device or nebulizer, either continuously or intermittently. When compared to nebulized medication, studies have demonstrated that MDI with spacer is equivalent or superior regarding improvement of pulmonary function

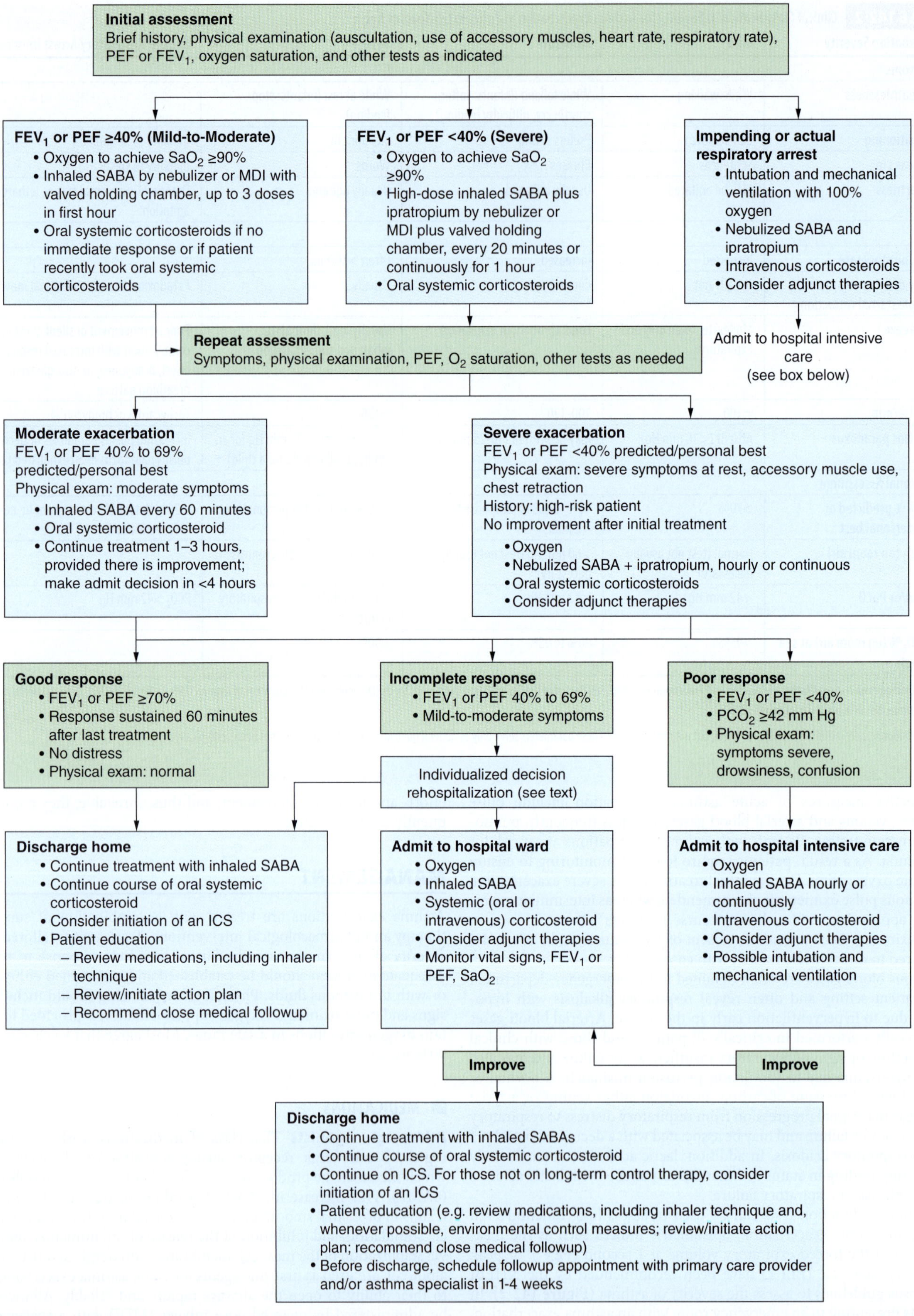

FIGURE 142-2. Management of asthma exacerbations: emergency department and hospital-based care. This figure does not include the 2020 Focused Updates including Single Maintenance and Reliver Therapy (SMART) (*Source:* Reproduced from National Asthma Education and Prevention Program: Full Report of the Expert Panel: Guidelines for the Diagnosis and Management of Asthma (EPR-3). Bethesda, MD, National Heart, Lung, and Blood Institute, National Institutes of Health, 2007.)

TABLE 142-3 Dosages of Bronchodilators Commonly Used for Asthma Exacerbations

Medications	Adult Dose	Child Dose (<12 y of age)	Onset of Action	Duration	Comments
Inhaled Short-Acting β-$_2$ Agonists					
Albuterol nebulizer 5.0 mg/mL 2.5 mg/3 mL 1.25 mg/3 mL 0.63 mg/3 mL	2.5-5.0 mg every 20 minutes for 3 doses then 2.5-10 mg every 1-4 hours as needed or 10-15 mg/hour continuously	0.15 mg/kg (minimum dose 2.5 mg) every 20 minutes for 3 doses then 0.1-5 to 0.3 mg/kg up to 10 mg every 1-4 hours as needed, or 0. mg/kg/hr by continuous nebulization	5-15 minutes	3-4 hours	Only selective β-2 agonists are recommended. For optimal delivery, dilute aerosols to minimum of 4 mL at gas flow of 6-8 L/min. As effective as nebulized therapy if patient is able to coordinate.
Albuterol or Levalbuterol metered-dose inhaler (MDI) (90 mcg/puff)	4-8 puffs every 20 minutes up to 4 hours, then every 1-4 hours as needed	4-8 puffs every 20 minutes for 3 doses, then every 1-4 hours inhalation maneuver Use VHC; add mask in children <4 years			
Levalbuterol nebulizer 1.25 mg/0.5 mL 1.25 mg/3 mL 0.63 mg/3 mL	1.25-2.5 mg every 20 minutes for 3 doses, then 1.25-5 mg every 1-4 hours as needed	0.075 mg/kg (minimum dose 1.25 mg) every 20 minutes for 3 doses, then 0.075-0.15 mg/kg up to 5 mg every 1-4 hours as needed			Levalbuterol administered in one-half the mg dose of albuterol provides comparable safety, without demonstrated benefit in efficacy.
Anticholinergics					
Ipratropium bromide nebulizer solution (0.25 mg/mL)	0.5 mg every 20 minutes for 3 doses then as needed	0.25-0.5 mg every 20 minutes for 3 doses, then as needed	20-30 minutes Peak 60-90 minutes	Duration 3-6 hours	May mix in same nebulizer with albuterol. Should not be used alone as first-line therapy, should be added to SABA therapy for severe exacerbations. The addition of ipratropium has not been shown to provide further benefit once the patient is hospitalized.
Ipratropium MDI (18 mcg/puff)	8 puffs as needed up to 3 hours	4-8 puffs as needed up to 3 hours			

Source: Modified from National Asthma Education and Prevention Program: Full Report of the Expert Panel: Guidelines for the Diagnosis and Management of Asthma (EPR-3). Bethesda, MD, National Heart, Lung, and Blood Institute, National Institutes of Health, 2007.

MDI, metered dose inhaler; SABA, short-acting bronchodilator; VHC, valved holding chamber.

parameters, clinical outcomes, and cost-effectiveness. Dosing information is provided in **Table 142-3**; however, please refer to institution recommendations and/or pharmacist for guidance.

Paradoxical worsening of hypoxemia due to increased ventilation-perfusion mismatching can be seen with the administration of β_2-adrenergic agents. This common adverse effect is secondary to pulmonary arteriolar vasodilation and perfusion of under- or unventilated areas of the lung and is treated with supplemental oxygen. Other side effects include sinus tachycardia, tremor, palpitations, headache, agitation, and ventricular irritability (e.g., ventricular premature contractions, ventricular tachycardia). In addition, prolonged continuous dosing with adrenergic agents can lead to hypokalemia, therefore patients receiving prolonged treatment should have serum potassium levels monitored. There is no clear consensus as to what constitutes prolonged, though one study demarcated 24 hours as the 75th percentile of continuous duration as prolonged therapy. Nonselective adrenergic agents (e.g., epinephrine) can cause transient hyperglycemia and elevations in neutrophil counts due to demargination.

Albuterol is a racemic mixture of R-albuterol and S-albuterol, with a 50:50 ratio of the two stereoisomers. Levalbuterol (Xopenex™) consists of the R-isomer, which is thought to be the active component of the racemic product. However, most clinical studies and in vitro pharmacology data have shown no significant differences in the bronchodilator effects or cardiopulmonary and tremor side effects when comparing racemic to R-isomer albuterol.

Subcutaneous or intravenous terbutaline, a selective β_2-adrenergic agonist, and subcutaneous or intramuscular epinephrine, a nonselective adrenergic agonist, are used in children with asthma who are not ventilating sufficiently to deliver inhaled beta-agonists to the bronchioles. Bronchodilation is seen within 5 minutes of administration and can persist for 3 to 4 hours. Terbutaline can also be given by continuous IV infusion starting with a bolus and titrating the dose to the desired effect. Dosing of β_2-adrenergic and bronchodilator agonists are shown in **Tables** 142-3 and **142-4**.

Corticosteroids Corticosteroids are indicated in the initial treatment of status asthmaticus. They are potent anti-inflammatory medications that have been shown to hasten recovery, prevent recurrence, and prevent hospitalizations. Due to their mechanism of action, the effect of corticosteroids is not immediate. Steroids bind to the intracytoplasmic glucocorticoid receptor and translocate to the nucleus thereby affecting RNA transcription in both a positive and negative fashion through the transcription factors NF-κB and AP-1. In general, corticosteroids lead to downregulation of inflammatory cytokines. Corticosteroids also activate histone deacetylase that inhibits DNA transcription. This change in transcription leads to increased numbers of β_2-adrenegeric receptors at the cell surface, leading to a synergistic effect when given with β_2-adrenergic agonists. Benefits are typically seen within 4 hours after corticosteroids are given. Studies comparing oral and intravenous corticosteroids have found no significant differences in efficacy; however, oral steroids are preferred for cost-effectiveness since IV access is not required.

Dexamethasone has a longer half-life compared to oral steroids. A single or two-dose regimen of dexamethasone has demonstrated noninferiority in the outpatient setting when compared to oral steroids. Similarly, retrospective studies in the inpatient setting have demonstrated equivalence of dexamethasone in place of oral steroids, though no randomized trials have been performed in severe exacerbations requiring hospitalization. Dosing of corticosteroids is shown in **Table 142-5**.

Inhaled Anticholinergic Agents Anticholinergic agents work by competitively inhibiting the neurotransmitter acetylcholine at the muscarinic junction to relieve cholinergic-mediated bronchoconstriction. Ipratropium bromide, when used in combination with inhaled albuterol in the emergency department, has demonstrated a decreased risk of admission and provides improved lung function. However, routine use of ipratropium bromide has not been found to be efficacious in the inpatient setting. Dosing is listed in Table 142-3.

TABLE 142-4 Systemic Bronchodilators for Acute Asthma Exacerbations

Medications	Adult Dose	Child Dose	Onset of Action	Duration	Comments
Systemic (Injected)					
β_2-Agonists					
Epinephrine 1:1000 (1 mg/mL) IV Infusion	0.3-0.5 mg every 20 minutes for 3 doses subcutaneous	0.01 mg/kg up to 0.3-0.5 mg every 20 minutes for 3 doses subcutaneously	1-3 minutes	30 minutes	No proven advantage of systemic therapy over aerosol, but indicated when a patient is not ventilating sufficiently to deliver inhaled beta-agonists to the small airways.
Terbutaline (1 mg/mL) IV Infusion	0.25 mg every 20 minutes for 3 doses subcutaneous	0.01 mg/kg every 20 minutes for doses then every 2-6 hours as need subcutaneously			

NONSTANDARD THERAPIES

If initiation of the above standard therapies does not improve the level of respiratory distress or if symptoms progress, additional interventions may be necessary. The clinical experience and expertise available at the institution should be considered. When necessary, transfer to a facility able to provide critical care management should be anticipated and expedited.

Magnesium Sulfate Magnesium is thought to inhibit mast cell degranulation and increase bronchial dilatation due to a decrease in calcium uptake by bronchial smooth muscle. Its use is considered when the patient fails to improve or worsens despite treatment with continuous inhaled β_2-agonist, systemic corticosteroids, and inhaled anticholinergic agents. While a meta-analysis of several small randomized trials of administration in the ED setting has demonstrated efficacy in preventing hospitalization, a retrospective study of magnesium sulfate has not demonstrated significantly improved hospital outcomes.

Heliox Heliox is a mixture of helium and oxygen used for inhalation. This agent is thought to improve airflow by creating a gas with a similar viscosity to air but with a lower density, which in turn can increase ventilation and decrease work of breathing. Heliox is a therapeutic option in patients with a refractory asthma exacerbation. Patients with significant oxygen requirements, however, are generally unable to tolerate heliox because they need a higher FiO_2 than a helium-oxygen mixture can provide. Heliox can also lower body temperature due to the high thermal conductivity of the mixture. Patients need to have their temperature monitored closely.

Methylxanthines Intravenous methylxanthines, such as aminophylline, were commonly used in the past due to their ability to act directly on β-adrenergic receptors and relax bronchial smooth muscle. Concerns regarding toxicity and efficacy of this class of medication and the availability of newer agents limit its use. Life-threatening events such as cardiac arrhythmia and seizures are associated with toxic levels of theophylline (>30 μg/mL).

Medication adverse effects are listed in **Table 142-6**.

INITIAL TREATMENT

The initial therapy of status asthmaticus has been outlined by the NHLBI guidelines (Figure 142-2). In brief, patients are first treated with short-acting inhaled β_2-adrenergic agonists (SABA) (e.g., inhaled albuterol), inhaled anticholinergics (e.g., ipratropium bromide), and corticosteroids either orally or intravenously. Patients who demonstrate significant improvement after these initial interventions may not require hospitalization.

Patients with moderately severe symptoms who are stable or are showing signs of improvement and patients with severe symptoms who are demonstrating clear signs of improvement should be hospitalized and treated with inhaled albuterol, either every 1 to 2 hours by MDI-spacer (preferred) or nebulizer, or delivered continuously via nebulizer. Corticosteroid therapy is continued orally, or if not tolerated, intravenously.

If patients continue to deteriorate, they must be monitored for respiratory insufficiency and failure. Pulse oximetry alone remains a poor monitoring device for respiratory failure since a patient may develop hypercarbia without significant hypoxemia, especially when patients are receiving supplemental oxygen. Therefore, venous or arterial blood gases should be obtained if clinically appropriate. Patients with impending respiratory failure often need mechanical ventilatory support either noninvasively with bilevel or continuous positive airway pressure administered via a mask or invasively with endotracheal intubation.

TAPERING HOSPITAL THERAPY

After patients are stabilized and demonstrate improvement, the therapies can be gradually reduced and withdrawn. If the patient remains

TABLE 142-5 Systemic Corticosteroids in the Setting of Asthma Exacerbations

Medication	Adult Dose	Child Dose (< or = 12 y of age)	Onset of Action	Duration	Comments
Corticosteroids					
Oral: Prednisone/ Prednisolone	40-80 mg/day in 1 or 2 divided doses until PEF reaches 70% of predicted or personal best	1-2 mg/kg in 2 divided doses (maximum = 60 mg/day) until PEF 70% of predicted or personal best		12-36 hours	For outpatient burst for 3-10 days: Adult: use 40-60 mg in single or 2 divided doses
IV: Methylprednisolone				12-36 hours	Children: use 1-2 mg/kg/day with maximum of 60 mg/day.
Oral, IM, IV: Dexamethasone	Oral: 12-16 mg daily for 1 to 2 days only	0.6 mg/kg once daily as a single dose or once daily for 2 days (maximum = 16 mg/dose)		72 hours	

Source: Modified from National Asthma Education and Prevention Program: Full Report of the Expert Panel: Guidelines for the Diagnosis and Management of Asthma (EPR-3). Bethesda, MD, National Heart, Lung, and Blood Institute, National Institutes of Health, 2007.

TABLE 142-6 Common Side Effects of Pharmacologic Therapies

Side Effect	Possible Causative Agent	Comment
Hypokalemia	Adrenergic agonists	Patients on prolonged hourly or continuous inhaled therapy (>24-48 hours), or intravenous therapy should have serum potassium levels monitored
Tremor/Agitation	Adrenergic agonists	Dose-dependent
Hypertension	Corticosteroids, adrenergic agonists	May require reduction of dose, discontinuation of therapy, or addition of antihypertensive medication
Tachycardia, palpitations, VPCs	Adrenergic agonists, aminophylline, theophylline	Usually dose-dependent Serum levels of methylxanthines should be monitored
		The risk is increased with hypoxemia or acidemia
Hyperglycemia/ Glucosuria	Corticosteroids, adrenergic agonists	Resolves with completion or discontinuation of therapy
Emotional lability	Corticosteroids	Resolves with completion or discontinuation of therapy
Hyperphagia	Corticosteroids	Resolves with completion or discontinuation of therapy
Seizure	Theophylline, aminophylline	Serum levels of methylxanthines should be monitored
		Risk is increased in the presence of acidosis
Elevated peripheral neutrophil count	Corticosteroids, adrenergic agonists (in particular epinephrine)	May interfere with utility of the white blood count in assessing for infection

comfortable with minimal signs of respiratory distress, the dosing of inhaled β-agonists is decreased. While not validated specifically for this use, respiratory scoring algorithms (e.g., PASS, PRAM) may be used in the inpatient setting to support treatment decisions regarding the weaning of β-agonists. For patients on continuous inhaled β-agonist therapy, the dose may be reduced and then subsequently transitioned to intermittent treatments, usually every 2 hours. As the patient continues to improve, the interval between treatments can be extended further. Similarly, the amount of supplemental oxygen is titrated to maintain oxygen saturations above the desired level, and eventually discontinued.

Many hospitals use clinical pathways, which are tools that detail a sequence of assessments and treatments for patients with various conditions. Studies have shown that asthma clinical pathways shorten hospitalization and decrease the need for readmission for up to 2 weeks after discharge. An asthma clinical pathway allows multiple caregivers, including nurses, respiratory therapists, and doctors to modify treatment based on structured assessments. The 2007 NHLBI guidelines (see Figure 142-2) outline specific criteria that can be used to determine a patient's severity and frequency of therapy. It also provides criteria to assist in weaning treatments.

THERAPY AFTER DISCHARGE TO HOME

The duration of oral corticosteroids depends upon the length and severity of illness and the patient's frequency of exacerbations. An acute asthma exacerbation may be treated with corticosteroids for 3 to 10 days. However, if a patient was admitted to the hospital for an extended period, they may require a prolonged course of corticosteroids (>10 days) and then tapering doses. A taper is prescribed to prevent a relapse of symptoms as well as to prevent risk of Addisonian crisis from adrenal suppression.

Patients who require admission to the hospital may not have an adequate outpatient treatment plan and a hospitalization offers the opportunity to assess the overall treatment regimen. Upon admission, the patient's chronic asthma impairment should be assessed. If indicated, patients should have their outpatient preventive treatment adjusted in a stepwise approach as outlined in the 2020 Focused Updates to the Asthma Management Guidelines. These guidelines include Single Maintenance and Reliever Therapy (SMART) for eligible individuals. Specific drug choices are outlined in Table 142-3.

ADMISSION AND DISCHARGE CRITERIA

ADMISSION CRITERIA

Admission to the hospital is individualized. Factors to consider for hospitalization include:

- Poor response to initial treatment
- Oxygen saturation <92% on room air
- Severe asthma with relapsing course despite prolonged corticosteroid therapy
- Prior emergency visits during current flare
- Concern for nonadherence to prescribed outpatient exacerbation treatment

Admission to an intensive care unit should be considered for patients with:

- Life-threatening or severe asthma that is unresponsive to initial therapy
- Inability to maintain oxygen saturations >90% requiring >40% FiO_2 of supplemental oxygen
- Evidence of hypercarbia and impending respiratory failure
- Inability to provide adequate monitoring outside of an intensive care setting

DISCHARGE CRITERIA

A patient is ready to go home when they are successfully weaned to albuterol treatments every 4 hours. Prior to receiving a treatment, they should be able to breathe comfortably during ambulation or speaking. The Pediatric Dyspnea Scale (PDS) is useful when evaluating patients aged six or older for discharge and may assist with the prediction of relapse, activity limitation, and asthma-related quality of life outcomes 14 days after discharge. Wheezing may persist on examination. A plan of care should include ongoing management of the current acute exacerbation and transition to maintenance therapy. Efforts should be coordinated with the primary care clinician, and, if involved, the asthma specialist.

Prior to discharge, it is important to consider the environment in which the patient will return. Potential triggers (e.g., tobacco smoke exposure, mold, pests) in the environment should be identified and addressed. Community resources (e.g., community health worker, integrated pest management, etc.) should be reviewed and provided to the patient and caregiver.

CONSULTATION

Outpatient referral to an asthma specialist (e.g., pulmonologist, allergist) should be considered for patients with the following scenarios:

- Patient has had a life-threatening asthma exacerbation.
- Patient is not meeting goals of asthma therapy after 3 to 6 months of treatment with earlier referral or consultation appropriate if physician concludes patient is unresponsive to therapy.
- Signs and symptoms are atypical, or there are problems in differential diagnosis.

- Patient requires step 4 care or higher (step 3 for children 0-4 years of age) and consider referral if the patient requires step 3 care (step 2 for children 0-4 years of age)

SPECIAL CONSIDERATIONS

PREVENTION

Educating patients and caregivers about the pathogenesis of asthma, triggers, and medications is crucial to preventing exacerbations and admissions to the hospital. Factors including gastroesophageal reflux, allergic rhinitis, and others that might exacerbate asthma should be explored and treated if possible (**Table 142-7**). For children experiencing symptoms daily, controllable environmental factors such as exposure to allergens and tobacco smoke exposure (includes cigarette and e-cigarette) can contribute to asthma exacerbations. Both tobacco use and tobacco smoke exposure significantly increase the risk of asthma and worsen asthma symptoms. Adolescent patients (11 years and older) and caretakers should be screened for tobacco use, including e-cigarettes. Those who use tobacco should be counseled to quit and provided cessation resources such as the 1-800-QUIT-NOW line. If cessation is not a short-term realistic goal, counseling on home and vehicle bans should be discussed. Additional tobacco cessation resources are available at the CDC and American Academy of Pediatrics.

TABLE 142-7 Factors That Worsen Asthma Severity and Control Measures

Factors That Worsen Asthma Severity	Control Measures
Animal dander	Remove animal from the environment At minimum, remove animal from the bedroom Appropriate medications: Histamine-1 antagonist
House dust mites	Encase mattress and pillows in an allergen-impermeable cover Wash bedding in hot water weekly >130°F Remove carpets from the bedroom
Cockroaches	Exterminate Do not leave garbage and food exposed
Pollens	During pollen season, stay indoors with windows closed, especially in the late afternoon Appropriate medications: Histamine-1 antagonist
Molds	Fix leaks, eliminate water sources Clean moldy surfaces
Adolescent tobacco use, including e-cigarette/vaping	Cessation counseling with motivational interviewing, refer for outpatient follow-up and 1-800-QUIT-NOW and text-based cessation resources (text ditchvape to 88709)
Tobacco smoke exposure (parents and caretakers)	Cessation counseling, prescribe nicotine replacement therapy for those ready to quit, and referral to local resources (1-800-QUIT-NOW)
Sinusitis	Promote sinus drainage Antibiotic therapy when appropriate
Gastroesophageal reflux	No eating 3 hours before bedtime Elevate head of bed 6-8 inches Appropriate medications: Histamine-2 antagonist
Medications	No beta-blockers Avoid aspirin and NSAIDS in patients with severe persistent asthma, nasal polyps, and aspirin sensitivity
Viral infections	Annual influenza vaccination, COVID-19 vaccination
Irritants	Decrease exposure to wood-burning stoves, fireplaces, unvented stores or heaters, perfumes, cleaning agents, sprays

An assessment of adherence to therapy and review of relevant drug delivery systems is important as well. For children with persistent disease on Step 2 or higher therapy, appropriate preventative medications should be maintained daily. These medications are essential for the prevention of asthma flares. Multiple studies have shown a strong negative correlation with asthma admission and daily inhaled corticosteroids or ICS/LABA medications. Suggested doses and regimens have been established in national and worldwide collaborations between pediatricians, allergists, pulmonologists, internists, and others. The 2007 NHLBI Expert Panel Report 3 (EPR3) focused assessment of asthma severity based on two domains: risk and impairment. The risk domain includes frequency and severity of exacerbations and the occurrence of treatment-related adverse effects. The impairment domain is multifactorial and assesses symptoms, SABA use, pulmonary function, and uses validated questionnaires. For each patient, the more severe of these two categories dictates the level of preventive medications a patient requires. A consideration for reduction of controller therapy can be considered after at least 3 months of good control of asthma.

Additional sources of support for caregivers include the Asthma and Allergy Network Mothers of Asthmatics, www.asthmacommunitynetwork.org/, and the Asthma and Allergy Foundation of America, www.aafa.org/.

BIOLOGICAL THERAPIES

As our understanding of the various mechanisms underlying different phenotypes of asthma evolves, several targeted biological therapies for the chronic management of severe asthma have entered the market for various age groups. FDA-approved therapies target various mediators of atopy and inflammation, including IgE (omalizumab, mepolizumab), IL-4 and IL-13 (dupilumab), IL-17 (benralizumab), and, most recently, thymic stromal lymphopoietin (tezepelumab). These agents currently have no role in the management of patients hospitalized for exacerbations and are generally the purview of allergists and asthma specialists. However, hospitalists may care for children on these therapies or be asked by asthma consultants to send laboratory testing to assess for eligibility and appropriateness, as the evidence base is rapidly expanding for their use and differential effectiveness in children with severe persistent asthma (Steps 5 or 6).

KEY POINTS

- Asthma is a chronic disorder that results in airway inflammation and smooth muscle dysfunction and manifests as recurrent episodes of wheezing, breathlessness, and chest tightness.
- Exacerbations can be triggered by a variety of stimuli including respiratory infections, exposure to allergens or irritants, exercise, or cold.
- Treatment of flares must be directed at decreasing airway inflammation and relieving bronchospasm while providing supportive care.
- The mainstay of pharmacologic therapy includes inhaled short-acting β_2-adrenergic agonist therapy and systemic corticosteroids. Supportive care includes supplemental oxygen if needed and maintenance of hydration.
- Many pharmacologic agents have significant side effects and therefore appropriate monitoring is required.
- Patients with severe symptoms or those with moderately severe symptoms that fail to demonstrate improvement on initial therapy are candidates for admission to an intensive care setting.
- At the time of discharge, patients should have a clear plan for ongoing treatment of the acute exacerbation and transition to controller therapy via a stepwise approach. In addition, an asthma action plan for subsequent exacerbations should be in place.
- Asthma disparities in the United States are well documented and multifactorial. Hospitalists must address gaps in the implementation of guideline-consistent care for at-risk populations as they risk perpetuating asthma disparities.

SUGGESTED READINGS

Akinbami LJ, Simon AE, Rossen LM. Changing trends in asthma prevalence among children. *Pediatrics*. 2016;137(1). doi:10.1542/peds.2015-2354.

Akinbami LJ, Moorman JE, Simon AE, Schoendorf KC. Trends in racial disparities for asthma outcomes among children 0 to 17 years, 2001-2010. *J Allergy Clin Immunol*. 2014;134(3):547-553.e5. doi:10.1016/j.jaci.2014.05.037.

Antoon JW, Hall M, Mittal V, et al. Intravenous magnesium and hospital outcomes in children hospitalized with asthma. *Hosp Pediatr*. 2021;11(8):785-793. doi:10.1542/hpeds.2020-004770.

Castro-Rodriguez JA. The Asthma Predictive Index: a very useful tool for predicting asthma in young children. *J Allergy Clin Immunol*. 2010;126(2):212-216. doi:10.1016/j.jaci.2010.06.032.

CDC. Most Recent National Asthma Data. Published May 26, 2022. Accessed August 4, 2022. https://www.cdc.gov/asthma/most_recent_national_asthma_data.htm

Ducharme FM, Chalut D, Plotnick L, et al. The pediatric respiratory assessment measure: a valid clinical score for assessing acute asthma severity from toddlers to teenagers. *J Pediatr*. 2008;152(4):476-480, 480.e1. doi:10.1016/j.jpeds.2007.08.034

Dunn NM, Katial RK, Hoyte FCL. Vocal cord dysfunction: a review. *Asthma Res Pract*. 2015;1:9. doi:10.1186/s40733-015-0009-z

Global Initiative for Asthma - GINA. https://ginasthma.org/gina-reports/

Gopal SH, Mukherjee S, Das SK. Direct and second hand cigarette smoke exposure and development of childhood asthma. *J Environ Health Sci*. 2016;2(6). doi:10.15436/2378-6841.16.1122.

Gorelick MH, Stevens MW, Schultz TR, Scribano PV. Performance of a novel clinical score, the Pediatric Asthma Severity Score (PASS), in the evaluation of acute asthma. *Acad Emerg Med Off J Soc Acad Emerg Med*. 2004;11(1):10–18. doi:10.1197/j.aem.2003.07.015.

Griffiths B, Ducharme FM. Combined inhaled anticholinergics and short-acting beta2-agonists for initial treatment of acute asthma in children. *Cochrane Database Syst Rev*. 2013;(8):CD000060. doi:10.1002/14651858.CD000060.pub2.

Griffiths B, Kew KM. Intravenous magnesium sulfate for treating children with acute asthma in the emergency department. *Cochrane Database Syst Rev*. 2016;(4). doi:10.1002/14651858.CD011050.pub2.

Hsu J, Qin X, Beavers SF, Mirabelli MC. Asthma-related school absenteeism, morbidity, and modifiable factors. *Am J Prev Med*. 2016;51(1):23-32. doi:10.1016/j.amepre.2015.12.012.

Irwin RS, Glomb WB, Chang AB. Habit cough, tic cough, and psychogenic cough in adult and pediatric populations: ACCP evidence-based clinical practice guidelines. *Chest*. 2006;129(1 Suppl):174S-179S. doi:10.1378/chest.129.1_suppl.174S.

Jat KR, Khairwa A. Levalbuterol versus albuterol for acute asthma: a systematic review and meta-analysis. *Pulm Pharmacol Ther*. 2013;26(2):239–248. doi:10.1016/j.pupt.2012.11.003.

Johnston SL, Pattemore PK, Sanderson G, et al. The relationship between upper respiratory infections and hospital admissions for asthma: a time-trend analysis. *Am J Respir Crit Care Med*. 1996;154(3 Pt 1):654-660. doi:10.1164/ajrccm.154.3.8810601.

Keeney GE, Gray MP, Morrison AK, et al. Dexamethasone for acute asthma exacerbations in children: a meta-analysis. *Pediatrics*. 2014;133(3):493-499. doi:10.1542/peds.2013-2273.

Kenyon CC, Fieldston ES, Luan X, Keren R, Zorc JJ. Safety and effectiveness of continuous aerosolized albuterol in the non-intensive care setting. *Pediatrics*. 2014;134(4):e976-982. doi:10.1542/peds.2014-0907.

Khan FI, Reddy RC, Baptist AP. A Pediatric Dyspnea Scale for use in hospitalized patients with asthma. *J Allergy Clin Immunol*. 2009;123(3):660-664. doi:10.1016/j.jaci.2008.12.018.

Kozyrskyj AL, Kendall GE, Jacoby P, Sly PD, Zubrick SR. Association between socioeconomic status and the development of asthma: analyses of income trajectories. *Am J Public Health*. 2010;100(3):540-546. doi:10.2105/AJPH.2008.150771.

NHLBI, NIH. 2020 Focused Updates to the Asthma Management Guidelines. Accessed August 27, 2022. https://www.nhlbi.nih.gov/health-topics/asthma-management-guidelines-2020-updates

NHLBI, NIH. Guidelines for the Diagnosis and Management of Asthma 2007 (EPR-3). Accessed August 27, 2022. https://www.nhlbi.nih.gov/health-topics/guidelines-for-diagnosis-management-of-asthma

Pappas G, Hadden WC, Kozak LJ, Fisher GF. Potentially avoidable hospitalizations: inequalities in rates between US socioeconomic groups. *Am J Public Health*. 1997;87(5):811-816. doi:10.2105/ajph.87.5.811.

Suehs CM, Menzies-Gow A, Price D, et al. Expert consensus on the tapering of oral corticosteroids for the treatment of asthma. A Delphi Study. *Am J Respir Crit Care Med*. 2021;203(7):871-881. doi:10.1164/rccm.202007-2721OC.

Tyler A, Cotter JM, Moss A, et al. Outcomes for pediatric asthmatic inpatients after implementation of an emergency department dexamethasone treatment protocol. *Hosp Pediatr*. 2019;9(2):92-99. doi:10.1542/hpeds.2018-0099.

CHAPTER 143

Aspiration

Valerie Jurgens, MD and Neha H. Shah, MD, MPH

BACKGROUND

The term *aspiration* refers to the entry of foreign material into the lungs. The consequences of aspiration encompass a variety of respiratory syndromes. Many medical conditions can predispose a pediatric patient to aspiration. The aspiration of oropharyngeal secretions or gastric contents may lead to the development of pulmonary symptoms. Accurate and timely diagnosis of an acute or chronic aspiration syndrome in a pediatric patient requires a careful history and physical examination because highly sensitive and specific diagnostic tests are lacking.

When aspiration leads to acute injury to the airways and lung parenchyma, two specific types of aspiration syndromes can be identified: aspiration pneumonitis and aspiration pneumonia. These aspiration syndromes are distinct entities, but considerable overlap exists. Attempts to distinguish between them may be important because the appropriate evaluation, management, treatment, and prevention strategies differ.

Aspiration pneumonitis may occur after gastric contents, which are typically acidic, are inhaled into the lower respiratory tract. Aspiration pneumonitis may also occur due to chemical inhalation or near-drowning. A prompt and intense inflammatory reaction, or pneumonitis, ensues, but bacterial infection is not a significant part of this immediate reaction. *Aspiration pneumonia* occurs after inhalation of oropharyngeal secretions or, less commoly gastric contents, which contain colonizing bacteria, into the lower airways. The infectious process that develops accounts for the clinical features of aspiration pneumonia. Preemptively identifying patients at risk for aspiration can aid in distinguishing between both types of aspiration syndromes.

PATHOPHYSIOLOGY

Even healthy adults and children may aspirate small amounts of oropharyngeal contents during sleep; however, pulmonary host defense mechanisms usually prevent the development of infection and mitigate the inflammatory response. There is a relatively low burden of virulent organisms colonizing the mouth and the naso- and oropharynx in healthy children; thus, aspiration of small amounts of normal flora rarely culminates in a clinically significant pulmonary infection. Additionally, there are protective mechanisms at all levels of the respiratory system; these include the anatomic design of the airway, functional cough reflexes, the mucociliary clearance system, and the innate antibacterial and anti-inflammatory properties of surfactant and airway surface liquid (**Table 143-1**). Impairment of any of these protective barriers places a child at risk for the development of an aspiration syndrome.

TABLE 143-1 Major Airway Defenses Protecting Against Aspiration

Type of Defense	Mechanism
Upper airways	Mechanical trapping of bacteria in nasal passages and larynx, and frequent branching of upper bronchial tree
Mucociliary transport	Prevents most particulate matter in inspired air from reaching lung parenchyma
Cough and gag reflex	Aspiration of large amounts of oropharyngeal material, including flora of the upper respiratory tract, may be prevented by cough and laryngeal reflexes
Humoral and cellular defenses of the upper respiratory tract	Immunoglobulin (primarily IgA), complement, and glycoproteins such as fibronectin in airway secretions prevent colonization of the oropharynx by virulent organisms such as *Streptococcus pneumoniae*, *Pseudomonas aeruginosa*, and *Klebsiella pneumoniae*, which can readily cause lower respiratory tract infection after scant aspiration of oropharyngeal contents
Humoral and cellular defenses of lower respiratory tract	Nonspecific antibacterial activity of surfactant and airway surface fluid Immunoglobulin-mediated opsonization Opsonization or direct lysis by complement activation Phagocytosis and intracellular killing by alveolar macrophages Cell-mediated immunity (effector functions of T lymphocytes) Recruitment of polymorphonuclear leukocytes for phagocytosis and intracellular killing

TABLE 143-2 Risk Factors for Aspiration Syndrome

Anatomic
Tracheoesophageal fistula
Gastrostomy or nasogastric enteral tube
Tracheostomy
Endotracheal tube
Cleft palate or other craniofacial syndrome
Pulmonary
Asthma
Bronchopulmonary dysplasia
Bronchiolitis
Respiratory distress
Impaired Airway Reflexes
Sedation
General anesthesia
Toxic ingestion
Medication
Central Nervous System
Cerebral palsy
Neuromuscular disease
Cerebrovascular accident
Seizure
Intracranial bleed
Head injury
Mass lesions
Miscellaneous
Impaired gastric motility
Swallowing disorder, dysphagia
Poor oral hygiene, gingivitis

The association between gastroesophageal reflux (GER) and the development of chronic respiratory symptoms that may result in an aspiration syndrome is not entirely understood. These disorders coexist, and the influence of GER on respiratory function as well as the influence of respiratory conditions on GER, continues to be explored. Some literature suggests that reflux of gastric contents into the esophagus, as measured by pH probe, is associated with respiratory symptoms in children. Likewise, chronic microaspiration may explain some chronic respiratory symptoms. Many chronic medical conditions are associated with an increased risk of aspiration syndromes (**Table 143-2**).

Although there is clearly a relationship among GER, recurrent aspiration, and respiratory disease, the specific interactions have not been fully elucidated. Nevertheless, acute and chronic respiratory disease related to aspiration accounts for much of the morbidity and mortality in children with impaired gastric motility and swallowing disorders as well as in children with anatomic abnormalities of the aerodigestive tract, including tracheoesophageal fistula.

ASPIRATION PNEUMONITIS

Any condition that depresses a child's level of consciousness and impairs airway reflexes predisposes them to aspiration. This includes drug and alcohol use, sedating medications, paralytic agents, and other anesthetic agents. Loss of airway protective reflexes may also occur in children with medical complexity (CMC), particularly those with central nervous system disorders (see Table 143-2). Infants and children with dysphagia and even respiratory distress are at increased risk of aspiration as well.

Aspiration pneumonitis may occur after a witnessed episode of vomiting in a patient at risk and in such instances, a sudden change in respiratory status is often noted. However, aspiration pneumonitis may also present in a subacute fashion. It may exacerbate a preexisting condition such as cerebral palsy, or it may be a complication of a primary condition such as tachypnea in an infant with bronchiolitis. Aspiration pneumonitis should also be considered when there is a change in the respiratory status of a patient who is at risk for aspiration (**Figure 143-2**).

Chemical injury to the lung may occur as a result of the inhalation of gastric acids, which are usually sterile due to their low pH. Lung damage is related to the acidity of the aspirate, with a more pronounced inflammatory response occurring at lower levels of pH. Additionally, aspirates containing large amounts of particulate food matter increase the inflammatory response. With aspiration of acidic gastric contents, the fluid may be sterile, so bacterial infection is not a significant part of the early process. However, children receiving acid-suppressing or acid-blocking therapy (e.g., antacids, proton pump inhibitors) as well as children fed through gastrostomy or nasogastric tubes, often have an elevated gastric pH which results in bacterial colonization of the stomach.

Aspiration pneumonitis may also occur in children who have ingested hydrocarbons, such as mineral oil (**Figure 143-2**), which can cause severe respiratory compromise. Hydrocarbons are present in many household products such as lighter fluid, furniture polish, paint remover, and motor oil. The inhalation may occur during ingestion or during regurgitation. The risk of aspiration and the severity of the lung injury are related to the viscosity and volatility of the ingested hydrocarbon. Higher-viscosity liquids (e.g., oils) are less volatile and less likely to cause acute injury than lower-viscosity liquids (e.g., furniture polishes), which have greater volatility. In addition to hydrocarbons, aspiration pneumonitis may also be caused by freshwater or salt water in near-drowning victims. Pneumonitis in near-drowning victims occurs primarily by disrupting the alveolocapillary barrier and decreasing pulmonary surfactant activity.

ASPIRATION PNEUMONIA

Aspiration pneumonia is an infectious process that results when the aspirated material has the presence of oral or enteric bacteria. GER may predispose to the development of aspiration pneumonia; however, in a neurologically normal child, intact airway defenses such as the gag and

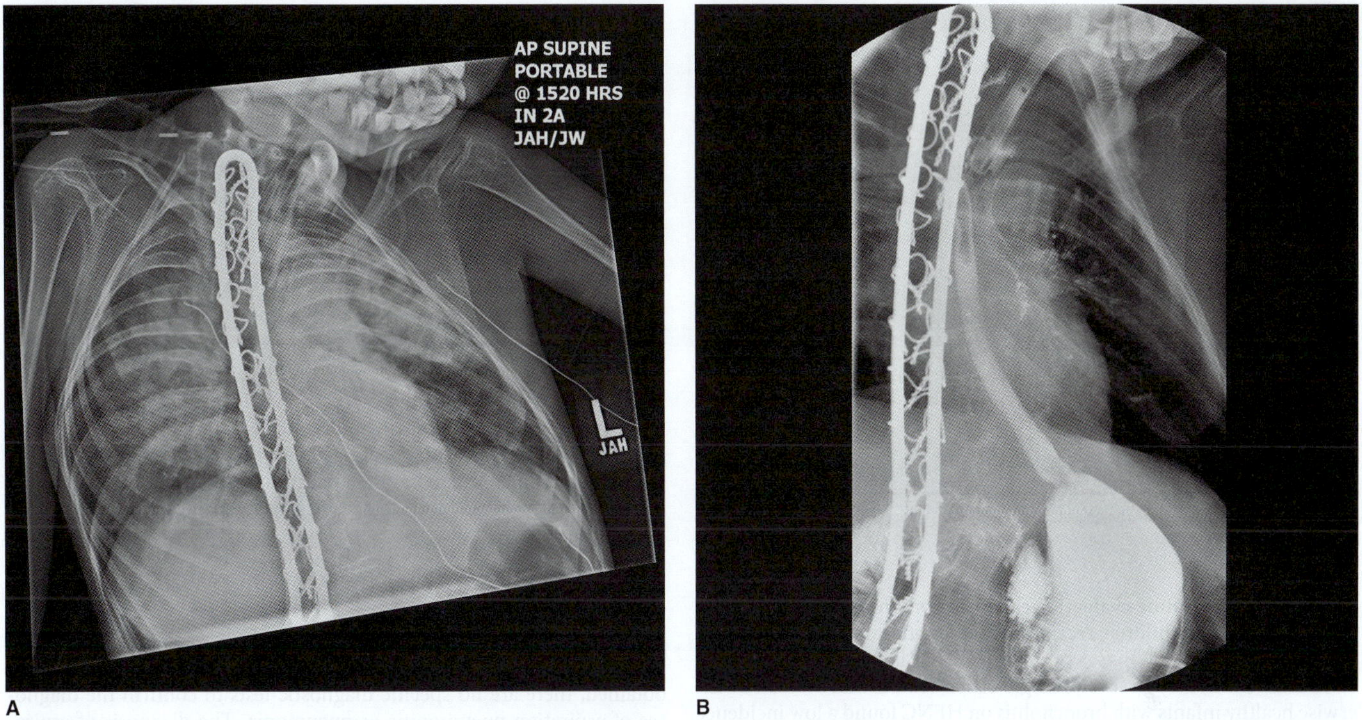

FIGURE 143-1. Acute multifocal pneumonia (A) in a medically complex patient presenting with acute-on-chronic respiratory failure. As part of a comprehensive evaluation, the patient underwent an upper gastrointestinal study via the gastrostomy tube (B), which revealed a recurrent tracheoesophageal fistula in addition to an incompetent fundoplication. (Images used with permission of A. Chidekel, MD.)

cough reflexes usually prevent this complication. Children with medical complexity who are neurologically impaired are at significant risk of aspiration pneumonia, particularly those with dysphagia, poor dental hygiene, and impaired gastric motility. Enteral feeding through gastrostomy and nasogastric tubes also increases the likelihood of aspiration pneumonia. As with aspiration pneumonitis, aspiration pneumonia may also have either an acute or a gradual onset of symptoms.

Critically ill children and children with severe neurologic impairment who are nonambulatory often have multiple factors that predispose to the development of aspiration pneumonia. Endotracheal intubation may also increase the risk of bacterial colonization and transmigration of bacteria from the upper to lower airway. The period immediately following removal of an endotracheal tube is also critical because patients have depressed or impaired protective airway reflexes in the postextubation

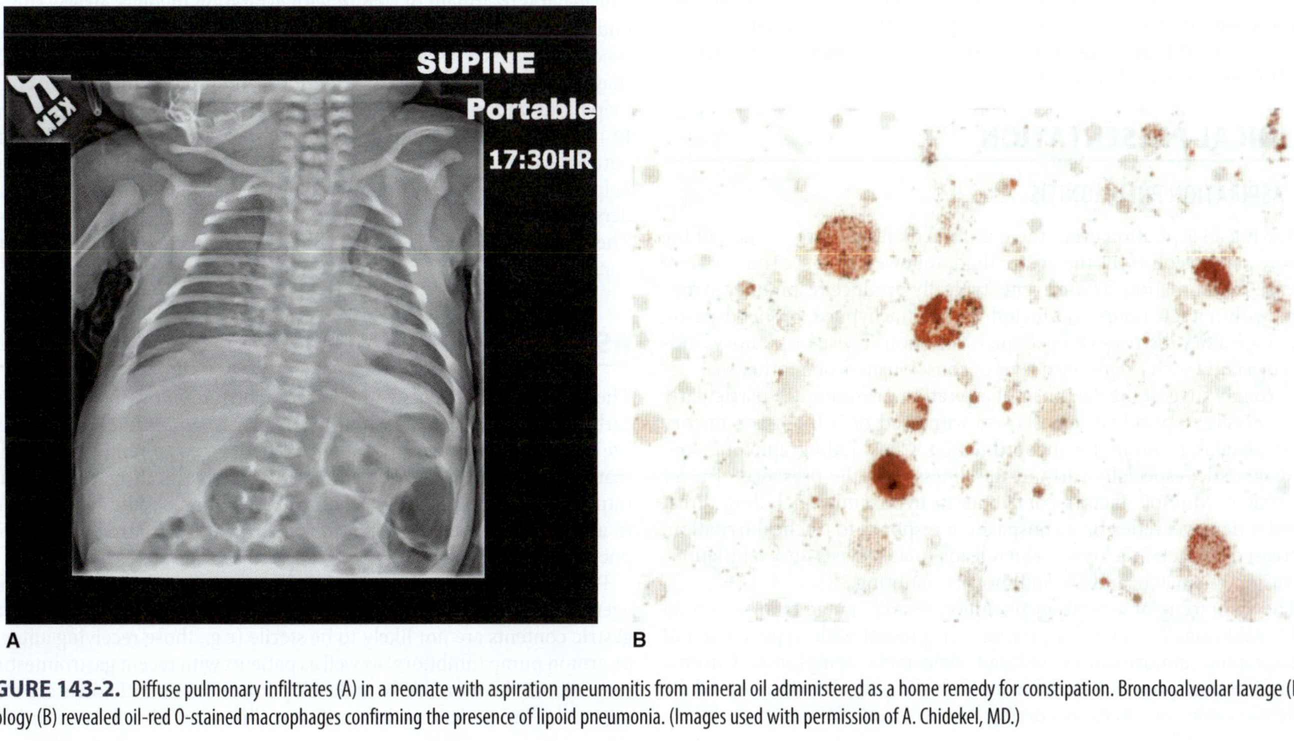

FIGURE 143-2. Diffuse pulmonary infiltrates (A) in a neonate with aspiration pneumonitis from mineral oil administered as a home remedy for constipation. Bronchoalveolar lavage (BAL) cytology (B) revealed oil-red O-stained macrophages confirming the presence of lipoid pneumonia. (Images used with permission of A. Chidekel, MD.)

TABLE 143-3 Organisms Causing Aspiration Pneumonia

Gram-positive
*Streptococcus pneumoniae**
*Staphylococcus aureus**
Alpha-Hemolytic Streptococci
Gram-negative
*Haemophilis influenzae**
Pseudomonas aeruginosa
Acinetobacter species
Escherichia coli
Klebsiella pneumoniae
Anaerobic
Bacteroides species
Peptostreptococcus
Fusobacterium species

*Most common community-acquired pathogens.

period. Recent literature evaluating risk of aspiration related to oral feeding in infants and children receiving nasal continuous positive airway pressure and high flow nasal cannula (HFNC) is insufficient to draw conclusion from, though several single-center studies that evaluated otherwise healthy infants with broncholitis on HFNC found a low incidence of adverse feeding events or aspiration. Gastroparesis and delayed gastric emptying are commonly observed among critically ill patients, including those with burns, significant trauma, and sepsis; all these conditions may increase a child's risk of developing aspiration pneumonia.

Much of the literature regarding the microbiology of aspiration pneumonia is based on adult data from the 1970s and involved transtracheal sampling. These studies observed a predominance of anaerobic pathogens among adults with aspiration pneumonia, which differs from the typical pathogens responsible for community-acquired pneumonia. A similar study conducted in children hospitalized with aspiration pneumonia observed both aerobic and anaerobic species (**Table 143-3**). More recent data, however, suggest that *Streptococcus pneumoniae*, *Haemophilis influenzae*, and *Staphylococcus aureus* account for most cases of aspiration pneumonia. Regardless, at present, the available evidence suggests that anaerobic antibiotic coverage is important in the treatment of children with aspiration pneumonia. Patients residing in long-term care facilities or those with frequent or prolonged hospitalization are at greater risk for colonization with gram-negative organisms; *Pseudomonas aeruginosa* is an etiologic agent in this population.

CLINICAL PRESENTATION

ASPIRATION PNEUMONITIS

Following an aspiration event there is immediate and direct injury of the airway and alveoli from the acidic fluid, followed by a second phase of intense inflammation. These events typically produce respiratory symptoms within a few hours and include cough, tachypnea, bronchospasm, and respiratory distress. Hypoxemia is common. These respiratory findings in a child with a depressed level of consciousness or another risk factor strongly suggest the diagnosis of aspiration pneumonitis, particularly if a preceding episode of emesis was witnessed or if there is a history of dysphagia or oral motor incoordination. Chest radiography may not be diagnostic, especially early in the illness, and the presence of fever is variable. Multiple factors contribute to hypoxemia, including direct alveolar damage; reflex bronchospasm in response to tracheal irritation; decreased surfactant activity, which leads to atelectasis and ventilation-perfusion mismatch; and intrapulmonary shunting.

The symptoms of aspiration pneumonitis may range from severe to mild. Additionally, "silent" aspiration can present with hypoxemia and radiographic abnormalities without detectable symptoms. Chronic aspiration may present in a subacute fashion, with deterioration of the patient's respiratory status occurring over a period of time.

ASPIRATION PNEUMONIA

Aspiration pneumonia may be clinically indistinguishable from community-acquired (nonaspiration) pneumonia; both typically present with fever, cough, and tachypnea, and consolidation may be detected on auscultation or chest radiography. Aspiration pneumonia is one predisposing cause of empyema caused by gram-negative bacteria. When compared to children with community-acquired pneumonia, children with aspiration pneumonis are more likely to have an associated complex chronic condition.

DIFFERENTIAL DIAGNOSIS

Other respiratory processes that overlap clinically with pneumonia, such as bronchiolitis, acute asthma exacerbation (especially with an inciting febrile viral respiratory illness), and bronchospasm unrelated to asthma (e.g., inhaled chemical exposure), should be considered. Aspiration pneumonia is uncommon in otherwise healthy, noncritically ill children without predisposing circumstances (e.g., general anesthesia).

DIAGNOSTIC EVALUATION

The diagnosis of acute aspiration syndromes is established by careful history and physical examination. Although a chest radiograph is often obtained, there are no specific diagnostic tests to confirm the diagnoses of aspiration pneumonitis or pneumonia. The diagnosis of aspiration pneumonia should be considered when a child at risk for aspiration develops new respiratory signs or symptoms especially if it coincides with a witnessed or suspected aspiration episode.

Typical location of aspiration pneumonia varies depending on the patient. In a supine patient, the dependent portions of the lung are the posterior segments of the upper lobes; in an upright patient, the dependent portions are the basal segments of the lower lobes. Other radiographic findings of aspiration pneumonia include abscess formation or cavitations. Radiographic findings are not always present in patients with aspiration pneumonia, and thus, the lack of radiographic findings should not exclude the diagnosis.

MANAGEMENT

The general treatment of a child with aspiration involves airway support and the maintenance of gas exchange. Airway clearance with inhaled medications such as albuterol, chest physiotherapy, or other devices may help open airways, clear secretions, and prompt an effective cough, helping to improve gas exchange and work of breathing. It is important to note that there is limited evidence for airway clearance in pediatric patients but devices such as cough-assist machines may be particularly helpful in children with underlying neurologic or neuromuscular disorders, in whom airway clearance may be impaired at baseline (**Table 143-4**). These supportive therapies should be individualized to the patient's clinical condition and needs.

ASPIRATION PNEUMONITIS

The treatment of patients with aspiration pneumonitis (including hydrocarbon aspiration and drowning) is primarily supportive. Suctioning of the mouth and oropharynx should be performed to remove particulate matter and gastric acid following a witnessed aspiration. Endotracheal intubation and the use of mechanical ventilation should be considered in any child with severe respiratory distress in the setting of aspiration pneumonitis.

Prophylactic antibiotics are generally not indicated in the initial management of a patient with aspiration pneumonitis. Patients in whom the gastric contents are not likely to be sterile (e.g., those receiving antacids or proton pump inhibitors) as well as patients with recent gastrointestinal surgery, may be more likely to develop infection, so antibiotics are often initiated. Any patient with significant illness or who fails to improve

TABLE 143-4 Examples of Commonly Used Airway Clearance Techniques

Manual chest physiotherapy	Chest is clapped and vibrated to loosen secretions. Performed with or without postural drainage.
Mechanical percussion	Pneumatic or electrical devices are used to vibrate the chest to loosen secretions.
High-frequency chest wall oscillation	An inflatable vest is donned by the patient. The vest is inflated and vibrated to loosen secretions.
Vibratory positive expiratory pressure (PEP) therapy	The patient is instructed to exhale against a variable resistor that generates pulsations in the airway to loosen secretions.
Mechanical in-exsufflation (cough-assist)	A device is used to provide pulses of positive pressure to expand the lungs and loosen secretions followed rapidly by pulses of negative pressure to clear secretions from the airway. Most often used in patients with neuromuscular disorders with a mask or mouthpiece.
Intrapulmonary percussive ventilation	A device that provides vibratory pulses of air into the lungs to loosen secretions.

within 48 hours should be placed on antibiotics as recommended for aspiration pneumonia. Obtaining bronchoalveolar lavage samples allows for targeted antibiotic therapy, particularly among patients with significant respiratory distress, other comorbidities, or those who fail to respond to initial therapy. There are insufficient data to recommend the use of corticosteroids in children with aspiration pneumonitis.

ASPIRATION PNEUMONIA

In contrast to the treatment of aspiration pneumonitis, antibiotics are an important component of therapy for children with aspiration pneumonia. Because pathogens are rarely recovered outside the research setting, antibiotic therapy is usually empirical. There is a paucity of prospective literature comparing antibiotic regimens among children with aspiration pneumonia. One randomized controlled trial conducted in 1997 by Jacobson et al found penicillin and clindamycin to be equally effective for the treatment of hospitalized children with aspiration pneumonia. Because studies have identified *S. pneumoniae*, *S. aureus*, and *H. influenzae* as the most common pathogens, ampicillin-sulbactam or a third-generation cephalosporin are reasonable first-line treatment for community-acquired aspiration pneumonia; alternatively, clindamycin can be used. For patients with uncomplicated aspiration pneumonia, the typical treatment duration is 7 to 10 days, although recent evidence has shown no difference in treatment failure for courses less than 7 days. The same study also showed no difference in treatment failure between PO and IV treatment courses.

For patients at increased risk for infection from *Pseudomonas aeruginosa,* gram-negative coverage should be adjusted to include this organism. In this population, piperacillin-tazobactam or cefepime are examples of appropriate choices. Anaerobic coverage is particularly important in children with severe periodontal disease, in children with neurologic impairment, and in those with evidence of lung abscess or necrotizing pneumonia on chest radiograph. In these cases, if a third-generation cephalosporin is used, the addition of clindamycin or metronidazole is recommended. Systemic corticosteroids are not indicated for aspiration pneumonia.

ADMISSION CRITERIA

- Hypoxia
- Moderate to severe respiratory distress or airway instability
- Failure of outpatient management strategies (e.g., inability to tolerate oral antibiotics, or need for increased respiratory support in CMC who are already on home airway clearance plans, oxygen, noninvasive positive pressure ventilation [NIPPV], or ventilation.)
- Dehydration with inadequate or unsafe nutritional strategy

DISCHARGE CRITERIA

- Respiratory stability
- Ability to complete the required therapeutic regimens
- Optimization of airway defenses, with careful attention to airway maintenance and clearance
- Safe and adequate nutritional plan

CONSULTATION

When the clinical picture is uncertain or a significant underlying disorder is contributing to an acute or chronic aspiration syndrome, subspecialty consultation should be considered. Acutely, pulmonology consultation may provide guidance for airway care in a patient with impaired airway clearance as well as bronchoscopy if the diagnosis is unclear. Infectious disease input may be required to tailor antimicrobial therapy. Finally, a child with medical complexity may have other acute and chronic conditions that are exacerbated by an acute illness due to aspiration pneumonia. They may require a multidisciplinary approach to manage worsening of chronic conditions, such as status epilepticus in a child with epilepsy.

PREVENTION

Because aspiration syndromes most often occur in patients with temporary or chronic impairment of airway protection, swallowing difficulties, gastrointestinal dysmotility, or altered gastric acidification, a targeted approach should be utilized. Optimizing the safe delivery of nutrition and airway clearance should be major clinical goals. Speech and occupational therapy can help to evaluate and identify children at risk of aspiration. For example, in children who can cooperate, a modified barium swallow study, a type of videofluoroscopic evaluation, can be used to visualize swallowed material through the upper aerodigestive tract. This study can help to identify children at risk of aspiration syndromes and allow for an alternative therapeutic feeding and treatment plan. In children with neurologic impairment and dysphagia who already have a gastrostomy tube in place, a Nissen fundoplication or transition to gastrojejunostomy tube feeding may be considered. Additionally, aspiration precautions, such as appropriate nil per os (NPO) status, should be in place for children undergoing sedation, general anesthesia, and removal of an endotracheal tube.

KEY POINTS

- Aspiration syndromes represent distinct but difficult to differentiate pulmonary disorders; they include aspiration pneumonitis and aspiration pneumonia.
- Aspiration pneumonitis is a sterile inflammatory process that most commonly follows inhalation of gastric contents.
- Aspiration pneumonia is a bacterial process that most commonly follows inhalation of infectious oropharyngeal secretions.
- The diagnosis of aspiration syndrome is generally clinical, though radiographs may show an infiltrate consistent with pneumonia.
- Treatment is supportive, but antibiotics play a key role in the management of aspiration pneumonia.
- Optimizing airway defenses, careful attention to airway maintenance and clearance, and a safe nutritional strategy may help prevent this condition in susceptible patients.
- There is a significant need for more sensitive and specific methods of diagnosing pulmonary aspiration. Similarly, evidence-based evaluation of supportive measures, such as inhaled medications and airway clearance devices for patients with chronic aspiration, is lacking.

SUGGESTED READINGS

Bierens JJ, Lunetta P, Tipton M, Warner DS. Physiology of drowning: a review. *Physiology*. 2016;31(2):147-166.

Canning A, Clarke S, Thorning S, Chauhan M, Weir KA. Oral feeding for infants and children receiving nasal continuous positive airway pressure and high flow nasal cannula: a systematic review. *BMC Pediatrics*. 2021;21:83.

Conway TP, Halaby C, Akerman M, Asuncion A. The use of high flow nasal cannula and the timing of safe feeding in children with bronchiolitis. *Cureus*. 2021;13(6):e15665.

Healy F, Panitch HB. Pulmonary complications of pediatric neurological diseases. *Pediatr Ann*. 2010;39:216-224.

Hirsch AW, Monuteaux MC, Fruchtman G, Bachur RG, Neuman MI. Characteristics of children hospitalized with aspiration pneumonia. *Hosp Pediatr*. 2016;6(11):659-666.

Jacobson SJ, Griffiths K, Diamond S, et al. A randomized controlled trial of penicillin vs clindamycin for the treatment of aspiration pneumonia in children. *Arch Pediatr Adolesc Med*. 1997;151:701-704.

Martin-Harris B, Canon CL, Bonilha HS, Murray J, Davidson K, Lefton-Greif MA. Best practices in modified barium swallow studies. *Am J Speech Lang Pathol*. 2020;29(2S):1078-1093.

Pavithran J, Puthiyottil IV, Narayan M, Vidhyadharan S, Menon JR, Iyer S. Observations from a pediatric dysphagia clinic: Characteristics of children at risk of aspiration pneumonia. *Laryngoscope*. 2019; 129 (11):2614-2618.11.

Simons JP, Rubinstein EN, Mandell DL. Clinical predictors of aspiration on radionuclide salivagrams in children. *Arch Otolaryngol Head Neck Surg*. 2008;134:941-944.

Slain KN, Martinez-Schlurmann N, Stormorken A. Nutrition and high flow nasal cannula respiratory support in children with bronchiolitis. *Hospital Pediatrics*. 2017;7(5):256-262.

Sochet A, McGee J, October T. Oral nutrition in children with bronchiolitis on high flow nasal cannula is well tolerated. *Hospital Pediatrics*. 2017;7(5):249-255.

Stone B, Hester G, Jackson D, et al. Effectiveness of fundoplication or gastrojejunal feeding in children with neurologic impairment. *Hosp Pediatr*. 2017;7(3):140-148.

Streck HL, Goldman JL, Lee BR, Sheets JM, Wirtz AL. Evaluation of the treatment of aspiration pneumonia in hospitalized children. *J Pediatric Infect Dis Soc*. 2022;11(3):102-107.

Thomson J, Hall M, Ambroggio L, et al. Antibiotics for aspiration pneumonia in neurologically impaired children. *J Hosp Med*. 2020;15(7):395-402.

Weir KA, McMahon S, Taylor S, Chang AB. Oropharyngeal aspiration and silent aspiration in children. *Chest*. 2011;140:589-597.

CHAPTER 144 Bronchopulmonary Dysplasia and Chronic Lung Disease of Infancy

Rebecca Steuart, MD, MS and Jennifer Henningfeld, MD

BACKGROUND

Bronchopulmonary dysplasia (BPD) is a chronic lung disorder that affects newborns born prematurely and results in chronic respiratory insufficiency often necessitating treatment with long-term supplemental oxygen therapy. It is one of the most common sequelae of preterm birth. BPD is caused by a combination of disrupted neonatal alveolar development and postnatal alveolar injury. BPD is manifested predominantly by chronic respiratory insufficiency secondary to alveolar simplification and abnormally developed pulmonary vasculature. In contrast, chronic lung disease of infancy (CLDI) is a broader term that includes various chronic conditions seen in both preterm and full-term infants that lead to chronic respiratory insufficiency, such as pulmonary hypoplasia, congenital diaphragmatic hernia, and persistent pulmonary hypertension of the newborn (**Figure 144-1**).

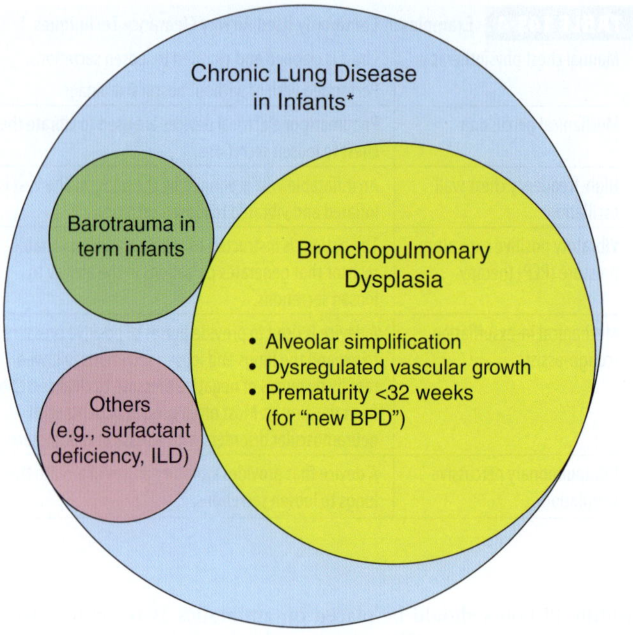

FIGURE 144-1. Framework for Disease Terminology. *Interchangeable with the term chronic lung disease of infancy (CLDI). After infancy, children with ongoing disease are re-categorized as the broader chronic lung disease (CLD). The term chronic lung disease of prematurity (CLDP) is sometimes used interchangeably with BPD. Abbreviations: BPD, bronchopulmonary dysplasia; ILD, interstitial lung disease.

Despite the differences between these disease entities, both BPD and the broader CLDI have the common clinical presentation of requiring chronic respiratory support, such as supplemental oxygen or mechanical ventilation, during and after the neonatal period to support growth and development. After the neonatal period, children with BPD and CLDI typically have persistent respiratory symptoms, recurrent respiratory illness especially due to RSV and other viruses, respiratory fragility during illness, and in most cases, the long-term need for respiratory support which often continues into early childhood. Although there is no discrete medical cure for BPD or CLDI, both diseases are generally anticipated to improve with time and lung growth. **The focus of this chapter is on BPD; however, due to the overlap in terminology, much of this information is also applicable to CLDI.**

Most children with BPD have multisystem disease and are predisposed to adverse neurodevelopmental, cardiovascular, and growth outcomes which may not present until after the neonatal period. These nonrespiratory comorbidities can complicate respiratory management and affect lung development and healing. Thus, this population can have substantial hospital and resource use and high medical costs. The pediatric hospitalist can expect to encounter infants and children with BPD and CLDI and will be called on to address the problems unique to this complex group of children. The hospitalist's detailed and thoughtful evaluation, proactive medical management, and collaborative care with the infant's multidisciplinary medical team and caregivers are imperative to ensuring excellent care and outcomes.

CLINICAL PRESENTATION

In practice, BPD is most simply defined by chronic respiratory insufficiency with an ongoing requirement of supplemental oxygen and/or mechanical ventilation persisting either at 28 days postnatal age or 36 weeks postmenstrual age; this broad definition is most consistent with the original definitions of BPD. Some experts would add a requirement for clinical and radiographic evidence of parenchymal lung disease to this chronic hypoxemia. Regardless, BPD is identified during the birth hospitalization and would be diagnosed prior to neonatal intensive care unit (NICU) discharge.

DIAGNOSTIC CRITERIA

Various definitions of BPD and grading/severity scales have been used over the last 50 years to categorize the disease manifestations and predict clinical outcomes. Definitions differ due to their individual clinical and research goals and each has its own recognized limitations. The *Eunice Kennedy Shriver* National Institute of Child Health and Human Development (NICHD) 2001 Diagnostic Criteria of Mild, Moderate, and Severe BPD (**Table 144-1**) are descriptive and thus useful for incidence and prevalence studies, but these criteria have poor association with long-term respiratory outcomes.

The more recent 2019 NICHD Diagnostic Criteria were developed with the goal of improving predictive outcomes through about 2 years of age (**Table 144-2**). This simplified definition is based only on the *mode* of respiratory support required at 36 weeks postmenstrual age, regardless of supplemental oxygen use. It more accurately identifies the highest-risk infants as those with BPD grade III. Note that with these updated 2019 criteria, infants breathing room air at 36 weeks postmenstrual age do not meet criteria for BPD.

While the newer diagnostic criteria are superior in simplicity and prediction of clinical outcomes, both the 2001 and 2019 definitions may be used in clinical practice, among other less common definitions. The hospitalist is encouraged to work within the local clinical context and use the nomenclature common to specialty groups treating this population to ensure the most consistent communication. As research advances in the study of BPD pathophysiology, the diagnostic criteria may move toward a more pathophysiologic approach.

TABLE 144-1 2001 NICHD Diagnostic Criteria for BPD

	Gestational Age	
	<32 weeks	≥32 weeks
Time point of assessment	36 weeks PMA or discharge to home, whichever comes first	>28 days but <56 days postnatal age or discharge to home, whichever comes first
	Treatment with oxygen >21% for at least 28 days ***plus***	
Mild BPD	Breathing room air at 36 weeks PMA or discharge, whichever comes first	Breathing room air by 56 days postnatal age or discharge, whichever comes first
Moderate BPD	Need* for <30% oxygen at 36 weeks PMA or discharge, whichever comes first	Need* for <30% oxygen at 56 days postnatal age or discharge, whichever comes first
Severe BPD	Need* for ≥30% oxygen and/or positive pressure (PPV or nCPAP) at 36 weeks PMA or discharge, whichever comes first	Need* for ≥30% oxygen and/or positive pressure (PPV or nCPAP) at 56 days postnatal age or discharge, whichever comes first

BPD: bronchopulmonary dysplasia; L/min: liters per minute of oxygen flow; nCPAP: nasal continuous positive airway pressure; NICHD: *Eunice Kennedy Shriver* National Institute of Child Health and Human Development; NIPPV: noninvasive positive pressure ventilation; PMA: postmenstrual age; PPV: positive pressure ventilation including full mechanical ventilation.

*Persistence of clinical features of respiratory disease (tachypnea, retractions, rales) are considered common to the broad description of BPD and have not been included in the diagnostic criteria describing the severity of BPD. Infants treated with oxygen >21% and/or positive pressure for nonrespiratory disease (e.g., central apnea or diaphragmatic paralysis) do not have BPD unless they also develop parenchymal lung disease and exhibit clinical features of respiratory distress. A day of treatment with oxygen >21% means that the infant received oxygen >21% for more than 12 hours on that day. Treatment with oxygen >21% and/or positive pressure at 36 weeks PMA, or at 56 days postnatal age or discharge, should not reflect an "acute" event, but should rather reflect the infant's usual daily therapy for several days preceding and following 36 weeks PMA, 56 days postnatal age, or discharge.

TABLE 144-2 2019 NICHD Diagnostic Criteria for BPD

BPD Disease Grade	Mode of Respiratory Support at 36 weeks PMA
I (mild)	Nasal cannula flow of 0.1-2 L/min
II (moderate)	Nasal cannula flow of >2 L/min or nCPAP or NIPPV
III (severe)	Invasive PPV

BPD: bronchopulmonary dysplasia, L/min: liters per minute of oxygen flow; nCPAP: nasal continuous positive airway pressure; NICHD: *Eunice Kennedy Shriver* National Institute of Child Health and Human Development; NIPPV: noninvasive positive pressure ventilation; PMA: postmenstrual age; PPV: positive pressure ventilation including full mechanical ventilation.

EPIDEMIOLOGY: INCIDENCE AND PREVALENCE

Depending on the definition used, as many as 48,000 infants annually develop BPD in the United States, with 10,000 of those infants having severe BPD. Additionally, an estimated 12,000 infants are discharged with home supplemental oxygen. In total, approximately 2,000 children with severe BPD use home ventilation in the United States. The prevalence of BPD is likely increasing, due in part to the increased survival of prematurely born infants.

BPD is a disease predominantly affecting extremely preterm and/or low birthweight infants. The incidence rate and severity are inversely related to gestational age and birthweight, as shown in **Table 144-3**. Infants with gestational age ≤28 weeks have an approximately 40% incidence of BPD grades I or II and a 4% incidence of BPD grade III. Among those with BPD, 97% have birthweight <1250 g.

PATHOPHYSIOLOGY

Pathology Fetal lung development proceeds through multiple stages starting at 3 weeks gestation (**Table 144-4**). By the time of fetal viability (Saccular Stage, 26-36 weeks), the fetal lung has begun developing alveolar saccules and preparing to produce surfactant. True alveoli begin developing around 36 weeks gestational age (alveolar stage). Postnatally, alveolarization and alveolar septation continue until around 6 to 8 years of age, and the larger airways will continue to increase in diameter through adolescence.

The physiology resulting in the development of BPD is multifactorial; a major contributing factor is the stage of fetal lung development at the time of birth. Delivery during the late Canalicular or Saccular Stages of lung development leads to physiological alterations in lung mechanics (increased compliance), structural immaturity of the airways, surfactant deficiency, atelectasis, and pulmonary edema. Postnatally, the lungs then experience ventilator-induced barotrauma and

TABLE 144-3 Incidence of BPD by Gestational Age

Gestational Age	Grade I or II BPD	Grade III BPD
22 weeks	70.4%	20.3%
23 weeks	73.6%	18.1%
24 weeks	68.5%	16.8%
25 weeks	65.8%	9.7%
26 weeks	55.6%	7.5%
27 weeks	45.1%	5.6%
28 weeks	36.2%	2.4%
29 weeks	--	0.8%

Incidence seen among surviving infants; mortality rates are inversely proportional to gestational age.

Source: Jensen EA, Edwards EM, Greenberg LT, et al. Severity of bronchopulmonary dysplasia among very preterm infants in the United States. *Pediatrics*. 2021;148(1):e2020030007; and Bell EF, Hintz SR, Hansen NI, et al. Mortality, in-hospital morbidity, care practices, and 2-year outcomes for extremely preterm infants in the US, 2013-2018. *JAMA*. 2022;327(3):248–263.

TABLE 144-4 Stages of Fetal Lung Development

	Embryonic Stage	Pseudoglandular Stage	Canalicular Stage	Saccular Stage	Alveolar Stage
Gestational Age	3-6 weeks	6-16 weeks	16-26 weeks	26-36 weeks	36 weeks to lung maturity
Developing Structures	Lung buds, Trachea, Large bronchi, Separation of trachea and esophagus	Subsegmental bronchi, Bronchioles, Mucous glands, Cartilage, Smooth muscle	Bronchioles, Acinus, Vascularization, Type I and II cell differentiation	Alveoli dilate and subdivide, Surface area grows, Surfactant begins	Mature alveolarization, Mature alveolar capillary network, Mature surfactant

Source: Adapted from Wilmott RW, Boat TF, Bush A, et al, eds. *Kendig and Chernick's Disorders of the Respiratory Tract in Children*. 8th ed. Philadelphia, PA: Elsevier Saunders; 2012.

oxygen toxicity, side effects of mechanical ventilation and oxygen support necessary to overcome the disrupted alveolar-capillary barrier, and interstitial and alveolar edema. Pulmonary edema can be exacerbated by the presence of a persistent ductus arteriosus leading to pulmonary overcirculation. Additionally, the severe lung inflammation results in increased fibroblast activity and collagen production. As a result, instead of developing new healthy lung tissue, the premature lungs experience progressive lung injury from the lifesaving measures used as respiratory support.

While the structure of the large and small airways of an infant with BPD can be abnormal, the primary pathology is in the distal airways and parenchyma. There are also changes in the pulmonary vascular development that directly impact gas exchange, morbidity, and mortality. Histologically, BPD has the following pathologic characteristics (**Figure 144-2**):

- Airway:
  - Hypoplastic and simplified alveoli from decreased septation reducing the surface area available for gas exchange
  - Larger airways with weaker cartilaginous structures leading to tracheomalacia or bronchomalacia
- Parenchyma:
  - Interstitial fibrosis (increased elastic tissue and thickening of the interstitium)

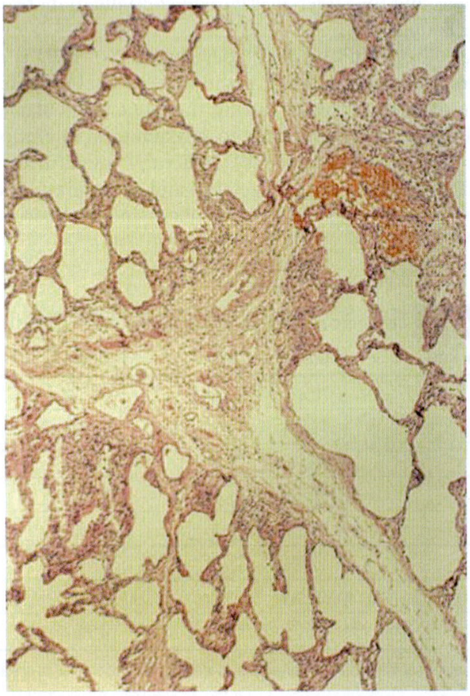

FIGURE 144-2. Lung pathology from an infant with severe BPD and intractable respiratory failure, demonstrating overdistented and simplified alveoli, interstitial scarring, and both interstitial and interlobular inflammation.

- Vasculature:
  - Capillary bed with abnormal morphology, distribution, and decreased density
  - Pulmonary arteries and arterioles develop smooth muscle cell hypertrophy contributing to pulmonary hypertension

CLASSIC BPD VERSUS NEW BPD

The invention of exogenous surfactant changed the physiology and clinical picture of BPD dramatically, prompting a differentiation between the pre-surfactant lung disease ("classic BPD") and the post-surfactant era BPD ("new BPD"). Preterm infants have transient surfactant dysfunction or deficiency, limiting the ability to actively or passively inflate the alveolar units resulting in atelectasis and difficulty with gas exchange. Delivery of exogenous surfactant improves lung volumes and compliance.

Originally termed the more pathologically descriptive "hyaline membrane disease," BPD was first defined by Northway et al in 1967 describing preterm infants suffering the adverse effects of aggressive mechanical ventilation and oxygen therapy needed to manage surfactant deficiency and respiratory distress syndrome. This "classic BPD" occurred primarily in relatively mature infants with an average birth weight of nearly 2 kg and a gestational age of 32 weeks. Classic BPD had a specific pattern of lung injury observed after barotrauma, toxic hyperoxygenation, and the resulting chronic inflammatory changes (**Table 144-5**). This entity had >50% neonatal mortality rate and survivors had a prolonged healing phase. With improvements in prenatal care, the availability of exogenous surfactant, newer ventilator technology, and recognition of the harmful effects of aggressive oxygenation, very few mature infants of greater than 30 weeks gestation now develop classic BPD.

Concurrent with a decline in incidence of classic BPD, increasing numbers of infants born at less than 28 weeks gestation began surviving and developing a new form of BPD. In these extremely premature infants, respiratory failure occurs at birth due to both surfactant deficiency and severe lung immaturity with unformed alveoli and peripheral airways. The oxygen therapy and mechanical ventilation necessary for survival in this "new BPD" premature population cause alveolar growth arrest, resulting in pulmonary hypoplasia, peripheral airway damage, and chronic inflammation.

Each form of BPD has distinct radiographic findings, as shown in **Table 144-5**.

Risk Factors BPD occurs primarily in premature infants. However, any neonate requiring prolonged respiratory support, such as with sepsis, congenital diaphragmatic hernia, or persistent pulmonary hypertension of the newborn, is at risk for BPD.

The risk of an infant developing BPD is related to prenatal environment, infant specific risk factors, and postnatal management strategies. Prenatally, maternal variables such as chorioamnionitis, fetal growth restriction, receipt of maternal antenatal steroids and maternal smoking are important risk factors. Infant-specific factors include gender, race, genetic predilection, nutritional status, pulmonary hypoplasia, patent ductus arteriosus, pulmonary hypertension, and neonatal sepsis. Postnatal lung injury can also occur from ventilation-induced trauma, oxygen toxicity, and inflammation or scarring secondary to critical respiratory illness. These factors often result in significantly different clinical courses and outcomes in infants despite apparently similar NICU care.

TABLE 144-5 Features of Classic BPD Versus New BPD

"Classic BPD"	"New BPD"
"Classic BPD" 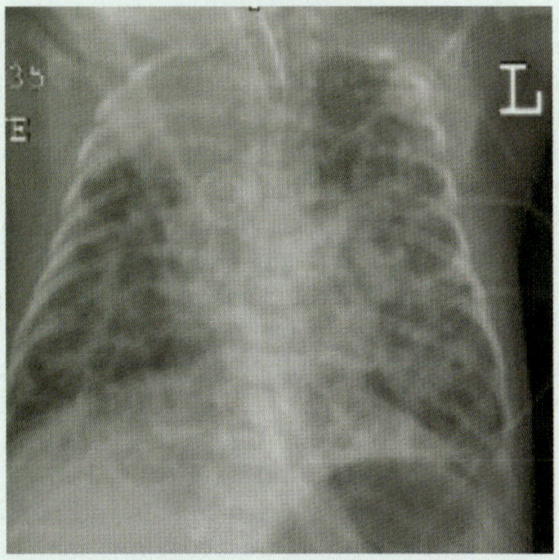	"New BPD" 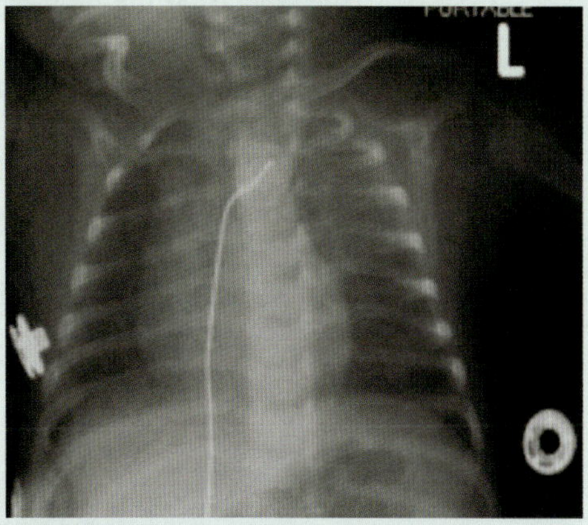
Radiography demonstrates diffuse groundglass opacification, coarse interstitial markings, and cystic changes	Radiography demonstrates diffusely hazy lung fields in a homogeneous pattern
Pre-Surfactant Era	Post-Surfactant Era
Average 32 weeks gestation Surfactant deficiency with atelectasis Hyperoxygenation injury Ventilation leads to severe inflammation and alveolar scarring	Majority ≤ 29 weeks gestation Severe lung immaturity - Unformed alveoli - Immature pulmonary vasculature Ventilation leads to alveolar growth arrest and peripheral airway damage
Alternating areas of atelectasis and hyperinflation Decreased alveolarization, low surface area Airway epithelial hyperplasia Airway smooth muscle hyperplasia, severe Diffuse fibroproliferation Pulmonary artery hypertensive remodeling	Less regional heterogeneity and patchiness Fewer, larger, and simplified alveoli Rare airway epithelial lesions Mild airway smooth muscle thickening Fewer pulmonary arteries Dysmorphic pulmonary arteries

Source: Adapted from Wilmott RW, Boat TF, Bush A, et al, eds. *Kendig and Chernick's Disorders of the Respiratory Tract in Children*. 8th ed. Philadelphia, PA: Elsevier Saunders; 2012.

CLINICAL FEATURES

PHYSICAL EXAM

The respiratory examination is variable among infants and children with BPD or CLDI and can even vary within the same child at different time points. Vital signs will demonstrate tachypnea and hypoxia on room air (see "**Persistent hypoxemia**" below). The physical examination will demonstrate mild to severe retractions at baseline; auscultation findings may include scattered crackles (from pulmonary edema, if present), diminished aeration (from atelectasis), and/or intermittent expiratory wheezing (from tracheobronchomalacia, overt bronchoconstriction, mucous retention, or airway narrowing due to scar formation).

IMAGING

Chest imaging in children with BPD will evolve throughout their lifespan and eventually improves with growth. Findings that can be seen on radiography can include atelectasis, pulmonary edema, low or normal lung volumes, and areas of air trapping (**Figure 144-3**). In severe cases there can be significant hyperinflation. The image can evolve over time to include cystic lesions and fibrosis.

LAB VALUES

No laboratory marker or value is independently associated with BPD diagnosis. However, infants and children with BPD often have the following changes on laboratory evaluation:

- Hypoxemia (see below "**Persistent hypoxemia**")
- Hypercapnea (see below "**Hypercapnia and chronic hypoventilation**")
- Electrolyte derangements, including hyponatremia, hypokalemia, hypocalcemia (see below "**Electrolyte abnormalities**")

DISEASE MANIFESTATIONS AND MANAGEMENT

Persistent Hypoxemia Hypoxia in BPD is caused by ventilation-perfusion mismatch secondary to alveolar simplification and lung scarring, resulting in areas of hyperinflation and atelectasis (**Figure 144-3**). The ongoing ventilation-perfusion mismatch results in continuous or intermittent hypoxemia. The American Thoracic Society defines hypoxemia in children ages 1 year old and older as:

- Spo_2 ≤ 93% for at least 5% of recorded continuous pulse oximetry readings, or
- At least three separate recordings of Spo_2 ≤ 93% obtained intermittently when measured near sea level.

In the NICU, maintaining oxygen saturations above 95% has not been shown to confer any advantage over targeting oxygen saturations of 91% to 94%; rather, this may simply prolong the duration of oxygen therapy. Targeting saturations below 90% reduces the rate of retinopathy of prematurity and BPD, but has an increased rate of death. These saturation goals are extrapolated to older infants with established BPD. Oxygen saturations should be measured both daytime and nighttime because nocturnal desaturation is frequent and may correlate poorly with daytime desaturation.

Persistent hypoxemia places children at risk for deleterious pulmonary circulation, neurodevelopmental, sleep, and growth outcomes, which limited evidence suggests improves with chronic supplemental oxygen therapy. Hypoxemia may also be associated with hypoxemic bronchoconstriction and sudden death. This hypoxemia is expected to persist for 6 months to 3 years of life (median 10.5 months), as it slowly

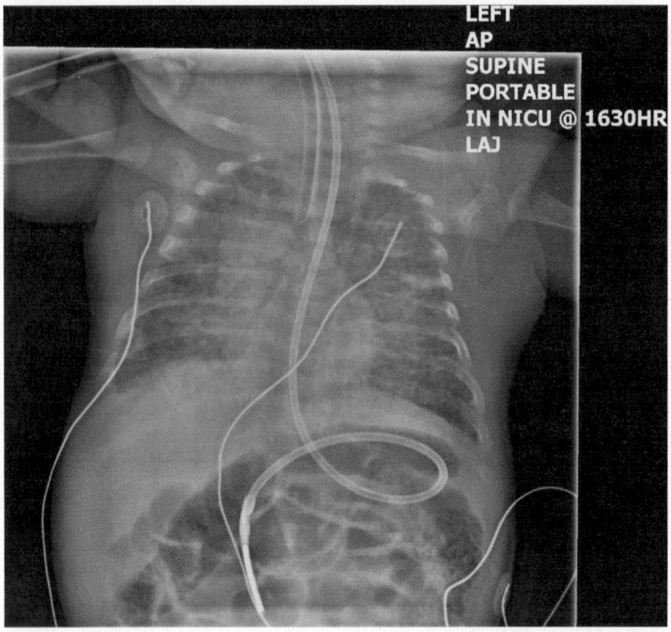

A

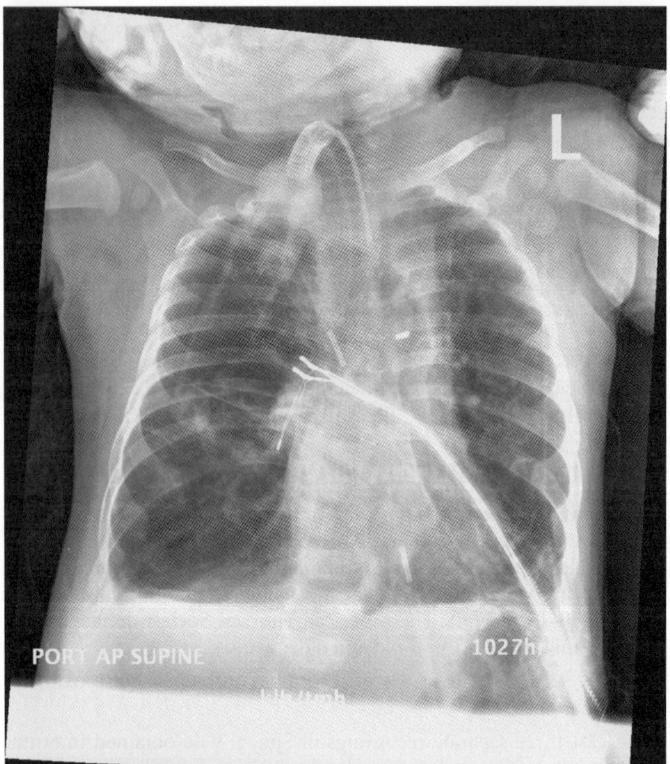

B

FIGURE 144-3. Chest radiographs from infants with established, severe BPD. (A) Intubated infant with coarse interstitial markings, and areas of overinflation and atelectasis. (B) Tracheostomy-dependent child with severe diffuse overinflation and cystic changes.

improves with lung growth, healing, and remodeling. Therefore, in 2019 the American Thoracic Society issued a strong recommendation for the administration of long-term, home oxygen therapy to treat chronic hypoxemia in children with BPD who are otherwise ready for hospital discharge, a recommendation which reaffirmed chronic oxygen as the mainstay of treatment.

In addition to supplemental oxygen, respiratory support with non-invasive or invasive positive pressure or ventilation may be indicated. Early exogenous surfactant therapy as a treatment for respiratory distress syndrome has the effect of reducing mechanical ventilation and oxygen required, both of which are risk factors for future development of BPD.

Hypercapnia and Chronic Hypoventilation In addition to chronic hypoxemia, infants with BPD may have chronic respiratory insufficiency with mild respiratory acidosis and hypercapnia related to the alveolar simplification and an inability to maintain sufficient alveolar ventilation to achieve normal carbon dioxide levels. With lung growth and reparative alveolar maturation, carbon dioxide levels do eventually return to normal; until that occurs any additional stress or insult can result in overt respiratory failure characterized by an acute increase in CO_2 above the patient's chronic hypercapnia and worsening respiratory acidosis. When mechanical ventilation is required, the ventilation strategy of "permissive hypercapnia," effectively limiting tidal volume by allowing pCO_2 to rise to 55 to 65 mm Hg, has been shown to reduce barotrauma and subsequent incidence and severity of BPD.

In the most severely affected infants with BPD, long-term invasive mechanical ventilation (via tracheostomy) may be required to achieve adequate growth. The decision to initiate long-term invasive ventilation is individualized, based on the infant's clinical status, comorbidities such as bronchomalacia or persistent pulmonary hypertension, and social situation; tracheostomy is most often considered in those with refractory respiratory failure, failure to thrive, or extreme cardiorespiratory instability. For infants with severe BPD or CLDI, chronic mechanical ventilation can provide stability, reduce acute respiratory events, reduce work of breathing and energy expenditure, and allow a path to discharge home. With comfortable, adequate ventilation, these infants have improved growth, toleration of therapies, and neurodevelopmental outcomes.

For those infants expected to require chronic, home mechanical ventilation, the shift in ventilation strategies from acute to chronic management is undertaken, which focuses on oversupporting the lungs to allow for better growth. For severe BPD, the ventilation strategy of "permissive hypercapnia" (limiting tidal volume and allowing pCO_2 to rise to 55-65 mm Hg) may be indicated beyond the NICU period. Diuretics, inhaled steroid therapy, and bronchodilators are also frequently used.

Airway Hyperreactivity and Obstructive Disease Wheezing presentations are one of the most common causes of unplanned hospital admission in the first years following NICU discharge. Although all children with history of preterm birth or low-birthweight are at risk of childhood wheezing, older infants and young children with BPD have increased risk for persistent, nonspecific airway hyperreactivity. Most infants with BPD are thought to have residual, chronic lung inflammation, and subsequent hyperreactivity at baseline. In the presence of an airway irritant such as a respiratory virus, tobacco smoke, or allergenic exposure, the inflamed airways may easily react, resulting in episodic bronchospasm and wheezing on auscultation. This airway hyperreactivity and resulting obstructive lung disease may develop or persist into late childhood or even early adulthood. Unlike the alveolar, hypoxemic manifestation of BPD disease, obstructive lung disease is less likely to resolve with time, lung growth, and alveolarization.

It is not clear how the diagnoses of childhood asthma and post-BPD obstructive lung disease overlap, intersect, or influence one another; however, the severity of hypoxemia in a child's BPD does not consistently correlate with the severity of wheezing and obstructive lung disease; indeed, it is possible that some children grow to be misdiagnosed/concurrently diagnosed as complicated asthma in future years. The consequences of airway hyperreactivity in BPD also include exercise and therapy intolerance, prolonged lung healing, and poor growth.

The differential diagnosis of wheezing in an infant with BPD is like that of any infant with chronic wheezing, including asthma, tracheobronchomalacia, dysphagia, acute viral infection, and gastroesophageal reflux (GER). These specific comorbidities occur more frequently in this group and a high index of suspicion is prudent. When wheezing is due to bronchoconstriction, infants with BPD typically demonstrate a positive response to inhaled β-agonist agents. The hospitalist may consider a therapeutic trial of β-agonist bronchodilators if there is evidence of persistent or acute bronchospasm, increased airway resistance, and gas trapping. Treatment with inhaled bronchodilators for BPD management is variable between hospitals but overall is common among children with severe BPD. Inhaled albuterol and levalbuterol are the most frequently used bronchodilators, but these may worsen malacia if present due to β-agonist relaxation of the airway smooth muscles; in children with severe malacia, the anticholinergic ipratropium bromide may provide bronchodilation without this side effect. Bronchodilators should not be used routinely in the neonatal period or in the absence of a therapeutic response.

Although inhaled corticosteroids are frequently used in infants with BPD and CLDI, there is debate both about their efficacy as well as their potential toxicity during the neonatal period. However, older infants with overt airway hyperreactivity likely benefit from long-term inhaled corticosteroids. Adherence to inhaled corticosteroid medications has been associated with fewer activity limitations, fewer emergency department visits, and less rescue β-agonist use. The potential risk of adrenal suppression, hyperglycemia, and inhibition of somatic growth should limit their use to infants who have a therapeutic response.

Poor Tolerance of Respiratory Infections Depending on the severity of residual lung disease, infants with BPD have up to a 50% chance of requiring readmission to the hospital within the first 2 years of life, usually secondary to viral respiratory tract infections. To minimize risk, parents of infants with BPD are advised to obtain all routine pediatric vaccinations on schedule, to receive the influenza vaccination for themselves, and to minimize the infant's exposure to respiratory viruses; this includes rigorous hand washing and avoidance of anyone who is potentially infectious. Eliminating tobacco smoke exposure, including counseling and providing resources to caregivers for tobacco cessation, is also critical.

Respiratory syncytial virus (RSV) is of particular concern to children with BPD in the first 5 years of life. Infected children have a likelihood of hospital admission for acute severe infection associated with oxygen supplementation and/or mechanical ventilation, and have high complication rates. For preventive therapy against RSV, intramuscular monoclonal antibodies (monthly palivizumab and the newer, long-acting nirsevimab) can provide partial passive immunity to children against this virus. While not completely effective at preventing infection, these monoclonal antibodies do reduce both the incidence and the severity of RSV infection in children. Additionally, RSV vaccination during the third trimester of pregnancy can provide robust transplacental immunity to infants, however the infants with BPD resulting from premature birth may less likely able to benefit from this vaccine. Further discussion of bronchiolitis and its management is provided in Chapter 97.

Fluid Intolerance Infants and young children with BPD and CLDI have fluid sensitivity due to the effect of pulmonary edema on lung mechanics. In the neonatal period, the lung inflammation that is associated with early, evolving BPD leads to pulmonary vascular leak.

In some children, chronic pulmonary edema can be successfully managed with fluid restriction from 130 to 140 mL/kg/day. In other children, diuretic medications are necessary. High-quality studies demonstrating acute improvement in pulmonary mechanics and oxygenation after diuresis have led to the use of as-needed and scheduled diuretic medications. However, chronic diuretic use has not been associated with faster weaning of respiratory support and other outcomes remain understudied. The diuretic medications used most often include thiazides, such as hydrochlorothiazide with or without spironolactone, and loop diuretics including furosemide. Ensuring adequate caloric intake in infants with BPD (see section on "**Inadequate Nutrition**") without excessive fluid loading requires close attention to weight changes and fluid intake and output. A sudden, unexplained weight gain, particularly if associated with acute illness or respiratory deterioration, may warrant a therapeutic trial of a diuretic. Persistent pulmonary edema should prompt further evaluation of an infant's protein status or testing for cardiac disease such as pulmonary hypertension, pulmonary vein stenosis, or pulmonary overcirculation.

When ongoing milder inflammation presumably persists into older infancy, this vascular leaking may also persist even after NICU discharge. This chronic fluid intolerance, and resulting respiratory distress from pulmonary edema, often worsens with acute illness. However, the expected course is to slowly improve over time, in concurrence with resolution of the hypoxemic component of BPD.

RESPIRATORY COMORBID CONDITIONS

Upper Airway Injury Infants with BPD frequently have a history of repeated or prolonged intubation, and therefore are at risk for associated subglottic stenosis complicating lower airway disease. Vocal cord injury, including vocal cord paresis or paralysis, and laryngeal webs or cysts are other possible postintubation complications. These airway injuries result in partial upper airway obstruction, increase the inspiratory work of breathing, and can interfere with gas exchange. Airway protective mechanisms may be impaired as well. Partial upper airway obstruction also increases the risk of respiratory failure during an acute illness. Persistent upper airway symptoms, dysphonia, or stridor should prompt an evaluation for subglottic stenosis and laryngeal injury. If the upper airway lesion is severe enough, tracheostomy or airway reconstructive surgery may be indicated.

Tracheomalacia, Bronchomalacia, and Laryngomalacia As many as 50% of infants with BPD have concomitant tracheomalacia, bronchomalacia, and/or laryngomalacia. These disorders represent abnormal or exaggerated airway collapse due to defects in the cartilaginous rings of the airway. They have various respiratory manifestations but often result in chronic wheezing (tracheomalacia and/or bronchomalacia) or stridor (laryngomalacia) with clinical features of increased work of breathing. They may result in partial or intermittently complete airway obstruction, especially during events associated with increased force of breathing, such as crying or a respiratory illness. At worst, this can lead to severe cyanotic episodes with apnea, bradycardia, or both. Airway growth and healing over time leads to an improvement in symptoms and respiratory mechanics. Although tracheomalacia and bronchomalacia may be congenital, they are usually acquired due to intubation and mechanical ventilation, which cause injury to the immature neonatal trachea and bronchi. Malacia responds poorly to bronchodilators or other medical therapy. Bronchoscopy can be used to diagnose these airway lesions, which, if severe enough, may result in a critical airway requiring tracheostomy and positive-pressure ventilation.

Sleep Disordered Breathing Infants with BPD are at high risk for sleep disordered breathing with altered gas exchange. Infants with normoxia during the daytime can have persistent, unrecognized nocturnal hypoxia. This sleep disordered breathing requires monitoring and treatment because nocturnal hypoxia can interfere with growth. A more complete discussion of obstructive sleep apnea is provided in **Chapter 141**.

Infants with BPD are also at risk for apnea of prematurity that may persist beyond 40 weeks gestational age. This is typically identified using cardiorespiratory and pulse oximetry monitors in the NICU, but may also be reported by caregivers and parents following discharge when pauses in breathing are observed. As in other populations, the routine use of apnea monitors in children with BPD is discouraged given the absence of any proven impact on the incidence of sudden infant death syndrome and caregiver's stress from associated repetitive false alarms.

NONRESPIRATORY COMORBID CONDITIONS

Pulmonary Hypertension While all infants with BPD have a component of pulmonary vascular disease due to disrupted pulmonary vascular growth, the most severe manifestation is pulmonary hypertension. With improved recognition and screening, pulmonary hypertension is estimated to coexist in 14% to 37% of infants with BPD. Infants with comorbid pulmonary hypertension and BPD have longer NICU courses and higher mortality (up to 48% within 2 years) compared with BPD alone.

Echocardiography is the recommended screening tool for pulmonary hypertension but has limited ability to classify severity of disease. All infants with BPD and persistent oxygen needs should be screened. Measures of right ventricular systolic pressure derived from the tricuspid regurgitant jet velocity are measured with echocardiography and compared to systemic blood pressures; these measures can be limited in the absence of significant tricuspid regurgitation. Cardiac catheterization is the gold standard for confirmation of diagnosis and determining severity of pulmonary hypertension but is invasive and not without risk.

Pulmonary hypertension usually responds to the pulmonary vasodilator effect of supplemental oxygen. Additionally, pulmonary vasodilator medications such as sildenafil and bosentan are frequently used. Infants with pulmonary hypertension are at risk of "crises," or episodes of acute worsening of pulmonary hypertension and circulation, particularly during physiologic stress including induction of anesthesia and respiratory infections. These crises can be severe and life-threatening if not emergently addressed.

Pulmonary hypertension generally improves or resolves by early childhood as alveoli and lung vasculature grow and heal. Sequential echocardiography and outpatient management by cardiology are important as there are rare infants with persistent or worsening pulmonary hypertension. The long-term implications of pulmonary hypertension on right ventricular function are unclear.

Gastroesophageal Reflux Disease Gastroesophageal reflux and reflux disease (GERD) is common in children born prematurely with a poor correlation between GERD and the severity of BPD. GERD can compound nutritional difficulties, regardless of oral or enteral tube feeding, because the regurgitation associated with GERD diminishes the net caloric intake. GERD may also be associated with oral aversion and dysphagia. Oropharyngeal incoordination, especially when associated with an inability to protect the airway, increases the risk of aspiration, which may further damage the lungs. Providers should have a low threshold to consider GERD when managing infants with BPD.

Inadequate Nutrition Nutrition is essential to promote lung growth and repair, and thus plays an important role in both the development of BPD in early postnatal life and the resolution of BPD over time. Infants with BPD often have some degree of growth failure and malnutrition. Insufficient postnatal nutrition and growth restriction have been associated with development and severity of BPD in preterm infants. Human milk has been associated with lower risk for development of BPD in neonates in several studies and should be encouraged as a partial or complete nutrition source whenever possible.

Infants with BPD often have high caloric requirements, up to 130% of normal, owing to the increased work of breathing as well as the need for catch-up growth. Critical illnesses including concern for sepsis, respiratory instability, and necrotizing enterocolitis, may limit the ability to provide enteral nutrition for periods of time. Oral feeding difficulties may further contribute to inadequate caloric intake; dysphagia from neurologic impairments, GERD, oral aversion, and respiratory status may all impact oral feeding skills.

Infants with BPD who cannot grow with oral feedings alone require supplemental feeding via nasogastric tube, percutaneous gastrostomy, or gastrojejunostomy tube. Concentrated infant formulas (24-30 kcal/ounce) can be used to increase calories both orally and via tube feedings. Collaboration with nutritionists and feeding specialists can assist in providing sufficient calories to optimize growth. If poor growth persists despite maximized enteral caloric intake, investigations into the cause of failure-to-thrive should include evaluation for hypoxia or hypercapnia requiring long-term mechanical ventilation.

During hospital admissions, the hospitalist should evaluate the growth of each infant or young child with BPD for signs of failure-to-thrive.

Neurologic Impairment The degree to which BPD contributes to neurologic disease is unclear; however, the two conditions often coexist. Neurologic changes seen among children born prematurely may include mild to severe intellectual disabilities, seizure disorders, and variable degrees of neuromotor disease (cerebral palsy). There is an increasing risk of neurologic differences associated with severity of prematurity and severity of BPD. Dysfunction of bulbar muscles increases the risk of swallowing dysfunction and aspiration (see Chapter 143).

Electrolyte Abnormalities, Nephrolithiasis Diuretic therapy used to manage BPD results in urinary losses of electrolytes and subsequent hyponatremia, hypokalemia, hypophosphatemia, hypocalcemia, and alkalosis. Dietary supplementation can be used to manage electrolyte derangements. Furosemide has additional side effects of nephrocalcinosis, ototoxicity, poor growth secondary to hypocalcemia, and renal injury. The effects of hypocalcemia and hypophosphatemia on long-term bone mineralization are unknown.

There is wide practice variation among institutions for weaning chronic diuretic therapy, and many infants and children with BPD or CLDI use these medications beyond the NICU. Clinicians caring for infants and children using chronic diuretics should have a high suspicion for side effects of diuretic therapy; in particular, acutely ill infants may have insidious but rapid electrolyte changes.

LONG-TERM DISEASE MANIFESTATIONS

While the hypoxemia and hypoventilation of BPD is expected to improve with lung growth, long-term follow-up studies have shown pulmonary dysfunction after BPD recovery that persists into adolescence. This may be characterized by airway hyperreactivity with bronchospasm, exercise intolerance, or persistent pulmonary hypertension in young adults. Children with BPD, especially those with cystic disease, have a higher risk of developing chronic obstructive pulmonary disease (COPD) later in life. Tobacco use is also associated with a higher prevalence or earlier onset of COPD and avoidance is critical to prevent lung irritation and hyperactivity.

DIAGNOSTIC EVALUATION

Chest radiography can demonstrate a range of findings, including diffuse ground glass opacification, coarse interstitial markings, pulmonary edema, and cystic changes (see Figure 144-3). Additional multidisciplinary diagnostic evaluations for common comorbidities should be considered for infants and children with BPD as listed in **Table 144-6**.

MANAGEMENT

PRENATAL MANAGEMENT

During pregnancy, optimizing maternal health with prenatal care, nutrition, and avoidance of nicotine and tobacco use is important to prolong gestation and avoid premature birth. When preterm birth is a risk, maternal steroid administration should be given whenever possible to stimulate lung maturation in the fetus. A 2-dose series of betamethasone has strong efficacy data; however, three or more series of prenatal steroids is associated with an increased risk of adverse neurodevelopmental outcomes, especially cerebral palsy, in the infant.

NICU MANAGEMENT

The mainstay of NICU management is supportive care. From a respiratory standpoint, this includes administration of supplemental oxygen, CPAP, or intubation with mechanical ventilation as indicated. Early exogenous surfactant therapy as a treatment for respiratory distress syndrome has the effect of reducing mechanical ventilation and oxygen required, both of which are risk factors for future development of BPD.

TABLE 144-6 Diagnostic Testing Considerations for Infants and Children with BPD

Screening for Comorbidities	
Chest CT with contrast	Assess for parenchymal disease, cystic disease
Echocardiography	Evaluate for pulmonary hypertension
Polysomnography	Evaluate for sleep-disordered breathing
Airway endoscopy	Evaluate for upper airway injury, airway malacia(s)
Clinical swallowing evaluation	Evaluate for aspiration risk
Preventive Care	
Avoidance of secondhand smoke exposure and air pollution	
Electrolyte monitoring	
Avoidance of aspiration	
Pavilizumab	
Influenza immunization	
Nutrition and promotion of linear growth	
Preoperative anesthesia consults	
Physical, Occupational, and Speech therapies as indicated	
Multidisciplinary team-based care	
Care coordination support	

Source: Adapted from Collaco JM, McGrath-Morrow SA. respiratory phenotypes for preterm infants, children, and adults: bronchopulmonary dysplasia and more. *Ann Am Thorac Soc.* 2018;15(5):530-538.

When mechanical ventilation is needed, the ventilation strategy of "permissive hypercapnia" (see above "**Hypercapnia and chronic hypoventilation**") has been shown to reduce volutrauma and subsequent incidence and severity of BPD.

Adequate nutrition to support growth and lung development is critical in the neonatal period and beyond (see section on "**Inadequate Nutrition**"). Additionally, careful fluid management, typically including fluid restriction to 130 or 140 mL/kg/day, is also important during the neonatal period to assist with adequate ventilation and pulmonary mechanics (see section on "**Fluid Intolerance**"). Fluid management may be augmented by thiazide or loop diuretic therapy, particularly for infants requiring positive pressure ventilation that fails to wean despite conservative fluid restriction.

Bronchodilators are less commonly used in the early neonatal period. Older infants with BPD, however, may develop acute episodes of bronchoconstriction, in which inhaled beta-2 agonists might prove beneficial (see section on "**Airway Hyperreactivity**").

CHRONIC MANAGEMENT

Following the initial injury and inflammatory response, BPD is not a progressive disorder. The expected disease course is one of slow, steady improvement. Following NICU discharge, the treatment of BPD and CLDI continues to be primarily supportive, aimed at maximizing lung growth and healing over time while preventing any further pulmonary damage. Owing to the heterogeneity of clinical disease in infants with BPD, there is no standard therapy protocol. Treatment must be individualized, depending on each infant's pattern and disease severity. The process for weaning chronic oxygen therapy, diuretics, and mechanical ventilation are also individualized, and also unique to the institution, local resources, clinician's experience, and family's comfort.

ADMISSION AND DISCHARGE CRITERIA

CAUSES OF HOSPITALIZATION

Common causes of hospitalization include:

- Respiratory infections, particularly with RSV
- Respiratory exacerbations
- Pulmonary hypertension
- Malnutrition/Failure to thrive
- Neurologic concerns

DISCHARGE GOALS DURING READMISSION

Infants with BPD constitute a high-risk and high-needs group of patients and place significant burdens on families and caregivers in the home. Careful discharge planning, either after the initial hospitalization or following readmission, ensures that adequate resources are in place for these infants and their families. Resolution of the acute events that prompted admission must be achieved before discharge. In addition, short-term or long-term setbacks in the infant's clinical status may require changes in the care plan or the institution of additional resources in the home environment.

CONSULTATION

Following NICU discharge, infants and young children with BPD and CLDI often require a team of specialists to manage their care in both the outpatient and inpatient settings. This is particularly true of infants with technology dependence or chronic medical problems associated with BPD and CLDI. Involving specialists in the care of these medically complex infants is important and can help the hospitalist facilitate a smoother and potentially earlier transition back home.

Aside from the assistance required for the management of acute issues, consultants can assess newly recognized conditions or reassess ongoing conditions. Common subspecialties involved include the following:

- Pulmonology
- Neonatology (many centers have a specific NICU follow-up program)
- Otolaryngology
- Gastroenterology
- Developmental medicine
- Neurology
- Nutrition
- Physical, occupational, or speech therapy
- Case management and/or social work
- Primary care provider
- Complex care provider (many centers have clinics or programs dedicated to primary or consultative care of children with medical complexity)

A physician-led outpatient team providing comprehensive care coordination is essential, whether provided by the primary care physician, pulmonology team, neonatology follow-up program, or complex care pediatrician. Communication with this team is important throughout any hospital stay and beyond.

SPECIAL CONSIDERATIONS

PREVENTION

The primary treatment of BPD is prevention, which involves optimizing maternal prepartum health and reducing the incidence of premature birth. Surfactant therapy and improved ventilator management are also recognized factors that reduce the severity and incidence of BPD. Once this respiratory damage has occurred the aim is to allow the child to grow and heal from the initial insult, primarily by supportive care. A secondary aim is, where possible, to prevent any further lung damage, using evidence-based NICU practices, ensuring appropriate vaccinations, minimizing respiratory infections, and eliminating tobacco smoke exposure.

KEY POINTS

- BPD and CLDI are chronic lung disorders affecting newborns and resulting in chronic respiratory insufficiency and need for long-term supplemental oxygen therapy.
- BPD affects infants born prematurely with immature lung development, which is complicated by injury from postnatal insults.
- BPD is characterized by the combination of simplified alveolar structure, airway malacias, and abnormal pulmonary vasculature.
- Readmission rates among infants with BPD and CLDI are high, especially in those with a history of extreme prematurity.
- Acute respiratory illness, especially viral illness, accounts for the majority of readmissions in this population.
- The lung disease may be associated with persistent hypoxemia, hypercapnia, and hyperreactive airways with bronchospasm.
- Infants with BPD and CLDI may demonstrate fluid intolerance and may require long-term diuretics with resulting electrolyte derangements.
- Providing adequate nutrition is a challenge owing to increased caloric needs and difficulties with oral feeding.
- These infants often have complex medical concerns, both short and long term, that are best served by a multidisciplinary team coordinated by a primary care physician. The hospitalist has a key role in managing acute medical issues and coordinating care during the hospital stay and after discharge.
- BPD and CLDI are evolving disorders. Advances in neonatal care and technology will continue to affect the outcomes of premature infants with respiratory failure, and others with critical respiratory illnesses.
- The long-term outcome of infants with BPD and CLDI is evolving as well. Older children with a history of BPD may have an increased risk of asthma and exercise intolerance, but in the absence of significant neurologic injury, the outcome of this fragile group of infants is quite good.

SUGGESTED READINGS

Abman SH, Collaco JM, Shepherd EG, et al. Interdisciplinary care of children with severe bronchopulmonary dysplasia. *J Pediatr.* 2017;181:12-28.e1.

Baker CD. Mechanical ventilation during chronic lung disease. *Clin Perinatol.* 2021;48(4):881-893.

Berkelhamer SK, Mestan KK, Steinhorn R. An update on the diagnosis and management of bronchopulmonary dysplasia (BPD)-associated pulmonary hypertension. *Semin Perinatol.* 2018;42(7):432-443.

Chaw PS, Hua L, Cunningham S, Campbell H, Mikolajczyk R, Nair H. Respiratory syncytial virus-associated acute lower respiratory infections in children with bronchopulmonary dysplasia: systematic review and meta-analysis. *J Infect Dis.* 2020;222(Suppl 7):S620-s627.

Clouse BJ, Jadcherla SR, Slaughter JL. Systematic review of inhaled bronchodilator and corticosteroid therapies in infants with bronchopulmonary dysplasia: implications and future directions. *PloS One.* 2016;11.

Davidson LM, Berkelhamer SK. Bronchopulmonary dysplasia: chronic lung disease of infancy and long-term pulmonary outcomes. *J Clin Med.* 2017;6(1).

DeMauro SB. Neurodevelopmental outcomes of infants with bronchopulmonary dysplasia. *Pediatr Pulmonol.* 2021;56(11):3509-3517.

Gallini F, Coppola M, De Rose DU, et al. Neurodevelopmental outcomes in very preterm infants: the role of severity of bronchopulmonary dysplasia. *Early Hum Dev.* 2021;152:105275.

Hayes D, Jr., Wilson KC, Krivchenia K, et al. Home oxygen therapy for children. An Official American Thoracic Society Clinical Practice Guideline. *Am J Respir Crit Care Med.* 2019;199(3):e5-e23.

Hines D, Modi N, Lee SK, et al. Scoping review shows wide variation in the definitions of bronchopulmonary dysplasia in preterm infants and calls for a consensus. *Acta Paediatr.* 2017;106(3):366-374.

Jensen EA, Dysart K, Gantz MG, et al. The diagnosis of bronchopulmonary dysplasia in very preterm infants. an evidence-based approach. *Am J Respir Crit Care Med.* 2019;200(6):751-759.

Kao LC, Warburton D, Cheng MH, Cedeño C, Platzker AC, Keens TG. Effect of oral diuretics on pulmonary mechanics in infants with chronic bronchopulmonary dysplasia: results of a double-blind crossover sequential trial. *Pediatrics.* 1984;74(1):37-44.

Lagatta J, Murthy K, Zaniletti I, et al. Home oxygen use and 1-year readmission among infants born preterm with bronchopulmonary dysplasia discharged from Children's Hospital Neonatal Intensive Care Units. *J Pediatr.* 2020;220:40-48.e5.

Mac S, Sumner A, Duchesne-Belanger S, Stirling R, Tunis M, Sander B. Cost-effectiveness of palivizumab for respiratory syncytial virus: a systematic review. *Pediatrics.* 2019;143(5).

Poindexter BB, Feng R, Schmidt B, et al. comparisons and limitations of current definitions of bronchopulmonary dysplasia for the prematurity and respiratory outcomes program. *Annals Am Thorac Soc.* 2015;12(12):1822-1830.

Rocha G, Guimarães H, Pereira-da-Silva L. The role of nutrition in the prevention and management of bronchopulmonary dysplasia: a literature review and clinical approach. *Int J Environ Res Public Health.* 2021;18(12).

Ryu J, Haddad G, Carlo WA. Clinical effectiveness and safety of permissive hypercapnia. *Clin Perinatol.* 2012;39(3):603-612.

Su YT, Chiu CC, Lai SH, et al. Risk factors for tracheobronchomalacia in preterm infants with bronchopulmonary dysplasia. *Front Pediatr.* 2021;9:697470.

CHAPTER 145

Cystic Fibrosis

Jennifer S. Hall, MD, FAAP and
Sandra Gage, MD, PhD, FAAP, SFHM

BACKGROUND

Cystic fibrosis (CF) is a multisystem disease affecting the gastrointestinal tract, lungs, reproductive tracts, and sweat glands. It is the most common life-limiting autosomal recessive disorder, affecting approximately 1 in 4000 newborns in the United States, with higher rates in some European countries. CF occurs among persons of all races and ethnicities. Although the classic CF triad is chronic obstructive lung disease, exocrine pancreatic insufficiency, and sweat gland abnormalities, CF can mimic many other common pediatric conditions. The presentation can vary from severe manifestations early in life to later presentations with mild or atypical symptoms. With the advent of newborn screening (NBS) for CF, clinical care guidelines have been developed to aggressively identify and address respiratory and nutritional problems prior to the development of symptoms. In addition, modulators affecting the abnormal protein in CF are becoming increasingly available, and patients now routinely undergo genetic testing to select targeted proactive daily care.

Pediatric hospitalists often evaluate and treat patients with chronic respiratory or gastrointestinal symptoms where CF is considered in the differential diagnosis or manage disease-related complications of CF in affected individuals.

PATHOPHYSIOLOGY

CF is caused by mutations in a single gene on the long arm of chromosome 7 that encodes for the cystic fibrosis transmembrane conductance regulator (CFTR) protein. The *CFTR* gene is primarily expressed in the respiratory and intestinal epithelia, pancreatic ducts, hepatobiliary tract, polymorphonuclear leukocytes (PMNs), and sweat ducts. Following the discovery of this gene in 1989, more than 2,000 variants and their impact on the amount and function of the CFTR protein have been reported; ~400 of these variants cause symptoms of CF. Six functional classifications categorize the implications of specific gene abnormalities (**Table 145-1**). Despite the number of CFTR mutations that lead to clinical disease, the class 2, F508del variant is most common, with at least one copy present in 86% of patients that have been genotyped. CF has been considered a disease affecting those with two CFTR mutations, but recent literature suggests that heterozygous carriers may be at increased risk for CF-related conditions, including chronic pancreatitis, atypical mycobacterial infections, and bronchiectasis.

The CFTR protein functions as a chloride and bicarbonate channel in the apical membrane of cells. The loss of function of the CFTR ion channel in CF results in abnormal ion and fluid movement across epithelial membranes, which leads to abnormal cell surface pH and secretion

TABLE 145-1 CFTR Mutations

Class	CFTR Defect	Examples
1	No CFTR protein synthesis	W1282X, G542X
2	Block in processing of CFTR	ΔAF508, N1303K
3	Improper regulation of CFTR	G551D, G551S
4	Abnormal conduction through CFTR	R117H, R334W
5	Reduced synthesis and/or mistargeting of CFTR	A455E, Q1412X
6	Increased turnover of CFTR at the cell surface	N287Y

viscosity in affected organs. These abnormalities lead to inspissated mucus and obstruction of glandular ducts, inflammation, and eventual organ destruction. In the lung, alterations in mucous viscosity result in slower clearance of microorganisms and decreased cell surface pH inhibits bacterial killing. In PMNs, CFTR function optimizes phagocytosis by aiding the movement of chloride into phagosomes. In individuals with CF, PMNs are impermeable to chloride, thereby limiting the killing of phagosome-ingested microbes. When the microbial load exceeds local efforts to respond, the host CF mucosa drives a strong chemotactic response. This causes robust and sustained inflammation characterized by neutrophil-dominated secretions and increased free neutrophil elastase activity and cytokine concentrations. Together, these factors predispose patients to specific bacterial infections that promote a cycle of inflammation, abnormal secretions, and, over time, lung damage in the form of bronchiectasis, cyst formation, and loss of parenchyma.

CLINICAL PRESENTATION

As CF is caused by numerous mutations diversely affecting multiple organ systems, the presentation can be quite variable. Historically, failure to thrive and pulmonary manifestations in infancy have been the most common presenting features; however, variable forms of CF may not present until adolescence or even adulthood (**Table 145-2**). Since universal NBS has been implemented throughout the United States, at least 63% of new CF diagnoses are made in asymptomatic infants (mean age 3 months) following a positive NBS result. However, not all mutations are detected by the NBS, and NBS, genetic, and sweat chloride testing results can be indeterminant.

TABLE 145-2 Clinical Features Consistent With Cystic Fibrosis

Clinical Features
Respiratory
Chronic cough and sputum production
Persistent chest radiograph findings, including atelectasis, bronchiectasis, hyperinflation, infiltrates
Chronic airflow obstruction, which can present as wheezing and air trapping
Persistent airway colonization with organisms such as *Staphylococcus aureus*, *Pseudomonas aeruginosa*, *Burkholderia cepacia*, and nontypeable *Haemophilus influenzae*, MRSA, *Stenotrophomonas maltophilia*
Nasal polyps
Digital clubbing
Chronic pansinusitis
Gastrointestinal
Meconium ileus
Distal intestinal obstruction syndrome
Rectal prolapse
Focal biliary cirrhosis
Multi-lobar cirrhosis
Pancreatic insufficiency
Recurrent pancreatitis
Failure to thrive
Other
Hypoproteinemia
Hypoalbuminemia
Hyponatremic, hypochloremic dehydration
Chronic metabolic alkalosis (pseudo-Bartter syndrome)
Male infertility (congenital bilateral absence of the vas deferens)

DIAGNOSIS

NBS for CF in the United States has been universally applied since 2009, however, testing protocols vary from state to state. The test is performed by measuring immunoreactive trypsinogen (IRT) levels in neonatal blood spots, which are elevated in most infants with CF. If elevated, most state laboratories perform confirmatory *CFTR* gene variant testing, while some repeat IRT levels. Screening is positive if the IRT level remains elevated or at least one deviant CFTR variant is identified. A positive screen triggers notification of the primary physician for referral to a Cystic Fibrosis Foundation (CFF) accredited center for further evaluation. These centers may be found on the CFF website (**http://www.cff.org/ccd/**).

NBS for CF is not definitive. For example, IRT levels may be low in infants with meconium ileus, and follow-up CFTR genetic tests are less sensitive in detecting mutations in newborns that are not of Scandinavian descent. Despite a negative screen, clinicians must maintain a high index of suspicion in symptomatic patients.

In 2017, the CFF published consensus guidelines for the diagnosis of CF. Diagnosis may be made if the patient has a presentation consistent with the disease, including a positive NBS result, clinical features consistent with the disease (Table 145-2), and/or a positive family history of CF and evidence of CFTR dysfunction. However, quantitative pilocarpine iontophoresis measuring the chloride concentration of sweat remains the gold standard for diagnosis. Sweat testing results are either diagnostic, intermediate, or unlikely. A sweat chloride concentration of >60 mmol/L is diagnostic of CF. To confirm the diagnosis, a second sweat test or genetic studies identifying two disease-causing mutations is needed. Sweat chloride values between 30 and 59 mmol/L are considered intermediate; levels should be repeated intermittently, patients monitored for clinical features of CF, and genetic testing considered. A sweat chloride concentration of <30 mmol/L is considered normal and a diagnosis of CF is unlikely; however, if 2 CF-causing genetic variants are identified via gene analysis, a diagnosis of CF may still be made.

While genetic testing has aided in diagnosis of CF for many, it remains imperfect as a final determinant of disease as there are asymptomatic children with known CF-causing mutations, children with phenotypical disease without a known variant, and over 1700 *CFTR* gene variants of unknown significance. The limitations of all available testing modalities may require that several be performed and clinical correlation applied to determine the diagnosis of CF.

COURSE OF ILLNESS

RESPIRATORY

CF causes abnormal secretions in the airway that lead to difficulty clearing and killing pulmonary pathogens. Early in the course of CF airway disease, the respiratory tract is colonized with bacterial pathogens and subjected to persistent infections with an abnormal inflammatory environment. This sets the stage for the development of chronic, progressive obstructive lung disease and the resulting symptoms, morbidity, and mortality. Airways of CF patients are susceptible to colonization with several specific pathogens, including *Staphylococcus aureus*, *Haemophilus influenzae*, *Pseudomonas aeruginosa*, *Stenotrophomonas maltophilia*, and *Burkholderia cepacia*. Although these microbes may infect healthy patients, colonization with these pathogens is a hallmark of CF.

Viral upper respiratory tract infections tend to evolve into lower tract infections and pulmonary exacerbations in CF patients. These infections last longer, are more severe, and lead to increased hospitalization rates when compared to the non-CF population. Viral illness may also enable *Pseudomonas* infection. The SARS-CoV-2 pandemic elicited concern that CF patients would be severely affected; however, it appears that CF comorbidity is protective compared to the general population. One theory implicates the CF community's familiarity with infection control measures, while another cites the tendency for CF patients to be underweight as advantageous. Additionally, the lower sputum IL-6 and higher ACE2 mRNA levels seen in CF patients are thought to attenuate the course of SARS-CoV-2. Risk factors for severe disease from SARS-CoV-2 specific to the CF population include CF-related diabetes, older

TABLE 145-3 Signs and Symptoms of a Pulmonary Exacerbation of Cystic Fibrosis
Increased cough (duration, frequency, intensity)
Increased or new onset of sputum production
Change in sputum appearance
Increased or new onset of hemoptysis
Increased shortness of breath, wheezing
Decrease in exercise tolerance
Increase in fatigue, weakness, poor appetite, and malaise
Increased work of breathing manifested by use of accessory muscles and intercostal retractions
Increased respiratory rate
New findings on chest examination, such as crackles
Air trapping
Weight loss
Decrease in FEV1 of 10% or more compared with baseline
Chest radiograph changes (increased air trapping, atelectasis, infiltrates)
Leukocytosis
Decreased oxygen saturation

FEV_1, forced expiratory volume in 1 second.

age, transplant status, and lower forced expiratory volume in 1 second (FEV_1).

Eventually, the persistence of bronchiolar inflammation leads to destruction of airway integrity, and proteolysis and chondrolysis of support tissues lead to airway dilation and bronchiectasis. Atelectasis, pneumonia, and, eventually, chronic respiratory failure and death follow. The course of respiratory deterioration in CF is variable, but one study demonstrated an average of ~2% loss/year in FEV_1 for children between ages 6 and 18 years.

CF pulmonary exacerbations are characterized by increased work of breathing, a decrease in FEV_1 of 10% or more from baseline, and changes in cough, sputum production, and/or lung examination (see **Table 145-3** for a comprehensive list). Exacerbations are a common reason for hospitalizations among patients with CF. Even in patients with severe disease, acute CF manifestations may be reversible enough to allow for meaningful return to baseline.

To extend and improve quality of life for individuals with CF, bilateral lung transplantation is often discussed once their FEV_1 reaches 50% of predicted or is demonstrating a rapid decline (>20% in 1 year). Early referral to a lung transplant center may be made for interested and eligible patients. Transplantation is usually considered once the FEV_1 nears 30%. Although CF affects many organ systems, more than 50% of patients ultimately die of respiratory failure. Currently, the median age of survival is 46 to 47 years.

GASTROINTESTINAL

Gastrointestinal (GI) manifestations of CF are common (see Table 145-2). GI complaints range from symptoms of steatorrhea, reflux, and constipation to life-threatening distal intestinal obstruction syndrome (DIOS) and liver failure. Additionally, the important relationship between excellent nutrition and the maintenance of lung health makes careful attention to nutrition and GI health a priority. GI manifestations can begin in utero, with up to 20% of newborns with CF suffering from inspissated, tenacious meconium obstructing the distal ileum and leading to meconium ileus. When meconium ileus is diagnosed in the newborn nursery, it usually requires transfer to a higher level of care, but recurrent obstruction in infancy is uncommon.

Eighty-four percent of CF patients have exocrine pancreatic insufficiency. This can present in the newborn period with steatorrhea resulting in failure to thrive. Approximately 60% of infants with CF diagnosed by the NBS have evidence of pancreatic exocrine insufficiency at birth. Other early GI manifestations include nonspecific feeding difficulties and irritability during feedings. Poor growth, rectal prolapse, and fat-soluble vitamin (A, D, E, K) deficiencies are all signs of fat malabsorption that should prompt an evaluation for CF in undiagnosed patients and intervention in those with known disease.

Exocrine pancreatic dysfunction can lead to carbohydrate intolerance and ultimately diabetes, most commonly during adolescence (5.1% of CF patients < 18 years; with an incidence of 18.6% in all CF patients). CF-related diabetes (CFRD) results from obstructive damage from thick secretions leading to fatty infiltration of the pancreas and islet cell destruction. CFRD most often results in nonketotic hyperglycemia, which is exacerbated by acute illness and the concurrent use of corticosteroids. CFRD is associated with increased morbidity and mortality due to poor nutritional status and secondarily diminished lung function. Aggressive management, often with insulin therapy, is required to optimize glycemic control. Annual diabetes screening with a 2-hour glucose tolerance test is recommended for all CF patients starting at age 10 years. Due to increased red blood cell turnover, hemoglobin A1c levels are not sensitive enough for diagnosis. CFRD is associated with the same secondary complications as diabetes mellitus, including retinopathy, microalbuminuria, and neuropathy. The management of carbohydrate intolerance in this population can be challenging due to comorbid delayed gastric emptying, malabsorption, and increased caloric needs.

In the hepatobiliary tree, the *CFTR* gene is thought to promote bile flow. Dysfunction in CF patients leads to cholestasis, inflammation, and biliary fibrosis with focal destruction. Approximately one-third of patients develop CF liver disease, with the highest incidence in those under 10 years. Clinical features include elevated liver enzymes, hepatomegaly, cholestasis, cholelithiasis, and fibrosis. Annual liver assessment should include laboratory markers of function and ultrasound evaluation. CF-related biliary cirrhosis develops in approximately 5% to 10% of patients, with a mean age at diagnosis of 10 years. Associated complications include portal hypertension, hypersplenism, and variceal bleeding. In some patients, cirrhosis can progress to frank liver failure, requiring liver transplantation.

TREATMENT

PROACTIVE DAILY CARE

The goal of CF management is to slow the rate of pulmonary decline and thus preserve respiratory function. A comprehensive multidisciplinary approach to patient care has been instituted at CF centers worldwide. While clinical approaches may vary between centers, the Cystic Fibrosis Foundation has established clinical practice guidelines that are followed by most centers in the United States. These guidelines emphasize the need for frequent monitoring at a CFF-accredited center where interdisciplinary care and patient and family education are provided.

While past treatments solely provided symptomatic care, the focus of current and future therapies is on modifying and curing the disease. First introduced in 2012, CFTR modulators work to improve the production, intracellular processing, and function of the defective CFTR protein. There are currently many modulators available in 1-to-3 drug combinations that address several gene mutations, with some approved for children as young as 4 months. As new modulators targeting different mutations have been found, treatment eligibility has increased from 6.3% in 2014 to approximately 90% in 2021. Most of the remaining 10% of CF patients currently not on modulators are ineligible due to their mutation type. Modulators can normalize sweat chloride concentrations, improve CFTR function in nasal and intestinal epithelia, and improve baseline FEV_1, respiratory quality of life, and body mass index (BMI). Modulators have also been shown to decrease the frequency of pulmonary exacerbations, acute pancreatitis hospitalizations, and overall hospitalizations in those under 20 years of age. They can also decrease the need for other CF therapies, including chronic antibiotics, frequent airway clearance, and supplemental feedings.

NUTRITION

Adequate nutrition is important in CF patients due to the strong association between nutritional health and preservation of pulmonary function and the link between malnutrition and increased morbidity and mortality. Patients with CF have much higher caloric requirements than healthy individuals secondary to increased metabolic demand from chronic infection, inflammation, and increased respiratory effort, as well as intestinal malabsorption. An unrestricted high-calorie, high-fat diet is encouraged, with a goal of maintaining a weight for length (<2 years) or BMI (>2 years) at or above the 50th percentile. Pancreatic enzyme replacement therapy is necessary for all pancreatic-insufficient patients. Enzymes are administered as enteric-coated tablets or microspheres, at doses ranging from 2000 to 2500 U/kg of lipase per meal or snack, with a daily maximum of 10,000 U/kg per day. Fat-soluble vitamin supplements are also required.

PULMONARY CARE

To maintain lung health, patients require individualized daily preventive care based on chronic symptoms, age, airway microbiology, and pulmonary function. **Table 145-4** summarizes CFF recommendations for respiratory care. Airway clearance and nebulized hypertonic saline to aid in the removal of viscous secretions are recommended twice daily. Common modalities include manual percussion, high-frequency chest wall oscillation, and positive expiratory pressure devices. Patients may also benefit from additional nebulized medications to thin secretions, such as recombinant human rhDNase. Chronic lung inflammation is typically managed with high-dose ibuprofen or azithromycin. The use of oral or inhaled steroids is avoided unless a comorbid condition, such as asthma or allergic bronchopulmonary aspergillosis (ABPA) exists.

Aggressive management of chronic airway infections delays decline in lung function. Therefore, frequent sputum cultures are done to monitor for pathogens of concern. As knowledge of the effect of CFTR channel abnormalities on lung mucosa and the killing abilities of PMNs has expanded, colonization by prevalent pathogens has become better understood. Prophylactic antibiotic therapy to prevent bacterial airway colonization with *S. aureus* is no longer recommended. Studies show unclear clinical significance of decreased infection with *S. aureus* and that prophylactic treatment may increase the risk of *P. aeruginosa* infection.

Infection with *P. aeruginosa* is highly clinically significant in CF patients. Initial infection is treated aggressively with 28 days of inhaled tobramycin in the hope of achieving eradication. While nebulized antibiotics are not recommended to prevent acquisition of *P. aeruginosa,* they are routinely prescribed as suppressive therapy for patients with chronic infection or colonization with *P. aeruginosa* or another gram-negative pathogen.

Because CF patients may be colonized with antibiotic-resistant organisms, infection control measures utilizing contact and droplet precautions are required during hospitalization to prevent the nosocomial spread of organisms such as MRSA and multiresistant gram-negative rods. Emerging pathogens associated with pulmonary exacerbations and secondary hospitalizations include the often, multidrug-resistant *S. maltophilia.*

ACUTE COMPLICATIONS

The most notable pulmonary complications of CF are pulmonary exacerbations, hemoptysis (**Figure 145-1**), and pneumothorax (**Figure 145-2**). A pulmonary exacerbation is a clinical diagnosis combining worsening symptoms with clinical signs, such as increased respiratory rate and effort, weight loss, and change in lung examination, as well as a decline in pulmonary function tests (PFTs) (**Table 145-3**). The most highly predictive factors of a CF exacerbation include increased cough, change in sputum, decreased appetite or weight loss, change in the lung examination, and increased respiratory rate. The causes of these exacerbations include bacterial or viral infections, clonal expansion of an existing bacterial strain (i.e., *P. aeruginosa*), exposure to air pollutants, and reactive airway disease. Regardless of etiology, exacerbations impact a patient's quality of life and can lead to permanent decline in lung function.

TABLE 145-4 Summary of Cystic Fibrosis Foundation Recommendations for Respiratory Therapy in Cystic Fibrosis

Airway Clearance (AC)
• AC is recommended for all patients with CF for assistance with cough, clearance of sputum, maintenance of lung function, improved quality of life.
• No form of AC is better than others and the method of AC should be tailored to the patient.
• Aerobic exercise is recommended in addition to (not in place of) AC.
Bronchodilators
• Evidence is insufficient to recommend for or against chronic use of B2 agonists and anticholinergics.
Inhaled Antibiotics for Patients with Pseudomonas on Sputum Culture
• Mild lung disease: There is evidence of benefit of inhaled Tobramycin or Aztreonam and their use is recommended.
• Moderate to severe lung disease: There is evidence of benefit of inhaled Tobramycin or Aztreonam and their use is strongly recommended.
• Insufficient evidence to recommend for or against other inhaled antibiotics.
Oral Antibiotics
• Evidence is insufficient to recommend for or against anti-*Staphylococcus aureus* or anti-*Pseudomonal* oral antibiotics for chronic use.
• There is evidence to recommend against the use of oral anti-Staphylococcus aureus antibiotics for prophylactic use.
Mucolytics for Daily Care
• Hypertonic saline is recommended for all patients with CF regardless of disease severity.
• Mild lung disease: There is evidence of benefit of dornase alfa and use is recommended.
• Moderate to severe lung disease: There is evidence of benefit of dornase alfa and use is strongly recommended.
Anti-Inflammatory Medications
• Recommend against using inhaled corticosteroids or oral corticosteroids unless there is also a diagnosis of asthma or allergic bronchopulmonary aspergillosis.
• For patients under 18 years old and FEV_1 >60%, ibuprofen use is recommended. For those over 18 years old, evidence is insufficient.
• Azithromycin is recommended for patients with and without chronic *Pseudomonas aeruginosa* infections.
• Evidence is insufficient to recommend for or against use of leukotriene modifiers, N-acetyl cysteine, or inhaled glutathione.
Acute Pulmonary Exacerbations
• Recommends against treatment with IV antibiotics in a non-hospital setting.
• Recommends continuing chronic medications and that airway clearance should be increased during an exacerbation.
• Evidence is insufficient to recommend for or against continuing chronic inhaled antibiotics when undergoing treatment with IV antibiotics.
• Evidence is insufficient to recommend that one antibiotic is as efficacious as using more than one antibiotic for *Pseudomonas* infection.
• When using IV aminoglycosides, recommend once-daily dosing over multiple-times daily dosing.
• When beta-lactam antibiotics are indicated, evidence is insufficient to recommend for or against continuous infusion.
• Evidence is insufficient to recommend an optimal duration of antibiotics.
• Evidence is insufficient to recommend for or against oral corticosteroids for an acute pulmonary exacerbation.

Source: Data from Cystic Fibrosis Foundation. Respiratory Care Guidelines. https://www.cff.org/medical-professionals/clinical-care-guidelines#respiratory-care-guidelines. Accessed July 25, 2022.

Patients with mild pulmonary exacerbations can be treated outpatient with oral and inhaled antibiotics. The choice of antibiotics should be based on recent sputum cultures (**Table 145-5**). Airway clearance therapy, mucolytics, and anti-inflammatory treatments may be increased to maximize secretion clearance and nutritional support optimized. Patients who fail to improve with outpatient management or present with severe symptoms usually require hospitalization and intravenous

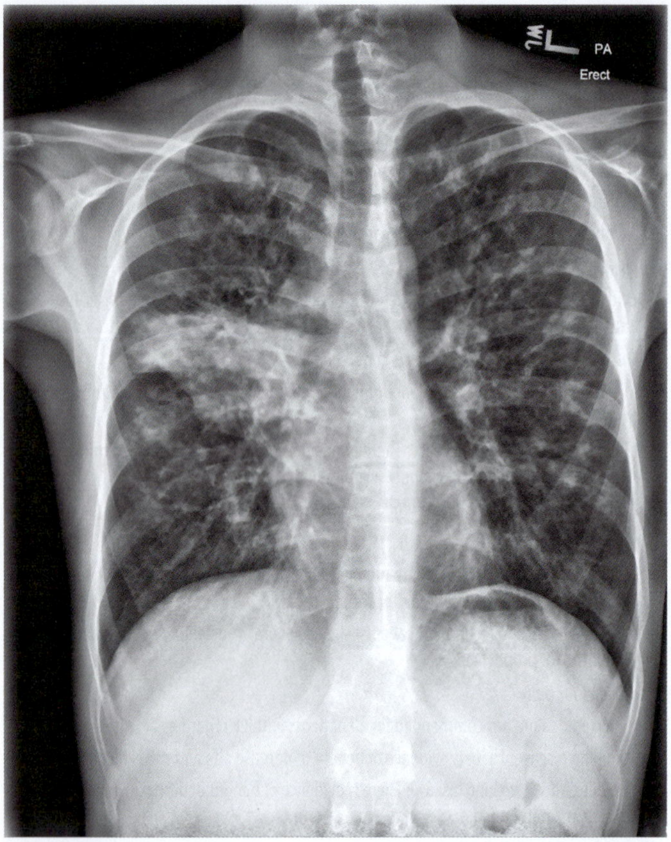

A

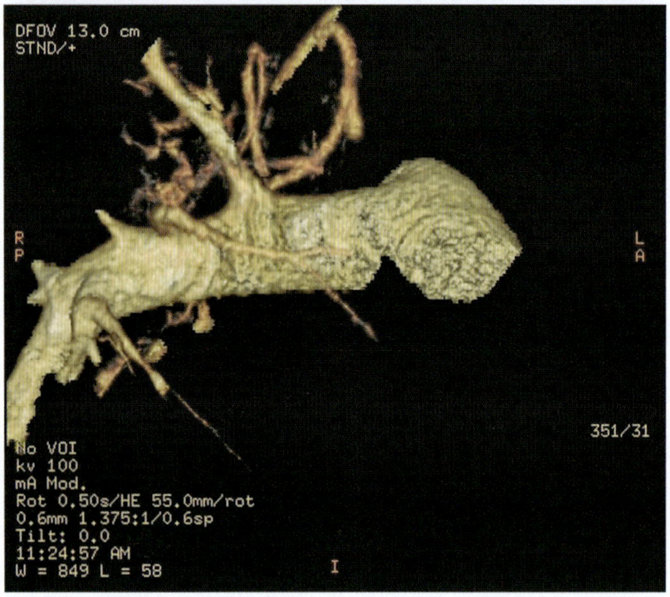

B

FIGURE 145-1. A. Right upper lobe consolidation in a 16-year-old male with CF and hemoptysis. B. Bronchial artery collateral vessels seen on CT angiography in the same patient. (Images used with permission of A. Chidekel, MD.)

antibiotics, often for 10 to 14 days (**Table 145-6**). For patients who improve during the first week of hospitalization, a 10-day course is recommended. Prolonged (21 day) courses of intravenous antibiotics have no benefit and incur an increased risk of adverse events, increased cost, and toxicity. Addition of inhaled antibiotics to an IV antibiotic treatment regimen has not been shown to improve outcomes or increase time to the next acute pulmonary exacerbation.

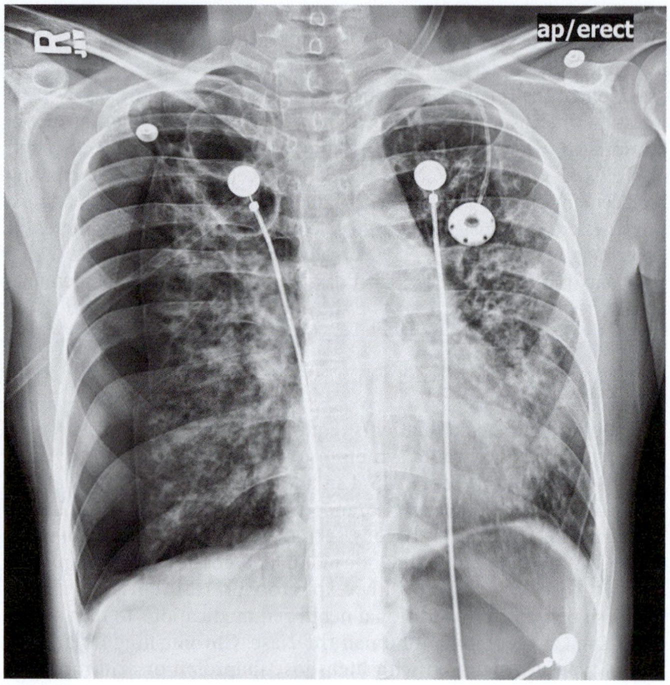

FIGURE 145-2. Large right-sided pneumothorax in a 19-year-old female with CF and severe lung disease. Note additional apical lung cysts and extensive scarring throughout both lungs. (Image used with permission of A. Chidekel, MD.)

Once hospitalized, psychosocial support should be offered, and the patient's outpatient health maintenance plan reinforced. For adults demonstrating clinical improvement, antibiotic therapy may be transitioned to home; however, studies have demonstrated that children have shorter duration of IV antibiotics and significantly greater improvement in FEV_1 when treated in the hospital.

If pulmonary exacerbations fail to improve with standard therapy, unusual infections such as fungi, atypical mycobacteria, and/or ABPA should be considered.

Hemoptysis is a concerning complication of CF airway disease that can accompany a pulmonary exacerbation or occur as an isolated event. Scant hemoptysis is <5 mL, mild to moderate is 5 to 240 mL, and massive or major hemoptysis is defined as >240 mL of blood loss in 24 hours or 100 mL/day over several days. Scant hemoptysis can be managed outpatient. Mild-to-moderate hemoptysis care should include antibiotics, holding nonsteroidal anti-inflammatory medications, and possible modification of airway clearance. This low-pressure bleeding is usually due to airway inflammation with subsequent airway wall erosion and generally resolves with treatment of the underlying infection.

Massive hemoptysis requires hospitalization as it may be life-threatening due to asphyxiation or hypotension. Massive hemoptysis is caused by bleeding in the collateral circulation (bronchial arterial vessels), which develops over time in CF lung disease due to pulmonary inflammation and infection. These abnormal vessels are subject to systemic arterial pressures. Massive hemoptysis occurs most commonly in patients with advanced lung disease but may occur at any stage of disease progression. The management of massive hemoptysis includes intravenous antibiotics, holding airway clearance, airway maintenance as indicated, and specialized interventions, such as bronchial artery embolization or lung resection, when required.

Pneumothorax in CF occurs due to the rupture of subpleural apical blebs, which form as emphysematous changes progress. Pneumothorax occurs more commonly in CF patients with advanced lung disease and may manifest acutely as chest pain or shortness of breath. Pneumothorax is an indication for hospital admission, and management is like that for non-CF patients. Although observation alone may be appropriate,

TABLE 145-5 Enteral Antibiotics to Treat Pulmonary Exacerbations of Cystic Fibrosis on an Outpatient Basis

Organism	Medication	Dose (mg/kg/day)	Dosing Interval	Maximum Dose (mg/day)
Pseudomonas aeruginosa	Ciprofloxacin	40	bid	2000
	Levofloxacin	<5 years: 20 ≥5 years: 10	<5 years: bid ≥5 years: daily	750
	Inhaled aztreonam	75 mg/dose*	tid	
	Inhaled tobramycin (solution)	300 mg/dose*	bid	
	Inhaled tobramycin (capsules)	112 mg/dose*	bid	
	Inhaled colistin	150 mg/dose*	bid	
Methicillin-Sensitive Staphylococcus aureus	Amoxicillin-clavulanate	45-90†	bid or tid	3000
	Cephalexin	50-100	tid or qid	4000
	Dicloxacillin	50-100	qid	2000
Methicillin-Resistant Staphylococcus aureus	Clindamycin	20-40	tid	2400
	Doxycycline	5	bid	200
	Linezolid	30-45	tid	1800
	Minocycline	4 mg/kg × 1 load, then 4	bid	400
	Trimethoprim-sulfamethoxazole	15-20††	bid or tid or qid	960
Stenotrophomonas maltophilia	Ciprofloxacin	40	bid	2000
	Levofloxacin	<5 years: 20 ≥5 years: 10	<5 years: bid ≥5 years: daily	750
	Minocycline	4 mg/kg × 1 load, then 4	bid	400
	Trimethoprim-sulfamethoxazole (preferred)	15-20††	bid or tid or qid	960
Haemophilus influenzae	Amoxicillin-clavulanate	45-90	bid or tid	3000
Achromobacter sp.	Ciprofloxacin	40	bid	2000
	Minocycline	4 mg/kg × 1 load, then 4	bid	400
	Trimethoprim-sulfamethoxazole	15-20††	bid or tid or qid	960
Burkholderia cepacia	Doxycycline	5	bid	200
	Minocycline	4 mg/kg × 1 load, then 4	bid	400
	Trimethoprim-sulfamethoxazole	15-20††	bid or tid or qid	960

*Not based on weight.

†Amoxicillin component.

††Trimethoprim component.

bid, twice daily; tid, three times daily; qid, four times daily.

References

1. Chmiel JF, Aksamit TR, Chotirmall SH, et al. Antibiotic management of lung infections in cystic fibrosis. I. The microbiome, methicillin-resistant Staphylococcus aureus, gram-negative bacteria, and multiple infections. *Ann Am Thorac Soc.* 2014;11(7):1120-1129.
2. Gibson RL, Burns JL, Ramsey BW. Pathophysiology and management of pulmonary infections in cystic fibrosis. *Am J Respir Crit Care Med.* 2003;168:918-951.
3. Epps QJ, Epps KL, Young DC, Zobell JT. State of the art in cystic fibrosis pharmacology optimization of antimicrobials in the treatment of cystic fibrosis pulmonary exacerbations: III. Executive summary. *Pediatr Pulmonol.* 2021;56(7):1825-1837.
4. Stockmann C, Sherwin CM, Zobell JT, et al. Optimization of anti-pseudomonal antibiotics for cystic fibrosis pulmonary exacerbations: III. fluoroquinolones. *Pediatr Pulmonol.* 2013;48(3):211-220.
5. Zobell JT, Young DC, Waters CD, et al. Optimization of anti-pseudomonal antibiotics for cystic fibrosis pulmonary exacerbations: VI. Executive summary. *Pediatr Pulmonol.* 2013;48(6):525-537.

Acknowledgment: Many thanks to David Seto, PharmD at Phoenix Children's Hospital for his assistance in creating this table.

chest tube placement with drainage is often indicated. Antibiotics are only indicated if there is evidence of a pulmonary exacerbation. Airway clearance therapies should be held, and patients should not perform PFTs for at least 2 weeks after pneumothorax resolution. Pneumothorax in individuals with CF is associated with a high rate of recurrence and, in children with CF, death prior to age 30.

Abdominal pain is a common reason for hospitalization in patients with CF secondary to numerous causes, some of which are CF-specific (**Table 145-7**). Complications such as acute cholecystitis, pancreatitis, bowel obstruction, and GI hemorrhage may represent GI emergencies and require prompt evaluation and treatment.

Recurrent obstruction due to dehydrated intestinal contents can occur in older patients and is referred to as distal intestinal obstruction syndrome (DIOS) (**Figure 145-3**). DIOS presents with symptoms of intestinal obstruction, including abdominal pain, vomiting, and distention. A history of obstipation, or inability to pass stool or gas, is often elicited. Nonadherence to pancreatic enzyme replacement therapy (PERT) recommendations increases risk of DIOS, as unabsorbed fat slows gut motility, promoting fecal dehydration and accumulation of densely packed mucus.

Cholelithiasis is also common, occurring in up to 25% of CF patients. Other potential causes of abdominal pain include pancreatitis,

TABLE 145-6 Intravenous Antibiotics to Treat Pulmonary Exacerbations of Cystic Fibrosis

Organism	Medication	Dose (mg/kg/day)	Dosing Interval (hr)	Maximum Dose (mg/day)
Pseudomonas aeruginosa	Combination therapy with one beta-lactam plus one aminoglycoside may be reasonable			
	Beta-lactam:			
	Cefepime	150-200	6-8	6000-8000
	Ceftazidime	200-400	6-8	8000-12000
	Ciprofloxacin	30	8	1200
	Levofloxacin	<5 years: 20 ≥5 years: 10	<5 years: 12 ≥5 years: 24	750
	Ticarcillin-clavulanate*	400-750†	6	24000-30000
	Piperacillin-tazobactam	350-600††	4-6	18000-24000
	Doripenem	90	8	6000
	Imipenem	100	6	4000
	Meropenem	120	8	6000
	Aztreonam	200-300	6	8000-12000
	Aminoglycoside:			
	Tobramycin	10	24	
	Amikacin	30-35	24	
	Colistimethate	8	24	480
Methicillin-Sensitive Staphylococcus aureus	Cefazolin	150	8	8000
	Nafcillin or Oxacillin	150-200	4-6	12000
Methicillin-Resistant *Staphylococcus aureus*	Clindamycin	20-40	6-8	1800-2700
	Doxycycline	5	12	200
	Linezolid	30-45	8	1800
	Trimethoprim-sulfamethoxazole	15-20§	6-8	960
	Vancomycin	60-80	6	4000
Stenotrophomonas maltophilia	Combination therapy with trimethoprim-sulfamethoxazole plus additional antibiotic may be reasonable			
	Trimethoprim-sulfamethoxazole	15-20§	6-8	960
	Additional:			
	Ampicillin-sulbactam	200-400¶	6	8000
	Ceftazidime	200-400	6-8	8000-12000
	Ciprofloxacin	30	8	1200
	Levofloxacin	<5 years: 20 ≥5 years: 10	<5 years: 12 ≥5 years: 24	750
	Doxycycline	5	12	200
	Minocycline	4 mg/kg × 1 load, then 4	12	400
Haemophilus influenzae	Ampicillin-sulbactam	200-400¶	6	8000
	Ceftriaxone	50-100	24	2000
Achromobacter sp.	Combination therapy with one carbapenem plus additional antibiotic may be reasonable			
	Meropenem	120	8	6000
	Imipenem	100	6	4000
	Additional:			
	Ceftazidime	200-400	6-8	8000-12000
	Ciprofloxacin	30	8	1200
	Minocycline	4 mg/kg × 1, then 4 mg/kg/day	12	400
	Piperacillin-tazobactam	350-600††	4-6	18000-24000
	Trimethoprim-sulfamethoxazole	15-20§	6-8	960

(Continued)

TABLE 145-6 Intravenous Antibiotics to Treat Pulmonary Exacerbations of Cystic Fibrosis (*Continued*)

Organism	Medication	Dose (mg/kg/day)	Dosing Interval (hr)	Maximum Dose (mg/day)
Burkholderia cepacia	Combination therapy with meropenem plus additional antibiotic may be reasonable			
	Meropenem	120	8	6000
	Additional:			
	Amikacin	30-35	24	
	Aztreonam	200-300	6	8000-12000
	Ceftazidime	200-400	6-8	8000-12000
	Chloramphenicol	60-80	6	4000
	Minocycline	4 mg/kg × 1, then 4 mg/kg/day	12	400
	Trimethoprim-sulfamethoxazole	15-20§	6-8	960

*No longer available in the United States.

†Ticarcillin component.

††Piperacillin component.

§Trimethoprim component.

¶Ampicillin component.

References

1. Chmiel JF, Aksamit TR, Chotirmall SH, et al. Antibiotic management of lung infections in cystic fibrosis. I. The microbiome, methicillin-resistant Staphylococcus aureus, gram-negative bacteria, and multiple infections. *Ann Am Thorac Soc.* 2014;11(7):1120-1109.
2. Epps QJ, Epps KL, Young DC, Zobell JT. State of the art in cystic fibrosis pharmacology optimization of antimicrobials in the treatment of cystic fibrosis pulmonary exacerbations: III. Executive summary. *Pediatr Pulmonol.* 2021;56(7):1825-1837.
3. Epps QJ, Epps KL, Zobell JT. Optimization of anti-pseudomonal antibiotics for cystic fibrosis pulmonary exacerbations: II. Cephalosporins and penicillins latest update. *Pediatr Pulmonol.* 2021;56(6):1784-1788.
4. Flume PA, Mogayzel PJ Jr, Robinson KA, et al. Cystic fibrosis pulmonary guidelines: treatment of pulmonary exacerbations. *Am J Respir Crit Care Med.* 2009;180(9):802-808.
5. Gibson RL, Burns JL, Ramsey BW. Pathophysiology and management of pulmonary infections in cystic fibrosis. *Am J Respir Crit Care Med.* 2003;168:918-951.
6. Stockmann C, Sherwin CM, Zobell JT, et al. Optimization of anti-pseudomonal antibiotics for cystic fibrosis pulmonary exacerbations: III. fluoroquinolones. *Pediatr Pulmonol.* 2013;48(3):211-220.
7. Young DC, Zobell JT, Stockmann C, et al. Optimization of anti-pseudomonal antibiotics for cystic fibrosis pulmonary exacerbations: V. Aminoglycosides. *Pediatr Pulmonol.* 2013;48(11):1047-1061.
8. Zobell JT, Young DC, Waters CD, et al. Optimization of anti-pseudomonal antibiotics for cystic fibrosis pulmonary exacerbations: VI. Executive summary. *Pediatr Pulmonol.* 2013;48(6):525-537.
9. Zobell JT, Young DC, Waters CD, et al. Optimization of anti-pseudomonal antibiotics for cystic fibrosis pulmonary exacerbations: I. Aztreonam and carbapenems. *Pediatr Pulmonol.* 2012;47(12):1147-1158.

Acknowledgement: Many thanks to David Seto, PharmD at Phoenix Children's Hospital for his assistance in creating this table.

nephrolithiasis, antibiotic-associated colitis, and fibrosing colonopathy. The etiology of fibrosing colonopathy is unclear but thought to be associated with high-dose PERT. Symptoms include pain, constipation, obstruction, and lower GI bleeding. Findings include submucosal fibrosis and stiffening, edema, and mucosal ulceration of the proximal colon.

CONSULTATION

Most patients with CF are managed by an accredited CF center, and this team should be involved in the care of any hospitalized patient. If admitted to a non-CF center, the patient's center care team should be contacted for management support. There are over 130 CF centers in the United States; contact information for these centers may be found at **http://www.cff.org/ccd/**. The center care team is comprised of a physician (usually a pulmonologist), nurse, dietician, respiratory therapist, social worker, and program coordinator. Other specialties involved in the care of CF patients include gastroenterology, infectious disease, endocrinology, psychiatry, psychology, physical therapy, pharmacy, palliative care, and surgical specialties, such as otolaryngology. As life expectancy increases for CF patients, it is important to ensure smooth transition to adult care, which the CFF recommends should coincide with high school graduation. In CF patients, the transition period from pediatric to adult care is associated with a high risk of hospitalization, highlighting the importance of transition support. The CF Foundation website provides resources to support patients through this transition, but the availability of providers equipped to manage the healthcare needs of adults with CF varies across the country.

ADMISSION CRITERIA

- Pulmonary exacerbation, severe or unresponsive to outpatient management
- Massive hemoptysis, consider with mild-moderate hemoptysis if persistent
- Pneumothorax
- Failure to thrive not improving with outpatient management
- Intestinal obstruction
- Acute cholecystitis or pancreatitis
- GI bleed
- New onset or poorly controlled diabetes

DISCHARGE CRITERIA

- Control of the acute process
- Return to baseline condition or significant improvement with outpatient treatment plan in place

TABLE 145-7 Causes of Abdominal Pain in Cystic Fibrosis

Upper abdominal pain
Gastroesophageal reflux
Gastritis
Gallbladder disease
Pancreatitis
Mid-abdominal pain
Obstipation
Distal intestinal obstruction syndrome
Appendicitis
Irritable bowel syndrome
Steatorrhea
Intussusception
Lower abdominal pain
Irritable bowel syndrome
Steatorrhea
Obstipation
Distal intestinal obstruction syndrome
Antibiotic-associated colitis (*Clostridium difficile*)
Intussusception
Other
Renal stones
Fibrosing colonopathy
Colon cancer
Rectal prolapse

Source: Data from Gabel ME, Galante GJ, Freedman SD. Gastrointestinal and hepatobiliary disease in cystic fibrosis. *Semin Respir Crit Care Med*. 2019;40(6):825-884.

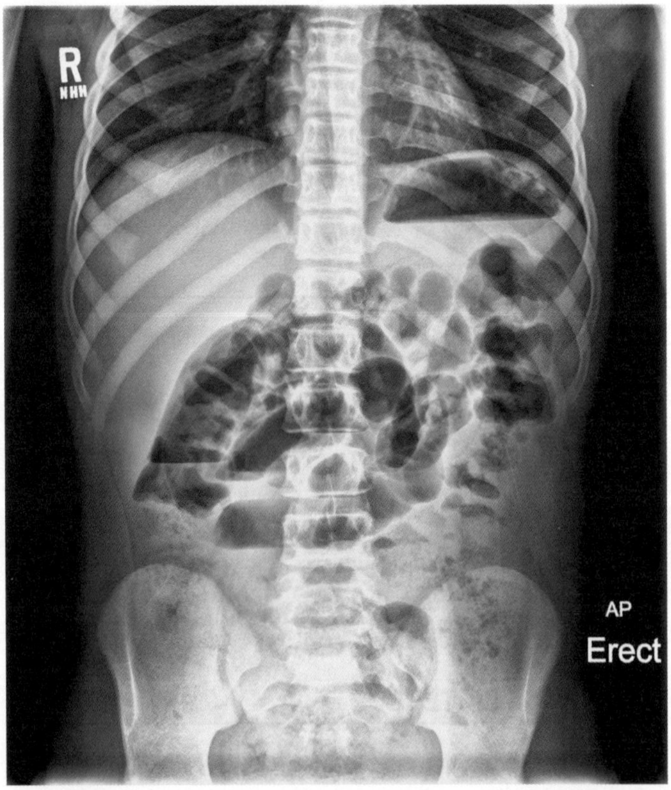

FIGURE 145-3. Dilated loops of small bowel, air fluid levels, and obstipation are seen in this 15-year-old male presenting with distal intestinal obstruction syndrome. (Image used with permission of A. Chidekel, MD.)

KEY POINTS

- CF is a common multisystem disorder with various presentations that should be considered in the differential diagnosis of patients with chronic respiratory or gastrointestinal symptoms.
- Common reasons for the hospitalization of CF patients include pulmonary exacerbation, pneumothorax, and hemoptysis.
- Acute cholecystitis, bowel obstruction, failure to thrive, and new-onset diabetes are other complications of CF that warrant hospitalization.
- Infection control measures are important as highly resistant organisms may colonize CF patients, and prevention of transmission to other immunocompromised hosts is essential.
- CF centers provide primary, extensive, long-term, multidisciplinary care, and these teams should be involved early in the care of CF patients, especially when hospitalized.
- CFTR modulators are available for most CF patients and improve the function of the CFTR protein. Genetic testing is required to select the appropriate modulator for the individual patient's gene defect.
- Although CF is a life-limiting disease, average life expectancy is now into the late 40s and will continue to increase with advances in proactive care.

SUGGESTED READINGS

Bergeron C, Cantin AM. Cystic fibrosis: pathophysiology of lung disease. *Semin Respir Crit Care Med*. 2019;40:715-726.

Blanchard AC, Waters VJ. Microbiology of cystic fibrosis airway disease. *Semin Respir Crit Care Med*. 2019;40(6):727-736.

Cabrini G, Rimessi A, Borgatti M, et al. Role of cystic fibrosis bronchial epithelium in neutrophil chemotaxis. *Front Immunol*. 2020;11:1438.

Cohen-Cymberknoh M, Shoseyov D, Kerem E. Managing cystic fibrosis: strategies that increase life expectancy and improve quality of life. *Am J Respir Crit Care Med*. 2011;183(11):1463-1471.

Cystic Fibrosis Foundation. Respiratory Care Guidelines. https://www.cff.org/medical-professionals/clinical-care-guidelines#respiratory-care-guidelines. Accessed July 6, 2022.

DeSimone E, Tilleman J, Giles ME, Moussa B. Cystic fibrosis: update on treatment guidelines and new recommendations. *US Pharm*. 2018;43(5):16-21.

Dickinson KM, Collaco JM. Cystic fibrosis. *Pediatr Rev*. 2021;42(2):55-67.

Flume PA, Mogayzel PJ Jr, Robinson KA, et al. Clinical Practice Guidelines for Pulmonary Therapies Committee. Cystic Fibrosis Foundation Pulmonary Therapies Committee. Cystic fibrosis pulmonary guidelines: treatment of pulmonary exacerbations. *Am J Respir Crit Care Med*. 2009;180:802-808.

Flume PA, Mogayzel PJ Jr, Robinson KA, et al. Cystic fibrosis pulmonary guidelines: pulmonary complications: hemoptysis and pneumothorax. *Am J Respir Crit Care Med*. 2010;182:298-306.

Goss CH, Heltshe SL, West NE, et al. A randomized clinical trial of antimicrobial duration for cystic fibrosis pulmonary exacerbation treatment. *Am J Respir Crit Care Med*. 2021;204(11):1295-1305.

Granger E, Davies G, Keogh RH. Treatment patterns in people with cystic fibrosis: have they changed since the introduction of ivacaftor? *J Cyst Fibros*. 2022;21(2):316-322.

Kramer-Golinkoff E, Camacho A, Kramer L, Taylor-Cousar JL. A survey: understanding the health and perspectives of people with CF not benefiting from CFTR modulators. *Pediatr Pulmonol*. 2022;57(5):1253-1261.

McClenaghan E, Cosgriff R, Brownlee K, et al. The global impact of SARS-CoV-2 in 181 people with cystic fibrosis. *J Cyst Fibros*. 2020;19(6):868-871.

Mogayzel PJ Jr, Naureckas ET, Robinson KA, et al. Cystic Fibrosis Foundation Pulmonary Clinical Practice Guidelines Committee. Cystic Fibrosis Foundation pulmonary guideline. Pharmacologic approaches to prevention and eradication of initial *Pseudomonas aeruginosa* infection. *Ann Am Thorac Soc*. 2014;11(10):1640-1650.

Nguyen N, Crealey G, O'Neill C. The impact of modulator therapy in cystic fibrosis on patterns of hospitalization related to age. Results from an analysis of US inpatient episodes 2006-2016. *J Cyst Fibros.* 2021;20(6):e114-e117.

O'Sullivan BP, Freedman SD. Cystic fibrosis. *Lancet.* 2009;373(9678):1891-1904.

Pique L, Graham S, Pearl M, Kharrazi M, Schrijver I. Cystic fibrosis newborn screening programs: implications of the CFTR variant spectrum in nonwhite patients. *Genet Med.* 2017 Jan;19(1):36-44.

Polgreen PM, Comellas AP. Clinical phenotypes of cystic fibrosis carriers. *Annu Rev Med.* 2022;73:563-574.

Ramsey ML, Lara LF, Gariepy CE, et al. National trends of hospitalizations in cystic fibrosis highlight a need for pediatric to adult transition clinics. *Pancreas.* 2021;50(5):704-709.

Sabharwal S. Gastrointestinal manifestations of cystic fibrosis. *Gastroenterol Hepatol* (NY). 2016;12(1):43-47.

Sosnay PR, White TB, Farrell PM, et al. Diagnosis of cystic fibrosis in nonscreened populations. *J Pediatr.* 2017;181S:S52-S57.e2.

Stallings VA, Stark LJ, Robinson KA, et al. Evidence-based practice recommendations for nutrition-related management of children and adults with cystic fibrosis and pancreatic insufficiency: results of a systematic review. *J Am Diet Assoc.* 2008;108(5):832-839.

CHAPTER 146 Choking and Foreign Body Aspiration

Alexandra M. Clark, MD and Janice Tsai, MD

BACKGROUND

Public health interventions over the past 54 years have led to a significant reduction in the number of choking-related injuries. Despite these interventions, choking and foreign body aspiration (FBA) will continue to be a risk because children remain curious and explore their world orally. As such, practitioners in the ambulatory clinic space, urgent care, emergency department, and inpatient wards must be knowledgeable about the full range of potential presentations of choking-related injuries. While the act of choking disrupts respiration due to a constricted or obstructed airway, it can be temporary, and a child might dislodge the object causing the choking event. Aspiration is when the foreign material descends into the trachea beyond the vocal cords which can lead to partial or full airway obstruction. Airway obstruction from external compression should be considered in certain clinical presentations. For any aspiration event leading to partial or full obstruction, children may present in full or impending cardiopulmonary arrest, they may be stable but symptomatic, or they may have chronic symptoms that have not been previously linked to an aspiration event.

The United States sees thousands of emergency room visits annually due to FBA, which accounts for more than 100 pediatric deaths per year. FBA has a slight predominance in males, and infants and toddlers are at higher risk of FBA at a younger age when there are older siblings in the home who can place food/objects into their younger sibling's mouth. In a review of the Nationwide Inpatient Sample from 2009 to 2011, children admitted with FBA had a mortality rate of 1.8% and an additional 2.2% suffered anoxic brain injury with long-term consequences, with an annual overall inpatient cost associated with pediatric FBA estimated in 2015 around $12.8 million.

PATHOPHYSIOLOGY

Children under 3 years of age account for the greatest burden of aspiration events in children both in the United States and worldwide, and organic material accounts for as much as 80% of foreign bodies in these children.

TABLE 146-1 Common Objects With a High Risk for Causing Choking

Foods
Hot dogs
Grapes
Peanuts
Other nuts
Popcorn
Raw carrots
Apples
Toys
Latex balloons
Small balls
Marbles
Toys containing small parts
Jewelry
Watch batteries

Children have narrow airways with less secondary alveolar connections, so even partial obstructions are more likely to be symptomatic. Developmentally, young children have less oral coordination with fewer primary teeth for mastication along with high respiratory rates which all lead to increased risk. Children with intellectual disability, anatomic airway malformations, or hypotonia carry an increased risk of aspiration past their young childhood years. Both food and non-food objects are choking, aspiration, and ultimately obstruction hazards in pediatric patients due to anatomic features and developmental maturity with organic material more likely to be aspirated than inorganic. Common choking hazards are classically small, smooth, or slippery, but can be spherical or asymmetric if the object can conform to the child's airway, such as small balls or balloons (**Table 146-1**). Medical providers should specifically ask about food and classic choking hazards when concerned about FBA.

Foreign bodies create variable degrees of airway obstruction and therefore disrupt the ability of oxygenation to occur distal to the obstruction. This makes the location and severity of the obstruction a critical element in the viability of the child after an aspiration event with proximal and more complete obstructions having the greatest risk for immediate anoxic brain damage and cardiopulmonary arrest. All foreign bodies cause an inflammatory reaction and delayed removal causes an increase in granulation tissue and atelectasis in response to the foreign body. Peanuts, seeds, and nuts are the most common organic material aspirated, and are high in oil which triggers a more intense inflammatory response causing further narrowing of the airway and distal consolidation which may be seen on chest radiographs. Mucus production and edema from the inflammatory response further narrows the airway and worsens obstruction. The longer a foreign object remains in the airway, the greater the risk for secondary bacterial infections, granuloma formation, and mucosal edema. These elements complicate removal and lead to increased risk during bronchoscopy of bleeding, airway trauma, bronchospasm, incomplete removal, and subsequent need for partial lung resection.

CLINICAL PRESENTATION

The clinical presentation of FBA is primarily respiratory, and since the symptoms can mimic other pediatric pulmonary diagnoses, including asthma, croup, and community-acquired pneumonia, a clinician must keep the differential diagnosis of FBA in mind. Acute complete airway obstruction at or above the level of the carina will always be symptomatic and poses the highest risk of morbidity and mortality. In the field, these patients can present with aphonia, absence of cough, and agitation, but will progress rapidly to cardiopulmonary arrest if the obstruction is not at least partially relieved. Partial obstructions have great variability in presentation, but infants younger than 1 year have cough and dyspnea as the most prevalent symptoms with rales as the most common physical examination finding. In contrast, children older than 1 year have decreased breath sounds followed by wheezing as the most common physical sign. If a partial obstruction occurs as a result of obstruction above the thoracic inlet, symptoms of stridor or cough will be worse during inspiration as the effect of atmospheric pressure compresses the trachea below the site of obstruction while intrathoracic obstruction is most severe during expiration.

Obstructions in the distal airway cause less immediate respiratory symptoms and are more likely to have normal physical examination findings; patients are more likely to present with chronic findings or have a delayed diagnosis since families may not recall a choking event. Conversely, proximal airway obstructions will present with increased respiratory effort as indicated by nasal flaring, use of accessory muscles, or retractions, and are likely to present with cough, localized wheezing, or asymmetric breath sounds depending on the level of obstruction. Cardiopulmonary arrest can occur from prolonged partial obstruction or due to movement from partial to complete airway obstruction so careful monitoring of these children is required while awaiting bronchoscopy. Particular attention should be paid to both lung fields as the propensity for aspiration to the right side is less pronounced in children.

Children with witnessed aspiration associated with a choking episode (penetration syndrome) have the highest likelihood of finding a foreign body on bronchoscopy while children without a witnessed choking event are more likely to have delayed diagnosis. The chest radiograph (CXR) in children with a witnessed aspiration and choking episode is more likely to be abnormal with atelectasis being the most common finding, followed by pneumonia. In addition, children younger than 2 years make up the majority of children with a delayed diagnosis of FBA. Thus, children in this age range with persistent pulmonary symptoms that are not responsive to traditional therapy should be evaluated for FBA in addition to uncommon findings such as monophonic wheezing or recurrent pneumonia in the same lobe, as well as unexplained lung abscesses. Children with prolonged retention of a foreign body generally present with persistent or recurrent fever, cough, or unilateral wheezing due to the granulation tissue, recurrent pulmonary infections, atelectasis, or bronchiectasis that develops. Other significant predictors of FBA include self-reporting in older children, children younger than 3 years old, children with developmental delay or neurological impairment, children with behavioral concerns, hypotonia, presence of anatomical abnormalities of the aerodigestive tract, or history of dysphagia. FBA must remain high on the differential in these populations when presenting with otherwise unexplained respiratory symptoms.

EVALUATION

FBA is less common than foreign body ingestion, but the diagnosis of FBA requires a strong index of clinical suspicion, as only 50% to 60% of cases present and are diagnosed within 24 hours of an aspiration event. The classic triad of cough, wheezing, and dyspnea/diminished aeration is not universally present, but instead only present in 31% of early diagnoses (within 24 hours of the aspiration event) compared to 47% in late diagnosis (after 24 hours of the aspiration event). Delays in diagnosis have been attributed to unwitnessed events, interval asymptomatic phases after mucosal cough receptors accommodate, or misdiagnoses with other respiratory illnesses. History remains the most reliable indicator of FBA, with 80% to 90% of FBAs having a reported choking episode, and a history of a choking episode reported to have sensitivity up to 97% and specificity up to 63%.

A patient who self-reports a choking episode or has a witnessed choking episode and does not self-expulse the foreign body does not need imaging studies and should proceed to definitive evaluation and management with bronchoscopy. For patients with a suspected FBA, radiographs can provide additional information, are widely available, relatively inexpensive, and can be obtained quickly. However, only 10% of FBAs are radiopaque, and up to 80% of laryngotracheal and 50% of bronchial foreign bodies have normal radiographs, with radiographs more likely to be positive after 24 hours. The odds of having an abnormal CXR increases if there are both clinical symptoms and physical examination findings consistent with FBA, but since organic material is mostly radiolucent and most abnormalities are suggested by nonspecific secondary changes, a normal X-ray does not rule out FBA. Symptoms of cough, inspiratory stridor, hoarseness, and throat pain suggest a laryngotracheal foreign body for which an airway radiograph can be obtained. This should be obtained as posteroanterior and lateral views with the arms and shoulders positioned inferiorly and posteriorly to optimize the image of the larynx and trachea. As most foreign bodies are radiolucent, secondary findings of a subglottic density, prevertebral soft tissue swelling, or overdistension of the hypopharynx may suggest the diagnosis.

Compared to laryngotracheal foreign bodies, bronchial foreign bodies are more commonly misdiagnosed on initial evaluation and lead to delayed diagnosis. Symptoms of cough, tachypnea, dyspnea, wheezing, and diminished aeration suggest a bronchial foreign body for which a chest radiograph can be obtained. In children, anteroposterior chest radiographs with inspiratory and expiratory films can help lateralize the foreign body by emphasizing air trapping on the ipsilateral side of the aspiration, causing mediastinal shift contralateral to the side of aspiration. Some obstructions have a check valve effect, where air is inhaled but cannot be fully expelled during exhalation leading to hyperinflation of the ipsilateral lung. Check valves have partial obstruction while ball valve or stop valves have complete obstruction. Given that 75% of FBA occurs in children younger than 3 years of age, CXR should be obtained as bilateral lateral decubitus views because this age group is unlikely to cooperate with inspiratory and expiratory films. Usually, the mediastinum shifts to the left on a left lateral decubitus and to the right on a right lateral decubitus due to gravity, but the check valve effect leads to hyperinflation of the ipsilateral lung, without the expected mediastinal shift (**Figure 146-1**). Other obstructions can have a ball valve effect or stop valve effect with impeded air passage, leading to atelectasis and consolidation of the involved bronchopulmonary segment with subsequent collapse. Therefore, secondary findings of focal air trapping, local airspace disease, or pneumothorax may suggest the diagnosis. While adults are more likely to have FBA in the right mainstem bronchus, the propensity for aspiration to the right side is less pronounced in children. Children have more symmetrical bronchial angles until their aortic knob fully develops in adolescence, which then displaces the left mainstem bronchus to create a more obtuse angle compared to the right.

Fluoroscopy is not indicated as it can be normal in 53% of cases, and difficult to obtain in uncooperative children, while also highly operator dependent. High-resolution multidetector computed tomography cannot differentiate FBA from mucous plugs and should only be used on rare occasions as a last resort as it contradicts the contemporary approach of minimizing unnecessary ionizing irradiation exposure. It can be considered in patients with differential diagnoses confounding or mimicking FBA such as tracheobronchial congenital anomalies, extrinsic compressions, or vascular anomalies, but can be impractical as high-quality scans require movement restriction necessitating sedation which can lead to diagnostic delay. In addition, sedation alters the forces of breathing and may result in a partial obstruction becoming a full obstruction. Magnetic resonance imaging is not indicated as it also most often requires sedation and can lead to diagnostic delay.

MANAGEMENT

Acute management often begins before a child arrives at the hospital and requires rapid assessment for airway patency and respiratory status. Many patients will manifest a forceful cough by reflex to clear the airway, and patients who can cough, speak, or cry should be allowed to spontaneously expulse the foreign body. Patients who are unable to make sounds or exchange air require immediate emergency action either by the caregiver or emergency medical technicians. If the object can be visualized in the posterior pharynx, then an attempt can be made to remove it, otherwise blind oropharyngeal finger sweeps should not be performed as they can further lodge the foreign body and lead to worsened occlusion. For patients 12 months of age or less, back slaps alternating with chest thrusts in head-down position is the treatment of choice, with

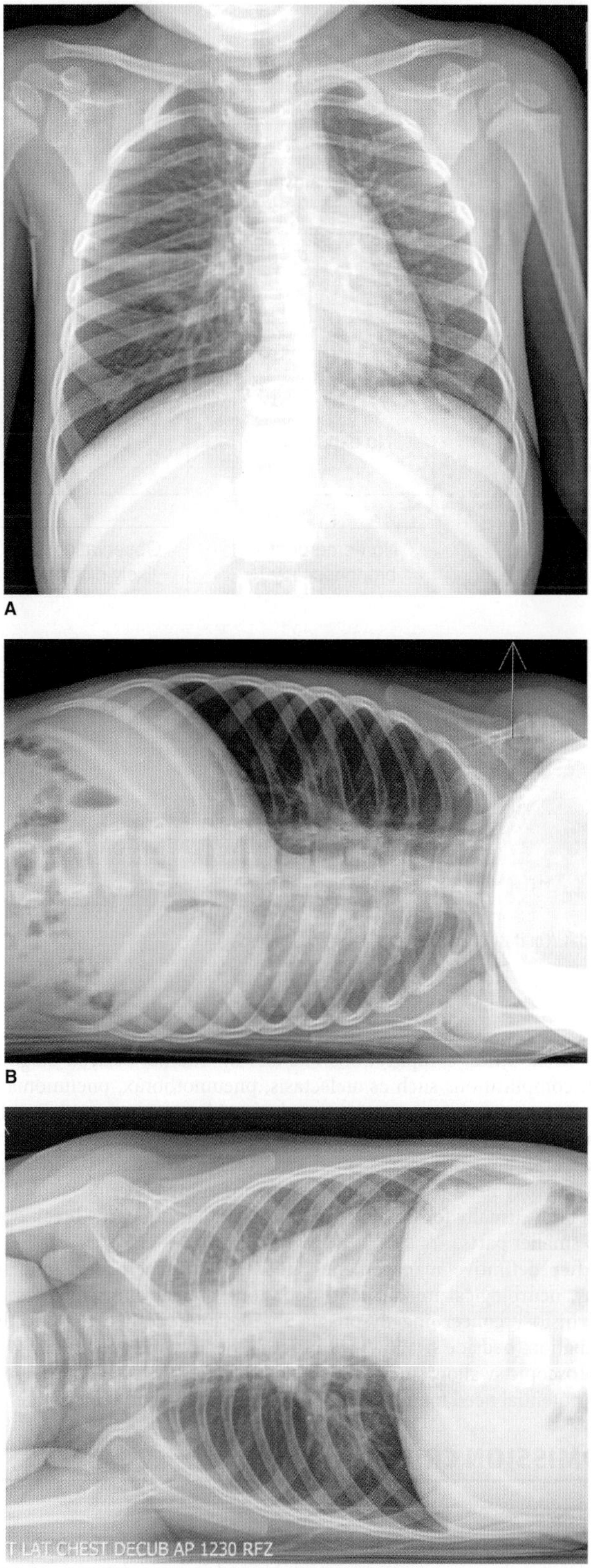

FIGURE 146-1. A. Frontal chest X-ray in a 21-month-old with witnessed choking event (aspiration of a peanut M&M). No radiopaque foreign body along the airway, however asymmetric hyper-expansion of the right lung with right middle lobe opacity suggests possible airway obstruction. B. Left lateral decubitus X-ray in the same patient showing left lung is under-expanded from expected dependent position (normal), while the right lung is hyper-expanded, suspicious for radiolucent foreign body (abnormal). C. Right lateral decubitus X-ray in the same patient showing left lung is re-expanded from expected non-dependent position (normal), while the right lung remains hyper-expanded, suspicious for radiolucent foreign body (abnormal).

abdominal thrusts being the treatment of choice for children older than 12 months of age. In children older than 12 months of age, 80% of normal respirations occur using the diaphragm so abdominal thrusts create abdominal pressure to compress the diaphragm upward, which raises intrathoracic pressure to help expel the obstructing object. If the patient becomes hypoxic, the muscle tone diminishes so abdominal thrusts that may have initially been ineffective may later become effective. Patients should be kept as calm and comfortable as possible. In patients who are unable to breathe and become unresponsive, cardiopulmonary resuscitation should be initiated. Prompt, effective first aid may often prevent morbidity and mortality.

If the patient has hypoxia, supplemental oxygen should be provided in the least invasive method possible such as with simple nasal cannula or simple mask. Positive pressure ventilation should be avoided unless the foreign body is confirmed to be bronchial or the patient is undergoing bronchoscopy, as this can wedge the foreign body further into the airway and could lead to a partial obstruction progressing to a complete obstruction or can lead to worsening hyper-expansion and subsequent pneumothorax.

Patients with high suspicion for FBA should proceed straight to bronchoscopy for definitive management rather than delaying care with imaging, while those with mild to moderate suspicion for FBA should receive imaging with a screening radiograph (**Figure 146-2**). Depending on the institution, this will require coordination between the emergency department, anesthesiology, and either pulmonology or otolaryngology teams, and occasionally respiratory therapy, surgery, hospital medicine, or intensive care teams. For those with a stable airway (usually bronchial foreign bodies), bronchoscopy should be scheduled during optimal operating room staffing conditions with trained professionals of the interdisciplinary team after the routine preoperative fasting time to minimize complications, but if there is risk of acute deterioration (usually laryngotracheal foreign bodies) then bronchoscopy should not be delayed and should be performed emergently. Patients with either abnormal imaging or abnormal physical examination findings should also proceed to bronchoscopy once optimal operating room staffing conditions are available. Bronchoscopy is not a mandatory recommendation for patients with normal imaging and normal physical examination but as this does not rule out FBA joint decision-making should be made with the patient, caregivers, and medical professionals regarding balancing the risks of bronchoscopy with those of a missed aspiration, which may vary on a case-by-case basis. The complication rate is twice as high for patients with delayed diagnoses or undergoing bronchoscopy after 24 hours of diagnosis.

Definitive diagnosis and management can only be made with bronchoscopy. The American Thoracic Society states that "rigid instruments are superior for detailed anatomic assessment of the larynx and cervical trachea and for operative manipulation, principally foreign body extraction." Rigid bronchoscopy performed under general anesthesia currently remains the gold standard of care, however, studies over recent years have varied suggesting the utility of flexible bronchoscopy. During bronchoscopy, both sides should be evaluated to ensure complete removal of any residual food or objects. Before bronchoscopy in the early 1900s, the mortality rate was approximately 50%, but with the improvement in techniques, instruments, and modern anesthesia, bronchoscopy is effective in >95% of patients in removal of the FB, with less than 1% complication rate. The remaining ~5% of patients may need further management including surgical retrieval and open thoracotomy with bronchotomy or lobectomy.

For patients with low suspicion or low risk for FBA who do not undergo bronchoscopy, anticipatory guidance should be provided to the caregivers on signs and symptoms of FBA, particularly later findings as in delayed diagnoses, caregivers often do not report the choking event. Patients with delayed diagnoses can later present with complications of a retained foreign body such as inflammation, atelectasis, bronchiectasis, focal pneumonia, pneumothorax, pneumomediastinum, abscess, or with partial obstruction progressing to total obstruction due to swelling and liquid absorption. These patients may have granulation tissue growing around the object, making the retrieval more difficult. They may also be vulnerable to the adverse effects from prior treatments such as repeat courses of steroids and antibiotics. Aspirated foreign bodies can lead to

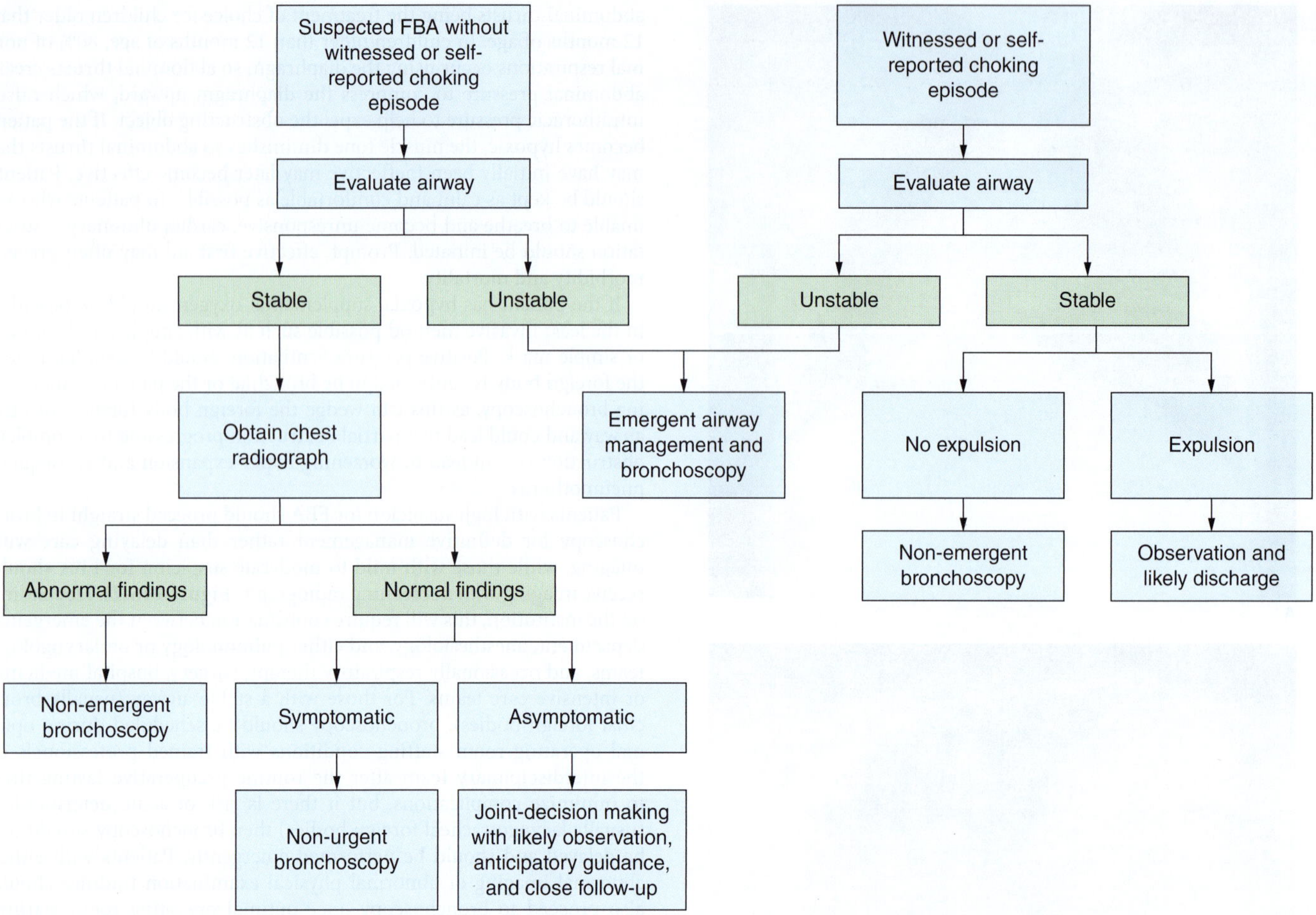

FIGURE 146-2. Management algorithm for suspected, witnessed, or self-reported choking episodes. (Courtesy of Drs. Alexandra Clark and Janice Tsai.)

superimposed focal pneumonias due to retained secretions and subsequent bacterial overgrowth and thus cultures should be obtained during bronchoscopy for patients showing signs or symptoms of aspiration pneumonia. The most common organisms isolated from tracheobronchial samples are oropharyngeal flora, *Streptococcus pneumoniae*, *Haemophilus influenzae*, and *Moraxella catarrhalis*. Amoxicillin-Sulbactam if not tolerating enteral medications, or Amoxicillin-Clavulanic acid if tolerating enteral medications (Clindamycin if anaphylactic penicillin allergy) should be first-line empiric therapy for patients with suspected aspiration pneumonia, with culture- and local antibiogram-directed narrowing of antibiotics once tracheobronchial culture results. Antibiotics are not indicated or recommended for patients without signs or symptoms of aspiration pneumonia.

For early diagnoses, symptoms usually resolve once the object is removed. Since prolonged retained foreign bodies result in inflammatory and parenchymal changes, removal of the object may not always result in immediate resolution of this inflammation; therefore, bronchodilators may improve lower airway ventilation and oxygenation when edema or bronchospasms are present. Bronchodilators and steroids have sometimes been administered intraoperatively, or postoperatively, but no studies to date have specifically evaluated the role of these medications in aspirated foreign bodies.

For early diagnoses of FBA, most patients who undergo uncomplicated removal shortly after the aspiration are discharged within 4 hours of bronchoscopy. Specifically for nonorganic FBA, over 80% of children are released from the emergency department the same day, with only approximately 11% requiring admission or transfer to a facility with advanced care available. Patients more likely to require admission following bronchoscopy are those with longer bronchoscopy and anesthesia times, complications like airway trauma, delayed diagnosis with complications such as atelectasis, pneumothorax, pneumonia, or those requiring postoperative supplemental oxygen, especially children who already have underlying respiratory diseases such as asthma or chronic lung disease. A small subset, approximately 1% to 3%, of patients may need repeat bronchoscopy for complete removal of a foreign body, usually for organic food material that can easily break down into smaller parts.

After definitive management, patients with severe developmental delay, neurological impairment, poor tone or neuromuscular disease, and history concerning dysphagia should undergo a clinical feeding evaluation (bedside swallow) with speech therapy, and a follow-up video fluoroscopic swallow study as indicated to assess the safety of oral feeds and potential need for adjustment in current diet prior to discharge.

ADMISSION CRITERIA

Pre-bronchoscopy criteria:

- Stable airway for which bronchoscopy is required but the decision to perform during regular operating hours has been determined to be the safest
- Unstable airway for which inpatient care must occur while awaiting bronchoscopy

Post-bronchoscopy criteria:

- Unstable airway after removal of foreign body
- Persistent hypoxia
- Need for additional diagnostic workup prior to safe feeding

DISCHARGE CRITERIA

- Removal of the foreign body without residual respiratory compromise
- Baseline home oxygen need level
- Safe transition to ambulatory care has been ensured, including specialist follow up if needed
- Safety education has been provided to the family to prevent recurrence

PREVENTION

Legislation related to FBA started in 1969, when the Child Protection and Toy Safety Act was created to regulate the size of product parts designed for children, choking hazard warning labels, and public awareness campaigns. In 1979, the Federal Hazardous Substances Act (FHSA) banned toy products with small parts intended for use in children under age 3. In 1972, Congress enacted the Consumer Product Safety Act to develop further safety standards presenting risk of injury or death. The Consumer Product Safety Commission developed the small parts test fixture in 1980, which is a 3.175 cm diameter (1.25 inches) cylinder with a slanted bottom, with depth ranging from 2.54 to 5.71 cm (1-2.25 inches) meant to test for objects that could slip into the posterior pharynx and cause obstruction. Any products that fit through this cylinder were banned for children under age 3. Balls intended for age under age 3 were also required to be greater than 4.44 cm (1.75 inches) in diameter. In 1994, the FHSA was amended to require choking-hazard warning labels on packages for small balls, balloons, marbles, and certain toys/games with small parts intended for use by children in defined age groups. More recently, the FHSA was amended in 2008 to require choking hazard warnings not just on the actual product, but to also be displayed on or adjacent to any product advertisements on websites, catalogs, and printed materials.

Over the 50 years since the Child Protection and Toy Safety Act, object-related aspiration deaths decreased from 1.02 per 100,000 children in 1968, to 0.25 per 100,000 children in 2017. Still, objects that pass the small parts test fixture evaluation account for more than 20% of both non-fatal as well as fatal aspiration incidences, suggesting that more stringent parameters could prevent more morbidity and mortality. Legislation to standardize the depth and increase the diameter of the small parts text fixture cylinder could further prevent injuries and fatalities in children. Public education campaigns can also better target toy rubber balloons, as they account for 43% of childhood deaths related to non-organic FBA, as well as round, ovoid, or cylindrical objects that have high elasticity, high lubricity, or pliability/ability to conform as they pose the greatest risk of choking death due to the ability to completely occlude the airway with a snug fit, as well as being difficult to dislodge with rescue maneuvers.

Caregivers should receive anticipatory guidance education that part of normal development includes infants and toddlers exploring by seeing, touching, and tasting the environment around them, before they have developed molars or mature coordinated chewing and swallowing skills. Caregivers should be counseled on the most common aspiration risks no later than the 6-month well child check, when children start developing the fine motor dexterity required to pick up small objects and place them into their mouths, as well as becoming more mobile.

The American Academy of Pediatrics (AAP) recommends cutting up raw fruits and vegetables into small bite-sized pieces, avoiding hard candy and gum before age 6, keeping small objects out of the child's reach while child-proofing the home, having young children seated and supervised while eating with minimal distractions (ensuring they are not walking, running, or lying down while eating), and ensuring caregivers are familiar with or trained on choking-related rescue maneuvers as well as toy safety and labeling. The AAP Committee on Injury, Violence, and Poison Prevention recommends for the CPSC to work on safer toy storage in stores, more stringent choking hazard warnings, for manufacturers to improve the effectiveness of product recalls, and increase efforts to prevent the resale of recalled products. The committee also calls for the Food and Drug Administration to create a systematic institutionalized process for examining and addressing hazards related to food aspirations because while food items are the most commonly aspirated objects in infants and toddlers, they are not regulated by the FHSA or subject to any testing for aspiration risk.

KEY POINTS

- Choking still presents a significant safety risk to children, particularly under 3 years of age, and aspiration events are life-threatening.
- Children are more likely to aspirate organic foreign bodies and counseling parents and caregivers starting no later than 6 months of age on food safety is recommended to decrease this risk.
- Infants and toddlers are at higher risk of FBA at a younger age when there are older siblings in the home who can place food/objects into their younger sibling's mouth.
- Toy rubber balloons account for 43% of childhood deaths related to nonorganic FBA.
- Aspiration of a foreign body creates an inflammatory process which compounds the obstruction, leading to worsening hypoxia and respiratory distress.
- The signs and symptoms of an aspiration event can mimic common childhood respiratory illnesses so FBA should be considered in the differential for respiratory illnesses as early recognition and definitive treatment is key.
- Clinical presentation varies widely from complete cardiopulmonary arrest to chronic cough based on proximity of the foreign body to the trachea and percentage of obstruction.
- Unlike adults, where FBA is more likely on the right, children can aspirate into either lung field so radiographic findings on the left should still prompt consideration of FBA.
- Chest radiograph is commonly used but since most foreign bodies are radiopaque, a normal chest radiograph does not exclude the diagnosis.
- Lateral decubitus X-rays are helpful diagnostically for young children who cannot cooperate with inhalation/exhalation films to observe for air trapping.
- Early removal of the foreign body is correlated with excellent outcomes, while delayed removal significantly increases the risk of chronic conditions or even lobectomy.
- Bronchoscopy (flexible or rigid) without CXR is indicated in witnessed choking/aspiration events (penetration syndrome).
- Admission after successful removal of the foreign body is based on the clinical stability of the child, and whether they need further work-up.

SUGGESTED READINGS

Committee on Injury, Violence, and Poison Prevention. prevention of choking among children. *Pediatrics*. 2010;125(3):601-607.

Cramer JD, Meraz T, Lavin JM, et al. Object-related aspiration deaths in children and adolescents in the United States, 1968-2017. *JAMA*. 2019;322(20):2020-2022.

Goyal S, Jain S, Rai G, et al. Clinical variables responsible for early and late diagnosis of foreign body aspiration in pediatrics age group. *J Cardiothoracic Surg*. 2020;15:271.

Green, S. Ingested and aspirated foreign bodies. *Pediatr Rev*. 2015;36(10):430-437.

Laya BF, Restrepo R, Lee EY. Practical imaging evaluation of foreign bodies in children. *Rad Clinics of North Amer*. 2017;55(4):845-867.

Serser SI, Rick WH, El Diasty MM, et al. Inhaled foreign bodies: presentation, management and value of history and plain chest radiography in delayed presentation. *Otolaryngol–Head Neck Surg*. 2006;134:92-99.

CHAPTER 147 Pulmonary Function Testing

Bridget C. Allard, DO and Parisa Kaviany, MD

BACKGROUND

Pulmonary function testing encompasses a variety of techniques and noninvasive tests to assist in the diagnosis and management of many respiratory conditions in pediatric patients. The indications for pulmonary function testing include: (1) documenting the presence of obstructive or restrictive ventilatory defects in the course of establishing a diagnosis, (2) monitoring the course of a known pulmonary disease (e.g., cystic fibrosis, asthma), (3) monitoring for pulmonary toxicity related to treatment (e.g., amiodarone, radiation, chemotherapy), and (4) monitoring response to therapy.

PULMONARY FUNCTION LABORATORY

The pulmonary function tests described herein require specialized equipment and experienced personnel. The equipment and laboratory should conform to the standards published by the American Thoracic Society, including daily calibration, biologic controls, and infection control practices. A stadiometer for accurate height measurement is required. The personnel should be patient, have the appropriate training, and be comfortable working with children of a variety of ages, who often require different coaching strategies. The space for testing should be quiet and free of distractions. During the COVID-19 pandemic, the American Thoracic Society released guidelines for the safe operation of pulmonary function testing labs. In addition to monitoring community prevalence of COVID-19 and prioritizing essential tests, staff should wear appropriate personal protective equipment. It is recommended to use in-line filters and to clean the equipment and the room after each use. A negative-pressure room and high-efficiency particulate air (HEPA) filter can improve room ventilation and air filtration. If bronchodilator testing is needed, use of a metered-dose inhaler (MDI) is preferred to nebulizer.

The values measured in the laboratory are usually normalized with the use of reference equations, most commonly based on the subject's height, gender, and age. With these equations, a predicted value can be calculated for each parameter, and the measured flows can be reported as a percentage of the predicted value or as a standardized deviation score (Z-score). Predicted values from different pulmonary function laboratories may not be directly comparable if different reference equations are used.

SPIROMETRY

Spirometry is the measurement of airflow during a maximally forced exhalation and is most commonly used for the evaluation of pediatric obstructive lung diseases such as asthma and cystic fibrosis (**Table 147-1**). Airflow rate is inversely proportional to the fourth power of the radius of the airway, therefore small or obstructed airways result in reduced airflow rates. The parameters measured by spirometry are considered to be reproducible in subjects, making them useful for assessing response to treatment over time.

Most children by the age of 6 years are able to follow directions and perform spirometry maneuvers. Some children as young as 3 to 4 years are able to perform spirometry. To perform spirometry, the subject breathes through a mouthpiece connected to a pneumotachometer while wearing nose clips. After maximal inhalation to total lung capacity (TLC), the subject is coached through a rapid and maximal exhalation for a minimum of 6 seconds until the lungs have emptied. Testing must meet criteria for reproducibility and acceptability. At least three efforts are required, with two efforts having an exhaled volume within 5% of each other to meet the criteria for reproducibility. Common errors that limit the acceptability of the study include coughing during the maneuver, early termination of exhalation, and leak at the mouthpiece. Due to the detailed nuances, review of the results by a trained professional is necessary for interpretation.

TABLE 147-1 Summary of Clinical Indications and Applications of Pulmonary Function Tests

Test Type	Clinical Indication	Examples of Clinical Application
Spirometry	Evaluation of an obstructive ventilatory defect	Diagnostic tool for asthma Response to treatment of cystic fibrosis exacerbation
Lung volumes (plethysmography, dilution techniques)	Evaluation of a restrictive ventilatory defect	Diagnostic tool for pulmonary involvement in systemic rheumatologic disease
Diffusing capacity for carbon monoxide (DLCO)	Evaluation of a gas transfer defect	Diagnostic tool for diffuse alveolar hemorrhage
Maximum expiratory pressure (MEP), maximum inspiratory pressure (MIP)	Evaluation of strength of muscles of respiration	Prognostic tool for neuromuscular respiratory disease
Cardiopulmonary exercise test (CPET)	Evaluation of exercise tolerance	Diagnostic tool for pulmonary or cardiac limitations to exercise
Exercise-induced bronchospasm (EIB) test	Evaluation of etiology of exercise intolerance	Diagnostic tool to differentiate between extrathoracic and intrathoracic etiologies
6-minute walk test (6MWT)	Evaluation of functional status in a patient with known pulmonary disease	Prognostic tool for patients with advanced lung disease

Several parameters can be calculated from these spirometry maneuvers. First, the total exhaled volume is termed the forced vital capacity (FVC). It is important to note that the volume remaining in the lungs after maximal exhalation (residual volume) is not measured with spirometry (**Figure 147-1**). The forced expiratory volume in the first second is the FEV_1. The forced expiratory flow in the mid-expiratory phase (i.e., the airflow rate between 25% of the exhaled volume and 75% of the exhaled volume) is the $FEF_{25\%-75\%}$ (or occasionally referred to as the maximal mid-expiratory flow). The patterns of these parameters can suggest an obstructive or a restrictive defect (**Table 147-2**). Low FEV_1/FVC ratio along with low FEV_1 is suggestive of an obstructive ventilatory defect. FEV_1 is reduced due to a decrease in the elastic recoil of the lung and is considered to be a reproducible metric. A normal FEV_1/FVC ratio along with low FVC and low FEV_1 is suggestive of a restrictive ventilatory defect, although the additional test of lung volume measurements is required to accurately diagnose restrictive lung disease (RLD). However, in some cases of RLD with increased residual volume (RV), flow rates can be abnormally high in late exhalation due to an increase in elastic recoil and radial traction holding airways open.

If an obstructive defect is observed on spirometry testing, reversibility can also be assessed using spirometry. A bronchodilator is administered, and the test is repeated in 15 to 20 minutes. Commonly, a 12% increase in the FEV_1 is considered indicative of a significant response.

When spirometry-measured flow is plotted against exhaled volume (**Figure 147-1A**), the resultant curve can help locate the site of any flow limitation. Intrathoracic obstructive defects such as asthma and cystic fibrosis usually result in a curve that is concave to the volume axis (**Figure 147-1B**), whereas restrictive defects such as pulmonary hypoplasia or neuromuscular weakness usually have a normally shaped but narrow curve (**Figure 147-1C**). Airway obstruction can manifest as flattening of the inspiratory limb of the flow volume curve if the lesion is variable and extrathoracic (e.g., laryngomalacia or vocal cord paresis), flatting of the expiratory limb of the flow volume curve if the lesion is variable and intrathoracic (e.g., compressible tracheal malignancy),

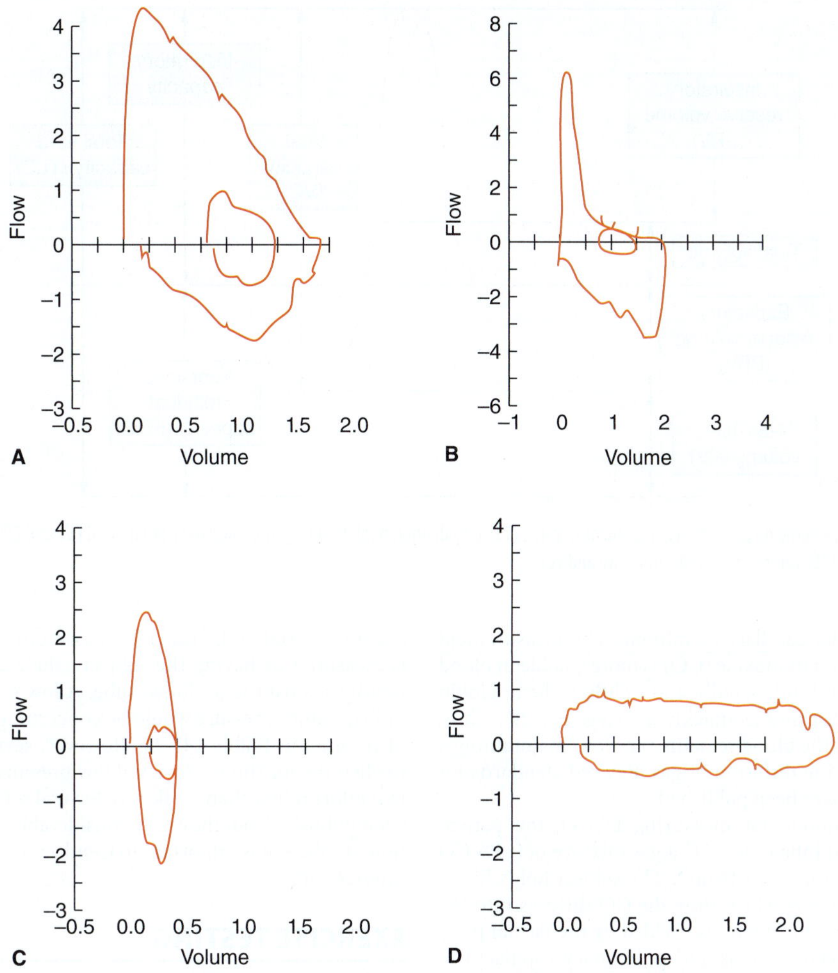

FIGURE 147-1. Flow-volume curves. The normal curve (A) has a smooth, linear decrease in flow from near total lung capacity (to the left) to residual volume (to the right). Note that time is not represented in these curves but is recorded in a separate volume-time curve (not shown). In a patient with obstructive lung disease (B), the curve is concave toward the volume access, such that for any given lung volume, measured flow is lower than predicted. Restrictive lung diseases (C) result in a curve that has a small, exhaled lung volume and is narrow, but without concavity. Fixed airway obstruction (D) results in a curve that is flattened in both inspiration and exhalation.

or flattening of both the inspiratory and expiratory portions of the curve (**Figure 147-1D**) if the lesion is fixed (e.g., subglottic stenosis).

LUNG VOLUMES

Although decreased FVC or high expiratory flow rates on spirometry may suggest RLD, lung volume measurements are necessary to confirm the diagnosis. In RLD, the inspired lung volume is limited due to a decrease in compliance. Disease states that affect lung growth alter both airway caliber and lung volume. These diseases include pulmonary hypoplasia due to severe oligohydramnios or space-occupying lesions (e.g., diaphragmatic hernia, cystic adenomatoid malformation), bronchopulmonary dysplasia, and conditions that alter the growth of the rib cage (e.g., thoracic dystrophies, scoliosis, radiation). Restriction may also be due to interstitial lung diseases (e.g., systemic juvenile idiopathic arthritis, primary antibody deficiencies), neuromuscular weakness, or obesity. The volume of gas in the lung can be measured using two techniques: dilution and plethysmography (Table 147-1).

A patient's lung capacity is the sum of two or more lung volumes; in the case of functional residual capacity (FRC), it is the sum of residual volume (RV; the amount of gas remaining in the lung after maximal exhalation) and expiratory reserve volume (ERV; the amount of gas exhaled from resting lung volume [FRC] until the lung cannot be emptied further). In combination with spirometry, other lung volumes and capacities can be calculated (**Figure 147-2**).

The pattern of lung volumes can also assist in diagnosis. Typically, patients with obstructive diseases have an increased RV, especially as a fraction of TLC. The TLC may be normal or elevated. In contrast, low lung volumes are the hallmark of RLD, and these patients have a reduced TLC and residual volume.

TABLE 147-2 Patterns of Obstructive and Restrictive Lung Disease

Parameter	Obstructive	Restrictive
FVC	Normal (may be low)	Low
FEV_1	Low	Low
FEV_1/FVC	Low	Normal
$FEF_{25\%-75\%}$	Low	Low

$FEF_{25\%-75\%}$, forced expiratory flow, mid-expiratory phase; FEV_1, forced expiratory volume in 1 second; FVC, forced vital capacity.

DIFFUSING CAPACITY

The diffusing capacity for carbon monoxide (DLCO) is usually obtained in conjunction with lung volumes and may be useful in evaluating patients with diffuse lung diseases or those with pulmonary vascular obstruction (Table 147-1). DLCO is an integrative measurement that describes the transfer of oxygen from the alveolus into the red blood cell. This transfer is (1) proportional to the surface area of the alveolar-capillary membrane, (2) proportional to the pressure gradient for oxygen between the alveolus and the blood, and (3) inversely proportional

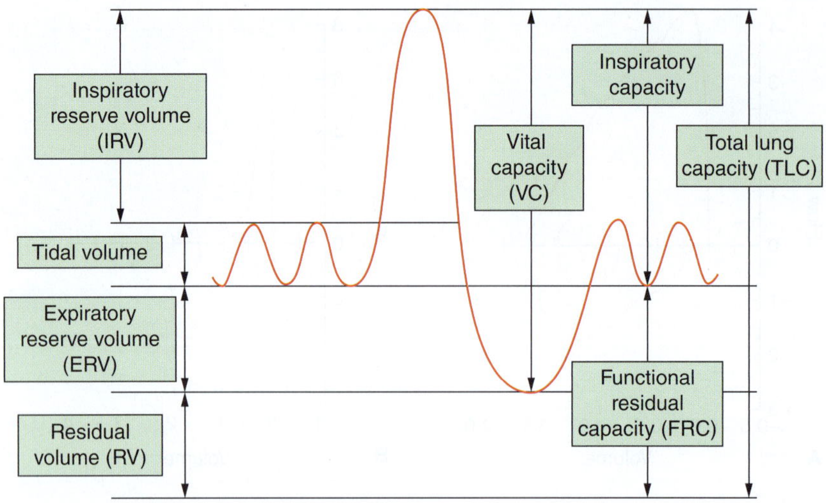

FIGURE 147-2. Fractional lung volume measurements. After measurement of FRC by dilution or plethysmography, and measurement of FVC and ERV by spirometry, RV can be calculated (difference between FRC and ERV) and TLC can be calculated (sum of RV and VC).

to the thickness of the alveolar-capillary membrane. The measurement depends on the fact that carbon monoxide (CO) is more soluble in blood than in lung tissue because it binds rapidly and tightly to hemoglobin in the blood (more than 200 times as quickly as oxygen does). Thus, the partial pressure of CO in the blood remains very low, maintaining a partial pressure gradient for the diffusion of gas. Revised standards for the measurement of DLCO have been published.

In the single-breath technique for measuring DLCO, the patient exhales completely to RV and inhales to TLC a gas mixture of 0.3% CO and an inert gas (usually helium or methane). The subject holds his or her breath for 10 seconds, during which time the CO diffuses into the blood. The uptake of CO (in mL/minute) is divided by the partial pressure gradient for CO (between alveolus and pulmonary capillary) to calculate DLCO (in mL/mm Hg per minute). Alveolar volume (VA) is calculated from the inspired and expired concentrations of the inert gas, and this is used to calculate a dilutional factor for the inspired CO concentration and to normalize the DLCO according to the lung volume in which the CO is diluted (DLCO/VA in mL/mm Hg per minute/L, where VA is the alveolar volume). DLCO is typically adjusted for the patient's hemoglobin to account for the effect of anemia.

Diseases that decrease the surface area for diffusion (emphysema, pulmonary emboli, resection of lung tissue, RLD), increase the thickness of the alveolar-capillary membrane (fibrosis, pulmonary edema, proteinosis), or decrease the amount of available hemoglobin (sickle cell anemia, blood loss) can decrease the diffusing capacity of the lung. The measured diffusing capacity can also be decreased if there is increased carboxyhemoglobin (which can occur in smoke inhalation or heavy tobacco smoking). Increased DLCO is much less common but can be seen in patients with alveolar hemorrhage (hemoglobin in the air space appears to make the uptake of CO very high) polycythemia, or during exercise (via recruitment of more pulmonary capillaries).

RESPIRATORY MUSCLE STRENGTH

The diaphragm, internal and external intercostal muscles, abdominal muscles, and the accessory muscles of inspiration are essential for breathing. Many diseases can affect the strength of these muscles, putting patients at risk for hypoventilation, impaired airway clearance of secretions, and respiratory insufficiency. These conditions include primary muscular disorders (muscular dystrophy, myopathy), conditions affecting nerve transmission to the muscles (neuropathies, disorders of the neuromuscular junction), malnutrition, and stretch of the muscles beyond their optimal length-tension relationship (which can occur in hyperinflation).

Typically, maximum expiratory pressure (PEmax) is measured by having the subject inhale maximally to TLC and blow out as hard as possible into a mouthpiece connected to a pressure transducer with an occluded distal end. Similarly, maximum inspiratory pressure (PImax) is measured by having the subject exhale completely to RV and inhale rapidly against the occluded tube. A low maximum expiratory pressure or inspiratory pressure would be concerning for weakness of the muscles of respiration (Table 147-1). However; several maneuvers are required to elicit the maximal effort and low pressures can often reflect submaximal effort rather than weakness. Several sets of standardized values have been published, but they vary considerably. In addition to the interpretation of values, it is important to trend values over time to monitor disease progression.

EXERCISE TESTING

Exercise tests assess the respiratory and cardiac systems during states of increased demand and can be performed using a variety of techniques.

Cardiopulmonary Exercise Test (CPET) Maximum cardiopulmonary exercise tests are performed to assess exercise tolerance and functional capacity, and to better understand the etiology of exercise intolerance (Table 147-1). This test can help to determine the factors contributing to exercise intolerance including cardiologic, respiratory, myopathic (such as mitochondrial disease), deconditioning, or psychological factors. Patients exercise on a treadmill or stationary bicycle while breathing into a gas analyzer while the work required for exercise is gradually increased by the technician. Treadmill ramp elevation and speed, or bicycle pedal resistance are increased in a graded fashion until the individual cannot continue, aiming for a heart rate near the maximum predicted heart rate for age. Heart rate, electrocardiography (ECG), respiratory rate, minute ventilation, oxygen uptake, and carbon dioxide output are measured. For example, individuals with significant cardiopulmonary disease would be expected to have low peak oxygen uptake, increased heart rates, and a decreased anaerobic threshold. Poor effort might be reflected with decreased peak oxygen uptake, maximal heart rate, and decreased respiratory quotient. The test should be aborted if the patient develops chest pain, ECG changes, cyanosis, or unstable vital signs.

Exercise Induced Bronchospasm (EIB) Exercise-induced bronchospasm tests can also be performed in patients with a history of wheezing and/or dyspnea with exercise. This study can help differentiate between exercise-induced bronchospasm and upper airway obstruction such as that due to vocal cord dysfunction (Table 147-1). Similar to maximal exercise tests, the exercise-induced bronchospasm test involves running on a treadmill, although the work of exercise is rapidly increased within the first few minutes. Submaximal exercise (heart rate of 85% of predicted maximum heart rate) is sustained for at least 4 minutes. Inspiratory flow-volume loops can be obtained during exercise to look for evidence of extrathoracic airflow obstruction (which can be seen in vocal cord dysfunction). Spirometry is performed before exercise starts and at 5-minute intervals (up to 30 minutes) after exercise ceases. In normal individuals, FEV_1 will increase during exercise. In individuals with exercise-induced bronchospasm, the FEV_1 will decrease 10% to 15% or more following exercise. A bronchodilator can be given at the end of the postexercise spirometry measurements to assess for reversible airflow obstruction. Flow-volume curves generated with each effort should be reviewed to look for evidence of distal airway obstruction or possible upper airway obstruction. Some centers may also perform a bedside flexible nasolaryngoscopy at the time that symptoms are elicited to assess vocal cord movement in patients with a history concerning vocal cord dysfunction.

FUNCTIONAL STATUS

A 6-minute walk test is a test of functional status most commonly performed in pediatric patients undergoing assessment for possible heart or lung transplantation (Table 147-1) and can be performed by a trained respiratory therapist (RT) or physical therapist (PT) using minimal equipment (stopwatch, pulse oximeter). For this test, the subject is asked to walk back and forth along a 100-foot path, as quickly as they can but self-paced, for 6 minutes. The primary outcome measurement is the walk distance, while heart rate, oxyhemoglobin saturation, and degree of dyspnea using the Borg Breathlessness Scale are also monitored. The walk test does not provide a specific diagnosis of what is causing exercise intolerance. The test can be repeated after an intervention to evaluate for change in clinical status. Standard predicted values have not been optimized and can vary with age.

PROVOCATIVE CHALLENGE TESTING

This is a type of testing done with spirometry to elicit airway hyperreactivity in patients with suspected asthma. Inhaled methacholine stimulates cholinergic receptors on airway smooth muscle, resulting in contraction and decreased airway caliber. Serial twofold increasing doses of methacholine (0.025-16 mg/mL) are delivered until a maximal dose is reached or there is a 20% decrease in FEV_1; this dose is termed the provocative dose required for a 20% decrease (PD_{20}). There is some controversy about what provocative dose constitutes an abnormal response, because even healthy controls may have decreased flows with high doses of methacholine. Following completion of the challenge, inhaled albuterol is given to document the reversibility of airflow obstruction. Similarly, graded exercise (using a treadmill or cycle ergometer) or hyperventilation with cold air (usually chilled to 4°C) can be used to provoke a bronchospasm response.

PEAK FLOW

Peak expiratory flow can be measured using a handheld flow-measuring device, which makes this readily available to providers without access to a pulmonary function lab. Subjects inhale maximally (to total lung capacity, TLC) and then exhale quickly with maximal force, and the resulting maximum or peak flow is indicated on the device. The convenience of this relatively inexpensive modality makes it potentially beneficial for monitoring daily symptoms in patients, especially those who are poor perceivers or in research studies. Peak flow can also be used to serially assess patients in the emergency department or hospital, to assist in monitoring recovery. However, peak expiratory flow is dominated by flows in large airways, and as such, it is very effort dependent. Additionally, peak expiratory flow can be preserved in the presence of significant small airway obstruction. Several studies have shown subjective reporting of symptoms to be as reliable as peak flow monitoring in identifying and treating asthma exacerbations.

INPATIENT APPLICATIONS OF PULMONARY FUNCTION TESTING

Pulmonary function tests complement other diagnostic studies in the evaluation of patients with respiratory symptoms and suspected lung disease. These tests have important uses in the evaluation of respiratory symptoms (shortness of breath, cough, wheeze) when there is no specific diagnosis.

Spirometry, a type of pulmonary function testing, is commonly used in the inpatient setting to monitor response to therapy. For example, patients with cystic fibrosis receiving intravenous antibiotics for a pulmonary exacerbation of their disease are usually monitored weekly with spirometry. The patient's prior baseline (or previous best) lung function is a helpful target when determining response to treatment and duration of therapy. Spirometry may also be helpful in characterizing the severity of an asthma exacerbation. Pulmonary function tests of lung volumes can be useful in preoperative planning to identify the severity of RLD for patients undergoing scoliosis repair. A less common use for pulmonary function testing would be use of maximal inspiratory and expiratory pressures to monitor the progression of muscle weakness in a patient with Guillain-Barre syndrome.

CONSULTATION

Consultation with a pediatric pulmonologist is suggested to guide selection of the appropriate pulmonary function test. Furthermore, interpretation of pulmonary function test results requires a fundamental understanding of patient effort and criteria for acceptability and reproducibility. Additionally, consultation is indicated for any test result that is inconsistent with the suspected clinical condition. For example, RLD would not be expected in a child with presumed asthma and should prompt an evaluation for other possible diagnoses. Flow-volume curves suggesting a fixed or variable airway obstruction should prompt consultation with a pulmonologist and/or otolaryngologist.

KEY POINTS

- Pulmonary function testing offers a noninvasive tool to assist in the diagnosis and management of a variety of respiratory and nonrespiratory conditions in pediatric patients. Trending values over time can be helpful for prognostic evaluations.
- Pulmonary function testing labs require specialized equipment run by trained and experienced personnel.
- Understanding of patient effort and criteria for a valid test are essential for accurate interpretation.
- Spirometry, lung volumes (plethysmography, dilution techniques), and DLCO have the most clinical use in the hospitalized patient, as they can help in diagnostic evaluation.

SUGGESTED READINGS

American Thoracic Society statement: guidelines for the six-minute walk test. *Am J Respir Crit Care Med.* 2000;166(1):111-117.

ATS/ACCP statement on cardiopulmonary exercise testing. *Am J Respir Crit Care Med.* 2003;167(2):211-277.

ATS/ERS statement on respiratory muscle testing. *Am J Respir Crit Care Med.* 2002;166:518-624.

Beydon N, Davis SD, Lombardi E, et al. An official American Thoracic Society/European Respiratory Society statement: pulmonary function testing in preschool children. *Am J Respir Crit Care Med.* 2007;175(12):1304-1345.

Loeb J, Blower W, Feldstein J, et al. Acceptability and repeatability of spirometry in children using updated ATS/ERS criteria. *Pediatr Pulmonol.* 2008;43(10):1020-1024.

Macintyre N, Crapo RO, Viegi G, et al. Standardisation of the single-breath determination of carbon monoxide uptake in the lung. *Eur Respir J.* 2005;26:720-735.

Miller MR, Crapo R, Hankinson J, et al. General considerations for lung function testing. *Eur Respir J.* 2005;26:153-161.

Miller MR, Hankinson J, Brusasco V, et al. Standardisation of spirometry. *Eur Respir J.* 2005;26:319-338.

Popa V. ATS guidelines for methacholine and exercise challenge testing. *Am J Respir Crit Care Med.* 2001;163:292-293.

Wanger J, Clausen JL, Coates A, et al. Standardisation of the measurement of lung volumes. *Eur Respir J.* 2005;26:511-522.

West JB, Luks AM. *West's Respiratory Physiology: The Essentials.* 10th ed. Wolters Kluwer; 2016.

Wilson K, Kaminsky D, Michaud G, et al. Restoring Pulmonary and Sleep Services as the COVID-19 Pandemic Lessens. From an Association of Pulmonary, Critical Care, and Sleep Division Directors and American Thoracic Society-coordinated Task Force. *Annal Am Thorac Soc.* 2020;17(11):1343-1351.

SECTION Q Rheumatology

CHAPTER 148 Kawasaki Disease

Diana S. Lee, MD

BACKGROUND

Kawasaki disease (KD), a vasculitis affecting small- and medium-sized blood vessels, is the second most common childhood vasculitis, and the most common cause of pediatric acquired heart disease in the developed world. It was first described in 1967 and initially called mucocutaneous lymph node disease because of the predominant clinical features. Affected children present acutely with fever, bilateral nonexudative conjunctivitis, erythema of the lips and oral mucosa, cervical lymphadenopathy, rash, and extremity changes. These findings are usually self-limited, but 15% to 25% of untreated children develop coronary artery abnormalities, putting them at risk for developing ischemic heart disease or sudden death later in life. Therapy with intravenous immunoglobulin in the acute phase is aimed at reducing inflammation, thereby minimizing the risk of coronary artery aneurysms and other late sequelae.

EPIDEMIOLOGY

Children under 5 years of age are most commonly affected, with a mean age of 3 years, and a male-to-female ratio of 1.5:1. Children of all ethnicities may be affected, although the incidence is higher among those of Asian and Pacific Islander heritage. The annual incidence of KD in children under 5 years of age in the United States and the United Kingdom is 20 and 8 per 100,000 children, respectively. The rates in Japan and Taiwan are 3 to 15 times higher. Adults also may develop KD but far less often; fewer than 100 cases have been reported worldwide to date. In the extratropical northern hemisphere, there is seasonal variation with KD being more common during the winter.

PATHOPHYSIOLOGY

The pathogenesis of KD remains unknown, though most hypotheses center on an infectious trigger. Several epidemiologic features of the disease support this theory. For example, the seasonality of KD incidence corresponds to peak seasons for infectious diseases. Studies showing a link between the seasonality of KD and tropospheric wind patterns suggest a possible wind-borne agent that triggers illness. Furthermore, KD exhibits "epidemics," as demonstrated by years with up to a tenfold spike in disease incidence in Japan in the 1980s and 1990s. Nonetheless, extensive testing using culture, serologic, and sequencing techniques has not implicated a specific transmissible agent as the cause. Additionally, anti-inflammatory medications such as intravenous immunoglobulins (IVIG) and TNF-inhibitors are clinically beneficial, while antibiotics are not. Taken together, these facts suggest that KD represents an exaggerated inflammatory response to one or more infectious agents.

Higher rates of KD in twins, siblings of index cases, parents of children with KD, and children of Japanese descent both residing in and outside of Japan support that this illness occurs when genetic predisposition interacts with a triggering agent. Genetic studies have identified genes and signaling pathways that influence susceptibility to KD, response to IVIG, and aneurysm formation.

CLINICAL PRESENTATION

The diagnosis of KD is a clinical one, with epidemiologic criteria as defined by Dr. Tomisaku Kawasaki in 1967 as follows:

Fever that persists for at least 5 days plus at least four of the following:

1. Bilateral nonexudative conjunctival injection
2. Changes of the lips and oral cavity
3. Cervical lymphadenopathy
4. Polymorphous exanthema
5. Changes in the peripheral extremities

These features may not occur in all KD patients, and their temporal sequence is very variable. Given that the clinical features may not all be present at the same time, it is necessary to assess whether there were symptoms prior to presentation that help establish the diagnosis. KD tends to occur in three phases: the initial acute febrile phases lasts up to 14 days, followed by a subacute phase of 2 to 4 weeks, with a convalescent phase that may extend to months or years.

ACUTE FEBRILE PHASE

The typical patient demonstrates a persistent high fever that responds minimally to antipyretics. The child can be very irritable during this stage, often out of proportion to the height of the fever. Without treatment, the fever lasts an average of 12 days, with the remaining mucocutaneous features evolving over the next 1 to 2 weeks. The sequence in which they appear varies among patients, highlighting the importance of repeated evaluation in young children with persistent unexplained fevers. KD is not excluded if the fever resolves spontaneously after 7 days.

Conjunctival injection is seen in 85% of children and is bilateral, painless, nonexudative, and tends to spare the limbal areas. Other less common ocular manifestations include anterior uveitis, keratitis, papilledema, vitreous opacities, and subconjunctival hemorrhages, often with accompanying photophobia.

Changes to the lips and oral cavity are seen in 90% of children. These manifest as diffuse erythema of the oropharynx, dry, cracked, and sometimes bleeding lips, and a strawberry tongue. Mucosal ulcerations and pharyngeal exudates are not typical of KD.

Cervical lymphadenopathy is the least common of the principal findings, affecting about 50% of children with KD. The enlarged lymph node is typically unilateral, 1.5 cm or larger in diameter, limited to the anterior chain, firm and nontender, and without significant overlying erythema. Patients with KD have been misdiagnosed with having infectious lymphadenopathy because of the prominence of the enlarged lymph node. Imaging with ultrasound or CT scan will reveal multiple enlarged nodes without suppuration, giving the appearance of a "bunch of grapes" similar to the lymphadenopathy seen in Epstein-Barr virus infections. Biopsies, though generally not necessary, reveal focal necrosis with an inflammatory infiltrate consisting of neutrophils and macrophages, and fibrin thrombi within the microvasculature. It is also possible to see retropharyngeal edema or phlegmon.

A *rash* is evident in 70% to 90% of affected patients and is polymorphous and nonspecific. A macular, targetoid, or morbilliform exanthem that is usually nonpruritic is most common. The rash may occasionally be urticarial, erythrodermic, or pustular. Bullous, vesicular, or petechial rashes are not consistent with KD and should prompt evaluation for other causes. In most cases, the rash is widespread, involving the trunk and limbs. In up to half of cases, it begins in the perineal region, typically desquamating after 2 to 3 days. Children with prior bacille

TABLE 148-1 Supplemental Clinical Findings in Kawasaki Disease

Cardiovascular	Shock, myocarditis, pericarditis, valvular regurgitation Coronary artery abnormalities Aneurysms of medium-sized noncoronary arteries Aortic root enlargement Peripheral gangrene
Central Nervous System	Extreme irritability Aseptic meningitis Sensorineural hearing loss Facial nerve palsy
Gastrointestinal	Diarrhea, vomiting, abdominal pain Hepatitis, jaundice Hydrops of gallbladder Pancreatitis
Genitourinary	Urethritis, meatitis Hydrocele
Musculoskeletal	Arthritis, arthralgia
Respiratory	Peribronchial and interstitial infiltrates on chest radiograph Pulmonary nodules
Other	Erythema, induration at bacille Calmette-Guérin (BCG) inoculation site Anterior uveitis (mild) Retropharyngeal phlegmon Desquamating rash in groin

Source: Data from McCrindle BW, Rowley AH, Newburger JW, et al. Diagnosis, treatment, and long-term management of Kawasaki disease: a scientific statement for health professionals from the American Heart Association. *Circulation*. 2017;135:e927-e999.

Calmette-Guérin (BCG) vaccination tend to have prominent erythema and induration over the BCG scar.

Changes in the extremities in the first week of KD appear as redness over the palms and soles, and/or swelling of the dorsum of the hands and feet. Periungual desquamation is a later finding that is usually seen within 2 to 3 weeks after fever onset.

Children with KD may have other clinical features, including anorexia, arthralgias/arthritis (initially involving large joints, then later, small joints), diarrhea, vomiting, abdominal pain, and tachycardia out of proportion to the fever, S3 gallop, and muffled heart sounds. These may assist in distinguishing KD from other childhood febrile exanthema, although they are not included among the diagnostic criteria. **Table 148-1** highlights the range of clinical findings in KD.

SUBACUTE PHASE

This phase begins as the fever resolves, typically by the end of the second week in patients not treated with IVIG. The affected child demonstrates periungual desquamation, beginning just under the nails and progressing to sheets of skin sloughing from the digits and at times from the palms and soles. Joint inflammation, typically a self-limited polyarthritis involving the small joints, may also develop during this period. Apart from these, the child treated with immunoglobulin tends to be asymptomatic. An untreated child may still have the mucocutaneous features, although these usually resolve spontaneously as well. At this stage, most coronary artery abnormalities that will develop are evident on echocardiography, though they may continue to expand for weeks due to both hemodynamic factors and ongoing inflammation, especially in untreated cases. Laboratory tests begin to return toward normal, particularly the white blood cell count and C-reactive protein (CRP). Other aberrations, however, including lymphocytosis, thrombocytosis, and elevated erythrocyte sedimentation rate (ESR) may persist for up to 2 months.

CONVALESCENT PHASE

Children tend to be asymptomatic during the convalescent phase, with normalization of all inflammatory markers and stabilization of coronary artery dilatation by about 2 months after the onset of the disease. Beau's lines—deep transverse grooves across the nails reflecting a nonspecific response to significant inflammation—may appear at this time.

INCOMPLETE OR ATYPICAL KAWASAKI DISEASE

The terms incomplete or atypical KD refer to children who only have some of the clinical features of KD and do not meet diagnostic criteria for the disease. Nonetheless, these children may develop coronary artery abnormalities, particularly infants under 6 months of age who are less likely to demonstrate the full spectrum of mucocutaneous manifestations. Because the diagnosis is not necessarily apparent, physicians must remain vigilant and should consider KD in children with unexplained fever for more than 5 days. An expert panel has developed guidelines for evaluating such children (**Figure 148-1**). Children under 6 months with persistent fever for 7 days and evidence of inflammation should have an echocardiogram to screen for atypical KD even in the absence of clinical criteria. Older children with two or three of the principal clinical features and supportive laboratory findings should be similarly evaluated. Findings such as perivascular brightness and ectasia or lack of tapering of the coronary arteries may represent early signs of vasculitis, though they are also reported in viral syndromes and systemic juvenile idiopathic arthritis. Decreased left ventricular contractility, mild valvular regurgitation (most commonly mitral regurgitation), and pericardial effusion also support a diagnosis of incomplete KD. Such patients should be treated no differently than those who fulfill traditional diagnostic criteria.

KAWASAKI SHOCK SYNDROME

A more severe and dangerous presentation of KD is characterized by sustained hypotension or clinical evidence of poor perfusion. Patients may present with more gastrointestinal symptoms, more severe perturbations of laboratory markers of inflammation, and an increased risk of cardiac involvement including coronary artery abnormalities, mitral regurgitation, and prolonged myocardial inflammation. Patients may also demonstrate less responsiveness to treatment with intravenous immunoglobulin and require additional anti-inflammatory treatment.

COMPLICATIONS

The most severe complications in KD primarily involve the cardiovascular system. Patients are at increased risk of developing coronary artery thrombosis and myocardial infarction. During the acute phase of the disease, such complications are caused by the combination of hypercoagulability from endothelial abnormalities and sluggish flow due to coronary artery dilatation. Later, coronary artery narrowing as a result of repair by myointimal proliferation combined with reactive thrombocytosis leads to a maximal risk of infarction during the first 6 months of convalescence. Control of inflammation using IVIG and other agents is essential to minimize these risks. Administration of IVIG early results in rapid clinical improvement, though not complete amelioration of any structural changes such as aneurysmal formation. After the first week, new myocardial dysfunction is usually due to ischemia or infarction. Electrocardiogram and measurement of inflammatory markers may be necessary to distinguish between inflammation and ischemia. Arrhythmias sometimes occur because of myocardial damage and are usually the cause of the rare deaths seen in KD. Peripheral artery disease may result in ischemia or gangrene of the involved limb.

DIFFERENTIAL DIAGNOSIS

KD is most often mistaken for an infectious disease such as scarlet fever, measles, or adenovirus. In fact, clinical features of KD may be indistinguishable from those of a variety of childhood illnesses, as outlined in **Table 148-2**, and KD may present concurrently with a variety of infections. Despite this difficulty, early diagnosis and treatment of KD is associated with an improved outcome and fewer cardiac sequelae, so a clinician may not have the luxury of waiting for results of serologic tests

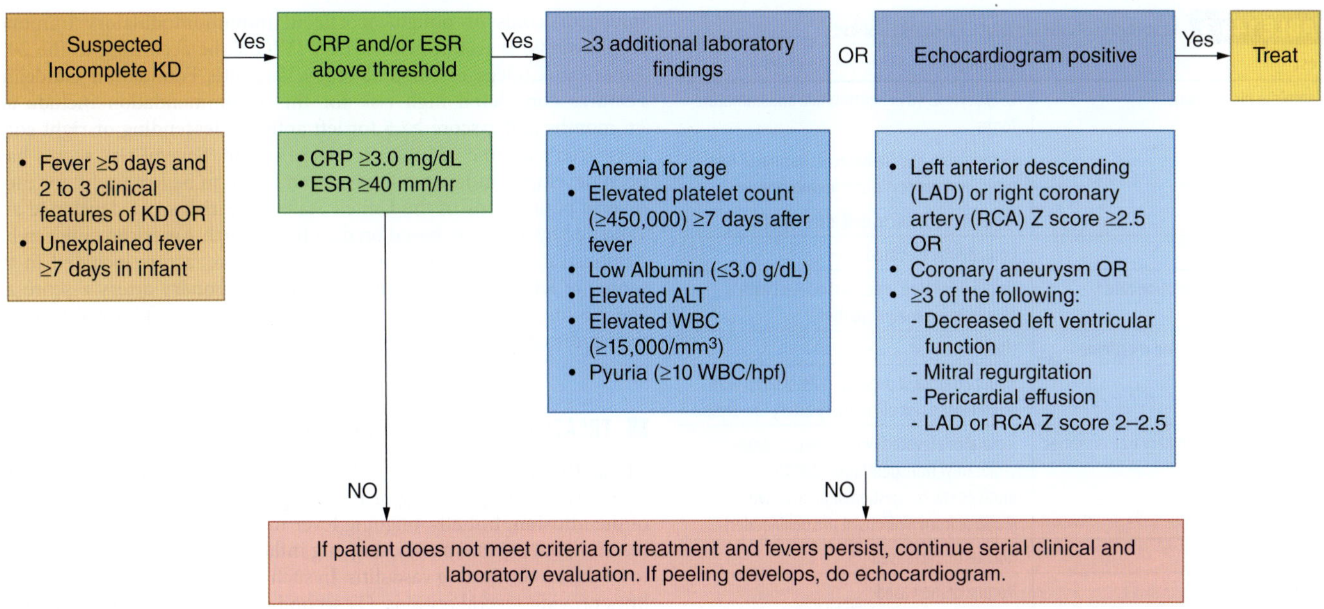

FIGURE 148-1. Diagnosis of incomplete Kawasaki Disease. CRP, C-reactive protein; ESR, erythrocyte sedimentation rate; ALT, alanine aminotransferase; WBC, white blood cells. (Adapted from McCrindle BW, Rowley AH, Newburger JW, et al. diagnosis, treatment, and long-term management of kawasaki disease: A Scientific Statement for Health Professionals From the American Heart Association [published correction appears in Circulation. 2019 30;140(5):e181-e184]. *Circulation*. 2017;135(17):e927-e999.)

or imaging studies. Burns et al. (1991) described findings more likely to be indicative of conditions other than KD, including exudative conjunctivitis, exudative pharyngitis, discreet intraoral lesions, bullous or vesicular rash, or generalized lymphadenopathy.

The multisystem inflammatory syndrome in children (MIS-C) associated with COVID-19 may present with clinical features similar to KD, making it challenging to distinguish between these entities. Epidemiologic differences may help to differentiate between them, with KD typically occurring in younger children (<5 years) with a higher incidence in children of Asian and Pacific Island heritage compared with MIS-C which more commonly affects older children (median age 6-11 years) and children of African and Hispanic heritage. Clinically, cardiac involvement, presentation with shock, need for critical care, gastrointestinal symptoms, and severe neurological symptoms are less common in KD than MIS-C. Laboratory parameters may also be useful in differentiating between KD and MIS-C. When compared to KD, children with MIS-C tend to have a lower platelet count, lower absolute lymphocyte count, higher C-reactive protein, higher N-terminal pro-B-type natriuretic peptide, higher troponin, higher ferritin, higher D-dimer, and higher fibrinogen (see Chapter 107: MIS-C).

TABLE 148-2 Differential Diagnosis of Kawasaki Disease

Infections
Viral infections (e.g., measles, adenovirus, enterovirus, echovirus, Epstein-Barr virus)
Toxin-mediated illnesses: Staphylococcal scalded skin syndrome, scarlet fever, toxic shock syndrome
Rocky Mountain spotted fever
Leptospirosis
Drug reactions
Stevens-Johnson syndrome
Serum sickness
Hypersensitivity reactions; e.g., mercury toxicity
Inflammatory conditions
Systemic-onset juvenile idiopathic arthritis
Polyarteritis nodosa
Multisystem inflammatory syndrome in children associated with COVID-19

DIAGNOSTIC EVALUATION

The diagnosis of KD is made clinically, with no definitive diagnostic test available. The underlying diffuse small and medium-sized vasculitis leads to systemic and mucocutaneous inflammation, with corresponding physical and laboratory findings. Unfortunately, clinical criteria have imperfect sensitivity and specificity, so the diagnosis and subsequent management of KD are often challenging. Not all children fulfilling all five principal criteria necessarily have KD, and conversely, children who do not meet classical criteria may be at risk of developing sequelae of the disease.

Laboratory studies were not included in the diagnostic criteria for classic KD but they may heighten or support the diagnosis in ambiguous cases (**Table 148-3**). An expert committee developed an evaluation algorithm for the diagnosis of incomplete KD which includes laboratory tests to improve clinicians' ability to accurately identify children at risk for developing coronary artery changes despite failing to meet diagnostic criteria (Figure 148-1). Uveitis on slit lamp examination may provide further evidence for the diagnosis, since inflammation of the anterior chamber is seen more often in KD than in mimics of KD.

MANAGEMENT

The main goal of treatment is to reduce inflammation and prevent the development of coronary artery abnormalities. The American Heart Association (AHA) recommends a single infusion of intravenous immunoglobulin at a dose of 2 g/kg along with moderate- (30-50 mg/kg daily) to high-dose (80-100 mg/kg daily, maximum 4 g/day) aspirin within the first 10 days of illness but as soon as possible after diagnosis. This therapy reduces the incidence of coronary artery aneurysms by up to 75%. Once the child has been afebrile for 48 hours, the aspirin dose may be reduced to 3 to 5 mg/kg daily. Children without evidence of coronary artery changes should continue this low-dose aspirin until 4 to 6 weeks after onset of illness. Children with coronary aneurysms should continue until resolution of the aneurysms.

The mechanism by which IVIG alleviates the signs and symptoms of KD is not known. In other conditions, it has been shown to downregulate pathologic autoantibodies, block inflammatory cytokine mRNA, and adsorb phlogistic complement fragments and toxins, among other actions.

Beyond 10 days of illness, IVIG may be administered to children with persistent fever without another explanation or coronary artery abnormalities plus ongoing systemic inflammation evidenced by an elevated

TABLE 148-3 Laboratory Studies in Acute Kawasaki Disease

Test	Finding
Complete blood count	Leukocytosis with neutrophilia and immature forms Hemoglobin and hematocrit: normal or low, typically normocytic and normochromic Platelet count: increased after week 1
C-reactive protein	Consistently elevated
Erythrocyte sedimentation rate	Usually elevated unless associated with a consumptive coagulopathy
Blood urea nitrogen and creatinine	Usually normal
Serum electrolytes	Hyponatremia, if present, is associated with an increased risk of coronary artery aneurysms
Transaminases and biliary tree enzymes	Normal or elevated with elevated serum γ-glutamyl transpeptidase (due to intrahepatic congestion or obstructive jaundice from hydrops of the gallbladder)
Albumin	Normal or decreased
Serum lipids	Normal or increased
Urinalysis	Sterile pyuria, due to urethritis (and hence not evident on urine samples obtained via suprapubic aspiration or catheterization)
Cerebrospinal fluid	Mononuclear pleocytosis with depressed glucose and elevated protein levels
Synovial fluid	Leukocytosis

ESR or CRP >3.0 mg/dL. IVIG is not recommended beyond the tenth day of illness in the absence of fever, coronary artery abnormalities, or significant elevation of inflammatory markers.

Despite its favorable risk-benefit ratio, IVIG nonetheless may cause a variety of side effects, particularly infusion reactions in children being exposed to the agent for the first time. **Table 148-4** provides a list of potential adverse effects of IVIG. Immediate reactions tend to occur during the infusion and are often rate-related. To prevent the occurrence or minimize the severity of these reactions, slow infusion rates with gradual stepwise increases are recommended. Premedication with acetaminophen, an antihistamine, and a nonsteroidal anti-inflammatory drug (these patients are usually on aspirin anyway) can help to reduce immediate infusion reactions as well. If a reaction does occur, slowing or stopping the infusion until symptoms subside is usually sufficient, after which the infusion may be restarted at a lower rate and then once again advanced as tolerated. It is important to remember that there is no substitute for IVIG in KD, so every effort must be made to continue the infusion whenever possible. True anaphylaxis may occur, particularly in IgA-deficient patients, but IgA measurement is not routinely recommended prior to giving IVIG. Delayed reactions may occur within hours to days after the end of the infusion.

In children at high risk for IVIG resistance or for developing coronary artery aneurysms, initial treatment with IVIG and another agent

TABLE 148-4 Adverse Effects of IVIG

Immediate Reactions	Delayed Reactions
Fever, chills, flushing	Headaches, aseptic meningitis
Urticaria	Hemolysis
Myalgia	Acute kidney injury
Malaise	Venous thrombosis
Nausea, vomiting	Transient ischemic attack, stroke
Headache	Myocardial ischemia
Anaphylactoid reactions (usually midway through the infusion): flushing, tachycardia, dyspnea, chest tightness or pain, nausea, vomiting, sudden anxiety, sense of impending doom; usually, hypertension	

(glucocorticoids or nonglucocorticoid immunomodulatory immunosuppressants) is recommended over IVIG alone according to the 2021 American College of Rheumatology/Vasculitis Foundation Guideline. Features considered high risk for this recommendation include age <6 months and z-score ≥2.5 for left anterior descending or right coronary artery at time of initial echocardiogram. Several risk scores have been developed in Japan but have been found to be less useful for more diverse populations in the United States. The risk score developed and validated by Son et al. based on data from North American children has demonstrated more predictive utility. The risk factors included in the score are left anterior descending or right coronary artery z-score ≥2, age < 6 months, Asian race, and CRP ≥13 mg/dL. Additional prospective studies are needed to assess the accuracy and generalizability of the score.

TREATMENT OF REFRACTORY DISEASE

About 10% to 15% of patients fail to respond to initial treatment with IVIG, with fever persisting or recurring within 36 hours of completion of the infusion. Initially, ongoing fever may be attributed to an infusion reaction, but as time passes, ongoing inflammation is increasingly likely to be due to continuing vasculitis. In such patients, the 2017 AHA guidelines provide several options: (1) second dose of IVIG (2 g/kg); 2) pulse steroids (20-30 mg/kg intravenously for 3 days) with or without subsequent taper; (3) IVIG plus longer steroid taper over 2 to 3 weeks; (4) infliximab (5 mg/kg). If these treatments fail, cyclosporine, non-TNF-α blocking monoclonal antibody therapy, cytotoxic agents (e.g., cyclophosphamide), and plasma exchange may be considered.

If coronary artery aneurysms develop, continuation of low-dose aspirin for its antiplatelet effects is warranted. Occasionally systemic anticoagulation with heparin or warfarin may be necessary to minimize the risk of arterial thrombosis. Should coronary artery thrombosis or ischemia occur, additional antiplatelet therapy, anticoagulation, and/or revascularization with thrombolysis or coronary angioplasty may be necessary. Management of such complex cases should preferentially occur in tertiary-care hospitals with considerable experience in treating complicated KD.

ADMISSION CRITERIA

- Probable or definite diagnosis of KD for which IVIG is indicated.
- Diagnosis of KD is in question and further evaluation and observation are necessary. This may include cardiology evaluation and an echocardiogram.

DISCHARGE CRITERIA

- Patient is clinically stable after completing IVIG. Fever and other signs of inflammation have been absent for 24 to 48 hours after completion of the IVIG infusion.
- Additional parenteral therapy is not deemed necessary.
- Family members and other caregivers are familiar with necessary monitoring and follow-up during the convalescent period.

CONSULTATION

Patients with KD may be managed by the general pediatric team with early consultation by pediatric cardiology for performance of a baseline echocardiogram and ongoing monitoring. Involvement by a pediatric rheumatologist may be helpful in patients who fail to resolve their fever after the first or second dose of IVIG, to assist in the consideration of advanced therapies for vasculitis.

OUTCOME AND FOLLOW-UP

In children with active varicella or influenza infection, high-dose aspirin should be discontinued or held given the risk for Reyes syndrome. Administration of high-dose IVIG without aspirin and use of alternative nonsalicylate antipyretics and a minimum of 2 weeks of an alternative antiplatelet agent should be considered. Low-dose aspirin used for antiplatelet effect has not been associated with the development of Reye syndrome. Children ≥ 6 months should receive the inactivated influenza vaccine if not yet immunized. Some physicians substitute another antiplatelet medication for aspirin for 6 weeks after administration of the influenza vaccine.

In most cases, the prognosis in KD is good and patients recover without long-term cardiovascular sequelae. The outcome is largely dependent on the presence or absence of coronary artery involvement and its attendant risk of myocardial ischemia. Mortality rates during the acute phase of KD are in the range of 0.1% to 0.3%, usually from myocardial infarction from coronary artery thrombosis, aneurysmal rupture, or arrhythmias. The highest mortality occurs in the first 2 months of disease, and in those with so-called "giant aneurysms" measuring more than 8 mm in diameter. On the other hand, coronary artery dilatation <8 mm generally regresses over time, and most aneurysms <6 mm in diameter fully resolve on echocardiographic follow-up. Children with persistent coronary artery changes have a small increase in mortality at 20 years, but to date, no definite effect on longevity has been demonstrated in others following KD.

The main long-term concern in children with KD is atherosclerosis, though the extent to which previous KD is an independent risk factor for its development is not known. Most children who do not have cardiovascular abnormalities on echocardiography up to 8 weeks after onset of disease appear to be asymptomatic 10 to 21 years later. However, there have been reports of late findings of impaired endothelial function and increased carotid media thickness, and these suggest that long-term vigilance is warranted. The AHA has published guidelines for subsequent therapy, physical activity, and follow-up visits based on the risk of myocardial infarction.

The recurrence rate has been reported to be between 1.5% and 3.5%, varying between countries and being higher in those of Asian and Pacific Islander heritage. Risks are also higher in younger children who had cardiac sequelae during the first episode and within 12 months of the initial KD. The risk of cardiac sequelae is increased in patients with recurrent KD.

VACCINATIONS

IVIG has immunomodulatory effects and is known to decrease the immunogenicity of vaccines. KD patients who have received IVIG should not receive any live vaccines 11 months after IVIG, except if they are exposed to any vaccine-preventable disease(s) where even reduced protection is important. Children who are immunized during this period should be reimmunized at least 11 months after having received IVIG. KD patients above the age of 6 months on aspirin therapy should receive the inactivated injectable influenza vaccine to minimize the risk of Reye syndrome. All their household contacts should also receive influenza vaccine, either inactivated or live attenuated.

KEY POINTS

- Kawasaki disease is a systemic inflammatory condition of childhood manifesting as prolonged fever and signs of mucocutaneous inflammation.
- KD is a vasculitis of the small and medium-blood vessels, and the leading cause of acquired heart disease in the developed world.
- Diagnosis of KD according to classification criteria is not always straightforward. Incorporation of laboratory features, echocardiographic findings, and results of slit-lamp examination may improve diagnostic accuracy.
- A high index of suspicion must be maintained for infants and younger children who are less likely to demonstrate classic clinical criteria for the disease but who are at increased risk of developing coronary artery abnormalities.
- IVIG therapy within the first 10 days of fever is associated with a significant decrease in the incidence of coronary artery aneurysms. All studies demonstrating efficacy of IVIG also employ aspirin.
- Persistent inflammation after IVIG therapy should be treated aggressively; prolonged fever is the single strongest predictor of coronary artery involvement in KD.

SUGGESTED READINGS

American Academy of Pediatrics. Kawasaki disease. In: Kimberlin DW, ed. *Red Book: 2021-2024 Report of the Committee on Infectious Diseases*. 32nd ed. Elk Grove Village, IL: American Academy of Pediatrics; 2021:457-464.

Benseler SM, McCrindle BW, Silverman ED, et al. Infections and Kawasaki disease: implications for coronary artery outcome. *Pediatrics*. 2005;116(6):e760-766.

Burns JC, Glodé MP. Kawasaki syndrome. *Lancet*. 2004;364:533.

Burns JC, Mason WH, Glode MP, et al. Clinical and epidemiologic characteristics of patients referred for evaluation of possible Kawasaki disease. United States Multicenter Kawasaki Disease Study Group. *J Pediatr*. 1991;118:680.

Franco A, Shimuzu C, Troulet AH, Burns JC. Memory T-cells and characterization of peripheral T-cell clones in acute Kawasaki disease. *Autoimmunity*. 2010;43:317-324.

Fujita Y, Nakamura Y, Sakata K, et al. Kawasaki disease in families. *Pediatrics*. 1989;84:666-669.

Fukushige J, Takahashi N, Ueda K, et al. Long-term outcome of coronary abnormalities in patients after Kawasaki disease. *Pediatr Cardiol*. 1996;17(2):71.

Godfred-Cato S, Abrams JY, Balachandran N, et al. Distinguishing multisystem inflammatory syndrome in children from COVID-19, Kawasaki disease, and toxic shock syndrome. *Pediatr Infect Dis J*. 2022;41(4):315-323.

Gorelik M, Chung SA, Ardalan K, et al. 2021 American College of Rheumatology/Vasculitis Foundation Guideline for the Management of Kawasaki Disease. *Arthritis Care Res (Hoboken)*. 2022;74(4):538-548. doi:10.1002/acr.24838

Henderson LA, Canna SW, Friedman KG, et al. American College of Rheumatology Clinical Guidance for Multisystem Inflammatory Syndrome in Children Associated With SARS-CoV-2 and Hyperinflammation in Pediatric COVID-19: Version 2. *Arthritis Rheumatol*. 2021;73(4):e13-e29.

Holman RC, Belay ED, Christensen KY, Folkema AM, Steiner CA, Schonberger LB. Hospitalizations for Kawasaki syndrome among children in the United States, 1997–2007. *Pediatr Infect Dis J*. 2010; 29:483-488.

Kanegaye JT, Wilder MS, Molkara D, et al. Recognition of a Kawasaki disease shock syndrome. *Pediatrics*. 2009;123(5):e783-789.

Kato H, Sugimura T, Akagi T, et al. Long-term consequences of Kawasaki disease: a 10- to 21-year follow-up study of 594 patients. *Circulation*. 1996;94:1379-1385.

Katz U, Shoenfeld Y, Zandman-Goddard G. Update on intravenous immunoglobulins (IVIg) mechanisms of action and off-label use in autoimmune diseases. *Curr Pharm Des*. 2011;17:3166-3175.

Kottek A, Shimuzu C, Burns JC. Kawasaki disease in monozygotic twins. *Pediatr Infect Dis J*. 2011;30:1114-1116.

Matsubara K, Fukaya T, Miwa K, et al. Development of serum IgM antibodies against superantigens of Staphylococcus aureus and Streptococcus pyogenes in Kawasaki disease. *Clin Exp Immunol*. 2006;143:427-434.

McCrindle BW, Rowley AH, Newburger JW, et al. Diagnosis, treatment, and long-term management of Kawasaki disease: a scientific statement for health professionals from the American Heart Association [published correction appears in Circulation. 2019 30;140(5):e181-e184]. *Circulation*. 2017;135(17):e927-e999.

Newburger JW, Takahashi M, Beiser AS, et al. A single intravenous infusion of gamma globulin as compared with four infusions in the treatment of acute Kawasaki syndrome. *N Engl J Med*. 1991;324:1633-1639.

Onouchi Y. Genetics of Kawasaki disease: what we know and don't know. *Circ J*. 2012;76:1581-1586.

Rowley AH, Baker SC, Shulman ST, et al. Ultrastructural, immunofluorescence, and RNA evidence support the hypothesis of a "new" virus associated with Kawasaki disease. *J Infect Dis*. 2011;203:1021-1030.

Son MBF, Gauvreau K, Tremoulet H, et al. Risk model development and validation for a prediction of coronary artery aneurysms in Kawasaki disease in a North American population. *J Am Heart Assoc*. 2019;8(11):e011319.

Uehara R, Yashiro M, Nakemura Y, Yanagawa H. Kawasaki disease in parents and children. *Acta Paediatr*. 2003;92:694-697.

CHAPTER 149

IgA Vasculitis (Henoch-Schönlein Purpura)

Mollie Wasserman, MD

BACKGROUND

IgA vasculitis (IgAV), formerly known as Henoch-Schönlein purpura (HSP), and also known as anaphylactoid purpura or purpura rheumatica, is a leukocytoclastic vasculitis affecting small blood vessels in virtually any organ system, but the skin, joints, and kidneys are most often involved. IgAV is the most common type of childhood systemic vasculitis, with an annual incidence of 10 to 20 per 100,000 children less than 17 years of age with a slight male predominance. Most patients are between the ages of 3 and 10 years, with the peak age of onset 4 to 6 years. The clinical course is usually benign and self-limited, although a small proportion of patients may have significant long-term sequelae, mainly as a result of renal involvement.

PATHOPHYSIOLOGY

IgAV is characterized by IgA deposition, complement deposition, and neutrophil recruitment in a variety of organs. In addition, immunoglobulin A (IgA) levels are elevated in the condition, though the pathophysiologic effect of this is not understood. Environmental, infectious, and chemical triggers, along with genetic factors, seem to play a role in the development of IgAV.

IgAV often follows infections, most commonly streptococcal upper respiratory tract infections, explaining the increased number of cases in the fall, winter, and spring. Other triggering factors may include immunizations such as the MMR vaccine, though data are mixed; and medications, such as biologics. From a genetics perspective, polymorphisms in the human leukocyte antigen (HLA) alleles, as well as other vascular and immunologic genes, are associated with IgAV. Further, the incidence is also higher in patients with certain complement deficiencies and those with a mutation in the gene associated with familial Mediterranean fever, the *MEFV* gene.

While biopsy of the affected organs is not routinely pursued in pediatric patients, it is sometimes required in the setting of atypical features or with significant renal involvement (see section Diagnostic Evaluation). Tissue biopsy in IgAV shows leukocytoclastic vasculitis with IgA immune complexes deposited within the affected organs, and a perivascular predominance of neutrophils and monocytes around necrotic small blood vessels. Immunofluorescence and electron microscopy may reveal deposits of IgA, C3, and fibrin within the walls of the involved vessels, and the endothelial and mesangial cells of the kidney. If the biopsy is delayed, findings will be nonspecific, as prolonged compromise of vascular integrity allows leakage of all plasma elements.

CLINICAL PRESENTATIONS

IgAV is marked by the classic tetrad of nonthrombocytopenic palpable purpura with normal coagulation studies, arthritis, abdominal pain, and renal involvement. Renal involvement may be reflected by the presence of hematuria or proteinuria, which is often mild. In rare cases, renal involvement may progress to chronic renal failure.

The typical history is of an otherwise well child with a recent upper respiratory infection in the preceding weeks, who presents with rash, arthralgia, and colicky abdominal pain. There may be a reported history of low-grade fever. Symptoms may occur concurrently or develop within days, and occasionally weeks, of each other. The classic rash and joint pain alone, or rash and abdominal pain, may be sufficient to make the diagnosis.

RASH

Rash is commonly the initial presenting feature of IgAV. It is characteristically a symmetric, dark red or purple, non-blanching palpable exanthema in the setting of normal platelet count and coagulation studies. The lesions are usually not painful but occasionally may be pruritic (**Figure 149-1**). They begin as urticarial wheals or petechiae, evolving later to form the typical purpura or ecchymoses, most prominent in pressure-dependent areas. Sometimes the rash may take the appearance of deep bruises or even bullous or hemorrhagic lesions.

In non-ambulatory children, the rash is classically noted on the face, trunk, and upper limbs, whereas the extensor surfaces of the legs and buttocks are involved in older patients. This pattern of distribution is thought to result from deposition of large IgA-immune complexes that activate the alternative complement pathway in gravity-dependent areas, disrupting vascular integrity and leading to extravasation of red blood cells. Cutaneous involvement may take the form of tender, localized subcutaneous edema affecting the forehead, periorbital region, or dorsum of the hands and feet.

Complete resolution of skin findings usually occurs in a week, with the rash fading to a yellow or purple-brown. Successive crops of lesions may develop over the course of the illness, leading to a polymorphous appearance. A recurrent rash is seen in about one-third of patients, usually within the first month of onset. Rarely recurrences may be seen for up to 2 years, although they tend to become milder over time.

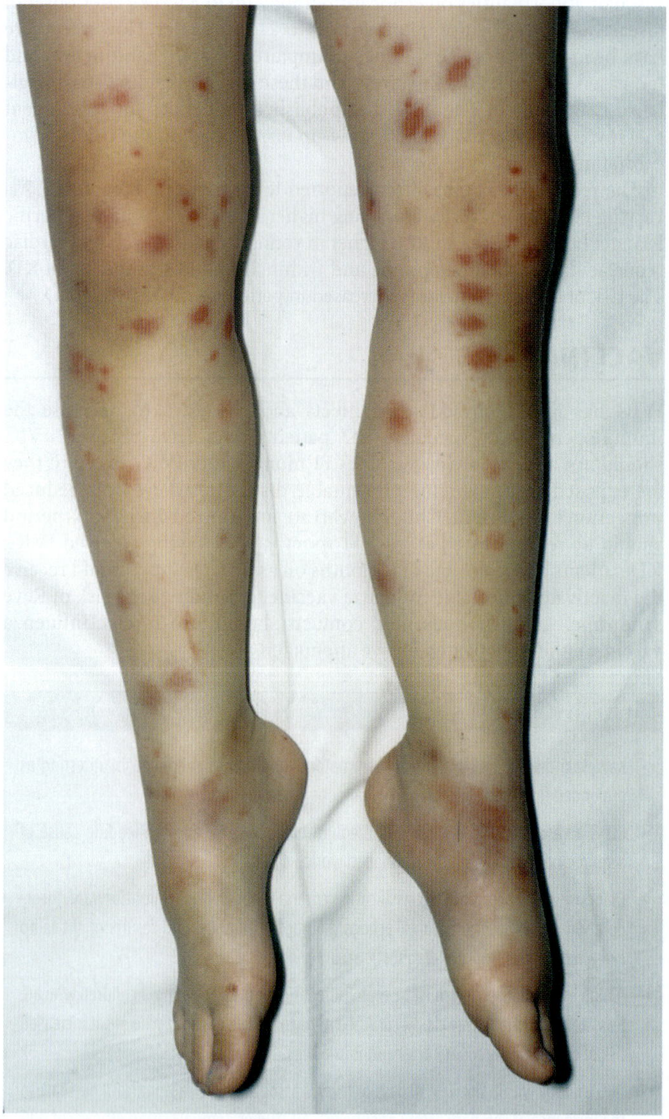

FIGURE 149-1. Characteristic palpable purpuric rash on the lower extremities in a child with IgAV. (From Knoop KJ, Stack LB, Storrow AB, Thurman RJ, eds. *The Atlas of Emergency Medicine*. 5th ed. New York: McGraw-Hill; 2021, Figure 14.67. Reproduced with permission from photo contributor: Lawrence B. Stack, MD.)

ARTHRALGIA/ARTHRITIS

Joint inflammation is the second most common manifestation of IgAV, seen in up to 82% of patients, though it is rarely the sole presenting symptom. The arthralgia is usually nondeforming, and characterized by periarticular swelling and tenderness without erythema, warmth, or joint effusion. Knees and ankles are the most frequently affected, while elbows, wrists, and hands may be involved as well. Usually, one to three joints are affected, with sparing of the small joints, although edema of the hands and feet may give the appearance of synovitis. The arthritis can be exquisitely painful and may severely limit the patient's range of motion, but it does not cause chronic or permanent joint damage. The characteristic accompanying rash of IgAV can help distinguish this entity from other forms of inflammatory joint disease, like reactive arthritis and transient synovitis.

GASTROINTESTINAL TRACT INVOLVEMENT

Colicky abdominal pain affects over 50% of patients with IgAV. Gastrointestinal (GI) symptoms usually occur within a week of the rash but can also present up to 4 weeks later or might precede the dermatologic manifestations. When the abdominal pain precedes the rash, it may be challenging to differentiate it from other causes of an acute abdomen, particularly appendicitis.

The abdominal pain in IgAV is caused by submucosal hemorrhage and edema stemming from vasculitis of the GI tract, like the vasculitis observed in the skin. The pain has an episodic waxing and waning nature. It may be associated with vomiting and may share features of a paralytic ileus. Complications such as intussusception, bowel infarction, or perforation may occur.

Intussusception occurs in 1% to 5% of patients and is ileo-ileal in up to 60% of cases, thus distinguishing it from the typical ileocolic intussusception associated with mesenteric adenitis or viral infections in young children. Hemorrhage and edema in a portion of the GI tract provide a lead point for the intussusception in IgAV.

GI mucosal injury might be present even without the characteristic abdominal pain, and is denoted by guaiac-positive stools, painless melena, hematochezia, increased stool alpha-1-antitrypsin, and/or hypoalbuminemia without proteinuria. Massive GI hemorrhage is rare. Less common GI manifestations are acute pancreatitis, cholecystitis, and protein-losing enteropathy.

RENAL INVOLVEMENT

Kidney disease is seen in 20% to 54% of children and is the fourth classical manifestation of IgAV, usually in the form of asymptomatic hematuria or proteinuria detected on urinalysis within the first 6 weeks of disease. Most patients will have some evidence of renal involvement within the first 6 months of disease, though it is often mild and evident on urinalysis only. In such cases, the risk of progression to chronic renal failure is less than 1%, with the risk increasing to 15% if the child has nephritic or nephrotic features and as much as 40% with evidence of both hematuria and high-grade proteinuria. The progression to renal failure is higher in older patients. Renal biopsies reveal histological features similar to IgA nephropathy. Urologic manifestations of IgAV may also be present, including scrotal swelling and tenderness secondary to epididymitis or orchitis, mimicking testicular torsion.

PULMONARY INVOLVEMENT

IgAV is a systemic vasculitis and thus may involve virtually any organ system, including the lungs. Rarely, interstitial pneumonia and diffuse alveolar hemorrhage (DAH) may occur, usually in male adolescents or in adults. DAH may present as hemoptysis, anemia, or chest infiltrates on radiographs. Imaging findings may be present in the absence of significant respiratory symptoms.

NEUROLOGIC INVOLVEMENT

Clinical neurologic involvement is uncommon and often transient. Mental status changes, headaches, ataxia, focal neurologic deficits, and peripheral neuropathies have all been described. The neurologic disturbances of IgAV may arise from a variety of causes other than cerebral vasculitis, including severe hypertension, electrolyte abnormalities due to renal or GI involvement, stroke, or intracranial hemorrhage.

DIFFERENTIAL DIAGNOSIS

The diagnosis of IgAV is straightforward in children presenting with the classic features, but can be more difficult in children with atypical presentations. Before concluding that a child has IgAV, other causes of palpable purpura should be considered. The differential diagnoses for the dermatologic features of IgAV include septicemia, idiopathic thrombocytopenic purpura, hemolytic-uremic syndrome, leukemia, and coagulopathies. Often, the overall clinical picture is sufficient to distinguish IgAV from these other conditions. If laboratory studies demonstrate thrombocytopenia and/or coagulation abnormalities, the diagnosis of IgAV is less likely.

When purpura is associated with normal platelet counts and coagulation studies, the differential diagnosis also includes other vasculitides, including hypersensitivity vasculitis, a small vessel vasculitis triggered by drug exposure or infection. In hypersensitivity vasculitis, the patient may present with fever, urticaria, arthralgias, lymphadenopathy, elevated inflammatory markers, and reduced serum complement. Histology reveals leukocytoclastic vasculitis without IgA deposition in the blood vessel walls, distinguishing it from IgAV. Other systemic and chronic vasculitides to consider include the cutaneous vasculitis associated with systemic lupus erythematosus (SLE), antineutrophil cytoplasmic antibody (ANCA)-associated vasculitides such as eosinophilic granulomatosis with polyangiitis (EGP, formerly known as Churg-Strauss syndrome) or granulomatosis with polyangiitis (GPA; previously known as Wegener granulomatosis), polyarteritis nodosa (PAN), and microscopic polyangiitis. These other vasculitides tend to have more significant systemic involvement, and they may be associated with supporting laboratory findings such as elevated autoantibodies and the presence of ANCAs, which are typically not seen in IgAV.

In children under 2 years of age, acute hemorrhagic edema of infancy (also known as Finkelstein or Seidlmayer disease) is a consideration. This is a self-limited, immune complex-mediated vasculitis characterized by rash, fever, and generalized edema. In acute hemorrhagic edema of infancy, the purpuric lesions tend to be larger (1-5 cm) and often involve the face, with the ears, cheeks, and eyelids most commonly involved. Visceral involvement is rare, and symptoms usually resolve spontaneously within 1 to 3 weeks. Biopsy reveals a leukocytoclastic vasculitis with occasional IgA deposition.

In children presenting with renal disease, the differential diagnosis is broad. Details are beyond the scope of this chapter, but consultation by a pediatric nephrologist should be considered.

DIAGNOSTIC EVALUATION

The diagnosis of IgAV is a clinical one, made after the appearance of the typical rash, with associated articular and/or GI involvement and possible renal involvement (**Table 149-1**). Laboratory investigations are nonspecific (**Table 149-2**) and are used mainly for assessing the extent of organ involvement or for excluding alternative diagnoses. A mild anemia may be the result of occult GI bleeding. Acute-phase reactants may be somewhat increased, with the degree of elevation often related to the triggering condition. Thus cases of IgAV triggered by bacterial infections, such as streptococcal pharyngitis, are more likely to present with increased ESR and CRP, while IgAV triggered by a virus may have no elevation in markers of systemic inflammation. Coagulation studies are not strictly necessary if the clinical picture is typical, though they may be helpful in excluding other diagnoses. Serum IgA is elevated in 50% to 70% of patients with IgAV, but not in many other causes of purpura, abdominal pain, hematuria, or arthritis, and serum complement levels can be transiently depressed. Autoantibodies are usually absent and therefore should not be routinely assayed unless alternative diagnoses are in question.

TABLE 149-1 EULAR/PRINTO/PRES Criteria for Classification of IgA Vasculitis

Clinical Feature	Description
Purpura (mandatory)	Purpura (commonly palpable and in crops) or petechiae, without thrombocytopenia. Often seen on lower limbs.
Abdominal pain	Acute onset diffuse abdominal colicky pain. Can present as intussusception and gastrointestinal bleeding.
Histopathology	Leukocytoclastic vasculitis with predominant IgA deposit or proliferative glomerulonephritis with predominant IgA deposit.
Arthritis/arthralgias	Acute onset arthritis (joint swelling, pain, decreased range of motion) or arthralgias (no joint swelling, preserved range of motion).
Renal involvement	Proteinuria >0.3 g/24 hr or >30 mmol/mg of urine albumin/creatinine ratio on a spot morning sample.
	Hematuria or red blood cell casts: >5 red blood cells/high-power field or red blood cell casts in the urinary sediment or ≥2+ on dipstick.

A patient is considered to have Henoch-Schönlein purpura if there is the classic purpura and at least one of the criteria 1 to 4 is present.

*For purpura with atypical distribution, a demonstration of an IgA deposit in a biopsy is required.

Source: Adapted from Ozen S, Pistorio A, et al. Paediatric Rheumatology International Trials Organisation (PRINTO). EULAR/PRINTO/PRES criteria for Henoch-Schönlein purpura, childhood polyarteritis nodosa, childhood Wegener granulomatosis and childhood Takayasu arteritis: Ankara 2008. Part II: Final classification criteria. *Ann Rheum Dis*. 2010;69(5):798-806.

All patients should have urinalysis for cells, casts, and proteinuria at diagnosis. Blood indices for renal function should be obtained in patients with abnormal urinalysis and/or hypertension. All adults should have a serum creatinine measured at presentation, as they are at increased risk for significant renal disease. Renal involvement typically follows other manifestations of IgAV by days or weeks, thus screening should be continued in all patients with IgAV for 6 months even if urinalysis is normal at presentation (see section Outcome and Follow-Up). Children with recurrent episodes of purpura, arthralgias, or abdominal pain require longer-term monitoring for renal involvement.

TABLE 149-2 Laboratory Studies in IgA Vasculitis

Test	Finding
Complete blood count	White blood cell count: normal or elevated Hemoglobin and hematocrit: normal or low Red blood cell indices: normal Platelet count: normal or increased
Serum electrolytes	Usually normal except for children with renal insufficiency or renal failure
Blood urea nitrogen and creatinine	Elevated in dehydration or renal insufficiency
Erythrocyte sedimentation rate and C-reactive protein	Normal or elevated
Transaminases and biliary tree enzymes	Normal or elevated with gallbladder or small bowel involvement
Albumin	Normal or decreased due to inflammation or nephrotic syndrome
Serum lipids	Triglyceride, cholesterol, and very-long-chain fatty acids may all be increased in patients with nephrotic syndrome
Immunoglobulins	May see polyclonal elevation; IgA and IgM elevated in 50% of patients
Antineutrophil cytoplasmic antibody (ANCA), antinuclear antibody, rheumatoid factor	All usually negative; may have "atypical" ANCA due to production of IgA ANCA
Coagulation profile	Prothrombin time, partial thromboplastin time, international normalized ratio all normal; D-dimer, fibrin split products may be increased
Complement	Clq, C3, C4 usually normal; properdin, factor B, CH50 may be decreased
Urinalysis	May contain red blood cells, white blood cells, protein, and casts, depending on degree of renal disease

In cases of diagnostic uncertainty, a biopsy of an affected organ may be performed. Most commonly, a skin biopsy of a lesion less than 24 hours old is sufficient for diagnostic purposes. Characteristic findings are a leukocytoclastic vasculitis with IgA deposits in the postcapillary venules. A renal biopsy is indicated in cases of continued diagnostic uncertainty and in patients with significant proteinuria, glomerulonephritis (hematuria and/or hypertension), or renal impairment. Histology is useful for delineating the extent and severity of kidney involvement, which would determine prognosis and guide management.

When abdominal symptoms are persistent, imaging should be considered if there is clinical concern for complications such as intussusception, ileus, or bowel perforation. Abdominal ultrasonography is the imaging modality of choice for suspected intussusception. Ultrasound may also reveal bowel wall thickening, abnormal peristalsis, or hematomas. An abdominal radiograph may show dilated small bowel loops from obstruction or ileus. However, findings of intussusception are not always evident on the plain film. A contrast enema will not be able to detect an ileo-ileal intussusception, as the contrast does not reach the ileum.

Imaging may be necessary in patients with IgAV who develop scrotal pain. Doppler flow studies will help distinguish testicular torsion, in which blood flow is decreased or absent, from the epididymitis or orchitis of IgAV, characterized by normal or increased perfusion caused by inflammation.

MANAGEMENT

In more than 90% of cases, IgAV is benign and self-limited. Outpatient care is adequate in the majority of the cases, with therapy aimed at providing symptomatic relief and supportive care. See section on Admission Criteria.

The arthropathy of IgAV tends to improve with acetaminophen, while more severe symptoms respond to nonsteroidal anti-inflammatory drugs (NSAIDs); for example, naproxen 10 to 20 mg/kg/day (maximum 1500 mg; 1000 mg if used beyond a week) in two divided doses. There is no evidence that NSAIDs increase the risk of GI hemorrhage in IgAV, so they are not contraindicated in children with normal renal function and/or urinalysis. Nevertheless, they may cause gastritis when taken on an empty stomach and should not be used in patients with active GI bleeding or glomerulonephritis. Adequate hydration can minimize potential adverse renal effects if NSAIDs are used. Where joint involvement is severe and interferes with ambulation and activities of daily living, a short course of steroids may be useful.

Abdominal pain may also be treated with acetaminophen and/or NSAIDs. Patients with physical findings concerning for peritonitis or obstruction should undergo urgent evaluation for concerns of bowel intussusception, infarction, or perforation. The physical examination alone is often insufficient to diagnose GI vasculitis and its complications.

For patients with more significant abdominal discomfort, corticosteroids may be helpful. Although steroids have not been shown to shorten the duration of abdominal involvement or reduce the risk of intussusception, they may be indicated in patients who have not responded to NSAIDs and whose abdominal pain is severe enough to preclude adequate oral intake. Steroids should not be given until abdominal complications such as intussusception or perforation are definitively excluded, as they may mask signs of peritonitis. The typical dose of prednisone or methylprednisolone is 1 to 2 mg/kg/day in two divided doses. Parenteral administration may be necessary until acute GI vasculitis improves, as bowel edema may compromise the absorption of oral medications.

It is important to note that steroids do not change the natural history of the disease but only ameliorate associated inflammation. Thus in a condition that typically resolves over 4 to 6 weeks, steroids should be tapered gradually by no more than 25% per week and the taper should be undertaken over 4 to 6 weeks. Symptoms recur when the steroid taper is more rapid than the speed with which pathologic immune complexes are cleared from the circulation, and aggressive steroid tapering is one of the major causes of readmission of children with IgAV. Symptoms may also worsen as children advance their diet and increase their level of physical activity (i.e., after discharge from the hospital), so families should support a gradual return to full activity.

Steroids have not been definitively shown to prevent long-term sequelae or alter the prognosis of IgAV. In particular, early treatment with steroids does not reduce the incidence and severity of nephropathy. For patients with more severe renal involvement (nephrotic-range proteinuria, renal impairment, or biopsy-proven crescentic glomerulonephritis) or organ- and/or life-threatening complications such as pulmonary hemorrhage or central nervous system vasculitis, early and aggressive management is essential. This typically includes steroids and often more potent immunosuppressive agents such as azathioprine, mycophenolate mofetil, or cyclophosphamide.

ADMISSION CRITERIA

- Diagnosis is in question and further evaluation or observation is necessary.
- Severity of abdominal symptoms prevents adequate enteral hydration.
- Joint pain precludes ambulation or activities of daily living despite oral medication.
- GI complications such as hemorrhage, intussusception, or perforation.
- Uncontrolled hypertension or significant renal involvement or insufficiency.
- Significant central nervous system or pulmonary involvement.
- Lack of appropriate outpatient follow-up.

DISCHARGE CRITERIA

- Clinically stable patient with resumption of oral intake and ambulation if previously impaired.
- Adequate pain control on a safe oral regimen.
- Sufficient caregiver education regarding outpatient plan and follow-up.

CONSULTATION

Involvement of a pediatric nephrologist is indicated when significant IgAV nephritis is present (see section on Special Considerations). Consultation with a pediatric rheumatologist is useful in patients with recalcitrant, recurrent, or steroid-resistant IgAV, or in patients with severe joint or significant other organ involvement.

OUTCOME AND FOLLOW-UP

Overall, the prognosis of IgAV in children is excellent. Aside from renal disease, the mean duration of symptoms is 3 to 4 weeks. Recurrence is seen in approximately one-third of children, usually within 4 months of the initial episode, but at times up to 2 years later. Recurrences are more likely in those who have a more severe course of IgAV. Subsequent episodes tend to be successively milder and of shorter duration. The long-term outcome is dependent on the presence and degree of renal involvement.

Patients with IgAV should have urinalysis and blood pressures checked weekly to biweekly for the first 2 months after presentation with ongoing but less frequent evaluation thereafter for up to a year from initial presentation. After 1 year, monitoring may be limited to urinalysis and measurement of blood pressure during annual physical examinations. In any patient with persistent or significant urinary abnormalities or hypertension, serum creatinine should be monitored more closely, in consultation with a nephrologist (see section on Special Considerations).

SPECIAL CONSIDERATIONS

Late renal deterioration can occur, even in patients with complete resolution of acute findings. A poor renal prognosis is associated with patients presenting with nephrotic syndrome, hypertension, kidney function impairment, and specific findings on biopsy including crescentic glomerulonephritis and tubulointerstitial fibrosis. Thus consultation with a pediatric nephrologist is indicated in patients presenting with significant renal involvement. Individuals who have a history of even mild renal symptoms at onset of IgAV should also be carefully observed during and after pregnancy, as a history of IgAV in childhood is associated with an increased risk of gestational hypertension and proteinuria.

KEY POINTS

- IgAV is the most common childhood vasculitis, with the classic tetrad of palpable purpura, joint pain, abdominal pain, and renal involvement.
- The prognosis of IgAV is excellent, even in the presence of recurrences.
- The long-term outcome is dependent on the presence of renal involvement.
- Steroids are useful in children with significant joint or GI involvement but there is no evidence that they alter the long-term prognosis of the GI or renal disease.
- Full recovery after IgAV typically requires at least 1 month, thus the resumption of normal activities and diet and the tapering of medications (especially steroids), should be very gradual.

SUGGESTED READINGS

Bayram C, Demircin G, Erdoğan O, Bülbül M, Caltik A, Akyüz S. Prevalence of MEFV mutations and their clinical correlations in Turkish children with Henoch-Schönlein Purpura. *Acta Paediatr.* 2011;100:745-749.

Branski D, Gross V, Gross-Kieselstein E, Roll D, Abrahamov A. Pancreatitis as a complication of Henoch–Schonlein purpura. *J Pediatr Gastroenterol Nutr.* 1982;1(2):275-276.

Brogan PBA. Leukocytoclastic vasculitis. In: Cassidy JT, Petty RE, Laxer RM, et al, eds. *Textbook of Pediatric Rheumatology.* Saunders Elsevier; 2011.

Calabrese LH, Michel BA, Bloch DA, et al. The American College of Rheumatology 1990 criteria for the classification of hypersensitivity vasculitis. *Arthritis Rheum.* 1990;33(8):1108-1113.

Chang WL, Yang YH, Lin YT, Chiang BL. Gastrointestinal manifestations in Henoch-Schönlein purpura: a review of 261 patients. *Acta Paediatr.* 2004;93(11):1427-1431.

Cho CS, Min JK, Park SH, et al. Protein losing enteropathy associated with Henoch-Schönlein purpura in a patient with rheumatoid arthritis. *Scand J Rheumatol.* 1996;25(5):334-336.

Choong CK, Beasley SW. Intra-abdominal manifestations of Henoch-Schönlein Purpura. *J Paediatr Child Health.* 1998;34(5):405-409.

Coppo R, Andrulli S, Amore A, et al. Predictors of outcome in Henoch-Schönlein nephritis in children and adults. *Am J Kidney Dis.* 2006;47(6):993-1003.

Dudley J, Smith G, Llewelyn-Edwards A, Bayliss K, Pike K, Tizard J. Randomised, double-blind, placebo-controlled trial to determine whether steroids reduce the incidence and severity of nephropathy in Henoch-Schönlein Purpura (HSP). *Arch Dis Child.* 2013;98(10):756-763.

Feldt RH, Stickler GB. The gastrointestinal manifestations of anaphylactoid purpura in children. *Proc Staff Meet Mayo Clin.* 1962;37:465-473.

Garzoni L, Vanoni F, Rizzi M, et al. Nervous system dysfunction in Henoch–Schönlein syndrome: systematic review of the literature. *Rheumatol.* 2009;48(12):1524-1529.

Goldstein AR, White RH, Akuse R, Chantler C. Long-term follow-up of childhood Henoch-Schönlein nephritis. *Lancet.* 1992;339(8788):280-282.

Gómez S, Pérez M, Pellegrini M, et al. Henoch-Schonlein purpura in pediatrics: ten years of experience at a moderate risk office of a general hospital. *Arch Argent Pediatr*. 2020;118(1):31-37.

Hahn D, Hodson EM, Willis NS, Craig JC. Interventions for preventing and treating kidney disease in Henoch-Schönlein Purpura (HSP). *Cochrane Database Syst Rev*. 2015;2015(8).

Jauhola O, Ronkainen J, Koskimies O, et al. Clinical course of extrarenal symptoms in Henoch-Schonlein purpura: a 6-month prospective study. *Arch Dis Child*. 2010;95(11):871-876.

Jennette JC, Falk RJ, Bacon PA, et al. 2012 Revised International Chapel Hill Consensus Conference Nomenclature of Vasculitides. *Arthritis Rheum*. 2013;65(1):1-11.

Kumon Y, Hisatake K, Chikamori M, et al. A case of vasculitic cholecystitis associated with Schönlein-Henoch purpura in an adult. *Gastroenterol Jpn*. 1988;23(1):68-72.

Leung AKC, Barankin B, Leong KF. Henoch-Schönlein Purpura in children: an updated review. *Curr Pediatr Rev*. 2020;16(4):265-276.

Lin Q, Min Y, Li Y, et al. Henoch-Schönlein purpura with hypocomplementemia. *Pediatr Nephrol*. 2012;27(5):801-806.

López-Mejías R, Genre F, Pérez BS, et al. Association of HLA-B*41:02 with Henoch-Schönlein Purpura (IgA Vasculitis) in Spanish individuals irrespective of the HLA-DRB1 status. *Arthritis Res Ther*. 2015;17(1).

Nadrous HF, Yu AC, Specks U, Ryu JH. Pulmonary involvement in Henoch-Schönlein purpura. *Mayo Clin Proc*. 2004;79(9):1151-1157.

Narchi H. Risk of long term renal impairment and duration of follow up recommended for Henoch-Schönlein purpura with normal or minimal urinary findings: a systematic review. *Arch Dis Child*. 2005;90(9):916.

Pittet LF, Siebert JN, Lacroix LE. Striking but benign: acute haemorrhagic oedema of infancy. *Lancet*. 2022;399(10336):e41.

Ronkainen J, Nuutinen M, Koskimies O. The adult kidney 24 years after childhood Henoch-Schönlein purpura: a retrospective cohort study. *Lancet*. 2002;360(9334):666-670.

Saraclar Y, Tinaztepe K, Adaliolu G, Tuncer A. Acute hemorrhagic edema of infancy (AHEI)–a variant of Henoch-Schönlein purpura or a distinct clinical entity? *J Allergy Clin Immunol*. 1990;86(4 Pt 1):473-483.

Stewart M, Savage JM, Bell B, McCord B. Long term renal prognosis of Henoch-Schönlein purpura in an unselected childhood population. *Eur J Pediatr*. 1988;147(2):113-115.

Trapani S, Micheli A, Grisolia F, et al. Henoch Schonlein Purpura in childhood: epidemiological and clinical analysis of 150 cases over a 5-year period and review of literature. *Semin Arthritis Rheum*. 2005;35(3):143-153.

Trygstad CW, Stiehm ER. Elevated serum IgA globulin in anaphylactoid purpura. *Pediatrics*. 1971;47(6):1023-1028.

Weiss PF. Pediatric vasculitis. *Pediatr Clin North Am*. 2012;59(2):407.

Zaffanello M, Brugnara M, Franchini M. Therapy for children with Henoch-Schonlein purpura nephritis: a systematic review. *Sci World J*. 2007;7:20-30.

CHAPTER 150 Juvenile Dermatomyositis

Susan Kim, MD, MMSc

BACKGROUND

Juvenile dermatomyositis (JDM) is the most common pediatric acquired inflammatory myopathy. It is a diffuse vasculopathy and multisystem condition that primarily involves inflammation in skin and striated muscle and often leads to significant weakness. Pathognomonic cutaneous features of JDM include heliotrope rash and Gottron papules, which aid in the diagnosis of this rare condition. JDM has an estimated incidence of 1 to 3 in 1 million children, with an approximate 2:1 female predominance. Affected children are typically between 4 and 10 years of age with an average age of onset of 7 years. Outcomes in JDM may vary, but historically there was significant morbidity and mortality; without adequate treatment, one-third of affected children will have moderate to severe disability, and another third will succumb to disease.

PATHOGENESIS

Despite extensive research, the pathogenesis of JDM remains unknown. There is often seasonal clustering of new cases of JDM, suggesting an environmental or infectious trigger. Ultraviolet radiation (UVR) has been found to be associated with JDM, and a higher UVR index has been associated with the presence of specific myositis-specific antibodies (i.e., anti-TIF-1) in patients with JDM compared to polymyositis patients. Maternal toxic exposures have also been implicated as a risk factor in the development of JDM. An association with specific infectious processes raises the possibility of molecular mimicry as a mechanism in JDM, but no single agent has been identified.

There appears to be genetic susceptibility to develop JDM, with one study suggesting nearly half of the families with JDM had at least one family member with another autoimmune condition. Other studies have described HLA associations in patients with JDM, and the TNF-α-308A allele has been associated with a prolonged disease course.

Abnormalities in humoral-mediated immunity, cell-mediated immunity, and immune complex disease have also been implicated in the pathogenesis, but these results have been varied. Some research suggests a role of major histocompatibility complex (MHC)-I, where there is overexpression in JDM and myositis-associated antibodies. Elevated immunoglobulin levels and myositis-specific autoantibodies, which have been identified in most patients with JDM, suggest a humoral component to the pathogenesis of JDM. Type 1 interferons have also been implicated and are thought to contribute to enhanced MHC-I expression, cell cytotoxicity, and activation of T cells. Additional research suggests a possible role of maternal microchimerism, where maternal cells trigger an immune response akin to graft-versus-host disease in the child.

CLINICAL PRESENTATION

Children with JDM are diagnosed at 18 years of age or younger, and typically present with proximal muscle weakness and a pathognomonic rash that includes Heliotrope rash and/or Gottron papules. There is a heterogeneous presentation of JDM, which can vary from mild to severe skin involvement and mild to severe weakness, and the presentation may be acute or insidious. The weakness of JDM may have variable clinical presentations including nonspecific or mild malaise, myalgia, decreased general stamina and endurance with activities, difficulty in climbing stairs and getting up out of bed, and difficulty with combing hair or brushing teeth.

The formal diagnosis of JDM had historically been based on the Bohan and Peter criteria from the 1970s, and in 2017 updated classification criteria for myositis were accepted by the European League Against Rheumatism (EULAR) and the American College of Rheumatology (ACR) (**Table 150-1**; www.imm.ki.se/biostatistics/calculators/iim).

TABLE 150-1 Bohan and Peter's Criteria of Dermatomyositis*

1. Symmetrical weakness of the proximal muscles
2. Characteristic skin changes consisting of heliotrope rash and Gottron papules
3. Elevation of the serum level of one of the muscle enzymes
4. Electromyography demonstrating denervation and myopathy
5. Muscle biopsy displaying necrosis and inflammation

Bohan and Peter's Criteria for Dermatomyositis are used to diagnose children with JDM.

*Patients with the characteristic skin changes and three additional criteria are considered to have definite JDM, and with two additional criteria are considered to have probable JDM.

Source: Data adapted from Bohan A, Peter JB. Polymyositis and dermatomyositis. *N Engl J Med*. 1975;292:344-347.

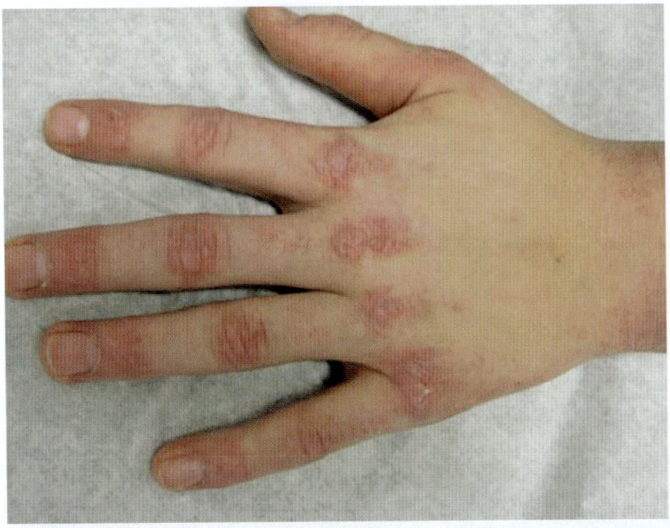

FIGURE 150-1. Gottron papules are typically found over the extensor surfaces of the hands, elbows, knees, or ankles and are typically described as erythematous, raised papules.

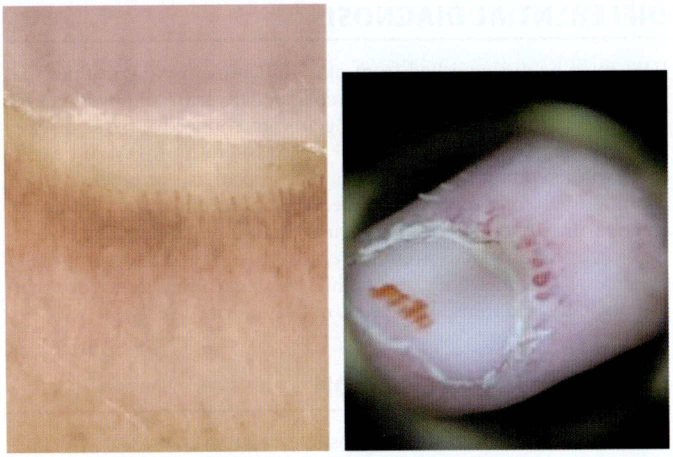

A B

FIGURE 150-3. Nail-bed capillaroscopy in juvenile dermatomyositis. Top panel shows a normal patient without evidence of vasculopathy on capillaroscopy. Bottom panel shows vasculopathy in a patient with juvenile dermatomyositis with thickening of capillaries and drop out of capillaries, as well as decreased number.

The pathognomonic rashes of JDM include Gottron papules and heliotrope rash. Gottron papules are typically found over the extensor surfaces of the interphalangeal joints, elbows, knees, or ankles and are described as erythematous, raised papules (**Figure 150-1**). Heliotrope rash is a periorbital red-purplish discoloration associated with periorbital edema (**Figure 150-2**). Other rashes associated with JDM include periungual erythema and nail-bed capillary abnormalities best seen with capillaroscopy (**Figure 150-3**), and a macular violaceous erythematous rash with distribution in the neck and upper chest (V-sign), nape of the neck, upper back, and posterior aspect of the shoulders (shawl sign), or lateral surfaces of the hips (holster sign).

All organ systems may be involved in JDM, including the gastrointestinal tract, heart, lungs, joints, and central and peripheral nervous systems, which can be a source of significant morbidity and mortality and should be monitored for throughout the disease course. Systemic features can include cardiac conduction abnormalities, diminished ventilatory and lung diffusion capacity, esophageal, gastric, and gastrointestinal dysmotility, ulcers, hemorrhage, and perforation. Ulcerative skin disease in JDM suggests a more aggressive disease course with extensive systemic vasculopathy that is potentially life-threatening and requires more aggressive therapy and closer monitoring.

Based on the severity and duration of muscle weakness, patients may present with muscular atrophy due to disuse as well as contractures around the joints of disuse that can lead to irreversible physical limitations if untreated. It is not uncommon for children to report myalgia. In addition, more than half of children with JDM are reported to have associated arthritis.

Long-term cutaneous sequelae may include calcinosis and lipodystrophy. Calcinosis occurs in up to 40% of children with JDM; findings may include small subcutaneous nodules and large tumorous deposits. Calcinosis typically occurs at sites of trauma (e.g., elbows, knees), especially in later phases of disease, severe cases, and cases where treatment is insufficient or delayed. Calcinosis may lead to physical limitations and contractures, as well as infections related to ulceration with significant cosmetic sequelae (**Figure 150-4**). Lipodystrophy occurs in up to 40% of children with JDM. It is an acquired loss of subcutaneous fat in a localized or generalized distribution that is cosmetically disfiguring. Lipodystrophy commonly results in metabolic abnormalities such as insulin resistance and hyperlipidemia.

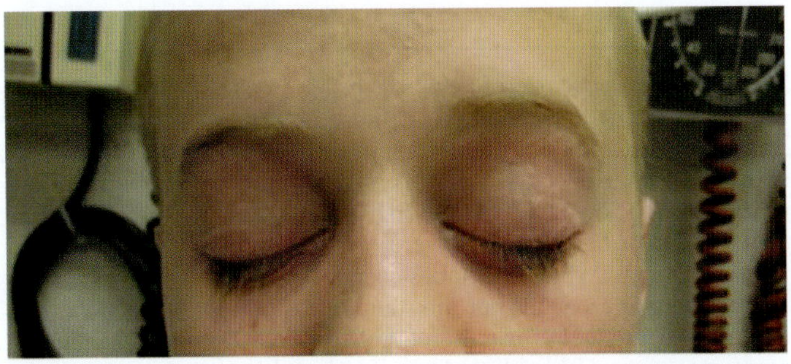

FIGURE 150-2. Heliotrope rash is a periorbital red-purplish discoloration associated with periorbital edema. (Photo used with permission from Dr. Fatma Dedeoglu.)

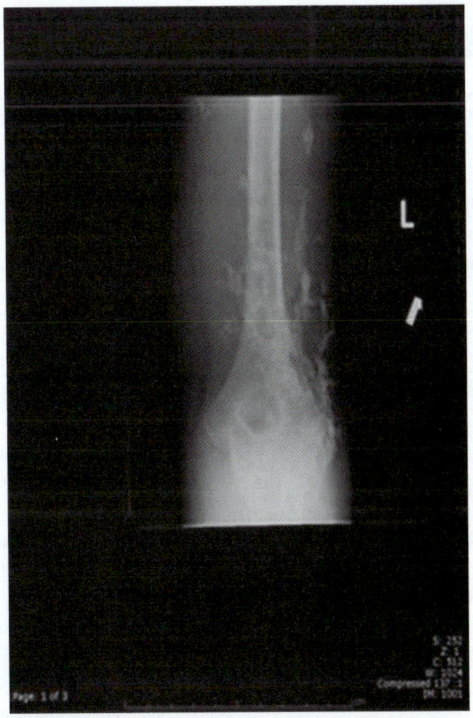

FIGURE 150-4. Calcinosis can be seen on plain film easily in this patient with juvenile dermatomyositis.

DIFFERENTIAL DIAGNOSIS

JDM must be distinguished from other inflammatory myopathies that cause muscle weakness, such as juvenile polymyositis and overlap syndromes with associated myositis (e.g., mixed connective tissue disease, scleroderma). It is also common for the classic rash of JDM to be confused with common skin conditions such as psoriasis or eczema. Other conditions to consider include infectious myopathies (e.g., influenza, enterovirus, coxsackievirus, parvovirus) and noninflammatory myopathies such as muscular dystrophies (e.g., Duchenne and Becker muscular dystrophy) and metabolic myopathies (e.g., carnitine deficiency syndromes, fatty acid transport defects, mitochondrial defects).

DIAGNOSTIC EVALUATION

The pace and extent of the diagnostic evaluation in a child with suspected JDM depends on the severity of disease. A comprehensive history and thorough physical examination with detailed strength and skin assessment are essential. Standardized methods of assessing and monitoring function and strength in JDM may include manual muscle testing (MMT) and the Childhood Myositis Assessment Scale which may be used to follow each child's clinical trajectory.

Further evaluation for JDM includes comprehensive laboratory analysis for myositis, as not all values may be elevated (**Table 150-2**). This testing typically includes creatine kinase, lactate dehydrogenase, aspartate aminotransferase, alanine aminotransferase, and aldolase. We often include Factor 8-related antigen, a marker of endothelial damage, which may be elevated in vasculopathies, including JDM. Autoantibodies such as antinuclear antibody may be positive but are not diagnostic for JDM, and rheumatoid factors are typically negative. Nonspecific markers of inflammation are typically normal (e.g., erythrocyte sedimentation rate and C-reactive protein). Myositis-specific and myositis-associated antibodies (MSAs and MAAs) may be found in most patients with JDM but are not used to confirm the diagnosis because they are not commonly available for commercial testing and the reliability in many labs is not confirmed. MSAs and MAAs are areas of active research and play a role in identifying specific phenotypes and subsets of inflammatory myopathies, and may help to inform response to therapy and prognosis.

TABLE 150-2 Initial Evaluation of Patients Suspected of Having Juvenile Dermatomyositis

Test	Comment
Creatinine kinase	Elevated in myositis; infrequent involvement of other organs that can generate creatinine kinase (e.g., brain, cardiac muscle)
Lactate dehydrogenase	Elevated in myositis
Aspartate aminotransferase (AST) and alanine aminotransferase (ALT)	Often elevated in myositis
Aldolase	Elevated in myositis
Factor 8–related antigen	A marker of endothelial damage, which may be elevated in vasculopathies such as JDM
Myositis-associated antibodies	These include Mi-2, Jo-1, anti-p155, anti-MDA 5 and anti-MJ Elevated in up to 40% of patients with JDM but do not have a role in confirming the diagnosis
Chest radiograph	To identify complications such as interstitial lung disease or dilated cardiomyopathy
Electrocardiogram	To identify complications such as tachyarrhythmias and dilated cardiomyopathy
Swallowing study	Consider this test in patients with changes in voice or difficulties with swallowing to assess aspiration risk and esophageal dysmotility

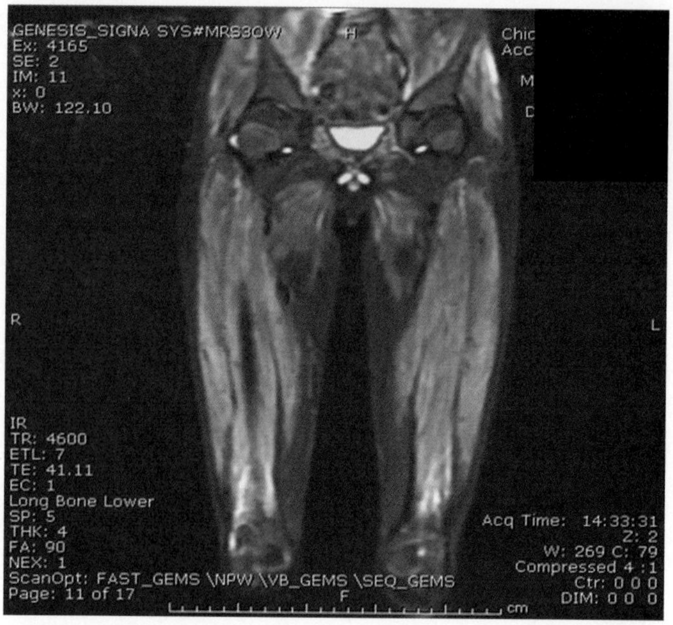

FIGURE 150-5. MRI imaging of a patient with juvenile dermatomyositis. MRI with short tau inversion recovery (STIR) technique shows extensive bright signal throughout the musculature in the left panel, with normalization of this signal several years later (right panel).

A baseline chest X-ray and electrocardiogram are reasonable for most patients (Table 150-2). Patients with changes in voice or with limitations in deglutition should have a baseline swallowing evaluation and modification of diet if abnormalities are found.

In cases where there is a classic JDM rash and weakness with elevated muscle enzymes, magnetic resonance imaging (MRI) is typically utilized in lieu of invasive procedures such as muscle biopsy and electromyography. MRI is typically ordered as T2-weighted images with fat suppression or MRI with short tau inversion recovery (STIR) technique that can demonstrate the edema associated with the inflammation in the muscles of JDM (**Figure 150-5**).

In cases that are not classic (e.g., atypical or no rash), skin biopsy, muscle biopsy, and/or electromyography (EMG) are necessary. The skin biopsy in JDM most often shows perivascular lymphocytic infiltrate in the dermis typically referred to as an interface dermatitis. Muscle biopsy in JDM usually reveals degeneration of types I and II muscle fibers, perivascular mononuclear infiltrate, and perifascicular atrophy. It is important that the biopsy site is an area of active inflammation and weakness, typically the deltoid or quadriceps muscles. When performed, an EMG shows short, polyphasic, small motor-unit potentials, insertional irritability, spontaneous fibrillations, and high-frequency repetitive discharges.

MANAGEMENT

Therapy with corticosteroids, which began in the 1960s, revolutionized the treatment and improved the prognosis of JDM. There are limited clinical trials in the treatment of JDM, but in general, retrospective case series suggest that the prompt and aggressive treatment of JDM is associated with better long-term outcomes. Treatment decisions should be based on the severity and extent of disease, and initial treatment for JDM often includes corticosteroids. There is variability in treatment approaches but the standard of care for JDM includes a steroid-sparing agent, usually methotrexate. Protocols and management recommendations have been developed in an attempt to make the treatment and study of outcomes in JDM more uniform. Patients diagnosed with JDM should be referred to a pediatric rheumatologist or neurologist with experience in the treatment and management of this uncommon condition.

In general, our approach for children with JDM who present with moderately severe weakness and limitations in activities of daily living includes initial therapy with high-dose intravenous immunoglobulin (IVIG) and parenteral pulse-dose corticosteroids. Following three sequential daily doses of intravenous steroids, we typically continue monthly IVIG with intravenous steroids until there is normalization of muscle enzymes and strength. Oral daily steroids are added concomitantly and weaned over the course of months based on normalization of rash, muscle enzymes, and strength. IVIG doses are typically 2 g per kilogram, often with a maximum dose of 70 g, parenteral pulse doses of methylprednisolone are typically 30 mg per kilogram with a maximum dose of 1 g, and initial oral doses of prednisone are typically 2 mg per kilogram with a maximum dose of 60 mg. In less severe cases, IVIG could be reserved for later use. Patients who fail to respond sufficiently to therapy are treated with additional steroid-sparing medications.

Steroid-sparing agents are normally administered along with corticosteroids, in hopes of weaning and limiting steroid exposure and associated side effects over time. The most used first-line steroid-sparing agent is methotrexate, but other second-line treatments may include cyclosporine, tacrolimus, intravenous immunoglobulin, azathioprine, mycophenolate mofetil, cyclophosphamide, abatacept, and rituximab. Medications are gradually tapered with close follow-up of strength and skin exams as well as laboratory markers of myositis. In general, only when there is significant or complete clinical and laboratory improvement of JDM markers are medications tapered. Escalation of therapy is necessary if patients fail to improve or worsen in terms of both their rash and muscle involvement.

Supportive care is very important to the recovery of JDM and should include adequate nutrition and physical therapy. Physical therapy and rehabilitation are very important in patients with severe weakness who are unable to ambulate and in patients who develop joint contractures.

ADMISSION AND DISCHARGE CRITERIA

We recommend that any patients with significant limitations in activities of daily living be admitted to the hospital to expedite evaluation and treatment. Any patient with changes in voice, difficulty swallowing liquids or solids, choking, abdominal pain, and/or melena or hematochezia requires prompt admission and treatment.

It is reasonable to discharge patients once severe weakness and ability to ambulate and function are improved. In severe cases, it may be necessary for patients to be discharged to a rehabilitation center during the initiation of treatment, as it may take some time for the treatment to take effect and for patients to regain muscle strength and stamina.

CONSULTATION

If JDM is suspected, a pediatric rheumatologist, dermatologist, or neurologist can help in making the diagnosis and in long-term management of this disease. Additional support may be needed with physical and occupational therapy based on the level of disability. If there is any significant dermatologic, gastrointestinal, pulmonary, or cardiac involvement, the appropriate subspecialists should be involved in the care of these patients. Patients receiving long-term corticosteroids or hydroxychloroquine should see an ophthalmologist regularly to monitor for toxicity. Patients and families benefit from formal mental health support and monitoring from a dietician.

SPECIAL CONSIDERATIONS

Sun protection is vital in children with JDM because sun exposure contributes to worsening skin disease. Sun protection should include avoidance of outdoor activity during peak hours and using high SPF sunscreens as well as protective clothing. Dietary considerations include optimizing caloric intake as well as calcium and vitamin D intake to maintain bone health.

KEY POINTS

- JDM is an autoimmune condition that most commonly affects the skin and muscle.
- JDM is a systemic condition that affects multiple organ systems and can have significant morbidity and mortality without prompt treatment.
- The rash of JDM can often be confused with common dermatologic conditions such as eczema or psoriasis, as well as systemic lupus erythematosus.
- Treatment for JDM is diverse and depends on the severity of disease.

SUGGESTED READINGS

Batthish M, Feldman BM. Juvenile dermatomyositis. *Curr Rheumatol Rep*. 2011;13: 216-224.

Bellutti Enders F, Meunier BB, Baildam E, et al. Consensus-based recommendations for the management of juvenile dermatomyositis. *Ann Rheum Dis*. 2017;76:329-340.

Bilgic H, Ytterberg SR, Amin S, et al. Interleukin-6 and type I interferon-regulated genes and chemokines mark disease activity in dermatomyositis. *Arthritis Rheum*. 2009;60:3436-3446.

Bohan A, Peter JB. Polymyositis and dermatomyositis: (First of Two Parts). *N Engl J Med*. 1975;292:344-347.

Bohan A, Peter JB. Polymyositis and dermatomyositis: (Second of Two Parts). *N Engl J Med*. 1975;292:403-407.

Enders FB, Meunier BB, Baildam E, et al. Consensus-based recommendations for the management of juvenile dermatomyositis. *Ann Rheum Dis*. 2017;76(2):329-340.

Fisler RE, Liang MG, Fuhlbrigge RC, Yalcindag A, Sundel RP. Aggressive management of juvenile dermatomyositis results in improved outcome and decreased incidence of calcinosis. *J Am Acad Dermatol*. 2002;47:505-511.

Gitiaux C, Latroche C, Gayet MW, et al. Myogenic progenitor cells exhibit Type I interferon-driven proangiogenic properties and molecular signature during juvenile dermatomyositis. *Arthritis Rheumatol*. 2018;70:134-145.

Greenberg SA. Dermatomyositis and type 1 interferons. *Curr Rheumatol Rep*. 2010;12:198-203.

Hinze CH, Oommen PT, Dressler F, et al. Development of practice and consensus-based strategies including a treat-to-target approach for the management of moderate and severe juvenile dermatomyositis in Germany and Austria. *Pediatr Rheumatol*. 2018;16:40.

Huber AM, Kim S, Reed AM, et al. Childhood arthritis and rheumatology research alliance consensus clinical treatment plans for juvenile dermatomyositis with persistent skin rash. *J Rheumatol*. 2017;44:110-116.

Huber AM, Giannini EH, Bowyer SL, et al. Protocols for the initial treatment of moderately severe juvenile dermatomyositis: results of a Children's Arthritis and Rheumatology Research Alliance Consensus Conference. *Arthritis Care Res*. 2010;62:219-225.

Huemer C, Kitson H, Malleson PN, et al. Lipodystrophy in patients with juvenile dermatomyositis–evaluation of clinical and metabolic abnormalities. *J Rheumatol*. 2001;28: 610-615.

Khanna S, Reed AM. Immunopathogenesis of juvenile dermatomyositis. *Muscle Nerve*. 2010;41:581-592.

Kim S, Hallak ME, Dedeoglu F, Zurakowski D, Fuhlbrigge RC, Sundel RP. Complete and sustained remission of juvenile dermatomyositis resulting from aggressive treatment. *Arthritis Rheum*. 2009;60:1825-1830.

Li CKC, Varsani H, Holton JL, et al. MHC Class I overexpression on muscles in early juvenile dermatomyositis. *J Rheumatol*. 2004;31:605-609.

Lundberg IE, Tjärnlund A, Bottai M, et al. 2017 European League Against Rheumatism/American College of Rheumatology Classification Criteria for Adult and Juvenile Idiopathic Inflammatory Myopathies and Their Major Subgroups. *Arthritis Rheumatol*. 2017;69:2271-2282.

Mamyrova G, O'Hanlon TP, Monroe JB, et al. Immunogenetic risk and protective factors for juvenile dermatomyositis in Caucasians. *Arthritis Rheum*. 2006;54:3979-3987.

Manlhiot C, Liang L, Tran D, Bitnun A, Tyrrell PN, Feldman BM. Assessment of an infectious disease history preceding juvenile dermatomyositis symptom onset. *Rheumatol.* 2008;47: 526-529.

Massa M, Costouros N, Mazzoli F, et al. Self epitopes shared between human skeletal myosin and Streptococcus pyogenes M5 protein are targets of immune responses in active juvenile dermatomyositis. *Arthritis Rheum.* 2002;46:3015-3025.

McCann LJ, Juggins AD, Maillard SM, et al. The Juvenile Dermatomyositis National Registry and Repository (UK and Ireland)–clinical characteristics of children recruited within the first 5 yr. *Rheumatol.* 2006;45:1255-1260.

Mendez EP, Lipton R, Goldman RR, et al. US incidence of juvenile dermatomyositis, 1995-1998: results from the National Institute of Arthritis and Musculoskeletal and Skin Diseases Registry. *Arthritis Rheum.* 2003;49:300-305.

Miller FW, Rider LG, Chung YL, et al. Proposed preliminary core set measures for disease outcome assessment in adult and juvenile idiopathic inflammatory myopathies. *Rheumatol.* 2001;40:1262-1273.

Moneta GM, Marafon DP, Marasco E, et al. Muscle expression of type I and type II interferons is increased in juvenile dermatomyositis and related to clinical and histologic features. *Arthritis Rheumatol.* 2019;71:1011-1021.

Niewold TB, Kariuki SN, Morgan GA, Shrestha S, Pachman LM. Elevated serum interferon-alpha activity in juvenile dermatomyositis: associations with disease activity at diagnosis and after thirty-six months of therapy. *Arthritis Rheum.* 2009;60:1815-1824.

Niewold TB, Wu SC, Smith M, Morgan GA, Pachman LM. Familial aggregation of autoimmune disease in juvenile dermatomyositis. *Pediatrics.* 2011;127:e1239-e1246.

Olson NY, Lindsley CB. Adjunctive use of hydroxychloroquine in childhood dermatomyositis. *J Rheumatol.* 1989;16:1545-1547.

Orione MAM, Silva CA, Sallum AME, et al. Risk factors for juvenile dermatomyositis: exposure to tobacco and air pollutants during pregnancy. *Arthritis Care Res.* 2014;66:1571-1575.

Pachman LM, Jonasson O, Cannon RA, Friedman JM. Increased frequency of HLA-B8 in juvenile dermatomyositis. *Lancet.* 1977;2:1238.

Pachman LM, Khojah AM. Advances in juvenile dermatomyositis: myositis specific antibodies aid in understanding disease heterogeneity. *J Pediatr.* 2018;195:16-27.

Pachman LM, Liotta-Davis MR, Hong DK, et al. TNFalpha-308A allele in juvenile dermatomyositis: association with increased production of tumor necrosis factor alpha, disease duration, and pathologic calcifications. *Arthritis Rheum.* 2000;43:2368-2377.

Pachman LM, Lipton R, Goldman RR, et al. History of infection before the onset of juvenile dermatomyositis: results from the National Institute of Arthritis and Musculoskeletal and Skin Diseases Research Registry. *Arthritis Rheum.* 2005;53:166-172.

Ramanan AV, Feldman BM. Clinical features and outcomes of juvenile dermatomyositis and other childhood onset myositis syndromes. *Rheum Dis Clin North Am.* 2002;28:833-857.

Ramanan AV, Feldman BM. Clinical outcomes in juvenile dermatomyositis. *Curr Opin Rheumatol.* 2002;14:658-662.

Ramanan AV, Webster NC, Ota S, et al. The effectiveness of treating juvenile dermatomyositis with methotrexate and aggressively tapered corticosteroids. *Arthritis Rheum.* 2005;52:3570-3578.

Reed AM, Pachman L, Ober C. Molecular genetic studies of major histocompatibility complex genes in children with juvenile dermatomyositis: increased risk associated with HLA-DQA1 *0501. *Hum Immunol.* 1991;32:235-240.

Reed AM, Peterson E, Bilgic H, et al. Changes in novel biomarkers of disease activity in juvenile and adult dermatomyositis are sensitive biomarkers of disease course. *Arthritis Rheum.* 2012;64:4078-4086.

Rider LG, Nistala, K. The juvenile idiopathic inflammatory myopathies: pathogenesis, clinical and autoantibody phenotypes, and outcomes. *J Intern Med.* 2016;280:24-38.

Sallum AME, Pivato FCMM, Filho UD, et al. Risk factors associated with calcinosis of juvenile dermatomyositis. *J Pediatr.* (Rio J.) 2008;84:68-74.

Shah M, Mamyrova G, Targoff IN, et al. The clinical phenotypes of the juvenile idiopathic inflammatory myopathies. Medicine (Baltimore) 2013;92:25-41.

Stringer E, Bohnsack J, Bowyer SL, et al. Treatment approaches to juvenile dermatomyositis (JDM) across North America: The Childhood Arthritis and Rheumatology Research Alliance (CARRA) JDM Treatment Survey. *J Rheumatol.* 2010;37:1953-1961.

Sullivan DB, Cassidy JT, Petty RE, Burt A. Prognosis in childhood dermatomyositis. *J Pediatr.* 1972;80:555-563.

Symmons DP, Sills JA, Davis SM. The incidence of juvenile dermatomyositis: results from a nation-wide study. *Br J Rheumatol.* 1995;34:732-736.

Tse S, Lubelsky S, Gordon M, et al. The arthritis of inflammatory childhood myositis syndromes. *J Rheumatol.* 2001;28:192-197.

Wu J-Q, Lu M-P, Reed AM. Juvenile dermatomyositis: advances in clinical presentation, myositis-specific antibodies and treatment. *World J Pediatr.* 2020;16:31-43.

CHAPTER 151

Juvenile Idiopathic Arthritis

Anthony Cooley, MD and Sampath Prahalad, MD, MSc*

BACKGROUND

Arthritis is inflammation of synovial tissue within a diarthrodial joint. Idiopathic arthritides are distinct from infection-related arthritides (see Chapter 153). Because the pathogenesis of the idiopathic forms is not completely understood, a variety of schemes have been devised to classify childhood arthritides according to the pattern of joint involvement, associated symptoms, and genetic factors. The classification criteria for juvenile idiopathic arthritis (JIA) proposed by the International League of Associations for Rheumatology (ILAR) is the most current and is followed in this chapter. Based on the number of inflamed joints, laboratory features, family history, and extra-articular features, seven categories are recognized: oligoarticular arthritis, rheumatoid factor (RF)-positive polyarthritis, RF-negative polyarthritis, systemic JIA (sJIA), enthesitis-related arthritis (ERA), psoriatic arthritis, or undifferentiated arthritis (**Table 151-1**).

The diagnosis of JIA is clinical, defined as joint swelling or limitation of joint range of motion with joint pain or tenderness. These signs must be present consistently for at least 6 weeks in a patient younger than age 16 years. The annual incidence of JIA is estimated at 10 per 100,000 children, and the prevalence of JIA in the United States is about 1 in 1000 children younger than 16 years.

CLINICAL PRESENTATION

Children with arthritis typically demonstrate stiffness after prolonged periods of inactivity, such as upon arising in the morning or after naps, long car rides, or sitting in class. Conversely, children with arthritis typically feel better after a warm bath or several minutes of activity. Cold, damp weather or swimming in cool water tends to be more difficult for children with arthritis, whereas warm weather generally relieves symptoms. Thus, a child with arthritis may suffer joint stiffness in the morning but may be quite comfortable exercising strenuously later in the day. Pain is an uncommon complaint in a child with JIA, and nighttime awakening is unexpected as well.

Systemic JIA, or Still's disease, accounts for about 10% to 15% of all children with JIA. This is the subtype of JIA that most closely resembles an infectious disease and is now thought to represent an autoinflammatory disorder. Although sJIA can occur at any age, the peak age of onset is between 1 and 6 years. Boys and girls are equally affected. As its name implies, this is a systemic illness characterized by fever, rash, and arthritis. These children are often admitted to the hospital for evaluation of

*Supported in part by the Marcus Foundation Inc., Atlanta, GA.

TABLE 151-1 Clinical Features of Juvenile Idiopathic Arthritis

Type	Peak Age of Onset	Frequency (%)	Typical Features
Oligoarthritis	2-4 years	27-56	Arthritis of ≤4 joints in the first 6 months Few or no complaints of pain, but swelling is noticeable, especially in large joints Morning limp or refusal to walk Girls >> boys
Polyarticular, RF negative	2-4 years	11-28	Arthritis of ≥5 joints for at least 6 weeks Insidious onset of joint symptoms Symmetrical distribution Small joints of hands and feet are commonly involved Girls > boys
Polyarticular, RF positive	Late childhood or adolescence	2-7	Arthritis of ≥5 joints for at least 6 weeks Symmetrical distribution Small joints of hands and feet are commonly involved Early joint erosions Subcutaneous nodules Girls >> boys
Systemic	Throughout childhood	5-15	Quotidian spiking fever Transient, salmon-colored rash Systemic features may precede arthritis Pericarditis and macrophage activation syndrome are potential complications Girls = boys
Enthesitis-related arthritis	Late childhood or adolescence	3-11	Arthritis, more often in lower extremity joints Enthesitis involving heels, ankles, and knees Inflammatory spinal pain At risk for acute iritis Often positive for HLA B27 Boys >> girls
Psoriatic arthritis	Biphasic 2-4 years, 9-11 years	2-11	Arthritis and psoriasis Dactylitis, nail pitting, or family history of psoriasis Girls > boys
Undifferentiated		11-21	Variable

HLA, human leukocyte antigen; RF, rheumatoid factor.

fever of unknown origin. The fever of systemic JIA is described as quotidian or double quotidian; children typically have one or two spikes of fever greater than 39°C at about the same time every day. In between episodes of fever, the temperature returns to the baseline level or may be below normal. The fever must be present for at least 2 weeks to be considered a diagnostic criterion. Although characteristic, the rash of systemic JIA can be elusive, appearing late in the course and transiently (lasting minutes to a few hours). The most typical rash is salmon pink, nonpruritic, and migratory. Discrete macules 2 to 5 mm in size appear mostly on the trunk and proximal extremities. Other rashes, including urticarial rashes, have also been described. The rash often accompanies fever spikes, and it is typically seen after a shower. Rubbing or lightly scratching the skin elicits erythema (Koebner phenomenon) and might be followed by the appearance of transient macular lesions. Fever and rash may precede the onset of arthritis by days to months. These symptoms are found in sJIA but are not part of the clinical picture of other subtypes of JIA, thus distinguishing it. Most children with sJIA develop chronic polyarthritis over time. Joint involvement is variable at disease onset, with anywhere from no joints to numerous joints being involved. Children with sJIA also have laboratory evidence of systemic inflammation. The white blood cell count is usually elevated, with a predominance of neutrophils, accompanied by anemia and thrombocytosis; both the C-reactive protein (CRP) and erythrocyte sedimentation rate (ESR) are moderately to significantly elevated. Hepatosplenomegaly, lymphadenopathy, and serositis can also be seen in sJIA. Children with sJIA are at risk for a serious and potentially life-threatening complication, macrophage activation syndrome (MAS), that is characterized by severe and dysregulated immune activation. (MAS is discussed in detail in Chapter 152).

Polyarticular JIA is characterized by the presence of arthritis of at least 6 weeks' duration in five or more joints. Polyarticular JIA accounts for 30% to 40% of cases of JIA and typically affects more girls than boys. Two distinct subtypes are recognized, based on the presence or absence of rheumatoid factor (RF). If the onset occurs during the first peak, at age 1 to 3 years, patients are generally RF negative. Girls affected during the second peak, just before puberty, have a disease that is essentially indistinguishable from adult rheumatoid arthritis, are RF positive, and have early erosions and often subcutaneous nodules. In both types of polyarticular JIA, the onset is generally insidious, with children gradually accruing additional involved joints over time. Typically, the arthritis is symmetrical above and below the waist, and it often involves the small joints of the hands and feet. Fever is generally absent, but children may complain of fatigue, malaise, and anorexia. Polyarticular JIA may be accompanied by mild anemia and a modest elevation of the ESR. Synovitis in multiple joints may lead to chronic joint changes and bony erosions. Up to 50% of those with polyarticular JIA show radiographic abnormalities within 2 years of onset if not treated aggressively.

Oligoarticular JIA, the most common type, accounts for about 40% of all children with JIA. It is characterized by the presence of arthritis in four or fewer joints during the first 6 months of disease. Oligoarticular JIA is more common in girls, and the onset age peaks between 2 and 4 years. Large joints are often involved, with the knee most commonly affected. The arthritis can be asymmetric, and often only one joint is affected at presentation. Inflammatory markers are often normal or mildly increased. Antinuclear antibodies (ANAs) are detected in about 60% of patients with oligoarticular JIA. In this clinical context, the presence of an ANA is clinically significant as it indicates an increased risk of uveitis for which frequent ophthalmologic screening is indicated. The ILAR classification distinguishes two subcategories of oligoarticular JIA depending on the number of joints involved after the first 6 months of disease. In persistent oligoarthritis, the arthritis is limited to four or fewer joints, and in extended oligoarthritis, the arthritis extends to more than four joints. About one-third of children with oligoarticular JIA go on to have extended oligoarthritis. In younger children, oligoarticular JIA often presents insidiously with refusal to walk or a limp in the morning that typically improves as the day goes on. Children seldom complain of pain, although parents may notice swelling of a knee or other large joint. This arthritis subtype is not associated with systemic signs such as fever.

Enthesitis-related arthritis (ERA), affects ~10% of children with JIA. This subtype is characterized by arthritis and enthesitis (inflammation of tendon and ligament attachments). Most often the heels (at Achilles tendon insertion site) and knees (at patellar tendon insertion site) are involved with enthesitis. The arthritis is more likely to involve the lower extremities. Inflammatory spinal pain and sacroiliac joint involvement can also be seen with this subtype. ERA typically affects boys after the age of 6. Most children are also positive for HLA-B27. In some cases, children present with just arthritis but have a positive family history of spondyloarthropathies in a first-degree relative. Children with ERA are at risk for painful acute anterior uveitis.

Psoriatic arthritis (PsA) is characterized by the presence of arthritis and psoriasis; however, the diagnosis of juvenile psoriatic arthritis may be made in the absence of rash. In children without a characteristic rash of psoriasis, the diagnosis requires any two of the following: family history of psoriasis in a first-degree relative, dactylitis (swelling of a digit extending beyond joint margins), and nail pitting or onycholysis. PsA comprises 2% to 11% of all JIA. There can be a biphasic distribution of presentation, with an early peak at 2 to 4 years and a later one at 9 to 11 years. This subtype is more common in girls. Chronic asymptomatic uveitis can be seen with this subtype.

Undifferentiated arthritis includes patients with JIA who either do not satisfy criteria for inclusion in any of the other categories or fulfill criteria for more than one category. As such, they do not have a characteristic pattern of arthritis. The ILAR criteria define several stringent exclusion criteria, which make it difficult to accurately classify some children with chronic arthritis. For example, a boy with 2 weeks of fever and the classic evanescent rash of systemic JIA but with a history of psoriasis in a first-degree relative would be placed in the "undifferentiated" category. In such cases, clinical management depends on the features of the disease in the individual patient.

COMPLICATIONS

MAS is rare, but it is a life-threatening complication of systemic JIA. MAS resembles hemophagocytic lymphohistiocytosis, which occurs as a familial form because of genetic abnormalities in natural killer T lymphocytes. It also occurs sporadically as a complication of malignancy or infection. In sJIA, MAS most commonly occurs during the first 6 months of disease, during periods of active systemic inflammation that are often associated with a change in medication. MAS manifests as unremitting fever, unlike the spiking fevers of the underlying illness. Activation of macrophages results in phagocytosis of erythrocytes, platelets, and leukocytes, so MAS should be suspected when patients with JIA present with a sudden drop in platelets, hematocrit, and white blood cells accompanied by an elevation of hepatic transaminases. Children may demonstrate bruising and mucosal bleeding from the consumptive coagulopathy seen in MAS, as well as mental status changes, hepatosplenomegaly, and diffuse lymphadenopathy. Laboratory studies also demonstrate elevated ferritin and newer diagnostic criteria focus on hyperferritinemia (Ravelli). In addition, one may see elevations in triglycerides, D-dimers, prothrombin time and partial thromboplastin time, and a fall in fibrinogen, ESR, and serum albumin. In particular, a paradoxical decrease in ESR with an increased CRP should be prompt consideration of MAS in a child with sJIA. Other subtypes of JIA are not usually associated with MAS.

Pericarditis is seen in about 3% to 9% of children with JIA, almost always in association with sJIA. Older children are more likely to develop pericarditis, which may present as precordial chest pain, dyspnea, or discomfort referred to the back, shoulder, or neck, or it may be noted incidentally on chest imaging. Physical examination findings include tachycardia, cardiomegaly, or a pericardial friction rub at the lower left sternal border. Cardiac tamponade is a rare but serious complication of constrictive pericarditis. It is characterized by venous distention, hepatomegaly, and peripheral edema. Urgent evaluation and management are necessary to avoid progressive cardiovascular instability.

JIA seldom causes parenchymal lung disease, but pleuritic chest pain due to a pleural effusion may accompany pericarditis or occur in isolation. Over the past decade, there has been a recognition that chronic lung disease can occur in some children with systemic JIA. Reports indicate that prior histories of MAS or treatment with IL-1 or IL-6 inhibitors may be associated, though causality has not been established. Some of these children also appear to fulfill criteria for Drug Rash with Eosinophilia and Systemic Symptoms (DRESS) or Drug-Induced Hypersensitivity Syndrome (DIHR).

Anterior uveitis, or iridocyclitis, is a well-recognized and potentially serious complication of JIA. Uveitis in JIA is usually asymptomatic and chronic; it is most common in children with oligoarticular JIA (approximately 10%) and seen to a lesser extent RF-negative polyarticular JIA. A younger age, female gender, and positive ANA test increase the risk of iritis in most studies, although boys are at risk as well. Uveitis is rare in sJIA, occurring in less than 1% of cases. Acute uveitis, accompanied by pain and redness, may be associated with ERA. The detection of acute uveitis in a child suspected of having sJIA should prompt a consideration of other causes of fever and rash, such as Kawasaki disease and acute viral infections.

Children with longstanding polyarticular or sJIA may develop involvement of the joints of the cervical spine. This can result in instability or fusion of the posterior elements, so care should be exercised when these children undergo procedures that require sedation or anesthesia. Preoperative flexion and extension views of the cervical spine may aid in the detection of cervical involvement and the avoidance of subluxation and injury to the spinal cord or brainstem with hyperextension.

DIFFERENTIAL DIAGNOSIS

JIA is a clinical diagnosis made by history and physical examination. Care must be exercised in labeling a child with JIA before symptoms have been present for more than 6 weeks because infectious arthropathies may be prolonged but ultimately transient. Although chronic inflammatory synovitis is seldom an emergency, acutely dangerous conditions must be excluded urgently in all cases. For instance, a child with an acute febrile monoarthritis must be considered to have septic arthritis or osteomyelitis until proved otherwise, especially in the presence of elevated inflammatory markers. A new monoarthritis in an otherwise healthy-appearing child may represent an acute postinfectious arthritis (see Chapter 153).

Systemic JIA may be difficult to distinguish from severe infections, particularly when children present with fever before the onset of arthritis. The fevers of infectious diseases usually spike less predictably than the fevers of sJIA, and the fevers due to infections often do not return to or dip below baseline between spikes. Additional studies are essential in most cases to exclude other causes of prolonged unexplained fever such as infections, malignancies, and other inflammatory conditions, like inflammatory bowel disease. When migratory arthritis and arthralgias accompany fever, acute rheumatic fever and serum sickness should be considered. Children with either dermatomyositis or systemic lupus erythematosus can present with polyarthritis and fevers, but additional clinical or laboratory features of the underlying disease are typically present.

Vasculitides such as Kawasaki disease and IgA vasculitis often include arthritis among their symptoms. Other entities to consider are transient synovitis of the hip, slipped capital femoral epiphysis, and traction apophysitis (e.g., Osgood-Schlatter syndrome).

EVALUATION

Laboratory tests may help rule out alternative diagnoses and classify the form of arthritis, but they are insufficient to confirm a diagnosis. Expected results from the complete blood count, ESR, CRP, and ANA are provided in **Table 151-2**. A positive ANA increases the risk for chronic uveitis. However, ANA is not a feature of JIA and its presence or absence is not helpful in the diagnosis of any form of JIA. RF is seen in about 5% to 10% of children with JIA, primarily in adolescent girls with RF-positive polyarticular JIA; hence, most children with JIA are RF negative, and again its presence or absence does not aid in diagnosis of JIA. Children with RF-positive polyarticular JIA are also often positive for anticyclic citrullinated peptide antibodies (anti-CCP antibodies) which are more specific than the RF.

In healthy-appearing patients with a new monoarthritis, parvovirus B19 titers, Lyme titers and antistreptococcal antibodies are generally included in the initial evaluation. Evaluation for a septic joint is pursued if clinically indicated.

At disease onset, imaging studies are usually normal, or they can show soft tissue swelling or effusions. Periarticular demineralization, narrowing of joint spaces, subchondral cysts, or bony erosions on plain radiographs are indicative of longstanding inflammatory arthritis and can be useful in assessment of disease duration and disease-related damage. Plain radiographs are also helpful for identifying children with cervical spine abnormalities. Imaging is particularly useful when other diagnoses must be excluded. For example, lucent metaphyseal bands in the long bones of a child older than 2 years suggest a diagnosis of leukemia, especially when unexpectedly severe anemia or thrombocytopenia is also present. Similarly, magnetic resonance imaging is often not necessary to make a diagnosis of JIA in child with arthritis, although MRI

TABLE 151-2 Key Laboratory Features of Juvenile Idiopathic Arthritis

Type	CBC	ESR and CRP	Likelihood of Positive ANA (%)	RF/CCP
Oligoarthritis	Normal	Normal or mildly elevated	70	Negative
RF-negative polyarthritis	Mild anemia, mild thrombocytosis	Normal or mildly elevated	40	Negative
RF-positive polyarthritis	Mild anemia, mild thrombocytosis	Mildly to moderately elevated	40	Positive for RF About 80% positive for CCP
ERA	Normal to mild anemia	Normal to mild elevation	5-10	Negative
Systemic	Leukocytosis, anemia, thrombocytosis	Elevated	5-10	Negative
Psoriatic	Normal	Normal or mildly elevated	30-60	Negative

ANA, antinuclear antibody; CBC, complete blood cell count; ESR, erythrocyte sedimentation rate; RF, rheumatoid factor.

may confirm the presence of synovitis that is not clearly demonstrable on physical examination and assist in diagnosis. When periarticular disorders are under consideration, MRI may be useful because it provides clear images of adjacent soft tissues and bone.

Arthrocentesis can be helpful in diagnosing JIA and excluding other causes of arthritis. Typically, synovial fluid in JIA is yellowish and cloudy, with white blood cell counts between 15,000 and 20,000 and a predominance of neutrophilic forms (75%). In septic arthritis, the fluid is usually serosanguineous and turbid, and the cell count is higher, often between 50,000 and 300,000, with more than 75% neutrophilic forms. Unlike in JIA, in septic arthritis the fluid has a low glucose level, and bacteria may be observed on Gram stain.

COURSE OF ILLNESS

All subtypes of JIA tend to be characterized by remissions and relapses. In addition, it is not unusual for children with JIA to experience a flare of symptoms triggered by intercurrent infection. Systemic JIA may follow a systemic course in which the fever, rash, and laboratory abnormalities persist. More commonly, it follows a polyarticular course, with arthritis persisting after resolution of the other systemic symptoms. Children with ERA may develop features of spondyloarthritis or inflammatory bowel disease. All subtypes of JIA have the potential to develop erosions or joint space narrowing after 2 to 5 years of persistent synovitis. Active synovitis can be detected in 30% to 55% of children with JIA 10 years after disease onset. Estimates of mortality in JIA range from 0.29 to 1.1 per 100 patients, severalfold higher than the standardized mortality rate for a similarly aged US population.

TREATMENT

Children with JIA are best served by a comprehensive interdisciplinary team of healthcare providers that includes the primary care provider, pediatric rheumatologist, rheumatology nurse, social worker, and physical and occupational therapists. The aims of management in all types of JIA are to control pain, prevent and restore loss of motion in affected joints, improve overall functioning, and minimize the effects of inflammation on normal growth and development. Nonpharmacologic modalities such as moist heat can be especially helpful for relieving morning stiffness.

The first line of pharmacologic management for all forms of JIA traditionally has been a nonsteroidal anti-inflammatory drug (NSAID), though the field is moving toward the prompt initiation of immune modulatory therapy. Naproxen is preferred by most rheumatologists for its ease of administration and pediatric labeling. It is usually administered at a dose of 10 to 20 mg/kg per day in two to three divided doses; as with all NSAIDs, 2 to 4 weeks of therapy is necessary before a child's response to naproxen can be assessed. NSAIDs should be administered with food to minimize gastrointestinal side effects such as abdominal pain, nausea, heartburn, or anorexia. Because extended H_2 blocker use prompts tachyphylaxis, proton pump inhibitor therapy is the preferred choice in conjunction with NSAID therapy greater than 2 weeks. Naproxen is associated with pseudoporphyria (small blisters that scar) or skin fragility in up to 10% of children; fair skin and blue or gray eye color are reported to be risk factors. Other NSAIDs are associated less often with increased skin fragility. Bruising or bleeding can also be seen with NSAIDs. In patients with sJIA, indomethacin can be particularly helpful in treating fever and pericarditis. Acetaminophen can be used occasionally for fever or breakthrough pain relief. Children on NSAIDs need a complete blood count, urinalysis, and levels of serum liver transaminases, blood urea nitrogen, and serum creatinine checked at baseline and every 3 to 6 months.

It is important to note that all forms of JIA usually require additional therapy beyond the use of NSAIDs. For children with oligoarticular JIA, arthrocentesis and injection of corticosteroids is often the second line of therapy. For children with other forms of JIA, medical management frequently requires aggressive escalation of therapy using multiple immune modulatory agents.

Corticosteroid therapy is often used as an adjunct to anti-inflammatory therapy in patients with JIA. The high frequency of side effects and lack of objective evidence that corticosteroids alter the long-term articular outcome weigh against the prolonged use of systemic corticosteroids in JIA. However, oral corticosteroids used at the lowest possible doses to minimize side effects may be useful in children with systemic disease and significant and persistent systemic features such as fever. Because corticosteroids can mask other diagnoses and worsen infections, they should be used only after the diagnosis has been clearly established. Intra-articular steroid therapy in the form of triamcinolone hexacetonide or triamcinolone acetonide is often effective in treating oligoarticular JIA and can be used in other subtypes as well when there is persistent pain or inflammation in a few joints amenable to therapy. Topical corticosteroid ophthalmic preparations are used in the treatment of uveitis.

Second-line or disease-modifying antirheumatic drugs (DMARD) are generally instituted by pediatric rheumatologists or others experienced in their use. However, the hospitalist is likely to encounter patients with an established diagnosis of JIA who are on these medications and are hospitalized for a flare of arthritis or other unrelated conditions. The following is a brief synopsis of some of the more commonly used medications.

NONBIOLOGIC DMARDS

Methotrexate, a folate antagonist, is the most commonly used DMARD to treat polyarticular, systemic JIA, and refractory oligoarticular JIA. Methotrexate is administered weekly by oral or subcutaneous routes; the latter is associated with better absorption and fewer gastrointestinal adverse effects. Although well tolerated in the majority of children, methotrexate may be associated with headache, nausea, or fatigue, usually within 1 or 2 days of administration. Oral mucosal ulcers are common unless children receive concurrent folic acid. More serious but less frequent side effects of methotrexate include leukopenia, hypersensitivity pneumonitis, and elevation of transaminases. These side effects may require modification of the dose or discontinuation of the drug. In some children intolerant to methotrexate, leflunomide may be administered. Older second-line medications such as hydroxychloroquine and sulfasalazine are used infrequently because more effective agents are now available.

BIOLOGIC RESPONSE MODIFIERS

The availability of biologic agents in particular has increased the therapeutic options for children with JIA. The most frequently used are directed against the cytokines tumor necrosis factor (TNF), interleukin 1, interleukin 6, or interleukin 17A. In addition, agents targeting T-cell costimulation and B-cells are also options for some children with JIA. All biological agents increase the risk of infection, including viral illnesses, severe bacterial infections, and reactivation of latent tuberculosis. A tuberculosis test should be performed before initiating treatment with a biologic agent and repeated annually. Biological agents can also exacerbate other serious bacterial or opportunistic fungal infections. Hence if a serious infection is suspected in a child on a biological agent, the medication should be withheld until the child is evaluated and appropriate antimicrobial treatment has been instituted. There is also concern that biological agents might increase the risk of malignancy in children with JIA.

ANTI-TNF AGENTS

TNF is a proinflammatory cytokine known to be elevated in children with JIA. There are many agents targeting TNF, but three of them are currently used widely in children with JIA. Etanercept (Enbrel) is a soluble TNF receptor that binds TNF, thereby blocking its binding to cell surface receptors. It is given by subcutaneous injection once or twice weekly. The most frequent side effects are injection site reactions. Usually these are mild, manifesting as erythema, and do not warrant discontinuation of etanercept. Infliximab (Remicade) is a chimeric anti-TNF monoclonal antibody that binds to TNF, thereby neutralizing its biologic activity. The antibody is administered by intravenous infusion every 4 to 8 weeks. These infusions may be accompanied by fever, chills, myalgia, or headache. Premedicating with acetaminophen and diphenhydramine is often helpful. Adalimumab (Humira) is a fully humanized anti-TNF antibody given subcutaneously every other week. The most common adverse effect is a mild injection site reaction manifested by a self-limited red rash or swelling. Cold compresses can be helpful in providing symptomatic relief. Several biosimilar agents are now available for these anti-TNF agents with the choice often dictated by payors.

OTHER BIOLOGIC AGENTS

Anakinra (Kineret) is an interleukin-1 receptor antagonist. It is used primarily in the treatment of sJIA. Anakinra is given as a subcutaneous injection daily. Common side effects include injection site reactions. Recently, Anakinra has been increasingly used in the treatment of MAS where it is administered either subcutaneously or intravenously. Other less commonly used anti-interleukin 1 agents include rilonacept and canakinumab. Tocilizumab (Actemra) is a monoclonal antibody against interleukin-6, which is elevated in systemic JIA. Actemra is given as an intravenous infusion every 2 weeks in systemic JIA. Infusion reactions might occur and are minimized by premedicating with acetaminophen and diphenhydramine. Periodic monitoring is required to detect abnormal liver function tests, leukopenia, and thrombocytopenia or abnormal cholesterol. Abatacept (Orencia) targets T-cell activation via blockade of the costimulatory signal needed for T-cell proliferation. It can be administered either intravenously monthly, or by subcutaneous formulations. Rituximab (Rituxan) is a chimeric anti-CD20 antibody that binds and destroys CD20-positive B cells. It is used in the treatment of adults with RA and might be an option for some children with RF-positive polyarticular JIA. It is given as a set of intravenous infusions. Recently Secukinumab (Cosentyx), a humanized monoclonal antibody directed against IL-17a, has been approved for the treatment of psoriasis and psoriatic arthritis in children.

MANAGEMENT

Ongoing pediatric rheumatology evaluation is important in the care of children with JIA. In addition, periodic evaluation by an ophthalmologist is needed to detect and treat chronic anterior uveitis. Uveitis in most patients with JIA is often asymptomatic, especially when it occurs in children with oligoarticular or RF-negative polyarthritis. The exception is the uveitis associated with ERA which presents with eye pain, redness, and photophobia. If undetected and untreated, JIA-associated uveitis can result in significant and irreversible loss of vision. For this reason, there is a recommended schedule of screening for uveitis based on the subtype of JIA, age of onset, and ANA status. These guidelines should be strictly adhered to and can be found in the published policy statement of the American Academy of Pediatrics.

Generally, children with JIA do well at school, and arthritis per se seldom accounts for absences. Nonetheless, children with significant arthritis might need special accommodations at school. Usually there is no need to restrict physical activity apart from avoiding direct trauma to joints, but children should be allowed to limit their activities as needed. Follow-up with a physical or occupational therapist should also be arranged to initiate a home exercise program to prevent or treat contractures, or splints.

JIA is a chronic illness, and families often have many concerns about the long-term consequences of the disease. The treatment of JIA should include education that addresses important issues such as peer relations, family dynamics, social adjustment, and vocational planning. The American Juvenile Arthritis Organization, a branch of the Arthritis Foundation, is an excellent source of information for newly diagnosed patients with JIA and their families; its link can be found at the Arthritis Foundation website (www.arthritis.org). Other sources of information include the National Institute of Arthritis, Musculoskeletal and Skin Diseases at the National Institutes of Health, (www.niams.nih.gov) and the American College of Rheumatology (www.rheumatology.org).

CONSULTATION

The diagnosis of JIA is a clinical diagnosis that requires the exclusion of other causes of acute and chronic arthritis. The long-term management of children with JIA can be challenging, often involving the use of medications that suppress the immune system and require monitoring for adverse effects. Consultation with a pediatric rheumatologist, when available, can facilitate an early diagnosis and the prompt institution of appropriate medical management. Subspecialty consultation may also be helpful in the diagnostic evaluation and treatment of patients with JIA (**Table 151-3**).

TABLE 151-3 Subspecialty Consultation to Consider in the Evaluation of Patients With Juvenile Idiopathic Arthritis

Subspecialty	Potential Role
Infectious diseases	To assist in evaluation of patients when fevers secondary to infectious disorders are suspected or in diagnostic evaluation when septic arthritis or osteomyelitis are included in the differential diagnosis
Cardiology	To assist in evaluation and management of chest pain, pericarditis, and pericardial effusions
Hematology/Oncology	To assist in the evaluation of MAS or when malignancy is suspected
Orthopedic surgery	To assist with diagnostic evaluation to exclude septic arthritis or osteomyelitis
Physical/Occupational therapy	To preserve and improve range of motion and strength
Ophthalmology	To screen for chronic (and clinically silent) anterior uveitis
Social services	To assist in locating financial, educational, and social assistance
Mental health services	To assist in the management of affective disorders associated with chronic disease and to improve coping skills needed to manage a chronic disease and long-term medication therapy

MAS, macrophage activation syndrome.

ADMISSION CRITERIA

- Evaluation of patients with suspected systemic JIA for persistent fever and progression of disease, while screening for serious infection or potential malignancy.
- Management of serious flares of disease associated with pain, disability, or nonarticular organ system complications.
- Monitoring for and management of complications of disease such as MAS.
- Intercession and education for patients with chronic disease who struggle with adherence therapeutic regimens.

DISCHARGE CRITERIA

- Completion of evaluation for possible malignancy or serious infection.
- Resolution of fever and evidence of improving inflammatory markers.
- Establishment of a therapeutic regimen, including medication, physical or occupational therapy, ophthalmology consultation, and social services.
- Discharge planning, including patient and family education as well as general pediatric and pediatric rheumatology follow-up.
- If on steroids, a plan for tapering the medication and monitoring for side effects, including measuring blood pressure and following urinalyses for glycosuria, should be considered.

KEY POINTS

- JIA is among the most prevalent chronic diseases of childhood, affecting 1 in 1000 children younger than 16 years.
- Children with arthritis typically complain of joint swelling or morning stiffness; pain is unusual and suggests a mechanical rather than an inflammatory process.
- Although NSAIDs are first-line treatment, aggressive management with disease-modifying agents such as methotrexate and biologic agents such as anti-TNF monoclonal antibodies effectively controls arthritis and prevents long-term complications in most children.
- Periodic ophthalmic evaluation is an essential component of the care of children with JIA.
- Further refinement of biologic response modifiers, including targeted B- and T-cell monoclonal antibodies, will continue to improve the safety and efficacy of therapy for JIA.
- Identification of genetically determined disease subsets will allow therapy to be individualized.
- Improved understanding of the pathophysiology of systemic-onset JIA may necessitate its reclassification as an autoinflammatory rather than an autoimmune disorder.

SUGGESTED READINGS

Beukelman T, Patkar NM, Saag KG, et al. 2011 American College of Rheumatology Recommendations for the treatment of Juvenile Idiopathic Arthritis; initiation and safety monitoring of therapeutic agents for the treatment of arthritis and systemic features. *Arthritis Care Res*. 2011;63:465-482.

Case SM, Nigrovic PA. Implications of evolving disease classification for drug approval in juvenile idiopathic arthritis. *Paediatr Drugs*. 2022;24(3):185-191.

Cassidy JR, Petty RE. Chronic arthritis in childhood. In: *Textbook of Pediatric Rheumatology*. 5th ed. Philadelphia, PA: WB Saunders; 2005:206-260.

Clarke SL, Sen ES, Ramanan AV. Juvenile idiopathic arthritis-associated uveitis. *Pediatric Rheumatol online J*. 2016;14(1):27.

Foster CS. Diagnosis and treatment of juvenile idiopathic arthritis-associated uveitis. *Curr Opin Ophthalmol*. 2003;14:395-398.

Grom AA. Natural killer cell dysfunction: a common pathway in systemic-onset juvenile rheumatoid arthritis, macrophage activation syndrome, and hemophagocytic lymphohistiocytosis? *Arthritis Rheum*. 2004;50:689-698.

Hashkes PJ, Laxer RM. Medical treatment of juvenile idiopathic arthritis. *JAMA*. 2005;294:1671-1684.

Horneff G. Update on biologicals for treatment of juvenile idiopathic arthritis. *Exp Opin Biol Ther*. 2013;13:361-376.

McGhee JL, Burks FN, Sheckels JL, Jarvis JN. Identifying children with chronic arthritis based on chief complaints: absence of predictive value for musculoskeletal pain as an indicator of rheumatic disease in children. *Pediatrics*. 2002;110:354-359.

Oen K, Malleson PN, Cabral DA, et al. Early predictors of long term outcome in patients with juvenile rheumatoid arthritis: subset-specific correlations. *J Rheumatol*. 2003;30:585-593.

Petty RE, Laxer RM, Lindsley CB, Wedderburn L. *Textbook of Pediatric Rheumatology*. 7th ed. Philadelphia, PA: Elsevier; 2016.

Petty RE, Southwood TR, Manners P, et al. International League of Associations for Rheumatology classification of juvenile idiopathic arthritis: second revision, Edmonton, 2001. *J Rheumatol*. 2004;31:390-392.

Prahalad S, Glass DN. Is juvenile rheumatoid arthritis/juvenile idiopathic arthritis different from rheumatoid arthritis? *Arthritis Res*. 2002;4(Suppl 3):303-310.

Ravelli A, Martini A. Juvenile idiopathic arthritis. *Lancet*. 2007;369:767-778.

Section on Rheumatology and Section on Ophthalmology. Guidelines for ophthalmologic examinations in children with juvenile rheumatoid arthritis. *Pediatrics*. 1993;92:295-296.

Weiss JE, Ilowite NT. Juvenile idiopathic arthritis. *Pediatr Clin North Am*. 2005;52:413-442.

CHAPTER 152 Hemophagocytic Lymphohistiocytosis and Macrophage Activation Syndrome

Chloë E. Nunneley, MD and Melissa M. Hazen, MD

BACKGROUND

Hemophagocytic lymphohistiocytosis (HLH) and macrophage activation syndrome (MAS) are clinically related life-threatening immune dysregulatory processes characterized by fever, systemic inflammation, organomegaly, coagulopathy, and hematologic cytopenias. Both conditions may also include neurologic symptoms, often accompanied by cerebrospinal fluid and brain imaging abnormalities. HLH and MAS are defined histologically by the phagocytosis of hematopoietic cells by normal-appearing macrophages. This hemophagocytosis is most typically seen on samples from bone marrow aspirates, but it can also be seen in the spleen and in other lymphatic tissue.

HLH may be inherited, as in the case of familial hemophagocytic lymphocytosis (FHL), or acquired. FHL is caused by genetic defects in proteins that mediate cytotoxicity in natural killer (NK) cells and cytotoxic T cells. These abnormalities lead to the impaired functioning of these cells, triggering cytokine storm and often cardiovascular collapse. Acquired HLH is typically triggered by viral infections, but it may also be associated with malignancies, acquired immunodeficiencies, and rheumatologic disorders. Historically, the diagnosis of FHL was made in infancy based on clinical criteria. With the discovery of several genetic mutations that lead to familial HLH, however, inherited cases have been identified in older children and even adults, suggesting that HLH presenting at any age may be due to both inherited and acquired factors. This finding may have important implications for treatment.

MAS typically exists in the context of severe rheumatologic diseases, most commonly systemic juvenile idiopathic arthritis (sJIA). Systemic lupus erythematosus (SLE) and Kawasaki disease are also associated with the development of MAS, though at times MAS may be the presenting manifestation of the underlying rheumatologic disorder, greatly complicating diagnosis. MAS is considered a form of acquired HLH occurring in a specific population, though the strict diagnostic criteria for HLH may not be met. More recently, diagnostic criteria for MAS in the context of rheumatic disease have been proposed. The diagnosis of either HLH or MAS should be considered in an ill child with prolonged fever, organomegaly, elevated inflammatory markers, cytopenias, coagulopathy, neurologic symptoms, and/or evidence of liver dysfunction. A significantly elevated ferritin greater than 10,000 μg L^{-1} has been demonstrated to be a sensitive and specific marker of these hemophagocytic processes, though many children with HLH and MAS demonstrate more modestly elevated ferritin levels.

PATHOPHYSIOLOGY

FAMILIAL HLH

To date, four FHL-associated genetic mutations have been identified. These mutations affect the ability of cytotoxic cells, such as NK cells and cytotoxic T lymphocytes, to carry out the effective killing of target cells. Mutations in perforin vitiate the cytotoxic granules of cytotoxic cells, while the other genes associated with FHL affect cytotoxic granule exocytosis. Of note, HLH has also been associated with heritable primary immunodeficiencies, including Griscelli syndrome, Chediak-Higashi syndrome, X-linked lymphoproliferative syndrome (XLP), and mutations in the *ITK* gene. HLH associated with XLP and ITK mutations is often triggered by Epstein-Barr virus (EBV) infection.

ACQUIRED HLH/MAS

Acquired HLH occurs in children without the described genetic mutations associated with familial HLH and is often triggered by infection, especially EBV. Children with some degree of acquired or iatrogenic immunocompromise, including those taking immunosuppressive drugs, infected with human immunodeficiency virus (HIV), or status-post stem-cell transplant, are at risk for developing HLH.

Acquired HLH in the setting of autoimmune disease, most commonly sJIA and adult-onset Still disease, is known as MAS. Approximately 10% of patients with sJIA develop MAS, though as many as 30% to 50% of these patients have subclinical HLH.

Several models seek to explain the manner in which known triggers interact with immunologic or inflammatory conditions to precipitate acquired HLH. The first parallels the model proposed for FHL in which the dysfunction of cytotoxic cells leads to the persistence of stimulated $CD8^{+}$ T cells, driving interferon-gamma production and attendant cytokine-mediated toxicity. However, not all patients with MAS have defects in these cytotoxicity pathways, leading to hypotheses that alternative pathways may also lead to HLH, including repeated stimulation of Toll-like receptors and decreased production of IL-10. In both the acquired and familial forms of HLH, self-sustaining feedback of numerous proinflammatory substances, including cytokines and chemokines, leads to a dysregulated immune response and the characteristic clinical presentation.

While details of the specific cytokines, chemokines, and signaling pathways implicated in HLH/MAS are beyond what the hospitalist needs to know, understanding of the pathophysiology of these disease processes, including the roles played by IL-18, CXCL9, and interferon-gamma, has recently expanded and led to the development of novel therapeutic options.

CLINICAL PRESENTATION

The diagnosis of HLH/MAS begins with first considering these processes as a possible cause of persistent fever in a very ill child with organomegaly, systemic inflammation, cytopenias, liver function abnormalities, and/or neurologic symptoms such as seizures, meningismus, or cranial nerve palsies. In addition, while many of these findings are nonspecific and can be associated with other disease processes, HLH and MAS are characterized by the severe and persistent nature of these findings. While most pediatric cases of FHL are diagnosed within the first year of life, new understanding of the spectrum of disease has led to diagnoses later in life. Acquired HLH/MAS may present at any point in childhood and may occur either in the context of a known autoimmune disease or as the presenting event.

DIFFERENTIAL DIAGNOSIS

Because the clinical characteristics of HLH and MAS are nonspecific, the differential diagnosis of these syndromes includes other systemic inflammatory processes, including infections, malignancies, metabolic disorders, and autoimmune diseases. It may be especially challenging to make the diagnosis of HLH or MAS in the setting of infection, as infection often triggers HLH/MAS in susceptible hosts. COVID-19 is also known to be a potential trigger for a postinfectious hyperinflammatory state in children, which may be difficult to distinguish from HLH/MAS (see Chapters 106 [COVID-19] and 107 [MIS-C]). However, the isolation of an infectious agent does not rule out the possibility of HLH/MAS, as these entities may coexist. Similarly, the inability to improve the condition of a sick child with a systemic autoimmune disorder such as sJIA or SLE should raise the possibility of MAS rather than exclude it. In light of lymphadenopathy associated with HLH and MAS, lymphoma remains on the differential diagnosis. Other considerations, especially in the neonatal period, include metabolic abnormalities that may present with CNS involvement as well as hepatic dysfunction and enlargement.

DIAGNOSTIC EVALUATION

As patients in whom HLH is suspected are typically admitted to general hospital medicine services, the early recognition of symptoms by hospitalists is critical to an expeditious diagnosis as well as for the assembly and coordination of a multidisciplinary team. A hospitalist may be uniquely positioned to mediate and mitigate the challenges of disparate approaches taken by subspecialty teams while driving a patient's evaluation and treatment forward. To further aid in this process, algorithms that outline a clinical pathway toward diagnosis, as well as delineate the responsibilities of various subspecialists, have proved effective in the care of patients with suspected HLH/MAS. Utilization of such pathways could be considered in settings in which similar resources are available.

The preliminary laboratory assessment includes a complete blood count with differential to assess for cytopenias as well as evaluation for hypertriglyceridemia, hypofibrinogenemia, and hyperferritinemia. More specific immune assays, including evaluation of NK cell numbers and function, as measured in a cytotoxicity assay, can assist in identifying this disorder. Perforin, soluble CD25 (a.k.a. soluble IL-2 receptor alpha) and soluble CD107a expression can be measured by flow cytometry and may be helpful in making the diagnosis. As the pathophysiology of these processes has been further illuminated, the role of additional proinflammatory cytokines and chemokines has been elucidated, and assays for IL-18 and CXCL9 may also aid in the diagnosis. The criteria for the diagnosis of HLH have been formalized (**Table 152-1**). These criteria were designed to identify children with FHL who need a bone marrow transplant to survive, so they are quite restrictive. In an appropriate clinical setting, MAS may be diagnosed even when HLH 2004 criteria are not met, and there are now formal diagnostic criteria for MAS (**Table 152-2**).

TREATMENT

Treatment of HLH and MAS is aimed at damping the hyperactive immune response, and delays in the initiation of immunosuppression can lead to significant patient morbidity. In the setting of acquired HLH or MAS, targeting the presumed trigger is the first step. When the diagnosis of HLH is made according to the HLH 2004 criteria, there is an associated treatment algorithm that is followed, usually under the guidance of a hematologist/oncologist, including administration of systemic corticosteroids, cyclosporine, and etoposide. In spite of these regimens, survival rates for FHL are only around 50% to 55%; use of

TABLE 152-1 HLH 2004 Diagnostic Criteria

The diagnosis of HLH can be established if one of either 1 or 2 is fulfilled:

1. A molecular diagnosis consistent with HLH
2. Diagnostic criteria for HLH fulfilled (5 out of 8 criteria below)
   A. Initial diagnostic criteria (*to be evaluated in all patients with HLH*)
      - Fever
      - Splenomegaly
      - Cytopenias (affecting ≥2 of 3 lineages in the peripheral blood):
        - Hemoglobin <90 g/L (in infants <4 weeks: hemoglobin <100 g/L)
        - Platelets <100 × 10^9/L
        - Neutrophils <1.0 × 10^9/L
      - Hypertriglyceridemia and/or hypofibrinogenemia:
        - Fasting triglycerides ≥3.0 mmol/L (i.e., ≥265 mg/dL)
        - Fibrinogen ≤1.5 g/L
      - Hemophagocytosis in bone marrow, spleen, or lymph nodes
      - No evidence of malignancy
   B. New diagnostic criteria
      - Low or absent NK-cell activity (according to local laboratory reference)
      - Ferritin ≥500 mg/L
      - Soluble CD25 (i.e., soluble IL-2 receptor) ≥2400 U/mL

If hemophagocytic activity is not proven at the time of presentation, further search for hemophagocytic activity is encouraged. If the bone marrow specimen is not conclusive, material may be obtained from other organs. Serial marrow aspirates over time may also be helpful.

The following findings may provide strong supportive evidence for the diagnosis: (a) spinal fluid pleocytosis (mononuclear cells) and/or elevated spinal fluid protein; (b) histological picture in the liver resembling chronic persistent hepatitis (biopsy).

Other abnormal clinical and laboratory findings consistent with the diagnosis are cerebromeningeal symptoms, lymph node enlargement, jaundice, edema, skin rash, hepatic enzyme abnormalities, hypoproteinemia, hyponatremia, VLDA elevated, HDL decreased.

Source: Reproduced with permission from Henter JI, Horne AC, Arico M, et al.; Histiocyte Society. HLH-2004: Diagnostic and therapeutic guidelines for hemophagocytic lymphohistiocytosis. *Pediatr Blood Cancer.* 2007;48:124-131.

an evidence-based guideline or clinical pathway can, however, expedite treatment and diminish practice variation that contributes to poor outcomes. In patients with FHL and those failing this treatment regimen, hematopoietic stem cell transplantation (HSCT) is indicated. Because HSCT may be curative in FHL, the considerable risks of the procedure may be accepted. Reduced-intensity conditioning, as opposed to the previously relied upon myeloablative conditioning, has led to improved rates of survival for these patients.

The treatment of acquired HLH is also aimed at quelling the immune response. Systemic steroids, often administered parenterally in the hospitalized child, are the mainstay of therapy. Historically, cyclosporine A was often used in conjunction with corticosteroids in this context; however, its use has diminished in the face of more targeted and better-tolerated therapies. As our understanding of the pathophysiology of HLH/MAS has become clearer, agents to halt the inflammatory response by blocking the implicated chemokines, cytokines, and their signaling pathways have demonstrated promise in treating HLH/MAS. Specifically, IL1-R antagonists, such as anakinra (Kineret), have demonstrated efficacy in

TABLE 152-2 Classification of Macrophage Activation Syndrome in Systemic Juvenile Idiopathic Arthritis

Essential Criteria *(all must be present)*	Additional Criteria *(any 2 of the following must also be present)*
Fever	Platelet count ≤181 × 10^9 L
Known or suspected systemic juvenile idiopathic arthritis	Aspartate aminotransferase >48 units/L
Ferritin >684 ng/mL	Triglycerides >156 mg/dL Fibrinogen ≤360 mg/dL

the treatment of MAS and can lead to rapid improvement even in children who have not responded to corticosteroids and cyclosporine A. Interferon-γ is now understood to be particularly important in driving the inflammatory response in HLH/MAS, making it and its downstream signaling pathway, Janus kinase (JAK)-signal transducer and activator of transcription (STAT), critical targets of newer therapeutic agents. Emapalumab, an anti-interferon-γ antibody, has recently been approved to treat familial HLH, with an open trial underway for its use in MAS showing promising preliminary results. As the JAK-STAT pathway plays a central role in the cellular response to interferon-γ as well as other cytokines, JAK inhibitors (such as ruxolitinib) are currently being explored as therapeutic options for the treatment of sJIA, MAS, and HLH.

ADMISSION AND DISCHARGE CRITERIA

HLH and MAS are severe life-threatening immune dysregulatory syndromes that typically escalate without aggressive interventions. Patients suffering from these entities are often quite ill with fever and other systemic symptoms. Prompt admission, often to the intensive care unit, is essential for monitoring hemodynamic and mental status and expediting diagnosis and treatment. As the process progresses, patients may develop sepsis-like physiology with cytokine storm and ultimately cardiopulmonary collapse. Thus, they often require hemodynamic and respiratory support in addition to treatment for potential infectious complications related to both treatment with immunosuppressive medications and the underlying illnesses. Recovery tends to be prolonged, and discharge from the hospital cannot be considered until fever and other vital sign abnormalities normalize and laboratory values confirm marked improvement if not normalization. Finally, to consider safe discharge, a careful outpatient plan including medications, many of which require prior authorization from insurance carriers, and close follow-up with primary care as well as subspecialty providers needs to be established.

CONSULTATION

Consultation with a pediatric rheumatologist is recommended to assist in the diagnosis and treatment of hemophagocytic disorders, as familiarity with these disease processes and with immune modulatory agents is essential to expertly manage these patients. If a patient is suspected of having FHL, consultation with a hematologist/oncologist is recommended to initiate treatment according to the HLH protocol as well as to prepare for bone marrow transplant if indicated. If HLH in the context of primary immune deficiency is suspected, immunology should be involved. Infections may trigger or complicate these disease processes; further, it may be difficult to distinguish HLH/MAS from systemic infection. As such, involvement of an infection disease specialist may be indicated to assist with evaluation for infection and possible anti-microbial therapy. Finally, if there are neurologic symptoms, then consultation with neurology or neuroimmunology if available is recommended. As noted above, in the case of severely ill patients, transfer to a higher level of care may be indicated, and consultation by an intensivist may be necessary.

KEY POINTS

- HLH and MAS appear to be related and often under-recognized severe immune dysregulatory syndromes characterized by fever, organomegaly, systemic inflammation, coagulopathy, and hematologic cytopenias.
- HLH can be acquired or inherited, whereas MAS is acquired and occurs in the setting of autoimmune disease.
- The diagnosis of MAS may be made even if the diagnostic criteria of HLH are not fully met and there are new diagnostic criteria specifically for MAS.
- Significant elevation of serum ferritin is a sensitive and specific marker of HLH/MAS.
- Treatment rests on damping the immune response and may include both broad (i.e., corticosteroids) and targeted (i.e., specific IL-1 receptor blockade) therapies.
- HSCT may be curative in the setting of FHL, and outcomes have improved in the era of reduced-intensity conditioning.

SUGGESTED READINGS

Allen CE, Yu X, Kozinetz CA, McClain KL. Highly elevated ferritin levels and the diagnosis of hemophagocytic lymphohistiocytosis. *Pediatr Blood Cancer*. 2008;50(6):1227-1235.

Behrens EM, Beukelman T, Paessler M, Cron RQ. Occult macrophage activation syndrome in patients with systemic juvenile idiopathic arthritis. *J Rheumatol*. 2007;34(5):1133-1138.

Bleesing J, Prada A, Siegel DM, et al. The diagnostic significance of soluble CD163 and soluble interleukin-2 receptor alpha-chain in macrophage activation syndrome and untreated new-onset systemic juvenile idiopathic arthritis. *Arthritis Rheum*. 2007;56(3):965-971.

Cooper N, Rao K, Goulden N, Webb D, Amrolia P, Veys P. The use of reduced-intensity stem cell transplantation in haemophagocytic lymphohistiocytosis and Langerhans cell histiocytosis. *Bone Marrow Transplant*. 2008;42(Suppl 2):S47-50.

Halyabar O, Chang MH, Schoettler ML, et al. Calm in the midst of cytokine storm: a collaborative approach to the diagnosis and treatment of hemophagocytic lymphohistiocytosis and macrophage activation syndrome. *Pediatr Rheumatol Online J*. 2019;17(1):7.

Henderson LA, Cron RQ. Macrophage activation syndrome and secondary hemophagocytic lymphohistiocytosis in childhood inflammatory disorders: diagnosis and management. *Paediatr Drugs*. 2020;22(1):29-44.

Henter JI, Samuelsson-Horne A, Aricò M, et al.; Histocyte Society. Treatment of hemophagocytic lymphohistiocytosis with HLH-94 immunochemotherapy and bone marrow transplantation. *Blood*. 2002;100(7):2367-2373.

Janka G. Hemophagocytic lymphohistiocytosis: when the immune system runs amok. *Klin Pediatr*. 2009;221(5):278-285.

Janka GE. Familial and acquired hemophagocytic lymphohistiocytosis. *Eur J Pediatr*. 2007;166(2):95-109.

Locatelli F, Jordan MB, Allen C, et al. Emapalumab in children with primary hemophagocytic lymphohistiocytosis. *N Engl J Med*. 2020;382(19):1811-1822.

Loh NK, Lucas M, Fernandez S, Prentice D. Successful treatment of macrophage activation syndrome complicating adult Still disease with anakinra. *Intern Med J*. 2012;42(12):1358-1362.

Marsh RA, Vaughn G, Kim MO, et al. Reduced-intensity conditioning significantly improves survival of patients with hemophagocytic lymphohistiocytosis undergoing allogeneic hematopoietic cell transplantation. *Blood*. 2010;116(26):5824-4831.

Miettunen PM, Narendran A, Jayanthan A, Behrens EM, Cron RQ. Successful treatment of severe paediatric rheumatic disease-associated macrophage activation syndrome with interleukin-1 inhibition following conventional immunosuppressive therapy: case series with 12 patients. *Rheumatology* (Oxford). 2011;50(2): 417-419.

Nagafuji K, Nonami A, Kumano T, et al. Perforin gene mutations in adult-onset hemophagocytic lymphohistiocytosis. *Haematologica*. 2007;92(7):978-981.

Ravelli A, Grom AA, Behrens EM, Cron RQ. Macrophage activation syndrome as part of systemic juvenile idiopathic arthritis: diagnosis, genetics, pathophysiology and treatment. *Genes Immun*. 2012;13(4):289-298.

Ravelli A, Minoia F, Davì S, et al. 2016 Classification Criteria for Macrophage Activation Syndrome Complicating Systemic Juvenile Idiopathic Arthritis: A European League Against Rheumatism/American College of Rheumatology/Paediatric Rheumatology International Trials Organisation Collaborative Initiative. *Arthritis Rheumatol*. 2016;68(3):566-576.

Risma K, Jordan MB. Hemophagocytic lymphohistiocytosis: updates and evolving concepts. *Curr Opin Pediatr*. 2012;24(1):9-15.

Taylor ML, Hoyt KJ, Han J, et al. An evidence-based guideline improves outcomes for patients with hemophagocytic lymphohistiocytosis and macrophage activation syndrome. *J Rheumatol*. 2022 Sep;49(9): 1042-1051.

Ueda I, Kurokawa Y, Koike K, et al. Late-onset cases of familial hemophagocytic lymphohistiocytosis with missense perforin gene mutations. *Am J Hematol*. 2007;82(6):427-432.

Verweyen EL, Schulert GS. Interfering with interferons: targeting the JAK-STAT pathway in complications of systemic juvenile idiopathic arthritis (SJIA) [published correction appears in Rheumatology (Oxford). 2023;62(5):2022]. *Rheumatology* (Oxford). 2022;61(3):926-935.

Zhang K, Jordan MB, Marsh RA, et al. Hypomorphic mutations in PRF1, MUNC13-4, and STXBP2 are associated with adult-onset familial HLH. *Blood*. 2011;118(22):5794-5798.

CHAPTER 153 Infection-Associated Arthritis

Lisa M. Rickey, MD and Melissa M. Hazen, MD

BACKGROUND

Many bacteria and viruses can cause arthritis without directly invading the joint space. The diseases that result are highly varied and are the focus of this chapter. These processes include reactive arthritis, which occurs after genitourinary or enteric bacterial infections, poststreptococcal reactive arthritis (PSRA), Lyme disease, and viral and post-viral arthritis (including transient synovitis).

Bacterial infection of the joint (septic arthritis) is addressed in Chapter 101. Acute rheumatic fever (ARF), which can also cause arthritis, is addressed separately (Chapter 55).

PATHOPHYSIOLOGY

REACTIVE ARTHRITIS

Reactive arthritis is the name given to an aseptic arthritis that follows a gastrointestinal or genitourinary infection. It is associated with certain bacteria; specifically, *Chlamydia trachomatis*, *Shigella*, *Salmonella*, *Yersinia*, or *Campylobacter*, but recent reports have also implicated atypical organisms as diverse as *Giardia lamblia* and *Clostridium difficile*. Although by definition reactive arthritis is a sterile arthritis, modern PCR techniques have identified bacterial DNA in synovial tissue. The significance of this finding is unclear.

Reactive arthritis is part of a group of diseases called spondyloarthritides (arthritis that affects primarily the axial skeleton), which includes psoriatic arthritis, enthesitis-related arthritis, and ankylosing spondylitis. They have a strong association to human leukocyte antigen B27 (HLA-B27) and share common extra-articular features including enthesitis, uveitis, and inflammatory bowel disease.

The pathogenesis of reactive arthritis is still not well understood. Evidence suggests that the resultant arthritis is caused by an abnormal innate immune response to bacterial antigens in the joint space, or to mechanical trauma.

POSTSTREPTOCOCCAL REACTIVE ARTHRITIS

Poststreptococcal reactive arthritis (PSRA) may be caused by antistreptococcal antibodies that cross-react with proteins expressed in the joint cartilage and synovial lining.

LYME ARTHRITIS

Lyme disease is the most common vector-borne infection in North America. It is caused by the spirochete *Borrelia burgdorferi* and transmitted to humans by infected *Ixodes scapularis* and *I. pacificus* ticks. The disease is endemic in the northeast and north-central regions of the United States and its incidence is increasing dramatically.

Although it cannot be cultured from the synovium of patients with Lyme arthritis, *B. burgdorferi* DNA is detectable in the synovial fluid via PCR. The spirochete does not secrete any toxins but is thought to cause a strong host inflammatory response that leads to arthritis. Phagocytosis of live *B. burgdorferi* by monocytes appears to stimulate the release of proinflammatory cytokines such as type I interferons that induce joint inflammation.

VIRAL ARTHRITIS

Viruses cause arthritis by various mechanisms, including the stimulation of proinflammatory cytokines, inducing the formation of antibodies that cross-react with joint structures, increasing the activation of lymphocytes that are autoreactive, or via direct infection of synovial cells.

CLINICAL PRESENTATION

Consideration for infection-associated arthritis first requires the presence of arthritis; that is, inflammation of the joints. The presenting history of inflammatory joint disease is that of a child with significant morning stiffness that improves with activity and worsens with rest. This contrasts with mechanical joint pain, which is worsened with activity and relieved with rest. Examination of an arthritic joint reveals the cardinal features of inflammation including swelling, warmth, tenderness, and limited range of motion. The timing of symptom onset, number, and pattern of joints involved as well as extra-articular signs and symptoms, provide clues that help to differentiate among these infection-associated arthritides. Clinical features of infection-associated arthritis are shown in **Table 153-1**.

REACTIVE ARTHRITIS

Reactive arthritis occurs 1 to 4 weeks after gastrointestinal or genitourinary infections. Not all infections are symptomatic and the inciting event may not be readily identified, so the diagnosis of reactive arthritis may be difficult to make in some cases. Chlamydial infection, the most common cause of reactive arthritis in adults, tends to be asymptomatic in most patients that develop reactive arthritis. Reactive arthritis usually presents as an acute, painful, sometimes erythematous oligoarthritis (four or fewer joints involved), usually of the lower extremities, most typically in the knees and ankles. A characteristic of reactive arthritis is enthesitis, or inflammation of the attachment of ligaments and tendons to bone. This commonly occurs in the patellar and Achilles tendons as well as in the plantar fascia. Dactylitis, or sausage digits, may also be present. As a form of spondyloarthritis, stiffness and pain of the back and neck may be present. Systemic features may include fever, weight loss, and fatigue during the disease course. Extra-articular features may include painless oral ulcers, urethritis, and conjunctivitis. Patients with reactive arthritis will often have a relapsing course, especially in the setting of repeated infections with the same organism. Although rare, reactive arthritis following SARS-CoV2 infection and vaccination has been reported.

POSTSTREPTOCOCCAL REACTIVE ARTHRITIS

Poststreptococcal reactive arthritis represents a heterogeneous group of diseases that occurs 1 to 2 weeks after streptococcal infection in the setting of incomplete diagnostic criteria for ARF. It occurs with equal frequency in males and females, and commonly affects children ages 8 to 14. Joint involvement is usually not migratory, in contrast to the arthritis that occurs in ARF. PSRA primarily affects the large joints of the lower extremities, and there is an equal incidence of patients with mono-, oligo-, and polyarthritis. The arthritis typically resolves within a few weeks, although it can last several months. Pharyngitis may be present in two-thirds of patients, and one-third report low-grade fever or rash. Glomerulonephritis, a recognized complication of streptococcal infection, occurs in some patients. Around 8% of children with PSRA subsequently develop valvular heart disease, which raises the questions of whether PSRA is a distinct entity from ARF and if antibiotic prophylaxis is indicated in this population. In contrast, carditis is not seen in adults with PSRA.

LYME ARTHRITIS

Most patients infected with *B. burgdorferi* are asymptomatic, but in symptomatic patients, Lyme disease may affect the skin, joints, nervous system, and heart. Lyme disease is most common in children ages 5 to 9 years, a finding likely related to the frequency and intensity of tick exposure. Historically, most patients have onset of disease in June, July, or August, but they may present throughout the year.

Most symptomatic children present with early Lyme disease, manifested as erythema migrans (EM), an enlarging, erythematous, painless rash at the site of the tick bite. The rash expands peripherally and may have central clearing. This usually appears days to weeks after infection. EM may be accompanied by flu-like symptoms including chills, fevers, arthralgias, headaches, myalgias, and fatigue. Early Lyme disease may also be accompanied by a lymphocytic meningitis and Bell's palsy. Lyme carditis is uncommon in children but can present with atrioventricular block.

Another common presentation of Lyme disease is arthritis, a late manifestation of the disease. Lyme arthritis occurs months to years after infection, with an average of 4 months between infection and presentation. Most patients do not recall a tick bite. Of children who present with Lyme arthritis, 90% have knee involvement, although the hip and ankles may be involved in a minority of patients. Arthritis may present as a single episode of mildly painful swelling that may resolve without treatment. Untreated, half of children with Lyme arthritis may have recurrent episodes of arthritis lasting weeks to months. However, even after appropriate antibiotic treatment, arthritis may recur within a year; most of these recurrences can be treated with nonsteroidal anti-inflammatory agents (NSAIDs) alone.

VIRAL AND POST-VIRAL ARTHRITIS

Most viral infections cause arthralgias (joint pain in the absence of inflammation) rather than arthritis, although a few viruses demonstrate a propensity for joint inflammation. Parvovirus B19 usually

TABLE 153-1 Clinical Presentation of Infection-Associated Arthritis

Disease	Timing	Joint Involvement	Typical Age of Presentation	Associated Features
Reactive arthritis	1-4 weeks after GI or GU infection	Acute painful oligoarthritis of lower extremities	8-12 y	Enthesitis, dactylitis, fever, weight loss, HLA-B27
Poststreptococcal reactive arthritis	1-2 weeks after streptococcal infection	Mono- oligo- or polyarthritis of the lower extremities	8-14 y	Pharyngitis
Acute rheumatic fever	2-3 weeks after streptococcal infection	Painful migratory arthritis of large joints	6-15 y	Carditis, chorea, erythema marginatum, subcutaneous nodules, fever
Lyme arthritis	Weeks to months after infection	Oligoarthritis of the knee	5-9 y	Residence in or travel to endemic areas
Viral (e.g., parvovirus B19)	Concurrent with infection or up to 2 weeks later	Varied	Any	Fever, "slapped cheek" rash, other viral symptoms
Transient synovitis	Follows URI	Painful hip with limp	3-10 y (male-to-female ratio 2:1)	Afebrile or low-grade fever, appear well

GI, gastrointestinal; GU, genitourinary; HLA, human leukocyte antigen; URI, upper respiratory infection.

causes erythema infectiosum, or fifth disease. Although most often an asymptomatic infection, this pathogen may cause fever and nonspecific influenza-like symptoms during viremia. Two weeks later, a cutaneous eruption is seen on the cheeks (slapped cheeks), thought to be due to the formation and deposition of immune complexes in the skin. The arthritis that sometimes occurs in this disease is also thought to be related to immune-complex deposition within joints. Adults often develop arthritis after parvovirus infection, with the sudden onset of symmetric swelling of the small joints of the hands, mimicking rheumatoid arthritis. However, only a few children with parvovirus B19 infection will develop joint symptoms, usually manifested as mild and transient arthralgias. A small minority will develop a symmetric arthritis similar to what occurs in adults, but they can also develop oligoarthritis of large joints such as knees and ankles. Symptoms usually resolve within weeks to months, though treatment directed against the arthritis may be necessary.

Several case reports have described a postinfectious arthritis following SARS-CoV2 infection, most commonly presenting with mono- or oligoarticular arthritis of the lower extremity joints days after the onset of viral symptoms with response to NSAIDs. The pathogenesis of arthritis in these cases is still not well understood, though is likely a consequence of the highly immunogenic properties of the virus.

Rubella infection, either naturally acquired or occasionally after vaccination with MMR, can cause arthralgias and arthritis, especially in girls. The distribution of involved joints is usually symmetric, appearing 2 weeks after infection or vaccination, or around the onset of the rash. The hands and knees are most often affected, and the arthritis usually resolves within 2 weeks.

Arthritis can also be seen in the setting of other common viral infections, including hepatitis C virus (HCV) infection, especially with the presence of cryoglobulins, with hepatitis B virus (HBV) infection in the presence of polyarteritis nodosa, and in HIV.

TRANSIENT SYNOVITIS

Transient synovitis of the hip usually follows a viral upper respiratory infection. It occurs most commonly in boys ages 3 to 10 years and presents with the sudden onset of hip pain and limp. The hip is held flexed and externally rotated, and weight bearing may be avoided, often raising concern for septic arthritis. In contrast to a septic joint, children with transient synovitis are usually afebrile or have low-grade fevers and otherwise appear well. Up to 25% of children with transient synovitis of the hips will have bilateral hip involvement.

DIFFERENTIAL DIAGNOSIS

The timing of onset of arthritis in relation to the onset of infection, the pattern of joints involved, and the presence of extra-articular signs and symptoms can help to differentiate among the different causes of infection-associated arthritis. As a caveat, however, one must be aware that infections may trigger an underlying chronic arthritis, such as juvenile idiopathic arthritis (JIA). Therefore, if the clinical course of a suspected infectious or postinfectious arthritis is atypical, referral to a rheumatologist is recommended.

An acute onset of arthritis with the presence or history of infection raises the index of suspicion for an infection-associated arthritis. On the other hand, JIA usually presents as indolent joint swelling and morning stiffness and is diagnosed after symptoms have been present for more than 6 weeks. The differential diagnosis of a swollen joint also includes trauma or injury as well as joint effusions related to malignancy. Typically, history, examination findings, radiographs, and laboratory data can differentiate among these entities.

Fever and monoarthritis should prompt strong consideration for a septic joint or osteomyelitis. The rapid and accurate diagnosis of septic arthritis is of paramount importance to avoid irreversible joint damage (see Chapter 101). Algorithms to differentiate septic arthritis from transient synovitis have been established and are shown in **Table 153-2**.

If fever is present when several joints are affected, other diagnoses should be considered, as shown in **Table 153-3**.

TABLE 153-2 Factors Suggesting a Diagnosis of Septic Arthritis Rather Than Transient Synovitis

History of fever
Inability to bear weight
ESR greater than 40 mm/g
WBC count greater than 12,000

Source: Data from Kocher MS, Zurakowski D, Kasser JR. Differentiating between septic arthritis and transient synovitis of the hip in children: an evidence-based clinical prediction algorithm. *J Bone Joint Surg Am.* 1999;81(12):1662-1670.

ARF and PSRA are distinguished by the Jones criteria for ARF. In the setting of arthritis in the aftermath of group A Streptococcus (GAS) infection, if the Jones criteria cannot be met for the diagnosis of ARF, then the diagnosis of PSRA is made.

Distinguishing septic arthritis from Lyme arthritis in Lyme disease–endemic areas may be difficult, although in one study comparing the presentation of Lyme disease versus septic arthritis, no child with ANC ≤10,000/mm^3 and ESR ≤40 mm/hr had a septic joint. In addition, certain MRI features favor a diagnosis of Lyme disease including myositis, popliteal lymphadenopathy, and lack of subcutaneous edema.

Malignancies, especially leukemias, can present with joint swelling, and may be distinguished from inflammatory etiologies by the combination of inappropriately low white blood cell count, low or normal platelet counts, and nighttime pain.

DIAGNOSTIC EVALUATION

Arthrocentesis is useful to evaluate for septic arthritis when clinically indicated, but synovial fluid analysis is not necessary for the diagnosis of these other infection-associated arthritides. Instead, it may be used to evaluate for other causes of arthritis, particularly septic arthritis when clinically indicated, rather than to diagnose these entities.

REACTIVE ARTHRITIS

The criteria for the diagnosis of reactive arthritis are well established, and are presented in **Table 153-4**.

POSTSTREPTOCOCCAL REACTIVE ARTHRITIS

Evidence of streptococcal infection by positive serologies (elevated ASO and/or anti-DNAse B antibodies) must be documented in patients with suspected PSRA. Due to the short latency between infection and the onset of arthritis, throat cultures or rapid Strep testing may be

TABLE 153-3 Differential Diagnosis of Arthritis in the Presence of Fever

Category	Conditions
Rheumatologic	Systemic juvenile idiopathic arthritis Kawasaki disease IgA Vasculitis Vasculitis
Malignancy	Acute lymphoblastic leukemia Neuroblastoma Lymphoma Bone tumor
Autoinflammatory	Familial Mediterranean fever
Infectious	Acute rheumatic fever Septic arthritis Gonococcal arthritis Reactive arthritis
Gastrointestinal	Inflammatory bowel disease
Miscellaneous	Serum sickness

TABLE 153-4 Diagnostic Criteria for Reactive Arthritis

Typical peripheral arthritis
Predominantly lower limb, asymmetric oligoarthritis PLUS
Evidence of preceding infection
If there is a clear history of diarrhea or urethritis within the preceding 4 weeks, laboratory confirmation is recommended
If there is no clear infection, laboratory confirmation is essential
Exclusion criteria
Patients with other known causes of arthritis

Source: Sieper J, Rudwaleit M, Braun J, van der Heijde D. Diagnosing reactive arthritis: role of clinical setting in the value of serologic and microbiologic assays. *Arthritis Rheum*. 2002; 46:319-327.

positive as well. The ESR is elevated in 75% of patients. In contrast, systemic inflammatory markers are rarely elevated in patients with JIA.

LYME ARTHRITIS

The diagnosis of Lyme arthritis hinges on the presence of positive serologies found in the appropriate clinical setting, most classically a marked mono- or oligoarthritis, typically involving the knee. Given their inherent limitations and the presence of clinically unrelated, chronically positive IgG antibodies directed against *B. burgdorferi* in endemic regions, tests for Lyme should be sent only if there is a high suspicion for Lyme arthritis.

The Centers for Disease Control and Prevention (CDC) recommends a two-tiered process for laboratory diagnosis of Lyme disease. The first recommended screening test is for *B. burgdorferi* antibodies with a sensitive test such as enzyme immunoassay (EIA) or immunofluorescence assay (IFA). As in any other disease, an antibody response to *B. burgdorferi* requires several weeks to develop, so this test may be negative early in the disease course (such as with the presentation of EM), but will be positive in Lyme arthritis, a late finding. Confirmatory testing with Western blot is required for positive or equivocal screening tests. Western blot IgM and IgG bands should be present when signs or symptoms have been present for fewer than 30 days, while IgG bands alone should be present for symptoms of longer durations. Since arthritis is a late presentation of Lyme disease, EIA or IFA as well as IgG Western blot must be positive to make the diagnosis of Lyme arthritis.

VIRAL AND POST-VIRAL ARTHRITIS

To diagnose viral and post-viral arthritis, the diagnosis of a preceding or concurrent viral infection is necessary. This may be done clinically, or for specific viral-associated arthritides, serologies demonstrating current infection are supportive. For example, parvovirus infection is diagnosed by the presence of IgM antibodies to parvovirus, or through DNA assays. Anti-rubella IgM and IgG antibodies are usually present at the onset of joint symptoms in the case of rubella-mediated arthritis.

TRANSIENT SYNOVITIS

The diagnosis of transient synovitis of the hip is typically made clinically by corroborating history and physical examination findings. Ultrasound can be used to confirm the presence of effusion, though this does not rule out other causes of arthritis.

MANAGEMENT

REACTIVE ARTHRITIS

Treatment of reactive arthritis involves NSAIDs in most patients, and some may require oral corticosteroids. If reactive arthritis becomes chronic, disease-modifying antirheumatic drugs (DMARDs), such as methotrexate or sulfasalazine should be added. A randomized trial has suggested that antibiotic therapy may be effective for Chlamydial reactive arthritis but not for the other causative organisms. Small studies of adult patients have shown that TNF inhibitors appear to be safe and effective in treating reactive arthritis.

TABLE 153-5 Infectious Diseases Society of America Guidelines for Treatment of Lyme Arthritis in Children

Drug	Dosage for Children
Preferred oral regimens	
Amoxicillin	For children <8 years, 50 mg/kg in 3 divided doses (maximum 500 mg per dose)
Doxycycline	For children ≥8 years, 4.4 mg/kg in 2 divided doses (maximum 100 mg per dose)
Cefuroxime axetil	30 mg/kg per day in 2 divided doses (maximum 500 mg per dose)
Alternative oral regimen (lower efficacy)	
Macrolides	Azithromycin 10 mg/kg once daily (maximum 500 mg per dose)
Preferred parenteral regimen	
Ceftriaxone	50-75 mg/kg intravenously daily (maximum 2g)
Aleternative parenteral regimens	
Cefotaxime	150-200 mg/kg daily in 3-4 divided doses (maximum 6 g daily)
Penicillin G	200,000-400,000 U/kg per day divided every 4 h (not to exceed 18-24 million U daily)

Source: Krause PJ, Auwaerter PG, Bannuru RR, et al. Clinical Practice Guidelines by the Infectious Diseases Society of America (IDSA): 2020 Guideline on Diagnosis and Management of Babesiosis. *Clin Infect Dis*. 2021;72(2):185-189.

POSTSTREPTOCOCCAL REACTIVE ARTHRITIS

It is unclear whether treatment with antibiotics for PSRA is beneficial for the acute episode. However, the use of antibiotic prophylaxis has been shown to prevent recurrence of arthritis, which may occur with subsequent streptococcal infections. NSAIDs are the mainstay of therapy; however, in refractory cases DMARDs or biologic agents may be necessary. Unlike ARF, there is not a dramatic improvement of symptoms with the administration of aspirin or other NSAIDs. The American Heart Association recommends prophylaxis for 1 year after the onset of symptoms; however, there is disagreement among rheumatologists regarding the utility of prophylaxis after a single episode of PSRA. If cardiac disease is detected, the patient should be classified as having ARF and should be managed accordingly, including with long-term antibiotic prophylaxis.

LYME ARTHRITIS

The Infectious Diseases Society of America has recommended antimicrobial guidelines for children with Lyme arthritis, as shown in **Table 153-5**. In light of the significant inflammation associated with Lyme arthritis, concurrent use of standing NSAIDs, such as Naproxen sodium 10 mg/kg/dose twice daily (up to 500 mg per dose), is recommended throughout the duration of antibiotic therapy. If the diagnosis of Lyme disease is confirmed via clinical and laboratory findings and the patient continues to have joint swelling after a first 28-day course of enteral antibiotics, a second course of enteral or intravenous antibiotics may be attempted. However, arthritis after appropriate antibiotic treatment is likely due to an alternate diagnosis, including a more chronic inflammatory arthritis unmasked by infection.

VIRAL AND POST-VIRAL ARTHRITIS

For most cases of viral arthritis, treatment is symptomatic. Ibuprofen 10 mg/kg/dose every 6 hours or naproxen sodium 10 mg/kg/dose (up to 500 mg per dose) twice daily can be used for pain and swelling. Treatment may be discontinued upon resolution of symptoms. If symptoms do not resolve as expected, or if they recur, then consideration for an underlying inflammatory arthritis may be made.

ADMISSION AND DISCHARGE CRITERIA

Most patients with arthritis do not need a hospital admission unless there is concern for septic arthritis, which may require operative debridement by an orthopedic surgeon. If a previously ambulatory child is not able to bear weight, then admission may be necessary to expedite evaluation and optimize treatment. Finally, if there are considerable systemic features that raise the concern of a systemic disease process of which arthritis is a part, then admission may be warranted to expedite evaluation and provide timely treatment.

Discharge criteria depend on the reasons for admission, but include improvement in function, specifically regaining the ability to bear weight or use the affected joint(s), ability to tolerate oral medications, and the arrangement of appropriate outpatient follow-up.

CONSULTATION

- Rheumatology: For help in determining the cause of arthritis, aspiration and injection of joints, creation of treatment plan, and for long-term outpatient follow-up.
- Orthopedics: For help with aspiration of joints, and with the management of septic arthritis.
- Cardiology: To help in the diagnosis of ARF.
- Ophthalmology: For evaluation of uveitis, which can be seen in reactive arthritis and other types of juvenile idiopathic arthritis.
- Oncology: For assistance with the evaluation of malignancy.

SPECIAL CONSIDERATIONS

There is ongoing disagreement among practitioners regarding whether PSRA lies on the spectrum of ARF or is its own discrete entity, and debate regarding the need for antibiotic prophylaxis among patients who do not fulfill Jones criteria. Hospitalists may consider consultation with Rheumatology and Cardiology to guide medical decision-making in these cases. Communication with primary care providers during transitions of care is recommended to ensure appropriate outpatient surveillance, especially for monitoring of post-discharge symptom evolution.

PREVENTION

Prevention of infection-associated arthritis generally involves hand hygiene and other standard efforts to prevent the primary infections that trigger the arthritis.

The prompt treatment of Chlamydial infections has been shown to prevent the development of reactive arthritis caused by this pathogen, but not for other causes of reactive arthritis.

To prevent Lyme disease, avoidance of tick-infested areas, covering bare skin with clothing, using tick repellents, doing periodic "skin checks" for ticks, and rapidly removing ticks with a fine-tip forceps after identification may help to prevent infection. There is some evidence that antibiotic prophylaxis after a proven *I. scapularis* tick bite may be efficacious in preventing Lyme disease. Individuals weighing 45 kg or more may receive a single dose of doxycycline 200 mg, while children weighing less than 45 kg can be treated with a single dose of doxycycline 4.4 mg/kg.

KEY POINTS

- Bacteria and viruses can cause arthritis without directly invading the joint space via several different mechanisms.
- Reactive arthritis, poststreptococcal reactive arthritis, Lyme disease, and viral and post-viral arthritis have different clinical and laboratory presentations that allow them to be distinguished from one another.
- Arthritis presenting with fever has a differential diagnosis that includes autoimmune, autoinflammatory, infectious, malignant, and other systemic etiologies.
- Arthrocentesis is essential to diagnose septic arthritis but may not be helpful in differentiating among the infection-associated arthritides.
- First-line treatment for most types of infection-associated arthritis includes NSAIDs, and symptoms usually resolve spontaneously.
- Persistence of arthritis after a suspected infection may indicate an underlying idiopathic inflammatory arthritis rather than the persistence of the triggering infection.

SUGGESTED READINGS

An QJ, Qin DA, Pei JX. Reactive arthritis after COVID-19 vaccination. *Hum Vaccin Immunother.* 2021;17(9):2954-2956.

Bacon RM, Kugeler KJ, Mead PS, Centers for Disease Control and Prevention (CDC). Surveillance for Lyme disease–United States, 1992-2006. *MMWR Surveill Summ.* 2008;57(10):1-9.

Baird RW, Bronze MS, Kraus W, Hill HR, Veasey LG, Dale JB. Epitopes of group A streptococcal M protein shared with antigens of articular cartilage and synovium. *J Immunol.* 1991;146(9):3132-3137.

Bardin T, Enel C, Cornelis F, et al. Antibiotic treatment of venereal disease and Reiter's syndrome in a Greenland population. *Arthritis Rheum.* 1992;35(2):190-194.

Carter JD, Espinoza LR, Inman RD, et al. Combination antibiotics as a treatment for chronic Chlamydia-induced reactive arthritis: a double-blind, placebo-controlled, prospective trial. *Arthritis Rheum.* 2010;62(5):1298-1307.

Carter JD, Hudson AP. Reactive arthritis: clinical aspects and medical management. *Rheum Dis Clin North Am.* 2009;35(1):21-44.

Cassidy JT, Petty RE, Laxer R, Lindsley C. *Textbook of Pediatric Rheumatology.* E-Book. Saunders; 2010.

Cervantes JL, Dunham-Ems SM, La Vake CJ, et al. Phagosomal signaling by *Borrelia burgdorferi* in human monocytes involves Toll-like receptor (TLR)2 and TLR8 cooperativity and TLR8-mediated induction of IFN-beta. *Proc Natl Acad Sci U S A.* 2011;108(9):3683-3688.

Deanehan JK, Kimia AA, Tan Tanny SP, et al. Distinguishing lyme from septic knee monoarthritis in lyme disease-endemic areas. *Pediatrics.* 2013;131(3):e695-701.

Dougados M, Baeten D. Spondyloarthritis. *Lancet.* 2011;377(9783):2127-2137.

Ecklund K, Vargas S, Zurakowski D, Sundel RP. MRI features of Lyme arthritis in children. *AJR Am J Roentgenol.* 2005;184(6):1904-1909.

Franssila R, Hedman K. Infection and musculoskeletal conditions: viral causes of arthritis. *Best Pract Res Clin Rheumatol.* 2006;20(6):1139-1157.

Garcia-Monco JC, Benach JL. Lyme neuroborreliosis. *Ann Neurol.* 1995;37(6):691-702.

Gasparotto M, Framba V, Piovella C, et al. Post-COVID-19 arthritis: a case report and literature review. *Clin Rheumatol.* 2021;40(8):3357-3362.

Gerber MA, Baltimore RS, Eaton CB, et al. Prevention of rheumatic fever and diagnosis and treatment of acute Streptococcal pharyngitis. *Circulation.* 2009;119(11):1541-1551.

Gerber MA, Zemel LS, Shapiro ED. Lyme arthritis in children: clinical epidemiology and long-term outcomes. *Pediatrics.* 1998;102(4):905-908

Jones OY. A multicenter case-control study on predictive factors distinguishing childhood leukemia from juvenile rheumatoid arthritis. *Pediatrics.* 2006;117(5):e840-844.

Kingsley G, Sieper J. Third International Workshop on Reactive Arthritis. 23-26 September 1995, Berlin, Germany. Report and abstracts. *Ann Rheum Dis.* 1996;55(8):564-584.

Kocher MS, Zurakowski D, Kasser JR. Differentiating between septic arthritis and transient synovitis of the hip in children: an evidence-based clinical prediction algorithm. *J Bone Joint Surg Am.* 1999;81(12):1662-1670.

Kocyigit BF, Akyol A. Reactive arthritis after COVID-19: a case-based review. *Rheumatol Int.* 2021;41(11):2031-2039.

Mackie SL. Poststreptococcal reactive arthritis: what is it and how do we know? *Rheumatology.* 2004;43(8):949-954.

Meyer A, Chatelus E, Wendling D, et al. Safety and efficacy of anti-tumor necrosis factor α therapy in ten patients with recent-onset refractory reactive arthritis. *Arthritis Rheum.* 2011;63(5):1274-1280.

Morris D, Inman RD. Reactive arthritis: developments and challenges in diagnosis and treatment. *Curr Rheumatol Rep.* 2012;14(5):390-394.

Nadelman RB, Hanincová K, Mukherjee P, et al. Differentiation of reinfection from relapse in recurrent Lyme disease. *N Engl J Med.* 2012;367(20):1883-1890.

Nocton JJ, Miller LC, Tucker LB, Schaller JG. Human parvovirus B19-associatedarthritis in children. *J Pediatr*. 1993;122(2):186-190.

Perl L, Kvint I, Matitiau A, et al. Late cardiac assessment in children diagnosed with post-streptococcal reactive arthritis: a long term study. *Clin Exp Rheumatol*. 2015;33(4):578-582.

Radolf JD, Caimano MJ, Stevenson B, Hu LT. Of ticks, mice and men: understanding the dual-host lifestyle of Lyme disease spirochaetes. *Nat Rev Microbiol*. 2012;10(12):87-99.

Reid DM, Brown T, Reid TMS, Rennie JAN, Eastmond CJ. Human parvovirus-associated arthritis: a clinical and laboratory description. *Lancet*. 1985;325(8426):422-425.

Rich E, Hook EW, Alarcón GS, Moreland LW. Reactive arthritis in patients attending an urban sexually transmitted diseases clinic. *Arthritis Rheum*. 1996;39(7):1172-1177.

Sinaei R, Pezeshki S, Parvaresh S, et al. Post SARS-CoV-2 infection reactive arthritis: a brief report of two pediatric cases. *Pediatr Rheumatol Online J*. 2021;19(1):89.

van Bemmel JM, Delgado V, Holman ER, et al. No increased risk of valvular heart disease in adult poststreptococcal reactive arthritis. *Arthritis Rheum*. 2009;60(4):987-993.

Warshafsky S, Lee DH, Francois LK, Nowakowski J, Nadelman RB, Wormser GP. Efficacy of antibiotic prophylaxis for the prevention of Lyme disease: an updated systematic review and meta-analysis. *J Antimicrob Chemother*. 2010;65(6):1137-1144.

Wingstrand H. Transient synovitis of the hip in the child. *Acta Orthop Scand Suppl*. 1986;219:1-61.

Wormser GP, Dattwyler RJ, Shapiro ED, et al. The clinical assessment, treatment, and prevention of Lyme disease, human granulocytic anaplasmosis, and babesiosis: clinical practice guidelines by the Infectious Diseases Society of America. *Clin Infect Dis*. 2006;43(9):1089-1134.

Young NS, Brown KE. Parvovirus B19. *N Engl J Med*. 2004;350(6):586-597.

CHAPTER 154 Systemic Lupus Erythematosus

Mindy S. Lo, MD, PhD

BACKGROUND

Systemic lupus erythematosus (SLE) is a chronic, potentially serious systemic autoimmune disease. It is characterized biochemically by the presence of autoantibodies, in particular, antibodies directed against nuclear antigens. SLE is a heterogeneous disease in that clinical manifestations can vary significantly from patient to patient, ranging from mild presentations to severe organ dysfunction. Morbidity and mortality rates have improved dramatically over the past few decades due to advances in therapy.

EPIDEMIOLOGY

SLE primarily affects women of childbearing age, including adolescents, with a female:male ratio of 4-5:1. Approximately 10% to 20% of SLE is diagnosed before adulthood. Female predominance is less pronounced in patients with younger age of onset. It is extraordinarily rare for SLE to present before the age of 5 years, and female:male ratio is essentially equal in this group. Children tend to have more severe diseases as compared with adults, with increased rates of nephritis and long-term morbidity.

Overall prevalence rates in the United States are estimated at 40 to 150 per 100,000 with a trend toward increasing prevalence over time. Non-White populations are more significantly affected, with higher prevalence in Asians, Hispanics, and African Americans. African American and Hispanic groups also have higher morbidity and mortality but it is unclear if this is due to socioeconomic or other factors.

PATHOPHYSIOLOGY

The pathogenesis of SLE is complex and remains inadequately understood. Immune abnormalities have been described on multiple levels involving both the innate and adaptive immune systems. From the innate immune perspective, dysregulated apoptosis and clearance of cellular debris lead to improper antigen presentation and increased production of proinflammatory cytokines. In particular, overproduction of type I interferon is characteristic of SLE and can correlate with disease activity. Loss of self-tolerance allows the development of autoreactive T and B cells that mediate tissue damage.

Immune abnormalities in SLE are affected by genetic, hormonal, and environmental influences. Polymorphisms in many immune-related genes have been described in SLE patients, including *STAT4*, *PTPN22*, and *IRF5*. In most patients, variations in multiple genes are thought to contribute to the development of lupus. There are also rare cases of monogenic SLE developing in children. Examples include deficiencies in complement (especially C1q and C4) and mutations in *TREX1*, a gene encoding an exonuclease involved in DNA repair and apoptosis.

Hormonal influences are suggested by the strong female predominance in SLE. Flares of disease triggered by pregnancy or exogenous estrogen administration have been well described. However, the exact mechanisms by which sex hormones interact with the immune system to promote autoimmunity are not known.

Environmental triggers, particularly viral infections, are also thought to affect SLE. One example is Epstein-Barr virus (EBV), which infects B cells leading to B cell activation and proliferation. In one study of pediatric SLE patients, more than 99% had evidence of prior seroconversion to EBV, as compared to 70% in age-matched controls.

Drug-induced lupus can present in identical fashion to SLE; common triggers include hydralazine, procainamide, and minocycline. Antihistone antibodies are often observed in these patients. Symptoms generally resolve with discontinuation of the triggering medication, but immunosuppressive medications are sometimes needed to speed this process.

CLINICAL PRESENTATION

INITIAL PRESENTATION

SLE is quite variable in its presentation, involving different organ systems with varying degrees of severity. Symptoms may develop acutely or insidiously. The diagnosis of SLE may thus be made in both outpatient and inpatient settings. In pediatric patients in particular, new presentations are often severe and require hospitalization. At diagnosis, the most common clinical manifestations are arthritis, malar rash, cytopenias, fatigue, fever, and nephritis. Palatal ulcers are also common findings that can be painless and unnoticed by the patient (**Figure 154-1**).

Classification criteria revised in 1997 by the American College of Rheumatology (ACR) for the study of SLE have been commonly used for diagnosis and are a useful framework for recalling the most notable clinical manifestations (**Table 154-1**). In 2019, the ACR collaborated with the European League Against Rheumatism (EULAR) to develop new classification criteria (**Table 154-2**). These criteria have similar specificity but better sensitivity as compared to the 1997 ACR criteria. Neither have been validated in the pediatric population.

Additional symptoms not included in the classification criteria but often described by patients include weight loss, malaise, alopecia, myalgias, lymphadenopathy, and Raynaud phenomenon. It is important to remember that clinical manifestations may evolve over time, and patients who do not yet meet classification criteria may still have SLE and thus warrant treatment.

DISEASE COURSE AND PROGNOSIS

SLE is a chronic disease with an unpredictable remitting and relapsing course. In general, lupus that presents during childhood is more likely to have renal involvement, more severe onset, and require more aggressive therapy as compared to adult-onset SLE. After the first 1 to 2 years of disease, new organs tend not to be involved, with the exception of the central nervous system.

TABLE 154-1	1997 American College of Rheumatology (ACR) Classification Criteria for the Diagnosis of Systemic Lupus Erythematosus
Criterion	**Comments**
Malar rash	"Butterfly" rash: fixed erythematous symmetrical rash that crosses the nasal bridge and medial cheeks but spares the nasolabial folds; photosensitive; rarely scars Most common skin manifestation in children
Discoid rash	Discrete, erythematous raised plaques with scale and follicular plugging on the face, scalp, and limbs; photosensitive; atrophic scarring Isolated discoid lupus is rare in childhood; if isolated, rarely progresses to systemic disease
Photosensitivity	Any rash with an unusually dramatic reaction to sunlight
Oral lesions	Shallow, painless ulcers of the hard palate, oral mucosa, or nasopharynx
Arthritis	Requires at least 2 peripheral joints for criteria Usually symmetric polyarthritis, commonly fingers, wrists, and knees; unlikely to be erosive
Serositis	Pleuritis OR pericarditis (abdominal peritonitis is not sufficient)
Renal disorder	Proteinuria >0.5 g/day, or 3+ on dipstick OR cellular casts Seen in 85%-100% of patients, often during the first year following diagnosis; see Table 154-5 for nephritis classification
Neurologic disorder	Seizures OR psychosis Additional symptoms not part of criteria include headache, chorea, stroke, transverse myelitis, mononeuritis multiplex, and mood disorders
Hematologic disorder	Any of the following: • Hemolytic anemia • Leukopenia <4000 cells/mm^3 on ≥2 occasions • Lymphopenia <1500 cells/mm^3 ≥2 occasions • Thrombocytopenia <100,000 cells/mm^3 ≥2 occasions
Anti-nuclear antibody (ANA)	Positive ANA at any point in time
Immunologic disorder	Any of the following: • Anti-DNA antibody • Anti-Smith antibody • Anti-phospholipid antibodies (anticardiolipin IgG or IgM, lupus anticoagulant, false positive RPR test for syphilis for at least 6 mo)

RPR, Rapid plasma reagin.

The long-term prognosis is primarily related to renal disease and central nervous system involvement, which are the main causes of morbidity. Risk factors for poor renal outcome include hypertension, impaired renal function at diagnosis, and specific renal biopsy findings such as diffuse proliferative lupus nephritis. The 2-year mortality of SLE approached 100% in the early 1960s. With the use of immunosuppressive treatments and improved management of chronic renal failure, the 20-year survival rate is now >75%. These increased survival rates are accompanied by greater morbidity related to medication side effects and development of comorbid conditions. Children with lupus are at increased risk for accelerated atherosclerosis, cerebrovascular accident, and myocardial infarction as they age. Risk factors for cardiovascular disease include prolonged use of steroids, coronary vasculitis, obesity, hypertension, lupus nephritis, hyperlipidemia, lupus anticoagulant, and family history of cardiac disease.

Overwhelming infection is the most frequent cause of mortality among children with SLE, and those with active disease are at the greatest risk of developing an infection. Children with SLE are immunocompromised by the disease itself (i.e., neutropenia, lymphopenia, hypocomplementemia, functional asplenia) as well as by immunosuppressive medications used to treat the disease. These medications may also mask fever and other signs of infection, complicating the ability to distinguish between lupus flares and acute infection. Other major causes of mortality include renal failure, central nervous system disease, pulmonary hemorrhage, and myocardial infarction.

NEONATAL LUPUS

Neonatal lupus is a distinct, uncommon condition found in infants born to mothers with anti-SSA/Ro and/or anti-SSB/La antibodies. The mothers may or may not have other evidence of systemic autoimmune disease; many are asymptomatic. Transplacental passage of these autoantibodies can cause a range of symptoms in the infant including rash, congenital heart block, anemia or thrombocytopenia, and hepatitis. Congenital heart block is the most worrisome feature and can be detected as early as the second trimester (**Figure 154-2**). Congenital heart block associated with neonatal lupus is thought to occur when transplacental passage of maternal autoantibodies to the intracellular ribonucleoproteins Ro (SS-A) and La (SS-B) cross the placenta and injure the previously normal fetal heart. Even when detected early in pregnancy, studies have not shown benefit with immunosuppressive treatment. Complete heart block is not reversible and requires placement of a pacemaker after birth. These infants are also at risk of subsequent cardiomyopathy. In contrast, the other clinical manifestations generally resolve over several months as the maternal antibodies are cleared. Mothers of infants with neonatal lupus should be counseled on the use of hydroxychloroquine to reduce the risk of congenital heart block in future pregnancies.

DIFFERENTIAL DIAGNOSIS

Due to the multiorgan involvement and the wide range of clinical presentations, many illnesses must be considered in children manifesting signs or symptoms of SLE (**Table 154-3**).

DIAGNOSTIC EVALUATION

LABORATORY TESTING

Despite the wide heterogeneity of clinical manifestations, SLE patients are linked by the near-universal presence of antinuclear antibodies (ANA). Importantly, the ANA is a nonspecific test, occurring in higher frequency in other inflammatory conditions as well as in up to 15% of the overall adult population, making it a poor screening tool. Additional autoantibodies are also frequently present in patterns that are sometimes predictive of specific organ system involvement (**Table 154-4**). For example, anti-dsDNA antibodies correlate with increased risk for nephritis, and a rise in titer may signify increased disease activity. Antiphospholipid antibodies are associated with increased risk for thrombotic events and thrombotic microangiopathy.

Cytopenias, particularly lymphopenia and thrombocytopenia, are commonly seen in pediatric SLE (**Table 154-5**). High IgG and low complement C3 and C4 levels are also common laboratory findings. Hypocomplementemia results from immune complex deposition in target organs, usually kidney or skin. Thus, falling complement levels can be a marker of worsening renal disease.

Inflammatory markers are also helpful in the evaluation of SLE. Erythrocyte sedimentation rate (ESR) is typically high, in part due to hypergammaglobulinemia. C-reactive protein (CRP), on the other hand, may be normal or low despite active disease. The reason for this is unclear but may be due to decreased CRP production in SLE patients or the development of anti-CRP antibodies. Regardless, the presence of high CRP levels in the context of fever should prompt consideration of infection in addition to lupus flare.

For evaluation of renal involvement, urinalysis and serum creatinine levels should be followed closely. The presence of elevated serum creatinine, proteinuria, hematuria, or pyuria is suggestive of renal disease.

ADDITIONAL STUDIES

Renal biopsy is usually indicated if there is evidence of nephritis, and is ideally performed prior to initiation of therapy. In addition to

TABLE 154-2 2019 ACR/EULAR Classification Criteria for the Diagnosis of Systemic Lupus Erythematosus

Patients must have an **ANA titer of ≥1:80**, at least **one clinical criterion**, and **≥10 points** from the following:

Clinical	Weight	Laboratory	Weight
Constitutional		**Antiphospholipid antibodies**	
Fever	2	Anti-cardiolipin *(high titer)* OR positive anti-β2 glycoprotein OR lupus anticoagulant	2
Hematologic		**Complement proteins**	
Leukopenia *(WBC <4000/mm³)*	3	Low C3 OR low C4 *(below lower limit of normal)*	3
Thrombocytopenia *(platelets <100,000/mm³)*	4	Low C3 AND low C4	4
Autoimmune hemolysis *(Coombs'+ hemolysis)*	4		
Neuropsychiatric		**SLE-specific antibodies**	
Delirium *(acute, fluctuating change in consciousness, behavior, or cognition)*	2	Anti-dsDNA OR anti-Smith	6
Psychosis *(delusions, hallucinations)*	3		
Seizure *(generalized or partial/focal)*	5		
Mucocutaneous – *must be observed by clinician*			
Non-scarring alopecia	2		
Oral ulcers	2		
Subacute cutaneous OR discoid lupus	4		
Acute cutaneous lupus	6		
Serosal			
Pleural or pericardial effusion seen on imaging	5		
Acute pericarditis *≥2 of 1) pericardial chest pain, 2) pericardial rub, 3) EKG with widespread ST elevation, 4) new or worsened pericardial effusion*	6		
Musculoskeletal			
Joint involvement – *synovitis in ≥2 joints*	6		
Renal			
Proteinuria >0.5 g/24 hr *or equivalent spot protein*	4		
Renal biopsy Class II or V nephritis	8		
Renal biopsy Class III or IV nephritis	10		

demonstrating severity and type of nephritis (**Table 154-6**), renal biopsy may also detect microvascular thrombotic disease for which anticoagulation may be beneficial.

In patients with suspected pericarditis or endocarditis, echocardiogram is warranted. Patients with pleuritic pain or shortness of breath may also require further evaluation with pulmonary function testing and/or chest CT. For patients with concern for neuropsychiatric involvement, neuroimaging may be helpful. However, normal studies do not exclude the possibility of lupus cerebritis, for which diagnosis is sometimes confirmed by brain biopsy (typically not pursued due to the morbidity of this procedure) or response to empiric therapy. SLE patients are also at high risk for cerebrovascular infarction due to both hypercoagulability and atherosclerotic disease. There should thus be a low threshold for neuroimaging in patients with suspicion of stroke.

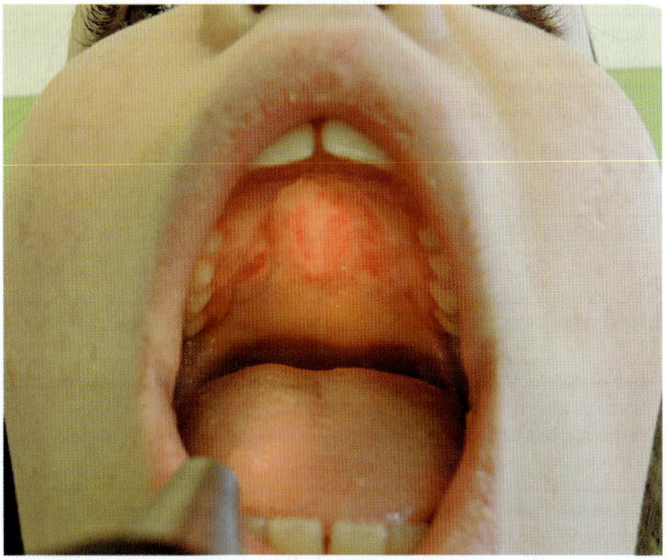

FIGURE 154-1. Oral ulcers in a patient with SLE. Note erythematous, macerated appearance of hard palate. (Used with permission from Dr. Mindy S. Lo.)

MANAGEMENT

The mainstay of SLE therapy is with glucocorticoids, usually prednisone or methylprednisolone. Steroids are effective in controlling inflammation, and it can be difficult to taper steroids in patients with more severe disease. Acute illness or severe flares are treated with high-dose steroids (oral prednisone 1-2 mg/kg/day or IV methylprednisolone 30 mg/kg/day × 1-3 pulses). Long-term steroids carry significant risks including adrenal suppression, osteoporosis, growth restriction, glaucoma and cataracts, glucose intolerance, mood disturbance, and myopathy. Chronic steroid and pulse-dose steroid use are associated with risk for avascular necrosis in SLE patients, especially those with hypercoagulability related to antiphospholipid antibodies. Additional side effects that may limit patient adherence to steroid regimens include weight gain, acne, striae, and Cushingoid facies.

Antimalarial medications such as chloroquine and hydroxychloroquine modulate the immune system through mechanisms that are not fully understood. They are not significantly immunosuppressive. Hydroxychloroquine has been shown to reduce the likelihood of SLE disease flares, and may also delay the accrual of additional autoimmune manifestations in patients with mild or early disease. In pregnant women

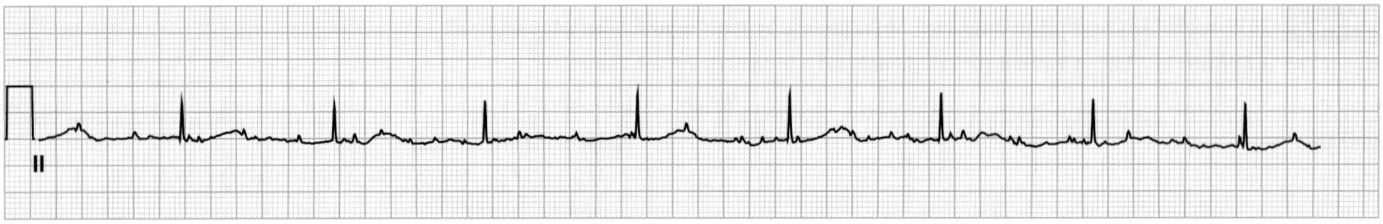

FIGURE 154-2. Electrocardiogram rhythm strip of an infant with neonatal lupus. This infant presented with symptomatic bradycardia. There is marked sinus bradycardia with atrioventricular dissociation and a junctional rhythm. The ventricular rate is 50 bpm and the atrial rate is 140 bpm. (Used with permission of Dr. Samir S. Shah, Cincinnati Children's Hospital Medical Center, Cincinnati, OH.)

TABLE 154-3 Differential Diagnosis of Systemic Lupus Erythematosus

Category	Condition
Other autoimmune conditions	Mixed connective tissue disease and other overlap syndromes Sjogren syndrome Juvenile idiopathic arthritis Systemic vasculitis Juvenile dermatomyositis
Infectious conditions	Epstein-Barr virus (EBV) and cytomegalovirus (CMV) Human immunodeficiency virus (HIV) Parvovirus B19
Malignant conditions	Leukemia Lymphoma

TABLE 154-4 Autoantibodies in Systemic Lupus Erythematosus

Autoantibody	Significance
Anti-nuclear antibody (ANA)	Sensitive (almost universally positive) but not specific (also found in other inflammatory conditions as well as 5%-15% of the overall population) Negative result suggests diagnosis other than SLE
Anti-double-stranded DNA (dsDNA)	Specific but not sensitive: positive in 50%-70% of children at presentation Associated with lupus nephritis; titer may correlate with disease activity
Anti-phospholipid antibodies	Includes lupus anticoagulant activity, anticardiolipin IgG and IgM, and anti-β2 glycoprotein IgG and IgM Seen in 65% of children with SLE; higher titers correlate with increased morbidity Associated with venous or arterial thrombosis, recurrent fetal loss, thrombocytopenia, transverse myelitis, and Libman-Sacks endocarditis
Anti-Ro/SSA Anti-La/SSB	Seen in 20%-30% of adults with SLE, as well as in Sjogren syndrome and neonatal lupus Also found in subacute cutaneous lupus (more common in adults)
Anti-Sm (Smith)	Very specific but not sensitive: positive in <50% of children with SLE
Anti-ribonucleoprotein (RNP)	Characteristic of mixed connective tissue disease; when seen in SLE, correlates with myositis, esophageal dysmotility, Raynaud phenomenon, interstitial lung disease, sclerodactyly
Anti-histone	Higher frequency in drug-induced lupus
Anti-ribosomal P, anti-neuronal antibodies	Associated with CNS disease of various causes, including SLE, schizophrenia, rheumatic fever

CNS, central nervous system; SLE, systemic lupus erythematosus.

with SLE, hydroxychloroquine may decrease the fetal risk for neonatal lupus. Antimalarial medications are generally well tolerated but are rarely associated with retinal toxicity and cardiomyopathy with cumulative exposure.

Steroid-sparing agents used for the treatment of SLE include mycophenolate mofetil (MMF) and azathioprine, both immunosuppressive agents that inhibit DNA synthesis. These medications are typically used

TABLE 154-5 Investigations to Consider in the Evaluation and Diagnosis of Systemic Lupus Erythematosus

Investigation	Significance
CBC with differential, Coombs test, smear review, reticulocyte count	Most SLE patients have at least one hematologic abnormality. Although autoimmune hemolytic anemia is classic, microangiopathic hemolytic anemia can also be seen Smear review is indicated if malignancy is on the differential diagnosis
ESR, CRP	Nonspecific markers of inflammation; ESR is typically elevated out of proportion to CRP. High CRP should raise concern for infection.
Immunoglobulins, C3 and C4	Immunoglobulins are elevated due to polyclonal activation of B lymphocytes Hypocomplementemia reflects immune complex deposition in target organs, usually kidney
Autoantibodies	See Table 154-4 for a list of autoantibodies
PT, PTT, INR	Prolongation of the PTT may indicate presence of lupus anticoagulant, which in vivo causes a hypercoagulable state
Liver function tests	Abnormalities more commonly due to medication toxicity than to SLE hepatitis
Serum BUN, creatinine, albumin, total protein; microscopic urinalysis; urine protein/creatinine ratio; renal biopsy	Type and severity of nephritis is classified according to histopathologic description (see Table 154-6)
Chest radiograph, pulmonary function tests	Pneumonitis can be asymptomatic. Other concerns include pulmonary hemorrhage, shrinking lung syndrome
Echocardiogram, ECG	Cardiac manifestations of SLE include pericarditis, myocarditis, endocarditis; also to evaluate complications such as atherosclerosis
Bone marrow biopsy	May be required to rule out malignancy or infection mimicking presentation of SLE
Brain CT; MRI, MRA/MRV; lumbar puncture (LP); electroencephalogram (EEG)	Neuroimaging to assess for infarction, inflammation, vasculitis LP to rule out infection (primary, opportunistic) EEG for patients with seizures

BUN, blood urea nitrogen; CBC, complete blood count; CRP, C-reactive protein; CT, computed tomography; ECG, electrocardiogram; ESR, erythrocyte sedimentation rate; INR, international normalized ratio; MRA, magnetic resonance angiography; MRI, magnetic resonance imaging; MRV, magnetic resonance venography; PT, prothrombin time; PTT, partial thromboplastin time.

TABLE 154-6 International Society of Nephrology-Renal Pathology Society (ISN-RPS) Histopathologic Classification of Renal Disease in SLE

Class	Description
I	**Minimal mesangial** • Normal light microscopy but mesangial deposits visible on electron microscopy • Minimal or no proteinuria
II	**Mesangial** • Mesangial hypercellularity and deposits visible by light microscopy • Microscopic hematuria and/or proteinuria
III	**Focal Proliferative** (<50% of glomeruli affected) • Focal subendothelial immune deposits • Glomerulonephritis is usually segmental (involves <50% of glomerular tuft)
IV	**Diffuse Proliferative** (>50% of glomeruli affected) • Most common form of lupus nephritis; high risk for renal failure • Class IV-S: primarily segmental lesions • Class IV-G: primarily global lesions
V	**Membranous** • Subepithelial immune deposits • Severe proteinuria
VI	**Advanced Sclerosing** • More than 90% of glomeruli are sclerosed and inactive • May represent end stage of class III, IV, or V nephritis • Refractory to further immunosuppressive therapy

for major organ system involvement (e.g., renal or cardiac) or systemic symptoms. MMF is more effective than azathioprine for the treatment of lupus nephritis. Both medications carry side effects including myelosuppression, hepatotoxicity, and immunocompromise.

Cyclophosphamide, a highly immunosuppressive DNA alkylating agent, is reserved for the treatment of severe disease, usually cerebritis or severe nephritis. Cyclophosphamide is given intravenously in monthly or biweekly doses for several months' duration. In addition to increased risk for opportunistic infection, short-term side effects include bladder and renal toxicity. Long-term cyclophosphamide can cause premature gonadal failure, infertility, and secondary malignancies; these effects are related to cumulative dose exposure.

Targeted therapies for SLE are being explored. In small studies, rituximab, a B cell-depleting agent originally developed to treat lymphoma, decreased disease activity scores, and improved serologic markers. Although not approved for the treatment of SLE, rituximab is commonly used in SLE and other autoimmune conditions mediated by autoantibodies. Belimumab, another monoclonal antibody, targets a B cell growth factor and is approved for use in adults and children when added to standard therapy. Newer agents such as those directed against type I interferon, plasmablasts, and plasmacytoid dendritic cells are in development.

Other treatments are useful for specific problems. Topical steroids are useful for treating inflammatory lupus rashes. Methotrexate is sometimes used to treat arthritis symptoms. Physical therapy is important for the treatment of arthritis and muscle weakness. Antipsychotics and anticonvulsants may be necessary as adjunctive therapy to control neuropsychiatric lupus. Hypertension must be treated aggressively because it accelerates the development of renal failure due to lupus nephritis. Vasodilators can be used to treat Raynaud phenomenon, and intravenous immunoglobulin can be helpful in patients with autoimmune cytopenias.

ADMISSION AND DISCHARGE CRITERIA

Hospitalization of a child with SLE may be necessary for any of the following reasons:

- Initial evaluation at presentation if the diagnosis is unclear or the patient is ill.
- Treatment of severe active disease, such as pulmonary hemorrhage, cerebrovascular accident or other thrombotic event, pericarditis, psychosis.
- Treatment of renal complications such as severe hypertension or renal failure.
- Intercurrent infection.

Discharge may be considered if:

- Diagnostic workup is complete, subspecialty consultations are obtained, and treatment is initiated.
- Any acute infection, lupus flare, or new end-organ involvement is stabilized and treated.
- Patient and family have been instructed regarding the disease, medications, and diet.
- Follow-up appointments have been arranged.

CONSULTATION

- Rheumatology: To provide follow-up by a subspecialist experienced in the recognition and management of the diverse manifestations of SLE.
- Nephrology: To monitor and treat renal involvement and hypertension.
- Hematology: To rule out other conditions; to treat significant cytopenias or coagulation dysfunction.
- Neurology: To treat neurologic consequences of SLE such as seizures and stroke.
- Ophthalmology: To monitor for complications of therapy, such as steroids (cataracts, glaucoma) and hydroxychloroquine (retinal damage).
- Psychiatry: To evaluate and treat psychosis due to neuropsychiatric lupus; to guide coping skills related to chronic illness

SPECIAL CONSIDERATIONS

There is no specific therapy known to prevent the development of SLE. However, once diagnosis has been made, preventive management is critical. This includes avoiding sun exposure, which is known to trigger lupus flares. Patients are advised to use the highest SPF, water-resistant, ultraviolet A- and B-protective sunscreen available. It is essential to promote a healthful lifestyle by discouraging smoking and encouraging exercise, weight control, and a balanced diet. Adolescent females must be counseled about the adverse effects that the disease and immunosuppressive medications may have on pregnancy, as well as the increased risks to pregnant women with active SLE. Vitamin D and calcium supplementation should be considered in patients on chronic steroids to prevent osteoporosis. Routine statin therapy for prevention of early atherosclerosis has been proposed, but as yet there is no clear evidence for its efficacy in children with SLE.

SLE patients are at increased risk of infection, due to their underlying disease as well as to immunosuppressive medications. For the most immunocompromised patients (severe lymphopenia, cyclophosphamide use, chronic high-dose steroids), antibiotic prophylaxis against *Pneumocystis jirovecii* is indicated. Patients should receive all indicated inactivated vaccines, including immunizations against *Pneumococcus*, hepatitis B, and influenza. Live vaccines should not be given to patients with active disease or those on high-dose steroids or immunosuppressive agents.

Adherence to therapy can be a problem in adolescent patients, as they often feel well despite having active disease. Poor adherence to steroid regimens in particular is common due to the cosmetic side effects. Regular follow-up by a pediatric rheumatologist is thus important, with regular monitoring of blood counts, inflammatory markers, renal function, and (if relevant) complement levels.

KEY POINTS

- SLE is a chronic multisystem autoimmune disease with widely varying manifestations.
- Children are more severely affected than adults with SLE.
- Diagnosis is usually conferred when a patient meets at least 4 of 11 established classification criteria.
- The prognosis of SLE is improving, but children with lupus continue to suffer significant morbidity and mortality related to infection and renal and central nervous system disease.
- Steroids and immunosuppressive steroid-sparing agents are the mainstays of treatment.
- Placental transfer of maternal autoantibodies can lead to neonatal lupus and congenital heart block.

SUGGESTED READINGS

Aringer M, Costenbader K, Daikh D, et al. 2019 European League Against Rheumatism/American College of Rheumatology classification criteria for systemic lupus erythematosus. *Ann Rheum Dis.* 2019;78(9):1151-1159.

Hersh AO, von Scheven E, Yazdany J, et al. Differences in long-term disease activity and treatment of adult patients with childhood- and adult-onset systemic lupus erythematosus. *Arthritis Rheum.* 2009;61(1):13-20.

Hiraki LT, Benseler SM, Tyrrell PN, Hebert D, Harvey E, Silverman ED. Clinical and laboratory characteristics and long-term outcome of pediatric systemic lupus erythematosus: a longitudinal study. *J Pediatr.* 2008;152(4):550-556.

Hochberg MC. Updating the American College of Rheumatology revised criteria for the classification of systemic lupus erythematosus. *Arthritis Rheum.* 1997;40(9):1725.

Izmirly P, Kim M, Friedman DM, et al. Hydroxychloroquine to prevent recurrent congenital heart block in fetuses of Anti-SSA/Ro-Positive mothers. *J Am Coll Cardiol.* 2020;76(3):292-302.

Ocampo-Piraquive V, Nieto-Aristizabal I, Canas CA, Tobon GJ. Mortality in systemic lupus erythematosus: causes, predictors and interventions. *Expert Rev Clin Immunol.* 2018;14(12): 1043-1053.

Singh S, Saxena R. Lupus nephritis. *Am J Med Sci.* 2009;337(6): 451-460.

Slater CA, Davis RB, Shmerling RH. Antinuclear antibody testing. A study of clinical utility. *Arch Int Med.* 1996;156(13): 1421-1425.

Tsakonas E, Joseph L, Esdaile JM, et al. A long-term study of hydroxychloroquine withdrawal on exacerbations in systemic lupus erythematosus. The Canadian Hydroxychloroquine Study Group. *Lupus.* 1998;7(2):80-85.

Weening JJ, D'Agati VD, Schwartz MM, et al. The classification of glomerulonephritis in systemic lupus erythematosus revisited. *J Am Soc Nephrol: JASN.* 2004;15(2):241-250.

SECTION R
Surgical Issues

CHAPTER 155 Gastrointestinal Obstruction: Infantile Hypertrophic Pyloric Stenosis, Malrotation and Volvulus, and Intussusception

Blair E. Simpson, MD and Rebeccah L. Brown, MD

BACKGROUND

Obstruction of the gastrointestinal (GI) tract can be due to a wide range of causes with many similarities in clinical presentation. Abdominal pain, early satiety or anorexia, and vomiting are common, with abdominal distention being more common with lower intestinal blockage. Nonbilious emesis is most commonly seen with obstruction or dysfunction of the stomach, pylorus, or duodenum proximal to the sphincter of Oddi but may also occur early in the course of more distal obstruction and become bilious as the obstruction progresses. Conversely, bilious emesis usually occurs with obstruction distal to the sphincter of Oddi in the duodenum (e.g., duodenal web, stenosis, atresia, or malrotation with or without volvulus) or beyond.

Obstruction can result from extrinsic compression, intrinsic blockage, or functional abnormalities leading to dysmotility, as detailed in **Table 155-1**. This chapter focuses on three of the more common causes of GI tract obstruction in children: pyloric stenosis, malrotation with and without volvulus, and intussusception.

PYLORIC STENOSIS

Infantile hypertrophic pyloric stenosis (IHPS) is one of the most common surgically correctable causes of vomiting in infants. While the overall incidence of IHPS appears to be decreasing, recent literature defines an incidence of 1 in 250 to 500 with a 4 to 5:1 male preponderance and a higher incidence in lower socioeconomic groups. The familial incidence of IHPS is remarkable: the highest incidence of pyloric stenosis occurs in the male children of mothers with a history of IHPS, and there is a 15-fold increase in siblings of affected patients.

IHPS results from hypertrophy of the pylorus muscle that results in progressive narrowing of the pyloric channel causing gastric outlet obstruction. The cause remains unclear, although multiple potential etiologies have been implicated, including hyperacidity leading to increased pyloric sphincter contractility, deficiency of nitric oxide synthesis, defective pyloric muscle innervation and pacemaker function, and infection. Perinatal risk factors may include first-born infants, bottle feeding, prematurity, cesarean section delivery, and young maternal age. Environmental factors may include maternal smoking during pregnancy (1.5-2× risk) and direct exposure (not perinatal or via breastfeeding) to macrolide antibiotics, especially in the first 2 weeks of life.

CLINICAL PRESENTATION

Most infants with IHPS present between the ages of 2 and 12 weeks (median age 6 weeks) with progressive nonbilious emesis in large quantities, often forceful ("projectile"), after every feeding. The infant usually remains eager to feed, and recognition of the condition typically occurs before the infant suffers from severe dehydration. However, if the obstruction remains incomplete and slowly progressive, severe dehydration with hypochloremic, hypokalemic metabolic alkalosis, and growth failure will develop. Ultimately, with progressive worsening of metabolic alkalosis, the infant may present with apnea in up to 5% of cases. Physical examination findings are often normal. However, infants may present with signs of dehydration (dry mucus membranes, poor skin turgor, tachycardia, low urine output), jaundice (unconjugated

TABLE 155-1 Causes of Gastrointestinal (GI) Obstruction in Children

Differential Diagnosis of GI Obstruction in Neonates
Extrinsic compression
Malrotation/volvulus
Incarcerated hernia
Intussusception
Annular pancreas
Intrinsic blockage
Pyloric stenosis
Gastrointestinal atresia (e.g., duodenal atresia, jejunal atresia, imperforate anus)
Meconium plug
Meconium ileus
Functional abnormality
Necrotizing enterocolitis
Hirschsprung disease
Gastroparesis
Ileus
Differential Diagnosis of GI Obstruction in Older Infants and Children
Extrinsic compression
Malrotation/volvulus
Incarcerated hernia
Intussusception
Adhesions
Appendicitis
Tumor
Hematoma
Annular pancreas
Intrinsic blockage
Fecal impaction
Polyp
Tumor
Hematoma
Stricture (e.g., Crohn disease)
Bezoar
Foreign body
Meckel diverticulum
Parasites
Functional abnormality
Hirschsprung disease
Gastroparesis
Ileus

hyperbilirubinemia due to inactivation of glucuronyl transferase from inadequate nutrition), gastric distention, visible peristaltic waves, and/or a palpable "olive" (the hypertrophied pylorus). The "olive" is along the lateral margin of the right rectus muscle, just below the liver edge, but gastric distention may make palpation difficult.

DIFFERENTIAL DIAGNOSIS

The differential diagnosis is broad and includes gastroesophageal reflux, gastroenteritis, constipation, necrotizing enterocolitis, acute renal failure, serious bacterial infection, trauma, allergy, or other causes of proximal intestinal obstruction, such as malrotation and volvulus.

DIAGNOSTIC EVALUATION

The hypertrophied pylorus may be apparent on either ultrasound or upper GI series. Ultrasound, with an available pediatric-trained technician, is preferred because of the lack of radiation exposure with this testing. Ultrasound is considered positive if the pyloric channel is longer than approximately 14 to 16 mm with muscular thickness greater than 3 to 4 mm (**Figure 155-1**). Upper GI series, though it exposes the patient to radiation, can show the "string sign," a thin line of barium visible as it passes through a thickened and elongated pylorus as well as compression of the gastric antrum and evidence of delayed gastric emptying.

Serum chemistry studies reveal hypochloremic and hypokalemic metabolic alkalosis when the emesis has been prolonged, but evidence of metabolic acidosis may also be seen when the dehydration is pronounced.

MANAGEMENT

Although definitive treatment of IHPS is surgical, initial management focuses on correction of the dehydration, electrolyte disturbances, and acid-base abnormalities which are often present at the time of diagnosis. The mainstay of rehydration is intravenous (IV) fluids, initially with the administration of an isotonic fluid bolus (20 mL/kg) followed by isotonic dextrose-containing fluids (e.g., 5% dextrose + 0.9% saline) at 1.5× maintenance rate. Serum potassium levels are often normal, but total body potassium is depleted because of gastric losses, alkalosis, and secondary aldosterone effects. Therefore, best practice includes prompt supplementation of IV fluids with potassium chloride (20 mEq/L), after the first urinary void confirms renal function. Serial serum electrolyte values are obtained until normalized. Goal electrolytes prior to surgery include bicarbonate <26 mmol/L, chloride ≥100 mmol/L, sodium ≥132 mm/L, and potassium ≥3.5 mmol/L. If IV access is not initially attainable, small volumes of oral electrolyte solution (e.g., Pedialyte) may be tolerated and provide some rehydration, ultimately allowing for the successful placement of a peripheral IV catheter. Alternate IV access may be necessary if vomiting persists and peripheral IV access is not successful. At times, gastric decompression with a nasogastric tube is indicated preoperatively though that is not standard practice.

IHPS is corrected surgically with a Ramstedt pyloromyotomy (longitudinal division of the pyloric muscle down to the submucosa) after correction of fluid and electrolyte abnormalities. Pyloromyotomy may be performed via an open approach, through either a right upper quadrant or supraumbilical incision, or laparoscopically. Though a debate remains about optimal surgical approach, open and laparoscopic pyloromyotomy both have low complication rates and high success. Overall, studies suggest that laparoscopy may be associated with a slightly shorter length of hospital stay, shorter time to full feeds, less pain, and better cosmetics; however, this approach may also be associated with slightly higher risk of mucosal perforation or incomplete myotomy. The preferred approach really depends on surgeon's preference and comfort level.

Post Management Complication(s) Complications are infrequent but may include surgical site infection (0.3%-12%), mucosal perforation (<1%), and incomplete myotomy (0%-5.5% for laparoscopic pyloromyotomy; 0%-1.9% for open pyloromyotomy). Perforation may be identified either intraoperatively and addressed at that time or postoperatively if the patient develops abdominal pain, distension, and sepsis.

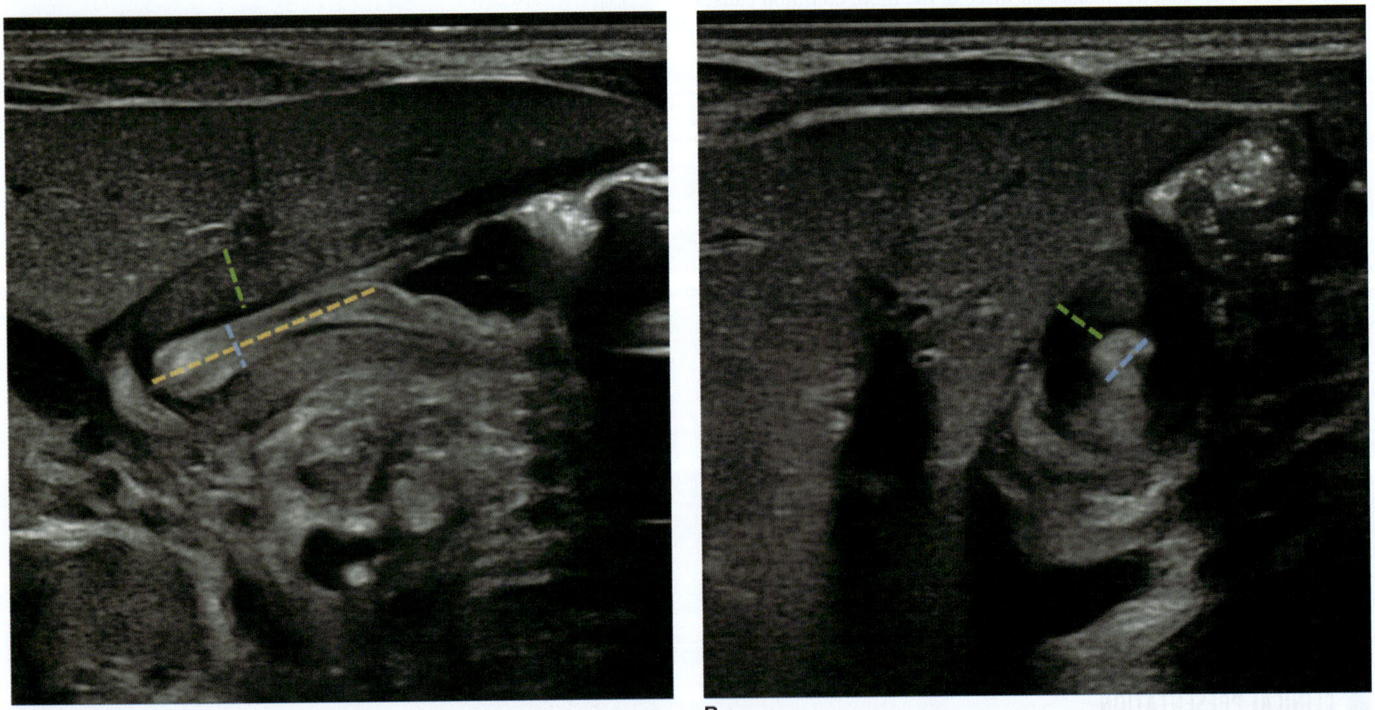

A B

FIGURE 155-1. Abdominal ultrasound of a 6-week-old boy with projectile vomiting shows the long-axis (A) and short-axis (B) views of the pylorus with elongated channel (2 cm, orange), increased single-wall thickness (4 mm, green), and thickened redundant echogenic mucosa (blue). Real-time and cine imaging showed minimal progression of gastric contents into the duodenum. Laparoscopic pyloromyotomy was performed the next day. (Images and caption courtesy of Dr. Adam Prasanphanich, Fellow, Department of Radiology, Cincinnati Children's Hospital Medical Center, Cincinnati, OH.)

Postoperative Care Postoperatively, feeding may be restarted a few hours after surgery. Early ad libitum refeeding with full-strength formula or breast milk (without an initial trial of clear oral electrolyte solution) has been demonstrated to be safe and cost effective, allowing prompt discharge home. Many patients experience some postoperative emesis, thought to be related to postoperative ileus or swelling of the incised portion of the pylorus, or both; however, persistent vomiting after 4 to 5 days is unusual and warrants further investigation for an incomplete pyloromyotomy.

ADMISSION AND DISCHARGE CRITERIA

All patients with IHPS should be admitted to correct fluid and electrolyte abnormalities in preparation for surgery.

The infant can be discharged once tolerating sufficient oral intake to maintain adequate hydration and growth after surgery, often in 1 to 2 days.

CONSULTATION

Early surgical consultation is recommended for definitive surgical intervention.

PREVENTION

Identification of patients with an increased risk for pyloric stenosis may lead to earlier recognition. Newborn exposure to erythromycin has been associated with an eightfold increased risk if the exposure occurs before 13 days of life. Exposure to erythromycin after 13 days of life or exposure to non-macrolide antibiotics is not believed to be associated with increased risk. Prenatal exposure to macrolides is not thought to increase the risk of IHPS. Breastfed babies may have a lower rate of IHPS than bottle-fed babies.

MALROTATION AND VOLVULUS

Prenatally, the midgut (distal duodenum to the transverse colon) extends into the umbilical cord during development and then rotates 270 degrees counterclockwise around the mesenteric vessels as it reenters the abdominal cavity. The distal third of the duodenum moves to the left of midline and is fixed at the ligament of Treitz, whereas the cecum elongates, descends, and eventually becomes fixed in the right lower quadrant. The entire midgut is thereby effectively fixed to the posterior abdominal wall preventing torsion around the mesentery. Malrotation occurs when there is failure of normal rotation and/or fixation which results in a narrow mesenteric pedicle, predisposing to volvulus and the development of Ladd's bands (adhesions from the cecum across the duodenum) which ultimately can cause duodenal obstruction. Malrotation is reported to occur in up to 1 in 500 births, although the true incidence is uncertain because it can be asymptomatic. The incidence of malrotation is higher in children with other congenital anomalies like heterotaxia syndromes associated with congenital heart disease and/or with multiple anomalies of the GI tract (intestinal atresia, Meckel diverticulum, intussusception, Hirschsprung disease, congenital diaphragmatic hernia, and abdominal wall defects).

Volvulus occurs when a loop of intestines twists leading to GI tract obstruction and bowel ischemia from disruption of mesenteric blood supply (**Figure 155-2**). Volvulus is usually associated with malrotation, although adhesions or other pathology may also lead to volvulus in a normally rotated GI tract. Most common is midgut volvulus, but gastric or cecal volvulus can occur and may also be associated with intestinal malrotation. Resultant bowel wall ischemia from the volvulus will lead to infarction or perforation, or both, which are life-threatening.

CLINICAL PRESENTATION

Malrotation can be asymptomatic. When it does present with symptoms, approximately one-third of patients present in the first year of life and another 20% present before age 18 years.

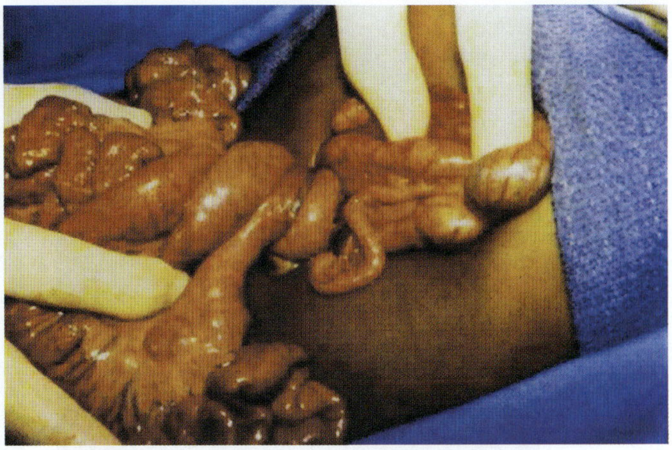

FIGURE 155-2. Intraoperative appearance of volvulus. Note that the intestine on the left of the picture is twisted around a very narrow mesenteric pedicle in the middle of the picture.

Malrotation often presents with signs of upper GI obstruction, including *bilious* vomiting and progressive dehydration. Obstruction can be caused from Ladd's bands compressing the duodenum or from volvulus. Findings on physical examination may be normal early in the course or may demonstrate a scaphoid abdomen secondary to the proximal obstruction. Volvulus as a complication of congenital malrotation often presents in the first month of life, most frequently in the first week. With volvulus, rapid deterioration occurs, resulting in progressive lethargy, tachypnea, grunting, abdominal distention, and shock.

Intermittent volvulus can occur in older children and be confused with cyclic vomiting or abdominal migraine. However, chronic symptoms, such as failure to thrive and malabsorption, are often present with an intermittent presentation.

DIFFERENTIAL DIAGNOSIS

In a neonate, *bilious emesis* is midgut volvulus until proven otherwise.

All etiologies of GI tract obstruction must be considered, including intussusception, incarcerated hernia, intra-abdominal adhesions, lymphoma, appendicitis, and chronic/severe constipation. In neonates, the differential also includes congenital GI malformations (e.g., intestinal/colonic atresia), gastroesophageal reflux, and gastroenteritis. Other, non-GI-specific diagnoses for progressive and nonremitting emesis include testicular or ovarian torsion, acute renal failure, central nervous system infection, and serious bacterial infection.

DIAGNOSTIC EVALUATION

In normal rotation, the duodenal-jejunal flexure, the marker for the ligament of Treitz, lies to the left of midline under the gastric antrum, usually near the second lumbar vertebra. In malrotation, the duodenum spirals down and the jejunum passes to the right of the vertebral column. Upper GI series reliably demonstrate these findings (**Figure 155-3**). Plain films can be evaluated for perforation and free air.

Ultrasound may have some limited utility in the diagnosis of malrotation. Ultrasound may be more useful in the diagnosis of volvulus if there is inversion of the superior mesenteric artery and vein or a demonstration of the "whirlpool sign" (wrapping of the superior mesenteric vein and mesentery around the superior mesenteric artery), with sensitivities ranging 83% to 96% and specificities ranging 89% to 100%. Barium enema may demonstrate malposition of the cecum, which is suggestive, but not reliably sufficient for definitive diagnosis.

In the setting of volvulus, laboratory tests likely will show acidosis secondary to lactate from bowel ischemia and dehydration. The white blood count is also typically elevated for similar reasons. Occult or gross blood in stool can suggest bowel ischemia or necrosis.

Plain films of the abdomen may show signs of obstruction, including air-fluid levels on upright or lateral decubitus views. If the obstruction

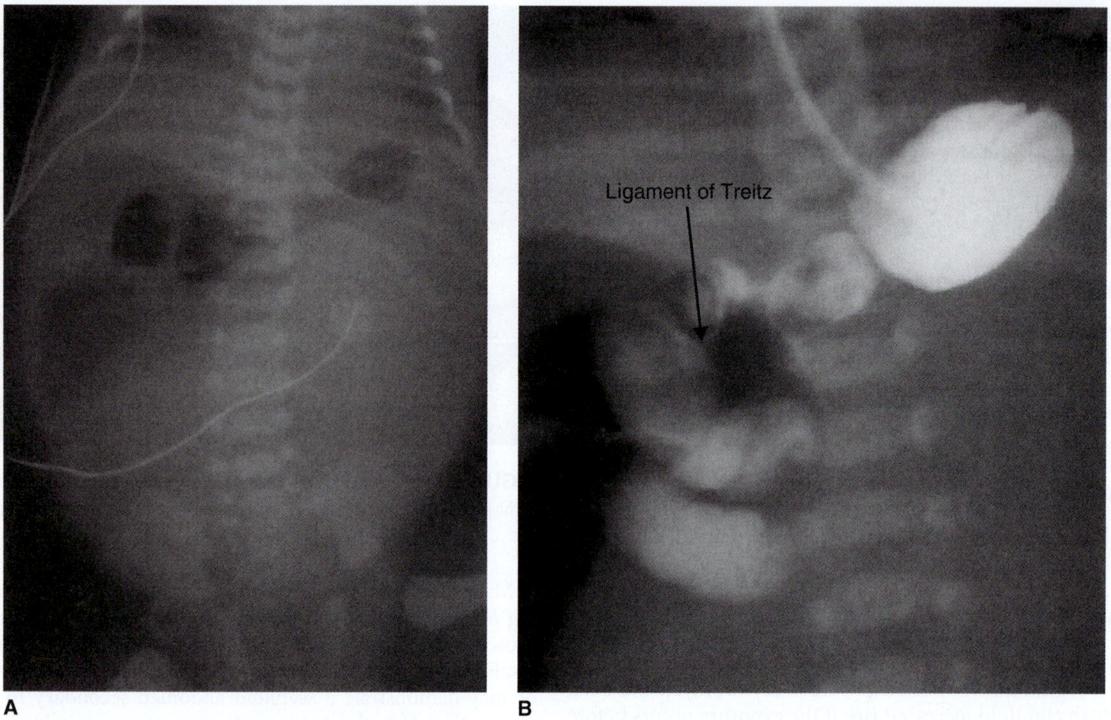

FIGURE 155-3. Radiographic appearance of malrotation. A. A kidney, ureter, bladder (KUB) radiograph from a 2-week-old infant with bilious vomiting shows proximal bowel obstruction, as evidenced by a few dilated bowel loops in the right upper quadrant and absence of bowel gas in the remainder of the abdomen. B. An upper gastrointestinal radiograph shows that the ligament of Treitz (arrow) denoting the duodenal-jejunal junction is abnormally located to the right of the spine below the duodenal bulb.

is proximal or incomplete, the film may show only a gasless abdomen or may even be normal. Free air in the peritoneal cavity is indicative of perforation. An upper GI series is usually diagnostic of volvulus and reveals the classic "beak" sign or "corkscrewing" at the obstructed point (**Figure 155-4**).

Note that when symptoms are severe with an abdominal source clearly identified, some children undergo emergent exploratory laparotomy without waiting for imaging studies.

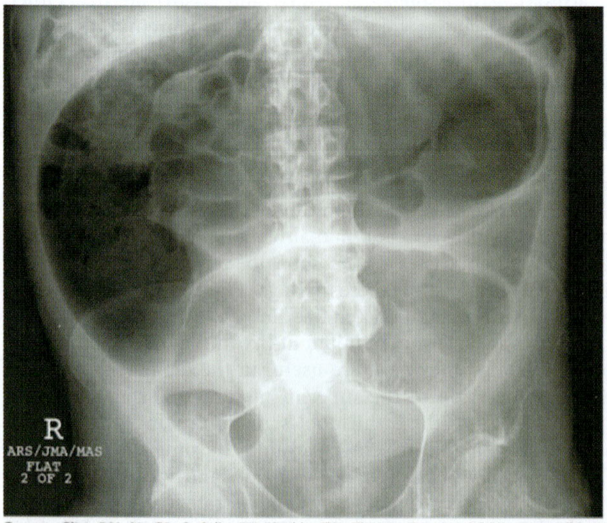

Source: Cline DM, Ma OJ, Cydulka RK, Meckler GD, Thomas SH, Handel DA: *Tintinalli's Emergency Medicine Manual, 7th Edition*: www.accessemergencymedicine.com

FIGURE 155-4. Sigmoid volvulus. Note that the open portion of the "C" formed by the twisted large bowel points toward the left side in the case of sigmoid volvulus. (Reproduced with permission from Cline DM, Ma OJ, Cydulka RK, Meckler GD, Thomas SH, Handel DA. *Tintinalli's Emergency Medicine Manual*, 7ed. New York: McGraw Hill; 2012.)

MANAGEMENT

Malrotation is corrected surgically with a Ladd procedure, which includes exploratory laparotomy with release of any Ladd's bands that may cause obstruction, widening of the mesentery to prevent volvulus, appendectomy to prevent future diagnostic dilemma, and positioning of the small bowel to the right and the colon to the left. The Ladd procedure is recommended both for relief of persistent or intermittent symptoms of bowel obstruction and for prevention of subsequent volvulus.

The Ladd procedure may be performed laparoscopically in select patients, although controversy remains regarding the efficacy and completeness of this approach. A laparoscopic approach may be better suited for elective rather than emergency cases, with a low threshold to convert to an open procedure with any difficulty assessing intestinal orientation and broadening the mesentery.

Volvulus is a surgical emergency. Decompression with a nasogastric tube on intermittent suction, aggressive fluid and electrolyte resuscitation, pain control, and administration of antibiotics empirically covering enteric pathogens are all indicated preoperatively. Commonly recommended antibiotic combinations include ampicillin, gentamicin, and metronidazole or a beta-lactam/beta-lactamase inhibitor with gentamicin to empirically cover for gram-negative bacilli, enterococci, and anaerobes. Prompt surgical intervention is warranted to reduce the volvulus, restore intestinal blood flow, and resect unsalvageable, necrotic gut. Placement of an ostomy may be indicated if there is ischemic bowel with perforation or severe abdominal contamination.

Post Management Complication(s) Even with surgical correction from the Ladd procedure, a low risk of recurrent volvulus exists, and patients should seek care immediately with recurrent bilious emesis or severe abdominal pain.

Postoperative adhesions can be a cause of subsequent bowel obstruction and may occur early or many years after surgery.

Postoperative Care Several postoperative clinical concerns need consideration, especially in patients requiring extended periods of bowel rest or requiring extensive bowel resection. Nutritionally, the amount and location of resected bowel as well as the functionality of the remaining intestine, determine the ability to eventually feed the child enterally. Parenteral nutrition is often indicated to sustain recovering infants. Infants with greater than 50 cm of remaining small intestine most likely will tolerate eventual transition from parenteral to enteral nutrition. Comparably, short gut syndrome is manifested by voluminous or malabsorptive stools and failure to thrive, and children with this condition are at risk for bacterial overgrowth and various nutritional deficiencies. Additionally, long-term parenteral nutrition can induce cholestasis, along with the additional risks associated with maintaining long-term IV access.

ADMISSION AND DISCHARGE CRITERIA

Patients with malrotation and persistent vomiting or dehydration require admission. The diagnosis of malrotation and volvulus must be considered in any infant who presents with bilious emesis, and prompt evaluation with an upper GI tract radiography (Upper GI) should be performed. Surgery is often performed at the time of initial diagnosis. All patients with volvulus need admission for rapid evaluation, resuscitation, and surgical management.

The patient should be well nourished and tolerating adequate nutrition prior to discharge.

CONSULTATION

Volvulus requires prompt resuscitative effort and surgical involvement. Intensive care support may also be necessary, especially in children with hemodynamic instability. Postoperative management, if the patient does not require intensive care support, may be handled collaboratively between the surgical and pediatric Hospital Medicine services.

Postoperatively, referral to gastroenterologists is indicated for children requiring prolonged parenteral nutrition or those at risk for short gut syndrome.

PREVENTION

Prevention of volvulus is accomplished by surgical correction of malrotation, whether symptomatic or asymptomatic. For patients without a known malrotation, a high index of suspicion allows prompt diagnosis of a volvulus and decreased bowel ischemia time, thereby decreasing post-ischemia complications.

INTUSSUSCEPTION

Intussusception is one of the most common causes of small bowel obstruction in the first 2 years of life. Telescoped bowel causes GI obstruction, compression of blood vessels to the gut, and eventual ischemia and necrosis (**Figure 155-5**). In younger children, intussusception generally involves the ileocolic region and is idiopathic, although invagination of the bowel at hypertrophied Peyer patches is frequently implicated. In approximately 5% to 10% of cases in older children, there is a pathologic lead point such as a Meckel diverticulum, hematoma, polyp, or lymphoma. Patients with cystic fibrosis, celiac disease, and IgA vasculitis are at increased risk.

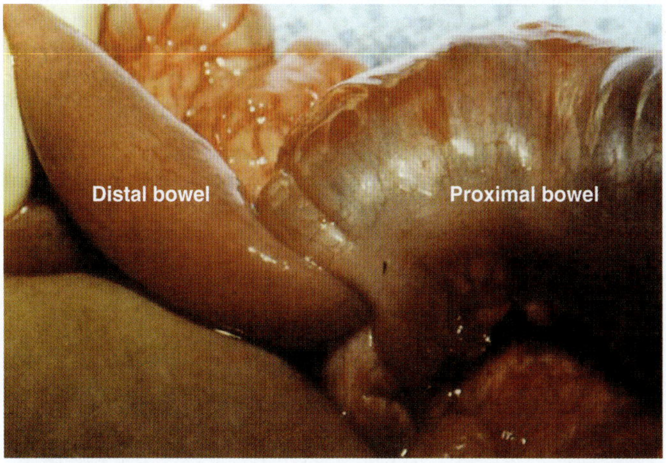

FIGURE 155-5. Intraoperative appearance of intussusception with the proximal bowel (right side of the picture) telescoping over the distal bowel (left side of the picture).

Most cases occur in the first year of life, with 80% occurring by 2 years of age. There is a slight male preponderance and an overall incidence of 3 to 5 per 10,000. A temporal association with viral gastroenteritis has been observed, and previously, intussusception was associated with early (now discontinued) forms of the rotavirus vaccine.

CLINICAL PRESENTATION

The classic signs of intussusception—intermittent abdominal pain ("colic") with vomiting, an abdominal mass, and currant jelly stools—are present concomitantly in less than 50% of patients. Currant jelly stools are evidence of bowel ischemia and necrosis and are a late finding. A clinician's goal should be to diagnose intussusception before currant jelly stools are produced. Occult blood in the stool is demonstrated in 75% of cases at presentation and can add to the diagnostic picture. Vomiting becomes bilious as the condition progresses. Fever can also be present but is not predictive. Some children with intussusception will have concurrent diarrhea.

Important symptoms in pediatric patients with intussusception are severe and include intermittent abdominal pain and lethargy. The pain is colicky in nature, often occurring every 20 to 30 minutes with normal, non-painful behavior between bouts of pain. Ten percent of young children with intussusception can present with intermittent bouts of lethargy and no other identifiable symptoms. Therefore, maintaining a high index of suspicion and a broad differential diagnosis is important for successful recognition of intussusception.

Abdominal examination is best performed between episodes of pain when the abdominal muscles tend to be more relaxed. The abdomen is often mild-moderately distended and bowel sounds are often high-pitched to normal. The Dance sign, palpation of a sausage-shaped mass in the right lower quadrant of the abdomen, and radiologic absence of bowel gas in the right lower quadrant (on plain abdominal x-ray) are considered pathognomonic of intussusception.

DIFFERENTIAL DIAGNOSIS

With symptoms of abdominal pain and vomiting, the differential diagnosis includes appendicitis, gastroenteritis, and other causes of GI obstruction (e.g., volvulus). Ureteral colic secondary to ureteropelvic junction obstruction or ureteral calculus can mimic these symptoms. Pneumonia in children may also present with abdominal pain and vomiting, but often respiratory symptoms and fever accompany this diagnosis. When lethargy is the sole or predominant feature, the differential diagnosis can be quite broad and includes sepsis, dehydration, nonaccidental trauma, toxic or metabolic abnormalities, central nervous system disorders or infections, and many other etiologies for altered mental status.

DIAGNOSTIC EVALUATION

Ultrasound has near-perfect sensitivity and specificity for the diagnosis of intussusception. Ultrasound also carries the advantage of lack of radiation exposure, better definition of potential lead points, consideration of perfusion to the area of intussusception, the ability to locate intussusception in atypical areas of the intestines, and the opportunity to evaluate other intra-abdominal and pelvic structures. The role of ultrasonography in treatment is evolving.

Contrast enema radiography provides a definitive diagnosis of intussusception as well as being a therapeutic intervention (**Figure 155-6** and see Management section) but does come with associated risks of exposure and contrast-induced toxicity. Air, or pneumatic, reduction is generally preferred to water-soluble or barium contrast agents.

For diagnosis, plain films of the abdomen with additional upright or cross-table lateral views are helpful initial studies and the presence of a soft tissue mass and evidence of bowel obstruction are highly suggestive of intussusception. Nonspecific findings of an abnormal bowel gas pattern or normal films do not exclude the possibility of intussusception.

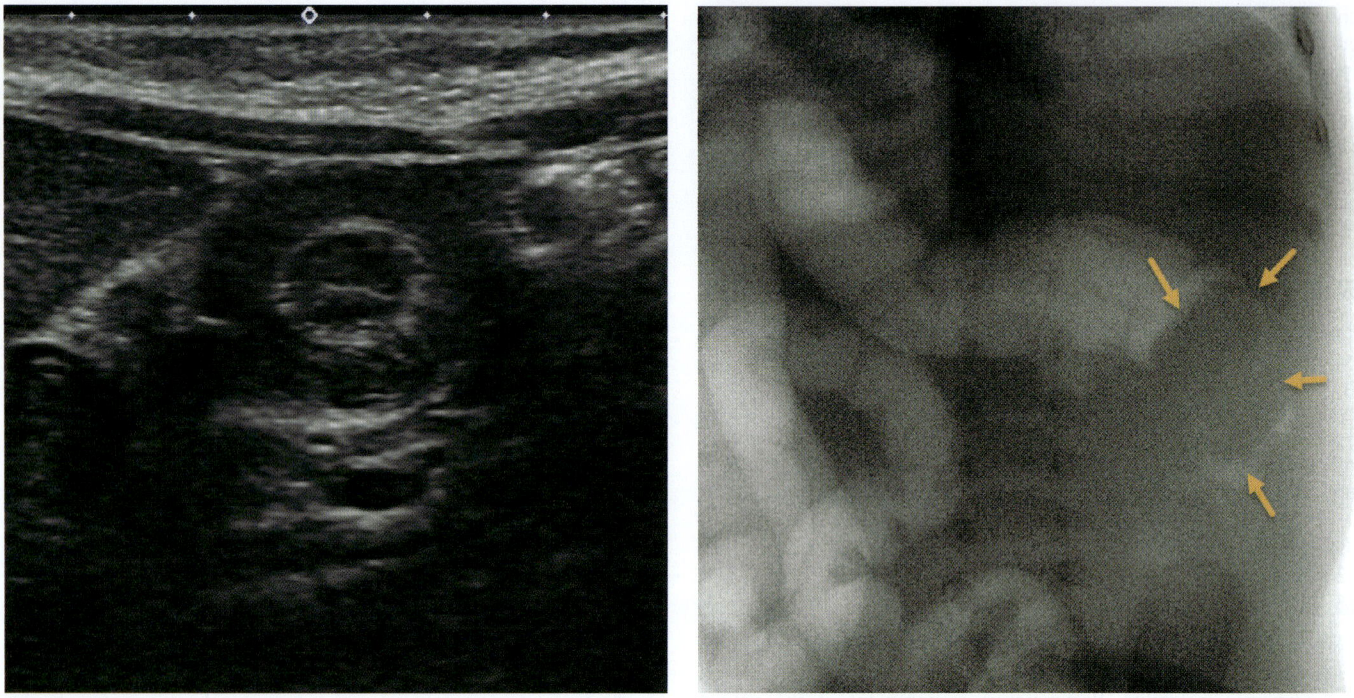

A B

FIGURE 155-6. Ileocolic intussusception A. Abdominal ultrasound short-axis view demonstrates the "target sign" measuring up to 2.2 cm in diameter (vertical line). B. Prone fluoroscopic images during air contrast enema shows reduction of mass-like colonic filling defect at the hepatic flexure. (Images and caption courtesy of Dr. Adam Prasanphanich, Fellow, Department of Radiology, Cincinnati Children's Hospital Medical Center, Cincinnati, OH.)

MANAGEMENT

Spontaneous resolution of intussusception can occur in up to 20% of cases. Similarly, intussusception can be found incidentally, be asymptomatic, and not require reduction.

Clinical stabilization, usually through fluid resuscitation and adequate pain control, should proceed until intussusception is suspected or confirmed. Oral or gastric intake should be withheld and, if bowel obstruction is present, nasogastric decompression should be considered. Although radiologists commonly perform the reduction, surgical involvement is required to provide operative management of unsuccessful reductions, perforation or peritonitis, or clinical deterioration. A concern for intestinal perforation or prolonged intussusception should prompt consideration for empiric antibiotics for enteric pathogens, as detailed earlier in the treatment section for volvulus. Perforation, if associated with intussusception, usually occurs at the time of reduction, and symptoms will appear within hours.

For a clinically stable patient without evidence of perforation, peritonitis, or sepsis, nonoperative management is preferred using an air or hydrostatic pressure (saline or water-soluble) contrast enema. Imaging guidance may be done via ultrasound or fluoroscopy and depends on the radiologist's proficiency with enema reductions. Ultrasound is also performed in some cases as a follow-up study to check for complete success of contrast enema reduction. If the initial attempt at ultrasound reduction is incomplete, a second or sometimes even a third attempt may lead to complete intussusception resolution.

If multiple enema attempts fail to resolve intussusception and/or if bowel ischemia is suspected, open or laparoscopic surgical reduction is required with resection of ischemic or perforated bowel as indicated.

Post Management Complication(s) Despite a high success rate with enema-directed reductions (60%-90% of all cases), perforations will occur in up to 2% of cases. Longer duration of symptoms (>48 hours), younger age (<1 year old), and rectal bleeding (concerning for bowel ischemia) have been associated with a decreased rate of success of nonsurgical reduction. Enema reduction can also be painful, so procedural analgesia should be provided as needed, including sedation as indicated.

A first recurrence of intussusception develops in approximately 10% of patients, with an increased risk for subsequent recurrences after the first recurrence.

Post Procedural Care Following nonoperative or surgical reduction of intussusception, pain control and nutritional advance are the most important factors. Most patients have relief of presenting symptoms quickly after reduction and can tolerate oral pain control and oral nutritional intake.

For patients requiring surgical reduction and/or bowel resection, pain and nutrition are similar mainstays of post-reduction care. The significance of postoperative pain management and nutritional advance is dependent on the intervention required and/or the extent of the bowel resection, similar to the postoperative care above following severe volvulus.

ADMISSION AND DISCHARGE CRITERIA

Symptomatic intussusception should be treated promptly, and care is often coordinated in the emergency department. However, if diagnosis is delayed or symptoms evolve later in presentation, therapeutic management after inpatient admission may also be required. Patients with unresolved intussusception, an identified lead point, evidence of perforation, or clinical instability should be admitted.

An otherwise well child following successful reduction of intussusception who demonstrates no signs of perforation, has no lead point identified, and is tolerating enteral feeding can be discharged home from the emergency department. Signs and symptoms of recurrence and other complications should be clarified with the caregivers, who should be instructed to return should they develop. Those without adequate follow-up or with abnormal or unreliable post-reduction findings may warrant more prolonged observation.

CONSULTATION

Intussusception is managed through the coordinated efforts of the emergency department or hospitalist provider, the surgeon, and the radiologist. If the patient becomes clinically unstable, intensive care involvement may be warranted.

PREVENTION

Prevention measures are not known for intussusception. However, early diagnostic recognition will result in improved pain recovery and outcomes.

SUGGESTED READINGS

Almaramhy HH, Al-Zalabani AH. The association of prenatal and postnatal macrolide exposure with subsequent development of infantile hypertrophic pyloric stenosis: a systematic review and meta-analysis. *Ital J Pediatr*. 2019;45:20.

Arshad S, Hebballi N, Hegde B, et al. Early discharge after nonoperative management of intussusception is both safe and cost-effective. *J Ped Surg*. 2022;57(1):147-152.

Danko ME, Asare-Afriyie B, Ayensu M, et al. Pyloric Stenosis: National trends in the incidence of rate and resource use in the United States from 2012 to 2016. *Hospital Pediatrics*. 2019;9(12):923-932.

Danko ME, Evans PT, Upperman JS. Current management of pyloric stenosis. *Semin Pediatr Surg*. 2022;31:151145.

Gluckman S, Karpelowsky J, Webster A, et al. Management for intussusception in children. *Cochrane Database Sys Rev*. 2017;6(6):CD006476.

Ismail I, Elsherbini R, Elsaied A, et al. Laparoscopic vs open pyloromyotomy in the treatment of IHPS. *Front Ped*. 2020;21:1-7.

Kelley-Quon L, Arthur L, Williams R, et al. Management of intussusception in children: a systematic review. *J Ped Surg*. 2021;56(3):587-596.

Lin-Martore M, Finberg M, Kohn M, et al. Diagnostic accuracy of point-of-care ultrasonography for intussusception in children: a systematic review and meta-analysis. *Am J Emerg Med*. 2022;58:255-264.

Murchinson L, De Coppi P, Eaton S. Post-natal erythromycin exposure and risk of HPS: a systemic review and meta-analysis. *Ped Surg International*. 2016;32:1147-1152.

Nguyen HN, Sammer MBK, Ditzler MG, et al: Transition to ultrasound as the first-line imaging modality for midgut volvulus: keys to a successful rollout. *Pediatr Radiol*. 2021;51(4):506-515.

Rich B, Dolgin S. Hypertrophic pyloric stenosis. *Peds in Review*. 2021;42(10):539-543.

Shah S, Zaoutis L, Catallozzi M, et al. *The Philadelphia Guide Inpatient Pediatrics*. 3rd ed. New York, NY: McGraw Hill Medical; 2021.

Sullivan KJ, Chan E, Vincent J, et al. Feeding post-pyloromyotomy: a meta-analysis. *Pediatrics*. 2016:137:1-11.

Svetanoff WJ, Srivatsa S, Diefenbach K, Nwomeh BC. Diagnosis and management of intestinal rotational abnormalities with or without volvulus in the pediatric population. *Semin Pediatr Surg*. 2022;31:151141.

van den Bunder FAIM, Hall JJ, van Heum LWE, et al. A Delphi analysis to reach consensus on preoperative care in infants with HPS. *Eur J Pediatr Surg*. 2020;30:497-504.

Wong K, Van Tassel D, Lee J, et al. Making the diagnosis of midgut volvulus: Limited abdominal ultrasound has changed our clinical practice. *J Pediatr Surg*. 2020;55912:2614-2617.

Zhu J, Zhu T, Lin Z, et al. Perinatal risk factors for infantile HPS. *J Ped Surg*. 2017;52(9):1389-1397.

CHAPTER 156 Appendicitis

Kathleen G. Brimsek, MD and Rabia A. Cheema, MD

BACKGROUND

Approximately 7% of all people will develop appendicitis over the course of their lifetime. Each year in the United States, about 60,000 to 80,000 children develop appendicitis. It is particularly common in the preteen and teenage years, with an average age of about 10 years. Before puberty, boys and girls are affected equally; after puberty, there is a slight male predominance.

PATHOPHYSIOLOGY

The appendix, whose function remains unknown, arises from the cecum. Roughly 5% to 15% of people have retrocecal appendices. In children, the appendix is relatively longer and thinner than in adults, which makes it more susceptible to perforation early in the course of the disease. The greater omentum remains thin, short, and fragile until about 10 years of age. It is therefore less likely to wall off a perforated appendix in a younger child, making generalized peritonitis more common in children than in adults.

The pathogenesis of appendicitis begins with obstruction of the appendiceal lumen. The most common cause of obstruction is enlargement of the lymphoid tissue (Peyer patches) in the wall of the appendix. The lymphoid follicles enlarge, probably in response to ingested microorganisms such as viruses associated with upper respiratory tract infections. Fecal material, undigested food, other foreign material, or pinworms may also lead to obstruction. Regardless of the initial trigger, the resultant obstruction causes dilation of the lumen of the appendix and thickening of its wall. Bacterial overgrowth leads to bacterial invasion of the appendiceal wall, inflammation, and ischemia. If unchecked, gangrene and eventual appendiceal perforation will occur. As the transmural appendiceal inflammation progresses, so does local peritoneal inflammation. With perforation, the peritonitis can become widespread.

The responsible bacteria are usually fecal flora, most commonly *Escherichia coli*, *Pseudomonas aeruginosa*, anaerobes, *Streptococcus anginosus*, *Enterococcus spp.*, and *Streptococcus viridans*. The process is usually polymicrobial.

CLINICAL PRESENTATION

CLASSIC PRESENTATION

The classic presentation of appendicitis is easy to recognize and occurs in approximately two-thirds of cases. Classically, a previously healthy child develops vague periumbilical pain that is uncomfortable but not debilitating. Shortly after the onset of pain, infrequent nonbilious emesis often develops. Over the next few hours, the poorly localized pain gradually increases in intensity before moving to the right lower quadrant. There may be associated anorexia and low-grade fever. A child with appendicitis prefers to remain still, such that jarring and shaking movements (during a car ride, for example) are painful. Diarrhea, if it occurs, is infrequent and consists of small stools caused by irritation of the sigmoid colon by the inflamed appendix (as opposed to large stools typical of gastroenteritis). Likewise, bladder irritation may produce dysuria or urgency.

ATYPICAL PRESENTATION

In atypical cases, the pain pattern may be quite different. Many preschool-age children present with an atypical clinical picture. Young children may not recognize or may be unable to verbalize the change in location of the pain, or they may not develop localized pain. In some, such as those with a retrocecal appendix, the pain may never shift in location, or it may originate in or migrate to the right upper quadrant or flank.

Up to 29% of children with appendicitis never develop vomiting, and while many patients with appendicitis have a low-grade fever, most are afebrile (83%). Finally, while anorexia is common (60%), some children may report being hungry.

PERFORATION

If appendicitis remains unrecognized, perforation will ultimately occur. About one-third to one-half of children with perforated appendices have been seen by medical providers before the diagnosis of perforation is made. With perforation, there is usually temporary relief of the pain, but within hours it becomes generalized and progressively more severe as the child develops diffuse peritonitis from spilled enteral and infectious material. However, if the contamination is well localized (walled off) by the omentum, the child develops a discrete abscess and may have localized tenderness without severe pain. A hunched-over posture, tentative gait, limp, or difficulty with climbing up and down are suggestive of peritoneal irritation. For nonambulatory patients, jarring the bed may produce evidence of pain.

PHYSICAL EXAMINATION

On physical examination, a patient with appendicitis (nonperforated) is usually hemodynamically stable but may exhibit tachycardia and fever. Reliable examination of the abdomen may require accommodations that ease the child's anxiety (e.g., examination on a caregiver's lap). Asking the child to point to the spot that hurts and examining that area last may also facilitate the examination. Classically, the abdomen appears flat with normal or hypoactive bowel sounds. Localized and reproducible tenderness at McBurney's point (one-third of the way between the umbilicus and the right anterior superior iliac spine) is virtually diagnostic, especially with a normally positioned appendix.

Many techniques are used to elicit signs of peritoneal irritation. For rebound tenderness, the examiner presses down on the tender area slowly, maintains pressure for a few seconds, and then abruptly removes his or her hand. The child experiences pain as the hand is withdrawn if there is peritoneal inflammation, but this maneuver may also be uncomfortable for anxious children without peritonitis. Additionally, many experts believe that this test is unduly distressing and recommend finger percussion throughout the abdomen, leaving the right lower quadrant for last. Pain limited to percussion of the right lower quadrant or referred pain to the right lower quadrant with percussion of other quadrants is suggestive of peritonitis (Rovsing sign). In older children in the supine position, tapping on the plantar surface of the heel or lateral aspect of the pelvis can elicit localized abdominal pain. Any of these maneuvers can produce pain if there is peritoneal irritation.

Voluntary muscle guarding is nonspecific and can be seen with abdominal pain from a myriad of causes or in ticklish or anxious patients. In contrast, involuntary muscle guarding is a powerful finding in a patient with appendicitis but can be subtle and difficult to appreciate.

The previously described signs are common when a normally positioned appendix is inflamed; however, with retrocecal appendicitis, these physical findings may be absent. When the inflamed appendix lies on the psoas muscle, use of this muscle causes pain. The examiner places his or her hand above the knee of the supine patient and asks him or her to raise the thigh against the resistance provided by the examiner. Alternatively, the child lies on his or her left side and the examiner extends the patient's right thigh at the hip. Pain with these maneuvers yields a positive psoas sign.

If the inflamed retrocecal appendix is adjacent to the internal obturator muscle, pain is elicited when it is stretched. With the patient supine, the examiner flexes the right lower extremity at the knee and hip and internally rotates it. If right lower quadrant pain is produced, the obturator sign is positive.

A rectal examination may sometimes be helpful. Suggestive findings include tenderness greater on the right side, fullness on the right, and heme-negative stools. Patient cooperation is needed for reliable rectal palpation. Grossly bloody stools are not found with appendicitis, and even occult blood should prompt a consideration of other diagnoses.

COURSE OF ILLNESS

By 24 hours after pain onset, about 15% of children have perforation. By 48 hours after the initial symptoms, roughly 75% have perforation. A child with pain of 4 days' duration has an approximately 90% risk of perforation. If perforation occurs, the mortality rate increases to as high as 5%, compared with less than 0.1% for nonperforated appendicitis. Those who die are predominantly very young children or those with perforated appendices and peritonitis who undergo surgery before adequate fluid resuscitation. The morbidity rate also rises appreciably in those with perforation.

DIFFERENTIAL DIAGNOSIS

Highest on the differential diagnosis for appendicitis is acute gastroenteritis, and in fact, many cases of acute appendicitis are initially misdiagnosed as such. Many other diseases can simulate appendicitis, including constipation, urinary tract infection, right lower lobe pneumonia, ovarian torsion or cyst, incarcerated inguinal hernia, testicular torsion, intussusception, hemolytic uremic syndrome, diabetic ketoacidosis, and abdominal trauma (**Table 156-1**). In sexually active female patients, pelvic inflammatory disease and ectopic pregnancy are also considerations.

TABLE 156-1 Appendicitis and Similar Conditions Presenting With Abdominal Pain and Vomiting

Similar Conditions	Distinguishing Characteristics of Appendicitis
Gastroenteritis	Pain precedes vomiting and fever Diarrhea, if it occurs, is small volume
Constipation	Pain progresses in intensity and is typically not fluctuating
Urinary tract infection	Pain usually not suprapubic or flank Urinalysis usually <10 WBCs/hpf
Pneumonia	Cough and tachypnea uncommon Fever typically low grade Abdominal tenderness
Pelvic inflammatory disease	Pain typically localized to right lower quadrant
Ectopic pregnancy	Gradual increase in pain Negative serum β-HCG
Ovarian torsion or ovarian cyst	Gradual increase in pain, which is initially periumbilical Elevated WBCs (>11,000/mm³)
Incarcerated inguinal hernia or testicular torsion	Normal testicular examination
Intussusception	Progressive, not colicky pain Uncommon in those younger than 2-3 y Stools typically heme negative
Hemolytic uremic syndrome	Diarrhea, if present, is nonbloody Normal platelets and hemoglobin Normal creatinine
Diabetic ketoacidosis	No polyuria or polydipsia Dehydration usually not severe Hyperglycemia or glucosuria
Abdominal trauma	Negative history of trauma No abdominal wall contusions

β-HCG, β-human chorionic gonadotropin; hpf, high-power field; WBC, white blood cell.

DIAGNOSTIC EVALUATION

Acute appendicitis is often a clinical diagnosis. With rare exceptions, it progresses gradually over several hours, which contrasts with the waxing and waning course of many other diseases. For equivocal cases, inpatient observation with serial abdominal examinations over a 6- to 12-hour period can be diagnostically valuable.

LABORATORY EVALUATION

A complete blood count (CBC) should be obtained to determine the peripheral white blood cell (WBC) count. Leukocytosis with WBC elevation over 10,000/mm^3, and more specifically neutrophilia with ANC (absolute neutrophil count) greater than 7500/mm^3, is commonly seen in appendicitis. However, both markers are nonspecific. Studies have shown that, in patients with nonperforated appendicitis, the WBC count was the most useful marker to predict appendicitis in those with fewer than 24 or more than 48 hours of pain, while the C-reactive protein (CRP) was most helpful between 24 and 48 hours. ANC does not appear to independently add additional diagnostic value. CRP is increased in the vast majority of patients with appendicitis who have been symptomatic for more than 12 hours. However, elevation in CRP is also nonspecific and therefore should be considered in the context of the patient's overall presentation.

Screening for pregnancy is indicated in all postmenarchal females to rule out pregnancy-related causes.

Urinalysis should be performed to rule out other conditions. Importantly, up to 25% of children with appendicitis have more than five white or red blood cells per high-power field, due to urethral or bladder irritation from the inflamed appendix.

RADIOGRAPHIC EVALUATION

Plain radiographs are often normal in appendicitis. In approximately 10% of cases, an abdominal plain film shows a calcified appendicolith, which is considered diagnostic. There may be right-sided scoliosis or an indistinct right psoas margin, although these findings are less specific. If a plain film is obtained, the chest should always be included to rule out pneumonia.

The use of ultrasonography (US) to evaluate appendicitis has been studied extensively. Although its specificity (88%-99%) and accuracy (82%-99%) are quite good, its sensitivity varies considerably (50%-100%). Appendiceal visualization rates also vary substantially, from as high as 98% to as low as 22%. Thus, negative findings by US are not helpful unless imaging unequivocally demonstrates a normal appendix. It should be noted that US is indicated in females when diagnoses such as ovarian torsion or ovarian cyst are being considered. For these conditions, US imaging is superior to computed tomography (CT).

A CT scan with IV and oral contrast has higher sensitivity for appendicitis in children (94%) than does ultrasound, and is far less operator dependent. In patients who present late with an abscess or inflammatory mass (phlegmon), CT is helpful in determining whether surgical intervention is warranted in addition to IV antibiotics. CT interpretation by radiologists with expertise in pediatrics further improves diagnostic accuracy.

A contrast enema may be useful if intussusception and appendicitis are both diagnostic considerations. Smooth and complete filling of the appendix without extrinsic compression of the cecum or terminal ileum is a reliable negative sign and occurs in about 80% to 90% of normal appendices. With both abdominal CT and contrast enema, radiation exposure is an important consideration and should be discussed with families.

Recently, fast magnetic resonance imaging (MRI) has become increasingly popular for the detection of appendicitis. Unlike CT, MRI has no radiation exposure. It is highly accurate for diagnosis in children, with a sensitivity and specificity of 96%. Logistically, fast MRI (with short duration and without oral or IV contrast) has not yet become widely available but this may become standard of care in the future given its high accuracy.

MANAGEMENT

Therapy is dependent on the stage of illness and the certainty of diagnosis of appendicitis. If the diagnosis of nonperforated appendicitis is equivocal or likely, management includes the following:

- Early consultation with a surgeon skilled in the evaluation and management of children with acute surgical abdomen.
- Nothing by mouth (NPO) and intravenous fluids as needed.
- In-hospital observation and monitoring with serial examinations, as indicated.
- Imaging studies as needed, depending on the institution's radiologic expertise with children.

To reduce the risk of perforation, many experts recommend that the decision whether to operate be made within 24 to 36 hours of pain onset.

In unequivocal appendicitis, options include surgical or medical (nonoperative) management. In select patients, a trial of medical management with IV antibiotics may be reasonable. Factors to consider include age, duration of illness, clinical stability, and presence of appendicolith. There is currently wide variability in individual institutional criteria for medical management.

Surgical management includes NPO status, appropriate pain control, assessment of hydration and administration of appropriate IV fluids if needed, and antibiotics which should be administered as soon as possible. Antibiotic prophylaxis reduces the incidence of wound infection and intra-abdominal abscess. In nonperforated appendicitis, the choice of preoperative antibiotics should provide broad-spectrum coverage of intraabdominal organisms. Regimens may include (1) ceftriaxone + metronidazole (or ciprofloxacin + metronidazole if cephalosporin allergy); (2) cefoxitin; or (3) piperacillin-tazobactam.

Postoperatively, pain control and adequate hydration are key. Oral pain medications are appropriate once the patient is awake and drinking well. In nonperforated appendicitis, oral fluids should be allowed when the child awakes postoperatively, and the diet should be advanced as tolerated. If oral intake is poor or if postoperative emesis persists, intravenous fluid support is continued with attention to maintenance and ongoing replacement needs. Antibiotics are continued only if the appendix is gangrenous or perforated.

The risk of postoperative complications is highest in those with a perforated appendix. If the patient has persistent fever, abdominal pain, or is unable to tolerate a regular diet by 5 to 7 days postoperatively, an intra-abdominal or wound abscess should be considered. Wound infections are treated by opening the wound, and most deep abscesses are treated by percutaneous drainage under US or CT guidance. For children unable to tolerate enteral feedings 1 week after surgery, consider parenteral nutrition.

Mechanical small bowel obstruction is an uncommon postoperative complication. Most patients who develop bowel obstruction more than 1 month after appendicitis require surgical intervention for lysis of adhesions.

ADMISSION AND DISCHARGE CRITERIA

Admission criteria include the following:

- Definite appendicitis requiring surgical intervention
- Abdominal pain of uncertain cause, particularly in preschool-age children, in whom the diagnosis of appendicitis is more difficult and perforation before diagnosis is more likely
- Lack of a reliable outpatient observer or inadequate follow-up

Postoperatively, children need to meet the following criteria for hospital discharge:

- Afebrile
- Reassuring abdominal examination
- Tolerating a regular diet
- Ambulating comfortably
- Pain well controlled on oral medications

CONSULTATION

Early consultation with a pediatric surgeon is recommended for any suspected case of appendicitis.

PREVENTION

If an incidental appendicolith is found on imaging, many authorities recommend an elective appendectomy. In cases of abdominal surgery for other indications, elective appendectomy is often performed at the same time.

KEY POINTS

- The classic presentation of appendicitis is gradually worsening periumbilical pain, followed by infrequent nonbilious emesis. After several hours, the pain shifts to the right lower quadrant.
- Atypical presentations are common.
- Appendicitis is often diagnosed by clinical assessment. Laboratory testing and imaging studies are useful in equivocal cases.
- Inpatient observation and early consultation with a surgeon are recommended for equivocal cases. Surgical or medical management is recommended for confirmed or highly suggestive cases. Preoperative antibiotics are recommended.

SUGGESTED READINGS

Becker C, Kharbanda A. Acute appendicitis in pediatric patients: an evidence-based review. *Pediatr Emerg Med Pract.* 2019;16(9):1-20.

Becker T, Kharbanda A, Bachur R. Atypical clinical features of pediatric appendicitis. *Acad Emerg Med.* 2007;14(2):124-129.

Bethell GS, Gosling T, Rees CM, et al. Impact of the COVID-19 pandemic on management and outcomes of children with appendicitis: The Children with Appendicitis during the Coronavirus pandemic (CASCADE) study. *J Pediatr Surg.* 2022;S0022-3468(22):00261-5.

Dabaja-Younis H, Farah H, Miron R, et al. The intraperitoneal bacteriology and antimicrobial resistance in acute appendicitis among children: a retrospective cohort study between the years 2007 and 2017. *Eur J Pediatr.* 2021;180(7):2091-2098.

Drapkin Z, Dunnick J, Madsen TE, Bryce M, Schunk JE. Pediatric appendicitis: Association of Chief Complaint With Missed Appendicitis. *Pediatr Emerg Care.* 2020;36(4):e204-e207.

Duke E, Kalb B, Arif-Tiwari H, et al. A systematic review and meta-analysis of diagnostic performance of MRI for evaluation of acute appendicitis. *AJR Am J Roentgenol.* 2016;206(3):508-517.

Fugazzola P, Coccolini F, Tomasoni M, Stella M, Ansaloni L. Early appendectomy vs. conservative management in complicated acute appendicitis in children: a meta-analysis. *J Pediatr Surg.* 2019;54(11):2234-2241.

Gonzalez DO, Deans KJ, Minneci PC. Role of non-operative management in pediatric appendicitis. *Semin Pediatr Surg.* 2016;25(4):204-207.

Kharbanda AB, Cosme Y, Liu K, et al. Discriminative accuracy of novel and traditional biomarkers in children with suspected appendicitis adjusted for duration of abdominal pain. *Acad Emerg Med.* 2011;18(6):567-574.

Lovell J. Calculated decisions: pediatric appendicitis score (PAS). *Pediatr Emerg Med Pract.* 2019;16(9):CD1-CD2.

Mushtaq R, Desoky SM, Morello F, et al. First-line diagnostic evaluation with MRI of children suspected of having acute appendicitis. *Radiology.* 2019;291(1):170-177.

CHAPTER 157 Hernias

Richard A. Falcone, MD, MPH, MMM and Dane C. Warner, MD, MPH

BACKGROUND

Hernias are common conditions that are among the most frequent indications for surgery in children. Although most hernias are identified in the outpatient setting, hospitalists may diagnose hernias from incidental subjective complaints or physical examination findings in patients who are admitted for other reasons. Hospitalists may more urgently diagnose an unrecognized incarcerated or strangulated hernia, for example, as the cause of an infant's fussiness or lethargy.

Hernia refers to any opening, congenital or acquired, in the abdominal musculature or fascia that allows all or part of an abdominal viscus to protrude beyond its usual boundaries. The term also sometimes refers to the protruding viscus itself. Most hernias include an extension of the peritoneum, the *hernia sac*, which encases the herniated viscus and may be excised as part of the surgical repair. An *incarcerated hernia* is one in which the herniated viscus cannot be reduced manually, usually because of edema. *Strangulated hernia* refers to an incarcerated hernia in which the vascular integrity of the herniated viscus is compromised. This usually involves venous and lymphatic congestion of the tissue but can progress to arterial insufficiency, ischemia, and eventually necrosis. *Sliding hernia* refers to a hernia in which the serosa of an intra-abdominal organ forms part of the hernia sac, which can make for a more difficult repair.

Essentially, all hernias in children are congenital defects and not the result of excessive straining or fascial disruption, which are often cited as causal factors in adults. Consequently, pain is rarely a symptom of an uncomplicated hernia in children. This also means that pediatric hernias rarely require fascial reconstruction or the use of prosthetic mesh, making the operation more straightforward and less painful than in adults.

The approach to hernias depends on their reducibility and location. Most hernias are spontaneous or easily reducible, so they can usually be repaired on an elective basis, depending on the preferences of the family. A hernia that is suspected to be incarcerated requires urgent surgical consultation. If it is unable to be reduced by someone skilled in the care of hernias through an attempted reduction with sedation, then it is truly incarcerated and can progress to a surgical emergency due to the risk for strangulation and bowel necrosis. Almost all hernias require operative repair, with the exception of asymptomatic umbilical hernias in children younger than 3 to 5 years of age, which often resolve spontaneously. However, a small percentage of umbilical hernias do become incarcerated, so monitoring and guidance for families are essential.

Most patients do not need to be admitted after surgical hernia repair, but postoperative admission is indicated for young infants at risk for apnea, for some children with complex medical conditions, and for patients who require urgent surgical repair for an incarcerated, strangulated, or otherwise complicated hernia.

This chapter reviews the two most common hernias in children, indirect inguinal hernias and umbilical hernias.

INDIRECT INGUINAL HERNIAS

In children, almost all hernias in the inguinal region are indirect inguinal hernias. Indirect inguinal hernias result from the persistence of the *processus vaginalis*, the remnant of an embryonic structure that plays a role in testicular descent in males but also exists in the embryonic development of females. The *processus vaginalis* normally closes before birth. When it does not close, an indirect inguinal hernia or a communicating hydrocele may develop (**Figure 157-1**). An indirect inguinal hernia occurs when an intra-abdominal viscus protrudes through a patent *processus vaginalis* and into the inguinal canal. A communicating hydrocele is essentially an indirect hernia, through which only fluid is transmitted because it is too small for any viscera to pass through it. Most inguinal hernias include the bowel, but they may involve other structures such as the omentum, ovary, bladder, or appendix. Sometimes only one wall of the bowel is involved, which can cause strangulation without obstruction and is known as a *Richter hernia*.

Estimates of childhood incidence of inguinal hernias vary by gestational age at 1% to 5% for full-term infants, 13% for premature infants, and as high as 30% for infants born at < 1000 g. The rate of inguinal hernia repair is 4 times higher for males than for females. It is highest for males in the first year of life. The epidemiology for *incarcerated* inguinal hernias is similar. Although incarcerated inguinal hernias occur throughout childhood, most happen during infancy with an overall median age of 8 months, demonstrating a significantly higher risk of incarceration for infants with inguinal hernias. The male-to-female ratio for incarcerated inguinal hernias is 7 to 1.

CLINICAL PRESENTATION

Most pediatric indirect inguinal hernias are uncomplicated and present as an asymptomatic mass in the inguinal region, lateral to the rectus sheath and superior to the pubic tubercle. In some cases, there may simply be asymmetry in the suprapubic fat pad. Because indirect inguinal hernias can extend into the scrotum or labia majora, there may be a difference in the size of the scrotal contents or labia. Inguinal hernias typically appear or become larger when the patient increases intra-abdominal pressure, such as during a Valsalva maneuver. The classic history is that of a painless groin bulge that appears during straining or crying, and there are typically no other symptoms.

Although some older children describe a vague discomfort when the inguinal hernia is "out," the vast majority of uncomplicated inguinal hernias in children are painless. Groin pain alone, without a mass in the inguinal canal, is rarely evidence of a hernia, and is more commonly due

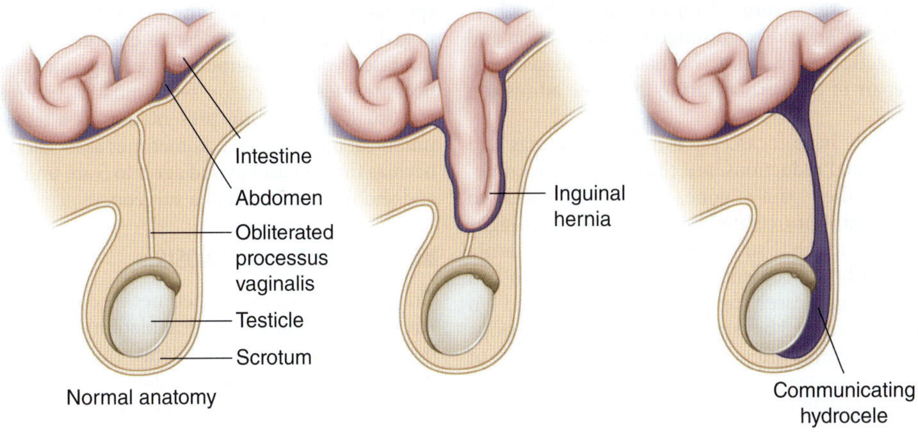

FIGURE 157-1. Indirect inguinal hernia versus communicating hydrocele.

to a muscle strain. However, the combination of a groin bulge from an apparent hernia and significant pain should raise the suspicion that a herniated viscus has become incarcerated. Infants with inguinal hernias can pose a particular diagnostic challenge because crying can cause a hernia to become larger and more tense, and it can be difficult to discern whether crying is due to pain from an incarcerated hernia or due to the myriad other reasons an infant may cry. In such situations, parents should be instructed to console the child in the usual ways, such as gentle rocking, feeding, and changing the diaper. If the tense protrusion persists for more than 20 to 30 minutes despite these measures or if other symptoms such as vomiting or fever develop, then the infant should be brought to the emergency department.

Incarceration occurs in 10% to 12% of pediatric patients with an indirect inguinal hernia. The presentation is rarely subtle. Children are typically in severe pain, very restless, and unable to find a comfortable position. Frequently there is vomiting, as a reflex secondary to visceral compromise or due to bowel obstruction. Fever, dehydration, and lethargy are usually late signs that suggest bowel ischemia. The hernia itself is usually quite prominent, tense, and tender on examination, and it may occur with or without overlying erythema. Concern for an incarcerated inguinal hernia is a true emergency requiring evaluation by a surgeon skilled in the management of hernias. Without early reduction or prompt surgical repair of the hernia, it can progress to a strangulated hernia with compromise of the trapped viscera.

DIFFERENTIAL DIAGNOSIS

A history of an asymptomatic bulge in the groin that enlarges with straining and promptly resolves spontaneously or with gentle manual pressure is diagnostic of a reducible inguinal hernia. It is sometimes difficult to distinguish incarcerated inguinal hernias from other, mostly benign congenital, inflammatory, or infectious processes (**Table 157-1**). Malignancies rarely present as groin swelling in children.

DIAGNOSTIC EVALUATION

The diagnosis of an indirect inguinal hernia is based solely on the history and physical examination. An excellent description by a parent with or without photos may be adequate to make the diagnosis in a young child. Ultrasonography is occasionally a useful adjunct to resolve clinical uncertainty. However, if there are no contents within the hernia sac at the time of imaging, a hernia can be missed. When the diagnosis is uncertain or imaging studies are equivocal, pediatric surgical consultation should be sought.

On physical examination, an inguinal hernia is diagnosed by the presence of an inguinal, labial, or scrotal bulge that can be manually reduced into the abdomen.

MANAGEMENT

Inguinal hernias do not resolve spontaneously, and they tend to enlarge or become more symptomatic over time. Incarceration can occur at any age and with any size hernia. As a result, all inguinal hernias should be surgically repaired.

Once the diagnosis of a reducible, uncomplicated hernia is confirmed, operative intervention is generally recommended within 2 to 3 months. Some recommend an earlier repair in children younger than 1 year old given their increased risk of incarceration. For premature infants less than 60 weeks postconception, the decision to operate must be weighed against the increased risk for anesthesia-related complications and postoperative apnea. The timing of the repair can be determined through shared decision-making by the surgeon and parents.

Activity restriction guidelines for patients awaiting surgery are based on expert opinion. Mild physical activities do not appear to increase the risk of incarceration for patients with asymptomatic and uncomplicated inguinal hernias. Extreme physical exertion that involves a great deal of straining or the potential for direct injury to the hernia should be avoided before and for at least 2 weeks after surgery.

If a patient presents with an inguinal hernia that does not reduce easily or spontaneously, manual reduction should be attempted by someone skilled in hernia care. This technique involves the application of constant pressure to the herniated bowel with one hand while using the thumb and first two fingers of the other hand to compress the neck of the hernia close to where it enters the abdomen. For males, gentle traction downward on the testicle should be applied to help straighten the inguinal canal as pressure is applied parallel to the canal. Constant, rather than increasing, pressure for more than 2 to 3 minutes is sometimes necessary. This technique requires patience and may benefit from analgesics or mild sedation. It likely enables reduction in part by reducing edema in the herniated bowel. Multiple attempts in the same session are sometimes necessary, allowing the hernia to be reduced incrementally with each attempt. As the contents reduce, you should appreciate a decrease in the resistance and a decrease in the mass in the inguinal canal. If you are unsure whether an adequate reduction has been achieved, an ultrasound can be helpful. Children with inguinal hernias that cannot

TABLE 157-1 Differential Diagnosis of Groin Mass or Swelling

Finding	Description and Comments
Hydrocele	• Collection of fluid along spermatic cord or in scrotum • Result of persistence of part of processus vaginalis • Size changes only gradually • May be either communicating or noncommunicating with peritoneal cavity • Distinguished from hernia by normal spermatic cord palpable in inguinal canal above hydrocele • Ultrasonography or surgery may be required for diagnosis
Lymph node	• Enlarges gradually and resolves slowly compared with hernia • Normal spermatic cord can be palpated separately from lymph node • Ultrasonography can aid in diagnosis
Tumor	• Extremely uncommon in pediatric population

be reduced manually require urgent surgical repair. Those whose hernias are reduced with difficulty should be admitted for observation and hydration. Institutional practices vary, but it is usually considered prudent to offer operative repair of the hernia during the same admission after a difficult reduction.

Most patients, who initially have incarcerated inguinal hernias and then undergo successful manual reductions, are clinically better immediately. They are more alert, their pain is gone, and they are ready to play and eat. Some patients with incarcerated hernias do not have signs or symptoms of a bowel obstruction. Usually, this is because the hernia opening is large enough that bowel contents continue to flow into and out of the herniated bowel. In rare cases, the bowel may be reduced "en masse," which means that it is reduced but stays kinked due to adhesions or irreversible injury. These patients often have persistent symptoms of bowel obstruction and require laparoscopy or laparotomy.

Although the repair of a pediatric inguinal hernia (herniorrhaphy) has traditionally been performed with an open approach, there is growing literature in support of the laparoscopic approach. Results of studies comparing laparoscopic and open inguinal hernia repairs show comparable short- and long-term outcomes.

COMPLICATIONS

Children with inguinal hernias are at risk for a variety of complications. The most serious is bowel ischemia requiring partial resection, which fortunately is rare even among children with incarcerated hernias. Intraoperatively, damage may occur to a viscus in the hernia sac, such as bowel, ovary, fallopian tube, or bladder. Significant bleeding is rare, though premature infants are more likely to have bruising and swelling. Hematomas and reactive hydroceles can occur postoperatively and almost always resolve spontaneously. Surgical site infections are uncommon. When they occur, they usually present within the first two weeks postoperatively, are almost always superficial, and can usually be treated on an outpatient basis with oral antibiotics. Postoperative pain that does not improve with over-the-counter medications should raise suspicion for injury to the gonadal blood supply or for postoperative testicular or ovarian torsion, though these are uncommon.

Recurrence rates vary based on patient age and other comorbidities. The rate of recurrence after inguinal hernia repair is only about 1% for elective cases, but it is much higher for premature infants (15%) and after incarcerated hernia repairs (20%-30%). Recurrences are also more common in children with a variety of chronic medical conditions including Ehlers-Danlos syndrome, seizure disorders, and conditions that increase intraabdominal pressure, such as bronchopulmonary dysplasia, ventriculoperitoneal shunts, and chronic coughing.

CONSULTATION

Surgical consultation is indicated whenever there is suspicion of an inguinal hernia. Any suspicion of an incarcerated hernia calls for immediate surgical consultation.

ANTICIPATORY GUIDANCE

When a child is suspected of having an inguinal hernia, caregivers should be told that if the child is inconsolable or complains of abdominal or scrotal pain and the hernia is visible or tender, they should proceed immediately to the emergency room.

UMBILICAL HERNIAS

Umbilical hernias result from persistence of the umbilical ring, the opening in the fascia that allows passage of the umbilical cord structures in the fetus. The umbilical ring usually closes spontaneously in the first few days or weeks of life.

CLINICAL PRESENTATION

An umbilical hernia presents as a painless bulge at the umbilicus during the neonatal period. The natural history of umbilical hernias is gradual spontaneous closure within the first few years of life. The size of the herniated contents may appear to enlarge over time, despite the fact that the fascial defect is gradually getting smaller. Umbilical hernias rarely become incarcerated or symptomatic. Incarcerated umbilical hernias are usually evident on presentation as a tense, tender, and irreducible umbilical mass, which is sometimes associated with vomiting. Umbilical hernias that persist beyond age 3 to 5 are unlikely to close spontaneously and should be referred to a surgeon.

DIFFERENTIAL DIAGNOSIS

Umbilical masses can sometimes be confused with an umbilical hernia. An umbilical mass with granulation tissue, especially if accompanied by drainage from the umbilicus, might represent a patent urachus or omphalomesenteric duct remnant. In newborns, a small omphalocele may be indistinguishable from a large umbilical hernia. Any suspicious umbilical lesion, especially in a newborn, should be evaluated by a pediatric surgeon.

DIAGNOSTIC EVALUATION

Umbilical hernias are usually quite evident on examination. If there is concern about an alternative diagnosis such as a patent urachus or omphalomesenteric duct remnant, an ultrasound may be performed. Once an umbilical hernia is diagnosed, the hernia contents should be gently reduced, and the fascial defect assessed for size by gentle palpation. Those with a defect less than 1.5 cm will likely close spontaneously, but even those of greater size have been observed to close and can generally be safely monitored. Reassurance is often all that is needed, followed by yearly re-examination for resolution until around age 3 to 5 years. In the older child whose umbilical hernia has resolved, there is sometimes residual redundant skin or scar tissue which can mimic a hernia. If there is no palpable fascial defect and no visible or palpable bulge with straining, this is of cosmetic importance only.

MANAGEMENT

Umbilical hernias that have not resolved by 3 to 5 years of age should be repaired electively. After age 5, umbilical hernias are very unlikely to close spontaneously and are more difficult and painful to repair, and they also present a risk later in life, especially during pregnancy.

Emergent surgical repair is necessary for incarcerated umbilical hernias. Children with umbilical hernias that were difficult to reduce should be admitted for hydration, monitoring, and subsequent surgical repair. They can be discharged when the risk of occult bowel obstruction or visceral ischemia has passed, and they are tolerating an oral diet and otherwise stable.

Currently, there is no role for laparoscopic repair of umbilical hernias in children. Similar to an inguinal hernia repair in children, and unlike in adults, umbilical hernias are repaired primarily with absorbable suture and without prosthetic mesh. The repair is performed under general anesthesia on an outpatient basis. Postoperative complications are uncommon and include hernia recurrence, wound infection, and hematoma.

CONSULTATION

It is generally safe to observe infants and toddlers with uncomplicated umbilical hernias and delay referral to a pediatric surgeon until age 3 to 5 years. In the rare case that an incarcerated umbilical hernia is suspected, emergent consultation should be sought. In addition, pediatric surgical consultation is indicated when considering an alternative diagnosis, such as an umbilical granuloma, patent urachus, or omphalomesenteric duct remnant.

ANTICIPATORY GUIDANCE

Parents of children with an umbilical hernia should be educated about the signs and symptoms of incarceration and the importance of seeking urgent medical care if they occur. It is also important to emphasize that there is no therapeutic benefit to placing tape or affixing a coin over an umbilical hernia and that doing so can induce local tissue damage and lead to an infection.

KEY POINTS

- Most hernias present as asymptomatic masses that can be evaluated on an outpatient basis and treated electively.
- The most common types in children are indirect inguinal hernias and umbilical hernias.
- All inguinal hernias require surgical repair in a timely fashion to avoid complications of incarceration, strangulation, and ischemia of the bowel, testis, or ovary.
- Umbilical hernias are safe to observe in infants; however, those that persist after age 3 or 5 years are unlikely to resolve spontaneously and should be repaired surgically.
- Parents should be educated about the signs and symptoms of incarceration and instructed to seek urgent medical attention, if they suspect an incarcerated hernia.

SUGGESTED READINGS

Aboagye J, Goldstein SD, Salazar JH, et al. Age at presentation of common pediatric surgical conditions: reexamining dogma. *J Pediatr Surg*. 2014;49(6):995-999.

Chong AJ, Fevrier HB, Herrinton LJ. Long-term follow-up of pediatric open and laparoscopic inguinal hernia repair. *J Pediatr Surg*. 2019;54(10):2138-2144.

Dreuning KM, Barendsen RW, van Trotsenburg AP, et al. Inguinal hernia in girls: a retrospective analysis of over 1000 patients. *J Pediatr Surg*. 2020;55(9):1908-1913.

Gholoum S, Baird R, Laberge JM, Puligandla PS. Incarceration rates in pediatric inguinal hernia: do not trust the coding. *J Pediatr Surg*. 2010;45(5):1007-1011.

Lautz TB, Raval MV, Reynolds M. Does timing matter? A national perspective on the risk of incarceration in premature neonates with inguinal hernia. *J Pediatr*. 2011;158(4):573-577.

Lee SL, Gleason JM, Sydorak RM. A critical review of premature infants with inguinal hernias: optimal timing of repair, incarceration risk, and postoperative apnea. *J Pediatr Surg*. 2011;46(1):217-220.

Masoudian P, Sullivan KJ, Mohamed H, Nasr A. Optimal timing for inguinal hernia repair in premature infants: a systematic review and meta-analysis. *J Pediatr Surg*. 2019;54(8):1539-1545.

Morini F, Dreuning KMA, Janssen Lok MJH, et al. Surgical management of pediatric inguinal hernia: A Systematic Review and Guideline from the European Pediatric Surgeons' Association Evidence and Guideline Committee. *Eur J Pediatr Surg*. 2022;32(3):219-232.

Pan ML, Chang WP, Lee HC, et al. A longitudinal cohort study of incidence rates of inguinal hernia repair in 0- to 6-year-old children. *J Pediatr Surg*. 2013;48(11):2327-2331.

Papagrigoriadis S, Browse DJ, Howard ER. Incarceration of umbilical hernias in children: a rare but important complication. *Pediatr Surg Int*. 1998;14(3):231-232.

Rasmussen SK, Haynes JH. Complications of herniorrhaphy. In: Caty MG, et al, ed. *Complications in Pediatric Surgery*. New York: Informa Healthcare USA; 2009:197-207.

Schier F, Danzer E, Bondartschuk M. Incidence of contralateral patent processus vaginalis in children with inguinal hernia. *J Pediatr Surg*. 2001;36(10):1561-1563.

Smith G, Wright JE. Reduction of gangrenous small bowel by taxis on an inguinal hernia. *Pediatr Surg Int*. 1996;11(8):582-583.

Strauch ED, Voigt RW, Hill JL. Gangrenous intestine in a hernia can be reduced. *J Pediatr Surg*. 2002;37(6):919-920.

Walther-Larsen S, Rasmussen LS. The former preterm infant and risk of post-operative apnoea: recommendations for management. *Acta Anaesthesiol Scand*. 2006;50(7):888-893.

Wang KS, Committee on F, Newborn AAoP, Section on Surgery AAoP. Assessment and management of inguinal hernia in infants. *Pediatrics*. 2012;130(4):768-773.

Yeap E, Pacilli M, Nataraja RM. Inguinal hernias in children. *Aust J Gen Pract*. 2020;49(1-2):38-43.

Zamakhshary M, To T, Guan J, Langer JC. Risk of incarceration of inguinal hernia among infants and young children awaiting elective surgery. *CMAJ*. 2008;179(10):1001-1005.

CHAPTER 158

General Trauma

Cori Grant, MD and Elizabeth Messer, MD

BACKGROUND

Traumatic injury remains the leading cause of death in adolescents and children older than 1 year of age and the fifth leading cause of death in newborns and infants in the United States. Motor vehicle injuries are the most common cause of unintentional death from ages 5 to 19. Providers must also consider nonaccidental trauma as a potential source of injury in children; child abuse is further discussed in Section A. Traumatic injuries can also result in long-term disability and remain a leading cause of emergency room, urgent care, and primary care visits. Childhood injuries cost billions of dollars annually and can lead to significant financial hardships for the patient's family.

Trauma is a public health issue that does not affect all groups equally. For example, higher rates of injury have been reported in males, individuals of lower socioeconomic status, and Native American/Alaskan natives. Many traumatic injuries in children are preventable. As such, traumatic injury should be a priority target for prevention efforts. Education for local providers is a vital first-line intervention and can be accomplished through teaching Advanced Trauma Life Support (ATLS). Availability of pediatric trauma centers can also lower pediatric injury mortality.

GENERAL ASSESSMENT

The evaluation of any trauma patient, regardless of age, is standardized and follows the ATLS method supported by the American College of Surgeons. The ATLS program begins with a primary survey, which follows the ABCDE mnemonic (Airway, Breathing, Circulation, Disability, Exposure). Each component of the primary survey is addressed before moving on to the next. The primary survey is followed by a secondary survey, which is a systematic, head-to-toe assessment to evaluate for other injuries. Important adjuncts to the primary and secondary survey include cervical spine X-ray, chest X-ray, Focused Assessment with Sonography in Trauma (FAST) examination, and pelvic X-ray. Once the trauma patient is stabilized, they may be admitted, sent to the operating room, or transferred to a different facility for a higher level of care.

Child physiology is distinct from that of adults and pediatric-specific issues must be considered during treatment. Children often display few external signs of trauma despite having sustained severe internal organ damage. Due to their small size, they can experience severe injury from forces that would not be significant to an adult and are susceptible to excessive heat loss during exposure and resuscitation. Children also have higher metabolic demands and oxygen consumption than adults, making early initiation of oxygen and glucose important. Finally, because children vary so greatly in body mass, knowledge of the child's weight is essential for the proper dosing of drugs, fluids, and blood products.

Special attention should be given at each level of resuscitation. Airway management is critical for children, as respiratory failure is the primary cause of cardiac arrest. Needle cricothyroidotomy is preferred over a surgical airway, which is considered unsafe due to the proximity of the vocal cords. For breathing, age-specific respiratory rates should be kept readily available. For circulation, if the practitioner is unable to obtain venous access, intraosseous access should be established. For disability, a modified Glasgow Coma Scale (GCS) is typically used to evaluate for neurologic deficits (**Tables 158-1** and **158-2**). It is imperative that cervical spine precautions are maintained during the primary and secondary survey until spinal injury can be ruled out.

HEAD AND NECK INJURIES

Head trauma is the most common pediatric injury. Healthcare utilization for head injuries has been increasing, with approximately 1100 emergency department visits, 31 hospitalizations, and 3.4 deaths per

100,000 children in the United States annually. The mechanism of head trauma varies by age. In children younger than 2 years, the most common causes are falls, followed by injuries suspicious for abuse. In older children, the most common causes are motor vehicle accidents, falls, and athletic injuries. Consequences of head injury include intracranial hemorrhage, cerebral contusion, diffuse axonal injury, skull fracture, concussion, long-term neuropsychological sequelae, and cervical spine injury. In this chapter, the discussion of head trauma is limited to minor head injuries. See Chapter 160 "Neurosurgical Issues" for more details on moderate to severe head injuries.

MINOR HEAD INJURY

Minor closed head injury is defined by the American Academy of Pediatrics (AAP) as an injury in a previously neurologically healthy child aged 2 years or older with normal mental status, no abnormal neurologic findings, and no evidence of skull fracture. Clinically important traumatic brain injury (ciTBI) resulting in death, neurosurgical intervention, prolonged hospitalization, or intubation occurs in less than 1% of children with minor head injury. Predictors of ciTBI include headache, vomiting, loss of consciousness, severe mechanism of injury, and nonfrontal scalp hematoma in children younger than 2 years of age. Children without any risk factors have a less than 0.05% risk of ciTBI, whereas the risk increases to 0.8% for those with multiple risk factors. Isolated headache, vomiting, or loss of consciousness are poor predictors of ciTBI in children.

Clinical Presentation Children with minor head injury may present with temporary loss of consciousness (<1 minute), vomiting, seizure, headache, or lethargy. Seizures are present in approximately 1% of children with minor head injury and most commonly occur on impact. While seizures alone do not predict intracranial injury, approximately 15% of children with posttraumatic seizures have evidence of TBI on head CT. Increased seizure duration and time from injury are associated with increased risk. Skull fracture may also occur in patients with minor head injury; the incidence is highest in those younger than 2 years. Scalp swelling or hematoma in a young child, especially parietal and temporal lesions, has been linked to the presence of an underlying skull fracture and intracranial hemorrhage. Skull fractures are associated with a 15% to 30% risk of intracranial injury.

Diagnostic Evaluation The Pediatric Emergency Care Applied Research Network (PECARN) clinical prediction rules may be utilized to identify patients with head injury who are at low risk for a clinically significant intracranial process. These rules were derived from a large, prospective multicenter study and can be applied to children either younger or older than 2 years of age (**Figure 158-1**). The decision to image, observe, or discharge a patient is based on the patient's presenting risk factors. Children with minor head injury who are observed in the emergency department are less likely to undergo CT imaging.

TABLE 158-1 Glasgow Coma Scale

Response	Description	Score (points)*
Eye opening	Spontaneous—open with blinking at baseline	4
	Opens to verbal command, speech, or shout	3
	Opens to pain not applied to face	2
	None	1
Verbal†	Oriented	5
	Confused but able to answer questions	4
	Inappropriate responses, words discernible	3
	Incomprehensible speech	2
	None	1
Motor	Obeys commands for movement	6
	Purposeful movement to painful stimulus	5
	Withdraws from pain	4
	Abnormal (spastic) flexion, decorticate posture	3
	Extensor (rigid) response, decerebrate posture	2
	None	1

*The total score is the sum of the scores in the three categories. Scores range from 3 to 15; patients with scores of 3 to 8 are usually said to be in a coma.

†For children younger than 5 years, the verbal response criteria are adjusted; see Table 158-2.

TABLE 158-2 Adjustment to Verbal Section of Glasgow Coma Scale for Children Younger Than 5 Years

Score	Age 2-5 Years	Age 0-23 Months
5	Appropriate words or phrases	Smiles or coos appropriately
4	Inappropriate words	Cries and consolable
3	Persistent cries or screams	Persistent inappropriate crying or screaming
2	Grunts	Grunts or is agitated or restless
1	No response	No response

Management Patients with a depressed skull fracture, intracranial blood, or cerebral contusion should be managed with the assistance of a neurosurgeon. Patients with amnesia or emesis despite normal imaging typically improve within 24 hours. Goals of inpatient admission are frequent neurologic examinations and hydration. Anticipatory guidance (including symptom management and the importance of cognitive and physical rest) as well as timely physician follow-up is paramount to enable recovery. Families should be counseled that a second injury prior to full recovery may cause greater morbidity and even mortality.

Consultation Obtain a neurosurgical consultation for patients with abnormal CT findings, depressed skull fracture, altered mental status, focal neurologic findings, or persistent emesis. Consult a general surgeon if the mechanism of injury is suspicious for occult thoracic or abdominal trauma.

Admission Criteria

- Persistent amnesia, lethargy, irritability, emesis, or seizures
- Inability to tolerate oral intake
- Focal neurologic deficits
- Abnormal CT findings

Discharge Criteria

- Normal mental status
- Normal neurologic examination
- Ability to tolerate oral intake
- Clearance by neurosurgical specialist

CERVICAL SPINE INJURIES

Cervical spine injuries are uncommon in children. They are found in 1% to 3% of children who sustain blunt trauma. The causes of cervical spine injuries vary by age. Overall, motor vehicle accidents are the most common cause of pediatric cervical spine injury. Falls and nonaccidental trauma are important mechanisms in younger children whereas sports injuries occur more frequently in older children. Children younger than 8 years are more susceptible to cervical spine injury than adults as the result of several anatomic factors. Due to their proportionally larger heads, the fulcrum of the spine is located at C2-C3 in young children and descends to C5-C6 by adolescence. Children also have increased ligamentous laxity, decreased muscle support, and physiologic anterior wedging of the vertebral bodies, resulting in spine hypermobility and a predisposition to upper cervical spine injury. Less than 30% of pediatric cervical spine injuries are below C3. In addition, younger children are at increased risk of ligamentous injuries and spinal cord injury without radiographic abnormality (SCIWORA); SCIWORA accounts for 30% to 40% of patients with traumatic myelopathy.

Clinical Presentation Patients with cervical spine injuries often experience focal pain, muscle spasm, and decreased range of motion. Additionally, transient or persistent neurologic findings such as weakness, numbness, or paresthesias may be present.

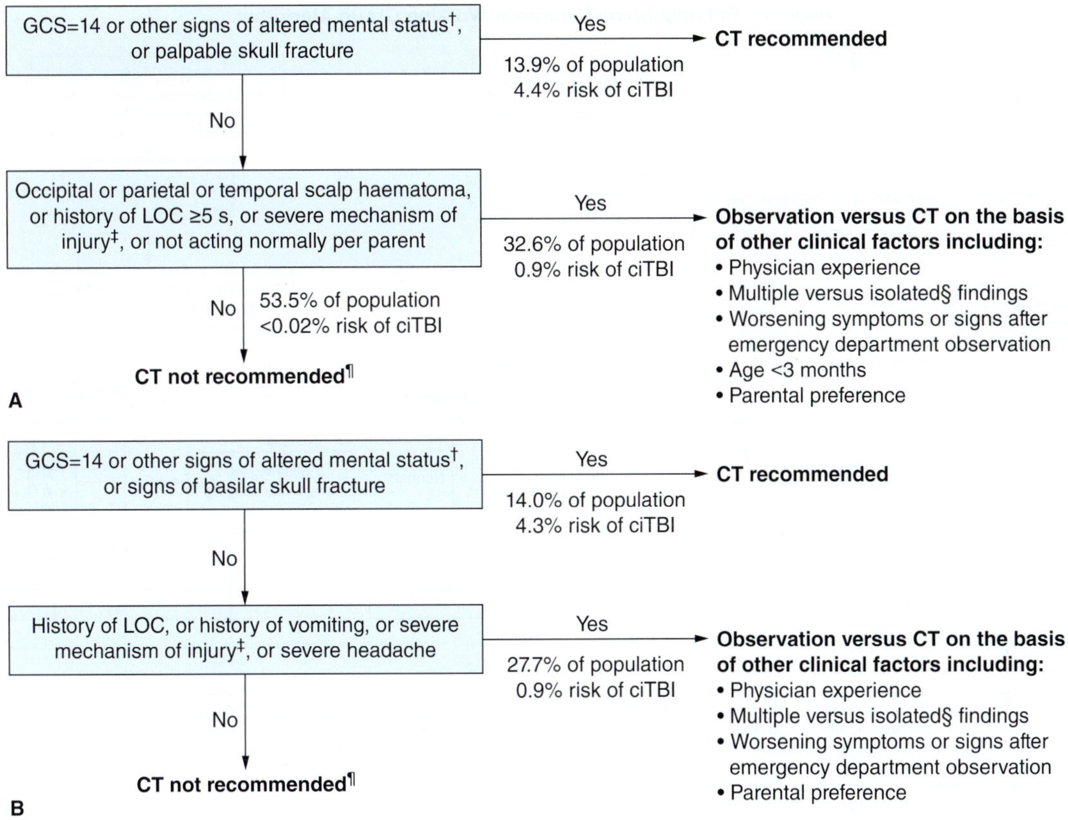

FIGURE 158-1. Suggested CT algorithm for children younger than 2 years (A) and for those aged 2 years and older (B) with GCS scores of 14-15 after head trauma. ciTBI, clinically important traumatic brain injury; GCS, Glasgow Coma Scale; LOC, loss of consciousness. *Data are from the combined derivation and validation populations. Other signs of altered mental status: agitation, somnolence, repetitive questioning, or slow response to verbal communication. Severe mechanism of injury: motor vehicle crash with patient ejection, death of another passenger, or rollover; pedestrian or bicyclist without helmet struck by a motorized vehicle; falls of more than 0.9 m (3 feet) (or more than 1.5 m [5 feet] for [B]; or head struck by a high-impact object. Patients with certain isolated findings (i.e., with no other findings suggestive of traumatic brain injury), such as isolated LOC,[1,2] isolated headache,[3] isolated vomiting,[3] and certain types of isolated scalp hematomas in infants older than 3 months,[4,5] have a risk of ciTBI substantially lower than 1%. Risk of ciTBI is exceedingly low, generally lower than risk of CT-induced malignancies. Therefore, CT scans are not indicated for most patients in this group. [1]Kuppermann N, Holmes JF, Dayan P, et al. Does isolated loss of consciousness predict traumatic brain injury in children after blunt head trauma? *Acad Emerg Med*. 2008;15:S82. [2]Palchak MJ, Holmes JF, Vance CW, et al. Does an isolated history of loss of consciousness or amnesia predict brain injuries after blunt head trauma? *Pediatrics*. 2004;113:e507-e513. [3]Dayan P, Holmes JF, Atabaki S, et al. Association of traumatic brain injuries (TBI) in children after blunt head trauma with degree of isolated headache or isolated vomiting. *Acad Emerg Med*. 2008;15:S175-S176. [4]Greenes DS, Schutzman SA. Clinical significance of scalp abnormalities in asymptomatic head-injured infants. *Pediatr Emerg Care*. 2001;17(2):88-92. [5]Dayan PS, Holmes JF, Schutzman S, et al. Association of traumatic brain injuries with scalp hematoma characteristics in patients younger than 24 months who sustain blunt head trauma. *Pediatr Emerg Care*. 2008;24:727. (Reproduced with permission from Kuppermann N, Holmes JF, Dayan PS, et al. Identification of children at very low risk of clinically-important brain injuries after head trauma: a prospective cohort study. *Lancet*. 2009;374(9696):1160-1170.)

Diagnostic Evaluation Any patient with midline cervical tenderness, decreased range of motion, focal neurologic findings, or a concerning mechanism of injury should remain immobilized with a cervical collar and undergo radiographic evaluation. At a minimum, this evaluation should include a cross-table lateral view of the cervical spine. Anteroposterior and open-mouth odontoid views may also be obtained, although there is evidence that additional views do not significantly add to the diagnostic sensitivity of plain radiographs. Further, it is challenging to obtain a high-quality odontoid view in young or uncooperative children. The ability of plain films to identify fractures varies by patient age, location of injury, type of immobilization, and position, with an overall sensitivity of approximately 90%.

Determining which pediatric patients would benefit from cervical spine imaging can be challenging and there is currently significant practice variability. The National Emergency X-Radiography Utilization Study (NEXUS) criteria can be safely applied to children older than 8 years. Factors associated with a low likelihood of cervical fracture include a normal mental status and the absence of midline cervical tenderness, focal neurologic findings, and distracting injury. Those who do not meet these low-risk criteria should undergo radiographic evaluation. Patients with persistent pain despite negative radiographs must remain immobilized and further imaging considered.

Adult clinical decision-making tools, including NEXUS and the Canadian C-Spine Rule, have not been validated in young children. A retrospective study conducted through the Pediatric Emergency Care Applied Research Network identified the following eight criteria as associated with cervical spine injuries: (1) altered mental status, (2) focal neurologic deficits, (3) complaint of neck pain, (4) torticollis, (5) substantial injury to the torso, (6) predisposing condition, (7) high-risk motor vehicle crash, and (8) diving injury. Having one or more of these criteria had a sensitivity of 98% (95% CI 96%-99%) and specificity of 26% (95% CI 23%-29%) for identifying cervical spine injuries in children under age 16. While subsequent studies have provided support for these risk factors, a validated pediatric clinical decision rule does not yet exist. Multiple institutions have created pediatric cervical spine clearance algorithms based on the available data and expert opinion; utilization of an algorithm has been shown to decrease the likelihood of missed injury while minimizing radiation exposure. The algorithm proposed by the Pediatric Cervical Spine Clearance Working Group is outlined in **Figure 158-2**.

Management If pain persists despite negative plain radiographs, CT or magnetic resonance imaging should be considered, along with pediatric neurosurgical consultation. The cervical spine can be cleared if the

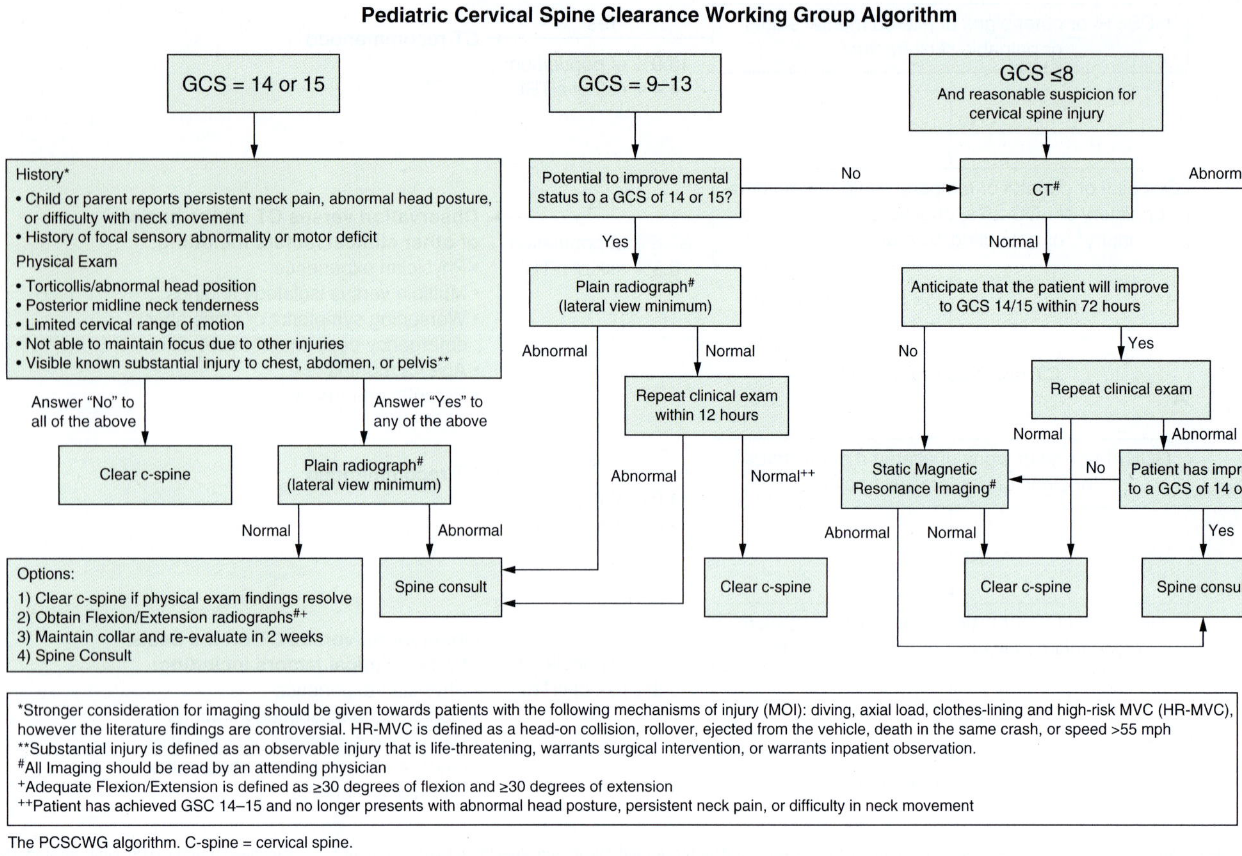

FIGURE 158-2. Pediatric Cervical Spine Working Group algorithm. (Reproduced with permission from Herman MJ, Brown KO, Sponseller PD, et al. PPediatric cervical spine clearance: A Consensus Statement and Algorithm from the Pediatric Cervical Spine Clearance Working Group. *J Bone Joint Surg Am.* 2019;101(1): e1.)

radiographs are negative, the neurologic examination is normal, there is no midline cervical tenderness or decreased range of motion, and the patient has no distracting injury.

Consultation Neurosurgical consultation should be obtained for patients with abnormal plain radiographs, persistent cervical tenderness, or focal neurologic deficits.

Admission Criteria

- Cervical fracture, subluxation, or ligamentous injury
- Focal neurologic deficits

Discharge Criteria

- Symptom improvement
- Clearance by neurosurgical subspecialist

THORACIC INJURIES

The thorax is comprised of the chest wall, mediastinum, and diaphragm. Thoracic trauma accounts for less than 10% of all pediatric injuries but is second only to head trauma as a cause of accidental death. The most common cause of thoracic injury is blunt force trauma from motor vehicle accidents, followed by falls. Penetrating thoracic trauma occurs less frequently. The most common thoracic injuries are pulmonary contusions, hemothorax/pneumothorax, and rib fractures. The most life-threatening injuries include injury to the heart, diaphragm, tracheobronchial tree, and great vessels. Thoracic injuries are frequently associated with trauma to the head, abdomen, and extremities. The initial treatment of thoracic injuries focuses on airway management and chest decompression.

Children are prone to different types of thoracic injury than adults as they have a more compliant chest wall with fewer ossified bones. This flexibility results in fewer rib fractures and more pulmonary contusions. The mediastinum is more mobile, allowing the heart and trachea to be displaced more easily. This displacement typically manifests as decreased venous return and cardiac output. In addition, the airway is smaller and more compressible. Children develop hypoxia more rapidly due to higher oxygen consumption and lower functional residual capacity relative to total lung volume. Children also have higher physiologic reserves so tachycardia may be the only sign of impending cardiopulmonary collapse.

PULMONARY CONTUSIONS

Pulmonary contusions are the most common thoracic injuries and are found even in the absence of rib fractures. They occur when there is damage at the level of the alveoli, resulting in hemorrhage or edema. This, in turn, leads to poor gas exchange, V/Q mismatch, and hypoxia. Pulmonary contusions can develop over several hours and may not be present on initial evaluation. Complications of pulmonary contusions include pneumonia, acute respiratory distress syndrome, and, in rare circumstances, death.

Clinical Presentation The clinical presentation depends on the degree of pulmonary involvement. Children may be asymptomatic or present with chest pain, shortness of breath, hemoptysis, hypoxemia, hypercarbia, acidosis, tachypnea, or respiratory failure.

Diagnostic Evaluation Pulmonary contusions should be suspected based on the mechanism of injury. Plain radiographs are the diagnostic method of choice. CT scan is not recommended if the chest X-ray is normal as it adds significant radiation exposure without changing patient management.

Management Most contusions are small and require only symptomatic treatment, although mechanical ventilation is sometimes necessary. Treatment includes supplemental oxygen, pain control, and incentive spirometry. The goals of therapy are to reduce atelectasis and prolonged immobilization, both of which can lead to the development of acute respiratory distress syndrome and pneumonia. Serial examinations are important to monitor symptom progression. The use of empiric antibiotics in patients with large pulmonary contusions remains controversial.

PNEUMOTHORAX/HEMOTHORAX

Pneumothorax is defined as the presence of air in the pleural space. Tension pneumothorax occurs when air accumulates within the pleural space through a one-way valve and is unable to escape. This collapses the affected lung and prevents venous return to the heart, leading to decreased cardiac output and obstructive shock. Tension pneumothorax is more common in children than adults due to the increased mobility of the mediastinum. Hemothorax is caused by bleeding into the pleural space, which can result from injuries to the tracheobronchial tree, blood vessels, pulmonary tissue, or heart. The pleura can hold a significant volume of blood, which can lead to both hemorrhagic shock and loss of lung volume. Hemothoraces and pneumothoraces may occur together.

Clinical Presentation The clinical presentation depends on the degree of pneumothorax or hemothorax. It can range from shortness of breath and tachypnea to respiratory failure. The physical examination is vital in the assessment of pneumothorax/hemothorax. The neck should be evaluated to ensure the trachea is midline and to look for jugular venous distension, which can be seen in tension pneumothorax. Signs of pneumothorax and hemothorax include chest wall bruising, subcutaneous emphysema, and asymmetric breath sounds. The affected lung will be hyperresonant on percussion in pneumothorax and dull in hemothorax.

Diagnostic Evaluation Chest X-ray is the diagnostic test of choice, although ultrasound has a high sensitivity and is being used more frequently.

Management For clinically ill patients, the first goal of treatment is to decompress the chest. This is accomplished primarily by chest tube thoracotomy, which is then connected to suction. In hemodynamically unstable patients, a chest tube may need to be placed before imaging is available. The chest tube should not be placed through an existing wound. Based on the size of the leak, multiple tubes may be necessary. Repeat chest X-rays are important to monitor disease progression. If mechanical ventilation is required, the pressure should be minimized to the extent possible. A small pneumothorax or hemothorax can simply be observed. Large hemothoraces require drainage as they can lead to empyema, lung entrapment, pneumonia, or scarring. Surgical intervention may be required if conservative treatment fails or if there is a large-volume hemorrhage. Blood transfusion should be administered if there is significant blood loss or hemodynamic instability.

RIB FRACTURES

Clinical Presentation The elasticity of the pediatric ribcage protects against rib fractures even in high-impact trauma. However, this means that force is frequently transmitted to internal organs. Upper rib fractures can be associated with upper airway, vascular, or cardiac injuries, while lower rib fractures can be associated with liver, spleen, or diaphragm injury. Patients can present with localized pain or shortness of breath regardless of injury location. Physical examination findings consistent with rib fracture are localized pain, palpable deformity, and crepitus. Clinicians should evaluate for flail chest, which is characterized by paradoxical chest wall movement with respiration and is indicative of multiple rib fractures. Flail chest is rare in children.

Diagnostic Evaluation The diagnosis can be made with plain radiographs. Chest CT should not be obtained if the chest X-ray appears normal.

Management Most rib fractures require only symptomatic treatment. This can be achieved through analgesics (NSAIDs and opiates) and, rarely, nerve blocks or epidurals. Incentive spirometry is also beneficial. Complications from rib fractures arise if ventilation is impaired secondary to pain and splinting of the thorax. This can lead to atelectasis and pneumonia from reduced clearance of secretions.

MEDIASTINAL INJURY (CARDIAC INJURIES, GREAT VESSEL INJURY, ESOPHOGEAL INJURY) AND DIAPHRAGMATIC RUPTURE

Both mediastinal and diaphragmatic injuries are rare. The clinical presentation can be subtle, and injuries are frequently missed on initial evaluation. Many patients with severe cardiac injuries die prior to arrival at the hospital and children who present to the emergency room already in shock tend to have worse outcomes.

THORACIC INJURY CONSULTATION

General or trauma surgery should be consulted for a concerning mechanism of injury, chest tube placement, surgical exploration, and evaluation for other injuries. Depending on the injuries identified, consultation with surgical subspecialists such as thoracic or vascular surgery may be necessary. Cardiology should be consulted for the evaluation of abnormal rhythms.

THORACIC INJURY ADMISSION CRITERIA

- Hemodynamic instability
- Oxygen requirement
- Respiratory distress
- Chest tube requirement or need for aggressive pulmonary clearance
- Flail chest or multiple rib fractures
- Abnormal rhythm on electrocardiography
- Pain control
- Need for surgical intervention
- Multiple associated traumatic injuries

THORACIC INJURY DISCHARGE CRITERIA

- Normal vital signs
- Stable or resolving symptoms
- No supplemental oxygen requirement
- Tolerating oral intake
- Pain controlled with oral medications
- Clearance by general surgery and/or cardiology

ABDOMINAL AND PELVIC INJURIES

Intra-abdominal injuries are the third leading cause of death in pediatric trauma patients. They occur in approximately 6% of children with blunt trauma to the torso and up to 25% of children with multisystem trauma. Blunt trauma from motor vehicle accidents, falls, and abuse is the most common mechanism of injury. Abdominal trauma most often leads to solid organ injury. Nonoperative management is the standard of care for the majority of abdominal injuries, with a greater than 90% success rate.

Trauma to the pediatric abdomen may be overlooked secondary to other injuries or decreased verbal ability related to a depressed level of consciousness or the patient's age. Suspicion of trauma should be based on the mechanism of injury and physical examination findings. Laboratory studies are not sensitive or specific screening tools for intra-abdominal injury but may be used in conjunction with the physical examination and imaging. Abdominal CT with intravenous contrast is the gold standard for imaging pediatric patients at high risk for intra-abdominal injury. Plain abdominal radiographs are of limited diagnostic utility. The Focused Assessment with Sonography for Trauma (FAST) examination is useful for identifying intra-abdominal injuries in adults, but the sensitivity is only 35% in hemodynamically stable children.

Multiple studies have attempted to determine which children require CT imaging following blunt abdominal injury. In 2009, Holmes and colleagues derived and validated an algorithm to identify patients with intra-abdominal injury after blunt trauma. A more recent study determined that patients with a GCS greater than 13, no abdominal pain or vomiting, and an unremarkable abdominal and thoracic examination are at very low risk of intra-abdominal injury. Normal chest X-ray, urinalysis, transaminases, and pancreatic enzymes further decrease the risk. Such patients likely do not require abdominal CT. Children with depressed mental status, evidence of abdominal wall trauma, and moderate to severe abdominal tenderness are at greatest risk of intraabdominal injury. Observation without imaging may be appropriate for some patients with one or more lower-risk variables, but this decision should be made in consultation with a pediatric surgeon.

SPLENIC INJURIES

Clinical Presentation Splenic injury often occurs from a direct blow to the left upper quadrant. Patients may complain of diffuse abdominal tenderness, left upper quadrant pain, or left shoulder pain (Kehr sign). The physical examination may reveal left upper quadrant abrasions, abdominal distention, or tenderness with or without peritoneal signs.

Diagnostic Evaluation Laparotomy should be considered for patients with persistent hemodynamic instability or those requiring more than 40 mL/kg of packed red blood cells to maintain stability. Angiographic embolization is a potential alternative to splenectomy and may preserve splenic function. Stable patients with suspected splenic injury should undergo a CT scan with intravenous contrast to determine the grade of injury and to look for other intra-abdominal injuries.

Management Most children with splenic injuries can be managed nonoperatively. Patients with splenic injuries should be hospitalized for serial abdominal examinations, close vital sign, and hematocrit monitoring. The majority of patients with isolated splenic injuries do not require intensive care unit observation, and only 10% to 20% of those treated nonoperatively require blood transfusion. Packed red blood cell transfusion should be considered for patients with symptomatic anemia or hemoglobin less than 7 g/dL. To avoid excessive hospitalization and bed rest, the American Pediatric Surgical Association (APSA) guidelines now recommend that the length of hospital stay and activity restriction be guided by hemodynamic status instead of grade of injury (**Figure 158-3**). One of the major goals of treatment is the preservation of splenic immune function. Patients undergoing splenectomy should be vaccinated against *S. pneumoniae*, *H. influenzae*, and *N. meningitidis*. Vaccination is recommended 14 days postoperatively; administration prior to discharge may be appropriate if there is concern for loss of follow-up. The approach to antibiotic prophylaxis remains controversial but is generally recommended for a minimum of 1 year post-splenectomy for all patients and until 5 years of age for young children.

LIVER INJURIES

Children have underdeveloped rib cages, decreased overlying soft tissue, and proportionally larger solid organs. As a result, liver injury often occurs by lower velocity mechanisms, including falls and sports. The liver's dual blood supply and close proximity to the inferior vena cava put patients with liver injuries at risk for severe bleeding after blunt trauma.

Clinical Presentation Patients with liver injuries may present with abdominal and right shoulder pain. Some children may report shortness of breath. On examination, they exhibit nonspecific abdominal tenderness that is commonly most severe over the right upper quadrant. Liver injuries should raise suspicion for associated rib fractures or trauma to other abdominal organs.

Diagnostic Evaluation In hemodynamically stable patients, elevated transaminases (aspartate transaminase >120; alanine transaminase >90) have been correlated with liver injury. CT should be obtained in high-risk patients to grade the extent of the liver injury and evaluate for associated injuries. However, it should be noted that the grade of liver injury on CT does not reliably predict patient outcome.

Management Most liver injuries (>90%) can be managed nonoperatively. Indications for laparotomy include persistent hemodynamic instability or a transfusion requirement of greater than 40 mL/kg of packed red blood cells. Hepatic artery embolization is an alternative to surgery in some cases. For hemodynamically stable patients, the goals of

Updated APSA Blunt Liver/Spleen Injury Guidelines 2019

Admission

- **ICU Admission Indicators**
  - Abnormal vital signs after initial volume resuscitation
- **ICU**
  - Activity - Bedrest until vitals normal
  - Labs - q6hour CBC until vitals normal
  - Diet - NPO until vital signs normal and hemoglobin stable
- **Ward**
  - Activity - No restrictions
  - Labs - CBC on admission and/or 6 hours after injury
  - Diet - Regular diet

Procedures

- **Transfusion**
  - Unstable vitals after 20 cc/kg bolus of isotonic IVF
  - Hemoglobin <7
  - Signs of ongoing or recent bleeding
- **Angioembolization**
  - Signs of ongoing bleeding despite pRBC transfusion
  - Not indicated for contrast blush on admission CT without unstable vitals
- **Operative exploration with Control of Bleeding**
  - Unstable vitals despite pRBC transfusion
  - Consider massive transfusion protocol

Set Free

- Based on clinical condition **NOT** injury severity (grade)
- Tolerating a diet
- Minimal abdominal pain
- Normal vital signs

Aftercare

- **Activity Restriction**
  - Restricting activity to grade plus 2 weeks is safe
  - Shorter restrictions may be safe but there is inadequate data to support decreasing these recommendations
- **Follow up Imaging**
  - Risk of delayed complications following spleen and liver injuries is low
  - Consider imaging for ***symptomatic*** patients with prior high grade injuries

FIGURE 158-3. Updated APSA Blunt Liver/Spleen Injury guidelines 2019. (Reproduced with permission from Williams RF, Grewal H, Jamshidi R, et al. Updated APSA Guidelines for the Management of Blunt Liver and Spleen Injuries. *J Pediatr Surg.* 2023;58(8):1411-1418.)

inpatient admission include fluid resuscitation, serial abdominal examinations, pain control, and evaluation for associated injuries.

SMALL AND LARGE BOWEL INJURIES

Clinical Presentation Intestinal injuries are uncommon, accounting for less than 5% of injuries in children presenting with blunt trauma, and their diagnosis can be challenging. The most common intestinal injury is perforation of the jejunum or ileum. The mechanism of injury is often a direct blow to the abdomen from a bicycle handlebar, child abuse, or motor vehicle accident. The physical examination may initially reveal only abdominal tenderness or ecchymosis. Over time, fever, peritoneal signs, abdominal distension, vomiting, or evidence of shock can develop due to obstruction or gradual leakage of intestinal contents. The "seatbelt syndrome" is the triad of abdominal wall bruising, intestinal and mesenteric contusions, and lumbar spine injury (Chance fractures) that can occur when a child is restrained with an improperly fitted lap belt in a motor vehicle collision. Bowel perforation and obstruction may present 24 to 48 hours after a lap-belt injury.

Diagnostic Evaluation Serial abdominal examinations are important for diagnosing intestinal injuries. CT may not detect intestinal perforations. The presence of a seatbelt or handlebar mark, abdominal tenderness, bowel wall edema, or free fluid in the abdomen (without other organ injury) should raise the suspicion of an intestinal injury. Patients with a seatbelt sign should be carefully evaluated for thoracolumbar spine injury and plain radiographs obtained if there is clinical concern for fracture.

Management Patients with a concerning history and physical examination in the absence of definitive imaging findings should be made NPO and admitted for inpatient observation with prompt pediatric surgery consultation for possible operative management.

Late Complications Duodenal hematoma is a rare injury that results from a blunt force trauma to the epigastrium. This injury may present several days after a traumatic event with signs and symptoms consistent with a bowel obstruction. Common clinical findings include abdominal pain, gastric distention, and bilious emesis. The diagnosis can be made by CT scan or an upper gastrointestinal series. Management includes nasogastric decompression and parenteral nutrition. Operative drainage of the hematoma is sometimes necessary.

PELVIC INJURIES

Pediatric pelvic fractures are relatively rare. Compared to adults, the pediatric pelvic skeleton is more flexible and has stronger ligaments. Avulsion fractures are more common and are primarily sports-related injuries. Ring disruption fractures are associated with high-impact trauma such as a motor vehicle accident. Overall, mortality is low and hemorrhage is the most concerning complication of a pelvic fracture. Hemorrhage is rare in children, however, as the pediatric vasculature vasoconstricts more readily than that of adults. Pelvic injury can be associated with genitourinary injury as well as other traumatic injuries throughout the body.

Clinical Presentation Clinicians should have a high index of suspicion for pelvic injury with high-impact mechanisms, altered mental status, or hemodynamic instability. Pelvic injury can present as pain, bruising, or inability to bear weight. The pelvis should be assessed on all trauma patients by visual inspection followed by palpation of all bony prominences. Rocking can elicit pain when pelvic fractures are present and increased mobility of the pelvic joints is concerning for severe fractures. Hemodynamic instability may be present if there is significant hemorrhage in the pelvis. In these patients, pelvic manipulation must be limited as it can dislodge a clot, worsening hemorrhage.

Diagnostic Evaluation Standard trauma imaging includes pelvic X-rays for all trauma patients. CT remains the gold standard but requires significant radiation exposure. CT is recommended if x-ray is suggestive of a pelvic ring fracture.

Management Most pediatric pelvic fractures are managed nonoperatively. Surgery is performed for unstable pelvic ring fractures. If there is a concern for hemorrhage into the pelvis or a volume-expanding fracture (anterior-posterior compression or vertical shear fracture), a pelvic binder is used until surgical intervention can be accomplished. If urethral injury is suspected, a retrograde urethrogram should be performed prior to catheterization. Children should be followed until skeletally mature to monitor for hip dysplasia and growth disturbances.

ABDOMINOPELVIC INJURY CONSULTATION

General surgery should be consulted for patients with pneumoperitoneum, persistent abdominal pain or vomiting, or evidence of liver, spleen, or intestinal injury on CT. Interventional radiology consultation should be considered for potential splenic or hepatic artery embolization.

Pelvic injuries may require orthopedic surgery, urology, and general surgery consultations based on the extent of injury.

ABDOMINOPELVIC INJURY ADMISSION CRITERIA

- Evidence of intra-abdominal injury on CT
- Persistent abdominal tenderness or vomiting despite normal imaging
- Low hematocrit
- Hemodynamic instability
- Unstable pelvic fracture
- Inability to tolerate oral intake
- Pain uncontrolled by oral analgesia
- Inability to bear weight
- Trauma with multiple injuries

ABDOMINOPELVIC INJURY DISCHARGE CRITERIA

- Stable or improving symptoms and examination
- Stable hematocrit
- Normalization of vital signs
- Able to maintain hydration by mouth
- Pain controlled by oral analgesia
- Clearance by surgical services

KEY POINTS

- Traumatic injuries are the leading cause of death in children.
- The initial evaluation of any trauma patient follows ATLS guidelines.
- The majority of traumatic injuries experienced by children can be managed nonoperatively in collaboration with a surgeon.
- The imaging modality is determined by the location and degree of injury.
- The goals of hospitalization are airway management, hemodynamic stability, serial examinations, intravenous hydration, pain control, and surgical management as indicated.

SUGGESTED READINGS

Alemayehu H, Aguayo P. Pediatric blunt thoracic trauma. *J Pediatr Intensive Care*. 2015;4(1):35-39.

American College of Surgeons. Advanced Trauma Life Support® ATLS® Student Course Manual. 10th ed. Chicago, IL: American College of Surgeons; 2018.

Badawy MK, Dayan PS, Tunik MG, et al. Prevalence of brain injuries and recurrence of seizures in children with posttraumatic seizures. *Acad Emerg Med*. 2017;24(5):595-605.

Centers for Disease Control and Prevention, National Center for Injury Prevention and Control. National Action Plan for Child Injury Prevention. Atlanta (GA): CDC, NCIPC; 2012.

Chatoorgoon K, Brown RL, Garcia VF, Falcone RA Jr. Role of computed tomography and clinical findings in pediatric blunt intestinal injury: a multicenter study. *Pediatr Emerg Care.* 2012;28(12):1338-1342.

Gates RL, Price M, Cameron DB, et al. Non-operative management of solid organ injuries in children: an American Pediatric Surgical Association Outcomes and Evidence Based Practice Committee systematic review. *J Pediatr Surg.* 2019;54(8):1519-1526.

Haarbauer-Krupa JK, Glang A, Kurowski B, Breiding MJ. Report to Congress: The Management of Traumatic Brain Injury in Children: Opportunities for Action. Atlanta, GA: Centers for Disease Control and Prevention; 2018.

Herman MJ, Brown KO, Sponseller PD, et al. Pediatric Cervical Spine Clearance: A Consensus Statement and Algorithm from the Pediatric Cervical Spine Clearance Working Group. *J Bone Joint Surg Am.* 2019;101(1):e1.

Kuppermann N, Holmes JF, Dayan PS, et al. Identification of children at very low risk of clinically-important brain injuries after head trauma: a prospective cohort study [published correction appears in Lancet. 2014;383(9914):308]. *Lancet.* 2009;374(9696):1160-1170.

Leonard JR, Jaffe DM, Kuppermann N, Olsen CS, Leonard JC; Pediatric Emergency Care Applied Research Network (PECARN) Cervical Spine Study Group. Cervical spine injury patterns in children. *Pediatrics.* 2014;133(5):e1179-e1188.

Liang T, Roseman E, Gao M, Sinert R. The utility of the focused assessment with sonography in trauma examination in pediatric blunt abdominal trauma: a systematic review and meta-analysis. *Pediatr Emerg Care.* 2021;37(2):108-118.

Lindholm EB, Malik A, Parikh D, et al. Single-lateral cervical radiograph in pediatric trauma is equivalent to multiple views. *J Trauma Acute Care Surg.* 2019;87(4):813-817.

Mikrogianakis A, Grant V. The kids are alright: pediatric trauma pearls. *Emerg Med Clin North Am.* 2018;36(1):237-257.

Nigrovic LE, Schunk JE, Foerster A, et al. The effect of observation on cranial computed tomography utilization for children after blunt head trauma. *Pediatrics.* 2011;127(6):1067-1073.

Notrica DM, Eubanks JW 3rd, Tuggle DW, et al. Nonoperative management of blunt liver and spleen injury in children: Evaluation of the ATOMAC guideline using GRADE. *J Trauma Acute Care Surg.* 2015;79(4):683-693.

Reynolds SL. Pediatric thoracic trauma: recognition and management. *Emerg Med Clin North Am.* 2018;36(2):473-483.

Shook JE, Chun TH, Conners GP, et al. Management of pediatric trauma. *Pediatrics.* 2016;138: e20161569.

Streck CJ, Vogel AM, Zhang J, et al. Identifying children at very low risk for blunt intra-abdominal injury in whom CT of the abdomen can be avoided safely. *J Am Coll Surg.* 2017;224(4):449-458.e3.

CHAPTER 159

Surgical Issues: Ear, Nose, and Throat

Rebecca E. Rosenberg, MD, MPH, FAAP and Megan M. Gaffey, MD

BACKGROUND

Maintaining a safe airway is one of the primary concerns when managing patients with otorhinolaryngology pathology. This includes not only ensuring adequate size and patency of the airway but also protecting against aspiration of blood, food, and secretions into the airway.

ANATOMIC REVIEW OF DEVELOPING AIRWAY

Because infants and children have disproportionately narrower airways, any additional structural impairment such as edema, inflammation, or mucus causes exponential decrease in airflow (**Figure 159-1**).

Although loss of a secure airway is one of the most feared complications in any pediatric patient, other disorders of the head and neck can have significant morbidity if not appropriately addressed. The head and neck have an abundant vascular supply, and blood loss can be brisk and substantial. Seemingly minor trauma can lead to significant cosmetic deformity if not promptly and appropriately treated. Localized infections can spread to the bloodstream or track along fascial planes to become life-threatening. The close proximity of head and neck structures to the brain, accompanied by the porous blood-brain barrier in young infants, facilitates easy intracranial spread of otolaryngologic disease or infection with potentially devastating results.

INDICATIONS FOR REFERRAL TO PEDIATRIC AIRWAY EXPERTISE

Most conditions that require otolaryngology referral can be safely and effectively managed in the outpatient setting. It is common for patients who are already hospitalized, especially postintubation or with respiratory diagnoses, to develop or have coexisting head and neck conditions.

Lastly, setting and capacity of providers and ancillary staff, radiology, and materials matter. While many otolaryngologic conditions can be managed successfully by general otolaryngologists, some conditions or situations merit timely including emergent referral or transfer to a pediatric otorhinolaryngologist. While not always immediately available outside of specialty settings, board-certified pediatric otorhinolaryngologists have the expertise and training for congenital airway conditions, airway reconstruction, and tracheostomy management. Medically complex patients are often optimally managed in multidisciplinary aerodigestive centers with subspecialists in pediatric airway surgery, pulmonology, and gastroenterology, along with sleep and swallowing specialists.

COMMON OTORHINOLARYNGOLOGY CONDITIONS IN INFANTS

INFANTS WITH NOISY BREATHING

A rapid preliminary assessment of the infant who presents with acute noisy breathing is essential and often transfer or timely referral to a pediatric subspecialist and center is indicated. The presence of retractions, change in work of breathing, vital sign instability, and gas exchange impairment provide a more accurate indicator of the patient's respiratory status than the quality of the noisy breathing. An infant with poor gas exchange and carbon dioxide retention will become lethargic and *less* noisy as obstruction worsens and airflow decreases. In such cases, the airway must be urgently secured in a controlled fashion by the most experienced pediatric provider available—this may be a neonatology provider in some settings, even for older infants.

However, many infants with subacute or chronic noisy breathing can be safely evaluated at bedside, without sedation or intubation. The history and physical examination will guide the initial management and workup of an infant with noisy breathing (**Tables 159-1, 159-2**). Careful history alone may suggest the diagnosis in more than 80% of cases.

A few components of the history are particularly important: age at onset of noisy breathing; quality of noisy breathing; quality of cry; duration of symptoms; and aggravating or alleviating factors. Bedside flexible fiberoptic laryngoscopy can often confirm the diagnosis by allowing examination of the entire upper airway as well as visualization of the larynx above the vocal cords.

In a stable infant with noisy breathing, the next step in the evaluation may include blood gases and plasma carbon dioxide to assess presence, duration, and type of airway compromise. Chest radiograph is the highest yield radiographic examination; focused anteroposterior and lateral neck films may be helpful in older infants. These imaging studies may assist with identification of the area of obstruction, asymmetry, or identify the presence of a foreign body or some pulmonary or even cardiovascular abnormalities. Guided by the index of suspicion and acuity, additional diagnostic information may be provided by airway fluoroscopy under sedation, esophagram, polysomnogram (PSG) also known as a "sleep study," echocardiogram, esophagram, computed tomography (CT), or magnetic resonance imaging (MRI) of the airway or neck.

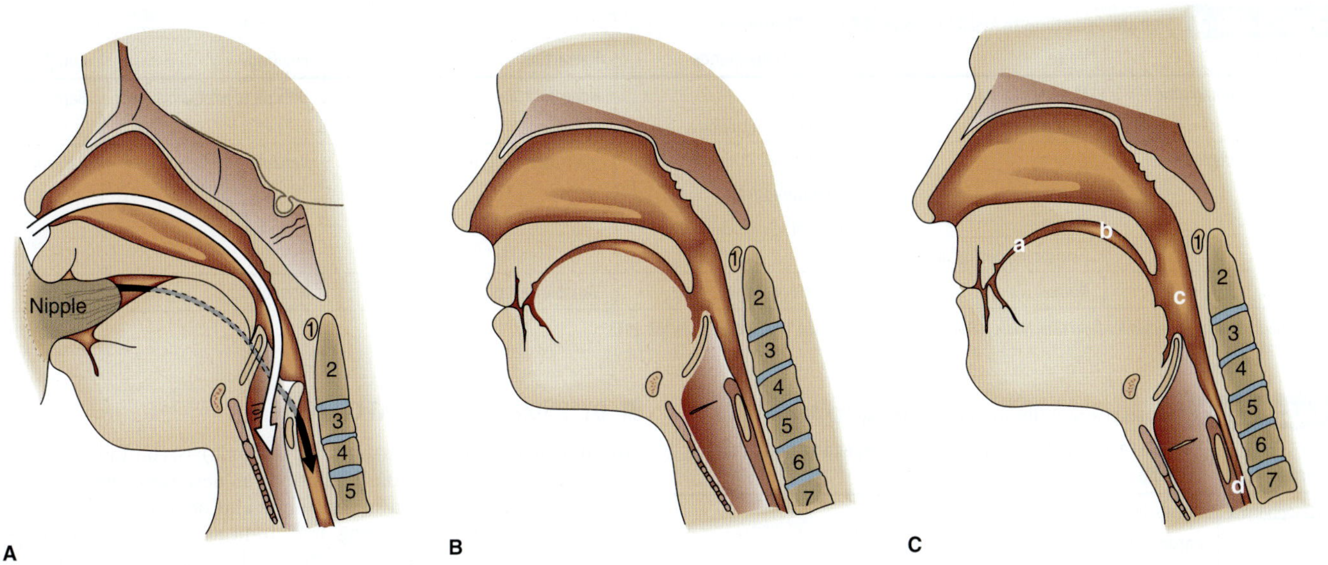

FIGURE 159-1. A: The infant oropharynx. The larynx is elevated, with the epiglottis touching the soft palate, creating a functional separation between the air passages (white arrow) and the food passages (black/gray arrow) in the pharynx. Food courses around the epiglottis, into the pharyngeal recess, and then to the esophagus. B: The toddler (2-3 years old) oropharynx. C: The adult oropharynx: (a) the oral preparatory phase, (b) the oral phase, (c) the pharyngeal phase, and (d) the esophageal phase. Note that the infant oral cavity is much smaller than the child or adult oral cavity, providing little space for manipulation of the food bolus. The larynx is elevated so that the epiglottis almost touches the soft palate, and the larynx is at the level of the first to third cervical vertebrae. The tongue is entirely within the oral cavity, with no oral region of the pharynx. In the toddlers, the larynx descends to the fifth cervical vertebra, and by adulthood, it descends to the sixth to seventh cervical vertebra. (Reproduced with permission from Kline MW, ed. *Rudolph's Pediatrics*. 23rd ed. New York: McGraw Hill; 2018.)

Any afebrile child admitted with acute noisy breathing should receive humidified air and be placed on continuous pulse oximetry monitoring. Supplemental oxygen can be reserved for situations with desaturations; overuse in patients who are saturating >90% will decrease respiratory drive and hide status changes. Systemic steroids and racemic epinephrine often provide effective first-line relief of acute airway obstruction.

The differential diagnosis of noisy breathing in the infant is extensive and includes pathology at all levels of the upper and lower airways (**Table 159-3**). Four of the more common causes are discussed below.

Laryngomalacia Laryngomalacia is the most common cause of stridor in young infants. It typically presents around 6 weeks of life with a high-pitched inspiratory stridor that is worse with supine position, feeding, and agitation. The majority of cases will resolve spontaneously by 12 to 18 months of age. The diagnosis is confirmed via flexible laryngoscopy which typically demonstrates short aryepiglottic folds, an omega-shaped epiglottis, and arytenoid prolapse (**Figure 159-2**). Patients with significant airway obstruction or failure to thrive require supraglottoplasty (division of the aryepiglottic folds and/or excision of the redundant arytenoid mucosa).

Vocal Cord Paralysis Vocal cord paralysis (VCP) is the second most common cause of stridor in infancy accounting for approximately 10% of all congenital laryngeal lesions. Unilateral VCP may be acquired from airway trauma or during surgery to correct congenital cardiac abnormalities. Bilateral VCP is usually neurogenic or idiopathic.

Infants with unilateral VCP typically have a weak, hoarse cry whereas infants with bilateral VCP commonly have airway obstruction that necessitates tracheostomy. Brain MRI is essential in patients with bilateral or suspicious unilateral VCP to rule out neurologic abnormalities (e.g., Arnold-Chiari malformation, hydrocephalus, congenital neuroblastoma). One of the biggest challenges in the surgical management of bilateral VCP paralysis is achieving an adequate airway without significantly compromising the quality of the voice or causing aspiration.

Subglottic Stenosis Subglottic stenosis is another common cause of stridor in infancy. Subglottic stenosis can be congenital due to congenital deformity of the cricoid cartilage or acquired because of prolonged or traumatic intubation. Severe cases present with stridor immediately after birth or failure to extubate. Milder cases can present as recurrent croup. Management is determined by the severity of the stenosis and the extent of respiratory distress and ranges from intermittent courses of steroids to laryngotracheal reconstruction or tracheostomy.

Subglottic Hemangioma Infants and toddlers with subglottic hemangiomas are typically asymptomatic at birth and present with biphasic stridor during the first few months of life as the hemangioma enters the proliferative phase. Approximately 50% of patients have a cutaneous hemangioma. Although the diagnosis is typically made via endoscopy, airway radiographs may show asymmetric narrowing of the subglottis. A variety of treatments have been utilized including systemic or injected corticosteroids, interferon alpha, laser excision, open excision, and tracheostomy. Oral propranolol is now the mainstay of therapy.

TABLE 159-1 History and Physical Examination for Airway Obstruction

History	Physical Examination
Time of onset: gradual, progressive, or sudden	Stridor, pitch, duration, and timing of the stridorous sound
Characteristics of cry	Careful inspection of the patient in the parent's arms
Relationship of stridor to feeding	Respiratory rate and degree of distress
Aspiration or reflux	Tachypnea and onset of fatigue
Cyanosis	Flaring of nasal alae and other signs of respiratory effort
Previous intubation	Auscultation of stridor
Careful, repeated questioning for possible foreign body aspiration	

Source: Reproduced with permission from Kline MW, ed. *Rudolph's Pediatrics*. 23rd ed. New York: McGraw Hill; 2018.

OLDER INFANTS AND CHILDREN WITH UPPER AIRWAY OR VOICE SYMPTOMS

As in young infants, a detailed, precise history with focus on chronicity of symptoms, especially regarding the timing and type of sound emitted, with precise examination findings, along with knowledge of patient's developmental skills, community infectious disease patterns, and past medical history can quickly narrow the differential of noisy breathing (see Tables).

TABLE 159-2 Sign and Symptoms to Assist With Site of Airway Obstruction

Location	Voice	Adventitious sounds	Retraction	Feeding	Cough
Laryngeal: supraglottic	Muffled "Hot potato"	Snoring Inspiratory fluttering	None until late	Difficult to impossible	Rare
Laryngeal: subglottic	Normal, hoarse, or absent (worsening obstruction)	Inspiratory-expiratory stridor Snoring	Intercostal early, then xiphoid	Variable	Barking
Tracheal	Normal	Expiratory and wheezing	Variable depending on severity	Normal	Brassy

Source: Reproduced with permission from Kline MW, ed. *Rudolph's Pediatrics*. 23rd ed. New York: McGraw Hill; 2018.

TABLE 159-3 Causes of Airway Obstruction in Infants and Children

Airway Area	Possible Causes of Obstruction, Likelihood Depending on Clinical Scenario
Nasopharynx	Adenoid hypertrophy Choanal atresia Encephalocele Nasal dermoid Nasal polyps Oropharynx Abscess (parapharyngeal, retropharyngeal, peritonsillar) Craniofacial anomalies (Apert, Robin) Cysts (branchial, thyroglossal) Foreign body Inflammatory Lingual thyroid Neoplasm (benign and malignant) Tonsillar hypertrophy
Larynx	Foreign body Inflammatory • Croup (bacterial and viral) • Epiglottitis (pending *Haemophilus influenzae* B vaccine receipt) • Miscellaneous; tuberculosis, diphtheria Laryngeal web Laryngocele Laryngomalacia Laryngospasm (extraesophageal reflux) Neoplasm • Laryngeal papilloma (see text) • Malignant (rhabdomyosarcoma, chondrosarcoma) • Vascular anomalies (lymphatic, hemangioma, venous) Posterior laryngeal cleft Trauma • Intubation (laryngeal or subglottic edema, subglottic stenosis) • External neck trauma Subglottic cyst (prominent after intubation) Subglottic stenosis Vocal fold paralysis
Trachea and bronchi	Complete tracheal rings (more prominent in trisomy 21) Compression by neoplasm of adjacent structure (thyroid, thymus, esophagus) Foreign body (tracheal or esophageal) Tracheal stenosis (congenital or secondary to intubation or tracheostomy) Trauma Vascular anomalies (rings and slings) Primary pulmonary disease (asthma/other reactive)

Source: Reproduced with permission from Kline MW, ed. *Rudolph's Pediatrics*. 23rd ed. New York: McGraw Hill; 2018.

DYSPHONIA AND THROAT CLEARING

Postviral or infectious hoarseness (dysphonia) is common, especially after upper airway infections. Persistent or new hoarseness, however, requires further evaluation for anatomic and/or functional pathology. Some persistent throat clearing may indicate psychological diagnoses (i.e., Tourette syndrome) or functional neurological disorder, also known as "habit cough." Asking about situational triggers and presence of cough or sound during sleep are important history elements. Referral to appropriate behavioral health and breathing clinics, in person or virtual, that use hypnosis, biofeedback, and other techniques can resolve such conditions surprisingly quickly.

Laryngeal papillomatosis, also known as recurrent respiratory papillomatosis (RRP), is the most common and typically benign neoplasm involving the pediatric larynx with 1000 new pediatric cases annually. In RRP, benign nonkeratinizing squamous papillomas caused by human papillomavirus types (HPV) 6 and 11 grow in the upper aerodigestive tract with a particular predilection for the larynx. Juvenile-onset RRP typically presents with subacute dysphonia (hoarseness) and/or intermittent stridor between the ages of 2 and 5 years. Risk factors for RRP include prolonged vaginal labor to a mother under age 20. Rates have been dropping due to uptake of the HPV vaccine.

Flexible laryngoscopy is often sufficient to make the diagnosis. Concurrent bronchoscopic evaluation is mandatory both to determine the extent of disease and to excise obstructing lesions. Treatment may

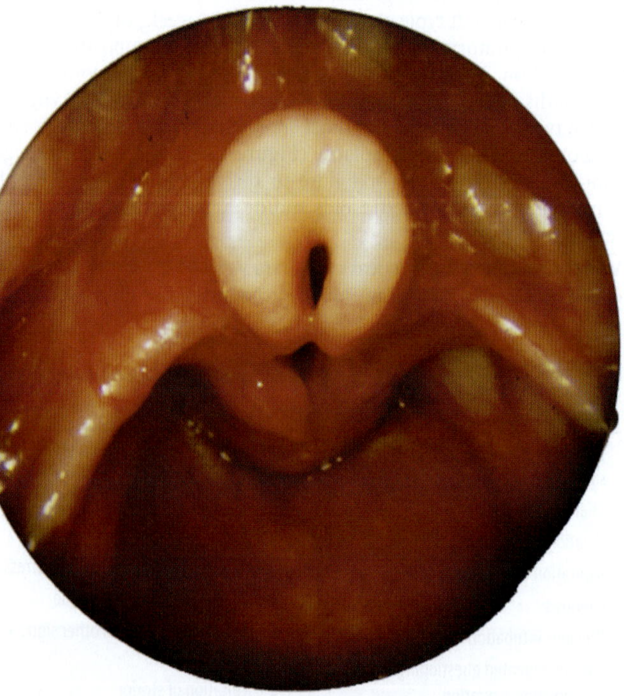

FIGURE 159-2. Laryngomalacia: Infantile appearing larynx with omega-shaped epiglottis and short aryepiglottic folds.

involve repeated surgical excision and adjuvant topical and intralesional and photodynamic therapies.

EPISTAXIS (NOSEBLEEDS)

Most spontaneous nosebleeds, or epistaxis, are self-limited, of benign etiology, and do not require further treatment or investigation. However, nosebleeds that are severe or recurrent require medical intervention. The anterior septum is particularly prone to nosebleeds with more than 90% originating from Little's area (Kiesselbach plexus), which is found along the anterior inferior septum approximately 1 cm from the nasal tip.

Epistaxis peaks between the ages of 3 and 8 years and has an extensive differential diagnosis. Minor trauma from nose picking or vigorous nose blowing and inflammation from upper respiratory infections or allergic rhinitis are the most common causes of epistaxis, along with exposure to heated dry air.

Intervention for epistaxis can be as simple as applying topical oxymetazoline and holding pressure just beneath the nasal bones, on the soft part of the nose. It is essential to hold pressure for a full 5 minutes without interruption. Silver nitrate cautery of prominent blood vessels on the anterior septum is often effective. If these measures are unsuccessful, packing may be required. Absorbable packing is ideal but not always effective. Patients with packing in place should be placed on prophylactic antibiotics to prevent toxic shock syndrome and considered for admission if they are not already inpatient. Surgical intervention is reserved for recalcitrant or life-threatening epistaxis.

Evaluation for and correction of an underlying condition such as tumor, coagulopathy (e.g., von Willebrand disease), or hereditary telangiectasia is essential for recurrent or severe epistaxis. Personal and family history of associated symptoms, such as menorrhagia, gum bleeding, telangiectasias, or epistaxis, suggest underlying hematological conditions requiring further management.

NECK MASS

Neck masses are common in children and rarely require admission. In cases of airway compromise, concern for malignancy, or serious illness, admission is warranted with both oxygen saturation and end-tidal carbon dioxide monitoring and careful positioning. Additionally, patients with a suspected infectious etiology who have failed outpatient therapy merit expert inpatient evaluation and management.

The differential diagnosis of a pediatric neck mass is extensive and varies by unilateral or bilateral presentation. It includes congenital anomalies, infectious and inflammatory conditions, traumatic lesions, and neoplasms. Key factors to assess on physical examination are: location of mass; consistency (solid, cystic, fluctuant); mobility; redness or changes to overlying skin and tenderness to palpation; and presence of co-occurring symptoms such as fever, weight changes, and night sweats.

In a child, bacterial cervical adenitis (see also Chapter 96) is the most common cause of a neck mass requiring admission. The most common superficial and deep neck spaces for infection are the submandibular and deep cervical nodes, and retropharyngeal and parapharyngeal spaces, respectively. The latter may lead to airway compromise or inability to take anything by mouth and often require admission for monitoring and management of airway, hydration, and pain.

Intravenous antibiotics are empirically started in many instances to cover presumed polymicrobial etiologies, including anaerobic pathogens. If the patient is nontoxic and naïve to any preadmission antibiotics and has no personal or family history of methicillin-resistant *Staphylococcus aureus* (MRSA), ampicillin/sulbactam or clindamycin often provides good coverage. Knowledge of local antibiograms is important since resistance prevalence greater than 10% renders an agent less effective for empiric use. Patients who have failed outpatient antibiotics, appear septic, are under- or unvaccinated, have implanted hardware such as cochlear implants or ventricular shunts, or have had recent surgery or hospitalization require broader empiric coverage. Agents typically include vancomycin, clindamycin, or linezolid for MRSA coverage and third/fourth-generation cephalosporin or equivalent for *Pseudomonas aeruginosa*.

Imaging is often useful for neck mass, especially for abscess evaluation. Sonography is a good initial test as it avoids radiation exposure and can be performed without sedation. If a deep neck space infection is suspected, contrast-enhanced computed tomography (CT) may be necessary to confirm the presence of a fluid collection versus inflammation as well as for surgical planning. Some small abscesses may be successfully treated with antibiotics alone, while large neck abscesses require incision and drainage. Serial monitoring by physical examination, clinical and radiographic findings will guide whether surgical intervention is warranted.

POSTOPERATIVE CARE OF OTORHINOLARYNGOLOGY PATIENTS

Although a variety of otorhinolaryngology patients may be admitted postoperatively to the acute care setting, two particular procedures warrant specific comment.

TONSILLECTOMY AND ADENOIDECTOMY

Tonsillectomy and adenoidectomy (T&A) are among the most frequently performed surgical procedures in children and adolescents and most are same-day surgeries. Current common indications include obstructive sleep apnea (OSA), recurrent tonsillitis, and associated airway malformations, though there are appreciable regional and center variations in practice. Shaving of this tissue may have fewer adverse effects than encapsular resection.

The 2019 American Academy of Otolaryngology–Head and Neck Surgery guidelines detail indications for surgery as well as preoperative diagnostic evaluation including polysomnography as well as perioperative and postoperative management. In properly selected patients, T&A may be safely performed as an outpatient procedure.

The main immediate postoperative risks of T&A include airway compromise, hemorrhage, dehydration, and suboptimally managed pain (odynophagia) leading to further dehydration. Most postoperative complications are attributed to the removal of the tonsils rather than the adenoids. Postoperative hemorrhage from adenoidectomy alone is 0.22% compared to 0.5% to 10% following tonsillectomy with or without adenoidectomy, respectively. Shaving may be employed rather than encapsulated resection.

Pain control can be challenging following T&A. Multimodal analgesia that "stays ahead of the pain" is effective and serves important purposes in reducing pain, increasing oral intake and preventing dehydration, and even decreasing inflammation. Standing acetaminophen and/or ibuprofen are safe, effective, and not associated with increased postoperative hemorrhage.

Certain pediatric patient populations are at higher risk for airway and respiratory complications. Overnight monitoring for reactive airway edema and other compromise after tonsillectomy is indicated if children are <3 years old, have severe presurgical obstructive sleep apnea (apnea-hypopnea index ≥10 obstructive events/hour, oxygen saturation nadir <80%, or both), or have any of the following comorbidities: obesity, hypotonia, Down syndrome, craniofacial abnormalities, neuromuscular disorders, sickle cell disease, or mucopolysaccharidoses. These patients have an increased risk for postoperative airway obstruction and respiratory insufficiency or failure.

Respiratory complications fall along a spectrum from mild oxygen desaturations requiring repositioning, gentle oral secretion clearance, and closer monitoring, to possible steroid administration if significant drooling and persistent airway concerns. In patients with pre-existing OSA who develop significant respiratory distress in the immediate postoperative period, clinicians must presume postobstructive pulmonary edema (POPE). POPE is typically managed with insertion of a stable airway, positive-pressure ventilation, and diuresis.

One rare subacute complication that is more often associated with adenoidectomy is inflammatory atlantoaxial subluxation (Grisel syndrome). The subluxation results from laxity of the transverse spinal ligaments, likely attributable to the use of monopolar cautery to remove the adenoid tissue and/or achieve hemostasis in the nasopharynx. Patients present with neck pain, torticollis, and C-spine tenderness. Diagnosis is confirmed via cervical spine CT scan and merits neurosurgical or orthopedic consultation, with conservative management including cervical collar, analgesia, and muscle relaxants.

KEY POINTS

- In an infant that presents with noisy breathing, history alone often identifies the diagnosis in up to 80% of cases.
- The top three causes of stridor in an infant are laryngomalacia, vocal fold paralysis, and subglottic stenosis.
- Subglottic hemangioma most commonly presents as biphasic stridor in an infant less than 6 months of age, with or without cutaneous hemangioma.
- Laryngeal papillomatosis should be considered in young children with subacute hoarseness and/or stridor.
- >90% of epistaxis originates from the anterior septum and can be managed conservatively with oxymetazoline and pressure or silver nitrate cautery.
- Neck mass is rarely an indication for admission unless there is resultant airway compression, risk for sepsis, failed outpatient management, or suspected malignancy.
- Airway management is one of the primary concerns in postoperative care of hospitalized otorhinolaryngology patients. Expectant management and appropriate bedside equipment are critical topics for communication among interdisciplinary teams especially familiarity with looming respiratory failure, worsening management of secretions, and team facility with intranasal trumpet and other artificial airways.

SUGGESTED READINGS

Barrette LX, Harris J, De Ravin E, Balar E, Moreira AG, Rajasekaran K. Clinical practice guidelines for pain management after tonsillectomy: Systematic quality appraisal using the AGREE II instrument. *Int J Pediatr Otorhinolaryngol.* 2022;156:111091.

Boesch RP, Balakrishnan K, Acra S, et al. Structure and functions of pediatric aerodigestive programs: a consensus statement. *Pediatrics.* 2018;141(3):e20171701.

Brook I. The increased risk of community-acquired methicillin-resistant *Staphylococcus aureus* in neck infections in young children. *Curr Infect Dis Rep.* 2012;14(2):119-120.

Bluestone CD, Simons JP, Healy GB, eds. *Bluestone and Stool's Pediatric Otolaryngology.* eBook, 2014, 5th ed. People's Medical Publishing House-USA, Shelton, Connecticut, 2014.

Cramer JD, Barnett ML, Anne S, et al. Nonopioid, Multimodal Analgesia as first-line therapy after otolaryngology operations: primer on nonsteroidal anti-inflammatory drugs (NSAIDs). *Otolaryngol Head Neck Surg.* 2021;164(4):712-719.

Houin P, Stillwell P, DeBoer EM, Hoppe J. Respiratory Tract & Mediastinum. In: Bunik M, Hay WW, Levin MJ, Abzug MJ. eds. *Current Diagnosis & Treatment: Pediatrics.* 26th ed. McGraw Hill; 2022. Available at: https://accesspediatrics-mhmedical-com.ezproxy.med.nyu.edu/content.aspx?bookid=3163&sectionid=266219189. Accessed August 28, 2022.

Hurvitz M, Weinberger M. Functional respiratory disorders in children. *Pediatr Clin North Am.* 2021;68(1):223-237.

Kaditis AG, Alonso Alvarez ML, Boudewyns A, et al. European Respiratory Society statement on obstructive sleep disordered breathing in 1- to 23-month-old children. *Eur Respir J.* 2017;50(6):1700985.

Mitchell RB, Archer SM, Ishman SL, et al. Clinical Practice Guideline: Tonsillectomy in Children (Update)-Executive Summary. *Otolaryngol Head Neck Surg.* Tonsillectomy and Adenoidectomy - Pediatr Clin North Am. 2022;69(2):247-259.

Tunkel DE, Anne S, Payne SC, et al. Clinical Practice Guideline: Nosebleed (Epistaxis). *Otolaryngol Head Neck Surg.* 2020;162(1_suppl):S1-S38.

Wootten CT, Belcher R, Francom CR, Prager JD. Aerodigestive programs enhance outcomes in pediatric patients. 2019. *Otolaryngol Clin North Am.* 2019;52(5):937-948.

CHAPTER 160

Neurosurgical Issues

Sarah F. Denniston, MD and Mirna Giordano, MD

INTRODUCTION

Pediatric hospitalists care for children with neurosurgical issues in many aspects of clinical practice. Whether in a primary, co-management, or consultative role, hospitalists should be familiar with the clinical presentation, diagnostic evaluation, and management of common pediatric neurosurgical problems. This chapter focuses on hydrocephalus, moderate and severe accidental head trauma, and the surgical management of drug-resistant epilepsy. While increased intracranial pressure (ICP) may be a feature of both hydrocephalus and head trauma, increased ICP is primarily covered in the hydrocephalus section.

HYDROCEPHALUS

BACKGROUND

Hydrocephalus is an abnormal increase in the volume of cerebrospinal fluid (CSF) in the cranial cavity caused by a disturbance in CSF flow due to obstruction, impaired absorption, and rarely, overproduction. Hydrocephalus can be acute, subacute, or chronic. The clinical features of hydrocephalus can be subtle, particularly with a subacute presentation, so it is important to understand the pathophysiology and clinical presentation to avoid a delay in diagnosis and management.

Pathophysiology CSF is produced primarily by modified ependymal cells in the choroid plexus in each cerebral ventricle, and a small amount is produced by cerebral tissue. CSF circulates from the pair of lateral ventricles, through the foramen of Monro to the third ventricle, then through the aqueduct of Sylvius to the fourth ventricle. CSF flow continues through the paired lateral foramina of Luschka and the foramen of Magendie to the subarachnoid space, to the arachnoid granulations, and finally to the dural sinuses and into the venous drainage system for absorption (**Figure 160-1**). Under normal conditions, daily production should approximately equal absorption to maintain a fairly constant volume of CSF.

Mechanisms of hydrocephalus include obstructed CSF circulation, compromised absorption of CSF, and overproduction of CSF. In obstructive hydrocephalus (or noncommunicating hydrocephalus), CSF accumulates due to a structural blockage within the ventricular system or its connections to the subarachnoid space. Obstruction of CSF circulation is the most common mechanism, with dilatation of the ventricular system often seen proximal to the obstruction. In communicating hydrocephalus, CSF accumulates due to impaired absorption or overproduction of CSF, which can dilate the entire ventricular system. An increased amount of CSF typically results in increased ventricular size and increased ICP.

Increased Intracranial Pressure According to the Monro-Kellie doctrine, the brain is a closed compartment, and its internal pressure is determined by the volume of the three intracranial components: blood, CSF, and brain tissue. If any of the three intracranial components increase in volume, a compensatory decrease in another component must occur, or ICP will rise. Increased ICP is an emergency that requires immediate evaluation and management. Physical compression of the brain leading to a shift across the midline or herniation through the base of the skull can result in death.

CLINICAL PRESENTATION

Signs and symptoms of hydrocephalus are mainly due to increased ICP as a result of increased CSF volume. The time to clinical presentation is variable since hydrocephalus can be acute, subacute, or chronic. Pediatric patients can tolerate gradual increases in ICP, but most increases beyond 20 mm Hg are likely to be symptomatic. The classic vital sign

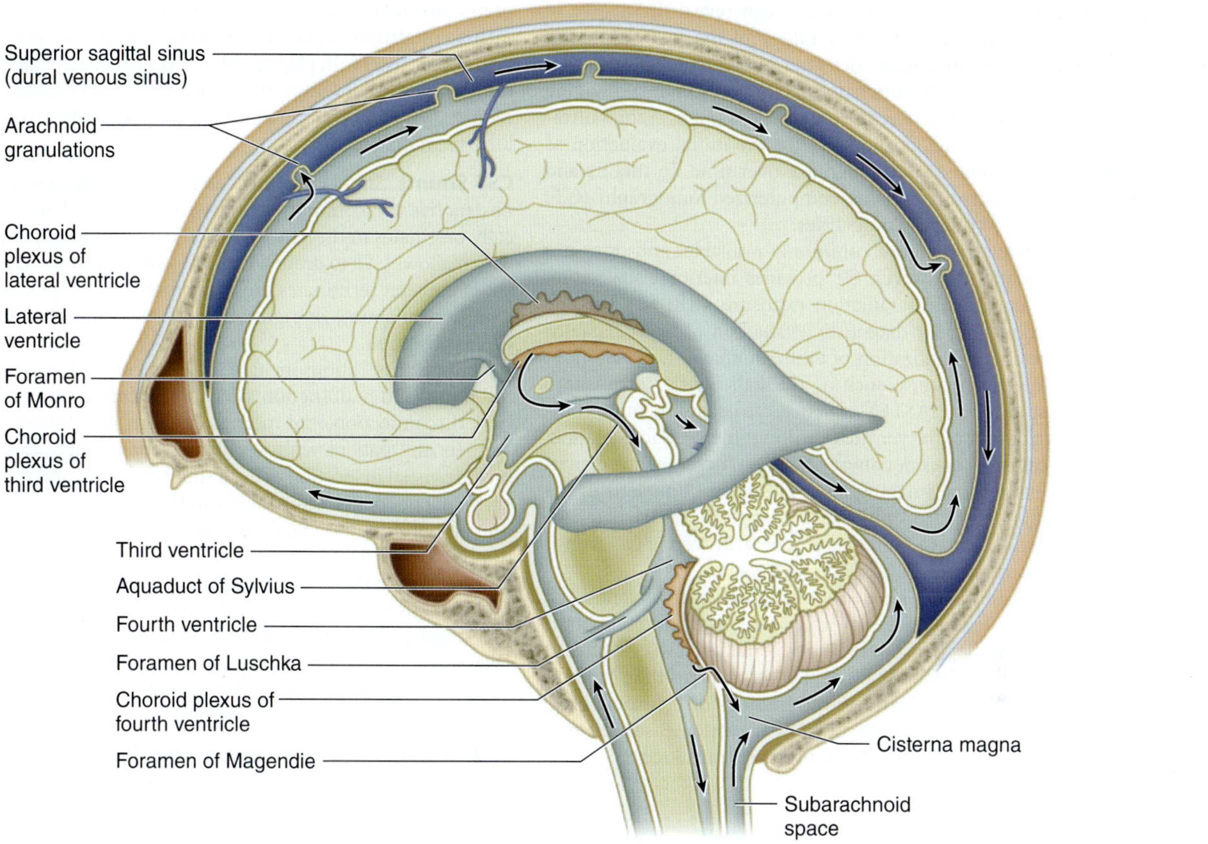

FIGURE 160-1. Illustration of cerebrospinal fluid circulation.

changes associated with increased ICP are known as Cushing triad and include hypertension (or less commonly, widening pulse pressure), bradycardia, and respiratory irregularity (or depression).

The symptoms of hydrocephalus are often nonspecific and vary by age. Infants may present with vague symptoms including poor feeding, vomiting, irritability, reduced activity, lethargy, and seizures. Since the cranial sutures have not fused, an enlarging head circumference is a common presentation in this population.

Older children with hydrocephalus can present with headaches as one of the earliest symptoms. The headaches classically occur in the morning, can be variable in intensity and location, and are often associated with nausea and vomiting. Other symptoms include vision changes (blurred or double vision), hearing symptoms (pulsatile tinnitus or hearing loss), change in personality or behavior, drowsiness, lethargy, dizziness, gait disturbance, and seizures. Developmental delays and cognitive decline can also occur in patients with hydrocephalus. In children with medical complexity, especially those who are non-verbal, an isolated behavior change can be a subtle but important presenting symptom that should not be overlooked.

Physical examination findings depend on age and may include:

- Vital signs: Hypertension, bradycardia, irregular respiratory rate
- Increased head circumference and/or frontal bossing
- Widening of cranial sutures
- Macewen sign ("cracked pot" sound with percussion of the head)
- Prominent and dilated scalp veins
- Tense, full, or bulging anterior fontanelle
- Setting sun sign (downward gaze, upward eyelid retraction revealing white sclera)
- Papilledema (can take a few days to develop)
- Cranial nerve III, IV, and VI nerve palsies, rarely VII
- Ataxia
- Hemiparesis, hyperreflexia, or hypertonia of extremities (late signs)

DIFFERENTIAL DIAGNOSIS

Hydrocephalus often presents in childhood as a result of many congenital and acquired etiologies (**Table 160-1**). The most common cause of congenital hydrocephalus is aqueductal stenosis, which obstructs CSF flow at the aqueduct of Sylvius. Common causes of acquired hydrocephalus are subarachnoid and intraventricular hemorrhage, which can lead to an inflammatory cascade and later fibrosis causing impaired absorption of CSF as well as possible obstruction of flow.

DIAGNOSTIC EVALUATION

The diagnosis of hydrocephalus is primarily based on a detailed patient history, presence of characteristic symptoms and physical examination

TABLE 160-1 Common Causes of Hydrocephalus

Congenital
Aqueductal stenosis
Arnold-Chiari malformation (Types I and II)
Dandy-Walker malformation
Neural tube defects (myelomeningocele, encephalocele)
Intrauterine infections (toxoplasmosis, cytomegalovirus, rubella, syphilis, zika virus)
Genetic disorders (X-linked hydrocephalus, Crouzon syndrome, Pfeiffer syndrome, Apert syndrome, Trisomy 13, Trisomy 18, mucopolysaccharidosis type VI)
Acquired
Subarachnoid hemorrhage
Intraventricular hemorrhage
Neoplasms (medulloblastoma, subependymal giant cell astrocytoma, ependymomas, Choroid plexus papilloma/carcinoma)
Infections (meningitis, mumps, cerebral abscess, neurocysticercosis)
Mass lesions (hematoma, intracranial cysts, neurocutaneous syndromes)

findings, and neuroimaging. Imaging studies can reveal the degree of ventricular enlargement and often the etiology of the hydrocephalus. Prenatally, ventriculomegaly can be detected by antenatal ultrasonography and further evaluated by antenatal magnetic resonance imaging (MRI) of the fetus. In infants where the fontanelle is open, cranial ultrasound is an appropriate imaging modality for the initial evaluation as well as a method to monitor ventricular size over time. In infants and children with suspected hydrocephalus, computerized tomography (CT) or MRI are the preferred imaging modalities.

Head CT is relatively fast, more commonly available, and does not typically require sedation. However, CT provides inferior visualization compared to MRI and involves radiation exposure. MRI has become the preferred neuroimaging for diagnostic evaluation of hydrocephalus and can provide detailed visualization of brain anomalies and CSF flow. Rapid-sequence MRI techniques, such as the half-Fourier acquisition single-shot turbo spin echo (HASTE) sequence, are becoming more commonly used for evaluation of the ventricles without the need for sedation.

Of note, hydrocephalus does not always cause an increase in ventricular size. Consequently, serial imaging must always be compared in the diagnostic evaluation of hydrocephalus. A change in ventricular size compared to a previous image could represent hydrocephalus, even if the ventricular measurements are appropriate for age.

Lumbar puncture (LP) is not needed to diagnose hydrocephalus. If a diagnostic LP is warranted in a patient with possible hydrocephalus and/or increased ICP, neuroimaging should be performed first to evaluate for a possible space-occupying lesion that could potentially result in cerebral herniation with an LP. In cases with subtle findings on neuroimaging, direct measurement of ICP may be obtained by LP with measurement of opening pressure or by a surgically placed pressure transducer.

MANAGEMENT

In most situations, hydrocephalus will result in progressive neurologic deterioration if left untreated. Temporizing procedures, particularly in premature infants or patients too unstable for definitive surgery, can include intermittent percutaneous removal of CSF through an implanted ventricular reservoir, placement of a ventriculosubgaleal shunt, or insertion of an external ventricular drain (EVD). Most cases of hydrocephalus require CSF shunt placement or endoscopic third ventriculostomy for long-term management.

CSF Shunts Shunt placement is the most common treatment of both obstructive and communicating hydrocephalus. The shunt catheter typically originates in the ventricles and connects to a one-way valve system which allows CSF to drain when pressure rises in the ventricle. The distal shunt catheter terminates most commonly in the peritoneum (ventriculoperitoneal shunt) or right atrium (ventriculoatrial shunt), where the CSF is absorbed.

Shunt complications include infection, often due to skin flora entering the shunt, and malfunction. Mechanical complications include obstruction, disconnection, and migration of any component of the shunt system. In any patient with a shunt, every physical examination should include visual inspection of each shunt reservoir and tract. Any overlying erythema or edema along the shunt tract could be a sign of a shunt infection or malfunction. The shunt tract should be palpated during examination for any kink, disconnection, or fluid collection along the shunt. In a shunted patient presenting with any symptom or examination finding discussed in the clinical presentation section above, hydrocephalus due to a shunt complication must be at the top of the differential diagnosis. Diagnostic evaluation of suspected shunt malfunction includes a head CT/MRI to evaluate ventricular size and plain radiographs of the tract (shunt series) to evaluate the integrity of the system.

Endoscopic Third Ventriculostomy Endoscopic third ventriculostomy (ETV) is a first-line treatment option for obstructive hydrocephalus, particularly for aqueductal stenosis. This procedure creates an outlet in the floor of the third ventricle that allows CSF to flow to the subarachnoid space, get absorbed into the superior sagittal sinus, and bypass the usual flow through the fourth ventricle (**Figure 160-2**). In certain

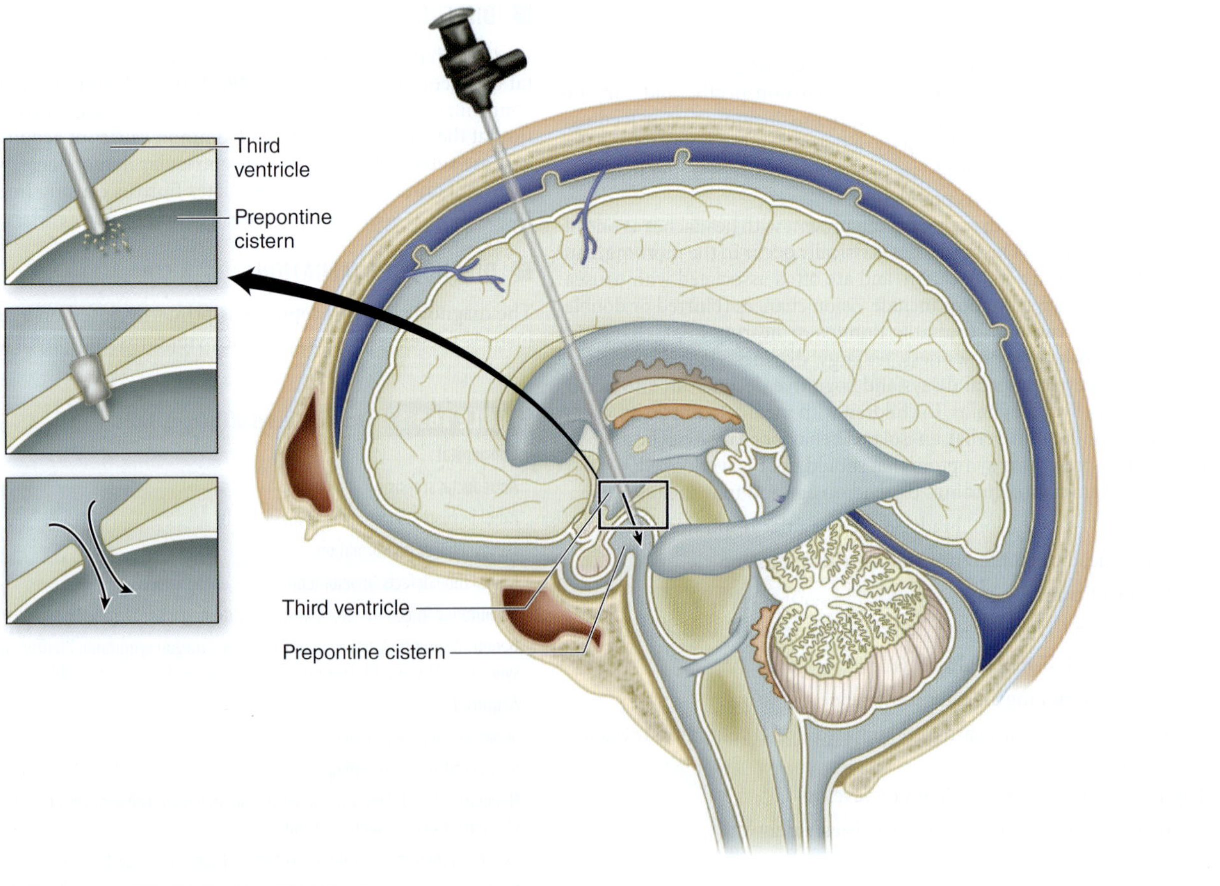

FIGURE 160-2. Illustration of endoscopic third ventriculostomy.

patients, ETV with/without choroid plexus cauterization can provide long-term treatment with fewer complications than shunts.

Increased Intracranial Pressure In a patient with signs or symptoms of increased ICP, medical management must begin immediately with initial stabilization. The goal of management is to minimize ICP elevation and maintain cerebral perfusion pressure to ensure adequate cerebral blood flow. The patient should be intubated via rapid sequence intubation if the Glasgow coma scale is ≤8 or if the patient is hypoventilating, as hypercapnia causes vasodilation.

While hyperventilation can reduce ICP through cerebral vasoconstriction and reduction in cerebral blood volume, hyperventilation can decrease cerebral oxygenation and induce brain ischemia. Therefore, prophylactic hyperventilation should be considered only in refractory increased ICP or impending herniation with advanced neuromonitoring to evaluate for ischemia. Cerebral perfusion should also be maintained with isotonic fluids to maintain euvolemia.

Multiple temporizing measures to manage increased ICP can be used, including control of position, temperature, pain, agitation, seizures, and bladder drainage. For example, the head can be elevated and positioned midline to promote venous drainage. Temperatures should be kept below 38°C with antipyretics and cooling blankets because the increased metabolic demands of hyperthermia increase ICP.

Intravenous administration of hyperosmolar agents such as hypertonic saline and mannitol are commonly used to manage acute increased ICP. Mannitol reduces ICP by (1) reducing blood viscosity, which allows cerebral blood flow to be maintained despite reduced cerebral blood volume, and (2) creating an osmotic gradient, which results in the gradual movement of fluid from the brain parenchyma into the systemic circulation. Hypertonic saline also creates an osmotic gradient by increasing serum osmolality. Additional management options to be considered when medical management fails and adequate cerebral perfusion pressure cannot be maintained include decompressive craniectomy, lumbar CSF drainage, and barbiturate coma.

Given various underlying causes of increased ICP (**Table 160-2**), management ultimately must include treatment of the underlying cause.

CONSULTATION

A diagnosis of hydrocephalus necessitates consultation with a neurosurgeon, which should be urgent if signs or symptoms of increased ICP are present. Consultation with other specialty services such as neurology, oncology, ophthalmology, and infectious diseases may be required depending on the underlying etiology of the presenting hydrocephalus.

SPECIAL CONSIDERATIONS

Children with medical complexity, especially non-verbal or developmentally delayed children with neurocognitive disabilities, are a high-risk population for developing hydrocephalus and CSF shunt malfunctions/infections. Subacute presentations of hydrocephalus and shunt malfunctions are often missed in this population, leading to a delay in diagnosis.

TABLE 160-2 Common Causes of Increased Intracranial Pressure
Head trauma/Intracranial hemorrhage (epidural hematoma, subdural hematoma, subarachnoid hemorrhage, intracerebral hematoma, diffuse axonal injury, cerebral edema)
Neoplasms (primary, metastatic)
Hydrocephalus
Intracranial infections (encephalitis, meningitis, cerebral abscess)
Venous sinus thrombosis
Vascular anomalies (arteriovenous malformation, vein of Galen malformation)
Hypoxic-ischemic encephalopathy
Diabetic ketoacidosis
Electrolyte abnormalities (hyponatremia, hypernatremia, hyperammonemia)
Status epilepticus
Craniosynostosis
Malignant hypertension
Pseudotumor cerebri (idiopathic intracranial hypertension)

HEAD TRAUMA

BACKGROUND

Head trauma is one of the most common childhood injuries. While many pediatric head injuries are minor, head injury is a leading cause of death and disability in children. Head trauma of variable severity can lead to traumatic brain injury (TBI), warranting hospitalization and possible surgical management. This chapter focuses primarily on moderate and severe accidental head injuries. See Chapter 158 "General Trauma" for an overview of minor head injuries. Various mechanisms can result in TBI, including falls, motor vehicle accidents, sports-related injuries, and abuse. Diffuse brain injury, usually due to acceleration and deceleration forces, is the most common type of TBI in children and ranges from concussion to diffuse axonal injury. More focal brain injuries include extracranial hematomas, skull fractures, and intracranial hemorrhage. Severity of TBI is classically characterized by the initial Glasgow coma scale (GCS) score: mild (GCS score 13-15), moderate (GCS score 9-12), and severe (GCS score ≤8). Moderate and severe TBI often have MRI or CT findings, whereas mild TBI typically does not have imaging findings.

Extracranial Hematomas Subgaleal hematomas are collections of blood in the loose tissue beneath the galea aponeurotica and above the periosteum. These hematomas can cross suture lines and are consequently in a potential space that can expand. In contrast, cephalohematomas are collections of blood between the periosteum and skull, and they are usually restricted from crossing suture lines. Subgaleal hematomas and cephalohematomas rarely require intervention, and needle drainage is contraindicated given the risk of infection.

Skull Fractures Skull fractures may be open (associated with overlying scalp injury) or closed. Major types include linear, comminuted (multiple branches), diastatic (bone edges split apart), depressed, and basilar. Linear fractures, the most common type of skull fractures in children, often have an associated hematoma and soft-tissue swelling, which may not have developed on early presentation. Depressed skull fractures are often the result of a more focal impact and have a higher likelihood of intracranial injury.

Intracranial Hemorrhage Epidural hematoma, subdural hematoma, and subarachnoid hemorrhage are typically due to blunt trauma. Epidural hematomas are more common in older children and develop when blood accumulates in the potential space between the dura mater and the skull. Bleeding may occur from a lacerated meningeal vessel, a dural venous sinus, or a diploic vein and is typically associated with a skull fracture. Acute subdural hematomas are more common in infants and younger children. They most often occur as a result of a high-velocity impact injury such as falls from great heights, motor vehicle accidents, and child abuse with acceleration-deceleration high-velocity trauma. Most subdural hemorrhages develop from tearing of the cortical bridging veins that drain into the dural venous sinuses with blood accumulating in the potential space between the dura mater and arachnoid layers. Subarachnoid hemorrhage arises from the tearing of the small blood vessels in the innermost meningeal layer, the pia mater.

Intraparenchymal hemorrhages can include focal contusions, diffuse axonal injury, and intracerebral hematomas. Deeper white matter hemorrhages may occur with severe angular forces. Brain stem, basal ganglia, and thalamus injuries may result from more severe acceleration injuries. Traumatic axonal injuries can also result from rapid acceleration-deceleration forces. Intraventricular hemorrhages may occur and, if large, may cause obstructive hydrocephalus.

Pathophysiology Brain injury from head trauma is a biphasic process. The primary injury is mechanical damage sustained immediately at the time of trauma from direct impact or shear forces when the gray and white matter travel at different speeds during deceleration or acceleration. Secondary injury refers to the ongoing disruption of cellular function from hypoxia, hypotension, inflammation, metabolic derangements, increased ICP, and cerebral edema. Early diagnosis and management are critical to address the primary injury, reduce the severity of secondary brain injury, and prevent subsequent injuries when the brain is vulnerable following a TBI.

CLINICAL PRESENTATION

At initial presentation, a detailed history should be obtained to help indicate potential complications from the trauma and guide the diagnostic evaluation and management. It is important to assess for any external evidence of head trauma that might suggest intracranial injuries. For example, several examination findings highly predictive of basilar skull fractures include hemotympanum, CSF rhinorrhea or otorrhea, mastoid ecchymosis (Battle sign), and periorbital ecchymoses (raccoon eyes).

Children with moderate and severe head trauma often have increased ICP. Signs and symptoms suggestive of increased ICP acutely following head trauma can indicate an acute epidural or large subdural hematoma. Symptoms of subdural hematomas may include depressed mental status, focal neurologic deficits, seizures, headache, vomiting, and other signs or symptoms of increased ICP. The presentation of subarachnoid hemorrhages is variable because they are often associated with other intracranial injuries. Subarachnoid hemorrhages in isolation may present with loss of consciousness, headache, and signs of meningeal irritation such as vomiting, photophobia, and nuchal rigidity.

Transient impairment in consciousness is common with minor head injuries, whereas more prolonged alterations in consciousness are more likely associated with severe head injuries. A detailed neurological examination should be performed at initial presentation. Focal neurologic deficits may help localize the brain injury. Motor and sensory function should be assessed to determine the integrity of the spinal cord in a conscious patient. Deep tendon reflexes should be evaluated because hyperactive reflexes could indicate head or spinal cord injury and asymmetric reflexes might suggest a unilateral lesion.

Examination of the pupil is an important part of the assessment of patients with head trauma. Size, shape, and reactivity to light can provide valuable information. For example, a fixed and dilated ipsilateral pupil due to compression of the ipsilateral oculomotor nerve is a hallmark of uncal herniation. Ocular movements can also help localize injury to the cranial nerves, brain stem, cerebellum, or cerebral hemispheres. Although papilledema can take up to 24 hours to develop in the setting of increased ICP, a funduscopic examination can give valuable information about the severity and mechanism of head injury and reveal signs of suspected abusive injury.

DIAGNOSTIC EVALUATION

The ultimate goal of evaluation is to determine if the child presenting with head trauma has TBI requiring further management while limiting unnecessary radiographic imaging. Initial laboratory studies to obtain and consider following serially include a complete blood count (CBC), chemistry studies, coagulation profile, blood type and crossmatch, blood gas, and toxicology screen.

An urgent, noncontrast head CT is warranted for initial evaluation of intracranial injury in patients with altered mental status, focal neurologic abnormalities, palpable skull fracture, signs of increased ICP, and/or other concerning findings on clinical presentation. Head CT is a quick, readily available study in most emergency departments to assess for skull fractures and acute hemorrhages. Epidural hematomas appear as a lens-shaped or biconcave high-density mass immediately under the skull (**Figure 160-3**). A CT scan of an acute subdural hematoma reveals a crescent-shaped or convex high-density collection directly overlying the convex surface of the brain (**Figure 160-4**). Unlike epidural hematomas, subdural hematomas are often associated with underlying brain injury, and the hemorrhages may be bilateral. On CT scan, diffuse axonal injury can appear as punctate hyperdensities at the gray-white matter junction.

MRI can offer a more complete evaluation of hemorrhage and can be used in dating the age of hemorrhage. Shearing injuries, more subtle parenchymal injuries, microhemorrhage, edema, and ischemia are best visualized on MRI sequences. MRI does not expose children to ionizing radiation, and rapid-sequence MRI protocols may offer a diagnostic imaging option that avoids sedation.

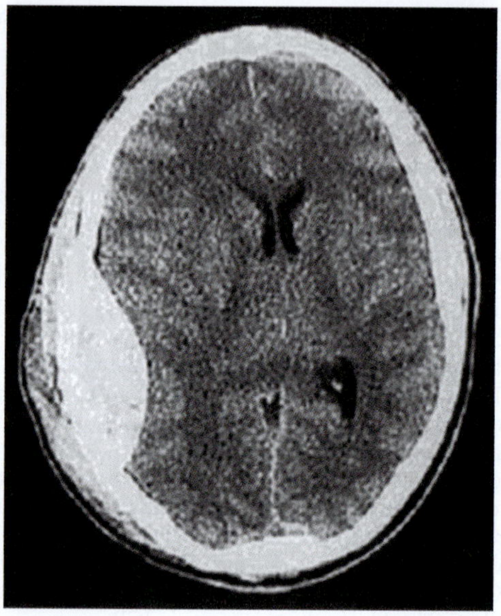

FIGURE 160-3. CT scan of an epidural hematoma with the characteristic lens shape.

MANAGEMENT

Management of moderate and severe head trauma focuses on preventing secondary injury by optimizing the delivery of oxygen and nutrients to the injured brain while minimizing metabolic demand. The priority is to evaluate and maintain an adequate airway, proper oxygenation and ventilation, and hemodynamic status. Many children with severe TBI will require prompt endotracheal intubation. The cervical spine needs to remain immobilized during intubation, and orotracheal intubation should be considered, particularly if there is suspicion of an anterior basilar skull fracture.

Following TBI, if suggested by the clinical presentation, acute management for increased ICP should be initiated. Sedation and pain control are required to achieve a level of anesthesia for invasive procedures, ICP control, and reduction of metabolic demand. Since seizures further increase ICP, immediate initiation of prophylactic antiepileptic medications following significant head injuries should be considered to mitigate the risk of posttraumatic seizures.

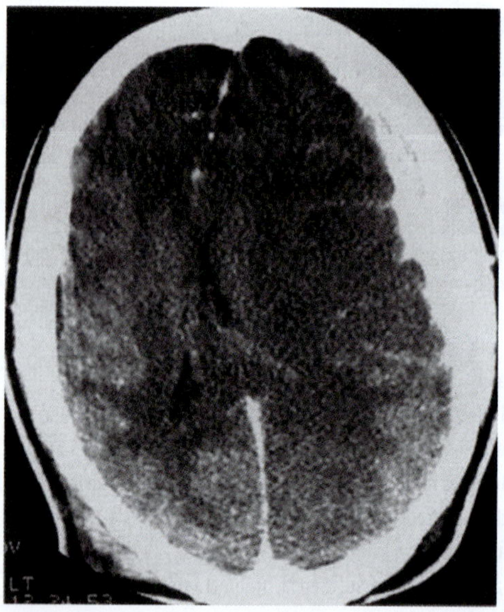

FIGURE 160-4. CT scan of a subdural hematoma with the characteristic crescent shape directly overlying the brain surface. (Reproduced with permission from Wilkins RH. Traumatic intracranial hematomas. In: Rengachary SS, Wilkins RH, eds. *Principles of Neurosurgery*. Philadelphia: CV Mosby; 1994:19.5. Copyright © Elsevier.)

In general, linear skull fractures heal without intervention. Basilar skull fractures require special consideration and management because of adjacent anatomic structures, an association with intracranial injury, and increased risk of meningitis. Leakage of CSF secondary to dural tears usually resolves spontaneously and should not require antibiotic therapy. There should be no attempt to stop the leakage with packing because packing may increase the chance of infection. Persistent leaks lasting longer than a week may need surgical intervention.

Any epidural hematoma requires prompt neurosurgical consultation. Many epidural hematomas require urgent surgical evacuation to prevent irreversible injury and death due to hematoma expansion and herniation. Epidural and acute subdural hematomas that are large and/or causing significant mass effect, focal neurologic deficits, and altered consciousness warrant urgent surgical intervention.

ADMISSION AND DISCHARGE CRITERIA

In general, patients with depressed skull fractures or any intracranial injury should be hospitalized. However, some small cerebral contusions may have little clinical significance. Patients with normal CT scans and resolution of symptoms typically do not warrant hospitalization. Patients with persistent symptoms, regardless of CT scan results, should be admitted. Admission or transfer to a pediatric trauma center is recommended if available, as treatment at pediatric trauma centers is generally associated with better outcomes. Prior to discharging any child following head trauma, symptoms indicative of intracranial injury requiring immediate return to medical care must be reviewed with caretakers.

CONSULTATION

Neurosurgical consultation should be obtained for most cases of moderate and severe TBI. All epidural hematomas and some subdural hematomas warrant neurosurgical consultation. Skull fractures that warrant neurosurgical consultation include depressed fractures, large diastatic fractures, fractures involving the frontal sinuses, and fractures involving tears in the dura.

Children who experience moderate and severe TBI can have medical disabilities, cognitive difficulties, neurodevelopmental deficits, and behavioral impairments. They should be referred for early intervention, rehabilitation services, and/or neuropsychiatric testing. Families and the child may benefit from psychosocial counseling.

SPECIAL CONSIDERATIONS

Multiple secondary short-term and long-term complications can arise following head trauma in children. Early posttraumatic seizures are more frequent in younger children and often present within 24 hours of injury. These immediate posttraumatic seizures seldom result in future complications or epilepsy. A range of medical, cognitive, developmental, emotional, and behavioral issues can present months and years after the injury. The severity of issues can change over time and may not be fully realized until years after the injury when higher-level functioning is required to meet milestones.

Prevention Prevention strategies for accidental pediatric head injury include educating parents and children on the proper use of car seats and vehicular restraints, and the importance of helmet use during certain activities. Education should also address safety in the home, such as the use of window guards and safety gates.

EPILEPSY SURGERY

BACKGROUND

Approximately 20% to 40% of children with epilepsy have persistent, frequent seizures refractory to antiepileptic medications. This can have neurodevelopmental, psychosocial, medical, and financial implications. For children who have drug-resistant epilepsy (DRE), surgical options should be considered in consultation with neurology and neurosurgery. The goal of surgical management of DRE is to resect or alter the epileptogenic tissue to eliminate the seizures (curative) or reduce the seizure burden (palliative) without causing neurological, behavioral, or other deficits. For children who are not surgical candidates or have not had successful surgical results, implantation of a vagal nerve stimulator (VNS) may be considered to improve seizure control.

DIAGNOSTIC EVALUATION

Presurgical evaluation for epilepsy surgery aims to identify the epileptogenic zone and correlate the area with function to determine the feasibility and safety of surgery. This comprehensive evaluation includes a clinical history, routine and long-term video electroencephalography (EEG), neuropsychological testing, high-resolution structural MRI, and other specialized neuroimaging studies such as magnetoencephalography and functional MRI. Of note, the intracarotid sodium amobarbital procedure (Wada test) was traditionally used to identify the laterality of the dominant language and memory areas in the brain. However, the Wada test has been largely supplanted by functional MRI testing for the presurgical evaluation. If the epileptogenic zone cannot be delineated with noninvasive testing, intracranial EEG may be conducted in the form of electrocorticography using subdural grid electrodes or stereotactic EEG using depth electrodes. Cortical stimulation mapping may then be used to localize the epileptogenic zone and functional zones (such as motor, sensory, and language) through direct electrical stimulation of the cerebral cortex.

MANAGEMENT

Epilepsy surgery originally focused on resecting or disconnecting the epileptogenic zone through procedures such as lobectomy, hemispherectomy, and corpus callosotomy. Less invasive surgical techniques such as ablation and neuromodulation are now additional surgical options to improve outcomes for management of DRE.

The surgical approach is based on the seizure type and epileptic lesion characteristics. Children with a well-localized, cortically based, single epileptic lesion can have high success rates with resection of the focal cortical lesion, called a lesionectomy. Lobectomy is a focal resection that removes the part of the brain where the seizure originates and is an excellent treatment option for seizures arising from one area of the brain. Specifically, temporal lobectomy is a common type of epilepsy surgery with high success rates and can be significantly more effective than medical management. If an entire cerebral hemisphere is diffusely involved, children can be considered for resection of the hemisphere (hemispherectomy) or tissue disconnection of the cortex of the involved hemisphere (functional hemispherectomy). Corpus callosotomy is a palliative surgical procedure that surgically divides the fibers of the corpus callosum to prevent synchronization of epileptic activity between hemispheres.

A variety of medical and neurologic complications can be associated with invasive monitoring during presurgical evaluation or after the surgical procedure. Potential complications include CSF leak, infection, intracranial hematomas, hydrocephalus, and new neurologic deficits. Apprehension to consider epilepsy surgery by families, patients, and referring physicians may deter appropriate candidates from being evaluated for epilepsy surgery.

DRE can impact neurodevelopment in children, and early surgical intervention has the potential to minimize cognitive delays, improve psychomotor function, and result in seizure freedom for some children. The greater plasticity of pediatric brains compared to adult brains contribute to favorable outcomes following even extensive surgical procedures.

SPECIAL CONSIDERATIONS

Children with refractory epilepsy who undergo surgical treatment can have significant reductions in healthcare utilization compared to children treated only with medication. A reduction in inpatient hospitalizations, emergency department encounters, ambulatory visits, and use of antiepileptic medications has been shown following surgery. Epilepsy surgery can significantly impact resource utilization, lower healthcare costs, and most importantly, improve the quality of life for children with DRE.

KEY POINTS

Hydrocephalus

- Hydrocephalus is an abnormal increase in cerebrospinal fluid (CSF) in the cranial cavity caused by a disturbance in CSF flow due to obstruction, impaired absorption, and overproduction.
- Signs and symptoms of hydrocephalus are mainly due to increased intracranial pressure (ICP) and vary by age. An isolated behavior change, particularly in children with medical complexity, can be the only presenting symptom.
- Long-term management of hydrocephalus usually requires shunt placement or endoscopic third ventriculostomy.

Head Trauma

- Early diagnosis and management of traumatic brain injury (TBI) are critical to address the primary injury, reduce the severity of secondary brain injury, and prevent subsequent injuries when the brain is vulnerable following a TBI.
- Head CT is warranted for initial evaluation of intracranial injury in patients with altered mental status, focal neurologic abnormalities, palpable skull fracture, and signs of increased ICP.
- Epidural hematomas, some subdural hematomas, and certain skull fractures warrant neurosurgical consultation for possible surgical intervention.

Epilepsy Surgery

- Children with drug-resistant epilepsy (DRE) should be considered for surgical management, to resect or alter the epileptogenic tissue to eliminate the seizures (curative) or reduce the seizure burden (palliative) without causing neurological, behavioral, or other deficits.
- Presurgical evaluation can include scalp/intracranial EEG, structural/functional MRI, and neuropsychological testing to identify the epileptogenic zone and correlate the area with function.
- Early surgical intervention has the potential to minimize cognitive delays, improve psychomotor function, and improve the quality of life for children with DRE.

SUGGESTED READINGS

Bauer DF, Baird LC, Klimo P, et al. Congress of Neurological Surgeons Systematic Review and Evidence-Based Guidelines on the Treatment of Pediatric Hydrocephalus: Update of the 2014 Guidelines. *Neurosurgery*. 2020;87(6):1071-1075.

Carney N, Totten AM, O'Reilly C, et al. Guidelines for the management of severe traumatic brain injury, fourth edition. *Neurosurgery*. 2017;80(1):6-15.

Dwivedi R, Ramanujam B, Chandra PS, et al. Surgery for drug-resistant epilepsy in children. *N Engl J Med*. 2017;377(17):1639-1647.

Gelineau-Morel RN, Zinkus TP, Le Pichon JB. Pediatric head trauma: a review and update. *Pediatr Rev*. 2019;40(9):468-481.

Haarbauer-Krupa J, Glang A, Kurowski B, Breiding M. *Report to Congress: The Management of Traumatic Brain Injury in Children: Opportunities for Action*. Centers for Disease Control and Prevention, National Center for Injury Prevention and Control, Division of Unintentional Injury Prevention. Atlanta, GA. 2018.

Kochanek P, Tasker RC, Bell MJ, et al. Management of Pediatric Severe Traumatic Brain Injury: 2019 Consensus and Guidelines-Based Algorithm for First and Second Tier Therapies. *Pediatr Crit Care Med*. 2019;20(3):269-279.

Kochanek PM, Tasker RC, Carney N, et al. Guidelines for the Management of Pediatric Severe Traumatic Brain Injury, Third Edition: Update of the Brain Trauma Foundation Guidelines. *Pediatr Crit Care Med*. 2019;20(3S):S1-S82.

Kulkarni AV, Riva-Cambrin J, Holubkov R, et al. Endoscopic third ventriculostomy in children: prospective, multicenter results from the Hydrocephalus Clinical Research Network. *J Neurosurg Pediatr*. 2016;18(4):423-429.

Kulkarni AV, Riva-Cambrin J, Rozzelle CJ, et al. Endoscopic third ventriculostomy and choroid plexus cauterization in infant hydrocephalus: a prospective study by the Hydrocephalus Clinical Research Network. *J Neurosurg Pediatr*. 2018;21(3):214-223.

Pan I, LoPresti MA, Clarke DF, Lam S. The effectiveness of medical and surgical treatment for children with refractory epilepsy. *Neurosurgery*. 2020;88(1):E73-E82.

Ryvlin P, Cross JH, Rheims S. Epilepsy surgery in children and adults. *Lancet Neurol*. 2014;13(11):1114-1126.

Tamber MS, Kestle JRW, Reeder RW, et al. Temporal trends in surgical procedures for pediatric hydrocephalus: an analysis of the Hydrocephalus Clinical Research Network Core Data Project. *J Neurosurg Pediatr*. 2020;27(3):269-276.

Wellons JC 3rd, Shannon CN, Holubkov R, et al. Shunting outcomes in posthemorrhagic hydrocephalus: results of a Hydrocephalus Clinical Research Network prospective cohort study. *J Neurosurg Pediatr*. 2017;20(1):19-29.

Whitehead WE, Weiner HL. Infantile and childhood hydrocephalus. *N Engl J Med*. 2022;387(22):2067-2073.

CHAPTER 161 Ophthalmologic Issues

Alison E. Niebanck, MD and Robin Ray, MD

OPHTHALMOLOGIC ISSUES

INTRODUCTION

Ophthalmic conditions can present to the pediatric hospitalist in several settings. They can be an incidental complaint or secondary finding during the evaluation of another presenting issue, for example, a red eye in a patient being treated for bronchiolitis; or the reason for admission as in orbital cellulitis. Other times ophthalmology consultation is required for supplemental information for a complicated systemic issue such as the need for a dilated fundus examination in the setting of presumed abusive head trauma.

This chapter will provide basic history taking and examination skills for the pediatric hospitalist. It will also provide information about the common ophthalmic conditions encountered by the pediatric hospitalist.

HISTORY AND EXAMINATION

As in most fields in medicine, the most important part of ophthalmologic assessment is the chief complaint and history. Many common ophthalmic diseases can be diagnosed from the history alone. Children present with eye conditions for three general reasons: visual changes, eye pain, and abnormal appearance; or some combination of the three. Eliminating one or more of these categories helps narrow the differential diagnosis.

If the child is old enough, it is important to ask if he or she has noticed a change or loss in vision. Most children will not differentiate one eye from the other and will simply say "things are blurry," or "I can't see." In preverbal children, eye complaints are often inferred by the caregiver, and history-taking will elicit information such as "He is sitting closer to the TV than he used to," or "She keeps closing her eyes around bright lights." It is imperative to ask about trauma to the eye. For example, children may not volunteer history related to impulsive or improper behavior.

Examination Essentials In addition to a good history, a focused and simple eye examination can help differentiate a minor issue from a vision- or life-threatening condition. If a near card is available, and the child can read numbers, the vision *in each eye individually* should be recorded. The vision with both eyes open is not useful. If this card is not available or the child cannot use it, documenting if the child can count fingers or blinks to light is necessary. If an objective assessment of vision cannot be obtained, it is necessary to obtain an accurate history regarding any change or loss in vision. Examination of the eyelids and skin around the eyes is helpful in settings of trauma and a red eye. The pediatric hospitalist should take note of any lacerations, foreign bodies, vesicles consistent with herpes simplex or zoster, or presence of a preauricular node. The conjunctiva, sclera, cornea, anterior chamber, iris, and lens compose the anterior segment of the eye. Evaluation with a penlight is useful for noting gross defects. When mild trauma is suspected, such as a corneal abrasion, fluorescein dye can be used to evaluate for an abrasion under cobalt blue light or Wood's lamp.

In a patient with a complaint of unilateral vision loss, perhaps the most important objective test is the presence or absence of a relative afferent pupillary defect (APD). The "swinging-flashlight test" is used to determine a defect in an eye's ability to sense light (**Figure 161-1**).

Two things should be noted with regard to motility. First, the extent of excursion (degree to which the eye moves in all positions of gaze) of each eye should be noted. Second, the alignment of the eyes in primary gaze is important. Gross misalignments can be assessed using the Hirschberg test. A stationary light is directed at the child's face from two to three feet away, and the position of the light reflex off the cornea is noted in both eyes. If the reflection is not in the same position of the cornea in both eyes, then a deviation is present (exotropia or esotropia).

COMMON OPHTHALMOLOGIC CONDITIONS

The Red Eye Perhaps the most common ophthalmologic complaint in an inpatient pediatric setting is a red eye. **Figure 161-2** presents a diagnostic algorithm of the red eye. Any red eye that is associated with eye pain should have an ophthalmology consultation. An exhaustive description of all causes of a red eye is beyond the scope of this chapter.

Preseptal and Orbital Cellulitis Bacterial infections of the periocular soft tissues are common in children and are differentiated by the

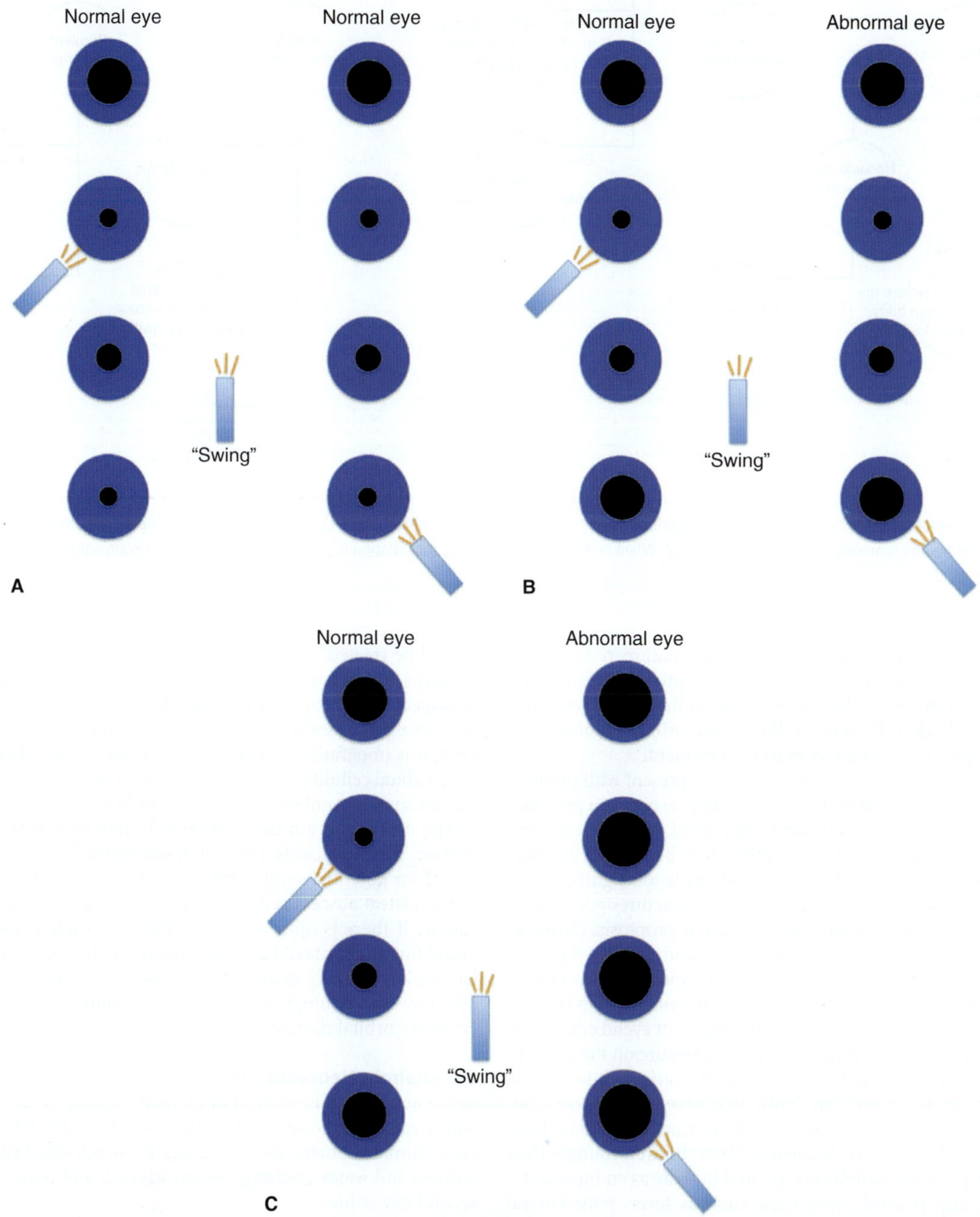

FIGURE 161-1. A. Intact direct and consensual light response. Both pupils react briskly to light and when the "swinging flashlight test" is performed, both pupils stay constricted. **B.** Left eye with a relative afferent pupillary defect (RAPD). As the light is swung from right eye to left, the left pupil shows a diminished direct response to light. The right eye has a similar diminished consensual response. **C.** Left eye with a RAPD in the setting of a fixed left pupil (i.e., traumatic pupil, left third nerve palsy, etc.). Though the left pupil has no direct response to light, the RAPD in the left eye can be ascertained by the swinging flashlight test. The right pupil dilates (from a previously constricted state) when the light swings from right eye to left eye. (Courtesy of Robin Ray, MD.)

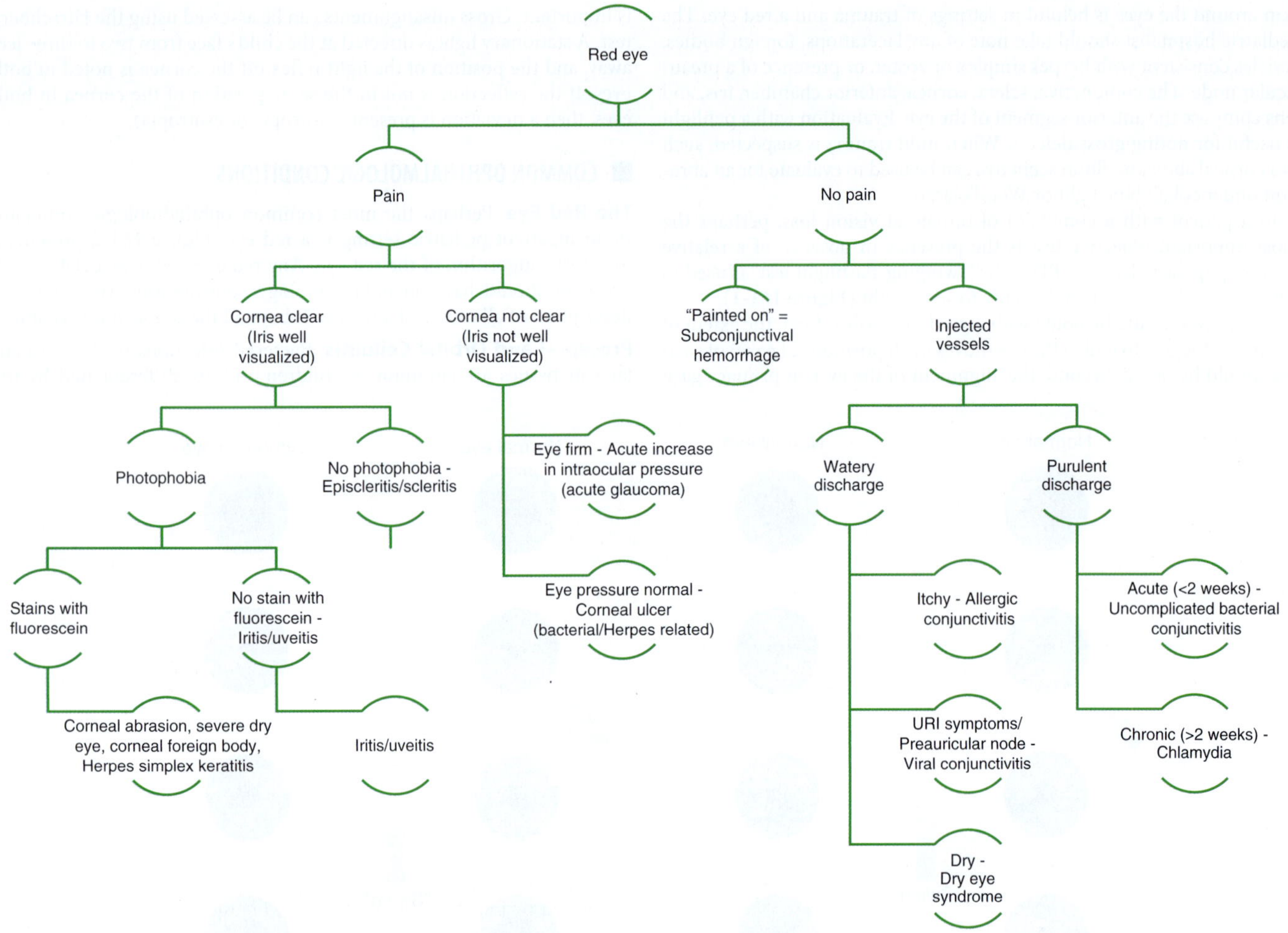

FIGURE 161-2. Diagnosis algorithm for a red eye. This algorithm covers broad spectrums of disease. Some conditions (i.e., herpes simplex infection) can fit into many of these categories. If a history of trauma is present, this algorithm is invalid. When in doubt, ophthalmology consultation is essential as more advanced examination techniques may be required. (Courtesy of Robin Ray, MD.)

anatomic location. Infection and resultant inflammation restricted to the eyelids and soft tissues anterior to the orbital septum is deemed *preseptal cellulitis.* Involvement of disease posterior to the orbital septum is considered *orbital cellulitis.* Preseptal cellulitis and orbital cellulitis have distinct ocular sequelae and differences in management.

For both of these conditions, children most often present with progressive edema and erythema of the eyelids. Differentiation between preseptal and postseptal disease can usually be made on clinical examination; however, computed tomography (CT) of the orbits may be needed to determine extent of disease in cases where eyelid edema is too significant for a good examination of the globe. Inflammation of structures posterior to the orbital septum can cause "orbital signs" such as proptosis, chemosis (edema of the conjunctiva), limited ocular motility, and an APD. A patient may complain of diplopia in cases of limited ocular motility. A complaint of decreased vision can be a sign of optic nerve inflammation but is unreliable as an indicator of posterior infection as significant eyelid edema can obscure the pupil and/or cause astigmatism with pressure on the cornea.

Treatment of preseptal cellulitis in a well-appearing child is oral antibiotics. Typically, an empiric antibiotic that covers Staphylococcus, Streptococci, and anaerobes is chosen, such as amoxicillin-clavulanic acid or clindamycin. It is often recommended that children younger than 1 year of age with preseptal cellulitis be treated initially as an inpatient.

Children with any systemic symptoms such as fever, poor enteral intake, severe upper respiratory infection/sinusitis, or who are failing outpatient management (worsening of eyelid edema despite antibiotics or development of orbital signs) should have a CT scan of the orbits and sinuses with contrast, have blood cultures obtained, and be admitted for intravenous antibiotics. The pediatric patient with orbital cellulitis should be treated with a broad-spectrum antibiotic that covers Staphylococcus, Streptococci, and gram-negative rods. If intracranial extension is suspected, metronidazole should be added to cover anaerobic organisms. Fungal causes should be considered in immunocompromised children. It is imperative to treat orbital cellulitis promptly as complications from orbital cellulitis include retinal artery occlusion, optic neuritis, cavernous sinus thrombosis, meningitis, or brain abscess.

The most common cause of orbital cellulitis is extension from sinus disease. If sinus disease is present, otolaryngology consultation is warranted for potential surgical intervention. Decision to drain an orbital or subperiosteal abscess is dependent on clinical presentation and disease course. If there is optic nerve involvement, such as signs of decreased visual function or an APD, surgical intervention may be indicated. Otolaryngology usually manages the sinus disease in cases of orbital cellulitis; however, oculoplastic surgeons are sometimes consulted for more extensive orbital disease.

Ophthalmia Neonatorum There are several causes of conjunctivitis in the newborn. Chemical conjunctivitis usually occurs within 24 hours and is caused by topical antibiotics used as prophylaxis for gonococcal ophthalmia neonatorum. Chemical conjunctivitis presents with mild redness and water discharge, is self-limited, and usually resolves by the second day of life.

Chlamydia trachomatis is the most common bacterial cause of neonatal conjunctivitis, followed by *Streptococcus viridans, Staphylococcus aureus,* and *Haemophilus influenzae.* Neisseria gonococcal conjunctivitis in the neonate is rare in industrialized countries due to routine prophylaxis with erythromycin ophthalmic ointment in newborns shortly following birth.

Signs of chlamydial conjunctivitis in the neonate usually occur around 1 week of life. Bilateral hyperemia with moderate discharge is common. Specimen collection for diagnostic tests (i.e., culture, DFA, NAAT) must contain conjunctival cells obtained from everted eyelid. The recommended treatment of chlamydial conjunctivitis in the neonate is oral erythromycin for 14 days or azithromycin for 3 days. A second course may be necessary for complete treatment, and thus close clinical follow-up is recommended. This treatment can be associated with infantile hypertrophic pyloric stenosis in infants younger than 6 weeks. Parents should be made aware of this risk and treated patients should be screened for this complication.

Neisseria gonococcal conjunctivitis presents 2 to 5 days after birth. The hallmark of gonococcal conjunctivitis is a serosanguinous drainage followed by a purulent discharge. Untreated disease can be complicated by keratitis (corneal infection), corneal perforation, and endophthalmitis, and thus all cases of gonococcal ophthalmia neonatorum should be comanaged with an ophthalmologist. Recommended treatment for uncomplicated gonococcal conjunctivitis is ceftriaxone 50 mg/kg/dose IV or IM for one dose, or cefotaxime 100 mg/kg/dose for one dose in infants under 28 days receiving calcium-containing intravenous products. Infants should be admitted for evaluation for disseminated disease. Hourly irrigation of the ocular surface with saline should also be performed until the discharge resolves. A white infiltration that obscures the view to the iris is a sign of corneal involvement. For these patients, ophthalmology consultation is also warranted for assistance with adjunctive topical antibiotics and monitoring for corneal thinning or perforation. Disseminated and/or resistant disease requires longer treatment.

Ocular Herpes Simplex Infection Both HSV-1 and HSV-2 can cause neonatal HSV infection, which may have eye involvement either in disseminated cases or in cases with skin, eyes, and/or mouth (SEM) disease. Ocular involvement may manifest as a superficial keratitis or conjunctivitis, and consultation with ophthalmology is indicated. Treatment consists of topical antivirals (in addition to parenteral antiviral therapy for neonates). Children risk having recurrence of eye lesions and may need long-term oral suppressive therapy.

Ophthalmic Care of the Obtunded Patient Intubated and sedated children are at risk of ocular surface disruption. The loss of corneal epithelium in this setting is known as exposure keratopathy and increases the risk of corneal infection (microbial keratitis). Eyes should be inspected daily by lifting the eyelids to ensure that the cornea is clear. If the details of the iris are obscured, corneal edema or infiltrate should be suspected. The most common sign is haziness of the tissue below the center cornea. Fluorescein dye can be used to highlight the loss of corneal epithelium. Incomplete closure (lagophthalmos) can occur for a variety of reasons including cranial nerve VII palsy or lax eyelids. More commonly seen in children on ventilators is chemosis (edema of the conjunctiva). This conjunctival edema prevents complete closure of the eyelids making it more likely the cornea will dry out. If there is incomplete eyelid closure, artificial tear ointment or gel should be applied several times a day. The eyes may also be taped shut for corneal protection, but it is important that they are inspected daily to evaluate the cornea for any signs of infection. It is prudent to ask family members of older children if they were wearing contact lens at the time of trauma, as these should be removed promptly.

Dacryocystocele and Dacryocystitis Dacryocystoceles are noticed soon after birth and may be encountered in the newborn nursery. They are characterized by a bluish swelling of the skin overlying the lacrimal sac. These patients should be referred promptly to ophthalmology due to risk of infection or nasal obstruction. Acute dacryocystitis, an infection of a dacryocystocele, is characterized by tender swelling of the inferior canthus area. These should be comanaged with ophthalmology and typically require nasolacrimal duct probing. Treatment includes empiric systemic antibiotics to prevent complications, which could include preseptal or orbital cellulitis, sepsis, meningitis, or brain abscess.

Papilledema Pediatric patients may be referred to the pediatric hospitalist service for admission and evaluation of a new diagnosis of papilledema. Commonly, the cause can be intracranial hypertension or brain tumors, and neuroimaging should be performed. If neuroimaging is unremarkable, a lumbar puncture with opening pressure should be obtained.

Ophthalmic Findings in Bartonella Henselae Infections (Cat-Scratch Disease) Ocular complications and manifestations occur in 5% to 10% of patients with Cat-Scratch disease.

One common presentation is parinaud oculoglandular syndrome, which includes conjunctivitis and preauricular lymphadenopathy. Additionally, *B. henselae* infections can cause neuroretinitis (inflammation of the optic nerve). Common chief complaints include acute vision loss, a blind spot, or visual field defects. The classic presentation is neuroretinitis with macular star, but can also include focal chorioretinitis. Treatment includes systemic antibiotics, often doxycycline and rifampin, and topical steroids, although visual recovery usually occurs regardless of treatment.

Optic Neuritis Optic neuritis is an inflammatory, demyelinating condition of the optic nerve that typically presents as eye pain with movement and acute monocular vision loss and/or abnormal color vision. It is classically associated with multiple sclerosis, but can also be caused by neuromyelitis optica (NMO), a condition that presents with optic neuritis, transverse myelitis, vomiting, cranial nerve defects, and brain lesions on MRI; acute disseminated encephalomyelitis (ADEM); or in other immune conditions such as lupus or sarcoidosis. Patients with optic neuritis should undergo magnetic resonance imaging of brain and orbits to determine underlying cause, treatment, and prognosis. Depending on diagnosis, children with optic neuritis may be treated with intravenous methylprednisolone.

Toxidromes With Ophthalmic Findings Ophthalmic findings can be common in toxic ingestions. Miosis (pupil constriction) can be seen in ingestions of clonidine, ethanol, opioids, organophosphates, and mushrooms. Mydriasis (pupil dilation) can be seen in ingestions of amphetamines, antidepressants, antihistamines, cocaine, LSD, marijuana, and methanol. Nystagmus can be seen with ingestions of phencyclidine, antiepileptics, ethanol, and sedatives.

Trauma Eye injury is the second leading cause of monocular vision loss in children after amblyopia. As in all trauma cases, signs/symptoms of life-threatening injury must be ruled out first. During initial assessment of the eye, the most important injury to rule out is an open globe (ruptured or penetrated eye). This can be especially difficult in young patients due to cooperation. If there is any suspicion of an open globe the treating pediatrician should stop the examination, put a shield on the eye (no patching), and an emergent ophthalmology consult should be obtained. No attempt to forcefully open the eyelids or patch the eye should be attempted in any scenario as this could cause further expulsion of the intraocular contents. Regardless of the initial sequelae of the initial injury, restoration of a clear pathway of light to the retina (i.e., removal of cataract, resolution of hyphema, or vitreous hemorrhage) is paramount to prevent deprivational amblyopia in children.

Open Globe Some open globe injuries are obvious, such as a penetrating fish hook to the eye, but occult penetrating injuries can occur commonly in children. New-onset eye pain or unilateral eyelid closure may be the only symptoms or signs of globe injury.

Signs that can indicate an open globe are severe eyelid laceration, visualization of a penetrating foreign body, extensive subconjunctival hemorrhage, hyphema (**Figure 161-3**), "peaked pupil" (pupil is not round—Figure **161-4**), uvea (pigmented tissue) extruding through the cornea or sclera (Figure 161-4), or traumatic cataract (white material in place of a normally black pupil).

If an open globe is suspected, the eye should be shielded immediately and emergent ophthalmology consultation obtained. Mechanism of injury should be determined and if foreign body is suspected (or if the history is not clear) computed tomography of the orbits should be obtained. Immunization status should be determined and tetanus booster given if required. In uncomplicated cases, a child who has had an open globe repair can usually be discharged 12 to 24 hours after surgery and managed by ophthalmology as an outpatient. A child with an open globe is at risk for endophthalmitis (internal eye infection), which presents as decreased vision, increase in pain, red eye, or hypopyon. Endophthalmitis requires emergent ophthalmologic consultation and intravitreal treatment.

Hyphema Blunt trauma to the eye can cause bleeding into the anterior chamber, known as a hyphema (Figure 161-3). Rupture of blood vessels in the iris root or ciliary spur are a common source of the bleeding. Symptoms of a hyphema are blurred vision and pain. As with all eye

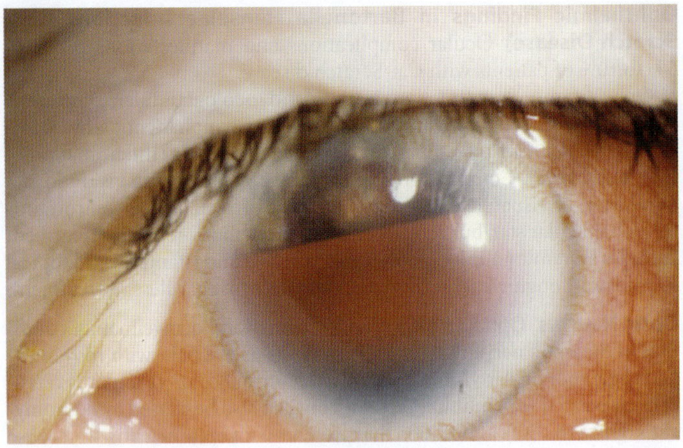

FIGURE 161-3. Large hyphema. (Reproduced with the permission from Maxine A. Papadakis, Stephen J. McPhee, Michael W. Rabow, Kenneth R. McQuaid, Monica Gandhi. *Current Medical Diagnosis & Treatment 2024*. New York: McGraw Hill; 2024.)

trauma, an open globe should be ruled out. All patients with hyphema should be comanaged with the ophthalmology service.

The intraocular pressure guides the management of a hyphema. If the intraocular pressure is normal, the child can be managed as an outpatient. The smaller the hyphema, the less likely the intraocular pressure will rise. Initial therapy consists of prednisolone acetate ophthalmic 1% four times a day (tapered upon resolution of the hyphema) and cycloplegic ophthalmic drops (i.e., atropine 1% twice a day). If the intraocular pressure is only mildly elevated (i.e., 21-25 mm Hg), a topical antiocular hypertensive may be added.

Initially, children with hyphema should be followed daily for intraocular pressure assessment and to evaluate for possible secondary hemorrhage. Patients who have a worsening hyphema (a "re-bleed") are more likely to have an increased intraocular pressure. High intraocular pressure can lead to decreased perfusion and ischemia of the optic nerve causing an optic neuropathy and glaucoma. Persistent hyphema, especially in the setting of a high pressure, can also lead to corneal blood staining (permanent discoloration and opacity of the cornea). Dense hyphema and blood staining can lead to deprivational amblyopia in young children. Should the intraocular pressure rise despite medical management, admission and surgical intervention (wash-out of the anterior chamber) may be necessary.

Children with hyphema and sickle cell trait or disease are more likely to have elevated intraocular pressure, experience a re-bleed, and have

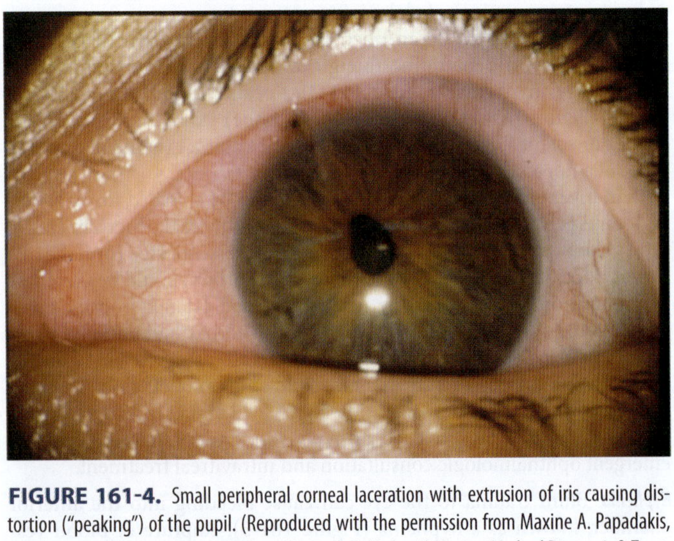

FIGURE 161-4. Small peripheral corneal laceration with extrusion of iris causing distortion ("peaking") of the pupil. (Reproduced with the permission from Maxine A. Papadakis, Stephen J. McPhee, Michael W. Rabow, Kenneth R. McQuaid, *Current Medical Diagnosis & Treatment 2023*. New York: McGraw Hill; 2023.)

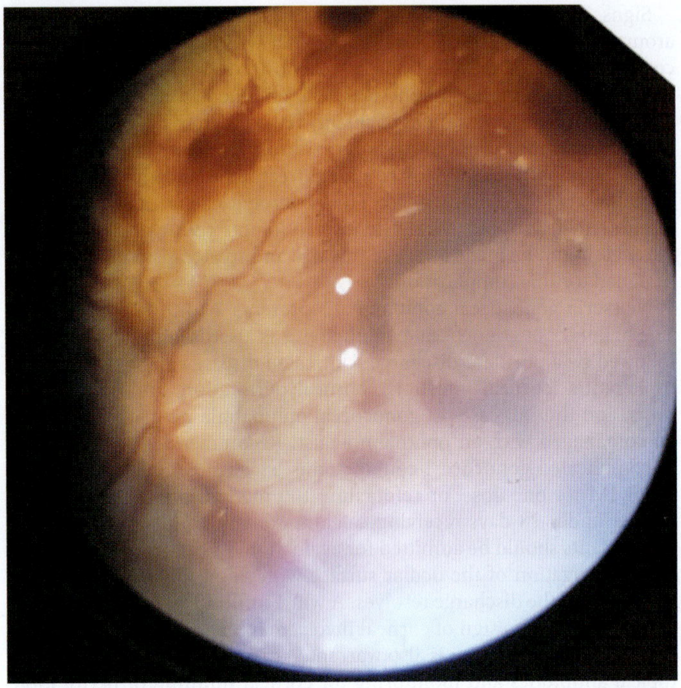

FIGURE 161-5. Diffuse multilayered retinal hemorrhages in a patient with nonaccidental injury (child abuse). (Reproduced with the permission from Gregg T. Lueder, Pediatric Practice: Ophthalmology, New York: McGraw Hill; 2011.)

a poorer visual outcome. All children with unknown history should be tested for sickle cell trait.

All children with a history of a hyphema need long-term ophthalmology follow-up as the eye is more likely to have chronic dysfunction of the angle (drainage system of the eye) and insidious visual loss from glaucoma.

Abusive Head Trauma Ophthalmology consultation is necessary in cases of suspected abusive head trauma (AHT) for children younger than the age of 5 years. Examination by an ophthalmologist is required to evaluate for presence of hemorrhage in the posterior segment of the eye, and is preferred to occur within first 24 hours following injury. Direct trauma to the eye does not cause diffuse retinal hemorrhages like those seen in a shaking injury.

Hemorrhage is usually most severe near the macula but can be seen throughout the retina in severe cases (**Figure 161-5**). Vitrectomy should be considered in cases of dense vitreous hemorrhage as these children are at risk for amblyopia. In abused patients with severe neurologic disability, vision loss is common and is usually due to cortical damage rather than retinal injury.

KEY POINTS

- Vision should be assessed in each eye individually.
- Any red eye associated with pain should generate an ophthalmology consultation.
- Orbital cellulitis may be distinguished by clinical features of proptosis, chemosis, limited ocular motility, and an afferent pupillary defect.
- Newborns with dacryocystocele and/or dacryocystitis should be referred promptly to ophthalmology.
- Obtunded patients should have their eyes inspected daily and protected with artificial tear ointment or gel.
- Trauma resulting in an open globe is an emergency requiring ophthalmology consultation.
- Ophthalmology consultation is required in suspected abusive head trauma in children under the age of 5.

SUGGESTED READINGS

Abdelhakim A, Rasool N. Neuroretinitis: a review. *Curr Opin Ophthalmol.* 2018;29(6):514-519.

Bartonella henselae. American Academy of Pediatrics. Committee on Infectious Diseases. *Red Book: Report of the Committee on Infectious Diseases.* Elk Grove Village, IL: American Academy of Pediatrics, 2021:226-229.

Chlamydia trachomatis. American Committee on Infectious Diseases. *Red Book: Report of the Committee on Infectious Diseases.* Elk Grove Village, IL: American Academy of Pediatrics, 2021:260-266.

Christian CW, Levin AV; Council on Child Abuse and Neglect, et al. The eye examination in the evaluation of child abuse. *Pediatrics.* 2018;142(2):e20181411.

Gise RA, Heidary G. Update on pediatric optic neuritis. *Curr Neurol Neurosci Rep.* 2020;20(3):4.

Gonococcal Infections. American Academy of Pediatrics. Committee on Infectious Diseases. *Red Book: Report of the Committee on Infectious Diseases.* Elk Grove Village, IL: American Academy of Pediatrics, 2021:338-344.

Habot-Wilner Z, Trivizki O, Goldstein M, et al. Cat-scratch disease: ocular manifestations and treatment outcome. *Acta Ophthalmol.* 2018;96(4):e524-e532.

Herpes Simplex. American Academy of Pediatrics. Committee on Infectious Diseases. *Red Book: Report of the Committee on Infectious Diseases.* Elk Grove Village, I: American Academy of Pediatrics, 2021:407-417.

Hyde RA, Mocan MC, Sheth U, Kaufman LM. Evaluation of the underlying causes of papilledema in children. *Can J Ophthalmol.* 2019;54(6):653-658.

Latham MD. Toxicology. In: *Harriet Lane Handbook.* 22nd ed. Philadelphia, PA: Elsevier, 2021:52-60.

Narang SK, Fingarson A, Lukefahr J; Council on Child Abuse and Neglect. Abusive head trauma in infants and children. *Pediatrics.* 2020;145(4):e20200203.

Singh S, Ali MJ. Congenital dacryocystocele: a major review. *Ophthalmic Plast Reconstr Surg.* 2019;35(4):309-317.

Tenembaum S, Chitnis T, Nakashima I, et al. Neuromyelitis optica spectrum disorders in children and adolescents. *Neurology.* 2016: 30;87(9 Suppl 2):S59-66.

Tolou C, Mahieu L, Martin-Blondel G, et al. Posterior segment involvement in cat-scratch disease: a case series. *J Fr Ophtalmol.* 2015; 38(10):974-982.

CHAPTER 162 Orthopedics

David I. Rappaport, MD, Rachna Kapoor, MD, MS and W.G. Stuart Mackenzie, MD

BACKGROUND

The care of children with musculoskeletal pathology often requires the collaboration of pediatric hospitalists and orthopedists. The approach to children with orthopedic conditions may vary greatly, including caring for young children with congenital anomalies, management of children with musculoskeletal trauma, postoperative care following elective procedures, and the evaluation of children with musculoskeletal pain or dysfunction. This chapter will review common forms of orthopedic pathology, with emphasis on the role of the pediatric hospitalist in optimizing timely, accurate diagnosis and high-quality care.

CONGENITAL CONDITIONS

Due to the synchronicity of fetal development, many apparent orthopedic congenital anomalies are associated with malformations of other organ systems. For example, congenital spine anomalies are frequently associated with renal and cardiac malformations due to disruptions in fetal development between weeks 6 and 8 of gestation. Any identified congenital pathology should prompt a thorough workup to identify any associated conditions.

DEVELOPMENTAL DYSPLASIA OF THE HIP

Background Developmental dysplasia of the hip (DDH) describes a spectrum of hip pathology in infants that includes hip dysplasia, subluxation, and frank dislocation. While DDH can be associated with orthopedic syndromes or neuromuscular disease, it is commonly idiopathic, and thought to be due to hip instability and capsular laxity.

Diagnostic Evaluation Screening for DDH is a routine part of the physical examination in the newborn nursery and involves testing hip range of motion and stability using the Ortolani and Barlow maneuvers. Any patient with a concerning physical examination should be referred to an orthopedic clinic within the first 2 weeks of life. Hip instability or asymmetry is evaluated using dynamic ultrasound due to the cartilaginous nature of the hip under 4 months of age. Ultrasound screening for DDH at 6 weeks is also recommended for infants with breech presentation or those with a first-degree relative with DDH.

Management Confirmed hip dislocations are treated immediately by positioning the patient in a "frog-leg" position using a Pavlik harness to encourage relocation and development of the dysplastic hip. Patients with hip subluxation or concern for dysplasia do not require treatment at this time; they typically undergo repeat ultrasound examination at 6 weeks of age, as many will spontaneously improve. Persistent DDH at 6 weeks of age is then treated with a Pavlik harness for a minimum of 6 weeks. The Pavlik harness is worn for more than 23 hours per day, can be removed for bathing in children with stable hips, and does not need to be removed for diaper changes. The Pavlik harness has been shown to be well tolerated, with up to 95% success in treating DDH, and low rates (2.4%) of avascular necrosis. For infants who fail nonoperative treatment with a Pavlik harness, several other semirigid braces can be considered, or the child can be taken to the operating room for hip arthrogram with either closed or open reduction, followed by immobilization in a hip spica cast for 12 weeks. Children with hip dysplasia beyond 18 months of age or with delayed diagnosis will often require open treatment with osteotomies of the proximal femur and acetabulum. The goal of treatment for DDH is to provide the child with a stable, concentric hip to delay or prevent the development of degenerative osteoarthritis in adulthood.

NEONATAL BRACHIAL PLEXUS PALSY

Neonatal brachial plexus palsy (NBPP) includes a range of neurologic injuries to the brachial plexus sustained by newborns. While brachial plexus palsies are more frequently associated with vaginal deliveries complicated by shoulder dystocia (up to 17%), it has been documented in up to 0.15% of cesarean deliveries. The mechanism is thought to be via stretch, and diagnosis is often made during the initial physical examination, which notes the limitation of motion in the affected upper extremity. Presentation can range from muscle weakness to paralysis, resulting from neuropraxia or nerve root avulsion. Common injury patterns are the Erb-Duchenne (C5-6) and Klumpke (C7-T1) palsies, which are characterized by the loss of affected motor groups. Initial treatment includes physical therapy to maintain passive range of motion and reduction of the glenohumeral joint, with splinting to limit contractures. Infants who regain antigravity strength in the arm by 2 months of age should have full function by 2 years of age, but those who have not regained antigravity strength by 6 months will likely experience permanent deficits. There is debate regarding the timing of intervention for children who do not regain function, and surgery can involve nerve transfers or grafting, soft tissue releases, tendon transfers, or osteotomies. Early referral to an upper extremity surgeon allows for a thorough evaluation of all potential treatment options. Perinatal trauma and infection should be ruled out with imaging and laboratory testing. Clavicle and humerus fractures are known complications of delivery and require supportive care only without true immobilization. Septic arthritis, most commonly of the glenohumeral joint, can present with shoulder pseudoparalysis or abnormal vital signs or lab values, and is definitively diagnosed by shoulder aspiration followed by treatment with irrigation, debridement, and intravenous antibiotics.

COMPARTMENT SYNDROME

Background Compartment syndrome is a feared complication of many pediatric injuries and fractures and may not only result in severe, permanent injury but may also be limb- or life-threatening. Early detection and prompt treatment are keys to avoiding complications from compartment syndrome.

Pathophysiology Compartment syndrome results from increased pressure within a muscular compartment of an extremity. Muscle groups in the extremities are contained within fibro-osseous compartments. When swelling occurs within the compartment (e.g., after an injury, from bleeding or reperfusion), the compartment may not be able to expand sufficiently to accommodate the structures residing within the compartment, leading to increased tissue pressure. Ischemia results when the pressure within the compartment is greater than the opening pressure of the venules traversing the compartment.

Risk factors for development of compartment syndrome include fractures of the tibia, forearm, and elbow; crush injuries; bleeding disorders such as hemophilia; ipsilateral forearm and elbow injuries; and open fractures. Compartment syndrome may arise from both extrinsic and intrinsic causes. Intrinsic causes include crush injury, reperfusion injury, fractures, and intraoperative positioning. Extrinsic causes include compression from a cast or bandages. Any injury may develop into compartment syndrome, including after elective surgery. There have also been reports of compartment syndrome after closed treatment of femur fractures with a spica cast. Patients with altered mental status (such as from a closed head injury) require particularly close evaluation because the most common symptom, increasing pain, may be undetected.

Diagnostic Evaluation The diagnosis of compartment syndrome is made via clinical assessment, sometimes supported by measurement of compartment pressures. Signs and symptoms result from increased tissue pressure and subsequent ischemia. Classically, the diagnosis of compartment syndrome is based on "5 P's": pain (particularly with passive stretch), pallor, paresthesias, pulselessness, and paralysis. However, findings of pallor, paresthesias, pulselessness, and paralysis occur late and frequently indicate irreversible ischemia.

The earliest and most sensitive clinical finding of compartment syndrome is pain. Patients often describe the pain as severe, unremitting, out of proportion to the initial injury, and poorly controlled by an appropriate dosage of analgesics. Intense pain with passive stretch of the muscles in the affected compartment is also a sign, and the involved compartments are often tense to palpation. Diagnosis of compartment syndrome in younger children and those with neurologic impairment is often challenging. Recently, the "3 A's" of compartment syndrome have been used to diagnose compartment syndrome: agitation, anxiety, and increasing analgesia requirements. In situations where the clinical assessment is equivocal, the pressure within a compartment can be directly measured by one of several techniques. Compartment pressures within 30 mm Hg of diastolic blood pressure are considered suggestive of compartment syndrome.

Management Compartment syndrome is a surgical emergency. Treatment of compartment syndrome involves decompression of the affected compartments by fasciotomy, and wounds are left open until the swelling subsides, at which point they are surgically closed. A high index of suspicion, early diagnosis, and prompt treatment are key to the successful treatment of this potentially devastating condition.

ORTHOPEDIC POSTOPERATIVE CARE

Most patients with orthopedic conditions do not require a prolonged hospital stay. The hospitalist may be involved in postoperative medical management for patients who have undergone surgery where there is an increased risk of complication, such as spinal fusion patients, or those with underlying medical comorbidities.

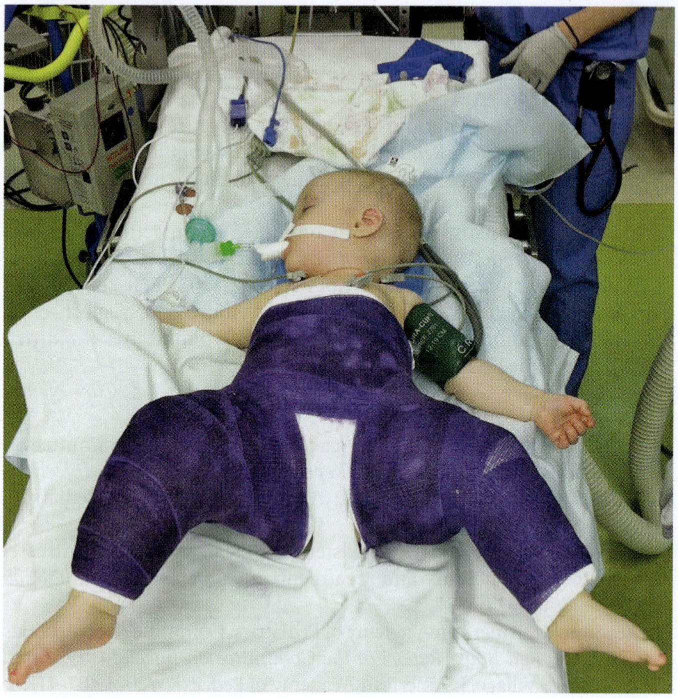

FIGURE 162-1. Appearance of a hip spica cast placed after closed reduction of bilateral hip dislocation in an 8-month-old with DDH.

CAST CARE

Casts and splints are used by orthopedic surgeons for a multitude of reasons (**Figure 162-1**). While both are constructed from a rigid material (usually plaster or fiberglass), casts are circumferential, while splints are noncircumferential, allowing for more swelling in the acute setting. After surgery, determining if a patient is experiencing pain due to the surgery or a constrictive cast may be difficult. Some casts are used to supplement fixation, while others are used to maintain alignment. The decision to split, bivalve, or remove a cast in a patient with an equivocal examination should be made by the operative team. In general, casts should stay clean and dry, must not have sharp edges, and should not have anything placed under the cast material.

POSTOPERATIVE SPINAL FUSION COMPLICATIONS

Background Although overall complication rates following spinal fusion are low in patients with idiopathic scoliosis, those with neuromuscular scoliosis (patients with cerebral palsy, muscular dystrophy, or similar conditions) have much higher complication rates. Comanagement of these patients between orthopedic and pediatric teams may improve the quality of care for these patients and may reduce their length of stay.

Neurologic Complications During spinal fusion surgery, implants (usually consisting of some combination of rods, hooks, screws, and wires) are used to correct the scoliosis, stabilize the spine, and facilitate fusion of the spine. Because of the risk of neurologic injury with placement of implants and the corrective maneuvers, most of these patients undergo intraoperative neurologic monitoring (somatosensory-evoked potentials with or without motor-evoked potentials). Patients who sustain prolonged or irreversible intraoperative changes will generally have their surgery aborted. The procedure is then usually completed 7 to 10 days later. All patients who have undergone spinal fusion surgery, even those in whom the surgery was uneventful, require careful postoperative neurologic monitoring via serial physical examinations. Late-onset neurologic deterioration due to spinal cord ischemia or compression is rare but serious. In these cases, return to the operating room may be indicated for implant removal and exploration.

Anemia Patients who undergo spinal fusion surgery often lose a significant amount of blood. Despite intraoperative transfusions and the use of cell savers, these patients require close monitoring of their intravascular volume status and hemoglobin postoperatively. Pediatric hospitalists should monitor for signs of symptomatic anemia postoperatively, including sustained tachycardia, hypoxemia, decreased urine output, and poor feeding/feeding intolerance. Thresholds for postoperative transfusion may depend on the specific clinical circumstances and should include surgical team input.

Nausea and Vomiting Postoperative nausea and vomiting may be due to a variety of causes, including anesthetic or narcotic medications or postoperative bowel dysmotility that has evolved into an ileus. For these reasons, oral intake (or enteral feeds in patients with feeding tubes) is usually advanced slowly. Some centers use standing antiemetics such as ondansetron in these patients for the first 24 to 48 hours after surgery. In patients with prolonged nausea, vomiting, or feeding intolerance, other causes must be considered. Bowel dysmotility secondary to narcotic use for pain control is common and may be managed by weaning narcotics and preventing constipation. Laxatives and stool softeners are sometimes used proactively prior to surgery to prevent constipation and help avoid bowel dysmotility, feeding intolerance, and pain; a general suggestion is to double the patient's standing constipation regimen for several days before surgery.

Less common causes of nausea and vomiting are superior mesenteric artery (SMA) syndrome and pancreatitis. SMA syndrome (or cast syndrome) is an upper intestinal obstruction caused by obstruction of the third part of the duodenum by the SMA. Patients with SMA syndrome present with abdominal pain, distention, nausea, vomiting with oral intake, and sometimes bilious emesis. Symptoms can be nonspecific and resemble those due to other causes of nausea/vomiting, so including it in the differential diagnosis is important. The diagnosis is confirmed with an upper gastrointestinal series demonstrating obstruction of the duodenum, though it may be diagnosed via ultrasound with Doppler or CT scan. SMA syndrome is treated with placement of a nasojejunal tube to provide feeds that bypass the obstruction, though persistent cases may require parenteral nutrition. Pancreatitis has also been reported after spinal fusion for scoliosis, though the mechanism is unclear. Patients with postoperative pancreatitis may present with abdominal pain, nausea, and vomiting after the initiation of oral intake or enteral feeds. In children with cerebral palsy and other comorbidities such as seizures, pancreatitis should be considered with postoperative feeding intolerance. The diagnosis is confirmed by two of the following: levels of serum lipase or amylase greater than 3 times normal, abdominal pain, or abdominal imaging demonstrating pancreatitis. Historical treatment of postoperative pancreatitis included bowel rest; however, more recent evidence suggests that earlier enteral feeds and aggressive (IV) hydration can improve outcomes. Serial monitoring of lipase is generally not recommended.

Respiratory Complications Postoperative hypoxia commonly occurs due to anesthesia, especially in children with medical complexity and ineffective airway clearance. This hypoxia is usually transient. Increased airway clearance measures may be implemented in some patients with medical complexity, along with early mobility as tolerated to help reduce requirement of respiratory support and prevent atelectasis and pneumonia. Despite historical dogma, atelectasis does not cause postoperative fever.

Fever Postoperative fever after orthopedic surgery is typically due to the inflammatory nature of the surgery itself and does not require significant evaluation. Possible exceptions include fever more than 4 to 5 days after surgery or in patients with evidence of surgical site infection, central lines, prolonged urinary catheter requirement, or other risk factors.

SIADH A surge in antidiuretic hormone release is common after spinal surgery, though only a minority of patients will develop the syndrome of inappropriate antidiuretic hormone (SIADH). This complication is important to recognize due to the risk of severe untreated hyponatremia (i.e., cerebral edema and herniation), although this is rare if recognized early. Symptoms of hyponatremia, which may include headache, mental status changes, or seizures, are more common. SIADH is diagnosed by noting serum hyponatremia, decreased urine output, serum hypo-osmolality, and increased urine osmolality. Monitoring urine output and electrolytes closely in the first 72 hours postoperatively is therefore important. SIADH is managed by fluid restriction until the problem spontaneously corrects, usually within 1 week.

Surgical Site Infections Surgical site infection occurs in up to 10% of neuromuscular scoliosis surgeries, and often requires additional surgical procedures and a prolonged treatment course including the use of vacuum-assisted wound closure and prolonged antibiotics. Some cases will require complete removal of the implants to resolve the infection. Standardized operative protocols have been found to reduce the incidence of surgical site infections. The Centers for Disease Control and Prevention (CDC) has published guidelines to prevent surgical site infections including appropriate preoperative bathing, use of prophylactic antibiotics, and wound care.

Postoperative Pain Control Patients who undergo spinal fusions and other major orthopedic surgeries typically benefit from a multimodal approach to pain control. This approach can often reduce the requirement for postoperative opioid use and help avoid side effects such as respiratory depression, sedation, and constipation. Medications include acetaminophen (IV or PO/enteral/rectal), nonsteroidal anti-inflammatory drugs (NSAIDs) such as ketorolac, benzodiazepines (diazepam) for muscle spasms, and opioids if needed for breakthrough pain. NSAIDs have historically been used sparingly in children after orthopedic injuries and surgery given concerns in adults of impaired bone healing. Newer evidence, however, suggests that NSAIDs can be used safely for postoperative pain control to help reduce opioid use. A full discussion of postoperative pain control lies beyond the scope of this chapter.

BACK PAIN

BACKGROUND

Acute back pain occurs frequently in adults and is uncommonly due to underlying serious pathology. Historical dogma has taught that back pain in children, in contrast, is rare and always pathologic. However, more recent data suggest that while back pain in children should be taken seriously, it is not uncommon and is often due to a benign cause. Pediatric hospitalists should recall that because most children with back pain are treated in the outpatient setting, they will often see patients whose back pain is atypical or requires further evaluation. In patients of all ages, back pain that is activity related and improves with rest is typically mechanical in origin. Nonmechanical back pain or pain that is constant or increasing or wakes the patient from sleep is more likely to be associated with an underlying pathologic diagnosis.

HISTORY/PHYSICAL EXAMINATION

In children or adolescents with back pain, several aspects of the history are important.

- Did the patient suffer any trauma?
- Does the patient have systemic signs of illness (fever, weight loss, or others)?
- Are there signs of neurologic involvement including bowel/bladder function?
- Is the pain relieved or worsened by any maneuver or intervention?

A thorough physical examination is especially important and includes palpation, assessment of range of motion and alignment, and a thorough neurologic assessment. The musculature should be evaluated for bulk, tone, and strength. Provocative tests are helpful as well. For example, forward flexion stresses the anterior elements of the spine, increasing pain if the pathology is anterior; a child with discitis will avoid bending down to pick up a toy. Hyperextension stresses the posterior elements and will reproduce the pain of symptomatic spondylolysis or spondylolisthesis. Neurologic examination should include deep tendon and Babinski reflexes, anal tone, Hoffman sign, anal wink, cremasteric reflexes (in boys), and evaluation of sensation.

DIFFERENTIAL DIAGNOSIS

Most serious causes of acute back pain can be divided into three major categories: traumatic, infectious/postinfectious, and neoplastic. Chronic back pain is often caused by etiologies such as amplified pain syndrome (AMPS) and will not be discussed here. Back pain may also be caused by nonorthopedic etiologies such as pyelonephritis, pelvic inflammatory disease, sacroiliitis, or constipation.

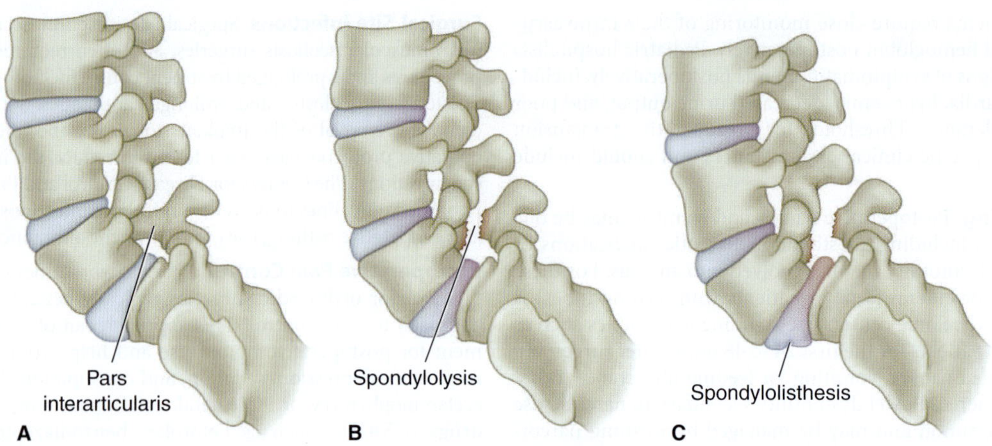

FIGURE 162-2. Pars interarticularis (A), spondylolysis (B), and spondylolisthesis (C). (Reproduced with permission from OrthoInfo. © American Academy of Orthopaedic Surgeons. https://orthoinfo.org/)

Traumatic Causes Pediatric hospitalists will uncommonly evaluate patients with traumatic back pain, whether due to acute injury or repetitive stress, because these patients do not often require emergency or inpatient care. In these patients, history and physical examination should determine which imaging studies, if any, are required. When a formal diagnosis can be established, spondylolysis (**Figure 162-2B**) and spondylolisthesis are the most common causes of mechanical back pain in adolescents. Spondylolysis is caused by repetitive compression of the posterior elements of the spine, often associated with activities such as weightlifting, football, and gymnastics, while spondylolisthesis represents one vertebra (most commonly L5-S1) slipping forward on the one below. Plain X-rays are often sufficient for establishing these diagnoses, with advanced imaging sometimes required. Higher grades of spondylolisthesis may require surgical intervention (**Figure 162-2C**). Spinal epidural hematoma, a rare and serious cause of back pain, may result from trauma or lumbar puncture and may cause spinal cord compression. Cases of spontaneous spinal epidural hematomas in children have also been described and should probably prompt evaluation for coagulopathy or vascular malformation.

Infectious and Postinfectious Causes Infections with many different agents may cause back pain, and patients may not present with systemic signs or symptoms such as fever. Common spinal infections include discitis, vertebral osteomyelitis, and epidural abscess (see Chapter 107). Advanced imaging such as MRI is often helpful in establishing a diagnosis; aspiration or biopsy may also be required to determine the causative organism, especially in patients with an unusual presentation and/or imaging findings or who have not responded to empiric antibiotics. Transverse myelitis, inflammation of a segment or segments of the spinal cord, may represent a postinfectious process or may be idiopathic. Symptoms can develop over several weeks or as rapidly as several hours. Patients with transverse myelitis often present with back pain, weakness, sensory disturbance, and bladder or bowel dysfunction. These patients' neurologic symptoms usually depend on the level of involvement.

Neoplastic Causes Patients with both benign and malignant tumors may present with back pain. Focal pain awakes a child from sleep and is constant and/or increasing should raise the hospitalist's suspicion for a neoplastic etiology. Benign tumors of the spine can be divided into those with a favorable course (Langerhans cell histiocytosis, osteochondroma, and osteoid osteoma) and those that are benign but locally aggressive (osteoblastoma, giant cell tumor, and aneurysmal bone cysts). Patients with an osteoid osteoma often respond dramatically to NSAIDs. Patients with leukemia and lymphoma can also present with back pain. Ewing sarcoma can often be mistaken for an infectious process because patients often present with fever and leukocytosis.

DIAGNOSTIC EVALUATION

Because patients with back pain can have a broad range of pathologies, the evaluation should be tailored to the patient's individual needs. In those with a suspected infectious cause of back pain, a complete blood count (CBC) and inflammatory markers such as an ESR or C-reactive protein should be obtained. Blood culture should be considered as it may reveal an organism without requiring a biopsy. Plain films are a simple, easily obtainable initial study but are often not diagnostic. In these patients, advanced imaging such as MRI, CT scan, or bone scan should be considered. Occasionally an aspiration or biopsy may be required.

MANAGEMENT

Treatment for patients with back pain depends on the suspected underlying cause. Consultation with orthopedics, infectious disease, neurology, rehabilitation medicine, and/or physical therapy may be required. In general, hospitalists should concomitantly pursue pain management with identification and treatment of the underlying etiology.

SUGGESTED READINGS

Absoud M, Greenberg BM, Lim M, Lotze T, Thomas T, Deiva K. Pediatric transverse myelitis. *Neurology*. 2016;87(9 Supplement 2):S46-52.

American College of Obstetricians and Gynecologists, editor. Neonatal brachial plexus palsy. Washington, DC: The American College of Obstetricians and Gynecologists, Women's Health Care Physicians; 2014;103.

Bae DS, Kadiyala RK, Waters PM. Acute compartment syndrome in children: contemporary diagnosis, treatment, and outcome. *J Pediatr Orthop*. 2001;21(5):680-688.

Birch JG, Paley D, Herzenberg JE, et al. Amputation versus staged reconstruction for severe fibular hemimelia: assessment of psychosocial and quality-of-life status and physical functioning in childhood. *JB JS Open Access*. 2019;4(2):e0053.

Borkhuu B, Nagaraju D, Miller F, et al. Prevalence and risk factors in postoperative pancreatitis after spine fusion in patients with cerebral palsy. *J Pediatr Orthop*. 2009;29(3):256-262.

Cady R, Hennessey TA, Schwend RM. Diagnosis and treatment of idiopathic congenital clubfoot. *Pediatrics*. 2022;149(2):e2021055555.

Christian CW, Committee on Child Abuse and Neglect. The evaluation of suspected child physical abuse. *Pediatrics*. 2015;135(5):e1337-1354.

Fernandez M, Carrol CL, Baker CJ. Discitis and vertebral osteomyelitis in children: an 18-year review. *Pediatrics*. 2000;105(6):1299-1304.

Giannoudis PV, Giannoudi M, Stavlas P. Damage control orthopaedics: lessons learned. *Injury*. 2009;40 Suppl 4:S47-52.

Grill F, Bensahel H, Canadell J, Dungl P, Matasovic T, Vizkelety T. The Pavlik harness in the treatment of congenital dislocating hip: report on a multicenter study of the European Paediatric Orthopaedic Society. *J Pediatr Orthop*. 1988;8(1):1-8.

Jimah BB, Mensah TA, Ulzen-Appiah K, et al. Prenatal diagnosis of skeletal dysplasia and review of the literature. *Case Rep Obstet Gynecol*. 2021;2021:9940063.

Kawamura K, Chung KC. Constriction band syndrome. *Hand Clin.* 2009;25(2):257-264.
Laine JC, Novotny SA, Weber EW, Georgiadis AG, Dahl MT. Distal tibial guided growth for anterolateral bowing of the tibia: fracture may be prevented. *J Bone Joint Surg Am.* 2020;102(23):2077-2086.
Lam DJL, Lee JZJ, Chua JHY, Lee YT, Lim KBL. Superior mesenteric artery syndrome following surgery for adolescent idiopathic scoliosis: a case series, review of the literature, and an algorithm for management. *J Pediatr Orthop* Part B. 2014;23(4):312-318.
Lamb M, Brenner JS. Back pain in children and adolescents. *Pediatr Rev.* 2020;41(11):557-569.
Lieh-Lai MW, Stanitski DF, Sarnaik AP, et al. Syndrome of inappropriate antidiuretic hormone secretion in children following spinal fusion. *Crit Care Med.* 1999;27(3):622-627.
Loder RT, Feinberg JR. Orthopaedic injuries in children with nonaccidental trauma: demographics and incidence from the 2000 kids' inpatient database. *J Pediatr Orthop.* 2007;27(4):421-426.
Rappaport DI, Adelizzi-Delany J, Rogers KJ, et al. Outcomes and costs associated with hospitalist comanagement of medically complex children undergoing spinal fusion surgery. *Hosp Pediatr.* 2013;3(3):233-241.
Ravindra VM, Eli IM, Schmidt MH, Brockmeyer DL. Primary osseous tumors of the pediatric spinal column: review of pathology and surgical decision making. *Neurosurg Focus.* 2016;41(2):E3.
Rosenberg RE, Ardalan K, Wong W, et al. Postoperative spinal fusion care in pediatric patients: Co-management decreases length of stay. *Bull Hosp Jt Dis* (2013). 2014;72(3):197-203.
Schaffzin JK, Harte L, Marquette S, et al. Surgical site infection reduction by the solutions for patient safety hospital engagement network. *Pediatrics.* 2015;136(5):e1353-1360.
Shapiro G, Green DW, Fatica NS, Boachie-Adjei O. Medical complications in scoliosis surgery. *Curr Opin Pediatr.* 2001;13(1):36-41.
Siebert MJ, Karacz CM, Richards BS. Successful ponseti-treated clubfeet at age 2 years: what is the rate of surgical intervention after this? *J Pediatr Orthop.* 2020;40(10):597-603.
Simpson BE, Kara S, Wilson A, et al. Reducing patient length of stay after surgical correction for neuromuscular scoliosis. *Hosp Pediatr.* 2022;e2021006196.
Stroud S, Katyal T, Gornitzky AL, Swarup I. Effect of non-steroidal anti-inflammatory drugs on fracture healing in children: a systematic review. *World J Orthop.* 2022;13(5):494-502.
Surgical Site Infection (SSI) | HAI | CDC [Internet]. 2021 [cited 2023 Jan 27]. Available from: https://www.cdc.gov/hai/ssi/ssi.html.
Yang S, Zusman N, Lieberman E, Goldstein RY. Developmental dysplasia of the hip. *Pediatrics.* 2019;143(1):e20181147.
Yousef M, Dranginis D, Rosenfeld S. Postoperative fever in pediatric patients with neuromuscular disorders after deformity correction surgery: frequency and utility of diagnostic workup. *Pediatrics.* 2018;142(1_MeetingAbstract):303.
Zionts LE, Dietz FR. Bracing following correction of idiopathic clubfoot using the Ponseti method. *J Am Acad Orthop Surg.* 2010;18(8):486-493.

CHAPTER 163 Burns and Other Skin Injuries

Melinda S. Murphy, MD, FAAP and
Raymond Rios-Nieves, MD, FAAP

BACKGROUND

Injuries to skin and adjacent deeper tissues range in severity from minor insults that can be managed on an outpatient basis to much more complex injuries that require the expertise of surgeons, usually with specific training in plastic surgery, trauma, or burn care. Pediatric hospitalists are often involved in the initial evaluation, stabilization, and management of children when they present to the hospital or require admission for significant injuries. In this chapter, the general management of thermal burns will be reviewed in detail followed by an overview of chemical burns, electrical injuries, and intravenous infiltrates.

Burns cause significant morbidity and mortality in the pediatric population throughout the world. In the United States, fire and burn injuries account for approximately 100,000 hospital admissions or emergency room encounters with an estimated 300 children under age 18 dying from burn injuries each year. Twenty percent of all burn cases in the United States involve children 4 years and younger; scalds are the more common mechanism of burn injury in this age group. Burns due to thermal causes (flame, contact, scald, or steam) require similar but distinct management from chemical or electrical burns. Careful attention must be paid to both the acute and chronic phases of burn care because many injuries require long-term rehabilitation and an interdisciplinary approach to minimize their functional, cosmetic, and emotional impact.

THERMAL BURNS

PATHOPHYSIOLOGY

Following a thermal injury, the body responds locally and systemically. Locally, there are three zones of injury. The zone of coagulation necrosis is an eschar, with irreversible surface tissue injury from the direct heat insult. The zone of stasis is an area of reversible, salvageable cell injury due to a microvascular reaction in the dermis associated with vasoconstriction and thrombosis. Cell damage is not complete, but inflammatory mediators and injured microcirculation put viable tissue at risk. Beyond this is the zone of hyperemia, which lacks direct cell injury but exhibits vasodilation secondary to the surrounding inflammatory cascade. Full recovery in this zone is expected in the absence of additional insults. Systemically, the loss of an effective skin barrier leads to fluid losses, electrolyte imbalances, decreased resistance to infection, and the release of vasoactive mediators, affecting hemodynamic status and creating a hypermetabolic state.

CLINICAL PRESENTATION

The diagnosis of a thermal injury is usually evident; however, the details of the history and full extent of the injury may not be obvious initially. An increased level of suspicion for neglect or abuse is warranted. Additionally, the depth and degree of injury can evolve within the first few hours of presentation. Thermal injuries are typically divided into first-, second-, third- and fourth-degree burns (**Figure 163-1**).

First-degree burns are superficial burns involving only the epidermis. They are associated with erythema, mild edema, dryness, and pain; first-degree burns do not blister. Pain typically resolves in 2 to 3 days, and wounds heal in 3 to 6 days. Sunburns are common first-degree burns.

Second-degree burns are partial-thickness burns extending into the dermis, often caused by hot liquids. Superficial second-degree burns involve the epidermis and superficial dermis. Blisters are typically present; the wounds are erythematous, edematous, moist, and extremely painful due to exposed nerve endings. These burns heal in 2 to 3 weeks because the dermal appendages that regenerate epithelial cells are preserved. Deep second-degree burns penetrate deep into the dermal layer. Blisters with weeping exudates are usually present; the wounds are dark red or yellow-white, with a slightly moist surface. These burns are less painful because fewer viable nerve endings are present. They generally require more than 3 weeks to heal and are at risk for hypertrophic scar formation.

Third-degree burns penetrate through the dermis into the subcutaneous fat. They are insensate because cutaneous nerves are destroyed, although there is pain in the surrounding second-degree burns. They appear dry, leathery, and charred and are pearly white or parchment-like; superficial vessel thrombosis may be visible. These burns are often caused by flame or grease. Resurfacing and grafting are required for closure. Deep second- and third-degree burns may be difficult to distinguish clinically, and the presence of multiple burn types limits the utility of pain as a delineator.

Fourth-degree burns extend to underlying muscle or bone.

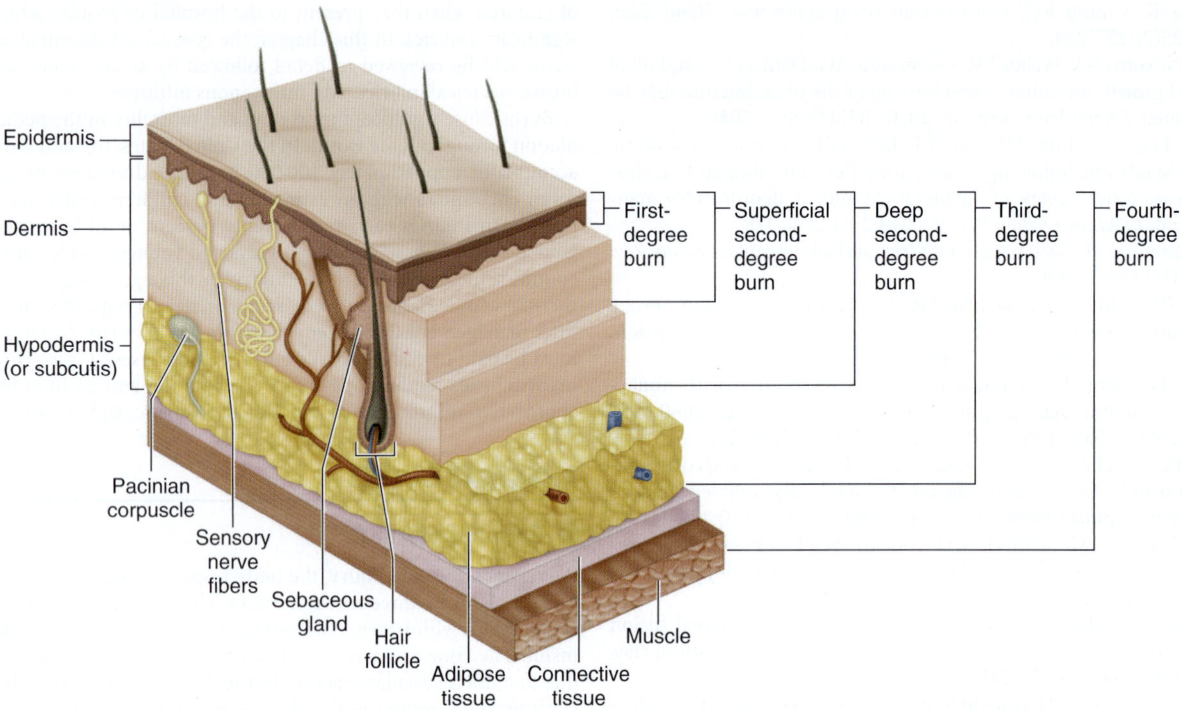

FIGURE 163-1. Depth of burn injury in relation to skin level. First-degree burns involve the epidermis, second-degree burns involve the epidermis and dermis, third-degree burns penetrate into the subcutaneous tissue, fourth-degree burns extend to the muscle layer. Key structures imbedded in each layer are indicated. (Reproduced with permission from Garner WL. Thermal burns. In: Achauer BM, Eriksson E, eds. *Plastic Surgery: Indications, Operations, and Outcomes*. St Louis, MO: Mosby, 2000.)

DIFFERENTIAL DIAGNOSIS

As with any injury in a child, vigilance for signs of abuse or neglect is essential. These include an inconsistent mechanism of injury, variation in historical details, delayed presentation, or a classic intentional injury pattern. A classic intentional scald injury pattern is buttock injury accompanied by perineal and foot injury that spares the flexion creases, suggestive of defensive posturing. Other intentional injury patterns include scald burns in a stocking or glove distribution and deep local contact burns, such as from a cigarette.

Certain skin conditions such as Stevens-Johnson syndrome or toxic epidermal necrolysis and staphylococcal scalded skin syndrome may mimic a diffuse burn injury but should be readily distinguished by the history and overall clinical picture.

DIAGNOSTIC EVALUATION AND MANAGEMENT

Initial Stabilization

Primary Survey The initial evaluation of a burned child should proceed in an organized and rapid manner with the first management priorities being airway, breathing, and circulation. The risk of inhalation injury, with associated airway edema and compromise, is high in victims of an indoor or chemical fire or a hot liquid ingestion. Clinical clues to airway injury include facial burns, hoarseness, stridor, oral lesions, soot in sputum or deposits in the nares, singed eyebrows or facial hair, and shortness of breath. In the case of airway injury, the risk of progressive airway edema warrants early intubation. The potential for carbon monoxide poisoning should be considered in all children who are rescued from house fires, any burn-injured patient with impaired thinking, syncope, or coma that is otherwise unexplained, or if there is a strong exposure history (e.g., kerosene or gas stove, automobile exhaust). Secure vascular access should be obtained as part of initial stabilization even if it requires intravenous or intraosseous access through burned areas.

Secondary Survey Following the primary survey, a complete, thorough examination should be performed to assess for any other injuries or conditions that may have been missed initially. A full history should be obtained from caregivers along with pertinent historical information from emergency personnel, including length of exposure and extrication time. Attention should be paid to any conflicting stories regarding the injury. Radiographs and laboratory studies should be obtained as indicated by history and physical examination. Tetanus status should be assessed and addressed, and tetanus immunoglobulin should be considered in patients with incomplete or unknown immunization status and large contaminated wounds.

Early Management

Evaluation of Wounds Following initial stabilization, the identification of the burn type and total surface area involved is imperative for appropriate management and disposition. For total burn surface area (TBSA) assessment, the "rule of 9s" is typically used in adults and children older than 15 years. In younger children, however, this is inaccurate because they have relatively larger heads and a different body size distribution. Further, children have an increased body surface area to mass ratio, increasing their risk of hypothermia and more profound fluid losses. For a rapid estimation of TBSA, a child's hand (palm plus digits) represents approximately 1% of the body surface area. For more precise estimates, charts that estimate burn area based on age can be used (**Figure 163-2**). First-degree burns are not included in surface area calculations for purposes of fluid resuscitation.

Pay particular attention to burns to vulnerable areas: the face, hands, feet, genitalia, perineum, and major joints, and evaluate for corneal injury in patients with facial burns. Be vigilant for circumferential burns that may compromise circulation or respiration.

Initial Wound Care For small superficial burns in children without any other injuries, outpatient management is generally appropriate. The burns should be cleansed thoroughly, and any thin, loose, blistered skin should be gently debrided. Affected areas should be covered with antimicrobial ointment and clean dressings or a commercially available burn dressing. Follow-up within 72 hours is preferred and caregivers should be instructed on monitoring for signs of infection. Pain control can generally be achieved with over-the-counter analgesics.

Children with large burns (>20% TBSA) are best managed by a pediatric burn center; early transfer improves survival and decreases morbidity. Adequate pain control with narcotics and/or sedatives is appropriate

Burn estimate chart and diagram
Age vs. Area

Area	Birth–1yr	1–4 yr	5–9 yr	10–14 yr	15 yr	Adult	2°	3°	Total	Donor areas
Head	19	17	13	11	9	7				
Neck	2	2	2	2	2	2				
Ant. trunk	13	13	13	13	13	13				
Post. trunk	13	13	13	13	13	13				
R buttock	2½	2½	2½	2½	2½	2½				
L buttock	2½	2½	2½	2½	2½	2½				
Genitals	1	1	1	1	1	1				
R U arm	4	4	4	4	4	4				
L U arm	4	4	4	4	4	4				
R L arm	3	3	3	3	3	3				
L L arm	3	3	3	3	3	3				
R hand	2½	2½	2½	2½	2½	2½				
L hand	2½	2½	2½	2½	2½	2½				
R thigh	5½	6½	8	8½	9	9½				
L thigh	5½	6½	8	8½	9	9½				
R leg	5	5	5½	6	6½	7				
L leg	5	5	5½	6	6½	7				
R foot	3½	3½	3½	3½	3½	3½				
L foot	3½	3½	3½	3½	3½	3½				
						Total				

Burn diagram

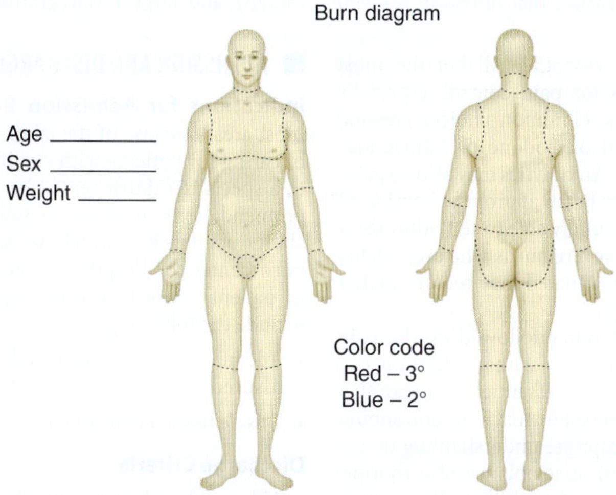

FIGURE 163-2. Lund and Browder burn estimate diagram, as modified by the US Army Institute of Surgical Research. (Reproduced with permission from Yowler CJ, Fratianne RB. Current status of burn resuscitation. *Clin Plas Surg.* 2000;27:1-10.)

given how severe burn pain can be. Fluid resuscitation should be initiated prior to transfer (see below). Children with large areas of compromised skin are at increased risk of hypothermia as well as are subject to more profound fluid losses compared to adults. Keep affected areas covered with clean dressings or a sheet while awaiting emergent transfer. Treatment rooms should be kept warm to decrease the risk of hypothermia for very small children.

In cases of superficial partial-thickness burns, the mainstay of management involves debridement followed by dressings designed to prevent wound infection and maintain a moist environment to facilitate healing. Dressings typically consist of a sterile ointment and nonadherent dressing. On the face, consider the use of ophthalmic bacitracin ointment. Deep second-degree burns similarly require debridement and dressing with topical antibiotics. Because they are at higher risk for infection, scarring, and contractures, these burns should be managed in consultation with a specialist. Early excision and grafting may be indicated. Temporary skin substitutes are used infrequently because the presence of necrotic material on the wound predisposes such applications to infection. Third-degree burns are debrided and treated with an appropriate topical antibiotics and dressings which will need to be frequently assessed and changed.

Decompression Procedures In cases of circumferential burns of extremities or the torso, early escharotomy may be necessary. The combination of edema and the decreased elasticity of burned tissue can result in compartment syndrome that will cause further injury. Chest wall escharotomy incisions are made along the anterior axillary lines, along the costal margins, and across the top of the chest. Extremity incisions should cross the joints because they are particularly vulnerable to constriction owing to the lack of subcutaneous tissue. It is important to remember that elevated pressures sufficient to cause muscle necrosis can exist in the presence of palpable pulses.

Fluid Resuscitation Patients with >15% TBSA have extensive fluid requirements, and early and aggressive fluid resuscitation is critical. In the first 24 hours, there are large fluid shifts owing to third-spacing of intravascular volume into injured tissue and injury-related histamine release. Most pediatric burn centers recommend fluid resuscitation according to the Parkland formula:

$$4\text{ mL} \times \text{Body weight (in kg)} \times \text{Total burn surface area} = \text{Total fluid replacement in first 24 hours}$$

The first half of the total fluid replacement is given over the first 8 hours, and the second half is given over the next 16 hours.

Most clinicians add maintenance fluids for children younger than 5 years. The goal is a urine output of at least 1 mL/kg per hour; placement of a transurethral bladder (Foley) catheter provides more accurate and continuous measurements.

Ongoing Care

Nutritional Considerations After early stabilization and initial management, continuing needs are addressed. Burn patients experience a hyperdynamic state with increased metabolic demands. Calorie requirements are based on burn surface area. Previous recommendations suggested delayed initiation of nutrition for the first 72 hours; however, recent findings suggest that early insertion of nasogastric tube and provision of enteral feeds is associated with improved mortality and morbidity associated with sepsis due to bacterial translocation. If the patient can tolerate oral intake, then weaning of continuous enteral nutrition can take place. Development of nutritional intolerance should be promptly investigated as a subset of patients can develop transient gastroparesis after a burn injury due to hormonal dysregulation. Parenteral nutrition should generally be avoided as it has been linked to increased mortality, therefore every effort should be made to ensure that nutrition is given enterally.

Pain Control Ongoing pain management is essential. All but the most minor wounds typically require narcotics for pain control, especially during debridement and dressing changes. Common choices are oral acetaminophen scheduled with either oral oxycodone or intravenous morphine as needed for breakthrough pain. Anxiolytics may also be helpful. Patient-controlled analgesia (PCA) may be an appropriate option in older children who are alert and developmentally able to self-administer pain medication as needed. Children with severe burns who are sedated due to being intubated and mechanically ventilated may require higher sedative doses during burn dressing changes.

The trauma associated with the initial injury followed by the pain and fear that many children experience during a hospitalization can heighten their pain. Appropriate pain control is essential to ensure that these stressors do not cause additional distress. Further, attention should be given to ensuring the child has an appropriate understanding of any procedures and that they are provided with a semblance of a routine, particularly during prolonged hospitalizations. A multidisciplinary team that includes child-life specialists and psychologists can help improve the child's immediate recovery and lessen the risk of developing long-term psychological problems.

Wound Care Dressing changes and wound checks should be performed daily to look for signs of infection, which is the most common cause of morbidity and mortality in burn patients. Assessment may be difficult because of the inflammatory changes seen with a healing burn. Burn wound infections are characterized by marked or painful erythema, lymphangitis, focal areas of discoloration within the eschar, discoloration or edema of unburned skin at the wound margin, conversion of partial-thickness wounds to full-thickness wounds, or accelerated separation of eschar. Infections are rare in properly treated partial-thickness burns. In extensive or deep burns, prevention of colonization is generally not achievable. The goal of topical antibiotics is to decrease bacterial colonization and prevent frank infection of the wound, bacteremia, and sepsis. The presence of large TBSA burns predisposes a patient to higher risks of infection or sepsis; however, infection can also occur in smaller burns, especially in those who are very young or with a history of immune dysfunction. When burned patients lose that primary barrier of defense, they are at risk for infection at site of injury, which can also progress to systemic illness. As the TBSA increases, the possibility for infection also increases necessitating frequent clinical evaluation of the patient. White blood cell count is not a reliable indicator of sepsis given that burned patients are constantly exposed to external environments; more reliable indicators include other signs that have to be addressed, such as vital sign alteration, oliguria, hyperglycemia, or acute thrombocytopenia.

Antibiotic Use Most centers reserve systemic antibiotics for systemic spread of infection rather than for prophylactic use. If antibiotics are used, consideration should be given to the common organisms found in burn wounds, including *Streptococcus pyogenes*, *Staphylococcus aureus*, gram-negative organisms (e.g., *Pseudomonas* species), and *Candida* species. Burn wound infection presents a high risk for systemic bacteremia and sepsis and may warrant surgical excision of the infected tissue.

Complications Children with underlying medical conditions and those with large TBSA burns (>15%) are more likely to undergo significant fluid shifts, which can lead to a wide array of complications. Pulmonary edema, acute respiratory distress syndrome, abdominal compartment syndrome, ileus, and extremity compartment syndrome can all occur. Patients with more extensive burns have an increased risk of acute kidney injury (AKI), especially if they are not fluid resuscitated adequately in the first 24 hours following injury. Management of AKI is not limited to fluid only but to correction of electrolyte imbalances and acid/base status. A rapid evaluation of the patient which includes a physical examination and review of objective findings such as intake/output and vital signs is warranted whenever there is a sudden deterioration in their clinical status that may warrant transfer to a higher level of care.

Any substantial burn carries a risk of hypertrophic scar formation and contractures, with resultant functional impairment and disfigurement. Burns involving joints, cosmetically significant areas, and growth regions are managed with a combination of compression and splinting; physical therapy; and surgical skin grafting, tissue expansion, and transposition.

ADMISSION AND DISCHARGE CRITERIA

Indications for Admission Regional burn centers have evolved in most areas because of the labor-intensive and highly specialized nature of caring for patients with significant burn injuries. Criteria for referral to a specialized burn center, based on American Burn Association recommendations, are listed in **Table 163-1**. Depending on resource availability, patients meeting these criteria should be transferred to a regional burn center for hospitalization. Additional reasons for hospitalization in patients who do not necessarily require burn center management include the following:

- Adequate wound care, including return for follow-up visits, cannot be assured
- Unsafe home environment

Discharge Criteria

- Able to take adequate nutrition and fluids by mouth
- Risk of wound infection is substantially diminished

TABLE 163-1 Criteria for Treatment at a Specialized Burn Facility
Second- and third-degree burns over more than 10% of body surface area.
Second- and third-degree burns posing a serious functional or cosmetic threat to the face, hands, feet, genitalia, perineum, or major joints.
Third-degree burns in any age group.
Electrical burns, including lightning injury.
Chemical burns posing a serious functional or cosmetic threat.
Concomitant inhalation injury.
Preexisting medical problems that could complicate burn management.
Associated trauma, when the burn injury poses the greater risk.
Injuries that will require special emotional or rehabilitative support.
Inadequate hospital facilities to provide burn care.

Data based on American Burn Association. Advanced *Burn Life Support: Burn Center Referral Criteria*. http://ameriburn.org/BurnCenterReferralCriteria.pdf. Accessed February 22, 2013. (Excerpted from Committee on Trauma, American College of Surgeons. Resources for Optimal Care of the Injured Patient. Guidelines for the Operation of Burn Center; 2006:79-86.)

- Appropriate wound coverage is in place
- All wounds of questionable viability have been demarcated
- Outpatient dressing changes can be accommodated by a combination of caregiver, visiting nurse, and clinic visits
- A safe home environment is available
- Ongoing follow-up for both immediate and long-term issues is assured

Outpatient care instructions should address acute wound care management and safety education. Instructions for long-term care should include the use of moisturizer and sunblock as well as long-term follow-up.

PREVENTION

Given the devastating injuries that can result from burns, prevention is key. Anticipatory guidance with regard to home safety should be part of routine health maintenance visits and should be re-explored and reemphasized for any patient with a burn injury. Decades of fire prevention education through public schools, education on smoke detectors, and increased availability of fire-retardant materials can be credited with improved rates of injuries from house fires over the past decade. Scald injuries, however, have increased in incidence. The American Academy of Pediatrics (AAP) recommends that water heaters be set at a maximum of 120°F.

Further, fire- and burn injuries are increasing in prevalence in children who come from lower socioeconomic classes. Further work should be devoted to improving education and decreasing the risks of burns in all children.

CHEMICAL BURNS

Chemical burns result from exposure to household or industrial products that are categorized as acids, alkalis, and other agents. Injury is usually due to direct chemical injury, but there may also be heat-related injury due to exothermic reactions. Chemical type, concentration, and quantity and the duration, size, and location of contact all influence the severity of a chemical burn. The potential for systemic absorption and toxicity must also be considered with any chemical exposure, especially hydrocarbons or chemicals associated with industrial use. Consider consulting a local poison control center in cases of chemical injury.

The mainstay of therapy for all chemical exposures is rapid and copious irrigation. A litmus paper test documenting a return to normal pH may help guide the duration of irrigation. Neutralization agents are generally not recommended because they may result in exothermic reactions and thermal injury. In cases of ingestion, emetics are not recommended owing to the risk of esophageal injury or aspiration.

Acids are found in household toilets and drain cleaners as well as in common industrial chemicals. Acids cause coagulation necrosis, thereby avoiding the deeper injury seen with alkali agents. Ingestion causes esophageal injury, and concentration at the pyloric valve may lead to pyloric strictures. Worthy of specific mention is the highly toxic hydrofluoric acid. It causes severe ongoing injury and systemic hypocalcemia due to ion trapping in cases of extensive tissue involvement. After irrigation, topical calcium gel should be applied to the affected area, and the patient should be monitored and treated as needed for systemic hypocalcemia.

Alkalis such as lye (sodium hydroxide) are found in many household cleaners and detergents, hair relaxants, bleach, cement, and fertilizers. A deeply penetrating liquefaction necrosis causes extensive tissue injury. Irrigation is recommended for extended periods until there is resolution of the soapy feeling representing saponification of fat and oils. In cases of ingestion, severe esophageal injury and perforation may occur, and there is a long-term risk of stricture formation. Early gastroenterology and pulmonary consultations for esophagoscopy and bronchoscopy, respectively, are indicated.

ELECTRICAL INJURY

Electricity traveling through the body meets resistance and generates thermal energy, causing tissue damage. Voltage drop and current flow are related to the cross-sectional area; thus, extremities with small cross-sectional areas are more vulnerable to injury.

Low-voltage injuries (<1000 volts) are typically from household currents. With these injuries, the severe tissue burn limits further flow and minimizes further damage. If contact is sustained, local injury can be substantial. A common electrical injury is the oral commissural injury sustained by a child chewing on an electrical cord. Although this is often managed conservatively with splinting, subspecialty consultation is indicated, because surgical reconstruction is sometimes required. Families should be advised about the possibility of a delayed labial artery bleed occurring before or with eschar separation at 2 to 4 weeks after injury. Systemic consequences are rare with low-voltage injuries, and in many cases, admission is not required if local wound care can be managed at home.

High-voltage injuries are those involving electrical currents of 1000 volts or greater, but they also include injuries sustained from contact with high-tension wires (10,000 to 1 million volts). In these injuries, there is no reduction of flow, and a small cutaneous burn may belie significant internal injury. Patients are at risk for cardiac arrhythmia, particularly ventricular fibrillation or asystole, and cardiac monitoring is recommended for 48 hours. Patients are often thrown by the current, so assessment for associated trauma is required. As with other burn injuries, adequate fluid resuscitation is essential; however, because the surface injury may be small, burn surface area calculations are inadequate. Fluid resuscitation should be titrated to a urine output of 1 to 1.5 mL/kg.

Because bone has a high resistance to electrical energy, deeper muscles may sustain greater injury than superficial muscles, and a high index of suspicion must be maintained for necrotic deep tissue. Muscle injury creates a risk for compartment syndrome, which may manifest as tense swelling and decreasing perfusion, with associated pain, pallor, paresthesias, or pulselessness. In these cases, immediate fasciotomy is required. Depending on the nature of the injury and the amount of energy involved, urinalysis, electrocardiogram monitoring, and creatine kinase levels may be considered. Damaged muscle may result in myoglobinuria, with resultant renal injury, especially if fluid resuscitation is inadequate. Forced diuresis with consideration of urine alkalinization in severe cases is indicated and is effective in decreasing this complication. Muscle injury can also lead to hyperkalemia.

As in third-degree burns, mafenide acetate is often used in electrical burns because of its deeper tissue penetration. However, antibiotics alone are often inadequate, and surgical debridement is often required. Close follow-up is required for all victims of significant electrical injury; late sequelae include neurologic problems such as neuropathy, depression, memory loss, and ophthalmic dysfunction due to cataracts.

INTRAVENOUS INFILTRATES

Infiltration of intravenous fluids or medications is a common complication of peripheral venous catheters; it is estimated to occur in 23% to 78% of patients with such devices. Children's tendency to be mobile leads to a high risk of intravenous line malfunction. Such malfunction may be difficult to detect in children owing to their decreased ability to communicate pain as well as their flexible subcutaneous tissue, which can distend without increasing infusion pressures and thereby alerting providers to the line malfunction.

A vesicant is a solution capable of causing tissue injury or destruction. Strictly speaking, infiltration is the inadvertent delivery of a nonvesicant solution, such as normal saline, into the subcutaneous tissue. Extravasation is the delivery of a vesicant to this layer. Here, we use the term *infiltration* to refer to both these processes.

PATHOPHYSIOLOGY

Infiltration occurs when a catheter dislodges or punctures a vein. Multiple mechanisms of injury have been proposed. Irritation from infusate may lead to vasoconstriction and decreased blood flow, creating an ongoing cycle of less dilution of infusate, increased pressure, and subsequent vessel rupture or exit of fluid from the catheter insertion hole. Alternatively, infiltration of infusate through the catheter insertion hole may occur when the flow becomes obstructed. Additionally, endothelial irritation can damage the vessel intima and allow diffusion of infusate into tissue.

Infusate osmolality, pH, and chemical properties play a role in the vascular injury that predisposes to infiltration, and they can mediate tissue injury after infiltration has occurred. Injury also occurs via ischemia and compression. Certain compounds are especially irritating, including electrolyte solutions (notably calcium, high concentrations of dextrose, and parenteral nutrition), antimicrobials (particularly oxacillin and amphotericin B), contrast media, antineoplastic agents, and pressor agents. Vasoactive medications cause intense vasoconstriction, which can lead to ischemia and necrosis.

Direct tissue damage can result in ulceration and tissue necrosis. Increased compartment pressures can lead to arteriolar compression, vascular spasm, pain, and muscle necrosis. Muscular changes can occur in 4 to 12 hours, and ischemic nerve damage can result in functional loss of an extremity within 24 hours. Finally, long-term complications such as complex regional pain syndrome can develop.

CLINICAL PRESENTATION

The hallmark of infiltration is edema, but mild edema may be difficult to detect. Comparison to the opposite side—either visually or by measurement—is the most reliable method of assessment. Other markers include induration, tenderness or pain, blanching or discoloration, blistering, temperature change, and decreased range of motion and sensation. Digital pressure at the tip of an intravenous catheter should occlude flow; if solution continues to infuse even with this pressure, the intravenous line is probably infiltrated. The catheter should be assessed for blood return; however, the presence of blood return does not always rule out infiltration, nor does the absence of blood return rule it in, especially in infants.

A small-volume infiltrate may be difficult to defect, but significant damage can occur if a vesicant is involved. With infusion of such an agent, frequent reassessment is needed, and a conservative approach is warranted, including the early removal of any line suspected of being infiltrated. Assessing the severity of injury may be difficult because cutaneous damage may not reflect evolving subcutaneous fat and fascial damage. Edema may resolve or progress to blistering or necrosis.

DIFFERENTIAL DIAGNOSIS

Infiltrated intravenous lines should be differentiated from other intravenous line complications such as phlebitis, restrictive taping, venous stasis, and infection.

MANAGEMENT

The first step in management is to stop the infusion and attempt to aspirate any remaining drug. Leave the catheter in place if an antidote is indicated; otherwise, remove the line, because the site can no longer be used. Supportive care, notably elevation, is the mainstay of therapy for most infiltrates; many resolve spontaneously. Although there is some controversy, ice applied for 20 minutes, four times a day, for 24 to 48 hours is sometimes recommended. Warm compresses may be indicated for certain chemotherapy drugs, such as the vinca alkaloids. Close and frequent reassessment is needed.

The indications for antidotes are limited and somewhat controversial, and typically best administered in consultation with a specialist. If an antidote is indicated, inject it through the line if the remaining infusate was aspirated; otherwise, avoid using the line, because that will simply infiltrate the remaining medication. An antidote for dopamine and other pressor agents is phentolamine, an adrenergic blocker. It is used to reverse peripheral ischemia in an attempt to avoid tissue necrosis. Phentolamine is given at a dose of 0.1 to 0.2 mg/kg (to an adult maximum of 5 mg) diluted in 10 mL of normal saline; doses as low as 1 mg are frequently sufficient. It is injected through the infiltrate catheter and subcutaneously around the entire area of infiltration with a 25-gauge needle as soon as the infiltration is detected, or within 12 hours at the latest. For other significant infiltrates, especially when compression is an issue, hyaluronidase may be indicated. It breaks down connective tissue around the area of infiltration, allowing medication reabsorption and decreasing fluid pressures. Hyaluronidase is administered subcutaneously and intradermally into the infiltration site. It is diluted to a concentration of 15 units/mL; a single 15-unit dose (1 mL) is then divided into five 0.2-mL doses. Other specific antidotes may be indicated for antineoplastic agents.

CONSULTATION

Any vesicant infiltration, particularly one that requires an antidote, necessitates an urgent surgical consultation. Early intervention with wound debridement can minimize the impact of severe infiltrations.

PREVENTION

Use the smallest catheter possible to avoid restriction of blood flow in the vein. Avoid the administration of vesicants at any site more than 24 hours old or sites that are difficult to immobilize. Vesicants should be administered through central venous access devices whenever feasible.

KEY POINTS

- Initial burn management involves methodical assessment, airway management, fluid resuscitation, and pain control.
- Ongoing burn therapy includes wound debridement, topical antimicrobials, and close observation to detect complications.
- Prompt surgical consultation is indicated for any deep or large surface area burn or any burn with functional or cosmetic significance.
- For infiltration, supportive care is the mainstay of treatment.
- Use vesicants with caution if there is any question about the patency or adequacy of the intravenous access.

SUGGESTED READINGS

Agency for Healthcare Research and Quality. (2021). Fire Burn Resource Guide. National Inpatient Sample (NIS), Healthcare Cost and Utilization Project (HCUP), 2016-2018. https://www.childrenssafetynetwork.org/resources/fire-burn-2021-resource-guide.

Bittner EA, Shank E, Woodson L, Martyn JA. Acute and perioperative care of the burn-injured patient. *Anesthesiology*. 2015;122(2):448-464.

Greenhalgh DG. Topical antimicrobial agents for burn wounds. *Clin Plast Surg*. 2009;36(4):597-606.

Greenhalgh DG, Saffle JR, Holmes JH 4th, et al. American Burn Association consensus conference to define sepsis and infection in burns. *J Burn Care Res*. 2007;28:776.

Herndon DN, Wurzer P, Culnan D, Cancio LC, Kramer GC. Chapter 8: Pathophysiology of Burn Shock and Burn Edema. In: Herndon DN, ed. *Total Burn Care*. 5th ed. Philadelphia: Saunders Elsevier; 2018:70-71.

Pardesi O, Fuzaylov G. Pain management in pediatric burn patients: review of recent literature and future directions. *J Burn Care Res*. 2017;38(6):335-347.

Partain KP, Fabia R, Thakkar RK. Pediatric burn care: new techniques and outcomes. *Curr Opin Pediatr*. 2020;32(3):405-410.

Richardson P, Mustard L. The management of pain in the burns unit. *Burns*. 2009;35:921.

Romanowski KS, Palmieri TL. Pediatric burn resuscitation: past, present, and future. *Burns Trauma*. 2017;5:26.

Saffle JR, Graves C, Cochran A. Nutritional support of the burned patient. In: Herndon DN, ed. *Total Burn Care*. 4th ed. Philadelphia: Saunders Elsevier;2012:333.

Sheridan RL. Burn care for children. *Pediatr Rev*. 2018;39(6):273-286.

Strobel AM, Fey R. Emergency care of pediatric burns. *Emerg Med Clin North Am*. 2018;36(2):441-458.

Wiechman Askay S, Patterson DR, Sharar SR, et al. Pain management in patients with burn injuries. *Int Rev Psychiatry*. 2009;21:522.

CHAPTER 164

Pneumothorax and Pneumomediastinum

Allison E. Williams, MD

BACKGROUND

Pneumothorax and pneumomediastinum are examples of air-leak syndromes in which air accumulates in the spaces outside the lung airways and alveoli. Pneumothorax refers to the abnormal presence of air in the pleural space, whereas pneumomediastinum describes accumulation of air in the mediastinum. Air leak can be traumatic, iatrogenic, or spontaneous.

Both pneumothorax and pneumomediastinum are subdivided into two categories—primary and secondary. Primary occurs in otherwise healthy children without trauma, underlying lung disease or iatrogenic etiology. Secondary pneumothorax occurs when a cause is known. Common secondary causes of air leak syndrome include trauma, iatrogenic (such as medical procedures or barotrauma from mechanical ventilation), and those with underlying lung diseases such as asthma or cystic fibrosis.

Over the past 10 years, there has been a surge of data on pediatric air leak syndromes. The most recent pediatric data suggest that the majority of patients present in the second decade of life and has a male predominance of 4:1. The overall incidence of spontaneous pneumothorax in patients less than 18 years of age is 3.4 to 4 per 100,000. For pneumomediastinum the incidence has a bimodal distribution, occurring most frequently in children between 6 months and 4 years and again in adolescents. The true incidence of spontaneous pneumomediastinum is unknown, however; it ranges from 1 in 800 to 1 in 42,000 pediatric cases.

PNEUMOTHORAX

PATHOPHYSIOLOGY

Although patients with primary spontaneous pneumothorax (PSP) do not have underlying lung disease, computed tomography (CT) and surgical findings show that the majority have subpleural bullae and/or pleural blebs. These findings are not fully understood but may be due to imbalances in protease and antiprotease enzymes leading to emphysema-like changes. Cigarette smoking increases the risk of the development of spontaneous pneumothorax by nearly 10 times, although the magnitude of the risk from secondhand exposure in pediatric patients is not known. Vaping, or the use of e-cigarettes, has also been associated with increased risk of spontaneous pneumothorax amongst other pulmonary pathologies.

Increased intra-alveolar pressure, often from inflammation of small airways, results in tension on the alveolar wall and, ultimately, rupture leading to pneumothorax. Alternatively, air leak occurring within the interstitium can track through the hilum and collect in the mediastinum (causing pneumomediastinum), or rupture into the pleural space leading to pneumothorax. When air entrapped within the pleural space leads to compression of essential organs within the cardiopulmonary system, this is defined as a tension pneumothorax.

CLINICAL PRESENTATION

Patients with primary spontaneous pneumothorax typically present with acute-onset pleuritic chest pain, usually described as sharp initially, becoming dull over time, and frequently resolving after 24 hours even without treatment. Onset frequently occurs while the patient is at rest. Many patients endorse dyspnea, though ipsilateral shoulder pain and dry cough are also common.

Physical examination findings vary depending on the size of the pneumothorax. Patients with small pneumothoraces (<15% of the hemithorax) may show only tachycardia, subjective dyspnea, or may have completely normal findings. In those with larger pleural air collections, examination findings include decreased chest wall movement and decreased or absent breath sounds on the affected side. Hyperresonance and decreased fremitus may also be appreciated. More severe cases demonstrate increased work of breathing with accessory muscle use. Isolated tachycardia is common. However, when accompanied by hypotension, cyanosis, jugular venous distention, or tracheal deviation then tension pneumothorax with tamponade physiology needs to be considered and immediate intervention is required.

DIFFERENTIAL DIAGNOSIS

The differential diagnosis for chest pain with or without associated respiratory symptoms includes cardiovascular, gastrointestinal, pulmonary/pleural, and chest wall diseases. The differential for *pleuritic* chest pain can be narrowed to include pneumonia, idiopathic or viral pleurisy, pulmonary embolism, pericarditis, costochondritis, or other chest wall pathology. Decreased breath sounds on physical examination may be secondary to pneumonia, severe bronchospasm, pleural effusion, foreign body aspiration, or poor respiratory effort. Primary psychological etiologies such as anxiety disorder, panic attack, and vocal cord dysfunction are also on the differential for patients with chest pain, tachycardia, and tachypnea. Radiographically, congenital lobar emphysema, skin folds, and overpenetrated films may be mistaken for pneumothoraces.

DIAGNOSTIC EVALUATION

Definitive diagnosis is made by chest radiograph. On posteroanterior or portable chest film, a linear shadow of thin visceral pleura is seen, along with absence of lung markings beyond the pleural line (**Figure 164-1**). Sensitivity of chest radiograph in the diagnosis of pneumothorax has been reported as high as 80%, though this is greatly reduced with supine views. When clinical suspicion is high but routine films are unrevealing, a lateral decubitus view can help reveal the pleural line. Chest radiographs allow for diagnosis of pneumothorax, but often are inaccurate for sizing, especially for those patients who experience trauma and are unable to have an upright film. In adults, validated formulas can be used to determine the size of pneumothoraces; however, they have not been shown to be accurate in children.

Given the limitation of chest radiography with traumatic pneumothoraces, CT has become the standard of care. These scans are often able to show underlying blebs and bullae much more accurately than with chest radiography; however, the significance of blebs and natural history of this disease is not fully established (**Figure 164-2**). They are also able to detect occult pneumothoraces, though again the clinical significance of these findings is unknown. The focused assessment with sonography in trauma (FAST) examination has recently gained more widespread acceptance and accuracy. Initial studies in pediatric trauma patients with suspected pneumothoraces show that ultrasonography is more accurate than supine chest radiography and equivalent to that of CT, reporting 86% to 98% sensitivity and 97% to 100% specificity.

Laboratory tests offer very little in the diagnosis or management of pneumothorax. In cases where clinical circumstances dictate the need for arterial blood gas analysis, an increased alveolar-arterial gradient proportional to the size of the pneumothorax is commonly seen. Hypercapnia is rare in patients without underlying lung disease. Conversely, many patients demonstrate respiratory alkalosis secondary to associated tachypnea.

MANAGEMENT

Patients presenting with signs and symptoms consistent with tension pneumothorax require immediate needle thoracostomy without delaying for radiographic confirmation. Such patients may include those with pulseless electrical activity without a clear underlying cause. Tube thoracostomy should follow needle decompression in these patients.

In patients with a clinical presentation consistent with pneumothorax without tension physiology, treatment depends on symptomatology and size of the pneumothorax. The two goals of management are to re-expand the affected lung and prevent recurrences. During the initial

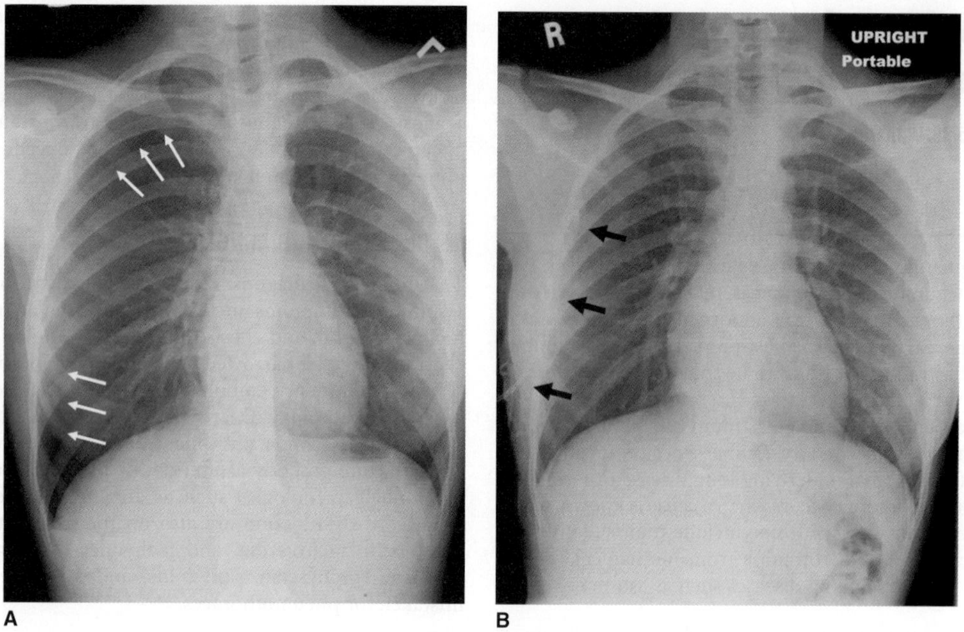

FIGURE 164-1. A. Simple pneumothorax. Note the lack of pleural markings along the right lateral and hemithorax and at the right apex (white arrows). B. Same patient after pigtail thoracostomy tube (black arrows) placement along the lateral wall of the hemithorax with re-expansion of the lung.

evaluation, children may require continuous cardiorespiratory monitoring and supplemental oxygen. High concentrations of oxygen should be avoided to prevent toxicity. In adults, clinical decision-making for management is supported by consensus statements; however, no such guidelines exist in pediatrics. Therefore, management depends on individual practice patterns, available resources, and patient or family preferences.

A wide variety of therapeutic options exist. **Figure 164-3** provides an algorithm for various management strategies.

Observation without intervention is a reasonable approach for first episodes of PSP in otherwise healthy patients with no or minimal symptoms and a small (<15%) pneumothorax by radiograph. Newer data support that this may be done with close outpatient follow-up. While adult data have shown improvement in rates of reabsorption with use of supplemental oxygen, these data are varied in pediatrics often showing no statistical differences or decrease in hospital length of stay or recurrence rates.

Patients with more severe symptoms or those with a large (>15%) pneumothorax require active re-expansion of the affected lung. The American College of Chest Physicians recommends the use of thoracostomy tube as opposed to needle aspiration alone due to high risk of recurrence and persistent air leak. Pigtail (6.5-10.5 French) catheters have been shown to be safe and as effective as large-bore surgical thoracostomy tubes (16-32 French) for pneumothoraces and are less painful. Low-level wall suction is indicated for patients with underlying lung disease or those who fail to show improvement with water seal setup alone. Serial chest radiographs should show re-expansion of the affected lung without a persistent air leak.

Once the affected lung is re-expanded, chest tubes should be clamped and the patient carefully monitored for a minimum of 6 to 8 hours. Patients with reaccumulation of air are likely to become symptomatic during this time. A repeat chest radiograph is recommended before discharge to document improvement.

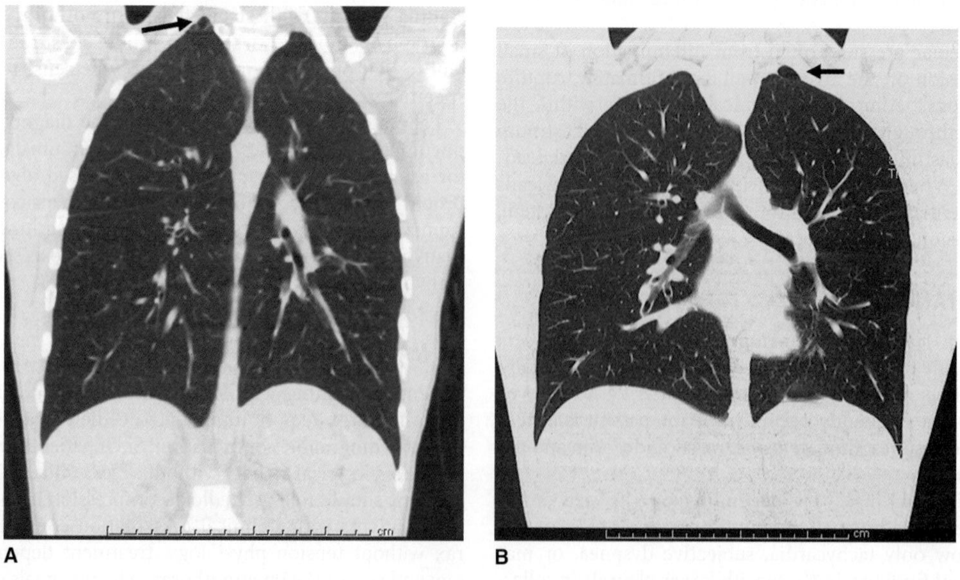

FIGURE 164-2. Coronal images of the chest using CT showing apical blebs (black arrows).

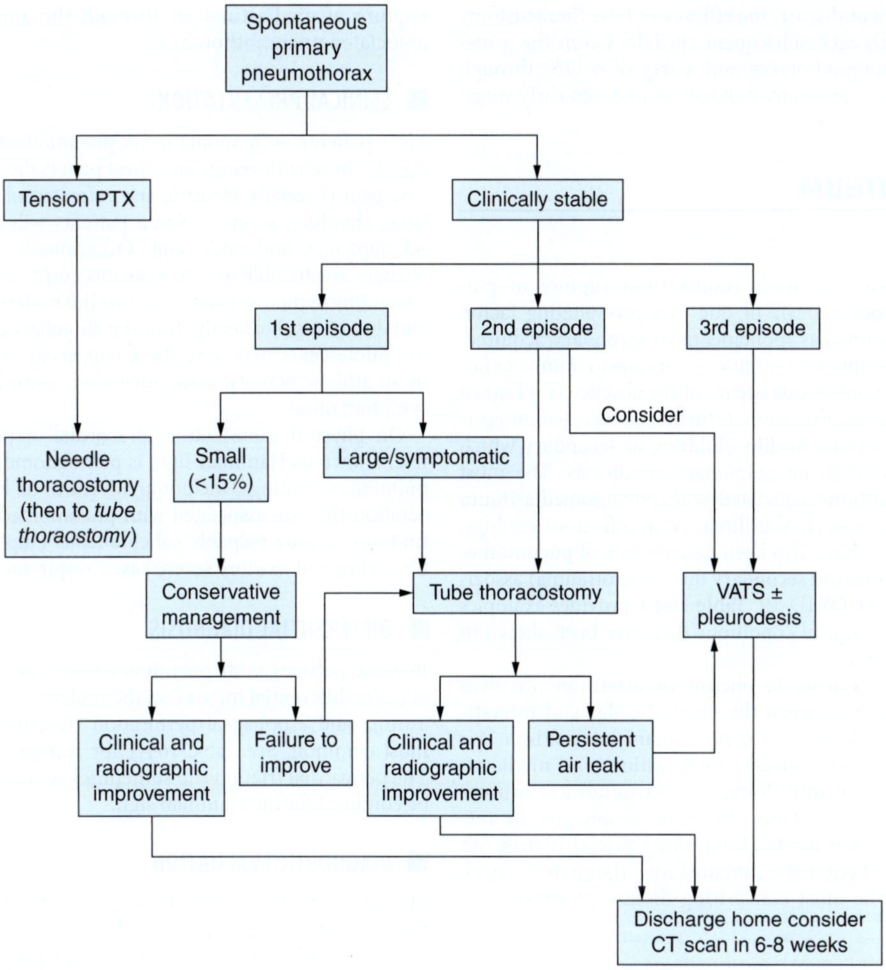

FIGURE 164-3. Management of pneumothorax. CT, computed tomography; PTX, pneumothorax; VATS, video-assisted thoracoscopic surgery.

If tube thoracostomy is not successful in re-expanding the affected lung or the patient has a persistent air leak after 3 to 5 days, surgical repair is indicated. Recent literature has suggested there may be benefit to early surgical intervention. VATS has been demonstrated to be safe and effective in children with pulmonary disease. Studies have indicated that surgical management often leads to lower rate of recurrence than with conservative management alone. In addition, early VATS may reduce length of hospitalization and the number of procedures children require due to failure of conservative management alone.

ADMISSION AND DISCHARGE CRITERIA

Hospitalization is indicated for any of the following reasons:

- Tension pneumothorax
- Hypoxia
- Respiratory distress
- Large (>15% of the hemithorax) primary pneumothorax
- Any secondary pneumothorax

Discharge criteria include:

- No supplemental oxygen requirement
- No increased work of breathing
- For patients being managed without intervention:
  - Complete or nearly complete resolution of pneumothorax on serial radiographs
- For patients treated with pigtail or surgical thoracostomy:
  - Re-expansion of the affected lung
  - No persistent air leak after 6 to 8 hours of observation with the tube clamped
  - No recurrence of pneumothorax on chest radiograph 4 to 6 hours after the tube is removed
- For patients with secondary pneumothoraces:
  - Adequate medical/surgical management of the underlying lung disease as well

CONSULTATION

- General surgery: For thoracostomy placement or VATS as indicated
- Interventional radiology: For pigtail catheter placement
- Pulmonology: Should be considered for patients with primary pneumothoraces that do not resolve rapidly or those with secondary pneumothoraces
- Thoracic surgery: For thoracotomy when clinically indicated

PREVENTION

Avoidance of cigarette smoke, vaping products, and even passive secondhand exposure is an important intervention to reduce the risk of pneumothoraces for all patients.

Recurrence of spontaneous pneumothorax has been estimated between 36% and 52% in otherwise healthy children; this risk is increased in those with secondary pneumothoraces. No currently known risk factors for the development of pneumothoraces can reliably identify patients at high risk for recurrence. Even findings of blebs or bullae on CT have not been shown to predict recurrence in case series.

For patients with recurrent disease, the efficacy of tube thoracostomy drops off significantly with each subsequent episode. Given the growing data on pediatric pneumothoraces and safety of VATS, through shared decision-making care teams may choose to undergo early surgical management.

PNEUMOMEDIASTINUM

PATHOPHYSIOLOGY

Pneumomediastinum most commonly results from rupture of pulmonary alveoli, either spontaneously or due to a precipitating factor. Pneumomediastinum is defined as spontaneous or secondary/acquired. Secondary or acquired pneumomediastinum occurs due to trauma or iatrogenic procedure while spontaneous occurs in the absence of a known cause. Spontaneous pneumomediastinum is further subdivided into primary, which occurs in otherwise healthy children, or secondary which occurs in patients with underlying pulmonary conditions. The most common pulmonary conditions associated with pneumomediastinum are obstructive lung diseases, such as asthma, or an infectious etiology, such as bronchiolitis. There have also been case reports of pneumomediastinum (both spontaneous and secondary due to barotrauma) associated with pediatric cases of COVID-19. **Table 164-1** provides examples of numerous medical and surgical conditions that have been shown to lead to pneumomediastinum.

The pathophysiology resulting in pneumomediastinum involves increased pressure gradient between the intra-alveolar and interstitial spaces that leads to air leak into the pulmonary interstitium. Air then dissects along the vascular sheaths to the hilum and mediastinum. In other cases, air from intrathoracic or extrathoracic sources can dissect along fascial planes from the neck, esophagus, or retroperitoneum. Similarly, such air tracking along fascial planes can leave the mediastinum and enter the subcutaneous tissue in the neck and upper extremities. The most concerning disease progression is rupture of mediastinal air through the adjacent pleura causing an associated pneumothorax.

TABLE 164-1 Conditions Causing Pneumomediastinum and Subcutaneous Emphysema in Children

Airway Obstruction
Bronchial occlusion, foreign body aspiration, space-occupying lesions
Iatrogenic
Adenoidectomy and tonsillectomy, air abrasion device, bronchoscopy, dental procedures, Heimlich maneuver, mechanical ventilation, surgery (abdominal, laparoscopic, thoracic), tracheostomy
Infections
Bacterial and viral pneumonia, laryngitis, *Pneumocystis carinii* pneumonia, retropharyngeal abscess
Obstructive Lung Disease
Asthma, bronchiolitis, bronchiolitis obliterans with organizing pneumonia, cystic fibrosis, lung emphysema
Toxic Effects
Inhaled drug abuse (cocaine, marijuana), paraquat intoxication, toxic gas
Trauma
Barotrauma (diving, flying, nose blowing), oral or blunt cervical trauma, chest trauma, child abuse
Valsalva Maneuvers
Coughing, defecation, postpartum status, vomiting
Weakness of Tissue
Anorexia nervosa, bone marrow transplantation and chemotherapy, dermatomyositis, diabetic hyperpnea, hypersensitivity pneumonitis, lymphangioleiomyomatosis, ulcerative colitis
Idiopathic

Source: Reproduced with permission from Gesundheit B, Preminger A, Harito B, et al. Pneumomediastinum and subcutaneous emphysema in an 18-month-old child. *J Pediatr.* 2002;141:116-120.

CLINICAL PRESENTATION

Most patients with spontaneous pneumomediastinum are asymptomatic. In those with symptoms, chest pain is the most common complaint. The pain is usually pleuritic and retrosternal and often radiates to the back, shoulder, or arms. Some patients will note dyspnea, dysphagia, odynophagia, and neck pain. Occasionally, patients will notice skin changes attributable to subcutaneous emphysema. More commonly, the presenting symptoms are related to the underlying illness (e.g., asthma) and do not result directly from the air collection in the mediastinal cavity. Adolescents may describe a triggering event such as participating in an athletic activity, eating/drinking, vomiting, or coughing prior to symptom onset.

On physical examination, precordial crepitus associated with systole, known as Hamman sign, is pathognomonic. There are no specific pulmonary findings, including adventitious lung sounds or decreased aeration that are associated with pneumomediastinum. Other possible findings include palpable subcutaneous emphysema, neck swelling or torticollis, and in more severe cases, respiratory distress.

DIFFERENTIAL DIAGNOSIS

Because patients with pneumomediastinum are generally asymptomatic, the differential focuses on the underlying cause of the air leak, with asthma and esophageal perforation (Boerhaave syndrome) being the most common. See Table 164-1 for recognized associated conditions. The pericardial friction rub sometimes appreciated with pericarditis can be confused for the Hamman sign.

DIAGNOSTIC EVALUATION

Pneumomediastinum may be suspected from description of a triggering event or findings on physical examination; however, more often it is found incidentally on a chest radiograph performed to evaluate for symptom etiology. Chest radiograph remains the gold standard for diagnosis of pneumomediastinum. Pneumomediastinum is seen as a vertical radiolucent line along the left side of the cardiac silhouette (see **Figure 164-4A**). In addition, subcutaneous emphysema can sometimes be seen as streaks or pockets of hypolucency in the soft tissue of the neck, shoulders, and upper extremities (see **Figures 164-4** and **164-5**). Lateral views may be helpful to document retrosternal air if the diagnosis is in doubt or for other clinical concerns. Chest radiography may also elucidate an underlying cause, including hyperinflation with asthma or widening of the inferior mediastinum with esophageal perforation. Evaluation for associated pneumothorax is similarly important. Forced expiratory films should be avoided because they may worsen the pneumomediastinum.

CT scans are not routinely recommended as the information they provide often will not change clinical management. Concern for foreign body aspiration may be an indication for bronchoscopy or esophagoscopy, or both, whereas pneumomediastinum in the setting of prolonged or violent vomiting requires investigation for Boerhaave syndrome with esophagoscopy, CT, or esophagram.

MANAGEMENT

Unlike air in the pleural space, pneumomediastinum rarely requires intervention. This generally benign condition resolves without sequelae, so conservative management with careful observation is the standard of care. Appropriate analgesia, rest, avoidance of Valsalva maneuvers (e.g., peak expiratory flow measurement in asthmatics), and careful control of underlying conditions are key to successful resolution. In patients with clinical stability and adequate analgesia, observation may occur in the emergency room for 2 to 4 hours, with further monitoring at home with appropriate primary care follow-up. Time until improvement is dependent on the size of the air collection and the severity of the underlying illness. Most patients require only a few days; however, up to 14 days may be needed in more severe cases.

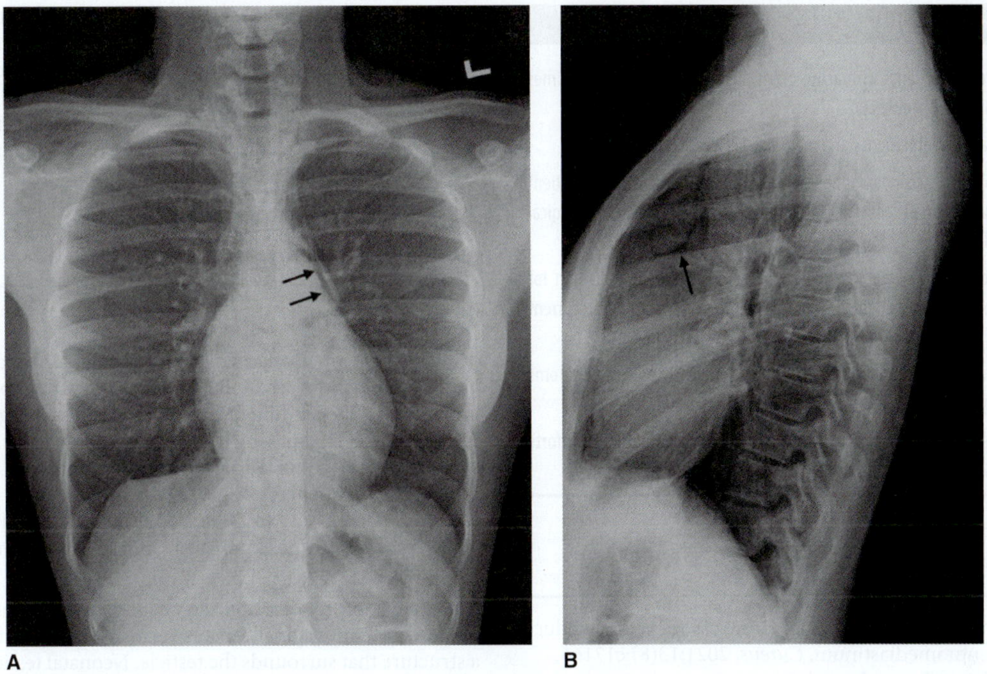

FIGURE 164-4. Posterior-anterior and lateral radiographs with pneumomediastinum and pneumopericardium. Note the line of air along the cardiac silhouette (black arrows) consistent with pneumopericardium as well as the air within the soft tissues of the neck.

Complications of pneumomediastinum are rare but include tamponade physiology, laryngeal compression, and mediastinitis in the setting of esophageal perforation. Because of the predictable benign course of this illness and the low incidence of recurrent disease, follow-up radiography is not routinely required in patients with isolated pneumomediastinum without pneumothorax. For clinically tenuous patients or those who fail to improve with conservative therapy, mediastinal drainage, and mediastinotomy have been described, but such measures are rarely required.

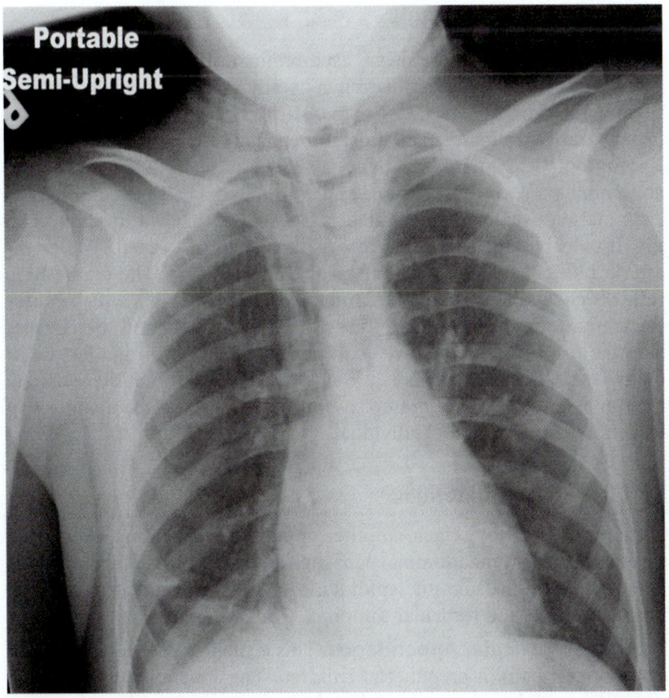

FIGURE 164-5. Portable chest radiograph showing air throughout the superior mediastinum extending into the soft tissues of the neck.

ADMISSION AND DISCHARGE CRITERIA

Hospitalization is indicated for any of the following reasons:

- Severely symptomatic patients—respiratory distress or uncontrolled analgesia
- Hypoxia
- Associated pneumothorax
- Medical/surgical management of the underlying illness as indicated
- Uncertainty regarding the cause of the pneumomediastinum, if potentially concerning etiologies for the air leak cannot be ruled out

Discharge criteria include:

- No respiratory distress
- No supplemental oxygen requirement
- Stable or resolving air collection
- Adequate management of relevant underlying medical conditions
- Adequate analgesia with oral medications

CONSULTATION

- Pulmonology: For management of severe, underlying lung disease
- Gastroenterology: For evaluation of esophageal perforation by esophagoscopy or esophagography, or both

PREVENTION

Prevention of pneumomediastinum is best accomplished with adequate management of the underlying disease and close monitoring of the risks during medical procedures and interventions (e.g., barotrauma during treatment of pulmonary disease with mechanical ventilation). In addition, avoidance of maneuvers that may exacerbate the air leak such as peak expiratory flow measurement in asthmatics, forced expiratory radiographs, other Valsalva maneuvers is important.

KEY POINTS

- Pneumothorax frequently presents with acute-onset pleuritic chest pain, oftentimes with associated breathing difficulties.
- Tension pneumothorax is an emergency and requires immediate decompression.
- Large spontaneous or any secondary pneumothoraces are managed by inpatient admission, often requiring small caliber thoracostomy tubes and potential for surgical intervention with VATS.
- Growing body of literature may support the early use of surgical intervention for pneumothoraces especially for patients with underlying lung disease or recurrent pneumothoraces.
- Patients with pneumomediastinum are usually asymptomatic, except for symptoms related to any underlying illness or injury.
- Management of pneumomediastinum is nearly always conservative, with efforts focused on diagnosing and treating any underlying medical conditions.

SUGGESTED READINGS

Adhikari R, Manduva D, Malayala SV, et al. A rare case of vaping-induced spontaneous pneumomediastinum. *Cureus*. 2021;13(8):e17166.

Dixit A, Uvaise M, Canet-Tarres A, et al. Spontaneous massive pneumomediastinum in a previously well infant with COVID-19. *Pediatrics*. 2021;148(6):e2021051904.

Enrica M, Lauriti G, Lisi G, Riccio A, Chiesa PL. Management of spontaneous pneumothorax in children: a systematic review and meta-analysis. *Eur J Pediatr Surg*. 2020;30:2-12.

Gariepy M, Beaunoyer M, Miron MC, Garvel J. Management and recurrence of spontaneous pneumothorax in children. *Paediatr Child Health*. 2020;25(2):86-92.

Goldman RD. Spontaneous pneumothorax in children. *Can Fam Physician*. 2020;66: 737-738.

Hung C-S, Chen Y-C, Yang T-F, Huang FH. Systematic review and meta-analysis on juvenile primary spontaneous pneumothorax: conservative or surgical approach first? *PLoS One*. 2021;16(4):e0250929.

Kuo HC, Lin YJ, Huang CF, et al. Small-bore pigtail catheters for the treatment of primary spontaneous pneumothorax in young adolescents. *Emerg Med J*. 2013;30(3):e17.

MacDuff A, Arnold A, Harvey J. Management of spontaneous pneumothorax: British Thoracic Society pleural disease guideline 2010. *Thorax*. 2010; 65(Suppl 2):ii18-31.

Noorbakhsh KA, Williams AE, Langham JJW, et al. Management and outcomes of spontaneous pneumomediastinum in children. *Pediatr Emerg Care*. 2021;37(12):e1051-e1056.

Rowan KR, Kirkpatrick AW, Kevin D, Forkheim KE, Mayo JR, Nicolaou S. Traumatic pneumothorax detection with thoracic US: correlation with chest radiography and CT - initial experience. *Radiology*. 2022;225(1):210-214.

CHAPTER 165 Urology

Joana Dos Santos, MD, MHSc, FRCPC,
Natasha Brownrigg, BScN, MN, NP-Pediatrics,
and Katie Meier, MD

BACKGROUND

Pediatric hospitalists encounter several urologic conditions in the care of hospitalized children. Primary urologic surgical emergencies such as testicular torsion and urinary obstruction require prompt diagnosis and intervention to limit morbidity. Other conditions, such as recurrent urinary tract infection (UTI) and vesicoureteral reflux (VUR), hydronephrosis, urolithiasis, and voiding dysfunction, may also benefit from urologic consultation. Although most surgeries in pediatric urology are same-day procedures with patients discharged a few hours postoperatively, newborn and young infants, children with complex urological conditions, or those who present with surgical complications (e.g., postoperative urinary retention) are hospitalized. In this chapter, we discuss the inpatient management of common urologic conditions requiring admission.

TESTICULAR TORSION

BACKGROUND

Testicular torsion is caused by the spontaneous twisting of the spermatic cord resulting in decreased blood flow and hypoxia to the testicular parenchyma. Depending on the mechanism and degree of torsion, there is a variable period in which the testis is salvageable, but studies suggest surgical repair within 4 to 8 hours after symptom onset may result in 90% to 100% testicular salvage rates, while only 10% of testicles are saved if surgery occurs in 12 to 24 hours. Although testicular torsion can occur at any age, it has a predominantly bimodal occurrence, in the neonatal and pubertal periods.

Pathophysiology Torsion can occur by two mechanisms: extravaginal torsion and intravaginal torsion, terms referring to the tunica vaginalis, a structure that surrounds the testicle. Neonatal testicular torsion is typically extravaginal (85%-90%), in which the spermatic cord twists outside the tunica vaginalis, carrying a higher risk of eventual contralateral torsion. It occurs during the descent of the testicle from the abdomen into the scrotum. Torsion may occur in the prenatal period (60%-75%), during delivery, or postnatally. Risk factors include breech presentation, prolonged labor, and babies large for gestational age. Testicular torsion in pubertal patients is more commonly intravaginal.

Twisting of the spermatic cord causes ischemia, and reperfusion of the testicle when torsion is released. Testicular ischemia-reperfusion is the main mechanism of injury, potentially leading to necrosis of the testicle and loss of function. The undescended testicle is at risk for testicular torsion, presumably because of abnormal mesorchial fixation. Any child with a nonpalpable testicle and abdominal pain should be evaluated for intra-abdominal testicular torsion. Other risk factors include underlying bell clapper deformity, prior torsion-detorsion, and trauma.

CLINICAL PRESENTATION

Neonatal torsion is almost always asymptomatic and discovered on routine examination. The examination generally shows an edematous, erythematous hemiscrotum with a firm testicle. The hemiscrotum does not usually transilluminate. In contrast to neonatal torsion, pubertal torsion is symptomatic. Patients experience a sudden onset of hemiscrotal pain, abdominal pain, or both. Nausea and vomiting may also occur. Physical examination usually demonstrates an elevated testicle within the scrotal sac. If palpable, the spermatic cord is thickened or twisted. The cremasteric reflex is generally absent on the affected side. The cremasteric reflex is elicited by stroking the inner aspect of the thigh, which causes the cremasteric muscle within the scrotum to contract and thereby elevate the testis and scrotum. It is important to perform this test bilaterally because asymmetry is key. Some individuals do not demonstrate this reflex and it is therefore not useful in establishing the diagnosis of testicular torsion in these individuals.

DIFFERENTIAL DIAGNOSIS

Differential diagnoses include other conditions presenting with acute scrotal and/or lower abdominal pain such as torsion of testicular appendages, epididymitis, orchitis, epididymo-orchitis, incarcerated inguinal hernia, trauma, and testicular tumor.

Torsion of Testicular Appendages This is the most common cause of acute scrotal pain in prepubertal children. The appendix testis and the appendix epididymis are two embryological remnants with no function that can twist and may cause scrotal pain and swelling. However, there are several characteristics that can help distinguish this diagnosis from testicular torsion. The onset of pain and swelling is usually gradual and is rarely associated with nausea or vomiting. Most boys continue with their activities, reporting discomfort only when the area is touched. Physical examination reveals tenderness of the upper pole of the superior aspect of the testicle or the epididymis. The cremasteric reflex is generally intact. Sometimes the necrotic appendage is visible through the scrotum, a finding called the "blue dot" sign. Scrotal ultrasound rarely identifies the necrotic appendages, but it does demonstrate normal blood flow to the testicle and increased blood flow to the epididymis. Treatment is conservative with rest and analgesics. The prognosis is excellent with no known long-term sequelae.

DIAGNOSTIC EVALUATION

The TWIST (Testicular Workup for Ischemia and Suspected Torsion) score is a validated clinical decision scoring system that helps estimate the risk of testicular torsion based on signs and symptoms (**Table 165-1**). A score of 0 to 2 is considered low risk, while a score ≥5 is classified as high risk with a 100% positive predictive value for testicular torsion. In addition to the clinical findings, scrotal Doppler ultrasound (when available) is the imaging test of choice as it can accurately determine the presence or absence of testicular blood flow in testicular torsion. However, ultrasound results and interpretation can vary due to operator experience and other technical factors, and therefore clinical judgment is paramount. In cases in which the diagnosis is not in question, proceeding directly to surgery is appropriate. Likewise, surgery should not be delayed when testicular torsion is suspected and ultrasound is not readily available.

MANAGEMENT

The viability of the testicle will be determined intraoperatively, and orchiectomy or orchidopexy will be performed. Viability is assessed after intraoperative manual detorsion and observation for a period. Contralateral scrotal fixation is often performed to prevent the small risk of similar occurrence on the unaffected side.

ADMISSION/DISCHARGE CRITERIA

Neonates may require admission due to age and postanesthesia monitoring. Typically, otherwise healthy children and adolescents who present with testicular torsion do not require postoperative admission and are discharged from the postanesthesia care unit.

Discharge criteria:

- Patient is alert with adequate oral intake.
- Adequate pain control with oral analgesics (e.g., acetaminophen and ibuprofen).

CONSULTATION

- Testicular torsion requires urgent surgical consultation and treatment.
- Transfer to a tertiary center is advisable only if anesthetic or surgical services are inadequate for treating the neonate or pediatric patient.

TABLE 165-1 The TWIST (Testicular Workup for Ischemia and Suspected Torsion) score—a validated clinical decision scoring system to estimate the risk of testicular torsion. A score of 0-2 is considered low risk, while a score ≥5 is classified as high risk with a 100% positive predictive value for testicular torsion.

Clinical criteria	Points
Testicular swelling	2
Hard testicle on palpation	2
Absent cremasteric reflex	1
Nausea/vomiting	1
High-riding testicle	1

HYDRONEPHROSIS

BACKGROUND

Hydronephrosis is a finding on ultrasound that describes the dilatation of the collecting system (renal pelvis and calyces) for various etiologies ranging from more benign to pathologic in nature. Each of these etiologies has its own unique pathophysiology and can be congenital (e.g., ureteropelvic junction obstruction) or acquired (e.g., nephrolithiasis). The more common etiologies will be described further in this chapter. Once hydronephrosis is detected, it is imperative to identify which cases need further investigation and expert consultation.

Prenatal hydronephrosis is common, and the vast majority of prenatal hydronephrosis (75%-80%) will resolve without surgical intervention.

CLINICAL PRESENTATION

Hydronephrosis can be detected as early as in utero, throughout childhood, and into adolescence.

It is a common prenatal anomaly occurring in up to 5% of pregnancies. Amniotic fluid is primarily composed of urine produced by the fetal kidneys after the 18th week of gestation. Hydronephrosis is usually detected with ultrasound but can be seen on other imaging modalities (e.g., MRI, CT scan) the latter usually as an incidental finding. If not detected prenatally, pathologic causes of hydronephrosis can present with failure to thrive, hematuria, hypertension, urinary tract infection, and abdominal/flank pain.

DIFFERENTIAL DIAGNOSIS

- Transient primary hydronephrosis
- Ureteropelvic junction obstruction (UPJO)
- Vesicoureteric reflux (VUR)
- Uretero-vesical junction obstruction (UVJO) or primary nonobstructive megaureter
- Ureterocele
- Ectopic ureter
- Causes of megacystis (dilated bladder)/bladder outlet obstruction: posterior urethral valves (PUV), Prune Belly syndrome, megacystis-megaureter syndrome, megacystis-microcolon intestinal hypoperistalsis syndrome (MMIHS), anterior urethral valves, megalourethra, urethral atresia, and cloacal anomalies.

DIAGNOSTIC EVALUATION

Evaluation of all hydronephrosis cases should include a thorough clinical examination that focuses on the genitalia, back/lumbosacral regions, and abdomen. Laboratory tests including chemistry, hematology, urinalysis, and urine culture should be considered when clinically relevant, such as bilateral involvement or solitary kidney.

Ultrasound is the primary diagnostic test used to evaluate hydronephrosis. There are several classification systems that can be used to describe the degree of hydronephrosis. One way is to describe hydronephrosis by the anterior-posterior diameter (APD) measured in the mid-transverse view. The Society for Fetal Urology (SFU) classification consists of four grades which relate to the amount of hydronephrosis visualized (grade 0: no hydronephrosis, grade 1: renal pelvis visualized, grade 2: renal pelvis and a few calyces, grade 3: all calyces seen, grade 4: all calyces seen + parenchymal thinning). The newest classification system is the Urinary Tract Dilatation (UTD) classification, and it incorporates APD, parenchymal characteristics, calyceal dilatation, ureter dilatation, and bladder abnormalities.

Voiding cystourethrogram (VCUG) is used to evaluate VUR, ureteroceles, and bladder outlet obstruction (i.e., PUV). The routine use of VCUG for all prenatal hydronephrosis cases is no longer standard of care. VCUG should be routinely performed in cases of dilated ureter(s), bladder abnormalities, febrile UTI, and suspected bladder outlet obstruction.

Diuretic renography is helpful in the evaluation of differential function, drainage, and renal scarring. The two most commonly used are MAG 3 (mercaptoacetyltriglycine) to assess drainage and DMSA (dimercaptosuccinic acid) to provide more accurate differential function and assess for renal scarring. MAG3 should not be performed prior to 8 weeks of age due to immature GFR. Other diagnostic tests that could be considered for more complex cases include magnetic resonance urography (MRU) and cystoscopy.

MANAGEMENT

In nearly all cases, prenatal hydronephrosis is monitored by serial ultrasonography until delivery. Babies suspected of lower urinary tract obstruction (e.g., PUV, urethral atresia, urethral stenosis) should be born at a high-risk center to facilitate neonatal intensive care, pediatric urology intervention, and nephrology care. These babies are at risk for postobstruction diuresis after bladder decompression, fluid/electrolyte disturbances, and may need dialysis. Oligohydramnios complications including lung hypoplasia, intrauterine growth restriction, and feeding difficulties must also be considered.

Renal/bladder ultrasound (RBUS) should be performed after 48 hours of life because of the relative oliguria that occurs during the early neonatal period except in cases that necessitate immediate intervention. Postnatal management includes prophylactic antibiotics (preferred agents: trimethoprim, amoxicillin, cephalexin), although the use of prophylaxis remains controversial, especially for isolated hydronephrosis. Trimethoprim-sulfamethoxazole and nitrofurantoin should not be used in the neonatal period due to the risk of kernicterus and hemolytic anemia, respectively. Prophylactic antibiotics should be considered for higher-risk hydronephrosis populations (hydroureter, VUR, female gender, uncircumcised males, lower urinary tract obstruction), while the use in lower-risk hydronephrosis populations (isolated hydronephrosis or low-grade hydronephrosis) may be optional. Due to the paucity of high-quality evidence, antibiotic prophylaxis remains a controversial topic.

ADMISSION CRITERIA

- Pediatric patients with symptomatic hydronephrosis necessitating investigation, IV antibiotics, fluid/electrolyte management, and surgical intervention.

DISCHARGE CRITERIA

- Improved symptoms
- Stable fluid/electrolytes
- Plan for further investigation/procedures
- Follow-up with specialty services (i.e., urology, nephrology) arranged

CONSULTATION

Pediatric urologic consultation is strongly advisable in patients with moderate-to-severe hydronephrosis (SFU grade 3/4; UTD 2/3; APD >7mm), VUR, bladder wall abnormalities, suspected lower urinary tract obstruction, evidence of renal asymmetry or renal scarring, symptomatic hydronephrosis (i.e., UTI, flank/abdominal pain). Pediatric urologic consultation should be considered for mild hydronephrosis.

OBSTRUCTION

PATHOPHYSIOLOGY

Obstruction within the urinary tract is a term that encompasses many different urologic conditions; the most common pediatric causes being UPJ obstruction, congenital megaureter or UVJ obstruction, PUVs, ectopic ureter, and ureterocele. In most cases, urinary tract obstruction does not involve complete obstruction of urinary flow but can still cause upper tract deterioration and symptoms. UPJ and UVJ obstructions refer to the anatomical narrowing of these two connection points which impair urine flow. PUVs are obstructive membranes of tissue in the urethra. An ectopic ureter is a ureter that inserts somewhere other than the bladder. A ureterocele is a cystic dilatation of the distal ureter within the bladder. Ectopic ureters and ureteroceles are associated with duplication anomalies. All of these anomalies occur during fetal development.

CLINICAL PRESENTATION

The vast majority of patients with obstruction are asymptomatic. Infants and children rarely present with an abdominal mass, but this presentation should prompt immediate evaluation. Most children with hydronephrosis are detected antenatally and monitored postnatally. Others will present with a febrile UTI or complaints of episodic abdominal pain.

The presentation of obstructive uropathy is dependent on where the obstruction occurs and the sequelae. In infancy, UPJ and UVJ obstructions are usually asymptomatic if unilateral, although the latter has a higher risk of UTI. UPJ obstruction presenting later in childhood can cause pain, nausea/vomiting, and UTI. Intermittent UPJ obstruction presents as episodic abdominal pain often associated with nausea/vomiting (also called Dietl's crisis). Diagnosis is challenging as ultrasound may not detect significant hydronephrosis because of the intermittent obstruction. Diuretic renography or MRU is helpful. The effect of bilateral obstructive uropathy requires more immediate intervention due to the risk of kidney dysfunction.

The spectrum of PUV presentation ranges from mild (responding well to bladder decompression and surgical intervention) to the most severe (requiring renal replacement therapy shortly after birth and renal transplantation). Fluid and electrolyte disturbances, growth and development impairment, and resulting failure to thrive, acid/base disturbances, hypertension, and anemia can occur as a result of kidney disease. Furthermore, some infants may require respiratory support due to lung hypoplasia related to oligohydramnios.

Large ureteroceles can potentially obstruct urethra resulting in symptoms similar to lower urinary tract obstruction. Obstructing ureteroceles can cause increased hydroureteronephrosis and UTIs. Ectopic ureters presenting later in life can cause urinary incontinence for girls as the ectopic ureter inserts below the bladder neck or into the vagina. For boys, the insertion of ectopic ureter is above the external sphincter and therefore not associated with urinary incontinence. Boys may present with recurrent epididymo-orchitis.

DIFFERENTIAL DIAGNOSIS

In addition to congenital anomalies of urinary tract obstruction, the following differential diagnosis should be considered: renal calculi, tumor, and urethral stricture.

DIAGNOSTIC EVALUATION

In most clinical settings, obstruction is suspected by the presence of hydronephrosis on renal ultrasound; however, confirmation by a functional study such as a nuclear medicine renal scan should be done. The two most common types of renal scans are the MAG3 Lasix renal scan and the DMSA renal scan. The MAG3 Lasix renal scan provides information on the differential function of the kidneys (how the kidneys function in relation to each other) as well as drainage time of the kidneys. The DMSA renal scan detects cortical defects (renal scars) and provides a more accurate differential function of the kidneys.

VCUG is performed if lower urinary tract obstruction such as PUV is suspected. In addition to providing information on VUR, the urethra, and the presence of other bladder abnormalities (trabeculations, ureteroceles, diverticuli), the contrast used in the VCUG can also delineate anatomical areas impeding urine flow. For suspected acquired conditions US, MRI, CT scan, X-ray, and cystoscopy can be considered.

MANAGEMENT

Treatment depends on the diagnosis established. Patients with clinically significant obstruction as determined by functional imaging studies, worsening trend of hydronephrosis on ultrasound, or symptoms, require surgery. The prognosis is excellent in most cases after surgical correction of UPJ obstruction, UVJ obstruction, ectopic ureter, and ureterocele. Patients with severe PUV can have long-term sequelae such as chronic kidney disease (CKD), bladder instability, myogenic bladder failure, urinary incontinence, hypertension, or progression to end-stage renal disease and renal replacement therapy. Consequently, these patients need long-term urologic follow-up and coordinated care with a pediatric nephrologist for optimal bladder and renal management. Management of acquired urinary tract obstruction is beyond the scope of this chapter except urolithiasis which will be reviewed later.

ADMISSION CRITERIA

- Pediatric patients with urosepsis due to obstruction must be admitted for treatment and management of obstruction.
- Asymptomatic patients can be managed with close monitoring in ambulatory settings and antibiotic prophylaxis should be considered for higher-risk populations.
- Pediatric patients considered at risk for postobstructive diuresis should be admitted for IV therapy and fluid/electrolyte management.

DISCHARGE CRITERIA

- Based on obstruction relief
- Renal function and fluid/electrolyte stability

CONSULTATION

- Infants with obstruction and sepsis require immediate surgical intervention by a pediatric urologist.

VESICOURETERAL REFLUX

PATHOPHYSIOLOGY

Vesicoureteral reflux (VUR) is a common childhood condition defined as the backflow of urine from the bladder to one or both ureters toward the upper urinary tract. VUR can be primary or secondary. Primary VUR is the result of a congenital anomaly at the ureterovesical junction (UVJ), whereas secondary VUR refers to reflux that occurs from increased bladder pressure (such as in PUV, neurogenic bladder). Normally, the position and functionality of the ureters within the bladder act as both passive and active anti-reflux mechanisms, respectively. In passive VUR, reflux occurs as the bladder fills. There is an alteration in the passive compression of the intravesical ureter against the detrusor which relies on the length and diameter of ureteral tunnel within the bladder wall. During active VUR, reflux occurs during the voiding phase. Alterations of smooth muscle configuration and loss of interstitial cells of Cajal at the ureterovesical junction create an uncoordinated detrusor contraction resulting in retrograde flow of urine.

CLINICAL PRESENTATION

Febrile UTI is a common presentation of VUR. VUR is usually diagnosed during work-up following UTI or during postnatal investigations of asymptomatic babies with a history of prenatal hydronephrosis. The prevalence of VUR in healthy children is estimated to be 1% to 3%. In contrast, Visuri et al. found the prevalence of VUR in children with one or more UTIs is much higher (overall 30%-50% and 70% in the first year of life). Because of this, renal ultrasound is recommended for all febrile UTIs. VUR may also present with CKD, and failure to thrive. Secondary VUR has a more varied clinical presentation.

DIFFERENTIAL DIAGNOSES

Secondary VUR: neurogenic cause (e.g., spina bifida, tethered cord, trauma, tumor), dysfunctional voiding (Hinnman Syndrome), constipation, urethral stricture.

DIAGNOSTIC EVALUATION

VUR is almost exclusively diagnosed with VCUG and less commonly radionuclide cystography. VCUG involves catheterization and filling of the bladder with contrast, followed by X-ray images during the filling and voiding phases. VUR is graded on a scale of 1 to 5 from least to most severe, as defined by the International Reflux Study Committee (**Figure 165-1**).

A DMSA renal scan can also be considered to evaluate differential function of the kidneys and assess for any cortical defects (renal scarring).

MANAGEMENT

The management is threefold:

- Prevent recurrent febrile UTIs
- Prevent renal injury
- Minimize the morbidity of treatment and follow-up

In children younger than 1 year of age with a history of febrile UTIs, continuous antibiotic prophylaxis is commonly recommended. In the absence of febrile UTIs, prophylaxis is still recommended for grades 3, 4, and 5 and may be considered/offered for grades 1 and 2. Circumcision may also be considered for male infants to decrease the risk of UTI in the first year of life.

In children older than 1 year, factors such as the presence of bowel and bladder dysfunction, renal scarring, VUR grade, parental preferences, and clinical context should be considered. Generally, prophylaxis is recommended in the presence of bowel and bladder dysfunction, recurrent febrile UTIs, or renal scarring. The RIVUR trial demonstrated a 50% reduction in the risk of UTIs with antibiotic prophylaxis in children with recurrent UTI and VUR but no significant change in renal scarring. Antibiotic prophylaxis continues to be a controversial issue.

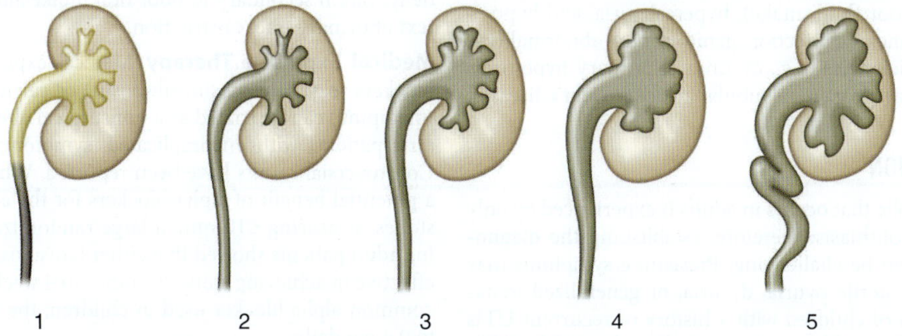

FIGURE 165-1. Classification of grades of VUR used by the International Reflux. Study Committee. Grade 1: Reflux is limited to the ureter, no dilation. Grade 2: Reflux that extends into the kidney, no dilation (normal fornices). Grade 3: Reflux that extends into the kidney with mild to moderate dilation of the ureter renal pelvis and calyces with minimal blunting of fornices. Grade 4: Reflux that extends into the kidney with ureter dilation and dilation of the renal pelvis and calyces. Grade 5: Dilation of the ureter with tortuosity, severe dilation of the renal pelvis and calyces.

Endoscopic treatment with hyaluronic acid/dextranomer (Deflux®) injections or ureteral reimplantation should be considered for cases of recurrent febrile UTIs, especially in the presence of renal scarring.

Follow-up care for a child with VUR should involve an annual assessment including blood pressure measurement, weight, height, urinalysis (to assess for proteinuria), and urine culture if urinalysis is suggestive of infection. Ultrasound to monitor renal growth and any parenchymal scarring is also recommended annually. Optimal treatment of bowel dysfunction is especially important in the older child. Repeat VCUG to reassess VUR is only recommended if recurrent UTIs persist despite antibiotic prophylaxis and/or bladder and bowel management.

Management of secondary VUR is based on treating the underlying cause. For example, patients with high-pressure bladders such as in PUV (after surgical resection of valves) or neurogenic bladder may benefit from medications to decrease bladder pressure (e.g., anticholinergics, beta-3 agonist, or intravesical botulinum toxin).

CONSULTATION

- Pediatric urology for initial evaluation, management, and follow-up
- Pediatric nephrology consultation for renal scarring, proteinuria, hypertension, elevated creatinine, or chronic kidney disease

UROLITHIASIS

BACKGROUND

Urolithiasis has been rising steadily in the pediatric population over the past 3 decades by approximately 10% annually. This rise is likely related to increasing rates of obesity in children, lifestyle and diet changes, and possibly more readily available imaging tests. The prevalence of urolithiasis varies widely in North American children from 1 in 1000 to 1 in 7600 according to geographic location. The presentation, evaluation, and management of stone disease is unique in pediatrics due to the following: 1) underlying metabolic abnormality occurs in up to 70% children with renal stones; 2) higher stone recurrence rates in children (16%-44%); 3) the association with congenital anomalies of the kidneys and urinary tract (CAKUT), such as hydronephrosis, UPJ obstruction or VUR, is more common; 4) variability in symptoms and normative values, which vary according to gender and age of the child.

Pathophysiology Stone formation is a complex process that involves a delicate chemical balance between substances that induce (supersaturation) and substances that inhibit stone formation. Clinically speaking, the most important factors include urinary volume, solute excretion (e.g., calcium, oxalate, uric acid), urinary pH, and inhibitors (citrate, magnesium).

For example, urinary pH can have a dramatic effect on the solubility of stone-forming ions. Acidic urine favors uric acid and cystine stones, while alkaline urine (pH >6.5) favors calcium phosphate stones. Struvite stones occur in alkaline urine because bacterial action on urea produces ammonia and thus results in alkaline urine. Free ions such as magnesium and citrate bind calcium and reduce the free ion concentration of calcium, which reduces the chance of crystal formation.

The most common causative factors for pediatric urolithiasis are low urinary volume (due to poor fluid intake), hypercalciuria, and hypocitraturia, but other factors include infection, genitourinary abnormalities, congenital enzymatic deficiencies (e.g., cystinuria, primary hyperoxaluria) and renal tubulopathies (e.g., renal tubular acidosis, Dent's disease).

CLINICAL PRESENTATION

The characteristic renal colic that occurs in adults is experienced by only half the children with urolithiasis; therefore, establishing the diagnosis in pediatric patients can be challenging. Presenting symptoms may include UTIs, hematuria, sterile pyuria, dysuria, or generalized irritability. Approximately 30% of children with a history of recurrent UTIs will develop urolithiasis. The incidence of hematuria varies widely (30%-90%), and it can be either microscopic or macroscopic. Sterile pyuria should trigger consideration of urolithiasis. Dysuria or urinary frequency (or both) may be due to bladder stones and the resultant local irritation to the bladder wall. Patients with congenital urinary tract anomalies or urinary diversions are also at increased risk for urolithiasis. Fifteen percent to 20% of children diagnosed with urolithiasis are asymptomatic, with stones incidentally found on abdominal imaging studies ordered for unrelated complaints.

DIFFERENTIAL DIAGNOSIS

Urolithiasis must be distinguished from other causes of flank or abdominal pain, gross or microscopic hematuria, nausea, and vomiting. Differential diagnosis includes acute pyelonephritis, symptomatic ureteropelvic junction obstruction (Dietl's crisis), renal papillary necrosis, Nutcracker syndrome (entrapment of the left renal vein between the aorta and superior mesenteric artery), and appendicitis.

DIAGNOSTIC EVALUATION

The initial evaluation includes a complete history and physical examination. A thorough history should investigate potential risk factors for urolithiasis such as prematurity, use of stone-inducing medications (e.g., furosemide, topiramate, corticosteroids, vitamin D supplementation), predisposing medical conditions and treatments (e.g., inflammatory bowel disease, short gut syndrome). Family history is essential, particularly regarding urolithiasis and inheritable metabolic abnormalities. A dietary history should be obtained to assess dietary excesses (especially sodium and oxalate-rich foods) and fluid intake. Urinalysis and urine culture should be performed. Findings on urinalysis include pH, specific gravity, hematuria, and sedimentary crystals. Further urinary studies include a 24-hour urine collection for volume, calcium, cystine, citrate, oxalate, uric acid, and creatinine. In non-toilet-trained children, spot urine samples (ratio with creatinine excretion, including nitroprusside which is a screening test for cystinuria) can be obtained. Serum studies include calcium, potassium, creatinine, bicarbonate, blood urea nitrogen, phosphorus, magnesium, uric acid, 25-OH-vitamin D, and serum intact parathyroid hormone level (PTH). The least invasive and oftentimes most expeditious method to evaluate the upper urinary tract is renal and bladder ultrasound. Current ultrasound technology has greatly improved the ability to image small stones in the kidney and ureter. The degree of hydronephrosis is also easily assessed with ultrasound. The most sensitive test is a noncontrast-enhanced computed tomography (CT) scan. Its disadvantages include ionizing radiation exposure and the occasional need for sedation in pediatric patients. Because of lack of radiation, ultrasound is the imaging study of choice to investigate urinary tract stones in pediatric patients, with CT reserved for cases when small stones could have been missed on ultrasound, but clinical suspicion is high for urolithiasis. Determining the composition of the stone can help determine optimal medical management strategies to prevent recurrence.

MANAGEMENT

Supportive Care Hydration and pain control are the mainstays of supportive care for nephrolithiasis. While pain can be well controlled with NSAIDS and/or opioids, NSAIDS must be avoided or used with caution in the setting of acute kidney injury (AKI), especially in the presence of dehydration secondary to poor oral intake and vomiting, or in the context of urinary tract obstruction.

Medical Expulsive Therapy Medical expulsive therapy with alpha-blockers (e.g., tamsulosin, silodosin) or calcium channel blockers (e.g., nifedipine) can be trialed as a nonsurgical alternative in adult and pediatric patients with uncomplicated, symptomatic small ureteric stones. Controversial results have been reported. While studies have suggested a potential benefit of alpha-blockers for the expulsion of distal ureteral stones measuring ≤10 mm, a large randomized controlled trial involving adult patients showed that either tamsulosin or nifedipine have been effective in achieving stone clearance in 4 weeks. Tamsulosin is the most common alpha blocker used in children; the recommended dose is 0.2 to 0.4 mg daily.

Surgical Therapy Surgical options for stone removal include extracorporeal shock wave lithotripsy, endoscopic surgery, or rarely, open versus laparoscopic surgery. Lithotripsy success rates in children are similar to adults, with complete stone clearance in about 50%. Endoscopic surgery involves fiberoptic instrumentation such as a ureteroscope or nephroscope. Ureteroscopy involves the use of a flexible fiberoptic scope that is passed up the urethra and into the bladder and ureter. It is now commonly used for ureteral stones and stones within the renal pelvis. Once visualized, the stone can be grasped by small flexible instruments passed through the working port of the ureteroscope. The trapped stone and ureteroscope are then removed. This therapy is highly effective in adults and also successful in children. In infants and some children, technical limitations because of the small-caliber ureter may limit access. Tamsulosin started 1 week prior to surgery may be considered to facilitate the passage of the flexible ureteroscope during elective procedures. Potential complications of ureteroscopy include perforation of the ureter, bleeding, and ureteral or urethral stricture formation. Open or laparoscopic surgery for stone removal is rarely indicated for infants and children. When needed for reserved, unique cases, these are well-established and effective methods of removal.

CONSULTATION

- Patients with UTIs and urinary tract stones require urologic consultation.
- Patients with solitary kidney and urinary tract stones require urologic consultation.
- Patients with any suggestion of obstruction require admission and immediate urologic consultation.
- A metabolic stone work-up and nephrology consultation are required for all children diagnosed with urolithiasis given the higher prevalence of underlying metabolic diseases and higher risk of recurrence.

ADMISSION/DISCHARGE CRITERIA

Pain control and hydration are common indications for admission. Optimal hydration, pain control, and management of urolithiasis (medical or surgical) completed or planned.

COMMON UROLOGY CONSULTATIONS

Pediatric hospitalists commonly encounter hospitalized children and adolescents with acute urinary retention or lower urinary tract symptoms.

ACUTE URINARY RETENTION

Acute urinary retention is relatively rare in pediatric patients. Most common causes are constipation, idiopathic urinary retention, trauma, urinary tract infection, and local inflammation from vulvovaginitis or balanoposthitis. In this chapter, we will limit the discussion to common causes of acute urinary retention in children and immediate management, meaning prompt relief, urgent investigations, and most appropriate next steps. However, it is important to rule out rare, but serious and potentially life-threatening causes. Rarely, spinal cord tumors (especially in children <1 year of age), CNS tumors, and other neurological conditions such as transverse myelitis, Guillain-Barré syndrome, and encephalitis, can cause acute urinary retention (**Table 165-2**).

Management The management of acute urinary retention will depend on the underlying cause (Table 165-2). Whenever possible, a child-friendly approach without catheterization must be attempted, especially in cases of functional or local inflammatory conditions.

Functional Causes Constipation is a common, but often underdiagnosed cause of urinary retention in children. History and physical examination are usually enough for the diagnosis, but an abdominal X-ray can confirm fecal impaction (**Figure 165-2**). Renal and bladder ultrasound may show a distended rectum (**Figure 165-3**). Typically, a transverse rectal diameter measuring ≥3 cm on ultrasound correlates with chronic constipation. In the presence of a large fecal load, fecal disimpaction with enemas and laxatives is recommended, after which maintenance therapy should occur with stool softeners such as polyethylene glycol (PEG 3350)

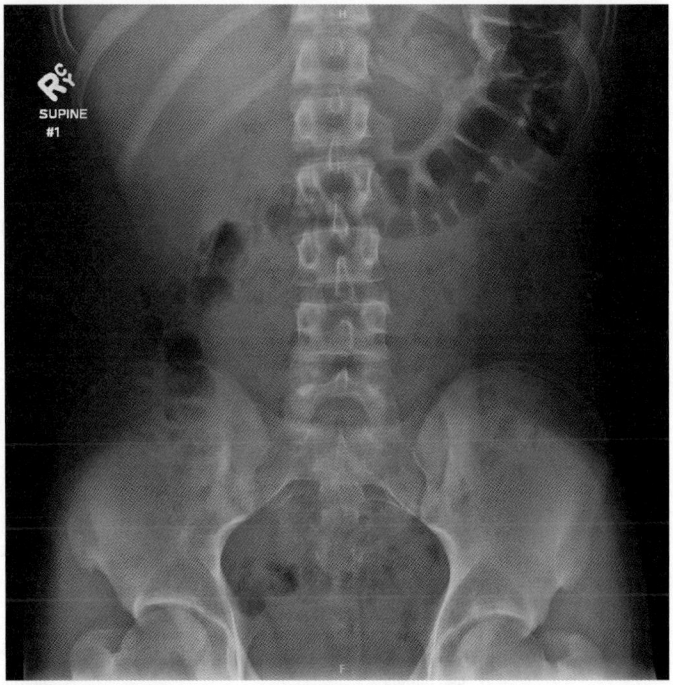

FIGURE 165-2. Abdominal X-ray showing large fecal loading throughout bowels. (*Source:* archive (unidentified image) of Joana Don Santos MD, MHSc, FRCPA.)

aiming for daily, soft, and painless bowel movements. Therapy may be required for at least 6 to 12 months.

Local Inflammatory Causes

1. Balanoposthitis: The inflammation of both the prepuce and glans penis. Local irritation, infection, or trauma are possible etiologies. It is a relatively common condition in boys, occurring more frequently between 2 and 5 years of age. Poor hygiene, physiologic adhesions, or phimosis are possible causes. Acute urinary retention secondary to balanoposthitis is rare. However, if the child is unable to void after a trial of warm or sitz bath, and in the presence of severe phimosis causing lower urinary tract obstruction, a straight (in and out) catheter must be inserted. If unable to place a catheter, urgent Urology consultation is warranted. Specific treatment typically involves topical steroids, antibiotic, or antifungal cream depending on etiology.
2. Vulvovaginitis: One of the most common gynecological conditions affecting females during childhood and adolescence. The etiology

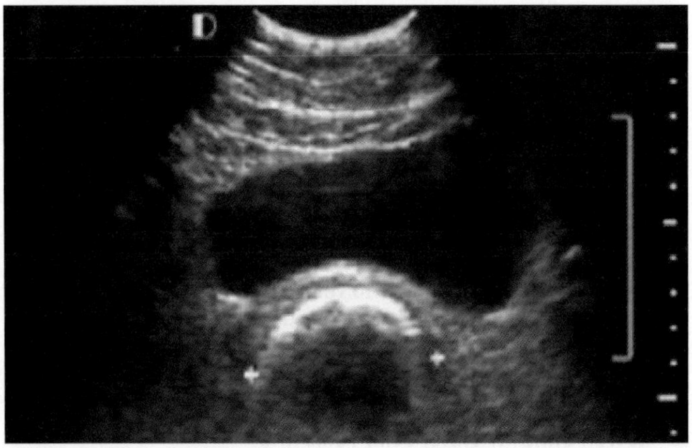

FIGURE 165-3. Bladder ultrasound image showing large rectal fecal loading pushing the bladder anteriorly. (*Source:* archive (unidentified image) of Joana Don Santos MD, MHSc, FRCPA.)

TABLE 165-2 Causes of Acute Urinary Retention in Children

Causes	Diagnosis	Investigations	Management
Inflammatory	Balanoposthitis Vulvovaginitis	History and physical examination	Sitz baths Warm baths Topical antibiotics/antifungal/steroids Oral antibiotics in severe cases
Functional	Constipation/Fecal impaction BBD Hinman syndrome	RBUS/pelvic US Abdominal X-ray	Bowel cleanout PEG 3350 Warm baths Alpha-blockers (e.g., tamsulosin) In and out catheterization*
Infectious	UTI Cystitis	UA Urine culture RBUS	Antibiotics Sitz baths Warm baths
Trauma	Spinal cord injury Bladder/urethral injury Straddle injury Catheter-related injury (traumatic false passage)	Spine MRI RBUS Cystoscopy/urethroscopy	CIC Indwelling catheter
Neurological	Tethered cord CNS tumors Spinal cord tumors (sacral teratoma, neuroblastoma, Ewing's sarcoma) Transverse myelitis Guillain-Barré syndrome Encephalitis	Brain/spine MRI Specific labs	CIC Indwelling catheter Alpha-blockers Specific treatment of underlying cause
Drug-induced	Post-anesthesia Opioids (morphine, hydromorphone) Anticholinergics (oxybutynin) Antihistamines (brompheniramine, diphenhydramine, pseudoephedrine) Neuroleptics (haloperidol, carbamazepine)	History and physical examination	In and out catheter Indwelling catheter Stop medication as soon as possible
Lower urinary tract obstruction	Phimosis/BXO Meatal stenosis Labial adhesions Genital cellulitis Urethral stone	History and physical examination Consider renal bloodwork	Urgent Urology consult (urgent dorsal slit, circumcision, meatotomy, lysis of adhesion, stone removal) Indwelling catheter when possible Specific treatment
Pelvic tumors	Rhabdomyosarcoma, Burkitt lymphoma	Pelvic/RBUS Abdominal/pelvic MRI	CIC Indwelling catheter Specific treatment

BBD: bladder and bowel dysfunction; BXO: balanitis xerotica obliterans; CIC: clean intermittent catheterization; PEG 3350: polyethylene glycol; RBUS: renal and bladder ultrasound; spine MRI: spine magnetic resonance imaging; UA: urinalysis; US: ultrasound; UTI: urinary tract infection.

in children is often nonspecific, with sitz baths and avoidance of irritants, and hygiene measures being the first line of treatment. Yeast and bacterial vaginosis are common etiologies in teenagers. Common symptoms include vulvar itchiness, discharge, burning, and irritation, but rarely urinary retention may occur secondary to pain during micturition in severe cases. If a child or adolescent with vulvovaginitis is unable to void, a trial of warm or sitz baths is recommended and only if this is unsuccessful, place an in and out catheter. Topical antibiotic treatment for specific pathogens may be indicated.

LOWER URINARY TRACT SYMPTOMS AND BLADDER AND BOWEL DYSFUNCTION

Pediatric hospitalists frequently manage children and adolescents complaining of other lower urinary tract symptoms as well, such as increased or decreased urinary frequency, urgency, incontinence, dysuria, hesitancy, straining, incomplete bladder emptying, or holding maneuvers. By far, the most common cause of these symptoms in children is bladder and bowel dysfunction (BBD). BBD refers to a multitude of lower urinary symptoms associated with functional constipation and/or encopresis. The large fecal load in the distended rectum directly pushes the bladder wall anteriorly leading to mechanical compression and changes in the neural stimuli of the bladder, ultimately affecting bladder emptying and/or storage. Bladder retraining and constipation management are the initial recommended treatment for BBD. Bladder retraining involves timed voiding, increased hydration, and education of the child and caregivers. Stool softeners are the mainstay of constipation treatment, which is often needed for at least 6 to 12 months. Children who do not respond to behavioral changes and optimal bowel management after 6 months should be referred to a urologist for further investigations and treatment.

KEY POINTS

- Testicular torsion is a surgical emergency. Doppler scrotal ultrasound is reliable in determining testicular blood flow, but surgical exploration should not be delayed when ultrasound is not readily available and whenever testicular torsion is highly suspected.
- Hydronephrosis is common and generally asymptomatic, resolving in approximately 75% to 80% of children without surgical intervention.
- Moderate to severe hydronephrosis requires a full evaluation and is more likely to represent a surgical etiology (VUR, UPJ, or UVJ obstruction).
- Consultation with a pediatric urologist is highly recommended as soon as urinary obstruction is suspected.
- All febrile UTIs warrant evaluation with renal/bladder ultrasound.
- Recurrent febrile UTIs and those with ultrasound findings that show hydronephrosis, scarring, and those with an atypical clinical circumstance warrant evaluation with a VCUG.
- Bowel and bladder dysfunction should be aggressively managed in the older child with VUR.
- Metabolic stonework-up, Nephrology and/or Urology consultations are recommended for all children admitted with urolithiasis.

SUGGESTED READINGS

Austin PF, Bauer SB, Bower W, et al. The standardization of terminology of lower urinary tract function in children and adolescents: update report from the standardization committee of the International Children's Continence Society . *Neurourol Urodyn.* 2016;35(4):471-481.

Dos Santos J, Varghese A, Williams K, Koyle M. Recommendations for the management of bladder bowel dysfunction in children. *Pediatr Ther.* 2014;04:1-11.

Hernandez JD, Ellison JS, Lendvay TS. Current trends, evaluation, and management of pediatric nephrolithiasis. *JAMA Pediatr.* 2015;169(10):964-970.

Keays M, Rosenberg H. Testicular torsion. *CMAJ.* 2019;191(28):E792.

Kylat RI, Ahmed MN. Neonatal testicular torsion. *Afr J Paediatr Surg.* 2022;19(1):1.

McGee LM, Sack BS, Wan J, Kraft KH. The effect of preoperative tamsulosin on ureteroscopic access in school-aged children. *J Pediatr Urol.* 2021;17(6):795.e1-795.e6.

Ming JM, Lopes RI, Harvey EA, et al. Cost effectiveness and impact in quality of care of a pediatric multidisciplinary stone clinic. *Pediatr Qual Saf.* 2021;6(5):e474.

Morello W, La Scola C, Alberici I, Montini G. Acute pyelonephritis in children. *Pediatr Nephrol.* 2016;31(8):1253-1265.

Peters CA, Skoog SJ, Arant Jr. BS, et al. (2017). Management and screening of primary vesicoureteral reflux in children (2010, amended 2017). American Urological Association. Retrieved online: auanet.org/guidelines/guidelines/vesicoureteral-reflux-guideline. Accessed date April 26 2023.

Pogorelić Z, Mustapić K, Jukić M, et al. Management of acute scrotum in children: a 25-year single center experience on 558 pediatric patients. *Can J Urol.* 2016;23:8594-8601.

Rickard M, Dos Santos J, Keunen J, Lorenzo AJ. Prenatal hydronephrosis: bridging pre-and post natal management. *Prenat Diagn.* 2022;42(9):1081-1093.

RIVUR Trial Investigators; Hoberman A, Greenfield SP, et al. Antibiotic prophylaxis for children with vesicoureteral reflux. *N Engl J Med.* 2014;370:2367-2376.

Robinson J, Finlay J, Lang M, Bortolussi R. Urinary tract infection in infants and children: diagnosis and management. *Paediatr Child Health.* 2014;19(6):315-319.

Santos JD, Lopes RI, Koyle MA. Bladder and bowel dysfunction in children: an update on the diagnosis and treatment of a common, but underdiagnosed pediatric problem. *Can Urol Assoc J.* 2017;11(1-2Suppl1):S64-S72.

Schlomer BJ. Urologic treatment of nephrolithiasis. *Curr Opin Pediatr.* 2020;32(2):288-294.

CHAPTER 166

Craniofacial Disorders

Cassi Smola, MD, Rene P. Myers, MD, and Kelly N. Evans, MD

BACKGROUND

Craniofacial conditions constitute a wide range of anatomic and functional disorders that impact hospital care. Swallowing, airway, and breathing problems are common among infants and children with craniofacial conditions. These differences range from mild to severe and can even be life-threatening.

Early recognition is important to facilitate accurate diagnosis, evaluation, treatment, and involvement of specialists to achieve optimal outcomes.

Given the range of syndromes and disorders that classify as craniofacial, this chapter focuses on three broad categories as each has their own surgical implications: Orofacial clefts, Robin Sequence (RS), and Craniosynostosis (CS).

OROFACIAL CLEFTS

PATHOPHYSIOLOGY

Orofacial clefts are among the most common congenital anomalies. They can be classified as cleft lip and palate, isolated cleft lip, or isolated cleft palate. See **Figures 166-1 and 166-2**. Clefts can be complete or incomplete as well as unilateral or bilateral. Submucous cleft palate is a subtype of cleft palate with bifid uvula and abnormally oriented palate muscles that can have symptoms of a true cleft. The most common form of cleft is a unilateral cleft of the lip, alveolus, and palate.

Causes of clefting are unknown and thought to be multifactorial from genetic and environmental factors. However, known risks include maternal tobacco and alcohol use, anticonvulsant treatment, and nutritional status. Routine genetic testing for individuals with an isolated cleft without a family history of clefting is not recommended.

CLINICAL PRESENTATION

Clefting occurs when there is failure of fusion of the medial and lateral nasal and maxillary processes, which is usually completed by the seventh week of gestation. The primary (lip, alveolus, anterior hard palate) or secondary palate (posterior hard palate and soft palate) can be affected. Digital examination of the palate can miss a posterior or submucous cleft palate. Therefore, obtaining visual examination of the uvula and palate is important to identify clefting.

DIAGNOSTIC EVALUATION

All children with clefts should undergo comprehensive and longitudinal evaluations focusing on feeding, growth, airway obstruction, speech development, hearing, and dentition.

An infant with an isolated cleft lip may be able to effectively breastfeed or bottle feed with a standard bottle. However, if any part of the palate is involved, infants often cannot form negative pressure and are unable to nurse or drink from a normal bottle efficiently. Increased work of eating can lead to difficulty gaining weight. Frequent weight checks are recommended during the first 1 to 2 months of life. A feeding specialist should be consulted to determine best bottle and feeding options. While most feeding challenges can be overcome with the proper bottle/nipple feeding system, swallow studies are considered for infants with concern for swallow dysfunction, aspiration, or continued poor growth. Babies with clefts can swallow more air which can potentiate increased reflux. Holding babies in an upright position can help decrease nasal regurgitation and improve feedings. Children with isolated clefts are expected to follow a typical growth chart. However, consultation with a dietician and

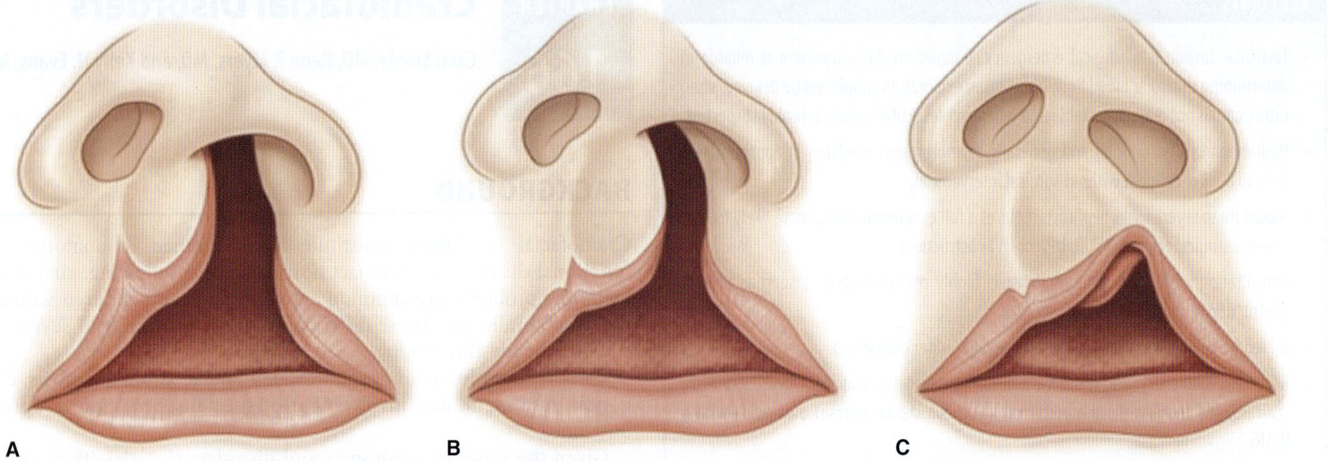

FIGURE 166-1. Examples of asymmetrical bilateral cleft lip with a contralateral lesser form. (A) Left complete and right minor-form; (B) left complete and right microform; (C) left incomplete and right mini-microform. (Reproduced with permission from Mulliken JB. Repair of bilateral cleft lip. In: Neligan P, Rodriguez ED, eds. *Plastic Surgery*, 3rd ed, vol 3. London: Elsevier Saunders; 2013.)

concentration of milk may be needed. Adequate weight gain is considered a marker for overall health and essential when assessing readiness for surgical repair.

Isolated clefting does not usually cause airway concerns. However, if there is micro or retrognathia, concern for a concurrent syndrome, or laryngeal cleft, the airway should be evaluated. This can be with a sleep study, imaging, or endoscopy, depending on the clinical concern and presenting symptoms.

Neonates with a cleft palate often fail the newborn hearing screen due to the presence of fluid in the middle ear space. A diagnostic hearing test can be pursued to detect sensorineural, conductive or mixed hearing loss, which can occur at a higher rate in cleft palate.

Most patients with clefts have normal language development and will start making sounds, babbling and produce words at the same time as children without a cleft. Many consonants will sound different due to nasal air escape and inability to build up the pressure in the mouth. Common sounds that are altered include the following: "p" "b" "t" "d" "k" "g" "s" "sh" and "f". Early speech therapy evaluation is imperative. Understandable speech is a desired outcome following cleft palate surgery.

Dentition can also be altered in clefting. Enamel hypoplasia can affect both primary and permanent teeth. Children can have missing teeth or abnormalities in timing of dental eruption. Craniofacial orthodontist referral is recommended at 5 to 6 years of age, when a child is entering mixed dentition. An alveolar bone graft may be needed between 6 and 9 years of age to fill the bony gap in the maxilla.

MANAGEMENT

Infants with clefts should be seen ideally within the first week after birth. Then followed with frequent weight checks until consistent weight gain is achieved. Cleft lip is typically repaired within the first 6 months and cleft palate surgery typically occurs between 9 and 12 months, although delays can occur if patients have comorbid conditions prompting poor growth, frequent infections, respiratory problems, or frequent hospitalizations. To address conductive hearing loss associated with Eustachian tube dysfunction, children with cleft palate frequently undergo tympanostomy and placement of tubes at the time of cleft surgery. The goal of ear tube placement is to normalize hearing to support communication development.

Depending on the degree of clefting and structures involved (lip, nose, gumline, bony, and soft palate), patients may require multiple surgeries (cleft lip, cleft palate, bone graft, midface advancement, speech surgery, revision surgeries). Therefore, individuals with cleft are often followed through teenage years or early twenties to complete comprehensive cleft care.

ROBIN SEQUENCE

PATHOPHYSIOLOGY

The triad of micrognathia, glossoptosis, and airway obstruction is known as Robin sequence (RS) or Pierre Robin Sequence. See **Figure 166-3**. Cleft palate, although not an obligatory feature, is often present and thought to be associated with the tongue positioned vertically obstructing the palatal shelves from closing. The cleft palate in RS is often wide and U-shaped. The cause of RS is multifactorial (genetic and/or environmental). The phenotypic spectrum and presentation of RS is heterogeneous and as a result, the prevalence is challenging to determine; average birth prevalence has been estimated at 1:24,500. RS occurs with associated anomalies or an associated syndrome about half of the time. The most common associated syndrome in RS is Stickler syndrome.

CLINICAL PRESENTATION

While the initial presentation of RS can vary, early recognition can facilitate timely initiation of treatments. Those with mild airway symptoms may never need intervention. However, when severe, micrognathia and glossoptosis can cause significant upper airway obstruction necessitating intubation or emergency tracheostomy. For most infants with RS, clinical symptoms develop over the first 1 to 2 months. Signs of tongue base airway obstruction include feeding difficulties, snoring, stertor, stridor, obstructive sleep apnea (OSA), and malnutrition. All infants with the RS triad should be evaluated for presence of a cleft palate and managed appropriately.

DIAGNOSTIC EVALUATION

Airway obstruction in RS is localized to the base of tongue. A detailed exam assessing the mandible for the maxillomandibular discrepancy, tongue position and listening for snoring, stertor and stridor, and observing inspiratory work of breathing/apneas can identify RS. Monitoring oxygen saturations and ventilation with blood gas and carbon dioxide (CO_2) levels is recommended for any signs of upper airway obstruction. A formal sleep study can be helpful to diagnose obstructive sleep apnea, guide interventions, and determine safety for discharge. Together, these measures will aid in determining if and when to escalate airway treatment. Diagnostic laryngoscopy and bronchoscopy under anesthesia can reveal distal levels of airway narrowing and collapse and is recommended prior to surgical intervention.

Airway obstruction can impact feeding and swallowing coordination, increase the risk for gastroesophageal reflux, aspiration and feeding intolerance, and lead to increased caloric expenditures impacting growth. Evaluation by a feeding therapist and objective evaluation of

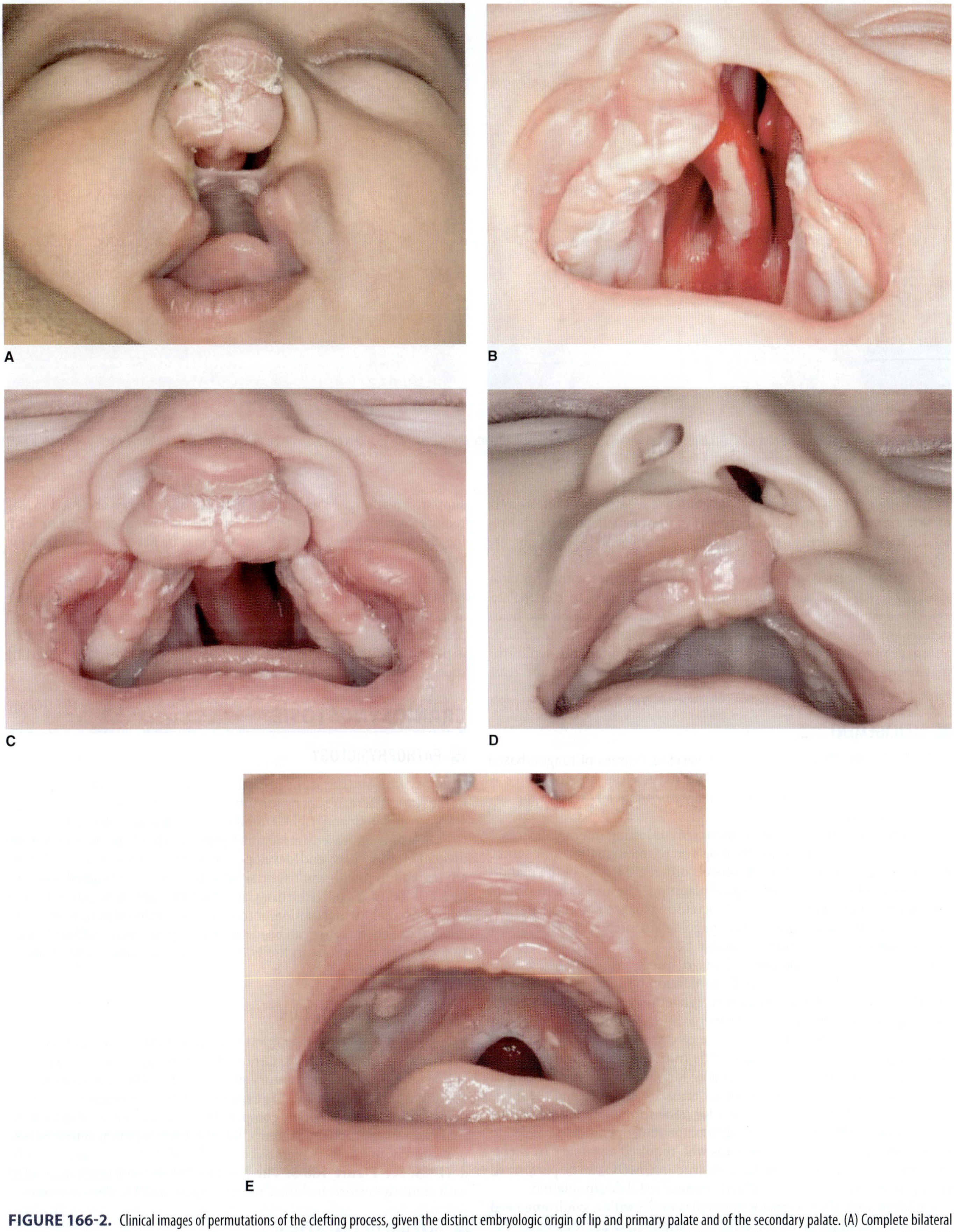

A B C D E

FIGURE 166-2. Clinical images of permutations of the clefting process, given the distinct embryologic origin of lip and primary palate and of the secondary palate. (A) Complete bilateral cleft lip and primary palate. (B) Complete/incomplete cleft lip and primary palate and complete cleft of secondary palate. (C) Complete bilateral cleft lip, primary and secondary palates. (D) Incomplete cleft lip and primary palate. (E) Incomplete cleft of secondary palate. (Reproduced with permission from Plastic Surgery - Principles and Practice 2022, Pages 212-231. Copyright 2022 Elsevier. Fig. 17.1.)

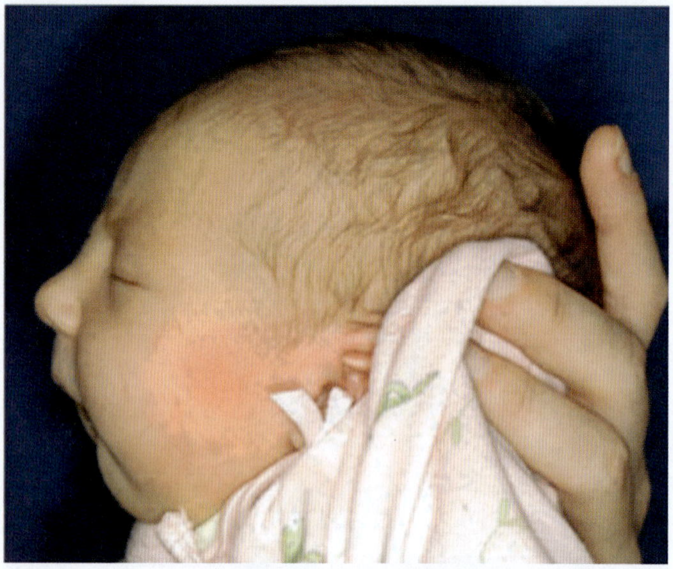

A

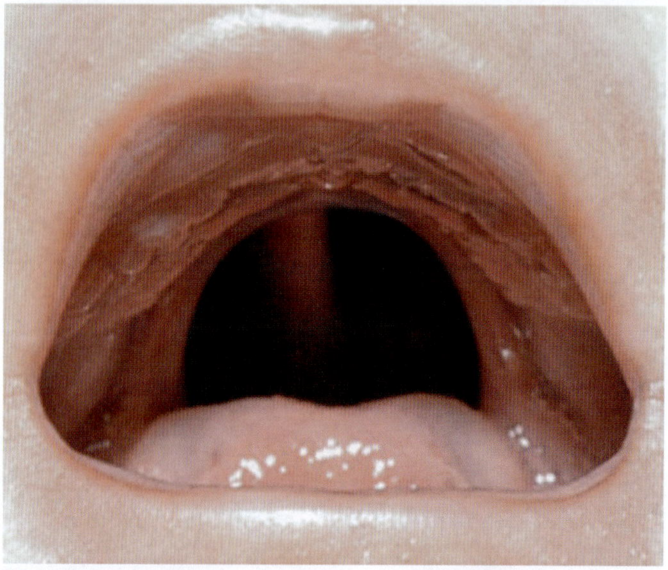

B

FIGURE 166-3. A. Example of micrognathia associated with RS. **B.** Example of cleft palate associated with RS. (Reproduced with permission from Kelly N. Evans, Anne V. Hing, Michael L. Cunningham *Avery Neonatology textbook* 9e , 2018, Pages 1417-1437.e2. Fig. 100.1.)

swallowing safety is common, while guidance from a dietitian on milk fortification to achieve optimal growth is often beneficial. After hospital discharge, reassuring oxygen saturations and normal weight gain are signs of respiratory stability.

RS can be isolated, associated with other anomalies without a clear syndrome (RS plus), or with a syndrome. In addition to cleft palate, associated anomalies include skeletal dysplasias, joint problems, heart defects, eye and vision issues, central nervous system (CNS) anomalies, and developmental delay. As the presence of an underlying syndrome may become apparent over time, initial genetics consultation and reassessment over time is needed.

MANAGEMENT

Individuals with RS can present with varying degrees of tongue-based airway obstruction. Prone position and oxygen can attenuate airway obstruction and hypoxia but are unlikely to completely resolve the airway obstruction.

Mandibular distraction osteogenesis (MDO) using internal devices is considered fairly standard for treating severe micrognathia and can be performed in neonates. While protocols differ, a CT scan of the mandible is often obtained to aid in surgical planning. The airway of the infant with severe micrognathia can be difficult to visualize and intubate, and involvement of anesthesia and otolaryngology to safely secure the airway for any surgical intervention is essential.

Risks of MDO include nerve damage, infections, asymmetry, nonunion, device failure, and damage to developing tooth buds. Benefits of MDO allow a safer upper airway, reduction or removal of oxygen and respiratory support in the supine position, comfortable breathing, improved oral feeding, and avoidance of a tracheostomy. After placement of devices, distractor pins outside of the skin are turned daily to lengthen the mandible, thereby bringing forward the tongue. Once goal advancement is reached, the distractor arms are removed and the internal devices are left in place to allow for bone formation and hardening (consolidation phase). A second, often outpatient, operation is needed to remove the devices. For some infants who required a primary tracheotomy surgery for severe tongue base obstruction, MDO can be performed to improve airway patency and facilitate successful decannulation.

Children with RS plus major anomalies or RS with a syndrome need thoughtful planning given the outcomes after MDO are less successful. The risks of both surgery and residual respiratory insufficiency after surgery need to be considered. For children with multilevel airway obstruction, the presence of lung disease or need for positive pressure ventilation, placement of a tracheostomy tube may be the optimal treatment to support breathing. Many infants with RS and airway obstruction will require supplemental tube feeding, and if swallowing concerns or feeding challenges persist, gastrostomy tube may be needed for secure delivery of nutrition.

Individuals with RS are followed by a craniofacial team through skeletal maturity (completion of growth) with specialists monitoring feeding, assessing for recurrent or residual OSA, monitoring hearing and speech production, and evaluating and treating malocclusion. If a cleft palate is present, timing of palate surgery must be balanced with supporting speech development and avoiding airway compromise.

CRANIOSYNOSTOSIS

PATHOPHYSIOLOGY

Craniosynostosis (CS) is the premature fusion of one or multiple sutures of the skull. There are six major sutures (metopic, sagittal, left and right coronal, and left and right lambdoid). See **Figure 166-4**. Untreated CS can cause increased intracranial pressure (ICP), brain injury, papilledema, vision loss, and developmental delay. These risks are higher among children with multisutural synostosis. CS is estimated to occur in 1 in 1400 to 2500 live births. Causes are thought to be multifactorial (chromosomal, twin gestation, intrauterine growth restriction, environmental). A genetic cause can be identified in approximately 25% of cases. In particular, mutations in the FGFR gene family have shown associations with syndromic CS.

CLINICAL PRESENTATION

Patent sutures allow the head to fit through the birth canal and the skull to expand as the brain grows. Fusion of a suture causes restricted growth at that suture with compensatory growth that produces a progressively abnormal and unique head shape for each of the presentations of CS. CS does not improve postnatally compared to an abnormal head from birth trauma or plagiocephaly. Sagittal CS is the most common suture to fuse prematurely, followed by metopic, coronal, and the least common, lambdoid CS. See **Figure 166-5**. The most common syndromes associated with craniosynostosis include Crouzon, Apert, and Pfeiffer syndrome.

DIAGNOSTIC EVALUATION

Diagnosis of CS can be made clinically by examination of the head shape, and assessment of patent sutures in a newborn or infant can occur by gently palpating the cranial bones across the suture and watching and

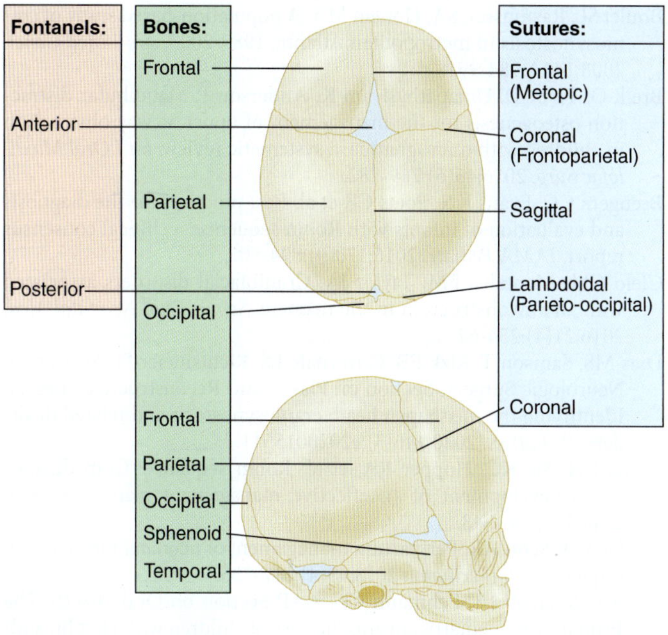

FIGURE 166-4. Reproduced with permission from J Biller, G. Gruener, P. W. Brazis. *DeMyer's The Neurologic Examination: A Programmed Text*, 7e. New York: McGraw-Hill Education; 2017.)

feeling them move freely. Often skull x-rays or CT scans are obtained prior to referral to a craniofacial center and can help confirm the diagnosis by illustrating closed or open sutures. When obtained, CT scans are also helpful in surgical planning.

Nonsyndromic CS is most often isolated without involvement of other systems or development. Based on the clinical presentation and suture(s) involved, the infant with CS should be evaluated for other anomalies that can include cardiac, urogenital, ophthalmologic, and otic malformations with low threshold for referral. For babies with multisuture fusion, or heightened risk of increased intracranial pressure, a dilated fundoscopic eye exam can evaluate for papilledema. Continued monitoring of the optic nerves, acuity, and eye alignment can be helpful in protecting vision. Development should be evaluated in infancy and followed over time as children with CS can have neurodevelopmental differences. Neuropsychological testing should be obtained for any concerns that arise.

Physical features of nonsyndromic or single-suture CS can be identified at birth, progress over time, and may take months to become evident. Single-suture CS (particularly lambdoid CS) can resemble deformational plagiocephaly given presentation with an asymmetric back of the head. Infants with deformational plagiocephaly tend to have a parallelogram head shape from the birds-eye view. Infants with lambdoid synostosis can have a trapezoid head shape when viewed from above. A head shape will improve with deformational plagiocephaly, whereas the head will become more asymmetric in growth deficiency caused by craniosynostosis.

Children with syndromic CS or multisuture CS often have additional craniofacial and extracraniofacial features. Additional screening evaluations may include assessing for involvement of the airway, cervical spine, limbs/hands, eyes, midface, cleft palate, hearing loss, brain and spine, and intestinal abnormalities. Some of the FGFR gene-associated craniosynostoses can be differentiated by looking at the patient's hands. For example, Apert syndrome involves syndactyly, Pfeiffer syndrome involves broad great toes and thumbs and fusions at the elbows, and Crouzon syndrome has typically formed extremities. Infants with multisuture craniosynostosis are often identified close to birth and hospitalized early to provide comprehensive care.

MANAGEMENT

Nonsyndromic or single-suture CS repair is encouraged prior to the first year of age as bony gaps created with surgery during this time period will easily fill in. There are three options offered for surgical correction: endoscopic strip craniectomy and helmeting, endoscopic strip craniectomy with spring-mediated cranioplasty, and open cranial vault remodeling. If CS is recognized by 2 months of age, families can discuss all the options. Risks for all surgeries include cerebrospinal fluid leak, damage to adjacent structures (eyes, periorbita, and sagittal sinus), life-threatening blood loss, air emboli, infection, scarring, asymmetries, and need for future surgery. Endoscopic release and helmeting can be performed at 2 to 4 months of age with wearing a molded helmet for 23 hours a day for up to a year of age with frequent visits for molding. Spring-mediated cranioplasty does not need a helmet and can be performed from 2 to 6 months of age but requires a second surgery for removal of springs. Open cranial vault expansion approach is generally performed between 6 and 12 months of age. Hospitalization will vary but endoscopic strip craniectomy or spring-mediated cranioplasty usually require a one to two night stay. Open approach generally requires 5 to 7 days that often includes time in the ICU and blood transfusions are often needed. Outcomes relating to head shape and increased skull volume are similar for all operations.

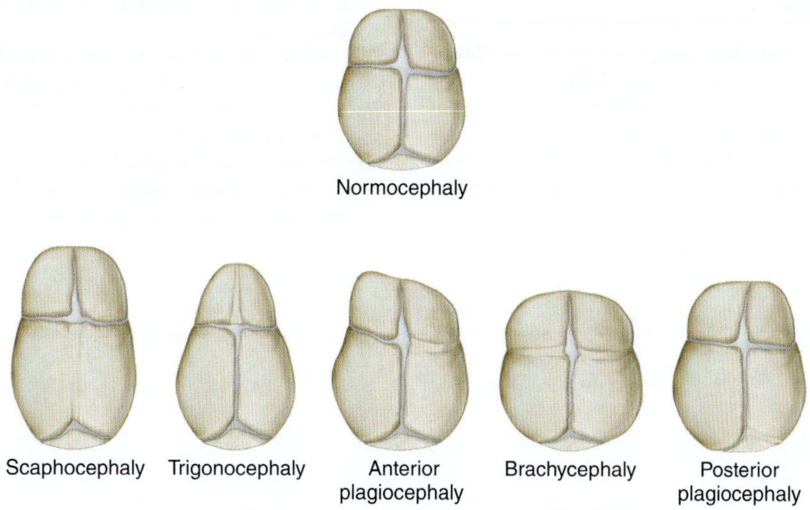

FIGURE 166-5. Patterns of single suture craniosynostosis. (Reproduced with permission from Chandawarkar RY, Miller MJ, Kellogg BC, Schulz SA, Valerio IL, Kirschner RE. Plastic and Reconstructive Surgery. In: Brunicardi F, Andersen DK, Billiar TR, Dunn DL, Kao LS, Hunter JG, Matthews JB, Pollock RE. eds. *Schwartz's Principles of Surgery*, 11e. New York: McGraw-Hill Education; 2019.)

Syndromic or multisuture CS often requires multiple surgeries. The first priority is evaluation and stabilization of the airway, spinal cord, heart, and other medical comorbidities that affect safety of cranial surgery. Once deemed safe, planning for CS repair begins. A primary goal in treating multisuture or syndromic craniosynostosis is to alleviate brain constriction. The surgical approach may include early suturectomy (especially in the presence of a cloverleaf skull) with the possible addition of low-Newton springs. Additional surgeries are often needed over time, for example to repair patients' orbits or address midface hypoplasia.

Individuals with craniosynostosis are generally followed through mid-adolescence to monitor for head growth, developmental delays, recurrence of increased ICP as well as any other concurrent issues identified from birth. Those with syndromes are often followed into early adulthood given additional craniofacial orthodontic and orthognathic needs.

CONSULTATION

The authors of this text recommend any patient born with a craniofacial condition to be referred to a craniofacial center where multidisciplinary care can be provided. The American Cleft Palate-Craniofacial Association (ACPA) has an up-to-date list of accredited cleft and craniofacial centers for each state that are recommended: https://acpacares.org/find-a-care-team. These teams vary in size and structure and can contain many subspecialties: craniofacial pediatrician, craniofacial plastic surgeon, orthodontist, oral surgeon, otolaryngologist, geneticist, genetic counselor, feeding therapist (occupational/Speech therapist), dietitian, audiologist, social worker, psychologist, and pulmonary or sleep medicine specialist. While most patients will not need every discipline, craniofacial centers have the ability to consolidate care into one center and more efficiently coordinate referrals as necessary for both high quality and complex care.

KEY POINTS

- Swallowing, airway, and breathing problems are common among infants and children with craniofacial conditions; both hospital and clinic providers should have a low threshold for testing and referral to cleft and craniofacial experts.
- Early recognition is important to facilitate accurate diagnosis, comprehensive and efficient workup, coordinated treatment, and involvement of specialist(s).
- Multidisciplinary care of individuals with craniofacial conditions is critical to ensure the best possible outcomes.

SUGGESTED READINGS

American Cleft Palate-Craniofacial Association. *Parameters for Evaluation and Treatment of Patients with Cleft Lip/Palate or Other Craniofacial Anomalies*. Revised edition, January 2018. https://acpa-cpf.org/team-care/standardscat/parameters-of-care/.

American Cleft Palate-Craniofacial Association. Feeding Your Baby. https://acpa-cpf.org/acpa-family-services/family-resources/feeding-your-baby/.

Boulet SL, Rasmussen SA, Honein MA. A population-based study of craniosynostosis in metropolitan Atlanta, 1989-2003. *Am J Med Genet*. 2008;146A:984-991.

Breik O, Tivey D, Umapathysivam K, Anderson P. Mandibular distraction osteogenesis for the management of upper airway obstruction in children with micrognathia: a systematic review. *Int J Oral Maxillofac Surg*. 2016;45(6):769-782.

Breugem CC, Evans KN, Poets CF, et al. Best practices for the diagnosis and evaluation of infants with Robin sequence: a clinical consensus report. *JAMA Pediatr*. 2016;170(9):894-902.

Cielo CM, Montalva FM, Taylor JA. Craniofacial disorders associated with airway obstruction in the neonate. *Semin Fetal Neonatal Med*. 2016;21(4):254-62.

Dias MS, Samson T, Rizk EB, Governale LS, Richtsmeier JT; Section on Neurologic Surgery, Section on Plastic and Reconstructive Surgery. Identifying the misshapen head: craniosynostosis and related disorders. *Pediatrics*. 2020;146(3):e2020015511.

Evans KN, Sie KC, Hopper RA, et al. Robin sequence: from diagnosis to development of an effective management plan. *Pediatrics*. 2011;127;936-948.

Insalaco LF, Scott AR. Peripartum management of neonatal Pierre Robin sequence. *ClinPerinatol*. 2018;45(4):717-735.

Lewis CW, Jacob LS, Lehmann CU, AAP Section on Oral Health. The Primary care pediatrician and the care of children with cleft lip and/or cleft palate. *Pediatrics*. 2017;139(5):e20170628.

Mai CT, Isenburg JL, Canfield MA, et al. National population-based estimates for major birth defects, 2010-2014. *Birth Defects Res*. 2019;111(18):1420-1435.

Massimi L, Bianchi F, Frassanito P, Calandrelli R, Tamburrini G, Caldarelli M. Imaging in craniosynostosis: when and what? *Childs Nerv Syst*. 2019;35(11):2055-2069.

Mathijssen IMJ. Working Group Guideline Craniosynostosis. Updated guideline on treatment and management of craniosynostosis. *J Craniofac Surg*. 2021;32(1):371-450.

McCarthy JG, Warren SM, Bernstein J, et al. Parameters of care for craniosynostosis. *Cleft Palate Craniofac J*. 2012;49(S1):1S-24S.

Mossey PA, Little J, Munger RG, Dixon MJ, Shaw WC. Cleft lip and palate. *Lancet*. 2009;374:1773-1785.

Paes EC, Mink van der Molen AB, Muradin MS, et al. A systematic review on the outcome of mandibular distraction osteogenesis in infants suffering Robin sequence. *Clin Oral Investig*. 2013;17:1807-1820.

Speltz ML, Collett BR, Wallace ER, et al. Intellectual and academic functioning of school-age children with single-suture craniosynostosis. *Pediatrics*. 2015;135(3):e615-e623.

Wenger T, Miller D, Evans K. FGFR Craniosynostosis Syndromes Overview. 1998 Oct 20 [Updated 2020 Apr 30]. In: Adam MP, Everman DB, Mirzaa GM, et al., editors. GeneReviews® [Internet]. Seattle (WA): University of Washington, Seattle; 1993-2022. Available from: https://www-ncbi-nlm-nih-gov.offcampus.lib.washington.edu/books/NBK1455/.

Wilkie AOM, Johnson D, Wall SA. Clinical genetics of craniosynostosis. *Curr Opin Pediatr*. 2017;29(6):622-628.

Worley ML, Patel KG, Kilpatrick LA. Cleft Lip and Palate. *Clin Perinatol*. 2018;45(4):661-678.

Yates D, Allareddy V, Caplin J, Yadav S, Markiewicz MR. An overview of timeline of interventions in the continuum of cleft lip and palate care. *Oral Maxillofac Surg Clin North Am*. 2020;32(2):177-186.

SECTION S

Toxins, Substance Abuse, and Environmental Exposures

CHAPTER 167 Stabilization and Hospitalization of the Poisoned Child

Laurie Seidel Halmo, MD, FAAP

BACKGROUND

Over 2 million xenobiotic exposures, or exposures to substances that are "foreign" or exogenous, are reported to the American Association of Poison Control Centers' National Poison Data System each year. Over half of these exposures occur in children and adolescents, primarily young children under 3 years of age. Although most reported exposures are benign with minimal to no associated toxicity, approximately 30% require treatment in a healthcare facility. While fatalities are uncommon, deaths due to drug overdose and poisoning in children increased dramatically in 2020 to become the third-leading cause of death in this population.

The epidemiology of pediatric poisoning is bimodal: the majority of cases occur in young children who are exposed via normal hand-to-mouth behavior, and a smaller peak occurs in older children and adolescents who more often intentionally expose themselves, either recreationally or in a self-harm attempt. Because exploratory ingestions in young children tend to be small volume, "lick/sip/taste" ingestions, the dose ingested is typically low. Consequently, hospitalization rates, morbidity, and mortality are lower than in the older age group, where the intentional nature of the exposure leads to higher ingested doses and more significant medical outcomes. Occasionally, young children do present with life-threatening toxicity despite ingesting only one or two tablets, capsules, or swallows of a xenobiotic in an exploratory fashion; **Table 167-1** reviews the so-called "one pill can kill" list. Both age groups are appropriate targets for preventive education in the hospital setting.

Poisoned children are frequently encountered by pediatric hospitalists. Typically, the poisoning scenario has been identified before inpatient hospitalization; however, children are occasionally admitted with an unknown underlying diagnosis that later turns out to be poisoning. Families of all children admitted to the hospital should be queried with regard to the child's medication use; use of vitamins, herbs, supplements, or ethnic remedies; and recreational drug use. Older children and adolescents should be directly asked about each of these in a private, confidential interview. Families of children admitted with concern for a toxicologic exposure should be asked about all medications present in the home, including old or expired medication and medication for pets, occupational drug and chemical exposures, and environmental drug and chemical exposures.

In the United States, regional poison control centers can be contacted by telephone at 1-800-222-1222. Poison control centers play an important public health role by triaging nontoxic exposures away from hospitals, assisting healthcare providers with medical decision-making when treating a poisoned or potentially poisoned patient, and providing regional and national epidemic surveillance.

TABLE 167-1 Xenobiotics Highly Dangerous to Young Children
Benzonatate
Beta blockers
Calcium channel blockers
Camphor
Chloroquine
Clonidine
Cyclic antidepressants
Diphenoxylate, atropine (Lomotil)
Methyl salicylate (oil of wintergreen)
Opioids
Phenothiazines
Quinidine
Sulfonylureas
Theophylline

INITIAL STABILIZATION

Respiratory failure, shock, cardiac dysrhythmias, and neurological insults are the most acute threats to life from poisoning. A standardized approach to initial life support is recommended (**Table 167-2**). It is important to identify hypoglycemia, hypoxemia, or hypercarbia as a cause of altered mentation early in the resuscitative process.

With critical life functions stabilized, attention should be given to decontamination of the patient from offending poisons. After dermal exposures, all clothing including diapers should be removed and skin should be washed with soap and copious water. Topical contamination of the eyes can be flushed with warmed normal saline; care should be taken to remove contact lenses if present.

Activated charcoal administration is the decontamination strategy of choice for most potentially toxic pediatric ingestions. Activated charcoal is typically administered as a slurry at a 10:1 charcoal:toxin ratio up to a maximum of 100 g if the ingested dose of the toxin is known. It is empirically dosed at 1 g/kg up to a maximum of 100 g when the ingested dose of the toxin is unknown. Charcoal should be regarded as a drug with its own set of indications, contraindications, cautions, and associated risks (**Tables 167-3** and **167-4**). Common adverse events associated with charcoal use include nausea, vomiting, and constipation. Some manufacturers combine activated charcoal with sorbitol to decrease the incidence of constipation; these combination products should not be used in children with hereditary fructose intolerance, as sorbitol is contraindicated for these patients. Charcoal pneumonitis is a rare but life-threatening complication of charcoal use which occurs after aspiration of gastric contents containing activated charcoal. The black color, gritty texture, unpleasant taste, and tendency to cake when in contact with mucus membranes all make charcoal unappealing to young children. Though charcoal may adsorb flavoring agents, mixing charcoal with flavored beverages improves palatability without significantly decreasing adsorptive capacity.

TABLE 167-2 Initial Resuscitation of a Poisoned Patient
A: Airway—maintain adequate airway
B: Breathing—ensure adequate oxygenation and ventilation
C: Circulation—support circulation and perfusion
D: Disability—altered consciousness merits resuscitation
Oxygen
Dextrose
Naloxone
Active cooling for hyperthermia if present

TABLE 167-3 Indications for Single-Dose Activated Charcoal[a]

Potentially injurious toxic ingestion
Toxicant can be adsorbed by activated charcoal
Charcoal can be given before the absorption of the drug is expected to be complete
Charcoal can be administered safely, with attention to the prevention of pulmonary aspiration

[a]All must apply.

TABLE 167-4 Poisons for Which Activated Charcoal Is Not Helpful

Poor adsorption
Alcohols and glycols
Most metals and inorganic salts
Most liquid preparations (due to rapidity of absorption compared to solid preparations)
May cause harm
Hydrocarbons (poor adsorption and high risk of aspiration)
Caustics/corrosive agents (poor adsorption and high risk of perforation)
Anticipated need for endoscopy (charcoal will obscure visualization of the mucosa)

TABLE 167-5 Indications for Gastric Lavage[a]

Suspected life-threatening toxic ingestion
Procedure can be performed early after ingestion when significant amount of drug remains in stomach
The suspected poison is not adsorbed by activated charcoal
Airway patency can be maintained
General supportive care, or antidotal therapy, expected to be ineffectual
Procedure can be performed with proper technique, including large bore orogastric tube, body positioned on left side with head lower than feet

[a]All must apply.

TABLE 167-6 Poisons for Which Whole-Bowel Irrigation Might Be Considered

Ingested packages of drugs of abuse
Iron pills
Lithium pills
Sustained-release drugs
Ingested medicinal patches
Pill concretions

Gastric decontamination of ingested poisons via induction of emesis with syrup of ipecac has not been shown to improve clinical outcomes and is therefore not recommended. Gastric lavage, once a mainstay of gastric decontamination, has also fallen out of favor, as studies of its clinical utility have demonstrated minimal to no added benefit over activated charcoal administration. As such, gastric lavage should be considered only in rare circumstances (**Table 167-5**). Whole-bowel irrigation with a polyethylene glycol-balanced electrolyte solution can also be used to prevent the absorption of ingested toxic substances (**Table 167-6**). It is typically administered via nasogastric tube at rates titrated to 500 mL/hr in young children and 2 L/hr in adolescents. It is continued until the rectal effluent is clear but should be discontinued for refractory vomiting, abdominal pain, or abdominal distention.

CLINICAL PRESENTATION

The clinical presentation after exposure to certain xenobiotics can be categorized into characteristic poisoning syndromes known as toxidromes. During a physical examination, careful attention should be paid to suspected poisoning patients' mentation, vital signs, pupil size and reactivity, bowel and bladder function, and skin moisture and color (**Table 167-7**). It is important to recognize, however, that the presentation after exposure to many poisons will not fit into a classic toxidrome, and some exposures leave a patient asymptomatic for an extended period of time before ultimately manifesting toxicity. While most patients who will become ill following a poisoning exposure develop symptoms or signs within 6 hours, several "toxic time bombs" are notorious for causing relatively late clinical deterioration (**Table 167-8**).

DIAGNOSTIC EVALUATION

Urine is the preferred specimen for most toxicology screens because many drugs and their metabolites are renally eliminated and become concentrated in the urine. Blood or serum testing is typically reserved for quantification of specific drug or chemical levels such as acetaminophen, salicylates, toxic alcohols, anticonvulsants, lithium, iron, and lead. Hair testing is sometimes used to determine the chronology of poison exposure.

Most hospitals offer a urine immunoassay for drugs of abuse, including amphetamines, barbiturates, benzodiazepines, cocaine, and opiates. Of note, semisynthetic and synthetic opioids such as fentanyl which are responsible for a significant proportion of poisoning morbidity and mortality are not detected on common, commercially available urine

TABLE 167-7 Common Toxidromes

Physical Findings	Sympathomimetics (Cocaine, Amphetamine)	Anticholinergics	Organophosphates/ Carbamates	Opioids, Clonidine	Barbiturates, Sedative-Hypnotics	Salicylates
Mental status	Agitation Delirium Psychosis Seizures	Somnolence Delirium Psychosis Seizures	Somnolence Delirium Fasciculations Seizures	Somnolence	Somnolence	Somnolence Seizures
Heart rate	↑	↑	↓(↑)	↓		—(↑)
Blood pressure	↑	↑	—(↑)	↓	↓	—
Temperature	↑	↑	—	↓	↓	↑
Respirations	—		↓	↓	↓	↑
Pupil size	↑ (reactive)	↑ (sluggish)	↓	↓↓	—	—
Bowel sounds	—	↓	↑	↓	—	—
Skin	Sweaty	Flushed, dry	Sweaty	—	Bullae (IV use)	Sweaty
Antidote(s) and Management	Benzodiazepines, active cooling if hyperthermic	Physostigmine	Atropine, pralidoxime, benzodiazepines for seizures	Naloxone*	Flumazenil for benzodiazepines**	Urine alkalinization, dialysis

*The data regarding the utility of naloxone for clonidine toxicity is mixed; if naloxone is used, higher doses may be necessary to achieve clinical effect in cases of clonidine toxicity

**Flumazenil should only be considered for patients who are not chronically using benzodiazepines. Benzodiazepine-dependent patients may experience precipitated withdrawal including refractory seizures if flumazenil is administered for reversal of toxicity.

Source: Reproduced with permission from Osterhoudt KC, Wiley J. Poisonings. In: Selbst SM, Cronan K, eds. *Pediatric Emergency Medicine Secrets*. 2nd ed. Philadelphia: Elsevier; 2006.

TABLE 167-8 Xenobiotics That Can Cause Delayed-Onset Toxicity After Acute Exposure

Acetaminophen
Antithrombotic agents, especially vitamin K antagonists
Buprenorphine
Colchicine
Hydrocarbons
Many plants and mushrooms containing toxic compounds
Methotrexate and other chemotherapeutic agents
Monoamine oxidase inhibitors
Oral hypoglycemic agents (e.g., sulfonylureas)
Rodenticides
Some envenomation syndromes
Sustained-release preparations
Thyroid hormones
Toxic alcohols, glycols

drug immunoassays. Because urine drug immunoassays are known to have both false-positive and false-negative results, results with significant medicolegal implications, such as positive screens for drugs of abuse in young children, should always be confirmed by another method such as gas or liquid chromatography coupled with mass spectrometry (GC/MS or LC/MS). Most hospitals do not perform confirmatory testing in-house but rather contract with reference laboratories, which adds substantially to the cost and turnaround time; as such, despite their limitations, urine drug immunoassays are clinically heavily utilized as an initial screen because they are fast and inexpensive. Some reference laboratories offer more comprehensive testing of urine or blood for drugs, chemicals, or metals; these also typically employ GC/MS or LC/MS and are thus prohibitively expensive and time-consuming for routine clinical use but may be considered in special circumstances.

When the poisoning exposure is well defined, as is common with exploratory ingestions in young children, laboratory analysis and diagnostic studies may be goal directed. When the exposure history is unreliable, as is often the case with adolescents' polypharmacy attempts at suicide, empirical testing is warranted. Acetaminophen and salicylate concentrations should be obtained in all patients with intentional self-harm ingestions as acetaminophen poisoning may be asymptomatic until hepatic failure ensues, and the nausea, vomiting, and tachypnea associated with early salicylism are nonspecific and easily attributable to other exposures. Measurement of the serum pH, serum electrolytes, serum ammonia, osmolar gap calculation, creatine kinase, hepatic and renal function, and hemoglobin co-oximetry are sometimes indicated depending on the patient's history and clinical presentation. An electrocardiogram should be obtained in any patient presenting with exposure to xenobiotics known to cause cardiotoxicity and should be considered in patients with unknown exposures or those who had plausible access to cardiotoxic drugs.

TABLE 167-9 Common Antidotes Used to Treat Poisoning and Envenomation

Antidote[a]	Indications
N-Acetylcysteine	Acetaminophen (Chapter 168)
Antivenom	Snake, spider, scorpion envenomation (Chapter 178)
Atropine	Organophosphates, carbamates
Benztropine	Drug-induced dystonia
Bicarbonate (sodium)	Sodium channel cardiotoxicity, salicylate poisoning (Chapter 168)
Bromocriptine	Neuroleptic malignant syndrome
Calcium	Calcium channel blockers, hydrogen fluoride
Carnitine	Valproate-induced hyperammonemia
Cyproheptadine	Serotonin syndrome
Dantrolene	Malignant hyperthermia
Deferoxamine	Iron
Digoxin-specific Fab	Digoxin, digitalis, other cardiac glycosides
Dimercaprol (BAL)	Lead, other metals (e.g., arsenic, mercury; Chapter 170)
Diphenhydramine	Drug-induced dystonia
Edetate calcium disodium	Lead (Chapter 170)
Flumazenil	Benzodiazepines
Folic acid	Methanol (Chapter 169)
Folinic acid (leucovorin)	Methotrexate
Fomepizole	Ethylene glycol, methanol (Chapter 169)
Glucagon	Beta-blocker-induced bradycardia and hypotension
Hydroxocobalamin	Cyanide
Insulin (high dose)	Beta blocker- or calcium channel blocker-induced hypotension
Lipid emulsion	Local anesthetic overdose
Methylene blue	Methemoglobinemia, vasodilatory shock
Naloxone	Opioids (Chapter 171)
Octreotide	Sulfonylurea-induced hypoglycemia (Chapter 168)
Penicillamine	Lead, other metals (e.g., copper; Chapter 170)
Physostigmine	Anticholinergic delirium
Pralidoxime (2-PAM)	Organophosphates
Pyridoxine	Isoniazid, ethylene glycol (Chapter 169)
Sodium nitrite, sodium thiosulfate	Cyanide
Succimer (DMSA)	Lead, other metals (e.g., arsenic, mercury; Chapter 170)
Thiamine	Wernicke encephalopathy, ethylene glycol (Chapter 169)
Vitamin K_1	Warfarin and other vitamin K antagonists (e.g., brodifacoum)

[a]Does not include gastrointestinal decontamination agents, routine supportive pressor agents, sedatives, and anticonvulsants.

MANAGEMENT

The physiologic derangements caused by acute poisoning are typically of finite duration, until the drug or chemical is eliminated from the body, and good supportive care suffices for the majority of patients. Children exposed to arrhythmogenic poisons such as antiarrhythmic drugs, chloroquine, cyclic antidepressants, and diphenhydramine merit telemetry monitoring when available. Children with impending or existing failure of the respiratory, cardiovascular, or neurologic systems or those children with special needs at baseline (e.g., hemodialysis-dependent) are good candidates for intensive care. Some poisons have specific or nonspecific antidotes (**Table 167-9**), and some poisons are amenable to methods that enhance their elimination from the body, such as urinary alkalinization for salicylates. Hemodialysis augments the clearance of many toxicants, particularly those with lower molecular weights, low protein binding, and a low volume of distribution such as lithium, methanol, ethylene glycol, and salicylates. Multiple doses of activated charcoal, typically given every 4 to 6 hours, enhance the elimination of xenobiotics that undergo enterohepatic recirculation by adsorbing the poison in the gut after its excretion in the bile, thus preventing reabsorption and hastening elimination. Examples of drugs that undergo enterohepatic recirculation include carbamazepine, colchicine, dapsone, phenobarbital, quinine, and theophylline. Once a patient is physiologically back to baseline, psychiatric care should be sought for patients presenting after a self-harm attempt, and addiction care should be sought for patients with substance use disorders. Poison prevention education should additionally be prioritized for all patients and their family members upon discharge after a toxic exposure.

SUGGESTED READING

Benson BE, Hoppu K, Troutman WG, et al. Position paper update: gastric lavage for gastrointestinal decontamination. *Clin Toxicol (Phila).* 2013;51:140-146.

Bond GR. Home syrup of ipecac use does not reduce emergency department use or improve outcome. *Pediatrics.* 2003;112:1061-4.

Chiew AL, Buckley NA. The serotonin toxidrome: shortfalls of current diagnostic criteria for related syndromes. *Clin Toxicol (Phila).* 2022;60:143-158.

Goldstick JE, Cunningham RM, Carter PM. Current causes of death in children and adolescents in the United States. *N Engl J Med.* 2022; 386:1955-1956.

Gosselin S, Hoffman RS. The management of agitated toxidromes. *Emerg Med Clin North Am.* 2022;40:223-235.

Gummin DD, Mowry JB, Beuhler MC, et al. 2020 Annual Report of the American Association of Poison Control Centers' National Poison Data System (NPDS): 38th Annual Report. *Clin Toxicol (Phila).* 2021;59:1282-1501.

Hoegberg LCG, Shepherd G, Wood DM, et al. Systematic review on the use of activated charcoal for gastrointestinal decontamination following acute oral overdose. *Clin Toxicol (Phila).* 2021;59:1196-1227.

Lowry JA, Burns M, Calello DP. Pediatric pharmaceutical ingestions. *Pediatr Ann.* 2017;46:e459-e465.

Parris MA, Calello DP. Found down: approach to the patient with an unknown poisoning. *Emerg Med Clin North Am.* 2022;40:193-222.

Tesfazghi MT, Bardelmeier R, Saunders AN, Riley SM, Roper SM, Dietzen DJ. Development and implementation of one-step, broad-spectrum, high-sensitivity drug screening by tandem mass spectrometry in a pediatric population. *J Appl Lab Med.* 2022;7:409-420.

CHAPTER 168 Toxicity of Over-the-Counter Medications and Oral Hypoglycemic Agents

Kristin Shadman, MD and Ann Allen, MD

BACKGROUND

The household medicine cabinet is commonly filled with over the counter and prescription products, including analgesics, iron, antihistamines, and oral hypoglycemics, that are potentially toxic to children and adolescents in unintentional and intentional ingestions. According to the 2020 American Association of Poison Control Centers' National Poison Data System (NPDS) Annual Report, analgesics, vitamins, antihistamines and cough and cold preparations account for approximately 18% of all exposures in children younger than 6 years. Although hospitalists may frequently encounter these ingestions, consultation with a medical toxicologist or regional Poison Control Center (1-800-222-1222) is indicated for all patients.

ACETAMINOPHEN

Acetaminophen, also known as paracetamol, is responsible for a substantial number of pediatric poisonings each year. Hepatic injury is the most frequent cause of morbidity and mortality after an overdose of acetaminophen. Extensive clinical research and experience have allowed clinicians to better predict and prevent the development of hepatotoxicity.

Most forms of acetaminophen are rapidly absorbed after ingestion. Although extended-release acetaminophen preparations have similar pharmacokinetics as the regular-release formulations, with peak levels occurring less than 4 hours after ingestion, elimination may be delayed in some patients. Intravenous acetaminophen presents a novel formulation of acetaminophen with potential for toxicity.

Acetaminophen is metabolized almost exclusively in the liver; approximately 90% is glucuronidated or sulfated, 5% is excreted unchanged in urine, and the remaining 5% is oxidized by liver cytochrome enzymes, specifically CYP2E1, CYP1A2, and CYP3A4. Oxidation produces the reactive electrophile *N*-acetyl-*p*-benzoquinone imine (NAPQI). In conditions of therapeutic dosing, NAPQI is detoxified by glutathione, whereas in conditions of decreased glutathione stores, large doses of acetaminophen, or induction of cytochrome enzymes, NAPQI overwhelms the capacity of glutathione. Free NAPQI binds to hepatocytes and causes hepatocellular damage.

The risk for hepatocellular injury can be assessed by the dose ingested, the acetaminophen level, or both. In acute ingestion, patients who take more than 200 mg/kg (children) or 7.5 g (adults) are at risk for acetaminophen toxicity. Some patients may be more at risk for hepatotoxicity including those with preexisting liver disease, children with acute febrile illness, and patients who chronically ingest drugs that induce CYP2E1, such as olanzapine, tizanidine, or ciprofloxacin.

CLINICAL PRESENTATION

Patients who have been exposed to toxic doses of acetaminophen may have a paucity of findings on physical examination. Acetaminophen toxicity is divided into four clinical stages, and the findings of each phase are presented in **Table 168-1**.

DIFFERENTIAL DIAGNOSIS

The early signs and symptoms of acetaminophen toxicity are nonspecific and represent a large toxic and nontoxicologic differential diagnosis of acute liver injury (e.g., viral hepatitis, Reye's syndrome, ischemic hepatitis).

DIAGNOSTIC EVALUATION

Initial laboratory analysis for a patient with a suspected acetaminophen overdose should begin with a serum acetaminophen level. Acetaminophen levels should be obtained in all cases of intentional overdose because acetaminophen is a frequent co-ingestant. Levels obtained prior to 4 hours after ingestion are difficult to interpret. The standard (Rumack-Matthew) acetaminophen nomogram may be used to predict the risk for acetaminophen toxicity in patients in whom levels were obtained 4 hours or longer after a single, acute ingestion **(Figure 168-1).**

TABLE 168-1 Stages of Acetaminophen Toxicity

Stage	Time After Ingestion	Clinical Findings
I	0.5-24 hr	Anorexia, nausea, vomiting, malaise, pallor, diaphoresis
II	24-48 hr	Resolution of early symptoms Right upper quadrant abdominal pain and tenderness Elevated hepatic transaminases, prothrombin time, bilirubin Oliguria
III	72-96 hr	Reappearance of anorexia, nausea, vomiting Onset of fulminant hepatic failure with metabolic acidosis, coagulopathy Changes in mental status progressing toward encephalopathy
IV	4 days to 2 wk	Either resolution of hepatic dysfunction or progression of liver failure, oliguric renal failure, and death

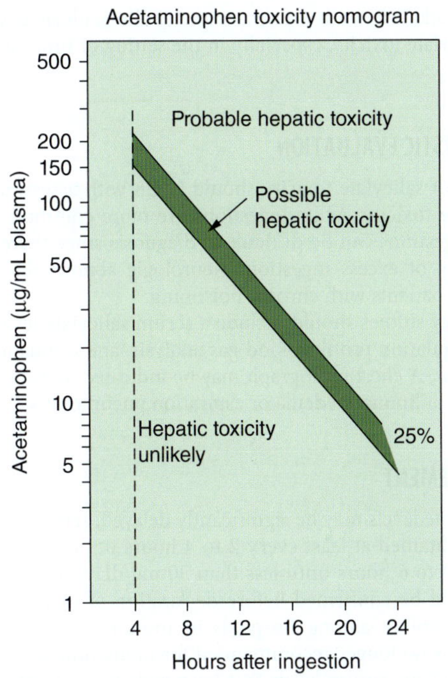

FIGURE 168-1. The Rumack-Matthew nomogram relating expected severity of liver toxicity to serum acetaminophen concentrations. (Reproduced with permission from Smilkstein MJ, Bronstein AC, Linden C, et al. Acetaminophen overdose: a 48-hour intravenous N-acetylcysteine treatment protocol. *Ann Emerg Med.* 1991; 20:1058.)

In the United States, the lower line of the nomogram is used as the clinical indicator to begin treatment. Additional laboratory evaluation should consist of measurement of hepatic transaminases and determination of liver synthetic function (coagulation studies) and renal function. Repeated supratherapeutic overdoses of acetaminophen cannot be plotted on the nomogram.

MANAGEMENT

Gastric decontamination with a single dose of activated charcoal is recommended in patients with an ingestion within the first 4 hours. *N*-acetylcysteine (NAC) is effective when administered by both the oral and intravenous routes. A 21-hour intravenous preparation is now widely used in the United States due to its ease of use and shorter treatment duration than the historic 72-hour oral course. Shorter intravenous treatment regimens are under investigation. The equally efficacious enteral therapy is more cost effective; however, adherence to the full treatment protocol may be limited by intolerance of enteral therapy. No deaths from hepatic injury have been reported in patients treated with NAC within 8 hours of overdose. While no serious complications have been reported after the use of oral NAC, intravenous NAC has been shown to cause urticaria, anaphylactoid reactions, and rarely, death, particularly in patients with asthma. Intravenous NAC is preferred in patients with intractable vomiting despite the use of antiemetics, fulminant hepatic failure (FHF), or pregnancy.

The treatment regimen for oral NAC is a loading dose of 140 mg/kg, followed by 70 mg/kg every 4 hours for a total of 17 doses (not including the loading dose). Patients with persistent laboratory abnormalities may benefit from NAC past the standard oral 72-hour regimen. NAC may be given intravenously as a 3% solution (in 5% dextrose) as 150 mg/kg over 1 hour, followed by an infusion over an additional 20 hours, at 12.5 mg/kg/hr. Various IV dosing regimens have been evaluated to reduce side effects including the use of the two-bag protocol.

Transaminases, liver synthetic function (coagulation studies), and renal function should be checked initially and daily during therapy in any patient with a serum acetaminophen concentration above the treatment nomogram line, until NAC is discontinued. Worsening hepatic function may necessitate more frequent laboratory studies. Patients who demonstrate hepatotoxicity despite treatment with NAC will need further clinical and laboratory monitoring, including the prothrombin time, international normalized ratio (INR) clotting measure, arterial pH, lactic acid, and serum creatinine. Patients with an INR greater than 2 at 24 hours, 4 at 48 hours, or 6 at 72 hours are at high risk for the development of FHF. Any patient in whom FHF develops should be referred for possible liver transplantation. Criteria for referral and transplantation are found in **Table 168-2**.

TABLE 168-2 Criteria for Transplantation

Prothrombin time >100 s or INR >6
and
Serum creatinine >3.3 mg/dL
and
Grade III or grade IV hepatic encephalopathy
or
Arterial pH < 7.3 any time after FHF that fails to correct with IV fluids
or
Lactic acid >3 mmol/L that fails to correct with IV fluids

FHF, fulminant hepatic failure; INR, international normalized ratio.

Source: Adapted from Makin AJ, Williams R. Acetaminophen-induced hepatotoxicity: predisposing factors and treatments. *Adv Intern Med.* 1997;42:453-483.

ADMISSION AND DISCHARGE CRITERIA

Treatment with NAC is the mainstay of acetaminophen poisoning and necessitates hospital admission. For a single, acute overdose taken at a known time, NAC should be administered to all patients with an acetaminophen level in the "possible and probable hepatotoxicity" range. When the time of ingestion is unknown or in cases of repeated supratherapeutic overdoses, NAC may be administered while the acetaminophen is eliminated, and hepatic transaminases should be monitored.

Demonstration of a normal serum aspartate transaminase (AST) level 36 hours after acetaminophen ingestion nearly eliminates the possibility of liver toxicity. In the face of hepatic toxicity, a decline in the serum AST level may indicate clinical recovery or complete hepatocellular death and must be interpreted in the context of liver function. Patients with hepatic toxicity may be discharged once hepatic recovery is clearly in progress.

SALICYLATES

From its introduction 100 years ago, aspirin (acetylsalicylic acid) has remained a mainstay of clinical medicine. Despite the development of newer and more specific nonsteroidal anti-inflammatory drugs (NSAIDs), aspirin continues to be widely used because of its multiple applications and benefits. Although reported cases of aspirin toxicity have declined in recent decades, aspirin still accounts for thousands of cases reported to poison control centers and approximately 50 deaths each year. In addition to aspirin, other salicylate-containing products and combination aspirin preparations are commonly used, including liniments for arthritis, acne creams, sunscreens, antidiarrheals, wart remover, and Chinese herbal medications.

The pathophysiology of salicylate toxicity is complex. Salicylates directly stimulate the respiratory center of the medulla and result in hyperventilation and hyperpnea. To compensate for respiratory alkalosis, the kidney excretes bicarbonate creating metabolic acidosis, which is exacerbated by the salicylate-driven uncoupling of mitochondrial oxidative phosphorylation, increased carbon dioxide production and accumulation of lactic and pyruvic acids. Additionally, disruption of Krebs cycle metabolism leads to gluconeogenesis, lipolysis, and increased ketone formation. The salicylate ion itself contributes very little to metabolic acidosis. The pathophysiology of the most common presenting symptoms in salicylate toxicity is described in **Table 168-3**.

TABLE 168-3 Pathophysiology of Symptoms in Salicylate Toxicity

Symptom	Pathophysiology/Etiology
Nausea, vomiting, and epigastric discomfort	Gastrointestinal irritation
	Stimulation of the medullary chemoreceptor trigger zone
Tinnitus and deafness	Vasoconstriction of the auditory microvasculature
Sweating, hyperpyrexia, and dehydration	Uncoupling of mitochondrial oxidative phosphorylation and increased metabolism of skeletal muscle
Dehydration	Decreased oral intake, vomiting, tachypnea, diaphoresis, and obligatory early diuresis
Hyperpnea and tachypnea	Direct stimulation of the medullary respiratory center
Disorientation, hallucinations, lethargy, agitation, coma, and seizures	Acidosis, cerebral edema
Noncardiogenic pulmonary edema	Leukotriene-induced increased permeability of the microvasculature
Renal failure	
Acid-base disorders (e.g., respiratory alkalosis, mixed respiratory alkalosis, and anion gap metabolic acidosis)	Combination of direct stimulation of the medullary respiratory center (respiratory alkalosis) with renal compensation (metabolic acidosis) and uncoupling mitochondrial respiration (metabolic acid acidosis)
Hypokalemia and hyponatremia or hypernatremia	Increased renal excretion of potassium/sodium because of the anion drag of bicarbonate
	Hypernatremia may ensue if free H_2O is lost in excess of salt in the kidneys and sweat
Hypoglycemia/hyperglycemia	Salicylates enhance insulin secretion from pancreatic islet cells (hypoglycemia); also decrease peripheral glucose utilization (hyperglycemia)
Hypoprothrombinemia	Acts as a vitamin K antagonist which results in disturbance in vitamin K-dependent clotting factors

CLINICAL PRESENTATION

Salicylates produce analgesic, antipyretic, and anti-inflammatory effects, mostly through inhibition of cyclooxygenase and a subsequent decrease in the production of prostaglandins. Therapeutic doses of acetylsalicylic acid, 10 to 20 mg/kg for children and 650 to 1000 mg every 4 to 6 hours for adults, produce a serum salicylate level of 3 to 6 mg/dL. Although aspirin is often avoided in children due to the risk of Reye syndrome, there are several circumstances, including Kawasaki disease, in which it is therapeutically used with a dose up to 80 to 100 mg/kg.

Evidence of toxicity usually appears around serum levels of 30 mg/dL. The potentially toxic acute dose is greater than 150 mg/kg, whereas chronic toxicity may occur with doses that exceed 100 mg/kg/day. Toxic doses for other salicylate formulations may be calculated by using known aspirin equivalencies.

Salicylates are absorbed in the stomach and proximal part of the intestine. Peak serum levels in therapeutic doses occur at 1 to 2 hours (4 to 6 hours for enteric-coated tablets) but may be delayed for 10 to 60 hours in cases of overdose. The most notorious reason for delayed absorption is an aspirin bezoar, but other causes include enteric-coated products, contraction of the pylorus, and delayed gastric emptying from coingestants. The elimination half-life of salicylate in therapeutic doses is 4 hours, but it increases to 15 to 29 hours with toxic plasma levels.

DIFFERENTIAL DIAGNOSIS

The signs and symptoms of salicylate toxicity are commonly found in other disorders and represent a large nontoxicologic differential diagnosis, such as diabetic ketoacidosis, sepsis, and pneumonia. Other possible toxicologic etiologies include agents that cause anion gap metabolic acidosis including toxic alcohols, iron, isoniazid, massive ibuprofen ingestions, and metformin toxicity. The metabolic profile of primary respiratory alkalosis with a primary metabolic acidosis is very suggestive of salicylate toxicity, especially in the setting of tinnitus, tachypnea, or emesis.

DIAGNOSTIC EVALUATION

Evaluation of salicylate toxicity should begin with assessment of chronicity of the toxicity. Acute ingestions are more common in children. Chronic ingestions can be difficult to diagnosis since there is often no clear history of excess ingestion. Neurologic abnormalities are more common in patients with chronic poisoning.

Laboratory studies should include a serum salicylate level, chemistry panels, coagulation profile, blood gas analysis, and evaluation for other co-ingestants. A chest radiograph may be indicated to evaluate for noncardiogenic pulmonary edema or aspiration pneumonitis.

MANAGEMENT

Peak salicylate levels may be significantly delayed; serial salicylate levels should be obtained at least every 2 to 4 hours until clearly decreasing, then every 4 to 6 hours until less than 30 mg/dL. Units (mg/dL versus mg/L) should be confirmed before declaration of toxic levels because there is variability among hospitals in units of measure. The Done nomogram is no longer recommended for prediction of the severity of salicylate toxicity. Serum levels that have wide vacillations or are rising despite treatment may indicate the presence of a bezoar.

There is no specific antidote; treatment of salicylate poisoning centers around supporting adequate respiration and circulation, gastrointestinal decontamination, and correction of fluid, electrolyte, and acid-base disturbances. Strict measurement of urine output is necessary. The various modalities for treatment of salicylate toxicity can be found in **Table 168-4**. Patients with salicylate-induced hyperpnea may be easily misdiagnosed as imminent respiratory failure. However, intubation and mechanical ventilation may contribute to mortality by impairing acid-base homeostasis by altering the primary respiratory alkalosis that counteracts the serum salicylate anions.

TABLE 168-4 Treatment of Salicylate Toxicity

Treatment	Method	Comments
Activated charcoal	1 g/kg PO initially Repeat doses of 25 g or 0.5 g/kg at 2-4 hr	MDAC useful in cases of prolonged absorption Uncertain whether MDAC adds benefit once urinary alkalinization is achieved
Urinary alkalinization	1-2 mEq/kg of $NaHCO_3$ by IV bolus, then D5W with 100-150 mEq/L $NaHCO_3$ at 1-2 times maintenance requirements	Traps ionized salicylate in proximal tubule Start when salicylate levels >30 mg/dL Goal is urine pH of 7.5-8.0 (should be monitored hourly) Monitor serum pH (should be 7.45-7.55) Correct hypokalemia or other electrolyte imbalances Watch for fluid overload
Hemodialysis		Indications include: Serum levels >100 mg/dL with acute ingestion Serum levels >60 mg/dL with chronic intoxication Pulmonary edema Renal failure Congestive heart failure No response to standard therapies Altered mental status and acidemia

D5W, 5% dextrose in water; MDAC, multiple-dose activated charcoal.

ADMISSION AND DISCHARGE CRITERIA

Patients who have a history of significant exposure (>150 mg/kg) should be admitted to the hospital. Other criteria for admission include rising salicylate levels, acidosis, coagulopathy, mental status changes, or persistent abnormalities in vital signs. Admission to an intensive care setting may be warranted for patients with abnormal mental status, severe acidosis, renal failure, or coagulation abnormalities. Discharge from inpatient medical care may occur when the patient has been asymptomatic and has serial falling salicylate levels below 30 mg/dL after cessation of bicarbonate therapy.

IRON

Historically, drug overdoses of iron preparations were a leading cause of pediatric mortality. In 1997, the Food and Drug Administration (FDA) issued a regulation requiring warning labels and childproof packaging for iron-containing products with 30 mg or more of iron per dosage unit, however, these regulations were repealed in 2003. The trend in NPDS data suggested that iron poisoning and fatalities were decreasing following implementation of warning labels and childproof packaging; updated trends have not been published following the reversal of regulations.

CLINICAL PRESENTATION

Different oral formulations of iron contain disparate amounts of elemental iron (**Table 168-5**). Acute mild toxicity, expressed in terms of milligrams of elemental iron per kilogram of body weight, is seen with doses as low as 20 mg/kg elemental iron, whereas systemic illness generally occurs with doses in the range of 40 to 60 mg/kg. Iron levels are thought to peak 2 to 6 hours after ingestion; however, this timing may be longer for time release formulations or enteric-coated preparations. Serum iron levels generally correlate with clinical severity: mild symptomatology (vomiting, diarrhea) is seen with levels less than 300 μg/dL, moderate symptoms with levels of 300 to 500 μg/dL, and severe manifestations (shock, acidosis, seizures, coma, death) with levels exceeding 500 μg/dL.

Acute iron toxicity is described in phases. Early toxicity results in local irritant effects, whereas later findings are thought to be due to mitochondrial damage, particularly in the liver (**Table 168-6**).

TABLE 168-6 Phases of Iron Toxicity

Phase	Time from Ingestion	Symptoms	Pathophysiology
1	0-6 hr	Abdominal pain, emesis, and diarrhea	Direct local irritant effect on gastrointestinal mucosa
2	6-12 hr	Improvement of phase 1 symptoms, also known as latent phase	Iron entering cells
3	12-24 hr	Hypovolemic shock (from gastrointestinal fluid losses) Wide anion gap acidosis Depressed myocardial function Increased pulmonary vascular resistance Hepatotoxicity with hypoglycemia and coagulopathy	Iron concentrates intracellularly in mitochondria and disrupts oxidative phosphorylation, resulting in free radical formation and lipid peroxidation; free iron may exhibit a direct inhibitory effect on the formation of thrombin and thrombin's effect on fibrinogen in vitro
4	2-6 wk and beyond	Emesis Liver failure	Emesis secondary to pyloric stricture leading to bowel obstruction, liver failure secondary to hepatic cirrhosis

DIFFERENTIAL DIAGNOSIS

The signs and symptoms of iron toxicity (nausea and vomiting, anion gap metabolic acidosis, acute liver injury, altered mental status) overlap with other disorders, including sepsis, gastroenteritis, and diabetic ketoacidosis. Other possible toxicologic etiologies that cause anion gap metabolic acidosis include toxic alcohols, salicylates, isoniazid, massive ibuprofen ingestions, and metformin toxicity. Acetaminophen toxicity causes acute liver injury in a similar pattern to iron.

DIAGNOSTIC EVALUATION

An abdominal radiograph is indicated to look for the presence and location of iron tablets. Completely dissolved iron tablets/capsules/liquid preparations may not be radiopaque; consequently, a negative radiograph does not eliminate the possibility of toxic iron ingestion. However, patients with negative abdominal radiographs may be discharged after a 6-hour period of observation if they remain asymptomatic. Baseline laboratory studies, including blood glucose, serum iron levels (4 to 6 hours after ingestion of regular iron and 8 hours after extended-release iron ingestion), hepatic studies (serum transaminases, albumin, and coagulation studies), and electrolytes including serum bicarbonate concentration should be obtained 4 to 6 hours after ingestion for any patient with symptoms of toxicity or a significant history of ingestion. Leukocytosis and hyperglycemia may be seen, however are neither sensitive nor specific to iron ingestion.

TABLE 168-5 Iron Formulations

Formulation	Elemental Iron (%)
Ferrous sulfate	20
Ferrous sulfate (anhydrous)	30
Ferrous gluconate	12
Ferrous fumarate	33
Ferrous lactate	19
Ferrous chloride	28

MANAGEMENT

Whole-bowel irrigation with a polyethylene glycol-balanced electrolyte solution may be considered as a means of gastrointestinal decontamination. Activated charcoal does not absorb iron and is not recommended. Further therapeutic guidelines, including deferoxamine chelation, are presented in **Table 168-7**.

Iron chelation with intravenous deferoxamine remains the mainstay of treatment following gut decontamination. Deferoxamine may be administered intramuscularly, however injections are painful and may cause local tissue inflammation. Oral deferoxamine is not recommended. Once therapy with deferoxamine is instituted, clinical monitoring should include serial measurements of blood pressure, serum iron concentration (if available), hepatic transaminases, electrolytes, and prothrombin time. Therapeutic end points for deferoxamine therapy include resolution of clinical symptoms and metabolic acidosis as well as narrowing of the anion gap, rather than serum iron level. Moreover, in the presence of deferoxamine, serum iron levels may be falsely low. Recurrent symptomatology may warrant reinstitution of deferoxamine, which should be undertaken carefully and at a lower dose. Additional treatment modalities such as continuous veno-venous hemofiltration and exchange transfusion have been described for the severely iron-poisoned patient.

Complications of deferoxamine may include dose-related hypotension and pulmonary toxicity manifested as tachypnea, hypoxemia, fever, eosinophilia, urticaria, and pulmonary infiltrates in patients receiving both prolonged (>24 hours) and high (>15 mg/kg/hr) doses of intravenous deferoxamine. Ocular and otic toxicity have also been reported. *Yersinia enteroeolitica* septicemia and mucormycosis infection are rare complications. Although the mechanism of this complication is unclear, deferoxamine may provide the iron siderophore complex growth factor needed to induce overgrowth.

TABLE 168-7 Treatment of Iron Toxicity (Ingestion >20 mg/kg Elemental Iron)

Symptom	Laboratory Finding	Treatment
Asymptomatic	Negative KUB	Observe for 6 hr—discharge home if no symptoms develop
Asymptomatic	Radiopaque pills on KUB	Whole bowel irrigation and repeat KUB Determine electrolytes and SI 4-6 hr after ingestion Start deferoxamine if peak SI > 500 μg/dL or metabolic acidosis
Symptomatic[1]	Radiopaque pills on KUB Or Peak SI >500 μg/dL Or Patient is symptomatic and SI cannot readily be obtained	Whole bowel irrigation and repeat KUB Determine electrolytes and SI 4-6 hr after ingestion Start deferoxamine by continuous infusion at a rate of up to 15 mg/kg/hr
Symptomatic[1]	Anion gap acidosis	Aggressive fluid resuscitation Consider hemodialysis if refractory acidosis
Hypotension, shock		Watch for cardiogenic pulmonary edema Dopamine and/or norepinephrine may be needed for refractory hypotension Consider exchange transfusion
Symptomatic[1]	Hypoglycemia	Watch for hypoglycemia and correct as needed
Acute liver failure	Coagulopathy	Fresh frozen plasma, cryoprecipitate as needed

KUB, abdominal radiograph; SI, serum iron concentration.

[1]e.g., nausea, vomiting, anion gap metabolic acidosis, acute liver injury, mental status changes.

ADMISSION AND DISCHARGE CRITERIA

Patients with signs of mild poisoning (e.g., vomiting, diarrhea) should be admitted for inpatient management. Those who demonstrate serious systemic signs of toxicity (e.g., shock, central nervous system depression) should be admitted to an intensive care setting. Discharge from inpatient medical care may occur when symptoms and laboratory abnormalities have resolved, and no clinical deterioration is noted following cessation of deferoxamine therapy.

ANTIHISTAMINES

Over-the-counter antihistamines are ubiquitous and used for cold and allergy symptoms and as sleep aids. Most of the toxicity associated with an overdose of antihistamines is due to their anticholinergic effects through inhibition of both central and peripheral muscarinic cholinergic receptors. First-generation antihistamines have a higher toxicity potential than second-generation antihistamines. While some discontinued non-sedating antihistamines (i.e., terfenadine, astemizole) demonstrated significant cardiac toxicity associated with drug interactions, cardiotoxicity is less likely with the second-generation antihistamines. A list of some common antihistamines is provided in **Table 168-8**.

CLINICAL PRESENTATION

Absorption of antihistamines from the gastrointestinal tract is rapid, with the peak drug effect usually seen in 1 hour. However, after large ingestions, symptoms may not occur for several hours and may last for days. Patients who have taken an overdose of antihistamines may present with the classic anticholinergic toxidrome (Chapter 169). In addition, seizures are common after large overdoses of antihistamines. Some antihistamines, especially diphenhydramine, can cause wide QRS tachyarrhythmias from sodium channel blockade as well as QT interval prolongation, placing patients at risk for malignant arrhythmias such as torsades de pointes. Antihistamines are often combined with other drugs in commercial products, so concomitant toxicity from sympathomimetic agents, acetaminophen, or dextromethorphan may be encountered.

TABLE 168-8 Common Histamine Receptor Antagonists

Azelastine (Astelin)
Bilastine (Bilaxten)
Brompheniramine (Dimetane)*
Cetirizine (Zyrtec)
Chlorpheniramine (Chlor-Trimeton)*
Cyclizine (Marezine)*
Dimenhydrinate (Dramamine)*
Diphenhydramine (Benadryl)*
Doxylamine*
Fexofenadine (Allegra)
Hydroxyzine (Atarax, Vistaril)*
Loratadine (Claritin)
Meclizine (Antivert)*
Promethazine (Phenergan)*

*Prominent anticholinergic symptoms.

DIFFERENTIAL DIAGNOSIS

Other toxicologic causes of an anticholinergic toxidrome as seen in antihistamine ingestion include poisoning from agents such as tricyclic antidepressants (i.e., amitriptyline, nortriptyline), atypical antipsychotic medications (i.e., quetiapine, olanzapine), skeletal muscle relaxants (i.e. cyclobenzaprine), antispasmodics (i.e., Donnatal [phenobarbital, hyoscyamine, atropine, and scopolamine], Lomotil [diphenoxylate and atropine]), or ingestion of anticholinergic alkaloid plants (i.e., Jimsonweed, Deadly nightshade, *Amanita muscaria* mushrooms).

DIAGNOSTIC EVALUATION

The diagnostic course for patients with a suspected overdose of antihistamines depends on the symptomatology and dose ingested. The mean dose in symptomatic children has been reported as 17.3 mg/kg and deaths have occurred with doses as low as 33 mg/kg. Initially, vital signs, including temperature, heart rate, respiratory rate, and blood pressure should be assessed. Electrocardiographic evaluation, specifically checking for widening of the QRS complex or QT interval, is warranted to look for signs of impending arrhythmia. Acetaminophen levels are of particular importance because many cold products contain both antihistamines and acetaminophen. Further diagnostic testing can be useful, although unreliable in some aspects. For example, diphenhydramine may result in a false-positive urine immunoassay for phencyclidine (PCP). Additional laboratory testing could be considered such as creatinine and blood urea nitrogen (BUN) or creatinine kinase.

MANAGEMENT

Activated charcoal may reduce the absorption of antihistamine drugs if administered soon after ingestion. Physostigmine should be considered for both diagnosis and symptom management. The benefits of physostigmine, which include restoration of gastrointestinal motility and improvement in mental status, must outweigh the potential risks (worsening of cardiac conduction delays). Physostigmine may be used safely when the patient has a narrow QRS complex on electrocardiography and no evidence of ingestion of other agents (e.g., class IA or IC antiarrhythmics, tricyclic antidepressants) that may cause intraventricular conduction delays. Intravenous access and cardiovascular monitoring must be established before the use of physostigmine. The initial dose of physostigmine, 0.02 mg/kg in children or 1 to 2 mg in adults, may be

TABLE 168-9 Treatment of Antihistamine Overdose

Symptom	Treatment	Comments
Agitation/delirium	Physostigmine IV over 5-min period (adults, 1-2 mg; pediatric, 0.02 mg/kg) Benzodiazepines IV	Electrocardiographic conduction delay (prolonged PR, wide QRS) is relative contraindication for physostigmine
Seizures	Benzodiazepines IV Physostigmine IV over 5-min period (adults, 1-2 mg; pediatric, 0.02 mg/kg)	In the setting of tricyclic antidepressant overdose, use of physostigmine has been associated with seizures and intractable cardiac arrest
Hyperthermia	Cool bath, fans, sedation	
Ventricular arrhythmia	Sodium bicarbonate bolus (1-2 mEq/kg), then drip (in D5W) Lidocaine bolus (1 mg/kg), then drip as needed (20-50 μg/kg/min)	Monitor electrocardiogram continuously; monitor serum electrolytes and arterial blood gases Goal serum pH, 7.45-7.55 Continue 24 hr past end points of cessation of dysrhythmias, normalization of QRS complexes
Other tachyarrhythmia	May consider beta-blocker (propranolol) May consider physostigmine if refractory	Supportive treatment if hemodynamically stable
Torsades de pointes	Cardioversion Magnesium sulfate IV (adults, 2-6 g; pediatric, 25-50 mg/kg) Overdrive pacing	
Rhabdomyolysis	Fluid resuscitation, urinary alkalinization, and maintenance of urine output at 1-2 mL/kg/hr	

D5W, 5% dextrose in water; IV, intravenous.

administered by slow intravenous infusion over 5 minutes with repeat doses every 10 to 15 minutes up to a maximum dose of 2 mg in children and 4 mg in adults until the anticholinergic symptoms are reversed. Additional physostigmine should not be administered if significant cholinergic symptoms develop, particularly bradycardia or excessive salivation. A dose of atropine should be readily available to reverse side effects. Patients considered at high risk for the development of seizures may be co-administered a prophylactic dose of benzodiazepine.

Inpatient care should be directed at symptoms (**Table 168-9**). Benzodiazepines may help decrease agitation and tachycardia.

ADMISSION AND DISCHARGE CRITERIA

Patients displaying persistent changes in mental status, abnormalities in vital signs, electrocardiographic changes, or seizures should be admitted to the hospital. The severity of symptomatology may warrant admission to an intensive care setting.

Discharge from inpatient medical care may occur when the patient has become asymptomatic and no further drug absorption is anticipated.

ORAL HYPOGLYCEMICS

Oral hypoglycemics are the mainstay of treatment of Type 2 diabetes. As more patients are diagnosed with diabetes and prescribed these medications, the risk of unintentional pediatric ingestions increases. A brief review of glycemic control is necessary to better understand the mechanism of toxicity after an overdose of oral hypoglycemics.

Glycemic control is achieved through the careful balance of hormonal, neural, and substrate mechanisms. In conditions of hyperglycemia, pancreatic beta cells secrete insulin. Insulin binds to the insulin receptor, which unleashes a signaling cascade. The biologic activity of insulin results in a decrease in plasma glucose that occurs by inhibition of hepatic glucose production, increased glucose uptake, and increased glycogen stores in insulin-sensitive tissues.

Hypoglycemia is corrected by the counterregulatory hormones glucagon, epinephrine, norepinephrine, cortisol, growth hormone, and adrenocorticotropic hormones. The initial response to hypoglycemia is the release of glucagon, secreted from pancreatic alpha cells. Glucagon acts on the liver to increase glycogenolysis and gluconeogenesis. Epinephrine, synthesized in the adrenal medulla, constitutes the bulk of circulating catecholamines released in response to hypoglycemia. Epinephrine works primarily through β_2-adrenergic receptors to increase plasma glucose by indirect stimulation of lipolysis. Cortisol is necessary for the liver to respond appropriately to glucagon and epinephrine. Long-standing hypoglycemia raises plasma cortisol levels, thereby reducing the autonomic adrenomedullary response to subsequent hypoglycemia.

Oral hypoglycemics work by either increasing insulin production, increasing insulin receptor sensitivity, or decreasing serum glucose levels. Sulfonylureas and thiazolidinediones can cause hypoglycemia in overdose and other oral hypoglycemics can further potentiate these effects. **Table 168-10** lists the most common oral hypoglycemics and their mechanism of action.

CLINICAL PRESENTATION

The clinical symptoms of hypoglycemia are variable and can include unstable vital signs, fixed and dilated pupils, dysrhythmias, diaphoresis, and altered mental status. Neurologic symptoms are often most prominent. Mild neurologic symptoms of hypoglycemia include weakness, fatigue, and behavioral and cognitive dysfunction, whereas severe hypoglycemia can result in hemiplegia, decerebrate posturing, ataxia, choreoathetosis, and seizures.

DIFFERENTIAL DIAGNOSIS

The nontoxicologic differential diagnosis of hypoglycemia is quite broad, including many metabolic and endocrine disorders (Chapter 78). The toxicologic causes of hypoglycemia include toxicity from a diverse group of agents including beta-blockers, ethanol, salicylates, insulin, intravenous quinine, and unripened Jamaican ackee fruit.

DIAGNOSTIC EVALUATION

The onset and duration of symptoms can be predicted if the type of oral hypoglycemic agent and the time of ingestion are known. Although hypoglycemia can occur early after the ingestion of oral hypoglycemic agents, hypoglycemia may be delayed up to 48 hours after ingestion. Recurrent hypoglycemia has been reported as long as 94 hours after ingestion. A combination of a history of ingestion and rapid bedside testing may be needed to confirm the diagnosis of exposure to oral hypoglycemic agents. Lactic acidosis from biguanide use should be suspected in patients presenting with lethargy, vomiting, diarrhea, and an elevated anion gap metabolic acidosis. It can present 4 to 6 hours after ingestion.

MANAGEMENT

Treatment of hypoglycemia is presented in **Table 168-11**. Intravenous dextrose is the mainstay of therapy. Delay in treatment may result in profound sequelae, including death. The most common sequelae are neurologic, and the risk increases with prolonged hypoglycemia. Recurrent, severe hypoglycemia is associated with electroencephalographic changes and cognitive impairment, particularly in children, with reported IQ deficiencies of 6 points. The possibility of hypoglycemia must be considered in any patient with an onset of central nervous system dysfunction; intravenous dextrose can be administered empirically if bedside testing is unavailable.

TABLE 168-10 Oral Hypoglycemics

Class	Examples	Mechanism of Action	Comments
Sulfonylureas (first generation)	Acetohexamide Chlorpropamide Tolazamide Tolbutamide	Increased insulin release Bind to the sulfonylurea receptor and inhibit the pore-forming unit of the adenosine triphosphate-sensitive potassium channel, which ultimately causes insulin secretion from the beta cell	High risk for hypoglycemia Many drug interactions Exhibit ionic protein binding and are displaced by various drugs, including phenylbutazone, salicylates, sulfonamides, and warfarin
Sulfonylureas (second generation)	Glipizide Glyburide Glimepiride	See above	100 times more potent than first generation, although better safety profile Increased risk for hypoglycemia in patients with renal insufficiency Should be avoided in patients with severe liver disease
Biguanides	Metformin Phenformin (not available in the United States)	No increase in insulin release Inhibit lipolysis, which causes increased glucose uptake, decreased hepatic glucose production, decreased intestinal absorption of glucose, and increased insulin receptor binding	Lactic acidosis: metformin > phenformin Does not cause hypoglycemia when taken alone Should not be used in patients with congestive heart failure, metabolic acidosis, drug hypersensitivity, and renal impairment Use of iodinated radiographic contrast dyes can also precipitate metformin-associated lactic acidosis Avoid using with other drugs that affect creatinine clearance or compete with renal tubular secretion, including vancomycin, trimethoprim, triamterene, quinidine, quinine, morphine, digoxin, amiloride, ranitidine, cimetidine, nifedipine, furosemide, nonsteroidal anti-inflammatory drugs, and loop diuretics
α-Glucosidase inhibitors	Acarbose Miglitol Voglibose	No increase in insulin release Reversible competitive inhibition of α-glucosidase on the brush border of the small bowel, delayed carbohydrate absorption, and lower postprandial glucose and insulin concentrations	Does not cause hypoglycemia when taken alone Effects by concomitant administration of intestinal-absorbing agents (charcoal) or carbohydrate-splitting enzymes (amylase, pancreatin) Flatulence, borborygmi, abdominal pain, and diarrhea are the most common side effects Transaminitis and decreased serum iron also reported
Gliptins	Linagliptin Sitagliptin Saxagliptin Vidagliptin	Increase insulin release in a glucose dependent manner Block dipeptidyl peptidase 4 (DPP-4), causing increase of glucagon-like peptide 1 (GLP-1), which is active in stimulating insulin release in presence of glucose load Delay gastric emptying	Unlikely to cause hypoglycemia in mild to moderate overdose Hypoglycemia can occur in very large overdoses and when ingested with other anti-diabetic agents
Incretin mimics	Exenatide	Increase insulin release in a glucose-dependent manner Glucagon-like peptide 1 (GLP-1) receptor agonist, which stimulates insulin release in presence of glucose load Delay gastric emptying	No hypoglycemia seen in limited number of case reports of overdose Nausea and vomiting common with therapeutic use
Thiazolidinediones	Troglitazone Rosiglitazone	Increase sensitivity to insulin Bind to nuclear peroxisome proliferator-activated receptors involved in the transcription of insulin-responsive genes and in the regulation of adipocyte differentiation and lipid metabolism	Hepatotoxicity Hypoglycemia can occur with repaglinide, although less frequently than with sulfonylureas No significant drug interactions have been reported; however, concomitant use of other agents that affect the CYP3A4 system should be done with caution
Meglitinides	Mitiglinide Repaglinide Nateglinide	Bind to nuclear peroxisome proliferator-activated receptors involved in the transcription of insulin-responsive genes and in the regulation of adipocyte differentiation and lipid metabolism	Hypoglycemia can occur with repaglinide, although less frequently than with sulfonylureas No significant drug interactions have been reported; however, concomitant use of other agents that affect the CYP3A4 system should be done with caution
Sodium-glucose cotransporter-2 (SGLT2) inhibitors/ Gliflozins	Canagliflozin Dapagliflozin	Reduces renal tubular glucose reabsorption, leading to glucosuria	Unlikely to cause hypoglycemia Ketoacidosis Bone fractures

*Withdrawn from the US market because of severe hepatotoxicity.

Octreotide is considered the first-line agent to suppress further insulin secretion. Prompt administration of octreotide to patients exposed to sulfonylureas leads to fewer dextrose boluses and fewer episodes of hypoglycemia. Octreotide should be administered intravenously or subcutaneously every 6 hours until hypoglycemia resolves.

Other metabolic abnormalities such as lactic acidosis may also need to be corrected. Sodium bicarbonate should be administered in severe metabolic acidosis. Hemodialysis may be necessary if the acidosis is refractory. Thiamine, 100 mg, should be administered to adults receiving glucose to prevent Wernicke encephalopathy.

ADMISSION AND DISCHARGE CRITERIA

A patient who ingests an oral hypoglycemic agent should be admitted if (i) hypoglycemia develops, (ii) it is an intentional overdose, or (iii) the patient is a child, even in the absence of hypoglycemia. While the

TABLE 168-11 Treatment of Hypoglycemia

Treatment	Mechanism of Action	Dose
Dextrose	Raises serum glucose	*Neonate*: 200 mg/kg (2 mL/kg of D10 by IV bolus) *Child*: 0.5 g/kg (2 mL/kg of D25 by IV bolus) *Adult*: 25 g (50 mL of D50 by IV bolus) Continuous infusion of D5, D10, or D20 can be used, but may contribute to fluctuating serum glucose levels due to stimulation of insulin release Bolus dosing of dextrose is preferred if needed for significant hypoglycemia
Octreotide	Inhibits insulin release from pancreatic beta cells	*Adult*: 50-100 µg q12h SC (preferred), IV *Child*: 1-1.5 µg/kg q6h SC (preferred), IV

D10, 10% dextrose; SC, subcutaneous; IV, intravenous.

absence of hypoglycemia within the first 8 hours of ingestion may be predictive of a benign outcome, multiple studies of sulfonylurea ingestion in children have shown that hypoglycemia can occur as late as 16 hours after ingestion. Ingestion of sulfonylureas can be life-threatening due to the ability to produce severe hypoglycemia, even with a single tablet. Because of the long half-life and duration of action of these drugs, clinicians should have a low threshold for admitting a patient with a suspected sulfonylurea exposure. Even though the non-sulfonylurea oral agents do not generally cause hypoglycemia, after an overdose, patients in whom hypoglycemia develops from these agents should be admitted. Patients who present with lactic acidosis secondary to biguanide ingestion should also be admitted.

If euglycemia is achieved in the emergency department and the patient is asymptomatic, the patient can be admitted to a general medical unit with the capability of frequent glucose monitoring. Patients with metabolic acidosis, continued neurologic symptoms/signs, or continued episodes of hypoglycemia despite treatment should be admitted to an intensive care setting.

Patients with suspected or evident sulfonylurea poisoning may be considered safe for discharge if they can tolerate a normal overnight fast without hypoglycemia. Children with biguanide-induced acidosis may be discharged once the acidosis has resolved.

CONSULTATION

Consultation with a medical toxicologist or regional Poison Control Center is recommended for all ingestions. The national toll-free and confidential number is 1-800-222-1222. Psychiatry consultation is indicated for any intentional overdose intended for self-harm.

Social Work consultation may be helpful in assessing the safety of the home, as well as strategizing with families to prevent recurrence of unintentional ingestions.

PREVENTION

Most ingestions in younger children are unintentional. Occasionally, childhood poisonings are the result of intended harmful behaviors by caregivers. Ingestions in teens are frequently intentional and may involve larger doses and higher risk of significant toxicity. Prevention is highly effective in reducing exposures and unintentional ingestions in small children. In all cases, parents, grandparents, guardians, and/or caregivers should be counseled about keeping medications "up and away" and in locked containers. Additional anticipatory guidance should include methods for safe disposal of prescription drugs that are no longer in use. One option includes the Drug Enforcement Administration's (DEA) National Prescription Drug Take Back Day which occurs twice a year across the United States and provides local drop-off locations for unwanted prescription drugs.

KEY POINTS

- Common over-the-counter medications account for nearly 20% of all toxic exposures in children younger than 6 years.
- Early consultation with a medical toxicologist or regional Poison Control Center is recommended for all poisonings.
- Iron chelation with intravenous deferoxamine remains the mainstay of treatment following whole bowel irrigation.
- Physostigmine should be considered both for diagnosis and symptom management of an antihistamine overdose, but the benefits must outweigh the potential risks, which include worsening of cardiac conduction delays, bradyarrhythmias, and asystole.
- Use of NAC for the treatment of acetaminophen toxicity is based on the clinical scenario and serum acetaminophen levels as guided by the Rumack-Matthew nomogram.
- Treatment of salicylate toxicity focuses on gastrointestinal decontamination and correction of fluid, electrolyte, and acid-base disturbances. Activated charcoal, urinary alkalinization, and hemodialysis may be considered.
- Children may have a prolonged risk for hypoglycemia after exposure to any amount of oral hypoglycemic, thus hospitalization and close monitoring of blood glucose and treatment with IV dextrose as needed are usually warranted.

SUGGESTED READINGS

Arens AM, Shah K, Al-Abri S, Olson KR, Kearney T. Safety and effectiveness of physostigmine: a 10-year retrospective review. *Clin Toxicol (Phila)*. 2018;56(2):101-107.

Chan TP, Rangan C. Iron poisoning: a literature based review of epidemiology, diagnosis, and management. *Pediatr Emerg Care*. 2011;27:978-985.

Chyka PA, Butler AY, Holley JE. Serum iron concentrations and symptoms of acute iron poisoning in children. *Pharmacotherapy*. 1996;16:1053-1058.

Dargan PI, Wallace CI, Jones AL. An evidence based flowchart to guide the management of acute salicylate (aspirin) overdose. *Emerg Med J*. 2002;19(3):206-209.

Glatstein M, Scolnik D, Bentur Y. Octreotide for the treatment of sulfonylurea poisoning. *Clin Toxicol (Philadelphia)*. 2012;50:795-804.

Lung DD, Olson KR. Hypoglycemia in pediatric sulfonylurea poisoning: an 8-year poison center retrospective study. *Pediatrics*. 2011;127:1558-1564.

Macarol V, Yawalkar SJ. Desferoxamine in acute iron poisoning. *Lancet*. 1992;339:1601.

Smilkstein MJ, Bronstein AC, Linden C, et al. Acetaminophen overdose: a 48-hour intravenous *N*-acetylcysteine treatment protocol. *Ann Emerg Med*. 1991;20:1058.

Thanacoody R, Caravati EM, Troutman B, et al. Position paper update: whole bowel irrigation for gastrointestinal decontamination of overdose patients. *Clin Toxicol (Phila)*. 2015;53(1):5-12.

Verdu E, Blanc-Brisset I, Meyer G, Le Roux G, Bruneau C, Deguigne M. Second-generation antihistamines: a study of poisoning in children. *Clin Toxicol (Phila)*. 2020;58(4):275-283.

Williamson K, Wahl MS, Mycyk MB. Direct comparison of 20-hour IV, 36-hour oral, and 72-hour oral acetylcysteine for treatment of acute acetaminophen poisoning. *Am J Ther*. 2013;20:37-40.

CHAPTER 169

Hazardous Household Chemicals: Hydrocarbons, Alcohols, and Caustics

Kirstin Weerdenburg, MD, FRCPC
and Yaron Finkelstein, MD, FACMT

BACKGROUND

Young children are frequently poisoned by visually appealing and readily available agents. The combination of curiosity, desire to mimic parental behavior (such as drinking from a bottle or can), newly acquired developmental milestones, and access to household products make children younger than 6 years particularly vulnerable to harm. In the United States, household cleaning substances represent the second most common poisoning exposure in young children.

Household chemicals highly likely to cause harm fall into three main categories: hydrocarbons, toxic alcohols, and caustics. Ingestion is the most common route of exposure in children seeking medical attention for poisoning from such agents. **Table 169-1** lists some common products and their potentially toxic components. Of note, the introduction of laundry detergent and dishwasher packets, commonly called "pods" or "capsules," into the North American market led to a surge of pediatric exposures, due in large part to their visually appealing packaging. Typically categorized as an alkaline caustic, the nature of their toxicity is not necessarily related to a single specific toxic substance, but rather to a variety of substances concentrated in a small and easy to consume form.

HYDROCARBONS

Hydrocarbon compounds include petroleum distillates (lighter fluid, kerosene, mineral oil, naphtha, gasoline, butane); plant extract oils, also referred to as terpenes (turpentine, lamp oil, menthol, eucalyptus oil); camphor; inhalants (toluene, chlorofluorocarbons); and organic solvents (toluene, xylene, benzene). Hydrocarbon ingestions are most often accidental and occur more often in males and younger (age 1-2 years) toddlers.

TABLE 169-1 Contents of Common Household Products

Product	Contents	Category
Toilet bowl and porcelain cleaners	Sulfuric, hydrochloric acid	Caustic/corrosive, acid
Drain/pipe cleaners/ openers	Sodium, potassium hydroxide	Caustic/corrosive, alkali
Detergent/laundry pods/ packets	Variety of ingredients	Caustic/corrosive, alkali
Lighter fluid (naphtha), gasoline, kerosene, butane	Petroleum distillates	Hydrocarbons
Pine oil, lamp oil, potpourri oil	Terpenes (plant extracts)	Hydrocarbons
Mouthwash	Ethanol	Alcohols
Sterno fuel, windshield wiper fluid	Methanol	Alcohols
Antifreeze	Ethylene glycol	Alcohols
Rubbing alcohol	Isopropyl alcohol	Alcohols
Airplane glue, inhalants	Toluene, xylene	Aromatic/halogenated hydrocarbons
Hair relaxer crème	Sodium hydroxide	Caustic/corrosive, alkali
"No-lye" hair relaxer crème	Calcium hydroxide	Caustic/corrosive, alkali
Mothballs	Camphor	Aromatic hydrocarbons

Kerosene ingestion is most common and often occurs due to inappropriate storage in drinking bottles or cups that children may access. Fortunately, calls to poison centers and rates of emergency department visits for hydrocarbon ingestions have decreased significantly, likely due to increased awareness and prevention efforts.

PATHOPHYSIOLOGY

After ingestion, hydrocarbon compounds enter the esophagus but also spread into the tracheobronchial tree; the lungs are the primary site of injury. The potential for a given compound to cause direct lung injury is influenced by its viscosity, surface tension, and volatility. Highly volatile liquids with low viscosity and surface tension have the highest potential for pulmonary injury. Highly viscous hydrocarbons (motor oil, paraffin) very seldom cause lung injury, whereas low-viscosity substances (gasoline, kerosene) readily enter the lungs causing injury. These chemicals can cause alveolar collapse and damage surfactant, which may lead to pneumonitis and in some cases progress to respiratory failure.

Other organ damage may result from a particular compound's inherent toxicity. **Table 169-2** offers a mnemonic, which lists the hydrocarbons and their specific systemic effects. For example, lipid-soluble hydrocarbons, such as terpenes and aromatics, can easily cross the blood-brain barrier causing central nervous system (CNS) depression. Importantly, inhalant abuse of organic solvents can cause sudden death syndrome, as they sensitize the myocardium to catecholamines. Chronic encephalopathy may also occur.

CLINICAL PRESENTATION

Children may be brought to medical attention for a witnessed or suspected ingestion, even if asymptomatic. More than half of patients present with at least one episode of vomiting and occasionally somnolence, but more often they are fully conscious. Patients with severe ingestion may have signs of chemical pneumonitis soon after ingestion, including dyspnea, tachypnea, hypoxemia, cough, wheezing, or increased work of breathing. The development of respiratory distress within the first hours after ingestion is very concerning as the child may quickly experience respiratory failure. Fever, which develops in about 50% of patients with chemical pneumonitis, reflects the inflammatory response to the noninfectious lung injury. An aroma of the hydrocarbon remaining on the skin, clothing, or breath may suggest ingestion or exposure. Some hydrocarbon compounds may irritate the mucosae (e.g., pharyngeal erythema).

DIAGNOSTIC EVALUATION

The respiratory status of a child after hydrocarbon ingestion or exposure is paramount. Assessment of respiratory rate, work of breathing, pulse oximetry, and lung auscultation should be performed promptly and repeated frequently. Breath sounds may be normal or decreased, with wheezing, rales, or rhonchi. Patients with abnormal breath sounds on admission, correlating with pneumonitis, often have longer hospital stays. Clinical factors associated with requiring a higher level of care include wheezing, altered level of consciousness, or a rapid respiratory rate for age within 2 hours of exposure.

A chest radiograph should be performed on initial assessment and repeated if the child clinically deteriorates or as part of a reassessment

TABLE 169-2 "CHAMP" Mnemonic for Hydrocarbons With Systemic Toxicity

C: *Camphor*	Seizures, CNS depression
H: *Halogenated* compounds (carbon tetrachloride, chloral hydrate)	Hepatic necrosis, arrhythmias
A: *Aromatic* compounds (benzene, toluene)	CNS depression, arrhythmias, white matter degeneration
M: Hydrocarbons that contain heavy *metals*	Heavy metal poisoning (multisystem)
P: Hydrocarbons as vehicles for *pesticides*, other toxic compounds	Organophosphate, other compound poisoning

CNS, Central nervous system.

(e.g., consideration for admission or discharge). Patients with abnormal chest radiographs usually require hospitalization and have longer hospital stays. Elevated white blood count (WBC) and neutrophil count may be seen in patients with significant pneumonitis. Such leukocytosis early after ingestion reflects the noninfectious inflammation associated with lung injury.

Further evaluation may be indicated, depending on the toxicities of the substance involved (see Table 169-2). For example, serum transaminase levels should be considered for patients exposed to halogenated compounds.

MANAGEMENT

The mainstay of treatment for these patients involves supportive care with careful monitoring of respiratory status with respiratory support, as indicated, and treatment of other concomitant organ dysfunctions if present.

Gastric lavage or inducing emesis should be avoided, as this can further increase the risk of aspiration. Corticosteroids do not improve the course of hydrocarbon pneumonitis and can increase the risk for secondary bacterial infection. Antibiotics for pneumonitis have also failed to show benefit and may increase the risk of infection with resistant organisms; antibiotics are only indicated for patients in whom fever and leukocytosis persist and secondary bacterial infection is likely. Endotracheal intubation and ventilation or extracorporeal membrane oxygenation may be needed if significant lung injury develops. Exogenous surfactant administered early during acute respiratory failure may improve the patient's course and should be considered.

CONSULTATION

- Critical care specialists should be consulted in patients who are deteriorating and when there is an anticipated need for increasing respiratory support or level of monitoring.
- Consultation with a regional poison control center is appropriate, especially for children with severe or atypical symptoms or with a highly toxic substance.
- Social services consultation may be indicated if the circumstances surrounding the ingestion raise suspicion of abuse or neglect.

ADMISSION CRITERIA

- Patients with respiratory symptoms should be admitted for monitoring and support. Those who remain asymptomatic for 6 to 8 hours after exposure may be candidates for outpatient follow-up with reliable parental supervision.

DISCHARGE CRITERIA

- Patients whose respiratory symptoms have resolved have no further risk from hydrocarbon pneumonitis and can be discharged.

ALCOHOLS

The term "toxic alcohols" refers to different short-chain alcohols that, when ingested, cause adverse effects related to their metabolites. The metabolites can lead to metabolic acidosis and/or specific end-organ damage. The major compounds involved in pediatric alcohol exposures include ethylene glycol, methanol, isopropanol, and ethanol. Ethylene glycol has a sweet taste and is found in antifreeze. Methanol is primarily found in windshield washer fluid and chafing fuel. Isopropanol is the active ingredient in rubbing alcohol. Ethanol is readily available for adult consumption in many households and in toiletries such as mouthwash and antibacterial soap.

PATHOPHYSIOLOGY

These alcohols are metabolized by the enzyme alcohol dehydrogenase. They act on the CNS to cause intoxication, CNS depression, and hypothermia. While the mechanism of hypothermia is complex and not entirely elucidated, it is believed to stem from the depth of CNS depression and resultant loss of behavioral responses to cold.

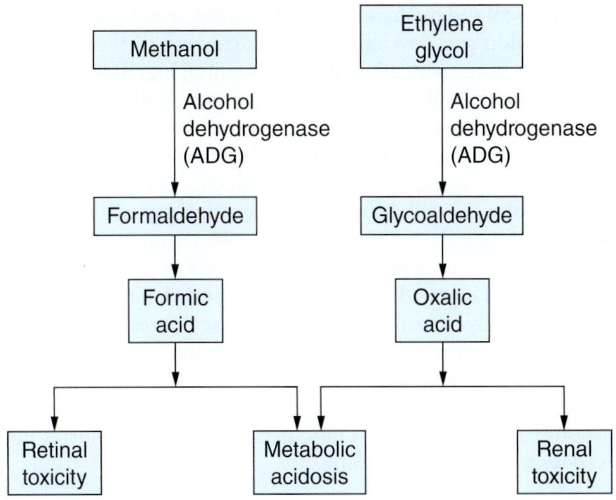

FIGURE 169-1. Methanol and ethylene glycol metabolism. Both methanol and ethylene glycol undergo transformation to toxic metabolites via the enzyme alcohol dehydrogenase (ADH). ADH is inhibited by ethanol and fomepizole therapy.

Ethylene glycol is metabolized to glycolic and oxalic acids, which cause profound acidosis and renal failure, partially because of oxalate crystalluria. In addition, oxalate forms complexes with calcium, which can lead to systemic hypocalcemia and its attendant complications (e.g., seizures, tetany, dysrhythmia). Methanol is metabolized to formic acid, which also causes severe metabolic acidosis, as well as retinal toxicity. **Figure 169-1** illustrates the metabolism and toxic metabolite effects of ethylene glycol and methanol. Isopropanol is metabolized to acetone, which causes ketonemia and ketonuria without acidosis, unlike other toxic alcohols; in addition, isopropanol irritates the gastrointestinal tract. In young children, ethanol metabolism suppresses gluconeogenesis and ingestion may cause hypoglycemia due to their reduced stores.

CLINICAL PRESENTATION

After any of these ingestions, patients may be intoxicated and have profound CNS depression and, in extreme cases, hypothermia. Alcohols are osmotically active and can lead to dehydration because of osmotic diuresis. Young children may become hypoglycemic 2 to 8 hours after alcohol ingestion and present with jitteriness, combativeness, obtundation, or seizures. Profound acidosis and metabolic derangements can lead to death.

Patients with ethylene glycol ingestions are at risk for anuria and renal failure. Those with ethylene glycol or methanol ingestions may initially appear intoxicated, accompanied by metabolic acidosis, and may develop organ failure within the next 24 hours. Children who ingest isopropanol can also become intoxicated and present with hematemesis, hemorrhagic gastritis, ketonuria, and a strong acetone odor from the mouth. Retinal injury secondary to the toxic metabolite of methanol can cause several visual abnormalities, including blurred vision, spots, and scotomas, a condition collectively described as "snowstorm" vision, which may progress to irreversible blindness.

DIAGNOSTIC EVALUATION

Alcohols are not part of routine urine toxicology screening due to their high volatility and evaporation. Serum levels of ethylene glycol, methanol, isopropanol, and ethanol should be obtained when poisoning is suspected; levels correspond well with toxicity. However, these tests are not readily available in all hospitals. Indirect evidence of their presence may be revealed through analysis of serum electrolytes, serum osmolality, and blood gas. Within an hour after ingestion, the presence of alcohols in serum may be detected by an elevated osmolar gap (difference between calculated serum osmolarity and measured serum osmolality).

As ethylene glycol and methanol are metabolized, metabolic acidosis with an elevated anion gap develops, with a narrowing of the osmolar gap, which does not occur with ethanol or isopropanol ingestions. Abnormalities in the osmolar and anion gap should appear within 12 hours after ingestion, so it is reassuring if derangements do not develop within this timeframe. A normal osmolar gap should be interpreted in the context of the anion gap and vice versa. As the toxic alcohol compound is metabolized, the osmolar gap will decrease and the anion gap will rise.

Additional testing should include urinalysis, serum creatinine, and an ophthalmologic exam, depending on the toxicities associated with the suspected alcohol ingested. Specifically, after ethylene glycol ingestion, oxalate crystals may be visible in urine. Because fluorescein is often used as an additive to antifreeze, Wood lamp examination of the urine can demonstrate fluorescence as a sign of ethylene glycol ingestion; however, it absence cannot rule out ethylene glycol ingestion. Ketonuria occurs with isopropanol metabolism. Optic nerve and retinal injuries may be observed with methanol poisoning.

MANAGEMENT

These patients require close observation and supportive care, along with careful blood glucose levels monitoring in young children, because of their increased risk of hypoglycemia. Although ethanol and isopropanol ingestions are associated with fewer complications, clinicians should closely monitor the patient's consciousness and respiratory status.

The antidotal treatment with either fomepizole or ethanol reduces the formation of toxic metabolites by inhibiting the action of alcohol dehydrogenase on the toxic alcohols until a more definitive treatment (e.g., hemodialysis) is available. Ethanol or fomepizole (4-methylpyrazole [4-MP]) compete with toxic alcohols in binding to alcohol dehydrogenase. Ethanol infusions (commonly 10% ethanol) are intoxicating and warrant frequent monitoring of CNS status, blood glucose, and ethanol levels (desired level 100 mg/dL), typically in the setting of a critical care unit. Fomepizole is superior to ethanol, if available, particularly in young children. Fomepizole does not cause obtundation or drowsiness, is easy to administer as a subcutaneous injection, which may be repeated, and the patient can be admitted to the pediatric ward. Fomepizole also has fewer adverse effects associated with its use, therefore, is safe and effective in children. In some children treated with fomepizole, hemodialysis may not be necessary despite metabolic acidosis. See **Table 169-3** for more details of ethanol and fomepizole therapy.

The use of ethanol or fomepizole slows the ongoing metabolism of alcohols to their toxic metabolites, but does not prevent further production, nor treat the toxic effects of metabolites already present. Several treatments may help prevent end-organ damage and reverse acidosis. Sodium bicarbonate therapy can treat acidosis and reduce further entry of toxic metabolites into target tissues. Pyridoxine (1 mg/kg intravenously, maximum of 100 mg, every 6 hours) and thiamine (50 mg intravenously every 8 hours) may help detoxify the acid metabolites of ethylene glycol, and folic acid (1 mg/kg intravenously, maximum of 50 mg, every 4 hours) may help detoxify metabolites of methanol. In children treated with fomepizole, these additional treatments may not be necessary.

Hemodialysis is highly effective in removing ethylene glycol, methanol, and their toxic metabolites. Hospitalists should consider hemodialysis when the serum ethylene glycol or methanol level is higher than 50 mg/dL, when there is evidence of end-organ damage, with a late presentation, refractory acidosis, or if there is a high osmolar gap without another cause. Some patients may require repeat hemodialysis for a significant ingestion. Many experts recommend that ethanol or fomepizole infusion accompany hemodialysis because the dialysis process is not instantaneous, and the residual toxic alcohol may still be metabolized.

TABLE 169-3 Antidotes for Toxic Alcohol Ingestion

Agent	Dosage/Administration	Comment
Ethanol	10% solution for IV use	Side effects: obtundation, hyperosmolarity, hypothermia, hypoglycemia
	Loading dose: 0.8 g/kg	
	Maintenance: 80-130 mg/kg/hr	Commonly requires intensive care unit admission
	Target level: 100 mg/dL	Frequent monitoring of levels
		May necessitate central venous access
Fomepizole (4-methylpyrazole)	Loading dose: 15 mg/kg IV over 15-min period	Fewer side effects and monitoring than ethanol
		Less availability
	Maintenance: 10 mg/kg q12h	Administer q 4 h during dialysis
	Increase to 15 mg/kg after 4 doses	Can be admitted to ward

CONSULTATION

- Consultation with a regional poison control center can aid with diagnosis and management decisions.
- Ophthalmology should be consulted in cases of methanol poisoning.
- Nephrology should be consulted if there is a history of ingestion of a toxic alcohol, particularly if hemodialysis is considered.
- Social services should be considered if circumstances surrounding the ingestion raise suspicion of abuse or neglect.

ADMISSION CRITERIA

- Patients with suspected ingestion of a toxic alcohol should be admitted unless they have undetectable alcohols in the blood or, if those tests are not available, the anion and osmolar gaps remain normal on serial measurements. Patients who exhibit CNS depression should be admitted regardless of acid-base status.
- Observe or admit all intoxicated children until the intoxication resolves.

DISCHARGE CRITERIA

- Patients may be discharged once the intoxication resolves, levels of toxic alcohols are undetectable, and end-organ toxicity recovers.

CAUSTICS

Caustic substances are found in many household products (see Table 169-1), including drain and oven cleaners, porcelain cleaners, and some detergents, including those in the packet form ("pods" or "capsules"). Of note, ammonia and bleach packaged for household use are significantly less concentrated than many commercial preparations and are, therefore, associated with a lower risk of injury.

The Federal Poison Prevention Packaging Act of 1970 mandates that alkaline caustics greater than 2% in concentration and other caustics greater than 10% in concentration be sold in child-resistant containers. As a result, the number of serious pediatric caustic injuries has greatly decreased. However, children are involved in most caustic ingestions in the United States, typically due to exploratory behaviors. Severe injuries in children occur, often with industrial-strength chemicals or products inappropriately stored in non-child-resistant containers.

PATHOPHYSIOLOGY

The degree of caustic injury depends on the properties of the substance (e.g., pH, concentration, ability to penetrate tissues); the nature of the exposure (e.g., eye splash, ingestion) including the volume and duration of contact; and the timeliness of initiating appropriate therapy. Severe or fatal caustic injuries are more likely to occur with a substance with pH of 0 to 2 or 12 to 14, and in the context of large-volume or intentional ingestions.

The two types of caustic ingestions are distinct in their pathophysiology. Bases (alkali) lead to liquefactive tissue necrosis, whereas acids lead to coagulation necrosis. Liquefactive necrosis causes tissue to dissolve quicker and infiltrates deeper than coagulative necrosis. In contrast, coagulation necrosis causes damage to superficial proteins, resulting in an eschar, which may prevent deeper penetration and tissue injury. Some hypothesize that acid ingestions are associated with greater morbidity and mortality than alkali ingestions, however significant tissue damage can occur with both.

Aside from injury from direct contact with the caustic agent, some compounds cause additional toxicity through systemic absorption of components. For example, acids may be absorbed and cause metabolic acidosis, and zinc and mercuric chloride ($ZnCl_2$, $HgCl_2$) may be associated with heavy metal toxicity.

The most common targets of caustic injury ingestion are the airways, esophagus, and upper gastrointestinal tract. Although acid and alkali substances produce different histopathologic patterns of injury, the clinical picture is often similar. On ingestion, the liquid traveling down the gastrointestinal tract encounters esophageal epithelium and causes damage ranging from edema and erythema to necrosis and perforation. Fluid reaching the stomach may also cause burns of varying degrees to the gastric mucosa, including perforation.

CLINICAL PRESENTATION

Since tissue damage from caustic ingestion manifests immediately, patients generally become symptomatic quickly. Signs and symptoms of esophageal injury predominate; early symptoms may include oropharyngeal, retrosternal, or epigastric pain, hoarseness, stridor, dysphagia, refusal to drink, hematemesis, drooling, and vomiting. It is important to note that the lack of visible injury to the cheeks, lips, and oropharynx does not rule out airway or gastrointestinal injury. In fact, one-third of children without visible injury have burns in visceral organs. Airway injury or impending collapse may cause stridor, respiratory distress, cough, and wheezing. Patients with severe injuries may develop life-threatening complications, including respiratory distress, upper gastrointestinal tract bleeding, esophageal or gastric perforation, mediastinitis, and peritonitis. Such complications may not occur until 72 hours after the ingestion. A patient with overwhelming tissue damage may be hemodynamically unstable with metabolic acidosis. Severe chest pain and shortness of breath may be a sign of esophageal perforation and mediastinitis. Perforation of the stomach with resultant caustic peritonitis usually causes severe abdominal pain, rigid abdomen, acidosis, and hemodynamic instability. Gastrointestinal hemorrhage from direct vessel injury can present with hematemesis, melena, or shock.

Late sequelae, such as esophageal strictures and gastric outlet obstruction, may develop over weeks to months after ingestion. Strictures should be suspected in a patient in whom dysphagia or failure to thrive develops after caustic ingestion. Patients with high-grade injuries are also at increased risk of developing esophageal cancer.

DIAGNOSTIC EVALUATION

Esophagogastroduodenoscopy (EGD) of the upper gastrointestinal tract can delineate the location and degree of injury to the hypopharynx, esophagus, and stomach. To reduce the risk of perforation, EGD should be performed within 12 hours and preferably not later than 24 hours post-ingestion; the greatest risk of perforation is between 48 hours and 14 days post-ingestion. **Table 169-4** provides a list of indications for this diagnostic procedure. Previous studies of exploratory ingestions of caustics in children showed that asymptomatic patients can be safely observed and discharged without an EGD, however, the safety of this practice is currently debated. Studies have demonstrated that having two or more findings of vomiting, drooling, and stridor are highly predictive of a significant esophageal injury, with stridor being nearly 100% specific. The absence of these findings has a high negative predictive value. Additionally, the asymptomatic toddler who has ingested an unknown quantity of a caustic substance presents a particular challenge. Several studies have demonstrated that children without symptoms or signs after 6 hours of observation will have no significant injury and, therefore, do not warrant endoscopy. Notably, young children who ingest thick cream hair relaxer products may have isolated oral burns, but episodes of more extensive injury are uncommon.

TABLE 169-4 Indications for Endoscopy After Caustic Ingestion

History of large-volume, intentional or suicidal ingestion, especially highly caustic products (e.g., drain cleaner)
Any *symptoms*, including vomiting, dysphagia, hematemesis, chest or abdominal pain, drooling, refusal to drink
Any *signs*, including stridor, respiratory distress, oropharyngeal burns, abdominal tenderness, peritoneal signs
Further evaluation reveals acidosis, anemia, coagulopathy, or radiographs suggestive of perforation or mediastinitis

TABLE 169-5 Endoscopic Zargar Classification of Esophageal Injury and Prognosis

Class	Characteristics	Prognosis
0	Normal mucosa	Complete recovery
I	Edema, hyperemia	Complete recovery
IIa	Hemorrhage, erosions, blisters, superficial ulcers	Stricture unlikely
IIb	Circumferential lesions	High risk of stricture, low risk of perforation
IIIa	Focal deep ulcerations	High risk of stricture, increased risk of perforation
IIIb	Extensive deep ulcerations	High risk of stricture and perforation
IV	Perforation	Often fatal

Source: Adapted from Zargar SA, Kohhar R, Mehta S, et al. The role of fiberoptic endoscopy in the management of corrosive ingestion and modified endoscopic classification of burns. *Gastrointest Endosc.* 1991;37:165-169.

Burns are frequently classified based on the Zargar classification (**Table 169-5**), which defines them as grade 0 (no injury), I (edema and hyperemia of the mucosa), IIa (superficial ulcerations and friability involving less than 75% of the esophageal circumference), IIb (superficial ulcerations and friability, involving 75% or more of the esophageal circumference), or III (deep gray or black ulcer). The endoscopic classification is prognostically important, as grade 0, I, or IIa burns typically recover without long-term complications, while grade IIb or III burns are frequently associated with esophageal or gastric strictures and may require long-term interventions.

Radiographs of the chest may be useful if there is a concern for aspiration with chemical pneumonitis, esophageal perforation, or mediastinitis. Abdominal radiographs may reveal intraperitoneal free air in patients with distal esophageal or gastric perforation. Lateral neck films may be useful to evaluate the upper airway in cases in which stridor or respiratory distress is present and may demonstrate airway narrowing or epiglottic swelling.

Laboratory studies may be warranted in some situations. For patients at risk for systemic absorption of caustic agents or with concern for severe injury, a complete blood count (CBC), coagulation studies, electrolytes, and blood gas analysis should be performed. A blood type and crossmatch should be obtained for patients with hemorrhage or peritonitis or for those in need of surgical intervention. Surgical exploration is typically reserved for patients with abdominal pain, tachycardia, and worsening acidosis, or radiographic evidence of catastrophic visceral perforation or mediastinitis.

MANAGEMENT

On initial presentation for medical care after ingestion, patients may require resuscitation, including endotracheal intubation, if airway collapse is imminent. Gastrointestinal decontamination is not routinely indicated. Tissue injury will have already occurred on arrival, so introducing either activated charcoal or a lavage tube into a potentially damaged esophagus incurs risk. Dilution, a process by which patients drink milk or water to decrease the concentration of the caustic substance, also has little benefit beyond the first 1 to 2 minutes after ingestion.

Systemic corticosteroid therapy to prevent stricture formation is controversial but sometimes used. Theoretically, corticosteroids prevent the collagen cross-linking that takes place during healing and stricture formation. Whereas patients with type I burns uniformly do well and patients with type III injury nearly always form strictures, patients with type II burns may be good candidates for this therapy. Few studies have attempted to evaluate the efficacy of this treatment, but the data is contradictory, therefore, there are no definitive recommendations. When used, most clinicians administer either methylprednisolone (2 mg/kg/day) or dexamethasone (1 mg/kg/day), for patients with circumferential type II esophageal burns. Antibiotics and H2-blockers are often given concurrently.

Consultation with specialists, usually a gastroenterologist, otolaryngologist, and/or a general surgeon, is recommended to aid in decisions, such as when to institute oral feeding and whether nasogastric tube placement is indicated. In general, patients with mild (type I, IIa) burns can be started slowly on a liquid diet as soon as tolerated, while in those with more advanced burns (IIb, III), the risk of perforation may require longer periods of restricted oral intake.

Swallowing difficulty, gastric outlet obstruction, or dysmotility may develop in patients with strictures, most often in the weeks to months after the ingestion. Alternative enteral feeding regimens may be needed and can include nasogastric, gastrostomy, or transpyloric feeding. Patients with severely narrowed or obstructing segments may require esophageal dilation or surgical resection of strictures. Those with significant esophageal injury require lifelong surveillance due to the increased risk of esophageal carcinoma.

CONSULTATION

- Gastroenterologists are often involved in assessing symptomatic children. They should continue to manage the care of children with mucosal injury, feeding difficulties, or gastrointestinal bleeding.
- Surgeons should be consulted early in children at risk for perforation, mediastinitis, or peritonitis. Further in the clinical course, surgical services may be needed to place gastrostomy feeding tubes or to evaluate strictures that may need resection.
- Critical care physicians should be consulted for patients with hemodynamic instability and those in need of airway management. Patients with injury to the upper or lower airways may warrant input from otolaryngology or pulmonology.
- Social services should be contacted if circumstances surrounding the ingestion raise suspicion of abuse or neglect.

ADMISSION CRITERIA

- Any patient with symptoms or abnormal physical examination findings after caustic ingestion.
- Any patient with a large-volume or intentional ingestion.
- Observation and discharge may be considered for an asymptomatic child after insignificant ingestion or for a patient with cream hair relaxer exposure with oral burns only. However, such management is advisable only with close follow-up and reliable caregivers.

DISCHARGE CRITERIA

- Patients may be discharged when asymptomatic and able to tolerate oral feeding. For patients unable to feed orally, alternative enteral nutritional therapy must be established.
- Appropriate outpatient follow-up is needed for ongoing evaluation of known complications, most commonly stricture formation.

PREVENTION

The advances in preventive legislation have already made a significant impact on household poisonings in the United States; however, exposures still occur and are largely preventable. Education by healthcare providers regarding the safe storage of household chemicals, both out of reach and out of attractive non-child-resistant containers, is still needed. Caregiver awareness of the national poison control centers system can be lifesaving, so each household should have contact information readily available.

KEY POINTS

- The risk for injury secondary to hydrocarbon ingestion is related to the nature of the substance (e.g., volatility, viscosity, surface tension).
- Aspirated hydrocarbons with high volatility, low viscosity, and low surface tension (e.g., gasoline, kerosene) can cause pneumonitis.
- After hydrocarbon ingestion, symptomatic patients should be monitored closely and have a chest radiograph performed.
- Toxic alcohol ingestions may be challenging to diagnose, therefore, the anion gap and osmolar gap should be calculated in intoxicated patients, as they help raise the suspicion of toxic alcohol ingestion.
- Ethylene glycol and methanol ingestions may be life threatening, and treatment includes inhibition of alcohol dehydrogenase with fomepizole (or ethanol), and potentially hemodialysis.
- Caustic ingestion may cause acute life-threatening injuries, including airway damage, gastrointestinal hemorrhage, and esophageal or gastric perforation with mediastinitis or peritonitis.
- Endoscopy, preferably within 12 hours and no later than 24 hours after caustic ingestion can delineate the location and severity of the injury.
- Children who remain asymptomatic for 6 hours after caustic ingestion are at low risk for injury and may be discharged without endoscopy and close observation.

SUGGESTED READINGS

Betalli P, Falchetti D, Giuliani S, et al. Caustic ingestion in children: is endoscopy always indicated? The results of an Italian multicenter observational study. *Gastrointest Endosc.* 2008;68(3):434-439.

Brent J. Fomepizole for the treatment of pediatric ethylene and diethylene glycol, butoxyethanol, and methanol poisonings. *Clin Toxicol (Phila).* 2010;48(5):401-406.

Cheng HT, Cheng CL, Lin CH, et al. Caustic ingestion in adults: the role of endoscopic classification in predicting outcome. *BMC Gastroenterol.* 2008;8:31.

Chirica M, Bonavina L, Kelly MD, et al. Caustic ingestion. *Lancet.* 2017;389:2041-2052.

Das S, Behera SK, Xavier AS, et al. Prophylactic use of steroids and antibiotics in acute hydrocarbon poisoning in children. *J Pharm Pract.* 2020;33(1):90-95.

Davis MG, Casavant MJ, Spiller HA. Pediatric exposures to laundry and dishwasher detergents in the United States: 2013-2014. *Pediatrics.* 2016:137(5):e20154529.

Fremont D, Berleur MP, Megarbane B. Loading dose of fomepizole is safe in children with presumed toxic alcohol exposure—a case series. *Basic Clin Pharmacol Toxicol.* 2014;115(3):229-230.

Gummin D, Mowry JB, Beuhler DA, et al. 2020 Annual Report of the American Association of Poison Control Centers; National Poison Data System (NPDS): 38th Annual Report. *Clin Toxicol.* 2021;59(12):1282-1501.

Gupta SK, Croffie JM, Fitgerald JF. Is esophagogastraduodenoscopy necessary in all caustic ingestions? *J Pediatr Gastroenterol Nutr.* 2001;32(1):50-53.

Hoffman RS, Burns MM, Gosselin S. Ingestion of caustic substances. *N Engl J Med.* 2020;382:1739-1748.

Jolliff HA, Fletcher E, Robert KJ, et al. Pediatric hydrocarbon-related injuries in the United States: 2000-2009. *Pediatrics.* 2013;131(6):1139-1147.

Lamireau T, Rebouissoux L, Denis D, et al. Accidental caustic ingestion in children: is endoscopy always mandatory? *J Pediatr Gastroenterol Nutr.* 2001;33(1):81-84.

Lepik KJ, Levy AR, Sobolev BG, et al. Adverse drug events associated with the antidotes for methanol and ethylene glycol poisoning: a comparison of ethanol and fomepizole. *Ann Emerg Med*. 2009;53(4):439-450.e410.

Makrygianni EA, Palamidou F, Kaditis AG. Respiratory complications following hydrocarbon aspiration in children. *Pediatr Pulmonol*. 2016;51(6):560-569.

Ngobese A, Govender S, Peer N, et al. Caustic ingestion in children treated at a tertiary centre in South Africa: can upper endoscopy be omitted in asymptomatic patients? *Pediatr Surg Int*. 2022;38(3):505-512.

Pelclová D, Navrátil T. Do corticosteroids prevent oesophageal stricture after corrosive ingestion? *Toxicol Rev*. 2005;24(2):125-129.

Poley JW, Steyerberg EW, Kuipers EJ, et al. Ingestion of acid and alkaline agents: outcome and prognostic value of early endoscopy. *Gastrointest Endosc*. 2004;60(3):372-377.

Rayar P, Ratnapalan S. Pediatric ingestions of household products containing ethanol: a review. *Clin Pediatr (Phila)*. 2013;52(3):203-209.

Ross JA, Borek HA, Holstege CP, et al. Toxic Alcohol Poisoning. *Emerg Med Clin North Am*. 2022;40(2):327-341.

Sen V, Kelekci S, Selimoglu Sen H, et al. An evaluation of cases of pneumonia that occurred secondary to hydrocarbon exposure in children. *Eur Rev Med Pharmacol Sci*. 2013;17 Suppl 1;9-12.

Sommer C, Johnson AB, Sam Wang G, et al. Surfactant for the management of pediatric hydrocarbon ingestion. *Am J Emerg Med*. 2018;36(12):2260-2262.

Tenenbaum A, Rephaeli R, Cohen-Cymberknoh M, et al. Hydrocarbon intoxication in children: clinical and sociodemographic characteristics. *Pediatr Emerg Care*. 2021;37(10):502-506.

Tormoehlen LM, Tekulve KJ, Nanaga KA. Hydrocarbon toxicity: a review. *Clin Toxicol (Phila)*. 2014;52(5):479-489.

Usta, M, Erkan T, et al. High doses of methylprednisolone in the management of accidental caustic esophageal burns in children. *J Pediatr Gastroenterol Nutr*. 2009;48:E49.

WHO EMRA Pediatric Hydrocarbon Study Group, Cairo, Egypt, Bond GR, Pieche S, Sonicki Z, et al. A clinical decision rule for triage of children under 5 years of age with hydrocarbon (kerosene) aspiration in developing countries. *Clin Toxicol (Phila)*. 2008;46(3):222-229.

Zargar SA, Kohhar R, Mehta S, et al. The role of fiberoptic endoscopy in the management of corrosive ingestion and modified endoscopic classification of burns. *Gastrointest Endosc*. 1991;37:165-169.

CHAPTER 170 Lead, Other Metals, and Chelation Therapy

Joseph D. Lynch, MD, FAAP, CHSE

LEAD

BACKGROUND

Lead is a highly toxic metal, which can produce a wide range of adverse health effects in children. It is soft and pliable and when ingested, has a sweet taste. Lead is a ubiquitous environmental containment found in water and soil. The most common cause of childhood lead poisoning is ingestion of lead-containing paint chips or lead-contaminated dust from normal hand-to-mouth activity. Until 1978, lead was commonly used in paints to provide pigment and color stability. According to the Centers for Disease Control and Prevention (CDC), 29 million housing units in the United States still contain significant lead-based paint hazards. Although intact lead paint does not pose an immediate concern, lead paint that is deteriorating or disturbed during repair or renovation activities creates a hazard. Other potential sources include water contaminated from lead pipes and soil contaminated by gasoline emissions. The Natural Resources Defense Council conducted a study between 2018 and 2020 that found multiple cities had high levels of lead in their tap water including: Baltimore, Chicago, Detroit, Milwaukee, Newark, New York, Pittsburgh, and Washington D.C. Exposure to elevated maternal lead levels in utero or while breastfeeding, parental occupational exposure, and contaminated food sources, also place children at risk for lead poisoning.

Accumulating evidence indicates lead poisoning is harmful at blood levels that were once thought safe. Sustained exposure can result in learning disabilities in children with lead levels as low as 5 μg/dL (0.24 μmol/L); there is no evidence of a safe lead level to avoid these effects. As of 2021, the CDC uses a blood lead reference value of 3.5 μg/dL (0.17 μmol/L) to identify children with lead toxicity. This value represents the 97.5th percentile of children in the United States aged 1 to 5 years from 2015 to 2016 and 2017 to 2018 National Health and Nutrition Examination Survey cycles. Children from low-income households, those who were born outside of the United States, and those living in housing built before 1978 more commonly have higher blood lead levels. Racial and social inequities in housing because of interpersonal, structural, and institutional racism, influence children's exposure to lead paint and contaminated plumbing.

TOXICOKINETICS

Ingested lead is subsequently absorbed by the gut. Children are more likely than adults to demonstrate hand-to-mouth and other behaviors that result in lead ingestion, and they absorb lead much more readily than adults. Effectiveness of lead absorption from the gut depends on age, recent food intake, and the makeup of the individual's diet. Recent food intake can decrease the uptake of water-soluble lead, as can younger age. Once absorbed, 99% of lead binds to erythrocytes, and the remaining 1% is free to diffuse into soft tissues and bone, where it equilibrates with blood lead. In the body, the total lead burden can be divided into four compartments: blood (half-life 35 days), soft tissue (half-life 40 days), trabecular bone (half-life 3 to 4 years), and cortical bone (half-life 16 to 20 years). Lead that is deposited in hair, teeth, nails, and bones is tightly bound and generally not harmful. However, as lead from bone deposition can redeposit in previously cleared blood, fetal exposure to resorbed maternal lead deposits is possible during skeletal construction.

Lead affects the heme synthetic pathway by inhibiting δ-aminolevulinic acid dehydrase and ferrochelatase (heme synthetase). As a result, δ-aminolevulinic acid cannot be converted into porphobilinogen. This prevents iron from being incorporated into the protoporphyrin ring, which is the final intermediate in the heme biosynthetic pathway. The heme precursor erythrocyte protoporphyrin (EP), commonly assayed as zinc protoporphyrin (ZPP; zinc substitutes for iron in the porphyrin moiety), increases, and heme synthesis is subsequently reduced.

Lead can negatively affect the release and/or transmission of neurotransmitters. This negatively affects developing nervous systems and may be one of the underlying causes of cognitive and behavioral problems seen in lead-poisoned children. The biologic dysfunction produced by lead appears to be associated with the metal's ability to mimic or inhibit the action of calcium, and to bind sulfhydryl ligands. Lead's ability to mimic or inhibit calcium during normal action potentials can block the release of neurotransmitters. Lead diminishes calcium entry into neurons and/or negates its effects. The binding of sulfhydryl ligands may alter enzyme activity, or protein receptor shape, negatively affecting neurotransmission.

CLINICAL PRESENTATION

Children are often asymptomatic at diagnosis of lead toxicity, highlighting the importance of routine screening. Changes in behavior or neurologic status can be the earliest manifestation of lead intoxication. The clinical presentation of lead poisoning varies widely, depending on blood lead level (BLL), age at exposure, and amount and duration of exposure. Children presenting with possible lead poisoning should be assessed for correlates of exposure and recognizable sequelae. These sequelae can include gastrointestinal complaints such as colicky pain, constipation, anorexia, and intermittent vomiting. Signs and symptoms suggestive of central nervous system (CNS) involvement include irritability, lethargy, alterations in sleep pattern, decreased attention span, and developmental delay.

Acute encephalopathy may be seen in children with BLLs greater than 70 to 90 µg/dL (3.4 to 4.4 µmol/L). These children can develop persistent vomiting, somnolence, and ataxia. As encephalopathy worsens, the level of consciousness deteriorates further, and seizures or even coma can occur.

DIAGNOSTIC EVALUATION

The initial evaluation of lead poisoning includes a venous BLL, detailed environmental and social histories, and systematic physical examination.

The following laboratory data should be obtained to aid in making the diagnosis and guide management.

- Repeat BLL—confirmatory test must be a *venous* BLL, specimens obtained by finger stick are less reliable
- Complete blood count with differential
- Serum iron studies: iron, ferritin, total iron binding capacity, C-reactive protein (CRP) or if available, reticulocyte hemoglobin content
- ZPP or EP level for moderate to severe poisoning, not to be used as a screening tool as not reliable in early or less severe lead poisoning
- If chelation is likely: electrolytes, calcium, magnesium, blood urea nitrogen (BUN), creatinine, alanine and aspartate aminotransferases, and a urinalysis

Note that lead measurement of hair, fingernail, and dentin is not recommended.

Table 170-1 details recommended laboratory studies for diagnosis and monitoring during therapy.

Radiographic studies should be considered; an abdominal radiograph is recommended for children with (i) symptoms or signs concerning for lead toxicity; (ii) a history of pica; or (iii) an acute ingestion of lead containing compounds. Radiopaque specks in the GI tract, particularly the stomach and small intestine, may represent lead-containing particles, leading to consideration of gut decontamination (**Figure 170-1**). The CDC does not recommend obtaining long-bone radiographs as they are not useful in guiding management of lead poisoning. However, if obtained, characteristic lead lines, radiodensities in metaphyseal plates of the long bones, are typically seen in children with BLL greater than 45µg/dL (2.17 µmol/L).

Developmental evaluation is of utmost importance as by the time children are found to have elevated BLLs on screening, neurodevelopmental harm may have already occurred. According to the World Health Organization the neurologic and behavioral effects are thought to be irreversible. Thus, it is important to screen children with BLL > 97.5th percentile (3.5 µg/dL, 0.17 µmol/L) for developmental delay. Children with abnormal screening tests should be referred for formal neuropsychological testing.

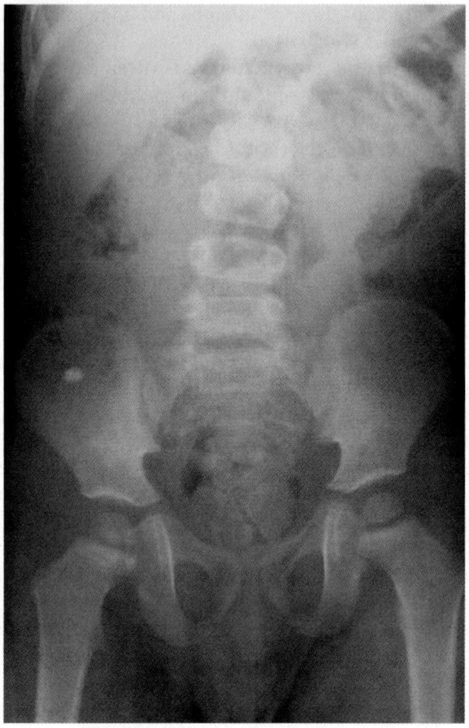

FIGURE 170-1. Child with paint chip in bowel.

All families warrant a complete social work assessment. The local health department's childhood lead poisoning prevention program should be notified of the child's admission and can advise pediatric care providers and families on obtaining environmental assessments. Local public health officials may be able to identify lead hazards when they make home visits. They can also provide risk-reduction education and make recommendations to the family about how to diminish the hazard.

MANAGEMENT

The treatment of childhood lead poisoning involves eliminating ongoing or additional exposure and providing adequate nutrition. If these

TABLE 170-1 Monitoring Laboratory Studies for Patients Receiving $CaNa_2EDTA$ and BAL

Baseline (Before Infusion)	Daily	Day 3	Day 5
Venous BLL, G6PD level[?]	Urinalysis with urine-specific gravity every day	Venous BLL*	Venous BLL*
Serum electrolytes (Na, K, Cl, CO_2, BUN, Cr, glucose, Ca, Mg, phosphate)	Plus Urine dip and urine-specific gravity every 8 hr	Serum electrolytes (Na, K, Cl, CO_2, BUN, Cr, glucose, Ca, Mg, phosphate)	Serum electrolytes (Na, K, Cl, CO_2, BUN, Cr, glucose, Ca, Mg, phosphate)
Liver enzymes (AST, ALT, alkaline phosphatase)		Liver enzymes (AST, ALT, alkaline phosphatase)	Liver enzymes (AST, ALT, alkaline phosphatase)
ZPP or EP (reference level ≤35 µg/dL whole blood)		ZPP or EP CBC with indices	ZPP or EP CBC with indices
CBC with indices		Iron studies: iron, ferritin, TIBC, if available CHr	Iron studies: iron, ferritin, TIBC, if available Chr
Iron studies: iron, ferritin, TIBC, if available CHr Urinalysis with urine-specific gravity			

ALT, alanine transaminase; AST, aspartate transaminase; BAL, British anti-lewisite (dimercaprol); BLL, blood lead level; BUN, blood urea nitrogen; $CaNa_2EDTA$, calcium disodium edetate; CBC, complete blood count; CHr, reticulocyte hemoglobin content; EP, erythrocyte protoporphyrin; G6PD, glucose-6-phosphate dehydrogenase; TIBC, total iron binding capacity; ZPP, zinc protoporphyrin.

*Stop infusion for 1 hour before drawing blood to avoid falsely elevated lead level.

[?]Consider in patients before receiving BAL.

conditions cannot be met, or venous blood levels do not decrease, chelation therapy should be considered.

Gut Decontamination When there is radiographic evidence of lead densities in the stomach or small intestine of children, the GI tract must be evacuated to eliminate further absorption. Gut decontamination should occur before chelation. Whole bowel irrigation with a polyethylene glycol (PEG) solution is the preferred method of GI decontamination. PEG solution is given orally or instilled by nasogastric tube at a dose of 20 to 40 mL/kg per hour, up to a maximum of 1000 mL/hr for a minimum of 4 hours, or until the rectal effluent is clear. PEG's effect of action is usually 30 to 60 minutes. Contraindications to polyethylene glycol solution include bowel perforation, adynamic ileus, significant GI hemorrhage, intestinal obstruction, and inability to protect the airway. A follow-up radiograph may be indicated to document removal or transit of any lead densities.

Nutrition Nutrition can play a pivotal role in the prevention and treatment of lead poisoning, especially in young children. To decrease their susceptibility to lead intoxication, children should be provided with balanced nutrition, including adequate amounts of foods rich in calcium (e.g., milk, cheese, yogurt), iron (e.g., beef, ham, beans, green leafy vegetables), and ascorbic acid (e.g., citrus fruit, tomatoes, broccoli). Lead can mimic or inhibit calcium, thus having adequate levels is thought to help protect against this effect. Proper levels of ascorbic acid also help iron uptake in the body. Lead-poisoned children should be assessed for iron deficiency because lead is more readily absorbed when iron stores are depleted. Lead-poisoned children who are iron deficient should receive oral elemental iron supplementation at a dose of 3 to 6 mg/kg per day following chelation therapy.

Chelation Therapy Table 170-2 provides a quick guide to chelation therapy.

Asymptomatic Patients With BLL 45 to 69 µg/dL Asymptomatic children with BLLs of 45 to 69 µg/dL should be treated with oral succimer. Parenteral calcium disodium edetate ($CaNa_2EDTA$) is an option if succimer cannot be tolerated or if patients are allergic to succimer or its components. Succimer and $CaNa_2EDTA$ are similar in terms of safety and efficacy. Before initiation of chelation therapy, consultation with a pediatric toxicologist is strongly advised.

Oral succimer is often preferred given ease of administration and the potential for outpatient treatment (although this is generally not advised for children with BLLs in this range). Succimer is rapidly absorbed from the GI tract, with a peak concentration at 3 hours and an elimination half-life in children of 3 hours. Succimer has a small volume of distribution, with 95% binding to albumin in blood, and the succimer-lead complex is excreted renally. Adverse effects include nausea, rash, and increased serum transaminases. Cardiac arrythmias may also manifest but are almost exclusively observed in adult patients.

Baseline laboratory studies that should be obtained before treatment with succimer include confirmation venous BLL, ZPP or EP level, complete blood count (with differential and platelets), electrolytes, and liver function tests (alanine transaminase, aspartate transaminase, alkaline phosphatase) (Table 170-1). Lead poisoning may create transaminitis and is not a contraindication to starting chelation therapy. Succimer is given orally at 10 mg/kg per dose (rounded to the nearest 100 mg) 3 times a day for 5 days, then twice a day for an additional 14 days. Initial laboratory studies should be repeated on days 6 and 20 of treatment to monitor for adverse effects. Treatment should be repeated as directed until BLL < 45 µg/dL (2.17 µmol/L).

Although formulated as a capsule, succimer may be opened and sprinkled on food or dissolved in juice for young children unable to swallow pills. The foul smell and taste of succimer, may present challenges to oral toleration and administration via nasogastric tube may be considered. The most common adverse effects in children are nausea, vomiting, diarrhea, and appetite loss. Hypersensitivity reactions have been reported in ~4% of patients, including chills, fever, urticaria, and rashes. Some skin rashes may necessitate the discontinuation of therapy; however, if a rash occurs, other causes should be considered before ascribing it to a drug reaction. Mild, transient elevations of serum transaminases have been observed in 6% to 10% of patients. Mild to moderate reversible neutropenia has also been noted. Therapy should be withheld or discontinued if the absolute neutrophil count falls below 1200/µL.

$CaNa_2EDTA$ must be administered by intravenous (IV) or intramuscular (IM) route, necessitating greater resource utilization. Because of the pain of IM administration, it should be given IV, when possible, which may require hospitalization. The half-life of $CaNa_2EDTA$ is 20 to 60 minutes. If given intramuscularly, $CaNa_2EDTA$ should be mixed with procaine to decrease injection site pain. $CaNa_2EDTA$ should not be confused with disodium edetate (sodium EDTA); use of the latter may result in severe hypocalcemia and possible death.

The baseline laboratory studies listed in Table 170-1 should be obtained before administering $CaNa_2EDTA$. After ensuring adequate urine output, chelation can be initiated with an intravenous infusion of $CaNa_2EDTA$

TABLE 170-2 Chelation Therapy Based on Clinical Presentation and Blood Lead Level

Clinical Presentation	Chelating Agent and Dose	Route	Duration
Asymptomatic patients with BLL <45 µg/dL (2.17 µmol/L)	Not routinely indicated	N/A	N/A
Asymptomatic patients with BLL 45-69 µg/dL (2.17 to 3.33 µmol/L)	Succimer (Chemet) 10 mg/kg/dose 3 times/day for 5 days, then twice/day for remaining 14 days or $CaNa_2EDTA$ 25-50 mg/kg/day if succimer cannot be tolerated or is contraindicated	PO or nasogastric tube; 100-mg capsules of medicated beads can be opened and sprinkled on food or dissolved in juice IM (with procaine) IV (24-hr infusion)	19 days; may repeat course, with a minimum of 2 week between courses 3-5 days; may repeat course, with 2-5 days between courses
Asymptomatic patients with BLL ≥70 µg/dL (3.38 µmol/L)	Succimer (Chemet) 10 mg/kg/dose 3 times/day for 5 days, then twice/day for remaining 14 days and $CaNa_2EDTA$ 25-50 mg/kg/day	PO or nasogastric tube; 100-mg capsules of medicated beads can be opened and sprinkled on food or dissolved in juice IV (24-hr continuous infusion)	19 days; may repeat course, with a minimum of 2 week between courses Begin 48 hours after the initiation of succimer for 5 days. 2 weeks between courses.
Symptomatic patients without encephalopathy with BLL > 45 µg/dL (2.17 µmol/L)	BAL 3-4 mg/kg/dose every 4 hr and $CaNa_2EDTA$ 25-50 mg/kg/day	IM IV (24-hr continuous infusion)	3-5 days Begin 4-5 hr after first dose of BAL and continue for 5 days. 2 week minimum between courses if BLL < 70. IF BLL > 100 may necessitate sooner treatment.
All patients with acute encephalopathy	BAL 3-4 mg/kg/dose every 4 hr and $CaNa_2EDTA$ 50-75 mg/kg/day	IM IV (24-hr continuous infusion)	5 days. 2 days between courses. Begin 4-5 hr after first dose of BAL and continue for 5 days. Treatment may be repeated.

BAL, British antilewisite (dimercaprol); BLL, blood lead level; $CaNa_2EDTA$, calcium disodium edetate; N/A, not applicable.

for 3 to 5 consecutive days. The dosage of $CaNa_2EDTA$ is 25 to 50 mg/kg per day and must be diluted to 2 to 4 mg/mL in either 5% dextrose or 0.9% saline solution. It is incompatible with high-concentration dextrose solution or lactated Ringer's solution. The rate of infusion is calculated to deliver the total dose over a 24-hour continuous infusion. If administered intramuscularly, the total daily dose is divided into two doses given 12 hours apart. Regardless of the route of administration of $CaNa_2EDTA$, vigorous hydration (intravenous or oral) should be provided to reduce the risk of nephrotoxicity; urine specific gravity should be maintained at less than 1.020 at all times. Total fluid intake should be 1.5 times the maintenance fluid requirements. The patient should receive strict input and output monitoring, with vital signs checked every 4 hours. Electrocardiogram monitoring is also recommended. The suggested schedule of laboratory monitoring studies is provided in Table 170-1.

$CaNa_2EDTA$ is excreted renally; as a result, the major adverse effects include acute necrosis of proximal tubules (exhibited by glycosuria, proteinuria, microscopic hematuria) and large epithelial cells in urinary sediment. Hypotension and cardiac rhythm irregularities have been documented and patients should be monitored with telemetry. Mild increases in serum transaminases are common, with a return to normal within 48 hours after cessation of therapy. Elevation of serum transaminases also occurs with lead poisoning so it may precede $CaNa_2EDTA$ chelation and is not a contraindication. $CaNa_2EDTA$ also increases the urinary excretion of zinc, but this is clinically insignificant unless therapy is continued for more than 5 days. Chelation should be repeated as directed until BLL < 45 μg/dL (2.17 μmol/L).

Asymptomatic Patients With BLL Greater Than 70 μg/dL and Symptomatic Patients Without Encephalopathy Asymptomatic patients with BLLs greater than 70 μg/dL require combination therapy with $CaNa_2EDTA$ and succimer. $CaNa_2EDTA$ should be started 48 hours after the initiation of succimer. Therapy for lead poisoning should be continued until BLL < 45 μg/dL (2.15 μmol/L), repeating as directed, if indicated.

Symptomatic Patients Without Encephalopathy With BLL Greater Than 45 μg/dL Symptomatic patients with BLL > 45 μg/dL (2.15 μmol/L) should receive a combination therapy of dimercaprol and $CaNa_2EDTA$.

Dimercaprol, or British antilewisite (BAL), is used for a wide variety of heavy metal poisonings because of its ability to form stable complexes with many metals, facilitating solubility and elimination. Peak BAL concentrations are reached in 30 to 60 minutes, with a duration of action of 4 hours. As a result, frequent doses at 3- to 4-hour intervals are necessary to maintain the therapeutic effect. The BAL-metal complex is eliminated via the renal and biliary tracts.

Table 170-3 lists the baseline laboratory studies that should be performed before chelation with BAL and during therapy. In addition, before beginning therapy, one must identify any allergy to peanuts, because BAL is suspended in peanut oil. BAL may also induce hemolysis in those with glucose-6-phosphate dehydrogenase (G6PD) deficiency; therefore, a G6PD assay should be obtained if the patient's G6PD status is not known. Withhold oral iron supplementation during BAL treatment to avoid potential toxic interactions. BAL is given by deep intramuscular injection in a dose of 3 to 4 mg/kg every 4 hours. $CaNa_2EDTA$ (50 mg/kg per day) is started 4 to 5 hours after the first dose of BAL and given as a continuous intravenous infusion (over 24 hours). The hemodynamic stability of severely lead-poisoned children as well as changes in neurologic status that may indicate encephalopathy, should be closely monitored. Just as when administering $CaNa_2EDTA$ alone, aggressive hydration is important to facilitate renal excretion. Dual therapy should be continued for a minimum of 72 hours, and a BLL should be repeated. If the BLL is greater than 50 μg/dL (2.42 μmol/L), BAL is continued for an additional 48 hours in conjunction with $CaNa_2EDTA$, for up to a total of 12 doses. If the BLL is less than 50 μg/dL (2.42 μmol/L), $CaNa_2EDTA$ alone is continued for a total of 5 days.

Approximately one-third of patients who receive BAL experience side effects. Mild febrile reactions and transient elevations in serum transaminases may be observed. Hypertension and tachycardia can also occur. Other minor adverse effects include, in order of frequency, nausea, vomiting, headache, lacrimation, rhinorrhea, and salivation. These side effects are transient and usually disappear with cessation of the drug.

Patients With Clinical Signs and Symptoms of Acute Encephalopathy Children with signs and symptoms of acute encephalopathy (usually seen with a BLL > 70 μg/dL [3.38 μmol/L]) should be admitted to an intensive care setting. The poison control center, toxicology consulting service, or pediatric environmental health service should be consulted immediately. Lead encephalopathy is a life-threatening emergency that should be treated using contemporary standards for the intensive care treatment of increased intracranial pressure, including appropriate pressure monitoring, osmotic therapy, and drug therapy in addition to chelation therapy. If the admitting hospital does not have intensive care services, toxicology or the local poison control center should be asked for advice on stabilizing the patient for transfer. A lumbar puncture should *not* be performed on any child suspected of having lead encephalopathy. The use of $CaNa_2EDTA$ alone is avoided in children with lead levels greater than 70 μg/dL (3.38 μmol/L) because it may precipitate encephalopathy by causing a redistribution of lead to the brain, resulting in a lethal increase in intracranial pressure.

Children with signs and symptoms of encephalopathy or a venous BLL greater than 100 μg/dL (4.83 μmol/L) should receive nothing by mouth (usually for the first 24 hours), and parenteral fluid therapy should begin immediately. Total volume should be restricted to basal requirements plus ongoing losses. Although it is desirable to evacuate residual lead from the gut, this should not delay the start of chelation therapy in severely lead-poisoned children. For acute encephalopathy or a BLL greater than 100 μg/dL (4.83 μmol/L), BAL and $CaNa_2EDTA$ are co-administered for a total of 5 consecutive days, as detailed earlier.

TABLE 170-3 Mercury Absorption and Target Organs

	EXPOSURE		
Mercury Form	***Inhalation***	***Oral***	**Target Organ**
Elemental (metallic) mercury Hg^0 liquid, Hg^0 vapor	Major	Minor	Acute: lungs Chronic: CNS/PNS, erethism Other: kidney, acrodynia
Inorganic mercury salts Hg^{+1} (mercurous), Hg^{+2} (mercuric)	Minor	Major	Acute: GI (caustic injury) Chronic: CNS/PNS, erethism, triad (tremor, neuropsychiatric disturbances, gingivostomatitis) Other: kidney, acrodynia
Organic (alkyl) mercury methylmercury, ethylmercury, dimethylmercury	Minor	Major	Acute and chronic: CNS/PNS, teratogen Other: kidney, liver

CNS/PNS, central nervous system/peripheral nervous system; erethism, irritability, excitability, decreased concentration; GI, gastrointestinal.

CONSULTATION

Consider consultation with toxicology or a poison control center for guidance in treatment and acute and long-term management. If encephalopathy is present, the inclusion of critical care specialists and neurology services is warranted. Contact local health department or lead abatement programs and referral for early intervention.

ADMISSION CRITERIA

The decision to admit a child for the treatment of lead poisoning is multifaceted and is never based solely on the BLL. In addition to the BLL, the medical evaluation, environmental history, social history, and laboratory facilities available in the outpatient and inpatient settings are all key factors. It is important that the laboratory has the capacity to run a BLL with a prompt turnaround of results. Asymptomatic patients with BLLs greater than 45 to 50 μg/dL (2.17 μmol/L) should have a confirmatory venous lead level within 48 hours. They should also have laboratory testing to assess for anemia, electrolytes, blood urea nitrogen, and creatine screening. These patients may benefit from hospitalization and chelation, which should be guided by the chronicity of the exposure, social situation, and the ability to isolate the lead source.

- All children with symptoms of toxicity, particularly encephalopathy (e.g., headache, ataxia, sleepiness) or evidence of raised intracranial pressure. Children with signs or symptoms suggesting lead encephalopathy should be evaluated for admission to the pediatric intensive care unit or transfer to a tertiary center where critical care can be provided if necessary.
- Asymptomatic children with venous BLLs of 45 to 69 μg/dL (2.17-3.33 μmol/L) who are not candidates for oral therapy with succimer (e.g., no lead-free housing available, unable to tolerate enteral therapy, concern about noncompliance, inadequate follow-up). Halting the child's exposure to the source of lead is the most important consideration and can help guide whether a patient needs admission when asymptomatic with a borderline BLL.
- Children with venous BLLs greater than 70 μg/dL (3.38 μmol/L)

DISCHARGE CRITERIA

- Children with BLLs less than 45 μg/dL (2.17 μmol/L) can be discharged home, with the understanding that outpatient chelation will most likely be required. Generally, children whose admission BLL is less than 70 μg/dL (3.38 μmol/L) will have an end-of-chelation BLL of less than 45 μg/dL (2.17 μmol/L), making them candidates for discharge after a single course of chelation.
- A repeat BLL obtained at the end of chelation determines the need for reinstitution of chelation therapy:
  - If the BLL is 45 to 69 μg/dL (2.17-3.33 μmol/L) at the end of the first course, a second course of chelation therapy is necessary, which is best done as an inpatient.
  - If, at the end of the first course of chelation, the BLL is 70 μg/dL (3.38 μmol/L) or greater, dual therapy with BAL and $CaNa_2EDTA$ should be reinitiated. A minimum of 2 days must elapse before restarting intravenous $CaNa_2EDTA$ (a chelation "honeymoon") to minimize the risk of nephrotoxicity and permit at least partial recovery from the urinary losses of zinc produced by $CaNa_2EDTA$.
- Referral to an early intervention program is advised for lead-poisoned children suspected of having developmental delay.
- Before the child is discharged, the home should be inspected to ensure it is a lead-safe environment and alternate housing secured (e.g., with friends or relatives or in designated transitional housing) if the child's residence remains contaminated. There should be plans for lead abatement in the home where the exposure occurred.

FOLLOW-UP CARE

The first follow-up visit should be scheduled for 7 to 14 days after chelation to allow for a period of re-equilibration. At this visit, a BLL and ZPP or EP level are repeated to determine whether subsequent outpatient chelation is needed. Many children require more than one round of outpatient chelation therapy. The time interval of follow-up care is detailed in the Centers for Disease Control and Prevention lead screening guidelines (http://www.cdc.gov/nceh/lead). During follow-up visits, pediatric care providers can assess the patient and family's ability to reduce lead exposure and encourage proper nutrition. These aims can be supported with the recommended risk-reduction practices, including the abatement or reduction of lead hazards as well as dietary counseling to ensure adequate intake of calcium, ascorbic acid, and iron. All children with significant lead exposure, and especially those who have undergone chelation, need routine screening for lead-induced developmental injuries such as speech or language impairments, learning disabilities, and behavioral disturbances. If at any time during follow-up a possible developmental delay is identified, the child should immediately be referred for a complete developmental evaluation and for neuropsychological testing, if older than 4 years.

ARSENIC

BACKGROUND

Arsenic, a known carcinogen, is the 20th most abundant element in the earth's crust; it is found worldwide as a pollutant. It is released into the environment by volcanoes, through the weathering and smelting of arsenic-containing minerals and ores, and by commercial and industrial processes. It is also found in some folk and naturopathic remedies. Children are commonly exposed to arsenic by the ingestion of contaminated well water or by contact with arsenate wood preservatives, such as copper chromium arsenate found in pressure-treated wood. Arsenic exists in organic and inorganic forms and is rarely found in its elemental form. Trivalent arsenic (As^{+3}) is considered the most toxic form, followed by pentavalent arsenic (As^{+5}). Organic arsenic is the nontoxic form that is commonly found in seafood, particularly shellfish. Arsenic is well absorbed by all routes. Once absorbed, arsenicals disrupt cellular metabolism by interacting with sulfhydryl groups and by inhibiting enzymatic pathways required to produce adenosine triphosphate. Arsenic is rapidly cleared from the blood (1-hour half-life), and excretion is almost entirely by the kidney.

CLINICAL PRESENTATION

The clinical presentation of arsenic poisoning depends on the route, dose, timing, and duration of exposure. Mild acute arsenic poisoning often manifests as dysphagia associated with a metallic taste. Severe exposures generally present with GI upset (e.g., nausea, vomiting, abdominal pain, diarrhea) and a garlic odor in the breath and stool. Within hours of severe exposure, diffuse capillary and endothelial cell damage results in vasodilation and leakage of plasma, which precipitates hemorrhagic gastroenteritis. In severe cases, extensive third spacing of fluids combined with fluid loss may lead to cardiovascular collapse consisting of hypotension, shock, and even death. Electrocardiogram findings may include nonspecific T-wave changes and a prolonged Q-Tc interval that may occur promptly or after a delay of several days. Acute tubular necrosis may also occur after a large ingestion. Acute poisoning can cause delirium, encephalopathy, seizures, and coma. A delayed sensorimotor peripheral neuropathy may appear within 3 weeks after acute ingestion along with pancytopenia.

Chronic arsenic poisoning develops insidiously and includes peripheral neuropathy and dermal changes. "Raindrop" lesions of the skin can take years to manifest and are characteristically described as hypo- and hyper-pigmentation with hyperkeratosis. Skin, bladder, and lung malignancies have been observed in adults. General manifestations of chronic arsenic toxicity can include malaise, weakness, anorexia, alopecia, headache, diarrhea, nausea, vomiting, leukopenia, and anemia.

DIAGNOSTIC EVALUATION AND MANAGEMENT

The diagnosis of arsenic poisoning is based on a history of exposure combined with a characteristic presentation. Arsenic levels can be obtained from urine, blood, hair, and nail samples. Blood arsenic levels are rarely useful because of the short half-life, and hair and nail samples are of limited value owing to external contamination. Urine concentration is the preferred biomarker for arsenic exposure and must be obtained as a timed (24-hour) urine collection. A "spot" urine sample is not accurate but may be helpful in acute poisoning because of arsenic's short half-life and urinary excretion. A spot urine is less useful in chronic poisoning because urinary levels will be low. There are two methods of measuring arsenic in urine samples: fractionated (speciated) measurement for inorganic plus organic arsenic, or total arsenic level (this must be done 48-72 hours after seafood abstinence to avoid false-positive results). Urine arsenic has a reference value of less than 50 mcg/L (0.67 μmol/day).

Because arsenic is readily excreted in urine, elimination of exposure is the most effective treatment. In patients with mild symptoms, BAL at a dose of 2.5 mg/kg/dose intramuscularly every 6 hours for 2 days, then every 12 hours on day 3, and every 24 hours after, can be administered and should continue until the urinary arsenic level is less than 50 μg/L per 24 hours (0.67 μmol/day). For patients with severe symptoms BAL at a dose of 3 mg/kg/dose every 4 hours for the first 2 days, every 6 hours on day 3, and every 12 hours after for 10 days should be administered. Nausea and vomiting are common side effects, but hypertension and lacrimation have also been described with multiple injections. Ampules of BAL in peanut oil may still exist, thus patients with peanut allergies should be monitored closely. Chelation is rarely needed outside the setting of symptomatic acute poisoning; however, if outpatient chelation is prescribed, succimer is the preferred agent at a dose of 10 mg/kg orally every 8 hours for 5 days, then every 12 hours for 14 days.

CONSULTATION

- Chelation should be undertaken only after consultation with a medical toxicologist

ADMISSION CRITERIA

- Symptomatic arsenic poisoning requiring parenteral chelation therapy

DISCHARGE CRITERIA

- Completion of parenteral therapy and resolution of symptoms
- Identification and elimination of source of arsenic exposure

MERCURY

BACKGROUND

Mercury, a naturally occurring metal, is present throughout the environment. It has been used in medications, disinfectants, thermometers, dental amalgams, and ethnic remedies. There have been concerted efforts to limit mercury exposure through policy changes in the United States and globally. Mercury exists in three primary forms, each with a different toxicity: elemental or metallic mercury (Hg^{o}), inorganic mercury salts (Hg^{+1} [mercurous], Hg^{+2} [mercuric]), and organic or alkyl mercury (e.g., methylmercury). Inorganic mercury is readily converted to methylmercury by aquatic microorganisms and can bioaccumulate in the tissues of large carnivorous fish. The toxicokinetics of mercury vary, depending on the route of absorption and chemical form. Elemental, inorganic, and organic mercury can all be absorbed after inhalation. Elemental mercury is poorly absorbed orally; conversely, organic mercury is well absorbed (Table 170-3). Dermal absorption is limited for all forms of mercury. Organic mercury may be transmitted to the fetus via the placenta. Elemental and inorganic mercury have a half-life of 40 to 60 days and are excreted via urine. Organic mercury has a half-life of 70 to 90 days and is eliminated via bile and feces. Within the central nervous system, the half-life can be significantly longer, of several years to a decade.

CLINICAL PRESENTATION

Acute inhalation of elemental mercury vapor is the main cause of toxicity. Proper cleanup is key to limiting exposure, as vacuuming has been shown to increase volatilization of spilled mercury. Symptoms may develop within a few hours and include nausea, vomiting, chills, metallic taste, tachypnea, dyspnea, abdominal pain, and diarrhea. These symptoms may subside in a few days or progress to interstitial pulmonary fibrosis, noncardiogenic pulmonary edema, interstitial chemical pneumonitis, and hemoptysis. Elemental liquid mercury can irritate the skin and cause hives and dermatitis. Chronic inhalation of elemental mercury vapor produces the classic triad of tremor, neuropsychiatric disturbances, and gingivostomatitis. Acrodynia (painful extremities) is a rare disease that affects primarily young children with exposure. Symptoms include irritability, photophobia, pink discoloration of the hands and feet, and polyneuritis.

Acute ingestion of inorganic mercury salts is caustic to the gastrointestinal tract and can produce a sudden onset of corrosive stomatitis, hemorrhagic gastroenteritis, and abdominal pain. Acute oliguric renal failure from acute tubular necrosis may also occur within days of exposure. Chronic manifestations of inorganic mercury toxicity are similar to those of elemental mercury.

Organic mercury affects primarily the central nervous system, causing paresthesias, ataxia, dysarthria, spasticity, hearing impairment, and progressive visual field constriction. Perinatal exposure to methylmercury, a known potent teratogen that easily crosses the placenta, can lead to micrognathia, cerebral palsy, and/or intellectual disability.

DIAGNOSTIC EVALUATION AND MANAGEMENT

The diagnosis of mercury poisoning depends on the integration of characteristic findings with a history of known or potential exposure and the presence of a positive biomarker. Whole blood or, preferably, urine can be used to determine metallic and inorganic mercury levels. Whole blood samples are preferred for organic mercury levels because that form is excreted in feces. Hair samples have limited value.

Removing the mercury source and preventing additional exposure are the best treatments. Chelation is reserved for symptomatic patients with 24-hour urine or whole blood levels ≥100 μg/L (50 μmol/L). Elemental and inorganic mercury poisoning can be treated with BAL, or preferably oral succimer. Succimer dosing under 5 years of age is 350 mg/m^2 every 8 hours for 5 days, then every 12 hours for 14 days. Dosing for children ≥5 years of age is 10 mg/kg/dose every 8 hours for 5 days, and then every 12 hours for 14 days. Alternatively, intramuscular BAL can be given initially at a dose of 5 mg/kg, then 2.5 mg/kg 1 to 2 times per day for 10 days. Organic mercury has been treated with oral succimer; however, data on its effectiveness are limited. Chelation therapy is rarely indicated and should be initiated only after consultation with a medical toxicologist.

KEY POINTS

Lead

- Lead poisoning remains common; no BLL is safe for children.
- BLL > 3.5 μg/dL (0.17 μmol/L) represents >97.5th percentile based on NHANES data and indicates children at risk for lead toxicity.
- Severe lead poisoning, defined as a BLL greater than 45 μg/dL (2.17 μmol/L), requires immediate intervention. Hospitalization is recommended for these children, with the goals of providing immediate environmental protection and the rapid institution of chelation therapy. In rare circumstances, children with BLLs of 45 to 69 μg/dL (2.17-3.33 μmol/L) can be considered for outpatient therapy if a safe, lead-free environment and 100% compliance with the outpatient chelation regimen can be assured.
- The chelation agents of choice for asymptomatic hospitalized children with BLLs of 45 to 69 μg/dL (2.17-3.33 μmol/L) are succimer or $CaNa_2EDTA$. For asymptomatic children with BLLs greater than 70 μg/dL (3.38 μmol/L), dual chelation therapy with $CaNa_2EDTA$ and succimer is recommended. For symptomatic children with BLL > 45 μg/dL (2.17 μmol/L) dual therapy with BAL and $CaNa_2EDTA$ is given until the BLL has fallen below 70 μg/dL (3.38 μmol/L), at which time $CaNa_2EDTA$ alone can be given.
- Children with symptoms of encephalopathy should be admitted to intensive care units and treated with BAL and $CaNa_2EDTA$.

Arsenic

- Arsenic exposure commonly occurs from ingestion of contaminated well water or by contact with arsenate wood preservatives (e.g., pressure-treated wood).
- Acute toxicity presents initially with dysphagia and metallic taste. Endothelial damage ensues, with vasodilation and leakage of plasma, which can lead to hemorrhagic gastroenteritis and progress to cardiovascular collapse. Neurotoxic effects can progress to coma. Evidence of chronic poisoning develops over years with peripheral neuropathy, dermal changes, and hair loss.
- Chelation therapy is indicated for symptomatic patients with acute poisoning and is best treated with BAL.

Mercury

- Elemental, inorganic, and organic mercury can all be absorbed after inhalation which is the main cause of toxicity.
- Symptoms may develop within a few hours and include nausea, vomiting, chills, metallic taste, tachypnea, dyspnea, abdominal pain, and diarrhea. These symptoms may subside in a few days or progress to interstitial pulmonary fibrosis, noncardiogenic pulmonary edema, interstitial chemical pneumonitis, and hemoptysis.
- Urine samples should be used to measure metallic and inorganic mercury levels.
- Removing the mercury source and preventing additional exposure are the best treatments; elemental and inorganic mercury poisoning can be treated with oral succimer or BAL.

SUGGESTED READINGS

Angle CR. Childhood lead poisoning and its treatment. *Ann Rev Pharmacol Toxicol.* 1993;33:409-434.

Jacobs DE, Clickner RP, Zhou JY, et al. The prevalence of lead-based paint hazards in US housing. *Environ Health Perspect.* 2002;110:A599-A606.

McLaine P, Navas-Acien A, Lee Robert, et al. Elevated blood lead levels and reading readiness at the start of kindergarten. *Pediatrics.* 2013;131:1081-1089.

Ettinger AS, Gurthrie Wengrovitz, A. Guidelines for the identification of and management of lead exposure in pregnant and lactating women. National Center for Environmental Health/Agency for Toxic Substances and Disease Registry; Centers for Disease Control and Prevention, Atlanta, GA 2010.

Centers for Disease Control and Prevention. *Sources of Lead Exposure: Lead in Paint.* Atlanta, GA; US Department of Health and Human Services; May 26, 2022. https://www.cdc.gov/nceh/lead/prevention/sources/paint.htm. Accessed July 11, 2022.

Dart RC. Succimer. In: Dart RC, ed. *Medical Toxicology*. 3rd ed. Philadelphia: Lippincott Williams & Wilkins; 2001:266-268.

American Academy of Pediatrics. *Lead Exposure in Children.* July 20, 2021. https://www.aap.org/en/patient-care/lead-exposure/lead-exposure-in-children/. Accessed July 11, 2022.

Centers for Disease Control and Prevention. *Childhood Lead Poisoning Prevention: Guidelines and Recommendations.* October 27, 2021. https://www.cdc.gov/nceh/lead/resources/guidelines.html. Accessed July 11, 2022.

Centers for Disease Control and Prevention. *Childhood Lead Poisoning Prevention: Blood Levels in Children.* Atlanta, GA; US Department of Health and Human Services; June 6, 2022. https://www.cdc.gov/nceh/lead/prevention/sources/paint.htm. Accessed July 11, 2022.

Radulescu A, Lundgren S. A pharmacokinetic model of lead absorption and calcium competitive dynamics. *Sci Rep.* 2019;9:14225.

Shannon MW, Graef JW. Lead intoxication in infancy. *Pediatrics.* 1992;89:87-90.

Hussain JH. Blood Lead Level in Children with Encephalopathy. *Indian Pediatr.* 2009;46:841-2.

Baum C, Hauptman M, Newman N, Woolf A. Recommendations on Management of childhood lead exposure: A resource for health professionals. Pediatric Environmental Health Specialty Units and the American Academy of Pediatrics. September 2021. https://www.pehsu.net/Lead_Exposure.html. Accessed July 11, 2022.

Bellinger D, Sloman J, Levitón A, et al. Low-level lead exposure and children's cognitive function in the preschool years. *Pediatrics.* 1991;87:219-227.

Liebelt EL, Shannon MW. Oral chelators for childhood lead poisoning. *Pediatr Ann.* 1994;23:616-619.

Watanabe T, Hirano S. Metabolism of arsenic and its toxicological relevance. *Arch Toxicol.* 2013;87:969-979.

World Health Organization. Exposure to arsenic: A major public concern. 2019. Available at https://apps.who.int/iris/bitstream/handle/10665/329482/WHO-CED-PHE-EPE-19.4.1-eng.pdf Accessed July 25th, 2022.

Hall AH. Chronic arsenic poisoning. *Toxicol Lett.* 2002;128:69-72.

Centers for Disease Control and Prevention (CDC). National Center for Health Statistics (NCHS). National Health and Nutrition Examination Survey Data. Hyattsville, MD: U.S. Department of Health and Human Services, Centers for Disease Control and Prevention.

Rooney JP. The retention time of inorganic mercury in the brain: a systemic review of the evidence. *Toxicol Pharm.* 2014;274:425-435.

Ozuah PO. Mercury poisoning. *Curr Probl Pediatr.* 2000;30:91-99.

Kosnett M. The role of chelation therapy in the treatment of arsenic and mercury poisoning. *J Med Toxicol.* 2013;9:347-354.

Dapul H, Laraque D. Lead poisoning in children. *Adv Pediatr.* 2014;61:313-333.

CHAPTER 171 Drugs of Abuse

Lauren L. Titus, MD and Vanessa McFadden, MD, PhD

BACKGROUND

Drugs of abuse have a significant impact on healthcare utilization in the pediatric population. With the current mental health crisis for youth and teens, pediatric hospitalists should consider that drugs of abuse may be used for self-harm, self-medication, or simply recreation. Ingestion of drugs of abuse should be considered in the differential diagnosis of any patient who presents with altered mental status (e.g., hallucinations, stupor, coma), abnormal motor activity (e.g., tremor, seizure), or behavioral disturbance (e.g., agitation, outburst, withdrawal, depression, suicidal, or homicidal ideation).

EPIDEMIOLOGY

Each fall, the American Association of Poison Control Centers publishes its annual summary of poisoning exposures reported to its member centers. In 2020, there were a total of 2.1 million exposures reported, 1434 of which led to a fatality. Of these fatalities, 64 (4.3%) involved a child (<20 years of age) who intentionally abused (alone or in combination with other substances) narcotics, analgesics, prescribed medications, cannabinoids, hallucinogens, or stimulants (**Table 171-1**).

Another annual resource is the National Institute on Drug Abuse's (NIDA) Monitoring the Future surveys of eighth-, tenth-, and twelfth-grade students conducted to gauge trends in drug use as well as levels of perceived risk and disapproval among these children. First performed in 1975, the most recent of these extensive studies is in the public domain and posted on the organization's website (https://nida.nih.gov/research-topics/trends-statistics/monitoring-future). The 2021 survey reached 32,000 students in 319 secondary schools. While the authors note significant limitations to their 2020 data due to the beginning of the COVID-19 pandemic and early completion of data collection, the data from the year 2021 revealed a widespread, atypical decline in all illicit drug use compared to previous years. The number of youth who reported using any drugs in the past year or in their entire lifetime decreased significantly, by 7.4% and 7.8%, respectively. There were particularly sharp declines in marijuana use (both self-described casual users and daily users), vaping (both nicotine and marijuana), cocaine, amphetamines, and tranquilizers. This study notes that prescription drugs used outside of a medical regimen are perceived by young people to be less dangerous because they are widely used for legitimate purposes. Despite this perception, their use amongst youth decreased, with a relative decline of 41% from 2020 to 2021. While the overall decline in casual or recreational drug use amongst youth during the COVID-19 pandemic is encouraging, this decline should be taken into context with the uptrend in intentional ingestions and fatalities involving drugs of abuse, suggesting that teens' impetus for using certain drugs may be shifting to more frequent instances of self-harm or self-medication.

Newer classes of drugs of abuse include synthetic opioids, synthetic cannabinoids ("K2" or "Spice"), and the synthetic cathinones, stimulants often referred to as "bath salts." Synthetic opioids, in particular fentanyl, were initially designed and produced with the intent of having stronger pain-reducing effect that was longer-lasting with fewer of the respiratory depression side effects of traditional opioids. Unfortunately, fentanyl's potency has given it a high abuse potential. National deaths associated with overdose of synthetic opioids (primarily fentanyl) have increased every year since 2014, making it by far the most common cause of deaths due to overdose in the country. Providers should realize synthetic opioids' pervasiveness and the danger they pose to teens' health.

While synthetic cannabinoids and cathinones were initially inexpensive and widely available over the internet and at local gas stations and convenience stores, use of these substances in the United States peaked around 2011, and recent studies suggests lifetime use of "bath salts" to

TABLE 171-1 Drugs of Abuse Involved in Pediatric Fatalities Reported to US Poison Centers, 2020

Age Range	Total Number of Fatality Cases	Number of Intentional Fatality Cases	Class	Substances Reported	Fatalities
≤ 5 years	37	0	Analgesics	Fentanyl, Methadone, Morphine	14
			Alcohols	Isopropanol, Ethanol	3
			Cold and Cough Preparations	Antihistamines, Dextromethorphan	3
			Stimulants and Street Drugs	Amphetamine, Methamphetamine	3
			Antidepressants	Bupropion	1
			Sedative/Hypnotics/Antipsychotics	Ketamine	1
6-12 years	9	2	Antidepressants	Bupropion, TCAs	2
			Analgesics	Acetaminophen, Codeine	1
13-19 years	90	62	Analgesics	Fentanyl, Oxycodone, Tramadol, NSAIDs, Salicylates	81
			Antidepressants	Bupropion, SSRIs, TCAs	11
			Stimulants and Street Drugs	Heroin, Cocaine, Methamphetamine, MDMA, LSD, Marijuana	10
			Cough and Cold Preparations	Antihistamines	2
			Muscle Relaxants	Methocarbamol, Baclofen	2
			Sedative/Hypnotics/Antipsychotics	Benzodiazepine, Clozapine, Benztropine, Clonidine	2

TCA, tricyclic antidepressant; SSRI, selective serotonin reuptake inhibitor; NSAID, non-steroidal anti-inflammatory drug; MDMA, methylenedioxymethamphetamine; LSD, lysergic acid diethylamide.

Source: Data from Gummin DD, Mowry JB, Beuhler MC, et al. 2020 Annual Report of the American Association of Poison Control Centers' National Poison Data System (NPDS): 38th Annual Report. *Clin Toxicol (Phila)*. 2021;59(12):1282-1501, Tables 8, 11, 17E, and 21.

be as high as 1% among high school seniors. Synthetic cannabinoid use is most strongly correlated with higher frequency marijuana use. Undetectable by commonly used serum and urine drug screens, users believed that these substances were effective as a "legal high." However, the Synthetic Drug Abuse Prevention Act of 2012 added both synthetic cannabinoids and cathinones to the Schedule I controlled substance list.

Additionally, while the previously mentioned NIDA survey results of declining cigarette, tobacco, and marijuana use among adolescents is encouraging, the CDC warns that pediatric tobacco and nicotine dependence continues to have high overall prevalence. Young adults are particularly vulnerable to developing dependence on nicotine, and almost 90% of adult tobacco users begin using before adulthood. Similar to the synthetic analogues of drugs previously mentioned, electronic cigarette use (i.e., "vaping") was initially seen as a "safer" alternative to cigarettes by the general population until the clinical syndrome of E-cigarette or Vaping Associated Lung Injury (EVALI) became public knowledge. The same public health measures that were effective for addressing tobacco use in youth (education, public policy, clinical practice, advocacy) will have to be implemented to abate e-cigarette use.

The 2019 Youth Risk Behavior Survey, a report by the CDC looking into the trends of substance use in high school students from 2009 to 2019, found that males had substantially higher rates of cocaine, methamphetamine, heroin, and intravenous drug use, whereas females had higher rates of alcohol use and binge drinking. They noted differences between racial/ethnic groups' substance use patterns, including higher alcohol misuse and binge drinking in White students and higher prescription opioid misuse in Black and Hispanic students. Universally higher rates of all types of substance use are seen among sexual and gender minority youth. These demographic differences reflect that marginalized groups are likely more vulnerable to substance use disorders due to exposure to chronic stressors. Known risk factors for adolescent substance use include child abuse or neglect, familial risk factors (parental or familial substance use, lower socioeconomic status, and perception that parents approve of child's substance use), physical or sexual abuse, and social factors (bullying, peer pressure, deviant peer relationships, and gang affiliation). Individual risk factors for substance use include mood disorders and attention-deficit hyperactivity disorder (ADHD). Results from the 2020 National Survey on Drug Use and Health emphasized an association between mental health issues and substance use, noting that adolescents who had a major depressive episode in the past year were more likely to use illicit drugs or marijuana. Stimulant medications, commonly used as treatment for ADHD (methylphenidate, dextroamphetamine, or mixed amphetamine formulations), are often abused as study aids by college students.

CLINICAL PRESENTATION

INITIAL ASSESSMENT AND HISTORY

Initial assessment of a patient who may have been exposed to any drugs of abuse follows the principles outlined in Chapter 169. Reassessment should occur periodically, even in patients who appear stable on initial evaluation. If drug absorption and distribution are not complete at the time of presentation, the clinical condition may worsen with the passage of time.

After the initial assessment, the hospitalist should attempt to elicit a complete history from the patient, if lucid and cooperative, or from a parent, guardian, or other companion who may be able to provide details of the exposure. Pre-hospital personnel may be able to shed additional light, particularly if pill containers or other items are available at the scene. A thorough history often elicits clues about specific drugs of abuse. Providers should ask what drugs and medications are in the patient's home. If patients are lucid enough to provide a history, youth will often be more comfortable discussing drug use among their friend group with clinicians as opposed to their own personal drug use; this may provide insight into potential substances the patient may be using. Exposure to drugs of abuse can occur at bars, parties, or rave dances, and in such cases "club" drugs such as MDMA or ketamine, and "date rape" drugs such as flunitrazepam (Rohypnol) or gamma hydroxybutyric acid (GHB) should be suspected.

TOXIDROMES

Patients suspected of intentional or unintentional exposure to drugs of abuse may present with symptom/sign complexes or toxic syndromes (toxidromes) that suggest a specific drug class. Commonly abused drugs and related symptoms and signs are listed in **Table 171-2**.

DIFFERENTIAL DIAGNOSIS

Although considerable symptom/sign overlap exists among the drugs listed above, a presenting toxidrome may refine the search to some degree.

A broad range of neurologic, infectious, or metabolic conditions, including seizures and postictal states, encephalitis, encephalopathy, cerebrovascular accidents, hypoglycemia (Chapter 26), and hyperammonemia can present with features of altered mental status (Chapter 18) similar to those

TABLE 171-2 Symptoms/Signs of Common Drugs of Abuse

Class	Symptoms/Signs
Alcohol	Slurred speech, ataxia, nystagmus, characteristic breath odor, lethargy, hypothermia, bradycardia, hypotension, respiratory depression, hypoglycemic seizures
Cannabinoids	
Classic cannabinoids (cannabis, THC, Delta 8 THC, CBD)	Conjunctival injection, slowed reflexes, tachycardia, xerostomia, increased appetite, sedation, distorted perception of time, paranoia
Synthetic cannabinoids (K2, Spice)	Intense psychoactive effect (including psychosis), tachycardia, agitation, anxiety, hypertension, acute kidney injury
Cough/Cold Medications (Dextromethorphan)	Ataxia, coma, drowsiness, dystonia, fever, hallucinations, miosis, respiratory depression, tachycardia, tremors
Date rape drugs	
GHB and precursors	Drowsiness, confusion, amnesia, apnea, arrhythmias, coma, respiratory depression, seizures
Rohypnol	Drowsiness, confusion, loss of motor coordination, unconsciousness, amnesia, bradycardia
E-cigarettes	EVALI: Shortness of breath, cough, chest pain, hypoxemia, hemoptysis, nausea, vomiting, diarrhea, abdominal pain, weight loss
Hallucinogens	
LSD	Visual hallucinations, distortion in perception of time and sounds, seizures, mydriasis, hyperthermia, tachycardia, hypertension, diaphoresis, sleeplessness
Psilocybin (mushrooms)	Euphoria, visual distortions, visual hallucinations, nausea, vomiting
MDMA (ecstasy)	Euphoria, empathy, talkativeness, increased sensitivity to touch, sexual arousal, muscle tension, tremors, nausea, chills, diaphoresis, dehydration
Inhalants	Arrhythmias, coma, drowsiness, encephalopathy, frostbite, paint stains, respiratory depression
Opioids	Bradycardia, coma, constipation, dizziness, histamine release, hypotension, miosis, respiratory depression
Sedatives	
Benzodiazepines, Barbiturates	Relief of anxiety, relaxed mood, sleepiness, CNS depression, respiratory depression, hypothermia
Ketamine	Dissociation from pain and sense of self, "out of body" experiences, hallucinations, hypersalivation, hypertension, nystagmus, tachycardia, amnesia, seizures
Stimulants (including prescribed stimulants, e.g., methylphenidate)	General: arrhythmias, euphoria, hallucinations, insomnia, mydriasis, nervousness, restlessness, seizures
Bath salts	Agitation, paranoia, psychosis, violent behavior
Methamphetamine	"Meth mouth" (dental decay)
Cocaine	Chest pain, nasal congestion, rhinitis

"Bath salts," synthetic cathinones; CBD, cannabidiol; EVALI, E-cigarette or Vaping Associated Lung Injury; GHB, γ-hydroxybutyrate; LSD, lysergic acid diethylamide; MDMA, methylenedioxymethamphetamine; THC, tetrahydrocannabinol.

Source: Data from Leikin JB, Paloucek FP, eds. *Poisoning & Toxicology* [electronic book for the PDA]. Hudson, OH: Lexi-Comp; 2004 and information from dea.gov.

of drug abuse. Primary cardiovascular dysfunction, including myocarditis, severe hypertension, and conduction abnormalities, can mimic some of the cardiac features of drug abuse. Acute psychiatric disorders can have overlapping signs and symptoms or may coexist with drug ingestions.

DIAGNOSTIC EVALUATION

Often initiated in the emergency department, the diagnostic evaluation may include a number of tests, including electrocardiogram, chemistry panels, and toxicology screens.

Though a cardiac rhythm strip may provide the first clues of a drug-induced arrhythmia, a 12-lead electrocardiogram should be obtained for diagnostic purposes. Urinalysis may reveal rhabdomyolysis or pregnancy. Alterations in blood chemistry, including serum glucose, electrolytes, renal and liver function tests, and cardiac enzymes, may provide additional if indirect evidence of drug toxicity, such as metabolic acidosis, hepatic failure, or cardiac ischemia.

Drugs of abuse may be detected in serum/plasma, gastric aspirates, and urine; most hospital laboratories offer a drugs-of-abuse panel to screen urine samples. A number of techniques may be used: thin-layer chromatography, high-pressure/performance liquid chromatography, immunoassay, and gas chromatography/mass spectrometry. In general, immunoassays offer high sensitivity, rapid turnaround time, low cost, and simple technical protocols, and are therefore often used to screen for drugs of abuse. Typical drugs-of-abuse immunoassay panels include amphetamines, barbiturates, benzodiazepines, cannabinoids, cocaine metabolites, methadone, opiates, oxycodone, and phencyclidine. Understanding which drugs of abuse are tested for in your institution's toxicology screen and having an index of suspicion for the toxidrome that fits your patient's clinical presentation will improve the toxicology screen's pre-test probability and lead to more meaningful results.

INACCURATE TEST RESULTS: FALSE NEGATIVE AND FALSE POSITIVE SCREENS

The hospitalist should consider the possibility of both false-negative and false-positive screening tests. False-negative results may arise because many of these immunoassay panels do not detect a number of common substances, including anabolic steroids, the benzodiazepines alprazolam, lorazepam, and flunitrazepam (Rohypnol), ethanol, β-hydroxybutyrate (GHB), ketamine, lysergic acid diethylamide (LSD), synthetic cannabinoids, "bath salts," and synthetic opioids such as fentanyl. Many of these not-detected substances have structurally similar drug analogs that are included in standard toxicology screens. For example, the screen for phencyclidine will not usually detect ketamine and the screen for opioids will not usually detect fentanyl. Thus, a "negative tox screen" may falsely reassure a hospitalist who is not familiar with the limitations of a particular laboratory's immunoassay. For this reason, clinical presentation is essential to an accurate interpretation of the toxicology screen. For instance, the presence of amnesia or coma should raise the possibility of exposure to common "date rape drugs" such as flunitrazepam, GHB, or ketamine, despite a likely negative result from the toxicology screen. Furthermore, a negative test may occur when the concentration of the metabolite falls below the federally mandated threshold or cutoff value established by the Substance Abuse and Mental Health Services Administration for that particular substance. Detection of synthetic drugs or substances that are otherwise not tested on typical toxicology screens often requires specialized laboratories using mass spectrophotometry methods.

In contrast, false-positive results may arise because immunoassays are intended to maximize sensitivity, so confirmatory testing with a highly specific technique, such as gas chromatography-mass spectrometry or high-performance liquid chromatography, should follow any positive result. Fluoroquinolones, for example, may cause a screen to be positive for opiates, whereas high concentrations of dextromethorphan may screen positive for phencyclidine. Screens may remain positive for days to weeks, depending on the drug and the pattern of use. Cocaine metabolites such as benzoylecgonine and ecgonine methylester typically persist for up to 72 hours, and cannabinoids may yield a positive test in the urine of a heavy marijuana user for weeks after the last use.

TESTING FOR CO-INGESTANTS

Plasma toxicology screens for coingestants, such as acetaminophen, acetylsalicylic acid (aspirin), alcohols (ethanol, isopropanol, methanol), barbiturates, ethylene glycol, and tricyclic antidepressants, are generally available and should be considered. For example, children may abuse easily available over-the-counter products, particularly dextromethorphan-containing cough-and-cold formulations, for their euphoric effects, but many combination products also contain acetaminophen, the toxicity of which may not be apparent on presentation.

AT-HOME DRUG TESTS

Parents or guardians who inquire about home kits that test breath, hair, saliva, or urine for drugs of abuse should be advised of the significant limitations of these products. It is important to emphasize that asymptomatic children should not be tested without their consent or assent.

MANAGEMENT

Stabilization and ongoing support of the respiratory, circulatory, and neurologic systems are fundamental management principles. An ABCDEF mnemonic, with DEF representing *d*econtamination/*d*iagnosis, *e*nhancement, and *f*ollow-up, helps guide further care of a drug-of-abuse patient (**Table 171-3**).

Enhancement is a reference to the use of drugs that serve as antidotes, including those that correct physiologic abnormalities, or to methods for enhancing elimination of the absorbed toxicant. Examples of these antidotes include naloxone (for opiates) and *N*-acetylcysteine (for acetaminophen). As an example of correcting physiologic abnormalities, dextrose should be administered to treat hypoglycemia. Enhanced elimination methods include hemodialysis, multidose activated charcoal (although indications are limited), urinary alkalinization, and whole-bowel irrigation. The latter technique uses non-absorbable polyethylene glycol in a balanced electrolyte solution, administered by mouth or via nasogastric tube, to clear the gastrointestinal tract of ingested substances. Whole-bowel irrigation may be particularly useful when the hospitalist encounters a body stuffer (drug packets hastily placed in body cavities to avoid police detection) or packer (drug packets sealed and ingested, often for transport across international borders). Specific treatment strategies are summarized in **Table 171-4**.

Follow-up refers to the importance of reviewing all consultations and laboratory investigations and ensuring appropriate disposition for a patient who has been exposed to drugs of abuse. Social workers and psychiatrists may have been consulted as part of the evaluation, and the results of some laboratory investigations, particularly "send-out" tests, may not be available immediately on admission to the hospital. Appropriate disposition may require inpatient detoxification services or follow-up with a primary care provider or toxicology clinic.

CONSULTATION

The hospitalist should consider regional poison control center (1-800-222-1222) and medical toxicology consultation, which may provide clinically relevant guidance about management and disposition of the patient and may be aware of local trends in the use or abuse of certain substances. Calls to the regional poison control center also help document exposures that contribute to the annual statistics reported to the American Association of Poison Control Centers.

TABLE 171-3 Priorities in the General Approach to a Poisoned Patient

	Priority	Examples of Interventions
A	*Airway*	Endotracheal intubation
B	*Breathing*	Supplemental oxygen, ventilatory support
C	*Circulation*	Antiarrhythmics, pressor support
D	*Decontamination*	Activated charcoal, whole-bowel irrigation
E	*Enhancement*	Dextrose Antidotes Enhanced elimination Hemodialysis Multidose-activated charcoal Urinary alkalinization Whole-bowel irrigation
F	*Follow-up*	Social work/Psychiatric consultations Laboratory and toxicology screen results Inpatient detox(ification) Toxicology clinic Outpatient follow-up Primary care provider

TABLE 171-4 Management Strategies for Drugs of Abuse

Class	Monitor for	Treatment
Alcohol	Respiratory depression Hypoglycemia	Supportive care
Cannabinoids (particularly synthetic)	Agitation AKI Seizures	Decreased stimulation, reassurance Fluid repletion Benzodiazepines
Cough/Cold Medications	Respiratory depression Dystonia	Naloxone Diphenhydramine
Date rape drugs (GHB & Rohypnol)	Apnea	Respiratory support
E-cigarettes (EVALI)	Hypoxemia	Systemic glucocorticoids Respiratory support
Hallucinogens MDMA (ecstasy)	 Dehydration Hyponatremia	 Fluid repletion
Inhalants	Apnea Arrhythmias	Respiratory support Avoid catecholamine stimulation of sensitized myocardium
Opioids	Apnea	Naloxone, respiratory support
Sedatives Benzodiazepines	 Respiratory depression	 Respiratory support Flumazenil (caution as this may precipitate seizures)
Barbiturates Ketamine	Respiratory depression Hypersalivation Hypertension/emergence reactions/seizures	Respiratory support Atropine Benzodiazepines
Stimulants	Arrhythmias Seizures	Lidocaine (caution if cocaine exposed) Sodium bicarbonate Benzodiazepines

AKI, acute kidney injury; EVALI, E-cigarette or Vaping Associated Lung Injury; GHB, γ-hydroxybutyrate; MDMA, methylenedioxymethamphetamine.

Source: Data from Leikin JB, Paloucek FP, eds. *Poisoning & Toxicology* [electronic book for the PDA]. Hudson, OH: Lexi-Comp; 2004.

ADMISSION CRITERIA

Hospitalization is indicated for either of the following reasons:

- Altered mental status or vital signs that do not return to baseline within 4 to 6 hours of presentation
- Exposures that require prolonged monitoring or therapy (e.g., acetaminophen coingestion, which presents a risk for hepatotoxicity and requires a course of *N*-acetylcysteine)

DISCHARGE CRITERIA

- Mental status and vital signs returned to baseline
- All pending laboratory investigations reviewed
- Social work/psychiatric consultations completed (if appropriate) and discussion and resolution of the need for an inpatient detoxification program
- Primary care provider contacted, and outpatient follow-up arranged

TABLE 171-5 Online Information and Prevention Resources (Accessed September 2022)

Organization	Internet Address (URL)
Al-Anon	*alateen.org*
American Academy of Pediatrics	*healthychildren.org*
American Association of Poison Control Centers	*aapcc.org*
Monitoring the Future	*monitoringthefuture.org*
National Institute on Drug Abuse	*drugabuse.gov*
Partnership for a Drug-Free America	drugfree.org
Substance Abuse and Mental Health Services Administration	*samhsa.gov*
U.S. Drug Enforcement Administration	*dea.gov*
World Anti-Doping Agency	*wada-ama.org*

PREVENTION

Preventive strategies should always be considered to prevent the morbidity and mortality associated with drug abuse. Many reliable online resources are available (**Table 171-5**) to provide accurate information about drugs of abuse and the risks associated with them. However, consumers should be aware that internet searches might direct children to websites, such as the Vaults of Erowid, that may contain disinformation about drugs of abuse.

KEY POINTS

- Suspicion of exposure to drugs of abuse should be prompted by signs and symptoms as well as by associated risk factors such as age (<25 years), smoking, social setting (dance clubs, bars), and alcohol ingestion.
- Toxicology screens should be ordered judiciously and interpreted cautiously because false-positive and false-negative results are important considerations and vary by the method of testing performed.
- Drugs of abuse are often ingested or inhaled along with other medications. Common coingestants include acetaminophen, aspirin, and alcohols.
- Consultation with a regional poison control center or medical toxicologist provides clinically relevant guidance about management and disposition of the patient; in addition, such resources may be aware of local trends in the use or abuse of certain substances.

SUGGESTED READINGS

Ahmad FB, Cisewski JA, Rossen LM, Sutton P. Provisional drug overdose death counts. National Center for Health Statistics. 2022. Designed by LM Rossen, A Lipphardt, FB Ahmad, JM Keralis, and Y Chong: National Center for Health Statistics.

Amaro H, Sanchez M, Bautista T, et al. Social vulnerabilities for substance use: stressors, socially toxic environments, and discrimination and racism. *Neuropharmacology*. 2021;188:108518. Available at: https://www.sciencedirect.com/science/article/pii/S0028390821000721.

Charach A, Yeung E, Climans T, et al. Childhood attention-deficit/hyperactivity disorder and future substance use disorders: comparative meta-analyses. *J Am Acad Child Adolesc Psychiatry*. 2011;50(1):9-21.

Gummin D, Mowry J, Beuhler M, et al. 2020 Annual Report of the American Association of Poison Control Centers' National Poison Data System (NPDS): 38th Annual Report. *Clin Toxicol (Phila)*. 2021;59(12):1282-1501.

Johnston L, Miech R, O'Malley P, et al. Monitoring the Future national survey results on drug use 1975-2021: Overview, key findings on adolescent drug use. Ann Arbor: Institute for Social Research, University of Michigan; 2022.

Jones C, Clayton H, Deputy N, et al. Prescription opioid misuse and use of alcohol and other substances among high school students—Youth Risk Behavior Survey, United States, 2019. *MMWR Suppl.* 2020;69(1):38-46.

Kann L, McManus T, Harris WA, et al. Youth Risk Behavior Surveillance—United States, 2017. *MMWR Surveill Summ*. 2018;67(8):1-114.

Reisner S, Greytak E, Parsons J, et al. Gender minority social stress in adolescence: disparities in adolescent bullying and substance use by gender identity. *J Sex Res*. 2015;52:243-256.

Substance Abuse and Mental Health Services Administration. Key substance use and mental health indicators in the United States: results from the 2020 National Survey on Drug Use and Health (HHS Publication No. PEP21-07-01-003, NSDUH Series H-56). Rockville, MD: Center for Behavioral Health Statistics and Quality, Substance Abuse and Mental Health Services Administration; 2021. Retrieved from https://www.samhsa.gov/data/.

Tobacco Use: Consideration for Clinicians. American Academy of Pediatricians. Last updated: Mar. 8, 2022. Accessed: Sept. 27, 2022. https://www.aap.org/en/patient-care/tobacco-control-and-prevention/youth-tobacco-cessation/tobacco-use-considerations-for-clinicians/.

Washio Y, Fairfax-Columbo J, Ball E, et al. A review of guidelines on home drug testing web sites for parents. *J Addict Med*. 2014;8(4):258-63.

Whitesell M, Bachand A, Peel J, et al. Familial, social, and individual factors contributing to risk for adolescent substance use. *J Addict*. 2013;2013:579310.

CHAPTER 172 Withdrawal Syndromes

Laura Piper, MD

BACKGROUND

Drug withdrawal is a physiologic response to an effectively lowered drug concentration in a patient tolerant to the drug in question. Withdrawal results in a predictable constellation of symptoms that are reversible if the drug is reintroduced. The symptoms of withdrawal are a phenomenon of altered neurochemistry most commonly affecting the central nervous system.

Clinicians may encounter withdrawal symptoms as the primary reason for hospitalization or as a consequence of hospitalization when intentional or unintentional interruption of drug use occurs. Withdrawal syndromes are well known to occur in hospitalized patients, particularly those admitted in intensive care units (ICUs). Many pediatric ICU patients who receive sedative infusions of opioids or benzodiazepines experience withdrawal symptoms, with a reported incidence of iatrogenic withdrawal as high as 73%. Patients who have received infusions for at least 48 hours or intermittent dosing of sedation and analgesia for 5 days are at higher risk for withdrawal. Avoidance of oversedation and appropriate medication tapering may reduce the incidence of drug withdrawal in hospitalized children who are receiving opioid and benzodiazepine sedation. Additionally, in recent decades overuse and abuse of prescription opioids have been epidemic in North America, Europe, and Australia, opioid withdrawal has become a recognized issue associated with prescription opioid abuse and may be encountered in hospitalized adolescents.

This chapter focuses on syndromes associated with withdrawal from the following classes of agents: ethanol, sedative-hypnotics (e.g., benzodiazepines, baclofen, barbiturates), opioids, and selective serotonin reuptake inhibitors (SSRIs).

CLINICAL PRESENTATION

The onset, progression, duration, and severity of withdrawal symptoms depend on the patient's degree of tolerance and the half-life of the drug involved. In general, drugs with shorter half-lives produce withdrawal

TABLE 172-1 Expected Onset and Duration of Withdrawal Symptoms by Agent in Children

	Symptom Onset	Duration
Alcohol	Hours	5-7 days
Alprazolam	12-48 hours	3-7 days
Baclofen	Hours to days	Resolves with treatment, without it results in high risk of mortality
Diazepam	4-48 hours	3-10 days
Lorazepam	12-48 hours	3-10 days
Heroin/morphine	Hours	3-5 days
Methadone	1-2 days	5-7 days
Phenobarbital	7-10 days	3-10 days
GHB/GBL	Hours	5-10 days

GBL, γ-butyrolactone; GHB, γ-hydroxybutyric acid.

symptoms sooner after discontinuation, and symptoms tend to be more severe (**Table 172-1**).

ETHANOL WITHDRAWAL

Ethanol, or alcohol, withdrawal, though rare in children, is one of the most common withdrawal syndromes in the general population, behind those of nicotine and caffeine. Pediatric alcohol withdrawal is most frequently seen in neonates born to alcohol abusing mothers. See section below on neonatal withdrawal syndromes for further details.

SEDATIVE-HYPNOTIC WITHDRAWAL

Sedative-hypnotic agents include benzodiazepines, baclofen, barbiturates, γ-hydroxybutyric acid (GHB), and γ-butyrolactone (GBL). Withdrawal from these drugs may be indistinguishable from alcohol withdrawal because the presenting symptoms are nearly identical. Sedative-hypnotic withdrawal symptoms include tremulousness, altered mental status, agitation, insomnia, hypertension, tachycardia, diaphoresis, and in severe cases seizures. Chronology may offer a clue to differentiating the cause of withdrawal between different sedative-hypnotics. Because of rapid metabolism and the lack of active metabolites, withdrawal from GHB or GBL generally occurs within 2 to 6 hours of cessation of use. In contrast, diazepam has active metabolites, and thus withdrawal symptoms may occur within several hours but might not be manifested for >24 hours.

Baclofen withdrawal can occur within hours to days of drug interruption for either oral baclofen or intrathecal baclofen and can rapidly progress. It has a high rate of morbidity and mortality; prompt recognition is imperative. The signs and symptoms of baclofen withdrawal are nonspecific and include pruritis, hyperthermia, psychiatric symptoms including hallucination, anxiety and paranoia, hyperreflexia, tremors, headache, paresthesias, seizures, altered mental status, bradycardia or tachycardia, hypotension or hypertension, nausea, vomiting, diarrhea, rhabdomyolysis, and respiratory failure. Typically, withdrawal from oral baclofen will have milder symptoms than withdrawal from intrathecal baclofen. Mild symptoms of baclofen withdrawal include worsening spasticity, fever, nausea, weakness, and autonomic instability. Severe symptoms include hallucinations, delirium, seizures, muscle rigidity, rhabdomyolysis, and severe autonomic instability. Left untreated baclofen withdrawal can rapidly progress to multisystem organ failure, cardiac arrest, respiratory failure, and death. While severe symptoms of baclofen withdrawal are more often seen with intrathecal baclofen because of human error, pump malfunction, migration of the intrathecal catheter, or removal of the pump, if mild symptoms of baclofen withdrawal are not recognized and treated severe symptoms may result.

OPIOID WITHDRAWAL

Opioid withdrawal can be divided into physical signs and symptoms and psychological symptoms. Physical signs and symptoms of opioid withdrawal include piloerection, yawning, lacrimation nausea, vomiting, and diarrhea; psychological symptoms may include dysphoria, emotional distress, sleep disturbances, drug cravings, anxiety, and restlessness. Infants may exhibit irritability, crying, insomnia, and poor feeding. Although there is no plausible pathophysiologic explanation for such, seizure has been well described in association with opioid withdrawal in infants. Opioid withdrawal in any other age patient is never associated with alteration of sensorium or seizure.

Withdrawing patients also have intense opioid craving associated with the feeling of being unwell. In contrast to sedative-hypnotic withdrawal, opioid withdrawal is associated with minimal autonomic instability. Patients may be tachycardic and have a slight elevation in blood pressure, but this is partly in response to the additional physical and emotional symptoms associated with opioid withdrawal (e.g., cravings, anxiety). In further contrast to withdrawal from sedative-hypnotics, opioid withdrawal is associated with normal mental status other than agitation.

Opioid withdrawal may occur in a gradual manner when discontinuation begins or may occur abruptly with severe symptoms if an opioid antagonist such as naloxone or naltrexone is administered to an opioid-tolerant patient. Opioid-tolerant adolescents with precipitated withdrawal secondary to naloxone or other opioid antagonists may exhibit extreme psychomotor agitation or become violent.

SELECTIVE SEROTONIN REUPTAKE INHIBITOR WITHDRAWAL

Withdrawal to SSRIs has also been described and is likely related to temporary and self-limited serotonin dysregulation. Signs and symptoms include dizziness, gastrointestinal disturbances, headaches, lethargy, anxiety, or agitation (or both), paresthesias, tremors, sweating, insomnia, irritability, and poor feeding. SSRI withdrawal symptoms usually begin within 1 week of abrupt cessation of treatment; symptoms generally resolve within 3 weeks. Most reports of SSRI withdrawal are specific to venlafaxine, but the syndrome, which occurs in both neonates and children, has also been reported with citalopram, fluoxetine, fluvoxamine, paroxetine, and sertraline.

NEONATAL WITHDRAWAL SYNDROMES

Maternal addiction can lead to neonatal withdrawal. The time to symptom presentation after birth varies with the agent in question and many of the withdrawal syndromes can have similar symptoms in neonates. Neonatal alcohol withdrawal and both opioid and sedative-hypnotic withdrawal are often very similar. Neonatal opioid withdrawal (abstinence) syndrome is discussed in Chapter 131.

Neonatal alcohol withdrawal typically begins within 3 days of parturition. The neonatal alcohol withdrawal syndrome should be considered a spectrum; the discrete symptoms of alcohol withdrawal can follow a progression or occur independently. Symptoms most typically include agitation, irritability, crying, tremors, tachycardia, hypertension, insomnia, diaphoresis, poor sucking, and poor feeding. Nystagmus, clonus, seizures, hypertonia, hyperactive or asymmetric reflexes, excessive rooting, diarrhea, vomiting, and inability to thermoregulate may also occur. Opisthotonos and abdominal distention rarely occur in opioid withdrawal and can help differentiate the two when the mother has abused multiple substances. Although initially thought to occur only as a complication of fetal alcohol syndrome (FAS), neonatal alcohol withdrawal can occur independently of FAS. The presentation of neonates withdrawing from sedative-hypnotics such as benzodiazepines or barbiturates would be clinically similar to neonatal alcohol withdrawal.

Withdrawal from caffeine, inhalants, and SSRIs has also been reported in neonates. It is estimated that 20% to 30% of newborns exposed in the third trimester are affected. Symptoms include jitteriness, agitation, crying, shivering, increased muscle tone, difficulty with breathing and sucking, and seizures.

DIFFERENTIAL DIAGNOSIS

The withdrawal symptoms described have some distinguishing and overlapping features (**Table 172-2**). Further, a number of nontoxic disorders may be mistaken for withdrawal (**Table 172-3**), and certain toxic agents

TABLE 172-2 Vital Signs and Mental Status Changes in Withdrawal

	Opioids	Sedative/Hypnotics	Alcohol
Heart rate	↑	↑↑	↑↑
Blood pressure	↑	↑↑	↑↑
Respiratory rate	↑	↑↑	↑↑
Hyperthermia	–	+	+
Altered mental status	–	+/–	+/–

TABLE 172-4 Poisoning Syndromes That May Mimic Withdrawal Syndromes

Amphetamines
Carbamates
Cocaine
Lithium
Organophosphates
Salicylates
Theophylline

can mimic withdrawal symptoms (**Table 172-4**). Organophosphate poisoning can result in constricted pupils, diaphoresis, vomiting, agitation, seizures, and altered mental status. This combination of symptoms could be confused for either opioid or sedative-hypnotic withdrawal. Similarly, sympathomimetic intoxication can present in a manner similar to sedative-hypnotic withdrawal and create the same diagnostic dilemma. Additionally, a patient with anticholinergic toxicity may present with hallucinations, tachycardia, and hyperthermia, a combination of symptoms that may be confused for sedative-hypnotic withdrawal.

Symptoms associated with SSRI withdrawal may be difficult to distinguish from features of the underlying anxiety or depressive disorder or side effects of the therapy, especially in patients with unreliable medication adherence. When the timing of SSRI discontinuation is known, it is easier to distinguish withdrawal symptoms (usually within 1 week) from relapse of depression (more commonly after 2 or more weeks). Withdrawal symptoms are uncommon in patients who have been taking SSRIs for less than 7 weeks.

MANAGEMENT

ETHANOL AND SEDATIVE-HYPNOTIC WITHDRAWAL

Different sedative-hypnotic agents often share enough common receptor or metabolic activity that one drug can be substituted for the other in treatment of withdrawal—a phenomenon known as cross-tolerance.

Mild to moderate ethanol or sedative-hypnotic withdrawal usually responds well to low-dose oral benzodiazepines. Benzodiazepines are also preferred to treat benzodiazepine withdrawal, and barbiturates are used for barbiturate withdrawal. Various treatment regimens exist, including fix-scheduled and symptom-triggered regimens. Studies demonstrate that "front-loading" benzodiazepines by giving diazepam in repeated doses on an hourly basis until the patient is asymptomatic relieves withdrawal symptoms more promptly than fixed-schedule treatment alone does. Additionally, symptom-triggered therapy has been demonstrated to be superior to fixed-dose regimens due to the wide variety in withdrawal severity and the amount of medication needed to control symptoms. Patients who experience benzodiazepine or barbiturate withdrawal in the setting of chronic or intensive care may be treated by reinstituting the infusion or dosing of the drug that they were taking before withdrawal symptoms and then tapering the dose of the drug, typically by 10% daily.

Propofol is effective in the treatment of alcohol, benzodiazepine, barbiturate, and GHB withdrawal in adults. Due to the infrequency of these withdrawal syndromes in children, there is little clinical experience with propofol treatment, and potential risk of propofol infusion syndrome in patients receiving prolonged infusions. Therefore, propofol should be considered only for ethanol or sedative-hypnotic withdrawal in adolescents. In particular for GHB withdrawal, which is severe and life threatening, propofol may be considered second-line therapy if benzodiazepine treatment is inadequate.

TABLE 172-3 Nontoxic Differential Diagnosis of Sedative-Hypnotic Withdrawal

Hypoglycemia
Encephalitis
Hypomagnesemia
Meningitis
Neuroleptic malignant syndrome
Pneumonia
Serotonin syndrome
Thyrotoxicosis

Baclofen withdrawal is unique because cross-tolerance between baclofen and benzodiazepines or barbiturates is much less than that of other sedative-hypnotics. Baclofen withdrawal, which is more frequently severe and life threatening than benzodiazepine withdrawal, should be treated with the same dosing of baclofen used before withdrawal symptoms. If baclofen cannot be administered immediately, such as in circumstances of a failed intrathecal pump or inability to take enteral medications, high-dose benzodiazepines should be used until baclofen can be restarted. Propofol and cyproheptadine have also been used in the treatment of baclofen withdrawal.

Dexmedetomidine is a sedative that exerts its effect by centrally acting α-adrenergic antagonism. Dexmedetomidine has been postulated to reduce withdrawal-related symptoms from opioids or clonidine due to the similarity in mechanism of action and the nonlethal nature of opioid withdrawal. However, studies to date have not found that it significantly modifies the prevalence of withdrawal symptoms in children. Due to its lack of GABA agonist activity, dexmedetomidine should not be considered safe or appropriate to treat withdrawal from ethanol, benzodiazepines, barbiturates, or other sedative-hypnotic drugs.

Specific dosing recommendations are provided in **Table 172-5**.

OPIOID

Opioid withdrawal is best treated with an opioid of similar potency and equal or longer duration of action. In neonates, a neonatal opiate solution containing an aqueous solution of morphine sulfate is often used, although older more traditional treatment uses tincture of opium or paregoric (Chapter 131).

Beyond the neonatal period, patients who experience opioid withdrawal in the setting of chronic use or intensive care may be treated by reinstituting the infusion or dosing of the drug that they were taking before withdrawal symptoms and then tapering the dose, typically by 10% daily. Oral opioids may also be used and can be dosed similarly by using morphine equivalents. In the treatment of withdrawal symptoms, medications with a longer half-life are expected to be more useful, with the understanding that inadvertent oversedation would also be of longer duration if it occurred. Oral morphine is the oral opioid with the most established record in treatment of opioid withdrawal. Although it is used extensively with physiologic success to treat adults and adolescents, use in younger children is not well established.

Methadone is a preferred treatment of withdrawal in adolescents and adults. It has also been examined as potentially useful to prevent or treat pediatric opioid withdrawal and recently has become a preferred opioid weaning agent. However, the comparative effectiveness of methadone to alternatives remains unknown due to a lack of studies.

Buprenorphine is an opioid receptor agonist-antagonist intended to ease withdrawal symptoms and encourage abstinence in a manner similar to methadone. However, as a partial agonist, buprenorphine users do not experience euphoria or the desired high associated with methadone or other opioids. Buprenorphine is administered by specially licensed dispensing physicians. It is safe and effective for treating adolescent opioid withdrawal.

TABLE 172-5 Pharmacologic Therapy for Withdrawal

Drug Causing Withdrawal	Therapeutic Agent Used	Dose
Alcohol	Diazepam	0.1 mg/kg IV q30min
		Double dose every third administration until sedate
Sedative-hypnotic drugs		Once sedate, continue last dose administered q1h as needed for agitation
Benzodiazepines		Taper dose by 10% daily
Barbiturates	Phenobarbital	Loading dose of 20 mg/kg IV, followed by maintenance dosing of 2-8 mg/kg/day
		Taper dose by 10% daily
Baclofen	Baclofen	Same dose and route used before withdrawal
	Benzodiazepine	Administer high-dose benzodiazepine until baclofen can be administered. Adult dosing: Diazepam IV 2mg-10mgq6h or Lorazepam 0.5-2mg q6h.
	Propofol	IV: 20–200 µg/kg/min
	Cyproheptadine	PO: 4-8 mg q6h, should not exceed 0.5mg/kg/day
Caffeine	Caffeine	Caffeine as a soft drink or tea taken to treat headache or agitation
		Neonates: no treatment
Opioid-neonatal	Paregoric	0.1 mL/kg of a 0.4-mg/mL solution q4h with feeding
		Dose may be doubled to control symptoms
		After 3-5 days, taper by decreasing the dose without altering the frequency of administration
	Tincture of opium	Diluted solution (1:25) at 0.1 mL/kg orally with feeding q4h
		Dosing may be doubled to control symptoms
		After 3-5 days, taper by decreasing the dose without altering the frequency of administration
	Methadone	0.05-0.1 mg/kg PO (max 20 mg) given q6h until symptoms are controlled
		Then dose daily, weaning dose to 0.05 mg/kg/day
		Discontinue drug at that point and self-taper will occur
	Morphine	Orally administered to deliver the same morphine-equivalent dose as paregoric
		Dosing may be doubled to control symptoms
		After 3-5 days, taper by decreasing the dose without altering the frequency of administration
Selective serotonin reuptake inhibitor (SSRI)		Children: Administer the same agent in the same dose used before withdrawal
		Taper by 10% daily
		Neonates: No consensus on treatment of neonates
		Diazepam may be used

Opioid withdrawal symptoms acutely precipitated by naloxone use require only supportive care. Although the patient may be uncomfortable or agitated, the duration of action of naloxone is brief, and symptoms typically improve within 10 to 45 minutes. If patients experience vomiting, parenteral ondansetron or other anti-emetics may be used. Under no circumstances should opioids be administered in an attempt to overcome the antagonist activity of naloxone. Due to the risk of oversedation when the naloxone effect has dissipated, it is recommended to simply wait for improvement.

Adolescents for whom an opioid-tapering plan is judged undesirable may be symptomatically supported through the withdrawal process. It is possible to control most of the unpleasant symptoms of opioid withdrawal using non-opioids. Clonidine (oral or transcutaneous patch) works by central α-adrenergic agonism to decrease sympathetic outflow and has a well-proven record of safety and moderate efficacy. Dexmedetomidine, another central α_2-adrenergic agonist, has been hypothesized to have similar usefulness in opioid withdrawal. However, the role of dexmedetomidine and its benefits are much less defined, so caution should be used until clinicians have gained familiarity and experience using this medication to treat withdrawal symptoms. Anti-emetics are needed to treat symptoms of significant opioid withdrawal, and ondansetron safety and efficacy make it preferred for this purpose.

SELECTIVE SEROTONIN REUPTAKE INHIBITORS

Primary prevention of withdrawal symptoms can often be accomplished by slowly tapering the SSRI. Recommended strategies for managing mild withdrawal symptoms include reassurance; patients may be relieved to understand that the symptoms are not related to relapse or reactions to coincidental life events and that resolution is likely within days. If withdrawal symptoms are not well tolerated, re-initiation of therapeutic doses followed by a more slowly tapered dosing regimen may be appropriate. In some cases, substitution of a longer-acting SSRI (e.g., fluoxetine) may be needed to complete a slow discontinuation program.

Neonatal SSRI abstinence syndrome is described with irritability, crying, shivering, insomnia, increased muscle tone, poor feeding, and seizures reported in association. Optimal treatment is undefined, and management may consist of supportive care only with no medications, or use of benzodiazepines or barbiturates. Administration of SSRI to an infant or neonate is not recommended. Chapter 131, Neonatal Abstinence Syndrome, contains more information.

ADMISSION CRITERIA

- Withdrawal symptoms in a neonate
- Initial presentation of withdrawal from a sedative-hypnotic agent, including benzodiazepines, baclofen, barbiturates, ethanol, GHB, or any similar drug
- Withdrawal associated with derangement of vital signs beyond acceptable limits that are not corrected with outpatient congruent therapy, such as oral medication or patch treatment

DISCHARGE CRITERIA

- Stability of vital signs and neurologic symptoms that can be maintained with outpatient congruent therapy, such as oral medication or patch treatment

KEY POINTS

- Withdrawal from substances that have γ-aminobutyric acid activity, including benzodiazepines, baclofen, barbiturates, alcohol, GHB, and similar drugs, can produce life-threatening withdrawal symptoms.
- Withdrawal from sedative-hypnotic drugs may progress rapidly from mild symptoms to severe or life-threatening withdrawal. Failure to estimate the potential severity of withdrawal because of initially mild symptoms, could be catastrophic.
- Withdrawal from opioids should not result in alteration of cognition, although changes in mood and behavior typically occur.
- A number of drug overdose syndromes (e.g., ethanol) may cause poisoning that mimics sedative-hypnotic withdrawal.
- Treatment of withdrawal varies but includes supportive care, tapering medications, and fixed dosing.

SUGGESTED READINGS

Coffey RJ, Edgar TS, Francisco GE, et al. Abrupt withdrawal from intrathecal baclofen: recognition and management of a potentially life-threatening syndrome. *Arch Phys Med Rehabil*. 2002;83:735-741.

Coles CD, Smith IE, Fernhoff PM, et al. Neonatal ethanol withdrawal: characteristics in clinically normal, nondysmorphic neonates. *J Pediatr*. 1984;105:445-451.

Conrad P, et al. Iatrogenic withdrawal syndrome in specialty pediatric critical care. *Appl Nurs Res*. 2020;55: 151284.

Dervan LA, et al. The use of methadone to facilitate opioid weaning in pediatric critical care patients: a systematic review of the literature and meta-analysis. *Paediatr Anaesth*. 2017; 27(3): 228-239.

Dyer JE, Roth B, Hyma BA. Gamma-hydroxybutyrate withdrawal syndrome. *Ann Emerg Med*. 2001;37:147-153.

Dyer JE, Roth B, Hyma BA. Gamma-hydroxybutyrate withdrawal syndrome. *Ann Emerg Med*. 2001;37:147-153.

Fenn NE 3rd, Plake KS. Opioid and benzodiazepine weaning in pediatric patients: review of current literature. *Pharmacotherapy*. 2017;37(11):1458-1468.

Fernandez-Carrion F, Gaboli M, Gonzalez-Celador R, et al. Withdrawl syndrome in the pediatric intensive care unit, incidence and risk factors. *Med Intensiva*. 2013;37:67-74.

Geven BM, et al. Dexmedetomidine and iatrogenic withdrawal syndrome in critically ill children. *Crit Care Nurse*. 2021;41(1): e17-e23.

Glue P, Nutt D. Overexcitement and disinhibition. Dynamic neurotransmitter interactions in alcohol withdrawal. *Br J Psychiatry*. 1990;157:491-499.

Grant MJ, Balas MC, Curley MA, RESTORE Investigative Team. Defining sedation-related adverse events in the pediatric intensive care unit. *Heart Lung*. 2013;42:171-176.

Haddad P. The SSRI discontinuation syndrome. *J Psychopharmacol*. 1998;12:305-313.

Jeffries SA, McGloin R, Pitfield AF, Carr RR. Use of methadone for prevention of opioid withdrawal in critically ill children. *Can J Hosp Pharm*. 2012;65:12-18.

Khan NA, Sullivan MA, Vitale MG, Tresgallo ME, Saroyan JM. Undetected Ultracet dependence in an adolescent with nonmalignant back pain. *J Opioid Manag*. 2013;9:225-230.

Manikant S, Tripathi BM, Chavan BS. Loading dose diazepam therapy for alcohol withdrawal state. *Indian J Med Res*. 1993;98:170-173.

Mayo-Smith MF. Pharmacological management of alcohol withdrawal. A meta-analysis and evidence-based practice guideline. American Society of Addiction Medicine Working Group on Pharmacological Management of Alcohol Withdrawal. *JAMA*. 1997;278:144-151.

Mondardini MC, et al. Dexmedetomidine for prevention of opioid/benzodiazepine withdrawal syndrome in pediatric intensive care unit: interim analysis of a randomized controlled trial. *Pharmacotherapy*. 2022;42(2):145-153.

Motamed M, Marsch LA, Solhkhah R, Bickel WK Badger GJ. Differences in treatment outcomes between opioid-dependent and heroin-dependent adolescents. *J Addict Med*. 2008;2:158-164.

Nordeng H, Lindeman R, Perminov KV, Reikvam A. Neonatal withdrawal syndrome after in utero exposure to selective serotonin reuptake inhibitors. *Acta Paediatr*. 2001;90:288-291.

Nordent H, Lindemann R, Perminov KV, Reikvan A. Neonatal withdrawal syndrome after in utero exposure to selective serotonin reuptake inhibitors. *Acta Paediatr*. 2001;90:288-291.

Oschman A, McCabe T, Kuhn RJ. Dexmedetomidine for opioid and benzodiazepine withdrawal in pediatric patients. *Am J Health Sys Pharm*. 2011;68:1233-1238.

Romito JW, Turner ER, Rosener JA, et al. Baclofen therapeutics, toxicity, and withdrawal: a narrative review. *SAGE Open Med*. 2021;9:20503121211022197.

Rosenbaum JF, Zajecka J. Clinical management of antidepressant discontinuation. *J Clin Psychiatry*. 1997;58(suppl 7):37-40.

Sanz EJ, De-las-Cuevas C, Kiuru A, et al. Selective serotonin reuptake inhibitors in pregnant women and neonatal withdrawal syndrome: a database analysis. *Lancet*. 2005;365:482-487.

Scott CS, Decker JL, Edwards ML, Freid EB. Withdrawal after narcotic therapy: a survey of neonatal and pediatric clinicians. *Pharmacotherapy*. 1998;28:1308-1312.

Tobias JD. Tolerance, withdrawal, and physical dependency after long-term sedation and analgesia of children in the pediatric intensive care unit. *Crit Care Med*. 2000;28:2122-2132.

Vet NJ, Ista E, de Weldt SN, et al. Optimal sedation in pediatric intensive care patients: a systematic review. *Intensive Care Med*. 2013;39(9):1524-34.

Zajecka J, Tracey KA, Mitchell S. Discontinuation symptoms after treatment with serotonin reuptake inhibitors: a literature review. *J Clin Psychiatry*. 1997;58:291-297.

CHAPTER 173 Fire-Related Inhalation Injury

Adriana Herrera, MD, MPH and Eric Zwemer, MD

BACKGROUND

Fire-related injury is the fourth leading cause of unintentional injury death among children of all races in the United States, killing about 500 children under the age of 14 each year. Injury to the skin can be just one facet of the potentially multisystem insults that occur. Inhalation injury and subsequent secondary pneumonia are the leading cause of death in house fires, with mortality rates of approximately 5% to 8%. The physiological mechanisms of inhalation-related injuries have not been well-defined. Few human studies have been conducted. As a result, reliable, proven concrete diagnostic criteria, directed therapeutic interventions, and prognostic indicators for survivors of fire-related inhalation injuries have not been developed. This chapter will review inhalation injury associated with fires and incomplete combustion, specifically, thermal airway injuries, smoke inhalation, carbon monoxide (CO), and cyanide poisoning. Dermal burns are discussed in Chapter 163.

PATHOPHYSIOLOGY

Smoke inhalation causes injuries through multiple mechanisms, and the high minute ventilation in children puts them at increased risk for smoke inhalation injury when compared to adults. Direct tissue injury, immune response, chemical exposure, and systemic sequelae of inhaled toxins need to be considered when addressing inhalation injuries. Complicating these injuries are the neurologic sequelae from hypoxic brain injury that can result from inhalation of oxygen-deprived gas, in addition to secondary lung infection and acute respiratory failure occurring days after the initial injury. Injury due to smoke inhalation can be categorized into three physiological types: thermal injury occurring predominantly in the supraglottic airway, chemical injury seen in the subglottic airway, and systemic sequelae of inhalation of toxic gases.

SUPRAGLOTTIC AIRWAY: DIRECT THERMAL INJURY

The upper airways and the trachea can dissipate heat very effectively, and direct thermal injury is uncommon. However, when it does occur, injury is often limited to structures above the carina. Swelling of these structures ensues in the hours following the injury and can result in critical upper airway obstruction.

SUBGLOTTIC AIRWAY: CHEMICAL INJURY

Even without dermal burns or upper airway injury, significant lower airway involvement can occur in a child who inhales toxic particles in smoke. Household items such as cleaning products and fabrics release smaller particles that can reach the lower airways and lung parenchyma and can cause delayed injury. These irritants and gases can cause direct mucosal injury, inflammation, edema, interference with surfactant production, and loss of normal protective ciliary action. Inhalation injuries can also trigger local reactive oxygen species, which in turn propagate the release of cytokines and pro-inflammatory molecules. This inflammatory cascade results in tissue-level effects including bronchorrhea-induced alveolar flooding, bronchial exudate, cast formation, bronchospasm, and vasospasm. The injuries to the respiratory epithelium, along with impaired ciliary clearance, lead to debris accumulation from mucosal sloughing. As a result, occlusions of the small airway and atelectasis lead to ventilation-perfusion mismatching and predispose lung tissue to infection. Acute respiratory failure can also occur due to development of Acute Respiratory Distress Syndrome (ARDS), which can be seen 4 to 8 days after initial burn injury. In addition, cytokine release can lead to distributive shock if the patient is not adequately fluid resuscitated. Despite surviving the initial stages of inhalation injury, these secondary effects of inhalation injury are what contribute the most to in-hospital mortality.

SYSTEMIC EFFECTS OF INHALED TOXINS

The cytokine-mediated inflammatory response to dermal and inhalation fire injury is further exacerbated by the inhalation of toxins. When inhalation of common household toxins, such as CO and cyanide, goes unrecognized or is not properly treated, the systemic effects can be lethal.

Carbon Monoxide CO is a colorless, odorless gas produced from the incomplete combustion of carbon-containing substances. Other important sources of CO exposure include car exhaust fumes, furnaces, and wood-burning stoves. Cases tend to rise in winter months or with natural disasters associated with power outages. Alternative methods of heating and cooking and snow-obstructed motor vehicle exhaust systems are more common under these conditions.

CO is rapidly absorbed and acts as a systemic toxin disrupting both hemoglobin's oxygen-carrying capacity and cellular metabolism. CO binds hemoglobin with an affinity 200 to 300 times greater than that of oxygen. The resultant carboxyhemoglobin (COHb) shifts the oxyhemoglobin dissociation curve to the left, thereby resulting in impaired oxygen delivery at the tissue level. CO also affects cellular metabolism by inhibiting mitochondrial cytochrome oxidase, which induces free-radical-mediated oxidative injury. This impaired oxygen delivery and oxidative injury places the brain at high risk of injury.

Cyanide Cyanide gas is produced from the burning and combustion of various nitrogen-containing and synthetic materials: cigarette smoke, wool, silk, nylon, polyurethane, resins, and plastics. Cyanide causes systemic asphyxia by inhibiting mitochondrial cytochrome oxidase, the terminal enzyme of the electron transport chain; this disrupts the Krebs cycle and leads to accumulation of lactic acid. Metabolic acidosis refractory to fluid resuscitation should raise suspicion for cyanide gas poisoning. Early death after inhalation injury is thought to result in part from impaired oxygen utilization from cyanide toxicity.

CLINICAL PRESENTATION

AIRWAY AND LUNG INJURY

Children who have suffered airway burns or have a history of smoke inhalation are at increased risk for airway compromise. Classic signs are facial burns, singed nasal or facial hairs, hoarseness, stridor, and carbonaceous sputum. Significant airway inflammation and edema, however, can occur even in the absence of these findings. In cases where physical signs of inhalation injury are not present, obtaining a more detailed history of the injury is essential. Duration of exposure to smoke, burned materials present, location of injury (industrial accident versus house fire), enclosed versus open spaces, and changes in mental status can assist in determining risk of fire inhalation injury.

Mucosal injury threatens airway patency by increasing capillary permeability, tissue swelling, and plugging of distal airways with sloughed, injured tissue. Progressive upper airway edema and bronchospasm are often responsible for deterioration within the first 12 hours. Signs of acute lung injury (e.g., cough, respiratory distress, tachypnea, wheezing, rales, rhonchi) may develop by the time of patient presentation but are often delayed up to 24 hours after the initial insult. The peak in mucosal changes with sloughing and mucopurulent membrane production may be delayed up to 72 hours.

CARBON MONOXIDE POISONING

There is a broad range of symptoms from acute CO exposure. Patients can have vague or mild symptoms including flu-like symptoms, headache, nausea, and ataxia. Patients with severe toxicity can have severe neurologic impairment with loss of consciousness, seizures, pulmonary edema, respiratory failure, myocardial ischemia, and cardiac arrest. A history of multiple affected family members is often a clue to CO toxicity. A cherry-red appearance of the skin has been classically described but is rarely seen and should not be used to determine CO toxicity.

CYANIDE POISONING

With lower levels of exposure, symptoms of cyanide poisoning can be similar to CO and include headache, dizziness, fatigue, shortness of breath, or altered mental status. After high levels of exposure, clinical effects can be quick and severe including hypotension, seizures, dysrhythmias, and cardiovascular collapse. Death can ensue rapidly.

DIAGNOSTIC EVALUATION

BRONCHOSCOPIC EXAMINATION

Bronchoscopy is the gold standard for diagnosing inhalation injury. Direct visualization can reveal carbonaceous debris, ulceration, erythematous tissue, and mucosal pallor. However, the airway may appear normal if bronchoscopy is performed early in the course of injury, and thus, the clinician should continue to use history and clinical suspicion to adequately address potential inhalation injury. Serial observation by fiberoptic laryngoscopy and bronchoscopy can be used in an intensive care setting to assess the degree and extent of injury.

IMAGING

Chest x-ray can be obtained but is often of low yield for smoke inhalation injury at the time of presentation. Clinical findings on lung auscultation often precede abnormalities seen on chest radiograph, such as atelectasis, edema, or interstitial infiltrates, by 12 to 24 hours. Computed tomography is used in some centers to assess the extent of lung injury when fiberoptic laryngoscopy is unrevealing or limited to proximal airway visualization. Ground-glass opacities have been described in some studies. Though not routinely recommended when assessing patients with suspected inhalation injury, some studies show promising use of CT scan to risk stratify patients' severity. However, because CT findings are unlikely to change management, the risks of unnecessary radiation exposure and cost outweigh potential benefits of obtaining CT scan routinely.

LABORATORY TESTS

Any patient who presents to the emergency room with suspected inhalation injury should have an arterial blood gas (ABG), electrolytes, and lactic acid sent. Blood gas measurement can help assess acid-base status, along with signs of poor ventilation and oxygenation from inhalation injury. Although arterial blood gas (ABG) measurement should be part of the diagnostic assessment of any patient with suspected toxin exposure, it is often found to be normal in pure CO toxicity. The partial pressure of oxygen (PaO_2) measured on ABG analysis is a measurement of the amount of oxygen dissolved in blood (not bound to hemoglobin). Because CO does not affect the amount of dissolved oxygen, PaO_2 may be normal in patients with CO poisoning. The calculated oxygen

TABLE 173-1 Symptoms of Acute Carbon Monoxide Poisoning Based on Carboxyhemoglobin Levels*

COHb%	Symptoms
10	Asymptomatic or headache
20	Dizziness, nausea, dyspnea, impaired cognition
30	Visual disturbances, muscle weakness
40	Confusion, syncope
50	Seizures, coma
≥60	Cardiopulmonary dysfunction, death

COHb%, carboxyhemoglobin percentage from CO-oximetry.

**Note:* COHb levels often do not closely correlate with symptoms, especially if there has been a delay in determining levels after exposure or if the patient has been pretreated with supplemental oxygen.

Source: Reproduced with permission from Varon J, Marik PE, Fromm RE, Gueler A. Carbon monoxide poisoning: a review for clinicians. *J Emerg Med.* 1999;17: 87-93.

saturation level on ABG analysis (SaO_2) and monitored oxygen saturation will also be "normal," even in the setting of substantial CO toxicity. Traditional pulse oximetry uses only two wavelengths of light to determine hemoglobin saturation and divides the molecules into oxyhemoglobin and deoxyhemoglobin. COHb is misread as oxyhemoglobin, thus giving a CO-poisoned patient a falsely elevated and often normal or low normal reading of oxygen saturation.

The diagnosis of CO poisoning is made through the history and detection of carboxyhemoglobin (COHb) by co-oximetry of venous or arterial blood. Peak levels less than 20% are often associated with mild toxicity, and those above 60% are associated with coma and death (**Table 173-1**). However, the COHb level does not accurately correlate with the severity of poisoning, especially in children. Carboxyhemoglobin levels rapidly decrease upon administration of 100% oxygen, which can obscure the initial clinical picture when assessing patients who received oxygen therapy prior to hospital arrival. Suspecting CO inhalation is important in such cases, as a low COHb cannot always be used to rule out CO poisoning.

Cyanide poisoning is a diagnosis made clinically based on suspicion of exposure, along with signs and symptoms. Cyanide levels can be obtained but rarely return in time to affect patient care. Arterial blood gas, electrolytes, and lactate can aid in the diagnosis of cyanide toxicity; they will show a high anion gap metabolic acidosis and elevated lactate concentration.

MANAGEMENT

INITIAL ASSESSMENT AND STABILIZATION

The initial evaluation and stabilization of a child with suspected airway or inhalation injury most often occurs in the field or in an emergency department and follows pediatric advanced life support guidelines and recommendations. Evaluation and management of life-threatening injuries are the first priorities. Immediate decompensation usually results from hypoxemia, airway obstruction, and CO or cyanide poisoning. In accordance with the "ABCs" (airway, breathing, circulation) of standard resuscitations, airway patency and the risk for upper airway injury should be evaluated (**Figure 173-1**). All patients should initially receive maximum oxygenation with a 100% concentration of inspired oxygen and assisted ventilation when necessary. In instances where intubation is not required, providing humidified air and raising the head of the bed are important while maintaining close surveillance of airway compromise. Hypotonic pharyngeal structures can obstruct the upper airway in unconscious patients, thus making a chin-lift maneuver critical in the preservation of airway patency. After adequate control of the airway and ventilation, assessment of circulation can proceed with appropriate interventions as needed. Systemic vasodilation should be addressed with fluid resuscitation, and vasopressors should be given when necessary. After initial stabilization, further assessment should concentrate on identifying potential inhalation injury and CO or cyanide poisoning.

AIRWAY AND LUNG INJURY

The airway should be protected early; any signs of airway compromise indicate the need for direct laryngoscopy and consideration of early elective endotracheal intubation. Indications for early endotracheal intubation and mechanical ventilation are provided in **Table 173-2**. In the setting of acute mucosal inflammation, intubation with a smaller endotracheal tube than expected for age may be necessary. Vigilant airway surveillance is critical when monitoring for early mucosal edema, as sequelae of initial injury may not present until after 48 hours after inhalation.

Treatment of smoke inhalation and parenchymal lung damage focuses on supportive care to maximize respiratory function. Supplemental oxygen can be weaned upon resolution of symptoms related to CO toxicity in conjunction with normal COHb level (by co-oximetry), and correction of ventilation-perfusion mismatch. It should be noted that the normal COHb levels in patients who have received appropriate treatment with improvement in symptoms contrast with the falsely reassuring low COHb levels in symptomatic patients that can be seen after oxygen supplementation during initial resuscitation.

In the setting of pulmonary edema from increased capillary leak, delivery of peak end-expiratory pressure support by endotracheal tube will maintain small-airway patency and improve alveolar gas exchange. Because airway obstruction is usually mechanical, adequate humidification and pulmonary toilet are the mainstays of supportive care. Particulate matter may cause hypersensitivity and bronchoconstriction, especially in children with previous reactive airway history. Bronchodilators such as nebulized albuterol may help alleviate lower airway obstruction. The use of steroids and prophylactic antibiotics is not indicated in the setting of acute lung injury from smoke inhalation. Corticosteroids have been associated with a significant increase in the risk for death and infectious complications and should not be used in the treatment of burn patients. Antibiotic use should be reserved for clinical signs of infectious pneumonia, which rarely occurs during the first 24 hours; prophylactic antibiotics are not recommended. The use of certain exogenous surfactants has been shown to effectively restore endogenous surfactant function after inhalation injury by wood smoke.

CARBON MONOXIDE POISONING

Patients suspected of suffering CO poisoning should have 100% oxygen therapy initiated and should be continued until the COHb has fallen below 5%. The half-life of COHb decreases from approximately 4 to 6 hours in patients breathing room air at sea level to 60 to 90 minutes with 100% inspired oxygen. Treatment with 100% oxygen at hyperbaric treatment pressures increases the oxygen concentration in blood and further shortens the half-life of COHb to 20 to 30 minutes. Patients with significant CO poisoning are at risk for delayed neurologic sequelae, including cognitive and memory difficulties, personality changes, peripheral neuropathies, and neurologic deficits. The role of hyperbaric oxygen (HBO) therapy in the prevention of delayed neurologic sequelae is controversial. HBO therapy can inhibit the leukocyte adherence that initiates the cerebral injury from severe CO poisoning. As evidence on HBO therapy is conflicting, routine use of HBO for treatment of patients with CO poisoning is not recommended. Instead, the decision to initiate HBO therapy should be made individually based on the history, clinical presentation, and degree of neurologic impairment in conjunction with the local poison center or hyperbaricist. Certain criteria that have been traditionally used as indications to consider HBO therapy include any history of loss of consciousness or syncope, focal or persistent neurologic symptoms, ischemic changes on electrocardiography, pregnant patients with COHb levels higher than 15% or any signs of fetal distress, significantly elevated COHb levels (>25%), seizure, and abnormal cerebellar function. HBO therapy should not delay resuscitative measures or addressing more acute sequelae or symptoms such as myocardial infarction or seizures. Relative contraindications to the use of HBO include the presence of airway debris and bronchospasm as these can result in gas embolism and pneumothorax. Given no empirical support for HBO in CO poisoning, long or potentially dangerous (e.g., helicopter) transport to an HBO facility should be discouraged.

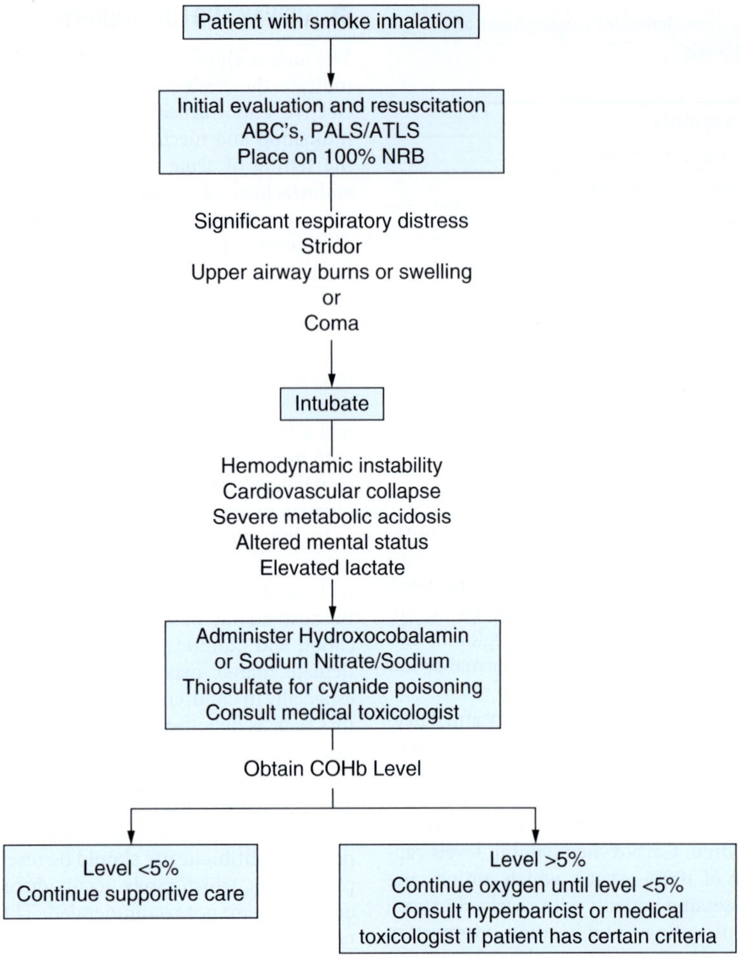

FIGURE 173-1. Fire inhalation injury resuscitation algorithm. (ABC, airway, breathing, circulation; PALS, pediatric advanced life support; ATLS, advanced trauma life support; NRB, non-rebreather; COHb, carboxyhemoglobin)

CYANIDE POISONING

Cyanide toxicity should be suspected in those who have altered levels of consciousness and hypotension, cardiovascular collapse, cardiac arrest, or persistent or worsening lactic acidosis not responsive to maximal oxygenation and fluid resuscitation. The preferred and more readily available antidote for cyanide toxicity is hydroxocobalamin, which combines with cyanide to form the non-toxic compound cyanocobalamin. If hydroxocobalamin is not available, the cyanide scavenger sodium thiosulfate can be given instead. Of note, sodium nitrite and amyl nitrite, two other possible antidotes for cyanide toxicity, are contraindicated in cases of confirmed or suspected CO poisoning. All antidotes should be given with close collaboration with poison control and pharmacy expertise. Dosing and adverse effects are summarized in **Table 173-3.**

ADMISSION CRITERIA

Hospitalization is indicated for patients with:

- Hemodynamic instability (intensive care setting)
- The need or potential need for endotracheal intubation and mechanical ventilation (consider intensive care setting)
- High risk for airway injury despite being asymptomatic during the initial period of observation (e.g., signs of airway erythema or edema, prolonged or severe exposure to smoke, other victims with similar exposure who have demonstrated clinical deterioration)
- Evidence of significant CO or cyanide poisoning, especially if symptoms persist after normalization of COHb levels

TABLE 173-2 Indications for Early Endotracheal Intubation

Signs of upper airway obstruction
Altered level of consciousness associated with loss of cough or gag reflex
Persistent hypoxia (PaO_2, 60 mm Hg on >60% inspired oxygen)
Need for aggressive pulmonary toilet

TABLE 173-3 Cyanide Toxicity Treatment*: Dosing and Adverse Effects of Hydroxocobalamin and Sodium Thiosulfate

Drug	Pediatric Dosing	Administration	Adverse Effects
Hydroxocobalamin	70 mg/kg (Max 5 g) IV	Dose can be repeated if necessary.	Red discoloration of secretions, urine, and mucous membranes, and hypertension
Sodium thiosulfate	250 mg/kg (max 12.5g) IV	Sodium thiosulfate should be given IV immediately following sodium nitrite administration though should not be given in same IV as they will bind and be ineffective.	Hypotension, nausea, and vomiting

*Sodium nitrite and amyl nitrite are contraindicated in any patient with suspected or confirmed concurrent carbon monoxide poisoning.

DISCHARGE CRITERIA

- Stabilization of all airway and pulmonary issues
- Normalization of COHb levels
- Resolution of all toxin-associated symptoms

CONSULTATION

- Critical care: For patients with a severe cardiopulmonary insult or instability
- Otolaryngology/pulmonology: For patients with evidence of airway injury
- Medical toxicology: For patients with significant CO or cyanide poisoning, or exposure to other inhaled toxins

SPECIAL CONSIDERATIONS

- The high minute ventilation characteristic of children puts them at increased risk for smoke inhalation injury as compared with adults.

PREVENTION

- Smoke alarms
- CO detectors
- Cook with care
- Attempt to quit smoking
- Safe space heater use
- Fire escape plan

KEY POINTS

- The airway should be protected early, and any signs of airway compromise indicate the need for direct laryngoscopy and early elective endotracheal intubation.
- Even without dermal or upper airway injury, significant lower airway involvement can occur in a child who inhales toxic particles in smoke. Lung injury and chest x-ray findings can be delayed.
- Exposure to combustion or smoke in a closed or partially closed space puts the patient at high risk for CO and/or cyanide poisoning. Obtain a COHb level and lactate concentration for evaluation.
- COHb levels following initial oxygen administration drop rapidly and should not be used to guide initial management when CO poisoning is suspected based on clinical symptoms. Clinical suspicion for CO poisoning warrants aggressive management with appropriate fluid resuscitation, ongoing oxygen administration, and workup.
- Hydroxocobalamin and sodium thiosulfate are treatments of choice for cyanide poisoning. Though included in cyanide toxicity kits, sodium nitrite and amyl nitrite are contraindicated in any patient with suspected or confirmed concurrent CO toxicity.

SUGGESTED READINGS

Annane D, Chadda K, Gajdos P, Jars-Guincestre MC, Chevret S, Raphael JC. Hyperbaric oxygen therapy for acute domestic carbon monoxide poisoning: two randomized controlled trials. *Intensive Care Med.* 2011;37(3):486-492.

Brooks DE, Lin E, Ahktar J. What is cherry red, and who cares? *J Emerg Med.* 2002;22(2):213-214.

Buckley NA, Juurlink DN, Isbister G, Bennett MH, Lavonas EJ. Hyperbaric oxygen for carbon monoxide poisoning. *Cochrane Database Syst Rev.* 2011(4):CD002041.

Carvajal HF, Griffith JA. Burn and Inhalation Injuries. In: Fuhrman BP, Zimmerman JJ, eds. *Pediatric Critical Care.* Philadelphia: CV Mosby; 2006:1565-1576.

Deutsch CJ, Tan A, Smailes S, Dziewulski P. The diagnosis and management of inhalation injury: an evidence based approach. *Burns.* 2018;44(5):1040-1051.

Duffy BJ, McLaughlin PM, Eichelberger MR. Assessment, triage, and early management of burns in children. *Clinical Pediatric Emergency Medicine.* 2006;7(2):82-93.

Fire Safety and Burns—Injury Statistics and Incidence Rates. Stanford Children's Health Web site. https://www.stanfordchildrens.org/en/topic/default?id=fire-safety-and-burns-injury-statistics-and-incidence-rates-90-P02978. Accessed June 2022.

Hamad E, Babu K, Bebarta VS. Case files of the University of Massachusetts Toxicology Fellowship: does this smoke inhalation victim require treatment with cyanide antidote? *J Med Toxicol.* 2016;12(2):192-198.

Henretig FM, Calello DP, Osterhoudt KC. More on carbon monoxide poisoning during major US power outages. *N Engl J Med.* 2022;386:1386-1387.

Kao LW, Nanagas KA. Carbon monoxide poisoning. *Med Clin North Am.* 2005;89(6):1161-1194.

Kuroda H, Fujihara K, Kushimoto S, Aoki M. Novel clinical grading of delayed neurologic sequelae after carbon monoxide poisoning and factors associated with outcome. *Neurotoxicology.* 2015;48:35-43.

Miller K, Chang A. Acute inhalation injury. *Emerg Med Clin North Am.* 2003;21(2):533-557.

Martin JD, Osterhoudt KC, Thom SP. Recognition and management of carbon monoxide poisoning in children. *Clin Pediatr Emerg Med.* 2000;1(3):244-250.

Rabinowitz PM, Siegel MD. Acute inhalation injury. *Clin Chest Med.* 2002;23(4):707-715.

Sheridan RL. Fire-Related Inhalation Injury. *N Engl J Med.* 2016;375(5):464-469.

Weaver LK, Hopkins RO, Chan KJ, et al. Hyperbaric oxygen for acute carbon monoxide poisoning. *N Engl J Med.* 2002;347(14):1057-1067.

CHAPTER 174

Heat Disorders

Tara N. Calhoun, MD, MS

BACKGROUND

Heat disorders such as heat exhaustion and heatstroke result from a failure of the body's regulatory mechanisms to maintain a constant body temperature. These are most commonly due to external sources. Individuals at the extremes of age and those with chronic diseases are the most vulnerable. Approximately 600 people die annually in the United States from heat-related illnesses. Malignant hyperthermia, another thermoregulatory disorder, results from a triggering exposure in a genetically susceptible individual. Fever is not addressed in this chapter as it is a normal physiologic response secondary to inflammation or infection (Chapter 24).

Heat disorders occur most commonly in the summer months or in tropical regions. Although elderly patients are most severely affected, healthy children are also susceptible. Young children have suboptimally developed thermoregulatory controls and are dependent on others to provide them with fluids and to keep them from unsafe environments (e.g., hot vehicles). Comorbid conditions such as obesity, physical disabilities that limit rapid egress from a warm environment, or cystic fibrosis increase a child's susceptibility to heat stress.

PATHOPHYSIOLOGY

The human body maintains a relatively constant body temperature despite wide swings in environmental temperature. Heat is acquired both endogenously (from basal metabolism, muscle activity, hormonal effects, and sympathetic stimulation) and exogenously (when environmental temperature exceeds body temperature). Heat is lost to the environment by radiation (up to 60% of losses), evaporation of sweat (22%-25%), conduction (3%), and convection (12%-15%).

The hypothalamus, the body's primary thermoregulator, maintains the core body temperature within a narrow range. Increases in body temperature result in sympathetically mediated peripheral blood vessel dilation (increased radiation losses), increased sweat gland activity (higher evaporative losses), and reduced endogenous heat production. Hyperthermia occurs when the body cannot adequately dissipate excess exogenous or endogenous heat.

Malignant hyperthermia is a group of genetic myopathies associated with a defect in the calcium channels of skeletal muscles. Patients are usually asymptomatic until exposed to the triggering agent, most commonly during a surgical or invasive procedure. Implicated triggers include inhaled anesthetics and neuromuscular blockers. Nitrous oxide is the only inhalation anesthetic that is not a possible trigger for malignant hyperthermia. A muscle biopsy is needed to confirm the predisposing defect. Physical stressors can, though rarely, precipitate malignant hyperthermia in susceptible individuals.

CLINICAL PRESENTATION

Heat-related illnesses are on a continuum; if the mild signs of a heat illness are not treated quickly and adequately, it can progress to a more severe presentation. **Table 174-1** describes the symptoms, clinical and laboratory findings, treatment, and prognosis of the three major types of heat-related illnesses: heat cramps, heat exhaustion, and heatstroke.

HEAT CRAMPS

Heat cramps are painful muscle spasms that typically occur several hours after vigorous exertion. They are thought to be due to water repletion without adequate salt repletion. The voluntary muscles of the calves, thighs, and shoulders are most affected. Symptoms typically last only a few minutes but may recur. The affected muscles feel hard to palpation. Laboratory abnormalities may include hyponatremia with very low or undetectable urine sodium.

TABLE 174-1 Descriptions of Heat Illnesses

	Heat Cramps	Heat Exhaustion	Heatstroke
Core body temperature	Normal	Elevated (≤39°C)	Very elevated (≥40°C)
Symptoms	Painful muscle spasms	Weakness Thirst Headache Nausea, vomiting Diarrhea	Confusion Delirium Seizures Coma
Physical examination	Hard knot in muscle belly	Tachycardia Orthostatic hypotension Diffuse sweating	Tachycardia Circulatory collapse Anhidrosis Central nervous system dysfunction
Laboratory studies	Hyponatremia Low urine sodium	Hypo- or hypernatremia Hemoconcentration Urinary concentration	Hypo- or hypernatremia Hemoconcentration Acute renal failure Rhabdomyolysis
Therapy	Oral rehydration Electrolyte solutions	Passive cooling IV rehydration	Active cooling Cardiorespiratory support
Prognosis	Excellent	Excellent	High mortality

HEAT EXHAUSTION

Heat exhaustion occurs secondary to water depletion, salt depletion, or both. Affected patients experience systemic complaints, including fatigue, weakness, nausea, vomiting, diarrhea, and headache. Irritability may be a prominent sign in infants and nonverbal children. Core temperature is mildly elevated (<39°C), and the patient often experiences tachycardia, orthostatic hypotension, profuse sweating, and flushed skin. Laboratory abnormalities may include hyponatremia or hypernatremia, hemoconcentration, and urinary concentration.

HEATSTROKE

Heatstroke is a life-threatening condition. Classic heatstroke, also referred to as non-exertional heatstroke, typically occurs in children when they are in environments with quickly rising temperatures. Common predisposing factors include children's limited ability to increase their fluid intake (e.g., young infancy, nonverbal status), remove themselves from a hot environment (e.g., immobility, car seat), or dissipate heat (e.g., overdressing, obesity, underlying medical condition). Exertional heatstroke usually occurs in otherwise healthy individuals who participate in vigorous activities when it is hot and humid, often with inadequate efforts to maintain hydration.

Patients present with a significantly elevated core body temperature or hyperpyrexia (>40°C) associated with central nervous system dysfunction. Anhidrosis is frequently but not universally observed. Neurologic symptoms include progressive lethargy, confusion, headache, delirium, seizures, and coma. On physical examination, patients are tachycardic, hypotensive, and tachypneic. Laboratory abnormalities may include hyponatremia or hypernatremia, hypokalemia, hemoconcentration and urinary concentration, acute renal failure, and elevated liver function tests. Hyperventilation may cause a respiratory alkalosis. Rhabdomyolysis may occur as a result of thermal injury to myocytes. Circulating myoglobin as well as thermal and ischemic insults can result in acute renal compromise.

MALIGNANT HYPERTHERMIA

When a susceptible individual is exposed to a triggering agent, the uncontrolled influx of calcium into the muscle cell results in muscle contraction, accelerated metabolism, and resultant hyperthermia. Initially, end-tidal carbon dioxide increases and arterial oxygen decreases, with muscle rigidity and a rapid rise in body temperature.

Laboratory evaluation reveals acidosis as well as hyperkalemia, hyperphosphatemia, hypocalcemia, and myoglobinuria from muscle breakdown. Although serum creatinine starts to rise almost immediately due to the rhabdomyolysis, peak levels are not seen until several days after the exposure.

DIFFERENTIAL DIAGNOSIS

Increased body temperature can occur secondary to a wide range of causes (**Table 174-2**). Encephalitis or other causes of encephalopathy, especially when accompanied by fever, can mimic heatstroke. Other causes of myositis or tonic muscle contractions can present with features similar to heat cramps, including viral or drug-induced myositis and electrolyte imbalances leading to tetany.

Many drug-induced hyperthermia syndromes exist. These include serotonin syndrome; neuroleptic malignant syndrome; acute drug withdrawal; and poisoning with sympathomimetic drugs, salicylates, thyroid hormones, or anticholinergics.

DIAGNOSTIC EVALUATION

Patient history should determine heat exposure, hydration status, and predisposing factors including problems with heat dissipation. The physical examination should focus on identifying the signs of heat illness as

TABLE 174-2 Causes of Hyperthermia
Sepsis
Central nervous system infection
Environmental exposure
Tetanus
Typhoid fever
Thyroid storm
Pheochromocytoma
Catatonia
Hypothalamic stroke
Status epilepticus
Cerebral hemorrhage
Dystonic reaction
Toxicologic ingestion

Source: Data from Lanken PN, Manaker S, Hanson CW III, eds. *The Intensive Care Unit Manual.* Philadelphia: Saunders; 2001.

well as determining the severity of the condition. A core temperature must be obtained with a rectal thermometer. Laboratory assessments and typical derangements are listed in **Table 174-3**. Additional studies such as imaging of the head; urine toxicology screen; cultures of blood, urine, or cerebrospinal fluid; and chest radiograph may be indicated depending on the suspicion for other diagnoses.

MANAGEMENT

HEAT ILLNESSES

Minor heat illnesses are typically managed with fluid and electrolyte replacement. Heat cramps can be effectively treated with rest as well as oral salt and water replacement. Passive stretching of the affected area can help resolve muscle cramps. Heat exhaustion requires intravenous rehydration with unrestricted dietary sodium. Electrolyte imbalances should be corrected slowly over 12 to 24 hours.

Heatstroke victims should be removed immediately from the hot environment and their clothing removed. Airway protection may be required to prevent aspiration, and patients need close cardiovascular monitoring. Patients with elevated core body temperatures should be aggressively cooled. Core body temperature should always be checked with a rectal or esophageal thermometer and monitored frequently. Active cooling should be initiated to bring core body temperature down to between 38.5°C and 39.0°C. Rapid cooling can begin either by immersion in cold water with ice or by evaporative cooling. Gastric or peritoneal lavage can be considered as a supplemental cooling method in severe cases. Cooled intravenous fluids are not used given the risk of an arrhythmia with an already stressed myocardium. Delays in the onset of treatment have been associated with higher cases of morbidity, mortality, and longer hospital stays.

Heatstroke victims require aggressive fluid resuscitation to maintain cerebral perfusion. If urine output cannot be maintained at greater than 1 mL/kg per hour with aggressive fluid repletion, the addition of diuretics (e.g., furosemide, mannitol) should be considered.

Hypotension refractory to intravenous fluids warrants vasopressor therapy. Dobutamine, a β_1-adrenergic agent, should be selected because it both increases cardiac contractility, raising blood pressure, and causes peripheral vasodilation allowing ongoing heat loss. Agents with α-adrenergic activity, such as dopamine, epinephrine, and norepinephrine, should be avoided because the resulting peripheral vasoconstriction minimizes heat dissipation. Isoproterenol, a β-adrenergic agent, may increase myocardial oxygen consumption beyond oxygen delivery capacity and should also be avoided.

Rhabdomyolysis may develop as a complication of heatstroke or malignant hyperthermia. Creatine kinase levels typically peak several days after the heat or drug exposure. Monitoring for electrolyte imbalances and renal injury (evidenced by urine myoglobin) is required. Ample hydration should be maintained, and some experts recommend alkalization (target urine pH > 6.5).

Disseminated intravascular coagulation, seizure, renal failure, hepatic dysfunction, and acute respiratory distress syndrome can complicate heatstroke and should be managed appropriately, typically in an intensive care setting.

MALIGNANT HYPERTHERMIA

The initial management of malignant hyperthermia requires discontinuing the offending agent. Hyperventilation with 100% oxygen and volume replacement with intravenous fluids should begin immediately. As soon as the diagnosis of malignant hyperthermia has been made, dantrolene should be given (up to every 5 minutes until muscle relaxation is achieved). Dantrolene causes muscle relaxation directly by blocking the release of calcium from the sarcoplasmic reticulum. External cooling measures should be initiated to treat hyperthermia. Benzodiazepines or paralysis should be considered for patients with persistent shivering. Cardiac arrhythmias resulting from malignant hyperthermia should be treated with procainamide and calcium chloride. Rhabdomyolysis, management discussed earlier, may also occur as a complication of malignant hyperthermia.

TABLE 174-3 Laboratory Studies for the Evaluation of Heat Disorders

Study	Common Abnormalities
Complete blood count	Leukocytosis, hemoconcentration, and, if DIC is present, thrombocytopenia
Serum electrolytes: sodium, potassium, chloride, bicarbonate	Variable derangements indicative of dehydration
Blood urea nitrogen, serum creatinine	Elevations consistent with dehydration or renal injury
Hepatic enzymes	Elevated if there is hepatic injury
Creatine kinase	Elevated with rhabdomyolysis
PT, INR, PTT, D-dimer	Elevated with DIC
Urinalysis	Elevated specific gravity, proteinuria, ketonuria, dipstick-positive for blood without red blood cells on microscopic examination

DIC, disseminated intravascular coagulation; INR, international normalized ratio; PT, prothrombin time; PTT, partial thromboplastin time.

ADMISSION AND DISCHARGE CRITERIA

Most otherwise healthy patients with heat cramps and heat exhaustion can be treated with cooling and rehydration in the primary care office or emergency department without hospital admission. Patients with heatstroke or other evidence of end-organ injury (e.g., rhabdomyolysis), drug-induced hyperthermia syndromes, coexisting chronic medical conditions, or malignant hyperthermia warrant inpatient stabilization. Children can be discharged once all the following have occurred: return to hemodynamic stability, return to baseline mental status, ability to maintain adequate hydration and resolution of rhabdomyolysis with decreasing levels of creatine kinase, and clearance of myoglobinuria.

CONSULTATION

Involvement of critical care specialists is indicated for patients who require or are anticipated to need intensive care support. Nephrologists may be helpful for patients at risk for or with evidence of renal injury, especially those with severe rhabdomyolysis. Emergency consultation for a patient thought to have malignant hyperthermia can be obtained by calling the hotline (800-MH-HYPER or 800-644-9737) or reviewing the website (https://www.mhaus.org/healthcare-professionals/).

TABLE 174-4 Recommendations for the Prevention of Heat Illness
Drink plenty of nonalcoholic fluids
Replace salts and minerals (e.g., salt-containing foods, sports drinks)
Dress in lightweight, light-colored, loosely fitted clothing
Avoid or limit sun exposure
Avoid outdoor activity, especially during midday and afternoon
Seek out air-conditioned environments
Check on individuals at increased risk for heat injury
Check the car for children prior to exiting

Source: Adapted from the Centers for Disease Control and Prevention website. *Extreme Heat: A Prevention Guide to Promote Your Personal Health and Safety.*

SPECIAL CONSIDERATIONS

PREVENTION

The best preventative approaches for heat illnesses are activity restriction and avoidance of environmental situations that put a child at risk (**Table 174-4**). The National Weather Service and the Centers for Disease Control and Prevention issue heat advisories through local broadcasting systems that can alert individuals and communities to dangerous conditions.

Early recognition of malignant hyperthermia and prevention of exposure to triggering agents are the most effective therapies for this life-threatening condition. Preoperative assessments should include careful questioning about reactions to anesthesia in the patient or family members. To prevent recurrences, patients should always carry malignant hyperthermia medical identification bands.

KEY POINTS

- Heat-related illnesses are preventable.
- Heat cramps are usually managed with rest and hydration.
- Features of heat exhaustion include weakness, irritability, vomiting, diarrhea, diaphoresis, elevated body temperature, and orthostasis.
- Heatstroke is a life-threatening condition that presents with a significant elevation in core body temperature, changes in mental status, and often, cardiovascular instability. Sweating may be absent. The difference in presentation of heat exhaustion and heatstroke is mental status changes.
- Rapid cooling and appropriate management of fluid and electrolyte derangements are the mainstays of therapy for heat disorders.
- Malignant hyperthermia results in susceptible individuals following exposure to a triggering agent and manifests with rapidly rising temperatures and muscle rigidity. Dantrolene is used for treatment.

SUGGESTED READINGS

Bergeron MF, Devore C, Rice SG. Policy statement—climatic heat stress and exercising children and adolescents. *Pediatrics*. 2011;128(3): e741-e747.

Denborough M. Malignant hyperthermia. *Lancet*. 1998;352(9134): 1131-1136.

Glazer JL. Management of heatstroke and heat exhaustion. *Am Fam Physician*. 71(11):2133-2140.

Halloran LL, Bernard DW. Management of drug-induced hyperthermia. *Curr Opin Pediatr*. 2004;16(2):211-215.

Mangus CW, Canares TL. Heat-related illness in children in an era of extreme temperatures. *Pediatr Rev*. 2019;40(3):97-107.

McLaren C, Null J, Quinn J. Heat stress from enclosed vehicles: moderate ambient temperatures cause significant temperature rise in enclosed vehicles. *Pediatrics*. Jul 2005;116(1):e109-112.

Rosenberg H, Davis M, James D, Pollock N, Stowell K. Malignant hyperthermia. *Orphanet J Rare Dis*. 2007;2:21.

Singleton KD, Wischmeyer PE. Oral glutamine enhances heat shock protein expression and improves survival following hyperthermia. *Shock*. 2006;25(3):295-299.

Von Duvillard SP, Braun WA, Markofski M, Beneke R, Leithauser R. Fluids and hydration in prolonged endurance performance. *Nutrition*. 2004;20(7-8):651-656.

CHAPTER 175 Hypothermia and Cold-Related Injuries

Courtney A. Gilliam, MD and Jeffrey P. Louie, MD

BACKGROUND

Maintaining the body's core temperature is essential for human life. The human body can lose heat by four mechanisms: (i) radiation, or transfer of heat through infrared energy; (ii) evaporation, which includes respiration; (iii) convection, or transfer of heat by the movement of air currents; and (iv) conduction, or heat loss through direct contact with another object. When conduction and convection are combined, heat loss may be as high as 10% to 15%, which is why removing cold and wet clothes is essential in initial management of hypothermia. Young infants and children are at risk of hypothermia (HT) and cold-related injuries given (i) their greater body surface area-to-mass ratio and less subcutaneous fat, which leads to greater heat loss; (ii) immature thermoregulation and an inability to shiver in infants; (iii) children with neurologic conditions are more prone to hypothermia due difficulty with thermoregulation; and (iv) children are active participants in outdoor sports, camping and hiking which puts them at risk for exhaustion, hunger, dehydration, and lack of adequate clothing.

Additional predisposing factors that increase the risk for hypothermia and cold-related injuries are listed in **Table 175-1.**

Hypothermia is preventable, yet over 1000 people per year in the United States die of excessive natural cold. Hypothermia and cold-related injuries in children are more common in boys, more prevalent in infants than in older children, and, within the United States, more common in the southern regions of the country.

Hypothermic patients are traditionally classified into three categories according to core temperature: mild (32°C-35°C), moderate (30°C-31.9°C), and severe (less than 30°C). The lower the core temperature, the more organ systems are affected and the greater the potential for morbidity and mortality. In the pre-hospital setting, obtaining an accurate core temperature is impractical. Thus, clinical criteria were developed by wilderness search and rescue teams and emergency medical services providers. The

TABLE 175-1 Risk Factors Predisposing to Hypothermia
General conditions
Malnutrition
Hypothyroidism
Hypoglycemia
Immobility
Extreme ages: neonates and geriatrics
Intoxications/ingestions
Trauma
Neuromuscular disorders
Infection
Sepsis

criteria are as follows: HT I—Conscious and shivering (estimated core temperature 35°C to 32°C); HT II—Impaired consciousness, not shivering (<32°C to 28°C); HT III—Unconscious, not shivering, vital signs present (<28°C to 24°C); HT IV—No vital signs (<24°C).

Localized hypothermia (cold injury) can be classified as (i) *frostbite*, the most common type of cold injury that occurs due to freezing of tissue; (ii) *frostnip*, a localized cold injury with paresthesias that reverse on warming; (iii) *pernio* or *chilblains*, localized inflammatory lesions due to damp cold exposure above freezing temperatures; and (iv) *trench foot*, a non-freezing cold injury associated with prolonged exposure to damp cold conditions leading to injury of the sympathetic nerves and vasculature of the feet. These four types of cold injury represent a continuum from tissue injury to irreversible tissue damage.

PATHOPHYSIOLOGY AND CLINICAL PRESENTATION

Two mechanisms are responsible for cold-related tissue injury. The first is cellular death at the time of cold exposure. Cold exposure leads to ice crystal formation in the extracellular space, inducing an osmotic shift and resulting in intracellular dehydration and cell death. The body's response to this localized trauma and cellular destruction is to alternate vasoconstriction and vasodilation as an attempt to rewarm the area. This process furthers the cellular damage. The second mechanism of injury, similar to thermal burns, is a result of prolonged, progressive dermal ischemia from cold exposure. This induces inflammatory mediators (thromboxanes, prostaglandins, histamine, and bradykinins) that promote edema and result in the formation of blisters.

The signs and symptoms of a hypothermic patient are inherently associated with the person's core temperature. **Table 175-2** outlines the core temperatures associated with clinical findings.

CENTRAL NERVOUS SYSTEM

Hypothermia results in decreased metabolism and blood flow to the brain. Brain function, thought processes, and motor skills decline as the body's core temperature drops below 35°C. Fine motor skills decline, which leads to frank clumsiness. Dysarthria and ataxia follow. As hypothermia worsens, a phenomenon known as "paradoxical undressing" may occur whereby victims undress themselves. It is thought that this phenomenon signifies impending thermoregulatory collapse. By 32°C, confusion and drowsiness become evident. Below 32°C, the person becomes unconscious.

CARDIOVASCULAR SYSTEM

The early cardiovascular response to hypothermia is tachycardia. However, as the body cools below 35°C, heart rate slows and cardiac output decreases. Hypotension may occur secondary to decreased cardiac output, cardiac contractility, and intravascular volume. Electrocardiographic findings are nonspecific and include prolongation of the PR, QRS, and QTc intervals as well as ST-segment and T-wave changes. As the core temperature drops to 32°C, roughly 30% of hypothermic victims will demonstrate the J wave or Osborn wave, on electrocardiograms. The Osborn wave is an upward deflection after the QRS complex (**Figure 175-1**). There are no arrhythmias specific to hypothermia, but atrial and ventricular fibrillations are well documented.

TABLE 175-2 Typical Clinical Findings Associated With Low Core Temperatures

Temperature	Finding
35°C	Confusion, dysarthria, shivering, cold diuresis
34°C	Impaired judgment
33°C	Apathy
32°C	Decreased level of consciousness, hallucinations, appearance of J (Osborn) wave
31°C	Stupor, loss of shivering
30°C	Onset of arrhythmias
28°C	Coma, loss of reflexes, decreases in blood pressure and heart rate
24°C	Apnea and asystole
19°C	Flat electroencephalogram

RESPIRATORY SYSTEM

Tachypnea is initially seen in mild hypothermia, but as the core temperature continues to decline, hypopnea will follow. Hypoxia and hypercapnia ensue and produce a mixed metabolic and respiratory acidosis. Ciliary function ceases as hypothermia intensifies, predisposing the victim to pneumonia.

MUSCULAR AND PERIPHERAL VASCULAR SYSTEM

Shivering produces heat to maintain core temperature. This mechanism of heat production stops when the core temperature drops below 32°C. Cessation of shivering signifies the body's inability to combat hypothermia.

Arteriolar vasoconstriction decreases blood flow to the skin. A slight increase in blood pressure may be noted. However, as the body's temperature drops, blood pressure also declines as a result of loss of sympathetic tone. Conversely, intense peripheral vasoconstriction leads to pallor. Facial puffiness may ensue secondary to increased capillary permeability with subcutaneous edema.

SKIN

Blisters may occur with prolonged cold exposure. Blisters may be superficial or deep dermal injuries. Superficial injuries portend a good prognosis and on examination include normal-colored skin and blisters filled with clear fluid. In addition, the skin will have the ability to deform with palpation. In contrast, the physical findings after deep dermal injury include dark, hemorrhagic blisters, and hard, non-deforming skin on palpation. Such injuries suggest long-term morbidity.

Frostbite is classified into four categories—first to fourth degree—based on severity. First-degree frostbite is characterized by an anesthetic central white area with peripheral erythema. Second-degree injury represents blisters filled with either clear or milky fluid, surrounded by erythema or edema, that appear in the first 24 hours (**Figure 175-2**). Third-degree frostbite is associated with hemorrhagic blisters that progress over a course of 2 to 4 weeks, resulting in a thick, black eschar (**Figure 175-3**). Fourth-degree frostbite produces complete tissue necrosis and autoamputation.

RENAL SYSTEM

Peripheral vasoconstriction increases blood flow to the kidneys, which induces diuresis. In addition, there is a decrease in circulating antidiuretic hormone. These two factors, along with insensible water loss (sweating and respiration) and tissue third spacing, lead to a decrease in intravascular volume and prerenal failure.

DIFFERENTIAL DIAGNOSIS

The clinical presentation, along with a clear history from first responders, witnesses, or family members, makes the diagnosis of hypothermia or frostbite straightforward. Underlying medical conditions that may predispose the patient to hypothermia (e.g., malnutrition) as well as intercurrent processes (e.g., trauma, overdose) are important to consider. Signs and symptoms of these coexistent conditions may overlap with those of hypothermia.

DIAGNOSIS AND EVALUATION

Hypothermia is a clinical diagnosis based on the patient's core body temperature. Patients presenting in extremis should have their core temperatures obtained by thermometer probe inserted into the distal esophagus. Rectal temperatures are useful for initial assessment, but once rewarming has begun, temperatures may be falsely low secondary to unintentional

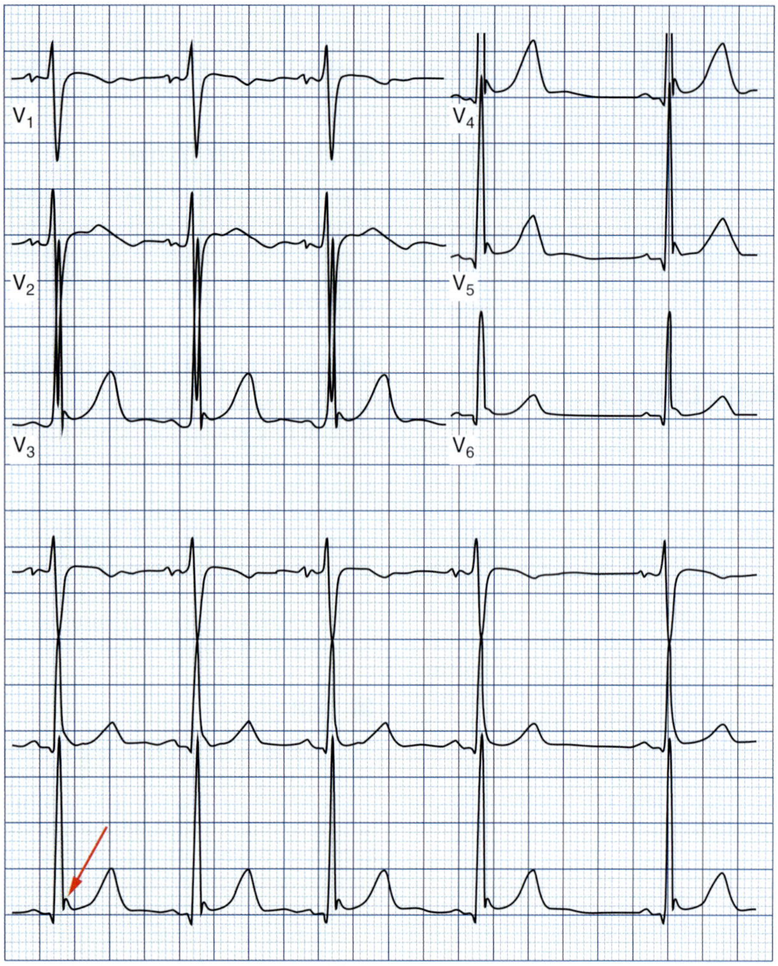

FIGURE 175-1. Osborn wave. Note the upward deflection following the QRS complex.

insertion of the probe into stool. Handheld, digital thermometers may not be capable of registering temperatures below 34°C and thus may be inaccurate. Cardiac and respiratory monitoring leads must be placed, but because the victim's skin is usually very slick, even after drying, proper placement may be difficult.

The initial evaluation of hypothermic patients focuses on cervical spine immobilization (if trauma is suspected); support of airway, breathing, and circulation; and removal of wet clothes. A secondary survey should also be performed, much like the secondary survey during trauma resuscitations. The skin should be thoroughly inspected and documented for sensation to light touch and noxious stimuli. Blister formation secondary

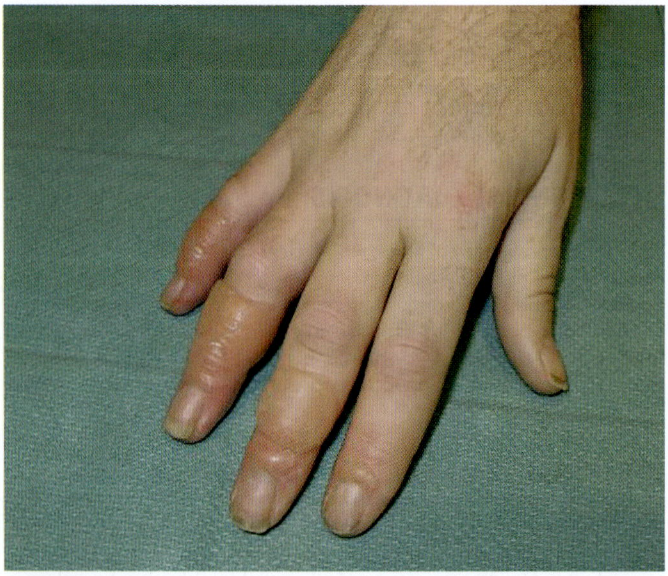

FIGURE 175-2. Second-degree frostbite is demonstrated by blisters filled with either clear or milky fluid. Tissue tends to be malleable. (Used with permission of Doug Brunette, MD.)

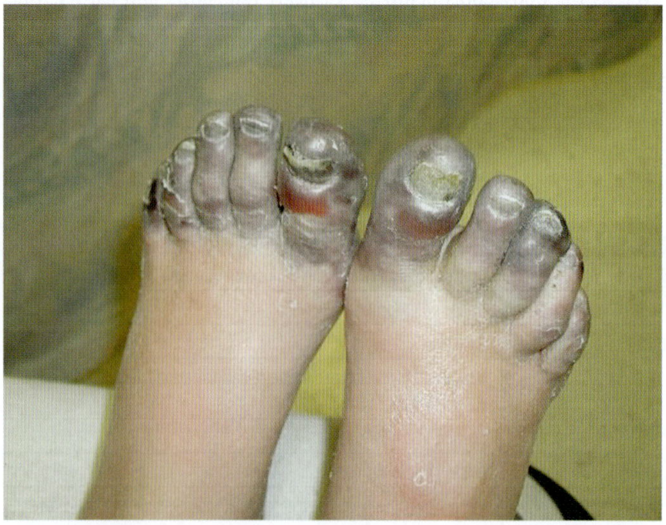

FIGURE 175-3. Third-degree frostbite. Hemorrhagic blisters can be seen on both feet, first digits. (Used with permission of Doug Brunette, MD.)

to frostbite may be found and should be categorized as either superficial or deep (second versus third degree). Lacerations, fractures, and bruises should all be noted and addressed appropriately. Laboratory data to be considered include serum electrolytes, complete blood cell count, coagulopathy studies (prothrombin time, partial thromboplastin time, fibrinogen), blood gas analysis, blood type and screen, and hepatic and pancreatic enzymes. Laboratory abnormalities clinicians can anticipate are decreased white blood cell and platelet count due to splenic sequestration; increased hemoglobin and hematocrit due to hemoconcentration; and elevated lipase due to hypothermia-induced pancreatitis. Urine and serum toxicology testing may be indicated in some scenarios. A bedside blood sugar quantification should also be obtained. Blood gas interpretation should not be corrected for core temperature. It is now believed that any metabolic and respiratory acidosis will resolve as core temperature rises and that management of acidosis is more successful with uncorrected gases.

Imaging studies should be performed if indicated. A chest radiograph is useful if pulmonary edema or aspiration pneumonia is suspected and to verify endotracheal tube placement. Head or abdominal computed tomography is indicated if trauma or abuse is suspected. An electrocardiogram should be performed if any arrhythmia is suspected. Likewise, it may be useful to document cardiac electrical activity, J waves, and cardiac ischemia.

MANAGEMENT

INITIAL RESUSCITATION

Prehospital management of hypothermic patients consists of evaluating the patient's ABCs (airway, breathing, and circulation) and providing basic or advanced life support as needed. During resuscitation, if there is an organized rhythm or pulses are noted, even in the face of profound bradycardia, most researchers argue to forgo chest compressions because of the possibility that external cardiac massage might induce arrhythmias. In addition, given the depressed metabolic demands of the brain and body, a slow pulsatile rate may be sufficient to sustain survival. The only true indication for chest compressions is asystole or unstable ventricular arrhythmias. Electrical defibrillation is warranted with ventricular fibrillation but may not be effective until core temperature rises. Likewise, resuscitation medications are rarely effective.

Patients who are rewarmed and resuscitated but continue to be pulseless should be declared dead only after core temperature rises above 35°C. Defibrillation and resuscitation medications are thought to be more effective at core temperatures higher than 30°C.

REWARMING IN HYPOTHERMIA

Mildly hypothermic patients will recover fully without any complications. Any mental confusion or dysarthria should resolve once normal core temperature returns. A rewarmed hypothermic patient with persistent altered mental status requires a "second look" as to the etiology: intracranial bleeding, intoxication, ingestion, sepsis, endocrinopathies, cardiac conditions, and so on. Moderate to severely hypothermic victims should always be rewarmed. The lowest core temperature to survive to full neurologic recovery was 13.7°C. Survival rates have ranged from 47% to 71%. Patients with chronic medical conditions tend to have a worse prognosis.

Rewarming any hypothermic patient, which typically begins in an emergency department setting, is divided into two methods: passive and active rewarming. Active rewarming is further differentiated into active core and active external. Passive rewarming is noninvasive and involves removing wet clothes, drying, and wrapping the patient in a blanket. This is suitable for mildly hypothermic patients who are stable. Active external rewarming requires the use of warm blankets or heating blankets (which can raise the body's temperature by up to 0.8°C per hour) and heat lamps or forced heat. Both passive and active external rewarming modalities are typically for moderate hypothermia victims who are not in shock.

Active core rewarming techniques are the most efficient and rapid methods of warming patients. In this phase, core body temperature can be expected to rise by 0.5°C to 2°C per hour. Intravenous administration of warmed crystalloid as a bolus to avoid volume overload is the initial step in the treatment of a profoundly hypothermic patient; portable intravenous warmers can warm any intravenous fluids to 40°C to 42°C. Hospital management also includes active core rewarming with a water bath at 40°C for 15 to 30 minutes.

If the patient is pulseless, cardiopulmonary bypass or extracorporeal membrane oxygenation (ECMO) are the methods of choice. Bypass can raise a patient's core temperature by 1°C to 2°C every 5 minutes. Indications for bypass are (i) cardiac arrest or instability with a temperature lower than 32°C; (ii) suboptimal response to other warming measures; (iii) frozen extremities; and/or (iv) severe hyperkalemia secondary to rhabdomyolysis. ECMO may show improved survival rates owing to its ability to manage severe respiratory failure, a well-documented complication of rewarming patients.

Patients with severe hypothermia may experience renal failure, coagulopathies, hyperglycemia or hypoglycemia, electrolyte disturbances, pulmonary edema, or aspiration pneumonia. Dialysis may be required for renal failure. Coagulopathies should be corrected with fresh frozen plasma (10 mL/kg). Electrolyte disturbances, hyperkalemia in particular, may resolve with rewarming. However, some authors suggest no resuscitation if an initial serum potassium is greater than 12 mmol/L. Patients who are hypothermic secondary to cold-water submersion may require seizure management related to a cerebral hypoxic-ischemic event.

FROSTBITE

Frostbite injuries may take as long as 4 weeks for definitive care. Decisions for debridement are rarely necessary in the acute phase of treatment because delineation of viable versus nonviable tissue is difficult to determine in the early phases. Treatment of frostbite is a three-phase approach.

The initial phase is the pre-thaw care, typically started by pre-hospital care providers. This phase involves using soft padding to protect the affected area. No other treatment should be initiated. No rubbing or rewarming of tissues is indicated because this may potentially do more damage.

The second phase, emergency department management, is the rewarming process. Rewarming should be done for 15 to 30 minutes or until thawing is complete by immersing the involved area in circulating water at a temperature between 40°C and 42°C. Tissue that has been adequately rewarmed will become supple and demonstrate capillary refill. Intravenous analgesics may be necessary during the rewarming phase because it can be severely painful. Blisters should be left intact, and a topical antibiotic ointment applied every 6 hours. Tetanus prophylaxis is indicated for potentially contaminated wounds. The post-thaw or third phase requires gentle handling of injured tissue. Areas of injury should be covered with dry, sterile dressings. The dressings should be loosely secured with noncompressive and nonadhesive material. If the hands or feet are involved, they should be splinted and placed in an elevated position. Digits must be separated with cotton gauze.

Patients successfully rewarmed in the emergency department may warrant observation. The need for hospital admission of frostbite should be assessed based on the severity of injury, comorbidities, medical history, and the need for in-hospital interventions (intravenous medication, radiology, surgery). Patients with frostbite beyond first degree typically require inpatient wound care, pain control, and rehabilitation. When stratifying the potential interventions needed in the inpatient setting, it is important to note that during the first 24 hours patients should be admitted to a facility capable of administering thrombolysis. Since one of the mechanisms of frostbite includes vascular thrombosis, literature has shown tissue plasminogen factor (tPA) can play an important role in salvaging digits. Further, adult literature has shown decreased risk of amputation in more severe grades of frostbite with iloprost, a prostacyclin analog. Thus, for adults with frostbite it is recommended that during the first 72 hours, patients be admitted to a facility capable of iloprost treatment; however, the long-term implications of iloprost therapy and its application in the pediatric population requires more investigation. Healing of frostbite can take from a few days up to several months. The decision for debridement or amputation is often delayed weeks to months to fully assess if the damaged or dead tissue can heal. If nonviable tissue continues to be present at the final demarcation stage (could be 1-3 months after injury) amputation is considered.

Most frostbite cases are due to exposure to cold in the urban setting, and can be seen in conjunction with substance use, trauma, hypothermia, physical disability, and psychosocial issues. Such issues can complicate long-term management and require attention during hospital admission.

ADMISSION CRITERIA

Hospitalization is indicated for any of the following criteria:

- Moderate to severe hypothermia
- Frostbite beyond first degree
- Altered mental status despite adequate rewarming
- Questions of abuse or neglect
- Suicide attempt

DISCHARGE CRITERIA

- Normal physical and mental examination
- Normal laboratory data
- Acceptable social environment
- Frostbite injuries suitable for outpatient follow-up

CONSULTATION

HYPOTHERMIA

- Critical care: For patients with cardiovascular instability, on ECMO or bypass, requiring bedside services or monitoring that exceed the capacity of general inpatient unit (frequent neurological checks, labs, etc.)
- Nephrology: For patients with or at risk for (e.g., rhabdomyolysis) renal failure
- Cardiology and cardiothoracic surgery: For patients in need of cardiopulmonary bypass or ECMO
- General or trauma surgery: All hypothermic patients admitted to the hospital should have a trauma consultation

FROSTBITE

- Interventional radiology: Thrombolytic interventions
- Pain team: To provide adequate short- and long-term analgesics
- General, plastic, or otolaryngology surgery: For debridement of open blisters and amputation of necrotic, dead tissue, from digits, limbs, nose, and ears
- Nutrition: For the caloric adjustment needed for recovery from severe frostbite
- Rehabilitation: For daily physical and occupational therapy
- Psychological services: For ongoing support, evaluation of social determinants and on-going risk factors, especially if extremities and digits are expected to be amputated

SPECIAL CONSIDERATIONS

WHEN TO TRANSFER TO A PEDIATRIC TRAUMA CENTER

Hypothermia Most hospitals should be able to provide adequate rewarming. For patients with severe hypothermia, transfer to a pediatric trauma center should be considered if serum potassium is less than 12 mmol/L and transfer time from "door to door" is reasonable. For example, a 6-hour transfer time in an ambulance for a patient with cardiac instability or in full arrest is not acceptable. It would be better to keep aggressive, noncardiac bypass/ECMO, rewarming techniques going until the patient's core temperature reaches 35°C.

Frostbite Inability to provide adequate care with appropriate services: surgical, physical, and occupational care. Regional burn centers are the referral centers of choice.

PREVENTION

Hypothermia Stay warm in cold weather by avoiding the outside or wearing layers of clothing. Wearing a hat and protective covering such as mittens are essential. Layers of clothing also help prevent heat loss. Avoid overexertion. Sweating increases heat loss. If clothes get wet from falling into water or from sweating, dry off skin and change into dry clothes.

Frostbite Limit time outdoors, wear a hat that covers ears. Mittens are better than gloves at keeping fingers warm. Be aware of the signs of frostbite: redness and skin sensation of numbness or "pins and needles."

KEY POINTS

- **Clinical Presentation of Hypothermia:** The spectrum of physical signs and symptoms is dependent on the victim's temperature and can be as simple as dysarthria and shivering to frank coma and cardiovascular collapse.
- **Management:** The initial management of hypothermia includes removal of all wet clothes, active and passive rewarming techniques, supportive care, and cardiopulmonary resuscitation (until the body is at least 35°C). A serum potassium of 12 mmol/L or greater and noncompatible injuries from trauma are considerations for not pursuing/continuing resuscitation.
- **Frostbite:** Frostbite treatment includes (i) pre-thaw care (use of soft padding to protect the affected area); (ii) rewarming (immersion in warm water, pain control, and tetanus prophylaxis); and (iii) post-thaw care (application of dry, sterile, noncompressive and nonadhesive dressings). Consider transfer to a burn center for extensive injury.

SUGGESTED READINGS

Brown D, Brugger H, Boyd J, et al. Accidental hypothermia. *N Engl J Med.* 2013;367:1930-1938.

Centers for Disease Control and Prevention (CDC). QuickStats: Death Rates Attributed to Excessive Cold or Hypothermia, by Urbanization Level and Sex-National Vital Statistics System, 2018-2020. *MMWR Morb Mortal Wkly Rep.* 2022;71:282.

Corneli HM. Accidental hypothermia. *Pediatr Emerg Care.* 2012;28(5):475-480.

Gilbert M, Busund R, Skagseth A, et al. Resuscitation from accidental hypothermia of 13.7°C with circulatory arrest. *Lancet.* 2000;355:375-376.

Hallam M, Cubison T, Dheansa B, et al. Managing frostbite. *BMJ.* 2010;341:1151-1156.

Lorentzen AK, Davis C, Penninga L. Interventions for frostbite injuries. *Cochrane Database Syst Rev.* 2020;12(12):CD012980.

Mallet ML. Pathophysiology of accidental hypothermia. *QJM.* 2002;95:775-785.

McDaniel L. Hypothermia and Cold Injury in Children. *Pediatr Rev.* 2022:58-60.

McIntosh SE, Freer L, Grissom CK, et al. Wilderness Medical Society clinical practice guidelines for the prevention and treatment of frostbite: 2019 update. *Wilderness Environ Med.* 2019;30:Suppl:S19-S32.

Paal P, Pasquier M, Darocha T, et al. Accidental hypothermia: 2021 update. *Int J Environ Res Public Health.* 2022;19(1):501.

Regli IB, Strapazzon G, Falla M, Oberhammer R, Brugger H. Long-term sequelae of frostbite—a scoping review. *Int J Environ Res Public Health.* 2021;18(18):9655.

Sheridan RL, Goverman JM, Walker TG. Diagnosis and treatment of frostbite. *N Engl J Med.* 2022;386(23):2213-2220.

Tisherman SA. Hypothermia and injury. *Curr Opin Crit Care.* 2004;10(6):512-519.

Urlich SA, Rathlev NK. Hypothermia and localized cold injuries. *Emerg Med Clin North Am*. 2004;22:281-298.

Walpoth BH, et al. Outcome of survivors of accidental deep hypothermia and circulatory arrest treated with extracorporeal blood warming. *N Engl J Med*. 1997;337(21):1500-1505.

CHAPTER 176 Drowning

Kristyn Jeffries, MD, MPH and Khoon-Yen Tay, MD

BACKGROUND

In the past, submersion events have been defined in various ways in the medical literature. The lack of consistency and standardization of terms makes research analysis and communication in the field difficult, confusing, and imprecise. In 2002, the International Liaison Committee on Resuscitation (ILCOR) approved guidelines for definitions and reporting of data related to drowning developed by international investigators and experts in the field. Many terms, such as, "near drowned" which previously referred to survival of a submersion victim for longer than 24 hours as well as "wet" and "dry drowning" were abandoned. According to ILCOR, the term *drowning* should refer to a process resulting in primary respiratory impairment from submersion/immersion in a liquid medium. *Drowning* can be further subcategorized as *nonfatal drowning* when the victim survives after submersion in a liquid medium.

EPIDEMIOLOGY

Drowning remains a significant pediatric problem. In the United States, drowning is the leading cause of death for children 1 to 4 years and the second leading cause of unintentional injury-related death in children 5 to 14 years. From 2001 to 2020, drowning represented over 10,000 deaths for children 0 to 4 years, accounting for nearly 75% of all child drownings in recent years. Toddlers and teenagers are particularly at risk given their unique developmental and behavioral stages. Toddlers are more likely to drown in pools, bathtubs, toilets, and buckets of water whereas older adolescents are more likely to drown in open water. Males are two times more likely to drown than females. Black children overall are nearly two times more likely to be hospitalized than White children, with the highest risk of hospitalization and death for Black children 10 to 12 years of age. This group of children may be particularly vulnerable to drowning for several reasons driven by systemic factors related to structural racism, including inequitable access to affordable swimming lessons and safe, well-supervised swimming pools in Black communities.

Overall, the incidence of hospitalization for children with nonfatal drowning has been decreasing over the past decade with most injuries being managed in the emergency department. Yet morbidity and mortality are high for those subsequently admitted to the hospital, with higher risk of mortality for children <5 years old and those with prolonged submersion times, who develop cerebral edema, who require cardiopulmonary resuscitation (CPR), and who require mechanical ventilation. Thus, it is important that providers have an enhanced knowledge of the pathophysiology of the drowning process to avoid secondary insults in the care of drowning victims and that the lay public has increased awareness of water safety and CPR.

PATHOPHYSIOLOGY

Hypoxemia is the final common pathway of injury in the drowning process which, if not interrupted, ultimately results in profound tissue hypoxia and multiorgan failure. While the lungs are the primary and initial site of injury in the drowning process, the heart and the brain are the most important organs affected, often permanently.

During the initial phases of submersion, victims hold their breath and struggle until they reflexively breathe, causing the aspiration of fluid. This aspiration results in laryngospasm; if it is sustained, the victims do not aspirate any more fluid. In most cases, however, the laryngospasm resolves, and the victims aspirate more fluid. Because of progressive neurologic failure and the swallowing of fluid, victims often vomit and may aspirate gastric contents as well. The aspiration of fluid results in acute impaired lung function and worsening hypoxemia due to loss of surfactant, caustic injury from aspirated contents, and pulmonary edema. Atelectasis, ventilation-perfusion mismatch, and acute respiratory distress syndrome (ARDS) may result. Pneumonia may develop, but usually occurs later in the course, in intubated patients who survive hospital admission.

Hypoxic injury may occur in any organ; however, the brain and the heart are particularly sensitive to even brief periods of hypoxia. Hypoxic-ischemic injury causes cerebral edema and increased intracranial pressure. The neurologic sequelae for hypoxic-ischemic injury are often the most devastating for submersion victims. The effects of hypoxemia on cardiovascular function include decreased cardiac output and increased systemic and pulmonary resistance. Arrhythmias may occur secondary to hypoxemia, hypothermia, or other metabolic derangements. Common arrhythmias include sinus bradycardia, pulseless electrical activity (PEA), and asystole; ventricular fibrillation occurs rarely. Less common end-organ sequelae include renal insufficiency or failure, acute tubular necrosis, and disseminated intravascular coagulopathy.

CLINICAL PRESENTATION

The initial presentation of a submersion victim can range from asymptomatic to critically ill. This initial presentation reflects the severity of injury sustained as well as the projected outcome. Children who present alert and without respiratory distress usually remain well with no deterioration in their clinical status. Critically ill patients often present with hypothermia and poor perfusion; despite heroic resuscitative efforts, the outcome is often poor. Body temperature rapidly decreases in submersion victims. Lung sounds may be coarse, clear, or absent. Pulses may be diminished or absent, and perfusion is usually decreased secondary to peripheral vasoconstriction from hypothermia.

The history focuses on identifying the life-threatening injury or insult, determining the details of the submersion and rescue, and obtaining the pertinent medical history (**Table 176-1**). It is important to determine any resuscitation efforts attempted following rescue, as bystander CPR appears to be critical to patient morbidity and mortality. The physical

TABLE 176-1 Focused History after A Drowning Event

Scene Events
When was the patient last seen alive? How long was he or she underwater?
Where did the event occur? Was the water excessively contaminated or stagnant?
What is the estimated water temperature?
Was the patient diving? Is head trauma suspected?
Did the patient vomit?
Is alcohol or drug use suspected, especially in teenagers?
Rescue Events
Was the patient responsive and breathing when rescued? Did he or she have a pulse?
Was the patient removed with cervical spine precautions (if necessary)?
What initial rescue maneuvers were done? Who performed these maneuvers? How long did it take for emergency technicians to arrive, and what steps did they take? What response did the patient have to these maneuvers?
Past Medical History
Underlying seizure disorder
History of syncope, long QT syndrome
Other History
Allergies
Last meal

examination consists of an immediate assessment of the patient's airway, breathing, and circulation (ABCs), followed by a full head-to-toe survey of other possible injuries.

DIFFERENTIAL DIAGNOSIS

For older children, the diagnosis of submersion is obvious. However, it is important to consider comorbidities that may have placed the patient at higher risk, such as long QT syndrome, alcohol or drug intoxication, autism spectrum disorder, attention-deficit hyperactivity disorder (ADHD), or a poorly controlled seizure disorder. Inflicted submersion, as in nonaccidental trauma, should be suspected when the reported history is not consistent with the child's developmental stage or physical examination. Inflicted submersions are seen predominantly in children younger than 2 years, and they often occur in the bathtub.

MANAGEMENT

INITIAL STABILIZATION

No prognostic factors reliably predict survival or good neurologic outcome for drowning patients managed in the emergency department. Additionally, there are many case reports of survival after prolonged downtimes and significantly abnormal physiologic parameters. Therefore, in the emergency department, all patients should undergo initial resuscitation as indicated by the patient's severity of injury at the time of presentation. Those who are critically ill are treated like any other critically ill or injured patient, focusing primarily on the immediate identification and treatment of life-threatening conditions. A stepwise approach begins with an assessment of the patient's ABCs.

For patients in asystole or PEA, endotracheal intubation with positive-pressure ventilation, initiation of chest compressions, and parenteral administration of epinephrine should occur immediately, following the Pediatric Advanced Life Support (PALS) algorithms. For patients who have a pulse, assuring an airway remains paramount, as the airway may be obstructed from secretions or water, or poorly protected due to an altered sensorium. Clear and maintain a patent airway with suctioning, positioning, and adjunctive airways (e.g., oropharyngeal or nasopharyngeal airway) as necessary. Institute cervical spine immobilization if there is suspicion of a cervical spine injury. Provide 100% oxygen as hypoxemia is the final common pathway of injury. Consider obtaining an arterial or venous blood gas to assess the patient's ventilatory status. If there is still ineffective ventilation or oxygenation after these airway maneuvers, endotracheal intubation should be performed. Other indications for intubation include apnea or significant neurologic injury. The use of rapid sequence intubation medications helps facilitate mechanical airway control, although is unnecessary for patients without a pulse. Pulmonary edema may be suspected with the presence of pink, frothy pulmonary secretions in the endotracheal tube or an inability to adequately oxygenate. In such cases, peak inspiratory pressures should be maximized and administration of a diuretic (e.g., furosemide) can be considered.

Circulatory assessment should focus on the patient's pulse, perfusion, and blood pressure. Bradycardic patients (heart rate <60 beats per minute) from prolonged hypoxia may require only simple airway maneuvers and/or bag-mask ventilation for a short period of time which will improve oxygenation, ventilation, and the declining heart rate. If the patient remains bradycardic, despite these interventions, and has evidence of poor perfusion, PALS guidelines should be instituted, including initiation of CPR and administration of epinephrine. Fluid resuscitation (e.g., 20 mL/kg of crystalloid fluid as an initial bolus) should be started if there is evidence of inadequate perfusion or hypotension, followed by frequent reassessments and administration of more fluid as needed. The patient should always receive cardiorespiratory and pulse oximetry monitoring.

The ABCs should be expanded to include an assessment of disability and exposure ("D" and "E"). A quick assessment of disability includes the patient's pupillary response and assignment of a mental status: alert (A), response to verbal stimuli (V), response to painful stimuli (P), or unresponsive (U) (AVPU). The Glasgow coma scale (GCS), more often used in trauma resuscitations and evaluations, can also provide a baseline measure of neurologic status. After managing the ABCDEs, a head-to-toe examination should be done to identify signs of coexisting trauma (whether intentional or unintentional) and toxidromes. The patient should be undressed completely to allow a full physical assessment and to minimize further heat loss secondary to wet clothing. The patient should then be covered with warm blankets and body temperature should be monitored. In children, the role and benefits of therapeutic hypothermia or targeted temperature management after a cardiopulmonary arrest and other new interventions are still being explored.

FURTHER MANAGEMENT

In the emergency department, patients should be triaged into one of two groups: those who have moderate to severe perturbations in their cardiorespiratory or central nervous system physiology, and those who are minimally symptomatic or asymptomatic. For the first group, the primary focus is the immediate identification and treatment of life-threatening conditions. Following the interventions described in the previous section, pulse oximetry, arterial blood gas measurement, chest radiograph, laboratory testing (e.g., glucose, electrolytes), and computed tomography (CT) of the brain, and electrocardiograms can provide important information. Increasing hypoxia as shown by continuous pulse oximetry can identify children who are developing pulmonary edema or ARDS. Consider serial arterial blood gas levels in patients who are hypoxemic, acidotic, deteriorating, or not responding to interventions. Chest radiographs are often normal initially but later reveal evidence of pulmonary injury or aspiration (**Figure 176-1**). Providers should not be falsely reassured by normal chest radiographs and continue to have a high index of suspicion for progressive pulmonary injury and worsening respiratory distress. Consider bedside glucose measurement to identify hypoglycemia in infants and young children, whose limited glycogen stores may be depleted by the increased demands associated with the event. Laboratory studies may be normal initially or may reflect derangements from initial fluid shifts (e.g., hypo- or hypernatremia) or sequelae of cardiovascular and respiratory compromise. Serum bicarbonate levels are often reduced when lactic acidosis develops secondary to shock, hypoxemia, and hypoperfusion. A complete blood cell count may reveal elevations in the neutrophil count likely secondary to demargination from the vascular endothelium. Serum liver transaminases or creatinine may be elevated due to end-organ hypoperfusion. A urine toxicology screen or serum alcohol level is indicated in the appropriate clinical setting. Noncontrast head CT, looking for intracranial hemorrhage, is useful in neurologically compromised patients or if the history suggests trauma as the cause of the drowning event. Additionally, cerebral edema from prolonged hypoxic injury may also be observed on CT, though magnetic resonance imaging (MRI) is the diagnostic imaging of choice when this is suspected. If there is a suspicion of syncope or a family history of syncope or early unexplained death, consider an electrocardiogram to determine the Q-Tc (increased in long QT syndrome) and P-R intervals (shortened with an accessory atrioventricular pathways) ECG interpretation is covered in Chapter 50.

After the initial stabilization, treatment is directed toward limiting further injury and identifying and managing disease progression. While novel therapies are currently being explored, goals of management should still focus on normothermia, normocapnia, normoglycemia, and normotension. Critically ill pediatric submersion victims, due to the multisystem involvement and complex airway management issues that arise, should be transferred to the nearest available facility with a pediatric intensive care unit (PICU) as soon as they are stabilized.

When hypoxemia persists despite adequate ventilation, pulmonary edema or ARDS should be suspected. Diuresis with furosemide may be beneficial for cases of pulmonary edema, although hypovolemia should be corrected before this is initiated. Fluid restriction to two-thirds of maintenance may be warranted if the patient is hemodynamically stable. Extracorporeal membrane oxygenation (ECMO) may be necessary in patients who progress to ARDS or when there is profound hypothermia requiring rewarming. Vasoactive agents, such as epinephrine and

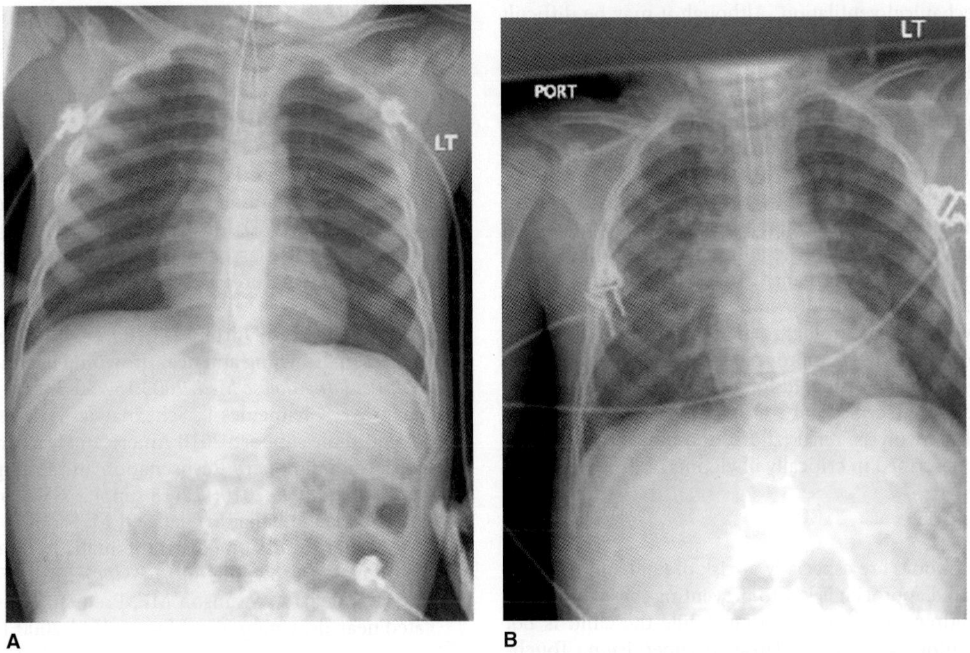

FIGURE 176-1. Initial chest radiograph (A) and radiograph taken 2 days later (B) in a 4-year-old boy who was found submerged in a bathtub after being left unattended for a few minutes. Note the initially clear lungs and the subsequent development of pulmonary edema, as evidenced by increased interstitial markings.

dopamine, are used when adequate perfusion cannot be established despite fluid resuscitation. Prophylactic antibiotics do not prevent the development of pneumonia, even in the setting of suspected aspiration of orogastric fluid, and are not recommended. Additionally, steroids do not improve outcome and should not be used routinely.

Moderately affected patients should be observed closely for progression of disease, particularly respiratory status, because signs and symptoms may be subtle and delayed. Delivery of supplemental oxygen can be decreased to maintain normal oxygen saturation levels. Wheezing may develop due to airway edema, increased airway debris or secretions, or bronchospasm. The inhalation of a β-agonist may help reduce the bronchospastic component.

In well-appearing patients with little or no disturbance in their respiratory and neurologic status, evaluation should consist of a careful history and physical examination, along with an initial and discharge pulse oximetry, respiratory exam, and a chest radiograph. Close observation for 6 to 12 hours after the event in the ED or the inpatient hospital setting should be sufficient to identify the small proportion of children who become progressively worse despite their reassuring appearance on initial presentation. It is unlikely that any laboratory studies, including an arterial blood gas measurement, will provide relevant data to assist in the evaluation of a well-appearing patient after a drowning event.

ADMISSION CRITERIA

- Critically ill patients or those with a deteriorating status should be transferred to an intensive care setting.
- Patients with mild to moderate symptoms should be admitted for close observation, including continuous pulse oximetry and cardiorespiratory monitoring. Observe mildly symptomatic patients until they have returned to baseline.
- The management of asymptomatic children is somewhat controversial due to limited data. Most reports show that for the vast majority of well-appearing children, observation for at least 6 to 12 hours after the event is prudent. Children who do not show development of respiratory distress, hypoxemia, or adventitious lung sounds, and have a reliable guardian who can return them to the hospital if needed, can be discharged after the period of observation.

DISCHARGE CRITERIA

- Patients should demonstrate normal heart and respiratory rates and oxygen saturation greater than 94% on room air.
- Patients should have no increase in the work of breathing, and breath sounds should be clear on auscultation.
- Caretakers should be available who are able to detect signs and symptoms of clinical deterioration and return the child to the hospital if necessary.
- For children with long-term sequelae, institution of appropriate home care and follow-up is needed.
- If an unintentional nonfatal drowning occurred, the caretakers should receive counseling for injury prevention.
- If nonaccidental injury is suspected, child protective services should be notified, and discharge to a safe environment must be assured.

CONSULTATION

- Critical care when cardiorespiratory support is needed
- Subspecialty medical consultation based on end-organ system involvement
- Rehabilitation medicine consultation when significant neurologic deficits necessitate coordination of multidisciplinary therapies after discharge
- Child protective services when there is suspicion of nonaccidental events or negligence

SPECIAL CONSIDERATIONS

COMPLICATIONS

Complications from drowning are common among critically ill patients and result from the initial hypoxic-ischemic insult or the primary lung injury. Pulmonary edema, ventilation-perfusion mismatch, pneumothorax, and ARDS are often encountered, especially among patients requiring mechanical ventilation. Although it may be difficult to determine which of these conditions coexist, the need for increased supplemental oxygen or ventilatory support may raise suspicion for pneumonia, especially if chest radiography shows a new infiltrate. Common pathogens are those aspirated from the body of water or the human oropharyngeal tract. Although antibiotics are not indicated for prophylaxis, patients with a clinical picture consistent with bacterial pneumonia warrant empiric antibiotic therapy covering suspected pathogens. An extended-spectrum penicillin-β-lactamase inhibitor combination (i.e., ampicillin-sulbactam) is reasonable to administer.

Cerebral edema and resultant permanent neurologic injury are the most feared complications following drowning. Hospitalists often provide care for patients with these neurologic deficits following a drowning event after stabilization in the PICU. Appropriate therapies and discharge care needs should be carefully considered for each patient based on the specific neurological deficits (see Section T Care of the Child with Medical Complexity). Rhabdomyolysis, renal failure, and multiorgan system failure have also been described in critically ill victims of drowning.

PREVENTION

Toddlers and adolescent boys are especially at risk of fatal and nonfatal drowning. A multilayered approach is key to preventing these drowning events. For young children, many events occur while the child is not expected to be swimming or during a lapse in supervision. Touch-supervision while in water and restrictive barriers to water access in and around homes, should be emphasized to all parents. To address the disproportionately higher rates of submersion injuries among Black children, providers should advocate for equitable access to swimming lessons at a young age and safe, well-supervised community swimming pools.

KEY POINTS

- Drowning events are predominantly events of childhood and adolescence.
- Rapid response and delivery of bystander basic life support at the scene are critical for survival.
- The most severe complications of drownings include pulmonary edema and ARDS secondary to direct lung injury as well as hypoxic-ischemic cerebral injury and cardiac arrest secondary to prolonged hypoxemia.
- Victims who are asymptomatic on presentation or who have minimal signs of respiratory compromise warrant a period of observation because their condition can deteriorate. Most do not usually show decompensation, however, and can be discharged after 6 to 12 hours of observation.
- Consider both medical and social comorbidities, such as child abuse in a toddler who nearly drowned in the bathtub or alcohol or drug use in a teenager.

SUGGESTED READINGS

Centers for Disease Control and Prevention (CDC). *Web-Based Injury Statistics Query and Reporting System (WISQARS)*. Atlanta, GA: US Department of Health and Human Services, CDC; 2021. http://www.cdc.gov/injury/wisqars/index.html. Last accessed on August 31, 2022.

Consumer Product Safety Commission. Pool or Spa Submersion: Estimated Nonfatal Drowning Injuries and Reported Drownings, 2020 Report. Washington, DC: Consumer Product Safety Commission; 2020. Available at: https://www.cpsc.gov/s3fs-public/2020-Submersion-Report-4-29-20_0.pdf?ghYmKOmkLBzmXo6Rjm96Qkn16JC%20pM1ir. Last accessed on August 31, 2022.

Denny SA, Quan L, Gilchrist J, et al. Prevention of drowning. *Pediatrics*. 2021;148(2):e2021052227.

Umapathi KK, Thavamani A, Dhanpalreddy H, Khatana J, Roy A. Incidence trends and predictors of in-hospital mortality in drowning in children and adolescents in the United States: a National Inpatient Database Analysis. *Clin Pediatr (Phila)*. 2020;59(2):134-141.

Jeffries K, Puls H, Hall M, et al. Racial and ethnic differences in pediatric unintentional injuries requiring hospitalization. *J Hosp Med*. 2022;17(1):19-27.

Felton H, Myers J, Liu G, Davis DW. Unintentional, non-fatal drowning of children: US trends and racial/ethnic disparities. *BMJ Open*. 2015;5(12):e008444.

Semple-Hess J, Campwala R. Pediatric submersion injuries: emergency care and resuscitation. *Pediatr Emerg Med Pract*. 2014;11(6):1-21.

Tobin JM, Ramos WD, Pu Y, Wernicki PG, Quan L, Rossano JW. Bystander CPR is associated with improved neurologically favourable survival in cardiac arrest following drowning. *Resuscitation*. 2017;115:39-43.

Hwang V, Shofer FS, Durbin DR, Baren JM. Prevalence of traumatic injuries in drowning and near drowning in children and adolescents. *Arch Pediatr Adolesc Med*. 2003;157:50-53.

Kleinman ME, Chameides L, Schexnayder SM, et al. Part 14: pediatric advanced life support: 2010 American Heart Association Guidelines for Cardiopulmonary Resuscitation and Emergency Cardiovascular Care. *Circulation*. 2010;122(18 suppl 3):S876-S908.

Cohen N, Capua T, Lahat S, Glatstein M, Sadot E, Rimon A. Predictors for hospital admission of asymptomatic to moderately symptomatic children after drowning. *Eur J Pediatr*. 2019;178(9):1379-1384.

Causey AL, Tilelli JA, Swanson ME. Predicting discharge in uncomplicated near-drowning. *Am J Emerg Med*. 2000;18:9-11.

CHAPTER 177 Human and Animal Bites

Eleanor A. Sharp, MD, MS and Elena C. Griego, MD

BACKGROUND

Animal and human bites are common, with approximately 5 million bite occurrences annually in the United States. Of these, between 400,000 and 500,000 patients seek care for human or animal bites in emergency departments each year, and up to 2% of those presenting to emergency departments require hospitalization. Of children presenting to an emergency department for injuries, approximately 1.5% of visits were related to dog bites and hospitalization rates were as high as 9%. Factors resulting in increased rates of hospitalization include location of injury (head, neck, and upper limb) and age younger than 5 years. Domesticated dogs and cats inflict most bites in the United States, together accounting for over 95% of all cases. While dog bites are most common, accounting for 60% to 90% of all bites, cat bites are disproportionately responsible for infectious complications. Rates of infection after cat bites are reported as high as 50%, while infection rates after dog or human bites are reported at 5% to 25%.

Bite wounds cause morbidity and mortality through both direct physical trauma and infection. Patients who present for care within 12 hours of injury typically have some form of crush injury, disfiguring wounds, ongoing bleeding, and/or the need for rabies or tetanus therapy. In contrast, patients presenting more than 12 hours after an injury often have swelling, erythema, and/or purulence at the bite site due to evolving infection. Bite wounds are typically contaminated with multiple strains of aerobic and anaerobic bacteria. Approximately 10% to 20% of all bite wounds become infected and require antibiotic treatment.

In this chapter, both mechanical injury and infectious complications from dog, cat, and human bites are discussed. Topics that warrant special consideration, such as other animal bites, clenched-fist injuries, bites to the face and hands, bites in immunocompromised patients, and rabies and other infection screening and prophylaxis, are also reviewed.

COMMON BITE TYPES

Human and animal bites present with a variety of injuries, ranging from superficial abrasions and lacerations to puncture, complex laceration, or crush injury.

Dog Bites Dog bites can cause a spectrum of injuries, from lacerations to avulsions and crush injuries. While adult canine teeth are not very sharp, they can exert a pressure of 200 to 450 psi, which is strong enough to perforate sheet metal. Thus, these bites commonly result in crush injuries surrounded by infection-prone, devitalized tissue. Children younger than 18 years of age account for between 50% and 60% of dog bite cases that seek medical attention. Dog bites to the head and neck region are common in younger children, occurring in 50% to 65% of bites in children younger than 5 years and between 30% and 40% of those 5 to 10 years old. Younger children are more likely to provoke or startle an animal accidentally, and due to their smaller stature, they are more frequently at eye level with dogs, increasing the risk of injury to the head and neck region. The thin and immature calvaria of a young child has little resistance to the pressure that can be exerted by a dog bite, and a small, minor cranial puncture can breach dural integrity, which carries a high risk of intracranial infection. The most common site of bite injury shifts to the extremities in children older than 10 years of age. Dog bites are rarely fatal; fatal injuries from dog bites typically involve injury to the neck with resultant hemorrhage.

Cat Bites Cat teeth are sharper than dog teeth; thus, cat bites are more likely to present with puncture wounds, rather than crush injuries. Most cat bites occur in the upper extremities. These puncture wounds inoculate bacteria, commonly anaerobes and *Pasturella multocida*, deeply into tissue. While cat bites result in less wound trauma than dog bites, they more commonly become infected and are associated with a higher likelihood of osteomyelitis and septic arthritis.

Human Bites Human bites, while less common than dog or cat bites, frequently become infected and often are polymicrobial in nature. Human bite marks with an intercanine distance of >3 cm (measured as the distance between the tips of the right and left canine teeth) are likely to have been inflicted by an adult and are therefore highly concerning for abuse. In young children, bites to the face, upper extremity, and trunk are common while in older children and teens, human bites often involve injury to the hand after fist-to-mouth contact.

Clenched-fist injuries are the result of a patient's fist encountering teeth, typically during a fight or sporting event, resulting in soft tissue, bone, tendon, and/or joint injury. The teeth may penetrate the extensor tendon, causing injury to the tendon and/or the metacarpal joint capsule. It is often not recognized as a bite, and patients may not seek medical care until the hand has become infected. Clenched-fist injuries have a high rate of complications, including infection and injury to a tendon, bone, joint, or cartilage.

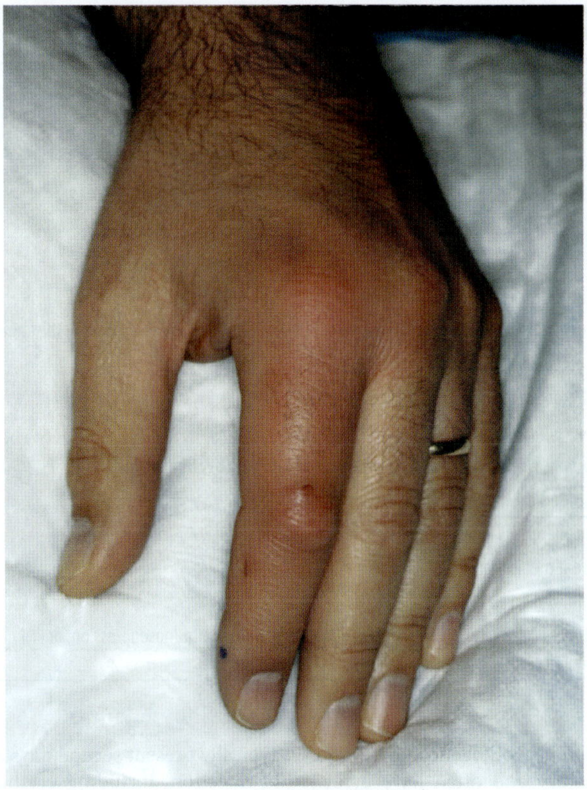

FIGURE 177-1. Cat bite. Note swelling and erythema to the index finger indicating infection. (From Knoop KJ, Stack LB, Storrow AB, Thurman RJ, eds. *The Atlas of Emergency Medicine.* 5th ed. New York, McGraw-Hill, 2021, Figure 18.26. Reproduced with permission from photo contributor: Kevin J. Knoop, MD, MS.)

INFECTIOUS COMPLICATIONS

The type of infection that develops depends on the nature of the bite injury and the proximity to and/or involvement of bones or joints. Infections can manifest as cellulitis (**Figure 177-1**), septic arthritis, osteomyelitis, tenosynovitis, or local abscesses in any potential anatomic space. Regional lymphadenopathy or lymphangitis may also develop. Penetrating skull wounds may result in meningitis or brain abscess. Septicemia is rare and occurs primarily in immunocompromised patients, particularly those who are asplenic. Endocarditis is likewise a rare complication. Important prognostic factors for the development of infection include the extent of tissue damage, the location and/or depth of the wound and compartments entered, the pathogenicity of the inoculated oral bacteria, and the immunocompetence of the host.

Bacteria recovered from infected bite wounds are most often reflective of the oral flora of the biting animal. However, bacteria may also originate from the victim's own skin or the physical environment at the time of injury. Therefore, bites should be considered polymicrobial infections including both aerobes and anaerobes. The organism most commonly implicated in dog and cat bites is *Pasteurella*, specifically *P. canis* in dogs and *P. multocida* in cats. Other species commonly isolated from dog and cat bites include *Streptococcus*, *Staphylococcus*, *Moraxella*, *Neisseria*, *Corynebacterium*, and *Enterococcus*. Common anaerobic isolates include *Bacteroides*, *Fusobacterium*, *Porphyromonas*, *Prevotella*, *Propionibacterium*, and *Peptostreptococcus* species. *Capnocytophaga* species have been implicated in endocarditis, septicemia, and other more severe infections, primarily in immunocompromised hosts such as those with asplenia. Cats are also the main reservoir of *Bartonella henselae*, the causative agent of cat scratch disease, which typically presents as tender regional lymphadenopathy, but can involve a myriad of other areas, including the liver, spleen, eyes, heart, and central nervous system. Other systemic illnesses that can be caused by animal bites include tularemia and tetanus (cats and dogs) and leptospirosis (dogs only).

In human bites, the most common aerobic organisms are *Streptococcus*, *Staphylococcus aureus*, *Eikenella*, and *Haemophilus* species. The most common anaerobic organisms are *Prevotella*, *Bacteroides*, *Peptostreptococcus*, *Fusobacterium*, and *Veillonella* species. Human bite injuries also represent a potential means of transmitting hepatitis B (HBV), hepatitis C (HCV), human immunodeficiency virus (HIV), and herpes simplex (HSV) infections if blood exposure also occurs.

EVALUATION

INITIAL STABILIZATION

Patients presenting for care after a bite wound should first be assessed for adequate airway, breathing, and circulation (ABCs), especially if the wound involves the head and neck. After stabilization of the ABCs, the secondary survey should focus on areas of devitalized tissue, possible neurovascular injuries, or penetrating injuries. Once life-threatening or catastrophic injuries have been stabilized, attention can be directed toward local wound assessment and care.

HISTORY AND PHYSICAL

Certain features of the history and physical examination warrant particular attention after a bite injury. The focus may vary by type of bite and time of presentation (**Tables 177-1** and **177-2**). Further evaluation focuses on determining the extent of injury and the extent or type of complicating infection.

TABLE 177-1 History

Description of the Event and Injury
Date and time of injury
Mechanism of injury
Circumstances and environment in which the bite occurred
History of discharge, redness, or increasing pain at the site of injury
For animal bites:
Type of animal
Provoked versus unprovoked attack
Assess risk for rabies immunization status of the animal, ability to observe the animal
For human bites:
Recognize clenched-fist injuries as possible bites
Recognize human bites as possible abuse
Assess risk of transmission of viruses, such as HIV, HBV, HCV, and HSV
Past Medical History
Drug allergies
Current medications
Immunization status
History of splenectomy, liver disease, diabetes mellitus, immunosuppression, or immunocompromise

Patients with clenched-fist injuries typically present several days after an injury and often have evidence of infection, including erythema, swelling and drainage, as well as pain and limited range of motion in the affected hand. Examination of the hand should include a musculoskeletal and neurovascular examination, with documentation of extensor tendon function. Pain with active or passive finger motion should raise the concern for deep compartment infection or tendonitis. Injuries to the extensor tendon and joint capsule can be overlooked, especially if the metacarpophalangeal (MCP) joint is examined in extension when the injury occurred with the joint in flexion.

RADIOGRAPHIC EVALUATION

Plain radiographs are helpful if a fracture, foreign body (teeth or teeth fragments), or bone penetration is suspected. For deep puncture wounds to the extremities, multiple views may be required to reveal small cortical defects of the adjacent bones. Such findings can serve as baseline information if concerns for osteomyelitis arise in the future. Radiographic evaluation, via plain radiography or computed tomography (CT) scan of dog bite injuries to the scalp, face, and neck in children can identify occult cranial puncture wounds. If performed, plain films of the skull should be taken in both the anteroposterior and lateral projections to assess for evidence of fracture.

TABLE 177-2 Physical Examination

Vital Signs
Fever
Tachycardia
Tachypnea
Hypotension or widened pulse pressure
Injury Assessment
Diagram or photograph the wound
Location, type, and depth of injury
Joint or bone penetration
Edema
Presence or absence of pain at rest and with movement
Erythema, including lymphatic streaking
Regional adenopathy
Presence of and odor of any exudates
For crush injuries—assess distal pulses, nerve and tendon function, and range of motion

LABORATORY EVALUATION

Because of the polymicrobial nature of bite wounds, aerobic and anaerobic cultures of the injury site are of paramount importance in the evaluation of suspected wound infections. Cultures of fresh (<12 hours since injury) wounds are not recommended. Blood cultures and inflammatory markers can be considered if fever or other systemic signs of sepsis are present, especially in immunocompromised children.

MANAGEMENT

WOUND MANAGEMENT

Initial management of bite wounds involves control of bleeding, irrigation, debridement, wound closure if indicated, and protection from infection. These management steps are usually completed before hospitalization, but pertinent aspects are presented briefly.

Bite wounds should be meticulously cleansed with sterile water or saline, but high-pressure irrigation should be avoided as this can result in infections deeper in the tissues. Debridement may be necessary to remove any devitalized or necrotic tissue as well as any debris or foreign bodies remaining after irrigation. Additionally, operative exploration may be needed if there is concern for muscle, nerve, or vascular injury, involvement of the MCP joint from a clenched-fist injury, or cranial injury from the bite of a large animal.

Infectious Diseases Society of America (IDSA) guidelines recommend against routine primary wound closure for animal bite wounds except in cases of bites to the face. Primary wound closure is not indicated for wounds at high risk of infection, including puncture wounds, bites to the hands or feet, bites near a prosthetic joint, bites with underlying venous or lymphatic compromise, wounds more than 12 hours old (except to the face where within 24 hours is acceptable), cat bites (including those to the face), wounds that are clearly infected, crush injuries, or bites in immunocompromised hosts. Wounds not undergoing primary closure are typically left to heal by secondary intention following cleaning and debridement. Small wounds not at high risk for infection can be treated by approximating the wound edges with adhesive strips; the use of tissue adhesive should be avoided.

Elevation of edematous wounds or wounds in dependent areas is an important aspect of successful treatment. Immobilization of extremity injuries, especially hand injuries, is essential to prevent spread of infection along tendon sheaths (**Figure 177-2**). These injuries should be splinted in a position of function.

ANTIBIOTIC THERAPY

Given concerns for infection following human and animal bites, it is important to assess if prophylactic antibiotics are indicated. A Cochrane analysis found that the use of prophylactic antibiotics may reduce the risk of infection after human bites and bites to the hand but did not impact the overall rate of infection after other dog or cat bites. Dog bites, puncture wounds, and wounds that were closed are associated with higher rates of infection. However, because there continues to be limited evidence to further determine the utility of antibiotic prophylaxis for animal bites, the IDSA currently recommends the use of antibiotics for moderate or severe injuries, puncture wounds, surgically closed facial wounds, wounds to the hands, feet, and genitals, and cat bites, as well as for bites in immunocompromised or asplenic patients. Additionally, wounds undergoing primary closure are often treated with antibiotic prophylaxis, although strong evidence is lacking for this recommendation. Antibiotics should cover both aerobic and anaerobic bacteria. The drug of choice for antibiotic prophylaxis is amoxicillin-clavulanic acid for 3 to 5 days. In penicillin-allergic patients, an extended-spectrum cephalosporin or trimethoprim-sulfamethoxazole *plus* clindamycin is an alternative regimen. Combination therapy is needed to ensure coverage of *Pasteurella* (cephalosporin or trimethoprim-sulfamethoxazole) and

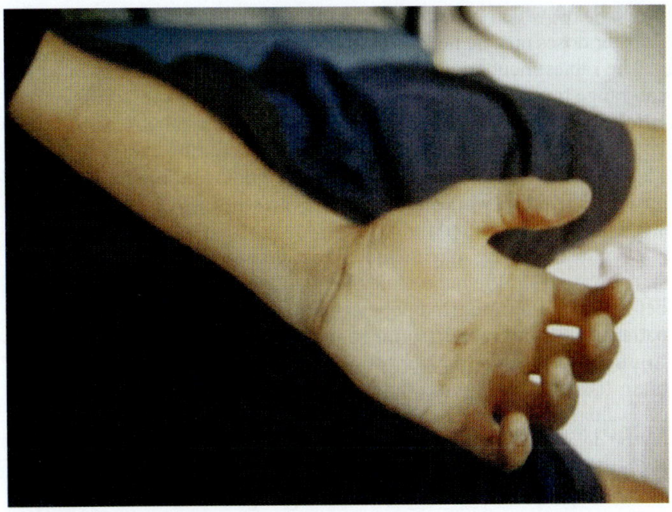

FIGURE 177-2. Tenosynovitis from cat bite. Note the streak of erythema extending proximally along the anterior forearm.

oral anaerobes (clindamycin). Patients should be re-evaluated within 48 hours to assess wound healing and examine for signs of infection.

Amoxicillin-clavulanic acid is also an ideal empiric choice for an infected wound as it will cover most animal and human bite pathogens. As noted above, alternatives in penicillin-allergic patients include an extended-spectrum cephalosporin or trimethoprim-sulfamethoxazole *plus* clindamycin to ensure adequate empiric coverage. Ampicillin-sulbactam is preferred for parenteral antibiotic coverage in both animal and human bites, with alternatives in penicillin-allergic patients including an extended-spectrum cephalosporin or trimethoprim-sulfamethoxazole *plus* clindamycin, or a carbapenem. Typically, a 5-day treatment course is sufficient to treat an infected bite wound, though duration of therapy should be individualized based on infection site and severity, culture results, and response to therapy. Infections involving other structures, such as tenosynovitis, osteomyelitis, and septic arthritis require a longer duration of treatment.

There is insufficient information to recommend routine coverage for methicillin-resistant *S. aureus* (MRSA). If the prevalence of community-acquired MRSA is high in the community, or if the infection is severe, then empiric therapy for MRSA should be considered while awaiting wound culture results.

PROPHYLAXIS

For animal and human bites, tetanus immunization status should be ascertained, and appropriate prophylaxis administered as detailed in **Table 177-3**. Patients who have not completed their primary tetanus series (≥3 doses) and those with unknown tetanus vaccination status should receive tetanus toxoid and human tetanus immune globulin. Tetanus toxoid is also recommended for patients with animal bites who have not been vaccinated within the last 5 years.

For human bites, additional considerations include HIV, HBV, and HCV. Baseline HIV testing should be performed on all persons seeking evaluation for potential HIV exposure. Based on assessment of the risk, postexposure prophylaxis should be initiated according to current recommendations from the US Department of Health and Human Services Working Group on Nonoccupational Postexposure Prophylaxis. For exposure to blood that contains (or might contain) hepatitis B surface antigen, the decision to give hepatitis B immune globulin prophylaxis and hepatitis B vaccine is based on the infectious status of the source of the exposure and the immunization status (including response to immunization) of the exposed person. Immunization is recommended for any person who was exposed but does not have evidence of immunity. If the source is unknown or not available for testing, the clinician should institute the hepatitis B series to individuals without evidence of immunity. No vaccine for hepatitis C is available, and prophylaxis with immune

TABLE 177-3 Guide to Tetanus Prophylaxis in Wound Management

	Clean, Minor Wounds		All Other Wounds*	
History of Absorbed Tetanus Toxoid	*Td, Tdap or DTaP*†	*TIG*‡	*Td, Tdap or DTaP*†	*TIG*‡
<3 doses or unknown	Yes	No	Yes	Yes
≥3 doses	No§	No	No¶	No

DTaP, diphtheria and tetanus toxoid booster, acellular pertussis; Td, adult-type diphtheria and tetanus toxoid vaccine; Tdap, booster tetanus toxoid, reduced diphtheria toxoid, and acellular pertussis; TIG, tetanus immune globulin (human).

*Such as, but not limited to, wounds contaminated with dirt, feces, soil, and saliva; puncture wounds; avulsions; and wounds resulting from missiles, crushing, burns, and frostbite.

†DTaP is used for children <7 yo. Tdap is preferred over Td for underimmunized children ≥7 years old who never received Tdap.

‡Intravenous immune globulin should be used when TIG is not available.

§Yes, if 10 or more years since the last tetanus-containing vaccine dose.

¶Yes, if 5 or more years since the last tetanus-containing vaccine dose. More frequent boosters are not needed and can accentuate adverse effects.

Source: Adapted from American Academy of Pediatrics: Tetanus. In: Kimberlin DW, Barnett ED, Lynfield R, Sawyer MH, eds. *Red Book: 2021–2024 Report of the Committee on Infectious Diseases*. 32nd ed. Elk Grove Village, IL. American Academy of Pediatrics; 2021.

globulin is not effective in preventing HCV infection after exposure. If possible, the HCV status of the source should be obtained and if positive or unable to be determined, the exposed person should have baseline HCV antibody testing within 48 hours of exposure, followed by either HCV RNA testing after 3 weeks or repeat anti-HCV testing after 6 months.

ADMISSION AND DISCHARGE CRITERIA

ADMISSION CRITERIA

Hospitalization following human or animal bites is typically related to the treatment of infected wounds complicated by fever, sepsis, or spreading cellulitis. On initial presentation, wounds with significant edema or crush injury causing loss of function, at high risk for cosmetic morbidity, at risk for joint infection or osteomyelitis, or occurring in an immunocompromised host or a noncompliant patient are best managed in the hospital setting. A small minority of patients require admission; those with injuries to the head and neck as well as children younger than 5 years of age have higher rates of prolonged observation or inpatient admission. Patients re-presenting after initial management may require hospitalization for signs of sepsis, rapid spread of erythema or induration, lack of improvement on oral antibiotics, or the development of deep infections requiring intervention. Some recommend hospitalization, surgical consultation, and surgical wound exploration for all clenched-fist injuries to the hand.

DISCHARGE CRITERIA

Discharge criteria are determined by initial indication for admission. For wounds on initial presentation, this includes completion of necessary surgical debridement and repair, as well as adequate pain control. For wounds presenting with concerns for infection, discharge should occur when there is clear improvement in signs of infection, after transition to oral antibiotics, and a plan for completing antibiotic therapy is in place. Outpatient follow-up with the primary care physician is important to assess continued wound healing and resolution of any infection. Additionally, follow-up with surgical specialists may be indicated.

CONSULTATION

Plastic surgery consultation is recommended for disfiguring or complex lacerations, especially those involving the face. Ophthalmologic consultation is indicated for the treatment of wounds involving the eye or orbit. Surgical (vascular, general, hand, orthopedic) consultation is needed for wounds affecting major blood vessels or concern for neurovascular compromise, abscesses or deep tissue infections, and deep wounds involving bones, tendons, and/or joints. Additionally, wounds at risk for compartment syndrome or with a potential for loss of function (as in clenched-fist wounds) also warrant subspecialty surgical consultation. An infectious disease specialist can provide guidance regarding antimicrobials, especially if the infection is not responding to initial antibiotic therapy. Neurosurgery should be consulted for penetrating wounds to the skull. Involvement of physical and occupational therapy may be helpful, especially with immobilization or when activities are limited. Psychology services should be solicited as appropriate, especially when the event was particularly frightening or when there is concern for disfigurement.

SPECIAL CONSIDERATIONS

REPORTING

Many counties and states have laws in place that require the reporting of animal bites to animal control and/or the state health department. It is important for physicians to be aware of local laws and to ensure appropriate reporting has occurred.

OTHER ANIMAL BITES

Although outside the scope of this chapter, it is worth noting that monkey and other simian bites are becoming more common. Other bites that may be seen include those caused by horses, pigs, aquatic animals, ferrets, and bird pecking and bites. Rodent bites carry a low risk of secondary infection. Rat-bite fever is a rare systemic infection manifested by fever, chills, headache, malaise, and rash 1 to 3 weeks after the bite.

RABIES

Rabies virus is a neurotropic RNA virus in the Rhabdoviridae family (*Lyssavirus* genus) that causes acute encephalitis with atypical focal neurologic signs or paralysis and is almost always fatal. Human rabies is rare, with only twenty-five cases of human rabies reported in the United States from 2009 to 2018, but approximately 60,000 individuals in the United States seek postexposure prophylaxis (PEP) per year to prevent rabies infections.

Rabies should be considered after any animal bite, but especially for bats, ferrets, foxes, and raccoons. Transmission is known to occur by bite, aerosolization of virus in laboratories, and organ transplantation from infected donors. However, it is still unclear how bat-variant rabies is transmitted as 76% of human cases of bat-variant rabies since 1990 do not have a record of a definitive bite. It is hypothesized that the bites may be minimized or unrecognized or that aerosol transmission may have taken place. Therefore, PEP should be considered for any direct contact between a human and a bat, regardless of bite history. Consultation with local and/or state public health officials for guidance with risk assessments and PEP administration is recommended.

For unvaccinated individuals, human rabies immune globulin (HRIG) is administered concomitantly with the first dose of the rabies vaccine to provide passive immunity until the vaccine induces active immunity. Ideally, prophylaxis is started within 24 hours of possible exposure. The recommended dose of HRIG is 20 IU/kg. As much of the dose as possible should be infiltrated into the wound(s), with the rest given intramuscularly. If more volume is needed for infiltration, the dose should not be increased, but HRIG may be diluted twofold or threefold with saline to provide more volume for large wounds.

The human rabies vaccine is a four-dose series and should be administered as soon as possible after exposure, with the first administration dose counted as day 0 and subsequent doses given on days 3, 7, and 14. Immunocompromised individuals should receive a fifth dose on day 28 and be tested 7 to 14 days after completion to document seroconversion. Although it has not been studied specifically, pregnancy is not a contraindication to giving rabies vaccine and RIG after exposure.

If an individual previously immunized against rabies has a rabies exposure, they should receive two doses of rabies vaccine on day 0 and 3; however, they should not receive HRIG. Those at high risk for rabies exposure, including veterinarians, animal handlers, laboratory workers, spelunkers, and travelers to endemic areas, should undergo preexposure prophylaxis, which includes a three-dose series (day 0, 7, and 21 or 28). Booster doses may be needed in high-risk groups as serum titers fall.

The rabies incubation period in humans averages 1 to 3 months but can range from days to years. Clinical presentation begins with nonspecific prodromal symptoms (such as fever, chills, malaise, nausea, and vomiting) followed by either encephalitic or paralytic rabies. Hydrophobia, aerophobia, autonomic instability, and agitation are features of encephalitic rabies while paralytic rabies presents with a flaccid paralysis starting from the injured limb.

Diagnostic testing may include direct fluorescent antibody testing of skin biopsy from the nape of neck, isolation of virus in saliva, antibody detection in unimmunized people and in cerebrospinal fluid of infected patients, and/or viral nucleotide sequencing of infected tissues or saliva. Confirmatory diagnosis is most often postmortem via examination of brain tissue using immunofluorescent evaluation, immunohistochemical evaluation, or examination of viral nucleotide sequences. PEP should not be delayed while awaiting diagnostic testing.

Once symptoms have developed, treatment is supportive and rabies infections are almost all fatal. Work is ongoing to determine the utility of sedation and other medical interventions. The use of the rabies vaccine or HRIG does not improve the prognosis once a patient is symptomatic, which highlights the importance of PEP when appropriate.

Prevention of human rabies transmission involves vaccinating animals, limiting exposure to potentially rabid animals, and immunoprophylaxis for exposure. Parents and children should be educated regarding behavior around animals, especially those that are unfamiliar to the child. Teasing animals and approaching them when sleeping, eating, or caring for their young is especially risky. Dogs that are spayed or neutered are less likely to bite, as are trained and socialized dogs. Encourage local leash laws and reporting of bites, and educate the public about responsible dog selection, ownership, and training. In the United States, most states have laws requiring that dogs and cats be vaccinated against rabies. However, if a bite is sustained and the animal's immunization status cannot be ascertained, post-exposure prophylaxis should be pursued.

KEY POINTS

- More than 5 million animal and human bites occur annually in the United States; approximately 1% to 2% require hospitalization.
- Dog bites are often associated with crush injury and local trauma, which can result in devascularized tissue and an increased risk for infection.
- Cat bites and resulting puncture wounds are associated with the highest rate of infection, as the puncture wound inoculates mouth flora deep into soft tissues, making decontamination of the wound difficult.
- Clenched-fist injuries are a type of human bite that result from a punch to the mouth and are often associated with delayed presentation to care. The penetrating tooth can cause laceration of the extensor tendon and result in infection of the skin, tendon, bones, or joints of the hand.
- Primary wound closure is generally deferred in the management of human and animal bites unless the risk for infection is low. In selected situations, especially those associated with a high risk for disfigurement, early wound closure may be considered. Subspecialty consultation is recommended.
- Although not routinely administered, prophylactic antibiotics may be appropriate for moderate to severe injuries less than 8 hours old; puncture wounds; suspected bone or joint penetration; wounds to the face, hand, foot, or genitals; cat bites; and immunocompromised patients.
- Empirical therapy for infected bites is amoxicillin-clavulanate or ampicillin-sulbactam or, for penicillin-allergic patients, an extended-spectrum cephalosporin or trimethoprim-sulfamethoxazole *plus* clindamycin.
- Tetanus immunization should be administered to unimmunized or underimmunized patients.
- Rabies postexposure prophylaxis is indicated for bites from raccoons, skunks, foxes and other carnivores, ill-appearing animals, or unvaccinated domestic animals, along with any exposure to bats. Contact local public health officials if rabies is suspected.

SUGGESTED READINGS

Ball V, Younggren BN. Emergency management of difficult wounds: part I. *Emerg Med Clin North Am.* 2007;25:101-121.

Basco AN, McCormack ER, Basco WT. Age- and sex-related differences in nonfatal dog bite injuries among persons aged 0-19 years treated in hospital emergency departments, United States, 2001-2017. *Public Health Reports.* 2020;135(2):238-244.

Bula-Rudas FJ, Olcott JL. Human and animal bites. *Pediatr Rev.* 2018;39(10):490-500.

Daniels DM, Ritzi R, O'Neil J, et al. Analysis of nonfatal dog bites in children. *J Trauma.* 2009;66:S17-S22.

Ellis R, Ellis C. Dog and cat bites. *Am Fam Physician.* 2014;90(4):239-243.

Gilchrist J, Gotsch K, Annest JL, et al. Nonfatal dog bite-related injuries treated in hospital emergency departments-United States, 2001. *MMWR Morb Mortal Wkly Rep.* 2003;52(26):605-610.

Holmquist L, Elixhauser A. Emergency department visits and inpatient stays involving dog bites, 2008. 2010 Nov. In: *Healthcare Cost and Utilization Project (HCUP) Statistical Briefs [Internet].* Rockville (MD): Agency for Healthcare Research and Quality (US); 2006 Feb-. Statistical Brief #101. Available from: https://www-ncbi-nlm-nih-gov.offcampus.lib.washington.edu/books/NBK52650/.

Holzer KJ, Vaughn MG, Murugan V. Dog bite injuries in the USA: prevalence, correlates, and recent trends. *Inj Prev.* 2019;25:187-190.

Jaindl M, Grunaer J, Platzer P, et al. The management of bite wounds in children—a retrospective analysis at level I trauma centre. *Injury.* 2012;43(12):2117-2121.

Kimberlin DW, Barnett ED, Lynfield R, Sawyer MH, eds. *Red Book: 2021-2024 Report of the Committee on Infectious Diseases.* 32nd ed. Elk Grove Village, IL. American Academy of Pediatrics; 2021. Chapters on Bite Wounds: 169-175, Rabies: 619-627, and Tetanus: 750-755.

Lyu C, Jewell MP, Piron J, et al. Burden of bites by dogs and other animals in Los Angeles County, California, 2009-2011. *Public Health Reports.* 2016;131(6):800-808.

Medeiros I, Saconato H. Antibiotic prophylaxis for mammalian bites. Cochrane Database Syst Rev. 2001;(2):CD001738.

Perron AD, Miller MD, Brady WJ. Orthopedic pitfalls in ED: fight bite. *Am J Emerg Med.* 2002;20(2):114-117.

Rothe K, Tsokos M, Handrick W. Animal and human bite wounds. *Dtsch Arztebl Int.* 2015;112:433-443.

Stevens DL, Bisno AL, Chambers HF, et al. Practice Guidelines for the Diagnosis and Management of Skin and Soft Tissue Infections: 2014 Update by the Infectious Diseases Society of America. *Clinical Infectious Diseases,* 2014;59(2):e10-e52.

Tabaka ME, Quinn JV, Kohn MA, et al. Predictors of infection from dog bite wounds: which patients may benefit from prophylactic antibiotics? *Emerg Med J.* 2015;32:860-863.

CHAPTER 178 Envenomation

Daniel Herchline, MD, MSEd

BACKGROUND

Terrestrial and marine envenomation events are responsible for thousands of medical visits each year in the United States. Venomous bites are of particular concern in the pediatric population with the potential for higher rates of morbidity and mortality in smaller patients. Diagnostic and management strategies for envenomation vary according to the type of animal, specific toxic properties of the venom, location and appearance of the bite or wound, elapsed time since exposure, systemic symptoms, and size of the child (**Table 178-1**). This chapter specifically addresses the presentation and management of common snake bites, and spider bites.

TABLE 178-1 Important Details to Elicit on History and Physical Examination

History
Description of animal (identification may not always be possible)
Time of exposure
Location of wound on the body
Changes in appearance of wounds before presentation
Pain
Local symptoms (paresthesia, weakness, swelling)
Systemic symptoms (dizziness, diaphoresis, respiratory compromise, seizures, muscle cramping, bleeding)
Physical Examination
Patient's weight
Wound characteristics (erythema, edema, target lesion, bleeding, necrosis, hemorrhagic blebs)
Local compromise (airway compromise, perfusion, neurovascular status)
Systemic compromise (vital signs and end-organ perfusion)

SNAKE BITES

In North America, the most common venomous snakes belong to the Viperidae family (Crotalinae subfamily), most commonly referred to as pit vipers. Members of crotaline group include rattlesnakes, copperheads, and water moccasins (also known as cottonmouths). These venomous snakes are generally distinguished from nonvenomous snakes by their triangular heads, vertically positioned elliptical pupils, heat-sensing nostril pits, and a single row of scales at the tail. Crotaline venom contains a mixture of multiple enzymes and toxic substances that are usually deposited subcutaneously but rarely can involve subfascial or intravascular deposition.

CLINICAL PRESENTATION

Snake bites occurring with envenomation are capable of producing both local and systemic toxicity. Although presentations among adult and pediatric populations are similar, children are at increased risk for morbidity and mortality given the larger venom load to patient size ratio. Local effects usually begin approximately 15 to 30 minutes following the bite and include pain, paresthesias, numbness, edema, ecchymosis, necrosis, bleeding, and hemorrhagic blistering. Edema can be extensive and is of particular concern if airway obstruction occurs from bites to the face or neck. Although the appearance of a swollen bite may mimic compartment syndrome, the subcutaneous location of envenomation makes compartment syndrome unlikely.

Systemic symptoms can involve a broad array of organ system involvement depending on the type of snake and location of the bite (**Table 178-2**). Generalized signs and symptoms may include diaphoresis, hypotension, lightheadedness, chills, nausea, and vomiting. Rhabdomyolysis is a rare complication. With crotaline snake bites, systemic effects primarily involve the hematologic system, with laboratory abnormalities suggestive of disseminated intravascular coagulation including decreased fibrinogen and platelets and increased prothrombin time, partial thromboplastin time, fibrin split products, and D-dimer. A select group of crotaline snakes (Mojave rattlesnakes) and coral snakes also produce venom with neurotoxic properties. Neurologic symptoms resulting from these bites can include fasciculations, paresthesias, cranial nerve deficits, and muscular weakness. Prolonged time between bite and provision of care, younger patient age, and larger snake size increase the likelihood of severe systemic symptoms.

DIAGNOSTIC EVALUATION

Primary diagnostic evaluation should include an assessment of the patient's airway, breathing, and circulation as well as characterization of the local wound. Although not always known, a description of the

TABLE 178-2 Severity of Snake Bite Envenomation			
	Mild	Moderate	Severe
Wound (all bites)	Pain, erythema, mild swelling	Increased pain, mild bleeding, moderate swelling	Hemorrhagic blisters and blebs, extensive swelling (at risk for compromising local structures)
Hematologic (most pit vipers)	Limited local bleeding, normal laboratory values	Mild abnormalities in laboratory values	Disseminated intravascular coagulation
Neurologic (Mojave rattlesnake, coral snakes, other neurotoxic envenomation)	Local paresthesias	Local extension of paresthesias and weakness	Systemic weakness

snake responsible for envenomation can be helpful in guiding management. For suspected crotaline envenomation, laboratory markers that should be obtained include complete blood count, prothrombin time, partial thromboplastin time, fibrinogen, fibrin split products, D-dimer, electrolytes, blood urea nitrogen, creatinine, creatine kinase, urinalysis, and type and screen.

MANAGEMENT

For every envenomation, initial management should include stabilization of respiratory and cardiovascular status. Local wound care should be performed with copious irrigation. Contrary to common belief, venom should not be removed by oral suction as it has not been proven effective and may increase the likelihood of wound infection. The use of tourniquets is not recommended, but the affected location should be immobilized to minimize the spread of toxins. Tetanus immunization status should be confirmed and toxoid administered, if indicated. Prophylactic antibiotics have not been proven to be effective.

Crotaline antivenom is indicated for edema that compromises local structures including the hands, neck, or face as well as for any neurologic or hematologic abnormalities. Crotalidae polyvalent immune fab-ovine is the primary commercially available ovine antibody preparation for treatment of crotaline snake envenomation in the United States and has been proven to be safe in pediatric populations. Recommended dosing is the same for both adult and pediatric populations; repeat dosing may be necessary if there is no clinical improvement following initial drug administration. The antivenom is generally well-tolerated with low rates of immediate hypersensitivity reactions and serum sickness though epinephrine should be readily available during administration as a precaution.

CONSULTATION

Antivenom administration is generally best guided by clinicians with experience in caring for snake envenomation and should ideally be completed in consultation with a toxicologist or poison control center given the nuances involved in determining when a patient requires treatment. However, initial administration of antivenom should not be delayed while seeking consultation. Consultation with a toxicologist is particularly key in cases of envenomation that are life-threatening, delayed or recurrent, or involve complicated wounds.

ADMISSION AND DISCHARGE CRITERIA

A patient may be discharged from the emergency department with close follow-up after a 6- to 8-hour period of observation that reveals no worsening local effects, laboratory abnormalities, or systemic involvement. Any patient with moderate or severe symptoms (Table 178-2) should be admitted for neurovascular assessment of the wound or hematologic and neurologic monitoring. Admitted children may be discharged when progression of the local injury has halted, coagulation abnormalities have resolved, pain is adequately controlled on an outpatient regimen, and no additional antivenom is indicated.

SPIDER BITES

The two most clinically relevant spiders in the United States include widow spiders (*Latrodectus*) and recluse spiders (*Loxosceles*). Both can be found over large territories within the United States though recluse spiders most commonly reside across the Midwestern and Southwestern US.

BLACK WIDOW SPIDER

Black widow spiders (*Latrodectus mactans*) are indigenous throughout North America. Envenomation by black widow spiders occurs with bites by females, which are identifiable by red hourglass-shaped markings on the abdomen. Symptoms of black widow bites arise from the activation of nerve cells when toxins cause the release of neurotransmitters via calcium channel modulation.

Clinical Presentation The most common symptom following a black widow spider bite is localized pain around the bite, which can be severe. The wound may develop a characteristic target appearance with blanching immediately surrounding the bite and an outer erythematous ring. Systemic symptoms develop between 1 and 8 hours after the bite and most frequently include muscle cramping and rigidity at the site of the bite and in large muscle groups such as the abdomen, thighs, and back. Other signs and symptoms are facial spasm, diaphoresis, vomiting, tachycardia, hypertension, and rarely, priapism. Toxicity occurs variably with most mild bites incurring only local effects, though severe envenomation can occasionally cause systemic symptoms (**Table 178-3**).

Management Initial management for black widow spider bites includes local wound care with irrigation as well as cardiopulmonary support, if necessary. Pain control can often be achieved with the use of opioids and benzodiazepines, which are particularly useful in managing associated muscle spasms. For severe cases of envenomation, a highly purified form of equine antivenom is available. Antivenom should be administered in consultation with a toxicologist.

Admission and Discharge Criteria Patients with moderate or severe toxicity should be hospitalized for symptom control and monitoring. Discharge is safe when symptoms have resolved, typically within 24 to 72 hours.

BROWN RECLUSE SPIDER

Recluse spiders (*Loxosceles*) are distributed throughout temperate regions of the United States with the most common species being the brown recluse spider (*Loxosceles reclusa*). Brown recluse spiders are frequently misidentified, particularly in nonendemic areas of the country. Clinical manifestations arise from a mixture of toxins that can induce an inflammatory response, dermonecrosis, coagulopathies, and renal injury.

Clinical Presentation While initial bites are often undetected, pain can develop around the site in the ensuing 6 to 8 hours. Local reactions with associated edema and erythema are common presenting symptoms in mild envenomation. Moderate-to-severe envenomation can lead to the development of blistering lesions that develop into necrotic ulcers over the course of 2 to 4 days. Systemic symptoms, while rare, include weakness, vomiting, and hematologic abnormalities (**Table 178-3**).

TABLE 178-3 Severity of Spider Bite Envenomation			
	Mild	Moderate	Severe
Black widow	Local pain, target lesion, erythema, normal vital signs	Muscular cramps at local bite and proximal muscles, normal vital signs	Generalized muscle cramps (abdomen, back, thighs), diaphoresis, tachycardia, hypertension
Brown recluse	Local pain, erythema	Extension of wound and blistering	Large necrosis and ulceration

TABLE 178-4 A Helpful Mnemonic to Avoid Overdiagnosis of Brown Recluse Bites

N – Numerous	Recluse bites are typically single lesions.
O – Occurrence	Recluse bites usually occur during an encounter with a secluded recluse spider.
T – Timing	Bites are unlikely to happen outside the months of April to October.
R – Red Center	The center of most recluse bites are pale, blue-white, or purple.
E – Elevated	Recluse bites are unlikely to be raised.
C – Chronic	Most recluse bites heal within 3 months. Lesions persisting after this time are unlikely to be recluse bites.
L – Large	Most recluse bites are smaller than 10 cm in diameter.
U – Ulcerates Too Early	Recluse bites do not typically ulcerate until 1-2 weeks following envenomation.
S – Swollen	Recluse bites typically do not cause significant swelling below the neck though facial bites can cause marked facial edema.
E – Exudative	Recluse bites are not purulent initially.

Adapted from Stoecker WV, Vetter RS, Dyer JA. NOT RECLUSE-A Mnemonic Device to Avoid False Diagnoses of Brown Recluse Spider Bites. *JAMA Dermatol*. 2017;153(5):377-378.

Diagnostic Evaluation Accurate diagnosis of brown recluse spider bites can be a challenge as most bites are unwitnessed. Overdiagnosis also remains a problem in dermonecrotic wounds, particularly in non-endemic areas, as a wide variety of illnesses can mimic necrotic arachnidism. A helpful mnemonic to avoid overdiagnosis of brown recluse spider bites is "NOT RECLUSE" (**Table 178-4**).

Management Initial management for brown recluse spider bites includes local wound care with irrigation followed by dry dressings as well as pain control. Large wounds with extensive necrosis may require skin grafting, although this is rare. Tetanus immunization should be addressed. Prophylactic antibiotics do not prevent infection; however, wound infection can often occur, and appropriate antibiotic therapy tailored toward typical skin flora should be initiated if secondary infection is suspected.

Admission and Discharge Criteria Patients with moderate or severe toxicity should be hospitalized for symptom control and monitoring. Discharge is safe when symptoms have resolved, typically within 24 to 72 hours.

KEY POINTS

- Crotaline snake envenomation may cause soft tissue destruction and coagulopathies; they can be treated with analgesics and antivenom in addition to supportive care.
- Black widow (*Latrodectus* sp.) spider bites may cause painful muscle cramping and hyperautonomicity; they are best treated with sedatives, analgesics, and antivenom (when necessary).
- Brown recluse spiders (*Loxosceles* sp.) may cause necrotic skin lesions, but clinicians are encouraged to consider a broad differential diagnosis for focal necrosis.

SUGGESTED READINGS

Holve S. Venomous spiders, snakes, and scorpions in the United States. *Pediatr Ann*. 2009;38(4):210-217.

Juckett G. Arthropod bites. *Am Fam Physician*. 2013;88(12):841-847.

Keating GM, Lyseng-Williamson KA. Crotalidae polyvalent immune Fab: a guide to its use in North American crotaline envenomation. *Clin Drug Investig*. 2012;32(8):555-560.

Li L, McGee RG, Isbister G, Webster AC. Interventions for the symptoms and signs resulting from jellyfish stings. *Cochrane Database Syst Rev*. 2013;2013(12):CD009688.

Monte AA, Bucher-Bartelson B, Heard KJ. A US perspective of symptomatic *Latrodectus* spp. envenomation and treatment: a National Poison Data System review. *Ann Pharmacother*. 2011;45(12):1491-1498.

Ruha AM, Kleinschmidt KC, Greene S, et al. The epidemiology, clinical course, and management of snakebites in the North American Snakebite Registry. *J Med Toxicol*. 2017;13(4):309-320.

Stoecker WV, Vetter RS, Dyer JA. NOT RECLUSE-A Mnemonic Device to Avoid False Diagnoses of Brown Recluse Spider Bites. *JAMA Dermatol*. 2017;153(5):377-378.

CHAPTER 179 Infant Botulism

Michael Del Vecchio, MD and Arsala Syed, DO, MS, MA

BACKGROUND

Infant botulism, the most common form of botulism encountered in the United States, has a unique pathogenesis. Unlike food-borne botulism, which results from the ingestion of preformed toxin, infant botulism occurs following the ingestion of *Clostridium botulinum* spores that germinate and colonize the infant gut. Botulinum neurotoxin is then produced in vivo and absorbed, producing clinical disease. This form of botulism occurs almost exclusively in children younger than 1 year.

PATHOPHYSIOLOGY

C. botulinum is a gram-positive, spore-forming, obligate anaerobe that is found worldwide in soil and dust. Approximately 90% of US cases of infant botulism are caused by toxin types A and B. However, cases due to toxin type E from *Clostridium butyricum* and toxin type F from *Clostridium baratii* have been reported. The relatively diminished intestinal microflora in infants has been hypothesized to play a critical role in the pathophysiology of infant botulism. Once the spores are ingested and colonized botulinum toxin is produced in the gut, it is absorbed into the bloodstream, and carried to peripheral cholinergic synapses where it blocks the release of acetylcholine. Autonomic effects such as swallowing difficulties, constipation, ptosis, reduced sweating, as well as the classic somatic muscle weakness or paralysis can occur. Botulinum toxin does not penetrate the central nervous system.

EPIDEMIOLOGY

While spores can be found on fresh fruits and vegetables, honey is the only food that has been unequivocally linked to specific cases of infant botulism. Corn syrup was implicated as a source of infection in the past; changes in the production process of corn syrup have largely eliminated this risk. With the decrease in the ingestion of honey by infants, the exact source of the spores is rarely found in individual cases though it is not uncommon to find recent soil disturbance near the living quarters of an infected infant. Although *C. botulinum* spores are ubiquitous, there is a clear geographic clustering of cases mirroring the geographic distribution of spores in California, eastern Pennsylvania, New Jersey, and Delaware. Toxin serotype also varies geographically. Type B toxin causes about 90% of cases in Pennsylvania, whereas most California cases are due to type A toxin.

All reported cases of infant botulism have occurred in patients younger than 1 year of age; 95% in the first 6 months of life. *C. baratii* toxin-type F causes disease in the youngest of infants; the youngest reported case occurring at 38 hours of life. No sex, race, or seasonal risk factors have been identified.

CLINICAL PRESENTATION

The paralysis of infant botulism is symmetrical, flaccid, and descending. The onset of symptoms may be gradual (days) or abrupt (hours) with a widely variable clinical severity. Some infants, regardless of treatment, never require respiratory support whereas others require prolonged endotracheal intubation. Constipation is present in approximately 95% of patients at the time of presentation. If the patient is evaluated early in the course of disease or has a slowly progressive course, abnormal physical findings may be limited to weakness of the muscles innervated by the cranial nerves, though weakness is detectable in all affected infants on presentation. Initial deep tendon reflexes may be normal, only to diminish later. Clinical assessment should include careful and repeated examination of pupillary constriction, extraocular movement, and gag, suck, and swallow reflexes. Repeated stimulation of a muscle is the most sensitive way to induce a clinically evident paralysis. Due to the nonspecific nature of botulism, it is a diagnosis that is infrequently considered upon presentation, particularly when there are concomitant viral infections. On the opposite spectrum when a patient presents in severe distress, diagnosis can be delayed due to prioritization of other diagnostic possibilities (e.g., sepsis, stroke).

DIFFERENTIAL DIAGNOSIS

Other diagnostic considerations can usually be eliminated by history and physical examination. Constipation and abnormal cranial nerve weakness are key features that distinguish infant botulism from other entities causing muscular weakness such as spinal muscular atrophy (SMA) type 1 and metabolic disorders, which are potential mimickers of infant botulism. As SMA is now included on the newborn screen in 47 states, allowing 97% of infants born in the United States to be screened for SMA at birth, checking the newborn screen results is prudent in working through the differential diagnosis for an infant with muscular weakness. Pursuit of a metabolic evaluation for consideration of diagnoses that present with hypotonia (e.g., mitochondrial disorders, glycogen storage diseases) could be undertaken as indicated per the clinical course of the infant. Other diagnoses to consider are Miller Fisher variant of Guillain-Barré syndrome, neuroblastoma, and viral infections. Sepsis is the most common clinical diagnosis at the time of hospital admission in patients later found to have infant botulism.

DIAGNOSTIC EVALUATION

Laboratory confirmation of the diagnosis requires the isolation of *C. botulinum* or the demonstration of botulinum toxin from the patient's stool. The mouse neutralization test is the preferred confirmatory method and is available from state health laboratories and from the Centers for Disease Control and Prevention (CDC) in Atlanta. Because of severe constipation, an enema with sterile, nonbacteriostatic water is often required to obtain a sample. The stool sample should be kept at 4°C during transport. Polymerase chain reaction testing, though promising, is not being used clinically. All other laboratory tests are typically normal. Electromyography (EMG) testing is rarely needed for initial diagnosis. While unpleasant and technically challenging, EMG may demonstrate brief, small, abundant motor unit potentials, and repetitive stimulation of peripheral nerves shows facilitation of neuromuscular transmission, though this is not found in all cases. Additional diagnostic testing for complications of botulism (including infections and respiratory failure) may be necessary.

MANAGEMENT

BIG-IV (botulism immune globulin), or BabyBIG, is a human-derived antitoxin used for treatment of infant botulism. BabyBIG is available through the California Department of Public Health Infant Botulism Treatment and Prevention Program (telephone number 510-231-7600; https://www.infantbotulism.org). Given that early treatment is crucial in the management of infant botulism, treatment should not be delayed while awaiting laboratory confirmation of disease. A single dose of BabyBIG is effective for both type A and type B toxins. Though the half-life of the immune globulin preparation, BabyBIG, is approximately 28 days, a single infusion is sufficient to neutralize ongoing toxin production or absorption for at least 6 months.

Because botulinum toxin has a prolonged duration of action following its binding to receptors, symptoms may persist for days to weeks even following administration of BabyBIG. Nutritional, airway, and respiratory support remain essential.

Nutritional support can be effectively accomplished by enteral tube feeding (e.g., nasogastric feeds). Enteral feeding should be initiated immediately on presentation, beginning with a low rate of continuous ("drip") feedings to reduce the risk of aspiration. Constipation does not quickly resolve but should not interrupt enteral feedings. Other than the initial removal of an inspissated fecal plug, constipation can be managed with routine measures.

Frequent assessment of the airway status and respiratory effort is required. Loss of protective airway reflexes is the primary indication for placement of an artificial airway in infant botulism. Patients who meet criteria for suspected infantile botulism should be monitored closely with continuous pulse oximetry, continuous measurement of carbon dioxide with end-tidal monitoring or transcutaneous CO_2, measurement of negative inspiratory pressures, as well as physical exam at least every 12 hours and more frequently if weakness is progressing rapidly. Physical exams should include careful physical examination of the airway reflexes including suck, gag, and cough. If patients develop weakness in their protective reflexes, intubation of the airway is indicated to protect them from aspiration. In general, patients will require airway protection before they develop blood gas abnormalities. Once intubated, ventilator management can be guided by blood gases and noninvasive measures of respiratory support (end-tidal carbon dioxide measurements and pulse oximetry). While it is tempting to use noninvasive ventilation to support the respiratory efforts of the patient, careful clinical judgment should be used when making this decision. The patient's gag, cough, and swallow are essential for handling normal secretions in the respiratory system and noninvasive support does not protect the airway between the episodes of suctioning which is required while these patients are weak. Meticulous attention to positioning can reduce the risk of aspiration.

Urinary retention is not uncommon, but catheter placement should be avoided due to increased risk of urinary tract infections. Gentle manual pressure over the suprapubic region (the Credé method) is usually sufficient to empty the bladder. With the widespread availability of bedside ultrasound, this can be used to assess urinary retention. Specific bladder management can be tailored to the individual patient.

SIADH is a rare complication, possibly due to venous pooling. Careful monitoring of urine-specific gravity is indicated, and; if rising, evaluation of electrolytes can be undertaken to monitor for SIADH. Treatment would be fluid restriction.

Antibiotics are not effective for the primary treatment of infant botulism but may be indicated for infectious complications (e.g., pneumonia, otitis media, urinary tract infection). Antibiotics with activity against *C. botulinum* can cause additional intraintestinal toxin release and absorption. For this reason, antibiotics for secondary infection should be initiated after BabyBIG has been administered, since it has the capacity to bind any additional toxin released. Infectious complications should be treated as appropriate; though aminoglycosides are contraindicated as they can potentiate the action of the botulinum toxin at the neuromuscular junction.

CLINICAL COURSE AND PROGNOSIS

The clinical time course can vary considerably; however, patients are expected to have a peak in paralysis, followed by a period of stability, and then gradual recovery. The use of BabyBIG has dramatically reduced the length of hospitalization to about 2 weeks. Early use of BabyBIG, that is within 3 days of hospitalization, leads to 1 week less of hospitalization compared to infants treated 4 days or later after hospitalization. As BabyBIG antitoxin does not remove toxin already bound to nerve synapses, full recovery from infant botulism requires regeneration of nerve endings and subsequent induction of new motor end plates. The entire process of regeneration takes several weeks.

In the absence of secondary complications, complete recovery can be expected. Relapses are rare, if they occur at all; deterioration after initial clinical improvement suggests a complication (e.g., pneumonia, hyponatremia due to SIADH). There have been no definite cases of reinfection of infants with *C. botulinum* reported in the literature. A comprehensive list of complications can be found at the infantbotulism.org website, though it should be noted that many "complications" are a part of the natural history of the illness or related to required interventions such as intubation and mechanical ventilation.

ADMISSION CRITERIA

Infants suffering from botulism are often hospitalized before consideration or confirmation of the diagnosis owing to their worrisome clinical presentation. All infants with suspected or confirmed botulism require hospitalization. The course of the illness is unpredictable at the time of presentation; therefore, close observation is required, and the admitting hospital should have the capacity to provide full cardiopulmonary support.

DISCHARGE CRITERIA

The infant must demonstrate unequivocal and sustained improvement in symptoms with resolution of requirement for respiratory support. Adequate ventilation must be demonstrated, and ability to self-protect the airway is essential. Safe and sufficient means for hydration and nutrition must be in place. While most patients can tolerate oral feedings at discharge, some may go home on a combination of oral and enteral tube feedings. Physical, speech, and occupational therapy may be warranted after discharge to speed recovery, maintain developmental skills, and avoid complications. Standard infection control measures are usually adequate, but ongoing shedding of spores in stools can continue for months.

CONSULTATION

Neurologists can provide guidance in terms of clinical evaluation and diagnostic testing. Input from critical care physicians can assist in the assessment of clinical status, including signs of deterioration that warrant transfer to an intensive care setting. Pulmonologists can offer management expertise if respiratory insufficiency develops. Infants with incomplete recovery at the time of discharge may benefit from neurology follow-up as well as pediatric rehabilitation medicine and/or speech, physical, and occupational therapy.

SPECIAL CONSIDERATIONS

Of special note is the change in immunizations after an infant has had infant botulism and has been treated with BabyBIG. The infant should not receive Measles, Mumps, and Rubella (MMR) or Measles, Mumps, Rubella, and Varicella (MMRV) vaccines for 5 months after receiving BabyBIG. Further, the live-virus vaccines for rotavirus should be delayed until there is persistent return of normal bowel function in patients who have received BabyBIG. Practitioners should consult the *Red Book* of the American Academy of Pediatrics for the most up-to-date information regarding immunization recommendations.

KEY POINTS

- Infant botulism is the most common form of botulism in the United States.
- Infant botulism has a unique pathogenesis. It is caused by colonization of the infant gut with *Clostridium botulinum*, whereas in adults, the disease is caused by ingestion of the preformed toxin.
- Diagnosis is based on the history and physical examination. Treatment should not be delayed for confirmation of diagnosis.
- Suspected cases should be treated with BabyBIG. Call the California Department of Public Health at 510-231-7600. The website is http://www.infantbotulism.org.
- Management consists of meticulous airway, respiratory, and nutritional support.
- Long-term prognosis is excellent.
- Attention to alteration of vaccine schedule must be noted.

SUGGESTED READINGS

Antonucci L, Locci C, Schettini L, Clemente MG, Antonucci R. Infant botulism: an underestimated threat. *Infectious Diseases*. 2021;53(9):647-660.

Panditrao MV, Dabritz HA, Kazerouni NN, Damus KH, Meissinger JK, Arnon SS. Descriptive epidemiology of infant botulism in California: The first 40 Years. *J Pediatr*. 2020;227:247-257.e3.

Payne JR, Khouri JM, Jewell NP, Arnon SS. Efficacy of human botulism immune globulin for the treatment of infant botulism: The first 12 years post licensure. *J Pediatr*. 2018;193: 172-177.

Rao AK, Sobel J, Chatham-Stephens K, Luquez C. Clinical Guidelines for Diagnosis and Treatment of Botulism, 2021. *MMWR Recomm Rep*. 2021;70(2):1-30.

Welcome to the infant botulism treatment and prevention program. Welcome to the Infant Botulism Treatment and Prevention Program. (n.d.). Retrieved July 29, 2022, from https://www.infantbotulism.org/.

SECTION T
Care of the Child With Medical Complexity

CHAPTER 180 Introduction to the Child With Medical Complexity

Erin Avondet, MD and Benjamin Kalm, MD, FAAP

BACKGROUND

Caring for children with medical complexity (CMC) is a principal component of Pediatric Hospital Medicine. The consensus definition for this population follows a conceptual framework with four key domains: high levels of family-identified needs, severe chronic conditions, significant functional limitations, and elevated health resource utilization. Children with medical complexity include children with static or progressive neurologic, neuromuscular, and genetic or acquired conditions that require the assistance of medical technologies such as gastrostomy or tracheostomy, necessitate care from multiple subspecialists and therapists, and have significant family-identified needs for care coordination across the continuum of care. Some diseases (quadriplegic cerebral palsy, muscular dystrophies, congenital myopathies) should invariably be considered medically complex. For some conditions with variable severity of manifestations, a subset of more severely affected patients, typically with multisystem involvement, would be considered medically complex. For instance, a child with sickle cell disease with multiple comorbidities (pulmonary hypertension, stroke) and/or medical fragility (e.g., frequent hospitalizations for vaso-occlusive events) would also be considered medically complex. Health services researchers use a variety of methods to identify such children from diagnostic (ICD-10) codes, such as the Complex Chronic Conditions, 3M Clinical Risk Groups (CRG), and Pediatric Medical Complexity Algorithm (PMCA)). Per data from 2016 to 2019, nearly 20% of children in the United States have a special healthcare need, and the prevalence of medical complexity ranges from 0.7% to 11.4%.

Although definitions of CMC and methods to administratively identify them evolve, children with complex chronic conditions or the highest CRG levels comprise a growing proportion of hospitalizations. Children with complex chronic conditions currently account for up to 50% of hospital days in US children's hospitals. Hospitals with comprehensive care programs for this population demonstrate lower utilization and cost. A complex chronic condition or use of medical technology is an independent risk factor for adverse patient safety events and readmission.

THE HOSPITALIST AND CHILDREN WITH MEDICAL COMPLEXITY

Pediatric hospitalists care for CMC in a variety of ways, including when admitted to hospitalist inpatient services for reasons as variable as aspiration pneumonia, exacerbations of asthma or chronic lung disease, feeding problems, complex wound care, elective surgical procedures, urinary tract infection, sepsis, and malfunction of technology assistance devices. Alternatively, hospitalists may provide consultations for CMC admitted to subspecialty services or presenting to emergency departments. Often, hospitalists who provide sedation services are consulted to advise on the suitability of sedative agents in multisystem disease.

Ideally, the care coordination of CMC is spearheaded by a patient-centered, team-based, comprehensive medical home focused on quality and safety. However, 43% of US children with special healthcare needs lack medical homes. Moreover, pediatric hospitalists are vital to the "medical neighborhood" for CMC who require frequent or prolonged hospitalizations. Hospitalists are often the first and last healthcare providers to interact with CMC and their families during hospitalizations, offering continuity and supportive care. Upon discharge, hospitalists must ensure that CMC are linked to their medical homes (or find the patient a medical home), knowing that having a medical home is associated with fewer emergency department visits, inpatient admissions, and unmet medical needs.

Hospitalists, like other healthcare providers, encounter obstacles in caring for CMC. Pediatric hospitalists' caring for CMC's top barriers include lack of time, post-discharge resources, evidence-based guidelines, reimbursement, and primary care engagement. Despite the challenges, hospitalists can enjoy long-term therapeutic relationships, intellectual challenges, and interdisciplinary interactions with other hospital-based providers as they care for CMC and their families.

APPROACH TO THE CARE OF CMC

CMC requires particular attention at all inpatient hospitalization phases, beginning at admission or transfer from another service. Pediatric hospitalists must take care to rely on something other than prior documentation when constructing current histories and physicals. Misinformation from previous encounters is easily propagated, patients may have data from many providers not readily available in the Electronic Health Record (EHR), and plans change rapidly. CMC presenting to the hospital will have a chief complaint, but thorough history taking may reveal a series of interdependent conditions requiring various attention levels, outlined in subsequent chapters. Attention to underlying conditions and differentiating among time-limited acute conditions, stable chronic conditions, and progressive and life-limiting conditions ensures that the care rendered is appropriate to the needs of each child. Triage is a crucial role of hospitalists who care for children with acute illnesses superimposed on chronic conditions.

PREHOSPITAL QUALITY OF LIFE AND FUNCTION

Many CMCs have intellectual and physical disabilities that affect their overall health and development; hospitalists must remember that they see CMC when sick and may lack context about quality of life and function when the child is well. The World Health Organization's International Classification of Function, Health and Disability (ICF) provides a framework for hospitalists who care for CMC. The ICF broadens the traditional organ–system approach to care by shifting focus to health rather than disease and ability rather than disability. The ICF can facilitate goal-setting during hospitalizations in partnership with CMC and their families. This approach involves careful documentation of each CMC's baseline level of functioning during the initial history with families. This information helps providers recognize when CMC are approaching their own "normal" and can resume communal activities or demonstrate a change in status. For example, sleep patterns, frequency of bowel movements, communication skills, mobility limitations, and general functional abilities should be reviewed on admission. Some CMC pass stool only once every 2 to 3 days; some might communicate yes and no responses via unique eye movements. Understanding these individual patterns is integral to recognizing illness and progression to wellness in CMC.

POLYPHARMACY

Medication reconciliation is a critical responsibility of hospitalists. Children with medical complexity often take a combination of medications prescribed by multiple providers with doses that may have been adjusted verbally and without documentation. Admission medication discrepancies are estimated to occur in 30% of admissions to pediatric tertiary care centers (some studies indicate up to 72%), and children who need four or more medications, particularly antiepileptic drugs, are at the most significant risk. Diligence ensures that complicated medication and feeding regimens are accurately communicated in electronic health records and to home caregivers. CMC may have detailed home routines that are difficult to replicate on hospital units because of policies, regulations, and nurse staffing ratios. These children may only avoid negative consequences by adhering to specific, seemingly idiosyncratic routines. Partnerships between providers, patients, and home caregivers can preserve routines during hospitalizations that promote healing environments that are satisfying and safe, particularly during transitions between home and hospital.

CARE COORDINATION

The hospitalist ensures that inpatient care coordination is effective and efficient. Adequate communication with the child's primary care provider (PCP) is essential. Establishing a line of communication with a patient's PCP can facilitate subsequent care management decisions and discharge planning. Similarly, communication with hospital-based specialists is critical to providing coordinated care. Specialists may be consulted for acute management questions; their multiple inputs must be integrated and, if conflicting, diplomatically adjudicated. Hospitalists must be active and resourceful in interacting with subspecialists, asking specific questions, and suggesting management approaches. CMC and their families are best served when the hospitalist advocates for their needs; for example, hospitalists may attempt to coordinate multiple procedures by multiple providers under a single anesthesia. Hospitalists can consult with subspecialists for acute illness management and develop a discharge care plan that minimizes readmissions as much as possible. Even when formal inpatient consultation is not indicated, keeping established subspecialists "in the loop" can contribute to effective discharge plans anticipating care needs at home. With CMC, communication and coordination with allied health professionals are as important as communication with other physicians. Guardians, home caregivers, therapists, care managers, discharge planners, social workers, home care medical providers, educators, and others play vitally essential roles in the care of CMC, and it is critical to incorporate their input into all stages of care planning.

COMMUNICATION

Hospitalists sometimes care for CMC and their families as they contend with major decisions such as choosing gastrostomy, tracheostomy, or other life-changing procedures or technologies. They often care for families making decisions regarding end-of-life care for their children with life-limiting conditions. Increasingly, families opt for end-of-life care at home rather than in hospitals, and discharge planning has become the highest priority. Family-centered, interdisciplinary communication is of utmost importance. The Pediatric Hospitalist must recognize the level of medical literacy for each situation and emphasize family-centered communication, including interpretation as needed, to decrease medical errors and ensure that all the patient's needs are met.

HOME CAREGIVER AND FAMILY WELLBEING

The presence of CMC in the family affects the physical and emotional health and well-being of the caregivers, siblings, and other family members. Caregivers of children with disabilities more likely to be in poorer physical and emotional health than caregivers of typically developing children. The physical and mental health of patients' caregivers is directly associated with their children's physical and psychological health and quality of life. Hospitalists should recognize family stress and engage in family support services as needed. Hospitalists must also be mindful of the particular social determinants of health affecting families and caregivers of children with medical complexity. These families are more likely to face barriers to equitable healthcare, such as poverty, housing, food and formula security, financial instability, etc. Furthermore, families with non-English preferring, Black or Hispanic, or household income below the federal poverty level are even more likely to face further health inequities. In the face of these challenges, many healthcare systems have begun screening for and developing processes to address caregiver social stressors upon admission to the hospital. The needs, preferences, and resources of families of CMC should be evaluated well before hospital discharge.

PATIENT HANDOFF

The typical patient handoff process is highly variable, unstructured, and at high risk for communication errors for all children, particularly for CMC. Patient safety is optimized when transitions between providers are deliberate, proactive, and interactive, emphasizing strategies to address ongoing acute issues and anticipated condition-specific problems that might arise. Hospitalist schedules in which inpatient attendings rotate frequently can frustrate families if plans change with each new attending. It is incumbent on hospitalists to communicate effectively with each other as a team, with documentation in the chart, verbal communication, and standardized, validated handoff tools to minimize adverse impact in such transitions.

DISCHARGE PLANNING

Hospitalists must proactively plan for hospital discharges of CMC, especially when home health nursing care and equipment must be in place for discharge. For CMC, sending a discharge summary to the patient's PCP is often insufficient; direct communication via telephone and/or electronic messaging facilitates a safe and efficient transition of care. As 40% of families of children with special healthcare needs (CSHCN) experience a financial burden related to their child's conditions, resources to fill prescriptions, purchase specialized diets, and contend with loss secondary to the need to reduce or eliminate employment should be explored. Home medication and feeding schedules should be developed considering family, school, and child needs to maximize opportunities for the child to participate in the community. Discharge documentation provided to the family should be complete, easy to understand, and in the family's preferred language.

FUTURE DIRECTIONS

With the increasing need for medical homes for CMC, residency training programs must ensure that future pediatricians demonstrate comfort and familiarity with devices and medications and have the knowledge and technical skills needed to address ambulatory-sensitive problems and minimize emergency department and hospital admissions. To date, pediatric residency programs offer little formal training regarding the lives and needs of CSHCNs and their families outside the hospital setting, particularly regarding identifying community resources and collaborating with community agencies and schools. Indeed, it has been suggested that the care of CMC, which demands that providers have specialized knowledge and expertise in indwelling catheters, seizure control, treatment of spasticity, management of home ventilators, tube feeding management, dealing with home nursing agencies, advocacy with payers, the care of healthy siblings, among many others, might be its own subspecialty.

Hospitalists, like all providers, must be increasingly focused on delivering high-value care. Advances that reduce information fragmentation will hopefully result in better care and outcomes for CMC. Specific examples of advances include informatics that make electronic health records more accessible to home caregivers and providers alike, privacy-protected health information exchanges that support the organization and real-time sharing of clinical information (including medication reconciliation and comprehensive care plans), telemedicine for immediate clinical assessments, and patient provider electronic communications. Readmission rates, shared accountability, and delivering the right amount of care in the right setting (inpatient vs. ambulatory settings) demand our attention. Fragmented care is not an option, and partnerships between guardians/caregivers, hospitalists, subspecialists, and generalists across the continuum are needed to ensure coordinated care. The critical roles of guardians/caregivers, social workers, care managers, home care providers, educators, and community health providers in coordinating care for CMC cannot be underestimated, and team-based care is necessary. Hospitalists are well-positioned to nurture these partnerships as they care for CMC.

SUGGESTED READINGS

Berry JG, Agrawal R, Kuo DZ, et al. Characteristics of hospitalizations for patients who use a structured clinical care program for children with medical complexity. *J Pediatr*. 2011;159(2):284-290.

Berry JG, Hall M, Cohen E, O'Neill M, Feudtner C. Ways to identify children with medical complexity and the importance of why. *J Pediatr*. 2015;167(2):229-237.

Berry JG, Hall M, Hall DE, et al. Inpatient growth and resource use in 28 children's hospitals: a longitudinal, multi-institutional study. *JAMA Pediatr*. 2013;167(2):170.

Berry JG. Hospital utilization and characteristics of patients experiencing recurrent readmissions within children's hospitals. *JAMA*. 2011;305(7):682.

Child and Adolescent Health Measurement Initiative. 2016-2017 National Survey of Children's Health (NSCH) data query. Data Resource Center for Child and Adolescent Health supported by the U.S. Department of Health and Human Services, Health Resources and Services Administration (HRSA), Maternal and Child Health Bureau (MCHB).

Cohen E, Berry JG, Sanders L, Schor EL, Wise PH. Status complexicus? the emergence of pediatric complex care. *Pediatrics*. 2018;141(Supplement_3):S202-S211.

Conkol KJ, Martinez-Strengel A, Coller RJ, Bergman DA, Whelan EM. Pediatric Hospitalists' Lessons Learned From an Innovation Award to Improve Care for Children With Medical Complexity. *Hospital Pediatrics*. 2020;10(8):694-701.

Dodds C, Rempel G. A quality of life model promotes enablement for children with medical complexity. *J Pediatr Rehabil Med*. 2016;9(4):253-255.

Elias ER, Murphy NA, Council on Children with Disabilities. Home care of children and youth with complex health care needs and technology dependencies. *Pediatrics*. 2012;129(5):996-1005.

Feudtner C, Feinstein JA, Satchell M, Zhao H, Kang TI. Shifting place of death among children with complex chronic conditions in the United States, 1989-2003. *JAMA*. 2007;297(24):2725-2732.

Gattari TB, Krieger LN, Hu HM, Mychaliska KP. Medication discrepancies at pediatric hospital discharge. *Hospital Pediatrics*. 2015;5(8):439-445.

Ghandour RM, Hirai AH, Kenney MK. Children and youth with special health care needs: a profile. *Pediatrics*. 2022;149(Supplement 7): e2021056150D.

Goudie A, Narcisse MR, Hall DE, Kuo DZ. Financial and psychological stressors associated with caring for children with disability. *Fam Syst Health*. 2014;32(3):280-290.

Identification of Caregiver-Reported Social Risk Factors in Hospitalized Children | Hospital Pediatrics | American Academy of Pediatrics. Accessed July 30, 2022. https://publications.aap.org/hospitalpediatrics/article/10/1/20/25937/Identification-of-Caregiver-Reported-Social-Risk.

Jette AM. Toward a common language for function, disability, and health. *Phys Ther*. 2006;86(5):726-734.

Khan A, Spector ND, Baird JD, et al. Patient safety after implementation of a coproduced family centered communication programme: multicenter before and after intervention study. *BMJ*. 2018;363:k4764.

Knighton AJ, Bass EJ. Implementing family-centered rounds in hospital pediatric settings: a scoping review. *Hosp Pediatr*. 2021;11(7):679-691.

Kuo DZ, Goudie A, Cohen E, et al. Inequities in health care needs for children with medical complexity. *Health Affairs*. 2014;33(12):2190-2198.

Kuo DZ. The medical home for children with medical complexity: back to basics. *J Pediatr*. 2019;206:8-9.

Lykens KA, Fulda KG, Bae S, Singh KP. Differences in risk factors for children with special health care needs (CSHCN) receiving needed specialty care by Socioeconomic Status. *BMC Pediatr*. 2009;9:48.

Murphy NA, Christian B, Caplin DA, Young PC. The health of caregivers for children with disabilities: caregiver perspectives. *Child Care Health Dev*. 2007;33(2):180-187.

Yu JA, McKernan G, Hagerman T, Schenker Y, Houtrow A. Identifying Children With Medical Complexity From the National Survey of Children's Health Combined 2016-17 Data Set. *Hosp Pediatr*. 2021;11(2):192-197.

CHAPTER 181 Acute Care of the Medically Complex Child With Severe Neurologic Impairment

G. Joy Walton, MD, David E. Hall, MD, and Laurie Glader, MD

BACKGROUND

Children with medical complexity (CMC) are growing in number in children's hospitals. They are at high risk for medical errors and for readmission after discharge. Characterized by chronic, severe health conditions, they have substantial health service needs, functional limitations, and high healthcare resource utilization. Severe neurologic impairment (SNI) is a frequent defining feature of this population. Multisystem chronic conditions often lead to dependence on medical technology, such as gastrostomy tubes, tracheostomies, ventilators, and ventriculoperitoneal (VP) shunts. Although the underlying conditions are frequently neurological, multiorgan comorbidities are common, and these do not fit into a single subspecialty, resulting in hospital-based pediatricians caring for them in ward or intensive care settings.

PATHOPHYSIOLOGY AND MANAGEMENT

Children with SNI comprise a diverse group from an etiological perspective. Yet, despite this diversity, commonalities exist in the comorbidities and complications they experience. Although these patients may be intimidating to providers, severe central nervous system dysfunction leads to a predictable set of problems with tendrils across multiple systems. **Figure 181-1** provides a proposed framework to anchor the clinician's understanding of the child with SNI and to anticipate complications, allowing for a systematic approach to care.

The range of comorbidities in children with underlying neurologic impairment is extensive, encompassing virtually every organ system. Therefore, medical issues that may not directly relate to the reason for admission often surface over the course of their hospitalization. The hospitalist who appreciates common comorbid conditions in children with SNI will be prepared to evaluate the child fully admitted with an acute illness for predisposing risk factors and potential complications.

An evidence-based approach to treatment is always desirable. However, the literature base for the clinical management of this population is often sparse. Thus, the recommendations in this chapter reflect a combination of evidence-based care and expert opinion. Despite the range of comorbidities and the lack of outcomes data, a systematic approach to assessment and management can enable the care provider to feel confident in monitoring and initiating treatment for likely complications.

PULMONARY

PNEUMONIA

Pneumonia or respiratory distress is a common reason for admission in children with SNI. Causes of lower respiratory infection reflect typical pathogens encountered in the hospital. Severe pulmonary complications of influenza are a particular risk for this population. Immunization to prevent acute infectious exacerbations from vaccine-preventable diseases remains critical. While children have largely been spared the grave

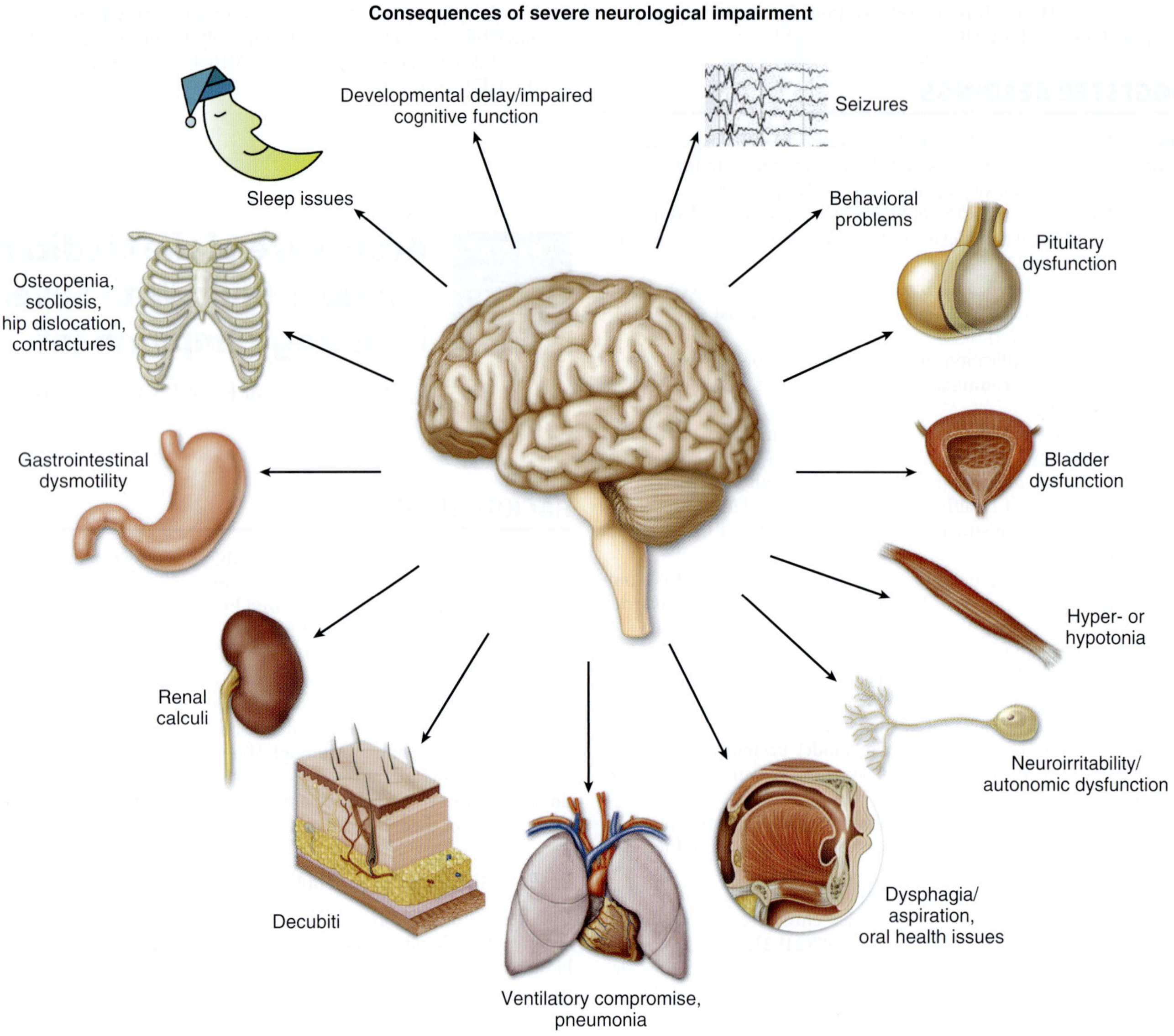

FIGURE 181-1. Consequences of severe neurological impairment.

consequences of COVID-19, children with SNI are at increased risk for serious illness. Children with severe COVID-19 may develop pneumonia, shock, and respiratory failure and risk developing multisystem inflammatory syndrome in children (MIS-C). Hospitalization may be an excellent opportunity to promote age-appropriate COVID-19 vaccination in this high-risk group.

Aspiration plays a prominent role in pneumonia among this population, specifically in recurrent pneumonia, and can affect the choice of antibiotics. However, the decision to treat aspiration pneumonia is often based on clinical judgment rather than clear-cut radiographic evidence, and antibiotic choice is controversial. If antibiotics are used, anaerobic coverage may be recommended, but evidence of its efficacy in the ill-hospitalized patient is limited to retrospective analyses.

AIRWAY CLEARANCE AND SIALORRHEA

Aggressive pulmonary clearance is important for managing acute, recurrent, and chronic infections and aspiration. Chest physiotherapy, manually or with high-frequency oscillating vests, can mobilize airway secretions in conjunction with nebulized therapies. Evidence for the impact of chest physiotherapy on outcomes is limited, but it remains an important treatment mainstay. In some patients with an ineffective cough, a cough-assist device may also be helpful to expectorate mobilized secretions. Many children with underlying neuromuscular weakness or altered chest mechanics hypoventilate. In these cases, positive pressure ventilation, such as BIPAP, may be used to decrease atelectasis. Due to the risk of reflux and aspiration, facial BIPAP should be avoided during feeding patients with gastrostomy tubes. Post-pyloric feeding with a gastrojejunostomy (GJ) tube is not contraindicated. (For further information, see Chapter 182.)

Oromotor dysfunction can contribute to sialorrhea as well as interfere with speech production. Particularly troublesome is the posterior pooling of secretions. Controlling sialorrhea may decrease the frequency of lower respiratory tract infections and recurrent aspiration pneumonia episodes.

Anticholinergic medications effectively reduce oral secretion volume, but side effects may limit their use. Glycopyrrolate is the only FDA-approved agent for the pharmacologic treatment of sialorrhea in children. Off-label treatments for sialorrhea include using a scopolamine patch, sublingual application of ophthalmic atropine, and trihexyphenidyl. Refractory oral secretions may be amenable to botulinum injections into the submandibular and parotid glands. Surgical ligation or removal of the salivary glands may ultimately provide a more permanent solution. Patients undergoing treatment to reduce sialorrhea require regular dental care to minimize the risk of dental caries and periodontal disease risk.

For persistent sialorrhea and difficulty with airway clearance, a tracheostomy can provide enhanced access for suctioning secretions. The most definitive procedure to avoid aspiration is a laryngotracheal separation, in which the trachea is brought out to a stoma, and the larynx is closed off. Effective ventilation occurs only at the tracheal stoma, as the upper airway ends in a blind pouch. This is a radical procedure reserved for children with persistent daily symptoms and recurrent pneumonias resulting in repeated hospitalizations, a decline in pulmonary baseline, and diminished quality of life. This procedure results in permanent tracheostomy placement and loss of phonation but can positively impact pulmonary health and quality of life.

TRACHEITIS

Bacterial tracheitis is unusual in children without medical complexity but not uncommon in children with tracheostomies. Patients with tracheitis or tracheobronchitis may present with increased, thickened, or purulent secretions. They may have symptoms consistent with pneumonia, such as decreased oxygen saturation and fever but no signs of pneumonia on chest X-ray. White blood cells are commonly increased on the gram stain of tracheal secretions. The trachea may be colonized with *Staphylococcus aureus*, *Moraxella catarrhalis*, *Streptococcus pneumonia*, *Haemophilus influenzae*, *Pseudomonas aeruginosa*, and other bacteria, making interpretation of cultures difficult. Although positive tracheal cultures alone do not indicate infection, they may be used to guide antibiotic treatment in the patient. Many clinicians treat for 7 to 10 days with systemic antibiotics; nebulized tobramycin could also be considered in some cases.

UPPER AIRWAY OBSTRUCTION

Upper airway issues include anatomic obstruction, such as choanal atresia or septal deviation, and functional obstruction, such as tracheomalacia and abnormal airway tone. Signs of upper airway obstruction can include snoring, stridor, stertor, and concerning respiratory patterns, such as pausing or gasping while asleep. Repositioning, nasal trumpet insertion, and positive airway pressure may improve upper airway difficulties. A tracheostomy may be indicated for severe upper airway obstruction.

Obstructive sleep apnea (OSA) is prevalent in children with SNI. If suspected, polysomnography can clarify the diagnosis. This test is best performed when the patient is at their baseline state. Surgical intervention is indicated if OSA is identified in adenotonsillar hypertrophy. If no anatomic abnormality or adenoidectomy and/or tonsillectomy do not improve the OSA, then a trial of positive pressure should be undertaken. Continuous positive airway pressure (CPAP) requires a child to wear a tight-fitting mask, which can be challenging. Bilevel-positive airway pressure (BiPAP) provides a backup rate and is helpful if an element of central sleep apnea is present. Other treatment options for upper airway obstruction include supraglottoplasty, uvulopalatoplasty, tracheostomy, or mandibular distraction, depending on the cause of the obstruction.

NEUROLOGY

Children with SNI, by definition, have underlying neurologic disorders (Figure 181-1). Delays are often identified across all development streams, including speech, gross and fine motor, and social/adaptive skills. Additionally, children with underlying neurologic conditions often have associated sensory impairment. Common visual concerns include cortical visual impairment, amblyopia, nystagmus, visual field cuts, refractory errors, and exposure keratosis. Hearing loss is also common and may be sensorineural or conductive, sometimes based on congenital malformation.

SEIZURES

Children with SNI have a predisposition to seizure disorders. They are often treated with multiple antiepileptic agents, sometimes resulting in detrimental side effects such as somnolence, behavioral change, hepatitis, pancreatitis, abnormal bone density, or kidney stones. For refractory seizure disorders, other treatment options include the ketogenic diet, vagal nerve stimulator, corpus callosotomy, and neurosurgical ablation or resection of the epileptic focus.

Many patients with SNI experience seizures during an acute illness. If anticonvulsant levels are appropriate and no other cause for the increased seizures is found, a bridge treatment is often provided of lorazepam or clonazepam, either enterally or intravenously, until the illness improves. Patients who are NPO/NPG may need modification of their anticonvulsant regimen if their maintenance medications are unavailable in an intravenous form. Consultation with pediatric neurology can facilitate short-term bridging and ongoing chronic management of seizures.

VENTRICULOPERITONEAL SHUNT DYSFUNCTION

Children with SNI may have hydrocephalus secondary to central nervous system (CNS) malformations, cysts, meningitis, tumors, or intraventricular bleeding. Ventriculoperitoneal, ventriculoatrial, and ventriculopleural shunts are often placed in this condition. However, these devices are prone to dysfunction, most commonly due to shunt obstruction, and less frequently by infection. Infections tend to cause early shunt failures, while catheter occlusions typically account for late shunt dysfunction.

Children with shunt malfunction can develop signs of increased intracranial pressure. Initially, they may experience headaches or irritability, then progress to lethargy and vomiting. Increased intracranial pressure may also cause Cushing triad of bradycardia, hypertension or widening pulse pressure, and irregular respirations. Less frequently, a stiff neck will be present, failure of upward gaze, or papilledema. A child with a shunt and these symptoms are presumed to have shunt malfunction until proven otherwise. Evaluation of shunt function and integrity includes a radiological shunt series to assess the tubing and a head CT (or, if available, a rapid sequence MRI) to evaluate changes in ventricular size.

Most shunt infections occur in the first 6 months postoperatively, with a peak incidence of around 2 to 3 weeks, although late shunt infections can be observed. Early shunt infections are often due to inoculation during shunt insertion, while late infections are often associated with peritonitis, abdominal pseudocyst, bowel perforation, and bacteremia. Despite improved sterile techniques, antibiotic-impregnated catheters, and programmable valves, VP shunt infections remain a common problem, leading to multiple and costly hospital admissions for revisions and replacements. If an infection is suspected, neurosurgery should be consulted and may obtain cerebrospinal fluid (CSF) for culture and analysis. Ventricular CSF from the shunt reservoir is an efficient means of diagnosis when a high index of suspicion exists. Skin organisms are the most common cause of infection, especially *Staphylococcus epidermidis* and *Staphylococcus aureus*.

SLEEP PROBLEMS

Sleep problems often go unrecognized in children with neurologic complexity, who experience longer-lasting and more complex sleep problems than their typically developing peers. They can be responsible for significant daytime irritability, behavioral dysregulation, altered cognitive function, and can cause familial disruption. There is growing support in the literature for using melatonin as a sleep aid for children with a primary neurologic etiology for their sleep disturbance. Dosing regimens still need more consensus, but a standard of 3 to 6 mg is often used. When this is not successful, gabapentin, clonidine, or trazodone can be helpful though the insufficient evidence base remains largely extrapolated from adult data.

IRRITABILITY OF UNKNOWN ORIGIN

Severe and persistent irritability in the child with SNI can lead to extreme parent frustration, exhaustion, and sometimes admission. These factors commonly impact the child and their family's quality of life and require advocacy for increased social support (see Special Considerations). Diagnostic work-ups center around looking for sources of pain, which is common and may be a source of behavioral dysregulation. However, assessment and therapeutic interventions can be challenging. A detailed history and physical exam should be conducted to evaluate the irritability, including a review of medications and the feeding regimen and a careful examination of tone and teeth (see **Table 181-1** for a list of conditions to consider). A reasonable initial laboratory evaluation without an apparent cause includes a complete blood count, acute phase reactants such as C-reactive protein or erythrocyte sedimentation rate, electrolytes, liver function tests, amylase, lipase, and urinalysis. Constipation is a common trigger of discomfort and can be difficult to detect by history due to the presence of overflow stools. Hints include painful or hard bowel movements, bloating, a large fecal mass on a rectal exam, a palpable stool mass, large diameter stools, and two or fewer stools/week (except overflow stools). An abdominal radiograph may provide additional information if the diagnosis is questionable. If some evidence supports the diagnosis of constipation, consider treatment. Ultrasound is another useful tool as cholelithiasis and nephrolithiasis are also in the differential. If pain is suspected to be secondary to spasticity, a trial of baclofen may be indicated. When pain behaviors persist despite treatment of an identified source or when no source is found after a thorough investigation, an empiric trial of gabapentin can be considered. Tricyclic antidepressants, alpha agonists, and serotonin-norepinephrine reuptake inhibitors have also been used. Parents may ask about cannabinoids as an adjunct treatment for irritability of unclear etiology, but little information is available regarding its use. A therapeutic intervention may address multiple problems, improving symptoms but diminishing the capacity to know the source with absolute certainty.

Paroxysmal sympathetic hyperactivity (PSH) is an entity on the end of the spectrum of irritability of unknown origin in patients with SNI. Common manifestations include irritability, fever, tachypnea, dystonic posturing, hyperhidrosis, seizure-like episodes, hypertension, tachycardia, vomiting, retching, and diaphoresis. In 2014, an international multidisciplinary consensus group developed an 11-point diagnostic scale to standardize the definition of PSH as a "syndrome, recognized in a subgroup of survivors of severe acquired brain injury, of simultaneous, paroxysmal transient increases in sympathetic and motor activity." The first step is to look for a trigger of the episodes, as in Table 181-1. Sometimes associated fevers can be very high, mimicking a severe infection. However, if no infection is present, acute phase reactants typically are not elevated (although the white blood cell count may be increased due to catecholamine release), and the fever tends to improve quickly with a resolution of the flare-up. If a source of pain is determined, treat the underlying problem. However, often no obvious trigger is found and additional pharmacological interventions may be required. Evidence as to the best treatment is mainly anecdotal. A useful approach in the hospital is to begin with daily controller medications, such as gabapentin, clonidine, or propranolol, alone or in combination, to control sympathetic overactivity, plus an order for as-needed medication, usually a benzodiazepine or opiate. Scheduled baclofen is helpful if the patient has severe muscle spasticity. In the most severe cases, patients may require heavy sedation with drugs such as dexmedetomidine in an intensive care setting. Nonpharmacological interventions such as swaddling, weighted blankets, creating a calm environment, and avoiding noxious stimuli should be considered staples of any treatment plan.

TABLE 181-1 Differential Diagnosis of Irritability in Children With Severe Neurologic Impairment

System or Disease Category	Conditions	Notes
Infection	Otitis media, sinusitis, pneumonia, pharyngitis, tracheitis, gastroenteritis, urinary tract infection, cellulitis, osteomyelitis, meningitis, endocarditis, hardware infection, and other sources	A history of fever, symptoms, and examination findings help corroborate the source of infection.
Pulmonary	Obstructive sleep apnea causing lack of sleep, mucus plugging, multiple infectious etiologies (see above)	
Gastrointestinal	Constipation, gastroesophageal reflux with esophagitis, gastritis, ulcer, pancreatitis, appendicitis, intussusception, gallstones, hepatitis, small intestinal bacterial overgrowth, feeding tube malfunction, irritation, or ill-fitted tube, ingested foreign body, intestinal distention due to motility issues, or pain due to visceral hyperalgesia	Constipation may not be obvious by history due to potential overflow stool. Consider KUB to assess stool burden. Obtain LFTs and amylase/lipase. Consider abdominal ultrasound for stones.
Genitourinary	Renal stones, urinary tract infection, urinary retention, testicular or ovarian torsion, dysmenorrhea, symptoms related to pregnancy	Consider KUB, U/A, and/or urinary catheterization if retention suspected (may be able to palpate enlarged bladder, bladder scan can verify findings). Abdominal CT or ultrasound are useful to look for stones and/or torsion.
Dermatologic	Decubitus ulcer, eczema, cellulitis (see above)	Conduct a full body skin assessment including sacral and ischial areas.
Musculoskeletal	Pathological or traumatic fracture, subluxed or dislocated hips, severe muscle spasms related to spasticity	Parents can be very helpful in localizing pain associated with pathological fracture. Subluxed or dislocated hips may be painful with movement such as diaper changes.
Neurologic	Ventriculoperitoneal shunt dysfunction, seizures	Look for lethargy, vomiting. Consider a shunt series, head CT, or rapid sequence MRI. Consider EEG as indicated.
Medications	Drug side effect or toxicity, withdrawal from missed doses, baclofen shunt malfunction	Missed doses of baclofen, benzodiazepines, narcotics, antiepileptic drugs, medications related to GERD and constipation should be considered.
Ophthalmologic	Corneal abrasion, glaucoma	Lagophthalmos increases the risk of abrasion.
Dental	Caries, abscess, gingivitis	
Cardiac	Supraventricular tachycardia	Consider EKG and/or cardiac monitoring during an acute episode.
Autoimmune illness	Rheumatoid arthritis, SLE	Clues are usually available by history and exam.
General	Change in home environment	New placement, change in home nursing or caretakers, and/or parental stress may contribute to agitation.
Other	Neuroirritability of unknown cause	After a detailed and thoughtful evaluation (or even during a prolonged evaluation), it is acceptable to treat pain empirically and continue to follow the patient closely for response or new developments.

NEUROPSYCHIATRIC

BEHAVIORAL ISSUES AND AGGRESSION

Children with SNI sometimes demonstrate dysregulated behavior, including aggression, when ill or in a strange environment. This can be exacerbated by communication impairment. Working with caregivers to employ techniques, using communicative aids, and rehearsing planned procedures with child-life specialists can be helpful when behavioral challenges arise. The hospitalist may be called upon to intervene when a child is biting or hitting caretakers, or pulling out lines or tubes. Adaptive clothing, protective beds, and patient care attendants may be required to keep patients safe. Medications such as clonidine or benzodiazepines may also be helpful in this situation. In the most urgent and severe situations, antihistamines such as diphenhydramine or hydroxyzine, or antipsychotics such as haloperidol, quetiapine, olanzapine, or risperidone can be utilized. Both typical and atypical antipsychotics can prolong the QT interval and require monitoring. Rarely, restraints may be needed. If necessary, standardized hospital policies should be followed carefully to ensure patient safety.

NEUROMUSCULAR AND ORTHOPEDIC CONCERNS

Differences in muscle tone, including spasticity and hypotonia, are associated with altered strength and stamina, mobility challenges, contractures, hip migration, and neuromuscular scoliosis. Children with neurologic impairment often have surgeries related to some of these complications and are hospitalized in the postoperative period. Knowledge of common comorbidities and complications can help navigate the postoperative course.

Neuromuscular interventions tend to progress from least to most invasive. Children with motor differences and delays should be involved in physical and occupational therapies from an early age: these target posture, positioning, strength, stamina, and coordination while encouraging motor development and independence. Orthotics and specialized equipment are integral additions to augment these therapeutic goals, from mobility aids, such as wheelchairs and gait trainers, to hospital beds and adaptive toileting systems. Often equipment needs can be anticipated and addressed during the hospitalization or at the time of discharge.

Management of tone abnormalities generally revolves around spasticity. Diazepam and baclofen are commonly used agents; other pharmacologic choices may include gabapentin or dantrolene. Side effects from systemic baclofen often limit its utility. In such cases, intrathecal baclofen may be an effective alternative. Patients with intrathecal baclofen pumps who present with hyperthermia, altered mental status, increased hypertonia or myoclonus, and/or evidence of rhabdomyolysis must be considered for baclofen withdrawal, either based on pump malfunction or an empty reservoir. Baclofen pumps require careful maintenance with clearly planned refills to avoid this situation. Once identified, baclofen withdrawal may be treated acutely with intravenous benzodiazepines and loading doses of enteral baclofen until further plans are devised to address the underlying cause for withdrawal.

For focal spasticity, children may receive targeted botulinum toxin injections. Over time, contractures (and often pain) progress despite a comprehensive approach to treatment involving therapies, stretching, orthotics, pharmacologic interventions, and botulinum toxin. Surgical intervention becomes an important consideration. Common surgeries the hospitalist will see include soft tissue releases (tenotomies); bony procedures, particularly regarding hip integrity (derotational osteotomies with or without acetabuloplasties); and spinal fusion to address progressive neuromuscular scoliosis. These surgeries may be associated with postoperative pneumonia, urinary tract infections, and skin or hardware infections, among other complications, and are often the focus of hospitalist care.

Pathologic fractures present another orthopedic problem the hospitalist caring for this population of children may encounter. Decreased mobility, limited weight-bearing, and polypharmacy contribute to osteopenia, which increases the risk for fractures, even with minimal and sometimes unidentified trauma. Taking care of transfers, positioning, routine hygiene, or other interventions should be encouraged by all team members. Patients may be monitored periodically with 25-hydroxy vitamin D levels and treated to maintain levels in a normal range. Although more of a longitudinal outpatient concern, this can be easily checked during an inpatient stay when labs are frequently drawn. Patients with pathologic fractures may benefit from bisphosphonate treatment to help accrue bone mass. This is usually administered intravenously in an outpatient venue, but occasionally there is an opportunity to consider infusion during an inpatient stay.

GASTROENTEROLOGY

FEEDING ISSUES AND DYSMOTILITY

Feeding issues are ubiquitous in patients with severe neurological impairment, and infantile feeding challenges may herald a central nervous system dysfunction diagnosis. It is often helpful to inquire how long a parent takes to feed a child. Excessive time spent feeding a child (more than 30 minutes per meal) is a red flag for feeding difficulties, whether mechanical or behavioral. Many caregivers may spend much of their day attempting to feed their child by mouth, yet the child can still appear malnourished on examination.

In children with SNI, oral feeding may pose an aspiration risk, and further assessment is often warranted. Many patients experience silent aspiration, so a history of coughing or choking with feedings is not a sensitive risk indicator. The evaluation may include a clinical feeding assessment, a radiographic video swallowing study performed in consultation with a feeding therapist, and/or a bedside flexible endoscopic swallowing study. Evaluation of possible dysphagia is generally best done when a child is at baseline. Nasogastric (NG) tube feedings can be helpful as an interim solution before considering a gastrostomy insertion, and home NG feedings are safe and effective when parents are instructed in their use. Gastrostomy tubes can lead to improved nutrition in severely neurologically impaired children (refer to Chapter 182). They can positively impact the entire family by reducing caregiver anxiety about achieving daily caloric goals and freeing time for other activities. Family values and preferences should be incorporated into a shared decision making framework when approaching decisions around feeding.

Once a gastrostomy tube is established, bolus feedings may allow for more time off a pump but increase the chance of gastroesophageal reflux compared to continuous feeds. If bolus feedings are not tolerated, one may provide continuous nighttime feedings with smaller or slower boluses during the day. Feeding intolerance often requires a trial-and-error approach. Some patients who do poorly with processed formulas will tolerate a blenderized diet preparation. Some commercial formulas have become available that offer a whole food or blenderized option. Many nonambulatory patients require surprisingly few calories. Weight gain trajectory must be monitored to avoid excessive weight, which can cause lifting, transfers, and mobility difficulty.

Feeding intolerance often requires more than adjustment of feeding routines since gastrointestinal dysmotility manifesting as GERD, poor gastric emptying, and gastroparesis is common in this population. Histamine type 2 receptor antagonists and proton pump inhibitors (PPIs) are frequently used in GERD or gastritis and should be monitored closely and tapered as tolerated. Agents that enhance gastric accommodation or emptying (cyproheptadine) or provide prokinetic effects (erythromycin, amoxicillin/clavulanic acid) can be useful. Small bacterial intestinal overgrowth (SIBO) is another etiology of feeding intolerance to consider with both gastrointestinal (abdominal distention, diarrhea, and flatulence) and nongastrointestinal manifestations (pain and irritability). Antibiotics targeting enteric aerobes and anaerobes are often used.

The family and physician may consider post-pyloric feeding with a gastrojejunostomy (GJ) tube in patients who cannot tolerate gastrostomy tube feedings. Placement of a GJ tube does not require surgery but does require continuous feedings. Usually, a 4- to 8-hour window without feedings can be created to give children a break from the pump. However, GJ tubes cannot be replaced at home and may require frequent hospital visits for replacement or repositioning with interventional radiology. Intussusception can also occur around the distal portion of the GJ tube, which can be further elucidated on ultrasound. If a patient with a GJ tube develops vomiting or persistent abdominal pain or distension, obtain an abdominal radiograph to check positioning; a contrast study may offer further verification (see Chapter 182).

Fundoplication surgery may also be considered in patients who do well with GJ tubes or those with significant GERD over time. A successful fundoplication allows for bolus feedings with a reduced risk of aspiration due to reflux (but not from aspiration of oral secretions, which sometimes pool above the area of surgery). Fundoplications are not always well-tolerated and may exacerbate gagging and retching. Ultimately, no clear consensus exists regarding which option—fundoplication with G tube or GJ tube placement—has better outcomes, and treatment should be individualized. Providers should work collaboratively with appropriate consultants and the care team to determine the best course of action based on both the available evidence and the values and preferences of the patient and caregivers.

CONSTIPATION

Constipation is prevalent in children with severe neurological impairment. Disturbances in neurologic modulation, physical inactivity, and decreased fluid intake contribute to the problem. Constipation is a frequent cause of pain and irritability, predisposes patients to urinary retention, leading to urinary tract infections, and can cause vomiting and feeding intolerance. Overflow diarrhea may also occur. An abdominal radiograph can help assess stool burden in cases of diagnostic uncertainty. In the inpatient setting, patients may require cleanout with a polyethylene glycol/electrolyte solution administered as a nasogastric or G-tube infusion. Most children with SNI require daily use of a stool softener and often a laxative or suppository to minimize complications of constipation.

GENITOURINARY

Children with SNI are at risk for associated underlying bladder dysfunction, and many patients have abnormally high residual urinary volumes after voiding, leading to recurrent urinary tract infections. In this setting, some children are on prophylactic antibiotics, either systemically or topically instilled, and some require scheduled clean intermittent catheterization. Bacterial colonization is common, and a positive urine culture alone is not always an indication for antibiotic treatment. Clinical signs of infection must also exist to avoid overtreatment and the development of resistant organisms.

ENDOCRINE

Patients with profound neurological impairment risk endocrinopathies when the hypothalamic-pituitary axis is disrupted. Unexplained hypoglycemia can be a clue to centrally mediated adrenal insufficiency. Hypotension and shock after even minor surgical procedures can occur when adrenal insufficiency goes unrecognized and untreated. Pituitary failure may be partial rather than complete, and signs may be subtle. Hypothyroidism, premature adrenarche, diabetes insipidus, and growth hormone deficiency may also occur.

SKIN

Decubitus ulcers are a common and often preventable problem for children with less mobility and decreased fat stores. Chronic in nature, skin challenges often lead to recurrent hospitalizations related to deeper infections such as chronic osteomyelitis. The skin should be examined carefully during all physical examinations, particularly over bony prominences such as the coccyx, ischium, greater trochanter, heels, occiput, lateral elbows, and ears. They may also be seen on pressure points of splints and wheelchairs. Attention should be paid to seating and mobility devices. Specialized cushioning can be ordered for wheelchairs. If there are problems with skin breakdown, an air mattress can reduce the risk of recurrence and promote healing.

SPECIAL CONSIDERATIONS

SHARED DECISION-MAKING

A child with SNI has an intricate web of medical concerns that impact development, autonomy, and virtually all aspects of daily living. Questions about the quality of life are important to raise with caregivers. Identifying the family's and child's goals is critical in carving out a care plan that will be most satisfying to all involved. The American Academy of Pediatrics provides a four-step framework for shared-decision making (SDM) to increase alignment of parent choice and values while improving medical outcomes for children.

An important variable to consider is the child's comfort. Families differ in the aggressiveness with which they seek interventions. Navigating those choices and supporting families in their decisions is one of the most important roles a provider can play. Care conferences can help provide a sense of team unity and work through difficult decisions. The notion that *not* doing every possible medical intervention should be discussed with families. Families need to be reassured that the patient will be cared for attentively regardless of their decision to pursue or not pursue major medical interventions. Bringing in palliative care specialists to specifically address physical and psychological comfort can be helpful for the family and child and the medical team.

CARE COORDINATION

Medically complex children with SNI and their caretakers need educational and therapeutic services, durable medical equipment, and assistance in care provision, such as home nursing or personal care attendants. The elaborate and endless coordination and uncertainty can be challenging, and the effects of having a child with complex medical needs on families are well-documented.

Hospital discharge requires a great deal of coordination and planning. The wise clinician proactively includes caregivers in discharge planning. Children with complex medical problems take multiple medications, providing opportunities for errors. The assistance of a care coordinator and social work support during hospitalization and discharge can be invaluable to ensure smoother transitions from hospital to home and help assess eligibility and access to essential resources. Children with SNI greatly benefit from the care of an experienced generalist and advocate who can assist in identifying care gaps, synthesizing information, and translating it into an actionable plan.

FAMILIAL EFFECTS

The care of children with SNI rests primarily on the shoulders of their parents and families. Assessing the need for additional psychosocial support for family members must be a routine part of evaluation as inadequate support may lead to challenges with home care, increase the risk for hospital admission, and create barriers to discharge. The impact on families caring for children with medical complexity is well-studied, and the effects can be profound. The cumulative impact of time and travel demands to receive specialty care and the financial strain on caregiver families creates tremendous stress, which has lifelong and serious implications on primary caregiver health, who are mothers most often. Marital relations may be strained. Siblings, too, are affected because they often receive less attention from caregivers than their brother or sister with significant and complex needs.

CONCLUSION

The inpatient care of SNI children can be incredibly challenging but also rewarding. Providing high-quality, coordinated care to a vulnerable population with complex conditions and limited evidence-based guidance creates a unique opportunity for the pediatric hospitalist. A basic framework for understanding common complications can have a profound impact, both short-term, on hospital utilization and medical outcomes, and long-term, on the quality of life for patients and their families.

KEY POINTS

- Children with severe neurologic impairment represent a growing and significant sector of the inpatient population of children's hospitals.
- Although neurologically impaired patients have a broad scope of etiologies for their presentation and are at risk for multiple comorbidities, predictable complications lead to most admissions.
- The provider who understands common comorbidities and complications will find it much easier to care for this population when they require hospitalization.

SUGGESTED READINGS

Baguley IJ, Perkes IE, Fernandez-Ortega JF, Rabinstein AA, Dolce G, Hendricks HT; Consensus Working Group. Paroxysmal sympathetic hyperactivity after acquired brain injury: consensus on conceptual definition, nomenclature, and diagnostic criteria. *J Neurotrauma*. 2014;31(17):1515-1520.

Berman L, Baird R, Sant'Anna A, et al. Gastrostomy tube use in pediatric: a systematic review. *Pediatrics*. 2022;149:e2021055213.

Berry JG, Difazio RL, Melvin P, Glader L, Casto E, Shore BJ. Hospital resource use after hip reconstruction surgery in children with neurological complex chronic conditions. *Dev Med Child Neurol*. 2021;63(2):204-210.

Berry JG, Poduri A, Bonkowsky J, et al. Impact of children with neurological impairment on the U.S. inpatient healthcare system. *PLoS Med*. 2012;9:e1001158.

Blackmore AM, Gibson N, Cooper MS, Langdon K, Moshovis L, Wilson AC. Interventions for the management of respiratory disease in young people with cerebral palsy: a systematic review. *Child Care Health Dev*. 2019;45:1-18.

Cohen E, Kuo D, Agrawal R, et al. Children with medical complexity: an emerging population for clinical and research initiatives. *Pediatrics*. 2011;127:529-538.

CohenE, Horváth-PuhóE, Ray JG, et al. Association between the birth of an infant with major congenital anomalies and subsequent risk of mortality in their mothers. *JAMA*. 2016;316(23):2515-2524.

COVID-19. Clinical Considerations for Special Populations. *Centers for Disease Control*. 2024, June 13. https: www.cdc.gov/covid/hcp/clinical-care/considerations-special-groups.html. Accessed 10/30/2024.

Depositario-Cabacar DF, Zelleke TG. Treatment of epilepsy in children with developmental disabilities. *Dev Disabil Res Rev*. 2010;16(33): 239-247.

Difazio RL, Shore BJ, Melvin P, Mauskar S, Berry JG. Pneumonia after hip surgery in children with neurological complex chronic conditions. *Dev Med Child Neurol*. 2023;65(2):232-242.

Fitzgerald K, Dugre J, Pagala S, Homel P, Marcus M, Kazachkov M. High frequency chest wall compression therapy in neurological impaired children. *Respir Care*. 2014;59:107-112.

Gburek-Augustat J, Krause M, Bernhard M, et al. Unusual mechanical failures of intrathecal baclofen pump systems: symptoms, signs, and trouble shooting. *Childs Nerv Syst*. 2021;37(8):2597-2604.

Gelfand YM, Duncan NO, Albright JT, Roy S, Montagnino B, Edmonds JL. Laryngotracheal separation surgery for intractable aspiration: our experience with 12 patients. *Int J Pediatric Otorhinolaryngology*. 2011;75(73):931-934.

Gitto E, Salvatore A, Russel JR, Barberi I, Pellegrino S. Update on the use of melatonin in pediatrics. *J Pineal Res*. 2011;50:21-28.

Gutierrez GM, Siqueira VL, Loyola-Rodriguez JP, et al. Effects of treatments for drooling on caries risk in children and adolescents with cerebral palsy. *Med Oral Patol Oral Cir Bucal*. 2019;24(2):204-210.

Hauer J, Houtrow A; Section on Hospice and Palliative Medicine, Council on Children with Disabilities. Pain assessment and treatment in children with significant impairment of the central nervous system. *Pediatrics*. 2017;139:e20171002.

Lawrence R, Bateman N. Surgical management of the drooling child. *Curr Otorhinolaryngol Rep*. 2018;6:99-106.

Morse BL, Solodiuk JC, Greco CD, Mauskar S, Hauer J. Initial validation of GRASP: a differential diagnoses algorithm for children with medical complexity and an unknown source of pain. *Hosp Pediatr*. 2020;10(8):633-640.

Novak I, Morgan C, Fahey M, et al. State of the Evidence Traffic Lights 2019: systematic review of interventions for preventing and treating children with cerebral palsy. *Curr Neurol Neurosci Rep*. 2020;20(2):3.

Oliver C, Richards C. Self-injurious behavior in people with intellectual disability. *Curr Opin Psychiatry*. 2010;23(53):412-416.

Opel DJ. A 4-step framework for shared decision-making in pediatrics. *Pediatrics*. 2018;142 (Supplement_3):S149–S156.

Ozel S, Switzer L, Macintosh A, Fehlings D. Informing evidence-based clinical practice guidelines for children with cerebral palsy at risk of osteoporosis: an update. *Dev Med Child Neurol*. 2016;58(9):918-923.

Paff M, Alexandru-Abrams D, Muhonen M, Loudon W. Ventriculoperitoneal shunt complications: A review. Interdisciplinary Neurosurgery. 2018; 13:66-70.

Parr JR, Todhunter E, Pennington L, et al. Drooling reduction intervention randomised trial (DRI): comparing the efficacy and acceptability of hyoscine patches and glycopyrronium liquid on drooling in children with neurodisability. *Arch Dis Child*. 2018;103(4):371-376.

Rabinstein AA, Benarroch EE. Treatment of paroxysmal sympathetic hyperactivity. *Curr Treat Options Neurol*. 2008;10:151-157.

Rappoport A. Sublingual atropine drops for the treatment of pediatric sialorrhea. *J Pain Symptom Manage*. 2010;40(5):783-738.

Stone B, Hester B, Jackson D, et al. Effectiveness of fundoplication or gastrojejunal feeding in children with neurologic impairment. *Hosp Pediatr*. 2017;7:140-148.

Thomson J, Hall M, Ambroggio L, et al. Antibiotics for aspiration pneumonia in neurologically impaired children. *J Hospital Med*. 2020;15:395-402.

Turchi RM, Zekerias B, Bethell C, Pomponio A, Antonelli R, Minkowvitz C. Care coordination for CSHCN: association with family-provider relations and family/child outcomes. *Pediatrics*. 2009;124(S4):S430-434.

CHAPTER 182 Technologic Devices in the Child With Medical Complexity

Michael Weinstein, MD and Jackie K. Chiang, MD, MA, FRCPC

ENTEROSTOMY TUBE FEEDING

If the gastrointestinal tract functions adequately, enteral nutrition is preferable to parenteral nutrition in a child with medical complexity. Enteral feeding is a normative experience for children and caregivers. Compared with parenteral nutrition, enterostomy tubes are easier to handle and less expensive, and several randomized trials have shown that complications (e.g., sepsis, thrombosis, liver dysfunction) are less common. Enteral feeding prevents mucosal atrophy, maintains gut flora, and plays an important role in preserving the enteral immune system. Supplementation can be complete or partial, depending on the child's ability to feed by mouth.

Gastrostomy (G), jejunostomy (J), and gastrojejunostomy (GJ) tubes are often preferred to nasogastric (NG) and nasojejunal (NJ) tubes when the anticipated length of enteral feeding exceeds 8 to 12 weeks.

Tubes through the nose, although simple to place, are not well tolerated in the long term and are cosmetically unappealing. They can lead to increased secretions, nasal ulceration, and sinusitis and predispose to gastroesophageal reflux, esophagitis, strictures, and irritation of the upper airway. They are easily displaced and may result in aspiration.

Concerns about the permanence of the tube, relinquishing of normalcy, loss of autonomy, and loss of the ability to feed orally often make this a difficult decision for caregivers. A series of discussions centered around the family's overall values and preferences and the potential benefits and harms of gastrostomy tube feeding versus long-term nasogastric feeding is essential before an informed decision can be made.

This first part of this chapter outlines the indications for enterostomy tube placement, the different techniques available, and the complications and outcomes reported.

INDICATIONS

There are several reasons to consider the placement of an enteral tube:

- Oral-motor feeding problems, which can result in aspiration of orally ingested food into the lungs or an inability to maintain hydration (especially in children with neurological impairment)
- Failure to thrive as a result of oral-motor feeding problems, malabsorption, or a specific disease process (e.g., congenital heart disease, cystic fibrosis, chronic renal failure, cancer)
- Need for an unpalatable elemental diet (e.g., inflammatory bowel disease, various metabolic diseases, ketogenic diet)
- Persistent feeding aversion
- Decompression ("venting") for functional or mechanical bowel obstruction

On occasion, a J or GJ tube may be more appropriate, for example, in managing severe gastroesophageal reflux disease (GERD) resistant to maximal medical therapy and still symptomatic with NG or G-tube feeding. Anatomic or mechanical issues, such as superior mesenteric artery syndrome or gastroparesis, would be another indication for a GJ or J tube (where the tip of the feeding tube is placed distal to the obstruction). In general, an upper gastrointestinal series is not required preprocedure unless unexplained emesis occurs.

METHOD OF PLACEMENT

There are three well-accepted techniques for the placement of enterostomy tubes in children: Surgical (open or laparoscopic), percutaneous endoscopic gastrostomy (PEG), and percutaneous radiologic gastrostomy (PRG).

Surgical gastrostomy is technically simple and has been performed since the late 1800s. Since the 1990s, an increasing number of these procedures are being performed laparoscopically. PEG, first performed in 1980, is a quick and low-cost method of placing a tube percutaneously under endoscopic guidance by the "pull" or "push" technique, according to the preference of the endoscopist. Percutaneous nonendoscopic or radiologic gastrostomy done under fluoroscopic guidance was first performed in 1981 and does not require endoscopy.

The technique used often depends on what is most readily available in the institution. Studies comparing rates of major complications (perforated viscous, hemorrhage, and need for a second procedure) between techniques are subject to substantial risk of bias. Studies are mainly retrospective and single institutional. A single randomized single institution trial found similar outcomes when comparing PEG and PRG techniques. However, certain conditions may be important to consider. In children with medical complexity avoiding general anesthesia may be of significant benefit, thus arguing against a surgically placed tube. However, patients requiring another surgical procedure, such as fundoplication, are better served through surgical tube placement simultaneously. In patients with portal hypertension and gastric varices, simultaneous endoscopy may be helpful to avoid puncturing a varix and causing bleeding. Unfavorable anatomies, such as previous gastric surgery or interposition of the liver resulting in the absence of a safe access route, are a relative contraindication to the PEG or PRG technique.

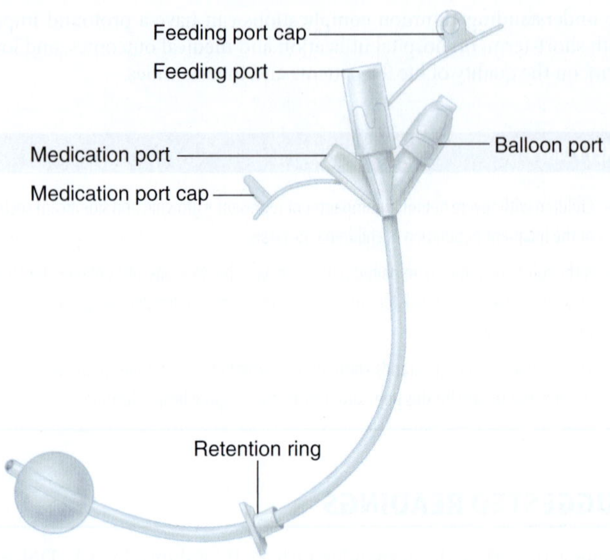

FIGURE 182-1. Typical gastrostomy tube. Note the inflated balloon at the tip, which helps prevent the tube from becoming dislodged.

Many types of G-tubes are available, and no single catheter is appropriate for all patients. Most are secured by a pigtail, balloon, or bulb in the stomach, which helps prevent accidental dislodgement (**Figure 182-1**). After 6 to 12 weeks, the tube can be changed to a low-profile device (e.g., MIC-KEY, Bard button) (**Figure 182-2**). They are more cosmetically appealing, tend to move less, and are more difficult to remove accidentally.

NEED FOR ANTIREFLUX SURGERY

Although G-tubes are often placed because of concern about the risk for direct aspiration with oral feeding, it is also possible to aspirate saliva and refluxed gastric contents. Many children requiring a G-tube (e.g., those with NI) are likely at high risk of having GERD in addition to their oral-motor feeding problems and failure to thrive. The risk of developing or exacerbating pre-existing GERD after G-tube placement is controversial and has been the subject of some studies with differing results. Unless the child's GERD symptoms are very severe despite maximal medical therapy, fundoplication at the time of G-tube insertion is not usually recommended. If severe GERD is present, another option would be to

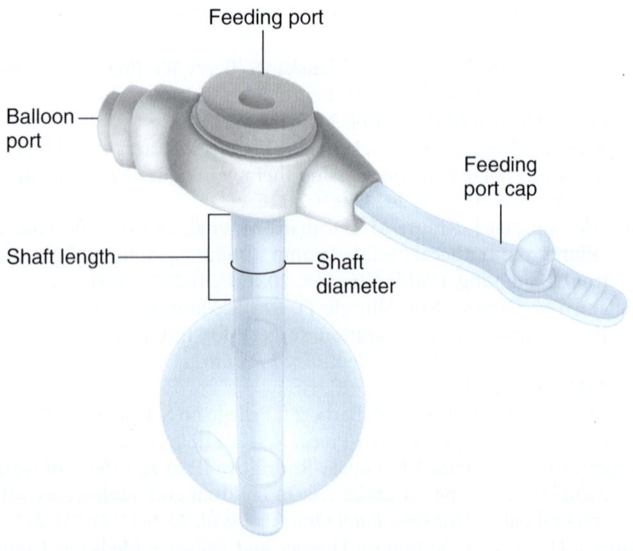

FIGURE 182-2. Typical low-profile gastrostomy tube device.

feed via a GJ or jejunal tube. Observational studies suggest that pulmonary outcomes, particularly aspiration pneumonia, may be comparable between fundoplication and jejunal feeding.

The ability of reflux testing, particularly in relatively asymptomatic patients, to predict the need for conversion to a GJ tube or fundoplication is not well established. Reflux can, of course, be clinically silent, and investigations for GERD are far from perfect. These factors make it difficult to decide what effect tube placement has on the child's reflux, and studies thus far remain inconclusive. Compared with standard commercial formula preparations, preliminary studies suggest that blended feeds administered through a gastrostomy tube may improve gastroesophageal reflux symptoms.

Chapter 181 explores in additional detail feeding issues and dysmotility including decision-making around the use of technology in children with severe neurologic impairment (SNI).

COMPLICATIONS

Complications can be classified as early (within 30 days of the procedure) or late (after 30 days). They may also be divided into major and minor complications. One clinically useful definition would be that major complications require a significant medical or surgical intervention (**Table 182-1**).

Peritonitis may result from leakage into the peritoneal cavity from around the G-tube site or from a dislodged or misplaced tube. Children in whom peritonitis develops after G-tube insertion may present with vomiting, fever, irritability, tachycardia, and progressive peritoneal signs, with progression to sepsis and death if not recognized. Early recognition is especially difficult in younger infants and those with neurologic impairment (NI). If peritonitis is suspected, feeding should be withheld, and an urgent contrast study should be performed through the tube to rule out leakage and confirm tube position. Peritonitis can usually be managed with bowel rest, total parenteral nutrition, empirical antibiotic therapy, and close observation, but surgical intervention is occasionally required. Intussusception of the small bowel is not uncommonly seen with certain types of GJ tubes, especially in young infants and in the presence of a tube with a distal pigtail. This complication should be suspected in patients with a GJ tube presenting with bilious vomiting and feed intolerance. The diagnosis of intussusception can be made by ultrasonography or fluoroscopy, and it is usually managed by changing the tube and/or shortening the tube.

While classified as minor in literature reviews, the most common complications (dislodgement, leak, and granuloma) can lead to considerable caregiver and patient burden (Table 182-1). Dislodged tubes should be replaced as promptly as possible. Caregivers can be taught to place a Foley catheter to keep the stoma open once the tract has matured. Patients can resume feeding through the Foley catheter if this is achieved without difficulty and gastric contents can be aspirated.

Pericatheter leakage can sometimes become a problem. If the leakage results from excessive external tube motion, external fasteners may successfully stabilize the tube. If the stomal site enlargement is due to skin breakdown due to infection, antibiotic therapy and replacement with a GJ tube (to minimize fluid contact at the stomal site) may be helpful.

Tubes can migrate into the duodenum or the esophagus (and in the case of GJ tubes, retrogradely into the stomach) and result in obstruction and vomiting. Migration is generally diagnosed using a contrast study through the tube.

Tube blockage usually results from failing to flush the tube after feeding or administration of medications or from certain medications (i.e., ciprofloxacin suspension) that are notorious for their ability to clog up G and GJ tubes. Flushing the tube with warm water or a carbonated beverage may unblock the tube. Alternatively, the blockage can sometimes be corrected with a guidewire, or the tube will need to be changed. Tubes should be flushed with a minimum of 5 to 20 mL of water after feeding or medications. Medications should be given in liquid format or, if not feasible, finely crushed and completely dissolved in water before administration through the tube.

Infections around the G-tube site can lead to cellulitis and occasionally a subcutaneous abscess. Infection can result in redness, swelling, tenderness, and increased discharge that may be foul-smelling. Children rarely have constitutional symptoms, and the infection usually resolves rapidly with local wound care and topical or oral antibiotics. G-tube site infections are often polymicrobial, but *Staphylococcus aureus* and β-hemolytic streptococci are commonly involved, as is fungal superinfection. It is important to distinguish infection from skin redness and irritation caused by sensitivity to acidic gastric contents. The latter may respond to a nonmedicated barrier cream or benefit from acid-suppressing agents. The skin can also become reddened because of a reaction to the tape used to hold the tube in place. Granulation tissue around the stoma is caused by an overgrowth of dark pink "cauliflower-like" tissue, which bleeds easily but generally responds to repeated applications of silver nitrate.

TABLE 182-1 Potential Complications of Gastrostomy Tubes

Major complications
- Aspiration (as a direct result of the procedure)
- Peritonitis
- Pneumoperitoneum
- Gastrointestinal bleeding
- Severe wound and abdominal wall infection
- Gastrocolonic fistula
- Sepsis
- Death (very rare)

Minor complications
- Tube dislodgement
- Tube leakage
- Tube migration
- Tube blockage
- G-tube site infection
- G-tube site granuloma
- Intussusception (around tip of GJ tube)

OUTCOMES

It is generally assumed that enterostomy feeding is a necessary, safe, and effective intervention in CMC with oral-motor feeding problems. The finding in some earlier cohort studies of a higher death rate and an increase in GERD in children with cerebral palsy (CP) who were fed by gastrostomy is cause for concern. It has been hypothesized that the increased mortality may be due to an increase in pulmonary disease secondary to overly vigorous nutritional maintenance and subsequent aspiration. Unfortunately, no randomized controlled trials of enterostomy tube feeding have been conducted in children with SNI, which raises the question of whether the control group was equally severely disabled before the intervention. This is supported by noting that the association between feeding and death was substantially reduced when other confounding factors were controlled. Most studies investigating the risks and benefits of tube feeding in neurologically impaired children are limited by methodologic weaknesses, thus making it difficult to draw any firm conclusions.

Based on the literature to date, children generally show improved weight gain and improved triceps skinfold thickness after initiation of G-tube feeding. Several case series have suggested that earlier intervention may be associated with greater nutritional benefits. Change in the linear growth rate and effects on bone mineralization and density are less predictable in the population of children with CP.

Caregivers of children with CP generally report an increase in the ease of feeding and a decrease in the time taken up feeding after enterostomy tube placement. They usually see an improvement in the child's disposition and nutrition and often report that they are pleased with the G-tube and the enhancement of the child's comfort and abilities. However, there may not necessarily be improvement in caregiver perception of their child's quality of life despite their improved nutritional status.

RESPIRATORY TECHNOLOGY

OXYGEN

In healthy children 1 year of age and older, median baseline oxygen saturation levels have been identified as 98% (5th percentile is 96%-97%). Hypoxemia is spending 5% of the time with a SpO_2 ≤93% or three independent measures of SpO_2 ≤93%. Chronic hypoxemia may be defined as a low SpO_2 for at least 2 weeks. In children with medical comorbidities, hypoxemia may occur for several reasons and is generally treated to avoid potential complications such as poor sleep quality, growth, development of pulmonary hypertension, and adverse effects on cognition and behavior. Suitability for home oxygen therapy should ideally be evaluated by a specialist with relevant experience, and patients assessed through continuous pulse oximetry for at least 6 to 12 hours, including a period of sleep and feeding. Target oxygen saturation for children with respiratory conditions is typically ≥93%. However, lower oxygen saturations for children with severe neurologic disabilities may be acceptable, particularly when the focus of care is on quality of life.

Home oxygen is commonly supplied through oxygen cylinders or concentrators. Oxygen concentrators are preferred with cylinders as backup devices to avoid the need to continually replace oxygen as concentrators work by filtering room air and removing nitrogen to increase the oxygen concentration that may be delivered to the patient. Oxygen via simple nasal cannulas is considered a low-flow oxygen delivery system. In contrast, high-flow oxygen delivery options include Venturi mask systems and heated high-flow devices, which are more prevalent in hospital settings. For flow rates of ≥4 L/min, humidification of oxygen is recommended.

INDICATIONS

The following are common indications for oxygen therapy in the pediatric population: respiratory infection, chronic lung disease of prematurity, interstitial lung disease, congenital heart disease, pulmonary hypertension, cystic fibrosis, end-stage lung disease, and palliation. In children with conditions that may result in hypoventilation, careful monitoring of carbon dioxide levels is required to ensure hypercapnia is not precipitated or exacerbated by the initiation of oxygen.

CARE CONSIDERATIONS

The use of a home pulse oximeter for long-term monitoring of home oxygen therapy is generally recommended. Such monitoring may help caregivers recognize clinical deterioration or the need for intervention such as suctioning. When facilitating safe discharge home with oxygen, families should be counseled on ensuring appropriate space for the oxygen equipment and adequate electricity. Smoking and open flames in the home should be discouraged, considering oxygen is highly flammable. During travel, portable cylinders must be securely attached to strollers or wheelchairs. It is also important to recognize that during air travel, patients will likely require higher oxygen concentrations as commercial flights generally pressurize cabins to altitudes of 8000 feet, which results in partial pressure of oxygen equivalent to inspiring 15% oxygen rather than 21% oxygen typically found at sea level.

POSITIVE AIRWAY PRESSURE

Children with medical complexity are at higher risk of sleep-disordered breathing due to the impact of their underlying medical conditions on the craniofacial anatomy, central nervous system, and neuromuscular tone. The use of noninvasive positive airway pressure (PAP) has significantly increased in the pediatric population over the span of a decade, related to advances in medical therapies and technology that have increased the life expectancy of children with medical complexity as well as greater awareness of children at high risk of sleep-disordered breathing. The two forms of PAP therapy are continuous positive airway pressure (CPAP), which provides a uniform level of pressure to prevent airway obstruction, and Bilevel positive airway pressure (BPAP), which cycles pressure from a lower expiratory positive airway pressure (EPAP) to a higher inspiratory positive airway pressure (IPAP). Noninvasive PAP therapy may be delivered via nasal, oronasal, or total face mask interfaces and with nasal pillows, which are inserted into the nares.

INDICATIONS AND CONTRAINDICATIONS

While CPAP is primarily indicated for obstructive sleep apnea (episodes of complete or partial airway obstruction), BPAP may be required when CPAP inadequately controls upper airway obstruction or is not tolerated, for severe central sleep apnea (absence of central respiratory drive resulting in pauses in respiratory effort), or nocturnal hypoventilation that is defined as a carbon dioxide recording >50 mm Hg for ≥25% of total sleep time. The latter mode of PAP is considered a form of ventilation as it supports respiratory effort to maintain adequate oxygenation and carbon dioxide clearance.

Although obstructive sleep apnea is the most common type of sleep-disordered breathing in typically developing children, all forms of sleep-disordered breathing may occur in children with medical complexity. Sleep-disordered breathing has been identified to be more prevalent in subsets of patients with medical complexity, such as children with Down syndrome, cerebral palsy, neuromuscular disease, and spina bifida. A formal polysomnogram is considered the gold standard for diagnosing and assessing the severity of sleep-disordered breathing. However, not all children identified with significant sleep-disordered breathing are suitable candidates for PAP therapy. The following are potential contraindications to therapy: hemodynamic instability, facial trauma or burns, recent upper airway surgery, pneumothorax, absent gag reflex/inability to protect own airway, significant sialorrhea/gastroesophageal reflux with high aspiration risk, and individuals requiring ≥16 hours of respiratory support per day.

CARE CONSIDERATIONS

There are no well-established criteria to measure PAP adherence in children; however, limited pediatric data suggest that adherence to therapy is suboptimal, with average usage in some studies reported to be only 3 to 4 hours per night. Higher rates of PAP usage have been noted when patients are initiated in dedicated pediatric noninvasive PAP units and when support and close follow-up is available for patients and caregivers. Caregivers should receive formalized education on the use of PAP and a detailed emergency plan (e.g., what to do in the event of a prolonged power failure and who to contact when issues arise with their device) before discharge.

Furthermore, assessment of appropriate mask fit before discharge is essential to avoid excessive air leak around the mask, which can adversely affect therapy efficacy and compliance due to discomfort and resulting side effects or complications listed below. At least half of PAP failure rates are attributable to suboptimal interface fit and/or discomfort.

COMPLICATIONS

- Skin irritation and breakdown
- Eye dryness
- Nasal mucosal irritation/epistaxis
- Pneumothorax
- Gastric insufflation/emesis and aspiration
- Midface hypoplasia

TRACHEOSTOMY

A tracheostomy is an artificial airway that consists of a tracheal tube surgically placed in the airway. The first pediatric report dates from 1808, with most subsequent uses of tracheostomy being in the setting of acute infections such as diphtheria. In the early twentieth century, tracheostomy was utilized to manage chronic respiratory failure due to polio. While the use of tracheostomy for managing respiratory complications due to acute infection has declined due to immunization and other advances, the last few decades have seen an increase in the utilization of tracheostomies to manage chronic respiratory failure, usually from underlying neurological conditions.

INDICATIONS

Children may require tracheostomy tubes for several reasons, including bypassing significant upper airway obstruction, pulmonary hygiene, or facilitating long-term mechanical ventilation. Obstruction may occur above, at, or below the level of the glottis or vocal cords. Obstruction above the level of the glottis may result from various craniofacial abnormalities (e.g., Treacher-Collins syndrome). Vocal cord palsy can obstruct the level of the glottis and may be congenital or acquired. Subglottic stenosis often results from prolonged intubation in the neonatal period, particularly in extremely premature infants. While infants and children are felt to tolerate longer periods of intubation than adults, tracheostomy is considered when it is thought that prolonged endotracheal intubation may interfere with normal development (feeding, expressive communication) and lead to progressive laryngotracheal trauma. A tracheostomy does not prevent acute infection and lung damage from aspiration; however, it does assist with suctioning and subsequent clearance of secretions. Furthermore, if prolonged invasive ventilation is desired, tracheostomy facilitates the care of children outside of an institutional setting.

COMPLICATIONS

Compared to adults with tracheostomy tubes, children have been reported to have higher rates of complications. The potential complications that may result from a tracheostomy can be categorized into intraoperative, early, and late complications. These are outlined in **Table 182-2**.

CARE CONSIDERATIONS

The use of tracheostomy care protocols and a multidisciplinary approach for individuals with tracheostomies has led to reduced morbidity and mortality for this complex population of patients. An alert, awake, fully trained caregiver is recommended to be always with the child with a tracheostomy. Thus, caregiver education is essential, and competency assessment in tracheostomy care procedures should be evaluated before discharge from the hospital. In addition, preparation of the home environment and coordination of home care services, such as home nursing, are also deemed important.

Although there is no consensus on how frequently to change pediatric tracheostomy tubes, infants and younger children with smaller diameter tubes are often changed weekly as they can be more prone to blockage from secretions or mucous. External humidification is recommended to reduce the risk of tube obstruction and ensure proper function of the lower respiratory tract. Passive humidification is provided via a heat-and-moisture-exchanger (HME) attached to the tracheostomy tube's proximal end. Active humidification can be provided as a high-output compressor, heated high-flow device, or ventilator. **Table 182-3** highlights the commonly encountered problems and actions for managing frequently observed tracheostomy-related concerns.

TABLE 182-2 Complications of a Tracheostomy

Intraoperative	Early Postoperative	Late
Loss of airway control	Stomal breakdown	Stomal or suprastomal granuloma
Bleeding	Neck skin erosion	Tube occlusion
Pneumothorax	Subcutaneous emphysema	Tracheal stenosis
Pneumomediastinum	Pneumothorax	Tracheoinnominate artery fistula/hemorrhage
Esophageal injury	Infection	Tracheomalacia
Damage to the recurrent laryngeal nerve	Accidental decannulation	Tracheitis or bacterial colonization
Death	Creation of a false passage	Accidental decannulation

TABLE 182-3 Troubleshooting Tracheostomy Problems

Problems	Potential Causes	Actions
Thicker secretions	Inadequate humidity	Increase humidity output from air/02 source Increase frequency of use of high humidity source
Change in color, consistency, or malodorous secretions	Infection	Send lower airway secretions for culture Consider antibiotic treatment if required
Blood-tinged secretions	Mucosal irritation from suctioning Granulation tissue Infection	Avoid suction pressure >100 mm Hg Ensure appropriate premeasured depth of suctioning with suction catheter Increase humidity as needed Consider antibiotic treatment if required Otolaryngology evaluation if persistent
Frank bleeding from tracheostomy site	Granuloma Vessel hemorrhage	Identify source of bleeding Apply pressure to site (inflate cuff of tracheostomy tube if available) Emergent otolaryngology involvement
Increasingly audible breathing	Increased secretions/obstruction	Clear secretions by suctioning If problem does not resolve, consider tracheostomy change
Shortness of breath during or post-suctioning	Prolonged suctioning	Limit suctioning to 5-10 seconds
Labored breathing	Possible tube occlusion Accidental decannulation	Suction Change or reinsert tracheostomy tube
Unable to pass suction catheter through tracheostomy tube	Suction catheter too large Secretions blocking tracheostomy tube	Try smaller suctioning catheter If inner cannula present, remove and clean otherwise perform tracheostomy change
Skin breakdown	Entrapment of moisture or irritation from tracheostomy ties	Use of barrier protection (e.g., gauze, duoderm) Treat potential skin infection

EMERGENT REPLACEMENT OF A TRACHEOSTOMY TUBE

While parents or home care nurses often replace tracheostomy tubes in the community regularly, hospital-based healthcare providers infrequently perform this procedure. When patients with tracheostomies are hospitalized, and the procedure is indicated, it is often carried out under urgent circumstances. Practitioners should acquire the skills to facilitate efficient replacement.

The two primary indications for an urgent replacement of tracheostomy tubes in pediatric patients are dislodged or obstructed tubes. If a tube accidentally dislodges, a replacement tube must be inserted immediately. Respiratory distress caused by clogging from thickened secretions sometimes develops in a child with a tracheostomy tube. If suctioning fails to clear the blockage, the tracheostomy tube must be rapidly removed and a new tube is inserted by a trained practitioner. If a tracheostomy tube dislodges or becomes obstructed, there are no absolute contraindications to replacement. However, extreme caution must be exercised when replacing a tracheal tube in a patient who has a fresh tracheostomy.

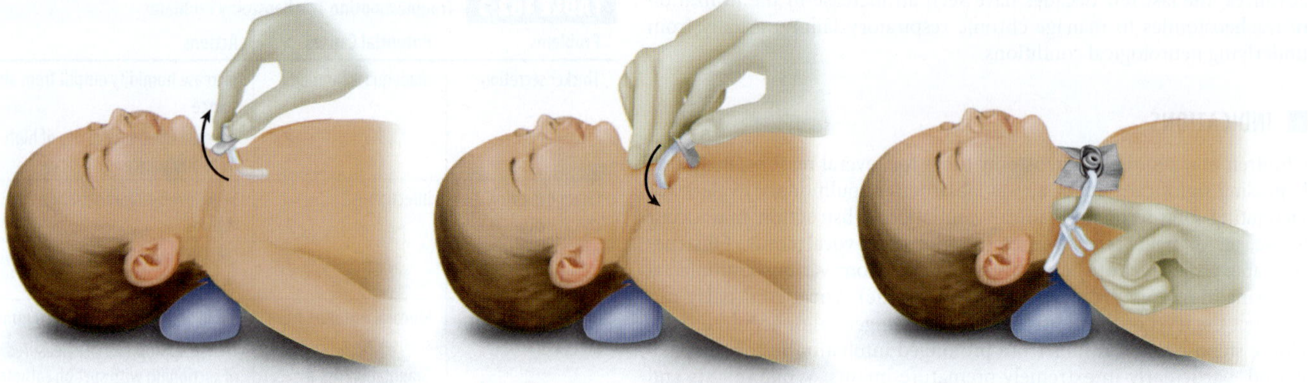

FIGURE 182-3. Tracheostomy tube and placement.

Patients should always have an emergency tracheostomy kit with them, including in the hospital, which includes a tracheostomy tube of the same size (with obturator in situ), a size smaller than the tracheostomy tube, lubricant, normal saline, tracheostomy gauze, scissors, and a manual suction device. Standard airway equipment should also be readily available in the hospital: laryngoscope and blade, endotracheal tube, suction equipment, oxygen, and bag-valve-mask device. All tracheostomy tubes have a 15-mm "universal" adaptor to allow bag ventilation in an emergency.

The equipment should be checked at the start of the procedure. The patient should be placed in a supine position with a towel roll under the shoulders (if needed) to allow extension of the head and neck. This permits the best access to the tracheostomy site. If not already present, vital sign monitoring should be established, particularly pulse oximetry. Before beginning the procedure, the patient may be preoxygenated with supplemental oxygen administered via the nose, mouth, or tracheal stoma. The airway and stoma should be suctioned to enable better visualization at the start of the procedure.

First, the original tracheostomy tube should be removed. This is accomplished by cutting sutures and ties, or undoing velcro while stabilizing the tube. If the indwelling tracheostomy tube is cuffed, an empty syringe should deflate the balloon. The old tracheostomy tube may then be removed. At this time, the new tube is ready to be inserted. The technique involves posterior and caudal insertion in one swift movement. It should be done gently to avoid trauma. The obturator is removed immediately, and the tracheostomy is secured with tracheostomy ties (**Figure 182-3**). Breath sounds should be evaluated.

If the stoma is constricted, it may be difficult to pass the tracheal tube, and resistance may be encountered. To avoid the creation of a false tract, one should not force the tracheostomy tube into the stoma. Instead, the insertion of a smaller tracheostomy tube should be attempted to allow oxygenation and ventilation. If this fails, insertion of an endotracheal tube or suction catheter into the stoma may be considered while seeking additional assistance. If successful recannulation is not possible, it may be necessary to provide bag-valve-mask ventilation via the mouth and nose while covering the stoma with a gloved finger while again seeking additional assistance.

SUGGESTED READINGS

Ahmedzai S, Balfour-Lynn IM, Bewick T, et al. Managing passengers with stable respiratory disease planning air travel: British Thoracic Society recommendations. *Thorax*. 2011;66:i1-i30.

American Academy of Sleep Medicine. *The International Classification of Sleep Disorders. Diagnostic and Coding Manual, ICSD-2*. 2nd ed. American Academy of Sleep Medicine; Darien, IL, USA, 2005.

American Thoracic Society. Care of the child with a chronic tracheostomy. *Am J Resp Crit Care Med*. 2000;161:297-308.

Amin R, MacLusky I, Zielinski D, et al. Pediatric home mechanical ventilation: A Canadian Thoracic Society clinical practice guideline executive summary. *Can J Resp Crit Care Sleep Med*. 2017;1(1):7-36.

Balfour-Lynn IM, Field DJ, Gringras P, et al. BTS guidelines for home oxygen in children. *Thorax*. 2009;64:ii1-26.

Chiang J, Amin R. Respiratory care considerations for children with medical complexity. *Children*. 2017;4(5):E41.

Deutsch, E. Tracheostomy: pediatric considerations. *Respir Care*. 2010;55(8):1082-1090.

Friedman JN, Ahmed S, Connolly B, et al. Complications associated with image-guided gastrostomy and gastrojejunostomy tubes in children. *Pediatrics*. 2004;114:458-446.

Hayes D, Wilson KC, Krivchenia K, et al. Home oxygen therapy for children: An official American Thoracic Society Clinical Practice Guideline. *Am J Resp Crit Care Med*. 2019;199(3):e5-23.

Mitchell RB, Hussey HM, Setzen G, et al. Clinical consensus statement: tracheostomy care. *Otolaryngol-Head Neck Surg*. 2012;148(1):6-20.

Parmar A, Baker A, Narang I. Positive airway pressure in pediatric obstructive sleep apnea. *Paediatr Resp Rev*. 2019;31:43-51.

Volsko TA, Parker SW, Deakins K, et al. AARC clinical practice guideline: management of pediatric patients with tracheostomy in the acute care setting. *Respiratory Care*. 2021;66(1):144-155.

White AC, Kher S, O'Connor HH. When to change a tracheostomy tube. *Respiratory Care*. 2010;55(8):1069-1075.

Wollman BS, Horacio BD, Walus-Wigle J, et al. Radiologic, endoscopic and surgical gastrostomy: an institutional evaluation and meta-analysis of the literature. *Radiology*. 1995;197:699-704.

CHAPTER 183

Palliative Care

Grace Slater, MD and Tammy I. Kang, MD, MSCE, FAAHPM

BACKGROUND

Palliative care seeks to optimize the quality of life for patients with serious illnesses through an interdisciplinary model of care. Palliative care services were once only considered appropriate for imminently dying children but are now recognized as vital to the care of those with complex, potentially life-threatening conditions, regardless of illness trajectory or prognostic certainty. Palliative care practice includes identifying and minimizing physical, emotional, and spiritual distress, supporting patients and families in establishing goals of care, and navigating complex medical decision-making to best align medical treatments with patient and family hopes and values. Despite progress in integrating palliative care into the care of patients with serious illness, the prevailing medical model continues to present palliative care as a mutually

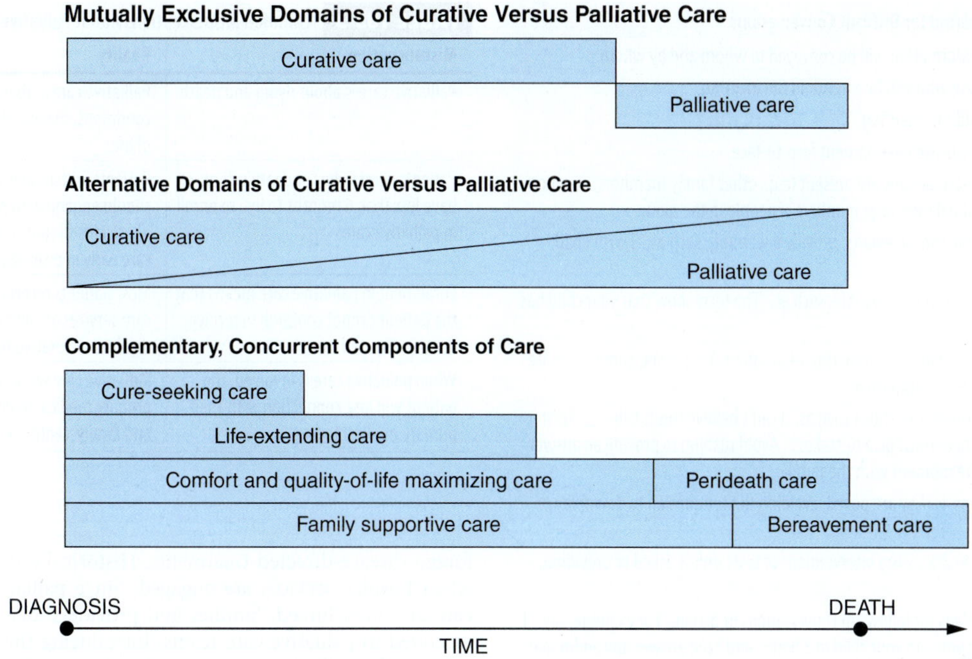

FIGURE 183-1. Palliative care as a complement to disease-directed care.

exclusive alternative to curative care. Best practice guidelines recommend that patients receiving care that seeks to cure disease or extend life should also receive complementary care that seeks to minimize bothersome symptoms and maximize the quality of life (**Figure 183-1**). Healthcare systems that care for medically complex children, adolescents, and young adults should provide excellent pediatric palliative care through access to subspecialty palliative care services and primary palliative care education and training for providers engaged in the care of seriously ill patients. Although access to specialty palliative care has become the standard of care in many hospitals, few eligible pediatric patients receive these services. Most hospitals caring for children have a pediatric palliative care program though the staffing and scope of programs vary widely. Additionally, there is often a lack of clarity as to which patients warrant subspecialty palliative care services versus those who are well served by a care team with training in domains of palliative care. This chapter addresses core challenges in providing palliative care and, to the extent possible, provides evidence-based and practical strategies for addressing these challenges.

IDENTIFYING PATIENTS WITH PALLIATIVE CARE NEEDS

Determining (1) which patients and families might benefit from palliative care and (2) when referral is appropriate can be challenging due in part to the varied clinical situations that occur in children with serious illnesses. Over 55,000 children die each year in the United States with several trajectories of dying, including:

1. Children who die suddenly, before any diagnosis is made (e.g., due to trauma or conditions such as sudden infant death syndrome or occult cardiac arrhythmias). These families warrant bereavement care.
2. Children whose conditions are inevitably fatal. This group can be subdivided into the following groups:
   a. Patients who will inevitably die relatively quickly after diagnosis (e.g., nonviable prematurity, inoperable brain tumor). All of these patients warrant palliative care immediately.
   b. Patients who will inevitably die, but years to decades after diagnosis (e.g., many neurodegenerative disorders). These patients warrant palliative care, but when to institute such care is variable. Along with life-extending care, complementary palliative care and advanced-care planning should be initiated at the time of diagnosis. Appropriately trained primary interdisciplinary teams could perform these palliative care domains.
3. Children who have conditions that make them extremely frail and vulnerable (e.g., severe spastic quadriplegia with swallowing dysfunction and risk of aspiration pneumonia; cancer that requires debilitating chemotherapy; sepsis that makes the child critically ill; some complex congenital heart diseases). Because of their fragile health, such children have an increased risk of dying on any given day; however, the risk is still low enough that although death is likely at some point, it is not inevitable in the next year or even the next decade. For these patients, complementary palliative care and advanced-care planning are warranted as early as possible, with a transition toward a more exclusive focus on palliative care if the condition progresses to the point where the benefits of life-extending care are outweighed by the suffering such care imposes.

COMMUNICATION AS A CORE COMPETENCY: DELIVERING DIFFICULT NEWS

Delivering difficult news to families is one of clinical medicine's most demanding and difficult communication tasks. Dividing the task into two major components—(1) what the patient and family are up against, and what can and will be done—and (2) having a distinct plan for each aspect of the conversation can be helpful. These will likely be multiple conversations that occur over time.

The first component focuses on delivering the difficult news itself, which may be a new diagnosis or the latest setback in a long series of illnesses and deteriorating health. This news threatens patients' and parents' goals, plans, and hopes, and the resulting emotions can make even the most seasoned clinician feel overwhelmed and desperate. It is, therefore, essential to prepare for the conversations (**Table 183-1**).

The second component of palliative conversations focuses on possible therapeutic actions and deciding which ones to pursue. Moving to this part of the conversation is often rushed by providers in an effort to reassure families that something can be done for their child. Instead, giving the family time to process the initial news is advisable. In urgent

TABLE 183-1 Preparing for Difficult Conversations

- A precise plan of what information will be conveyed to whom and by whom.
- Share this plan with those who will be attending the meeting.
- Allow ample time to hold this meeting.
- Hold the discussion in a private environment face-to-face.
- Ensure appropriate support persons are present (e.g., other family members, nursing staff, social workers) but balance large numbers of people in the room.
- After briefly reviewing the clinical events, provide a warning, such as, "I wish I had better news."
- State the information as simply as possible, such as, "The tests show that your child has cancer."
- STOP talking and let the family assimilate this information. Your quiet, compassionate presence will be perceived as supportive.
- Families often pose rhetorical questions such as, "I can't believe this is true.... He/she was doing so well.... There must be a mistake... Avoid rushing to provide an answer to these; rather, sit in the moment with the family.
- Answer specific questions as they are posed, avoiding the temptation to downplay or sugar-coat the news.
- Avoid pushing forward to discussing interventions or tests unless asked or providing false reassurances.
- Propose some specific plans for follow-up conversations or actions. For example, say, "I will be back to check on you and your child in 2 hours, and I can answer any additional questions that may have occurred to you and start to discuss plans at that point."

situations, this is not possible, but in most cases, this part of the conversation can wait until the family has had time to understand the situation's implications. The objective of this next conversation is to help formulate new goals, plans, and hopes considering the constraints imposed by the diagnosis and potential therapeutic options. Instead of focusing on dying and death per se, this conversation focuses on what the therapeutic alliance among the patient, family, and care team can strive to accomplish, even if death is likely to occur soon. For patients for whom cure is not possible, a useful way to proceed is along the following lines: "Learning that your child has an incurable condition that will shorten her [or his] life has been incredibly upsetting and difficult. Given the problems that the condition creates, I am wondering how we can best care for your child. What are your major hopes for her?" At this juncture, family members often both mourn the loss of hope for a normal life and mention the desire to keep pain or other forms of suffering to a minimum or quality-of-life goals, including social or spiritual concerns. These hopes provide the basic goals of all subsequent palliative and end-of-life care plans and are the compass by which the rest of clinical care is oriented. For patients where therapeutic interventions are possible and desired, it can be helpful to engage in steps to outline how to proceed if the intervention does not achieve the hoped-for goals (**Table 183-2**).

INTRODUCING PALLIATIVE CARE: DISPELLING THE MYTH THAT PALLIATIVE CARE MEANS GIVING UP

One of the most challenging aspects of providing palliative care to children and families has been overcoming the stigma that palliative care entails giving up; that to receive palliative care services, parents must forego disease-directed treatments. Historically this has been the case when hospice services are engaged. Since palliative care and hospice care are often linked, families and providers' bias toward hospice has extended to palliative care teams. Introducing the topic of involving a subspecialty palliative care team to families can therefore be challenging. It is important to dispel common misconceptions about palliative care (**Table 183-3**) and introduce palliative care using some of the following language:

- Palliative care is an added layer of support for patients and families facing challenging medical issues. We engage palliative care alongside other medical treatments.
- They work in conjunction with the primary teams to help in a variety of areas, including managing symptoms that come with serious illness or treatments, providing additional emotional and spiritual support, and working to ensure the care teams are communicating with you in the ways that are the most helpful to you.

TABLE 183-2 Discussing Possible Interventions

- Clarify with the family the goals of the intervention.
- Work with other medical teams to identify the likelihood that the intervention will achieve the desired goals.
- Understand the potential benefits and harms of the intervention.
- Engage in defining a time in which the intervention would likely show benefit.
- Most importantly, open the conversation to a plan if the desired benefits do not occur in the time period expected.

TABLE 183-3 Common Misperceptions About Palliative Care

Misconception	Reality
Palliative care is about dying and death.	Palliative care is about living with serious conditions, making the most of one's quality of life.
Patients need to be "at death's door" or have less than 6 months to live to enroll in palliative care.	Patients with longer life expectancies can and should engage with palliative care teams and physicians should consider referral to palliative care early in disease trajectory.
Enrollment in palliative care means that the patient cannot continue to receive disease-directed care.	Most patients receiving pediatric palliative care services are also receiving disease-directed or curative treatments
When palliative care is involved, the patient will lose connection with their primary medical teams.	Palliative care works in conjunction with primary medical teams in providing patient and family-centered care.

PATIENTS WITH MEDICAL COMPLEXITY

Pediatric patient care has become more complex, and an increasing proportion of hospitalizations are attributable to pediatric patients with complex chronic conditions (CCC). Many of these patients receive palliative care consults to help with symptom management, quality-of-life issues, longitudinal goals of care discussions, patient/family anticipatory grief support for patients with life-limiting illnesses, or end-of-life care. Despite the overlap of palliative care and the care for pediatric patients with CCC, these patients still require robust, dedicated primary and specialty care services and care coordination. Palliative care can be an essential adjunct to the treatment team; however, the patients require ongoing care coordination that is sometimes out of the scope and staffing abilities of a palliative care team. Many hospitals have developed specialized pediatric medical teams to help manage and coordinate care for this population.

CHILDREN WITH SEVERE NEUROLOGIC IMPAIRMENT

Palliative care is often involved in the treatment of children with severe neurologic impairment (SNI) due to their medical complexity, complex symptoms, and life-limiting diagnosis. This population has an increased risk for developing acute and chronic physical pain that is difficult to recognize and adequately treat given the complexity of identifying a source. Common triggers are often associated with underlying medical complexity and require thorough evaluation. Symptoms of pain are often dystonia and dysautonomia which in turn can also be triggers of each other. Pharmacologic management of these symptoms can be considered while thorough evaluation for common triggers is being completed. This is an evolving field that is best served with a collaborative team of Physical Medicine and Rehabilitation, Neurology, and Palliative care.

SYMPTOM MANAGEMENT

Children with serious or life-limiting illnesses often suffer with symptoms that severely decrease their quality of life. A brief overview of pharmacologic and nonpharmacologic management of common palliative physical symptoms is shown in **Table 183-4** and special considerations are discussed in the following sections. The experience of pain and other symptoms is well represented by the concept of "Total Pain" shown in **Figure 183-2**; this framework recognizes that a child's experience of pain is altered by the context of social, emotional/psychological, spiritual, and physical

TABLE 183-4 Pharmacologic and Nonpharmacologic Management for Common Palliative Care Symptoms

Nonpharmacologic Interventions	Pharmacologic Interventions	Comments
	Symptom Management	
	Nausea and Vomiting	
Optimize bowel regimen, small frequent meals, surgical intervention (G-tube for decompression, etc.), acupuncture, acupressure bands, aromatherapy	Target serotonin receptors: ondansetron, granisetron, palonosetron	Serotonergic medications can cause constipation in some patients.
	Target histamine H1 receptors: Benadryl, hydroxyzine, dramamine, meclizine	
	Target acetylcholine receptors: scopolamine	
	Target dopamine receptors: olanzapine, haldol, metoclopramide, prochlorperazine	Metoclopramide and haldol second-line treatments due to risk of extrapyramidal symptoms.
	Other: aprepitant, marinol, benzodiazepines, IV fluids, steroids	
	Anorexia—disease Related	
High-calorie foods, small frequent meals, avoid nagging/punishment, offer favorite foods, provide praise	Cyproheptadine, dronabinol, olanzapine, mirtazapine, steroids	
	Fatigue	
Energy-conservation therapies, scheduled activity, improved sleep hygiene, exercise therapy, optimize nutrition, pain control	Promote wakefulness with psychostimulants: methylphenidate, dextroamphetamine, amantadine, corticosteroids	
	Improve sleep: melatonin	
	Pain	
	Nociceptive	
Heat, ice, massage, acupuncture, acupressure, transcutaneous electrical nerve stimulation (TENS), biofeedback, mindfulness, physical therapy, music/art therapy	Topical: lidocaine patch, diclofenac	Medications should be selected based on best route of administration and need for long/short-acting coverage. If an opioid is needed it is often helpful to optimize regimen with nonopioid adjuvants.
	Nonopioids: acetaminophen, non-steroidal anti-inflammatory drugs, ketorolac, ketamine	
	Opioids: tramadol, oxycodone, morphine, hydromorphone, fentanyl, methadone	
	Neuropathic	
Same as nociceptive pain above	Gabapentin, pregabalin, serotonin-norepinephrine reuptake inhibitors, tricyclic antidepressants	Gabapentin and SNRIs are generally preferred in children given anticholinergic effects and risk of prolonged QTc with tricyclic antidepressants
	Pain Special Cases	
Radiation	Metastatic bone pain: steroids, bisphosphonates	
Surgical intervention	Spinal cord compression, increased intracranial pressure, bowel obstruction	
	Hepatic capsular distention: steroids	
	Dyspnea	
Positioning, fan, cooler room temperatures, oxygen therapy, treat underlying pathology	Opioids, benzodiazepines	Anxiety is a common comorbid symptom in patients with dyspnea; prompt evaluation and treatment are crucial.
	Terminal Secretions	
Repositioning, avoiding aggressive suctioning	Atropine, scopolamine, glycopyrrolate	Glycopyrrolate does not cross the blood-brain barrier reducing risk of systemic anticholinergic symptoms.
	Neurologic Issues	
	Seizures at end of life	
Discontinuing medications that lower seizure threshold, minimizing exposure to noxious stimuli	Lorazepam, midazolam, diazepam, levetiracetam, oxcarbazepine	Medications to terminate breakthrough seizures should be provided in addition to scheduled medications for patients who experience seizures at end of life.
	Dysautonomia	
Evaluation and treatment for pain triggers (i.e., feeding intolerance, fractures, pancreatitis, etc.)	Clonidine, gabapentin, propranolol	For difficult cases, collaboration with Neurology and/or Physical Medicine and Rehabilitation can be helpful.
	Dystonia & Spasticity	
Positioning, stretching, massage, splinting, orthoses, surgical interventions	Baclofen, botulinum toxin (botox), diazepam, clonidine, tizanidine, trihexyphenidyl	Recommend collaboration with Neurology and Physical Medicine and Rehab

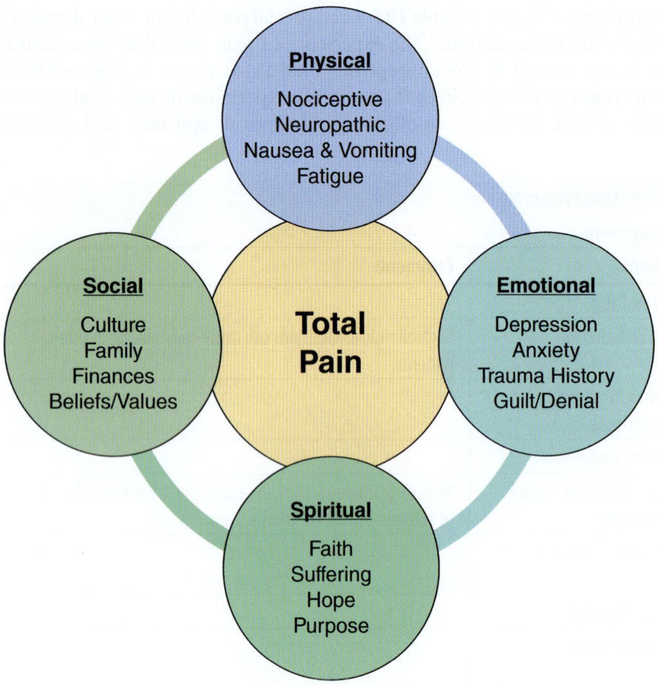

FIGURE 183-2. Concept of total pain encompasses the physical, social, emotional, and spiritual aspects of the child's experience.

environment. Failure to acknowledge and attend to any of the domains can make treatment of physical symptoms extremely challenging. Total pain is managed most effectively within a holistic framework that extends well beyond pharmacotherapy to a multidisciplinary team including therapists (i.e., psychology, occupational therapy, physical therapy, Massage), spiritual care, and social work.

PAIN

Most children experience pain at some point during their illness. Two of the essential components of good palliative care are to assess pain frequently and treat it aggressively. Pain is a subjective symptom that is physically and emotionally distressing for both the patient and caregivers. The type of pain may be nociceptive (somatic, visceral) or neuropathic and may be the result of a combination of disease-related, treatment-related, and psychological causes.

Evaluation of pain should begin with a detailed assessment of pain, including location, duration, and character. Additionally, assessment of the patient's ability to take oral medications and the family's reaction to the use of pain medications should also be considered.

Treatments should include a multidisciplinary team to address all the aspects of total pain including psychological, spiritual, and social influences as difficulties in these areas have been shown to amplify physical pain. Treatment must consider the developmental level of the child, stage of illness, living environment (home, hospital, or healthcare facility), and goals of care.

Pharmacologic treatment of nociceptive pain should begin with mild nonopioid and topical analgesics, based on the patient's response escalation to joint treatment with opioids. When opioids are initiated, patients should also be started on a bowel regimen to avoid constipation; bowel regimen should be titrated to achieve soft stools daily. Neuropathic pain treatment should also include topical and nonopioid agents in addition to medications focused on neuropathic etiologies as shown in Table 183-4.

Many parents are afraid to permit treatment with opioids owing to the widespread negative cultural perception of opiates as drugs of abuse. Education and reassurance of safety of properly prescribed opioids as well as a discussion of the risks and benefits should be completed prior to prescribing treatment. In the terminal phase of illness, there is no maximum dose for pain and symptom management and medications should be titrated appropriately with the goal of comfort.

There are specific special cases of pain encountered in palliative care that benefit from radiation or surgical intervention to relieve pain (spinal cord compression, increased intracranial pressure [ICP], bowel obstruction, metastatic bone lesions). In many of these cases, steroids are also helpful in treating pain associated with increased inflammation.

NAUSEA AND VOMITING

Many children experience nausea and vomiting for a variety of reasons, including chemotherapy, other drugs, metabolic disturbances, central nervous system tumors, vestibular or middle ear pathology, gastrointestinal pathology, and anxiety or other conditioned responses. Vomiting is triggered by a neuron cluster in the medulla called the vomiting center. The vomiting center receives input from the cerebral cortex, sensory organs, and vestibular apparatus in addition to indirect stimulation from the chemoreceptor trigger zone. The primary neurotransmitter receptors that are active in the chemoreceptor trigger zone are acetylcholine, dopamine, histamine H1, and serotonin. Initial therapy should target the receptors relevant to the primary cause of the nausea or vomiting. Medications should be titrated to a maximal dose, and if ineffective, additional agents that target different receptors should be added to gain therapeutic control. Often, symptom relief can be achieved only with multiple agents. Pharmacologic interventions can be augmented with the use of nonpharmacologic implements such as aromatherapy and acupressure.

ANOREXIA

Loss of appetite is common and often results from other symptoms, such as changes in taste, nausea, vomiting, constipation, pain, depression, gastritis, and weakness. It is important to assess and treat any underlying causes. As with nausea and vomiting, nonpharmacologic measures may be helpful, including giving small, frequent meals, removing unpleasant odors, and providing a relaxing atmosphere for meals. Many of the pharmacologic therapies have significant adverse effects (e.g., anxiety, dizziness, hypertension, hyperglycemia, adrenal insufficiency, fatigue, sedation, prolonged QTc) that can limit their usage. When able medications to increase appetite should be selected to also target concurrent symptoms (Steroids can also treat fatigue; olanzapine and mirtazapine have antidepressant properties). As end-of-life approaches anorexia is a natural part of the disease process; this can be very hard for families that view feeding their child as a form of showing love. During this time clinicians should guide families with education about the body's decreased calorie requirement at the end of life and help families identify nonfood methods of expressing love including gentle massage, reading aloud, and sharing stories.

FATIGUE

Fatigue is one of the most prevalent symptoms in children at the end of life. It can be associated with the disease process in addition to other underlying factors like depression/anxiety, pain, poor nutrition, medications, infection, or dehydration. Diagnosis is based on subjective reports by the patient or parent and assessment should include comprehensive screening for concurrent causes of fatigue. Treatment begins by addressing any possible underlying causes and maximizing the patient's rest with environmental changes (energy-conservation therapies, improved sleep hygiene) and sleep-promoting agents. Using psychostimulants to increase wakefulness can also be beneficial and should be selected based on synergistic treatment of comorbid conditions. Some medications (steroids, certain selective serotonin reuptake inhibitors and selective norepinephrine reuptake inhibitors) can have activating effects on patients, it is helpful to improve wakefulness and sleep by scheduling activating medications in the morning.

DYSPNEA

The sensation of breathlessness commonly occurs in conditions with respiratory insufficiency. Patients experiencing dyspnea typically breathe in a shallow, rapid pattern as they struggle with musculoskeletal or pleuritic pain, respiratory muscle weakness, poorly compliant lung tissue, and lung lesions that compromise the airway, fill airspaces, or occupy space in the chest cavity. Dyspnea treatment should prioritize correcting the underlying cause. The discomfort associated with hypoxemia can be ameliorated by administering supplemental oxygen. Fatigued respiratory muscles can often be supported using noninvasive ventilation through a nasal or oronasal interface. This can be offered at home or in a healthcare institution if in line with the goals of care. The sensation of dyspnea and the associated anxiety can be abated directly with opioids and anxiolytics, thereby reducing discomfort, and maximizing quality of life.

TERMINAL SECRETIONS

In the last days and hours of life, copious secretions can also be a distressing symptom to both the family and the patient. Pharmacological management is with anticholinergic medications (Table 183-4). Caution should be used when adding these medications as they can make secretions too thick and lead to mucus plugging. Often glycopyrrolate is preferred due to its lower deliriogenic effects and reduced anticholinergic-related systemic side effects. Nonpharmacologic interventions include positioning and avoiding deep suctioning as much as possible for terminal secretions. The stimulation for suctioning will often increase the amount of secretion due to irritation. Often in the dying process, the muscles around the larynx relax causing noisy breathing sometimes referred to as the "death rattle." This process is not uncomfortable for the patient; however, it can be extremely distressing for family to witness. The best course of action is to explain to the family the normal process of musculature relaxing and offer reassurance that the patient is comfortable.

SEIZURES

Convulsions may occur as patients approach the end of life, and they are often particularly distressing to patients and family members. In the context of end-of-life care, clinical decisions regarding the treatment of seizures are guided by the acuity of presentation, the presence of other organ damage or malfunction, and, most important, the wish to preserve or cloud the patient's consciousness. Benzodiazepines are the mainstay of treating seizures acutely, but they cause substantial sedation and may cause respiratory depression when used in conjunction with opioids. Newer oral anticonvulsants such as levetiracetam (Keppra) and oxcarbazepine (Trileptal) are options when sedation is undesirable. Chronic antiepileptics are often transitioned to benzodiazepine at the end of life to minimize volume of medication and optimize possible route of administration. For patients with long-standing seizure disorders collaboration with the patient's neurologist is helpful for a smooth transition. Patients with status epilepticus at the end of life should be considered candidates for a continuous infusion of benzodiazepines.

MAXIMIZING QUALITY OF LIFE

To support children nearing the end of life, as well as their families, healthcare professionals need to encourage them to maintain their normal lifestyles to the best of their ability and ensure that their philosophy of life is respected. In any discussion about quality of life, the healthcare team should take into consideration the family's cultural values and traditions.

In conversations with families, it is important to discern what is important for quality of life to the patient and family and support them fully in optimizing symptom management. It is important to consider that quality of life is subjective and can be interpreted differently by each family and culture. Because time is a paramount consideration, the focus should be on making each day meaningful. Healthcare providers should encourage the child and family to make memories out of big and small moments and to celebrate milestones—first tooth, first words, birthdays, graduations, religious ceremonies—while the child is still able to participate. Activities such as keeping a journal, making a photo album, videotaping special occasions, making imprints of the child's hands or feet, sharing stories, recording heartbeats, and keeping locks of hair all help create memories for the whole family.

EMOTIONAL AND PSYCHOSOCIAL PAIN

In the face of life-altering or serious news children commonly feel fear, sadness, anger, or confusion, regardless of if the diagnosis is shared with the child. Depression and anxiety have been found to be underrecognized and undiagnosed in children with serious illness. Screening both the parent and the child for social and psychological stressors is important for treating the child. Understanding the patient's and family's emotional and psychological processing can help the interdisciplinary team develop a well-rounded plan to decrease the burden of serious illness. Management of the patient's emotional and psychosocial pain through therapy and building of coping skills should include input from therapists, social workers, and behavioral health when needed. Concurrent pharmacologic treatment of anxiety, depression, or psychological diagnoses should be implemented as needed. Parents often are dealing with many of the same issues and should be encouraged to seek emotional and psychological care if needed.

SPIRITUAL AND PSYCHOSOCIAL ISSUES

Most have religious or spiritual beliefs of some kind. As mentioned, these factors can contribute to total pain especially when dealing with older children and adolescents. When people confront grave illness or death, their beliefs and associated rituals or practices are often of paramount concern. Accordingly, when caring for a critically ill or dying child, healthcare professionals should always ask patients or family members whether their religious or spiritual beliefs should be considered in the provision of care, and they should offer to arrange a meeting with the hospital's pastoral care service.

ADVANCE CARE PLANNING

Advanced care planning benefits patients, families, and healthcare providers. Ideally, advance care planning takes place during a period of clinical stability rather than in the context of a medical crisis. This is a critical aspect of caring for children with serious illness and medical complexity that all providers caring for these patients should be able to perform. When parents can discuss their child's end-of-life care plan, they feel more control over the situation, are more certain in their decisions, report improved communication with their child's healthcare team, and have more confidence that their child received the best care possible. Effective advance care planning increases the likelihood that a child will die in the families' preferred locations and can decrease levels of complicated grief after death. However, for patients, families, and providers, there are common barriers that result in these discussions occurring late in the illness trajectory and often in acute situations. Parents have reported hesitancy due to fear of death, fear of losing hope, worry that care from the medical teams will change, and uncertainty about the severity of the illness. Providers have reported barriers including lack of training, medical system issues, including time constraints, lack of supportive personnel, uncertain prognosis, and fear of taking away hope

Pediatric-focused advance care planning tools can assist the clinician in guiding discussions around preferences for care. These resources can be found at https://www.fivewishes.org *My Wishes*, for pediatric patients, and *Voicing My Choices*, for adolescents, use developmentally appropriate language and medical terms to cover the following themes:

- How I want people to treat me
- How I want to be comforted
- What I want my family and friends to know
- What I want my doctors and nurses to know

TRANSITIONS OF CARE

The decision about whether to have a child die at home or in the hospital is one of the most difficult that parents face. Not all families are comfortable having a child die at home; the choice depends on many factors, including medical resources, the child's condition, and the family's cultural belief system. Even when families decide to take a child home, they must be reassured that they can always return to the hospital. Going home is often a stressful time, especially for long-term patients, because it represents the first step toward separating from the acute medical facility and team and often symbolizes the beginning of the end-of-life journey. To make the transition as seamless as possible, the healthcare team needs to have a well-organized plan that is communicated to everyone involved.

The most important consideration in discharge planning is to honor the child's and family's wishes. Ideally, the conversation between the healthcare team and the family about going home should take place as early as possible so that referrals to hospice or home care services can be made and strategies for improving the quality of life can be implemented.

Transitioning a dying patient to home or to a hospice facility is best achieved through a concentrated, team approach. As an advocate for the child and family, the healthcare team can help identify appropriate services and providers, as well as clarify the treatment plan and the patient's needs with third-party payers to ensure maximum utilization of benefits. The healthcare team can facilitate the discharge planning process by working with its institutional system (e.g., case management, social work) to access all the necessary information and medical orders and to arrange the desired hospice or home care services.

Children and families choose to manage their end-of-life care in a variety of ways. Some continue with home care, others transition to home care with hospice services, and still others choose to end their life's journey in an inpatient hospice or hospital facility. Unfortunately, there are not always appropriate community-based resources available for children at the end of life. Hospice services for children can be scarce in many communities, making desired transitions difficult. The most important thing to remember is that the journey belongs to the child and the family, and their wishes should be supported if possible.

CONCURRENT CARE FOR CHILDREN

Pediatric patients can pursue parallel disease-directed care and palliative care at the same time. This is evidenced by studies showing the majority of patients being cared for by palliative care teams also are receiving treatments with curative intent. For a subset of patients who might also meet hospice criteria, there is the possibility of also engaging home-based hospice services to provide additional support for the patient and family.

Historically, families wishing for hospice services in the United States needed to forgo disease-directed treatments for their child. In 2010, this requirement changed with the passing of the Patient Protection and Affordable Care Act (PPACA). This act includes the "Concurrent Care for Children" provision which requires that programs for children in state Medicaid or CHIPs allow children younger than 21 years to receive hospice care while still receiving disease-directed treatments. Implementation of the provision has been challenging in many states and utilization of the provision has yet to be fully documented. However, concurrent care for children may open the doors for children requiring technology support at home that requires in-home nursing care to receive the addition of hospice services as their condition progresses. It has also allowed many parents to be able to use hospice services to help maximize quality time at home while still pursuing potentially life-extending treatments.

BEREAVEMENT

Families whose children have died need help to heal and find new ways to live. Family members will each experience the grief and pain of loss differently depending on their relationship with the child and the influences of their culture surrounding death. There are many individuals outside of the familial relationship that will also experience grief and loss with a child's death including those within their communities at school, church, and other peers.

With advances in diagnostic and therapeutic capabilities, the period between the diagnosis of a terminal illness and the moment of death is becoming longer, and people often have time to consider death and grief before the loved one dies. Known as anticipatory grief, this form of grieving may help families prepare for the loss and lower the degree and intensity of grief at the time of a child's death. Physicians and nurses who detect that parents or other family members are filled with anticipatory grief acknowledge and help families explore these emotions (with simple comments such as "I can see how sad you are"), helping them cope. If a family is experiencing significant anticipatory grief bereavement counselors can also be utilized prior to the patient's death to aid families in the grief process.

TABLE 183-5 Talking to Children About Death

- Provide calm reassurance.
- Understand the developmental stage of the child.
- Use clear language: "died" instead of "is gone now" or "in a better place."
- Repeat the information.
- Expect and support a variety of responses including no reaction.
- Be open to talking about feelings.
- Give the child space to process and opportunities to talk at later times.
- Include the sibling in funerals or memorial events.

A comprehensive bereavement program helps families start on the painful journey of grieving. The National Coalition for Hospice and Palliative Care recommends that an interprofessional team provide bereavement support to families through direct or indirect means for at least 13 months. A program should be tailored to meet the unique needs of each family, which includes providing a safe place to sit with sadness, acknowledging the many facets of grief, and helping the family glue the pieces of life back together over time. Parents who have experienced the loss of a child often report that joining a grief support group can increase a sense of peace, healing, and comfort, knowing they are not alone in their grief.

Siblings also benefit from guidance through the grief journey after loss. Bereaved siblings will cope differently depending on the cognitive and emotional developmental stage as well as the emotional and cultural environment of the family. Child-life therapists can be instrumental in guiding parents to provide sensitive, age-appropriate answers to vulnerable questions about the death and memory of their sibling (**Table 183-5**). Siblings can also benefit from guided support through bereavement camps, group therapy, counseling, and psychotherapy.

Extended family members such as aunts, uncles, cousins, and grandparents can also be greatly affected by the death of a child and may be left unrecognized and poorly supported as forgotten grievers. It is important to acknowledge that extended family members are grieving multiple losses. For example, a grandparent experiences both the loss of a grandchild and the grief of seeing their child grieving. Individuals from the child's greater support system in the community (church, school, extracurricular, etc.) are also forgotten grievers and may have decreased access to bereavement resources.

Although the journey is not easy, support, hope, and guidance should be offered to families who must begin the process of healing. Grieving families should be provided with bereavement and grief services and encouraged to choose which, if any, suit their needs. Bereavement follow-up services may include needs assessments and consultations, crisis intervention and referrals, individual counseling (in person or by telephone), support groups (for parents, siblings, and extended family), follow-up mailings and phone calls, written materials and resources, and memorial services.

DO-NOT-ATTEMPT-RESUSCITATION ORDERS

Do-not-attempt-resuscitation (DNAR) orders are considered at the end of this chapter because there is so much more involved in pediatric palliative care. Indeed, because DNAR orders require a discussion among the healthcare team and the patient and family members about values, preferences, and views regarding the quality of life—and about whether the patient's or family's therapeutic goals are best achieved through cardiopulmonary resuscitation (CPR) or other modes of care—hospitalists who participate in these discussions should thoroughly understand and be capable of providing the other forms of care outlined in this chapter. The conversation, in other words, should be as much about what will be done to promote comfort as about what will not be done. Ultimately, tailoring the DNAR order to fit the personal therapeutic goals set by the patient or family is an expression of the patient- and family-centered philosophy of care that lies at the core of excellent palliative care. However, hospitalists should be cautious about permitting families to pick and choose components of CPR. For example, administering medications while withholding chest compressions lacks a pathophysiologic rationale; the medications cannot be effective if they are not circulated.

The hospitalist should carefully document conversations with the patient and the patient's family in the medical record and understand how the documentation can be visible in both inpatient and outpatient settings. DNAR orders should be reviewed periodically and any time there is a significant change in the patient's medical condition. Hospitalists should communicate the substance of their discussions to primary care providers and complete out-of-hospital DNAR orders if appropriate at the time of discharge.

Hospitalists should be familiar with the policies of the hospitals and the laws of the country and or states where they practice. Hospitals may require the attending physician to write the initial DNAR order, prohibit verbal or telephone orders, and specify how frequently the order must be renewed. Renewal does not always require another discussion with the patient or guardian if the clinical situation has not changed. Parents have vocalized the distress of being required to repeat their desires for limited or no resuscitation multiple times.

Children with chronic or progressive conditions who are at risk of dying may also attend school and it is recommended that pediatricians work with school nurses to incorporate a specific action plan into the student's individualized healthcare plan.

SUGGESTED READINGS

American Academy of Pediatrics. Committee on Bioethics and Committee on Hospital Care. Palliative care for children. *Pediatrics.* 2000;106(2 Pt 1):351-357.

Council on School Health and Committee on Bioethics; Murray RD, Antommaria AHM. Honoring do-not-attempt-resuscitation requests in schools. *Pediatrics.* 2010;125(5):1073-1077.

Feudtner C, Kang TI, Hexem KR, et al. Pediatric palliative care patients: a prospective multicenter cohort study. *Pediatrics.* 2011;127(6):1094-1101.

Feudtner C, Nye R, Hill DL, et al. Polysymptomatology in pediatric patients receiving palliative care based on parent-reported data. *JAMA Netw Open.* 2021;4(8):e2119730.

Keim-Malpass J, Cozad MJ, R Svynarenko, Mack JW, Lindley LC. Medical complexity and concurrent hospice care: a national study of Medicaid children from 2011 to 2013. *J Spec Pediatr Nurs.* 2021;26(4):e12333.

Linebarger JS, Johnson V, Boss RD, et al. Guidance for pediatric end-of-life care. *Pediatrics.* 2022; 149(5):E2022057011.

Lord BT, Morrison W, Goldstein RD, Feudtner C. Parents as advocates for pediatric palliative care. *Pediatrics.* 2021;148(5):E2021052054.

National consensus project for quality palliative care: Clinical practice guidelines for quality palliative care. 2018.

Ragsdale L, Miller E. *Pediatric Palliative Care (What Do I Do Now Palliative Care).* 2nd ed. New York, NY: Oxford University Press; 2020.

Rogers MM, Friebert S, Williams CSP, Humphrey L, Thienprayoon R, Klick JC. Pediatric Palliative Care Programs in US Hospitals. *Pediatrics.* 2021;148(1).

Snaman J, McCarthy S, Wiener L, Wolfe J Pediatric palliative care in oncology. *J Clin Oncol.* 2020; 38(9):954-962.

Spraker-Perlman HL, Tam RP, Bradsley T, et al. The impact of pediatric palliative care involvement in the care of critically ill patients without complex chronic conditions. *J Palliat Med.* 2019;22(5):553-556.

Warlow TA, Hain RDW. 'Total Pain' in Children with Severe Neurological Impairment. *Children* (Basel). 2018;5(1):13.

Weaver MS, et al. Palliative Care Programs in Children's Hospitals. Pediatrics. 2022; 150(4):E2022057872.

Wiener L, Zadeh S, Battles H, et al. Allowing adolescents and young adults to plan their end-of-life care. *Pediatrics.* 2012;130(5):897-905.

Wolfe J, Hinds PS, Sourkes BM. *Textbook of Interdisciplinary Pediatric Palliative Care.* 2nd ed. Oxford University Press. New York, NY; 2022.

PART IV

Procedures

Part Editor
Alexander W. Hirsch, MD

CHAPTER 184

Procedural Sedation

Yasmeen N. Daud, MD and Mythili Srinivasan, MD, PhD

SEDATION AND ANALGESIA

The goals of sedation and analgesia are to allow diagnostic and therapeutic procedures to proceed with comfort, safety, efficacy, and efficiency. The specific goals of sedation are to provide analgesia, amnesia, anxiolysis, and/or relative immobility as indicated for the procedure with attention to patient safety. Adherence to the guidelines for the care of sedated patients developed by the American Academy of Pediatrics (AAP), the American Society of Anesthesiologists (ASA), and The Joint Commission (TJC) is essential. The information provided in this chapter is not sufficient guidance for the safe administration of procedural sedation. Each institution should have its own procedural sedation guidelines as well as training and certification requirements for maintaining competence in providing procedural sedation.

The following definitions for the depth of sedation have been adopted from the AAP, ASA, TJC, and the American College of Emergency Physicians (ACEP) (**Table 184-1**).

Sedation is a continuum and therefore healthcare sedation providers should be prepared to manage unintended deeper levels of sedation, including maintaining a patent airway, effective ventilation, and cardiovascular function. Providers should select a planned level of sedation that is determined by both patient and procedural factors.

PRESEDATION EVALUATION

The goal of the presedation evaluation is to evaluate the patient for factors that would put them at increased risk for complications from sedation. The evaluation includes examination of the airway for any potential difficulties in providing positive pressure ventilation or intubation, as well as assessment of cardiac, respiratory, renal, neurologic, or other systemic risk factors for sedation and contraindications to any sedation medications.

TABLE 184-1 Depth of Sedation

Minimal	A drug-induced state during which patients respond normally to verbal commands. Although cognitive function and coordination may be impaired, ventilatory and cardiovascular functions are usually maintained.
Moderate	A drug-induced depression of consciousness during which patients respond purposefully to verbal commands, either alone or accompanied by light to moderate tactile stimulation. No interventions are required to maintain a patent airway, and spontaneous ventilation is adequate. Cardiovascular function is usually maintained.
Deep	A drug-induced depression of consciousness during which patients cannot be easily aroused but respond purposefully following repeated or painful stimulation. The ability to maintain independent ventilatory function may be impaired. Patients may require assistance in maintaining a patent airway and spontaneous ventilation may be inadequate. Cardiovascular function is usually maintained.
Dissociative	Ketamine-induced state of consciousness in which the central nervous system is dissociated from external stimuli leading to a trance-like state characterized by analgesia, amnesia, and sedation. There is relative preservation of protective airway reflexes, spontaneous respirations, and cardiopulmonary stability.
General	A drug-induced loss of consciousness during which patients cannot be aroused, even by painful stimulation. The ability to maintain independent ventilatory function is often impaired. Patients often require assistance in maintaining a patent airway and positive-pressure ventilation may be required because of depressed spontaneous ventilation or depression of neuromuscular function.

TABLE 184-2 AMPLE History

A	Allergies to medications, latex, food
M	Medications–current
P	Past medical history, including sedation/general anesthesia history
L	Last meal, fluid intake
E	Events leading to procedure

HISTORY AND PHYSICAL EXAMINATION

All children scheduled to undergo sedation should be screened for factors that increase risk for potential adverse events during sedation and recovery. A presedation evaluation includes a focused history and physical examination, with attention to the airway and cardiorespiratory status. A focused history can be guided by the mnemonic AMPLE (**Table 184-2**).

The evaluation of a potentially difficult airway includes a history of previous problems with sedation or anesthesia, stridor, snoring, sleep apnea, and any recent respiratory illness. Patients with significant obesity, short neck, small mandible, dysmorphic facial features, small mouth opening, large tongue or tonsils, or nonvisible uvula are at increased risk of airway obstruction with sedation.

The patient's physical status, as classified by the ASA, can be useful in assessing sedation risk (**Table 184-3**). ASA class I and II children are at low risk for adverse events during sedation when they are carefully monitored. Anesthesiology consultation should be considered when planning the sedation of an ASA class III patient.

PRESEDATION FASTING

There is no proven relationship between the duration of fasting before sedation and the risk of aspiration in humans. However, the general consensus is that fasting likely reduces the risk of aspiration. For elective procedures, the ASA consensus recommendations should be followed (**Table 184-4**). For nonelective procedures, the patient should be fasted as soon as the potential need for sedation is identified. Although the risk of clinically significant aspiration is low, it should be weighed carefully against the need to perform a diagnostic or therapeutic procedure quickly.

SEDATION PLANNING

SELECTION OF AN AGENT

The selection of medications is guided by the desired effect: analgesia, anxiolysis, amnesia, relative immobility, or some combination. Desired depth of sedation must be considered carefully. Patient factors should also be considered including consideration of the degree of patient anxiety, comorbidities, and risks identified during the presedation assessment. The lightest effective sedation is preferred, but because of the wide variety of individual responses, clinicians should be trained and prepared to administer increasingly deeper sedation guided by the patient's response. The clinician should consider using effective nonpharmacologic techniques such as distraction, imagery, and parental involvement whenever possible.

PERSONNEL

All sedation providers should have Pediatric Advance Life Support (PALS) and advanced airway management training. A second support

TABLE 184-3 American Society of Anesthesiologists Physical Classification

Class	Disease State
I	No organic, physiologic, biochemical, or psychiatric disturbance
II	Mild to moderate systemic disturbance
III	Severe systemic disturbance
IV	Severe systemic disturbance that is life-threatening
V	Moribund patient with little chance of survival

TABLE 184-4 Fasting Guidelines for Elective Sedation

Type of Food/ Liquid	Time (hours)
Clear liquids	2
Breast milk	4
Fortified breast milk/Infant formula/solids	6

Clear liquids: Water, sugar water, Kool-aid, Pedialyte, soda, apple or grape juice without pulp, Gatorade.

Solids: All food, cow milk, unstrained fruit juices, tube feedings, candy, and gum.

person with PALS training is also required. The support person is responsible for monitoring the patient's cardiopulmonary status, recording these data on a sedation record, and may assist in brief, interruptible tasks once the level of sedation is stabilized.

The sedation provider should monitor the patient closely during sedation and should not be the person responsible for the procedure. Problems with ventilation and oxygenation are easily managed when they are recognized quickly.

MONITORING

Monitoring of the patient before, during, and after sedation should follow guidelines established by the AAP. A full set of vital signs should be documented prior to any sedation. For all levels of sedation, the patient should have continuous monitoring of heart rate and oxygen saturation. The child's color, airway patency, and rate and depth of respiration should be monitored by direct observation. Capnography should be used to assess ventilation if tolerated. Vital signs including heart rate, respiratory rate, blood pressure, oxygen saturation, and end-tidal carbon dioxide levels should be recorded at least every 10 minutes or more frequently depending on the level of sedation. For deep sedation, IV access should be obtained, and vital signs should be recorded every 5 minutes. Patients should be recovered by appropriate staff with access to rescue equipment, and medications and vital signs should be recorded every 5 to 10 minutes depending on the level of sedation until the patient is fully awake.

MEDICATIONS

There are many reasonable choices for safe sedation. It is best for clinicians to become familiar with a limited number of agents or combinations of agents to develop a more thorough understanding of their use. This allows healthcare providers to become more experienced with each drug's indications, pharmacokinetic and pharmacodynamic profiles, dosing, responses, drug interactions, and adverse effects. It is also important to use agents that best meet the needs of the individual patient and the procedure, based on whether the goal is anxiolysis, amnesia, immobility, analgesia, or some combination.

Concomitant administration of a second medication with sedation or analgesia effects can act additively or synergistically with the initial medication. It is important to be aware of the drug metabolism so that adverse events due to drug-drug interactions can be avoided.

PENTOBARBITAL

Pentobarbital is a short-acting barbiturate with sedative-hypnotic effects without analgesia.

Route: IV

Dose: IV: Initial dose of 2.5 mg/kg followed by increments of 1 mg/kg every 3 to 5 minutes to a maximum dose of 6 mg/kg. Maximum dose 150 mg.

Pharmacokinetics: The onset of action is less than 60 seconds. Recovery time is 50 to 75 minutes.

Side effects: Respiratory depression associated with pentobarbital is dose dependent. Significant agitation is often seen in patients during recovery. Contraindicated in patients with liver disease, moderate to severe renal impairment, and porphyria.

Reversal agent: None

Uses: Pentobarbital is used primarily for nonpainful radiologic procedures.

MIDAZOLAM

Midazolam is a benzodiazepine that provides anxiolysis, amnesia, and sedation.

Route: IV, intranasal (IN), PO.

Dose: IV

6 months-5 years: 0.05 to 0.1 mg/kg, may repeat dose every 2 to 3 minutes with a maximum single dose of 2 mg and maximum total dose of 6 mg.

6-12 years: 0.025 to 0.1 mg/kg, may repeat dose every 2 to 3 minutes with a maximum single dose of 2 mg and a maximum total dose of 6 mg.

>12 years: 1-2 mg/dose every 2 to 3 minutes with a maximum total dose of 10 mg.

IN: 0.2 to 0.5 mg/kg, maximum dose 10 mg (use the injectable form of the drug, may cause nasal irritation).

PO: 0.5 to 1 mg/kg, maximum dose 20 mg.

Pharmacokinetics: Onset of action is less than 1 minute, with a peak at 2 to 6 minutes when given IV, 5 to 15 minutes when given IN, and 15 to 20 minutes when given PO. Recovery time is 30 to 90 minutes.

Side effects: Can cause respiratory depression, bradycardia, hypotension, and agitation. Respiratory depression is more common when administered with opioids.

Reversal agent: IV flumazenil 0.01 mg/kg IV (max dose 0.2 mg) over 15 seconds, may repeat this dose every 1 minute as needed up to a total cumulative maximum dose of 1 mg.

Uses: Midazolam alone can be used to provide anxiolysis. It may also be combined with an analgesic (e.g., fentanyl, ketamine) for painful procedures.

DEXMEDETOMIDINE

Dexmedetomidine is a selective alpha-2 adrenergic receptor agonist that has sedative, anxiolytic, hypnotic, and some analgesic properties.

Route: IV

Dose: IV, Loading dose of 1 to 3 micrograms/kg over 10 minutes followed by maintenance infusion of 1 to 2 micrograms/kg/hr

Pharmacokinetics: Onset of sedation is usually by the end of the bolus dose. Mean recovery time can range from 30 to 60 minutes.

Side effects: There is generally no significant respiratory depression. Transient hypotension, bradycardia, or hypertension can be seen. It is contraindicated in patients with liver disease and moderate to severe renal impairment. It is also contraindicated in patients on digoxin, beta blockers, cardiac conduction abnormalities, cardiovascular compromise, moyamoya disease, arteriovenous malformations, or new-onset stroke.

Reversal agent: None

Uses: Dexmedetomidine alone is used for nonpainful radiological procedures. It may also be used in combination with an analgesic (e.g., fentanyl, ketamine) for painful procedures.

KETAMINE

Ketamine is a dissociative agent that provides sedation, amnesia, and analgesia.

Route: IV, IM. IV route is preferable due to faster recovery and less emesis.

Dose: IV: 0.5 to 1 mg/kg followed by repeat doses of 0.5 to 1 mg/kg as needed. IM: 2-4 mg/kg.

Pharmacokinetics: The onset of action is 30 to 60 seconds when given IV and 3-10 minutes when given IM. A return to coherence occurs in approximately 15 to 30 minutes.

Side effects: Respiratory depression can occur; however, effective spontaneous respirations are generally preserved and airway reflexes remain intact. Laryngospasm is a rare but potentially serious adverse reaction. Per the clinical practice guidelines by Green et al, absolute contraindications for ketamine are age less than 3 months and known or suspected schizophrenia. Relative contraindications per the guidelines are airway instability, cardiovascular disease, active pulmonary disease, major oropharyngeal procedures, increased intracranial or intraocular pressure, porphyria, and thyroid disease. Studies by Green et al have shown that co-administration of anti-cholinergics to decrease salivation or midazolam to decrease recovery agitation increases risk for adverse airway and respiratory events and thus are not recommended.

Reversal agent: None

Uses: The relative lack of respiratory depression and sparing of airway reflexes make ketamine a popular choice for short, painful procedures.

PROPOFOL

Propofol is a nonbarbiturate sedative-hypnotic agent that has no analgesic effect.

Route: IV

Dose: IV, 1 to 2 mg/kg can provide sedation for short procedures. For prolonged painless sedation, induction dose is 1 to 2 mg/kg and maintenance infusion is started at 100 to 150 micrograms/kg/min, can be titrated up to a maximum dose of 250 micrograms/kg/min.

Pharmacokinetics: The onset of action is less than 1 minute. Plasma levels fall quickly because of metabolic clearance and rapid redistribution, so a continuous infusion is needed to maintain sedation longer than a few minutes. Median recovery time when used for longer procedures such as MRI is 30 minutes.

Side effects: Propofol can cause respiratory depression, apnea, and hypotension. Owing to its extremely short half-life, it can be difficult to titrate its effect. Thus, propofol should be administered only by experienced providers with advanced airway skills. Propofol causes pain at the injection site. Administering lidocaine through the IV prior to propofol can reduce this side effect. Propofol is contraindicated in patients with severe allergies to egg or soy.

Reversal agent: None

Uses: The quick onset of action and short duration make propofol an attractive drug for brief, nonpainful procedures. It may also be used in combination with an analgesic for painful procedures.

FENTANYL

Fentanyl is a high-potency opioid that has minimal adverse hemodynamic effects.

Route: IV, IN

Dose: IV, 1 to 2 micrograms/kg with a maximum of 50 micrograms per dose, subsequent dose of 0.5 to 1 micrograms/kg with a maximum single dose of 25 microgram repeated every 3 to 5 minutes. IN: 1 to 2 micrograms/kg

Pharmacokinetics: The onset of action is 30 to 60 seconds IV and the duration of action is 30 to 60 minutes. The onset of action is 5 to 10 minutes when given IN.

Side effects: The major side effect of fentanyl is respiratory depression, which is dose related but can occasionally occur with low doses. The risk of respiratory depression is significantly increased when fentanyl is given with other sedation medications. Hypotension and chest wall rigidity are rare adverse events that can occur with rapid infusion of large doses.

Reversal agent: Naloxone < 20 kg: 0.1mg/kg/dose, ≥ 20 kg or > 5 years: 2mg/dose. May repeat every 2 to 3 minutes as needed. Reversal may result in severe pain, hypertension, tachycardia, etc.

Uses: As an analgesic, fentanyl is used for painful procedures. It is frequently combined with other sedation medications for procedural sedation.

NITROUS OXIDE

Nitrous oxide (N_2O) is a colorless, odorless gas which provides analgesia, sedation, amnesia, and anxiolysis.

Route: Inhalational agent

Dose: Administered with oxygen at a concentration of 50% to 70% nitrous.

Pharmacokinetics: Peak effect within 2 to 3 minutes. N_2O is not metabolized but instead exhaled by the patient resulting in rapid recovery of the patient within 5 to 10 minutes after discontinuation of the agent. It is recommended that 100% oxygen be administered for 2 to 3 minutes after discontinuation of N_2O to prevent diffusion hypoxia and improve scavenging of exhaled N_2O to reduce the environmental exposure.

Side effects: Common side effects are nausea/vomiting and in some cases hallucination, which can be disturbing to children causing agitation. N_2O is contraindicated in patients with any trapped air in a body cavity such as pneumothorax, recent tympanoplasty, bowel obstruction, or recent intraocular surgery, wherein gas bubbles may have been introduced during surgery. N_2O irreversibly inactivates vitamin B_{12} and is contraindicated in patients with a deficiency in vitamin B_{12} or the enzyme 5,10 methylenetetrahydrofolate reductase. Nitrous oxide is not recommended for use in pregnant patients.

Reversal agent: None

Uses: The rapid onset and recovery and the lack of need for an IV makes N_2O a useful agent for short, painful procedures. It can be combined with an opioid to achieve a deeper level of sedation.

SUGGESTED READINGS

American Society of Anesthesiologists Task Force on Sedation and Analgesia by Non-Anesthesiologists. Practice guidelines for sedation and analgesia by non-anesthesiologists. *Anesthesiology.* 2002;96(4):1004-1017.

Becker DE, Rosenberg M. Nitrous oxide and the inhalation anesthetics. *Anesth Prog.* 2008;55(4):124-130; quiz 131-122.

Cote CJ, Wilson S. American Academy of Pediatrics, American Academy of Pediatric Dentistry. Guidelines for monitoring and management of pediatric patients before, during, and after sedation for diagnostic and therapeutic procedures. *Pediatrics.* 2019;143(6).

Cravero JP, Beach ML, Blike GT, Gallagher SM, Hertzog JH, Pediatric Sedation Research Consortium. The incidence and nature of adverse events during pediatric sedation/anesthesia with propofol for procedures outside the operating room: a report from the Pediatric Sedation Research Consortium. *Anesth Analg.* 2009;108(3):795-804.

Godwin SA, Burton JH, Gerardo CJ, et al. Clinical policy: procedural sedation and analgesia in the emergency department. *Ann Emerg Med.* 2014;63(2):247-258 e218.

Green SM, Krauss B. Should I give ketamine i.v. or i.m.? *Ann Emerg Med.* 2006;48(5):613-614.

Green SM, Roback MG, Kennedy RM, Krauss B. Clinical practice guideline for emergency department ketamine dissociative sedation: 2011 update. *Ann Emerg Med.* 2011;57(5):449-461.

Green SM, Roback MG, Krauss B, et al. Predictors of airway and respiratory adverse events with ketamine sedation in the emergency department: an individual-patient data meta-analysis of 8,282 children. *Ann Emerg Med.* 2009;54(2):158-168 e151-154.

Green SM, Roback MG, Krauss B, et al. Predictors of emesis and recovery agitation with emergency department ketamine sedation: an individual-patient data meta-analysis of 8,282 children. *Ann Emerg Med.* 2009;54(2):171-180 e171-174.

Hathout L, El-Saden S. Nitrous oxide-induced B12 deficiency myelopathy: perspectives on the clinical biochemistry of vitamin B12. *J Neurol Sci.* 2011;301(1-2):1-8.

The Joint Commission. Comprehensive Accreditation Manual for Hospitals (CAMH): the official handbook. Oakbrook Terrace, IL: The Joint Commission 2014.

McMorrow SP, Abramo TJ. Dexmedetomidine sedation: uses in pediatric procedural sedation outside the operating room. *Pediatr Emerg Care.* 2012;28(3):292-296.

Practice Guidelines for Preoperative Fasting and the Use of Pharmacologic Agents to Reduce the Risk of Pulmonary Aspiration: Application to Healthy Patients Undergoing Elective Procedures: An Updated Report by the American Society of Anesthesiologists Task Force on Preoperative Fasting and the Use of Pharmacologic Agents to Reduce the Risk of Pulmonary Aspiration. *Anesthesiology.* 2017;126(3):376-393.

Roback MG, Wathen JE, MacKenzie T, Bajaj L. A randomized, controlled trial of i.v. versus i.m. ketamine for sedation of pediatric patients receiving emergency department orthopedic procedures. *Ann Emerg Med.* 2006;48(5):605-612.

Selzer RR, Rosenblatt DS, Laxova R, Hogan K. Adverse effect of nitrous oxide in a child with 5,10-methylenetetrahydrofolate reductase deficiency. *N Engl J Med.* 2003;349(1):45-50.

Srinivasan M, Turmelle M, Depalma LM, Mao J, Carlson DW. Procedural sedation for diagnostic imaging in children by pediatric hospitalists using propofol: analysis of the nature, frequency, and predictors of adverse events and interventions. *J Pediatr.* 2012;160(5):801-806 e801.

Vespasiano M, Finkelstein M, Kurachek S. Propofol sedation: intensivists' experience with 7304 cases in a children's hospital. *Pediatrics.* 2007;120(6):e1411-1417.

CHAPTER 185

Radiology for the Pediatric Hospitalist

Lindsay S. Baron, MD

BACKGROUND

The purpose of this chapter is to familiarize hospitalists with common pediatric imaging modalities so that they can order the most appropriate test for their patient and be able to properly inform and prepare the patient and family before the study. The techniques, indications, and patient preparation for common pediatric imaging examinations are described here.

Given the wide array of choices, it is sometimes difficult for clinicians to determine the best exam for a particular clinical situation. Discussion with a radiologist regarding available options is strongly encouraged. Many common clinical scenarios are addressed in the American College of Radiology Appropriateness Criteria, a regularly updated, evidence-based internet resource designed to assist clinicians in choosing the best test to answer their clinical question.

Following a discussion of radiation safety and contrast agents (for non-nuclear medicine studies), the chapter is divided into imaging studies that require ionizing radiation (conventional radiographs, fluoroscopy, computed tomography [CT], and nuclear medicine examinations) and those that do not (ultrasound [US] and magnetic resonance imaging [MRI]). Vascular and nonvascular interventional procedures are described at the end of the chapter.

With the exception of some interventional procedures, parents may remain with their child when any of these examinations are performed. Pregnant mothers and siblings under the age of 18 will be asked to wait in a separate area for studies utilizing radiation. Ionizing radiation exposure in the fetus is known to cause miscarriages and malformations and carries a small but real risk for the development of childhood cancers. Parents and other personnel who remain in the same room during x-ray or CT examinations must wear lead shielding for protection. For patients who are pregnant, studies with ionizing radiation are contraindicated unless the medical need (such as a ventilation-perfusion [V/Q] scan in a patient at high risk for pulmonary emboli) outweighs the medical risk. MRI is avoided in early pregnancy but is used for fetal assessment later in pregnancy.

RADIATION SAFETY

Whenever considering a radiographic examination for any patient, one must be cognizant of the amount of radiation that the patient will receive, especially if the patient has a chronic condition. The guiding principle behind radiation protection is that radiation exposures should be kept "as low as reasonably achievable (ALARA)." This principle must be especially adhered to in children because for the same dose, children are more susceptible to radiation effects than adults. As knowledge of the risks of medical radiation has grown in recent years, radiologists have responded by lowering the doses of common medical tests. Referring physicians have also responded by ordering fewer tests with ionizing radiation.

The clinician may find themselves confronted by a concerned parent regarding the necessity of a test that uses ionizing radiation. **Table 185-1** provides a real-world reference for clinicians and parents when discussing these risks. While appropriate indications for evaluation of a pediatric patient with an exam utilizing ionizing radiation cannot be stressed enough, the benefit of a clinically indicated exam far outweighs its potential risks. Other imaging modalities such as US or MRI should be considered as alternatives when appropriate, with the caveat that they are not necessarily superior for a given clinical condition, and there may be a need for sedation or general anesthesia with MRI. Studies performed in pediatric hospitals are much more likely to use the lowest possible radiation dose compared to adult counterparts.

TABLE 185-1 Ionizing Radiation Dose Estimates

Procedure	Average Estimated Effective Dose	Comparable Natural Background Radiation
KUB child	0.02-0.15 mSv	2-18 days background radiation
VCUG child	0.14 mSv	17 days background radiation
CT scan abdomen	0.8-2.7 mSv	3-11 months background radiation
RNC	0.5-2.9 mSv	2-12 months background radiation

Source: Reproduced with permission from Department of Radiology, Boston Children's Hospital, personal communication, Da Zhang, PhD, DABR.

RNC, radionuclide cystography.

CONTRAST MATERIALS

Natural variation in tissue density and water content is what makes radiographic diagnosis possible. Contrast agents are often used to enhance these differences. Contrast agents are given through the body's natural or surgically created orifices, intravenously, or both, depending on the goals of the exam. These agents aid in visualizing certain organ systems, such as the gastrointestinal (GI) tract or the genitourinary system, but they can also more accurately assess certain disease processes; for example, the presence of tumor or infection.

ENTERIC CONTRAST

Enteric contrast may be used during GI fluoroscopic exams, CT of the abdomen and pelvis, or MRI, for certain bowel indications. Several varieties of enteric contrast exist.

Barium sulfate suspension is an inert white liquid that attenuates the passage of x-rays and is commonly used during fluoroscopy. It comes in different consistencies, depending on its intended use. Barium has a chalk-like taste, but its palatability can be improved with mild flavoring. Double-contrast barium studies involve the use of barium and gas. These studies introduce gas into the intestines to distend the bowel and create a thin coat of barium on the bowel mucosal surfaces to assess mucosal detail. Because double-contrast studies require strict patient cooperation and are most useful for mucosal detail, they are not routinely performed in the pediatric population; more typically, single-contrast studies are performed. The main effect of barium is constipation, therefore additional hydration is recommended after barium studies. For this reason, barium is relatively contraindicated in those with cystic fibrosis or constipation. It is also contraindicated in those with bowel perforation, as excess barium within the peritoneal cavity causes barium peritonitis (**Figure 185-1**). Barium is commonly used to evaluate children for aspiration and tracheoesophageal fistula, as it is not inherently toxic to lung tissue.

Water-soluble low-osmolar non-ionic agents are used for enteric contrast in neonates and cases in which barium use is contraindicated. They are also commonly used for CT examinations. Enteric use of water-soluble high-osmolar contrast agents is generally limited to therapeutic enemas; for example, in a cystic fibrosis patient with meconium ileus equivalent, or in a neonate with meconium ileus. Many different iodinated contrast agents are available that can also be used to evaluate the GI tract.

Enteric contrast agents for MRI can be either positive (appear bright) or negative (appear dark) and are chosen based on the exam indication. Popular agents include water, Miralax, and blueberry juice (which contains manganese and causes T2 shortening). Gadolinium-containing enteric contrast is also available.

INTRAVENOUS CONTRAST

Iodinated contrast agents are used intravenously for CT. The osmolality of the available agents varies widely. Most hospitals now primarily use low-osmolar contrast, particularly in children, as these are far less likely to cause adverse effects such as fluid shifts or allergic reaction. If there has been a previous contrast reaction, premedication with

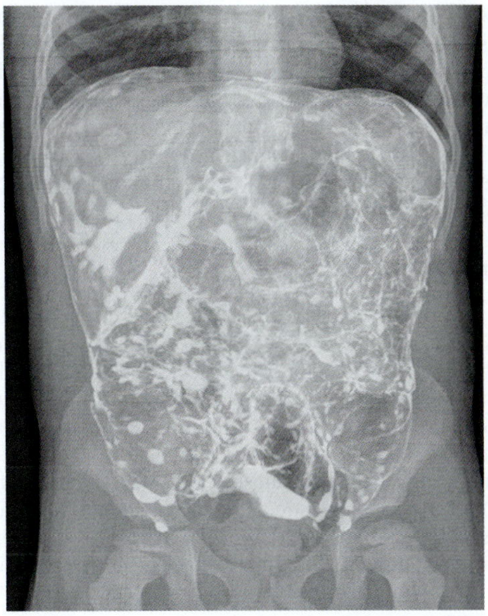

FIGURE 185-1. This AP radiograph of the abdomen shows the chronic residual of barium lining the peritoneal cavity after extravasation from perforated bowel.

steroids is mandatory, or an alternative examination should be sought (**Table 185-2**). Administration of contrast agents is generally safe but as with any medication, allergy may cause adverse reactions ranging from benign urticaria to death from fulminant anaphylaxis. Once intravenous contrast is administered, subsequent contrast administration is limited to a total of 7 mL/kg dose per 24 hours to limit nephrotoxicity. This should be kept in mind when scheduling examinations, particularly when done in a separate department (e.g., cardiac catheterization) or an outside institution.

There are no established guidelines for avoiding contrast-induced nephropathy in children. Children with renal dysfunction should be imaged with alternate modalities when possible. When an exam with intravenous contrast is required, children should be treated with similar caution as an adult in the same situation.

MRI contrast agents containing gadolinium are frequently used in the pediatric population, although as some agents have not yet been approved for use in children and few are approved for children under 2, use is often off-label. This contrast agent is administered intravenously. Some MRI contrast agents may also be administered parenterally. These agents have an extremely low incidence of adverse reactions and allergy is rare. Gadolinium chelates are not known to be nephrotoxic at approved doses. They must be used with caution in patients with severe renal dysfunction due to a potential risk of nephrogenic systemic fibrosis (NSF), although this risk has been dramatically minimized in recent years with the use of more stable gadolinium chelates.

Although US contrast agents are more widely used in adult patients, their use is rapidly expanding in the pediatric population in the United States.

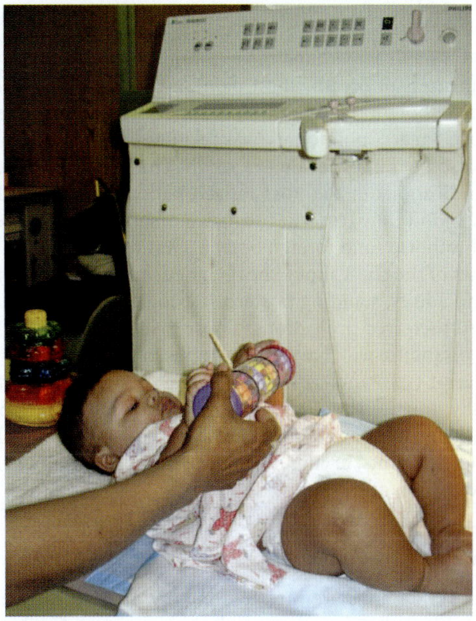

FIGURE 185-2. An infant lying on the fluoroscopy table prior to a voiding cystourethrogram. The patient is playing with a colorful toy that will be used to distract him throughout the procedure.

PATIENT COOPERATION

For most imaging examinations performed in children, sedation or general anesthesia is not necessary. With the advent of multidetector CT scanners increasing the speed with which information is obtained, far fewer patients need to be sedated to obtain diagnostic images than in prior decades. However, a small number of patients undergoing CT and a larger number undergoing MRI need to be sedated or even placed under general anesthesia. The benefit of information obtained from these studies must outweigh the risk of possible adverse events from sedation or general anesthesia.

During studies where occasional motion is less disruptive to the diagnostic quality of the exam, such as fluoroscopy, distraction can be an adequate alternative to sedation. Diversion techniques may be used by a child life expert or the parent. Exciting toys and portable electronics have proven their value in guiding children through exams that would otherwise have required sedation (**Figure 185-2**).

CONVENTIONAL RADIOGRAPHS

Plain radiographs, commonly known as x-rays, are produced when a beam of photons penetrates through a part of the body and strikes a film. Although more sophisticated imaging modalities exist, the conventional radiograph remains an invaluable means by which to evaluate certain organ systems. They provide a rapid, widely available, low-radiation means to diagnose and monitor a multitude of conditions.

TABLE 185-2

A. Sample Pediatric Corticosteroid and Antihistamine Premedication Regimen

	Dosage	Timing
Prednisone	0.5-0.7 mg/kg PO (up to 50 mg)	13, 7, and 1 hr prior to contrast injection
Diphenhydramine	1.25 mg/kg PO (up to 50 mg)	1 hr prior to contrast injection

B. Sample Pediatric Corticosteroid and Antihistamine Premedication Regimen for Urgent or NPO patients

	Dosage	Timing
Hydrocortisone	2 mg/kg IV (up to 200 mg)	5 and 1 hr prior to contrast injection
Diphenhydramine	1 mg/kg IV, IM, or PO (up to 50 mg)	1 hr prior to contrast injection

Source: ACR Manual on Contrast Media, 2024

CHEST

A chest radiograph is perhaps most commonly ordered for the evaluation of shortness of breath, chest pain, or pneumonia in the pediatric population. Although the lungs do occupy the majority of the chest, the mediastinum, heart, pulmonary vasculature, diaphragm, pleura, and bones can also be initially evaluated on the chest radiograph. Additional common indications in the hospitalized patient include evaluation for pulmonary blood flow pattern, cardiac anomalies, support device position, pneumothorax, and foreign body aspiration.

Two views of the chest should be obtained whenever possible. In older children and adults, standing posteroanterior (PA) and lateral views are the standard preferred projections. Those unable to stand or sit because of age or disability will have radiographs obtained while supine, in anteroposterior (AP) and cross-table lateral or lateral decubitus projections. Ideally, images should be obtained during inspiration, which is often a challenge in infants and young children who are unable to cooperate. In these patients, crying during the exam is actually beneficial, as it causes expansion of the lungs.

ABDOMEN

Abdominal radiographs are most commonly ordered for evaluation of the bowel gas pattern when there is clinical suspicion for ileus or bowel obstruction. The presence of increased stool burden, organomegaly, abnormal calcifications, or pneumoperitoneum (**Figure 185-3**) may also be assessed. In neonates, the course and position of umbilical arterial and venous lines is best assessed on an abdominal radiograph.

Supine and standing upright views are obtained in any radiographic evaluation of the abdomen for concern of bowel obstruction. If the patient is too young or sick to stand, a left lateral decubitus film is obtained in place of the upright view. If intussusception is suspected, a decubitus or prone view may be obtained to aid in filling the cecum with air, which would prove the absence of an ileocolic intussusception. The exception to the usual requirement for two views of the abdomen is for the evaluation of renal calculi or stool burden. In this case, a single kidneys, ureters, bladder (KUB) view usually suffices.

SKULL

Skull radiographs remain a required component of a skeletal survey in the setting of suspected non-accidental trauma. They are also useful for evaluation of the sutures in suspected cases of craniosynostosis (**Figure 185-4**). Generally, if there is a history of injury with sufficient force to suspect skull fracture, CT should be performed in order to allow simultaneous assessment for intracranial injury. However, skull radiographs may be complementary to CT in this setting, as occasionally a fracture can be very difficult to visualize on CT if the orientation of the fracture is in the same plane as image acquisition. Surface rendering of CT images creates a 3D reformat of the skull and can help avoid this error, but can be sensitive to motion artifact.

EXTREMITIES

When the area of abnormality can be localized to a particular joint or location, such as the forearm, a dedicated radiographic series coned down to that anatomic location is performed. AP and lateral views are the basic radiographs obtained when evaluating the musculoskeletal system. These projections are frequently supplemented with an oblique or specialized views, as required by the clinical situation. Although CT and MRI may evaluate the musculoskeletal system in greater detail, radiography alone can be diagnostic without the aid of additional imaging, and in most cases it provides additional important information essential to diagnosis. Therefore, radiography remains central to the diagnosis of bone lesions and should be the first imaging step in the evaluation of any bone pathology.

SPINE

In radiographic evaluation of the spine, the number of views obtained depends on which part of the spine is studied (i.e., cervical, thoracic, or lumbar) and the indication. As with most other locations, radiographs of the spine begin with PA and lateral views. Additional views are often obtained to better evaluate specific anatomy. For example, in the setting of trauma, additional views are obtained to visualize the dens and the C7-T1 junction. If the dens or the C7-T1 junction is not clearly visualized, the radiologist cannot "clear" the cervical spine. For further evaluation of these focal areas, CT is sometimes needed. Full cervical spine CT evaluation is not typically recommended in children, in keeping with the ALARA principle. The incidence of spinal fractures is relatively low in the pediatric population, so CT is reserved for further investigation of any focal area of tenderness that the patient may have, for more thorough evaluation of any region of abnormality seen on plain films, or for patients who have sustained major trauma and have resultant neurologic deficits. For the evaluation of lower back pain in an adolescent, bilateral oblique views are obtained in addition to the standard AP and lateral

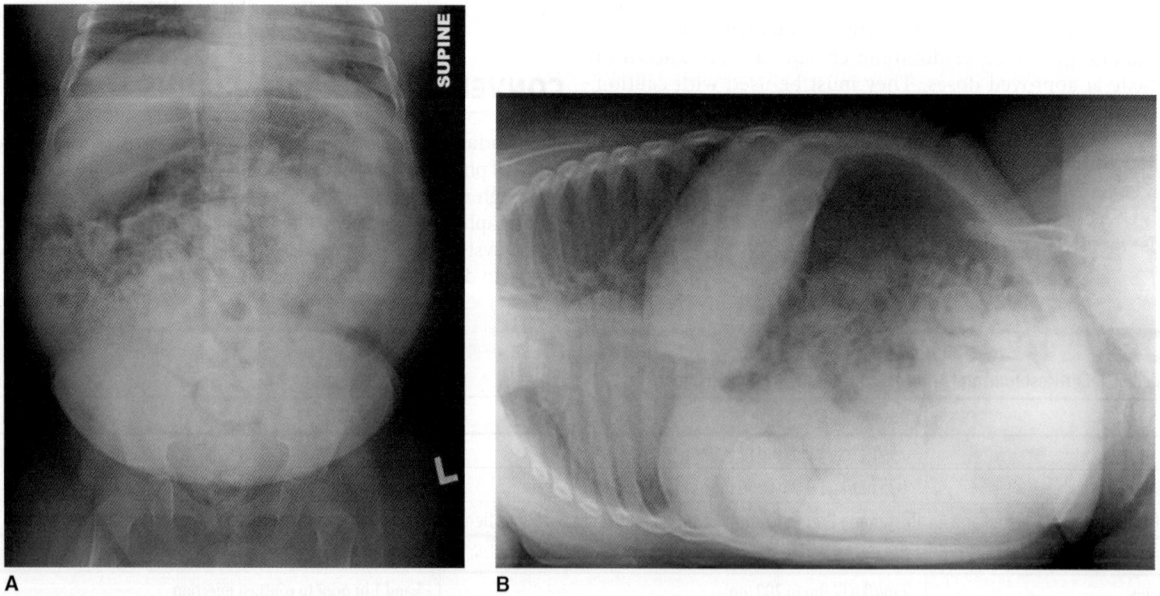

FIGURE 185-3. Supine (A) and left lateral decubitus (B) radiographs demonstrate massive pneumoperitoneum. Upright and decubitus radiographs are more sensitive than supine radiographs for detecting subtle free air.

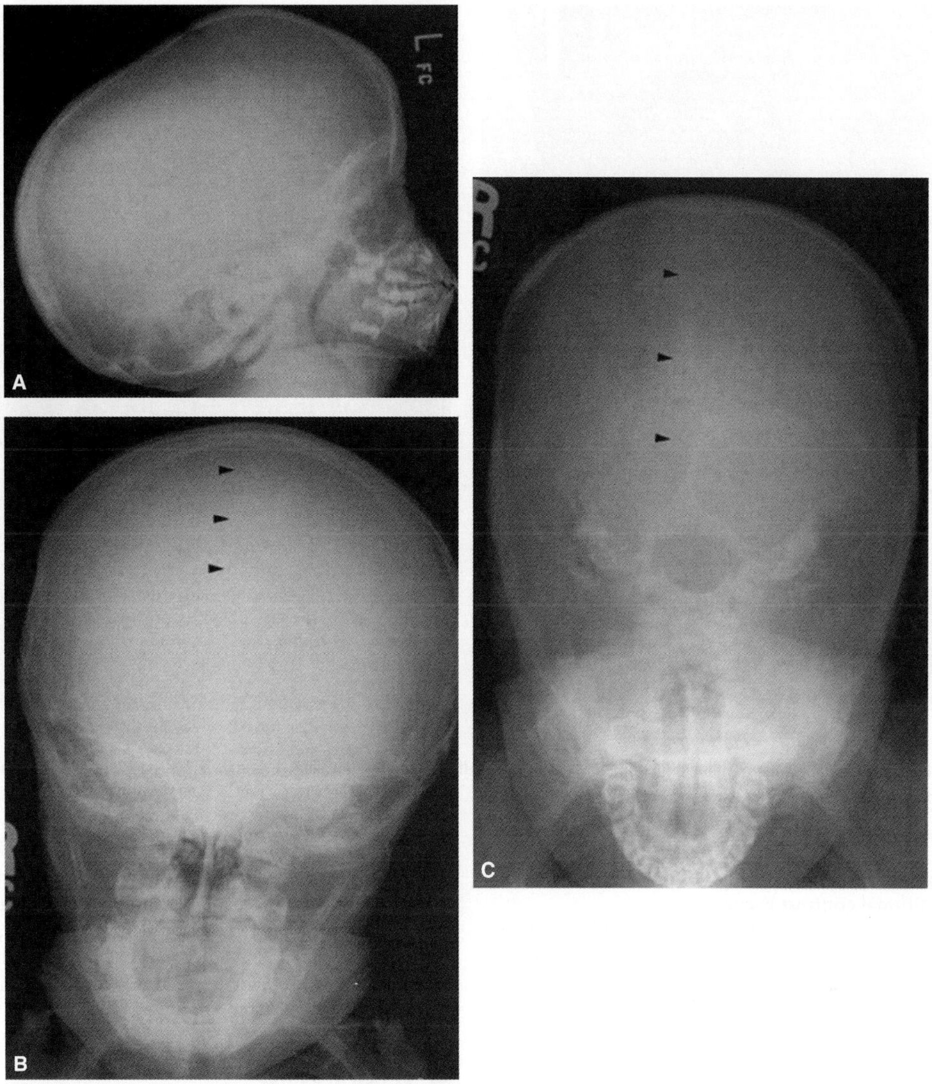

FIGURE 185-4. Lateral view of the skull shows an elongated calvarium, likely representing sagittal suture synostosis (A). Non-visualization of the sagittal suture on AP and Town's views of the skull (arrowheads) confirms the diagnosis (B, C).

views to better evaluate the pars interarticularis. If a fracture or spondylolysis is noted on plain films and grading of the pars defect is necessary, obtaining a focused CT scan limited to the region of abnormality is recommended to decrease the amount of radiation that the pelvis receives. This practice is especially important in females because the ovaries may be in the radiation field.

SOFT TISSUES OF THE NECK

Radiographic evaluation of the soft tissues of the neck is indicated in suspected cases of epiglottitis, croup, and retropharyngeal abscesses. AP and lateral radiographs are the typical projections obtained. In a case of suspected epiglottitis, a healthcare provider should accompany the patient to the radiology department in case the airway becomes obstructed. To prevent airway obstruction, placing the patient in a supine position to obtain radiographs is contraindicated.

PORTABLE RADIOGRAPHS

The radiographic examinations just described are best performed within the radiology department; however, sometimes the patient is too sick to leave the intensive care unit or emergency room, and thus portable radiographs may be obtained. There is sometimes temptation to order portable examinations for patient or staff convenience. This should be strongly discouraged as they often provide inferior diagnostic information when compared with standard radiographs. Portable series should be reserved for critically ill patients who cannot be transported, because suboptimal patient positioning and external conditions may limit the evaluation.

FLUOROSCOPY

Fluoroscopy uses continuous x-rays to allow evaluation of dynamic processes in the patient. Unlike many other types of imaging studies, a radiologist performs these exams and acquires the images, rather than a technologist. Most fluoroscopy studies also use a contrast material to better demarcate the anatomic area of interest.

Digital pulsed fluoroscopy units are now the standard of care in children. These units emit a beam of photons only a fraction of the time compared with traditional continuous units, thereby dramatically reducing the radiation dose. Gonadal shielding and careful image coning also significantly decrease patient radiation exposure.

NECK/AIRWAY

Fluoroscopy is very useful in the dynamic evaluation of the airway, glottis, and diaphragm. While CT and MRI are gradually replacing fluoroscopy in evaluation of the tracheobronchial tree and soft tissues of the neck, it should be remembered that fluoroscopy of these anatomic locations requires no patient preparation or sedation and may provide valuable information. The natural difference between the density of gas in

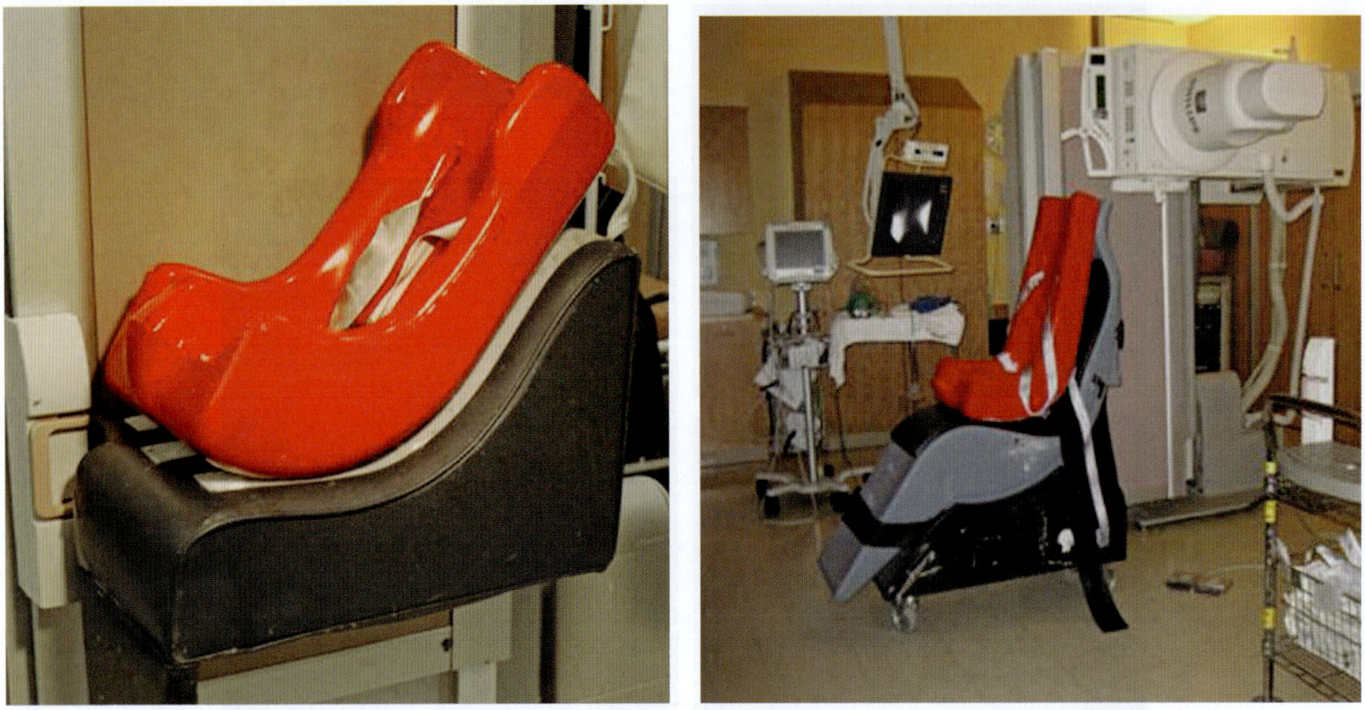

A B

FIGURE 185-5. During a modified barium swallow, children sit in special chairs affixed to the fluoroscopy table and consume various consistencies of solids and liquids mixed with barium. The infant (A) and child seat (B) are shown here.

the airways and lungs and the adjacent soft tissues provides the contrast for these studies; no additional contrast is necessary.

Fluoroscopy is a simple noninvasive test to evaluate children who are suspected of having aspirated a foreign body when plain radiographs are equivocal or further confirmation is necessary to look for air-trapping. In addition, fluoroscopy is frequently used for further evaluation after plain radiographs suggest a prevertebral soft tissue mass as well as to evaluate movement of the vocal cords and diaphragm.

MODIFIED BARIUM SWALLOW (SWALLOWING STUDY)

A swallowing study is performed to evaluate the oral and pharyngeal phases of swallowing and to detect the presence of aspiration with different consistencies of liquid and food. Often a radiologist and speech pathologist perform the exam jointly. All tested items are first mixed with barium, allowing their visualization with x-ray. Infants and young children sit in a specially designed chair affixed to the fluoroscopy table (**Figure 185-5**). Older children may stand during the exam. The parent or speech pathologist administers the various preparations to the child while the radiologist controls the fluoroscopy unit. Swallowing is observed with different consistencies of barium preparations, including solids, purees, and thick and thin liquids. The parent may provide favorite food items for testing, which has the dual benefit of replicating the child's home diet and increasing likelihood of patient cooperation.

ESOPHAGRAM (BARIUM SWALLOW)

Esophagrams evaluate the appearance and motility of the esophagus. Indications depend on the patient's age. Newborns are most commonly evaluated for symptoms of choking or wheezing—to look for a vascular ring or sling, esophageal stricture, or tracheoesophageal fistula. Older children with symptoms of dysphagia or a feeling that something is "stuck" in the throat may be assessed for abnormal esophageal motility, narrowing, or a foreign body obstructing the esophagus.

The examination is performed with the patient lying on the fluoroscopy table. In children, esophagrams are most often performed as single-contrast studies. In general, a child must be able to cooperate by drinking contrast and lying on the table. Infants can be fed barium via bottle or by injection into the mouth via syringe. In certain situations, such as evaluation for postoperative esophageal leak or tear, a nasoenteric tube can be inserted into the proximal esophagus to allow water-soluble contrast to be injected directly. This does not provide the same amount of information as a properly performed esophagram and is limited to use in specific clinical situations.

UPPER GI SERIES

An upper GI (UGI) examination studies the digestive system from the mouth to the duodenojejunal junction. This study is performed on an emergency basis in a child suspected of having malrotation with symptoms of obstruction (**Figure 185-6**), but it is more commonly ordered for evaluation of unexplained vomiting and detection of gastroesophageal reflux. It is useful for evaluating the esophagus, stomach, and duodenum and the location of the ligament of Treitz. Because the column of contrast is followed dynamically, peristalsis can be evaluated.

For patients suspected of having an obstruction at the level of the second portion of the duodenum (i.e. secondary to duodenal atresia, an annular pancreas, or a duodenal web), UGI examination may not be necessary; a plain film of the abdomen can be diagnostic when gas within the distended stomach and proximal duodenum serves as a contrast agent to delineate the level of obstruction.

The child must be able to drink oral contrast, or alternatively have contrast instilled via nasogastric tube or gastrostomy tube (this would preclude evaluation of the esophagus). The child must refrain from food or drink prior to the examination, as outlined in **Table 185-3**.

In general, a UGI series is performed with barium. Water-soluble contrast agents are preferred in recently postoperative patients or others where there is concern for intestinal perforation.

SMALL BOWEL SERIES

A small bowel series is used to evaluate the small intestine from the ligament of Treitz to the ileocecal valve. It is often performed in conjunction with a UGI series but can be performed separately. It is useful in evaluating the site of small bowel obstruction, small bowel masses, and inflammatory bowel disease.

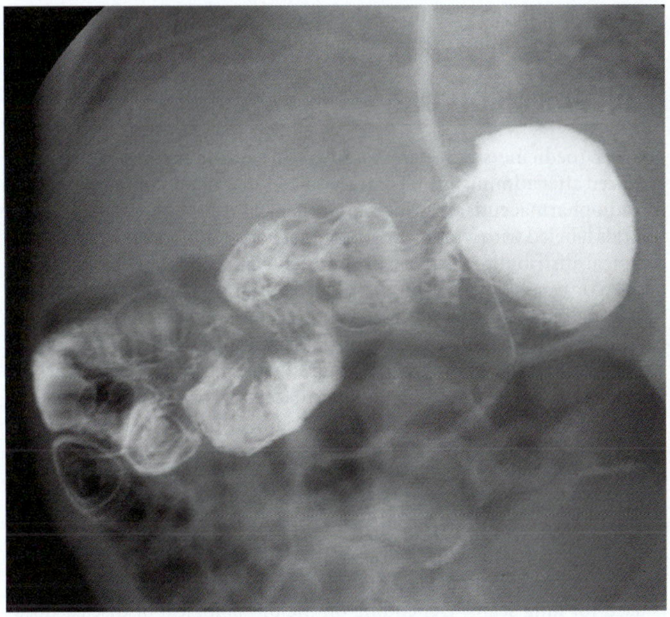

FIGURE 185-6. A single image from an upper GI in a patient with bilious vomiting demonstrates malrotation; the fourth portion of the duodenum does not reach the expected location of the ligament of Treitz to the left of the spine at the level of the pylorus.

The examination is performed almost exclusively with barium because water-soluble contrast tends to become diluted and lose its opacity before reaching the ileum. This examination requires a child to cooperate in consuming a large volume of barium in order to opacify the entire small bowel. Water-soluble contrast agents are used when the patient is recently postoperative or when there is concern for bowel perforation, to avoid barium peritonitis. The duration of this examination depends on the time needed for the contrast to pass through the small intestine, which can take many hours in some cases. Patients and families should be informed of the possibility that they may spend an extended period of time in the radiology department.

CONTRAST ENEMA

A contrast enema is most frequently indicated for the evaluation of distal intestinal obstruction in a newborn infant as occurs with Hirschsprung disease, ileal atresia, or meconium ileus. Older patients with a suspected mass, inflammatory bowel disease, or a stricture can likewise be evaluated with a contrast enema.

Bowel preparation is not required for most pediatric lower GI contrast studies. The exception is the rarely performed double-contrast (air and barium) lower intestinal study.

Prior to beginning the study, the radiologist will perform a brief rectal exam to exclude any obstructing mass or lesion, and then place a soft rectal catheter. Barium or water-soluble contrast is then instilled into the rectum by gravity technique through the catheter while fluoroscopic images are taken. At the conclusion of the study, contrast is drained from the patient.

INTUSSUSCEPTION REDUCTION

An important diagnostic and therapeutic use for GI fluoroscopy is diagnosis and reduction of ileocolic intussusception. Institutions may vary in the workup and management of suspected intussusception. Typically, an abdominal radiograph is performed as a screening examination. When the cecum is clearly identified or other causes of abdominal pain are revealed, further imaging may not be necessary. Alternatively, an abdominal radiograph may show definite evidence of intussusception. If plain films are unrevealing and additional imaging is needed, abdominal US is recommended. US can reliably demonstrate intussusception with high specificity and sensitivity. It can also evaluate for other causes of the patient's symptoms. Rather than obtaining a US examination, some pediatric radiologists prefer to proceed directly to an enema, which may both diagnose and reduce the intussusception (**Figure 185-7**).

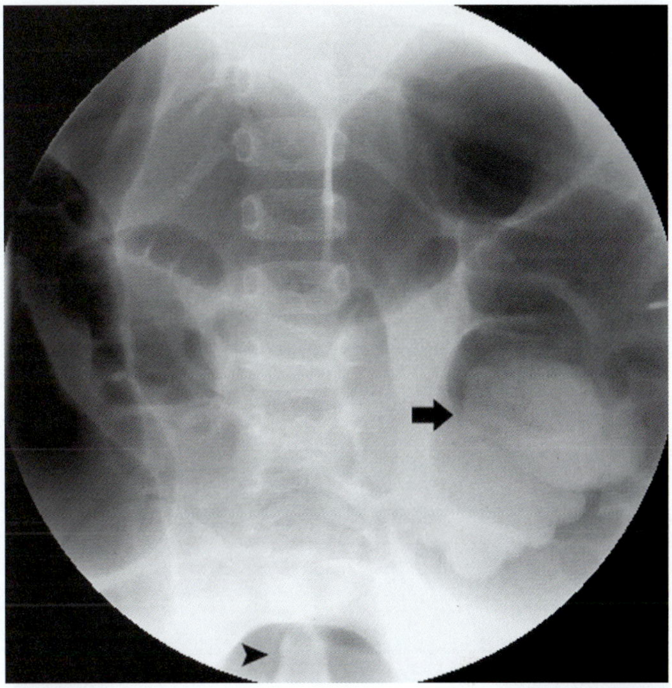

FIGURE 185-7. A single image from an air enema reduction of an intussusception demonstrates the intussusceptum as a soft tissue density within the colon (arrow). Air is being insufflated into the rectum via a soft catheter (arrowhead). This 2-year-old presented with intermittent abdominal pain and bloody stools.

A scout film of the abdomen is first obtained to evaluate for pneumoperitoneum. During the enema, a surgeon should be in attendance in the event of bowel perforation, tension pneumoperitoneum, and the need for emergency surgery.

The risks and benefits of the procedure are explained to the parents in detail before the examination, and informed consent is obtained. The patient should not be sedated because the instinctive Valsalva maneuver performed by a crying or agitated child provides both a natural protective mechanism to prevent bowel perforation as well as a higher pressure gradient to aid in reduction of the intussusception. Air or barium is instilled per rectum under fluoroscopic guidance. The pressure of the contrast or air reduces the intussusception. After the procedure, radiographs are obtained to assess for successful reduction and any complications. Contraindications to enema reduction are bowel perforation or signs of peritonitis. Ultrasound-guided hydrostatic reduction of intussusception is an acceptable alternative to fluoroscopic reduction, with the advantage of no radiation exposure, however the availability in the United States remains limited at this time.

TABLE 185-3 Timing for NPO Status Prior to Procedure

Newborn-6 months old	2 hours before the procedure
6 months-2 years old	3 hours before the procedure
2-4 years old	4 hours before the procedure
4 years or older	6 hours before the procedure

VOIDING CYSTOURETHROGRAM

The voiding cystourethrogram (VCUG) evaluates for vesicoureteral reflux (**Figure 185-8**) and the function and appearance of the bladder and urethra. This study is commonly performed in patients with a history of pyelonephritis or hydronephrosis. VCUG also can detail complex congenital anomalies such as ambiguous genitalia and anorectal malformations.

During the examination, the bladder is catheterized and dilute water-soluble contrast is instilled into the bladder through the catheter by

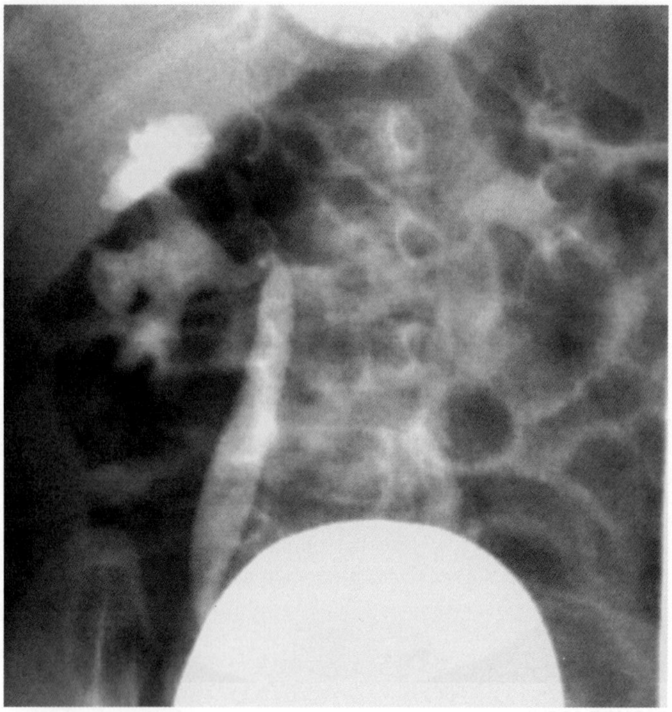

FIGURE 185-8. Voiding cystourethrogram image demonstrates bilateral vesicoureteral reflux, grade 3 on the right and grade 2 on the left. This child presented with a febrile urinary tract infection diagnosed by catheter specimen.

gravity. Fluoroscopy is performed during bladder filling and voiding. A cyclic study, when the bladder is refilled after voiding, is performed in infants. For older children, the bladder is typically filled one time only to its predicted capacity based on age.

When the study is performed in an environment comfortable for the patient, family, and physician and the parents and children are well informed and reassured, sedation can often be avoided. If sedation is used, midazolam and nitrous oxide can be administered without any negative outcome on the results of the examination.

Prophylactic antibiotics before VCUG, previously recommended for high-risk patients, are no longer recommended. Radionuclide cystography (RNC) is an alternative to VCUG for evaluating reflux and is discussed in the Nuclear Medicine section.

RETROGRADE URETHROGRAM

A retrograde urethrogram is performed in males to examine the anterior urethra only. The most common indication for this examination is evaluation for urethral trauma (**Figure 185-9**) or stricture. A catheter is gently placed in the very tip of the urethra, and contrast is then slowly introduced under fluoroscopic visualization.

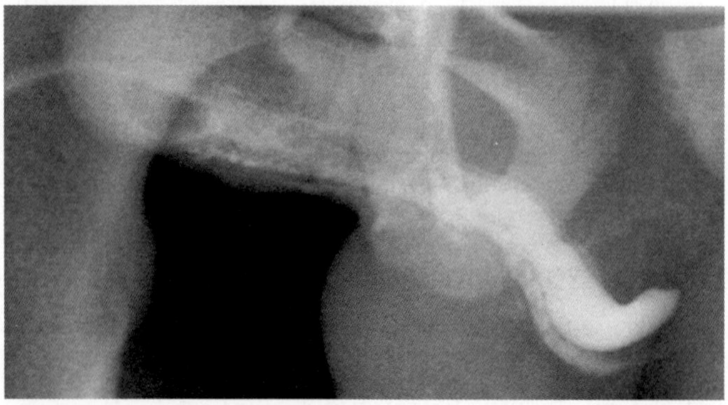

FIGURE 185-9. An oblique view of the urethra during a retrograde urethrogram demonstrates contrast extravasation along the course of the urethra due to a tear of the bulbar urethra. This boy suffered a skateboard injury.

NUCLEAR MEDICINE

Nuclear medicine studies are based on the tracer method. Images are acquired after administration of trace (picomolar or nanomolar) amounts of radiopharmaceuticals, which are organ- and function-specific compounds labeled with a radioactive isotope. Each radiopharmaceutical has a typical distribution pattern in the body, and alteration in either the pattern or time-course of this distribution can be a marker for disease or functional abnormality. Over 20 different radiopharmaceuticals are in routine use for imaging a wide range of conditions.

Nuclear medicine studies are acquired with a gamma camera, which can detect a wide variety of radiopharmaceuticals that emit low-energy gamma radiation. Most radiopharmaceuticals are labeled with the radioisotope technetium-99m, which has a half-life of 6 hours and a low-energy emission matched to the sensitivity of the gamma camera. Another common radioactive label is radioactive iodide (either iodine-123 or iodine-131), which is used to label some radiopharmaceuticals and also to image and treat thyroid diseases. Not all radiopharmaceuticals are administered via intravenous injection; xenon-133 gas is used for lung scans. Depending on the physiological or disease question, a nuclear medicine study can be performed as either a dynamic or intermittent static study. Images can be acquired of the whole body, of a specific region of the body, or as a magnified view of a small organ or body part. Single-photon emission computed tomography (SPECT) is an imaging method used to create three-dimensional images with a gamma camera. Occasionally additional drugs, such as furosemide or sincalide, are used as part of a nuclear medicine study. Another method of imaging nuclear medicine studies is positron emission tomography (PET). PET primarily is used to image radiopharmaceuticals labeled with fluorine-18, a positron emitter with a half-life of 110 minutes. Nearly all PET studies are performed with the radioactive glucose analog ^{18}F-fluorodeoxyglucose (^{18}F-FDG), which can be used to assess metabolic activity of tumors, the brain, and the heart.

Unlike many other imaging studies, nuclear medicine examinations provide both anatomic and functional information, but the anatomic resolution usually is not as high as with other radiological studies, such as CT or MRI. Co-registering nuclear medicine and either CT or MR images to create fusion images can provide additional information about both function and anatomy. Many nuclear medicine departments have hybrid cameras that can perform both a nuclear medicine study (SPECT or PET) and a CT during the same imaging study.

Most nuclear medicine studies require patient preparation specific to the study. This patient preparation is necessary to facilitate appropriate imaging of the physiological activity of interest. For example, many GI studies require a period of fasting. Most FDG-PET scans also require pre-test fasting to ensure appropriate physiological handling of the radiolabeled glucose. Other studies, such as renal studies, may require adequate hydration before the study is started. Overlying objects such as jewelry may interfere with imaging, but residual barium contrast from a prior radiographic study also can disrupt nuclear medicine imaging. Although nuclear medicine studies typically provide only low doses of radiation, the radiation exposure can be minimized by using radiopharmaceutical doses based on patient size and appropriate for children.

GENITOURINARY IMAGING

A variety of nuclear medicine studies demonstrate the form and function of the kidneys. These examinations may require venous access or bladder catheterization (or both) and hydration before the examination.

Dynamic Renal Scintigraphy Dynamic renal scintigraphy and diuresis renography are used to evaluate renal cortical function and the urinary collecting system. Dynamic renal scintigraphy is commonly used to assess hydronephrosis or hydroureteronephrosis, reflux nephropathy, and renal transplants. Occasionally, this study is used to evaluate acute renal failure or hypertension. Dynamic renal scintigraphy is performed with the radiopharmaceutical ^{99m}Tc- mercaptoacetyl-triglycine (^{99m}Tc-MAG3), which is excreted by active renal tubular transport.

^{99m}Tc-diethylene-triamine-pentacetic acid (^{99m}Tc-DTPA) is a less commonly used alternative to ^{99m}Tc-MAG3.

Dynamic renal scintigraphy depends on the rapid excretion of radiopharmaceutical through the kidney. This requires three steps: (i) renal perfusion and cortical uptake of ^{99m}Tc-MAG3, (ii) cortical transit of ^{99m}Tc-MAG3 into the renal collecting system, and (iii) excretion of ^{99m}Tc-MAG3 through the urinary collecting system. Imaging and quantitative measure of each of these steps provides information about renal function. The pattern of cortical uptake, which is measured during the first 2 minutes of the study, can identify regions of cortical hypoperfusion or scar as well provide a measure of differential (left vs. right) renal function. Although this provides an approximate differential function, a renal cortical scan will provide a more accurate indication of differential renal function. The rate of cortical transit, typically 3 to 6 minutes, is an indicator of renal function. The rate and pattern of ^{99m}Tc-MAG3 excretion is used to assess collecting system drainage. Delayed drainage may indicate collecting system obstruction but also may occur with low urine flow or in a markedly dilated collecting system. With diuresis renography, urine flow is increased, typically with intravenous saline infusion and intravenous administration of furosemide, to help distinguish collecting system obstruction from other causes of delayed collecting system drainage (**Figure 185-10**).

Several patient factors can confound interpretation of the studies. Infants, especially those younger than 1 month, have functionally immature kidneys, which may delay cortical uptake and excretion of radiopharmaceutical. In older children, impaired renal function can slow urinary excretion of radiopharmaceutical and limit evaluation of the urinary collecting system. Recent administration of radiographic contrast may transiently diminish radiopharmaceutical excretion.

Renal Cortical Scintigraphy Renal cortical scintigraphy is a static imaging study that provides both a visual and quantitated evaluation of renal cortical function. The main indications for cortical scintigraphy are evaluation of acute pyelonephritis or renal scarring and assessing differential (left vs. right) renal function. Renal cortical scintigraphy also is used to evaluate patients with renal ectopia or renal dysplasia.

Renal cortical scintigraphy is performed with the radiopharmaceutical ^{99m}Tc-dimercaptosuccinic acid (^{99m}Tc-DMSA), which is taken up and trapped in the cells of the proximal tubules. Images are acquired 3 to 4 hours after intravenous administration of ^{99m}Tc-DMSA. Images can be acquired in a variety of ways, including planar images, with a pinhole collimator, or by SPECT. These images can provide detailed function-structure information about the renal cortex. Cortical defects can be seen with cortical infarcts or scars as well as with other cortical lesions, such as tumors and cysts. Because ^{99m}Tc-DMSA is trapped in the renal cortex and excreted very slowly, renal cortical scintigraphy can provide a more precise measure of differential function than dynamic renal scintigraphy.

Radionuclide Cystogram RNC is performed to diagnose vesicoureteral reflux. Preparation and bladder catheterization of the patient are identical to that for VCUG, described earlier in this chapter. RNC usually is performed with the radiopharmaceutical ^{99m}Tc-pertechnetate, which is instilled through a urinary catheter into the bladder. In patients who have had bladder augmentation, the preferred radiopharmaceutical is ^{99m}Tc-pertechnetate–labeled sulfur colloid. Dynamic images are acquired by gamma camera to allow identification of vesicoureteral reflux of tracer.

The indications for deciding whether to perform RNC or VCUG to evaluate vesicoureteral reflux vary from institution to institution and from physician to physician. RNC is a very sensitive examination for determining the presence of reflux (**Figure 185-11**), and exposes the patient to a low dose of radiation. However, VCUG provides more detailed anatomic information about the bladder, sites of ureteral insertion, the male urethra, and the possibility of duplex collecting systems. The risks and benefits of each examination should be considered and the choice tailored to each patient.

Glomerular Filtration Rate Determination of glomerular filtration rate (GFR) uses the radiopharmaceutical ^{99m}Tc-DTPA, which is excreted solely by glomerular filtration. The patient should be well hydrated before the examination. After intravenous administration of ^{99m}Tc-DTPA, blood samples are obtained (usually at 2, 3, and 4 hours). The rate of radiopharmaceutical clearance is used to determine the GFR (mL/min). Alternative methods, such as 24-hour creatinine clearance, provide less precise measures of GFR. In children, GFR values may be expressed in terms of body surface area (mL/min/m^2) or in terms of the idealized adult body surface area (mL/min/1.7 m^2)

SKELETAL IMAGING

Bone Scintigraphy (Bone Scan) Bone scans are one of the most frequently performed nuclear medicine studies. One common indication for bone scan is osteomyelitis or evaluation for suspected bone infection in a child with fever. Sports medicine injuries, including possible stress fractures and lower back pain related to suspected pars interarticularis injury, are also common indications for a bone scan. Bone scans may be used to evaluate the skeleton in cases of suspected nonaccidental trauma (child abuse) (**Figure 185-12**). Other clinical indications for skeletal scintigraphy include avascular necrosis, osteoid osteoma, complex regional pain syndrome, and primary and secondary bone tumors.

Bone scintigraphy typically uses the radiopharmaceutical ^{99m}Tc-methylene diphosphonate. After intravenous administration of ^{99m}Tc-MDP, regional or whole-body scanning can be performed 2 to 3 hours later. ^{99m}Tc-MDP uptake is proportional to bone turnover or osteogenesis. Therefore, increased ^{99m}Tc-MDP uptake is seen at sites of

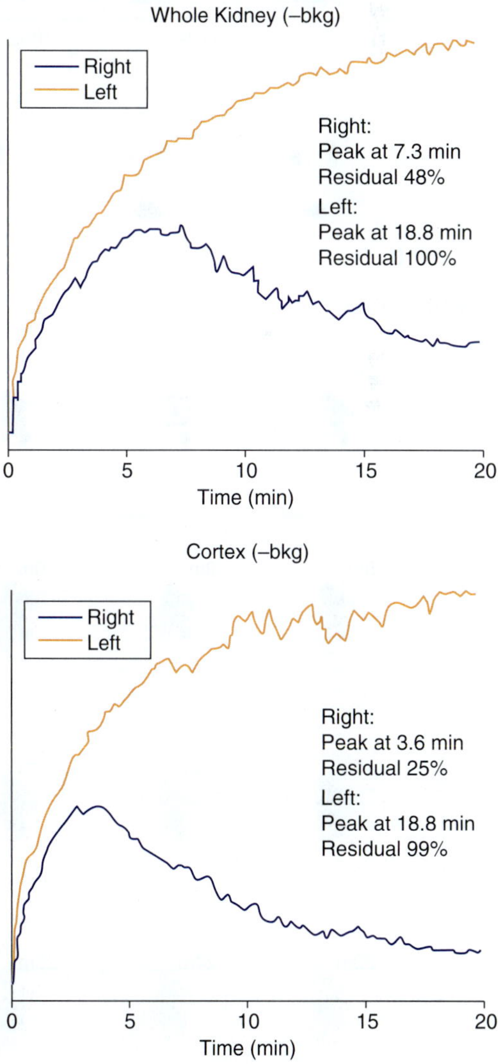

A

FIGURE 185-10. (A) Output results and (B) images from a MAG3 study demonstrate left-sided obstruction with a time activity curve showing that the half time of radiotracer excretion is greater than 20 minutes, or in the obstruction range. The curve for the right kidney is normal. It was known prenatally that the patient had left-sided pelvic dilatation.

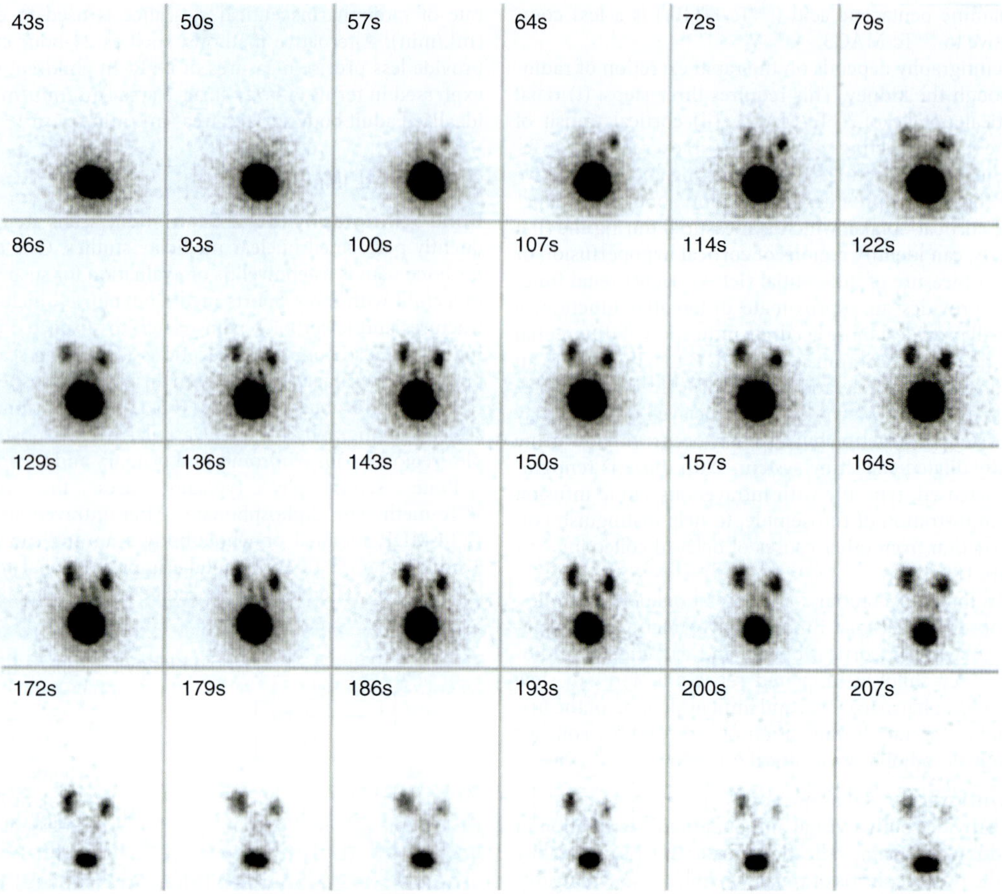

B

FIGURE 185-10. *(Continued)*

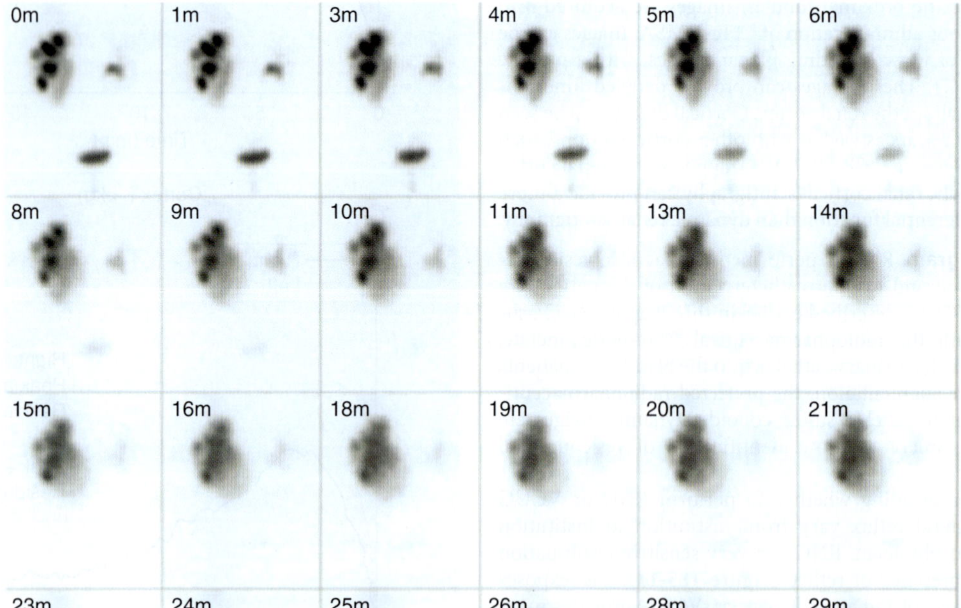

FIGURE 185-11. Selected images from a radionuclide cystography demonstrate bilateral grade 2 vesicoureteral reflux in a child whose sibling has reflux. The refluxed material drains promptly.

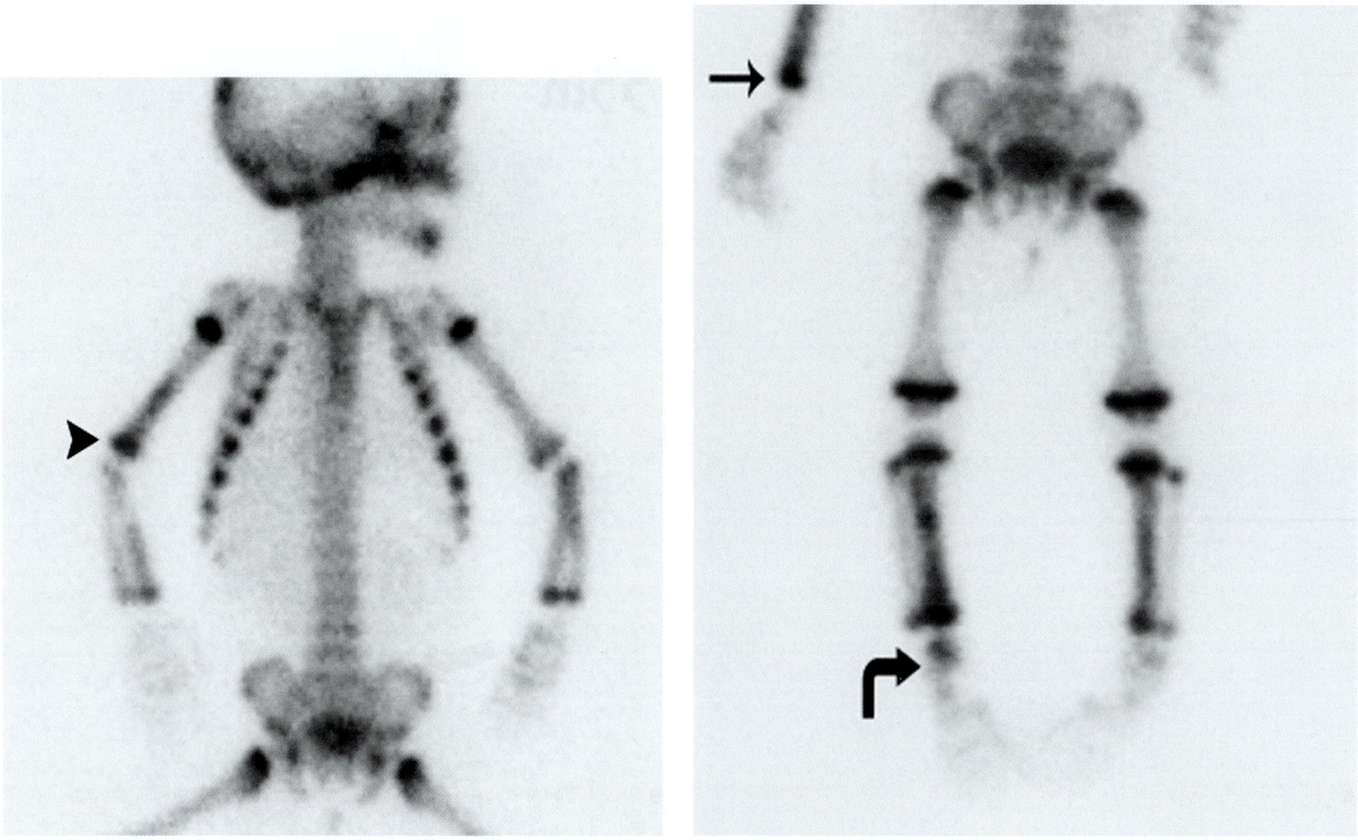

A B

FIGURE 185-12. Bone scan images of (A) torso and upper extremities and (B) pelvis, distal right upper extremity and lower extremities in a child who presented to the emergency room with lethargy. Increased radiotracer uptake is demonstrated in the (A) metaphysis of the right distal humerus (arrowhead) and (B) right radius (arrow), bilateral tibia and right talus (curved arrow).

increased bone turnover associated with bone stress, fracture, tumor, or infection. In children, increased uptake is seen at the physes (growth plates). Decreased bone uptake can be seen at sites of bone infarct/necrosis or lytic bone lesions.

A three-phase bone scan includes images acquired at three phases of bone uptake: (i) immediate perfusion, (ii) early soft tissue tracer accumulation, and (iii) skeletal-phase images acquired 2 to 3 hours after tracer administration. Typically, a three-phase bone scan is used to evaluate a specific bone site for possible osteomyelitis. Due to the increased local perfusion (hyperemia) associated with a bone infection, increased tracer is seen in images acquired at all three phases. Other causes of a positive three-phase bone scan can include tumors and acute fracture. Another indication for a three-phase bone scan is evaluation of complex regional pain syndrome (CRPS). CRPS is associated with regional changes in blood flow, the effects of which can be seen on all three phases of a three-phase bone scan. In adults, CRPS almost always is associated with regional hyperemia, with a three-phase bone scan showing increased perfusion, increased soft tissue accumulation of tracer, and diffusely increased skeletal uptake. Children with CPRS may have either increased or decreased regional perfusion in the affected limb.

Despite the examination's high sensitivity, bone scans are not highly specific because increased bone turnover is seen with many pathological processes, including bone stress, fracture, infection, and tumors. The pattern of abnormal uptake is important to determining the disease process. In some institutions, bone scans are performed using ^{18}F-sodium fluoride, which is imaged with a PET scanner. It is helpful to correlate findings on bone scan with the patient's age, clinical history, symptoms, and radiographs or other imaging studies. Additionally, the sensitivity and specificity of conventional radiographs can be increased with the addition of information from a bone scan. Abnormal findings on bone can guide a targeted evaluation with conventional radiographs.

HEPATOBILIARY IMAGING

Hepatobiliary Scan The hepatobiliary scan uses the radiopharmaceuticals ^{99m}Tc-disofenin or ^{99m}Tc-mebrofenin, which share the same hepatocyte uptake, transport, and excretion pathways as bilirubin. Therefore, hepatobiliary scans can be used to evaluate hepatocellular function and to assess excretion through the biliary tree and gallbladder. After intravenous administration of radiopharmaceutical, dynamic imaging of the liver and biliary system is performed for 1 hour.

In older children, a hepatobiliary scan is used to evaluate gallbladder function. In patients with typical acute calculous cholecystitis, cystic duct obstruction will prevent accumulation of radiopharmaceutical in the gallbladder. Gallbladder contraction will prevent filling, so patients must be fasting for at least 4 hours prior to hepatobiliary scan. However, prolonged fasting (greater than 24 hours) also may decrease gallbladder filling due to stasis of a filled gallbladder. Another cause of delayed gallbladder filling is chronic cholecystitis, so some departments will acquire additional images to evaluate for delayed gallbladder filling.

In pediatric patients, cholecystitis may not be associated with complete obstruction of the cystic duct. In patients with acalculous cholecystitis or with chronic cholecystitis, the gallbladder may fill with radiopharmaceutical, but will have impaired gallbladder contraction. Gallbladder function can be assessed by stimulating gallbladder contraction with a fatty meal or by slow intravenous administration of sincalide (an analog of cholecystokinin) and continuing gallbladder imaging for another 30 to 60 minutes.

In infants, hepatobiliary scans most commonly are used to evaluate suspected congenital biliary atresia or other congenital abnormalities of the hepatobiliary tree. Hepatobiliary excretion of radiopharmaceutical into the bowel demonstrates an intact biliary tree and essentially excludes the diagnosis of biliary atresia (**Figure 185-13**). Occasionally, hepatobiliary scans may be used to evaluate other abnormalities of the

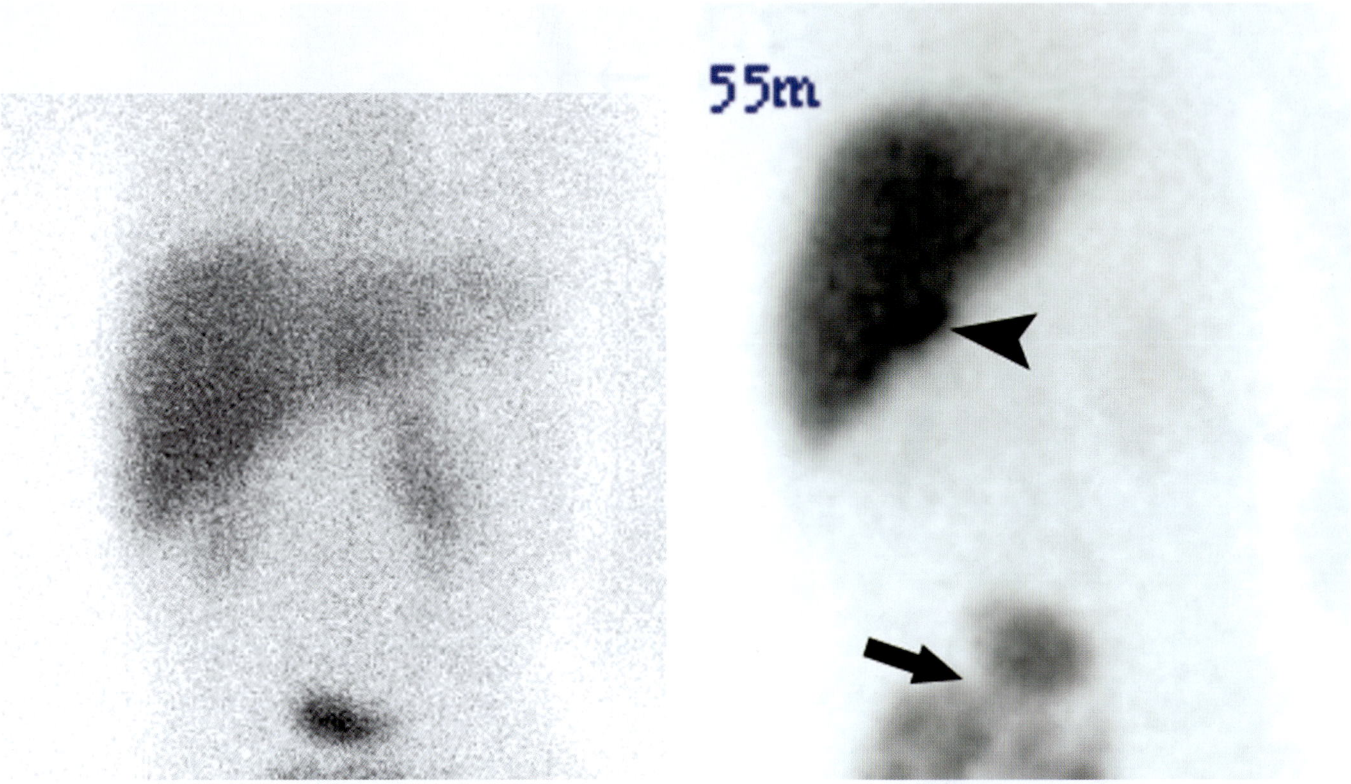

A B

FIGURE 185-13. (A) DISIDA scan of a 5-week-old with elevated direct bilirubin and non-visualization of the gallbladder on ultrasound demonstrates no radiotracer uptake in the gallbladder or bowel after 4.5 hours. The patient was pretreated with phenobarbital prior to the examination. Exploratory laporotomy demonstrated biliary atresia and the patient underwent a Kasai portoenterostomy. (B) In the example of a normal DISIDA scan, radiotracer is seen in the gallbladder (arrowhead) and within the bowel (arrow).

biliary tract, such as choledochal cysts. Patients undergoing evaluation for biliary atresia do not need to be fasting, but should be pretreated with phenobarbital for 3 to 5 days before the study to stimulate hepatocellular function, enhance biliary excretion, and increase the specificity of the study.

GASTROINTESTINAL IMAGING

A variety of nuclear medicine studies can be used to evaluate the GI system. For many studies the patient must fast for 4 hours before the examination. GI nuclear medicine studies should not be performed when there is residual barium contrast from prior radiographic studies.

Gastric Emptying Quantitative assessment of gastric function can be performed by observing the gastric emptying of a radiolabeled meal. A common meal is scrambled eggs labeled with ^{99m}Tc-labeled sulfur colloid, which will bind to egg proteins. Other suitable solid meals include foods with radiolabeled cheese. For adults, a standard mixed meal including radiolabeled eggs, bread, jelly, and water is now recommended. Infants and children with nasogastric or percutaneous gastric feeding tubes will require a radiolabeled liquid meal, such as milk or formula. The volume of feeding must be individualized and is determined in collaboration with the referring physician and family. A good rule of thumb is to provide a meal size similar to that typically associated with symptoms.

For pediatric gastric emptying studies, patients are encouraged to finish the radiolabeled meal within 10 minutes, and then dynamic imaging is performed for 1 hour. Region-of-interest analysis is used create a time-activity curve to quantify gastric emptying and evaluate the pattern of emptying. The pattern of gastric emptying is important, as rapid emptying or a lag-time with no gastric emptying may be abnormal. Solid meals typically show a linear pattern of gastric emptying, while with a liquid meal, the pattern of emptying should resemble an exponential decay curve. There are no generally applicable standard values for pediatric gastric emptying. This is due in part to the varieties of meal composition, patient positioning, and instrumentation among departments, but also reflects the difficulty in recruiting normal children for reference studies.

Gastroesophageal Reflux Gastroesophageal reflux can be assessed on a standard gastric emptying study. Gastroesophageal reflux may be identified by visual inspection or by region-of-interest analysis of the esophagus (**Figure 185-14**). If there is a high suspicion for tracheobronchial aspiration, it may be appropriate to perform a radionuclide salivagram before challenging the patient with a gastric emptying/gastroesophageal reflux study.

Radionuclide Salivagram A salivagram is the study of choice to assess for tracheobronchial aspiration of pharyngeal contents. Patients with difficulty handling their oral secretions or those suspected of aspiration are candidates for testing. The study is performed by placing a small drop of saline containing ^{99m}Tc-labeled sulfur colloid under or on the back of the tongue. Dynamic imaging is performed for up to 1 hour. Aspiration is demonstrated by tracer accumulation in the trachea or bronchial tree.

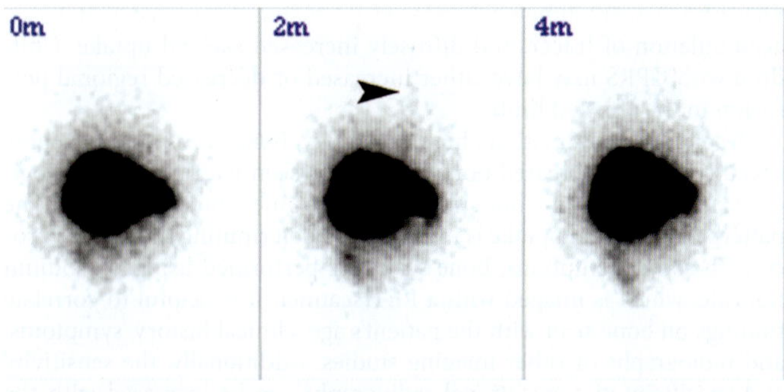

FIGURE 185-14. Selected images from a gastric emptying study demonstrate intermittent gastroesophageal reflux (arrowhead) in a patient with persistent vomiting after feeds.

Once aspiration is identified, continued imaging may demonstrate bronchial clearance of tracer.

Meckel Scan In children, the Meckel scan can be the first study of choice to evaluate GI bleeding. The Meckel scan is used to localize ectopic gastric mucosa that can be associated with intestinal ulceration and bleeding. Ectopic gastric mucosa typically is located in a Meckel diverticulum, but also can be found in intestinal duplication cysts. The scan is performed with ^{99m}Tc-pertechnetate, which accumulates in gastric mucosa. Uptake in ectopic gastric mucosa may be obscured by tracer accumulation in the urinary collecting system or by tracer excreted from the stomach into the duodenum. Tracer uptake also may be seen in inflamed intestinal mucosa. Rarely, active GI bleeding may be detected by accumulation of labeled blood within the intestinal lumen.

Gastrointestinal Bleeding Scan Active GI bleeding can be evaluated with a nuclear medicine bleeding study. The patient's own red blood cells can be labeled in vitro (outside the body) or in vivo (in the body). In vitro labeling is more specific and is associated with less background tracer activity, but requires handling and readministration of the patient's blood. With either technique, red blood cells are labeled with technetium-99m, and dynamic imaging is performed of the abdomen and pelvis. Typicalimaging time is 1 hour, but additional delayed imaging may be performed. Only areas of active bleeding during the time of imaging are revealed. In cases of intermittent bleeding, delayed imaging may help to identify a bleed up to 24 hours after injection. Delayed images will detect the presence of GI bleeding but will not be as useful in defining a location, due to normal movement of bowel contents.

PULMONARY IMAGING

Pulmonary nuclear medicine studies assess regional pulmonary blood flow and ventilation and are useful for a variety of clinical indications.

Lung Perfusion Scan A lung perfusion scan is performed after intravenous administration of ^{99m}Tc-labeled microaggregated albumin (^{99m}Tc-MAA), which is trapped in the capillary bed of the lungs. Particle accumulation is in proportion to pulmonary blood flow, which allows determination of differential lung perfusion (left vs. right) and regional perfusion within each lung. Transient capillary occlusion occurs in less than one in a thousand capillaries and is cleared within hours. The most common pediatric indication for a lung perfusion scan is the evaluation of children with congenital heart disease. If there is a right-to-left (pulmonary-to-systemic) cardiac shunt, a portion of the ^{99m}Tc-MAA particles will enter the systemic circulation. MAA particles will be trapped in proportion to perfusion. Because of this possibility of a cardiac shunt and due to the smaller number of pulmonary capillaries in the pediatric lung, fewer ^{99m}Tc-MAA particles are used in children, compared to adults.

Lung Ventilation Scan Ventilation scans usually are performed in conjunction with perfusion scans, but occasionally may be used to assess primary airway diseases, including cystic fibrosis, lobar emphysema, asthma, and pulmonary hypoplasia. A ventilation scan can be performed with inhalation of either xenon-133 gas or aerosolized ^{99m}Tc-DTPA. An advantage of Xe-133 is that, as a gas, dynamic imaging can be performed to assess regional ventilation, washout, and air trapping. Aerosolized ^{99m}Tc-DTPA clears too slowly for dynamic imaging, but does facilitate acquisition of multiple planar images to better localize ventilation defects.

Lung Ventilation/Perfusion Scan A combined V/Q scan of the lungs allows comparison between the patterns of perfusion and ventilation. In adults, this exam is most often performed to evaluate for pulmonary embolus. A pulmonary embolus will demonstrate a perfusion and ventilation mismatch, characterized by ventilation without perfusion. While this is a less common indication in children, the ventilation-perfusion scan is used to evaluate children with repaired congenital diaphragmatic hernia or complex congenital cardiopulmonary disease.

CARDIAC IMAGING

Pediatric cardiovascular nuclear medicine studies detect and quantify abnormal cardiac shunts, evaluate myocardial perfusion, determine cardiac output and ejection fraction, and demonstrate cardiac function and wall motion. Echocardiography and MRI are also used cooperatively in these indications.

Myocardial Perfusion Imaging In children with known heart disease, myocardial perfusion studies can provide useful clinical information. Myocardial perfusion is assessed with the radiopharmaceutical ^{99m}Tc-methoxyisobutyl isonitrile (^{99m}Tc-sestamibi; ^{99m}Tc-MIBI). Uptake of ^{99m}Tc-MIBI is relative to perfusion, so that regions of relative hypoperfusion will appear with decreased radiopharmaceutical uptake. Images are acquired with dynamic SPECT and with cardiac gating, which allows for assessment of possible abnormalities in cardiac wall motion. The usual approach is to perform gated cardiac SPECT during rest and then to repeat the study after a period of cardiac stress. The most common form of cardiac stress is exercise, using clearly defined protocols of treadmill exercise. Some patients, particularly younger children, may perform better with a bicycle exercise protocol. Pharmacological stress protocols are used in adults but are used very rarely in children. Regions of ischemia show decreased myocardial perfusion after stress compared to rest, while myocardial scars will have decreased perfusion with both studies. Using a gated study permits assessment of ventricular ejection fraction and cavity size at rest and after stress. Common indications for myocardial perfusion imaging include chest pain, trauma, cardiac transplantation, Kawasaki disease, and anomalous coronary arteries.

ENDOCRINE IMAGING

Thyroid Scintigraphy Thyroid scintigraphy can provide anatomic and physiologic information about the thyroid gland. The most common indication is evaluation of hyperthyroidism. Graves disease is characterized by increased autonomous iodine uptake, while subacute thyroiditis results in minimal iodine uptake. Other indications include evaluation of congenital hypothyroidism, localization of ectopic thyroid tissue, and rarely, evaluation of a thyroid nodule. For the most part, a thyroid scan should be used to evaluate a thyroid nodule only when it may be autonomous, as indicated by a suppressed serum TSH level. Thyroid scans can be performed with ^{99m}Tc-pertechnetate or radioactive isotopes of iodine, such as iodine-123 or iodine-131. Each radiopharmaceutical has potential advantages and disadvantages. Iodine isotopes have more specific thyroid uptake, with less uptake in tissues such as salivary gland. Iodine isotopes also permit quantitative assessment of iodine uptake, but ^{99m}Tc-pertechnetate usually provides a lower radiation dose. For most indications, iodine-123 provides the best balance of image quality and radiation dose.

Whole-body imaging with iodine-123 is used to evaluate patients with differentiated thyroid cancers, including papillary and follicular carcinomas. Whole-body scans are used to identify and localize remnant thyroid tissue in the neck and iodine-avid metastatic disease.

Appropriate patient preparation is necessary before performing thyroid scintigraphy. Patients with hyperthyroidism must discontinue antithyroid drugs, usually for 3 days before the study. Patients must avoid iodine uptake, both from foods and iodinated radiologic contrast. Iodine in a patient's body can lead to misleading results or interfere with thyroid scintigraphy. This is particularly important with thyroid cancer imaging. Most patients are placed on a strict low-iodine diet for 7 to 14 days and cautioned to avoid contrast-enhanced radiologic studies for 6 to 8 weeks prior to whole body imaging.

Parathyroid Gland Imaging Parathyroid scans are used to identify and localize abnormal parathyroid glands. Ultrasound also is used evaluate the parathyroid glands, and the most accurate localization of abnormal parathyroid tissue may be with the combined use of a parathyroid scan and US. Parathyroid imaging relies on the nonspecific uptake of ^{99m}Tc-methoxyisobutyl isonitrile (^{99m}Tc-sestamibi; ^{99m}Tc-MIBI) in mitochondrial-rich tissues such as adenomas. Because the adjacent thyroid gland also may take up ^{99m}Tc-MIBI, two strategies have been developed to increase the specificity for abnormal parathyroid glands. A dual-phase study images at two time points—typically 20 minutes and 2 hours after radiopharmaceutical administration. By 2 hours, ^{99m}Tc-MIBI will wash out of normal thyroid and parathyroid tissue but will be retained in most adenomatous tissue. This is the preferred method in most pediatric institutions. A second approach is the dual-isotope study, which combines a parathyroid scan with a thyroid scan. Image subtraction is used to identify abnormal parathyroid tissue. Both approaches have high sensitivity for parathyroid adenomas but will detect only about half of hyperplastic parathyroid glands. The most common indications for parathyroid imaging are evaluation for parathyroid adenoma in patients with primary hyperparathyroidism, and evaluation of patients with renal failure.

CENTRAL NERVOUS SYSTEM IMAGING

Nuclear medicine studies of the central nervous system are used in the evaluation of seizure disorders but also may be indicated for trauma and brain tumors.

Seizure Imaging Epileptogenic foci may be located using either brain SPECT or PET. Brain SPECT uses either ^{99m}Tc-ethyl cysteinate dimer (^{99m}Tc-ECD) or ^{99m}Tc- hexamethylpropyleneamine oxime (^{99m}Tc-HMPAO). For each, uptake is proportional to regional brain perfusion, which is increased during seizure (ictal) activity and relatively decreased during the interictal period. Uptake is rapid, and essentially occurs during the first pass after intravenous administration. When radiopharmaceutical is administered during an ictal event, increased perfusion leads to increased uptake and trapping of radiopharmaceutical in the region of the epileptogenic focus. Reliable imaging can be performed many hours after the seizure and radiopharmaceutical administration. Digital subtraction of ictal and interictal images may help to identify regions of increased ictal uptake (**Figure 185-15**).

PET is also used to evaluate children with refractory epilepsy who are being considered for surgical cure. Functional alterations related to ictal or interictal states can be detected with FDG-PET.

Brain Perfusion Brain SPECT using either ^{99m}Tc-ECD or ^{99m}Tc-HMPAO also can be used to assess cerebral perfusion in other conditions, such as moyamoya disease or in the determination of brain death. In some departments, brain perfusion is assessed with dynamic imaging after intravenous administration of ^{99m}Tc-pertechnetate. This approach provides a rapid and dynamic demonstration of brain perfusion but does not permit delayed brain SPECT.

Radionuclide Cisternography Normal and abnormal flow of cerebrospinal fluid (CSF) can be assessed by radionuclide cisternography. Indications for radionuclide cisternography include evaluation of communicating hydrocephalus, CSF leaks, and CSF shunt patency. This procedure also may be used to confirm normal CSF flow before intrathecal administration of chemotherapy. Imaging is performed after intrathecal administration of ^{111}In-DTPA either by lumbar puncture or through an indwelling intracranial catheter.

INFECTION IMAGING

Bone Scan Common indications for bone scans are osteomyelitis or evaluation for suspected bone infection in a child with fever (see Bone Scintigraphy).

White Blood Cell Scan The white blood cell scan images the accumulation of the patient's own white blood cells at a site of inflammation or infection. The white cells must be removed by phlebotomy, labeled with either technetium-99m or indium-111, and then reinfused into the patient's circulation. Depending on the radioisotope label, whole-body or regional scans may be acquired at 4 hours, 1 day, or 2 days after the labeled white blood cells are infused.

^{18}F-FDG PET or PET/CT PET or PET/CT with the radiopharmaceutical ^{18}F-FDG is becoming an alternative method of functional infection imaging. ^{18}F-FDG uptake by white blood cells at sites of inflammation and infection can provide a useful method for identifying sites of occult or multifocal infection. Patients must fast for at least 4 hours before radiopharmaceutical administration. In many children, intense uptake in brown adipose tissue (BAT) can interfere with interpretation of the study. Uptake in BAT is enhanced by cold exposure, and may

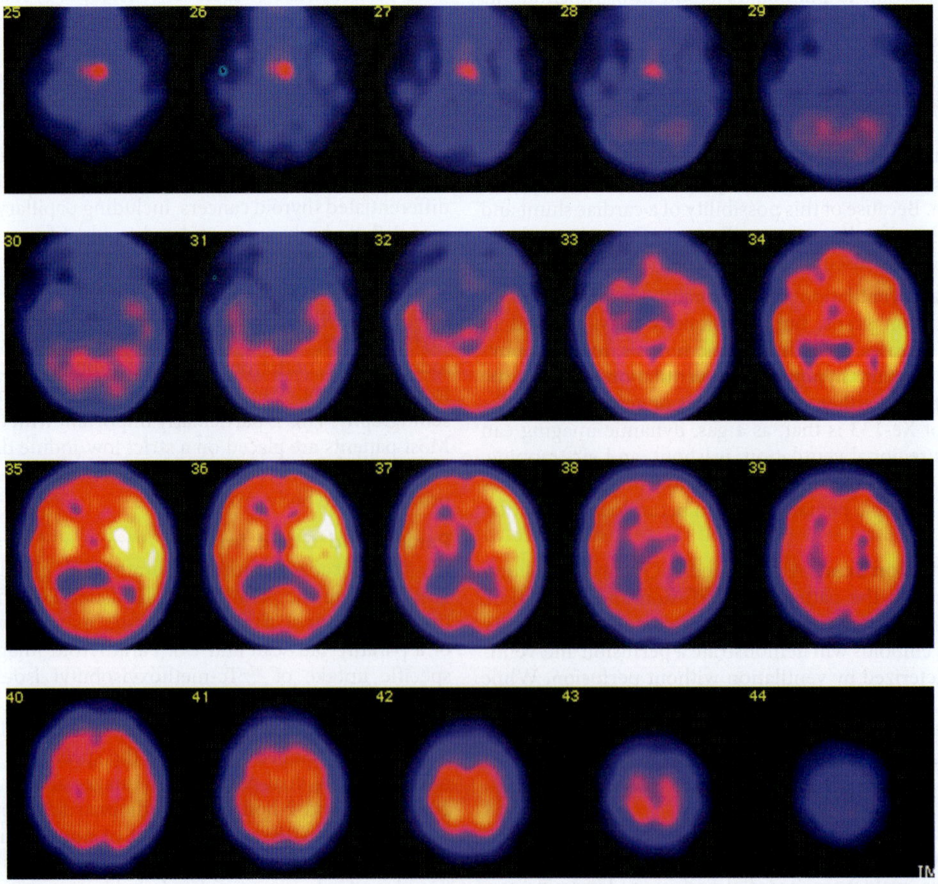

FIGURE 185-15. SPECT images from a brain scan obtained in the interictal state in a child with seizures demonstrates marked asymmetric uptake in the left temporal lobe.

be more prominent in children, females, and lean patients. BAT uptake can be decreased by having patients dress warmly while traveling to the department before the study, but this may not minimize the problem. Most pediatric nuclear medicine departments have protocols that heat the patient in a warm room or use pharmacological intervention to minimize interference from BAT.

TUMOR IMAGING

A variety of radiopharmaceuticals can be used for the evaluation of tumors based on the tumor type and location. Although many tumor-specific agents have been used in the past, the majority of pediatric tumor imaging now uses PET with ^{18}F-FDG.

^{18}F-FDG PET or PET/CT Most functional pediatric tumor imaging uses PET or PET/CT with the radiopharmaceutical ^{18}F-FDG. Tumor viability is assessed by using ^{18}F-FDG uptake as an indicator of tumor metabolic activity and may have a utility for imaging lymphomas, most solid tumors, and brain tumors. Depending on tumor type, FDG-PET may be most useful for staging, assessing response to therapy, and/or follow-up surveillance for tumor recurrence. Patients must fast for at least 4 hours before radiopharmaceual administration. In many children, intense uptake in BAT can interfere with interpretation of the study (see above for additional details).

MIBG Scan Metaiodobenzylguanidine (MIBG) is an analog of norepinephrine that can be radiolabeled with either iodine-123 or iodine-131 and used to image sympathochromaffin tissues. Due to better image quality, ^{123}I-MIBG usually is the radiopharmaceutical of choice. The primary pediatric indication for ^{123}I-MIBG imaging is neuroblastoma (**Figure 185-16**), but occasionally it may be used to identify or localize a pheochromocytoma or paraganglioma. I-MIBG is more specific than CT or MRI for preoperative and postoperative evaluation of neuroblastoma. Images are acquired 1 day after intravenous administration of ^{123}I-MIBG. Imaging typically includes a whole-body scan acquired either as a whole-body sweep or multiple static images. In most cases, SPECT is performed of the torso. Numerous medications can interfere with tumor uptake of MIBG, and the patient's medications must be evaluated carefully before MIBG imaging.

^{111}In-Pentreotide (Octreoscan) Scan Pentreotide is a ligand for somatostatin receptors that usually are located on neuroendocrine tumors, including carcinoid tumors and gastroenteropancreatic tumors. Imaging typically is performed 1 day after administration of ^{111}In-pentreotide and includes whole-body and SPECT imaging. Radiopharmaceutical excretion in the gut may interfere with imaging abdominal disease. Therefore, some departments also will acquire images of the torso at 4 hours or 2 days after ^{111}In-pentreotide administration. Another approach is to use a bowel preparation, such as an osmotic laxative or polyethylene glycol solution, to clear residual radiopharmaceutical from the bowel.

Bone Scan ^{99m}Tc-MDP (see Skeletal Imaging) is used for the evaluation of primary bone tumors, especially osteosarcomas and metastatic bone tumors. Tumors with increased osteogenic activity cause areas of increased radiotracer uptake on bone scans. Tumors that cause pure osteolysis demonstrate decreased uptake, but this is rarely encountered by bone scan. Occasionally, skeletal imaging will use ^{18}F-sodium fluoride, which is imaged with a PET scanner.

Gallium Scan In the past, gallium-67 scintigraphy frequently was used for tumor imaging. It was useful for evaluation of Hodgkin and non-Hodgkin lymphoma, infections, and nonmalignant conditions such as sarcoidosis. For the most part, gallium scans have been replaced by FDG-PET scans, which can provide higher image quality and lower radiation dose. Gallium scans are still used for tumor evaluation when PET or PET/CT is not available.

COMPUTED TOMOGRAPHY/COMPUTED AXIAL TOMOGRAPHY

CT or computed axial tomography (CAT) scans, like conventional radiographs and fluoroscopy, create images based on the variable absorption of x-rays by different body tissues. Differences in tissue density and

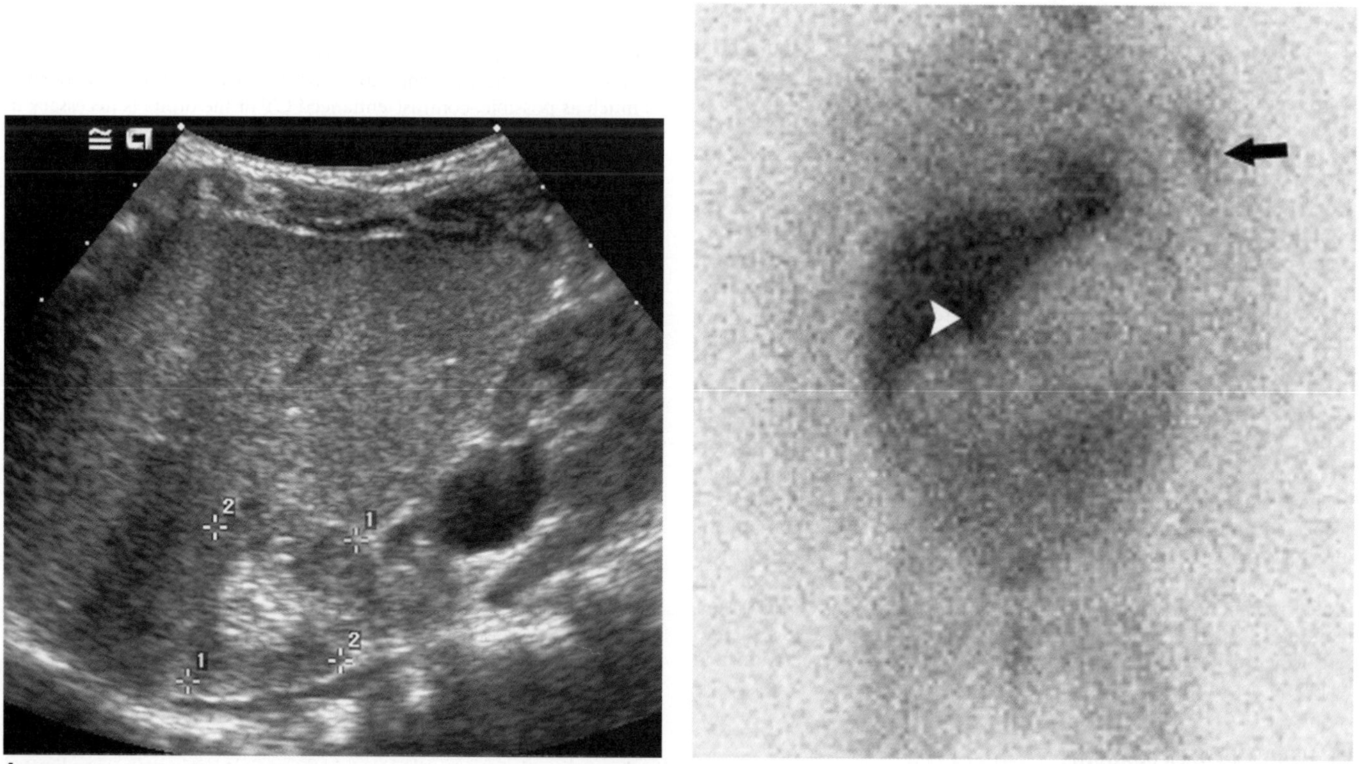

A B

FIGURE 185-16. This 6-month-old underwent a renal ultrasound for follow-up of prenatal renal pelvic dilatation. (A) US demonstrates an echogenic mass cephalad to the right kidney (marked). (B) An MIBG study demonstrates abnormal radiotracer uptake in the area seen on US (arrowhead), and in the left humerus (arrow). This patient had metastatic neuroblastoma.

composition affect the ability of x-rays to pass through the body, and ultimately create images.

CT is widely available, and image acquisition is rapid. In a critically ill patient, all life support systems are compatible with the CT scanner, unlike MRI, which has restrictions regarding metallic objects in the scanner area.

During a CT scan, the patient lies flat in the bore of the scanner while the x-ray tube rotates around. A ring of detectors replaces the film used in conventional radiography. In recent years, the number of rings or rows of detectors continues to increase, which has decreased scan time considerably while also potentially increasing the radiation dose if adjustments are not made.

During a CT examination, the patient must hold still, which with new-generation scanners can frequently be accomplished with minimal or no sedation. CT scan times are now often only seconds long, but any motion during the scan can degrade the imaging. Therefore, careful assessment of a child's ability to hold still before examination is recommended.

CT scans have excellent spatial resolution, and large areas of the body may be rapidly imaged. With the data acquired, images can be reconstructed in many planes and formatted to enhance the conspicuity of soft tissues, bones, or vascular structures. The ease and speed of obtaining this type of information need to be weighed against the patient's potential radiation risk and the cost of the examination.

The diagnostic accuracy of most CT scans is improved with contrast agents. The appearance of bowel without contrast may mimic or disguise pathology. Bowel contrast agents can be given by mouth or via stomas, nasogastric or gastric tubes, or rectum, according to the indication. The quantity depends on the patient's age. Patients may also receive intravenous contrast to enhance the conspicuity of vascular and soft tissue structures. Required contrast flow rate varies with the type of exam requested, and an IV of appropriate gauge must be placed prior to the study. Patients with previous contrast allergies need to be premedicated (see prior section on Contrast Agents), or other tests should be considered.

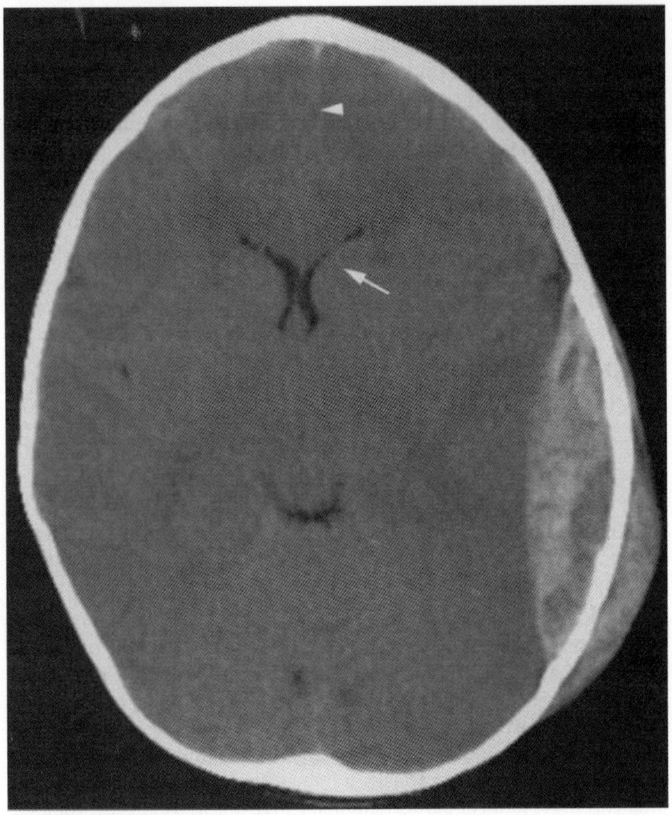

FIGURE 185-17. A large epidural hematoma is causing mass effect with minimal splaying of the falx to the contralateral side (arrowhead), and mild effacement of the left frontal horn (arrow). This hematoma was associated with a skull fracture. The patient was brought emergently to the operating room following the CT scan.

BRAIN IMAGING

Head CT is often requested in the pediatric population for the evaluation of acute change in neurologic status. For the evaluation of trauma, head CT is the imaging modality of choice. CT is excellent for the evaluation of intracranial hemorrhage (**Figure 185-17**). CT is also the preferred imaging modality for the evaluation of intracranial calcifications. With CT, beam-hardening artifact can limit assessment of the posterior fossa and temporal lobe regions.

In children with shunted hydrocephalus, head CT is often the most rapidly available imaging modality with which to assess ventricular size if shunt malfunction is suspected, although this has been supplanted in some institutions by rapid-sequence MRI. In the evaluation of these patients, it is imperative to compare the current examination with prior neuroimaging, and every effort should be made to acquire these studies from outside institutions if necessary.

Head CT may be performed with or without the administration of an intravenous contrast agent. Depending on the urgency of the examination, our practice is to administer contrast in cases in which treatment may be altered immediately based on the findings; for example, in the evaluation of an extra-axial abscess. In cases in which a lesion is suspected on CT and contrast would aid in further evaluation but the information is not going to change the immediate course of management (e.g., tumor requiring further characterization), administering contrast is deferred and instead, brain MRI is obtained. Increasingly, MRI is supplanting CT as the initial test for many neurologic indications such as sensorineural hearing loss, spondylolysis, hydrocephalus evaluation, and head and neck tumors.

HEAD AND NECK IMAGING

CT is particularly useful in the evaluation of trauma or infection involving the head and neck. The exam should be limited to the anatomic area of interest. Imaging data can and should be reconstructed in multiple anatomic planes. Three-dimensional models are now easily created and may help in surgical planning.

Contrast is administered in most cases of suspected infection. Although exposing the orbits to ionizing radiation should be avoided as much as possible, contrast-enhanced CT of the orbits is necessary in cases of suspected deeper extension of orbital cellulitis, where there is a potential risk for loss of vision (**Figure 185-18**).

Temporal bone CT is frequently part of the workup in cases of sensorineural or conductive hearing loss.

CT of the paranasal sinuses is indicated in cases of chronic or complicated sinusitis. The raw data obtained from the axial images is used intraoperatively to guide the surgeon during functional endoscopic sinus surgery.

Superficial neck masses can be easily evaluated by US, which is generally the initial study of choice. Following US, some surgeons may request neck CT because it allows easier assessment of the surrounding anatomic structures. Contrast-enhanced neck CT is useful for the evaluation of any neck mass and can distinguish the many reactive lymph nodes located in this region in a pediatric patient versus a mass lesion of another cause (**Figure 185-19**).

SPINE IMAGING

Spine CT is a vital adjunct in the workup of spinal trauma. To keep the radiation dose as low as reasonably achievable, only the area of clinical concern should be scanned. In the setting of trauma, images of the cervical spine obtained at our institution are limited to the area of concern. This same concept holds true for imaging the lumbar spine in cases of suspected trauma or spondylolysis. At times patients have previous plain radiographs or bone scans that can aid the radiologist in scanning a limited area of interest; if these are not available, relying on the referring clinician's assessment of the level of concern is necessary. Larger portions of the spine are sometimes imaged for preoperative planning in patients with severe

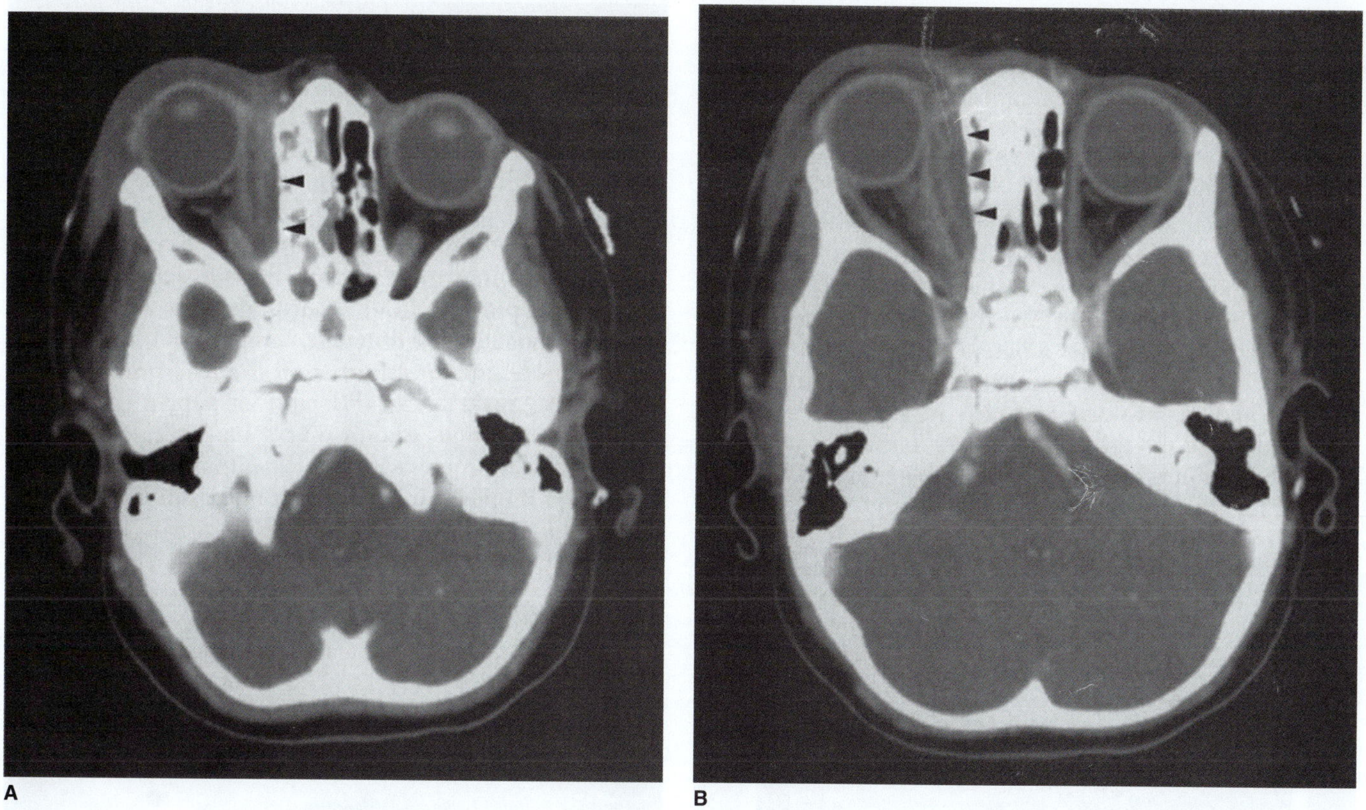

FIGURE 185-18. Contrast-enhanced axial images through the orbits demonstrate right-sided preseptal soft tissue inflammatory changes, proptosis, with mass effect on the globe from the adjacent subperiosteal abscess (arrowheads). These findings are secondary to spread of infection from adjacent sinusitis; note the opacification of the right-sided paranasal sinuses.

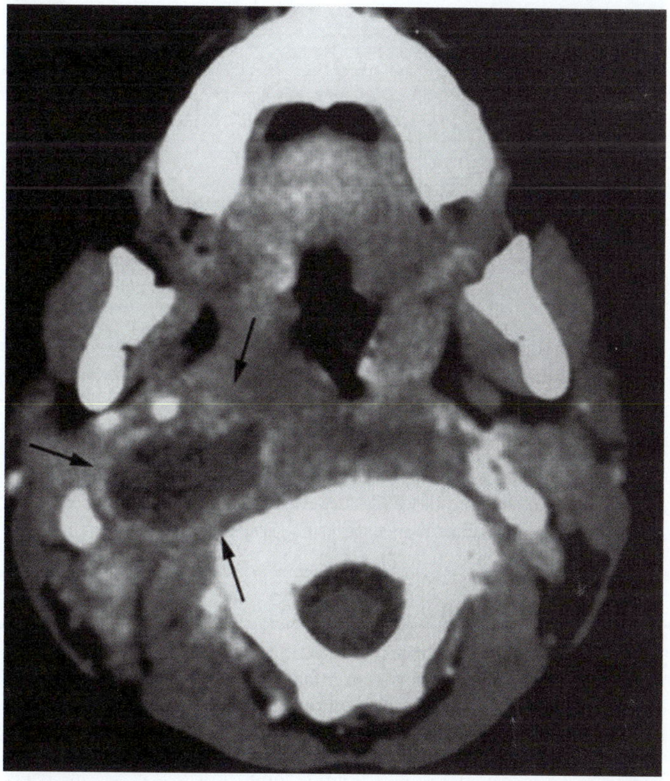

FIGURE 185-19. A contrast-enhanced axial image through the neck demonstrates a low-density lesion in the right lateral retropharynx with scalloping wall enhancement, consistent with an abscess.

scoliosis, where the formation of a three-dimensional model is very helpful to the surgeon. For evaluation of the intervertebral disks or paraspinal soft tissues, MRI should be performed (discussed later in this chapter).

CHEST AND CARDIOVASCULAR IMAGING

Indications for chest CT are evaluation of the lung parenchyma, mediastinum, pleural spaces, soft tissues, bones, and cardiovascular structures (**Figure 185-20**). Because of the natural density difference between normal lung parenchyma and abnormal soft tissues within the lung, studies to evaluate the lungs often do not require intravenous contrast. High-resolution images are useful to assess for interstitial lung disease. Evaluation of the mediastinum, great vessels, pulmonary masses, and pleural disease typically requires intravenous contrast administration. The use of CT to assess heart disease is controversial in children because of the high radiation dose, and is most commonly used when there are contraindications to MRI.

ABDOMEN/PELVIS IMAGING

Indications for abdominal and pelvic CT are numerous. However, because US is non-irradiating and does not require sedation, it is the study of choice for the initial investigation of most abdominal and pelvic abnormalities in children (**Figure 185-21**). US and MRI are superior to CT in evaluation of the uterus and ovaries. Administration of bowel and intravenous contrast is typically required for imaging the abdomen and pelvis, with the exception of evaluating renal stone disease.

EXTREMITY IMAGING

The ability to create multiplanar reconstructions makes CT ideal for the evaluation of complex fractures, especially before surgery as well as congenital anomalies (**Figure 185-22**). After surgery, metallic hardware

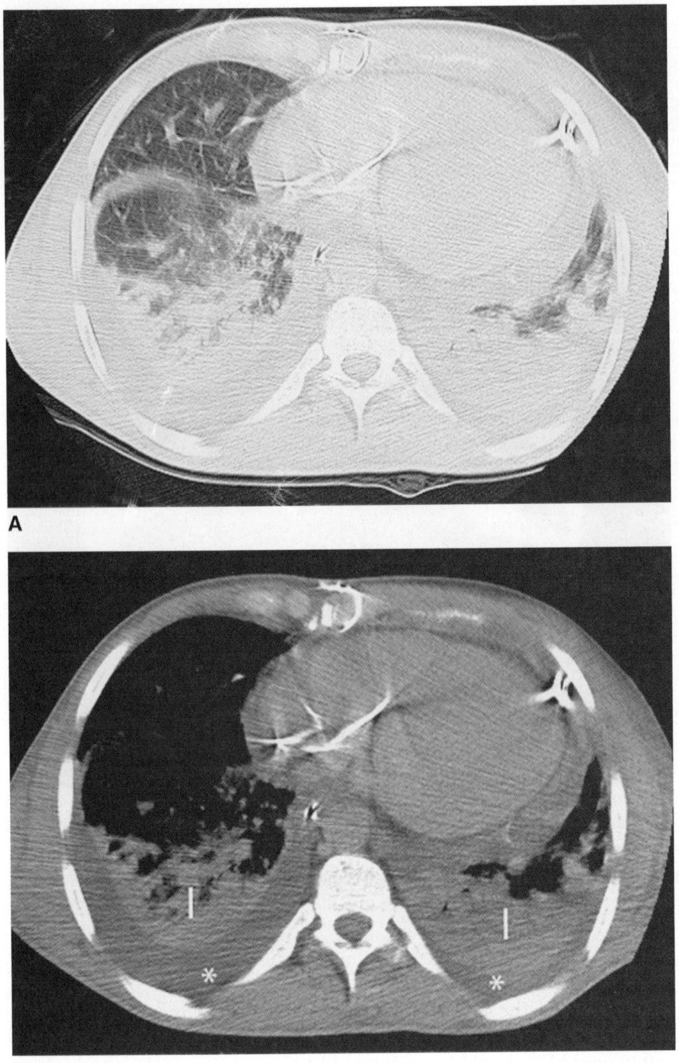

FIGURE 185-20. CT scan of the chest. These axial images of the lower chest demonstrate the difference in lung and soft tissue windows. This patient has a history of congenital heart disease and presented with sepsis from bilateral pneumonia. (A) The lung windows emphasize the lung parenchyma. (B) The soft tissue windows help to distinguish the different soft tissues, including the consolidated lung (l) and pleural effusions (*) bilaterally.

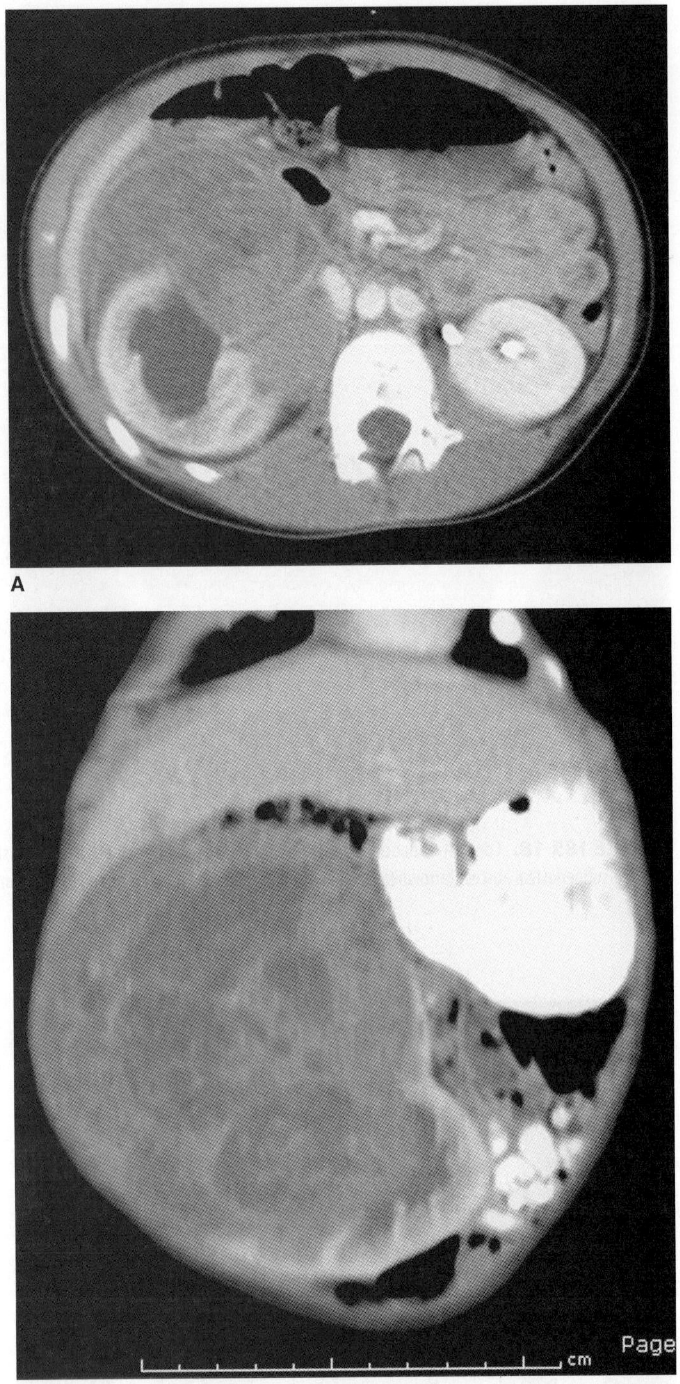

FIGURE 185-21. (A) An axial image of a large mass, likely renal in nature is seen here. With a reformatted image in the coronal plane (B), the tumor can be seen in its craniocaudal extent with a rim of renal parenchyma visualized at the inferior aspect of the mass, confirming its renal origin, consistent with a Wilms tumor in this young child.

artifact may obscure bony and soft tissue detail. CT and MRI may help better characterize bone lesions that do not have a typical plain film appearance. Masses within the soft tissues of the extremities are usually better characterized by US or MRI than by CT.

ULTRASOUND

Ultrasound is the most common cross-sectional imaging modality in children due to its wide availability, relative affordability, dynamic imaging, and lack of ionizing radiation. Rarely does a child need to be sedated for an US. US produces images based on the different reflectivity of sound waves that each tissue inherently possesses. This is the examination of choice for the pediatric abdomen and pelvis, gonads, infant hips, neonatal brain, and neonatal spine. US can be used to assess blood flow and is an excellent noninvasive test to evaluate the patency of arteries and veins throughout the body. US also provides images in real time, which is extremely useful in evaluation of the bowel and heart. Cardiac US, or echocardiography, is not discussed in this section. Most US examinations do not require patient preparation, with the exception of abdominal and pelvic US, which are discussed later in this section.

HEAD ULTRASOUND

Ultrasound plays a major role in evaluation of the neonatal brain, particularly in a premature or near-term infant who is critically ill and cannot be transported to radiology or cannot undergo a lengthy examination such as MRI. US may be performed at the bedside, is quick, and provides crucial information needed to manage some of these patients.

Sonography of the brain is possible until the anterior fontanelle is too small to image through; the age at which this occurs is variable. Although the fontanelle may not completely close until 18 to 24 months, image quality is significantly degraded much sooner secondary to the size of the

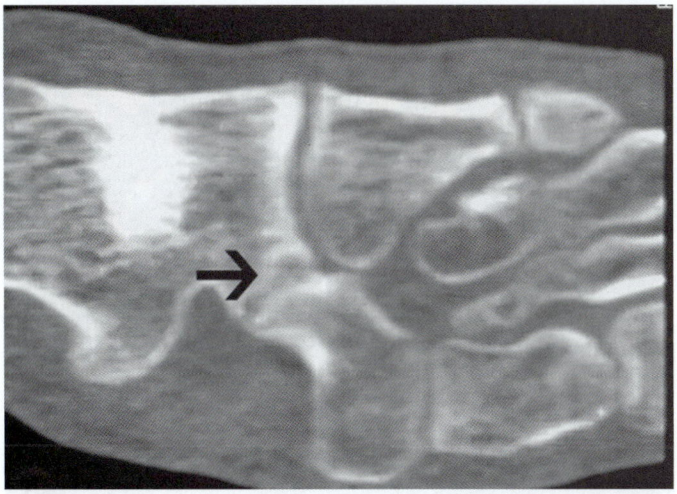

FIGURE 185-22. CT reconstruction. An oblique sagittal reconstruction of the tarsal bones demonstrates a membranous talonavicular coalition (arrow) in a patient who presented with a painful flatfoot.

transducer required to obtain images, often by 12 months. Imaging via the anterior fontanelle is used first and foremost because it is the largest nonossified membranous junction of the parietal bone. To better assess the posterior fossa, the sonographer may also attempt imaging through the posterior fontanelle or posterolateral (mastoid) fontanelle if these are patent.

Head US is mostly used to evaluate for the presence of intracranial hemorrhage at the germinal matrix (**Figure 185-23**) and periventricular leukomalacia in preterm infants. More definitive characterization of periventricular leukomalacia suspected on US may be made with MRI when the patient is stable. Serial US examination in a patient known to have an intracranial hemorrhage can be used to monitor ventricular size and spare the patient the exposure to ionizing radiation that would be incurred if head CT were used.

Head US may also be used for the evaluation of parenchymal calcifications or septations in a cyst, both of which may be too small to be seen with CT or MRI. US is useful in the evaluation of midline congenital anomalies, vascular malformations, and extra-axial collections.

Not only is a gray-scale index used to evaluate the brain parenchyma, but color Doppler imaging capabilities also make evaluation of intracranial arteries and veins possible. Color Doppler imaging plus real-time examination capability makes it possible to evaluate change in intracranial arterial parameters in response to increased intracranial pressure.

NECK ULTRASOUND

Ultrasound is an excellent initial tool for evaluation of neck masses. It is commonly used to distinguish lymphadenitis from other neck masses such as a congenital cyst, lymphatic malformation, or neoplasm. With color Doppler, increased or decreased vascularity of a neck mass may be demonstrated and can aid in determining the cause of the mass. If the initial US provides a diagnosis, further evaluation with CT or MRI could be avoided along with potential complications from sedation, contrast, or radiation exposure (in the case of CT).

SPINE ULTRASOUND

Ultrasound of the spine is performed until the posterior elements ossify, between 2 and 3 months of age. Beyond this age, full visualization of the contents of the canal may not be possible. Appropriate indications in a neonate include a suspected tethered cord, fatty filum, or distal thecal sac mass. US examination of the lumbar spine is frequently requested because a sacral dimple or pit or a hairy patch is found on neonatal physical examination. A study demonstrated that the vast majority of spinal US performed for sacral dimple were normal or revealed sonographic abnormalities that did not result in neurologic sequela. This study recommends that patients with physical exam abnormalities or any neurologic signs or symptoms associated with occult spinal dysraphism be evaluated with lumbar spine US due to its relative convenience and safety.

ABDOMEN AND PELVIS IMAGING

Abdominal Ultrasound A so-called "complete abdominal US" primarily evaluates the upper abdomen and includes images of the liver, gallbladder, pancreas, spleen, kidneys, bladder, portions of the aorta and

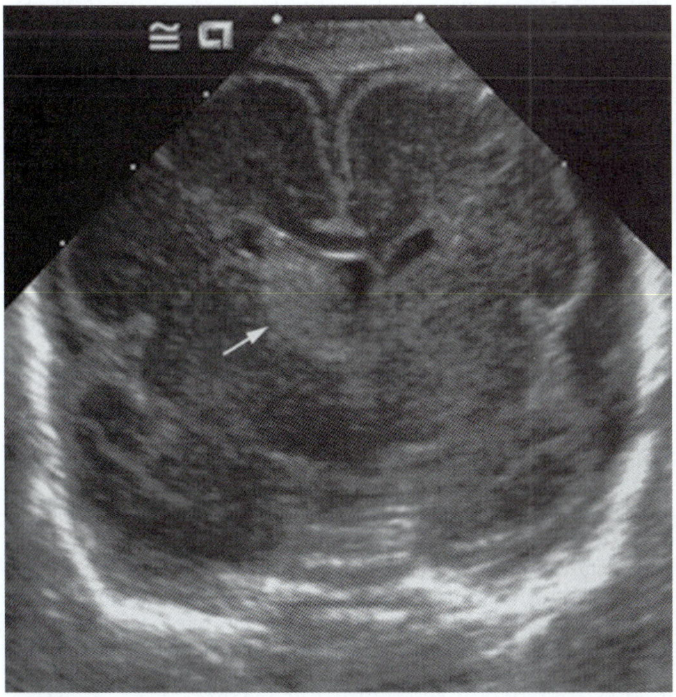

A

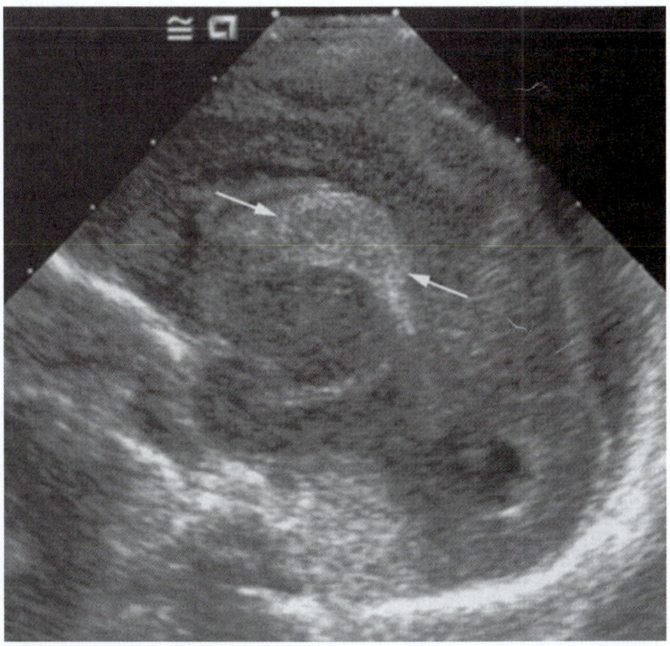

B

FIGURE 185-23. (A) Coronal and (B) sagittal views, respectively, from a head ultrasound show a relatively large bleed (white arrow) at the caudothalamic groove (2 white arrows).

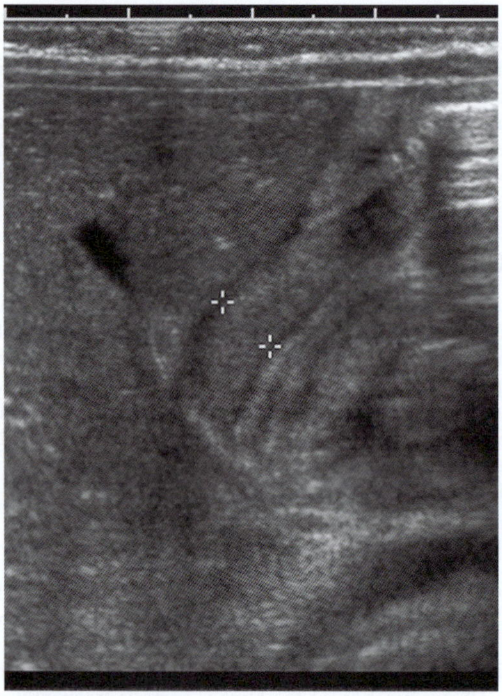

FIGURE 185-24. Ultrasound image of the right upper quadrant in a 4-week-old boy with projectile vomiting demonstrates pyloric stenosis. The thickened muscularis of the pylorus (marked) measures greater than 3 mm.

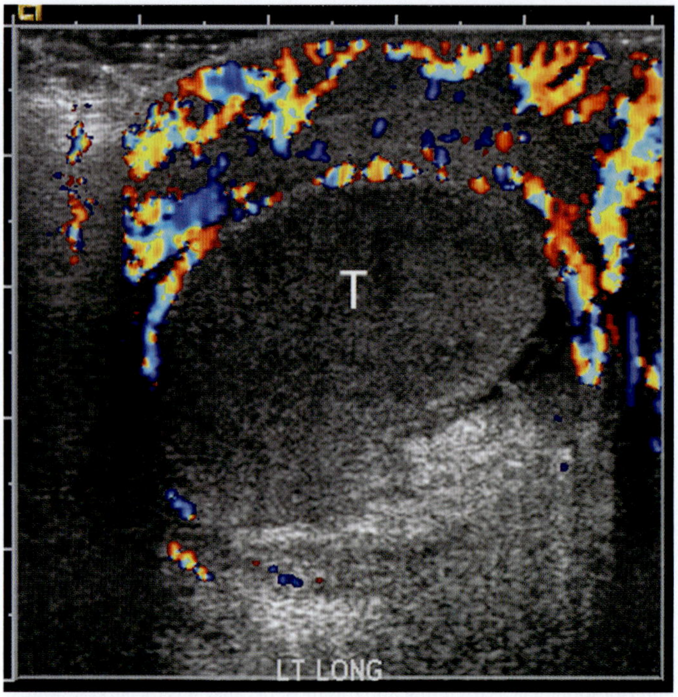

FIGURE 185-25. Ultrasound of the left scrotum in a boy who presented with acute left scrotal pain demonstrates skin thickening and hypervascularity surrounding the testicle, which shows no internal flow by color Doppler. At surgery, the patient was found to have testicular torsion.

IVC, and a general sweep of the abdomen and pelvis for ascites. The size and configuration as well as blood flow, of these organs is examined in real time, and masses can be excluded with this imaging modality.

More limited exams are also frequently obtained for particular clinical indications, with a focus only on the right upper quadrant or kidneys, for example. US can be useful in evaluation of the bowel, especially in the evaluation of pyloric stenosis (**Figure 185-24**), intussusception, appendicitis, and bowel wall thickening. Ultrasound also has an increasing role in the monitoring of inflammatory bowel disease in children.

Patients need to fast for 2 to 6 hours prior to an upper abdominal US, depending on the age and indication. The main deterrents to obtaining diagnostic-quality images are bowel gas, large body habitus, and difficulty positioning the patient.

Pelvic Ultrasound Ultrasound is useful in the initial evaluation of pelvic pain, pelvic mass, amenorrhea or dysmenorrhea, and müllerian duct anomalies. It is the best imaging modality for the evaluation of suspected ovarian torsion. MRI is also useful in evaluation of the female pelvic organs, and is discussed later.

For pelvic US in females, a full urinary bladder is the best way to view the pelvic organs. A full urinary bladder is also useful to evaluate the bladder itself. As with US of the upper abdomen, bowel gas, large body habitus, and difficulty with patient positioning may limit diagnostic yield. Additionally, in the pelvis, an underfilled urinary bladder may prevent adequate visualization of the pelvic organs.

The uterus and ovaries can be evaluated by transabdominal scanning, with a full urinary bladder used as the acoustic window, as discussed earlier. Additional transvaginal images are often obtained in sexually active females, as they provide more detailed images of the endometrium and adnexa. This is especially important in cases of early pregnancy when ectopic pregnancy is being considered.

EXTREMITY AND SUPERFICIAL ORGAN IMAGING

Ultrasound is useful in the evaluation of palpable soft tissue masses anywhere in the body, including the extremities, to determine whether they are solid, cystic, or vascular (or any combination) in nature. The use of US in evaluation of the musculoskeletal system has increased significantly in recent years. Ultrasound is also very useful to evaluate superficial organs such as the thyroid gland or testes. The combination of high-resolution imaging and no ionizing radiation makes US especially ideal in examining the testes. US is the best imaging modality for the evaluation of a painful scrotum and easily distinguishes testicular torsion (**Figure 185-25**) from other causes of pain.

MAGNETIC RESONANCE IMAGING

MRI creates images through the manipulation of magnetic fields. No ionizing radiation is required. Natural differences in water content cause various tissues to respond differently to an applied magnetic field and allow creation of detailed images.

MRI studies vary in length, but most take at least 30 minutes to complete, often longer depending on the sequences required. Individual sequence time varies widely, but is generally in the range of 2 to 8 minutes. During this time, the patient must lay still within the bore of the magnet. Even a small amount of motion may cause enough degradation of image quality that an entire sequence needs to be repeated. Depending on the age of the patient, sedation or even general anesthesia may need to be administered to obtain images of diagnostic quality. For a newborn, the "feed and wrap" method is an alternative to sedation. The bore of an MRI is smaller than that of CT and some with even mild claustrophobia have difficulty completing the exam. Sedation should be considered for these patients as well. Open-bore MRI machines are sometimes available; however, the image quality varies widely and discussion with the radiologist regarding the indication for the exam and the appropriate choice of magnet is recommended.

Metal within a patient's body, in the form of an implanted medical device, such as a pacemaker, or residua from prior injury, such as bullet fragments, can cause not only artifact on images and destruction of the device, but physical damage to the patient through superheating. Prior to scheduling a patient for MRI, one should carefully screen for the possibility of indwelling metal. In the case of medical devices, the device maker should have easily accessible information regarding MRI compatibility of the device. Prior successful completion of an MRI study is not evidence that the device is compatible and should not be taken as such. As the magnet is always on, a magnetic field exists around the MRI scanner even

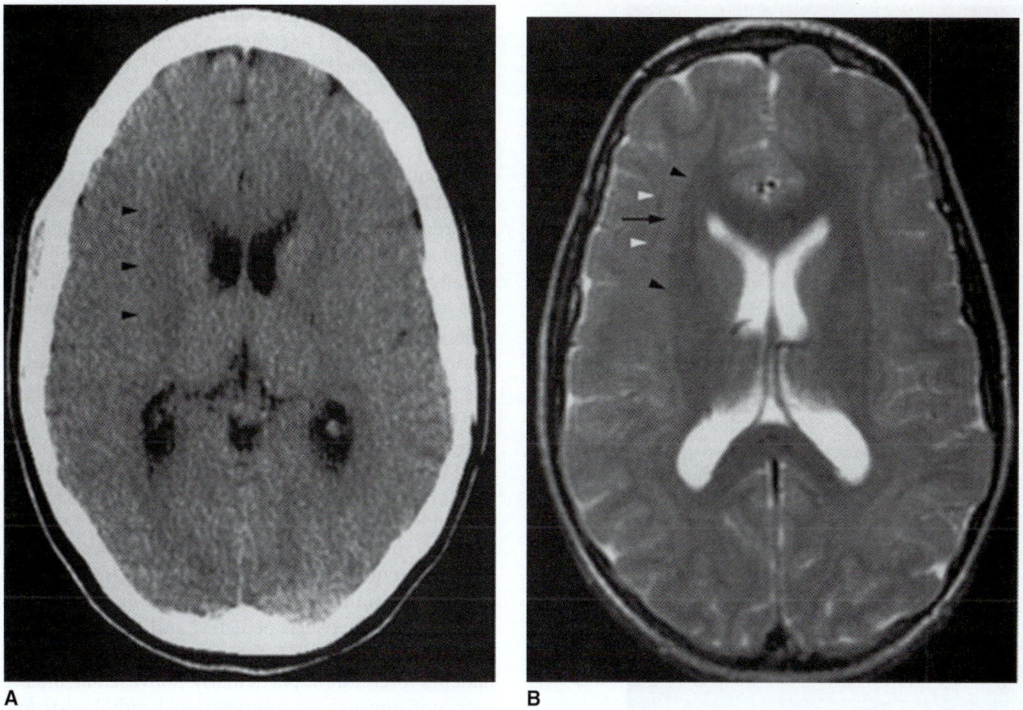

FIGURE 185-26. (A) Head CT of this child with seizures does not show the white matter to extend well into the periphery, as it should, but rather shows the low density of the white matter located more centrally (white arrowheads). This patient has band heterotopia, also known as double cortex, better depicted on brain MRI. (B) Shows white matter (black arrowheads) followed by a "band" of cortex (black arrow), followed by a thin layer of white matter (white arrowheads), followed by cortical gray matter as one proceeds peripherally.

when no exam is being performed. Every person who enters the examination room must be cleared before entering. This includes hospital staff as well as parents who might like to accompany their child during the exam.

BRAIN IMAGING

Brain MRI provides superb depiction of brain parenchyma, making it possible to diagnose subtle lesions and evaluate small structures that might be missed with CT. MRI also provides superior evaluation in regions where one is limited with CT because of beam-hardening artifact; specifically, the temporal lobe or posterior fossa. MRI diagnosis of ischemia and infarction is often straightforward. Because of the clear demonstration of myelination patterns, MRI exceeds any imaging modality for the evaluation of developmental delay. Almost any white matter abnormality is best evaluated with MRI. MRI is the gold standard for evaluation of the brain parenchyma when imaging is indicated in the workup of a patient with seizures (**Figure 185-26**). Although CT is useful in the acute management of any patient with new signs or symptoms that suggest the possibility of an intracranial lesion or mass, brain MRI is often necessary to better distinguish not only the lesion but also the lesion's effects on adjacent parenchymal structures.

FACE/NECK IMAGING

Face or neck lesions, or both, in the pediatric population are frequently examined with MRI because of its excellent soft tissue differentiation, especially when intracranial extension is suspected; for example, with skull base, nasal, or orbital lesions. In addition, if cross-sectional imaging of an isolated neck mass is needed and the patient has a contraindication to the administration of iodinated contrast for CT, MRI or US should be performed instead.

SPINE IMAGING

The indications for spine MRI are vast, and include evaluation of developmental abnormalities, neoplasm or, increasingly, scoliosis. Spine MRI is also used for the evaluation of any inflammatory process, whether it involves the vertebrae or is located deeper in the central canal (i.e., osteomyelitis or transverse myelitis, respectively) (**Figure 185-27**). In the evaluation of spinal ligamentous injury after trauma, MRI is also superior to CT despite the latter's superior ability to detect fractures. Certain sequelae of spine trauma such as nerve root avulsion can be depicted with MRI as well. Finally, for any pediatric patient with back pain, MRI may be indicated in the search for an intraspinal or paraspinal mass.

CARDIAC/CHEST/VASCULAR IMAGING

MRI is useful for the evaluation of cardiac, vascular, and soft tissue structures of the chest. CT currently remains superior to MRI in evaluating parenchymal lung disease.

Cardiovascular anatomy, cardiac function, perfusion and blood flow, and pulmonary vascular anatomy can be assessed with cardiac MRI, an examination that complements echocardiography. Cardiovascular imaging is performed with cardiac gating, which means that images are timed to the cardiac cycle. Because patient cooperation is crucial and breath holding is often required, young or uncooperative patients typically undergo general anesthesia for cardiovascular imaging.

Although CT scans are often the initial cross-sectional imaging modality for evaluating noncardiac anatomy of the chest, MRI is particularly useful for evaluating the mediastinum and soft tissues of the chest wall. Chest MRI is excellent in the evaluation of congenital abnormalities of this region, such as bronchopulmonary foregut malformations.

Vascular imaging throughout the body can be achieved with or without the use of gadolinium intravenous contrast. MR angiograms and MR venograms are excellent noninvasive studies for assessing vascular anatomy and patency.

EXTREMITY IMAGING

One of the most common indications for MRI is evaluation of the extremities. MRI is used to evaluate the joints for bony, ligamentous, tendinous, and cartilaginous injury. It is very useful in evaluating the composition and extent of soft tissue and bony masses and infections.

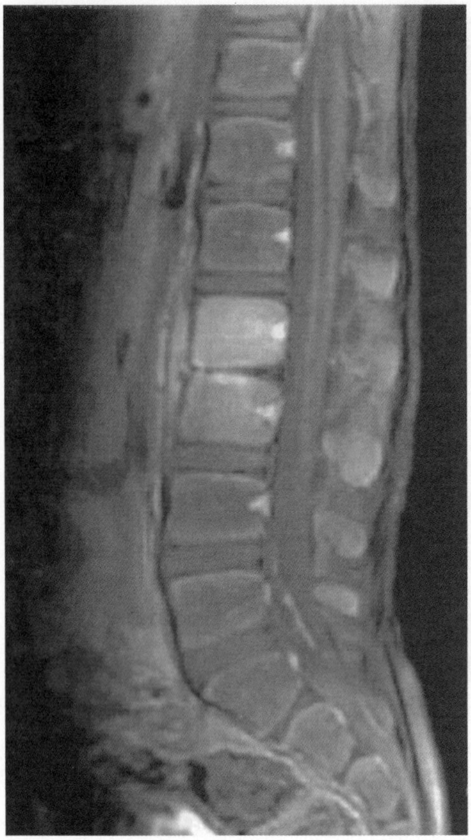

FIGURE 185-27. This sagittal T1-weighted post-contrast image of the lumbosacral spine shows abnormal enhancement involving the L2 and L3 vertebrae with abnormal enhancement involving the prevertebral soft tissues and a marked decrease in the disc height at this level. These findings are consistent with vertebral osteomyelitis/discitis. There is no evidence of epidural extent of the infection, but the disc minimally bulges posteriorly.

ABDOMEN AND PELVIS IMAGING

Like CT, MRI offers multiplanar evaluation of the abdominal and pelvic solid organs, the bowel, the peritoneal cavity, surrounding soft tissues, and bones. Abdominal imaging with MRI is well established and is particularly valuable in evaluation of the liver, biliary tree, and pancreas. MRI has also become a valuable method for evaluation of bowel disease in children, such as in the setting of Crohn's disease. MRI is superior to CT for evaluation of the female pelvic organs and is a useful adjunct to US of the pelvis. CT and US are often preferred over MRI because MRI is more time consuming and thus more often requires sedation, is more costly, and is less available.

INTERVENTIONAL RADIOLOGY

Image-guided therapy and interventions, which are minimally invasive, have a low risk for complications and morbidity. On an outpatient basis, interventional radiologists now perform many procedures previously done surgically and requiring a lengthier hospital admission. With new advances in this field, the radiologist can not only provide diagnostic information but also deliver primary therapy in many instances and frequently during the same visit. The possibility of diagnosis and treatment in one setting is important to consider, especially if the patient will need sedation under general anesthesia. Consultation with the interventional radiologist is important for comprehensive patient care. In the workup of complex cases, multiple subspecialty consultation along with the interventional radiologist may be needed.

There are important differences that arise when interventional radiology procedures are performed on pediatric versus adult patients. The first involves sedation and anesthesia. Many procedures, although minimally invasive, are painful. Certain procedures also stand a greater chance for success with a quiet, still patient. With this in mind, procedural sedation and anesthesia are far more frequently administered to pediatric patients. Not only does one need to administer the appropriate sedative in these cases so that the patient remains motionless as for other diagnostic imaging studies, but administration of an analgesic is also usually necessary. In general, the level of sedation is usually deeper for interventional radiology procedures, and general anesthesia is frequently administered, thereby increasing the overall risk associated with the procedure. In addition, patients in a hospital setting requiring an interventional radiology procedure have a far more complex medical history and usually have acute pathology, which in turn further increases the overall risk associated with the procedure when combined with the need for sedation. The overall risk should always be weighed against the benefits gained by performing the particular interventional procedure. Consulting the anesthesiologist and interventional radiologist during complex clinical scenarios cannot be stressed enough. In some children's hospitals, there is an anesthesiologist dedicated to the interventional division. This person is familiar with the various procedures performed and tailors the sedation to the particular case being performed.

In addition to differences in sedation between pediatric and adult patients, there are differences related to iodinated contrast administration, technique, and equipment needed to perform a given procedure, not to mention the overall differences in pathophysiology and differential diagnoses between pediatric and adult disease. Nonetheless, many of the interventional techniques are directly transferable from adult patients to children, particularly nonvascular interventions. It is, however, not unusual for interventional radiologists and surgeons trained and experienced with adults to refer pediatric patients to a pediatric specialist for image-guided procedures because of the aforementioned issues. Conversely, pediatric interventional radiologists may not be facile in all interventional radiology techniques, and collaboration with their adult counterparts is common. It should be noted that there are very few dedicated training programs in pediatric interventional radiology, and these specialists primarily practice at tertiary pediatric referral centers.

Another issue regarding pediatric interventional procedures relates to radiation exposure. Many adult interventional radiologists use fluoroscopy and CT as image guidance modalities for the sake of speed and ease of use; they tend to use US guidance less frequently. Typical radiation doses for an adult interventional procedure can sometimes be unacceptable for a pediatric patient. To avoid ionizing radiation, most pediatric interventional radiologists use US whenever possible. Altering the fluoroscopy and CT parameters during interventional procedures also helps in decreasing the overall radiation dose to the patient. Given the possibilities of extended exposure time during complex procedures, patients are counseled and occasionally consented for radiation exposure risk.

VASCULAR PROCEDURES

Diagnostic Angiography Diagnostic angiography is less commonly performed in the pediatric population because of the availability of less invasive modalities such as CT or MR angiography. Still, this procedure remains the gold standard for the diagnosis of vascular diseases. Some of the indications for conventional angiography in children include localization of hemorrhage, complications of organ transplantation, and the workup of vascular malformations. Important precautionary measures need to be taken during this procedure for a pediatric patient because the risk for complications, particularly those related to the puncture site (i.e., vasospasm with the potential for arterial thrombosis), is higher than in an adult patient. This procedure is contraindicated in a patient who is medically unstable. Relative contraindications include substantial electrolyte imbalance, cardiac arrhythmia, a documented serious reaction to contrast administration, impaired renal status, coagulopathy, inability to lie flat on the table, residual barium in the abdomen, and pregnancy. A comprehensive clinical history and physical examination, with special attention to the common femoral and more distal arterial pulses, should be obtained. Screening laboratory studies may include a complete blood count (CBC), chemistry, prothrombin time (PT), partial thromboplastin time (PTT), and international normalized ratio (INR). All patients require some form of sedation, particularly to reduce motion artifact during imaging. Previous imaging studies, when necessary, should be available. Informed consent for the procedure is necessary. The interventional radiologist performing the procedure should obtain this consent so that the procedure itself, its benefits and risks, and any questions can be fully discussed. Preprocedural medications such as antibiotics are not routinely used.

Angiography is performed in a dedicated angiography suite with sterile technique. Arterial access is typically gained via puncture of the common femoral artery. A vascular sheath is placed to lessen trauma to the vessel during catheter exchanges. Catheters and guidewires are placed under fluoroscopic guidance to access the desired vessels. Intravascular contrast is administered via a mechanical injector at a high flow rate through the catheter as serial radiographic images are obtained. Digital techniques are used to subtract background information, such as bony structures, so that only images of the blood vessels remain (**Figure 185-28**). It is essential that no motion be present during this process to avoid blurring of images. Typically, images are obtained during a breath hold. During abdominal imaging, glucagon is routinely given to slow bowel motility, which can also interfere with optimal imaging.

As mentioned earlier, vessels in children are particularly prone to vasospasm and thrombosis. The presence of a catheter and guidewire in the vessel may be enough to induce spasm. It is typical to heparinize a patient during this procedure, particularly infants. Induced hypercapnia during anesthesia is another strategy used to reduce the propensity for vasospasm.

After completion of the procedure, pressure on the arterial puncture site is typically held for 5 to 10 minutes, depending on the patient's coagulation status. It is suggested that patients attempt to limit activity for approximately 24 hours after arterial puncture, after which they may resume normal activity. Lower extremity pulses, particularly on the puncture side, are monitored for possible spasm or impending thrombosis. Hydration at one to two times maintenance is recommended to promote renal clearance of contrast.

There are maximum limits on the amount of contrast that can be administered to a patient because of nephrotoxicity. At our institution, this limit is 7 mL/kg in 24 hours, including any other contrast administration on the same day that may have been used for diagnostic imaging (CT, IVP, etc.). Monitoring of renal function by serum creatinine levels is not an absolute requirement after the procedure except in high-risk patients.

Primary Vascular Interventions In the vascular arena, primary interventions can be divided into restoring patency to blood vessels (angioplasty, stenting) or occluding them (embolization, sclerotherapy). One of the more common uses of angioplasty is for treatment of patients with renovascular hypertension secondary to either fibromuscular dysplasia or renal artery stenosis. Vessels may be occluded via particle embolization in a patient with massive hemoptysis. Embolization and sclerotherapy are used for the treatment of congenital vascular malformations (arteriovenous, venous, or lymphatic malformations). In general, preprocedural preparation is similar to that for diagnostic angiography. For certain procedures, corticosteroids may be administered to reduce the inflammatory response. Prophylactic antibiotics may also be administered during certain vascular interventions. Because treatment of vascular malformations may be complicated and require staged interventions, consultation with the interventional radiologist is essential before discussing these procedures and treatment options with the parents.

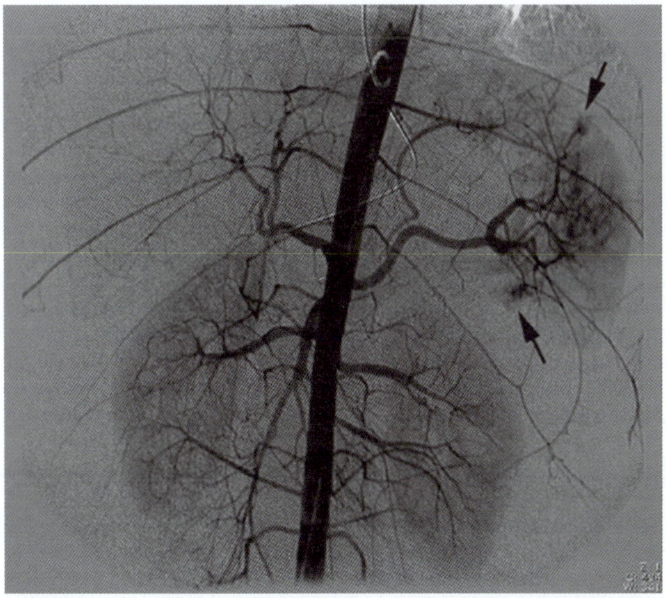

FIGURE 185-28. Abdominal aortogram performed with digital subtraction. This 13-year-old female was under general anesthesia, and breath hold and glucagon were utilized to reduce motion artifact. The patient was involved in a fall with a splenic laceration by CT. Multiple areas of contrast extravasation consistent with bleeding are noted (arrows).

Vascular Access Procedures Image-guided venous access, which includes peripherally inserted central catheter (PICC) and central venous line placement, is generally reserved for patients in whom multiple attempts at gaining venous access without image guidance have proved futile. Success rates for placement of PICCs and central venous catheters under US and fluoroscopic guidance are excellent. Preprocedural preparation usually involves fasting for sedation or anesthesia and is generally reserved for younger patients. Review of the patient's previous imaging examinations and history of previous line placement is essential before the procedure to assess whether there is any known venous obstruction, thrombosis, or stricture. Under US guidance, PICC placement is usually performed in the upper part of the arm with a basilic vein puncture. US guidance is also used for placement of central venous lines and is typically performed via an internal jugular vein approach. In theory, any vein that can be visualized with US can be punctured. This is particularly important in the patient where the more traditional routes of access are not suitable. Preservation of venous access, particularly in a pediatric patient with chronic disease, is important, so the smallest, least invasive catheters are used to reduce repetitive trauma to the veins. Most catheters placed under image guidance can be used immediately after the procedure.

NONVASCULAR INTERVENTIONS

Percutaneous Drainage of Fluid Collections and Abscesses Minimally invasive image-guided drainage of fluid collections and abscesses, such as those that might arise as a result of complications of appendicitis, is common (**Figure 185-29**). Indications for the procedure include: (i) reduction in size of collections causing symptoms (such as bowel or urinary obstruction), (ii) characterization of fluid (both chemical and microbiologic), and (iii) prevention of sepsis in patients with infected collections not responding to antibiotic treatment alone. Contraindications include a percutaneously inaccessible area, intervening bowel being the most common cause of an inaccessible area, and coagulopathy. Review of previous imaging studies and laboratory values, and consultation with the pediatric surgeon are needed before performing this procedure. Sedation or general anesthesia is needed in all age groups. The procedure can usually be performed under US guidance. CT guidance is occasionally used for more difficult collections. In most cases, after aspiration, a drainage catheter is left within the cavity for several days. Fluid output from these catheters is monitored daily. The catheters may become obstructed, which could require tube flushing, repositioning, or even tube replacement in certain cases. Drainage catheters are removed at the bedside without sedation in most instances.

Image-guided thoracentesis and paracentesis can be performed with similar techniques and preprocedural preparation as for the procedures described earlier. With regard to thoracentesis, consultation with a pediatric surgeon is recommended, particularly for complex effusions or empyemas because the patient may be a more suitable candidate for video-assisted thoracoscopic surgery (VATS) or large-bore chest tube drainage (or both). Use of tissue plasminogen activator through small-bore pigtail catheters has been very successful in draining complex collections that may be loculated. Given this, image-guided chest tube placement tends to be the first line of therapy at our institution in these situations (**Figure 185-30**).

Percutaneous Image-Guided Biopsy Minimally invasive biopsy of tumors and other lesions is gaining more acceptance as histologic techniques become more sophisticated. Imaging guidance not only increases the safety of the procedure but also affords the ability to be very precise in targeting specific abnormalities, even if they are small (**Figure 185-31**).

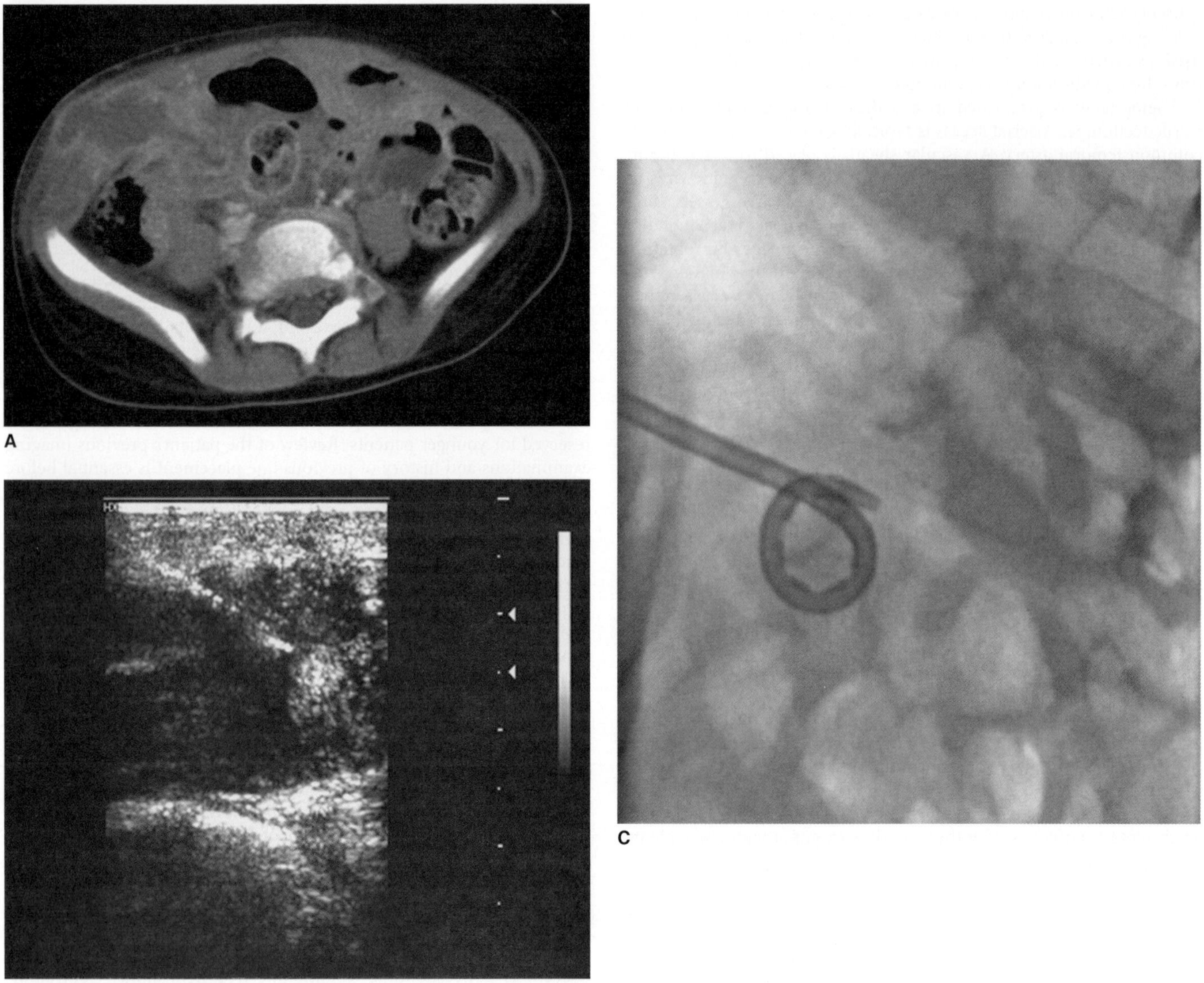

FIGURE 185-29. Ultrasound-guided drainage of superficial abscess. This 2-year-old male developed a superficial abscess after open appendectomy. (A) Preprocedure CT. (B) Ultrasound appearance with the access needle in position. (C) Fluoroscopic image after placement of a pigtail drainage catheter.

The vast majority of these biopsies can be performed on an outpatient basis under conscious sedation or with a short-lasting general anesthetic. Fine-needle aspirates as well as small-core biopsies can be obtained by the interventional radiologist. Preprocedural preparation is similar to that for other percutaneous techniques described earlier: fasting status for the patient before sedation/anesthesia, evaluation of the patient's history, imaging examinations, laboratory analysis (CBC, PT/PTT, INR), and cessation of anticoagulant medications. Open surgical biopsy remains necessary in certain cases, such as a large tumor that is partially necrotic, because fine-needle aspiration or even a small core biopsy may not yield adequate specimens. Similarly, in certain cases the patient may need to proceed to immediate surgical excision because of a deleterious mass effect on adjacent structures. Seeding of the biopsy tract is possible for certain tumors. It is best to consult with the oncologist and oncology surgeon when contemplating ordering a minimally invasive biopsy of a presumed tumor.

Percutaneous Gastrostomy/Gastrojejunostomy Placement The preferred route of gastrostomy placement, endoscopic or percutaneous, is institution and patient dependent. Percutaneous image-guided gastrostomy placement is increasingly common as it is less costly and quicker to perform and may be associated with fewer complications. In the pediatric population, gastrostomy placement is often considered if nutritional requirements for growth and development are not being met. In patients with severe reflux, who are at increased risk for aspiration, transgastric jejunal feeding tubes can be placed. Percutaneous feeding tube placement may use fluoroscopy or US guidance. In a pediatric setting, the procedure is routinely performed with general anesthesia. The stomach is insufflated with air via an NG tube. Ultrasound is used to delineate the solid organs. Barium enema can be performed to delineate the transverse colon. Once the stomach is distended with air, percutaneous needle puncture is made with both fluoroscopic and US guidance. Guidewire access is then obtained. The tract is then dilated and tube placed over the wire. Optionally, gastropexy with percutaneously deployed retention sutures can also be deployed. The procedure can be performed on an outpatient basis. The stoma is allowed to mature for about 8 to 12 weeks before attempting to place a transgastric jejunal tube. These tubes are placed under fluoroscopic guidance to ensure placement in the proximal jejunum. Getting the feeding tube to the proximal jejunum can be challenging in many instances, and it is not uncommon that radiation exposure is prolonged in both the patient and operator. These feeding tubes frequently need to be replaced because they can become obstructed or the patient inadvertently pulls the tube out, which in turn increases the cumulative radiation exposure. Consideration for this increased radiation dose must be balanced against the potential benefits/risks of surgical fundoplication for treating the reflux.

Percutaneous Cecostomy Many patients with chronic neurologic, developmental, or metabolic diseases are plagued with chronic constipation. In this group of patients, placement of a catheter within the cecum with the administration of regular antegrade enemas can be life

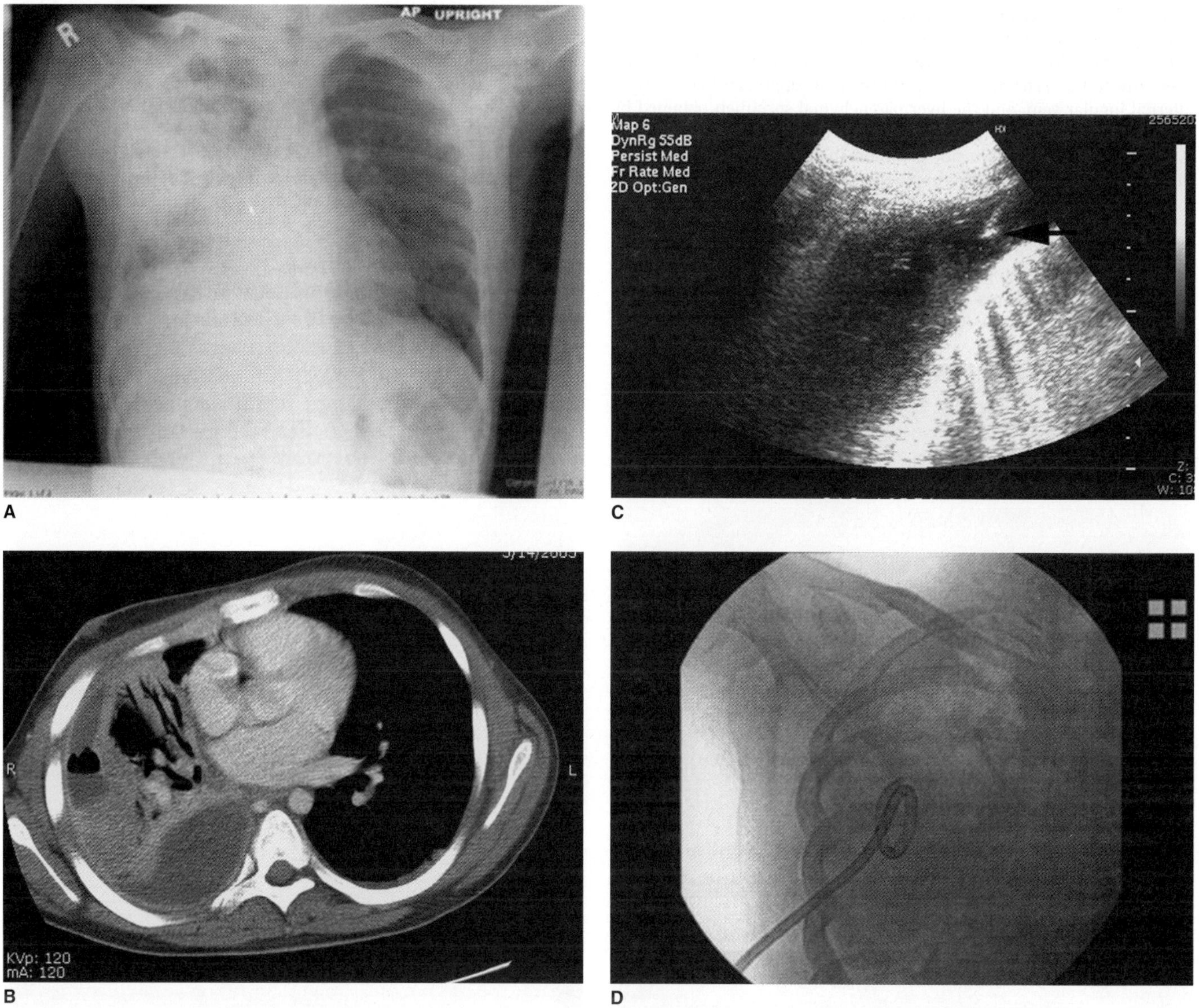

FIGURE 185-30. Ultrasound-guided thoracentesis and chest tube placement. This 18-year-old male with developmental delay developed a right lower lobe pneumonia with a complex pleural effusion. (A, B) Pre-procedure appearance under chest x-ray and CT, respectively. (C) Ultrasound appearance of the collection with a catheter needle in position. (D) Placement of a pigtail catheter in the collection under fluoroscopy.

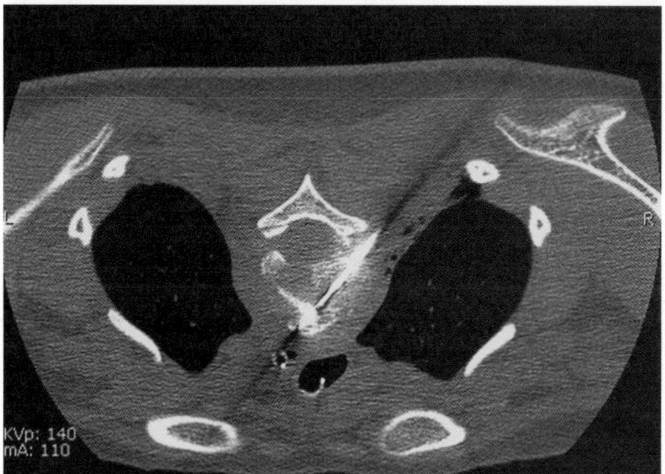

FIGURE 185-31. CT-guided biopsy of compressed T3 vertebral body. This 13-year-old female presented with scapular pain and a collapsed T3 vertebral body on MRI. This image demonstrates placement of a coaxial needle and trephine biopsy needle by CT guidance.

changing. Placement of a cecostomy tube is similar to placement of a gastrostomy tube, again performed under US and fluoroscopic guidance. Cecal air distension is performed via colonic insufflation via rectal tube, and direct percutaneous puncture is made with image guidance. Preprocedural preparation is similar to gastrostomy placement.

Hepatic and Biliary Interventions In the pediatric population, interventions involving the liver are common. Image-guided liver biopsy is now the preferred standard of care at many institutions, replacing blind biopsies. Liver biopsy is necessary for diagnosis of many metabolic and infectious diseases involving the liver, most commonly viral hepatitis as well as monitoring of therapy. Many patients taking hepatotoxic medications also require monitoring. At institutions that perform liver transplantation, biopsy is routinely performed to monitor for organ rejection. Percutaneous liver biopsy is performed with the same techniques as described earlier for image-guided biopsy, with careful attention to avoiding adjacent vessels or transgressing the liver capsule and inadvertently puncturing nearby structures. Performance of the procedure can be challenging in that many of these patients may be coagulopathic. A coagulation profile should be obtained prior to biopsy. If a coagulopathy exists, blood products should be available for correction or resuscitation as necessary. The biopsy is performed with sedation or anesthesia. A hematocrit level is obtained 4 hours after the procedure. A significant decrease in hematocrit or the presence of pain after the procedure warrants further workup and possible blood transfusion.

In patients with severe uncorrectable coagulopathy, liver biopsy can alternatively be performed with a transvenous approach via the right internal jugular vein, and the liver parenchymal specimen obtained by puncturing through the right or middle hepatic vein.

Biliary interventions are not common in the pediatric population. Most biliary procedures in this population are performed through endoscopic or surgical methods. Noninvasive methods for evaluation of the biliary system, such as magnetic resonance cholangiopancreatography (MRCP), are widely available, thus precluding the need for endoscopy and cholangiopancreatography in some cases. Interventional biliary procedures are sometimes performed in liver transplantation patients with complications involving the biliary-enteric anastomosis. Balloon cholangioplasty of strictures at these anastomoses is performed with good results (**Figure 185-32**). Other biliary interventions that are common in the adult population, such as biliary stone removal or common bile duct stenting, are performed rarely in children. Preprocedure preparation for biliary interventions includes the administration of prophylactic antibiotics to cover gram-negative organisms.

Urologic Interventions Percutaneous nephrostomy is performed primarily for relief of urinary tract obstruction. In the pediatric population, this is often performed in the setting of congenital obstruction of the ureteropelvic junction. Nephrostomy may also be indicated in the setting of postoperative edema of the ureterovesical junction after ureteral reimplantation surgery for vesicoureteral reflux. Relief of obstruction secondary to nephrolithiasis, the most frequent indication in the

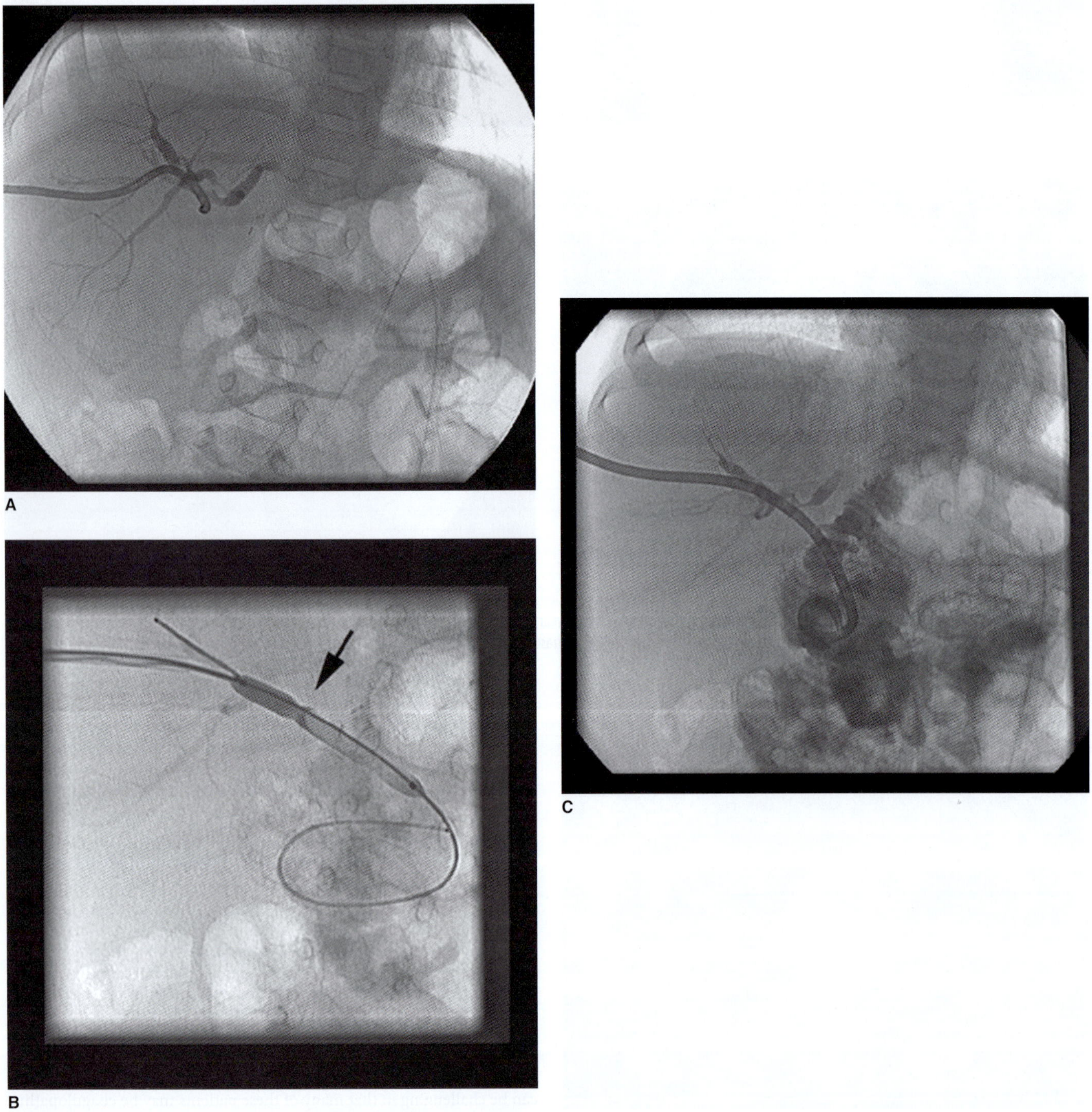

FIGURE 185-32. Balloon cholangioplasty of biliary duct structure after split liver transplant. (A) Cholangiogram demonstrating non-opacification of the bowel and common bile duct anastamosis. (B) Inflated angioplasty balloon with a "waist" at the point of structure (arrow). (C) External/internal biliary stent catheter post dilatation.

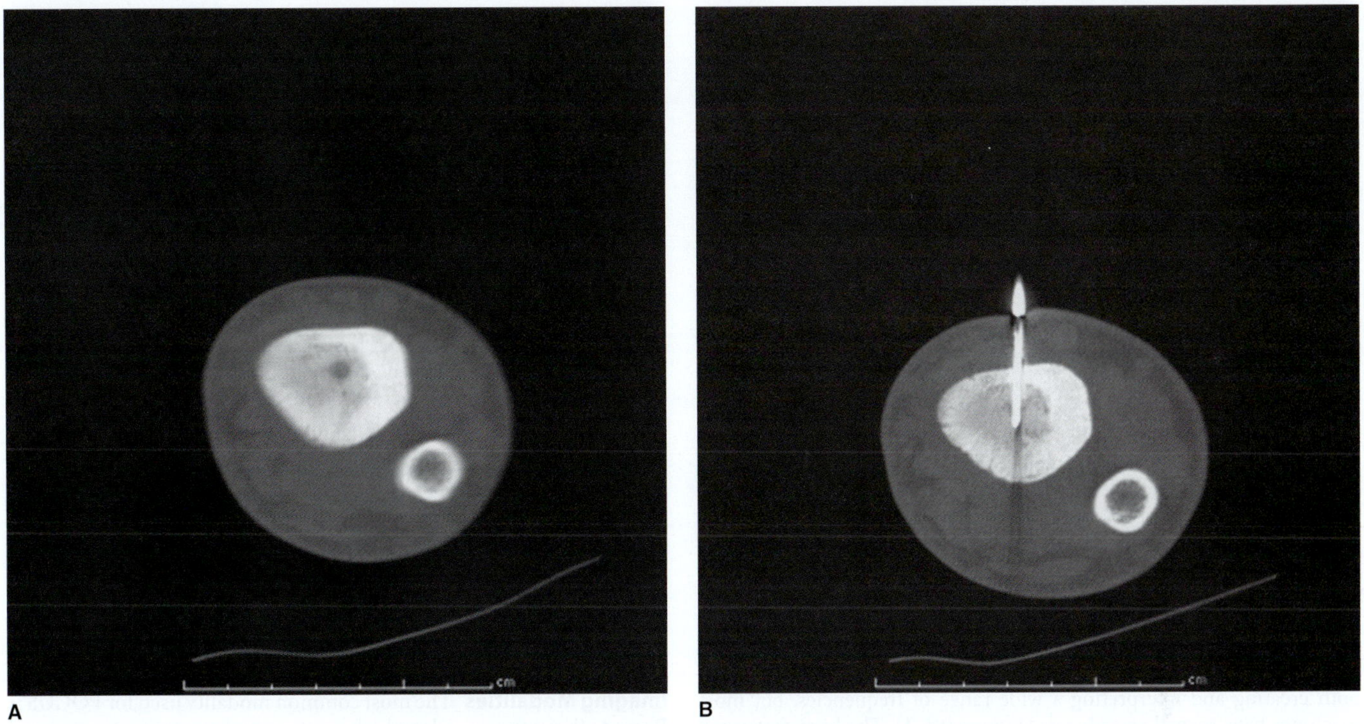

FIGURE 185-33. Radiofrequency ablation of radial osteoid osteoma. (A) Preoperative appearance on CT. (B) Radiofrequency probe traversing the nidus under CT.

adult population, is not as common in children. Techniques are similar to that for drainage of fluid collections, with the same preprocedure preparation of the patient. Prophylactic antibiotics are usually administered. Whereas in adult institutions the procedure is performed under fluoroscopic guidance, US guidance is more commonly used in children. Using US reduces the radiation dose to the patient, and having Doppler affords one the ability to locate an avascular plane to access the collecting system. A small pigtail catheter is placed within the renal pelvis after aspiration of urine. This catheter can form a mature tract, thus making the renal pelvis easier to access so that future interventions can be performed, such as balloon dilation or stent placement for a stricture. The catheter can remain within the renal pelvis for several weeks with proper care on an outpatient basis.

Musculoskeletal Interventions Musculoskeletal interventions account for a large portion of the nonvascular pediatric interventional radiology practice. Percutaneous bone biopsy under either fluoroscopic or CT guidance can be helpful in the diagnosis of both neoplastic and infectious disease. Therapeutic interventions are also becoming more commonplace as technology advances. Needle biopsy followed by treatment of osteoid osteomas with radiofrequency ablation under imaging guidance is well documented and highly effective (**Figure 185-33**). Percutaneous biopsy of presumed histiocytosis lesions can be followed by direct injection of a steroid into the lesion with good results. Preoperative embolization of aneurysmal bone cysts and tumors has significantly reduced the morbidity associated with these operations. Primary sclerotherapy for aneurysmal bone cysts is also being performed. General anesthesia for pain control is usually required with the same preprocedural preparation as for image-guided biopsy. Most of these procedures can be performed on a day surgery basis. Again, consultation with the orthopedic surgeon, oncologist, and interventional radiologist is essential.

SUGGESTED READINGS

American College of Radiology Appropriateness Criteria. https://www.acr.org/Clinical-Resources/ACR-Appropriateness-Criteria.

American College of Radiology. *ACR Manual on Contrast Media*. 2022.

Brenner D, Elliston C, Hall E, et al. Estimated risks of radiation-induced fatal cancer from pediatric CT. *AJR Am J Roentgenol*. 2001;176(2):289-296.

Choi JH, Lee T, Kwon HH, et al. Outcome of ultrasonographic imaging in infants with sacral dimple. *Korean J Pediatri*. 2018;61(6):194-199.

Cohen MD. Safe use of imaging contrast agents in children. *J Am Coll Radiol*. 2009;6(8):576-581.

Khun JP, Slovis TL, Haller JO, eds. *Caffey's Pediatric Diagnostic Imaging*. 10th ed. Philadelphia: Mosby; 2004.

Plut D, Phillips GS, Johnston PR, Lee EY. Practical imaging strategies for intussusception in children. *AJR Am J Roentgenol*. 2020;215(6):1449-1463.

Squires JH, McCarville MB. Contrast-enhanced ultrasound in children: implementation and diagnostic applications. *AJR Am J Roentgenol*. 2021;217:1217-1231.

Treves ST, et al. Treves ST ed. *Pediatric Nuclear Medicine*. 3rd ed. New York: Springer; 2007.

CHAPTER 186 Ultrasonography for the Pediatric Hospitalist

Erin Finn, MD, FAAP, William Kwan, MD, FAAP, and Ria Dancel, MD, SFHM, FACP, FAAP

INTRODUCTION

Point-of-care ultrasound (POCUS) refers to ultrasound performed by non-radiologist clinicians on their own patients. Rather than performing a comprehensive ultrasound exam, the POCUS sonographer uses ultrasound to answer a specific, focused clinical question or to aid in performing a procedure. POCUS delivers immediate results at the point of care, uses no ionizing radiation, and does not require sedation.

POCUS has been used by non-radiologists for decades and has made its way into pediatric emergency rooms and critical care settings. While many pediatric hospitalists are familiar with procedural ultrasound, diagnostic POCUS remains relatively new to the field of pediatric hospital medicine (PHM). The purpose of this chapter is to familiarize pediatric hospitalists with the basics of how to perform POCUS and some indications for which POCUS can be utilized.

BASIC ULTRASOUND PHYSICS

The methods by which ultrasound waves are created and translated into images are beyond the scope of this chapter. For most basic POCUS, we will describe findings seen in brightness mode, or B-mode, which displays structures as grayscale two-dimensional images. Structures that are dense are highly reflective of ultrasound waves and appear closer to white on the gray scale, or hyperechoic. Calcified structures such as bones reflect nearly all ultrasound waves, hindering visualization of deeper structures and leading to acoustic shadowing. Simple fluid does not reflect ultrasound waves and therefore appears black, or anechoic. Most structures appear gray due to their intermediate densities and are described as hyperechoic, hypoechoic, or isoechoic based on their brightness relative to each other. Air scatters ultrasound waves, resulting in the inability to image structures deep to air. Despite this, lung POCUS takes advantage of artifacts produced by air and air-fluid interfaces.

EQUIPMENT

Advances in ultrasound technology have resulted in more affordable ultrasound machines that are smaller in size, enabling greater portability. Some ultra-portable machines utilize a single transducer capable of both creating and interpreting a wide range of frequencies, but most machines have several transducers (**Figure 186-1**). The high-frequency linear array transducer provides high resolution images of superficial structures. The phased array transducer uses a lower frequency to image deeper structures, but at the expense of resolution. Its footprint (the part of the transducer in contact with the patient's skin) allows it to fit into smaller spaces, such as the intercostal spaces for cardiac imaging. The curvilinear transducer is also a low-frequency transducer used to image deeper structures but has a wider footprint that allows a wider field of view, making it useful for imaging intra-abdominal organs, for example. Additional transducers are available for more specialized POCUS exams that will not be covered in this chapter.

Basic Controls ("Knobology") Ultrasound machines typically have presets that optimize image quality for a particular exam (e.g., cardiac, lung, abdomen), but adjustments are still needed to optimize the image. Machines from various manufacturers allow a variety of adjustments by the user, but all allow adjustments of depth and gain.

The depth setting determines the maximum depth displayed on the image screen. Increasing the depth allows visualization of deeper structures. The depth should be adjusted such that the object of interest is in the center of the screen. This is especially important for machines whose focal zone (the area where the ultrasound waves are most concentrated) is fixed.

Gain refers to the ultrasound machine's amplification of reflected ultrasound waves. Increasing the overall gain results in brighter ultrasound images while decreasing the gain results in darker images. The gain should be adjusted until blood-filled structures are completely anechoic. Time gain compensation (TGC) allows the user to amplify the signal in the far field of an image to account for attenuation of the waves through tissue or alternatively to dampen posterior acoustic enhancement artifact that occurs deep to anechoic structures.

Orientation Each transducer has an indicator that corresponds to the ultrasound image screen orientation marker. For most POCUS exams in PHM, the image screen orientation marker is at the top left of the screen. The exception is cardiac POCUS, which is frequently performed with the screen orientation marker at the top right of the screen. We recommend following the convention used by your institution's cardiologists.

Most imaging in POCUS is obtained in one of three planes: transverse, sagittal, or coronal. Using radiology convention, scanning in the transverse plane is performed with the transducer marker to the patient's right. Scanning in the sagittal and coronal planes is performed with the transducer marker toward the patient's head (cephalad). Generally, structures of interest should be viewed in at least two planes.

Imaging Modalities The most common modality used for POCUS is B-mode (brightness mode) which creates a real-time two-dimensional grayscale image. M-mode (motion mode) follows the motion of a structure (such as a heart valve, for example) along a single vertical line through the two-dimensional image. The position of the structure is plotted vertically on the image screen while time is plotted horizontally. M-mode can be used to examine movement of a structure and to measure distances between two moving structures (such as the distance between the anterior mitral valve leaflet and interventricular septum).

Doppler ultrasound uses frequency shifts of moving objects to assess the presence of and direction of blood flow or tissue movement toward or away from the transducer. Conventionally, objects moving towards the transducer are displayed in red while objects moving away are displayed in blue. Though color Doppler is used often to detect blood flow, the colors used in color Doppler have nothing to do with oxygenation and were chosen due to being on opposite ends of the light spectrum.

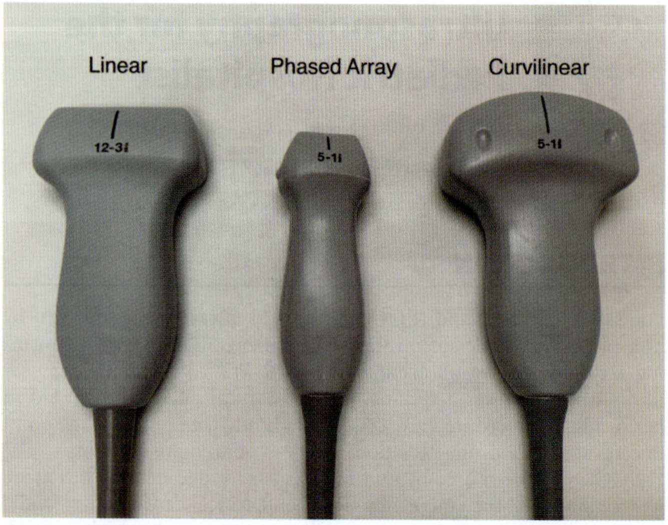

FIGURE 186-1. High-frequency linear array, low-frequency phased array, and low-frequency curvilinear transducers.

BASIC POCUS APPLICATIONS

FOCUSED CARDIAC ULTRASOUND

Introduction As with all POCUS exams, the cardiac POCUS exam (also called "FOCUS" for focused cardiac ultrasound) is used to answer simple, categorical questions at the bedside. Unlike a comprehensive trans-thoracic echocardiogram, the FOCUS exam is a limited exam involving three windows (parasternal, apical, and subcostal) and five cardiac views that will be discussed here. The phased array transducer with the cardiac preset is used for this exam. This preset increases the frame rate in order to image a rapidly moving object smoothly.

Parasternal Long Axis (PLAX)

Acquisition For the parasternal long axis (PLAX) view of the heart, positioning the patient in the left lateral decubitus position will usually improve the view by bringing the heart closer to the chest wall. If lung interference remains a problem, having the patient hold their breath at end-exhalation may help. The transducer is placed in the left second intercostal space close to the sternum with the transducer marker directed toward the patient's right shoulder (approximately 10 o'clock). The transducer may need to be moved into a more caudal intercostal space or laterally away from the sternum to locate the best view (**Figure 186-2**).

Normal view The structures that should be identified are shown in **Figure 186-3**.

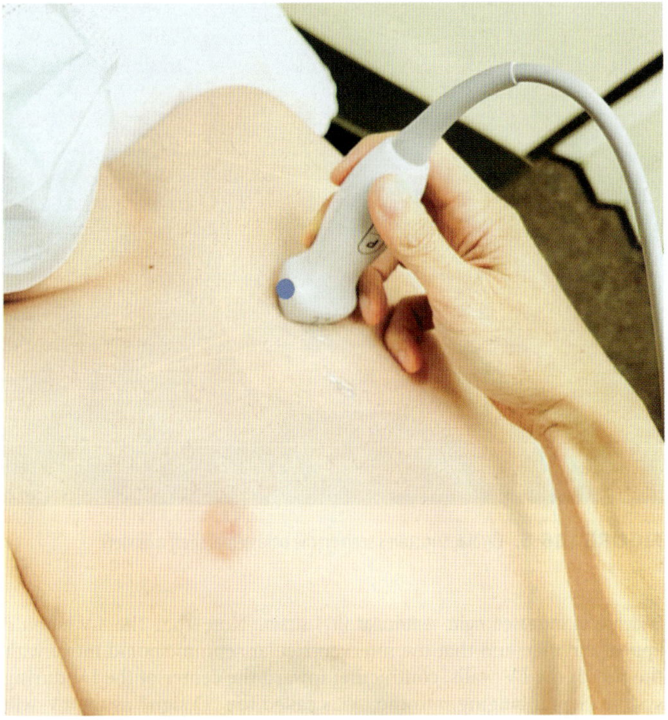

FIGURE 186-2. Phased array transducer positioned at the second intercostal space with the transducer marker (indicated by the blue dot) pointed toward the right shoulder (approximately 10 o'clock) for the parasternal long axis view.

Clinical Questions That Can Be Answered With This View

Left ventricular function. The goal of FOCUS is not to quantify left ventricular (LV) fractional shortening or ejection fraction but rather to qualitatively assess function as normal, mildly reduced, moderately reduced, or severely reduced. There are multiple ways to evaluate LV function:

- Excursion of the anterior leaflet of the mitral valve. The anterior leaflet of the mitral valve should approximate or touch the interventricular septum during diastole.
- Decrease in LV cavity size. The LV endocardium should symmetrically move inward toward the center of the LV cavity during ventricular contraction, decreasing the cavity size during systole.
- Pitfalls. Because the PLAX view typically demonstrates the function at the base and mid-portion of the LV, additional views are needed to evaluate apical function.

Presence of a pericardial effusion. An anterior pericardial effusion may be seen above the right ventricular outflow tract. A posterior pericardial effusion will appear as an anechoic stripe between the layers of the pericardium, tracking between the descending aorta and the left heart chambers.

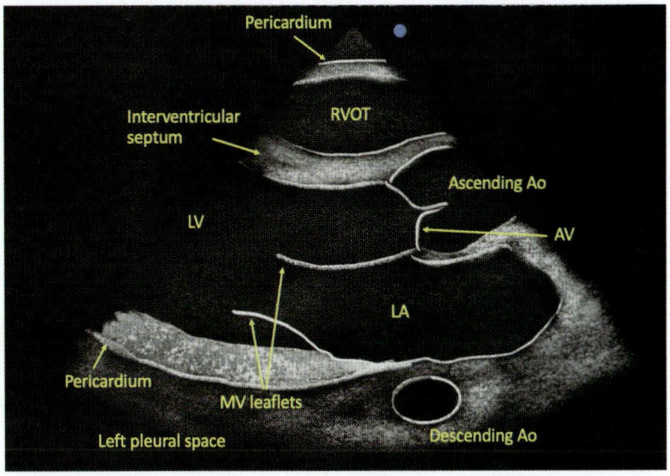

FIGURE 186-3. Cardiac structures seen on the parasternal long axis view (RVOT—right ventricular outflow tract, LV—left ventricle, LA—left atrium, AV—aortic valve, MV—mitral valve, Ao—aorta).

Presence of a left pleural effusion. The left pleural space is visualized deep to the left ventricle and left atrium. A pleural effusion in this space can be mistaken for a pericardial effusion; however, a left pleural effusion will be deep in to the descending aorta (**Figure 186-4**). This highlights the importance of increasing depth to visualize the descending thoracic aorta and left pleural space.

Parasternal Short Axis (PSAX)

Acquisition From the PLAX view, the transducer is rotated 90° clockwise so that the transducer marker is pointing toward the patient's left shoulder, or approximately 2 o'clock (**Figure 186-5**).

Normal views Starting from the base of the heart and fanning (changing the angle of the transducer while maintaining transducer contact with the patient's skin) toward the apex, the following levels will be seen: the aortic valve level, the mitral valve level, the papillary muscle level, and the apical level. The papillary muscle level marks the mid-ventricular level and provides the most reliable information regarding LV function, while also allowing evaluation for a pericardial effusion. Discussion of the anatomy and utility of the other levels in this window is outside of the scope of this chapter.

Papillary muscle/mid-ventricular level. Once the PSAX view is obtained, the transducer is fanned to visualize the papillary muscles at the mid-ventricular level. This level and the structures to visualize are shown in **Figure 186-6**.

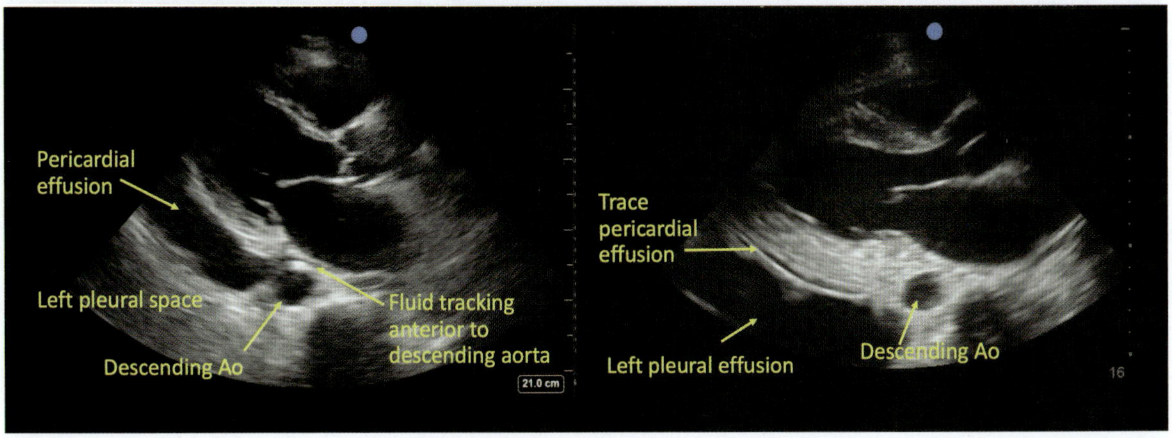

FIGURE 186-4. A pericardial effusion will track anterior to the descending thoracic aorta (left) whereas a pleural effusion will be seen posterior to the descending thoracic aorta (right).

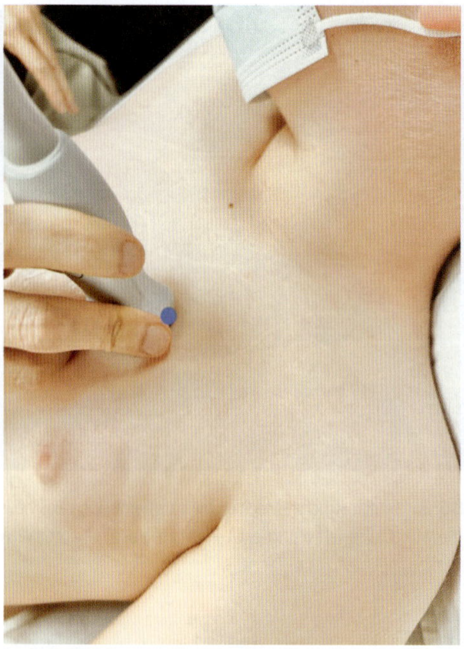

FIGURE 186-5. Phased array transducer positioned at the second intercostal space with the transducer marker pointed toward the left shoulder (approximately 2 o'clock) for the parasternal short axis view.

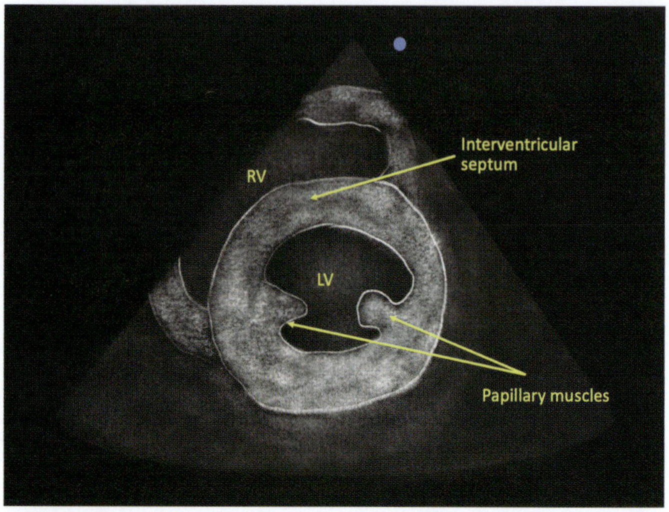

FIGURE 186-6. Cardiac structures seen on the parasternal short axis view.

Clinical Questions That Can Be Answered With This View

Left ventricular function.

- Decrease in LV cavity size. With normal LV function, the LV walls equally thicken and move toward each other, and the LV chamber cavity should decrease by roughly a third by end-systole.
- Wall segment thickening. The LV myocardium thickens during ventricular contraction, reaching its maximum wall thickness at end-systole.
- Pitfalls. While there is good concordance between pediatricians and cardiologists in assessing LV function using the "eyeball" technique, the subjective nature of this evaluation favors experience and assumes optimal technique, image quality, and normal LV anatomy and wall movements.

Presence of a pericardial effusion. A small, free-flowing pericardial effusion will appear as an anechoic stripe posterior to the left ventricle. A circumferential effusion will be seen surrounding both ventricles.

Evidence of increased right ventricular (RV) strain. Note that the LV should appear circular, and that the interventricular septum should move with the rest of the LV walls, contracting toward the center of the LV during systole. Septal bulging into the LV is called the "D sign," as the LV will resemble the letter D, signifying increased RV pressure and/or volume overload (**Figure 186-7**).

Apical Four Chamber View

Acquisition The apical view is best obtained by placing the patient in the left lateral decubitus position. The transducer is placed at the point of maximal impulse with the transducer marker pointed toward the patient's left, or about 2-3 o'clock (**Figure 186-8**). More depth will be needed for this view than for the parasternal views.

Normal View Once the apical four chamber view is located, the structures to visualize are shown in **Figure 186-9**.

Clinical Questions That Can Be Answered With This View

Left ventricular function.

- Decrease in LV cavity size. The LV endocardium should symmetrically move inward toward the center of the LV cavity as described in the PLAX and PSAX views.
- Wall segment thickening. The LV myocardium should symmetrically thicken as previously described in the PSAX view.
- Longitudinal shortening. During systole, the base of the heart moves toward the apex until the segment between the base and apex of the

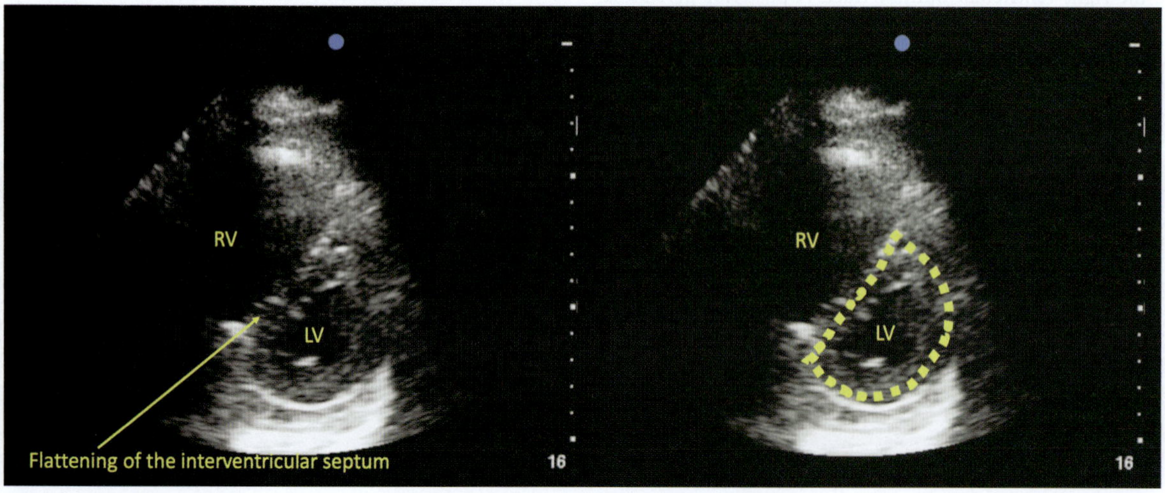

FIGURE 186-7. The "D-sign" caused by septal bulging into the LV, creating a D-shaped LV. This sign is suggestive of increased RV pressure and/or volume overload.

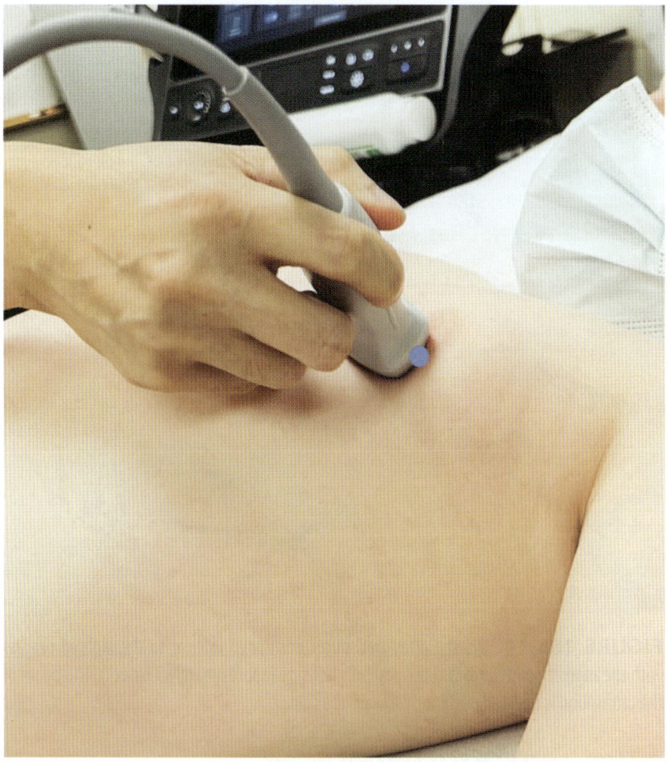

FIGURE 186-8. Phased array transducer positioned at the apex of the heart with the marker pointed toward the patient's left side (approximately 2-3 o'clock).

heart is at its minimum length at end-systole. This segment is at its maximum length at end-diastole. The difference between these two lengths is referred to as longitudinal shortening and should be at least 1 cm.

Presence of a pericardial effusion. While some effusions may be seen in this view, it is not as sensitive for detecting a pericardial effusion compared to the parasternal or subcostal views.

Relative size of the right ventricle to the left ventricle. The RV should be no more than two-thirds the size of the LV (**Figure 186-10**).

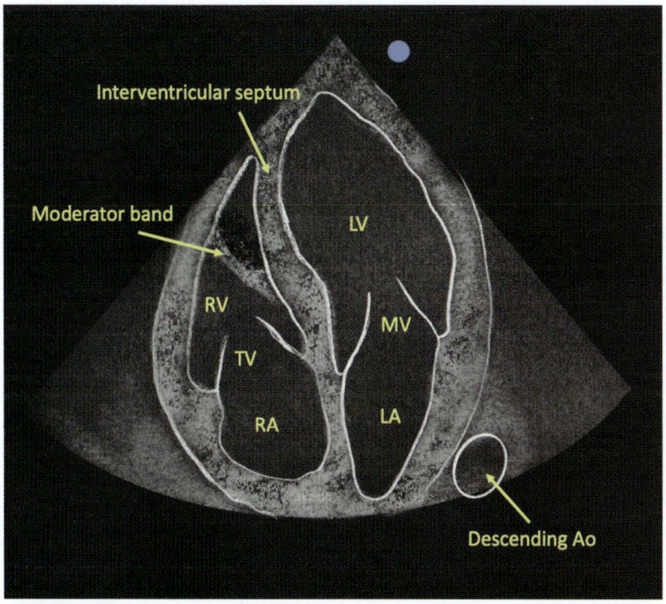

FIGURE 186-9. Cardiac structures seen on the apical four chamber view (RA—right atrium, TV—tricuspid valve).

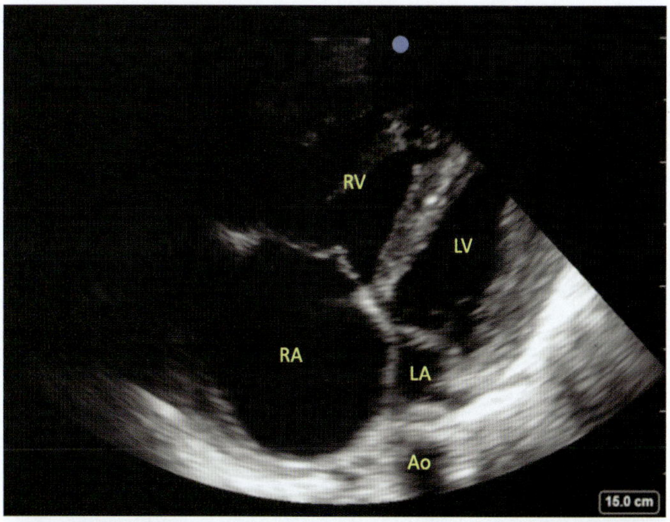

FIGURE 186-10. Apical four chamber view in a patient with right heart failure. Note that the RV is larger than the LV.

Subcostal Four Chamber View

Acquisition The patient is placed supine with knees flexed to relax the abdominal muscles and facilitate visualizing the heart. A breath hold at end-inhalation can improve visualization by moving the diaphragm down and the heart closer to the transducer. The transducer is placed just inferior to the xiphoid process with the transducer marker to the patient's left (around 2-3 o'clock) and flattened with an anterior fanning motion (**Figure 186-11**). Because the transducer is initially positioned inferior to the xiphoid process, this view is also called the subxiphoid view. However, if gas obscures the view in this position, the transducer can be moved toward the right along the costal margin in order to use the liver as an acoustic window.

Normal View Once the subcostal four chamber view is located, the structures seen are shown in **Figure 186-12**.

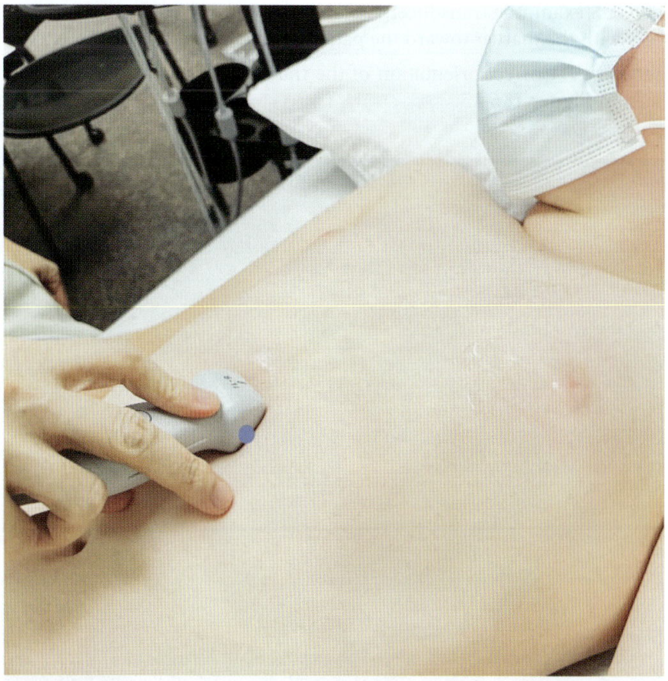

FIGURE 186-11. Phased array transducer positioned inferior to the xiphoid process with the marker pointed toward the patient's left side (approximately 2-3 o'clock). An overhand hold facilitates anterior fanning of the ultrasound beam.

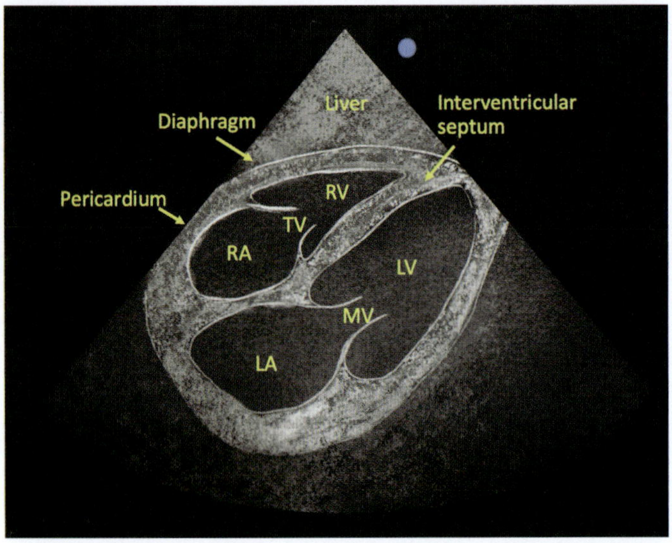

FIGURE 186-12. Cardiac structures seen on the subcostal four chamber view.

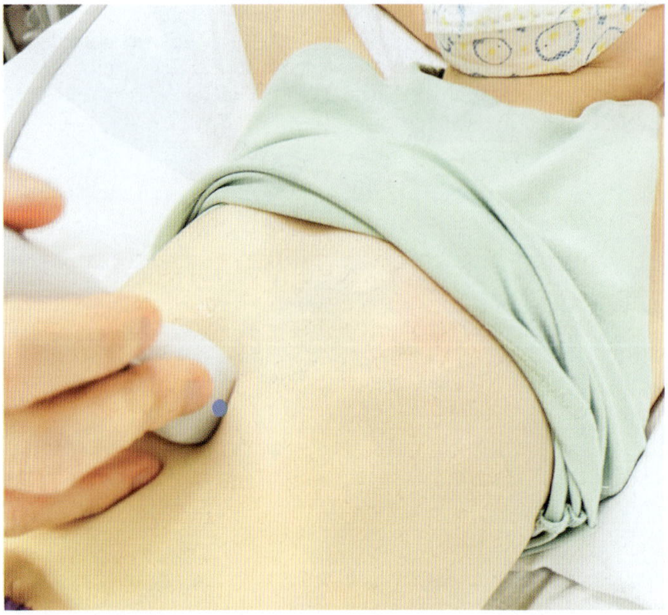

FIGURE 186-14. Phased array transducer positioned inferior to the xiphoid process with the marker pointed toward the patient's left side (approximately 3 o'clock). The beam of the ultrasound is directed posteriorly toward the spine.

Clinical Questions That Can Be Answered With This View

Left ventricular function. While the other views discussed previously are used more frequently for evaluating LV function, LV function can still be assessed in the subcostal view by applying the same principles.

Presence of a pericardial effusion and evidence of tamponade. This is the best view to identify a pericardial effusion and to evaluate its effects on the right side of the heart in cases of tamponade. Fluid will be seen accumulating in the space between the liver and the right heart chambers (**Figure 186-13**). Because the right heart is a lower-pressure system, the right heart will demonstrate evidence of collapse well before the left side of the heart. As a result, the core FOCUS findings suggestive of cardiac tamponade consist of a pericardial effusion, diastolic RV collapse (highly specific), systolic right atrial (RA) collapse (the earliest sign), and a plethoric inferior vena cava (IVC) with minimal respiratory variation (highly sensitive).

Subcostal Inferior Vena Cava

Acquisition When including the transverse view of the IVC as part of the FOCUS exam, the transducer is placed just inferior to the xiphoid process with the marker toward the patient's left (**Figure 186-14**).

Normal view Correct orientation of the transducer should yield the view seen in **Figure 186-15**.

Clinical Question That Can Be Answered With This View

Estimation of right atrial pressure. The most simplified evaluation of the IVC involves assessing its collapsibility. A normal right atrial pressure (RAP) will be reflected by an IVC that collapses >50% in diameter. An IVC with <50% collapse suggests an elevated RAP. Studies of pediatric patients with clinical signs of dehydration suggest that transverse imaging allows calculation of the ratio of the cross-sectional area of the aorta to the cross-sectional area of the IVC (Ao/IVCA). Kwon et al found that a ratio of 1.81 can predict dehydration requiring fluid resuscitation with a sensitivity of 72% and specificity of 89%.

Pitfalls. Evaluating the size and collapsibility of the IVC has previously been touted as a way to evaluate a patient's volume status and fluid-responsiveness; however, this is a far more nuanced topic, and caution must be exercised when integrating IVC findings into the management of patients. IVC size and collapsibility are not directly reflective of volume status but can provide information about the RAP. Similarly, the RAP does not provide

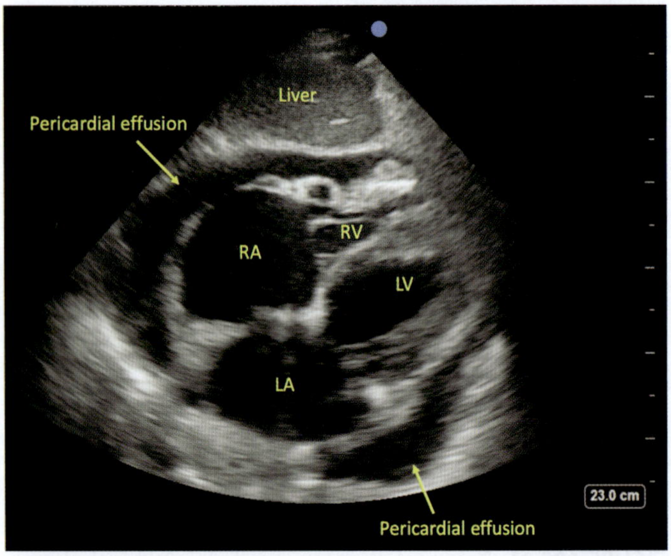

FIGURE 186-13. The subcostal four chamber view will show a pericardial effusion between the liver and the right side of the heart.

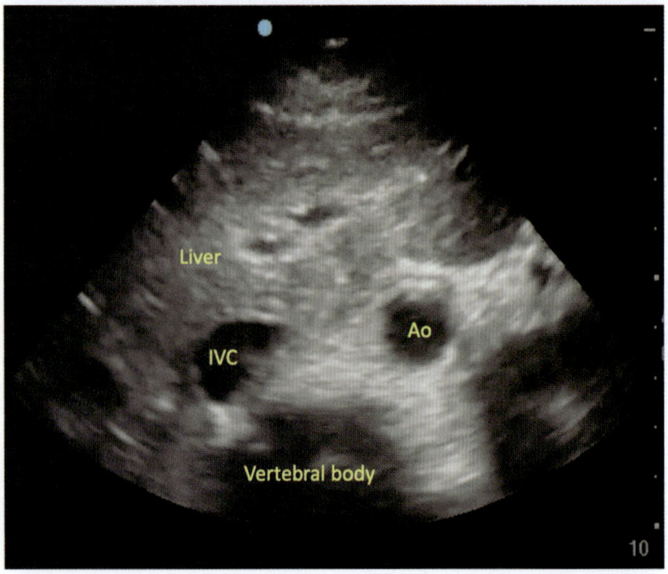

FIGURE 186-15. Transverse view of the IVC and aorta, which are superficial to the vertebral body (IVC—inferior vena cava).

information as to whether a patient will be "fluid-responsive" (i.e., whether infusion of fluids will lead to an increase in cardiac output). Existing studies both in adults and children have shown conflicting results. Consequently, it is important to consider history and other parts of the POCUS exam (e.g., cardiac and pulmonary) to put RAP into context.

PLEURA AND LUNG ULTRASOUND

Introduction There are two important components of lung ultrasound (LUS). The first involves evaluating the pleural line for associated pathology, and the second involves looking deeper for lung parenchymal pathology. The high-frequency linear array transducer can be used for both components in infants because the maximum depth of 6 to 9 cm allowed with most linear array transducers may provide sufficient depth. However, in most pediatric patients, a combination of high- and low-frequency transducers will be needed to image the pleura and parenchyma, respectively.

Pleural Ultrasound

Acquisition The pleura is best visualized using the high-frequency linear array transducer on the lung ultrasound preset. A low-frequency transducer may also be used, but we recommend using the linear array transducer if evaluating the pleura specifically (e.g., for a pneumothorax) due to the superior resolution of a superficial structure. The transducer is placed between two ribs with the marker cephalad in a sagittal plane (**Figure 186-16**). The pleural line should be seen between the ribs and about 0.5 cm deep to them (**Figure 186-17**).

Normal View The visualized single pleural line actually represents both the parietal and visceral pleura, which are normally apposed. The movement of the separate layers against each other causes the pleural line to shimmer and is referred to as lung sliding. With M-mode imaging, normal lung sliding creates the "seashore sign"—the dynamic, moving lung produces a granular sandy beach appearance deep to the pleural line, while the static soft tissue and musculature superficial to the pleural line create what look like waves (**Figure 186-18**).

Clinical Question That Can Be Answered With This View

Significance of absent lung sliding. The absence of lung sliding will result in a static pleural line without any evidence of shimmering. In M-mode, absent lung sliding produces the "stratosphere sign" or "barcode sign" where the grainy appearance of the "sandy beach" is replaced by straight horizontal lines that indicate lack of movement deep to the parietal pleura (**Figure 186-19**). The absence of lung sliding can be seen in various clinical scenarios, including but not limited to pneumothorax, apnea, history of pleurodesis or chest irradiation, blebs, and right mainstem intubation. The presence of a lung point, however, is 100% specific for a pneumothorax. A lung point is the point where the visceral pleura begins to separate from the parietal pleura at the margin of a pneumothorax. If seen on ultrasound, this appears as an area where lack of lung sliding alternates with the presence of lung sliding at the point on the chest wall where the lung contacts the chest wall during inhalation and falls away during exhalation.

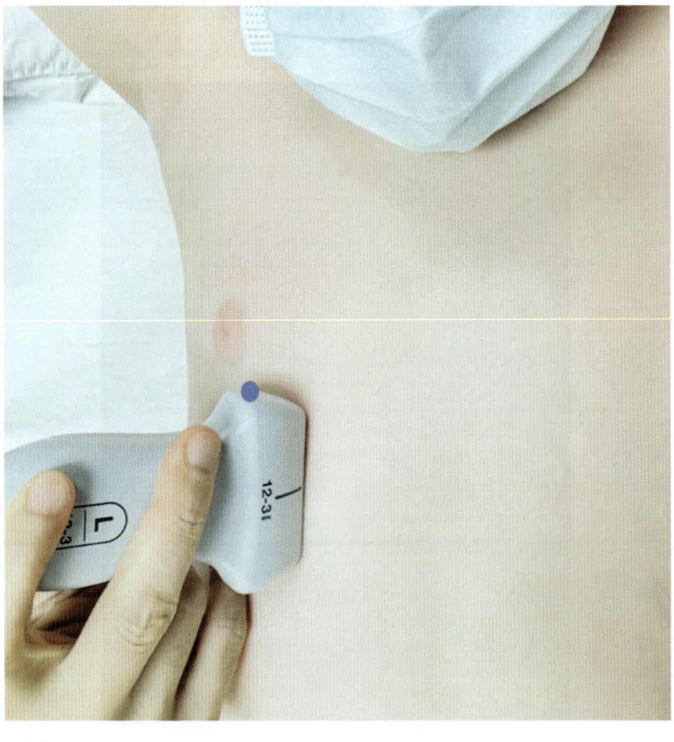

FIGURE 186-16. High-frequency linear array transducer positioned in a sagittal plane between 2 ribs to image the pleura.

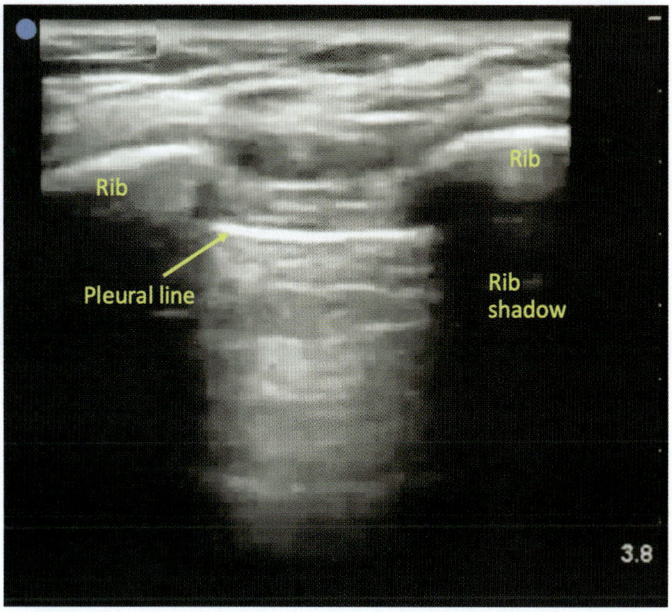

FIGURE 186-17. Two ribs and the pleural line between them are seen in this sagittal image.

Lung Ultrasound

Acquisition A low-frequency transducer is used to evaluate the lung parenchyma deep to the pleura. We recommend using the lung preset, if available. If not, LUS artifacts may be best seen with the focal zone at the pleural line, harmonics turned off, and far-field gain increased. As with pleural ultrasound, the transducer is placed in a sagittal plane between two ribs with the marker cephalad. The transducer is then fanned slightly toward the patient's mediastinum to direct the ultrasound waves perpendicular to the pleura.

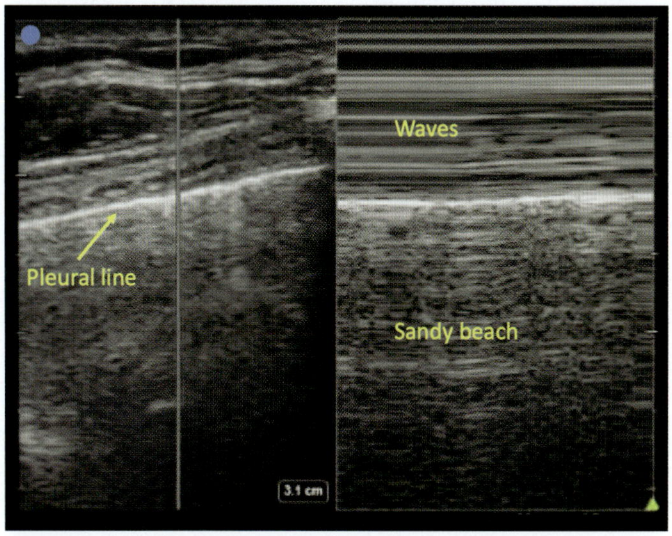

FIGURE 186-18. The "seashore sign" of lung sliding seen in M-mode.

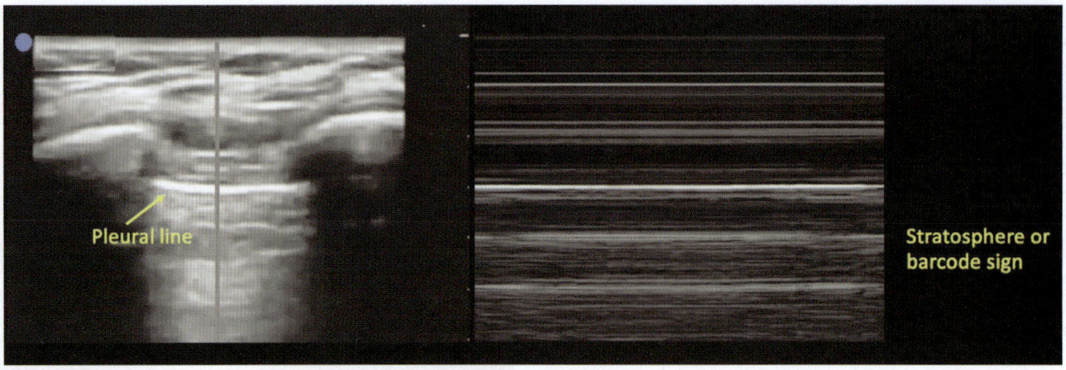

FIGURE 186-19. The "stratosphere sign" or "barcode sign" signifying lack of lung sliding.

Multiple areas of the lungs (called "lung zones") should be evaluated to ensure a comprehensive exam. There are different protocols for LUS that can be used, from an abbreviated 8-zone protocol to a comprehensive 28-zone protocol. At a minimum, 4 zones per hemithorax should be assessed (**Figure 186-20**).

Normal View

A-lines. When LUS is performed on normal, aerated lungs, the ultrasound waves cannot penetrate the air deep to the pleura and instead reverberate between the highly reflective pleura and the surface of the transducer on the skin. This reverberation creates a series of horizontal lines called A-lines at depths that are multiples of the distance between the transducer and the pleural line (**Figure 186-21**). Normally aerated lungs will demonstrate both lung sliding and A-lines in all zones.

Curtain sign. In the most posterolateral zone just cephalad to the diaphragm, the "curtain sign" is created by the inferior edge of the normally aerated lung moving caudally during inhalation and the air within the lung temporarily obscuring the diaphragm and the liver or spleen (**Figure 186-22**).

Absence of vertebral bodies cephalad to the diaphragm. In addition to identifying the diaphragm in this posterolateral zone, it is important to increase depth enough to visualize the spine. The vertebral bodies will be seen as hyperechoic humps deep to the liver, spleen, and kidneys. With fully aerated lungs, the spine should not be seen cephalad to the diaphragm, as air within the lungs will not allow ultrasound waves to penetrate down to the spine. If the spine is seen cephalad to the diaphragm, this "spine sign" suggests pathology above the diaphragm (**Figure 186-23**).

Clinical Questions That Can Be Answered With This View

Interstitial syndrome. B-lines are artifacts created by thickening of the interstitium between alveoli. They appear as hyperechoic vertical lines

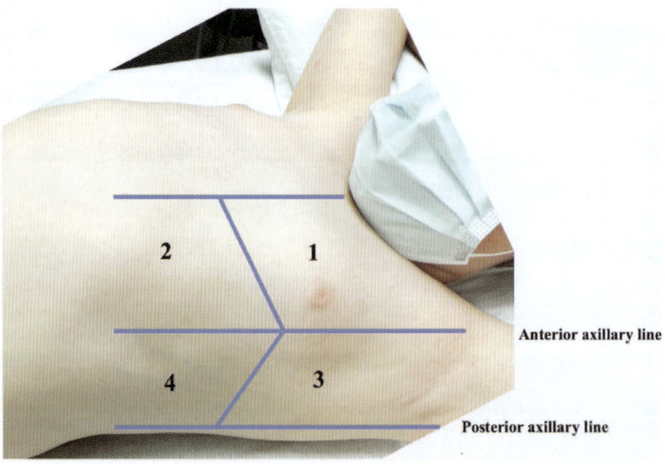

FIGURE 186-20. One lung ultrasound protocol divides the hemithorax into 4 lung zones.

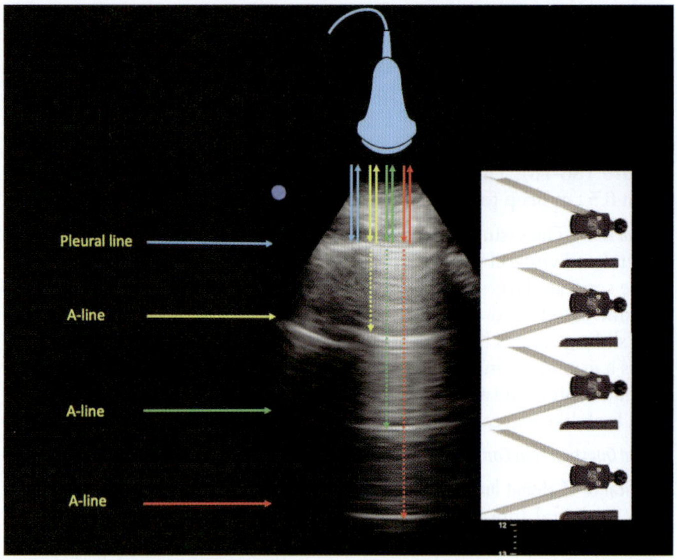

FIGURE 186-21. A-lines are reverberation artifacts that occur due to ultrasound waves bouncing between the highly reflective pleural line and transducer.

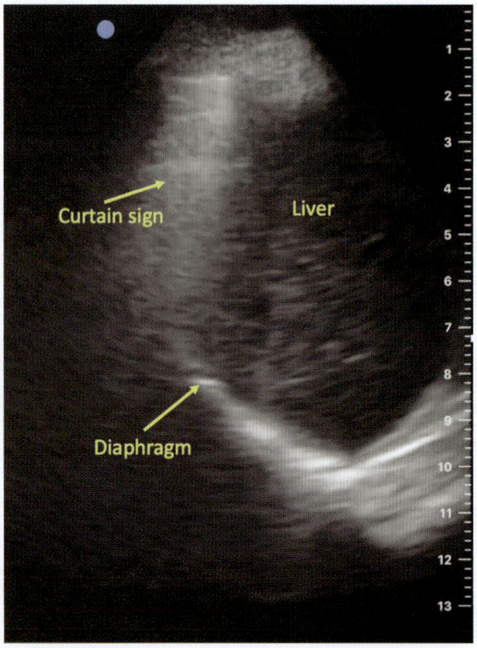

FIGURE 186-22. The curtain sign occurs when normally aerated lung obscures the diaphragm during inhalation.

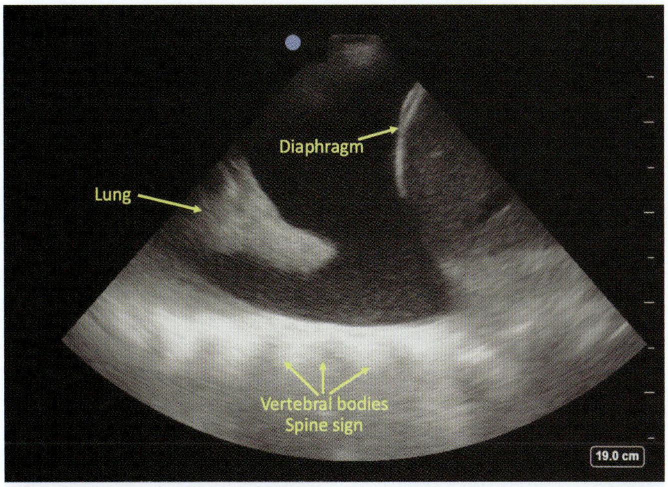

FIGURE 186-23. The vertebral bodies will be seen cephalad to the diaphragm only when there is lung pathology that allows passage of ultrasound waves deep enough to penetrate to the spine.

that originate from the pleural line and extend to the bottom edge of the ultrasound screen, obliterating normal A-lines (**Figure 186-24**). The presence of three or more B-lines in one lung zone is pathologic and is referred to as interstitial syndrome. The differential diagnosis of B-lines can be narrowed based on the distribution of B-lines across the lung zones as well as the patient's symptoms. For example, B-lines due to pulmonary edema are typically distributed bilaterally and may be associated with the presence of pleural effusions. Diffuse B-lines may also be seen in patients with pulmonary fibrosis or acute respiratory distress syndrome. B-lines in a patient with respiratory infection symptoms may be more indicative of pneumonia, as can be seen in patients with influenza or COVID-19, the latter of which classically causes posterior B-lines. It is not uncommon to see a few scattered B-lines at the bases of the lungs in the setting of atelectasis.

Pleural effusions. A pleural effusion appears as an anechoic or hypoechoic area cephalad to the diaphragm. Simple pleural effusions (**Figure 186-25**) are homogeneous and anechoic whereas complex pleural effusions (**Figure 186-26**) may have echogenic material within them ("plankton sign") or hyperechoic septations. LUS performs better than chest radiography (CXR) in detecting pleural effusions, with superior sensitivity, specificity, and positive and negative likelihood ratios.

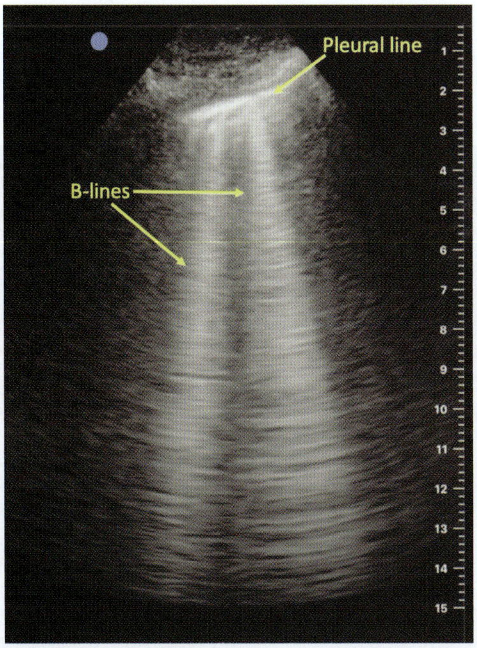

FIGURE 186-24. B-lines are vertical lines that extend from the pleural line to the bottom edge of the screen. More than three B-lines in a rib space indicate interstitial pathology.

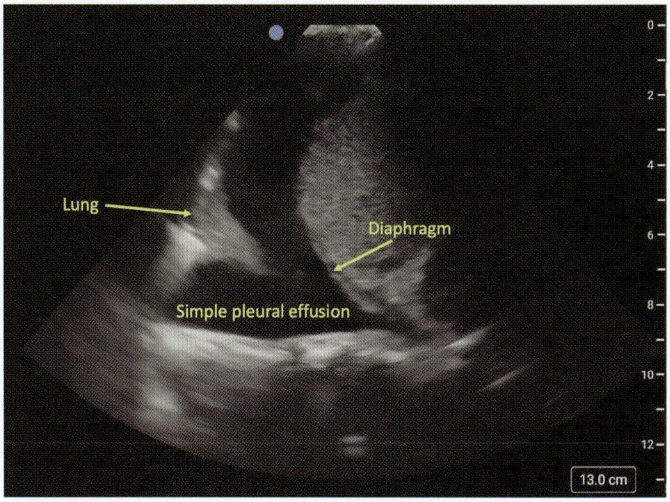

FIGURE 186-25. A simple, anechoic pleural effusion.

Consolidations. Consolidated lung has an appearance similar to that of the liver that is referred to as hepatization (**Figure 186-27**). The differential diagnosis for consolidation includes any process that fills the alveoli with fluid (e.g., pneumonia) or collapses the alveoli (e.g., atelectasis). Hyperechoic air bubbles may sometimes be seen moving in bronchioles with the patient's respirations in the background of consolidated lung. These are called dynamic air bronchograms and are more typically seen with pneumonia whereas static air bronchograms may be seen with atelectasis. In a 2015 meta-analysis performed by Pereda et al, LUS demonstrated excellent sensitivity and specificity (96% and 93%, respectively) for the diagnosis of pneumonia in children.

Bronchiolitis. Ultrasound findings that may be seen with bronchiolitis include pleural line anomalies (e.g., thickening or irregular-appearing surface), B-lines, and subcentimeter subpleural consolidations without air bronchograms. LUS findings in bronchiolitis may have prognostic value and can possibly guide treatment while decreasing use of chest radiography.

ABDOMINAL ULTRASOUND

Introduction Abdominal POCUS is performed using the abdominal ultrasound preset with any low-frequency transducer, although the high-frequency linear transducer may be used on infants. While ultrasound has long been used in pediatrics to diagnose conditions such as

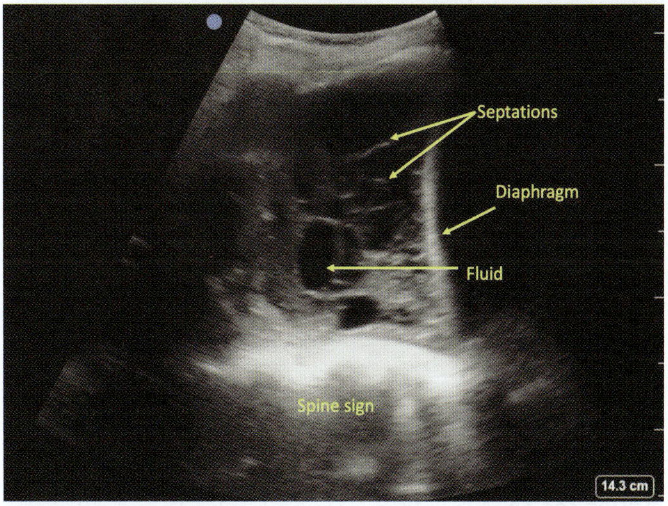

FIGURE 186-26. A complex pleural effusion with hyperechoic septations seen throughout.

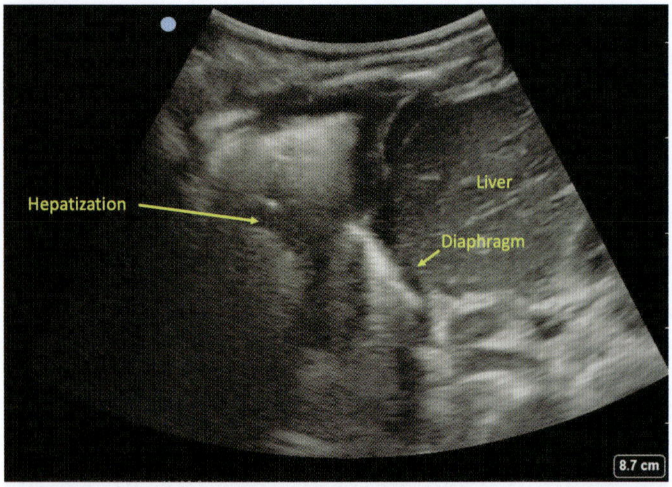

FIGURE 186-27. Hepatization of the lung gives the lung a tissular appearance similar to liver.

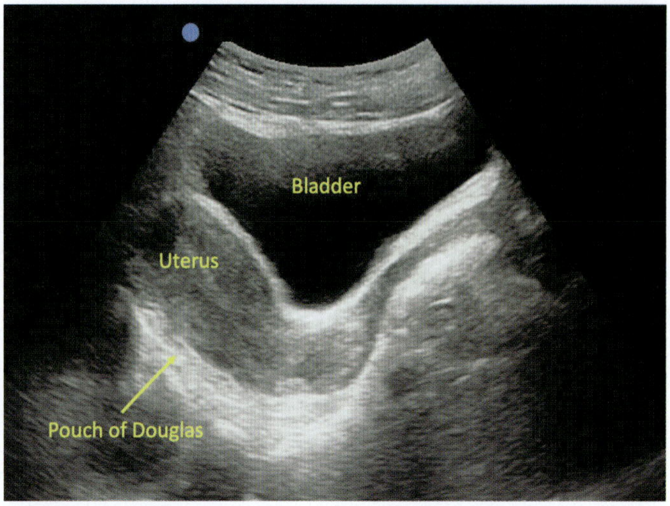

FIGURE 186-29. Sagittal view of the female bladder.

appendicitis and pyloric stenosis, making these diagnoses with POCUS requires advanced skills that are beyond the scope of this chapter. More basic applications of abdominal POCUS will be discussed here.

Bladder

Acquisition To image the bladder in transverse view, the transducer is placed just superior to the pubic symphysis with the transducer marker directed to the patient's right (**Figure 186-28**). Fanning into the pelvis may be necessary to visualize a decompressed bladder. From the transverse view, the transducer is rotated 90° clockwise so that the marker is cephalad to obtain the sagittal view.

Normal View The normal bladder will appear as an anechoic, fluid-filled structure. In a female, the uterus and vagina will appear just posterior to the bladder and anterior to the rectum (**Figure 186-29**). In males, the rectum will appear posterior to the bladder, and the prostate may be seen inferior to the bladder (**Figure 186-30**).

Clinical Questions That Can Be Answered With This View

Bladder volume. There are multiple formulas available to calculate bladder volumes based on the shape of the bladder. Measurements should be taken in both transverse and sagittal planes (**Figure 186-31**). Bladder volume is often estimated by multiplying the product of the bladder height, depth, and width by a correction coefficient that varies depending on the shape of the bladder (e.g., cuboid, ellipsoid, triangular prism) and ranges from 0.66 to 0.89. Age-adjusted bladder capacity in milliliters may be estimated using the following: bladder capacity = (years of age + 2) × 30 mL.

Malfunctioning indwelling urinary catheter. Bladder ultrasound is useful for evaluating patients with indwelling urinary catheters with poor urine output. If a catheter is functioning appropriately, the bladder should be completely decompressed with no fluid visible surrounding the circular catheter balloon. If the catheter is not draining, however, the bladder will be clearly visualized, filled with anechoic fluid surrounding the balloon (**Figure 186-32**).

Presence of free fluid. In females, there are two potential spaces where free pelvic fluid can accumulate: (i) the vesicouterine space between the bladder and uterus and (ii) the rectouterine or rectovaginal recess, also known as the pouch of Douglas. The pouch of Douglas is the most posterior and caudal reflection of the female peritoneal cavity and is therefore the location where free peritoneal fluid accumulates first in the female pelvis. In males, free fluid is likely to accumulate first in the rectovesicular space. Free fluid will appear as an anechoic stripe in these spaces. The pelvis is the most sensitive site of blood accumulation in pediatric trauma.

Right Upper Quadrant View (Liver and Kidney)

Acquisition To obtain a coronal view of the liver and right kidney, the transducer is placed on the patient's right mid-axillary line at the level of the xiphoid process with the marker cephalad (**Figure 186-33**). If the

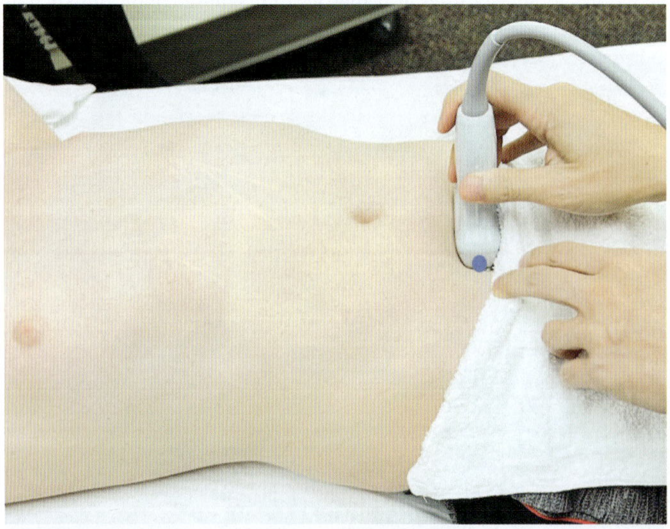

FIGURE 186-28. Position of the transducer just above the pubic symphysis to visualize the bladder.

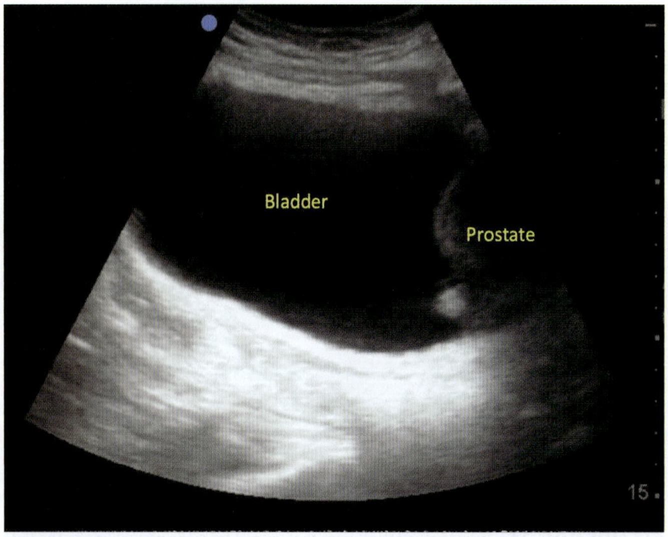

FIGURE 186-30. Sagittal view of the male bladder.

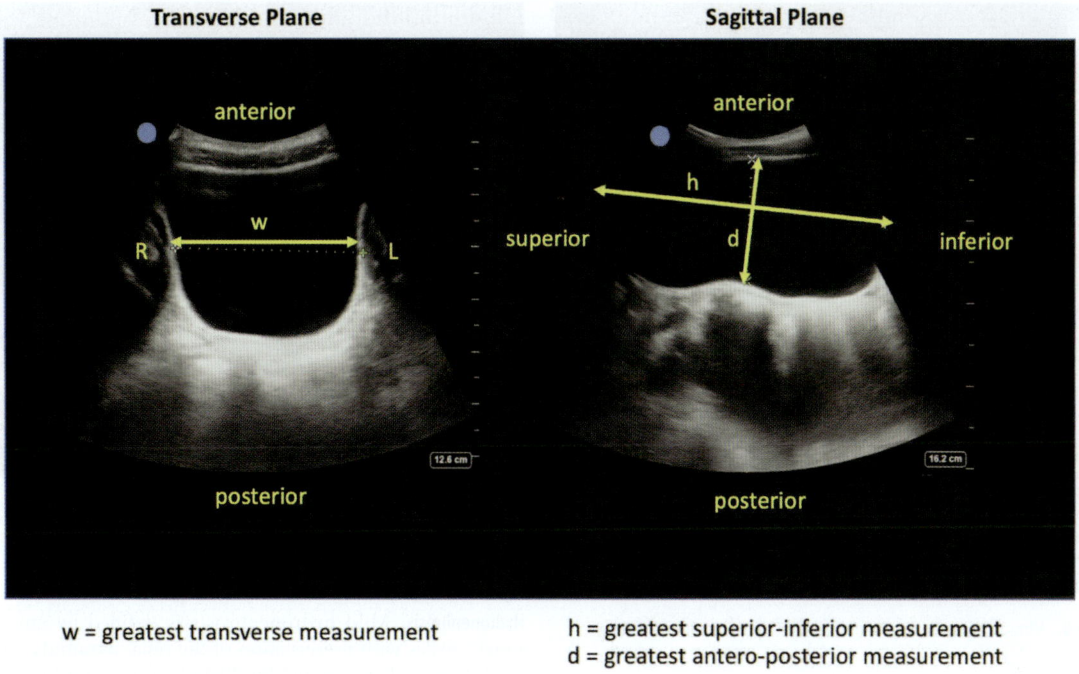

FIGURE 186-31. The width of the bladder is measured in the transverse view while the depth and height are measured in the sagittal view.

kidney is not immediately visualized, the transducer should be fanned posteriorly until it comes into view.

Normal View The liver will be seen superficial to the kidney with the hyperechoic curvilinear boundary between them representing the hepatorenal space or Morison's pouch (**Figure 186-34**).

Clinical Question That Can Be Answered in This View

Presence of free fluid. Free fluid may accumulate within the abdomen due to entities such as trauma, ascites, infection, and ruptured ectopic pregnancy or ovarian cysts. The hepatorenal recess and tip of the liver are also sensitive areas to evaluate for the presence of free fluid.

Left Upper Quadrant View (Spleen and Kidney)

Acquisition To obtain a coronal view of the spleen and left kidney, the transducer is placed on the patient's left posterior axillary line at the level of the xiphoid process with the marker cephalad (**Figure 186-35**). The spleen is typically smaller and more posterior compared to the liver so the transducer may need to be moved and/or fanned posteriorly if the spleen and kidney are not immediately visualized.

Normal View The spleen will be seen superficial to the kidney with the hyperechoic curvilinear boundary between them representing the splenorenal space (**Figure 186-36**).

Clinical Question That Can Be Answered With This View

Presence of free fluid. As with the right upper quadrant view, free abdominal fluid can be seen in this view as anechoic areas in the splenorenal space or between the diaphragm and spleen.

Kidneys

Acquisition The upper poles of the kidneys are identified using the techniques described earlier. Once the kidney is visualized, the transducer is moved caudally and slightly rotated to obtain a view of the whole kidney

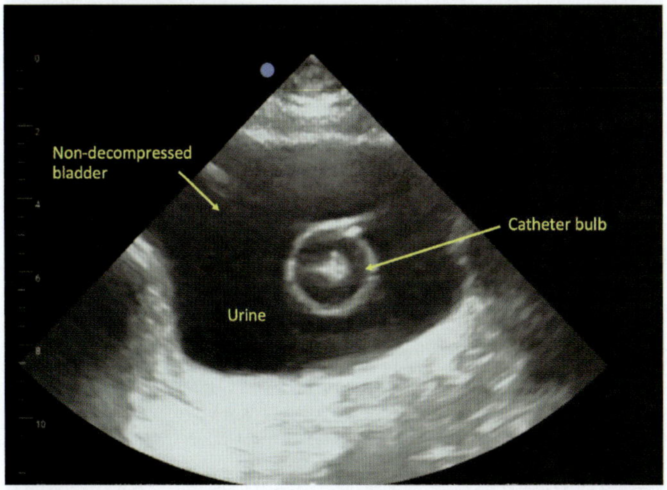

FIGURE 186-32. In this image of a malfunctioning indwelling urinary catheter, urine can be seen surrounding the catheter bulb.

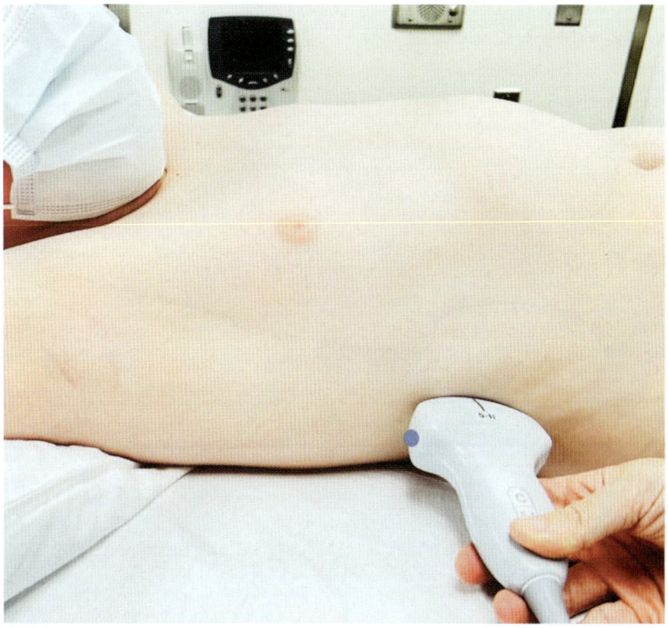

FIGURE 186-33. Transducer position to obtain a right upper quadrant view of the liver and kidney.

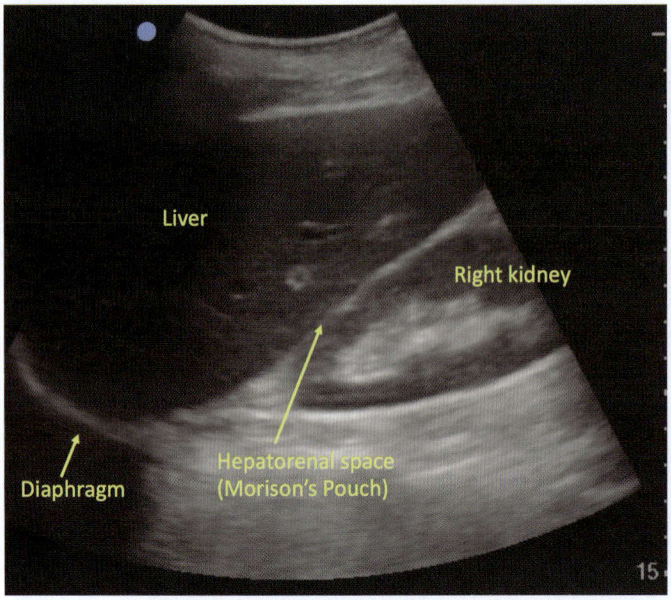

FIGURE 186-34. Ultrasonographic view of normal right upper quadrant anatomy.

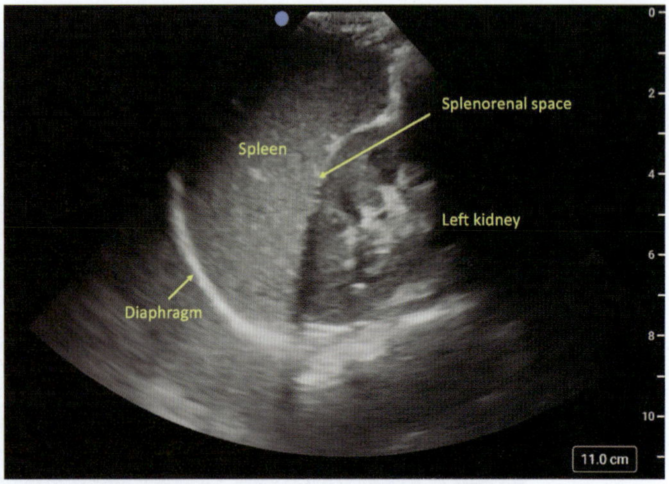

FIGURE 186-36. Ultrasonographic view of normal left upper quadrant anatomy.

in its longest axis. The transducer is then rotated 90° counterclockwise to image the kidney in its short axis.

Normal View A normal kidney on ultrasound has an iso- or hypoechoic cortex (relative to the nearby liver or spleen) surrounded by a hyperechoic renal capsule. The medulla contains the renal pyramids, which are triangular, hypoechoic, and more easily visualized in younger and well-hydrated patients. The renal sinus appears hyperechoic due to the presence of fat in this area and contains the anechoic renal pelvis that is formed by the convergence of the renal calyces (**Figure 186-37**).

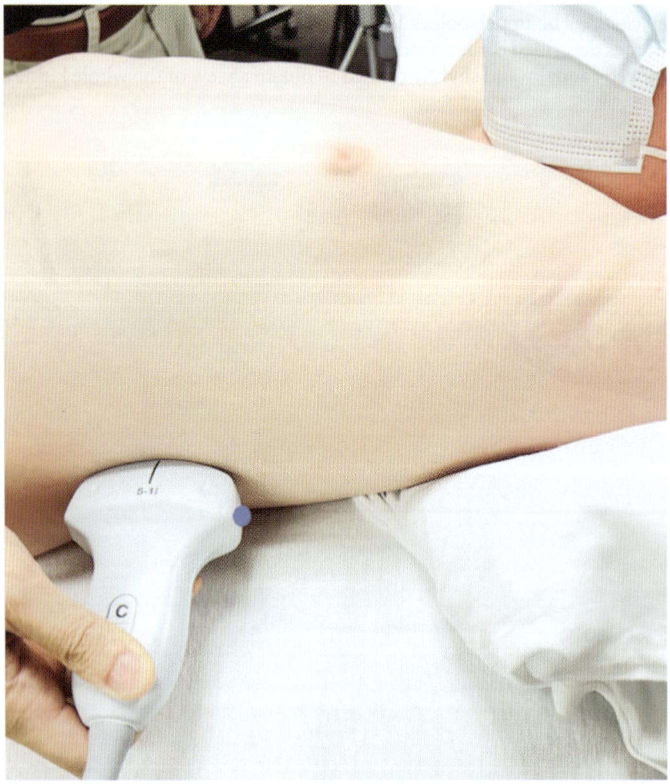

FIGURE 186-35. Transducer position to obtain a left upper quadrant view of the spleen and kidney.

Clinical Question That Can Be Answered With This View

Hydronephrosis. Mild hydronephrosis is defined by enlargement of the renal calyces with preservation of the renal pyramids. Moderate hydronephrosis is characterized by dilated calyces and blunting of the renal pyramids. Severe hydronephrosis is demonstrated by ballooning of the calyces and obliteration of the renal pyramids with cortical thinning. Renal cysts can mimic hydronephrosis; however, cysts are discrete, fluid-filled structures that do not connect with the renal pelvis. Hydronephrosis should prompt further evaluation for causes of obstruction.

SKIN AND SOFT TISSUE ULTRASOUND

Introduction POCUS is a useful adjunct to the physical exam for evaluating skin and soft tissue pathology, most commonly to distinguish uncomplicated cellulitis from abscess. Adams et al found that POCUS is superior to physical exam alone and leads to an appropriate change in management in 25% of cases.

Acquisition The high-frequency linear transducer is used and optimized using the skin or superficial preset. The transducer is placed on the abnormal area and scanned completely in orthogonal planes. POCUS examination of surrounding normal skin and soft tissue is often helpful for comparison when assessing for skin and soft tissue abnormalities.

Normal View The epidermis and dermis are the most superficial layers. Deep to the dermis is the subcutaneous tissue. Fascial layers are seen

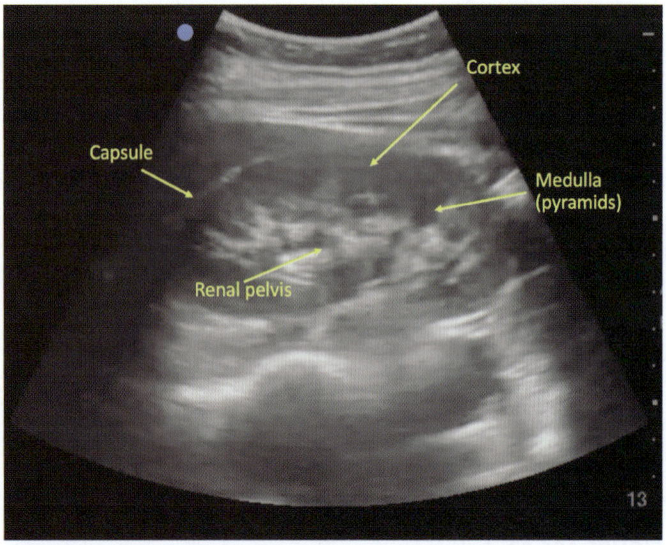

FIGURE 186-37. Normal renal anatomy.

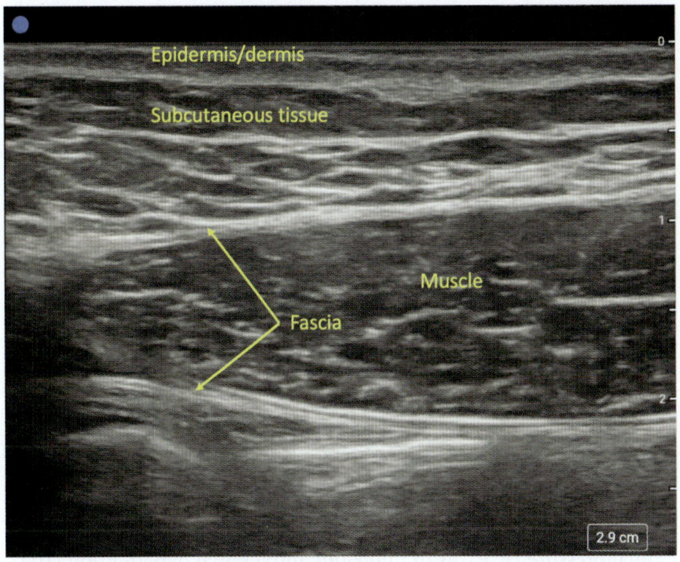

FIGURE 186-38. Normal skin and soft tissue.

as continuous hyperechoic stripes. Muscles have a characteristic striated appearance (**Figure 186-38**).

Clinical Questions That Can Be Answered With This View

Edema and Cellulitis Edema and cellulitis are both characterized by a "cobblestone" appearance of the subcutaneous tissue (**Figure 186-39**). This appearance is due to hypoechoic fluid surrounding bright fat lobules. Differentiating the two entities depends on clinical signs and symptoms as well as the typically generalized nature of edema versus the more focal inflammation seen with cellulitis.

Abscess An abscess appears as a larger fluid collection (**Figure 186-40**). The fluid collection may contain echogenic material that will swirl with compression which can help distinguish an abscess from soft tissue. Because anechoic abscesses can appear similar to blood vessels, color Doppler is applied to ensure lack of flow (**Figure 186-41**) and to map surrounding vasculature prior to any invasive intervention.

Necrotizing Fasciitis Necrotizing fasciitis is a rare but life-threatening entity for which POCUS may be vital given the potential delay in obtaining conventional imaging to support the diagnosis. The presence of subcutaneous air, which appears as bright echogenic foci with "dirty" acoustic shadowing, is highly suggestive of necrotizing fasciitis if there is already clinical suspicion (**Figure 186-42**). Thickened fascia and fluid collections between fascial layers may also be seen.

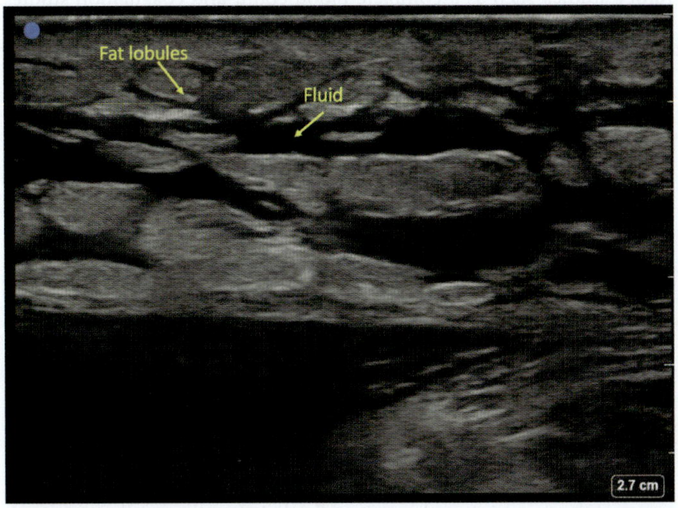

FIGURE 186-39. Fluid around fat lobules resulting in a cobblestone appearance of soft tissue can be seen with edema or cellulitis.

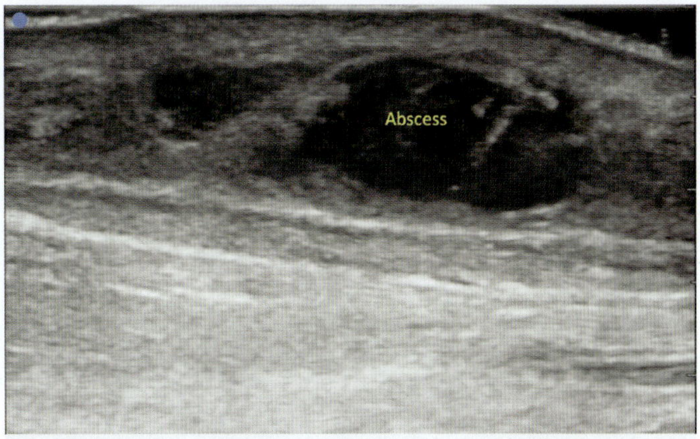

FIGURE 186-40. A collection of hypoechoic fluid representing an abscess.

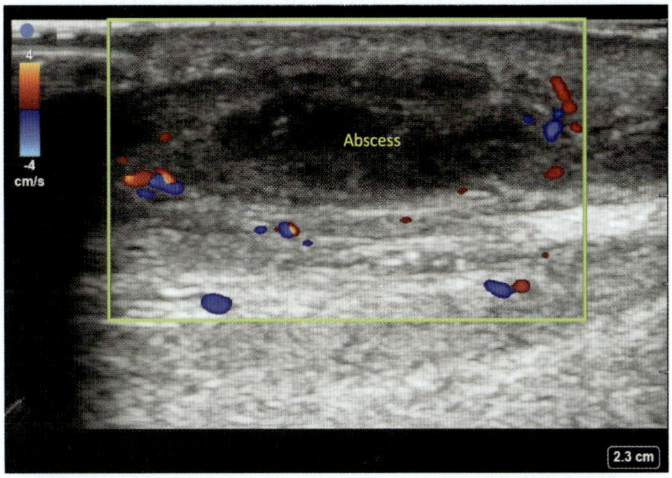

FIGURE 186-41. Color Doppler shows lack of flow within the abscess, maximizing safety of incision and drainage.

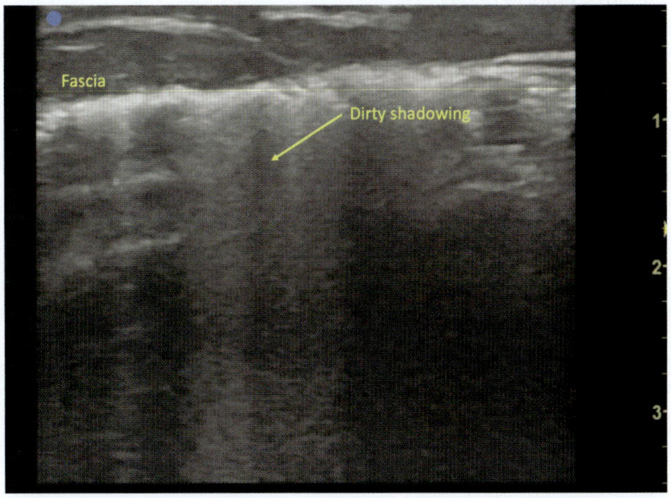

FIGURE 186-42. Air causing a "dirty shadowing" appearance at the fascial plane is seen in necrotizing fasciitis.

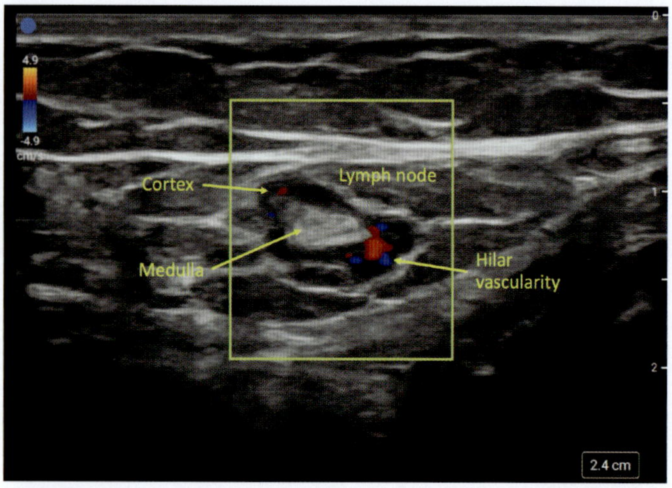

FIGURE 186-43. Lymph nodes have prominent hilar vascularity with color Doppler.

Lymphadenopathy Lymph nodes may sometimes be confused for abscesses. On ultrasound, a lymph node appears as a circular or oval structure with a hyperechoic central hilum and a hypoechoic cortex. When color Doppler is applied, flow can be seen in the hilum (**Figure 186-43**).

SUGGESTED READINGS

Adams CM, Neuman MI, Levy JA. Point-of-care ultrasonography for the diagnosis of pediatric soft tissue infection. *J Pediatr*. 2016;169:122-7.e1.

Basile V, Di Mauro A, Scalini E, et al. Lung ultrasound: a useful tool in diagnosis and management of bronchiolitis. *BMC Pediatr*. 2015;15:63.

Chao HC, Kong MS, Lin TY. Diagnosis of necrotizing fasciitis in children. *J Ultrasound Med*. 1999;18(4):277-281.

Hopkins A, Doniger SJ. Point-of-care ultrasound for the pediatric hospitalist's practice. *Hosp Pediatr*. 2019;9(9):707-718.

Kwon H, Jung JY, Lee JH, et al. Sonographic aorta/IVC cross-sectional area index for evaluation of dehydration in children. *Am J Emerg Med*. 2016;34(9):1840-1844.

Lichtenstein DA, Meziere GA. Relevance of lung ultrasound in the diagnosis of acute respiratory failure: the BLUE protocol. *Chest*. 2008; 134(1):117-125.

Long E, Oakley E, Duke T, Babl FE. Does respiratory variation in inferior vena cava diameter predict fluid responsiveness: a systematic review and meta-analysis. *Shock*. 2017;47(5):550-559.

Pereda MA, Chavez MA, Hooper-Miele CC, et al. Lung ultrasound for the diagnosis of pneumonia in children: a meta-analysis. *Pediatrics*. 2015;135(4):714-722.

Perera P, Mailhot T, Riley D, Mandavia D. The RUSH exam: Rapid Ultrasound in SHock in the evaluation of the critically ill. *Emerg Med Clin North Am*. 2010;28(1):29-56, vii.

Prada G, Fritz AV, Restrepo-Holguín M, Guru PK, Díaz-Gómez JL. Focused cardiac ultrasonography for left ventricular systolic function. *N Engl J Med*. 2019;381(21):e36.

Singh Y, Tissot C, Fraga MV, et al. International evidence-based guidelines on Point of Care Ultrasound (POCUS) for critically ill neonates and children issued by the POCUS Working Group of the European Society of Paediatric and Neonatal Intensive Care (ESPNIC). *Crit Care*. 2020;24(1):65.

Soni NJ, Arntfield R, Kory P. *Point of Care Ultrasound*. Elsevier; 2019.

Spencer KT, Kimura BJ, Korcarz CE, Pellikka PA, Rahko PS, Siegel RJ. Focused cardiac ultrasound: recommendations from the American Society of Echocardiography. *J Am Soc Echocardiogr*. Jun 2013;26(6):567-81.

Taus PJ, Manivannan S, Dancel R. Bedside assessment of the kidneys and bladder using point of care ultrasound. POCUS J. 2022;7(Kidney):94-104.

Volpicelli G, Elbarbary M, Blaivas M, et al. International evidence-based recommendations for point-of-care lung ultrasound. *Intensive Care Med*. 2012;38(4):577-591.

CHAPTER 187 Lumbar Puncture

Zia Bismilla, MD, MEd, FRCPC

Lumbar puncture (LP) is a frequently performed procedure by hospital-based physicians. Although its description may sound frightening to parents or other caregivers, in actuality, it is a fairly simple and straightforward procedure for most patients.

INDICATIONS

LP is performed whenever cerebrospinal fluid (CSF) is needed for evaluation or needs to be accessed for therapy. The most typical scenario for a pediatric hospitalist is a febrile patient in whom meningitis is a concern, including febrile infants. Other indications include evaluation of suspected central nervous system (CNS) bleeding, measurement of intracranial pressure (ICP), as in idiopathic intracranial hypertension (IIH), and investigation of suspected demyelinating or inflammatory conditions of the CNS. In patients with confirmed IIH, removal of CSF via LP is sometimes done to acutely lower ICP, providing symptom relief and preventing complications that may result from untreated increased ICP. LP may also be used to administer therapeutic agents such as antibiotics, anesthetics, chemotherapeutics, contrast agents, or muscle relaxants (e.g., baclofen), or to investigate for CNS malignancy; however, these are not commonly performed by pediatric hospitalists.

CONTRAINDICATIONS

The practitioner should always consider whether it is safe to perform an LP. LP is contraindicated in the hemodynamically unstable patient or patient with respiratory compromise. If a patient has increased ICP, such as from a cerebral mass, release of pressure during the LP may potentially precipitate shifting of intracranial contents from an area of high pressure to one of low pressure (i.e., cerebral herniation). If this is at all a possibility, the patient should have CNS imaging performed before a spinal tap is done. The risk is significantly less in infants who have an open fontanelle. The same is true for significant intracranial bleeding. In general, if the patient does not have focal neurologic findings on physical examination or demonstrate signs or symptoms of increased ICP by history or on physical examination, it is safe to perform LP before imaging. LP is relatively contraindicated in patients with underlying bleeding diatheses to avoid the formation of a hematoma around the spinal column or within the surrounding soft tissues. If this problem is suspected, laboratory studies such as a complete blood count and coagulation studies should be performed before LP is attempted. Local infection overlying the site of spinal needle insertion is also a relative contraindication to LP.

ANATOMY

CSF is produced in the choroid plexuses of the lateral ventricles. It circulates between the lateral ventricles and around the spinal cord and cerebrum in the subarachnoid space. The goal of LP is to obtain a sample of CSF in the safest possible manner, which is achieved by puncturing the dura mater in the lumbar region, below the termination of the spinal cord itself, where only the cauda equina is found. In young children, the inferior termination of the spinal cord is at the level of L3, and in older children it is even higher. Thus, LP can nearly always be performed safely, barring any anatomic anomaly, by inserting the spinal needle between the spinous processes of L4 and L5. To locate this interspace, palpate the posterior superior iliac crests; the L4-L5 interspace is located at the intersection between the top of the iliac crests and the lumbar spine midline (the supracristal line or Tuffier's line). You will feel the spinous processes of the vertebrae on the patient's back. When the needle is inserted, it will sequentially penetrate the skin, fascia and subcutaneous fat, and then the supraspinous ligament, the interspinous ligament, and the

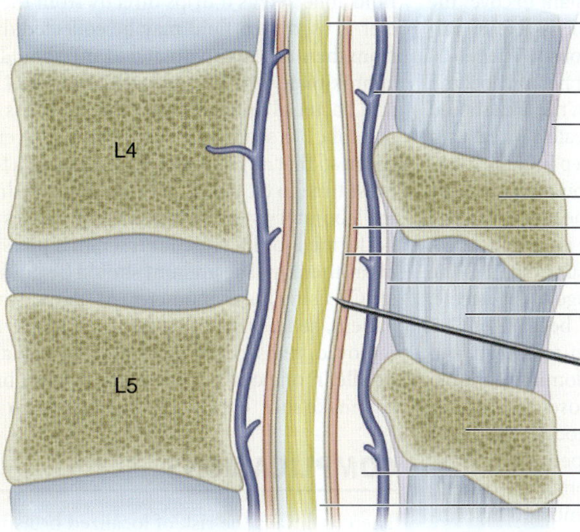

FIGURE 187-1. The spinal needle is inserted between the L4 and L5 vertebrae.

ligamentum flavum (entering the epidural space), before finally puncturing the dura mater to enter the subarachnoid space, where CSF is found (**Figure 187-1**). The depth of lumbar puncture of children younger than 3 months of age is roughly 1.0 to 1.5 cm. Many formulae exist to estimate the depth of needle insertion after 3 months old using the patient's height and/or weight; however, none of these are commonly used in practice.

EQUIPMENT

Virtually all hospitals will have a commercially made LP tray that contains most of the equipment needed to perform LP (**Table 187-1**). While some kits contain local anesthetic, most do not contain topical anesthetic (e.g., EMLA, ELA-Max). One will also need to obtain an appropriately sized spinal needle based on the age or size of the patient (**Table 187-2**). It should also be noted that some pediatric LP kits have no manometer; to measure opening pressure, a manometer must be obtained separately. Finally, labels to affix to specimens after collection should be prepped and ready to apply.

PROCEDURE

PREPARATION

Consent should be obtained prior to beginning the procedure. Before beginning, the practitioner should carefully consider issues of analgesia.

TABLE 187-1 Equipment Needed for Lumbar Puncture

Lumbar puncture tray
Spinal needle (see **Table 187-2**)
Sterile collecting tubes
Sterile drapes
Antiseptic (povidone-iodine or chlorhexidine swabs or sterile sponges and tray to pour antiseptic solution)
Gauze
Manometer (may need to be added)
Syringe and local anesthetic (1% lidocaine with or without epinephrine)
Sucrose (for neonates)
Antiseptic solution (e.g., chlorhexidine, povidone-iodine)
Additional spinal needle(s)
Sterile gloves
Face mask and eye protection
Bandage
Specimen labels

If LP is anticipated, the patient should have a topical anesthetic applied widely to the lower lumbar area in the midline. Topical anesthetics take approximately 35 to 50 minutes to take effect, so some foresight is needed. If it is anticipated that the patient may have difficulty staying still for the procedure, sedation can be considered. For neonates, sucrose may also be used for analgesia.

For positioning, the two options are to have the patient either sitting up or lying on their side. If opening pressure is required, the patient must be lying on their side. In either position, the goal is to get the patient to flex the back while drawing up the legs to maximize the size of the intervertebral space between L4 and L5. Studies using ultrasound to evaluate the size of the intervertebral spaces during various positions have shown that flexing the neck does not increase this size and is associated with more upper airway obstruction in infants being restrained. Older patients often prefer to be sitting, but infants are more often positioned on their side. The latter will be discussed because an infant requiring LP will be encountered much more frequently by the pediatric hospitalist.

TECHNIQUE

The patient is usually placed in the lateral decubitus position, on a bed of appropriate height for the practitioner. Some practitioners prefer to have the patient lying with the patient's head on the side of the practitioner's dominant hand and the feet to their non-dominant side. Others prefer the patient's head to the side of the practitioner's non-dominant hand. An important factor in determining the eventual success of LP is the skill of the person who restrains the patient. The holder should flex the spine by simultaneously holding the patient's shoulders and flexing the hips, pulling the knees to the chest while keeping the patient as still as possible. It is also important that the holder keep the back vertical, with an imaginary line between the posterior superior iliac crests lying perpendicular to the table. Open the LP tray in sterile fashion and place it close by so that you can reach the tray with one hand during the procedure. The kit has only one spinal needle. Not only should one make sure that it is an appropriate size, but it is also a good idea to have one or two extra needles on the tray in case they are needed. Once the patient is positioned, put on sterile gloves and use gauze or a swab stick soaked with anti-septic solution (e.g., povidone-iodine or chlorhexidine) to sterilize the area, starting at the desired entry site and moving out in a circular fashion, sterilizing most of the lumbosacral area. Place a fenestrated drape over the patient such that only this

TABLE 187-2 Spinal Needle Size Based on Age

Neonate-2 years	22-gauge, 1½-inch needle
2-12 years	22-gauge, 2½ inch needle
Older than 12 years	20- or 22-gauge, 3½ inch needle

sterilized area is visible. The drape is large enough in an infant to cover the posterior superior iliac spines and will be sterile; thus one is able to palpate the spines and locate the L4-L5 interspace simultaneously. The L3-L4 interspace is also acceptable. When the space is located, draw up 1 to 2 mL of lidocaine. With the use of topical anesthetics, the skin in the area should be blanched and anesthetized. After topical anesthesia, create a wheal with injectable lidocaine just below the skin, and proceed as deep into the intervertebral space as the thin ⅝-inch needle will allow. Aspirate back to be sure that there is not blood or CSF return. Then, pull the needle out slowly while injecting the lidocaine as you go. Once the lidocaine is administered, you are ready to insert the spinal needle, again making sure that it is the appropriate size. It should be noted that the larger the gauge of the needle, the more likely the patient will have a "spinal headache" because of CSF leakage after the procedure (see Complications). If the patient's head is to the same side as your dominant hand, place your non-dominant thumb over the lower of the spinous processes that you have chosen (i.e., L5 for the L4-L5 interspace). With your thumb on the spinous process, the rest of your non-dominant hand can still be on the posterior superior iliac crest, both to ensure landmarks and also to assist in stabilization of the patient. While holding the spinal needle with your dominant thumb and first finger close to its end, insert it, bevel up, through the skin pointing toward the umbilicus (slightly cephalad). Use your non-dominant thumb as a fulcrum to steady the needle as you insert it. Some practitioners find it easier to have the patient's head to the side of their non-dominant hand. With this technique, the natural extension of your dominant arm tends to direct the needle in a slightly cephalad direction as you insert it. If using this technique, the fingers of your non-dominant hand can rest on the iliac crest to ensure landmarks and help to steady the patient. The practitioner's non-dominant thumb should then palpate the more cephalad spinous process of the interspace that you are using (e.g., L4 for the L4-L5 interspace). The needle is slowly inserted in a slightly cephalad direction using the thumb over the spinous process as a fulcrum.

If there is immediate bony resistance, you are probably in contact with the spinous process, so pull the needle back and redirect it, most commonly more cephalad. Once you are past the superficial bony structures, insert the needle slowly. If you think that you may be in the subarachnoid space, remove the stylet and watch for CSF flow. Experienced practitioners may feel a "pop" as they penetrate the dura mater and a "give" as they enter the subarachnoid space. If there is no flow of CSF, it may help to rotate the needle 90 degrees. If there is still no flow of CSF, reinsert the stylet and advance the needle a few millimeters further. Literature has shown that removing the stylet after completely penetrating the epidermis and dermis (0.5-1 cm in most children) and advancing the spinal needle without the stylet leads to higher success rates, but there is concern that it may be associated with a higher incidence of intraspinal epidermoid tumors, presumably from introduction of dermis and epidermis into the spinal canal. The slow advancement of the needle is performed repeatedly until flow of CSF is obtained. If blood flows from the needle, the venous plexus just outside the epidural space (see **Figure 187-1**) may have been punctured, a so-called traumatic tap. Blood from a traumatic tap will clot, as opposed to bloody CSF, which will not. In addition, blood from a traumatic tap will gradually lessen as flow occurs, whereas bloody CSF will be homogenous throughout. If you are convinced the fluid is blood and not CSF, remove the needle completely and make another attempt in a different interspace (preferably a higher interspace e.g., L3-4). For this reason, it is recommended to start with the L4-5 interspace such that a second attempt may use a higher interspace and avoid potential blood from a puncture of the venous plexus below.

Once CSF flow has begun, opening pressure can be measured by attaching a manometer. This apparatus is a bit cumbersome, and attaching it often requires the help of an assistant. The patient must be still and not struggling, to obtain an accurate reading, which is often difficult in infants. The patient's legs must also be fully extended. Wait for the level of CSF to rise and then reach a steady height in the manometer. This takes approximately 1 to 2 minutes, and the level may continue to oscillate slightly with respiration.

Once CSF flow begins and opening pressure is measured, if necessary, collect specimens in the sterile tubes included in the kit. Fluid in the manometer may be collected if present. Once the manometer is empty it can be removed if no pressure measurement is no longer needed, and fluid collected as it drips directly from the spinal needle. If no manometer is used then fluid may be collected directly from the spinal needle from the start. Approximately 1 mL should be collected per tube (usually approximately 10-12 drops of CSF). Tube 1 is sent for culture, Gram stain, and bacterial antigen detection; tube 2 is sent for protein and glucose; and tube 3 is sent for cell count and differential. Tube 3 is selected for cell count so that any blood in the CSF from a traumatic tap will have had the most time to clear. It is good practice to draw off a fourth tube and have the laboratory store it in case other studies are desired later. If the LP was performed for increased intracranial pressure, more CSF can be drained off as therapy. The amount should be guided by frequent measurements of ICP using the manometer. As above, since this requires a cooperative patient, sedation is often required. Once the desired amount of CSF is removed, reinsert the stylet into the spinal needle and then remove the needle in one quick movement. Apply a bnadage over the puncture site and make sure that any excess antiseptic solution is wiped off the patient.

COMPLICATIONS

There is always the risk of localized bruising, bleeding and discomfort at the injection site when performing an LP, and this possibility should be discussed with the family in advance. The risk of herniation was discussed earlier. In small infants, respiratory compromise can occur, but more as a result of positioning and restraint than the LP itself. In general, young patients should be on a monitor while being tightly held. Some patients may experience transient paresthesias during the procedure. In the adult or older adolescent population, up to 30% will experience headache after LP. This is thought to be due to a small leak of CSF through the puncture in the dura. Post-LP headaches may be prevented by use of a smaller needle, directing a beveled needle parallel to the dural fibers, or use of an atraumatic pencil tip needle rather than a beveled cutting tip needle. These headaches usually respond to analgesics and fluids, with mixed evidence for the effectiveness of caffeine. Lying flat may be helpful, however routine bed rest is not required. For a prolonged headache, an epidural blood patch can be applied to stop the leak, but this is not generally necessary. Hematomas in the subdural or epidural space are reported but are rare. If the patient has neurologic deficits after LP, traumatic bleeding must be ruled out. Iatrogenic meningitis, nerve root injury or damage to other adjacent structures are possible but exceedingly rare. Finally, as noted above, there is a risk of pushing superficial dermal material into the subarachnoid space during LP, and subsequent risk for development of intraspinal epidermoid tumors. This can generally be avoided by having the stylet in the needle whenever it is advanced and when it is removed.

SPECIAL CONSIDERATIONS

In patients who have had unsuccessful attempts at LP because of body habitus, anatomic abnormality, an inability to obtain CSF, or a "traumatic tap," several radiologic modalities are available to assist the hospitalist. Fluoroscopy allows the radiologist, via serial spine x-rays while the needle is gradually inserted, to visualize penetration through the appropriate interspinal space, and can suggest that the needle is in the subarachnoid space. Computed Tomography (CT) gives greater detail but is associated with higher levels of radiation exposure. Ultrasound is increasingly used as the first-line option for image guidance, especially in neonates. Ultrasound can visualize the anatomy of the spine and spinal canal in real time and increases success rates of LP without associated radiation exposure. If there was a previous traumatic tap, ultrasound can also delineate the presence and extent of any epidural hematoma, and guide subsequent attempts away from the affected interspaces. Lastly, many pediatric tertiary care centers have pediatric neurosurgeons or interventional neuroradiologists who can be an invaluable consulting resource for difficult lumbar punctures.

SUGGESTED READINGS

Abo A, Chen L, Johnston P, Santucci K. Positioning for lumbar puncture in children evaluated by bedside ultrasound. *Pediatrics*. 2010;125(5):e1149-1153.

Bonadio W. Pediatric lumbar puncture and cerebrospinal fluid analysis. *J Emerg Med*. 2014 Jan;46(1):141-150.
Janssens E, Aerssens P, Alliet P, et al. Post-dural puncture headache in children. A literature review. *Eur J Pediatr*. 2003;162:117-121.
Muthusami P, Robinson AJ, Shroff MM. Ultrasound guidance for difficult lumbar puncture in children: pearls and pitfalls. *Pediatr Radiol*. 2017;47(7):822-830.
Nath S, Koziarz A, Badhiwala JH, et al. Atraumatic versus conventional lumbar puncture needles: a systematic review and meta-analysis. *Lancet*. 2018 4;391(10126):1197-1204.
Per H, Kumanda S, Gumus H, et al. Iatrogenic epidermoid tumor: late complication of lumbar puncture. *J Child Neurol*. 2007;22(3):332-336.

CHAPTER 188

Bladder Catheterization

Beth Harper, MD

BACKGROUND

Urinary bladder catheterization in children can serve as both a diagnostic and therapeutic intervention. Catheterization is a simple, sterile procedure that can be performed at the bedside in most circumstances. Ease of performing the procedure, ability of nursing to catheterize, and decreased pain are some reasons catheterization has largely replaced suprapubic aspiration as the primary method of urine collection in young children. Children usually tolerate the procedure well when it is done carefully, requiring only a topical anesthetic, if any. Success rates are usually high with this bedside procedure, although point of care ultrasound may increase the yield as well by ensuring there is enough urine in the bladder prior to catheterization.

INDICATIONS

The most common indication for urinary bladder catheterization is collection of urine for analysis and culture. A catheter specimen is recommended to rule out urinary tract infection in those children who are not yet toilet trained or who are unable to cooperate with a midstream clean-catch specimen. Catheterization is also indicated to relieve urinary retention or obstruction. This may be due to anatomic abnormalities such as posterior urethral valves, prolapsing ureterocele, inflammation of the urethra, or mechanical obstruction. Neurogenic bladder or medication effects may also cause retention requiring catheterization. In critically ill patients, urinary catheterization is used to monitor urine output and assess fluid status.

CONTRAINDICATIONS

Few contraindications exist for urinary catheterization. In certain specific situations, consultation with a urologist is recommended prior to attempting bladder catheterization. These include known or suspected urethral trauma or pelvic fracture; recent genitourinary surgery; or known urethral or genital abnormality such as hypospadias or bladder exstrophy.

ANATOMY

A catheter is placed into the bladder via the urethral meatus. In males, the meatus is located in the center of the glans of the penis. If the patient is uncircumcised, the foreskin may need to be gently retracted to expose the urethra. In females, the urethra is located between the clitoris and the vaginal introitus. The labia majora and minora obscure the urethra in most patients and will need to be spread in order to visualize the meatus (**Figure 188-1**).

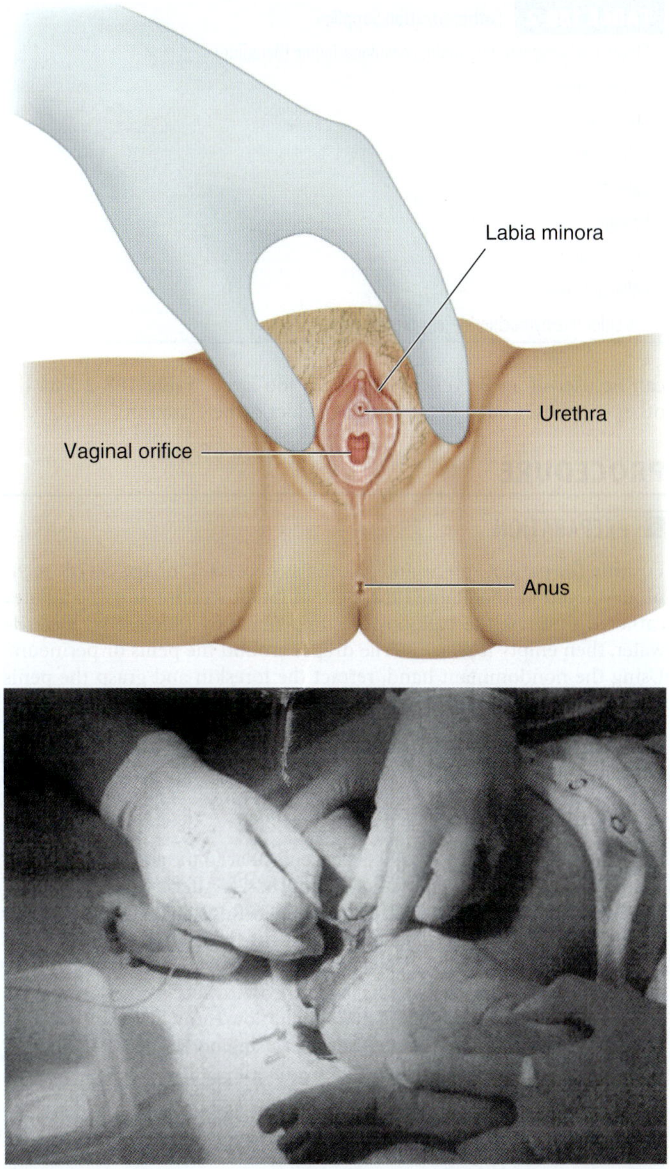

FIGURE 188-1. Transurethral bladder catheterization; anatomy and position in the female. (Reproduced with permission from Dieckmann RA, Fiser DH, Selbst SM, eds. *Illustrated Textbook of Pediatric Emergency and Critical Care Procedures*. St Louis: Mosby; 1997:415. Copyright © Elsevier.)

EQUIPMENT

Catheters come in many shapes and sizes. The most common sizes for age are listed in **Table 188-1**. The two most common catheters used in children are a straight catheter and a self-retaining Foley catheter. A straight catheter is used for one-time or intermittent catheterization. If long-term catheterization is anticipated, a Foley catheter is appropriate. Choose the smallest lumen possible to pass the catheter easily and accomplish the goals of catheterization. In a newborn or infant, a 5-French feeding tube

TABLE 188-1 Catheter Sizes

Age	Size (French)
Newborn	8
Young child	10
Adolescent	12
Adult	16

TABLE 188-2 Catheterization Supplies
Sterile cleansing solution (iodine, povidone-iodine [Betadine])
Sterile drapes
Sterile gloves
Lubricant
Catheter
Syringe
Sterile water
Collection device
2% Lidocaine hydrochloride jelly (optional)

can be used if an 8-French catheter is too large. **Table 188-2** lists the other supplies needed to perform a bladder catheterization.

PROCEDURE

PREPARATION

Position the patient supine and restrain as necessary for age. Sterile technique should be maintained throughout the procedure. If using a Foley catheter, first test the balloon for competency by filling it with sterile water, then empty it. Place sterile drapes around the penis or perineum. Using the nondominant hand, retract the foreskin and grasp the penis or spread the labia to expose the urethral meatus. Cleanse the urethral opening and surrounding tissue with sterile or antiseptic solution. If desired, slowly inject viscous lidocaine into the urethral opening.

TECHNIQUE

Extend the penile shaft so that it is perpendicular to the abdomen in order to straighten the urethra in males (**Figure 188-2**). After lubricating the tip, slowly advance the catheter into the bladder. Resistance in males is frequently the result of volitional constriction of the external sphincter and can usually be overcome with firm, steady pressure. For straight catheterization, stop advancing once urine is obtained. Advance a Foley catheter its entire length into the bladder. Urine should flow easily into the collection container. If no urine is obtained, consider using point of care ultrasound to confirm catheter location, or irrigating the catheter with sterile water to confirm urine return. In females, absence of urine return may indicate misplacement into the vagina or a bladder that is empty of urine. If the catheter is removed and additional attempts are necessary to obtain urine, the clinician should use a new, sterile catheter to reduce contamination. Once the Foley catheter is advanced its entire length, inflate the balloon with sterile water, and pull the catheter back until resistance is met, indicating that the balloon is at the bladder neck. If using a straight catheter, remove the catheter after the bladder is emptied. If the patient is an uncircumcised male, be sure to replace the foreskin to its original position. If a Foley catheter is to be left in place, secure the catheter by taping it to the child's leg.

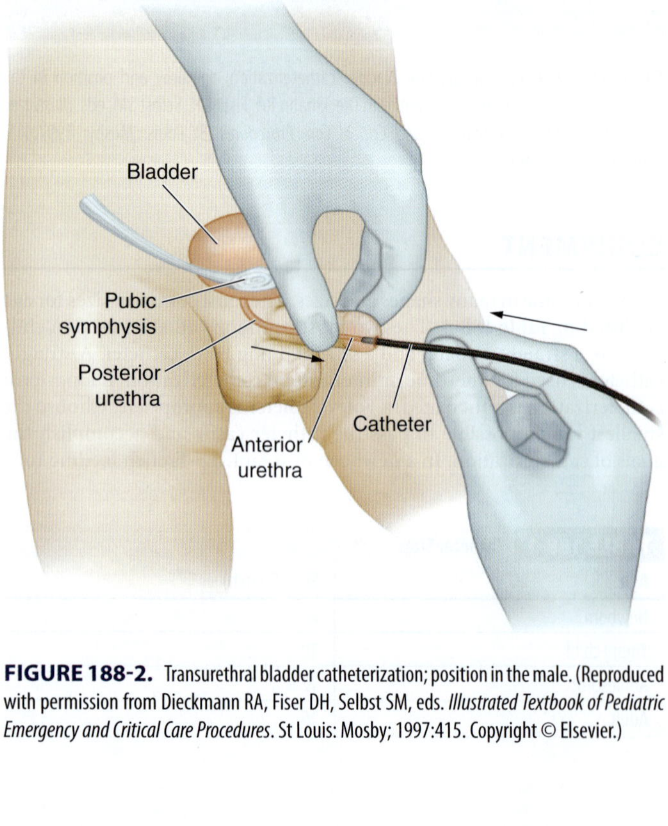

FIGURE 188-2. Transurethral bladder catheterization; position in the male. (Reproduced with permission from Dieckmann RA, Fiser DH, Selbst SM, eds. *Illustrated Textbook of Pediatric Emergency and Critical Care Procedures*. St Louis: Mosby; 1997:415. Copyright © Elsevier.)

COMPLICATIONS

If continued resistance is met while attempting catheterization, stop. Potential complications of catheterization include localized trauma, creation of a false passage, and future stricture formation. Other rare complications include urinary retention, bladder perforation, knotting of the catheter while in the bladder, and introduction of bacteria with resultant infection. The risk of catheter-associated urinary tract infection increases with the duration of indwelling time; therefore, Foley catheters should be removed as soon as clinically indicated.

SUGGESTED READINGS

Akca Caglar A, Tekeli A, Karacan C, Tuygun N. Point-of-care ultrasound-guided versus conventional bladder catheterization for urine sampling in children aged 0 to 24 months. *Pediatr Emerg Care*. 2021;37(8):413-416.

Al-Farsi S, Oliva M, Davidson R, Richardson SE, Ratnapalan S. Periurethral cleaning prior to urinary catheterization in children: sterile water versus 10% povidone-iodine. *Clin Pediatr*. 2009;48(6):656.

Desjardins MP, Gaucher N, Gravel J, Lebel D, Gouin S. A randomized double-blind trial comparing the effect on pain of an oral sucrose solution versus placebo in children 1-3 months old needing bladder catheterization. *Canadian J Emerg Med*. 2021;23(5):655-662.

Krozer E, Rosenbloom E, Goldman D, Lavy G, Rosenfeld N, Goldman M. Pain in infants who are younger than 2 months during suprapubic aspiration and transurethral bladder catheterization: a randomized, controlled study. *Pediatrics*. 2006;118:e51-e56.

Letica-Kriegel AS, Salmasian H, Vawdrey DK, et al. Identifying the risk factors for catheter-associated urinary tract infections: a large cross-sectional study of six hospitals. *BMJ Open*. 2019;9(2):e022137.

Subcommittee on Urinary Tract Infection, Roberts KB, Downs SM, et al. Reaffirmation of AAP Clinical Practice Guideline: the diagnosis and management of the initial urinary tract infection in febrile infants and young children 2-24 months of age. *Pediatrics*. 2016;138(6):e20163026.

Vaughan M, Paton EA, Bush A, Pershad J. Does lidocaine gel alleviate the pain of bladder catheterization in young children? A randomized controlled trial. *Pediatrics*. 2005;116(4):917.

Wingerter S, Bachur R. Risk factors for contamination of catheterized urine specimens in febrile children. *Pediatr Emerg Care*. 2011;27(1):1.

CHAPTER 189 Arterial Blood Gas

Joseph DiCara, MD, MPH

BACKGROUND

Arterial puncture or arterial blood gas sampling is a necessary procedure in the evaluation of any critically ill patient, especially those with significant respiratory distress or compromise. The ability to measure and interpret pH, PCO_2, PO_2, and HCO_3^- in these patients is an essential skill for the pediatric hospitalist. Arterial blood sampling is also essential when needing significant amounts of blood, particularly in newborns and preterm babies where venipuncture is challenging or impractical. Although the procedure itself is similar to venipuncture, there are significant differences and potential complications of which to be aware.

INDICATIONS

Arterial puncture is a common procedure in the management of critically ill and injured children. Arterial blood gas sampling provides information about lung ventilation through the interpretation of PCO_2 and tissue oxygenation through the interpretation of PO_2 for patients with respiratory distress and/or cardiovascular compromise. It is also often needed to clarify abnormal capnography or pulse oximetry readings. Quantification of the levels of dyshemoglobins such as carboxyhemoglobin and methemoglobin may be obtained as well. Acid-base problems are associated with a number of diseases, such as diabetic ketoacidosis, shock, dehydration, metabolic diseases, and certain toxic ingestions. They are also critical in the evaluation of newborns with potential hypoxic-ischemic encephalopathy. Both the diagnosis and treatment of these conditions are often based on the interpretation of arterial pH, PCO_2, PO_2, and bicarbonate (HCO_3) levels. Arterial blood draws are also essential when requiring larger samples of blood for workups in neonates and young children.

CONTRAINDICATIONS

Collateral circulation of the hand must be assessed when attempting radial artery puncture or catheterization. Hosokawa and Yano, in their study of the Allen test on 2940 arms, found it demonstrated consistent and valid results in the assessment of collateral blood flow to the hand. The correct procedure for an Allen test is shown in **Figure 189-1.** Arterial puncture should not be attempted at that site if return of perfusion takes longer than a few seconds, indicating inadequate collateral circulation. In a young, difficult, or unconscious patient, a modified Allen test can be performed.

Caution should be taken with patients receiving anticoagulants or those with bleeding disorders. Avoid arterial access when the patient has an infection or burn of the overlying skin.

ANATOMY

Arterial blood gas samples can be obtained from a number of sites, including the following:

- Radial artery at the wrist—the most common site for arterial blood sampling because of its easy accessibility, superficial location, and availability of collateral circulation.
- Posterior tibial artery at the foot between the medial malleolus and the calcaneal tendon while the foot is in dorsiflexion.
- Dorsalis pedis artery on the dorsal aspect of the midfoot between the extensor hallucis and extensor digitorum longus while the foot is in plantar flexion.
- Brachial artery at the antecubital fossa, right above the crease and medial to the biceps tendon.
- Femoral artery below the midpoint of the inguinal ligament. This site should be used only as a last resort in emergent situations because of the increased risk of complications.
- Umbilical artery in the neonate can be accessed for hours to days after delivery.

EQUIPMENT

Although prepackaged arterial puncture kits are commercially available, only minimal equipment is needed:

- Butterfly or regular needle (23 gauge is most commonly used; may also use 21 or 25 gauge)
- Heparinized syringe that can be sealed air-tight for blood gas; 3 or 5 cc syringe for blood draws.

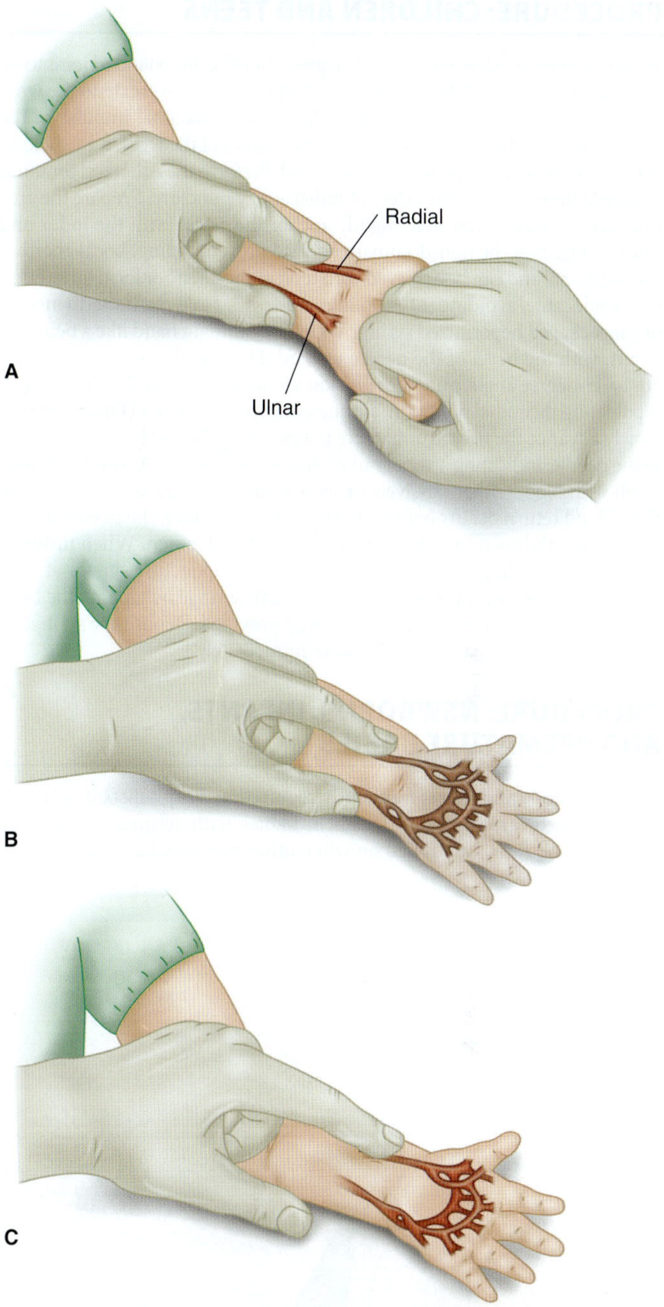

FIGURE 189-1. Modified Allen test. (A) Close the child's hand with firm pressure while simultaneously occluding the ipsilateral radial and ulnar arteries with the index finger and thumb of the opposite hand. (B) After a few seconds to allow an adequate reduction of blood volume in the hand, release the hand while maintaining point pressure on the radial and ulnar arteries. When this maneuver is performed properly, this hand should appear paler than the other one. (C) Release the pressure applied to the ulnar artery while maintaining point pressure on the radial artery. Reperfusion of the entire hand should occur within a few seconds if sufficient collateral circulation is present. (Reproduced with permission from Dieckmann RA, Fiser DH, Selbst SM, eds. *Illustrated Textbook of Pediatric Emergency and Critical Care Procedures*. St Louis: Mosby; 1997:166. Copyright © Elsevier.)

- Iodophor or other antiseptic solution to prepare the puncture site.
- Sterile drapes, gauze, and gloves.
- Optional—Local or topical anesthetic (in an awake or conscious patient)
- Transillumination or bedside ultrasound can be used to locate the artery.

An arterial catheter can be considered if it frequent arterial blood sampling will be required.

PROCEDURE: CHILDREN AND TEENS

Hold the wrist in extension 30 to 45 degrees, or affix the extended joint to an arm board with tape. While extension is helpful, do not overextend the wrist because this may occlude the pulse. The point of maximal impulse of the radial artery can be palpated on the palmar aspect of the wrist at the second transverse wrist crease proximal to the hand. Perform the Allen test for ulnar collateral flow to assess the safety of radial artery puncture. Prepare the area in a sterile fashion. You may slightly anchor the artery with the index and middle fingers of the non-dominant hand to prevent rolling. Local anesthesia is optional and can be achieved with topical anesthetic or local infiltration of 1% lidocaine, avoiding infusion into the vessel. Hold the butterfly needle or prepackaged heparinized syringe with the dominant hand like a pencil or a dart, with the bevel of the needle upward. Holding the needle at about a 30- to 45-degree angle, puncture the skin just distal to where the index finger is palpating the radial pulsation, aiming away from the hand **(Figure 189-2)**. Slowly advance the needle until there is a pulsating flash of blood in the hub of the needle, indicating arterial rather than venous access. Allow the syringe to fill with blood either passively or with aspiration to the amount desired. If no blood return occurs before meeting bony resistance, the needle should be slowly withdrawn in order to reenter the arterial lumen. When finished, remove the needle and apply firm pressure at the puncture site for at least 5 minutes. Expel any air bubbles in the upright syringe by tapping the bubbles to the top. Seal the syringe with the cap provided. Deposit the syringe in a bag of ice and send it to the laboratory immediately.

PROCEDURE: NEWBORNS, INFANTS, AND PREMATURE BABIES

Arterial blood sampling is frequently required by hospitalists in a NICU. In addition to arterial blood gases in babies with respiratory distress, arterial blood draws are relied on when other methods have failed or are impractical including a clotted CBC, hemolyzed potassium, and when venous or heel stick sampling of larger samples of blood in small babies is not practical. While the general technique is similar, the following are the important factors and adaptations to consider which increase the success of the procedure.

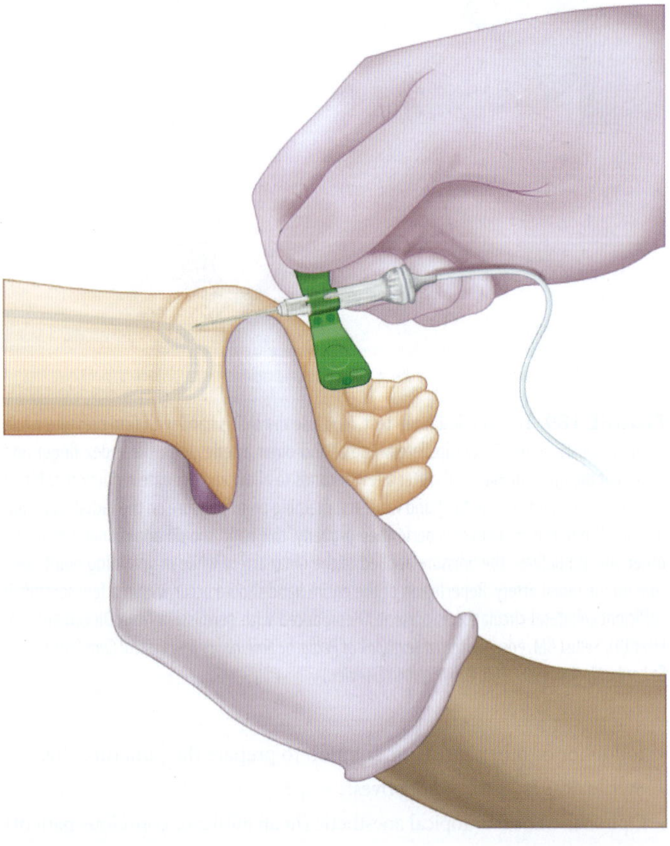

FIGURE 189-2. Technique for arterial blood draws. Secure the arm distally grasping the palm of the hand in case the child moves while slightly flexing the wrist; enter at an approximately 30 degree angle.

SITE SELECTION AND RESTRAINT

The most common sites used in neonates are the radial and posterior tibial arteries. The brachial and femoral arteries are rarely, if ever used. Since neonates and infants are likely to move, the non-dominant hand should be used to grasp the child's palm and straighten and secure the arm. Artery "rolling" is not a concern when grasping the wrist and straightening the arm.

NEEDLE GAUGE

You do not need to use smaller, 25-gauge needles. In even the smallest pre-term babies, we have found that 23-gauge needles have higher rates of success. In lower diameter needles, the resistance caused by the inner walls of the lumen will increase by the inverse square of the radius ($\frac{1}{r^2}$). Therefore, small changes in diameter can cause significant increases in resistance. In addition, the normal mean arterial blood pressure in premature babies is much lower—approximately equal to their gestational age. The combination of lower mean arterial pressure trying to push through a needle lumen with higher internal resistance makes the use of the smallest diameter needles questionable at best.

ASPIRATION

Neonates and young children have lower arterial pressures, and therefore cannot spontaneously push blood back against the resistance caused by the syringe's barrel with the plunger and air-tight gasket. Therefore, after the flashback, attach the syringe and be prepared to aspirate the blood back. When drawing a blood gas with a butterfly, do not attach the syringe until after the tubing completely fills with blood or this may falsely elevate the PO_2.

TRANSILLUMINATION

Transillumination is a very effective method of doing peripheral arterial blood draws in neonates and small toddlers. The human eye can see objects as small as 29 microns. Continuous visualization by sight is much more reliable than estimating exactly where you felt a pulse after removing your finger. In addition, transillumination will help you see the direction of the artery over a few centimeters, enabling you to align your needle with the exact trajectory of the artery. There are many ways to transilluminate using commercially available lights, or you can use a pen light or a typical fiberoptic transilluminator used to check for a pneumothorax. Generally, the larger the baby or infant, the stronger the light required. The preparation and angle of introduction is the same as previously noted. Lower the lighting in the room for better visualization. Use the transilluminator to make a flat table over which to drape the wrist, bending the hand to approximately 30 to 45 degrees **(Figure 189-3)**. It is important that the wrist surface is horizontal or else one can risk hitting the artery obliquely. Typically, the physician drawing the blood is holding or positioning the hand against the light with one hand, while directing the needle with the dominant hand, and a colleague is aspirating the blood into the syringe.

ADDITIONAL TIPS

Have an Assistant In babies and children who are likely to move, the physician will most likely use their dominant hand to direct the needle and their other hand to secure the arm. An assistant is therefore helpful to aspirate the blood, attach syringes especially when drawing additional blood, provide additional restraint to the child, and calm the patient including giving high sucrose solution orally to babies.

Don't Hold On! Once in the artery and experiencing blood return, it is not necessary to grasp the butterfly needle with two fingers. If the patient moves while the needle's being grasped, it will come out of the artery. There is

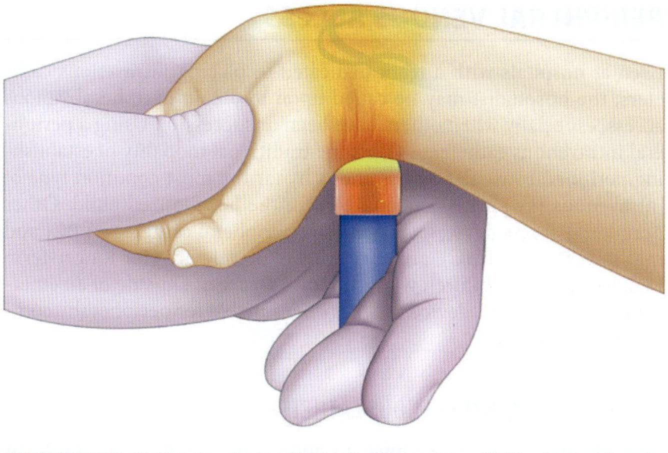

FIGURE 189-3. Technique for transillumination in neonates and babies. Grasp at the palm while draping the wrist over the light source; keep the wrist horizontal avoiding any rotation.

sufficient smooth muscle in the arterial wall to hold the needle in place with minimal support of the butterfly. (**Figure 189-4**) shows a method to support the needle with one finger underneath the butterfly. If the child moves, the needle will move with the child and not come out of the artery.

If Blood Return Pauses If an initial blood return stops, the first maneuver should not be to advance or retract the needle. Oftentimes, the bevel of the needle is against the upper wall of the artery. Instead of advancing or retracting the needle which may take your needle out of an artery, support the butterfly from below, and slowly lift the needle upward. This often reinitiates blood flow. If this does not work, then you can slowly retract or advance the needle (**Figure 189-5**).

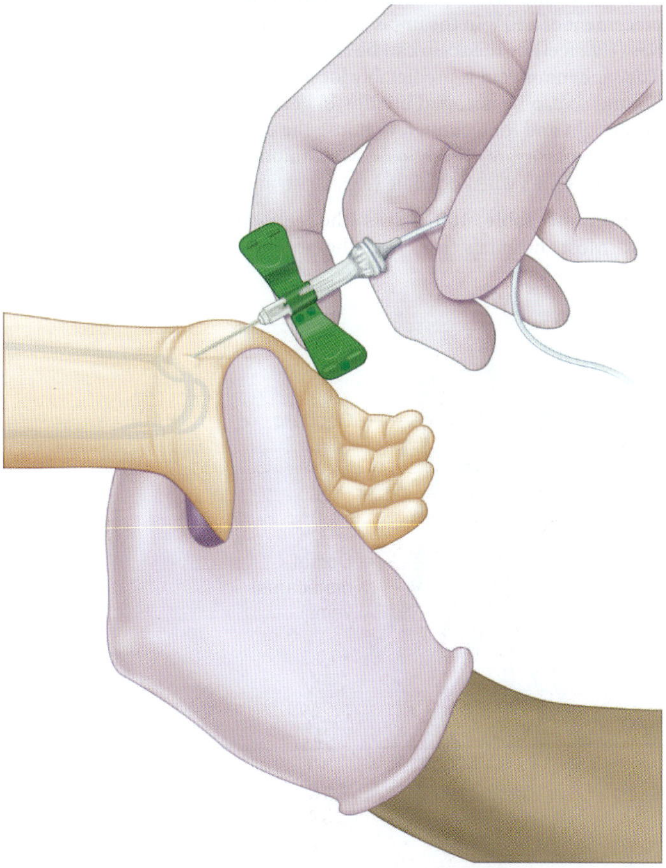

FIGURE 189-4. Supporting the needle. After flashback, support the butterfly or needle without grasping by placing your index finger below the needle. If the child moves, the needle is less likely to come out of the artery. This technique is particularly important when also drawing larger volumes of blood for studies.

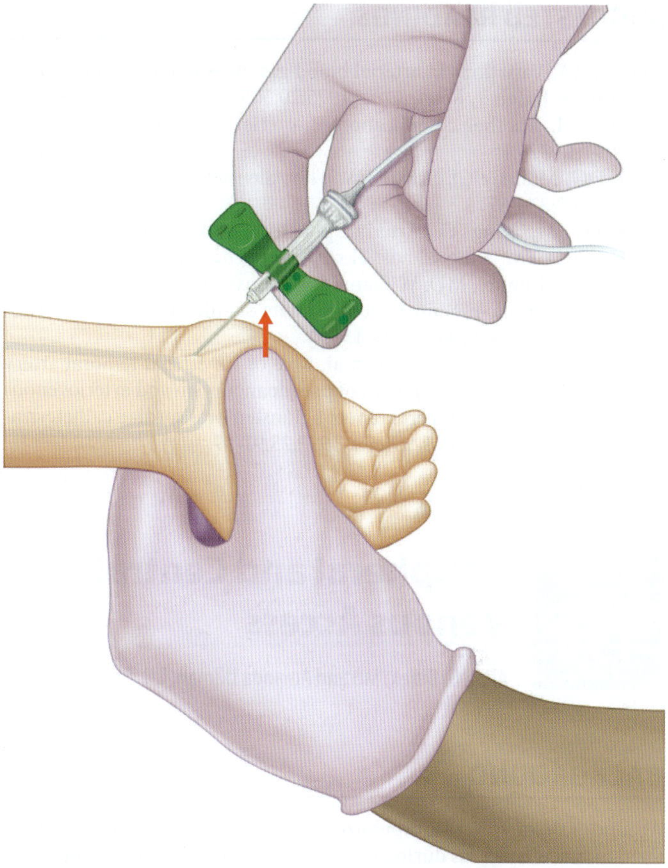

FIGURE 189-5. Troubleshooting a flashback that stops. The initial maneuver is to angle the needle up slightly. If this doesn't reinitiate blood return, then you can advance or withdraw the needle.

COMPLICATIONS

The most significant potential complication of arterial puncture is permanent damage to the artery that interferes with the arterial supply to the distal aspect of the extremity. This is especially serious in patients who have absent or reduced collateral circulation. Damage, which is rare, is more commonly seen as a result of repetitive punctures and can result from thrombus of the lumen, sheering of the intima, pseudoaneurysm, or arteriovenous fistula. A more common complication is hematoma formation, which can be reduced with the application of direct pressure. To reduce infection, one should always employ sterile technique and avoid using sites with overlying cellulitis. Bageant, in the journal Respiratory Care, lists a variety of sampling errors that may occur owing to the transport or timing of the blood gas sample or to the patient's underlying condition (**Table 189-1**).

TABLE 189-1 Blood Gas Sampling Errors
Air or air bubbles in the syringe: equilibration between blood and air causes PO_2 to be altered and PCO_2 to decrease
Delay in icing or analyzing blood gas sample: allows for metabolism, causing a decrease in PO_2 and pH and an increase in PCO_2
Venous or venous admixture sample: correlates with clinical presentation and oxygen saturation as measured by pulse oximetry (SpO_2)
Alterations in temperature (< or >37°C):
Fever: PO_2 and PCO_2 are increased and pH decreased
Hypothermia: PO_2 and PCO_2 are decreased and pH increased
Excess heparin in syringe: dilutional acidic effect causes alterations in PO_2, PCO_2, and pH
Leukocytosis and thrombocytosis may elevate PCO_2 and lower pH

SUGGESTED READINGS

Bageant RA. Variations in arterial blood gas measurements due to sampling techniques. *Respir Care*. 1975;20:565.

Brown MM. Another complication of arterial cannulation. *Anesthesia*. 1991;46:326.

Cable DG, Mullany CJ, Schaff HV. The Allen test. *Ann Thoracic Surg*. 1999;67:876-877.

Henretig FM, King C. Arterial puncture and catheterization. In: Henretig FM, King C, eds. *Textbook of Pediatric Emergency Procedures*. Baltimore, MD: Williams & Wilkins; 2008:715-725.

Hosokawa K, Hata Y, Yano K, et al. Results of Allen test on 2940 arms. *Ann Plast Surg*. 1990;24:149-151.

Kim D, Orron DE, Skillman JJ, et al. Role of superficial femoral artery puncture in the development of pseudoaneurysm and arteriovenous fistula complicating percutaneous transfemoral cardiac catheterization. *Cathet Cardiovasc Diagn*. 1992;25:91-97.

CHAPTER 190

Peripheral and Central Venous Access

Alina G. Burek, MD and Amanda Ullman, RN, PhD

BACKGROUND

Around 60% to 70% of hospitalized pediatric patients will need some form of vascular access during their initial evaluation or hospitalization. The child's severity of illness or injury, type of infusion needed, duration of therapy, and skill of the provider will often determine the type of vascular access device selected. The use of technology to guide vascular access insertion, including ultrasound, is an important advance in safety and efficacy. This chapter reviews the insertion and monitoring needed for peripheral intravenous access (including peripheral venous catheters, midline catheters, and long peripheral catheters) and central venous access (including peripherally inserted central catheters and central venous catheters). The following two chapters review the placement of the intraosseous catheters and umbilical artery and vein catheterization.

PERIPHERAL VENOUS ACCESS

Even at hospitals with a team dedicated to placing intravenous catheters, the hospitalist may be called upon to obtain peripheral venous access, especially when others have been unsuccessful. Using a peripheral intravenous catheter (PIV) is the traditional modality of establishing peripheral vascular access and is by far the most common type of intravenous (IV) access encountered in the hospitalized child. Other peripheral access devices, such as long peripheral catheters (LPC) and midline catheters (MC), are effective vascular devices for longer-term IV needs and for children with difficult IV access. Outside of an emergency situation, this device range is only suitable for peripherally compatible therapies.

PERIPHERAL INTRAVENOUS CATHETER

Indications A PIV is obtained to administer medications, fluids, or blood products when IV access need is immediate and/or therapy length is less than 5 days in duration as the average dwell-time for a PIV is about 3.5 days. It may also be used for frequent phlebotomy draws, but the appropriateness of this depends on patient and device characteristics, such as device location, catheter size, and flow.

Contraindications Avoid areas distal to a fracture, as there may be vascular disruption, and it may be difficult to assess for swelling associated with extravasated IV fluids or medications. When possible, avoid areas with edema, burns or cellulitis, or abnormal skin integrity. A vein that has been scarred from frequent use may be difficult to access.

Anatomy Common PIV sites include veins in the dorsum of the hand and the forearm (preferred). The cephalic vein that courses over the distal radius is a reliable site that is often overlooked and is affixed firmly to the underlying fascia. If the upper extremity is being used, the nondominant hand/arm is preferable. **Figure 190-1** shows common sites for placement of a PIV in the upper extremity. In infants, the lower extremities (e.g., feet) or the scalp can be considered as sites for PIV placement. The saphenous vein is predictably located anterior to the medial malleolus and so can be accessed blindly. In general, the vein of choice should be straight and long enough to house the catheter, and without bifurcations, tortuosity, or thrombosis. Most importantly, avoid areas of insertion near joints when possible (e.g., wrist, antecubital fossa).

Equipment Table 190-1 lists the equipment needed to place a PIV. Most hospitals use over-the-needle catheters that include a

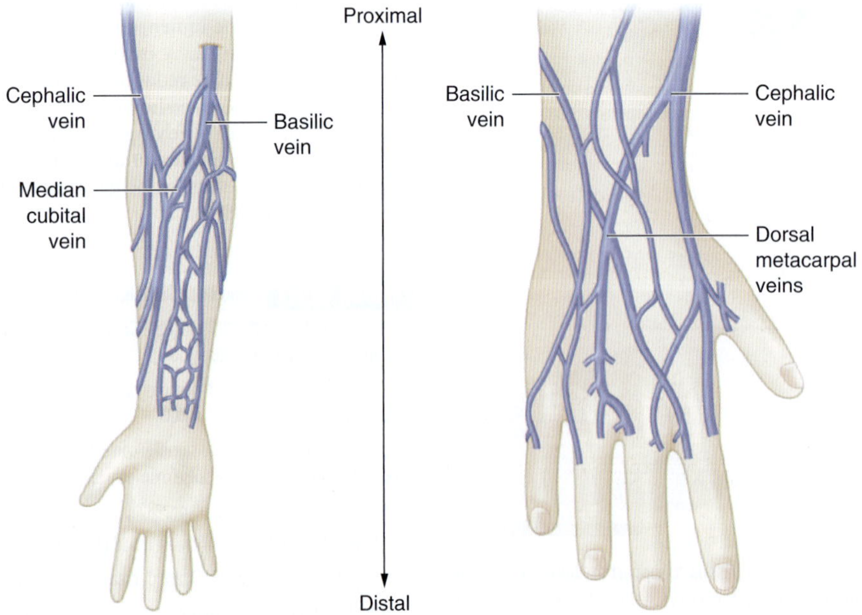

FIGURE 190-1. Venous anatomy of the upper extremity.

TABLE 190-1 Equipment Needed for Placement of an Intravenous Catheter

Appropriate-sized angiocatheter
Skin cleanser (e.g., 70% ethyl alcohol, povidone-iodine, chlorhexidine)
Tourniquet (or rubber bands if placing a scalp PIV)
T-connectors and needleless port
Normal saline flush and 3- or 5-mL syringe
Transparent dressing, securement device, arm board/splint, and other devices to secure catheter in place
Additional 3- or 5-mL syringes if blood is being drawn simultaneously or vacutainer blood transfer device to use with specimen tubes
Gauze
Gloves, nonsterile
Topical anesthetic—cream or spray (optional)
Laboratory specimen tubes when applicable

self-sheathing device. A 24- or 22-gauge catheter is usually suitable for infants and young children and 18-, 20-, or 22-gauge catheters are used for older children. In cases of emergency, when rapid administration of medication, fluids, or blood products is needed, the largest bore and shortest catheter possible should be placed.

Procedure • *Preparation* It is important to have your equipment assembled and easily available before starting the procedure. In children, IV access often requires a second healthcare provider to help hold the extremity and provide comfort to the child (see section "Interventions for needle-related procedural pain and distress").

Technique Universal precautions and aseptic non-touch technique (ANTT) should be used during the entire procedure. Hand washing should be performed before each patient interaction and prior to any procedure.

1. Identify possible sites. Near infra-red light may assist in direct visualization of a vein. Ultrasound visualization and placement should be used in children with difficult access.
2. Apply a topical anesthetic to numb the site.
3. Hot packs, tapping the vein, placing the extremity in a dependent position, or having the child open and close their hand may help with vasodilation and identification.
4. Prepare your equipment:
    a. Prepare securement device and sterile polyurethane transparent dressing
    b. Have any blood sampling tubes ready.
    c. Hook the extension tubing to the needleless access port. If no blood is being drawn, flush the tubing/port with saline.
5. Apply a tourniquet proximal to the site. Make sure not to make it so tight that it impedes arterial flow.
6. Don gloves and apply the antiseptic in a circular fashion, allowing it to dry the required time before attempting access.
7. Have an assistant restrain the limb proximally.
8. With the bevel of the catheter facing up, puncture the skin at a 30- to 45-degree angle and slowly advance the needle until you see flashback of blood in the needle hub (**Figure 190-2**).
9. Advance the needle/catheter only slightly more to make sure the catheter is in the vein (**Figure 190-3**).
10. Tilt the needle parallel to the skin, advance the plastic catheter, and activate the self-sheathing needle system (**Figure 190-4**).
11. Place your finger proximal to the catheter tip to staunch blood flow.
12. Connect your port/tubing to the catheter.
13. Clean and dry the area.
14. Secure the catheter in place prior to transparent dressing application (**Figure 190-5**).

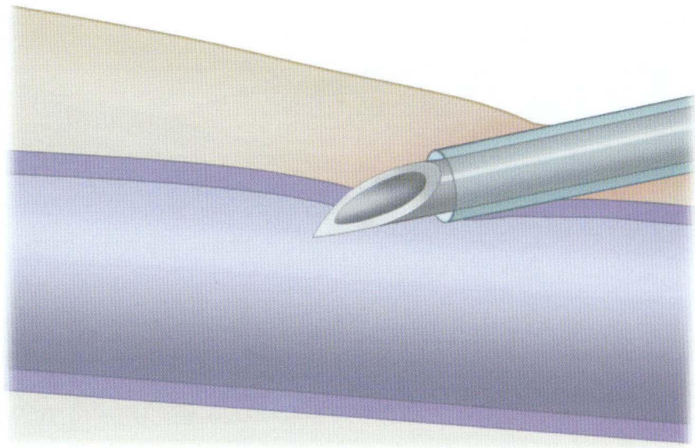

FIGURE 190-2. The needle punctures the vein before the catheter.

15. To collect blood samples, attach an empty syringe or vacutainer to the extension tubing.
16. Remove the tourniquet and flush with saline.
17. Consider the use of a splint if the PIV is inserted over a joint. Use of a soft circumferential arm restraint to further prevent IV dislodgement may be helpful in young children.

Common Problems

1. If there is no blood flow after an initial flashback, loosen the tourniquet, remove the metal stylet, and flush a small amount of saline. If it flushes easily without swelling subcutaneously you can continue to advance the catheter slowly into the vessel.
2. Once the metal stylet has been removed, it should not be reinserted into the catheter, as it may cause catheter shearing.

Follow-up The PIV should be checked by medical personnel to ensure the adequacy of the site (no signs of infection, no erythema) and that it is infusing without any problem (e.g., pain) using the "Touch, Look, Compare" policy for IV safety.

Complications PIV dislodgement and intravenous infiltrates are common complications. The amount and substance extravasated determine whether there will be local injury. Most infiltrates require only elevation and compression. However, hospital policy as well as consultation with your pharmacist and/or hospital vascular access team may help identify more specific therapies to prevent further tissue injury from certain vesicants (e.g., hyaluronidase). Serious complications are rare. Arterial puncture, phlebitis, cellulitis, thrombus formation, catheter fragment embolism or air embolism, and tendon/nerve injury are uncommon complications.

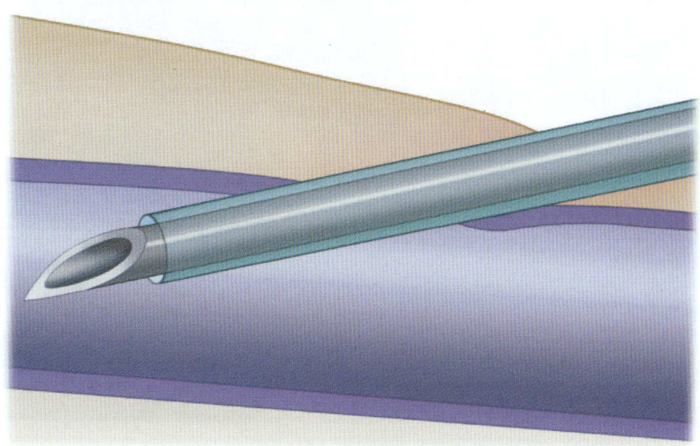

FIGURE 190-3. Advance the needle and catheter into the vein.

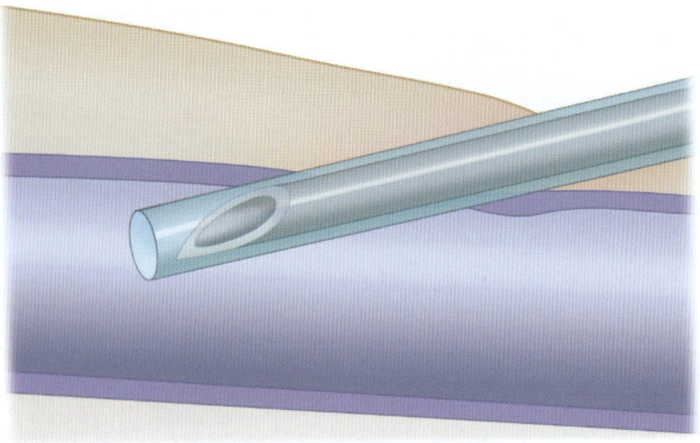

FIGURE 190-4. Withdraw the needle, leaving the catheter in place intravenously.

LONG PERIPHERAL CATHETER AND MIDLINE CATHETER

Indications Long peripheral catheters (LPCs) and midline catheters (MCs) are newer peripheral access devices, generally 6 to 15 cm in length, and made of polyurethane. They dwell longer than the traditional PIV and are therefore indicated for length of therapy that exceeds 5 days or in cases of difficult access. MCs are long peripheral devices in which the tip of the catheter ends specifically at the axilla ("at the midline"). Use of LPCs/MCs has been shown to reduce the use of central vascular access devices (e.g., PICCs) in adults.

Contraindications Avoid areas distal to a fracture, as there may be vascular disruption, and it may be difficult to assess for swelling associated with extravasated IV fluids or medications. When possible, avoid areas with edema, burns or cellulitis, or abnormal skin integrity. LPCs and MCs should not be used for therapies that are not peripherally compatible—vesicants, parenteral nutrition, extremes of pH, or osmolarity—since the tip of the catheter remains in a peripheral vein.

Anatomy The most common location for placement of an LPC or MC is the upper arm, including the basilic, brachial, and cephalic veins. Depending on the size of the child and length of catheter, LPCs can also be placed in the forearm similar to a traditional PIV. Less commonly, the lower extremity (e.g., saphenous vein), hand, or scalp is utilized.

Equipment Multiple prepackaged LPC/MC catheter kits are commercially available; however, catheters can also be purchased separately. It is important for a clinician who will be inserting an LPC/MC to be familiar with the kits that are used at their institution.

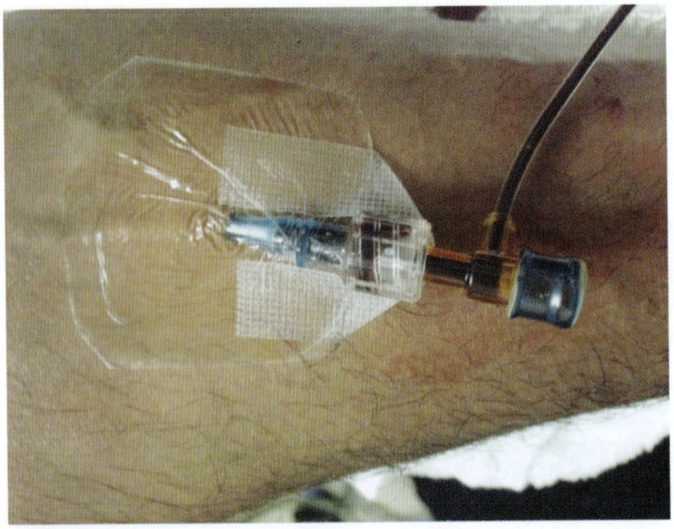

FIGURE 190-5. Occlusive adherent dressing with transparent tape in chevron configuration.

Procedure Depending on the type of catheter your institution has available, most LPCs/MCs are placed using the Seldinger or modified Seldinger technique with ultrasound guidance. Both of those techniques are reviewed in the Central Venous Access section. The device can be placed in a procedural room or at the bedside without need for sedation. Local anesthetics and other procedural support, as described in the "Interventions for needle-related procedural pain and distress" section, should be used to maximize patient comfort during procedure.

Complications The most common complications seen with LPC/MC are dislodgement, occlusion, and infiltration; similar to a traditional PIV. Rare cases of catheter-related thromboembolism have also been reported. The rate of catheter-related blood stream infections is zero in most pediatric studies.

Special Considerations When monitoring for infiltration and thrombus formation, the clinician should look at the site where the tip of the catheter ends (e.g., near the axilla) and not at the site of insertion.

CENTRAL VENOUS ACCESS

Few hospitalists will be expected to have the skills needed for obtaining central venous access; however, most hospitalists will need to be able to troubleshoot problems related to central vascular access devices. Understanding the basics of placement and maintenance of a central venous device is, therefore, an essential competency for a pediatric hospitalist.

PERIPHERALLY INSERTED CENTRAL CATHETERS

A peripherally inserted central catheter (PICC) is a vascular access device that is inserted percutaneously into a peripheral vein of the arm, leg, or scalp, depending on the age and size of the patient and vein availability, with the tip of the catheter ending in at the right atrial junction. PICCs are not considered an emergent vascular access option and are usually reserved for intermediate to long-term vascular access in non-emergent situations. In most settings, clinicians may have the opportunity to utilize an indwelling PICC for IV access or be called upon to troubleshoot problems when patients have an existing PICC. Clinicians who have had additional training may insert PICCs as well.

PICCs are primarily made of power-injectable polyurethane, can be coated/impregnated with a range of materials, and vary in diameter and length, ranging from 28 gauge and 1.9 French for neonates to 3 and 5 French single- and double-lumen sizes for older pediatric patients. Triple-lumen PICCs are also available, but the larger diameter often precludes use in children. Always choose the minimum number of lumens that would be clinically necessary as more lumens are associated with higher rates of catheter-related infections and thrombosis. An upper extremity PICC tip resides at the junction of the superior vena cava and right atrium. For lower-extremity insertions the PICC tip should reside in the thoracic inferior vena cava.

Indications PICCs are intended for intermediate to long-term use (weeks to months to years) for vascular access in a hospital, extended care facility, or home care setting. PICCs are most used for intravenous fluids or antimicrobial therapy with duration of at least 14 days or for parenteral nutrition. PICCs may be used for chemotherapeutic agents, blood products, and infusates classified as vesicants or with properties of irritating pH levels and osmolarities. Blood samples can be obtained from PICCs 3 French and larger.

Contraindications PICCs are not inserted in areas distal to a fracture or other injury or if a venous occlusion exists. PICCs should not be inserted through skin that appears infected or with signs of dermatologic disease that might increase the risk for the area to become infected. When possible, do not place a PICC in a patient with active bacteremia because of concern of catheter contamination. Avoid placing a PICC in children with chronic renal failure or end-stage renal disease in order to preserve veins for the potential need of a dialysis catheter. Similar to other vascular access devices, PICCs should not be inserted near a joint (e.g., antecubital fossa).

Anatomy The upper arm is the most common entry site for PICC placement, with the basilic and brachial veins typically used; however,

TABLE 190-2 Equipment List for PICC Insertion

Ultrasound and sterile probe sheath cover, ultrasound gel
Tourniquet
Sterile gloves, gowns, masks, and drapes; gauze
Tape measure
Catheter
Skin cleansing solution (chlorhexine/alcohol)
Sterile PICC kit: may contain 1-mL syringe for anesthetic, two 5-mL syringes for flush, scissors, threaded tape strips, drapes, finder needle, scalpel, dilator, guide wire, catheter
Sterile flush solution
Topical anesthetic cream
Buffered lidocaine
Peripheral IV safety catheter
29-gauge needle and syringe for intradermal lidocaine use
Securement device
Luer-locking microbore extension set (depending on PICC design)
Needle-less injection cap
Sterile labels for drugs/solutions on sterile field

other peripheral veins may be used as long as they have a large enough diameter, and the vein is continuous with a central vein and the right atrium. In neonates and infants, the saphenous and femoral veins may be used. Ideally, the placement of a PICC should be assisted by fluoroscopy and/or ultrasound guidance.

Equipment Virtually all hospitals use commercially available prepackaged kits that contain most of the necessary equipment; however, they may not contain local anesthetic or a scalpel blade. It is important for a clinician who will be inserting a PICC to be familiar with the kits that are used at their institution. A general list of equipment needed is found in **Table 190-2**. In addition, all the necessary items to provide maximum sterile barrier precautions should be obtained before beginning the procedure, including sterile drapes for the field as well as a sterile gown, hat, and mask for the clinician placing the PICC and any other clinicians who will be assisting with the procedure.

Procedure • ***Preparation*** Typically, younger children require procedural sedation and cardiorespiratory monitoring during insertion. The procedure usually occurs in the interventional radiology suite, procedure room, or at the bedside in critical care areas. As with any painful procedure, assessment of a child's activity, anxiety, and potential need for sedation prior to the procedure will help to improve success. Older children may only need a combination of topical and local anesthesia for PICC placement.

Technique Use maximum sterile barrier precautions for all PICC insertions (establish sterile field, sterile gown, hat, mask, sterile drapes for body of patient, and insertion site).

The Seldinger, modified Seldinger, micro-introducer technique is becoming the most popular technique for placing PICCs due to the ability to place a larger gauge catheter via a small gauge introducer needle or catheter, and is used in conjunction with ultrasound. See **Table 190-3** for a stepwise list of PICC insertion using this technique.

Care and Maintenance Once inserted, care and maintenance of the PICC should be performed according to institutional policies. Sites should be inspected frequently for signs of complications. Many institutions use the Infusion Therapy Standards of Practice as a guide.

Complications Central venous access devices in pediatric patients are not without risks of complications. Review the patient's vascular access device history and past complications in planning for the appropriate central venous access device. Central venous catheter complications are usually divided into insertion complications and post-insertion complications. The most frequently reported neonatal and pediatric PICC complications are:

TABLE 190-3 Stepwise Insertion of a PICC Using Ultrasound Guidance and a Modified Seldinger Technique

Vascular Assessment (Non-Sterile)

1. Instruct the patient on the purpose of the ultrasound and how it will feel.
2. Wash hands.
3. Place the patient with the arm to be accessed extended at 45 degrees to the trunk of the body. Apply liberal amount of ultrasound gel to the probe or patient arm where you want to visualize a vein.
4. Position the probe with the ridge down toward the user and probe 90 degrees to the skin surface.
5. Identify fluid filled structures and vessels as dark circles. Locate arteries and veins by moving the probe over the vessels and analyzing the compression quality of the vessel walls. Arteries do not compress easily.
6. Move the ultrasound probe and follow basilic vein distally up the arm, compressing the vein and noting its characteristics of increasing size and tributaries. Note the arteries in relation to the veins through compression and pulse. Note approximate size and depth.
7. Note the position of the probe and vein for later reference. You may mark the area with a skin marker so that you can more readily return there for placement.
8. Remove ultrasound gel from subject and clean probe head with compatible disinfectant

PICC Placement Using Ultrasound

1. Complete preliminary steps for PICC insertion (orders, consent, identify patient, time out, etc.).
2. Assemble equipment and prep patient, and set up maximum sterile barrier as per protocol for PICC placement using modified Seldinger technique.
3. Apply sterile ultrasound gel to the probe.
4. Cover probe and probe cord with sterile plastic sheath, removing all air, and secure with rubber bands/strap to keep gel on face of probe.
5. Have assistant place tourniquet on extremity.
6. Apply sterile ultrasound gel to probe or selected insertion site. Place ultrasound probe on selected area and revisualize vein. Move probe to center vein in the ultrasound screen.
7. Instill local anesthesia intradermally at insertion site.
8. Insert peripheral catheter or needle just through the skin.
9. Watch the ultrasound screen and proceed to advance needle toward vein.
10. Once through the vein, you should be able to visualize the bevel of the needle in approximately the center of the vein. Observe for flashback in catheter needle or flashback chamber.
11. Remove ultrasound probe from site without disturbing position of needle in the vein. Remove peripheral catheter stylet, if appropriate.
12. Carefully insert wire partway into the access device. Slowly advance wire to below axilla. Do not force the wire. Wire should advance freely in the vein. If using fluoroscopy, wire may be inserted to desired location in the superior vena cava.
13. Enlarge the insertion site opening using a needle or scalpel to make a small (2 mm) opening for dilator to pass easily.
14. Thread dilator peel-away assembly over wire into vessel.
15. Remove wire and dilator, leaving peel-away in place.
16. Thread PICC into peel-away to premeasured length and verify tip location in vena cava or at cavoatrial junction.
17. Remove peel-away sheath (see **Figure 190-6**).
18. Secure, apply dressing, and flush PICC (see **Figure 190-7**) per institutional protocol.
19. Document insertion in medical record, indicating size, length of PICC, tip location, and related details.

Insertion related complications:

- Cardiac tamponade
- Arrhythmias
- Nerve injury
- Malposition of the tip of the catheter, which can often be adjusted post-insertion or via rewire of the device.

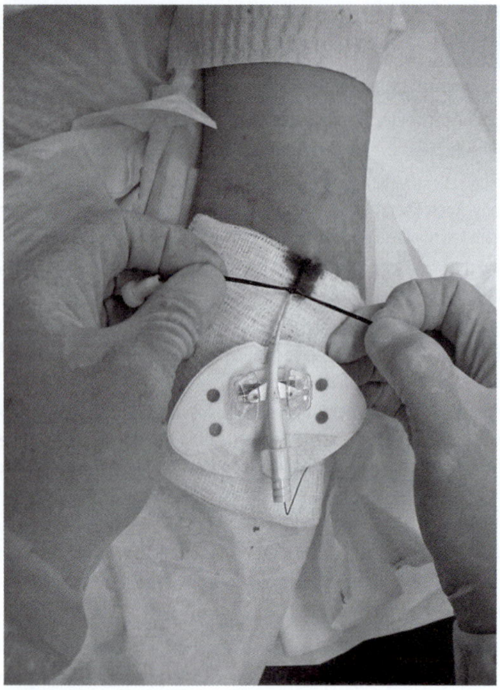

FIGURE 190-6. Peel-away sheath with PICC in place.

Post-insertion complications:

- Blood stream infection
- Venous thromboembolism
- Phlebitis
- Dislodgement
- Occlusion, with consideration of different possible etiologies: mechanical occlusion (e.g., dysfunctional needleless connector, tip placement), infusate-related occlusion (e.g., lipids), thrombotic occlusion (thrombolytic agent can be used)
- Other mechanical malfunction (e.g., catheter fracture or migration)

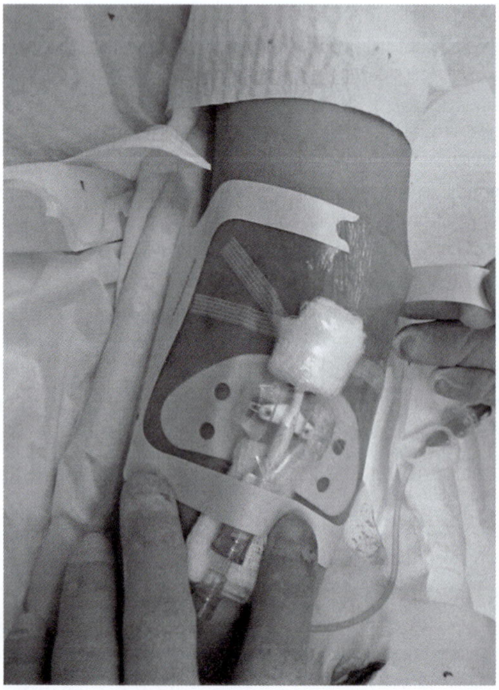

FIGURE 190-7. PICC with gauze and transparent dressing.

CENTRAL VENOUS CATHETER

Central venous cannulation involves percutaneously placing a vascular catheter into a high-flow vein located in either the thorax or the abdomen. It is an essential skill for the resuscitation and stabilization of critically ill or injured children. The main sites of access include the femoral, internal and external jugular veins, and subclavian veins.

Indications Central venous catheters (CVCs) are placed for a variety of reasons, primarily in the critically ill patient. Consider some of the following factors when deciding the need for a CVC:

Patient factors:

- Urgent need for vascular access when peripheral access is unobtainable (e.g., hemodynamic instability)
- Critically ill patient with difficult peripheral access

Infusate factors:

- Infusion of vasoactive medications, blood products, or large volumes of fluid when rapid distribution and onset of therapy are vital
- Delivery of hypertonic fluids such as total parenteral nutrition and chemotherapy
- Long-term vascular access for repeated medication administration

Other factors:

- Frequent blood sampling
- Insertion of devices such as transvenous pacemakers or Swan-Ganz catheters
- Ongoing measurements of venous pressures or mixed venous blood gases

Contraindications CVCs should not be attempted at sites with abnormal vasculature. Relative contraindications include a bleeding diathesis or hypercoagulable state as well as overlying cellulitis, acute inflammation, or skin injury at the planned site of entry. Other contraindications specific to the individual sites are discussed with each approach.

Equipment **Table 190-4** lists the equipment needed for central venous catheter placement. Use of ultrasound is recommended whenever possible. Virtually all hospitals use commercially available, prepackaged kits that contain most of the necessary equipment; however, they may not contain local anesthetic or a scalpel blade. Squirt some sterile saline onto the tray for flushing after access is obtained.

TABLE 190-4 Equipment Needed for Central Venous Catheter Placement

Equipment
Catheter
Ultrasound and sterile probe sheath cover, ultrasound gel
Flexible guidewire
Finder needle
Sterile gloves, gowns, masks, and drapes
Sterile gauze
Antiseptic solution
Syringes
Heparinized saline
Silk suture on straight needle, needle holder
Transparent dressing
Tissue dilator
Number 11 scalpel
Topical anesthetic

TABLE 190-5 Catheter Choice for Pediatric Patients

Age	AVERAGE CATHETER DIAMETER (FRENCH) AND LENGTH (CM)					
	Femoral		Internal Jugular		Subclavian	
1 mo	3	15.7	3	6.0	3	5.5
3 mo	3	17.3	3	6.6	3	6.0
6 mo	3/4	19.1	3	7.3	3	6.6
9 mo	3/4	20.1	3	7.6	3	6.9
12 mo	3/4	21.1	3	8.0	3	7.3
18 mo	3/4	22.9	3	8.7	3	7.9
2 yr	3/4	24.2	3	9.2	3	8.3
4 yr	4	28.1	4	10.6	4	9.6
6 yr	4	31.4	4	11.8	4	10.7
8 yr	4/5	34.2	4/5	12.9	4/5	11.7
10 yr	4/5	36.8	4/5	13.8	4/5	12.5
12 yr	4/5	39.9	4/5	15.0	4/5	13.5
14 yr	5	44.0	5	16.5	5	14.9
16 yr	5	46.3	5	17.3	5	15.7

Source: Reproduced with permission from Lavelle J, Costarino A Jr. Central venous access and central venous pressure monitoring. In: Henretig FM, King C, eds. *Textbook of Pediatric Emergency Procedures*. 2nd ed. Baltimore: Lippincott Williams & Wilkins; 2008:256.

It is important to note that the equipment in each kit is size-specific. If one has opened more than one kit of different sizes, it is extremely important to ensure that the equipment is not mixed up. For example, a guidewire from one kit may not be long enough to accommodate a catheter from another.

Procedure Several different catheters and techniques have been used for percutaneous central venous cannulation, with each involving a slightly different technique. By far the most common is the Seldinger technique, which is based on passing a catheter over a guidewire. This technique is discussed here.

It is important to recognize that different patients need varying amounts of sedation and analgesia for this procedure, based on their age and clinical condition. The success of the procedure can be greatly enhanced by immobilization and proper positioning as well as ensuring that all necessary equipment is available and ready before beginning.

Use the ultrasound to identify the target vein. The chosen site is sterilely prepared, draped, and anesthetized with local anesthetic. Then puncture the skin and blood vessel with a small-gauge needle attached to a syringe while applying gentle negative suction until there is free flow of blood. Remove the syringe, placing your thumb over the hub, and thread the guidewire through the needle into the vein. Remove the needle used for entry, leaving the wire in place. Make a small incision, using a number 11 scalpel, at the entry site to facilitate insertion of a larger catheter. Advance the catheter of choice (**Table 190-5**) over the guidewire into the desired vessel and remove the wire. It is vitally important to always hold the end of the wire to prevent inadvertently losing it in the vessel. Different kits have different sizes of catheters. Some will require dilation of the vessel before insertion. When dilation is necessary, insert the dilator over the wire after the skin incision has been made. Once the dilator is removed, the catheter can be easily advanced over the wire into the vessel. The catheter is then secured in place (e.g., suture, subcutaneous anchor) and the site is dressed with a transparent occlusive dressing. There is evidence that chlorhexidine-impregnated dressings may decrease CVC colonization and bloodstream infections, but mainly in the ICU setting.

Site-Specific Considerations *Femoral vein* This is the most popular approach for pediatric central venous access (**Figure 190-8**). Advantages include (i) distance from the head and chest, and thus minimal interference with the evaluation and treatment of critically ill children; (ii) the requirement of less technical expertise; and (iii) the easily exposed anatomy. Disadvantages include contamination risk, difficulty securing the device, and difficulty in obese patients. Relative contraindications include abnormal vascular anatomy, abdominal trauma, tumor, or ascites, femoral hernia, and future need for cardiac catheterization.

The entry point is identified 1 to 2 cm medial to the femoral artery and 1 to 2 cm below the inguinal ligament. If pulses are weak or absent, the site can be estimated to be halfway between the pubic symphysis and the anterior iliac spine, still 1 to 2 cm below the inguinal ligament. Optimal patient positioning requires abduction and external rotation of the hip, often facilitated by placing a towel beneath the ipsilateral buttock. Perform needle entry at a 45-degree angle, taking care not to puncture the inguinal ligament or above to avoid causing a bowel perforation or retroperitoneal hematoma.

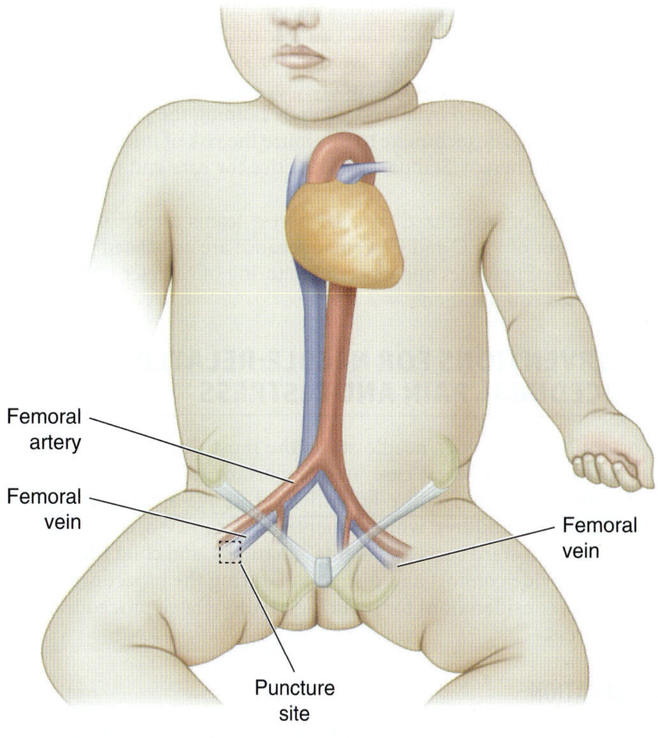

FIGURE 190-8. Femoral venous anatomy.

Internal jugular vein Internal jugular venous access is less common than the femoral approach but is considered the entry site of choice by many experienced clinicians because of the inherent advantages of increased stability, patient comfort, and more accurate central venous pressure measurements. The complication rate is somewhat higher than with a femoral catheter and includes inadvertent laceration of the carotid artery, thoracic duct, or stellate ganglion as well as pneumothorax. Of the three approaches (median, anterior, and lateral) used in cannulating the internal jugular vein, the median approach is the most popular. All methods require the patient's head to be turned 30 degrees away from the puncture site while in the Trendelenburg position. Landmarks for the median approach involve locating the midpoint between the sternal notch and the mastoid process at the apex of the triangle formed by both heads of the sternocleidomastoid muscle. The internal jugular vein is lateral to the carotid artery. Insert the needle at a 30-degree angle and aim toward the ipsilateral nipple.

External jugular vein Although the external jugular vein can be readily identified most of the time, the chance of successful CVC placement is low. However, complications such as pneumothorax, carotid artery puncture and hematoma, and injury to the sympathetic chain are lower than in the internal jugular vein site. The patient should be in 15 to 30 degrees of Trendelenburg, with the head turned 45 degrees to the contralateral side. Puncture the skin where the external jugular vein crosses over the sternocleidomastoid muscle.

Subclavian vein This is a less common site for percutaneous CVC placement in children; however, it is becoming more popular and safer due to the use of ultrasound guidance. Complications of pneumothorax and subclavian artery puncture are considered traditionally highest with this approach. Access the subclavian vein from either a supraclavicular or infraclavicular site. The patient should be supine in 10 to 25 degrees of Trendelenburg. The entry site for the supraclavicular approach is one finger-width lateral to the clavicular head of the sternocleidomastoid muscle superior to the clavicle. Direct the needle so it bisects the angle formed by the clavicle and the sternocleidomastoid, aiming toward the contralateral nipple, and advancing the needle two to three times the width of the clavicle. The entry site for the infraclavicular approach is just lateral to the midclavicular line below the clavicle. Advance the needle 2 to 4 cm toward the sternal notch parallel to the chest wall.

Complications Site-specific complications have been addressed above. Other general complications include thrombosis, infection (cellulitis, bacteremia), air embolus, vascular or cardiac perforation, and cardiac arrhythmia (see PICC section for more details). Guidewires have been lost in the central circulation, requiring surgical removal. This can be prevented by always securely holding the proximal end of the wire. Use sterile technique to minimize the risk of infection. Follow the Infusion Therapy Standards of Practice for care and maintenance best practices.

Utilization of specialized vascular access teams for PICC insertion and oversight of PICC and CVC maintenance are associated with standardization of practices and closer monitoring of catheter sites leading to decreased complications.

INTERVENTIONS FOR NEEDLE-RELATED PROCEDURAL PAIN AND DISTRESS

Most children consider needle sticks the most distressing and painful part of their hospital care. It is important to prepare the family and child for the procedure honestly and in age-appropriate terms. The families of children who frequently undergo IV access may have helpful hints toward success. Parents, guardians, and child life specialists can provide comfort and distraction during the procedure. Below are several considerations for reducing needle-related procedural pain and distress.

SEDATION

Consider use of sedation in children undergoing central venous access device placement based on their level of alertness, developmental age, anxiety/distress level, and length of procedure. In general, peripheral vascular access can be obtained quickly and is well tolerated without sedation, using other interventions discussed below.

LOCAL ANESTHETIC

There are many topical anesthetic preparations that can be used in conjunction with nonpharmacological methods to reduce the pain and distress of vascular access device insertion. These anesthetics are applied directly to the potential IV site(s). Onset of numbness varies between products and may take up to 30 to 60 minutes to work. A small bleb of lidocaine buffered with sodium bicarbonate in a 9-to-1 ratio can be superficially injected over the vein for more immediate anesthesia, but it may obscure visualization and palpation of the vein. In recent years, the use of the J-tip™, a needle-free injection system, has been adopted by many children's hospitals. The J-tip™ deliveres lidocaine into the subcutaneous tissue using compressed CO_2 gas instead of a needle.

PSYCHOLOGICAL INTERVENTIONS

Distraction, hypnosis (deep relaxation, imagery), specific breathing, and combining multiple strategies are effective interventions for reducing pain and distress in children and adolescents. Ways to distract them include reading, watching a movie, listening to music, and playing video games. Other examples of strategies that can be used in combination with the above are positive thoughts, learning the steps of the procedure, and coaching parents on ways to support their child.

SUGGESTED READINGS

Birnie KA, Noel M, Chambers CT, Uman LS, Parker JA. Psychological interventions for needle-related procedural pain and distress in children and adolescents. *Cochrane Database Syst Rev*. 2018; 2018(10).

Bozaan D, Skicki D, Brancaccio A, et al. Less lumens-less risk: A pilot intervention to increase the use of single-lumen peripherally inserted central catheters. *J Hosp Med*. 2019;14(1).

Burek AG, Liljestrom T, Dundon M, Shaughnessy EE, Suelzer E, Ullman A. Long peripheral catheters in children: a scoping review. *J Hosp Med*. 2022;17(12):1000-1009.

Clark E, Giambra BK, Hingl J, Doellman D, Tofani B, Johnson N. Reducing risk of harm from extravasation: a 3-tiered evidence-based list of pediatric peripheral intravenous infusates. *J Infus Nurs*. 2013; 36(1).

Gorski LA, Hadaway L, Hagle ME, et al. Infusion Therapy Standards of Practice. 8th ed. *J Infus Nurs*. 2021;44.

Grewal S, Towbin R, Schaefer C, Aria D. How We Do It : Peripherally Inserted Central Catheter Placement. Applied Radiology. 2020. https://appliedradiology.com/articles/how-we-do-it-peripherally-inserted-central-catheter-placement-picc.

Hill S. Insertion. In: Moureau NL, ed. *Vessel Health and Preservation: The Right Approach for Vascular Access*. Cham: Springer; 2019.

Kleidon TM, Schults J, Rickard CM. Techniques and technologies to improve peripheral intravenous catheter outcomes in pediatric patients: systematic review and meta-analysis. *J Hosp Med*. 2021;16(12):742-750.

Kleidon TM, Schults JA, Wainwright C, et al. Comparison of midline catheters and peripherally inserted central catheters to reduce the need for general anesthesia in children with respiratory disease: A feasibility randomized controlled trial. *Pediatr Anesth*. 2021;31:985-995.

Knue M, Doellman D, Rabin K, Jacobs BR. The efficacy and safety of blood sampling through peripherally inserted central catheter devices in children. *J Infus Nurs*. 2005;28(1):30-35.

Marie Frey A. Peripherally inserted central catheters in neonates and children: modified Seldinger (microintroducer) technique. *J Vasc Access Devices*. 2002;7(2).

Qin KR, Ensor N, Barnes R, Englin A, Nataraja RM, Pacilli M. Long peripheral catheters for intravenous access in adults and children: A systematic review of the literature. *J Vasc Access*. 2021;22(5).

Qin KR, Ensor N, Barnes R, Englin A, Nataraja RM, Pacilli M. Standard versus long peripheral catheters for multiday IV therapy: A randomized controlled trial. *Pediatrics*. 2021;147(2):e2020000877.

Ullman AJ, Bernstein SJ, Brown E, et al. The Michigan appropriateness guide for intravenous catheters in pediatrics: miniMAGIC. *Pediatrics*. 2020;145(Suppl 3):S269-S284.

Ullman AJ, Cooke ML, Mitchell M, et al. Dressing and securement for central venous access devices (CVADs): a Cochrane systematic review. *Int J Nurs Stud*. 2016;59.

CHAPTER 191 Intraosseous Catheters

Ellen Szydlowski, MD and Maria Quidgley-Martin, MD

BACKGROUND

Intraosseous (IO) cannulation is an effective and reliable means of rapidly accessing the central circulation for the administration of fluids, medications, and blood products. The non-collapsible intramedullary venous sinuses offer great stability during states of profound vasoconstriction and circulatory failure, such as shock and cardiac arrest, when peripheral access is emergently needed but untenable. Highly vascular marrow spaces are capable of absorbing large volumes of fluids, medications, and blood products with rapid distribution to the rest of the body. The procedure can be safely performed with minimal training by pre-hospital providers as well as by staff skilled in pediatric hospital, emergency, or critical care medicine. Power-assisted devices for IO placement have made this procedure even more accessible to providers of all skill levels.

INDICATIONS

IO access is indicated for pediatric patients requiring resuscitative efforts in whom placement of a peripheral intravenous catheter is unsuccessful or cannot rapidly be established. For patients in cardiac arrest, IO placement should be performed before all other means of securing access and should be considered early as an alternative to central venous access in the resuscitative efforts of patients with sepsis in whom peripheral access cannot be readily obtained. The procedure can be attempted in patients of any age in whom peripheral access is unsuccessful. Manual IO cannulation is generally successful in 30 to 60 seconds. Access with powered devices can be achieved in as little as 5 to 10 seconds with success rates of >90%. IO catheters are intended to be used during immediate resuscitative efforts only. Once a patient has been stabilized, peripheral IV or central venous access should be secured for long-term use.

IO lines can deliver any medication, fluid, or blood product prepared for intravenous administration. A strong evidence base supports IO use for neuromuscular blockade as well as for resuscitative medications such as catecholamines (bolus preparations and continuous infusions), lidocaine, calcium, and sodium bicarbonate. In general, the onset of action and drug levels in the central circulation following IO delivery are comparable to those achieved with intravenous administration. Boluses of crystalloids, colloids, blood products, and viscous medications must be delivered under pressure, either manually with a large-caliber syringe or with the assistance of a pressure bag to overcome the resistance of the emissary veins running through the bony cortex which are responsible for transporting materials from the intramedullary space to the central circulation.

Blood samples obtained from the marrow space can be sent for culture and type and cross-match, and can be used to analyze pH, glucose, hemoglobin, chloride, bicarbonate, blood urea nitrogen, creatinine, and serum drug levels with accuracy comparable to venous blood samples. Importantly, blood obtained from the medullary cavity does not reflect accurate values for white blood cells, platelets, CO_2, potassium, aspartate aminotransferase, alanine aminotransferase, or ionized calcium. Sodium from an IO draw is within 5% of venous values. Labs should be obtained prior to IO drug administration as they may alter subsequent laboratory values.

CONTRAINDICATIONS

Few contraindications to the use of IO catheters exist. Absolute contraindications include a recent fracture in the bone to be used for the procedure, recent unsuccessful IO attempt in the same bone, or underlying bone disease such as osteopenia or osteogenesis imperfecta given the high risk of fracture in these patient populations. Relative contraindications include overlying cellulitis or burn at the site of puncture.

EQUIPMENT

Needles used for IO cannulation should be sturdy enough to penetrate bone and long enough to reach the marrow cavity. Several catheters can be used to establish IO access: the Jamshidi bone aspiration-infusion needle, the Cook IO infusion needle, or a wide-gauge spinal needle with an internal stylet. There are also several semiautomatic devices available for IO insertion including the battery-powered EZ-IO drill (Teleflex, Morrisville, NC), and the spring-loaded Bone Injection Gun (BIG) (PersSys Medical, Houston, Tx). All function effectively, but the evidence base suggests that the EZ-IO may be placed most rapidly. The Jamshidi infusion needle may be placed with greater ease than the Cook infusion needle and the BIG.

Table 191-1 lists the other equipment needed for IO placement.

ANATOMY

IO needles can be placed into any intramedullary space, but the distal lower extremities are preferred given their large marrow cavities, low potential for injury to surrounding tissues, and distance from the airway and chest where resuscitative measures may be ongoing. The proximal tibia (1-2 cm inferior and medial to the tuberosity) has been identified as the most appropriate initial site for placement. The distal femur (1-2 cm above the superior border of the patella) is an alternate insertion site in infants, while the distal tibia (1-2 cm superior to the medial malleolus) may be used in older children. (**Figure 191-1**) The proximal humerus is an option for IO cannulation in adults, but is not recommended in children. IO infusion may also be successful in bones without medullary cavities, including the calcaneus and radial styloid.

PROCEDURE

PREPARATION

The following discussion describes placement in the proximal tibia, the preferred site for IO cannulation in children.

Place the patient in the supine position and prop the knee over a rolled towel or blanket at 30 degrees of flexion, allowing the patient's heel to rest on the stretcher. Palpate along the anteromedial surface of the bone, 1 to

TABLE 191-1 Equipment Needed for Intraosseous Catheter Placement
Appropriate personal protective equipment
Antiseptic solution (per institutional protocol)
1% lidocaine for topical anesthesia
3- or 5-mL syringe for collecting blood
Sterile saline flushes
Gauze and tape to secure device
Pump or pressure-bag

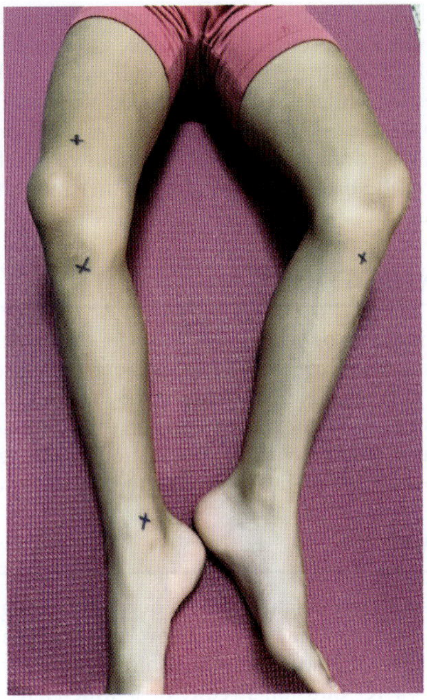

FIGURE 191-1. Intraosseous catheter placement landmarks. The preferred location for IO placement in a pediatric patient is the proximal tibia. Other locations include the distal femur and the distal tibia. (Photo credit: Ellen Szydlowski, MD.)

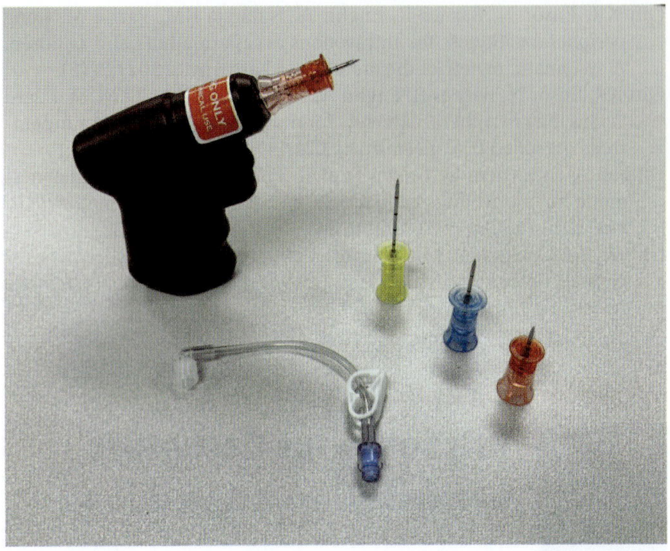

FIGURE 191-2. EZ-IO intraosseous driver and needles. The EZ-IO needles are available in three sizes: 15 mm for 3-40 kg (pink), 25 mm for >40 kg (blue), and 45 mm for >40 kg and extra subcutaneous tissue (yellow). (Photo credit: Ellen Szydlowski, MD.)

2 cm (or approximately 1 finger breadth) below the tibial tuberosity and up to 1 cm medially to identify a smooth, flat surface for needle placement. Using sterile technique, clean and drape the area. In conscious or awake patients, anesthetize the skin and underlying periosteum with 1% lidocaine (without epinephrine). Using a small needle, place a wheal of lidocaine in the skin, and then slowly direct the anesthetic along the path of the IO needle. Alternately pull back on the syringe while advancing the needle to confirm that the vascular space has not been entered.

TECHNIQUE

Manual Firmly grasp the patient's lower extremity over the distal anterior thigh with one hand. With the other hand, hold the hub of the IO catheter in the palm, and grasp the IO needle close to the tip with the thumb and index finger. The operator should avoid placing any part of his or her hand behind the site of insertion to prevent inadvertent puncture should the needle pass through the bone and posterior soft tissues. Ensure that the stylet is in place and that the bevels are aligned. Direct the bevel distally and introduce the IO needle at a 90-degree angle through the skin. Use continuous rotary motion with steady, firm downward pressure at a 45- to 60-degree angle away from the growth plate to enter the cortex. A significant drop in resistance indicates successful penetration of the marrow space.

Power-Assisted The EZ-IO is a battery-powered driver that can drill a needle through bone. To begin, select an appropriate needle size based upon the patient's weight. There are three sizes available: 15 mm for 3 to 40 kg, 25 mm for >40 kg, and 45 mm for >40 kg and extra subcutaneous tissue. **(Figure 191-2)** Ensure that the needle is securely inserted into the needle driver. As with manual IO placement, use one hand to firmly stabilize the patient's lower extremity by holding the distal anterior thigh. Position the drill at a 90-degree angle to the site of insertion. Pierce the skin prior to engaging the drill and advance the needle down through the soft tissue to the level of the bone. Ensure that one black line on the IO needle is visible prior to engaging the trigger. Squeeze the trigger and use slow and steady pressure to penetrate the bone, allowing the driver to do the work. Once a drop in resistance is detected, release the trigger. Holding the needle in place, pull the driver completely off the needle and remove the stylet. Attach the EZ-connect extension tubing.

Securing an IO Catheter A correctly placed IO needle should remain upright without support. To confirm placement, remove the stylet and attempt to draw back bone marrow contents with a 3- or 5-mL syringe. Send blood for laboratory analysis if indicated and then instill 0.5 mg/kg of 2% lidocaine if the patient is awake, followed by a 10 mL normal saline power flush to displace the marrow. Despite successful insertion, blood may not always be aspirated. However, a correctly placed catheter should flush easily with saline. Due to the intrinsic high resistance of the medullary cavity, high pressures may be required. Monitor closely for evidence of extravasation into the surrounding tissues manifesting as increased circumference of the extremity proximate to the infusion site, increased resistance to product infusion through the needle, or tense soft tissues in the area surrounding the needle. Once appropriate placement of the IO needle has been confirmed, secure it in place.

COMPLICATIONS

Serious complications associated with IO catheters are rare. The most common complications observed are local edema or extravasation of fluid. Perhaps most significant are through-and-through penetration of the bone and failure to perform the procedure satisfactorily. Infrequently, osteomyelitis and subcutaneous abscess have been associated with this procedure and may been seen in patients where the IO was in place for more than 24 hours. Additional serious complications include tibial fracture, compartment syndrome, and cerebral arterial air embolism. Despite evidence of bone marrow and fat emboli in patients after IO infusion, this appears to be of no clinical significance. IO catheter use has minimal effects on the long-term growth and health of the bone and bone marrow.

SUGGESTED READINGS

Advanced Trauma Life Support for Doctors: Student Course Manual. Chicago, IL: American College of Surgeons; 2018.

Buck ML, Wiggins BS, Sesler JM. Intraosseous drug administration in children and adults during cardiopulmonary resuscitation. *Ann Pharmacother*. 2007;41(10):1679-1686.

Gazin N, Auger H, Jabre P, et al. Efficacy and safety of the EZ-IO™ intraosseous device: out-of-hospital implementation of a management algorithm for difficult vascular access. *Resuscitation*. 2011; 82(1):126-129.

Hansen M, Meckler G, Spiro D, et al. Intraosseous line use, complications, and outcomes among a population-based cohort of children presenting to California hospitals. *Pediatr Emerg Care*. 2011;27(10): 928-932.

Hartholt KA, van Lieshout EMM, Thies WC, et al. Intraosseous devices: a randomized controlled trial comparing three intraosseous devices. *Prehosp Emerg Care*. 2010;14(1):6-13.
Horton MA, Beamer C. Powered intraosseous insertion provides safe and effective vascular access for pediatric emergency patients. *Pediatr Emerg Care*. 2008;24(6):347-350.
King C, Henretig F, King B, Loiselle J, Ruddy R, Wiley J II. *Textbook of Pediatric Emergency Procedures*. 2nd ed. Blackwell Publishing; 2009.
McCarthy G, O'Donnell C, O'Brien M. Successful intraosseous infusion in the critically ill patient does not require a medullary cavity. *Resuscitation*. 2003;56(2):183-186.
Miller LJ, Philbeck TE, Montex D, Spadaccini CJ. A new study of intraosseous blood for laboratory analysis. *Arch Pathol Lab Med*. 2010;134(9):1253-1260.
Nagler J, Krauss B. Videos in clinical medicine. Intraosseous catheter placement in children. *N Engl J Med*. 2011;364(8):e14.
Orlowski JP, Porembka DT, Gallagher JM, et al. Comparison study of intraosseous, central intravenous, and peripheral intravenous infusions of emergency drugs. *Am J Dis Child*. 1990;144(1):112-117.
Pediatric Advanced Life Support. American Heart Association, 2020.
Roberts JR, Hedges JR. *Clinical Procedures in Emergency Medicine*. Philadelphia, PA: Saunders/Elsevier; 2017.
Tobias JD, Ross AK. Intraosseous infusions: a review for the anesthesiologist with a focus on pediatric use. *Anesth Analg*. 2010;110:391-401.
Topjian A, Raymond T, Atkins D, et al. Part 4: Pediatric basic and advanced life support: 2020 American Heart Association Guidelines for Cardiopulmonary Resuscitation and Emergency Cardiovascular Care. *Circulation*. 2020;142:S469-S523.

CHAPTER 192 Umbilical Artery and Vein Catheterization

Anne Daley Ryan, MD and Blair Simon, MD

BACKGROUND

Umbilical artery and vein catheterization is a common procedure in the neonatal intensive care unit (NICU) and offers lifesaving central access to neonates. Placement of an umbilical artery catheter often occurs in the first 24 hours of life and may occasionally be placed in an infant up to 1 week of age. Umbilical vein catheterization is frequently used in an emergency setting after birth and feasible up to 2 weeks of age.

INDICATIONS

Indications for central access include volume expansion, blood transfusion, infusion of resuscitative medications, administration of hypertonic solutions including parenteral nutrition, and frequent laboratory draws. Peripheral access should be attempted first, but one should not delay central access in a critically ill infant.

Arterial catheters are indicated in newborns requiring frequent arterial blood gases and/or invasive blood pressure monitoring. An umbilical artery catheter has the advantage of rapid insertion and may also be used to deliver fluids, medications, and blood products.

CONTRAINDICATIONS

Overlying soft tissue infection (e.g., omphalitis), peritonitis, possible necrotizing enterocolitis, and abdominal anomalies (e.g., omphalocele) are contraindications to placing an umbilical vessel catheter. Umbilical lines should not be placed in infants greater than 2 weeks of age and should be avoided in patients with known thrombotic disease. Finally, one must remember that these are central lines and are not placed for routine blood sampling or administration of fluids or medications.

EQUIPMENT

NONSTERILE

- Radiant warmer with light source
- Cardiorespiratory monitor
- Pulse oximeter
- Measuring tape
- Surgical mask with face shield, surgical cap
- D5W, D10W, or 0.45% NaCl infusion setup with heparin 1 unit/mL (unless medications are incompatible with heparin)
- Soft infant restraints
- Adhesive tape

STERILE

- Povidone-iodine solution
- Sterile drapes, gauze, gloves, gown
- Scalpel (number 11 or 15)
- Curved hemostats (2)
- Straight forceps
- 3-0 silk suture
- Needle driver
- Scissors
- Umbilical tape
- Umbilical catheters (3.5 or 5 french)
  - Umbilical vein catheter size = 5 Fr if >500 g; 3.5 Fr if <500 g
  - Umbilical artery catheter size = 5 Fr if >1500 g; 3.5 Fr if <1500 g
- Three-way stopcock
- Curved, toothless forceps or pointed, solid metal dilator
- 10-mL syringe filled with sterile normal saline (with heparin 1 unit/mL if available)

PROCEDURE

PREPARATION

Preparation for the insertion of the umbilical catheter is key to a successful catheterization. Arranging the materials prior to patient arrival is preferred. The first 60 minutes after birth is referred to as the Golden Hour, a key period of time in which effective stabilization of the neonate helps prevent irreversible damage, increasing the likelihood of survival. Studies have shown that proper preparation leading up to and during the Golden Hour leads to decreased incidence of hypoglycemia and hypothermia. The first step is to prepare the infant for the procedure. Infants should have a peripheral intravenous catheter (PIV) placed prior to beginning umbilical catheterization for infusion of dextrose containing fluids. This will minimize the risk of hypoglycemia. Infants should be under a radiant warmer with the arms and legs restrained in the supine, frog-leg position (see **Figure 192-1**).

Attach cardiorespiratory, temperature, and oxygen saturation sensors for monitoring throughout the procedure.

Prior to insertion, you should determine the proper length of insertion of the catheter. For **arterial catheter** placement, an estimated length can be calculated using the formula (birth weight [kg] × 3) + 9 cm. **Venous catheter** placement can be estimated by dividing the arterial catheter length by 2 and then adding 1 (UAC length/2 + 1). Venous catheter diameters are typically 5 French unless the infant is <1500 gm. Arterial catheters are 5 French for infants weighing more than 1.5 kg and 3.5 French for smaller infants.

Next, you will need to set up the umbilical catheterization tray. A sturdy surface (i.e., Mayo tray) is best to lay out your supplies on a sterile field. Hair covering, face mask, sterile gown, and gloves should be worn by all members of the team working in the sterile field. The practitioner

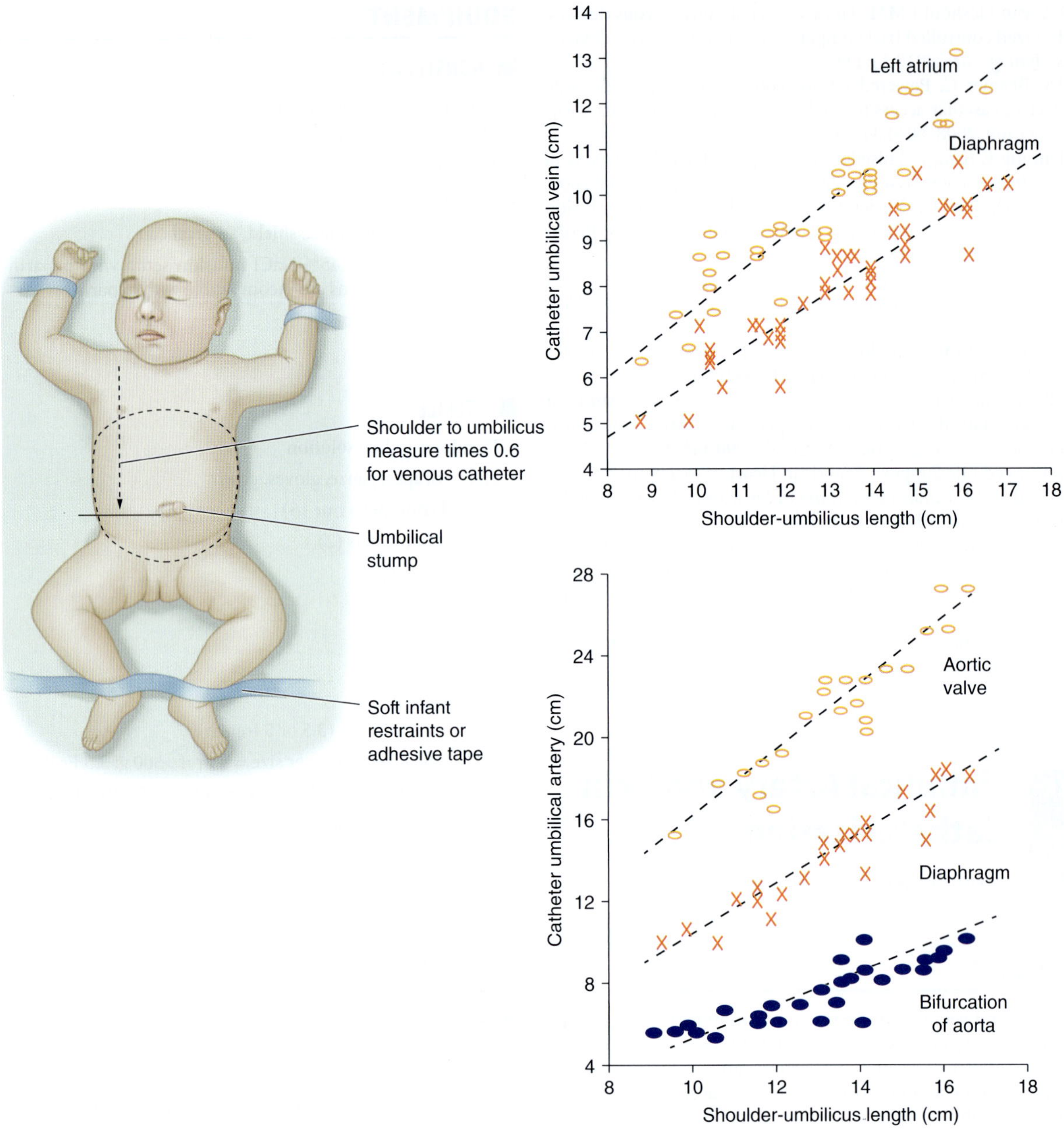

FIGURE 192-1. Infant placement and catheter lengths.

performing the procedure should have a nonsterile assistant deposit the heparinized flushes inside an open well in the catheter kit. Heparinized flushes are not sterile; thus, the syringe itself should not touch the sterile field. Attach the three-way stopcock to the umbilical catheter, and flush both ports and the catheter with sterile solution. Care should be taken while flushing each port with heparinized saline to avoid air bubbles within the catheter system. If you identify any air bubbles, flush them out of the catheter before insertion. Turn off the stopcock to all ports. Repeat these steps to flush all remaining ports.

Once you have your supplies prepped and infant prepared, you are now ready to move forward with umbilical catheter insertion. Your assistant should stand on the opposite side of the bed from where you are working. The assistant should hold the umbilicus up with an umbilical clamp. Use the iodine solution provided within the umbilical catheter kit, and scrub the area using a circular motion beginning near the umbilical stump and moving outward. The scrubbing radius should range from the umbilical stump to the pubic symphysis inferiorly and the xiphoid process superiorly. The umbilical clamp your assistant is holding is now nonsterile and should be placed separate from your sterile supplies. Drape the umbilical region in a sterile manner, using additional sterile surgical towels to create a comprehensive sterile field. Apply either umbilical tape with a loose overhand tie or a purse-string suture around the base of the umbilicus. Use forceps to grasp the umbilical cord 1 to 2 cm from the skin. Cut the cord transversely at the top of the forceps using the scalpel with a single clean incision (**Figure 192-2A**). Slowly release the forceps to watch for bleeding. Adjust the umbilical tape or purse string suture if necessary. Use two hemostats to grasp and evert the edges of the umbilicus and expose the umbilical vessels (**Figure 192-2B**). A normal umbilicus has paired umbilical arteries and a single larger umbilical vein. The umbilical artery can be differentiated from the umbilical vein by its thick muscular wall and smaller caliber.

UMBILICAL VEIN CATHETER PLACEMENT

Emergent Prepare the cord as described and identify the umbilical vein. Remove any visible clot. Gently insert a 5 French flushed catheter into the vein lumen, aiming the tip toward the right shoulder. Advance 1 to 2 cm beyond the point when good blood return is obtained. Do not insert further than 5 cm (see **Figure 192-2B**). This allows blood draws and infusion of high-osmolarity solutions while minimizing the risk of

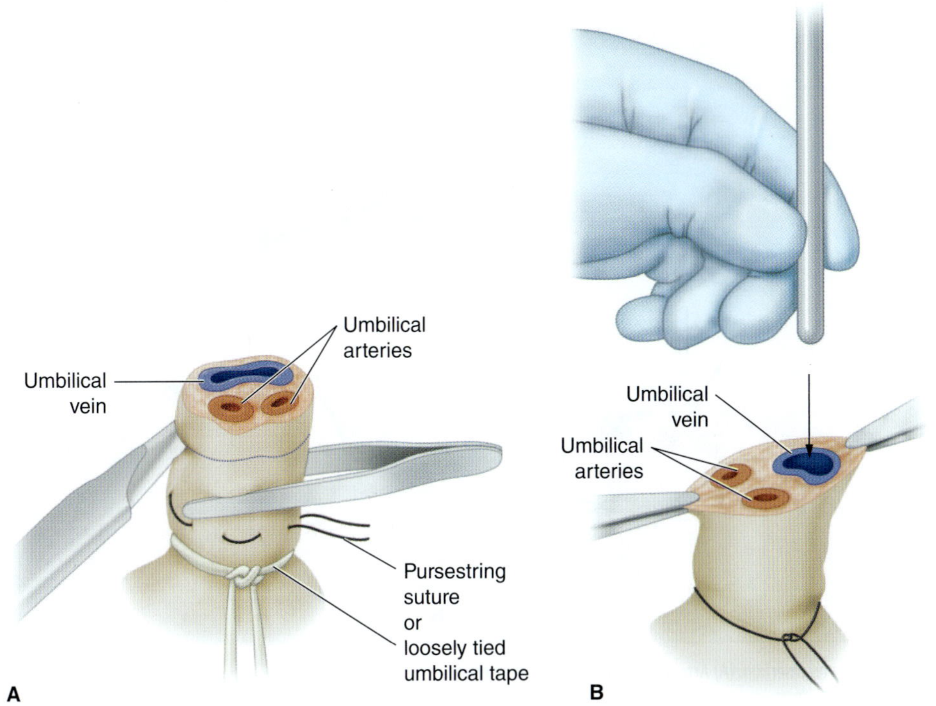

FIGURE 192-2. Preparing the umbilical cord. (A) Cutting the cord. (B) Exposing the vessels and inserting the umbilical vein catheter.

hepatic injury. Radiographic confirmation of placement is not necessary in the emergent setting. Remove the catheter once fluid resuscitation is achieved and replace the umbilical clamp.

Non-emergent Determine the appropriate catheter depth. The equation ((birth weight [kg] × 3) + 9 cm)/2) + 1 may be used. Ideal placement is above the diaphragm at the junction of the inferior vena cava and right atrium (about T7-T9). Proceed as described earlier, but continue to advance the catheter to the desired length. If resistance is felt at 5 to 10 cm, the catheter may have passed into a branch of the portal vein and must be repositioned. If this occurs, withdraw the catheter to a depth of 1 to 2 cm and try again. A clockwise twisting motion can help avoid the liver. In addition, passing a second catheter beside the malpositioned catheter may allow the second catheter to transverse the ductus venosus. Infusion of solutions through a catheter suspected to be in the liver risks hepatic necrosis. Confirm placement with a radiograph, adjust if necessary, and secure as detailed later. Remember that the catheter may be pulled back but cannot be advanced once sterile technique is broken.

UMBILICAL ARTERY CATHETER PLACEMENT

Ideal placement is in the descending aorta above the diaphragm between the ductus arteriosus and the celiac root (thoracic spine level T6-T10). The equation (birth weight [kg] × 3) + 9 cm may be used to estimate the correct placement depth of the catheter. A recent meta-analysis advises against the use of low-placed umbilical artery catheters (UAC) because of increased risk of ischemic complications, possibly aortic thrombosis, as well as shorter duration of catheter usability. If the catheter is initially placed too low (below T9), it can be withdrawn to the level between the inferior mesenteric artery and the aortic bifurcation (lumbar spine level L3-L4) and used temporarily in this low position.

Identify the umbilical artery as described earlier, and dilate the lumen gently by repeatedly inserting a closed, curved forceps and opening the tips in the lumen (**Figure 192-3A**). The artery should be dilated to a depth of approximately 1 cm. Many catheter setups contain a pointed metal dilator that can be used for this purpose. Gently introduce the tip into the lumen of the artery and apply countertraction to the cord in the cephalad direction so that the catheter is directed inferiorly along the natural course of the artery (**Figure 192-3B**). Resistance may be felt at 1 to 2 cm as the artery courses inferiorly and at 5 to 6 cm at the junction with the internal iliac artery. A twisting motion can help overcome this resistance. If resistance is felt at 4 to 5 cm, strongly consider the creation of a false tract and try the other artery. Once the catheter has been advanced to the desired location, obtain a radiograph to confirm its placement. More than one radiograph may be necessary to correctly confirm placement after adjustments are made. If the line is too high, measure on the radiograph and adjust the length accordingly. If it is too low, it can be converted temporarily into a low-lying position at L3-L4. Observe for blanching, cyanosis, or mottling of lower extremities or buttocks after placement (see Complications, later).

SECURING THE CATHETER

Secure the catheter with the ends of the previously tied purse-string suture or the ends of another suture placed at the skin margin of the umbilical stump. Be careful to avoid the umbilical vessels when suturing. Wrap each end of the suture in opposite directions one or two times around the catheter and tie a square knot. For added security, repeat the knot 2 cm from the stump. Secure the catheter and suture it to the body using a tape bridge (**Figure 192-4**). Fluids should be run through the catheter continuously at a low rate to minimize the risk of thrombus formation and to extend the life of the catheter.

RADIOGRAPHICALLY CONFIRMING POSITION OF CATHETERS

Many complications arise from malpositioned catheters. Unless in an emergency setting, catheter placement should be confirmed radiographically prior to use for anything except blood draws or intravenous fluids. It is straightforward to distinguish an umbilical venous catheter from an umbilical artery catheter on x-ray. The umbilical venous catheter enters the abdomen at the umbilicus and travels cephalad in the umbilical vein, through the portal vein and ductus venosus, and enters the IVC, terminating near the right atrium. The optimal position for a venous catheter is above the diaphragm at the IVC and right atrial junction between T7 and T9. Umbilical artery catheters also enter the abdomen at the umbilicus but initially extend inferiorly and posteriorly into the iliac artery before coursing superiorly into the aorta. The optimal position for umbilical artery catheters is T6-T10 to prevent thrombotic complications. Ultrasound is an increasingly viable option for obtaining imaging of an umbilical line to monitor for movement of the line.

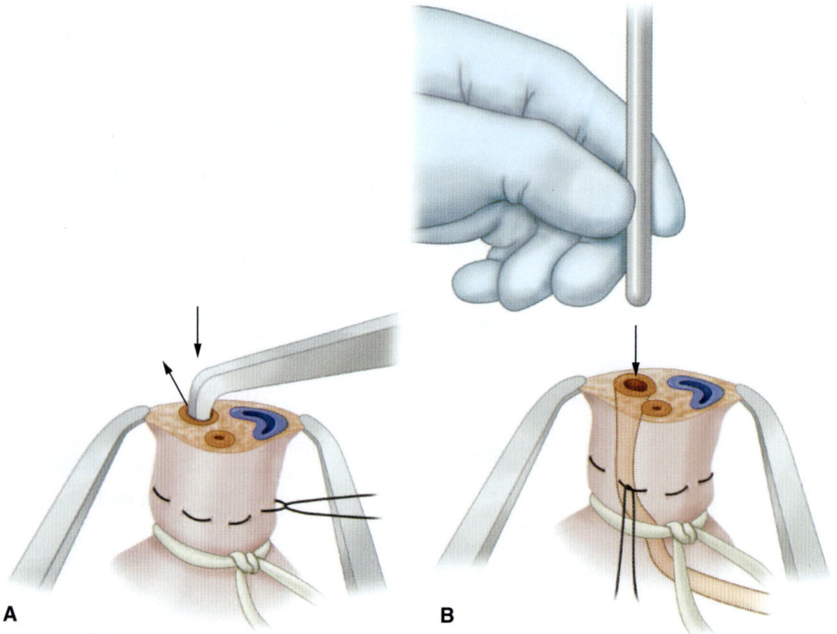

FIGURE 192-3. Umbilical artery catheter insertion. (A) Artery dilation. (B) Catheter insertion.

COMPLICATIONS

Possible complications of umbilical catheter placement include thrombosis, bacteremia, sepsis, and peripheral vasospasm. Thrombosis may present as limb ischemia, renal infarct, bowel ischemia, pulmonary embolus, or stroke, and may result in septic emboli. Removing the catheter as soon as possible, especially a UAC, can also decrease the risk of complications. Thrombosis is rarely seen if the UAC is removed within 5 to 7 days.

Ischemia to the limbs or organs can result from improper catheter positioning. Lower extremity and buttocks ischemia can also be caused by vasospasm. If ischemia of the buttocks or lower extremity is suspected, apply warm compresses to the contralateral lower extremity; this results in reflex vasodilation of the ipsilateral extremity. If no improvement in limb color or pulse is seen within 15 minutes, remove the catheter.

Bacterial colonization or sepsis is always a concern with central line placement. Using sterile technique will decrease but not eliminate this risk. There is currently insufficient evidence to support the use of prophylactic antibiotics in patients with umbilical artery catheters. To help prevent sepsis and bacterial colonization, remove central access as soon as possible.

Malpositioned catheters increase the risk of complications. Umbilical vein catheters that are improperly placed in the main portal vein can result in hepatic hematoma, and infusion of high osmolarity solutions into an improperly placed umbilical vein catheter in the liver can cause hepatic necrosis. Catheters that are advanced too far can result in arrhythmias, or more rarely in pericardial tamponade from perforation of the right or left atrial wall. Cardiac arrhythmias should alert the practitioner to the possibility of a catheter in the right atrium. The catheter should be withdrawn immediately in the setting of arrhythmia. Renal or bowel ischemia can result from improper placement of the arterial catheter in a branch of the aorta. If there is concern for ischemia, it is best to remove the catheter promptly. Proper measurement prior to placement and radiographic confirmation before use are important ways to prevent these complications. Other rare complications include peritoneal, vessel, or organ perforation; aneurysm formation; air embolus; significant blood

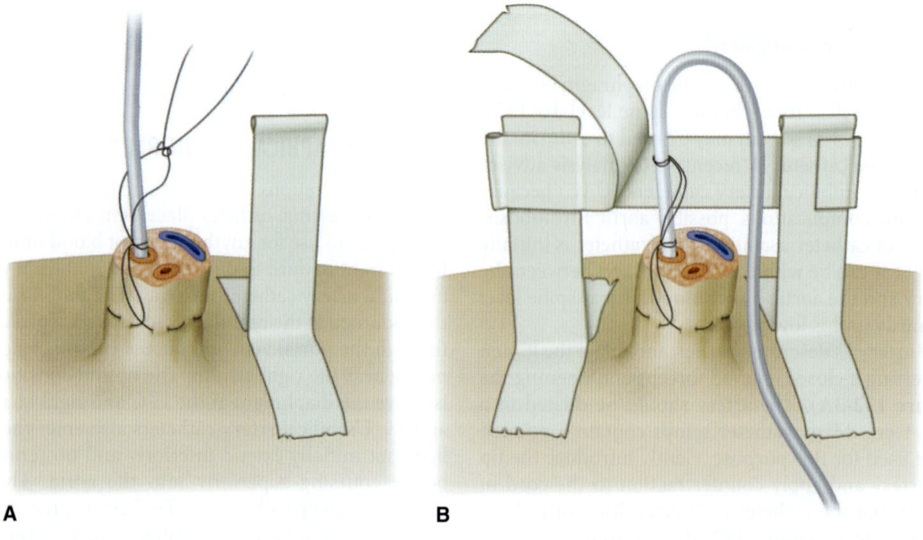

FIGURE 192-4. Securing the catheter. (A) Suture anchor. (B) Tape bridge.

loss; and portal hypertension. Organ, vessel, pericardial, and peritoneal perforation are rare complications but require emergent surgical consultation. The risk of significant blood loss or air embolism is reduced by flushing all catheters before insertion, using a three-way stopcock, and taking care to secure the catheter with sutures and tape.

SUGGESTED READINGS

Ashmeade TL, Haubner L, Collins S, Miladinovic B, Fugate K. Outcomes of a neonatal Golden Hour Implementation Project. *Am J Med Qual.* 2016;31(1):73-80.

Croop SEW, Thoyre SM, Aliaga S, et al. The Golden Hour: a quality improvement initiative for extremely premature infants in the neonatal intensive care unit. *J Perinatol.* 2020;40:530-539.

Kishigami M, Shimokaze T, Enomoto M, Shibasaki J, Toyoshima K. Ultrasound-guided umbilical venous catheter insertion with alignment of the umbilical vein and ductus venosus. *J Ultrasound Med.* 2020;39(2):379-383.

Lewis GC, Crapo SA, Williams JG. Critical skills and procedures in emergency medicine: vascular access skills and procedures. *Emerg Med Clin N Am.* 2013;77-80.

CHAPTER 193 Noninvasive Positive-Pressure Ventilation

Alla Lescure Smith, MD

BACKGROUND

This chapter will discuss the use of noninvasive positive pressure ventilation (NIPPV) in the pediatric inpatient setting by pediatric hospitalists. Noninvasive ventilation augments alveolar ventilation by providing airflow under pressure, with or without supplemental oxygen, for gas exchange via an external interface. One of the primary goals of NIPPV in the management of acute respiratory failure is avoidance of intubation and the risks associated with invasive mechanical ventilation and sedation. The use of NIPPV in pediatrics has significantly increased, both as a tool to support acute respiratory failure in several commonly encountered pediatric diagnoses like bronchiolitis and asthma, and as a support for chronic respiratory failure in patients with underlying chronic medical conditions. While the initiation of NIPPV for acute respiratory failure remains largely the purview of the intensive care unit (ICU), pediatric hospitalists may be called on to initiate NIPPV while awaiting ICU transport and may occasionally manage these patients on the inpatient floor or in pediatric intermediate care units. The evidence supporting the use of NIPPV for pediatric acute and chronic respiratory failure is mounting, but lags behind clinical practice. Nevertheless, given the increasing prevalence of these modalities in the pediatric inpatient space, hospitalists should familiarize themselves with the indications for and management of NIPPV in both acute and chronic respiratory failure.

MODES OF NONINVASIVE VENTILATION

CONTINUOUS POSITIVE AIRWAY PRESSURE

Devices for continuous positive airway pressure (CPAP) provide a continuous flow of air to generate a preset pressure throughout the entire respiratory cycle. As illustrated in **Figure 193-1**, CPAP provides a constant airflow at a set supra-atmospheric pressure, superimposed on a patient's spontaneous breaths. The additional airflow raises inspiratory pressures and applies a positive end-expiratory pressure, overall increasing mean airway pressure, preventing airway collapse/atelectasis, and increasing the patient's functional residual capacity. These effects have been shown to improve oxygenation and reduce work of breathing. CPAP does not directly increase tidal volume, and as such it provides respiratory support but not truly assisted ventilation. Given this, some textbooks and articles do not consider CPAP to be a form of NIPPV. Although CPAP does not provide ventilation per se, it is commonly used to support patients in respiratory failure, and we will review indications for its use and key management principles in this chapter.

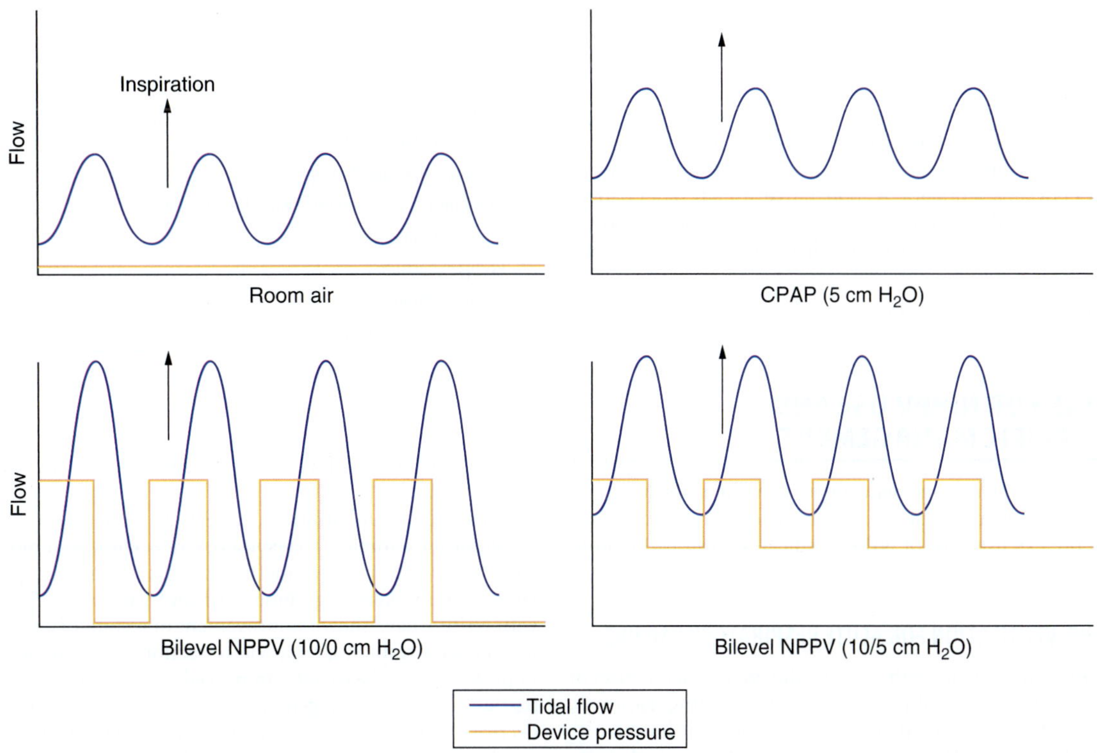

FIGURE 193-1. Respiratory air flow with various modes of noninvasive ventilation. CPAP, continuous positive airway pressure; NPPV, noninvasive positive pressure ventilation.

BILEVEL POSITIVE AIRWAY PRESSURE

Bilevel positive airway pressure devices (e.g., BiPAP) can provide different set pressures during inspiration and expiration. The pressure difference between expired positive airway pressure (EPAP) and inspired positive airway pressure (IPAP) serves to increase tidal volume and hence minute ventilation (**see Figure 192-1**). When the EPAP is set at >0 cm H_2O, BiPAP provides continuous PEEP, like CPAP, but with the IPAP adding support for ventilation.

BiPAP is commonly delivered in either the spontaneous (S) or spontaneous-timed (S/T) mode. In S mode, each patient breath is assisted by machine delivered IPAP when the machine senses the change in airflow triggered by the inspiratory effort of the patient. Because there is no background respiratory rate set on the machine, a child must initiate each breath on his or her own. In S/T mode, a respiratory rate can be set to provide a backup rate if the child slows or ceases respiratory efforts. In this mode, the device responds to inspiratory and expiratory flow rates to cycle machine-initiated breaths between the patient's inhalation and exhalation.

HIGH-FLOW NASAL CANNULA

High-flow nasal cannula provides heated, humidified air with titratable FiO_2 (0.21-1), typically at flows of greater than 4 liters per minute. HFNC facilitates improved gas exchange via dead-space wash-out and humidification of the airways. In addition, it may provide flow-dependent PEEP, although there is conflicting evidence about this. Even among studies that do demonstrate flow-dependent PEEP, the intrathoracic pressures generated by HFNC are smaller and more variable compared with other forms of NIPPV (largely a product of its non-occlusive interface with fixed, rather than responsive air flow). And, like CPAP, HFNC is not classically thought of as assisting in ventilation. However, it has gained popularity in the past decade, particularly for the management of patients with bronchiolitis. HFNC is more comfortable and generally better tolerated compared to NIPPV. There may also be fewer issues with skin breakdown when using HFNC compared to some NIPPV interfaces.

OTHER MODALITIES

- Volume-Controlled Ventilation: While most NIPPV encountered by pediatric hospitalists will be pressure-controlled modalities, like CPAP and BiPAP, certain ventilators can deliver volume-controlled NIPPV as well. In these modes, a goal tidal volume is set and the ventilator adjusts delivered pressure (often within set parameters) to achieve these tidal volumes.
- Sip and Puff Ventilation: This describes intermittent patient-triggered positive pressure ventilation delivered through a straw-like device connected to a portable ventilator. A cooperative, usually older patient can place the straw in their mouth and "pull" a breath from the portable ventilator— which, when triggered, delivers a pressure-supported breath.
- NIPPV use in the NICU involves other modes of ventilation that are beyond the scope of this chapter.

TABLE 193-1 Selected Indications for Noninvasive Positive-Pressure Ventilation

Acute Indications
Predominantly hypoxemia-related
• Neonatal respiratory distress syndrome
• Meconium aspiration syndrome
• Acute lung injury and pediatric acute respiratory distress syndrome
• Bronchiolitis
• Pneumonia
• Parapneumonic effusion
• Acute chest syndrome in sickle cell disease
• Cardiogenic pulmonary edema
• Postoperative atelectasis
Lower airway diseases
• Status asthmaticus
• Bronchiolitis
• Bronchomalacia*
Upper airway obstruction
• Post-extubation stridor
• Croup
• Status post tonsillectomy and adenoidectomy
• Tracheomalacia*
Avoidance of invasive ventilation
• Immunocompromised state
• Post-extubation sedation
• Thoracic insufficiency and chest wall abnormalities*
• Neuromuscular diseases*
• DNR/DNI
Post-extubation weaning of support
Chronic Indications
Severe chronic lung disease
Central hypoventilation syndrome
Upper airway obstruction
• Obstructive sleep apnea syndrome
• Craniofacial abnormalities and syndromes
• Pharyngeal hypotonia
• Tracheomalacia/bronchomalacia*
Neuromuscular diseases
• Spinal muscular atrophy
• Duchenne muscular dystrophy
Thoracic insufficiency and chest wall abnormalities*
• Scoliosis/kyphoscoliosis
• Pectus excavatum
• Poland syndrome
• Obesity/abdominal competition

*May be an acute or chronic indication.

INDICATIONS FOR NIPPV USE AND DISEASE-SPECIFIC MANAGEMENT

NIPPV can be used for the management of both acute and chronic respiratory failure. We will review some commonly encountered indications for NIPPV. A more extensive list of NIPPV indications can be found in **Table 193-1**.

NONINVASIVE VENTILATION FOR ACUTE RESPIRATORY FAILURE

Initiation of NIPPV for patients with an acute illness or exacerbation of subacute disease processes typically occurs in an ICU setting. However, some pediatric wards and intermediate care units allow for hospitalist-led initiation of CPAP and BiPAP for acute respiratory failure, with nursing and respiratory therapy support. In addition, many institutions offer HFNC to patients with acute respiratory failure from bronchiolitis outside the ICU.

The initiation and titration of NIPPV in the acute setting can be guided by physical examination (respiratory rate, chest wall movement, breath sounds), bedside monitoring (e.g., pulse oximetry or capnography), and laboratory markers (e.g., blood pH and gas levels). Studies of success with NIPPV have shown improvement in respiratory rate, improvement in accessory respiratory muscle retractions and paradoxical breathing, improvement in heart rate, improved gas exchange, improved ratio of partial pressure of oxygen to inspired oxygen level (PaO_2/FiO_2), and decreased partial pressure of carbon dioxide ($PaCO_2$). Lack of improvement in these parameters in the first hour after initiation has been correlated with NIPPV failure.

Oxygen saturation monitoring is a helpful tool, but adequate saturations may not represent normal ventilation when supplemental oxygen is being used. Some children with central blunting of their respiratory drive or with impending respiratory arrest may appear comfortable with supplemental oxygen in place but have an elevated or climbing $PaCO_2$. Care must also be taken in the use of any sedating drugs (including some over-the-counter cough medicines), which may, by reducing respiratory drive, interfere with a child's ability to trigger BiPAP. Children who require sedation to tolerate NIPPV interfaces may be more optimally managed in an ICU setting.

In terms of enteral intake, children with acute respiratory failure who require NIPPV are generally made NPO and given intravenous hydration. There is significant variation in the practice of when and how to initiate feeds in patients on CPAP/BiPAP. Both gastric and post-pyloric feeding regimens have been described in the patient who has been stabilized on NIPPV. Several studies suggest that the risk of clinically significant aspiration in previously healthy patients on HFNC for bronchiolitis is low, and so clinicians may choose to have children on HFNC eat by mouth.

Patients with acute respiratory failure who require HFNC or NIPPV often benefit from additional medical management including frequent suctioning (including nasopharyngeal suctioning with a catheter), pulmonary toileting, and chest PT. The availability of trained and experienced nursing and respiratory staff is integral for the safe management of these patients outside the ICU. These patients benefit from a reduced nursing ratio. In addition, a close relationship with an ICU, with clear guidelines on when to initiate ICU consultation or transfer is an important component of safe management.

Bronchiolitis Bronchiolitis makes up a significant proportion of pediatric admissions to the general wards and ICUs. While NIPPV use remains relatively uncommon, the percentage of patients admitted with bronchiolitis who receive some sort of NIPPV has dramatically increased in the past decade. The widespread increase in HFNC for bronchiolitis—driven partially by its use outside the ICU on the general wards—is responsible for much of this change.

Given its relative safety and comfort, HFNC is a reasonable choice for hospitalized patients with bronchiolitis who have failed standard therapies, and have persistent moderate to severe tachypnea, dyspnea or hypoxia despite low flow nasal canula oxygen. HFNC, when delivered using weight-based flows of 2L/kg/minute, reduces tachypnea and dyspnea in patients with bronchiolitis. HFNC may provide some PEEP (3-5 cm H_2O) at these flow rates. However, it is not clear whether HFNC impacts clinical trajectory in patients with bronchiolitis—including key outcomes such as hospital length of stay, critical care length of stay, need for escalation to CPAP/BiPAP, and invasive mechanical ventilation.

Patients with persistent tachypnea and dyspnea on HFNC, or those who require high FiO_2 to prevent hypoxia should be considered for CPAP/BiPAP initiation. For patients who require initiation of CPAP/BiPAP, initial settings should be patient specific, but may be in the range of 5 to 7 cm H_2O when using CPAP. BiPAP should be considered in patients with hypercapnia. NIV should be titrated to support adequate gas exchange and ensure appropriate oxygenation, often in consultation with the ICU.

Asthma Asthma remains one of the most common chronic pediatric conditions. While the overall number of hospital admissions for asthma is declining, the proportion of admissions for critical asthma with status asthmaticus requiring ICU admission has increased. Management of this patient population remains highly variable. Historically, use of NIPPV in asthma had been tempered by concerns of exacerbating air-trapping and dynamic hyperinflation. However, the use of NIPPV for patients in status asthmaticus has dramatically increased in the past 10 years. In this population, NIPPV is administered with continuous albuterol running in-line through the device. In addition to the usual respiratory support that NIPPV provides, the airway stenting it affords allows better distal delivery of bronchodilators. There is a paucity of robust randomized trials that support the use of NIPPV in status asthmaticus. However, there are many descriptions of safe and effective use of NIPPV in this patient population. BiPAP is a commonly reported modality, often with starting pressures of 10/5 (IPAP/EPAP) or 12/6. Recent literature has described HFNC use for status asthmaticus as well.

Pneumonia Management of children with mild to moderate acute hypoxic respiratory failure from pneumonia with NIPPV is increasing, based on evidence that NIPPV may reduce the need for intubation in this population. Therefore, children with pneumonia and mild hypoxic or hypercapnic respiratory failure could be considered for initiation of NIPPV, often in consultation with the ICU. HFNC has also been used successfully for pneumonia. Success of NIPPV in these patients is manifested by decreased respiratory rates and heart rates as well as improved gas exchange. However, this remains a high-risk group, and some studies have suggested that NIPPV may not impact the need for intubation, particularly in children with more severe disease who meet criteria for pediatric acute respiratory distress syndrome.

Upper Airway Obstruction Acute upper airway obstruction can occur in the setting of multiple clinical scenarios including critical croup, deep neck infections, acute post-surgical changes (e.g., following tonsillectomy), and post-extubation. While NIPPV can be useful in the treatment of acute airway obstruction, these patients are generally critically ill and are often managed in an ICU setting.

Neonatal Support Some of the most common indications for NIPPV use in the neonatal period include support in the delivery room, primary therapy for respiratory distress syndrome (surfactant deficiency) or meconium aspiration syndrome, post-extubation support and weaning, avoidance of reintubation, and treatment of apnea. One of the important goals of introducing noninvasive ventilation has been to decrease the need for intubation and mechanical ventilation, theoretically limiting the risk of barotrauma and volutrauma to newborn lungs. Management of NIPPV in the neonatal population, particularly amongst premature infants, is usually done in consultation with a neonatologist.

Other NIPPV has also been successfully used in the treatment of other conditions affecting the lower airways and lung parenchyma, such as the acute chest syndrome in sickle cell disease, cardiogenic pulmonary edema, and postoperative atelectasis.

NIPPV FOR CHRONIC RESPIRATORY FAILURE

Many pediatric hospitalists will encounter children with chronic respiratory failure admitted to inpatient wards for non-respiratory indications who rely on NIPPV for support at baseline. Familiarity with common indications for and management of NIPPV for chronic respiratory failure allows for effective patient care.

The initiation of chronic NIPPV is sometimes undertaken in an inpatient setting, where physiologic and laboratory data can be closely monitored. For patients whose chronic respiratory failure is sleep-related, initiation and titration can be done with the help of polysomnography. Different disease pathophysiologies require different ventilatory strategies, which can be chosen in consultation with the involved subspecialty service—often pulmonology or neurology. Poor respiratory system compliance, such as in restrictive lung disease or scoliosis, may require higher pressures (e.g., IPAP in excess of 12). In contrast, patients with neuromuscular disease often require minimal EPAP, and IPAP should be adjusted to ensure adequate ventilatory support. Once NIPPV has been established, pressures can be adjusted after a period of use, as the patient adapts to the equipment, the condition changes, and the patient grows.

The decision to initiate long-term NIPPV for out-of-hospital use often requires input from the medical team, case management, social work, respiratory therapy, and the home care agency. A family should have access to the appropriate equipment and supplies, undergo rigorous training, and demonstrate mastery of device use. The family should also have access to trained personnel who are available to help troubleshoot technical and clinical problems that may arise. Consideration should be given to home nursing when it is appropriate and available. A pre-discharge plan should be developed for routine follow-up and contingencies.

Obstructive Sleep Apnea During sleep, relative hypotonia develops in upper airway muscles, which causes an increase in upper airway resistance. Partial collapse of the upper airways results in vibration of the pharynx, manifested as snoring. Complete obstruction of the upper airways can also occur, resulting in obstructive apnea. Obstructive sleep apnea syndrome (OSAS) includes a spectrum of disorders ranging from snoring alone to complete obstruction of the upper airways, resulting in cessation of airflow (see Chapter 141). Adenotonsillar hypertrophy is most common cause of OSAS, making surgical adenoidectomy and tonsillectomy (T&A) first-line treatment and curative in many cases. Surgical failure to relieve OSAS is seen in some patients, and those with obesity, craniofacial abnormalities, hypotonia, and more severe OSAS initially are at highest risk. CPAP, or in severe cases (when CPAP pressure greater than 12 cm H_2O is needed), BiPAP, has been shown to help decrease symptoms of OSAS and on nocturnal polysomnography (PSG) leads to decreases in the apnea-hypopnea index. Therefore, NIPPV should be considered for OSAS in patients who are not surgical candidates, patients who have had T&A but continue to have OSAS, and in perioperative management of severe obstructive sleep apnea or obstructive sleep apnea complicated by pulmonary hypertension and cor pulmonale.

Chronic Respiratory Insufficiency Chronic respiratory insufficiency will eventually develop in a number of children with progressive diseases, such as severe chronic lung disease, respiratory muscle weakness secondary to neuromuscular diseases, and pharyngeal hypotonia related to various syndromes or chronic static encephalopathies. In such patients, hypoventilation that is initially present only during sleep can become prevalent throughout the day as the disease progresses. Respiratory failure typically develops insidiously, although this varies by disease pathophysiology. Pulmonary function tests can be helpful but are not always reliable in predicting which children may be at risk for significant nocturnal hypoventilation. Laboratory testing can begin to show increasing bicarbonate levels as the body chronically adapts to hypercapnia. Patients with neuromuscular disease may be candidates for noninvasive positive pressure ventilation when vital capacity is less than 50% predicted.

In patients with neuromuscular diseases such as Duchenne muscular dystrophy or spinal muscular atrophy, decreasing muscle strength leads to alveolar derecruitment, and patients ultimately are unable to generate adequate tidal volumes. In such patients, BiPAP support leads to improved minute ventilation and work of breathing, leading to improved gas exchange, decreased respiratory effort, and reduced sleep fragmentation. In selected populations, long-term BiPAP has demonstrated improvement in nocturnal respiratory parameters and daytime functioning as well as significant improvement in nutritional status. BiPAP use has been linked to improved perceived quality of life, reduction in the frequency and duration of healthcare utilization, and is associated with significant cost savings in the year after BiPAP in comparison to the preceding year.

In patients with severe restrictive lung disease such as that related to kyphoscoliosis or thoracic insufficiency, insidious onset of hypoxia may indicate progressive hypercapnia and failure of the patient's compensation efforts. Similar to patients with neuromuscular diseases, initial nighttime hypoventilation will progress, and initiation of NIPPV can be helpful. Depending on the degree of restrictive lung disease, NIPPV either during sleep or around the clock may be needed to help maintain necessary lung recruitment and provide sufficient tidal volume breaths. As with neuromuscular disorders, a patient's disease severity determines whether NIPPV is sufficient or if there is need for tracheostomy.

Cardiac Effects By increasing intrathoracic pressure, NIPPV reduces left ventricular afterload. This effect can be helpful in some acute and chronic cardiac conditions and in cardiogenic pulmonary edema. NIPPV decreases right ventricular return and preload, and so should be used with caution in patients with preload-dependent lesions.

INTERFACES

Essential to the successful delivery and effectiveness of noninvasive ventilation is selection of the proper interface. Experienced respiratory therapists can offer support in the selection and fit of the appropriate mask for individual patients, several of which are pictured in **Figure 193-2**. It is important to ensure adequate venting through the mask.

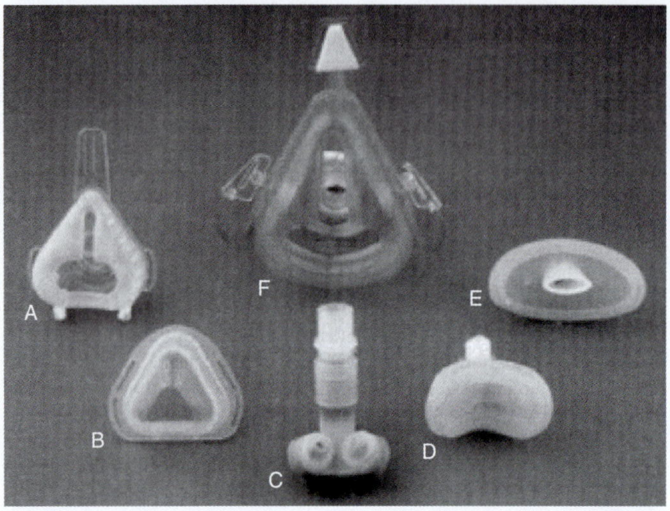

FIGURE 193-2. Noninvasive mechanical ventilation masks. (A) Standard nasal mask (Respironics Inc., Murrysville, PA); (B) Sullivan nasal mask (Sullivan Bubble Mask, ResCare, San Diego, CA); (C) nasal pillows (ADAM circuit, Nellcor Puritan Bennett, Pleasanton, CA); (D) mini mask (Respironics Inc.); (E) lip seal (Nellcor Puritan Bennett); (F) total face mask (Spectrum, Respironics Inc.). (Reproduced with permission from Lobato S, Alises S. Modern non-invasive mechanical ventilation turns 25. *Arch Bronconeumol*. 2013;49(11):475-479. Copyright © SEPAR. Figure 3, pg 477.Elsevier.)

TOTAL FACE MASK "HOCKEY MASK"

These masks cover the entire face, including the eyes, and span from the forehead to the chin. Different pressure points allow these masks to be used in patients with skin breakdown caused by other mask types. This mask can also fit some patients with craniofacial abnormalities. Disadvantages of this mask include the theoretical risk of aspiration with emesis or excessive secretions, so it must be used with caution in a patient who cannot remove the mask himself or herself. The area this mask covers also increases dead space significantly, which may render it less useful in carbon dioxide elimination.

FULL FACE MASK

This mask covers the mouth and nose, and its ideal fit should be from the bridge of the nose to just below the lower lip. The full-face mask helps to minimize air leak by covering both nose and mouth. As with the total face mask, the full-face mask should be used with caution in the setting of increased aspiration risk.

NASAL INTERFACES

Nasal masks cover the nose only, leaving the mouth uncovered. These are commonly used in the hospital as well as chronically by patients at home. Originally, these masks spanned from the bridge of the nose to the upper lip, but newer designs have covered just the nares or made use of large-bore nasal prongs (nasal pillow and nasal prong masks). Nasal masks do not cover the mouth, which decreases the risk of aspiration, but this can also lead to a large amount of leak and affect pressure delivery. Many nasal masks exist, each offering slightly different fits and pressure points on the face. HFNC is administered by non-occlusive prongs that are manufacturer specific and largely determined by a combination of patient weight and nares size.

CONTRAINDICATIONS FOR NIPPV USE

BiPAP is not capable of providing guaranteed ventilation and is therefore contraindicated when this is required (e.g., in patients with severe acute hypoxic and hypercarbic respiratory failure). In patients with pneumothorax, applying positive pressure can worsen air leak and compound the initial problem. NIPPV requires that the patient have a patent upper airway without choanal atresia/stenosis or significant fixed airway compression such as from vascular rings, hemangiomas, or neoplasms. Mask fit and compliance are essential for successful NIPPV; if these cannot be assured, an artificial airway is likely a better option in these patients. Impairment or loss of airway protective reflexes, commonly represented by Glasgow coma scale of eight or lower, is an indication for intubation for airway protection, and the use of NIPPV is generally not appropriate in these patients. Patients with rapidly progressive neuromuscular diseases or ascending paralysis require very careful consideration, and often intubation is preferred over noninvasive support.

LIMITATIONS AND RISKS OF NIPPV

NIPPV has significant practical limitations that curtail its clinical use:

- The connection at the mask interface is insecure. Leaks may be both uncomfortable (especially into the eyes) and make control of ventilation parameters unreliable and unsafe in certain circumstances.
- There are limitations to the maximal pressure that can be delivered, particularly when using a nasal mask in children who may have difficulty keeping their mouth closed.
- With increasing pressure, there is a risk of gastric distention and gastroesophageal reflux. In children using a full or total face mask, particularly those who lack adequate upper limb control, there is a risk of aspiration of stomach contents or excessive secretions. If a gastrostomy tube is in place, it should be vented when NIPPV is initiated to relieve gastric distention.
- Although NIPPV can be used on a continuous (24 hr/day) basis for short periods, it limits patient mobility. With long-term use, BIPAP and nasal CPAP have been associated with facial remodeling, particularly in smaller children.
- The prolonged or inappropriately fitted use of NIPPV interfaces can lead to skin breakdown. Techniques for addressing this problem include trying a different mask or nasal pillows and using foam or gel dressings (e.g., Mepilex or Duoderm) at the mask interface.
- Nasal obstruction from mucus plugs (which can occur with viral respiratory infections) can limit NIPPV effectiveness. Frequent suctioning (including nasopharyngeal suctioning with a catheter) is an important part of successful NIPPV use in this patient population.
- NIPPV reduces right ventricular return and preload (see Cardiac Effects above) and can cause hemodynamic compromise in patients with preload-dependent conditions.
- Barotrauma such as pneumothorax can occur, especially with increased pressure settings and in patients with high lung compliance.

KEY POINTS

- NIPPV is a technique of augmenting alveolar ventilation without requiring an artificial airway. It is a safe and effective tool for managing acute and chronic respiratory failure in select pediatric patients.
- CPAP delivers a continuous flow or air at a preset pressure throughout the respiratory cycle. It increases mean intrathoracic airway pressure and helps maintain end-expiratory lung volume and airway patency.
- BiPAP can provide set, specific pressures during inspiration and expiration and serves to increase tidal volume and minute ventilation. It can be used in the spontaneous mode to support patient-initiated breaths. Alternatively, it can be used in the spontaneous-timed mode to supply machine-initiated breaths in addition to support of patient-initiated breaths.
- HFNC delivers heated and humidified air mixed with oxygen via nasal prongs and can be used to treat many different etiologies of acute respiratory failure. It is often better tolerated compared to other forms of NIPPV but generally offers lower and less consistent positive pressure.
- Indications for the use of NIPPV include acute respiratory failure in bronchiolitis, status asthmaticus, pneumonia and premature birth. In addition, it can be used in chronic respiratory failure due to obstructive sleep apnea, restrictive lung disease, and neuromuscular weakness.
- Selection of the appropriate NIPPV interface is crucial to device success. Options include total face masks, masks that cover the mouth and nose, those that cover the nose only, and newer devices that cover only the nares or use large-bore nasal prongs.
- NIPPV requires application by skilled and knowledgeable staff. Initiation of NIPPV for acute respiratory failure is frequently done in an ICU, or in consultation with intensivists. However, safe initiation and management of NIPPV, particularly HFNC but also CPAP and BiPAP, by pediatric hospitalists for select patients with acute respiratory failure has been described. Initiation and titration can be guided by physical examination and laboratory studies.
- Initiation and titration of chronic NIPPV is best done in consultation with the managing outpatient service—often pulmonary or neurology—and may be accomplished with the aid of polysomnography. Appropriate settings and management are disease specific.
- NIPPV has a variety of contraindications and carries significant risks, which are important to consider prior to initiation.

SUGGESTED READINGS

Amaddeo A, Frapin A, Fauroux B. Long-term non-invasive ventilation in children. *Lancet Respir Med.* 2016;4:999-1008.

Chisti MJ, et al. Bubble continuous positive airway pressure for children with severe pneumonia and hypoxaemia in Bangladesh: an open, randomised controlled trial. *Lancet.* 2015;386:1057-1065.

Franklin D, et al. A randomized trial of high-flow oxygen therapy in infants with bronchiolitis. *New Engl J Med.* 2018;378:1121-1131.

He H, et al. A multicenter RCT of noninvasive ventilation in pneumonia-induced early mild acute respiratory distress syndrome. *Crit Care.* 2019;23:300.

Kopp W, et al. The Impact of Preintubation Noninvasive Ventilation on Outcomes in Pediatric Acute Respiratory Distress Syndrome*. *Crit Care Med.* 2021;49:816-827.

LoMauro A, D'Angelo MG, Aliverti A. Assessment and management of respiratory function in patients with Duchenne muscular dystrophy: current and emerging options. *Ther Clin Risk Manag.* 2015; 1475-1488.

Lyager S, Steffensen B, Juhl B. Indicators of need for mechanical ventilation in Duchenne muscular dystrophy and spinal muscular atrophy. *Chest.* 1995;779-785.

Marcus CL, Brooks LJ, Davidson Ward S, et al. Diagnosis and management of childhood obstructive sleep apnea syndrome. *Pediatrics.* 2012;130(3):e714-755.

Mayordomo-Colunga J, et al. Non-invasive ventilation practices in children across Europe. *Pediatr Pulm.* 2018;53:1107-1114.

Morley SL. Non-invasive ventilation in paediatric critical care. *Paediatr Respir Rev.* 2016;20:24-31.

Munshi L, Mancebo J, Brochard LJ. Noninvasive respiratory support for adults with acute respiratory failure. *N Engl J Med.* 2022;387:1688-1698.

Philips MF, Quinlivan RC, Edwards RH, Calverley PM. Changes in spirometry over time as a prognostic marker in patients with Duchenne muscular dystrophy. *Am J Respir Crit Care Med.* 2001;2191-2194.

Ramnarayan P, et al. Effect of high-flow nasal cannula therapy vs continuous positive airway pressure following extubation on liberation from respiratory support in critically ill children. *JAMA.* 2022;327:1555-1565.

Rubin S, et al. Effort of breathing in children receiving high-flow nasal cannula. *Pediatr Crit Care Med.* 2014;15:1-6.

Sahni AS, Wolfe L. Respiratory care in neuromuscular diseases. *Respir Care.* 2018;63:601-608.

Simonds AK. Home mechanical ventilation: an overview. *Ann Am Thorac Soc.* 2016;13(11):2035-2044.

CHAPTER 194

Emergent Airway Management

Thomas Guggina, MD and Timothy Gibson, MD

INDICATION

Emergent airway management is an essential skill for the pediatric hospitalist, enabling life-saving efforts and preventing untimely morbidity or mortality. It is indicated in cases of acute respiratory failure or other causes of respiratory depression or shock when the ability to maintain normal airway tone or oxygen saturation is compromised. The use of noninvasive treatment of respiratory distress has expanded markedly, with high-flow nasal cannula (HFNC) continuous positive airway pressure (CPAP) and bilevel positive airway pressure (BiPAP) all allowing for management of respiratory failure without intubation. When airway integrity is compromised or if noninvasive ventilation fails, intubation is necessary. Most hospitals will have an airway management team or in-house anesthesiologists, so knowing how to access more specialized practitioners is the most important first consideration in managing an airway. If not rapidly available, the proper steps for emergent airway management are covered in this chapter.

CONTRAINDICATIONS

In an emergency, there is no absolute contraindication to performing an endotracheal intubation. There are several factors that make intubation more challenging. In a controlled setting, patients are kept NPO to reduce the likelihood of vomiting, which could potentially lead to aspiration. This is often not possible in an emergent situation. Trauma also presents a challenge with even bag mask ventilation. Facial trauma can make placement of an alternate airway difficult or impossible, and in the case of significant trauma, the cervical spine should be immobilized before any airway manipulation.

ANATOMY

There are several unique aspects to the pediatric airway which bear special consideration. Depending on the age of the child, anatomic considerations for the pediatric airway when compared to adults include the following:

- Large occiput
- High tongue to mouth opening ratio
- Superior and anterior location of the glottis
- Large and floppy epiglottis
- Proper head positioning varies depending on the age of the child

EQUIPMENT

Once the decision to manage a patient's airway has been made, the importance of preparation cannot be overstated. Any piece of equipment that could potentially be necessary should be readily available (see **Table 194-1**), with attention paid to the size of the equipment based on the patient's age or size. Many pediatric code carts are topped by the Broselow Pediatric Emergency Tape, a color-coded tape measure that helps spell out sizes of airway management equipment, such as face masks, laryngoscope blades, and endotracheal tubes.

TABLE 194-1 Equipment Needed for Emergent Airway Management

Airway equipment
Laryngoscope handles and blades
Appropriate size endotracheal tubes (cuffed or uncuffed, with or without stylets) and laryngeal mask airways
Oral or nasal airways
Tape to secure tube in position
Oxygen
Positive-pressure delivery system, including manometer
Tubing
Appropriately sized face masks, self-inflating bag or infant T-piece system for bag-mask ventilation
Suction
Flexible catheter or Yankauer suction device
Nasogastric or orogastric tube to decompress the stomach
Medications
Intravenous access
Sedatives, analgesics
Other medications (e.g., atropine, lidocaine) as clinically warranted
Monitoring
Cardiac monitor
Pulse oximeter
End tidal carbon dioxide monitor and color-coded CO_2 detector

PROCEDURE

PREPARATION

To allow for ease of intubation and to prevent psychological and physical trauma to the patient, in addition to mitigating the risk of laryngospasm, sedation of the patient is recommended prior to intubation. Atropine is often used to counteract the prominent vagal response in pediatric patients less than 1 year of age. For sedatives, etomidate, ketamine, dexmedetomidine, propofol, opiates, and benzodiazepines are commonly used in emergency settings. Since hospitalists are generally not licensed to prescribe paralytic agents, we do not recommend their use.

TECHNIQUE

Because practitioners with more extensive airway skills are often called on to definitively manage an airway, the importance of a hospitalist having excellent bag-mask ventilation (BMV) skills is paramount. Indeed, an overwhelming percentage of the "airway management" done by hospitalists entails effective BMV until either the patient improves (as in the stunned neonate), or until additional resources arrive.

For BMV, the physician should stand at the head of the bed. The patient's head should be placed in the so-called "sniffing" position, a slight extension at the neck in an attempt to align the oropharynx with the trachea. In older patients, sometimes a neck roll is helpful to achieve this position. The practitioner should hold an appropriately sized face mask with their nondominant hand in the "C3" grasp, with the thumb and forefinger grasping the stem of the face mask (the "C") while the third, fourth, and fifth fingers are under the angle of the patient's jaw, lifting the airway toward the mask. Once a seal is made, the practitioner should hold the resuscitation bag or infant "T piece" mask system (**Figure 194-1**) with their dominant hand and administer a breath while looking for chest rise. If there is an audible leak around the mask or if there is no chest rise with ventilation attempts, the patient needs to be repositioned, which can often be done with an assistant. If there is still no chest rise after repositioning, insertion of an oral airway may be helpful. This is a plastic instrument placed in the mouth to follow the curve of the oropharynx that allows the bypass of any oral obstruction, such as secretions or a large tongue. A manometer should be attached to the bag or dialed into the T piece, and care must be taken to avoid high pressures. Once a seal has been ensured and chest rise established with reasonable pressures, the patient should be bagged until spontaneous respirations return or a more definitive airway can be placed. Care should be taken to only provide the pressure required to raise the chest well to avoid barotrauma.

If mechanical ventilation is required, however, placement of a secure airway will be necessary. For intubations intended to be short-term or

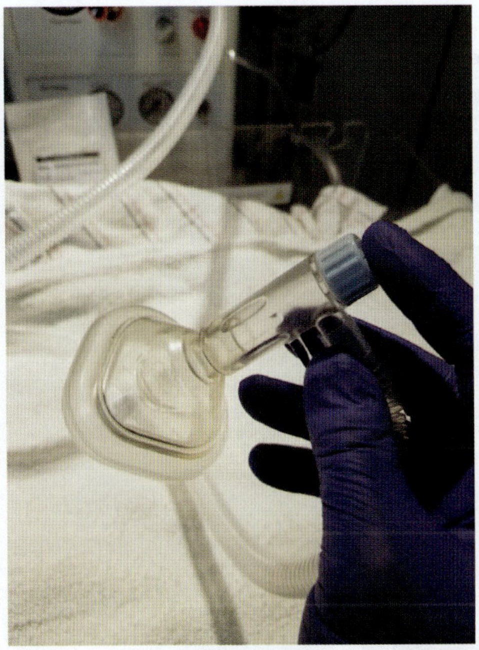

FIGURE 194-1. Infant T-piece resuscitator system. (Photo provided by Timothy Gibson, MD.)

temporizing, the placement of a laryngeal mask airway (LMA) is often considered, which takes far less skill to place than an endotracheal tube (ETT). The physician stands at the head of the bed and holds the LMA between thumb and forefinger of the dominant hand. The ventilating end of the LMA is guided into the mouth and along the palate until it cannot be advanced further, then its cuff is inflated. At this point the ventilating end sits on top of the larynx. Successful ventilation happens much more readily, especially with practitioners who have relatively little experience with ETT placement. An LMA does not protect against aspiration, however, so for longer-term ventilation, subsequent change to an ETT is often performed.

When intubating with an ETT, cuffed tubes should always be placed, with recognition that the pediatric airway is not, in fact, tunnel shaped but more elliptical. Care must be taken to assure proper placement and avoidance of overinflation of the cuff.

For placement of the ETT, alignment of the airway, the mouth opening, and the operator's visual field is the key to success. Strategies for successful visual alignment vary based on age. For infants a shoulder roll or folded blankets under the shoulders often compensate for the large occiput. Video laryngoscopy, if available, can allow for a wider and improved view of the glottis. The laryngoscope blade should be held in the left hand while the right hand should be used to place the ETT. We advocate for a midline approach with progressive visualization of anatomic structures—uvula, then epiglottis, then glottic opening. A straight (Miller) blade can be advanced to directly lift the epiglottis, or a curved (Macintosh) blade can be slid to the base of the tongue to the hyoepiglottic ligament in the vallecula to indirectly lift the epiglottis out of the visual field. In general, use of the Miller blade is useful until age of 2, then Macintosh blade is used at age 2 ("switch to a Mac 2 at 2"). It is important not to "crank" the laryngoscope back into the patient's teeth or palate to avoid improper visual alignment or injury to teeth, lips, or gums. The endotracheal tube should be inserted along the right side of the mouth so that the visual field is not obstructed, and the tip of the ETT is guided through the vocal cords and advanced to an age-appropriate depth and the stylet removed. A CO_2 colorimeter should be used to verify ventilation by turning from purple to yellow. The tube is held into place by pressing against the hard palate until taped into place. Appropriate depth and placement should be confirmed by chest X-ray.

COMPLICATIONS

Failed attempts at intubation can result in hypoxemia, increased vagal tone, and oropharyngeal trauma. To minimize these risks, the most experienced provider should attempt intubation and attempts should be limited to 30 seconds each, with no more than two per provider before an alternate approach is made. Laryngospasm may occur if sedation is inadequate or an attempt is prolonged. Inadequate stabilization of the ETT after placement can lead it to become dislodged. Copious airway secretions or blood can lead to obstruction of a properly placed ETT. Complications of ventilation after a successful intubation include barotrauma and pneumothorax.

SPECIAL CONSIDERATIONS

The hospitalist should anticipate when the airway may be difficult to manage and request assistance accordingly. As with any skill, frequent practice remains the key to an ultimately successful real-life procedure. The fidelity of simulation equipment has increased significantly, and many hospitalists will have ready access to high-quality simulation experiences which can improve skill with airway management.

SUGGESTED READINGS

Engelhardt T, Fiadjo JE, Weiss M, et al. A framework for the management of the pediatric airway. *Paediatr Anaesth.* 2019;29(1):985-992.

Miller KA, Nagler JN. Advances in emergent airway management in pediatrics. *Emerg Med Clin North Am.* 2019;37(3):473-491.

CHAPTER 195

Thoracentesis

Tonia Branche, MD, MPH and Jacqueline Guay, MD

BACKGROUND

Thoracentesis is the evacuation of fluid or air from the pleural space. This discussion encompasses the evacuation of fluid (effusion) and air (pneumothorax) from the pleural space in patients who have not suffered traumatic injuries. In the setting of trauma and concern for hemothorax, appropriate surgical consultation should be obtained and tube thoracostomy should be performed.

INDICATIONS

The indications for thoracentesis can be either therapeutic, to remove fluid or air that is causing pain or respiratory distress, or diagnostic, to determine the etiology in the case of a pleural effusion. The diagnosis of pleural effusion should be established by clinical examination and chest radiograph or ultrasonography. Lateral decubitus films or ultrasonography are useful in identifying small effusions and determining whether the pleural fluid is free-flowing or loculated. Clinical examination, chest radiograph, transillumination, and point of care ultrasound (US) can all be used to identify pneumothorax. In the case of tension pneumothorax, where the pleural air is causing hemodynamic compromise, there may not be adequate time to obtain a chest radiograph, and the clinician must rely on clinical examination, US, and transillumination for diagnosis. Tension pneumothorax is a clinical emergency and requires swift needle decompression for resolution.

CONTRAINDICATIONS

The following are *relative* contraindications to thoracentesis:

- Uncooperative patient (consider procedural sedation)
- Skin infection at the site of needle or catheter insertion
- Thrombocytopenia, bleeding, or clotting disorder, disseminated intravascular coagulation (consider transfusion or Hematology consultation to reduce bleeding risk with procedure)

- Small collection of fluid or pleural adhesions (increased danger of causing iatrogenic pneumothorax; consider doing the procedure under US guidance)
- Small collection of air not causing significant clinical decompensation (increased danger of causing iatrogenic tension pneumothorax; consider following clinically without intervention)
- Prior pleurodesis or other surgical intervention to pleura (consider discussion regarding patient's eligibility for procedure with surgery team)

ANATOMY AND PHYSIOLOGY

The pleural space is the potential space that exists between the visceral and parietal pleura in the lung. Normally, there is only a small amount (15 mL) of fluid in this space. Excess pleural fluid can accumulate when there is a systemic change in the forces that govern fluid production and drainage. Effusions can be classified as transudates (ultrafiltrates of plasma with a low protein concentration) or exudates (due to increased capillary permeability and the resulting accumulation of larger molecules). Common causes of transudative effusions in children are congestive heart failure, nephrotic syndrome, cirrhosis, and hypoalbuminemia. Exudative pleural effusions are usually caused by pneumonia (parapneumonic effusion), empyema, connective tissue disease, malignancy, pancreatitis, trauma, or pulmonary infarction.

Air accumulates in the pleural space when a connection develops to the pleural space from within the lung or from outside of the thoracic cavity. This can happen slowly over time with no symptoms or rapidly with hemodynamic changes. Pneumothoraces often occur without known cause as well as in patients with history of high-pressure positive pressure ventilation, surfactant deficiency or lung disease of prematurity, cystic lung disease, pleural blebs, porous pleural disease, and traumatic chest injury. In the case of tension pneumothoraces, the air rapidly enters the pleural space causing increased intrathoracic pressure, mediastinal shift of organs and structures, and decreased venous return and cardiac output, which leads to hemodynamic collapse.

EQUIPMENT

Virtually all hospitals carry a commercially or locally made kit that contains most of the equipment needed for thoracentesis (**Table 195-1, Figure 195-1**). In addition, the appropriate chest tube equipment (e.g., pigtail catheters, argyle catheters, etc.) should be available at the start of thoracentesis, in case chest tube placement becomes necessary to permit continued drainage of fluid or air.

PROCEDURE

The following method can be used when there is a significant amount of free-flowing pleural fluid or air. Many medical organizations, including the British Thoracic Society, American College of Emergency Physicians,

TABLE 195-1 List of Equipment Typically Included in Thoracentesis Kit

Sterile gloves
Povidone-iodine solution
Sterile gauze, sterile dressing, tape to secure bandage
Sterile towels and drapes
Syringes: 5mL, 15-30 mL
25-, 22-gauge needles
14-22-gauge angiocatheter
1%-2% lidocaine
Three-way stopcock (may also use 4-way stopcock)
T-connector or intravenous tubing
Sterile specimen collection bottles, blood gas syringe

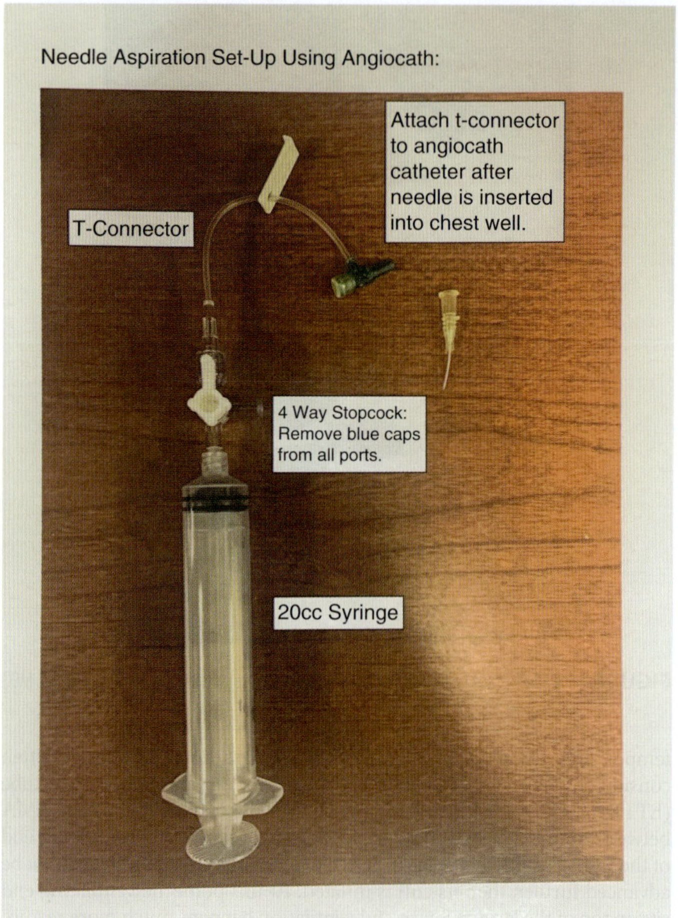

FIGURE 195-1. Example of assembled thoracentesis equipment.

and Society of Hospital Medicine recommend performing thoracentesis under US guidance. Evidence shows that complications of thoracentesis are significantly reduced with real-time US guidance performed by experienced providers. Evaluation using US enhances the preprocedural, intraprocedural, and postprocedural assessment of the pleural space. As the availability of point of care US equipment within emergency, inpatient, and intensive care units has increased, it has become the standard of care to use US guidance when performing thoracentesis if available.

PREPARATION

- Before commencing the procedure, obtain a proper informed consent from the parent and assent from the patient as indicated, explain the procedure to the patient, identify the patient and procedure, mark the site, verify the medical images, and conduct a time-out.
- Place an intravenous line, if not already established, in case of the need for emergent resuscitation. For pleural effusions, draw blood for complete blood count, INR, protein, lactate dehydrogenase (LDH), glucose, and other studies as indicated. Elective thoracentesis in patients with coagulopathy should be discussed to determine the necessity; however, a recent study has shown that thoracentesis and tube thoracostomy in patients with uncorrected coagulopathy can be done safely. Thus, obtaining coagulation labs prior to the procedure may not be necessary.
- Continuously monitor heart rate, respiratory rate, oxygen saturation, and blood pressure.
- Administer supplemental oxygen as needed. Avoid positive pressure in the case of pneumothorax to avoid reaccumulation of air or additional pneumothoraces.
- Use procedural sedation as needed.

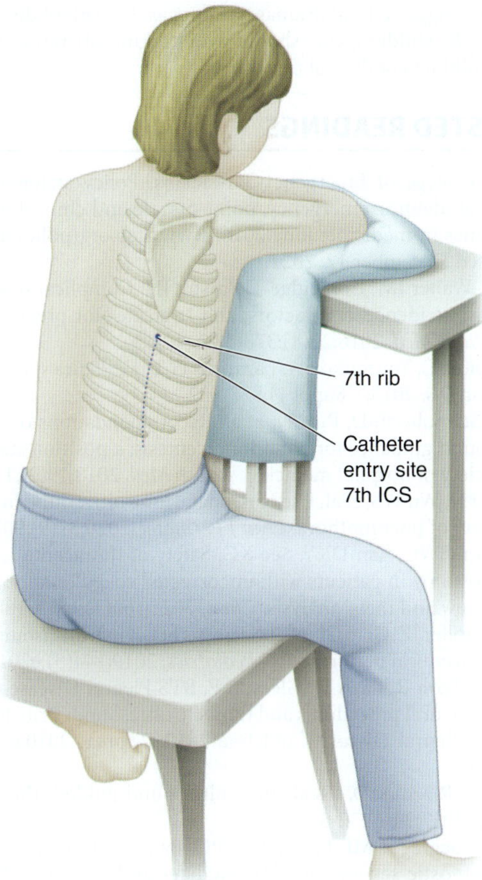

FIGURE 195-2. Patient position for thoracentesis for pleural effusion. ICS, intercostal space.

Pleural Effusion Thoracentesis for pleural effusion is best performed with the child in the sitting position. The upright position ensures that the diaphragm is dependent and facilitates the removal of fluid that localizes at the base of the chest. Have the child lean over a pillow placed on a bedside table or over the back of a chair (**Figure 195-2**). The patient's arms should be abducted and resting on the table. If the child is an infant or point-of-care US is being used to guide thoracentesis, the procedure may be done with the patient in supine or lateral recumbent position (with the affected side down) with head and chest elevated to 30 to 45 degrees so the pleural fluid will accumulate in the deepest part of the pleural space.

The thoracentesis site is determined based on the chest radiograph and physical findings, with attention to the site of maximal dullness on percussion. A reasonable site is in the midscapular line in the intercostal space immediately below the tip of the scapula if the procedure is being done with the patient sitting or in lateral recumbent position. This usually corresponds to the seventh intercostal space. If the procedure is performed with the patient supine, the mid-axillary line in the same intercostal space is a reasonable site.

Pneumothorax For evacuation of pneumothorax, the patient is best positioned supine with the head and neck slightly elevated at about 30 degrees or side-lying with the affected side up to allow air to rise and collect against the chest wall for evacuation (**Figure 195-3**). Thoracentesis location is selected based on chest radiography showing the location of the pneumothorax. The two sites used for thoracentesis are the 2nd intercostal space at the midclavicular line and the 4th intercostal space at the anterior axillary line.

TECHNIQUE

Pleural Effusion The area is prepared with povidone-iodine solution and draped with sterile towels. Raise a wheal of local anesthetic with a 25-gauge needle over the rib below the desired intercostal space. Remove

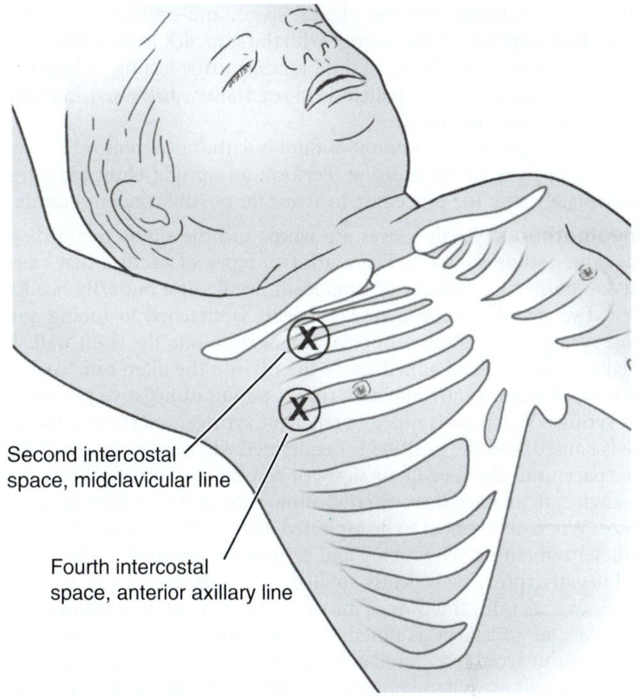

FIGURE 195-3. Patient position for thoracentesis for pneumothorax. (Reproduced with permission from Goodman DM, Green TP, Unti SM, Powell EC. *Current Procedures: Pediatrics*. New York: McGraw Hill; 2007, Figure 20-3.)

the 25-gauge needle and substitute a 22-gauge needle. Enter perpendicular to the skin, injecting lidocaine into the periosteum. Slowly walk the needle above the rib and toward the pleural space while aspirating and injecting lidocaine (**Figure 195-4**). Avoid the inferior rib area to prevent injury to the neurovascular bundle (intercostal artery, vein, and nerve), which runs in the groove in this location. Once pleural fluid is aspirated, mark the needle at the skin surface by clamping with a hemostat. Withdraw the needle and syringe.

Connect the 30-mL syringe to a 16- to 18-gauge angiocatheter using a three-way stopcock. Determine the depth of insertion from the hemostat mark on the previously used needle and enter the pleural space through the anesthetized area of the skin, with gentle negative pressure on the syringe. Once fluid is obtained, advance the needle by 1 to 2 mm to ensure that the catheter is in the pleural space, withdraw the needle,

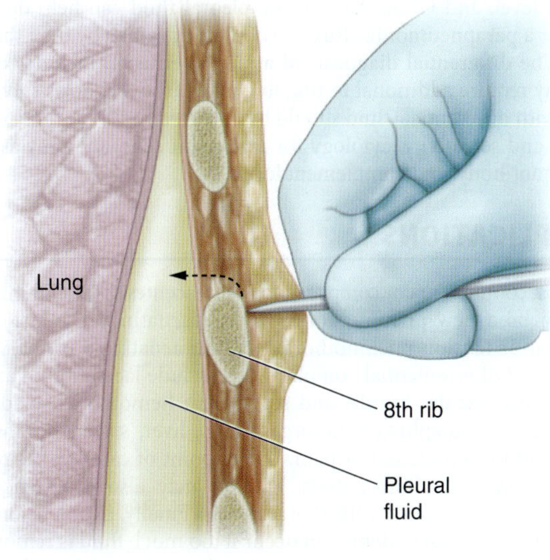

FIGURE 195-4. Technique of thoracentesis.

advance the catheter into the pleural space, and occlude the catheter with a fingertip. Attach the syringe with the stopcock to the catheter and withdraw about 20 to 30 mL of fluid for diagnostic testing. A larger volume can be drained if the patient is in respiratory distress, using tubing attached to a vacuum bottle.

Once the appropriate amount of fluid is withdrawn, remove the catheter and apply a sterile dressing. Perform an upright chest radiograph immediately after the procedure to assess for possible pneumothorax.

Pneumothorax Sterile gloves are worn, and the site is prepped with povidone-iodine solution. There are two types of needles that can be used: a butterfly needle or an angiocath needle. If a butterfly needle is used, two people are needed. The needle is attached to tubing and a large syringe (e.g., 20-50 mL) prior to insertion into the chest wall. The needle is inserted and aimed above the rib into the intercostal space, as another clinician gently applies a small amount of negative pressure on the syringe. When air is noted to enter the syringe, insertion of the needle is paused, and the position is maintained while air is evacuated from the space until the flow of air slows or resistance is noted. When using an angiocath, the needle is inserted aiming above the rib into the pleural space. When air is noted to be aspirated, the needle is removed with the catheter remaining. The tubing and syringe are attached to the catheter and negative pressure is gently applied as air fills the syringe. Continue to remove air until the flow of air slows, the patient's respiratory status improves, or resistance is noted. It is important not to remove all the pleural air to avoid reaccumulation of the pneumothorax on completion of the procedure. When enough air is removed, the needle or catheter with tubing apparatus is retracted and the site is dressed immediately with Vaseline gauze and Tegaderm. The site must be dressed with an occlusive dressing to avoid entry of air into the pleural space from the environment and recurrence of the pneumothorax. All sharp instruments should be disposed of in the designated receptacles.

PLEURAL FLUID TESTING

If pleural fluid is obtained for diagnostic purposes, the most important step is to decide whether the effusion is exudative or transudative. Light's criteria have traditionally been used to make this distinction. Pleural fluid analysis should include measurement of the following:

- Protein level (pleural to plasma protein ratio >0.5 implies exudate)
- LDH level (pleural to plasma LDH ratio >0.6 implies exudate)
- Other tests appropriate to the clinical situation (e.g., Gram stain and cultures if concern for infection, or cytology if concern for malignancy).

Treatment of a transudative pleural effusion is directed at the underlying cause. If the fluid is exudative, additional tests must be considered based on the history and physical examination findings. The pH, glucose level, and Gram stain of the pleural fluid can help determine whether a parapneumonic effusion should be drained by tube thoracostomy. The differential diagnosis of a pleural effusion includes diseases that may require additional testing to confirm the diagnosis such as cell count with differential (fluid should be collected in EDTA tube for this), culture and sensitivity, cytology for malignant cells, and amylase, antinuclear antibody, and complement levels.

COMPLICATIONS

The most common major complication of thoracentesis is pneumothorax—this can be a new pneumothorax when evacuating an effusion, or a recurrent or tension pneumothorax when evacuating a primary pneumothorax. Other potential complications include laceration of an intercostal neurovascular bundle and subsequent hemothorax, inadvertent puncture of subdiaphragmatic organs (e.g., liver, spleen) or the heart (rare), and local infection or pain. Use of point of care US has reduced organ injury with thoracentesis. Patients may also experience transient hypoxia associated with thoracentesis. Finally, hypotension or reexpansion pulmonary edema can occur if too much fluid is removed too quickly. In an adult-sized patient, the traditional recommendation has been to remove no more than 1000 to 1500 mL of fluid at a time. Newer studies have suggested full drainage as long as the patient does not have discomfort. In children, one should avoid taking off more than a few hundred milliliters of fluid at one time.

SUGGESTED READINGS

American College of Emergency Physicians. Policy statement. Ultrasound guidelines: emergency, point-of-care and clinical ultrasound guidelines in medicine. June 2016. www.acep.org/policystatements. Accessed December 12, 2022.

Cantey EP, Walter JM, Corbridge T, Barsuk JH. Complications of thoracentesis: incidence, risk factors, and strategies for prevention. *Curr Opin Pulm Med.* 2016;22(4):378-385.

Charalampidis C, Youroukou A, Lazaridis G, et al. Pleura space anatomy. *J Thorac Dis.* 2015;7(Suppl 1):S27-S32.

Dancel R, Schnobrich D, Puri N, et al. Recommendations on the use of ultrasound guidance for adult thoracentesis: a position statement of the society of hospital medicine. *J Hosp Med.* 2018;13(2):126-135.

Deng BY, Li N, Wu WS, et al. Use of neonatal lung ultrasound for the early detection of pneumothorax. *Am J Perinatol.* 2020;37(9):907-913.

Fong C, Tan CWC, Tan DKY, See KC. Safety of thoracentesis and tube thoracostomy in patients with uncorrected coagulopathy: a systematic review and meta-analysis. *Chest.* 2021;160(5):1875-1889.

Fraga MV, Stoller JZ, Glau CL, et al. Seeing is believing: ultrasound in pediatric procedural performance. *Pediatrics.* 2019;144(5):e20191401.

Havelock T, Teoh R, Laws D, Gleeson F; BTS Pleural Disease Guideline Group. Pleural procedures and thoracic ultrasound: British Thoracic Society Pleural Disease Guideline 2010. *Thorax.* 2010;65 Suppl 2: ii61-ii76.

Krackov R, Rizzolo D. Real-time ultrasound-guided thoracentesis. *JAAPA.* 2017;30(4):32-37.

Light RW, Macgregor MI, Luchsinger PC, Ball WC Jr. Pleural effusions: the diagnostic separation of transudates and exudates. *Ann Intern Med.* 1972;77(4):507-513.

Liu J, Kurepa D, Feletti F, et al. International expert consensus and recommendations for neonatal pneumothorax ultrasound diagnosis and ultrasound-guided thoracentesis procedure. *J Vis Exp.* 2020;(157):10.3791/60836.

Williams JG, Lerner AD. Managing complications of pleural procedures. *J Thorac Dis.* 2021;13(8):5242-5250.

CHAPTER 196 Circumcision

Kimberly Monroe, MD, MS

Male circumcision is the surgical removal of the foreskin (or prepuce) from the penis. Typically, circumcisions are performed in the neonatal period by pediatricians, obstetricians, and neonatologists. Approximately 55% of all newborn males in the United States are circumcised in the neonatal period, ~30% are circumcised in Canada, with lower rates in Europe, Australia, Asia, South America, and Mexico. An understanding of the indications, methods, and risks is essential for counseling parents and will be evaluated in this chapter.

INDICATIONS

Circumcisions performed in the newborn period are based on parental desire, as it is not medically required for the newborn male to be circumcised. Parents generally give consent based on cultural, religious, personal reasons (i.e., circumcision status of the father) and perceived health benefits. The, now retired, American Academy of Pediatrics (AAP) 2012 Technical Report and Policy Statement state that the health benefits of circumcision outweigh the risks, but these benefits are not enough to recommend universal newborn circumcision. The AAP, along with the Centers for Disease Control and Prevention (CDC), state that parents should be offered the option of a circumcision for their newborn and receive non-biased information on the health risks and benefits of circumcision.

Both the AAP and CDC list the health benefits of circumcision as reductions in urinary tract infections (UTIs), a decrease in acquisition of HIV and other sexually transmitted infections, penile cancer, phimosis, paraphimosis, balanitis, and lichen sclerosis. UTI prevention is mainly seen in the first year of life with the estimated number needed to treat to prevent one UTI being 111. For boys with recurrent UTIs or high-grade vesicoureteral reflux, the risk of UTI recurrence is 10% and 30% and the numbers needed to treat in these populations are 11 and 4, respectively, making this population one with a more robust health benefit. However, a Cochrane Review concluded there is no reliable evidence from randomized-controlled clinical trials (RCTs) proving that circumcision reduces the incidence of UTIs.

CONTRAINDICATIONS

The following abnormalities are contraindications to performing an elective circumcision:

ANATOMY

The foreskin is a complex structure of skin that protects and moisturizes the head of the penis. It is the most densely innervated and sensitive portion of the penis playing an important role in the mechanical function of the penis during sexual acts. For boys who are uncircumcised, it is important for the pediatric hospitalist to know that preputial retraction can occur at variable ages, with the mean age being approximately 10.4 years. As the foreskin becomes retractable, gentle retraction and cleaning of the glans with soap and water is recommended. Retraction of the foreskin should never be forced. This may lead to bleeding, adhesions, scarring, or paraphimosis, which is a medical emergency.

PREPARATION/EQUIPMENT/PROCEDURE/TECHNIQUE

Consent Parental consent must be obtained before the circumcision is performed. (See complications section for risks.) It is important to include that circumcisions are not medically necessary, and the alternative to delay the circumcision till the newborn is older and can decide for himself is an option that allows for patient autonomy. Adverse events secondary to circumcisions performed in the adult age group are slightly higher than in the neonatal period but are still minimal and mainly include bleeding and infection. Given male newborn circumcision is a controversial topic with a wide spectrum of views and no medical requirement for the procedure, the pediatric hospitalist may feel they are in a challenging position. The important task of providing accurate non-biased information to the parent often rests solely on our conversations. Therefore, it is critical that pediatric hospitalists stay up to date on the topic. Engaging parent(s) in a well-informed and thorough consent process including the risks, ethical issues, and potential benefits is as important as properly performing the procedure.

Screening It is important to inquire about a family history of bleeding disorders. If maternal thrombocytopenia, Von Willebrand Disease, hemophilia, or platelet function disorders are present in the family history, laboratory studies may be needed before a circumcision can be safely performed. Hematology should be consulted as needed. In addition, it is necessary to confirm confirmation that intramuscular vitamin K was given. Oral vitamin K is not sufficient to limit the amount of bleeding from a circumcision. Newborns who have significant bruising, excessive bleeding from injection sites or petechiae may need further evaluation before circumcision.

NPO Time Period Some providers recommend an NPO time period before circumcision to reduce the risk of aspiration or regurgitation. However, there currently is not enough evidence on this topic to support an NPO time period.

Void Newborns do not need to void prior to being circumcised. Nor is there evidence supporting a delay in discharge while waiting for a post circumcision void unless there is a complication noted with the meatus.

PAIN CONTROL

Sucrose Sucrose is used to help with analgesia throughout the procedure and should be given 2 minutes before the initial nerve block to take full effect. Providers typically use SweetEase™ (24% sucrose and water) (0.5-2 mL) which is applied either via a needleless syringe or via a pacifier dipped into the Sweetease™ and then placed in the child's mouth. It is the neonate's detection of a sweet substance, not the volume, which produces the analgesic effect. Nonpharmacologic techniques alone are insufficient to prevent procedural and postprocedural pain and should be used as adjuncts in addition to a nerve block.

Nerve Block Providers may use a ring block or dorsal nerve block. For both blocks, 1 mL of 1% lidocaine without epinephrine is drawn up using a 27-gauge needle and the area is prepped with an alcohol swab. The penile ring block (RB) was first described by Broadman et al in 1987 and is a circumferential subcutaneous injection at the base of the penile shaft. Injections (0.2 mL) are made superficial to Buck's fascia at the base of the penis at the 8, 10, 2, 4, and 6 o'clock positions and result in a bleb. However, to reduce the number of needle insertions by two, injections at 8 and 4 o'clock may be done first with advancement of the needle through to the 10 and 2 o'clock positions. The dorsal nerve block is an injection made deep to Buck's fascia. Two injections are made over the inferior edge of the pubic bone at approximately 10 o'clock (0.4 mL) and 2 o'clock (0.4 mL) relative to the base of the penis with the depth of the needle not more than 0.25 to 0.5 cm. For both blocks, it is important to pull back on the syringe prior to injecting lidocaine to ensure you are not in a vessel. A third subcutaneous injection (0.2 mL) is made at the 6 o'clock position. In a 2020 systematic review, the combination of a ring block, EMLA (1 g of EMLA cream applied to the penis of the newborn and wrapped with Tegaderm dressing 1 hour prior to the circumcision) and sucrose appeared to be the analgesic combination superior to other approaches. EMLA cream is a eutectic mixture of 2.5% lidocaine and 2.5% prilocaine and is a topical anesthetic. Pereira et al demonstrated that it is ideal to place EMLA between the internal surface of the foreskin and the glans of the penis for optimum analgesia. In addition, the integration of sensorial saturation during male circumcision may improve current analgesic practices. Sensorial saturation is a validated method to reduce newborns' stress response to nociception and is based on the so-called gate-control theory by which the brainstem can filter and reduce the transmission of pain to the brain if the person is concentrated on something else. By attracting babies' attention with positive stimuli (tactile, auditory, gustatory, and visual), it is possible to reduce and even nullify the perception of painful stimuli.

Acetaminophen A dose of oral acetaminophen may be offered once post procedure for pain.

PRE/POST PROCEDURE CARE

Betadine Circumcisions are performed under sterile conditions. Betadine is applied to the penis and surrounding area and sterile drapes are placed accordingly.

Petroleum Jelly For circumcisions performed with a Gomco clamp and Mogen techniques, petroleum jelly is to be applied to the penis with every diaper change for one to two weeks or until all the granulation tissue has fully healed. Circumcisions performed with a Plastibell can apply petroleum jelly after the device falls off until it heals. It is important that both the ventral and dorsal surfaces of the penis are covered with petroleum jelly. Petroleum jelly helps prevent adhesions from developing and the penis from sticking to the diaper as it heals. Antibiotic ointment is generally not needed.

Post Procedure Monitoring The newborn is monitored for 2 hours post circumcision for bleeding. Typically, the penis and surrounding area is evaluated every 15 minutes twice, post procedure.

SURGICAL DEVICES

Three surgical devices are commonly used to perform circumcisions: the Gomco clamp, the Plastibell device, and the Mogen clamp. Each of these devices produces a crush injury or tissue strangulation such that there is no need for sutures.

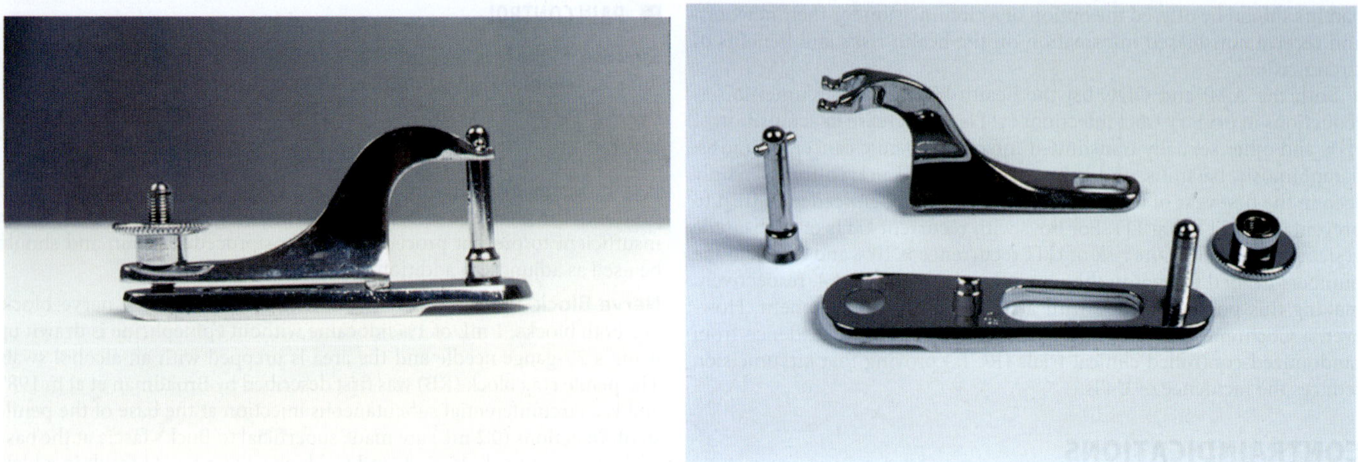

FIGURE 196-1. Gomco clamp. (Photos courtesy of Julian Wan, MD.)

Gomco Clamp (Figure 196-1) The Gomco clamp, acronym for Goldstein Manufacturing Company is an instrument introduced in 1934. Advantages include protection of the glans during the procedure and absence of a remaining foreign body. However, because the Gomco clamp is made of three major parts, there is a chance that pieces can be incorrectly assembled from differently sized units or those produced by different manufacturers. Using mismatched parts results in a device that might not sufficiently crush the foreskin, potentially resulting in bleeding. The Gomco contains a base plate, top plate, bell (size dependent on glans size and not penis length), and a nut. These parts fit together allowing the bell to protect the glans of the penis during the procedure and the nut to achieve skin hemostasis between the bell and base plate where the foreskin will be removed by the operator with a scalpel. First, adhesions are lysed by gentle blunt dissection to the level of the corona with care to keep the tip of the dissecting hemostat tenting the skin at all times. This ensures the hemostat does not enter the urethra. A crush injury is made at the 12 o'clock position with a hemostat one-third to one-half the distance from the coronal margin followed by an incision to expose the glans. When making the dorsal slit the blunt edge of the scissors should be used. The foreskin is then retracted, and any remaining adhesions are lysed such that the coronal ridge is completely free of adhesions. The bell is then placed over the glans at the level of the corona, the foreskin is pulled over the bell, the top plate is then placed over the bell, trapping the foreskin between the bell and the base plate. The clamp is then tightened, crushing the foreskin between the bell and the base plate. A minimum clamp time length is not needed. However, turning the nut as tightly as you are able is recommended. Next, the flared bottom of the bell fits tightly against the hole of the base plate, so the foreskin may be cut away with a scalpel from above the base plate. If difficultly unscrewing the nut, place gauze over the nut to improve your grip or use pliers. The provider may remove the bell, top and base plate once the foreskin is adequately removed. A video demonstrating a circumcision using a Gomco clamp is available at https://med.stanford.edu/newborns/professional-education/circumcision/gomco-clamp-technique.html.

Plastibell (Figure 196-2) The Plastibell was introduced in 1950. Infection risk is more common than with the Gomco clamp or Mogen techniques. In addition, incorrectly sized Plastibells may lead to glans and/or shaft incarceration and significant pain. The Plastibell technique begins similarly to the Gomco clamp technique but instead of bell placement, the Plastibell is inserted and the foreskin is pulled over the Plastibell stabilized by clamping it to the handle of the Plastibell. Device size is dependent on glans size and not penis length. Suture material is then looped around the groove and tied tightly to prevent blood supply to the prepuce distal to the groove. Excess foreskin past the outer edge is removed and the handle is broken off, leaving the ring in place. The Plastibell ring will fall off on its own within 1 to 8 days. A video demonstrating a circumcision using the Plastibell technique is available at https://med.stanford.edu/newborns/professional-education/circumcision/plastibell-technique.html.

Mogen (Figure 196-3) The Mogen clamp, created by a Jewish mohel in 1954, gives the advantages of not leaving a foreign body at the circumcision site and the ability for it to be rapidly performed. The disadvantage is that the device does not directly protect the glans during the procedure. The Mogen technique begins similarly to the Gomco clamp and Plastibell techniques up to and including the dorsal slit, glans inspection, and returning the foreskin back over the glans. However, it is also optional to retract the foreskin and lyse adhesions without making a dorsal slit. A hemostat is then placed along the dorsal midline with its tip about 3 mm short of the corona. A key step in Mogen circumcision is the safe placement of the clamp. To push the glans out of the way, the thumb and index finger pinch the foreskin below the dorsal hemostat. The fully opened Mogen clamp is then slid across the foreskin from dorsal to ventral following along the same angle as the corona to avoid removing excess skin ventrally. The hollow side of the clamp faces the glans. Before locking the clamp shut, the glans is manipulated to be sure it is free of the clamp's jaw. If it is, the clamp is locked. Once locked, the foreskin is removed flush with the flat surface of the clamp with a

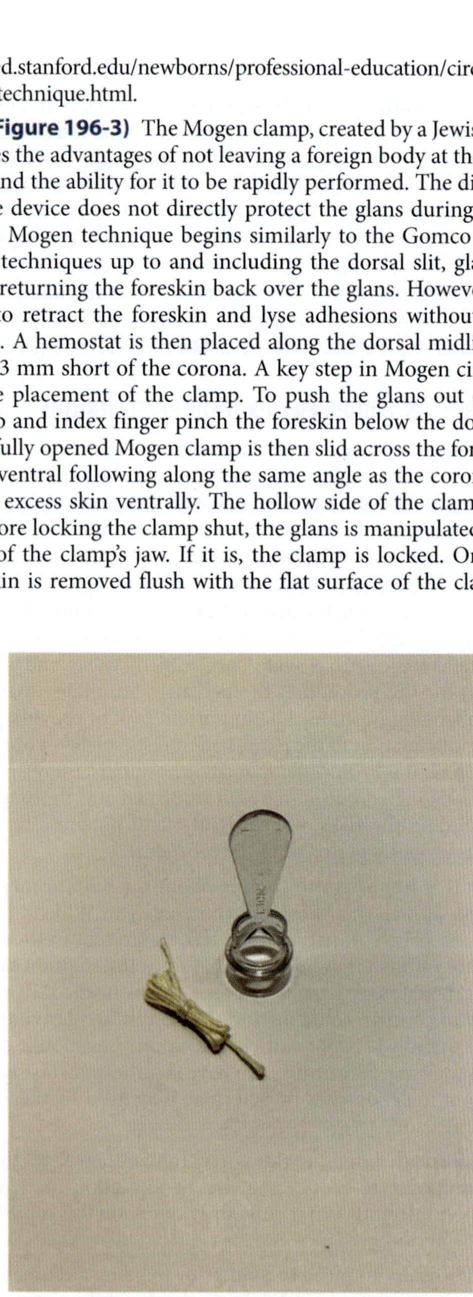

FIGURE 196-2. Plastibell. (Photo provided by Kim Monroe, MD, MS.)

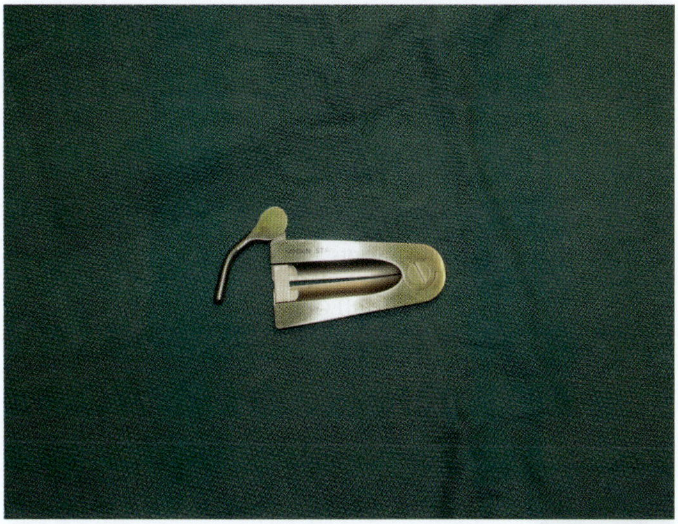

FIGURE 196-3. Mogen. (Photo courtesy of Janelle L. Aby, MD.)

#10 blade scalpel. The Mogen device is then unlocked and removed. After removal of the clamp, the seal between the skin and the mucosa is separated, downward pressure is applied until the glans is fully visualized. Any remaining adhesions are removed, and the penis is covered with petroleum jelly. The procedure usually takes 3 to 4 minutes. A video demonstrating a **circumcision** using a Mogen clamp is available at https://med.stanford.edu/newborns/professional-education/circumcision/mogen-clamp-technique.html.

TABLE 196-1 Contraindications

- Hypospadias—If after retracting the foreskin, it is noted that the meatus is either dorsal or ventral to the tip, but still located on the glans or if there is a megameatus, the circumcision may be completed as any urologic surgical repair would not involve use of foreskin.
- Epispadias
- Chordee
- Penoscrotal webbing
- Buried/Concealed penis
- Large hydroceles or inguinal hernias that encroach on the penile shaft
- Bleeding disorder
- Medically unstable
- Size < 1.9 cm stretched penile length
- Torsion greater than 90 degrees
- Incomplete foreskin
- Ambiguous genitalia

COMPLICATIONS

Per the AAP, the true incidence of complications after newborn circumcision is unknown. This is in part due to differing definitions of "complication," differing standards in timing of when a complication has occurred (i.e., early or late) and which provider performed the circumcision. The medical complication rate can be as high as 20%. See **Table 196-1** for a detailed list of complications.

Early

Bleeding is the most common complication with rates 0.6% to 9.6% range. If more than a few drops of blood are noticed, pressure may be applied and held in place for 1 to 2 minutes. Avitene™ Microfibrillar Collagen Hemostat or a Gelfoam® wrap can be applied. Gelfoam® is an absorbable gelatin sponge that promotes blood clot formation. Instructions should be given to leave the Avitene™ in place as the circumcision heals, letting it absorb naturally. If continued bleeding occurs, sutures may be needed and concern for a bleeding disorder should be considered. Urology should be consulted as needed. As hemophilia can occur via a genetic spontaneous mutation, newborn males with hemophilia may first present post circumcision. If significant bleeding or bleeding that continues despite pressure, etc. consider sending the following labs to test for bleeding disorders: CBC with platelets, Factors XIII and IX, Von Willebrand Factor Antigen, PT, and PTT.

Infection is a potential but infrequent complication of circumcision when performed under sterile conditions. The risk of actual infection is thought to be increased with use of the Plastibell device, due to the presence of a foreign body at the surgical site. When infection does occur, it should be recognized and treated promptly. Although rare, meningitis, necrotizing fasciitis, gangrene, and sepsis have all been reported as complications of infected circumcision sites.

Insufficient foreskin removal can occur and increases the likelihood for penile adhesions. If parents desire, a circumcision revision can be performed to remove the redundant foreskin. However, if secondary phimosis or skin bridges develop, surgical repair may be recommended.

Excessive foreskin removal or ventral slippage can occur, and the denuded area will epithelialize and may produce a poor cosmetic result. Although unlikely, it can also result in a buried penis or require skin grafting.

Iatrogenic hypospadias can occur from injury by a clamp device that results in avulsion or splitting of the ventral glans.

Iatrogenic epispadias can occur if a hemostat or scissors is inserted into the urethra inadvertently.

Glanular amputation is a rare complication of circumcision but has been reported with inappropriate placement of the Mogen clamp. If recognized promptly with both the amputated piece (in a saline-soaked sponge) and the patient transported immediately to a pediatric urologist, successful reattachment of the glans may be possible.

Death is an extremely unlikely complication of neonatal circumcision, but it has been reported secondary to blood loss or infection.

Late

Adhesions can develop if redundant foreskin slides back onto the glans and forms an adhesion or from inadequate lysis of natural adhesions prior to circumcision. Petroleum jelly application can help prevent this from happening as well as regular follow up with a physician. For patients at higher risk of adhesions, compression of the suprapubic area (fat pad) to make the penis protrude can help with prevention. Minor adhesions can often be lysed in a pediatrician's office by using gauze to gently push away the adhesions from the glans after administering a topical anesthetic cream such as EMLA. Use of sucrose is also recommended if this is performed. If adhesions or skin bridges develop that cannot be easily lysed in the outpatient setting, surgical repair is necessary.

Secondary phimosis is more likely if the newborn has a penile web or buried penis and is related to insufficient removal of the inner mucosal layer of the foreskin. Surgical repair may be necessary.

Meatal stenosis is the narrowing of the urethral meatus. It is thought to be secondary to glans irritation causing meatitis or ischemia from damage to the frenular artery during circumcision. It is a complication that is usually asymptomatic until toilet training, if it ever becomes symptomatic. It presents as a urinary stream deviation, dysuria, narrow stream, and potentially urinary retention if severe. Surgery is recommended if the patient is symptomatic.

Iatrogenic chordee can develop due to uneven amounts of foreskin removal from the ventral and dorsal surfaces. Surgical correction may be necessary.

Urethrocutaneous fistula occurs when there is injury to the urethra from aggressive clamping or suturing on the ventral surface of the glans or penile shaft. Surgical correction is necessary. (Please note that sutures are not used in any of the above-described techniques).

Glanular necrosis can occur in the setting of infection or use of an electrocautery device to control bleeding. The Plastibell ring technique has caused necrosis when it is inappropriately sized. (Please note that electrocautery devices are not used in any of the above-described techniques).

Epidermal inclusion cysts can occur and can lead to infection.

SUGGESTED READINGS

Abdulwahab-Ahmed A, Mungadi IA. Techniques of male circumcision. *J Surg Tech Case Rep*. 2013;5(1):1-7.

Amir M, Raja MH, Niaz WA. Neonatal circumcision with Gomco clamp—a hospital-based retrospective study of 1000 cases. *J Pak Med Assoc*. 2000;50(7):224-227.

Bellieni CV, Alagna MG, Buonocore G. Analgesia for infants' circumcision. *Ital J Pediatr*. Jun 13 2013;39:38.

Brady MT. Newborn male circumcision with parental consent, as stated in the AAP circumcision policy statement, is both legal and ethical. *J Law Med Ethics*. 2016;44(2):256-262.

British Medical Association. Non-therapeutic male circumcision (NTMC) of children—practical guidance for doctors 2019.

Bronselaer GA, Schober JM, Meyer-Bahlburg HF, T'Sjoen G, Vlietinck R, Hoebeke PB. Male circumcision decreases penile sensitivity as measured in a large cohort. *BJU Int*. 2013;111(5):820-827.

Earp BD, Mishori R, Rotta AT. Newborn Circumcision Techniques and Medical Ethics. *Am Fam Physician*. 2021;103(2):69-70.

Feinberg AN, Brust RA, Walker TA. Bleeding at circumcision: patient or operator issue? *Clin Pediatr (Phila)*. 2010;49(8):760-763.

Gologram M, Margolin R, Lomiguen CM. Need for increased awareness of international male circumcision variations and associated complications: a contemporary review. *Cureus*. 2022;14(4):e24507.

Jacobson DL, Balmert LC, Holl JL, Rosoklija I, Davis MM, Johnson EK. Nationwide circumcision trends: 2003 to 2016. *J Urol*. 2021;205(1): 257-263.

Jagannath VA, Fedorowicz Z, Sud V, Verma AK, Hajebrahimi S. Routine neonatal circumcision for the prevention of urinary tract infections in infancy. *Cochrane Database Syst Rev*. 2012;11.

Krill AJ, Palmer LS, Palmer JS. Complications of circumcision. *ScientificWorldJournal*. 2011;11:2458-68.

Many BT, Rizeq YK, Vacek J, et al. A contemporary snapshot of circumcision in US children's hospitals. *J Pediatr Surg*. 2020;55(6): 1134-1138.

McPhee AS, McKay AC. Dorsal Penile Nerve Block. [Updated 2022 Nov 28]. In: StatPearls [Internet]. Treasure Island (FL): StatPearls Publishing; 2022 Jan. Available from: https://www.ncbi.nlm.nih.gov/books/NBK535389/.

Monroe KK, Razoky P, Murphy S, et al. The length of Gomco clamp timing and its effect on bleeding. *Hosp Pediatr*. 2021;11(9): 1003-1010.

Morris BJ, Wamai RG, Henebeng EB, et al. Estimation of country-specific and global prevalence of male circumcision. *Popul Health Metr*. 2016;14:4.

Myers A, Earp BD. What is the best age to circumcise? A medical and ethical analysis. *Bioethics*. 2020;34(7):645-663.

Okeke LI, Asinobi AA, Ikuerowo OS. Epidemiology of complications of male circumcision in Ibadan, Nigeria. *BMC Urol*. 2006;6:21.

Omole F, Smith W, Carter-Wicker K. Newborn circumcision techniques. *Am Fam Physician*. 2020;101(11):680-685.

Peleg D, Steiner A. The Gomco circumcision: common problems and solutions. *Am Fam Physician*. 1998;58(4):891-898.

Pereira EG BL, Driver RP. EMLA, dorsal penile nerve block, and iontophoresis for analgesia during newborn circumcision. *Reg Anesth Pain Med*. 1998;23(3):S8.

Phili R, Abdool-Karim Q, Ngesa O. Low adverse event rates following voluntary medical male circumcision in a high HIV disease burden public sector prevention programme in South Africa. *J Int AIDS Soc*. 2014;17:19275.

Pieretti RV, Goldstein AM, Pieretti-Vanmarcke R. Late complications of newborn circumcision: a common and avoidable problem. *Pediatr Surg Int*. 2010;26(5):515-518.

Prabhakaran S, Ljuhar D, Coleman R, Nataraja RM. Circumcision in the paediatric patient: a review of indications, technique and complications. *J Paediatr Child Health*. Dec 2018;54(12):1299-1307.

Reynolds RD. Use of the Mogen clamp for neonatal circumcision. *Am Fam Physician*. 1996;54(1):177-182.

Rossi S, Buonocore G, Bellieni CV. Management of pain in newborn circumcision: a systematic review. *Eur J Pediatr*. 2021;180(1):13-20.

Sharara-Chami R, Lakissian Z, Charafeddine L, Milad N, El-Hout Y. Combination analgesia for neonatal circumcision: a randomized controlled trial. *Pediatrics*. 2017;140(6).

Simpson E, Carstensen J, Murphy P. Neonatal circumcision: new recommendations & implications for practice. *Mo Med*. 2014;111(3): 222-230.

Task Force on Circumcision. Male circumcision. *Pediatrics*. 2012;130(3): e756-85.

Weiss HA, Larke N, Halperin D, Schenker I. Complications of circumcision in male neonates, infants and children: a systematic review. *BMC Urol*. 2010;10:2.

World Health Organization & JHPIEGO. (2010). Manual for early infant male circumcision under local anaesthesia. World Health Organization. https://apps.who.int/iris/handle/10665/44478.

CHAPTER 197

Nasogastric Tube Insertion

Nicholas A. Lunig, MD

INTRODUCTION

Nasogastric (NG) tube insertion is a common procedure used in the pediatric population for many reasons, including enteral feeding, medication administration, and gastric decompression. This chapter will provide an overview of the indications, contraindications, and technique for NG tube insertion in pediatric patients.

INDICATIONS

NG tube insertion is indicated in pediatric patients for a number of reasons. One of the most common is as an alternative to oral feedings in instances where a patient is not safe to feed by mouth due to aspiration risk, anatomical abnormalities, or neurological deficits. It may also be indicated in children who need enteral nutritional support or supplemental hydration. Other indications for NG tube placement include medication administration, delivering a large volume of fluid as in constipation treatment or radiographic contrast administration, or for gastric decompression or to empty stomach contents.

CONTRAINDICATIONS

NG tube insertion may be contraindicated in certain pediatric patients, including those with:

- Severe nasal obstruction or nasopharyngeal anatomical abnormalities
- Known or suspected esophageal or gastric perforation or recent surgical manipulation
- Recent oropharyngeal facial surgery or trauma
- Unstable airway, or inability to protect airway
- Coagulopathy or other bleeding disorders

ANATOMY

The NG tube passes through multiple structures en route to the stomach. The NG tube is inserted into one nare and then is advanced into the nasal cavity, traveling through the nasopharynx, followed by the oropharynx, hypopharynx, esophagus, and finally terminating in the stomach. Another important anatomic structure is the epiglottis, which the NG tube passes by and serves to cover the trachea and protect the airway during swallowing.

It is important to note that pediatric patients have smaller nasal passages and a shorter distance from the nostrils to the stomach compared to adults. Careful attention and skillful insertion technique are necessary to minimize discomfort and trauma during NG tube insertion.

EQUIPMENT (TABLE 197-1)

The nasogastric tube is a flexible tube made of polyurethane or silicone. Typical diameters of tube used are 6 french for newborns, 8 to 10 french for infants through toddlers, 10 french for school age children, and 10 to 12 french for adolescents. Considerations for the length of the tube should involve the purpose of the tube. For example, in a patient receiving continuous feeds a longer tube may be used to prevent tension of the tube between the child and the feeding pump, while a shorter, less cumbersome tube may be used for a more active child who only uses the tube intermittently for medications. Ultimately, the provider should base the tube length and diameter based on the size of the child and the rationale for insertion.

PROCEDURE

PREPARATION

Before starting the insertion, be sure to explain the procedure to the patient/family, including risks, benefits and alternatives to the procedure, perform hand hygiene, and appropriately identify the patient. Ensure all supplies are present at bedside. Apply the pulse oximetry sensor prior to feeding tube insertion to establish a baseline reading.

TECHNIQUE

The following is a general guide for NG tube insertion in pediatric patients. Please note that the specifics of the procedure may vary depending on the patient's age, size, and clinical condition.

1. Place patient in a sitting or semi-sitting position (minimum of 30-45 degree angle) with the head slightly tilted forward if patient's age and clinical condition allows.
2. Measure the length of the NG tube from the nostril to the earlobe and then the midway point between the xiphoid process and umbilicus, and mark the tube with a piece of tape or a marker. The NEMU mnemonic is sometimes used to help guide measurement- measure from the tip of the patient's **N**ose to the **E**arlobe and then to a point **M**idway between the xyphoid process and the **U**mbilicus (**Figure 197-1**).
3. Apply water-soluble lubricant to the tip of the NG tube.
4. Insert the tube through one nostril and gently advance it in a posterior direction while instructing the patient to swallow or take sips of water to help facilitate passage if possible. If resistance is encountered, withdraw the tube slightly and reposition the patient's head slightly and attempt advancing again.
5. Once the tube has passed the pharynx and esophagus and entered the stomach at the distance marked on the tube, check the placement of the tube by aspirating gastric contents (2-5 mL), and confirming the pH. A pH of less than or equal to 5 typically indicates that the tube is in the acidic environment of the stomach.
6. Cut the tape or adhesive to an appropriate size and secure the tube across the patient's cheek toward the ear. Ideally, the adhesive should secure the tube as close to the nostril as possible to minimize the length of unsecured tube and thus the chance of dislodgement.
7. If indicated, confirm the placement of the tube by X-ray.
8. Provide care and maintenance of the tube as appropriate, including checking the placement, flushing the tube, and monitoring for complications per institutional protocol.

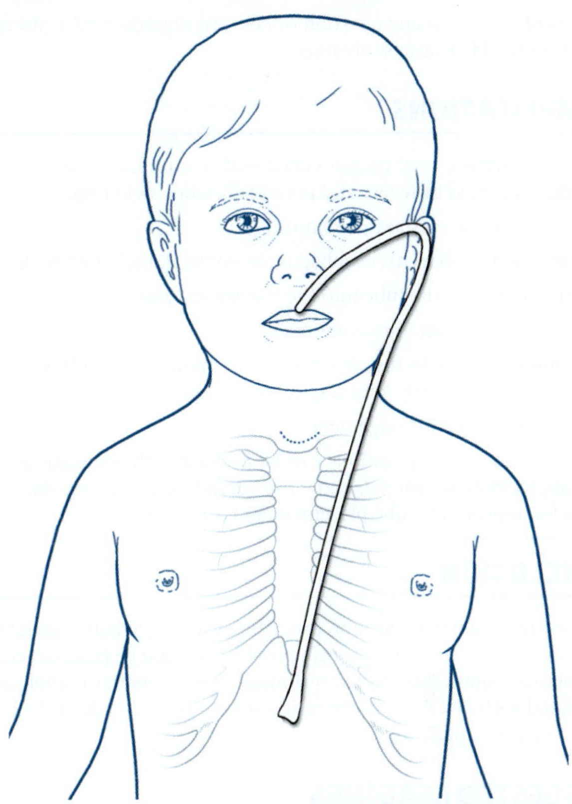

FIGURE 197-1. Measuring the NG tube. Prior to insertion, the length of the NG tube is estimated by running the tube from the tip of the nose to the earlobe to the midpoint between the xiphoid process and umbilicus. (Reproduced with permission from Goodman DM, Green TP, Unti SM, Powell EC. *Current Procedures: Pediatrics*. New York: McGraw Hill; 2007, Figure 25-1.)

One of the most important aspects of the procedure is accurately assessing the tube's location in a timely fashion. The two most common methods to do so are testing the pH of the fluid aspirated from the tube or via X-ray. An X-ray should be obtained if patient has impaired cough or gag reflex, has any neurologic impairment, is sedated, or is critically ill. It is also recommended that an X-ray be obtained if the tube met significant resistance while advancing or required multiple attempts to place. Finally, the patient should be closely observed both during and after the placement for any of the concerning clinical changes (**Table 197-2**).

Many pediatric institutions now have a dedicated X-ray protocol to confirm NG tube placement which utilizes a more focused and lower resolution image, allowing for less radiation exposure. Ultimately, given the risk of severe complications that can arise from inappropriate tube

TABLE 197-1 Equipment Needed for NG Tube Insertion
Nasogastric tube
Water Soluble Lubricating Gel
10 or 20 mL Syringe
pH Strips
Tape or Adhesive
Sterile water for Flushing
Non-sterile gloves
Marker for measuring

TABLE 197-2 Concerning Clinical Change Following NG Tube Insertion
Prolonged or persistent cough, gagging or choking
Color change
Vomiting
Change in respiratory status, including decrease in pulse ox reading
Increased fussiness or inconsolability
Change in voice or quality of cry
Caregiver concern

placement, if there is any question or concern regarding tube placement an X-ray should always be obtained.

COMPLICATIONS

NG tube insertion may be associated with a number of complications ranging from mild to severe and potentially fatal, including:

- Nasal irritation, epistaxis, or sinusitis
- Trauma to the pharynx, esophagus, or stomach, including perforation
- Misplacement of the tube into the trachea or bronchus
- Infective or aspiration pneumonia
- Chemical damage to the airway or lung parenchyma leading to pneumonitis or potentially fatal respiratory compromise
- Tube blockage or dislodgement

Many of these complications can be avoided with adequate preparation, appropriate technique, and close surveillance and ongoing monitoring for appropriate tube placement and function.

CONCLUSION

NG tube insertion is a common procedure used in pediatric patients for a variety of indications. Healthcare providers should be familiar with the indications, contraindications, technique, and potential complications associated with NG tube insertion in order to provide safe and effective care to pediatric patients.

SUGGESTED READINGS

Blumenstein I, Shastri YM, Stein J. Gastroenteric tube feeding: techniques, problems and solutions. *World J Gastroenterol.* 2014;20(26):8505-8524.

Irving SY, Rempel G, Lyman B, et al. Pediatric nasogastric tube placement and verification: best practice recommendations from the NOVEL project. *Nutr Clin Pract.* 2018;33(6):921-927.

Metheny NA, Meert KL, Clouse RE. Complications related to feeding tube placement. *Curr Opin Gastroenterol.* 2007;23(2):178-182.

Vadivelu N, Kodumudi G, Leffert LR, et al. Evolving therapeutic roles of nasogastric tubes: current concepts in clinical practice. *Adv Ther.* 2023;40(3):828-843.

CHAPTER 198 Incision and Drainage

Joseph Lazar, MD

INDICATIONS

For superficial skin abscesses, incision and drainage (I&D) is the primary mode of treatment, as antibiotic treatment alone is usually insufficient for larger abscesses. Incision and drainage is a procedure that can be performed safely and effectively in office or emergency department settings by the pediatric hospitalist.

CONTRAINDICATIONS

Abscesses less than 5 mm should not typically be drained as they are unlikely to be drained effectively and are often managed well with oral antibiotics. Other relative contraindications that should prompt consideration of consultation with a general or subspecialty surgeon include:

- Abscesses >5 cm, deep abscesses, or interconnected abscesses that may represent connected networks of fistulas

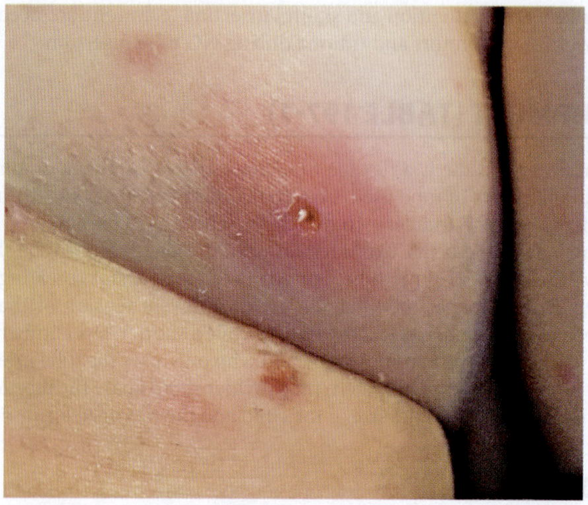

FIGURE 198-1. An abscess is a localized, usually loculated, collection of purulent fluid. Clinical exam findings may include swelling, erythema, fluctuance, and spontaneous purulent drainage. Abscesses can occur almost anywhere in the body. Common areas for development of cutaneous abscesses include the buttocks, axillae, groin, and extremities. (Reproduced with permission from Prose NS, Kristal L. *Weinberg's Color Atlas of Pediatric Dermatology*. 5th ed. New York, NY: McGraw Hill; 2017, Figure 3-18.)

- Abscesses of areas that are anatomically sensitive or have higher rates of complications such as palms, soles, breasts, the area between the nasolabial folds, genitalia, perirectal area, areas near vascular or neurologic structures, anterior, and lateral neck abscesses potentially arising from congenital cysts

ANATOMY

Abscesses are localized collections of pus in the dermis or subcutaneous tissues (**Figure 198-1**). Abscesses are caused by bacterial infection, which can result from disruption of the skin barrier and inoculation of bacteria into these spaces. Fighting the infection, the body forms an abscess when pus and other cellular debris are walled off and loculated. These loculations form separate compartments of purulent fluid within the larger abscess. While abscesses can occur virtually anywhere in the body, the most common sites of abscess formation include the groin, buttocks, axillae, and extremities. The diagnosis of skin abscess should be confirmed by physical exam. Ultrasound has also been shown to improve diagnostic accuracy (**Figure 198-2**).

EQUIPMENT

After making a decision to proceed with I&D, a clinician should gather the following materials:

- Universal precautions to protect provider, including gloves, face covering, and eye shield, as abscess contents are likely under pressure
- Skin cleansing agent like povidone-iodine or chlorhexidine solution
- Sterile gauze
- Sterile gloves
- Local anesthetic (e.g., 1% lidocaine)
- 5 to 10 mL syringe with 25 to 30-gauge needle
- Scalpel with #11 blade
- Small curved hemostat
- Forceps
- Normal saline in sterile bowl
- 30 to 60 cc Syringe with 19-gauge intravenous catheter or needleless irrigation device and splash protector
- Swabs for culture

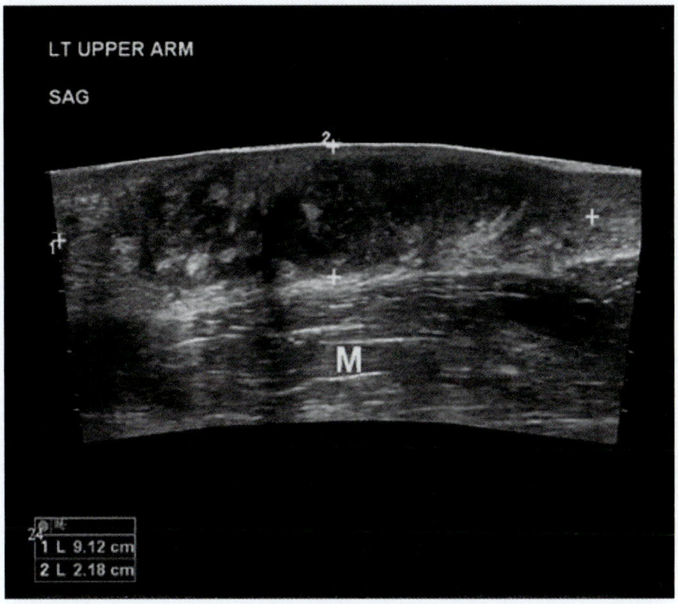

FIGURE 198-2. Longitudinal ultrasound image of a cutaneous abscess of the upper arm, showing a fluid-filled collection with variable echogenicity, corresponding to multiple areas of loculated pus. Ultrasound imaging can assist in diagnosis of cutaneous abscesses but is not required. (Reproduced with permission from McCulloch JM, Kloth LC, eds. *Wound Healing: Evidence-Based Management*. 4th ed. Philadelphia, PA: FA Davis Company; 2010, Figure 9.26.)

- Wound packing material (e.g., iodoform or plain gauze packing tape)
- Scissors
- Tape

PROCEDURE

(SUB-HEADING)—PREPARATION

It is important to ensure a patient's tetanus vaccination is up to date. Tetanus vaccine can be provided if indicated.

Informed written consent must be obtained from the patient or guardian.

Clean the skin overlying and surrounding the abscess with povidone-iodine or chlorhexidine solution, swabbing in a circular motion, extending outward in concentric circles, extending to margins beyond the area that the abscess can be palpated.

Anesthesia is provided with intradermal injection of 1% lidocaine into the top of the wound, infiltrating in a number of different directions to provide a "field" of anesthesia. Alternatively, a regional block can be used, depending on the area of the body, as the acidic pH of the infected abscess tissue can theoretically reduce the proportion of active, uncharged anesthetic.

Some patients, especially younger children, may require anxiolysis or procedural sedation for further comfort and to reduce the risk of patient movement, which can make the procedure less effective or less safe.

(SUB-HEADING)—TECHNIQUE (FIGURE 198-3)

1. With an #11 blade, make an incision at the center of the lesion, parallel to the long axis of the lesion
2. Extend the incision outward in both directions, parallel to the long axis of the lesion, and if possible, parallel to existing skin tension lines. Ensure that the incision is large enough to allow for complete exploration of the interior of the abscess and subsequent drainage.
3. Swab for culture from the inside of abscess. While culture results may not change management in many cases, it is recommended to send infected material for culture.

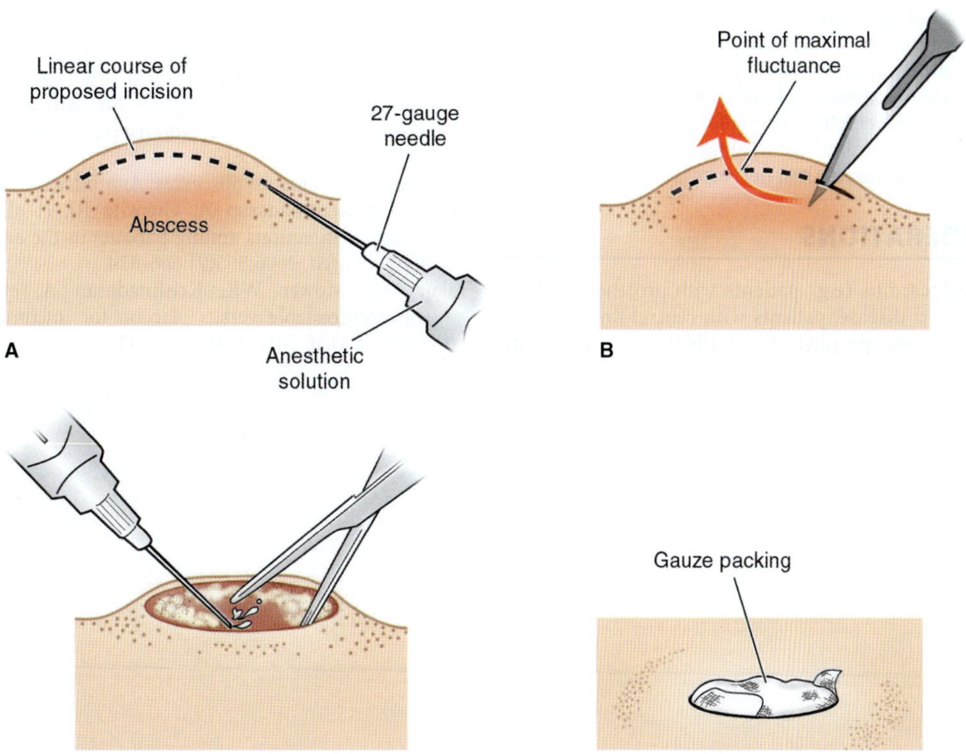

FIGURE 198-3. Incision and drainage of a superficial abscess. A. Infiltration of local anesthetic above the abscess, which may require multiple points of entry. B. Incision made at center, extending along parallel axis in both directions. C. Loculations within the wound are broken up with blunt dissection. Wound is irrigated using an IV catheter and sterile saline. D. In large abscesses, wound is gently packed with ¼ or ½ inch gauze with a tail left to assist in removal in 2-3 days. (Reproduced with permission from Reichman EF, ed. *Reichman's Emergency Medicine Procedures*. 3rd ed. New York: McGraw Hill; 2019.)

4. Allow wound to drain spontaneously and then apply pressure from the outside. This may require additional anesthetic into the wall of the abscess for additional pain control.
5. Break up loculations by blunt dissection with a curved hemostat that has been inserted into the incision. Do this in a circular motion until the entire wound cavity has been explored in all directions. Failure to sufficiently break up loculated pockets will lead to higher failure rates.
6. Irrigate inside the wound with sterile saline, using a 30-60 cc syringe with a 19-gauge intravenous catheter or needleless irrigation device and splash protector. Continue irrigation until effluent is clear.
7. Wounds should heal by secondary intention. Some controversy exists in the literature regarding the need for packing of abscesses. We recommend wound packing for abscesses >5cm. If packing is indicated, gently pack with ¼ or ½ inch packing strips with or without iodoform, beginning in one quadrant and moving in circular motion until all areas of the space are packed. Take care not to overpack as this can cause tissue ischemia. Leave a 1 cm tail outside of the incision, which will facilitate removal of packing at follow-up.
8. Cover the wound with an absorbent dressing.
9. If wound was packed, ensure that the patient can make an appointment for removal and wound check in 2 to 3 days. Packing can usually be removed at this time. If there is significant continued wound drainage at this time, there may be need for repacking and scheduling of another follow-up visit 2 to 3 days later.

COMPLICATIONS

Common risks of the procedure include pain, bleeding, scar formation, and abscess reaccumulation if incompletely drained. It is important for the clinician to review symptoms to observe for with the patient and family before discharge. In general, patients should be encouraged to seek medical attention if any of the following symptoms arise: fever or chills, increased swelling or increased drainage of pus, increased pain, surrounding redness, or red streaking.

One of the main complications to alert families to be aware of is local or systemic extension of the infection. Inadequate drainage can lead to reaccumulation of abscess or extension of infection, including development of osteomyelitis, thrombophlebitis, fistula formation, and cellulitis.

Overly aggressive drainage or drainage in areas near important neurologic or vascular structures can result in nerve or blood vessel injury.

SPECIAL CONSIDERATIONS

Patients at risk for endocarditis (e.g., patients with prosthetic valves, history of rheumatic heart disease, patients with central lines) should be treated with appropriate prophylactic antibiotics with activity against staphylococci and beta-hemolytic strep, as incision and drainage procedures are often accompanied by transient bacteremia from these species.

If the decision is made to prescribe a course of antibiotics, it is important to consider the likely bacteria species that cause abscesses in different areas of the body, as well as local antibiotic resistance patterns. *Staph aureus* accounts for the majority of abscesses on the body, and beta-hemolytic strep accounts for a much smaller fraction. Abscesses in the perineal, genital, perianal areas, on the other hand, are caused by anerobic enteric bacteria, so antibiotic therapy for these patients should be directed accordingly.

We recommend a 7-day course of cephalexin *and* metronidazole for perineal area abscesses including pilonidal abscesses. For nonperineal abscesses, a 7-day course of mono-therapy with trimethoprim-sulfamethoxazole *or* clindamycin *or* doxycycline is prescribed in the following cases:

- Abscesses >2 cm
- Rapid progression in presence of cellulitis
- Signs/symptoms of systemic illness
- Associated co-morbidities or immunosuppression
- Abscess in area difficult to drain
- Lack of response to previous I & D

SUGGESTED READINGS

Daum RS, Miller LG, Immergluck L, et al. A Placebo-Controlled Trial of Antibiotics for Smaller Skin Abscesses. *N Engl J Med.* 2017;376(26):2545-2555.

Fitch MT, Manthey DE, McGinnis HD, Nicks BA, Pariyadath M. Abscess Incision and Drainage. *N Engl J Med.* 2007;357(19):e20.

Frazee BW, Lynn J, Charlebois ED, Lambert L, Lowery D, Perdreau-Remington F. High prevalence of methicillin-resistant *Staphylococcus aureus* in emergency department skin and soft tissue infections. *Ann Emerg Med.* 2005;45(3):311-320.

Gaspari RJ, Resop D, Mendoza M, Kang T, Blehar D. A randomized controlled trial of incision and drainage versus ultrasonographically guided needle aspiration for skin abscesses and the effect of methicillin-resistant *Staphylococcus aureus. Ann Emerg Med.* 2011;57(5):483-491.e1.

Meislin HW. Cutaneous abscesses. *Ann Intern Med.* 1977;87(2):145.

Moran GJ, Krishnadasan A, Gorwitz RJ, et al. Methicillin-resistant *S. aureus* infections among patients in the emergency department. *N Engl J Med.* 2006;355(7):666-674.

Talan DA, Mower WR, Krishnadasan A, et al. Trimethoprim–sulfamethoxazole versus placebo for uncomplicated skin abscess. *N Engl J Med.* 2016;374(9):823-832.

Index

Page numbers followed by "f" denote figures, "t" denote tables, and "b" denote boxes.

I

N

O

P

W